Hazzard's

Geriatric Medicine
and Gerontology

Eighth Edition

Hazzard's
Geriatric Medicine
and Gerontology

Editors

Jeffrey B. Halter, MD
Professor Emeritus
Department of Internal Medicine
Division of Geriatric and Palliative Medicine
University of Michigan
Parkway Visiting Professor in Geriatrics
Department of Medicine
Yong Loo Lin School of Medicine
National University of Singapore
Ann Arbor, Michigan

Joseph G. Ouslander, MD
Professor of Geriatric Medicine
Senior Advisor to the Dean for Geriatrics
Charles E. Schmidt College of Medicine
Professor (Courtesy), Christine E. Lynn College of Nursing
Florida Atlantic University
Boca Raton, Florida
Editor-in-Chief, *Journal of the American Geriatrics Society*

Stephanie Studenski, MD, MPH
Professor Emeritus
University of Pittsburgh School of Medicine
Pittsburgh, Pennsylvania

Kevin P. High, MD, MS
President, Atrium Health—Wake Forest Baptist
Professor of Internal Medicine–Infectious Diseases
Wake Forest School of Medicine
Winston-Salem, North Carolina

Sanjay Asthana, MD, FACP
Associate Dean for Gerontology
Professor and Head, Division of Geriatrics and Gerontology
Director, NIA/NIH Wisconsin Alzheimer Disease
Research Center (ADRC)
Director, Madison VAMC Geriatric Research,
Education and Clinical Center (GRECC)
Duncan G. and Lottie H. Ballantine Endowed Chair in Geriatrics
University of Wisconsin School of Medicine and Public Health
Madison, Wisconsin

Mark A. Supiano, MD
D. Keith Barnes, MD and Dottie Barnes Presidential
Endowed Chair in Medicine
Professor and Chief, Division of Geriatrics
University of Utah School of Medicine
Executive Director, University of Utah Center on Aging
Salt Lake City, Utah

Christine S. Ritchie, MD, MSPH
Kenneth L. Minaker Endowed Chair in Geriatric Medicine
Director, Mongan Institute Center for Aging and Serious Illness
Professor of Medicine
Massachusetts General Hospital and
Harvard Medical School
Boston, Massachusetts

Kenneth Schmader, MD
Professor of Medicine-Geriatrics
Co-Director, Pepper Older Americans Independence Center
Duke University Medical Center
Director, Geriatric Research Education and Clinical Center
Durham VA Health Care System
Durham, North Carolina

Editor Emeritus and Senior Advisor

William R. Hazzard, MD
Professor Emeritus, Internal Medicine—Gerontology and
  Geriatric Medicine
J. Paul Sticht Center on Aging and Rehabilitation
Wake Forest School of Medicine
Winston-Salem, North Carolina

Senior Editorial Assistant

Nancy F. Woolard
Senior Manager for Clinical Research
Section on Gerontology & Geriatric Medicine
Wake Forest School of Medicine
Winston-Salem, North Carolina

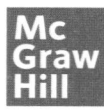

New York Chicago San Francisco Athens London Madrid Mexico City
New Delhi Milan Singapore Sydney Toronto

Hazzard's Geriatric Medicine and Gerontology, Eighth Edition

1 2 3 4 5 6 7 8 9   LWI   27 26 25 24 23 22

ISBN 978-1-260-46445-0
MHID 1-260-46445-8

This book was set in Minion Pro by KnowledgeWorks Global Ltd.
The editors were Leah Carton and Kim J. Davis.
The production supervisor was Richard Ruzycka.
Project management was provided by Radhika Jolly of KnowledgeWorks Global Ltd.
The designer was Janice Bielawa.
The cover designer was W2 Design.

This book is printed on acid-free paper.

Library of Congress Cataloging-in-Publication Data

Names: Halter, Jeffrey B., editor.
Title: Hazzard's geriatric medicine and gerontology / editor, Jeffrey B.
   Halter, Joseph G. Ouslander, Stephanie Studenski, Kevin P. High, Sanjay
   Asthana, Mark A. Supiano, Christine Ritchie, Kenneth Schmader.
Other titles: Geriatric medicine and gerontology
Description: Eighth edition. | New York : McGraw Hill, [2022] | Includes
   bibliographical references and index. | Summary: "This textbook has
   become a mainstay of the rapidly developing field of geriatric
   medicine"—Provided by publisher.
Identifiers: LCCN 2021059323 (print) | LCCN 2021059324 (ebook) | ISBN
   9781260464450 (hardcover ; alk. paper) | ISBN 9781260464467 (ebook)
Subjects: MESH: Geriatrics | Health Services for the Aged
Classification: LCC RC952 (print) | LCC RC952 (ebook) | NLM WT 100 | DDC
   618.97—dc23/eng/20220106
LC record available at https://lccn.loc.gov/2021059323
LC ebook record available at https://lccn.loc.gov/2021059324

McGraw Hill books are available at special quantity discounts to use as premiums and sales promotions or for use in corporate training programs. To contact a representative, please visit the Contact Us pages at www.mhprofessional.com.

Contents

Part III

Geriatric Conditions 573

Part IV

Principles of Palliative Medicine and Ethics 1043

Contributors

CHAPTER AUTHORS

Numbers in brackets refer to the chapters written or cowritten by the contributor.

Andres Acosta, MD, PhD
Assistant Professor of Medicine
Division of Gastroenterology and Hepatology
Mayo Clinic
Rochester, Minnesota [87]

Owoicho Adogwa, MD, MPH
Associate Professor of Neurosurgery
Department of Neurological Surgery
University of Cincinnati School of Medicine
Cincinnati, Ohio [102]

Kathleen M. Akgün, MD, MS
Associate Professor of Medicine
Section of Pulmonary, Critical Care and Sleep Medicine
Yale University School of Medicine
New Haven, Connecticut
Director, Medical Intensive Care Unit
VA Connecticut Healthcare System
West Haven, Connecticut [81]

Asrar Alahmadi, MBBS MAS-CR
Assistant Professor of Medicine
Division of Oncology, Department of Medicine
The Ohio State University Comprehensive Cancer Center
Columbus, Ohio [91]

Steven M. Albert, PhD, MS, FGSA, FAAN
Editor-in-Chief, *Innovation in Aging*
Professor and Hallen Chair
Department of Behavioral and Community
    Health Sciences
Graduate School of Public Health
University of Pittsburgh
Pittsburgh, Pennsylvania [4]

Cathy Alessi, MD
Director, Geriatric Research, Education and Clinical
    Center; VA Greater Los Angeles Healthcare System
Professor, Department of Medicine
University of California, Los Angeles
Los Angeles, California [44]

Karen P. Alexander, MD
Professor of Medicine/Cardiology
Duke University and Duke Clinical Research Institute
Durham, North Carolina [74]

Bradley D. Anawalt, MD
Professor and Vice Chair
Department of Medicine
University of Washington School of Medicine
Chief of Medicine, University of Washington
    Medical Center
Seattle, Washington [97]

Hidenori Arai, MD, PhD
President
National Center for Geriatrics and Gerontology
Obu, Aichi, Japan [13]

Muhammad S. Ashraf, MBBS
Associate Professor
Division of Infectious Diseases, Department of
    Internal Medicine
University of Nebraska Medical Center
Omaha, Nebraska [106]

Tara Asokan, BS
Graduate Intern
The John A. Hartford Foundation
New York, New York [12]

Sanjay Asthana, MD, FACP
Associate Dean for Gerontology
Professor and Head, Division of Geriatrics and
    Gerontology
Director, NIA/NIH Wisconsin Alzheimer Disease
Research Center (ADRC)
Director, Madison VAMC Geriatric Research,
Education and Clinical Center (GRECC)
Duncan G. and Lottie H. Ballantine Endowed Chair
    in Geriatrics
University of Wisconsin School of Medicine and
    Public Health
Madison, Wisconsin [59]

Steven N. Austad, PhD
Protective Life Endowed Chair in Healthy Aging Research
Department of Biology
University of Alabama at Birmingham
Birmingham, Alabama [5]

x **Thilinie D. Bandaranayake, MBBS**
Assistant Professor of Medicine
Section of Infectious Diseases
Yale School of Medicine
New Haven, Connecticut [3]

Steven Barczi, MD FAASM
Director of Clinical Services, Division of Geriatrics,
    Department of Medicine
Director of Clinical, Geri-PACT & GRECC Connect
Madison VA Geriatric Research, Education and
    Clinical Center
Professor of Medicine, Geriatrics/Sleep Medicine
University of Wisconsin-Madison School of Medicine and
    Public Health
Madison, Wisconsin [31]

Roxanne Bavarian, DMD
Orofacial Pain Fellow
Department of Oral and Maxillofacial Surgery
Massachusetts General Hospital
Boston, Massachusetts [68]

Christina L. Bell, MD, PhD
Clinical Associate Professor
Department of Geriatric Medicine
John A. Burns School of Medicine
University of Hawaii
Hawaii Permanente Medical Group
Honolulu, Hawaii [72]

Mark Benson, MD
Associate Professor
Department of Medicine
Division of Gastroenterology and Hepatology
University of Wisconsin
Madison, Wisconsin [86]

Amy Berman, BS, RN, LHD (hon), FAAN
Senior Program Officer
The John A. Hartford Foundation
New York, New York [12]

Cheryl D. Bernstein, MD
Associate Professor
Departments of Anesthesiology and Perioperative
    Medicine and Neurology
University of Pittsburgh School of Medicine
Pittsburgh, Pennsylvania [103]

John Best, MD
Behavioral Neurology Clinical Fellow
Weill Institute for Neurosciences
Memory and Aging Center
University of California San Francisco
San Francisco, California [63]

Nirav R. Bhatt, MD
Assistant Professor of Neurology
Marcus Stroke and Neuroscience Center at Grady
    Memorial Hospital and Emory University
    School of Medicine
Atlanta, Georgia [62]

Jawad Bilal, MD
Clinical Assistant Professor
Division of Rheumatology, Department of Internal Medicine
University of Arizona Arthritis
Tucson, Arizona [52]

Ellen F. Binder, MD
Professor of Medicine
Program Director, Geriatric Medicine Fellowship Program
Washington University in St. Louis, School of Medicine
St. Louis, Missouri [53]

Joyce M. Black, PhD, RN, FAAN
Florence Niedfelt Professor
College of Nursing
University of Nebraska Medical Center
Omaha, Nebraska [46]

Caroline S. Blaum, MD, MS
Senior Research Scientist
National Committee for Quality Assurance
Washington, DC
Adjunct Professor Geriatric Medicine and Palliative Care
NYU Grossman School of Medicine
New York, New York [25]

Laura Block, BS, BSN, RN
Nurse, PhD Student
School of Nursing
University of Wisconsin-Madison
Madison, Wisconsin [6]

Nicolaas I. Bohnen MD, PhD
Professor of Radiology (Division of Nuclear Medicine)
    and Neurology
University of Michigan
Staff Neurologist & GRECC Investigator
VA Ann Arbor Healthcare System
Ann Arbor, Michigan [61]

Alice F. Bonner, PhD, RN, FAAN
Adjunct Faculty and Director of Strategic Partnership
CAPABLE Program
Johns Hopkins School of Nursing
Baltimore, Maryland [16]

Cynthia Boyd, MD, MPH
Professor of Medicine, Epidemiology and Health Policy
    and Management
Division of Geriatric Medicine and Gerontology
Center for Transformative Geriatric Research
Johns Hopkins University School of Medicine
Baltimore, Maryland [41]

Jennifer S. Brach, PT, PhD, FAPTA
Professor
Department of Physical Therapy
Associate Dean for Faculty Affairs and Development,
  School of Health and Rehabilitation Sciences
University of Pittsburgh
Pittsburgh, Pennsylvania [50]

Francesca Brancati, BS
Johns Hopkins University School of Medicine
Baltimore, Maryland [41]

Amber K. Brooks, MD
Associate Professor, Department of Anesthesiology
Wake Forest University School of Medicine
Winston Salem, North Carolina [68]

Cynthia J. Brown, MD, MSPH, FACP
Charles V. Sanders, MD Endowed Chair in
  Internal Medicine
Professor and Chair
Department of Medicine
Louisiana State University Health Sciences Center
New Orleans, Louisiana [55]

William Bryson, MD, MPH
Assistant Clinical Professor
Department of Psychiatry and Behavioral Sciences
University of Washington
Seattle, Washington [65]

Nitin Budhwar, MD
Associate Professor of Internal Medicine
Division of General Internal Medicine
Section Chief Geriatric Medicine
University of New Mexico
Albuquerque, New Mexico [83]

Daniel C. Butler, MD
Assistant Professor, Director of UCSF Aging Skin and
  Geriatric Dermatology Clinic
Department of Dermatology
University of California, San Francisco
San Francisco, California [93]

Mandy L. Byers, MD, CMD
Assistant Professor
Division of Geriatrics, Gerontology, and Palliative
  Medicine, Department of Internal Medicine
University of Nebraska Medical Center
Omaha, Nebraska [106]

Joseph M. Calabrese, DMD
Clinical Professor
Director of Geriatric Dental Medicine
Associate Dean of Students
Henry M. Goldman School of Dental Medicine
Boston University
Boston, Massachusetts [32]

Gerardo Calderon, MD
Physician Resident
Department of Medicine
Indiana University School of Medicine
Indianapolis, Indiana [87]

Brook Calton, MD, MHS
Division of Palliative Medicine and Geriatrics
The Massachusetts General Hospital
Boston, Massachusetts [71]

Anne R. Cappola, MD, ScM
Professor of Medicine
Division of Endocrinology, Diabetes, and Metabolism
Director, Penn Medical Communication Research Institute
Perelman School of Medicine at the University of
  Pennsylvania
Philadelphia, Pennsylvania [98]

Whitney L. Carlson, MD
Clinical Associate Professor
Department of Psychiatry and Behavioral Sciences
University of Washington
Seattle, Washington [65]

Cynthia M. Carlsson, MD, MS
Professor of Medicine
Division of Geriatrics and Gerontology
University of Wisconsin School of Medicine and
  Public Health
Madison, Wisconsin [59]

Christopher R. Carpenter, MD, MSc
Professor of Emergency Medicine
Department of Emergency Medicine
Washington University in St. Louis School of Medicine
St. Louis, Missouri [15]

Carol K. Chan, MBBCh, MSc
Clinical Assistant Professor
Department of Psychiatry
Case Western Reserve University School of Medicine
Cleveland, Ohio [60]

Elizabeth N. Chapman, MD
Associate Director, Education and Evaluation
Geriatrics Research Education and Clinical Center
William S. Middleton Memorial VA Medical Center
Madison, Wisconsin
Clinical Associate Professor
Department of Medicine – Division of Geriatrics and
  Gerontology
University of Wisconsin School of Medicine and
  Public Health
Madison, Wisconsin [18]

CONTRIBUTORS

xii **Nathaniel A. Chin, MD**
Assistant Professor of Medicine
Division of Geriatrics and Gerontology
University of Wisconsin School of Medicine and
    Public Health
Madison, Wisconsin [59]

Brenna Cholerton, PhD
Senior Research Scientist/Neuropsychologist
Department of Pathology
Stanford University School of Medicine
Stanford, California [57]

Monica Christmas, MD, NCMP
Associate Professor
Department of Obstetrics and Gynecology
University of Chicago
Chicago, Illinois [35]

Jacqueline C. T. Close, MBBS, MD, FRCP, FRACP
Geriatrician and Conjoint Professor
Prince of Wales Clinical School
University of New South Wales
Sydney, Australia [13]

Harvey Jay Cohen, MD
Walter Kempner Professor of Medicine
Director Emeritus, Center for the Study of Aging and
    Human Development
Chair Emeritus, Department of Medicine
Duke University Medical Center
Durham, North Carolina [88]

Jessica Colburn, MD
Assistant Professor of Medicine
Division of Geriatric Medicine & Gerontology
Johns Hopkins University School of Medicine
Baltimore, Maryland [17]

Lisa Cooper, MD
Division of Aging
Brigham and Woman's Hospital
Boston, Massachusetts
Department of Geriatric Medicine, Rabin Medical Center
Petach Tikva, Israel
Instructor of Medicine, Sackler Faculty of Medicine
Tel Aviv University
Tel Aviv, Israel [70]

Suzanne Craft, PhD
Professor of Medicine
Director, Wake Forest Alzheimer's Disease
    Research Center
Co-Director, Sticht Center on Healthy Aging and
    Alzheimer's Prevention
Wake Forest School of Medicine
Winston-Salem, North Carolina [57]

Alfonso J. Cruz-Jentoft, MD, PhD
Jefe del Servicio de Geriatría
Hospital Universitario Ramón y Cajal (IRYCIS)
Madrid, Spain [49]

Juan González del Castillo, MD, PhD
Head of the Infectious Disease Group
The Spanish Emergency Medicine Society
Head of Emergency Department
Clínico San Carlos Hospital
Madrid, Spain [105]

Shannon Devlin, MD
Instructor of Medicine
Department of Internal Medicine, Division of
    Palliative Medicine
Washington University in St. Louis School of Medicine
St. Louis, Missouri [67]

Maryama Diaw, MPH
Graduate Intern
The John A. Hartford Foundation
New York, New York [12]

Nikola Dobrilovic, MD
Assistant Professor of Surgery
Boston University School of Medicine
Boston, Massachusetts [75]

Liang Dong, MD
Post-doctoral Research Fellow
Brady Urological Institute
Johns Hopkins University School of Medicine
Baltimore, Maryland [90]

Margaret A. Drickamer, MD
Professor, Division of Geriatric Medicine & Palliative
    Care Program
Medical Director, UNC Home Hospice & Hospice Home
School of Medicine
University of North Carolina at Chapel Hill
Chapel Hill, North Carolina [10]

Catherine E. DuBeau, MD
Professor of Medicine
Department of Medicine
Section of General Internal Medicine – Geriatrics
Dartmouth-Hitchcock Medical Center
Lebanon, New Hampshire [38]

Ruth E. Dunkle, PhD
Wilbur J. Cohen Collegiate Professor of Social Work
School of Social Work
University of Michigan
Ann Arbor, Michigan [20]

Gustavo Duque, MD, PhD, FRACP, FGSA
Geriatrician, Chair of Medicine and Director of the
    Australian Institute for Musculoskeletal Science (AIMSS)
The University of Melbourne and Western Health
St Albans, Australia [51]

Katharina V. Echt, PhD
Associate Director Education and Evaluation
Veterans Affairs Birmingham/Atlanta Geriatric Research
    Education and Clinical Center (GRECC)
Associate Professor
Department of Medicine, Geriatrics and Gerontology
Emory University School of Medicine
Atlanta, Georgia [33]

Niloo M. Edwards, MD
Chief Cardiothoracic Surgery
Professor of Surgery
Boston University
Boston, Massachusetts [75]

Kristine M. Erlandson, MD
Associate Professor of Medicine and Epidemiology
Department of Medicine
Divisions of Infectious Diseases and Geriatric Medicine
University of Colorado—Anschutz Medical Campus
Aurora, Colorado [107]

Sara E. Espinoza, MD, MSc
Professor
Barshop Institute for Longevity and Aging Studies
University of Texas Health Science Center at San Antonio
Director, Geriatrics Research, Education and
    Clinical Center
South Texas Veterans Health Care System
San Antonio, Texas [40]

Timothy W. Farrell, MD, AGSF
Professor of Medicine
Geriatrics Division Associate Chief for Age-Friendly Care
Spencer Fox Eccles School of Medicine at the
    University of Utah
Physician Investigator, VA Salt Lake City Geriatric
    Research, Education, and Clinical Center
Salt Lake City, Utah [72]

Mizhgan Fatima, MBBS, FRACP
Geriatrician, Department of Geriatric Medicine,
    Western Health
Australian Institute for Musculoskeletal Science (AIMSS)
The University of Melbourne
St Albans, Australia [51]

Cynthia Felix, MD, PhD
Postdoctoral Associate
Department of Epidemiology
University of Pittsburgh
Pittsburgh, Pennsylvania [4]

Luigi Ferrucci, MD, PhD
Scientific Director
National Institute on Aging
National Institutes of Health
Baltimore, Maryland [42]

Tamara G. Fong, MD, PhD
Associate Professor of Neurology,
    Harvard Medical School
Staff Neurologist, Beth Israel Deaconess Medical Center
Assistant Scientist, Aging Brain Center, Institute for
    Aging Research, Hebrew SeniorLife
Boston, Massachusetts [58]

Laura Frain, MD, MPH
Director of Outpatient Geriatrics
Division of Aging
Brigham and Women's Hospital
Instructor of Medicine, Harvard Medical School
Boston, Massachusetts [70]

Marilisa Franceschi, MD, PhD
Endoscopic Unit, Department of Medicine
Azienda ULSS 7 Pedemontana - Alto Vicentino Hospital
Via Garziere, Santorso (Vicenza), Italy [85]

Kaitlyn Fruin, MD
Resident Physician
Department of Internal Medicine
University of California Los Angeles
Los Angeles, California [35]

Terry Fulmer, PhD, RN, FAAN
President
The John A. Hartford Foundation
New York, New York [12]

Ajeet Gajra, MD, FACP
Clinical Professor
Department of Medicine
SUNY Upstate Medical University and Hematology-
    Oncology Associates of Central New York
Syracuse, New York [91]

James E. Galvin, MD, MPH
Professor of Neurology
Chief, Division of Cognitive Neurology
Director, Comprehensive Center for Brain Health
University of Miami Miller School of Medicine
Miami, Florida [9]

Chandrika Garner, MD, FASE
Clinical Assistant Professor
Section on Cardiothoracic Anesthesiology
Department of Anesthesiology
Wake Forest School of Medicine
Winston Salem, North Carolina [28]

Kathleen M. Gavin, PhD
Assistant Professor
Department of Medicine, Division of Geriatric Medicine
University of Colorado Anschutz Medical Campus
Aurora, Colorado [54]

Sudeep S. Gill, MD, MSc, FRCPC
Associate Professor
Department of Medicine Division of Geriatric Medicine
Queen's University
Kingston, Ontario, Canada [22]

Andrea Gilmore-Bykovskyi, PhD, RN
Deputy Director, Center for Health Disparities Research
Associate Professor, School of Nursing
University of Wisconsin
Madison, Wisconsin [6] [18]

Carey E. Gleason, PhD
Associate Professor of Medicine
Division of Geriatrics and Gerontology
University of Wisconsin School of Medicine and
    Public Health
Madison, Wisconsin [59]

Parag Goyal, MD, MSc
Assistant Professor of Medicine
Director, Heart Failure with Preserved Ejection Fraction
    and Cardiac Amyloidosis Program
Weill Cornell Medicine
New York Presbyterian Hospital
New York, New York [76]

Len Gray, MBBS, MMed, PhD, FRACP, FACHSM, FAAG, FANZSGM
Director: Centre for Health Services Research
Faculty of Medicine
The University of Queensland
Brisbane, Australia [13]

Leanne Groban, MS, MD
Professor
Department of Anesthesiology
Wake Forest School of Medicine
Winston Salem, North Carolina [28]

Matthew E. Growdon, MD, MPH
Geriatrician and Aging Research Fellow
Division of Geriatrics
University of California, San Francisco
San Francisco, California [58]

Daniel Guidot, MD, MPH
Fellow
Division of Pulmonary and Critical Care
Duke University Medical Center
Durham, North Carolina [80]

Jerry H. Gurwitz, MD
The Dr. John Meyers Professor of Primary Care Medicine
Professor of Medicine, Family Medicine and Community
    Health, and Population & Quantitative Health Sciences
Chief, Division of Geriatric Medicine
Executive Director, Meyers Health Care Institute
UMass Chan Medical School
Worcester, Massachusetts [22]

Karen E. Hall, MD, PhD
Emeritus Professor of Medicine
Division of Geriatric and Palliative Medicine
University of Michigan
Ann Arbor, Michigan [84]

Jeffrey B. Halter, MD
Professor Emeritus
Department of Internal Medicine
Division of Geriatric and Palliative Medicine
University of Michigan
Parkway Visiting Professor in Geriatrics
Department of Medicine
Yong Loo Lin School of Medicine
National University of Singapore
Ann Arbor, Michigan [99]

Benjamin H. Han, MD, MPH
Assistant Professor
Division of Geriatrics, Gerontology, and Palliative Care
University of California, San Diego
La Jolla, California [23]

Lauren Hartman, MD
Assistant Professor
Gerontology and Geriatric Medicine
Atrium Health Wake Forest Baptist
Winston-Salem, North Carolina [108]

Jennifer Hayashi, MD
Assistant Professor of Medicine
Division of Geriatric Medicine & Gerontology
Johns Hopkins University School of Medicine
Baltimore, Maryland [17]

Kevin P. High, MD, MS
President, Atrium Health—Wake Forest Baptist
Professor of Internal Medicine–Infectious Diseases
Wake Forest School of Medicine
Winston-Salem, North Carolina [104]

Kerry L. Hildreth, MD
Assistant Professor
Division of Geriatrics, Department of Medicine
University of Colorado Anschutz Medical Campus
Aurora, Colorado [54]

Wendy Huang, MPH
Graduate Intern
The John A. Hartford Foundation
New York, New York [12]

Scott L. Hummel, MD, MS
Associate Professor of Medicine
Director, Heart Failure with Preserved Ejection
    Fraction Program
University of Michigan
Section Chief, Cardiology
VA Ann Arbor Healthcare System
Ann Arbor, Michigan [76]

CONTRIBUTORS

Ula Hwang, MD, MPH
Professor, Vice Chair for Research
Department of Emergency Medicine
Yale School of Medicine
New Haven, Connecticut
Core Physician Investigator
Geriatric Research, Education and Clinical Center
James J. Peters VA Medical Center
Bronx, New York [15]

Sharon K. Inouye, MD, MPH
Director, Aging Brain Center
Marcus Institute for Aging Research, Hebrew SeniorLife
Milton & Shirley F. Levy Family Chair
Professor of Medicine, Harvard Medical School
Staff Physician, Beth Israel Deaconess Medical Center
Boston, Massachusetts [58]

Nelia Jain, MD, MA
Director of Inpatient Adult Palliative Care Consultation
Department of Psychosocial Oncology and Palliative Care
Dana-Farber Cancer Institute/Brigham and
    Women's Hospital
Instructor of Medicine, Harvard Medical School
Boston, Massachusetts [70]

Dilip V. Jeste, MD
Senior Associate Dean for Healthy Aging and Senior Care
Estelle and Edgar Levi Chair in Aging
UC San Diego Center for Healthy Aging
Distinguished Professor of Psychiatry and Neurosciences
Director, Sam and Rose Stein Institute for
    Research on Aging
Department of Psychiatry, University of California,
    San Diego
San Diego, California [66]

Jason M. Johanning, MD, MS
Professor of Surgery
Vice Chair for Surgery: Quality and Compliance
Medical Director, VA Surgery Quality Improvement
    Program
University of Nebraska Medical Center
Omaha, Nebraska [78]

Larry E. Johnson, MD, PhD
Central Arkansas Veterans Healthcare System
Associate Professor of Geriatrics, and Family and
    Preventive Medicine
University of Arkansas for Medical Sciences
Little Rock, Arkansas [30]

Theodore M. Johnson, II, MD, MPH, AGS-Fellow
Paul Seavey Chair and Chief, General Internal Medicine
Chair, Family and Preventive Medicine
Investigator, Birmingham/Atlanta VA GRECC
Atlanta, Georgia [47]

Judith A. Jones, DDS, MPH, DScD
Professor
University of Detroit Mercy School of Dentistry
Detroit, Michigan [32]

Jamie N. Justice, PhD
Assistant Professor
Department of Internal Medicine
Section on Gerontology & Geriatrics, Sticht Center on
    Healthy Aging and Alzheimer's Prevention
Wake Forest School of Medicine
Winston-Salem, North Carolina [40]

Robert Kalayjian, MD
Professor of Medicine
Department of Medicine, MetroHealth System
Case Western Reserve University School of Medicine
Cleveland, Ohio [94]

Jennifer M. Kapo, MD
Associate Professor of Palliative Medicine
Chief, Palliative Medicine, Palliative Care Program
Section of Palliative Medicine
Division of Geriatrics
Yale University School of Medicine
New Haven, Connecticut [81]

Marshall B. Kapp, JD, MPH
Professor Emeritus
Center for Innovative Collaboration in Medicine and Law
Florida State University, College of Medicine and
    College of Law
Tallahassee, Florida [26]

Jay Kayser, MSW, LCSW
PhD Student
School of Social Work and Department of
    Developmental Psychology
University of Michigan
Ann Arbor, Michigan [20]

Dae Hyun Kim, MD, MPH, ScD
Associate Professor of Medicine
Harvard Medical School
Hinda and Arthur Marcus Institute for Aging Research
Hebrew SeniorLife
Boston, Massachusetts [75]

Amy J. H. Kind, MD, PhD
Associate Dean for Social Health Sciences and Programs
Director, UW Center for Health Disparities Research
Professor, Department of Medicine
University of Wisconsin School of Medicine and
    Public Health
Madison, Wisconsin [6] [18]

xvi Daniel Kirsch, BA
MD/PhD Candidate
Boston University School of Medicine
Jamaica Plain VA Medical Center
Boston, Massachusetts [64]

Dalane W. Kitzman, MD
Professor of Internal Medicine
Sections on Cardiovascular Medicine and
    Geriatrics/Gerontology
Wake Forest School of Medicine
Winston-Salem, North Carolina [73]

Heidi D. Klepin, MD, MS
Professor
Department of Medicine
Section on Hematology and Oncology
Wake Forest School of Medicine
Winston-Salem, North Carolina [95]

Nway Le Ko Ko, MD
Cardiology Fellow
Mayo Clinic College of Medicine
Department of Cardiovascular Diseases
Mayo Clinic Arizona
Phoenix, Arizona [77]

Vikas Kotagal, MD, MS
Associate Professor of Neurology
University of Michigan
Staff Neurologist & GRECC Investigator
VA Ann Arbor Healthcare System
Ann Arbor, Michigan [61]

Ashwin A. Kotwal, MD, MS
Assistant Professor of Medicine
Division of Geriatrics
UCSF and San Francisco VA Medical Center
San Francisco, California [11]

George A. Kuchel, MD CM, AGSF
Professor and Travelers Chair in Geriatrics and
    Gerontology
Director, UConn Center on Aging
Chief, Geriatric Medicine
University of Connecticut and UConn Health
Farmington, Connecticut [39] [40]

Alexis Kuerbis, LCSW, PhD
Associate Professor
Silberman School of Social Work
Hunter College
New York, New York [23]

Jeffrey T. Kullgren, MD, MS, MPH
Research Scientist
VA Center for Clinical Management Research
VA Ann Arbor Healthcare System
Associate Professor
Department of Internal Medicine
Division of General Medicine
University of Michigan
Ann Arbor, Michigan [21]

Anita J. Kumar, MD, MSc
Assistant Professor
Department of Medicine
Tufts University School of Medicine
Boston, Massachusetts [95]

Hiroko Kunitake, MD, MPH
Assistant Professor, Harvard Medical School
Department of Surgery
Massachusetts General Hospital
Boston, Massachusetts [29]

C. Kent Kwoh, MD
Professor of Medicine and Medical Imaging
Division of Rheumatology, Department of Medicine, and
    University of Arizona Arthritis Center
University of Arizona College of Medicine and Banner
    University Medical Center
Tucson, Arizona [52]

Mark S. Lachs, MD, MPH
Psaty Distinguished Professor of Medicine
Weill Cornell Medicine
Director of Geriatrics
New York Presbyterian Health System
New York, New York [48]

Jeffrey Lam, BA
Warren Alpert Medical School of Brown University
Providence, Rhode Island [66]

Ellen E. Lee, MD
Assistant Professor of Psychiatry
University of California, San Diego
Staff Psychiatrist
Veterans Affairs San Diego Healthcare System
San Diego, California [66]

Jiha Lee, MD, MHS
Assistant Professor
University of Michigan
Ann Arbor, Michigan [101]

Patty J. Lee, MD
Professor of Medicine, Cell Biology & Pathology
Division of Pulmonary, Allergy and Critical Care
Duke University School of Medicine
Durham, North Carolina [80] [81]

Pearl G. Lee, MD
Clinical Associate Professor
Department of Internal Medicine
Division of Geriatric and Palliative Medicine
University of Michigan
Geriatric Research Education and Clinical Center
  (GRECC)
VA Ann Arbor Healthcare System
Ann Arbor, Michigan [99]

Sei J. Lee, MD, MAS
Professor of Medicine
Division of Geriatrics
UCSF and San Francisco VA Medical Center
San Francisco, California [11]

Bruce Leff, MD
Professor of Medicine
Division of Geriatric Medicine & Gerontology
Johns Hopkins University School of Medicine
Baltimore, Maryland [17]

Bernardo Liberato, MD
Assistant Professor of Neurology
Marcus Stroke and Neuroscience Center at Grady
  Memorial Hospital and Emory University
  School of Medicine
Atlanta, Georgia [62]

Ming Y. Lim, M.B.B.Chir
Associate Professor
Department of Internal Medicine
Division of Hematology and Hematologic Malignancies
University of Utah
Salt Lake City, Utah [96]

Stacy Tessler Lindau, MD, MAPP
Professor
Departments of Obstetrics and Gynecology and
  Medicine-Geriatrics and Palliative Medicine
University of Chicago
Chicago, Illinois [35]

Lewis A. Lipsitz, MD
Professor of Medicine, Harvard Medical School
Chief Academic Officer and Director, Marcus Institute for
  Aging Research, Hebrew Senior Life
Chief, Division of Gerontology, Beth Israel Deaconess
  Medical Center
Editor-in-Chief, *Journal of Gerontology Medical Sciences*
Boston, Massachusetts [45]

Julia Loewenthal, MD
Instructor in Medicine
Harvard Medical School
Division of Aging
Brigham and Women's Hospital
Boston, Massachusetts [24]

David B. Lombard, MD, PhD
Associate Professor
Department of Pathology
University of Michigan
Ann Arbor, Michigan [1]

Stephen R. Lord, PhD, DSc
Professor
Senior Principal Research Fellow
Falls Balance and Injury Research Centre
Neuroscience Research Australia
University of New South Wales
Sydney, Australia [43]

Michael R. Lucey, MD, FRCPI, FAASLD
Professor of Medicine
Chief, Division of Gastroenterology and Hepatology
Co-Medical Director, UW Digestive Health Center
Medical Director, UW Liver Transplant Program
University of Wisconsin School of Medicine and
  Public Health
Madison, Wisconsin [86]

Hillary D. Lum, MD, PhD
Division of Geriatric Medicine
Department of Medicine
University of Colorado School of Medicine
Aurora, Colorado [7]

Constantine G. Lyketsos, MD, MHS
Chair, Department of Psychiatry and
  Behavioral Sciences, Johns Hopkins Bayview
Elizabeth Plank Althouse Professor, Johns
  Hopkins University
Director, Richman Family Precision Medicine Center of
  Excellence in Alzheimer's Disease
Director, Johns Hopkins Memory and
  Alzheimer's Treatment Center
Baltimore, Maryland [60]

Tanya Mailhot, RN, PhD
Researcher, Montreal Heart Institute Research Center
Assistant Professor, Faculty of Nursing
Université de Montréal
Montréal, Canada [58]

Una E. Makris, MD, MSc
Assistant Professor
Department of Internal Medicine, Division of
  Rheumatic Diseases
UT Southwestern Medical Center
Dallas, Texas [102]

Preeti N. Malani, MD, MSJ
Chief Health Officer
Professor of Medicine
University of Michigan
Ann Arbor, Michigan [21]

CONTRIBUTORS

CONTRIBUTORS

Michael L. Malone, MD
Medical Director, Aurora Senior Services &
    Aurora at Home
Geriatrics Fellowship Director, Aurora Sinai Medical Center
Clinical Adjunct Professor of Medicine
University of Wisconsin School of Medicine &
    Public Health
Co-Editor, *Journal of Geriatric Emergency Medicine* (JGEM)
Section Editor, *Journal of the American Geriatrics
    Society* (JAGS)
Models of Geriatric Care, Quality Improvement and
    Program Dissemination
Milwaukee, Wisconsin [14]

Mark C. Markowski, MD, PhD
Assistant Professor
Department of Oncology
Johns Hopkins University School of Medicine
Baltimore, Maryland [90]

Michelle M. Marrero, MD
Instructor of Neurology
Division of Cognitive Neurology
Department of Neurology
University of Miami Miller School of Medicine
Miami, Florida [9]

Finbarr C. Martin, MD, MSc, FRCP
Emeritus Geriatrician and Professor of Medical
    Gerontology
Population Health Sciences, Faculty of Life Sciences and
    Medicine
King's College London
London, United Kingdom [13]

Kedar S. Mate, MD
President and Chief Executive Officer
Institute for Healthcare Improvement
Boston, Massachusetts
Department of Medicine
Weill Cornell Medical College
New York, New York [12]

Daniel D. Matlock, MD, MPH
Division Head (Interim), Division of Geriatrics
Director, Colorado Program for Patient Centered
    Decisions
Associate Professor of Medicine
University of Colorado School of Medicine
Aurora, Colorado [7]

Alvin M. Matsumoto, MD
Professor Emeritus, Department of Medicine
Division of Gerontology and Geriatric Medicine
University of Washington School of Medicine
Clinical Investigator, Geriatric Research, Education and
    Clinical Center
VA Puget Sound Health Care System
Seattle, Washington [37] [97]

Mathew S. Maurer, MD
Arnold and Arlene Goldstein Professor of Cardiology
Professor of Medicine
Director, Clinical Cardiovascular Research Laboratory
    for the Elderly
Columbia University Irving Medical Center
New York Presbyterian Hospital
New York, New York [76]

Nadine J. McCleary, MD, MPH
Assistant Professor of Medicine, Harvard Medical School
Senior Physician, Dana-Farber Cancer Institute
Boston, Massachusetts [92]

Shelley R. McDonald, DO, PhD
Associate Professor
Department of Medicine
Division of Geriatrics
Duke University Medical Center
Durham, North Carolina [27]

Ann C. McKee, MD
William Fairfield Warren Distinguished Professor of
    Neurology and Pathology
Director of Neuropathology VA Boston
Director of the BU Chronic Traumatic Encephalopathy
    (CTE) Center
Boston University School of Medicine
Boston, Massachusetts [64]

Simon Mears, MD, PhD
Professor of Orthopedic Surgery
University of Arkansas for Medical Sciences
Little Rock, Arkansas [53]

Darshan H. Mehta, MD, MPH
Assistant Professor of Medicine
Harvard Medical School
Education Director
Osher Center for Integrative Medicine
Brigham and Women's Hospital and
    Harvard Medical School
Boston, Massachusetts [24]

Jasmine C. Menant, PhD
Research Fellow
Falls Balance and Injury Research Centre
Neuroscience Research Australia
University of New South Wales
Sydney, Australia [43]

David J. Meyers, PhD, MPH
Assistant Professor
Department of Health Services, Policy, and Practice
Brown University School of Public Health
Providence, Rhode Island [19]

Christine Miaskowski, RN, PhD, FAAN
Professor of Physiological Nursing
School of Nursing, University of California
University of California San Francisco School
of Nursing
San Francisco, California [69]

Bruce Miller, MD
A.W. and Mary Margaret Clausen Distinguished Professor
of Neurology
Director, Memory and Aging Center
University of California, San Francisco
San Francisco, California [63]

Richard A. Miller, MD, PhD
Professor
Department of Pathology
University of Michigan
Ann Arbor, Michigan [1]

Alison A. Moore, MD, MPH, FACP, AGSF
Professor of Medicine
Larry L. Hillblom Chair in Geriatric Medicine
Chief, Division of Geriatrics, Gerontology,
and Palliative Care
University of California, San Diego
La Jolla, California [23]

Kerrie L. Moreau, PhD
Professor
Department of Medicine, Division of Geriatrics
University of Colorado Anschutz Medical Campus
Aurora, Colorado [54]

Hyman B. Muss, MD
Mary Jones Hudson Distinguished Professor of
Geriatric Oncology
Professor of Medicine
Director of Geriatric Oncology, Lineberger
Comprehensive Cancer Center
University of North Carolina
Chapel Hill, North Carolina [89]

Vivek Nagaraja, MD
Clinical Associate Professor
Division of Rheumatology
Department of Internal Medicine
University of Michigan
Ann Arbor, Michigan [100]

Aanand D. Naik, MD
Professor and Nancy P. & Vincent F. Guinee, MD
Distinguished Chair
Department of Management, Policy and Community
Health, University of Texas School of Public Health
Executive Director, UTHealth Institute on Aging
University of Texas Health Science Center
Houston, Texas
Investigator, Houston Center for Innovations in Quality,
Effectiveness and Safety
Michael E. DeBakey VA Medical Center
Houston, Texas [25]

Abhijit S. Naik, MD, MPH, FASN
Assistant Professor of Internal Medicine
Division of Nephrology
University of Michigan
Ann Arbor, Michigan [82]

Michael G. Nanna, MD, MHS
Assistant Professor of Medicine/Cardiology
Yale School of Medicine
New Haven, Connecticut [74]

Anne B. Newman, MD, MPH
Distinguished Professor and Chair
Department of Epidemiology, Graduate School of
Public Health
University of Pittsburgh
Pittsburgh, Pennsylvania [2]

John C. Newman, MD, PhD
Assistant Professor
Buck Institute for Research on Aging
Division of Geriatrics
University of California San Francisco
Novato, California [40]

Ryan D. Nipp, MD
Assistant Professor of Medicine
Medical Oncology at Stephenson Cancer Center
University of Oklahoma Health Sciences Center
Oklahoma City, Oklahoma [92]

Stephanie Nothelle, MD
Assistant Professor of Medicine and Health Policy and
Management
Division of Geriatric Medicine and Gerontology
Center for Transformative Geriatric Research
Johns Hopkins University School of Medicine
Baltimore, Maryland [41]

Michele R. Obert, MD
Internal Medicine Resident
Department of Medicine
University of Arizona
Tucson, Arizona [52]

xx **Michelle C. Odden, PhD**
Associate Professor
Department of Epidemiology and Population Health
Stanford School of Medicine
Stanford University
Stanford, California [2]

Suzanne Olbricht, MD
Chief of Dermatology
Beth Israel Dermatology, Beth Israel Deaconess
  Medical Center
Associate Professor of Dermatology
Harvard Medical School
Boston, Massachusetts [93]

Christopher D. Ortengren, MD
Senior Resident Physician
Department of Surgery
Section of Urology
Dartmouth-Hitchcock Medical Center
One Medical Center Drive
Lebanon, New Hampshire [38]

Joseph G. Ouslander, MD
Professor of Geriatric Medicine
Senior Advisor to the Dean for Geriatrics
Charles E. Schmidt College of Medicine
Professor (Courtesy), Christine E. Lynn
  College of Nursing
Florida Atlantic University
Boca Raton, Florida [16] [19]

Ambarish Pandey, MD, MSCS
Assistant Professor of Internal Medicine
Division of Cardiology
University of Texas Southwestern Medical Center
Dallas, Texas [73]

Changsu Park, MD
Department of Medicine, MetroHealth System
Case Western Reserve University School of Medicine
Cleveland, Ohio [94]

Jino Park, PhD
Assistant Professor
Division of Hematology/Oncology
Department of Medicine, MetroHealth System
Case Western Reserve University School of Medicine
Cleveland, Ohio [94]

Sanjeevkumar R. Patel, MD, MS
Associate Professor
Department of Internal Medicine
University of Michigan
Ann Arbor, Michigan [82]

Leslie Pelton, MPA
Vice President
Institute for Healthcare Improvement
Boston, Massachusetts [12]

Angela K. Perone, PhD, JD, MSW, MA
Assistant Professor
University of California, Berkeley
School of Social Welfare
Berkeley, California [20]

Kenneth J. Pienta, MD
Professor
Brady Urological Institute
Johns Hopkins University School of Medicine
Baltimore, Maryland [90]

Robert J. Pignolo, MD, PhD
Chair, Division of Geriatric Medicine & Gerontology
Robert and Arlene Kogod Professor of Geriatric Medicine
Mayo Clinic College of Medicine
Rochester, Minnesota [40]

Alberto Pilotto, MD
Director Geriatrics Unit
Director Department Geriatric Care, OrthoGeriatrics
  and Rehabilitation
Galliera Hospital
Genova, Italy
Full Professor in Geriatrics
Department of Interdisciplinary Medicine
University of Bari "Aldo Moro"
Bari, Italy [85]

Scott D. Pletcher, PhD
Professor
Department of Molecular and Integrative Physiology
University of Michigan
Ann Arbor, Michigan [1]

Jennifer D. Possick, MD
Associate Professor of Medicine
Section of Pulmonary, Critical Care and Sleep Medicine
Yale University School of Medicine
New Haven, Connecticut
Medical Director, Winchester Center for Lung Disease
  and Director, Post-COVID Recovery Program
Yale-New Haven Hospital
North Haven, Connecticut [81]

Bayard L. Powell, MD
Professor, Department of Medicine
Section on Hematology and Oncology
Wake Forest School of Medicine
Winston-Salem, North Carolina [95]

Thomas Clark Powell, MD, MPH
Fellow, Division of Urogynecology and Pelvic
  Reconstructive Surgery
Instructor, Department of Obstetrics and Gynecology
University of Alabama at Birmingham
Birmingham, Alabama [36]

W. Ryan Powell, PhD, MA
Scientist, UW Center for Health Disparities Research
(CHDR)
University of Wisconsin School of Medicine and
Public Health
Madison, Wisconsin [6]

Aishwarya Pradeep, BS
Medical Student
Mayo Clinic Alix School of Medicine
Rochester, Minnesota [103]

Carolyn J. Presley, MD, MHS
Assistant Professor, Associate Medical Director
Oncogeriatrics Program
Division of Medical Oncology, Department of
Internal Medicine
The Ohio State University Comprehensive Cancer Center
Oncogeriatrics Program
Columbus, Ohio [88] [91]

Luigi Puglielli, MD, PhD
Professor of Medicine
Division of Geriatrics and Gerontology
Professor of Neuroscience
Waisman Center
University of Wisconsin School of Medicine and
Public Health
Geriatric Research, Education and Clinical Center (GRECC)
William S. Middleton Memorial Veterans Hospital
Madison, Wisconsin [56] [59]

M. Carrington Reid, MD, PhD
Professor of Medicine
Department of Medicine
Weill Cornell Medical College
New York, New York [102]

Christina Reppas-Rindlisbacher, MD, FRCPC
Clinical Associate
Department of Medicine, Division of Geriatric Medicine
University of Toronto
Toronto, Ontario, Canada [22]

David B. Reuben, MD
Archstone Professor of Medicine/Geriatrics
David Geffen School of Medicine at UCLA
Los Angeles, California [8]

Holly E. Richter, PhD, MD
The Endowed Chair of Obstetrics and Gynecology
Professor of Obstetrics and Gynecology, Urology and
Geriatrics
Research Director, Division of Urogynecology and Pelvic
Reconstructive Surgery
Associate Director, Gynecologic Research, Center for
Women's Reproductive Health
Medical and Quality Officer, Ambulatory OBGYN Clinics
University of Alabama at Birmingham
Birmingham, Alabama [36]

Christine S. Ritchie, MD, MSPH
Kenneth L. Minaker Endowed Chair in Geriatric Medicine
Director, Mongan Institute Center for Aging and
Serious Illness
Professor of Medicine
Massachusetts General Hospital and
Harvard Medical School
Boston, Massachusetts [69]

JoAnne Robbins, PhD
Professor Emerita
Department of Medicine
University of Wisconsin-Madison School of Medicine and
Public Health
Madison, Wisconsin [31]

Ria Roberts, MD
Clinical Instructor in Medicine, Harvard Medical School
Director, GME Diversity Inclusion and Advocacy
Director, Diversity Recruitment & Retention, BIDMC
Internal Medicine Residency Program
Boston, Massachusett [45]

Luis Miguel Gutierrez Robledo, MD, PhD
Founding Director
National Institute of Geriatric Medicine at the National
Institutes of Health Mexico
Mexico City, Mexico [13]

Carolyn L. Rochester, MD
Professor of Medicine
Director, Yale COPD Program
Section of Pulmonary, Critical Care and Sleep Medicine
Yale University School of Medicine
New Haven, Connecticut
Director, Pulmonary Rehabilitation Program
VA Connecticut Healthcare System
West Haven, Connecticut [81]

Paula A. Rochon MD, MPH, FRCPC
Founding Director, Women's Age Lab
Women's College Hospital
Professor, Department of Medicine, Division of Geriatric
Medicine and Dalla Lana School of Public Health
RTO/ERO Chair in Geriatric Medicine
University of Toronto
Toronto, Ontario, Canada [22]

Nicole Rogus-Pulia, PhD, CCC-SLP
Assistant Professor
Division of Geriatrics and Gerontology,
Department of Medicine
University of Wisconsin-Madison School of Medicine and
Public Health
Director of Swallowing and Salivary Bioscience Lab
Geriatric Research Education and Clinical Center (GRECC)
William S. Middleton Memorial Veterans Hospital
Madison, Wisconsin [31]

CONTRIBUTORS

Caterina Rosano, MD, MPH
Professor and Vice Chair of Research in Epidemiology
School of Public Health
University of Pittsburgh
Pittsburgh, Pennsylvania [50]

Howie Rosen, MD
Professor of Neurology
Weill Institute for Neurosciences
Memory and Aging Center
University of California San Francisco
San Francisco, California [63]

Tony Rosen, MD, MPH
Associate Professor of Emergency Medicine
Department of Emergency Medicine, Division of Geriatric
    Emergency Medicine
Program Director, Vulnerable Elder Protection Team
    (VEPT)
Weill Cornell Medicine / New York-Presbyterian Hospital
New York, New York [48]

Jeanette S. Ross, MD, FAAHPM, AGSF
Clinical Professor
University of Texas Health Sciences Center at
    San Antonio
Medical Director for GEC Transitions of Care
South Texas Veterans Health Care System
San Antonio, Texas [67]

Matthew L. Russell, MD
Instructor of Medicine
Division of Palliative Care and Geriatric Medicine
Massachusetts General Hospital/Harvard Medical school
Boston, Massachusetts [71]

Armand Ryden, MD
Assistant Professor
Division of Pulmonary, Critical Care, and Sleep Medicine
Veterans Affairs Greater Los Angeles Healthcare System
University of California Los Angeles
Los Angeles, California [44]

Bonnie C. Sachs, PhD, ABPP
Associate Professor
Departments of Neurology
Department of Internal Medicine – Section of
    Gerontology & Geriatric Medicine
Wake Forest School of Medicine
Winston-Salem, North Carolina [57]

Jane S. Saczynski, PhD
Professor
Department of Pharmacy & Health System Sciences
Northeastern University
Boston, Massachusetts [58]

Francisco Javier Martín Sánchez, MD, PhD
Associate Professor of Medicine
Complutense University
Emergency Department
Clínico San Carlos Hospital
Madrid, Spain [105]

Jochen Schacht, PhD
Professor of Biological Chemistry in Otolaryngology
Department of Otolaryngology - Head & Neck Surgery
University of Michigan Medical School
Ann Arbor, Michigan [34]

Kenneth Schmader, MD
Professor of Medicine-Geriatrics
Duke University Medical Center
Director, Geriatric Research Education and Clinical
    Center (GRECC)
Durham VA Health Care System
Durham, North Carolina [107]

Kara C. Schvartz-Leyzac, AuD, PhD
Assistant Professor
Department of Otolaryngology - Head & Neck Surgery
Medical University of South Carolina
Charleston, South Carolina [34]

Mina S. Sedrak, MD, MS
Assistant Professor
Medical Oncology & Therapeutics Research
City of Hope
Duarte, California [88] [89]

Su-Hua Sha, MD
Professor
Department of Pathology and Laboratory Medicine
Medical University of South Carolina
Charleston, South Carolina [34]

Jay P. Shah, MD
Physiatrist/Associate Research Physician
Rehabilitation Medicine Department
National Institutes of Health
Bethesda, Maryland [103]

Albert C. Shaw, MD, PhD
Professor of Medicine
Section of Infectious Diseases
Yale School of Medicine
New Haven, Connecticut [3]

Win-Kuang Shen, MD
Professor of Medicine
Mayo Clinic College of Medicine
Mayo Clinic Arizona
Phoenix, Arizona [77]

CONTRIBUTORS

Valerie Shuman, PT, DPT
Board-certified Clinical Specialist in Geriatric
    Physical Therapy
University of Pittsburgh
Pittsburgh, Pennsylvania [50]

Kendra D. Sims, PhD
Postdoctoral Scholar
Department of Epidemiology and Biostatistics
Stanford University
San Francsico, California [2]

Alexander Smith, MD, MPH, MS
Professor of Medicine
School of Medicine
University of California San Francisco
San Francisco, California [69]

Laurie D. Snyder, MD, MHS
Associate Professor of Medicine
Duke University
Durham, North Carolina [80]

Erica S. Solway, PhD, MSW, MPH
Manager, Signature Initiatives and Partnerships
Institute for Healthcare Policy and Innovation
University of Michigan
Ann Arbor, Michigan [21]

Shreya A. Sreekantaswamy, BS
Geriatric Dermatology Research and Clinical
    Student Fellow
Department of Dermatology
University of California San Francisco
San Francisco, California
Medical Student
University of Utah
Salt Lake City, Utah [93]

Nathan M. Stall, MD, FRCPC
Geriatrics and Internal Medicine
Sinai Health System and the University Health Network
    Hospitals
Departments of Medicine and Health Policy, Management
    and Evaluation
Women's College Research Institute
University of Toronto
Toronto, Ontario, Canada [22]

Dylan Stanfield, MD
Fellow, Division of Gastroenterology and Hepatology
Department of Medicine
University of Wisconsin School of Medicine
    and Public Health
Madison, Wisconsin [86]

Russell Stanley
Instructor/Fellow
Division of Urogynecology and Pelvic Reconstructive
    Surgery
Department of Obstetrics and Gynecology
University of Alabama at Birmingham
Birmingham, Alabama [36]

Sarah Stoneking, MD
Clinical Geriatric Fellow
Division of Geriatric Medicine
University of North Carolina at Chapel Hill
Chapel Hill, North Carolina [10]

Stephanie Studenski, MD, MPH
Professor Emeritus
University of Pittsburgh
Pittsburgh, Pennsylvania [13]

Dennis H. Sullivan, MD
Director, Geriatric Research Education and
    Clinical Center
VISN 16/Central Arkansas Veterans Healthcare System
Professor and Vice Chairman, Donald W. Reynolds
    Department of Geriatrics
University of Arkansas for Medical Sciences
Little Rock, Arkansas [30]

Mark A. Supiano, MD
D. Keith Barnes, MD and Dottie Barnes Presidential
    Endowed Chair in Medicine
Professor and Chief, Geriatrics Division, University of
    Utah School of Medicine
Executive Director, University of Utah Center on Aging
Salt Lake City, Utah [79]

Christine M. Swanson, MD, MCR
Assistant Professor
Division of Endocrinology, Metabolism and Diabetes
University of Colorado Anschutz Medical Campus
Aurora, Colorado [54]

George E. Taffet, MD
Professor of Medicine
Sections of Geriatrics and Cardiovascular Research
Baylor College of Medicine
Houston, Texas [73]

H. Keipp Talbot, MD, MPH
Associate Professor
Departments of Medicine and Health Policy
Vanderbilt University Medical Center
Nashville, Tennessee [108]

Shaida Talebreza, MD, AGSF, FAAHPM
Professor, Division of Geriatrics, University of Utah
Associate Chief of Staff, Geriatrics, Palliative, &
    Extended Care Service
George E. Wahlen Veterans Affairs Medical Center
Salt Lake City, Utah [67]

CONTRIBUTORS

Paul Tatum, MD, MSPH, CMD, FAAPM, AGSF
Associate Clinical Professor of Medicine
Department of Internal Medicine
Washington University School of Medicine
St. Louis, Missouri [67]

Jonny Macias Tejada, MD, AGSF
Medical Director, Acute Care for Elders (ACE) Program
    and AGS CoCare: Hospital Elder Life Program (HELP)
Aurora St. Luke's Medical Center
Clinical Adjunct Associate Professor
University of Wisconsin School of Medicine and
    Public Health
Milwaukee, Wisconsin [14]

J. Lisa Tenover, MD, PhD
Clinical Professor of Medicine/Geriatrics (Affiliated)
Stanford University School of Medicine, Stanford, CA
GRECC (182B)
VA Palo Alto Health Care System
Palo Alto, California [37]

Stephen Thielke, MD, MS
Professor
Psychiatry and Behavioral Sciences
University of Washington
Seattle, Washington [65]

Jonathan R. Thompson, MD, RPVI, FACS
Assistant Professor of Surgery
Program Director, Vascular Surgery Fellowship
Department of Surgery
University of Nebraska Medical Center
Omaha, Nebraska [78]

Bruce R. Troen, MD, AGSF
Professor and Chief, Division of Geriatrics and
    Palliative Medicine
Physician-Investigator, Veterans Affairs Western
    New York Healthcare System
Director, Center for Successful Aging
Director, Center of Excellence for Alzheimer's Disease
Jacobs School of Medicine and Biomedical Sciences
University at Buffalo
Buffalo, New York [51]

William Tse, MD, FACP
Professor of Medicine
Division of Hematology/Oncology
Department of Medicine, MetroHealth System
Case Western Reserve University School of Medicine
Cleveland, Ohio [94]

Mark Unruh, MD, MS
Professor and Chair of Internal Medicine
Division of Nephrology
New Mexico VA
University of New Mexico
Albuquerque, New Mexico [83]

Bharathi Upadhya, MD
Associate Professor of Internal Medicine
Section on Cardiovascular Medicine
Wake Forest School of Medicine
Winston-Salem, North Carolina [73]

Ryan J. Uyan, MD
Clinical Instructor
David Geffen School of Medicine at UCLA
Los Angeles, California [8]

Victor Valcour, MD, PhD
Professor
Department of Neurology and Division of
    Geriatric Medicine
University of California San Francisco
San Francisco, California [63]

Camille P. Vaughan, MD, MS
Atlanta Site Director, Birmingham/Atlanta VA GRECC
Assistant Professor
Division of Geriatrics & Gerontology,
    Department of Medicine
Emory University School of Medicine
Atlanta, Georgia [47]

Elizabeth K. Vig, MD, MPH
Associate Professor of Medicine
Division of Gerontology and Geriatric Medicine
University of Washington
Staff Physician
VA Puget Sound Health Care System
Seattle, Washington [72]

Ernest R. Vina, MD, MS
Associate Professor of Medicine
Section of Rheumatology
Lewis Katz School of Medicine
Temple University
Philadelphia, Pennsylvania [52]

Caroline A. Vitale, MD
Professor of Internal Medicine
Division of Geriatric and Palliative Medicine
University of Michigan & VA Ann Arbor
    Healthcare System
Ann Arbor, Michigan [72]

Jeffrey I. Wallace, MD, MPH
Professor of Medicine
Division of Gerontology and Geriatric Medicine
University of Colorado Denver
Aurora, Colorado [30]

Jeremy D. Walston, MD
Raymond and Anna Lublin Professor of
    Geriatric Medicine
Johns Hopkins University School of Medicine
Baltimore, Maryland [42]

Jiasheng Wang, MS, MD
Department of Medicine, MetroHealth System
Case Western Reserve University School of Medicine
Cleveland, Ohio [94]

Gale R. Watson, MEd, CLVT
Director, National Blind Rehabilitation Service (Retired)
Department of Veterans Affairs
Washington, DC [33]

Peter M. Wayne, PhD
Associate Professor of Medicine
Harvard Medical School
Director, Osher Center for Integrative Medicine
Brigham and Women's Hospital and Harvard Medical School
Boston, Massachusetts [24]

Debra K. Weiner, MD
Professor of Medicine, Psychiatry, Anesthesiology and
    Clinical & Translational Science
University of Pittsburgh School of Medicine
Associate Director for Research
VA Pittsburgh Healthcare System Geriatric Research,
    Education & Clinical Center
Pittsburgh, Pennsylvania [103]

Jonathan Weiss, MD
Dermatologist
Department of Dermatology
Beth Israel Deaconess Medical Center
Boston, Massachusetts [93]

Sarah J. Wherry, PhD
Assistant Professor
Division of Geriatric Medicine
University of Colorado Anschutz Medical Campus
Aurora, Colorado [54]

Eric Widera, MD
Professor of Clinical Medicine
Division of Geriatrics
University of California San Francisco (UCSF)
Director, Hospice and Palliative Care, San Francisco VA
San Francisco, California [67]

Jocelyn Wiggins, MA, BM, BCh, MRCP
Professor of Internal Medicine
Division of Geriatrics and Palliative Care
University of Michigan
Ann Arbor, Michigan [82]

Tanya M. Wildes, MD, MSCI
Associate Professor of Medicine Division of Oncology,
    Section of Medical Oncology
Washington University School of Medicine
St. Louis, Missouri [95]

Heidi Wold, MSN, APRN, ANP-BC
Chief Clinical Officer
Longevity Health Plans
Palm Beach Gardens, Florida [19]

Valerie S. Wong, MD
Clinical Instructor
David Geffen School of Medicine at UCLA
Los Angeles, California [8]

Gloria Y. Yeh, MD, MPH
Associate Professor of Medicine, Harvard Medical School
Director of Clinical Research, Osher Center for
    Integrative Medicine
Department of Medicine
Beth Israel Deaconess Medical Center
Boston, Massachusetts [24]

Simge Yonter, MD
Physiatrist
Rehabilitation Medicine Department
National Institutes of Health
Bethesda, Maryland [103]

Raymond Yung, MB, ChB
Jeffrey B. Halter M.D. Collegiate Professor of Geriatric
    Medicine
Director, Geriatrics Center and Institute of Gerontology
Chief, Division of Geriatric and Palliative Medicine
University of Michigan
Ann Arbor, Michigan [101]

Jesse Zanker, MBBS, BMedSci, MPHTM, DipPallMed, FRACP
Geriatrician, Research Fellow, Australian Institute for
    Musculoskeletal Science (AIMSS)
The University of Melbourne and Western Health
St Albans, Australia [51]

Chaoli Zhang, MPA
The John A. Hartford Foundation
New York, New York [12]

Jinghan Zhang, MPH
Medical Student
UT Southwestern Medical School
Dallas, Texas [12]

Foreword

"My inspiration and my passion will always come from my older patients. One day I hope to be like them; when that day comes, I hope that my doctor will be a geriatrician."[1]

It has been my privilege as Editor Emeritus of this latest edition to follow its progress over the past 2 years from design at the first meeting of the editorial board in September 2019 to publication. I am pleased to predict that the eighth edition of *Hazzard's Geriatric Medicine and Gerontology* will solidify its reputation as the leading "go to" source for readers seeking the latest, most comprehensive, in-depth, and reliable treatise in research and practice that optimizes the care of our aging and older patients. Moreover, this edition will continue to expand its influence toward worldwide enhancement in the care of those patients, whose numbers are expanding dramatically as population aging becomes a global phenomenon.

Especially gratifying in my association with this textbook has been its widespread use as core material in geriatric fellowship training programs. I am frequently flattered to be asked to autograph the latest volume for fellows who have come to value the book highly during their training for its accessibility, breadth, depth, and authenticity as a single source for their scholarly education in our field.

Their appreciation brings me special satisfaction. A focused approach on geriatrics fellows in training as our primary target audience was adopted by Reubin Andres, Ed Bierman, and me when, in 1983, we were charged by McGraw Hill to collaborate as editors of the first edition of a new textbook in the field, *Principles of Geriatric Medicine*. We envisioned our textbook as complementing the prior education that physicians received in medical school, graduate training in residency, and then maintained in continuing education programs, education that forms the foundation of physician care for all patients. In retrospect, that thoughtful, deliberate approach to defining our project generated the most important and enduring attribute of our series as it grew and matured through its successive editions: specifically, that our textbook should focus on the needs of future leaders in this new field, those who would choose to undergo training at the post-graduate level—that is, fellows in Gerontology and Geriatric Medicine.

Through our textbook we have hoped that physicians will be enriched and continuously kept current from its concentration upon the special needs of their older patients. Clinical topics have been integrated with chapters summarizing the aging process across the lifespan from conception to death (gerontology), but honing down on those older than 65, 75 (my personal definition as the threshold to old age), and, perhaps most germane to our special contributions as geriatricians, the "oldest old," those older than 85 (the group to which I now belong!) in whom the art and science of caring for the most complex and vulnerable can be most appreciated. And with the "Aging Tsunami" of retiring baby-boomers upon us, our mission to enhance the practice of all professionals and caregivers in managing such patients through our textbook is all the more urgent. Thus, it has been gratifying to observe the

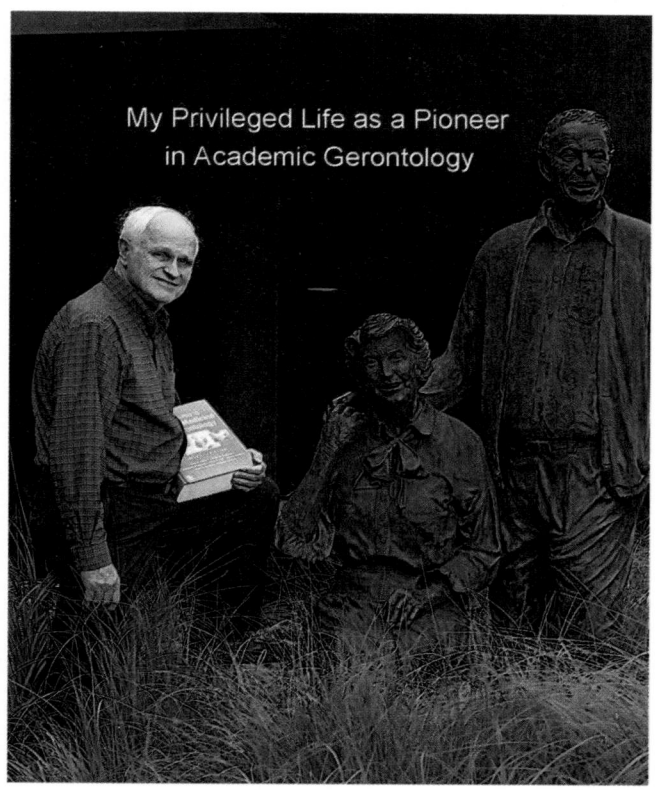

My Privileged Life as a Pioneer in Academic Gerontology

[1]Hazzard WR. I am a geriatrician. *JAGS*. 2004; 52:161.

expansion of our original focus on physicians training in geriatrics to encompass the educational needs of trainees in the wide range of health professions that are required to meet the clinical challenges presented by older adults with complex health care problems.

I am especially pleased that one of the editors of the eighth edition, Stephanie Studenski, has worked with other leaders in the field to document the range of geriatrics training experiences for physicians and other health professionals as summarized in the new chapter, Geriatrics Around the World. This special expertise will serve them well as future leaders in health care as it becomes progressively skewed toward caring for older patients. Thus, it will be incumbent upon editors of future editions of this textbook to remain abreast of leading edge developments in our field, which promises to become ever more sophisticated and challenging as aging citizens continue to enjoy increasing healthspan as well as lifespan.

This textbook remains the most enduring icon of my career in the field of Gerontology and Geriatric Medicine. It is with pride and confidence that I predict that the education of future generations of all clinicians and researchers who focus on the care of older patients will be enhanced by the eighth edition and future editions of this textbook.

William R. Hazzard, MD

Preface

On behalf of the editors, it is an honor and privilege to provide this preface to *Hazzard's Geriatric Medicine and Gerontology*, Eighth Edition. This textbook has become a mainstay of the rapidly developing field of geriatric medicine. Building on the textbook's already rich history since it was first published in 1985, the eighth edition emerges renewed and vibrant. This is the third edition of this textbook to carry the name of its founding editor Bill Hazzard in its title. We are pleased that Bill has contributed a foreword to the eighth edition, providing his view of the critical importance of fellowship training in geriatrics to the future of our field.

Planning for the eighth edition began in 2019, but the chapters were written and revised during the height of the COVID-19 pandemic. Thus, we are even more grateful than usual to the many contributors who found time to do their work on the book despite the stresses imposed on both work and personal time by the pandemic. One new editor has played a critical role in the revitalized eighth edition of this textbook: Kenneth Schmader. We recruited Ken to join us in 2019 because of his leadership in the field and many academic accomplishments. Little did we know then how timely that choice was, as Ken is a world leader in infectious diseases in the older adult population, especially viral illnesses and in vaccines to prevent them. As a result, the eighth edition includes extensive coverage of the COVID-19 pandemic and its especially devastating impact on vulnerable older adults. Chapter 108, Influenza, COVID-19, and Other Respiratory Viruses, is primarily focused on the pandemic. As summarized in Table 1, COVID-19 is covered in 25 other chapters as well, including many with a specific section devoted to it.

TABLE 1 ■ COVID-19 COVERAGE IN THE EIGHTH EDITION

Extensive Coverage

Chapter 2 Demography and Epidemiology

Chapter 3 Immunology and Inflammation: Entire section—SARS-CoV-2 (COVID-19) Vaccines

Chapter 8 Principles of Geriatric Assessment

Chapter 16 Institutional Long-Term and Post-Acute Care: Entire section—Impact of the Coronavirus-19 (COVID-19) Pandemic in Nursing Homes

Chapter 17 Community-Based Long-Term Services and Support, and Home-Based Medical Care: Multiple mentions

Chapter 21 The Patient Perspective: Multiple mentions

Chapter 53 Hip Fractures: Entire section—Changes in Hip Fracture Care: Bundled Care for Hip Fracture and COVID

Chapter 58 Delirium

Chapter 66 General Topics in Geriatric Psychiatry: Entire section—Impact of COVID-19 Pandemic

Chapter 72 Ethical Issues

Chapter 81 Chronic Obstructive Pulmonary Disease: Entire section—COVID-19 (SARS-CoV-2) and COPD

Chapter 85 Upper Gastrointestinal Disorders: Entire section—PPIs and COVID-19

Chapter 101 Rheumatoid Arthritis and Other Autoimmune Diseases: Entire section—COVID-19 and Rheumatic Diseases

Chapter 108 Influenza, COVID-19, and Other Respiratory Viruses: Bulk of chapter about COVID-19

Moderate Coverage

Chapter 5 Sex Differences in Health and Longevity

Chapter 26 Legal Issues

Chapter 67 Palliative Care and Special Management Issues

Chapter 80 Respiratory System and Selected Pulmonary Disorders

Minor Coverage

Chapters 1, 15, 22, 25, 32, 40, 104, 105, and see Index

In addition to Ken, the eighth edition's editorial team includes me (my sixth edition); Joe Ouslander (his fifth edition); Sanjay Asthana, Kevin High, and Stephanie Studenski (their third edition); and Christine Ritchie and Mark Supiano (their second edition). Fortunately for all of us, Bill Hazzard has stayed actively involved as Editor Emeritus and senior advisor. The eighth edition acknowledges and recognizes the worldwide growth of the field of geriatric medicine. Overall, our authors are not only a large and diverse group including many geriatricians but also a substantial number of subspecialists from a range of medical and surgical disciplines. In addition, multiple health profession disciplines are represented among the authors.

The eighth edition is substantially different from its predecessors, reflecting the continued growth and increasing sophistication of geriatrics as a defined medical discipline. Vitality and continued rejuvenation have been enhanced through the addition of seven chapters (see Table 2). In addition to the new chapters, we have carried out a major restructuring of the book to put more emphasis on the growing knowledge base for key topics in the field, Parts I–IV: Principles of Gerontology, Principles of Geriatrics, Geriatric Conditions (those health problems occurring almost exclusively in older people), and Principles of Palliative Medicine and Ethics. In parallel we have deemphasized the subspecialty-oriented Part V: Organ Systems and Diseases by combining many of the topics and focusing them more on geriatric aspects of these age-related diseases. Thus, for the first time in this book's history, more than half of the chapters (in fact, two-thirds, 72 of 108) are in Parts I–IV and only one-third are in Part V. The revised structure aligns closely with the geriatric "M's" of Age-Friendly Care—notably in Part II, Section B: Age-Friendly Care Across Settings (Chapters 12–21), Medications (Chapter 22), Mobility (Part III, Section B, Chapters 49–55), Mentation (Part III, Section C, Chapters 56–66), and What Matters Most (Chapters 7, 24, 25, 41, and 67–72). Furthermore, total number of chapters has been reduced from 130 in the seventh edition to 108, and the total pages of text have been reduced by 13% despite increasing the number of tables and figures.

As a result of these changes, many more chapters have been written by geriatricians and fewer by subspecialists with a geriatrics interest. In addition, a growing number of authors are women. In the eighth edition, nearly half of all chapters have a woman first author (52/108) and 70% have at least one female author (73/108), up from 60% in the seventh edition. Contrast these numbers with the first edition of the book (7/84 with a woman first author and 11/84 with at least one female author). On a personal note, as I reviewed the contributors to that first edition, I realized that the only one left of those authors who has contributed to the eighth edition (in fact to all editions) is me! We do take seriously the goal of recruiting new authors and transitioning out the older ones.

This is the second edition of the book to be published in full color, thereby greatly enhancing the many illustrations and figures included. To promote and facilitate the book's utility as an educational resource for Geriatric Medicine fellows in training and others, each chapter includes learning objectives and key clinical points. These have been linked to one or more of the Geriatric Fellowship Curriculum milestones to allow easy access by readers. This educational emphasis is highly relevant to Bill Hazzard's comments in the Foreword. A major step forward for this textbook is the electronic version, which is now widely available online and will continue to be available as the eighth edition. One of the original goals of working with McGraw Hill as the publisher of this textbook was to provide a link with *Harrison's Principles of Internal Medicine*. This link was greatly strengthened with the electronic version of *Hazzard's Geriatric Medicine and Gerontology*, which became part of McGraw Hill's *AccessMedicine.com* collection with publication of the sixth edition. Access Medicine includes not only our textbook and *Harrison's Principles of Internal Medicine*, but also multiple other important books in the clinical library of McGraw Hill. We are especially pleased that students of the health professions, both undergraduate and postgraduate, have full access to our textbook through the electronic version if they are at an institution that subscribes to *AccessMedicine*.

Thus, just as our population is inexorably aging, and medicine is faced with an ever-growing number of older patients with multiple and complex problems, we have been able to bring together the best minds and leaders in the field to provide authoritative guidance. Our authors present a highly diverse and dynamic range of thinking that has not previously existed in our textbooks of geriatric medicine. We are now reaching a broader audience through the availability of the electronic version of the textbook. We have kept it a living and growing document that encompasses the rapid stream of new information, which is helping us to provide more compassionate and effective care to the rapidly growing population of older adults.

The strong and effective working relationship that we have with McGraw Hill is made possible by the outstanding efforts of Leah Carton, Associate Editor for the McGraw Hill geriatrics publishing program; Kim J. Davis, Managing Editor; and their McGraw Hill colleagues who have

TABLE 2 ■ NEW CHAPTERS IN THE EIGHTH EDITION
Chapter 6: Social Determinants of Health, Health Disparities, and Health Equity
Chapter 12: Age-Friendly Care
Chapter 13: Geriatrics Around the World
Chapter 21: The Patient Perspective
Chapter 23: Substance Use and Disorders
Chapter 40: Applied Clinical Geroscience
Chapter 41: Managing the Care of Patients with Multiple Chronic Conditions

ensured the progress of the publication and the important next steps in the textbook's evolution. We are grateful for the help of Karen G. Edmonson, who managed the seventh edition of the book and initiated planning for the eighth edition before leaving McGraw Hill, and for the continued support of James F. Shanahan, publisher at McGraw Hill, who was instrumental in the initial publication of this textbook and served as its Managing Editor for the first six editions. We especially appreciate the efforts of Nancy Woolard from Wake Forest University School of Medicine, who has served as a senior editorial project manager for multiple previous editions. Her role for the current edition has been critical to provide a strong link to our past history and as the final common pathway for assembly of the eighth edition. We thank Drs. Rachel Brenner and Celia Pena Heredia, Geriatric Medicine fellows at the University of Utah, for their helpful advice mapping the fellowship curricular milestones to relevant chapters in the textbook.

Jeffrey B. Halter, MD

Part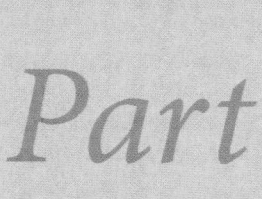

Principles of Gerontology

Chapter 1

Biology of Aging and Longevity

David B. Lombard, Richard A. Miller, Scott D. Pletcher

Aging is the process that converts young adults, most of them healthy and in no need of assistance, into older adults whose deteriorating physiologic fitness leads to progressively increasing risks of illness and death. The effects of aging are so familiar to health professionals and aging adults that they are viewed as immutable, taken for granted, an arena in which diseases and their treatments take place, but not subject to intervention or modulation. The major discovery in biogerontology is that this old-fashioned viewpoint is wrong, and that the aging process can be delayed or decelerated in mammals like us by simple manipulations of nutritional signals and genetic circuits similar to those already well-documented in people. It is now routine to extend lifespan, in rats and mice, by about 40%. This effect is, remarkably, 10 times greater than the increase in active life expectancy that would ensue from elimination of all neoplastic illnesses, or all heart attacks, in a human population. As importantly, genetic and pharmacologic interventions that increase longevity typically delay or even prevent many classes of age-associated diseases, such as cancer, metabolic decline, and neurodegeneration. It thus seems likely that a more detailed understanding of the factors that determine aging and the processes by which aging increases the risk of such a wide range of lethal and nonlethal illnesses and disabilities could, in the foreseeable future, have a profound impact on human health and preventive medicine.

Aging is a mystery, in the same sense that infectious disease was once a mystery, and consciousness still is an area of investigation in which well-informed researchers cannot be certain that they have selected a line of investigation bound to be productive. For a long time, most published papers in biogerontology journals consisted of descriptions of the ways in which young mice, rats, or people differed from older ones. This descriptive era has been superseded by one focused on specific molecular hypotheses about the key factors that regulate aging and on specific genes, drugs, and nutritional manipulations that could delay aging.

WHAT IS AGING?

This question—what is aging?—is posed not as an invitation to semantic quibbling, but to initiate reexamination of facts so familiar that they are seldom examined. A case

Learning Objectives

- Describe how biological aging induces progressive functional decline and loss of homeostatic capacity.
- Understand how diet, genetics, and pharmacologic intervention can affect the rate of aging.
- Explain how genetic or pharmacologic interventions affect intracellular signaling pathways such as insulin/insulin-like growth factor (IGF), mammalian target of rapamycin (mTOR), and sirtuins to extend mammalian lifespan.

Key Clinical Points

1. **Biological aging predisposes older individuals to disease and increased mortality risk.**
2. **Dietary restriction (DR) extends lifespan and promotes late life health in diverse taxa, including mammals.**
3. **Interventions that slow the aging rate also delay or even prevent multiple age-associated pathologies simultaneously, such as cancer, neurodegeneration, metabolic syndrome, renal dysfunction, and many others.**

history of an individual who has mild arthritis, some loss of hearing acuity, some evidence of incipient cataract, loss of muscle mass and strength, a progressive decline in capacity for aerobic exercise, troubles with learning and remembering, and an increased vulnerability to infectious illness would lead any physician to assume that the individual described is a man or woman age 60 or older. But the list of signs and symptoms refers with equal accuracy to a 20-year-old horse, a 10-year-old dog, or a 2-year-old mouse. The specific list of deficits and impairments shifts a bit from person to person, and from species to species, but it is extremely rare to find an 80-year-old person, a 3-year-old mouse, or a 14-year-old dog that has avoided all of these age-associated problems. The aging process is synchronized, in that it is common to see all of these difficulties in older people, horses, dogs, and mice, but rare to encounter any of them in young adults just past puberty. This synchrony is the central challenge in biological gerontology: How is it that such a process affects so many cells, tissues, organs, and systems at a rate that varies, even among mammals, over a 100-fold range from the shortest-lived shrews to the longest-lived whales? Structural features of shrews, mice, dogs, and people are remarkably similar at scales from the arrangement of DNA and histones in the nucleus, to the architecture of most tissues, to the role of the central nervous system (CNS) and endocrine systems in regulating responses to heat and cold, hunger and thirst, infection, and predators. Why, then, in molecular terms, will the eye, kidney, immune system, brain, and joints of a mouse last only 2 to 3 years under optimal conditions, while the same cells and organs and systems persevere for 50 or more years in people, and longer still in some species of whales?

The definition proposed at the beginning of this chapter—aging as a process for turning young adults into distinctly less healthy old ones—is straightforward enough to appear simple-minded, but in practice draws some prominent distinctions. In this view, aging is not a disease. Diseases are certainly among the most salient consequences of aging, but aging produces many changes not classified as diseases, and many diseases also affect young people. Similarly, lifespan and mortality risks are influenced by many factors besides aging. Thus, evidence that a gene or diet or public health measure has altered life expectancy, upwards or downwards, does not imply that the effects have been achieved by an effect on aging. In the context of the whole organism definition of aging used in this chapter, the sequence of changes that affect the quality of a fine burgundy wine or mature cheddar cheese, or changes that cell lines undergo in culture, do not qualify as aging.

From a biological standpoint, it is critical to see the distinction between aging and development. Development creates a healthy young adult from a fertilized egg and is strongly molded by natural selection. Genetic mutations that impair development, creating a clumsy falcon, a nearsighted chipmunk, or a chimpanzee uninterested in social cues, are rapidly weeded from the gene pool. But the force of natural selection diminishes dramatically at ages beyond those typically reached by members of a given species. Mice, for example, typically live only 6 months or so in the wild, before they succumb to predation, hypothermia, starvation, or other natural hazard. There is therefore strong selective pressure against mutations that cause cataracts in the first few months of mouse life, but little or no pressure against genotypes that postpone cataract formation for 2 years, an age seldom reached by mice in their natural environment. Mice protected, in a laboratory setting, against predation, starvation, and other risks typically do develop cataracts in their second or third year. In wolves, however, a genotype that delayed cataracts for only 2 years would be a disaster; natural selection favors wolf genes that preserve lens transparency for a decade or more. A similar process, working on our ancestors in environments where survival to 15 was common, but survival to 55 distinctly uncommon, has filled our own genome with alleles that postpone cancer, osteoarthritis, coronary disease, Alzheimer disease, presbycusis, cataracts, sarcopenia, immune senescence, and many other familiar maladies, for about 50 to 60 years. Thus, although aging and development seem, superficially, to be similar processes in that both lead to changes in form and function, they are different in a fundamental and critical way: Development is molded directly by the forces of Darwinian selection, and the changes of aging are the consequence of the failure of these selective processes to preserve function at ages seldom reached by individuals in any given species.

Aging as a Coordinated, Malleable Process

The definition of aging as a process that turns young adults into old ones conflicts with a view of aging as instead a collection of processes, some that lead to arterial disease, some that affect endocrine function, some that impair cognition or cause neoplastic transformation, etc. Each of these ailments is itself the outcome of a complex interaction among many factors, including genes, diet, accidents, viruses, toxins, and the environment. Furthermore, each of these diseases, and many others, seems an inextricable part of aging. As a result, it originally seemed implausible to regard aging as less complex than its (apparent) constituents. Considering aging as a unitary process, potentially susceptible to modulation, rather than as a collection of complex processes, has thus seemed, to some, to be an oversimplification.

However, two lines of evidence support the merits of the view of aging as a unitary process, with its own (still incompletely defined) physiologic and molecular basis, which underlies and tends to synchronize the multiple changes seen in older individuals. The first of these discoveries was caloric restriction (CR): The observation that rodents allowed to eat only 60% of the amount of food they would voluntarily consume live 40% longer than controls permitted free access to food, discussed in greater depth subsequently. This observation, first made in the 1930s, has been repeated in more than a dozen species in scores of laboratories. Studies in rhesus monkeys have produced suggestive evidence that similar benefits may accrue in our own order of mammals. The key point is not merely that lifespan is extended, but that nearly all of the consequences of aging are coordinately delayed. CR delays changes in cells that proliferate continuously (such as gut epithelial cells), cells that can be triggered to proliferate when called upon (such as lymphocytes), and those that never proliferate (such as most neurons), as well as on tissues that are extracellular or acellular (such as lens tissue and extracellular collagen fibrils). CR delays aspects of aging characterized by excess proliferation, such as neoplasia, and also those characterized by failure to proliferate (such as immune senescence). It delays or decelerates age change at the tissue level (such as degradation of articular cartilage) and those involving complex interplay among multiple cells and tissues (such as loss of cognitive function and endocrine control circuits). Because CR alters, in parallel, so vast an array of age-associated changes, it seems inescapable that these many changes, distinct as they are, must be in some measure coordinately timed, that is, synchronized or delayed by a mechanism altered by caloric intake. This synchrony does not reflect a "clock" that turns on molecular and cellular damage at a set time, producing programmed changes of the sort common in development. Synchrony reflects, instead, processes that can, through unknown links, delay and decelerate age-associated damage in multiple cells and tissues in parallel, to an extent that varies widely across species.

A second, more recent, set of experiments leads to the same inference. In 1996, Bartke and his colleagues reported that Ames dwarf mice, in which a developmental defect in the pituitary impairs production of growth hormone (GH), thyrotropin, and prolactin, show an increase of more than 40% in both mean and maximal lifespan compared to littermates with the normal allele at the same locus. Since then, studies of this mutant, and the closely similar Snell dwarf mouse, have documented delay in kidney pathology, arthritis, cancer, immune senescence, collagen cross-linking, cataracts, and cognitive decline, making a strong case that these genetic changes in endocrine levels do indeed modulate the aging process as a whole, with consequent delay in a very wide range of age-synchronized pathology. Since 1996, mouse researchers have documented increased lifespan in dozens of other genetically altered mouse strains, some of which show lower levels of or responses to GH, and/or its downstream mediator IGF-1.

Studies such as these justify a paradigm shift in thinking about aging and its relationship to disease. The new framework includes three key tenets: (1) the aging process, despite the complexity of its many effects, can be postponed by a single, coordinating mechanism; (2) the rate at which aging progresses can be decelerated in mammals as well as in other taxa; and (3) the time of onset and pace of many age-associated diseases are closely linked to the aging rate. From this perspective, a fundamental challenge to biogerontologists is to develop and test models of how age-dependent changes can be delayed, during middle age, to maintain relatively healthy people or mice or worms. Studies of aged individuals, as opposed to studies of aging, are relevant to this challenge only insofar as they are exploited to generate or test ideas about coregulation and synchrony, rather than disease-specific pathogenesis. The key resource for meeting the challenge is not comparisons between young and old donors, but rather comparisons between young or middle-aged adults who are known to be aging at different rates because of genetic differences or exposure to dietary or pharmacologic intervention. Fortunately, the same experiments that have documented the malleability of aging rate have produced sets of animals that do indeed age at slower-than-normal paces. With luck, future studies may produce at least tentative answers to the

two key questions in biogerontology: How does aging produce the signs and symptoms of aging, and what controls the rate of this process in mammals?

MODERN STUDIES OF AGING USING ANIMAL MODELS

Modern aging biology might be considered to begin in the early 1990s, when studies of genetically tractable invertebrate models, principally the budding yeast *Saccharomyces cerevisiae*, the nematode roundworm *Caenorhabditis elegans*, and the fruit fly *Drosophila melanogaster*, began to identify ways in which the lifespan of these simple organisms can be extended. Two decades of work in these systems have led to a set of guiding principles: (1) single-gene mutations—lots of them—can extend lifespan, (2) groups of genes with related functions often influence lifespan through common mechanisms, thereby revealing defined biological pathways that modulate aging, (3) many biological processes regulate aging in a conserved manner, in diverse phyla separated by billions of years of evolutionary time, and (4) consequently, aging studies in simple model organisms—with all of their advantages in terms of facile genetics and rapid experimental turnaround—are a valuable "breeding ground" for directed studies of similar processes in vertebrate animals such as mice.

Diet

One of the earliest manipulations to prolong healthy lifespan involved diet. Mice or rats fed approximately 30% or 40% less food than they would ordinarily consume typically live up to 40% longer than freely fed animals. Fruit flies intermittently starved are also long-lived. Remarkably, rodents and flies exposed to CR stay healthy and active, with intact physical, sensory, and cognitive function, at ages at which most of the controls have already died. In mice, CR extends lifespan if initiated at very young ages (eg, at weaning), or when started early in adulthood (eg, at 6 months, in a species where puberty occurs at 2 months and median survival is normally about 28 months). Whether CR diets extend lifespan when initiated in animals already older than half the median lifespan is controversial, with some early studies suggesting little or no response, and some more recent experiments showing a beneficial effect. Lifespan extension by dietary manipulations appears to represent an evolutionarily conserved effect, and it occurs in taxa as diverse as daphnia, worms, flies, spiders, and rodents.

Historically, the beneficial effects of dietary manipulations have been attributed to a reduction in the caloric content of the food. Indeed, most of the early rodent and fly studies were performed by reducing availability of all dietary components (eg, protein, carbohydrates, and lipids). More recently, however, comprehensive experiments in flies and mice that cover a broad dietary landscape suggest that individual macronutrients do not act independently,

6 nor is caloric value the primary predictor of dietary effects on lifespan. Nutrients interact, and it is their balance that appears to be critical (**Figure 1-1**). A diet containing relatively low protein (in relation to other macronutrients) commonly results in the longest lifespan. This broader view of dietary composition as a major determinant of health and lifespan had led to the term "dietary restriction" largely replacing the traditional term "caloric restriction."

While comprehensive analysis of the dietary landscape is prohibitively expensive in primates, diminished food intake in rhesus monkeys can delay many indices of aging and age-related disease. Results on lifespan extension have been inconsistent between studies, perhaps due to subtle differences in diet composition, food intake by control animals, and the intensity of veterinary intervention. In humans, DR leads to dramatic improvements in lipid profile, blood pressure, and other cardiovascular parameters. Whether or not DR without malnutrition would extend longevity in humans is unknown, though population studies hint that the answer is likely to be yes.

How DR promotes longevity mechanistically remains uncertain and so is the subject of active investigation. Invertebrate models have revealed that the health and lifespan benefits associated with DR require coordinated changes in specific signaling pathways and in gene expression. Biological processes that have been implicated in the response include stress resistance, mitochondrial respiration, and protein synthesis. Some of the effects of DR also appear to be in part independent of actual nutrient consumption, suggesting that animals may respond to the perception of nutrient availability in a way that promotes survival.

Some of the candidate mechanisms of DR identified in invertebrates may also be active in mammals. The effects of severe DR on rodent lifespan do not depend solely on avoidance of obesity. Although DR rodents have far lower adiposity than control animals, this is not due simply to a global reduction in the overall metabolic rate. In fact, in some tissues, mitochondrial respiration actually increases in response to DR. DR does, however, increase the efficiency of the mitochondrial electron transport chain, and reduces levels of damage attributable to reactive oxygen species (ROS) in certain tissues such as the liver. Possible mechanisms of DR effects in rodents, which are not mutually exclusive, include alterations in nutrient-responsive signaling pathways, increases in stress-resistance pathways including resistance to oxidative injury, diminished inflammatory responses, changes in stem cell self-renewal, alterations in the ratio of visceral to subcutaneous fat, alterations in cellular properties related to protein metabolism, and many others, each plausible, but none of them proven at this point.

The benefits of specific nutrient manipulations have been highlighted by experiments that alter the availability of individual amino acids, either acutely or throughout the lifespan. Rats fed a diet containing much reduced levels of

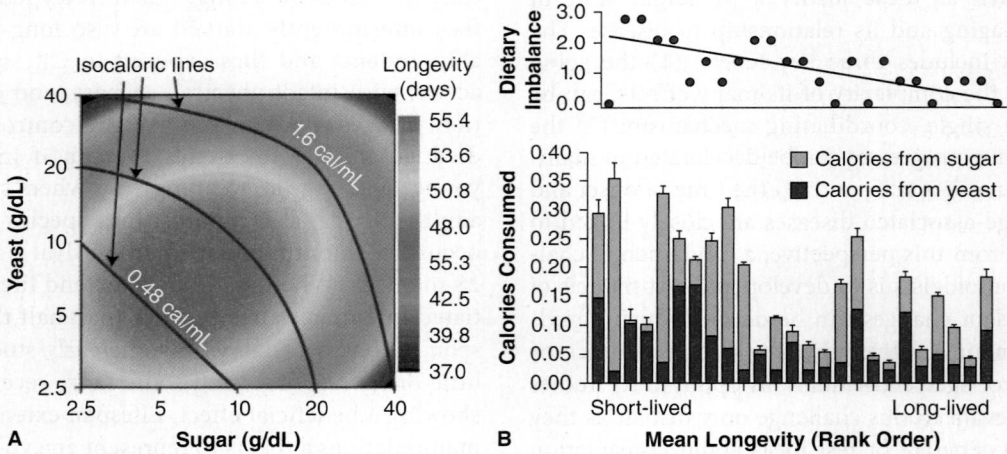

FIGURE 1-1. Dietary composition, not caloric value, specifies lifespan in *Drosophila*. (**A**) A diet response surface that characterizes the lifespans of female fruit flies across a range of 25 different diets composed of different concentrations of sugar and yeast, which are the two macronutrients in the *Drosophila* diet. Longevity is maximized at intermediate concentrations of both nutrients, and trends in lifespan are not coincident with differences in the caloric value of the food, as evidenced by the significantly different lifespans observed in isocaloric diets. (**B**) When lifespans from each of the 25 diets are rank-ordered, there is little association with amount of calories the flies consume (bottom panel), but there is a significant negative correlation between lifespan and a measure of dietary imbalance, which is proportional to the difference in nutrient concentrations (top panel). (Adapted with permission from Skorupa DA, Dervisefendic A, Zwiener J, et al. Dietary composition specifies consumption, obesity, and lifespan in Drosophila melanogaster. *Aging Cell.* 2008;7[4]:478–490.)

the essential amino acid methionine live 40% longer than rats on a standard diet, and there is a similar, though smaller, effect in mice. The lifespan effect in mice is seen even when methionine restriction (MR) is not begun until the mice are well into adulthood, roughly the equivalent of a 35-year-old person. These animals are not calorically restricted—they eat more calories, per gram of lean body mass, than control rats, and rats pair-fed normal food to match the total caloric intake of an MR rat show a much smaller degree of lifespan extension. Diets in which amino acids are restricted could, in principle, affect tissue health and organism aging by causing changes in protein translation or rate of protein turnover, by changes in DNA methylation (which depends on metabolites of methionine), by alterations in levels or distribution of the antioxidant glutathione (also a metabolite of methionine), by changes in hormone levels (MR mice show low levels of insulin, glucose, and IGF-1), by changes in hydrogen sulfide production, and/or by induction, through hormesis, of augmented stress response pathways at the cellular level. Work in flies suggests that methionine might be more influential than other amino acids in this context, though parallel studies in mammals have not been attempted. Comparisons of similarities and differences between amino acid restriction and full DR in rodents are likely to prove highly informative. Restriction of food, or of protein alone, for a period of several days prior to ischemic or surgical injury, or prior to chemotherapy, leads to better outcomes in rodents, but the extent to which such benefits reflect the same pathways through which long-term DR extends lifespan is not yet clear.

Broadly speaking, mice and rats on DR diets show delay or deceleration in a very wide range of age-dependent processes, including neoplastic and nonneoplastic diseases, changes in structure and function of nearly all tissues and organs evaluated, endocrine and neural control circuits, and ability to adapt to metabolic, infectious, and cardiovascular challenges. Mouse stocks that have been engineered for vulnerability to specific lethal diseases, such as models of lupus or early neoplasia, also tend to live longer when placed on DR.

Insulin/IGF Signaling

In the 1990s, the Kenyon and Ruvkun laboratories led research showing that loss of function in key components of the nematode *C elegans* insulin/IGF receptor homolog signaling pathway, including insulin-like receptor *daf-2*, results in large increases in lifespan in this organism, and that this benefit is dependent on a FoxO transcription factor. Conserved elements of this pathway were soon shown to have similar effects on lifespan in the fly, in brewer's yeast, and eventually in mice (**Figure 1-2**). FoxO proteins regulate expression of genes involved in stress resistance, DNA repair, cell cycle arrest, apoptosis, metabolism, and other processes, in a cell- and tissue-specific manner. Over subsequent decades, dozens of studies in worms and flies have revealed that signaling

by invertebrate insulins play a major, evolutionarily conserved role in limiting longevity.

The observation that longevity in mice could be improved by reduction of hormones in the insulin/IGF family provided a key foundation for exploiting comparative cell biology in biogerontology research. Subsequent work then showed that the lifespan benefit seen in Ames dwarf mice is also present in Snell dwarf mice, whose endocrine defects are very similar to those of Ames dwarfs, and in mice that lack the GH receptor (GHR-KO mice). This last observation, together with documented lifespan extension in mice producing low levels of GH-releasing hormone (GHRH), the hypothalamic factor that stimulates GH secretion by the pituitary, and in mice lacking the receptor for GHRH, suggests that longevity of the Snell and Ames dwarf mice is due mainly to loss of GH and/or IGF-1 signals. Studies of Snell and Ames dwarf mice, and of GHR-KO mice, have shown that the exceptional longevity of these mice is accompanied by a delay or deceleration of age-dependent changes in T lymphocytes, skin collagen, renal pathology, lens opacity, cognitive function, and neoplastic progression. Taken with the lifespan data, these observations suggest strongly that these mutations, like DR, act to slow the aging process itself (**Figure 1-3**). These mutations increase healthy lifespan in both male and female mice, with some evidence for stronger effects in females.

It is uncertain whether longevity in these mutant or engineered mice reflects loss of GH signals per se, or a decline in levels of IGF-1, whose production by the liver is GH-dependent. Mice with lower levels of the receptor for IGF-1 have inconsistent findings, ranging from a lifespan benefit in female mice, to little or no benefit in either sex.

Perhaps the strongest evidence for a direct role of IGF-1 comes from reports of increased lifespan in mice lacking the protease pregnancy-associated plasma protein A (PAPP-A). PAPP-A is thought to increase levels of free, active IGF-1 in many tissues by removal of binding proteins that ordinarily sequester IGF-1 and inhibit its activity. Thus genetic deletion of PAPP-A would be expected to diminish IGF-1 action in some tissues, without an effect on circulating or local GH levels. Clarifying details of local control of GH and IGF-1 action could have important implications for human applications, if it proves possible to target inhibition of GH or IGF-1 signals specifically to cell types that modulate aging rate, and thus avoid side effects that might occur if GH or IGF-1 signals were blocked throughout the body. Suppression of IGF-1 signaling in female mice using a neutralizing antibody can extend lifespan in older animals, highlighting the therapeutic potential of targeting this pathway.

Some of the longevity effects in Ames and Snell dwarf mice appear to reflect adjustments to limits in GH levels in the first few weeks of life, between birth and weaning 3 weeks later. Ames dwarf mice injected daily with GH, starting at 2 weeks, fail to show the increased lifespan characteristic of

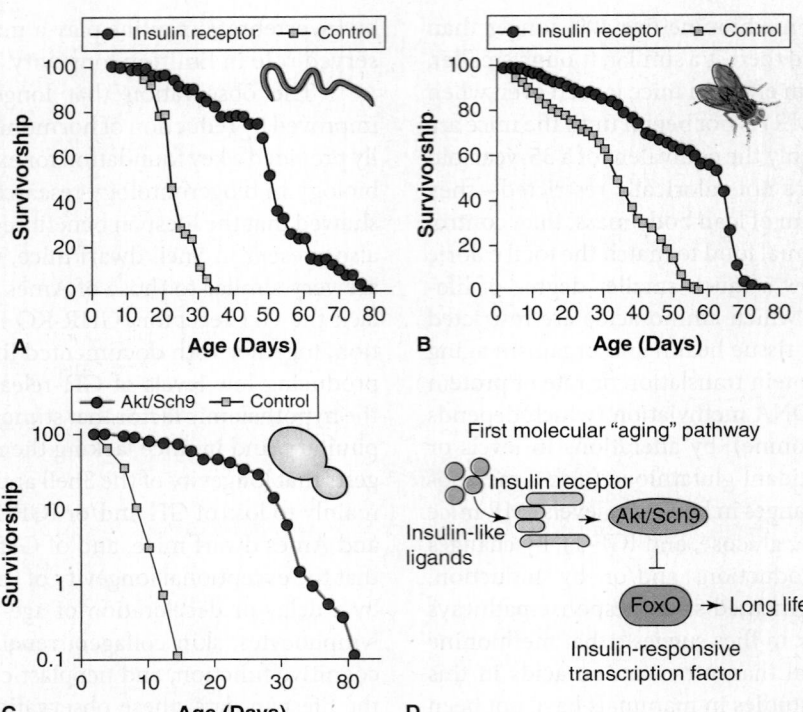

FIGURE 1-2. Research in simple model systems reveals the first molecular pathway that modulates aging. (**A**) One of the first single-gene manipulations capable of significantly extending the lifespan of an organism was discovered in the nematode worm, *Caenorhabditis elegans*. When a mutation was introduced into the gene *daf-2*, which encodes the only insulin-like growth factor (IGF) receptor in the worm, the animals lived over twice as long as the control animals. (**B, C**) Subsequent studies in (**B**) the fruit fly, *Drosophila melanogaster*, which also targeted its sole insulin-like receptor, and in (**C**) the brewer's yeast, *Saccharomyces cerevisiae*, which targeted the insulin-responsive Akt protein kinase, revealed that disruption of insulin/IGF-like signaling extended the lifespan of these organisms as well. (**D**) A member of the FoxO transcription factor family was soon found to be required for these life-extending effects, thus establishing the first evolutionarily conserved molecular pathway that influences aging. (A, Data from Kenyon C, Chang J, Gensch E, et al. A C. elegans mutant that lives twice as long as wild type. *Nature* 1993;366[6454]:461–464; B, Data from Tatar M, Kopelman A, Epstein D, et al. A mutant Drosophila insulin receptor homolog that extends life-span and impairs neuroendocrine function. *Science*. 2001;292[5514]:107–110; C, Data from Fabrizio P, Pozza F, Pletcher SD, et al. Regulation of longevity and stress resistance by Sch9 in yeast. *Science*. 2001;292[5515]:288–290; D, Reproduced with permission from Scott Pletcher.)

this mutation and also resemble nonmutant control mice in other ways, including lowered cellular stress resistance and diminished hypothalamic inflammation. GH injections started at 4 weeks, however, do not produce such an effect. Conversely, restricting the amount of milk available to normal mice, in their first 3 weeks of life, can lead to a 10% to 20% increase of lifespan; such mice show lower than normal levels of IGF-1 at the end of the nursing period. Thus it appears that the availability of nutrients, perhaps reflected as higher levels of circulating GH and IGF-1 in the first few weeks of life, may produce long-lasting changes in cellular and hormonal properties that persist throughout adult life and affect mortality risks in old age (**Figure 1-4**).

Target of Rapamycin (TOR)/Proteostasis

A second nutrient-sensing pathway, the amino acid–sensing TOR pathway, interacts extensively with insulin and IGF signaling in complex ways, some of which are diagrammed in **Figure 1-5**. TOR plays a major role in regulating protein

translation rates and other key target pathways in response to both external cellular stress, the available supply of amino acids and carbohydrate fuels, and hormonal signals. Downregulation of TOR signaling was initially shown to extend lifespan in flies, with evolutionary conservation later demonstrated in nematode worms and then in yeast. It is likely that many dietary interventions that extend lifespan recruit TOR-related mechanisms to affect aging, and inhibition of TOR function by the drug rapamycin can extend longevity in rodents and invertebrates (as discussed subsequently). TOR exists in two distinct molecular complexes, called mTORC1 and mTORC2, which have a wide range of effects on cell size and shape, responses to stress and nutrient levels, as well as protein synthesis and responses to glucose and insulin. Experimental work to distinguish the distinct, but interacting, effects of mTORC1 and mTORC2 activation in specific cell and tissue types is now under way. Signals mediated by the TOR complexes interact with those generated through insulin action.

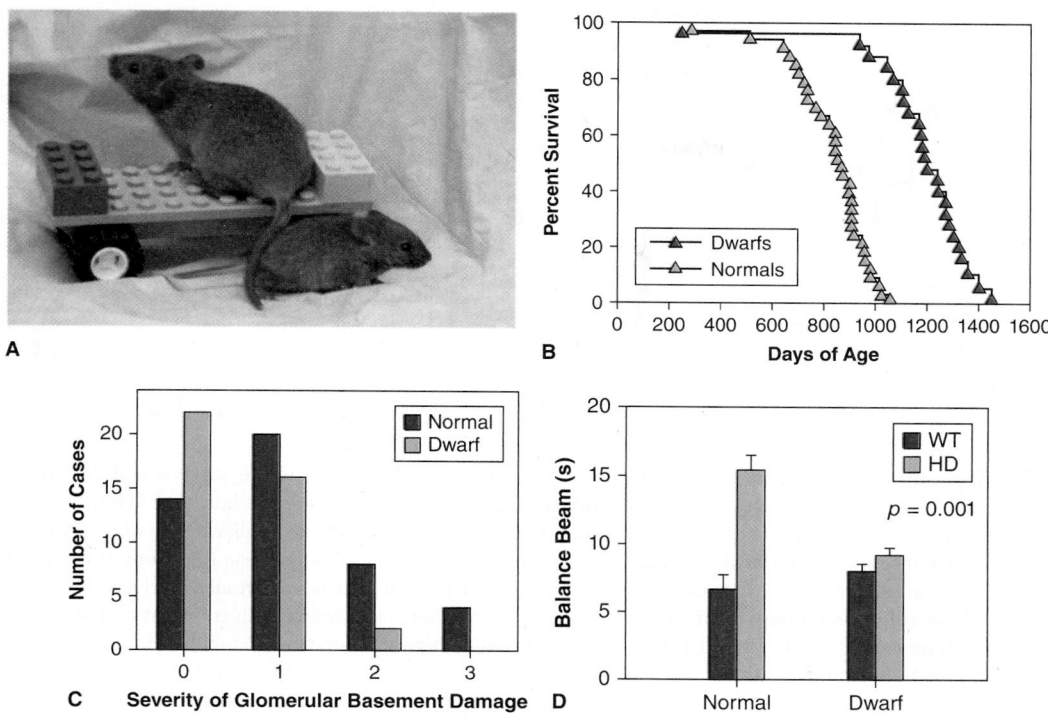

FIGURE 1-3. Mice carrying the Snell dwarf mutation are one-third of the size of their normal littermates, because the mutation diminishes production of growth hormone by the pituitary (**A**). This mutation increases mean and maximum lifespan by about 40% (**B**), and reduces the severity of kidney lesions at death among many other forms of late-life illness (**C**). Mice carrying a dominant mutation for Huntington disease (HD) perform less well than wild-type (WT) control mice on a balance beam task (**D**), but the HD gene does not produce corresponding symptoms when it is placed on a Snell dwarf background. (A, Reproduced with permission from Richard Miller; B, Reproduced with permission from Flurkey K, Papaconstantinou J, Miller RA, Harrison DE. Life span extension and delayed immune and collagen aging in mutant mice with defects in growth hormone production. *Proc Natl Acad Sci U S A*. 2001;98[12]:6736–6741; C, Data from Vergara MM, Smith-Wheelock JM, Harper R, et al. Hormone-treated Snell dwarf mice regain fertility but remain long-lived and disease resistant. *J Gerontol A Biol Sci Med Sci*. 2004;59[12]:1244–1250; D, Data from Tallaksen-Greene SJ, Sadagurski M, Zeng L, et al. Differential effects of delayed aging on phenotype and striatal pathology in a murine model of Huntington disease. *J Neurosci*. 2014;34[47]:15658–15668.)

Building on interest in TOR signaling and its effects on protein translation, work in invertebrates and increasingly in mammals has revealed fundamental links between the maintenance of proteostasis and longevity. Proteostasis refers globally to the processes that improve the quality and function of cellular proteins, collectively termed the proteome. It includes regulation of protein translation, folding, damage repair, and degradation. Autophagy is a process by which damaged cellular proteins and even whole organelles such as mitochondria are degraded in lysosomes. In invertebrates, intact autophagy systems are required for longevity extension by essentially all interventions that increase lifespan. Increased expression of the autophagy protein ATG5 extends mouse lifespan and improves neuromuscular function and glucose tolerance in old mice. Rapamycin, which extends lifespan in many different organisms, decreases translation of many cellular proteins, while promoting increased autophagic function. Snell and GHR-KO mice show augmented levels of a specific form of autophagy, "chaperone-mediated autophagy,"

which can affect levels of proteins involved in cell cycling, fat synthesis, and mRNA translation. Collectively, these findings indicate that maintenance of proteostasis is a key requirement of longevity.

Sirtuins

Sirtuin proteins, which play a major role in aging in yeast, have captured the public interest and sparked robust debate in aging circles. The sirtuins are a family of protein deacylases that consume the metabolic cofactor NAD+ during catalysis. Cellular NAD+ levels increase under conditions of fasting or DR, in a tissue-type specific manner. In light of their NAD+ requirement, sirtuins have been implicated as energy sensors and potentially as mediators of some of the benefits of DR. In yeast, worms, and flies, sirtuin overexpression extends longevity, albeit more modestly in worms and flies than initial reports suggested. Mammals possess seven distinct sirtuins; these are a diverse protein family, from the standpoint of biochemical activity, protein targets, and localization. Mammalian sirtuins target their protein

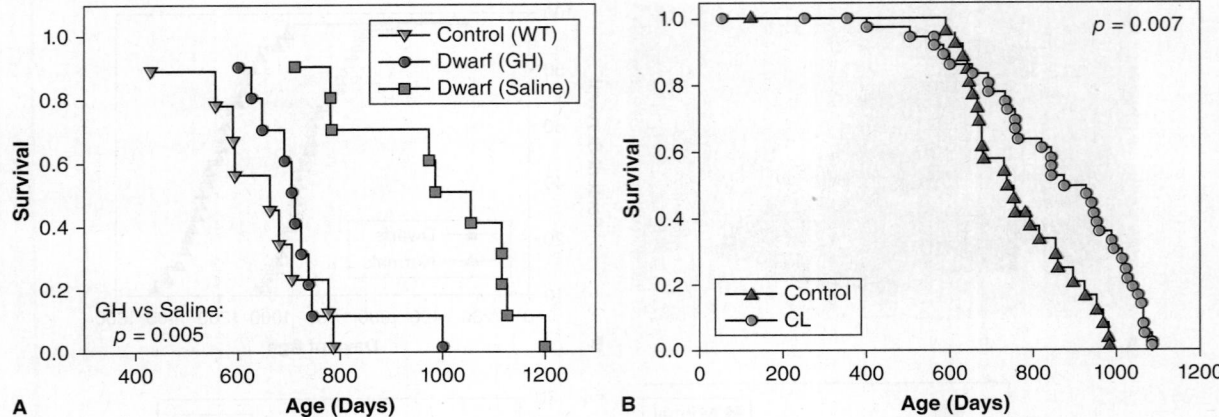

FIGURE 1-4. Early-life hormonal and nutritional status can have major effects on late-life survival and disease. The left panel shows an experiment in which Ames dwarf mice were given injections of growth hormone (GH) for an 8-week period beginning at 2 weeks of age. These hormone-injected mice had survival patterns similar to that of normal mice (WT controls), and therefore much shorter than Ames mutant mice (green) that had only saline injections at early ages. The right panel shows a complementary experiment, in which genetically normal mice were partially deprived of milk ("CL" for "crowded litter") by adding extra pups during the suckling phase, from birth to 3 weeks. This transient milk deprivation led to a substantial increase in lifespan in the CL mice. (A, Reproduced with permission from Panici JA, Harper JM, Miller RA, et al. Early life growth hormone treatment shortens longevity and decreases cellular stress resistance in long-lived mutant mice. *FASEB J.* 2010;24[12]:5073–5079; B, Adapted with permission from Sun L, Sadighi Akha AA, Miller RA, et al. Lifespan extension in mice by preweaning food restriction and by methionine restriction in middle age. *J Gerontol A Biol Sci Med Sci.* 2009;64[7]:711–722.)

substrates via deacetylation, or removal of other posttranslational modifications, to regulate a wide range of proteins involved in gene expression, DNA repair, metabolism, and many other processes. Three sirtuins are present in the mitochondrial matrix, where they regulate intermediary metabolism and other aspects of mitochondrial function.

In mammals, most studies have focused on SIRT1, the closest homolog of the yeast SIR2 protein. Whole-body overexpression of SIRT1 does not increase overall lifespan in mice, although it is protective against age-associated metabolic dysfunction and certain forms of neoplasia. Overexpression of SIRT1 in the brain only, however, does extend mouse lifespan. Overexpression of the sirtuin SIRT6 throughout the body also extends lifespan in male mice. SIRT6 promotes metabolic homeostasis and enhances genomic stability; it will be important to elucidate which of SIRT6's many functions are most important in its pro-longevity role. For example, sequence variations among SIRT6 homologs across different mammalian species may contribute to altered DNA repair efficiencies, and even to differences in lifespan.

Beginning with resveratrol, a series of small molecule activators of SIRT1 have been developed. In mice, these drugs show some beneficial effects, particularly in the context of dietary challenge such as high-fat feeding. There are continued controversies regarding these agents, particularly focused on the extent to which they target SIRT1 directly, versus exerting indirect effects through other signaling molecules, such as AMPK. Nevertheless, these or similar agents could conceivably find utility in treating age-associated metabolic dysfunction in humans.

Stress Response

Mutations that extend lifespan in invertebrates typically render the animals resistant to multiple forms of lethal injury, whether the threat comes from oxidative agents, heat, heavy metals, or irradiation. Genetic dissection of the relevant pathways—which must have evolved very early in the evolutionary tree, that is, prior to the common ancestor shared by worms, flies, and humans—has shown, surprisingly, that in normal, non-mutant worms, the levels of stress resistance, and thus resistance to aging, are actively diminished by inhibition of specific DNA-binding transcription factors, members of the FoxO family (see **Figure 1-5**). These pathways are retained by evolutionary pressures because they provide reproductive advantages in the natural environment, in which animals must be able to quickly take advantage of transient access to nutrients. Activation of FoxO proteins in the laboratory produces mutant animals that are not ideally suited for natural conditions, but which are resistant to many kinds of stress and which age more slowly than normal. Studies of gene expression patterns in the long-lived mutant worms have shown that the FoxO proteins can regulate transcription of over 100 genes that together protect against many different forms of cellular damage. The list includes enzymes that destroy free radicals, heat shock proteins, and other chaperones that guard against misfolded proteins, proteins that protect against infection, and chelating agents that bind toxic metal ions, among others.

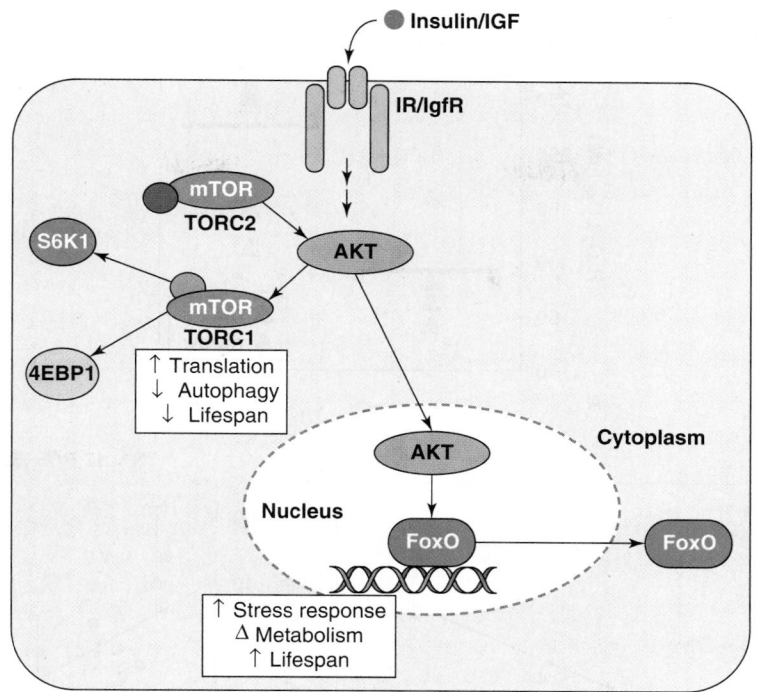

FIGURE 1-5. Insulin–IGF (insulin-like growth factor) signaling and mTOR (mammalian target of rapamycin) signaling regulate lifespan. Insulin and IGF binding to their cognate receptors (R) activates the intracellular kinase AKT. AKT in turn phosphorylates a large number of cellular substrates, including members of the FoxO transcription factor family, leading to their nuclear export and inactivation. Nuclear FoxO family members regulate stress responses and lifespan in multiple organisms, including mammals. mTOR kinase is found in two distinct cellular complexes, TORC1 and TORC2. TORC1 inhibits autophagy and promotes protein translation through its downstream effectors, 4EBP1 and S6K1. Inhibition of TORC1 has been most closely linked to longevity, although TORC2 may play a role as well. (Reproduced with permission form David Lombard.)

Induction of these stress-resistance pathways may be linked to late-life diseases. For example, worms with genetic variants leading to protein aggregation and neurodegeneration, as in human Huntington disease, show neurological dysfunction that can be delayed, and in some cases prevented entirely, by augmentation of the FoxO-dependent stress-resistance pathways. Similarly, age-dependent increases in susceptibility to stress-induced cardiac arrhythmias in *Drosophila* can be significantly postponed by activation of FoxO-dependent protective pathways.

Figure 1-6 shows some of the evidence linking stress resistance to lifespan in worms, mice, and cells from longer-lived mammalian species. DR and at least some of the long-lived endocrine mutant stocks show elevated levels of enzymes with antioxidant action, heavy metal chelators, and intracellular chaperone proteins, and also have lower levels of oxidative damage to DNA, proteins, and lipids. Cells grown in tissue culture from long-lived Snell and Ames dwarf mutant mice, or from mice lacking GH receptor, are resistant to lethal injury caused by cadmium, peroxide, heat, a DNA alkylating agent, ultraviolet light, and paraquat (which induces mitochondrial damage by free radical generation). Mice prepared by CR or MR diets are resistant to liver damage induced by the oxidative

hepatotoxin acetaminophen, and long-lived mutant mice are somewhat more resistant to death induced by paraquat injection. Stress resistance also seems to play a role in evolution of long-lived species. For example, cells from long-lived rodents and other mammals are resistant in culture to several forms of oxidative and nonoxidative damage, have high levels of an enzyme that protects mitochondria from oxidative injury, and high levels of molecular complexes that degrade damaged proteins. Cells from longer-lived species also employ a range of approaches, some involving control of telomere length and some unrelated to telomere biology, to diminish the likelihood of neoplastic transformation. This work suggests that variations in aging rate may be due in part to differences in stress-resistance pathways, but many questions remain unanswered.

Genome Maintenance and Reactive Oxygen Species (ROS)

A long-standing model posits that chronic accumulation of unrepaired damage to nuclear and/or mitochondrial DNA contributes to the effects of aging. ROS, generated via normal cellular metabolism, have been hypothesized to represent a major source of this damage. In support of this

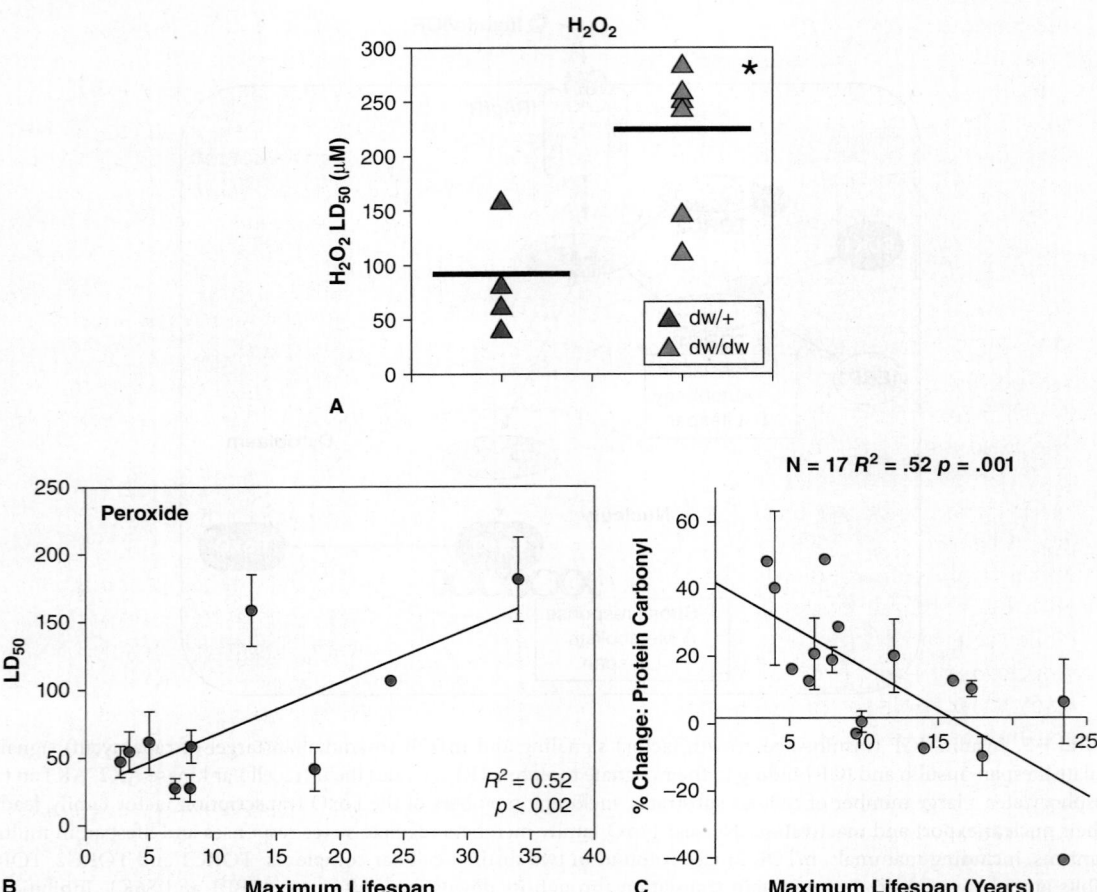

FIGURE 1-6. Links between exceptional longevity and resistance to stress. (**A**) Skin-derived fibroblasts from long-lived mutant (red symbols, dw/dw, Snell dwarf) mice are resistant to the lethal effects of hydrogen peroxide, H_2O_2. Each symbol is an individual mouse, and the Y-axis shows the amount of H_2O_2 needed to kill 50% of the cells. (**B**) Skin-derived fibroblasts from long-lived species are relatively resistant to lethal injury induced by H_2O_2. Each symbol represents a different rodent or bat species with the indicated maximum lifespan. Species, left to right, are laboratory mouse, wild-caught mouse, rat, red squirrel, white-footed mouse, deer mouse, fox squirrel, porcupine, beaver, and little brown bat. LD_{50} is the amount of hydrogen peroxide that kills 50% of the cells. (**C**) Cells from long-lived rodent species are resistant to changes in oxidized proteins ("protein carbonyl" on Y-axis) induced by 1-h exposure to H_2O_2. Each symbol is a different species, with the species' lifespan indicated on the X-axis. (A, Adapted with permission from Murakami S, Salmon A, Miller RA. Multiplex stress resistance in cells from long-lived dwarf mice. *FASEB J.* 2003;17[11]:1565–1566; B, Reproduced with permission from Harper JM, Salmon AB, Leiser SF et al. Skin-derived fibroblasts from long-lived species are resistant to some, but not all, lethal stresses and to the mitochondrial inhibitor rotenone. *Aging Cell.* 2007;6[1]:1–13; C, Reproduced with permission from Pickering AM, Lehr M, Kohler WJ, et al. Fibroblasts from longer-lived species of primates, rodents, bats, carnivores, and birds resist protein damage. *J Gerontol A Biol Sci Med Sci.* 2015;70[7]:791–799.)

idea, DNA lesions, mutations, and aneuploid cells (cells with incorrect chromosomal number or rearranged chromosomes) accumulate with age in mammalian tissues. Because such events occur stochastically on a cell-by-cell basis, it has proven difficult to rigorously identify and quantitate such events. Aging leads, in mice and humans, to increased incidence of aneuploidy. Although evidence that accumulation of DNA damage contributes to aspects of aging other than neoplasia is currently modest, elevated levels of a protein involved in repair of DNA damage, SIRT6, can increase mouse lifespan in males and delay cancer and metabolic dysfunction. Further work in

this and similar models may help to clarify the possible role of genome maintenance in aging and nonneoplastic diseases.

The role of ROS in inducing age-associated genetic damage, or in aging more generally, remains controversial. Resistance to many forms of stress, including oxidative injury, is a common feature of long-lived mutants, as described above. However, many mouse mutations that impair resistance to ROS damage have no detectable effect on lifespan and show no obvious acceleration of age-related pathology. Furthermore, administration of antioxidants to mice or people does not extend lifespan and may under some circumstances actually increase mortality. Conversely, for the most part mouse strains with increased activity of ROS defense systems show protection from specific toxins that cause oxidative injury, but do not show extended lifespan. The only current exception is a mouse strain overexpressing the antioxidant enzyme catalase in mitochondria. These animals show increased lifespan, and, by some measures, improved health in old age.

Cellular Senescence, Telomeres, and Cancer

The famous observation of Hayflick that human diploid fibroblasts cease to grow in culture after a limited number of population doublings sparked a line of experimentation that continues to yield important insights into the molecular control of cell growth, differentiation, and neoplastic transformation. Human fibroblasts placed in tissue culture will divide until approximately 50 cell doublings have occurred, after which the remaining cells survive indefinitely in a healthy but nondividing state. In the 1970s and 1980s, this "clonal senescence" model seemed to be an attractive approach to study the genetics and cell biology of aging. It is now clear that growth cessation of continuously passaged human fibroblasts is caused principally by the progressive loss of telomeric DNA at the ends of each chromosome at each mitosis, which occurs in cells that lack a specialized enzyme complex called telomerase. Critically shortened telomeres induce a DNA damage response in the cell, leading to senescence or cell death. Short telomeres can influence intracellular signaling to hamper mitochondrial function, thereby impairing cellular metabolism, suggesting that damaged telomeres might exert effects even in tissues such as the liver that are largely postmitotic.

Telomeres and cancer (also see Chapter 82) Telomere-dependent clonal senescence clearly plays a critical role in the protection of humans from many forms of cancer. Telomerase is turned on, and telomere attrition prevented, in approximately 90% of malignant tumors in humans. Genomic sequencing efforts have revealed that individuals with mutations that chronically elevate telomerase activity, or increase the accessibility of telomeres to telomerase, are at increased risk for a variety of cancers.

Studies of the role of telomeres and telomerase in the biology of aging in mice have produced controversial findings. Mice have much longer telomeres than humans, but live much shorter lives. The rate at which telomeres shorten, however, is more rapid in mice than in humans, and mouse strains engineered to have elevated telomerase show increased cancer rates, consistent with a role for telomere length as a contributor to malignancy in mice, as in humans. Paradoxically, elevated telomerase function may improve some aspects of health in mice carrying other alleles that block many forms of neoplasia, though with no effect on maximum lifespan, a provocative observation worth further exploration. As indicated in **Figure 1-7,**

telomere erosion can, in different settings, lead to cellular senescence, or to changes in cell properties related to DNA damage, genomic instability, or neoplastic transformation. The potential role of these changes in late-life human disease is an area of active investigation. Genetic disruption of telomerase can also produce lines of mice with shortened telomeres. These mice are short-lived, but the spectrum of pathology, featuring skin ulceration, infertility, increased frequencies of specific forms of neoplasia, and frequently lethal gastrointestinal lesions, does not closely resemble the pattern of illnesses seen in normal aging mice or humans. Thus telomere attrition, except for its major role in oncogenesis, does not seem likely to represent a major contributor to aging in rodents.

Senescent Cells Early work based on histologic assays suggested that senescent cells were rare (< 0.1%), even in biopsies from very old donors, although new methods for detecting other aspects of the senescent phenotype have led to upward revisions of this estimate. Senescent cells in vitro express a suite of secreted enzymes and inflammatory cytokines (not produced by dividing fibroblasts), which may facilitate the growth of cancer cells and could in principle contribute to other aspects of aging at the tissue or organ level. The *p16/INK4a* protein serves to maintain a balance between senescence and oncogenic transformation. P16 is induced as part of the process during which cellular senescence halts cell proliferation. An increase in levels of P16 is observed in many tissues of aging mice, but particularly in stem cells, suggesting that senescent stem cells may indeed accumulate as a consequence of normal aging and may represent an evolved mechanism to prevent early-life neoplasia. P16 accumulation leads to diminished stem cell function in the aging bone marrow, brain, and pancreas. Mice engineered to have reduced levels of p16 retain stem cell activities at ages at which these cells proliferate poorly in normal animals, though these mice are somewhat more cancer-prone than normal controls. In humans, genetic polymorphisms near the *p16/INK4a* gene have been linked to age-associated conditions such as type 2 diabetes, coronary artery disease, and frailty. Interventions that prevent age-related induction of p16 might be an attractive approach to diminishing many forms of late-life illness in parallel, if the intervention did not simultaneously increase cancer risk.

Several research groups have developed genetic methods to delete senescent cells from adult mice, and there is current interest in the possible therapeutic potential of pharmacologically targeting senescent cells. However, thus far there is little evidence for beneficial effects of these drugs, termed senolytics, in humans and little data on possible negative effects of such treatment. A series of ongoing clinical trials will evaluate the possible efficacy of senolytic drugs in the context of many age-associated diseases in humans, including osteoarthritis, Alzheimer disease, and others.

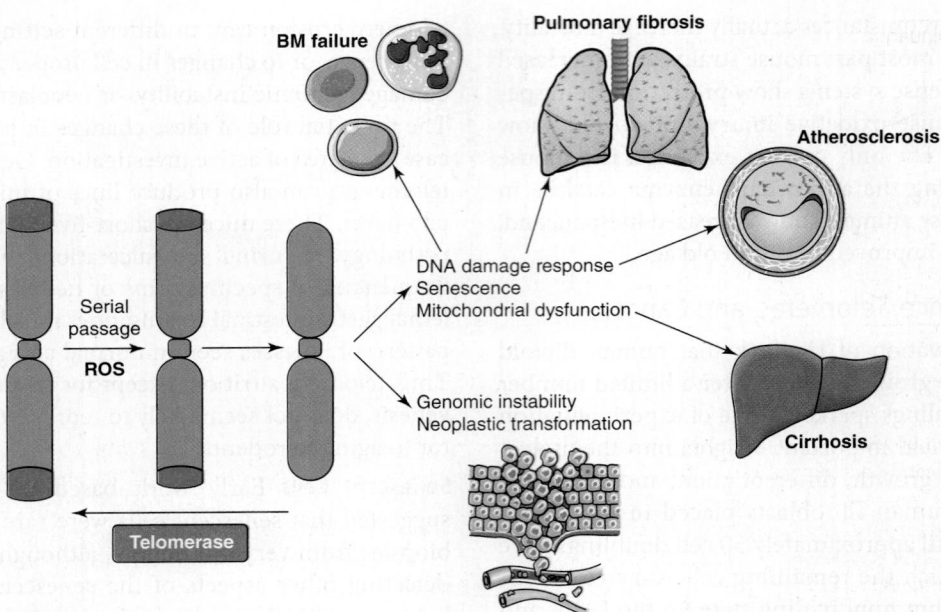

FIGURE 1-7. Two possible pathways by which telomere shortening can affect aging and diseases. The distal tips of mammalian chromosomes are "capped" by numerous copies of a hexanucleotide repeat (TTAGGG, designated in red). During serial cell division, or in response to genomic insults such as reactive oxygen species (ROS), telomeres progressively shorten. **Pathway 1 (senescence).** When they reach a critical threshold of attrition, loss of telomere binding proteins and telomere unfolding ("uncapping") occurs, provoking a DNA damage response and leading to permanent cell cycle arrest (ie, senescence). Critically shortened telomeres can also cause mitochondrial dysfunction in vulnerable tissue types like the liver. Telomere uncapping and senescence can promote age-related pathologies such as bone marrow (BM) failure, pulmonary fibrosis, atherosclerosis, and hepatic cirrhosis. **Pathway 2 (neoplasia).** In contrast, in cells that lack checkpoint control proteins like p53, shortened telomeres can provoke genomic instability, such as chromosomal end-to-end fusions, eventually culminating in neoplastic transformation. In stem cells and most cancer cells, telomerase is expressed and opposes telomere shortening by adding telomeric repeats back to the ends of chromosomes, thereby stabilizing telomere length. (Reproduced with permission form David Lombard.)

Other Genes and Processes That Influence Mouse Aging

Complementing the mechanisms of aging discussed earlier, there are many more engineered mouse strains for which increased longevity has been reported in at least one laboratory. For some mutants, lifespan extension is sex-specific, as with SIRT6 overexpression, which increases male longevity specifically. In other cases, for example, the Ames and Snell dwarf strains, extended lifespan is observed in both sexes. Long-lived mouse mutants often show protection against important classes of age-associated pathologies, such as cancer, kidney disease, cataracts, immune failure, and glucose intolerance. This finding underscores the close connection between aging and age-associated disease. As noted previously, several of these long-lived mutants show reduced GH signaling, typically with lower IGF-1 levels, and some also feature increased insulin sensitivity or alterations in insulin responses by specific cell types. Other mutants show impaired mTOR function or reduced activity of TOR's downstream effectors, although these changes are often seen in one sex only, and typically produce less increase in lifespan than alterations in GH

and IGF-1 signals. Other long-lived genetically engineered mouse strains highlight particular cellular functions that are important for longevity, such as genome integrity. For example, mice overexpressing the BUBR1 mitotic checkpoint protein show improved maintenance of the proper chromosomal number (euploidy) during age, along with protection from cancer, and extended longevity. Similarly, mice overexpressing the ATG5 protein show increased levels of autophagy, a cellular process for recycling damaged proteins and organelles, and increased lifespan. As a cautionary note, the majority of these studies have been performed in one laboratory, mostly in a single mouse strain. It will be important to replicate such studies in different genetic backgrounds and in multiple laboratories, to see whether the findings are reproducible and robust. Mutations that produce a specific form of pathology on one mouse strain often have no effect, or even the opposite effect, on other backgrounds, highlighting the dangers of forming general conclusions from work on a single inbred stock.

More work is needed to determine to what extent these mutations influence common pathways, to see whether they do or do not influence aging through the

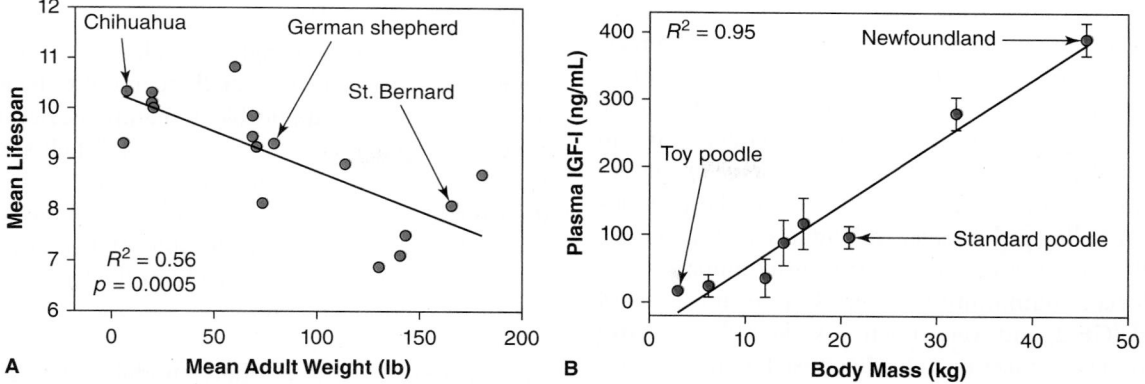

FIGURE 1-8. Longevity, size, and insulin-like growth factor 1 (IGF-1) levels among breeds of purebred dogs. Left panel (**A**) shows mean breed lifespan as a function of mean breed weight for each of 16 breeds of dogs; three breeds are indicated by arrows. Right panel (**B**) shows mean plasma IGF-1 levels as a function of body mass in eight breeds of purebred dogs. (A, Data from Li Y, Deeb B, Pendergrass W, et al. Cellular proliferative capacity and life span in small and large dogs. *J Gerontol A Biol Sci Med Sci.* 1996;51[6]:B403–B408; B, Reproduced with permission from Masoro EJ, Austad SN, eds. *Handbook of the Biology of Aging*, 6th ed. New York, NY: Academic Press; 2006.)

same mechanism. It is possible, for example, that some of these mutations diminish risk of cancer, a common cause of death in many inbred mouse strains, without effect on any other age-dependent trait, while others may modulate the effects of aging on multiple organ systems, thus diminishing both neoplastic and nonneoplastic diseases, lethal and nonlethal. In this regard, it will be useful to determine how these pathways may intersect with the DR response. In invertebrates, genetic studies have revealed that reduced mTOR signaling appears to overlap mechanistically with the response to DR. Analogous studies of DR have given ambiguous results: DR enhances lifespan effects in the Ames dwarf mouse, but has no such effect when administered to long-lived GHR KO mice. Some proteins may be required only for specific aspects of the response to DR, but dispensable for others. For example, in mice, SIRT1 is required for the increased skeletal muscle insulin sensitivity that occurs during DR, but dispensable for many other DR-associated effects.

As mentioned earlier, diminution of GH or IGF-1 levels can create mice that are long-lived compared to controls. Similarly, mouse stocks bred by selection for slow early-life growth trajectory are smaller than controls and also longer-lived. There is also highly suggestive evidence for a similar relationship between IGF-1, body size, and lifespan in dogs and horses. For dogs, small-size breeds have greater longevity than large breeds, and there is a strong relationship between body size and life expectancy among mixed-breed dogs as well (**Figure 1-8**). Pony breeds of horses are also substantially longer-lived than horses of full-sized breeds. The relationship between body size and life expectancy in humans is complicated by the strong effects of socioeconomic status on both endpoints; wealthier people tend to be both taller and longer-lived than poor people. On the whole, tall stature is associated

with lower mortality risks from cardiovascular diseases, which are a major cause of mortality in developed countries. In contrast, a remarkably consistent set of studies (**Table 1-1**) show that tall stature is associated with higher

TABLE 1-1 ■ POPULATION-BASED ASSOCIATION BETWEEN SHORT STATURE AND LOWER MORTALITY RISK FOR MULTIPLE NEOPLASTIC DISEASES		
TEST POPULATION	**TALL PEOPLE DO BETTER**	**SHORT PEOPLE DO BETTER**
15,000 Scots	All-cause mortality Stroke Coronary disease	Colorectal, prostate, hematopoietic cancers
12,000 NHANES (United States) men		Cancers; 40%–60% effect; adjusted for race, smoking, income
NHANES women		Breast and colorectal cancer
22,000 US male physicians		Cancer; adjusted for age, BMI, exercise, smoking
570,000 Norwegian women		Breast cancer
400,000 American women		Breast cancer, postmenopause
1.1 million Norwegians		Esophageal cancer
England and Wales (by county)	All-cause mortality Ischemic heart disease	Breast, prostate, ovarian cancer

BMI, body mass index; NHANES, National Health and Nutrition Examination Survey. *Data from Masoro EJ, Austad SN: Handbook of the Biology of Aging, 6th ed. New York, NY: Academic Press; 2006.*

mortality risk from a wide range of neoplastic diseases. There is also limited data that centenarians, on average, were shorter as mature adults than those who do not attain centenarian status. Testing the idea that short midlife stature is associated with delayed or decelerated aging in humans will depend on measuring a wide range of age-dependent traits, rather than merely lifespan, on large populations of middle-aged people. Individuals with a genetic abnormality in GH receptor ("Laron dwarf mutation") in an Ecuadorian community had very low serum levels of IGF-1 and IGF-2, and were much less likely than control subjects to die of cancer or to be diagnosed with adult-onset diabetes, findings consistent with the low age-adjusted cancer incidence and excellent insulin sensitivity of the corresponding long-lived, mutant mouse stock.

Connections to Molecular Pathobiology

Integration of findings from invertebrates (including yeast cells), rodents, and cultured human cells has substantially enhanced understanding of the molecular pathogenesis of many diseases and continues to provide the driving engine for experimental therapeutics leading to clinical trials. A similar strategy focusing on pathways that regulate the aging process, and through altered rates of aging, could lead to the coordinated postponement of the wide array of age-dependent diseases. Thus, pathways that clearly deserve deeper scrutiny have been delineated, usually because investigations in invertebrates, or, more rarely, mice, have revealed that genetic or chemical alteration of the target molecules can slow aging, preserve health, and extend maximal lifespan. Elucidation of the links between these biochemical pathways and hormonal signals, neoplastic transformation, stem cell homeostasis, and the balance between cell growth and cell death is likely to provide both rationale and direction for translational work aimed at slowing the aging process and retarding age-related disease and dysfunction.

Many of these pathways are interconnected, either within cells or through neuroendocrine connections, often making it difficult to draw simple, unidirectional maps discriminating causes from effects. Making the leap from convenient invertebrate organisms to the added physiologic complexity of rodents and humans also poses major challenges. **Figure 1-5** illustrates connections among many of the molecular targets and intercellular pathways, potentially involved in the control of aging rate in mammals, which have attracted experimental attention and continue to be sources of controversy and new ideas. None of these has yet been proven to be a central regulator of aging and multiple age-related illnesses; none of those shown has yet been ruled out. Research in the coming decade should expand the list of interesting candidates, refine our knowledge of how these molecules control one another within the cell, and start to delineate the specific cell types, and tissues, through which these pathways influence aging rate and age-related diseases in mammals.

Looking to the Future

Seminal discoveries of aging regulatory mechanisms in simple model systems repeatedly turn out to be evolutionarily conserved and applicable to mammals. Because of the time required to create mutant mice and their significantly longer lifespan, it normally takes 5 to 10 years for initial discoveries to be repeated in vertebrate systems. Nevertheless, it is worth pondering the importance and potential impact of ideas that are currently in the "pipeline," two of which are mentioned here:

1. **Sensory systems** strongly modulate aging in nematodes and fruit flies, and this modulation is evolutionarily conserved. Exposure of worms or flies to food-based odorants is sufficient to reduce lifespan and limit the beneficial effects of dietary restriction, while mutations that largely abolish olfactory function result in long life. It has become clear that some sensory neurons enhance longevity while others suppress it and that even the well-known relationship between body temperature and lifespan may have a sensory component. All organisms share similar goals: the need for food and mates, and the desire to avoid danger. While the specific smells, tastes, etc., that are associated with these goals are different among species, the biological responses to what those cues represent are much the same. Flies and humans both produce insulin-like peptides when they smell food, for example, suggesting deeper biological responses to sensory input should be targets for studies of aging in mammals. Encouragingly, the first instance of sensory modulation of lifespan in mice, involving a pain-sensing TRP channel, has been described. Similarly, alterations in pain nerve sensitivity have been noted in an exceptionally long-lived (and cancer-resistant) rodent species, the naked mole rat.

2. **Interactions among tissues.** In worms and flies there is mounting evidence that the aging process of the entire organism is coordinated nonautonomously by ongoing communication among specific tissues. Signaling from the germline controls aging of nonmitotic tissues. A few sensory neurons that detect food, danger, or mates can increase or decrease a fly's lifespan, and a similar number control the DR response in worms. Similar results are emerging from rodent studies where the hypothalamus has become a focus point through its influence on global energy homeostasis and inflammation. Long-lived mice, produced by mutation or drug treatment, have lower hypothalamic inflammation, and conversely interventions that diminish hypothalamic inflammation can extend mouse lifespan. Surgical removal of visceral fat, though not of subcutaneous fat, extends lifespan in rats, suggesting that some adipose tissue depots may modulate aging rate through metabolic or endocrine factors. Similarly, mutations

that extend mouse lifespan by lowered GH/IGF-1 signals lead to reduced levels of visceral fat, with relative sparing of subcutaneous fat depots. Inducible genetic recombination systems can now knock out genes in specific tissues and at specific times. These tools, together with the ability to activate or inhibit specific neurons with light (optogenetics), will likely permit delineation of cell- and tissue-specific control of aging as a major focus of mammalian studies in the coming years.

DRUGS THAT EXTEND LIFESPAN IN MODEL SYSTEMS

Characterizing genetic mutants with increased lifespan is one means to elucidate pathways important in regulating longevity. A different, complementary strategy is to identify small molecules that extend lifespan. Work in this direction is being carried out by a consortium of three laboratories, funded by the US National Institute on Aging as the Interventions Testing Program (ITP). The ITP consortium evaluates three to six new drugs or nutritional supplements each year for possible benefits to mouse lifespan, using a genetically heterogeneous mouse stock to diminish the chances of detecting, or missing, results that would apply only in mice carrying a single, potentially idiosyncratic, genotype. There is now evidence that at least four drugs—rapamycin, canagliflozin, acarbose, and 17-α-estradiol—can improve survival and increase maximal longevity in mice. Rapamycin, an inhibitor of the intracellular enzyme mTOR, increases lifespan in both males and females, with increases as high as 26% at the highest dose so far tested. Acarbose, which slows the intestinal digestion of starches to sugars and thus blunts postprandial surges in blood glucose, increases male lifespan by 22%, and has smaller, though still significant, effects in females. Similarly, canagliflozin, a widely prescribed drug for diabetes that primarily inhibits glucose reabsorption by the kidney, extends the median lifespan of male mice by 14%, but had no benefit in females. 17-α-Estradiol, a nonfeminizing isoform of estrogen (17-β-estradiol), increases lifespan of male mice by 19%, but does not extend lifespan in females. Another agent, nordihydroguaiaretic acid (NDGA), which has both antioxidant and anti-inflammatory actions, improves lifespan of male mice only, and a significant survival benefit was also reported for male and female mice given food supplemented with high levels of the amino acid glycine. **Figure 1-9** illustrates lifespan extension in mice given rapamycin or acarbose, and shows the delay in several forms of midlife pathology in rapamycin-treated mice.

Studies of this kind can establish, as proof of principle, that drugs added to food can increase mammalian lifespan. From this perspective they help support the evidence from studies of diets and single-gene mutations that the aging process in mammals can be delayed or decelerated

sufficiently to have an important effect on survival, and overall health, at older ages. **Figure 1-10** compares the extent of lifespan extension achieved, so far, in drug-treated mice, in parallel to effects produced by single-gene mutations, both spontaneous and targeted.

These studies point to specific drugs, and classes of drugs, that might deserve further, more intensive analysis, as tools to learn more about the biology of aging and late-life diseases. The benefits of rapamycin on lifespan seem to be equivalent whether the drug is initiated in young adult mice or in mice already more than half the age of median survival, suggesting that inhibition of TOR function may be beneficial even if started at relatively late ages. Moreover, this result hints that mTOR signaling may increase in older individuals and contribute to the degenerative effects of aging. Strikingly, pharmacologic mTOR inhibition in older adult humans improves responses to influenza vaccination, hinting that drugs identified as having beneficial effects on lifespan and late-life health in rodents may have similar effects in humans.

The striking acarbose and canagliflozin results should prompt additional studies of the role of transient glucose surges in the control of aging rate. Although the effects of both drugs on peak glucose levels make them useful for the treatment of diabetes in humans, it is noteworthy that diabetes is quite rare in the mouse stock used by the ITP, and that most of the ITP mice die because of some form of neoplasia. More work will be needed to discover how acarbose and canagliflozin slow cancer progression, whether they slow the pace of other age-related changes, such as cataracts, sarcopenia, immunosenescence, and cognitive decline, and why the lifespan benefit is so much stronger in male than in female mice. The male-specific benefits of 17-α-estradiol will prompt new work on the routes by which steroids can modulate cancer and other late-life diseases. Both acarbose and 17-α-estradiol produce significant lifespan and functional benefits even when started in midlife; parallel studies on canagliflozin are now under way. Obstacles related to translation of these experimental results into clinical trials are discussed later.

GENETIC APPROACHES TO ANALYSIS OF AGING IN HUMANS

Attempts to find genetic variations that influence aging in humans have been plagued with practical and conceptual problems. For one thing, heritability calculations show that only 15% to 20% of the variation in lifespan among humans can be attributed to genetic factors. However, the magnitude of the influence of genetics on longevity may rise with increasing age. Furthermore, an unknown but potentially large fraction of this genetic variation probably reflects genetic variants that influence susceptibility to diseases of childhood, infectious agents, and specific common illnesses of old age. For example, genetic variants that cause Huntington disease or type 1 diabetes or that triple

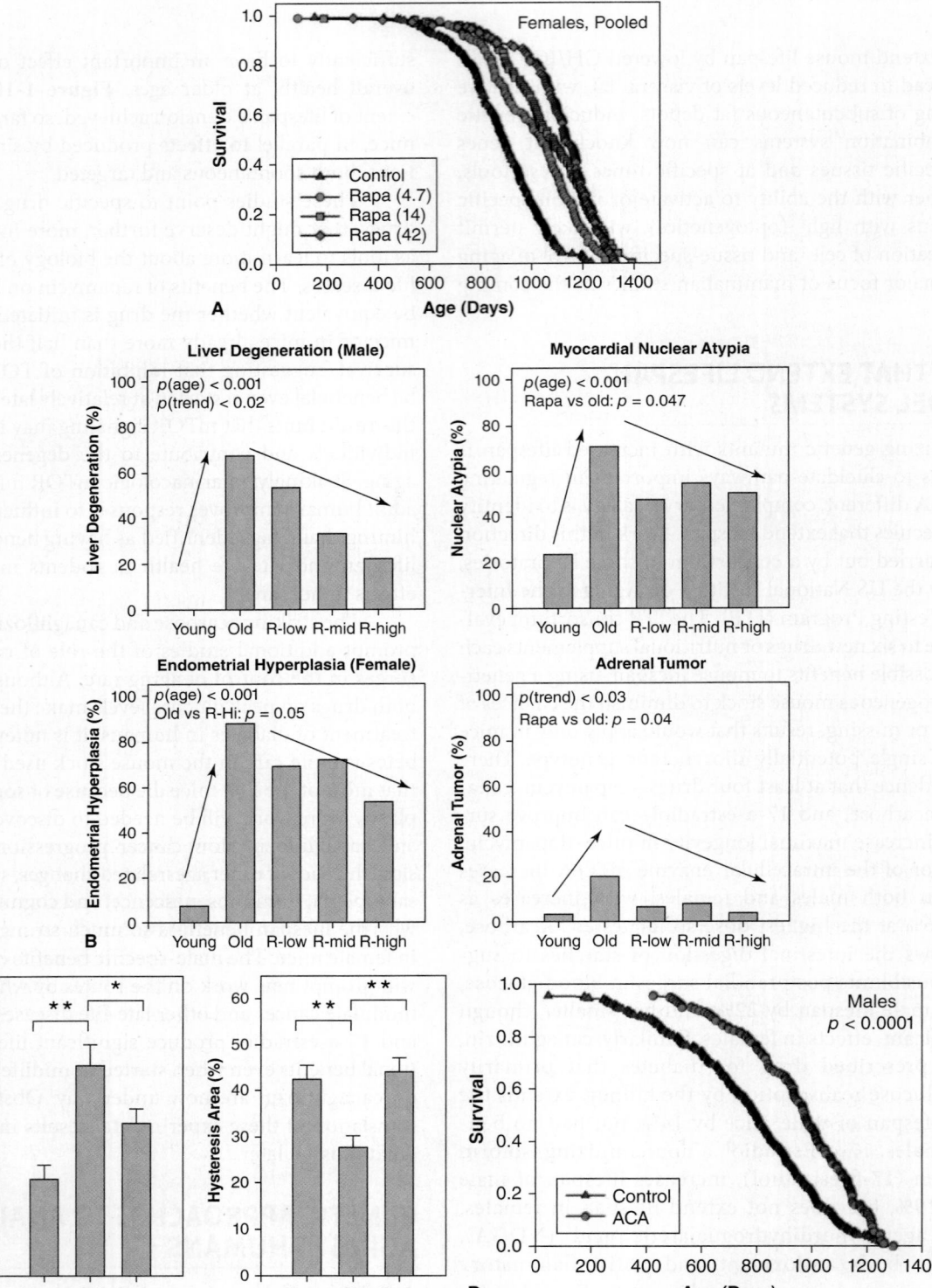

FIGURE 1-9. Increased lifespan and improved late-life health in mice treated with rapamycin (R, or Rapa) or acarbose (ACA). (**A**) Increased mean and maximal lifespan in female mice exposed to varying doses of rapamycin (4.7, 14, or 42 mg drug per kg food) from 9 months of age. (**B**) Four forms of age-related pathology seen in 22-month-old mice that are less frequent in mice treated with rapamycin. (**C**) Rapamycin treatment delays the effects of aging on the properties of an extracellular tissue, in this case elasticity of collagen fibers from the tail tendon. (**D**) Extension of lifespan in male mice treated with acarbose (1000 mg per kg food) from 4 months of age. (A, Reproduced with permission from Miller RA, Harrison DE, Astle CM, et al. Rapamycin-mediated lifespan increase in mice is dose and sex dependent and metabolically distinct from dietary restriction. *Aging Cell.* 2014;13[3]:468–477; B & C, Reproduced with permission from Wilkinson JE, Burmeister L, Brooks SV, et al. Rapamycin slows aging in mice, *Aging Cell.* 2012;11[4]:675–682; D, Reproduced with permission from Harrison DE, Strong R, Allison DB, et al. Acarbose, 17-α-estradiol, and nordihydroguaiaretic acid extend mouse lifespan preferentially in males. *Aging Cell.* 2014;13[2]:273–282.)

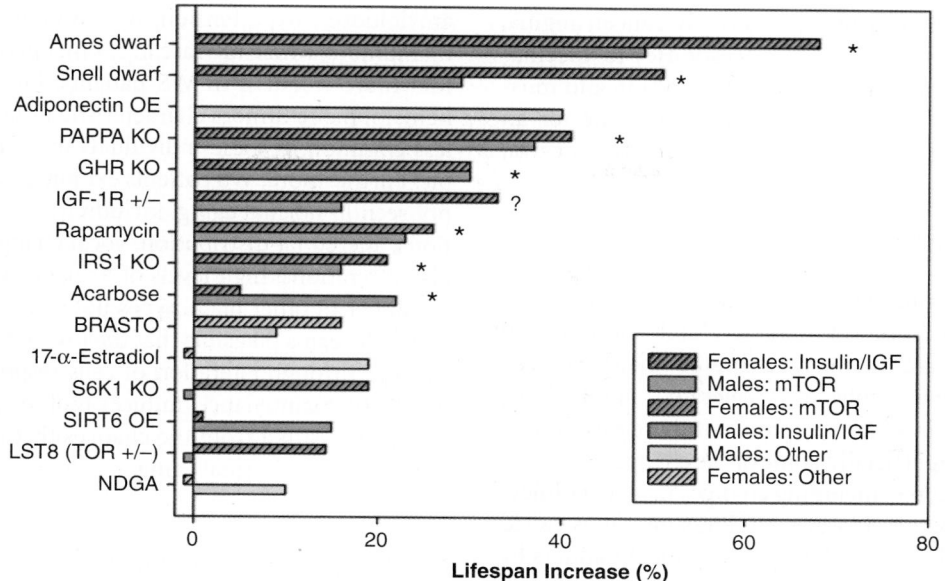

FIGURE 1-10. Selected reports for mouse lifespan extension mediated by mutations or drugs. Colors indicate functional groupings: pink for alteration of GH (growth hormone), insulin, or IGF-1 (insulin-like growth factor 1), green for mTOR (mammalian target of rapamycin), yellow for unknown or other pathways. (∗) indicates confirming reports from at least one other laboratory group and/or in at least two independent cohorts. (?) indicates that substantially smaller results were obtained in another laboratory. Effects that were reported as "zero" are illustrated, as a convention, at −1 to allow the bar to be visible. BRASTO: brain-specific SIRT1-overexpressing; IRS1: insulin receptor substrate 1; KO: knockout; LST8: lethal with SEC13 protein 8; OE: overexpressor; PAPP-A: pregnancy-associated plasma protein A; s6K1: S6 kinase 1. (Reproduced with permission from David Lombard and Richard A. Miller.)

the normal risk of myocardial infarction by the age of 50 would all contribute to the measured heritability of lifespan but do so by altering mortality risks from a specific form of illness rather than by alteration of aging with its effects on multiple late-life traits. Thus, genetic variants that mold lifespan by effects on aging per se, if they exist at all, are likely to influence only a small fraction of variation in how long people live.

Formal analyses of the genetics of human aging have so far relied mostly on candidate gene approaches, in which long-lived and control populations are evaluated for variations at one or a small number of genetic loci selected on theoretical grounds as most likely to be involved in aging or disease processes. In such studies, polymorphisms near the *FOXO3A*, *APOE*, and *SIRT3* genes have been identified as enriched in long-lived individuals. The *FOXO3A* transcription factor is a FoxO protein, modulated by insulin and IGFs. Apolipoprotein E (*APOE*) polymorphisms are well-known to affect the risk of developing cardiovascular disease and Alzheimer dementia. SIRT3 is a sirtuin family member; this protein resides in mitochondria, where it regulates multiple metabolic processes. An alternative approach is whole genome screening of large populations for association of longevity with hundreds of thousands of genetic variants. Thus far, only *APOE* polymorphisms have been identified in multiple studies, while other potential genetic associations have proven difficult to replicate. There are several possible explanations for these

discrepancies, including lack of a consistent definition of longevity between studies, different ethnic backgrounds of study populations, inadequate sample sizes leading to insufficient statistical power, differing living conditions, lack of ideal control populations, and other confounding factors.

A major problem with all these approaches, from the perspective of biological gerontology, is the lack of a defensible phenotype: a measure of aging better than lifespan. There are now several dozen reports of candidate loci at which particular alleles are overrepresented among centenarians or near-centenarians, and advocates of this strategy hope that among this collection are some loci that control aging rate. But skeptics note that alleles that increase risk of cardiac disease, Alzheimer disease, stroke, various common forms of cancer, or severe osteoporosis are likely to have contributed to disease and death before the age of 90 or 100, and thus to have been eliminated or greatly reduced among very old people. Thus, it should be assumed that a collection of genetic loci whose frequency discriminates very old people from others of the same birth cohort will include many genes with influence over common forms of lethal illnesses rather than genes that modulate aging per se. This problem is not one that can be solved by technological innovation or larger numbers of tested subjects; it requires development of a phenotype that provides more information about health in old age than merely a record of the age at death. For example, a genetic allele that identified, among 70-year-old people, those most likely to have excellent eyesight and hearing, no history of cancer, angina, diabetes, or arthritis, above-average responses to vaccination, and retention of baseline levels of cognition and muscle strength would be a much stronger candidate for an authentic "antiaging" gene than one that predicted survival to the age of 100.

MODELS OF ACCELERATED AGING

There are a small number of rare inherited diseases, of which Werner syndrome (WS) and Hutchinson-Gilford syndrome (HGPS) are the most celebrated, that have been mooted as possible examples of "accelerated" aging. Some of the physical features and symptoms of these diseases do resemble, at least superficially, some of the changes that typically affect older people, including changes in skin, connective tissues, and the vasculature. HGPS, sometimes called "progeria," is now known to be caused in most patients by mutations in the gene encoding Lamin A, a component of the nuclear membrane. WS patients usually have mutations in an enzyme (WRN) that functions as a DNA helicase (unwinding coiled DNA) and as an endonuclease.

It is debatable whether either of these diseases provides strong clues about the molecular or cellular basis for age-related changes in normal individuals. WS patients do resemble older people in some ways: They frequently suffer from cataracts and premature graying of the hair, and by their early thirties often develop osteoporosis, diabetes, and atherosclerosis. On the other hand, many features of normal aging are not seen in WS patients and many features of WS are not seen in normal old individuals. WS patients, for example, do not show signs of Alzheimer disease or other

amyloidoses, hypertension, or immune failure. Mesenchymal tumors, which are rare in normal people, are about 100-fold more frequent in WS patients, but the epithelial and hematopoietic tumors characteristic of normal aging are far less common in these individuals than in normal old people. Furthermore, WS patients exhibit many features that are not seen in normal aging, including subcutaneous calcifications, altered fat distribution, vocal changes, flat feet, malleolar ulcerations, high levels of urinary hyaluronic acid, and a number of other phenotypes not seen commonly in older adults. It seems plausible that the loss of the *WRN* mutation, perhaps through alteration of cells responsible for connective tissue maintenance, induces multiorgan failure through processes distinct from the changes that impair some of the same organs in normal aging.

AGING RESEARCH AND PREVENTIVE MEDICINE

The central rationale for biological gerontology is the hope that discoveries in this field will lead to innovations in preventive medicine. Mice subject to DR, or with genetic manipulations that increase lifespan, show protection from a wide array of diverse age-associated pathologies, and there is growing evidence that multiple signs of aging occur more slowly in mice treated with rapamycin. An authentic antiaging drug that produced the same demographic changes in humans seen in rodents on DR or MR diets would yield about 10-fold greater improvement in mean life expectancy than would the complete elimination of cancer or of myocardial infarction (**Figure 1-11**). A detailed understanding

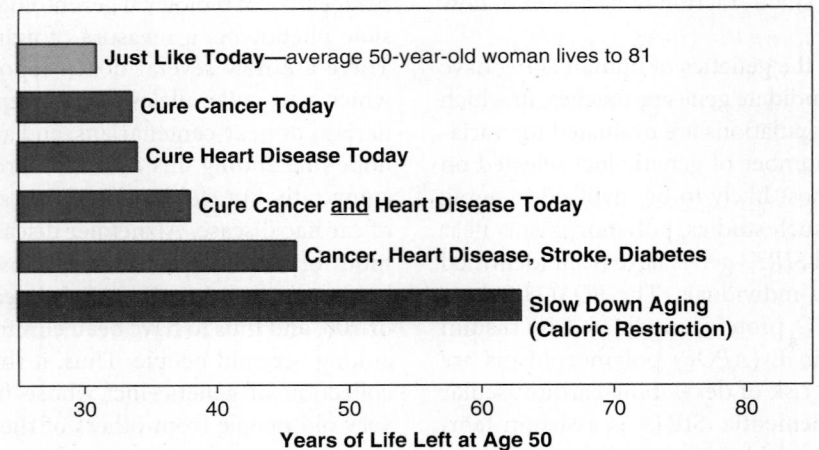

FIGURE 1-11. Theoretical remaining life expectancy of a 50-year-old White woman in the United States under a variety of demographic assumptions. The top bar shows remaining life expectancy with disease-specific mortality rates that prevailed in 1985. The four middle bars show projected life expectancy under the assumption that mortality risks for the indicated diseases were in fact zero. The bottom line shows projected longevity if it were possible to retard human aging to the same degree that is obtained in the typical study of caloric restriction in rats or mice. (Data from Olshansky SJ, Carnes BA, Cassel C. In search of Methuselah: estimating the upper limits to human longevity. *Science.* 1990;250[4981]:634–640.)

of the molecular pathways that lead to coordinated stress resistance in cells of dwarf mice, or of the adjustments that render DR rats resistant to autoimmune, neoplastic, and degenerative diseases, or of the evolutionary changes that permit large animals to survive cancer-free and cataract-free for many decades should in principle suggest avenues to preventive medical care that could dramatically postpone disability and lethal illnesses.

But the pathway connecting discovery in this area of basic science to intervention is strewn with obstacles, some scientific, and others political, economic, and legal. Testing directly whether an agent that dramatically increases healthy longevity in other species is able to safely extend human lifespan would require vast resources and treatment of young or middle-aged adult subjects for many decades. Neither pharmaceutical firms nor governmental agencies are likely to be able to support such an ambitious long-term undertaking. Nor are many scientists eager to devote their careers to an experiment whose conclusions are unlikely to emerge until the time of their own retirement. A hypothetical agent that is active in those already old could, in principle, be tested with a relative short follow-up, that is, over a period of 5 to 10 years. Such agents might be evaluated in the context of discrete age-associated pathologies or well-defined markers of the rate of aging, rather than in lifespan extension. In this regard, the demonstration that an mTOR inhibitor enhances the response to the influenza vaccine in older individuals represents a significant step forward. Many of the interventions tested so far in mice, including rapamycin, acarbose, 17-α-estradiol, and a diet low in methionine, lead to lifespan extension even when initiated in mice already well into the second third of their lifespan, and they provide some hope that interventions that slow aging could in principle be effective when administered to middle-aged people as well. A current clinical trial will test the ability of metformin to inhibit development of multiple age-associated diseases (Alzheimer or other dementias, cancer, heart disease, and diabetes) in healthy older individuals.

Introduction of authentic antiaging compounds into the practice of health care may involve relatively unconventional pathways. Some people appear willing to consume compounds and mixtures, labeled as "nutritional supplements" to render them exempt from laws that govern prescription and nonprescription drugs, which are purported to oppose the effects of aging. Thus far, there is no evidence that any of the agents so touted, including melatonin, dehydroepiandrosterone, resveratrol, homeopathic remedies, and many others, can retard, delay, or reverse aging in humans. Intervention studies in pet dogs that provide evidence that a drug extended healthy lifespan could help to shape the discussion about ways to introduce such interventions into human preventive medicine, and one such study, using rapamycin, has already been initiated. If a promising agent can be shown through typical short-term clinical tests to be useful for the treatment or prevention

of a specific disease or condition, further study of broader disease prevention and enhanced survival may ensue.

ANTIAGING RESEARCH: SOCIAL OBSTACLES AND ETHICAL CONCERNS

Serious research into the basic biology of aging and proposed translational research to turn gerontological discoveries into antiaging medicines have long been hobbled by pessimism, specifically the assumption that aging is immutable, and by stigma, arising from claims made for allegedly effective antiaging potions promoted unscrupulously for commercial gain. For these reasons, many political and scientific leaders have been understandably shy of lending support for research efforts whose goal is to develop antiaging interventions for human use. Journalists, who are often aware of promising discoveries in biological gerontology, are nonetheless often drawn ineluctably toward promotion of extreme claims, which, while entertaining, go well beyond scientific evidence and thus further impair the credibility of the antiaging research enterprise. Although several decades of evidence has now clearly refuted the commonly held assumption that the aging process is too complex or too stable to be altered, the attitudes and expectations of opinion leaders and the lay public greatly undermine and complicate efforts to attract support for this area of research.

A related concern is often posed as a question of ethics: If the goal of antiaging research is to help keep people alive and healthy for several decades beyond their current "natural" lifespan, would not realization of this goal greatly complicate efforts to solve the current set of Malthusian dilemmas? In a world where resource depletion, food and water shortages, and environmental degradation already consign billions to great suffering, would not methods that delay aging and death lead to unacceptable exacerbations of these and related problems? Arguments along these lines are often influenced by the unstated assumption that old people are typically ill, unhappy, and unproductive, and by a desire to avoid creating a society in which an ever-increasing proportion of the population has the problems that can afflict people at the very end of life.

The concern that development of antiaging medicines would be unethical is easy to refute. Most of modern medical research is designed to help prevent or treat diseases with a high risk of mortality and thus to increase the likelihood that patients will enjoy additional years or decades of good health. Efforts to develop vaccines for COVID-19, or to eradicate residual tumor burden by adjuvant chemotherapy, or to correct arrhythmias, or to alleviate the symptoms of diabetes or gallstones are all designed to allow patients to remain healthy and active as long as possible. These research efforts are appropriately considered ethical and indeed heroic, even though patients so treated are quite likely to encounter additional illnesses, often associated with suffering, at later ages. A similar motivation and justification underlies translational research in biological gerontology. Clearly, there is no pressing need for agents that merely prolong life in people who are in the final stages of a dementing illness or nearing death in great pain, and developing drugs that extend lifespan without improvements in health would not be an attractive goal. Fortunately, each of the dietary, pharmacological, and genetic manipulations shown in rodent models to extend longevity does so by an increase in the length of healthy lifespan; postponement of death goes hand in hand (and is almost certainly caused by) postponement of a very wide range of diseases and forms of disabilities.

A society in which many people remain active and productive at ages of 80 to 100 or so would indeed require economic adjustments and alterations of assumptions about retirement ages and family structure, just as adjustments of this kind have been required as societies have experienced reductions in infant and childhood mortality that greatly increase the proportion of newborns that reach the ages of 20 to 50. Such adjustments are not trivial, but such fears have not raised concerns about the ethical merit of insulin therapy, vaccination programs, smoking cessation clinics, or adjuvant chemotherapy. Thus, success in antiaging research should be considered highly desirable rather than pernicious.

ACKNOWLEDGMENTS

Preparation of this chapter was supported by NIH grants AG022303, AG023122, and AG024824 (RAM), R01GM101171 and R21ES032305 (DL), and R01AG030593, R01AG043972, and R01AG023166 (SP), and by a grant from the Glenn Foundation for Medical Research. We appreciate the willingness of several colleagues, mentioned in the figure legends, to share with us some of their own data for inclusion in this chapter.

FURTHER READING

Austad SN. *Why We Age: What Science Is Discovering About the Body's Journey Through Life*. Chichester, UK: Wiley; 1999.

Bartke A, Wright JC, Mattison JA, Ingram DK, Miller RA, Roth GS. Extending the lifespan of long-lived mice. *Nature*. 2001;414:412.

Brooks-Wilson AR. Genetics of healthy aging and longevity. *Hum Genet*. 2013;132:1323–1338.

Harper JM, Salmon AB, Leiser SF, Galecki AT, Miller RA. Skin-derived fibroblasts from long-lived species are resistant to some, but not all, lethal stresses and to the mitochondrial inhibitor rotenone. *Aging Cell*. 2007;6:1–13.

Harrison DE, Strong R, Sharp ZD, et al. Rapamycin fed late in life extends lifespan in genetically heterogeneous mice. *Nature*. 2009;460(7253):392–395.

Kapahi P, Boulton ME, Kirkwood TB. Positive correlation between mammalian life span and cellular resistance to stress. *Free Radic Biol Med*. 1999;26(5–6):495–500.

Kenyon C, Chang J, Gensch E, Rudner A, Tabtiang R. A *C. elegans* mutant that lives twice as long as wild type. *Nature*. 1993;366(6454):461–464.

Kirkwood T. *Time of Our Lives: The Science of Human Aging*. Chichester, UK: Oxford University Press; 2000.

Lombard DB, Miller RA. Aging, disease, and longevity in mice. In: Sprott Richard L, ed. *Annual Review of Gerontology and Geriatrics*. Vol. 34. New York, NY: Springer Publishing Company; 2014.

Lopez-Otin C, Blasco MA, Partridge L, Serrano M, Kroemer G. The hallmarks of aging. *Cell*. 2013;153:1194–1217.

Miller RA. Cell stress and aging: new emphasis on multiplex resistance mechanisms. *J Gerontol A Biol Sci Med Sci*. 2009;64(2):179–182.

Miller RA. "Dividends" from research on aging—can biogerontologists, at long last, find something useful to do? *J Gerontol A Biol Sci Med Sci*. 2009;64(2):157–160.

Miller RA. Extending life: scientific prospects and political obstacles. *Milbank Quart*. 2002;80:155–174.

Miller RA. Genes against aging. *J Gerontol A Biol Sci Med Sci*. 2012;67(5):495–502.

Morimoto RI. Stress, aging, and neurodegenerative disease. *N Engl J Med*. 2006;355:2254–2255.

Olshansky SJ, Hayflick L, Perls TT. Anti-aging medicine: the hype and the reality. *J Gerontol Ser A Biol Sci Med Sci*. 2004;59:B513–B514.

Olshansky SJ, Perry D, Miller RA, Butler RN. In pursuit of the longevity dividend: what should we be doing to prepare for the unprecedented aging of humanity? *Scientist*. 2006;20:28–36.

Stipp D. *The Youth Pill: Scientists at the Brink of an Anti-Aging Revolution*. New York, NY: Penguin Books; 2010.

Tatar M, Bartke A, Antebi A. The endocrine regulation of aging by insulin-like signals. *Science*. 2003;299:1346–1351.

Weindruch R, Sohal RS. Caloric intake and aging. *N Engl J Med*. 1997;337:986–994.

Chapter 2

Demography and Epidemiology

Michelle C. Odden, Kendra D. Sims, Anne B. Newman

INTRODUCTION

The aging of a population reflects the health of the population. The changes in life expectancy over the past century have varied tremendously throughout the world, with losses in some regions due to the epidemic of human immunodeficiency virus (HIV) and war, and gains in life expectancy in politically stable countries with low infant mortality. Improvements in the control of infectious disease, largely through sanitation but also through the development of antimicrobials and vaccines, account for the majority of gain in life expectancy worldwide. As a result, many developing countries have transitioned to having a larger proportion of the population reaching old age within one or two generations. This shift toward greater longevity has been accompanied by higher rates of chronic disease and a need for more chronic health care. The simultaneous decline in birth rates has left a smaller proportion of young to old. This change in the dependency ratio makes the prevention of disability in old age a public health priority.

Older adults develop multiple chronic health conditions that contribute to physical and cognitive decline. Many of these conditions are driven by age itself, with age representing the sum of time-dependent exposures and the biologic response to damage. This damage is both extrinsic, from behavioral and environmental insults, and intrinsic due to imperfect cell maintenance and repair. With time, these processes lead to distinct chronic conditions with hypertension, degenerative arthritis, coronary artery disease, cancer, and dementia among the most common. Though patterns of onset and duration vary widely, multimorbidity drives much of the disability that occurs in late life. Recent epidemiologic research regarding how chronic conditions combine and interact suggests that multimorbidity is an informative outcome for clinical trials of therapies designed to improve overall health in older adults.

In the twentieth and twenty-first centuries, gains in life expectancy have resulted from reductions in infant mortality and prevention of chronic diseases, especially cardiovascular disease and chronic lung disease, which is largely related to a decline in smoking. More recently, gains have been made after age 65, with better survival after the onset of chronic illness. While many projections continue to show continued large increases in the numbers and

Learning Objectives

- Describe and interpret key demographic features of aging and life expectancy, including birth cohort and secular trends in the United States and globally.
- Identify major conditions leading to death and disability, including patterns of multimorbidity and polypharmacy.
- Understand major biological and social determinants of health, disability, aging, and longevity.

Key Clinical Points

1. Improvements in the last century in life expectancy and the increasing proportions of populations reaching old age are threatened by counterpoising trends in obesity, health inequities, and the current COVID-19 pandemic.
2. Most older adults have multiple chronic health conditions, and the co-occurrence of multiple conditions, or multimorbidity, drives increasing disability and mortality in older adults.
3. Prevention of disability is informed by targeting its many contributors including sensory, motor, cognitive, social, and emotional impairments, multimorbidity, and environmental factors.

proportions of older adults in countries around the world, the current pandemic of COVID-19 is already showing an impact. The earliest outbreaks in China, Italy, and the United States were most prominent in the oldest and frailest, especially those living in congregate setting such as nursing homes. Since longevity projections are based on mortality rates across the lifespan and since children and young adults have not been greatly impacted by COVID-19 mortality, we might anticipate that the gains in life expectancy will be slowed or reversed in the oldest old. However, current threats to education and employment have the potential to adversely impact health across the lifespan, and particularly in marginalized populations such as racial and ethnic minorities. Therefore, our discussion of trends in the numbers and survival of older adults must be viewed with the changing environment in mind.

In this chapter, we will review the current estimates for population aging and demography including the leading causes of death in older adults and the role of birth cohort and period effects in interpreting aging trends. We will address rates and risk factors for the most common chronic conditions as well as patterns of multimorbidity and shared risk factors. We will also review trends in disability, including physical and cognitive disability and several novel risk factors under study that may tell us about the epidemiology of the biology of aging itself.

DEMOGRAPHICS

Aging of the US Population

Table 2-1 summarizes the actual and projected aging population of the United States over 150 years. At the turn of the twentieth century, adults aged 65 and older made up only 4.1% of the population, and this percentage tripled over the following 100 years to 12% at the turn of the millennium. The US Census Bureau projects this number will continue growing to over 20% by the year 2050. The numbers of *oldest old* adults, aged 85 and older, are growing at an even more dramatic rate. In the twentieth century, the number of adults aged 65 and older grew 11-fold, whereas the number of adults aged 85 and older grew 42-fold. The number of

TABLE 2-1 ■ ACTUAL AND PROJECTED GROWTH OF THE OLDER US POPULATION, 1900 TO 2050 (MILLIONS)

	TOTAL POPULATION (ALL AGES)	65 YEARS AND OLDER		85 YEARS AND OLDER	
		NUMBER	% OF TOTAL	NUMBER	% OF ≥ 65
1900	76	3.1	4.1	0.1	3.3
1950	151	12	8.1	0.6	4.9
2000	281	35	12	4.2	12
2050	400	84	21	18	22

Data from Population Division, US Census Bureau, Washington, DC, 20233.

oldest old adults is projected to continue to grow and is projected to comprise over a fifth of the population age 65 and older. This aging of the population has important implications for family structures, the labor market, economy, medicine, and long-term care; moreover, it ensures that older adults will be an increasingly influential segment of our population.

Global Aging

The aging of the population is a global phenomenon. **Figure 2-1** illustrates the increase in the percentage of the population age 65 and older from 2010 to 2050 in all six regions of the world. The highest current and projected percentage of 65 and older adults is in Europe, with North America, Latin America/Caribbean, Asia, and Oceania not far behind. Africa has the lowest percentage of older adults, but this number is expected to nearly double

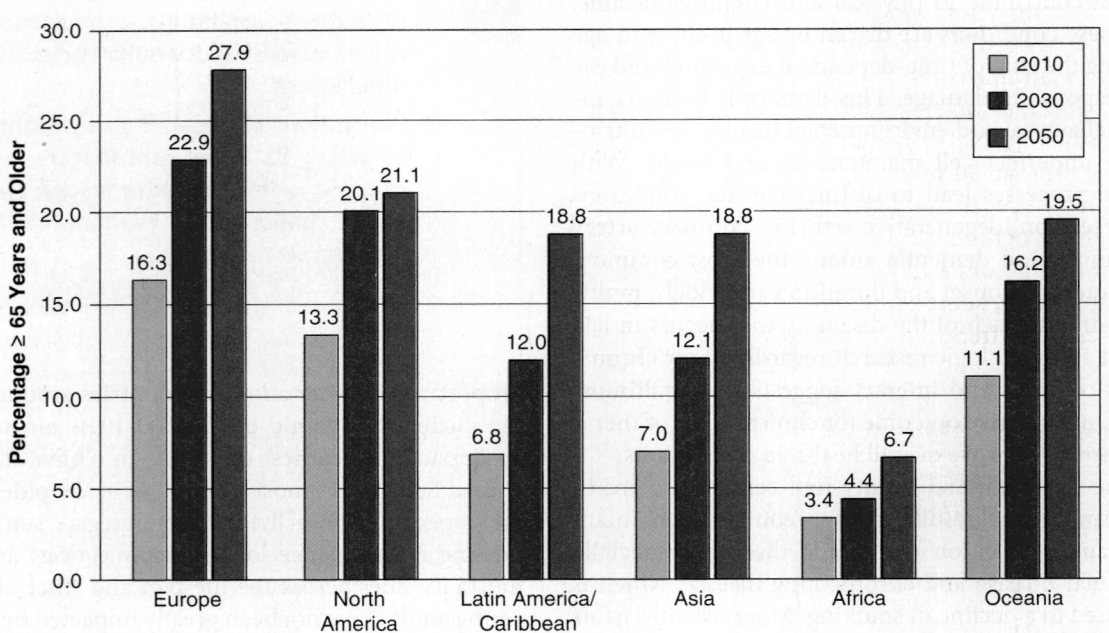

FIGURE 2-1. Percentage of population age 65 and older in 2010 and projected for 2030 and 2050. (Data from US Census Bureau, International Data Base.)

from 2010 to 2050. Latin America/Caribbean and Asia also have high projected growth in the population age 65 and older; the percentage is expected to double from 2010 to 2050. Nine of the top 10 countries with the oldest populations are in Europe, although Japan tops the list. The percentage of the population that is aged 65 and older depends on both the change in life expectancy as well as the fertility rate. Life expectancy is increasing globally, and fertility rates are falling. Older adults are living longer and thus comprise a larger proportion of the population. Dropping fertility rates can also lead to a relatively greater proportion of older adults by decreasing the number of children entering the population. Europe has the lowest fertility rate of 1.6 children per woman, whereas Africa has the highest fertility rate of 4.7 children per woman.

Life Expectancy at Different Ages

Survival curves are commonly used to illustrate the proportion of a population that survives to specified ages. **Figure 2-2** illustrates the changes in the survival curves in the United States since 1900. In 1900, the steep drop in the survival curve between birth and 5 years demonstrates the high burden of infant and early-childhood mortality. In this era, there was a modest slope of the proportion surviving across adulthood, with less than half of the population reaching age 65. By the mid-twentieth century, there had already been substantial improvements in early life mortality, and survival increased for those in mid-life due to sanitation and availability of antimicrobials and vaccines. Although the greatest gains in the proportion surviving were for those in mid-life, there were gains in the proportion surviving across the age-spectrum. Survival continued to increase for older adults through the latter half of the twentieth century and into the twenty-first century. These gains have been largely due to improved therapies for people with chronic conditions, such as cardiovascular disease and cancer, as well as reductions in some risk factors, such as smoking. Notably, these gains extended even to those above 80 or even 90 years. The change in the shape of the survival curve over the past century is referred to as the rectangularization of the survival curve and some have proposed that this will continue until full rectangularization is achieved. However, some question this outcome. There are adverse temporal trends, such as the increasing obesity

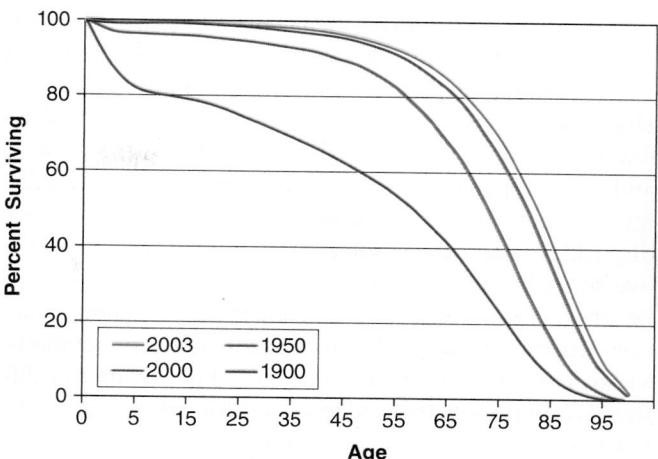

FIGURE 2-2. Survival curves for US population. (Data from Arias E. United States life tables, 2009. *Natl Vital Stat Rep*. 2014;62[7]:1–63.)

epidemic, that threaten the gains in life expectancy, as well as emerging risk factors such as the COVID-19 pandemic.

While the above survival curves are based on observed data, life tables project the life expectancy for a given birth cohort. These projections assume that period-specific death rates apply to the future. While there may be deviations from this assumption, this method evaluates the long-range implications of the contemporary death rates. **Table 2-2** illustrates the life expectancy projections at birth, 65, 75, and 85 years for men and women, and across race and Hispanic ethnicity. Notably, the older age groups in 2017 have a higher expected age at death compared with those born in 2017. This is because survival to older age represents a selected group of individuals who are more likely to continue to survive. For example, those who are 85 years in 2017 represent a selected group who have already exceeded the median life expectancy for the population, so it is not surprising that this group represent a healthy survivor group with an additional life expectancy of another 5.9 years for men and 7 years for women. In developed countries, women have a greater projected life expectancy than men. At any given age, including preconception, women have lower mortality rates than men. Many explanations for the female survival advantage have been proposed including genetics, hormones, lower rates of smoking and alcohol

TABLE 2-2 ■ LIFE EXPECTANCY IN 2017 (YEARS)								
	MALE				FEMALE			
AGE	ALL	WHITE	BLACK	HISPANIC	ALL	WHITE	BLACK	HISPANIC
At birth	76	76	72	79	81	81	79	84
At 65 years	18	18	16	20	21	21	20	23
At 75 years	11	11	11	13	13	13	13	15
At 85 years	5.9	5.9	6.1	6.7	7	6.9	7.3	8

Data from Arias E. United States Life Tables, 2017. Natl Vital Stat Rep. 2019;68(7):1–66.

use, greater health-seeking behavior, differences in occupational hazards, and others. Also apparent in **Table 2-2** are the striking disparities in life expectancy by race; non-Hispanic Black men born in 2017 are projected to live 4.5 fewer years than their non-Hispanic White counterparts, and non-Hispanic Black women are projected to live 2.7 fewer years than non-Hispanic White women. These disparities reflect the unequal conditions in which people live, as well as the related racial disparities in chronic conditions. Hispanic adults have a longer life expectancy than non-Hispanic White and non-Hispanic Black populations. Various hypotheses have been proposed to explain this difference, commonly referred to as the *Hispanic paradox*. The most common potential explanations are (1) the healthy migrant effect, which suggests that Hispanic immigrants are in better health compared with their non-migrating peers; (2) the "salmon effect", which posits that US residents of Hispanic origin may return to their birth country to die or when ill; and (3) differences in culture, including family structure, lifestyle behaviors, and social networks.

Extreme Longevity

Exceptional longevity has been of interest in both the scientific and lay communities. Scientists have studied extreme longevity to gain insight into mechanisms of healthy aging and survival. Several centenarian studies have emerged across the world in parallel to a growing prevalence of people living to at least 100. When the New England Centenarian Study began in 1994, the estimated prevalence was one centenarian per 10,000 people; in 2012, this prevalence had doubled to 1 in 5000. This means that most geriatricians will encounter centenarians in their practice. However despite this interest from the popular and scientific communities, little is known about the factors that predict survival to very old age as well as determinants of morbidity, disability, and mortality among the very old.

Scientists have long been interested in areas of the world where people appear to live longer than average, first termed "Blue Zones" by Dan Buettner in a 2005 *National Geographic* cover story. Some have proposed that a lack of validated birth certificates could play a primary role in apparently longer life expectancy. However, certain regions, such as Sardinia, Italy, have verified records and can confirm that residents live among the longest in the world. Hypotheses behind these concentrated geographic areas of long life expectancy include engagement in moderate physical activity as a part of life, plant-based diet, social engagement, a focus on family, and life purpose. However, there is currently no validated explanation about why centenarians are concentrated in such geographic areas.

There is emerging evidence that genetics influence extreme longevity. The New England Centenarian Study has reported that siblings of centenarians have between 8 and 17 times the likelihood of living to 100 compared with others from the same birth cohort. Based on these estimates the heritability of extreme longevity to 100 years is expected to be between 0.33 and 0.48. Notably, this is larger than the estimates of survival to the mid-80s. Apolipoprotein E (*APOE*) and forkhead box O-3 (*FOXO3*) have polymorphisms that have been consistently shown to have associations with extreme longevity.

In 1980, Jim Fries proposed the "compression of morbidity" hypothesis that posits that as life expectancy increases, the years lived free of morbidity and disability (often termed the health span) will increase. Although there is substantial debate on whether we are observing the compression of morbidity in the general population, the evidence points toward a compression of morbidity as one reaches the limits of the human lifespan. For example, the majority of centenarians do not experience disability until their 90s, although a substantial proportion accumulate one or more chronic condition. However, supercentenarians, those reaching age 105 or older, have a marked decrease in disability and disease compared with those who die at younger ages. Previous studies that found no evidence of compression of morbidity may have been evaluating individuals who did not survive long enough to display this phenomenon.

Age, Period, and Cohort Effects

The difference in life expectancy based on year of birth, highlights an important epidemiologic phenomenon known as cohort effects, where people have some common experience based on their year of birth, or another shared temporal experience. This is to be distinguished from age effects, which are effects common to people of a given age. Another time effect is known as period effects, in which people share some common effect due to the occurrence of an event defined by chronologic time. These three effects—age, period, and cohort effects—confound one another and can be difficult to disentangle in epidemiologic studies.

Conceptual differences in age, period, and cohort effects are illustrated in **Figure 2-3**. In this figure, three birth cohorts are illustrated: those born in 1930, 1940, and 1950. The first panel demonstrates pure age effects—the event rate of some disease increases with age. Age effects are familiar to many in health care, as the incidence of many conditions, such as cardiovascular disease, increases with age. The second panel illustrates pure period effect. Each birth cohort has a spike in event rates at the year 2020. An example of a period effect is the 2020 SARS-CoV-2 pandemic, which increased the rate of pneumonia across persons in all three birth cohorts. The third panel illustrates pure cohort effects; those born in 1930 have the highest event rate, and the rate decreases with each decade of birth year. An example of a cohort effect is that children born during the Great Depression may have suffered from malnutrition, and be more likely to develop adult-onset diseases compared with those born in more prosperous times. One can observe how this would confound age effects, by evaluating the rate of disease in 2020 (indicated

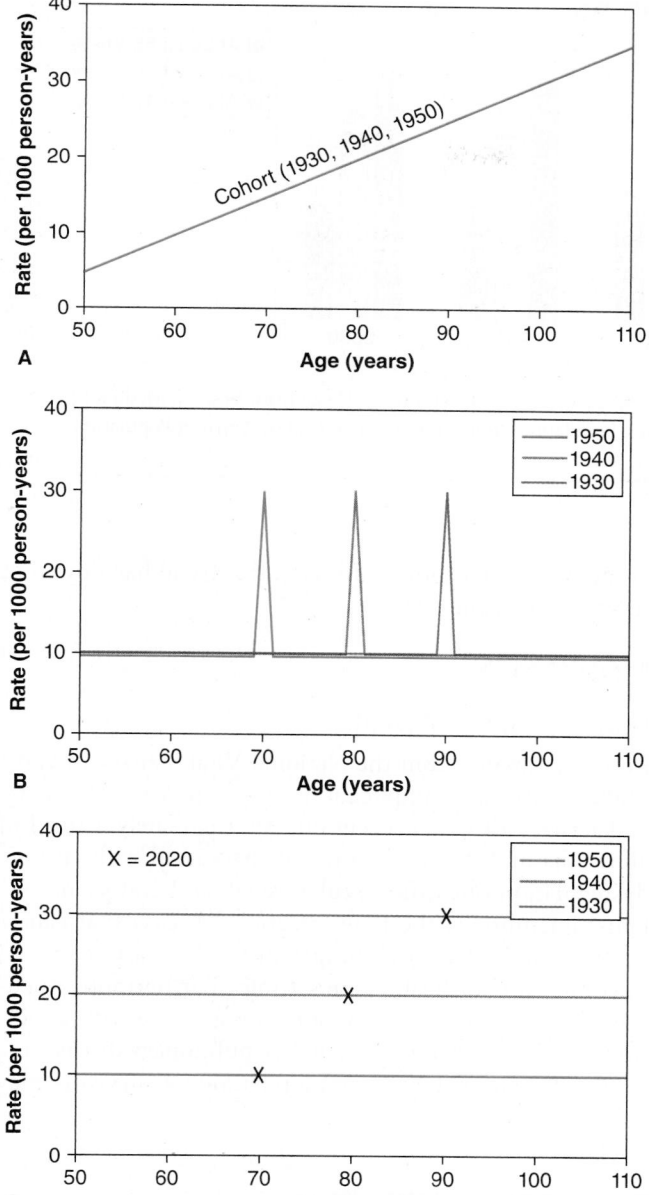

FIGURE 2-3. Illustration of hypothetical age, period, and birth cohort effects.

27

to outnumber similarly aged men, though as shown in **Figure 2-4** the sex differences in life expectancy will modestly narrow over the next four decades. For every 100 women aged at least 65, there will be 82 men in 2030 and 86 men in 2060. The sex ratio among centenarians will remain 2:5 (40 to 100) in favor of women for the next 40 years. These sex ratios reflect sex assigned at birth, and not gender identity.

The majority of men, but not women, aged 65 and older are married. Among men aged 65 and older, 70% are married, 12% are divorced, and 12% are widowed. Among women aged 65 and older, 44% are married, 15% are divorced, and 34% are widowed. Women are more likely to outlive their husbands because of the longer life expectancy of women; 72% of women aged 85 and older are widowed. Living situation is determined by health, financial factors, and widowhood. The majority (68%) of adults aged 65 and older live with family, and about a quarter (26%) live alone.

Minority Aging

The older population is becoming more diverse in the United States. Non-Hispanic White adults made up 77% of those aged at least 65 in 2017, but are expected to make up only 55% of older adults by 2060 as seen in **Figure 2-5**. All racial/ethnic groups are expected to increase proportional to non-Hispanic White older adults, with the greatest increases projected among Hispanic adults age 65 and older. Black and Hispanic populations tend to shoulder a disproportionate burden of morbidity and disability compared with their White counterparts. For example, among adults aged 65 and older, 46% of Black adults had a disability compared with 33% of Asian and 38% of White adults. Among those who reported Hispanic origin, 42% had a disability compared with 38% of those who were not Hispanic. The higher burden of poor health in these communities reflects the unequal conditions in which Black and Hispanic populations live. Only 7.2% of White adults aged 65 and older live in poverty, compared with 13% of Asian and 16% of Black Americans. Among those who report Hispanic origin, 18% fall below the poverty line. Educational attainment follows similar patterning, with only 73%, 74%, and 52% of Asian, Black, and Hispanic adults age 65 and older reporting a high school education, compared with 89% of White older adults.

Employment

The growth of the older population has led to an increase in the non-working-age population (0–14 and 65 and older) relative to the working-age population (aged 15–64). The ratio of non-working-age to working-age people, which demographers term the dependency ratio, has grown from 49 in 2010 to 54 in 2019. Dependency ratios offer a unique perspective on the nation's aging. However, this statistic provides limited insight into the economic repercussions, as many older adults remain in the labor force well past 65. Moreover, many older adults have accumulated financial

by X's on the figure). The older age groups have higher disease rates in 2020, which could be inappropriately attributed to the aging process. These simplified figures illustrate what can be complex to disentangle with real world data, which generally contain a mix of age, period, and cohort effects.

Demographic Characteristics of the Aging Population

In the past decade, the 65-and-older population has grown by 34% (14 million people), in large part due to the aging Baby Boomer generation, the first of whom turned 65 in 2011. Older adult women have and will continue

PART I   PRINCIPLES OF GERONTOLOGY

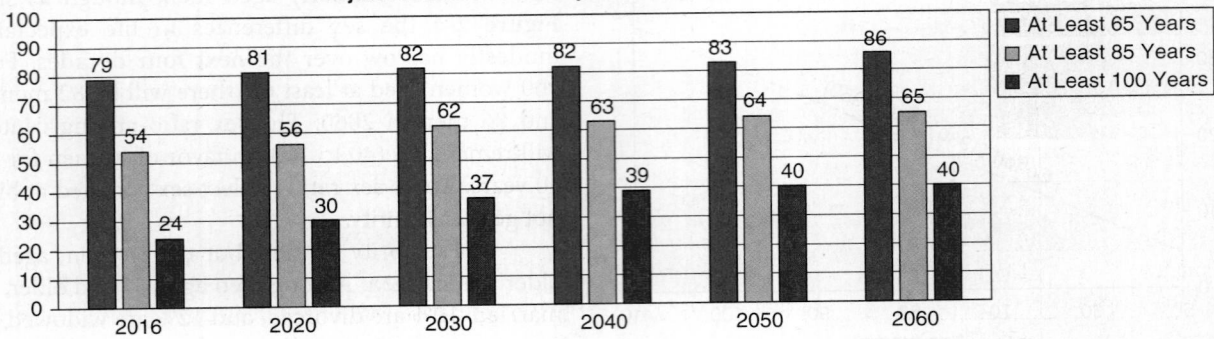

Projected Number of Men per 100 Women

FIGURE 2-4. Protected number of men living per 100 women at 65, 85, and 100 years and older. (Data from Vespa J, Medina L, Armstrong DM. Demographic Turning Points for the United States: Population Projections for 2020 to 2060. Current Population Reports, P25-1144. Washington DC: US Census Bureau; 2020.)

assets and asset transfer may mitigate this dependency ratio. Among those 65 and older, 22% of men, and 14% of women remained in the labor force in 2016 in the United States. These numbers decreased with age; only 3.7% of men and 1.5% of women age 85 and older remained in the labor force.

Temporal trends demonstrate that the years spent working and in retirement have changed dramatically. Based on estimates from the Organization for Economic Cooperation and Development (OECD), in 1960, men in developed countries could expect to spend 46 years in the labor force and about 1 year in retirement. By 2005, years in the labor force had decreased to 36, whereas years in retirement had increased to 14. The striking increase in the number of years people can expect to live after retirement are primarily driven by the gains in life expectancy. There was a trend toward earlier retirement near the end

of the twentieth century, although this trend has slowed or reversed in recent years.

MORTALITY

Leading Causes of Death

Recent estimates from the National Vital Statistics Report (**Table 2-3**) have implications for primary, secondary, and tertiary disease prevention. Approximately a third of all deaths in 2017 can be directly associated with chronic dysregulation of cardiovascular, renal, and endocrine systems. Pneumonia, the lone infectious disease that causes death, includes bacterial, fungal, or viral diseases acquired in community or health care settings. Furthermore, pneumonia has a higher fatality rate among those with conditions including chronic obstructive pulmonary disease; the resultant organ damage among pneumonia survivors may

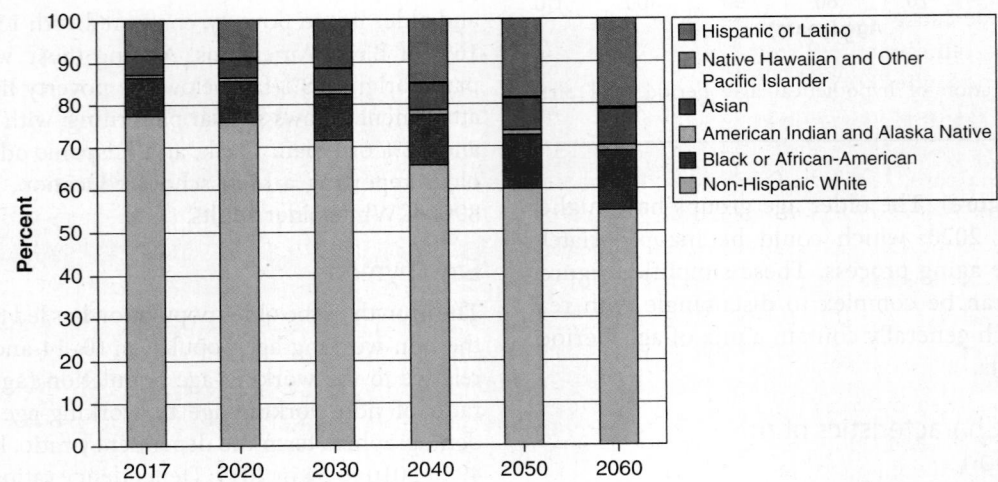

FIGURE 2-5. Percent distribution of the U.S. population aged 65 and older by race and ethnicity, 2017, 2020, 2030, 2040, 2050, 2060. (Data from the US Census Bureau, 2017 National Populations Projections Tables: Main Series. https://www.census.gov/data/tables/2017/demo/popproj/2017-summary-tables.html.)

TABLE 2-3 ■ LEADING CAUSES OF DEATH AMONG PERSONS 65 YEARS AND OLDER IN 2017

CAUSE OF DEATH	NUMBER OF DEATHS	DEATH RATE (PER 100,000 POPULATION)	% OF ALL DEATHS IN PERSONS ≥ 65 YEARS
Heart disease	519,052	1021	25
Malignant neoplasms	427,896	841	21
Chronic lower respiratory disease	136,139	268	6.6
Cerebrovascular disease	125,653	247	6.1
Alzheimer disease	120,107	236	5.8
Diabetes mellitus	59,020	116	2.9
Unintentional injuries	55,951	110	2.7
Influenza and pneumonia	46,862	92	2.3
Nephritis, nephrotic syndrome, and nephrosis	41,670	82	2.0
Parkinson disease	31,177	61	1.5
All other causes (residual)	503,877	24	24
Total	**2,067,404**	**4,065**	**100**

Data from Heron M. Deaths: Leading Causes for 2017. Natl Vital Stat Rep. 2019;68(6):1–77.

precipitate further life-threatening health events. The risk of nonintentional accidents and falls that result in death can be partially a consequence of sensory and functional decline. Thus the leading causes of death have overlapping and underlying causal risk factors.

Notably, a quarter of older adult deaths could not be ascribed to a single cause. This highlights the challenges of mortality ascertainment among the segment of the population with the highest burden of chronic conditions. Additionally, the all-other cause category includes deaths subject to social stigma, such as "diseases of despair": alcohol-related liver disease, controlled substance overdose, and suicide. The rate of diseases of despair among adults aged 65 increased from 45 to 57 deaths per 100,000 from 2009 to 2019, according to Centers for Disease Control and Prevention data.

Mortality Rates

Mortality rates declined by 21% among all ages between 1935 and 2017. The reduction in death is even more pronounced among older adults. Among adults between 65 and 74 years, mortality rates were 60% lower in 2017 compared to the period of the Great Depression. Comparing people aged at least 85 over time reflects these gains in population health; though there is a higher absolute number of deaths among the oldest old, the mortality rate was 40% lower in 2017 than 1935.

The elevated prevalence of chronic conditions in older adults corresponds to the patterning of older adult mortality. As observed in **Figure 2-6**, the mortality rates increase for the leading causes of death with advancing age. As the most striking example, the estimated Alzheimer's mortality is less than 1 per 100,000 among people younger than 65 and 350 per 100,000 among people between the ages of 80 and 84. The only leading cause not following a consistent age-gradient is death related to accidents. Fatal accidents appear highest among people in their early to mid-80s and second highest among people in their mid to late 50s, with modest declines between the sixth and seventh decades. The most common type of accident also varies between the middle aged (vehicular) and the oldest old (falls).

Figure 2-7 illustrates how cancer mortality rates peaked among the oldest old of both sexes at the turn of the twenty-first century. Men were disproportionately affected. In 1990, there were more than 500 cancer-related deaths per million men among both the 75 to 84 and 85+ age groups. Partially a consequence of better prevention of fatal events such as heart failure and stroke, more men seem to be surviving until oldest age in order to die from advanced-stage cancer. This is among the many factors, now partially understood, that account for the 33% increase in cancer mortality among men aged at least 85 between 1950 and 2016. More research is needed to determine much of this disparity is due to sex hormone differences or to gender differences in health behaviors such as preventative screening.

CHRONIC HEALTH CONDITIONS

Prevalence of Common Diseases

The most common chronic conditions among Medicare beneficiaries aged 65 and older are presented in **Table 2-4**. Hypertension is the most common chronic condition and a risk factor for cardiovascular disease, and is prevalent in over half of older adults. Hyperlipidemia, another risk factor for cardiovascular outcomes, is the second most chronic condition and impacts 41% of older men and women. Ischemic heart disease, arthritis, diabetes, and chronic kidney disease affect over one-fifth of older men and women. There are important gender differences in the prevalence of many conditions. Arthritis, depression, and osteoporosis are more common among women, whereas ischemic heart disease is more common among men.

It is important to note that these prevalence estimates were based on Medicare claims, and thus would not capture undiagnosed conditions. Discrepancies between claims-based estimates and true prevalence of conditions are highest for asymptomatic conditions, such as hypertension and hyperlipidemia, and in marginalized populations,

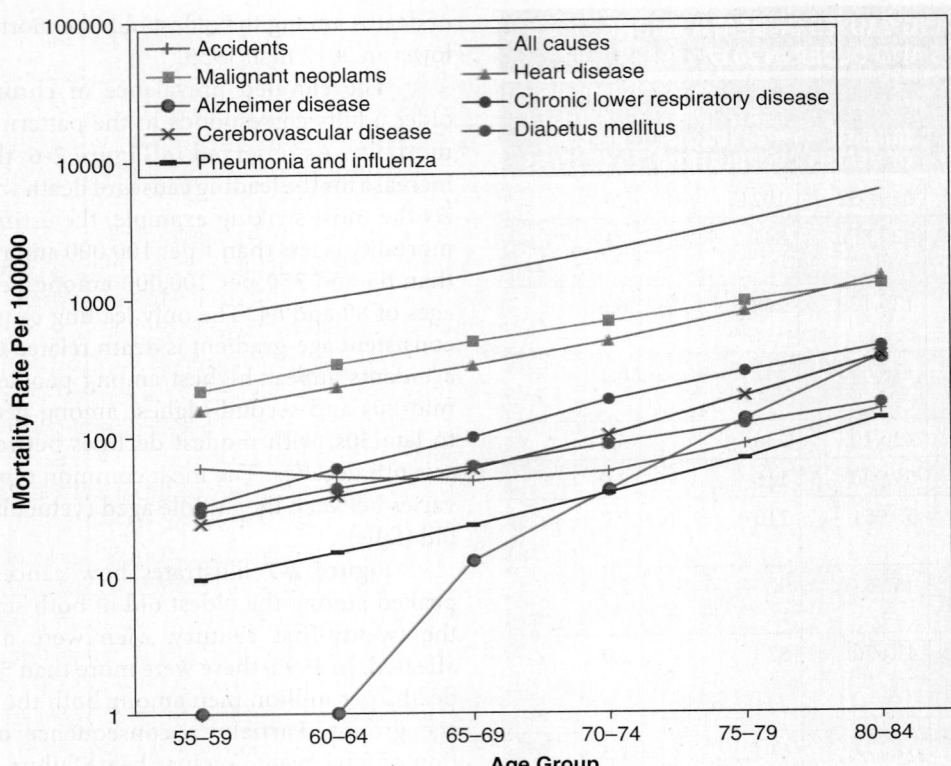

FIGURE 2-6. Age-specific death rates for leading cause of death in the older population, United States, 2017. (Data from CDC/NCHS, National Vital Statistics System, Mortality 2017. National Center for Health Statistics; 2018. https://www.cdc.gov/nchs/data/dvs/lcwk/lcwk1_hr_2017-a.pdf.)

such as individuals experiencing homelessness, those who are incarcerated, and those who reside in long-term care. Population-based surveys and epidemiologic cohort studies can provide more accurate estimates. These types of

studies may use a combination of testing, examinations, and medical record review to more accurately diagnose chronic conditions. However, even these studies do not reach marginalized populations.

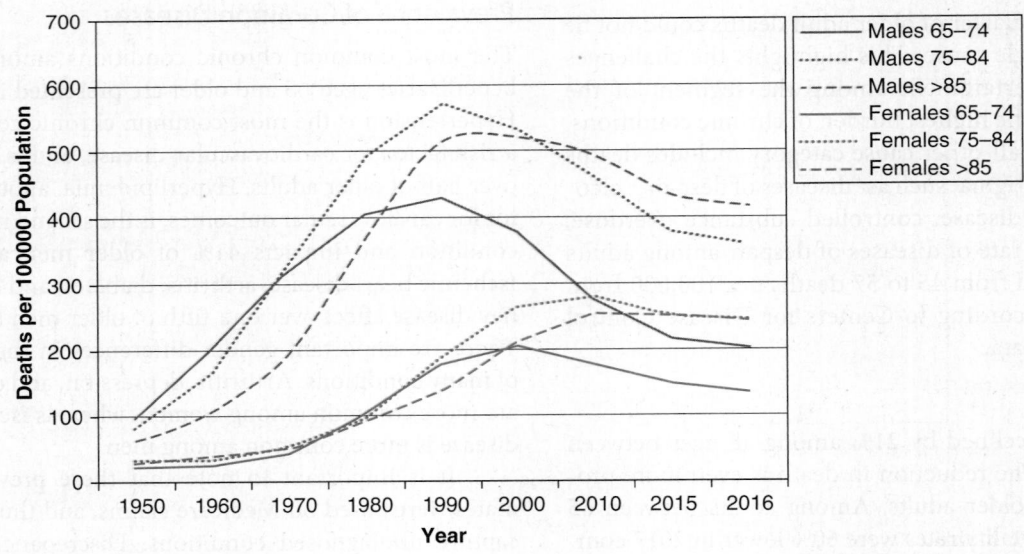

FIGURE 2-7. Mortality rate for malignant neoplasms by age, sex, and year: United States, 1950–2016. (Data from National Center for Health Statistics; 2017. https://www.cdc.gov/nchs/data/hus/2017/024.pdf.)

TABLE 2-4 ■ MOST COMMON CHRONIC CONDITIONS PER 100 MEDICARE BENEFICIARIES 65 YEARS AND OLDER IN 2017		
CONDITION	MALE	FEMALE
Hypertension	56	58
Hyperlipidemia	41	41
Ischemic heart disease	32	22
Arthritis	27	38
Diabetes	29	26
Chronic kidney disease	26	23
Depression	13	22
Heart failure	14	13
Chronic obstructive pulmonary disease	12	12
Alzheimer disease	9	12
Atrial fibrillation	9	8
Cancer	9	7
Osteoporosis	0	11
Asthma	3	6
Stroke	4	4

Data from chronic conditions among Medicare beneficiaries, 2017. https://www.cms.gov/Research-Statistics-Data-and-Systems/Statistics-Trends-and-Reports/Chronic-Conditions/CC_Main.

Co-Occurrence of Multiple Chronic Conditions

A core principle of geriatric medicine is that chronic conditions often occur in combination among older adults. Multiple chronic conditions are common among older adults. In 2018, 33% of adults 45 to 64 years had two or more chronic conditions, compared with 64% of adults 65 years and older. When one or more chronic conditions occur in relation to an index condition, this is often termed comorbidity; whereas when multiple chronic conditions occur together, this is termed multimorbidity. Multimorbidity accumulates with time, varies by ethnicity, and accelerates in later life. African-Americans have substantially higher levels of multimorbidity at every age, with similar age acceleration (**Figure 2-8**). Multimorbidity is a risk factor for multiple outcomes that include hospitalization, disability, and death, and comorbidity can increase the risk of outcomes associated with an index condition. For example, comorbidity can increase the risk of all-cause mortality among women with breast cancer, compared with women with breast cancer and no comorbid conditions. Moreover, comorbidity can complicate the treatment of a given condition, and certain therapies may be contraindicated, such as the use of diuretics to treat hypertension in the presence of comorbid gout.

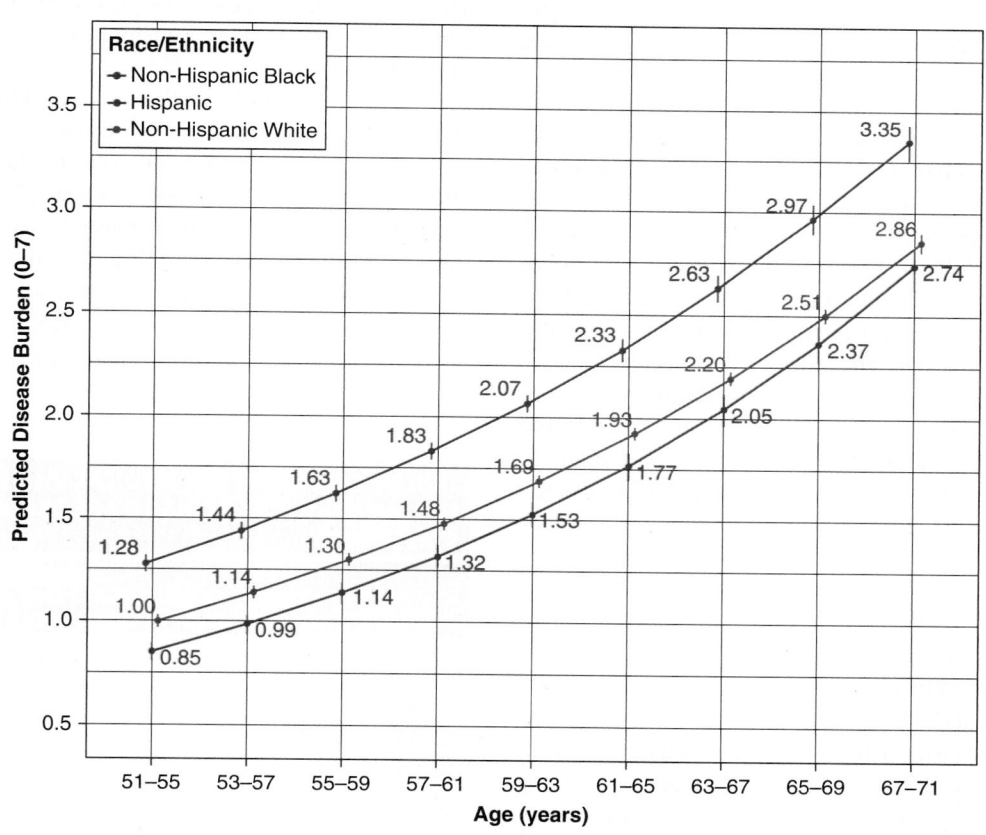

FIGURE 2-8. Multimorbidity trajectories: non-Hispanic Black, non-Hispanic White, and Hispanic trajectories of chronic disease accumulation over time, HRS 1998–2014. (Reproduced with permission from Quiñones AR, Botoseneanu A, Markwardt, et al. Racial/ethnic differences in multimorbidity development and chronic disease accumulation for middle-aged adults. *PLoS One.* 2019;14[6]:e0218462.)

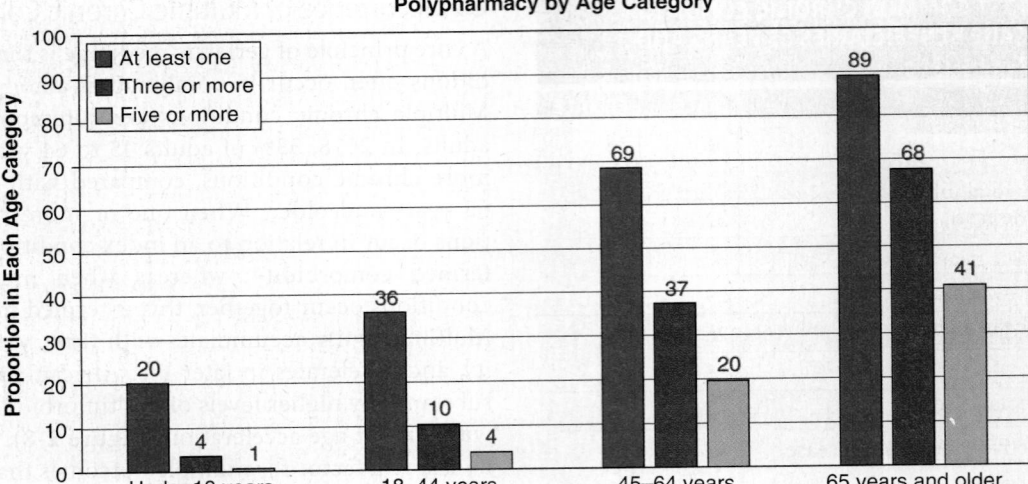

FIGURE 2-9. Prescription medication use in the past 30 days by age, United States: 2013–2016. (Data from National Center for Health Statistics; 2018. National Health and Nutrition Examination Survey. National Health and Nutrition Examination Survey (NHANES) https://www.cdc.gov/nchs/data/hus/2018/038.pdf.)

A common consequence is that people with multiple chronic conditions are often given multiple medications to treat those conditions. Most medications are evaluated one at a time in a single disease setting. While the benefit of treatment may be clear in this setting, the long-term benefits and harms associated with the combination of medications that are taking as a result of disease-specific treatment are less clear. Polypharmacy, or the use of multiple medications, is frequently associated with adverse outcomes including poor physical function, cognitive problems, and even death. Data on prescription drug use are shown in **Figure 2-9**. The number of prescription drugs used increases with age. Two-thirds of adults 65 years and older use three or more drugs, and 40% of this age group uses five or more. In response to concerns about medication overuse in older adults, many clinicians are considering *deprescribing* medications when the benefit of a medication no longer outweighs the harms. Deprescribing is the planned and supervised process of dose reduction or stopping of medication.

Health Care Utilization

Another way to appreciate the burden of chronic conditions in older adults is to examine health care utilization. **Table 2-5** illustrates that adults 75 years and older have the highest rate of ambulatory care visits of any age group based on data from the 2016 National Ambulatory Medical Care Survey. Among every 100 adults 75 years and older, there is an average of 547 outpatient medical visits per year, or between five and six visits per person. This is about double what is observed in midlife, where the average rates are 205 per 100 persons per year for adults aged 25 to 44, and 302 per 100 persons per year for adults aged 45 to 64. Also notable is that over half of

visits in adults 75 years and older are for a chronic condition, whereas this proportion is progressively smaller in younger age groups. The most common conditions reported at ambulatory care visits are hypertension, hyperlipidemia, arthritis, diabetes, and cancer.

Based on data from the National Hospital Discharge Survey, heart disease is the top cause of hospitalization in persons aged 65 and older and accounts for nearly 600 hospitalizations per 10,000 people per year (**Table 2-6**). Among the different types of heart disease, heart failure results in the highest burden of hospitalizations, due to the recurrent nature of this condition. After heart disease, the most common causes of hospitalization are cerebrovascular disease, pneumonia, cancer, fractures, osteoarthritis, septicemia, and

TABLE 2-5 ■ OUTPATIENT MEDICAL VISITS AND REASONS FOR THE VISIT[a] ACCORDING TO AGE GROUP, UNITED STATES, 2016

AGE GROUP	NUMBER OF VISITS PER 100 PERSONS PER YEAR[b]	PERCENT VISITS FOR CHRONIC PROBLEMS (ROUTINE OR FLARE-UP)
< 15	257	16
15–24	153	31
25–44	205	33
45–64	302	44
65–74	465	49
75+	547	54

[a]Table does not account for pre- or postsurgery/injury follow-up, nonillness care, or unknown reason for visit.
[b]Per person estimates utilizing 2010 census numbers.
Data from National Ambulatory Medical Care Survey: 2016 National Summary Tables. https://www.cdc.gov/nchs/data/ahcd/namcs_summary/2016_namcs_web_tables.pdf.

TABLE 2-6 ■ THE 10 LEADING CAUSES OF HOSPITALIZATION IN PERSONS AGED 65 AND OLDER, FIRST LISTED DIAGNOSIS IN UNITED STATES, 2010

	DISCHARGE RATE PER 10,000 POPULATION
1. Heart disease	582
Acute myocardial infarction	87
Coronary atherosclerosis	92
Other ischemic heart disease	11
Cardiac dysrhythmias	124
Congestive heart failure	178
2. Pneumonia	153
3. Cerebrovascular disease	164
4. Malignant neoplasms	146
5. Fractures, all sites	145
Fractures, neck of femur	64
6. Osteoarthrosis and allied disorders	141
7. Septicemia	129
8. Urinary tract infection	104
9. Chronic bronchitis	98
10. Psychoses	52

Data from National Hospital Discharge Survey: 2010 annual summary with detailed diagnosis and pocedure data. National Center for Health Statistics. Vital Health Stat. 2012;13(151). http://www.cdc.gov/nchs/data/nhds/3firstlisted/2010first3_rateage.pdf.

urinary tract infections, which all have rates that exceed 100 hospitalizations per 10,000 people per year. These statistics not only represent a high burden of morbidity for patients, but a high cost to the health care system, which highlights the importance of prevention for these conditions.

Cardiovascular Disease

The prevalence of cardiovascular disease, which includes heart failure, stroke, and coronary heart disease, rises sharply with age. **Figure 2-10** illustrates the age-specific prevalence of these conditions among men and women. All increase with age, with coronary heart disease demonstrating the sharpest increase, reaching over 30% in men and 25% in women.

Cancer

The incidence rate for most cancers rises with age, although some, such as prostate, breast, uterine, and lung cancer, decline in the oldest age groups as seen in **Figure 2-11**. Incidence data are available nationally from the Surveillance, Epidemiology, and End Results (SEER) survey of cancer registries. In both men and women, sex-specific cancers, prostate in men and breast in women, have the highest incidence rates, peaking in adults in their early 70s.

Sensory Impairments

Sensory impairments are often overlooked when assessing the burden of chronic conditions but can contribute importantly to the quality of life and the ability to remain independent. Sensory impairments are often classified as a

geriatric syndrome because their incidence increases with age and is often due to multiple different pathophysiologic causes. According to data from the National Health and Nutrition Examination Survey, one out of six Americans aged 70 and older has a visual impairment, one out of four has a hearing impairment, and three out of four have abnormal testing for postural balance. These numbers continue to increase with age and the prevalence of vision and hearing impairments in those aged 80 and older are over double that in adults in their 70s. Unfortunately, many older adults are undertreated for their impairments, and almost 60% of older persons with vision problems could benefit from new or improved glasses, and 70% of older persons with hearing problems could benefit from a hearing aid. These statistics represent a missed opportunity for treatment to attenuate the detrimental effects of hearing and vision loss.

DISABILITY AND FUNCTIONAL HEALTH

Older adults frequently report preservation of functional and cognitive health as their highest priorities for care. Maintenance of health in these domains allows older adults to engage in activities that enhance meaning in their lives. For some, this could mean being able to go for long walks or play with their grandchildren. For others, it could be the ability to continue working in their careers or engaging in volunteerism. Moreover, functional health is not only an important outcome on its own, but poor functional health is predictive of disability, loss of independence, institutionalization, and ultimately death. For these reasons, geriatric medicine has always prioritized preservation of functional health as a goal of care. In parallel, the epidemiology of aging has evolved as a discipline to study the distribution of functional health in older age, as well as risk and protective factors with the goal of informing interventions.

Measurement of Disability and Function

The terminology used to describe functional health is complex, so we begin with a brief overview. *Functional health* is a broad term that is often defined as an individual's ability to perform activities in their daily lives, including both simple and complex activities. *Disability* is defined as difficulty completing usual activities, and is frequently assessed through difficulty or inability to complete one's *activities of daily living* (ADLs): activities essential for self-care (eg, bathing, dressing oneself, using the toilet) (see Chapter 42). The distinction between difficulty and inability is meaningful and has led to variation in disability estimates across studies. *Instrumental activities of daily living* (IADLs) refer to the activities that allow an individual to remain independent in the community (eg, driving, shopping, preparing food). Preceding the onset of a disability is often a *functional limitation*, which refers to a restriction in basic physical action, such as difficulty crouching or kneeling. *Mobility limitation* refers to difficulty in walking or climbing stairs and is often measured by self-report. However,

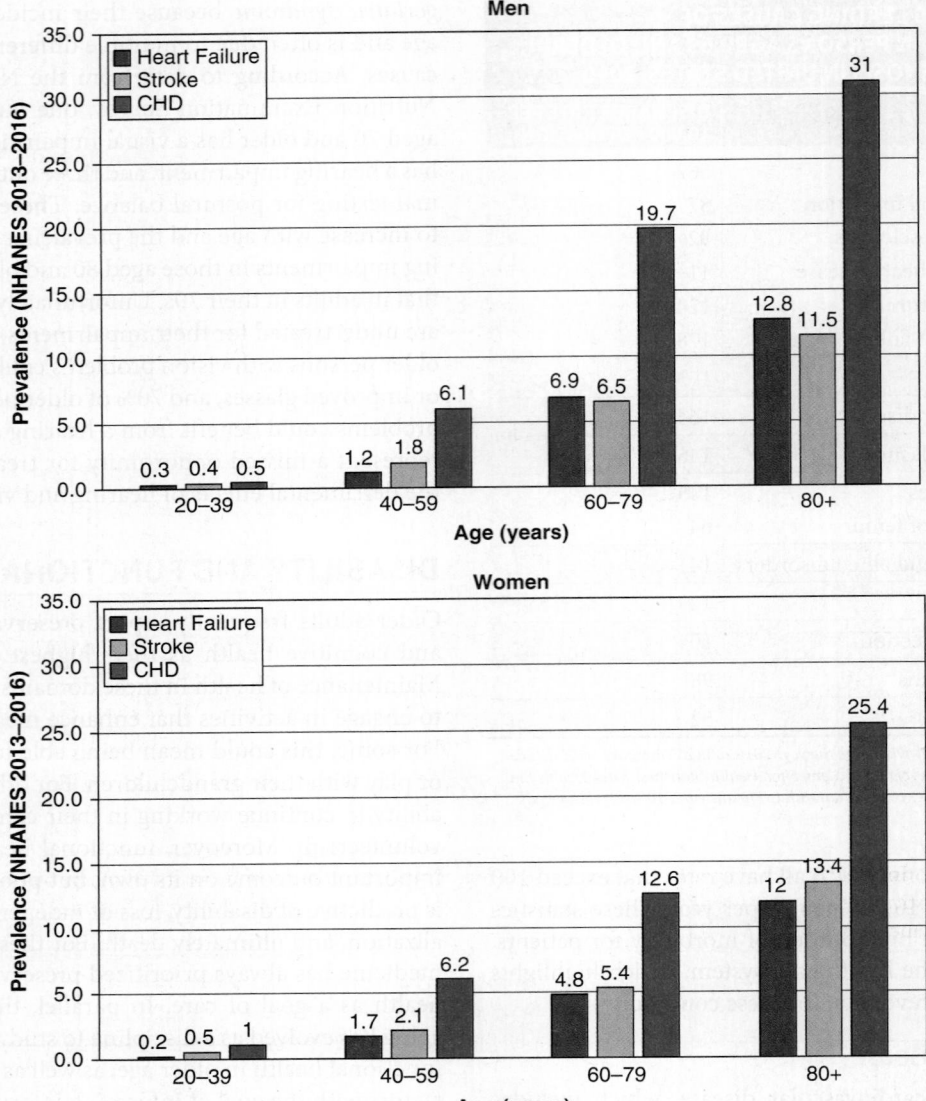

FIGURE 2-10. Prevalence of heart failure, stroke, and coronary heart disease (CHD) by sex and age in the United States. (Data from the National Health and Nutrition Examination Survey, 2013–2016. https://wwwn.cdc.gov/nchs/nhanes/Default.aspx.)

some experts have defined *dismobility* as a measured gait speed less than 0.6 m/s or inability to walk 400 meters. *Physical performance* measures include objective measures of physical function such as walking, balance, and strength. One of the most common tools for evaluating physical performance is the Short Physical Performance Battery (SPPB), which includes a 4-meter gait speed test, chair stands as a measure of lower body strength, and balance.

Epidemiology of Disability

Data from Medicare beneficiaries demonstrate the striking impact of age on the prevalence of disability and residence in a long-term care facility (**Figure 2-12**). With each decade

of ascending age, the proportion of those with no disability drops from 66% in adults 65 to 74 years old to only 27% in adults 85 years and older. In this survey, disability was defined as serious difficulty hearing, seeing, concentrating, remembering, or making decisions, walking or climbing stairs, dressing or bathing, or with errands. Moreover, the prevalence of two or more disabilities increases from 15% to 38% in the same age groups, respectively. Notably, the prevalence of adults living in a long-term care facility reaches 13% among those aged 85 and older. These same data show modest sex differences, with women being more likely to have prevalent disability than men. **Figure 2-12** also demonstrates disparities by race/ethnicity, with White

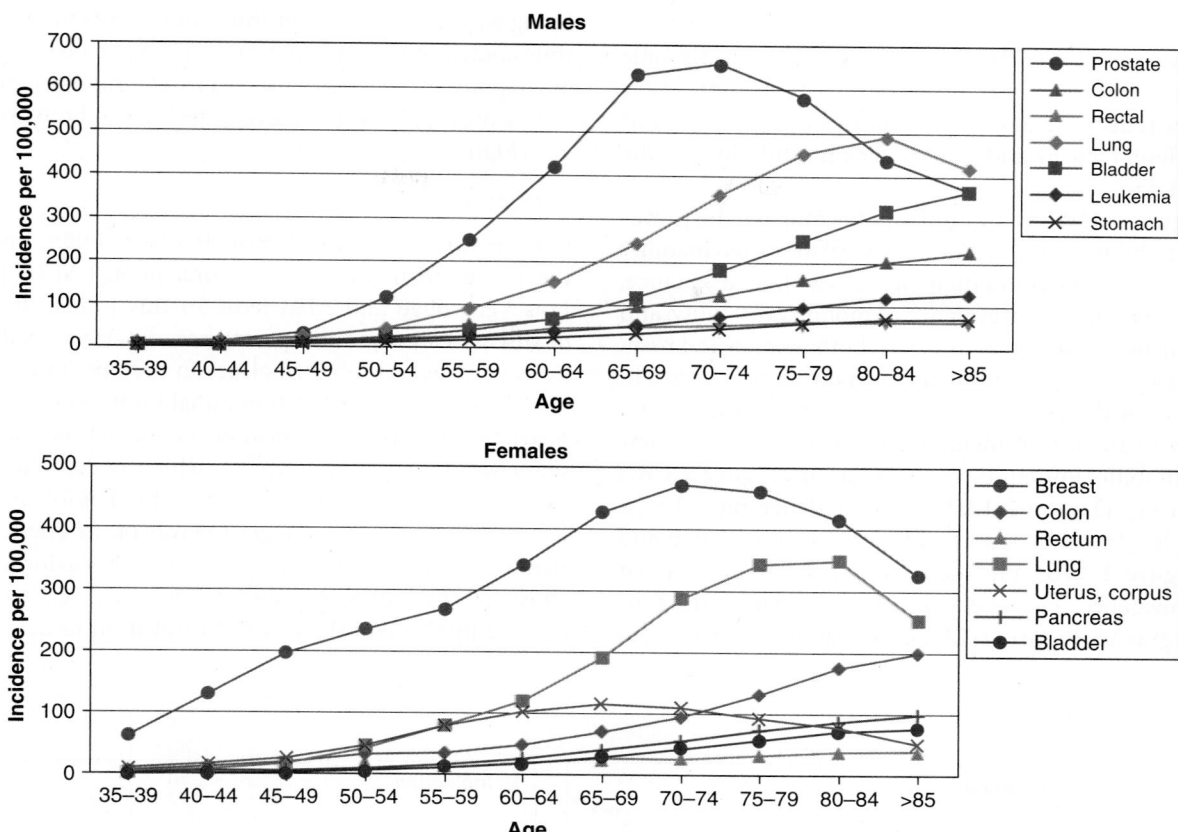

FIGURE 2-11. Incidence rates of specific cancers in men (top panel) and women (bottom panel) by age. (Data from SEER Cancer Statistics Review 1975–2017. Surveillance, Epidemiology and End Results Program, National Cancer Institute. https://seer.cancer.gov/csr/1975_2017/.)

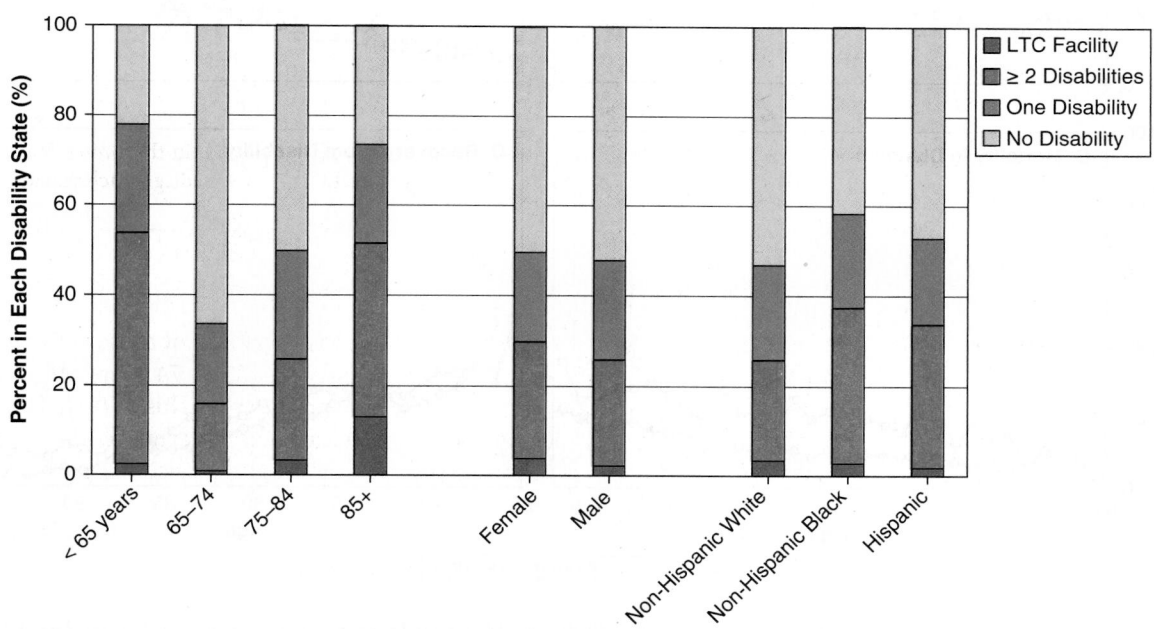

FIGURE 2-12. Disability status among all Medicare beneficiaries by age, sex, and race/ethnicity. LTC, long-term care. (Data from Centers for Medicare and Medicaid Services. https://edit.cms.gov/Research-Statistics-Data-and-Systems/Downloadable-Public-Use-Files/MCBS-Public-Use-File/index.)

PART I · PRINCIPLES OF GERONTOLOGY

non-Hispanic adults having the lowest prevalence of disability compared to Black non-Hispanic and Hispanic adults, yet the highest prevalence of long-term care. These inequities reflect the unequal conditions in which persons from different racial and ethnic backgrounds live in the United States.

Figure 2-13A shows similar patterning for the prevalence of mobility disability, defined as self-reported inability to walk 1/2 mile or climb a flight of stairs without assistance. Women have a higher prevalence of mobility disability, and the prevalence increases with age for both women and men. The subsequent panels allow us to examine prevalence in the setting of the dynamics of disability and death. Prevalence is a function of incidence (**Figure 2-13B**), or new cases of mobility limitation, as well as death (**Figure 2-13C**) and recovery (**Figure 2-13D**). The incidence rate of new mobility limitation increases with age for both women and men (**Figure 2-13B**), but the differences are not as great as for prevalence. This is explained by evaluating the subsequent graphs; **Figure 2-13C** demonstrates that women

living with a disability have lower mortality rates than men, thus contributing to greater prevalence at a given age. Men are slightly more likely to recover from mobility disability than women, although recovery declines in both groups by age (**Figure 2-13D**).

Dynamics of Disability

One of the foundational models of disability, known as the Disablement Process, was first published in 1994 by Lois Verbrugge and Alan Jette. In this model, pathology or disease can lead to impairments, described as dysfunctions or structural abnormalities in specific body systems. This, in turn, can lead to functional limitations, which is a restriction in a basic physical or mental action. Last in the sequence of events is disability, which is defined as difficulty doing activities of daily life. This Disablement Process model also acknowledges the role of the environment, risk factors, and person factors such as behavior and psychosocial attributes. An alternative model was presented in 2002 by the World Health Organization to describe the

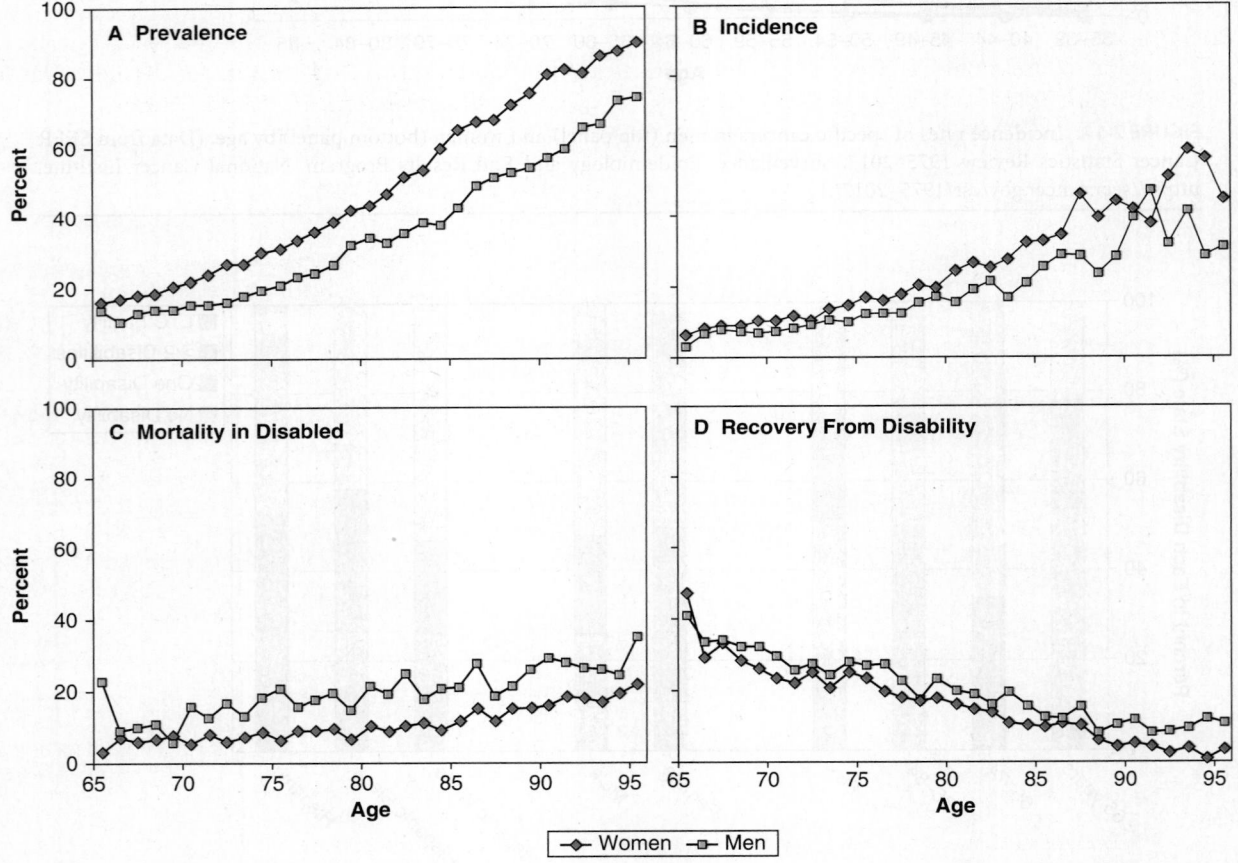

FIGURE 2-13. Women's and men's prevalence of mobility disability (**A**), 1-year incidence among nondisabled persons (**B**), and 1-year mortality (**C**) and recovery (**D**) among disabled persons, by age. Established populations for the epidemiologic study of older persons. (Reproduced with permission from Leveille SG, Penninx BW, et al. Sex differences in the prevalence of mobility disability in old age: the dynamics of incidence, recovery, and mortality. *J Gerontol B Psychol Sci Soc Sci.* 2000;55[1]:S41–S50.)

International Classification of Functioning, Disability, and Health (ICF). This model presents a biopsychosocial model of disability, which is viewed as an interaction between the features of a person and the context in which they live. Much like the Disablement Process, the ICF model also posits levels of functioning that encompass health conditions, impairments, activity limitations, and participation restriction. However, there is increased focus on level of health, as well as a distinction between an individual's capacity and performance, which is what a person does in their environment.

Regardless of the model used, it is important to understand that disability is not a fixed state, but a dynamic and bidirectional process. Many adults recover from disability and may report the onset and recovery of disability multiple times throughout their life course. One study in the United States found that impairment in ADLs developed in one-fifth of adults aged 50 to 64. Among this population with impairment, 2 years later, 4% had died, 9% had further declined, 50% had persistent impairment, and 37% had recovered. In another study of a population of African-American adults residing in Jackson, Mississippi, found that 32% had an incident mobility limitation, but nearly half had recovered within a year. The important takeaway for geriatric care is that, although avoiding an incident limitation is preferred, recovery after limitation or disability is likely. Interventions to facilitate recovery, prevent persistent disability, or further loss can help older adults to stay independent and actively engaged in their communities.

Finally, the dynamic process of disability can occur over different timescales. Often there is a distinction made between catastrophic disability, with the sudden onset of disability, such as after an acute event such as a stroke, and progressive disability, which can develop slowly over time. The Precipitating Events Project is one study that has illuminated the time scale of disability onset by contacting participants aged 70 and older monthly. By assessing individuals frequently, study investigators were able to describe disability onset using a more granular timescale than is usually evaluated in large-scale epidemiologic investigations. The investigators reported five different trajectories of disability in the last year of life, illustrated in **Figure 2-14**, highlighting the heterogeneity of this process: persistent severe disability, progressive disability, accelerated disability, catastrophic disability, and no disability.

Risk Factors for Disability

Data from earlier discussion illustrate differences in disability by age, sex, and race/ethnicity. We next turn to risk factors for disability and poor functional health. Many chronic conditions are risk factors for disability, including cardiovascular disease, heart failure, osteoarthritis, chronic

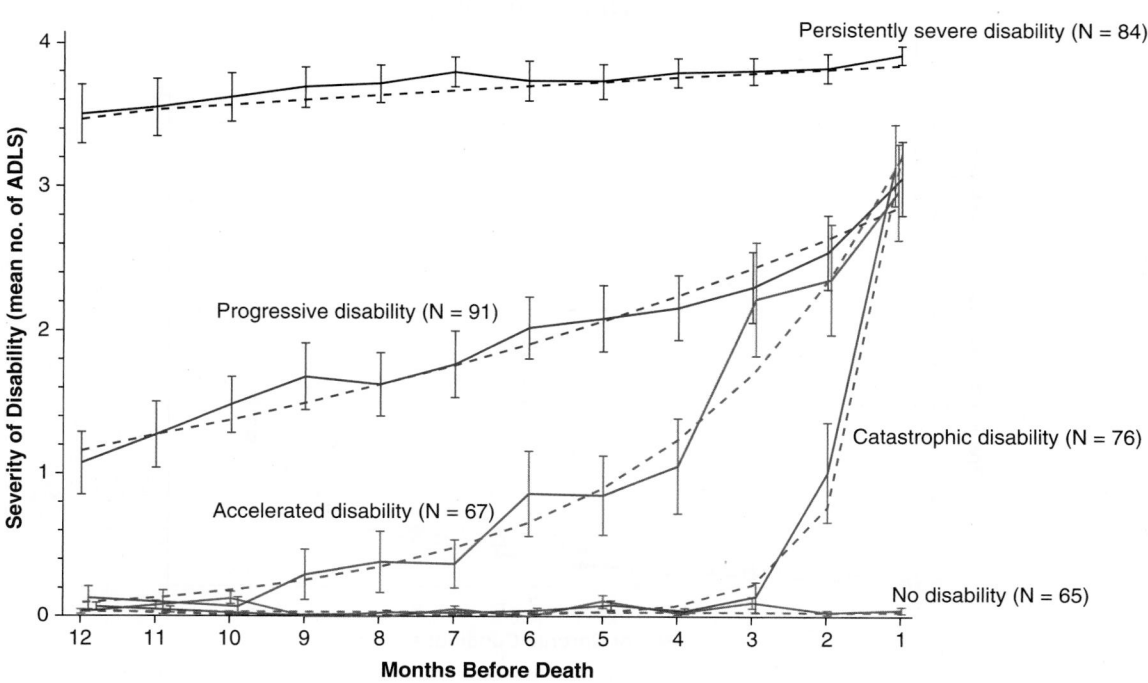

FIGURE 2-14. Trajectories of disability in the last year of life among 383 decedents. The severity of disability is indicated by the mean number of activities of daily living in which the subjects had disability. (Reproduced with permission from Kurrle S, Cameron ID, Maier AB. Trajectories of disability in the last year of life. *N Engl J Med*. 2010;363[3]:294.)

obstructive pulmonary disease, diabetes, cancer, depression, dementia, and sensory impairments. Moreover, the presence and burden of disability and functional limitations increases notably with the number of chronic conditions (**Figure 2-15**). This figure demonstrates the prevalence of up to 19 functional limitations (**Figure 2-15A**) and 7 ADL/IADL (**Figure 2-15B**) rises sharply with the number of chronic conditions. This graph also illustrates the higher

burden of functional limitation and disability among women and those aged 75 and older.

A healthy lifestyle can not only prevent disease but disability as well. There is a substantial body of work that has demonstrated that no smoking, healthy diet, and physical activity can all reduce the risk of disability. In 2014, investigators in the Lifestyle Interventions and Independence for Elders (LIFE) study found that

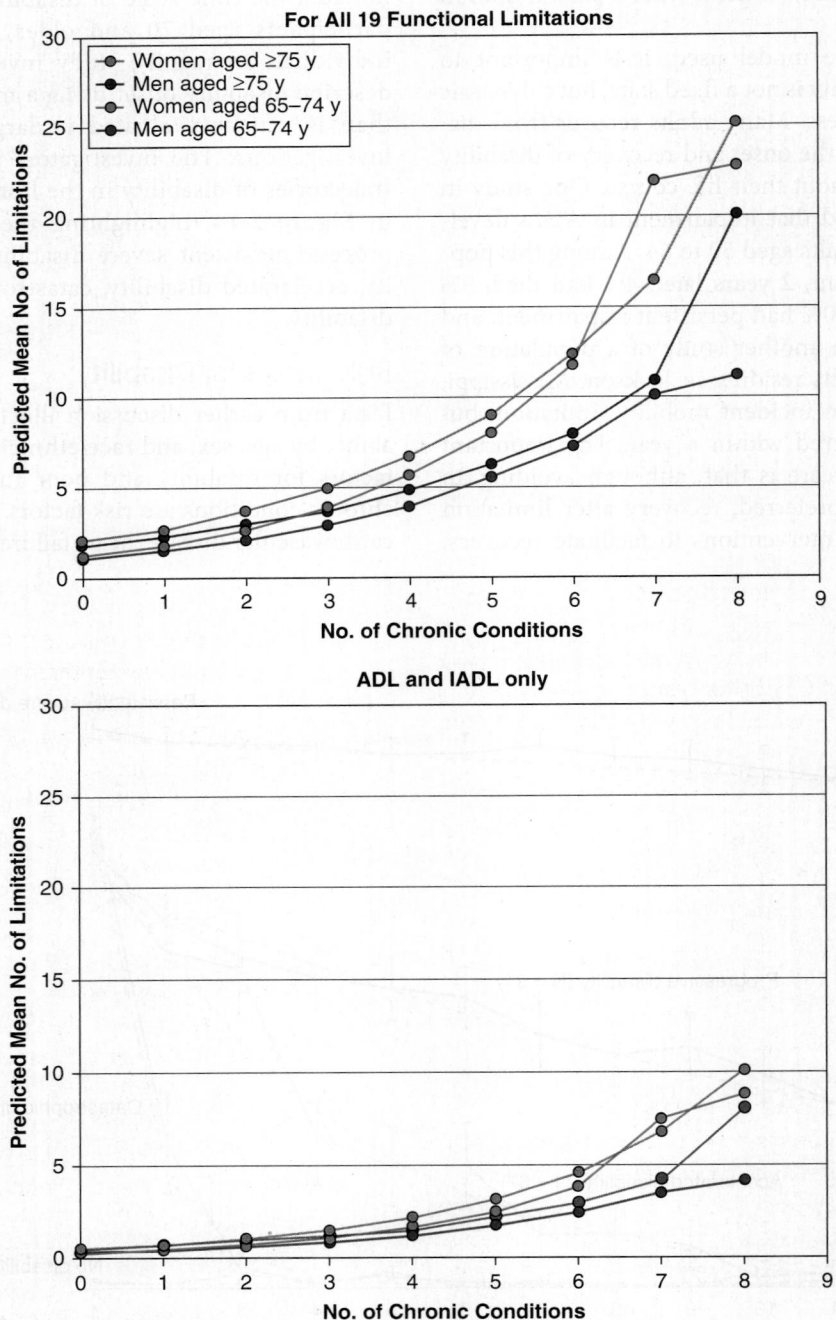

FIGURE 2-15. Predicted mean number of limitations by the number of chronic conditions, stratified by sex and age group. Abbreviations: ADL, activities of daily living; IADL, instrumental activities of daily living. (Reproduced with permission from Jindai K, Nielson CM, Vorderstrasse BA, et al. Multimorbidity and Functional Limitations Among Adults 65 or Older, NHANES 2005–2012, *Prev Chronic Dis.* 2016;13:E151.)

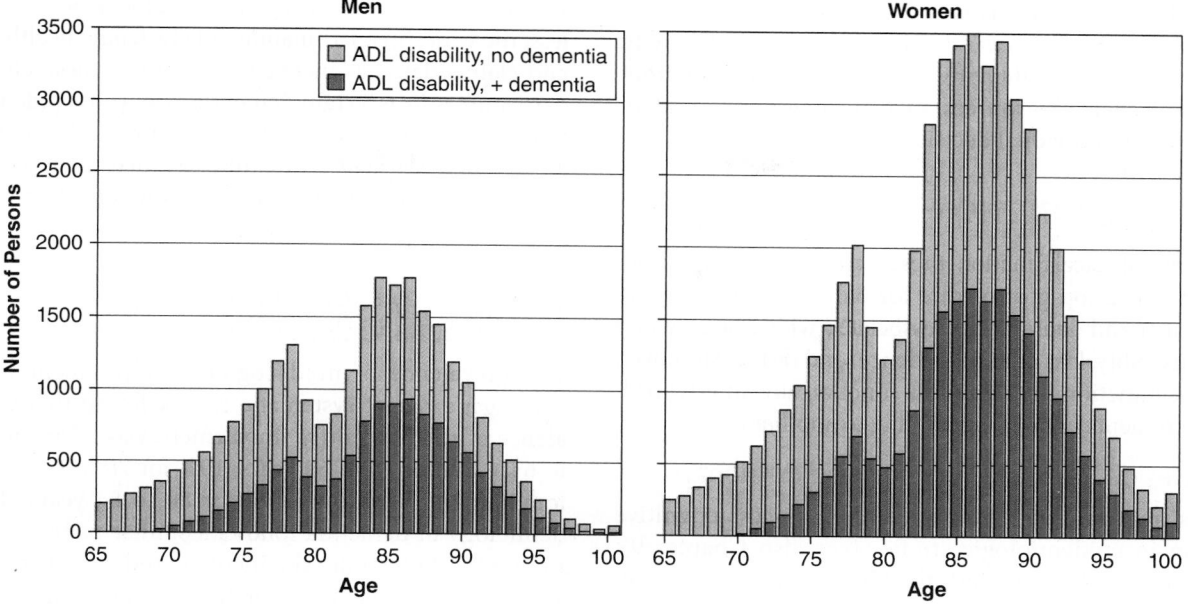

FIGURE 2-16. Estimated number of men and women with activities of daily living (ADLs) disability (need for help of another person) with and without an additional diagnosis of dementia according to age, Tuscany, Italy, 1999. (Data from three large population-based epidemiologic studies in the Tuscany population, the Italian Longitudinal Study on Aging, JCARE Dicomano, and InCHIANTI. The original analyses and population estimates are from Istituto Nazionale di Statistica: National Statistical Institute of Italy, 1999, www.istat.it.)

a structured, moderate-intensity physical activity program reduced the risk for major mobility disability by about 20% over 2.6 years. The intervention included aerobic, resistance, and flexibility training activities in a center and at home. The study targeted adults at risk for disability, demonstrating that disability is to some extent preventable.

Cognitive impairment and poor functional health are interrelated and often follow similar epidemiologic patterns. **Figure 2-16** illustrates the number of men and women with disability with and without dementia in three population-based studies in the Tuscany region of Italy in 1999. One can see that these conditions are similarly distributed across the age spectrum in men and women. The dip in the number of people living with a disability in these studies with and without dementia among persons around 80 years of age is due to the low birthrate during and shortly after World War I. Dementia is a determinant of limitations in IADLs, such as paying bills or shopping, where problems in memory can limit an individual's ability to complete these tasks. Dementia is also a risk factor for other types of functional limitations and disability, and conversely, functional limitation is also a risk factor for dementia. The bidirectional relationship between cognitive and physical function is an important active area of research. The potential clinical implication is that patients with limitations in one domain may be more likely to develop limitations in another.

Trends in Disability

Disability is commonly considered a key indicator of older adult health; it is patient-centered outcome, and also tightly connected to an individual's ability to remain independent and age in place. The prevalence of disability is also a measure of caregiving required by a population, either in the form of at-home or institutionalized care. For these reasons, researchers have monitored trends in disability, through large-scale nationally representative surveys. Monitoring temporal trends is challenging due to confounding by age and birth cohort effects, as well as trends that vary by characteristics of the population (ie, age, sex, geography) and the measurement tools used.

In general, there have been declines in disability prevalence over the past several decades, although this decline appears to have slowed or stopped around the turn of the millennium. Freedman et al. pooled results from five large surveys from 2000 to 2008: the Health and Retirement Study, the Medicare Current Beneficiary Survey, the National Health Interview Survey, the National Health and Nutrition Examination Survey, and the National Long Term Care Survey. The researchers found that disability prevalence was relatively stable for those aged 65 to 84, and appeared to be increasing among 55 to 64 years and decreasing among 85 years and older. These findings likely reflect the converging influences of advances in the care of older adults, especially the oldest old, as well as temporal increases in disability risk factors such as obesity and inactivity. Research has demonstrated physical activity, a cornerstone of disability prevention and requires environmental and societal resources, such as sidewalks and safety, in addition to individual decision-making.

COGNITIVE FUNCTION

Along with physical function, preservation of cognitive function remains a top goal of care for older adults. Cognitive impairment and dementia are associated with worse quality of life, disability, loss of independence, and death. Moreover, cognitive function and physical function are intertwined, with decrements in one contributing to another.

Measures of Cognitive Function and Dementia

Various instruments have been used to assess cognitive function in epidemiologic studies (see also Chapter 9). Commonly used tests include the Mini-Mental State Exam, Modified Mini-Mental State Exam, and the Montreal Cognitive Assessment, which are measures of global cognitive function, and the Digit Symbol Substitution Test, a measure of processing speed, and others. Some tests are better at detecting low function than high function such that highly educated older adults may perform at the test ceiling in spite of early cognitive decline. Moreover, tests may be insensitive for small declines in cognitive function.

The gold standard for clinical Alzheimer disease and dementia diagnosis is through a neuropsychological evaluation with a full battery of cognitive tests, a neurologic examination, and brain imaging. However, many epidemiologic studies use other data sources such as medical record review including ICD codes, medication use, death certificates, and brief cognitive tests to define dementia. Each of these sources is subject to misclassification and thus the incidence and prevalence of dementia may be biased, as well as any associations with risk factors. For example, one systematic review found that the positive predictive values of codes for dementia diagnosis ranged from 33% to

100% and sensitivities ranged from 21% to 86%. Nonetheless, the widespread availability of electronic health records and claims data has increased the use of these alternative data sources to ascertain dementia. Rigorous epidemiologic analyses that incorporate these measures will include sensitivity analyses such as quantitative bias analysis to evaluate the potential impact of the misclassification on study findings.

Epidemiology of Cognitive Impairment and Dementia

The prevalence of mild cognitive impairment increases with age; a recent systematic review found that the prevalence of mild cognitive impairment was 6.7% for ages 60 to 64, 8.4% for 65 to 69 years, 10% for 70 to 74 years, 15% for 75 to 79 years, and 25% for 80 to 84 years. The epidemiology of dementia follows a similar pattern with age. **Figure 2-17** illustrates the increase in dementia cases with age. Notably, women have more dementia than men after the mid-70s. These data were obtained from a pooled study of 11 European population-based studies. Incidence rates of dementia were 2.4 per 1000 person-years in adults aged 65 to 69, 5.5 in 70 to 74 years, 16 in 75 to 79 years, 31 in 80 to 84 years, 49 in 85 to 89 years, and 70 per 1000 person years in those aged 90+. Risk factors for cognitive impairment and dementia include lower educational attainment, cardiovascular disease, hypertension, diabetes, obesity, and apolipoprotein ε-4 genotype.

BIOMARKERS

Biomarkers measure aspects of biologic processes in blood or urine or with physiologic monitoring or imaging. Associations of biomarkers with outcomes can indicate the level of risk or inform on biologic underpinnings. While many biomarkers have been studied for specific diseases, interest is turning to biomarkers of the aging process itself. A biomarker of aging is conceptualized along two main

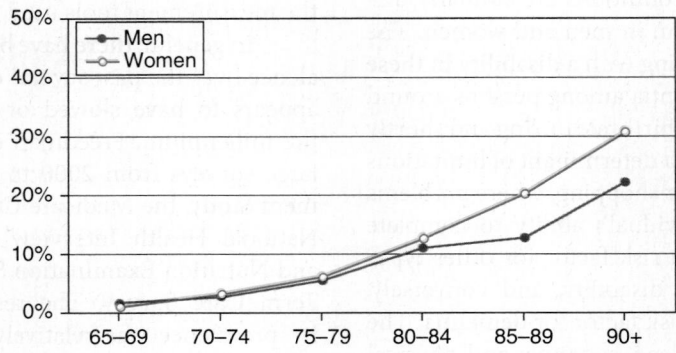

FIGURE 2-17. Pooled prevalence of dementia by sex and age in 11 pooled cohort studies in eight European countries. (Reproduced with permission from Lobo A, Launer LJ, Fratiglioni L, et al. Prevalence of dementia and major subtypes in Europe: a collaborative study of population-based cohorts. Neurologic Diseases in the Elderly Research Group. *Neurology.* 2000;54[11 Suppl 5]:S4–S9.)

dimensions: first as a marker or set of markers that captures the state of one or more fundamental aging hallmarks and second, markers that can predict outcomes at least as well, if not better than, chronological age. Hallmarks of aging include inflammation, mitochondrial dysfunction, protein misfolding, impaired autophagy, and telomere shortening, among others. These have proven to be challenging to measure in epidemiologic studies, as they often require fresh blood or tissue. However, there is hope that new markers that more closely reflect aging biology could be useful to track aging over time and ultimately to assess responses to preventive measures that promote healthy aging.

Interleukin-6 (IL-6), a marker of inflammation, is one of the most robust biomarkers of aging, predicting many adverse aging outcomes. Interleukin-6 is a cytokine produced by activated immune cells, muscle, and fat, signaling the liver to induce C-reactive protein. An IL-6 level of 2.5 pg/dL may appear to fall in the upper normal range for community-dwelling older adults, but levels in this range robustly predict decline in strength, walking speed, and mortality in observational studies of older adults. Along with experimental studies in animal models, these studies support the hypothesis that directly lowering IL-6 could prevent age-related disability. Based on this hypothesis, a clinical trial, ENRGISE tested whether IL-6 could be reduced with either fish oil or losartan. While there was no change in either IL-6 levels or walking speed with either intervention, the study provided a roadmap for translating biomarker associations in epidemiologic studies to targeted intervention clinical trials in aging. Another biomarker is telomere length, which is thought to mark biologic age as the length of the telomeres shortens with each cell division. When critical shortening is reached, cell senescence ensues. Epidemiologic studies of telomere length have been inconsistent, perhaps because most studies use mixed populations of white cells from peripheral blood. Telomere length is also quite variable and difficult to track over time. Nevertheless, telomere biology is clearly important in cell senescence and cancer biology, warranting continued interest in the biology of telomere loss and maintenance.

Increasingly, panels of biomarkers are being used to detect hundreds or thousands of unique molecules circulating in the blood, ranging from single nucleotide polymorphisms in the DNA (genomics), metabolites (metabolomics), proteins (proteomics), or the composition of microbes in body fluids (microbiome). By harnessing these "-omics" technologies to study population aging, new pathways or targets for healthy aging might be identified.

Genomics and epigenetics are well-established among the "-omics" methods. Genome-wide association studies (GWAS) have linked specific risk alleles to a broad array of aging outcomes such as walking speed and muscle strength or longevity. Prior to the GWAS era, the *APOE4* genotype had already been established as a risk factor for cardiovascular disease and dementia. More recently, polymorphisms in this region of the genome have been found to

predict longevity. The methylation of DNA, which controls transcription, clearly changes across the lifespan. By correlating methylation patterns with chronologic age, "methylation clocks" have been developed. The mechanisms of these associations are not well understood, yet changes in methylation age have been proposed as a potential agnostic marker of interventions purported to impact biologic aging.

Proteomic studies evaluate proteins that serve as enzymes or transcription factors in cellular processes. Growth differentiation factor 15 (GDF-15) has been identified in proteomic analysis as strongly related to mobility disability disease and frailty. Groups of proteins can be evaluated for the degree to which they fall into a pattern for a particular biologic pathway. For example, pathway analysis has revealed that signaling pathways of inflammation and phagocytosis are related to mobility disability.

Metabolomics include the circulating products of metabolism, such as lipids, alcohols, and amino acids. Several different platforms are needed to assess lipophilic and hydrophilic molecules. Many of the molecules that can be measured are as yet unknown or are adducts or other byproducts that are artifacts. Early studies have examined obesity and frailty, which are thought to have distinct metabolic fingerprints that may better define the underlying biology. More studies are needed that assess metabolic changes with specific interventions and diets.

Composite Biomarkers

Summary measures of health have been used to approximate biologic age by validating scores of deviation of multiple laboratory tests and physiologic measures against mortality risk. Many of these measures do not seem to have substantial correlation with telomere length or methylation age, although neither of these would be considered as gold standards. Currently, composite measures of biologic age are more accessible than blood measures as most rely on clinically available information. In a study of caloric restriction (CALERIE), a composite measure of biologic age increased less in calorically restricted adults. Such studies illustrate the potential utility of understanding the global impact of interventions on health and aging.

Physiologic Tests and Imaging

Whole person physiologic measures can also be biomarkers. One of the most well-validated is gait speed, which can be viewed as summarizing aging in multiple systems. Longer endurance walks and treadmill stress tests can also be considered as biomarkers as loss of exercise capacity is clearly age-related, even among the most fit master's athletes. Blood pressure and pulse wave velocity can detect vascular stiffening, a strongly age-related physiologic process. Some of the composite measures of biologic age use such measures in combination with or without blood laboratory tests.

Imaging has been used to assess many systems. Brain aging can be defined by the degree of overall brain atrophy and increases in white matter hyperintensities on brain MRI. Such measures have been validated as biomarkers in that they are strongly age-associated and predict future morbidity and mortality in epidemiologic studies. Imaging has also been used to describe the age-related loss of muscle mass and the central infiltration of body fat. Fat infiltration of muscles and organs is clearly related to worse metabolic health and appears to progress with aging, even without overall obesity or disease. Whether body composition can serve as a biomarker of aging per se is still controversial as muscle mass has been more difficult to measure precisely. New imaging or isotope tracer methods may better define the role of these measures as biomarkers.

Epidemiology and Population Biology

Epidemiology can support the study of aging by identifying modifiable risk factors for accelerated aging and/or longevity and their biologic pathways. Beyond individual biomarkers, multi-omics studies can link genes to proteins to metabolites and these factors to biomarkers of intermediate-aging phenotypes. Physiologic measures and imaging can summarize the state of aging at the level of individual organs. Together these can create a deeper understanding of the aging process in population studies and identify new opportunities for prevention and treatment of the adverse effects of aging.

BEHAVIORAL, SOCIOECONOMIC, AND ENVIRONMENTAL RISK FACTORS

Behavioral Risk Factors

Health behavior can precipitate or slow functional decline among older adults. Studies conducted among twins and family members indicate that, for the first eight decades of life, environmental factors are stronger predictors than genetics of health and survival. Surveillance from the Centers for Disease Control and Prevention (**Table 2-7**) indicates that adults aged at least 65 have a lower likelihood of reported binge drinking and smoking compared with middle-aged adults. Potentially due to increased need of medical care, older adults are the age group that reports regular routine checkups and immunization. Over the life course, the effect of behavior on disability and lifespan appears to attenuate. The updated framework for biomedical research involves contextualizing patterns of health behavior with social circumstances. Further research needs to identify the ideal interplay of modifiable lifestyle and environmental factors that grant older adults more disability-free life-years.

A plurality of randomized controlled trials among older adult populations target specific health behaviors to slow disease progression or reduce the incidence of functional decline. Smoking abstention or cessation,

TABLE 2-7 ■ BEHAVIORAL RISK FACTORS IN MIDDLE-AGED AND OLDER PERSONS, UNITED STATES, 2018

	PERCENTAGE OF AGE GROUP	
	45–64	65+
Alcoholic beverages		
≥ 1 within the past 30 days	53	42
Men > 14/wk Women > 7/wk	35	14
Men ≥ 5 / Women ≥ 4 at one time within the past 30 days	8.9	4.1
BMI		
Overweight (25.0–29.9)	37	39
Obese (≥ 30.0)	36	29
Any physical activity within past 30 days	32	19
Smoking status		
Everyday	13	6.3
Some days	4.6	2.5
Former	26	40
Never	56	52
Immunization		
Flu in past year	34	54
Pneumonia ever	25	71
Use of seatbelts		
Always	89	90
Nearly always	5.3	2.1
Sometimes	2.2	0.6
Seldom	0.8	2
Never	1.8	0.5
Length of time since last routine checkup		
Past 12 mo	80	92
1–2 y ago	9.8	4.9
2–5 y ago	5	1.5
> 5 y ago	4.6	1.6
Never	0.5	0.3

Reproduced with permission from Centers for Disease Control and Prevention (CDC). Behavioral Risk Factor Surveillance System Survey Questionnaire. Atlanta, Georgia: US Department of Health and Human Services, Centers for Disease Control and Prevention, 2018.

regular physical activity, and healthy diet are certainly recommended for the preservation of older adult health and independence. However, the associations between individual behaviors and health outcomes appear to weaken among older adult populations in observational data as well as in randomized trials. Compared to those assigned to health education control groups, older adult participants engaging in behavioral intervention arms commonly experience modest reduction in the incidence of transient or permanent impairment over follow-up. The smaller than expected differences in incident mobility limitation between trial groups may be attributable to the community benefit that the control participants receive. Additionally, the long-term effect of such interventions remains understudied among older adults, whose average risk of functional decline increases due to the concurrent accumulation of chronic conditions and loss of social resources. The research into the determinants of healthy aging accordingly incorporates factors that influence and eventually supersede the effects of individual behavior.

Socioeconomic Status

Low socioeconomic status (SES) has been associated with higher rates of disability and mortality. Whether operationalized as educational attainment, income, or main occupation, higher SES can provide the resources (eg, time, information, money) necessary to engage in positive health behaviors over the lifespan. Higher parental SES both determines adult SES and is associated with better cognitive reserve (good cognition in the face of brain pathology) in observational studies of dementia. In a nationally representative sample of US older adults, attainment of a high school degree or equivalent was associated with greater cognitive function, while late-life income was a more deterministic of cognitive decline. Compared to current individual income, household wealth may better characterize the finances available to adults at retirement age. Wealth is the net value of assets, investments, businesses, and property value minus debts. Older adults lacking wealth may be reliant on state-funded pensions far below their earnings during working years. Belonging to the lowest versus highest quartile of wealth was associated with greater 8-year declines in grip strength and gait speed among English older adults. Furthermore, the socioeconomic differentials in healthy aging appear to be widening over time. Wealthy adults born in 1960 have fewer reported functional impairments and better cognitive performance than their same-age counterparts born in 1915. The influence of SES on older adult health is cumulative, complex, and may be subject to cohort effects.

Marginalization, Acculturation, and Social Stratification

Access to more economic and political resources facilitates successful avoidance of premature morbidity and mortality. The unequal distribution of resources has historically been drawn along racial and ethnic lines. Biomedical research is shifting from treating racial or ethnic identity as a homogenous and innate, instead understanding self-assigned background as a proxy for aggregated elements including cultural norms and discriminatory treatment. Discrimination includes both interpersonal experiences including harassment and police brutality, as well as structural inequality including redlining and biased bank loan practices. Forms of discrimination, such as racism, can also be internalized, that is, members of marginalized groups accepting as fact the stereotypes

propagated by the majority. Beyond inducing psychological stress and physiologic dysregulation, discrimination motivates adverse coping mechanisms, reduces the likelihood of engaging in health-promoting behaviors, and restricts socioeconomic mobility. David Williams has developed one of the earliest psychometric scales to assess discrimination. Initially used to characterize racism experienced by Black Americans, these measures have been implemented and validated among diverse groups to assess discrimination attributable to gender, class, sexual orientation, and age. Analogous to discrimination based on race or ethnicity, cultural prioritization of younger people devalues older adults in the health care and employment spheres. Ageism manifests as detrimental treatment of older adults along with the negative aging stereotypes held by the society, health care providers, and older adults themselves. Compared to older adults reporting no discrimination due to age and after controlling for baseline health status, more experiences of ageism are associated with lower preventative health care use, greater stress, poor balance, and impaired cognitive performance. Conversely, even older adult carriers of ε4 variant of the *APOE* gene who expressed positive aging beliefs scored better on the telephone interview for cognitive status than carriers who expressed negative aging beliefs. Understanding the impact that various forms of discrimination have on older adult health improves the equity of medical care.

Acculturation involves both maintaining attitudes and beliefs from the culture from which a person originates and developing new ties with a dissimilar and usually dominant culture. Strategies for acculturation include integrating these new cultural beliefs with original ideas, entirely assimilating the attitudes of the new culture to replace original ones, separating from the attitude of the new culture by remaining in original cultural enclaves, and being marginalized by not identifying with either their original or new culture. Though acculturation can be crudely approximated by immigration status, language use, and duration of residence in new country, culturally specific tools such as the Acculturation Rating Scale for Mexican Americans–Version II have been developed to better assess how individuals perceive identity, utilize language, and engage in interpersonal interactions. Context as individualized as immigration experience or as system-level as discriminatory legislation can influence both acculturation patterns as well as health outcomes. Highly acculturated people tend to smoke, consume more alcohol, and have unhealthier diets; they are also more likely to exercise, have higher SES, and have greater health care access as well as utilization.

Built Environmental Risk Factors

The built environment is comprised of the buildings, public spaces, roads, and infrastructure where communities live, work, and socialize. After retirement, people spend more time near their area of residence, making the built environment increasingly deterministic of older adult health outcomes. Features of the built environment that facilitate independence among community-dwelling older adults include proximity to health-promoting resources, including medical providers as well as healthy food options. Meanwhile, extreme weather conditions, high ambient noise, poor street conditions, and heavy traffic can prevent independent mobility. A strengthening evidence base continues to reframe health policy around positive neighborhood features: for example, low crime, cleanliness, adequate street lighting, and land use consisting of a diverse mix of residential, commercial, and natural locations.

Social Environmental Risk Factors

A positive-built environment can promote community engagement among older adults; this can counteract the tendency of social networks to shrink with age due to personal functional decline as well as life stage changes including retirement, widowhood, and the death of peers. Older adults increasingly rely on interpersonal resources and networks called social capital to maintain their mental and physical health. Researchers use psychometric scales such as those developed by the Chicago Neighborhood and Disability Study and the Chicago Health and Aging Project to survey about neighborhood disorder, such as vacancies and low safety, along with social cohesion, which involves a perception of a neighborhood that promotes a sense of belonging.

The Administration for Community Living estimates that a quarter of people aged at least 65 live alone. Scales such as the UCLA Loneliness Scale assess subjective isolation with items such as "I feel isolated from others" and "I am unhappy doing so many things alone." The Berkman-Syme Social Network Index assesses the type of support received from partners, friends, family members, religious as well as community groups. Expressions of empathy, tangible aid, and advice all comprise distinct forms of interpersonal contact whose absence indicates social isolation. Among Framingham Heart Study participants, perceived social isolation was cross-sectionally associated with lower levels of serum brain-derived neurotrophic factor (BDNF), while higher levels of emotional support corresponded with lower rates of stroke and dementia over the subsequent 11 years. The health benefits vary by intensity and frequency of support, independent of network size; not all social contacts are beneficial. Older adults can experience loneliness, irrespective of the objective size of their social network, making the subjective indicators of isolation interrelated but not mutually exclusive.

Older adult health outcomes are nested within multilevel determinants at the individual and societal level. Features of the built and social environment can increase the likelihood of engaging in health-promoting behaviors. Neighborhoods rich in resources are associated with better subjective and objective measures of health. Beyond promoting positive health behaviors, intrapersonal and interpersonal resources appear to influence each other as well as promote meaningful participation in society. Insufficiently supportive social networks, resource-poor environments, and social stratification render older adults vulnerable to excess morbidity and disability.

FURTHER READING

Freedman VA, Spillman BC, Andreski PM, et al. Trends in late-life activity limitations in the United States: an update from five national surveys. *Demography*. 2013; 50(2):661–671.

Fried LP, Tangen CM, Walston J, et al. Frailty in older adults: evidence for a phenotype. *J Gerontol A Biol Sci Med Sci*. 2001;56(3):M146–156.

Fries JF. Aging, natural death, and the compression of morbidity. *N Engl J Med*. 1980;303(3):130–135.

Gill TM, Gahbauer EA, Han L, Allore HG. Trajectories of disability in the last year of life. *N Engl J Med*. 2010; 362(13):1173–1180.

Gill TM, Robison JT, Tinetti ME. Difficulty and dependence: two components of the disability continuum among community-living older persons. *Ann Intern Med*. 1998; 128(2):96–101.

Jani BD, Hanlon P, Nicholl BI, et al. Relationship between multimorbidity, demographic factors and mortality: findings from the UK Biobank cohort. *BMC Med*. 2019;17(1):1–13.

Lobo A, Launer LJ, Fratiglioni L, et al. Prevalence of dementia and major subtypes in Europe: a collaborative study of population-based cohorts. Neurologic diseases in the elderly research group. *Neurology*. 2000;54(11suppl 5): S4–9.

Marden JR, Tchetgen Tchetgen EJ, Kawachi I, Glymour MM. Contribution of socioeconomic status at 3 life-course periods to late-life memory function and decline: early and late predictors of dementia risk. *Am J Epidemiol*. 2017;186(7):805–814.

Newman AB, Kritchevsky SB, Guralnik JM, et al. Accelerating the search for interventions aimed at expanding the health span in humans: the role of epidemiology. *J Gerontol A Biol Sci Med Sci*. 2020;75(1):77–86.

Newman AB, Murabito JM. The epidemiology of longevity and exceptional survival. *Epidemiol Rev*. 2013;35(1): 181–197.

Newman AB, Sachs MC, Arnold AM, et al. Total and cause-specific mortality in the cardiovascular health study. *J Gerontol A Biol Sci Med Sci*. 2009;64(12):1251–1261.

Pahor M, Guralnik JM, Ambrosius WT, et al. Effect of structured physical activity on prevention of major mobility disability in older adults: the LIFE study randomized clinical trial. *JAMA*. 2014;311(23):2387–2396.

Revelas M, Thalamuthu A, Oldmeadow C, et al. Review and meta-analysis of genetic polymorphisms associated with exceptional human longevity. *Mech Ageing Dev*. 2018;175:24–34.

Salomon JA, Wang H, Freeman MK, et al. Healthy life expectancy for 187 countries, 1990-2010: a systematic analysis for the Global Burden Disease Study 2010. *Lancet*. 2012;380(9859):2144–2162.

Verbrugge LM, Jette AM. The disablement process. *Soc Sci Med*. 1994;83(1):1–14.

Chapter 3

Immunology and Inflammation

Albert C. Shaw, Thilinie D. Bandaranayake

OVERVIEW OF IMMUNOSENESCENCE

Immunosenescence refers to the changes in the immune system that occur with aging. These changes affect virtually all cell lineages of the immune system, and result in alterations in diverse innate immune responses mediating the earliest interactions of the immune system with pathogens or vaccines, as well as slower onset, highly specific adaptive immune responses in B cells and T cells. Indeed, these changes extend to hematopoietic stem cells (HSC) in the bone marrow that give rise to all cell lineages of the immune system. These immunological alterations are manifested in changes in cellular signal transduction or function that may arise from intrinsic mechanisms with a genetic component, but also reflect the complex interactions of the aged immune system with factors such as chronic or repetitive infection (such as with herpesvirus family reactivation or HIV), hormonal changes, and endogenous cellular damage as a potential result of chronic medical conditions. Immunosenescence has profound clinical consequences in older adults, who are at increased risk for morbidity and mortality from infectious diseases. For example, older adults are at increased risk for the development of reactivation tuberculosis and varicella zoster virus (VZV) infection; age is also an independent risk factor for mortality and impaired functional outcome from sepsis and infection with the severe acute respiratory syndrome coronavirus 2 (SARS-CoV-2), the cause of COVID-19. Immune system aging also contributes to impaired responses to vaccines against influenza and other pathogens. The protean manifestations of immunosenescence provide insights into clinically important problems that disproportionately affect older adults and potential interventions to improve immunologic responses. Here, we provide an overview of aging of the human immune system.

EFFECTS OF AGING ON HEMATOPOIESIS

HSCs in the bone marrow give rise to all blood cell lineages (**Figure 3-1**) and as a result must maintain their ability to both differentiate and self-renew so that hematopoiesis can continue throughout life. The effects of aging on HSCs are complex; for example, HSC numbers appear to increase with age, rather than the decrease that might be

Learning Objectives

■ Recognize the relationship of immunosenescence with impaired vaccine responses and increased risk of infections such as zoster, influenza, and SARS-CoV-2.

■ Understand the age related changes in the immune system that lead to "inflammaging."

Key Clinical Points

1. Immunosenescence—the cumulative effect of aging on immune function—affects all cell types and many molecular pathways at all levels of the immune response. The resulting general phenotype is one of low-level inflammation at baseline, but impaired innate and adaptive immune responses to an acute stimulus. Reponses to naïve antigens are often more impaired than memory responses.

2. Increased levels of proinflammatory cytokines such as interleukin-6 (IL-6) and tumor necrosis factor-α (TNF-α), acute phase reactants such as C-reactive protein (CRP), and clotting factors are found in the plasma of older adults, compared to younger adults, a phenomenon called "inflammaging," and thought causal links have not yet been demonstrated, is associated with cardiovascular events, Alzheimer disease, decreased muscle mass/strength, and mortality risk in cohorts of older adults.

3. Cumulative immune changes render many vaccines less effective in seniors. Specific changes in vaccine formulation (eg, high-dose influenza vaccine, conjugated pneumococcal vaccine, recombinant Zoster vaccine) attempt to address this concern, and clinical efficacy trials demonstrate benefit versus standard vaccines in some (eg, high-dose influenza).

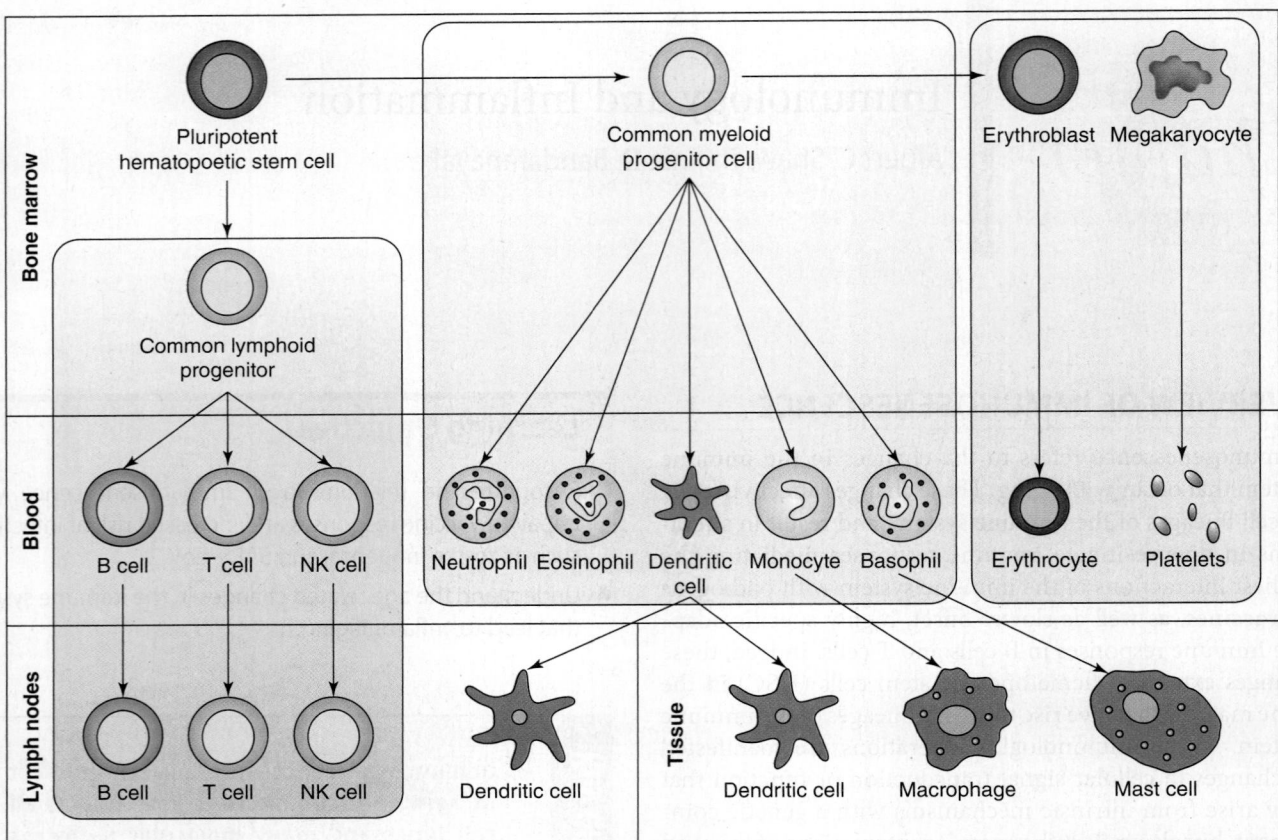

FIGURE 3-1. Schematic representation of hematopoiesis. Hematopoietic stem cells (HSCs) differentiate into lymphoid progenitors in the bone marrow that give rise to T cells (which develop in the thymus) and B cells, and myeloid progenitors that differentiate to monocytes, dendritic cells, neutrophils, basophils, eosinophils, as well as erythroid and megakaryocytic lineages. Aging is associated with impaired HSC differentiation and repopulation function and with a bias toward myeloid at the expense of lymphoid progenitors.

expected. Aging is associated with impaired differentiation and repopulation of blood cell lineages upon transplantation; this has been most clearly demonstrated in model mouse systems, although the substantial effect of donor age on outcomes from HSC transplantation suggests a similar effect in humans. Notably, there appears to be a significant bias favoring development of progenitor stem cells for the myeloid lineage (which give rise to granulocytes, monocytes, macrophages, erythrocytes, and platelets) and diminished numbers of lymphoid progenitors responsible for B and T lymphocyte development. This likely contributes to the impairment in B and T cell development found in older adults, and it is attractive to speculate that increases in myeloid progenitors could contribute to age-associated myeloproliferative disorders. The mechanisms underlying these alterations in hematopoiesis remain incompletely understood, but likely involve stem cell-intrinsic changes such as the accumulation of cellular and DNA damage (with age-related chronic inflammation likely playing a contributing role) and telomere shortening in HSCs with age, as well as inefficient DNA replication and alterations in signaling pathways mediating the response to DNA

damage. In addition, changes in the bone marrow microenvironment that interacts with HSCs to facilitate their maintenance, renewal, and differentiation are also likely to contribute; one example of this is the increased fat cell content of bone marrow with age, which may alter the production of cytokines, chemokines, and other factors influencing HSC function.

OVERVIEW OF THE INNATE IMMUNE SYSTEM

The earliest onset responses to pathogens or vaccines are mediated by the innate immune system. Innate immune responses are mediated by a network of cells including epithelial cells, neutrophils, monocytes, dendritic cells (DCs), natural killer (NK) cells, basophils and eosinophils, and by biochemical factors including complement, antimicrobial peptides (defensins), proinflammatory cytokines, and antiviral interferon responses (**Table 3-1**). Such responses include pathogen clearance via intracellular killing (in neutrophils and macrophages/monocytes), killing of virus-infected or

TABLE 3-1 ■ COMPONENTS AND FUNCTIONS OF THE INNATE IMMUNE SYSTEM

COMPONENT	FUNCTION
Epithelial barriers of skin, mucus membranes	Prevent entry of microbes, mucosal immunity (mucociliary clearance)
Complement	Coat microbes to facilitate phagocytosis (opsonization), killing of microbes, activation of leukocytes
Cytokines	Recruit phagocytic cells to site of infection, inflammation
Neutrophils	Phagocytosis, killing of pathogens
Eosinophils	Antiparasitic, allergic (Th2) responses
Mast cells and basophils	Release of granules containing histamine and active agents, induction of inflammation and tissue responses
Macrophages	Phagocytosis, killing of pathogens, cytokine release, antigen presentation
Dendritic cells	"Professional" antigen-presenting cells, cytokine release
Natural killer cells	Destroy tumor cells and virus-infected cells, antibody-dependent cellular cytotoxicity

malignant cells (by NK cells), and complement fixation and lysis of extracellular organisms.

Pattern Recognition Receptors of the Innate Immune System

Another crucial function of the innate immune system is to activate proinflammatory cytokine and chemokine production, particularly in cells such as DCs or monocytes, which present peptides derived from pathogens in conjunction with a host major histocompatibility antigen for recognition by T cell antigen receptors. Activation of such antigen-presenting cells (APCs) results in the expression of so-called costimulatory molecules such as CD80 and CD86—proteins that interact with a ligand on the surface of T cells to provide a critical additional signal (in conjunction with that provided by engagement of the T cell receptor [TCR]) for T cell activation. This innate proinflammatory response and upregulation of costimulatory protein expression are mediated by a series of invariant innate immune pattern recognition receptors (PRRs). Toll-like receptors (TLRs) are one family of PRRs that are associated with either extracellular or intracellular membranes and recognize highly conserved, so-called pathogen-associated molecular patterns (PAMPs) found in bacteria, mycobacteria, fungi, and viruses. Examples of PAMPs recognized by TLRs include lipopolysaccharide (LPS) and flagellin on gram-negative bacteria (TLR4 and TLR5, respectively), lipopeptides found in bacteria, mycobacteria, and yeasts (recognized by the TLR1/2 and TLR2/6 heterodimers, respectively). While these TLRs are expressed as membrane-associated receptors on the cell surface, other TLRs recognizing nucleic acids are localized to intracellular endosomal plasma membranes; such TLRs are activated by single-stranded RNA (TLR7 and TLR8) and double-stranded RNA (TLR3) produced during viral infections, as well as unmethylated CG-rich DNA (TLR9). Activation of TLRs on APCs engages signal transduction pathways employing myeloid differentiation primary response gene 88 (*MyD88*) or a pathway including the toll-interleukin-1 receptor (TIR)-domain-containing adapter-inducing interferon-β (TRIF) protein and TRIF-related adaptor molecule (TRAM), resulting in not only upregulation of costimulatory proteins but also production of proinflammatory cytokines such as IL-6 and TNF-α via activation of the NF-κB transcription factor, or production of type I interferons via interferon regulatory factor (IRF) engagement (eg, IRF3 and IRF7). By activating APCs presenting antigen to T cells, such TLR signaling links the innate immune response to adaptive immunity.

Recent studies have also identified families of PRRs localized to the cytoplasm (in contrast to the membrane localization of TLRs) that also include receptors recognizing viral RNAs (retinoic acid-inducible gene-I [*RIG*-I] and melanoma differentiation antigen-5 [*MDA*-5]) that interact with a mitochondria-localized signaling intermediate (mitochondrial antiviral signaling protein [MAVS]) are particularly important for antiviral interferon responses. Cytosolic DNA (that can arise in the context of infections—such as with DNA viruses—or DNA damage, such as in cancer) is recognized by numerous innate immune sensors including cyclic GMP-AMP synthase, gamma interferon inducing protein (IFI)-16, and others; the stimulator of interferon genes (STING) protein plays a central role in inducing type I interferon production following activation by such a DNA sensor. A member of the nucleotide-binding oligomerization domain (NOD)-like receptor family, NLRP3, has emerged as an example of an innate immune PRR that responds to not only bacterial and viral motifs but also so-called damage-associated molecular patterns (DAMPs). NLRP3 activation results in assembly of a multiprotein complex termed the inflammasome, a multiprotein complex containing the adaptor protein ASC (apoptosis-associated speck-like protein containing a CARD [caspase activation and recruitment domain]) polymerized into helical filaments that can be visualized using immunofluorescence as a protein "speck" within cells. The CARD domains of these multimerized ASC proteins then mediate the activation of caspase-1 and the consequent proteolytic processing of immature forms of proinflammatory cytokines such as IL-1β and IL-18 to their mature, active forms. DAMPs activating NLRP3 include exogenous factors such as silica and asbestos, and endogenous factors such as uric acid, extracellular ATP, and necrotic cells. The activation of innate immune inflammatory responses by such endogenous DAMPs is hypothesized to be a contributing factor to the increased levels of inflammation found in older adults, as discussed below.

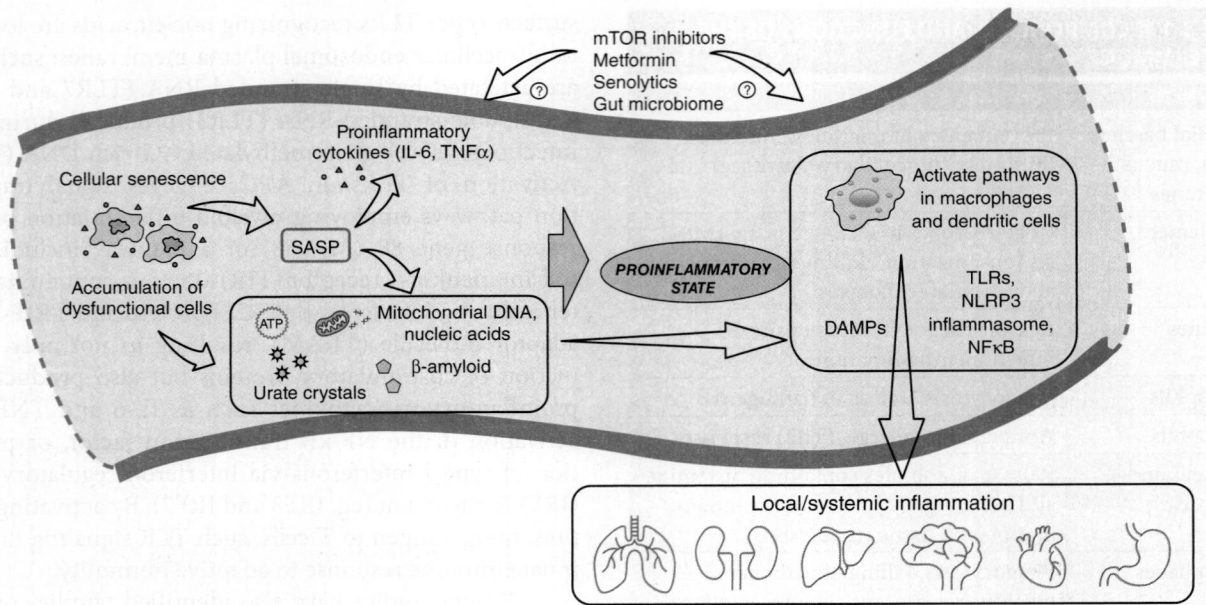

FIGURE 3-2. Depiction of potential factors that contribute to age associated chronic inflammation. SASP, senescence-associated secretory phenotype.

A Heightened Proinflammatory Environment in Older Adults

The effects of age on innate immunity are complex, and reflect the diversity of innate immune responses. Increased levels of proinflammatory cytokines such as IL-6 and TNF-α, acute phase reactants such as C-reactive protein (CRP), and clotting factors are found in the plasma of older, compared to young adults; this age-associated chronic inflammatory state was first referred to by Franceschi as "inflammaging." Inflammaging, as manifested by such elevated cytokine levels, is associated with mortality risk in cohorts of older adults, and is also correlated with decreased muscle mass and strength. In this regard, it is also notable that several diseases of aging, such as cardiovascular disease, diabetes, Alzheimer disease, and osteoporosis, are reported to have an inflammatory component that contributes to pathogenesis. The mechanisms underlying inflammaging remain incompletely understood, but are hypothesized to include activation of innate immune PRRs by PAMPs arising from chronic infections (such as viral infections with herpesvirus family members, or HIV infection, which is associated with increased inflammatory parameters even in individuals with nondetectable viral loads); in addition, age-associated accumulation of DAMPs such as noncell-associated nucleic acids, mitochondria, ATP, urate crystals, heat shock proteins, ceramide, hyaluronan, amyloid, and others resulting from cellular or tissue damage leads to activation of innate immune PRRs such as TLRs and the NLRP3 inflammasome. Defects in autophagy with aging may result in reduced ability to dispose of damaged cellular elements, exacerbating the chronic inflammatory state. In this regard, Campisi and colleagues have described the senescence-associated secretory phenotype (SASP), a secretome of proteins released by damaged cells that includes chemokines and proinflammatory cytokines such as IL-6 and IL-8—another link between cell damage and inflammation (**Figure 3-2**). The inflammatory environment in older adults can also be influenced by additional factors; for example, both testosterone and estrogen suppress IL-6 production, with reduced sex hormone levels of menopause and andropause associated with increased cytokine levels. Finally, increased mitochondrial function with aging and associated uncoupling of oxidative phosphorylation could result in increased levels of reactive oxygen species that may also increase proinflammatory cytokine production.

Age-Associated Alterations in Innate Immune Cell Function (Table 3-2)

Neutrophil function in older adults In cells of the innate immune system, age-associated changes include both impaired responses and inappropriate persistence of inflammation that may result from alterations in signal transduction. For example, neutrophils from older adults show diminished signaling via the granulocyte-macrophage colony-stimulating factor (GM-CSF) receptor that usually mediates antiapoptotic cell survival. Impaired age-associated signaling via the triggering receptor expressed on myeloid cells-1 (TREM-1) may also contribute to functional alterations in cytokine or reactive oxygen species (ROS) production. Human neutrophils also show an age-associated decline in migration toward a chemical stimulus (chemotaxis) and in phagocytosis and intracellular killing of engulfed pathogens. In addition, the

TABLE 3-2 ■ AGE-RELATED CHANGES IN INNATE IMMUNE CELLS

	AGE-RELATED DECREASE	AGE-RELATED INCREASE
Neutrophils	Phagocytosis and intracellular bacterial killing	
	NET formation	
	Chemotaxis	
	Signal transduction (eg, via GM-CSF, TREM-1)	
Monocytes	TLR-1/2-induced cytokine production	LPS-induced cytokine production by CD14+ CD16+ monocytes
	Expression of TLR-1	
	TLR-induced costimulatory molecule expression	IL-10 production
	RIG-I-induced type I interferon production	
	TNF production (skin macrophages)	
	Clearance of neutrophils by efferocytosis	
NK cells	Cytotoxic killing	CD56low population (cytotoxic activity)
	CD56hi population (cytokine production)	
	Secretion of proinflammatory cytokines	
	Recruitment of perforin to the cell membrane	
Dendritic cells	TLR-induced cytokine production (myeloid and plasmacytoid DCs)	Basal cytokine production
	Type I interferon production following viral infection (monocyte-derived DCs and plasmacytoid DCs)	LPS and self-DNA induced Cytokine production (monocyte-derived DCs)

release of neutrophil extracellular traps (NETs), complexes of DNA, histones, and antimicrobial proteins released from the neutrophil that facilitate pathogen capture and killing, is also decreased in neutrophils from older compared to young adults. While alterations in specific signaling pathways as discussed above have been linked to some of these findings, how age influences these functions remains unclear, particularly in view of the short lifespan of human neutrophils in vivo (approximately 5 days). It should be noted that alterations in function such as chemotaxis that may influence migration to sites of infection or injury could result in not only impaired migration to sites of infection or wound healing, but also impaired egress of neutrophils from these sites—potentially resulting in an inappropriate prolongation of the inflammatory response. In this regard, the clearance of apoptotic neutrophils by macrophages (a process termed efferocytosis) in a skin blister model of sterile inflammation was diminished in older, versus young adults, and was associated with elevated activation of macrophage p38 mitogen-activated protein (MAP) kinase; in vivo administration of an orally administered p38 inhibitor restored efferocytosis and inflammatory resolution, suggesting an additional approach to modulating age-related inflammatory dysregulation.

NK cell function in aging Age-associated decline in function has also been reported for NK cells, a class of innate immune lymphocyte sensitive to cytokine activation, which plays an important role in killing virus-infected cells and in immunosurveillance against malignant cells. Critical proteins for the killing function of NK cells include proteases known as granzymes (for their storage in cytoplasmic granules), and perforin, a protein that forms a pore or channel in the target cell through which granzymes may be introduced. Inhibitory NK cell surface receptors recognize host class I major histocompatibility complex (MHC) protein expression and prevent apoptosis, but with loss of MHC class I expression—as frequently occurs on tumor cells to facilitate evasion of antitumor T cell responses—NK-dependent killing via apoptosis of target cells ensues. NK cells also express surface receptors recognizing the so-called Fc constant region of antibodies, and may thereby also mediate killing of targets bound to immunoglobulin—a process termed antibody-dependent cytotoxicity. With age, the proportion of NK cells specialized for cytotoxicity (as assessed by low expression of the surface CD56 adhesion protein) increases at the expense of NK cells specialized for cytokine production (which express high levels of CD56). However, the cytotoxic function of aged NK cells is decreased on a per cell basis, likely in part resulting from diminished recruiting of perforin to the target cell. Studies of NK cell function in the context of aging are likely to have future clinical impact; notably, NK cell counts and measures of NK function have been associated with mortality from sepsis and other critical illness, and with increased infection and mortality rates in older nursing home residents.

Age-associated alterations in PRR function The effects of aging on human innate immune PRR function such as TLRs show evidence for an age-associated impairment in TLR-dependent expression of costimulatory proteins on monocytes, likely influencing the ability of these cells to serve as APCs that can maximally engage T cells. In addition, TLR-induced production of proinflammatory cytokines such as IL-6 and TNF-α in APCs such as monocytes and DCs is also diminished in cells from older adults. In particular, TLR1/2-induced cytokine production (in response to triacylated lipopeptides such as those found in many gram-positive organisms) appears diminished in monocytes from older compared to young adults. TLR function has also been evaluated in human DC populations, which may be predominantly divided into myeloid DCs, which express a wide range of TLRs and mediate production of IL-12 for activation of T cell immunity, and plasmacytoid DCs, which express a narrower range of TLRs but are particularly adept at type I interferon production in response to viral infection. For both of these DC subtypes, a generalized age-associated decrease in TLR-induced cytokine production has been observed. At the same time, it is important to recognize that these studies largely represent in vitro assessments of TLR function. In vivo tissue context is likely to be an important factor; for example, evaluation of TLR function in monocyte-derived DCs showed an age-associated increase in cytokine production; such DCs are derived from monocytes using growth factors and cytokines (GM-CSF and IL-4), and could model DCs generated in the context of inflammation. LPS (recognized by TLR4)-induced cytokine production also appears increased in so-called CD14+CD16+ monocytes (as opposed to CD14+CD16– conventional monocytes) that arise in the setting of inflammation-associated conditions such as sepsis, HIV infection, and myocardial infarction. As a final example, TNF-α production by macrophages in human skin was diminished in the setting of a delayed-type hypersensitivity response to purified protein derivative (PPD)—yet TNF-α production in vitro by such macrophages was preserved, arguing for the importance of local factors (such as the potential influence of regulatory T cells in the skin of older adults, in this case) in assessing innate immune function.

The mechanisms underlying these age-related changes remain incompletely understood; some changes in expression of specific TLRs have been reported in APCs (including an age-associated decrease in surface TLR1 in monocytes), but such decreases in protein expression alone do not appear sufficient to explain the observed findings and it is likely that both transcriptional (ie, gene expression) and posttranscriptional (eg, protein stability, modification, localization, or damage) mechanisms contribute. Moreover, these effects are not uniform for all cell types and must be reconciled with age-related increases in circulating cytokine levels. In this regard, there is evidence for increased basal cytokine production, for example in DCs in the absence of in vitro TLR stimulation. Thus, age-associated impairment in cytokine production could reflect inflammatory dysregulation and an inability to further increase cytokine levels beyond a basal level in response to a newly encountered antigen (such as a PAMP from a pathogen or vaccine). In addition, the wide range of TLR expression on nonblood-derived cells—including cells of epithelial, endothelial, and neuronal origin—represents an additional, largely unexplored source of complexity in the integration of TLR activity in older adults. The function

of cytoplasmic PRRs in older adults remains to be definitively evaluated; however, the demonstration that "specks" of multimerized ASC and inflammasome components can be released from the cell, where they may cause extracellular inflammatory activation and activate inflammation in neighboring cells, suggests a potential source for endogenous immune activation that could contribute to an age-related inflammatory environment.

OVERVIEW OF ADAPTIVE IMMUNITY

The term adaptive immunity refers to highly specific immune responses mediated by lymphocyte-specific antigen receptors: in B cells, immunoglobulins (Ig) or antibodies, which are both membrane-bound as the B cell antigen receptor (BCR) and secreted antibodies that are effectors of humoral immunity; or in T cells, the exclusively membrane-associated TCR, mediating cell-mediated immunity. Humoral and cell-mediated immunity are both characterized by immunologic memory, in which the response to previously encountered antigens is enhanced upon repeat exposure.

Both the BCR and TCR are comprised of two polypeptide chains. The BCR contains two antigen-binding sites, each comprised of one heavy chain and one light chain; the TCR contains a single α chain complexed with a β chain that recognizes a host MHC protein bound to a peptide derived from enzymatic processing of a protein antigen on the surface of an APC (such as a monocyte, macrophage, DC, or even in some cases a B cell) (**Figure 3-3**). The specificity of the humoral or cell-mediated immune response results from a highly diverse repertoire of BCRs on B cells and TCRs on T cells, respectively, that can recognize millions of different antigenic specificities. This diversity results from a lymphocyte-specific gene rearrangement program that acts on the genetic loci for Ig heavy chains or the β TCR subunit, which contain clusters of variable (V regions), diversity (D regions), and joining (J regions), or V and J regions only for Ig light chains or the α TCR subunit. All BCR or TCR chains contain a constant or invariant region (C region). For the BCR Ig heavy chain, several different C regions are present, which denote the Ig isotype and functional implications—such as the Cμ region found in IgM, Cγ1-Cγ4 regions found in IgG subclasses, Cα found in IgA secreted at mucosal surfaces, and Cε denoting IgE, a critical component for allergic responses or immune responses to parasitic infections. The BCR light chain locus contains two C regions, encoding sequences specific for either the κ or λ light chains.

The state of BCR or TCR gene rearrangement denotes specific maturation stages of B or T lymphocyte development, respectively. A rearranged Ig heavy chain or β TCR locus contains a single V, D, and J region linked together to form the variable region of the heavy chain or β TCR protein, while VJ gene rearrangement is found for the

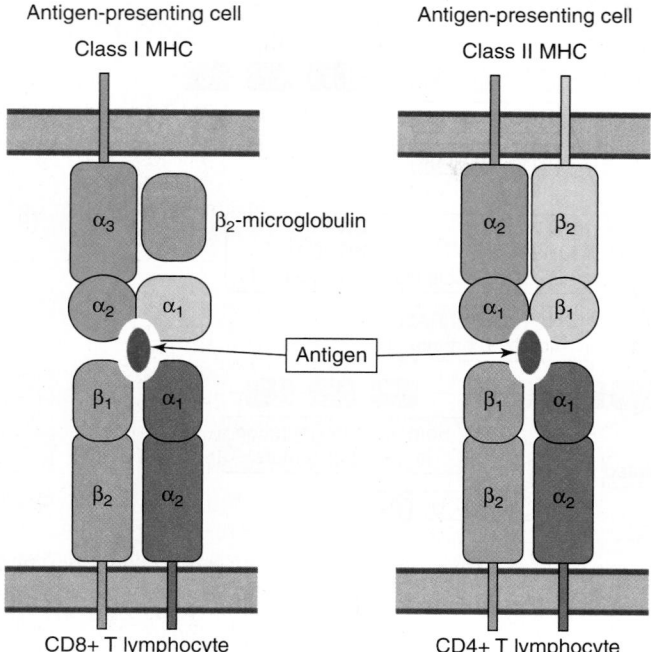

FIGURE 3-3. Depiction of presentation of a peptide (red) resulting from proteolytic processing of a protein antigen in antigen-presenting cells (APCs) such as monocytes, dendritic cells, or B cells. The peptide is bound to host MHC protein, and this combination of peptide and class I or peptide and class II MHC is recognized by T cell receptors on CD8+ cytotoxic or CD4+ helper T cells, respectively.

Ig light chain and α TCR rearranged loci. To accomplish this, the lymphocyte-specific recombinase activating genes (RAG) mediate site-specific DNA cleavage at unrearranged V, D, and J regions. The subsequent joining of these gene segments to form a rearranged antigen receptor gene utilizes proteins responsible for DNA repair (nonhomologous end joining) that are generally expressed in all cell types as part of the response to DNA damage; such proteins include Ku70, Ku80, DNA-dependent protein kinase (DNA-PK), Artemis nuclease, X-ray repair cross-complementing protein 4 (XRCC4), DNA ligase IV, and others. Recombinatorial gene rearrangement of V regions to a more limited number of D and/or J segments, combined with imprecision in the rejoining of cleaved gene segments, results in the tremendous antigenic diversity found in B and T lymphocytes at birth (**Figure 3-4**). Substantial changes in this diversity occur with age, as described below.

In B cells, additional genetic steps are required for the evolution of a humoral immune response. Following gene rearrangement, an IgM BCR is generated (with surface IgM on B cells that can differentiate to a plasma cell secreting IgM with the same antigenic specificity), since the Cμ constant region is most proximal to the rearranged VDJ region. Following initial VDJ gene rearrangement and expression of a mature IgM BCR containing the Cμ

constant region, a B cell–specific process known as heavy chain class switching results in the replacement of the C region exon with that of another isotype, and deletion of the intervening DNA (in this case, containing the previous Cμ region) while preserving the rearranged variable region gene. This process is the mechanism by which evolution of the humoral immune response occurs, from initial expression of IgM early in infection to subsequent expression of IgG and other isotypes. A B cell–specific protein, activation-induced cytidine deaminase (AID), is essential for heavy chain class switching. The mechanism of heavy chain class switching is still a subject of investigation, but is facilitated by transcription at highly repetitive regions of DNA found upstream of each C region exon, termed switch regions. Current models suggest that AID targets single-stranded regions of DNA exposed by transcription, and deaminates cytosine DNA residues to induce a mutation to uracil residues. These mutations are then subjected to generally expressed DNA excision repair proteins to generate double-stranded DNA breaks, which are then repaired by similar nonhomologous end-joining repair mechanisms utilized for VDJ recombination. The ability of AID to induce C to U mutations that are resolved by DNA repair processes also plays an essential role in another function critical to the memory B cell response—somatic hypermutation, the process by which rearranged variable region genes in mature B cells undergo additional mutation, resulting in improved affinity of the encoded immunoglobulin molecule for antigen (**Figure 3-4A**). Thus, mechanisms associated with maintaining the integrity of genomic DNA such as DNA repair pathways—which are likely affected by aging—play crucial roles in these fundamental processes in adaptive immunity.

Overview of T Cell Development and Function

The generation of mature T cells occurs in the thymus, a bilobed organ located in the anterior mediastinum (**Figure 3-5**). Each lobe is comprised of a capsule, a cortex with abundant numbers of developing T cells and a deeper medulla region with sparser quantities of lymphocytes. In addition to developing T cells, several other cell types are present in the thymus to carry out crucial functions related to selection of T cells and clearance of apoptotic cells resulting from thymic selection processes (described below), such as cells of the thymic epithelium, DCs, and macrophages. The thymic cortex is colonized by early thymic progenitor cells originating from the bone marrow. Subsequent developmental steps are driven by rearrangement of TCR genes and are linked to specific regions of the thymus; in general, more mature T cell subsets are found in deeper layers of the cortex, with the most mature cells occupying the medulla. The TCR β chain locus is the first to undergo rearrangement, with subsequent incorporation of the β chain protein in a pre-TCR complex that signals for

Ig heavy chain

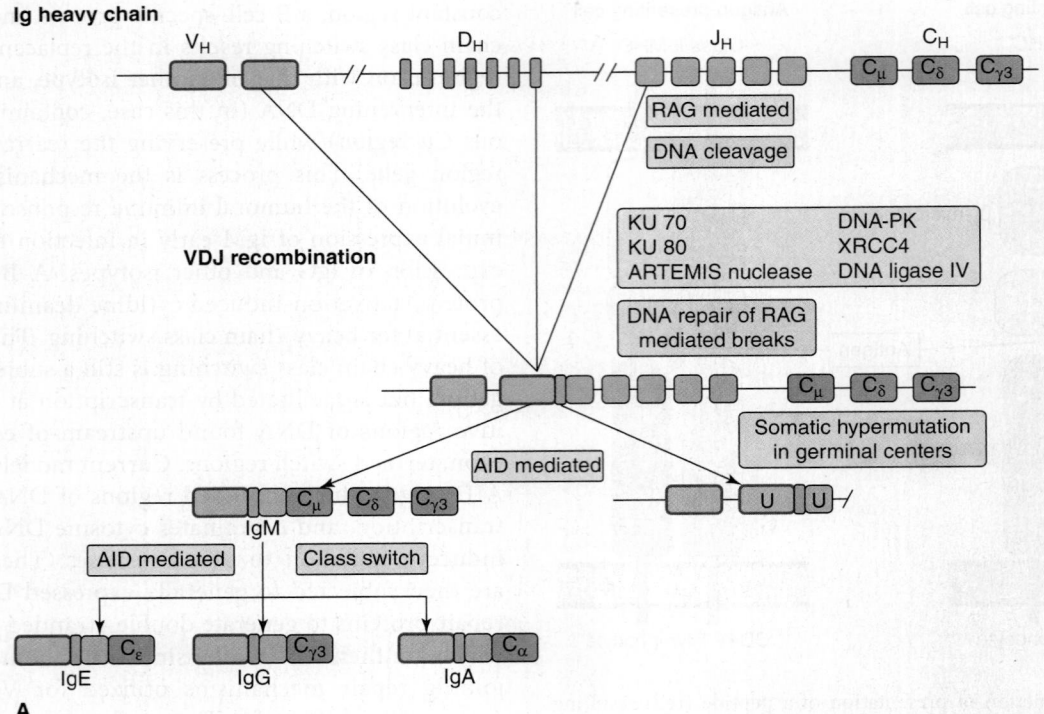

FIGURE 3-4A. Depiction of DNA rearrangement events occurring in B cells. The immunoglobulin (Ig) heavy chain locus is shown. VDJ recombination is initiated by lymphocyte-specific recombinase activating gene (*RAG1* and *RAG2*)-induced breaks at specific sequences upstream of V, D, and J gene segments, with joining of breaks using generally expressed DNA nonhomologous end joining repair proteins. D to J gene rearrangement occurs first, followed by a V to DJ gene rearrangement to yield the complete heavy chain variable region gene recognizing antigen. IgM (expressing the μ constant region gene) is first expressed during an initial antibody response, with subsequent expression of additional Ig isotypes such as IgG subtypes, IgE, and IgA resulting from class switch recombination that deletes previously expressed constant region genes in mature B cells. Somatic hypermutation also occurs in mature B cells, a process where the Ig V region undergoes mutation to enhance affinity of antigen recognition. Both class switch recombination and somatic hypermutation require the B cell–specific protein activation-induced cytidine deaminase (AID), as well as generally expressed DNA repair proteins.

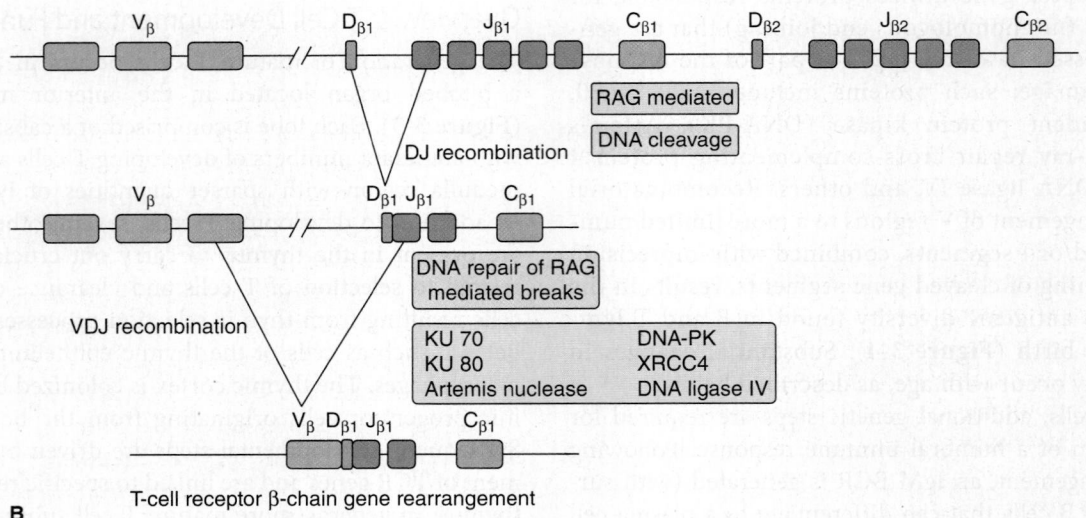

FIGURE 3-4B. Depiction of T cell receptor (TCR) gene rearrangement. The TCR β chain genetic locus is shown. As in the immunoglobulin loci, RAG-1- and RAG-2-dependent cleavage at specific sequences upstream of TCR β V, D, and J segments, with D to J gene rearrangement occurring first, followed by V to DJ gene rearrangement. Joining of DNA breaks is accomplished by DNA nonhomologous end joining repair proteins.

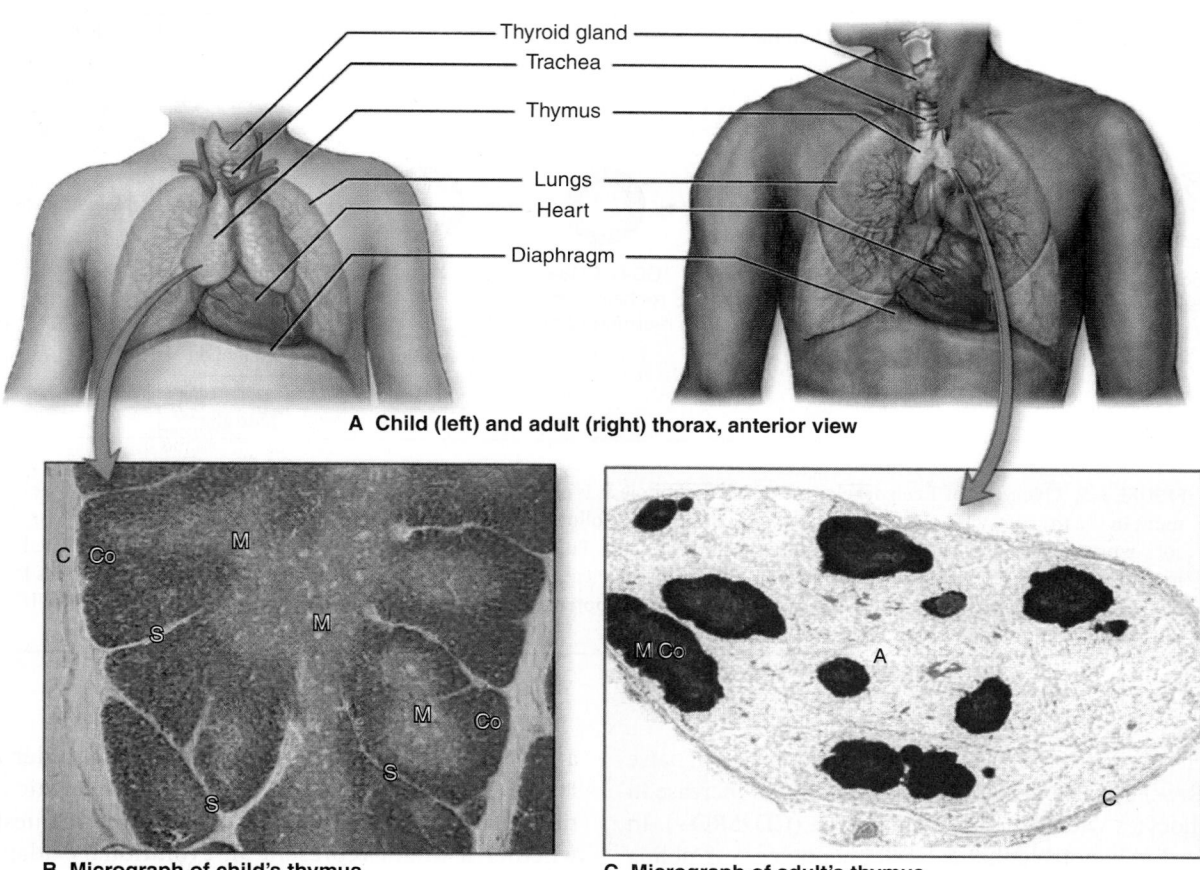

- Thyroid gland
- Trachea
- Thymus
- Lungs
- Heart
- Diaphragm

A Child (left) and adult (right) thorax, anterior view

B Micrograph of child's thymus

C Micrograph of adult's thymus

FIGURE 3-5. Histologic examination of the thymus in a child (left) and adult (right). The thymic capsule (C) is indicated, with the thymic cortex (Co) (which is initially colonized by T cell progenitors originating in the bone marrow) and medulla (M) (containing mature T cell subsets) indicated. With age, marked thymic involution occurs, with increased replacement of thymic epithelium with adipose tissue (A). (Reproduced with permission from Mescher AL. *Junqueira's Basic Histology*, 13th ed. New York, NY: McGraw Hill; 2013.)

survival of precursors with a successful β chain gene rearrangement. Subsequent rearrangement of the TCR α chain genes corresponds to upregulation of both CD4 and CD8 expression (such CD4+ CD8+ cells are referred to as "double-positive" thymocytes), and if a productive gene rearrangement occurs (ie, one able to encode for an α chain protein), the mature αβ TCR is expressed. These developing cells subsequently undergo so-called positive selection, in which cells bearing TCRs that recognize host class MHC class I or class II proteins survive, while those that do not undergo apoptosis. This step coincides with differentiation to "single-positive" CD4+ cells recognizing MHC class II proteins, and cytotoxic CD8+ T cells recognizing MHC class I. Another process of negative selection eliminates those T cells carrying αβ TCRs with high affinity for self-peptide/MHC complexes that could result in autoimmunity. Additional lineage specification for development of regulatory T cells (Treg), which inhibit T cell activation, and γδ T cells expressing two distinct classes of TCR proteins that may play a role in the recognition of lipid antigens, also occurs in the thymus (**Figure 3-6**).

Aging and T Cell Development and Function (Table 3-3)

Thymic involution The human thymus is at its maximal size in infancy, and begins to decrease in size and cellularity in childhood. The thymic epithelium begins to diminish, particularly after puberty, and is replaced by adipose tissue that may be a source of cytokines and chemokines that interfere with thymopoiesis (**Figure 3-5**). The T cell generation capacity of the thymus is substantially diminished by young adulthood, to around 10% of the capacity seen in infancy. T cell lifespan can be assessed by in vivo metabolic labeling, and the generation of new T cells may be measured via the detection of T cell receptor excision circles (TRECs), the excised products of VDJ recombination of DNA that are only detectable in recently matured T cells, since they cannot undergo replication and are diluted by cell division. Such analyses have revealed minimal thymic activity in older adults, and indicate that maintenance of the T cell pool occurs instead via cell division and expansion of preexisting T cells. Not surprisingly, this absent thymic

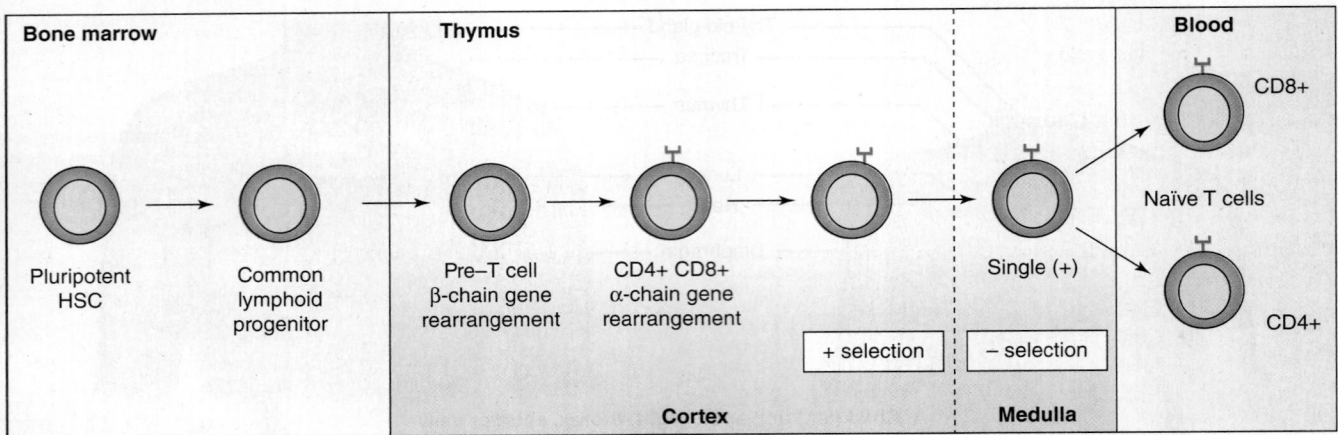

FIGURE 3-6. Overview of T cell development. T lymphopoiesis is closely linked to the state of T cell receptor gene rearrangement in the thymus, with initial β chain gene rearrangement followed by TCR α chain gene rearrangement in T cell precursors expressing both CD4 and CD8 ("double-positive" T cells). Following expression of a TCR on the cell surface (indicated in red), positive selection (+ selection), which selects for survival of T cells bearing TCRs that recognize host MHC class I or class II, and negative selection (– selection), which deletes potentially autoreactive T cells, occur in single-positive T cells (Single [+]) expressing CD4 or CD8.

activity results in decreased numbers and proportion of naïve (CD45RA+) T cells in peripheral blood, with an increase in T lymphocytes with a memory phenotype (CD45RO+). In this regard, it is notable that a T cell phenotype resembling that seen in aged adults was found in young adults who had undergone thymectomy in childhood. The mechanisms underlying thymic involution remain a subject of active study; alterations in thymic epithelial cells that facilitate the developmental expansion and selection steps of T cell development, such as changes in expression of the master transcriptional regulator FoxN1, are thought to play an important role. There is interest in developing interventions that can stabilize or reverse thymic involution and thereby improve T cell production in older adults. However, the widespread conservation of thymic involution in most mammals raises the speculative question of whether it might represent an evolutionary adaptation, perhaps protecting the host from lymphocytic malignancies in older age.

Influence of CMV infection on T cell repertoire The lack of generation of new (naïve) T cells in older adults as a result of thymic involution also results in marked changes in the diversity of the TCR repertoire, which decreases substantially with age. Notably, cytomegalovirus (CMV) infection is associated with such profound alterations in diversity (**Figure 3-7**). Like other herpesviruses, following primary infection CMV establishes a state of latency in the host, with reactivation to productive infection throughout life, often in the setting of stress or non-CMV–associated illness that is usually asymptomatic and not associated with CMV-dependent end organ disease. However, such reactivations result in marked expansion of CMV-specific CD4+ and CD8+ memory T cell populations, and resultant decreases in TCR diversity with expansion of nonmalignant T cell clones—many of which recognize CMV peptides. Such oligoclonal T cell expansions may comprise a large proportion (even in some cases the majority) of CD4+ or CD8+ T cells, and are also found in CMV seronegative older adults; in such individuals, it is likely that other herpesviruses associated with latent infection, such as EBV or HHV-6, other viruses such as hepatitis C virus, or other sources of chronic immune system activation may contribute to loss of repertoire diversity. Notably, the extent of diversity loss has been linked to decreased lifespan in older adults, though the underlying mechanisms or associated factors remain incompletely understood.

TABLE 3-3 ■ AGE-RELATED CHANGES IN THE ADAPTIVE IMMUNE SYSTEM

	AGE-RELATED DECREASE	AGE-RELATED INCREASE
T cells	T cell lymphopoiesis (thymic involution) Naïve T cells Mitogen-associated proliferation Signal transduction Diversity of T cell repertoire Expression of CD28 on CD8+ T cells	Antigen-experienced memory T cells (effector memory)
B cells	Antibody-secreting cells (eg, responding to vaccination) Class switch recombination Expression of AID Diversity of B cell repertoire	Autoantibody titer (eg, rheumatoid factor)

Aging and alterations in T cell phenotype and signal transduction The age-related increase in memory phenotype T cells, with decreased naïve T cells is also associated with several additional findings. For example, aged human T cells show a substantial loss of expression of the costimulatory protein CD28 from the surface of CD8+ cytotoxic T cells (**Figure 3-7**). CD4+ T cells show a much lesser degree of CD28 loss with aging, although marked increases

in CD4+ CD28− cells can be found in adults with rheumatologic disease. CD28 associates with ligands (CD80 and CD86) on the surface of APCs such as activated macrophages or DCs, and this interaction provides a second signal, in addition to that provided by the TCR interaction with peptide bound to host MHC, that is critical for optimal T cell activation. Thus, this loss of CD28 would be expected to influence T cell activation in CD8+ T cells.

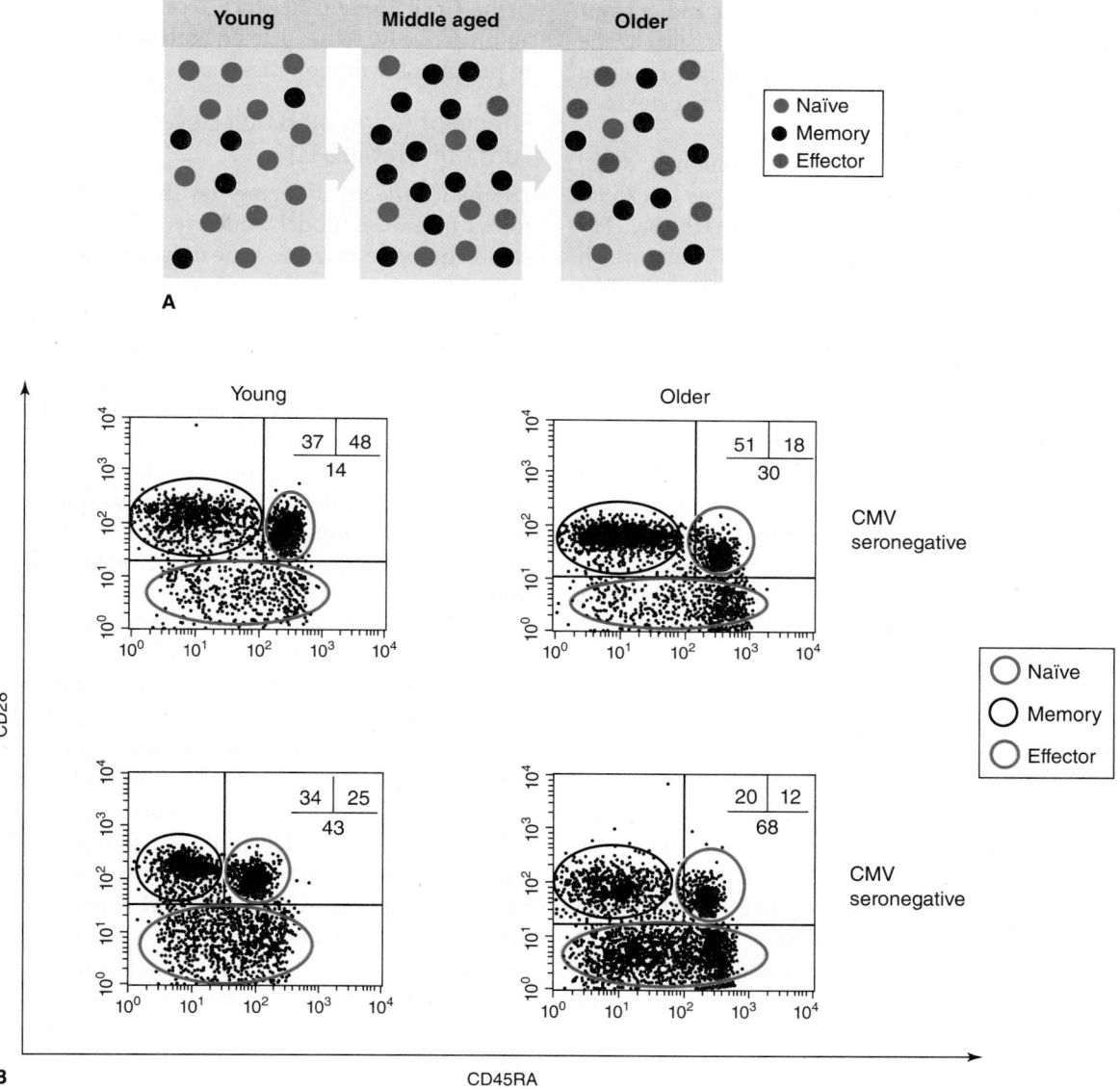

FIGURE 3-7. A. Graphical depiction of age-associated decrease in naïve T cells and increased proportion of memory and effector T cells, reflecting thymic involution and proliferative expansion of preexisting T cells. **B.** Flow cytometric plots of CD28 expression (Y-axes) versus expression of CD45RA (a marker of naïve T cells) in CD8+ T cells from representative young and older subjects stratified by CMV seroreactivity. Note the increased proportion of CD8+ T cells expressing low or absent levels of CD28 and decreased proportion of CD45RA expressing naïve T cells in older adults; these changes are enhanced in CMV-seropositive older adults. (Modified with permission from Almanzar G, Schwaiger S, Jenewein B, et al. Long-term cytomegalovirus infection leads to significant changes in the composition of the CD8+ T-cell repertoire, which may be the basis for an imbalance in the cytokine production profile in elderly persons. *J Virol.* 2005;79[6]:3675–3683.)

In this regard, signal transduction by the TCR is also diminished in the context of aging—in general, nonreceptor tyrosine kinase–dependent pathways downstream of the TCR are inhibited in T cells from older adults, with potential mechanisms for impaired signaling including increased expression of phosphatases that are negative regulators of MAP kinase–dependent signaling. Though the mechanisms underlying diminished signaling in human T cells remain incompletely understood, both cell-intrinsic mechanisms, such as mitochondrial dysfunction in T cells resulting in increased levels of reactive oxygen species (ROS), and cell-extrinsic mechanisms, such as the inhibition of TCR signaling and engagement of inhibitory cytokine signaling pathways (such as the suppressor of cytokine signaling [SOCS] proteins) resulting from increased systemic levels of TNF-α and other cytokines, appear to be important contributing factors.

It is likely that such signaling alterations may differ among different T cell populations and lineages to extend beyond the dichotomy of CD8+ and CD4+ T cells to CD4+ T cell subtypes. These include T_{H1} helper T cells, which develop in response to IL-12 produced by activated APCs and the transcriptional regulator T-bet to produce interferon-γ and facilitate intracellular immunity against bacteria, viruses, and fungi; T_{H2} helper cells developing in response to the GATA3 transcription factor that produce IL-4, IL-5, and IL-13 and mediate allergic and antiparasitic T cell responses; T_{H17} cells, a heterogeneous lineage in humans that are named for their production of IL-17 and are associated with inflammatory responses in the context of bacterial and fungal infections, autoimmunity, and malignancy; follicular helper T cells providing critical help for B cells in lymphoid follicles of lymph nodes and other secondary lymphoid organs; regulatory T cells (Treg) expressing the FoxP3 transcription factor that inhibit immune responses; and resident memory T cells (T_{RM}) present in specific tissues or organs such as lung, skin, or gut that do not recirculate and appear critical for rapid responses to pathogens (both Treg and T_{RM} cells may be either CD4+ or CD8+ single positive). The functional consequences of aging on these human T cell subsets remain incompletely understood, but are likely to be complex; for example, current evidence suggests that human CD4+ and CD8+ Treg cells are found in increased numbers in the blood of older, compared to young adults, but the ability to induce Treg cell development (particularly CD8+ Treg cells) with cytokine treatment is diminished with age. The consequences of these opposing effects on the regulation of T cell responses remain to be determined.

OVERVIEW OF B CELL DEVELOPMENT

In contrast to T lymphopoiesis, where T cell progenitors migrate from the bone marrow to the thymus, B cells arise from HSC that differentiate to a common lymphoid progenitor. However, as with the T cell lineage, antigen receptor gene rearrangement (in this case, of immunoglobulin [Ig] heavy and light chain genes) is intimately linked to B cell development, with Ig heavy chain gene rearrangement occurring in early B cell progenitors (pro-B cells). The Ig heavy chain protein in conjunction with an invariant surrogate light chain protein forms the pre-B cell receptor complex that links to signal transduction pathways to mediate expansion and progression to the pre-B cell stage, when light chain gene rearrangement occurs to generate the mature Ig BCR (**Figure 3-8**). Through this process, a library of B cells is developed with a repertoire of millions of specificities. Notably, an incompletely understood mechanism of negative selection occurs in the B cell lineage (as in the T cell lineage) by which B cells expressing potentially autoreactive BCRs are deleted both in the bone marrow and in peripheral lymphoid tissues.

Effects of Aging on B Cell Development and Function (Table 3-3)

Dramatic effects of aging on B cell development are found in mouse models; however, human B lymphopoiesis in the bone marrow appears generally preserved with age, although the total number and percentage of B cells diminish in the blood of older compared to young adults. Moreover, B cell production of antibodies in response to infection or vaccination is impaired with age, and is associated with diminished production of antibody-secreting B cells termed plasmablasts, which generally appear approximately 7 days following immunization. In part because of the use of varying definitions of B cell subsets, it has proven difficult to determine whether, as in the T cell lineage, memory B cells are expanded with age. Notably, the proportion and number of memory B cells that have undergone heavy chain class switching do decrease with age; it is likely that age-associated alterations in T cell function contribute to such differences, since B cell responses are intimately associated with helper T cell activity. However, B cell–intrinsic changes have been identified in older adults, such as the decreased expression of AID (essential for heavy chain class switching—**Figure 3-4A**) in B cells from older adults that is linked to decreased levels of the E47 transcription factor. Though age-related developmental changes in the B cell lineage remain completely understood, functional alterations are manifested for example by the age-associated increase in monoclonal gammopathy, which has been estimated to affect as many as 3% of adults 50 years or older and 5% of adults 70 years or older. In addition, titers of autoantibodies such as rheumatoid factor are generally increased with age, suggesting additional dysregulation and in particular, possible alterations in the negative selection steps mediating deletion of autoreactive B cell clones. The persistence of autoreactive B cell clones may also be reflected in age-related changes in the B cell repertoire; repertoire diversity appears to be diminished with age, with marked increases in nonmalignant clonal expansions of B cells. As with T cells, there is evidence that such expansions could be associated with the control of reactivation of chronic herpesvirus infections with CMV or EBV. In addition,

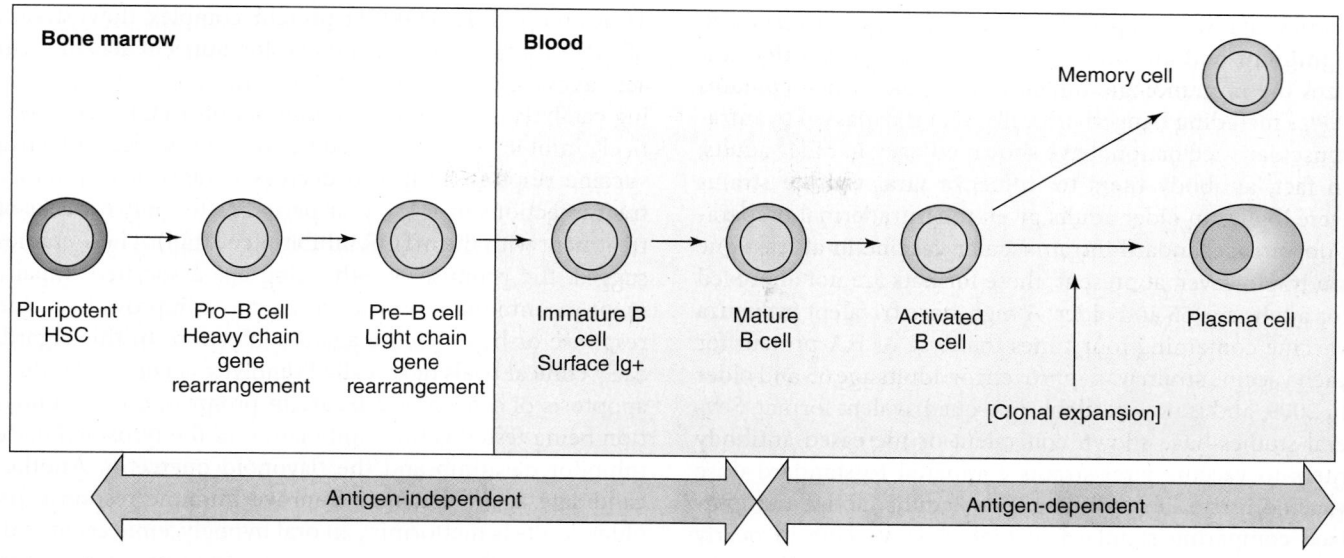

FIGURE 3-8. Depiction of B cell development. Immunoglobulin gene rearrangement (first of the heavy chain genes, followed by light chain gene rearrangement) is crucial to B lymphopoiesis, resulting in generation of a library of mature B cells collectively expressing a highly diverse repertoire of surface immunoglobulin (the B cell antigen receptor). Encounter with a specific antigen results in expansion of a clone of B cells recognizing that antigen, and generation of memory B cells and plasma cells secreting immunoglobulin of the same specificity.

profound loss of B cell repertoire diversity has been associated with alterations in health or functional status, such as frailty; the effects of functional alterations or multimorbidity on the immune system in older adults is an emerging area of significant research and clinical interest.

EFFECTS OF AGE ON VACCINE RESPONSES

Impaired responses to vaccines represent perhaps the clearest examples of the consequences of immunosenescence, and have important clinical consequences reflected in the increased susceptibility to infectious diseases found in older adults. Mechanisms discussed in this chapter contribute to this impaired response, but multiple additional host factors including gender, age-associated changes in body composition (eg, changes in adipose tissue), and associated comorbid medical conditions or medication use all contribute. Here, we provide an overview of three vaccines—against influenza, VZV, and *Streptococcus pneumoniae*—currently recommended for older adults and briefly discuss vaccines against SARS-CoV-2 infection.

Influenza Vaccine

Over 90% of the approximately 30,000 annual deaths from influenza in the United States occur in adults 65 years or older, and older adults are at increased risk for morbidity arising from complications of influenza, such as viral pneumonia or bacterial superinfection. Although the incidence of influenza infection decreased substantially with the advent of SARS-CoV-2 disease, it is virtually certain that influenza outbreaks will resume following the pandemic.

The seasonal vaccine in wide use is an inactivated vaccine containing defined doses of the hemagglutinin (HA) protein, one of the surface glycoproteins of the influenza virus; anti-HA antibodies are associated with protection against disease. However, because of a high mutation rate in the HA protein, the composition of viral strains in the vaccine is adjusted annually based on surveillance of circulating strains. Currently, four (quadrivalent) influenza strains are present in the vaccine, with two influenza A strains (typically one H1N1 and one H3N2 subtype) and two B strains.

The efficacy of the standard dose seasonal influenza vaccine in older adults has been estimated at approximately 40% for the prevention of an influenza-like illness, and approximately 60% for confirmed influenza, and is lower in older individuals with increased comorbid conditions (such as residents in long-term care facilities). Demonstration of a mortality benefit for influenza vaccination has proven to be difficult; it has been hypothesized that many studies may be influenced by selection bias in which a subset of frail adults who are undervaccinated because of poor health disproportionately contribute to mortality from influenza. However, a history of revaccination, as opposed to first vaccination against influenza, has been associated with decreased mortality in at least one study.

Evidence for poor vaccine efficacy, combined with the demonstration of impaired antibody responses to vaccination reflected in decreased levels of antibody-producing cells following influenza immunization have led to interest in alterative vaccine formats to improve response in older adults. Both the live attenuated influenza vaccine, which uses a cold-adapted virus that replicates in nasal mucosal tissues (at lower temperature than in the lungs) to establish immunity, and an intradermal influenza vaccine that utilizes the immunologic milieu of the skin (which contains APCs including Langerhans cells) that is bypassed by intramuscular vaccination, have shown efficacy in older adults; in fact, antibody titers to influenza viral vaccine strains were higher in older adults given the intradermal preparation versus standard intramuscular vaccine in at least one study. However, at present, these formats are not approved for adults age 65 and older. A high-dose trivalent influenza vaccine containing four times the dose of HA protein for each vaccine strain was approved for adults age 65 and older in 2009, and is now available in a quadrivalent format. Several studies have shown equivalent or increased antibody titers to vaccine viral strains compared to standard dose vaccine in studies enrolling older adults, and a randomized comparing standard to high-dose vaccine in nearly 32,000 older adults revealed a modest benefit for the high-dose vaccine (with a 24% relative efficacy for prevention of influenza-like illness compared to standard dose vaccine). A second vaccine approved for use in adults 65 years and older is a standard-dose quadrivalent vaccine combined with MF59, a squalene-derived adjuvant that appears to enhance antigen presentation. A cluster-randomized trial comparing the MF59 adjuvanted vaccine to unadjuvanted, standard-dose vaccine in 823 nursing homes revealed a 17% reduction in suspected or laboratory-confirmed influenza outbreaks and a 20% reduction in hospitalization for pneumonia or influenza for the adjuvanted vaccine. Ongoing work to further improve influenza vaccines includes the use of adjuvants, including those activating the innate immune system such as TLR agonists. An additional research direction is the development of a "universal" influenza vaccine, which would not require annual revision. The immune response to current HA-based vaccines is dominated by antibodies to the highly variable head region of HA; approaches to a universal vaccine include the use of viral antigens that are highly conserved across influenza strains, such as the HA stalk region or neuraminidase protein. Such vaccines are in early clinical trials, and their efficacy in eliciting strong immune responses in older adults remains to be studied. Finally, biochemical pathways implicated in vaccine response may be pharmacologically modulated to enhance vaccine protection. An example of this possibility came from the demonstration in a placebo-controlled trial that low doses of the immunosuppressive agent rapamycin enhanced antibody response to influenza vaccination by about 20% in older adults. This study implicated the mechanistic target of rapamycin (mTOR) pathway, which is inhibited by rapamycin, in vaccine response. Notably, in addition to its effects on T cell signal transduction (relevant particularly for prevention of transplant rejection), rapamycin administration to mice late in life resulted in significant lifespan extension (14% for female and 9% extension for male mice). These increases in lifespan and vaccine response are principally mediated by the TOR complex 1 (TORC1) protein complex downstream of mTOR, which appears crucial for nutrient sensing and activation of protein translation. Additional studies utilizing catalytic and allosteric inhibitors of mTOR that selectively inhibit TORC1 showed not only improved influenza vaccine response, but also decreased rates of respiratory tract infections over a 1-year period (after only 6 weeks of treatment with the mTOR inhibitor cocktail). These studies suggest the promise of enhancing age-associated impairment in immune responses to promote improved vaccine response or host defense against infection. In this regard, early clinical trials of so-called senolytic agents that induce apoptosis of senescent cells are in progress; one combination being tested is the combination of the tyrosine kinase inhibitor dasatinib and the flavonoid quercetin. Another candidate agent that may improve immune responses in older adults is metformin, an oral hypoglycemic agent with pleiotropic effects that result mainly from its activity as an AMP kinase activator, with inhibition of TORC1, decreased oxidative stress resulting from inhibition of complex I of the mitochondrial electron transport chain, and decreased age-related chronic inflammation through inhibition of the transcription factor NF-κB. The upcoming TAME (Targeting Aging by Metformin) trial represents a new paradigm for clinical trials in specifically targeting aging phenotypes; improving age-related deficits in immune response will be an important direction for these and other future trials designed to improve human health span (**Figure 3-2**).

Varicella Zoster Vaccine

Herpes zoster (shingles), resulting from reactivation of VZV, frequently affects older adults—usually manifesting as a painful cutaneous vesicular eruption in a dermatomal distribution that could also present as multidermatomal or disseminated zoster in the setting of immunosuppression or malignancy. The incidence of herpes zoster increases markedly with age, and the CDC estimates that approximately one-third of Americans will have an episode of zoster infection during their lifetime. Studies in immunosuppressed adults have established that defects in T cell immunity, like those associated with aging, are essential for maintaining VZV in a state of latency in ganglia associated with peripheral and cranial nerves—although the precise mechanisms involved in maintaining VZV latency remain incompletely understood. Notably, studies to quantify VZV-specific CD4+ T cells have revealed that approximately 30% to 40% of adults 55 years and older have no detectable CD4+ VZV responses, a potential correlate for the increased risk of older adults for zoster infection; in an effort to boost this defective cell-mediated immunity the first-generation zoster vaccine (Zostavax) was a live attenuated viral preparation containing 10- to 40-fold higher viral plaque forming units compared to the VZV vaccine given to prevent primary infection in childhood. Based on a large placebo-controlled efficacy trial enrolling over 38,000 adults age 60 and older, the vaccine reduced the incidence of zoster by 51%, but a substantial decrease in efficacy was seen as a function of age: protection against zoster was estimated at 64% in individuals 60 to 69, 41% for those 70 to 79, and 18% for individuals over 80. This reduced efficacy in adults 70 years and older, limited the utility of the vaccine, particularly as it became clear that repeat vaccination would be necessary to maintain protection against shingles outbreaks. This first-generation vaccine is no longer available in the United States, and has been replaced by a second-generation, recombinant vaccine (Shingrix) containing VZV glycoprotein E and the AS01B adjuvant consisting of monophosphoryl lipid A (a TLR4 agonist) complexed with a saponin derivative (QS-21) in liposomal form. This vaccine reduced the incidence of shingles by 97% in a trial of adults 50 years and older and by 90% in a second trial of adults 70 years and older. This last trial also found an 89% decrease in the incidence of postherpetic neuralgia. In contrast to the first-generation live attenuated vaccine, no age-related decrease in efficacy was reported for this second-generation vaccine, suggesting that the AS01B adjuvant could potentially overcome age-related alterations in vaccine-immune response and would be a candidate for use in other vaccines used in older adults.

Pneumococcal Vaccine

Adults 65 years and older and children under age 2 are at greatest risk for the development of invasive pneumococcal disease (eg, bacteremia, endocarditis, meningitis), but the highest mortality rates (of 15%–20%) are found in adults 65 years and older. For decades, vaccination against *Streptococcus pneumoniae* utilized the 23-valent polysaccharide vaccine, which contains purified pneumococcal capsular polysaccharides from 23 (of at least 90) strains that are commonly associated with infection in the United States. In most studies, this polysaccharide vaccine appears to reduce the risk for invasive pneumococcal disease, but at the same time most studies have not shown a benefit for this vaccine in prevention of noninvasive disease (such as pneumococcal pneumonia) or all-cause pneumonia in older adults. From an immunologic perspective, the polysaccharide vaccine is generally considered to be a so-called "T-independent" vaccine, as the pneumococcal polysaccharides stimulate B cells directly, inducing activation and differentiation to antibody-secreting cells. While it appears possible that some T-dependent responses may arise from this vaccine (for example from copurifying pneumococcal protein components in the vaccine), there remains concern regarding the potential defect in T cell–dependent immunologic memory—a potential limitation given the importance of the memory response in facilitating more rapid responses mediated by higher affinity antigen receptors resulting from processes such as somatic hypermutation in B cells.

For this reason, pneumococcal conjugate vaccine offered the possibility of improved efficacy, since in these vaccines polysaccharides are conjugated to a carrier protein, CRM197—a nontoxic mutant of diphtheria toxin.

This step allows the polysaccharide conjugate to undergo antigen processing for presentation in the context of host MHC to T cells, allowing a full memory response to be generated (with the resulting generation of memory B and T cells). While T cell function and memory responses are clearly diminished in older adults (as discussed above), there is biological plausibility to the hypothesis that immunologic memory, even diminished, is preferable to a complete absence of memory. The CAPiTA study specifically evaluated the 13-valent conjugate pneumococcal vaccine in a randomized, placebo-controlled trial of more than 80,000 adults 65 years and older in the Netherlands who had never previously received a pneumococcal vaccine. The conjugate vaccine was found to diminish the risks of both noninvasive and invasive pneumococcal infection arising from vaccine-related strains, and the protective effect extended for the duration of the study (~4 years). While this was the first study to show a benefit to vaccination in decreasing the incidence of pneumococcal pneumonia, it remains unclear whether a similar benefit for older adults in the United States would be found. Because the CAPiTA trial began in the Netherlands prior to the general use of conjugate vaccine in Dutch children, it has been speculated that the benefits of vaccinating older adults may be less clear in the United States, where the general use of pneumococcal conjugate vaccine in children has led to a substantial decrease in invasive disease in older adults. Currently, the 23-valent polysaccharide vaccine remains the mainstay of recommendations for the prevention of pneumococcal disease in older adults, while for adults with immunocompromising conditions a series of vaccination with the 13-valent conjugate vaccine followed by the polysaccharide vaccine in 8 weeks or later is suggested. However, newer generation conjugate vaccines with increased numbers of strains may further modify these recommendations for older adults.

SARS-CoV-2 (COVID-19) Vaccines

As with other infectious diseases, the COVID-19 pandemic has had a disproportionate impact on older adults, with approximately 80% of deaths from COVID-19 occurring in adults 65 years and older; outbreaks in nursing homes have been particularly devastating, and it is estimated that nearly 1 in 10 nursing home residents in the United States died of COVID-19 during the pandemic. The specific immunologic mechanisms contributing to COVID-19 pathophysiology in older adults remain an area of active investigation; however, many aspects of the aging immune system appear to be manifested in COVID-19, such as increased levels of proinflammatory cytokines such as IL-6 and TNF-α, alterations in innate immune activation such as those responsible for the type I interferon response, and expansion of activated T cell populations with features of terminal differentiation. Such studies in patients with COVID-19 are challenging to interpret because of substantial heterogeneity resulting from differences in treatment regimens, comorbid medical conditions, and variability in timing of sample acquisition

CHAPTER 3 IMMUNOLOGY AND INFLAMMATION

relative to disease course, and this remains an active area of investigation.

The first vaccines against SARS-CoV-2 to show efficacy in older adults were RNA vaccines—BNT162b2 and mRNA-1273—both containing messenger RNA (mRNA) encoding the full-length SARS-CoV-2 spike protein, with specific nucleoside modifications to minimize activation of host innate immune PRR pathways recognizing RNA. Such mRNAs were packaged in a lipid-containing nanoparticle, and upon intramuscular administration are translated in the cytoplasm of host cells to generate SARS-CoV-2 spike protein. Both vaccines elicit spike protein-specific neutralizing antibody and T cell responses, and initial data indicate excellent efficacy (92% for BNT162b2 and 86% for mRNA-1273) in adults 65 years and older. Additional vaccine platforms are also likely to find clinical use, using replication-deficient adenoviral-based vectors and recombinant protein vaccines. Many unanswered questions remain for all of these vaccines, such as duration of protection for B and T cell–dependent immunity, need for repeat of vaccinations/booster doses, and protection against emerging SARS-CoV-2 variants.

FUTURE PERSPECTIVES

Understanding of the mechanisms underlying age-associated immune dysfunction has implications not only for morbidity and mortality from infectious diseases and vaccine response, but also for the age-related increase in malignancy (perhaps reflecting age-related changes in tumor surveillance and DNA repair or genome stability) and for emerging fields of research such as wound healing and organ transplantation. Studies of immune system aging have begun to utilize multidimensional data from whole-genome analyses of gene expression, including evaluation of small microRNAs whose expression has been implicated in the regulation of many genes. The analysis of age-related epigenetic changes, such as methylation or histone modification, that are linked to the regulation of gene expression has also advanced and will soon be routinely done at the single-cell level. In addition, the emerging interface of immunity and metabolism, as manifested for example by mitochondrial alterations or engagement of the mTOR pathway, suggests the utility of metabolic pathway analyses (metabolomics) using mass spectroscopy platforms. Immunologic studies increasingly will also include high dimensional data from mass cytometry (CyTOF) platforms that should be able to substantially exceed the number of analytic channels available using conventional flow cytometry. An additional area of ongoing research will evaluate the components of intestinal commensal organisms (the intestinal microbiome) or those at other tissue sites, and their interaction with the immune system in modulating inflammation, metabolic activity, and other parameters; initial studies have already found age-related differences in content of the intestinal microbiome that are associated with factors such as nutritional status, diet, and functional status such as frailty. In view of the high degree of heterogeneity found in older adults, encompassing medical comorbidities, medication use, as well as gender and race, future research on the aged immune system should provide new biological insights into how this heterogeneity is translated into changes in functional status—with the hope of identifying methods to improve quality of life in older adults.

FURTHER READING

Anderson EJ, Rouphael NG, Widge AT, et al. Safety and immunogenicity of SARS-CoV-2 mRNA-1273 vaccine in older adults. *N Engl J Med.* 2020;383:2427–2438.

Black S, Gregorio ED, Rappuoli R. Developing vaccines for an aging population. *Sci Transl Med.* 2015;7(281):281ps8.

Bonten MJ, Huijts SM, Bolkenbaas M, et al. Polysaccharide conjugate vaccine against pneumococcal pneumonia in adults. *N Engl J Med.* 2015;372(12):1114–1125.

Cunningham AL, Lal H, Kovac M, et al. Efficacy of the herpes zoster subunit vaccine in adults 70 years of age or older. *N Engl J Med.* 2016;375:1019–1032.

DiazGranados CA, Dunning AJ, Kimmel M, et al. Efficacy of high-dose versus standard-dose influenza vaccine in older adults. *N Engl J Med.* 2014;371(7):635–645.

Franceschi C, Garagnani P, Parini P, Giuliani C, Santoro A. Inflammaging: a new immune-metabolic viewpoint for age-related diseases. *Nat Rev Endocrinol.* 2018; 14(10): 576–590.

Frasca D, Blomberg BB. B cell function and influenza vaccine responses in healthy aging and disease. *Curr Opin Immunol.* 2014;29:112–118.

Goronzy JJ, Weyand CM. Mechanisms underlying T cell ageing. *Nat Rev Immunol.* 2019;19:573–583.

Hazeldine J, Lord JM. Immunesenescence: a predisposing risk factor for the development of COVID-19? *Front Immunol.* 2020;11:573662.

Kirkland JL, Tchkonia T. Senolytic drugs: from discovery to translation. *J Intern Med.* 2020;288:518–536.

Kulkarni AS, Gubbi S, Barzilai N. Benefits of metformin in attenuating the hallmarks of aging. *Cell Metab.* 2020;32(1):15–30.

Liu GY, Sabatini DM. mTOR at the nexus of nutrition, growth, ageing and disease. *Nat Rev Mol Cell Biol.* 2020;21(4):183–203.

Mannick JB, Morris M, Hockey H-U P, et al. TORC1 inhibition enhances immune function and reduces infections in the elderly. *Sci Transl Med.* 2018;10(449): eaaq1564.

McConeghy KW, Davidson HE, Canaday DH, et al. Cluster-randomized trial of adjuvanted vs. non-adjuvanted tri-valent influenza vaccine in 823 U.S. nursing homes. *Clin Infect Dis.* 2021;73(11);e4237–4243.

Nikolich-Zugich J. The twilight of immunity: emerging concepts in aging of the immune system. *Nat Immunol.* 2018;19:10–19.

Partridge L, Fuentealba M, Kennedy BK. The quest to slow ageing through drug discovery. *Nat Rev Drug Discov.* 2020;19(8):513–532.

Shaw AC, Goldstein DR, Montgomery RR. Age-dependent dysregulation of innate immunity. *Nat Rev Immunol.* 2013;13(12):875–887.

Chapter 4

Psychosocial Aspects of Aging

Steven M. Albert, Cynthia Felix

OVERVIEW

As people age they experience changes in physical and cognitive capacities, such as gait speed and reaction time, and also changes in emotional experience and social interests. Cultures impose an order on this continuum of change in widely shared understandings of the life course, which partition the lifespan into different stages. One of the most famous is Shakespeare's seven ages of man (*As You Like It*, II, 7). The Elizabethan stages of life include infancy, "whining school boy … creeping unwillingly to school," lover, soldier ("seeking the bubble reputation even in the cannon's mouth"), judge, and then two stages of decline: initial loss of capacities ("big manly voice, turning again toward childish treble"), and finally "second childishness and mere oblivion … *sans* teeth, *sans* eyes, *sans* taste, *sans* everything." Other cultures are more charitable in their ideas about advanced age. The Samia people of Kenya describe old age as a pleasant time to sit before the fire and be fed. Such differences in thinking about the life course remind us that psychosocial aging is governed both by biological and sociocultural elements. A major focus of developmental approaches to psychosocial aging is to distinguish between invariant biological change and cultural constructions that selectively emphasize particular transitions across this continuum of change.

Life Course Developmental Perspective

There is no single age at which we can say that people cross the threshold into "old age" and become an "older adult." People age at different rates; hence, for any given age, there will be great variation in proposed biomarkers of aging or phenotypes of healthy aging. In the United States, establishment of the Social Security system linked old age to age 65, but research on the start of aging and its pace suggests that adults with the same chronologic age differ in proposed aging biomarkers and that accelerated aging may have social determinants, such as experience of adverse childhood events and poverty.

But people do have an idea of when they become old. A number of surveys have asked at what age someone is old. The start of "old age" can be assigned to a wide range of chronological ages. Choices of an age for "old age" tell us the decade when people are expected to slow down, retire, and focus on self-maintenance rather than new careers

Learning Objectives

- Apply the life course perspective to show how psychosocial changes with age depend on cultural factors as well as lifespan developmental changes in affective experience.

- Identify core psychosocial factors, including resilience, that affect well-being across aging-related challenges, such as increasing disability, declining health, and the end of life.

- Identify current trends in common old-age transitions, such as retirement, widowhood, and caregiving, and sociocultural factors that make these transitions more or less stressful.

- Examine psychosocial factors that affect decision making and quality of life at the end of life.

Key Clinical Points

1. Lack of support (social isolation and loneliness) has a negative effect, and social engagement (volunteering, lifelong learning, and involvement in intergenerational programs) has a positive effect, on health and well-being in old age.

2. Social environments that promote aging in place support psychosocial health.

3. The aging services network is important in promoting engagement across diverse domains.

4. Hospice and palliative care promote involvement of older people in decision making at the end of life and the psychosocial health of family caregivers.

or goals. **Figure 4-1** shows the age at which respondents consider women to be old. These data are drawn from the National Council on Aging *Myths and Realities of Aging* survey, conducted in 2000. The data are weighted to reflect the sampling scheme and overrepresentation of older people and minorities. The figure plots the mean age "the average woman" is said to be "old" by respondent's age and sex.

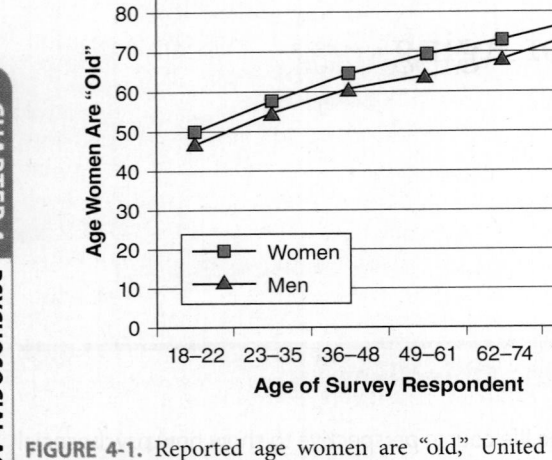

FIGURE 4-1. Reported age women are "old," United States, 2000. (Data from National Council on Ageing.)

Note the strong relationship between the survey respondent's age and his or her report of when women are old. Young people consider the start of old age to be much earlier than older people. For people around age 20, women become old at age 45 or 50. By the time respondents reach their sixth or seventh decades, old age is pushed back to the late 60s and early 70s. Note the strong gender difference in reports of when a woman is old. Female respondents date the start of old age to a later age than men, whatever the respondent's age. Women consider old age to begin 2 to 4 years later than men. These differences suggest a need to consider social elements when examining perceived age-related changes.

Cultural Variation in Definitions of the Life Course

The relevance of social or cultural factors in conceptions of the life course is evident in the "infantilization" of older adults, such as use of baby talk or saccharine language applied to frail or very old people. Cognitive anthropological studies show that cultural dimensions, such as productivity, vulnerability, and reproductive potential, underlie judgments of "young," "middle-aged," and "old." In one study, respondents were asked to group hypothetic age-linked social statuses according to similarity. Multidimensional scaling analyses revealed that respondents grouped old people and children together as opposed to people of middle age. This cultural logic may explain why baby talk is often applied to older people with cognitive impairment or other disabilities and terms typically reserved for children are often applied to older people. The reverse is also true: younger adults who are not active, not interested in new experiences or travel, not willing to switch careers, or who are slow, deliberate, or risk averse, are often called "old" or "old before their time." We are enjoined "to act our age."

Even this brief discussion of the use of age criteria to label behaviors suggests that attitudes toward aging and old age are mostly negative. Old age is usually seen as a time of decline, withdrawal, vulnerability, and even reversion

to childhood. In this view, aging is not welcome and little should be expected of older people, except perhaps to ease decline, provide care, and protect people from exploitation or danger related to their increased vulnerability. These are the elements of "ageism": assumptions of disability or vulnerability (and hence need for protection) based on age, rather than actual competencies. A goal of developmental approaches to psychosocial aging is to avoid such oversimplifications and cultural biases to determine the range of changes in social, affective, and cognitive experience associated with aging.

DEVELOPMENTAL CONSTRAINTS ON RESILIENCE AND THE STRESS PROCESS

Understanding the role of psychosocial factors in late life requires that we first take a high-altitude view of human development to identify the basic biological and social forces that fundamentally shape the development of people as they age and the ways they respond to challenges associated with aging. These forces are typically viewed as constraints and can be briefly summarized in four propositions.

The first is that biological development follows a sequential pattern. Although there is considerable interindividual variability in biological development, overall biological resources across the lifespan resemble an inverted U-function. During childhood and adolescence, cognitive and physical abilities increase and provide the basis for the development of complex motor and cognitive skills. Physical development plateaus during adulthood and then later declines. Cognitive function, especially "fluid" capacities, decline in old age even apart from dementing disease.

Second, societies impose age-graded structural constraints on development. Lifespan psychologists and sociologists emphasize that all societies impose age grades. These roles provide predictability and structure at both individual and societal levels. A prototypical case is childbearing in women, which is shaped by both social institutions and biological constraints.

Third, life is finite. Whatever is to be achieved or experienced in life has to be done in a limited period of time, typically fewer than 80 to 90 years. At any given point in an individual's life, the anticipated amount of time left to live may shape behavior and affect in important ways.

Fourth, genetic endowment is a limiting factor on biology and behavior. Although the potential behavioral repertoire of humans is vast, function in a given domain is often constrained by genetic makeup.

In this view of development, the accumulated resilience or adaptive capacity of individuals will vary as a function of the individual's location in the life course. Behavioral resources and psychological reserves may be greater at older ages because of accumulated life experiences, acquisition of skills, and increased knowledge. The type and intensity of biological pathways activated by stressful encounters as well as the manifestation of overt disease will also vary as a function of the individual's position in the life course.

PSYCHOSOCIAL FACTORS, HEALTH, AND QUALITY OF LIFE

Psychosocial aspects of aging are involved in changes in many domains, including work, retirement, residence, sexuality, stress, widowhood, emotion, mental health, social support, and friendship, to name just a few. A broad conceptual framework identifying key psychosocial factors is presented in **Figure 4-2**. At the far left, the model identifies a broad array of *sociodemographic characteristics* that directly and indirectly shape individual development, quality of life, and health throughout the life course. For example, many of the health disparities in our society, such as differences in life expectancy or risk of low birth weight, have been linked to socioeconomic status (SES), race and ethnicity, and gender.

Environmental and social resources and constraints include multiple indicators known to affect health outcomes, including physical and social characteristics of environments. Discrimination, negative life events, and existing comorbidities can be major sources of constraint, while religious involvement and social support are often important protective resources.

Psychological influences include positive factors, such as optimism, self-esteem, mastery, and control, as well as negative effects, such as depressive symptoms and perceived stress. The effects of psychological and social/environmental factors on health are mediated by *health behaviors* and *biological pathways*, such as the central nervous system and endocrine response. Although the causal links between these groups of variables are still debated (hence no arrows are shown in the figure), all are clearly important contributors to health and quality of life.

The Biology of Psychosocial Aging

Biological changes are relevant to psychosocial aging. Late-life depression (LLD) may stem from inflammatory and hormonal abnormalities. LLD is often associated with greater chronicity, relapse, resistance to treatment, and suicide risk,

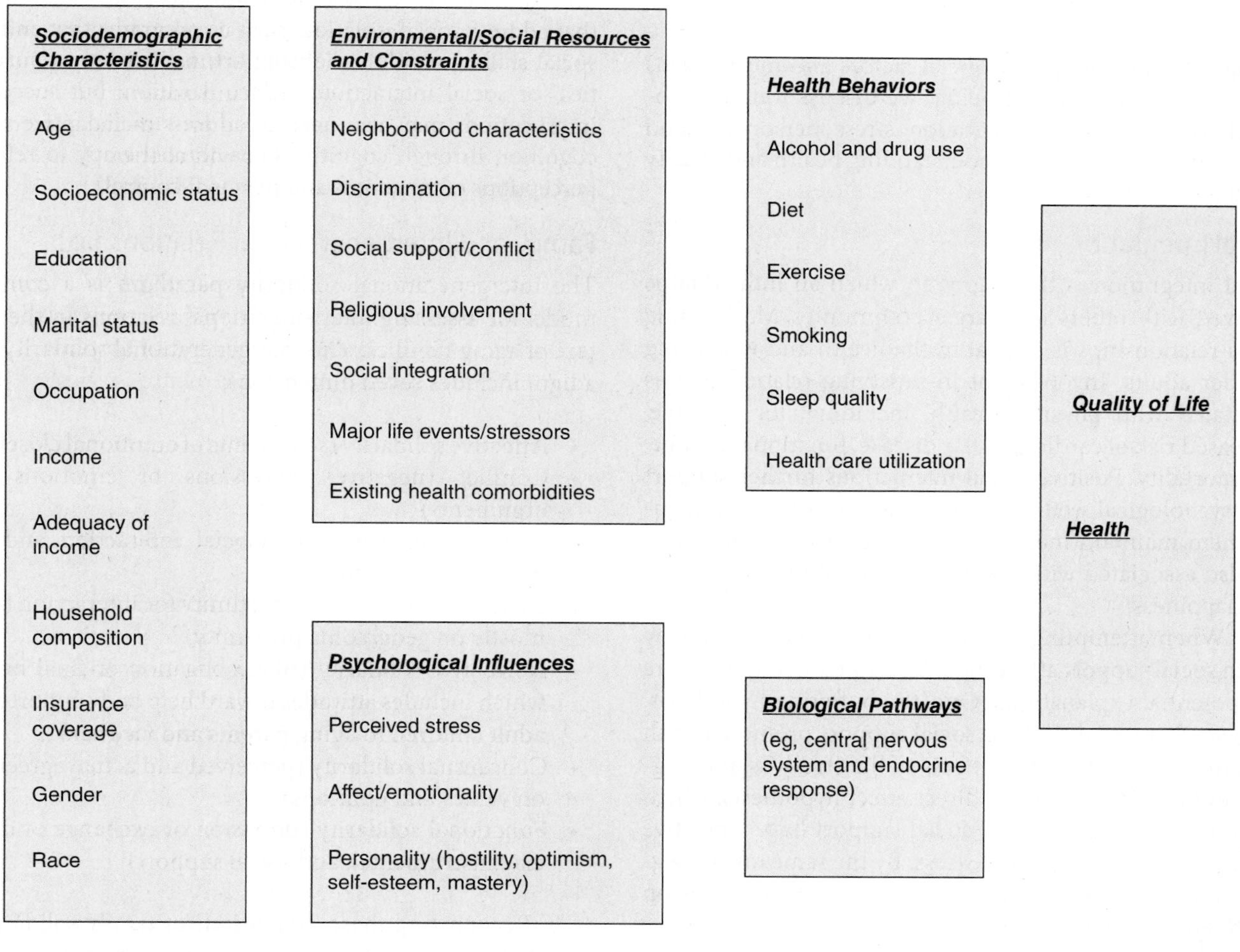

Sociodemographic Characteristics	Environmental/Social Resources and Constraints	Health Behaviors	
Age	Neighborhood characteristics	Alcohol and drug use	
Socioeconomic status	Discrimination	Diet	
Education	Social support/conflict	Exercise	
Marital status	Religious involvement	Smoking	Quality of Life
Occupation	Social integration	Sleep quality	
Income	Major life events/stressors	Health care utilization	
Adequacy of income	Existing health comorbidities		Health
Household composition			
Insurance coverage	Psychological Influences		
Gender	Perceived stress	Biological Pathways	
Race	Affect/emotionality	(eg, central nervous system and endocrine response)	
	Personality (hostility, optimism, self-esteem, mastery)		

FIGURE 4-2. Psychosocial factors and health and quality of life.

as compared to depression in younger adults. It may also be comorbid with dementia and hence points to the need to evaluate cognitive status. In women, the perimenopausal transition, but not necessarily the postmenopausal stage, can be associated with depression, resulting from declining and fluctuating estrogen levels. Among people undergoing chronic stress, chronically elevated serum cortisol can generate a proinflammatory milieu and accelerate the aging process, a phenomenon known as *inflammaging*.

Age-related decline in melatonin secretion from the pineal gland at night may explain sleep disturbances among older adults. Poor sleep hygiene may contribute to increased irritability, poor mood, and elevated dementia risk in this population. The declining functional status of organ systems associated with the aging process, including, for example, diastolic heart failure, may limit activities and therefore socialization. Reduced vision and hearing may also contribute to reduced social interaction.

Purposeful efforts at social engagement may aid in dementia prevention by maintaining brain cellular integrity before gross atrophy sets in. Recent research has shown that greater social engagement among older adults is associated with greater microstructural integrity of brain cells.

SOCIAL RELATIONSHIPS

In highlighting core psychosocial factors and mechanisms linked to health and well-being, we discuss four psychosocial domains—social integration, stress, personality, and affect—that are critical to understanding health and quality of life in old age.

Social Integration

Social integration is the degree to which an individual is involved with others in a larger community. Maintaining social relationships is critical to the health and well-being of older adults. Involvement in satisfying relationships is associated with physical health, including, for example, decreased risk of cardiovascular disease, functional decline, and mortality. Positive social interactions further support the psychological well-being of older adults through helping them maintain meaning in life, and such interactions are also associated with increased sense of life satisfaction and happiness.

When attempting to understand the mechanisms by which social support affects health and well-being, there are two potential explanations. One, the buffering hypothesis, suggests that social ties and social support promote health by acting as buffers to the effects of life stressors and negative events. Another is the direct effect hypothesis, which suggests that social ties and social support have a positive impact on health apart from stress. By the same token, negative social interactions may have detrimental effects on health and well-being.

It is important to consider the composition of social networks, which includes the number of family members, friends, neighbors, and acquaintances, and the density of social ties. Research indicates age differences in the size and composition of social networks, with networks shrinking at greater ages. A countervailing force is the larger proportion of well-known social partners in these smaller networks. According to socioemotional selectivity theory, discussed later, these changes serve an emotional regulatory function for older adults. Smaller networks with well-known social partners allow older adults to increase predictability in social interactions and maximize positive and minimize negative interactions. Based on this theory, the smaller size of networks in old age, therefore, does not necessarily indicate lack of support but may instead serve a protective function.

Social Isolation and Loneliness

Research suggests that a low level of social activity and social contacts is associated with poor functional outcomes. Loneliness, or perceived social isolation, may be most important for health effects. Population-based studies show that loneliness is associated with increased morbidity, including cardiovascular illness, coronary heart disease, and depressive symptoms, as well as mortality. Loneliness has also been associated with personality disorders and psychoses, suicide, impaired cognitive performance and cognitive decline over time, and increased risk of Alzheimer disease. Interventions that address social isolation, such as programs that enhance social skills, provide social support, or increase opportunities for social interaction, reduce isolation; but successful interventions may also need to address maladaptive social cognition through cognitive behavioral therapy to reframe perceptions of loneliness and personal control.

Family and Intergenerational Relationships

The intergenerational solidarity paradigm is a common model for assessing intergenerational relations in the context of aging families. The intergenerational solidarity paradigm includes seven dimensions:

- Affective solidarity (sentiments of emotional closeness)
- Conflict (negative expressions of emotions and arguments)
- Associational solidarity (social interaction and frequency of communicating)
- Structural solidarity (opportunity for interaction based mostly on geographic proximity)
- Normative solidarity (filial obligation or filial norms, which includes attitudes toward help and support from adult children to aging parents and vice versa)
- Consensual solidarity (perceived and actual agreement on values and opinions)
- Functional solidarity (provision or exchange of financial, instrumental, and social support)

Recognizing these dimensions of family solidarity is essential for understanding how families provide support to older adults.

Social Support and Family Caregiving

The widely held belief that contemporary families do not provide care for their aging members has been disproved by years of research. In fact, families continue to be the mainstay of long-term care and social support to older adults. While the majority of older adults in the United States live in independent households, older adults rely on children when they need support. Policymakers consider families the key source of support for meeting the growing needs of the older population. While spouses, mainly wives, provide most family caregiving support, adult children provide the bulk of care when a spouse is absent or unable to care.

Four forms of support are exchanged across generations: (1) *emotional support*: the expression of empathy, caring, concern, and love; (2) *instrumental support*: provision or direct assistance in instrumental activities (eg, transportation, shopping, cooking, cleaning, yard work, and house repair) or personal self-maintenance care, such as help with bathing, dressing, and feeding; (3) *informational and organizational support*: support in decision making, care coordination and management, and financial management; and (4) *financial support*: income transfers.

Overall, the exchange of support has a positive effect on a care recipient. However, receiving instrumental support may have a mixed effect on functional status.

Greater frequency of instrumental support may increase the risk of subsequent disability. Furthermore, receipt of instrumental support may lead to feelings of helplessness, perceptions of low mastery and autonomy, and reduced self-efficacy and sense of control.

The extent to which support is given, received, or exchanged between adult children and aging parents depends on several factors, some related to the adult children, others to the aging parents, others to the relationship between adult children and aging parents, and still others to the larger contexts governing relationships. **Figure 4-3** displays the many factors involved in predicting parental support, described here.

Characteristics of the adult child Findings regarding gender differences in filial norms toward older parents are mixed. While sons and daughters seem equally committed to provide care to aging parents, gender differences are apparent for specific types of support. Adult sons are more likely to provide financial and instrumental support, while adult daughters are more likely to provide personal care, complete household chores, and offer social support.

Another predictor is income or more generally, social class, as it affects both the need and the availability of support. Financially and educationally advantaged families can more easily purchase care on the private market, thereby

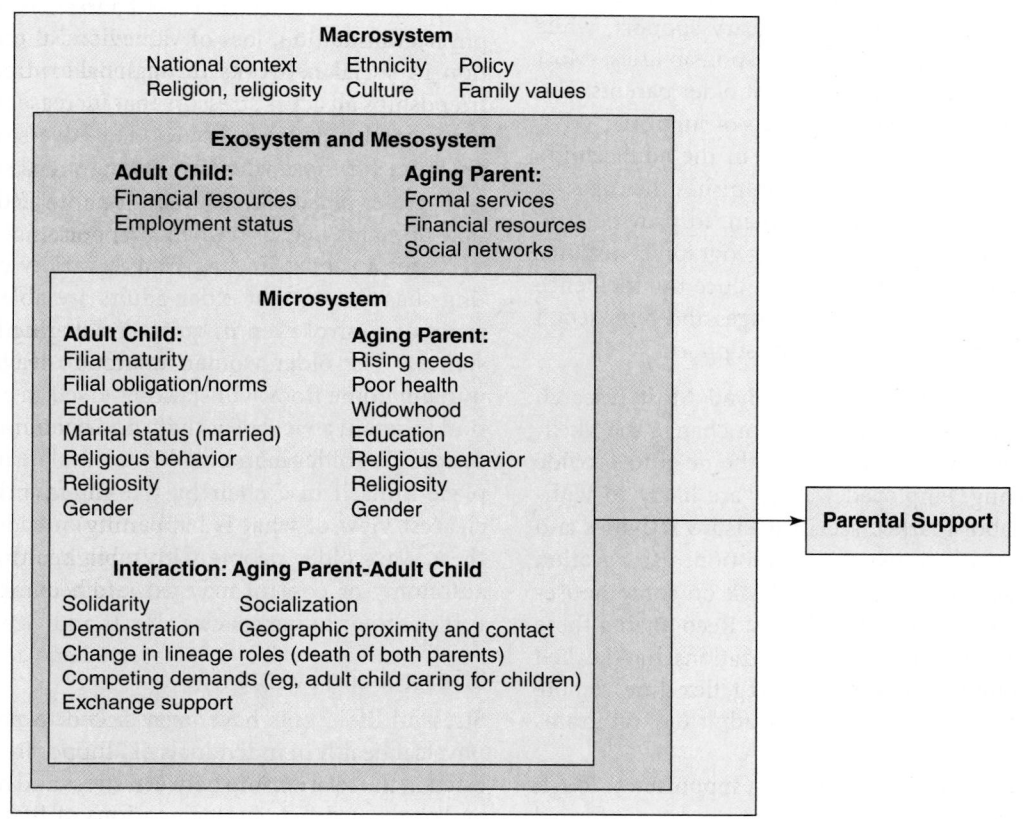

FIGURE 4-3. Conceptual framework for understanding factors affecting parental support.

diminishing their sense of obligation to provide care themselves. Lower-income families are less likely to purchase services and express stronger filial obligation.

Marital disruption and remarriage have a major impact on parental support and filial obligation. Divorce disrupts the exchange of support between parents and children. Some research suggests that divorced children feel less filial obligation. Additionally, divorce affects the amount of resources available to help family members and breaks ties that may be important for the needs of their parents. In addition, divorces and remarriages may increase the number of potential care recipients per adult child by adding stepparents and other step relatives. Having more kin as potential care receivers may diminish the amount of care given by each one. Widowed and divorced parents receive more help than married parents.

Financial factors also play a role. Aging parents with higher financial resources can purchase services and may access services of higher quality, thereby diminishing the need for some types of informal care from children.

Interrelationship between the adult child and the aging parents Affectual solidarity between parents and their children is a major factor in the exchange of intergenerational support. Adult children who witnessed their parents care for their own parents are more likely to provide support, emphasizing the role of social learning on the likelihood of parental caregiving. The presence of siblings in the family is also a predictor of intergenerational assistance. Only children are relied upon for all necessary support, while individuals with siblings can share responsibilities. Most research in the United States shows that older parents who have more children receive higher levels of support.

The presence of young children in the adult child's house is a competing demand that diminishes the capacity of adult children, and especially women, to provide support to their aging parents. Greater geographic distance and limited face-to-face contact also reduce the incidence of all types of intergenerational exchanges and represent a significant barrier to intergenerational support.

Effects outside caregiver-care-receiver dyad Most research shows that women's paid work does not change the likelihood of caregiving. When faced with the need to provide parental caregiving, employed women are likely to withdraw from the labor market, sacrifice leisure activities and sleep, pass up opportunities for promotion, use vacation and sick days for parental care, cut back on some housework activities, and reduce work hours. Recognizing these pressures, caregiving advocacy organizations have called for greater flexibility in the workplace (eg, flex time, remote work, employee assistance programs, adult day programs on site).

The availability of formal services, supported through public sector investment, will affect the need for informal support. Advocates of small government fear that such services will "crowd out" families and lead to less efficient service provision. An alternative view suggests that families and formal services complement each other in an efficient division of labor. For example, formal organizations are optimal in managing technical tasks in caregiving, while primary groups, such as families, are optimal for managing nontechnical support. As a result, a partnership between formal organizations and primary groups may be the best approach to negotiate informal and formal care.

Race and ethnicity also influence filial norms and parental support. Traditionally, African-American and Latinx cultures were viewed as giving greater emphasis to family ties ("familism"). However, recent research suggests type of support rather than level of support may best differentiate variation in caregiving.

STRESS AND DISTRESS

Stress is a common response to physical, cognitive, and emotional challenges. The stressed person will experience adverse physiologic effects (primarily in the pituitary-adrenal axis and immune system) but also clinically appreciable effects on decision making, problem-solving, vigilance, social inference, and perceptual and motor skills. In this case, stress, a normal feature of interaction with an environment, becomes *distress*, prolonged stress that overwhelms physiologic and psychological regulatory mechanisms. Prolonged stress may be associated with accelerated aging.

For older adults, the rising prevalence of chronic disease and disability, increased awareness of cognitive or physical limitation, loss of valued social roles, and reduction in social networks through widowhood and loss of friendships all act as stressors that increase the risk of negative mental and physical states. The adverse effects of stress are lower for those who have strong social support systems and greater personal resources, but repeated losses in multiple domains may overwhelm supports.

Yet a robust finding from a variety of research settings has shown that older adults are able to maintain a sense of control even in quite challenging health circumstances. The older woman unable to leave the home or nursing home floor will station herself in a strategic position to retain a view of activity and encourage social interaction. The older man unable to ambulate in his home will place himself in a chair by the window that affords the clearest view of what is happening outside the home. In these ways older people with poor health and threats to autonomy or control may yet retain command over features of their living space.

Stressful Life Events

Stressful life events have been linked to poor mental and physical health in individuals of all ages. Researchers interested in the relationship between stress and health have generally pursued two strategies to assess life event stressors. Major life events such as illness and death of a loved one are often assessed using checklists or interviews to gauge the frequency and intensity of these types of experiences. Daily hassles, on the other hand, are the bothers and challenges of day-to-day living and are measured with structured self-report or interviewer-administered instruments.

Compared to younger persons, older individuals experience fewer life events overall, although they experience more events involving loss, particularly those associated with declining health and deaths of friends and loved ones. Younger individuals report more hassles in the domains of finances, work, home maintenance, personal life, and family and friends, whereas older men and women report more hassles in domains reflecting social issues, home maintenance, and health. Overall, for both younger and older individuals, daily hassles are more potent determinants of physical and psychological well-being than major life stressors.

Older individuals demonstrate remarkable ability to adapt successfully to major life stressors. One important exception to this general observation occurs when older individuals are exposed to unrelenting chronic stressors, such as having to care for a spouse with Alzheimer disease. Under these circumstances the chronicity, intensity, and variety of stressors impinging on the caregiver exact a high price in physical and psychiatric morbidity, including increased risk of substance abuse, and in rare cases murder-suicide.

The considerable variability in response to major life stressors reflects resilience associated with aging. Resilience is the ability to recover from or benefit from adversity. Individuals able to overcome adversity are thought to have high levels of resilience, a combination of internal personality traits such as hardiness, self-efficacy, mastery, and optimism, along with a strong external support system. However, the empirical and clinical utility of the concept of resilience remains to be determined.

Biological Consequences of Stress

Because increasing age is associated with significant alterations in the functioning of many physiologic systems, old age has become a fertile ground for examining the relation between stress, biological mediators, and disease. For example, a significant body of research views family caregiving as a chronic stressor with the ability to disrupt immune and neuroendocrine function. Compared to noncaregiver older adults, older caregivers have higher antibody titers for latent viruses, poor immune control over latent viral infections, reduced responsiveness of natural killer (NK) cells to cytokine signals, slower healing of wounds, poorer antibody responses to vaccination, and higher levels of basal cortisol. Physical health effects of caregiving include greater risk of infectious disease, hypertensive changes, increased prevalence of cardiovascular disease, and mortality. These findings suggest a strong link between stress, biological mediators, and illness; however, few studies have examined the progression of stress as a biological mediator of disease over time.

Personality and Health

Personality is defined as psychological characteristics and attributes and associated behavioral patterns that differentiate one person from another. Personality has long been of interest to researchers, especially with respect to how it develops and may change across the lifespan. The five-factor model (FFM) of personality has been influential among gerontologists and claims that personality can be defined by five broad traits—openness to experience, conscientiousness, extraversion, agreeableness, and neuroticism—that remain relatively fixed into old age. Other important traits include mastery or control, the belief that important outcomes in life are under one's own control, as well as optimism and hostility. Despite the relative stability of key traits, functional declines in late life may erode one's sense of mastery, extraversion, or optimism.

An important emerging area of research is focused on the link between two distinct dispositional attributes and health. Enduring negative effects, such as anger, depression, and anxiety, increase the risk of morbidity and mortality, while positive effects have been linked to lower morbidity, decrease in symptoms and pain, and increased longevity. Multiple mechanisms account for the relation between dispositional affect and morbidity and mortality, including health practices such as diet, exercise, and sleep quality, biological processes such as cardiovascular reactivity, and the effects of the stress hormones epinephrine, norepinephrine, and cortisol. Inasmuch as individuals with positive affect are typically more pleasant to be around, they may also accrue health benefits through more positive social interactions and more attentive and higher-quality health care from health care providers.

AFFECTIVE PROCESSES OVER THE LIFESPAN

Emotional life changes across the lifespan. If one talks to older people and asks about the emotions, one is likely to hear statements about the decline of emotion: "the highs are not so high anymore, but the lows are not so low either." Older people speak wistfully of their more intense emotional life at younger ages but also report a good deal of relief at getting off that treadmill.

Population surveys, such as the General Social Survey (GSS) and Eurobarometer, track the prevalence of reported effects by age and across birth cohorts and confirm this broad pattern. "Hot emotions," such as feeling excited about something or feeling overjoyed, decline in age cross-sections. For example, in the GSS the proportion reporting they were overjoyed about something at least 1 day in the last month was 71% in people aged 18 to 29, 56% in people aged 40 to 49, and 47% in people aged 70+. By contrast, the proportion reporting they were fearful about something was 47%, 45%, and 30% in the same age groups. The contrast confounds developmental and birth cohort effects, but

TABLE 4-1 ■ AGE AT WHICH LIFE SATISFACTION IS LOWEST

	MALES	FEMALES
Western Europe	45	47
Eastern Europe	47	48
Developing countries	43	44
Latin America	50	43
Asia	47	39

Data from Blanchflower DG, Oswald AJ. Is well-being U-shaped over the life cycle? Soc Sci Med. 2008;66(8):1733–1749.

such changes have been reported as well for longitudinal cohorts.

The GSS and Eurobarometer surveys (which cover 72 countries and over a half million respondents) show that "life satisfaction" and depressed mood follow a U-shape distribution over the lifespan. Life satisfaction is assessed with subjective global appraisals, such as "Taken all together, how would you say things are these days—Would you say that you are very happy, pretty happy, or not too happy?" **Table 4-1** shows the age at which life satisfaction is lowest in cross-sectional surveys, adjusted for a number of important covariates, such as income, health indicators, marital status, and education. Life satisfaction is lowest at age 40 to 50 in both men and women and remarkably stable across continents.

Self-reported depressed mood follows the same pattern. Using the same surveys, depressed mood is also most common at ages 40 to 50, as shown in **Figure 4-4**.

If we turn to changes at older ages, we find that variation in emotional experience is related less to age than to disability, as shown by results drawn from the Women's Health and Aging Study, WHAS-I. The sample included the most disabled third of older women living in the community. The sample of over 1000 women was divided into three age groups (65–74, 75–84, 85+) and three disability groups: women with "moderate disability" (limitations in

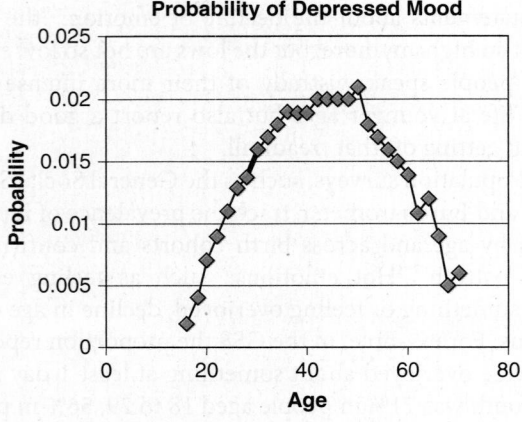

FIGURE 4-4. Depressed mood over the lifespan. (Adapted with permission from Blanchflower DG, Oswald AJ. Is well-being U-shaped over the life cycle? *Soc Sci Med.* 2008;66[8]:1733–1749.)

upper extremity, lower extremity, or instrumental activities of daily living [IADLs] but no difficulty with the basic activities of daily living [ADLs], such as bathing or dressing), those with ADL difficulty who were able to manage without personal assistance, and those with ADL difficulty who received personal assistance.

Tables 4-2 and **4-3** report the affective experience of these older women. **Table 4-2** shows little variation by age group; mental health and emotional experience were quite similar across the age groups. **Table 4-3**, by contrast, shows the very strong association between disability and virtually all the indicators. For example, the proportion with depressed mood was 13% in women with moderate limitations, 16% in women with ADL difficulty not receiving help, and 29% in women with ADL difficulty who received personal assistance. The corresponding proportions by age group for depressed mood were 19% (age 65–74), 17% (age 75–84), and 14% (age 85+).

Results from WHAS-I show the strong effects of disability and poor health on mood, yet also great resiliency in the face of health limitation. About three-quarters of women with the most severe disability reported satisfaction with help. Over half the sample with the most severe disability still reported they were able to provide assistance to others to a satisfying degree. "Satisfaction with variety in life" declined from 70% to 51% across categories of disability, but again more than half of the women with severe disability reported satisfaction. By contrast, "satisfaction with the meaning and purpose of your life" was stable across age and disability categories; about three-quarters of these women, whatever their age or level of disability, reported such satisfaction.

Finally, this sample of women on the whole reported relatively low self-efficacy. Less than half reported confidence they could accomplish "anything I really set my mind to do." However, only a minority reported "helplessness," under 10% in the less severe disability groups and 20% in women receiving assistance with ADL tasks.

This inquiry suggests that disability has only a minor impact on mental health and general well-being. This is an important result. Most of the women in this sample were able to maintain well-being despite disability.

One theory advanced to explain these changes in emotional experience with age and disability involves "socioemotional selectivity." The theory begins with recognition of the effect of limited time. Aging, health limitation, losses, and disability give time a different significance. Present-oriented goals are given greater value. Thus, older people will be more content with ongoing satisfying social experiences rather than novel experiences that may be emotionally "risky" (because they may be unsatisfying). This awareness of limited time leads to motivational changes that promote well-being and social adjustment and a skew in attention toward positive information. These theoretic predictions have been confirmed in a variety of experimental settings and may have a neural substrate. An unfortunate consequence may be greater susceptibility to financial scams.

TABLE 4-2 ■ AFFECTIVE EXPERIENCE, WOMEN'S HEALTH AND AGING STUDY I, BY AGE GROUP

	AGE GROUP		
	65–74	75–84	85+
High level of depressive symptoms, % GDS > 13	19	17	14
High level of anxiety, %	2.8	4.0	5.1
Satisfied with help received from family and friends, %	79	81	78
Satisfied with help you give to family and friends, %	78	70	68
Satisfied with amount of variety in your life, %	66	62	62
Satisfied with the meaning and purpose of your life, %	76	76	76
I can do just about anything I really set my mind to do, % strongly agree	49	45	44
I feel helpless in dealing with the problems of life, % strongly agree	8.8	10	12

Data from Guralnik JM, Fried LP, Simonsick EM, et al. The Women's Health and Aging Study: Health and Social Characteristics of Older Women with Disability. Bethesda, MD: National Institute on Aging; 1995; NIH Pub. No. 95-4009.

A related theory of psychosocial aging suggests that emotional change is part of a more general "selection, optimization, compensation" process. Older people become expert in managing depleted resources. Successful aging requires selecting domains to focus limited resources, optimizing investments of time, energy, and emotion to maximize gains, and compensating for losses. Minimizing losses in the emotional domain is consistent with socioemotional selectivity.

ENVIRONMENTS TO SUPPORT PSYCHOSOCIAL HEALTH

Aging in Place

Aging in place refers to the ability to remain in one's home and community even when facing health and challenges in function. Surveys show that the majority of older adults with deteriorating health prefer staying in their home rather than moving to an institutional setting, and research suggests a positive relationship between aging in place and the well-being of older adults. The familiarity of the surroundings and the embedded social network and social support of neighbors may support well-being. Beyond the benefits to older adults and their families, opportunities to age in place also contribute to the community as a whole. Older adults remaining in the community may support others through volunteering or caregiving activities. Furthermore, aging in place is superior to institutional care because of lower costs to families and government-funded long-term care. However, residence in skilled nursing facilities may be cost-effective relative to home care in the case of older adults who require 24-hour care or advanced medical technologies.

Successful aging in place relies on the availability of supportive physical, social, and economic elements within the infrastructure of cities, towns, and communities. Since such elements may benefit other age groups, it is common to refer to communities that make a focused effort to increase safety and accessibility as *age-friendly cities* or *livable communities*. A report from the Stanford University Center on Longevity and MetLife Mature Market Institute provides a summary of the most important elements of a livable community required for successful aging in place. These elements, depicted in **Figure 4-5**, identify the

TABLE 4-3 ■ AFFECTIVE EXPERIENCE, WOMEN'S HEALTH AND AGING STUDY I, BY DISABILITY STATUS

	DISABILITY STATUS		
	MODERATE[a]	ADL DISABILITY: NO HELP[b]	ADL: HELP[c]
High level of depressive symptoms, % GDS > 13	13	16	29
High level of anxiety, %	2.1	4.4	4.7
Satisfied with help received from family and friends, %	84	79	75
Satisfied with help you give to family and friends, %	84	71	56
Satisfied with amount of variety in your life, %	70	64	51
Satisfied with the meaning and purpose of your life, %	80	75	72
I can do just about anything I really set my mind to do, % strongly agree	51	45	40
I feel helpless in dealing with the problems of life, % strongly agree	9.3	6.8	20

[a]Moderate = IADL disability, no ADL disability.
[b]ADL disability: No help = Difficulty with ADL, not receiving help.
[c]ADL: Help = Difficulty with ADL, receiving help.
Data from Guralnik JM, Fried LP, Simonsick EM, et al. The Women's Health and Aging Study: Health and Social Characteristics of Older Women with Disability. Bethesda, MD: National Institute on Aging; 1995; NIH Pub. No. 95-4009.

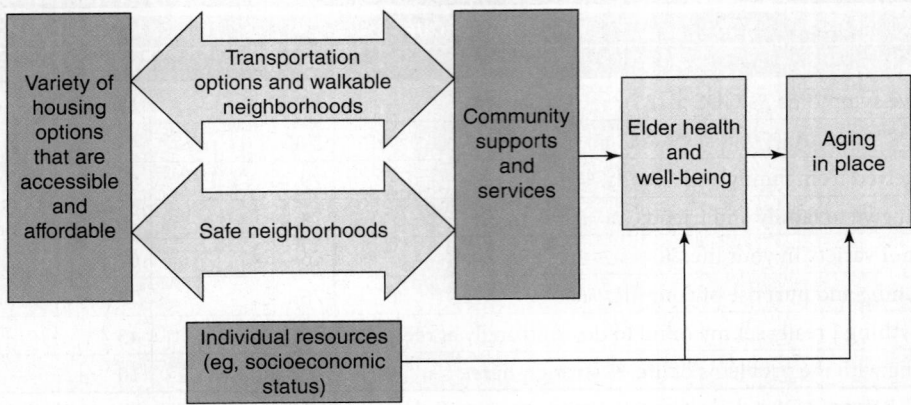

FIGURE 4-5. Aging in place, characteristics of livable communities. (Reproduced with permission from Liveable Community Indicators for Sustainable Aging in Place. March, 2013. MetLife Mature Market Institute.)

economic, social, and environmental supports that sustain older adults in their communities, including:

- Accessible and affordable housing options and availability of home modification services to adapt the home environment to the needs of an aging individual.
- Availability of appropriate transportation options to ensure accessibility to and from the community and mobility within the community, along with safe walking conditions (ie, well-maintained sidewalks, benches, and parks). Communities ensure safe driving by providing protected left-turns, reasonable signage, and adequate lighting. Safe walking and driving conditions promote independence of older adults, an important contributor to health and well-being.
- Availability of a wide range of supports and services and opportunities to participate in community life, including health care services, supportive services, groceries with healthy food options, and opportunities for flexible employment, volunteering, recreation, and socialization.

The World Health Organization (WHO) has developed a guide for age-friendly cities, which includes similar elements, as depicted in **Figure 4-6**. Both the MetLife and WHO models recognize that the physical, social, and economic environment is critical, but that successful aging in place also requires adequate individual resources, such as availability of supportive care, either through paid in-home services or from family or other informal caregivers.

Long-Term Care: In-Home and Community-Based Services and Supportive Housing

Long-term care encompasses a wide spectrum of personal care services provided to individuals who need continual support. One end of the spectrum of services is informal care provided at home by a family member, typically a spouse or adult child. On the other end is around-the-clock care provided by trained clinical teams in a skilled nursing facility. Between the two we find a variety of services that vary in the intensity, location, and cost of care.

The different options available to an older adult at home, in the community, and if needed, in residential settings are shown in **Figure 4-7**. Options for supportive care in the home include paid in-home health care, provided by nurses and allied health professionals, as well as homemaker and personal assistance services, provided by paraprofessionals. Other in-home services include home-delivered meals, social visiting from neighborhood organizations or programs such as the Senior Corps Companions, and support for medical equipment, such as oxygen, lymphedema

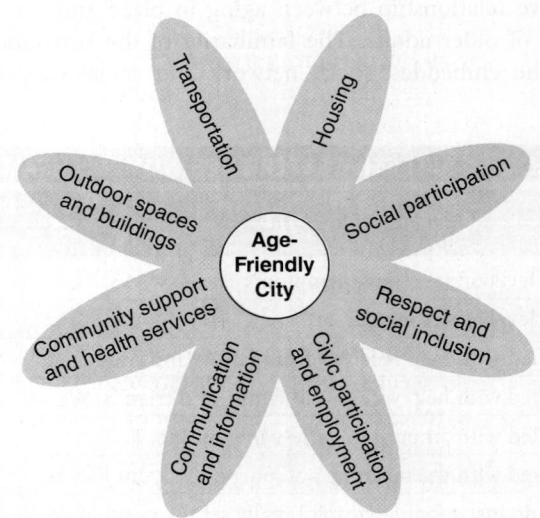

FIGURE 4-6. Aging in place: age-friendly domains. (Reproduced with permission from World Health Organization, 2007. *Global Age-Friendly Cities: A Guide*. Geneva, Switzerland: WHO Press; 2007.)

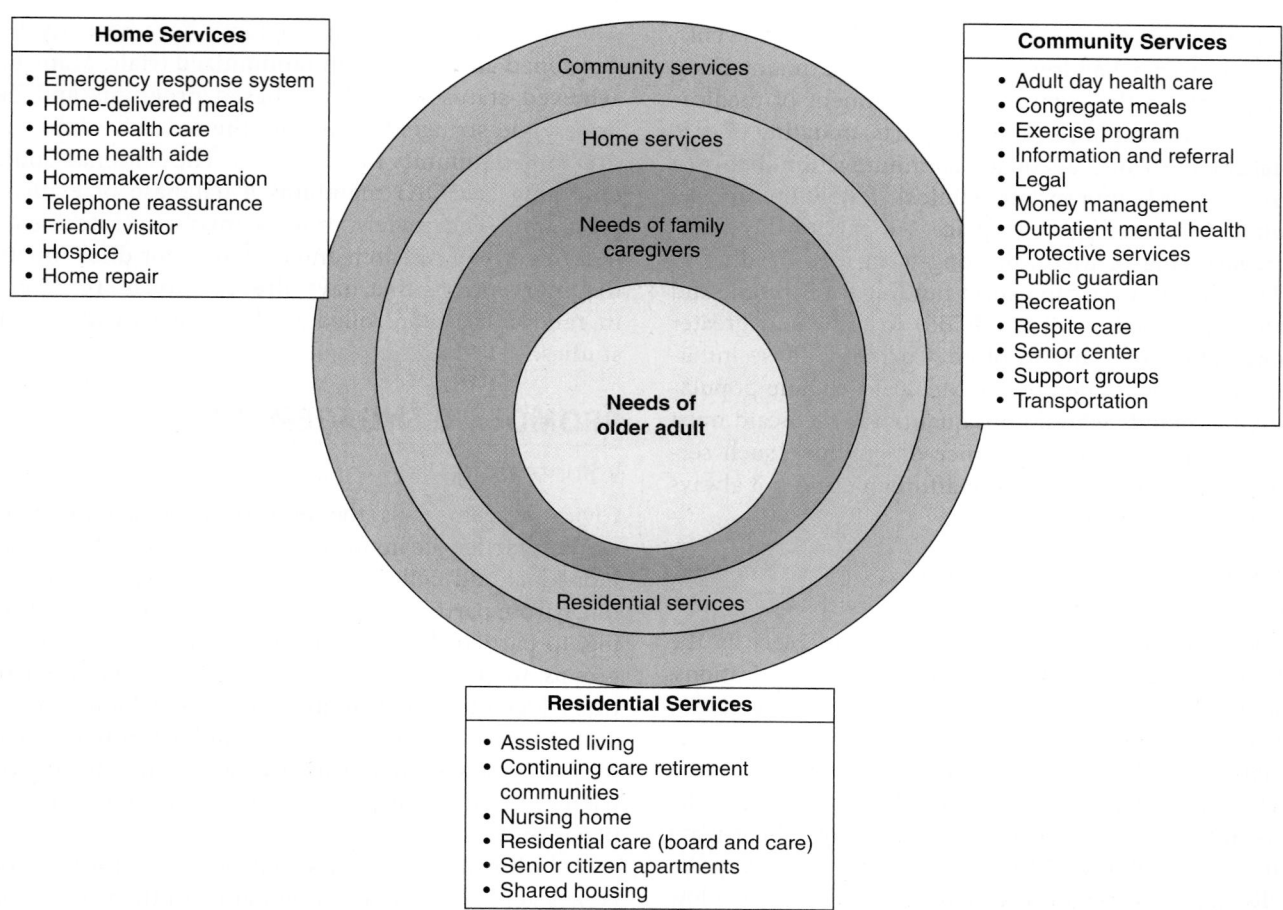

Home Services
- Emergency response system
- Home-delivered meals
- Home health care
- Home health aide
- Homemaker/companion
- Telephone reassurance
- Friendly visitor
- Hospice
- Home repair

Community Services
- Adult day health care
- Congregate meals
- Exercise program
- Information and referral
- Legal
- Money management
- Outpatient mental health
- Protective services
- Public guardian
- Recreation
- Respite care
- Senior center
- Support groups
- Transportation

Community services
Home services
Needs of family caregivers
Needs of older adult
Residential services

Residential Services
- Assisted living
- Continuing care retirement communities
- Nursing home
- Residential care (board and care)
- Senior citizen apartments
- Shared housing

FIGURE 4-7. Long-term care: home, community, and residential settings.

support, adjustable beds and chairs, lifts, and respiratory devices. Home modification to address mobility limitation may also be considered an in-home service. Community supports for aging in place include adult day care, congregate meals, senior center programming, and transportation services. These services in the home and the community are designed to help older adults to age in place by addressing their needs as well as the needs of informal family caregivers.

The services range in intensity and frequency. Some provide a solution to a specific problem and thus support older adults who are otherwise independent. For example, home-delivered meals, or "Meals on Wheels," cover one-third of the daily nutrition needs of older adults. Subsidized transportation services may allow otherwise independent adults to get to and from medical appointments. Other services may provide a more intensive level of services for individuals who need a more comprehensive set of supports, such as home health aides for personal care or adult day programs for people with mild to moderate dementia. Given adequate assessment and care management, individuals with nursing home-equivalent needs can be maintained in their homes. Indeed, care management services

provided through Medicaid and Administration on Community Living Title IIID funds often require that these older adults be "nursing facility clinically eligible" (NFCE).

Similarly, residential services offer varying degrees of support based on the continuum of care. These range from independent living residences with occasional nursing or social service support (as in naturally occurring retirement communities, or NORCs), to assistive living communities and personal care homes (residences integrated with health services and communal meals and housing services), to skilled nursing facilities. Some of these residential services offer the full continuum of care whereby residents can move from more independent living settings to more supportive settings as their needs change.

It is important to note variability in the functional trajectory of older adults. This variability is important for targeting services to support aging in place. Older adults often face a health crisis, such as a hip fracture, which will require that they be temporarily placed in a restrictive environment, such as a skilled nursing home or rehabilitative setting. Once they regain functioning, they may go back to a less supportive environment, either in a residential setting or in the community.

Well-planned transitions after such health events, so-called "warm handoffs," are critical for maintaining older people in the community. Adjustment of medication, reassessment of in-home supports, updating of care management plans, adequate communication between providers, and appropriate clinical follow-up are all required to ensure aging in place. As part of the ongoing rebalancing of Medicaid long-term care funding in the United States, we can expect funding for in-home and community-based services (HCBS) to grow and greater opportunities for aging in place. Currently, these initiatives are mostly limited to the Medicaid-eligible population. Older adults who do not qualify for Medicaid must rely on long-term care insurance or purchase such services, which is in many cases unaffordable and not always available and appropriate.

Villages and Naturally Occurring Retirement Communities

A new and growing approach to aging in place is the "Village" model. Developed as grassroots organizations, these villages provide older adults living in the community with a combination of supportive services, such as transportation, housekeeping, and companionship, and a referral service for vetted community services, potentially at a reduced rate using their bargaining power. Villages are similar to the NORC with Supportive Services Program (NORC-SSP), as they provide supportive services to allow for successful aging in place, yet are initiated, governed, and funded (through membership fees) by the consumers they serve rather than by an agency. While each village operates with autonomy as a response to the local needs, the village to village (VtV) network provides help in establishing and managing villages.

SUPPORTING PSYCHOSOCIAL HEALTH THROUGH THE AGING SERVICES NETWORK

A productive way to support psychosocial health among older adults is to harness community-based agencies that provide aging services. These agencies have regular contact with vulnerable elders and are sometimes the only source of such contact. For example, virtually all aging services providers provide social visiting or other "check-in" services, in which agency staff or volunteers call seniors who receive services to stay in contact and unobtrusively determine new needs. These kinds of contact may uncover mental health needs and could be explicitly harnessed for assessment of depressive or anxiety symptoms and, when needed, referral. But the challenges of developing such programs are not trivial. How should staff or volunteers, who often lack mental health training, be trained? What kind of supporting staff needs to be attached to agencies for mental health services? What kind of referral pipeline would best link aging services providers to mental health services?

A number of such programs have recently been developed and assessed in randomized trials. Many have achieved status as evidence-based programs and have undergone stringent review by the federal Administration for Community Living (ACL). The National Council on Aging (NCOA) maintains a database of evidence-programs. The review process involves assessment of both quality of research and readiness for dissemination for interventions that have already shown effectiveness in randomized-controlled trials or quasi-experimental studies.

PROMOTING ENGAGEMENT

Volunteering

Civic engagement is the process by which individuals actively participate in the life of their communities through individual and collective activities. The engagement can range from participating in collective activities such as voting, to participation in religious, spiritual, or community groups, to volunteering time in unpaid productive activities. Older adults commit more hours to volunteering than any other age group, although recent birth cohorts are less likely to volunteer than earlier cohorts. Volunteering contributes to the community and is associated with a variety of personal benefits.

Volunteering is associated with positive outcomes across a number of domains. In the psychosocial domain, volunteering is associated with a reduction in depressive symptoms and improvements in life satisfaction and social support. Volunteering is also associated with better overall health, reduced functional limitations, and lower mortality risk. *Experience Corps* was a major randomized controlled trial to assess the health effects of volunteering. This program places groups of older adults in public elementary schools to work with children in kindergarten through third grade as tutors and teacher's aids. Each volunteer serves about 15 hours per week, usually over 3 to 4 days, throughout the school year. Volunteers work with students to promote reading and arithmetic skills, as well as problem-solving and conflict resolution. The program aims to improve children's academic performance, for example, by boosting school attendance, graduation rates, and performance on standardized tests; but it also aims to improve older adult outcomes by simultaneously enhancing psychosocial, physical, and cognitive well-being. Experience Corps was hypothesized to promote these outcomes through specific pathways, as shown in **Figure 4-8**, and demonstrated benefit in a number of domains.

While less research is available on the effects of volunteering for cognitive functioning, a randomized controlled trial of group volunteering in elementary schools, Experience Corps, showed improvements in cognitive function. While postretirement volunteer activities show positive effects on health and well-being, these activities are also

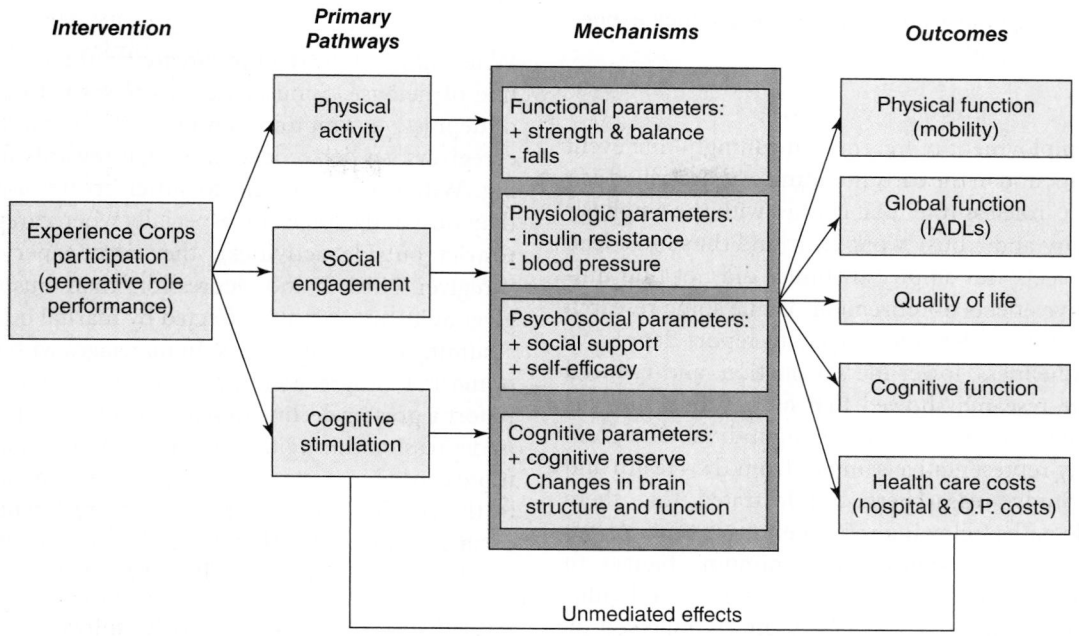

| Intervention | Primary Pathways | Mechanisms | Outcomes |

FIGURE 4-8. Causal pathways through which volunteering may support psychosocial, physical, and cognitive functioning. (Reproduced with permission from Fried LP, Carlson MC, Freedman M, et al: A social model for health promotion for an aging population: initial evidence on the Experience Corps model. *J Urban Health.* 2004;81(1):64–78.)

important for generative reasons: While helping those in need, this kind of engagement taps into broader prosocial or altruistic interests, which in itself is satisfying and may offer psychological reward (the so-called "positive glow" associated with helping others). Benefits to older volunteers increased if volunteer opportunities have a prosocial component and if people feel they are appreciated for their contribution.

Another important effort to promote volunteerism among older adults is the *Senior Corps* program. Senior Corps, funded by the US Corporation for National and Community Service, provides aid to senior citizens while promoting a sense of community. There are about 360,000 volunteers in the program nationwide each year. Senior Corps focuses on helping individuals aged 55+ to become mentors, coaches, or companions to people in need, and in this way contribute their job skills and expertise to the community. Senior Corps has three flagship programs, including (1) *Senior Companions*, in which volunteers provide assistance and friendship to adults who have difficulty with daily living tasks, as well as support to family caregivers by providing respite; (2) *RSVP*, which connects interested seniors to service opportunities, such as organizing neighborhood watch programs, tutoring or mentoring disadvantaged children, and teaching English to immigrants; and (3) *Foster Grandparents*, in which older volunteers tutor children, serve as mentors to at-risk teenagers and young mothers, help with care for premature infants and children with disabilities, and work with abused or neglected children.

Lifelong Learning

Much like volunteer activity, continued learning in old age has been associated with positive effects in psychosocial, physical, and cognitive health. One of the leading organizations in this area is Road Scholar educational adventures, formerly known as Elderhostel, a not-for-profit world organization facilitating lifelong learning in various locations in the United States and internationally. Some of these learning opportunities allow for a grandparent-grandchild combined learning experience, thus including an intergenerational component.

Another important model is the Osher Lifelong Learning Institutes (OLLI). The Osher Foundation supports lifelong-learning programs on US university and college campuses, with one or more programs in each of the 50 states and the District of Columbia. The Foundation also supports a National Resource Center to enhance programming and outreach. These efforts involve a membership-based community of adults, "age 50 and better," who take classes on campus, both traditional classes with undergraduates but also classes taught by members, who, in many cases, are retired academics and teachers.

LIFE EVENTS AND TRANSITIONS

Older adults face many life transitions or changes in roles related to age and declining health. A key age-related transition is retirement. Major health-related transitions include bereavement due to loss of a spouse or partner and the onset of caregiving when a spouse or partner experiences declines in health.

Retirement

The loss of employment represents a meaningful life event for older adults, and in the early literature was described as a transition to a "roleless role" that clashes with the emphasis on productivity and a busy work ethic and thus must lead to negative effects. Yet empirical studies did not find uniformly negative effects of retirement. While some research showed that retirees were more likely to report depressive symptoms, loneliness, lower life satisfaction, and reduced activity, other research showed that older adults are satisfied following retirement. Using longitudinal data from two nationally representative samples from the Health and Retirement Study, researchers demonstrated that there were multiple paths following retirement over time. About two-thirds of people experienced minimum changes in psychological well-being, about a quarter of individuals showed initial negative well-being effects followed by improvement, and a small group of people showed immediate positive changes.

Current retirement trends suggest that older people are now maintaining full employment to later ages (in 2019, about 17% of men aged 70+ and 10% of women aged 70+ were employed). More importantly, retirement is no longer an abrupt transition from a full-time career to no employment. Instead, current retirement behavior suggests that many older adults remain in work in later years, choose partial retirement through reducing work hours, take bridge jobs if their long-term career ends, or even start their own businesses. It is also clear that volition and choice are important in adjustment to retirement, with those choosing to retire reporting greater satisfaction than those who felt obligated to retire. Good health and adequate income are also important determinants of post-retirement adjustment.

Widowhood, Bereavement, and Grieving

The transition to widowhood is among the most stressful transitions in later life. The well-being of the surviving spouse depends on features of the end-of-life period. Strains associated with bereavement are ameliorated if physical discomfort is kept to a minimum and families provide support. Research suggests that men and women who report greater independence are better able to adjust to loss of a spouse or partner. This may suggest that successful coping in widowhood may require altering traditional gender roles.

Widowhood is a transition that leads to the reconfiguration of family roles and functions. While less likely than their married counterparts to have a confidant, widowed individuals are more likely to receive support from children, friends, and relatives. Widows are also more likely than their married counterparts to pursue volunteer roles, which in turn can lead to improved health and well-being.

Caregiving

When older adults require caregiving, the spouse is the first line of defense. Spousal caregivers seem to exhibit levels of depressive symptoms similar to adult children who are caregivers yet derive less emotional rewards from caregiving. Wife caregivers tend to suffer greater adverse effects than husband caregivers (especially when caregiving duties restrict outside activities); they also experience greater caregiver burden and depression than husbands. Caregiver adjustment is also affected by marital quality prior to assuming caregiving duties. In marriages with higher levels of marital disagreement pre-caregiving, spousal caregivers report a greater decline in happiness and a greater increase in depression during the caregiving period than spouses in more cordial marriages. A caregiver's well-being is sensitive to the condition of the spousal care recipient, with those caring for spouses with dementia experiencing higher levels of negative effects on well-being.

Grandparents Raising Grandchildren

Older adults are the first of line of recourse for caregiving support when the parental generation is unavailable due to incarceration, disease, substance abuse, or other conditions. Caregiving grandparents typically face challenges beyond their role as caregivers. They tend to live in poverty and rely on public assistance, are less educated, and in many cases do not have access to adequate health care.

The demands of caring for grandchildren have negative effects on the well-being of custodial grandparents. Cultural expectations for care arrangements in this case also have mental health consequences. For example, a cross-cultural comparison found that African-American grandmothers who were sole providers for their grandchildren were less distressed than comparable White grandmothers. In cultures that rely on extended families, caregiving stresses associated with grandparent care for grandchildren may have less negative effects.

PSYCHOSOCIAL ASPECTS OF PARTICIPATING IN HEALTH CARE DECISIONS

Cognitive, physical, and sensory limitations in older adults often limit informed decision making in medical encounters. Yet older adults continue to show interest in making informed health care choices, and patient-centered care will require innovations that promote engagement of older adults in care decisions. It is valuable to ask if older adults feel they are adequately informed about their health care choices and to identify the psychosocial correlates of "informed care."

In one large cohort of very old adults (mean age 86), participants were considered "informed" about their health-care choices if they reported that (1) a health care professional checked to see that they understood their condition and care, and (2) the health care professional gave them enough or more than enough information about their medical condition. Participants reported on their most recent medical encounter. By this standard, three-quarters of participants met criteria for informed care. Participants who met criteria for informed care were less likely to report depressed mood.

PSYCHOSOCIAL ASPECTS OF QUALITY OF LIFE AND VALUATION OF LIFE

Quality of life (QOL) includes two overlapping domains. *Health-related quality of life* specifies elements of daily function and well-being that change as a result of disease or therapeutic intervention. A satisfactory QOL measure in this sense allows researchers to rank different health conditions (and treatments) according to their impact on domains of health, such as mobility, independence in bathing and dressing, sensory acuity, mood, and absence of pain. The more negative the impact in these areas, the greater the quality of life impact of the health condition. *Environment-based quality of life*, by contrast, is not a health impact measure but rather registers the effect of personal resources or environmental factors on daily experience. Environment-related QOL domains include features of the natural and built environment (such as economic resources, housing, air and water quality, community stability, access to the arts and entertainment), as well as personal resources (such as the capacity to form friendships, appreciate nature, or find satisfaction in spiritual or religious life).

Health-related QOL can be assessed as the difference between a population norm and mean value for patient samples, or more directly as a "utility" rating, that is, a numeric rating of how preferred (and thus how much better) one health state is relative to another. One common way to derive utilities for health states is to ask how many years of life people would be willing to give up to live without a health condition or disability.

The psychological analog to quality of life is valuation of life (VOL), the extent to which the person is attached to his or her present life. VOL can be measured by reports of hope, the sense that life has meaning, and continued commitment to personal projects, that is, goal-driven activity. VOL is independent of many factors associated with health-related QOL, such as health state, cognitive capacity, and mental health. VOL was a significant independent correlate of the wish to live under a great range of severe health limitations, including states of mobility impairment and severe pain.

However it is measured, health-related QOL declines with age. This is a central, inescapable consequence of the increased prevalence of chronic disease with greater age and the effects of senescent changes in many physiologic domains. As we have seen, older people adjust their daily lives to accommodate these decrements, and adjustment strategies may reduce the effects of such decrements on health-related QOL. Still, cross-sectional studies show strong declines in health-related QOL with increasing age. VOL may not show so clear a pattern. Here we need to ask when the wish to hasten dying is an expression of discouragement based on depression, and when it is an expression of discouragement based on a judgment that life no longer has intrinsic value because impaired health does not allow meaning, purpose, or desired personal projects.

In contrast to health-related QOL, environment-related QOL may remain high throughout life and may even improve with greater age. With retirement, for example, older people have greater leisure time; and with children gone, houses paid for, and successful investments, they may have greater disposable income as well. As a result, older people have increased opportunities to develop interests and create satisfying environments. These freedoms and opportunities counterbalance declines in health-related QOL and may be responsible for the great resiliency older people show in the face of declining health.

PSYCHOSOCIAL ASPECTS OF THE END OF LIFE

Dying in America has changed markedly in the past quarter century and continues to evolve as the population ages, treatment of chronic disease becomes more effective, and clinicians, policymakers, and the public refine practices related to end-of-life care. "Dying" can be considered a new, emerging stage of the life course: Unlike dying in the past, dying now can be protracted (as with cancer), planned, involve new awareness and self-definition, and require particular developmental psychosocial tasks and challenges. Older adults with life-limiting illness and their caregivers face an increasing array of treatment choices at the end of life as well as an expansion in settings for receiving care, including hospice (which mostly involves in-home services). Half of the deaths in the United States involve hospice care, with the predominant arrangement involving hospice services delivered in homes. However, this care is usually implemented only a few days before death, preventing patients and families from receiving the full benefit of hospice. In 2015, 1.6 million people received hospice care in the United States, and 33% were age 85 and older.

As hospice becomes the predominant model for end-of-life care, it is important to monitor its psychosocial costs and benefits. Use of hospice services is associated with greater satisfaction with quality of dying, better quality of care at the end of life, and less conflict in decisions regarding care and treatment. On the other hand, use of hospice also involves greater investment of time and effort on the part of family members, as evidenced by the higher proportion of caregivers who administer medications and report taking time off from work during end-of-life care compared to caregivers who do not make use of hospice. Despite this greater involvement in end-of-life care, caregivers who make use of hospice do not report a greater prevalence of depressed mood, anxiety, or postdeath persistent grief, suggesting that involvement in hospice buffers the negative impact of greater involvement in end-of-life care.

Aggressive treatment at the end of life remains common among older adults. An analysis of nearly 30,000 Surveillance, Epidemiology, and End Results (SEER) patients aged 65+ (all with a cancer diagnosis), for example, showed an increase in aggressive cancer care near the end of life, as indicated by the proportion starting a new chemotherapy regimen within 30 or 14 days of death; the proportion with more than one emergency department visit, more than 14 days in hospital, or an intensive care unit (ICU) admission in the last month of life; or the proportion of hospice patients with length of stay fewer than 3 days. Nearly 20% continued to receive chemotherapy in the last 2 weeks of life. More generally, analyses of Medicare claims show a decline in the likelihood of dying in an acute care hospital but a high prevalence of 30% for use of the ICU during the last month of life.

Aggressive interventions before death are declining in people with advanced dementia, as shown by decreases in rates of hospitalization, emergency room admission, and feeding tube placement in the last 3 months of life among residents of skilled care facilities. For some therapies with no clear benefit for this population, such as parenteral feeding tube placement, clinicians have recommended that this choice no longer appears as an option in advance care planning documents, such as the Physician Orders for Life-Sustaining Therapies (POLST). The difficulty of preparing for end-of-life treatment is visible as well in recent discussions on the best way to deprescribe medications that are no longer appropriate.

Defining advance care planning is challenging. A consensus statement did not emerge until 2017: "Advance care planning is a process that supports adults at any age or stage of health in understanding and sharing their personal values, life goals, and preferences regarding future medical care. The goal of advance care planning is to help ensure that people receive medical care that is consistent with their values, goals and preferences during serious and chronic illness." In partnership with health care professionals, families face the challenge of limiting inappropriate care for older adults who are dying or who are unlikely to benefit from aggressive hospital interventions because of frailty or multimorbidity. The high risk of death in late ages (8%–10% per year in people age 85+ and over 30% per year for people aged 90+) suggests that clarifying preferences for end-of-life treatment should be a priority for the very old. Yet "the talk," discussion of end-of-life treatment preferences among older people and their families, is often difficult. Older people are more likely to initiate such discussions than their adult children. Adult children may resist such discussions and are often more in favor of aggressive treatment at the end of life than parents. Older adults completing POLST are less likely to receive aggressive treatment at the end of life in nursing homes but not in admissions through the emergency room.

Deaths are challenging for survivors as well. Estimates suggest that 9% to 25% of older people are unable to recover from the emotional challenges of the death of a loved one and develop persistent or complicated grief. *DSM-V* has defined this complex bereavement disorder as a trauma or stress-related condition lasting 6 or 12 months after the death. In older adults, complicated grief is associated with disability, cognitive impairment, and suicidal thinking. New measures are available now to assess persistent grief, such as the Inventory of Complicated Grief, and a number of trials have shown that psychotherapy targeted to complicated grief is more effective than standard grief-focused interpersonal psychotherapy.

A final consideration is distress and regret at the end of life, which may be impairing even if not accompanied by frank depression or anxiety. Such distress often reflects active questioning of the meaning of life, such as whether a person has made good use of a life and left an appropriate legacy. Since patients with a higher sense of meaning experience less distress at the end of life, interventions that bolster meaning may reduce this existential distress and accordingly lower the risk of poor mental health at the end of life. One promising approach to supporting meaning at the end of life is dignity therapy, a short-term psychotherapy that has been shown to improve well-being in people with life-limiting illnesses. In dignity therapy, patients complete a guided elicitation of the major accomplishments of their life, which, after editing and revision, is shown to family and placed in the medical chart as a statement of the value of the life lived.

PSYCHOSOCIAL EVALUATION DURING COMPREHENSIVE GERIATRIC ASSESSMENT

Assessment of psychosocial domains is an integral component of the comprehensive geriatric assessment (CGA) in an older adult. Geriatric syndromes such as malnutrition may be multifactorial in origin, including psychosocial causes like substance abuse, social isolation, and psychiatric disturbances.

A detailed psychosocial history is very important in the evaluation of any geriatric patient. The CGA in older adults includes ascertainment of social support, depressive symptoms, mood, financial concerns, whether one has durable power of attorney for health care, religious and spiritual beliefs, availability of caregivers to support ADLs, home safety, and caregiver burden. It can give information on a need to change the living situation or to consider placement.

Patient-centered goal setting is very important in the management of any patient and this is particularly so in an older adult patient. He or she may prefer quality of life or the ability to attend a major family event over even survival.

CONCLUSION

Psychosocial factors are critical contributors to the health and quality of life of older individuals. We have focused on factors that appear to be most potent for explaining variability in health outcomes using a broad conceptual model that shows how psychosocial factors contribute to behaviors and biological processes linked to illness and quality of life. These effects do not occur in a vacuum but rather are set within the larger social and cultural contexts in which people live. The life course perspective shows how the experience of aging depends on cultural factors, such as the conceptualization of the lifespan, as well as biologically driven developmental changes in social and affective experience. A significant advance of the last decades is research showing how psychosocial factors get "under the skin" to affect the physiology and functioning of the organism, and hence health and quality of life. Continued advances in mind-body science along these lines will enhance our understanding of the relationships between biology, psychology, and social experience and will provide new opportunities for intervention.

A second theme of this chapter is the remarkable resilience of older individuals. Despite significant declines in multiple functional domains in late life, most older individuals adapt well to the challenges they face and maintain high quality of life. Depression and dissatisfaction with life do not come in late life, but earlier, in mid-life. While psychosocial health is clearly affected by disability, it is remarkable that majorities of older people with substantial disability report high levels of positive affect and involvement in daily life. This resilience reflects finely tuned adaptive mechanisms that maximize the ability to cope with major life challenges. Common old-age transitions such as retirement, widowhood, health decline, and caregiving, are challenging; but older people are able to navigate these changes through selection, optimization, and compensation to maximize function and well-being. Consistent with the greater socioemotional selectivity of old age, the landscape of affective and social experience changes and may look narrow to younger people; but the greater reports of satisfaction and happiness typical of old age suggest that these processes help buffer more challenging features of aging.

Finally, a third theme is the strong association between social engagement and well-being. Lack of support (social isolation and loneliness) has a negative effect, and social engagement (volunteering, lifelong learning, and involvement in intergenerational programs) has a positive effect. Beyond these social factors, many kinds of intervention support psychological health. For example, the aging services network is important in promoting engagement across diverse domains, with clear benefit. Social environments that promote aging in place, involvement of older adults in their care and in health decision making, and supporting family caregivers who provide end-of-life care all offer benefits and show it is possible to promote engagement across multiple levels and domains. New models of engagement, such as school-based volunteering and intergenerational programs, suggest that engaging older adults may be good for older adults as well as other age groups. This kind of programming will likely become more important as increasingly larger cohorts of older people reach old age in better health.

FURTHER READING

Albert SM, Freedman VA. *Public Health and Aging: Maximizing Function and Well-Being.* New York, NY: Springer Publishing Company; 2010.

Albert SM, Logsdon RG, eds. *Assessing Quality of Life in Alzheimer's Disease.* New York, NY: Springer Publishing Company; 2000.

Aldwin CM, Park CL, Spiro AS III, eds. *Handbook of Health Psychology and Aging.* New York, NY: Guilford Press; 2007.

Anderson ND, Damianakis T, Kröger E, et al. The benefits associated with volunteering among seniors: a critical review and recommendations for future research. *Psychol Bull.* 2014;140(6):1505–1533.

Carstensen LL, Mikels JA, Mather M. Aging and the intersection of cognition, motivation and emotion. In: Birren J, Schaie KW, eds. *Handbook of the Psychology of Aging.* 6th ed. San Diego, CA: Academic Press; 2006.

Chochinov HM, Kristjanson LJ, Breitbart W, et al. Effect of dignity therapy on distress and end-of-life experience in terminally ill patients: a randomised controlled trial. *Lancet Oncol.* 2011;12(8):753–762.

Cohen S. Social relationships and health. *Am Psychol.* 2004;59:676–684.

Cohen S, Pressman SD. Positive affect and health. *Curr Dir Psychol Sci.* 2006;15(3):122–125.

Epel E, Burke HM, Adler N, Wolkowitz O, Sidney S, Seeman T. Socio-economic status and the anabolic/catabolic neuroendocrine balance. *Ann Behav Med.* 2006;31:50–80.

Felix C, Rosano C, Zhu X, Flatt JD, Rosso AL. Greater social engagement and greater gray matter microstructural integrity in brain regions relevant to dementia. *J Gerontol B Psychol Sci Soc Sci.* 2021;76(6):1027–1035.

Fried LP, Carlson MC, Freedman M, et al. A social model for health promotion for an aging population:

initial evidence on the Experience Corps model. *J Urban Health*. 2004;81(1):64–78.

Gans D. The nexus of informal and formal elder care. *J Comp Fam Stud*. 2013;44(4):415–424.

Gans D, Silverstein M, Lowenstein A. Do religious children care more and provide more care to older parents? A study of filial norms and behavior across five nations. Response to Comment. *J Comp Fam Stud*. 2010;41(4):632–637.

Hawkley LC, Cacioppo JT. Loneliness matters: a theoretical and empirical review of consequences and mechanisms. *Ann Behav Med*. 2010;40:218–227.

Lawton MP, DeVoe MR, Parmelee P. Relationship of events and affect in the daily life of an elderly population. *Psychol Aging*. 1995;10(3):469–477.

Lawton MP, Kleban MH, Dean J. Affect and age: cross-sectional comparisons of structure and prevalence. *Psychol Aging*. 1993;8(2):165–175.

Lawton MP, Moss M, Hoffman C, Grant R, Ten Have T, Kleban MH. Health, valuation of life, and the wish to live. *Gerontologist*. 1999;39:406–416.

Lawton MP, Moss MS, Winter L, Hoffman C. Motivation in later life: personal projects and well-being. *Psychol Aging*. 2002;17(4):539–547.

Levine C, ed. *Family Caregivers on the Job: Moving Beyond ADLs and IADLs*. New York, NY: United Hospital Fund; 2004.

Seaman JB, Bear TM, Documet PI, Sereika SM, Albert SM. Hospice and family involvement with end-of-life care: results from a population-based survey. *Am J Hosp Palliat Care*. 2016;33(2):130–135.

Shear K, Frank E, Houck PR, Reynolds CF III. Treatment of complicated grief: a randomized trial. *JAMA*. 2005;293(21):2601–2608.

Sudore RL, Lum HD, You JJ, et al. Defining advance care planning for adults: a consensus definition from a multidisciplinary Delphi panel. *J Pain Symptom Manage*. 2017;53(5):821–832.

Wang M. Profiling retirees in the retirement transition and adjustment process: examining the longitudinal change patterns of retirees' psychological well-being. *J Appl Psychol*. 2007;92:455–474.

World Health Organization. *Global Age-Friendly Cities: A Guide*. Geneva, Switzerland: WHO Press; 2007. http://www.who.int/ageing/publications/Global_age_friendly_cities_Guide_English.pdf. Accessed February 3, 2021.

Chapter 5

Sex Differences in Health and Longevity

Steven N. Austad

THE ROBUSTNESS OF SEX DIFFERENCES IN LONGEVITY

Women live longer than men in every country and in every historical epoch for which reliable information exists. This fact is documented in the Human Mortality Database (www.mortality.org), which compiles historical demographic information from 41 countries over periods for which data are particularly dependable. Accordingly, the length of these records varies. Sweden has the longest period of reliable birth and death records of any country. Beginning in 1751 these records are moderately reliable, and they are very reliable from 1860 to the present day. Sweden's life expectancy over this 250+-year period dipped as low as 18 years during periods of famine or pestilence and has risen as high as today's 83 years. However, in each and every year, regardless of overall life expectancy, women have outlived men (**Figure 5-1**). The same is true for each of the 41 countries in the Human Mortality Database for every year on record!

Understanding Life Expectancy

To interpret sex differences in longevity—call it the "life expectancy gender gap"—it is useful to understand the meaning of two demographic parameters. The first of these is life expectancy itself. Life expectancy, unlike its name suggests, does not measure the expectation of future life, which is by its nature not really knowable. Life expectancy, as typically used in describing human longevity, measures past life. That is, as most commonly reported, life expectancy is equivalent to the average age of death of all individuals who died during a specific period—usually 1 year. So life expectancy in the United States in 2017—76 years for men, 81 years for women—is equivalent to the average age of all people who died during 2017. More technically, such a measure is called the *period* life expectancy *at birth* because it is the average of deaths at any age from birth during a defined *period*. Unless otherwise specified, life expectancies reported in this chapter (as they are in the literature generally) will be period life expectancies at birth. Life expectancy can be calculated for any other age as well. Life expectancy at age 50, for instance, is the average age of death of those who survived for at least 50 years. Such a measure is useful for eliminating the impact of infant

Learning Objectives

- Understand the demographic metrics that define the female longevity advantage.
- Identify disease patterns that differentially affect men and women.
- Describe the health impacts of hormone transitions and replacement therapies for men and women.

Key Clinical Points

1. Women live longer than men in every country and in every historical epoch for which reliable information exists.
2. Women appear more resistant than men to multiple fatal diseases, acquiring them at lower rates and/or later in life.
3. Despite their broad survival advantage, women are more likely to suffer from physical ailments than men later in life.

mortality or other early-life events such as military combat, therefore providing better comparisons on the health of older populations. Life expectancy from age 50, as at birth, uniformly favors women not only in Sweden (**Figure 5-1B**) but in all other countries and at all times recorded in the Human Mortality Database.

Prior to the middle of the twentieth century, most deaths worldwide occurred in infancy. Consequently life expectancy at birth was not particularly informative about the health of the older population. For example, in 1773, the year in which Swedish life expectancy at birth fell dramatically to 18 years (**Figure 5-1A**), about half of all deaths occurred before age 5. Most adults died in their 40s and 50s, however. Thus the 18-year life expectancy at birth would be highly misleading if used as an indicator of typical ages of adult deaths. Life expectancy at age 50 is considerably more informative about survival of older adults and shows that in the same year, there was a relatively small life expectancy difference (1 year) between men and women. However, as

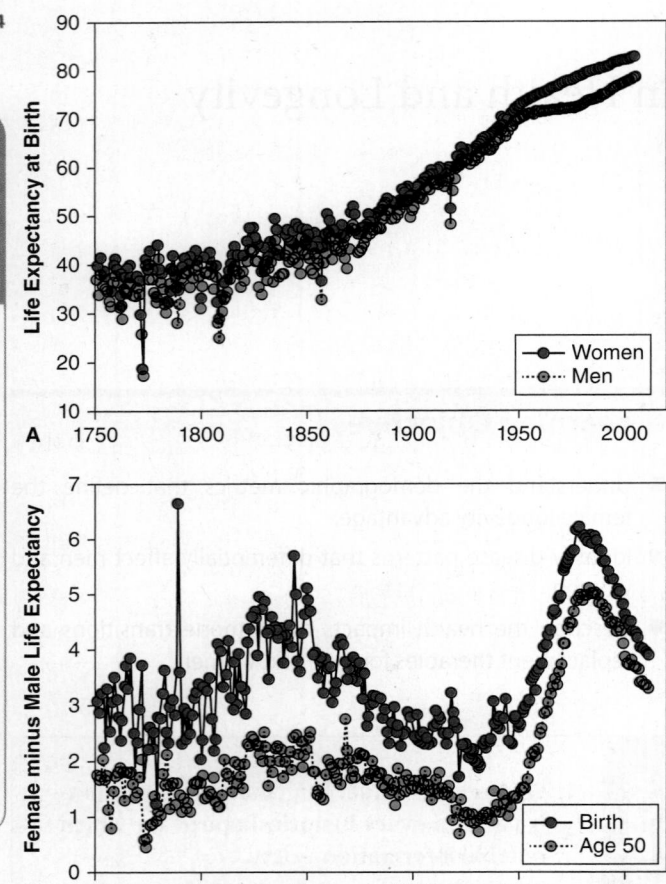

FIGURE 5-1. Demographic data from Sweden from 1751 to the present. **A.** Male and female life expectancies at birth show a steady increase after 1800 with occasional brief decreases due to war, famine, or infectious disease. **B.** Sex difference (female minus male) in life expectancy at birth and at age 50 is always positive, indicating greater female survival in all years for both ages. (Reproduced with permission from Human Demographic Database.)

infant and early-life mortality in developed countries has plummeted in recent decades (only 5% or fewer of deaths now occur before age 50 in most industrialized countries), life expectancy—even life expectancy at birth—has become an increasingly useful measure of health in old age because virtually all deaths occur in older adult age groups.

Note that these "period" life expectancies combine deaths from people who were born at different times. That is, a 50-year-old who died in 2010 would have lived through a considerably different health environment than a 90-year-old who died in the same year. For instance, antibiotics and vaccinations against a number of common infectious diseases did not become widely available until the latter half of the twentieth century, so people born earlier in the century survived threats to health not faced by later generations. Sometimes it is useful to compare survival of people who were *born* during the same period—thus lived in similar health environments from birth—rather than

who *died* during the same period. Life expectancy of people born during the same period is called *cohort* life expectancy. Cohort life expectancy can be dramatically different from period life expectancy because it records deaths that occur after—often many decades after—rather than during the eponymous year. Compared to the 18-year period life expectancy in Sweden in 1773, cohort life expectancy was 39 years for women, 36 years for men, and at age 50 it was 21 years for women, 19 years for men. A disadvantage of cohort life expectancy is that it can only be calculated precisely when all the people born at a certain time have died. Therefore, it can only tell us about the relatively distant past. Cohort life expectancies can also fluctuate wildly with events like wars or epidemics where people of a certain age are particularly prone to die. French men from the 1895 birth cohort, for instance, had a 16-year life expectancy disadvantage compared to women, due to the massive war casualties among 19- to 24-year-old men during World War I. Regardless of how it is calculated, life expectancy of women always exceeds that of men wherever records are reliable. The gender gap in life expectancy may be one of the most robust features of human biology known.

The accumulated effects of women's lifelong survival advantage means that with advancing age there is a progressive excess of women compared to men. Again, using Sweden with its precise, historical birth and death records as an example, there are currently 105 women born per 100 men. By age 80, there are roughly 150 women per 100 surviving men, by age 90 there are 200 women per 100 men, and by age 100 there are nearly 350 women per 100 men. The Gerontology Research Group (https://gerontology.wikia.org/wiki/Oldest_Validated_supercentenarians_All-Time) is a global e-group of researchers in gerontology that tracks and seeks to validate reports of supercentenarians (age 110 or older). According to their records, about 95% of supercentenarians are women.

Impact of Age-Specific Mortality on the Gender Gap in Longevity

Life expectancy differences are the product of survival differences over the life course. A reasonable question is whether women survive better than men at all ages or whether their survival advantage is confined to certain periods of life. Using the United States as an example, during a period in which the gender gap in life expectancy was particularly small (the year 1900 when the gap was 2.6 years), and a period during which it was larger (the year 2000 when it was 5.4 years), several patterns appear (**Figure 5-2**). First, age-specific mortality, the probability of dying in a specific year, drops sharply from birth to age 10 for both sexes during both historical periods, then climbs at varying rates thereafter. Second, from age 35 on, that climb is log-linear, the so-called Gompertz mortality pattern—a pattern of aging in which mortality accelerates at a constant rate. From age 50, mortality rate doubling, which is determined by the slope of the line, is virtually the same—about

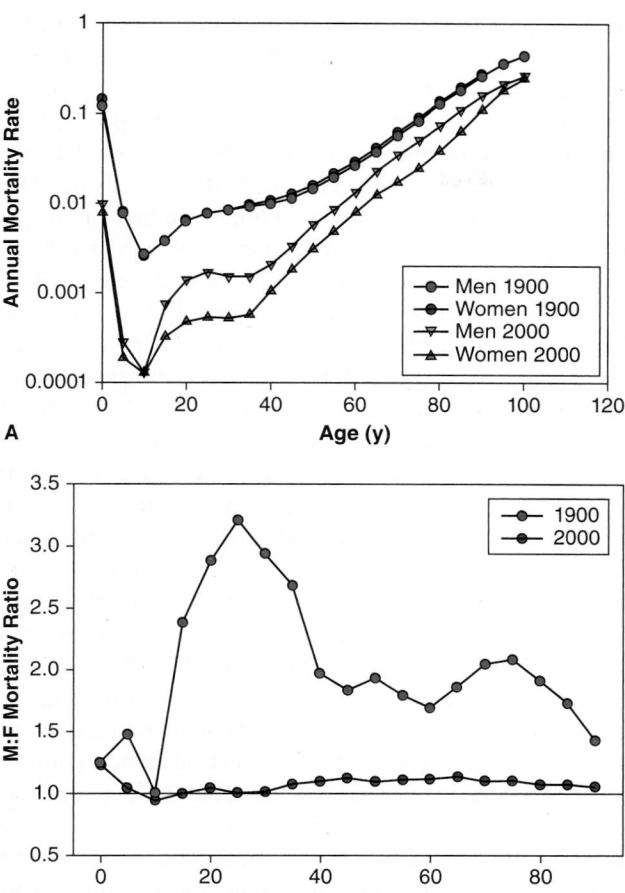

FIGURE 5-2. A. Age-specific mortality in men and women in the United States in the years 1900 and 2000. Note the logarithmic scale for mortality. In 1900, life expectancy at birth in the United States was 46 years for men and 49 years for women; in 2000, the analogous numbers were 74 years for men and 79 years for women. **B.** Ratio of male-to-female age-specific mortality. The reference line at 1 marks where male and female mortality is equivalent. (Reproduced with permission from US Social Security Administration, 2005.)

around 50 years, although in both these cases female mortality slightly exceeded male mortality through the teenage years. It is apparent that as mortality fell and life expectancy increased throughout the twentieth century, women benefited more than men. In particular, men died at much higher rates than women at all ages from age 20 onward. The huge peak in mortality difference shown in **Figure 5-2B** through the 20s and 30s is as a result of excess male deaths from accidents, homicides, and suicides. This pattern is seen in many, but not all countries. In current Japan, for instance, although male mortality is roughly double that of females through their 20s and 30s, the largest mortality differences are at ages 60 to 80.

Special attention should be paid to lower female than male mortality in the first years of life. A gender gap favoring females in survival from birth to 1 year appears to be as universal as greater female life expectancy, being found in every year of every country in the Human Mortality Database. Given that female babies less than 1 year are unlikely to receive better care than male babies, particularly in the distant past, this survival difference likely reflects an important biological difference between the sexes. The gender gap in survival even extends to prematurely born infants. Neonatologists consistently report that response to therapy and survival among prematurely born infants also favors female over male babies. Thus females appear better designed for survival than males perinatally and even prenatally.

A similar pattern of increasing mortality differences between the sexes over the course of the twentieth century has also been observed in analyses of cohort mortality. An examination of birth *cohorts* from 1800 to 1935 across 13 developed countries found that the gender gap in adult (ages 40–90) mortality rates widened dramatically among those born in the late nineteenth and early twentieth centuries (thus typically dying in the latter half of the twentieth century). This widening gap—termed excess male mortality by the authors—was particularly noticeable at ages 50 to 70 years. The causes for these changes are examined below.

Temporal Trends in the Gender Gap

There is considerable variability in the magnitude of the sex difference in life expectancy across time and countries. It may be difficult to avoid biological explanations for the seemingly universal advantage that women have over men in terms of life expectancy. However, the magnitude of the gender difference above a certain irreducible biological minimum is likely to be affected by cultural, environmental, and behavioral factors. Investigation into this variation might provide insight into how some of these factors affect health. For instance, in Sweden between 1750 and about 1950, variability in the gender gap is considerably more pronounced in life expectancy at birth than at age 50 (see **Figure 5-1B**), indicating that the magnitude of the gap was largely driven by sex differences in survival in early and midlife. However, since the middle of the twentieth

8 years—in the year 2000 as it was in 1900. It is just that mortality declined by a nearly equivalent amount at all ages. Finally, although survival was markedly improved at all ages, the largest gains over this 100-year time span were those prior to age 50. Women clearly gained significantly more than men.

The logarithmic scale of **Figure 5-2A** makes it difficult to distinguish sex differences in mortality pattern particularly in 1900 where the differences were small, so the ratio of male-to-female mortality is shown in **Figure 5-2B**. This analysis shows that in 1900 when overall mortality was high, women survived better during the first years of life, there was little sex difference during childhood, adolescence, and the early reproductive years, then women gained a small but consistent survival advantage throughout the rest of life. Similar patterns are seen in 1900 Sweden and 1947 Japan which also had life expectancies of century when early-life deaths became a much smaller contributor to life expectancy calculations, the gap has changed in parallel fashion whether measured from birth or from age 50. During this time a striking pattern has emerged. Between 1950 and about 1980, the gender gap rose from near its lowest magnitude to its highest sustained level, then plummeted at its most rapid historical level to its current 3.5-year difference. Such a clear pattern demands explanation.

First, though, it should be pointed out that **Figure 5-1B** is misleading in one sense. It depicts the gender gap as absolute difference in number of years. Between 1750 and 1950, the period during which the differences appear consistently lower than they became later on, Swedish life expectancy climbed from about 40 years to more than 70 years. An absolute difference of 3 years in life expectancy is arguably more meaningful if overall life expectancy is 40 years rather than 70 years. If the difference is expressed as a percentage of male life expectancy (**Figure 5-3A**), a somewhat different picture emerges. The gender gap was actually larger for

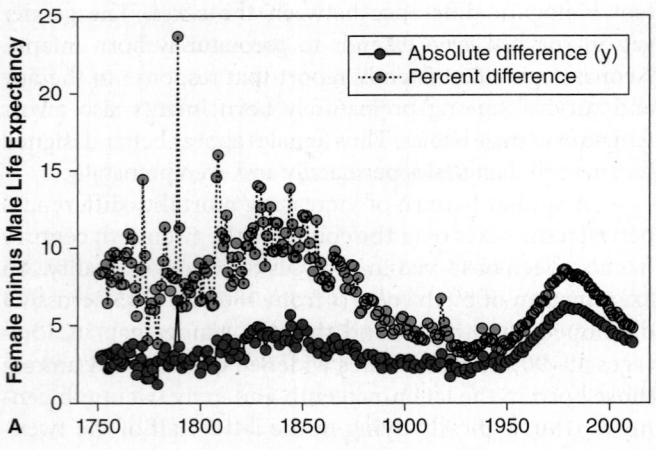

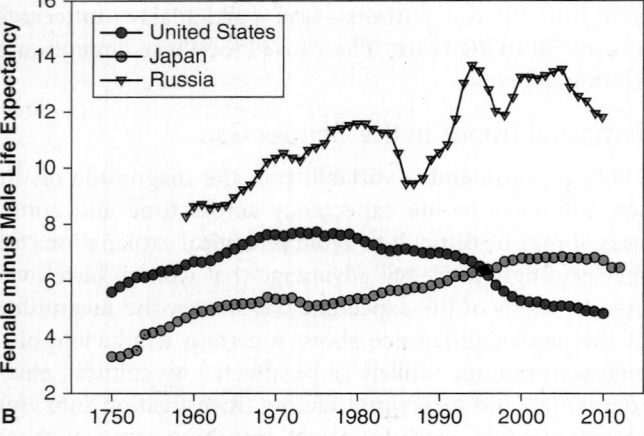

FIGURE 5-3. Gender gap in life expectancy. **A.** Sweden since 1751 expressed in absolute difference versus as a percentage of male life expectancy. **B.** Absolute differences in three countries. Note that when Japan's difference was little more than 3 years (early 1950s), overall life expectancy in Japan was still low by modern standards (60–63 years).

the most part prior to 1850, then declined until the 1930s after which it rose abruptly, although never reaching earlier levels, and then it declined rapidly.

Before discussing possible reasons for this pattern, it might be revealing to look at patterns in several other representative countries (**Figure 5-3B**). For some time countries of the former Soviet Union have had the world's largest gender gap in life expectancy. In Russia that difference now approaches 12 years. This large difference is not due to exceptionally long-lived women, but to exceptionally short-lived men. Russian women are in fact among the shortest-lived women in the industrialized world—their current life expectancy of 77 years is only marginally higher than it was in the 1960s. But health and longevity of Russian men is abysmal. Their life expectancy of 65 years is a consequence of poor diet, poor sanitation, a virtual absence of preventative medical care, and dreadful health habits. As a result, 25% of Russian men die by age 55 compared with less than 10% of women. To place this statistic in an international perspective, only 5% of Swedish or Japanese men die by age 55. The main factors driving the Russian gender gap in life expectancy are smoking and alcoholism. Russian men have traditionally had among the highest smoking prevalence in the world. Fluctuations in the life expectancy gap has also marched in lock step with the availability of vodka. Specifically, in 1985 vodka production was drastically cut and vodka was not allowed to be sold before lunch-time. The gender gap abruptly shrunk as men began living longer. When alcohol availability was later liberalized, the gap expanded again just as abruptly. Since 2006 when new restrictions were implemented, the gap has again begun to shrink.

Has there been a consistent pattern of change in the gender gap as overall life expectancy has rocketed upward in most industrialized countries in recent decades? Again using Sweden as an example, the life expectancy gap both at birth and at age 50 rose dramatically after World War II, but has fallen steadily since the 1980s (see **Figure 5-1B**). This is the most common pattern among high-income countries. Similar patterns of rapid increase in the gender gap after World War II, followed by a rapid decrease beginning in the 1980s or 1990s and continuing to the present have been seen in the United States, Canada, Australia, Iceland, and most European countries. The life expectancy gender gap is not declining everywhere, however. In Japan, where life expectancy at birth has grown explosively—nearly 5 years per decade—since the end of World War II, the sex difference also steadily increased until the 2000s where it appears to have stabilized at about 7.5 years (see **Figure 5-3B**).

The major reason for these various patterns—at least after World War II when causes of death were more reliably recorded—appears to be largely the delayed impact of historical smoking habits. In the United States and most of Europe women's deaths from lung cancer and respiratory diseases have declined slowly if at all, compared to a relatively rapid decline among men. Smoking of course adversely affects multiple aspects of health in addition to its effects on the lungs, but lung cancer and respiratory diseases serve as convenient indicators of smoking's impact on general health. As noted previously, women in most western countries took up smoking in large numbers more recently than men and have been slower to stop. In Sweden, smoking is now more prevalent among women than men. An example of the delayed effect of smoking can be seen in data from the United States (**Figure 5-4**). As with smoking itself, deaths due to respiratory diseases and lung cancer (now the number one cause of cancer deaths in women) peaked among women somewhat later and have so far declined more slowly than among men. In Japan where the gender gap in life expectancy has not closed appreciably, smoking prevalence among women has always been—and continues to be—very low compared with men. Importantly, both history and biology suggest that despite the recent contraction of the gender gap in life expectancy across most high-income countries, there is likely to be an irreducible floor to the gap of probably about 3 to 4 years.

The gender gap is now playing a role in the US declining rank in life expectancy among countries internationally: from 12th in the world in 1950, sexes combined, to 39th for women and 40th for men in 2010—near the bottom of all industrialized countries. The US National Research Council investigated the reasons for this pattern and concluded that American women began smoking in large numbers earlier and more intensively than women in Europe and Japan. Damage from smoking was estimated to account for nearly four-fifths of the sluggish improvement in US women's life expectancy relative to Europe and Japan. As US women also began reducing smoking earlier than women in many other high-income countries, it is expected that

their life expectancy rank may begin to rise over the next several decades.

DO WOMEN AGE MORE SLOWLY THAN MEN?

Does the universal difference in life expectancy between men and women suggest that men age more rapidly than women? This is not an easy question to answer as it requires defining aging—a task that defies simplicity.

Demographic Evidence

One definition often favored by demographers is that aging in a population can be measured by the rate of increase in age-specific mortality. By this definition, men and women age at surprisingly similar rates (see **Figure 5-2A**). Note in the figure that in the United States whether one considers data from 1900 when life expectancy was 46 years and 49 years for men and women, respectively, or data from 2000 when life expectancy reached 74 years for men and 79 years for women, age-specific mortality increases from age 40 in almost perfectly parallel fashion in the two sexes. Women simply die at lower rates throughout later life. The same general pattern is seen in almost all countries with reliable death statistics. So at least by this metric, women do not age more slowly than men. They are simply better designed for survival regardless of age.

Causes of Death

Another way to define relative aging rates might be to compare the ages at which they get major diseases of later life. Do women tend to die of the same diseases as men, they just get them later? If so, then plausibly women age more slowly than men. Alternatively, maybe women are more resistant than men to only one or a few major causes of death such as cardiovascular diseases and stroke; except for that difference, perhaps they would age at the same rate as men. This latter hypothesis seems unlikely given that the major causes of death have changed historically, while women have always lived longer. It is also not supported by available evidence. Men die at higher rates than women from a broad swathe of diseases with one particularly interesting exception (**Table 5-1**).

Comparing causes of death between the sexes and even within a sex over time requires some careful thinking. One common metric of comparison is the simple percentage of deaths caused by a disease. Using this metric, some causes of death have decreased over the past 50 years (eg, heart disease, stroke) while others have increased (eg, cancer, diabetes). This metric can be seriously misleading though. For instance, in 2017 roughly 24% of all men's deaths in the United States were due to heart diseases, whereas for women the analogous figure was about 22%. Thus, at first glance heart disease seems to be roughly an equivalent health problem for men and women. Similarly, cancer causes a higher percentage of deaths today (23%)

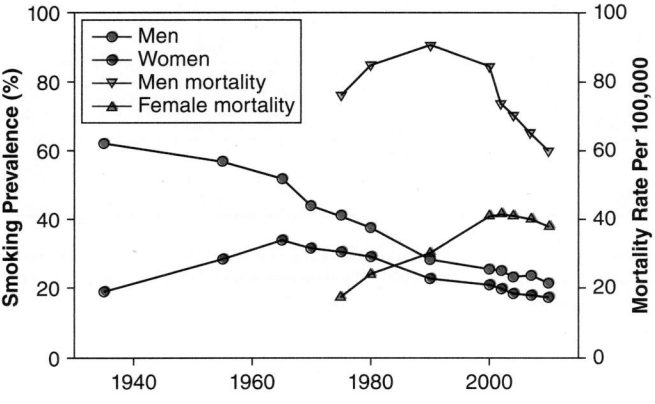

FIGURE 5-4. Historical changes in smoking prevalence and mortality rate from lung and bronchial cancer in the United States. Note that smoking among women reached its peak later and declined more slowly than among men and lung cancer death rates followed suit with a delay of several decades. (Reproduced with permission from United States Centers for Disease Control and Prevention and National Cancer Institute SEER Database.)

TABLE 5-1 ■ SEX DIFFERENCES IN TOP CAUSES OF DEATHS IN THE UNITED STATES OVER THE 50-YEAR PERIOD BETWEEN 1960 AND 2017

DISEASES	1960		2017	
GENDER (LIFE EXPECTANCY)	MEN (67)	WOMEN (73)	MEN (76)	WOMEN (81)
Heart disease (1)				
Percent of all deaths	40	37	24	22
Age-adjusted rate	376	206	209	130
Age-adjusted ratio (male to female)	**1.8**		**1.6**	
All cancers (2)				
Percent of all deaths	15	17	21	23
Age-adjusted rate	143	111	181	131
Age-adjusted ratio	**1.3**		**1.4**	
Chronic lower respiratory disease (3)				
Percent of all deaths	0.7	0.4	5.2	6.2
Age-adjusted rate	6.8	4.8	45	38
Age-adjusted ratio	**1.4**		**1.2**	
Stroke (4)				
Percent of all deaths	9.5	14	4.3	6.2
Age-adjusted rate	85	75	38	37
Age-adjusted ratio	**1.1**		**1.0**	
Alzheimer disease (6)				
Percent of all deaths	0.01	0.04	2.6	6.1
Age-adjusted rate	0.2[a]	0.3[a]	25	35
Age-adjusted ratio	**0.7[a]**		**0.7**	
Diabetes mellitus (7)				
Percent of all deaths	1.2	2.4	3.2	2.7
Age-adjusted rate	12	15	27	17
Age-adjusted ratio	**0.8**		**1.6**	
Chronic kidney diseases (8)				
Percent of all deaths	1.2	1.3	1.8	1.8
Age-adjusted rate	6.8	4.8	19	13
Age-adjusted ratio	**1.4**		**1.4**	
Influenza and pneumonia (9)				
Percent of all deaths	3.9	3.9	1.8	2.1
Age-adjusted rate	35	22	17	13
Age-adjusted ratio	**1.6**		**1.3**	

[a]Standardized to 100,000 population, not age-adjusted rates.
Numbers in parentheses represent rank in percent of total deaths in 2017. Causes among top 10 not listed are unintentional accidents (#5) and suicides (#10), both heavily male-biased. The 1960 age-adjustment used the 1940 US standard population, whereas the 2017 adjustment used a different—year 2000—standard population. Therefore, comparisons of age-adjusted values cannot meaningfully be made across years.
Data from US National Vital Statistics Reports.

than it did 57 years ago (16%). Does this mean that we are getting progressively worse at preventing and treating cancer?

Obviously not. The occurrence of heart disease or cancer, like 9 of the 10 top causes of death (excluding only cause #10—suicide) in the United States today, accelerates with age. Today, we live roughly 9 years longer than we did in 1960, sexes combined. Thus, we are more frequently succumbing to cancer today compared with 50 years ago simply because we are not dying of other things first. We are also *less* frequently succumbing to heart diseases *despite* not dying of other things first *and despite* living longer. This is truly one of the signature accomplishments of modern medicine.

A critical limitation of using percent of deaths caused by specific diseases is that it masks information on the ages at which death occurs. Presumably, heart disease or cancer should be considered a more serious health problem if it kills earlier in life rather than later. In addition, delaying the onset or progression of these diseases should be considered a sign of medical progress. There is a meaningful health difference in other words between dying of a heart attack at age 50 versus age 80.

The confounding impact of age in the interpretation of health trends can be removed by using *age-adjusted mortality rate*. This metric gives the relative probability of dying from a disease while controlling for age. If the percent of deaths caused by a particular disease is similar, but the age-adjusted rate is lower for women than men, it indicates that women are contracting the disease later in life or are surviving longer with the disease. For instance, there is currently minimal difference between sexes in percent of deaths due to heart disease (24% for men, 22% for women), but a major difference in the age-adjusted rate (209 vs 130 per 100,000 for men vs women, respectively), indicating that women typically have heart diseases later in life or are better at surviving them. The former appears to be true. For example, US women have their first heart attack 8 years later than men on average, but are in fact *less* likely to survive (probably because they are 8 years older when it occurs).

Sex-specific profiles of deaths can be compared as they were reported over a 57-year interval using the 1960 and 2017 US Vital Statistics Reports (see **Table 5-1**). Because the age-adjustment for 1960 was calculated based on a different standard population than in 2017, comparison of age-adjusted rates between years is not meaningful. Age-adjustment in this case is useful for making comparisons within years. However, the ratio of male-to-female age-adjusted rates does allow comparison of gender bias in death rates across years.

Note that across this 57-year time interval, life expectancy increased by 9.5 years for men, but only 7.8 years for women. Also note the dramatic reduction in percent deaths due to heart diseases, stroke, and respiratory infections. As might be expected with the much older population in 2017, percentage of total deaths from a range of diseases of aging such as cancers, chronic lower respiratory disease, diabetes, chronic kidney disease, and especially Alzheimer disease (AD) increased fairly dramatically as well.

In 1960, males died at higher age-adjusted rates for 8 of the top 10 causes of death. Males died at 80% higher rates from heart diseases and 60% higher rates from influenza and pneumonia. Not shown in the table for 1960 are accidents, cirrhosis of the liver, and tuberculosis, all of which were male-biased as well (male/female age-adjusted ratios: 1.3, 2.1, and 2.8, respectively). The comparative female resistance to dying of infectious diseases such as pneumonia, influenza, and tuberculosis is not specific to the United States. In Japan in 1960, men

died of tuberculosis at twice the age-adjusted rate of women. Such resistance in fact may help explain the historical female survival advantage. In 1900 and presumably earlier, pneumonia/influenza was the leading cause of death, followed closely by tuberculosis. Not shown for 2017 are deaths from accidents, cause #5 (age-adjusted sex ratio: 2.0), and cause #10, suicides (age-adjusted sex ratio: 1.4). By 2017, 9 of the 10 top causes of death were male-biased, although only slightly so for stroke. Thus across a span of 50 years despite better overall improvement in health and survival among men than women, men still died at higher age-adjusted rates from virtually all of the top causes of death.

Note that the same pattern holds true for COVID-19. When the data are in from 2020 and 2021, COVID-19 will rank among the top causes of death. In fact from mid-November 2020 to the current time (February 2021), COVID-19 killed roughly twice as many Americans as either of the previous top two causes of death, heart disease and cancer. As with influenza and pneumonia, men died at higher rates than women from this emerging disease.

The trend for men to die at greater age-adjusted rates from a diversity of causes is by no means unique to the United States. Among the 28 countries of the European Union, in which life expectancy ranges from 74 years (Latvia, Lithuania) to 83 years (Iceland), men die at higher age-adjusted rates than women of nearly every top cause of death as well. The same is true in Japan, the country with the highest life expectancy in the world.

In sum, as women do seem to contract multiple diseases of aging (fatal diseases anyway) later in life than men, it is at least arguable that despite the demographic evidence, women age more slowly than men.

It is important to note the source and limitations of the US national statistics as presented in **Table 5-1**. These data are compiled from causes of death listed on US Standard Death Certificates filled out by a physician, medical examiner, or coroner at the time of death. Determining cause of death is an inexact process and frequently opens to interpretation even with a complete autopsy; complete autopsies are infrequently done today. Even in cases where the cause of death would be clear upon autopsy, for example myocardial infarction, studies have found that death certificates frequently misattribute the cause. This is particularly an issue for chronic diseases.

Diabetes mellitus is one chronic disease for which death reporting may be problematic. In the United States, diabetes deaths were female-biased by 25% in 1960 but male-biased by 57% in 2017. In fact, over the 57-year period between these two reports, there has been a steady gradual shift from female-to-male bias. (Other studies both from the United States and Europe reported female bias in deaths from diabetes in the first half of the twentieth century as well.) Now, however, similar male biases to those found in the United States are reported across the European Union as well as in Japan. Changing diagnostic criteria for diabetes and variable death certificate reporting are likely contributors to these differences.

Women and dementia An outlier in the pattern of virtually complete female dominance in resistance to lethal disease appears to be AD, which according to 2017 US national statistics is our sixth leading cause of death and which kills women at substantially higher rates than men whether raw percentages or age-adjusted rates are used (see **Table 5-1**). That is, US women currently die more than twice as often as men from AD *both* because they live longer *and* because they are generally more susceptible. In comparing the 2017 to the 1960 data in **Table 5-1**, the percentage of total deaths reported due to AD (called senile psychosis in 1960) increased more than 250-fold for men and more than 150-fold for women over this 57-year period. As diagnostic criteria for AD were not well established in 1960, AD was dramatically underdiagnosed then and so very few deaths were attributed to AD. Thus, the 1960 data are not interpretable. A more accurate portrayal of what AD means at present on American death certificates is probably "AD and other dementias," which is how causes of death are categorized in the United Kingdom. For UK women, AD and other dementias have now surpassed heart disease as the number one cause of death, whereas for men it is now number five.

The current female bias in US deaths from AD is consistent with a large body of data from the rest of the developed world. In Japan and across Europe, the age-adjusted sex ratio of AD deaths is similar to the United States. **Figure 5-5**, which summarizes 31 independent studies from across Europe, shows the relative prevalence of AD as it accelerates with age in each gender. Thus, as populations become older, AD will likely become more and more female-biased.

Sex hormones, health, and disease The pattern of women's increased susceptibility to dementias in addition to their consistently increased resistance to most other fatal diseases relative to men, provokes speculation about the role of sex hormones in health and disease. This has been a fraught topic in aging research at least since the late nineteenth century when French-American physiologist Charles-Édouard Brown-Séquard began injecting himself with a cocktail of macerated dog and guinea pig testicles and subsequently proclaimed that he was rejuvenated in both mind and body.

Sex hormones such as testosterone, estrogens, and progestins decline with age in both sexes, although male testosterone decline is considerably more gradual than the relatively abrupt change across the menopausal transition in women. That restoring these hormones to youthful levels will have a generalized rejuvenating effect is a plausible hypothesis. Hormone replacement for women is reviewed in Chapter 36. Data from observational epidemiology and laboratory rodent studies suggested that replacing female hormones might lead to multiple health benefits. However, such hormonal therapy does not enhance longevity and has mixed effects on various age-related diseases. Hormone replacement for men is reviewed in Chapter 97. It has limited benefits on age-related conditions in normal older men.

The reverse is also plausible. That is, one could equally reasonably speculate that declining hormone levels with age are an adaptive response to reduce hormonally-induced adverse health effects with increasing age. Returning hormones to youthful levels, according to this hypothesis, may actually cause harm. Indeed, some historical information from the complete removal of gonadal hormones is provocative. For instance, a review of longevity records for 81 eunuchs employed as guards or servants of the royal court of Korea during the seventeenth and eighteenth centuries found that eunuchs lived on average 20 years longer than intact men of similar rank and status—a result notable mainly for the magnitude of the difference. These findings echo a previous study comparing nearly 300 castrated men with more than 700 intact controls who lived in the same institution for the intellectually disabled in the United States in the early twentieth century. This study found not only a large (> 13-year) difference in life expectancy favoring the castrated men but also a bigger survival advantage the earlier-in-life surgery was performed. Whether these studies have any relevance to men living with modern hygiene, diets, and medical monitoring is of course not clear.

HEALTH DISPARITIES AND GENDER

The United States has been particularly well studied regarding how gender interacts with nonbiological determinants of health such as income, education, race, health habits, or access to medical care to influence longevity. This work has been motivated by a desire to understand why despite spending far more on health care than any other country, US life expectancy—especially among women—increasingly lags behind most other high-income countries.

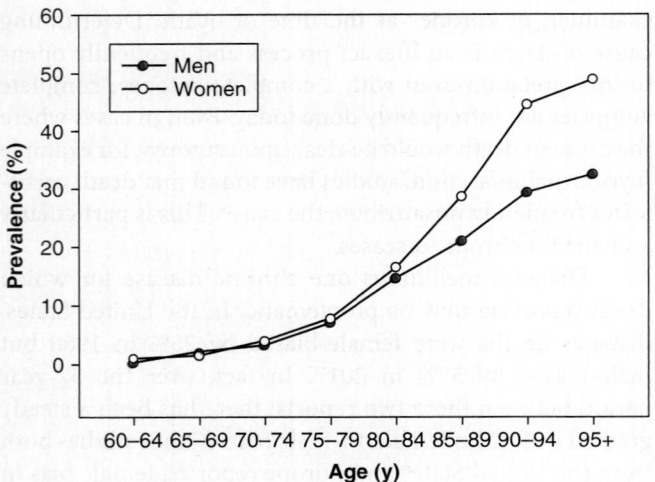

FIGURE 5-5. Relation of age and gender to prevalence of Alzheimer disease. Summarized from 31 studies from across Europe. (Data from Alzheimer's Europe.)

As noted earlier, the gender gap in life expectancy in the United States grew rapidly from about 1950 to around 1980 and has been steadily shrinking since the early 1980s (see **Figure 5-3**). This pattern is due to a more rapid gain in women's life expectancy relative to men's prior to the early 1980s followed by a slower gain thereafter. Specifically, between 1985 and 2017, life expectancy of US women increased by only 3.2 years compared with 5.2 years for men. Although life expectancy of neither gender grew as rapidly as in many other high-income countries, the growth for women was particularly slow—only 50%, 55%, and 73% the rate of Japanese, French, and Swedish women, respectively. Compare that with the equivalent figures for men. US men's life expectancy grew 13% *faster* than Japanese men's, 78% and 88% as fast as French and Swedish men.

A useful tool for assessing whether this national pattern could be due to inequalities in health within the United States is a county-by-county analysis. Not only are life expectancies and mortality rates available for each of the 3143 counties in the United States, so are data on income, racial composition, education level, and a host of other variables potentially informative for understanding the reasons underlying observed health disparities. There is tremendous variability among counties across the United States in all these variables. For instance, per capita income varies by more than sixfold from the poorest to the richest county, and the life expectancy gap between the longest- and shortest-lived counties is nearly 18 years for men and 13 years for women. This gap is greater than the life expectancy gap between Sweden and Nicaragua. Reiterating the larger historical and international perspective presented earlier, despite this striking variation among US counties, female life expectancy exceeded male life expectancy in every county for every year between 1960 and the present.

Several interesting patterns appear in such an analysis. First, variability among county life expectancies has been consistently greater for men than women since at least 1960. Second, life expectancy inequalities *within* each gender were smallest in the early 1980s when the gap *between* genders was at its maximum. Since then, within-in-gender inequalities have steadily risen for both sexes.

The period between 1985 and 2010 has been particularly well studied. An astonishing finding has been that while the most advantaged counties have continued a steady increase in life expectancy for both sexes, there has been little change in life expectancy over the past 25 years for the least advantaged counties. This is particularly true for women for whom more than 42% of counties in the United States showed no increase in women's life expectancy whatsoever across the entire 25-year period. Furthermore, nearly 10% of counties showed a significant *decrease*. Analogous figures for men reveal that fewer than 5% of counties showed no increase and fewer than 1% showed a decrease. A separate county-by-county study traced mortality rates (rather than life expectancy) from the early 1990s through 2006 and found similar results. Average mortality rates fell by 9.8% over that period for men and only 1.5% for women. Male mortality rate actually increased in only 3.4% of counties, whereas women's mortality rate increased in almost 43% of counties! In sum then, although national US averages continue to show steady gains in life expectancy during the past 25 years, for a significant fraction of women there have been no gains—or even losses—in life expectancy over that time period.

Two additional patterns emerge from an inspection of the causes of death. First, mortality due to cardiovascular disease has been falling steadily for both sexes for over 60 years. As mentioned previously, this should be considered a major medical and public health triumph. During the period—roughly 1960 to 1980—when the gender gap in life expectancy was increasing, men were more frequently dying from lung cancer and chronic respiratory diseases than women. Since then as the gender gap has been shrinking, reduction in cardiovascular disease has continued although at a slower rate for women relative to men, and the relative rate of increase in deaths from lung cancer and chronic respiratory diseases has risen. Second, that pattern was particularly marked in counties in which women lost life expectancy in recent years. Clearly these patterns, as with the international patterns, reflect differences in current and past smoking behavior.

Beyond that, there is a puzzling geographic component above and beyond obvious socioeconomic factors. Most counties with increased women's mortality were in the South, or in counties in the West with a significant proportion of Native American residents. Local diets would be one obvious place to look for clues to the reasons for this geographic component. Possibly more interesting than what variables were associated with decreasing life expectancy, are variables that were not. No simple correlations were found, for instance, between change in life expectancy and per capita income, educational attainment, percent of adults who were obese, availability of primary care providers, or proportion of the population lacking health insurance.

If instead of focusing on the counties that did worse over time, we focus on the ones that did better, which after all was the overwhelming number of counties for men and the majority for women, we find more of the expected explanatory factors. The two most significant associations with improved men's survival were percent of adults with a college degree and percent of Hispanic residents. The Hispanic effect is due to the so-called Hispanic paradox, the observation that Hispanic people of both sexes live longer than White people of equivalent socioeconomic status. Still significant, but somewhat less strongly associated, were population density (the higher, the better), and median household income. Similarly, in counties in which women's health improved over these study years, significant associations were seen with higher proportion of Hispanic people, higher proportion with college degrees, higher population density, and higher median household income. For neither sex was obesity or obvious medical care factors, such as percent of the population with health insurance or number of primary care physicians, statistically involved.

It is important to understand that the lack of statistical association between a socioeconomic or behavior factor and increasing versus declining survival in a county-by-county study does not indicate that a particular factor is unimportant for health or survival. For example, many studies have identified obesity as a significant contributor to poor health. The lack of association with obesity described above just means that a county-by-county analysis is too crude a tool to pick up a likely obesity effect.

The trend in the United States for women to gain less than men in life expectancy over time is particularly apparent if one examines differing education levels and ethnicities. Education generally can be considered almost a miracle drug for improved health and life expectancy regardless of ethnicity. For instance, among White Americans, the impact of having 16 years or more of education compared with having not completed high school was a difference in life expectancy of 10 years for women and 13 years for men. To emphasize the magnitude of this education effect, it is comparably greater than the magnitude of life expectancy difference between Sweden and Paraguay. Education is hypothesized to exert its impact via better health habits, better ability to deal with stress, and more effective management of chronic conditions. More disturbing is the impact of low education. White women and men with less than a high school diploma actually lived about 5 and 3 years less, respectively, in 2008 than they did in 1990! Puzzlingly, this temporal decline in life expectancy for poorly educated Americans was not seen in African-American or Hispanic populations. In fact, in those ethnic groups life expectancy rose over that time period for all education levels, including those not completing high school.

In sum, health disparities within the United States are generally larger for men than women, but a substantially larger fraction of women than men are showing worse health now compared with 25 years ago.

THE HEALTH-SURVIVAL PARADOX

As robust and widespread as is women's survival advantage over men, equally robust, widespread, and puzzling, is men's health advantage over women. Although women live longer than men everywhere, women also display greater overall rates of physical illness and functional limitations than men from adolescence throughout life. In the United States, for instance, women make more doctor visits, spend more days in hospital, miss more work due to illness, and take more medications than do men. Women also self-report more functional limitations and are overrepresented relative to their proportion of the population in residential care facilities.

This health-survival paradox is a worldwide phenomenon. In most of the world's 187 countries, unlike in the United States, women's life expectancy is increasing slightly faster than men's. Also, increasing faster in women than men is the number of unhealthy years they live. One measure of ill health is "years living with disability (YLD)," which is the severity-adjusted prevalence of disability. Across countries of the world per capita YLD is generally higher for women than for men, particularly at young and middle ages. Thus the additional unhealthy years lived by women compared to men are not just those at the end of life. Additionally, self-reported health surveys of people over 50 years from the US and Europe revealed that despite more men than women being overweight and currently smoking, women in all countries were more likely to have functional difficulties or disabling conditions. Similarly consistent differences were found in a comparative study of the United States, Jamaica, Malaysia, and Bangladesh, in which participants were asked about their ability to perform a variety of tasks, such as walk a certain distance, bend over, or climb stairs (**Figure 5-6**).

One hypothesis to explain the health-survival paradox is that women are more attentive to physical discomfort and more willing to seek medical attention when they perceive it. However, empirical evidence to support such an explanation is uneven and sometimes contradictory. Also, if this hypothesis is valid, it would have to be a worldwide phenomenon rather than a cultural feature of wealthy, Western countries. **Figure 5-6** shows that the same patterns obtain in poor, culturally diverse countries such as Jamaica, Malaysia, and Bangladesh. A second plausible hypothesis is that because men die at higher rates than women throughout life, ill men are more likely to die than ill women. Thus the surviving men will be more highly selected for health and vigor than surviving women. If this sex-selection hypothesis is valid, one would predict that the sex differences in various health metrics would increase with age as more and more ill men die while more and more ill women survived. As intriguing as is this hypothesis, several large cross-national studies have failed to find such predicted divergence in health status with age. They find instead a relatively constant male health superiority throughout life.

The ubiquity of these health differences between the sexes begs for a biological explanation. One of the most consistent findings among dozens of studies investigating sex-based morbidity differences is that women are subject to more bone and joint diseases, including idiopathic back pain and osteoarthritis. Chronic pain can limit activities and cause sufferers to seek medical attention. In addition, it can have more far-reaching, secondary health consequences from sequelae such as sleep deprivation and chronic stress. So, a plausible, if partial, biological hypothesis for the health-survival paradox may be sex differences in joint components such as cartilage and ligaments. Uterine connective tissue undergoes extensive remodeling and increasing elasticity during pregnancy under the influence of various reproductive hormones. Could it be that a side

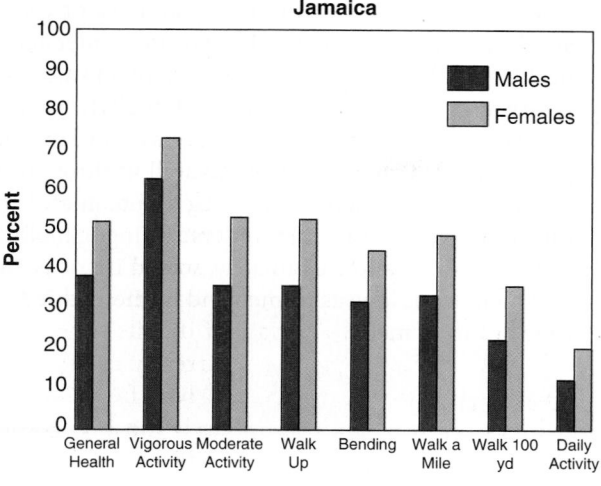

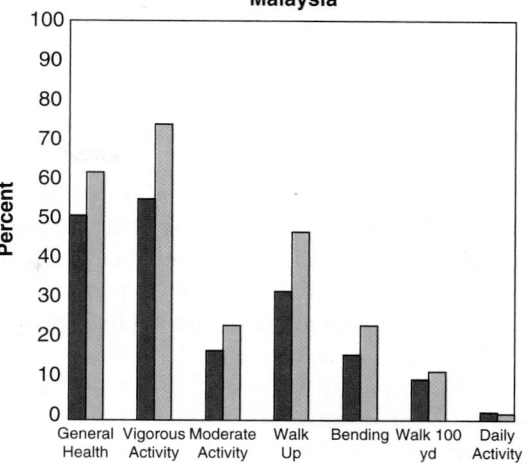

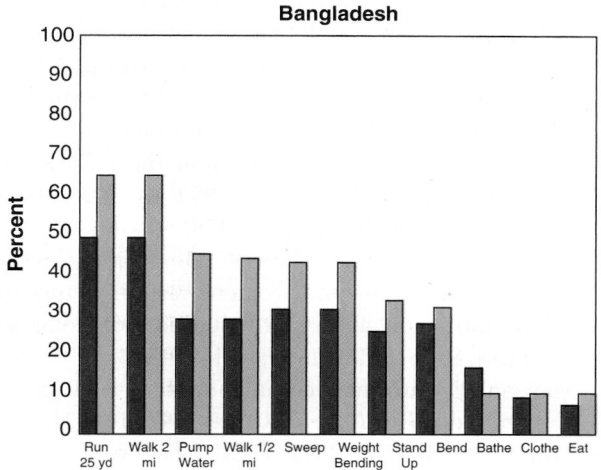

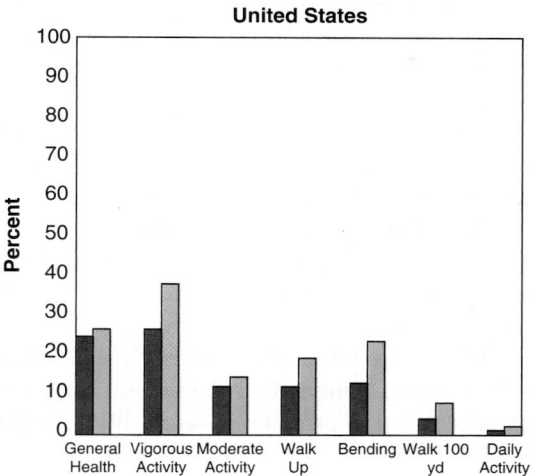

FIGURE 5-6. Self-reported health across several countries. Proportion of respondents reporting fair-to-poor ability to perform these tasks. (Reproduced with permission from Rahman O, Strauss J, Gertler P, et al: Gender differences in adult health: an international comparison. *Gerontologist.* 1994;34(4):463–469.)

effect of the responsiveness of women's cartilage, tendons, ligaments, and muscle to female reproductive hormones is an increased susceptibility of women to joint instability and resultant inflammation and pain? Provocatively, female athletes in sports such as soccer and basketball are 5 to 10 times more likely to suffer anterior cruciate ligament knee injuries than male athletes, and most are from noncontact events. Also, the prevalence of idiopathic knee osteoarthritis is similar in men and women prior to menopause, but much greater in women after menopause, again suggesting a hormonal influence on joint health. Women also tend to have more robust inflammatory and immune responses than men, perhaps helping to account for their greater resistance to infectious diseases, and also greater susceptibility to autoimmune and inflammatory joint diseases such as osteo- and rheumatoid arthritis. Taken together, these sex differences may contribute to the health-survival paradox.

CONCLUSION

Several robust features of human biology emerge from considering sex differences in health and longevity. Most particularly, women appear more resistant than men to multiple fatal diseases, acquiring them at lower rates and/or later in life. Women also appear to be more resistant to a range of infectious diseases from early in life. A notable exception to this pattern is AD and other dementias, to which women are more susceptible than men worldwide. Despite the broad survival advantage, women are more likely to suffer from physical ailments than men later in life even controlling for age effects. It is tempting to hypothesize that differential lifetime exposure to sex hormones contributes to both the positive and negative sex differences. Yet to date, no simple answers on how lifetime sex hormone exposure relates to diseases and disabilities of later life have materialized. In the United States, there is a puzzling trend over the past several decades for women to gain life expectancy at a slower rate than men, and some groups of disadvantaged women are even shorter-lived today than they were decades ago. Learning more about sex difference in health and longevity will be critical to determining how to reduce health disparities in both sexes.

Since the US National Institutes of Health (NIH) Revitalization Act of 1993, women have been required to be adequately represented in NIH-funded clinical studies. Today, roughly half of clinical research participants are women. However, similar attention has not been paid to sex balance in studies with laboratory animals or cells, which are heavily male-biased. Mechanistic understanding of health and disease relies to a large extent on studies of laboratory animals or cells. In May 2014, the NIH issued a policy statement promising to redress this imbalance through program oversight and review, as well as through collaboration with publishers. One desired outcome of this new direction would be a better understanding of biological sex differences in health. Ultimately, would it not be desirable that men live as long as women and women achieve the lifetime health of men?

FURTHER READING

Austad SN. Sex differences in longevity and aging. In: Masoro EJ, Austad SN, eds. *Handbook of the Biology of Aging*. 7th ed. San Diego, CA: Academic Press; 2011: 479–496.

Beltrán-Sanchez H, Finch CE, Crimmins EM. Twentieth century surge of excess adult male mortality. *Proc Natl Acad Sci U S A*. 2015;112(29):8993–8998.

Boyan BD, Hart DA, Enoka RM, et al. Hormonal modulation of connective tissue homeostasis and sex differences in risk for osteoarthritis of the knee. *Biol Sex Differ*. 2013;4(1):3.

Bronikowski AM, Altmann J, Brockman DK, et al. Aging in the natural world: comparative data reveal similar mortality patterns across primates. *Science*. 2011;331(6022): 1325–1328.

Clayton JA, Collins FS. NIH to balance sex in cell and animal studies. *Nature*. 2014;509(7500):282.

Crimmins EM, Kim JK, Solé-Auró A. Gender differences in health: results from SHARE, ELSA, and HRS. *Eur J Public Health*. 2010;21(1):81–91.

Crimmins EM, Preston, SH, Cohen B, eds. *International Differences in Mortality at Older Ages: Dimensions and Sources*. Washington, DC: National Academies Press; 2011.

Ezzati M, Friedman AB, Kulkani SC, Murray CJ. The reversal of fortunes: trends in county mortality and cross-county mortality disparities in the United States. *PLoS Med*. 2008;5(4):e66.

Hamilton JB, Mestler GE. Mortality and survival: a comparison of eunuchs with intact men and women in a mentally retarded population. *J Gerontol*. 1969;24(4):395–411.

Human Mortality Database. University of California, Berkeley (USA), and Max Planck Institute for Demographic Research (Germany). www.mortality.org or www.humanmortality.de. Accessed November 2014.

Kindig DA, Cheng ER. Even as mortality fell in most US counties, female mortality nonetheless rose in 42.8 percent of counties from 1992 to 2006. *Health Aff (Millwood)*. 2013;32(3):451–458.

Macintyre S, Ford G, Hunt K. Do women 'over-report' morbidity? Men's and women's responses to structured prompting on a standard question on long standing illness. *Soc Sci Med*. 1999;48(1):89–98.

Manson JE. Current recommendations: what is the clinician to do? *Fertil Steril*. 2014;101(4):916–921.

Min K-J, Lee C-K, Park H-N. The lifespan of Korean eunuchs. *Curr Biol*. 2012;22(18):R792–793.

Rahman O, Strauss J, Gertler P, Ashley D, Fox K. Gender differences in adult health: an international comparison. *Gerontologist*. 1994;34(4):463–469.

Saloman JA, Wang H, Freeman MK, et al. Healthy life expectancy for 187 countries, 1990–2010: a systematic analysis for the Global Burden Disease Study 2010. *Lancet*. 2012;380(9867):2144–2162.

Stanczyk FZ, Bhavnani BR. Current views of hormone therapy for management and treatment of postmenopausal women. *J Steroid Biochem Mol Biol*. 2014;142:1–2.

Wang H, Schumacher AE, Levitz CE, Mokdad AH, Murray CJ. Left behind: widening disparities for males and females in US county life expectancy, 1985–2010. *Popul Health Metr*. 2013;11:8.

Chapter 6

Social Determinants of Health, Health Disparities, and Health Equity

Laura Block, W. Ryan Powell, Andrea Gilmore-Bykovskyi, Amy J. H. Kind

INTRODUCTION

Scientific progress in aging and geriatrics has led to longer life expectancy, improved quality of life, and many advancements in geriatric medicine. Unfortunately, these benefits are not equally distributed across populations. Lower life expectancy, higher age-related disease incidence including Alzheimer disease, chronic disease burden, and worse health care quality and access disproportionately affect historically disenfranchised groups in the United States—which include but are not limited to racial and ethnic minorities, persons living in rural areas or who are socioeconomically disadvantaged, and sexual and gender minorities. Such health differences are broadly referred to as health disparities, and across the life course these negative health impacts are often compounded, exerting a cumulative influence on age-related health outcomes in older adults.

Getting to the root causes of health disparities requires a well-rounded understanding of the social/environmental, behavioral/psychological, and biological processes involved and how they interrelate. We often have a better understanding of geriatric conditions from a biological and sometimes behavioral vantage point, yet less often do we understand how unequal exposure to disadvantaged social and environmental contexts drives health disparities. Frailty risk, for example, is shaped by biological (female sex) and behavioral (physical activity level and cognitive status) factors along with social and environmental factors, such as access to safe spaces within which to exercise or financial resources to wear proper footwear for safe exercise. However, social and environmental factors are frequently overlooked in key clinical and research domains.

Social determinants of health are the conditions within which we live, grow, work, play, and age that impact health. They are particularly salient in the development and reinforcement of health disparities, playing a role in an estimated 80% of health outcomes. They include factors related to financial wealth and stability, education, the social and community context, the neighborhood and built environment, and health care access and quality. Social determinants of health exert influence at individual, family, community, organizational, and policy levels.

Laura Block and W. Ryan Powell contributed equally and are co-first authors of this chapter.

Learning Objectives

- Define social determinants of health, health disparities, and health equity.
- Understand historical and contemporary contributing factors to health disparities in older adults within historically disenfranchised groups.
- Apply a life course perspective to health equity and its role in older adult health.
- Describe features of effective interventions to foster health equity.

Key Clinical Points

1. Social determinants of health reflect the educational, economic, health care, neighborhood/environmental, and social and community context of everyday life. Social determinants of health play a key role in approaches to prevent and address adverse health outcomes.

2. Health disparities are common among older adults and are often rooted in unfavorable exposure to social determinants, for example, disparate access to health opportunities and barriers.

3. Multiple factors, including biological, health behavior–related, sociocultural, and environmental, *interact* and operate across the life course to influence later-life health outcomes.

4. Individualized assessments are needed to understand opportunities and barriers to older adult health, and to avoid biased assumptions about individuals.

5. Consideration of social determinants and their contribution to age-related health disparities requires increasing levels of collaboration among members of the care team, including geriatrics, mental health, and community-based supports and services (CBSS).

It is important to recognize that social determinants of health affect the health of older adult populations. Having an awareness of the mounting evidence on these complex factors, along with being equipped with a strong conceptual, will help geriatricians and other clinicians to recognize and respond effectively to social factors that drive health disparities later in life. This chapter provides a practical foundation for defining and understanding social determinants, health disparities, and health equity as they relate to the health of older adults. While this chapter provides many examples pertaining to the United States, the underlying themes apply globally even if their manifestation and consequences are unique by country and region. Both a historical lens and a life course approach are applied to deepen understanding of the fundamental causes of health disparities. Interventions to foster health equity across individual, community, and policy levels are presented to illustrate real-world approaches to applying this knowledge.

DEFINITIONS

Understanding the key concepts of social determinants of health, health disparities, and health equity, and how they are interrelated is necessary for untangling the historical and contemporary forces that shape health for older adults and the multilevel interventions sought to foster equitable outcomes.

Social Determinants of Health

Social determinants of health are the conditions in daily life that impact health. They include the social, economic, physical, and environmental factors that shape everyday lives, and the opportunities and barriers to health older people may experience. Examples of social determinants of health can include the lack of access to quality education; economic stability commonly tied to employment and income; neighborhood and built environment factors like housing, safety, and access to healthy food options; and the social and community context such as challenges due to discrimination. Social determinants of health can also influence the nature of care delivery, and care delivery can further influence health outcomes—creating a compounding effect. Domains of the social determinants of health are shown in **Figure 6-1**, as adapted from the Centers for Disease Control and Prevention Model.

Some social determinants, such as air pollution contributing to asthma and related exacerbations, have a clear, direct pathway to health outcomes. However, many social determinants operate indirectly to affect health; for example, chronic exposure to social and environmental stressors can be linked to disproportionate rates of respiratory and cardiovascular conditions. Thanks to new targeted funding efforts, an understanding of these indirect pathways is an active area of investigation, with the hopes of making new mechanistic discoveries that explain the link between social determinants and adverse health outcomes.

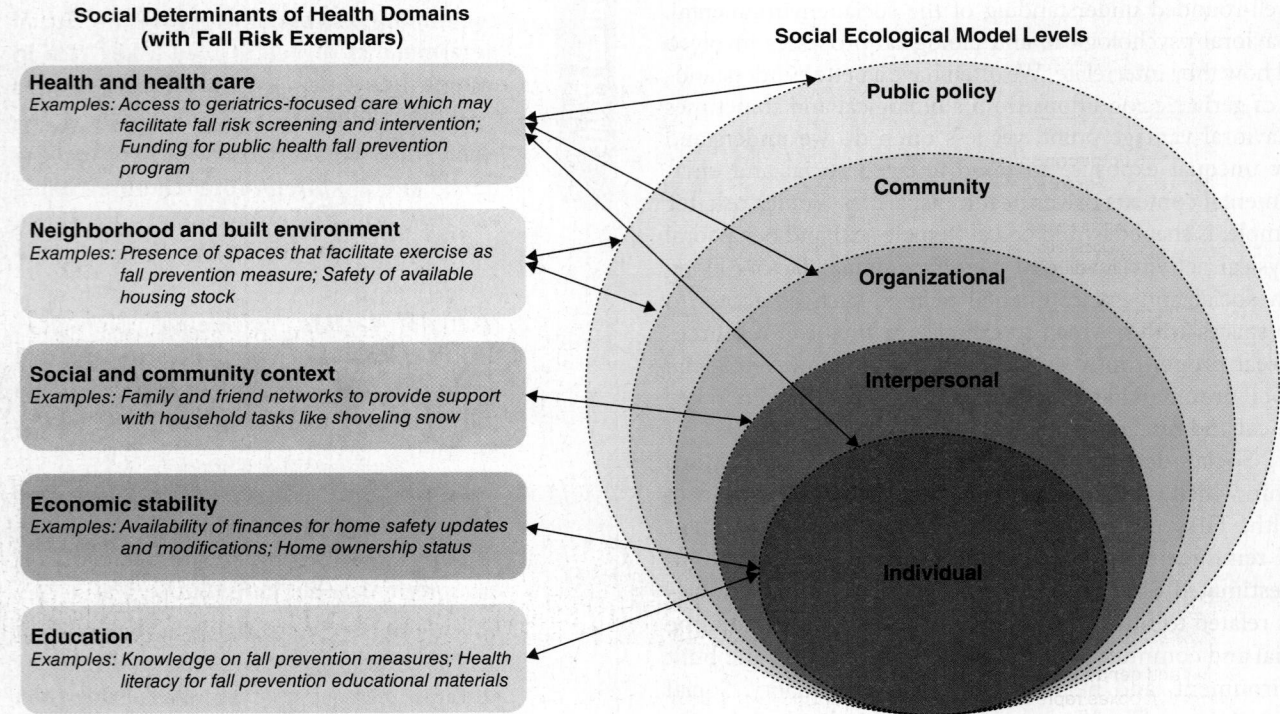

Social Determinants of Health Domains (with Fall Risk Exemplars)

Health and health care
Examples: Access to geriatrics-focused care which may facilitate fall risk screening and intervention; Funding for public health fall prevention program

Neighborhood and built environment
Examples: Presence of spaces that facilitate exercise as fall prevention measure; Safety of available housing stock

Social and community context
Examples: Family and friend networks to provide support with household tasks like shoveling snow

Economic stability
Examples: Availability of finances for home safety updates and modifications; Home ownership status

Education
Examples: Knowledge on fall prevention measures; Health literacy for fall prevention educational materials

Social Ecological Model Levels

Public policy

Community

Organizational

Interpersonal

Individual

Note: Each of these social determinants of health domains can operate at all levels of the social ecological model. This figure shows just some of the social determinants of health operating at different levels when considering fall prevention strategies. Additionally, social determinants of health may interact with each other.

FIGURE 6-1. Social determinants of health operate within and interact across all levels of the social ecological model.

Social determinants of health can often originate from systems and structures, yet they influence persons and families. The social ecological model provides a helpful visual for appreciating that individuals are situated within a larger context and shaped by these cross-cutting social determinants of health. Social determinants of health can operate within and interact across levels of society (the individual, organization, community, public) as depicted in **Figure 6-1**. For example, when considering fall prevention strategies for older adults, home modifications may not be an affordable or feasible option for persons who are not home-owners; and though conversations on fall prevention may be operating on a person or individual level, consideration of rental agreements may function at an interpersonal and organizational level, access to affordable housing may occur at a community level, and patterns in home-ownership may be impacted by public policy.

Health Disparities

Health disparities are differences in health outcomes driven by unjust, inequitable causes that negatively affect a population or groups of individuals. The presence and persistence of health disparities require understanding their sources and addressing their occurrence. Though health disparities have long existed in the United States, groundbreaking reports, including the 1984 Department of Health and Human Services Report, "Health, United States, 1983," and the 2003 Institute of Medicine Report "Unequal Treatment: Confronting Racial and Ethnic Disparities" brought broader attention to these inequities by highlighting the social and structural health system factors involved.

Older adults may experience age-related health disparities that result from unjust, inequitable access to aging-specific care, supports, and services. They may experience the accumulation of health disparities across the lifespan, resulting in long-standing and new negative health outcomes. Within the context of aging, the National Institute on Aging (NIA) provides a framework for understanding the environmental, sociocultural, behavioral, and biological factors that shape health and lead to health disparities across the lifespan (**Figure 6-2**). The NIA framework

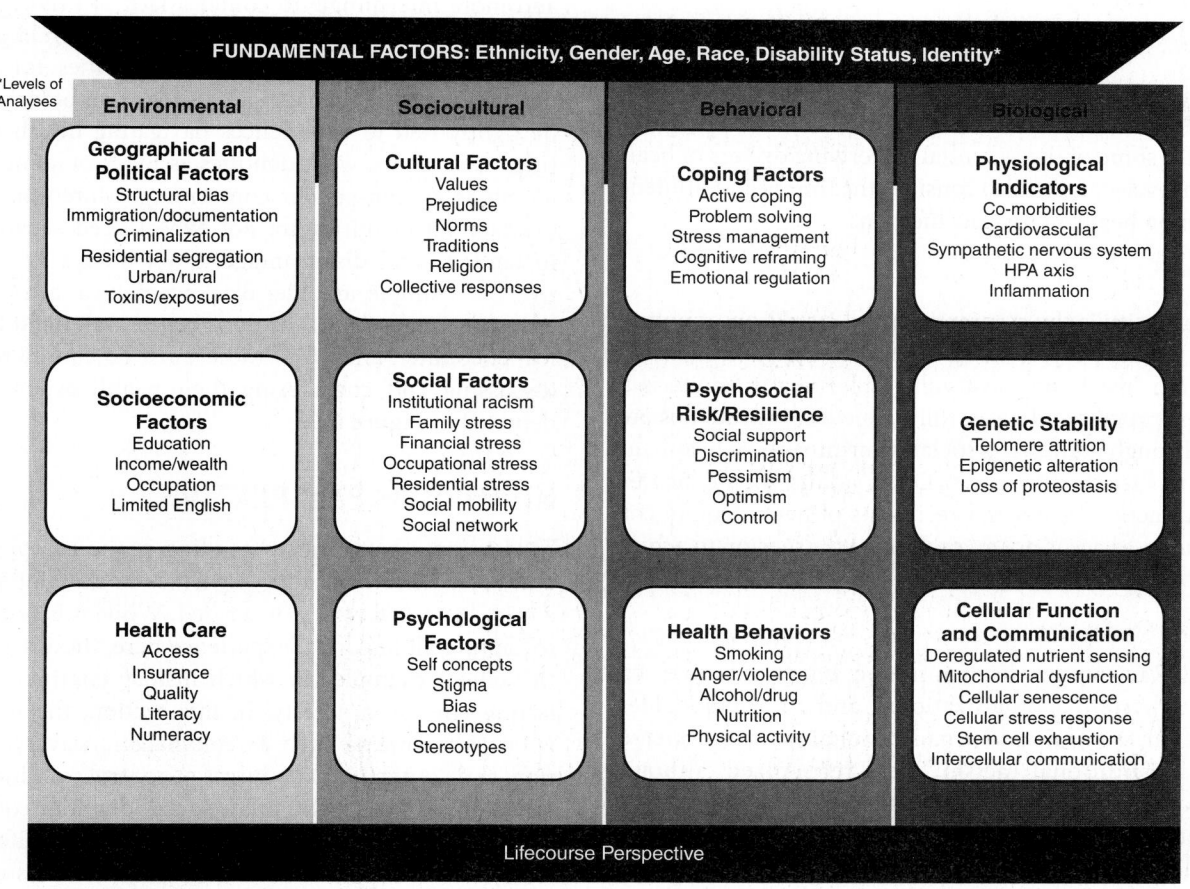

*Sexual and gender minorities.
**Text within boxes represents examples of related factors.

FIGURE 6-2. The National Institute on Aging health disparities framework helps to recognize the variety of reasons why health disparities exist. (Reproduced with permission from Hill CV, Pérez-Stable EJ, Anderson NA, et al: The National Institute on Aging Health Disparities Research Framework. *Ethn Dis.* 2015;25(3):245–254.)

Note:

Though health disparities often exist for historically disenfranchised populations (eg, Indigenous, Black, or rural populations), a person's group membership or identity itself does not create health disparities. However, these individuals may be disproportionately impacted or intentionally targeted by systemic, contextual, and relational forces that result in health disparities. To illustrate this point, a common misconception is that race is a risk factor for poor health—for example, that Black identity directly leads to early mortality. However, the true driver in this association is the systemic racism operating at multiple levels that results in the development and perpetuation of a health disparity, for example, shaping access to resources needed for health. Race is a social construct. It is not a biological construct. Yet, this erroneous perception of race as a biological construct remains pervasive across a wide array of venues. Such flawed interpretations support the need for better medical education and training, and the need for wider efforts to address the structural factors that promulgate such errors.

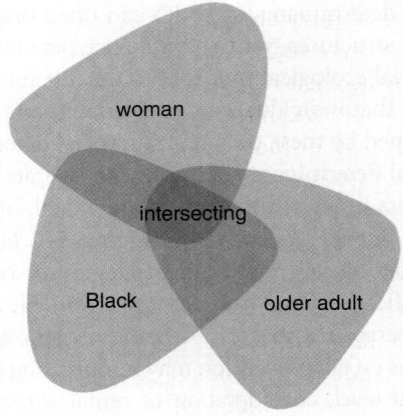

FIGURE 6-3. An intersectional lens helps to understand the overlapping nature of identities.

provides nested classifications for each factor, helping us to consider some of the potential underlying drivers of health at each level—and to also consider the timing and influence of each on health across the lifespan.

Health Equity

Health equity is the assurance of the condition of optimal health for all people, centering those who are historically disenfranchised and most vulnerable. Health equity is an ongoing process and never fully achieved; instead, it is pursued through addressing social determinants of health and reducing health disparities. Older adults should be centered as active agents and recipients of health equity conversations, as age is not an exclusionary criterion to achieve health potential.

Related Concepts

Racism Racism, or discrimination based on race, can occur at systemic, organizational, and interpersonal levels. Often, systemic and organizational racism is referred to as "institutional racism." Less recognized, although insidious, is "internalized racism" or the biases people carry due to larger narratives about race. Racism is experienced by many older adults of color and can often be intertwined and compounded with experiences of ageism.

Intersectionality The confluence of lifelong experiences and social identities interact in specific and individual ways that contribute to older adults' health in late life. An intersectional lens emphasizes a more nuanced and accurate understanding of how health is shaped by the many ways people experience disadvantage. Avoiding oversimplifications, intersectionality instead takes into account that the experiences and identities of race, social class, gender, age, and more intermingle to confer a lack of privilege. It can also facilitate an understanding of how health experiences are inseparable from their multiple identities; for example, the experience of managing diabetes as an older adult will be tightly tied to experiences navigating health care settings as someone who identifies as Black or someone who identifies as non-gender conforming. Moreover, multiple overlapping identities are not experienced separately but in tandem, and disadvantage is not always simply additive. For example, an older Black woman cannot leave their age, race, or gender at the door before walking into a clinical encounter, and all of these must be considered when discussing and considering their health experiences, as depicted in **Figure 6-3**.

HISTORICAL PERSPECTIVE

To develop a better understanding of the complex nature and persistence of health disparities in the United States, a brief historical review is needed. While it is not possible to capture all historical experience here, these are some of the salient examples in which history continues to have lasting effects on society. In this section, the manner in which phenomena such as colonialism, slavery, segregation, and contemporary sources of control over individuals based on skin color and other social identities continue to deny key resources to populations, affecting life, opportunity, and health is reviewed. A historical lens allows us to understand the manner in which social identities have been constructed over time. The lasting effects of these historical and contemporary forces, although described in the United States context, are perpetuated across multiple axes (eg, race, sex, gender, disability, immigrant status) and worldwide. Though manifestations and impacts may be unique by country and region, the resultant health disparities often share similar features.

Colonialism has resulted in ongoing repercussions on Indigenous health and may be considered a distal or underlying determinant of Indigenous health—in other words, a cause of the causes of health determinants. Not only can colonialism be linked to Indigenous health, as an underlying determinant and source of historical trauma, but it paved the way for the continued displacement and marginalization of Indigenous persons, systemic underfunding of health resources (including the Indian Health Services), failure to recognize Indigenous health traditions, and erasure of the successes of Indigenous communities, including self-governance and self-determination.

For African-Americans, a history of slavery followed by sharecropping, segregation, and state-sponsored oppression (eg, redlining and lending bias) have shaped the opportunities for housing, employment, education, and health across families and neighborhoods. For example, notably yet often overlooked is the intense violence against and systematic removal of supports for freed slaves during the post-Civil War Reconstruction era followed by 10 decades of subservience and segregation. This, in part, fueled the Great Migration of African-Americans out of Southern States from approximately 1916 to 1970 for risky jobs in other areas of the country with little to no family wealth or education. Some narratives portray slavery, segregation, and racism as a thing of the past, or if present, a rare interpersonal occurrence. These narratives forget recent history along with contemporary events that demonstrate persistence and long-lasting harms of racist and often state-sponsored tools that oppress opportunity and health.

Disadvantage is perpetuated by a history of discriminatory practices (including in the workplace and community), and denial of rights and certain protections against many groups including women, persons with disabilities, persons from immigrant backgrounds, and lesbian, gay, bisexual, and transgender (LGBT+) people, generating health disparities over the lifespan. For example, LGBT+ people have long-faced legal discrimination: the ways in which family and partnerships have been defined block access to health insurance in safety net programs like Medicaid as well as social security, employment, and veteran benefits. Home equity is often the main source of family wealth, yet discriminatory lending practices contribute to widening wealth gaps. These lending practices have often discriminated based on place, race or ethnicity, and immigrant status. For example, mortgage discrimination in the form of redlining or denying credit, has origins which trace back to the 1930s, dispersing and segregating communities in addition to damaging home equity. Furthermore, the practice of reverse redlining during the housing crisis of the 2000s has garnered attention, where risky, high-cost subprime loans were disproportionately offered to borrowers in Black and Latinx neighborhoods. Given the allocation of

resources by place, and the manner in which neighborhood and health are tied together, not only does displacement, redlining, and mortgage bias impact opportunity, but it also hurts health.

While concentration of populations within certain regions and neighborhoods may not be, in itself, a negative phenomenon, restriction of movement of these persons based on their social identity represents discriminatory policies and practices. Moreover, these regions and neighborhoods are more likely to be zoned in manners that allow industrial and mixed environments, resulting in poorer air and water quality, less access to food and green space, and greater likelihood of highway construction. Another modern phenomenon is the mass incarceration of disproportionately non-White populations, which can contribute to family separation, poverty and trauma, and subsequent poor health.

Additionally, in a disturbingly persistent manner, health care professionals have wielded medicine as a tool of oppression against specific groups. For example, there is a long history of people with disabilities being involuntarily sterilized, a practice which was upheld in a 1927 Supreme Court ruling and after which resulted in forcible sterilization of roughly 70,000 people, often disproportionately women, racial minorities, and poorer people.

> **Note:**
>
> A historical lens can help us understand that the "mistrust" toward health care systems is in fact the absence of *earned trust.*

POPULATION TRENDS

The United States is undergoing major population shifts. In less than 20 years, people 65 years and older will outnumber those under the age of 18. Soon after, groups considered to be racial and ethnic minorities will outnumber White populations. And by 2060, persons 65 years and older will have grown nearly 69% larger and represent 23% of the total population, with White persons representing half of the entire population 65 years and older (see Chapter 2).

Other notable trends include the rising numbers of adults 65 years and older remaining in the labor force and the decrease in poverty rates among older adults. However, poverty rates remain around 10% and are nearly double for racial and ethnic minorities. The US population is becoming more diverse, and correspondingly so are older adults. This diversity can be seen in the growing number of older adults who identify as Black, Indigenous, Latinx, for example—all identities which have experienced historical disenfranchisement and therefore may experience corresponding consequences on health. A nonexhaustive review of population trends for historically disenfranchised groups and unique health considerations is presented below; yet further investigation is merited with caution to the harms that can occur with assuming individuals may conform to and experience wider phenomena.

- Indigenous populations (Native American, American Indian, and Alaska Native) are growing and expected to be 1.4% of the total population by 2060, with corresponding growth in numbers of older adults. Nearly half of older Indigenous adults have one or more disabilities, and twice as many experience poverty compared to counterparts.
- There are an estimated 1.5 million older adults who identify as lesbian, gay, or bisexual, with poorly established numbers for transgender older adults. This number is expected to nearly double by 2030. LGBT+ older adults are more likely to be single and without children and to experience poverty as compared to non-LGBT+ counterparts. There has also been a history of systemic denial of services and benefits based on LGBT+ identity and same-sex marriage status. LGBT+ older adults often face discrimination and ignorance by health care providers, lesser health insurance coverage, delays in seeking and receiving care, and sexual and mental health stigma.
- An often-overlooked group of older adults includes those living in federal and state prisons. A growing number of incarcerated persons are 50 years and older. Incarceration may accelerate aging by 10 to 15 years, with age 50 often cited as the cutoff point for older age among persons who are incarcerated. Incarcerated older adults are at greater risk for mental and chronic health conditions, cancer, dementia, and HIV/AIDS; have higher rates of disability; experience more substance abuse and addiction; and have higher rates of prior trauma. Prisons are often underprepared and under-resourced for supporting medical and mental health needs, particularly for older adults who may be experiencing higher disease burden.
- There are also unique challenges faced by older adults upon release from prison—a trend which may increase with compassionate release laws—due to barriers and discrimination in accessing CBSS. Additionally, some of these adults require nursing home-level care, yet these facilities are often unequipped to support individuals in successful reentry.
- Older adults who identify as immigrants or foreign-born are growing in number, representing long-term and recent migration patterns. These populations have specific economic, familial, cultural, and language-related needs—all of which may be moderated by social supports, education, and literacy levels. Integrated translation services, accessible materials, and culturally responsive services that flexibly integrate family and friend supports are important in the care of older adult immigrants. Today, a majority of US immigrants come from the following origin countries: Mexico, China, India, Philippines, and El Salvador. When considering culturally responsive services for older adult immigrants, it is imperative to consider the heterogeneity of immigrant populations rather than broad classifications of older adults as Latinx or Asian, as these categorizations do not account for the rich diversity in language and culture of subpopulations. Status as a naturalized citizen, lawful permanent resident, unauthorized immigrant, and refugee can also affect an older adult's health status and interaction with health care services, for example, impacting resource eligibility.
- Older adults living in rural areas often face extreme barriers in access to health care that can negatively influence their health outcomes and lead to increased mortality. Older adults living in rural areas are also more likely to experience poverty and chronic health conditions exacerbated by a lack of updated built infrastructure. Adults identifying as Indigenous, Latinx, and Black and living in rural areas may experience compounded barriers to health access and care. In rural areas, not only are health outcomes shaped by poor health care access, but also by limited options to access healthy food and safe places for exercise.

LIFE COURSE PERSPECTIVE

Applying a life course perspective to health disparities among older adults allows us to understand how experiences throughout the lifetime and across generations may differentially influence health opportunities and outcomes. As experiences are often shaped by the social and physical environment, a life course perspective recognizes the accumulation of social determinants of health across time. There are two major schools of thought regarding life course perspectives:

- A developmental life course perspective emphasizes critical periods or developmental windows with adaptation in response to adversity. These factors across the life course affect health in later life. Exposure during these windows or periods can result in acute and chronic adverse health outcomes. Critical periods can include fetal and infant developmental stages, where exposures may result in irreversible health consequences.
- A structural life course perspective emphasizes the historically and socially influenced nature of health. It also emphasizes that health-promoting or harming exposures may be disproportionally and cumulatively experienced differently by different groups. This perspective gives way to the weathering hypothesis, where structural inequalities create chronic exposure to disadvantage that can result in disproportionate rates of disease.

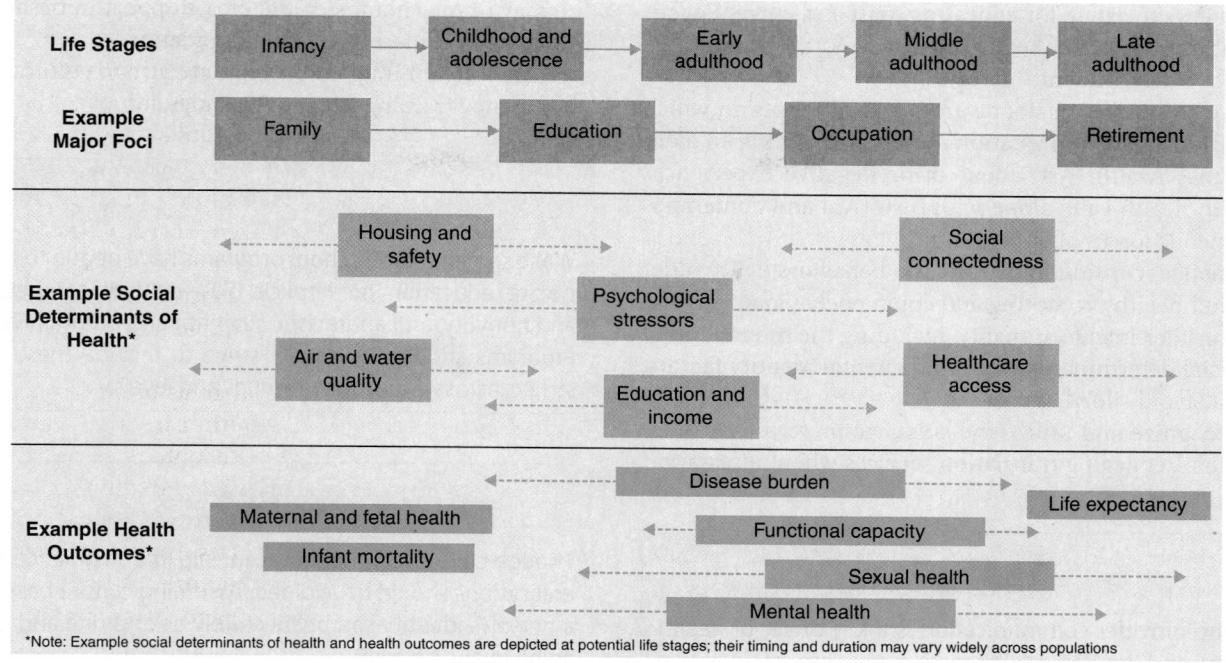

*Note: Example social determinants of health and health outcomes are depicted at potential life stages; their timing and duration may vary widely across populations

FIGURE 6-4. Social determinants of health and health outcomes interact across life course stages and foci. (Data from 2017 National Population Projections Tables: Main Series https://www.census.gov/data/tables/2017/demo/popproj/2017-summary-tables.html.)

Life course perspectives have been applied to and investigated in common chronic health conditions, including diabetes, cardiovascular disease, respiratory disease, and specific cancers. Life course perspectives also examine trajectories in both exposures and health, and the intergenerational transmission of exposure-related health determinants. As historical and social structures remain in place across generations, exposures and related health impacts may be experienced across time.

Applied to geriatrics, a life course perspective requires assessment of early life and cumulative exposures to adverse social and environmental stressors, and their consideration in care approach design to maximize health. Practical considerations toward this end are presented later in the chapter.

Figure 6-4 depicts major life stages and accompanying foci at each life stage. Example social determinants of health are depicted; these may occur and shape health at specific critical periods and may accumulate longitudinally across the lifespan. Example health outcomes that may be particularly sensitive to social determinants are also portrayed.

HEALTH EQUITY AND GERIATRICS INTERVENTIONS

Understanding health disparities—including their root causes, impact on health across the lifespan, and nature in geriatrics populations—is an important first step toward being able to realize health equity.

Health care providers are poised to deliver multilevel health equity interventions that can accelerate the elimination of health disparities. The Social Ecological Model and NIA Disparities Framework can help inform targeting of health equity interventions at multiple levels (individual, interpersonal, community, organizational, and public policy) and social determinant domains (environmental, sociocultural, behavioral, and biological). Though intervening at the highest level of the Social Ecological Model (public policy) may hold potential to influence the most persons, meaningful change must also occur at the interpersonal level, such as during provider–patient interactions.

There are numerous interventions providers can utilize before, during, and after the delivery of care to promote health equity. As a prerequisite, a comprehensive understanding of population and area-specific social determinants of health can equip providers with knowledge to inform assessment and tailored recommendations. From there, a life-story perspective that considers the potential life course impact of social determinants for an older adult can promote understanding of factors influencing presentation and help tailor recommendations to maximize effectiveness. A systematic, non-biased approach to assessment of social determinants is key, with suggestions presented later in the chapter.

Sample Individual Health Equity Interventions

- Screen for social determinants of health by conducting thorough psychosocial assessments and life-story reviews to assess for education, past and current occupations, income, health care access, and additional social determinants of health.

- Create an open dialogue around the manner in which racism and discrimination may be influencing an older adult's health. Ask about prior negative experiences with health care, along with historical and contemporaneous forces of oppression.
- Balance consideration of risk behaviors with older adult health promoting and coping behaviors.
- Consider intersectionality, including the interaction of social determinants with fundamental identity factors, and avoid siloed approaches.
- Recognize and utilize the language preferred by older adults, engaging translation services when necessary.

> **Note:**
>
> Patient–provider communication is a key driver of health quality and outcomes. Promoting the use of inclusive language, can be a step toward strengthening patient–provider relationships. Use preferred pronouns and terminology, acknowledging that there is at times no general consensus, and always seek the terms your patients prefer to self-identify. For example, some patients from Indigenous American groups may identify as Native Americans while others might use the term American Indian to self-identify.

Sample Interpersonal and Community Health Equity Interventions

- Involve older adult support systems as identified by that individual, including family and friends; avoid restrictive definitions of support systems.
- Consider ways in which health behaviors may be rooted in family and cultural practice; avoid bias, labeling, stigmatization, and imposing your own preferences or values.
- Realize the trauma that lifelong family, financial, occupational, and residential stress can create for individuals and families across generations.
- Recognize that racism and discrimination is a *lived experience* that impacts older adults' support systems and that this may lead to additional stress.

Sample Organizational and Public Policy Health Equity Interventions

- Advocate for expanded funding of programs that promote older adult health.
- Promote integration of health services and community-based services and supports.
- Appreciate that a diverse workforce is a strength and reflects on organizational practices and policies that

may or may not foster and create opportunities for historically underrepresented populations.
- Advocate for implicit bias, antiracist, and cultural competency training for your organization.

> **Note:**
>
> While some medical school programs have begun to incorporate education on implicit bias, cultural competency and humility, and antiracism, such training is not universal. Programs should universally strive to include these constructs across educational venues and levels.

> **Note:**
>
> Though cultural competency can help inform practice, generalizations should be avoided. Assuming culture based on a person's identity can be incredibly error prone and damaging in and of itself.

SOCIAL DETERMINANTS OF HEALTH SCREENING

Provider-older adult interactions create opportunity for social determinants of health screening. At a minimum, this should include: self-identified race and ethnicity, employment and education, use of tobacco/alcohol/drugs, car and firearm safety, domestic violence history, marital and children status, housing status, social supports, and information on neighborhood and built environment.

Geriatricians and teams have opportunities to identify unmet needs and provide immediate resources or act as a bridge to community-based services that have the potential to create meaningful change in the health and quality of life of older adults. Social determinants of health screening also has the potential to encourage person-centered, trauma-informed care; improve diagnosis and reduce missed diagnosis; provide resources that increase medication adherence; and potentially avoid unnecessary health care utilization.

When conducting assessments that consider social determinants of health, there are important considerations to prevent common errors and maximize organizational efficacy:

- While some clinics conduct social determinants of health screening through use of structured templates and tools, an open-ended, life-story approach may be better suited to older adults. Several visits may be required for a thorough life story and social determinants of health screening in order to promote greater buy-in and reduce burden on both the older adult and clinician. Allow the older adult to disclose the manner in which they identify with different social categories;

TABLE 6-1 ■ LIFE STORY PROMPTS WITH SOCIAL DETERMINANTS OF HEALTH SCREENING TAILORED TO OLDER ADULTS

EXAMPLE LIFE STORY PROMPTS	SOCIAL DETERMINANTS OF HEALTH EXAMPLES
"Tell me about your childhood." *"Could you share more about your early adulthood?"*	• Education • Neighborhood/built environment context • Residential segregation • Family and social support • Employment and work environment
"Can you tell me more about your family?" *"Do you provide care for any family or friends?"*	• Family and friend network • Social support, loneliness • Family stress • Caregiving status
"Can you describe your house?" *"Tell me more about your neighborhood."*	• Accessibility to health care, healthy foods, and transportation • Housing quality, stability, and safety • Neighborhood disadvantage • Environmental conditions
"What does your day-to-day life right now look like?" *"Is there anything that you would like to be doing in your day-to-day life that you are not doing right now? Why might that be?"*	• Neighborhood safety • Housing instability and quality • Poverty • Food insecurity • Caregiving status • Social network
"How easy or hard is it for you to care for your health right now?" *"What might be getting in the way?"*	• Access to affordable insurance, primary care provider, transportation • Poverty • Language and literacy needs • Health beliefs and cultural factors
Additionally, if not routinely collected, asking open-ended questions around the items to the right can also provide crucial information to inform intervention.	• Self-identified race, ethnicity, gender, and sex identities • Immigration • Religious or spiritual beliefs/practices • Coping style • Health behaviors

match the language they use. **Table 6-1** includes example life-story prompts that may allow for probing of social determinants of health and unmet needs impacting older adult health.

- Comprehensive assessment of social determinants of health and use of a life-story approach may heighten awareness of barriers that older adults may face to their health and of lifelong stressors that may be shaping current status. Be ready to meet newly identified older adult needs by:
  - Partnering with community-based organizations to streamline referrals
  - Integrating mental health services to address lifelong stressors and trauma
- Do not assume a person's social identities based on their visible characteristics, or previously recorded responses. Not only are social identities self-constructed, but some can shift over time.
- Do not withhold treatment or therapy based on the potential that someone's social determinants of health may make access or implementation more challenging. Rather, gauge the client's preferences for treatment or therapy and find individualized, tailored resources that will make that preference possible.
- Do not commit attribution error in associating a health issue with someone's identity or background, which could contribute to invasive, inappropriate questioning, or escalation of care. Rather, recognize that social determinants of health often work in concert with other factors to shape health outcomes.

To initiate social determinants of health screening and intervention, begin a conversation within your organization on the timing and location for social needs screening and intervention delivery; determine team process for conducting assessment and intervention; tailor screening tools to the local older adult population and known unmet needs; determine process for matching older adults with local resources based on their self-identified unmet needs and establish relationships with corresponding community-based organizations; and develop a process for documentation and follow-up.

TABLE 6-2 ■ EXAMPLES OF ORGANIZATIONS PROVIDING COMMUNITY-BASED SERVICES AND SUPPORTS

Key Organizations Providing Community-Based Services and Supports

- Area Agencies on Aging represent over 600 state-designated centers that focus on meeting the needs of older adults 60 years and older at a local or regional level.
- Aging and Disability Resource Centers (ADRCs) are present in a growing number of states and territories and serve as resource hub to connect adults with long-term care services and benefits like Medicaid.
- Meals on Wheels programs provide home-delivered meals in many areas across the United States with some programs also supporting congregate meals at senior centers. They may also incorporate important foci on social contact and safety.
- Senior Centers located in many sites throughout the nation can act as direct providers of services designated by the Older Americans Act. These centers often rely on federal, state, and local funding alongside grants and donations.
- Adult Day Services provide a community-based care option for persons who may rely on frequent care of a family member or friend. Centers often function during regular business hours, providing respite for the caregivers. Additionally, centers function at distinct levels, providing social care, medical/health care, or specialized care. Frequently, private pay is required to access these services.
- Promising home-based care models focused on functional goals and safety, like the Community Aging in Place, Advancing Better Living for Elders (CAPABLE) program address medical and home environment related needs for low-income older adults.
- Programs of All-Inclusive Care for the Elderly (PACE) are Medicare and Medicaid funded programs that provide community-based, coordinated care for adults 55 years and older who would otherwise require nursing home-level of care. PACE requires use of designated providers, cares, and services. They are only located in select, typically urban areas of the United States.

Example Tools for Finding Area-Specific Organizations

- To search for general supports and services and/or locate local Area Agencies on Aging (AAAs) and Aging and Disability Resource Centers (ADRCs), use the Eldercare Locator of the Administration on Aging: https://eldercare.acl.gov/Public/Index.aspx
- To search for resources for caregivers of people living at home or in residential settings, use the Family Caregiver Alliance Services by State tool: https://caregiver.org/family-care-navigator
- To search for local Meals on Wheels services, use the tool available at: https://www.mealsonwheelsamerica.org/
- To search for adult day services centers, follow guidance from the National Adult Day Services Association: http://nadsa.org/consumers/choosing-a-center/
- Recommend use of United Way's 2-1-1 service for broad needs around food, housing, health, for example. Dial 2-1-1 or search online here: https://www.211.org/about-us/your-local-211

COMMUNITY-BASED SUPPORTS AND SERVICES

A preliminary understanding of available community-based supports and services (CBSS) is needed prior to making recommendations, with examples specific to the United States context provided in **Table 6-2**. CBSS aim to meet educational, wellness, nutritional, counseling, financial, safety, and housing needs, yet CBSS availability and quality vary greatly. For example, CBSS in rural areas may provide services to older adults across several counties, requiring providers and older adults to drive long distances for access. While more than 20% of older adults regularly access CBSS, there may be unmet needs among these adults and those not yet connected to CBSS.

CBBS for older adults were first expanded by the 1965 passage of the Older Americans Act (OAA). Funding is allocated to services in at least these areas: supportive services, congregate and home-delivered meals, preventive health, caregiver support, abuse prevention, and ombudsman. The OAA made possible the Administration on Aging (AoA) and corresponding state-specific Area Agencies on Aging (AAAs). AAAs operate on federal, state, and municipal funding, though they also rely on private funding sources.

Over 3 million older adults rely on meal services, caregiver supports, home care, adult day services, and transportation on a regular basis, with over 9 million receiving these services intermittently. These services result in less meals skipped and greater nutrition, social contact, decreased caregiver burden, delays to institutionalization, among other outcomes. Resources vary by state and region. In some areas, waiting lists for these services are long.

A CASE STUDY

A 75-year-old veteran, Marshall, who self-identifies as African-American is being evaluated in a memory clinic for cognitive concerns. Upon evaluation in clinic, Marshall is found to have significant visuospatial and short-term memory impairment. He also shared that he recently had several, "fender benders", raising concerns regarding his driving safety. Dr. M., the geriatrician evaluating Marshall, asks if he has any family that could be contacted as they have determined that Marshall can no longer drive safely. Marshall says there is only one person he knows they could call. Dr. M. reviews Marshall's social history, sees that he is married, and asks if Marshall knows his wife's number, assuming this is the individual he would like to have called. Marshall grabs his car keys off the desk, yells "No!", and storms out of the office. Security cannot locate Marshall in a timely manner. On his way home, Marshall suffered minor injuries in a motor vehicle accident and is admitted to the hospital for treatment.

Several days later, on rounds, Dr. M. swings by Marshall's room. While Marshall is getting a CT scan, there is a visitor in the room. Dr. M. asks if he is a friend of Marshall's, and the visitor informs Dr. M. that he is Marshall's partner. Dr. M. learns that although Marshall was married and had several children, he identified as queer his entire life and suffered considerable discrimination and harm during his years of service in the military over questions of his sexual orientation. Due to the discrimination he encountered, he limited his social circle, made very few friends, and lost contact with much of his family, leaving him isolated. About 5 years ago, he decided to come out to his children as he wanted to spend the end of his life with his partner, but this resulted in him losing contact with all of his children. The visitor asks Dr. M. why he was not called when Marshall had his first visit, so he could come and take him home.

Reflection questions: (1) How does intersectionality play a role in this case study, specifically in the way Marshall may interact with the health care system? (2) When providing care to older adults, what are the risks of labels or assumptions?

FURTHER READING

Bailey ZD, Krieger N, Agénor M, Graves J, Linos N, Bassett MT. Structural racism and health inequities in the USA: evidence and interventions. *Lancet.* 2017;389(10077):1453–1463.

Ben-Shlomo Y, Kuh D. A life course approach to chronic disease epidemiology: conceptual models, empirical challenges and interdisciplinary perspectives. *Int J Epidemiol.* 2002;31(2):285–293.

Bharmal N, Derose KP, Felician MF, Weden MM. *Understanding the Upstream Social Determinants of Health.* Santa Monica, CA: RAND Corporation; 2015.

Braveman P. What are health disparities and health equity? We need to be clear. *Public Health Rep.* 2014;129 (Suppl 2): 5–8.

Carbado DW, Crenshaw KW, Mays VM, Tomlinson B. Intersectionality: mapping the movements of a theory. *Du Bois Rev.* 2013;10(2):303–312.

Czyzewski K. Colonialism as a broader social determinant of health. *Int Indig Policy J.* 2011;2(1):5.

Hammonds EM, Reverby SM. Toward a historically informed analysis of racial health disparities since 1619. *Am J Public Health.* 2019;109(10):1348–1349.

Hill CV, Pérez-Stable EJ, Anderson NA, Bernard MA. The National Institute on Aging Health Disparities Research Framework. *Ethn Dis.* 2015;25(3):245–254.

Jones NL, Gilman SE, Cheng TL, Drury SS, Hill CV, Geronimus AT. Life course approaches to the causes of health disparities. *Am J Public Health.* 2019;109(Suppl 1): S48–S55.

National Academies of Sciences, Engineering, and Medicine. Integrating social care into the delivery of health care: moving upstream to improve the Nation's health. Washington, DC, National Academies of Sciences, Engineering, and Medicine, 2019.

Phelan JC, Link BG, Tehranifar P. Social conditions as fundamental causes of health inequalities: theory, evidence, and policy implications. *J Health Soc Behav.* 2010; 51 Suppl:S28–40.

Tsai J, Cerdeña JP, Khazanchi R, et al. There is no 'African American Physiology': the fallacy of racial essentialism. *J Intern Med.* 2020;288(3):368–370.

US Department of Health and Human Services, Office of Disease Prevention and Health Promotion: Healthy People 2030. https://health.gov/healthypeople/objectives-and-data/social-determinants-health. Accessed March 23, 2021.

Part II

Principles of Geriatrics

Chapter **7**

Decision Making and Advance Care Planning: What Matters Most

Daniel D. Matlock, Hillary D. Lum

OVERVIEW: A COMMENT ON PERSPECTIVE

The importance of perspective is the basis of any discussion of decision making. All decisions are viewed through the lens of the decision maker. In medicine, decisions can be viewed from many perspectives including the patients, families, the clinicians, the health care system, and even society. This array of lenses with differing motivations and incentives can lead to widely disparate decisions. For example, a doctor may recommend an expensive medication such as a new chemotherapy in the interest of helping a patient live longer. The patient on the other hand may not be singularly focused on survival and/or may find the side effects intolerable. The family caregiver may be overwhelmed in coordinating medical care. The health care system in which the physician works may be eager to reap the reimbursements of an infusion associated with the medicine. Meanwhile, society may be concerned that the high costs and marginal benefits of the medication provides relatively little value (higher costs relative to the benefits) to society as a whole.

This chapter is not meant to be an exhaustive discussion of the science of decision making. As such, a detailed discussion of the contemporary politics and economics of cost effectiveness, insurance design, cost sharing, and other issues essential to understanding decision making at the health care system or societal level are beyond the scope of this chapter. Rather, this chapter will take a clinical perspective focusing on the challenges and opportunities for patients, surrogate decision makers, clinicians, and others involved in the complicated decision making with older adults.

Learning Objectives

- To understand the modern legal and ethical framework of clinical decision making.
- To describe how and why decision making is different and more challenging for older adults.
- To recognize the importance of incorporating patients' and families' outcome goals as the drivers of medical decision making.
- To understand the process of advance care planning and clinical tools available for it.

Key Clinical Points

1. Patients' and families' perspectives, goals, and values should be the major drivers of medical decision making.
2. Age-related changes, multiple chronic conditions, multifactorial symptoms, changing accuracy of diagnostic tests, changing patient goals, and family perspectives all sum in making decision making more challenging for older adults.
3. The history and physical examination should include a detailed assessment of the person's social/living situation, functional status, mood, and cognition.
4. Ascertainment of patients' preferences for current or future medical decisions, which are known to vary among older patients and patients with multiple health conditions, should occur early and often.

THEORETICAL FOUNDATION OF MODERN MEDICAL DECISION MAKING

Modern medical decision making sits largely on an ethical foundation. Grounded firmly on the ethical principle of autonomy, emphasis on a patient-centered approach has been rising since the early twentieth century when courts began charging physicians with battery for performing operations to which patients did not consent. While judges have softened this to negligence over time, court cases in the United States, including those involving Karen Ann Quinlan, Nancy Cruzan, and Terri Schiavo, and acts of US Congress such as the Patient Self-Determination Act continue to affirm a patient's and/or surrogate's right to determine their medical treatment plan.

The movement, often called "patient-centered care" is based on an underlying assumption that people make decisions in a normative and rational way. Normative decision theories, such as expected utility theory, are based on an ideal that people can approach decisions rationally and are able to cognitively weigh the risks and benefits of various interventions to make a good decision. However, there is a disconnection between the rhetoric of "good" decision making and the reality of decision making. Descriptive theories of decision making demonstrate that humans are subject to cognitive biases that cause decisions to deviate from what would be predicted by the normative/rational approach. One famous descriptive theory is prospect theory developed by Dan Kahneman and Amos Tversky. One aspect of this theory demonstrates that the way options are framed influences the decisions that are made. In a classic example, respondents were asked to imagine that an unusual flu-like disease is expected to kill 600 people. They were given the choice of two alternative programs which were mathematically identical according to the normative expected utility theory. In option A 200 people will be saved, and in option B there is one-third probability that 600 people will be saved and two-thirds probability that no one will be saved. When the options are presented as gains ("people will be saved"), 72% of the respondents chose to save the 200 people rather than take riskier option B. However, if options were presented as a loss ("400 people dying"), 78% of the respondents chose the riskier option B. This experiment elegantly demonstrates how decisions can change drastically simply based on framing; that when options are presented as gains, people tend to be risk averse, and when options are presented as losses, people tend to be risk seeking. Of note, the respondents to that survey were medical professionals highlighting the point that clinicians and patients alike are equally susceptible to these biases. Prospect theory is just one example from the growing field of behavioral economics (also referred to as cognitive psychology). The influences and applications of these theories to modern medical decision making is an active area of research.

The challenge for all clinicians and patients making decisions at the bedside is in finding ways to build a bridge between the legal and ethical mandate to promote patient-centered care and informed consent and the behavioral aspects where decision making, including related to future decision making, is not always rational. Ultimately, good decision making involves elicitation of the patients' priorities among general, often competing health outcome domains—such as longevity versus comfort/symptom relief—to assure that these preferences drive all evaluation and management decisions.

DECISION MAKING AND OLDER ADULTS: UNIQUE CHALLENGES

Clinical decision making for older adults, including diagnosis, treatment, and desired outcomes, is different and more challenging than it is for younger patients. Generally, the primary goal of medical care in younger adult patients is diagnosis of the disease causing the presenting symptoms, signs, and/or laboratory abnormalities. Treatment is targeted toward the pathophysiologic mechanisms deemed responsible for the disease. Survival is generally paramount. Relevant clinical outcomes are determined by the specific diseases and often include cure if the disease is acute.

In older adults, the conventional disease-specific approach is not optimal for several reasons. First, age-related physiologic changes in most organ systems affect diagnostic test interpretation and responses to treatments. Additionally, the average 75-year-old suffers from 3.5 chronic diseases. With multiple coexisting chronic diseases, there is a less consistent relationship between the pathology, the disease, and the clinical manifestations. One disease may obscure the presentation of another and treatment of one may increase the severity of another. With multiple coexisting diseases, it becomes difficult, and often impossible, to assess the severity of individual diseases and to ascribe health and/or functional status to specific disease processes.

Second, many distressing symptoms or impairments among older persons, such as pain, dizziness, fatigue, sleep problems, sensory impairments, and gait disorders cannot be ascribed to a single disease; instead, they result from the accumulated effect of physical, psychological, social, environmental, and other factors. A clinical focus solely on diagnosing and treating discrete diseases may lead to expensive diagnostic testing with inconclusive results. Worse, it may even harm if unnecessary and invasive interventions are not aligned with patient preferences. While clinicians may be reluctant to treat symptoms in younger and middle-aged patients without a specific diagnosis, treatment focused on improving symptoms in older patients with multimorbidity is often appropriate, because comfort and function are often the primary goals among this population.

Third, diagnostic test characteristics may be altered by age and comorbidity, making selection and interpretation of tests more complicated than for younger patients. Furthermore, both the benefits and harms of treatment regimens may differ in the face of age-related physiologic changes and multimorbidity. A good example of this is found in cancer screening where the false positive rate of many tests often increase as people age. Further, the true positives may be detecting things (eg, low-grade prostate cancer) that might have been better left undiagnosed. Consequently, more consideration needs to be taken regarding the individual patient characteristics and their treatment goals.

Fourth, older patients vary in the importance they place on potential health outcomes. When asked, older persons can prioritize among competing goals of increased survival, comfort, cognitive function, and physical function, and in certain instances may opt for comfort or function over survival. Optimal clinical decision making in the care of older patients includes (a) the articulation of patient preferences or goals of care; (b) the estimation of prognosis based on disease and non-disease factors; and (c) clarification of the role that impairments (ie, cognitive, mobility, sensory) and non-disease-specific factors have on the attainment of these preferences and goals. The multiplicity of impairments and diseases; the contribution of psychological, social, cultural, and environmental factors to health conditions; the enhanced likelihood of harm as well as benefit from many interventions; and the variability in goals and preferences all combine to make clinical decision making in the care of older persons very complex.

Fifth, clinical decision making is further complicated in older patients because other persons, including the spouse/partner, adult children, other relatives, and significant others, are often actively involved, particularly when cognitive impairment is present. Involvement of family of choice is helpful and often crucial, since they may provide additional sources of information, facilitate adherence to treatment recommendations, and offer both emotional and instrumental support. Up to 70% of older adults lose the capacity to make decisions prior to death and require surrogates. Conflicts may arise, however, when goals of the patient and family differ. Navigating the need for patient confidentiality and family involvement, between independence and support, and between patient and family goals is a constant challenge. When based on an understanding of these factors, however, the clinical care of older persons is both effective and immensely gratifying.

DECISION MAKING: THE CLINICIAN'S PERSPECTIVE

Clinicians are tasked with evaluating a patient including performing a history and physical examination, initiating a diagnostic workup when appropriate, and determining what medically reasonable options are appropriate given the patient's unique situation. Clinicians must then explore the patient's goals and share in the decision making to assure that the chosen treatments align with the patient's goals. Especially if a family member or care partner is a part of the clinical encounter, the clinician should identify preferences for who and how other individuals should be involved in decision making.

Evaluation: The History

The clinical interview is an important element of the decision-making process. It can be used to establish a diagnosis and monitor treatment and prognosis. The altered, often attenuated, presentation of diseases, the coexistence of multiple processes, and the underreporting of symptoms in older patients mandate a reordering of the importance of various components of the history. The chief complaint, the cornerstone of history-taking in younger patients, has decreased relevance in older persons.

Social history is of paramount importance in the care of older adults. Knowing a person's living arrangements and financial situation as well as how they make decisions is essential. Especially as older adults experience cognitive or functional impairment that increasingly involves caregiver support, it is critical to identify preferences or need for a surrogate medical decision maker.

The clinical history of older persons should also include assessments of cognitive function, affect, and mood (depressive symptoms). It is particularly important to observe for concerns related to undiagnosed dementia or cognitive impairment that may affect the person's decision-making capacity. These topics are discussed in detail in Chapters 9 and 10. Briefly, mood and affect can be screened for easily with tools such as the two-question depressive screen. (In the past month, have you been sad, blue, or down in the dumps? Have you lost interest in most things or been unable to enjoy them?) More formal, systematic assessments should be undertaken if there is any question of depression (see Chapter 65).

Evaluation: The Physical

The physical examination in older persons differs from younger persons as well. The purpose of the physical examination in younger persons is primarily to diagnose specific diseases. The physical examination in older persons, however, also serves to identify treatable impairments such as muscle weakness, gait instability, or sensory impairments, and to directly observe the performance of key functional tasks.

While the content of the physical examination will be much the same for older, as for younger patients, given time constraints, high-yield, relevant, but less traditional, examination items should take precedence. For example, during day 5 of a hospitalization, it is likely more important to see if a patient can sit up or stand than to listen to the heart sounds. Other high-yield examination elements might include postural blood pressure, cognitive status, hearing and vision limitations including inspection of ear canal for cerumen, visual acuity, and foot examination.

Diagnostic testing is often used to support decision making. However, even this poses additional challenges among older adults. The value of a diagnostic test is best determined by considering whether the test is accurate, the target disorder is dangerous if left undiagnosed, the test has acceptable risks, and effective treatment exists. All of these criteria are relevant as older patients often have multiple health conditions and limited life expectancy changing both the accuracy and value of diagnostic testing. Also, because older adults vary in the emphasis they place on outcomes other than mortality, even a good diagnostic test may not be appropriate for an individual patient.

Deciding whether a diagnostic test is important requires consideration of its ability to change the probability of disease prior to test completion (called the pretest probability of the target disorder) to a probability of the disease after test completion (called the posttest probability). As for the physical examination, the coexistence of diseases and age-related changes may affect the sensitivity, specificity, predictive value, and interpretability of laboratory, imaging, and other ancillary tests. Consequently, most tests have lower value among older adults. In addition, age-referenced normal values and ranges have been developed for some, albeit, not most laboratory tests.

In older persons, there are additional issues to consider including the ability of the patient to complete the test and whether the test does more good than harm. A patient with significant gait impairment, for example, is not going to be able to complete an exercise stress test. And, it may not be appropriate to consider a particular diagnostic test in someone with multiple comorbidities and poor quality of life if the purpose of that testing does not align with the patient's goals. For example, a diagnosis of dyslipidemia is not clinically relevant in someone with advanced cancer.

In deciding whether to perform laboratory, imaging, or other ancillary tests, the clinician should consider the issues outlined in **Table 7-1** and the principles described in this chapter. This decision process is illustrated for the example of noninvasive imaging for carotid stenosis. Consider for example, an 80-year-old patient who presents with a transient ischemic attack. A carotid Doppler ultrasound is ordered and reveals greater than 70% stenosis of the carotid artery on the affected side. Magnetic resonance angiography (MRA) is ordered and the patient's family wants to discuss whether to proceed with the test. Before the MRA is done, several issues should be considered in addition to ensuring that surgery is available and effective in your setting. Would the patient consider carotid endarterectomy? If the answer is no, further diagnostic testing is not warranted. Are there significant comorbidities or contraindications to the surgery? For example, if a patient has advanced dementia and poor functional status, the benefits of surgery would be questionable both because of their competing morbidities limiting the time through which they might benefit and

the greater difficulty they might have in participating in the perioperative care and rehabilitation. If surgery might be contemplated, then it is appropriate to determine whether there are accurate and reliable tests for diagnosing carotid stenosis available in your setting.

A recent systematic review of the accuracy of noninvasive imaging tests compared with intra-arterial angiography for significant carotid stenosis in symptomatic patients can help with the last question noted above. Forty-one studies including 2541 patients were included in this review. The accuracy of the four imaging techniques for diagnosing significant carotid stenosis is provided in **Table 7-2**. For diagnosing 70% to 99% stenosis, the specificity was lowest for MRA and Doppler ultrasonography. Thus, MRA may result in inappropriate surgery in up to one in seven patients. This systematic review suggests that noninvasive testing cannot appropriately be used to recommend carotid

---

TABLE 7-1 ■ ISSUES TO CONSIDER IN DECIDING WHETHER TO PERFORM A DIAGNOSTIC TEST AND HOW TO INTERPRET RESULTS

- How will the results be used?
  - Establish a diagnosis
    - Is there a safe and effective treatment?
    - Do comorbid conditions preclude treatment or make it ineffective?
    - Will the patient accept the treatment?
  - Establish prognosis
    - Does patient want the information?
    - Monitor disease progression or response to therapy
  - Definition and interpretation of normal (see **Table 7-2**)
- Is the test accurate in the patient for whom it is being considered?
- Can the test distinguish persons with and without the targeted condition?
- Do the potential consequences of the test justify its cost and inconvenience?
- Can the test be performed and interpreted in a competent fashion?

TABLE 7-2 ■ ACCURACY OF NONINVASIVE IMAGING TECHNIQUES FOR DIAGNOSING 70% TO 99% CAROTID STENOSIS COMPARED WITH INTRA-ARTERIAL ANGIOGRAPHY

IMAGING TECHNIQUE	SENSITIVITY (95% CI)	SPECIFICITY (95% CI)	+LR	−LR
CEMRA	95% (88–97)	93% (89–96)	13	0.06
DUS	89% (85–92)	84% (77–89)	5.6	0.13
MRA	88% (82–92)	84% (76–97)	5.5	0.14
CTA	77% (68–84)	95% (91–97)	15	0.24

CEMRA, contrast-enhanced magnetic resonance angiography; CTA, computed tomographic angiography; DUS, Doppler ultrasonography; LR, likelihood ratio; MRA, magnetic resonance angiography.
Adapted with permission from Kelly AG, Holloway RG. Review: noninvasive imaging techniques may be useful for diagnosing 70% to 99% carotid stenosis in symptomatic patients. ACP J Club. 2006;145(3):77.

endarterectomy. Patients should be made aware that they will likely require intra-arterial angiography, which does carry a small but real risk of complications. Unless the clinician considers patient outcome goals and risk preferences as well as the accuracy of the diagnostic tests, some patients will have surgery who do not need or desire it and some medically treated patients will have preventable strokes.

DECISION MAKING—INCORPORATING THE PATIENT'S PERSPECTIVE

Patient-centered care dictates that clinical decision making should occur within the context of individual preferences and goals. Ascertainment of these preferences, which are known to vary among older patients and among patients with multiple health conditions, should occur early and often (see Chapter 7). Older persons rarely volunteer their preferences. Active solicitation of priorities and preferences, therefore, needs to be an integral part of the patient and family interview. Good patient-centered care does not mean that the doctor tells the patient what to do. This is the paternalism that modern ethics and Western legal systems have largely overturned. At the same time, good patient-centered care does not entail putting a smorgasbord of options in front of a person and telling them to choose—an approach that has even been called patient abandonment. Rather, decisions should be shared between the clinicians and their patients. Clinicians bring expertise in the medical information and patients bring expertise in themselves and what is important to them. Then, a shared decision is less about information provision and more about a conversation between two experts.

Matching Treatments to Patients' Goals

A body of research suggests that patients are not adequately informed when receiving medical interventions. A large national survey across nine different medical conditions demonstrated that patients scored low on their knowledge, even if they had received those procedures. Perhaps even more concerning is the literature that patients often receive care that they would not want. Many patients, especially older patients, have difficulty in choosing among a set of treatment options. Rather than having patients make every specific treatment choice, which is difficult and often not feasible for the large number of medical decisions that older adults face, encouraging patients to prioritize among different outcome domains allows them to express directly what is most important to them regarding their health care. The elicitation of priorities among general, often competing health outcome domains, including longevity, comfort/symptom relief, cognitive functioning and physical functioning should ideally drive all evaluation and management decisions.

The process of goal elicitation can be complicated and requires a clinician adept in handling the communication challenges that will arise. First, the setting for the discussion may need to be adapted to the specific impairments of some older persons. Impairments in hearing, visual acuity, and cognition, each prevalent among older persons, mandate a quiet, well-lit, and unhurried setting in order to have a meaningful discussion. Multiple encounters may be required to complete the history and to gather the necessary information. While the patient remains the key informant, the discussion often needs to be supplemented by information obtained from the patient's family of choice, and/or other care providers, particularly if the older person has cognitive impairment.

Second, the process of goal elicitation can be emotional. Sometimes, a patient or family may articulate a goal that is just not feasible given their situation (eg, continuing to live alone in their home). Here, the task of the clinician is in helping the patient redefine goals that are feasible. This can be a difficult and emotional conversation for all involved. Often, to help patients define their goals, they must enter into the complicated discussion of prognosis. An area of active research is in improving clinicians' communication skills with patients to facilitate these patient-centered discussions.

ADVANCE CARE PLANNING: DECISION MAKING FOR FUTURE MEDICAL DECISIONS

An important aspect of decision making with older adults is planning for future medical decisions. This is often done through a process referred to as advance care planning (ACP). ACP is a process that supports adults at any age or stage of health in understanding and sharing their personal values, life goals, and preferences regarding future medical care. The goal of ACP is to help ensure that people receive medical care that is consistent with their values, goals, and preferences when they cannot speak for themselves. ACP is a multistep and iterative process that involves having conversations that explore the individual's values, identifying a surrogate decision maker, and translating those values and preferences into current and/or future medical care plans through shared decision making. Conversations and care plans may be documented in advance directives, portable medical orders, and/or clinical documentation as part of the patient's medical record. For patients who are at risk for a life-threatening event because they have a serious life-limiting medical condition, which may include advanced frailty, it may be appropriate to offer voluntary shared decision making related to specific life-sustaining treatment preferences (ie, CPR, ICU level care, hospitalization, comfort care) and then complete a POLST form, which is a portable medical order set that is available in many states (www.POLST.org).

Practical Approaches to Advance Care Planning Conversations

ACP and goals of care conversations can occur in various settings, including ambulatory care, emergency departments,

TABLE 7-3 ■ ADVANCE CARE PLANNING IS A MULTISTEP PROCESS

STEP	EXAMPLES OF QUESTIONS TO ENGAGE PATIENTS IN ACP DISCUSSIONS
Explore the person's readiness and identify barriers to advance care planning.	• "Advance care planning helps me work with you and your family to understand how to plan your medical care in case you lose the ability to make decisions. Can we talk about this today?" • "Have you ever completed an advance directive, like a living will? What did it say? Is it up-to-date?"
Identify a trusted person as a medical decision maker to help clinicians apply overarching care goals to specific clinical situations in the event that the person loses decisional capacity.	• "Is there someone you trust to be involved in making medical decisions on your behalf, if you are not able to do so?" "It is important to include her in these conversations so she knows what is important to you. Do you think she could come with you to your next clinic visit?" • "What have you talked about?" or "What would you tell him is important about your medical care?
Explore the person's values and priorities in life, and discuss what constitutes an acceptable quality of life.	• "Have you had any previous experience with making decisions about medical care during a serious illness? Can you tell me about that?" • "When (eg, you were hospitalized; a loved one died), did this situation change your thoughts about what is important to you in the future or what would be unacceptable, where you wouldn't want to live like that?"
Document care preferences in an advance directive document (eg, medical power of attorney, living will) or the electronic medical record; and ensure that written plans are communicated, stored, and retrievable.	• "Since you've chosen (someone) to help make decisions on your behalf if you are very sick and unable to speak with me, I recommend that you complete the medical power of attorney form to make it official." • "Can you bring in your advance directives? It helps me, the clinic, and the hospital, know what is important to you if you are very sick."

inpatient hospitalization, post-acute care, and long-term care. ACP conversations often involve patients, individuals serving as surrogate decision makers, and health care practitioners. While some ACP conversations are brief, other conversations may benefit from the structure and preparation in family meetings. For older adults, the ACP process is well-suited to outpatient, longitudinal care and should unfold over time; however it also often occurs around changes in medical conditions, new diagnoses, changes in functional or cognitive status, or care transitions such as hospitalization or admission to residential care.

Health care providers should have phrases for introducing a desire to discuss ACP, such as, "We're taking a step back to talk about the big picture with your care. I do this with all my patients so I can provide you with the kind of care you would want." The introduction should aim to normalize the process and emphasize to the patient and family the goal of providing medical care that is aligned with their goals. Then, clinicians and teams can engage individuals and their families by introducing key concepts over time, as outlined in **Table 7-3**. Each concept can be discussed individually and often in 5 minutes or less, based on time constraints and patient needs.

Many clinicians provide comprehensive care for older adults with multiple chronic conditions and functional limitations. Throughout an individual's journey of living with advanced illness, there are opportunities for ongoing conversations. Developed by the Ariadne Labs, the Serious Illness Conversation Guide helps clinicians conduct successful conversations in an intentional sequence. The guide is readily available and provides patient-tested language.

Given that discussing ACP may bring up strong emotions, there are communication training programs (ie, brief videos from VitalTalk) to help clinicians navigate these emotions to best support their patients (see **Table 7-4**).

Person- and Family-Centered Tools to Prepare Individuals

Person and family-centered tools can assist patients with knowledge and decision making related to ACP. Because ACP conversations can be a personnel- and time-intensive process, helping patients and families begin this process on their own is useful. Health care teams can systematically incorporate the use of patient-centered tools to help engage patients before meeting to have these conversations. **Table 7-4** summarizes resources that are available for practical use by patients and their families. For example, the Stanford Letter Project has videos of diverse individuals sharing their wishes with family or their doctor. The PREPARE website demonstrates multiple steps of ACP, such as deciding on flexibility in decision making for surrogate decision makers (see **Table 7-4**).

Incorporating Cultural, Religious, and Spiritual Values

ACP conversations will be more successful with consideration of the individual's family, cultural, spiritual, and religious norms. In a study of patient-reported barriers to high-quality end-of-life care, patients from multiethnic backgrounds identified: (1) finance/health insurance barriers, (2) doctor behaviors, (3) communication chasm between doctors and patients, (4) family beliefs/behaviors,

TABLE 7-4 ■ ADVANCE CARE PLANNING RESOURCES

RESOURCE	DESCRIPTION	WEB ADDRESS
ACP Decisions	ACP videos describing overall goals of care, CPR, and mechanical ventilation have been shown to influence patients' and surrogates' preferences for end-of-life care.	http://www.acpdecisions.org/
American Bar Association: Consumer's Toolkit for Health Care Advance Planning	Toolkit for patients regarding all aspects of advance care planning and state-specific advance directives.	www.abanet.org/aging (select under Resources & Research)
The Conversation Project	Written toolkit with values-based questions to help individuals start conversations with loved ones.	http://theconversationproject.org/
GO WISH Card Game	A card game that supports thinking and talking about what's important to individuals and their family members if someone becomes seriously ill.	http://codaalliance.org/go-wish/
National POLST	Resources for health care practitioners about shared decision-making conversations and appropriate use of portal medical orders for life-sustaining treatments.	www.polst.org
PREPARE	A website with video stories in English or Spanish that focuses on preparing people through a five-step process for exploring personal preferences and discussing with doctors and family.	https://www.prepareforyourcare.org
Respecting Choices	National training for medical professionals in advance care planning, using a facilitator-based approach.	https://respectingchoices.org/
Serious Illness Care Program	Resources for teams and health systems to develop a scalable serious illness care program.	http://ariadnelabs.org
Stanford Letter Project	An online template that creates an Advance Directive as a letter to the doctor; written at a fifth grade level, available in multiple languages.	http://med.stanford.edu/letter.html

(5) health system barriers, and (6) cultural/religious barriers. While the clinician should never assume that all members of a group have the same beliefs, knowledge of some of the norms can aid in the future medical care planning discussions and decision making. Additionally, literacy and language-appropriate documents may enhance ACP. Clinicians cannot predict what an individual patient wants or is even willing to discuss. The only way to know is to ask in a nonjudgmental, patient-centered manner. Questions to help understand an individual's perspective could include: "Are there any cultural, spiritual, or religious factors that I should know about as we talk about the care you would want if you got sicker?" and "How do your religious or spiritual beliefs influence your wishes for your medical care near the end of your life?"

CONCLUSION—THE ART

As noted above, decision making with older adults is challenging in many ways. For most, life comes with multimorbidity and functional decline and the traditional disease-focused models do not work. While a lucky few have truly compressed morbidity, the majority of older adults experience gradual decline, mounting morbidity, and frailty. However, underneath the challenge is a deep richness. Helping patients and families clarify their outcome goals and assuring that treatments align with those goals will never be automated by a machine. Perhaps more than anywhere else, the art and humanity of the sacred practice of medicine thrive when caring clinicians engage in decision making with older adults.

FURTHER READING

Beauchamp TL, Childress JF. *Principles of Biomedical Ethics.* 6th ed. New York, NY: Oxford University Press; 2008.

Bernacki RE, Block SD, Force ACoPHVCT. Communication about serious illness care goals: a review and synthesis of best practices. *JAMA Intern Med.* 2014; 174(12):1994–2003.

Boockvar KS, Lachs MS. Predictive value of nonspecific symptoms for acute illness in nursing home residents. *J Am Geriatr Soc.* 2003;51:1111–1115.

Boyd CM, Darer J, Boult C, et al. Clinical practice guidelines and quality of care for older patients with multiple comorbid diseases: implications for pay for performance. *JAMA*. 2005;294:716–724.

Fried TR, Bradley EH, Towle VR, et al. Understanding the treatment preferences of seriously ill patients. *N Engl J Med*. 2002;346:1061–1066.

Guyatt GH, Oxman AD, Ali M, et al. Laboratory diagnosis of iron-deficiency anemia: an overview. *J Gen Intern Med*. 1992;7:145–153.

Hirsch C. The Mini-cog had high sensitivity and specificity for diagnosing dementia in community-dwelling older adults. *ACP J Club*. 2001;74.

Ilic D, Neuberger MM, Djulbegovic M, et al. Screening for prostate cancer. *Cochrane Database Syst Rev*. 2013;(1):CD004720.

Kelly A, Holloway RG. Noninvasive imaging techniques may be useful for diagnosing 70 to 99% carotid stenosis in symptomatic patients. *ACP J Club*. 2006;145(3):77.

Kim S, Goldstein D, Hasher L, et al. Framing effects in younger and older adults. *J Gerontol*. 2005;60:P215–P218.

King JS, Moulton BW. Rethinking informed consent: the case for shared medical decision-making. *Am J Law Med*. 2006;32(4):429–501.

Lum HD, Sudore RL, Bekelman DB. Advance care planning in the elderly. *Med Clin North Am*. 2015;99(2):391–403.

Periyakoil VS, Neri E, Kraemer H. Patient-reported barriers to high-quality, end-of-life care: a multiethnic, multilingual, mixed-methods study. *J Palliat Med*. 2016;19(4):373–379.

Quill TE, Cassel CK. Nonabandonment: a central obligation for physicians. *Ann Intern Med*. 1995;122(5):368–374.

Scanlan J, Borson S. The Mini-cog: receiver operating characteristics with expert and naïve raters. *Int J Geriatr Psych*. 2001;16:216–222.

Silveira MJ, Kim SYH, Langa KM. Advance directives and outcomes of surrogate decision making before death. *N Engl J Med*. 2010;362(13):1211–1218.

Sudore RL, Fried TR. Redefining the "planning" in advance care planning: preparing for end-of-life decision making. *Ann Intern Med*. 2010;153(4):256–261.

Sudore RL, Lum HD, You JJ, et al. Defining advance care planning for adults: a consensus definition from a multidisciplinary Delphi panel. *J Pain Symptom Manage*. 2017;53(5):821–832.e821.

Teno JM, Fisher ES, Hamel MB, Coppola K, Dawson NV. Medical care inconsistent with patients' treatment goals: association with 1-year Medicare resource use and survival. *J Am Geriatr Soc*. 2002;50(3):496–500.

Tinetti ME, Bogardus ST Jr, Agostini JV. Potential pitfalls of disease-specific guidelines for patients with multiple conditions. *N Engl J Med*. 2004;351:2870–2874.

Tinetti ME, Fried T. The end of the disease era. *Am J Med*. 2004;116:179–185.

Tversky A, Kahneman D. The framing of decisions and the psychology of choice. *Science*. 1981;211(4481):453–458.

US Preventive Services Task Force. Screening for dementia: recommendation and rationale. *Ann Intern Med*. 2003;138(11):925.

Wardlaw JM, Chappell FM, Best JJ, et al. Non-invasive imaging compared with intra-arterial angiography in the diagnosis of symptomatic carotid stenosis: a meta-analysis. *Lancet*. 2006;367:1503–1512.

Widera E, Anderson WG, Santhosh L, McKee KY, Smith AK, Frank J. Family meetings on behalf of patients with serious illness. *N Engl J Med*. 2020;383(11):e71.

Zikmund-Fisher BJ, Couper MP, Singer E, et al. Deficits and variations in patients' experience with making 9 common medical decisions: the DECISIONS survey. *Med Decis Making*. 2010;30(suppl 5):S85–S95.

Chapter 8

Principles of Geriatric Assessment

David B. Reuben, Ryan J. Uyan, Valerie S. Wong

Geriatric assessment describes the health evaluation of the older patient and emphasizes components and outcomes different from that of the standard medical evaluation. This approach recognizes that the health status of older persons is dependent upon influences beyond the manifestations of their medical conditions. Among these are social, psychological, and mental health, and environmental factors. Geriatric assessment also places high value upon functional status, both as a dimension to be evaluated and as an outcome to be improved or maintained. Frailty is a related construct that is increasingly being measured for prognostic and occasionally for outcome purposes.

Although in the strictest sense geriatric assessment is a diagnostic process, many use the term to include both evaluation and management. Moreover, geriatric assessment is sometimes used to refer to evaluation by the individual clinician and at other times is used to refer to a more interdisciplinary process, comprehensive geriatric assessment (CGA) and adaptations by various specialties.

This chapter is divided into four components: (1) geriatric assessment by the individual clinician, with an emphasis on the outpatient setting; (2) a strategic approach to geriatric assessment for the practicing clinician; (3) CGA and evidence for its effectiveness; and (4) lessons learned from geriatric assessment that have been applied to health care delivery of older persons.

GERIATRIC ASSESSMENT BY THE INDIVIDUAL CLINICIAN

Geriatric assessment (**Figure 8-1**) by the individual clinician extends beyond the traditional disease-oriented medical evaluation of older persons' health to include assessment of cognitive, affective, social, economic, environmental, spiritual, functional, and frailty status, as well as a discussion of patient preferences regarding advance care planning. Assessment instruments can be used to guide these evaluations but do not substitute for clinical skills and judgment, including the skill of eliciting important items from the patient's history and physical examination. Systematic assessment of the multiple domains noted above ensures that the evaluation is comprehensive. Some clinicians may prefer to rely on less formal questions to probe

Learning Objectives

- To distinguish between geriatric assessment and comprehensive geriatric assessment.
- To identify the core components of geriatric assessment by individual clinicians.
- To learn practical approaches to geriatric assessment that can be administered within the constraints of a busy office practice.
- To understand the core components of comprehensive geriatric assessment.
- To know the evidence-based strengths and limitations of comprehensive geriatric assessment.
- To recognize how some important components of comprehensive geriatric assessment have been integrated into new health care innovations.

Key Clinical Points

1. Geriatric assessment extends beyond the traditional disease-oriented medical evaluation of older persons' health to include assessment of cognitive, affective, social, economic, environmental, spiritual, functional, and frailty status, as well as a discussion of patient preferences regarding advance directives.

2. Observing patients walking and performing balance maneuvers best assesses balance and gait disorders. Qualitative gait assessment can be performed while the patient is entering or leaving the examining room and can be augmented by measuring gait speed.

3. Although in 2020, the US Preventive Services Task Force (USPSTF) concluded that there is insufficient evidence on the balance of benefits and harms of screening

(Continued)

(Cont.)

for cognitive impairment, clinicians should assess cognition when there is suspicion of impairment or when conducting a Medicare Annual Wellness Visit.

4. Much of the germane information of the medical history can be obtained from old records, other professional or nonprofessional staff, or by self-report from patients or family members completing forms prior to office visits.

5. By delegating the administration of screening instruments for many of the important geriatric problems to trained office staff, the clinician may spend a short period of time reviewing the results of these screens and then decide which dimensions, if any, need greater evaluation.

6. In virtually all studies of comprehensive geriatric assessment, the process itself has resulted in improved detection and documentation of geriatric problems. However, such identification of problems has not always led to improved outcomes.

7. The best evidence for effectiveness of comprehensive geriatric assessment is for inpatient geriatric units and home assessments of young-old patients.

8. Concepts of comprehensive geriatric assessment have been incorporated into new successful models of care, specialty care, and disease management programs.

9. Geriatric comanagement programs for older patients with hip fractures have shown to shorten length of stay and reduce complications and discharge to an increased level of care compared to their prehospitalization living situation.

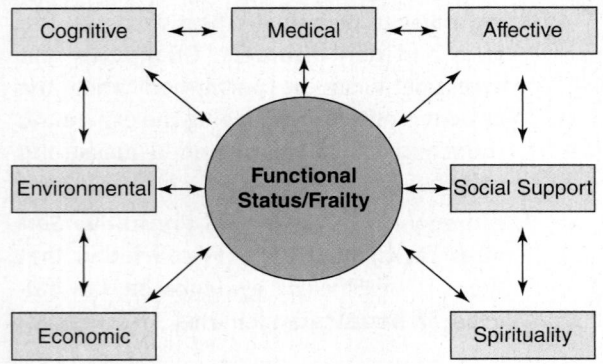

FIGURE 8-1. Components of geriatric assessment.

into potential problems but the responses to these should be documented in the patient's record.

Geriatric assessment differs according to the setting where the patient is being evaluated. In the hospital setting, the initial assessment is usually directed at the acute medical problem that precipitated the hospitalization and change from baseline. As the patient begins to recover and plans are initiated for discharge, other components (eg, social support, environment) assume increasing importance in the assessment. The inpatient setting can be problematic for geriatric assessment because of the rapidly changing status of several key dimensions. For example, a patient may temporarily become "dependent" on all measures of functional status when acutely ill and gradually improve prior to discharge. Because patients may overestimate their functional status based on their previous level of functioning, direct observational methods (eg, by nurses or rehabilitation therapists) provide a more accurate assessment. The patient's full potential to participate in rehabilitation may not be known until near the time of discharge.

Nursing home geriatric assessment requires that attention be directed to selected aspects of assessment such as nutritional status and self-care activities. Other components such as functional status at the instrumental activities of daily living level (eg, shopping, meal preparation) are less relevant in this setting. Geriatric assessment conducted in the patient's home provides an opportunity for assessment of environmental factors (eg, home safety) and may yield different insights into functional status (eg, cleanliness of the home).

Because the primary site of most clinicians' practices is the office setting, assessment techniques are described primarily for this setting. When appropriate, differing or particularly important information about assessment in other settings is added.

Components of the Geriatric Assessment

In addition to the standard medical history and physical examination, the clinician should systematically search for specific conditions that are common among older persons and that might have considerable impact on function. In the course of the traditional medical evaluation, these problems may go unnoticed because older patients fail to report them spontaneously. For example, they may not recognize that falling is a treatable medical problem. They may also be embarrassed to mention problems with maintaining urinary continence. Finally, they may believe that some symptoms, such as hearing loss, are normal aspects of aging that cannot be helped.

Visual Impairment

Visual impairment is a common and often underreported problem in the older population. The four major eye diseases (cataract, age-related macular degeneration, diabetic retinopathy, and glaucoma) increase in prevalence with age. Moreover, developing presbyopia is virtually universal and the vast majority of older persons require eyeglasses. Visual impairment has been associated with increased risk of falls, functional and cognitive decline, immobility, and depression. The high rates of vision disorders and their associated sequelae, the brevity of the screening process, and the treatments available for visual impairment justify screening for visual impairment. However, the revised 2016 US Preventive Services Task Force (USPSTF) guidelines concluded that there is insufficient evidence to determine whether screening older adults for vision impairment improves functional outcomes.

The standard method of screening for problems with visual acuity is the Snellen eye chart, which requires the patient to stand 20 ft from the chart and read letters, using corrective lenses. Patients fail the screen if they are unable to read all the letters on the 20/40 line with their eyeglasses (best corrected vision). A home-printable vision screening test for telemedicine has been validated.

Hearing Impairment

Hearing impairment is among the most common medical conditions reported by older persons, affecting approximately one-third of those age 65 or older. Hearing impairment is associated with reduced cognitive, emotional, social, and physical function, leading to increased hospitalizations and delirium. The use of amplification devices has led to improved functional status and quality of life in older persons.

Screening for hearing loss can be accomplished by several methods (**Table 8-1**). The most accurate of these is the Welch Allyn AudioScope 3 (Welch Allyn, Inc., Skaneateles Falls, NY), a handheld otoscope with a built-in audiometer. The AudioScope 3 can be set at several different levels of intensity, but should be set at 40 dB to evaluate hearing in older persons. A pretone at 60 dB is delivered and then four tones (500, 1000, 2000, and 4000 Hz) at 40 dB are delivered. Patients fail the screening if they are unable to hear either the 1000- or 2000-Hz frequency in both ears or both the 1000- and 2000-Hz frequencies in one ear, indicating the need for formal audiometric testing.

A simple alternative is based on the patient's own subjective report of hearing loss. A self-reported hearing loss question involves asking patients a single question of "Do you have difficulty hearing?" An affirmative answer is then considered to be a positive test for hearing loss, and patients should be referred to an audiologist.

Another alternative is the whispered voice test, which is administered by whispering three to six random words (numbers, words, or letters) at a set distance (6, 8, 12, or 24 inches) from the person's ear and then asking the patient to repeat the words. The examiner should be positioned behind the person to prevent speech reading and the opposite ear should be covered or occluded during the examination. Patients fail the screening if they are unable to repeat half of the whispered words correctly.

There are several screening questionnaires for hearing loss including the Hearing Handicap Inventory for the Elderly—Screening Version (HHIE-S), the Hearing Self-Assessment Questionnaire (HSAQ), and the Revised Five Minute hearing test. These screening tests are all self-administered and contain about 10 to 15 items. Although these questionnaires are brief and easy to administer, their accuracy for detecting mild hearing loss is inferior to audiometry.

A 2011 review of the evidence on screening of hearing loss in older adults found that inquiring about self-perceived hearing loss or the whisper test at 2 ft had similar rates of detecting hearing loss as the tone-emitting otoscope or formal hearing questionnaire. The most recent USPSTF review of screening concluded that there is insufficient evidence to formally recommend hearing screening for this population.

Malnutrition/Weight Loss (See Also Chapter 30)

Malnutrition is a global term that encompasses many different nutritional problems that are associated with diverse health consequences. Both extremes of body weight place older people at risk for subsequent functional impairment, morbidity, and mortality. Among community-dwelling older persons, the most common nutritional disorder is obesity. In addition, a small percentage of community-dwelling older persons have energy or protein energy undernutrition, which places them at higher risk for death and functional decline. Protein energy undernutrition is defined by the presence of clinical (physical signs such as wasting, low body mass index) and biochemical (albumin or other protein) evidence of insufficient intake.

TABLE 8-1 ■ SIMPLE TESTS OF HEARING LOSS

QUESTION/TEST	TIME TO ADMINISTER	LIKELIHOOD RATIO			
		POSITIVE		NEGATIVE	
		For 25 or > 30 dB loss	For > 40 dB loss	For 25 or > 30 dB loss	For > 40 dB loss
Audioscope	1–2 min	3.1–5.8	3.4	0.20–0.40	0.05
Single question: "Do you think you have a hearing loss?"	< 1 min	2.5	3.0	0.40	0.26
Whisper test	1 min	5.1	N/A	0.03	N/A
Hearing Handicap Inventory for the Elderly	2 min	3.5	3.1	0.52	0.43

On their initial visit, patients should be asked about weight loss within the previous year (> 4% should trigger further evaluation) and patients should be weighed at every subsequent office visit. Height should also be measured on the initial visit to allow calculation of body mass index (weight in kg/[height in meters]^2). Although screening for specific nutrients and vitamins is not recommended, older persons should be asked about intake of calcium and vitamin D, which are recommended for prevention of osteoporosis.

In hospitalized older persons, malnutrition has been associated with higher mortality rates, delayed functional recovery, and higher rates of nursing home use. The simplest and most practical method is for the nursing staff to report daily on the percentage of the diet that the patient is eating. Intake can be also measured through formal calorie counts. Laboratory monitoring is less likely to be useful. Although serum albumin levels can drop acutely during inflammatory states, physiologic stress, and in response to trauma or surgical conditions, this protein has a long half-life (approximately 18 days) and may provide an idea of the patient's baseline nutritional status. Prealbumin, which has a much shorter half-life (approximately 2 days) may be a better means of monitoring response to nutritional treatment. In the nursing home, weight loss or gain of greater than or equal to 5% in the past 30 days or greater than or equal to 10% in the last 180 days are Medicare Minimum Data Set triggers for malnutrition.

Urinary Incontinence

Urinary incontinence is common and estimated to affect 11% to 34% of older men and 17% to 55% of older women. Despite its high prevalence, incontinence is often under-recognized. Patients may find it embarrassing to raise the issue or they regard it as a normal aspect of aging. Urinary incontinence has been associated with depressive symptoms in older adults and is a major factor in nursing home placement. Moreover, effective treatments are available for incontinence. As a result, screening for urinary incontinence has been recognized as an indicator of quality of care.

Screening for urinary incontinence can be done with two questions: (1) "In the last year, have you ever lost your urine and gotten wet?" and if so, (2) "Have you lost urine on at least six separate days?" In a research setting, those who answered positive to both questions had high rates (79% for women and 76% for men) of urinary incontinence as determined by a clinician's evaluation (see Chapter 47).

The 3IQ questionnaire is another brief interviewer-administered instrument with high sensitivity and specificity that has been developed to distinguish between urinary stress and urge incontinence in women in primary care settings (**Table 8-2**).

The Women's Preventative Screening Initiative (WPSI) recommends annual screening for urinary incontinence, which should not be limited based on age, parity, or weight.

TABLE 8-2 ■ THE THREE INCONTINENCE QUESTIONS (3IQ)

1. During the last 3 mo, have you leaked urine (even a small amount?)

        Yes   No → [Questionnaire completed]

2. During the last 3 mo, did you leak urine:
   (Check all that apply.)
   a. When you were performing some physical activity, such as coughing, sneezing, lifting, or exercise?
   b. When you had the urge or the feeling that you needed to empty your bladder, but you could not get to the toilet fast enough?
   c. Without physical activity and without a sense of urgency?

3. During the last 3 mo, did you leak urine *most often*:
   (Check only one.)
   a. When you were performing some physical activity, such as coughing, sneezing, lifting, or exercise?
   b. When you had the urge or the feeling that you needed to empty your bladder, but you could not get to the toilet fast enough?
   c. Without physical activity and without a sense of urgency?
   d. About equally as often with physical activity as with a sense of urgency?

Definitions of type of urinary incontinence are based on response to question 3:

Response to Question 3	Type of Incontinence
a. Most often with physical activity	Stress only or stress predominant
b. Most often with the urge to empty the bladder predominant	Urge only or urge predominant
c. Without physical activity or sense of urgency cause	Other cause only or other predominant
d. About equally with physical activity and sense of urgency	Mixed

Balance and Gait Impairments and Falling

Over one-third of community-dwelling persons older than 65 fall every year. Falls are independently associated with functional and mobility decline.

Three screening questions, administered at the initial visit and annually, can identify older persons at subsequent risk for injurious falls: "Have you fallen and hurt yourself in the past year?", "Have you fallen two or more times in the past year?" (the best predictor of falls-related injury), and "Do you fear falling because of balance or gait?" The Centers for Disease Control and Prevention's 12-item Stay Independent Questionnaire (http://proptrehab.com/wp-content/uploads/2018/09/document9.pdf) is also a useful screening tool.

For those who fail the screen, a multifactorial falls assessment is indicated including testing balance, gait, and lower extremity strength; vision evaluation; medication review; measurement of orthostatic blood pressures; assessment of feet and footwear; and a home safety evaluation. Their risk of osteoporotic fracture should also be assessed using the FRAX, the WHO Fracture Risk Assessment Tool (http://www.shef.ac.uk/FRAX/), which can be completed with or without bone mineral density data.

Observing patients walking and performing balance maneuvers best assesses balance and gait disorders. Once the clinician is trained to assess gait, this evaluation can be performed while the patient is entering or leaving the examining room. Several simple tests of balance and mobility (**Table 8-3**) can also be performed quickly in the office setting, including the ability to maintain a side-by-side, semi-tandem, and full-tandem stance for 10 seconds; resistance to a nudge; and stability during a 360-degree turn. Quadriceps strength can be briefly assessed by observing an older person arising from a hard armless chair without the use of his or her hands. The timed "up and go" test is a timed measure of the patient's ability to rise from an arm chair, walk 3 m (10 ft), turn, walk back, and sit down again; those who take longer than 12 seconds to complete the test should receive further evaluation. Gait speed is also a helpful marker for recurrent falls. Patients who take more than 13 seconds to walk 10 m are more likely to have recurrent falls. The Short Physical Performance Battery incorporates

chair stands; side-by-side, semi-tandem, and full-tandem stance; and gait speed to calculate a summary score that assesses quadriceps strength, balance, and gait speed.

Polypharmacy (See Also Chapter 22)

Polypharmacy in older patients is associated with adverse drug reactions, reduced adherence, and inappropriate medication usage. Older persons often receive care from multiple providers and fill prescriptions at several pharmacies. Patients should be instructed to bring in all current medications—both prescription and nonprescription medications—to each visit for a thorough medication reconciliation and to check for potential drug-drug interactions.

Given the burden of complex comorbid disease in many older adults, it is important to balance guidelines for chronic disease management with the individual's goals of care, as well as risk factors for adverse drug events such as cognitive impairment, frailty, and renal impairment. A "prescribing cascade" can occur when additional pharmacotherapy is initiated to treat side effects of a prescription. Each new symptom should prompt a medication review and a trial of discontinuation of the suspected agent. The Beer's Criteria has been developed and periodically updated by the American Geriatrics Society to assist clinicians with identifying and avoiding potentially inappropriate medications for the older adults.

Cognitive Assessment

Because the prevalence of Alzheimer disease, other dementias, and cognitive impairment rises considerably with advancing age, the yield of screening for cognitive impairment increases with age. Although in 2020, the USPSTF concluded that there is insufficient evidence on the balance of benefits and harms of screening for cognitive impairment, clinicians should assess cognition when there is suspicion of impairment or when conducting a Medicare Annual Wellness Visit. Several screens are available for clinical use (**Table 8-4**) and some can be performed in 5 minutes or less (eg, the Mini-Cog, which combines three-item recall and clock drawing; the Memory Impairment Screen [MIS]; and the General Practitioner Assessment of Cognition [GPCOG]). Longer screens that are commonly used include the Mini-Mental State Examination (MMSE), which takes 7 to 10 minutes to administer and must be purchased for use, the Montreal Cognitive Assessment (MoCA), which takes 10 to 15 minutes to administer and requires paid certification, and the Rowland Universal Dementia Assessment Scale (RUDAS), which takes 10 minutes to administer.

Although normal results on these tests vastly reduce the probability of dementia and abnormal results increase the likelihood that the patient has dementia, these tests are not diagnostic for dementia and normal results do not exclude the possibility of this disorder. Patients who have abnormal findings on a cognitive screening test should

TABLE 8-3 ■ SIMPLE TESTS OF LOWER EXTREMITIES: STRENGTH, BALANCE, GAIT, AND FALL RISK

QUESTION/TEST	TIME TO ADMINISTER	COMMENTS
Timed up and go	<1 min	Sensitivity 88%, specificity 94% compared to geriatrician's evaluation using cutpoint > 15 s
Gait speed over 10 m	< 30 s	> 13 s predicts recurrent falls (likelihood ratio: 2.0; 95% CI, 1.5–2.7)
Office-based maneuvers Observed gait Resistance to nudge Tandem/semitandem stand Rising from chair 360° turn	2–3 min	Some are part of performance-oriented assessment of mobility
Functional reach	2 min	Adjusted odds ratios for > 2 falls within 6 mo 8.1 if unable to reach 4.0 if reach ≤ 6″ 2.0 if reach ≥ 6″ but < 10″
Short physical performance battery	5–7 min	Combines quadriceps strength, standing balance, and gait speed to generate a score from 0 (worst) to 12 (best)

TABLE 8-4 ■ COMMONLY USED COGNITIVE SCREENS

INSTRUMENT	TIME TO ADMINISTER (MINUTES)	SENSITIVITY	SPECIFICITY	STRENGTHS	LIMITATIONS
Mini-Cog™	2–4	76%	89%	• Developed for and validated in primary care and multiple languages/cultures • Little education/language bias • Short administration time	• Use of different word lists may affect failure rates • Requires in-person administration because of clock drawing
Montreal Cognitive Assessment (MoCA)	10–15	94%	94%	• Designed to test for mild cognitive impairment • Multiple languages accessible at www.mocatest.org • Tests many separate domains	• Lacks studies in general practice settings • Education bias when ≤ 12 y of education • Longer than many screens • Requires in-person administration, though blind and telephone versions are available • Requires paid certification at https://www.mocatest.org/training-certification/
Brief Alzheimer Screen (BAS)	< 5	92%	97%	• Short administration time • Does not require visual tasks	• Difficult for clinicians to remember items • Insensitive to mild cognitive impairment
Memory Impairment Screen (MIS)	4	87%	97%	• Verbal memory test (no writing/drawing) • Little education bias	• Does not test executive function or visuospatial skills
Mini-Mental State Exam (MMSE)	7–10	88%	94%	• Most widely used and studied worldwide • Often used as reference for comparative evaluations of other assessments • Required for some drug insurance reimbursements	• Education/age/language/culture bias • Ceiling effect (highly educated impaired subjects pass) • Requires in-person administration • Proprietary—unless administered from memory, test needs to be purchased at www.parinc.com
General Practitioner Assessment of Cognition (GPCOC) • Patient • Informant	• 2–5 • 1–3	96%	62%	• Developed for and validated in primary care • Informant component useful • Little education bias • Multiple languages accessible at www.gpcog.com.au	• Patient component scoring has an indeterminate range that requires an informant score to determine pass or fail • Informant component alone has low specificity • Requires in-person administration to draw clock
Rowland Universal Dementia Assessment Scale (RUDAS)	10	89%	98%	• Developed for culturally and linguistically diverse population • User friendly and can be translated in various languages	• Requires in-person administration for visuospatial orientation • Cube drawing task requires an education adjustment in individuals with limited or no education

receive more in-depth evaluation of memory, language, visual–spatial, and executive function.

Among hospitalized patients, mental status should be assessed at the time of hospital admission and then periodically because older persons are especially prone to develop delirium during the hospital stay. Abnormal findings on the mental status examination in hospitalized patients must be interpreted in the context of change from baseline and the clinical situation. The Confusion Assessment Method, which has an Intensive Care Unit version, provides a guide to interpreting such changes and assesses acute change or fluctuating course, inattention, disorganized thinking, and altered level of consciousness. The Ultra Brief two-item bedside screen asks patients to list the days of the week backward and what day of the week it is. Older persons who develop delirium should have their cognition reassessed several weeks later (see Chapter 58).

Affective Assessment (See Also Chapter 65)

Major depression and other affective disorders are common among the older persons and are likely underdiagnosed owing to underreported symptoms, atypical presentations, or comorbid cognitive impairment or other neurologic diseases such as Parkinson disease. These treatable disorders are associated with increased disability, health care utilization, morbidity, and mortality, and decreased quality of life. A brief two-item screening inquiry, the Patient Health Questionnaire-2 (PHQ-2), asks about the frequency of depressed mood and anhedonia over the past 2 weeks, and, if positive, can prompt further screening by completing the full nine-item survey, PHQ-9. The PHQ-9 is commonly used to detect and monitor depression symptoms in older adults and provides a reliable and valid measure of depression severity. A score of more than 10 has a sensitivity of 88% and a specificity of 88% for major depression. In patients with underlying cognitive impairment who may lack insight into their mood, caregivers can be asked to complete the Cornell Depression Scale for Dementia. A score of greater than or equal to 6 has a sensitivity of 93% and a specificity of 97% for depression in dementia.

Assessment of Function

Measurement of functional status is an essential component of the assessment of older persons. The patient's ability to function can be viewed as a summary measure of the overall impact of health conditions in the context of his or her environment and social support system. In older persons, the ability to function consistent with their personal lifestyle values should be an important consideration in all care planning. Therefore, changes in functional status should prompt further diagnostic evaluation and intervention. An early indicator of impending functional disability is self-perceived difficulty with performing functional tasks. Measurement of functional status is also valuable in monitoring response to treatment and may provide prognostic information that will help plan for long-term care.

Functional status can be assessed at three levels: basic activities of daily living (BADLs), instrumental or intermediate activities of daily living (IADLs), and advanced activities of daily living (AADLs). BADLs refer to self-care tasks such as bathing, dressing, toileting, continence, grooming, feeding, and transferring. Instrumental activities of daily living refer to the ability to maintain an independent household such as shopping for groceries, driving or using public transportation, using the telephone, meal preparation, housework, home repair, laundry, taking medications, and handling finances. AADLs refer to the ability to fulfill societal, community, and family roles as well as participate in recreational or occupational tasks. These advanced activities vary considerably from individual to individual but may be valuable in monitoring functional status prior to the development of disability.

Questions that ask about specific BADL and IADL functions have also been incorporated into a variety of more generic health-related quality-of-life instruments (eg, the Medical Outcomes Study Short-Form 36 and its shorter version, the SF-12). Some AADLs (eg, exercise and leisure time physical activity) can also be ascertained by using standardized instruments, but open-ended questions about how older persons spend their days might provide a better assessment of function in healthier older persons.

Physical function can also be assessed by directly observing the performance of functional tasks. Instruments have been developed for use in ambulatory, nursing home, and hospital settings, and predictive validity has been demonstrated for many. Some studies have demonstrated that combining self-reported functional with performance-based measures can provide more refined prognostic information than either method alone.

Frailty

Frailty is a clinical syndrome where dysregulation of multiple physiologic systems reaches a critical threshold which results in a physiologic state of heightened vulnerability. Frailty has been conceptualized as physical (phenotypic or syndromic) or as deficit accumulation (due to cumulative comorbidities). Frail patients are at higher risk of adverse clinical outcomes including falls, fractures, hospitalizations, surgical complications, disability and dependency, and mortality.

More than 60 frailty instruments have been developed and used for a variety of purposes, most commonly for risk assessment for adverse clinical outcomes. These instruments variably assess the following domains: physical function/disability, physical activity, cognition, comorbidity, weight loss, and other domains (eg, social, sensory, demographic). The Clinical Frailty Scale (CFS) (**Figure 8-2**) is an effective and rapid way to assess frailty in older adults. There are nine levels of functionality described ranging from "very fit" or level 1 to "terminally ill" or level 9. The CFS utilizes criteria such as activity levels, ADL/IADL dependence, and life expectancy. Other commonly used instruments include the Physical Frailty Phenotype (**Table 8-5**) and the Vulnerable Elders Survey-13 (**Table 8-6**).

Effective preventative strategies for decreasing frailty have been identified including interventions geared toward maintaining muscle mass and strength and consuming a Mediterranean diet. When frailty is identified, it is important to review advance care planning to ensure patient's goals and values will be considered moving forward.

CLINICAL FRAILTY SCALE

1 **VERY FIT** People who are robust, active, energetic and motivated. They tend to exercise regularly and are among the fittest for their age.

2 **FIT** People who have **no active disease symptoms** but are less fit than category 1. Often, they exercise or are very **active occasionally**, e.g., seasonally.

3 **MANAGING WELL** People whose **medical problems are well controlled**, even if occasionally symptomatic, but often are **not regularly active** beyond routine walking.

4 **LIVING WITH VERY MILD FRAILTY** Previously "vulnerable," this category marks early transition from complete independence. While **not dependent** on others for daily help, often **symptoms limit activities**. A common complaint is being "slowed up" and/or being tired during the day.

5 **LIVING WITH MILD FRAILTY** People who often have **more evident slowing**, and need help with **high order instrumental activities of daily living** (finances, transportation, heavy housework). Typically, mild frailty progressively impairs shopping and walking outside alone, meal preparation, medications and begins to restrict light housework.

6 **LIVING WITH MODERATE FRAILTY** People who need help with **all outside activities** and with **keeping house**. Inside, they often have problems with stairs and need **help with bathing** and might need minimal assistance (cuing, standby) with dressing.

7 **LIVING WITH SEVERE FRAILTY** **Completely dependent for personal care**, from whatever cause (physical or cognitive). Even so, they seem stable and not at high risk of dying (within ~6 months).

8 **LIVING WITH VERY SEVERE FRAILTY** Completely dependent for personal care and approaching end of life. Typically, they could not recover even from a minor illness.

9 **TERMINALLY ILL** Approaching the end of life. This category applies to people with a **life expectancy <6 months, who are not otherwise living with severe frailty.** (Many terminally ill people can still exercise until very close to death.)

SCORING FRAILTY IN PEOPLE WITH DEMENTIA

The degree of frailty generally corresponds to the degree of dementia. Common **symptoms in mild dementia** include forgetting the details of a recent event, though still remembering the event itself, repeating the same question/story and social withdrawal.

In **moderate dementia**, recent memory is very impaired, even though they seemingly can remember their past life events well. They can do personal care with prompting.

In **severe dementia**, they cannot do personal care without help.

In **very severe dementia** they are often bedfast. Many are virtually mute.

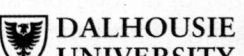

DALHOUSIE UNIVERSITY
www.geriatricmedicineresearch.ca

FIGURE 8-2. Clinical Frailty Scale. (Clinical Frailty Scale ©2005–2020 Rockwood, Version 2.0 (EN). All rights reserved. For permission: www.geriatricmedicineresearch.ca Rockwood K et al. A global clinical measure of fitness and frailty in elderly people. *CMAJ.* 2005;173:489–495.)

Assessment of Social Support

The composition of the older patient's social support structure can be assessed by asking about their relationships, such as with family, friends, neighbors, and caregivers, as well as the quality of these relationships in the social history. For frail older persons, the availability of assistance from family and friends is frequently the determining factor of whether a functionally dependent older person remains at home or is institutionalized. If dependency is noted during functional assessment, then the clinician should inquire as to who provides help for specific BADL and IADL functions and whether these persons are paid or voluntary help. Even in healthier older persons, it is valuable to raise the question of who would be available to help if the patient becomes ill. Early identification of social support needs may prompt planning to develop resources when the necessity arises. For vulnerable older adults, clinicians should be mindful of signs of elder abuse, neglect, or exploitation, and if suspected, are mandated to report cases to Adult Protective Services.

During the COVID-19 pandemic, social isolation played a more profound role in decreasing the quality of life, increasing mood symptoms, and worsening cognitive function of many older adults. While widespread adoption of a single tool for assessing for social isolation has not been applied clinically, research tools including the Lubben Social Network Scale (12-item instrument to assess for social isolation in older adults) as well as the UCLA Loneliness Scale (20-item scale designed to measure feelings of loneliness and social isolation) can be considered. However, the time needed to administer these tools has limited their widespread use in clinical medicine.

Economic Assessment

Many older adults live on fixed incomes, and the rising costs of medical expenses coupled with that of paid caregivers and residential facilities can cause financial hardship that may manifest as medication nonadherence, weight loss, or the appearance of self-neglect. Although some

TABLE 8-5 ■ PHYSICAL FRAILTY PHENOTYPE

CHARACTERISTIC	MEASUREMENT	MEETS CRITERIA IF:	
Shrinking • Unintentional weight loss • Sarcopenia (loss of muscle mass)	Weight changes	> 10 lb or 5% body weight unintentional weight loss in the past year Or BMI < 19 kg/m²	
Weakness	Grip strength ªRequires hand dynamometer	Lowest 20% (by gender, BMI) **Males** BMI ≤ 24 ≤ 29 BMI 24–26 ≤ 30 BMI 26–28 ≤30 BMI > 28 ≤32	**Females** BMI ≤ 23 ≤ 17 BMI 23–26 ≤ 17 BMI 26–29 ≤ 18 BMI > 29 ≤ 21

Poor Endurance
• Exhaustion
	"Exhaustion"	Subjective patient report to following:
		I felt that everything I did was an effort
		    (Answers: Yes, No, Refused, Don't Know)
		If Yes, how often in the last week did you feel this way?
		    3 - Most of the time
		    2 - Moderate amount of time (3–4 d)
		    1 - Some of the time (1–2 d)
		    0 - Rarely/none of the time (< 1 d)
		I could not get going
		    (Answers: Yes, No, Refused, Don't Know)
		If Yes, how often in the last week did you feel this way?
		    3 - Most of the time
		    2 - Moderate amount of time (3–4 d)
		    1- Some of the time (1–2 d)
		    0 - Rarely/none of the time (< 1 d)
		Answers of 2 or 3 to either question meet criteria for exhaustion	

Slowness	Gait speed per 15 ft distance	Slowest 20% by gender, height **Males** ≤ 0.7 s for height ≤ 173 cm ≤ 6 s for height > 173 cm	**Females** ≤ 7 s for height ≤ 159 cm ≤ 6 s for height > 159 cm
Low Activity	Based on short version of the Minnesota Leisure Time Activity Questionnaire to determine Kcals per week expended	Lowest 20% • **Males:** < 383 Kcals/wk expended • **Females:** < 270 Kcals/wk expended	

Frailty: ≥ 3/5 of the following characteristics present.
Intermediate or Prefrail: 1–2/5 of the following characteristics present.
Robust: 0/5 characteristics present.

clinicians feel uncomfortable assessing the economic status of their patients, inquiring about financial stress including food insecurities may prompt referral to social work or other agencies and help prevent the associated poor health outcomes.

Furthermore, insurance status is routinely collected by office staff and a patient's income can be assessed and eligibility determined for state or local benefits (eg, in-home supportive services through Medicaid or Veteran's benefits). For the frail and functionally impaired older adult, clinicians should partner with patients and families to provide anticipatory guidance regarding the resources that may be required to pay for care at home or in a residential facility.

Environmental Assessment

Environmental assessment encompasses two dimensions, the safety of the home environment and the adequacy of the patient's access to needed personal and medical services. Particularly among frail individuals and those with mobility and balance problems, the home environment should be assessed for safety with particular attention

TABLE 8-6 ▪ VULNERABLE ELDERS SURVEY (VES 13)

QUESTION	RESPONSES	SCORING
Age	75–84 ≥ 85	1 point 3 points
Health Self-Evaluation	Excellent Very Good Good Fair Poor	1 point for "fair" or "poor"
On average, how difficult are the following physical activities? a) Stooping, crouching, kneeling b) Lifting or carrying objects as heavy as 10 lb c) Reaching or extending arms above shoulder level d) Writing, or handling and grasping small objects e) Walking a quarter of a mile f) Heavy housework such as scrubbing floors or washing windows	No difficulty A little difficulty Some difficulty A lot of difficulty Unable to do	1 point for each answer of "a lot of difficulty" or "unable to do" **Max:** 2 points
Because of your health, do you have any difficulty: a) Shopping for personal items? b) Managing money? c) Walking across the room? (cane or walker use is OK) d) Doing light housework? e) Bathing or showering?	Yes No	4 points for one or more "Yes" responses

Score ≥ 3 considered vulnerable.

to fall risk. Although most physicians do not personally conduct environmental assessments, the Centers for Disease Control and Prevention has developed a home safety checklist (https://www.cdc.gov/steadi/pdf/check_for_safety_brochure-a.pdf) that patients and their families can complete. For those receiving home health services, in-home safety inspections can be performed, including recommendations for installation of adaptive devices such as shower bars and raised toilet seats. The benefits of such services was further supported by the CAPABLE trial, which showed that home visits provided by occupational therapists and registered nurses and home modifications to address functional goals led to decreases in disability in low-income community-dwelling older adults compared to those who received home visits solely for social purposes by a research assistant.

Older persons who begin to develop IADL dependencies should be evaluated for the geographic proximity of necessary services such as grocery shopping and banking, their need for use of such services, and their ability to use these services in their current living situations. Increasingly, some of these services are available online though many older persons, particularly those who are frail, do not feel comfortable using the Internet to purchase services. Older drivers are at increased risk for motor vehicle accidents secondary to functional impairments, medications, and medical conditions. The National Highway Traffic Safety Administration (NHTSA) has produced materials to help physicians talk with older drivers about safe driving (https://www.nhtsa.gov/road-safety/older-drivers).

Spirituality

Spirituality, whether affiliated with a formal religious denomination or nonreligious intangible elements, has been recognized as an important influence on health and quality of life. Frequent attendance of religious services has been associated with lower health care utilization and mortality rates. Formal instruments for assessing spirituality have been developed, such as the FICA or the HOPE questions for spiritual assessment, but these are not widely used in clinical practice. Simply asking older persons whether religion or spirituality is important to them may provide insights that may tailor their individual care. Especially in hospital settings, involvement of pastoral care may be valuable in supporting the patient and in framing medical decisions in the context of the patient's personal belief system.

Goals of Care and Advance Directives

Although goals of care and advance directives both solicit patient preferences, they are conceptually different. Goals of care are patient-directed wishes for either a state of well-being to be attained (eg, sleep through the night without being awakened by pain) or maintained (eg, continue volunteer work) or specific accomplishments (eg, being able to walk again after a stroke). Goals may be short term or long term but should be realistic with potential for attainment. Particularly in frail older persons and those with multimorbidity, goals are overarching, spanning multiple diseases, and are often nonmedical (eg, spending quality time with family, attending a grandchild's wedding). When goals are elicited by health care professionals, care planning can be focused toward attaining them, and attainment can be measured. For goals that are not attained, alternative strategies can be employed, or goals can be modified or discarded in favor of new goals.

In contrast, advance directives focus on wishes for care in the context of serious, usually acute, illness. An Advance Health Care Directive enables patients to ensure that their health care wishes are known in advance and considered if for any reason they are unable to speak for themselves. It also allows a patient to appoint a Durable Power of Attorney, or health care proxy, who will have legal authority to make health care decisions in the event that patient is incapacitated or whereupon the patient grants such authority. Discussions of advance directives are especially important for older patients and should be initiated early on, to discuss the patients' goals and preferences for care should they experience progressive cognitive impairment or acute illness. Physicians can assist patients by focusing on patients' overall goals of care, rather than specific detailed interventions, and incorporating these goals into the patients' current clinical situation. A particularly important time to discuss such preferences is prior to surgery because of the possibility of surgical complications or postoperative delirium, which may preclude discussions following the procedure. Such discussions should be revisited any time there are significant changes in a patient's medical condition and a better understanding about prognosis becomes available, as patients often revise their thoughts about the burdens and benefits of treatment. Cultural differences regarding preferences for advance directives and end-of-life care should be recognized and respected. Overall, patients are receptive and grateful for discussion of their goals and preferences for care, and increasingly advanced directive counseling discussions have been incentivized and recognized in quality of care measures, with various tools being developed to support advanced care planning in practice. Online tools, such as prepareforyourcare.org, have also allowed patients and families to take a proactive approach to reflecting on their goals and wishes.

A Strategic Approach to Geriatric Assessment

Much of the information needed to assess older persons can be obtained from old records, other professional or nonprofessional staff, or by self-report from patients or family members completing forms, rather than from direct clinician interview. This efficiency allows the clinician to spend more time following up on issues that are detected, conducting the physical examination, discussing treatment, and providing health education.

Pre-visit questionnaires can be completed by the patient or proxy before the clinical encounter. These questionnaires typically gather information on past medical history, medications, preventive measures, and functional status, including information on who helps when the patient is functionally dependent. As a result, they can markedly reduce the time needed to conduct an initial assessment and can ensure a consistent level of comprehensiveness for every patient. By including validated screening instruments, they can also be used to case-find individuals with common geriatric syndromes. With the advance of technology and electronic health records, there is the potential for patients, families, or caregivers to complete such questionnaires electronically, and the information obtained can be seamlessly integrated into the electronic health record.

A second method of streamlining the office visit is to delegate the administration of screening instruments for many of the important geriatric problems to trained office staff. Thus, the clinician may spend a short period of time reviewing the results of these screens and then decide which dimensions, if any, need greater evaluation. However, office staff must be properly trained to administer these instruments, which can be quite time-consuming (10–20 minutes). This time must be taken from other office tasks and the cost of screening may be considerable.

One approach integrates screening for geriatric conditions into the office workflow and then uses structured electronic health record templates to guide more detailed assessment and guide the clinician toward appropriate management steps. This approach has been demonstrated to improve the quality of care for falls, dementia, and urinary incontinence as well as patient-reported outcomes for falls and incontinence. Portions of the structured visit note can be delegated to office staff, further increasing efficiency.

This approach to increasing efficiency can be applied to many geriatric conditions. **Table 8-7** shows a strategy that optimizes the clinician's time by employing the most efficient methods to obtain assessment information. The initial step provides the clinician with basic information that can quickly be processed and followed with more extensive data gathering, when appropriate. Such a strategy begins with the pre-visit questionnaire and then is supplemented by information obtained by office staff. These two data sources are reviewed by the clinician and additional information is obtained from the patient and family at the time of the visit.

Telehealth

During the COVID-19 pandemic, most health care systems transitioned to telehealth services to continue providing care for older patients while decreasing their potential exposure to the virus. In 1 year, telehealth services increased by over 20% among older adults including telephone calls,

TABLE 8-7 ■ STRATEGY FOR EFFICIENT OFFICE-BASED ASSESSMENT

ASPECT BEING ASSESSED	METHOD AND DEPTH OF ASSESSMENT[a]				
	PREVISIT QUESTIONNAIRE	OFFICE STAFF ADMINISTERED	CLINICIAN ROUTINE	CLINICIAN AS NEEDED	REFERRAL[b] AS NEEDED
Past medical history	D		R		
Geriatric syndromes/health conditions					
Visual impairment	B	B	R		Ophthalmologist or optometrist
Hearing impairment	B	B (if needed)	R		Audiologist
Urinary incontinence	B	B	R	D	Urologist, gynecologist, or geriatrician
Malnutrition	D		R		Dietitian or social worker
Sexual dysfunction	B		R		Urologist or geriatrician
Polypharmacy	B		R		Pharmacist or geriatrician
Dental problems	B		R		Dentist
Gait, balance, falls	B	B	B	D	Physical therapist
Affective problems	D		R	D	Psychiatrist
Cognitive problems		B	R	D	Geriatrician, psychiatrist, or neurologist
Functional disability	D		R	D	Physical or occupational therapist, social worker
Environmental problems	D		R		Home health
Preventive services	D		R		

[a]B, brief screen (eg, less than 2 min); D, detailed evaluation (usually 5 min or more); R, review of collected information.
[b]Examples of referrals to specific health professional or comprehensive geriatric assessment might be used.

video visits, and digital messaging. Yet, approximately 38% of older adults are simply not ready for telehealth.

Many older adults have difficulties with technology including not having adequate access to telephones or internet, poor hearing and vision, as well as having dementia or cognitive impairment. Thus, it is important to screen for the capabilities to utilize telehealth. A social work referral may provide additional state or locally funded resources such as a free phone or cellphone plan.

Often, a family member or hired caregiver needs to assist the older adult in setting up telehealth visits. In assisted-living facilities, staff may need to obtain the right equipment and ensure preparedness for the appointment.

In situations where a physical examination and other diagnostic studies are required to obtain a diagnosis, telehealth visits are not recommended. Additionally, it is a challenge to observe ambulatory status and detect subtle gait abnormalities. Thus, telephone or video visits may be more appropriate as subsequent rather than initial visits.

Medicare, state-funded Medicaid, and various private insurances have expanded services and coverage for telephone or video visits during COVID-19 but their future reimbursement is still uncertain.

COMPREHENSIVE GERIATRIC ASSESSMENT

CGA is a systematic evaluation of frail older persons by a team of health professionals that may uncover treatable health problems and lead to better health outcomes. This evaluation typically includes four dimensions: physical health; functional status; psychological health, including cognitive and affective status; and socioenvironmental factors. Early randomized clinical trials provided convincing evidence that such programs conducted in hospital-based and rehabilitation units, which typically required several weeks of treatment, could lead to better survival rates, improved functional status, and more desirable placement (eg, home rather than nursing home) following discharge from the hospital. Conceptually, CGA is a three-step process: (1) screening or targeting of appropriate patients, (2) assessment and development of recommendations, and (3) implementation of recommendations, including clinician and patient adherence with recommendations. Each of these steps is essential if the process is to be successful at achieving health and functional benefits.

Within this broad conceptualization, CGA has been implemented using many different models in various health care settings (**Table 8-8**). Because of changes in length of hospital stays, many CGA programs rely on post-discharge

TABLE 8-8 ■ SPECTRUM OF COMPREHENSIVE GERIATRIC ASSESSMENT–LIKE INTERVENTIONS		
	MOST INTENSIVE ⟵———————————————⟶ **LEAST INTENSIVE**	
Setting	CGA, GEM, and rehabilitation units	CGA consultation and comanagement inpatient or outpatient	Community-based and in-home outreach programs
Targeting	Most restrictive		Least restrictive
Process	Large team, extensive evaluations		Screening and referral
Cost	Very expensive		Relatively inexpensive

CGA, comprehensive geriatric assessment; GEM, geriatric evaluation and management.

and community-based assessment. Furthermore, most of the early programs focused on restorative or rehabilitative goals (tertiary prevention), whereas many newer programs are aimed at primary and secondary prevention.

The purpose of the first step, targeting, is to distinguish older patients who are appropriate and will benefit from CGA, rather than those who are either too sick or well to benefit. To date, no easily administered targeting criteria have been demonstrated and validated to readily identify patients who are likely to benefit from CGA in different settings. Specific strategies used by CGA programs to identify older persons who are most appropriate for CGA have included chronological age, functional disability, physical illness, geriatric conditions, psychosocial conditions, and previous or predicted high health care utilization. All of these criteria have randomized clinical trial support for their effectiveness in identifying older persons likely to benefit from CGA. However, the definitions of these criteria and the interventions that have followed have varied from study to study.

Most CGA programs exclude patients who are unlikely to benefit because of terminal illness, severe dementia, complete functional dependence, and inevitable nursing home placement. Exclusionary criteria have also included identifying older persons who are "too healthy" to benefit.

The second step of CGA, the assessment process, continues to be highly variable across programs. The types of health care professionals included in the assessment team, the content of information collected, and the types and intensity of services provided have differed in studies of the effectiveness of CGA. In many settings, the CGA process relies on a core team consisting of a physician, nurse, and social worker and, when appropriate, draws upon an extended team of various combinations of physical and occupational therapists, nutritionists, pharmacists, psychiatrists, psychologists, dentists, audiologists, podiatrists, and opticians. Although these professionals are usually on staff in hospital settings and are available in the community, access to and reimbursement for these services have limited the effectiveness of the CGA process. Frequently, the composition of the team is determined by local expertise and availability of resources rather than programmatic needs. Some CGA programs use a "virtual team" concept in which members are included as needed,

assessments are conducted at different locations on different days, and conferencing is completed via telephone or electronically.

Traditionally, the various components of the evaluation are completed by different members of the team. There is considerable variability in which professional conducts the assessments. For example, the medical assessment of older persons may be conducted by a physician, nurse practitioner, or physician's assistant. The core team may conduct only brief initial assessments or screens for some dimensions. These may be subsequently augmented with more in-depth evaluations by additional professionals. For example, a dietitian may be needed to assess dietary intake and provide recommendations; an audiologist may need to conduct a more extensive assessment of hearing loss and evaluate an older person for a hearing aid.

Components of Comprehensive Geriatric Assessment

The process of care rendered by CGA teams can be divided into six key elements: (1) data gathering; (2) discussion among the team; (3) development of a treatment plan; (4) implementation of the treatment plan; (5) monitoring response to the treatment plan; and (6) revising the treatment plan.

Data gathering Standardized assessments can either use instruments developed specifically for clinical purposes or assemble standard instruments that have previously been studied for validity and reliability. The advantage of the former is that teams can customize the information being gathered to best suit the clinical needs of the program. The advantage of the latter is that patients in the program can be compared to those in other programs. Frequently, however, these instruments were developed for research purposes and may not provide information that is helpful in the care of patients.

Discussion among team Following initial data gathering, the team meets to discuss the patient's geriatric needs. Each conference typically begins with short discipline-specific presentations followed by interactive discussions among professionals. Sometimes additional information will need to be obtained before final recommendations can be made.

The team then identifies problems that need action and might be responsive to treatment.

Development of the treatment plan Based upon this discussion, the team develops an initial treatment plan and goals for the patient. Whenever possible, the patient and appropriate family members should be included in the development of the treatment plan. Through techniques such as motivational interviewing, patients can be asked to identify their priorities and willingness to make changes. Based on these, care plans can be created with patients as active partners.

Some CGA programs use protocols that are triggered by specific geriatric conditions whereas others rely on the experience and clinical judgment of the team. If the number of recommendations resulting from CGA is large, they should be prioritized to focus on the major recommendations, those that are most likely to produce the desired outcomes. The urgency of recommendations must also be determined. Although some recommendations may need to be implemented immediately to confer short-term benefit such as stopping a medication that may be the cause of delirium, others may be better implemented once the patient is more stable.

At the time of the assessment, a plan for implementation of each recommendation must be developed. It needs to be determined who will assume responsibility for initiation and completion of the recommendation. Similarly, the team must establish a plan for monitoring the patient's progress as treatment is being delivered.

Implementation of the Treatment Plan Options for implementation are available and include direct implementation of recommendations by the team, merely advising physicians and patients verbally or by a note in the chart, and coaching patients to approach their physicians to discuss CGA recommendations.

Monitoring To ensure that recommendations are implemented and to follow a patient's progress, patients must be monitored directly by the CGA team or by the primary care physician. During this phase, key issues to consider are how frequently and for how long this monitoring should occur. The more intensively and the longer patients are followed, the more resource intensive the consultation becomes. In some models, the CGA team may temporarily assume primary care for several months before returning the patient to the primary care physician for ongoing care.

Revising the treatment plan By monitoring the patient, CGA teams can continually assess the patient's progress toward meeting the goals established by the team. If progress is not proceeding according to expectations, the team may need to reevaluate the patient and resume the team discussion. Treatment recommendations and implementation plans may need to be revised. Again, engaging the patient is important as readiness to change or the patient's goals may have changed. Any modifications require additional monitoring.

Effectiveness of Comprehensive Geriatric Assessment

In virtually all studies of CGA, the process has resulted in improved detection and documentation of geriatric problems. However, such identification of problems has not always led to improved outcomes. Meta-analysis has been used to evaluate models of CGA in several settings.

Inpatient Units and Services

Geriatric Evaluation and Management Units (GEMUs), also referred to as Acute Care of the Elderly (ACE) units, are designed to be environment friendly to older persons. Two main benefits of these units are: (1) physicians staffing the unit generally assume primary care of the patient, thus facilitating the implementation of recommendations; and (2) the availability and experience of a dedicated team of providers (eg, nurses and therapists) increase the consistency and geriatric orientation of hospital and post-acute care. Similar in concept to Cardiac Care Units (CCUs) and Stroke Units, these units assemble resources for a specific patient population. A meta-analysis of 29 trials published through 2016 found that recipients of care on inpatient units were slightly more likely (relative risk [RR] 1.06) to be living at home and less likely to be admitted to a nursing home (RR 0.80) at 3 to 12 months compared to usual care. There were benefits on mortality, functional dependence, cognitive function, or length of stay in the hospital. Of note, earlier studies demonstrated more favorable outcomes than more recent studies suggesting that usual care for older persons in the hospital may be improving. Some programs have attempted to recreate the core elements of ACE units for hospitalized older persons who are not located on a single unit (mobile ACE services) due to logistical barriers of a dedicated physical unit.

Outside of the traditional geriatric units, many of the principles of CGA have been integrated into comanagement models. These models usually involve a geriatrician and a surgeon who share responsibility and decision making. In a meta-analysis of eight randomized trials, geriatric comanagement programs for older patients with hip fractures have shown reduced discharges to an increased level of care compared to their pre-hospitalization living situation. There was a nonsignificant trend for reduction of inpatient mortality. In another meta-analysis of 12 studies, the comanagement model had reduced length of stay and fewer complications; however, the evidence was considered to be low quality.

Posthospital Discharge Assessment and Management

Studies of CGA have found inconsistent benefits for posthospital discharge programs. In one randomized trial of posthospitalization, patients who received CGA versus usual care did not show any differences in reducing functional decline, post-discharge acute care visits, or depression after 24 weeks. However, patients assigned to the intervention group were less likely to be readmitted to the hospital. A systematic review found that many of the components of CGA were parts of care transition interventions that were effective in reducing rehospitalizations and emergency department visits. CGA programs for patients discharged to home from the emergency department were found to be effective at reducing emergency room visits and hospital admissions.

Outpatient CGA

The evidence for outpatient CGA has been inconsistent. Some individual studies have shown benefit on quality of care and functional decline. There have not been benefits on hospitalization and nursing home placement. Moreover, a meta-analysis of controlled trials found no benefit of outpatient CGA on survival.

In-Home Assessment

Home assessment programs are a variation of CGA that focus primarily on preventive rather than rehabilitative services and are aimed at patients at low rather than high risk of nursing home admission. Multiple meta-analyses have found home assessments to be consistently effective in reducing functional decline (if a clinical examination is performed) as well as overall mortality among younger patients (73–78 years).

Lessons Learned From Comprehensive Geriatric Assessment

Despite unresolved issues regarding the effectiveness of CGA, the principles of CGA have been incorporated into a number of programs that have been demonstrated to be effective. These models adopt various components of CGA including targeting, assessment, and interventions.

CGA with geriatric comanagement of frail patients on nongeriatric inpatient units has shown some promise with meta-analyses demonstrating decreased length of stay and improved functional status with geriatric comanagement of frail patients on nongeriatric wards. In addition,

CGA has been adapted to specialty treatment of older persons including oncology, cardiology, emergency department post-discharge management, inpatient orthopedic care, and the preoperative evaluation of older patients. As an example, CGA has been applied to patients with aortic stenosis undergoing evaluation for transcatheter aortic valve replacement (TAVR) and cancer patients undergoing chemotherapy. Elements of CGA have also been incorporated into disease management programs, including stroke and heart failure.

In summary, geriatric assessment continues to evolve as an integral component of the care of older persons. As assessment techniques become better standardized and validated, more efficient yet comprehensive approaches are possible. To date, implementation of such strategies has not occurred on a widespread basis in part due to barriers including cost, logistical implementation, training issues, and unique circumstances of different health care systems. However, as national initiatives to improve quality move forward, screening for geriatric conditions and appropriate assessment of patients who screen positive will likely gain more acceptance. Advances in technology and newer approaches to data collection have increased the ability to integrate geriatric assessment and management that could not have been possible a decade ago and further advances are likely on the horizon. In addition, principles developed in CGA models have now been incorporated into the care of many specialties, either through geriatric comanagement models or structured geriatric assessments.

ACKNOWLEDGMENTS

Sonja Rosen, MD, and Heather B. Schikedanz, MD, contributed to this chapter in the 7th edition and some material from that chapter has been retained here.

FURTHER READING

Borneman T, Ferrell B, Puchalski CM. Evaluation of the FICA tool for spiritual assessment. *J Pain Symptom Manage.* 2010;40:163.

Boureau AS, Trochu JN, Colliard C, et al. Determinants in treatment decision-making in older patients with symptomatic severe aortic stenosis. *Maturitas.* 2015; 82(1):128–133.

Brown JS, Bradley CS, Subak LL, et al. The sensitivity and specificity of a simple test to distinguish between urge and stress urinary incontinence. *Ann Intern Med.* 2006;144(10):715–723.

Buta BJ, Walston JD, Godino JG, et al. Frailty assessment instruments: systematic characterization of the uses and contexts of highly-cited instruments. *Ageing Res Rev.* 2016;26:53–61.

Chou R, Dana T, Bougatsos C, Fleming C, Beil TSO. Screening adults aged 50 years or older for hearing loss: a review of the evidence for the U.S. Preventive Services Task Force. *Ann Intern Med.* 2011;154(5):347.

Crossland MD, Dekker TM, Hancox J, Lisi M, Wemyss TA, Thomas PBM. Evaluation of a home-printable vision screening test for telemedicine. *JAMA Ophthalmol.* 2021;139(3):271–277.

Deschodt M, Flamaing J, Haentjens P, Boonen S, Milisen K. Impact of geriatric consultation teams on clinical outcome in acute hospitals: a systematic review and meta-analysis. *BMC Med.* 2013;11:48.

Eamer G, Taheri A, Chen SS, et al. Comprehensive geriatric assessment for older people admitted to a surgical service. *Cochrane Database Syst Rev.* 2018;1(1): CD012485.

Ellis G, Gardner M, Tsiachristas A, et al. Comprehensive geriatric assessment for older adults admitted to hospital. *Cochrane Database Syst Rev.* 2017;9(9):CD006211.

Fick DM, Inouye SK, Guess J, et al. Two-item bedside test for delirium. *J Hosp Med.* 2015;10:645–650.

Fried LP, Tangen CM, Walston J, et al. Frailty in older adults: evidence for a phenotype. *J Gerontol A Biol Sci Med Sci.* 2001;56(3):M146–156.

Ganz DA, Latham NK. Fall prevention in community-dwelling older adults. Reply. *N Engl J Med.* 2020;382(26): 2581–2582.

Hemmy LS, Linskens EJ, Silverman PC, et al. Brief cognitive tests for distinguishing clinical Alzheimer-type dementia from mild cognitive impairment or normal cognition in older adults with suspected cognitive impairment. *Ann Intern Med.* 2020;172(10):678–687.

Jennings LA, Reuben DB, Kim SB, et al. Targeting a high-risk group for fall prevention: strategies for health plans. *Am J Manag Care.* 2015;21(9):e519-526.

Reuben DB, Jennings LA. Putting goal-oriented patient care into practice. *J Am Geriatr Soc.* 2019;67(7): 1342–1344.

Reuben DB, Magasi S, McCreath HE, et al. Motor assessment using the NIH toolbox. *Neurology.* 2013;80(11 Suppl 3):S65–75.

Rodda J, Walker Z, Carter J. Depression in older adults. *BMJ.* 2011;343:d5219.

Shimura T et al; OCEAN-TAVI Investigators. Impact of the Clinical Frailty Scale on outcomes after transcatheter aortic valve replacement. *Circulation.* 2017;135(21): 2013–2024.

Szanton S, Xue QL, Leff B, et al. Effect of a biobehavioral environmental approach on disability among low-income older adults: a randomized clinical trial. *JAMA Intern Med.* 2019;179(2):204–211.

Van Grootven B, Flamaing J, Dierckx de Casterlé B, et al. Effectiveness of in-hospital geriatric co-management: a systematic review and meta-analysis. *Age Ageing.* 2017;46(6):903–910.

Mental Status and Neurologic Examination

James E. Galvin, Michelle M. Marrero

THE NEUROLOGY OF AGING

What Is Normal Neurologic Aging

The diagnosis of neurologic disease in the older adult requires recognition not only of abnormal signs and symptoms but also an understanding of what changes are expected as part of the normal aging process. To distinguish neurologic dysfunction related to disease from the neurologic changes associated with normal aging, the clinician must conduct a comprehensive mental status and neurologic examination. When establishing a neurologic diagnosis, the clinical history (ie, history of the present illness, past medical history, social habits, occupational experience, family illness, and disorders) assists the clinician in generating a differential diagnosis that can be further explored and refined by pertinent observations documented on the mental status and neurologic examinations. One of the most vital tools for the diagnosis of neurologic disorders is to perform a comprehensive neurologic examination.

The mental status assessment should evaluate cognition, emotion, and behavior. Because cognitive and affective disorders occur commonly in older adults, historical information should be obtained not only from the patient but a reliable informant such as the spouse, adult child, or caregiver. The neurologic examination should be performed on all older adults regardless of the chief complaint as up to 60% of older patients have either a primary or secondary neurologic sign or symptom. A complete mental status and neurologic examination provides the necessary data to develop reasonable diagnostic hypotheses and drive the necessary laboratory, imaging, or specialized assessments to care for the patient.

Age-Related Changes in the Neurologic Examination

Before discussion of the individual components of the examination, it would be useful to discuss changes that are expected as part of the aging process (**Table 9-1**). Normal age-related changes are due to progressive and irreversible changes associated with tissue senescence and the inability of nervous system to repair and regenerate secondary to the ravages of time. The frequency and qualitative characteristics of these changes vary from individual to individual but

Learning Objectives

- Learn about normal neurologic aging and aging-associated changes in neurologic examination.
- Recognize the significance of focused history taking and accurate bedside techniques to examine older adults with neurologic diseases.
- Understand the rationale and learn new skills to assess mental status, memory, attention, orientation, visuospatial, language, and executive function in the older population.
- Learn correct ways to examine cranial nerves, motor and sensory system, coordination, gait, and higher cortical functions in older adults.

Key Clinical Points

1. An extensor plantar response is not a normal aging-associated change and is always associated with some pathology in the upper motor neuron.

2. Comprehensive mental status examination includes observational, cognitive, functional, and neuropsychiatric evaluations.

3. Altered level of alertness is always associated with cognitive deficits and an underlying medical illness that is almost always treatable.

4. Language assessment involves evaluation of all aspects of communication, including spontaneous speech, comprehension, repetition, naming, reading, and writing.

5. Reduced hearing for high-pitched sounds and lack of perception of background noise are common findings in older adults and do not suggest a pathologic finding.

6. Mild muscular wasting without weakness or focal neurologic signs can be encountered in normal aging and commonly affect hand and foot muscles, calf, and shoulder girdle muscles.

7. Ocular motility is commonly limited in older adults and can exhibit restricted convergence and limitation of conjugate upward gaze.

TABLE 9-1 ■ NEUROLOGIC CHANGES ASSOCIATED WITH NORMAL AGING

Psychomotor slowing

Decreased visual acuity

Smaller pupil size

Reduced pupillary reactivity

Presbyopia

Slowed pursuit movements

Decreased ability to look upward

Decreased auditory acuity, especially for spoken language

Decreased muscle bulk

Mild motor slowing

Decreased vibratory sensation

Mild swaying on Romberg test

Mild lordosis and restriction of movement in neck and back

Depression of Achilles tendon reflex

are present in many older adults. It is important to note that these findings are not pathologic in nature and are considered to be part of the normal aging process.

Cognitive changes There continues to be a debate regarding the extent of cognitive changes associated with aging due largely to differences between cross-sectional and longitudinal study designs. When comparing older adults to young adults on similar cognitive tasks such as the Wechsler Adult Intelligence Scale, older adults generally score lower on both performance and verbal subtests. However, when differences in performance are considered in light of motor slowing and educational attainment, these changes are less apparent. Results from cross-sectional studies imply that normal cognitive aging is characterized by nearly linear declines from early adulthood in processing speed. Longitudinal evaluation of older adults has generally demonstrated little change in verbal intelligence with aging while performance is influenced significantly by motor and processing speed. Forgetfulness therefore is *not* a part of normal aging. While it may take longer to process new information and retrieve well-learned information, new learning and memory formation occurs in older adults. This is one reason why delayed recall of word lists is effective in discriminating older adults with cognitive impairment from those without.

Changes in cranial nerve function Visual and hearing changes are common in older adults. Visual acuity declines due to a number of ophthalmologic (cataracts, glaucoma) and neurologic (macular degeneration) causes. Pupillary size is typically smaller with age and pupils are less reactive to light and accommodation, forcing many older adults to use glasses for reading. There is also a restriction in eye movement in upward gaze. Also associated with aging is a decline in speech discrimination due to presbycusis, a progressive elevation in the frequency threshold for hearing. There are also age-related degenerative changes in inner ear

including loss of hair cells, atrophy of stria vascularis, and thickening of the basilar membrane.

Changes in motor function There is a progressive decline in muscle bulk and strength associated with aging. Most of the muscle loss is found in the intrinsic muscles of the hands and feet, and around the shoulder. There is a weakening of the abdominal muscles which may accentuate spinal lordosis and contribute to low back pain. Muscle loss is associated with denervation on electrophysiologic studies and with type II atrophy on muscle biopsy. In addition to loss of strength and muscle bulk, changes in the speed and coordination of movement increases with advancing age. These changes may interfere with activities of daily living (dressing, putting away the dishes, getting out of a chair) and recreation activities (golfing, shuffleboard). On examination, these changes may manifest as mild bradykinesia and dysmetria on finger-nose-finger and heel-shin tests.

Changes in sensory function By far the most common change will be the loss of vibration perception in the lower extremities and to a lesser extent position sense may be affected as well. As vibration sensation becomes impaired in lower extremities, there is an ascending pattern, from toe to ankle and knee. Pain and temperature sensation is also diminished in the older adult, but in the absence of a pathologic cause, usually does not elicit much symptomatology. The mild impairment in position sense often manifests as a mild swaying during the Romberg test.

Changes in gait and station Changes in gait and station in old age may be attributed in part to decreased muscle strength, weakening of abdominal muscles, arthritis and degenerative joint disease, diminished vibration and position sense, impairment in motor speed, and coordination. These changes make it more difficult for older adults to tandem, heel or toe walk for extended periods of time. Despite this, many older adults have adequate postural righting reflexes and are not likely to spontaneously fall (distinct from what is seen in Parkinson disease). Instead, polypharmacy, drug-drug interactions, and adverse effects from medications are significant risk factors for falls.

Changes in deep tendon reflexes The most common age-associated change is the depression or loss of the Achilles tendon reflex. Other reflexes usually remain present but are diminished in response. An extensor plantar response (Babinski sign) is *not* a normal age-related change but instead is always associated with some underlying pathology in the upper motor neuron. In patients in which a Babinski cannot be elicited (eg, patient with lower extremities amputation), an alternative test would be to elicit a Hoffman's sign. To elicit this sign, the examiner has to flick the fingernail of the middle finger down. A "positive" sign is obtained when there is involuntary flexion and adduction of the thumb and or flexion of the index finger. This can also be seen in upper motor neuron disease (ie, amyotrophic lateral sclerosis).

THE NEUROLOGIC HISTORY

There is no substitution for a carefully elicited history detailing the onset, duration, quality, and location of symptoms. The history helps the clinician develop a differential diagnosis and focus on the neurologic examination. The history will also guide the formulation of diagnostic evaluations and develop a treatment plan. In addition, a compassionate clinician will be able to build a trusting relationship with the patient that will enhance patient adherence to medical recommendations. As a general comment, to avoid bias, it is often useful to gather historical facts de novo and not read other records or review laboratory studies such as imaging before taking the history and performing the physical examination. Here we discuss two aspects of neurologic history taking—from the patient, and when available from an informant.

The Neurologic History From the Patient

An accurate history requires that absolute attention is paid to detail, both verbal (what the patient is saying) and nonverbal (what the patient is doing). This is critical to match the chief complaint with the patient's body language. For example, someone complaining about severe low back pain that appears to be sitting comfortably in the chair may raise suspicion. Likewise, the older adult who offers no complaints but is noted to have a rest tremor should prompt more detailed questioning. One of the most important attributes of a skilled clinician is the ability to be a good listener and to focus in on critical historical points. The most effective historians gather information by a combination of open-ended and structured questions. After asking the patient why they are in office and offer a chance to express concerns or worries in their own words, specific topics can be addressed by focused questioning.

Another important aspect of the history is to elicit qualitative and quantitative aspects of the chief complaint. It is not enough to elicit a history of a "headache" or "pain." What are the characteristics of the complaint, when did it start, what makes it better, what makes it worse? Has this happened before, and if so, did it present in the same fashion? Use simple scales to quantify the extent of the complaint by asking, "On a scale of 1 to 10, with 10 being the worst (symptom)...." These qualities can help focus a differential diagnosis and help to build trust with the patient. For example, the onset and characteristics of the headache might guide the clinician in the diagnosis and workup of headaches that may need an emergent intervention. For instance, a "thunderclap" severe headache associated with meningeal signs on examination may be suggestive of a subarachnoid hemorrhage or reversible cerebral vasoconstriction syndrome while a chronic headache with no "red flags" on history or examination might be a primary benign headache that needs no emergent intervention.

The Neurologic History From an Informant

In many instances, gathering information from a third party will be invaluable in determining the onset, duration, and extent of the neurologic problem. In cases where there are problems with cognition or alertness, this may be the only reliable way to gather information. Again, using both open-ended and structured questions will often provide the clinician with important information about the chief complaint and assist in the development of a differential diagnosis. If possible, interviewing the informant in an area separate from the patient may provide a true picture of what is transpiring.

MENTAL STATUS EXAMINATION

The elements of a comprehensive mental status examination include observational, cognitive, functional, and neuropsychiatric assessments. Although each of these elements is presented separately, they are interrelated and collectively characterize the neurobehavioral function of the patient. The initial contact with the patient affords the opportunity to assess whether a cognitive, attention, or language disorder is present. Questioning of an informant may bring to light changes in cognition, function, and behavior that the patient either is not aware of or denies.

Observational Assessment

Observation of a patient's level of arousal or alertness, appearance, emotion, behavior, movements, and speech provides insight into their mental status.

Level of consciousness An accurate assessment of a patient's mental status and neurologic function must first document the patient's alertness or level of arousal. Altered levels of consciousness can directly impact the patient's cognitive performance on mental status testing and influence the examiner's interpretation of the test results and may be indicative of a medical or neurologic condition requiring immediate medical intervention (eg, cardiopulmonary intervention, neurosurgical evaluation).

Abnormal patterns of arousal include hypoaroused or hyperaroused states. Decreasing levels of arousal include lethargy, obtundation, stupor, and coma. The lethargic patient is drowsy or fatigued and falls asleep if not stimulated, however while being interviewed, the patient will usually be able to attend to questioning. Obtundation refers to a state of moderately reduced alertness with diminished ability to consistently engage the environment. Even in the presence of the examiner, if not stimulated, the obtunded patient will drift off. The stuporous patient requires vigorous stimulation to be aroused. Responses are usually limited to simple "yes/no" responses or may consist of groans and grimaces. Coma, which represents the end of the continuum of hypoarousal states, is a state of unresponsiveness to the external environment. In older adults, hypoarousal states can be associated with systemic infection, cardiac or pulmonary insufficiencies, meningoencephalitis, increased intracranial pressure, toxic-metabolic insults, traumatic brain injury, seizures, or cerebrovascular disease. Coma requires either bilateral hemispheric dysfunction or brain stem dysfunction. Another important consideration is the role of polypharmacy. Drug interactions are more common in the older adult and can significantly impair consciousness.

Hyperarousal states, on the other hand, are characterized by anxiety, autonomic hyperactivity (tachycardia, tachypnea, and hyperthermia), agitation or aggression, tremor, seizures, or exaggerated startle response. In older adults, hyperarousal states are most often encountered in toxic-metabolic disorders including withdrawal from alcohol, opiates, or sedative-hypnotic agents. Other causes include tumors (both primary and metastatic), viral encephalitis (particularly herpes simplex), cerebrovascular, and hypoxemia. Some patients may experience fluctuating periods of both hypo- and hyperarousal.

Appearance Assessment of a patient's physical appearance should acknowledge body size and type, apparent age, posture, facial expressions, eye contact, hygiene, dress, and general activity level. A disheveled appearance may indicate dementia, delirium, frontal lobe dysfunction, schizophrenia or severe depression with psychotic features. Wearing excessive makeup or flamboyant grooming or attire in an old individual should raise the suspicion of a manic episode or frontal lobe dysfunction. Patients with unilateral neglect may fail to dress, groom, or bathe one side of their body. Patients with Parkinson disease may display a flexed posture, whereas patients with progressive supranuclear palsy have an extended, rigid posture. The overall appearance of an individual should also provide information regarding their general health status. The cachectic patient may harbor a systemic illness (eg, cancer) or have anorexia or depression.

Emotional state and affect Affect describes the mental representation of external reality and the patient's internal feelings about external reality, while emotional state describes the objective display of emotion through facial grimaces, vocal tone, and body movements, and the subjective component of how the patient reports what he or she feels internally: "I feel sad, happy, apprehensive, cynical."

Depression is the most frequent mood disturbance in older adults and occurs in a variety of neurologic disorders (**Table 9-2**). Euphoria or full-blown mania occurs less often than depression in the course of neurologic illness. Euphoria is most common with frontal lobe dysfunction (trauma, frontotemporal degenerations, and infections) and with secondary mania. Anxiety occurs in a variety of neuropsychiatric conditions including anxiety disorders, metabolic encephalopathies (eg, hyperthyroidism, anoxia), toxic disorders (eg, lidocaine toxicity), and degenerative diseases (eg, Alzheimer disease, Parkinson disease). Objective and subjective emotional components may be incongruent in

TABLE 9-2 ■ POSSIBLE CAUSES OF DEPRESSION IN OLDER ADULTS

Idiopathic
Secondary to life situation (loss of spouse, child, friends)
Cerebrovascular accident
Hypothyroidism
Alzheimer disease
Parkinson disease
Frontotemporal dementia
Dementia with Lewy bodies
Head injury
Drug withdrawal
Drug intoxication (alcohol, barbiturates, sedative-hypnotics)
Medications (β-blockers, reserpine, clonidine)
Multiple sclerosis
Epilepsy
Insomnia

certain psychiatric disorders (eg, schizophrenia and schizotypal personality disorder) and in neurologic conditions such as pseudobulbar palsy.

The range and intensity of the observable component of emotion should be noted. Constriction or flatness is observed in apathetic states, for example, in the context of negative symptoms of schizophrenia, severe melancholic depression, or in demented patients with apathy. Increased intensity, on the other hand, is seen in mood disorders such as bipolar illness, and in personality disorders such as borderline personality.

Lability is a disorder of emotional regulation. Patients with marked lability are irritable and shift rapidly among anger, depression, and euphoria. The emotional outbursts are usually short-lived. Labile mood is seen in mood disorders such as bipolar illness and in certain personality disorders such as borderline personality. It also may occur in frontotemporal dementia and pseudobulbar palsy.

Behavior Behavioral observations can reveal important information regarding the mental status and neurologic function of the patient. A variety of personality alterations can be encountered with focal brain lesions. Orbitofrontal dysfunction may be characterized by impulsiveness or undue familiarity with the examiner, lack of judgment or lack of social anxiety, and antisocial behavior. Individuals with dorsolateral frontal lobe dysfunction may be inattentive and distractible. Apathy (lack of motivation, energy, emotional reciprocity, social isolation) may be caused by medial frontal dysfunction. Dementias are associated with increased rigidity of thoughts, egocentricity, diminished emotional responsiveness, and impaired emotional control.

Movement Observation of patient's movements may provide evidence of parkinsonism, chorea, myoclonus, or tics (**Table 9-3**). Psychomotor retardation (ie, slowed central

TABLE 9-3 ■ COMMON MOVEMENT DISORDERS AND SIGNS

SIGN	DESCRIPTION	ETIOLOGY
Bradykinesia	Slowed initiation and sustained movements	Parkinson disease, drug-induced, may be normal variant
Dyskinesia	Abnormal involuntary movements either slow or fast	Drug-induced, Huntington disease, Parkinson disease, idiopathic
Action or postural tremor	Fast frequency (10–15 Hz) associated with movement (action) or sustained posture (postural), may improve with small amount of alcohol	Benign, essential tremor, drug-induced
Rest tremor	Low frequency (3–5 Hz) with pill rolling quality, may involve extremities or chin	Parkinson disease, drug-induced
Intention tremor	High frequency (10–15 Hz), worsening as approaching target	Cerebellar disease
Myoclonus	Lightning-fast movements from brief muscle contractions	Stroke, sleep, Huntington disease, epilepsy, Creutzfeldt-Jakob
Asterixis	Sudden loss of limb tone during sustained muscle contraction, sometimes considered "negative" myoclonus	Hepatic, renal, or pulmonary disease, drug-induced, encephalopathy, bacterial infection
Chorea	Brief, rapid, irregular contractions	Huntington disease, Sydenham chorea, drug-induced
Ballismus	Large-amplitude, jerky movements with flinging of extremities	Subthalamic nucleus lesions
Tics	Sequenced coordinated movements or vocalizations that appear suddenly	Tourette, drug-induced
Dystonia	Sustained muscle contraction with twisting or repetitive movements, may be painful	Idiopathic, infarcts, drug-induced
Athetosis	Slow, writhing movements predominantly proximal	Huntington disease, infarcts
Akathisia	Internalized restlessness with urge to move	Drug-induced, encephalopathy, Parkinson disease, restless legs syndrome

processing and movement) may be indicative of vascular dementia, subcortical neurologic disorders, parkinsonism, medial frontal syndromes, or depression. Psychomotor agitation may be indicative of a metabolic disorder, choreoathetosis, seizure disorder, mania, or anxiety.

Speech and communication Observation of spontaneous speech is the first step in formal language testing and can be assessed during history taking as well as in the course of the mental status examination. The examiner first observes spontaneity of speech as well as the timber, pitch, and modulation of voice. Mutism may be encountered in several neurologic conditions such as akinetic mutism, vegetative state, locked-in syndrome, catatonic unresponsiveness, or large left hemispheric lesions. Akinetic mutism is characterized by absent speech in the setting of alert-appearing immobility. The patient's eyes are open, and the individual may follow environmental events. The patient exhibits regular sleep-wake cycles but may be completely inert or display brief movements or postural adjustments spontaneously or in response to vigorous stimulation. Akinetic mutism may be seen with large frontal lobe injuries, bilateral cingulate gyrus damage, or midbrain pathology. Akinetic mutism should be distinguished from a vegetative state where the patient exhibits sleep-wake cycles with open eyes. A vegetative state can occur after severe brain injury. Locked-in syndrome occurs with bilateral pontine lesions, rendering the patient mute and paralyzed. Intellectual function, however, is not impaired and the patients can communicate by eye movements or eye blinks.

Spontaneous speech is characterized by its rate, rhythm, volume, response latency, and inflection. Accelerated speech may be encountered in mania, disinhibited orbitofrontal syndromes or festinating parkinsonian conditions, whereas a reduced rate of speech output can occur as a component of psychomotor retardation. Response latencies may be prolonged or the patient may impulsively interrupt the examiner, anticipating the question. Perturbed speech prosody (loss of melody or inflection) can be encountered in brain disorders affecting the right hemisphere or the basal ganglia. Empty speech with hesitations or circumlocutions can be exhibited in patients with word-finding difficulties. Word-finding impairment may occur in aphasias, metabolic encephalopathies, physical exhaustion, sleep deprivation, anxiety, depression, or dorsolateral frontal lobe damage in the absence of an anomia.

Aphasia is characterized by impairment in oral and/or written communication. Deficits will vary depending on the location and extent of anatomic involvement. Aphasias are generally characterized as nonfluent or fluent (**Table 9-4**). Nonfluent aphasias are characterized by a paucity of speech, often with a hesitant quality. There is impairment in word searching and writing. The patient

TABLE 9-4 ■ CHARACTERISTICS OF APHASIAS

FEATURE	BROCA APHASIA	WERNICKE APHASIA	CONDUCTION APHASIA	GLOBAL APHASIA	TRANSCORTICAL MOTOR	TRANSCORTICAL SENSORY	TRANSCORTICAL MIXED	PURE ANOMIA	THALAMIC
Anatomic localization	Inferior frontal (Broca area)	Superior temporal (Wernicke area)	Arcuate fasciculus	Middle cerebral artery distribution	Supplemental motor areas	Inferior parietal	Watershed areas	Angular/supramarginal gyrus	Dorsomedial or ventral anterior nuclei
Fluency	Nonfluent	Fluent	Fluent	Nonfluent	Nonfluent	Fluent	Nonfluent	Fluent	Nonfluent
Repetition	Impaired	Impaired	Impaired	Impaired	Normal	Normal	Normal, may be only preserved language function	Normal	Normal
Rhythm of speech	Effortful with dysarthria	Quickened, long-winded, effusive	Normal	Severely impaired, mute	Slightly effortful	May appear normal	Effortful, slow	Normal	Effortful, slow
Content	Agrammatical, telegraphic	Mispronunciation and neologism (nonsense words)	Occasional use of wrong words	Abnormal	Agrammatical	Circumlocution, tangential	Variable impairment	Often normal, but uses descriptive language	Variable
Paraphasias	Common	Common	Common	Common	Variable	Variable	Variable	Common	Variable
Comprehension—spoken	Good	Abnormal	Variable	Poor	Good	Abnormal	Abnormal	Normal	Abnormal
Comprehension—written	Worse than spoken	Better than spoken	May be normal	Poor	Good	Fair	Fair	Abnormal	Good
Writing	Impaired, with grammatical and spelling errors	Preserved, but inaccurate	Variable	Severely impaired	May be impaired	Preserved	Variable	Abnormal with spelling errors	Good
Naming	Poor	Poor	Fair	Poor	Poor	Good	Variable	Poor	Poor
Other findings	Hemiparesis, apraxia	Visual field deficits, hemisensory loss, apraxia	Mild hemiparesis, neglect	Hemiplegia, visual field deficits	Hemiparesis	Neglect, sensory loss	Variable with mild motor and sensory findings	Gerstmann syndrome (acalculia, agraphia, finger agnosia, left-right confusion)	Cognitive impairment, hemiataxia, hemiparesis, hemisensory loss

may appear frustrated or depressed because of awareness of the language deficit and the inability to communicate with family and health care providers. Fluent aphasias are characterized by empty speech. Word production is normal or may be increased but there is a lack of comprehension about what words mean, often associated with impairment in reading ability. The patient often displays little insight to the language deficit and instead may become agitated because others are not following the conversation.

Cognitive Assessment

The assessment of cognitive function should be conducted methodically and should assess comprehensively the major domains of neuropsychological function (attention, memory, language, visuospatial skills, executive ability). The patient's age, handedness, educational level, and sociocultural background may all influence cognitive function and should be determined prior to initiating or interpreting the evaluation.

Attention Two tests are useful in assessing attention: digit span forward and continuous performance tests. In the digit span forward test, the patient is asked to repeat increasingly long series of numbers (eg, 1, 3-7, 4-6-3, 5-1-9-2, etc). The examiner says the numbers at a rate of one per second. A normal forward digit span is seven digits; fewer than five is abnormal. Concentration is evaluated by a continuous performance test. An example would be to say the months of the year in reverse order, starting with the last month of the year (December). Distractible patients tend to lose track and skip 1 or 2 months. Serial subtraction can also be used to test concentration but heavily dependent on educational attainment and mathematical abilities. Confusional states such as delirium are characterized by impaired attention.

Memory Learning, recall, recognition, and memory for remote information are assessed in the course of mental status examination. Asking the patient to remember three words and then asking him or her to recall the words 3 minutes later can help assess learning, recall, and recognition. However, the shorter the list, the easier it is to remember, particularly in high-functioning individuals. When told to remember items, patients will often remember the first two items heard (known as "primacy") and the last two items heard (known as "recency"); therefore, longer lists of 10 words may be preferable. After a delay, recall of fewer than five words is considered abnormal. Patients having difficulty with recall may be given clues (eg, the category of items to which the word belongs or a list of words containing the target) to distinguish between storage and retrieval deficits. Prompting and clues will not aide patients with storage deficits (eg, amnesia); patients with intact storage but poor recall (eg, retrieval-deficit syndrome) may be aided by clues. Amnestic deficits are thought to be caused by lesions in the hippocampal-thalamic circuit while retrieval deficits are likely due to lesions of frontal-basal ganglia circuitry.

Information is gathered on the patient's remote memory function while taking a history of the patient's illness, inquiring about the patient's life events (marriage, births of children, etc), and asking about important historical events. An informant may also be helpful here to verify these events. The temporal profile of remote memory may be diagnostically important. Amnestic syndromes such as dementias usually feature normal, nonmemory cognitive functions, a period of retrograde amnesia following the onset of the disorder, variable periods of anterograde amnesia, and intact remote memory beyond the period of the retrograde amnesia. Psychogenic memory loss may include variable patterns of amnesia particularly in long-term events (eg, not recall birth of children, not recall being married).

Language Language assessment entails the evaluation of all aspects of communication including spontaneous speech, comprehension, repetition, naming, reading, and writing. Aphasic disturbances are characterized as fluent or nonfluent. Fluent aphasias are characterized by normal or excessive amounts of speech, preserved phrase length, intact speech melody, usually in combination with a paucity of information. Phonemic paraphasias (substitution of one phoneme for another); semantic paraphasias (the replacement of one word with another); or neologistic paraphasias (the construction of new words) may occur. Wernicke, transcortical sensory, conduction, and anomic aphasias are fluent aphasic syndromes.

Nonfluent aphasias feature reduced verbal output, short or one-word replies, agrammatism, poor speech initiation, reduced speech prosody, and dysarthria. There are few paraphasias. Broca, transcortical motor, global, and mixed transcortical aphasias are nonfluent aphasic disorders. Interestingly, nonfluent aphasic patients may have preserved abilities to curse fluently and sing well-learned songs (eg, "Happy Birthday") with few errors.

Primary progressive aphasia is a disorder seen in patients with asymmetric frontotemporal degeneration that involves dominant hemisphere. Progressive nonfluent aphasia involves primarily unilateral left frontal, left frontoparietal, or left frontotemporal degeneration and is characterized by agrammatism, paraphasias, and anomia. Bilateral temporal lobe atrophy and hypoperfusion with more pronounced involvement of the left anterior temporal lobe may cause semantic dementia that is characterized by progressive loss of knowledge about objects, people, facts, and words; it is often accompanied by visual agnosia (inability to name or recognize objects presented visually).

Language comprehension is tested by asking the patient to follow increasingly complex linguistic constructions. The easiest commands are one-step orders such as "stand up" and "turn around," "open your mouth," and "stick out your tongue." Asking the patient to point to room objects or body parts is the next level of comprehension difficulty. Finally, more complex questions, such as "If a lion is killed by a tiger, which animal is dead?" are asked. Impaired comprehension usually implies dysfunction of parietotemporal regions of the left hemisphere. Comprehension is abnormal in most fluent and global aphasic syndrome but may be preserved in nonfluent syndromes. In older adults, it is important to establish that hearing is intact before testing comprehension. Failure to comprehend commands may reflect the inability to hear as opposed to impaired comprehension.

Repetition is assessed by asking the patient to repeat increasingly long phrases or sentences. Generally, it is best to begin with simple phrases such as salutations ("Hello") and progress to more complex phrases ("Around the rugged rock, the ragged rascal ran"). Omissions and paraphasic substitutions may disrupt accurate repetition. Repetition is impaired in Wernicke, Broca, conductive, and global aphasia but is generally preserved in transcortical aphasias.

Naming tests involve asking the patient to name objects, parts of objects, and colors. Errors include paraphasias, circumlocutory responses, and simply making no response. Aphasic patients may use descriptive terms rather than giving the proper name. For example, a "watch" becomes "the thing you tell time with." Anomia occurs in aphasia, dementia, delirium, and can sometimes be seen as a consequence of head trauma. Adequate vision and object recognition must be ensured before errors are ascribed to naming deficits.

When assessing reading, the patient's ability to read aloud and to comprehend what is read must both be tested. Adequate vision must be ensured before failures are ascribed to an alexia. Most aphasias have concomitant alexias, however the converse may not be true. In alexia with agraphia and alexia without agraphia, reading abnormalities may occur in the absence of other signs of aphasia.

Mechanical or aphasic abnormalities may cause agraphia. Micrographia is a characteristic aspect of parkinsonism in which the script becomes progressively smaller as the patient writes a sentence or extended series of numbers or letters, and mechanical agraphias occur in patients with limb paresis, limb apraxia, or movement disorders such as tremor and chorea. Aphasic agraphias accompany aphasic syndromes and errors similar to those noted in verbal output are present in written form. In Gerstmann syndrome (agraphia, acalculia, right-left disorientation, finger agnosia), alexia with agraphia, and disconnection agraphia (occurring with injury of the corpus callosum), agraphia occurs without aphasia. Agraphia also occurs in dementia and delirium.

Orientation Orientation to time is tested by asking the patient to identify the correct day of the week, date, month, and year. Although some patients may make excuses (eg, they are retired, they don't need to know, etc.), only correct answers should be counted. This should be followed by asking the patient to guess the correct time of day without looking at a watch or clock. The patient should be within 1 hour of the correct time. Orientation to place is assessed by asking about city, county, state, and current location. If the patient is from out of town, major landmarks may be substituted for less well-known information such as county. Lastly, orientation to situation can be assessed by asking the patient why they are in the office today.

Abstraction Similarities, differences, idioms, and proverb interpretation can all be used to assess abstracting capacity. These tests are heavily influenced by culture and educational attainment. Abstraction abnormalities are a nonspecific indicator of cerebral dysfunction. Patients with frontal lobe disorders have disproportionately severe abstracting disturbances.

Judgment and problem-solving abilities Assessing judgment assists in exploring the patient's interpersonal and social insight. Judgment is impaired in many neurologic conditions. Damage to orbitofrontal subcortical circuit (eg, in frontotemporal dementia, trauma, or focal syndromes) produces marked alterations in social judgment. Problem-solving can be assessed by giving a scenario "If in a strange town, how would a person locate a friend they wished to see?" Correct answers might include use of phone book, the Internet, or city directory.

Visuospatial skills There are a number of visuospatial abilities including spatial attention, perception, construction, visuospatial problem-solving, and visuospatial memory. Constructional tasks are most widely used to assess visuospatial ability. In the clock-drawing test, the patient is asked to draw a clock and draw the hands of the clock to indicate a specific time. The hands should be of different lengths. Watching the patient complete the clock is sometimes as informative as the finished product.

Patients with executive dysfunction may draw a clock face that is too small to contain the required numbers (poor planning), whereas patients with unilateral neglect will ignore half of the clock face.

Tests of copying involve having the patient reproduce figures such as a circle, intersecting circle and triangle, overlapping pentagons, cube, or more complex figures. Abnormalities include failures to reproduce the shapes accurately, perseveration on individual elements, drawing over the stimulus figure, or unilateral neglect. Drawing disturbances are common with many types of neurologic conditions including focal brain damage, degenerative disorders, and toxic and metabolic encephalopathies.

Calculation In assessing calculation skills, patients are asked to add or multiply one or two digits mentally or to execute more demanding problems with pencil and paper. Calculation abilities are related to education and occupation. Acalculias may occur in association with a number of aphasic syndromes while visuospatial disorders lead to incorrect alignment of columns of numbers. Primary anarithmetias (inability to do math) are produced by damage to the posterior left hemisphere.

Executive function Executive function is assessed by asking the patient to perform tasks mediated by frontal-subcortical systems. Frontal-subcortical systems are complex neural circuits that include the dorsolateral prefrontal cortex, striatum, globus pallidus/substantia nigra, thalamic nuclei, and connecting white matter tracts. Patients with executive dysfunction manifest perseveration; motor programming abnormalities; reduced word list generation (left dorsolateral dysfunction); reduced nonverbal fluency (right dorsolateral dysfunction); poor set shifting; abnormal recall with intact recognition memory; loss of abstraction abilities; poor judgment; and impaired mental control. These abnormalities are common following head trauma, frontal lobe degenerations, frontal lobe neoplasms, multiple sclerosis, Huntington disease, and other basal ganglia disorders, subcortical infarctions, and in some brain infections such as syphilis.

Digit span backward is a test of mental control and complex attention, as well as executive dysfunction. It entails saying increasingly long series of numbers and asking the patient to say them backward (give 2-5-8, response should be 8-5-2). A normal digit span in reverse is five digits; fewer than three is abnormal.

Word list generation Word list generation is a very useful test and involves asking the patient to think of as many members of a specific category (most commonly animals) as possible within 1 minute. Normal individuals can name approximately 18 animals within 1 minute; fewer than 14 is considered abnormal. Word list generation deficits occur with anomia, frontal-subcortical systems dysfunction, and psychomotor retardation. It is a highly sensitive test but lacks specificity.

Informant assessment In many instances, asking questions of the informant will provide a wealth of information regarding the baseline abilities of the patient. There are several structured interviews that are short, easy to administer, and do not require specific training. Functional abilities and activities of daily living can be assessed with the Functional Activities Questionnaire, the Physical Self-Maintenance Scale, Instrumental Activities of Daily Living Scale, or the Barthel index. Baseline cognitive abilities can be assessed with brief informant interviews such as the Quick Dementia Rating System (QDRS), AD8, or the IQCODE. The AD8 was developed in a research sample and validated in a clinic population and asks eight questions regarding change in the patients' memory, orientation, judgment and problem-solving abilities, executive function, and interest level. Endorsement of two or more items suggests cognitive dysfunction and should trigger a more formal evaluation.

Neuropsychiatric Assessment

The neuropsychiatric interview of the patient includes the evaluation of thought form, thought content, and insight. The new onset of disturbances in any of these domains in older patients is unusual in the absence of a brain disease. Their emergence should trigger the search for a neurologic or psychiatric condition.

Thought form Formal thought disorders such as tangentiality, circumstantiality, loose associations, illogicality, derailment, and thought blocking are much less common than disturbances of thought content as a manifestation of psychosis in neurologic diseases. Thought disorders have been observed in the psychoses accompanying epilepsy, Huntington disease, and idiopathic basal ganglia calcification.

Perseveration and incoherence are disorders of the form of thought that are common in neuropsychiatric conditions. Perseveration refers to the inappropriate continuation of an act or thought after conclusion of its proper context. Intrusions are a special case of perseveration with late recurrences of words or thoughts from an earlier context. Perseverations and intrusions are seen in aphasias and dementing illnesses. Incoherence refers to the absence of logical association between words or ideas. It is observed in delirium, advanced dementias, and as part of the output of fluent aphasia.

Thought content Several types of disorders of thought content occur in neurologic diseases. Delusions are the most common manifestation of psychosis in neurologic disorders and are characterized by false beliefs based on incorrect inference about external reality. Common types of delusions encountered involve being followed or spied on, theft of personal property, spousal infidelity, or the presence of unwelcome strangers in one's home. Theme-specific delusions such as the Capgras syndrome (the belief that someone has been replaced by an identical-appearing impostor) may also be observed in neurologic illnesses. Delusions are common in a number of dementia etiologies including Alzheimer disease and dementia with Lewy bodies, and may occur in vascular dementia, frontotemporal dementia, and Huntington disease.

Hallucinations occur in many neurologic disorders. Hallucinations are sensory perceptions that occur without stimulation of the relevant sensory organ. Hallucinations and delusions occur together in psychosis; hallucinations are nondelusional when the patient recognizes the sensory experience to be unreal. Hallucinations may involve any sensory modality (visual, auditory, tactile, gustatory, olfactory) and may be formed (eg, people or things) or unformed (flashing lights or colors). Hallucinations occur with ocular and structural brain disorders as well as Charles Bonnet syndrome, epilepsy, narcolepsy, and migraine. Well-formed visual hallucinations (children, furry animals) are a prominent early sign in dementia with Lewy bodies. Less well-formed visual hallucinations occur in the moderate to severe stages of Alzheimer disease. Gustatory or olfactory hallucinations are most common in seizure disorders, bipolar disorder, and schizophrenia, and with tumors located in the medial temporal lobe. Tactile hallucinations are most commonly associated with schizophrenia, affective disorders, or drug intoxication or withdrawal.

Insight Patients with neuropsychiatric disease may display limited insight and be unaware of their medical conditions or limitations in function; thus assessment of a patient's insight into the severity of their illness can yield useful diagnostic information and assist in developing a therapeutic plan. For example, Alzheimer disease patients have impaired insight into their memory and cognitive difficulties, whereas patients with vascular dementia and dementia with Lewy bodies often exhibit more appropriate concern regarding their cognitive dysfunction. Lesions of the right parietal lobe are associated with unawareness, neglect, or denial of the abnormalities of the contralateral side.

Behavior and personality A variety of changes in personality and behavior have been described in neuropsychiatric disease in the older adult. Personality changes may include increased egocentricity and thought rigidity, impaired emotional control and diminished emotional responsiveness, loss of interest and apathy, and lack of concern for the feelings of others. No brief personality rating scales are available but in the proper setting the Neuroticism-Extroversion-Openness Five-Factor Inventory (NEO-FFI) can be used to evaluate personality. Behavioral changes including irritability, depression, anxiety, hallucinations, delusions, and vegetative changes can be assessed with the Neuropsychiatric Inventory (NPI). Both long and short forms of the NPI are available.

NEUROLOGIC EXAMINATION

The neurologic examination includes assessment of cranial nerve function, strength, coordination, sensation, muscle stretch reflexes, pathologic/primitive reflexes, and neurovascular status. Examination of head and neck may provide additional important information.

Cranial Nerve Examination

Cranial nerve I: olfactory In normal aging, loss of olfaction may be a nonspecific or clinically insignificant finding. Olfaction may be impaired following head trauma, infection, zinc deficiency, vitamin A deficiency, frontal lobe dysfunction, vitamin B_{12} deficiency, and frontal lobe tumors (olfactory groove meningioma). Olfaction is tested by asking the patient to identify a variety of odors. When testing, it is important to use simple and familiar odors (coffee beans, vanilla, or cinnamon). Complex scents such as perfumes and noxious agents (ie, ammonia) should not be used. Ideally, the patient should close their eyes and each nostril should be tested separately.

Cranial nerve II: optic Examination of the optic nerve includes visual inspection of the nerve head, testing of visual acuity, and mapping of the visual fields. In aging, visual acuity may be impaired and can be due to a number of neurologic and ophthalmologic causes. First, casual inspection of the corneal, sclera, and mucosal tissue should be carried out to evaluate structural abnormalities. Visual acuity can be evaluated with a Snellen visual chart or Rosenberg card held 14 in from the eye. Screening should be done in a well-lit environment and to the patient's advantage allowing them to use their corrective lenses. If they do not have their glasses with them, refractive errors can be partly corrected by using a pinhole. Visual fields are tested at the bedside by confrontation. The examiner should face the patient, sitting or standing at a similar height and each eye should be tested independently. The patient is asked to look at the examiner's nose and the examiner's arms are extended laterally. The patient is asked to differentiate between one or two fingers. Each quadrant should be tested separately. After testing each eye individually, both eyes should be tested simultaneously for visual neglect. Monocular visual field deficits can be associated with glaucoma. Abrupt changes in visual fields or acuity should alert the clinician to potential vascular etiologies. Homonymous field deficits reflect disruption of the optic pathway posterior to the optic chiasm.

Pupillary examination should include evaluation of size and shape. Up to a 1-mm difference in size is generally considered normal. Pupillary responses are tested with a bright flashlight (not the ophthalmoscope). A normal pupil reacts to light by constricting; the contralateral pupil should also constrict. The pupils also constrict when shifting focus from a distant object to a near object (accommodation) and during convergence such as when patients are asked to look at their nose. Abnormalities of pupillary responses are associated with a number of neurologic disorders (**Table 9-5**). A review of medications is also important as a number of drugs can affect pupillary size. Mydriasis (pupillary dilation) can be caused by atropine-like drugs, while miosis (pupillary constriction) can be caused by parasympathomimetic drugs.

A careful examination of the optic nerve should be performed in all patients. It is not always necessary to do a dilated examination, but the room should be darkened to increase pupillary size. The sharpness of optic disc margins, the ratio of optic cup to disc, venous pulsations, the caliber of blood vessels, and the presence of exudates, hemorrhages, emboli, and retinal pallor should be noted. Papilledema is characterized by blurring or elevation of the disc margins with the loss of normal venous pulsations and reflects raised intracranial pressure. As pressure increases, hemorrhages may be found adjacent to the disc. Glaucoma increases the size of the optic cup relative to the disc.

Cranial nerves III, IV, and VI: oculomotor, trochlear, and abducens The oculomotor, trochlear, and abducens nerves mediate ocular motility, pupillary responses, and eyelid position. The trochlear nerve innervates the superior oblique muscle, the abducens nerve innervates the lateral rectus muscle, while the oculomotor nerve innervates the remainder of the extraocular muscles. The oculomotor nerve also innervates the levator muscles of the eyelid and carries parasympathetic nerves to the pupil. Testing each eye individually helps to identify ocular motility dysfunction. In aging, ocular motility may be reduced. Normal older adults can exhibit restricted convergence and limitation of conjugate upward gaze. Other nonspecific concomitants of normal aging include the evolution of small sluggishly reactive pupils, loss of Bell phenomenon (upward eye deviation on eye closure), and the inability to dissociate ocular movements from head movements.

TABLE 9-5 ■ CAUSES OF PUPILLARY CHANGES IN OLDER ADULT

MIOSIS (PUPILLARY CONSTRICTION)	MYDRIASIS (PUPILLARY DILATATION)
Pontine lesion	Dorsal midbrain syndrome (Parinaud)
Organophosphates	Amphetamines and sympathomimetics
Cholinergic agents	Anticholinergic agents
Opioids (except meperidine)	Meperidine
Pilocarpine-like agents	Atropine-like agents
Barbiturates	Cocaine
Phenothiazines	Phenothiazines
MAO inhibitors	Antihistamines
Phencyclidine (PCP)	Lysergic acid diethylamide (LSD)
Argyll-Robertson (syphilis)	Seizures/postictal state
Horner syndrome (usually unilateral)	Thyrotoxicosis
Hypothermia	Hypermagnesemia
	Third nerve compression (usually unilateral)

SITE OF LESION	PUPIL SIZE	DIRECT RESPONSE	CONSENSUAL RESPONSE		ACCOMMODATION
			IPSILATERAL	CONTRALATERAL	
Retina	Normal	Impaired	Impaired	Normal	Normal
Optic nerve	Normal	Lost	Lost	Normal	Normal
Optic chiasm	Normal	Normal	Normal	Normal	Normal
Optic tract	Normal	Normal	Normal	Normal	Normal
Optic radiation	Normal	Normal	Normal	Normal	Normal
Oculomotor nerve or nucleus	Dilated	Lost	Normal	Lost	Lost
Argyll-Robertson	Constricted	Lost	Normal	Lost	Normal
Sympathetic	Constricted	Normal	Normal	Normal	Normal

The clinician should be concerned when an older patient exhibits new-onset diplopia, pupillary asymmetry, nystagmus (**Table 9-6**), or extraocular movement disorders. Ptosis (drooping of the upper lid) can be caused by a number of disorders (**Table 9-7**). Isolated abducens palsies may be a sign of elevated intracranial pressure since the sixth nerve has the longest intracranial course.

Cranial nerve V: trigeminal The trigeminal nerve is divided into three divisions: ophthalmic, maxillary, and mandibular. The first two divisions are pure sensory nerves mediating facial and corneal sensation. The third division carries both sensory fibers and innervates the muscles of mastication. The corneal reflex is mediated by the ophthalmic division and can be tested by lightly stimulating the cornea with a wisp of cotton. When the cornea on one side is stimulated, both eyes should close. Facial sensation is tested with a safety pin or cold handle of a tuning fork. Motor function is tested by asking the patient to bite down or open the jaw against resistance. Tumors of the middle fossa and in the cerebellopontine angle may compress the fifth cranial nerve and produce a cranial nerve syndrome with decreased corneal reflex and sensory loss on the ipsilateral face. Tic douloureux (trigeminal neuralgia) is a paroxysmal pain disorder triggered by touching sensitive zones usually within the mandibular division. The cause may be idiopathic, due to compressive lesions or demyelination at the root entry zone.

Cranial nerve VII: facial The facial nerve supplies the facial musculature, lacrimal and salivary glands, and taste fibers of the anterior tongue. The motor function is tested by asking the patient to wrinkle their forehead, close their eyes, and smile. Unilateral weakness may cause a flattening of the nasolabial fold. If very weak, the patient may experience drooling. The eyelid is usually not severely affected with central lesions and the upper forehead is spared. In peripheral lesions such as Bell palsy (**Table 9-8**), patients are unable to close their eye or wrinkle their forehead. The facial nerve also innervates the stapedius muscle of the middle ear which helps to modulate tympanic membrane vibration. This motor branch can be damaged during closed head trauma leading to hyperacusis, an increased perception of sound. The sense of taste is not often tested, but can be done at the bedside using sugar, salt, or lemon juice. The patient is asked to stick their tongue out and a small amount of solution is placed on one side of the tongue. The patient is asked to describe the taste, and then allowed to drink some water before the next solution is applied.

TABLE 9-6 ■ TYPES OF NYSTAGMUS AND OCULAR OSCILLATIONS

MOVEMENT	DESCRIPTION	LOCALIZATION
Physiologic end-stage	Fine, regular horizontal jerking at extremes of lateral gaze	No pathologic significance
Jerk	Horizontal and rotary	Vestibular disorder
Vertical	Jerk movements in vertical plane	Posterior fossa disease, sedatives, anticonvulsants
Downbeating	Rhythmic, horizontal gaze still possible	Cervicomedullary junction lesion
Upbeating	Rhythmic, horizontal gaze still possible	Lesion in pons, cerebellar vermis or medulla
Ocular bobbing	Arrhythmic, coarse movement with horizontal gaze palsy	Pontine lesion
Seesaw	Vertical dysconjugate movements with rotary component	Lesion by optic chiasm
Periodic alternating	Horizontal nystagmus with periodically alternating direction	Lower brain stem
Rebound	Horizontal jerk nystagmus transiently after sustained gaze to opposite side	Cerebellar pathways
Convergence-retraction	Eyes converge and move rhythmically back into the orbits on attempted upgaze	Periaqueductal gray (midbrain)
Ocular dysmetria	Overshoot or terminal oscillation of saccadic movements	Cerebellar pathways
Hypometric saccades	Slowed movements	Parkinson disease, basal ganglia
Opsoclonus	Chaotic multidirectional conjugate saccades	Paraneoplastic syndrome (neuroblastoma, breast, lung)
Square-wave jerks	Small saccades interfering with visual fixation	Progressive supranuclear palsy
Ocular myoclonus	Rhythmic oscillations, usually vertical	Associated with palatal myoclonus, brain stem lesion

Cranial nerve VIII: cochlear and vestibular Hearing and vestibular function are mediated by the eighth cranial nerve. Evaluation of hearing at the bedside is sometimes difficult. Use of a 512-Hz tuning fork can help discriminate conduction from sensorineural hearing loss. The Rinne test is done by placing a vibrating tuning fork on the mastoid process. As soon as the patient is unable to detect sound, the tuning fork is moved to a position near the external auditory canal. If the patient has normal hearing, air conduction should be better than bone conduction. If the patient has conduction deafness, the sound will not be heard because of pathology in the middle ear. In nerve deafness, air conduction is better than bone conduction, but both will be reduced. The Weber test looks for lateralization. The tuning fork is placed in the middle of the skull and the patient is asked to decide where they best hear the sound. In normal hearing, the sound is heard equally in both ears. In conduction deafness, vibrations are best heard in the abnormal ear. In nerve deafness, the sound is best appreciated in the normal ear. Decreased hearing for high-pitched sounds and lack of perception of background noise are common findings in normal aging and by themselves should not be considered a pathologic finding. Sensorineural deafness

TABLE 9-7 ■ CAUSES OF PTOSIS IN THE OLDER ADULT

Congenital

Myopathic causes
  Myasthenia gravis
  Oculopharyngeal muscular dystrophy
  Myotonic dystrophy
  Polymyositis
  Hypothyroidism

Horner syndrome

Vasculitis

Diabetes mellitus

Third nerve lesions (ptosis is rarely isolated finding)
  Nuclear lesion in mesencephalon
  Third nerve compression

TABLE 9-8 ■ CAUSES OF BELL PALSY

Idiopathic
Pregnancy
Guillain-Barré syndrome
Lyme disease (may present as bifacial weakness)
Herpes zoster (Ramsay Hunt syndrome)
Neoplasms
Sarcoidosis
Head trauma
Acute intermittent porphyria
Lead poisoning
Brain stem infarction (rare)

TABLE 9-9 ■ DIFFERENTIAL DIAGNOSIS OF TINNITUS

TONAL TINNITUS	NONTONAL TINNITUS
Otitis media	Contraction of muscles in eustachian tube
Disorder of tympanic membrane	Contraction of stapedius muscle
Inner ear disorder (hair cells, organ of Corti)	Contraction of tensor tympani muscles
Cochlear nerve lesion	Palatal myoclonus
Acoustic schwannoma	Carotid bruit
Meningioma	Arteriovenous malformations
Neurofibroma	Glomus jugulare tumor
Ménière disease	
Head trauma	

is characterized by loss of high-pitched sounds while conduction deafness is characterized by loss of low-pitched sounds. Tinnitus or ringing in the ears is a common symptom in adults. Tonal tinnitus is subjective and heard only by the patient. Nontonal tinnitus is more objective because in certain circumstances, the tinnitus can be heard by the examiner. The differential diagnosis of tinnitus is presented in **Table 9-9**.

Vestibular lesions produce nystagmus and vertigo. Vestibular nystagmus is horizontal or combined horizontal-rotatory and is typically accompanied by vertigo and nausea, whereas lesions disrupting vestibular connections in the central nervous system can produce nystagmus in any direction but are usually not associated with vertiginous or nauseous sensations. When characterizing nystagmus, only the fast component should be described. The complaint of dizziness in older adults is not uncommon; however, the examiner must determine whether the dizzy patient is experiencing light-headedness or true vertigo. If true vertigo is present, then the clinician should further discern whether it is peripheral (vestibular) or central (brain stem) in origin as well as associated features (**Table 9-10**). Causes of vertigo associated with vestibular disease include benign positional vertigo, Meniere syndrome, and trauma.

Cranial nerves IX and X: glossopharyngeal and vagus The ninth and tenth cranial nerves control pharyngeal and laryngeal function, taste, and the gag reflex. Glossopharyngeal lesions cause asymmetric elevation of the palate and deviation of the uvula. Hoarseness, aphonia, and dysphagia occur with vagus nerve lesions. In normal aging, the gag reflex can be reduced and, when accompanied by a decrease in the cough reflex, can result in difficulty handling bronchial secretions. Glossopharyngeal neuralgia is a rare paroxysmal pain syndrome involving the posterior pharynx or tonsils usually triggered by excessively hot or cold foods or liquids.

TABLE 9-10 ■ CAUSES OF VERTIGO AND ASSOCIATED FINDINGS

ANATOMIC LOCATIONS	CAUSES	OTOSCOPIC EXAMINATION	OTHER NEUROLOGIC FINDINGS	TESTS OF EQUILIBRIUM	NYSTAGMUS	HEARING LOSS
Labyrinth	Benign positional, trauma, Ménière, drug toxicity, viral infection	Usually negative	None	Ipsilateral past pointing, lateral pulsion to side of lesion	Horizontal or rotary to side opposite lesion, paroxysmal, positional	May be normal, sensorineural or conduction deafness
Vestibular	Vestibular neuronopathy, herpes zoster	Zoster vesicles in auditory canal, tympanic membrane, and palate	7th and 8th cranial nerves	Ipsilateral past pointing, lateral pulsion to side of lesion	Positional	Sensorineural
Cerebellopontine angle tumor	Acoustic neuroma, meningioma, glioma, glomus jugulare	Normal	Ipsilateral 5th, 7th, 9th, and 10th cranial nerves, ataxia, increased intracranial pressure	Ataxia	Gaze paretic, positional, coarser to side of lesion	Sensorineural
Brain stem and cerebellar lesions	Infarct, gliomas, encephalitis	Negative	Multiple cranial nerves, sensory or motor tract signs, ataxia, dysmetria	Ataxia	Horizontal and/or vertical, gaze paretic	Normal
Cortical lesions	Infarct, glioma, trauma	Negative	Fluent aphasia, visual field cuts, hemimotor/sensory findings, seizures	Usually no change, mild ataxia	Usually absent	Normal

Cranial nerve XI: accessory nerve The spinal accessory nerve innervates the upper half of the trapezius and the sternocleidomastoid muscle. In normal older adults, frank weakness of the trapezius or sternocleidomastoid muscle is not a typical finding and, if present, should be investigated further. A delayed shrug may be an indication of a mild ipsilateral hemiparesis.

Cranial nerve XII: hypoglossal The hypoglossal nerve innervates the tongue. Patients are asked to stick their tongue out; deviation to either side implies a lesion on the side of deviation. The tongue should also be examined for atrophy and spontaneous muscle contractions (fasciculation) suggesting upper motor neuron disease. Fasciculation is best detected on the lateral aspects of the tongue. Tongue weakness is also common in pseudobulbar palsy.

Motor System Examination

Muscle bulk, strength, tone, and coordination are assessed as part of the motor system examination.

Muscle bulk Muscle bulk is examined by visual inspection and palpation. Muscle wasting may occur with disuse; muscle, nerve, or spinal disease; and in generalized weight loss secondary to malnutrition, systemic illness, or advanced brain diseases. Mild muscular wasting without associated weakness can be encountered in normal aging most commonly involving the intrinsic hand and foot muscles, calf, and shoulder girdle muscles.

Muscle tone Muscle tone may be increased or decreased in neurologic disorders. Muscle tone is decreased in muscle and peripheral nerve disease, with cerebellar disorders, early in the course of many choreiform disorders, and acutely following an upper motor neuron lesion. Increased muscle tone is encountered in spasticity with pyramidal tract lesions and rigidity with extrapyramidal disorders. Cogwheel rigidity of Parkinson disease is best palpated when manipulating the distal limbs, usually in a circular motion. "Gegenhalten" refers to the active resistance to movement encountered in advanced brain diseases. In order to optimize the diagnostic yield of the muscular tone examination, the clinician should distract the patient while the examination is performed. For example, the clinician could ask the patient to perform circulatory movements with the right hand as if he "is washing a window" while he is examining the muscular tone on the left arm. By this means, a more accurate representation of the tone is obtained. This is particularly useful in patients with Parkinson disease, when the examiner is testing for cogwheel rigidity. Since rigidity is recognized as one of the cardinal motor symptoms in Parkinson disease, performing an optimal muscular tone examination increases the diagnostic yield of this disease.

Strength Strength is graded as 0 (no evidence of muscle contraction), 1 (muscle contraction without movement of the limb), 2 (limb movement after gravity eliminated), 3 (limb movement against gravity), 4 (limb movement against partial resistance), or 5 (normal strength). Distal weakness is most indicative of peripheral neuropathies, whereas proximal weakness is more consistent with primary muscle disease. In aging, mild generalized weakness may occur; however, focal weakness is indicative of a neuropathologic process. Focal weakness often is subtle and may be detected only with careful examination. Hemiparesis occurs with lesions of the pyramidal system. When testing strength, the examiner should attempt to isolate individual muscles (thumb abduction) rather than testing whole groups (hand grip) to detect subtle signs of weakness. A pronator drift is seen with mild forms of weakness. When testing for muscular strength, the examiner should be familiarized with functional motor weakness. Known as the "Hoover test", this sign is the most useful to examine for functional weakness. When performing this test, the clinician should ask the patient to raise the affected leg without resistance. If a discrepancy is observed between voluntary hip extension (which is weak) and involuntary hip extension when the opposite hip is being flexed against resistance (which is normal), this finding would point toward a diagnosis of functional weakness.

Abnormal movements During the interview and examination, the clinician should be observant for any movement that is not purposeful including tremor, chorea, dyskinesias, and ballismus. Tremor is usually described as action (associated with a movement) or rest (disappears with movement of affected extremities). "Essential" tremor is a usually benign hereditary condition associated with movement or sustained posture and may involve arms, legs, head, chin, or voice. Essential tremors often improve after drinking small amounts of alcohol.

Sensory Examination

Primary modalities, including light touch and temperature are tested to assess sensory function. Sensory examination is quite subjective, and it is important to consider the consistency of responses and how sensory complaints relate to other signs and symptoms. Peripheral causes of sensory loss typically present bilaterally and are largely symmetric. Unilateral sensory loss occurs with lesions of primary sensory cortex or its projections.

Light touch Evaluation of light touch is not particularly helpful in discriminating pathology but is useful in defining the presence or loss of sensation. Lightly stroking the fingers or a wisp of cotton across the skin may help elicit dermatomal patterns of sensory loss for further evaluation.

Pain and temperature Pain and temperature sensation is carried by small unmyelinated fibers. Pain can be assessed with the use of a disposable safety pin while temperature can be assessed with the handle of the reflex hammer or tuning fork. The loss of pain sensation due to a metabolic or toxic peripheral neuropathy typically follows a stocking glove pattern, while lesions due to a radiculopathy follow a defined dermatome.

Vibration Vibration is carried by large, myelinated fibers and is assessed with a 128-Hz tuning fork. The tuning fork should be struck and placed on a bony prominence. Causes of pathologic decreased vibratory sensation include peripheral neuropathies, diabetes, tabes dorsalis, vitamin B_{12} deficiency, and myelopathies.

Position Proprioception is assessed by having the patient close their eyes and the examiner gently moves toes or fingers in the vertical plane. Skin proprioception can be assessed by lightly stroking the skin in an up or down fashion. The Romberg sign is performed to assess the integrity of the dorsal columns. The patient is asked to stand with their feet together and eyes closed. The presence of a sway suggests a positive test. If the problem is due to a proprioceptive deficit, the patient is able to correct themselves with their eyes open. Position sense loss can be caused by peripheral neuropathies, diabetes, tabes dorsalis, vitamin B_{12} deficiency, and myelopathies.

Cerebellar Examination

Cerebellar function and coordination may be disrupted by many types of motor and sensory abnormalities. Tests of coordination include rapid alternating movements, fine finger movements, finger-to-nose movements, and heel-knee-shin maneuvers. During aging, there is an overall decrease in speed of coordinated movements that is of no pathologic consequence. However, gross abnormalities in cerebellar function are not anticipated and should be evaluated thoroughly (**Table 9-11**).

When unilateral cerebellar dysfunction is present, patient will overshoot target but may improve after a few trials. Dysdiadochokinesis occurs when the patient is asked to rapidly change hand or finger movements; difficulties in maintaining smooth movements are characteristic. Cerebellar lesions can also affect muscle tone causing hypotonia. Cerebellar tremors tend to be coarse and irregular, worsening in the terminal one-third of a movement.

Gait and Station

Gate and posture depend on motor, sensory, and cerebellar function. In normal aging, posture becomes more flexed, slowed, and may have a slightly unsteady quality. When assessing gait in the older adult, it is important to recognize gait abnormalities that may be secondary to joint pain and arthritic conditions. Gait is assessed by having the patient walk straight for at least 10 yd, making a turn, and maneuvering in a tight corridor. It is important to note the presence of arm swing and the distance of the stride. The patient should also be asked to tandem walk, walk on their toes and heels and if possible, walk up a few steps. Postural stability is assessed by asking the patient to stand with their shoulder-width apart. A forceful pull is given to their shoulders and the righting response is assessed. The clinician should be prepared to catch the patient. One or two steps of retropulsion are considered normal. **Table 9-12** lists common causes of gait disturbance in the older adult.

Muscle Stretch Reflexes

Decreased muscle stretch reflexes are found in muscle, peripheral nerve, and nerve root disorders, while increased reflexes occur with upper motor neuron lesions. Lateralized hyperactive reflexes in conjunction with spasticity and the Babinski sign are indicative of a contralateral lesion of the pyramidal system. In aging, deep tendon reflexes tend to become hypoactive. Ankle reflexes may be absent in normal aging, but knee reflexes persist. Reflexes are initially hyperactive in cervical and lumbar spondylosis; however, in advanced cases, absent or diminished reflexes may be found as nerve roots become compromised.

Pathologic and Primitive Reflexes

The Babinski sign is dorsiflexion of the great toe with plantar stimulation. It is produced by upper motor neuron lesions. The grasp reflex (involuntary gripping of objects in or near the patient's hand) occurs in patients with advanced brain disease and with lesions restricted to the medial frontal lobes. The sucking reflex (sucking movements of the lips, tongue, and jaw elicited by stimulation of the lips) occurs in patients with frontal lobe and diffuse brain dysfunction.

The palmomental reflex (ipsilateral contraction of the mentalis muscle in response to stroking of the thenar eminence of the hand) can be seen in normal-aged individuals and may be regarded as pathologic when it is unilateral or when it does not fatigue with repeated palmar stimulation. The glabellar reflex (Myerson sign) is elicited by tapping the patient between the eyes. After a few blinks the patient should suppress further blinking. Patients with Parkinson disease and other basal ganglia disorders will continue to blink.

Higher Cortical Function

Cortical sensory modalities, including two-point discrimination, graphesthesia, and stereognosis should be assessed. Two-point discrimination is best performed with calipers. Graphesthesia is performed with the patient's eyes closed

TABLE 9-11 ■ ELEMENTS OF ATAXIA AND CEREBELLAR DYSFUNCTION

SIGN	DESCRIPTION
Dysmetria	Overshooting or undershooting a target
Dysdiadochokinesia	Impairment in rapid-alternating movements
Tremor	Coarse, rhythmic movement on action
Ataxic speech	Abnormal variability of volume, rate, and phonation
Dysarthria	Slow and slurred speech
Gait ataxia	Wide-based, unsteady

TABLE 9-12 ■ GAIT ABNORMALITIES IN THE OLDER ADULT

GAIT	CAUSE	DESCRIPTION	ASSOCIATED SIGNS
Festinating	Parkinson disease	Slow, shuffling picks up speed and may require wall or furniture to stop	Postural instability, rest tremor, bradykinesia, decreased arm swing, masked face, rigidity
Antalgic	Joint pain	Slow, gingerly pace	Facial grimaces
Spastic	Stroke	Stiff extremity, may require circumduction or scissor movements	Scuffing toe of affected leg across ground, weakness
Ataxic	Cerebellar disease	Wide-based	Dysmetria, dysdiadochokinesis
Sensory ataxia	Peripheral neuropathy	Wide-based, high steps with foot slapping	Sensory loss, weakness
Apraxic	Normal pressure hydrocephalus	Feet appear "nailed" to floor, lower extremity bradykinesia	Dementia, urinary incontinence
Stooped	Lumbar stenosis	Forward flexion	Pain, lordosis, kyphoscoliosis
Myopathic	Proximal myopathy, myasthenia gravis	Uses arms to help push themselves up stairs or out of a chair (Gowers sign)	Muscle cramps, weakness, myoglobinuria
Astasia-abasia	Psychosis, malingering	Wildly lurching, "herky-jerky" movements; however, patient does not fall	Signs of intoxication, delusions, hallucinations, secondary gain

and numbers are traced onto the palm with the back of the reflex hammer. Stereognosis is also performed with the patient's eyes closed. Common objects are placed into the patients' hand and they are allowed to move them about without using the other hand. Deficits imply dysfunction in the contralateral parietal lobe. Cortical sensory function should be assessed independently for each upper extremity. It is important to first assess primary sensory modalities. In the presence of prominent sensory loss, cortical sensory function cannot be assessed.

Neurovascular Assessment

Examination of the vascular system, including auscultation for cranial and carotid bruits, palpation of peripheral pulses, and assessment of blood pressure (lying, sitting, and standing), complements the neurologic examination and should be performed on every patient.

CONCLUSION

A variety of neurologic disorders (eg, stroke, Parkinson disease, Alzheimer disease) preferentially present in older adults. A comprehensive mental status and neurologic examination should be performed in every patient to document changes in neurologic function (ie, memory/cognition, behavior/personality, cranial nerves, motor function, and sensory perception) associated with pathologic conditions that affect the nervous system and distinguish them from the functional changes associated with normal aging. Limited memory and cognitive function changes occur as one age. Subtle changes in memory that do not interfere with normal functioning in society and that do not impair activities of daily living occur in normal aging. More significant declines in memory and cognitive function can be encountered in dementia (**Table 9-13**).

Altered cognitive function in the setting of a clear sensorium is consistent with dementia secondary to a neurodegenerative process or medical illness. Dementias (eg, Alzheimer disease, frontotemporal dementias, dementia with Lewy bodies) are characterized by a specific constellation of signs and symptoms. In Alzheimer disease the individual typically exhibits limited insight into their cognitive deficits that involve memory, language, and visuospatial skills. Patients with frontotemporal dementias present with a predominance of features consistent with frontal and/or temporal degeneration. These individuals exhibit early changes in behavior and personality, such as social inappropriateness, disinhibition, apathy, perseveration, and oral/dietary changes. Other accompanying features may include language/speech impairment, executive dysfunction, and preserved posterior functions (eg, visuospatial ability, calculations). In dementia with Lewy bodies, patients may exhibit fluctuating cognition, recurrent well-formed and detailed visual hallucinations, and extrapyramidal signs consistent with parkinsonism. Dementia can occur as a consequence of other neurologic and medical illnesses such as cerebrovascular disease, vitamin B_{12} deficiency, hypothyroidism, Parkinson disease, and meningoencephalitis.

Delirium on the other hand causes alteration in sensorium and level of consciousness and is usually due to medications (**Table 9-14**), infection, head injury, or metabolic derangements. Associated features include disruption of sleep-wake cycle, intermittent drowsiness and agitation, restlessness, emotional lability, and frank psychosis (hallucination, illusions, delusions). Symptoms of delirium are often worse at night and occur in up to 20% of hospitalized patients. The risk increases in the older adult and the longer the hospital stay. Predisposing factors include advanced

TABLE 9-13 ■ DIFFERENTIAL DIAGNOSIS OF DEMENTIA

Neurodegenerative Disease
  Alzheimer disease
  Dementia with Lewy bodies/Parkinson disease
  Frontotemporal dementia
  Huntington disease
  Progressive supranuclear palsy
  Corticobasal degeneration
  Creutzfeldt-Jakob and other prion diseases
  Wilson disease
  Neuronal ceroid lipofuscinosis

Vascular Disease
  Vascular contributions to cognitive impairment and dementia
  Cerebral amyloid angiopathy
  CADASIL
  Vasculitis

Hydrocephalus

Demyelinating Disorders
  Multiple sclerosis
  Leukodystrophies

Traumatic Brain Injury

Metabolic Disorders
  Hepatic encephalopathy
  Hypothyroidism
  Storage disorders
  Electrolyte disorders (sodium, calcium)

Nutritional Disorders
  B_{12} deficiency
  Wernicke-Korsakoff syndrome (thiamine)

Mitochondrial Disorders

Toxic Disorders
  Alcoholism
  Drugs
  Heavy metals

Neoplasia
  Primary brain tumors (meningiomas, gliomas)
  Metastatic disease
  Paraneoplastic syndromes

Infection
  HIV
  Neurosyphilis
  Progressive multifocal leukoencephalopathy
  Subacute sclerosing panencephalitis
  Whipple disease

Epilepsy

CADASIL, cerebral autosomal dominant arteriopathy with subcortical infarcts and leukoencephalopathy.

TABLE 9-14 ■ EXAMPLES OF MEDICATIONS CAUSING DELIRIUM IN THE OLDER ADULT

α-Methyldopa
Amantidine
Anticholinergics
Antihistamines
Antipsychotics
Atropine
Barbiturates
Benzodiazepines
Bromides
Chlordiazepoxide
Chloral hydrate
Cimetidine and other H_2 blockers
Clonidine
Codeine and other opioids
Cocaine
Dextromethorphan
Digoxin
Dopamine agonists
Dopamine antagonists
Ethanol
Furosemide
Lithium
Levodopa
Nifedipine
Opioids
Phencyclidine (PCP)
Phenytoin
Prednisone and other steroids
Propanolol
Reserpine
Theophylline
Tricyclic antidepressants

age, dementia, impaired physical or mental health, sensory deprivation (poor vision or hearing), and placement in intensive care units.

A functional decline in some aspects of cranial nerve function (eg, vision, hearing, vestibular function, taste, and smell) can be anticipated in normal aging and should be distinguished from pathologic conditions afflicting the nervous system. Similarly, older individuals experience decreased mobility as they age. Subtle changes in gait, posture, coordination, and strength are expected concomitants of aging. However, more profound changes that significantly alter mobility and/or present as focal weakness or impaired coordination should alert the clinician to the possibility of a neuropathologic disorder.

Alterations in sensory perception can be indicative of neuropsychiatric dysfunction. Subtle deficits in vibration and other primary sensory modalities may be encountered in normal aging. However, marked deficits in sensory function are suggestive of neurologic disease and require further diagnostic testing.

In conclusion, neurologic findings of normal aging include subtle declines in cognitive function, mildly impaired motor function, and altered sensory perceptions. However, exaggerated impairments in cognitive, behavioral, motor, and sensory function suggest the onset of neurologic diseases that commonly afflict the older adult. A comprehensive mental status and neurologic examination is the foundation for identifying neuropathologic conditions that necessitate further laboratory and imaging investigation.

ACKNOWLEDGMENTS

This chapter was supported by grants from the National Institute on Aging (R01 AG071514, R01 NS101483, and R01 AG069765), the Anne and Leo Albert Charitable Trust, and the Harry T. Mangurian Foundation.

FURTHER READING

Aminoff MJ, Josephson SA. *Neurology and General Medicine.* 5th ed. New York, NY: Academic Press; 2014.

Burns A, Lawlor B, Craig S. *Assessment Scales in Old Age Psychiatry.* 2nd ed. London, UK: Martin Dunitz; 2004.

Claussen CF, Pandey A. Neurootological differentiations in endogenous tinnitus. *Int Tinnitus J.* 2009;15:174–184.

Cummings JL. *The Neuropsychiatry of Alzheimer's Disease and Related Dementias.* London, UK: Martin Dunitz; 2003.

Galvin JE, Powlishta KK, Wilkins K, et al. Predictors of preclinical Alzheimer disease and dementia: a clinicopathologic study. *Arch Neurol.* 2005;62:758–765.

Galvin JE, Roe C, Coats M, et al. The AD8: a brief informant interview to detect dementia. *Neurology.* 2005; 65:559–564.

Galvin JE. The Quick Dementia Rating System (QDRS): a rapid dementia staging tool. *Alzheimer Dem (DADM).* 2015;1:249–259.

Galvin JE. Using informant and performance screening methods to detect mild cognitive impairment and dementia. *Curr Rep Gerontol.* 2018;7:19–25.

Goodwin VA, Abbott RA, Whear R, et al. Multiple component interventions for preventing falls and fall-related injuries among older people: a systematic review and meta-analysis. *BMC Geriatr.* 2014;14:15.

Graff-Radford J, Jones DT, Graff-Radford NR. Pathophysiology of language, speech and emotions in neurodegenerative disease. *Parkinsonism Relat Disord.* 2014;20(suppl 1): S49–S53.

Jones HR, Srinivasan J, Allman GJ, Baker RA. *Netter's Neurology.* 2nd ed. Philadelphia, PA: Elsevier Saunders; 2011.

Karantzoulis S, Galvin JE. Distinguishing Alzheimer's disease from other major forms of dementia. *Expert Rev Neurother.* 2011;11:1579–1591.

Massano J, Bhatia KP. Clinical approach to Parkinson's disease: features, diagnosis, and principles of management. *Cold Spring Harb Perspect Med.* 2012;2(6):a008870.

Nelson PT, Alafuzoff I, Bigio EH, et al. Correlation of Alzheimer disease neuropathologic changes with cognitive status: a review of the literature. *J Neuropathol Exp Neurol.* 2012;71:362–381.

O'Brien M. *Aids to Examination of the Peripheral Nervous System.* London, UK: Saunders Ltd; 2010.

Posner JB, Saper CB, Schiff N, Plum F. *Plum and Posner's Diagnosis of Stupor and Coma.* 4th ed. New York, NY: Oxford University Press; 2007.

Robins Wahlin RB, Byrne GJ. Personality changes in Alzheimer's disease: a systematic review. *Int J Geriatr Psychiatry.* 2011;26:1019–1029.

Ropper A, Samuels M. *Adams and Victor's Principle of Neurology.* 10th ed. New York, NY: McGraw-Hill Professional; 2014.

Salthouse TA. Trajectories of normal cognitive aging. *Psychol Aging.* 2019;34(1):17–24.

Seraji-Bzorgzad N, Paulson H, Heidebrink J. Neurologic examination in the elderly. *Handb Clin Neurol.* 2019; 167:73–88.

Stone J, Zeman A, Sharpe M. Functional weakness and sensory disturbance. *J Neurol Neurosurg Psychiatry.* 2002;73:241–245.

Weiner RD, Blazer DG, Steffens DC. *Essentials of Geriatric Psychiatry.* 2nd ed. Arlington, VA: APA Publishing; 2012.

Chapter 10

Assessment of Decisional Capacity and Competencies

Margaret A. Drickamer, Sarah Stoneking

INTRODUCTION

All clinicians should be sufficiently familiar with the principles and processes to manage common situations requiring a judgement of decisional capacity that arise in their practice. The purpose of this chapter is to explain some of the ethical underpinnings to this responsibility, to highlight the strengths and weaknesses of approaches to assess decisional capacity, and to describe the role of the clinician in decision making.

Autonomy is defined as self-determination (see also Chapter 72). Respect for individual autonomy is understood to be an elemental principle of western society. Nonetheless, there are limitations on how autonomous each of us is, including, but not limited to, limitation of resources and opportunity, societal and legal prohibitions, and the limits imposed by the rights of others not to have their autonomy infringed upon. We are not just independent rational creatures devoid of context; decision making encompasses emotion, relationships (individual and community), as well as other enriched interpretations of autonomy that will be discussed further in this chapter.

Paternalism is defined as limiting an individual's autonomy in order either to prevent that individual from doing harm to themselves (or others) or to prevent the person from missing a substantial benefit. The circumstances under which paternalism is acceptable are not defined by the action the individual may wish to undertake, or by the probable untoward consequences of an action, but rather by the individual's ability to make decisions. In other words, our wish to protect an individual from doing themselves harm does not justify paternalism; we cannot prevent an individual from doing things that may cause them harm (ie, drinking alcohol in excess, hang gliding). We can only justify intervention if we judge that an individual lacks the capacity to make decisions. In such a case, we are responsible for protecting the person and society from the possible harm of a decision made by an individual who lacks the ability to understand the consequences.

This chapter will focus on those individuals who have cognitive impairment or a clouded sensorium (fixed brain lesions, dementia, or delirium) and will not discuss the competence of individuals whose decisional capacity may be impaired by psychiatric illness. When patients

Learning Objectives

- To review the elements of decisional capacity.
- To describe ways to determine capacity.
- To understand special instances where knowledge of decisional capacity should be applied.

Key Clinical Points

1. There are four necessary elements to making a capable decision: understanding, appreciation, reasoning, and expressing a choice.
2. Critical cortical functions involved in decision making include immediate memory, language, and executive function.
3. Decisional incapacity is task-specific and may be time-limited. Therefore, decision-making capacity may fall along a spectrum and the ability of an individual to make decisions often needs to be thought of in flexible terms.
4. An assent-consent model of surrogate decision making is key to decision making in patients who retain the ability to participate in decisions but do not have full decision-making capacity.

are cognitively impaired, clinicians have an obligation to respect their rights, to protect their persons, and to consider the safety of the public. This often requires careful balancing of conflicting imperatives.

ELEMENTS OF DECISIONAL CAPACITY

In the broadest sense of the word, for an individual to be competent, that individual must be well qualified to do whatever task they are doing. For decision making, competence is often viewed as a legal term, that is, a judge's ruling as to whether an individual has been deemed competent to make their own decisions. An individual adjudicated to be incompetent must have a guardian appointed to make the decisions for the area (or areas) in which the person has been found to be incompetent. Although guidelines vary from state to state, it is generally accepted that a ruling of incompetence cannot be made solely on the basis of a medical diagnosis, age, level of education, or personal eccentricity. An adjudication of competence or incompetence is based on an assessment of the individual's decisional capacity and that individual's demonstrated ability or inability to carry out a plan. Therefore, the assessment of decisional capacity should include not just the patient's cognitive ability, but other factors that may be influencing the process of making a capable decision.

The four elements of making a capable decision are understanding, appreciation, reasoning, and expressing a choice (**Table 10-1**). First, the individual must be able to comprehend the information being considered sufficiently well to understand the relevant facts. That information must have been presented in a clear and concise manner with special attention taken to ensure that barriers such as hearing impairment, illiteracy, or language difference do not constitute the sole reasons that the person is unable to understand the information. Other issues, such as aphasia, delirium, or depression, may also interfere with the individual's ability to comprehend and retain information.

Second, the individual must have the conceptual ability to appreciate the consequences of the decision that he or she is making. This includes both an appreciation of the risks and benefits of options and the ability to identify the consequences the decision will have on his or her life.

TABLE 10-1 ■ FOUR ELEMENTS THAT CONSTITUTE DECISION-MAKING ABILITIES

ABILITY	DESCRIPTION
Understanding	1. Comprehension of appropriately communicated information 2. Retention of information long enough to be able to recall it in discussion 3. Perception of the relationship between interventions and outcomes
Appreciation	1. Recognition of how the information relates to his or her own circumstances 2. Insight into the advantages and disadvantages of a proposed solution
Reasoning	1. Manipulation of information to generate comparisons between different alternatives and their consequences 2. Justification of a rationale as a context for making these comparisons
Expressing a choice	Articulation of a clear choice with regard to a specific decision

Beginning and ending a discussion by asking the individual what their understanding of the situation is and what the consequences are of the choice that they have made is an important method of assuring that they were able to comprehend the information and that they appreciate the consequences of the decision they are making.

Individuals must be able to reason, within their own frame of reference, why they are choosing a course of action. This is different from saying that a decision seems "reasonable" or "rational," but rather it refers to the cognitive processing of values and beliefs in view of the information provided. Even if we feel—and even if most of society would feel—that an individual's decision is irrational, it does not give us grounds to negate the person's right to self-determination. Nonetheless, an individual's ability to give a plausible rationale for his or her decision is sometimes used as secondary evidence of decisional capacity. That is, demonstrating justification for one's choices (eg, religious belief, personal value, etc.) provides another level of assurance that the patient's decision rests on intact reasoning, rather than a set of delusional or incoherent beliefs that may exist in the setting of cognitive impairment or psychiatric illness.

Finally, the person must be able to make a choice and communicate the decision. This is the lowest bar for decision-making capacity but one that may be impaired by specific damage in language or frontal lobe function as well as in severe global cognitive impairment.

The inconsistency of an individual's decision with past decisions made by that person provides a red flag to possible underlying cognitive or psychiatric problems that deserve exploration. But, in and of itself, inconsistency does not negate the person's right to make decisions. Inconsistency of a specific decision over time may indicate that the individual has had difficulty with remembering or understanding the information provided.

Individuals may choose to forego making their own decision and delegate that responsibility to someone else even though they retain decisional capacity (waiver of informed consent). Their wish to forego hearing medical information or participating in making a choice (the right to delegate informed consent) may rest on individual, family, societal or cultural difference in decision making.

LEGAL AND PRACTICAL ASPECTS IN DETERMINING DECISIONAL CAPACITY

In protecting an individual who is incapable of making decisions, one action that may become necessary is the application to a local probate court to ask that the individual be adjudicated to be incompetent and to have someone else appointed to make decisions. Although specifics of probate statutes vary among states, most follow a general pattern articulated in the Uniform Probate Code. Once an individual has been adjudicated incompetent, another person is appointed to represent his or her interests. This person is variably referred to as a guardian, conservator, or legal surrogate. Although there are movements toward "limited guardianship" that restrict the powers of the guardian to decision making in more specific areas where a person has been shown to be incapable, there are two broad categories of guardianship that are commonly used, those of finance and of person. Guardianship of finance is a self-evident term. Guardianship of person grants a more global responsibility for assuring that the individual is kept safe and that decisions are made either as substituted judgment or based on the individual's best interests (see Chapter 72). These decisions may involve medical care, where a person will live or what help the person will receive to maintain himself or herself.

It should be emphasized that not all incapacitated individuals need to be conserved. There are no statistics available to say how many incapacitated individuals have informal care management by relatives and never require probate action. Personal experience would lead us to believe that most adults with cognitive deficits fall into this category. Probate adjudication of a conservator may not be needed if financial management has been allocated to a family member by a Power of Attorney (POA) prior to the individual becoming incapacitated, and if there is a general agreement among concerned and interested parties that decisions should be made either by a specific individual or group consensus. If the individual involved has granted someone a durable POA for health affairs (see Chapter 26), there may not be a need for court action.

Even when the court has been asked to act, 75% to 85% of the time the court appoints a family member as conservator. The ability of an appointed conservator to act as an appropriate surrogate varies considerably. One advantage of having a court-appointed conservator is that the probate court has some oversight responsibilities for the management of the individual's affairs. If the need for complex medical decision making does not arise, then the ability of an individual to make those types of decisions is not questioned. If the individual is in a situation where others are managing household affairs and looking out for the person's needs, then the person's ability to care for self may not be examined. It is only when a problem arises that the individual's ability to make these types of decisions becomes an issue.

PROCESS OF DETERMINING CAPACITY

The clinician's assessment of an individual's ability to make decisions is conducted in two different ways; specific testing can measure cognitive dysfunction and observing the person's decision-making process can demonstrate his or her inability to complete the decision-making task capably. The clinician needs to first understand the cognitive processes involved in decisional capacity. These processes can be understood both as discrete neuropsychiatric functions and as contributors to the holistic process of making decisions.

Cortical functions involved in decision making include immediate memory and language. Immediate

memory is defined as the ability to remember rehearsed or consolidated materials. Language abilities are those that affect comprehension and the ability to produce the intended words when expressing one's thoughts in both spoken and written communication. The ability to understand language is highly correlated with an individual's ability to comprehend the information needed to make a decision. Problems with expressive language ability from cortical lesions can lead to statements by the individual that misrepresent his or her thoughts (ie, through misuse of words, word substitutions, or paraphasic errors).

Frontal lobe functions involved in the process of making capable decisions include the abilities to concentrate, express oneself, use abstract reasoning, initiate actions, solve problems, monitor one's behavior, and use judgment. The frontal lobe is responsible for filtering out both internal and external stimuli that interfere with the individual's ability to concentrate and to understand instructions or explanations. It helps the individual organize information, apply it to themselves and initiate action as well as to self-monitor. Frontal lobe problems can interfere with all four steps in decision making; understanding, applying reasoning, and the ability to make a decision.

Traditional Mental Status Tools

Tools commonly used for the assessment of cognition in patients serve as important triggers to further investigation of the individual's decisional capacity, but no single cut off score can determine capacity. Looking at performance on individual items and extrapolating to predict how performance will affect the processes necessary for decision making helps the clinician to evaluate a patient. Looking at individual items on these tests and having knowledge of how the cognitive function tested may influence the individual's ability to make decisions is useful. We recommend tests that look at cortical and frontal lobe function, such as the St Louis University Mental Status (SLUMS) or the Montreal Cognitive Assessment (MoCA). Evaluating the elements of decision making while discussing a decision with the patient and documenting their ability in one's note will enhance clinician comfort and skill in assessing and addressing decision making. There are more complex neuropsychological tests that can be done to test the same areas of function in more detail that are applied by neuropsychologists or in research.

Voluntarism, Coercion, and the Context of the Decision Making

The Nuremberg Code of Ethics states that individuals involved "should [have] the power of choice without the intervention of any element of force, fraud, deceit, duress, overreaching, or other ulterior form of constraint or coercion."

The legal definition of voluntarism is when there is no evidence that the individual was "unduly" influenced by shared values, inducements, persuasion, or force. Clinicians may be required to judge whether they feel that there is coercion Asking an individual *why* they are making the decision that they can help to clarify inducements, but the problem of "undue" influence is still a judgement.

Psychologically based influences on decision making include emotional distress, life history, pain and suffering, genuineness, coherence with other life decisions, and experiences of power relationships. Any of these may influence a person in the moment of decision making in ways that can change their decision. Their choice might be different if these issues were to be directly addressed.

Of profound importance is the context of and quality of the interaction during the decision-making process. Components of this interaction include trust, cultural competence, information quality, provider competence, and the quality of communication. These influence the individual's ability to understand and appreciate the personal impact of information before they can incorporate their own personal and cultural context and come to a decision. For medical decision making there is often a feeling of subtle or sometimes blatant coercion for a specific decision felt to be most appropriate by the medical personnel. There can be feelings of mistrust and poor-quality communication that lead to misunderstandings. Taking a lesson from narrative ethics, clinicians ought to help the patient answer the how and why of where they are with a particular decision and aid the patient in making a decision that resonates with their context and values.

CAPACITY TO MAKE SPECIFIC DECISIONS

Decisional incapacity is task-specific and may be time-limited. Although one may be adjudicated to be either incompetent or competent in the two broad legal categories of person and finance, the ability of an individual to participate in decisions needs to be thought of in more flexible terms. We will discuss incapacity in matters of person (medical decisions and ability for self-care), finance, wills, advance directives, and research.

Medical Decisions

Because patients have the right to decline medical interventions and they have the right to be informed before consenting to medical treatments, the need to make a medical decision frequently prompts the first assessment of decisional capacity.

Documentation of a formal cognitive test score is not necessary in most cases; a thoughtful interview with the patient and a written description of the areas in which the patient is unable to function is usually sufficient. It may be helpful to specifically comment on the individual's ability to understand the condition, the treatment alternatives (including no treatment), and their possible outcomes; demonstrate their appreciation of how they apply this information to their current situation; explain how their reasoning and values have helped them form their thinking; and document their choice.

Problems of Self-Care

Geriatricians are often confronted with situations where a patient demonstrates an inability to care for self or to accept the help needed to remain be safe in their present environment. To differentiate issues of cognitive impairment versus denial, a formal assessment of decision-making ability may be necessary. A person's tendency to be "eccentric" is not always easily distinguishable from dangerous behaviors stemming from increasing cognitive impairment and an inability to make decisions around self-care. Gross impairment of cortical function, especially short-term memory, can pose problems for day-to-day function. More subtle, but of high impact, is frontal lobe dysfunction. The inability to plan, initiate action, monitor one's behavior, and self-correct are essential to being able to care for oneself. A combination of findings on frontal lobe testing and demonstrated inability to care for oneself is often sufficient evidence for action, especially in combination with an inability to accept a level of care that would keep them safe. Patients who demonstrate an inability to perform functions such as organizing their medications or safely preparing meals (IADL functions) and have the need for the help that will obviate these problems (eg, home care, Meals-on-Wheels) may be regarded as having intact decision making with respect to resolving these issues.

A reasonable approach in this scenario would involve a structured assessment where the patient must demonstrate an ability to understand and appreciate a known functional problem; understand and appreciate the practicality, risks, and benefits of potential options; choose an option; and explain how this choice is preferable to the other options not chosen.

Problems of Finances

There are times when an individual remains able to make medical decisions and decisions related to self-care but is no longer capable of managing finances. When bills are going unpaid or gross mistakes are made in handling money, someone else will need to take over financial management. A demonstrated problem with finances is usually sufficient to warrant supervision, but an occupational therapist or a neuropsychologist can also assess this function. If the individual has enough insight to understand the problem and a reliable person is available to help, granting that person a POA for finances is sufficient. If the incapacitated person is reluctant to relinquish control, or court monitoring is deemed advisable, then the family or other concerned party should seek a guardian of finance.

OTHER ISSUES OF DECISIONAL CAPACITY AND CONSENT

Legal Documents

The ability to make a last will and testament is felt to be retained even after the ability to handle finances and make decisions has been lost. An individual's ability to remember what he or she is doing with the estate and to express some logic behind choices is usually sufficient evidence of capability.

The ability to grant someone durable POA for health is similar, in that a patient can indicate who they would be best for this and why they have chosen that person. A Living Will, on the other hand, deals with hypothetical situations that can often be hard even for cognitively intact individuals to fully understand and conceptualize. The clinician must also recognize that even very cognitively impaired individuals may still be able to portray wishes and desires (see "Consent Versus Assent")

Temporary Loss of Decisional Capacity

Individuals may be transiently incapacitated for decision making or their ability to recover their cognition may not be known, such as when a patient is delirious or has had a recent stroke. In these situations, the clinician should seek an interim solution. An informal surrogate, the person granted durable POA for health affairs, or a temporary guardian can make decisions while the clinician clarifies the prognosis for decisional capacity. The decisions needed during a time of uncertainty should follow the individual's prior wishes unless they are unknown and then treatment should fall on the side of aggressive protection of the individual's life or continued function until the person can make his or her wishes known, or the permanence and extent of the impairment becomes clear.

Consent Versus Assent

Even when an individual is no longer able to give informed consent to a procedure or a change in living situation, he or she should still participate in the decision-making process.

Substituted judgment is the process that a surrogate (legally appointed or informal) is supposed to apply as the basis for a decision. Substituted judgment enjoins one to consider the patient's prior wishes and long-held beliefs as the basis for one's decision, "deciding as they would have decided" (see Chapter 72). Assent refers to the impaired individual's willingness to cooperate with a plan of care. It is, in essence, a way to take into consideration the individual's present desires when making a decision. In cognitively impaired adults, there is a continuum of incapacity. An individual who is incapable of understanding the complexities of a situation or decision may retain high levels of understanding around specific aspects of the process and be able to express their opinions. Even very cognitively impaired patients can give indications of what brings them pleasure and what gives them pain.

Clinicians obtaining consent for medical treatment or research protocols may wish to use a combination of surrogate consent and patient assent (shared decision making). This may be essential in some cases where the patient's ability to cooperate will be necessary in order to carry out the treatment or procedure.

Informed Consent in Research

An individual's ability to consent to participate in research is complex. Because the risks and benefits of being in a research study are more abstract, decisional capacity must be even greater than that for accepting or declining an established medical treatment. This is an important time for dual decision making as outlined in the earlier section. It is also important to establish the voluntarism of the consent. Asking why an individual is volunteering (or a surrogate is volunteering the individual) for a research protocol is vital.

FURTHER READING

Applebaum PS. Assessment of patient's competence to consent to treatment. *N Engl J Med*. 2007;357:1834–1840.

Dunn LB, Nowrangi MA, Palmer BW, Jeste DV, Saks ER. Assessing decisional capacity for clinical research or treatment: a review of instruments. *Am J Psychiatry*. 2006;163:1323–1334.

Dy SM, Tanjala SP. Key concepts relevant to quality of complex and shared decision-making in health care: a literature review. *Soc Sci Med*. 2012;74:582–587.

Edwards A, Elwyn G, Covey J, Matthews E, Pill R. Presenting risk information—a review of the effects of "framing" and other manipulations on patient outcomes. *J Health Comm*. 2001;6:61–82.

Holzer JC, Gansler DA, Moczynski NP, et al. Cognitive functions in the informed consent evaluation process: a pilot study. *J Am Acad Psychiatry Law*. 1997;25:531–540.

Marson DC. Loss of competency in Alzheimer's disease: conceptual and psychometric approaches. *Int J Law Psychiatry*. 2001;24:267–283.

Montello M. Narrative ethics. *Hastings Cent Rep*. 2014;44: S2–S6.

O'Connor D, Hall MI, Donnelly M. Assessing capacity within a context of abuse or neglect. *J Elder Abuse Negl*. 2009;21:156–159.

Peisah C, Sorinmade OA, Mitchell L, Hertogh CM. Decisional capacity: toward an inclusionary approach. *Int Psychogeriatr*. 2013;25:1571–1579.

Pennington C, Davey K, ter Meulen R, Coulthard E, Kehoe PG. Tools for testing decision-making capacity in dementia. *Age Ageing*. 2018;47(6):778–784.

Roberts LW. Informed consent and the capacity for voluntarism. *Am J Psy*. 2002;159:705–712.

Wendler D, Prasad K. Core safeguards for clinical research with adults who are unable to consent. *Ann Int Med*. 2001;135:514–523.

Prevention and Screening

Ashwin A. Kotwal, Sei J. Lee

INTRODUCTION

Prevention and screening hold the promise of maintaining health by intervening before an illness can cause symptoms. Some preventive interventions, such as influenza vaccination, have truly minimal risks and clear public health benefits. However, many other interventions, such as cancer-screening tests, impose risks and burdens on patients, complicating the decision on who should (and should not) receive the intervention. For interventions with minimal risks, targeting is less important since many patients will benefit and few (or none) will be harmed. In contrast, for interventions with some risks or burdens, targeting is critical since some patients may be more likely to be harmed than helped by the preventive intervention.

In this chapter, the authors will present the evidence for several preventive interventions in older patients. First, the authors will focus on preventive interventions that impose some risks and burdens on patients, starting with a framework for targeting these preventive interventions and then focusing on the benefits and risks for each preventive intervention in greater detail. These interventions include cancer screening as well as treatment for asymptomatic chronic conditions such as hypertension or diabetes. Second, the authors will review the evidence for interventions with minimal risks. These interventions include behavioral and lifestyle modification as well as immunizations.

Screening for geriatric syndromes such as falls and incontinence are discussed in detail in their respective chapters.

FRAMEWORK FOR INDIVIDUALIZING PREVENTION

One challenge of appropriately targeting prevention in older adults is that few studies of preventive interventions have enrolled persons older than 75 years. The absence of age-specific data requires clinicians to extrapolate data about the benefits and harms of preventive interventions in younger persons and apply it to older persons. Furthermore, even if trials suggest that the effectiveness of a preventive intervention is similar in younger and older populations, challenges remain about how to apply data from trials to an individual older person. Trials show the

Learning Objectives

- To understand and apply a framework for individualized decision making to preventive medical interventions among older adults, including those with serious illness or residing in skilled nursing facilities.

- To understand the time-to-benefit, overall benefit, and potential harms of breast, prostate, lung, cervical, and colon cancer screening among older adults in the context of current national guidelines.

- To review recommendations for screening for asymptomatic chronic conditions, age-appropriate vaccinations, encouraging healthy behaviors, and counseling against behaviors with adverse health consequences.

Key Clinical Points

1. A framework for individualized decision making for preventive medical interventions should include an understanding of patient values and preferences, overall health and life expectancy, the potential harms of the intervention, and the expected time-to-benefit of the intervention.

2. The benefits of cancer screening are uncertain in older adults due to lack of inclusion of adults older than 75 years in the majority of randomized controlled trials. Cancer screening should be primarily considered in older adults with more than 10-year life expectancy after considering the risks and benefits of each test.

3. Treatments for many asymptomatic chronic medical conditions such as hypertension, diabetes, and hyperlipidemia impose immediate risks and burdens on patients with the promise of delayed benefits, and so should only be considered in patients whose life expectancy exceeds the expected time-to-benefit.

(Continued)

4. The risks associated with immunizations, healthy behavior counseling, and counseling against unhealthy behaviors are much lower than the benefits. Thus, targeting is less important and nearly all older adults should receive these preventive medical interventions.

5. Older adults with serious illness, advanced dementia, or those who are residing in skilled nursing facilities have limited life expectancy and are more likely to experience adverse effects from interventions, decreasing the likelihood of net benefit for many preventive interventions. Eliciting patient and family values and preferences can help clinicians align available preventive interventions with the goals of individual patients.

average effectiveness of an intervention, but they generally do not address individual patient characteristics, such as comorbid conditions or functional status, which may change the likelihood of receiving benefit or harm from a preventive intervention. Given these challenges, the need to individualize prevention and screening decisions is especially important for older people, because individuals become increasingly heterogeneous in their particular combination of health, function, remaining life expectancy, and values with advancing age.

The following framework can help individualize prevention and screening decisions so that patients who are most likely to benefit receive the intervention while patients who are more likely to be harmed avoid the intervention and avoid being harmed, and is summarized in **Figure 11-1**.

First, estimate life expectancy. By definition, prevention involves an intervention in the present to avoid illness in the future. Many preventive interventions expose patients to risks and burdens immediately for the promise of improved health later. However, older patients with a limited life expectancy may be unlikely to survive to benefit from prevention. For example, finding an asymptomatic cancer in a person who will die of something else before the cancer would become symptomatic does not benefit the person and may cause considerable harm. Thus, the first step in determining whether a preventive intervention may help an older person is to determine their overall life expectancy.

In estimating life expectancy, it is useful to have a general idea of the distribution of life expectancies at

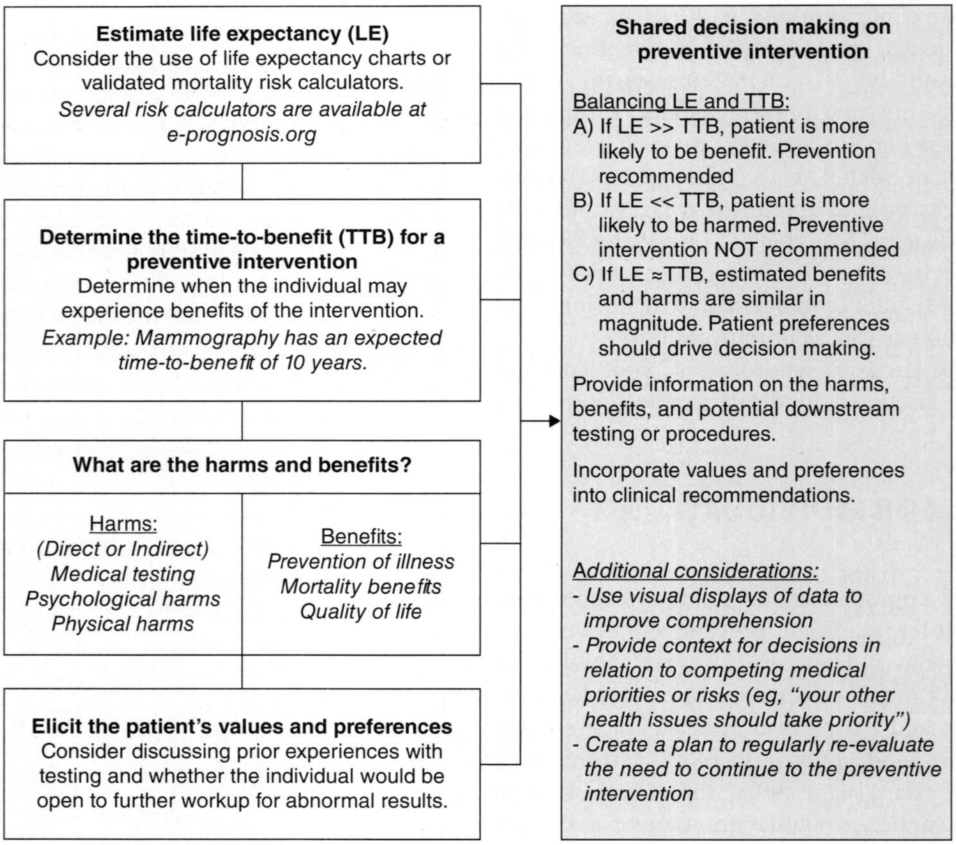

FIGURE 11-1. Algorithm for decisions on preventive medical interventions in older adults.

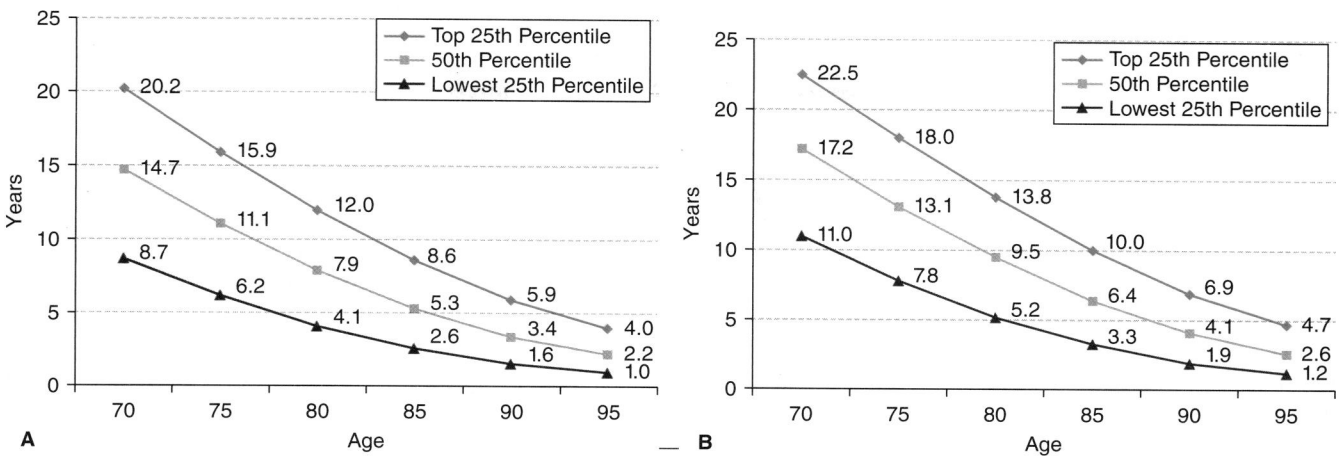

FIGURE 11-2. Upper, middle, and lower quartiles of life expectancy for men (**A**) and women (**B**) at selected ages. (Data from Arias E. United States Life Tables, 2017. *Natl Vital Stat Rep.* 2019;68[7]:1–66.)

various ages. For example, when estimating the life expectancy of an 80-year-old woman, it is useful to know that approximately 25% of 80-year-old women will live more than 13 years, 50% will live at least 9 years, and 25% will live 5 years or less. **Figure 11-2** presents the upper, middle, and lower quartiles of life expectancy for the US population according to age and sex, and illustrates the substantial variability in life expectancy that exists at each age. Although it is impossible for clinicians to predict the exact life expectancy of an individual person, it is possible to use clinical judgment to make reasonable estimates of whether a person is likely to live substantially longer or shorter than an average person in his/her age cohort. Such estimates, while not perfect, would allow for better estimations of potential benefits and harms of screening than focusing on age alone.

In addition, validated mortality risk calculators may help clinicians estimate the life expectancy of individuals better than clinical judgment alone. A systematic review found 16 general mortality risk calculators that have been developed and validated for older adults, and there are numerous risk calculators specific to life-limiting conditions (eg, cancer, dementia, or severe heart or lung disease). These mortality risk calculators have been gathered at https://eprognosis.ucsf.edu/index.php, allowing users to input a given patient's data such as age, comorbidities, and functional limitations to obtain an evidence-based estimate of mortality risk and life expectancy.

Second, determine the time-to-benefit for a preventive intervention. For preventive interventions that expose patients to immediate risks or burdens with delayed benefits, the time-to-benefit can be defined as the time between the intervention (when harms are most likely) to the time when improved health outcomes are seen. Just as different interventions have different magnitudes of benefit, different preventive interventions have different times to benefit. Unfortunately, although there are numerous widely accepted measures of the magnitude of benefit (eg, relative risk, odds ratio, and absolute risk reduction) there are no standardized measures of the time-to-benefit. Studies have focused on answering the questions, "Does it help?" (ie, $p < 0.05$?) and "How much does it help?" (ie, what is the relative risk reduction), generally ignoring the question, "When does it help?"

Because studies have generally focused on the magnitude of benefit, the time-to-benefit for many preventive interventions is unclear. Survival meta-analyses of screening trials have estimated the time-to-benefit for a few cancer-screening interventions. For preventive interventions where survival meta-analyses have not been conducted, the time-to-benefit can be estimated by reviewing Kaplan-Meier survival curves for the intervention and control groups. The point at which the curves last clearly separate provides a reasonable estimate of the time-to-benefit for a preventive intervention.

Third, review the most likely benefits of prevention. If a patient is likely to live long enough to benefit from a preventive intervention, the next step is to consider the potential benefits. For example, the main benefit of cancer screening is the reduction in cancer mortality experienced by a few people whose early-stage disease is detected and treated, which otherwise would have been lethal during their remaining lifetime. While the impact of cancer screening on quality of life or functional decline has not been studied, there is good evidence that mammography, fecal occult blood testing (FOBT), and Papanicolaou (Pap) smears are effective in reducing cancer-specific mortality. However, the strength of the evidence that these tests are effective in older adults is limited by the small number of older patients included in screening trials. In addition, even screening tests likely to be effective in older populations may not provide survival benefit to individuals with life expectancies that are shorter than the time-to-benefit from screening.

Fourth, review the most likely harms of prevention. Since many preventive tests pose both direct and indirect harms, the potential benefits of interventions, such as cancer screening, must be weighed against the potential harms of screening. Harms that would be accepted to treat a symptomatic person with known disease are less acceptable when they are caused by screening tests, which benefit only a few individuals but expose all screened individuals to the potential harms.

Individuals who are found not to have cancer after work-up of an abnormal screening result (false-positive result) clearly have experienced harm from screening, as they were subjected to physical and psychological distress from additional testing and procedures that would not have been necessary had they not been screened. However, what is often forgotten is that in older persons some of the greatest harms from screening occur by finding and treating cancers that would never have become clinically significant. The risk of identifying an inconsequential cancer (ie, over-diagnosis) increases with decreasing life expectancy as well as with the increasing likelihood that screening will detect certain neoplasms that are unlikely to progress to symptoms in older persons, such as ductal carcinoma in situ (DCIS). Fewer than 25% of DCIS lesions progress to invasive cancer within 5 to 10 years, yet because of the inability to distinguish which lesions will progress, many older women with DCIS will undergo surgery. Women who have surgery for DCIS that would never have become symptomatic in their lifetime have suffered serious harm from screening.

In addition to physical harms, the psychological distress caused by preventive interventions should be considered. For cancer screening, the potential psychological harms range from the emotional pain of a diagnosis of cancer in persons whose lives were not extended by screening, through the alarm of false-positive results to the stress of undergoing the screening test itself. Many older persons may have cognitive, physical, or sensory problems that make screening tests and further work-up particularly difficult, painful, or frightening. Considering factors that increase the likelihood of harm is vital to making appropriate preventive decisions.

Finally, review benefits and harms with each patient, integrating the patient's values and preferences into the decision. The final step of the framework for individualizing preventive decisions is to assess how individuals value the potential harms and benefits of a preventive intervention and to integrate their preferences into the decision. Because many cancer-screening decisions in older persons will not be answered solely by quantitative assessments of benefits and harms, talking to older persons about their values and preferences is especially important. The value placed on different health outcomes will vary among older people, as will preferences for screening. For example, some women undergoing screening mammography value "peace of mind" after a negative screening result, whereas women with dementia likely receive no such comfort.

In considering the benefits versus harm of screening, clinicians must elicit how individuals value the tradeoffs among longer survival, comfort, and functional status.

Clinicians should consider a person's usual approach to medical decision making to decide how to approach the discussion of preventive interventions. In some cases, clinicians will need to learn a person's values, apply them to the known benefits and harms of a preventive intervention, and make a formal recommendation. For other people, the clinician will want to discuss the benefits and harms with the person and allow the person to apply his/her values to the outcomes and come to a decision together. For people with dementia, discussion about preferences should be held with an involved caregiver. However, it should be remembered that despite being unable to articulate consent, many persons with dementia can still effectively communicate refusal. Assent from a person with dementia is essential if invasive or potentially harmful testing or treatments are being considered. If a person with dementia is likely to be frightened or agitated by a preventive test, the caregiver and clinician should forgo the test. Also, for screening tests there should be a general discussion prior to screening about the possible procedures and treatments that may be required after an abnormal screening result. Persons who would not want further workup or treatment of an abnormal result should not be screened.

In summary, the authors recommend estimating patient's life expectancy and then comparing that life expectancy to the time-to-benefit for a specific preventive intervention. The benefits and harms of prevention, such as cancer screening, should be reviewed to determine whether specific patient factors are present (such as excellent health or cognitive impairment) which suggest that a patient is more likely to benefit or be harmed by screening than the average patient. The benefits and harms should be incorporated into a discussion with the patient regarding his/her values and preferences. If the life expectancy is more than the time-to-benefit, the patient has a substantial chance of benefit and thus a preventive intervention should be encouraged. If the life expectancy is less than the time-to-benefit, the patient is more likely to be harmed than helped by a preventive intervention and thus should not be offered. If the life expectancy approximates the time-to-benefit, a patient's values and preferences are especially important and should play the dominant role in the decision whether to perform a preventive intervention or not.

APPLICATION OF SCREENING PRINCIPLES TO SPECIFIC CANCERS

Breast Cancer

Time-to-benefit for screening mammography A survival meta-analysis of randomized trials of screening mammography suggested that it takes 11 years to prevent 1 breast cancer death after screening 1000 women. Since the rate of serious complications after screening mammography appears to be approximately 1 in 1000, screening mammography may be most appropriate for women with a life expectancy greater than 10 years. Further, modeling studies suggest it is cost-effective to conduct biennial screening mammography as long as an older woman has a life expectancy of at least 9.5 years.

Benefits of breast cancer screening Mammography is the only screening modality that has been shown in randomized controlled trials to decrease breast cancer mortality. Mammography may detect cancers more frequently and accurately in older women. A pooled meta-analysis of trials demonstrated an overall relative risk reduction in breast cancer-related mortality of 27% for women between the ages of 50 and 69. Only one randomized trial examining mammography included a small number of women age 70 to 74 and found no breast cancer-specific mortality reduction in this age group, and no trials have included women older than 75 years. Consequently, data from trials in younger people must be extrapolated to older people.

Harms of breast cancer screening Among women aged 75 and older who undergo biennial screening mammography, the cumulative probability of a false-positive mammogram over 10 years ranges from 14% to 27% and this risk nearly doubles if women are screened annually. False-positives can cause anxiety and uncomfortable downstream testing such as breast biopsies, which can be distressing to older women with cognitive impairment who do not understand what is being done to them. The risk for overdiagnosis (finding a malignancy in a patient who would never have been affected clinically by the malignancy in the absence of screening) increases with age because life expectancy decreases and there is a higher proportion of slower growing cancers in older women. One study estimated the rates of overdiagnosis to be 12% to 29% for women who stop biennial screening at 74 years, 17% to 41% for women who stop at 80 years, and 32% to 48% for women who stop screening at 90 years. Frail older women are at increased risk for experiencing harms from screening. One study of frail community-living women found that 17% experienced burden from screening mammography as a result of work-up refusals, false-positive results, or overdiagnosis. Women with multiple comorbid conditions are also likely to experience adverse effects from surgery, radiation, and chemotherapy.

Recommendations The US Preventive Services Task Force (USPSTF) recommends mammography every 2 years for women age 50 to 74, stating that the evidence is insufficient to assess the additional benefits and harms of screening in women 75 years and older (**Table 11-1**). The American Cancer Society recommends annual screening among women 45 to 54 years old, and biennial screening among women 55 years or older and a life expectancy of greater than 10 years. The authors do not recommend screening

for breast cancer if a woman has an estimated life expectancy of less than 10 years. For women who have a life expectancy around 10 years the decision to screen is a close call, and patient preferences should play a major role in the decision to screen. For healthy older women who have a life expectancy greater than 10 years, biennial screening mammography, regardless of age, is a reasonable recommendation based on the data available. Publicly available decision aids and the ePrognosis Cancer Screening guide (http://cancerscreening.eprognosis.org/) compares a patient's life expectancy with the time-to-benefit for screening mammography to help clinicians determine whether mammography is likely to help a patient.

Colorectal Cancer

Time-to-benefit for colorectal cancer screening A survival meta-analysis of randomized trials of screening fecal occult blood testing for colorectal cancer suggested that it takes 10 years to prevent 1 colorectal cancer death after screening 1000 persons. Since the rates of serious complications after colorectal cancer screening also appear to be approximately 1 in 1000, colorectal cancer screening may be most appropriate for persons with a life expectancy greater than 10 years. Randomized trials of screening flexible sigmoidoscopy show similar times to benefit. Ongoing trials of screening colonoscopy will provide additional information about whether time to mortality benefit with screening colonoscopy is similar to screening fecal occult blood testing and screening sigmoidoscopy.

Benefits of colorectal cancer screening Methods for screening for colorectal cancer include FOBT, fecal immunochemical testing, flexible sigmoidoscopy, and colonoscopy. Guaiac-based fecal occult blood testing has the strongest evidence for screening efficacy based on three European randomized controlled trials showing reductions in colorectal cancer-specific mortality of 11% to 16%, and a large US trial showing reductions of 22% to 32% overall, and a 53% reduction among adults 70 to 80 years old. Randomized trials of screening sigmoidoscopies every 3 to 5 years suggest similar mortality benefits. Polypectomy during colonoscopies can prevent colorectal cancer in addition to early detection of colorectal cancers.

Harms of colorectal cancer screening Approximately 1 of 10 older adults who submit a screening guaiac-based fecal occult blood testing will have a false-positive result. Colonoscopy is the standard work-up following a positive fecal occult blood testing and may have serious complications, such as perforation (1/1000), serious bleeding (3/1000), cardiorespiratory events (12/1000), and death (1/1000). Complications may be higher if polypectomy is performed or if persons are in poor health. Discomfort from flexible sigmoidoscopy or colonoscopy may occur, and many older persons may experience substantial distress from the bowel preparation, including dizziness, nausea, and fecal incontinence.

TABLE 11-1 ■ GUIDELINE RECOMMENDATIONS FOR CANCER SCREENING IN OLDER ADULTS

CANCER SITE	TEST	FREQUENCY	USPSTF GUIDELINE[a]	ACS GUIDELINE[b]	ACP GUIDELINE[c]
Colorectal	Fecal occult blood test or fecal immunochemical test (FIT) or Sigmoidoscopy or Colonoscopy	Annual; Every 5 y; Every 10 y	Screen all adults 45–75 y. Individualized decisions about continued screening in individuals 76–85 y. Screening is not recommended for adults older than 85 y.	Screen all adults 45–75 y if life expectancy > 10 years. Individualized decisions in adults 76–85 y based on preferences, life expectancy, health status, and prior screening history. Discourage screening in adults > 85 y.	Screen all adults 50–75 y. Persons with life expectancy < 10 years should not be screened.
					ACOG GUIDELINE[d]
Breast	Mammography	Every 1–2 y	Biennial screening of all women 50–74 y. Evidence of benefits and harms is insufficient for women 75 y and older.	Annual screening for women 45–54 y old, biennial screening for women > 55 y with life expectancy of > 10 y	Annual or biennial screening starting at 40 y until age 75. Screening beyond 75 y should be a shared decision based on a woman's health status and longevity.
Cervical	Pap smear HPV test	Pap only, every 3 y; HPV + Pap, every 5 y	Screening in women 21–65 y. Discontinue at age 65 if adequate prior screening.	Screening in women 21–65 y. Discontinue at age 65 if regular screening with normal results.	Screening in women 21–65 y. Co-testing (Pap + HPV) every 5 y is the preferred screening method for women 30–65 y. Screening should stop at age 65 if evidence of negative adequate prior screening.
					ACCP GUIDELINE[e]
Lung	Low-dose CT scan	Annual	Screen 55–80-y-old current and former smokers with a 30+ pack-year smoking history and either currently smoke or quit within the past 15 y. Discontinue screening once a person has not smoked for 15 y or develops a health problem that limits their ability or willingness to have curative surgery.	Screen 55–74-y-old current and former smokers in fairly good health with a 30+ pack-year smoking history and either currently smoke or quit within the last 15 y.	Asymptomatic smokers and former smokers 55–77 y who have smoked 30+ pack-years and either currently smoke or quit within the past 15 y.
					AUA GUIDELINE[f]
Prostate	PSA	1–2 y	Individualized decision making about screening in men 55–69 y old. Men should have an opportunity to discuss the benefits and harms of screening with clinicians and incorporate their values and preferences. Consider family history, race/ethnicity, comorbid medical conditions, and patient values. Do not screen in men > 70 y old.	Men age 50 and older with a life expectancy > 10 y can consider screening after discussion about the risks, benefits, and uncertainties of PSA screening.	Shared decision making for PSA screening in men 55–69 y with life expectancy > 10–15 y based on patient's values and preferences. Recommend against routine screening for men older than age 70.

[a]USPSTF = United States Preventive Services Task Force.
[b]ACS = American Cancer Society.
[c]ACP = American College of Physicians.
[d]ACOG = American College of Obstetricians and Gynecologists.
[e]ACCP = American College of Chest Physicians.
[f]AUA = American Urological Association.

Recommendations The USPSTF recommends colorectal cancer screening for all older adults age 45 to 75 and that screening decisions should be selectively offered to persons 76 to 85 years based on overall health and prior screening history. The American Cancer Society recommends screening begin at age 45, continue until age 75 for individuals with greater than a 10-year life expectancy, individualized decisions for adults age 76 to 85, and screening be discouraged if older than 85. Most guidelines recommend annual screening fecal occult blood testing or fecal immunochemical testing and/or flexible sigmoidoscopy every 5 years or colonoscopy every 10 years for average risk (see **Table 11-1**). There is no evidence available to determine which screening method is preferable or when screening should stop. However, prior to FOBT or FIT testing, it is important to discuss the risk of false positives and whether individuals would be willing to undergo a colonoscopy if the test returns positive. In addition, individuals should receive information on procedural risks of colonoscopies, sedation, and the need to arrange transportation. The authors recommend against screening for colorectal cancer if a person has an estimated life expectancy of less than 10 years. For persons with life expectancies around 10 years, the decision to screen is a close call, and patient preferences should play a major role in the decision to screen. Notably, colorectal screening may have a larger benefit among older adults if they have never been screened before. For healthy older people who have a life expectancy greater than 10 years, colorectal cancer screening regardless of age, is a reasonable recommendation based on available data. The ePrognosis Cancer Screening guide (http://cancerscreening.eprognosis.org/) compares a patient's life expectancy with the time-to-benefit for colorectal cancer screening to help clinicians determine whether colorectal cancer screening is likely to help a patient.

Cervical Cancer

Time-to-benefit for cervical cancer screening A cluster randomized trial of younger women (age 30–59) suggests that cervical cancer screening with HPV testing leads to mortality reductions in 2 to 3 years. In contrast, screening with cervical cytology appears to lead to mortality benefits in 6 to 7 years. There are no data about the time-to-benefit for cervical cancer screening in women 65 years and older. The main consideration for cervical cancer screening is whether an older woman has received screening during her reproductive years because the likelihood an older woman will die of cervical cancer is remote if she has had normal screens in the past. Routine vaccination for human papilloma virus (HPV) strains related to cervical cancer occurrence in younger adults is expected to lower the incidence of cervical cancer in future generations.

Benefits of cervical cancer screening The principal method for screening for cervical cancer is through the use of cervical cytology. Since screening with Pap smears was initiated,

population studies in the United States show a 20% to 60% decline in mortality rates from cervical cancer. Decision models suggest that older women who have had repeated normal Pap smears during their reproductive years do not benefit from continued Pap testing beyond age 65 or 70. However, these models make variable recommendations about the number of normal Pap smears required prior to stopping screening.

Harms of cervical cancer screening False positives are common among older postmenopausal women. In one study of 2561 older women with a normal prior Pap smear, 110 women had an abnormal pap smear within the subsequent 2 years and only 1 was a true positive; the positive predictive value of an abnormal cervical smear is less than 1%. Harms of false-positive results include needless patient concern and invasive procedures, such as colposcopy or biopsy. Discomfort and anxiety during Pap smears also occurs as does the identification and treatment of clinically unimportant cervical lesions given the slow growing nature of cervical cancers and the possibility of regression of low-grade cervical lesions.

Recommendations Guidelines recommend cervical cancer screening with cytology every 3 years for women age 21 to 65. Combining cytology testing with HPV testing every 5 years may provide added benefit (see **Table 11-1**). Guidelines recommend that Pap smears be discontinued in women older than age 65 who have had adequate prior screening, defined as three consecutive negative cytology results or two consecutive negative HPV co-tests within 10 years of stopping screening, with the most recent test occurring within 5 years of stopping. The authors recommend cervical cancer screening in women older than age 65 who have not had adequate prior screening and are healthy enough to undergo cervical cancer treatment if cancer is found.

Lung Cancer Screening

Time-to-benefit for lung cancer screening Two large trials of low-dose lung CT scans show reductions in lung cancer-specific mortality after 6 years. For chest x-rays, one large trial found no lung cancer mortality benefit.

Potential benefits The National Lung Screening Trial (NLST) found that among current and former heavy smokers age 55 to 74, low-dose lung CT scans decreased lung cancer mortality by 20%. Specifically, for 1000 persons screened, 4 lung cancer deaths would be avoided in 6 years. The Dutch-Belgian Lung Cancer Screening (NELSON) Trial of low-dose lung CT scans among current and former heavy smokers found a 24% reduction in lung cancer-specific mortality at 10-year follow-up, and 3.3 lung cancer deaths avoided per 1000 participants.

Potential harms False positives are common with low-dose CT scans of the lung; in one trial 39% of people who received a CT scan had at least 1 positive test result and 96% of positive results were false positives. False positives may lead to unnecessary invasive testing, including surgical procedures and biopsies. Complications after invasive lung procedures may occur in 1 in 5 older adults, and rates may be higher for older adults in worse health compared to those who are younger or healthier. Reported rates of overdiagnosis range from 3% to 9%, although this is an active area of study. Additional harms include anxiety from false-positive results, frequent need for follow-up and repeat imaging, financial strain, and radiation exposure.

Recommendations The American Cancer Society and USPSTF recommend annual low-dose CT scans for lung cancer screening in adults 55 to 74 years old (or up to 80 in USPSTF guidelines) who have a 30-pack-year history and currently smoke or quit within the last 15 years. Guidelines suggest avoiding screening in older adults with a short life expectancy (< 10 years) or comorbidities that would make curative surgery or cancer-directed therapies not a reasonable option (see **Table 11-1**). The authors recommend low-dose CT scans when older adults are at high risk of lung cancer, are current or former heavy smokers, and have a low risk of a competing cause of death. Older adults considering screening should be counseled on the possibility of false positive results (including in the thyroid and other organs), potential downstream interventions, and the need for frequent follow-up for nodule tracking.

Prostate Cancer Screening

Although prostate-specific antigen (PSA) testing is frequently performed, there is conflicting evidence and guidelines regarding the benefits and harms of PSA testing. The mortality benefit is small and takes over 10 years to be realized. In contrast the harms from testing can include anxiety, unneeded prostate biopsies (associated with hematuria, pain, and infections), and overdiagnosis and unnecessary treatments of screen-detected cancers (associated with urinary incontinence, sexual dysfunction, and premature death). The USPSTF and American Cancer Society recommend that men age 55 to 69 make an individualized decision about PSA screening after discussion with a clinician

and consideration of life expectancy (typically greater than 10–15 years), and recommend against screening in men older than 70 years old (see **Table 11-1**). The authors do not recommend routine screening for prostate cancer in older men based on the available evidence.

TARGETING TREATMENT FOR ASYMPTOMATIC CHRONIC CONDITIONS

Treatment of asymptomatic chronic conditions such as hypertension and diabetes also impose immediate risks and burdens on patients for the promise of delayed benefits. More intensive glycemic control appears to decrease the risk of microvascular complications many years later. However, more intensive glycemic control clearly increases the risk for serious hypoglycemia immediately. Similarly, improved blood pressure control appears to decrease the risk of heart failure and stroke. However, initiating antihypertensive medications appears to increase the risk of hip fracture in the first 45 days. Thus, for asymptomatic chronic conditions, the risks and burdens of treatment often occur immediately while the benefits are not observed for years. This suggests that *treatment* for asymptomatic conditions can also be viewed as *prevention*, and should be targeted toward patients with an extended life expectancy who have a reasonable chance of benefiting from the delayed benefits.

Unfortunately, there is tremendous uncertainty surrounding the time-to-benefit for various interventions. Long-term follow up studies of more intensive glycemic control suggests that it take 8 to 15 years for the clinical benefits to be seen (**Table 11-2**). Studies of more intensive blood pressure control suggests that it take 1 to 3 years for clinical benefits to be seen. For HMG-CoA Reductase inhibitors ("statins"), the time-to-benefit appears to be dependent on clinical situation, with nearly immediate (< 3 months) benefit in patients with recent myocardial infarction and increasing to several years for primary prevention of major adverse cardiovascular events (see **Table 11-2**).

TABLE 11-2 ■ ESTIMATED TIMES TO BENEFIT FOR THE TREATMENT OF COMMON CHRONIC CONDITIONS					
TIME-TO-BENEFIT[a]	**CONDITION**	**INTERVENTION**	**IMMEDIATE RISK**	**DELAYED BENEFIT**	**DATA SOURCES**
8–15 y	Diabetes mellitus	Intensive glycemic control	Hypoglycemia	Decreased vascular complications	UKPDS, long-term follow-up
1–5 y	Hypertension	Hypertension treatment	Orthostatic hypotension, falls and fracture	Decreased stroke and cardiovascular mortality	HYVET, EWPHE, and MRCOA trials
3 mo–2.5 y	Hypercholesterolemia	Treatment with HMG-CoA reductase inhibitors ("statins")	Myalgias, rhabdomyolysis, and cost	Decrease cardiovascular events including death	WOSCOPS, AFCAPS/TexCAPS, MEGA trials

[a]The first number represents the time point when the event rates between the control and intervention groups diverge, representing the time at which population benefits are first seen. The second number represents the time point when event rates between the control and intervention groups reach near-maximal separation, representing the time at which maximal benefits are seen.
AFCAPS/TexCAPS = Air Force/Texas Coronary Atherosclerosis Prevention Study; EWPHE = European Working Party on Hypertension in the Elderly; HYVET = Hypertension in the Very Elderly Trial; MEGA = Management of Elevated cholesterol in primary prevention Group of Adult Japanese; MRCOA = Medical Research Council trial of treatment of hypertension in Older Adults; UKPDS = United Kingdom Prospective Diabetes Study; WOSCOPS = West of Scotland Coronary Prevention Study.

In summary, treatments for many asymptomatic chronic medical conditions impose immediate risks and burdens on patients with the promise of delayed benefits. Thus, the framework of individualizing prevention also applies to the treatment of these asymptomatic conditions, and treatment of these asymptomatic conditions should be targeted to those older adults whose life expectancy exceeds the time-to-benefit.

IMMUNIZATIONS

In contrast to screening interventions, the risks associated with immunizations are much lower than the benefits. Thus, targeting is less important and nearly all older adults should receive the pneumococcal vaccination, annual influenza vaccination, and zoster vaccination.

Pneumococcal Vaccination

Pneumococcal infections represent a major cause of morbidity and mortality in older adults. The US Advisory Council on Immunization Practices (ACIP) recommends all adults older than age 65 sequentially receive both the Pneumococcal Conjugate Vaccine (PCV13) followed in 6 to 12 months by the Pneumococcal Polysaccharide Vaccine (PPSV23). Minor local reactions such as pain or erythema are common with both vaccines; more serious side effects are rare. The ACIP also recommends pneumococcal vaccination for adults younger than 65 who have certain risk factors such as cigarette smoking, diabetes mellitus, or chronic lung disease.

Influenza Vaccination

The influenza virus causes annual epidemics of acute respiratory illnesses every winter that disproportionately affects older adults. Vaccination has been shown to decrease the morbidity and mortality associated with influenza and is recommended for all persons older than 6 months. There is some evidence that a high-dose influenza vaccine may be more effective in eliciting immunogenic response in adults older than age 65. The most common adverse events include local soreness. The risk of Guillain-Barre syndrome after influenza vaccination appears small, with estimates of 1 to 2 excess cases per 1 million persons vaccinated.

Tetanus/Diphtheria/Pertussis

Tetanus is cause by the neurotoxin expressed by *Clostridium tetani* when the ubiquitous bacteria spores are inoculated into tissues with trauma or deep puncture wounds. Tetanus toxoid vaccine is effective, but waning immunity has led to the large proportion of cases to occur in adults older than 60 years. Diphtheria is a rare, acute respiratory illness caused by a toxin expressed by *Corynebacterium diphtheria*. National serosurvey between 1988 to 1994 suggested that only 30% of adults age 60 to 69 had appropriate diphtheria antitoxin concentrations. ACIP recommends tetanus/diphtheria (Td) or Tdap revaccination every 10 years for all older adults.

Pertussis or whooping cough is a highly contagious respiratory illness that is underdiagnosed and underreported, especially in older adults. Studies suggest that acellular pertussis vaccination is equally effective among older adults as younger adults with similar low rates of adverse events and high rates of pertussis antibodies. ACIP recommends a one-time booster dose of pertussis vaccination after age 65.

In summary, the ACIP recommends that all adults receive Td (tetanus/diphtheria) or Tdap booster every 10 years. In addition, adults older than age 65 should receive a one-time dose of Tdap (tetanus/diphtheria/acellular pertussis) if they have not received pertussis revaccination after age 19 in lieu of Td vaccination.

Zoster Vaccination

Reactivation of herpes zoster is common (30% lifetime risk) and can result in significant morbidity from complications such as postherpetic neuralgia and ophthalmic zoster. The two-dose recombinant zoster vaccination (RZV) appears to be quite effective in persons 70 years or older, with an efficacy for prevention of herpes zoster of 91% and prevention of postherpetic neuralgia of 91%. In comparison, the one-dose live zoster vaccine (ZVL) has an efficacy of 38% among adults 70 years or older and prevention of postherpetic neuralgia of 67% (0.1% vaccine vs 0.4% control). The most common adverse reactions to zoster vaccinations are local injection site reactions (9% in RZV and 1% in ZVL); serious adverse reactions are rare. The ACIP recommends the two-dose RZV vaccination for adults age 50 and older, including those who have previously received the ZVL vaccination. The ZVL remains a recommended vaccine in adults age 60 or older.

BEHAVIORS TO MAINTAIN HEALTH

Like immunization, healthy behaviors have few, if any, adverse outcomes, meaning that they can be recommended to nearly all older adults. However, unlike immunizations which are initiated and provided by the health care system, healthy behaviors require a personal commitment from individual patients. While the advice and encouragement from health care professionals are important, the effectiveness of any behavioral modification requires the individual patient to accept primary responsibility for initiating and maintaining healthy behaviors. A summary of recommendations in healthy behavior counseling for older adults is included in **Table 11-3**.

Nutrition

A healthy diet can contribute to an increase in life expectancy, better health, and quality of life as meals can be a source of pleasure and social engagement. Healthy diets have shown the potential to lower blood pressure and blood cholesterol. Optimal diets have also been associated with lower risk of chronic diseases, notably CAD, diabetes, obesity, and some forms of cancer. National Health and

TABLE 11-3 ■ HEALTH BEHAVIOR SCREENING AND INTERVENTIONS IN OLDER ADULTS

HEALTH BEHAVIOR	SCREENING TOOLS OR QUESTIONS	INTERVENTION
Nutrition counseling	Mini-nutritional assessment; malnutrition screening tool; food insecurity screens	Healthy diet counseling, including the Mediterranean diet when appropriate. Prevention of malnutrition can include addressing polypharmacy, dental health, food insecurity, depression, reducing mealtime isolation, and avoiding restrictive diets when not needed.
Physical activity	Frequency of walking, light sports or recreational activity, stretching or balance activities, and housework. Frequency of sedentary behavior.	30 min or more of moderate-intensity exercise 5 d a week. Flexibility, stretching, and balance exercise can complement strength and endurance training. Provide individualized guidance for older adults with pain, arthritis, cardiovascular disease, or at risk of falling. Consider starting with light-intensity, low-impact physical activity if needed.
Social connection	Abbreviated Berkman-Syme social network index; UCLA 3-item loneliness questionnaire; frequency of engagement in community activities; availability of friends, relatives, and children	Ask if individuals would like more social contact, what types of contact they prefer, and connect individuals to community programs. Identify and address barriers to interacting with others such as hearing impairment, functional impairment, or cognitive impairment.
Depression	Patient Health Questionnaire 2-item or 9-item screen (PHQ-2 or PHQ-9)	Further assessment of older adults screening positive for depression to ensure accurate diagnoses, effective treatment, and follow-up.

Nutrition Examination Survey (NHANES) III data show potentially important decreases with age in median protein and zinc intakes as well as intakes of calcium, vitamin E, and other nutrients. Malnutrition can often be undetected and subclinical nutrient deficiencies can adversely affect health and physical functioning. Screening for nutritional status should therefore occur routinely and include measuring body weight, weight loss, and considering screening tools such as the Mini Nutritional Assessment (MNA) or Malnutrition Screening Tool (MST).

Older adults can be counseled on the traditional Mediterranean diet, dominated by consumption of olive oil, vegetables, nuts, and fruits, which meets criteria for a healthy diet and is associated with prevention of progression of cardiovascular disease and reversal of the metabolic syndrome. Either antioxidants or fiber may affect a reduction in the transient oxidative stress associated with macronutrient intake. Prevention of malnutrition may require addressing polypharmacy or medications that can contribute to changes in taste or anorexia, monitoring dental health, addressing food insecurity, addressing depression, reducing isolation at mealtimes, and avoiding unnecessarily restricted diets (limiting salt, fat, or sugar), which can contribute to inadequate eating. The latest edition of *Nutrition and Your Health: Dietary Guidelines for Americans*, available online at http://www.health.gov/dietaryguidelines/, can serve as a reference for providers in counseling adults about healthful eating patterns.

Physical Activity

Physical activity and physical fitness can help prevent or delay the onset of chronic illnesses such as CAD, type II diabetes, osteoporosis, obesity, and cognitive impairment; protect against the development of functional decline; improve mood; reduce stress; and, perhaps, increase life expectancy. Physical activities that improve endurance, strength, and flexibility will delay impairments in mobility and may preserve the ability to perform tasks of daily living. Regular, moderate-intensity physical activity increases muscle mass and oxidative capacity, improves immune function, increases antioxidant defense against oxygen free radicals, and reduces oxidative stress. The current recommendation that every American exercise at least 30 minutes on most, and preferably all days, derives from evidence that even moderate physical activity is associated with a substantial drop in all-cause mortality. The cumulative, lifetime activity pattern may be the most influential factor in terms of providing protection from most diseases, especially those with a long developmental period, as well as mediating secondary disease complications associated with CAD, diabetes, and hypertension. The benefits of physical activity appears to outweigh the risks for nearly all older adults, including older adults at high risk for falling. For older adults with joint pain, arthritis, or cardiovascular disease, individualized guidance from clinicians may help patients to safely start a physical activity regimen.

Despite an enormous amount of information about the positive effects of exercise in preventing disease and increasing life expectancy, the majority of adults do not engage in regular, sufficient physical activity. Furthermore, aging appears to be associated with a rise in the prevalence of inactivity, especially among women, such that by age 75, one in three men and one in two women engage in *no* regular physical activity. Societal changes over the past 50 years, including increased dependence on cars for transportation, the advent of television and computers, and rise in number of desk jobs, have virtually engineered physical activity out of the daily routines of many Americans. Thus, encouraging and prescribing physical activity for adults of all ages is imperative and can be viewed as a central tenet of preventive gerontology.

Individualized activity plans should be considered in all older adults. Regular participation in activities of moderate intensity (such as brisk walking, climbing stairs, scrubbing floors, yard work), which increase caloric expenditure and maintain muscle strength, is recommended, as it is activity of moderate intensity that appears to allow health benefits to accrue. Current national guidelines suggest at least 30 minutes of moderate-intensity exercise on 5 or more days per week (Centers for Disease Control and Prevention [CDC]) or vigorous-intensity exercise (such as swimming laps, bicycling more than 10 miles per hour, jogging, or running) for 20 or more minutes on 3 or more days per week. The CDC, American College of Sports Medicine, and Surgeon General further state that daily physical activity requirements may be accumulated over the course of the day in short bouts of 10 to 15 minutes. The authors recommend that older adults who are unable to participate in moderate-intensity exercise should be started on light-intensity, low-impact exercise (eg, 5–10 minutes) with gradual progression over time. Flexibility, stretching, and balance exercise should be additionally considered to complement strength and endurance training. Helpful, patient-centered information about how to become more active can be found at the CDC's Physical Activity for Everyone (http://www.cdc.gov/physicalactivity/).

Several psychological and environmental factors determine physical activity behavior throughout the life span. Self-efficacy, or confidence in one's ability to perform a particular behavior (in this case, regular exercise), is strongly associated with both adoption of and adherence to physical activity among adolescents, young adults, and older adults. Strategies suggested to enhance self-efficacy, such as assessing readiness for exercise using a behavior change philosophy, using motivational interviewing techniques, weekly action planning and feedback, collaborative problem-solving, and addressing barriers to exercise may all enhance self-efficacy for exercise. These techniques can be learned and implemented by health care providers. Affective disorders such as depression and anxiety are inversely associated with physical activity participation at any age. Thus, evaluation for the presence of these conditions and institution of treatment may be necessary before adoption of an exercise program can occur. Social influences on physical activity appear to be strong throughout the life span. Peer reinforcement is particularly important in youth, while social support from spouses, friends, and community organizations (eg, Silver Sneakers program) is correlated with vigorous activity in younger and older adult populations. Finally, environmental factors, particularly safety and accessibility, influence activity participation across the age span. These latter factors are increasingly becoming a focus of community intervention efforts.

Social Connection

Ongoing involvement in a social network permits social contact (integration), the provision of social support, and the opportunity for social influence, and is associated with positive health outcomes and self-assessed well-being. Through opportunities for social engagement, such as attending social functions, getting together with friends and family, and going to church, meaningful social roles are defined and reinforced, creating a sense of belonging and identity. Measures of social integration or "connectedness" are powerful predictors of mortality likely because ties give meaning to an individual's life by enabling and obligating them to be fully involved in their community and thereby to feel attached to it. Social connections have been further linked to reduced risks of cognitive impairment.

There are several pathways by which social networks are thought to influence health: (1) a health behavioral pathway; (2) a psychological pathway; and (3) a physiologic pathway. Regarding the health behavioral pathway, social ties have been shown to influence the likelihood that certain behaviors will be adopted and that behavior will change (see also Chapters 4 and 25). For example, marriage and friendship ties have been shown in several studies to promote a healthier diet, more regular exercise, less smoking and drinking, and more cancer screening. Notably, not all social ties are positive, and some can negatively impact health, for example, the presence of a smoker in one's social network has been associated with greater relapse in efforts to quit and family members can be involved in emotional, physical, or financial elder mistreatment. A second mechanism by which social networks influence health is via psychological pathways. Loneliness is the emotional distress that arises from a perception that one's social relationships are inadequate. Loneliness has been independently linked to psychological distress, physical symptoms such as pain, and mortality. In addition, social ties can provide emotional support to protect against depression or anxiety, moral support in a crisis, or reduce day-to-day stress through social connection (eg, calling a friend about an odd symptom to get advice). Just knowing one has support to call on in times of need can reduce stress. A third mechanism by which social networks influence health is via physiologic pathways. Social relationships may influence health via effects on the hypothalamic–pituitary–adrenal axis, altering immune responses and cardiovascular reactivity. For example, a low number of contacts with acquaintances is associated with high resting plasma levels of epinephrine, and people with low social support have been found to have higher levels of urinary norepinephrine, regardless of their level of stress.

The authors recommend that clinicians should ask individuals about their social connections and if they feel lonely. Clinicians can directly address social needs by asking if individuals would like more social contact, what types of contact they prefer, and connecting individuals to programs to enhance social connections or support. Clinicians can facilitate social connections by identifying and addressing barriers to interacting with others such as hearing impairment, functional impairment, or cognitive impairment. Preventive strategies that encourage maintaining or enhancing existing relationships may in certain cases be more effective than trying to develop new relationships when an individual is already isolated or lonely.

Depression

Depression in older adults is common, underdiagnosed, and often inadequately treated. Rates of depression vary according to the diagnostic criteria used, but 2% of adults older than age 55 meet criteria for major depression while 14% report depressive symptoms. Most depression is recognized and treated in primary care; however, studies suggest that depression is often undiagnosed. Further, depression treatment has been shown to improve outcomes. The USPSTF recommends screening adults for depression in clinical practices that have systems in place to ensure accurate diagnosis, effective treatment, and follow-up.

BEHAVIORS WITH ADVERSE HEALTH CONSEQUENCES

Tobacco Use

Tobacco use is the largest single preventable cause of illness and premature deaths in the United States. Illnesses related to tobacco use (coronary artery disease [CAD]; cancers of the lung, larynx, oral cavity, esophagus, pancreas, and urinary bladder; stroke and chronic obstructive pulmonary disease) account for one in every five deaths in the United States. Evidence from NHANES indicates that tobacco use predicts shorter survival time for middle-aged (45–54 years) and older (65–74 years) men. Tobacco use can also multiply the risk associated with other carcinogenic agents; for example, heavy alcohol consumption, associated with esophageal cancer, carries an even greater risk when combined with cigarette smoking.

Tobacco dependence should be viewed as a chronic condition requiring ongoing assessment and repeated intervention. However, effective treatments are available that can lead to long-term, and in some cases, permanent abstinence. Studies have shown that individuals at any age can benefit from quitting the tobacco habit. Benefits include reduction in the risk of CAD, malignancy, stroke, and even hearing loss, along with improved pulmonary function, arterial circulation, and pulmonary perfusion.

Studies have found that only about 35% of adults are routinely asked about their tobacco habits or counseled to quit if they use tobacco. If providers do advise patients not to use tobacco, as many as 25% will quit or reduce the amount they use. Thus, providers should ask all patients at each clinic visit about tobacco use and advise all tobacco users about the importance of quitting, emphasizing factors that have been found to contribute most to successful attempts to quit: health concerns (symptoms); a desire to set an example for children; the expense of the habit; odor of breath, home, and clothing; and loss of taste for food. Providers should then assess a patient's willingness to attempt to quit. Patients who are unwilling to attempt to quit should be provided with a brief intervention designed to increase their motivation to quit.

Patients who are willing to quit should be provided with treatments that have been identified as effective. First-line pharmacotherapies that have been shown to increase smoking cessation include nicotine replacement (gum, inhaler, nasal spray, or patch), varenicline, and bupropion. Varenicline and bupropion appear to lead to increased rates of neuropsychiatric side effects including suicidal ideation. Thus, patients started on either medication should be monitored for neuropsychiatric symptoms including changes in behavior, agitation, depressed mood, hostility, and suicidal ideation.

Alcohol

Epidemiological studies support a survival benefit associated with moderate (up to two 8-ounce drinks per day) alcohol consumption, primarily through reduction of cardiovascular risk, including elevation of high-density lipoprotein (HDL) cholesterol. Although initial studies suggested that red wine may be especially beneficial, more recent studies suggest that the type of alcohol is not as important as the amount of alcohol intake and the pattern of use.

However, consumption of alcohol beyond a moderate level can induce adverse effects on every organ system, including increased risk of hypertension; breast, colon, esophageal, liver, and head and neck cancer; cirrhosis; gastrointestinal bleeding; pancreatitis; cardiomyopathy; seizures; cerebellar degeneration; peripheral neuropathy; cognitive dysfunction; insomnia; depression; and suicide. Nearly 15% of adults older than age 65 drink more than the recommended moderate level (> 7 drinks/week or binge-drinking). Counseling about problem drinking following a few screening questions is a high-impact, cost-effective intervention. Screening can be accomplished by taking a careful history of alcohol use or by using a standardized screening questionnaire. All adults should be counseled on the health risks associated with excess alcohol consumption as well as the risk of injury (ie, motor vehicle crashes or other equipment-related injury) after drinking alcohol. Nondependent heavy drinkers as well as those with alcoholism (a chronic illness involving a state of dependency) should be counseled about the benefits of decreasing alcohol intake. Brief counseling by primary care providers can result in a significant reduction in alcohol use. Dependent drinkers should be referred to formal alcohol treatment programs and considered for a trial of naltrexone, an opioid antagonist that reduces the pleasurable effects of alcohol and may reduce relapse to heavy drinking.

Obesity

In adults, obesity is defined as a body mass index (BMI) of 30 kg/m^2 or more; overweight is a BMI of 25 to 30 kg/m^2 or more. Research suggests that although obesity and underweight are associated with increased mortality, being overweight (BMI 25–30) is not associated with increased mortality at any age. Further, increasing evidence suggests that being obese may not be as dangerous for older adults as younger adults. NHANES data suggest that for adults age 25 to 59, BMI more than 35 compared to BMI 19 to 25 nearly doubles the risk of all-cause mortality with a relative risk of 1.8. In contrast, for adults older than age 70, the all-cause mortality risk with BMI more than 35 is not statistically different from BMI 19 to 25 with a relative risk of 1.2. In fact, for adults older than age 70, being underweight (BMI < 19) was associated with higher mortality than being obese (BMI > 35). Thus, the optimal BMI for older adults appears to be slightly higher than the optimal BMI for younger adults.

For older adults, obesity is also a risk factor for impaired mobility and other functional limitations, disabling conditions such as osteoarthritis; sleep apnea; gallbladder disease; nonalcoholic fatty liver disease; and cancers of the breast, endometrium, and colon. Moreover, those who are obese may suffer from social stigmatization, impaired social interaction, depression, and low self-esteem. Thus, regardless of the relationship between obesity and mortality in older adults, counseling obese patients to lose weight is likely to be beneficial.

Because treatment and reversal of obesity is challenging, primary prevention is warranted. Efforts to maintain a healthy weight should start early in life and continue throughout adulthood, as this is likely to be more successful than efforts to lose substantial amounts of weight and maintain weight loss once obesity has developed. Data from NHANES I suggest that getting adequate rest may be important in obesity prevention. Sleeping less than 7 hours a night was shown to be a risk factor for subsequent obesity. This may be related to altered levels of leptin and ghrelin, two appetite-regulating hormones. Leptin is associated with appetite suppression and ghrelin is an appetite stimulant that is thought to play a role in long-term regulation of body weight. During sleep deprivation, leptin levels fall and ghrelin levels rise.

Adults who are trying to maintain a healthy weight after weight loss are advised to get even more physical activity than the 30 min/d (described above) that is currently recommended; the US Department of Agriculture has recommended at least 60 min/d to manage weight. Weight management leading to a slow, steady weight loss is more beneficial that a pattern of weight cycling, which actually contributes to an elevated risk of mortality. The basal metabolic rate decreases with age, in parallel with a decline in lean body mass, and body fat increases proportionally. Thus, in order to most readily achieve normalization of body weight and body composition, an energy-sufficient (but not excessive) diet should be combined with a program of regular physical activity to permit maintenance of basal metabolic rate.

Recreational Drugs

The prevalence of injection drug use among older adults is unknown. Injection drug users typically initiate injection drug use during late adolescence (younger than age 21);

however, a sizable subgroup begins injecting during early and late adulthood. Persons with a history of recreational drug use on only one or a few occasions are unlikely to self-identify; thus, clinicians should probe for such a pattern of usage.

Noninjection drug use (crack smokers, methamphetamine, intranasal heroin, or cocaine, etc.) contributes to development of gastroduodenal ulcers, chest pain and myocardial infarction, and increased risk of death. Higher levels of drug involvement also were associated with increased age-adjusted mortality. The normalization of recreation drug use through marijuana legalization laws and the aging of the baby boomer generation, which has had greater experience with recreational drugs, are widely expected to increase the rates of recreational drug use in older adults.

Prescription Drug Misuse

Prescription drug misuse is poorly described in the medical literature but is currently a more prevalent problem than illicit drug use among older adults. Misuse of prescription medications may be related to insomnia, chronic pain, depression, and anxiety. The potential misuse of benzodiazepines is well recognized and has led to prescribing recommendations that suggest only short-term use and use only for intended indications. Amphetamine-like stimulants have abuse potential, but addiction to these drugs is seldom documented. Other medications that are often misused are sedative hypnotics, opioid analgesics, and barbiturates. Chronic use of such agents may lead to physical dependency and the development of withdrawal symptoms with attempts to discontinue use. Treatment may require detoxification followed by rehabilitation.

PREVENTION AMONG NURSING HOME OR SERIOUSLY ILL POPULATIONS

The majority of older adults residing in nursing homes have significant physical impairments, with over half requiring assistance in toileting, bathing, and/or transferring. Nearly half have a diagnosis of Alzheimer disease or other dementias, and more than half receive 9 or more routine medications. Consequently, preventive medical interventions should carefully consider (1) the time-to-benefit of each intervention as life expectancy may be limited, (2) short-term harms, and (3) how to prioritize competing medical needs. In this respect, the framework for preventive care in most nursing home residents is analogous to the framework for preventive care for palliative care patients with serious, life-limiting illness (eg, cancer, end-organ failure, or neurodegenerative diseases).

In these populations, clinicians should consider early on whether screening tests might require downstream invasive testing for positive tests, and if individuals would be willing and able to undergo such testing. Seemingly simple testing or additional clinical visits may be overly burdensome to patients already managing multiple medical conditions. Moreover, individuals with dementia and their family members require careful counseling and consent prior to testing. Medications for asymptomatic conditions should be regularly reevaluated to determine if deprescribing is appropriate (eg, de-intensifying glycemic control). Behavioral counseling might involve managing expectations about reasonable goals, for example, with maintaining moderate physical activity or community engagement. Moreover, serious illness and multimorbidity may themselves lead to unavoidable changes in health behaviors. For example, dementia can lead to the loss of interest in eating and malnutrition, and so families should be provided anticipatory guidance on what can be "prevented" and what may be expected as part of the disease trajectory. In general, eliciting patient and family values and preferences can help clinicians align available preventive interventions with the goals of individual patients.

FURTHER READING

Advisory Committee on Immunization Practices. Vaccine recommendations of the ACIP. http://www.cdc.gov/vaccines/hcp/acip-recs/index.html. Accessed Feb 15, 2021.

American Cancer Society. Guidelines for the early detection of cancer. https://www.cancer.org/healthy/find-cancer-early/cancer-screening-guidelines/american-cancer-society-guidelines-for-the-early-detection-of-cancer.html. Accessed Feb 15, 2021.

Artaud F, Dugravot A, Sabia S, Singh-Manoux A, Tzourio C, Elbaz A. Unhealthy behaviours and disability in older adults: three-city Dijon cohort study. *BMJ*. 2013; 347:f4240.

Berkman LF, Kawachi I. *Social Epidemiology*. New York, NY: Oxford University Press; 2000.

Burns DM. Cigarette smoking among the elderly: disease consequences and the benefits of cessation. *Am J Health Promot*. 2000;14(6):357–361.

de Koning HJ, van der Aalst CM, de Jong PA, et al. Reduced lung-cancer mortality with volume CT screening in a randomized trial. *N Engl J Med*. 2020;382(6):503–513.

DiPietro L. Physical activity in aging: changes in patterns and their relationship to health and function. *J Gerontol A Biol Sci Med Sci*. 2001;56 Spec No 2:13–22.

Flegal KM, Graubard BI, Williamson DF, Gail MH. Excess deaths associated with underweight, overweight and obesity. *JAMA*. 2005;293(15):1861–1867.

King AC, Guralnik JM. Maximizing the potential of an aging population. *JAMA*. 2010;304(17):1944–1945.

Lee SJ, Boscardin WJ, Stijacic-Cenzer I, Conell-Price J, O'Brien S, Walter LC. Time lag to benefit after screening for breast and colorectal cancer: meta-analysis of survival data from the United States, Sweden, United Kingdom and Denmark. *BMJ*. 2013;346:e8441.

Nelson ME, Rejeski WJ, Blair SN, et al. Physical activity and public health in older adults: Recommendations from the American College of Sports Medicine and American Heart Association. *Circulation*. 2007;116(9):1094–1105.

Nichol KL, Nordin JD, Nelson DB, Mullooly JP, Hak E. Effectiveness of influenza vaccine in the community-dwelling elderly. *N Engl J Med*. 2007;357(14):1373–1381.

Rollnick S, Mason P, Butler C. *Health Behavior Change: A Guide for Practitioners*. Philadelphia, PA: Churchill Livingstone; 1999.

Schoen RE, Pinsky PF, Weissfeld JL, et al. Colorectal-cancer incidence and mortality with screening flexible sigmoidoscopy. *N Engl J Med*. 2012;366(25):2345–2357.

Schonberg MA, Hamel MB, Davis RB, et al. Development and evaluation of a decision aid on mammography screening for women 75 years and older. *JAMA Intern Med*. 2014;174(3):417–424.

Shaukat A, Mongin SJ, Geisser MS, et al. Long-term mortality after screening for colorectal cancer. *N Engl J Med*. 2013;369(12):1106–1114.

US Preventive Services Task Force. Recommendations for Primary Care Practice. October 2014. http://www.uspreventiveservicestaskforce.org/Page/Name/recommendations. Accessed Jan 27, 2015.

Van Ravesteyn NT, Stout NK, Schechter CB, et al. Benefits and harms of mammography screening after age 74 years: model estimates of overdiagnosis. *J Natl Cancer Inst*. 2015;107(7):djv103.

Walter LC, Covinsky KE. Cancer screening in elderly patients: a framework for individualized decision making. *JAMA*. 2001;285(21):2750–2756.

Walter LC, Lewis CL, Barton MB. Screening for colorectal, breast and cervical cancer in the elderly: a review of the evidence. *Am J Med*. 2005;118(10):1078–1086.

Welch HG. *Should I be Tested for Cancer? Maybe Not and Here's Why*. Berkeley, CA: University of California Press; 2004.

Wiener RS, Schwartz LM, Woloshin S, Welch HG. Population-based risk for complications after transthoracic needle lung biopsy of a pulmonary nodule: an analysis of discharge records. *Ann Intern Med*. 2011;155(3):137–144.

Wilson SR, Knowles SB, Huang Q, Fink A. The prevalence of harmful and hazardous alcohol consumption in older U.S. adults. *JGIM*. 2014;29(2):312–319.

Zauber AG, Winawer SJ, O'Brien MJ, et al. Colonoscopic polypectomy and long-term prevention of colorectal-cancer deaths. *N Engl J Med*. 2012;366:687–696.

Age-Friendly Care

Terry Fulmer, Maryama Diaw, Chaoli Zhang, Jinghan Zhang, Wendy Huang, Amy Berman, Tara Asokan, Kedar S. Mate, Leslie Pelton

INTRODUCTION

With an unprecedented acceleration of the population living successfully into old age, the reimagining of the health care system is an imminent and compelling responsibility. There is an urgency to reform the fragmented delivery of health care to improve continuity across care systems as well as to adopt a unifying framework that is readily understood and implemented universally by providers and patients alike. Patients and families want respect and compassion, to learn about what to expect about their health and health care, and to be able to have a strong sense of trust in their caregivers and institutions.

Reliable team approaches are essential, given the complexity of our systems. Interprofessional team (IPT) care is essential to providing effective care for older adults with multiple conditions and functional decline. Research has demonstrated that IPT care is associated with enhanced functional and cognitive status, reduced depression, and improved subjective well-being. IPT care has also been shown to reduce hospital readmissions and outpatient service use. Specialized IPTs focusing on specific conditions such as congestive heart failure, stroke, myocardial infarction, or dementia have also demonstrated improved patient outcomes in older adults.

The current and projected health care workforce shortage, coupled with the aging of the population, mandate that care models be measurably efficient and effective. The increasing number of frail older adults with complex needs demands widespread adoption of geriatric IPTs. In this chapter, the Age-Friendly Health Systems (AFHS) movement, coupled with the essential elements of team-based care, are discussed as a way forward and new standard of care.

Learning Objectives

- Articulate the importance of the 4Ms in health care for older adults.
- Discuss the evidence and approaches for acting on each of the 4Ms: What Matters, Medication, Mentation, and Mobility.
- Understand the intersection of team care required in the 4Ms approach.

Key Clinical Points

1. Team-based geriatric care is critical to the delivery of comprehensive, coordinated health care to older adults, their families, and caregivers.
2. The Age-Friendly Health Systems movement is an evidence-based approach to care that when implemented reliably, improves quality, improves health, and reduces costs.
3. The 4Ms set, What Matters, Mentation, Medications, and Mobility, provides a framework that addresses the multiple intersections of each of the 4Ms.

High-Functioning Teams as a Prerequisite to AFHS and 4Ms Care

Through the collaborative efforts of The John A. Hartford Foundation (JAHF) and the Institute for Healthcare Improvement (IHI), in partnership with the American

Age-Friendly Health Systems

We are helping health systems become Age-Friendly:

Age-Friendly Health Systems is an initiative of The John A. Hartford Foundation and the Institute for Healthcare Improvement in partnership with the American Hospital Association and the Catholic Health Association of the United States.

FIGURE 12-1. Age-Friendly Health Systems logo.

Hospital Association (AHA) and the Catholic Health Association of the United States, the AFHS initiative has had strong momentum (**Figure 12-1**). Already established in over 2,600 sites of care across the country, this progress indicates a willingness to adopt the 4Ms model and study the impact. The AFHS movement has the goal of reaching 25% of hospitals and primary care settings by 2025.

The IHI Triple Aim is the basis for the AFHS approach that focuses on improving the patient experience of care (including quality and satisfaction), improving the health of populations; and reducing the per capita cost of health care. The four evidence-based facets of care known as the 4Ms (What Matters, Medication, Mentation, and Mobility) have evolved from the tenets of the Triple Aim.

However, achieving specific health outcomes of at-risk populations also requires the combined skills of a wide range of professionals operating as a team. Team members possess extensive professional knowledge of their individual discipline but often have limited knowledge of other disciplines on the team. Beyond varied technical knowledge among team members, teams may be characterized by different values across professional disciplines. These differences are becoming less pronounced with the evolution of IPTs in most health care settings and with many populations. The 4Ms set, described in this chapter, provides every team member with the same elements of care that each member will see through their own clinical lens, which helps ensure a holistic approach to the care plan. The Veterans Health Administration characterizes high-functioning teams as those that excel in both function (effectiveness) and relationships (engagement). Effectiveness refers to the team's purpose and methods, role clarity, communication, awareness, and responsiveness (eg, how the team uses and shares information). Engagement is a function of the level of civility, respect, psychological safety, and cohesiveness of the team. There is a balance in the nature and function of relationships on the team. Limited attention to developing professional relationships may impede the development of trust and collaboration, which can impair team function.

However, excess focus on cohesion and collaboration may limit communication and prevent different opinions from being openly discussed.

Professional disciplines vary significantly in how they characterize problems and their etiology. For instance, more medically oriented disciplines may focus on conducting diagnostic tests and explaining findings in biological terms, whereas the social sciences (eg, psychology, social work) may emphasize psychosocial issues and consequences. In addition to differences in understanding and formulating plans of care, team members of different disciplines vary substantially in the nature of treatments they typically prescribe and in the length and frequency of patient visits. These differences in perspectives and approaches can be overcome when a 4Ms approach is used and all team member input is recognized and respected. While teams work toward a patient-centered outcome, individual team member competency remains essential. Teamwork requires discipline-specific clinical knowledge and skills and methods that allow all members to be heard—involving processes to communicate clearly, meet routinely, and understand the individual clinician's role in the care plan. Older adults with multiple chronic conditions or advanced illnesses stand to benefit most from a shift from a disease-centered care delivery system to the AFHS model of care.

The 4Ms Framework

An AFHS means being able to reliably provide a set of four elements of evidence-based, high-quality care, known as the 4Ms: What Matters, Medication, Mentation, and Mobility, shown in **Figure 12-2**. When the four elements are consistently implemented together as a set, they allow for a shift in focus from disease to function that accelerates the ability to better serve the needs and preferences of older adults. The 4Ms make the care of older adults more manageable and reduce the cognitive burden on care teams that is often felt in the delivery of complex clinical care. Focus is placed on the overall wellness and capabilities of older patients rather than siloed diagnostic assessments that often overlap and can create contradictions in care planning.

This approach guides the care of older adults irrespective of the location of care, and the 4Ms approach is most impactful when the team communicates progress in the 4Ms at every handoff. There is a strong evidence base for each of the 4Ms that is leading to improvement in health systems and creating sustainable change.

What Matters

What Matters is what truly drives patient-centered care and is essential to addressing the unique needs of older adults, eliminating harm, and maximizing the efficiency of health care delivery. What Matters supports the values and activities that each person wishes to prioritize. The AFHS initiative defines What Matters as knowing and aligning care with each older adult's specific health outcome goals and

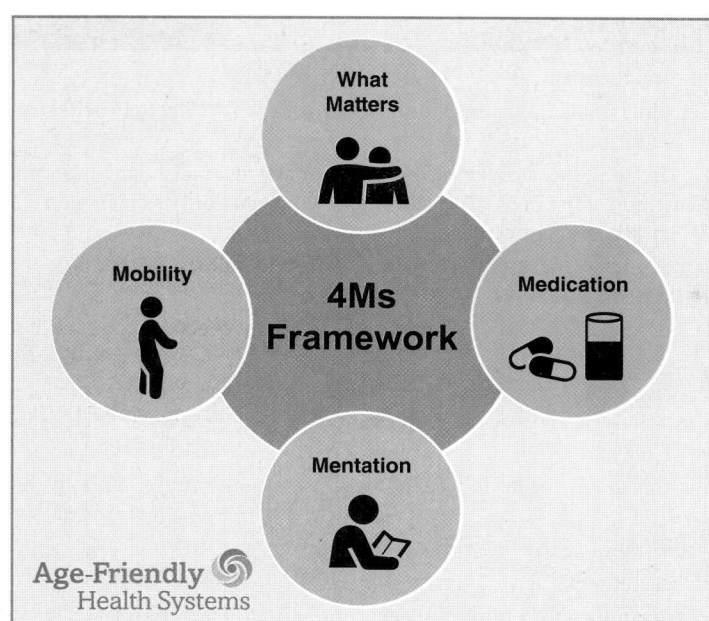

What Matters

Know and align care with each older adult's specific health outcome goals and care preferences including, but not limited to, end-of life care, and across settings of care.

Medication

If medication is necessary, use Age-Friendly medication that does not interfere with What Matters to the older adult, Mobility, or Mentation across settings of care.

Mentation

Prevent, identify, treat, and manage dementia, depression, and delirium across settings of care.

Mobility

Ensure that older adults move safely every day in order to maintain function and do What Matters.

FIGURE 12-2. 4Ms interaction. (An initiative of The John A. Hartford Foundation and the Institute for Healthcare Improvement [IHI] in partnership with the American Hospital Association [AHA] and the Catholic Health Association of the United States [CHA].)

care preferences, including, but not limited to, end-of-life care, across settings of care.

Beyond the scope of disease-specific outcomes and survival statistics, an age-friendly infrastructure considers What Matters and consistently documents the same care priorities among health care providers, families, and patients. Shared decision-making, which directly involves the patient in the care conversation, has been shown to increase trust and satisfaction within health care systems and with care delivery, while also reducing fragmentation among clinicians and supernumerary demands on clinicians. A network-wide clinical trial conducted by a team of researchers at Yale has shown this through the utilization and analyses of patient preference data collected from three surveys, including the Treatment Burden Questionnaire (TBQ). Older patients who were given the opportunity to express what mattered to them, compared to those who received usual, unprioritized care, were more likely to have unnecessary medications deprescribed and had fewer diagnostic tests, referrals, and procedures. After being explicitly asked to identify their values-based health priorities and speaking to their primary care physicians concerning these priorities, TBQ measurements collectively demonstrated a 5-point decrease in treatment burden score after a 6-month follow-up period, compared to baseline. As connoted in the 4Ms framework, health care that prioritizes older patients' health preferences can significantly decrease clinical harm and simultaneously have a positive impact on patient satisfaction. **Table 12-1** provides a checklist for culturally appropriate "What Matters" conversations.

The topic most sensitive to older adults' wishes and priorities is decision making related to end-of-life care and serious illness. In efforts to honor the bioethical principles of autonomy and informed consent, the development of advance care planning (ACP) has been a critical aspect of What Matters in the 4Ms framework. ACP is the process of intentional solicitation of decisions from patients and families regarding their preferences for health care. If nurses, physicians, and other health care professionals ask and document decisions based on older patients' health priorities, goals, and preferences, health systems can honor What Matters to older adults and avert potentially unwanted care. In a randomized controlled trial (RCT) conducted at a large university hospital, patients receiving formal, coordinated ACP from trained facilitators were found to have their end-of-life wishes known and respected significantly more than the control group, indicating increased patient and family satisfaction with the care provided in discharge questionnaires. Patients saw the benefits of ACP to include the informal communication of future wishes, preparation for end-of-life care and death, avoidance of prolongation of dying, strengthening of personal relationships, and relieving burdens placed on family.

Documenting and incorporating What Matters information is a reliable, timely nonpharmacologic intervention that, when deployed, benefits the older adult involved and participating health systems. It enables the leveraging of interdisciplinary team resources and serves to stand as a quantifiable process measure. Beneficial care in congruence with reductions in the incidence and duration of

TABLE 12-1 ■ CHECKLIST FOR CULTURALLY APPROPRIATE "WHAT MATTERS" CONVERSATIONS

- Learn the older adult's preferred term for his or her cultural identity.
- Determine the appropriate degree of formality. Learn the older adult's preference for how he or she would like to be addressed and use this title and the surname (eg, Mrs. Smith), unless a less formal address is requested.
- Determine the older adult's preferred language. If the older adult has basic or below basic literacy or English language proficiency, seek permission from the person to have a medical interpreter assist in the "What Matters" conversation, or determine if a trusted individual who is literate can be present during the "What Matters" conversation.
- Be respectful of nonverbal communication. Watch for body language cues that might be linked to cultural norms. Adopt conservative body language, use a calm demeanor, and avoid expressive gestures.
- Address issues linked to culture such as a lack of trust, fear of medical experimentation, fear of side effects, and unfamiliarity with Western biomedical belief systems.
- Review the medical records to determine if there has been a history of trauma, including refugee status, survivors of violence, genocide, and torture. These are very sensitive issues and must be approached with caution. Reassure the older adult of the confidentiality of the clinician–patient relationship.
- Determine the level of acculturation and recognize that this is a factor for individuals who are recent immigrants, as well as for those who are not recent immigrants.
- Recognize health beliefs that include the use of alternative therapies.
- Consider how gender or gender identity might affect decision making.
- Consider an approach to decision making that recognizes family and community decisions and does not automatically exclude them in favor of individual autonomy

Data from Laderman M, Jackson C, Little K, et al. "What Matters" to Older Adults? A Toolkit for Health Systems to Design Better Care with Older Adult. Copyright ©2019. Institute for Healthcare Improvement.

unwanted and avoidable hospital stays, procedures, emergency department visits, medications, etc., stand to improve quality and efficiency across the board for older adults and health systems alike.

Medication

Managing medications to ensure that they are only prescribed when necessary, are financially accessible, and well-understood and safely adhered to is central to the health of older adults who need them. Deprescribing may be even more important. In 2015, an estimated 29% of Medicare beneficiaries filled a prescription for at least one medication included in the 2015 American Geriatrics Society Beers Criteria list of drugs to avoid in older adults. The risk of dangerous side effects in older adults is high. The 4Ms framework, and medication management specifically, includes attention to age-friendly medications that do not interfere with What Matters to an older adult, Mobility, or Mentation across settings of care.

IHI's Guide to Using the 4Ms in the Care of Older Adults emphasizes the importance of proper prescription protocol for older adults. Clinicians need to be alert to inappropriate medications and polypharmacy (multiple medications). In research assessing polypharmacy's impact on delirium, polypharmacy was found to be a risk factor for delirium in older patients after emergency admission. One measure that health systems must prioritize is safely deprescribing or abstaining from prescribing high-risk medications.

An evidence-based approach to limiting the overprescription of high-risk medications and reducing the negative impacts of polypharmacy is the use of computerized decision support (CDS) systems. The Screening Tool of Older Person's potentially inappropriate Prescriptions (STOPP) and the Screening Tool of Alert doctors to the Right Treatment (START) have been used across systems to alert providers of potential problems with medications. Risks associated with prescribing a medication may outweigh the potential benefits. STOPP/START has been found to be beneficial in addressing inappropriate prescribing in older adults. When used, the criteria significantly improved prescribing methods, resulting in a lower prevalence of falls and all-cause mortality.

The impact of CDS systems on potentially inappropriate prescriptions (PIP) and potential drug-drug interactions has been positive. Avoiding drug-drug interactions is a critical aspect of providing medication services to older populations due to increased comorbidities in older adults.

The 4Ms framework ensures that medications are continuously reviewed, that high-risk medications are avoided, dose adjusted, or deprescribed when clinically appropriate, to improve the probability that medications are safe, appropriate, and well understood by the older adult and their caregivers. It should be noted that primary care physicians express a lack of time, poor awareness of the harms of medications, and fear of withdrawal symptoms or patient criticism as barriers to deprescribing. A team approach, where all members are empowered to do a medication assessment can help alleviate these concerns on the part of any one team member. Clinicians across the board must be proactive in deprescribing and improving medication management for older adults.

In a study designed to showcase the role of all health care settings in decreasing the negative impacts of polypharmacy through deprescribing, pharmacists were placed at the forefront of providing patients a role in the decision-making process to deprescribe. Pharmacists in the intervention arm were given educational brochures to distribute to both patients and prescribers, while those in the control group provided the usual standard of care. Those in the intervention arm experienced a discontinuation of medication in almost half the cases, compared to 39% of cases for those in the control group.

The benefits of desprescribing are also evident when complex medication plans contribute to poor medication adherence. The primary barriers affecting medication adherence have been characterized as patient factors, medication factors, prescriber factors, system-based factors, and other factors. Each play a key role in either enhancing or complicating the medication protocols/schedules found to negatively affect medication adherence. In alignment with the 4Ms framework, medication plans need to be person-centered and simplified whenever possible for all involved. Cost-related medication nonadherence in older adults is also a serious problem and can lead to skipped or reduced doses due to costs, as noted by an analysis of the 2017 National Health Interview Survey (NHIS). Knowing that approximately 20% of older adults take 10 drugs or more, eliminating medication overload can improve the outcomes of care.

Mentation

Assessment and care planning for optimal mentation, which includes mood and memory, helps prevent, identify, treat, and manage dementia, delirium, and depression across all settings of care. Dementia, delirium, and depression are covered in detail in other chapters in this text (see Chapters 58, 59, and 65, respectively). When health care providers reliably assess and create appropriate care plans for these three common conditions, qualitative and quantitative gains are evident for patients and health systems alike.

Dementia is more prevalent with advanced age but should not be conflated with normal aging. It is a neurodegenerative syndrome characterized by accelerated cognitive decline that interferes with activities of daily living. Dementia can compromise the independence of older adults and increase caregiving needs. Person-centered care (PCC) for older adults with dementia is a sociopsychological intervention that has been proven to significantly improve the overall quality of life and neuropsychiatric symptoms (NPS) when applied directly to clinical practice and care settings. **Table 12-2** highlights the philosophy of PCC, which revolves around six fundamentals in line with the Alzheimer's Association Dementia Care Practice Recommendations. A meta-analysis and systematic review drawing results from several RCTs favored PCC interventions by reducing agitation and decreasing the severity.

PART II PRINCIPLES OF GERIATRICS

TABLE 12-2 ■ PRACTICE RECOMMENDATIONS FOR PERSON-CENTERED CARE FOR PEOPLE LIVING WITH DEMENTIA

1. Know the person living with dementia	The individual living with dementia is more than a diagnosis. It is important to know the unique and complete person, including their values, beliefs, interests, abilities, likes, and dislikes—both past and present. This information should inform every interaction and experience.
2. Recognize and accept the person's reality	It is important to see the world from the perspective of the individual living with dementia. Doing so recognizes behavior as a form of communication, thereby promoting effective and empathetic communication that validates feelings and connects with the individual's in their reality.
3. Identify and support ongoing opportunities for meaningful engagement	Every experience and interaction can be seen as an opportunity for engagement. Engagement should be meaningful to, and purposeful for, the individual living with dementia. It should support interests and preferences, allow for choice and success, and recognize that even when the dementia is most severe, the person can experience joy, comfort, and meaning in life.
4. Build and nurture authentic, caring relationships	Persons living with dementia should be part of relationships that treat them with dignity and respect, and where their individuality is always supported. This type of caring relationship is about being present and concentrating on the interaction, rather than the task. It is about "doing with" rather than "doing for" as part of a supportive and mutually beneficial relationship.
5. Create and maintain a supportive community for individuals, families, and staff	A supportive community allows for comfort and creates opportunities for success. It is a community that values each person and respects individual differences, celebrates accomplishments and occasions, and provides access to and opportunities for autonomy, engagement, and shared experiences.
6. Evaluate care practices regularly and make appropriate changes	Several tools are available to assess person-centered care practices for people living with dementia. It is important to regularly evaluate practices and models, share findings, and make changes to interactions, programs, and practices as needed.

Reproduced with permission from Institute for Healthcare Improvement (IHI).

In the fifth edition of the American Psychological Association's *Diagnostic and Statistical Manual of Mental Disorders* (DSM-5), delirium is clinically classified as a "disturbance in attention (ie, reduced ability to direct, focus, sustain, and shift attention) and awareness (reduced orientation to the environment)…[that] develops over a short period of time (usually hours to a few days), represents an acute change from baseline attention and awareness, and tends to fluctuate in severity during the course of the day." It is especially important to note that mental status change in delirium appears as a direct psychological consequence of another etiology, especially preexisting medical conditions (excluding dementia) and medication toxicity. While its underlying pathophysiologic mechanisms can be elusive, delirium is a dangerous clinical condition. In hospitalized patients, an episode of delirium leads to detrimental sequelae, including major complications after surgeries, prolonged length-of-stay, loss of functional autonomy, decreased cognitive abilities, and increased mortality. These effects contribute to rising costs for health systems. In all settings of care including care by family members in the home, delirium poses a frightening and dangerous situation. With advanced education and assessment skills appropriate to the setting, every care provider can detect potential signs and symptoms of delirium and get the requisite care for the older adult in a timely manner.

The Tailored, Family-Involved Hospital Elder Life Program (t-HELP), which centers on family involvement for those older adults at risk for experiencing delirium, has been shown to improve detection and prompt early treatment. Postoperative delirium (POD) is associated with increased morbidity and mortality, and can be reduced or prevented. The improved mental and physical recovery after surgery and shorter hospitalizations are indicative of t-HELP's efficacy, which harbors the potential to save health care systems untold millions of dollars. In AFHS, the use of evidence-based protocols to assess and attend to modifiable risk factors of delirium (eg, mobilization, orientation, sensory adaptation, social interaction, assistance with meals and hydration, etc.) help ensure Triple Aim care. Hartford Hospital is an example of an organization that has made a commitment to rigorous delirium screening in the context of 4Ms care and is discussed in a later case study.

Depression is a potentially life-threatening condition for older adults and is encompassed in the 4Ms framework as a part of the Mentation assessment. Prevalence of depression is estimated to range from 10% to 30% (see Chapter 65). There are several types of depression, and the most common include: major depression with severe symptoms that interfere with the ability to work, sleep, concentrate, eat, and enjoy life; persistent depressive disorder, also known as dysthymia with symptoms that are less severe than those of major depression, but last a long time (at least 2 years); and minor depression with symptoms that are less

severe and shorter in length than those of major depression and dysthymia. In a 4Ms assessment of Mentation, depression screens are important to determine if depression is present and if so, making an appropriate referral to a provider who can follow up with a treatment plan. The older adult may also describe a grief event that is at the root of the depression and here as well, follow-up is important for the well-being of the older adult. Screening for depression is recommended annually or when symptoms arise. Evidence supports using one of the following four screening tools: Patient Health Questionnaire-2 (PHQ-2), Patient Health Questionnaire-9 (PHQ-9), Geriatric Depression Scale (GDS), and Geriatric Depression Scale - short form (GDS - short form).

Mobility

The positive effects of physical activity on mobility from improved muscle strength and balance as well as the protective effects against falling are well-documented. As older adults age, having the ability to move independently and safely plays an increasingly important role in how an older adult's quality of life is defined. Living with any disease puts additional burden on an older person's mobility. For example, diabetes mellitus increases the risk of falls in older adults, and clinicians must be attentive to the likelihood of older adults with diabetes needing education related to this risk and offer a mobility program that can be guided by physical therapy. Most chronic conditions play a role in reducing physical, cognitive, and social functioning. The 4Ms approach is especially effective in addressing function in a holistic manner that is readily understood by older adults and their families.

Medication, visual deficits, cognitive and mood impairment, and environmental hazards can all limit mobility. For instance, use of benzodiazepines, which are hypnotic sedatives prescribed to treat conditions such as anxiety and insomnia, correlates to an increased risk of falls in older adults and should be avoided. Preventative measures for maintaining mobility include regular vision and hearing examinations, continuous assessment of medications and provision of exercise protocols to increase balance, gait, and strength are recommended. Encouraging exercise in older adults is a recognized method for increasing the mobility of older adults and is recommended to be incorporated in their care. The role of exercise in decreasing the risks of falls is well-documented (see Chapter 43). However, as with any age group, motivation for maintaining exercise regimens can be a challenge. AFHS approaches strive to create person-centered, context-dependent care plans such as group exercise classes for some or caregiver education and strategies to ensure Mobility for others.

The Value of the 4Ms Approach

The value of becoming an AFHS and implementing the 4Ms framework (also referred to as financial benefits) is detailed in IHI's "The Business Case for Becoming an Age-Friendly Health System." When implemented properly, AFHS can ultimately lead to reduced hospital length of stay and fewer hospital readmissions.

Annual Wellness Visits (AWV), covered by Medicare Part B since 2016, are designed to engage older adults in What Matters conversations as a part of the annual benefit. An AFHS approach can improve value by systematically using the AWV to review the 4Ms. In fact, fee-for-service claims data from 2013 to 2018 demonstrated that AWV users had a reduction in Medicare spending over 12 months. St. Vincent Medical Group (Indianapolis, IN), an institution in the Ascension system, which represents one of the five pioneering health systems that spearheaded the AFHS initiative, also demonstrated value. When revenue from ACP and associated gross benefits from AWV are considered, St. Vincent showed an annual net income of nearly $3.6 million. When asking What Matters, clinical teams enhance value for patients and families.

Nonfatal falls account for almost 99% of the estimated health care costs for fatal and nonfatal falls, which amounted to a total of $50 billion in 2018. This number for just nonfatal falls was estimated at $38 billion in 2013. Beyond the key purpose of leveraging the 4Ms framework to improve quality of care, creating AFHS and ensuring that older adults can afford their medications and avoid medication overload can result in long-term savings that will benefit all sectors.

Case Studies At Hartford Hospital in Connecticut, age-friendly initiatives have led to resounding impacts in value and care. The ADAPT (Actions to enhance Delirium Assessment Prevention and Treatment) program was started in 2012 as an interprofessional team effort across various disciplines and departments, with support from the hospital administration and vital resource allocation for positive reinforcement and opportunities for improvement. A delirium care pathway was developed to ensure that delirium prevention, treatment, and management remained an interprofessional priority throughout the length of an older patient's stay and transitions. This included the implementation of delirium screenings three times a day, in addition to an initial screen. Adjunct support was provided through various means, from volunteer programs to therapeutic activities focusing on mobilization, nutrition, sleep/rest, and cognitive connection. A registry was also created for gathering data and analyzing quality outcome measures.

As seen in **Table 12-3**, delirium was shown to have serious consequences leading to poorer health outcomes, with the length of hospital stay averaging 4 days and $8,900 for those without delirium, and 12 days and $31,284 for those with delirium. Seventy percent of those without delirium were discharged home, compared to only 30% for those with delirium. And while mortality was less than 1% for patients without delirium, it was 10% for patients with

TABLE 12-3 ■ HARTFORD HOSPITAL PER-PATIENT COSTS ASSOCIATED WITH DELIRIUM[a]

	WITH DELIRIUM	WITHOUT DELIRIUM	DIFFERENCE
Hospital length of stay (LOS)	12 d	4 d	8 d
Daily cost	$2,798	$2,225	$573
Total cost of stay	$31,284	$8,900	$22,384

[a]Data is from July 2015 to June 2016.
Reproduced with permission from Hartford Hospital.

delirium. The implementation of the ADAPT program led to decreased hospital stays for delirium patients (16–10.6 days) and reduced delirium attributable days. This resulted in annual savings averaging $6.5 million from 2012 to 2019. Hartford Health care has now taken steps to scale up the program, with potential expansion to other care settings (post-acute and home care) and a focus on population health in primary care clinics for underserved community-dwelling older adults.

Another example that has exhibited beneficial results has been Providence St. Joseph Health in Oregon, one of the original five locations chosen to take place in the development of AFHS. Beginning in 2017, changes in care included coordinating fall-risk screening and management, developing an outpatient mobility program, creating a dementia care pathway, educating clinical staff on polypharmacy and high-risk medication, and utilizing a What Matters Discussion Guide to direct communication. To implement these changes on a greater scale, Providence St. Joseph Health formed the Geriatric Mini-Fellowship in 2018, training providers at 12 primary care clinics.

The training resulted in a myriad of improved outcomes at these clinics. In terms of mobility, the move toward more comprehensive and coordinated preventative measures and care led to a doubling in screening for fall risk and cognitive impairment and quadrupling of fall-risk interventions being administered. Older patients were also more likely to engage in What Matters conversations with their providers, and the prescribing of high-risk medication decreased by 3% when seen by a fellow. Finally, these clinics where providers received training on AFHS experienced a reduction of 2% to 7% in hospitalizations for patients.

SUMMARY

In a world where populations are aging more rapidly than ever before, the need to shape health systems to deliver quality care to older adults becomes an increasingly pressing health priority. The Triple Aim clearly points to the need for AFHS and 4Ms care, which improves the health and well-being of older adults through ensuring that families, caregivers, and health care provider teams all work synergistically. The 4Ms framework is driven by patient-centered care and prioritizes the older adult's preferences to simultaneously include medication management, prevention and treatment of dementia, delirium, and depression, and safe physical activity. The cost-effective practices and teaming of this approach can guide a higher quality of care for an aging population and significantly reduce unnecessary hospitalizations, saving health systems billions in health care spending. The evidence-based benefits of 4Ms care are clear and thus, emphasize the need for AFHS across health care settings.

FURTHER READING

American Hospital Association: The Value Initiative Issue Brief: Creating Value with Age-Friendly Health Systems; 2020. https://www.aha.org/system/files/media/file/2020/08/value-initiative-issue-brief-10-creating-value-with-age-friendly-health-systems.pdf [aha.org]. Accessed February 7, 2022

Chung GC, Marottoli RA, Cooney LM Jr, Rhee TG. Cost-related medication nonadherence among older adults: findings from a nationally representative sample. *J Am Geriatr Soc.* 2019;67(12):2463–2473.

Diaz-Gutierrez MJ, Martinez-Cengotitabengoa M, Saez de Adana E, et al. Relationship between the use of benzodiazepines and falls in older adults: a systematic review. *Maturitas.* 2017;101:17–22.

Fazio S, Pace D, Maslow K, Zimmerman S, Kallmyer B. Alzheimer's Association dementia care practice recommendations. *Gerontologist.* 2018;58(suppl_1):S1–S9.

Ganz DA, Latham NK. Prevention of falls in community-dwelling older adults. *N Engl J Med.* 2020;382(8): 734–743.

Hill-Taylor B, Sketris I, Hayden J, Byrne S, O'Sullivan D, Christie R. Application of the STOPP/START criteria: a systematic review of the prevalence of potentially inappropriate prescribing in older adults, and evidence of clinical, humanistic and economic impact. *J Clin Pharm Ther.* 2013;38(5):360–372.

Hshieh TT, Yang T, Gartaganis SL, Yue J, Inouye SK. Hospital elder life program: systematic review and meta-analysis of effectiveness. *Am J Geriatr Psychiatry.* 2018;26(10):1015–1033.

Institute for Healthcare Improvement: Age-Friendly Health Systems: Guide to Using the 4Ms in the Care of Older Adults; 2019. http://www.ihi.org/Engage/Initiatives/Age-Friendly-Health-Systems/Documents/IHIAge-FriendlyHealthSystems_GuidetoUsing4MsCare.pdf. Accessed February 7, 2022

Kim SK, Park M. Effectiveness of person-centered care on people with dementia: a systematic review and meta-analysis. *Clin Interv Aging.* 2017;12:381–397.

Lown Institute: Medication Overload and Older Americans; 2020. https://lowninstitute.org/projects/medication-overload-how-the-drive-to-prescribe-is-harming-older-americans/ [lowninstitute.org]. Accessed February 7, 2022

Martin P, Tamblyn R, Benedetti A, Ahmed S, Tannenbaum C. Effect of a pharmacist-led educational intervention on inappropriate medication prescriptions in older adults: the D-PRESCRIBE randomized clinical trial. *JAMA.* 2018;320(18):1889–1898.

Misra A, Lloyd JT. Hospital utilization and expenditures among a nationally representative sample of Medicare fee-for-service beneficiaries 2 years after receipt of an Annual Wellness Visit. *Prev Med.* 2019;129:105850.

Monteiro L, Maricoto T, Solha I, Ribeiro-Vaz I, Martins C, Monteiro-Soares M. Reducing potentially inappropriate prescriptions for older patients using computerized decision support tools: systematic review. *J Med Internet Res.* 2019;21(11):e15385.

Shah RC, Supiano MA, Greenland P. Aligning the 4Ms of age-friendly health systems with statin use for primary prevention. *J Am Geriatr Soc.* 2020;68(3):463–464.

Stacey D, Legare F, Col NF, et al. Decision aids for people facing health treatment or screening decisions. *Cochrane Database Syst Rev.* 2014(1):Cd001431.

Tinetti ME, Naik AD, Dindo L, et al. Association of patient priorities-aligned decision-making with patient outcomes and ambulatory health care burden among older adults with multiple chronic conditions: a nonrandomized clinical trial. *JAMA Intern Med.* 2019:1688–1697.

Wang YY, Yue JR, Xie DM, et al. Effect of the tailored, family-involved hospital elder life program on postoperative delirium and function in older adults: a randomized clinical trial. *JAMA Intern Med.* 2020;180(1):17–25.

Yang Y, Hu X, Zhang Q, Zou R. Diabetes mellitus and risk of falls in older adults: a systematic review and meta-analysis. *Age Ageing.* 2016;45(6):761–767.

Chapter 13

Geriatrics Around the World

Hidenori Arai, Jacqueline C. T. Close, Len Gray, Finbarr C. Martin, Luis Miguel Gutierrez Robledo, Stephanie Studenski

INTRODUCTION

Throughout the world, the aged proportion of the population is increasing. The number of older persons has tripled over the past 50 years and will more than triple again over the next 50 years. In contrast with the slow process of population aging experienced by the more developed countries, population aging in most of the less developed countries is taking place in a much shorter time period and is occurring in a larger population. Such rapid growth will require far-reaching economic and social adjustments in most countries. Effective and efficient health care for the chronic health problems facing this growing population of older adults will be a daunting challenge for all countries.

INCREASING LIFE EXPECTANCY

Notwithstanding some heterogeneity, life expectancy is increasing across the globe. In most industrialized countries, this increase in life expectancy has mostly occurred over the past century. However, in the most recent decades, its pace has progressed at an unprecedented speed, reaching estimates far beyond those predicted by most international organizations such as the United Nations. The increase in life expectancy has resulted in an increased proportion of individuals reaching the eighth and ninth decades of life. Aged individuals are consistently found to be the fastest growing segment of the population, and the rate of growth is more rapid in developing compared to developed countries (**Figure 13-1**). As life expectancy increases, there has been a wide decline in fertility rates, resulting in a decreasing dependency ratio: a smaller number of working age adults for each aged person. This trend has great and challenging implications for national approaches to support services for older adults. Since wealth and resources vary greatly across countries, priorities for health and social services vary as well. Many developing countries previously focused on infectious diseases and maternal-child health, but as they too face rapidly aging populations, they are now confronting the same challenges to health care as have developed countries in recent decades.

Learning Objectives

- Become familiar with similarities and differences in postgraduate (or post basic medical qualification) geriatrics training and clinical practice around the world.
- Learn about age-related health care policy initiatives in different nations.

Key Clinical Points

1. Since the backgrounds and training of geriatricians vary widely, so do skillsets and professional roles.
2. In most countries, there are still not enough geriatricians to serve the special needs of vulnerable older people.

DECLINE OF THE DISEASE MODEL

As age increases, there is a progressive, exponential increase in the occurrence of most chronic, degenerative, and progressive diseases, including cardiovascular disease, cancer, chronic obstructive pulmonary disease, dementia, and other degenerative conditions (see Chapter 2). Furthermore, there is an increase in the co-occurrence of these diseases, resulting in multimorbidity (see Chapter 41).

Health care systems around the world have been based on a disease model. Diagnosis and treatment focuses on eliminating or ameliorating the underlying pathology; health outcomes are determined by the disease. Also, functional impairment and quality of life are assumed to be improved by treating the "causative" disease. The disease model resulted in the creation of health systems centered on acute care hospitals and disease (or organ)-based specialists. This model informed the way we developed and accrued knowledge. Consequently, physicians and health

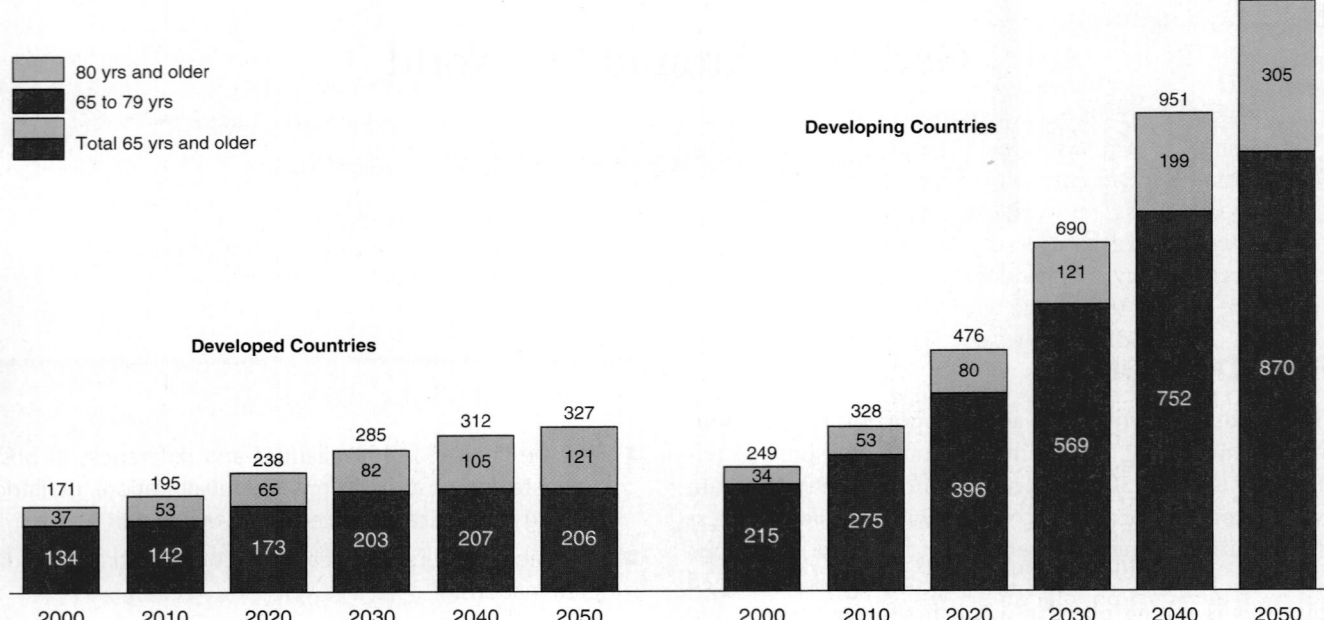

FIGURE 13-1. Growth over time in the aged population in developed and developing countries. All numbers are millions of people. (Reproduced with permission from US Census Bureau, Current Population Reports: 65+ in the United States.)

personnel are now facing a "new" and less familiar type of patient who presents with an array of concomitant clinical conditions. These combinations of conditions result in varying degrees of functional deficits, cognitive deterioration, nutritional problems, and geriatric syndromes (delirium, falls, incontinence), often in the face of inadequate social support and financial resources.

This "new" older patient presents a degree of complexity not previously considered by the traditional understanding of medicine and its role. The traditionally envisioned health care system, whether operating under universal coverage or private mechanisms, is challenged by this complex patient.

The response to the challenge of the complex older patient has been heterogeneous around the world; differences in resource availability and economic and cultural issues resulted in different organizations of health care systems. In addition, the methodological approaches adopted by systems to evaluate the needs of such complex patients have been highly variable and not standardized. In particular, the organization of services to care for geriatric patients, including geriatric assessment and management, remains highly variable. This variation is seen among nurses, physicians, therapists, nursing homes, home care services, and health systems.

EMERGENCE OF GERIATRIC MEDICINE

Geriatric Medicine emerged as a medical specialty in the mid-twentieth century—somewhat later than the majority of organ- and procedure-oriented specialties. This emergence was initially inspired by the realization that among older people living in institutions, there was a substantial prevalence of diagnoses and functional impairments that could be resolved by careful diagnostic review and implementation of rehabilitation techniques. However, ultimately Geriatric Medicine approaches were found relevant to all older people, regardless of the care setting. In addition, there was a growing body of evidence that disease presentations and responses to treatment may differ among very old people compared to middle-aged adults. As this awareness was applied to hospitalized patients and older people living in the community, there was an appreciation that the social and physical context of older people also influences functional status and outcomes.

Despite a growing body of knowledge pertaining to illness in old age and a strong evidence base for its practice, the specialty has not been uniformly adopted across, or even within, nations. Moreover, even where it is established, practice is often restricted to particular settings—hospitals, nursing homes, or ambulatory clinics. This may be a product of the overall configuration of specialty practice, funding and financial incentives, lack of leadership, or perceived lack of need at professional or government levels. In many jurisdictions, geriatric medical specialists are only present in large academic or metropolitan settings. In some developing nations, the discipline may not exist at all.

Within hospitals, a variety of practice models have emerged. Acute geriatric units, supervised by geriatricians, may admit acutely ill patients directly from the emergency department or community. Alternatively (or in addition),

Geriatric Medicine may be restricted to post-acute units, where patients are transferred after initial assessment and triaging in an acute unit. These post-acute services may be based on a separate subacute ward within an acute hospital, or co-located within a long-term care facility.

Outside of hospitals, Geriatric Medicine may have a presence in long-term care, where geriatricians might act as the primary physician workforce. In other jurisdictions, they may act primarily as specialists, consulting for patients who are referred by primary care practitioners, with or without any special training in care of older people.

In most jurisdictions, a shortage of geriatricians is perceived. Even where the specialty is firmly entrenched and available in a particular setting, there may be inadequate availability in other care settings. Situations where a geriatrician is available to consult about patients across the entire care spectrum are probably relatively rare.

Geriatric medical practice and its availability should reflect the needs of the oldest members of a society. As such, with near-universal population aging, it would be reasonable to anticipate that Geriatric Medicine should emerge progressively throughout the present century.

STANDARDIZED ASSESSMENT

Consistent assessments can provide a mechanism to draw comparisons among like services in different nations and, if configured appropriately, even across care settings within and among nations. The interRAI suite of assessment systems was designed to meet this requirement. It has been used to draw comparisons across nations and jurisdictions within them. Two important multination research projects in Europe in home care and long-term care have been influential in identifying different patterns of service use, clinical outcomes, medication use, and quality issues which, in turn, influenced policy in several nations. Data extracted from large databases (in some cases millions of assessments) enabled similar examinations among nations and jurisdictions and organizations within them. These systems have been adopted at an organizational level (eg, a nursing home) or by state or nations (eg, the interRAI Home Care and Long-Term Care systems in New Zealand). Several nations and states adopted multiple suite instruments (eg, Belgium and Ontario, Canada). These early suite adopters are exploring the utility of multiple compatible instruments to facilitate cross-setting continuity of care (a clinical benefit) and comparisons of caseloads across settings (a policy benefit).

CHAPTER GOALS

In this chapter, we provide an overview of geriatrics training and certification, clinical practice, and institutional support in 63 countries. While many countries have active aging research programs, this chapter does not address those. We are exceptionally grateful for the information provided by national leaders from each country through an online survey. Among the 63 countries, based on the current classification of countries by the World Bank, 42 were high income (national income per capita >US$ 12,536 in 2019) of a total of 59, 17 were upper middle income (of a total of 55), and 4 were lower middle income, of a total of 44. There were no respondents from low-income countries, of a total of 28. There are a few countries, mainly very small, that were not classified by WHO.

Please see the Acknowledgment section for a list of survey respondents. All respondents provided their best estimates about geriatrics in their countries; however, given the great variability in how health care is organized and geriatrics is defined, some of the information is likely to be inexact. We regret that we were not able to identify national leaders for every country and hope to include others in future versions of the chapter.

TRAINING AND CERTIFICATION OF GERIATRIC SPECIALISTS

Geriatrics training and certification vary among responding countries. Some countries with early emerging roles for geriatrics specialists largely import trained geriatric professionals from other countries. Nearly 90% of the countries surveyed reported the presence of formal training programs in geriatrics (**Figure 13-2A**). However, the timing and requirements vary considerably. For example, many countries train physicians in geriatrics through individual certified training programs offering 1 to 4 years of advanced geriatrics training after residency in Internal Medicine or Family Medicine, or combined Internal Medicine and geriatrics training lasting 4 to 5 years after medical school (**Figure 13-2B**). Many of these programs are operated independently by hospitals and academic health systems. Other countries have a single national training program which has been implemented in multiple health care systems. Many countries offer a national certification examination, while others provide certification through national societies using a range of metrics (**Figure 13-2C**). Some countries do not offer a formal path to certification, so the definition of a geriatrician can depend on national or regional standards. Many countries offer educational programs regarding care of older people to a wide range of trainees: some occur during professional training while others are designed for practicing health care providers. For the most part, this chapter focuses on formally trained geriatrics specialists.

In some countries, formal training and certification is offered to health professionals other than physicians. Most common is geriatrics specialization for nurses, followed by physical and occupational therapists and social workers.

While definitions vary for who is a geriatrician, our national respondents reported a very wide range of numbers of geriatricians per 100,000 persons age 65 or older (**Table 13-1**). A proposed criterion from the Royal College of Physicians (RCP) is that there should be 2 geriatricians for every 100,000 persons age 75 or older. This estimate is based on a consultative, not primary care, model of medical

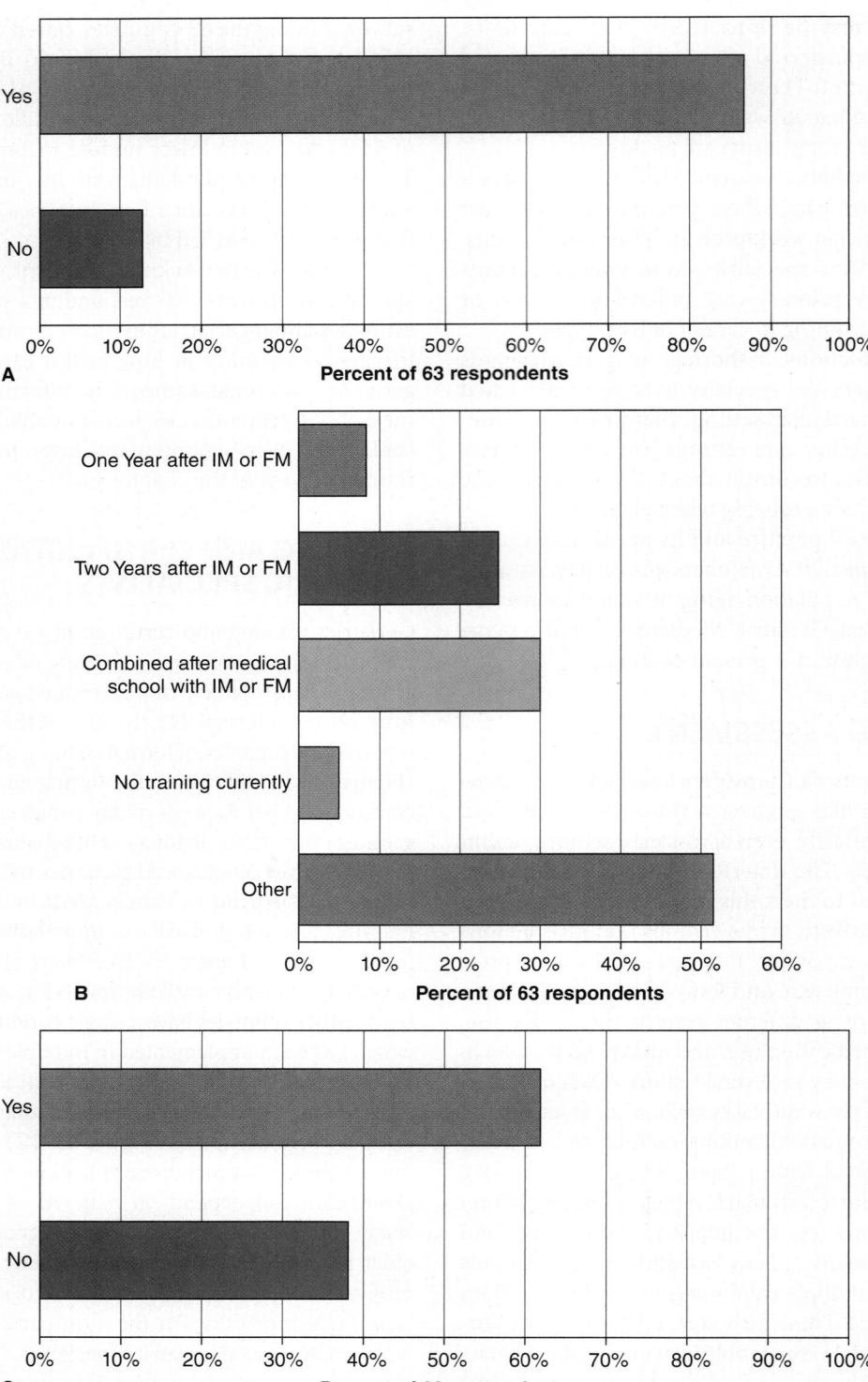

FIGURE 13-2. **A.** Does your country require a defined period in a certified training program to be qualified as a geriatrician? **B.** Types of training programs in geriatric medicine in 63 countries. Other includes some programs that are transitioning between types of training or are starting a formal training program, some geriatric training programs are longer than 2 years, and some are 18 months after Internal Medicine. FM, Family Medicine, IM, Internal Medicine. **C.** My country requires a successful score on a standardized certification examination to be qualified as a geriatrician.

TABLE 13-1 ■ TRAINING AND CERTIFICATION IN GERIATRICS IN DIFFERENT COUNTRIES

	COUNTRY	REQUIRES CERTIFIED TRAINING	TYPE OF TRAINING	REQUIRES SCORE ON STANDARD EXAM	NUMBER OF CERTIFIED TRAINING PROGRAMS	OTHER DISCIPLINES WITH CERTIFICATION	NUMBER OF GERIATRICIANS TRAINED PER YEAR	NUMBER OF GERIATRICIANS PER 100,000 AGE 65+
1	Argentina	Yes	2 y after IM or FM	Yes	10	Nursing, PT, OT, SW	80	> 100
2	Armenia	No	N/A	No	0	Nursing	0	< 1
3	Australia	Yes	3 y as advanced trainee in geriatric medicine after IM	No	1 (250 positions in multiple sites)	N/A	250 all years	24
4	Austria	Yes	2 y after IM, FM, Psychiatry, Neurology, or Rehabilitation Medicine	No	1	Nursing	5	14
5	Belarus	Yes	Combined IM/geriatrics	No	4	Nursing, PT	75	< 1
6	Belgium	Yes	Combined IM/geriatrics	Yes—varies regionally	N/A	Nursing, PT	20	> 100
7	Brazil	Yes	2 y after IM or FM OR combined IM/geriatrics	Yes	50	Gerontology training in many other disciplines	100	< 1
8	Canada	Yes	2 y after IM OR separate "care of the elderly: COE" certificate for FM after 1–2 y of geriatric training	Yes	11	Psychiatry	Geriatrics: 28–29 COE: 16–24	5
9	Chile	Yes	1 y after IM or FM	Yes	5	Nursing, PT	70 total all years	< 1
10	China	Yes	2 y after IM or FM	Yes	N/A	Other medical specialties	100	2.6
11	Colombia	Yes	2 y after IM or FM OR 4 y of direct training	Yes	4	None	60	2
12	Costa Rica	Yes	3 y after 2-y IM	Yes	N/A	Gerontology masters available	10	33
13	Croatia	Yes	Combined IM/geriatrics	Yes	3	None	30	< 1
14	Cuba	Yes	Combined IM/geriatrics	Yes	1 program with multiple sites	Nursing, PT, OT, SW	> 270	24
15	Czech Republic	Yes	18 mo after IM or FM	Yes	43—mainly specialties including geriatrics	None	120 at all levels	20
16	Denmark	Yes	Combined IM/geriatrics	No	N/A	None	N/A	15

(Continued)

TABLE 13-1 ■ TRAINING AND CERTIFICATION IN GERIATRICS IN DIFFERENT COUNTRIES (CONTINUED)

	COUNTRY	REQUIRES CERTIFIED TRAINING	TYPE OF TRAINING	REQUIRES SCORE ON STANDARD EXAM	NUMBER OF CERTIFIED TRAINING PROGRAMS	OTHER DISCIPLINES WITH CERTIFICATION	NUMBER OF GERIATRICIANS TRAINED PER YEAR	NUMBER OF GERIATRICIANS PER 100,000 AGE 65+
17	El Salvador	Yes	1 year after IM or FM	Yes	0	Gerontology certificate for other disciplines	2	1.8
18	Estonia	Yes	IM can take geriatrics as subspecialty	No	1	PT	2–3	< 1
19	Finland	Yes	5 y after medical school	Yes	5	N/A	50	2.5
20	France	Yes	Combined geriatrics with IM, emergency medicine, neurology, cardiology, rheumatology	No	1 (national program with multiple sites)	N/A	200 geriatric residents, about 500 geriatric specialists	32
21	Germany	Yes	18 mo after IM, FM, neurology, or psychiatry	Yes	> 200 (training in any hospital with a qualified geriatrics department)	Nursing, PT, OT	100–150	8
22	Greece	No	0 (geriatrics not recognized; efforts ongoing)	No	0	0	0	< 1
23	Guatemala	No	0	No	0	PT	N/A	< 1
24	Hungary	Yes	5 y in geriatrics OR 2–3 y after IM	Yes	9	Nursing, PT, SW	2–3	7.5
25	Iceland	Yes	2 y after IM or FM	No	1	Nursing	4	38
26	India	Yes	3 y after internship	Yes	8	None	30	< 1
27	Indonesia	Yes	2 y after IM or FM	Yes	50	PT	10	< 1
28	Ireland	Yes	4-y combined IM/geriatrics	No	1	Nursing	15	2.5
29	Israel	Yes	2 y after IM or FM OR combined IM/geriatrics	Yes	20	N/A	50	> 100
30	Italy	Yes	4 y includes residency	Yes	36	N/A	160	60
31	Japan	Yes	2–3 y after IM and other specialties	Yes	273	None	60	5
32	Korea	No	0 (geriatrics not formally recognized but some sites have training)	No	3	Nurse practitioner	0–1	< 1
33	Lithuania	Yes	4 y after medical school	Yes	59	Nursing, PT, OT	9	7.2
34	Luxembourg	Yes	Combined IM/geriatrics—most come from other countries	Yes	No full programs but 4 hospitals have 6–12 mo programs	None but may accept training from other countries	< 5, but partially trained	2

(Continued)

TABLE 13-1 ■ TRAINING AND CERTIFICATION IN GERIATRICS IN DIFFERENT COUNTRIES (*CONTINUED*)

	COUNTRY	REQUIRES CERTIFIED TRAINING	TYPE OF TRAINING	REQUIRES SCORE ON STANDARD EXAM	NUMBER OF CERTIFIED TRAINING PROGRAMS	OTHER DISCIPLINES WITH CERTIFICATION	NUMBER OF GERIATRICIANS TRAINED PER YEAR	NUMBER OF GERIATRICIANS PER 100,000 AGE 65+
35	Macedonia	No	None	No	0	Nursing	N/A	N/A
36	Malaysia	Yes	3 y after IM	No	1	Nursing, PT, OT, FM	5–6	2
37	Malta	Yes	Combined IM/geriatrics—2 y IM and 4 y geriatrics	Yes	1	N/A	14	23
38	Mexico	Yes	2 y after IM or FM OR 4 y direct entry geriatrics	Yes	33	Nursing	92	11
39	Netherlands	Yes	3 y combined IM/geriatrics/psychiatry/neurology	Yes	50–100	Nursing, PT, OT, SW	38	10
40	New Zealand	Yes	3 y as advanced trainee in geriatric medicine after IM	No	1	N/A	45	10
41	Nicaragua	Yes	2 y after IM or FM OR combined IM/geriatrics	No	0 (accepts certification from other countries)	0	2	3
42	Norway	Yes	2 y after IM or FM, combined IM/geriatrics	No	46	N/A	N/A	3
43	Panama	Yes	2 y after IM or FM, combined IM/geriatrics	No	2	Nursing	24	7
44	Paraguay	No	2 y after IM or FM	Yes	2	None	4	8.5
45	Peru	Yes	3–4 y in a university residency program	Yes	5	Nursing, OT	20–30	8.1
46	Poland	Yes	2 y after IM or FM, combined IM/geriatrics	Yes	3	Nursing, PT	116	7.5
47	Portugal	No	A competence attribution is made by the Geriatrics College	No	2	Nursing	30	> 100
48	Romania	Yes	Combined IM/geriatrics	Yes	6	None	38	6.3
49	Russia	Yes	1 y residency after medical school or 2–4 mo after qualified in IM or FM	Yes	50	FM, neurology, endocrinology cardiology	1349	5.8
50	Serbia	Yes	1 y after IM or FM	No	1	None	2	< 1
51	Singapore	Yes	3 y after IM or FM	Yes	3	Nursing, PT, OT	30	20
52	Slovenia	No	None	No	0	None	0	1
53	South Africa	Yes	2 y geriatrics after IM	Yes	3	Psychiatry	1	< 1
54	Spain	Yes	4 y geriatrics	No	N/A	Nursing	70	27

(*Continued*)

TABLE 13-1 ■ TRAINING AND CERTIFICATION IN GERIATRICS IN DIFFERENT COUNTRIES (*CONTINUED*)

	COUNTRY	REQUIRES CERTIFIED TRAINING	TYPE OF TRAINING	REQUIRES SCORE ON STANDARD EXAM	NUMBER OF CERTIFIED TRAINING PROGRAMS	OTHER DISCIPLINES WITH CERTIFICATION	NUMBER OF GERIATRICIANS TRAINED PER YEAR	NUMBER OF GERIATRICIANS PER 100,000 AGE 65+
55	Sweden	Yes	Combined IM/geriatrics	No	200	Nursing	200	N/A
56	Switzerland	Yes	3 y after IM	Yes	1	Nursing	20–25	18
57	Taiwan	Yes	1 y after IM or FM	Yes	21	Nursing	38	24.5
58	Thailand	Yes	2 y after IM or FM transitioning to 2–3 y of geriatrics after IM and other specialties	Yes	2	None	7	< 1
59	Turkey	Yes	3 y after IM	No	11 give licenses—in process of developing certification	None	50	1.4
60	United Kingdom	Yes	Combined IM/geriatrics (many not in formal geriatrics certified programs)	Yes	1	Nursing, PT, OT, paramedics	750	11
61	United States	Yes	1 y after IM or FM	Yes	158	Nursing, PT, OT, SW, pharmacy, psychology, psychiatry	262	14
62	Uruguay	Yes	3 y in geriatrics	Yes	1	None	18	16
63	Venezuela	Yes	N/A	Yes	1	Nursing	3	1

FM, family medicine, IM, internal medicine, OT, occupational therapy, PT, physical therapy, SW, social work.

care, so it is difficult to relate the RCP estimate to the findings of our survey. Some countries report national efforts to increase the number of trained geriatricians, but others do not.

GERIATRICS PRACTICE

Geriatricians practice in many settings (**Figure 13-3A**). The most common setting is the hospital, followed by outpatient clinics. Geriatricians tend to work in larger hospitals, academic centers, and cities. In many countries, medical aspects of long-term care are managed by general practitioners, not geriatricians. Practice varies widely within countries; many only have special geriatric services in a few health care settings, while other countries have somewhat greater geographical spread of services. Geriatricians practicing in hospitals usually work on dedicated geriatrics wards (**Figure 13-3B**), but also in collaboration and consultation with many other services, most commonly orthopedics, oncology, and emergency wards (**Figure 13-3C**). Similarly, general geriatrics is the most common outpatient service, but many other specific services are offered, including treatment for dementia, falls/balance/mobility,

and incontinence (**Figure 13-4A**). Over half of respondents reported that geriatricians in their country provide home services such as home visits or home care coordination. Similarly, over half of respondents reported that geriatricians worked in rehabilitation settings, more often in acute hospital compared to long-term care settings.

SUPPORT FOR GERIATRICS

Some geriatricians are salaried in almost all participating countries, while about half of countries report that geriatricians also receive individual payment for services (**Figure 13-4B**). Salaries come from governments, hospitals, and other institutions. Payments for services come from health insurance and directly from private payers. Somewhat less than half of countries report that geriatrician assessment is sometimes required for paid services such as long-term or home care (**Figure 13-4C**).

Quite a few countries have evolving policies and practices related to geriatrics. For example, in Israel, geriatricians can be paid by the Social Security System to assess people age 90 or older for eligibility for home services for those with functional impairment. The United Kingdom has

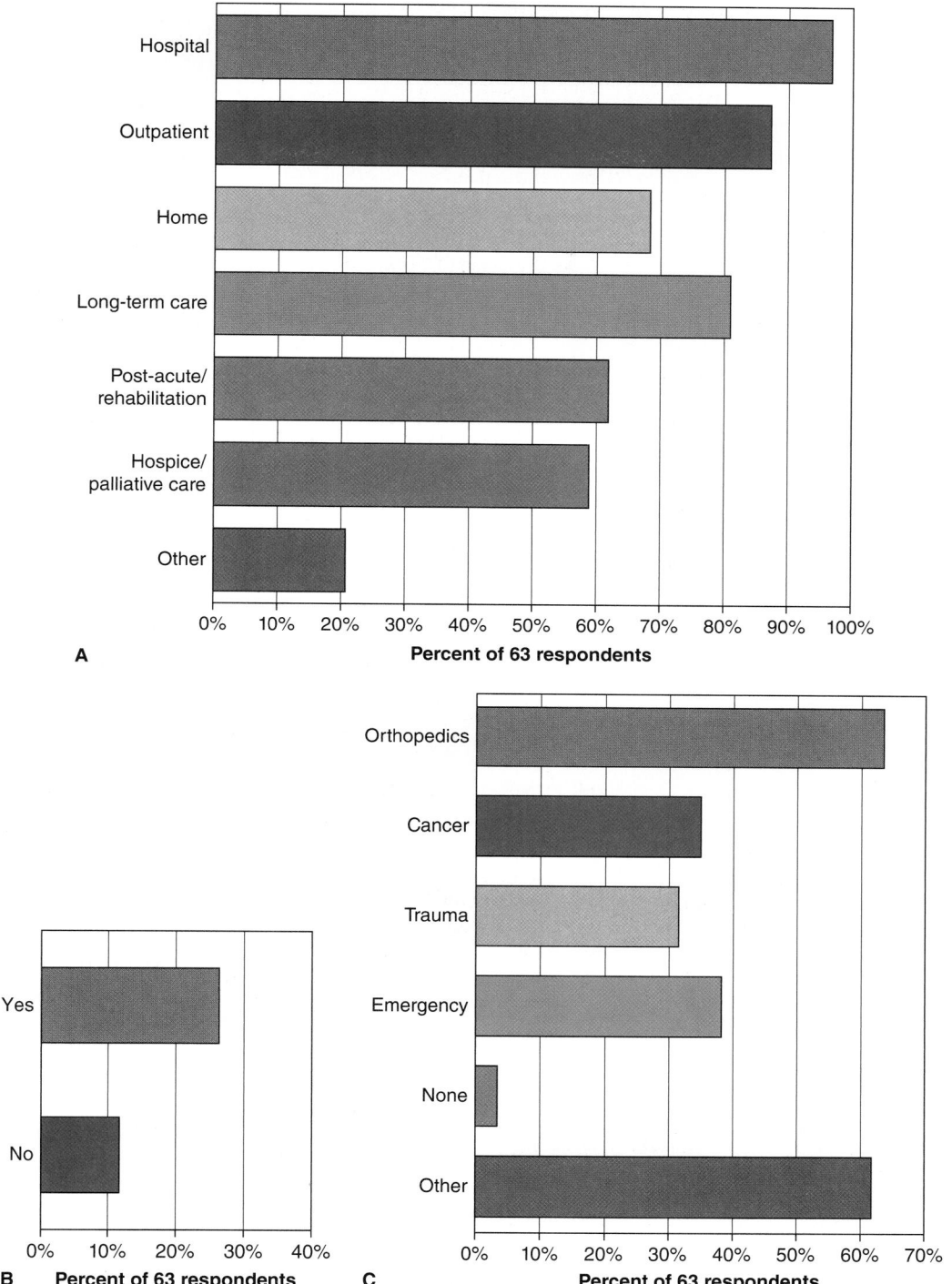

FIGURE 13-3. **A.** Where do geriatricians practice in your country? Respondents can select multiple sites. Other includes public health, regional variability in sites of practice, emergency room, mobile teams, life care communities, and PACE-type programs. **B.** Are there designated hospital beds for geriatrics in your country? **C.** Are there formally established collaborative teams with geriatrics on specialty hospital services in your country? Respondents can choose more than one. Other includes general and specialties of surgery, neurology, stroke, dermatology, psychiatry, rehabilitation, palliative care, COVID-19, and CGA screening for 75+. CGA, Comprehensive geriatric assessment; PACE, Program of All-Inclusive care of the Elderly.

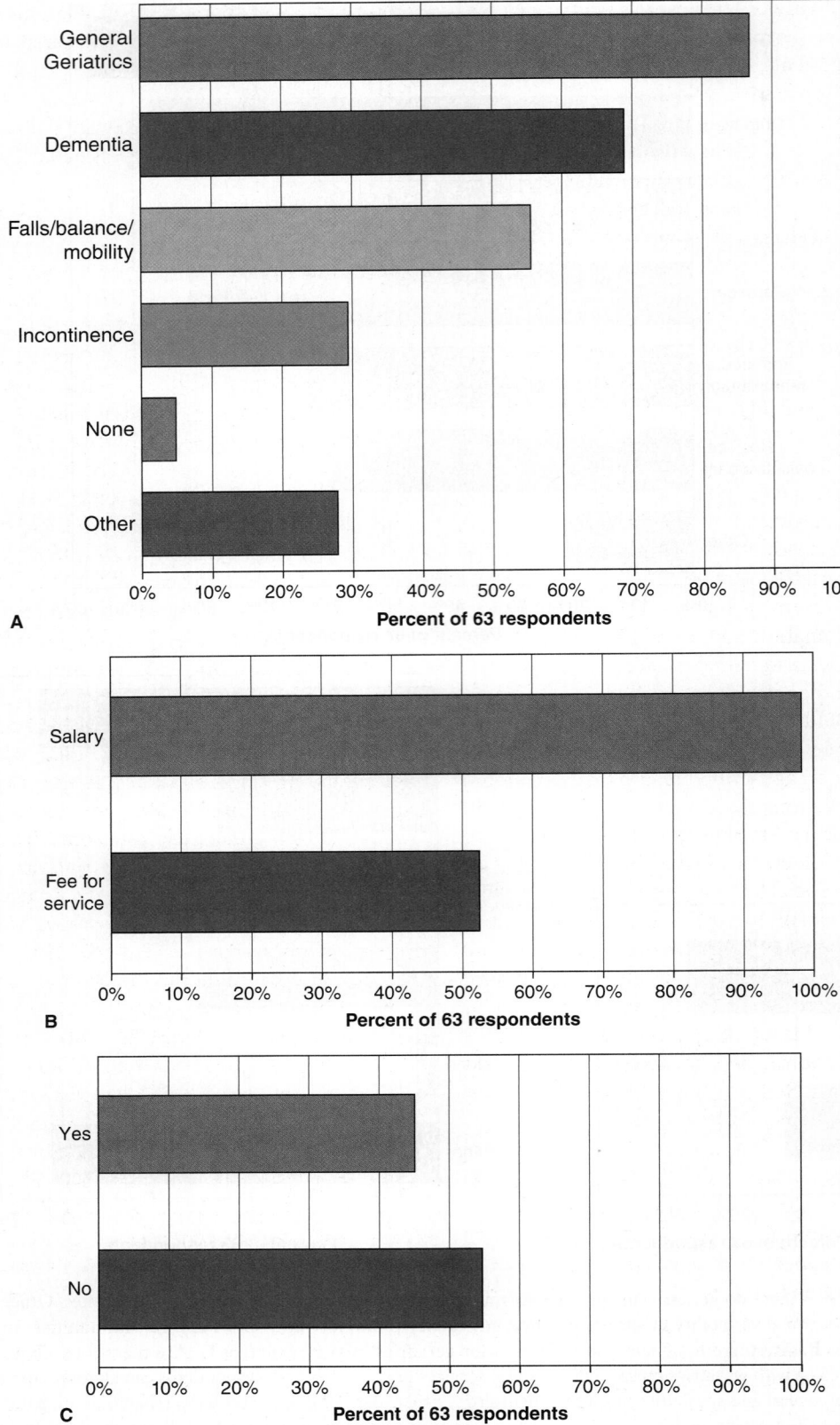

FIGURE 13-4. A. Types of geriatric outpatient services in 63 countries. Other includes frailty, polypharmacy, oncogeriatrics, geropsychiatry, osteoporosis, preoperation, movement disorders, and day hospital. **B.** How are geriatricians paid in your country? **C.** Does your country ever require a geriatrician assessment for eligibility for services or other benefits?

had a National Health Service framework for aging services and requires specialist geriatricians to participate in care for all hip fracture patients. Japan provides incentives for comprehensive geriatric assessment on hospital admission and for evaluating and deprescribing for polypharmacy. In Germany, geriatricians are obligatory providers in the care of hip fracture patients age 70 or older. In Australia, the Royal Commission is requesting an increased role for geriatricians in long-term care. Australia is also working to increase availability of geriatricians for indigenous older people and those in correctional settings. In Norway, there is an expectation that all large acute care hospitals have geriatricians. In Malta, geriatricians mostly work outside acute care, particularly in specialized post-acute/rehabilitation settings; they assess acute care patients for eligibility for transfer to the post-acute setting. In Turkey, there is an aim to increase the number of geriatricians, who have an obligatory service requirement to work in areas determined to have an unmet need. In France, nursing home care is provided by general physicians with specific training in geriatrics. North Macedonia is in the process of organizing a geriatrics specialty.

More broadly, several countries report other developments in the coordination and management of care for older people. New Zealand uses a national approach for assessment based on the interRAI tool. Taiwan is using an Integrated Care for Older People (ICOPE) assessment for screening older people. The government of Thailand has set a national agenda on aging and created the Association of Southeast Asian Nations Center on Active Aging and Innovation. Nicaragua has created a program *Todos con Vos* for persons age 60 or older. Nicaragua also has a program in collaboration with Social Security for retired people that partners with Public Health to provide health care, rehabilitation, and other services. Peru has created laws addressing issues of dementia. Singapore organizes health care among four Regional Healthcare Systems with a population health focus and efforts to address aging issues. Panama offers a home care system coordinated between the Health and Social Security Systems. Serbia has a national program for health care of older people, and Luxembourg is developing such a national plan. China offers special geriatrics services in certain hospitals, but is working to extend these services to geriatric wards more widely. Ireland is directing more care to community settings via the Sláintecare program. Belgium is expecting to implement the bel-RAI soon and offers comprehensive assessment through a day clinic. Costa Rica has laws addressing integrated care for older persons. Mexico has a National Institute of Geriatrics which is developing a national action plan for older adults in conjunction with the Ministry of Health. It is promoting the development of Departments of Geriatrics nationwide.

SUMMARY

Despite global aging, geriatrics remains a small field almost everywhere, although it is more advanced in developed countries compared to developing ones. There are clear signs that some nations are working to increase the training and availability of geriatricians and geriatric services in their countries. Some countries have integrated geriatricians into program eligibility standards or oversight. Most clearly, there exists a worldwide community of dedicated geriatricians working to improve care for older people in their countries.

ACKNOWLEDGMENTS

We especially recognize the exemplary support provided by Leah Carton of McGraw Hill who developed and managed the web-based survey. Survey participants: Edgar Aguilera Gaona, MD, Paraguay; Vidmantas Alekna, MD, PhD, Lithuania; Hidenori Arai, MD, PhD, Japan; Prasert Assantachai, MD, Thailand; Gülistan Bahat, MD, Prof, Turkey; Melba de la Cruz Barrantes Monge, MD, MsC, Nicaragua; Sylvie Bonin-Guillaume, MD, PhD, France; Carlos Cano, MD, Colombia; Liang-Kung Chen, MD, PhD, Taiwan; A. Mark Clarfield, MD, FRCPC, Israel; Jacqueline Close, MBBS, MD, Australia; Jacqueline Close, MBBS, MD, FRCP, New Zealand; Luis Manuel Cornejo MD, MSc, Panama; A.B. Dey, MD, India; Rebecca Dreher, Medical Doctor, Switzerland; John Ellul, MD, DM, Greece; Predrag Erceg, MD, PhD, Serbia; Helga Eyjólfsdóttir, MD, PhD, Iceland; Alberto Ferrari, MD, Italy; Pablo Garcia Aguilar, MSc, MD, Guatemala; Deon Greyling, MBChB, M Fam Med, M Med, South Africa; Luis Miguel Gutierrez Robledo, MD, PhD, México; Margarita Henriquez, MD, El Salvador; Susanne Hernes, MD, PhD, Norway; Andrei Ilnitski, MD, PhD, Belarus; José Jauregui, MD, PhD, Argentina; Peter Johnson, MD, Sweden; Shahrul Kamaruzzaman, MBBCh, PhD, Malaysia; Lin Kang, MD, China; Ana Kmaid Riccetto, MD, Uruguay; Helgi Kolk, MD, PhD, Estonia; Yulia Kotovskaya, MD, PhD, DMs, Russia; Adam Lelbach, MD, PhD, Hungary; Jean-Claude Leners, MD, Luxembourg; Wee-Shiong Lim, MBBS, MRCP (UK), MMed (Int Med), MHPEd, AGSF, FAMS, Singapore; Roberto Lourenço, MD, MPH, PhD, Brazil; Lia Marques, MD, Portugal; Nicolás Martínez-Velilla, MD, PhD, Span; Francesco Mattace- Raso, MD, PhD, Netherlands; Jesús Menéndez Jiménez, MD, MPH, Cuba; Manuel Montero Odasso, MD, PhD, Canada; Fernando Morales-Martínez, MD, Costa Rica; Hanna Öhman, MD, PhD, Finland; Shane O'Hanlon, MB, BCh, BAO, MRCPI, Ireland; Jose F. Parodi, PhD, Perú; Tajana Pavic, MD, PhD, Croatia; Biljana Petreska-Zovic, MD, Macedonia; Karolina Piotrowicz, MD, PhD, Poland; Gabriel-Ioan Prada, MD, PhD, Romania; Rupert Puellen, MD, Germany; Regina Roller-Wirnsberger, MD, MME, Austria; Irma Ruslina Defi, Sp.KFRs(K), Indonesia; Jesper Ryg, MD, PhD, Denmark; Dra. Juana Silva, Medical Doctor, Geriatrician, Chile; Stephanie Studenski, MD, MPH, United States; Artur Torosyan, MD, Armenia; Milagros Torres, MD, Venezuela; Nele Van Den Noortgate, MD, PhD, Belgium; Hana Vankova, MD, PhD, Czech Republic; Mark Anthony Vassallo MD(Melit.) DGM(Lond.) MA(Melit.) in Bioethics FRCP(Edin.) FRCP(Lond.), Malta; Michael Vassallo, FRCP, PhD, England; Gregor Veninsek, MD, Slovenia; Sol-Ji Yoon, MD, MPH, Korea.

FURTHER READING

Bates T, Kottek A, Spetz J. Geriatrician Roles and the Value of Geriatrics in an Evolving Health Care System. San Francisco, CA: UCSF Health Systems Workforce Center on Long-Term Care; 2019.

Fisher JM, Garside M, Hunt K, Lo N. Geriatric medicine workforce planning: a giant geriatric problem or has the tide turned? *Clin Med (Lond)*. 2014;14(2):102–106.

Habot B, Tsin S. Geriatrics in the new millennium, Israel. *Isr Med Assoc J*. 2003;5:319–321.

InterRAI. https://www.interrai.org. Accessed May 17, 2021.

Lester PE, Dharmarajan TS, Weinstein E. The looming geriatrician shortage: ramifications and solutions. *J Aging Health*. 2020;32(9):1052–1062.

Pitkälä KH, Martin FC, Maggi S, Jyväkorpi SK, Strandberg TE. Status of geriatrics in 22 countries. *J Nutr Health Aging*. 2018;22(5):627–631.

Royal College of Physicians. Consultant physicians working with patients: the duties, responsibilities and practice of physicians in medicine. London: RCP, 2013. https://www.rcplondon.ac.uk/projects/outputs/consultant-physicians-working-patients-revised-5th-edition. Accessed May 5, 2012.

Saka S, Oosthuizen F, Nlooto M. National policies and older people's healthcare in Sub-Saharan Africa: a scoping review. *Ann Glob Health*. 2019;85(1):91.

Tan MP, Kamaruzzaman SP, Poi PJH. An analysis of geriatric medicine in Malaysia-riding the wave of political change. *Geriatrics (Basel)*. 2018;3(4):80.

Ungureanu M, Brînzac MG, Paina AFL, Avram L, Crişan DA, Donca V. The geriatric workforce in Romania: the need to improve data and management. *Eur J Public Health*. 2020;30(Suppl 4):iv28–iv31.

Won CW, Kim S, Swagerty D. Why geriatric medicine is important for Korea: lessons learned in the United States. *J Korean Med Sci*. 2018;33(26):e175.

World Health Organization. https://www.who.int/publications/i/item/WHO-FWC-ALC-19.1. Accessed January 18, 2022.

Chapter 14

Models of Hospital and Outpatient Care

Jonny Macias Tejada, Michael L. Malone

INTRODUCTION

Over the past four decades, geriatrics models of care have emerged to address the unique needs of older adults. These models deliver evidence-based practices to this growing segment of our population. Some of these programs have been evaluated in randomized clinical trials. Other models have been evaluated as quality improvement projects. Identifying the needs of vulnerable older adults as they receive health care will allow geriatrics leaders the opportunity to respond to our patients' needs with programs that improve care. Geriatrics models of care use interdisciplinary approaches to address the needs of patients with multiple comorbid conditions. This chapter with describe models based in the hospital setting and in the outpatient setting. Approaches and models related to transitions in care are discussed in Chapter 18, Transitions of Care.

Common goals of these geriatrics models of care include engaging patients and families in their plan of care, enabling patients to remain safely in the least restrictive site of care, and focusing on prevention strategies that optimize patients' functional status and quality of life.

Geriatrics models of care commonly address a specific population of older patients. Models can exemplify how hospitals and health systems fulfill their mission within their community. Geriatrics leaders commonly need to build a case for geriatrics models of care to fit with the hospital/health system priorities, emphasizing efforts to continuously improve care. Working with key stakeholders in health care organizations, geriatrics leaders seek to identify the resources that are available to support a new model, define where the model fits within other programs, and create a strategy to implement the model.

A Background to Geriatric "Best Practice" Models

Table 14-1 provides several key components to geriatrics models of care. This chapter will help guide the reader to approach the framework of models of care and understand the key aspects of the design of various models. Further, the reader will appreciate how to choose a model to deploy in their hospital or outpatient setting.

Geriatrics models of care are standard approaches to the care of older adults. They are often deployed by geriatric medicine and gerontological nursing leaders in efforts to

Learning Objectives

- Describe the common goals of geriatrics models of care in the hospital and outpatient setting.
- Understand how to prepare for a geriatrics practice model.
- Describe how geriatrics models fit into the context of various payment mechanisms.
- Describe the key components of hospital-based models and outpatient models of care.
- Outline key strategies in sustaining and disseminating geriatrics models of care.

Key Clinical Points

1. Multiple, evidence-based practice models are available to help interdisciplinary teams to improve care for populations of vulnerable older individuals.

2. Choosing the geriatrics model that best fits into your practice setting depends on the challenges that your team is trying to address, your ability to make the case for a change, and your skills to lead an interdisciplinary team toward improved care.

3. Measuring key outcomes at baseline and over time can assist the team in efforts to improve care.

4. Assessing the fidelity of the key components of the model intervention is important to implementing and sustaining geriatrics models of care.

5. Disseminating geriatrics models may require novel strategies to incorporate the key components of geriatrics models into the workflow and processes of routine care of older patients.

TABLE 14-1 ■ KEY COMPONENTS TO SUCCESSFUL GERIATRIC BEST PRACTICE MODELS

1. Enable older adults to remain safely at home
2. Prevent functional disability
3. Preserve patient quality of life
4. Respect patient values, preferences and goals
5. Consider patient safety
6. Address the needs of family caregivers
7. Appreciate and address patient's psychosocial needs

address the needs of populations of vulnerable older adults. Many were developed in response to common challenges of older patients (eg, functional decline or new onset of delirium during an acute illness). Most models are set within a single context of care (eg, the hospital or the clinic setting). Some models continue care beyond a single setting. Most models provide key screens and assessments for patients, as well as appropriate interventions in response to the unique needs of each individual. Models of care require interdisciplinary team members who work together as opposed to health professionals who work independently. Models are commonly targeted to address a vulnerable patient population during a specific context of care.

We will highlight a few important aspects to choosing a geriatrics model. First is to clearly define the local problem or challenge which you are trying to solve. This will require you to tell the story of the challenge in care and the implications for individuals. You likewise will need to describe the scope of the problem and implications for older adults and the costs. Second is to get support from key leaders and stakeholders because they are critical in efforts to improve care. Third in choosing a model is finding one that has good evidence that it will work. We will describe the outcomes of various models later in this chapter. Next is knowing if the model is feasible in your setting. This means that you have the team and the resources to implement and sustain the program. Fourth is getting input from older adults and their family caregivers to guide choosing the model. Lastly is the ability to measure if the model will make a difference.

Additional details on implementing, sustaining, and dissemination models of care will be highlighted later in this chapter.

Over the past decade, new concepts and strategies have emerged globally and nationally to incorporate the unique needs of our aging population. The World Health Organization (WHO), introduced the "age-friendly systems and communities," a policy framework designed to address outdoor spaces and public building, transportation, housing, social participation, respect and social inclusion, civic participation and employment, communication and information, community support, and health services.

The John A. Hartford Foundation, in partnership with the Institute for Healthcare Improvement conceptualized the idea of "Age-Friendly Health Systems" (AFHS) (see Chapter 12 on Age-Friendly Care). The AFHS uses existing geriatrics evidence-based models of care to lessen iatrogenic adverse events to older adults, deliver the best care conceivable to older adults across all care settings (emergency departments, inpatient, post-acute, in home, and ambulatory), and effectively optimize value for all involved stakeholders. This concept was summarized as the 4Ms: (1) What <u>M</u>atters to the older person; (2) <u>M</u>edication; (3) <u>M</u>entation; and (4) <u>M</u>obility. Integrating the 4Ms into the design of geriatric models will help teams be more effective in addressing the needs of older patients. The AFHS approach uses regular meetings of key stakeholders toward implementing practice changes to improve care. National leaders help local teams to measure their care and improve outcomes. Geriatrics models of care can be the framework of these practice improvement activities.

Geriatrics Models of Care and Quality Improvement Projects

Some geriatrics models of care have been evaluated in clinical trials while others have been described as rigorous quality improvement projects (**Table 14-2**).

Quality improvement projects and geriatrics practice models each identify a clinical challenge. In both strategies, an institutional review board (IRB) waiver is required, a specific intervention is deployed, and outcomes are measured

TABLE 14-2 ■ KEY FEATURES OF STRATEGIES TO IMPROVE CARE FOR OLDER PATIENTS

	PRIMARY GOAL	FUNDING REQUIRED	IRB REVIEW	OUTCOMES
Quality improvement	Change performance	Hospital or health system quality department or patient safety department	Protection of participants is essential; IRB exemption is required	How the relevant outcomes change over time
Geriatrics models	Change performance for a unique population in the context of their care	Grants or philanthropy support initially, then incorporated in yearly budgets	Protection of participants is essential; IRB exemption is required to record and share outcomes	Predetermined outcomes change over time and unique lessons learned
Research	Discovery of new knowledge	Grant support or organizational support	Systematic investigations require IRB review	Predetermined clinical outcomes compared to nontreatment group

IRB, institutional review board.

to see if it has worked. In each approach there is no new science defined. Usually the results are never made available in peer-reviewed journals. The work is often limited to one practice site. Both strategies are intended to improve the quality, safety, and value of health care. Both are unlikely to be disseminated, unless the model represents a unique improvement to health care. In summary, both geriatrics models and quality improvement programs use systematic efforts to improve care.

We would like to highlight some differences between geriatrics models and quality improvement. First, geriatrics models target specific interventions for older patients. They usually replicate prior work (eg, Acute Care for Elders [ACE] or Hospital Elder Life Program [HELP]), striving to get the same outcomes of the original model. Quality improvement projects, on the other hand, define the needs that fit their unique problems. Quality improvement projects allow the team to design their own approach to the problem commonly using "Plan-Do-Study-Act" cycles. These projects use experiential learning strategies. Second, quality improvement programs often have a shorter time frame whereas geriatrics models of care are commonly deployed over long periods of time. In summary, geriatrics models deploy a specific intervention to address a problem, while quality improvement projects allow more freedom to develop and implement an intervention.

Some geriatrics models integrate quality improvement strategies to improve their outcomes. An example of this is in the HELP program. The leaders who implemented the HELP program in a local community noted that the outcomes for their program fell short of the original model. The leaders used simple quality improvement strategies to assess and manage the fidelity of the key ingredients of the model to eventually improve the outcomes. Hence, geriatrics models of care may integrate quality improvement techniques into their project.

Geriatric Models of Care in the Context of Different Payment Mechanisms

The financial incentive of the health system is a critical part of the environment in which models are developed and deployed (**Table 14-3**).

Most geriatrics models have been developed over the past 20 years in the Medicare fee for service payment system. The fee for service payment system provides reimbursement based on the use of services, hence more care provided results in additional payment to providers and health systems. Models that work in these systems may rely on increasing downstream revenues to the health system from the care of patients. The fee for service payment system provides reimbursement to the hospital through diagnosis-related groups. In short, the Medicare fee for service payment system pays for services provided for the beneficiary.

The value-based purchase payment system provides reimbursement that spans unique episodes of care (see Chapter 19 on Value-Based Care). This payment system promotes optimal health outcomes with more efficient use of resources. An example of a value-based purchase systems are in accountable care organizations (ACOs), where optimal quality of care is rewarded along with the efficient use of resources. Examples of models that could be beneficial to the patients and to the health system in the context of value-based purchasing payment models include Geriatric Resources for Assessment and Care of Elders (GRACE), ACE, and the HELP program. Models that could work better in these ACO systems would avoid hospitalization, readmission, and emergency department visits, and improve patients' coordination of care.

Models deployed in a Medicare Advantage program provide care for the beneficiary and attempt to optimally use resources. The cost savings help keep the insurance premiums lower and may improve benefits offered to the beneficiaries. Models deployed in this payment system focus on avoiding hospitalizations. The economic benefit may result in lower total costs of care. Models that could be deployed in this payment system include GRACE and Hospital at Home. Some Medicare Advantage plans create an opportunity for geriatric leaders and health care leaders to implement geriatric models that would not have been possible in standard Medicare fee for service reimbursement care.

Trying to deploy a model that could save money in a fee for service payment system may not be endorsed by the health system, because such a model would not make

TABLE 14-3 ■ EXAMPLES OF GERIATRIC MODELS OF CARE IN THE SETTING OF DIFFERENT PAYMENT SYSTEMS			
GERIATRIC MODEL	**MEDICARE FEE FOR SERVICE**	**MEDICARE VALUE-BASED PURCHASING (EG, ACCOUNTABLE CARE ORGANIZATION—ACO)**	**MEDICARE HMO**
Acute Care for Elders	Payment to the hospital is based on the diagnosis-related group (DRG).	Payment to the hospital will be based on the DRG; however, if overall costs for a group of patients are lower than predicted, savings may be shared with the ACO based on quality measures achieved.	Payment to hospital within a network based on DRG and reviewed by HMO.
GRACE model	Beneficiaries will not have access to this model and may hence use more acute-care (hospital and emergency department) services.	Beneficiaries may use more prevention/care coordination services to avoid hospitalization and decrease costs. Savings are shared between Medicare and the ACO.	Beneficiaries may use more prevention/care coordination services to avoid hospitalization and decrease costs to the HMO.

enough money to be sustainable. Geriatrics leaders need to work with their health system leaders to review models that provide excellent clinical care and fit in a payment system that rewards such care. To prepare for value-based purchasing (while in the fee for service payment model), systems may need pilot programs which assess both quality outcomes and costs of care. Piloting these models can allow the hospital to study the economic benefit, while the clinicians assess the patient outcomes (**Table 14-4**).

HOSPITAL-BASED MODELS

Acute Care for Elders

The ACE model is designed to prevent functional decline and to restore independent physical functioning in hospitalized, medically ill patients. The intervention merges principles of geriatric assessment with continuous quality improvement to prevent dysfunctional syndrome that results from hostile physical environments and processes of care and negative expectations of caregivers and patients (**Figure 14-1**).

Essential components of the ACE program include a prepared environment to enhance patient safety and independent functioning; patient-centered guidelines for patient assessment and management by nurses; medical care review to assure appropriate and safe medical care; and interdisciplinary team (IDT)-based care, which includes planning the patient's transition to home or post-acute care setting. Daily IDT rounds briefly review each admission, with attention to the patient's functional status, principal diagnoses and treatments, anticipated hospital length of stay, and post-acute care needs and expectations. The original model's intervention was targeted at patients admitted to an ACE unit for any general medical illness.

The ACE program also pays attention to patients' needs throughout their hospitalization and coordinates transitions of care based on function, cognition, and social situation. The IDT includes a geriatrician as medical director, geriatrics clinical nurse specialist (CNS), trained registered nurses, social worker, dietitian, and physical and occupational therapists. In the initial ACE unit model, attending physicians and internal medicine residents were welcomed to participate in IDT rounds or, if unable, to review their plan of care with the bedside nurses. In select situations, the team arranges for family/patient conferences to review diagnoses, therapies, advanced directives, and anticipated date of transition from hospital to home. Later iterations of the ACE unit include clinical pharmacists, chaplains, hospitalists, and case managers in the IDT. Geriatricians who participate in this model are paid by the sponsoring hospital administration through legal contracts.

The ACE model was initially studied on a medical-surgical nursing unit (the ACE unit). Three randomized clinical trials confirm the benefits of the ACE unit compared to usual care. Compared to patients receiving usual care those admitted to the ACE units were discharged with less disability and a shorter hospital length of stay. They were also less likely to transition to a skilled nursing facility. Total costs of hospitalization were slightly lower on the ACE unit. Trends toward less hospital-associated disability at discharge were shown in one study, with lower rates of disability or nursing home placement 1 year later. Caregivers, nurses, and physicians report higher satisfaction with patient care on the ACE unit compared to usual care. Other benefits of ACE demonstrated in the clinical trials and programs with elements similar to ACE included fewer patients falls and use of physical restraints, better performance-based mobility, and reduced 30-day hospital readmissions. The most consistent outcomes of trials of ACE are significant reductions in length of hospital stay and costs. These findings provide compelling evidence that ACE units present health care systems an opportunity to realign the goals of improving the patient experience, providing high-quality care, reducing costs, and avoiding hospital-acquired conditions (consistent with the "triple aim").

The strength of ACE units is their scalability in a health care system or large hospital. Clinicians have found it most feasible to define which older adults should *not* be admitted to the ACE unit (eg, those who need intensive care or those with unstable vital signs). Patient care is more efficient than usual care and additional costs for startup of the unit are modest compared to usual care once a unit is mature and necessary environmental alterations have been completed.

The major limitations of an ACE unit include the limited number of older patients who can be admitted to a small unit; the costs of initial model rollout, including training of nurse and team members; assembly and maintenance of the IDT; and the need to capture important metrics that demonstrate the "value proposition."

Where an ACE unit is not feasible or unable to meet the needs of many older patients, the ACE program is modifiable as a "virtual ACE unit," ACE without walls, or a mobile ACE program. The concept of an ACE unit is preserved, despite loss of unique environmental adaptations, as long as these programs attempt to maintain fidelity to the four core components: safe environment, patient-centered care, interdisciplinary team rounds to review medical care, and preparing for transitions.

The Mobile Acute Care of the Elderly (MACE) model consists of a mobile interdisciplinary team that includes a geriatrician, social workers, and clinical nurse specialists who consult on and provide care for older adult patients on medical-surgical units. The physical therapist, occupational therapist, and dietitian often are consulted to collaborate and coordinate care with the MACE team. The MACE team goals are to decrease the hazards of hospitalization, facilitate transitions of care, and provide patient and family education. In a clinical trial the MACE model was associated with lower rates of adverse events, shorter hospital stays, and improved satisfaction with transitions of care. Where a geriatrician is not available in a hospital, a quality

TABLE 14-4 ■ GERIATRIC MODELS OF CARE

MODEL OF CARE	GOAL	KEY COMPONENTS	FINDINGS THAT SUPPORT THIS INTERVENTION
HOSPITAL-BASED MODELS			
Acute Care for Elders (ACE)	Lessen the chance of functional decline for hospitalized older adults	• Interdisciplinary team assessment and care • Prepared environment • Early planning to go home • Medical care review (using ACE Tracker report)	• Less disability • Decreased falls • Shorter hospital length of stay • Reduction in total hospital costs • Reduced mortality

NICHE
https://nicheprogram.org
	Prepare nursing staff in care of older adults
	Train a cohort of geriatric resource nurses to become experts for other nursing staff
		• Nursing skills and competencies
		• Promotes geriatric quality of care
		• Patient safety across the care continuum
		• Benchmarking service
			• Improved clinical quality at multiple NICHE sites:
			  ○ Improved patient satisfaction
			  ○ Decreased falls
			  ○ Decreased use of high-risk medications
			  ○ Improved use of senior friendly protocols
			  ○ Improved cultural competency
			  ○ Improved care for older patients who developed delirium during hospital care

AGS CoCare: Hospital Elder Life Program https://help.agscocare.org	Lessen the chance of new development of delirium in hospital	• Screening of vulnerable older patients at risk for delirium • Trained and supervised volunteers deploying protocols	• Decreased delirium • Decreased readmissions to hospital • Decreased rate of hospital falls • Decreased hospital length of stay • Decreased sitter use
VA-Based STRIDE Program https://www.research.va.gov/research_in_action/STRIDE-program-to-keep-hospitalized-Veterans-mobile.cfm	Maintain musculoskeletal strength and mobility of hospitalized older adults	• Early gait and balance assessment • Supervised ambulation	• Participants are less likely to be discharged to a skilled nursing facility • Safe and feasible intervention
AGS CoCare: Ortho https://ortho.agscocare.org	Improved the perioperative care of older adults with hip fractures	• Trained physicians and advanced practitioners to co-manage hospitalized older adults with the orthopedic team during the perioperative period	• Shorter time to surgery • Reduced length of stay • Decreased re-hospitalization • Lower complication rates • Lower mortality • Institutional cost savings
ACS Geriatric Surgery Verification Program https://www.facs.org/quality-programs/geriatric-surgery	This program sets standards to improve geriatric surgical care	• Evidence-based principles of geriatric care to optimize perioperative care for older adults	• Better management of medications • Geriatric friendly rooms • Establishing goals of care • Discharge planning coordination • Effective transitions of care
Duke Perioperative Optimization of Senior Health (POSH) https://medicine.duke.edu/divisions/geriatrics/patient-care/duke-perioperative-optimization-senior-health	Interdisciplinary approach for preoperative assessment	• Coordinate the expertise of geriatrics, general surgery, and anesthesia teams	• Management of multimorbidity • Reduction of polypharmacy • Encourage mobility • Emphasis on nutrition • Delirium prevention

PART II

PRINCIPLES OF GERIATRICS

(Continued)

TABLE 14-4 ■ GERIATRIC MODELS OF CARE (CONTINUED)

MODEL OF CARE	GOAL	KEY COMPONENTS	FINDINGS THAT SUPPORT THIS INTERVENTION
COMMUNITY-BASED MODELS			
Program of All-Inclusive Care for the Elderly (PACE) https://www.medicaid.gov/medicaid/long-term-services-supports/pace/programs-all-inclusive-care-elderly-benefits/index.html	Comprehensive primary care for individuals age 55 and older	• Day health center • Medical care • Nursing services • Therapy • Meals • Personal care • Social worker	• Lower rates of hospital use • Lower rates of nursing home use • Higher use of adult day care services • Better reported health status • Lower rates of emergency department use
Stopping Elderly Accidents, Death and Injuries (STEADI) https://www.cdc.gov/steadi/index.html	Fall prevention initiative	• Coordinated care plan • Screen patients at risk for falls • Assess modifiable risk factors for falls • Reduce risk factors	• Reduced falls • Improve health outcomes • Reducing health care expenditures
Strategies to Reduce Injuries and Develop Confidence in Elders (STRIDE) Program https://www.stride-study.org	Multifactorial intervention risk assessment and individualized plans administered by trained nurses	• Assesses risk factors for falls • Deploys standardized protocols	• Significantly lower rate of a first adjudicated serious fall injury
GRACE Program http://graceteamcare.indiana.edu/home.html.	Improve quality of care for low-income seniors in the community	• Medical and psychosocial evaluation • Medication review • Functional assessment • Advance directives	• Reduced acute care utilization. • Fewer ED visits
UCLA Dementia Care Program https://www.uclahealth.org/dementia/about-us	Health system–based comanagement model for patients with Alzheimer disease and related dementias (ADRDs)	• Maximize patient function • Minimize caregiver burnout • Reduce unnecessary costs through improved care	• Improved quality care • Lower-cost expenditures • Better clinical outcomes
Gerofit https://www.va.gov/GERIATRICS/pages/gerofit_Home.asp	Exercise and health-promotion program for older veterans	• Targets older adults at risk for functional decline with chronic medical problems	• Improved health and mental and physical function • Delayed need for institutional care • Lower mortality
HOME CARE MODELS OF CARE			
Home-Based Primary Care (HBPC) https://www.va.gov/GERIATRICS/pages/Home_Based_Primary_Care.asp	Primary care and care coordination at home	• Geriatrician, nurse practitioner (NP), and social worker working together • Periodic follow-up	• Studies demonstrate improved quality of life without added cost
Independence at Home https://innovation.cms.gov/innovation-models/independence-at-home	Primary care and care coordination at home for frail older adults	• Assessment 24–72 hours of hospital discharge • NP • Home health agency	• Decrease in the use of hospital resources
Community Aging in Place Advancing Better Living for Elders (CAPABLE) https://nursing.jhu.edu/faculty_research/research/projects/capable/index.html	Help older adults remain in their homes longer	• Nursing care assessment • Occupational therapy assessment • Handyman for home repairs based on above	• Improve ADLs and IADLs • Improved quality of life • Lower hospitalization rates • Reduction in fall rates

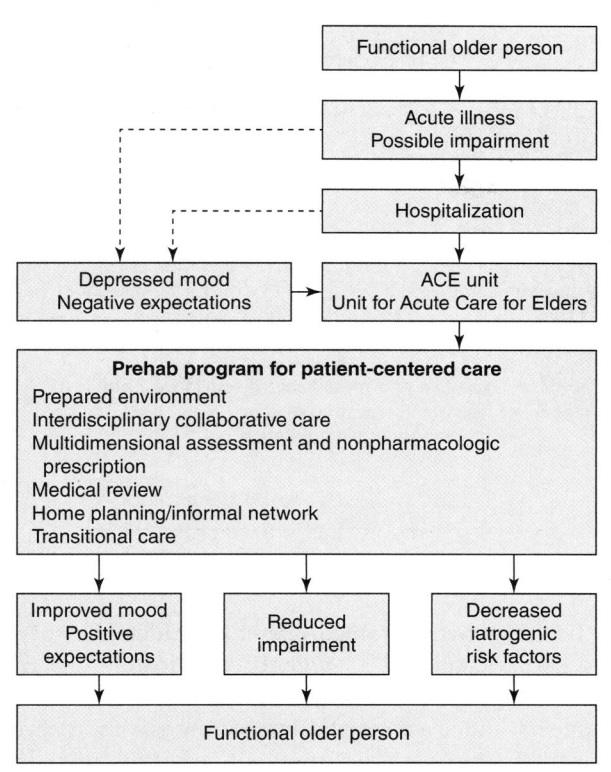

FIGURE 14-1. Acute Care for Elders (ACE).

improvement approach is the e-geriatrician consultation and an automated electronic medical record spreadsheet of relevant items, called the ACE Tracker (**Figure 14-2**). Consultation can be offered off campus and the ACE Tracker provides a spreadsheet of quality measures, geriatric conditions, and risk factors for adverse outcomes, such as falls and pressure ulcers. The ACE Tracker is a tool that can guide the development of the care plan and has been helpful in disseminating the principles of geriatrics to remote and rural hospitals.

ACE Consult Service

In the ACE consult service, the consultation model applies the same core principles as ACE without the unique environment. Consultation is performed by a geriatrician who often utilizes the expertise of the interdisciplinary team to comprehensively assess the patient's overall medical and functional status and post-discharge care needs. Inpatient geriatric consultations focus on clarifying diagnoses, identifying goals of care, and addressing polypharmacy, delirium, dementia, cognitive impairment, frailty, elder abuse, neglect, malnutrition, dementia with behavioral and psychological symptoms, falls, functional decline, and depression. Through a detailed review of the medical record and by obtaining key information from caregivers and family,

PART II — **PRINCIPLES OF GERIATRICS**

- **ACE Tracker: A real-time, simple, brief electronic health records report of the unique needs of older patients.**

QUA1000 ACE Tracker

Nursing Unit in Rural Hospital

Patient Room/Bed	Age	LOS/ICU	Cog	Help	Denm Sx	Delnm Rx	Meds	Beers	HX Morse	Mobility Falls Lst 24h	Therapy /Swiw	Sit/Res /VNPM ADL	CVC CATH	Pres Injury/ Stage	Wind Care	B/Cr R/ Braden H	BMI/ Alb	GOC Node	SS/ CM	Adv Dir	Pain Score	Readmit 30 days	Risk%
Patient A					F				10225560198					02/24/2021 9:54					02/28/2021 23:37				
K487/A	98	5	Y	VH	Y	A:H	13	A	75	3/R	POSCd	6			Y	16	30	21.4		Y	*	0	16%
Patient B					M				10223486708					02/15/2021 13:23					02/27/2021 17:12				
K488/A	87	14	Y	V	AMS		8		70	5/R	POSd		Y* II	Y	11*	11/H	28.7	2/19	Y	Y P	0	13%
Patient C					M				10226071489					02/25/2021 21:11					02/27/2021 18:20				
K489/A	86	4	Y		AMS		7		60*	1/U	POS	S			14	23/H			Y	Y G*	0	12%
Patient D					M				10226363908					02/27/2021 8:45					02/28/2021 11:45				
K491/A	66	2		V	AMS		6	O	45	2/B	POS	10			20	11	18.5		N		0	
Patient E					M				10226417812					02/28/2021 3:20					02/28/2021 9:25				
K492/A	82	1		V	Y		14		50	4/T	PO	6	Y III	Y	15	6/H	29.6				0	
Patient F					M				10226451978					02/28/2021 16:18					No BM Since Admit - 1 day(s)				
K494/A	84	1		V			11	O		Rb		12	Y II		19/H	30.8			Y P	0		
Patient G					M				10219273395					02/03/2021 11:34	02/10/2021				02/28/2021 23:20				
L472/01	69	26*		V	Y		15	A	95	Y	5/T	POSd	3	Y	Y* IV	Y	12	23	29.9			5	20%
Patient H					M				10222788411					02/11/2021 12:45	02/22/2021				02/28/2021 18:27				
L473/01	71	18		V	AMS		18	A	110*	Y*	3/U	POSd	V	12		15*	23		Y	Y P*	0	18%
Patient I					F				10225712621		Oc6			02/24/2021 16:49					02/27/2021 18:48				
L474/01	71	5		V			11		60*	2/U	PO	12			18	14/H	39.4		Y	N	0	
Patient J					F				10223169942					02/12/2021 20:30					02/28/2021 18:30				
L475/01	74	17		V	Y		11		100	Y	3/U	POSd	2	Y		Y	12*	17/H-	27.5	2/17	Y	Y G*	0	14%

FIGURE 14-2. The ACE Tracker.

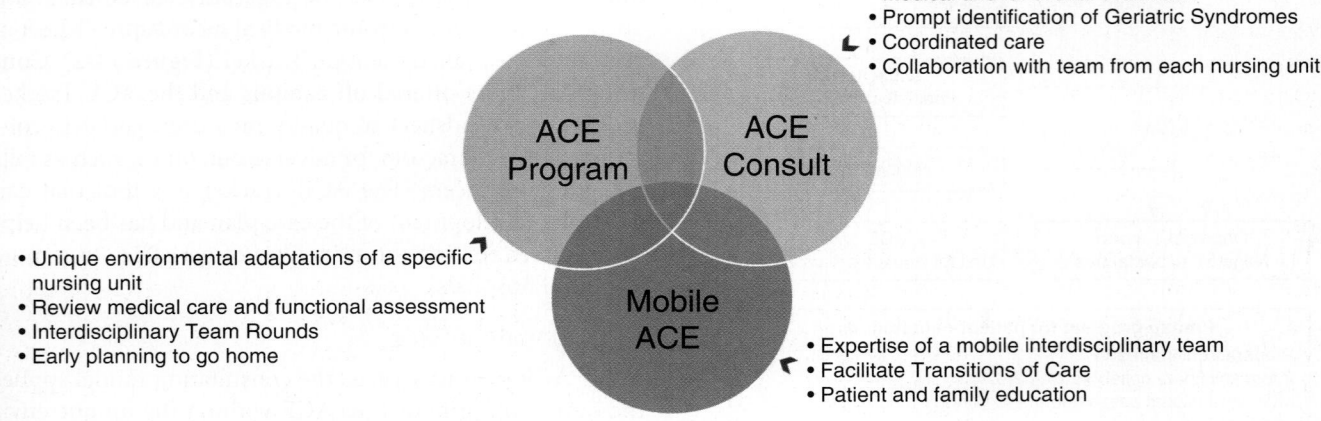

- Medical and functional evaluation
- Prompt identification of Geriatric Syndromes
- Coordinated care
- Collaboration with team from each nursing unit

- Unique environmental adaptations of a specific nursing unit
- Review medical care and functional assessment
- Interdisciplinary Team Rounds
- Early planning to go home

- Expertise of a mobile interdisciplinary team
- Facilitate Transitions of Care
- Patient and family education

FIGURE 14-3. Acute Care for Elders (ACE) principles.

geriatric consultations provide recommendations to the primary team. Geriatric consultation can be performed in multiple clinical settings in the hospital (**Figure 14-3**). Geriatricians and nurse practitioners who see patients in this model bill Medicare Part B for their services. In some sites, the consultation is performed by nurse practitioners under the supervision of a geriatrician.

AGS CoCare: HELP

The HELP is a multicomponent intervention designed to prevent incidents of delirium in hospitalized older patients. The intervention consists of six standardized protocols for reducing specific risk factors for delirium: cognitive impairment, sleep deprivation, immobility, visual impairment, hearing impairment, and dehydration. The intervention (**Figure 14-4**) is targeted at patients aged 70 and older with at least one risk factor for delirium.

The HELP intervention is conducted by an interdisciplinary HELP team. The team includes an advanced

practice or geriatric-trained nurse, the Elder Life specialist, a geriatrician, and a program coordinator—the Elder Life Nurse specialist. The Elder Life Nurse specialist trains volunteers and oversees the interventions. The delirium prevention strategies are carried out by highly trained and supervised volunteers. The HELP team collaborates with a unit-based interdisciplinary team that includes nursing, medicine, physical therapy, occupational therapy, pharmacy, nutrition, and chaplaincy care. The HELP team assesses and enrolls patients who meet specific criteria and designate the delirium prevention strategies based on each patient's needs. The HELP prevention strategies include a daily visitor program, therapeutic activities, an early mobilization program, nonpharmacologic sleep protocol, oral volume repletion, and a feeding assistance program.

The effectiveness of HELP was demonstrated in a prospective, individual-matching strategy, the Delirium Prevention Trial. The incidence of delirium was reduced by 40% among patients receiving the HELP intervention

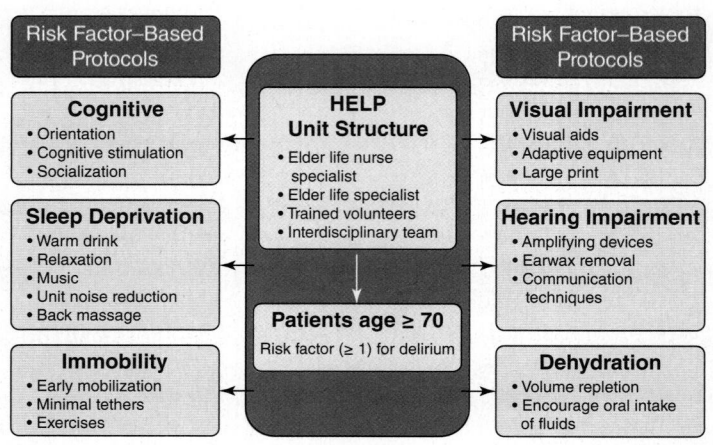

FIGURE 14-4. Hospital Elder Life Program (HELP).

compared to the control group receiving usual care. The days spent delirious and the total episodes of delirium were significantly lower in the intervention group, although the severity of delirium and delirium recurrence rates were not lower. The individual attention given to each patient by the volunteers and HELP team results in improved quality of care and reduced risks of hospital-associated conditions. The HELP program has been widely disseminated and integrated with other models, such as ACE units and Nurses Improving Care for Health System Elders (NICHE). The HELP model allows some flexibility in fidelity to the original model design. The national HELP program assists individuals to launch HELP by gaining support of hospital administration and staff. Hospitals that register for HELP assistance gain access to HELP manuals, training videos, handouts for families and caregivers, and information about national and local conferences.

HELP can be replicated and successfully implemented in medical units, surgical units, telemetry units, intensive care units, emergency departments, nursing home settings, and home care. HELP has been demonstrated to be both effective and cost-effective for patients at moderate risk of delirium. HELP has also shown to improve quality of care of hospitalized older patients and patient and family satisfaction with care.

In multiple studies, HELP has been consistently associated with lower rates of delirium, functional decline, and cognitive decline, and decreased hospital length of stay and decreased rate of hospital falls. The effectiveness of HELP is directly related to adherence to the interventions and protocols. Limitations of the original HELP program include the need for trained volunteers. Recent adaptations of HELP give hospitals the option of using non-volunteers.

The most successful HELP programs have seen expansion of the program to many medical-surgical units and have documented substantial cost savings to their hospital. Geriatricians in HELP programs are paid through legal contracts with the sponsoring hospital for their time in completing specific job functions. HELP offers geriatricians superb opportunities: (1) to transform quality and safety of patient care at their hospital, (2) to be an expert consultant to the HELP team, and (3) to be a leader in interdisciplinary team care.

Nurses Improving Care for Health System Elders

NICHE is a nursing care model designed to help hospitals and other health care organizations to improve quality of care for older adult patients and nurse competence in geriatric practice. NICHE principles and resources are consistent with professional nursing practice models. The program has several approaches to infuse evidence-based geriatric best practices into hospital care. At the foundation of NICHE is the model of the Geriatric Resource Nurse (GRN). The GRN prepares staff nurses to serve as the clinical resource on geriatric issues to other nurses on a medical-surgical unit. Through education and modeling by a NICHE coordinator, educational protocols and tools enable nurses to implement best practices. NICHE focuses on improving nursing skills and knowledge when caring for older adults by providing training tools to hospitals and health care organizations. NICHE promotes the use of interdisciplinary teams and helps nursing staff to apply evidence-based concepts to care for older adults. NICHE provides tools for best practices to manage pain and prevent pressure ulcers, adverse medication events, delirium, falls, and the management of urinary incontinence. At a system level NICHE provides a structure for nurses to collaborate with other disciplines and coordinate geriatrics models of care. Hospitals can achieve NICHE designation to demonstrate the hospital's commitment to improving quality and enhancing the patient experience. Nearly 500 hospitals in the United Sates and several other countries are NICHE-designated. Many ACE units and HELP programs are based in hospitals with NICHE designation.

NICHE can be implemented in hospitals, long-term care facilities, and home health care practices. The NICHE program provides geriatricians the opportunity to collaborate with GRNs to promote geriatric quality of care and patient safety across the care continuum. Hospitals pay an annual fee to the NICHE program to receive all components of this model and educational resources.

STRIDE Programs

There are two geriatric models called "STRIDE." One is hospital-based and was studied in Veterans Affairs Medical Centers. The second is a falls prevention intervention that was deployed in outpatient primary care practices. The latter program is described in the section on Community-Based Models.

VA-Based STRIDE Program

STRIDE (Assisted Early Mobility for Hospitalized Older Veterans) is a supervised walking program for hospitalized older adults focused on maintaining musculoskeletal strength and mobility during hospitalization. STRIDE's main features include: early assessment within 24 hours of admission, supervised ambulation, and education for the patient and their families that highlight the importance of daily ambulation. Patients admitted from a nursing home, planned surgery, bed rest order, chest pain, angina pectoris, new neurologic deficit, unable to follow a one-step command or cannot walk are excluded from the intervention. Patients are referred to this program by their treating physician.

The STRIDE intervention includes gait and balance assessment by a physical therapist, followed by supervised daily walks by a therapy assistant. The walk assistant follows specific protocols to ensure safety and monitoring of patient's vital signs.

Initial studies have demonstrated that this supervised walking program for hospitalized older adults is feasible and safe, and program participants were less likely to be discharged to a skilled nursing facility than a demographically and clinically similar comparison group. A key aspect of this model is the emphasis on early mobility of hospitalized older adults. The premise that a nurse or physical therapist is not required makes this model compelling. Some sites have used physical therapy aides to implement this program.

American Geriatrics Society CoCare: Ortho

Older adults with hip fractures generally have other comorbidities and geriatric syndromes that make them more vulnerable to experience complications when hospitalized.

Preexisting conditions and the risk of these patients to experience a complication postoperatively have generated the need to create geriatrics models of care that address the unique needs of older adults with hip fractures and multimorbidity.

AGS CoCare: Ortho is a Geriatrics-Orthopedics Co-Management model in which a geriatrician or specially trained clinicians work with orthopedic surgeons to coordinate and improve the perioperative care of older adults with hip fractures. This unique model of care focuses on training physicians, advanced practitioners such as nurse practitioners, and physician assistants to co-manage hospitalized older adults with the orthopedic team during the perioperative period. The training provided by this model covers a variety of topics relevant to older adults recovering from hip fractures. AGS CoCare: Ortho optimizes perioperative care in older adults. This model has demonstrated improved outcomes, such as shorter time to surgery, reduced length of stay and 30-day re-hospitalization, lower complication rates, lower mortality, and institutional cost savings. Hospitals pay a fee to the AGS for access to this model. Geriatricians who work in this model bill Medicare when they consult on individual patients.

American College of Surgeons Geriatric Surgery Verification Program

The American College of Surgeons (ACS) Geriatric Surgery Verification (GSV) Program is designed to take into account the surgical needs of older adults. The program establishes standards to improve geriatric surgical care and better outcomes. The GSV Program provides a foundation for hospitals to take an interdisciplinary approach to augment perioperative care for older adults.

The standards set by the GSV Program are the result of the combination of rigorous evidence-based principles of geriatric care and empowering the interdisciplinary team to participate, coordinate, and monitor the quality of surgical care of this vulnerable population.

This program outlines standards in multiple areas with the ultimate goal to improve the quality of care for older surgical patients. These standards include, but are not limited to: improving communications with patients before surgical procedures to focus on outcomes that matter most to the patient, screening for geriatric vulnerabilities, better management of medications, providing geriatric-friendly rooms, revisiting goals of care for patients admitted to the intensive care unit, discharge planning coordination, and effective transitions of care.

Duke Perioperative Optimization of Senior Health

The Perioperative Optimization of Senior Health (POSH) program was developed at Duke Health as a quality improvement initiative to coordinate the expertise of geriatrics, general surgery, and anesthesia teams. The POSH program provides integrated care coordination for older adults undergoing elective surgeries.

Patients are referred by the surgical team to an interdisciplinary team for preoperative assessment. The POSH preoperative team includes a geriatrician, geriatric resource nurse, social worker, program administrator, and nurse practitioner. This team focuses on targeted interventions such as management of multimorbidity, reduction of polypharmacy, improvement of mobility and nutrition, and delirium prevention. POSH team physicians are also available as consultants to ensure the implementation of recommendations made preoperatively. The POSH team collaborates with the surgical team, assisting with the optimizing medications, pain control, treatment and management of chronic medical conditions, and postoperative complications.

The main objective of the POSH program is to improve postoperative outcomes for high-risk population. Studies have demonstrated that patients who participate in this interdisciplinary perioperative care intervention had shorter hospitals stays, lower readmission rates, and a greater likelihood of discharge home without a nursing home stay or need for home health care. Patients in the POSH program also had overall fewer complications during their hospitalization.

COMMUNITY-BASED MODELS

Geriatric Resources for Assessment and Care of Elders

The GRACE model of care of primary care was developed specifically to improve the quality of care for low-income seniors. The model integrates geriatric and primary care services across the continuum of care in expectation that patients will receive the recommended care. In the original model, eligible patients for the GRACE program are aged 65 or older, have an established primary care physician, are patients in the community-based health centers of a large health system, and have an income less than 200% of the federal poverty level. The intervention includes a support team of advanced practice nurse and social worker who help provide care for seniors in collaboration with the patient's primary care provider and a geriatrics interdisciplinary team led by a geriatrician. The nurse practitioner and social worker support team performs an initial and annual in-home comprehensive geriatric assessment. The assessment includes medical and psychosocial history, medication review, functional assessment, and review of social supports and advanced directives. Their findings and recommendations are reviewed by the interdisciplinary team and discussed with the primary care physician. The interdisciplinary team also includes a pharmacist, physical therapist, mental health social worker, and community-based services liaison from the primary care practice. Based on the assessment and interdisciplinary team meeting, one or more of 12 GRACE protocols are recommended. The protocols target common geriatric conditions: advance care planning, health maintenance, medication management, difficulty walking/falls, chronic pain, urinary incontinence, depression, hearing loss, visual impairment, malnutrition or weight loss, dementia, and caregiver burden. Relevant features of the intervention also include use of an integrated electronic medical record and a web-based care management tracking tool. GRACE collaborates with an affiliated pharmacy, mental and home health services, and community-based and inpatient geriatric care services.

A randomized controlled trial of the GRACE intervention was conducted with patients who met eligibility criteria and were assigned to either usual care by their primary care physician or to the support team and geriatrics interdisciplinary team in collaboration with the primary care physician. High-risk patients enrolled in GRACE had fewer visits to emergency departments, fewer hospitalizations and readmissions, and reduced hospital costs compared to the control group. The 2-year program significantly reduced costs per enrolled high-risk patient by the second year. In addition, GRACE was rated highly by primary care physicians compared to usual care. GRACE-enrolled patients also reported higher quality of life compared to those in the control group for general health, vitality, social function, and mental health. The interdisciplinary team meeting occurred within 30 days of enrollment for 85% of patients, an average of 5.3 GRACE protocols were activated for each patient, and adherence to GRACE interdisciplinary team suggestions was very high.

The GRACE model of care appears to be cost-effective for low income patients who are at high risk for hospital readmission, and who receive medical care in a health care system that provides a wide array of supportive services. A barrier to greater implementation of the GRACE model is that only 10% of its costs are covered by fee for service Medicare. However, it appears to be ideal for managed-care practices and for ACOs who care for similar populations.

Several other hospitals, academic medical centers, and Department of Veterans Affairs Medical Centers have adopted the GRACE model of care. The GRACE model has been expanded to chronically ill homebound older patients as a home visitation program that includes physicians, nurse practitioners, and social workers. GRACE has been used successfully as a care transitions program for older adults who are discharged home from a hospital or skilled nursing facility. GRACE has the potential to provide coordinated care management of enrolled patients across the care continuum with shared responsibility between patients, medical care providers, and the core team. It provides geriatricians an opportunity to serve in a consultative role to the interdisciplinary team and to be the primary care physician in various settings. The geriatrician's expertise in chronic care management, interdisciplinary team care, knowledge of geriatric conditions, and training in system-based practice brings value to the health care system and insurance plans.

Program of All-Inclusive Care for the Elderly

The Program of All-Inclusive Care for the Elderly (PACE) provides comprehensive primary care for participants who are aged 55 or older, certified by their state to be eligible for nursing home care, able to safely continue living in the community with services, and living in a PACE service area. The goal of PACE programs is to enable the participants to remain living in the community for as long as it is safe and feasible. Each PACE site receives capitated payments from Medicare and Medicaid, with funds covering health-related services required by participants. The services are primarily provided at a day health center, which in addition to medical care, provides nursing services, physical and occupational therapy, recreational therapies, meals, nutrition services, social work, and personal care. In addition, comprehensive services are provided at each PACE site ranging from primary care, specialty consultation, hospital and emergency services, and long-term nursing home care. PACE also covers home health and personal care costs, necessary prescription drugs, social services, respite care, and specific medical services, primarily at the day health center. An interdisciplinary team of professional and nonprofessional staff review goals of care with participants and family members; and meet frequently to review health status of participants to identify additional services or equipment that could enable the enrollees to remain living at home and to support caregivers' needs. As a capitated program that is financially responsible for all Medicare and Medicaid-related services, the PACE site is incented to provide services that enable the enrollees to remain living in the community and to avoid unnecessary hospitalizations or medical interventions and therapies. PACE and the interdisciplinary team have flexibility for deciding how to pay for a participant's medical and nonmedical expenses that enable them to remain living at home. This flexibility enables PACE programs to provide services or durable medical equipment under the capitation model that are not typically covered by either Medicare or Medicaid. Nationally, most participants are older and have multiple morbidities and deficits in activities of daily living (ADLs), and about 50% have dementia.

As of 2021, 131 PACE programs were operational in 31 states. Although PACE programs serve primarily to dual-eligible participants, the Patient Protection and

Affordable Care Act created an optional long-term care insurance plan that could be used to pay for community services such as PACE, creating the potential for an increasing enrollment in programs. More than 54,000 Medicare beneficiaries are enrolled in the PACE program. Current barriers to enrollment in PACE programs include delays in enrollment of participants, limited number of sites in rural communities, lack of awareness of the program, and the requirement that enrollees transfer primary care to the PACE program.

Cross-sectional and cohort studies generally demonstrate that PACE programs enable enrollees to remain living in the community. Especially in mature programs, health care costs, hospitalization and readmission rates, and survival are better among enrollees in PACE compared to usual medical care settings that include case management and local community services. With its focus on chronic disease management, interdisciplinary care, and system-based practice, PACE is an attractive model of care for geriatricians.

Fall Prevention Programs: STEADI and STRIDE

Stopping elderly accidents, death and injuries Stopping Elderly Accidents, Death and Injuries (STEADI) is a fall prevention initiative for health care providers designed by the Centers for Disease Control and Prevention (CDC). This is a coordinated care plan that focuses on older adults at risk for falls or those who already have a history of multiple falls. This model has three core elements: (1) screen patients at risk for falls, (2) assess modifiable risk factors, and (3) intervene to reduce risk factors. The intervention creates strategies to address gait, balance, and strengthening, optimize medications, and discontinue medications that increase fall risk. These strategies also include collaboration with other disciplines to evaluate sensory impairment (ophthalmologist), footwear issues (podiatrist), and home safety evaluations.

This coordinated approach has been demonstrated to reduce falls, improve health outcomes, and reduce health care expenditures.

Strategies to reduce injuries and develop confidence in elders program Strategies to Reduce Injuries and Develop Confidence in Elders (STRIDE) is a multifactorial intervention to prevent serious fall injuries. The STRIDE program is a patient-centered intervention delivered by nurses that partner with patient's primary care physicians. (Note there is another program for older people named STRIDE [assiSTed eaRly mobIlity for hospitalizeD older vEterans].) This intervention assesses risk factors for fall injuries such as gait impairment, postural hypotension, vitamin D deficiency, home safety hazards, sensory impairment, and high-risk medications. This program deploys standardized protocols for management of specific risk factors. The care plans are individualized and reviewed by primary care physicians. Follow-up care conducted by phone or in person

and a review of care plans are other essential components of this intervention. A recent pragmatic, cluster-randomized trial that evaluated the effectiveness of this intervention did not show a significant lower rate of a first adjudicated serious fall injury. Nevertheless, clinicians can use these interventions to care for community-dwelling older adults, understanding the limitations of the evidence.

HOME CARE MODELS OF CARE

Home-Based Primary Care

Home-Based Primary Care (HBPC) focuses on the frailest subset of older adults, those with severe and disabling chronic illnesses who receive primary care in their homes. The model is implemented in over 150 sites of the Veterans Affairs Medical Centers. Common conditions or illnesses of HBPC recipients include dementia, congestive heart failure, diabetes mellitus, chronic obstructive pulmonary disease (COPD), stroke, and severe arthritis. The program delivers care coordination at home with a team of geriatricians, nurse practitioners, social workers, licensed practical nurses, and office coordinators. Periodic follow-up by members of the team is complemented by on-call telephone coverage. Studies demonstrate improved quality of life of enrolled patients.

Independence at Home

A Center for Medicare and Medicaid Innovation program, with similarities to HBPC, Independence at Home (IAH) is currently being implemented at multiple sites. IAH involves a mobility interdisciplinary team that rests on three pillars: targeting the highest-risk high-cost beneficiaries with limited mobility, longitudinal HBPC with accountability for care received across all settings, and aligned quality metrics and payment incentives.

The IAH model has potential value for frail older patients who may be unable to make follow-up visits with a primary care physician in office due to disease complexity or frailty. To be eligible, beneficiaries must be enrolled in Fee for Service Medicare, have two or more chronic medical conditions, need assistance with two or more basic ADLs, and have had a nonelective hospitalization and received acute or subacute rehabilitation services within the preceding 12 months. The patient is seen for a first home visit within 24 to 72 hours of hospital discharge. A comprehensive evaluation of their physical, medical, and functional needs, and of their caregiver's needs, is included in this first visit. Follow-up visits involve close contact between the nurse practitioner and home health agency. Analysis of administrative data demonstrates that the model is associated with a decrease in the use of hospital resources and cost reduction. In a case-controlled study of Medicare patients enrolled in a home care intervention, total costs were 17% lower over a mean of 2 years of follow-up. With the aging of the very old population and financial incentives favoring home care versus hospital or institutional treatment of frail patients, IAH offers opportunities for geriatricians to become both directors of programs and providers of home care.

Community Aging in Place—Advancing Better Living for Elders (CAPABLE)

CAPABLE is a program developed for low-income seniors to safely age in place and improve physical function. This interprofessional program includes an occupational therapist, a registered nurse, and a handyman.

The CAPABLE interdisciplinary team focuses on identifying daily activity goals in a community dwelling for older adults (eg, taking a shower and walking to the bathroom), evaluating barriers to achieving those goals, and monitoring outcomes collaboratively. The occupational therapist assesses patient's ADLs and instrumental ADLs (IADLs), and pays attention to activities that are challenging at home, such as functional mobility, meal preparation, bathing, and dressing. The registered nurse targets underlying issues that can potentially affect ADLs or IADLs, such as pain and mood. A registered nurse will also address fall prevention, medication review, incontinence management, sexual health, and smoking cessation. She communicates concerns to the primary care physician. The main goals of CAPABLE are to increase mobility, functionality, and ability for older adults to age in place, using their strengths to maximize safety and independence. CAPABLE has been demonstrated to improve ADLs and IADLs and quality of life, lower hospitalization rates, and reduce fall rates.

UCLA Dementia Care Program

The UCLA Alzheimer's and Dementia Care (ADC) Program is designed to assist patients with Alzheimer disease and related dementias (ADRDs). This program is a health system-based co-management model that uses a nurse practitioner supervised by a physician dementia specialist who works with primary care and specialty physicians to ensure the care of these patients is comprehensive and coordinated. The goals of this program are to maximize patient function, minimize caregiver burnout, and reduce unnecessary costs through improved care.

Patients are referred to the UCLA ADC Program by primary care physicians or specialty physicians. Key components of this program include structured needs assessment of patients and their caregivers; creation and implementation of individualized dementia care plans; ongoing dementia care management (caregiver education and training, coordination of care with neurology, geriatric psychiatry, psychology, or geriatrics, caregiver support groups, referral to community-based organizations for services); and access to a geriatrician for assistance and advice. The UCLA ADC Program monitors and revises care plans, as needed, including active monitoring via phone call or in person visit (a minimum of a telephone interaction every 4 months). The UCLA ADC Program has demonstrated outcomes of improved quality care, lower-cost expenditures, and better clinical outcomes.

Gerofit

Gerofit is an exercise and health-promotion program for older veterans. Gerofit program targets deconditioned older adults with chronic medical problems who use assistive devices and are at risk for functional decline. Patients are referred to this program by their primary care provider. Individuals eligible for this program must be aged 65 and older and able to function independently in a group setting. Patients with inability to perform basic activities of daily living, inability to transfer, oxygen dependence, unstable cardiac disease, and moderate to severe cognitive impairment are excluded from the program.

Participants enrolled in the program have demonstrated improved health, mental health, physical function, and well-being. A recent dissemination study showed that Gerofit has better long-term outcomes, such as a delayed need for institutional care, sustained improved functional abilities, improved well-being, and lower mortality, than usual care.

MODELS OF CARE: LESSONS LEARNED

Lessons Learned in Implementing Models of Care

There are several important lessons to share as the field moves from studying a geriatrics model of care to the actual implementation of the model. Some leaders describe multiple efforts to propose different models over a period of several years without getting hospital "buy in" for their ideas. Other models are championed by the health system as a priority in fulfilling a key aspect of their mission. The implementation of a geriatrics practice model can be an exciting and fulfilling aspect of a geriatrician's career. An understanding of implementation science and the ability to work with teams are two important principles in leading geriatric practice models.

First, geriatrics models must be deployed to address the local problems in the health care delivery system. An example would be if the nursing staff is struggling with a high rate of delirium among their older patients. Describing the problem with a patient story can help communicate the need for the program. In this context, the geriatrics leader could propose the development of a structured intervention (eg, the HELP program) with the engagement of the nursing administration. Identifying and addressing the contextual issues will increase the chance of successfully launching the model of care. The context further includes the culture of your organization and the economics of payment for health care at your site.

Second, to start a geriatrics model, the leaders will need to study their practice and measure their current performance as compared to other sites. This assessment defines the scope of the problem and the need for the new model of care. The Institute for Healthcare Improvement has multiple tools and strategies to measure outcomes, http://www.ihi.org. Consider partnering with your hospital administration to measure outcomes. Such a partnership with the administration provides a good working relationship and increases the validity of the information.

Third, your planning team needs to develop a business plan and a communication plan with the hospital administration, to get approval to proceed with model implementation. This plan outlines the costs and the potential savings of the geriatrics model. The philanthropy (or development) office can assist in launching your model by reaching out to prospective donors and securing grant funds to cover startup costs. Often the geriatrics leaders present a description of the new model and the business plan to an administrative executive team to get input and buy-in. The geriatrics leaders should make sure that the administration has agreed to the model before moving forward with full implementation. Once the planning team has gotten the agreement from the administration, one needs to define the roles of each team member and determine what the exact intervention entails. Finally, your team will need a communication plan to make sure that all stakeholders understand the model and their roles. In summary, there are key steps to the implementation of a geriatric model that can assure that the program has been successfully launched.

Lessons Learned in Efforts to Sustain and Manage Models of Care

While it is exciting to launch a geriatrics model, it is difficult to sustain that model over a long period of time. Six key points deserve some attention in this regard. First, your geriatrics model "planning team" can be converted to an "advisory committee" charged with reviewing outcomes and guiding the project over time. This group can identify challenges and find resources to address the identified needs. The advisory committee is not charged with personnel decisions or day-to-day management of the model. A patient should serve on this committee to help keep the team patient-centered. An annual report should be provided from the advisory committee to the hospital or funding organization to describe key outcomes and number of lives touched by the program.

Second, geriatric models may not initially improve outcomes. The hospital leadership should be able to define the key outcome measures benchmarked over time and explain if the program worked. If it appears that the outcomes are not being achieved according to the benchmarks, the leadership team will need to assess the fidelity of the model and the reliability of the measures. Leaders may be able to use baseline outcome measures prior to the implementation of the interventions in making these determinations. The post-intervention measures can help explain if the model is improving outcomes. Validated and endorsed quality measures should be used whenever appropriate to benchmark against national performance. The leadership

and the advisory team can guide the program, even if initial improvement is not achieved. In advising how to move forward, we have learned to pay careful attention to (1) the communication of the model to key stakeholders, (2) the training of the professionals who are key personnel in the model, and (3) the assessment/maintenance of the fidelity of the models.

Third, yearly personnel goals should be used to align individual employee goals with the goals for your geriatrics model. As an example, the Elder Life Specialist of the HELP model could have as his/her annual goal with the consistent use of all six of the delirium prevention protocols. This effort of using yearly personnel goals helps keep the leaders and the employees focused on achieving full implementation of the geriatrics model. This effort further rewards the employees for their contributions.

The fourth point in sustaining a geriatrics model is to make sure that model leaders continue to communicate with key stakeholders. Physicians and nurses who are providing clinical care will need to understand the importance of excellent care of older individuals in their community. Likewise, other health care professionals will need to understand the program and their role in the geriatrics model. Further, community leaders from the department on aging and the local Alzheimer's Association will need to understand the geriatrics model and how they can partner with your programs.

Fifth, careful attention to the funding of your geriatrics model is critical. The costs and savings of the geriatrics model will be important to sustaining the hospital support for the model. Billing and reimbursement from Medicare and other insurers should be carefully tracked, as should compliance with billing requirements. By following these outcomes, your team can responsibly manage resources. You can determine the direct variable costs per patient in your model and compare these costs with those of a matched cohort of patients receiving standard care. This effort can help make the case for further expansion of your program. Partnering with administrative colleagues who can help prepare these reports and can assist with program budgets will result in accurate and trusted reports.

Sixth and finally, compare your outcomes with other sites to try to find "best practices." This assessment may help your team to define what exactly is being done at each site and adjust processes to further improve outcomes. Again, using standardized outcome measures is essential in order to compare outcomes across sites.

Lessons Learned in Disseminating Models of Care

A few key points are important for "scaling up" geriatrics practice models. We have learned that the geriatrics leaders must articulate a clear message about how the model will be implemented broadly into practice. Your team must get agreement that the goal of spreading the geriatrics model broadly in the hospital or health system is consistent with the organization's mission. The geriatrics team must mobilize across a wide area to communicate the new model to "early adopters," so that the effort is implemented at new sites. The message will need to address: Exactly what will be done? Who is eligible for the model and who is not? What outcomes will be measured to know we have made a difference? The practice model must be communicated to the opinion leaders in the field, so that their input is considered as the model is rolled out. The University of New Mexico Project ECHO has developed effective methods to disseminate best practice. The four key components of Project ECHO include: (1) using technology to leverage scarce resources, (2) sharing best practices to reduce disparity, (3) deploying case-based learning to master complexity, and (4) monitoring outcomes using a web-based database. In summary, one of the most challenging aspects of implementing geriatrics models is the broad dissemination of that model into standard practice. The role of the geriatrician in this work is to lead a broad coalition of health providers toward a common goal of better care for older patients.

FURTHER READING

Allen K, Hazelett S, Martin M, et al. An innovation center model to transform health systems to improve care of older adults. *J Am Geriatr Soc.* 2020;68:15–22.

American College of Surgeons. Geriatric Surgery Verification Program. https://www.facs.org/Quality-Programs/geriatric-surgery.

American Geriatrics Society. CoCare: HELP. https://help.agscocare.org.

American Geriatrics Society. CoCare: Ortho. https://ortho.agscocare.org.

Bhasin S, Gill TM, Reuben DB, et al. A randomized trial of a multifactorial strategy to prevent serious fall injuries. *N Engl J Med.* 2020;383(2):129-140.

Boltz M, Capezuti E, Bower-Ferres S, et al. Changes in the geriatric care environment associated with NICHE. *Geriatr Nurs.* 2008;29(3):176–185.

De Jonge KE, Jamshed N, Gilden D, et al. Effects of home-based primary care on Medicare costs in high-risk elders. *J Am Geriatr Soc.* 2014;62:1825–1831.

Flood KL, Booth K, Vickers J, et al. Acute Care for Elders (ACE) team model of care: a clinical overview. *Geriatrics (Basel).* 2018;3(3):50.

Friedman SM, Mendelson DA, Kates SL, et al. Geriatric co-management of proximal femur fractures: total quality management and protocol-driven care result in better outcomes for a frail patient population. *J Am Geriatr Soc.* 2008;56:1349–1356.

Fulmer T, Mate KS, Berman A. The age-friendly health system imperative. *J Am Geriatr Soc.* 2018;66:22–24.

Fulmer T, Patel P, Levy N, et al. Moving toward a global age-friendly ecosystem. *J Am Geriatr Soc.* 2020;68:1936–1940.

Ganz DA, Latham NK. Prevention of falls in community-dwelling older adults. *N Engl J Med.* 2020;382(8):734–743.

Gill TM, McGloin JM, Shelton A, et al. Optimizing retention in a pragmatic trial of community-living older persons: the STRIDE Study. *J Am Geriatr Soc.* 2020;68:1242–1249.

GRACE. http://graceteamcare.indiana.edu/home.html.

Hastings N, Sloane R, Morey MC, et al. Assisted early mobility for hospitalized older veterans: preliminary data from the STRIDE Program. *J Am Geriatr Soc.* 2014;62:2180–2184.

Hastings SN, Choate AL, Mahanna EP, et al. Early mobility in the hospital: lessons learned from the STRIDE Program. *Geriatrics* 2018;3:61.

Hospital at Home. http://www.hospitalathome.org/about-us/history.php.

Hung WW, Macias Tejada, Soryal S, et al. The Acute Care for Elders Consult Program. In: Malone ML, Capezuti EA, Palmer RM, eds. *Geriatric Models of Care: Bringing 'Best Practice' to an Aging America.* Switzerland: Springer International Publishing; 2015:39-49.

Hung WW, Ross JS, Farber J, Siu AL. Evaluation of the mobile acute care of the elderly (MACE) service. *JAMA.* 2013;173:990–996.

Independence at Home. http://innovation.cms.gov/initiatives/independence-at-home/.

Jennings LA, Laffan AM, Schlissel AC, et al. Health care utilization and cost outcomes of a comprehensive dementia care program for Medicare beneficiaries. *JAMA Intern Med.* 2019;179(2):161–166.

Jennings LA, Tan Z, Wengner NS, et al. Quality of care provided by a comprehensive dementia care comanagement program. *J Am Geriatr Soc.* 2016;64:1724-1730.

Landefeld CS, Palmer RM, Kresevic DM, et al. Randomized trial of care in a hospital medical unit especially designed to improve the functional outcomes of acutely ill older patients. *N Engl J Med.* 1995;332:1338–1344.

Leff B, Burton L, Mader SL, et al. Hospital at Home: feasibility and outcomes of a program to provide hospital-level care at home for acutely ill older patients. *Ann Intern Med.* 2005;143:798–808.

Malone ML, Vollbrecht M, Stephenson J, et al. Acute care for elders (ACE) tracker and e-geriatrician: methods to disseminate ACE concepts to hospitals with no geriatricians on staff. *J Am Geriatr Soc.* 2000;58:161–167.

McDonald SR, Heflin MT, Whitson HE, et al. Association of integrated care coordination with postsurgical outcomes in high-risk older adults: The Perioperative Optimization of Senior Health (POSH) Initiative. *JAMA Surg.* 2018;153(5):454–462.

Morey MC, Lee CC, Castle S, et al. Should structured exercise be promoted as a model of care? Dissemination of the Department of Veterans Affairs Gerofit Program. *J Am Geriatr Soc.* 2018;66:1009–1016.

Naylor MD, Brooten D, Campbell R, et al. Comprehensive discharge planning and home follow-up of hospitalized elders: a randomized clinical trial. *JAMA.* 1999;281:613–620.

PACE. http://www.npaonline.org/website/article.asp?id=12&title=Who,_What_and_Where_Is_PACE?

Reuben DB, Ganz DA, Roth CP, et al. Effect of a nurse practitioner comanagement on the care of geriatric conditions. *J Am Geriatr Soc.* 2013;61:857–867.

Reuben DB, Tan ZS, Romero T, et al. Patient and caregiver benefit from a comprehensive dementia care program: 1-year results from the UCLA Alzheimer's and Dementia Care Program. *J Am Geriatr Soc.* 2019;67:2267–2273.

Rotenberg J, Kinosian B, Boling P, et al. Home-based primary care: beyond extension of the independence at home demonstration. *J Am Geriatr Soc.* 2018;66:812–817.

Rubin FH, Bellon J, Bilderback A, et al. Effect of the Hospital Elder Life Program on risk of 30-day readmission. *J Am Geriatr Soc.* 2018;66:145–149.

Schubert CC, Parks R, Coffing JM, et al. Lessons and outcomes of mobile acute care for elders consultation in a Veterans Affairs Medical Center. *J Am Geriatr Soc.* 2019;67:818–824.

Simpson M, Macias Tejada J, Driscoll A, et al. The Bundled Hospital Elder Life Program—HELP and HELP in Home Care—and its association with clinical outcomes among older adults discharged to home healthcare. *J Am Geriatr Soc.* 2019;67:1730–1736.

Sinvani L, Goldin M, Roofeh R, et al. Implementation of hip fracture co-management program (AGS CoCare: Ortho®) in a large health system. *J Am Geriatr Soc.* 2020;68:1706–1713.

Smith PD, Boyd C, Bellantoni J, et al. Communication between office-based primary care providers and nurses working within patients' homes: an analysis of process data from CAPABLE. *J Clin Nurs.* 2016;25(3–4):454–462.

Spoelstra SL, Sikorskii A, Gitlin LN, et al. Dissemination of the CAPABLE Model of Care in a Medicaid Waiver program to improve physical function. *J Am Geriatr Soc.* 2019;67:363–370.

Summary of the Updated American Geriatrics Society/British Geriatrics Society Clinical Practice Guideline for Prevention of Falls in Older Persons. *J Am Geriatr Soc.* 2011;59:148–157.

Szanton SL, Thorpe RJ, Boyd C, et al. Community aging in place, advancing better living for elders: a bio-behavioral-environmental intervention to improve function and health-related quality of life in disabled older adults. *J Am Geriatr Soc.* 2011;59:2314–2320.

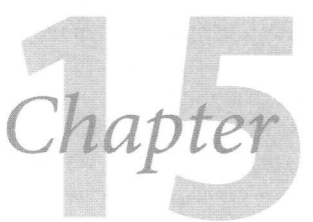

Chapter 15

Emergency Department Care

Christopher R. Carpenter, Ula Hwang

As populations worldwide age, older adults seek emergency care with increasing frequency. Based on current population projections in the United States, the number of individuals over age 65 will more than double while those over age 85 will triple by 2060. Emergency departments (EDs) already functioning as society's health care safety net will evaluate and disposition more complex older adults than in prior decades, often serving as the front porch of the hospital with expectations to cost-effectively manage admission rates and maintain patient flow. Unfortunately, the rapid evaluation model of emergency medicine that generally serves younger populations efficiently (**Figure 15-1A**), is an ineffective model for geriatric emergency care (**Figure 15-1B**). Recognizing this demographic shift, emergency medicine and geriatric professional societies responded over the past decade with core competencies for emergency medicine residency trainees, clinical practice guidelines, and pragmatic quality indicators.

The aforementioned Geriatric Emergency Department Guidelines, endorsed by the American College of Emergency Physicians (ACEP), American Geriatrics Society, and Society for Academic Emergency Medicine in 2013, provided the requisite framework for ACEP's Geriatric Emergency Department Accreditation (GEDA) program that launched in 2018 and has accredited nearly 300 EDs worldwide (https://www.acep.org/geda/). In order to attain accreditation, hospitals (not just EDs) must demonstrate a commitment to focused geriatric care processes via quality improvement efforts and their associated metrics that often require transdisciplinary coordination between geriatrics, emergency medicine, physiotherapy, nutrition services, hospitalists, primary care teams, and outpatient services. In addition, the Geriatric Emergency Department Collaborative (GEDC) arose to provide a transdisciplinary learning network of geriatric ED teams to share innovative ideas, solutions, and common lessons around the cost-effective improvement of older adult emergency care (https://gedcollaborative.com/). Internationally, the Silver Book II synthesizes best practices for the acute care of frail older adults from a multidisciplinary perspective. This chapter will review components of the Geriatric Emergency Department Guidelines and Silver Book II, as well as facilitators and barriers to widespread implementation of these guidelines.

Learning Objectives

- Geriatric emergency medicine has emerged internationally as a subspecialty with fellowship training, resident core competencies, guidelines, and research priorities for patient-centered transdisciplinary care.

- Resources such as the Geriatric Emergency Department Collaborative exist to share innovations around older adult-appropriate health care during times of emergency.

- The components of age-friendly emergency care include infrastructural modifications and protocols focused on geriatric syndromes such as delirium, dementia, and falls.

- While some geriatric screening such as vulnerability assessment currently lacks acceptable accuracy or obvious actionable next steps, a pragmatic approach emphasizes continued assessment for common older adult syndromes while concurrently ongoing research strives to improve prognostic accuracy and efficacy.

Key Clinical Points

1. Delirium, predominantly hypoactive delirium, is frequently encountered in geriatric emergency care, and multiple screening instruments for this cognitive disorder have been validated in emergency department (ED) settings.

2. Possible dementia frequently coexists with delirium, but is also identified without delirium in up to one-third of older adults when evaluated in the ED using valid screening instruments.

3. Elder abuse is a hidden epidemic impacting up to 10% of older adults in the ED—but usually unrecognized without coordinated communication between social work, nursing, physicians, and law enforcement.

4. Falls and injurious falls are a threat to many older adults following an episode

(Continued)

(Cont.)

of emergency care, and effective fall prevention requires coordination between emergency medicine, physiotherapy, pharmacology, home health, and primary care.

5. Multiple measures exist to predict post-ED vulnerability to adverse outcomes, such as preventable returns or functional decline, but currently lack sufficient accuracy to identify either high-risk or low-risk subsets.

INFRASTRUCTURE, STAFFING, AND TRAINING

The concept of an ED specializing in older adult processes and outcomes of care was first broached in 2007. Adapting the physical environment to a more geriatric-friendly space was noted at that time (**Table 15-1**). Improving the ED infrastructure alone, however, is inadequate to optimize older adult health care delivery and outcomes. Geriatric-focused continuing medical education, appropriate staffing, and protocols aligned with local resource availability are more important than the physical space in which emergency care occurs. Education and protocols should focus on the detection, prevention, or management of geriatric syndromes that frequently present to the ED (**Table 15-2**). Continuing medical education that uses the case of an octogenarian acute myocardial infarction or cerebrovascular accident to highlight the latest pharmaceutical or biomedical device is not considered geriatric in this context. Essential components of older adult-relevant medical education in the Geriatric Emergency Department Guidelines should incorporate the identification and management of aging-related syndromes such as delirium, falls, frailty, or polypharmacy in the setting of emergency care. Similarly, for ACEP's GEDA program, a general hospital-wide policy to reduce unnecessary urinary catheters regardless of age would not necessarily be considered a geriatric-emergency medicine focused protocol unless adapted to evaluate measures in **Table 15-2**. GEDA emphasizes an interdisciplinary staffing approach corresponding to the specific quality improvement efforts. If those efforts include reducing polypharmacy to promote medication safety then including a pharmacist in the ED (or readily available to the ED round-the-clock) with geriatric medication safety expertise or interest is encouraged. Because the ED will continue to be a societal safety net for all populations, geriatric-centered care, design, staffing, and continuing medical education may differ from that used in clinic settings or hospital wards.

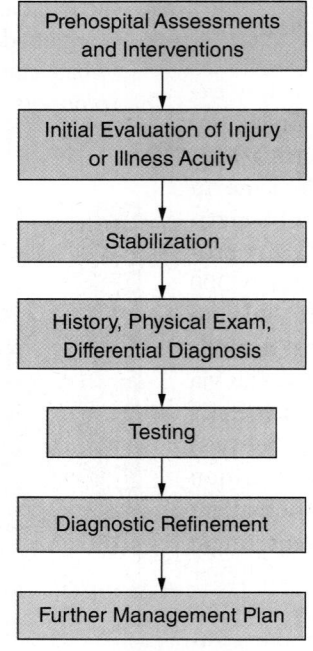

Settings Where Processes Occur

Green = Home, Clinic, Accident-Scene or Nursing Home Environment
Blue = Waiting Room or Triage station
Red = ED Patient Room or Hallway
Purple = Observation Unit, Inpatient or Outpatient Setting

A

FIGURE 15-1. (**A**) Traditional emergency medicine management pathway. (**B**) Geriatric emergency care model.

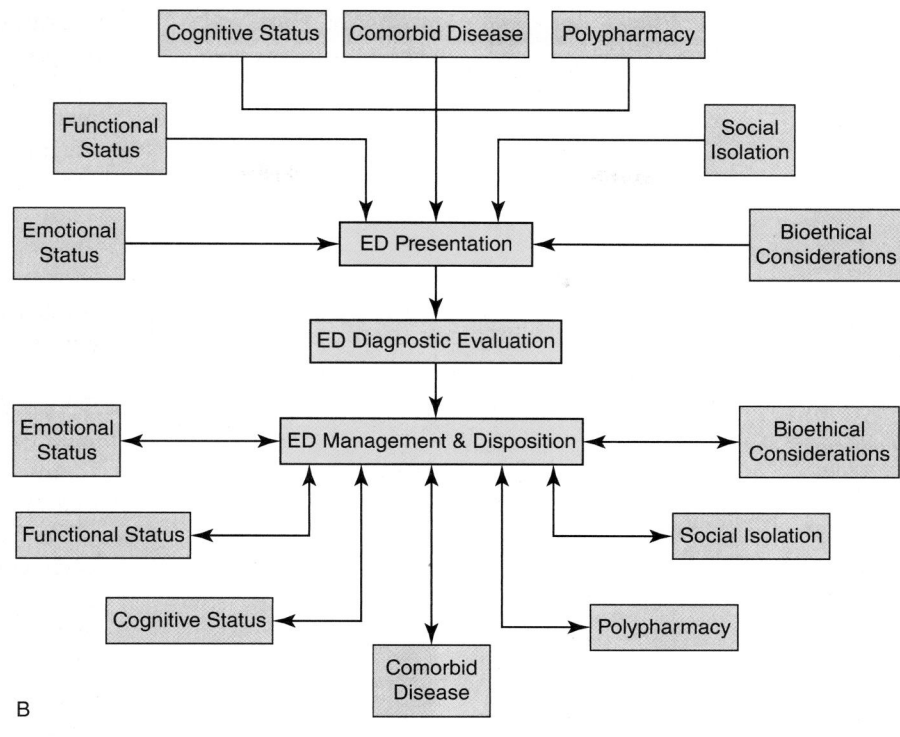

B

FIGURE 15-1. (Continued)

DELIRIUM

A range of 6% to 38% of ED adults over age 65 present with (prevalent delirium) or develop (incident delirium) delirium. Hypoactive delirium is more common than hyperactive delirium, yet has been identified by ED nurses and physicians far less frequently. Delirium is a transient symptom precipitated by an acute stressor or physiological insult, but is associated with an increased hospital length of stay, cognitive and functional decline, and post-hospital depression. Common precipitating factors are summarized in **Table 15-3**. ED nurse or physician judgment alone is inadequate to identify delirium accurately, so over 20 delirium screening instruments have been evaluated in this setting. Although the Confusion Assessment Method has been studied more frequently, the brief Confusion Assessment Method (bCAM), Richmond Agitation Sedation Scale, and the 4AT more favorably balance brevity, accuracy, and emergency provider acceptability (**Figure 15-2**). Since delirium is a symptom of an underlying physiological stressor, geriatric emergency care should

TABLE 15-1 ■ GERIATRIC EMERGENCY DEPARTMENT INFRASTRUCTURE

MODIFICATION	OBJECTIVE
Soundproof curtains	Diminish delirium risk by minimizing ambient noise
Hearing assist devices	Improve communication if hearing impaired
Reclining chairs or padded stretchers	Enhance comfort, reduce pressure ulcers and incident delirium
Large faced clocks and signage, boards with hospital staff names	Optimize patient orientation to reduce anxiety and delirium
Non-skid floors, hallway handrails, aisle lighting, commode	Reduce risk of falls
Sky light or diurnal lighting changes	Facilitate sleep cycles and reduce delirium risk

TABLE 15-2 ■ GERIATRIC EMERGENCY DEPARTMENT SYNDROME

GERIATRIC SYNDROME	SAMPLE POLICY/PROTOCOL
Delirium	Identification of delirium risk, prevalent or incident delirium
Dementia	Recognize dementia and caregiver capacity, link to resources
Elder abuse	Pattern recognition for many forms of abuse or neglect
Falls	Link high-risk fallers to available prevention resources
Frailty	Document physiological reserve visit-to-visit
Polypharmacy/ medication safety	Evaluate risk/benefit of medications and interactions
Vulnerability	Screen for increased risk of short-term returns, functional decline

TABLE 15-3 ■ RISK FACTORS FOR DELIRIUM

PATIENT VULNERABILITY

Demographic (advanced age, education attained, male)

Comorbid illness (dementia, depression, renal insufficiency, cirrhosis, terminal illness)

Functional issues (restricted ADLs, immobility)

Pharmacological (alcohol or substance abuse, polypharmacy, psychoactive medication use)

Sensory (hearing or visual impairment)

Dietary (dehydration, malnutrition)

PHYSIOLOGICAL STRESSORS

Systematic (infection, oligoanalgesia, hypo- or hyperthermia)

Central nervous system (cerebrovascular accident, intracranial hemorrhage, meningitis or encephalitis, seizure, mass)

Medication changes, drug use or withdrawal

Metabolic (sodium or calcium disorders, thyroid dysfunction, acute hepatic or renal failure)

Cardiopulmonary (acute coronary syndrome, congestive heart failure, hypoxia, hypercarbia, hypertensive encephalopathy, shock)

Other (serotonergic syndrome, paraneoplastic, anti-N-methyl-D-aspartate (NMDA) encephalitis

Data from Han JH, Suyama J. Delirium and dementia. Clin Geriatr Med. 2018;34(3):327–354.

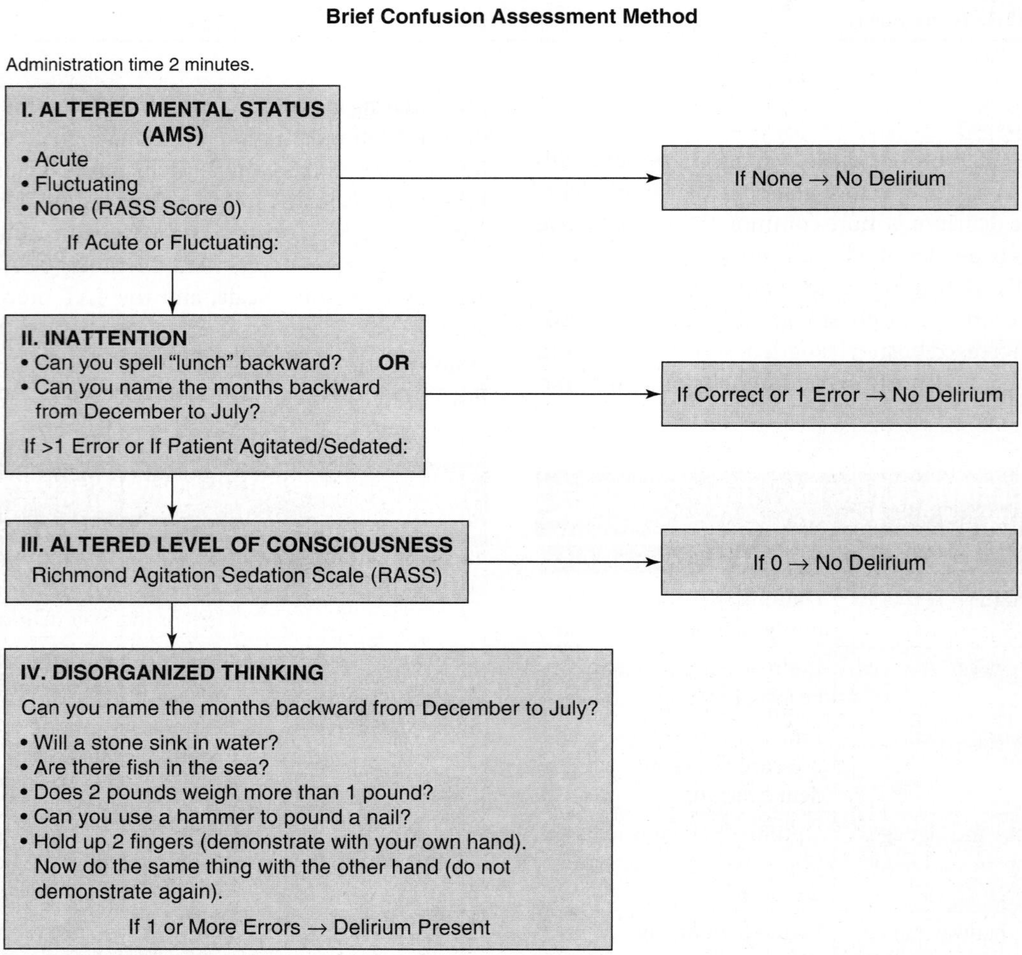

FIGURE 15-2. Delirium screening instruments in the emergency department (ED).

CIRCLE

[1] ALERTNESS
This includes patients who may be markedly drowsy (eg, difficult to rouse and/or obviously sleepy during assessment) or agitated/hyperactive. Observe the patient. If asleep, attempt to wake with speech or gentle touch on shoulder. Ask the patient to state their name and address to assist rating.

Normal (fully alert, but not agitated, throughout assessment)	0
Mild sleepiness for < 10 seconds after waking, then normal	0
Clearly abnormal	4

[2] AMT4
Age, date of birth, place (name of the hospital or building), current year.

No mistakes	0
1 mistake	1
2 or more mistakes/untestable	2

[3] ATTENTION
Ask the patient: "Please tell me the months of the year in backward order, starting at December."
To assist initial understanding, one prompt of "What is the month before December?" is permitted.

Months of the year backward Achieves 7 months or more correctly	0
Starts but scores < 7 months/refuses to start	1
Untestable (cannot start because unwell, drowsy, inattentive)	2

[4] ACUTE CHANGE OR FLUCTUATING COURSE
Evidence of significant change or fluctuation in: alertness, cognition, or other mental function (eg, paranoia, hallucinations) arising over the past 2 weeks and still evident in past 24 hours.

No	0
Yes	4

4 or above:	Possible delirium ± cognitive impairment
1–3:	Possible cognitive impairment
0:	Delirium or cognitive impairment unlikely (but delirium still possible if [4] information incomplete)

Administration time 1–2 minutes.

Richmond Agitation Sedation Scale (RASS)

+3	**Very agitated**	= pulls or removes tube(s) or catheter(s); aggressive.
+2	**Agitated**	= frequent nonpurposeful movement, fights ventilator.
+1	**Restless**	= anxious but movements not aggressive or vigorous.
0	**Alert & calm**	= no issues, all appearances and interactions appear normal.
–1	**Drowsy**	= not alert, but awake; eye opening/voice contact is > 10 seconds.
–2	**Light sedation**	= briefly awakens with eye contact to voice (< 10 seconds).
–3	**Moderate sedation**	= movement or eye opening to voice (but no eye contact).
–4	**Deep sedation**	= no response to voice, but moves/opens eyes to physical stimulation.
–5	**Unarousable**	= no response to voice or physical stimulation.

Score other than 0 = Delirium.   Administration time 30–60 seconds

FIGURE 15-2. (Continued)

try to identify the precipitant(s) of delirium (**Table 15-3**). Accurately identifying and treating the cause of delirium will require collaboration with inpatient services because patients with delirium who are discharged home without treating the delirium will return to the ED.

At least three pragmatic barriers exist to improving the detection, prevention, and management of delirium in the ED. First, simply publishing research or synthesizing recommendations into guidelines will not modify clinician behavior. Implementation Science or local quality improvement efforts are required, which is the rationale for GEDA and GEDC to

catalyze uptake of these principles. Second, even if ED teams incorporate one or more of the delirium screening instruments into routine practice, hospital providers often use different delirium detection tools and are unfamiliar with those used in emergency settings. Unfamiliarity breeds skepticism, which impedes efficient communication and harmonization of efforts to align diagnostic testing priorities, disposition decisions, and immediate management steps. Incorporating instruments used in non-emergency medicine settings may reduce reliability and/or accuracy. While awaiting research to harmonize dissimilar screening tools, clinicians should proactively communicate about delirium concerns and management with other health care teams and settings. Third and perhaps the most challenging scant proof-of-concept currently exists to guide actionable next steps for the prevention or treatment of delirium in the ED. While diurnal lighting and frequent reorientation described in **Table 15-2** seem appropriate, these strategies remain untested in ED or geriatric ED settings. Whether pharmacologic or nonpharmacologic strategies can reduce the incidence, duration, or severity of delirium remains to be proven.

DEMENTIA

Delirium and dementia frequently overlap in older adults in ED settings. When delirium is excluded as the cause of cognitive dysfunction in older ED patients, approximately 31% of all patients over age 65 still have a concern for cognitive dysfunction, specifically dementia. Whether recognized or not, ED patients with dementia (or possible dementia as many lack additional neuropsychiatric evaluation in the weeks to months after an episode of emergency care), this non-delirium cognitive dysfunction is associated with prolonged length of stay, fall risk, admission rates, return visits and readmissions, and patient/care partner dissatisfaction with the care provided. When features concerning for dementia are missed in ED settings, inpatient services also frequently miss subtle findings and opportunities to improve care transitions are neglected.

While eight dementia screening instruments have been evaluated in ED settings, those that balance brevity and accuracy are favored by clinicians, including the Abbreviated Mental Test (AMT-4), Ottawa 3DY (O3DY), and caregiver-administered Alzheimer's Disease-8 (cAD8) summarized in **Figure 15-3**. The cAD8 has the advantage

---

Caregiver AD8

If the patient has an accompanying reliable informant, they are asked the following questions.

Has this patient displayed any of the following issues? Remember a "Yes" response indicates that you think there has been **a change in the last several years** caused by thinking and memory (cognitive) problems.

1) Problems with judgment (example, falls for scams, bad financial decisions, buys gifts inappropriate for recipients)?
2) Reduced interest in hobbies/activities?
3) Repeats questions, stories, or statements?
4) Trouble learning how to use a tool, appliance, or gadget (VCR, computer, microwave, remote control)?
5) Forgets correct month or year?
6) Difficulty handling complicated financial affairs (for example, balancing check book, income taxes, paying bills)?
7) Difficulty remembering appointments?
8) Consistent problems with thinking and/or memory?

Each affirmative response is 1 point. A score of ≥ 2 is considered high risk for dementia.

Abbreviated Mental Test-4

1) How old are you?
2) What is your birthday?
3) What is the name of this place?
4) What year is this?

Any error is considered high-risk for dementia.

Ottawa 3DY

1) What day is today?	**Correct**	**Incorrect**
2) What is the date?	**Correct**	**Incorrect**
3) Spell "world" backward	Number correct	

0	1	2	3	4	5

4) What year is this?	**Correct**	**Incorrect**

A single incorrect response on any of these four items is consistent with dementia.

FIGURE 15-3. Emergency department (ED) dementia screening instruments.

of not relying upon an available, communicative, or cooperative patient in the ED where patients are often undergoing various tests and consultant evaluations. In addition, whereas AMT-4, O3DY, and most other dementia screening instruments often yield false-negative findings for more highly educated individuals, the cAD8 does not because it employs a knowledgeable care partner to report a cognitive change from baseline rather than a memory or performance test of the patient.

The recognition of possible dementia in an older ED patient affects clinical decision-making. While dementia may not be viewed as a medical emergency, the psychosocial model depicted in **Figure 15-1B** necessitates that effective geriatric emergency care contemplate cognitive capacity. If otherwise medically stabilized, is this patient safe to be discharged? Does the patient understand the discharge instructions, medications prescribed or deprescribed, and follow-up plan? Will the patient remember those factors after discharge? Although reflexive hospital admission is probably not the appropriate management option, transitions of care must be adapted for patients with suspected cognitive dysfunction.

Pragmatic and unanswered barriers exist to widespread dementia screening for older adults in the ED. First, these screening tools are not diagnostic for dementia. Most have positive likelihood ratios ranging from 1 to 4 and negative likelihood ratios from 0.17 to 0.39 when defining "dementia" using imperfect criterion standards such as the Mini Mental Status Exam. Clinicians and diagnosticians need to balance the theoretical value of non-delirium cognitive dysfunction screening against the possible harm of eliciting preventable anxiety for patients and families around the diagnosis of dementia. Second, inpatient and outpatient providers may be unfamiliar with ED dementia screening instruments, which can impede efficient between-clinician communication. Third and similar to delirium screening, the "so what?" implications of dementia screening remain poorly defined. Since dementia is incurable, screening has no direct therapeutic response for ED teams and dementia screening alone does not identify a cohort more likely to benefit from admission. Additionally, the impact of dementia screening on patient and family satisfaction ratings is uncertain and the cost of training/maintaining ED staff to evaluate for dementia and provide follow-up resources to higher risk individuals remains undefined.

ELDER ABUSE

Abuse of the older adult can take many forms, including physical or psychological harms, financial exploitation, or neglect. Although up to 10% of older adults in the United States experience some form of abuse each year, as few as 1 in 14 cases are reported. Screening for elder abuse in ED settings is frequently fraught with challenges, including a paucity of research to guide screening protocols and

effective interventions as well as the ethical quandary of patient denial motivated by fear of retribution by the perpetrator. Nonetheless, the clinical and forensic science of detecting and preventing elder abuse continues to evolve. The Senior Aid Tool (**Figure 15-4**) is a sensitive and reasonably specific screening instrument for elder abuse, but awaits external validation, feasibility assessment, and impact analysis demonstrating benefits beyond improved detection rates.

Preventing elder abuse requires a team-based approach that begins in the pre-hospital environment and continues through the ED into the post-ED setting with coordinated communication between social work, nursing, physicians, and law enforcement. Some hospitals have established "Vulnerable Elder Protection Teams" to standardize and coordinate the detection, comprehensive evaluation, and treatment for potential victims of elder abuse. ED elder abuse experts recommend simplifying data collection forms that include photographic evidence of visible injuries as well as documented and coordinated communication with radiologists when common injury patterns appear.

FALLS

Individuals over age 65 comprise one-fourth of trauma admissions with ground-level falls becoming an increasing proportion of those cases as populations age. Among community-dwelling older adults over age 65, one-third experience a fall each year, which increases, to 50% for those over age 80. An ED evaluation for a fall is often the only medical contact these patients have and an opportunity to prevent future fall injuries. Yet 36% to 50% of these patients experience a recurrent fall, ED revisit, or death within 1 year of an initial fall.

ED nurses and physicians acknowledge a role in proactively preventing future fall injuries for frail older adults, but cite pragmatic barriers to routine fall prevention secondary to inadequate training around risk stratification, insufficient emergency medicine-specific fall assessment tools, and uncertain access to downstream fall prevention resources. Part of the problem is that falls are often complex and multifactorial with predisposing fall risks (**Figure 15-5A**), diminished physiological factors to avoid fall injuries (**Figure 15-5B**), and an increased risk of injuries from ground-level falls (**Figure 15-5C**). Furthermore, there is no widely accepted post-ED fall risk assessment instrument. Another barrier to routine fall prevention initiatives is the perception of therapeutic nihilism since complex and individualized interventions often fail to reduce fall-related injuries. For example, the Strategies to Reduce Injuries and Develop Confidence in Elders pragmatic randomized controlled trial utilized risk assessments to formulate individualized fall prevention interventions, yet failed to effectively prevent the first injurious fall. Similarly, an ED-based randomized controlled trial to deprescribe

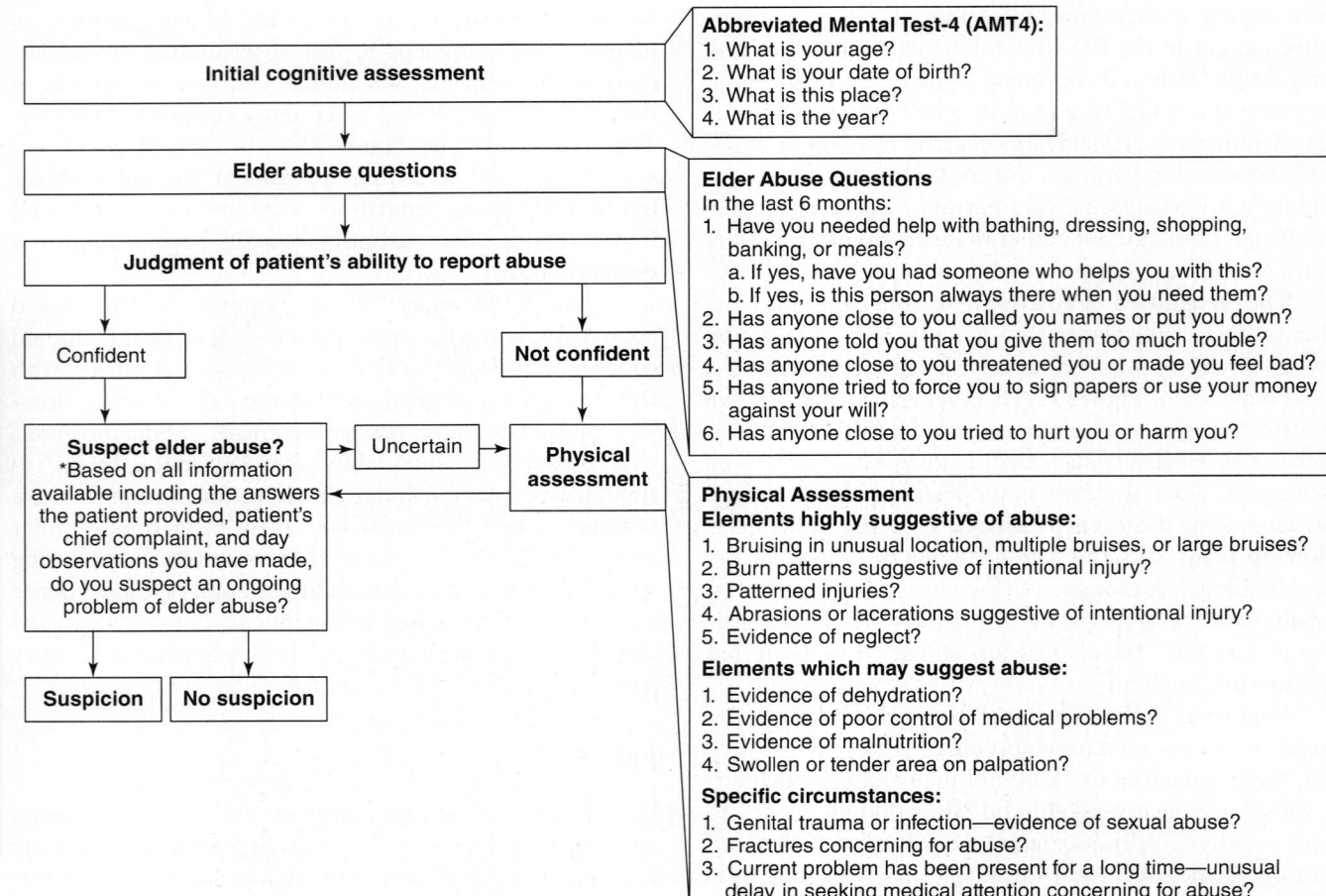

FIGURE 15-4. Emergency department (ED) Senior Aid Tool to screen for elder abuse.

medications associated with increased fall risk did not reduce falls at 1 year. However, another academic ED protocol that incorporated physical therapy and pharmacy to formulate a brief and individualized intervention during a visit for a fall reduced both overall and fall-related revisits at 6 months. Feasible approaches for ED initiated secondary falls prevention undoubtedly require a local champion, transdisciplinary coordination, and accessible resources to promote patient cooperation (**Figure 15-6**).

Figure 15-6 illustrates the real-world settings of falls prevention research moving forward: the outpatient clinic, the ED, the homes of older patients, the practice sites of nurse case managers and physical therapists, and the community. Identifying effective falls prevention strategies in post-STRIDE research necessitates a multipronged approach incorporating Implementation Science principles and an evolving understanding of impactful shared decision-making. Transdisciplinary alignment and harmonization of fall-related definitions, screening instruments, and outcome measures while catalyzing impactful change can promote healthy skepticism while avoiding therapeutic nihilism and advance patient-centric falls prevention. Rapidly learning

health systems can integrate incremental improvements from multiple settings to improve their research and clinical practice.

VULNERABILITY AND FRAILTY

As the proportion of older adults presenting to EDs increases in coming decades, health care systems will seek screening processes to identify subsets more or less likely to experience preventable short-term adverse outcomes, such as return visits, functional decline, institutionalization, or death. Many instruments exist to quantify such "vulnerability" (**Table 15-4**), but currently none accurately identifies either a high-risk or low-risk subset. Reasons underlying inadequate accuracy of these instruments include between-study variability in processes, definitions, interventions, outcomes, and objectives. One approach to align finite resources with populations most likely to benefit is depicted in **Figure 15-7**. Researchers continue efforts to derive more accurate instruments, while clinicians focus low intensity and widely available interventions on commonly harmful scenarios such as falls and delirium as previously discussed.

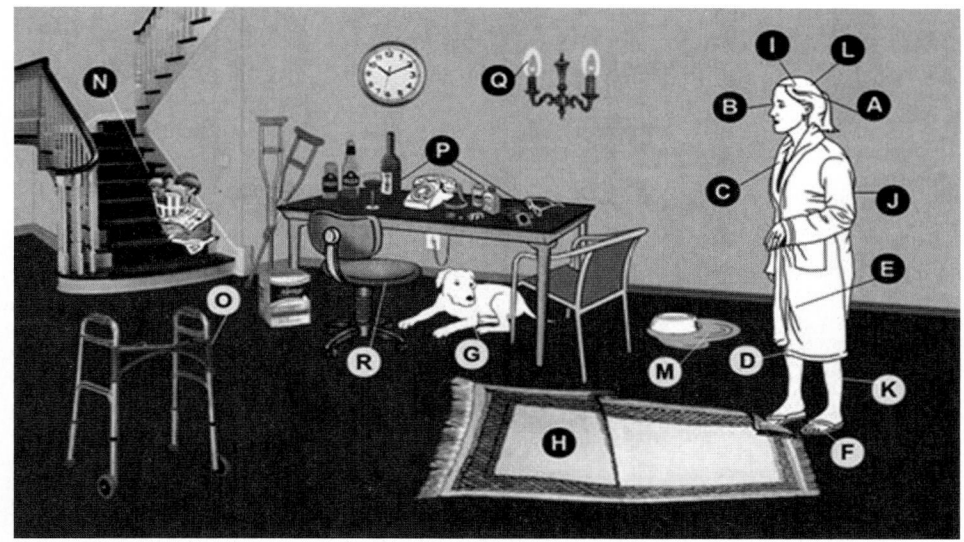

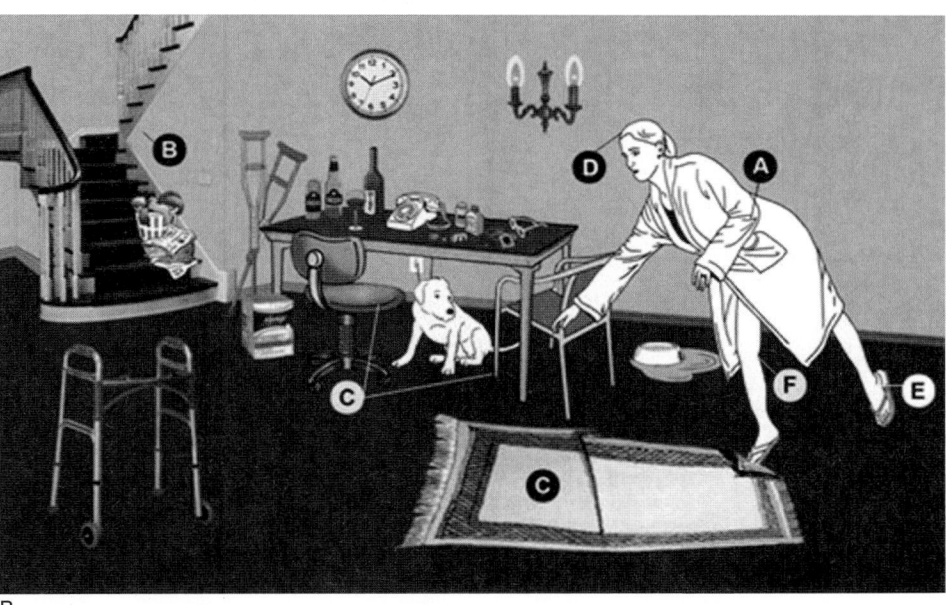

FIGURE 15-5. Understanding geriatric fall risks and factors related to injurious falls. **Figure 15-5A** depicts the older adult prior to a fall and illustrates the intrinsic (physiological attributes of the individual) and extrinsic (environmental surroundings) that can be related to a fall. Some of these factors are evidence-based from epidemiological studies (denoted with "*"), while others are recognized by the clinician authors of this review. These risk factors include (A) disequilibrium*, (B) visual deficits, (C) dysrhythmia, orthostatic hypotension, (D) degenerative joint disease and rheumatic disease*, (E) loose fitting clothing, (F) poorly fitting footwear or foot sores, (G) pets, (H) rugs or loose mats, (I) dementia, Parkinson disease*, (J) malnutrition, (K) deconditioning, frailty, muscle wasting, (l) preexisting stroke or other motor deficit*, (m) slippery surface, (N) stairs, (O) walker or crutches, (P) medications (sedatives)*, alcohol, (R) inadequate lighting, (S) transfers from sitting to standing, and (T) urinary incontinence*. **Figure 15-5B** depicts intrinsic and extrinsic factors that render older adults more likely to suffer a fall than a near-fall. Whereas younger populations sometimes suffer near-falls, they rarely fall to the ground and when they do the kinetic energy of the fall is usually disrupted by a variety of adaptive protection responses that are slowed, diminished, or absent in frail elderly persons. These factors include (A) impaired reflexes to ease fall, (B) lack of handrails, (C) cluttered furniture, (D) diminished awareness of falling, (E) impaired proprioception, and (F) diminished core body strength. **Figure 15-5C** illustrates the physiological, pharmacological, anatomical, and environmental factors that increase the probability of the primary fall injury severity for the mechanism and energy of a fall becoming more pronounced and for secondary injuries to ensue. These factors include (A) osteoporosis = fractures with minor trauma, (B) spinal cord stenosis and cervical spine degenerative disc disease = spinal cord contusion (anterior cord syndrome), (C) cerebral wasting = subdural hematoma, (D) medications (anticoagulants, antiplatelet agents) = increased risk of intracranial (and other) bleeding, (E) muscle wasting = inability to rise and "long lies," (F) diminished body fat/ padding = more force to brittle bones, and (G) frail skin = tears and lacerations. (Reproduced with permission from Michael L. Malone, Christopher Carpenter. Graphic artist: Brian Miller. Aurora Health Care. Copyright 2017.)

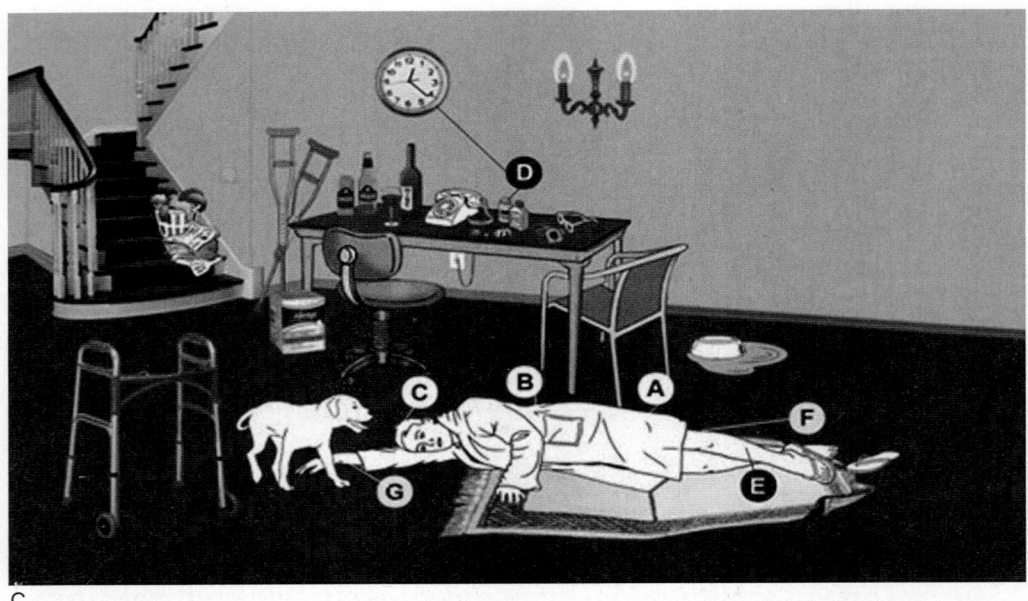

C

FIGURE 15-5. (Continued)

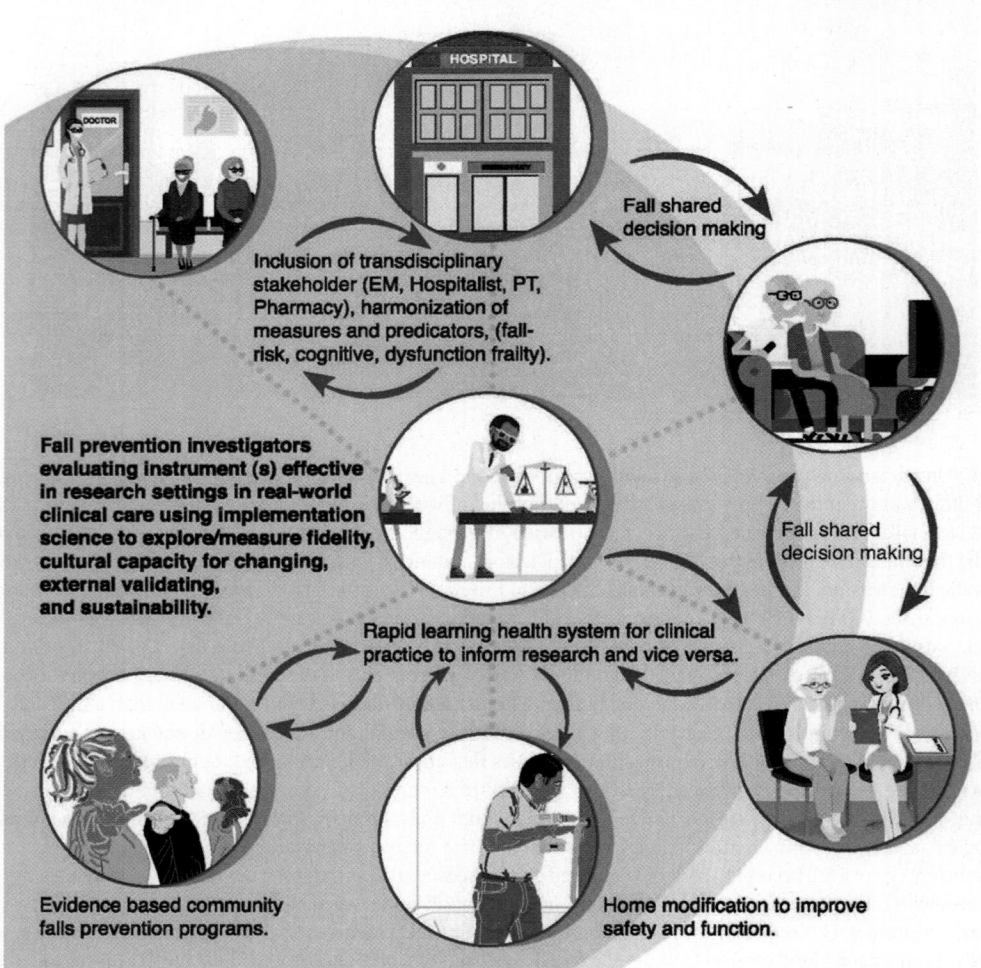

FIGURE 15-6. Transdisciplinary approach to falls prevention.

TABLE 15-4 ■ CURRENT STATE OF GERIATRIC ED "VULNERABILITY" INSTRUMENTS

INSTRUMENT	YEAR DERIVED	LANGUAGES EVALUATED	PUBLISHED ACCURACY STUDIES	OUTCOMES PREDICTED	LR+ RANGE	LR– RANGE
Pro-Age	2020	English	1	Hospitalization, prolonged length of stay, in-hospital mortality	2.4	0.39
Clinical Frailty Scale	2020	English, German	1	**30-day** mortality, ICU admission, hospitalization	NR	NR
APOP	2018	Dutch	1	**90-day** functional decline or mortality	3.3	0.71
interRAI	2017	English, French Flemish, German, Icelandic, Portuguese	1	**30-day** readmission **90-day** readmission	1.1 1.1	0.63 0.68
ISAR	1999	English, Spanish, Flemish	20	**30-day** ED returns Decline Readmission **90-day** ED returns Decline Readmission	 0.67–1.52 1.09–1.45 0.86–1.18 0.84–1.34 1.15–1.30 1.04–1.30	 0.13–1.47 0.45–0.62 0.38–1.32 0.49–1.47 0.41–0.73 0.24–0.92
Rowland	1990	English	1	**6-month** ED returns Readmission	 1.28 1.35	 0.94 0.93
Runciman	1996	English	1	**6-month** ED returns Readmission	 0.97 0.96	 1.19 1.28
Silver Code	2010	English	1	**6-month** ED returns Readmission	 1.15 1.19	 0.73 0.65
TRST	2003	English	14	**30-day** ED returns Decline Readmission **90-day** ED returns Decline Readmission	 1.25–1.51 1.11–1.58 0.94–1.57 1.01–1.23 0.94–1.58 1.16–1.22	 0.43–0.72 0.46–0.74 0.48–1.13 0.75–0.98 0.42–1.10 0.51–0.73
Variables Indicative of Placement	2008	English	4	**30-day** Decline Readmission	 1.11–3.55 0.93–1.12	 0.58–0.65 0.77–1.48

Frailty is an increased vulnerability to incomplete homeostasis after a physiological stressor. While early constructs of frailty failed to identify ED older adults at increased risk of preventable short-term adverse outcomes to the same extent as the instruments described in **Table 15-4**, the Clinical Frailty Scale appears to be a feasible, accurate, and reliable instrument to predict 30-day mortality. Whether the Clinical Frailty Scale can stratify older adults into higher or lower risk of return visits or functional decline, or if such identification can be linked to interventions that alter that trajectory, remains to be determined.

MEDICATION SAFETY

The ACEP Geriatric Emergency Department Guidelines and emergency medicine resident core curriculum both emphasize the importance of identifying and deprescribing high-risk medications primarily guided by Beers Criteria. However, Beers Criteria generally apply to the longer duration prescriptions provided in long-term care or outpatient clinic settings. The short time frame prescriptions commonly provided in the ED may represent a unique risk–benefit profile that remains relatively untested. Therefore, Beers Criteria are not unquestionably accepted

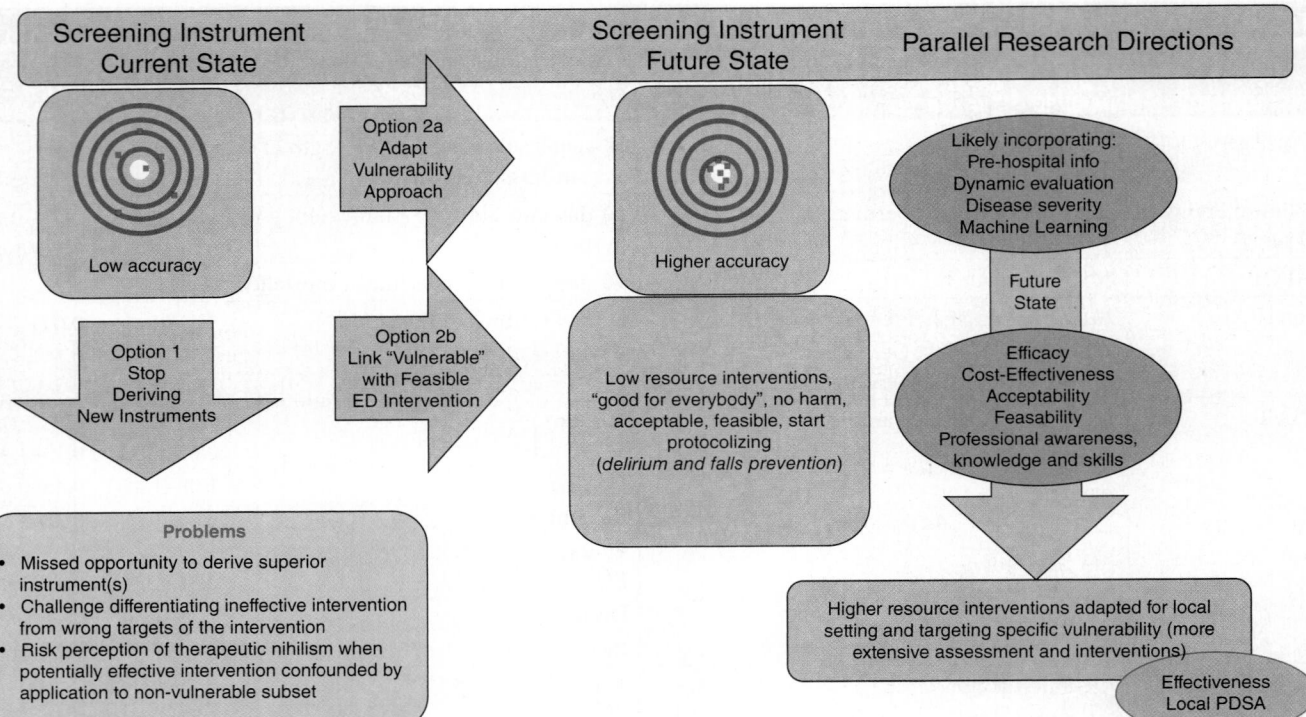

FIGURE 15-7. Approaches to advancing geriatric emergency department "vulnerability" screening research. Option 1, proposed by Heeren et al. would cease efforts to derive more accurate instruments than currently exist in order to focus on hybrid-effectiveness research. Alternatively, Option 2a would adapt prior methods to derive "vulnerability" instruments that incorporates pre-emergency department data, dynamic re-evaluations throughout emergency department episode of care, social and system factors, and current disease severity – perhaps using disruptive innovation such as machine learning. Option 2b could occur simultaneously with 2a, while responding to risk identified by current imperfect instruments with widely available and generally acceptable interventions. More labor-intensive interventions like Comprehensive Geriatric Assessment would be reserved for high-resource settings or clinical research like Plan-Do-Study-Act (PDSA) cycles.

as an indication of high-risk medications by ED teams. Nonetheless, Beers Criteria are frequently used in research and guidelines as one component of inappropriate medication prescribing for older adults. The Enhancing Quality of Provider Practices for Older Adults in the Emergency Department (EQUiPPED) protocol combines education with personal provider feedback and electronic clinical decision support to improve medication safety. Across four Veteran's Affairs hospitals, EQUiPPED demonstrated a significant and sustained reduction of potentially inappropriate medication prescribing at 1 year. EQUiPPED implementation kits for accelerated uptake of this medication safety initiative have also been developed in non-Veterans Affairs EDs.

Apart from these protocols, ED clinicians should be continuously aware of the potential of drugs to cause or exacerbate symptoms and interact with each other or with underlying diseases. In addition, many older adults are overtreated with hypoglycemic and antihypertensive medicine, which can result in ED visits. In these circumstances ED clinicians should initiate a deprescribing effort and communicate their findings and recommendations to the patient's physicians either through the patient or directly.

GERIATRIC EMERGENCY MEDICINE: THE NEAR FUTURE

As clinical researchers unravel the science of efficacious and cost-effective geriatric emergency care, others continue to expand the realm of possibilities with disruptive innovation. The original vision to enhance the process, experience, and outcomes of older adult emergency medicine depicted a dedicated location in the department distinct from sites where care for other populations occurred. Improving older adult emergency care need not rely upon a localized geriatric ED because many hospitals will lack the resources for this investment. Instead, alternative approaches include a geriatric observation unit, a focused practitioner model, or simply a site opinion leader to facilitate continuing medical education and local quality improvement initiatives. Adults over age 65 already represent over 30% of observation unit admissions, which is disproportionate to their overall ED volume. The observation unit can serve as another option to hospital admission by providing time to evaluate therapeutic response, obtain additional testing or consultations, and facilitate care transitions. The focused practitioner model can include a physician-led, trained geriatric emergency medicine (GEM) nurse or transitional care nurse, as well as lesser-trained personnel such as a "geriatric technician"–based volunteer model. In two observational studies across three academic hospitals, transitional care nurses reduced admission and readmission rates, but increased 72-hour returns. The GEM nurse model requires a significant investment in extra training and appears to increase geriatric syndrome screening rates. Establishing a qualified volunteer-based program in the ED requires an institutional commitment, continual onboarding and quality control processes, and a health care provider leader, but has been successfully implemented at two large academic centers with reasonable acceptance by nurses and physicians.

The twenty-first century technology revolution will inevitably affect geriatric emergency medicine as well. During the COVID-19 global pandemic when patients shunned EDs for fear of exposure to the life-threatening virus, telemedicine emerged as a viable alternative for acute care. Potential (and untested) applications of telemedicine for geriatric emergency care include evaluation of stable long-term care facility, rehabilitation unit, homebound, or rural patients who have a change in condition prior to transfer to an ED. This can be done in collaboration with the patient's primary care providers and/or paramedics. In addition, more resourced geriatric EDs with personnel available to screen for geriatric syndromes described in **Table 15-2** could remotely assess patients via telemedicine. Other emerging technologies that can catalyze improved geriatric emergency care without adding work for ED staff include pad-based screening for delirium and machine learning approaches to detect individuals at risk for dementia, delirium, falls, or other geriatric syndromes.

CONCLUSION

Sustainable and measurable geriatric emergency medicine advancement requires a village that extends beyond one specialty, discipline, or hospital locale. It must incorporate collaborative, transdisciplinary personnel and adapt around the infrastructure of the local ED to be successful. Ultimately, widely implementable improvements in the process, experience, or outcomes of geriatric emergency care must be cost-neutral and patient-centered. As clinical research expands around geriatric emergency medicine assessment accuracy and intervention effectiveness, guidelines and accreditation will continue to catalyze health care systems to engage in process redesign. Emergency care must become more adept at addressing the needs of an aging population and not allow perfection to impede necessary but incremental improvements.

FURTHER READING

Beach SR, Carpenter CR, Rosen T, Sharps P, Gelles R. Screening and detection of elder abuse: research opportunities and lessons learned from emergency geriatric care, intimate partner violence, and child abuse. *J Elder Abuse Negl.* 2016;28(4-5):185–216.

Berning MJ, Silva LOJE, Espinoza-Suarez N, et al. Interventions to improve older adults' emergency department patient experience: a systematic review. *Am J Emerg Med.* 2020;38(6):1257–1269.

Carpenter CR, Avidan MS, Wildes T, Stark S, Fowler SA, Lo AX. Predicting geriatric falls following an episode of emergency department care: a systematic review. *Acad Emerg Med.* 2014;21(10):1069–1082.

Carpenter CR, Banerjee J, Keyes D, et al. Accuracy of dementia screening instruments in emergency medicine: a diagnostic meta-analysis. *Acad Emerg Med.* 2019; 26(2):226–245.

Carpenter CR, Cameron A, Ganz DA, Liu S. Older adult falls in emergency medicine: 2019 update. *Clin Geriatr Med.* 2019;35(2):205–219.

Carpenter CR, Émond M. Pragmatic barriers to assessing post-emergency department vulnerability for poor outcomes in an ageing society. *Neth J Med.* 2016;74(8): 327–329.

Carpenter CR, Hammouda N, Linton EA, et al. Delirium prevention, detection, and treatment in emergency medicine settings: A Geriatric Emergency Care Applied Research (GEAR) Network Scoping Review and Consensus Statement. *Acad Emerg Med.* 2021;28(1):19–35.

Carpenter CR, Malone ML. Avoiding therapeutic nihilism for complex geriatric intervention 'negative' trials: STRIDE lessons. *J Am Geriatr Soc.* 2020;68(12): 2752–2756.

Carpenter CR, Mooijaart SP. Geriatric Screeners 2.0: time for a paradigm shift in emergency department vulnerability research. *J Am Geratr Soc.* 2020;68(7): 1402–1405.

Carpenter CR, Shelton E, Fowler S, Suffoletto B, Platts-Mills TF, Rothman RE, et al. Risk factors and screening instruments to predict adverse outcomes for undifferentiated older emergency department patients: a systematic review and meta-analysis. *Acad Emerg Med.* 2015;22(1):1–21.

Conroy S, Carpenter C, Banerjee J. Silver Book II: Quality Urgent Care for Older People, British Geriatrics Society, 2021. Available at https://www.bgs.org.uk/resources/resource-series/silver-book-ii.

Dresden SM, Hwang U, Garrido MM, et al. Geriatric emergency department innovations: the impact of transitional care nurses on 30-day readmissions for older adults. *Acad Emerg Med.* 2020;27(1):43–53.

Goldberg EM, Marks SJ, Resnik LJ, Long S, Mellott H, Merchant RC. Can an emergency department-initiated intervention prevent subsequent falls and health care use in older adults? A randomized controlled trial *Ann Emerg Med.* 2020;76(6):739–750.

Hwang U, Dresden SM, Rosenberg MS, et al. Geriatric emergency department innovations: transitional care nurses and hospital use. *J Am Geratr Soc.* 2018;66(3):459–466.

Hwang U, Dresden SM, Vargas-Torres C, et al. Association of a Geriatric Emergency Department Innovation Program with cost outcomes among Medicare beneficiaries. *JAMA Netw Open.* 2021;4(3):e2037334.

Hwang U, Morrison RS. The geriatric emergency department. *J Am Geriatr Soc.* 2007;55(11):1873–1876.

Kaeppeli T, Rueegg M, Dreher-Hummel T, et al. Validation of the Clinical Frailty Scale for prediction of thirty-day mortality in the emergency department. *Ann Emerg Med.* 2020;76(3):291–300.

Lee JS, Tong T, Tierney MC, Kiss A, Chignell M. Predictive ability of a serious game to identify emergency patients with unrecognized delirium. *J Am Geriatr. Soc* 2019;67(11):2370–2375.

Lo AX, Carpenter CR. Balancing evidence and economics while adapting emergency medicine to the 21st century's geriatric demographic imperative. *Acad Emerg Med.* 2020;27(10):1070-1073.

Rosen T, LoFaso VM, Bloemen EM, et al. Identifying injury patterns associated with physical elder abuse: analysis of legally adjudicated cases. *Ann Emerg Med.* 2020;76:266–276.

Rosenberg M, Carpenter CR, Bromley M, et al. Geriatric emergency department guidelines. *Ann Emerg Med.* 2014;63(5):e7–e25.

Sanon M, Baumlin KM, Kaplan SS, Grudzen CR. Care and Respect for Elders in Emergencies program: a preliminary report of a volunteer approach to enhance care in the emergency department. *J Am Geriatr Soc.* 2014;62(2):365–370.

Southerland LT, Hunold KM, Carpenter CR, Caterino JM, Mion LC. A National dataset analysis of older adults in emergency department observation units. *Am J Emerg Med.* 2019;37(9):1686–1690.

Southerland LT, Lo AX, Biese K, et al. Concepts in practice: geriatric emergency departments. *Ann Emerg Med.* 2020;75(2):162–170.

Stevens M, Hastings SN, Markland AD, et al. Enhancing Quality of Provider Practices for Older Adults in the Emergency Department (EQUiPPED). *J Am Geriatr Soc.* 2017;65(7):1609–1614.

Institutional Long-Term and Post-Acute Care

Joseph G. Ouslander, Alice F. Bonner

The focus of this chapter is the clinical care and support of nursing home (NH) residents. In this chapter we use the term "nursing home." However many terms are used in the US to describe the same types of facility, including "nursing facility," "skilled nursing facility or SNF," long-term care facility or LTCF, and "rehab facility." In the US there are approximately 15,500 NHs with approximately 1.5 million beds. The vast majority are certified as SNFs (approximately 90%) and provide both short and long-term care, and the rest provide long-term care only (see **Figure 16–1**).

Many older people who previously would have been in NHs now reside in assisted living residences or in their own homes. Support for older people with multiple chronic conditions in the NH setting is challenging for a number of reasons. Although many NHs provide excellent care, the poor quality of care provided in some NHs has been recognized for decades. Since the Institute of Medicine issued its critical report in 1986 and the Resident Assessment Instrument (RAI) was mandated in 1987, the overall quality of care has improved. The Centers for Medicare and Medicaid Services (CMS) has instituted several strategies that are designed to improve the quality of NH care. These include: the NH Compare website (http://www.medicare.gov/nhcompare/home.asp), which shows consumers (and NHs) how individual homes perform on surveys and specific quality indicators; a revised federal survey process (https://www.cms.gov/files/document/qso-19-03-nh.pdf); the CMS Five-Star Quality Rating System (https://www.cms.gov/Medicare/Provider-Enrollment-and-Certification/CertificationandComplianc/FSQRS); and the requirement in the Affordable Care Act that all NHs must have a Quality Assurance and Performance Improvement (QAPI) program (https://www.cms.gov/Medicare/Provider-Enrollment-and-Certification/QAPI/qapidefinition). Despite all of these efforts, the US Office of Inspector General issued a report documenting the high frequency of adverse events among NH residents during the first 1 to 2 months after admission (https://oig.hhs.gov/oei/reports/oei-06-11-00370.asp). The report documented that about one in three residents suffer an adverse event (including medication-related side effects; conditions such as falls or electrolyte disturbances; and infections). Thus, much remains to be done to improve NH care in the United States.

Learning Objectives

- List two or more goals of nursing home (NH) care.
- Understand the complexity of caring for residents/patients in NHs, including differences between short and long stayers.
- Identify the roles and responsibilities of different professionals and workers in NH care.
- Describe strategies to improve nursing care.
- Summarize key ethical issues in NH care.

Key Clinical Points

1. The goals of NH care include addressing social determinants of health and are different than traditional medical care in other settings.

2. NH care is provided by a team of health professionals and direct care workers such as certified nursing assistants (CNAs), all of whom provide critical input to the resident/patient's care plan.

3. Screening and preventive practices are relevant for many NH residents, but may be irrelevant for those with life-limiting illness who are near the end of life.

4. Several strategies, including collaborative practice among physicians and nurse practitioners (or physician assistants) and innovative use of health information technology, can help improve NH care.

5. Determination of decision-making capacity, appropriate use of advance directives, and proxy decision makers are critical aspects of NH care.

As older NH residents suffer from multiple underlying conditions, high quality clinical care is especially important. [Note: in this chapter we use the term "residents." However, many short-stay individuals are termed "patients" by many providers of NH care.] Despite the logistical and economic

TABLE 16-1 ■ GOALS OF NURSING HOME CARE

1. Provide a safe and supportive environment.
2. Restore and maintain the highest practicable level of functional independence.
3. Preserve individual autonomy.
4. Maximize quality of life, perceived well-being, and life satisfaction.
5. Provide effective rehabilitative, medical, nursing, and psychosocial care to individuals discharged from an acute hospital in order to facilitate their transition to their previous or desired living environment.
6. Provide comfort and dignity for terminally ill residents and their care partners.
7. Stabilize and delay progression of chronic conditions.
8. Prevent acute medical and iatrogenic illnesses and identify and treat them rapidly when they occur.

barriers that can foster inadequate care in NHs, many basic principles and strategies can improve the quality of care for NH residents. Fundamental to achieving these improvements is a clear perspective on the goals of NH care, which differ in some respects from the goals of medical care in other settings and populations.

GOALS OF NURSING HOME CARE AND SUPPORT

The modern NH supports residents in multiple ways. **Table 16-1** lists the key goals of NH care and support. While the prevention, identification, and treatment of chronic, subacute, and acute conditions are important, these goals are undergirded by a focus on functional independence, autonomy, quality of life, comfort, and dignity of residents. Physicians, nurse practitioners, physician's assistants, and other clinicians must consider these comprehensive, person-centered goals and at the same time address the more traditional goals of medical care.

The heterogeneity of the NH population results in diverse goals set by or with NH residents. There are five

basic categories of NH residents (**Figure 16-1**). Subgrouping NH residents in this manner will help clinicians and the interdisciplinary team focus the care-planning process on the most critical and realistic goals that matter most to individual residents. The "short-stay" population is largely in the NH for post-acute care after a hospitalization and requires a combination of skilled nursing care, rehabilitation therapy, adequate nutrition and hydration, and careful medical management in order to achieve a higher level of function and discharge home or to a less intensive care setting.

The underlying social contract implied by NH admission is quite different for each of the five groups of NH resident goals illustrated in the figure. Ideally, a NH should be able to provide what the name implies: high-quality nursing (and medical) care, in a home-like environment. In some cases, access to treatment takes precedence over the living environment; in other circumstances, the environment may be the most critical element of care. Those admitted to a NH with the intent of active treatment and discharge home may be willing to accept a living situation akin to that of a hospital with the expectation that the benefit they receive from treatment will offset any discomfort or inconvenience. For terminally ill residents receiving palliative or hospice care, the living environment should be as flexible and supportive as possible. Efforts are directed toward supporting these residents to be comfortable and permitting them to enjoy, to the extent possible, their last days. For the other groups in the middle of this distribution, attention to making their living situation comfortable and providing active primary care are important. There is in fact considerable overlap in the clinical characteristics of the short and long-stay populations in terms of multimorbidity, complexity, medication issues, among others. Some short-term patients become long-term residents because they do not have access to family or other caregiver support, limited availability of home-based service programs in their community, and the inability to pay for needed services and supports in the home versud spending down to qualify for Medicaid (which does cover the costs of institutional long-term care).

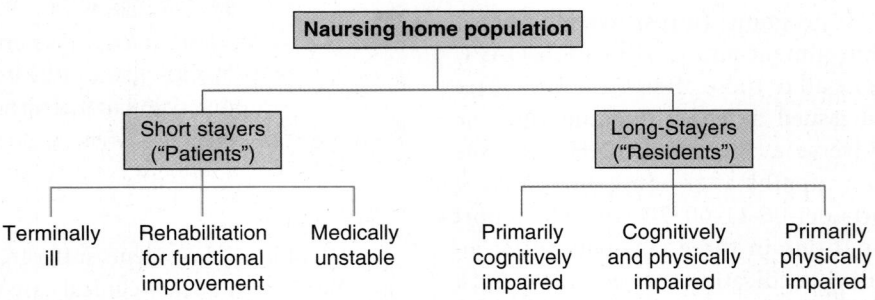

FIGURE 16-1. Characteristics of different types of nursing home residents.

1. The goals of care are often different (see **Table 16-1**).
2. Specific clinical disorders are prevalent among nursing home residents (see **Table 16-3**).
3. The approach to health maintenance and prevention may differ (see **Table 16-6**).
4. Mental and functional status are just as important, if not more so, than medical diagnoses.
5. Assessment must be interdisciplinary, including:
   a. Nursing
   b. Psychosocial
   c. Rehabilitation
   d. Nutritional
   e. Pharmacy
   f. Other (eg, dental, podiatry, audiology, ophthalmology, spiritual)
6. Sources of information are variable:
   a. Residents often cannot give a precise history.
   b. Family members and CNAs with limited assessment skills may provide the most important information.
   c. Information is often obtained over the telephone.
7. Administrative procedures for record keeping in both nursing homes and acute care hospitals can result in inadequate and disjointed information.
8. Clinical decision making is complicated for several reasons:
   a. Many diagnostic and therapeutic procedures are expensive, unavailable, or difficult to obtain and involve higher risks of iatrogenic illness and discomfort than are warranted by the potential outcome.
   b. The potential long-term benefits of "tight" control of certain chronic illnesses (e.g., diabetes mellitus, congestive heart failure, hypertension) may be outweighed by the risks of iatrogenic illness in many very old and functionally disabled residents.
   c. Many residents are not capable (or are questionably capable) of participating in medical decision making, and their personal preferences based on previous decisions are often unknown (see **Table 16-7**).
9. The appropriate site for and intensity of treatment are often difficult decisions involving medical, emotional, ethical, economic, and legal considerations that may be in conflict with each other in the nursing home setting.
10. Logistic considerations, resource constraints, and restrictive reimbursement policies may limit the ability of and incentives for clinicians to carry out optimal medical care of nursing home residents.

CLINICAL ASPECTS OF CARE FOR NURSING HOME RESIDENTS

In addition to the different goals for care in the NH, several factors make the assessment and treatment of NH residents different from those in other settings (**Table 16-2**). Many of these factors relate to the process of care (see the following section). A fundamental difference in NH care compared to care in other settings is that medical evaluation and treatment is one component of an assessment and care-planning process involving staff from multiple disciplines. The integral involvement of certified nursing assistants (CNAs) in the development and implementation of care plans is crucial to high-quality NH care. Data on clinical conditions and their treatment are integrated with assessments of the functional, mental, nutritional, and behavioral status of the resident in order to develop a comprehensive database and individualized plan of care.

Medical evaluation and clinical decision making for NH residents are complicated for several reasons. Unless the clinician has cared for the resident before NH admission, it may be difficult to access a comprehensive medical database that provides the background and context for their current status. Residents may be unable to relate their medical histories accurately or to describe their symptoms, and medical records are frequently unavailable or incomplete, especially for residents transferred between NHs and acute care hospitals. When acute changes in a condition occur, initial assessments are often performed by NH staff with limited skills and are communicated to clinicians (physicians, nurse practitioners, physician assistants) by telephone. Even when the diagnoses are known or strongly suspected, many diagnostic procedures and treatments among NH residents are associated with an unacceptably high risk–benefit ratio. For example, an imaging study may require sedation with its attendant risks; nitrates and other cardiovascular drugs may precipitate syncope or disabling falls in frail ambulatory residents with baseline postural hypotension; and adequate control of blood sugar may be extremely difficult to achieve among diabetic residents with marginal or fluctuating nutritional intake. Further compounding these challenges is the inability of many NH residents to participate effectively in important decisions regarding their medical care. Their previously expressed wishes are often not known, and an appropriate or legal surrogate decision maker has often not been appointed. These issues are further discussed in Chapters 7, 10, 26, and 72.

Table 16-3 lists the most commonly encountered clinical disorders in the NH population. They represent a

TABLE 16-3 ■ COMMON CLINICAL DISORDERS IN THE NURSING HOME POPULATION

MEDICAL CONDITIONS

Congestive heart failure

Degenerative joint disease

Diabetes mellitus

Gastrointestinal disorders

  Reflux esophagitis

  Constipation

  Diarrhea

  Gastroenteritis

Infections

  Respiratory

  Urinary

  Skin

  Conjunctivitis

Kidney disease (chronic kidney disease, renal failure)

Lung disease (chronic obstructive, emphysema, asthma)

Malignancies

Neuropsychiatric conditions

  Dementia

  Depression

  Psychosis

Behavioral disorders associated with dementia

  Anxiety

  Aggression

  Depression

Neurologic disorders other than dementia

  Stroke

  Parkinsonism

  Multiple sclerosis

  Brain or spinal cord injury

Pain: musculoskeletal conditions, neuropathies, malignancy

Geriatric conditions and syndromes

  Delirium

  Incontinence

  Gait disturbances, instability, falls

  Malnutrition, feeding difficulties, dehydration

  Pressure sores

  Insomnia

Functional disabilities necessitating rehabilitation

  Stroke

  Hip fracture

  Joint replacement

  Amputation

Iatrogenic disorders

  Adverse drug reactions

  Falls

  Nosocomial infections

  Induced disabilities

  Restraints and immobility, catheters, unnecessary help with basic activities of daily living

Palliative care and end-of-life care

broad spectrum of chronic illnesses; neurologic, psychiatric, and behavioral disorders; and problems that are especially prevalent in frail older adults (eg, incontinence, falls, nutritional disorders, chronic pain syndromes). The management of many of the conditions listed in **Table 16-3** is discussed in some detail in other chapters of this book.

PROCESS OF CARE IN THE NURSING HOME

The process of care in NHs is strongly influenced by numerous state and federal regulations, the highly interdisciplinary nature of NH residents' clinical issues, and the training and skills of the staff that delivers most of the hands-on care. Federal rules and regulations contained in the Omnibus Budget Reconciliation Act of 1987 (OBRA, 1987) and implemented in 1991 place heavy emphasis on assessment through use of the Resident Assessment Instrument (RAI) and care planning as a means of achieving the highest practicable level of functioning for each resident. The minimum data set (MDS) 3.0, is the foundation of clinical assessment and care planning for individual residents. In addition to the MDS, each resident or responsible health care proxy should be assisted in articulating the goals for their NH care (ie, short-term rehabilitation and/or medical and nursing management of unstable clinical conditions with the goal of returning home; long-term care of chronic conditions; or palliative or hospice care). Detailed guidance for state and federal surveyors is available for several clinical care areas, such as unnecessary drugs and urinary incontinence. Failure to adhere to the clinical recommendations contained in the regulations and related surveyor guidance can result in citations and, in some instances, financial penalties or other enforcement actions. In addition, failure to manage clinical conditions appropriately puts the NH and clinicians at risk for legal action.

Physician involvement in NH care and the nature of medical assessment and treatment offered to NH residents may be limited by logistic and economic factors. Few physicians have offices based either inside the NH or in close proximity to it. Many physicians who do visit NHs care for relatively small numbers of residents, often in several different NHs. Many NHs, therefore, have numerous physicians who make rounds once or twice per month, who are not generally present to evaluate acute changes in resident status, and who attempt to assess these changes over the telephone. Practice patterns are shifting to a model of physician-nurse practitioner practices caring for large numbers of residents in several NHs. Such physician-nurse practitioner teams have been shown to improve care, increase resident and family satisfaction, and reduce hospitalization rates. Value-based care programs such as intensive special needs plans (iSNPs) and bundled payments financially incentivize this approach to care. (iSNPs and other value-based programs are discussed in Chapter 19.)

Many NHs do not have ready availability of laboratory, radiologic, and pharmacy services with the capability of rapid response, further compounding the logistics of evaluating and treating acute changes in medical status. Thus, NH residents are often sent to hospital emergency rooms, where they are evaluated by personnel who are generally not familiar with their baseline status and who frequently lack training in the care of older adults.

Medicare and Medicaid reimbursement policies also dictate certain patterns of NH care. While physicians are required to visit NH residents only every 30 to 60 days, many residents require more frequent evaluation and monitoring of treatment, especially with the shorter acute care hospital stays brought about by the prospective payment system (PPS). While Medicare reimbursement for physician visits in NHs has improved, reimbursement for a routine visit is sometimes inadequate for the time that is required to provide good medical care in the NH, including travel to and from the NH; assessment and treatment planning for residents with multiple problems; communication with the resident, members of the interdisciplinary team and the resident's family; and proper documentation in the medical record. Activities often essential to good care in the NH, such as attendance at interdisciplinary conferences, family meetings, complex assessments of decision-making capacity, and counseling residents and proxy decision makers on treatment plans, are often not reimbursable. The coronavirus pandemic has led to increased use of telehealth, which may facilitate accomplishing some of this direct care more efficiently (see below). Medicare intermediaries sometimes restrict reimbursement for rehabilitative services for residents not covered under Part A skilled care, thus limiting treatment options for many residents. Although Medicaid programs vary considerably, many provide minimal coverage for ancillary services that are critical for optimal care and may restrict reimbursement for certain types of drugs that may be especially helpful for NH residents.

Amid these logistic and economic constraints, expectations for the care of NH residents are high. **Table 16-4** outlines the various types of assessment generally recommended for the optimal care of NH residents. Physicians are responsible for completing an initial assessment within 72 hours of admission and for monthly visits thereafter for the next 90 days. More frequent visits are often necessary for residents admitted on a Medicare Part A skilled nursing benefit. Licensed nurses assess new residents when they are admitted, on a daily basis, and summarize the status of each resident weekly. The nationally mandated MDS must be completed within 14 days of admission and updated when a major change in status occurs. Several sections of the MDS must be updated on a quarterly basis. The MDS is intended to assist NH staff in identifying important clinical problems that need care plans that include further evaluation, management, and monitoring. The MDS is also used as the basis for calculating daily reimbursement rates for residents on the Medicare Part A skilled benefit and as the basis for calculating various quality measures, including those on the NH Compare website and those used for the CMS Five-Star Quality Rating System.

The extent of involvement of other disciplines in the assessment and care-planning process varies depending on the residents' conditions, the availability of various professionals, and state regulations. Representatives from nursing, social services, dietary, therapeutic recreation (activities), and rehabilitation therapy (physical, occupational, speech) participate in an interdisciplinary care-planning meeting. Residents are generally discussed at this meeting within 2 weeks of admission and quarterly thereafter. Residents and family members or care partners are usually invited to participate in this initial care planning meeting. The product of these meetings is an interdisciplinary care plan that lists physical and psychosocial or behavioral conditions (eg, restricted mobility, incontinence, unstable gait, diminished food intake, poor social interaction, depression), goals set by or with the resident, approaches to achieving those goals, target dates for achieving the goals, and responsibilities for working toward the goals among the various disciplines. These care plans are important in supporting what matters to each resident and should be reviewed by the primary provider.

STRATEGIES TO IMPROVE CARE IN NURSING HOMES

Better medical care of NH residents should lead to fewer exacerbations of chronic illnesses, iatrogenic conditions, and other adverse events, and hence lower use of emergency rooms and hospitals. Several strategies might improve the process of medical care delivered to NH residents. Four strategies are briefly described: (1) improved documentation practices; (2) a systematic approach to screening, health maintenance, and preventive practices; (3) collaborative care with nurse practitioners or physician assistants; and (4) practice guidelines and related quality improvement activities.

In addition to these strategies, strong leadership of a medical director (and in some cases associate medical director) who is appropriately trained and dedicated to improving the NH's quality of medical care is essential in order to develop, implement, and monitor policies and procedures for medical services. Certification through the American Medical Directors Association (AMDA)–The Society for Post-Acute and Long-Term Care Medicine should be encouraged (https://paltc.org/). The medical director should set standards for medical care and serve as an example to the medical staff by caring for some of the residents in the NH. He/she should also be involved in various committees (eg, quality, infection control), and should try to involve interested medical staff in these committees, as well as in educational efforts through formal

TABLE 16-4 ■ IMPORTANT ASPECTS OF VARIOUS TYPES OF ASSESSMENT IN THE NURSING HOME

TYPE OF ASSESSMENT	TIMING	MAJOR OBJECTIVES	IMPORTANT ASPECTS
Medical initial	Within 72 h to 1 wk after admission	Verify medical diagnoses Medication reconciliation Document baseline physical findings, mental and functional status, vital signs, and skin condition Attempt to identify potentially remediable, previously unrecognized medical conditions Get to know the resident and family (if this is a new resident) Establish goals for the admission and a medical treatment plan	A thorough review of medical records and physical examinations is necessary Relevant medical diagnoses and baseline findings should be clearly and concisely documented in the patient's record Medication lists should be carefully reviewed and only essential medications continued Request for specific types of assessment and input from other disciplines should be made A database should be established (see example in **Figure 16-2**)
Periodic	Monthly or every other month	Monitor progress of active medical conditions Update medical orders Communicate with patient and nursing home staff	Progress notes should include clinical data relevant to active medical conditions and focus on changes in status Unnecessary medications, orders for care, and laboratory tests should be discontinued Mental, functional, and psychosocial status should be reviewed with nursing home staff and changes from baseline noted The medical problem list should be updated
As needed	When acute changes in status occur	Identify and treat causes of acute changes	Onsite clinical assessment by the physician (or nurse practitioner or physician's assistant), as opposed to telephonic consultations, will result in more accurate diagnoses, more appropriate treatment, and fewer unnecessary emergency room visits and hospitalization Vital signs, food and fluid intake, and mental status often provide essential information Infection, dehydration, and adverse drug effects should be at the top of the differential diagnosis for acute changes in status
Major reassessment	Annual	Identify and document any significant changes in status and new potentially remediable conditions	Targeted physical examination and assessment of mental, functional, and psychosocial status and selected laboratory tests should be done (see **Table 16-6**)
Nursing	On admission, and then routinely with monitoring of daily and weekly progress Minimum data set on admission; update when major change in status occurs and annually; update selected sections quarterly	Identify biopsychosocial and functional status, strengths, and weaknesses Develop an individualized care plan Document baseline data for ongoing assessments	Particular attention should be given to emotional state, personal preferences, and sensory function Careful observation during the first few days of admission is important to detect effects of relocation Potential problems related to other disciplines should be recorded and communicated to appropriate members of the interdisciplinary care team

Domain	Timing	Tasks	Comments
Psychosocial	Within 1–2 wk of admission and as needed thereafter	Identify any potentially serious psychosocial signs and symptoms and refer to mental health professional if appropriate Determine past social history, family relationships, and social resources Become familiar with personal preferences regarding living arrangements	Getting to know the family and their preferences and concerns is critical to good nursing home care Relevant psychosocial data should be communicated to the interdisciplinary team Discharge potential should be assessed
Rehabilitation (physical and occupational therapy)	On admission and daily or weekly thereafter (depending on the rehabilitation care plan)	Determine functional status as it relates to basic activities of daily living Identify specific goals and time frame for improving specific areas of function Monitor progress toward goals Assess progress in relation to potential discharge	Small gains in functional status can improve chances for discharge as well as quality of life Not all residents have areas in which they can reasonably be expected to improve; strategies to maintain function should be developed for these residents Assessment of and recommendation for modifying the environment can be critically important for improving function and discharge planning
Nutritional	Within days of admission and then periodically thereafter	Determine nutritional status and needs Identify dietary preferences Plan an appropriate diet	Restrictive diets may not be medically necessary and can be unappetizing Weight loss should be identified and reported to nursing and medical staff
Pharmacy	Within days of admission and periodically	Medication reconciliation and drug regimen review	Check for high-risk medications, appropriate indications, drug-drug and drug-disease interactions, stop dates, monitoring parameters
Interdisciplinary care plan	Within 1–2 wk of admission and every 3 mo thereafter	Identify interdisciplinary problems Establish goals and treatment plans Determine when maximum progress toward goals has been reached	Each discipline should prepare specific plans for communication to other team members based on their own assessment
Capacity for medical decision making	Within days of admission and then whenever changes in status occur	Determine which types of medical decisions the resident is capable of participating in A resident who is still capable of making decisions independently should be encouraged to identify a surrogate decision maker in the event the resident later loses this decision-making capacity If the resident lacks capacity for many or all decisions, appropriate surrogate decision makers should be identified (if not already done)	Residents with varying degrees of dementia may still be capable of participating in many decisions regarding their medical care Attention should be given to potentially reversible factors that can interfere with decision-making capacity (eg, depression, fear, delirium, metabolic and drug effects) Concerns of the family and health professional should be considered, but the resident's desires should be paramount The resident's capacity may fluctuate over time because of physical and emotional conditions
Preferences regarding treatment intensity and nursing home routines	Within days of admission and periodically thereafter	Determine residents' wishes as to the intensity of treatment they would want in the event of acute or chronic progressive illness	Attempt to identify specific procedures the resident would or would not want This assessment is often made by ascertaining the resident's prior-expressed wishes (if known), or through surrogate decision makers (legal guardian, durable power of attorney for health care, family)

presentations, teaching rounds, and appropriate documentation procedures. Federal quality measures, as well as other quality indicators, developed through literature review and expert consensus should be used to track improvements in overall care in the NH setting. Medical directors should use these indicators and other approaches in their quality improvement programs and assisting the NH with meeting CMS requirements for Quality Assurance and Performance Improvement ("QAPI").

Documentation Practices

Electronic health records (EHRs) specific for NHs are now widely available, and when used properly can greatly improve clinical documentation. Critical aspects of a NH resident's health status should be recorded on a clinical "face sheet" of the medical record. **Figure 16-2** shows an example of the elements of and a format for such documentation. Additional standardized documentation should contain social information, such as individuals to contact at critical times (health care proxy, durable power of attorney for health care, legal guardian) and information about the resident's treatment status in the event of acute illness (advance directives). These data are essential to the care of the resident and should be readily available in one place in the record, so that when emergencies arise, when medical consultants see the resident, or when members of the interdisciplinary team need an overall perspective, they are easy to locate. The face sheet should be sent to the hospital or other health care facilities when the resident is transferred. Time and effort are required in order to keep the face sheet updated. EHRs can facilitate incorporating the face sheet into a database and updating it periodically.

Many NHs currently use blended records with nursing and administrative documentation in the EHR. Handwritten medical documentation in progress notes for routine visits and assessments of acute changes is frequently scanty, uninformative, and/or illegible. Statements such as "stable" or "no change" are frequently the only documentation for routine visits. While time constraints may preclude extensive notes, certain standard information should be documented. The SOAP (*subjective, objective, assessment, plan*) format for charting routine notes is especially appropriate for NH residents (**Table 16-5**). Simple forms, flow sheets, or databases with word-processing capabilities can be used to enable physicians to efficiently produce legible, concise, comprehensive progress notes. Some EHRs include these capabilities.

Another area where medical documentation is often inadequate relates to the residents' decision-making capacity and treatment preferences. These issues are discussed briefly at the end of this chapter as well as in Chapters 7, 10, 26, and 72. In addition to placing critical information in a standardized format in readily accessible locations, it is essential that physicians thoroughly and legibly document all discussions they have had with the resident, designated family member, legal guardian, or durable power of attorney for health care about these issues. Failure to do so may result not only in poor communication and inappropriate treatment, but also in substantial legal liability. Notes about these issues should not be removed from the EHR or the paper medical record and are ideally kept in a separate advance care planning section.

As NHs increasingly use health information technology, these recommendations for improved documentation can eventually be incorporated into the NH EHR. AMDA (https://paltc.org/) and the Interventions to Reduce Acute Care Transfers (INTERACT) quality improvement program (https://pathway-interact.com/) have examples of tools that can help improve documentation of clinical care in the NH and that can be integrated into EHRs. Documentation in the EHR using discrete items will facilitate using them in a relational database that can be used for quality improvement and research.

Screening, Health Maintenance, and Preventive Practices

A second approach to improving medical care in NHs is developing and implementing selected screening, health maintenance, and preventive practices in order to delay or prevent exacerbations of chronic conditions. **Table 16-6** lists examples of such practices. With few exceptions, the efficacy of these practices has not been well studied in the NH setting. In addition, not all the practices listed in this table are relevant for every NH resident. For example, some of the annual screening examinations are inappropriate for short-stay residents or for many long-stay residents with end-stage dementia or other life-limiting illness in which the time to benefit from the screening exceeds life expectancy. Thus, the practices outlined in **Table 16-6** must be tailored to individual residents and must be creatively incorporated into routine care procedures as much as possible in order to be time-efficient, cost-effective, and reimbursable by Medicare. The Annual Wellness Visit is now supported by Medicare and can include individualized plans for screening and preventive health.

Advanced Practitioners (Nurse Practitioners, Clinical Specialists, and Physician Assistants)

A third strategy that may help improve care in NHs is partnering with or employing nurse practitioners and physician assistants. This approach appears to be cost-effective in both managed care and fee-for-service settings. These health professionals may be especially helpful in providing comprehensive care in the NH setting. Physician assistants and nurse practitioners can bill for services under fee-for-service Medicare and NHs and/or physician groups can hire them on a salaried basis. Nurse practitioners may have an especially helpful perspective in interacting with nursing staff about the non-medical aspects of care for NH residents. Nurse practitioners and physician's assistants can be very helpful in implementing some of the screening, monitoring, and preventive practices outlined

Health Summary for Long-Stay Nursing Home Residents

Active Medical Problems

1. ___
2. ___
3. ___
4. ___
5. ___
6. ___

Hospitalizations (last 12 months)

1. ___
2. ___
3. ___
4. ___

Major Past Surgical Procedures

Year
1. ___
2. ___
3. ___
4. ___

Allergies

1. ___
2. ___

Functional Status

A. Ambulation
__ Independent
__ With cane
__ With Walker
__ Unable
Transfer: __ Ind __ Dep

B. Continence

	Cont	Inc
Urine	___	___
Stool	___	___

C. Vision
__ Adequate for regular print
__ Impaired, can see large print
__ Severely impaired

D. Hearing
__ Adequate
__ Minimal Difficulty
__ Hears only with amplifier or aid

Date Updated — **Name of updating clinician**
__/__/___ ___
__/__/___ ___
__/__/___ ___
__/__/___ ___

Cognitive Status

1. Dementia? ___ Yes ___ No
a. If yes, type:
___ Alzheimer's ___ Lewy Body
___ Multi-infarct ___ Other
___ Parkinson's ___ Uncertain
b. If yes, behavioral symptoms?
___ Yes ___ No
If yes, describe:
___
___
___
___

2. Usual mental status
___ Alert, oriented, follows simple instructions
___ Alert, *dis*oriented, but *can* follow simple directions
___ Alert, *dis*oriented, *cannot* follow simple directions
___ Not alert (lethargic, comatose)

3. Most recent mental status test score if available:
Test ___ Score ___

Advanced Care Planning/Directives

1. Date of most recent relevant progress note, if available __/__/___

2. Decision Making Status
___ Capable of making health decisions
___ Can participate with proxy involvement
___ Proxy makes decisions

3. Care limiting orders
a. Refer to POLST, MOLST, POST if available
b. Specific orders
__ DNR __ Do not hospitalize
__ Other ___

4. Proxy Health Care Decision Maker
Name ___
Relationship ___
Contact No. ___

FIGURE 16-2. Example of a "face sheet" for a nursing home medical record. (Reproduced with permission from Kane RL, Ouslander J, Resnic B, et al. *Essentials of Clinical Geriatrics.* 8th ed. New York, NY: McGraw Hill; 2018.)

229 · PART II PRINCIPLES OF GERIATRICS

TABLE 16-5 ■ SOAP FORMAT FOR PROGRESS NOTES ON NURSING HOME RESIDENTS

Subjective	New complaints
	Symptoms related to active medical conditions
Objective	General appearance and mood
	Weight
	Vital signs
	Physical findings relevant to new complaints and active medical conditions
	Laboratory data
	Reports from nursing staff
	Progress in rehabilitative therapy (if applicable)
	Reports of other interdisciplinary team members
	Consultant reports
Assessment	Presumptive diagnosis(es) for new complaints or changes in status
	Stability of active medical conditions
	Responses to psychotropic medications (if applicable)
Plans	Changes in medications (optimal prescribing or deprescribing when appropriate) or diet
	Nursing interventions (e.g., monitoring of vital signs, skin care)
	Assessments by other disciplines
	Consultants
	Laboratory studies
	Discharge planning (if relevant)

in **Table 16-6**, and in communicating with interdisciplinary staff, residents, and family members or care partners at times when the physician is not available. One of the most appropriate roles for nurse practitioners and physician assistants is in the initial assessment of acute or subacute changes in resident condition. They can perform a focused history and physical examination and can order appropriate diagnostic studies. The INTERACT quality improvement program has several care paths for this purpose that address 10 of the most common conditions associated with hospital transfers, one of which is shown in **Figure 16-3**. Use of such care paths and other tools available through the INTERACT website (https://pathway-interact.com/), as well as through AMDA, enables onsite assessment of acute change, detection and treatment of new problems early in their course, more appropriate utilization of acute care hospital emergency rooms, and rapid identification of residents who need to be hospitalized.

Clinical Practice Guidelines and Quality Improvement Activities

Several clinical practice guidelines relevant to NH care have been developed by AMDA (https://paltc.org/). In addition, quality indicators for a number of conditions have been developed. While these guidelines and quality indicators are largely based on expert opinion rather than on controlled clinical trials, they are helpful as a basis for standards of practice that will improve care. Implementation and maintenance of clinical practice guidelines can be challenging in NHs, as it is in other practice settings. NHs are required to have an ongoing quality assessment and assurance (QAA) committee, and as mentioned above, federal regulations now require an active Quality Assurance Performance Improvement (QAPI) program. Principles of continuous quality improvement (CQI) and rapid-cycle performance improvement projects (PIPs) engage direct care staff to monitor objective outcomes (such as the frequency of falls, severity of incontinence, adverse drug reactions, and skin problems) and to identify work processes that can be modified to continuously improve these outcomes. NH administrators, directors of nursing, and medical directors must create an environment that provides incentives for ongoing quality activities in order to maintain these programs over time. The Medicare Quality Improvement Organization/Quality Innovation Network (QIO/QIN) program as well as AMDA and its journal have substantial free or low-cost resources for assisting NH providers with quality improvement initiatives. In addition, CMS provides educational resources and tools for NHs to help them meet QAPI requirements (https://www.cms.gov/Medicare/Provider-Enrollment-and-Certification/QAPI/qapidefinition).

POSTACUTE CARE AND THE NURSING HOME–ACUTE CARE HOSPITAL INTERFACE

As a result of the increasing acuity and clinical complexity of the NH resident population, transfer back and forth between the NH and one or more acute care hospitals is common. About one in five NH residents admitted from a hospital are readmitted to the hospital within 30 days. Transfer to an acute care hospital is often a disruptive process for a NH resident, and is especially hazardous for NH residents with dementia. In addition to the effects of the acute illness, NH residents are subject to acute mental status changes and a myriad of potential iatrogenic problems. The most prevalent of these iatrogenic problems are related to immobility, including deconditioning with resulting difficulty regaining ambulation and/or transfer capabilities, hospital-acquired infections, incontinence and catheter use, polypharmacy and adverse drug effects, delirium, and the development of pressure ulcers.

Because of the risks of acute care hospitalization, the decision to transfer a resident to the emergency room or hospitalize a resident must carefully balance a number of factors. A variety of medical, administrative, logistic, economic, and ethical issues can influence decisions to hospitalize NH residents. Decisions regarding hospitalization often boil down to the capabilities of medical care providers

TABLE 16-6 ■ SCREENING, HEALTH MAINTENANCE, AND PREVENTIVE PRACTICES IN THE NURSING HOME FOR LONG-STAY RESIDENTS

PRACTICE	RECOMMENDED FREQUENCY[a]	COMMENT
SCREENING		
History and physical examination	Yearly	Focused examination including rectal, breast, and, in some women, pelvic examination
Weight	Monthly	Generally required
		Persistent weight loss should prompt a search for treatable medical, psychiatric, and functional conditions
Functional status assessment, including gait and mental status testing and screening for depression	Yearly	Functional status assessed periodically by nursing staff using the minimum data set (MDS)
		Systematic global functional assessment done at least yearly using MDS to detect potentially treatable conditions (or prevent complications) such as early dementia, depression, gait disturbances, urinary incontinence
Visual screening	Yearly	Assess acuity, intraocular pressure, identify correctable problems
Auditory	Yearly	Identify correctable problems
Dental	Yearly	Assess status of any remaining teeth, fit of dentures, and identify any pathology
Podiatry	Yearly	More frequently in diabetics and residents with peripheral vascular disease
		Identify correctable problems and ensure appropriateness of shoes
Tuberculosis	On admission and yearly (may vary by state)	All residents and staff should be tested. Booster testing recommended for nursing home residents
Laboratory tests	Yearly	Not all tests are appropriate for individual residents
Stool for occult blood		
Complete blood count		
Fasting glucose		
Electrolytes		
Renal function tests		
Albumin, calcium, phosphorus		
Thyroid function tests		
MONITORING IN SELECTED RESIDENTS		
All residents		
Vital signs, including weight	Monthly	More often if unstable or ill
Diabetes Fasting and postprandial glucose, glycosylated hemoglobin (HgbA$_{1C}$)	Every 1–2 mo when stable (fasting) Every 4–6 mo (HgbA$_{1C}$)	Sliding scale insulin should be avoided. Periodic glucometer testing can be useful, but should not be overused for stable residents
Residents on diuretics or with renal insufficiency: electrolytes, BUN, creatinine	Every 2–3 mo	Nursing home residents are more prone to dehydration, azotemia, hyponatremia, and hypokalemia
Anemic residents who are on iron replacement or who have hemoglobin <10: hemoglobin/hematocrit	Monthly until stable, then every 2–3 mo	Iron replacement and/or erythropoietin should be discontinued once hemoglobin value stabilizes
Blood level of drug for residents on specific drugs, for example:	Every 3–6 mo	More frequently if drug treatment has just been initiated
Anticonvulsants		
Digoxin		
Lithium		

(Continued)

TABLE 16-6 ■ SCREENING, HEALTH MAINTENANCE, AND PREVENTIVE PRACTICES IN THE NURSING HOME FOR LONG-STAY RESIDENTS (CONTINUED)

PRACTICE	RECOMMENDED FREQUENCY[a]	COMMENT
PREVENTION		
Influenza vaccine	Yearly	All residents and staff with close resident contact should be vaccinated
Oseltamivir, zanamivir	Within 24–48 h of outbreak of suspected influenza	Residents and staff should be treated throughout outbreak
Zoster vaccination	Once	Selected residents
Pneumococcal vaccine	Once	All residents who have not had the vaccine
Tetanus booster	Every 10 y, or every 5 y with tetanus-prone wounds	Many older people have not received primary vaccinations; they require tetanus toxoid, 250–500 units of tetanus immune globulin, and completion of the immunization series with toxoid injection 4–6 wk later and then 6–12 mo after the second injection
Tuberculosis Isoniazid 300 mg/d for 9–12 mo	Skin-test conversion in selected residents	Residents with abnormal chest film (more than granuloma), diabetes, end-stage renal disease, hematologic malignancies, steroid or immunosuppressive therapy, or malnutrition should be treated
Antimicrobial prophylaxis for residents at risk	Generally recommended for dental procedures, genitourinary procedures, and most operative procedures	Chronically catheterized residents should not be treated with continuous prophylaxis
Body positioning and range of motion for immobile residents	Ongoing	Frequent turning of very immobile residents is necessary to prevent pressure sores
		Semi-upright position is necessary for residents with swallowing disorders or enteral feeding to help prevent aspiration
		Range of motion to immobile limbs and joints is necessary to prevent contractures
Infection-control procedures and surveillance	Ongoing	Policies and protocols should be in effect in all nursing homes Surveillance of all infections should be continuous to identify outbreaks and resistance patterns
Environmental safety	Ongoing	Appropriate lighting, colors, and the removal of hazards for falling are essential in order to prevent accidents Routine monitoring of potential safety hazards and accidents may lead to alterations that may prevent further accidents

[a]Frequency may vary depending on resident's condition. Not all recommendations are relevant to every resident. Some recommendations are not appropriate for residents with life-limiting illnesses in whom the time to benefit exceeds life expectancy or the risks and discomforts outweigh the potential benefits.

and the NH staff to provide services in the NH, the preferences of the resident and, when indicated, the family, and the logistic and administrative arrangements for hospital care. If, for example, the NH staff has been trained and has the personnel to institute intravenous therapy without detracting from the care of other residents, or if it has arranged for an outside agency to oversee intravenous therapy and there is a nurse practitioner or physician's assistant to perform follow-up assessments, the resident with an acute infection who is otherwise stable may best be managed in the NH. Better advance care planning and advance

directive use can also help to avoid unnecessary hospitalization of NH residents when the palliative or hospice care may be more appropriate than hospital transfer.

AMDA has developed a clinical practice guideline and related tools on care transitions (https://paltc.org/topic/transitions-care). The INTERACT program includes educational resources and tools that have been developed and have shown promise in reducing unnecessary hospital transfers. The INTERACT program uses several basic strategies to improve the management of acute changes in condition and prevent unnecessary

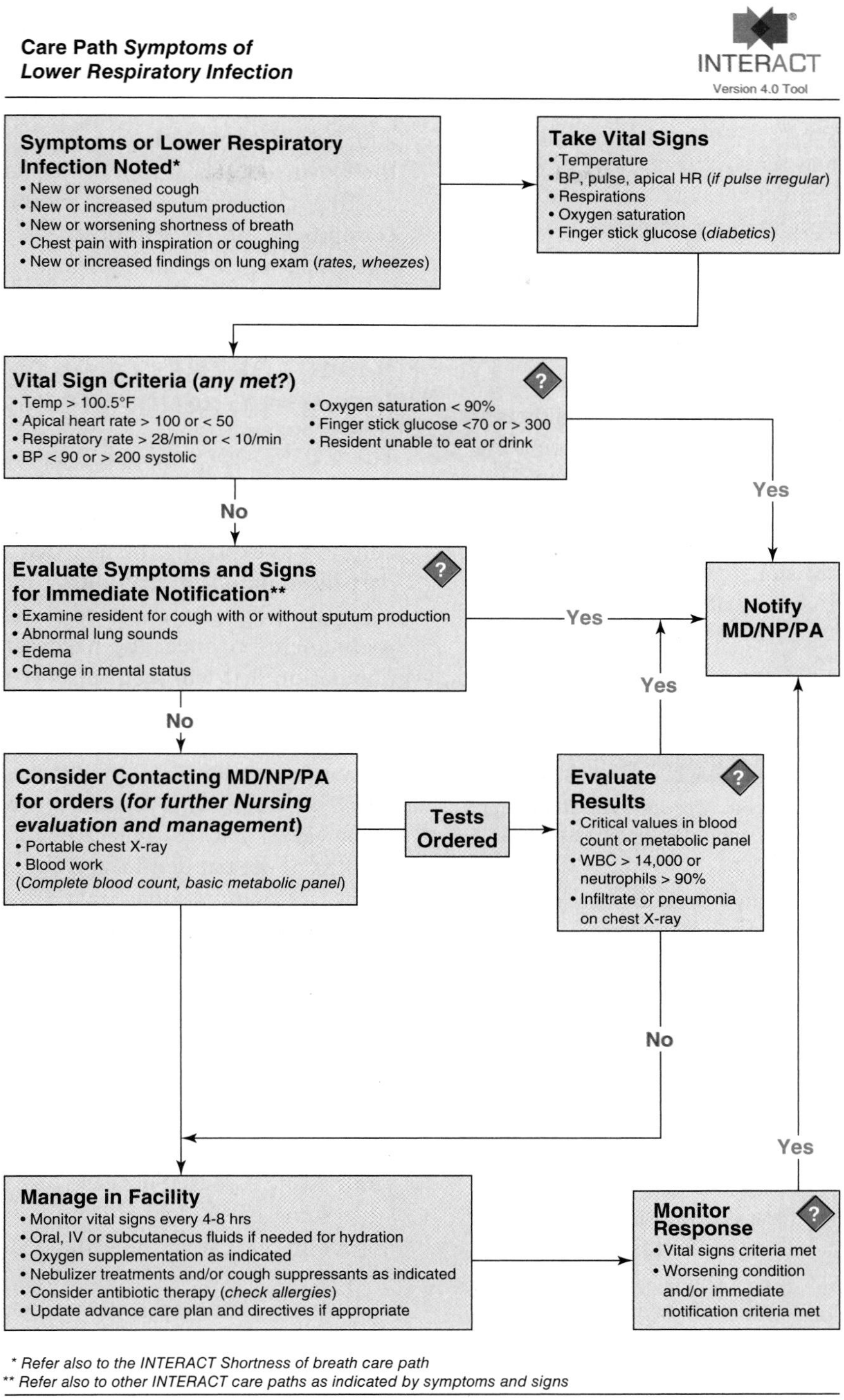

Care Path *Symptoms of*
Lower Respiratory Infection

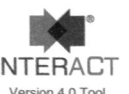
INTERACT®
Version 4.0 Tool

Symptoms or Lower Respiratory Infection Noted*
- New or worsened cough
- New or increased sputum production
- New or worsening shortness of breath
- Chest pain with inspiration or coughing
- New or increased findings on lung exam (*rates, wheezes*)

Take Vital Signs
- Temperature
- BP, pulse, apical HR (*if pulse irregular*)
- Respirations
- Oxygen saturation
- Finger stick glucose (*diabetics*)

Vital Sign Criteria (*any met?*) ?
- Temp > 100.5°F
- Apical heart rate > 100 or < 50
- Respiratory rate > 28/min or < 10/min
- BP < 90 or > 200 systolic
- Oxygen saturation < 90%
- Finger stick glucose <70 or > 300
- Resident unable to eat or drink

→ **Yes**

No

Evaluate Symptoms and Signs for Immediate Notification* ?
- Examine resident for cough with or without sputum production
- Abnormal lung sounds
- Edema
- Change in mental status

— **Yes** →

No

Notify MD/NP/PA

Yes

Consider Contacting MD/NP/PA for orders (*for further Nursing evaluation and management*)
- Portable chest X-ray
- Blood work
(*Complete blood count, basic metabolic panel*)

→ **Tests Ordered** →

Evaluate Results ?
- Critical values in blood count or metabolic panel
- WBC > 14,000 or neutrophils > 90%
- Infiltrate or pneumonia on chest X-ray

Yes

No

Manage in Facility
- Monitor vital signs every 4-8 hrs
- Oral, IV or subcutaneous fluids if needed for hydration
- Oxygen supplementation as indicated
- Nebulizer treatments and/or cough suppressants as indicated
- Consider antibiotic therapy (*check allergies*)
- Update advance care plan and directives if appropriate

→ **Monitor Response** ?
- Vital signs criteria met
- Worsening condition and/or immediate notification criteria met

Yes

* Refer also to the INTERACT Shortness of breath care path
** Refer also to other INTERACT care paths as indicated by symptoms and signs

FIGURE 16-3. Example of one of 10 INTERACT. (Reproduced with permission from Pathway Health Services, Inc. Lake Elmo, MN http://interact-pathway.com.)

hospital transfers including: (1) proactive identification of conditions before they become severe enough to require hospital care (eg, dehydration, delirium); (2) management of some conditions (eg, pneumonia, congestive heart failure) without transfer when safe and feasible; (3) improving advance care planning in order to consider palliative or comfort care as an alternative when the risks of hospitalization may outweigh the benefits; (4) improved documentation practices; (5) improved communication within the NH and between the NH and the hospital; and (6) embedding these strategies within everyday care, including within EHRs.

Ethical issues arise as much or more in the day-to-day care of NH residents as in care in any other setting. These issues are discussed in Chapter 72. **Table 16-7** outlines several common ethical dilemmas that occur in the NH. Although most attention has been directed toward those with limited ability to express their preferences, important daily ethical dilemmas also face those who are capable of decision-making. These more subtle problems are easily overlooked. Physicians, nurse practitioners, and physician assistants providing primary care must serve as strong advocates for the autonomy and quality of life for NH residents.

NHs care for a high concentration of individuals who are unable or are questionably capable of participating in decisions concerning their current and future health care. Among these same individuals, functional disabilities and terminal illnesses are prevalent. Thus, questions regarding individual autonomy, decision-making capacity, surrogate decision makers, and the intensity of treatment arise on a daily basis. These questions are both troublesome and complex and must be managed in a straightforward and systematic manner in order to provide optimal care to NH residents within the context of ethical principles and state and federal laws. NHs should be encouraged to develop their own ethics committees or to participate in a local existing committee within another organization. Ethics committees can be helpful in educating staff; developing, implementing, and monitoring policies and procedures; and providing consultation in difficult cases.

IMPACT OF THE CORONAVIRUS-19 (COVID-19) PANDEMIC IN NURSING HOMES

The COVID-19 pandemic has had profound effects on NHs in the United States that have already and continue to work toward major changes over the coming years. In addition to exposing the fact that NHs were for the most part unprepared to deal with a pandemic of this nature, it has shed light on the need to restructure NH care and its financing to meet the needs of a growing vulnerable population that will require short-term or long-term care over the next several decades. Many NHs have suffered devastating COVID-19 outbreaks that led to high mortality rates among NH residents and staff as well. Many NHs did not have adequate personal protective equipment (PPE) and testing capability throughout the first months of the pandemic, and some still do not, especially in the face of increasing viral positivity rates and influenza season. Staffing shortages have been severe in many NHs because a substantial number of staff have had positive viral tests and/or close exposure to an infected individual and have to undergo a minimum 14-day quarantine period off work. The federal government has promulgated waivers, guidance, and new regulations that have been helpful. It has also provided considerable financial relief for NHs, but it was not enough to support all the PPE and viral testing essential for care.

Some of the key issues that may have an enduring impact on NH care in the United States include:

1. Intensive development of education and oversight of infection control programs, including the requirement for an infection preventionist in each NH.
2. Rapid increase in the use of telemedicine for routine visits as well for evaluating acute changes in condition. If the federal government continues to reimburse providers for this method of care, it could greatly increase the ability to provide efficient care coordination among disciplines and interactions with residents' families and/or other proxy decision makers.
3. Further efforts to reduce unnecessary emergency department visits, hospitalizations, and hospital readmissions because of the risk of viral infection. These efforts can pay strong dividends in the future as value-based programs further penetrate NH care.

TABLE 16-7 ■ COMMON ETHICAL ISSUES IN THE NURSING HOME[a]

ETHICAL ISSUE	EXAMPLES
Preservation of autonomy	Choices in many areas are limited in most nursing homes (eg, mealtimes, sleeping hours)
	Families, physicians, and nursing home staff tend to be paternalistic
Decision-making capacity	Many nursing home residents are incapable or are questionably capable of participating in decisions about their care
	There are no standard methods of assessing decision-making capacity in this population
Surrogate decision making	Many nursing home residents have not clearly stated their preferences or appointed a surrogate before becoming unable to decide for themselves
	Family members may be in conflict, have hidden agendas, or be incapable of or unwilling to make decisions
Quality of life	This concept is often entered into decision making, but it is difficult to measure, especially among those with dementia
	Ageist biases can influence perceptions of nursing home residents' quality of life
Intensity of treatment	A range of options must be considered, including cardiopulmonary resuscitation and mechanical ventilation, hospitalization, treatment of specific conditions (eg, infection) in the nursing home without hospitalization, enteral feeding, comfort, or supportive care only

[a]See Chapter 72 for further information.

4. Renewed focus on polypharmacy and deprescribing of unnecessary medications has been recommended to not only decrease adverse effects and costs, but to avoid unnecessary contacts between staff and residents, as well as the time of administration and documentation for these medications.

5. More proactive discussions of advance directives, beyond "Do Not Resuscitate" to include "Do Not Hospitalize" orders have been recommended because of the potential for very rapid deterioration of residents with life-limiting illnesses among whom the discomforts and risks of hospitalization outweigh the potential benefits. Several organizations produced advance care planning tools with specific language about the pandemic which were useful and will continue to be in the future. The INTERACT website has examples of such tools and links to several other organizations that have developed imilar tools.

6. The need for health systems to evolve so that organizations providing post-acute and long-term care are more closely aligned with local hospitals and home health agencies in order to share learnings, trained staff, and other resources.

7. Continuing evolution of NHs into smaller more homelike facilities, and consideration of separating some types of short vs. long-stayers with appropriate reimbursement, staffing, and education for the different populations.

8. The need for the development of NH research networks with the capability to carry out robust clinical trials, quality improvement research, educational interventions, and epidemiological studies to continue to develop the evidence base for improving NH care with respect to pandemics as well as other areas of care and support.

ACKNOWLEDGMENTS

This chapter is based on and adapted from Chapter 16 of the eighth edition of *Essentials of Clinical Geriatrics* (McGraw Hill, 2018).

Dr. Ouslander is a full-time FAU employee and has received support through FAU to conduct research evaluating the INTERACT program from the National Institutes of Health, the Centers for Medicare and Medicaid Services, the Commonwealth Fund, the Retirement Research Foundation, PointClickCare, Medline Industries, and PatientOrderSets (now Think Research). Dr. Ouslander is a paid medical advisor to Pathway Health which holds the exclusive license from FAU for training and sublicensing of INTERACT, and he and his wife receive royalties related to INTERACT. Works on projects related to INTERACT are subject to terms of Conflicts of Interest Management plans developed and approved by the FAU Division of Research Financial Conflict of Interest Committee.

Alice Bonner is an Adjunct Faculty at the Johns Hopkins University School of Nursing and Director of Strategic Partnerships for the CAPABLE Program. She is also Senior Advisor for Aging at the Institute for Healthcare Improvement (IHI). From 2011 to 2013, Bonner was the Director of the CMS Division of Nursing Homes.

FURTHER READING

American Medical Directors Association. *Transitions of Care in the Long-Term Care Continuum Clinical Practice Guideline*. Columbia, MD: AMDA; 2010.

American Medical Directors Association. *Health Maintenance in the Long-Term Care Setting Clinical Practice Guideline*. Columbia, MD: AMDA; 2012.

Department of Health and Human Services Office of the Inspector General. Adverse Events in Skilled Nursing Facilities: National Incidence among Medicare Beneficiaries. February, 2014. OEI-06-11-00370.

Institute of Medicine. *Improving the Quality of Nursing Home Care*. Washington, DC: National Academy Press; 2000.

Jump RLP, Crnich CJ, Mody L, et al. Infectious diseases in older adults in long-term care facilities: update on approach to diagnosis and management. *J Am Geriatr Soc*. 2018;66:789–803.

Kane RL. Assuring quality in nursing homes care. *J Am Geriatr Soc*. 1998;46:232–237.

Mor V. Defining and measuring quality outcomes in long-term care. *J Am Med Dir Assoc*. 2006;7:532–540.

Morley J, Tolson D, Ouslander J, Vellas B. *Nursing Home Care: A Core Curriculum for the International Association for Gerontology and Geriatrics*. New York, NY: McGraw Hill; 2013.

Ouslander JG, Berenson RA. Reducing unnecessary hospitalizations of NH residents. *N Engl J Med*. 2011;365: 1165–1167.

Ouslander JG, Bonner A, Herndon L, Shutes J. The INTERACT quality improvement program: an overview for medical directors and primary care clinicians in long-term care. *J Am Med Dir Assoc*. 2014;15:162–170.

Ouslander JG, Naharci I, Engstrom G, et al. Root cause analyses of transfers of skilled nursing facility patients to acute hospitals: lessons learned for reducing unnecessary hospitalizations. *J Am Med Dir Assn*. 2016;17:256–262.

Ouslander JG, Grabowski DC. Rehabbed to death reframed: in response to "rehabbed to death: breaking the cycle". *J Am Geriatr Soc*. 2019;67:2225–2228.

Ouslander JG, Grabowski DC. COVID-19 in nursing homes: calming the perfect storm. *J Am Geriatr Soc.* 2019;68:2153–2162.

Saliba D, Schnelle JF. Indicators of the quality of nursing home residential care. *J Am Geriatr Soc.* 2002;50:1421–1430.

Saliba D, Solomon D, Rubenstein L, et al. Feasibility of quality indicators for the management of geriatric syndromes in nursing home residents. *J Am Med Dir Assoc.* 2005;6:S50–S59.

Saliba D, Solomon D, Rubenstein L, et al. Quality indicators for the management of medical conditions in nursing home residents. *J Am Med Dir Assoc.* 2004;5: 297–309.

Zarowitz B, Resnick B, Ouslander JG. Quality clinical care in nursing facilities. *J Am Med Dir Assn.* 2018;19: 833–839.

SELECTED WEBSITES

Interventions to Reduce Acute Care Transfers (INTERACT). https://pathway-interact.com/. Accessed June 1, 2021.

Long-Term Care Focus. http://ltcfocus.org. Accessed June 1, 2021.

The Society for Post-Acute and Long-Term Care Medicine/American Medical Directors Association. https://paltc.org/. Accessed June 1, 2021.

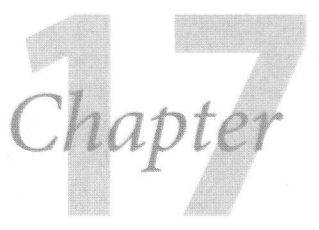

Community-Based Long-Term Services and Support, and Home-Based Medical Care

Jessica Colburn, Jennifer Hayashi, Bruce Leff

INTRODUCTION

Seventy percent of people turning age 65 will need some type of long-term care (LTC) services in their lifetime. While some of those people will be cared for in a nursing home, the majority will choose to remain in the community and require services to help them stay in their homes. These home-based care services come in the form of two general categories—community-based long-term services and support (LTSS) and home-based medical care services. Unfortunately, no coherent national policy drives LTSS in the United States, which leaves a "system" that is difficult to access, bewildering to navigate, unable to fully meet the needs of many patients, and exacerbates health disparities. Much of what is done to meet these needs is provided by unpaid family caregivers at great personal and economic cost. Among the many long-term sequelae of the COVID-19 pandemic, one that is most likely to persist is the preference for non-facility-based health care delivery. This preference, as well as the COVID-19-induced acceleration of telehealth approaches, is likely to create even greater demand for home-based services of all types in the future. This chapter addresses LTSS and home-based medical care for older adults in the United States. We outline the semantic challenges in understanding the scope and nature of LTSS and the heterogeneity of LTSS and home-based medical care models that comprise it; describe who receives, provides, and pays for it; and review the evidence for its effectiveness. We also discuss important public policy issues and identify emerging innovations and trends in this arena.

SPECTRUM OF CARE OF LTSS AND HOME-BASED MEDICAL CARE

Community-based long-term services and support (LTSS) and home-based medical care cover the spectrum of home-based care that exists to support and care for older adults living at home. The term "community-based long-term services and support" overlaps with several other terms in the medical and social sciences literature, including *home care, personal care services, home- and community-based services, home visits,* and others. In general, these terms refer to non-physician, nursing, personal care, or social services provided to older persons with an explicit goal of filling unmet needs or maintaining them in the community.

Learning Objectives

- Recognize the semantic challenges, scope, nature, and heterogeneity of community-based long-term services and support (LTSS) and home-based medical care in the United States.
- Identify the common models of LTSS and home-based medical care.
- Describe the evidence base and reimbursement mechanisms for common models of LTSS and home-based medical care.

Key Clinical Points

1. The vast majority of care for older people at home is provided by friends and family as unpaid informal caregivers, at enormous indirect cost to society in the form of lost wages, lost productivity, and future social insurance costs.

2. There is a substantial body of evidence suggesting that various models of LTSS and home-based medical care are effective; cost-effectiveness and outcomes associated with these models depend on targeting of services to appropriate populations.

3. Innovative home-based care delivery models hold promise for aligning payment incentives with health outcomes to improve care for older adults.

Unpaid family members or friends provide a majority of this care, sometimes with support from a variety of paid formal caregivers. Home-based medical care includes models that involve direct care by a physician or advanced practice provider (nurse practitioner or physician assistant). These may include longitudinal care models, such as home-based primary care, or may include episodic care, such as preventive home-based geriatric assessment visits, home-based rehabilitation, and hospital at home (HaH). LTSS and home-based medical care often overlap to such an extent that important aspects of a given intervention are not accurately reflected in a single label. For example, a program in which an interdisciplinary team provides comprehensive geriatric assessment followed by home-based primary care, inpatient management as needed, and continuing longitudinal care after hospital discharge does not fit neatly into any one category. Several forms of LTSS integrate housing arrangements with personal care and home-based medical care, further blurring the distinction between community-based and institutional LTSS. **Table 17-1** depicts the heterogeneity and scope of services and settings that fall under the rubric of LTSS.

Home health care encompasses a spectrum of care including long-term social services, informal and formal paid care in the home, and skilled home health care. Home and community-based services usually refers to LTSS provided under the Medicaid program. Informal care refers to services provided by unpaid caregivers, most commonly female family members. The estimated 48 million informal caregivers in the United States provide the majority of all home care and LTSS at an estimated economic value of $470 billion. Formal paid care includes paid home health aides for personal care services in the home (bathing, dressing, etc) and typically is covered via private pay by the patient, though also may be covered through state Medicaid waiver programs or Department of Aging Social Services programs. Paid care in assisted living facilities (ALFs), sheltered housing, and group homes is variable and may include medication administration and monitoring of vital signs as well as access to physicians when needed, such as domiciliary care visits or a clinic housed within a senior apartment building. Skilled home health care refers to formal services delivered by professional providers, such as nurses or physical, occupational, or speech therapists. Medicare certifies and reimburses home health care agencies (HHAs) to provide this type of care when a patient is homebound and has a skilled need (see "Who Provides and Pays for LTSS and Home-Based Medical Care" later in the chapter). HHAs may also provide formal personal care services (bathing, dressing, etc) under the Medicare home health care benefit while a patient is receiving skilled care. Referrals for Medicare skilled home health care are placed for patients who have a skilled need, such as physical therapy or nursing care, and may originate from the hospital, rehabilitation setting, or from outpatient or home-based primary care. For example, an older patient who suffers an acute exacerbation of chronic obstructive pulmonary disease may spend several days in bed (at home or in the hospital), and may need nursing to monitor her respiratory status and physical therapy to help her regain her baseline functional mobility. It is important to note that the effectiveness of skilled home care often relies on services provided by an informal caregiver who, if available, can help implement a home exercise program, clean and dress pressure ulcers, or bathe, dress, and toilet a dependent patient.

Models of home-based medical care include a spectrum of options, including both longitudinal and episodic care options: home-based primary care, home-based primary care co-management, home-based integrated medical and social care, home-based palliative care and hospice care, preventive home-based geriatric assessment, rehabilitation at home, and HaH. Home-based primary care, in which physicians, nurse practitioners, and physician assistants provide ongoing longitudinal medical care at home, can play an important role in providing access to routine and urgent care for older adults who have difficulty getting to a medical office. Home-based primary care programs have been increasing in prevalence in recent years and have been shown to be effective (see **Table 17-2** later in this chapter). In 2013, approximately 5000 individual health care providers made 1.7 million home visits in the United States, accounting for 70% of home-based medical visits. Some models include home-based primary care as part of their continuum of care, such as the Program of All-Inclusive Care for the Elderly (PACE), which relies heavily on a "day health center" in which dually eligible (ie, Medicare and Medicaid eligible) nursing home–eligible participants receive comprehensive medical, hygienic, social, and rehabilitative care. Home-based primary care co-management models involve the use of an interdisciplinary care team to help care for patients with complex needs in collaboration with a patient's primary care provider. Home-based integrated medical and social care models provide integrated medical and social services for patients with significant medical, behavioral health, and social needs with an interdisciplinary team that typically includes behavioral health specialists. Home-based palliative care may be embedded within home-based primary care models, or may be provided by hospice agencies as a continuum of care prior to home hospice care. Home hospice care provides end-of-life care to patients within the last 6 months of life, with home-based support focused on comfort care. Hospital-at-home is a care model that provides hospital-level care in a patient's home as a substitute for an acute hospital admission that has been shown to be associated with better care quality and lower costs than typical hospital care. Rehabilitation-at-home provides subacute rehabilitation at home posthospitalization.

Other home-based approaches offer one-time visits or assessments or care focused on specific diseases or conditions. Preventive home visits and home-based geriatric assessment typically aim to identify older adults in the community who have hidden risks for developing illness or functional decline, and modify those risks to prevent poor outcomes. These visits may be provided as part of Medicare Advantage programs, such as through Medicare Annual Wellness Visits provided at home, or may be done by community health workers as a geriatric assessment visit to assess risk. Home-based disease management programs target patients known to have specific diseases or conditions that require significant care coordination, such as diabetes or heart failure, for formal support in managing

TABLE 17-1 ■ LONG-TERM SERVICES AND SUPPORTS AND HOME-BASED MEDICAL CARE MODELS

TYPE OF LTSS/HBMC	DESCRIPTION/SERVICES	FUNDING
EPISODIC		
Home-based geriatric assessment	Multidisciplinary evaluation of medical, social, functional, and cognitive issues	Variable depending on evaluator and context
Preventive home visits	Health maintenance visits by health care professionals (physicians, nurses, social workers) or trained "health visitors"	National insurance (Europe/United Kingdom), research grants (United Kingdom, US), Medicare Advantage programs (US)
Home-based disease management programs	Disease-specific teaching and support provided by nurses	Medicare (as part of skilled home care) or private insurance
Hospital at Home	Acute-level care at home with daily nurse/physician in-person and/or virtual visits	Variable depending on system implementing the model. Recent Medicare payment waiver
Rehabilitation at home	Post-hospitalization subacute care, usually for patients requiring skilled therapy as a substitute for skilled nursing facility admission	Not currently reimbursed; episodic home nursing and physical therapy is reimbursed by Medicare Part A for homebound people who require these services (see below under Home Health Care)
Community paramedicine-mobile integrated health	Community-based care delivery via Emergency Medical Services. Two main models: (1) urgent, unplanned pre-hospital triage and care to avoid unnecessary emergency department or hospital use; and (2) non-urgent, planned post-hospital discharge care to prevent readmissions.	Mostly subsidized by health systems or risk arrangements between providers and health plans
Community Aging in Place, Advancing Better Living for Elders (CAPABLE)	Interprofessional team (occupational therapist, nurse, handyperson) to help achieve patient-centered goals; focus on improving functional status	Medicaid, private insurance
Maximizing Independence (MIND) at Home	Home-based dementia care coordination, uses community health workers as liaison between patients with dementia and team with dementia expertise	Medicare managed care, private pay
Home health care (usually episodic, may be longitudinal) Formal (agency or consumer-directed) • Skilled care • Personal care Community resources Informal	Home health care agency or client provides and pays personnel • Nursing, occupational and physical therapy • ADL assistance Meals on Wheels, Department of Social Services, Agency on Aging case management, pastoral care ADL/IADL assistance as needed	Medicare/Medicaid or private long-term care insurance/private pay (if no skilled need) Community agencies, local jurisdictions, local faith-based organizations None/opportunity cost of caregivers
LONGITUDINAL		
Home-based primary care	Medical care and visits in patient's home	Medicare, private insurance, private pay
Home-based primary care co-management	Provides patient assessment, coordination, and wrap-around services in the home in collaboration with patients' office-based primary care providers	Mostly subsidized by health systems or risk arrangements between providers and health plans
Home-based integrated -medical and social care	Integrated wraparound services for patients with significant medical, behavioral, health, and social needs in the home	Capitated payments from Medicare and Medicaid; a Medicare shared savings model (eg, Medicare ACO) can coordinate with LTSS services
Program of All-Inclusive Care for the Elderly (PACE)	Comprehensive medical, social, and functional care for dually eligible, nursing home-eligible patients	Medicare and Medicaid dual-capitated payments
Home-based palliative care and hospice	Provides basic or specialist palliative care in the home to alleviate physical symptoms and emotional distress	Medicare FFS for provider services; some Medicare Advantage, Medicaid managed care, or commercial plans use per-member per-month payments and shared savings arrangements

(Continued)

TABLE 17-1 ■ LONG-TERM SERVICES AND SUPPORTS AND HOME-BASED MEDICAL CARE MODELS *(CONTINUED)*

TYPE OF LTSS/HBMC	DESCRIPTION/SERVICES	FUNDING
LOCATION-BASED		
Adult day care • Medical • Social	Supervised congregate activities, 1–7d/wk for several hours/day • Includes medication administration and basic monitoring • Limited to social interaction	Private pay, Medicaid (this is a component of the PACE Program)
Assisted living	Apartment-style living with skilled and/or unskilled (personal care) services available on site	Long-term care insurance, private pay
Sheltered housing	"Senior apartments" with varying social services on site (eg, friendly visitors, congregate meals, transportation, social work)	Private pay, subsidized by federal and local governments
Adult foster care	Older adult who needs assistance or supervision moves in with "foster" family	Private pay, subsidized by federal and local governments
Group home	Group of adults who need assistance or supervision live in one building with skilled and/or unskilled services available on site (can be similar to assisted living)	Subsidized by federal and local governments
Continuing care retirement communities (CCRC)	Geographically localized and self-contained spectrum of living arrangements from independent housing to nursing home care	Private pay

ACO, accountable care organization; ADLs, activities of daily living; FFS, fee-for service; IADLs, instrumental activities of daily living.

those conditions, with the goal of delaying disease progression and avoiding hospitalization. Community paramedicine programs use emergency medical services to deliver hospital triage or assessment. They typically target high utilizers of emergency department or hospital services, or may work collaboratively with home-based primary care programs. Home-based urgent care programs provide urgent care options, sometimes through apps that help locate a local home-based care provider or to connect via telemedicine; these are typically urgent, one-time visits and not longitudinal, ongoing care. Additional short-term home-based interventions have been shown more recently to support older adults who continue to live in their homes. Community Aging in Place, Advancing Better Living for Elders (CAPABLE) is an intervention that involves an interprofessional team (occupational therapist, nurse, and handyperson) to help patients achieve goals they set and has been shown to reduce disability as well as costs for inpatient care and long-term support services. Maximizing Independence (MIND) at Home is a home-based dementia care coordination program that uses community health workers as a liaison between patients with dementia and a team with dementia expertise, and also has been shown to reduce costs of inpatient care and LTSS.

Still other forms of LTSS provide care outside the home or may require older adults to relocate to a new living situation. Adult day care generally includes transportation to a day care center, and can provide both structured social activities and basic medical monitoring and treatment. For patients who cannot continue to live in their own homes, assisted living, sheltered housing (also known as senior apartments), adult foster care, and group homes all provide varying levels of functional assistance and access to some medical services. Continuing care retirement communities (CCRCs), as the name suggests, are self-contained organizations that allow people to move within the community to increasing levels of care as their needs dictate. At one end of the continuing care spectrum, a fully independent older adult lives in a single-family home or apartment, but over time may transition first to an assisted-living apartment, then to the skilled nursing facility within the same CCRC. There are several variations of this model, but most charge an entrance and monthly fee that provides lifelong care in the event that the participant develops some kind of functional impairment.

This array of models can be framed as a quasi-continuum of care services for older adults, as shown in **Figure 17-1**. While some forms of home-based care are designed to address the needs of older adults through a variety of health or disease states, such as home health care, CCRCs, or post-acute disease management programs, others are targeted to specific populations based on levels of impairment or disability, such as home-based primary care or PACE. Again, many patients and programs do not fit neatly into a single category and patients do not usually move across the continuum in a straight line, as the use of services depends not only on the fit between the needs of an older adult and the care model, but also on the preferences of older adults and local availability of care models. For example, skilled home health care may be used by a healthy older adult after elective joint replacement surgery or a frail chronically ill patient recovering from a recent episode of community-acquired pneumonia treated at home by a

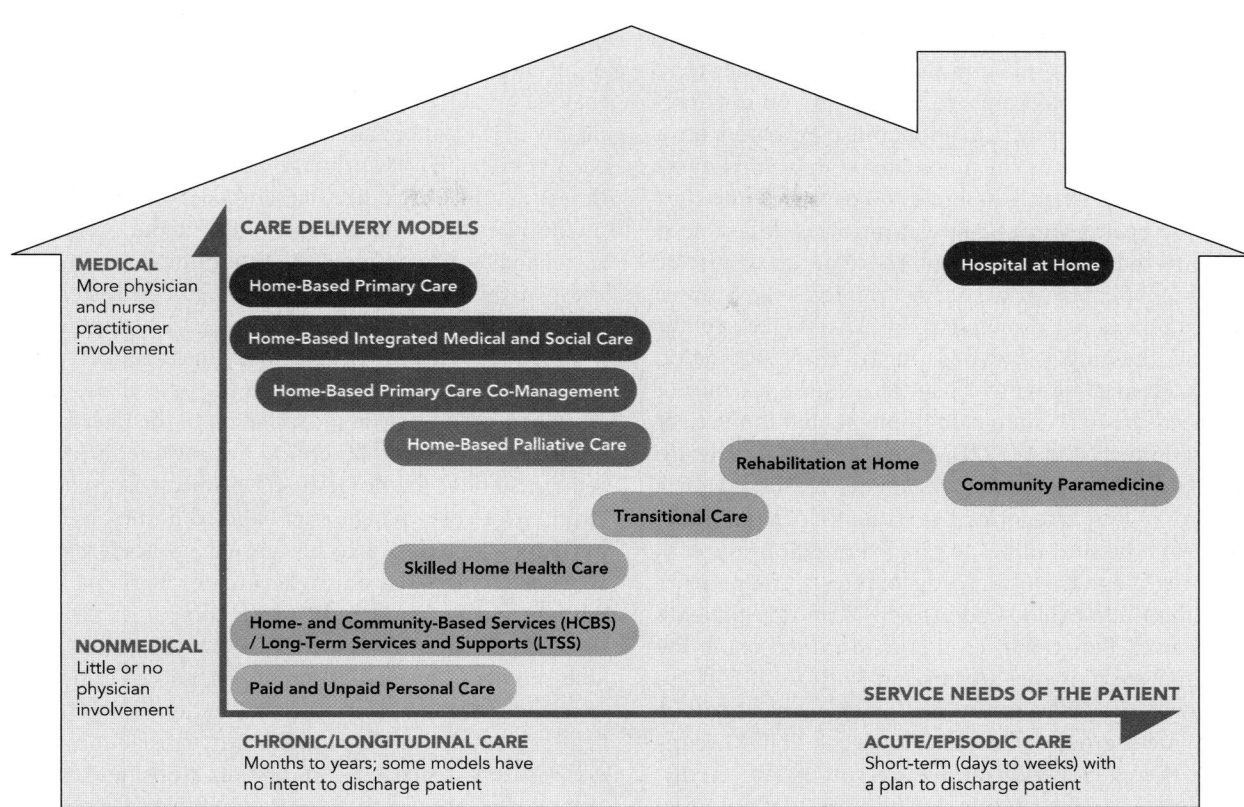

FIGURE 17-1. Home-based care delivery models across the continuum of care for older adults.

home-based primary care program. However, the concept of a continuum is a useful construct for organizing categories of LTSS and home-based medical care.

WHO RECEIVES LTSS AND HOME-BASED MEDICAL CARE?

Health maintenance strategies such as preventive home visits and geriatric assessment tend to target patients who are relatively robust and functionally independent, while PACE and home-based primary care address the needs of patients who are more frail and impaired. CCRCs explicitly transition patients from the robust state through functional decline. Post-acute home health care, home-based primary care, rehabilitation at home and HaH may be used by both robust and frail older adults in specific circumstances, but the primary intended users of most LTSS and home-based medical care remain those who have chronic and complex medical illness accompanied by some level of functional disability, and thus require care for a prolonged or even indefinite time. The likelihood of receiving formal care is generally lower for men, people of color, married individuals, those with lower socioeconomic status, and those who are less dependent for assistance with activities and instrumental activities of daily living (ADLs), but one particular diagnosis profoundly affects these demographics. In the

2015 National Health and Aging Trends Study (NHATS), 25% of patients with dementia and 48% of patient with advanced dementia received paid care, and the likelihood of paid care increased for men, unmarried patients, those on Medicaid (lower socioeconomic status), and those with more functional impairment. The racial disparities documented in outpatient offices and hospitals are also present in LTSS, with a 2017 systematic review demonstrating that minority of patients consistently had more adverse events, less functional improvement, and worse patient experiences than White patients.

WHO PROVIDES AND PAYS FOR LTSS AND HOME-BASED MEDICAL CARE?

The role of unpaid informal caregivers cannot be overemphasized. The work they perform is not directly reimbursed or financially rewarded by the health care system. The indirect costs are enormous when lost wages, lost productivity, health care costs related to caregiver burden, and future social insurance losses are calculated for caregivers who may sacrifice paid employment to provide informal care for a parent or other relative. For formal care, the provider varies with the type of care. In the most common model of skilled home health care, an HHA certified to provide care under Medicare reimbursement rules employs nurses, therapists, aides, and social workers, and assigns them to individual patient cases. A physician must certify that the patient is homebound and has a skilled need in order for a Medicare-certified HHA to provide care for a 60-day "certification period." This certification must be based on a face-to-face encounter by the physician or associated nurse practitioner within 90 days before or 30 days after the start date of home health services. By definition, a skilled need requires care that is part-time, intermittent, and must be provided by a person with special training (eg, a nurse or therapist). Personal care assistance with ADLs such as bathing and dressing is covered during the certification period, but Medicare does not pay for it in the absence of a skilled need. In 2021, Medicare implemented the Patient Driven Groupings Model (PDGM) to pay for home health care. Under this model, reimbursements are based on a combination of four categories: the patient's location in the 14 days before the start of home care ("admission source"), the admitting diagnosis ("clinical grouping"), the patient's comorbidities ("comorbidity adjustment"), and the patient's functional level. Functional level is determined using the Outcome and Assessment Information Set (OASIS). These four categories are then used to assign the patient to one of 432 "payment groups" that determine the PDGM reimbursement the agency will receive for the 60-day certification period. The certification period is divided into two 30-day payment units, and each 30-day period has a separate admission source determination, based on the patient's health care setting in the 14 days before the start of that period. Periods with "institutional" admission sources, when the patient has been in an acute or post-acute facility within the 14 days prior to the start of care, are reimbursed at a higher rate than periods with "community" admission sources, when there is no acute or post-acute stay in the preceding 14 days. A patient can be "recertified" for multiple 60-day periods as long as a skilled need exists. The settlement of the *Jimmo v Sebelius* case, in 2013, clarified that Medicare reimbursement for skilled home health services is allowed for people whose potential to improve may be limited, as long as there is a skilled need focused on preventing further deterioration or maintaining current level of function. LTSS can also be privately purchased by the care recipients. Additionally, a "consumer-directed" or "cash and counseling" model allows selected patients to choose, train, and pay their personal care providers directly with designated state funds (usually from Medicaid programs), instead of using an agency as an intermediary. In these programs, care providers can be family members or other previously unpaid caregivers. This model has had positive results, showing increased patient empowerment and satisfaction, and fewer unmet needs, although unmet needs persist, and new needs emerge as patients are required to function as employers.

Interdisciplinary teams are critical in coordinating and delivering care in home-based medical care, including skilled home health care ordered by physicians, home-based geriatric assessment, PACE, home-based primary care, and HaH (see Chapter 14). Such teams typically include physicians or advanced practice providers, although the provider's role may vary in different settings depending on the medical complexity of the patient and the setting. For example, in PACE, the provider delivers primary care services, manages acute illness during hospitalization, and coordinates the activities of the interdisciplinary team, often in the patient's home. In rehabilitation at home, the interdisciplinary team drives most of the management with a focus on restoring function and following up medical issues. In hospital-at-home interventions, the provider actively manages acute illness at home, so that medical house calls (in-person and/or virtual) complemented by close coordination of the interdisciplinary team are crucial in this setting. Improvements in Medicare reimbursement for home-based primary care and demonstrations of cost savings with targeted home-based services have contributed to a recent growth in academic and private sector home-based medical care programs. Emerging co-management models, in which companies provide coordinated and comprehensive telemedicine services, in-person assessments from medical providers, and/or social services, may reduce unnecessary hospitalization, lower costs, and improve health outcomes and patient satisfaction. Commercial insurers, managed care organizations, and health systems at risk for total costs for their populations are currently the main drivers developing these models.

Other forms of home-based care rely less on medical providers and more on specialized nurses or trained lay visitors. Disease management, post-acute home health care, and medical day care are often based on protocols driven by nurses. In transitional care interventions, specially trained registered nurses (RNs) provide a combination of telephone or video support, remote in-home monitoring of parameters such as weight, blood pressure, and pulse oximetry, and communication with primary care providers to reduce the risk of hospital readmission during the transition from acute care to home. Home-based geriatric assessment is usually performed by geriatric nurses or nurse practitioners and then discussed as needed with physicians, while preventive home visits have been successful in using "health visitors," or specially trained community health workers, in screening for health risks. The CAPABLE program is a time-limited intervention of nurse, occupational therapist, and handypersons targeted at community-dwelling older adults with functional impairment with the goal of improving their functional status. A small number of older adults carry privately funded long-term care (LTC) insurance, and in recent years, some businesses have added this option to their employees' benefit packages. Older adults with higher LTSS needs have higher Medicare and out-of-pocket costs, increased credit card debt attributable to health care expenses, and more difficulty paying for food, rent, utilities, medications, and medical care. Ultimately, many of these people exhaust their retirement savings and home equity to pay for LTSS, becoming eligible for Medicaid through this "spend-down" process.

IS HOME-BASED CARE EFFECTIVE?

Studies of home-based care can be challenging to interpret because of the semantic difficulties outlined above, the heterogeneity of home care interventions, difficulties in controlling for severity of disability or morbidity burden of patients, patient attrition issues, changes in regulation over time, and examination of a disparate range of outcome measures.

However, it is clear that the evidence base for home-based care has becoming increasing robust over the recent years. Key studies and their findings are summarized in **Table 17-2.** We discuss the current evidence by separating home-based medical care models into two broad categories by the time frames over which they provide care: (1) longitudinal models that provide care and follow patients over an extended period of time, and (2) episodic models that provide care that is limited to a single incidence or time-limited episode of care. **Figure 17-1** arrays the services and models along the axes of care from nonmedical (little or no physician involvement) to medical (more physician and nurse practitioner involvement) and from chronic/longitudinal models (those that may follow patients for months to years with no intent to discharge a patient) to models that are acute/episodic (short-term with a plan to discharge the patient).

Longitudinal Models

As described above, home-based primary care provides longitudinal primary care to homebound older adults with multiple chronic conditions and functional impairments who commonly face socioeconomic challenges. Medical care is a core component and interdisciplinary care is commonly provided. Systematic reviews demonstrate reductions in emergency department visits, hospitalizations, LTC admissions, and costs of care, and improvements in patient and caregiver quality of life and satisfaction with care. Home-based primary care co-management models have emerged in the recent years and provide wraparound care to high-need, high-cost populations often in risk arrangements between providers of such care and payers who seek to provide value-based care to this population. In collaboration with the primary care provider an interdisciplinary team addresses the patient's complex care needs. Randomized controlled trials of some models show reduced health care utilization and increased care coordination and patient/caregiver satisfaction. Home-based integrated medical/social care models provide multifaceted, longitudinal, wraparound medical and social services for high-need high-cost patients with complex medical, behavioral health, and social needs within interdisciplinary care team that often includes behavioral health specialists. Reimbursement is usually through shared savings mechanisms. Observational and case-control studies demonstrate lower health care utilization and institutionalization and higher patient satisfaction. Home-based palliative care provides interdisciplinary, longitudinal or episodic, specialist palliative care in the home to patients with serious illnesses. Providers usually focus on clarifying goals of care, symptom management of patients and families. There is evidence for improved quality of life and reduction in health care utilization and costs. The comprehensive management strategies of the PACE programs are effective at reducing institutionalization of at-risk patients.

Episodic Models

Transitional care focuses on patients at high risk of poor outcomes during the transitions from hospital back to home. Transitional care focuses on care coordination, education, follow-up, and medication management. Meta-analyses and systematic reviews demonstrate improved outcomes including reductions in mortality and reductions in emergency department visits and hospital readmissions in the 30 days after hospital discharge. Mobile Integrated Health–Community Paramedicine is an episodic care delivery model that has emerged recently. The model targets high utilizers of emergency department and hospital services via two main models: (1) urgent, unplanned pre-hospital triage and care to avoid unnecessary emergency department or hospital use; and (2) non-urgent, planned posthospital discharge care to prevent readmissions. Early evidence demonstrates reduced utilization and improved patient satisfaction. HaH provides hospital-level care in a patient's home as a substitute for care provided in the traditional acute care hospital. Substitution HaH admits patients to their home directly from the emergency department. Transfer HaH admits patients who require ongoing hospital-level care from the traditional hospital to their home. Reimbursement exists mainly through Medicare Advantage and Veterans Affairs health systems currently. During the COVID-19 pandemic, the Centers for Medicare and Medicaid Services provided a waiver to pay hospital-level reimbursement for HaH care for fee-for-service Medicare beneficiaries. HaH care has been demonstrated in multiple randomized controlled trials, systematic reviews, and meta-analyses to be associated with lower costs, lower complications and mortality, and improved patient/caregiver satisfaction and experience. Rehabilitation at Home is an emerging care delivery model that provides episodic care delivered at home to people requiring care at time of hospital discharge that would otherwise would be provided in a skilled nursing facility. Care is provided by an interdisciplinary care team with skilled therapists supported by doctor, nurse, social worker, and other team members as needed. Early evidence suggests good functional outcomes and lower costs of care. CAPABLE, described earlier, has demonstrated improvements in ability to perform ADLs and to reduce hospital utilization and costs of care with decreased annual health care costs to Medicaid by about $10,000 per patient, with a 5-month intervention at a cost of $2,825 per patient. It has been adopted by several state Medicaid plans.

TABLE 17-2 ■ EVIDENCE FOR EFFECTIVENESS OF LONG-TERM SERVICES AND SUPPORTS (LTSS) AND HOME-BASED MEDICAL CARE (HBMC) MODELS

AUTHOR/YEAR	MODEL	SETTING	TARGETED POPULATION	MAJOR FINDINGS
Huss 2008	Preventive home visits	Meta-analysis	Community-dwelling older adults	Functional decline reduced in trials with multidimensional assessment including clinical examination Mortality reduced in younger (< 77 y) but not older (> 80 y) populations Favorable but nonsignificant heterogenous effects on nursing home placement
LaBerre 2017	Transitional care	Systematic review	Older adults transitioning from hospital to primary care	Lower mortality Lower rate of emergency room visits Lower rate of hospital readmissions
Caplan 2012	Hospital at home	Meta-analysis	Acutely ill patients > 16 y randomized to hospital admission or hospital-at-home services	Significantly reduced mortality, readmission rates, and cost Significantly increased patient and caregiver satisfaction
Shepperd 2016	Hospital at home	Systematic review	Acutely ill adults > 18 y	Hospital-at-home models that substituted for inpatient admission reduced 6-mo mortality and cost, despite a nonsignificant increase in hospital transfer or readmission within 3 mo
Augustine 2020	Rehabilitation at home	Retrospective review	Adults qualifying for SNF-based rehabilitation services	SNF-level care at home is feasible and associated with functional improvement
Gregg 2019	Community paramedicine and mobile integrated health	Systematic review	Hospital, ED, or EMS users; "high-risk" or chronically ill patients	Decreased utilization of ED and hospital
Szanton 2018	CAPABLE	Clinical trial	Older adults with ADL impairment	Decreased hospital and long-term care utilization Lower Medicaid costs
Samus 2014	MIND at Home	Clinical trial	Older adults with cognitive disorders	Delay in time to transition from home; reduction in unmet needs; improved quality of life
Stall 2014	Home-based primary care	Systematic review	Homebound community-dwelling older adults	Decreased utilization (ED visits, hospital admissions/days of care, long-term care admissions/days of care) Positive influence of interprofessional team with regular team meetings and after-hours support
Valluru 2019	Home-based integrated medical and social care	Case-cohort study	Patients receiving HBPC integrated with long-term support services	HBPC integrated with medical and social care delays NH placement
Assistant Secretary for Planning and Evaluation 2014	PACE	Review of literature	Dually eligible, nursing home–eligible frail older adults	Increased life expectancy Decreased use of hospital Lower mortality rates No significant effect on Medicare costs Increased Medicaid costs
Gomes 2013	Home-based palliative care	Meta-analysis	Adults with advanced illness receiving home palliative care services	Increased chance of dying at home Reduced symptom burden No impact on caregiver grief

(Continued)

TABLE 17-2 ■ EVIDENCE FOR EFFECTIVENESS OF LONG-TERM SERVICES AND SUPPORTS (LTSS) AND HOME-BASED MEDICAL CARE (HBMC) MODELS *(CONTINUED)*

AUTHOR/YEAR	MODEL	SETTING	TARGETED POPULATION	MAJOR FINDINGS
Totten 2019	Telehealth	Systematic review	Use of any technology to facilitate consultations for inpatient, emergency, or outpatient care	Generally better outcomes or no difference from comparators in settings and clinical indications Reduced mortality from ICU teleconsultations Reduced patient time in ED from specialty teleconsultations Reduced heart attack mortality from EMS prehospital teleconsultations Improved access and clinical outcomes from outpatient specialty teleconsultations
Wysocki 2015	LTSS	Comparative effectiveness review of HCBS vs NH care	Older adults served by HCBS (including ALFs and NH)	Outcomes similar for ALF and NH residents Harms differed between HCBS recipients and NH residents Insufficient evidence for cost comparison

ADL, activities of daily living; ALF, assisted living facility; CAPABLE, Community Aging in Place, Advancing Better Living for Elders; ED, emergency department; EMS, emergency medical services; HBPC, home-based primary care; HCBS, home and community-based services; ICU, intensive care unit; MIND, Maximizing Independence; NH, nursing home; PACE, Program of All-Inclusive Care for the Elderly; SNF, skilled nursing facility.

As **Table 17-2** indicates, an extensive home care literature includes a wide variety of interventions and target populations. While this heterogeneity creates significant difficulty in drawing conclusions about the effectiveness and cost-effectiveness of home care, the overall body of evidence suggests that specific models when appropriately targeted are probably effective.

This issue of targeting care to appropriate patient populations is a major determinant of the cost-effectiveness of specific interventions. A related factor that complicates discussions of cost-effectiveness is the notion of paid care inappropriately substituting for informal care at a cost to society, or the "moral hazard" or "woodwork" effect. In theory, if LTSS are made widely available, functionally impaired patients will "come out of the woodwork" to utilize them, even though most of these patients would never enter an institution even without using LTSS. Thus, the cost of providing care will overwhelm the potential savings of avoiding institutionalization. Targeting services to patients who are at high risk for LTC placement is generally accepted as an important way to optimize cost-effectiveness, but no practical, precise, and accurate targeting tools have been developed and tested. This is because the need for LTC placement is multifactorial, and a highly person-centered decision. Greater state expenditures on LTSS are associated with lower rates of LTC placement of older adults who do not have significant impairment in "late-loss" ADLs (bed mobility, toileting, transferring, and eating). Cost-effectiveness also depends on the economic features of the health systems in which various forms of LTSS have been studied; findings from European programs in which the government is the payer for LTSS, institutional LTC, and acute care are difficult to apply to the United States fee-for-service environment with multiple public and private payers and complex cost-shifting pressures. The evidence base for home-based medical care models more clearly demonstrates effectiveness.

Innovations

Telemedicine and virtual care, accelerated by the COVID-19 pandemic, has emerged as a major innovation in health service delivery and has the potential to accelerate the development of home-based care for older adults and for the general population. Until the COVID-19 pandemic, telemedicine was used at some scale mostly in rural populations or in systems with particular needs for it such as the Veterans Affairs health system for certain types of specialized care. Use cases such as dermatology, ophthalmology, and wound care have been widely studied in small clinical trials and appear to allow accurate diagnosis and management through both real-time interactions and "store-and-forward" applications in which clinical data including video images are collected and stored for later review by a clinician. In addition, they have been used in disease management interventions to enhance communication between patients and providers and facilitate closer monitoring of overall health when conducted in settings with specialized equipment and dedicated staff. Although the evidence is limited by methodologic variability, lack of comparison with in-person evaluation, and absence of clinical outcome measures, a 2019 systematic review by the Agency for Healthcare Research and Quality (AHRQ) concluded that in some situations, the results of telemedicine vary by setting and condition and that remote consultations for outpatient care likely improve access and clinical outcomes.

In the early phases of the COVID-19 pandemic, ambulatory care came to a grinding halt. The Centers for Medicare and Medicaid Services (CMS) provided regulatory relief in their "Hospital Without Walls" regulatory guidance that allowed for reimbursement of non-in-person outpatient visits to help patients maintain care with their outpatient and home-based primary care and specialty physicians. Health systems, ambulatory, and home-based medical care practices implemented virtual visits at a scale and speed thought impossible. In addition, the CMS provided a hospital-based waiver to provide a hospital diagnosis-related group payment for fee-for-service Medicare beneficiaries for hospital at home care.

Point-of-care diagnostic and therapeutic technology including electrocardiography, ultrasound, blood analysis, and intravenous treatment holds promise for health care delivery in home care and house calls. Wireless telephone and Internet applications that allow secure, high-speed broadband connections between portable electronic medical records (EMR) systems and acute care or office information systems can provide safe and seamless continuity of care with immediate data access and entry for providers caring for complex older patients with multiple medical issues, medications, sites of care, and consultants.

Remote patient monitoring on intermittent and continuous basis is now feasible. It has been used in multiple contexts including hospital discharges, specific disease management programs for conditions such as heart failure, COPD, home-based dialysis, Parkinson disease, postoperative care, diabetes, blood pressure management, and others. Few randomized controlled trials have been conducted. Wireless and smartphone applications are the most commonly used strategies. Models also commonly employ teleconsultation approaches.

Trends and the Future

Several emerging trends in health care and the growing recognition of home-based care and the population it serves are driving innovation in health service delivery that will expand significantly for years to come. There is a growing recognition of the role of social, cognitive, and functional risk factors, as well as that a significant portion of health care spending on frail older adult populations are preventable. Further, there is recognition that home-based care can address these issues, as well as provide acute on primary geriatric medical care, in ways that facility-based care cannot.

The Affordable Care Act established the Medicare Shared Savings Program to promote the formation of accountable care organizations (ACOs). ACOs can be hospital or clinician group led and work to coordinate care for the defined population of Medicare beneficiaries they serve. ACOs emphasize value-based care over volume-driven care and reward or penalize clinicians based on their performance on cost and quality measures. The Medicare Shared Savings Program (MSSP) for ACOs was associated with modest cost savings while maintaining or improving patient quality of care. There are examples of home-based primary care-only-focused ACOs that have been among the ACOs that have saved the most money for the Medicare program.

In addition, the recognition of the importance of assessing and addressing social determinants of health has accelerated home-based care in the context of other financially at-risk delivery models. Several home-based medical co-management commercial entities that contract with Medicare Advantage plans to provide co-management services in collaboration with patients' primary care physician have emerged in the health care marketplace. These entities seek to improve patient engagement in care, address social determinants of health, improve care transitions, and care coordination, often with an underlying shared-savings model as the financial engine. Similarly, home-based palliative care has emerged as a specialized service utilized by Medicare Advantage plans and other financially at-risk health systems to address the needs of patients with palliative care needs and functional impairments with the goal of reducing hospital utilization.

Interdisciplinary team-based models of care providing medical care, nursing, and social work at home for older adults with multiple chronic illnesses, once seen only in academic medical centers, are being adopted more widely by health care delivery systems. These teams focus not on single-disease management, but on coordination of care, integration of patient goals and preferences, and improvement of patient outcomes relevant to this particularly frail and vulnerable group.

Over the past several decades, multiple home-based care models as described above have been developed and evaluated, often with clear advantages over traditional care approaches. The opportunity to start to align these models into a true and full continuum of home and communit-based care that also integrates social supports now exists. In the coming years, this continuum will be realized.

CONCLUSION

LTSS and home-based medical care are a varied collection of services and models aimed at allowing functionally impaired older adults to age in place and receive care in the home setting. Overall, these models are effective when appropriately targeted; older adults continue to prefer living in the community to living in institutions, and social pressures from an aging generation will only increase demand for such care in the future. The current fragmented system of LTSS will be untenable in the coming years as the number of older adults with complex multimorbidity and functional disability increases. Emerging models of home-based medical care including home-based primary care, hospital at home, and others hold promise for improving health care for these patients, although systematic barriers exist to their widespread implementation. Creative economic, technological, and clinical solutions that focus on quality and cost-effectiveness will be critical in reforming the system to affirm and fulfill the public trust.

FURTHER READING

Augustine MR, Davenport C, Ornstein KA, et al. Implementation of post-acute rehabilitation at home: a skilled nursing facility-substitutive model. *J Am Geriatr Soc.* 2020;68(7):1584–1593.

Caplan GA, Sulaiman NS, Mangin DA, Aimonino Ricauda N, Wilson AD, Barclay L. A meta-analysis of "hospital in the home." *Med J Aust.* 2012;197(9):512–519.

Counsell SR, Callahan CM, Clark DO, et al. Geriatric care management for low-income seniors: a randomized controlled trial. *JAMA.* 2007;298(22):2623–2633.

Evaluating PACE: A review of the literature. Office of the Assistant Secretary for Planning and Evaluation (ASPE). https://aspe.hhs.gov/sites/default/files/private/pdf/76976/PACELitRev.pdf. Accessed December 14, 2021.

Farias FAC, Dagostini CM, Bicca YA, Falavigna VF, Falavigna A. Remote patient monitoring: a systematic review. *Telemed J E Health.* 2020;26(5):576–583.

Gomes B, Calanzani N, Curiale V, McCrone P, Higginson IJ. Effectiveness and cost-effectiveness of home palliative care services for adults with advanced illness and their caregivers. *Cochrane Database Syst Rev.* 2013;(6):CD007760.

Gregg A, Tutek J, Leatherwood MD, et al. Systematic review of community paramedicine and EMS mobile integrated health care interventions in the United States. *Popul Health Manag.* 2019;22(3):213–222.

Hughes SL, Weaver FM, Giobbie-Hurder A, et al. Effectiveness of team-managed home-based primary care: a randomized multicenter trial. *JAMA.* 2000; 284(22): 2877–2885.

Huss A, Stuck AE, Rubenstein LZ, Egger M, Clough-Gorr KM. Multidimensional preventive home visit programs for community-dwelling older adults: a systematic review and meta-analysis of randomized controlled trials. *J Gerontol A Biol Sci Med Sci.* 2008;63(3):298–307.

Le Berre M, Maimon G, Sourial N, Guériton M, Vedel I. Impact of transitional care services for chronically ill older patients: a systematic evidence review. *J Am Geriatr Soc.* 2017;65(7):1597–1608.

Long-Term Services and Supports Expenditures on Home and Community-Based Services. https://www.medicaid.gov/state-overviews/scorecard/ltss-expenditures-on-hcbs/index.html. Accessed December 14, 2021.

Narayan MC, Scafide KN. systematic review of racial/ethnic outcome disparities in home health care. *J Transcult Nurs.* 2017;28(6):598–607.

Ornstein KA, Leff B, Covinsky KE, et al. Epidemiology of the homebound population in the United States. *JAMA Intern Med.* 2015;175(7):1180–1186.

Reckrey JM, Morrison RS, Boerner K, et al. Living in the community with dementia: who receives paid care? *J Am Geriatr Soc.* 2020;68(1):186–191.

Samus Q, Johnston D, Black B, et al. A multidimensional home-based care coordination intervention for elders with memory disorders: the Maximizing Independence at Home (MIND) Pilot Randomized Trial. *Am J Geriatr Psychiatry.* 2014;22(4):398–414.

Shepperd S, Iliffe S, Doll HA, et al. Admission avoidance hospital at home. *Cochrane Database Syst Rev.* 2016;9(9):CD007491.

Stall N, Nowaczynski M, Sinha SK. Systematic review of outcomes from home-based primary care programs for homebound older adults. *J Am Geriatr Soc.* 2014;62(12):2243–2251.

Szanton SL, Alfonso YN, Leff B, et al. Medicaid cost savings of a preventive home visit program for disabled older adults. *J Am Geriatr Soc.* 2018;66(3):614–620.

Totten AM, Hansen RN, Wagner J, et al. Telehealth for acute and chronic care consultations. Comparative Effectiveness Review No. 216. (Prepared by Pacific Northwest Evidence-based Practice Center under Contract No. 290-2015-00009-I.) AHRQ Publication No. 19-EHC012-EF. Rockville, MD: Agency for Healthcare Research and Quality; April 2019. Posted final reports are located on the Effective Health Care Program search page. https://doi.org/10.23970/AHRQEPCCER216. Accessed December 14, 2021.

Valluru G, Yudin J, Patterson C, et al. Integrated home- and community-based services improve community survival among independence at home Medicare beneficiaries without increasing Medicaid costs. *J Am Geriatr Soc.* 2019;67(7):1495–1501.

Willink A, Kasper J, Skehan ME, Wolff JL, Mulcahy J, Davis K. Are older americans getting the long-term services and supports they need? *Issue Brief (Commonw Fund).* 2019;2019:1–9.

Wysocki A, Butler M, Kane RL, Kane RA, Shippee T, Sainfort F. Long-term services and supports for older adults: a review of home and community-based services versus institutional care. *J Aging Soc Policy.* 2015;27(3):255–279.

Zimbroff RM, Ritchie CS, Leff B, Sheehan OC. Home-based primary and palliative care in the medicaid program: systematic review of the literature. *J Am Geriatr Soc.* 2021;69(1):245–254.

Chapter 18

Transitions of Care

Elizabeth N. Chapman, Andrea Gilmore-Bykovskyi, Amy J. H. Kind

INTRODUCTION

Older adults regularly experience changes in health status that contribute to frequent transitions between different levels and settings of care. These movements within and across care settings are commonly referred to as "transitions of care," and typically involve the management of a patient's care passing from one team of providers to another. Transitions of care are widely recognized as a point of heightened vulnerability for lapses in patient safety, as patients are at risk of "falling through the cracks" due to inadequate care coordination, preparation, and support prior to, during, and after the transition period. Inadequate care coordination and management of transitions of care contribute to $25 to $45 billion in unnecessary care costs resulting from hospital readmissions and other avoidable complications. Poor-quality transitions of care also contribute to substantial patient and caregiver stress and dissatisfaction. For these reasons, there is a sense of urgency in the United States to improve care management and coordination during transitions of care.

Older adults are at particularly high risk for experiencing adverse events during transitions of care. This is likely due to a number of factors, including their disproportionately higher rates of utilization of a range of different acute and postacute health services, increasing rates of multiple chronic conditions, and greater burden of conditions resulting in cognitive impairments, which may limit their ability to recognize or communicate important care needs.

This chapter provides an overview of transitions of care commonly experienced by older adults in the United States and discusses "transitional care," which is defined as a set of actions designed to ensure the coordination and continuity of health care as patients transfer between different locations or different levels of care in the same location. Transitional care is increasingly recognized as fundamental to ensuring safe and effective management of both chronic and acute illness in older adults. It also necessitates the involvement of all members of the interdisciplinary team working together across care settings. This chapter will provide an understanding of effective approaches to improving the management of transitions of care for older adult populations.

Learning Objectives

- Describe what a care transition is and identify different types of transitions of care commonly experienced by older adults.
- Understand how health system fragmentation and communication failures lead to poor-quality transitions of care.
- Identify outcomes of poor-quality transitions of care and how these outcomes affect patients, caregivers, and the health delivery system.
- Describe features of effective transitional care and transitional care interventions.

Key Clinical Points

1. Older adults are at increased risk for experiencing adverse outcomes following poor-quality transitions of care.
2. Effective communication lies at the core of safe transitions, especially for vulnerable older adults including those with cognitive impairment.
3. Providers managing transitions of care should actively engage both the patient and their identified caregiver in decision making about and in preparing for transitions of care.
4. High-quality transitional care programs can improve posthospital outcomes.

OVERVIEW ON TRANSITIONS OF CARE

Care System Fragmentation

Numerous factors pose barriers to the provision of high-quality transitional care, but one of the most important is health system fragmentation. The higher rates of acute and chronic illness in older adults predispose them to require care across multiple settings or fragments within the US health system, yet the health system fragmentation they experience is a newer phenomenon that has emerged and evolved over the past half-century.

Decades ago, most health care was provided within just a few settings by a small provider team that accompanied the patient across all settings. However, following the implementation of US payment structures that incentivized services, settings, and practices that reduced acute care utilization and length of stay, there was substantial growth in subacute, postacute, hospice, and rehabilitative services. Concurrently, providers became more specialized, with clinical practice increasingly restricted to specific settings (eg, hospitalist, skilled nursing facility specialist, emergency medicine physician, etc). While this ideally enabled more cost-effective use of resources at different stages in care, the rapid growth of single-site physician specialists and new service settings represented a fundamental change in the nature of care delivery in the United States.

In the mid-twentieth century, physicians commonly followed their patients across settings of care and specialist services were more often delivered following close communication with a patient's primary provider. It is now common for patients to travel between different settings of care and specialty providers without accompaniment of a consistent provider. For patients, this shift in care delivery has led to large gaps in care during the time after discharge from one setting and prior to being seen in the next, where it is unclear who is responsible for the patient's care.

With a shift away from acute care delivery, patients discharge from hospital settings sooner and generally more ill, yet they are often not adequately prepared to follow increasingly complex posthospital care plans. Minimal and often inadequate communication between care teams across settings compound these gaps, leading to confusion and delays in necessary follow-up care. Additionally, systems have been slow to develop infrastructures capable of meeting patients' needs in this new fragmented care delivery model. However, the need for high-quality transitional care to support patients during these system gaps is increasingly recognized.

Consequences of Poor-Quality Transitions of Care

Adverse consequences associated with poor-quality transitions have been well documented and include a range of undesirable outcomes for patients as well as their caregivers. Communication failures during the posthospital period are common and may involve the omission of vital elements of a care plan, such as information regarding mobility restrictions, medications, or diet orders. This may lead to inappropriate, disjointed, and/or harmful care in the next setting. For example, approximately one-third of patients discharge with pending laboratory tests that are not communicated to the next setting of care, and at least 10% of these could have led to actionable changes in patient care plans. Medication errors and/or discrepancies, which may be the result of poor-quality medication reconciliation or insufficient patient/caregiver education or support, occur in 30% to 50% of patients in the posthospital

period. When serious, they can lead to a number of adverse events, including avoidable rehospitalization, emergency department utilization, and death. Rehospitalization within 30 days of discharge occurs in 20% to 25% of Medicare beneficiaries and is more likely among certain vulnerable populations, such as older adults with functional or cognitive impairments. Research suggests that nearly half of these rehospitalizations could be avoided if better care were provided during transition periods.

Policies Surrounding Transitions of Care

Policy makers in the United States have long recognized poor-quality transitions of care as a dangerous and costly health delivery problem. The 2001 Institute of Medicine (IOM) report, *Crossing the Quality Chasm*, described the US health delivery system as complicated, poorly organized, and decentralized, resulting in "layers of processes and handoffs that patients and families find bewildering." The 2010 Patient Protection and Affordable Care Act includes multiple provisions aimed at improving transitions of care, including financial penalties for hospitals with higher than projected rehospitalization rates. The legislation also includes financial incentives for the development of care models that enhance coordination, such as the Medicare Shared Savings Program for accountable care organizations (ACOs). ACOs consist of a group of providers who are responsible for providing care for a group of patients across settings. The law authorizes financial incentives for ACOs that successfully keep patients out of acute care while maintaining high-quality care. The legislation also permits payment for care transition services to providers operating as medical home practices, which aim to manage and coordinate care for patients with chronic conditions. Following these policy changes, health systems have shown increased interest in adopting programs, policies, and interventions that improve transitions of care and decrease health system fragmentation.

More recently, policy changes from the Improving Medicare Post-Acute Care Transformation (IMPACT) Act of 2014 have sought to improve transitions by standardizing patient assessment data in postacute settings and better matching patients' clinical needs with the right postacute care environment (**Table 18-1**), which may have implications for discharge planning. Historically, provision of rehabilitation services drove Centers for Medicare and Medicaid Services reimbursement of skilled nursing facilities (SNFs) and home health agencies (HHAs), but documentation of patients' progress varied from setting to setting and focused on amount of service provided rather than the outcomes of those services on patients' function. Beginning in 2019, the Patient-Driven Payment Model (PDPM) for SNFs and Patient-Driven Grouping Model (PDGM) for HHAs adjust payment based on patients' clinical needs and utilize a single, standardized system for assessment and documentation. This shift in data collection has stewarded new opportunities to create a clinically meaningful record of a patient's longitudinal progress through the postacute setting.

TABLE 18-1 ■ POSTACUTE CARE CONTINUUM OF SERVICES				
DOMAIN	**CHARACTERISTICS OF SETTING**	**AVERAGE LOS**	**MANDATED PROVIDER AVAILABILITY**	**QUALIFYING FEATURES FOR MEDICARE COVERAGE**
Long-term care hospital (LTCH)	• Extended multidisciplinary care for patients with clinically complex problems • RN, OT, PT, ST, SW available	27 d	Daily physician visits	• Transfer directly from acute care hospital or admit within 60 d of discharge from inpatient hospitalization • Require care with mean LOS of 25+ d • Higher reimbursement for those with 3+ d in ICU prior to transfer and those requiring 96+ h of respiratory ventilation services in LTCH
Inpatient rehabilitation facility (IRF)	• Intense rehabilitation therapy, typically for acute orthopedic or neurologically injured patients • RN, OT, PT, ST, SW available	12 d	Physician visits at least 3 d/wk	• Patient must require intensive rehabilitation at least 3 h/d, 5 d/wk
Skilled nursing facility (SNF)	• Constant nursing care for patients with significant deficiencies with ADLs • RN, OT, PT, ST, SW available (limited), RN ratios much higher than in acute care settings	< 100 d; highly variable depending on patient needs and their primary insurance. In many SNFs average LOS now is 14–25 d	Physician visits at least once every 30 d for the first 90 d and at least once every 60 d after	• Medicare Part A provides partial coverage if patient had prior inpatient hospital stay of at least 3 d and admitted to SNF within 30 d of hospital stay • Requires skilled nursing care • Medicare fee-for-service pays fully for the first 20 d after which there is a daily copayment close to $200. The maximum benefit period for an episode is 100 d
Institutional long-term care (nursing home)	• Provides health care and services (above the level of room and board) not available in the community and needed regularly due to mental or physical impairment • RN/CNA provide daily supportive nursing cares	26 mo	Physician visit requirements vary by state	• Most long-term care facilities perform custodial care and thus are not covered by Medicare • Medicare Part B may cover therapy services in the facility even when Part A does not cover room and board
Home health agency (HHA)	• In-home care services for homebound individuals • RN, PT, OT, ST, SW, CNA available • Disciplines visit once daily or less	N/A	Physician or NPP visit no more than 90 d prior to or 30 d after home health start of care date	• Must be homebound • Requires intermittent skilled nursing care or other health services such as PT, OT, ST, SW • Short term coverage (60-d episodes of care; can be renewed if continues to meet criteria)
Assisted living	• Communities of group living arrangements with minimal professional nursing staff; wide spectrum of care • Staffed by resident assistants (no formal training); RN often not present on-site	28 mo	No physician on staff or requirement for physician involvement	• Medicare does not pay for assisted living facilities
Hospice	• Palliative care for terminally ill; • Care occurs in home or inpatient unit (IPU) • Does not provide custodial care outside IPU	72 d	Nursing and/or physician services available or on call on 24-h/d, 7 d/wk	• Must be terminally ill, life expectancy < 6 mo • Generally not available to those pursuing rehabilitation services (LTCH, IRF, SNF, HHA) • Medicare does not pay for the room and board fee when a person is on the Medicare Part A Hospice benefit while in the SNF.

LOS, length of stay; NPP, nonphysician practitioner; OT, occupational therapy; PT, physical therapy; RN, registered nurse; ST, speech therapy; SW, social work; CNA, certified nursing assistant; ADLs, activities of daily living.

Limited clinician training in transitional care The subfield of transitional care continues to grow, yet it remains a relatively new concept that has not been emphasized in clinical training programs until recently. As a result, many clinicians are unprepared to manage transitions of care successfully or even to recognize the consequences of health system fragmentation. Additionally, clinical training often takes place primarily in acute care settings. Many clinicians may have little to no exposure to other settings of care such as postacute care or home-based services. Postacute care services vary substantially in available resources, level of physician contact, and acuity of patient populations. **Table 18-1** provides an overview of the continuum of postacute care settings. A lack of exposure to these various settings may contribute to a limited understanding of the unique needs/resources outside of hospital settings, leading to communication failures between hospital-based and postacute providers and inappropriate care plans. As a result, patients may receive inadequate services in the postacute period, causing distress for the patient/caregiver and potentially avoidable rehospitalizations. In some cases, rehospitalizations may arise from clinical deterioration, but in others, patients/families may lose confidence in the setting's ability to provide care and choose to return to the hospital. Even when patients discharge to a more intensive level of care than necessary, they may face risks for rehospitalization. In addition to occupying beds better utilized by others, they may quickly discharge to a lower acuity setting, facing the attendant risks of yet another handoff.

Patient/caregiver underprepared for transitions Limited or inadequate preparation of patients and caregivers regarding what to expect at the next setting of care is also a common problem. Patients and their caregivers are often unaware of what to expect following hospital discharge or transitions of care. They often are not empowered to take part in their plan of care sufficiently. Patients' and caregivers' sense of underpreparation may not necessarily be due to a lack of discharge information, but more so due to the complexity and amount of information communicated are overwhelming. These vast quantities of information would be challenging for anyone to encode and retain in the short time frame for discharge teaching that is typically provided. It is also common for patients and their caregivers not to recognize that they are unprepared to succeed in their next setting of care until they arrive and experience a care failure in that setting.

Poor-quality communication among provider teams High-quality communication between care teams at points of patient transition across settings is essential to patient safety, particularly at hospital discharge. More than half of all avoidable events following hospital discharge relate to poor communication among providers. Physicians have traditionally played the key role in communicating a patient's care plan to the next setting provider at hospital discharge, typically in the format of a discharge summary. The discharge summary is the only form of communication at hospital discharge mandated by The Joint Commission (TJC) and must be completed within 30 days of discharge, according to TJC standards. In this new era of health system fragmentation, most experts believe that this 30-day time frame is much too long. While TJC has minimal standards for the content of discharge summaries, these are widely considered by experts to be insufficient. Despite the importance of discharge summaries in facilitating coordinated care, physicians receive little to no training in discharge summary creation, and there is no mandated standard format for these documents. Perhaps unsurprisingly, research examining the quality and content of discharge summaries has found that they routinely omit the most important care plan components, such as code status, diet, warfarin instructions, and pending laboratory tests.

While a physician has historically been the recipient of hospital discharge summaries, patients now discharge to a range of postacute care facilities with varying multidisciplinary clinician teams who may require different information than what has been traditionally included within discharge summaries. Poor-quality discharge communication is particularly problematic for transitions to SNFs. SNF staff rely heavily on written discharge communication, which may serve as the only source informing a patient's care plan for up to 30 days postdischarge. In focus groups, SNF nurses have reported regularly receiving discharge information that is untimely, incomplete, inaccurate, or conflicting. Because discharge summaries often dictate a patient's plan of care for a significant period of time postdischarge and clarifying the confusing information in discharge summaries often takes several days, nurses in SNF settings have identified a list of discharge summary components that they require to safely transition patients to posthospitalization care (**Table 18-2**).

Special Considerations for Transitions of Care among Older Adults

Older adults are heavy users of a range of health care services, including acute care stays, postacute care, subacute care, and home health care services. Those with one or more chronic conditions see an average of eight different physicians annually. **Figure 18-1** depicts the experience of an older adult receiving care in a series of fragmented systems, where the patient often serves as the only link between providers, and communication and integration between providers are commonly infrequent.

Older adults experience a variety of transitions of care. Hospital discharge is a particularly vulnerable care transition for older adults and results in an adverse event for approximately one in five adult medical patients within 3 weeks of discharge. Furthermore, nearly 20% of Medicare beneficiaries age 65 and older experience rehospitalization within 30 days of discharge, accounting for over $17 billion in health care spending annually. Patients increasingly discharge to a range of settings following hospitalization,

TABLE 18-2 ■ HOSPITAL DISCHARGE INFORMATION THAT SKILLED NURSING FACILITY NURSES NEED TO DEVELOP AND IMPLEMENT A SAFE PLAN OF CARE

Contact information
Discharging unit and telephone number
Attending doctor and telephone number
Other providers who will manage specific conditions (eg, infectious disease, anticoagulation) and contact information
Registered nurse who cared for individual and telephone number
Spouse or partner and telephone number
Family member(s) involved in care and telephone number
Power of attorney, if activated, and telephone number

Past medical history and hospital stay
Remarkable medical history
Remarkable events during hospital stay
Comorbidities
Code status

Medications
Discharge medication list
  Drug name
  Dose
  Diagnosis and rationale for every medication
  Start and stop dates and last dose administered
Opioid prescriptions (signed hard copy)
Significant medication changes
  Change in psychiatric medications during stay
  Change in opioid medication at discharge
  Withdrawal of medication because of side effects

Allergies and intolerances
Medications
Food
Latex

Functional status
Ability to perform and assistance required for activities of daily living
Sensory aids (dentures, glasses, hearing aids)
Mobility status
  Level of assistance needed
  Equipment requirements
  Fall risk

Psychosocial and behavioral concerns
Personal interests/communication preferences
Cognitive status
Behavioral symptoms related to dementia
  Type and severity
  Need for personal safety attendant during stay
  Effective comforting and reorientation strategies

Treatments
Wound care
  Dressing type
  Dressing schedule
Peripherally inserted central catheter line care
  Dressing type
  Dressing schedule
  Flushing schedule

Elimination status
Bladder or bowel incontinence and use of absorbent pads
Perineal skin concerns
Last bowel movement
  Type and amount of medication administered for bowel-related problems before discharge
Use of indwelling urinary catheter and if and when discontinued

Nutritional status
Swallowing or feeding concerns
Special eating devices
Appetite
Weight
Dentures

Follow-up care
Scheduled appointments
  Who
  When
  Where
  Telephone number
Laboratory results
  Pending results
  Follow-up laboratory tests that need to be done
  Name and number of insurance policy

PART II

PRINCIPLES OF GERIATRICS

with approximately 25% of older adults being discharged to a different institution and 12% being discharged to their homes with home health care services. **Table 18-3** includes examples of different types of transitions in the level of care or setting that older adults may experience. Older adults who may be at increased risk for rehospitalization include those with difficulty with activities of daily living (ADLs), socioeconomic disadvantage, depression, substance abuse disorders, a history of previous hospitalization, difficulty with treatment adherence or medication compliance, or cognitive impairment.

While patients do not always transition between institutional settings, transitions to community settings may still include a range of other care provider teams who may manage medical needs following hospitalization, including home health teams and primary care providers.

Patient and Caregiver Perspective on Transitions of Care

High levels of stress and dissatisfaction often characterize experiences of transitions for patients and families. In addition to poor communication between hospital providers,

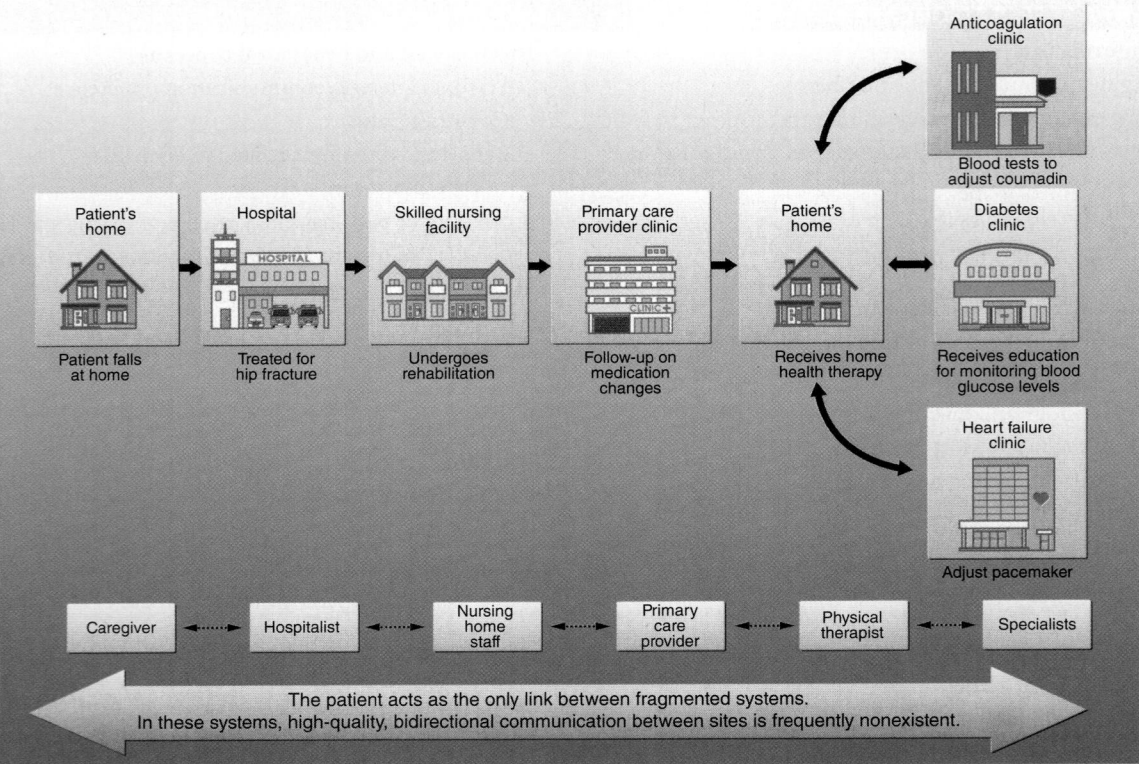

FIGURE 18-1. System fragmentation example.

TABLE 18-3 ■ TYPES OF TRANSITIONS IN LEVEL OF CARE OR CARE SETTING COMMONLY EXPERIENCED BY OLDER ADULTS

TRANSITIONS WITHIN ACUTE CARE SETTING

Emergency department to intensive care unit

Intensive care unit to medical unit

TRANSITIONS OUT OF ACUTE CARE SETTING

Medical/surgical unit to skilled nursing facility

Medical/surgical unit to community setting[a]

Medical/surgical unit to community setting[a] with home health services

Medical/surgical unit to inpatient hospice

Acute rehabilitation hospital, long-term acute hospital, or psychiatric hospital to any of the above referenced settings

Emergency room to community setting[a]

TRANSITIONS FROM NURSING FACILITIES

Skilled nursing facility to community setting[a]

Nursing facility[b] to emergency room

Nursing facility[b] to medical/surgical unit

Nursing facility[b] to urgent care office

Nursing facility[b] to primary care office

Nursing facility[b] to inpatient hospice

[a]Examples of community settings are home or assisted living facilities.
[b]Examples of nursing facilities are nursing homes or skilled nursing facilities.

postacute providers, and primary care physicians (PCPs), ineffective physician-patient communication likely contributes to patients' underpreparation for managing their care following transitions, particularly after hospitalization. Various communication failures involving and surrounding patients during transitions also lead to the lack of appropriate follow-up care (eg, visit with PCP following hospitalization), which likely increases risk for rehospitalization. Failure to receive follow-up care and the resulting subsequent negative sequelae may incorrectly be attributed to the patient's noncompliance rather than other factors, such as inadequate preparation or education prior to discharge, leading patients and their caregivers to feel frustrated and unsupported.

Little research has examined patients' and caregivers' preferences surrounding transitional care. Some qualitative research has found that patients and caregivers struggle with hospital discharges. Patients report feeling anxious and reluctant to ask clarifying questions about posthospital care needs when hospital discharge occurs quickly or with little notice, leading to patients discharging without a clear understanding of their posthospital care needs. Patients and caregivers also expressed insecurities about their ability to ask questions of the care team. **Table 18-4** includes quotations provided by patients and caregivers in research studies that illustrate their experiences surrounding transitions of care.

TABLE 18-4 ■ THE EXPERIENCE OF CARE TRANSITIONS FROM THE PERSPECTIVE OF PATIENTS AND THEIR CAREGIVERS

PATIENT EXPERIENCE	
"They put it in their technical words and then they [primary care physicians] will understand what happened to me … I can't express what is written in this paper."[a]	Difficulty understanding discharge documentation, which is written for the primary care provider
"I needed some serious education about some things…I didn't know if they were not explaining things to me because I was not going to live much longer and it was just not worth it…how do I know?"[b]	Sense of underpreparation and inadequate education prior to discharge
"…to ask a question would be right but I have no clue what to ask…It's like you don't know what you don't know."[b]	Uncertainty regarding how to ask questions prior to discharge
CAREGIVER EXPERIENCE	
"They prescribed her over $1000 in medicines…The discharge paper was blank… They didn't give her what she needed. They changed what was working to other medicines. It seemed like we had never spoken to those people at all…"[c]	Medication changes made during hospitalization that were poorly communicated with caregiver Lack of medication reconciliation
"Several times we didn't know what was out there to help us…She wanted to come home and we wanted to provide care for her at home…But we didn't know what other type of care there was…We finally got some of that information but…We had to struggle to search it out, and answers weren't readily available."[c]	Lack of involvement of caregiver in decision making surrounding transition
"The medical system, if you are not part of it, is a pretty foreign thing…If you find a person that will work with you, whether it be a doctor, a nurse…the scheduler… They are there to help guide you through the system. But finding them and really cultivating that relationship makes a huge difference."[c]	Difficulty connecting with clinical team to ask questions regarding transition

[a]Groene RO, Orrego C, Suñol R, Barach P, Groene O. It's like two worlds apart: an analysis of vulnerable patient handover practices at discharge from hospital. *BMJ Qual Saf.* 2012;21(suppl 1): i67–i75.

[b]Fuji KT, Abbott AA, Norris JF. Exploring care transitions from patient, caregiver and health-care provider perspectives. *Clin Nurs Res.* 2013;22(3):258–274.

[c]Benzar E, Hansen L, Kneitel AW, Fromme EK. Discharge planning for palliative care patients: a qualitative analysis. *J Palliat Med.* 2011;14(1):65–69.

HIGH-QUALITY TRANSITIONAL CARE

High-quality transitional care can combat system fragmentation to better support patients in bridging the gaps during transitions of care. One central component of effective transitional care is identifying and engaging caregivers for patients whenever possible. This is particularly important during hospitalization. Prior to experiencing a transition, such as hospital discharge, patients are often overwhelmed and acutely ill. Furthermore, navigating care needs following transitions often places patients in situations where they must rely on social supports and resources beyond themselves. These social supports (eg, caregivers) are more likely to be effective if they are engaged in and prepared for the posthospital period along with patients. This is critical for patients with cognitive impairments, such as dementia or delirium, who may struggle to retain information about the transition period. Effective transitional care also merits the involvement of the entire interdisciplinary team.

While most transitional care programs have focused on transitions from hospital to community settings, the common elements of these programs are applicable to supporting patients across any range of transitions. Multicomponent interventions, which address more facets of a transition, have the ability to tailor their care responses to an individual patient's needs and fully integrate with both the sending and receiving setting and are likely the most effective. Some specific elements of effective and high-quality transitional care include, but are not limited to: (1) involvement of the patient/caregiver in care plan decisions prior to and during the transition to ensure that their goals are addressed and that the plan is feasible, (2) patient and caregiver empowerment and preparation for necessary care in the posttransition period that is reinforced through a series of contacts before, during, and after the transition, (3) timely, complete, and accurate communication with the next care team with mechanisms for the receiving team to ask questions and obtain clarifications, and (4) high-quality medication reconciliation. Examples of activities that fulfill the definition of high-quality transitional care are provided in **Table 18-5** and are contrasted with typical, less-optimal care activities that may facilitate a discharge but do not necessarily support a high-quality, coordinated transition.

Patient/Caregiver Involvement in Decision Making

Involving patients and their caregivers in decisions about care plans prior to transitions addresses several important barriers to effective transitions. First, it enables patients to gain an idea of what to expect at the next setting of care, which may ultimately help them prepare for their needs. Early involvement in decision making also provides patients with the opportunity to express their goals and values, which may impact placement decisions.

TABLE 18-5 ■ HIGH-QUALITY TRANSITIONAL CARE AS COMPARED TO LESS-OPTIMAL TYPICAL CARE

Transitional care is defined as a set of actions designed to ensure the coordination and continuity of health care as patients transfer between different locations or different levels of care in the same location. The following list is not comprehensive, but is meant to provide examples of the intensity of activity necessary to support high-quality transitional care.

EXAMPLE OF LESS-OPTIMAL TYPICAL CARE ACTIVITIES	EXAMPLE OF HIGH-QUALITY TRANSITIONAL CARE ACTIVITIES
Example of less-optimal discharge planning activity: • Identify at least one nursing home that will accept the patient prior to hospital discharge to ensure a short hospital length of stay.	More optimal: • Involve patient/caregiver in ongoing discharge planning throughout hospitalization to ensure that the posthospital plan for a site of care is acceptable, feasible, and optimal for the patient and caregiver.
Example of less-optimal discharge education: • On the day of discharge, provide the patient with an extensive and comprehensive paper binder that includes their medication list, recommended posthospital care, and information on all acute and chronic conditions. No limit to the number of pages offered.	More optimal: • Provide patient-tailored, reinforced, consistent, simple, goal-directed, education-based messaging over time (within and posthospitalization) for key care principles including medication management, follow-up care, and when/whom to contact with questions/problems. Actively engage the patient in care activities and observe performance over time (within and posthospital) to ensure understanding. Engage caregivers in all teaching.
Example of less-optimal postdischarge support/contact: • Routine 1–5 min postdischarge phone calls made to all hospital patients that ask a few general yes/no questions about satisfaction or concerns, with little tailoring to the patient's condition or needs or to their ability to recognize disease worsening.	More optimal: • Intensive postdischarge contacts that follow structured, evidence-based protocols and assess for medication discrepancies, signs of worsening condition, and presence of /adherence with follow-up care, typically with in-depth discussions and in-depth medication reconciliation. Depending on the program and patient, these contacts could be made via phone and/or home visit.

Patient/Caregiver Empowerment, Preparation, and Support

Providing patients and their caregivers with the necessary empowerment, preparation, and support to manage their needs in the next setting of care successfully is critical. In successful transitional care programs, this preparation generally includes the following components: (1) education and empowerment in medication management, ideally using either in-person assessments or patient-/caregiver-led medication reconciliation techniques, (2) ensuring adequate follow-up care is in place and that the patient/caregiver is prepared to actively participate in that follow-up, (3) education of the patient/caregiver about signs of a worsening condition (often referred to as "red flags") and empowerment to act upon those signs, and (4) ensuring that patient/caregiver understands who to contact with follow-up questions and how to make these contacts. These core areas should be reinforced in the early discharge period through a series of contacts over time to adhere to standard principles of adult learning.

High-Quality Communication Between Sending and Receiving Care Teams

High-quality communication is central to achieving safe transitions. While ongoing, bidirectional communication between the sending and receiving health care team would be ideal, typically, most communication between care settings occurs in a written format at one point in time.

Written discharge communication, primarily the discharge summary, is the primary and often only form of communication that accompanies a patient following hospitalization. For patients discharged to nursing homes, the orders received concurrently with or contained in the discharge summary can dictate a patient's care for up to 30 days, so high-quality written communication is especially a key for these patients. Yet, as noted earlier in this chapter, the quality of written communication tends to be poor.

Several strategies can improve the quality of written discharge communication. First, whenever possible, a provider who is familiar with the patient should create, complete, and sign the discharge summary. In current practice, discharge summaries are sometimes iteratively modified by multiple rotating providers until the time of discharge. In such cases, the posthospital care setting may receive several versions of discharge summaries with conflicting information. It is important to recognize that many of these settings, such as SNFs, are not capable of implementing last-minute changes in orders and may face long delays in responding to medication changes or special equipment orders due to the lack of on-site pharmacies and central supply services. Consequently, last-minute changes in discharge orders should be minimized and, when they do occur, should be communicated to the admitting facility using another method (eg, via phone) prior to patient transport. Because many postacute care settings require information about care plan elements that are not immediately available to the physician, engaging the interdisciplinary team in creating certain components of the document or providing recommendations for the document in the electronic medical record (EMR) may be advantageous. Some examples of these care plan elements may include information about behavioral symptoms in patients with dementia such as agitation, that are critical for staff in the next setting of care to be aware of in order to arrange appropriate staffing and supportive care. A care system can use a standard format for discharge summary creation to reduce omission of key information. A list of recommended discharge summary components required by nurses in SNF settings can be found in **Table 18-2**.

While written discharge communication is the primary form of communication for physician providers, other members of the care team should also consider verbal handoffs with providers in the next setting of care. Nurses in SNFs have identified high-quality verbal handoff with hospital nurses to be very helpful in preparing for patient transitions. This contact also provides an opportunity for both the sending and receiving end of the transition to identify and resolve relevant questions that may not have been recognized until patient transfer.

High-Quality Medication Reconciliation

Medication reconciliation is an essential component of transitional care programs in which the patient, members of the health care team, and other caregivers can collaborate to improve medication safety as the patient transitions between health care settings (eg, hospital admission or discharge) or other care units. Medication reconciliation is the formal process recognized by TJC of creating the most accurate medication list by comparing, or reconciling, the patient's current list of medications with the medications ordered by providers upon admission, transfer, and discharge. TJC recommends five steps in the medication reconciliation process (**Table 18-6**). This process is intended to identify and resolve any medication discrepancies or errors, such as omissions, additions, duplications, and frequency or dosing errors, with the goal of preventing adverse drug events (ADEs) and subsequent patient harm. Since medication discrepancies are a major contributor to ADEs,

TABLE 18-6 ■ PRIMARY COMPONENTS OF A MEDICATION RECONCILIATION

1. Develop a list of current medications (also known as the medication history).
2. Develop a list of medications to be prescribed.
3. Compare the medications on the two lists.
4. Make clinical decisions based on the comparison.
5. Communicate the new list to appropriate caregivers and to the patient.

TABLE 18-7 ■ INFORMATION FOR THE PREADMISSION MEDICATION HISTORY

- Which medications taken at which times
- Identities of prescribing providers
- Identities of pharmacies dispensing medications
- Nonoral medications used (eye drops, suppositories, patches, inhalers, creams, etc)
- Assessment of patient's (or caregiver's) understanding of drug indications
- OTCs[a] and herbals/vitamins/supplements
- Allergies and adverse drug reaction history
- Assessment of adherence (eg, number of doses missed per week)
- How patient (or caregiver) manages the regimen at home (eg, use of pill box)

[a]OTCs, over-the-counter medications.

TJC has made medication reconciliation a National Patient Safety Goal and requires all of its accredited institutions to have a process implemented at their site for reconciling medications. Despite these efforts, however, medication reconciliation processes have been challenging to perform effectively and consistently as evidenced by a continuing high prevalence of medication discrepancies for patients transitioning between health care settings and levels of care.

The medication reconciliation process starts by obtaining the patient's medication history. Often, a physician, pharmacist, or nurse will obtain the patient's medication history by (1) interviewing the patient and their caregivers, (2) accessing the patient's past medical records, and (3) contacting other providers involved in the patient's care and the patient's community pharmacy for recently dispensed medications (**Table 18-7**). When creating the patient's list of current medications, it is important to identify all medications the patient is taking, including prescription drugs, over-the-counter medications, herbal remedies, and supplements. The patient's medication histories are then reconciled with medications to be ordered to ensure that the new medications and doses are appropriate for the patient. Changes to the patient's medication regimen are documented in their medical chart, and a complete medication list is communicated to the patient, caregiver, and next provider/team. Reconciling medications applies to all health care settings, including ambulatory care, inpatient services, emergency and urgent care, long-term care, and home care.

EXAMPLES OF HIGH-QUALITY TRANSITIONAL CARE INTERVENTIONS

Transitional care interventions support patients as they move between different settings of care and generally emphasize medication management, empowerment/support with self-care management, and posthospital contact with a care provider. Many of these interventions

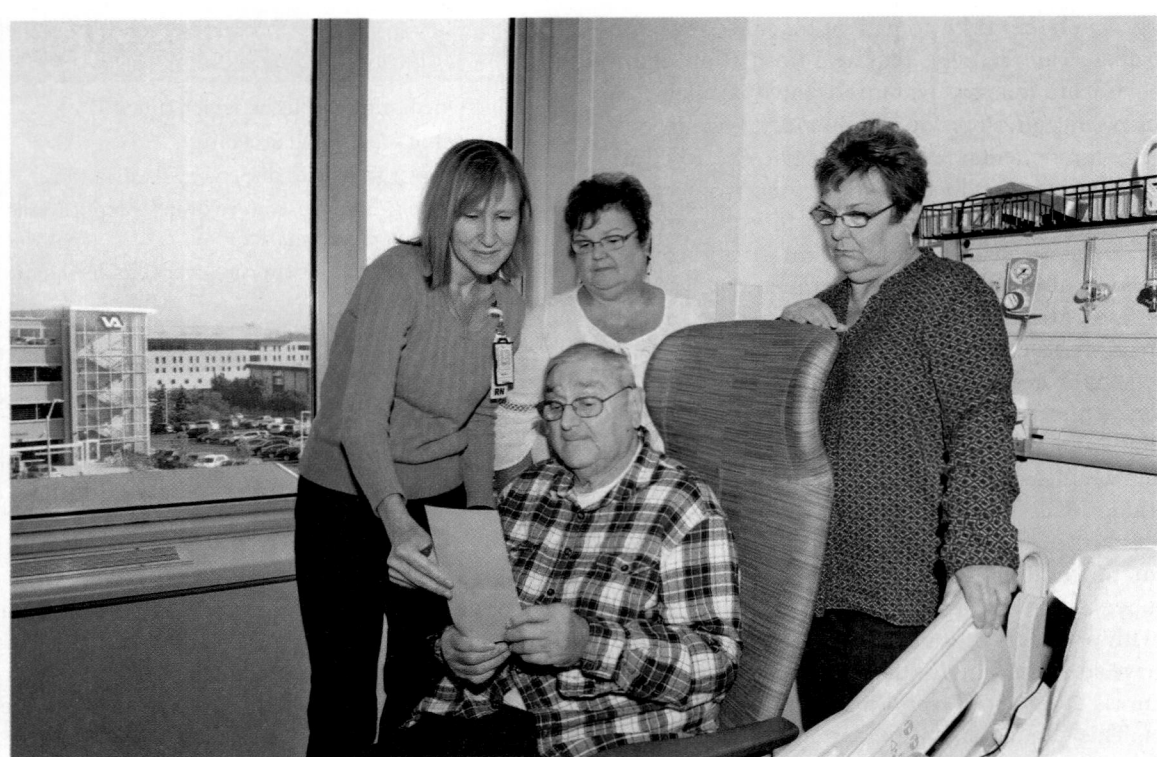

FIGURE 18-2. Transitional care nurse working with a patient and his family.

recognize nurses as clinical leaders for supporting patients and their families as they navigate transitions **(Figure 18-2)**. They engage nurses as well as other members of the interdisciplinary team in developing care plans, performing medication reconciliation, and supporting medication adherence and self-care in the early discharge period. Most transitional care interventions focus on transitions from hospital to community settings; however, emerging care models continue to be developed to support patients during a range of unique transitions. Some examples of specific transitional care interventions are noted below.

Interventions to Improve Hospital-to-Community Transitional Care Quality

Home visit–based transitional care interventions that have been tested in randomized controlled trials include Coleman's Transitions of Care Intervention (CTI) and Naylor's Transitional Care Model (TCM). These interventions reduce rehospitalizations by about one-third. Both programs utilize posthospital in-home visits with a nurse practitioner to educate high-risk patients about their medications, medical follow-up, signs of condition worsening, and provider's contact information. While contact with patients in these programs only lasts for a few weeks, the effect on rehospitalization has been shown to last up to 180 days—likely due to improved self-management. Both of these interventions, however, are limited to patients who

agree to in-home supports and live within geographic reach of a home visit.

Transitional care interventions utilizing similar steps as CTI and TCM have recently emerged to target vulnerable patients, including those with cognitive impairment, and those who refuse home visits or live too far from discharging hospitals to receive home visits. One of these, the Coordinated-Transitional Care (C-TraC) program, developed within the US Department of Veterans Affairs, is a low-cost, telephone-based program. It uses a nurse case manager to coordinate the patient's transition via a series of protocol-driven in-hospital visits, intensive posthospital phone calls, and integration with in-hospital and posthospital clinical teams. In preliminary testing, the C-TraC intervention reduced 30-day rehospitalizations by one-third among enrollees, leading to a substantial cost avoidance. However, more rigorous testing is needed to better understand its impact.

Project Re-Engineered Discharge (RED) is an intervention based within the acute care setting that involves enhanced in-hospital discharge processes and education. A randomized controlled trial of Project RED showed a decrease in 30-day emergency room visits but no significant effect on rehospitalizations. The average age of the population tested in the study was 50 years, much younger than the typical older adult population at most risk for rehospitalization. Given this and the limited posthospital support available within this program, its role in high-risk and older patient populations remains unclear.

The success of a care transition relies not only on adequate preparation of patients/caregivers and effective communication between health care teams but also on the selection of the most appropriate setting for subsequent care. Development of clinical decision support tools could assist in directing clinicians to the best postacute setting for patients' needs. Such tools have shown promise in identifying patients in need of postacute care and, when used to develop the discharge plan, may reduce inpatient rehospitalizations. More investigation is necessary to determine whether these tools could be incorporated broadly into routine practice and whether the reductions in rehospitalization can be replicated.

Interventions to Improve Nursing Home–to–Hospital Transition Quality

Nursing home patients experience a high degree of costly transfers to the hospital setting that may be avoidable through earlier recognition of changes in condition by nursing home staff. These transfers are burdensome for nursing home residents, many of whom may be physically frail and have some degree of cognitive impairment. Interventions to Reduce Acute Care Transfers (INTERACT) is a program that was developed to reduce the frequency of transfers to acute care for nursing home patients by supporting nursing home staff's ability to identify, assess, and communicate changes in condition. The program consists of a toolkit composed of: (1) a Situation-Background-Assessment-Recommendation (SBAR) tool to support effective communication between nurses and physicians, (2) an early warning tool designed to promote early recognition changes in condition, (3) a hospital transfer review tool to support review of hospitalizations and potentially avoidable causes, and (4) a standardized patient transfer form to communicate key patient information during transfer. INTERACT tools are available for no cost for clinical and educational use at www.interact-pathway.com and consist of a toolkit that supports both education for nursing home staff as well as implementation and data collection support. Data suggest that INTERACT tools can decrease rehospitalizations in engaged facilities that implement the interventions fully.

Several other resources and programs are also available. The Society for Post-Acute and Long-Term Care Medicine/American Medical Directors Association has several relevant tools on its website. A CMS demonstration program involving 7 sites and over 140 nursing homes demonstrated significant reductions in all-cause hospitalizations among long-stay nursing home residents. All of the interventions involved components of the INTERACT program and provided additional on-site personnel to help implement the interventions. Examples of additional interventions included a focus on advance care planning, medication reconciliation, oral health care, and telemedicine. One site that provided on-site nurse practitioners to implement core components of the INTERACT program showed a 30% reduction in all-cause hospitalizations.

SPECIAL POPULATIONS

Patients with Cognitive Impairment and/or Nearing End of Life

Older adults with cognitive impairments, such as dementia, are at increased risk for experiencing negative outcomes associated with transitions. Research suggests that dementia may increase care rehospitalization risk by an alarming 40%. While little research has examined reasons for this increased risk, it is apparent that the limited capacity to learn, recall, and effectively communicate elements of their care plan among those with dementia may result in an inability to compensate for poor communication across clinical teams and may play a role in subsequent rehospitalizations. Persons with dementia also have difficulty adapting to stressors and responding to change. They generally benefit from consistency in caregiver teams and environment, making transitions across care settings particularly burdensome. Considerable changes in surroundings (eg, transitioning from nursing home to the hospital) for a person with dementia may result in increased behavioral symptoms, such as agitation or increased depressive symptoms.

While most people with dementia spend most of their life in community settings, they also experience transitions into permanent care (eg, placement in a nursing home) more often than non-cognitively impaired older adults. Transitions into permanent care represent considerable changes for both the individual with dementia and their family/caregivers. Persons with dementia have expressed a desire to be involved in the transition process and to have their family members engaged to offer support. However, research also suggests that persons with dementia may be excluded from the decision-making surrounding transitions of care. The lack of inclusion of people with dementia of care decisions may result from the incorrect assumption that people with dementia are unable to contribute to decision-making conversations or that these conversations will result in distress due to a lack of comprehension. Though some individuals with more advanced cognitive impairment may be unable to participate in their care at this level, many individuals with mild to moderate impairment could benefit from this opportunity, as providing input into the decision to transition into a nursing home for permanent care has been shown to lead to a greater sense of acceptance with the decision. Developing a longitudinal care plan may help incorporate the wishes and values of people with dementia into transitions of care more effectively. Early discussion about preferences regarding settings of care and whether the benefits of seeking acute care for an illness outweigh the harms of the transition to an unfamiliar

TABLE 18-8 ■ EDUCATIONAL RESOURCES FOR PATIENTS AND FAMILIES DURING TRANSITIONS OF CARE

RESOURCE	DESCRIPTION
Family Caregiver Alliance, Hospital Discharge Planning: A Guide for Families and Caregivers (https://caregiver.org/hospital-discharge-planning-guide-families-and-caregivers)	Includes explanations of important transition elements and suggestions for improving the process, and provides checklists/questions to ask to ensure caregivers provide the best care for their loved ones in the transition process.
Centers for Medicare and Medicaid Services, Your Guide to Choosing a Nursing Home or Other Long-Term Care (http://www.medicare.gov/pubs/pdf/02174.pdf)	Includes resources on the following: how to find and compare nursing homes and other long-term care options, how to pay for nursing home care, your rights as a nursing home resident, and alternatives to nursing home care.
The National Consumer Voice for Quality Long-Term Care (http://theconsumervoice.org/uploads/files/general/Consumer-Voice-brochure.pdf)	A platform of resources to advocate for public policies that support quality care and quality of life in all long-term care settings. The Consumer Voice advocates for a strong, sufficient direct-care workforce and promotes best practices in delivering quality care.
Center for Advancing Health, Be a Prepared Patient (http://www.cfah.org/prepared-patient/plan-for-your-end-of-life-care/choosing-a-nursing-home)	A collection of trusted resources, tips, and stories from patients, caregivers, and health care experts about finding good care and making the most of it.
American Geriatrics Society's Health in Aging Foundation (http://www.healthinaging.org/)	Provides consumers and caregivers with up-to-date information on health and aging. Highlighted resources include easy-to-understand tip sheets on managing health and a series that provides practical questions to help direct conversations with health care providers.

environment can guide surrogates' choices in later stages of dementia. Dementia-specific advance directives have been suggested as one means of conveying these wishes.

Transitions near the end of life are common in those with and without dementia. Such end-of-life transitions may not improve quality of life, instead adding to suffering and burden, and may be preventable. More than 80% of individuals experience at least one transition between health care settings in the past 6 months of life, with about one-third experiencing four or more transitions. Despite the substantial burden associated with transitions for persons with dementia, they experience more transitions within the past 3 months of life than those without dementia. Advance care planning may reduce the likelihood of burdensome transitions, particularly when completed earlier in the course of illness.

Patients with dementia also benefit from inclusion in transitional care interventions that emphasize empowerment and preparation of caregiver and adapt patient education strategies to meet the needs of individuals with

TABLE 18-9 ■ CASE EXAMPLE OF A POOR-QUALITY TRANSITION FROM HOSPITAL–TO–NURSING HOME FOR A PERSON WITH DEMENTIA

Genevieve is an 87-year-old woman with a history of Alzheimer disease who was recently hospitalized for pneumonia. According to family who accompanied Genevieve to the hospital, she has been struggling with managing at home alone ever since her husband of 60 y passed away 2 mo ago. Genevieve has had four hospital admissions for exacerbations of congestive heart failure and pneumonia in the past 2 y. During her hospital stay, she had dysphagia and she was placed on a thickened liquid diet to avoid further aspiration, which likely contributed to her recurrent pneumonia. She had experienced functional decline during her hospital stay and was discharged to a skilled nursing facility for rehabilitation. The physician writing the hospital discharge orders did not include any information for her diet, and dietary information was also omitted from her discharge summary. Genevieve had a score of 23/30 on a global cognitive test (mild impairment). However, because she had a diagnosis of Alzheimer disease in her medical record, the discharging nurse decided that it was not necessary to review changes in her care plan with her prior to discharge as she thought it was unlikely that Genevieve would understand. Although he did discuss her antibiotics with her in detail, the physician did not review dietary changes with Genevieve under the assumption that others on the care team would perform that activity.

When sent to the nursing facility, Genevieve told the nurses there that her hospital doctors and nurses did not give her any special instructions regarding her diet, and that she was eating normally while at home. The nursing facility nurses did not have a diet order and could not reach any of Genevieve's hospital providers when they tried to call to clarify her diet, as the hospital providers had all rotated off-shift for the evening. When called, Genevieve's outpatient physician was surprised to hear that she had been in the hospital and had not yet received any information regarding Genevieve's hospital stay. Therefore, Genevieve was started on a regular diet at the nursing facility. While in the nursing facility, Genevieve seemed to tolerate her regular diet well; however, 5 d later she was noted to have a persistent cough, a low-grade fever, and to be short of breath. Genevieve was transported to the emergency department and ultimately was readmitted for recurrent aspiration pneumonia.

cognitive impairment. The C-TraC program previously described is one example of a transitional care program that actively engages caregivers and uses methods of spaced retrieval to aid in information retention in persons with dementia.

Most community-dwelling older adults with dementia live with or receive frequent support from informal caregivers, who are often but not always family members. Because caregivers of people with dementia experience considerable burden and negative health outcomes related to the caregiving role, it behooves clinicians overseeing transitions of care for persons with dementia also to be responsive to the needs of their family/caregivers. Caregivers often experience guilt and frustration surrounding transitions into nursing home settings and are rarely prepared to manage these emotional conflicts and sense of bereavement during placement. Caregivers also generally express a desire to continue to participate in care following the transition. Enhanced support and counseling surrounding transitions to nursing home placement have been shown to have both short- and long-term benefits for caregivers. Providers may wish to refer caregivers to these or similar programs and may also refer caregivers to website resources provided at end of this chapter (**Table 18-8**). **Table 18-9** illustrates a case example of the experience of transitional care for an older adult with dementia that illustrates a life-threatening complication and hospital readmission because of poor communication between the hospital and the SNF.

ACKNOWLEDGMENTS

The authors would like to acknowledge Jacquelyn Mirr, Brian Mirr, and Michael Gehring for assistance with formatting/graphics.

FURTHER READING

Aaltonen M, Rissanen P, Forma L, et al. The impact of dementia on transitions in care during the last two years of life. *Age Ageing*. 2012;41:52–57.

Callahan CM, Arling G, Tu W, et al. Transitions in care for older adults with and without dementia. *J Am Geriatr Soc*. 2012;60:813–820.

Coleman EA. Falling through the cracks: challenges and opportunities for improving transitional care for persons with continuous complex care needs. *J Am Geriatr Soc*. 2003;51:549–555.

Coleman EA, Berenson RA. Lost in transition: challenges and opportunities for improving the quality of transitional care. *Ann Intern Med*. 2004;141:533–536.

Coleman EA, Mahoney E, Parry C. Assessing the quality of preparation for post-hospital care from the patient's perspective: the transitions in care measure. *Med Care*. 2005;43:246–255.

Coleman EA, Parry C, Chalmers S, Min SJ. The transitions in care intervention results of a randomized control trial. *Arch Intern Med*. 2006;166(17):1822–1828.

Dimant J. Roles and responsibilities of attending physicians in skilled nursing facilities. *J Am Med Dir Assoc*. 2003;4:231–243.

Fakha A, Groenvynck L, de Boer B, van Achterberg T, Harners J, Verbeek H. A myriad of factors influencing the implementation of transitional care innovations: a scoping review. *Implement Sci*. 2021;16:21–44.

Forster AJ, Murff HJ, Peterson JF, et al. The incidence and severity of adverse events affecting patients after discharge from the hospital. *Ann Intern Med*. 2003;138:161–167.

Fuji KT, Abbott AA, Norris JF. Exploring transitions in care from patient, caregiver, and health-care provider perspectives. *Clin Nurs Res*. 2013;22(3):258–274.

Gleason KM, Brake H, Agramonte V, Perfetti C. Medications at Transitions and Clinical Handoffs (MATCH) Toolkit for Medication Reconciliation. http://www.ahrq.gov/professionals/quality-patient-safety/patient-safety-resources/resources/match/match.pdf. Accessed March 31, 2015.

Gozalo P, Teno JM, Mitchell SL, et al. End-of-life transitions among nursing home residents with cognitive issues. *N Engl J Med*. 2011;365:1212–1221.

Jencks SF, Williams MV, Coleman EA. Rehospitalizations among patients in the Medicare fee-for-service program. *N Engl J Med*. 2009;360:1418–1428.

Joint Commission. *Improving America's Hospitals: A Report on Quality and Safety*. Oakbrook Terrace, IL: Joint Commission; 2006.

Kind AJ, Jensen L, Barczi S, et al. Low-cost transitional care with nurse managers making mostly phone contact with patients cut rehospitalization at a VA hospital. *Health Aff (Millwood)*. 2012;31:2659–2668.

King BD, Gilmore-Bykovskyi A, Roiland R, et al. The consequences of poor communication during hospital-to-skilled nursing facility transitions: a qualitative study. *J Am Geriatr Soc*. 2013;61(7):1095–1102.

Moore C, McGinn T, Halm E. Tying up loose ends: discharging patients with unresolved medical issues. *Arch Intern Med*. 2007;167:1305–1311.

Moore C, Wisnivesky J, Williams S, et al. Medical errors related to discontinuity of care from an inpatient to an outpatient setting. *J Gen Intern Med.* 2003;18: 646–651.

Naylor MD, Brooten DA, Campbell RL, et al. Transitional care of older adults hospitalized with heart failure: a randomized, controlled trial. *J Am Geriatr Soc.* 2004;52:675–684.

Ouslander JG, Bonner A, Herndon L, Shutes J. The Interventions to Reduce Acute Care Transfers (INTERACT) quality improvement program: an overview for medical directors and primary care clinicians in long term care. *J Am Med Dir Assoc.* 2014;15(3):162–170.

Rantz MJ, Popejoy L, Vogelsmeier A, et al. Successfully reducing hospitalizations of nursing home residents: results of the Missouri Quality Initiative. *J Am Med Dir Assoc.* 2017;18:960–966.

Tena-Nelson R, Santos K, Weingast E, Amrhein S, Ouslander J, Boockvar K. Reducing potentially preventable hospital transfers: results from a thirty nursing home collaborative. *J Am Med Dir Assoc.* 2012;13(7):651–656.

Chapter 19

Value-Based Care

David J. Meyers, Heidi Wold, Joseph G. Ouslander

The purpose of this chapter is to provide an overview of value-based care as it currently exists in the United States, and to highlight aspects of common value-based care models that are most relevant to the care of older adults. In many respects, geriatricians and other geriatric health professionals are in a position to make these value-based care models successful and to assume leadership roles in them. Value-based care requires health professionals to work as interprofessional teams and participate in care coordination across settings of care, to understand evidence-based care and as well as its limitations in older adults, and to practice person-centered care in the context of evidence and many other factors important to patients—all skills that geriatricians and other geriatric health professionals have developed.

At the same time, older adults with multiple comorbidities and related health care needs are likely to benefit from being in one or more value-based care models when implemented effectively. These individuals are especially susceptible to the potential for excess diagnostic testing, therapeutic intervention, and related complications and costs that are common in the Medicare fee-for-service system. Value-based care mitigates the incentives that create this situation and can therefore result in better outcomes and lower costs for the vulnerable older population.

DEFINING VALUE-BASED CARE

In most industries, value can be defined as the output achieved relative to the cost incurred. In health care, the most common definition of value is the patient health outcomes achieved per dollar spent. Central to the concept is that the value should be to the patient. Importantly, value is defined by both the quality of outcomes and the costs incurred. Cost-containment efforts without a focus on improving value may negatively impact patient health outcomes. Efforts devoted to improving quality metrics alone may not be sustainable or may not meet the needs or preferences of patients.

In the Porter model of value-based care, the outcomes that a patient experiences can be considered the numerator, while the cost of providing those outcomes can be considered the denominator. To improve the value of care, a provider can try to address either factor. However, in practice, addressing both simultaneously is often necessary. Value-based care can be seen as a direct response

Learning Objectives

- Understand the basic definitions of value-based care
- Explain the key elements of value-based care models
- Discuss the value-based care issues particular to older adults
- Identify different value-based care and alternative payment models

Key Clinical Points

1. There are substantial efforts in process to shift toward value-based care models and these types of arrangements are likely to become more common in the future.
2. Several alternative payment models are relevant to care for older adults. Examples include the Medicare Advantage (MA) program, accountable care organizations (ACOs), Programs of All-Inclusive for the Elderly (PACE), Institutional Special Needs Plans (ISNPs), the Merit-Based Incentive Payment System, and the Skilled Nursing Facility Value-Based Purchasing Program (SNF VBP).
3. There is no silver bullet in achieving value-based care. Rather, each initiative has strengths and drawbacks and forms a part of the greater whole.

to more traditional models of fee-for-service medicine. In fee-for-service, providers are simply paid a set amount for each unit of care they provide. Under fee-for-service, there is no incentive to improve on patient outcomes and there is a strong incentive to provide more care than is necessary. Engaging in value-based care should be an aspirational goal of many health systems as it puts the care of the patient first and the profit or provider second. A well-designed value-based care system will ideally maximize value for patients while at the same time providing value and potential cost savings for providers and payers as well.

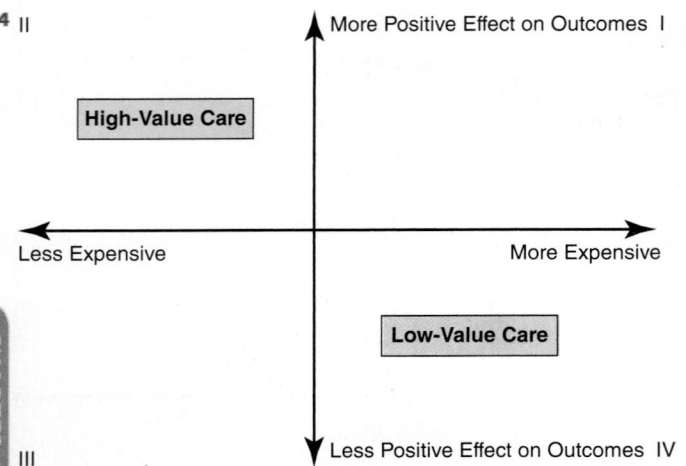

FIGURE 19-1. High- and low-value care.

Low-Value Care

In a simple model, we can consider care on two axes (**Figure 19-1**). On the x-axis we can consider a spectrum from the least expensive to the most expensive care. On the y-axis we can consider treatments that provide minimal benefits to patients to treatments that provide a large benefit for outcomes. If the upper left quadrant can be considered high-value care—delivering positive outcomes for low cost, then its inverse is in the lower right quadrant: low-value care. Low-value care is often defined as "services that provide little or no benefit to patients, have potential to cause harm, incur unnecessary cost to patients, or waste limited healthcare resources." Prior work has found that as much as $300 billion is spent annually on services that can be considered low value. As health systems and providers try to embrace concepts of value-based care, finding ways to maximize the use of high-value care and minimize the use of low-value care are often both necessary.

While there are many initiatives underway that aim to reduce the use of low-value care in clinical practice, one initiative that has grown in prominence is Choosing Wisely. Originally a project of the American Board of Internal Medicine, over 90 medical societies now publish lists of services that are deemed to be low value that clinicians should seek to avoid. The American Geriatrics Society published a list of 10 treatments that should be avoided (**Table 19-1**). While some work has found that the introduction of these lists are an important first step in addressing low-value care, they are a single component of a larger constellation of interventions that can help move delivery closer to value-based care.

KEY FEATURES OF VALUE-BASED CARE MODELS

While models of value-based care are variable and there are no one-size-fits-all approaches, there are several features that tend to be included as a component of most models.

TABLE 19-1 ■ AMERICAN GERIATRICS SOCIETY CHOOSING WISELY GUIDELINES

1. Don't recommend percutaneous feeding tubes in patients with advanced dementia; instead offer oral assisted feeding.
2. Don't recommend percutaneous feeding tubes in patients with advanced dementia; instead offer oral assisted feeding.
3. Avoid using medications other than metformin to achieve hemoglobin A1c < 7.5% in most older adults; moderate control is generally better.
4. Don't use benzodiazepines or other sedative-hypnotics in older adults as first choice for insomnia, agitation or delirium.
5. Don't use antimicrobials to treat bacteriuria in older adults unless specific urinary tract symptoms are present.
6. Don't prescribe cholinesterase inhibitors for dementia without periodic assessment for perceived cognitive benefits and adverse gastrointestinal effects.
7. Don't recommend screening for breast, colorectal, prostate or lung cancer without considering life expectancy and the risks of testing, overdiagnosis and overtreatment.
8. Avoid using prescription appetite stimulants or high-calorie supplements for treatment of anorexia or cachexia in older adults; instead, optimize social supports, discontinue medications that may interfere with eating, provide appealing food and feeding assistance, and clarify patient goals and expectations.
9. Don't prescribe a medication without conducting a drug regimen review.
10. Don't use physical restraints to manage behavioral symptoms of hospitalized older adults with delirium.

Data from https://www.choosingwisely.org/societies/american-geriatrics-society/.

First, they tend to feature some type of financial risk sharing between the payer (eg, a health plan) and the provider (eg, a hospital). Second, there is almost always effort devoted to quality measurement. Third, there is often increased care coordination than might be traditionally included in a fee-for-service model. Fourth, many models also embrace concepts of population health management.

Financial Risk Sharing

Financial risk sharing can take many forms and exists along a spectrum (**Figure 19-2**). Risk can be understood as the possibility of losing or gaining money on an investment. In health care, there can be substantial heterogeneity in the patients' experiences and care needs. When a provider assumes more risk, they are making themselves more responsible for that variation. In traditional fee-for-service health care, a provider does not bear any risk financially. A provider is paid a fixed amount for providing patient services, and is not liable to losing financially if the patient requires more care or does not achieve desired outcomes. In fee-for-service there is an incentive for providing excess care that may not be beneficial to patients or the US health care system as a whole. In value-based care, providers take

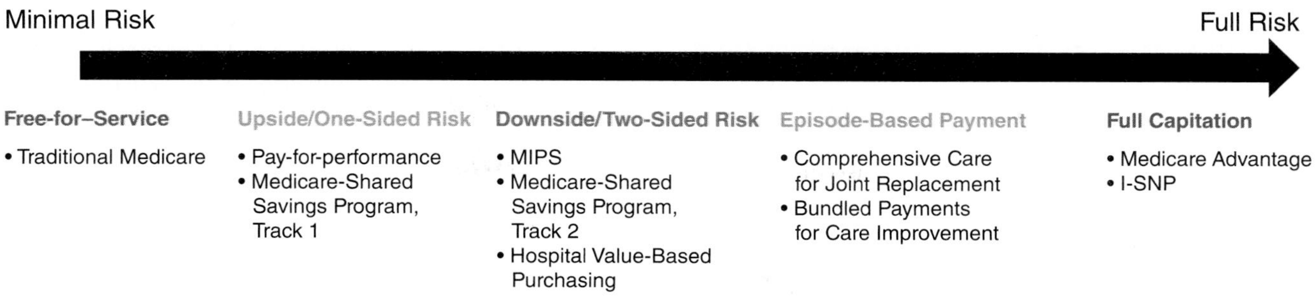

Free-for–Service	Upside/One-Sided Risk	Downside/Two-Sided Risk	Episode-Based Payment	Full Capitation
• Traditional Medicare	• Pay-for-performance • Medicare-Shared Savings Program, Track 1	• MIPS • Medicare-Shared Savings Program, Track 2 • Hospital Value-Based Purchasing	• Comprehensive Care for Joint Replacement • Bundled Payments for Care Improvement	• Medicare Advantage • I-SNP

FIGURE 19-2. Spectrum of risk sharing.

on more risk, which incentivizes the provision of higher quality services.

When a provider takes on risk, it can take the form of upside risk or downside risk. Upside risk is the ability to benefit financially for delivering high value care and is also sometimes called one-sided risk. In the most basic iteration of upside risk, a provider may be "paid for performance"; receiving financial bonuses for delivering certain levels of quality. Another example of upside risk is in the early Medicare shared savings accountable care organization (ACO) models. If providers were able to meet quality standards and provide care under a financial benchmark, they could "share" some of those savings with the Medicare program. The upside risk models provide the least uncertainty to providers as they are not liable to repay any financial loses, however the ability to benefit in these models are typically more limited.

In downside risk models, a provider who does not meet a financial benchmark for their patients may be liable to refund a payer for the losses they incur. Downside risk may provide a stronger financial incentive to deliver on high value care. An example of downside risk is payment penalties under the hospital value-based purchasing program. If a hospital does not meet specific quality benchmarks, the Medicare program may withhold payments by 2%. Models that include both upside and downside risk are called two-sided risk models.

The next level of risk is episode-based payments. Under episode-based payment models, a provider may be paid a lump sum to cover all services a patient may need related to a specific condition. The Medicare program has launched several episode-based payment models, such as the Comprehensive Care for Joint Replacement (CJR) model. In the CJR model, providers are paid a single amount to cover all the care a patient needs for a lower extremity joint replacement, for up to 90 days postdischarge. If, for instance, a patient is readmitted to the hospital unnecessarily, the provider stands to lose financially; however, if care is delivered in an efficient matter, then they may benefit financially.

The highest level of risk a provider may take on is full capitation. Under full capitation, a provider or health plan may be paid "per capita" or per person. These payments are typically "risk-adjusted," paying a higher amount for patients who have more complex care needs. The most prominent example of full capitation in the US health care system is the Medicare Advantage (MA) program, where private plans are paid per capita for their enrollees. If a plan is successful in reducing unnecessary care and preventing adverse events such as hospitalizations, they may benefit substantially; however, if patients are repetitively hospitalized, the plan may lose substantially on that patient. While under full capitation, the payer or provider assumes the highest level of risk, they also stand the benefit the most if they provide high value care.

Quality Measurement

Quality measurement is vital in value-based care for two primary reasons. First, if value-based aims to deliver maximal outcomes for minimal costs, it is imperative to measure quality to ensure that patients experience beneficial outcomes. Second, in the presence of a risk-sharing model, without quality thresholds there would be an incentive for providers to "stint" on care or to save money by cutting back on services to the detriment of a patient. In a fully capitated model, without the assurance of a baseline level of quality, a provider could deny all services to a patient in order to retain all of the payment they received for that patient. We describe quality measurement in value-based care in greater detail later in this chapter.

Care Coordination

Care coordination is defined by the Agency for Healthcare Research and Quality as the "deliberate organizing of patient-care activities and sharing information among all of the participants concerned with a patient's care to achieve safer and more effective care." While this definition focuses on clinical care processes, other definitions also include a focus on the coordination of social and community-based services that might be beneficial to patients with advanced care needs. Despite varying definitions, care coordination can be an important tool for achieving value-based care. **Table 19-2** lists common care coordination activities. If the two primary inputs into value-based care are reduced costs

TABLE 19-2 ■ EXAMPLES OF CARE COORDINATION ACTIVITIES

Examples of broad care coordination approaches include:

- Teamwork
- Care management
- Medication management
- Health information technology
- Patient-centered medical home

Examples of specific care coordination activities include:

- Establishing accountability and agreeing on responsibility
- Communicating/sharing knowledge
- Helping with transitions of care
- Assessing patient needs and goals
- Creating a proactive care plan
- Monitoring and follow-up, including responding to changes in patients' needs
- Supporting patients' self-management goals
- Linking to community resources
- Working to align resources with patient and population needs

Data from the Agency for Healthcare Research and Quality https://www.ahrq.gov/ncepcr/care/coordination.html#:~:text=Care%20coordination%20involves%20deliberately%20organizing,safer%20and%20more%20effective%20care.

and improved patient outcomes, care coordination has the potential to address both.

On the efficiency and cost side of the equation, care coordination can play an important role in organizing a patient's care and preventing unnecessary additional visits and complications. After a hospitalization some patients, particularly those with advanced care needs, may have difficulties in making it to follow-up appointments. A provider who successfully coordinates a patient's care, perhaps through the use of a patient navigator or community health worker, may be able to aid patients in receiving all of their necessary follow-up care, thus reducing the risks of an adverse event and a preventable hospital readmission. Other patients may see providers from different health systems and receive duplicative care across sites such as extra blood tests or imaging. These studies can result in false-positive or abnormal, but clinically insignificant findings that often result in repeat or follow-up testing. A system that is able to coordinate a patient's care across providers, potentially through the use of electronic health records, may be able to prevent unnecessary services and invasive procedures by communicating results between providers rather than duplicating them.

Care coordination approaches can also be used to potentially improve upon patient outcomes. Some patients may have challenges in understanding and successfully taking their medications. Inappropriate medications and poor adherence to necessary medications may have downstream negative health effects. Successful care coordination could include regular medication reviews and reconciliation by the patient's care team to ensure that the patient has access and is taking the

medication that they need. In other instances, a patient may benefit by being connected to social services in their communities such as meal services or transportation to their specialty visits, which may both lead to improved patient outcomes.

Population Health Management

Population health can be defined as the health outcomes of groups of individuals including the distribution of such outcomes within the group. Population medicine acknowledges that many of the outcomes that patients face are driven in part by what occurs in the community. As such, population health management has become a key feature of value-based care. If providers are going to be held accountable for the outcomes their patients experience, there can be a strong incentive to promote positive outcomes through community-wide interventions and public health efforts. Examples of population health interventions for older adults include those targeted toward lifestyle behavior change, fall risk, polypharmacy, psychosocial interventions, and disease management programs. Common population health problems that lead to adverse health for older adults can include physical inactivity, unhealthy diets, and smoking. To address these concerns, patient-centered medical homes (PCMHs) often provide nutritionist services for patients and many MA plans cover smoking cessation services. To address concerns around fall risk, MA plans have recently started covering the costs of in-home safety modifications, such as the installation of handles in showers and hallways, exercise, and other fall prevention interventions. To address concerns of loneliness and depression among older adults, some hospitals and Program of All-Inclusive Care for the Elderly (PACE) programs have invested in friendly visitor services to ensure that older adults living in the community are able to socialize. Many ACOs and health plans also provide patients with disease management tools, such as remote glucose monitors, in order to ensure that the needs of their patients are being met. While each of these value-based models may need to cover the upfront costs of these services for their patients, over time, they may be beneficial in improving patient outcomes and reducing the risk of costly events such as hospitalizations.

Population health strategies can also be helpful to value-based practices to identify patients at highest risk for complications and health care costs. In heterogeneous populations of older adults, some will be relatively healthy and others will have multiple comorbidities requiring considerable medical care. We know that in such populations, a relatively small proportion of patients can account for the majority of costs. Various models, such as for hospitalizations, readmissions, injurious falls, and other expensive events, can assist in identifying those at highest risk and developing targeted and tailored interventions that can improve care and reduce morbidity and related costs.

VALUE-BASED CARE MODELS RELEVANT TO THE CARE OF OLDER ADULTS

In recent years there has been a dramatic shift toward embracing different models of value-based care in the US health care system. Many of these new models have been developed by the Centers for Medicare and Medicaid Services Innovation Center (CMS CMMI) and focus on addressing the needs of older adults. Below and in **Table 19-3** we present an overview of several of these new value-based care models.

MEDICARE ADVANTAGE

Medicare Advantage (MA) or Medicare Part C is a privately run segment of the Medicare program. While in traditional Medicare, the federal government is the primary payer for patient services; in the MA program private insurance plans are paid by the government to cover the needs of their enrollees. MA is a fully capitated program—plans are paid a single risk-adjusted amount by CMS to cover all enrollee needs each year. While MA plans need to cover at least the same benefits available in traditional Medicare, they may also provide additional supplemental benefits such as fitness programs, meal delivery services, and dental coverage, which are not available in traditional Medicare. Plans also have flexibility in the premiums and other cost-sharing that they require, and can limit patients to specific provider networks and require prior authorization for services. Enrollment in MA is rapidly growing and, as of 2019, included over 22 million enrollees representing 34% of all Medicare beneficiaries.

Institutional Special Needs Plans

Institutional Special Needs Plans (I-SNPs) are MA Special Needs Plans that restrict enrollment to individuals who, for 90 days or longer, have had or are expected to need the level of services provided in an institutional environment (skilled nursing facility [SNF], long-term care nursing facility [NF], a SNF/NF, intermediate care facility for individuals with intellectual disabilities [ICF/IDD], or an inpatient psychiatric facility). There is strict enrollment marketing guidance from CMS, and the I-SNP does not have direct access to institutionalized long-term residents unless they express an interest to be contacted by the I-SNP sales team.

Institutional Equivalent Special Needs Plans

Institutional Equivalent Special Needs Plans (Ie-SNPs) care for individuals who are living in the community, but qualify for an institutional level of care (LOC). For an I-SNP to enroll MA eligible individuals living in the community, but requiring an institutional LOC, the following two conditions must be met:

1. A determination of institutional LOC that is based on the use of a state assessment tool. The assessment tool used for persons living in the community must be the same as that used for individuals residing in an institution. In states and territories without a specific tool, I-SNPs must use the same LOC determination methodology used in the respective state or territory in which the I-SNP is authorized to enroll eligible individuals.

2. The I-SNP must arrange to have the LOC assessment administered by an independent, impartial party (ie, an entity other than the respective I-SNP) with the requisite professional knowledge to identify accurately the institutional LOC needs. Importantly, the I-SNP cannot own or control the entity.

I-SNPs/Ie-SNPs are full risk-bearing value payment models. The I-SNP/Ie-SNP health plans must submit bids that demonstrate the ability to perform within CMS FFS established benchmarks each year to continue its contract with CMS. All Medicare premiums paid to these health plans are based on the hierarchical condition category (HCC) payment model, which adjusts payments for the presence of specific chronic conditions. All medical, behavioral, special supplemental benefits and prescription drug costs are paid out of the plan premium amounts on a per member per month basis. I-SNPs must manage member costs of care within the plan premium payments amounts.

Each I-SNP/Ie-SNP health plan must submit an SNP Model of Care document along with their CMS application. This document is reviewed and approved by the National Committee for Quality Assurance (NCQA) on behalf of CMS. The SNP Model of Care describes the specific targeted population, provider network, care coordination, quality program, and quality metrics and targets to be achieved. In most instances each member of an I-SNP has an assigned care coordinator (mostly nurse practitioners or physician assistants) supported by an interdisciplinary care team that coordinates members' care and services and delivers all the specific activities outlined in the I-SNP Model of Care. These include annual comprehensive evaluation, individualized plan of care with advanced care planning, interdisciplinary care team meetings, transitions of care, closing quality gaps in care, use of evidenced-based care guidelines, and accurate clinical documentation.

Many I-SNPs have special supplemental benefits beyond traditional Medicare to support the unique needs of the special population. These typically include routine eye examinations, glasses, hearing examinations, hearing aids, transportation, and/or music therapy.

Providers have a variety of payment options in an I-SNP. These include fee for service, a value-based payment model, or a combination. In the value-based payment model, a monthly per member per month capitation is granted where the provider can earn a performance and quality bonus in addition to the capitation payment.

Program of All-Inclusive Care for the Elderly

The PACE model serves nursing home eligible seniors' chronic care needs and their families in the community

TABLE 19-3 ■ MODELS OF CARE

MODEL NAME	CARE SETTING	KEY FEATURES	TYPE OF RISK	EVIDENCE OF SUCCESS
Medicare Advantage	Health insurance	• Private plans are responsible for covering all enrollee needs. • Can offer supplemental benefits not available in traditional Medicare. • Can enforce provider networks and prior authorization requirements for patients. • Most plans include patient care coordinators. • Plans are rated using a 5-star rating system and can be paid bonuses if they are high performing.	Full capitation	• Plans may lead to a reduction in hospital admissions and readmissions and postacute care use. • Plans are associated with some improvements in patient reported outcomes and quality screenings, however, enrollees at the end-of-life report worse quality care. • Patients with complex care needs disenroll at higher rates and evidence of success in complex patients is mixed. • Cost savings are ambiguous.
Institutional Special Needs Plans (I-SNPs)	Nursing homes	• Medicare Advantage plans that restrict enrollment to individuals who, for 90 d or longer, have had or are expected to need the level of services provided in an institutional environment. • I-SNPs are paid under full capitation to care for their enrollees. • Many I-SNPs have special supplemental benefits beyond traditional Medicare to support the unique needs of the special population. These typically include routine eye examinations, glasses, hearing examinations, hearing aids, transportation, and/or music therapy.	Full capitation	• Early evidence finds I-SNPs may be associated with lower costly utilization and an increase in hospice use. • More evidence is needed to understand the long-term outcomes of these programs.
Program of All-Inclusive Care for the Elderly (PACE)	Community	• PACE serves individuals who are age 55 or older, certified by their state to need nursing home care, able to live safely in the community at the time of enrollment, and live in a PACE service area. • PACE can provide a wide range of services including adult day care, medical care, home health care, social services, respite care, hospital, and nursing home care.	Full capitation	• May be associated with some reductions in hospitalizations and readmissions.
Hospice	Hospitals, facilities, and community	• Medicare hospice is a program where the hospice provider is paid a per member per day premium to provide all hospice-related care and services. • Medicare hospice covers items and services needed for symptom relief, social services, drugs for pain management, durable medical equipment for pain relief, aid and homemaker services, spiritual and grief counseling. • Hospice does not cover curative treatments, custodial room and board, or other nonterminal illness-related medical costs. • CMS has recently launched a value-based insurance design model for hospice through Medicare Advantage	Partial capitation-per day payments	• Medicare hospice use is often associated with reductions in spending at the end of life.
Patient-Centered Medical Homes (PCMH)	Outpatient clinics	• Primary care practices are oriented around patient-centered care, which typically includes comprehensive team-based care, care coordination, and a focus on patient quality outcomes. • In many cases PCMHs receive per-beneficiary per-month payments to incentivize coordination of care. • Prominent examples of PCMHs for older adults include Medicare's Comprehensive Primary Care and Comprehensive Primary Care Plus programs (CPC+).	Upside/one-sided risk	• PCMHs have been linked to modest improvements in cancer screenings and reductions in unnecessary emergency department care. • Effects on cost savings are still ambiguous. • Evaluations of the CPC+ program are still ongoing.

Program	Applies to	Description	Risk	Evidence
Accountable Care Organizations (ACOs)	Hospitals and outpatient providers	• Patients are attributed either at the beginning or the end of the year to ACOs, which are accountable to their care. • Depending on the track selected, ACOs in the Medicare Shared Savings Program may opt into one-sided or two-sided risk. • ACOs are also evaluated on a set of quality indicators that must be met in order to be eligible for savings.	Either one-sided or two-sided risk	• ACOs in the MSSP have been associated with modest reductions in Medicare spending and minimal effects on quality outcomes. • ACOs that are based in physician organizations tend to perform better than ACOs based out of hospitals. • ACOs have been associated with large reductions in the use of postacute care.
Hospital Value-Based Purchasing and the Readmissions Reduction Program	Hospitals	• In the HBP, hospitals are rewarded or penalized on the basis of 20 measures of mortality, hospital-acquired infection, spending, and patient satisfaction. • In the HRRP, hospitals are penalized for poor performance on several metrics of hospital readmissions. • Neither program includes other value-based care features such as care coordination; however, many hospitals embrace value-based care practices to improve outcomes on these metrics. • Both programs are mandatory for most acute care hospitals nationally.	Two-sided risk	• The HRRP has been linked to a reduction in readmissions since its implementation. • The HBP has been linked to modest improvements in patient experience. • There are concerns that both programs disproportionately penalize safety-net hospitals and those that treat more complex patients. • There is ambiguous evidence that the HRRP may be associated to increased mortality.
Merit-Based Incentive Program (MIPS)	Outpatient providers	• Individual or group practices may select 6 quality measures to be evaluated on. Practices are also assessed on interoperability standards and spending benchmarks. • Providers that perform poorly under the program may be penalized up to 9% of their payments, while high-performing providers may receive a payment boost. • Participation is mandatory for all providers that meet a minimum number of patients and that are not participating in other value-based models.	Two-sided risk	• Given the recent introduction of the program, evidence is limited on if it improves patient outcomes or reduces spending. • Early evidence suggests that providers with more complex patient panels may face steeper penalties.
Skilled Nursing Facility Value-Based Purchasing	Skilled nursing facilities	• SNFs that receive Medicare payments are evaluated on their readmission rates. • If SNFs have a readmission rate above a certain threshold, they are liable to be penalized up to 2% of their Medicare payments. SNFs that perform exceptionally well have the potential to receive a payment bonus.	Two-sided risk	• Given the recent introduction of the program, evidence is limited on if it improves patient outcomes or reduces spending. • Early findings indicate that as many as 72% of SNFs nationally were penalized in the first year of the program.
Bundled Payment Programs (Bundled Payments for Care Improvement, Comprehensive Care for Joint Replacements)	Hospitals and postacute care	• In bundled payment models, providers are given a set payment to cover all the care needs of an enrollee during an episode of care. • In the BPCI program, hospitals could voluntarily participate for up to 48 different clinical conditions. • In the CJR program, all hospitals within specific markers were required to bundle their care for hip and knee replacement surgeries.	Episode-based payment partial capitation	• Both the CJR and BPCI have been found to lead to significant reductions in spending for joint replacements without impacts to quality. • Evidence on other clinical conditions is mixed. • Most savings under bundling appear to come from large reductions in SNF use and substitution for less costly PAC care.

whenever possible. Members enrolled in PACE receive both Medicare services and Medicaid home and long-term care support services. PACE serves individuals who are age 55 or older, certified by their state to need nursing home care, able to live safely in the community at the time of enrollment, and live in a PACE service area. While all PACE participants must be certified to need nursing home care to enroll in PACE, only about 7% of PACE participants nationally reside in a nursing home. If a PACE enrollee needs nursing home care, the PACE program pays for it and continues to coordinate the enrollee's care.

The PACE model of care can be traced to the early 1970s, when the Chinatown-North Beach community of San Francisco saw the pressing needs for long-term care services by families whose elders had immigrated from Italy, China, and the Philippines. William Gee, DDS, a public health dentist, headed the committee that hired Marie-Louise Ansak in 1971 to investigate solutions. Along with other community leaders, they formed a nonprofit corporation called On Lok Senior Health Services to create a community-based system of care. On Lok is a Cantonese term for "peaceful, happy abode."

The PACE program is able to provide the entire continuum of care and services to seniors with chronic care needs, while maintaining their independence in their homes for as long as possible. Services include:

- Adult day care that offers nursing; physical, occupational, and recreational therapies; meals; nutritional counseling; social work and personal care;
- Medical care provided by a PACE physician familiar with the history, needs, and preferences of each participant;
- Home health care and personal care;
- All necessary prescription drugs;
- Social services;
- Medical specialties, such as audiology, dentistry, optometry, podiatry, and speech therapy;
- Respite care; and
- Hospital and nursing home care when necessary

Similar to an Ie-SNP, the PACE model is a full risk-bearing program that receives premium payments for both Medicare and Medicaid services rendered to members using the HCC model by CMS blended with Medicaid waiver program funding by the states. These services are typically provided in a defined geographical location and are paid for through the full risk-reimbursement model.

Like I-SNPs/Ie-SNPs, PACE programs are also required to define a Model of Care and execute the activities outline in the Model of Care. Providers working in PACE programs are reimbursed in either a fee-for-service model of value-based capitation model.

Hospice Services Under Medicare

Medicare hospice is a program where the hospice provider is paid per member per day premium to provide all hospice-related care and services. In this context it is a form of a value-based program. Hospice services covered under the daily payment include:

- All items and services needed for pain relief and symptom management
- Medical, nursing, and social services
- Drugs for pain management
- Durable medical equipment for pain relief and symptom management
- Aide and homemaker services
- Other covered services needed to manage pain and other symptoms, as well as spiritual and grief counseling

Other related medical services are paid for under the original Medicare fee-for-service program. Medicare beneficiaries become eligible for hospice services after being certified by a provider as terminally ill (life expectancy 6 months or less), if they choose to participate in a comfort care not curative care, AND only if they sign a hospice election form with the selected hospice organization.

Typically, patients on Medicare hospice do not access acute care services and have a hospice plan of care. Original Medicare will still pay for covered benefits for any health problems that are not part of the patient's terminal illness and related conditions, but this is unusual. Hospice does not cover curative treatments, custodial room and board, or other nonterminal illness-related medical costs.

While Medicare pays hospice agencies a daily rate for each day a beneficiary is enrolled in the hospice benefit, regardless of the amount of services provided on a given day and on days when no services are provided. The daily payment rates are intended to cover costs that hospices incur in furnishing services identified in patients' care plans. Payments are made according to a fee schedule that has four different levels of care: routine home care (RHC), continuous home care (CHC), inpatient respite care (IRC), and general inpatient care (GIC). The payment rates are updated annually based on the hospital market index.

The four levels of care are distinguished by the location and intensity of the services provided. Currently, when an enrollee in an MA plan elects hospice, Fee-for-Service (FFS) Medicare becomes financially responsible for most services, while the MA plan retains responsibility for certain services (eg, supplemental benefits).

Primary care providers are reimbursed for approved hospice services typically as fee for service. Medicare is shifting hospice services to full value-based payment models by testing the administration of those services in 2021 through the Primary Cares Initiatives program, one of which focuses on those with serious illness.

Through the MA Value-Based Insurance Design (VBID) Model, CMS is testing a broad array of complementary MA health plan innovations designed to reduce Medicare program expenditures, enhance the quality of care for Medicare beneficiaries, including those with low incomes such as those dual-eligible, and improve the coordination and efficiency of health care service delivery. Overall, the VBID Model contributes to the modernization of MA and tests whether these model components improve health outcomes and lower expenditures for MA enrollees. For plan year 2021, 19 Medicare Advantage Organizations (MAOs) offering MA benefits to plan benefit packages (PBPs) with 4.6 million projected enrollees will provide tailored model benefits and rewards and incentives to over 1.6 million projected enrollees in 45 states, the District of Columbia, and Puerto Rico. Out of the 19 MAOs, 9 are participating in the Hospice Benefit Component.

Under the Hospice Benefit Component of the VBID Model, participating MAOs retain responsibility for all original Medicare services, including hospice care. The Hospice Benefit Component of the Model implements a set of changes recommended by the Medicare Payment Advisory Commission (MedPAC), the Health and Human Services (HHS) Office of Inspector General (OIG), and other stakeholders.

Patient-centered medical homes PCMH is a model of primary care where a patient engages in a relationship with a provider who seeks to center the patient's need through the whole care process. While there is no one model that constitutes a PCMH, the common functions and attributes of a PCMH include comprehensive care, patient-centeredness, coordinated care, accessible services, and a focus on quality and safety. Comprehensive care typically involves including a team of care providers across disciplines such as mental health professionals, social workers, and nutritionists to come together to create a care plan for a patient that addresses all of their needs. Patient-centeredness includes a focus on ensuring that patients or their caregivers are directly involved in the processes of care. Coordinated care includes ensuring that patients have smooth transitions between sites of care. Accessible services typically include longer in-person hours, and the creation of different channels the patient can use to communicate with providers. Quality and safety includes the use of registries to track disease and pay-for-performance in an effort to improve patient outcomes.

An example of a PCMH in the Medicare program is the Comprehensive Primary Care (CPC), and Comprehensive Primary Care Plus (CPC+) models. In the CPC programs, participating provider groups are paid a care management fee, which is per patient per month payment to incentivize care coordination activities. Practices that perform well on quality metrics may receive bonus payments. Otherwise, most other payment follows the fee-for-service risk schedule.

Accountable care organizations Accountable care organizations (ACOs) are groups of doctors, hospitals, and other healthcare providers that come together in an effort to coordinate care and share risk. ACOs differ from PCMHs in that PCMHs typically focus on single outpatient clinics,

while ACOs encompass a wider range of providers. In an ACO there is typically some degree of coordination and integration between different provider types, often facilitated by a shared electronic health record. While most ACOs still operate under a fee-for-service pay schedule, there is typically some degree of either upside or two-sided risk.

The primary example of ACOs that care for older adults is the Medicare Shared Savings Program (MSSP). Under the MSSP, organizations voluntarily come together as ACOs to care for the needs of Traditional Medicare beneficiaries. While there are different tracks within the MSSP, they typically include several key features. First, patients are attributed to specific ACOs that are accountable for their care through the year. Attribution can either be retrospective, when patients are assigned after seeing which ACO provided for the majority of their care at the end of the year, or prospective, when patients are assigned to an ACO for the upcoming year based on prior year care use. ACOs may also decide whether to take on one-sided risk, receiving payment bonuses for hitting quality and efficiency benchmarks, or two-sided risk, which provides a greater opportunity to save money, but also exposes the ACO to a greater potential for financial loss. ACOs also must typically meet certain scores on a set of quality metrics if they are to be eligible for shared savings. Despite the voluntary nature of the program, participation in ACOs are steadily increasing over time, although most ACOs still prefer to engage in the one-sided risk track.

Hospital value-based purchasing and the readmissions reduction program After the Affordable Care Act, CMS implemented two new value-based programs for acute care hospitals nationally: the Hospital Value-Based Purchasing Program (VBP) and the Hospital Readmissions Reduction Program (HRRP). Under the VBP, hospitals are evaluated on a number of quality metrics including preventable hospital acquired infections, mortality rates for acute myocardial infarction (AMI), heart failure, and pneumonia, spending per beneficiary, and patient rating of care experience. If a hospital performs well on these metrics, they may receive a bonus payment from CMS at the end of the year. If a hospital performs poorly, then it may receive a financial penalty up to 2% of payments. Similarly, in the HRRP, hospitals are evaluated on readmissions rates for select health conditions. If a hospital has readmission rates higher than a benchmark, they may be penalized up to 3% of Medicare payments. Neither of these models includes a stated care coordination or population health component, but are intended to reduce adverse events through strong financial incentives. Outside of the payment adjustments, hospitals subject to these programs are paid using the fee-for-service fee schedule.

Merit-based incentive program The Merit-Based Incentive Program (MIPS) was implemented by CMS in 2017 to add a value-based care focus to most outpatient providers who see Medicare patients. Under MIPS, individual providers or group practices select from a set of possible quality measures that they would like to be evaluated on. The MIPS program also evaluates whether providers meet certain interoperability standards for their health records as well as certain spending benchmarks. Each of these metrics is combined together into an overall score. Very low performing providers may be subject to a 9% payment reduction; however, most penalties that have occurred in the program so far have been around 1%. Very high performing practices may also receive a small increase to their payments. All provider groups that meet a minimum number of patients are subject to MIPS unless they participate in an Alternative Payment Model (APM), such as the MSSP or the CPC. As a result, virtually all providers that receive Medicare payments are subject to at least some form of value-based care.

Skilled nursing facility value-based purchasing In 2018, CMS implemented the Skilled Nursing Facility Value-Based Purchasing (SNF VBP) program. All SNFs that receive Medicare payments were required to participate in the program, which evaluates SNF performance on hospital readmissions. SNFs that performed poorly on the readmission's metric could be subject to a 2% reduction in Medicare payments, while top performing SNFs could receive bonus payments of up to 2% of Medicare payments. In 2019, SNFs with readmission rates above 18% were penalized. Similar to the hospital VPB programs, there are no other structural components that facilities subject to this model needed to implement, but the strong financial incentive is designed to encourage SNFs to change their practices to reduce adverse outcomes.

Bundled payment programs The Bundled Payments for Care Improvement (BPCI) and the Comprehensive Care for Joint Replacement (CJR) programs are two examples of episode-based payment models. In bundled payments, providers or a group of providers are paid a single set amount to cover all of the care needs a patient requires during a specific procedure and typically 90 days post procedure. The Medicare prospective payment system, which pays hospitals for patient care on the basis of an assigned Diagnosis-Related Group (DRG), is in essence a bundled payment for the hospital care a patient requires. The newer episode-based bundle models expand on that concept and cover all costs related to the episode of care which may include postacute care use following a procedure and rehabilitation services. If a patient has an unnecessary readmission following a procedure, the bundle would need to cover that care as well. If a provider is efficient in delivering care, bundles present an opportunity for them to save substantially; however, if a provider is not efficient, then they may lose money on a patient's episode. Bundled payment programs typically involve substantial care coordination and partnerships between hospitals and postacute care providers in order to deliver patients the most efficient care possible.

The BPCI program is a voluntary bundled payment program that providers can choose to participate in for up to 48 different clinical conditions, the most common of which was lower joint replacement. Under the program, depending on the selected tracks, a spending benchmark was set for each condition and adjusted for patient complexity. If the hospital performed under the benchmark, they were permitted to keep all the savings during an end-of-year adjustment. If they performed above the threshold, their payments would be reduced at the end of the year. Given the voluntary nature of the program, the providers who tended to participate already performed well for those episodes of care. In 2016, CMS launched the CJR program for hip or knee replacement. While the program operates similarly to the BPCI, it was a mandatory program for providers who operated in randomly assigned service areas.

QUALITY MEASUREMENT FOR VALUE-BASED CARE

Achieving high-quality outcomes for patients is central to the goals of value-based care. The traditional framework for understanding how quality of care can be measured is one proposed by Donabedian. The underpinning of this framework is that high-quality medical care is defined as care that is expected to achieve the best balance of health benefits and risks, in other words, medical care that does the best job at improving health or preventing health decline. Within this framework, quality is conceptualized as pertaining to technical and interpersonal care, each of which may influence the other. Technical care can be measured in three domains: structure, process, and outcomes. *Structure* refers to the relatively stable characteristics of the providers, the tools and resources available to them, and the physical environment and organizational characteristics of the health system. Examples of structural measures of quality include board certification of physicians and accreditation of health organizations such as hospitals and health plans; the use of electronic health records or computerized provider order entry; and designation as a level 1 trauma center, which requires several structural requirements be met, including but not limited to, 24-hour in-house coverage by general surgeons, a minimal annual volume of severely injured patients and a comprehensive quality assessment program. The validity of structural measures depends on the evidence to support a relationship between the structure and a health outcome. An advantage of structural measures is that they are relatively easy to measure. However, given the stability of most health care structures, structural measures are generally not suitable for continuous quality assessment/improvement activities, but rather for periodic assessment.

Process refers to what health care providers do for patients. Examples of process measures include the prescription of β-blocker medications to patients following an AMI, the offering of annual influenza vaccinations for certain classes of patients, screening for colorectal cancer with a fecal occult blood test or colonoscopy, and providing yearly examinations of the feet in patients with diabetes. As with structural measures, the validity of process measures depends on demonstrated evidence that the process is associated with a favorable health outcome. For example, there is good evidence that β-blockers given after a myocardial infarction will reduce future myocardial infarctions, cardiac arrhythmias including sudden death, and mortality. An advantage of process measures is that they can be used in real time, or over relatively short periods of time, to identify and correct process of care gaps that can be closed to improve health outcomes. While data for some process measures can be collected with relative ease from health plan administrative data, many process measures require detailed clinical data available only from medical record abstraction or clinical registries designed specifically to capture those data.

Outcome refers to a person's health state and is commonly divided into two categories: *indirect* (or *intermediate* or *proxy*) *outcomes*, and *patient health outcomes* (or sometimes *patient-centered outcomes*). Patient health outcomes include specific clinical events that are ascertained or diagnosed by clinicians such as myocardial infarction, stroke, or death. Patient health outcomes also include "patient-reported outcomes" or "PROs," which are things patients can feel or observe for themselves such as pain, function, or urinary incontinence. Indirect outcomes refer to outcomes that lead to, or act as a proxy for, patient health outcomes that are otherwise difficult to measure. Indirect outcomes include measures of *clinical parameters* such as blood pressure, blood sugar, and lipid levels, and of *utilization* such as hospital admissions, readmissions, and emergency room visits. Blood pressure is one of the most well-known clinical parameters used as an indirect outcome. The vast majority of patients with elevated blood pressure have no symptoms attributable to it, but the presence of persistent high blood pressure is known to be a contributing cause to many patient health outcomes, such as stroke, myocardial infarction, and kidney failure. It takes many years for these outcomes to develop, and it is proven that lowering elevated blood pressure can reduce the risk of stroke, myocardial infarction, etc. Thus, we accept that the control of blood pressure—a condition most patients can't feel—is a valid indirect measure of patient outcome. Other examples of commonly used indirect clinical measures of patient outcome include the value of hemoglobin A_{1c} in patients with diabetes and various lipid measurements in patients with (or at risk for) cardiovascular disease. Similarly, certain types of health care utilization are used as proxies for poor or worsened health. For example, it is presumed that the health of a patient with asthma had declined if the patient visited an emergency room (ER). Likewise, it is presumed that the health of patient is poor if the patient requires a readmission to a hospital within 30 days of discharge.

Outcome measures are often considered the "gold standard" of quality measures as they directly measure the health that the medical system is intended to improve. However, many other factors outside the control of the health system may also impact health outcomes. Additionally, underlying patient health status may impact achievable outcomes. Hence, outcome measures must be risk-adjusted as appropriate for factors beyond the health system that may impact the outcome.

Quality measures operationalize the concepts of interpersonal and technical care quality for measurement in different settings. Quality measures specify in great detail the specific structures, processes, outcomes, or consumer experiences to be measured, the specific population in which these should be measured, and the time frame over which measurement should occur. Types of data (eg, patient report, medical records, administrative data from health plans or other sources) are also explicitly defined for a quality measure. Quality measures in the United States are developed by a number of different types of entities with interest in the health care quality including accreditation organizations, government, provider organizations, health delivery systems, specialty societies, and academic institutions. The same quality concept could be developed into several different measures, generally in order to measure quality at different levels within the health care system.

Measuring the quality of care in older adults has many similarities, but also some important differences, to measuring quality of care in younger adults that make quality measurement challenging in the older population. Many health conditions—pneumonia, myocardial infarction, stroke, diabetes, etc—occur with equal or greater frequency in older adults, and have similar or identical process and outcome measures that are relevant to assessing quality of care. However, there are a number of health care conditions that are far more common in older adults than in younger adults, and for which (in the past) many existing quality measurement schemes had few or no measures. Dementia, falls, urinary incontinency, hearing impairment, and end-of-life care are a few such conditions. In addition, even for conditions such as hypertension, AMI, stroke, and diabetes, the goals of care may not be the same in older adults as in younger adults. One of the best examples of this is in tight control of glucose in patients with diabetes. The benefits of tight control only manifest themselves after many years of treatment, and while this may make sense for a patient aged 50, with 25 years or more of life expectancy, it may make less sense for patient age 75, for whom the benefits of tight control in terms of fewer complications in 5 to 10 years may be offset by the immediate risks of hypoglycemia as a result of tight control. Moreover, younger adults have fewer health care conditions than do older adults, and multimorbidity is the rule in older adults. Determining what constitutes quality care may be very different when it occurs as a single condition, such as diabetes or heart failure, than when it occurs in a patient who also has many other health conditions such as osteoporosis, osteoarthritis, ischemic heart disease, and mild cognitive impairment. Attention has to be given to interactions between drugs and diseases, drug-drug interactions, and the potential for recommending multiple nonpharmacologic interventions that may be impractical in a vulnerable older person.

Improving quality and safety for older adults Robust methods for improving quality and safety remain an elusive goal. There is no cookbook that can be followed that will produce consistent results in all settings. Quality improvement interventions depend on implementation and are frequently context-sensitive, meaning that their success depends on a host of local factors, such as leadership support and other factors both internal and external to the organization. The Consolidated Framework for Implementation Research lists five major domains important to an understanding of quality improvement interventions: intervention characteristics, the outer setting, the inner setting, characteristics of the individuals involved, and the process of implementation. Various constructs for each major domain are listed in **Table 19-4**.

CURRENT CHALLENGES IN VALUE-BASED CARE

As the health care delivery moves toward value-based care approaches, it is inevitable that challenges with these approaches will continue to arise. Two of the more pressing issues facing value-based care today are the burdens that measurement may have and how to best risk-adjust performance measures.

Burdens and challenges of measurement One potential concern that has arisen in value-based payment models is the number of different measurement schemes that a single provider may be subject to. A single hospital for instance may be subject to the value-based purchasing, may be organized as an ACO, and may participate in bundled payment programs. Each of these programs brings its own success metrics, spending targets, and quality measures. As such providers may need to spend considerable amounts of time devoted to meeting each of these different administrative requirements. One study of four common specialties estimates that physicians in the United States may spend more than $15 billion a year in quality reporting. Another study found that CMS itself may have spent $1.3 billion alone in the development of quality measures for value-based care models. Despite these burdens, value-based care may have the potential to substantially impact patient care positively; however, this challenge may call for a greater harmonization of success metrics across models of care. In addition, measures that are appropriate, and not counterproductive, for older adults with multiple comorbidities and those with life-limiting illness are essential to improving the quality of care for this population. For example, tightly controlling diabetes or hypertension in these patients is not evidence-based. Quality measures that do not consider

TABLE 19-4 ■ CONSOLIDATED FRAMEWORK FOR IMPLEMENTATION RESEARCH

Intervention characteristics
- Intervention source
- Evidence strength and quality
- Relative advantage
- Adaptability
- Trialability
- Complexity
- Design quality and packaging
- Cost

Outer setting
- Patient needs and resources
- Cosmopolitanism
- Peer pressure
- External policies and incentives

Inner setting
- Structural characteristics
- Networks and communications
- Culture
- Implementation climate

Characteristics of individuals
- Knowledge and beliefs about the intervention
- Self-efficacy
- Individual stage of change
- Individual identification with organization
- Other personal attributes

Process
- Planning
- Engaging
- Executing
- Reflecting and evaluating

Data from Damschroder LJ, Aron DC, Keith RE, Kirsh SR, Alexander JA, Lowery JC. Fostering implementation of health services research findings into practice: a consolidated framework for advancing implementation science. Implement Sci. 2009;4:50.

the many patient-centered factors related to treatment decisions in vulnerable older patients could result in more harm than good in terms of driving episodes of hypoglycemia and their consequences, and hypotension and near syncope and falls.

Risk adjustment The issue of risk adjustment is central to the success of value-based care. Risk adjustment is a statistical process that considers the underlying health status and spending of enrollees when setting quality and spending benchmarks. In a value-based model that takes quality and spending into consideration, without risk adjustment there may be an incentive not to provide care for patients with more complex care needs. Under capitation for instance, a patient with advanced needs will almost definitely cost more money to take care of than a healthy patient, so a health plan or a hospital would have a strong incentive to

TABLE 19-5 ■ COMMON HIERARCHICAL CONDITION CATEGORY CONDITIONS

HCC	DESCRIPTION	ADJUSTMENT WEIGHT
HCC17	Diabetes with acute complications	0.37
HCC18	Diabetes with chronic complications	0.37
HCC19	Diabetes without complication	0.12
HCC84	Cardiorespiratory failure and shock	0.33
HCC85	Congestive heart failure	0.37
HCC106	Atherosclerosis of the extremities with ulceration or gangrene	1.0
HCC107	Vascular disease with complications	0.41
HCC108	Vascular disease	0.30
HCC134	Dialysis	0.48
HCC135	Acute renal failure hematological disorders	0.48
HCC136	Chronic kidney disease stage 5	0.22
HCC137	Chronic kidney disease stage 4	0.22
HCC111	Chronic obstructive pulmonary disorder	0.35
HCC114	Aspiration and specified bacterial pneumonias	0.67
HCC115	Pneumococcal pneumonia, empyema, lung abscess	0.2
HCC58	Major depressive, bipolar, and paranoid disorders	0.33
HCC22	Morbid obesity	0.37

High adjustment weights lead to higher payments during risk adjustment.

"cherry-pick" healthier patients who will save them money. Risk adjustment takes account of a patient's underlying risk of adverse outcomes and high spending, and will lead to higher payments for their care than a healthier patient. One example of risk adjustment that the Medicare program uses is Hierarchical Condition Categories, which assign risk scores to patients on the basis of specific chronic conditions and are used to adjust payments in MA. A list of common HCC codes and the adjustment factor attributed to each is in **Table 19-5**.

If perfectly implemented, risk adjustment will make it no more expensive to care for complex patients and ensure that the outcomes of complex patients are taken account of when evaluating quality. In practice however, risk adjustment is unlikely to be perfect. There are several studies that find that despite the use of risk-adjustment methods across all CMS value-based payment models, in many cases the providers who treat more complex patients are still disproportionately penalized, meaning the risk adjustment did not adequately account for their higher care needs. Other studies have found benefits from incorporating social risk factors into risk adjustment as well. While traditional risk-adjustment approaches adjust for age, sex, and chronic conditions, there is growing evidence that these algorithms may benefit by also adjusting for factors such as socioeconomic status. An additional concern with current risk-adjustment efforts is the potential for upcoding, or administratively making a patient appear more ill in an effort to boost payments or performance on quality scores. As value-based care continues to evolve, risk adjustment will continue to be a key area of focus.

SUMMARY

The shift from fee-for-service toward value-based care models is likely to continue for the next several years in the United States. Value-based care programs mitigate the financial incentives in the Medicare fee-for-service system to perform tests and procedures that may cause more harm than good in vulnerable older patients with multiple comorbidities, as well as those near the end of life. There are many current value-based payment models relevant to the care of older adults, including the MA program, ACOs, bundled payments, the PACE, and I-SNPs, among others. Robust and clinically valid quality measures are critical to the success of these programs, so that financial considerations do not result in less care than is appropriate and lower quality. While the specific names and structures of value-based models of care are likely to evolve over time, the underlying principles will provide substantial benefit for the older population. Geriatricians and other geriatric health professionals have the training and experience to help make these programs successful and to assume leadership roles in them.

FURTHER READING

Agency for Health Care Policy and Research. (2014). *Care Coordination Measures Atlas*. https://www.ahrq.gov/ncepcr/care/coordination/atlas.html. Accessed December 14, 2021.

Barnett ML, Wilcock A, McWilliams JM, et al. Two-year evaluation of mandatory bundled payments for joint replacement. *N Engl J Med.* 2019;380(3):252–262.

Centers for Medicare and Medicaid Services. (n.d.). *CMS Innovation Center*. https://www.cms.gov/Medicare/Health-Plans/SpecialNeedsPlans/I-SNPs. Accessed December 14, 2021.

Centers for Medicare and Medicaid Services. (n.d.). *Institutional Special Needs Plans (I-SNPs)*. Retrieved

January 13, 2021. https://www.cms.gov/Medicare/Health-Plans/SpecialNeedsPlans/I-SNPs.

Choosing Wisely. (2019). *American Geriatrics Society: Ten Things Clinicians and Patients Should Question.* https://www.choosingwisely.org/societies/american-geriatrics-society/. Accessed December 14, 2021.

Daras LC, Vadnais A, Pogue YZ, et al. Nearly one in five skilled nursing facilities awarded positive incentives under value-based purchasing. *Health Aff.* 2021;40(1):146–155.

Dhingra L, Lipson K, Dieckmann NF, Chen J, Bookbinder M, Portenoy R. Institutional special needs plans and hospice enrollment in nursing homes: a national analysis. *J Am Geriatr Soc.* 2019;67(12):2537–2544.

McGarry BE, Grabowski DC. Managed care for long-stay nursing home residents: an evaluation of institutional special needs plans. *Am J Manag Care.* 2019;25(9):438–443.

McWilliams JM, Hatfield LA, Chernew ME, Landon BE, Schwartz AL. Early performance of Accountable Care Organizations in Medicare. *N Engl J Med.* 2016;374(24):2357–2366.

National PACE Association. (n.d.). *The History of PACE.* Retrieved January 13, 2021. https://www.npaonline.org/policy-advocacy/value-pace.

Neuman P, Jacobson GA. Medicare Advantage checkup. *N Engl J Med.* 2018;379(22):2163–2172.

Peikes D, Dale S, Ghosh A, et al. The comprehensive primary care initiative: effects on spending, quality, patients, and physicians. *Health Aff.* 2018;37(6):890–899.

Porter ME. What is value in health care? *N Engl J Med.* 2010;363(26):2477–2481.

Rosenthal MB. Beyond pay for performance—emerging models of provider-payment reform. *N Engl J Med.* 2008;359(12):1197–1200.

Segelman M, Szydlowski J, Kinosian B, et al. Hospitalizations in the Program of All-Inclusive Care for the Elderly. *J Am Geriatr Soc.* 2014;62(2):320–324.

Sinaiko AD, Landrum MB, Meyers DJ, et al. Synthesis of research on patient-centered medical homes brings systematic differences into relief. *Health Aff (Project Hope).* 2017;36(3):500–508.

Teisberg E, Wallace S, O'Hara S. Defining and implementing value-based health care: a strategic framework. *Acad Med.* 2020;95(5):682–685.

Tkatch R, Musich S, MacLeod S, Alsgaard K, Hawkins K, Yeh CS. Population health management for older adults: review of interventions for promoting successful aging across the health continuum. *Gerontol Geriatr Med.* 2016;2:1-13.

Zuckerman RB, Stearns SC, Sheingold SH. Hospice use, hospitalization, and Medicare spending at the end of life. *J Gerontol B Psychol Sci Soc Sci.* 2016;71(3):569–580.

The Role of Social Workers

Ruth E. Dunkle, Jay Kayser, Angela K. Perone

Social workers provide services to older patients across a continuum of care needs that range from supporting community living to providing palliative care services at the end of life. This occurs in many different health care arenas including institutional settings, such as acute care hospitals, nursing homes, and other long-term institutional settings, as well as in patients' homes in the community. Given the multiple settings that social workers function within, the way that they refer to those they work with can vary. In more formal and medical settings (eg, hospitals) the term "patient" is most frequently used. In long-term settings (eg, nursing homes and assisted-living facilities), the term "resident" is often used. In community settings, the terms "client" or "consumer" are favored as they emphasize agency and autonomy. Social workers support and enhance the adaptive capacities of patients within their living environments and are knowledgeable about interviewing, assessment, and intervention in social problems faced by individuals, couples, families, and groups. Using negotiating skills, social workers also mediate conflicts and obtain resources for clients and their families. Knowledge of group process makes social workers effective in forming natural helping networks and serving as members of interdisciplinary teams. Their expertise in coordinating services within a single organization or across different agencies or settings helps to ensure appropriate and adequate care for older patients. Social workers often work on interdisciplinary teams in health care settings benefiting physicians, nurses, and other health care workers as well as the patients they serve.

While 76% of social workers in health care settings work with older patients, not all social workers have specialized training in geriatrics. Proper care provided by gerontologically trained professionals including social workers can reduce the cost of care by 10% each year in hospitals, nursing homes, and patients' homes as well as improve psychosocial outcomes and reduce mortality.

This chapter describes the key roles for geriatric social workers, the practice issues they face, and the settings in which they work.

Learning Objectives

- Understand the roles that social workers play in various health care settings, including direct service work, linkage roles, and support services.
- Determine health care settings where social workers practice and some of the issues they may face in nursing homes, community mental health facilities, hospitals and health care facilities, hospice and palliative care, and home care.
- Identify key populations that social workers serve and some of the practice issues that arise with older adults in these groups.

Key Clinical Points

1. There are unique practice issues and considerations in older populations that face particular vulnerability because of oppression and/or poverty due to race, ethnicity, immigration status, sexual orientation, gender identity, or HIV/AIDS diagnosis.
2. Several core issues emerge when working with people who face abuse, neglect, mental health concerns, cognitive impairment, and substance or alcohol misuse.

KEY ROLES FOR GERIATRIC SOCIAL WORKERS

The roles social workers play vary within health care settings (**Tables 20-1** and **20-2**). Social workers provide direct service to older adults and facilitate linkages between service workers and agencies.

Direct Service Provision

Social workers meet face to face with patients and consumer groups to provide services as caseworkers, therapists, group workers, or educators. Individual casework and counseling services help older adults who have mental health problems or need help with resolving issues in areas such as housing,

TABLE 20-1 ■ THE ROLES SOCIAL WORKERS PERFORM

ROLES	DESCRIPTION	EXAMPLES
Group worker	Social worker plans and conducts group activities for clients to help understand themselves better through a variety of methods; can be therapeutic, educational, social, or for support.	Worker organizes a group for grandparents raising grandchildren to share information and provide support.
Advocate	Social worker fights for, defends, and promotes patient's perspectives and rights.	Social worker helps a patient destined for a nursing home receive home health care rather than be institutionalized.
Case manager	Social worker assesses patient needs, connects patient to resources, and coordinates and oversees delivery and participation of services.	The case manager coordinates the services. A patient might need rehabilitation therapy, psychotherapy, and home health care as well as transportation services.
Educator	Social worker offers knowledge regarding health care information, processes, and procedures with patients and provides knowledge of patient with the team.	In hospice, the social worker provides information regarding the dying process, pain management, stages of grief, and option for burial services.
Discharge planner	Social worker prepares patient for next phases of departure from facility by designing a course of action.	When patient leaves the hospital and goes home, the social worker may arrange transportation services, meal delivery, home care services, and assessment of home for safety.
Therapist	Social worker engages clients in interpersonal interactions regarding client's behavior, feelings, attitudes, and perceptions.	Social worker works with an older couple who is having marital problems resulting from stress of caregiving.
Team member	Social worker collaborates with health professionals to provide efficient delivery of services.	Social worker shares information with physicians and nurses and provides insight into the patient's cultural and personal life.
Broker	Social worker connects patients to most relevant resources.	Social work brokers help African-American elders overcome the racial and ethnic disparities they face in receiving health care, by building trust between the patient and health care professionals.
Information and referral	Social worker has knowledge of community resources and offers connection to these agencies.	Social worker has knowledge of respite care services and links caregiver of Alzheimer patient to the respite care agency.
Mediator/ arbitrator/ advocate	Social worker facilitates conflict resolution.	The social worker advocates for the older patient in a guardianship hearing.

finances, or interpersonal problems. Therapy includes meeting with individual older adults, with partners, as well as with groups of older adults who are experiencing concerns related to their families. Such therapies could involve helping grandparents with resources and tools for raising grandchildren, aiding families in coping with an aging parent with dementia, or supporting older couples as they struggle with debilitating health problems that can create emotional and financial strain on the relationship. Group work services include support groups for older adults with a variety of health concerns, such as cancer, low vision, or early-stage dementia. Support groups have been particularly helpful to caregivers of patients with such diseases as Alzheimer, diabetes, and Parkinson. These groups, run by social workers, help caregivers better understand the disease process and provide information that helps them cope with problems of caregiving more effectively and thus improve the disease outcome. Groups can also focus on self-help issues, where older adults learn to deal with such problems as alcoholism, obesity, or smoking. Psychotherapy groups work to resolve such concerns as abuse (as victim or perpetrator), depression, and marital problems. Social workers also work directly with older adults and their families as educators and disseminators of information. For example, social workers provide educational sessions on caregiving, stress management, and various aspects of mental and physical health care.

Linkage Roles

Social workers link older adults to the services they need. This may be necessary because agencies fail to meet older persons' needs, because older adults lack knowledge of available resources or ability to access those resources, or because older adults and their families need help in overcoming fears and concerns about using services. For example, family members struggling to provide home care to a mother with Alzheimer disease may be reluctant to participate in a support or educational group used by other family members in similar circumstances due to fear of revealing personal problems they and their mother face. Social workers can help overcome these fears by assisting family members in realizing that families coping with dementia face similar problems and have similar reactions to their circumstances. Social workers also work as case managers to help older adults receive services in a timely fashion. In

TABLE 20-2 ■ SETTINGS WHERE SOCIALWORKERS WORK AND ROLES THEY PERFORM

SETTINGS	ROLES
Home	Support patients' adjustment to health status, provide emotional support, address barriers in access to medical care (ie, transportation), provide education so that patient can make informed decisions, assess social support and referral to resources, and case management
Primary care	Plan and implement safety and illness prevention programs, identify social factors that support prevention of illness and causes of diseases, provide emotional and social support, facilitate support groups around a specific disease or mental illness, and provide education, information, and referral
Community agencies	Case management, oversee and evaluate programs, community outreach, advocacy, development of services, income assistance, protective services, support parents raising grandchildren
Community mental health setting	Perform client assessments, conduct support groups, provide emergency and crisis services to older mental health clients and their families; referral to other resources in the community such as adult day care, respite services, and partial day treatment programs
Adult day care/respite program	Assess clients' mental and physical abilities, plan and facilitate activities to maximize physical and cognitive functioning, facilitate support groups, provide information and support for Alzheimer and other disease processes, and referral to community resources
Assisted living facility	Negotiate placement and transition, support in navigating decision making and emotions regarding changes in autonomy, financial planning, and fostering communication
Nursing home	Financial planning; psychosocial assessment and addressing emotional needs; care planning; mediation between residents, staff, and family; linking residents and families to resources
Hospital	Assessment; discharge planning; prevention and treatment of mental and physical health; promotion of psychosocial health, advocacy in relation to aspects of human diversity; mediate between patients, families, and the health care team; group work; psychotherapy
Hospice	Liaison between care settings; case manager; address psychosocial needs of families and patients; support for adjustment to setting, treatment, illness, and death; educator, advocate, broker, and mediator between family members, patient, and medical professionals; team member; information and referral; group worker; and counselor

general, case management involves screening, assessment, care planning, implementation, monitoring, and reassessment to evaluate ongoing service needs. Case management meets a variety of goals in numerous settings. The social worker assesses problems and needs to determine eligibility for services and financial resources. The social worker also links older adults to needed services. Family and friends may provide collateral information to help the social worker determine their capacity for support. Goals for a care plan are determined by discussing older adults' perceptions of their needs. Social workers then identify interventions and resources designed to meet these goals. Subsequently, the social worker monitors the delivery of the services. When an older adult requires care over a longer period of time, a social worker will reevaluate needs and necessary interventions and resources. Ultimately, a social worker will conduct an outcome evaluation to determine if the patient's goals were achieved.

Social workers also work as mediators and advocate for their clients/patients. As mediators, social workers determine the issues behind a conflict. Social workers facilitate family discussion of issues identified by the family and older adults as important. For example, adult guardianship mediation can inform how the family can best help older adults preserve autonomy (or to maximize one's greatest level of independent functioning).

WHERE SOCIAL WORKERS PRACTICE

Medical social workers serve important roles across the care continuum, from in-home services to acute care. Medical social workers perform roles such as patient advocate and counselors, providing psychosocial assessments, referring patients and families to medical resources, and providing patient and family assistance in obtaining financial and legal help. They provide education and support to link clients to resources. **Table 20-2** lists a broader range of practice settings. Several of the central practice arenas are reviewed below.

Home Care

Home care is a term that encompasses a variety of services, including home health agencies, homemakers, home health aides and assistance, medical equipment and supplies, visiting nurses, caregiver respite, and other medical services provided in the home. One agency may provide one or several of these services to older adults. Social workers in home care address a wide range of issues including adaptation to illnesses and chronic conditions, decisions regarding end of life, dementia and behavior management, caregiving, issues of abuse and neglect, prescription drug misuse, and family discord. In addition, they provide financial management, address unsafe living conditions, connect to resources to provide safe living quarters, address social support, mental health, and legal issues, and support compliance with medical treatments.

Community Health and Mental Health Agencies

Social workers work in direct practice and leadership roles in community health and mental health agencies. They work in nonprofit settings (eg, Alzheimer Association) as well as state and federal agencies (eg, Administration on Aging, Centers for Medicare and Medicaid Services). Aside from issues related to psychosocial support and education, social workers can also develop policy and practice standards. Social workers who work in community mental health agencies are part of a team of mental health practitioners, which includes nurses, psychologists, and psychiatrists. Social workers conduct client assessments, run support groups, provide emergency and crisis services to older mental health clients and their families, and refer these people to other resources in the community such as adult day care, respite services, and partial day treatment programs. They often provide therapeutic interventions in the form of brief psychotherapy and behavior modification to individuals or groups and provide indirect services through community education and consultations in long-term care facilities. Social workers assist with supportive housing, daily living skills, transitional employment, and counseling needs.

Nursing Homes and Assisted-Living Facilities

Social workers in nursing homes and assisted-living facilities have diverse responsibilities to residents and their families, facility staff, and the overall institutional environment. Their assistance begins when residents move into the facility. Adjustment to a new living environment is faced by not only the older person, but their family as well. The social worker provides direct services to residents and their families as part of an interdisciplinary team. They assess the psychosocial needs of the resident and aid in the development of a care plan, guided by federal requirements of maintaining a minimum data set (MDS). The MDS is part of the US federally mandated process for clinical assessment of all residents in Medicare or Medicaid-certified nursing homes. This process provides a comprehensive assessment of each resident's functional capability that helps nursing home staff (physicians, social workers, and nurses) identify health problems and develop strategies to address them. Social workers also facilitate psychosocial well-being among residents and their families, linking the resident and family members to services inside and outside the facility, helping with discharge planning, and serving as advocates for appropriate care and treatment for all patients and their families. Because social workers are often the only staff members focused on the psychosocial needs of residents and their families, they are well positioned to identify and address mental health issues. Often, they complete the cognitive, mood, behavioral, and psychosocial portion of the MDS along with the resident assessment protocol, which can identify the mental health needs of residents. Assisted-living facilities are not required to have a social worker on staff and the roles of social workers in these facilities are less uniform when compared to skilled nursing facilities.

Hospitals and Health Care Facilities

Social workers practice in all areas of hospitals, from the emergency departments to intensive care units. Social work practice with older adults in health care settings is focused on adaptation and coping with chronic illness, crisis management, adjustment to disability and physical limitation, decisions about end-of-life care, compliance with medical regimens, wellness, long-term care, quality of life, and discharge planning. Social workers also provide mental health services that address depression, substance abuse, management of long-term mental health issues, cognitive deficits, suicide prevention, and adjustment to changes in life by patients and families. Medical social workers take on many roles such as patient advocate and counselor and perform psychological assessments, refer patients and families to medical resources, and provide patient and family assistance in obtaining financial and legal assistance.

In hospital settings, social workers are members of an interdisciplinary team, providing services to patients and families regarding assessments of a patient's cognitive, emotional, and behavioral status, and connection to social support networks. Social workers counsel patients and families, assisting them in adjustment to illness and providing crisis intervention and connection to community resources. Additionally, social workers identify interpersonal aspects of patients' lives that contribute to positive outcomes in relation to their illnesses. They also address obstacles to medical compliance and financial concerns. Social workers advocate and affirm the cultural, linguistic, sexual, ethnic, religious, and other aspects of diversity present in their patients' lives and advocate on behalf of patients with the health care team when patients face barriers to receiving care. For example, social workers can aid in the care of abused and neglected older adults by documenting and reporting instances of abuse and neglect and testifying in court with regard to these matters.

In acute care settings, where patient stays are very short, social workers focus on high-risk screening, brief counseling, bereavement services, discharge planning, collaboration, information, referral, follow-up, and emergency services on-call programs. Social workers are typically assigned to specific medical or psychiatric departments in hospitals where patients are screened to determine whether they need social work services. Need for services is also conveyed to other health care professionals by having social workers attend team meetings and discharge planning conferences, by referrals from nurses or physicians, or by requests from patients and families. A social worker's presence, when a diagnosis, death, or other unpleasant news is communicated, can ease shock and help individuals

TABLE 20-3 ■ SOCIAL WORKERS IN HOSPICE SETTINGS

OVERVIEW	SETTING	PATIENT PROFILE
Though the setting of patients receiving hospice services may differ, social workers provide similar services in all levels of care. The core services of hospice social workers involve providing psychosocial support to families and patients, advocacy for patient wishes, activating available social supports, and locating services and resources. Social workers can also facilitate transitions between levels of care as medically appropriate and necessary.	Home	Able to either receive care from family members or caregivers or function independently. This is the preferred setting for most patients (80% of patients endorse wishing to die at home).
	Assisted living and nursing homes	Skilled nursing facilities and some assisted living facilities offer round-the-clock access to nurses and nursing assistance, though 1:1 support is not provided. Hospice recipient is still responsible for paying room and board of facility.
	General inpatient	Ideal for patients requiring more involved care that cannot be safely provided outside of an inpatient setting (eg, aggressive pain management, uncontrolled nausea or vomiting or shortness of breath).
	Hospice home	Similar requirement for entry as general inpatient. This setting is generally for patients very near to the end of their lives.

address the emotional loss and face forthcoming decisions. Additionally, the social worker can provide information regarding aspects of diseases, care options, and assistance in meeting patient and family needs.

Discharge planning is particularly important for older adults who are transitioning from the hospital to other facilities or their homes. Addressing older adults' needs during discharge is necessary in order to allow the older adult the best possible scenario for recovery from illness. Social workers assess caregiving needs, the availability of social supports, family support, financial barriers, and home and community environment in facilitating the discharge.

Hospice and Palliative Care

Hospice social workers practice in a variety of end-of-life care settings, such as hospitals, nursing homes, assisted-living facilities, outpatient practices, residential hospice facilities, and in residential homes. Please review **Table 20-3** for an overview of these settings. Palliative care requires an interdisciplinary team, where the social worker is a crucial member providing psychosocial support and referral to resources, easing transitions between settings, and addressing issues of loss for patients and families.

Social workers help those who are approaching death. Their work begins when patients enter into hospice or palliative care and continues with families and loved ones after death. Social workers provide a variety of services to address the needs of patients, families, and caregivers serving in a variety of roles such as liaison, educator, mediator, advocate, broker, and counselor. As patients face debilitating illness in palliative care, social workers help with the transition between care facilities, assessing readiness for palliative care and beginning to address the emotional and psychological aspects of nearing death. Social workers are pivotal in assessing and supporting patients, families, and caregivers in their psychological, spiritual, social, financial, and cultural needs at the end of life. Addressing loss is essential, as individuals and families may have difficulty communicating and accepting their feelings regarding the losses they face. Identifying social support for patients and families is important, as discord can arise when families come together at the end of life, and social workers can assist families to communicate and understand decisions, emotions expressed, and relationships.

Social workers act as brokers for resources and services to address the needs of patients who are dying and their families. They arrange services, facilitate communication among family members, provide services to fulfill last wishes, and provide assistance with funeral plan arrangements. As an advocate, the social worker supports and represents patients' and families' needs, wishes, and desires to the health care team and recognizes the dying person as a social person during the end-of-life stages. As a counselor, the social worker addresses the psychological, emotional, and spiritual needs of the family in addressing losses and illness and reconciling relationships. Grief support to families, friends, and caregivers is also provided after death through individual counseling sessions with family members, support groups, grief camps for children, and formal ceremonies and services for families who have lost loved ones. Social workers help patients and families understand their options, identify services they need, and fill out the necessary paperwork to secure these services. They also help them fill out other important forms like advance directives.

PRACTICE ISSUES WITH POPULATIONS SERVED

Geriatric social workers strive to meet the basic human needs of all older adults, with a particular emphasis on those who are vulnerable due to discrimination, oppression and poverty. With health care provided in a myriad of public and private settings, the social worker acts as a broker, a mediator, and an advocate for clients.

This section reviews key populations served by social workers and some of the practice issues that come into play with older adults in these groups. Social workers identify barriers to seeking help, such as stigma, denial, and financial and access barriers resulting from service fragmentation and gaps in health care. For some older racial, ethnic, and cultural minorities, health problems are rooted in historic experiences of discrimination that prevent access to the social service system. Therefore, culturally specific interventions should consider the unique background, context, and resources of the individual.

Racial, Ethnic, and Cultural Diversity

Social workers are uniquely situated to respond to the needs of older adults across racial and ethnic groups because of their skills in training and cultural awareness in service delivery. Attention to cultural diversity includes sensitivity to differences in cultural history, language, values, religion, ethnicity, nationality, and regionality, as well as recognition of within-group variation. For example, social workers use cultural assessment strategies to understand clients' definition of a problem. During the assessment process, social workers working with culturally diverse groups evaluate attitudes toward health care and the clients' belief about the causes of illness and benefits of health care services. As social workers attempt to understand clients' problems, they evaluate the language skills, educational level, and degree of acculturation of the older person. In addition, determining the surrogate decision maker who has the authority to make care decisions is important for the health care team to know. For females, in some cultures, a male decides how care proceeds. In some Native American cultures, generational standing predominates in care decision making. The patient's use of language to label and categorize a problem, the availability and use of indigenous community resources, the decision making involved in problem intervention strategies, and the patient's cultural criteria for determining problem resolution are important issues for the social worker and other health care workers to consider in working effectively with older adults and their families.

While there are common themes that are relevant to people of color and other minority groups, each group has its own cultural history relevant to care. This cultural history often contributes to health disparities that social workers must address. For example, racial and ethnic minorities have poorer access to care than the White population, and research suggests that this gap is not narrowing. Despite these collective findings, it is important to remember that racial, ethnic, and cultural groups are not homogenous. Individuals and families have their own themes, caregiving patterns, and stories of access to and discrimination in social service and health care delivery.

Poverty

While government programs such as Social Security, Medicare, unemployment insurance, and welfare have reduced the extent of poverty in the older population, poverty remains a significant problem. This results, in part, from the cumulative effects of lifelong discrimination, particularly for older adults of color, LGBT older adults, adults older than the age of 75, older adults residing in rural areas, and women. Underutilization of health and mental health services by older adults in poverty makes these groups a target for social work intervention. One significant barrier to meeting the needs of older adults in poverty is lack of knowledge about their problems and needs. Another barrier is that some older adults in poverty may lack resources, such as transportation, to access to care. Social workers aim to understand and eradicate these barriers that impede the development and delivery of appropriate services and connect older adults to formal and informal resources to aid impoverished older adults in rural communities, women, LGBT older adults, and racial/ethnic minorities.

Immigration and Refugee Status

Since the early twentieth century, rising numbers of older adults have arrived to the United States from Mexico, Cuba, and various countries in South America and Asia. As of 2018, one out of seven US residents is foreign born representing 14% of the population. Half of older immigrants have limited English proficiency with more than 40% of these older adults speaking Spanish. Older immigrants are also more likely to have lower incomes than nonimmigrants.

Older immigrants are more likely to live in households with extended family, children, and nonbiological family than are nonimmigrants. Families are often central to caregiving for aging relatives. However, demand for family caregiving often occurs in the context of limited coping resources, limited knowledge of services, misperceptions of eligibility requirements of government programs, and beliefs that children must provide caregiving. Unfortunately, multiple roles may result in greater caregiving strain and increased neglect and abuse of older family members.

Older immigrants also encounter cultural and linguistic barriers to service use. Immigrants who migrated after age 60 face additional challenges, including little or no US work experience, limited ties to social institutions, and potentially limited English proficiency. Older immigrants comprise a diverse population, reflected in race and ethnicity, as well as age, length of residence in the United States, English language proficiency, and reasons for immigration.

Sexual Orientation and Gender Identity

LGBT older adults often comprise an invisible population that has special needs and face social service barriers based on individual and collective experiences of discrimination. Many LGBT older adults came of age at a time when failure to conform to gender or sexual norms resulted in job termination, involuntary hospitalization, cessation of parental rights, and criminal punishment. A fear of discrimination by health providers prompts many older LGBT adults who were once open about their sexual orientation and/or gender identity to return to the "closet" when entering long-term care facilities; and, some LGBT older adults fail to disclose their sexual orientation and gender identity to health care providers who have treated them throughout their life. Fear of differential or discriminatory treatment also precludes LGBT older adults from seeking health care and social services at all, unless absolutely necessary. Discrimination and delays in accessing care lead to higher rates of disability, mental distress, excessive drinking, and poorer physical health outcomes for LGBT older adults. Intersections of various identities (eg, race, ethnicity, sexual orientation, and gender identity) can create even higher health risks for particular communities. For example, one study found that African-American LGBT older adults had higher lifetime LGBT-related discrimination compared to Whites, which was linked to a decrease in their physical and psychological health-related quality of life (ie, vitality, mobility, pain, dependence on medical treatment, satisfaction with sleep, daily living activities, and work capacity). Transgender older adults have a higher risk of poor physical health, disability, depressive symptoms, and stress than cisgender (non-transgender) peers.

While the legal landscape for LGBT older adults is rapidly changing, ambiguity in state and federal laws often limits access to services and rights for LGBT older adults. LGBT older adults continue to experience discrimination from health care providers, and recent court battles about whether the Affordable Care Act protects LGBT people from discrimination have not helped. After courts affirmed marriage equality for same-sex couples, some health care providers began refusing care to LGBT older adults based on religious and moral reasons. Transgender older adults have reported particularly high rates of discrimination in health care. Many transgender older adults seeking medical services to affirm their gender identity also encounter obstacles in insurance coverage, which means many medical services are financially inaccessible.

Despite social, health care, and legal barriers for service delivery, many LGBT older adults have extensive support networks through partners and friends of similar age and rely on them for informal caregiving. Social workers can directly provide or connect LGBT clients to inclusive services and service providers and provide LGBT-friendly resources, such as physicians, living facilities, and attorneys to assist with health care documents.

HIV/AIDS

Older adults can encounter HIV/AIDS either as patients with the disease or as caretakers for loved ones with HIV/AIDS. More than 50% of all Americans living with HIV are age 50 or older, facing the same risk factors as younger people. Many newly diagnosed older people are "late testers," meaning that they likely had HIV for years before their diagnosis and may face more immediate challenges than someone who is diagnosed early. LGBT older adults and transgender people of color have particularly high rates of HIV/AIDS. Although older adults visit doctors more often than younger people, they are less likely to discuss sexual behavior with their physicians. Social workers can help to identify older HIV/AIDS patients and improve access to services and informal care that is necessary for successful treatment. Social workers offer educational information and coordinate services such as caregiver respite services, home health care and hospice care, individual and group supportive counseling, and financial assistance.

Abuse and Neglect

The abuse or neglect of older adults often surfaces in a health care setting. Many types of maltreatment, such as physical abuse, sexual abuse, and neglect (including self-neglect), result in injury, pain, and physical and psychological harm. Please review **Table 20-4** for an overview. Other types of abuse such as financial and identity theft are more difficult to detect in health care settings. The assessment of mistreatment, which may require several contacts, involves an interview with the older adult to better understand risk. Cognitively impaired older adults who present with concerning complaints or who express concern for abuse and neglect should be taken especially seriously.

TABLE 20-4 ■ ELDER ABUSE AND NEGLECT		
TYPE OF ABUSE	**RED FLAGS**	**ADDITIONAL INFORMATION**
Neglect (and self-neglect)	Pressure wounds, poor access to medical care, inadequate nutrition, poor personal hygiene, unsanitary living conditions	Older adults in long-term care facilities can also be victims of elder neglect. The failure of a facility to provide a reasonable and proper level of care can be negligence. Neglect can also be self-neglect.
Physical abuse	Abrasions, contusions, fractures, or lacerations that suggest intentional harm	Abuse victims residing in settings where guns are present are at especially high risk.
Psychological abuse	Fear or distrust of caregivers or family members, becoming withdrawn around particular caregivers	Typically, abuser is well-known to victim.
Financial exploitation	Sudden and unexplained financial difficulty, transfer of property or other assets	Financial abuse can be further complicated when the alleged victim lacks capacity.
Sexual abuse	Contusions on breasts or genital area, unexplained vaginal or anal bleeding	Though uncommon, this form of abuse has especially serious physical and psychological consequences.

While all states have mandatory or voluntary reporting laws, the older adult's willingness to receive help, provided they have capacity, is voluntary. When a report of elder abuse is made to local authorities, additional personnel may be involved in safety planning. Social workers can be instrumental in helping older adults recognize the power imbalance in abusive relationships and devise strategies for protection. One of the biggest challenges that health professionals face consists of identifying and helping abused or neglected older adults who do not realize that they are victims of mistreatment. All forms of elder abuse can also occur when an older adult is residing in an institutional setting. Further details regarding elder abuse and neglect can be found in Chapter 48.

Cognitive Impairment

Social workers are involved with assessing older adults with dementia and their caregivers. These assessments consider the client's social and medical history, including a physical and mental status examination, an evaluation of the individual's living environment, functional ability including both instrumental activities of daily living (IADLs) and activities of daily living (ADLs), social service needs and family dynamics, service and resource needs, and legal issues such as power of attorney and health care proxy, advance care planning, and end-of-life planning. Social workers also play a variety of roles on the interdisciplinary team used when an older adult and his/her family experience dementia. In the early stages of dementia, social workers can support the older adult with dementia and provide cognitively stimulating programs. In some cases, the older adult is able to plan for his/her own future physical and financial needs, which the social worker can facilitate. Social workers also help family members struggling with the physical and emotional changes in their loved one with dementia as it progresses. Social workers assist family members in navigating multiple caregiving responsibilities through therapy, resources, and support groups and

TABLE 20-5 ■ COMMON MENTAL HEALTH CONDITIONS AND DEVELOPMENTAL DISABILITIES IN OLDER ADULTS

CONDITION	RISK FACTORS	PREVALENCE AND OTHER CONSIDERATIONS
Dementia	Age, poverty, family history, mild cognitive impairment, heart disease, educational attainment, diabetes, smoking and alcohol use	Older adults with high cognitive reserve may be functionally intact with some activities while impaired in others. When cognitive impairment is detected, formal screening is beneficial for providing an accurate clinical picture. The general prevalence is approximately 7% for those older than 65 years. Risk factors, such as age and poverty, can elevate chance of developing dementia significantly.
Depression	Poverty, poor physical health, history of depression, low cognitive function, loss of spouse	Can present differently than in younger adults. Older adults more frequently endorse cognitive and affective concerns. Older adults who have received care for depression previously tend to have more favorable responses to treatment. General prevalence is 5%, though in some populations (eg, homebound and socially isolated older adults) depression rates can be as high as 44%.
Anxiety	Similar to depression, with a particularly strong relationship between clinically significant early life experiences	Similar to depression, often presents differently in older adults. May present as "problems with nerves," restlessness, or difficulty concentrating. Anxiety is highly comorbid with depression. Prevalence is approximately 5%.
Substance use	Physical disabilities, poverty, chronic pain, chronic illness, grief, early life history of substance use	Substance use disorders are often unrecognized and undertreated in older adults. As with younger adults, the patient may not recognize that behaviors are problematic. In older adults, secondary harm (eg, falling) is of high concern. Prevalence is approximately 4%.
Bipolar disorder (I and II)	Family history, high-stress environment, substance abuse	Bipolar disorder that is untreated or undertreated tends to worsen with age. Comorbidity with anxiety disorders and substance use disorders is very common. Older men with bipolar disorder, especially if untreated, are at especially high risk for suicide. Prevalence is less than 1% of older adults.
Schizophrenia	Family history, complications during birth, early-life substance abuse	Initial diagnosis is typically in 20s and 30s. A diagnosis after age 40 is rare. Late-onset schizophrenia is believed to be more common in women and to be characterized by lower severity of positive symptoms. Late-onset patients generally have less impairment than adult-onset patients. Comorbidities, such as depression and substance use disorder, are common. Prevalence is approximately 1%.
Intellectual disabilities and autism	Family history, parental health and behavior, complications during birth (intellectual disabilities). Family history and being born to an older mother (autism)	Onset is in childhood, though diagnosis may not be present for those who are more functionally independent, especially with autism spectrum disorder, making prevalence estimates difficult. Linkage to community services, promoting involvement of family members and advocates, and close monitoring of health conditions are important in these populations.

can function as case managers for individuals experiencing cognitive impairment.

Mental Illness

The Centers for Disease Control and Prevention (CDC) reports estimate that nearly 20% of people 55 years or older experience a mental health problem. The most common forms of mental health conditions include anxiety and depression. **Table 20-5** provides an overview of common conditions. Older White men have the highest suicide rate of any age group. Individuals with severe and persistent mental health conditions (a long-standing diagnosis that is disabling) require specialized attention, especially if their mental health condition interferes with their ability to function independently. Care planning for these individuals typically involves an interdisciplinary team that includes a social worker. Stigma toward mental illness leaves many older adults suffering in silence and too fearful or ashamed to seek help. Language barriers and the lack of racial, ethnic, or culturally appropriate services also hinder older adults from seeking assistance. Social workers collaborate with a health care team to assess mental health issues and identify appropriate treatment and services. They can provide structured cognitive-behavioral, interpersonal, and problem-solving treatments that are effective mental health approaches, often in conjunction with prescribed medication. Pharmacologic interventions and psychosocial treatments are effective for older adults.

Substance and Alcohol Misuse

Substance and alcohol misuse often remain unrecognized by health care professionals who sometimes mistake symptoms for other age-related problems such as depression and dementia. Risk factors for substance and alcohol misuse include social isolation, living alone, chronic pain, and a variety of losses such as retirement, widowhood, and impaired mobility. Research suggests that a growing number of older adults misuse alcohol and other substances, including prescription medication and at a higher rate than previous generations. The National Survey on Drug Use and Health found that among individuals age 50 and older, over 12% were heavy drinkers, over 3% were binge drinkers, and nearly 2% used illicit drugs. Men older than age 65 had even higher rates of binge drinking at 14%. While misuse of individual substances or alcohol remains an important concern, another growing trend among older adults consists of mixing alcohol with psychoactive medications, which can have dangerous impacts for many older adults. Because older adults frequently suffer from chronic pain, and serious adverse effects of nonsteroidal anti-inflammatory drugs are common, older adults frequently use opioids on a chronic basis. There is a fine balance between appropriate use and transitioning into opioid use disorder. Moreover, a substantial number of older adults simultaneously use opioids and benzodiazepines, increasing the risk of serious adverse events such as falls and car crashes. Social workers aid other health care professionals in assessing substance and alcohol misuse and providing the necessary treatment. Social workers also provide successful educational interventions with older adults who are unaware that they are consuming too much alcohol or misusing medications.

SUMMARY

Social workers with training and experience in geriatrics and gerontology are integral members of the health care team serving older patients. Their wide range of skills, as well as their knowledge of available services in a variety of settings, makes social workers highly valuable members of the inter-professional team serving older patients by identifying, evaluating, prioritizing and providing or arranging for the support services they need.

With ongoing efforts to further cost containment and effectively deal with treatment, models of health care delivery will continue to evolve (see Chapters 19 and 14). Innovations such as the patient-centered medical home, accountable care organizations (ACOs), and other forms of value-based care population health management, which combine new payment arrangements that reward for health outcomes achieved rather than paying a fee for each service rendered will further highlight the critical role of social workers in the care of older adults. Social workers are integral to these service delivery models. In team-based care, social workers play an important role in recognizing and addressing social determinants of health that drive both health care needs and costs. As health care delivery models evolve, social workers will continue to play a critical role in assisting older patients, their families, and other caregivers in navigating the complexities involved in receiving care.

FURTHER READING

Administration on Aging. *A Profile of Older Americans.* Washington, DC: Administration on Aging; 2019. https://acl.gov/sites/default/files/Aging%20and%20Disability%20in%20America/2019ProfileOlderAmericans508.pdf. Accessed December 10, 2020.

Anthony S, Traub A, Lewis S, et al. Strengthening Medicaid Long-Term Services and Supports in an Evolving Policy Environment: A Toolkit for States. Center for Health Care Strategies, Inc. March 2019. http://allh.us/x3mK.

Barry KL, Blow FC. Drinking over the lifespan: focus on older adults. *Alcohol Res.* 2016;38(1):115–120.

Beaulieu EM. *A Guide for Nursing Home Social Workers.* New York, NY: Springer; 2013.

Berkman B, ed. *Handbook of Social Work in Health and Aging.* New York, NY: Oxford Press; 2015.

Buch ED. *Inequalities of Aging: Paradoxes of Independence in American Home Care.* New York, NY: New York University Press; 2018.

Fredriksen-Goldsen KI, Hoy-Ellis CP, Goldsen J, Emlet CA, Hooyman NR. Creating a vision for the future: key competencies and strategies for culturally competent practice with lesbian, gay, bisexual, and transgender (LGBT) older adults in the health and human services. *J Gerontol Social Work.* 2014;57(2–4):80–107.

Gehlert S. *Handbook of Health Social Work.* 3rd ed. New York, NY: John Wiley & Sons, Inc; 2019.

Han BH, Moore AA, Sherman S, Keyes KM, Palamar JJ. Demographic trends of binge alcohol use and alcohol use disorders among older adults in the United States, 2005–2014. *Drug Alcohol Depend.* 2017;170:198–207.

HIV Among People Aged 50 and Over, Centers for Disease Prevention and Control. https://www.cdc.gov/hiv/group/age/olderamericans/index.html. Accessed December 6, 2021.

Kadushin G, Egan M. *Gerontological Home Health Care: A Guide for the Social Work Practitioner.* New York, NY: Columbia University Press; 2008.

Kcomt L. Profound health-care discrimination experienced by transgender people: rapid systematic review. *Soc Work Health Care.* 2019;58(2):201–219.

Kim H-J, Jen S, Fredriksen-Goldsen K. Race/ethnicity and health-related quality of life among LGBT older adults. *Gerontologist.* 2017;57(Suppl 1):S30–S39.

Mpondo BCT. HIV infection in the elderly: arising challenges. *J Aging Res.* 2016;2016:2404857.

National Association of Social Workers. NASW standards for palliative and end of life care (2015). https://www.socialworkers.org/Practice/Practice-Standards-Guidelines. Accessed December 6, 2021.

National Association of Social Workers. NASW guidelines for social work practice in healthcare settings (2016). www.socialworkers.org/practice/standards/NASWHealthCareStandards.pdf.

Rodriguez J. *Labors of Love: Nursing Homes and the Structure of Care Work.* New York, NY: New York University Press; 2014.

Standards and Indicators for Cultural Competence in Social Work Practice, NASW, 2015. https://www.socialworkers.org/LinkClick.aspx?fileticket=7dVckZAYUmk%3D&portalid=0. Accessed December 6, 2021.

Weaver RH, Roberto KA. Home and community-based service use by vulnerable older adults. *Gerontologist.* 2017;57(3):540–551.

World Health Organization. Suicide in the world, 2019. https://www.who.int/publications/i/item/suicide-in-the-world. Accessed January 5, 2022.

Zerden L, Lombardi B, Jones A. Social workers in integrated health care: improving care throughout the life course. *Soc Work Health Care.* 2019;58(1):142–149.

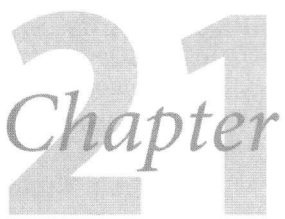

Chapter 21

The Patient Perspective

Preeti N. Malani, Erica S. Solway, Jeffrey T. Kullgren

INTRODUCTION

One often talks about wanting to hear the perspectives of everyday people, to inform gaps in knowledge that cannot be addressed through traditional research methods. The University of Michigan National Poll on Healthy Aging (NPHA) grew out of a desire to identify and fill some of those gaps through learning about issues that affect the day-to-day lives and experiences of older adults in the United States to improve their health and health care.

Launched in 2017, the NPHA examines older adults' knowledge and attitudes on timely topics related to healthy aging through a recurring nationally representative household survey. Surveys are fielded two to three times per year with a sample of approximately 2000 individuals aged 50 to 80, and completion rates are typically 60% to 80% (**Table 21-1**). The NPHA is directed by the University of Michigan Institute for Healthcare Policy & Innovation and sponsored by AARP and Michigan Medicine, the University of Michigan's academic medical center.

As of June 2021, the NPHA has released nearly 40 reports on a wide range of topics related to healthy aging, including the impact of the COVID-19 pandemic on the health and well-being of older adults. While these reports reach diverse audiences including the public, policymakers, and advocates, they offer unique insights into the perspectives and experiences of older adults that can be particularly helpful for geriatricians and other clinicians caring for patients in this age range. In this chapter, key findings and messages for clinicians are highlighted from a selection of past NPHA reports that can be organized into three broad categories: (1) health and health care (2) health care-related access and decision making, and (3) social aspects of health and well-being.

HEALTH AND HEALTH CARE

Brain Health

As the number of older adults in the United States increases, so does interest in strategies to promote "brain health" and ways to reduce the risk or slow the progression of dementia. In October 2018, the NPHA asked adults aged 50 to 64 about their memory, their concerns about developing dementia, and whether they would participate in dementia research.

Learning Objectives

- Describe older adults' knowledge and attitudes about healthy aging through a selection of past reports from the National Poll on Healthy Aging.
- Highlight specific interventions that can help improve health and well-being among older adults.
- Examine the impact of the COVID-19 pandemic on the health and well-being of older adults.

Key Clinical Points

1. Primary care providers are trusted sources of information and guidance for older adults.
2. The poll results highlight topics that are important to many patients but not always discussed by health care providers, such as sexual health, emergency preparedness, and the cost of prescription medications.

Being worried about developing dementia was more pronounced among adults aged 50 to 64 with a family history of dementia compared to those without (66% vs 28%). Likewise, the 18% who had been a caregiver of a person with dementia were more likely to worry about developing dementia than those who had not been caregivers (65% vs 39%).

More than half of respondents (55%) reported doing crossword puzzles or other brain games, and 48% reported taking some type of vitamin or supplement to help their memory. About one in three (32%) said they took fish oil or omega-3 supplements. Overall, 73% of adults aged 50 to 64 reported engaging in at least one of these strategies to help maintain or improve their memory. About half of adults aged 50 to 64 reported being open to participating in research related to dementia, and those with a family history of dementia were more likely to participate in research.

Despite widespread concerns about developing dementia and engagement in strategies aimed at preventing

TABLE 21-1 ■ NATIONAL POLL ON HEALTHY AGING, RESPONDENT DEMOGRAPHICS (n = 2023)[a]

Age	
50–59 (n = 650)	32%
60–69 (n = 792)	39%
70–80 (n = 581)	29%
Gender	
Male (n = 950)	47%
Female (n = 1073)	53%
Race/Ethnicity	
White, non-Hispanic (n = 1530)	76%
Black, non-Hispanic (n = 187)	9%
Hispanic (n = 181)	9%
Other, non-Hispanic (n = 125)	6%
Marital Status	
Married or partnered (n = 1437)	71%
Not married or partnered (n = 586)	29%
Lives Alone	
Yes (n = 423)	21%
No (n = 1600)	79%
Physical Health (Self-reported)	
Excellent/Very good (n = 914)	45%
Good (n = 816)	40%
Fair or poor (n = 292)	14%
Mental Health (Self-reported)	
Excellent/Very good (n = 1353)	67%
Good (n = 510)	25%
Fair or poor (n = 154)	8%
Education	
High school or less (n = 668)	33%
Some college (n = 668)	33%
Bachelor's degree or higher (n = 687)	34%
Current Employment Status	
Employed (n = 813)	40%
Retired (n = 939)	46%
Not working at this time (n = 169)	8%
On disability (n = 99)	5%
Total Household Income (Annual)	
< $30,000 (n = 243)	12%
$30,000–$59,999 (n = 434)	21%
$60,000–$99,999 (n = 511)	25%
$100,000 or more (n = 835)	41%

[a]Some items included nonresponse and percentage may not add to 100 due to rounding.

it, just 5% of all adults aged 50 to 64, and 10% among those with a family history of dementia, reported having ever discussed dementia prevention with their physician. Such conversations could be vital opportunities for older adults to have their concerns addressed by using more evidence-based approaches to preventing or delaying cognitive decline. For example, there is such evidence for regular physical activity, controlling diabetes, quitting smoking, managing hypertension, and addressing hearing loss. In contrast, no major research studies support the effectiveness of supplements to enhance memory. The poll findings suggest that many adults aged 50 to 64 could benefit from discussing these strategies with their doctors to address their concerns about future memory loss.

Medication Review

Older adults often have complex medication regimens involving multiple prescription and nonprescription medications. An NPHA poll from April 2017 found that 69% of older adults had seen two or more doctors in the past year and 21% of older adults had used more than one pharmacy over the past 2 years. Both findings suggest that their doctors and pharmacists may not be aware of all the medications the person is taking. In addition, 27% of adults aged 50 to 80 reported that the cost of their prescription drugs was a burden for them. One way to maximize the benefits and minimize the harms of medications is through a comprehensive medication review (CMR). A CMR is an in-person, telephone, or video appointment, often with a pharmacist and a patient or caregiver, at which medications are reviewed, including how they are taken, their indications, side effects, potential for interactions, and costs. In December 2019, the NPHA asked adults aged 50 to 80 about their medication use and experiences having CMRs with pharmacists.

Two in five adults aged 50 to 80 (41%) reported taking two to four prescription medications, and 23% said they take five or more in addition to any nonprescription medications or supplements they may also take. Among those taking two or more prescription medications, 24% had ever had a CMR. A similar proportion of older adults who were enrolled in Medicare Part D prescription drug plans, which cover CMRs for eligible members, reported ever having a CMR (25%). Among adults aged 50 to 80 who had not had a CMR, the majority (86%) were unaware that their insurance might cover one, including 85% of those enrolled in a Medicare Part D prescription drug plan.

This poll shows that CMRs are an underutilized opportunity to help ensure medication regimens are as effective, safe, and affordable as possible. Clinicians can increase awareness about the benefits and availability of CMRs among older adults, including as a potential opportunity to address high health care costs, particularly those enrolled in Medicare Part D plans for whom such services may be covered.

Antibiotics

As a treatment for bacterial infections, antibiotics can save lives. However, inappropriate use can reduce their effectiveness and lead to other harms. In May 2019, the NPHA asked adults aged 50 to 80 about their experiences with and opinions about antibiotics. Nearly half of adults aged 50 to 80 (48%) reported filling a prescription for antibiotics in the last 2 years. Among those who filled a prescription for an antibiotic in the last 2 years, 13% reported having leftover medication.

Among those who kept leftover antibiotics, 60% said they did so in case they got another infection. A smaller proportion (6%) kept leftover antibiotics in case a family member got an infection, 4% were not sure how to dispose of the leftovers, and 2% forgot to dispose of them. In addition, among all respondents, 19% reported ever taking antibiotics without talking to a health care professional (17% took their own leftover medication and 3% took someone else's medication).

While patients should be counseled to take all the antibiotics that are prescribed in order to appropriately treat their infection and minimize the emergence of resistance, some stop taking them. Across the population, this represents several million doses of leftover antibiotics. Use of these leftover antibiotics without medical supervision could result in serious drug interactions and other side effects, and could also contribute to increased antibiotic resistance.

To help ensure that antibiotic use is appropriate, safe, and effective, clinicians should give careful consideration to the number of pills given, so that excess medication does not contribute to misuse. Patients should be counseled about the risks of taking antibiotics without consulting a health care professional, and patients and family members should be encouraged to bring leftover antibiotics to community "take back" events or follow other guidelines for disposal.

Opioids

Health conditions and procedures that result in pain are more common as people age. In March 2018, the NPHA asked adults aged 50 to 80 about their use of opioids for pain management, the education they received, how they disposed of unused medications, and perceptions of current and proposed policies related to opioid disposal and prescribing.

Overall, 29% of respondents said they filled a prescription for an opioid pain medication for themselves within the past 2 years. As summarized in **Figure 21-1**, 90% said they talked with the prescribing health care provider about how often to take the pain medication. However, fewer said they talked about side effects, when to reduce the amount of medication, risk of addiction, risk of overdose, and what to do with leftover pills. Among those who were prescribed an opioid, half said they had medication left over (49%). When asked what they did with extra pain medication, 86% said they kept it in case they had pain again.

Health care providers who prescribe and dispense medications should discuss how and why to safely use and dispose of medications in language that patients understand. In addition to providing recommendations for safe storage and disposal, they should help patients in identifying where and how they will dispose of extra medication.

A quarter of older adults did not try to take less pain medication and half did not switch to a non-opioid medication as soon as possible, illustrating missed opportunities to reduce opioid use that should be addressed. Therefore, it is critically important that clinicians work with patients to identify pain management strategies that will address pain

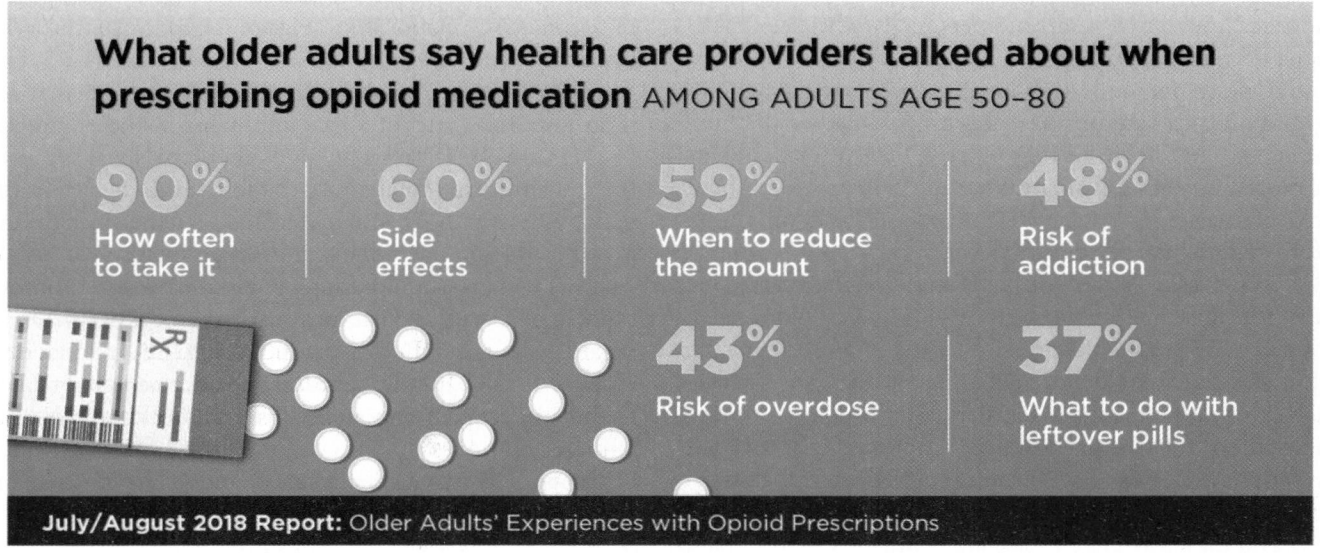

FIGURE 21-1. Opioids. (Courtesy from National Poll on Healthy Aging. University of Michigan https://www.healthyagingpoll.org/reports-more/report/older-adults-experiences-opioid-prescriptions.)

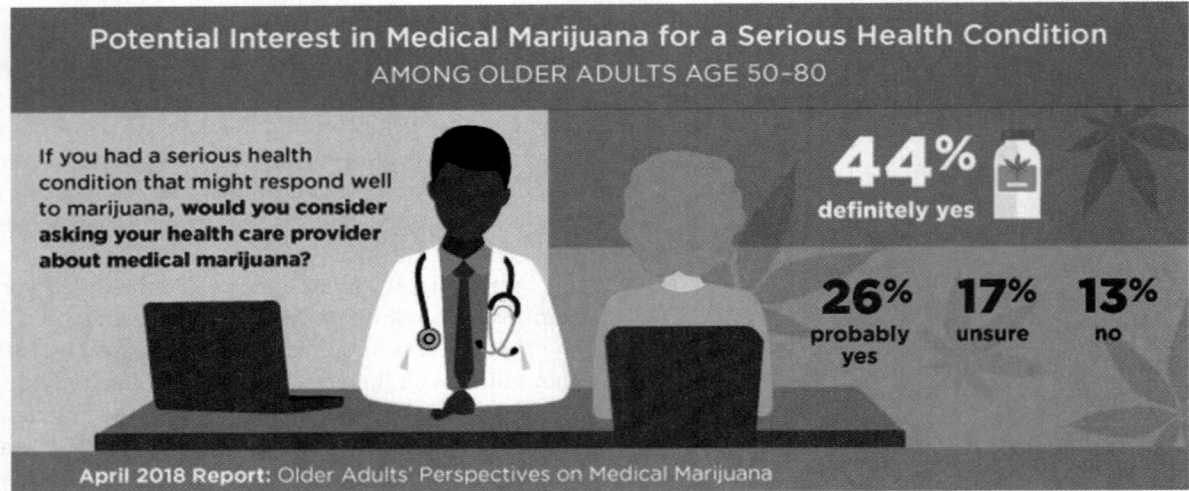

FIGURE 21-2. Marijuana. (Courtesy from National Poll on Healthy Aging. University of Michigan https://www.healthyagingpoll
.org/reports-more/report/older-adults-perspective-medical-marijuana.)

while minimizing the risks of opioid medications. Since there are effective nonopioid medication and nonmedication strategies to treat pain for a variety of conditions, the opioids should not be the first-line treatment for most pain conditions.

Medical Marijuana

As an increasing number of US states have legalized marijuana, there has been an upward trend in marijuana use among older adults. In October 2017, the NPHA asked adults aged 50 to 80 about marijuana use for medical purposes, its perceived benefits, perception of how marijuana compares to prescription pain medicine, and support for marijuana-related policies. Overall, 6% of poll respondents reported using marijuana for medical purposes and 18% indicated they know someone personally who uses marijuana for medical purposes.

One in five older adults (21%) reported that their primary health care provider has asked whether they use marijuana. As shown in **Figure 21-2**, 70% of respondents expressed an interest in speaking to their provider about uses of marijuana for medical purposes and only 13% expressed no interest in doing so.

When asked about the benefits of medical marijuana, 31% felt that marijuana definitely provides pain relief, another 38% believed it probably does, 27% were unsure, while 4% said they believed marijuana does not provide pain relief. When comparing marijuana with prescription medications for treating pain, 48% indicated that they felt prescription pain medication was more effective than marijuana, 14% thought marijuana was more effective, and 38% said they considered marijuana and prescription pain medication to have about the same effectiveness. About half of respondents (53%) thought the government should develop rules to standardize medical marijuana dosing and

64% felt the government should fund research to study the health effects of marijuana.

These findings suggest that more screening as well as rigorous studies on the health effects and safety of marijuana use may be needed, especially in older adults.

Sexual Health

Romantic relationships are important to well-being and quality of life at any age. While sex is an integral part of the lives of many older adults, this topic remains understudied and infrequently discussed. In October 2017, the NPHA asked adults aged 65 to 80 about their perspectives on relationships and sex and their experiences related to sexual health.

Two in five (40%) adults aged 65 to 80 indicated that they are currently sexually active, and 54% of those are in a romantic relationship (**Figure 21-3**). Sexual activity decreased with age (46% age 65–70, 39% age 71–75, and 25% age 76–80). Most older adults (76%) agreed that sex is an important part of a romantic relationship at any age (see **Figure 21-3**). Yet only 17% reported speaking with their health care provider about their sexual health in the past 2 years. Of those who had talked with their health care provider, 60% initiated the conversation themselves.

Clinicians should inquire about and offer opportunities to discuss sexual health with their older patients, regardless of age or health status. Raising the topic can help older adults to better understand and address issues related to this important component of overall health and quality of life. A more detailed discussion of this topic is provided in Chapter 35 (women's sexuality) and Chapter 37 (men's sexuality).

Urinary Incontinence in Women

Although urinary incontinence is common among older women, embarrassment about urine leakage or the belief

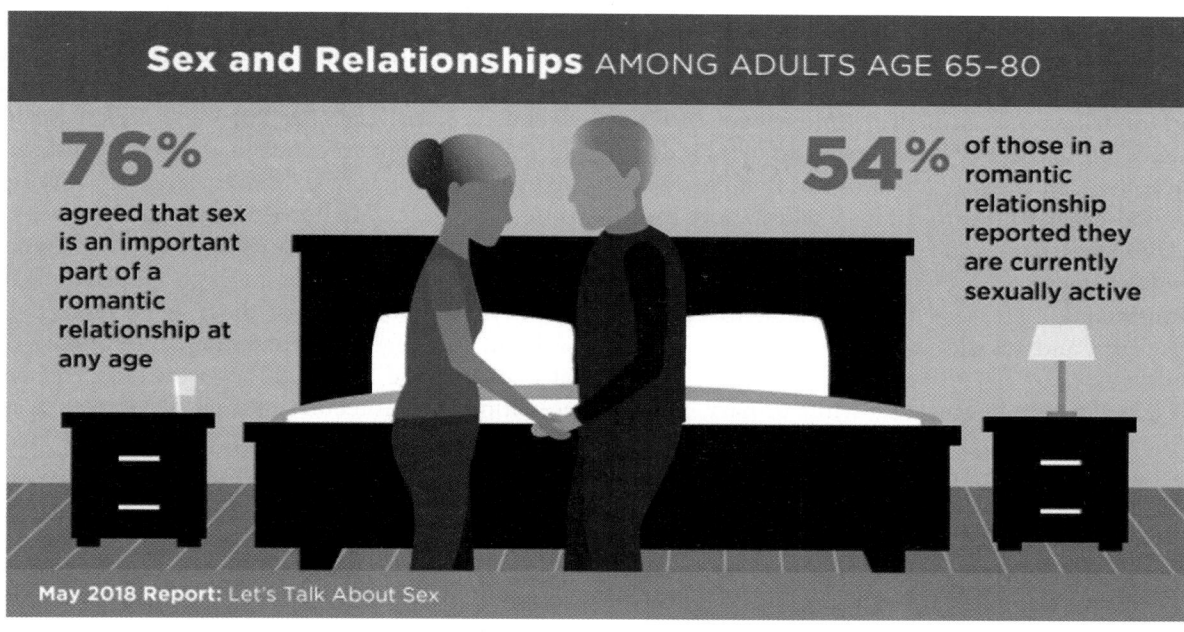

FIGURE 21-3. Sexual health. (Courtesy from National Poll on Healthy Aging. University of Michigan https://deepblue.lib.umich .edu/bitstream/handle/2027.42/143212/NPHA-Sexual-Health-Report_050118_final.pdf?sequence=1&isAllowed=y.)

that incontinence is a normal part of aging may prevent women from seeking treatment. In March 2018, the NPHA asked women aged 50 to 80 about their experiences with urinary incontinence and related discussions with their doctors.

Nearly half of older women (46%) reported urinary incontinence in the past year. Of women reporting urinary incontinence, 41% described leakage as a problem, and 31% had leakage episodes almost daily. The most common strategies used to manage urinary incontinence are summarized in **Figure 21-4**. Overall, 34% of older women who experienced incontinence said they spoke to their doctor about urinary leakage (28% for those aged 50–64 and 44% among those aged 65–80). Women who viewed incontinence as a

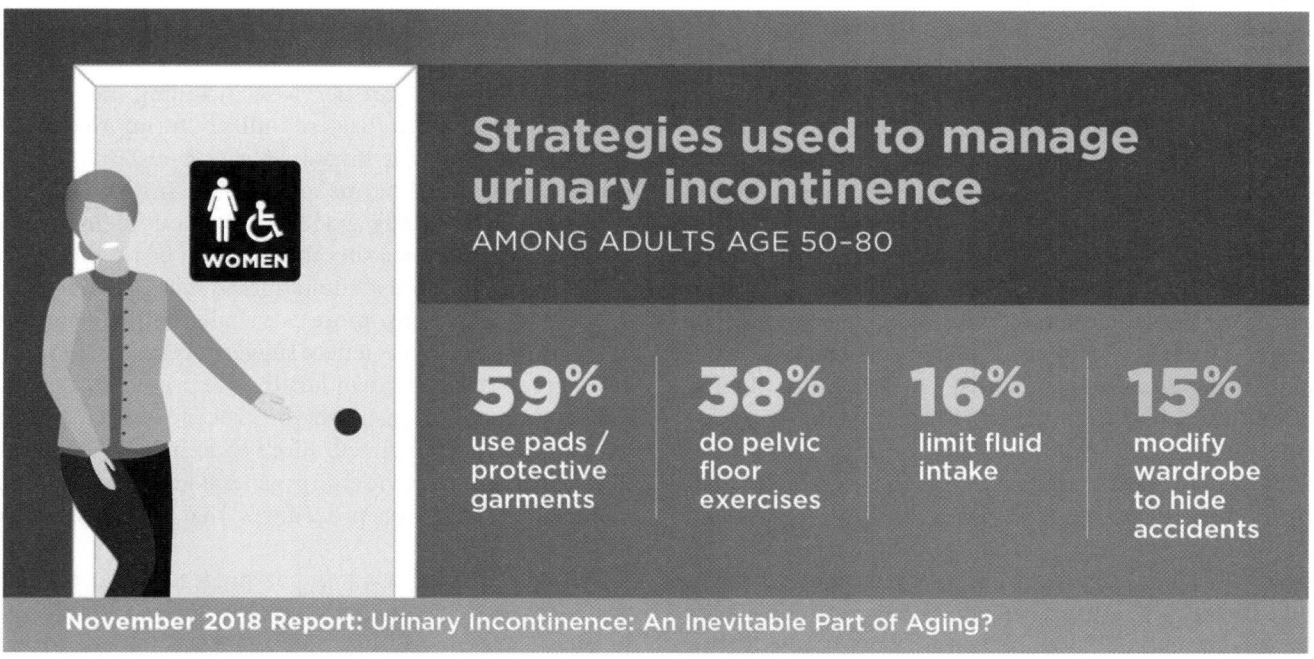

FIGURE 21-4. Urinary incontinence. (Courtesy from National Poll on Healthy Aging. University of Michigan https://www .healthyagingpoll.org/reports-more/report/urinary-incontinence-inevitable-part-aging.)

problem or felt embarrassed by it were more likely to have sought medical advice.

What prevented women from seeking medical treatment for urinary incontinence? Among women with incontinence, 66% said they had not spoken to their doctor because they felt the problem was not that bad, 23% said they had other things to discuss, and 22% did not see urinary incontinence as a health problem. Another 15% of women said their doctor had not asked about urinary incontinence, 10% were uncomfortable discussing urinary leakage, and 4% did not think the doctor could help.

These poll results suggest that while urinary incontinence is experienced by nearly half of older women, most manage their symptoms without support or input from their health care providers and many do not seek treatment because they prioritize other medical issues or they do not consider urinary incontinence to be a health problem. Yet, any urine leakage can diminish quality of life, and incontinence that prevents women from participating in health-promoting behaviors such as exercise can have a negative impact on overall health. Screening for urinary incontinence can help to identify patients who may benefit from education or services to address their urinary incontinence which can have important implications for health and quality of life.

Dental Care and Oral Health

Oral health is an integral part of overall health. Keeping teeth healthy involves a combination of good oral hygiene and routine preventive dental care with prompt attention to dental problems before they become severe. In April 2017, the NPHA explored oral health and experiences with dental care and coverage among adults aged 50 to 64.

More than one in four adults (28%) reported that their oral health was fair or poor. One in three (34%) said they were embarrassed about the condition of their teeth, and a similar percentage reported that they have experienced dental pain or problems in the past 2 years. One in five (19%) said it had been more than 5 years since their last preventive dental visit. More than one in four respondents (27%) reported that they needed dental care in the past 2 years but either delayed or did not get care. Among those with unmet dental needs, 69% cited cost as a major factor. Being afraid of the dentist (20%), finding time to go (18%), and finding a dentist (14%) also contributed to unmet dental needs.

Overall, 28% of adults aged 50 to 64 indicated they did not currently have dental coverage. Many respondents expressed uncertainty about their insurance coverage for dental care when they turn 65: 51% did not know how they will get dental insurance when they turn age 65 and 13% thought that traditional Medicare would provide their dental coverage even though traditional Medicare's coverage of dental services is limited to narrowly defined medically necessary dental services only.

Recognizing that oral health is integral to good health at every age and that adults in older age groups can have unique oral health needs and barriers to accessing dental care, in December 2019, the NPHA asked adults aged 65 to 80 about oral health, dental care utilization and access, dental coverage, and their perspectives on proposed changes to Medicare to cover dental care.

Overall, 25% of adults aged 65 to 80 rated their oral health as fair or poor and 24% reported having dentures. In addition, 46% of those age 65 to 80 said they were missing teeth for which they did not have dentures or implants, and 27% said they were embarrassed by the condition of their teeth. In the past 2 years, 20% said they had experienced dental pain and the same percentage reported problems with eating and chewing. Nearly half (47%) of respondents reported that they do not have dental coverage.

The condition of one's teeth can affect self-esteem, social relationships, job seeking and retention, ability to maintain good nutrition, and overall health. Both polls found poorer oral health status and lower use of dental services among those with self-reported fair or poor physical or mental health. People with chronic health conditions and disabilities may face challenges maintaining oral hygiene and getting dental care, and medications can contribute to dry mouth which can negatively affect oral health. Oral health problems can also negatively affect physical and mental health. For example, dental pain or problems with eating and chewing may lead to difficulty maintaining a healthy diet. Clinicians should encourage patients to prioritize their oral health and be aware of accessible, lower cost options for dental care in their communities.

Overuse of Health Care Services

"Low value" health care services, including medications, tests, and procedures that are unlikely to improve health outcomes, are not only unnecessary and wasteful, but may also create potential harms for patients. In October 2017, the NPHA asked adults aged 50 to 80 about their perspectives on health care services that may not be needed.

Only 14% of older adults agreed that "when it comes to medical treatment, more is usually better." However, older adults' own experiences suggest overuse is common: 25% agreed that their own health care provider often recommends medications, tests, or procedures that they do not think they really need. More than half (54%) agreed that health care providers in general often recommend medications, tests, or procedures that patients do not really need.

Conventional wisdom has suggested that patients' preferences drive overuse of low-value health care services. Results of this poll suggest that health care providers may be making incorrect assumptions about their patients' desire for services that have limited clinical value.

HEALTH CARE-RELATED ACCESS AND DECISION MAKING

Telehealth

As COVID-19 began to spread across the United States in early 2020, health systems made rapid and sweeping changes to how care was delivered. These changes and the risk of COVID-19 required many older adults to have appointments with their health care providers through telehealth rather than in-person visits. In May 2019 and June 2020, the NPHA asked adults aged 50 to 80 about their use of and perspectives on telehealth.

In May 2019, 14% of older adults said that their health care providers offered telehealth visits, compared to 62% in June 2020. Similarly, the percentage of older adults who had ever participated in a telehealth visit rose dramatically from 4% in May 2019 to 30% in June 2020.

In June 2020, 30% of older adults with a telehealth visit said that video or phone visits were the only options available when scheduling their appointment. Nearly half (46%) indicated that in-person visits were canceled or rescheduled to telehealth visits by their health care provider. Fear of COVID-19 led 15% to request or reschedule an in-person appointment as a telehealth visit.

Poll results demonstrate that the availability, use, and interest all increased substantially over 1 year, as did the personal use of and comfort with video-conferencing technologies commonly used in telehealth visits. As more older adults experienced telehealth visits, some perceived concerns, including privacy and communication with health care providers, diminished. Perceptions about the overall convenience of telehealth visits also increased.

As use of telehealth continues to increase, clinicians should be aware of the challenges and concerns some older patients have with virtual visits, as summarized in **Figure 21-5**. Importantly, while the vast majority of older adults who had a telehealth visit reported that the technology was easy to use, some older adults have limited experience and comfort with technology and may need additional support. Furthermore, some older adults were concerned about the quality of care compared to in-person visits and about not being able to get a physical examination. Until these concerns are addressed, some older adults may be hesitant to seek health care in this format.

Patient Portals

Patient portals have become the preferred form of communication with patients for many health care practices. In March 2018, the NPHA asked older adults aged 50 to 80 about their experiences with patient portals. About half of older adults (51%) reported they have set up a patient portal. There were demographic differences, with higher proportions setting up a patient portal among women versus men (56% vs 45%), among adults with some college versus high school only (59% vs 40%), and among those with higher versus lower annual household income (59% for ≥ $60,000 vs 42% for < $60,000).

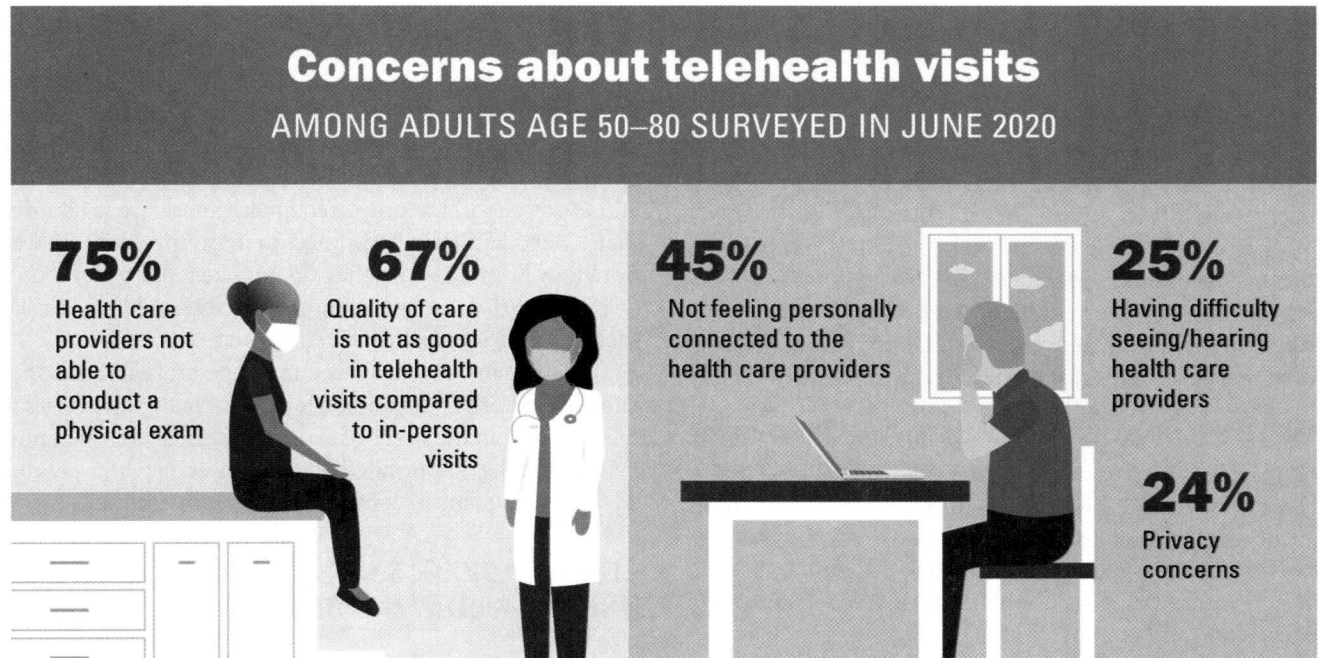

FIGURE 21-5. Telehealth. (Courtesy from National Poll on Healthy Aging. University of Michigan https://www.healthyagingpoll .org/reports-more/report/telehealth-use-among-older-adults-and-during-covid-19.)

Interestingly, there were similar rates of portal use for those aged 50 to 64 (52%) and 65 to 80 (49%). Older adults aged 65 to 80 identified technology barriers and lack of comfort as key reasons for not setting up a portal. In contrast, adults aged 50 to 64 report few specific barriers, but simply reported not taking the time to set one up. Eliminating barriers to setup and use of patient portals, while maintaining the option to continue telephone communication, may be the appropriate strategy to meet the varied needs of older adults.

Emergency Department Use

Each year in the United States, adults aged 50 and older make more than 40 million visits to an emergency department (ED). In June 2020, the NPHA asked adults aged 50 to 80 about their ED experiences. Overall, 26% of adults aged 50 to 80 reported having an ED visit in the past 2 years (32% for respondents aged 65–80 and 23% for those aged 50–64). Almost half of adults with self-reported fair or poor mental (46%) or physical (45%) health had an ED visit in the past 2 years.

When deciding whether to go to the ED, most aged 50 to 80 reported that they would be concerned about wait times (91%), exposure to COVID-19 (86%), out-of-pocket costs (79%), and being admitted to the hospital (77%); 37% said they would be concerned about transportation home. Nearly two in three older adults (63%) said they would first ask their health care provider or office staff before going to the ED. One in eight (13%) said they went to the ED because they could not get a timely primary care or specialty care appointment.

When considering where to go for ED care, older adults reported that their insurance coverage (86%), the reputation of the ED (69%), location (68%), and a recommendation by a health care provider (61%) were very important factors. Overall, 80% of adults aged 50 to 80 were concerned about the costs of a future ED visit and 18% were not confident about being able to afford out-of-pocket costs for a future ED visit. Seven percent of older adults reported that they did not go to the ED when they thought they needed to due to concerns about their out-of-pocket costs.

These poll results could help hospitals, emergency and other health care providers, and insurers improve the ways they advise older adults on seeking emergency care, treat them once they arrive at the ED, address their cost-related concerns, and assist them in receiving follow-up care.

Health Insurance Decision-Making Near Retirement

As Americans approach retirement age and eligibility for Medicare coverage, many face difficult decisions about their health insurance and its associated costs. In October 2018, the NPHA asked adults aged 50 to 64 about their current and future plans for their health insurance coverage, medical care, and employment.

Overall, 27% had little or no confidence in being able to afford the cost of their health insurance over the next year and 45% had little or no confidence in being able to afford the cost of their health insurance when they retire.

In the previous year, 11% of adults aged 50 to 64 reported thinking about going without health insurance, and an additional 5% decided to go without health insurance. In the previous year, 13% of adults aged 50 to 64 did not get medical care because of its high cost.

Adults aged 50 to 64 also reported making decisions about the timing of their retirement based on health insurance–related considerations. In the past year, 14% reported keeping a job specifically to have health insurance through their employer and 11% delayed or considered delaying retirement specifically to have employer-sponsored health insurance. Overall, 19% either kept a job, considered delaying retirement, or delayed retirement to keep their employer-sponsored health insurance.

Clinicians and patients should discuss the out-of-pocket costs of health care which can help to inform decisions about health insurance options and the timing, choice, and appropriateness of health care services.

Advance Care Planning

Advance care planning, which often includes legal documentation of a medical durable power of attorney and an advance directive, helps ensure people receive medical care that is consistent with their values, goals, and preferences. In June 2020, the NPHA asked adults aged 50 to 80 about their advance care planning before and during the early months of the COVID-19 pandemic.

Overall, 59% said they have talked to someone (ie, a spouse, adult children, other family, or friends) about the types of medical care they want or do not want if they become seriously ill (**Figure 21-6**). People aged 65 to 80 were more likely than those aged 50 to 64 (70% vs 51%) and women were more likely than men (62% vs 55%) to have talked to someone about their care preferences.

Also shown in **Figure 21-6**, nearly half of older adults (46%) reported they had completed at least one advance care planning legal document (ie, a medical durable power of attorney or advance directive). Among the 54% of older adults who had not completed an advance care legal document, 62% said they had not gotten around to it, 15% did not know how, 13% said they do not like talking about these things, 13% did not think it necessary, 9% said no one asked them to, and 7% were deterred by cost.

Clinicians can help to encourage and facilitate these vital discussions about and documentation of preferences for medical care in the event of serious illness, as well as remind patients of the importance of regularly reviewing previous advance care plans to confirm they remain accurate.

SOCIAL ASPECTS OF HEALTH AND WELL-BEING

Ageism

Ageism is prevalent, and older adults may experience ageism in their day-to-day lives. In December 2019, the NPHA asked adults aged 50 to 80 about their experiences with

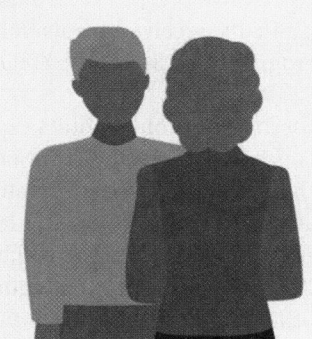

Advance care planning
AMONG ADULTS AGE 50–80

59%
have talked with someone about medical treatment they want or do not want if seriously ill

Of those,
29% did so in the first 3 months of the pandemic

46%
have a medical durable power of attorney and/or advance directive

Of those,
7% completed them in the first 3 months of the pandemic

FIGURE 21-6. Advance care planning. (Courtesy from National Poll on Healthy Aging. University of Michigan https://www.healthyagingpoll.org/reports-more/report/older-adults-experiences-advance-care-planning.)

different forms of everyday ageism, positive views on aging, and health. The nine forms of ageism explored through this poll were organized into three categories: (1) exposure to ageist messages, (2) ageism in interpersonal interactions, and (3) internalized ageism (personally held beliefs about aging and older people), as summarized in **Table 21-2**.

Two in five older adults (40%) reported often or sometimes experiencing three or more (out of the nine) forms of everyday ageism. Experiencing three or more forms was more common among those aged 65 to 80 as compared to those aged 50 to 64 (49% vs 35%), women compared to men (43% vs 38%), and those with annual household incomes below $60,000 compared to those with higher incomes (50% vs 33%). Being retired and living in a rural area were also associated with experiencing more forms of ageism.

Older adults who reported experiencing three or more forms of everyday ageism in their day-to-day lives had worse physical and mental health than those who reported fewer forms of ageism. For example, older adults who reported three or more forms of ageism were less likely to rate their overall physical health as excellent or very good compared to those reporting fewer forms (34% vs 49%). Older adults who experienced more forms of ageism were also more likely to have a chronic health condition such as diabetes or heart disease than those reporting fewer forms (71% vs 60%). Those who regularly experienced three or more forms of ageism were less likely than people who reported fewer forms to rate their mental health as excellent or very good (61% vs 80%) and more likely to report symptoms of depression (49% vs 22%).

Notably, older adults with positive views on aging reported experiencing fewer forms of everyday ageism and

better physical and mental health. Clinicians should be aware of how negative stereotypes, prejudice, and discrimination toward older people affect health and well-being and be part of efforts to challenge it and highlight

TABLE 21-2 ■ NINE FORMS OF EVERYDAY AGEISM AND THEIR PREVALENCE AMONG ADULTS AGED 50–80[a]

Exposure to ageist messages (65%)
- I hear, see, and/or read jokes about old age, aging, or older people (61%)
- I hear, see, and/or read things suggesting that older adults and aging are unattractive or undesirable (38%)

Percentage reporting that this sometimes or often happens to them in their day-to-day lives

Ageism in interpersonal interactions (45%)
- People assume that I have difficulty with cell phones and computers (22%)
- People assume I have difficulty hearing and/or seeing things (17%)
- People assume I have difficulty remembering and/or understanding things (17%)
- People assume I do not do anything important or valuable (15%)
- People insist on helping me with things I can do on my own (15%)

Percentage reporting that this sometimes or often happens to them in their day-to-day lives

Internalized ageism (36%)
- Feeling lonely is part of getting older (29%)
- Feeling depressed, sad, or worried is part of getting older (26%)

Percentage reporting that they strongly agree or agree with these statements

[a]NPHA report from July 2020.

positive views. Addressing everyday ageism may have far-reaching benefits for the health and well-being of older adults.

Food Security

Food insecurity, defined as difficulty in acquiring or accessing food due to a lack of money, affected an estimated one in nine US households in 2018. Although trends in food insecurity are tracked through surveys of the general US population, few surveys specifically focus on food insecurity among older adults. In December 2019 (prior to the COVID-19 pandemic), the NPHA surveyed adults aged 50 to 80 about household food insecurity and participation in food-assistance programs.

As summarized in **Figure 21-7**, 14% of respondents reported experiencing household food insecurity in the past year. Among older adults who experienced household food insecurity in the past year, 42% reported severe food insecurity, meaning individuals in their household reduced the quality or quantity of foods they consumed due to limited resources. Household food insecurity was higher among adults aged 50 to 64 (17%) than adults aged 65 to 80 (10%), and higher among non-Hispanic Black adults (22%) and Hispanic adults (22%) compared to non-Hispanic White adults (12%). It was also more common among older adults with lower levels of education and lower household income.

As shown in **Figure 21-7**, household food insecurity was associated with lower self-reported physical and mental health. Nearly half of adults ages 50 to 80 who were food insecure rated their physical health as fair or poor (45%), compared to 14% of those who were food secure. Almost a quarter of those who were food insecure reported fair or poor mental health (24%) compared to 5% of those who were food secure.

During the past year, 10% of respondents aged 50 to 80 reported receiving Supplemental Nutrition Assistance Program (SNAP) benefits. Adults aged 60 and older are eligible to receive home-delivered or congregate meals (eg, meals delivered in community or group settings) through the Older Americans Act. Yet among adults 60 and older, only 2% reported participating in meal programs through a community or senior center, and 1% received meals delivered to their home from a program like Meals on Wheels in the past year.

These poll results suggest that some older adults experiencing food insecurity may not be benefitting from programs designed to support them. Barriers to participating in SNAP or other community programs can include lack of knowledge or misinformation about services or eligibility, complex application procedures, waitlists, inadequate transportation, stigma, and other factors.

Improved communication about the benefits of participating in SNAP and community meal programs, as well as increased screening in clinical settings and referrals to community resources, may help to improve participation rates in nutrition programs and help alleviate food insecurity among older adults.

Emergency Planning

When natural disasters and other emergencies occur, some older adults, including those with chronic health conditions and impaired mobility, may be particularly vulnerable to adverse effects. In May 2019, the NPHA asked adults aged 50 to 80 about their experiences with disasters, emergency planning, and their preparedness for such events.

More than one in five of older adults (22%) had experienced an emergency or disaster such as a power outage lasting more than a day, severe weather, evacuation from their home, or a lockdown in the past year, while 73%

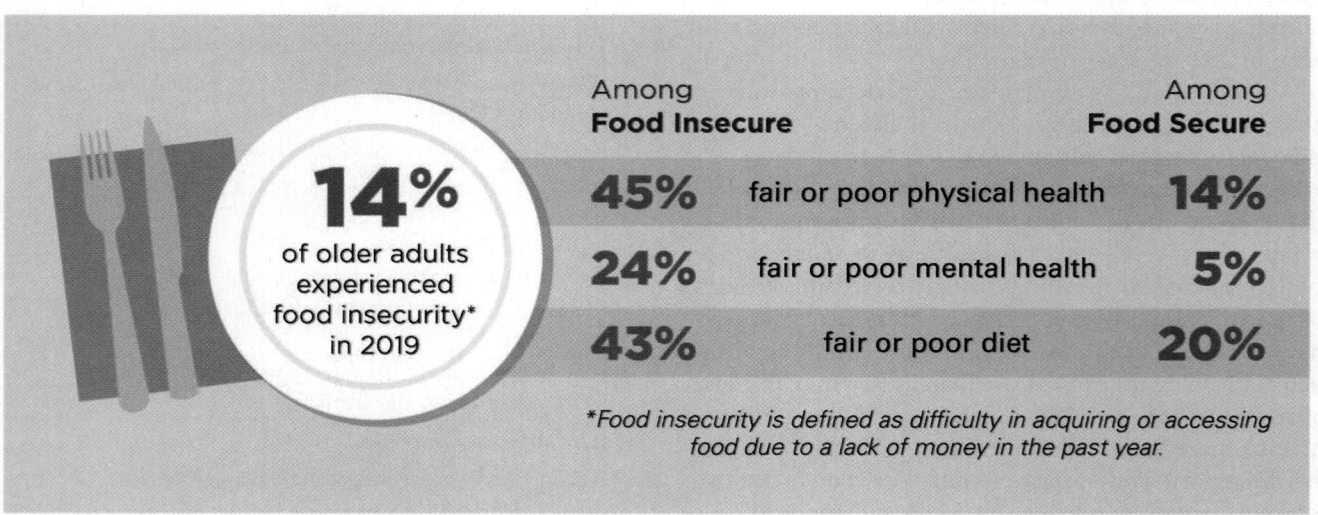

FIGURE 21-7. Food insecurity. (Courtesy from National Poll on Healthy Aging. University of Michigan https://www .healthyagingpoll.org/reports-more/report/how-food-insecurity-affects-older-adults.)

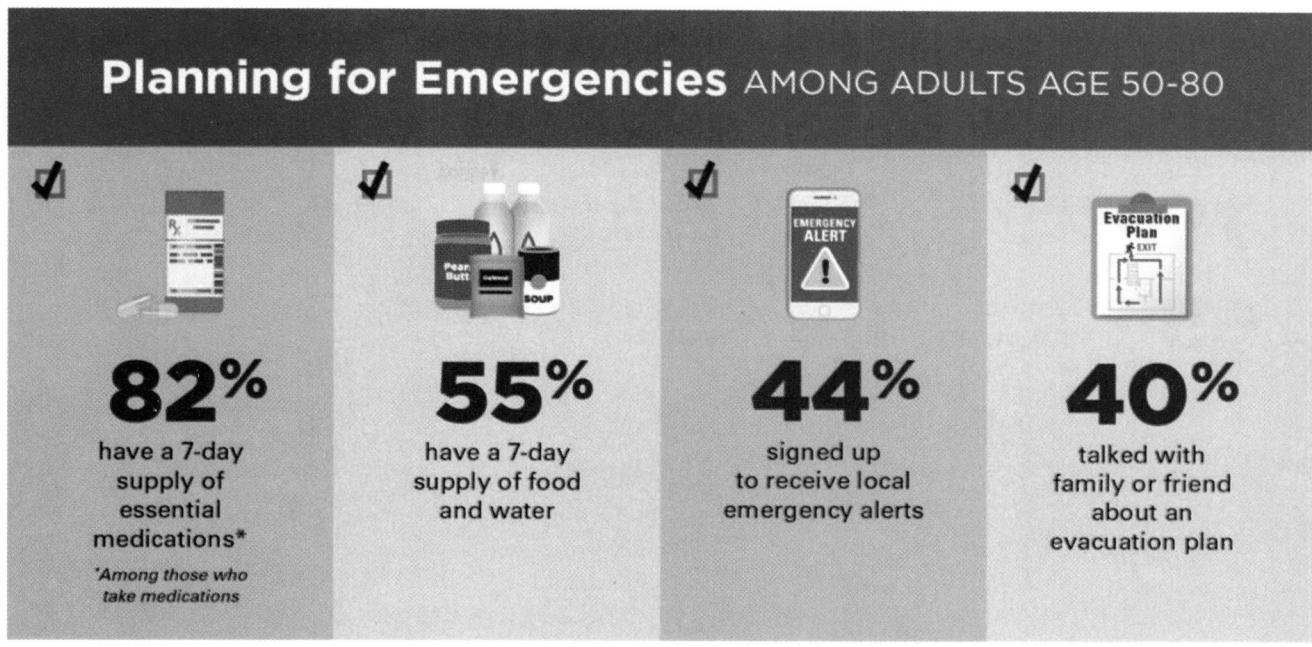

FIGURE 21-8. Emergency planning. (Courtesy from National Poll on Healthy Aging. University of Michigan https://www
.healthyagingpoll.org/reports-more/report/emergency-planning-among-older-adults.)

reported experiencing at least one such event during their lifetime. As shown in **Figure 21-8**, among older adults who required essential medications or health supplies, 82% had a 7-day supply of medication and 72% had a 7-day supply of health supplies, but only half reported having a 7-day supply of food and water. Among the 9% of respondents who used essential medical equipment that requires electricity, 25% had an alternative power source. Less than half had signed up for emergency alerts or had spoken to family or friends about an evacuation plan (see **Figure 21-8**).

More than half of older adults believed they will likely experience some type of natural disaster or emergency in the coming year and the majority generally felt confident in their ability to manage through them, yet these poll results suggest that many older adults have not taken key steps recommended by disaster preparedness agencies. Clinicians should discuss disaster preparedness with their older patients, particularly in areas that routinely face natural disasters.

Pets

Many older Americans live with pets and consider them part of the family. Pets can offer companionship and have a positive impact on health and well-being. In October 2018, the NPHA asked adults aged 50 to 80 about their pets and the benefits and challenges of owning a pet.

More than half of older adults (55%) reported having a pet. Among pet owners, the majority (68%) had dogs, 48% had cats, and 16% had a small pet such as a bird, fish, or hamster. More than half of pet owners (55%) reported having multiple pets.

Some possible health benefits of pets are included in **Figure 21-9**. Pet owners said that their pets help them enjoy life (88%), make them feel loved (86%), reduce stress (79%), provide a sense of purpose (73%), and help them stick to a routine (62%). Respondents also reported that their pets connect them with other people (65%), help them be physically active (64% overall and 78% among dog owners), and help them cope with physical and emotional symptoms (60%), including taking their mind off pain (34%). Among those who lived alone and/or reported fair or poor physical health, 72% said pets help them cope with physical or emotional symptoms.

While most pet owners reported positive experiences with their pets, some noted challenges. About one in five (18%) indicated that pet care puts a strain on their budget. One in six (15%) said that their pet's health takes priority over their own health, and 6% reported that their pets caused them to fall or otherwise injure themselves.

These results suggest that pets can provide a myriad of benefits for older adults, including boosts to emotional and physical health while also potentially contributing to challenges for some people. Health care professionals should be aware of the important role that pets play in the lives of many older adults, as pets have the potential to help, or hinder, self-care and adherence to treatment plans.

Caregiving

Family caregivers play a vital role in providing support to older adults living with dementia and other cognitive impairments. In April 2017, the NPHA asked adults aged 50 to 80 who identified as caregivers about their experiences caring for a person with dementia.

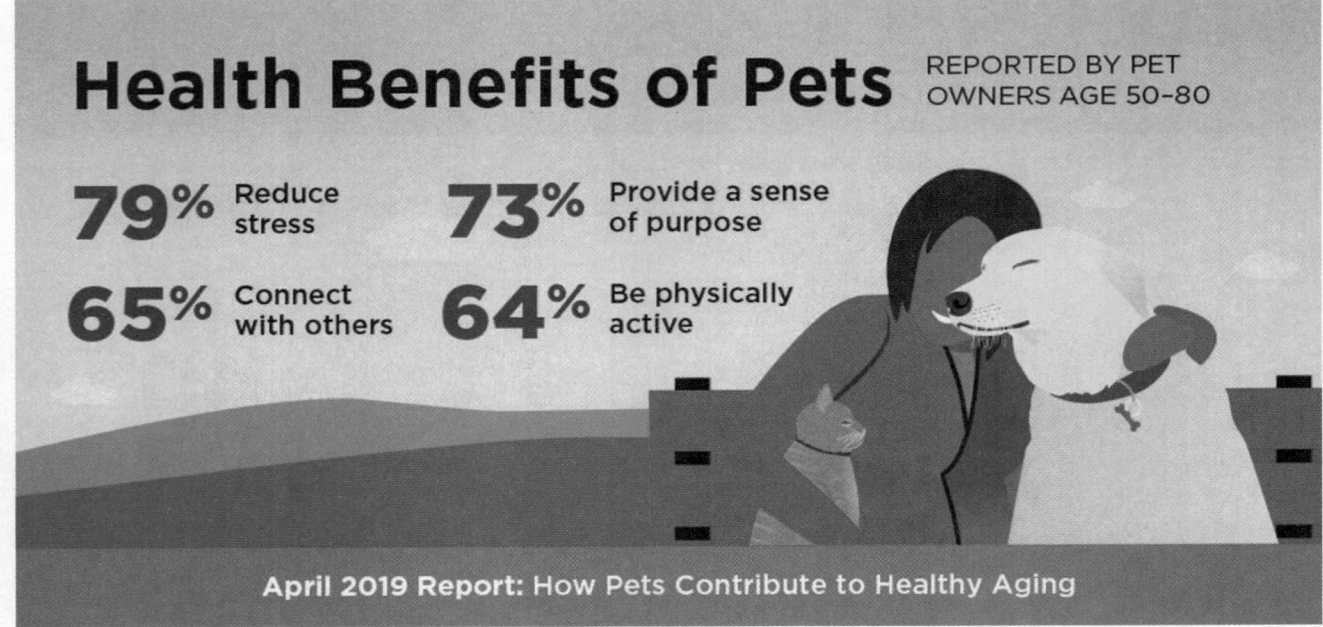

FIGURE 21-9. Pets. (Courtesy from National Poll on Healthy Aging. University of Michigan https://www.healthyagingpoll .org/reports-more/report/how-pets-contribute-healthy-aging.)

Overall, 7% of poll respondents (n = 148) identified as a caregiver of a person age 65 or older with dementia, Alzheimer disease, or another cognitive impairment. The majority of caregivers (62%) were women; 60% provided care to a parent, 19% to a spouse, and 21% to another relative, friend, or neighbor. Most caregivers (60%) have been providing care for 1 to 5 years and 29% have been doing so for 5 years or more. Nearly half of caregivers (45%) were employed in addition to having caregiving responsibilities.

Most caregivers (85%) reported they find caregiving rewarding (45% very rewarding and 40% somewhat rewarding). A slightly lower percentage (78%) said they find caregiving to be stressful (19% very stressful and 59% somewhat stressful) and 62% reported they find caregiving both stressful and rewarding. Overall, 27% of caregivers had used caregiving resources in the past year such as self-help resources, family therapy, classes or trainings, support groups, and/or respite care; 41% of those who had not used any caregiving resources indicated an interest in using them.

More than a quarter of caregivers (27%) reported delaying or not doing things they should do for their health; 66% said caregiving interferes with their ability to take good care of themselves, go to the doctor when they have a health problem, spend time with family and friends, take care of everyday responsibilities, and/or keep up with work duties. Nearly three in four dementia caregivers (73%) had not used caregiving resources in the past year, and among those, 41% expressed an interest in using them.

These findings suggest that there are opportunities to provide more support to dementia caregivers. A first step in meeting their needs is that health care providers should ask about caregiving responsibilities as a routine part of clinical care. As the population ages and the number of available caregivers is unlikely to keep pace, it is critically important to ensure that resources to support dementia caregivers are readily available and accessible.

Loneliness

Chronic loneliness can adversely affect memory, mental and physical health, and longevity. The NPHA asked adults aged 50 to 80 about their feelings of lack of companionship and isolation (loneliness), social interactions, and health behaviors in June 2020 as a follow-up to a similar NPHA survey conducted in October 2018 among a different national sample. The follow-up survey showed a substantial increase in loneliness among older adults from before the COVID-19 pandemic to the early months of the pandemic (March–June 2020).

As shown in **Figure 21-10**, two in five adults aged 50 to 80 reported feeling a lack of companionship (32% some of the time, 9% often) during the early months of the pandemic, compared to one-third (26% some of the time, 8% often) in 2018. In June 2020, 35% of older adults said they felt less companionship compared to before March 2020, 12% felt more, and 53% felt the same amount of companionship.

As shown in **Figure 21-10**, in June 2020, more than half of older adults reported feeling isolated from others (43% some of the time, 13% often) compared to one-quarter (22% some of the time, 5% often) in 2018. Nearly half of older adults in June 2020 reported infrequent social contact

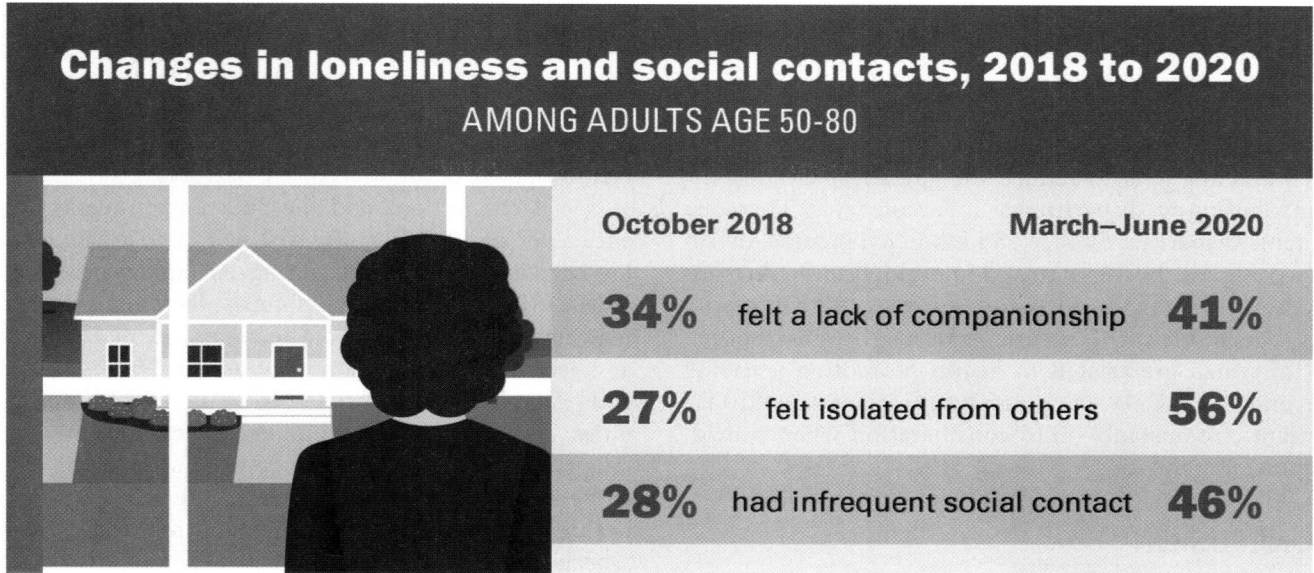

FIGURE 21-10. Loneliness. (Courtesy from National Poll on Healthy Aging. University of Michigan https://www.healthyagingpoll.org/reports-more/report/loneliness-among-older-adults-and-during-covid-19-pandemic.)

(once a week or less) with family, friends, or neighbors from outside the home, compared to one-quarter in 2018. When comparing their feelings in June 2020 to before the pandemic, about half of adults age 50 to 80 (48%) felt more isolated, 8% felt less isolated, and 44% reported feeling the same level of isolation.

Feeling a lack of companionship some of the time or often during the first 3 months of the pandemic was more common among women (47% vs 35% of men), people who lived alone (50% vs 39% who lived with others), and those who were unemployed, disabled, or not working (52% vs 39% of those employed or retired). Others more likely to report a lack of companionship included those from households with annual incomes less than $60,000 (46% vs 38% of those with higher incomes) and caregivers (48% vs 40% of non-caregivers). In addition, feeling a lack of companionship was more common for those who reported fair or poor physical health (52% vs 39% of those reporting excellent, very good, or good physical health) or fair or poor mental health (68% vs 39% of those reporting excellent, very good, or good physical health), and more common for those reporting more symptoms of depression (84% vs 36% among those with fewer symptoms).

This poll demonstrates that a greater proportion of adults aged 50 to 80 felt a lack of companionship, felt socially isolated, and had infrequent contact with others from outside their home during the early months of the pandemic than in 2018 when those numbers were already worrisomely high. Loneliness and limited social contact during the pandemic were strongly associated with depressive symptoms and overall mental health among older adults. In addition, these results suggest that those who engage in healthy behaviors less frequently experience more loneliness than those who have a healthier lifestyle (eg, get regular exercise and enough sleep). Supporting patients in maintaining connections and initiating or maintaining healthy behaviors can have wide ranging health benefits and can be protective during times of stress and uncertainty.

Built Environment

Recommendations to slow the spread of COVID-19 included staying home when possible, isolating from others if symptoms develop, and getting outdoors to safely connect with other people and exercise. Yet where a person lives, their home and neighborhood, could influence peoples' ability to follow these recommendations. In June 2020, the NPHA asked adults aged 50 to 80 about their living environments and behaviors during the pandemic.

Nearly one in five older adults who lived with others (18%) reported they do not have a place where they live to safely isolate if they were to contract COVID-19. Most adults ages 50 to 80 (85%) reported having an outdoor space (such as a balcony, patio, porch, or yard) to safely engage with their neighbors and community during the pandemic. Three in four older adults (72%) said they have a view of nature from inside their home. Two in three (68%) noted they have a greenspace (such as a garden, park, or woods) within walking distance of their home.

Older adults who had access to an outdoor space to engage with their neighbors and community, a view of nature, or nearby greenspaces were more likely to engage in outdoor activities. In addition, older adults who did not have access to outdoor spaces, a view of nature, or nearby greenspaces were more likely to report feelings of loneliness, including a lack of companionship and feeling isolated from others, than those who had access to these features in their environment.

The characteristics of homes and neighborhoods can affect an individual's ability to carry out public health recommendations to reduce the spread of COVID-19, contributing to disparities in infection rates. There are notable disparities by race and ethnicity, income, dwelling type, and health status. Some older adults are less likely to have access to outdoor spaces to engage with neighbors, views of nature, and nearby greenspaces, all of which are related to health-promoting activities beyond COVID-19. As a result, clinicians should take patient circumstances into consideration when providing recommendations.

CONCLUSION

Since 2017, the University of Michigan NPHA has provided a unique vehicle to amplify the voices of US adults aged 50 to 80 and identify and share opportunities to improve their health and health care. The findings summarized in this chapter come from a selection of prior NPHA reports. Several common themes emerge from these reports, such as the vital importance of older adults' primary care providers as trusted sources of information and guidance. While there are many existing time constraints during clinical encounters, particularly in geriatric medicine, the poll results highlight topics that are important to many patients but not always discussed by health care providers, such as sexual health, emergency preparedness, and the cost of prescription medications. Additionally, a number of factors outside of the walls of the health care system, such as social connections and the built environment, influence older adults' day-to-day well-being and are important for clinicians to consider during encounters with older patients. In these and other contexts, there remain persistent disparities by education, income, and race/ethnicity, and recent trends in technology use (eg, patient portals and telehealth) have the potential to increase health inequities. Taken together, the findings of the NPHA highlight critically important and timely opportunities for clinicians and policymakers to improve health care delivery, support health care access and decision making, and address social aspects of health for older US adults to optimize their overall well-being.

ACKNOWLEDGMENTS

We acknowledge the support of Dianne Singer, MPH (production manager), and Matthias Kirch, MA (lead data analyst), of the University of Michigan National Poll on Healthy Aging. We also acknowledge Emily Smith, MA (multimedia designer).

FURTHER READING

Agochukwu-Mmonu N, Malani PN, Wittmann D, et al. Interest in sex and conversations about sexual health with health care providers among older U.S. adults. *Clin Gerontol.* 2021;44(3):299–306.

Bell SA, Singer D, Solway E, Kirch M, Kullgren J, Malani P. Predictors of emergency preparedness among older adults in the United States. *Disaster Med Public Health Prep.* 2020;1:1–7.

Chen J, Malani P, Kullgren J. Patient Portals: Improving the health of older adults by increasing use and access. *Health Affairs Blog.* Electronically published September 6, 2018.

Feldman SJ, Solway E, Kirch M, Malani P, Singer D, Roberts JS. Correlates of formal support service use among dementia caregivers. *J Gerontol Soc Work.* 2021; 64(2):135–150.

Harbaugh CM, Malani P, Solway E, et al. Self-reported disposal of leftover opioids among US adults 50-80. *Reg Anesth Pain Med.* 2020;45(12):949–954.

Institute for Healthcare Policy & Innovation. https://ihpi.umich.edu/. Accessed June 23, 2021.

Kullgren JT, Malani P, Kirch M, et al. Older adults' perceptions of overuse. J Gen Intern Med 2020;35:365–367.

Leung CW, Kullgren JT, Malani PN, et al. Food insecurity is associated with multiple chronic conditions and physical health status among older US adults. *Prev Med Rep.* 2020;20:101211.

Malani P, Solway E, Kirch M, Singer D, Kullgren J. Use and perceptions of antibiotics among US adults aged 50–80 years. *Infect Control Hosp Epidemiol.* 2021;42(5):628–629.

Maust DT, Solway E, Langa KM, et al. Perception of dementia risk and preventive actions among US adults aged 50 to 64 years. *JAMA Neurol.* 2020;77(2):259–262.

National Poll on Healthy Aging. https://www.healthyaging-poll.org/. Accessed June 23, 2021.

Scherer AM, Solway E, Malani PM, et al. Factors associated with health insurance affordability concerns among U.S. adults age 50–64: a cross-sectional, nationally representative study. *J Gen Intern Med.* 2021;36:546–548.

Tipirneni R, Solway E, Malani P, et al. Health insurance affordability concerns and health care avoidance among US adults approaching retirement. *JAMA Netw Open.* 2020;3(2):e1920647.

Chapter 22

Medication Prescribing and De-Prescribing

Paula A. Rochon, Sudeep S. Gill, Christina Reppas-Rindlisbacher,
Nathan M. Stall, Jerry H. Gurwitz

INTRODUCTION

Prescribing for older adults presents special challenges. Older people take about three times as many prescription medications as do younger people, mainly because of an increased prevalence of chronic medical conditions among the older population. Taking several drugs together substantially increases the risk of drug interactions and adverse events, and older women are more likely than men to experience an adverse drug event (ADE).

While a provider can usually do little to alter the characteristics of individual older adults to affect the kinetics or dynamics of drugs, the decision whether to prescribe any drug, the choice of drug, and the manner in which it is to be used (eg, dose and duration of therapy) are all factors that are largely under the control of the provider. This chapter discusses ways to optimize prescribing of drug therapy for older women and men.

EPIDEMIOLOGY OF DRUG THERAPY

Writing a prescription is the most frequently employed medical intervention. Yet, creating optimal drug regimens that meet the complex needs of older adults requires careful thought and planning. Multiple factors contribute to inappropriate drug prescribing, including lack of adequate training of providers in safe prescribing practices, and in prescribing for older adults. Further, a lack of routine use of safe medication prescribing practices, such as checking drug allergies, confirming appropriate drug doses, adjusting doses for renal impairment, and potential drug–drug interactions and medication reconciliation, also contribute to prescribing errors. Avoidable ADEs are the most serious consequences of inappropriate and unsafe drug prescribing. The possibility of an ADE should always be borne in mind

Learning Objectives

- Understand the current problems with drug prescribing in older adults.
- Recognize the importance of applying a sex and gender lens to drug prescribing.
- Consider the importance of polypharmacy.
- Describe approaches to identifying inappropriate prescribing.
- Understand the importance of the deprescribing process, including utilizing tools such as the DRUGS guide to optimizing medication safety for older adults.

Key Clinical Points

1. Prescribing for older adults presents unique challenges as they are at higher risk for drug-related adverse events.
2. When prescribing medications to older adults, consider the pharmacokinetic and pharmacodynamic changes that are observed with aging and differences by sex.
3. Criteria and frameworks, developed by experts internationally to assess the quality of drug prescribing in older adults, can be applied in clinical practice.
4. Prescribing cascades are common and important to consider in older adults with multiple chronic conditions who are likely to be prescribed multiple drug therapies.

(Continued)

5. Incorporating an individual's goals of care is critical to optimizing prescribing for older adults. It is essential that the risks are balanced against the benefits of each medication. An important tension exists between avoiding inappropriate medications and avoiding underuse of potentially beneficial drugs.

6. Special considerations are needed when prescribing for long-term care residents, the majority of whom are older women and live with dementia.

7. Assessing medication safety in older adults using real-world data is critical. This process encompasses the evaluation of the safety and effectiveness of medications in large populations of older adults who may have been excluded from randomized trials. These studies also provide the opportunity to explore important sex, gender, and age-based considerations.

8. Considerations in drug prescribing in older adults range from cost-related barriers to adherence, medication review and reconciliation, the use of nonpharmacologic approaches, and the risks and benefits of deprescribing.

9. The DRUGS guide to optimize medication safety for older adults outlines steps to follow in order to optimize drug prescribing for older adults and incorporates sex and gender considerations into each step. These steps include:
   - DISCUSS goals of care
   - REVIEW medications
   - USE tools and frameworks to guide decision making
   - GERIATRIC medicine approach
   - STOP the medication where appropriate

when evaluating an older individual. A valuable maxim in geriatric medicine posits that when evaluating virtually any new symptom in an older patient, the possibility of an ADE should be considered in the differential diagnosis. Female sex, advanced age, frailty, cognitive impairment, and increased drug utilization are all factors that contribute to an individual patient's risk for developing a drug-related problem. US data indicate that older adults in the community are up to three times more likely to have an ADE that requires evaluation in an outpatient setting or in an emergency department and are seven times more likely

to require a hospital admission. In the inpatient setting, older adults account for more than 50% of hospitalizations complicated by an ADE. In the nursing home setting, the incidence of ADEs approaches 10 per 100 resident-months, of which over half may be preventable. These estimates are probably conservative because preventable ADEs were strictly defined and it was assumed that, in many cases, the prescription of the offending drug was indicated, and the ADE was therefore not preventable.

Herbal medicines are frequently used by older adults, and physicians often do not question patients about such use. An estimated 22% of the US adult population takes an herbal medicine or supplement such as ginseng, ginkgo biloba extract, and glucosamine. In one survey, almost 75% of patients did not inform their physician that they were using unconventional treatments including herbal medicines. Herbal medicines may interact with prescribed drug therapies leading to adverse events, underscoring the importance of routinely questioning patients about their use of these therapies. Examples of herbal–drug therapy interactions include warfarin in combination with ginkgo biloba extract leading to an increased risk for bleeding and serotonin-reuptake inhibitors in combination with St. John's Wort leading to serotonin syndrome.

PHARMACOKINETICS AND PHARMOCYNAMICS

When prescribing medications to older adults, it is important to consider pharmacokinetic and pharmacodynamic changes observed with aging and differing by sex. Age-related pharmacologic changes combined with sex related changes, and medical conditions that are more common in older adults can impact the pharmacokinetics of drug therapies. Understanding these issues can help to guide prescribing decisions.

Pharmacokinetics relates to the way the body handles a drug. Traditionally, pharmacokinetics involves consideration of drug absorption, distribution across body compartments, metabolism, and elimination. Drug absorption is largely unchanged with aging. Changes in drug distribution, metabolism, and excretion can impact the clearance of a medication from the body in older adults. Age-related changes in body composition can affect the volume of distribution of a drug. With advancing age, older people have less lean body mass and greater fat stores relative to younger people. These age-related changes may affect women more than men. As such, drug therapies such as benzodiazepines which are highly lipid-soluble have an increased volume of distribution in older people relative to those who are younger.

Much of the literature on age-related changes in drug metabolism has focused attention on reduced oxidative metabolism by the family of cytochrome P450 (CYP450) isoenzymes in the liver. The activity of various CYP450 isoenzymes can be inhibited or induced by a wide range of medications, which contributes to numerous drug-drug interactions. In addition, elimination of many drug therapies occurs through renal clearance, and renal function declines with age. Taken together, these age-related changes in pharmacokinetics have substantial impact on the clearance of many medications commonly used in older adults. Conventional wisdom and prudent prescribing practice warrants that special care be taken in drug dosing for older patients, particularly in the case of highly lipid soluble drugs, medications metabolized via reactions catalyzed by CYP enzymes, and renally excreted drugs. It is important to consider both age- and sex-related issues.

In contrast to pharmacokinetics, pharmacodynamics relates to the effect that a drug has on the body. Age and female sex are associated with enhanced sensitivity to a number of drug therapies. For example, older people may be more sensitive to the effects of benzodiazepines, opioids, and warfarin, exclusive of age-related pharmacokinetic changes that might exist. Older women may be even more sensitive to men to some drug therapies. This highlights the importance of integrating sex and age information when exploring pharmacodynamics and pharmacokinetics and making prescribing decisions for older women and men.

The science of geriatric pharmacology remains to be fully elucidated. A dogmatic approach to applying currently accepted principles of geriatric pharmacology in prescribing medications to older adults is not ideal. For example, the risk of fall-related injuries in older adults prescribed short half-life benzodiazepines and so-called "Z-drugs" (eg, zolpidem) may actually be similar to that of long-half-life benzodiazepines. These observations are clearly at odds with what would be expected based on the pharmacologic changes that occur with aging. Schwartz has written that "clinical factors such as disease, concomitant medications, lifestyle, diet, and nutraceutical intake may have greater effects and lead to greater variability in drug clearance and effects than would be estimated based on investigations of pure aging or sex effects in animal or human studies."

Various strategies may assist in formulating the most appropriate and individualized drug dose for older patients. These approaches may include weight-based and renal-based dosing. Individualized dosing of renally cleared medications, particularly those with a narrow therapeutic index, is facilitated by the provision of estimates of glomerular filtration rates now routinely added to the results of laboratory panels. In addition, clinical decision support tools are commonly incorporated into electronic health records to assist in the choice of medication dose when ordering for patients with reduced renal function. Finally, while controversy remains concerning the clinical utility and practicality of applying pharmacogenetic data to the direct care of older patients (eg, to guide warfarin dosing), pharmacogenetic-dosing holds both the promise and potential for enhancing the safety and effectiveness of geriatric pharmacotherapy in the future.

MEASURING THE QUALITY OF DRUG PRESCRIBING IN OLDER ADULTS

Various criteria and frameworks have been developed by experts internationally to assess the quality of medication use in older populations. These criteria generally comprise a list of drugs that are potentially inappropriate for use in older adults or highlight medications that should be considered in older people with certain indications. Criteria such as Beers and STOPP/START are designed to assist with clinical decision making and should be applied while considering patient preferences and using other tools such as clinical pharmacy interventions and computerized alerts.

One of the most widely employed approaches for the assessment of inappropriate prescribing are the Beers Criteria. These criteria, initially developed in 1991 by a consensus panel of experts in geriatric medicine, geriatric psychiatry, and pharmacology, have been updated and revised a number of times over the years and most recently in 2019. Use of drug therapies considered inappropriate according to the Beers Criteria has been identified as an ongoing issue of widespread concern across all clinical settings. The 2019 Beers Criteria update was sponsored by the American Geriatrics Society and involved a panel of 13 experts in geriatric care and pharmacology following an evidence-based approach. The aim of the 2019 update was to use a comprehensive, systematic review and grading of the evidence on drug-related problems and adverse events in older adults. The 2019 update retained each of the five criteria from 2015: (1) medications that are potentially inappropriate in most older adults, (2) those that should typically be avoided in older adults with certain conditions, (3) drugs to use with caution, (4) drug-drug interactions, and (5) drug dose adjustment based on kidney function.

A different approach to facilitating medication review in older adults is the STOPP (Screening Tool of Older Persons potentially inappropriate Prescriptions) and START (Screening Tool to Alert to Right Treatment) criteria. The STOPP criteria were initially developed in 2008 in Ireland using a Delphi consensus method with experts in geriatric medicine, clinical pharmacology, clinical pharmacy, geriatric psychiatry, and primary care. These criteria identify common instances of potentially inappropriate prescribing including drug-drug and drug-disease interactions, drugs that adversely affect those at risk for falls and duplicate drug class prescriptions. The criteria are organized by organ system, and the reason for each of the prescribing concerns is explained. The prevalence of older patients with at least one potentially inappropriate prescription identified using the STOPP criteria ranges from 21% to 39% in the primary care setting, from 26% to 77% in the hospital setting, and from 23% to 70% in nursing homes. The STOPP criteria's potentially inappropriate medications have been associated with avoidable ADEs in older people that contributed to acute care hospitalization. Version 2 of the STOPP

TABLE 22-1 ■ SCREENING TOOL OF OLDER PERSONS' PRESCRIPTIONS (STOPP) VERSION 2

Section A: Indication of medication

1. Any drug prescribed without an evidence-based clinical indication.
2. Any drug prescribed beyond the recommended duration, where treatment duration is well-defined.
3. Any duplicate drug class prescription, eg, two concurrent NSAIDs, SSRIs, loop diuretics, ACE inhibitors, anticoagulants (optimization of monotherapy within a single-drug class should be observed prior to considering a new agent).

Data from O'Mahony D, O'Sullivan D, Byrne S, et al. STOPP/START criteria for potentially inappropriate prescribing in older people: version 2. Age Ageing. 2015;44(2): 213–218.

criteria was published in 2015 and provides guidance on prescribing indicators (**Table 22-1**) along with a list of 80 evidence-based potentially inappropriate prescriptions for older adults, categorized by body system.

It is important to consider the cumulative burden of prescribing a combination of drugs with anticholinergic effects rather than view them individually. Drugs with anticholinergic effects are commonly prescribed to patients with conditions ranging from depression to urinary incontinence to neuropathic pain and migraine headaches. These therapies raise concerns for older patients because they are associated with serious adverse events including confusion, urinary retention, and constipation. The cumulative burden of anticholinergic agents may more accurately reflect the risk for development of these adverse events. A number of scales have been identified to measure anticholinergic burden. These scales assign points to commonly prescribed anticholinergic drug therapies based on the risk for developing anticholinergic adverse events. In a recent review of these scales, the *Drug Burden Index* was the most commonly used scale or tool in community and database studies, while the *Anticholinergic Risk Scale* was used more frequently in care homes and hospital settings. In a study of geriatric evaluation and management in the primary care setting, it was found that higher Anticholinergic Risk Scores were associated with an increased risk for anticholinergic-related adverse events including falls, confusion, dry mouth, and constipation.

A concern with using a limited list of "inappropriate" drug therapies like the Beers Criteria relates to the extent that such a list fully captures the spectrum of drug-related problems likely to befall older patients. For example, studies of older patients presenting to US emergency departments for ADEs or of ADEs in older patients recently discharged from the hospital have suggested that the Beers Criteria drugs capture only a very small fraction of the medications implicated in these events. The majority of these agents are not included among Beers Criteria medications. Furthermore, only a minority of Beers Criteria and STOPP/START criteria

recommendations are based on high-quality evidence, attesting to the dearth of pharmacologic and drug safety and effectiveness research that directly focuses on the older population. A 2013 report issued by the US Department of Health and Human Services on the creation of a national action plan for ADEs prevention highlighted the need to explore strategies to improve medication prescribing more broadly. This report identified older adults as one of the most vulnerable groups for the development of ADEs. The action plan identified three classes of drug therapies that were associated with the highest risk for the development of ADEs. These were anticoagulants leading to bleeding, opioids leading to delirium and mental status changes, and insulin leading to hypoglycemia.

Ultimately, many different factors contribute to making the best prescribing decisions for the individual patient. In order to remain clinically valid, prescribing appropriateness criteria must be regularly updated to keep up with the evolving clinical evidence and ever-increasing number of new medications. Appropriate prescribing also needs to consider time-to-benefit, which takes into account a patient's life stage and frailty and goes well beyond simply knowing the patient's chronologic age. What remains essential is the need for ongoing assessment of the medication regimen in light of the individual's clinical status, goals of care, and balancing of the risks and benefits of each medication.

PRESCRIBING CASCADES

A particularly concerning aspect of suboptimal medication use in older adults relates to the occurrence of prescribing cascades. The prescribing cascade concept was created by Rochon and Gurwitz in 1997 and updated in 2017. A prescribing cascade begins when a drug side effect is misinterpreted as a new medical condition. An additional drug therapy is prescribed, and the patient is placed at risk for the development of additional side effects relating to this potentially unnecessary treatment (**Figure 22-1**). Prescribing cascades and other risks associated with drug therapy are particularly important for older adults with multiple chronic conditions who are likely to be prescribed multiple drug therapies. Prescribing cascades are now part of the definition of potentially inappropriate prescribing and have been included in numerous deprescribing processes.

Selected examples of prescribing cascades are described below and summarized in **Table 22-2**.

Calcium Channel Blockers, Edema, and Diuretic Initiation

There has been concern that calcium channel blockers (CCB) used for the management of hypertension may lead to the development of edema. This drug-related side effect may in turn be misdiagnosed as a new medical condition and treated with a further drug therapy.

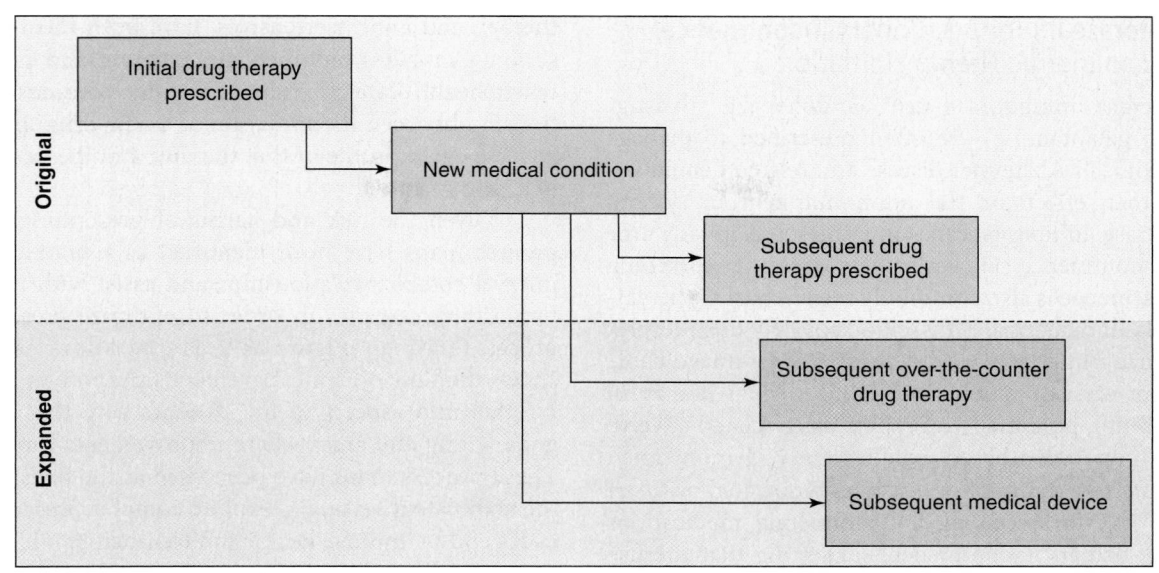

FIGURE 22-1. The prescribing cascade. (Reproduced with permission from Rochon PA, Gurwitz JH. The prescribing cascade revisited. *Lancet.* 2017;389[10081]:1778–1780.)

This association was explored in a cohort of more than 41,000 older adults with hypertension who were 66 years or older in a population-based study in Canada's most populous province of Ontario. The population-based association between the initiation of a CCB and the initiation of a diuretic therapy was demonstrated. Those who were newly dispensed a CCB had an increased risk for being dispensed a loop diuretic compared to those who were newly dispensed other antihypertensive medications or an unrelated drug therapy. This is an important prescribing cascade given that CCBs are so widely prescribed, and it highlights the importance of raising awareness of this prescribing cascade to clinicians.

Antipsychotics, Parkinsonism, and Anti-Parkinson Therapy Initiation

Antidopaminergic-related adverse effects associated with antipsychotic agents have long been recognized, including the development of extrapyramidal signs and symptoms. This drug-related symptom may be potentially misdiagnosed as a new medical condition (ie, Parkinson disease).

The association between antipsychotic drug exposure and subsequent treatment of parkinsonism was identified among 3512 adults aged 65 to 99 who were enrolled in a Medicaid program and initiated on a drug therapy for the treatment of parkinsonian symptoms. Patients dispensed a typical antipsychotic therapy or clozapine in the 90 days prior to the initiation of anti-Parkinson therapy were more than five times more likely to begin anti-Parkinson therapy relative to control patients who were not dispensed antipsychotic therapy. Furthermore, a dose–response relationship was demonstrated.

Antipsychotic therapy is widely used in older adults for the management of the behavioral and psychological symptoms of dementia. One of the initial studies to explore the association between atypical antipsychotic drug therapy and the development of parkinsonism demonstrated that these newer agents were also associated with parkinsonism and that this was in a dose-related fashion. Patients who are placed on anti-parkinsonian therapy then become vulnerable to the adverse events associated with this added therapy, including orthostatic hypotension and delirium. A better approach may be to discontinue or reduce the dose of the antipsychotic therapy. If an antipsychotic is deemed essential, it may be prudent to try to select a therapy with less potent anti-dopaminergic blockade and to use this therapy at the lowest possible dose.

Drug-induced parkinsonism has also been reported with other anti-dopaminergic therapies, including metoclopramide. Such drug-induced symptoms in an older adult can be misinterpreted as indicating the presence of a new disease or be attributed to the aging process rather than to the drug therapy. This misinterpretation is particularly likely when the symptoms are indistinguishable from an illness, such as Parkinson disease, which has a greater prevalence in older adults.

TABLE 22-2 ■ EXAMPLES OF PRESCRIBING CASCADES

INITIAL DRUG THERAPY PRESCRIBED	NEW MEDICAL CONDITION	SUBSEQUENT DRUG THERAPY PRESCRIBED
Calcium channel blockers	Edema	Diuretic
Antipsychotic (typical and atypical)	Parkinsonism	Anti-Parkinson therapy
Cholinesterase inhibitor	Urinary incontinence	Anticholinergic bladder therapy

Cholinesterase Inhibitors, Urinary Incontinence, and Anticholinergic Therapy Initiation

Cholinesterase inhibitors (such as donepezil, rivastigmine, and galantamine) are often prescribed to manage the symptoms of Alzheimer disease and related dementias. Through their effects on the autonomic nervous system, cholinesterase inhibitors can sometimes precipitate urge urinary incontinence. However, new-onset or worsening urge incontinence is also commonly seen as part of the natural history of dementia. Thus, clinicians may misinterpret incontinence in patients with dementia as an unavoidable progression of their underlying disease, when it may in fact represent a potentially reversible drug-related adverse event. A population-based cohort study demonstrated that cholinesterase inhibitor use was associated with an increased risk for receiving anticholinergic medications to manage urinary incontinence, suggesting that the use of anticholinergic drugs in patients with dementia may sometimes represent an unrecognized ADE related to cholinesterase inhibitor use. In addition, the use of anticholinergic drugs by older adults with dementia may expose them to anticholinergic adverse effects (such as urinary retention and postural hypotension) and may also counter the potential neurocognitive benefits of cholinesterase inhibitor treatment.

Other prescribing cascade scenarios, such as the association between the use of hydrochlorothiazide therapy and the initiation of anti-gout therapy or the use of NSAID therapy and antihypertensives, have been identified. Prescribing cascades only become apparent and preventable when health care providers carefully consider the relationship between the initiation of a new drug therapy, the adverse event profile of that therapy, and the development of a new symptom.

Given the risk and harms of prescribing cascades, process maps have been identified as a practical way to unravel complex relationships and assist with identifying prescribing cascades in order to optimize prescribing. A process flow map (**Figure 22-2**) is a workflow diagram that shows the flow of clinical events. Its purpose is to provide insights into aspects of the patient's care that may have gone wrong and areas where improvements can be made. These process maps have been used at the bedside and in the ambulatory setting to explore complex prescribing cascades and to improve health and well-being.

UNDERUSE OF POTENTIALLY BENEFICIAL THERAPY

Appropriate prescribing is also a highly dynamic process that changes with time, incorporating considerations of age-related physiological changes (eg, changes in renal and hepatic function), disease-related factors, and shifts in the older individual's goals of care. An important tension also exists between avoiding inappropriate medications ("errors of commission") and avoiding the underuse of potentially

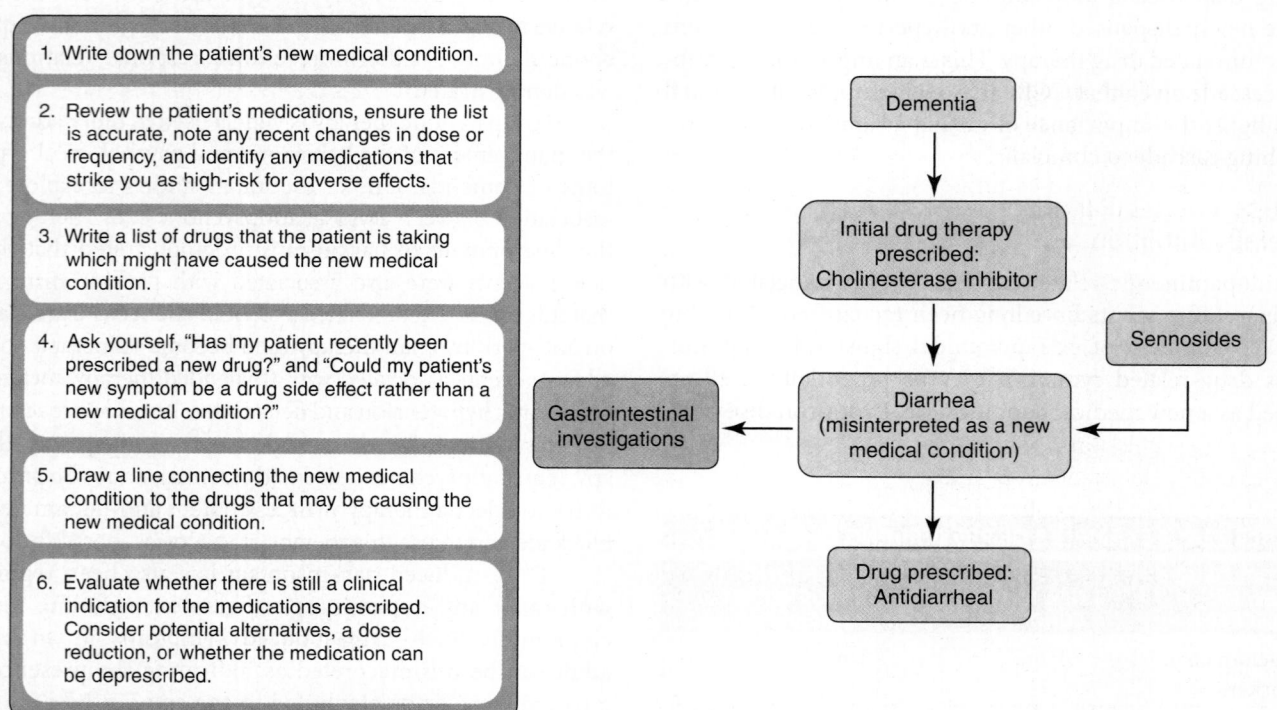

FIGURE 22-2. How to create a clinical process map of a prescribing cascade, and an example of a clinical process map investigating a prescribing cascade. (Modified with permission from Piggott KL, Mehta N, Wong CL, et al. Using a clinical process map to identify prescribing cascades in your patient. *BMJ.* 2020;368:m261.)

beneficial drugs ("errors of omission"). As a result of these many influences, appropriate prescribing for older adults represents a complex and ever-shifting balancing act for clinicians.

Polypharmacy may be necessary and appropriate in some patients to permit the optimal management of their multiple chronic conditions. Underuse of beneficial therapy must be carefully balanced against inappropriate overprescribing. The tension between these two aspects of prescribing is complex. Interestingly, overprescribing of inappropriate medications and underprescribing of beneficial medications are correlated, with both simultaneously present in more than 40% of older adults in some studies.

Conceptual Definition of Underuse

Underuse of medications is conceptually defined as the absence of initiation of an effective treatment in an individual with a condition for which there exists one or more medications with a favorable benefit-to-risk ratio. Frail older adults are often underrepresented in pivotal clinical trials evaluating medications and the true benefit-to-risk ratio may be different from that observed in younger and healthier study participants. Thus, determinations of underuse require a careful assessment of whether randomized clinical trial results are truly generalizable to the older adult being cared for in real-world settings of care. Analyses focusing on older participants and post-marketing pharmacosurveillance studies can provide a more complete picture of the likely benefits and risks of medications that may not be initially apparent.

Operational Definition of Underuse

Attempts have been made to operationally define medication underuse in older adults. Analogous to the development of tools designed to define potentially inappropriate prescribing or "errors of commission"; there are now tools available to assist with the operational definition of underuse of potentially beneficial medications.

The START criteria represent an explicit tool to identify underuse of potentially beneficial medications. The START criteria include 34 evidence-based prescribing indications for older adults and also categorize medications according to organ system. The prevalence of potential prescription omissions, according to START criteria, was 23% among older adults in primary care, from 42% to 66% in hospitalized older adults, and from 42% to 44% among nursing home residents.

Assessing Underuse: Implications of Clinical Practice Guideline Recommendations

Different approaches to profiling underuse of potentially beneficial medications have been applied. A common approach to characterizing underprescribing is to assess the use of medications that clinical practice guidelines suggest should be prescribed to treat or prevent a condition in the absence of contraindications. This approach has been used in a number of studies to demonstrate underuse of specific drug therapies in the care of patients with heart failure, myocardial infarction, osteoporotic fractures, atrial fibrillation, and depression. Unfortunately, most clinical guidelines do not incorporate considerations such as life expectancy and time needed to derive clinical benefit as legitimate justifications to forego prescribing a "beneficial" medication to a patient. In addition, several studies have emphasized that caution should be exercised when applying disease-specific clinical practice guidelines to older adults with multiple chronic diseases.

Striking the Right Balance in Prescribing

Incorporating an individual's goals of care and preferences is critical to making optimal prescribing decisions relating to older patients. Holmes and colleagues have proposed a practical strategy whereby life expectancy, time to realization of treatment benefit, primary goals of care (eg, prevention, cure, or palliation), and validity of specific treatment targets (eg, blood pressure) are integrated to decide on appropriate treatments for older individuals with the aim of minimizing unwarranted polypharmacy. Information about estimating remaining life expectancy in older adults can inform decision making around prescribing a new medication, as an understanding of the lag time until benefit is achieved for a specific medication under consideration. In individuals with advanced dementia for whom the primary goal is focused on quality of life, there may be opportunities to deprescribe medications that were previously considered essential (eg, lipid-lowering therapy with statins) to help reduce the overall pill burden, cost, and the potential for drug-drug interactions and ADEs.

An important example of striking the right balance is the case of antihypertensive treatment regimens in older adults. In 2015, a landmark trial titled SPRINT evaluated the benefits of intensive versus standard blood pressure control and concluded that among patients at high risk of cardiovascular disease (eg, > 75 years), a systolic blood pressure target of less than 120 mmHg resulted in decreased death from any cause. However, applying this intensive target to all adults over the age of 75 without considering comorbidities, the risk of falls and frailty status may have unintended harmful results. Prescribers should be cognizant of the potential for increased harm from a systolic blood pressure target of less than 140 mmHg in the following patient groups: older than 80 years, moderate to severe frailty, cognitive impairment or functional limitations, history of orthostatic hypotension or labile blood pressure, syncope and falls. Intensifying blood pressure medications in hospitalized older adults is particularly problematic and can lead to adverse outcomes such as syncope and falls. Maximizing the net benefit of blood pressure treatment in older patients requires applying the guidelines in an individualized manner while considering the setting, patient values and preferences, and level of comorbidity and frailty.

SPECIAL CONSIDERATIONS REGARDING DRUG THERAPY IN LONG-TERM CARE SETTINGS

Long-term care residents include a disproportionate number of women, people of advanced age, and those with multiple chronic conditions including dementia. Medications are the most commonly used therapeutic intervention in the nursing home setting. Nearly half of all nursing home residents take nine or more medications every day, placing this group at particularly high risk for ADEs.

Antipsychotic Therapy in the Long-Term Care Setting

In long-term care homes, excess use of antipsychotic therapy for the management of the behavioral and psychological symptoms of dementia continues to be a focus of great concern. Atypical antipsychotic medications are among the drugs most frequently associated with adverse events in long-term care homes. While recent data suggest that use of antipsychotic therapy has declined in US nursing homes over recent years, nearly one in five long-stay nursing home residents continue to be prescribed antipsychotic medications. Further, there is substantial variation in the use of antipsychotic therapy by geographic region and between nursing homes in the same region. A study of antipsychotic therapy in provincially regulated Canadian nursing homes found that antipsychotic prescribing rates were more than double in those with the highest rates of antipsychotic prescribing compared to those with the lowest rates of antipsychotic prescribing. Compared with individuals residing in nursing homes with the lowest mean antipsychotic prescribing rates, those residing in homes with the highest rates were three times more likely to be dispensed an antipsychotic therapy irrespective of their potential clinical indication. There is accumulating evidence that the benefit from atypical antipsychotics for the management of behavioral and psychological symptoms in Alzheimer-type dementia may be offset by the increased risk for ADEs. There is also evidence that antipsychotic use is associated with an increased risk of death with both conventional and atypical antipsychotic drug therapy in older adults with dementia-related behavioral disorders. Health Canada and the US Food and Drug Administration (FDA) have issued strong warnings about their use. Given these important safety concerns, the use of antipsychotic therapy should generally be reserved for situations where the benefit clearly outweighs the risk, such as in situations where the behavior poses a risk to the resident or others. Additionally, antipsychotic therapy should be frequently reassessed, with consideration for lower the dose or discontinuing the therapy altogether in favor of superior non-pharmacological approaches.

Risk of Adverse Drug Events in the Long-Term Care Setting

The occurrence of preventable ADEs is among the most serious concerns regarding suboptimal medication use in the nursing home setting. Few studies have systematically examined the incidence of ADEs in the nursing home population. In a study conducted in two academic long-term care homes in Ontario and Connecticut over a 9-month period, drug-related incidents were detected by computer-generated signals from a computerized physician order entry system, clinical pharmacist investigators, and periodic review of medical record.

In this study, residents using anticoagulants, atypical antipsychotics, diuretics, anti-infectives, and anticonvulsants were at greatest risk for ADEs. Psychoactive drugs (ie, antipsychotics, antidepressants, and sedatives/hypnotics), cardiovascular and anticoagulants were the most commonly implicated drug categories associated with the occurrence of preventable ADEs (**Table 22-3**). Confusion, oversedation, delirium, and hemorrhagic events were the most commonly identified preventable ADEs. Errors resulting in preventable ADEs occurred most often at the stages of ordering and monitoring. Among the prescribing errors, the most common were wrong dose, wrong drug choice, and known drug interaction. Dispensing and administration errors were less commonly identified. Independent risk factors for experiencing a preventable ADE included using medications in several drug categories, such as antipsychotic agents, anticoagulants, diuretics, and antiepileptics. Extrapolating from the results of this research, 1.9 million ADEs per year may occur among the 1.6 million US nursing home residents and more than 40% may be preventable. There are almost 86,000 fatal or life-threatening ADEs per year, of which 70% may be preventable. Drug-related morbidity and mortality is one of the most important areas to target in efforts to both improve the quality of medical care for older adults and reduce the costs of health care for this population.

Failures in the design of systems of care are considered the most important contributor to the occurrence of medical errors, as well as the injuries that result from some of those errors. Enhanced surveillance and reporting systems for ADEs occurring in the nursing home setting are required as are continued educational efforts relating to the optimal use of drug therapies in the frail older patient population. However, as Leape et al. concluded in regard to the occurrence of serious medication errors, "preventive efforts that focus solely on the individual provider or which rely on inspection alone have limited impact. Analysis and the correction of underlying systems faults is much more likely to result in enduring changes and significant error reduction." Ordering and monitoring errors in the nursing home setting may be particularly amenable to prevention strategies that use systems-based approaches. The benefits

TABLE 22-3 ■ FREQUENCY OF ADVERSE DRUG EVENTS AND POTENTIAL ADVERSE DRUG EVENTS IN LONG-TERM CARE FACILITIES BY DRUG CLASS[a]

DRUG CLASS	ADVERSE DRUG EVENTS NO. (%) (N = 815)	PREVENTABLE ADVERSE DRUG EVENTS NO. (%) (N = 318)	NONPREVENTABLE ADVERSE DRUG EVENTS NO. (%) (N = 497)
Atypical and typical antipsychotics	110 (11)	52 (16)	58 (12)
Antibiotics/anti-infectives	106 (13)	5 (2)	101 (20)
Antidepressants	77 (9)	41 (13)	36 (7)
Sedatives/hypnotics	61 (8)	43 (14)	18 (4)
Anticoagulants	167 (21)	65 (20)	102 (21)
Antiseizure	40 (5)	22 (7)	18 (4)
Cardiovascular	195 (24)	98 (31)	97 (20)
Hypoglycemics	49 (6)	26 (8)	23 (5)
Nonopioid analgesics	26 (3)	16 (5)	10 (2)
Opioids	51 (6)	26 (8)	25 (5)
Antiparkinsonians	11 (1)	4 (1)	7 (1)

[a]Drugs in more than one category were associated with some events. Frequencies in each column sum to greater than the total number cited.
Data from Gurwitz JH, Field TS, Judge J, et al. The incidence of adverse drug events in two large academic long-term care facilities. Am J Med. 2005;118(3):251–258.

of these approaches to error reduction have been reported in the hospital setting with computerized order entry. A computer-based decision aid reduced in-hospital inappropriate dosing of psychotropic medications for geriatric inpatients. Successes in the hospital setting pave the way for similar efforts in long-term care. For instance, clinical decision support at the time of medication ordering has been shown to improve the quality of prescribing to long-term care home residents with renal insufficiency.

DEFICIENCIES IN INFORMATION ABOUT DRUG THERAPY IN OLDER ADULTS

Selecting the right medication and the right dose to prescribe for an older adult is difficult because so little evidence is available to guide choices. Decision making often has to draw on information obtained from study participants who are different from those encountered in real world settings, where patients often have several medical conditions and are taking more than one drug. The results of clinical trials of treatments for conditions commonly affecting older people often cannot be directly extrapolated to individual patients, as older adults, particularly women, frail persons and those with multiple illnesses, have often been excluded from participation in clinical trials. This poses challenges to the adoption of clinical practice guidelines developed to improve the quality of health care for many chronic conditions. A review of clinical practice guidelines for nine common chronic diseases promulgated by national and international medical organizations found that they did not modify or discuss the applicability of their recommendations for older patients with multiple comorbidities. Most did not comment on medication burden, short- and long-term goals, and the quality of the underlying scientific evidence, nor give guidance for incorporating patient preferences into treatment plans. Boyd and colleagues have reported that if relevant guidelines were followed, a hypothetical 79-year-old patient with osteoporosis, osteoarthritis, type 2 diabetes mellitus, hypertension, and chronic obstructive pulmonary disease would be prescribed 12 medications. The doses of those drugs may be inappropriately high, particularly for older women who are commonly underrepresented in clinical trials. There are several ways in which the quality and availability of information about the use of drugs in older adults might be improved. These include enhancing the inclusion of older adults in drug trials, and using observational studies and systematic reviews to provide information to guide clinical decision making.

Inclusion of Older Adults in Clinical Trials

In 1989, the US FDA published "Guidelines for the Study of Drugs Likely to be Used in the Elderly." The guideline was intended to encourage routine and thorough evaluation in older populations of the effects of new drugs being proposed for federal approval so that physicians would have sufficient information to use such drugs properly. The guidelines state "there is no good basis for the exclusion of patients on the basis of advanced age alone, or because of the presence of any concomitant illness or medication, unless there is a reason to believe that the concomitant illness or medication will endanger the patient or lead to confusion in interpreting the results of the study." It was not until 1993 the US National Institutes of Health (NIH) created guidelines for the inclusion of women and minority groups in the studies that they funded. Further, it was only in 2019 that the NIH Inclusion Across the Lifespan policy was put in place

310

CHAPTER 22 MEDICATION PRESCRIBING AND DE-PRESCRIBING

to address the underrepresentation of older adults in their studies. The concern is that when policies focus separately on sex and age, the intersection required to identify older women who are most at risk for drug-related adverse events will be missed. Drug trials should include study subjects that reflect the group that would eventually be prescribed the therapy, but this is often not what happens.

A case in point are trials in cardiovascular disease, which is overwhelmingly a disease of old age. A recent study of NIH-funded trials before and after the introduction of the new Inclusion Across the Lifespan policy showed that despite the implementation of new safeguards, older adults continue to be underrepresented where 30% of trials had explicit age limits and 70% excluded participants due to factors which disproportionally impact older adults (functional status, cognitive impairment, or decreased life expectancy). Meanwhile, outcomes relevant to geriatric populations, such as measures of function, mobility, or quality of life, were usually lacking. Another study examining NIH-funded phase III clinical trials since the introduction of the policy found that 67% of studies reported mean or median ages that skewed younger than expected for the disease or condition of interest. As with the cardiovascular trials, older adults were often implicitly excluded based on polypharmacy/concomitant medication (37%) or cardiac issues (30%). Ongoing evaluation of enrollment by age group and reasons for exclusions will be critical to monitoring the success of the policy and improving the collection of evidence for drug therapies in older adults.

The underrepresentation of older individuals in clinical trials can be considered from a variety of perspectives. Even in the absence of explicit age limits or criteria that preclude eligibility based on clinical or functional grounds, older adults may be excluded. Often large numbers of older patients need to be screened to enroll just one eligible study participant, with an adverse impact on costs and the ability to meet study timelines. In addition, participation in a clinical trial by an older adult may never even be considered, relating to a confluence of factors, including bias, value judgments, and rationalization. The dynamics of the patient-physician relationship may confuse legitimate clinical concerns with subjective feelings regarding what is best for the older adult.

ASSESSING MEDICATION SAFETY IN OLDER ADULTS

Pharmacoepidemiology uses the science of clinical epidemiology to measure patterns of medication use and outcomes in large populations. Pharmacoepidemiology allows assessment of the safety and efficacy of medications in large populations, which are often more diverse than the participants in randomized trials, over long periods of time.

Advantages of Pharmacoepidemiologic Studies

The advantages of pharmacoepidemiology over randomized controlled trials include (1) detection of adverse events that are too rare or too delayed to be detected in randomized trials; (2) assessment of efficacy over longer periods in a broader population; (3) correlation of medication use with outcomes that may not have been assessed in randomized trials; (4) assessment of safety and efficacy of medications beyond the stringent monitoring of a randomized trial.

Pharmacoepidemiology is a particularly useful tool to assess medications in older adults. Older adults are often excluded from randomized trials, either on the basis of age alone, or because of comorbidities, co-medications, or functional impairment. Observational pharmacoepidemiologic studies can assess patterns of medication use, safety, and efficacy in frail individuals. It is particularly important to understand safety and efficacy over many years when deciding whether to continue or cease medications in older adults who have often been taking their medicines for decades. Many randomized trials only assess disease and mortality outcomes, and pharmacoepidemiologic studies can correlate medication exposure with functional and quality-of-life measures that may be more relevant to older adults. Pharmacoepidemiology assesses the effects of medications in the presence of medication management issues that occur in real clinical settings, for example, limited adherence and monitoring.

Limitations of Pharmacoepidemiologic Studies

Pharmacoepidemiologic studies can be limited by confounding and bias. Interpretation of studies is limited by variable prescribing patterns, variable comorbidities, confounding by indication, severity and prognosis, and controlling for the time dependency of drug use. Studies that rely on large epidemiologic databases often contain very limited clinical information, including the exact indication for prescribing a given medication. There are several emerging approaches to manage confounders, including restricting study populations to more homogeneous groups, creating a propensity score to predict the probability of receiving a drug based on baseline covariates, and examining within-patient variability of drug exposure using crossover designs.

Sex and Gender-Based Considerations

Age-based exclusions may also have important secondary effects on the participation of women in clinical trials. A number of studies have demonstrated a strong association between the average age of participants in a clinical trial and the enrollment of women, because women account for a substantially greater proportion of the older adult population than do men. Many of the ongoing concerns regarding the enrollment of women in clinical trials are intimately related to the exclusion of older participants.

The underrepresentation of older women and lack of sex and age disaggregated data in clinical research are concerning. The case of zolpidem dosing is just one example where increased harms for women were not discovered until post-marketing surveillance. A growing body of research highlights the influence of sex on drug-related adverse events and other clinically relevant health outcomes. Sex and gender factors are still largely neglected in research, and this has become starkly evident in the case of COVID-19 related studies, where less than 5% of investigators had planned for sex disaggregated data analysis in their studies. In the case of SGLT-2 inhibitors for diabetes, current guidelines do not reflect the fact that these drugs appear to be less effective in reducing major adverse cardiac events in women compared to men. Funding agencies must set analysis guidelines for drug trials to report sex disaggregated adverse events and outcomes for all therapeutics including vaccines and devices. Understanding the sex and gender factors that influence efficacy and adverse events will help regulatory bodies and providers provide safe, evidence-based, and equitable care.

ADDITIONAL ISSUES RELATED TO DRUG THERAPY IN OLDER ADULTS

Cost-Related Non-Adherence

A prescription may be written but not dispensed, or dispensed but not taken regularly. A common barrier to appropriate medication use relates to financial considerations. The use of drug therapy has been shown to be directly related to coverage of drug costs. It is estimated that more than 40% of all Medicare enrollees in the United States had no coverage for outpatient drug expenditures prior to the implementation of the 2003 Medicare Modernization Act. In the United States, cost has been identified as an important reason that patients do not take medication that are prescribed by their health care provider. Specifically, among older adults and prior to the implementation of Medicare Part D, 13% of a national sample of 13,869 noninstitutionalized Medicare enrollees reported cost-related underuse of medications. Those in fair to poor health, with multiple comorbidities, and without coverage were most at risk.

Following the implementation of Medicare Part D, there were incremental improvements in medication affordability for older Americans. Recent concerns have been raised that these trends, especially for Medicare beneficiaries with multiple chronic conditions, have plateaued or even reversed, indicating that high drug costs remain a persistent barrier for this vulnerable population. Practical strategies available to optimize pre- and post-discharge medication management have been reviewed and can aid in improving outcomes in vulnerable older patients.

Limited Manufacturing of Low-Dose Formulations of Recommended Drug Therapy

Limited manufacturing of low-dose formulations of drug therapy may make it more difficult or expensive for patients to take their prescribed drug therapy. Low-dose therapy is often recommended for older adults but may not be manufactured or available from publicly funded drug programs in the prescribed low dose. For example, there is considerable evidence supporting the efficacy and greater safety of low doses of thiazide diuretic therapy in the treatment of hypertension in the older patient population. The Joint National Committee on Detection, Evaluation, and Treatment of High Blood Pressure Guidelines suggest starting antihypertensive therapy at low doses. Specifically, these guidelines suggest that therapy could be initiated with a thiazide diuretic. Low doses of thiazide diuretics often produce as large an antihypertensive effect as larger doses, with a reduced risk for metabolic abnormalities.

Women are more likely than men to require a lower dose of drug therapies. Despite this there are only a very few drug therapies used by women that are manufactured with a dose for women and another for men. Zolpidem, a widely used sleep aid, was on the market for more than 20 years before data became available showing that next morning drowsiness interfering with the ability to drive was greater in women than men. As a result, the dose for women is now half of the dose that is recommended for men.

Medication Review and Reconciliation

Medication review is required on a regular basis to determine if the medications prescribed to an older adult are appropriate for them. Randomized controlled trials examining the effect of medication reviews report mixed results. All studies have reported that medication review leads to recommendations for different types of changes, including elimination of drugs, increasing the number of drugs, therapeutic substitutions, or better dosing. There are few reported statistically significant changes in patient drug use and drug expenditures. Studies that involved direct contact between the consulting pharmacist and the patient appeared to be more effective than interventions aimed at recommending drug changes to the patient's physician. One intervention study found that patients were resistant to reducing medications to recommended levels, particularly psychoactive drugs.

Medication reconciliation determines if the prescribed drugs are taken as they have been prescribed and intended. In the United States, the Joint Commission has required accredited facilities to implement a system of medication reconciliation to reduce medication errors at transitions of care. Medication reconciliation is defined as the process of identifying the most accurate list of all medications that the patient is taking, including name, dosage, frequency, and route, by comparing the medical record to an external list of medications obtained from a patient, hospital, or other provider (**Table 22-4**). Patients and responsible physicians, nurses, and pharmacists should be involved in the medication reconciliation process. This reconciliation is done to avoid medication errors such as omissions, duplications, dosing errors, or drug interactions. Changes in medication (different dose, discontinued therapies, additional therapies), common during care transitions,

TABLE 22-4 ■ FIVE STEPS OF MEDICATION RECONCILIATION

1. Develop a list of current medications.
2. Develop a list of medications to be prescribed.
3. Compare the medications on the two lists.
4. Make a clinical decision based on the comparison.
5. Communicate the new list to the patient and appropriate caregivers.

Data from Hospital: 2022 National Patient Safety Goals. National Patient Safety Goals®. The Joint Commission, January 1, 2022.

are a frequent source of medication errors and confusion. ADEs attributed to medication changes occurred in 20% of patients on transfer from hospital to a nursing home, happening most commonly for patients on readmission to the nursing home. One study found that discharged patients understood the potential side effects of their medications less frequently than their attending physicians believed. One Canadian multisite study found that 25% of 325 older adults experienced an ADE after discharge home from the hospital; half of these events were considered preventable. Medication reconciliation systems and processes have successfully reduced medication errors in many health care organizations. Pharmacy technicians at one hospital reduced potential ADEs by 80% within 3 months by obtaining medication histories of patients scheduled for surgery.

In the United States, policy efforts to promote the use of new health care information technology serve to encourage medication reconciliation as patients transition from one setting of care (eg, hospital, ambulatory primary care, ambulatory specialty care, nursing home, home health, rehabilitation) to another or from one health care provider to another. For example, the Health Information Technology for Economic and Clinical Health (HITECH) Act and Meaningful Use criteria (stage 1) require that health professionals who receive a patient from another setting of care or provider of care should perform medication reconciliation.

Medication reconciliation has been recognized as a key component of patient safety, but there remains a lack of consensus and evidence about the most effective methods of implementing reconciliation. Reviews suggest that this lack of consensus stems in part from the low certainty of the evidence. Targeting specific vulnerable patient populations for medication reconciliation may be more effective than widescale nontargeted reconciliation efforts.

Consider Nonpharmacologic Approaches

Physicians should limit prescribing a new drug therapy to situations in which benefits clearly outweigh risks and to use drug therapy only after potentially safer alternatives have been attempted. For example, the use of NSAIDs to manage pain in older adults with osteoarthritis may be inappropriate because safer options are available. Epidemiologic and clinical studies have characterized the adverse consequences of NSAID use in older adults, particularly the association between NSAID use and gastrointestinal bleeds and renal impairment. Thus, alternative approaches should be considered before NSAIDs are prescribed for indications such as osteoarthritis. Possible nonpharmacologic approaches, such as gentle exercise and weight reduction, may be beneficial alternatives to treatment with NSAIDs. When pharmacologic therapy is required, a drug therapy with a more favorable adverse event profile, such as acetaminophen, should be tried first.

Another example is the use of nonpharmacologic approaches to manage behavioral and psychological symptoms of dementia. Behavioral symptoms such as wandering and agitation are common and represent a major source of disability and caregiver distress. These symptoms frequently result in prescriptions for psychotropic medications such as antipsychotic drugs, but these drugs are on average only modestly effective and can provoke serious adverse effects. Thus, nonpharmacologic strategies are increasing emphasized to manage behavioral symptoms in dementia, and are usually recommended as first-line treatments. The evidence base has grown recently to support a wide variety of nonpharmacologic treatments for the behavioral and psychological symptoms of dementia. Examples of effective nonpharmacologic treatment strategies include caregiver education and support, training in problem solving, and targeted interventions directed at the underlying causes for specific behaviors (eg, introduction of structured nighttime routines to reduce sleep disturbances). Nonpharmacologic management can improve both patient and caregiver quality of life and can help to reduce the inappropriate use of potential harmful psychotropic medications such as antipsychotic drugs.

Deprescribing

Deprescribing has been defined by Scott as the process of "identifying and discontinuing drugs in instances in which existing or potential harms outweigh existing or potential benefits within the context of an individual patient's care goal, current level of functioning, life expectancy, values, and preferences." Medication review and reconciliation may indicate the need for changes to currently prescribed drug therapies, especially if new evidence has emerged about the benefits and risks of these drug therapies. These changes may include discontinuation of a therapy prescribed for an indication that no longer exists or reduction in dosage of a drug that the patient still needs to take.

Physicians are often reluctant to deprescribe, for example, reduce or stop medications, especially if they did not initiate the treatment and the patient seems to be tolerating the therapy. Sometimes, medications only expose the patient to the risks for an adverse event with limited or no therapeutic benefit. The use of chronic digoxin therapy among older adults with normal systolic function is one such example. Use of digoxin therapy by older adults is not without risk. Renal impairment that progresses over time or dehydration associated with a gastrointestinal or respiratory illness or a urinary tract infection may predispose older adults to digoxin toxicity. Often, digoxin therapy has been prescribed for years for reasons that were not well-documented. In a small study of 23 nursing home residents with normal sinus rhythm, normal ejection fraction, and no clinical evidence of heart failure, digoxin was discontinued in 14 residents. One patient developed a decreased ejection fraction (from 60% to 50%) and digoxin therapy was restarted even though the patient remained clinically asymptomatic. At 2 months following the discontinuation of digoxin therapy, all patients with digoxin therapy discontinued remained clinically stable. These findings suggest that digoxin can be safely discontinued in select nursing home residents. Other investigators, however, have found that discontinuation of digoxin therapy in patients with impaired systolic function can have a detrimental effect.

Scott and colleagues have commented on the dangers of *therapeutic inertia*—whereby drugs continue to be prescribed in the absence of periodic review of net benefit—and *therapeutic momentum*, where more drugs are added in response to new but questionable indications, including unrecognized side effects arising from preexisting medications, potentially resulting in a prescribing cascade. Therapeutic inertia can also be avoided by periodically repeating the process of comprehensive medication review, with this process triggered in particular at times when the patient experiences an important health transition (eg, development of a new medical condition and/or changes in their preferences or overall goals of care).

PRACTICAL APPROACH TO OPTIMIZING MEDICATIONS IN OLDER ADULTS

The DRUGS guide to optimize medication safety for older adults was created by an international group of eight geriatricians from six countries. This guide outlines steps for prescribers to follow to optimize drug prescribing for older adults (**Figure 22-3**). These steps are DISCUSS goals of care, REVIEW medications, USE tools and frameworks to guide decision making, follow a GERIATRIC medicine approach, and STOP medications where appropriate, all while integrating critical sex and gender considerations.

DISCUSS goals of care and what matters most to the patient. It is essential to tailor the prescribing approach to the individual patient and emphasize the importance of taking primary goals of care (eg, prevention, cure, or palliation) into consideration, an approach described by Holmes and colleagues. Others have also emphasized the importance of incorporating patient preferences and what represents meaningful health outcomes for the individual and their family. For example, the Canadian Geriatrics Society 5M model highlights "Matters Most" as one of the pillars to optimizing geriatric care. Taking into consideration the health goals and care preferences of the patient and their family is a critical component of comprehensive care. With the patient's overall goals of care in mind, it becomes easier to

balance potential tensions between clinical practice guideline recommendations and the inappropriate generation of problematic polypharmacy.

REVIEW medications. To conduct a medication review, the prescriber should ask the patient to bring all the bottles of pills, dosettes, and/or blister packs that they are using to their visit. For example, patients may not consider over-the-counter (OTC) products, ointments, vitamins, ophthalmic preparations, or herbal medicines to be drug therapies and thus, need to be specifically told to bring these therapies to the visit. In addition, patients should be instructed to keep a complete, accurate, and up-to-date medication list including over-the-counter medications and herbal preparations. A patient-generated list is particularly important as they are frequently prescribed medications from several physicians and patients may receive their medications from several pharmacies.

A periodic comprehensive review of the drug regimen that a patient is taking is an essential component of the medical care of an older adult; this process is referred to as medication reconciliation with the development of the best possible medication history, including OTC and herbal/nutraceutical products as detailed earlier. In addition to an accurate and complete medication list, details regarding the patient's medical history and the clinical indications for each medication, sociodemographic information (ie, gender considerations) previous ADEs including drug sensitivities and allergies should also be obtained and documented.

Although there are an increasing number of effective medications for preventing or controlling a range of illnesses and for alleviating many symptoms, several studies show that adherence decreases, and adverse medication effects increase, with the complexity of the medication regimen. The goal should thus be to implement the simplest regimen that controls the patient's symptoms and illnesses, and optimizes disease prevention. A medication grid, which displays each medication with dosage and frequency, has been found effective at facilitating the reduction in medication complexity. Where appropriate, nonpharmacologic approaches should be considered as first-line treatment.

It is important to emphasize that prescribing is a dynamic and iterative process and thus, the determination of appropriate prescribing needs should be periodically repeated, especially when the patient experiences an important health transition. Assessment for changes to a patient's medication regimen should be conducted as the patient's health evolves and also as newer evidence emerges about the benefits and harms of existing drug therapies and the introduction of newer treatments.

USE tools and frameworks. When reviewing medications, it is important to utilize available tools and frameworks to help guide decision making. Well-known tools used to identify potentially inappropriate prescribing include the Beers Criteria and the STOPP criteria. To identify drugs with strong anticholinergic effects, consider consulting the

		DRUGS Guide to Optimising Medication Safety for Older Adults	Sex and Gender Considerations
D		**DISCUSS goals of care and what matters most to the patient** • Include patients and caregivers in deprescribing discussions to ensure decisions focus on goals of care	Women are more likely than men to be caregivers, and might not have a caregiver to advocate for them.

R		**REVIEW medications**
		• Encourage patients to bring all prescribed and over-the-counter medications to their appointment
		• Review medications on an ongoing basis and when clinical conditions or goals of care change
		  • Discontinue potentially unnecessary drugs
		  • Consider drug side-effects as a potential cause for a new symptom
		  • Consider nonpharmacological options
		  • Change for safer alternatives
		  • Lower the dose
		• To identify possible prescribing cascades, determine when the medication was started and why
			Women use more prescribed and over-the-counter medications than men.

U		**USE tools and frameworks**
		• Identify drugs from the inappropriate prescribing tools, including Beers Criteria or STOPP criteria
		• Use the STOPPFrail list when the individual is extremely frail and approaching the end of life
		• Consider whether the new or existing medical condition could be the result of a prescribing cascade and ask:
		  • Is a new drug being prescribed to manage a side-effect from another prescribed drug?
		  • Could the initial drug be replaced with a safer drug or could the dose be reduced?
		  • Does the patient need the first drug or could this drug be stopped?
		• Pay attention to older people who are receiving so-called good drugs with narrow therapeutic windows that might no longer be needed or for whom dose reduction might be beneficial
			Women are more often prescribed psychoactive drugs, whereas men are more often prescribed secondary prevention drugs; women might require lower doses; men receive more aggressive medical therapy.

G		**GERIATRIC medicine approach** • Geriatricians carefully consider how multiple medical problems, frailty, cognitive impairment, and limited life expectancy reduce medication benefit, increase adverse events, or interfere with medication adherence	Women are more likely than men to have multiple medical problems, frailty, and adverse drug events; men are more likely than women to adhere to drug therapies; women might be less able than men to pay for medicines, decreasing adherence.
S		**STOP the medications** • Consider the algorithm created by Scott or the Good Palliative–Geriatric Practice algorithm to guide deprescribing	Women are more likely to discuss deprescribing with providers than men.

FIGURE 22-3. DRUGS guide to optimising medication safety for older adults. (Reproduced with permission from Rochon PA, Petrovic M, Cherubini A, et al. Polypharmacy, inappropriate prescribing, and deprescribing in older people: through a sex and gender lens. *Lancet Healthy Longev.* 2021;2[5]:E290–E300.)

Drug Burden Index and the Anticholinergic Risk Scale. Frameworks that can guide medication reviews are the prescribing cascade and the US National Action Plan for Adverse Drug Event Prevention, which provides helpful guidance to inform prescribing. These tools do not consider sex and gender. It will be important for clinicians to consider how sex and gender may impact their prescribing.

GERIATRIC medicine approach. When considering medication change, one approach described by Steinman and Hanlon is to match the patient's conditions to each of the medications. Through this process, areas where there is a mismatch can be identified. For example, situations where a drug is used with no indication, conditions that may benefit from a therapy where a therapy is not currently being offered, and drugs that are being given for an appropriate indication but where there is room for improvement (eg, dose adjustment or substitution with a drug therapy with a better risk-to-benefit profile). Further, the match between the medical condition and the medications should be directed not only by clinical guidelines but should also take into consideration the patient's goals of care and sociodemographic/sociocultural factors.

STOP medications. In some cases, there will be a need to deprescribe drug therapy by reducing the dose or stopping the medication entirely. The CEASE deprescribing protocol outlined by Scott provides excellent guidance of the factors to evaluate when considering discontinuing or reducing the dose of a medication.

Many ADEs are dose related, so it is critical to prescribe the minimal dose required to obtain clinical benefit. A classic example of a dose-related adverse event is the association between use of long elimination half-life hypnotic-anxiolytics, antipsychotics, and tricyclic antidepressants and the development of hip fractures. A dose-related association has been found for each class of drug.

Another clinically important example of the benefit of reducing the dose involves the intensity of diabetes treatment. The doses of oral hypoglycemic agents and insulin therapy should not result in overly tight glycemic control, as there is little evidence that using medications to achieve tight glycemic control in older adults with type 2 diabetes is beneficial. Tight glycemic control has been consistently shown to produce higher rates of hypoglycemia in older adults. Realizing this point, the American Geriatrics Society (AGS) has recommended in the Choosing Wisely campaign (an initiative of the ABIM) that physicians should generally avoid using medications to achieve hemoglobin A1c less than 7.5% in most older adults. The AGS suggests hemoglobin A1c targets should reflect the individual older adult's treatment goals, health status, and remaining life expectancy. The AGS suggests that reasonable glycemic targets would be 7% to 7.5% in healthy older adults with long life expectancy, 7.5% to 8% in those with moderate comorbidity and a life expectancy less than 10 years, and 8% to 9% in those with multiple comorbid conditions and a shorter life expectancy.

SUMMARY

Optimizing use of drug therapy is a critical priority for older adults and involves achieving the balance between overuse (over prescribing of inappropriate therapy), underuse (under prescribing of beneficial therapy), and misuse (eg, inappropriate dose or duration of therapy). Sex, gender, age, and frailty considerations are important to inform optimal prescribing decisions for all older adults. There are additional considerations that are needed when making prescribing decisions for older adults living in long-term care settings or with limited life expectancy. Prescribing cascades should be avoided and managed by deprescribing when noticed. Particular attention should be given to using all drug therapies only when required and at the minimum effective dose. Practical approaches that integrate patient's values and preferences should be followed to ensure that older adults are receiving optimal drug therapy.

FURTHER READING

Abrahamsen B, Hansen RN, Rossing C. For which patient subgroups are there positive outcomes from a medication review? A systematic review. *Pharm Pract (Granada)*. 2020; 18(4):1976.

Boyd CM, Darer J, Boult C, Fried LP, Boult L, Wu AW. Clinical practice guidelines and quality of care for older patients with multiple comorbid diseases: implications for pay for performance. *JAMA*. 2005;294(6):716–724.

Budnitz DS, Lovegrove MC, Shehab N, Richards CL. Emergency hospitalizations for adverse drug events in older Americans. *N Engl J Med*. 2011;365(21):2002–2012.

By the 2019 American Geriatrics Society Beers Criteria® Update Expert Panel. American Geriatrics Society 2019 Updated AGS Beers Criteria® for Potentially Inappropriate Medication Use in Older Adults. *J Am Geriatr Soc*. 2019;67(4):674–694.

Christensen M, Lundh A. Medication review in hospitalised patients to reduce morbidity and mortality. *Cochrane Database Syst Rev*. 2013;2:CD008986.

DeJong C, Covinsky K. Inclusion across the lifespan in cardiovascular trials-a long road ahead. *JAMA Intern Med*. 2020;180(11):1533–1534.

Duerden M, Avery T, Payne R. Polypharmacy and medicines optimisation—Making it safe and sound. The King's Fund. 2013. https://www.kingsfund.org.uk/sites/files/kf/field/ field_publication_file/polypharmacy-and-medicines-optimisation-kingsfund-nov13.pdf.

Gurwitz JH, Field TS, Judge J, et al. The incidence of adverse drug events in two large academic long-term care facilities. *Am J Med*. 2005;118(3):251–258.

Holmes HM, Hayley DC, Alexander GC, Sachs GA. Reconsidering medication appropriateness for patients late in life. *Arch Intern Med*. 2006;166(6):605–609.

Molnar F, Frank CC. Optimizing geriatric care with the GERIATRIC 5Ms. *Can Fam Physician*. 2019; 65(1):39.

O'Mahony D, O'Sullivan D, Byrne S, O'Connor MN, Ryan C, Gallagher P. STOPP/START criteria for potentially inappropriate prescribing in older people: version 2. *Age Ageing*. 2015;44(2):213–218.

Piggott KL, Mehta N, Wong CL, Rochon PA. Using a clinical process map to identify prescribing cascades in your patient. *BMJ*. 2020;368:m261.

Rochon PA, Gurwitz JH. The prescribing cascade revisited. *Lancet*. 2017;389(10081):1778–1780.

Rochon PA, Petrovic M, Cherubini A, et al. Polypharmacy, inappropriate prescribing, and deprescribing in older people: through a sex and gender lens. *Lancet Healthy Longevity*. 2021;2(5):E290–E300.

Rudolph JL, Salow MJ, Angelini MC, McGlinchey RE. The anticholinergic risk scale and anticholinergic adverse effects in older persons. *Arch Intern Med*. 2008;168(5): 508–513.

Schwartz JB. The current state of knowledge on age, sex, and their interactions on clinical pharmacology. *Clin Pharmacol Ther*. 2007;82(1):87–96.

Scott IA, Hilmer SN, Reeve E, et al. Reducing inappropriate polypharmacy: the process of deprescribing. *JAMA Intern Med*. 2015;175(5):827–834.

Tinetti ME, Bogardus ST Jr, Agostini JV. Potential pitfalls of disease-specific guidelines for patients with multiple conditions. *N Engl J Med*. 2004;351(27):2870–2874.

US Department of Health and Human Services, Office of Disease Prevention and Health Promotion. (2014). National Action Plan for Adverse Drug Event Prevention. Washington, DC: Author.

US Food and Drug Administration. Risk of next-morning impairment after use of insomnia drugs; FDA requires lower recommended doses for certain drugs containing zolpidem (Ambien, Ambien CR, Edluar, and Zolpimist). 2013. https://www.fda.gov/media/84992/download.

Chapter 23

Substance Use and Disorders

Benjamin H. Han, Alexis Kuerbis, Alison A. Moore

INTRODUCTION

In the United States there is an increasing prevalence of substance use (eg, alcohol, tobacco products, cannabis, illegal drugs, and nonmedical use of prescription drugs) among older adults. The combination of population aging and increasing use of substances has created a growing public health problem; rising numbers of older adults are at risk for and experiencing unhealthy use, including SUDs. This public health problem is serious because older adults are more susceptible to the harms of substance use due to age-associated biological changes, social factors, increases in comorbidity, and the use of medications that may interact with substances. Therefore, it is critical to understand the age-related epidemiology, risk factors, unique vulnerabilities, and approaches to addressing and managing the spectrum of unhealthy substance use, including at-risk use and SUDs.

DEFINITIONS

Unhealthy substance use is typically defined as use that increases the risk for health consequences (hazardous or at-risk use) or has already led to adverse health or social consequences (harmful use and SUDs). For alcohol, at-risk use is typically defined as the use of alcohol at more than low-risk levels. In the United States, a standard drink contains 14 g or about 0.6 fluid ounces of pure ethanol (12 oz of beer, 5 oz of table wine, 1.5 oz of distilled spirits, 86 proof). The National Institute on Alcohol Abuse and Alcoholism (NIAAA) previously recommended that adults age 65 or older who are healthy and do not take medications should not have more than three drinks on a given day or seven drinks per week. This recommendation is now replaced by the US Department of Health and Human Services and US Department of Agriculture's 2020–2025 *Dietary Guidelines* that recommend all adults limit alcohol use to two drinks or less in a day for men and one drink or less in a day for women, on days when alcohol is consumed. The guidelines also recommend that older adults avoid drinking alcohol entirely if planning to drive or operate machinery, take certain medications, have certain medical conditions, or are recovering from AUD or cannot control the amount they drink. While the

Learning Objectives

- Understand the definitions and epidemiology of substance use and substance use disorder (SUD) among older adults.
- Recognize that substance use and addiction treatment is highly stigmatized in the United States and learn what stigmatizing language to avoid when discussing drug and alcohol use with patients.
- Learn about the unique vulnerabilities to the harms of substance use among older adults.
- Understand how to approach and screen older adults for unhealthy substance use.
- Recognize how identifying SUDs in older adults can be challenging.
- Learn about treatment approaches including evidence-based pharmacological treatments for older adults with SUDs.

Key Clinical Points

1. Substance use among older adults is increasing nationally.
2. Unhealthy substance use is often unrecognized in older adults due to lower rates of screening by health care providers and challenges in diagnosing SUDs in older populations.
3. Due to the presence of age-associated biological changes, social factors, increases in comorbidity, and the use of medications that may interact with substances, older adults are at higher risk for harm from psychoactive substances.
4. There are several screening tools to assess substance use and unhealthy substance use; tools focused on alcohol specifically for older adults are available.
5. Evidence-based pharmacologic treatments should be offered to older adults for the treatment of alcohol use disorder (AUD) and opioid use disorder (OUD).

amount of cannabis use considered at-risk among adults is not clear in light of increasing legalization, cannabis potency, social acceptability, and subsequent increasing use among adult populations, any use could be considered at-risk for older adults. *The Diagnostic and Statistical Manual of Mental Disorders 5th Edition* (DSM-5) outlines criteria for diagnosing SUDs, which are medical illnesses causes by repeated misuse of a substance or substances. According to DSM-5, SUDs are characterized by clinically significant impairments in health and social function and impaired control over substance use **(Table 23-1)**.

Prevalence Rates

Alcohol Alcohol continues to be the most commonly used substance among older adults in the United States. While generally, older adults reduce alcohol use as they age, alcohol use is increasing within this population in the past decade. Data from the National Survey on Drug Use and Health (NSDUH) estimate that the past-year use of alcohol increased among adults age 65 and older nationally from 52% in 2010 to 56% in 2019. For adults age 65 and older, the prevalence of binge drinking in the past 30 days (defined

TABLE 23-1 ■ DIAGNOSTIC AND STATISTICAL MANUAL OF MENTAL DISORDERS 5TH EDITION (DSM-5) CRITERIA FOR SUBSTANCE USE DISORDERS (SUD) WITH CONSIDERATION FOR OLDER ADULTS

DSM-5 CRITERIA FOR SUD[a]	CONSIDERATION FOR OLDER ADULTS
A substance is often taken in larger amounts or over a longer period than was intended.	Cognitive impairment can prevent adequate self-monitoring. Substances themselves may more greatly impair cognition among older adults than younger adults.
There is a persistent desire or unsuccessful efforts to cut down or control substance use.	It is the same as the general adult population.
A great deal of time is spent in activities necessary to obtain the substance, use the substance, or recover from its effects.	Consequences from substance use can occur from using relatively small amounts.
There is craving or a strong desire to use the substance.	It is the same as the general adult population. Older adults with entrenched habits may not recognize cravings in the same way as the general adult population.
There is recurrent substance use resulting in a failure to fulfill major role obligations at work, school, or at home.	Role obligations may not exist for older adults in the same way as for younger adults because of life-stage transitions, such as retirement. The role obligations more common in late life are caregiving for an ill spouse or family member, such as a grandchild.
There is continued substance use despite having persistent or recurrent social or interpersonal problems caused or exacerbated by the effects of the substance.	Older adults may not realize the problems they experience are from substance use.
Important social, occupational, or recreational activities are given up or reduced because of substance use.	Older adults may engage in fewer activities regardless of substance use, making it difficult to detect.
There is recurrent substance use in situations in which it is physically hazardous.	Older adults may not identify or understand that their use is hazardous, especially when using substances in smaller amounts.
Substance use is continued despite knowledge of having a persistent or recurrent physical or psychological problem that is likely to have been caused or exacerbated by the substance.	Older adults may not realize the problems they experience are from substance use.
Tolerance is developed, as defined by either of the following: 1. A need for markedly increased amounts of the substance to achieve intoxication or the desired effect 2. A markedly diminished effect with continued use of the same amount of the substance	Because of the increased sensitivity to substances as they age, older adults will seem to have lowered rather than increase in tolerance.
Withdrawal, as manifested by either of the following: 1. The characteristic withdrawal syndrome for the substance 2. The substance or a close relative is taken to relieve or avoid withdrawal symptoms	Withdrawal symptoms can manifest in ways that are more "subtle and protracted." Late-onset substance users may not develop physiologic dependence; or nonproblematic users of medications, such as benzodiazepines, may develop physiologic dependence.

[a]SUD is defined as a medical disorder in which two or more of the aforementioned listed symptoms are occurring in the last 12 months. The severity of the SUD diagnosis is defined by the number of the criteria met: mild 2–3, moderate 4–5, and severe 6 or more.
Data from Barry KL, Blow FC, Oslin DW. Substance abuse in older adults: review and recommendations for education and practice in medical settings. Subst Abus. 2002;23(Suppl 3): 105–131 and American Psychiatric Association. Diagnostic and Statistical Manual of Mental Disorders. 5th ed. Arlington (VA): American Psychiatric Publishing; 2013.

as five or more drinks on the same occasion for men and four or more for women) was estimated nationally in 2019 at 11%, with the prevalence of meeting DSM-5 criteria for AUD at 2%. However, the prevalence of AUD may be underestimated as the DSM diagnostic criteria for AUD are not ideal for older adults (see **Table 23-1**).

Tobacco Tobacco is the second most commonly used substance among older adults and is used primarily via smoking cigarettes. While over the last decade, cigarette smoking rates have gone down in the general adult population, they have remained stable in older adults. Data from NSDUH show the past-year use of tobacco has remained stable over the past 10 years among adults age 65 and older, with the past-year prevalence estimated to be 13% in 2019.

Cannabis While cannabis is federally illegal and remains a Schedule I drug under federal law, there has been a marked increase in the number of states that have legalized cannabis for medical and recreational use. Reflecting the changing laws and attitudes regarding cannabis, data from NSDUH indicate past-year use of cannabis increased from a national prevalence of 0.3% among adults age 65 and older in 2007 to 5% in 2019 and is likely to rise further as more states legalize cannabis. With the overall increase in cannabis use, there has also been an increase in cannabis use among older adults who also use alcohol. In 2015, 2.9% of adults age 65 and older who use alcohol also used cannabis, while in 2018, this prevalence increased to 6.3%.

Other substances Data from the 2019 NSDUH reveal that the prevalence of other illegal drug use such as cocaine, methamphetamine, heroin, and hallucinogens remains low (< 1%) among older adults, but such use may be hazardous for older adults, especially among those with comorbid conditions. The prevalence of SUDs as defined by DSM-5 criteria also remains low among older adults, with a 2019 national prevalence of 0.5% for all SUDs, not including AUD. While SUDs and AUDs both have a low prevalence among older adults nationally in the general population, it is crucial to recognize that several subpopulations of older people experience SUDs at much higher rates. Due to long-standing discrimination and vulnerabilities, older criminal justice-involved adults, older adults experiencing homelessness, and older persons living with HIV have a higher prevalence of SUDs than national populations.

Non-medical use of prescription drugs Because of increases in comorbidities, older adults take more prescribed and over-the-counter medications than younger adults and are therefore at increased risk for harmful drug interactions and misuse. Nonmedical or misuse is typically defined as use in a way a prescriber did not direct, including use without a prescription, taking the medication for longer or in higher amounts than intended, or taking the medication for reasons other than prescribed. Misuse of psychoactive prescription medications, including opioids, benzodiazepines,

hypnotics, and stimulants, are of particular concern and may indicate undertreated symptoms. Among adults age 65 and older, the national prevalence of past-year prescription psychotherapeutic misuse was 2.1% in 2019, with prescription opioids being the most commonly misused with a prevalence of 1.6%. The prevalence of misuse is likely higher than these reported rates as older adults prescribed these psychoactive medications may not view any use, even if for longer or in higher amounts or for reasons other than intended, as being misuse. Further, older adults who misuse psychoactive medications are much more likely to rely on physician sources for the medications compared to younger adults.

Despite contraindications for older adults, benzodiazepines are disproportionately prescribed to older adults. The estimated prevalence of benzodiazepine use among older adults is 13%, with up to a third using them long term. Therefore, prescription drug misuse is complicated in older adults as it is affected by overprescription, misdiagnosis (ie, symptoms of misuse being mistaken for other conditions like depression and dementia), accidentally taking more a prescribed medication than intended, mixing up of medications (eg, not knowing what medication is prescribed for or combining prescription and nonprescription drugs and dietary supplements), and potentially inappropriate prescribing, rather than intentional misuse.

Factors Associated With Unhealthy Substance Use and Substance Use Disorders

The data on risk factors for unhealthy substance use in later life are most robust for alcohol use. While it is reasonable to extrapolate factors related to unhealthy alcohol use among older adults to other substances, the unique characteristics that may contribute to substance use and SUDs for specific drugs other than alcohol are not as well studied (**Table 23-2**).

Demographic factors Several demographic characteristics are associated with unhealthy drinking among older adults. Male gender and Caucasian race are those most strongly associated with late-life drinking. It is important to note that unhealthy alcohol use has increased sharply among older women over the past decade. In addition, adults age 65 to 74 are more likely to engage in unhealthy alcohol use compared to adults age 75 and older. For other substances, female gender is consistently associated with misuse of prescription benzodiazepines, while male gender is associated with tobacco and cannabis use among older adults.

Social factors Generally, divorce, separation from a spouse, or being single are associated with increased drinking in late life, particularly among men. Affluence is associated with alcohol use. Within a retirement community, having a more active social life with friends and family may increase one's risk of unhealthy drinking in later life. Having sustained or increased social interactions from midlife into older age, mainly postretirement, tends to increase alcohol use.

TABLE 23-2 ■ FACTORS ASSOCIATED WITH UNHEALTHY SUBSTANCE USE AND SUBSTANCE USE DISORDERS

Demographics
Younger age
Male sex (alcohol, tobacco, cannabis)
Female sex (prescription medications)
Caucasian race (alcohol)

Social Factors
Being single, divorced, separated
High socioeconomic status
Having a social network of substance users
Transitions in living arrangement
Retirement
Bereavement

Health-Related Factors
Physical and/or psychiatric comorbidity
Chronic pain
Multiple prescription drugs
Insomnia
Cognitive impairment
Avoidance coping style (eg, drinking to cope with stressful events)
History of unhealthy substance use
Loneliness
Boredom

Late-life transitions and events may also increase an older adult's vulnerability to unhealthy substance use. Loss in many forms is associated with unhealthy substance use among older adults. Loss can take the form of bereavement, living arrangement transitions, declining overall health, and loss of function. Caregiving for a chronically or terminally ill loved one may increase the stress and subsequent vulnerability to unhealthy substance use. Preretirement job satisfaction, involuntary retirement, and workplace stress can negatively impact how the older adult copes with retirement and has been shown to increase alcohol use in general and drinking problems.

Health-Related Factors

In general, as the population ages, hospitalizations, disabilities, and physical and mental comorbidities increase, as substance use decreases. Among older drinkers, heavy drinkers have worse physical and mental health compared to moderate drinkers. Further, in most observational studies among adults, including older adults, being a drinker is associated with having fewer comorbidities and overall better health. This association of alcohol use and better health is likely due to selection biases common in observational studies of alcohol use as people with illness tend to stop drinking. This is referred to as the "sick quitter" hypothesis. Because of this selection bias, a population of healthy older drinkers is compared to unhealthy older nondrinkers.

Though data are sparse, those who continue to use substances other than alcohol in older age (eg, tobacco, opioids, cannabis, and methamphetamine) are more likely to have physical and psychiatric comorbidities. Specific conditions that older adults commonly use psychoactive substances to treat include chronic pain and insomnia. Alcohol, benzodiazepines, and cannabis are used as sleep aids. Alcohol, cannabis, and opioids are also used to treat chronic pain. Prior history of SUDs, cognitive impairment, an avoidance coping style, loneliness, and boredom are also risk factors for unhealthy substance use. Undertreated insomnia and anxiety symptoms are risk factors for prescription tranquilizer or sedative misuse among older adults. For prescription opioid misuse, the motive for misuse is overwhelmingly for pain relief. Loneliness is a risk factor for cannabis, alcohol, and prescription drug misuse among older adults.

Unique Vulnerabilities to Harms of Substance Use

Even with low amounts of substance use, there is potential for harm due to physiologic and biological aging (**Table 23-3**). However, the nature and severity of many health risks may vary by type, amount, and frequency of the substances used, medical and psychiatric comorbidities, medications used, and functional status. Our understanding of potential harms among older adults is strongest for alcohol and sedating medications (eg, opioids and benzodiazepines), and what we do know about the health impacts of other substances is primarily from data in younger age groups.

Aging affects drug and alcohol metabolism and distribution in the body. The liver and kidneys' ability to metabolize alcohol, other substances, and medications decreases. Cognitive function also evolves, including changes in the dopaminergic, glutaminergic, and serotoninergic systems. Changes in brain structure and function (eg, diminished white matter and increased permeability of the blood-brain barrier) can increase sensitivity to the psychoactive effects of substances. Body composition also changes; lean body mass and total body water decrease while total body fat increases. Because alcohol is water-soluble, older adults who drink a given amount of alcohol have a higher blood alcohol level compared to younger adults who drink the same amount. Drugs that are fat-soluble, such as benzodiazepines, have a longer duration of action in older adults compared to younger adults. Therefore, substances with long half-lives, such as diazepam, can be excessively sedating. All these factors result in older adults who consume a variety of substances having more significant impairment, lower tolerance, and less awareness of their impairment than younger adults. This contributes to an increased risk of harm including confusion or delirium,

TABLE 23-3 ■ UNIQUE VULNERABILITIES TO HARMS OF SUBSTANCE USE

Physiological and Biological Changes
Increased permeability of the blood-brain barrier
Diminished liver function
Reduction in renal function
Decreases in total body water
Increase in total body fat
Less lean muscle mass

Chronic conditions and symptoms[a]
Cardiovascular disease
Chronic obstructive lung disease
Gout
Liver disease
Gastroesophageal diseases
Cognitive impairment
Mood disorders
Insomnia
Gait impairment

Medications[a]
Antihypertensive agents
Antiplatelets
Blood thinners (eg, warfarin)
Central nervous system (CNS) depressants
Nonsteroidal anti-inflammatory drugs
Serotonin reuptake inhibitors

Improper Use of Medications
Multiple prescribers
Medication errors–intentional and unintentional

[a]Partial list.

falls, intoxicated driving, injuries or accidents, impaired functioning, and an increased risk for substance use–related emergency visits, hospitalizations, and nursing home admissions.

Older adults are also vulnerable to the harms of substance use as even low levels of substances may exacerbate existing comorbidities (eg, alcohol worsens gout) and cause other conditions (eg, tobacco worsens chronic obstructive lung disease). Substances can worsen symptoms of insomnia (eg, alcohol, stimulants) and memory impairment (eg, benzodiazepines, cannabis). They can also interact with many medications, increase medication side effects, or lessen their efficacy. For example, alcohol and niacin can cause flushing and itching, alcohol and nitrates increase risk of hypotension, and opioids and other sedating medications can cause excessive sedation. These interactions are magnified when multiple substances are used. For example, concurrent use of alcohol and benzodiazepines increases further the risk for injury and cognitive impairment.

Other factors that increase risks for harm among older adults are the common practice of seeing multiple prescribers, each of whom may prescribe medications without full knowledge of other prescribed and over-the-counter medications, and nonmedication substances used by the older adult. Older adults may borrow medications from other household members, use medications for reasons other than intended, unintentionally take the wrong medication, take more than intended, and stockpile medications. Older adults may not be aware that their use of the substance exceeds recommended limits or is risky when combined with other substances.

Addressing Unhealthy Substance Use and Substance Use Disorders

Avoiding stigmatizing language In the United States, drug use and addiction treatment are heavily stigmatized. Stigma and stigmatizing language can adversely affect the quality of medical care and prevent patients from receiving the care they need. Earlier cohorts of older adults, those born before or during World War II and those who grew up during Prohibition and the Temperance Movement, are more likely to consider substance use as a moral failure. This group will need a particularly sensitive approach to substance use screening. The Baby Boomers, born between 1946 and 1964, grew up when substance use was more acceptable and may have more permissive attitudes about substance use. They also may be more willing to engage in substance use screening and assessment. Health care providers often address alcohol and drug use differently from other health risks, contributing to continued stigma. The American Society of Addiction Medicine, along with other national organizations, have published policy statements on terminology and advise against using potentially stigmatizing terms, including "abuse or abuser," "user," "addict," "junkie," or the terms "clean versus dirty." Instead, language should place substance use in a health context and focus on the medical nature of SUDs and its treatment. The National Institute on Drug Abuse (NIDA) emphasizes that SUDs are a chronic brain disease, often with periods of recurrence, and a strong genetic component that can produce profound brain structure and function changes. Thus, providers must talk with patients about substance use in the same way they discuss other chronic medical conditions such as cardiovascular disease or diabetes. Therefore, the discussion surrounding alcohol and other substance use should occur in the context of an older adult's overall health with the goals of optimizing health, function, independence, and quality of life.

Screening

Unique issues Despite the increasing prevalence of substance use among older adults, this population is less likely to be screened for unhealthy substance use than younger adults. The US Preventive Services Task Force (USPSTF) recommends screening all persons age 18 and older for unhealthy alcohol, tobacco, and drug use. The Substance Abuse and Mental Health Services Administration (SAMSHA) recommends screening all older persons at least annually. Screening for substance use faces many barriers, including lack of time, competing health issues, and the challenges of integrating screening into regular clinical care. Patients, their families, and providers may be uncomfortable discussing and reporting stigmatized behavior such as substance use, especially among older adults. Further, signs and symptoms of unhealthy substance use may be mistaken for manifestations of other chronic diseases (eg, weight loss, depression, insomnia, cognitive impairment). A common perception among older adults is that symptoms of unhealthy substance use are due to aging or other diseases and not to the substance itself. Regardless of its difficulties, universal screening helps identify patients at risk or who are currently engaging in unhealthy substance use behaviors.

Approaches to screening When assessing individuals of any age regarding substance use, it is vital to understand that stigma is a significant barrier for people with SUDs from seeking and receiving help. Therefore, as discussed earlier, it is imperative that the language used when discussing issues of substance use with patients is not stigmatizing. As part of overall health promotion, one can reduce stigma by asking questions about quantity and frequency of drinking, medications (prescription and over-the-counter), and other drugs, including various forms of cannabis and illegal drugs, in a nonconfrontational and supportive manner.

Diagnostic challenges for SUDs When screening older adults for unhealthy substance use, it is also important to recognize that specific physiologic, biological, and social factors unique to older adults may pose challenges in the accurate diagnosis of SUDs. **Table 23-1** presents several DSM-5 criteria for SUDs and lists special considerations for older adults. Due to the physiologic and biological changes of aging that may increase the effects of substances, older adults generally experience a reduction of tolerance as they age—eliminating one of the hallmarks of DSM-5's criteria for SUDs. Additionally, changes in social and vocational roles, such as retirement or loss of peers, may mask problems related to substance use. Another challenge is the criterion of continued use despite persistent or recurrent problems may not apply to older adults who may mistake their problems related to substance use for normal aging. Therefore, given the diagnostic challenges, many older adults are "diagnostic orphans," individuals who qualify for only one diagnostic criterion for SUD and are therefore subthreshold.

Screening instruments Several screening instruments for unhealthy substance use are available for various substances (alcohol, tobacco, illegal drugs, and prescription drugs), but only a handful, focused on alcohol, were explicitly designed for and validated in older adults. The USPSTF and SAMSHA recommend the AUDIT-C and AUDIT for screening

for unhealthy alcohol use. Interviewer-administered one-item and two-item screening tests for unhealthy alcohol and other drug use have been validated in the general population and may be a way to start asking about substance use. An alternative are self-administered screening tools, which may help patients feel more comfortable reporting stigmatized behavior. It is important to note that many of the available screening tools use higher unhealthy alcohol use thresholds than what is recommended for older adults.

SELECTED SCREENING INSTRUMENTS

Alcohol

The Alcohol Use Disorders Identification Test (AUDIT) and AUDIT-C The World Health Organization (WHO) developed the AUDIT as a screening tool to assess excessive drinking. The AUDIT has been used in a variety of settings and diverse populations, including older adults. The AUDIT contains 10 items that assess alcohol consumption, drinking behaviors, and alcohol-related problems in the past year. Scoring on the AUDIT ranges from 0 to 40, with each item assigned 0 to 4 points. The cut-off for a potential AUD beginning with a score of eight. However, studies have shown a lower score of five is more accurate in identifying older adults with potential unhealthy drinking. The AUDIT-C is a shorter version of the AUDIT and consists of the first three questions of the AUDIT: How often do you have six or more drinks on one occasion? How often did you have a drink containing alcohol in the past year? How many drinks containing alcohol did you have on a typical day when you were drinking in the past year? A score of three or more is indicative of potential unhealthy drinking. These measures have high sensitivity and specificity in adult populations.

The Michigan Alcohol Screening Test-Geriatric Version The Michigan Alcohol Screening Test-Geriatric Version (MAST-G) was the first instrument designed to identify drinking problems among older adults. The MAST-G has 24 yes/no questions with five or more positive responses indicating problematic alcohol use. The questions focus more on potential stressors and behaviors that are common among older adults. The MAST-G has high sensitivity (95%) and specificity (78%) and generally has strong psychometric properties. The Short MAST-G or SMAST is a 10-item version; two or more positive responses indicate potential unhealthy alcohol use.

The Comorbidity Alcohol Risk Evaluation Tool (CARET) The CARET is a more comprehensive screening and assessment instrument for unhealthy alcohol use developed for older adults that assesses risk based on alcohol use behaviors, health-related conditions, and symptoms that may be caused or worsened by alcohol (ie, liver disease, gout, hypertension, stomach pain, memory issues), medications that may interact with alcohol or whose efficacy may be diminished by alcohol (eg, pain and sedating medications), and risky behaviors (ie, drinking and driving). It is scored using an algorithm that considers alcohol amount with the other factors to indicate potentially unhealthy alcohol use. It has a sensitivity of 91% and sensitivity of 68% in identifying older unhealthy drinkers.

The CAGE and CAGE-AID The CAGE questionnaire is one of the most commonly used screening tools for unhealthy alcohol use. It has four questions, and scoring ranges from 0–4 with a cut-off of 1 as the suggested threshold to identify unhealthy drinking in older adults and women. It has been studied in older adults with a sensitivity of 86% and a specificity of 78% to detect lifetime AUDs. The limitations of the CAGE are that it does poorly in identifying binge drinkers and does not distinguish between lifetime versus current use. The CAGE-AID consists of the CAGE questions that have been altered by expanding the scope of the questions to include drug use but has not been studied in older adults.

NIDA Quick Screen V1.0 This interviewer-administered brief screener asks about past year use of alcohol, tobacco, prescription drugs (nonmedical use), and illegal drugs. If respondents answer more than never, the interviewer is directed to substance-specific follow-up questions or resources to continue screening and assessment.

Tobacco, Alcohol, Prescription Medication, and Other Substance Use (TAPS) tool The TAPS tool combines screening and brief assessment. It consists of four-item screening questions about past-year frequency of use for tobacco, alcohol, illegal drugs, and nonmedical use of prescription drugs (similar to the NIDA Quick Screen), followed by a substance-specific assessment of risk level for individuals who screen positive. Scores on these questions generate a risk level per substance endorsed based on a range of possible scores per substance. The TAPS tool has the flexibility to be administered face-to-face or self-administered using a tablet computer. TAPS has been validated in a diverse population of adult primary care patients, but not specifically for older adults.

The Alcohol, Smoking, and Substance Involvement Screening Test (ASSIST) The ASSIST is another screening instrument developed by the WHO that screens for tobacco, alcohol, and illegal drug use. An interview is administered with eight questions that help assess the risk level and guide treatment decisions. The ASSIST, while widely used in research and clinical practice, has not yet been validated in older adults.

ASSESSMENT

If screening indicates unhealthy substance use, then an assessment for a SUD should occur using the DSM-5 criteria (see **Table 23-1**). Also, to guide advice given for both those with and without SUDs, older adults should be questioned about the circumstances of their substance use (eg, when and with whom they use substances, why they use substances), their medical and psychiatric history, prior and current substance use history, medications, symptoms that may be caused or exacerbated by substances, symptoms that are often treated by substances (eg, chronic pain, insomnia, anxiety, depression, loneliness), social support, and functional status. These assessments should be complemented by a physical examination that includes a cognitive assessment and fall-risk assessment.

INTERVENTIONS

Interventions to reduce substance use may include psychosocial interventions or medications. Screening for substance use, brief intervention, and referral to treatment (the SBIRT model) have been promoted to facilitate getting people into treatment. Brief interventions can be performed in almost any clinical setting and by nearly any trained medical staff. They are an approach best used for unhealthy substance users who do not meet the criteria for a SUD. For those with a suspected SUD, referral to more extensive treatment that includes more intensive psychosocial interventions and medical treatment may be warranted.

Psychosocial Interventions

Brief interventions Brief interventions, which range from 15 minutes of brief advice to up to four 1-hour long sessions of psychotherapy, are usually conducted in person. Common counseling techniques used in SBIRT programs are borrowed from motivational interviewing (MI) and cognitive-behavioral therapy (CBT). Brief interventions provide the older adult with information about potential harms and consequences of substance use, enhance motivation to change, identify goals, and, where needed, refer to more intensive services. Many older patients are unaware of low-risk drinking limits or that substances may worsen existing chronic diseases, contribute to symptoms, or interact with medications. Brief interventions that focus on alcohol and prescription medication misuse are effective for older adults.

Brief Advice

Brief advice by clinicians is recommended by NIAAA and NIDA when the initial screening of an older individual indicates they are engaging in unhealthy substance use. Similar recommendations are made by the USPSTF for tobacco users. Specifically, it is recommended that clinicians share the screening results and make clear recommendations. As an example, a provider might say: "Based on your responses to the screening questions, your current use is more than is medically safe." It is essential to relate the advice about substance use to the context of a patient's health and use nonjudgmental, non-stigmatizing language. This is an opportunity for providers to deliver a brief intervention that engages the patient in education about the substance, its potential health-related consequences, provides feedback and advice. It is also an opportunity to share how guidelines specifically relate to older adults and how substances may adversely impact other chronic diseases and function.

MI focuses on enhancing motivation and self-efficacy utilizing a shared decision-making approach. It can be implemented as part of a brief stand-alone intervention or a supplement to longer term or more intensive treatment of SUDs. It is a patient-centered intervention that encourages a nonconfrontational, supportive approach to promote healthy changes by eliciting and exploring the person's reasons for change. The focus is to reduce ambivalence to change. While older adults may have uniquely strong motivations related to their life stage to reduce unhealthy substance use, such as optimizing health and preserving function, such an intervention may be less influential on behavior than in younger counterparts. Substance use may be viewed as "one last pleasure," reducing the urgency among both older adults and their families for potential change. Additionally, low self-efficacy is associated with fewer health promotion behaviors among older adults due to perceiving the consequences of aging as nonmodifiable. Therefore, MI may be more challenging to implement with older adults compared to younger adults.

CBT helps individuals identify and correct unhealthy behaviors by applying a range of skills (eg, coping strategies, exploring positive and negative consequences of continued substance use) that can be used to stop unhealthy substance use. Ways to make CBT more beneficial for older adults are encouraging them to take notes, implementing sessions at a slower pace, and summarizing and repeating information. Other counseling strategies include problem-solving therapy (PST), which identifies the person's view of the problem, defines the problem, brainstorms possible solutions, reviews them, selects the best possible solution, uses the solution, and tracks and adjusts it as needed over time.

Referral to treatment for those with a suspected SUD Older adults identified as needing more treatment (eg, than brief interventions can deliver) should be referred for specialized SUD treatment focused on SUDs. Some studies suggest that older adults do better in specialized SUD treatment than do younger persons, especially those that have services are tailored to their age group. Due to various factors, including lower rates of SUDs, issues with diagnosis, screening, and stigma, there are many fewer older adults who seek treatment. The website, https://findtreatment.gov/, is useful to locate SUD treatment programs. It is important to develop a plan for seamless transitions between services and patient handoffs. During treatment, it is important to keep in touch with the older adult and the treatment program. Twelve-step recovery support groups such as Alcoholic Anonymous (A.A.) and Narcotics Anonymous (N.A.), typically in conjunction with other treatments for a SUD, help maintain abstinence, improve psychosocial functioning, and improve self-efficacy.

Medications Medications can be used in conjunction with or without psychosocial interventions to treat SUDs.

Despite the significant and robust evidence base for the benefit of several pharmacological treatments for SUDs, such treatments are severely underutilized, especially among older adults. Due to the higher risks for complications, older adults require inpatient or closely monitored specialty care for alcohol or benzodiazepine withdrawal or detoxification. However, as geriatric medicine providers care for patients across the clinical spectrum of care in various care settings, including long-term care, they should be comfortable initiating or maintaining medications for SUD treatment.

Alcohol Use Disorder

There are three FDA-approved medications for treating moderate to severe AUD: naltrexone, acamprosate, and disulfiram (**Table 23-4**). None of them have been studied in long-term randomized controlled trials (RCTs) of older populations, which limits understanding of their actual benefits and challenges to older persons.

Naltrexone is the only medication for AUD that has been tested in short-term RCTs among older adults. It reduces craving and the pleasurable effects of alcohol, is usually well tolerated by older adults, and can be started while a patient is still using alcohol. It is considered first-line therapy for many patients and can be safely given with medications for HIV; however, it is contraindicated in patients with acute hepatitis, liver failure, or patients taking prescribed opioid medications since it is an opioid antagonist and will precipitate opioid withdrawal. Naltrexone is given orally in daily dosing or a monthly injection.

Acamprosate reduces symptoms of protracted withdrawal from alcohol, such as sleep and mood problems. Like naltrexone, it can also reduce craving and the pleasurable effects of alcohol. In clinical trials in younger adults, it is most effective for patients after initial abstinence from alcohol. Acamprosate does require three times a day oral dosing and requires dose reduction for renal insufficiency, but can be used for patients with liver disease or patients needing opioid medications.

Disulfiram triggers an acute physical reaction to alcohol, including flushing, tachycardia, nausea, chest pain, dizziness, and changes in blood pressure. These adverse effects, when used with alcohol, are negatively reinforcing. Because these effects can be harmful to older people, disulfiram is generally not recommended for use in older adults and, if used, is done so only with great caution.

Opioid Use Disorder

While studies focused on older adults with opioid use disorder are limited, a large body of evidence demonstrates that medications for opioid use disorder (MOUD) decrease mortality. MOUD is often improved when combined with psychosocial treatment (counseling, mutual help groups), but MOUD should be the first-line treatment for opioid use disorder rather than psychosocial treatment alone. The number of adults age 55 and older who are on MOUD

TABLE 23-4 ■ FDA-APPROVED MEDICATIONS TO TREAT ALCOHOL USE DISORDER (AUD) AND OPIOID USE DISORDER (OUD)

MEDICATION (TYPICAL DOSAGE)	MECHANISM	PRECAUTIONS / SIDE EFFECTS	NOTES
MEDICATIONS TO TREAT AUD			
Naltrexone Oral: 50–100 mg daily IM: 380 mg gluteal injection monthly	Opioid antagonist; reduces reward in response to alcohol use.	Precipitates severe opioid withdrawal if concurrently taking opioids and therefore must be opioid-free 7–10 d. Hepatotoxicity at supratherapeutic doses. Avoid in patients with decompensated cirrhosis, acute hepatitis, or liver failure; use with caution with hepatitis, compensated cirrhosis. Nausea, vomiting, headache, fatigue, and somnolence. Injection site reactions.	Contraindicated with concurrent opioid use. Can be useful for patients with concurrent opioid-use disorder.
Acamprosate 666 mg oral three times a day If creatinine clearance (CrCl) 30–50 mL/min: 333 mg three times a day	Mechanism unknown, but may antagonize glutamate-mediated neuronal hyperexcitability and reduce prolonged withdrawal symptoms.	Nausea, vomiting, diarrhea, myalgia, rash, dizziness. Evaluate renal function: reduce for CrCl 30–50 mL/min, avoid CrCl < 30 mL/min.	Can be used in patients with alcohol-related liver disease. Can be combined with naltrexone. Medication adherence may be challenging.
Disulfiram 250 mg oral daily (range 125–500 mg)	Aldehyde dehydrogenase inhibition results in acetaldehyde accumulation with alcohol use, which can cause flushing, nausea, dizziness, and tachycardia if patient uses alcohol.	Potential for many drug-drug interactions. Patient must be abstinent at least 12 h before medication administration. Disulfiram-alcohol reaction, hepatotoxicity, drowsiness, rash. Avoid in patients with hepatic impairment or cardiovascular disease.	Must never be administered to a patient when they are in a state of alcohol intoxication or without their full knowledge. Most appropriate for patients with strong motivation to be abstinent without many chronic diseases and with support to promote medication adherence.
MEDICATIONS TO TREAT OUD			
Methadone	Full, long-acting opioid agonist.	Sedation, prolongation of the QTc interval, nausea, constipation, weight gain, edema, amenorrhea, decreased bone density, decreased libido. Risk for respiratory depression and overdose. Potential for drug interactions with inducers or inhibitors of P-450 system.	Schedule II medication. For outpatient addiction treatment, only available through state-licensed opioid treatment programs.
Buprenorphine-Naloxone Start 4 mg/1 mg of sublingual buprenorphine/naloxone, total of 8 mg/2 mg in first day. Typical maintenance dose between 16 and 24 mg daily.	Partial opioid agonist. Most common formulation includes naloxone, which discourages injection.	Constipation, dizziness, nausea and vomiting, headache. Hepatoxicity is rare, but monitoring of liver enzymes is recommended. Rarely associated with overdose given ceiling effect as a partial agonist, usually in combination with other sedating drugs (ie, benzodiazepines).	Schedule III medication. Providers currently need DEA "X-waiver" to prescribe. FDA approved for pain.
Naltrexone IM: 380 mg gluteal injection monthly	Opioid antagonist; reduces reward in response to alcohol use.	Precipitates severe opioid withdrawal if concurrently taking opioids and therefore must be opioid-free 7–10 days. Hepatotoxicity at supratherapeutic doses. Avoid in patients with decompensated cirrhosis, acute hepatitis, or liver failure; use with caution with hepatitis, compensated cirrhosis. Nausea, vomiting, headache, fatigue, and somnolence. Injection site reactions.	Can be useful for patients with concurrent alcohol use disorder. Limited clinical trial data.

sharply increased nationally over the past decade, and geriatric medicine providers will increasingly care for patients on MOUD.

Currently, there are three FDA-approved MOUD, including methadone (scheduled II), buprenorphine (scheduled III), and naltrexone (see **Table 23-4**). Like medications for AUD, those for OUD have not been tested in long-term RCTs among older adults.

Methadone, a full opioid agonist, is highly regulated in the United States and dispensed through licensed opioid treatment programs. It can prevent opioid withdrawal symptoms and reduce drug cravings. Methadone decreases opioid use and reduces all-cause mortality among people with OUD.

Buprenorphine is a partial opioid agonist. Like methadone, buprenorphine decreases opioid use and reduces all-cause mortality among people with OUD. Studies comparing the two medications suggest that methadone may be slightly more effective than buprenorphine for retaining patients in treatment. However, in the absence of studies focused on older adults, several factors suggest buprenorphine may be a safer choice for older adults initiating MOUD. The risk of overdose with buprenorphine is significantly lower than methadone since it is a partial opioid agonist with a lower potential risk for respiratory depression given its ceiling effect. Buprenorphine also has a shorter half-life and is likely safer for patients with ventricular arrhythmias compared to methadone. No dose adjustment is needed for renal impairment or dialysis, and while hepatoxicity is rare, dose reduction may be required for severe hepatic impairment.

Naltrexone is a full opioid antagonist and will block any euphoric effect of opioids and does not cause physiologic dependence or withdrawal when stopped, unlike opioid agonists. However, initiating naltrexone requires that patients are not taking opioids as it can precipitate withdrawal if opioids are present. Naltrexone, especially the long-acting injectable form, has been found to be more effective than placebo for OUD; comparisons with methadone or buprenorphine are limited. As described above, naltrexone is usually well tolerated by older adults and can be used for patients with both AUD and OUD. However, it is contraindicated for patients who require prescribed opioids for pain.

Reversal of opioid overdose Naloxone does not treat OUD, but it can reverse potentially fatal opioid overdoses, and low-dose naloxone is safe and effective in older adults. Intranasal naloxone kits and overdose prevention education should be prescribed to patients at increased risk for overdose, such as those taking daily doses of 50 morphine milligram equivalents per day or more, or concurrently with a benzodiazepine. Those with chronic obstructive pulmonary disease, obstructive sleep apnea, other SUDs, and mental health disorders are at increased risk for opioid-related death. Friends, family members, and caregivers may also receive prescriptions and training in naloxone use.

Tobacco

All smokers without contraindications should receive at least one of seven FDA-approved treatments for tobacco use disorder. Though none have been explicitly tested in older adults, in adult populations, varenicline is more efficacious than other treatments, and varenicline combined with nicotine replacement is the most effective therapy. Combining more than one type of nicotine replacement therapy (short-acting and long-acting) is more effective than a single treatment. Initiation of varenicline before smoking is stopped may increase quitting success rates.

Follow-Up

After patients with unhealthy substance use receive intervention and/or referral to specialty treatment, it is essential to maintain support and monitor progress by regularly checking in with patients and asking about substance use. For those older adults who are not ready to make a change, it is important to continue to be supportive and make it clear you are prepared to help if and when they are ready to make a change. For those who are making change, it is important to support their progress. Return to use is common, just as exacerbations occur for other chronic diseases that require changes in behavior to manage like congestive heart failure or diabetes. The focus should be on using nonjudgmental language and assisting patients in re-engaging with interventions to address unhealthy use.

CONCLUSION

Substance use and SUDs continue to increase among older adults and may present challenges for clinicians managing patients with multiple chronic diseases. Understanding that substance use and its treatment are highly stigmatized mandates that geriatric medicine providers use patient-centered and nonstigmatizing language when talking to their older patients. Screening for substance use can be challenging for older adults, and providers must consider unique aspects of aging to detect unhealthy use. Older adults with unhealthy substance use and SUDs must be offered evidence-based treatment and regularly monitored to support them.

FURTHER READING

Broyles LM, Binswanger IA, Jenkins JA, et al. Confronting inadvertent stigma and pejorative language in addiction scholarship: a recognition and response. *Subst Abus.* 2014;35(3):217–221.

Grant BF, Chou SP, Saha TD, et al. Prevalence of 12-month alcohol use, high-risk drinking, and DSM-IV alcohol use disorder in the United States, 2001-2002 to 2012-2013: Results from the National Epidemiologic Survey on Alcohol and Related Conditions. *JAMA Psychiatry.* 2017;74(9):911–923.

Han BH, Moore AA, Ferris R, Palamar JJ. Binge drinking among older adults in the United States, 2015 to 2017. *J Am Geriatr Soc.* 2019;67(10):2139–2144.

Han BH, Moore AA, Sherman S, Keyes KM, Palamar JJ. Demographic trends of binge alcohol use and alcohol use disorders among older adults in the United States, 2005 to 2014. *Drug Alcohol Depend.* 2017;170:198–207.

Han BH, Palamar JJ. Trends in cannabis use among older adults in the United States, 2015 to 2018. *JAMA Intern Med.* 2020;180(4):609–611.

Jonas DE, Amick HR, Feltner C, et al. Pharmacotherapy for adults with alcohol use disorders in outpatient settings: a systematic review and meta-analysis. *JAMA.* 2014;311(18):1889–1900.

Kuerbis A. Substance use among older adults: an update on prevalence, etiology, assessment, and intervention. *Gerontology.* 2020;66(3):249–258.

Kuerbis A, Sacco P, Blazer DG, Moore AA. Substance abuse among older adults. *Clin Geriatr Med.* 2014;30(3):629–654.

Lehrmann SW, Fingerhood M. Substance-use disorders in later life. *N Engl J Med.* 2018;379(24):2351–2360.

McNeely J, Saitz R. Appropriate screening for substance use vs disorder. *JAMA Intern Med.* 2015;175(12):1997–1998.

McNeely J, Wu LT, Subramaniam G, et al. Performance of the tobacco, alcohol, prescription medication, and other substance use (TAPS) tool for substance use screening in primary care patients. *Ann Intern Med.* 2016;165(10):690–699.

Qato DM, Manzoor BS, Lee TA. Drug-alcohol interactions in older US adults. *J Am Geriatr Soc.* 2015 63:2324–2331.

Saitz R, Brady KT, Levin FR, Galanter M, Kleber HD. *The American Psychiatric Press Textbook of Substance Use Disorders. Screening and Brief Intervention.* American Psychiatric Press, 2020.

Saitz R, Miller SC, Fiellin DA, Rosenthal RN. Recommended use of terminology in addiction medicine. *J Addict Med.* 2021;15(1):3–7.

Schepis TS, McCabe SE, Teter CJ. Sources of opioid medication for misuse in older adults: results from a nationally representative survey. *Pain.* 2018;159(8):1543–1549.

Schepis TS, Wastila L, Ammerman B, McCabe VV, McCabe SE. Prescription opioid misuse motives in US older adults. *Pain Med.* 2020;21(10):2237–2243.

Schepis TS, Wastila L, McCabe SE. Prescription tranquilizer/sedative misuse motives across the US population. *J Addict Med.* 2021;15(3):191–200.

Sordo L, Barrio G, Bravo MJ, et al. Mortality risk during and after opioid substitution treatment: systematic review and meta-analysis of cohort studies. *BMJ.* 2017; 357:j1550.

Substance Abuse and Mental Health Services Administration. Key substance use and mental health indicators in the United States: Results from the 2019 National Survey on Drug Use and Health (HHS Publication No. PEP20-07-01-001, NSDUH Series H-55). Rockville, MD: Center for Behavioral Health Statistics and Quality, Substance Abuse and Mental Health Services 185 Administration. https://www.samhsa.gov/data. Accessed November 15, 2020.

Substance Abuse and Mental Health Services Administration. Treating Substance Use Disorder in Older Adults. Treatment Improvement Protocol (TIP) Series No. 26, SAMHSA Publication No. PEP20-02-01-011. Rockville, MD: Substance Abuse and Mental Health Services Administration, 2020.

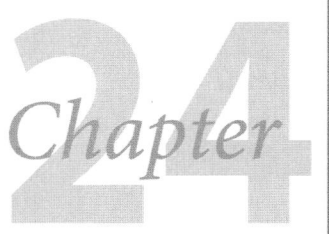

Integrative Medicine and Health

Julia Loewenthal, Gloria Y. Yeh, Darshan H. Mehta, Peter M. Wayne

INTRODUCTION

The National Center for Complementary and Integrative Health (NCCIH) defines complementary approaches as those that may have originated outside of conventional medicine. Integrative health care brings together both conventional and complementary approaches in a safe, coordinated way. Integrative health emphasizes a holistic, patient-focused approach to health care and wellness. These practices encompass dietary, psychological, and physical approaches, often in multimodal systems. In the past, the NCCIH was known as the National Center for Complementary and Alternative Medicine (NCCAM), but there has been a movement toward integrating complementary therapies with conventional care rather than using them as an alternative, so the term "alternative" has been deemphasized.

Both integrative and geriatric medicine aim to maximize health across an individual's life span, including those living with chronic conditions, disabilities, cognitive impairment, and/or frailty. In addition, both fields emphasize the importance of a larger biopsychosocial framework in the provision of clinical care. A common thread between integrative and geriatric medicine is the concept of whole person health. While medical specialization has resulted in the development of life-saving pharmaceuticals and procedures, this reductionist framework can overlook the rich interdependence of systems and factors contributing to whole person health. It is well recognized that social determinants of health and lifestyle behaviors can contribute to disease among multiple organ systems, such as cardiovascular disease and diabetes mellitus. However, there has been less progress made in the development of effective interventions to catalyze recovery from chronic, multisystem diseases, nor strategies that promote resilience and prevent their occurrence. Integrative medicine, by incorporating multimodal conventional and complementary health approaches, is well-situated to maximize whole-person care with the goal of promoting and restoring resilience.

The 2018 American Geriatrics Society White Paper on Healthy Aging stated: "Promotion of a realistic, dynamic, multidimensional view of healthy aging is an important goal obtainable through traditional and innovative models of health promotion and prevention." Integrative medicine, by

Learning Objectives

- Define integrative and complementary health approaches and describe current patterns of use among older adults.
- Apply the integrative health history to the comprehensive geriatric assessment.
- Describe integrative modalities (dietary supplements, mind-body practices, manual therapies, and traditional medicine systems), current evidence regarding clinical efficacy, and potential adverse effects.

Key Clinical Points

1. Approximately 30% of adults age 65 and over report use of a complementary health approach.

2. Of patients who use a complementary health approach, approximately half do not disclose use to their clinician, though this may be ameliorated by incorporating an integrative health history.

3. Older adults tend to be the highest consumers of herbal and dietary supplements, with nearly 70% taking a supplement in the past 30 days.

4. Mind-body practices encompass a diverse range of practices such as tai chi, yoga, seated meditation, and others; their multimodal nature may explain effectiveness in treating geriatric syndromes (eg, tai chi and fall prevention).

5. Manual therapies, such as acupuncture and chiropractic treatment, are effective in several prevalent conditions among older adults (eg, back pain).

incorporating nonpharmacologic, multimodal approaches, is poised to serve in both the promotion of healthy aging and prevention and management of geriatric syndromes (**Figure 24-1**). Furthermore, the inherent multimodal

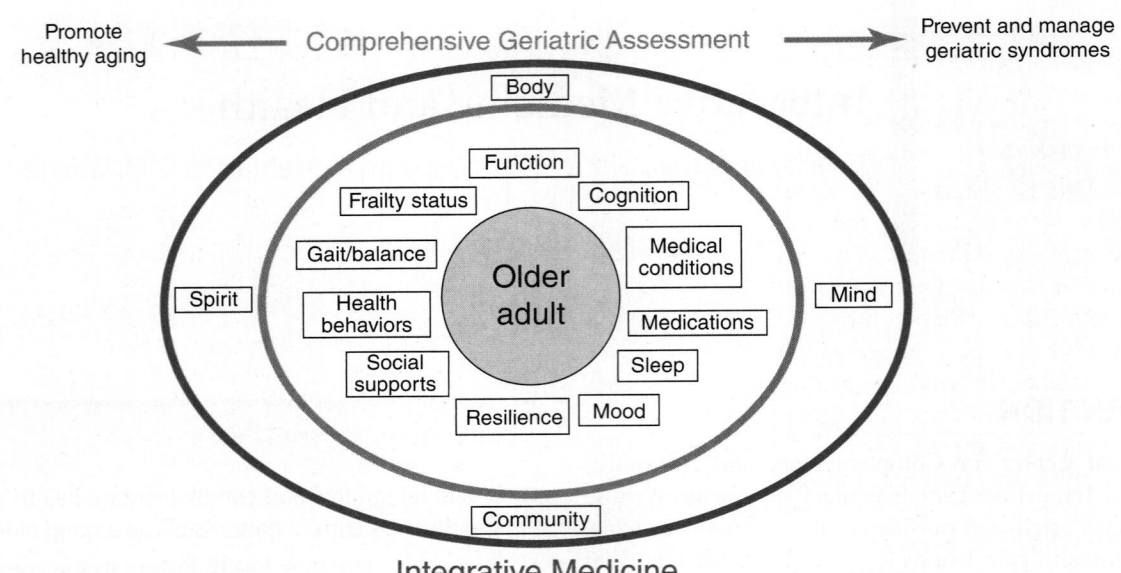

Promote healthy aging ← Comprehensive Geriatric Assessment → Prevent and manage geriatric syndromes

Integrative Medicine

FIGURE 24-1. Integrative geriatrics framework to promote healthy aging and prevent and manage geriatric syndromes.

approach is well-suited to preventing and managing complex geriatric syndromes, which extend beyond single organ systems and a traditional disease-based approach.

CURRENT PATTERNS OF USE

For the purposes of this chapter, complementary and integrative modalities are grouped into four major categories (**Figure 24-2**):

1. Dietary supplements, including herbal medicine, vitamins, and non-herbal, non-vitamin supplements.

2. Mind-body practices, including yoga, tai chi, qigong, and meditation.
3. Manual therapies, including chiropractic care, acupuncture, massage, and osteopathy.
4. Traditional medicine systems, including Ayurveda and Traditional Chinese Medicine (TCM).

The latest data regarding trends in the use of complementary health approaches among US adults comes from the 2012 and 2017 National Health Interview Surveys (NHIS). Approximately 30% of adults age 65 and over

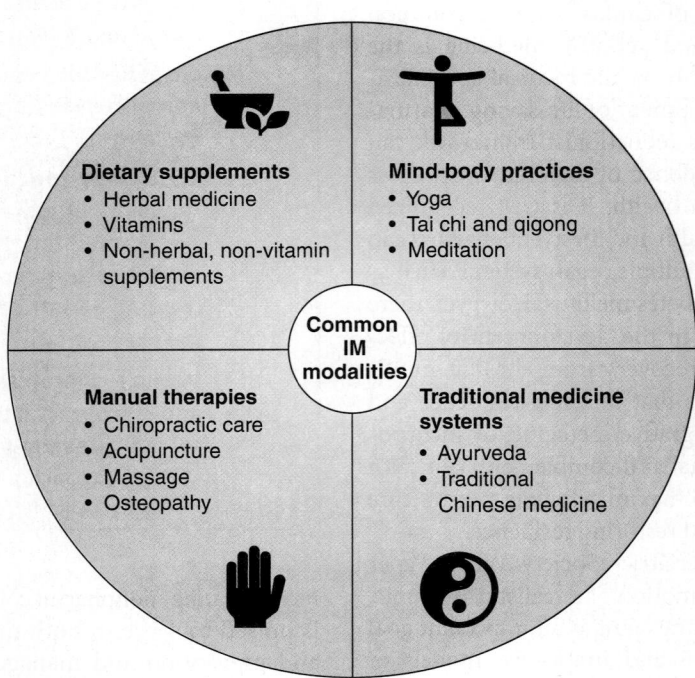

FIGURE 24-2. Integrative medicine (IM) modalities.

reported use of any complementary health approach in 2012. Older adults tended to use complementary health approaches less often than those aged 18 to 44 or 45 to 64, but consistent increases in use have been observed over time. In 2017, yoga was the most popular approach among all adults, but meditation use was more common among older adults as compared to yoga and chiropractic manipulation. In general, non-Hispanic White adults reported use of complementary health approaches more often than Hispanic and non-Hispanic Black adults.

Reasons for use of complementary health approaches are varied. US adults reported using these approaches most commonly for back and neck pain, joint pain or stiffness, colds, depression, and anxiety. Over half of adults believed complementary health approaches would help when combined with conventional medical approaches. Approximately half of patients who use complementary health approaches did not disclose this to clinicians involved in their care. Reasons for this include clinicians not asking about complementary and integrative health approaches and concerns about clinician knowledge regarding these approaches. Cost is another important factor in use of complementary health approaches, with many adults reporting high out-of-pocket expenditure. This has improved over time for certain modalities: in 2012 60% of adults who saw a chiropractor had some insurance coverage, versus 25% for acupuncture and 15% for massage therapy, but coverage was more likely to be partial than complete. Most recently in 2020, the Centers for Medicare and Medicaid Services finalized a decision to cover acupuncture for low back pain.

The Integrative Health History

There are several ways clinicians can improve disclosure of complementary therapy use to better care for their patients. An important strategy is to incorporate elements of the integrative health history into the comprehensive geriatric assessment (CGA) including: illness representation, patients' perceived sources of stress and support, complementary and integrative modality use and history, current health behaviors, and dietary supplement use in the medication history (**Table 24-1**).

CLINICAL CASE

Ms. S is an 81-year-old female with history of cerebrovascular accident (CVA) complicated by residual left-sided weakness, atrial fibrillation, heart failure (HF) with preserved ejection fraction, gout, lumbar spinal stenosis, mild cognitive impairment, falls, and depression who presents to the outpatient geriatrics consult clinic. Her goal is to live independently as long as possible. Since her stroke 1 year prior, she has struggled with her gait and ambulates with a rolling walker. She had one fall in the past 6 months and is afraid of falling. She is interested in integrative therapies she could use to improve her health and well-being.

Ms. S reports some fatigue but no other current symptoms. She lives alone in the community. Ms. S is

TABLE 24-1 ■ INCORPORATING AN INTEGRATIVE MEDICINE HISTORY INTO THE COMPREHENSIVE GERIATRIC ASSESSMENT (CGA)

Components of an Integrative Health History for the CGA:

- Illness representation:
  - How do you explain your current illness or symptoms?
  - What do you think is the cause of your current illness or symptoms?
- Ask patient to identify current sources of stress and support
- Ascertain current interprofessional team of conventional and complementary health care providers (see I-CAM-Q)
- Ask about health behaviors, such as nutrition, physical activity, sleep, and avoidance of substance use
- Assess motivational stage of patient
- Ask about spiritual or cultural beliefs that help patient cope with illness and maintain health
- Ask patient about current and past complementary therapy use (see I-CAM-Q)
- During medication history, ask patient about use of natural products (eg, herbal medicine, dietary supplements)

independent with activities of daily living (ADLs), but requires some assistance for instrumental activities of daily living (IADLs) such as shopping, heavy housework, and driving given physical limitations. She hired a homemaker to assist with cleaning and shopping; she relies on her daughter for transportation. She denies loneliness and reports receiving limited social support from her church group. Her medications include allopurinol, apixaban, atorvastatin, fluoxetine, furosemide, gabapentin, senna, and vitamin E. She drinks one glass of wine on holidays, but otherwise denies substance use. She completed the Timed Up and Go (TUG) test in 15 seconds ($\geq$ 12 seconds suggests increased risk of falls). Gait examination revealed decreased gait speed with uneven stride length and step height, but a normal base and no bradykinesia. Cognitive testing was notable for Montreal Cognitive Assessment (MoCA) score of 24 out of 30. She scored a 7 on the Patient Health Questionnaire-9 (PHQ-9), consistent with mild depression. A frailty screen was consistent with mild frailty.

In addition to tools from conventional medicine, what approaches might you recommend in the clinical care of this patient? How would you make this decision?

DIETARY SUPPLEMENTS

According to the World Health Organization, the use of herbal and dietary supplements (HDS) in the United States has increased significantly over the past two decades. Older adults tend to be the highest consumers of HDS, with nearly 70% taking an HDS in the past 30 days. Studies consistently show that women use HDS more than men, and family households with greater wealth also use more.

The Dietary Supplement and Health Education Act (DSHEA) was passed in 1994; it defined a dietary supplement as a product (other than tobacco) that is intended to supplement the diet; that contains one or more dietary ingredients (including vitamins, minerals, herbs or other botanicals, amino acids, and other substances) or their constituents; is intended to be taken by mouth as a pill, capsule, tablet, or liquid; and is labeled on the front panel as being a dietary supplement. Under this law, supplements can be marketed without proof of safety or efficacy if no claim is made for their use in the diagnosis, treatment, cure, or prevention of disease. Manufacturers can, however, make "structure and function" claims that a product enhances a normal body function or state. For example, saw palmetto can be marketed to support urinary tract health but not to treat benign prostatic hyperplasia. In contrast to prescription medications, which must be proven safe, the US Food and Drug Administration (FDA) must first prove that an HDS is unsafe before a product is taken off the market. In 2006, DSHEA was updated so that dietary supplement producers were responsible for reporting serious adverse events related to their products. In 2007, the FDA published current good manufacturing practice guidelines, including requirements for manufacturers to test products to ensure product quality, confirm the absence of some contaminants, verify accuracy of labeling, maintain minimum standards for manufacturing and packing, monitor adverse event reports, and make all records available for FDA inspection. However, these guidelines are nonbinding on the manufacturer. Since 2007, the FDA has increased inspections of HDS manufacturers and enforcement of regulations. In 2019, the FDA reported that they will be updating the regulation of HDS to continue to promote safety, quality, and efficacy.

When approaching the use of HDS in older adults, the clinician should carefully weigh the anticipated benefit of the dietary supplement with the risk of polypharmacy. Approximately half of prescription medication users also use dietary supplements on a regular basis. The number of drugs taken by a patient has been shown to be the single most important predictor of harm, and both drug-drug and drug-supplement interactions must be considered. Therefore, an integrative approach in the older patient should incorporate an assessment of polypharmacy and the practice of deprescribing to prevent harm and maximize health and well-being. **Table 24-2** includes resources for clinicians regarding HDS safety.

Multivitamins

For a discussion of multivitamins, please refer to Chapters 30, Nutrition Disorders, Obesity, and Enteral/Parenteral Alimentation and Chapter 46, Pressure Injuries.

Vitamin D

Vitamin D is a fat-soluble vitamin that has numerous roles in the body, including bone health, the maintenance of normal serum calcium and phosphate concentrations, reduction of inflammation, and others. Older adults are at risk of vitamin D deficiency because of increased time spent indoors, reduced synthesis in the skin, and inadequate dietary intake. There is evidence that vitamin D supplements increase bone mineral density and reduce fracture rates in institutionalized older adults. For further information about vitamin D status and falls, please refer to Chapter 43, Falls.

Studies of vitamin D supplements and muscle strength have had inconsistent results. There is mixed evidence regarding vitamin D supplements and cancer prevention. Vitamin D supplements do not appear to help prevent or treat mild depression, but there have not been any studies to date in older adults with vitamin D deficiency who are taking antidepressants. Observational studies have shown an association between vitamin D deficiency and poorer cognition, but it is not clear if there is cognitive benefit from vitamin D supplementation.

Magnesium

Magnesium is a mineral that is a cofactor in numerous enzyme systems in the body. Supplements are available in many forms, such as magnesium citrate, oxide, and chloride. Older adults are at risk for magnesium deficiency given lower dietary intake and reduced gut absorption with age. However, it is difficult to assess magnesium stores since serum magnesium levels do not necessarily correlate with intracellular or bone stores, which is where most magnesium is stored.

Low magnesium intake is strongly correlated with hypertension, but clinical intervention studies have not demonstrated a consistent benefit. Magnesium supplementation appears to be beneficial in the prevention of migraine. Though magnesium deficiency may be a risk factor for osteoporosis, it is not clear that magnesium supplementation is effective for the prevention and management of osteoporosis. There is some evidence that magnesium is effective for insomnia, stress, and constipation. For a more complete discussion of magnesium for constipation, please refer to the Chapter 87, Constipation.

Fish Oil

Eicosapentaenoic (EPA) and docosahexaenoic (DHA) acids are the two main omega-3 long-chain polyunsaturated fatty acids that have been extensively studied in the prevention and treatment of cardiovascular diseases. Dietary sources of EPA and DHA include fatty fish, such as salmon, anchovies, and sardines. Despite the large number of studies, the research has produced inconsistent results. The reasons for this are several, including differences in who is being treated, whether or not they are on statins, the formulation used (EPA+DHA or EPA alone), the dose or duration of treatment, the placebo arm (eg, olive oil versus mineral oil), and the end point measured. The recent Omega-3 Fatty Acids in Elderly Patients With Acute Myocardial Infarction (OMEMI) trial found no reduction in clinical events in older patients with recent acute myocardial infarction who were treated with 1.8 g EPA/DHA daily for 2 years.

TABLE 24-2 ■ INTEGRATIVE MEDICINE RESOURCES FOR THE GERIATRIC HEALTH PROFESSIONAL

AREA/DOMAIN	RESOURCE	DESCRIPTION
General information about integrative medicine	Textbook: *Integrative Medicine: Fourth Edition* by David Rakel	Written by physicians, this textbook is organized via a clinical, disease-oriented approach, providing evidence-based practical guidance for an integrative approach to patient care.
	National Center for Complementary and Integrative Health (NCCIH): nccih.nih.gov	Provides information oriented toward patients and health care professionals regarding complementary health products and practices.
	Cochrane Complementary Medicine: cam.cochrane.org	Access evidence-based information about complementary, alternative, and integrative medicine therapies.
	Academic Consortium for Integrative Medicine & Health	Membership of academic medical centers that disseminates information on research, education, and clinical models of integrative health.
Dietary supplements and natural products	*Natural Medicines* Database	Provided by the Therapeutic Research Center, the *Natural Medicines* Database is a comprehensive resource for dietary supplements, herbal medicines, and complementary and integrative therapies.
	National Institutes of Health Office of Dietary Supplements	Provides fact sheets that give a current overview of individual vitamins, minerals, and other dietary supplement ingredients. Fact sheets are available for both clinicians and consumers. https://ods.od.nih.gov/
	ConsumerLab.com	Provides independent test results and information to help consumers and health care professionals identify high-quality natural products.
Lifestyle medicine	American College of Lifestyle Medicine	Medical professional society for physicians and other health professionals dedicated to the practice of Lifestyle Medicine, or the use of evidence-based lifestyle therapeutic approaches (nutrition, physical activity, sleep, stress management, avoidance of risky substances, and social connection).
	VA Whole Health	US Department of Veterans Affairs program that supports health and well-being—centers around "what matters to you, not what is the matter with you." https://www.va.gov/wholehealth/
Physical activity	National Association of Area Agencies on Aging (AAAs)	More than 90% of AAAs deliver at least one program targeted toward healthy aging, including balance and tai chi classes.
	National Institute on Aging Exercise and Physical Activity resource	Includes a series of articles and resources oriented toward patients to support physical activity in older age.
Tai chi	NCCIH	Information about the evidence for tai chi for health professionals: https://www.nccih.nih.gov/health/tai-chi-and-qi-gong-in-depth
Yoga	Yoga Alliance	Locate registered yoga schools and teachers at yogaalliance.org/Directory.
	International Association of Yoga Therapists (IAYT)	Locate a C-IAYT certified yoga therapist at https://www.iayt.org/.
	SilverSneakers Yoga	Offers yoga classes oriented toward older adults: https://tools.silversneakers.com.
Acupuncture	National Certification Commission for Acupuncture and Oriental Medicine	Information on national and state regulations, licensure, and database to find practitioners: https://www.nccaom.org/.
Chiropractic care	American Chiropractic Association	Locate a licensed chiropractor in your state at https://www.acatoday.org/About/Related-Organizations/State-Licensing-Boards.
Integrative clinical care	Osher Collaborative for Integrative Medicine	An international group of seven academic centers funded by The Bernard Osher Foundation to study, teach, and practice integrative medicine. Locate clinical centers and other resources via https://www.oshercollaborative.org/.

In addition, the VITAL trial found that older individuals treated with 840 mg omega-3 fatty acids did not experience a lower incidence of major cardiovascular events or cancer than those treated with placebo in a 5-year follow-up. Two recent meta-analyses and reviews found fish oil slightly reduces risk of cardiovascular disease mortality and events (myocardial infarction, angina, stroke, HF, peripheral arterial disease, sudden death, and nonscheduled cardiovascular surgical interventions) and reduces serum triglycerides. However, with higher doses of EPA+DHA, there may be a reduction in myocardial infarction and coronary heart disease events. Fish oil supplements are relatively low cost and have benign side effect profiles. In addition, given the low drug-drug interactions with other standard therapies used in primary and secondary cardiovascular disease prevention, it is prudent to consider the potential benefits of omega-3 (EPA/DHA) supplementation, especially using 1000 to 2000 mg/d dosages. These levels are rarely obtained in most diets, even those including some routine fish consumption.

Fish oil has been extensively studied in the treatment of depression. Meta-analyses suggest that fish oil may be helpful, although there is quite a bit of debate. There is variability between doses, ratios of EPA to DHA, and other study design issues. The most effective preparations appear to have at least 60% EPA relative to DHA. In older adult populations, a 2018 meta-analysis found mixed findings in studies of fish oil for depression. It appears that doses greater than 1.5 g of EPA/DHA may have benefit. Current large-scale studies are underway and will hopefully inform future guidelines. There is no convincing evidence for the efficacy of fish oil supplements in the treatment of mild to moderate Alzheimer dementia, as well as age-related macular degeneration.

Coenzyme Q10

Coenzyme Q10, also known as ubiquinone or CoQ10, is endogenously produced and found throughout the body. It functions as a critical cofactor in the production of adenosine triphosphate (ATP), and its reduced form, ubiquinol, acts as an antioxidant. The majority of CoQ10 is in mitochondria where it serves as a critical cofactor in the electron transport chain and thus ATP production. CoQ10 can also be obtained through the diet or as a dietary supplement. Primary dietary sources of CoQ10 include oily fish (such as salmon and tuna), organ meats (such as liver), and whole grains. Most individuals obtain sufficient amounts of CoQ10 through a balanced diet.

As a dietary supplement, it is most well-known for its role in managing statin-associated muscle symptoms. While statins affect cholesterol biosynthesis, they also decrease the biosynthesis of CoQ10. Decreased circulating levels of CoQ10 are hypothesized to cause mitochondrial dysfunction, resulting in muscle pain, weakness, cramps, and tiredness. A 2018 meta-analysis of 12 RCTs found that CoQ10 supplementation decreased statin-associated muscle symptoms. This finding was independent of administration doses of CoQ10 (100–600 mg/d) or CoQ10 supplementation time (30 days to 3 months). Future studies will need to determine both optimal dose as well as duration of treatment.

CoQ10 supplementation may be beneficial for patients with HF, as HF is believed to be a low energy, reduced functional state due to metabolic alterations that affect both skeletal and cardiac muscle. The 2014 Q-SYMBIO study was one of the largest prospective RCTs of CoQ10 in the management of HF. Patients with moderate to severe HF (with reduced ejection fraction) were randomly assigned to receive either CoQ10 100 mg three times daily or placebo, in addition to standard therapy. At 2 years, there were significant reductions in major adverse cardiac events (ie, death, hospitalization) in patients receiving CoQ10. It was safe and well-tolerated.

CoQ10 has been purported to be beneficial in the treatment and management of numerous other conditions. This includes hypertension, diabetes, obesity, migraines, Parkinson disease, and kidney disease. In general, the data are limited due to heterogeneity in dosage, duration, and trial design.

Supplements for Memory

Gingko biloba The dried leaf of the ginkgo tree has been used medicinally for thousands of years. Multiple pharmacologically active compounds have been isolated, including flavonoids and terpene lactones, which increase the production of nitric oxide and activate certain central neurotransmitters, which may contribute to gingko's beneficial effects on memory and cognition. EGb761, the formulation that has been studied most extensively, is standardized to contain 24% flavonoid glycosides and 6% terpene lactones; it is approved by the German Commission E for the treatment of cognitive impairment and intermittent claudication. This was supported by a 2018 meta-analysis of randomized controlled trials studying EGb761 in the treatment of dementia; this study found that 22- to 24-week treatment with a standardized 240 mg EGb761 dose may lead to improvements in behavioral and psychological symptoms of dementia, as well as significant decreases in caregiver distress. In addition, another 2018 review found that this standardized extract also may alleviate tinnitus and dizziness that are often seen as concomitant symptoms in patients with dementia. A 2020 updated review noted that while ginkgo biloba may be able to improve the cognitive function in patients suffering from mild dementia/cognitive decline when given for more than 24 weeks and at appropriate dosage (240 mg per day), there is very little data on the long-term administration. In summary, there are conflicting data on the effect of ginkgo on cognition; however, with the paucity of options in the treatment of mild cognitive decline, ginkgo may be considered an option.

There are theoretical concerns about a risk of increased bleeding because higher antiplatelet activating factor activity has been demonstrated in vitro. Cases of increased bleeding in patients taking ginkgo have been reported, but establishing a causal relationship is challenging because many of these patients had other risk factors including age and medications such as aspirin, NSAIDs, or warfarin. Of note, there have been no reports of bleeding complications in clinical trials. Ginkgo should still be used cautiously in patients with bleeding disorders or who are taking aspirin, NSAIDs, warfarin or other anticoagulants, or other botanicals that may increase the risk of bleeding. Allergic skin reactions, gastrointestinal disturbances, and headaches occur in less than 2% of patients.

Vitamin E Vitamin E is a family of eight different lipid-soluble substances, namely α-, β-, γ-, and δ-tocopherol, and -tocotrienol. Vitamin E acts as a chain-breaking antioxidant, terminating lipid peroxidation. α-Tocopherol is the main vitamin E form found in the human body. It has important roles, including diminishing the rate of oxidative stress—an important component in the pathogenesis of atherosclerosis and nonalcoholic fatty liver disease. Although studies have suggested possible cardiovascular disease benefits, meta-analyses have not substantiated the protective effects of vitamin E. Furthermore, some meta-analyses have suggested increase in all-cause mortality when high doses are used. One reason for this has been the various forms and blends of vitamin E that have been studied. For example, it has been suggested that γ-tocopherol exerts a much more potent antioxidant, anti-inflammatory, and cardioprotective effect than α-tocopherol, the one present in most formulations. In cancer populations, including bladder, prostate, colorectal, and lung cancer, the benefits are inconclusive. Most meta-analyses of individuals with these cancers have found no benefit with vitamin E supplementation. A recent finding from the Women's Genome Health Study (WGHS, N = 23,294) in which participants received 10-years of alpha-tocopherol in a placebo-controlled trial reported a highly significant gene (COMT) by alpha-tocopherol interaction, such that alpha-tocopherol was beneficial for cancer prevention among rs4680 met-allele (28%), but not val-allele (23%) homozygotes. This and other studies suggest the full benefit of HDSs may not be understood until they are evaluated within a precision medicine framework. Studies of the α-tocopherol form of vitamin E in individuals with mild cognitive impairment found that it does not prevent progression to dementia, nor improve cognitive function in people with mild cognitive impairment or dementia due to Alzheimer disease. With the caveat that more research is needed, a 2017 Cochrane review concluded there is some evidence that it may slow functional decline in Alzheimer disease. There appears to be a benefit of α-tocopherol supplementation in nonalcoholic fatty liver disease, in that it improves hepatic steatosis and hepatic inflammation; however, there are inconsistent findings in its ability to improve liver fibrosis. The 2018 practice guidelines of the American Association of Liver Disease recommend 800 IU/d of α-tocopherol for the treatment of biopsy-proven, nondiabetic patients with nonalcoholic steatohepatitis.

Glucosamine and Chondroitin

Glucosamine and chondroitin are naturally occurring compounds in the body functioning as the principal substrates in the biosynthesis of proteoglycan. They are believed to relieve joint pain and slow the rate of joint destruction and cartilage loss by serving as chondroprotective agents and disease-modifying osteoarthritis drugs. However, the biology of both compounds is poorly understood. Results have been conflicting in clinical trials. This is largely due to differences in study designs and populations of patients, investigator bias, or the use of different drug formulations (eg, glucosamine sulphate vs glucosamine hydrochloride). Despite it being a commonly used dietary supplement, the American College of Rheumatology and the Arthritis Foundation (ACR/AF) do not recommend the use of glucosamine, chondroitin, or a combination product in hand, hip, or knee osteoarthritis. The one exception is chondroitin in the management of hand osteoarthritis, where the ACR/AF has provided a conditional recommendation. This is due to a single trial of chondroitin sulfate, which found improvements in pain in hand osteoarthritis with a daily dose of 800 mg. Glucosamine and chondroitin have been found to have low potential toxicity.

S-Adenosylmethionine (SAM-e)

S-Adenosyl-L-Methionine (commonly known as SAM-e) is a naturally occurring molecule that owns a chemically reactive methyl group, responsible for several physiological transmethylation reactions. It is ubiquitously present in cells, where it is involved in many cellular functions and takes part in several metabolic pathways—including synthesis of proteoglycans for cartilage along with myelination and synthesis of endogenous anti-inflammatory, neurotrophic, and antioxidant molecules. In addition, it has potential epigenetic effects involving synthesis, repair, and recombination of DNA.

SAM-e has been marketed for the treatment of depression and for other medical conditions such as osteoarthritis, fibromyalgia, liver disease, and migraine headaches. In general, the data are limited in interpretation with reference to high-quality randomized controlled trials. With that being said, there are encouraging results for SAM-e as a monotherapy or as an adjunctive therapy. Moreover, there appears to be clinical consensus that SAM-e may be useful in treatment-resistant depression, especially as an adjunctive therapy. Similarly, SAM-e has been shown to have promise in the treatment of osteoarthritis, with respect to function and pain management; data are sparse, and further studies are needed.

Recommended daily doses of SAM-e range from 200 mg to 1600 mg taken in divided doses, depending upon the condition for which it is being taken and its severity, and upon the route of administration. Most commonly, SAM-e is administered orally; it has a short half-life, undergoing first-pass effects and rapid metabolism. Oral doses of SAM-e at 1600 mg/d are significantly bioavailable and nontoxic. Because SAM-e is best absorbed on an empty stomach, it should be administered 30 to 60 minutes before meals or 2 hours after meals. One reported but uncommon adverse effect of SAM-e is that it may induce mania in some cases. However, this should be interpreted with caution as individuals may be misdiagnosed with major depressive disorder, when they in fact have bipolar disorder.

Supplements for Sleep

Melatonin Melatonin is a lipophilic hormone that is an important regulator of circadian and seasonal rhythms. In humans, its primary physiological function is to control sleep-wake cycles and reinforce sleep behavior. Endogenous melatonin is produced by the pineal gland and regulated tightly by visual light cues in the hypothalamic suprachiasmatic nucleus. Production is inhibited during the day and disinhibited at night. In a healthy, normal individual, serum levels start to rise in the evening hours, reaching peak concentration around 2 to 4 am, after which levels decline again until reaching low daytime levels.

Melatonin levels decline with age due to altered hormone regulation and secretion, changes in renal and hepatic clearance, and other neuroanatomical degeneration. The lower peak levels of endogenous serum melatonin may be due to decreased pineal gland melatonin synthesis or pineal gland calcification. Endogenous melatonin synthesis may be further reduced by drugs (eg, benzodiazepines, NSAIDs, and calcium channel blockers). Mean levels of excretion have been shown to be particularly low in multiple, chronic disease states, so that older adults with chronic comorbidities might be especially vulnerable to inadequate melatonin levels and impaired sleep. Studies suggest older adults are prone to disorders related to an altered circadian rhythm, including disorders of cognitive function, delirium, and sleep.

Exogeneous melatonin has been studied in various primary and secondary sleep disorders. It has been shown to induce phase shifts in the circadian pacemaker, synchronizing the sleep–wake cycle and restoring the circadian secretion pattern to normalize levels of melatonin. When administered acutely, it reduces core body temperature and lowers alertness, encouraging sleep propensity. Melatonin may have potential in treating disorders of sleep initiation, sleep maintenance, as well as circadian phase disturbance. In a recent meta-analysis of 12 randomized controlled trials the most convincing evidence was in reducing sleep-onset latency in primary insomnia, delayed sleep-phase syndrome, and regulating the sleep-wake patterns in blind patients compared with placebo. Much of the literature includes patients aged 55 to 80. Ramelteon is a selective melatonin receptor agonist used in the treatment of insomnia. Studies show that ramelteon is effective in improving sleep latency, sleep efficiency, and subjective total sleep time for individuals with insomnia.

Dose, formula (extended release or fast acting), and timing of administration appear to be important, although not well-studied. There may be decreased effectiveness in patients with neurological deterioration or comorbid clinical disorders such as Alzheimer disease. Other studies report efficacy of melatonin in improving sleep quality in older adults with underlying neurodegenerative disorders. Two studies investigated the treatment of primary insomnia of older people (aged 55+) with melatonin (2 mg 1–2 hours before bedtime orally) and concluded long-term use of melatonin (for 13–24 weeks) is well-tolerated. Initial recommended starting doses of melatonin in older adults are 0.3 to 2 mg of immediate-release formulation melatonin, taken 1 hour before bedtime to best mimic the normal physiological circadian rhythm of melatonin and to avoid prolonged, supra-physiological blood levels; a maximum dose is 9 to 10 mg. Little evidence is available regarding the potential adverse effects of long-term melatonin use. Uncommon side effects potentially include headaches, dizziness, vomiting, and nausea.

Valerian Historically, the therapeutic use of valerian is thought to date back to classical antiquity and the herb is touted as an anxiolytic and sleep aid. It was described by Hippocrates and prescribed by Galen in the second century for insomnia. While there are over 200 valerian species worldwide, *Valeriana officinalis L.* is the most well-known in Europe and North America. Valerian preparations are available in aqueous or dry hydroalcoholic extracts, or as whole or communitive herbal roots and stems.

Potential mechanisms and sites of action include modulation of GABA receptors and increasing the amount of GABA available in the synaptic cleft. Other sites of action include adenosine A1 receptor activation and serotonin (5-HT5a) receptor signaling. The active ingredient of valerian is not agreed upon, and different constituents including volatile oils like valerenic acid (giving a characteristically unpleasant odor), sesquiterpenes, or valepotriates have been used to standardize valerian extracts. Combination herb preparations have been studied such as valerian-Humulus lupulus (hops), valerian-Melissa officinalis (lemon balm), and valerian-Passiflora incarnata (passion flower).

Several reviews and meta-analyses have been published with inconsistent results and criticism regarding methodological quality. Most recently in 2020, a systematic review of 60 studies of valerian for sleep problems and associated disorders was conducted, with a subgroup meta-analysis on subjective sleep quality (10 randomized controlled trials). This analysis concluded that valerian could be a safe and effective herb to promote sleep and associated disorders. However, inconsistent outcomes may be due to variable quality of herbal extracts and that more reliable effects might be expected from the whole root/rhizome. The safety profile of valerian is good, although some note caution in severe liver disease. Importantly, valerian requires use for several weeks for effect. In contrast to prescription sedative hypnotics, valerian does not cause psychomotor retardation or impair cognitive performance and is non-habit forming with no reported withdrawal symptoms on discontinuation. A common dose is 300 to 900 mg of standardized extract (0.8% valerenic acid) or 2 to 3 g dried root taken as a tea 30 minutes to 2 hours before bedtime.

Black Cohosh

Black cohosh (*Cimicifuga racemosa* or *Actaea racemosa*), also known as bugbane, black snakeroot, or rattleweed, is a perennial plant from the buttercup family native to Canada and eastern US with a characteristic dark-colored rhizome. The rhizome extracts were traditionally used by Native Americans to treat multiple ailments including menstrual irregularity. Over the past 2 decades, there has been steady interest in black cohosh for the treatment of menopausal symptoms.

The rhizome of black cohosh contains several potential, biologically active constituents (including the triterpene glycosides actein and cimicifugoside, as well as fatty acids, resins, caffeic acids, isoferulic acids, and isoflavones). Black cohosh was originally thought to be a phytoestrogen with its isoflavone component exerting estrogenic effects selectively on the LH receptor; however, recent studies have not consistently demonstrated this. Instead, central neuromodulation through the triterpene glycosides may be the mechanism of action, including dopaminergic effects that oppose prolactin (possibly affecting libido and bone metabolism), serotonergic effects (much like SSRIs widening the thermoregulatory zone for vasomotor symptoms and mood), and GABAergic effects.

While popular among women seeking nonhormonal options, the literature has been inconsistent. A Cochrane review in 2012 reviewed 16 RCTS of peri-/postmenopausal women using oral mono preparations of black cohosh at a median daily dose of 40 mg for a mean duration of 23 weeks concluded that there was insufficient high-quality evidence to recommend black cohosh in improving frequency or intensity of vasomotor hot flashes, vulvovaginal symptoms, or overall menopause symptoms score (including insomnia, headache, paresthesia, and anxiety). Since then, higher-quality studies have reported improvements in composite menopausal symptoms with black cohosh over placebo. There is significant heterogeneity in studies with regard to herb preparation, but many have standardized to 27-deoxyactein (triterpene glycoside). The most studied commercial product is Remifemin® (contains 1 mg of 27-deoxyactein in one 20-mg tablet, to be taken 1–2 times daily).

The herb appears relatively safe with no known medication interactions. The most commonly reported side effects are mild and transient gastrointestinal upset and rashes. Most studies have examined black cohosh use for 6 months or less, so long-term safety is not known. Due to theoretical estrogenic effects, caution should be used in any patient (eg, with history of breast cancer) for which estrogen therapy would be contraindicated. There has also been a concern raised regarding hepatotoxicity; however, there is little evidence to support an adverse effect on liver function.

Saw Palmetto

Saw palmetto (*Serenoa repens*), from the berries of the American dwarf palm tree, is used for symptomatic benign prostatic hypertrophy. Available in multiple formulations including liquid extracts, tablets, capsules, and tea, the active components of palmetto extracts are not well understood but may include phytosterols, volatile oils, and free fatty acids. Purported mechanisms of action include weak inhibition of 5-alpha-reductase and the conversion of testosterone to dihydrotestosterone (DHT), inhibition of DHT binding in prostatic cells, anti-inflammatory effects, and inhibition of fibroblast and epithelial growth factors and induction of apoptosis.

Many earlier, smaller studies showed benefit of saw palmetto for mild to moderate lower urinary tract symptoms such as urinary frequency, nocturia, and dysuria as compared to placebo. Some studies suggested similar effects to finasteride or tamsulosin. Studies were unclear regarding an effect on urinary flow rate, but there is likely no effect of saw palmetto on prostate size or serum prostate specific antigen. The literature overall has been mixed. A 2011 multicenter RCT evaluated escalating doses beyond the standard dose (320 mg per day) up to 960 mg per day did not find that saw palmetto extract was better than placebo in ameliorating lower urinary tract symptoms of BPH. There was, however, also no difference in adverse effects suggesting overall safety. A 2012 Cochrane Review of 32 RCTs also concluded there was no difference between saw palmetto and placebo for BPH symptoms. Most recently, however, a 2018 meta-analysis which evaluated a particular European product of saw palmetto (hexanic extract Permixon®) at the standard dose (320 mg per day) concluded that saw palmetto reduced nocturia and improved flow rate compared with placebo with a similar efficacy to tamsulosin and short-term 5-alpha reductase inhibitors in relieving lower urinary tract symptoms. Other studies have suggested that the efficacy of saw palmetto is enhanced with selenium and lycopene (a common commercial formulation) or may be useful as an adjunct to conventional medication and safe to use in combination.

The usual dosing is 160 mg twice a day with an allowance of 8 weeks therapy to evaluate effects. Side effects are uncommon and mild and may include dizziness, headache, nausea, vomiting, constipation, and diarrhea. Rare case reports of liver enzyme elevations have occurred resembling viral hepatitis with resolution within 1 to 3 months.

MIND-BODY PRACTICES

Mind-body practices encompass a diversity of interventions including movement-based practices (eg, tai chi, yoga, contemplative dance, Pilates, Feldenkrais) and less physically oriented practices such as seated meditation. The multimodal nature of these practices, and especially movement-based ones, which coordinate motor, cognitive, and breath training, reflects, their inherent integrative nature, and may explain their effectiveness in treating complex geriatric syndromes such as falls, chronic pain, cognitive decline, and affective disorders, which often involve multiple physiological systems. Here we highlight three of the most evidence-based mind body practices—yoga, tai chi, and meditation—with a focus on application to geriatric conditions.

Yoga

Yoga is a multicomponent mind-body practice that incorporates physical postures, breath regulation, relaxation practices, and meditative techniques. Yoga has increased in popularity among US adults in recent years, from 9.5% reporting practice in 2012 to 14.3% in 2017. Most of this group were adults age 18 to 44, but interest and practice among older adults are expected to grow given baby boomers' increased knowledge, acceptance, and access to mind-body practices.

Yoga practice seems to positively impact aging on multiple levels, from cellular stress to improvements in overall physical and mental health. Some small studies have suggested that yogic meditative practice may reduce telomerase activity in dementia care partners. Yoga practices are thought to reduce inflammation by downregulating the sympathetic nervous system response and hypothalamic-pituitary adrenal axis, thereby decreasing cytokine release. There have been several studies of the impact of yoga on cardiovascular function, suggesting improved heart rate variability, improved baroreflex responsiveness, and slowing of age-related changes in cardiovascular function. In addition, yoga may increase respiratory muscle strength. However, data are incomplete and variable in these areas.

Beyond the cellular and organ systems levels, yoga positively impacts multiple aspects of physical function in older adults. There are several randomized controlled trials demonstrating improvements in measures such as the timed up and go test, gait speed, chair stand test, 6-minute walk test, functional reach, tests of standing balance, range of motion, flexibility, and muscle strength. These trials were conducted in a variety of populations, including the community, assisted-living facilities, and nursing homes. Interventions consisted of a variety of styles of yoga generally taught one to three times per week over 8 to 24 weeks. There are a few studies that showed improvements in higher level functional outcomes, such as ADLs or the ability to carry heavier objects. In one study yoga practice reduced the number of falls, but this was only seen in within-group analysis and was not significant in the yoga group as compared to an exercise control. In multiple studies yoga practices seem to improve fear of falling.

In terms of cognition, yoga likely has a positive impact, though the evidence is less robust than other areas. In a systematic review and meta-analysis of 12 studies including 912 older adults, about 70% of whom had preexisting cognitive impairment, yoga was beneficial for memory, executive function, attention, and processing speed. Neuroimaging of long-term versus naïve yoga practitioners has shown thicker gray matter in brains of long-term practitioners, including the hippocampus and those associated with attention, interoception, and sensory processing.

Yoga improves mood and quality of life in older adult populations. There are many randomized controlled trials demonstrating reduced depression and anxiety in older adults after a yoga intervention, and also many that demonstrate benefit for fatigue, quality of life, stress, and emotional well-being. Yoga interventions seem to improve social support, with at least one study demonstrating reduced loneliness.

There is consistent evidence to support the use of yoga for chronic low back pain—a 2017 Cochrane review found low- to moderate-certainty evidence that yoga resulted in small to moderate improvements in back-related function at 3 and 6 months. Many studies also suggest benefit for low back pain in addition to function. The American College of Physicians issued clinical practice guidelines in 2017 recommending yoga as one of many nonpharmacologic treatments to utilize as an initial approach in chronic low back pain (strong recommendation; low-quality evidence).

Adverse effects have been reported from yoga practice, though high-quality data are limited. In one study of approximately 2500 yoga class attendees with a mean age of 58 years, 27% of attendees reported an adverse event. These were mostly muscle and joint pain, followed by dizziness. People over age 70 reported fewer adverse events, but orthostasis was more common in this group as compared to younger participants. There have been case reports of vertebral compression fracture, particularly in postures with flexion or forward folding. There are some postures that should be avoided in certain medical conditions, such as inversions in participants with hypertension or glaucoma.

Clinicians who work with older adults should be aware of some basics of the yoga profession when referring patients. There are many styles and schools of yoga; all typically include an initial focus on physical posture (*asana*), breath control (*pranayama*), and sensory withdrawal (*pratyhara*), then moving to incorporate principles of ethics (*yamas* and *niyamas*) and meditation (*dharana, dhyana, samadhi*). Commonly utilized approaches for older adult populations, with focus on alignment and slower movements, include Iyengar yoga, chair yoga, and restorative yoga. However, most yoga styles can be suitably adapted for the needs of older adults under the guidance of an experienced teacher or therapist.

The majority of yoga teachers have a minimum of 200 hours of yoga teacher training and are typically certified by the Yoga Alliance. However, there is a large range of experience, with some teachers conducting classes right out of training and others having apprenticed with another teacher for many years. Yoga teachers may have additional expertise with specific populations, such as pregnant women or older adults. Yoga therapists are trained yoga teachers with a minimum of 800 additional hours of yoga therapy school through the International Association of Yoga Therapists. They are trained to work with people with medical conditions in a safe and effective way. A yoga therapy prescription typically looks more like a physical or occupational therapy referral. Older adults who are experiencing more medical complexity and/or geriatric syndromes may benefit from one-on-one work with a trained yoga therapist rather than engaging in a general yoga class conducted by a yoga teacher. Physical and occupational therapists are often knowledgeable about yoga resources in the area and can help guide the patient and clinician in selecting an appropriate path for referral.

Tai Chi

Tai chi is a multimodal mind-body exercise that originated in Asia, and is growing in popularity in the West, especially among older adults. Data from the 2012 and 2017 NHIS report prevalence of tai chi practice in the United States in the general population at less than 5%, substantially lower than yoga. However, it is thought that these numbers under-report growing use among older adults. Originally developed as a martial art, tai chi integrates training in balance, flexibility, and neuromuscular coordination with multiple cognitive components including heightened body awareness, focused attention, imagery, multi-tasking, and goal-oriented training. This may underlie its benefits to balance, cognition, gait health, and chronic pain, as compared to conventional unimodal exercise. High-quality meta-analyses support that tai chi reduces falls by 20% to 45%, and a Cochrane review concludes it is among the best available exercise options for fall prevention in ambulatory older adults. A recent study reported that a 24-week program of twice a week group tai chi led to a 58% reduction in falls among those at high risk for falls, as compared to a stretching exercise control. There is also sound evidence that tai chi can effectively reduce falls in people with Parkinson disease. Experimental research supports that tai chi reduces falls by positively impacting multiple fall-related risk factors including: reduced lower extremity strength and flexibility, reduced proprioception and postural awareness, poor neuromuscular coordination, impaired executive function, and fear of falling.

In addition to fall prevention, a growing body of evidence supports benefits of tai chi for a range of cardiopulmonary and metabolic issues including chronic HF, hypertension, hyperlipidemia, and COPD. Mixed evidence suggests tai chi training may reduce the risk of stroke. Meta-analyses also support potential cognitive benefits, including improved executive and global cognitive function in older adults that are cognitively intact as well as those with mild cognitive impairment. Evidence for pain conditions including knee osteoarthritis and chronic neck and back pain is also promising, and recent studies have begun to specifically evaluate the benefits of tai chi for chronic and multisite pain conditions specific to older and frail adults.

Tai chi is a safe and adaptable exercise, including for frail older adults. A 2014 systematic review including 153 RCTs concluded tai chi is unlikely to result in serious AEs, but it may be associated with minor musculoskeletal aches and pains. However, poor and inconsistent reporting of AEs limits the conclusions that can be drawn regarding the safety of tai chi. A 2019 review (256 RCTs) with an embedded meta-analysis (24 RCTs) also reported higher levels of minor AEs typical of any exercise program. Subgroup analyses in HF patients reported significantly more serious AEs for inactive control interventions compared with tai chi.

Community-based tai chi programs for fall prevention have been shown to be scalable, effectively implementable, and cost-effective. The majority of successful programs have included group based classes that meet 2 times per week over a period of 3 to 6 months. There are no national standards for tai chi instructor certification, and programs can vary considerably. Similar to yoga, there are many styles and forms of tai chi available. However, they all share common principles and typically include core elements of body awareness and mindful movement. A common approach for older adults is Yang style tai chi, although most programs can be adapted for older adults who are deconditioned or have other physical limitations. Practical considerations when looking for a class include: experience of instructors, program focus (health vs martial applications), and accessibility. For individuals with significant health concerns, choosing teachers with experience teaching in a health care setting or formal training (eg, physical therapists, nurses, physicians) is suggested. Observing a single class and talking with others already enrolled in any given program before formally enrolling is advisable.

Tai chi has reportedly been associated with improved exercise self-efficacy. In combination with its safety and adaptability to many conditions, it has been proposed as an excellent "gateway exercise" for sedentary or deconditioned adults wanting to become more physically active.

Meditation

Meditation is a broad term that incorporates features of self-regulation, awareness, attention, and presence that is typically cultivated through an intentional practice. It has increased tremendously in popularity. Compared to the 2012 NHIS, the 2017 NHIS survey noted that there was nearly a fourfold increase in the use of meditation (4.1%–14.2%). Meditation practices can be broadly categorized as focused attention and open monitoring practices. Focused attention practices, which improve concentration abilities, involve focusing one's full attention on a designated object of meditation, such as one's breath. When it is noticed that the mind has wandered from this object, attention is returned to the object. Training the mind, beginning with this basic exercise, has many effects including relaxation, metacognition, cognitive flexibility, uncoupling of painful physical sensations from maladaptive cognitive patterns, and revelation of previously subconscious content. In open monitoring practices, the individual improves the ability to monitor the contents of experience without any reactions or judgments. This can include other aspects of human experience, such as physical sensations (eg, pain) or mental and emotional states (eg, anxiety). In lay contexts, the word "mindfulness" is often interchanged with or joined to "meditation." This reflects the ambiguity in the interpretation of these words as well as their cultural origins.

There have been extensive cardiac, respiratory, metabolic, endocrine, and neurological studies of individuals during meditation. Though much remains unknown, it is clear that meditation involves modulation of the autonomic nervous system as well as the hypothalamic-pituitary-adrenal axis, as originally demonstrated in the late 1960s and early 1970s by Dr. Herbert Benson. At the physiologic level, studies of meditation have found effects on the immune system (reduction in pro-inflammatory cytokines), nervous system (enhanced cortical thickness in specific brain regions; neuroplastic changes in the anterior cingulate cortex, insula, temporo-parietal junction, and fronto-limbic network), and endocrine system (reduced cortisol levels). There are also epigenetic changes seen including telomere length and gene expression. From a psychological perspective, it is thought that meditation enables a stable field of awareness around one's emotions, thoughts, and physical sensations, without reactivity.

In health care settings, one popular application of mindfulness meditation is the mindfulness-based stress reduction (MBSR) program. Originally developed by Jon Kabat-Zinn, this program and its derivatives have been extensively studied in patient populations. It is an 8-week program that introduces mindfulness practice (with Buddhist origins) in a secular, practical form to participants in the context of their life circumstances. This program is intended to create a deliberate, sustained, nonjudgmental way of paying attention to one's experience in order to enhance self-awareness, change maladaptive thinking, increase the capacity for skillful response to challenges, and reduce suffering. There are now thousands of MBSR programs in the United States and other countries. A close derivative of MBSR, mindfulness-based cognitive therapy (MBCT), was developed exclusively for people with recurrent major depression and has been widely applied to other psychiatric populations.

Meditation-based interventions (MBI) have been found to be useful in the comprehensive treatment of anxiety and depression, along with stress-related conditions. A recent meta-review of meta-analyses supports the notion that MBIs hold promise as evidence-based adjunctive treatments in a wide range of mental disorders. MBIs show efficacy in treating common cancer-related side effects, including nausea and vomiting, pain, fatigue, anxiety, and depressive symptoms, and improving overall quality of life. A 2020 meta-analysis found that mindfulness-based interventions were associated with reductions in anxiety

for at least 6 months after the intervention in adults with a cancer diagnosis. Finally, in individuals with hypertension, meta-analyses have found that meditation can significantly reduce systolic and diastolic blood pressures by 7 mmHg and 4 mmHg, respectively. In subgroup analyses, these findings are particularly striking in patients over age 70. There is a fair amount of heterogeneity in the results; however, they continue to be statistically significant and clinically relevant. Many studies are limited by small numbers, heterogeneous design, and varied clinical outcomes. In addition, it is often unclear as to how adherent individuals are to the prescribed protocols. In meta-analyses very few adverse events have been reported. In summary, meditation can be thought of as a safe intervention, that can be used in a variety of medical conditions that have a stress-related component. While it may not be a primary treatment option in isolation, it can be used effectively as an adjunctive treatment as a part of an overall multidimensional treatment in any chronic medical condition.

MANUAL THERAPIES

Chiropractic Care

Chiropractic is a nationally licensed health care profession that focuses on the relationship between spinal function and general health. The profession was first recognized for its use of manually applied spinal manipulative therapy (SMT) in the treatment of musculoskeletal, as well as many nonmusculoskeletal, disorders. In fact, the word "chiropractic" comes from the Greek words cheir (meaning "hand") and praktos (meaning "done"), ie, done by hand. In addition to manually applied therapies, chiropractors administer soft tissue manipulation, recommend lifestyle changes, engage their patients in rehabilitation and fitness coaching, and provide nutritional counseling. The 2017 NHIS survey reported that 9.5% of adults in the United States over age 65 used chiropractic in the prior 12 months. Back and neck pain were the most prevalent conditions treated by chiropractors.

A significant body of research has focused on one component of chiropractic treatment, spinal manipulation, for a number of conditions ranging from back, neck, and shoulder pain to carpal tunnel syndrome, fibromyalgia, and headaches. Low back pain has received the most research attention and spinal manipulation appears to benefit some people with this condition. The 2017 clinical practice guidelines issued by the American College of Physicians strongly recommended spinal manipulation, based on low-quality evidence, as initial treatment for patients with chronic low-back pain. A systematic review supporting the 2017 clinical practice guidelines for low back pain evaluated 32 randomized controlled trials involving more than 6000 participants and found modest, short-term effects on pain.

The benefit of chiropractic for chronic neck pain is less clear. A 2015 Cochrane review of 51 randomized controlled trials involving a total of 2920 participants concluded that there is some evidence to support the use of thoracic manipulation versus another active control for neck pain, function, and quality of life; however, results for cervical manipulation and mobilization are few and diverse. There is some evidence to suggest that multiple cervical manipulation sessions may provide better relief of pain and improvement in function than certain medications at immediate-, intermediate-, and long-term follow-up. Because there is risk of rare but serious adverse events for cervical manipulation, more rigorous research is needed on manually applied therapies, and comparing mobilization and manipulation versus other treatment options. There are no high-quality studies that investigate the full scope of chiropractic care for neck pain and the aforementioned studies focus only on one component of chiropractic treatment.

Data on the benefits of chiropractic care for back and neck pain in older adults specifically is more limited. One trial in older adults over age 65 with chronic mechanical neck pain found that SMT combined with home exercise (HE) resulted in greater pain reduction after 12 weeks of treatment compared with both supervised rehabilitative plus HE and HE alone. A follow-up study including older adults with back and/or neck pain that compared a short (12 weeks) versus long (36 weeks) course of combined SMT and supervised rehabilitative exercise (SRE) concluded that extending management with SMT and SRE from 12 to 36 weeks did not result in any additional important reduction in disability; however, long-term management led to greater improvement in neck pain, self-efficacy, and functional ability and balance. Systematic adverse event monitoring in both studies revealed that no serious adverse events related to interventions occurred. However, nonserious musculoskeletal adverse effects were commonly related to SMT and exercise interventions. The authors concluded that these adverse effects may be regarded as normal reactions to SMT and exercise and should be anticipated and discussed by care providers with their patients. With respect to cervical manipulation, some studies have reported associations between chiropractic care and cervical artery dissection, a rare but serious event. However, the causal nature of this relationship has not been established and is questioned by other studies, which have reported associations between cervical artery dissection and primary care practitioner visits and biomechanical studies which demonstrated that cervical manipulation causes significantly less arterial strain than normal range of motion.

Acupuncture

Acupuncture is a therapy in which practitioners stimulate specific points on the body, usually by inserting thin needles through the skin. Acupuncture has origins in TCM, a holistic healing system that includes diet, herbal remedies, mind-body therapies (tai chi and qigong), massage, and acupuncture. From a traditional perspective, acupuncture is based on a system of acupoints, channels and meridians, and flow of vital energy (qi). Within biomedicine, clinical efficacy of acupuncture as well as biological basis and mechanisms of acupuncture have been studied extensively. In terms of acupuncture mechanism, there is no unified theory, although the neural model, most salient for acupuncture analgesia, is most common. Basic science research first reported that acupuncture stimulates the secretion of the endogenous opioid endorphin. Since that first discovery in the 1970s, a multitude of studies have continued to elucidate central and peripheral networks engaged with acupuncture, including those that affect serotonergic and dopaminergic systems, and influence nociceptive pathways and release of interleukins, adenosine, and substance P. For musculoskeletal pain, myofascial stretch, microinjury, increased local blood flow, and facilitated healing may be involved.

Acupuncture has modest evidence of efficacy for treatment or rehabilitation in a wide range of conditions; however much of the literature is inconsistent and has been limited by methodological challenges, including appropriate controls and acupoint specificity. For example, acupuncture may be a useful adjunct to stroke rehabilitation. Preclinical studies have suggested neurogenesis as a mechanism of acupuncture in ischemic stroke. Systematic reviews and meta-analyses of randomized controlled trials have reported that when added to standard stroke rehabilitation, acupuncture may impact balance function, reduce spasticity, increase muscle strength, and general well-being.

The most robust evidence base has been in acupuncture for pain management. From 1991 to 2009, there were almost 4000 studies of acupuncture, 41% of these for pain conditions. With the opioid epidemic and interest in nonpharmacological approaches to chronic pain, the number of studies has continued to grow. In an individual participant data meta-analysis in 2018 (N = 20,827 patients from 39 trials), investigators concluded that acupuncture is effective for the treatment of chronic musculoskeletal, headache, and osteoarthritis pain. Treatment effects of acupuncture persist over time and have effects above what is seen with placebo. Referral for a course of acupuncture treatment is a reasonable option for a patient with chronic pain. Several other reviews support the use of acupuncture for chronic low back pain. In 2020, the Centers for Medicare and Medicaid Services began coverage for acupuncture services for chronic low back pain.

Most states require a license, certification, or registration to practice acupuncture, and the vast majority of practitioners receive diplomas from the National Certification Commission for Acupuncture and Oriental Medicine for licensing. Some conventional medical practitioners—including physicians and dentists—also practice acupuncture. Practitioners can be identified through national acupuncture organizations, or through referral from physicians and allied health providers. A growing number of hospitals and medical centers now offer acupuncture services, often integrated within pain clinics and oncology programs. The typical course of treatment can vary with conditions, but for common pain conditions, can include 12 to 15 treatments over a 6 to 8 week period.

Ayurvedic Medicine

Ayurveda is the traditional medical system originating from the Indian subcontinent. The practice and education around Ayurvedic medicine were based upon ancient writings that promoted integration between diet, lifestyle, and stress reduction (including meditation and yoga). It is one of the world's oldest medical systems. In India, the practice of Ayurvedic medicine is considered part of the health system, and the education and practice of Ayurvedic medicine regulated is under the Ministry of AYUSH. Diagnoses and evaluation in Ayurvedic medicine are made using a systems-based interpretation through an intrinsic understanding of many factors involved in disease manifestation. This includes a constitutional evaluation as well as pathogenic factors, season, and a patient's entire course of action (diet, drug, and regimen compatible with the constitution) for the expression of the disease. An Ayurvedic clinical examination includes diagnostic methods through inspection, interrogation, and palpation. Ayurvedic treatment combines products (mainly derived from plants, but may also include animal, metal, and mineral), diet, exercise, and lifestyle. In the United States, there are practitioners of Ayurvedic medicine, along with schools and training programs; however, it is presently not an independently licensed profession.

Research in Ayurvedic medicine is limited to studies of individual herbs (eg, turmeric, ashwagandha); there are very few studies looking at it from a systems perspective. Of specific note, some Ayurvedic preparations include metals, minerals, or gems. Previous studies have shown that about one in four supplements tested had high levels of lead and almost half of them had high levels of mercury. The US Food and Drug Administration warns that the presence of these metals in some Ayurvedic products makes them potentially harmful.

Traditional Chinese Medicine

Traditional Chinese medicine (TCM) approaches include acupuncture, herbal medicine, moxibustion, and tai chi/qigong. Acupuncture and herbal medicine are two of the most commonly used integrative medicine therapies. While these therapies are covered elsewhere (ie, acupuncture, tai chi), TCM is a systems-based theory that integrates relationships between symptoms, as well as the human body's relationship with the natural environment. TCM practitioners will discern overall physiological and/or pathological patterns of the human body in response to a given internal and external condition. This is usually a pronouncement of internal disharmony defined by a comprehensive analysis of the clinical symptoms and signs gathered by a practitioner using inspection, auscultation, olfaction, interrogation, and palpation of the pulses.

In the United States, the National Certification Commission for Acupuncture and Oriental Medicine is the certification body that many states use to credential TCM practitioners. Often times, these may be individuals who are also licensed acupuncturists. In many states, the scope of practice for an acupuncturist can include the disbursement of herbal medicines.

Research for herbal medicines used in TCM is increasing. There is promise in TCM in part due to its theoretical framework around holism. Similar to Ayurveda, patient treatments are individualized through reinforcement of the body's immunity, elimination of pathogenic factors, and improvements in innate healing capacities. However, there have been TCM preparations that have been found to be adulterated as well as mislabeled. That is, they contain genetic material from animals or plants that were not listed on the packaging. Certain herbs have had serious health consequences. The most notable ones have been ma huang, or ephedra, and *Aristolochia*, or birthwort. Ephedra, which was marketed as a weight loss medication, was banned by the FDA, as it was associated with sudden cardiac death. *Aristolochia* plants contain aristolochic acid, which is a powerful nephrotoxin and human carcinogen associated with chronic kidney disease and bladder cancer.

Traditional Chinese Medicine has shown some promise in the treatment of temporomandibular disorders. In one study women ages 25–55 with temporomandibular disorders were randomized to receive TCM versus specialty care. Those who received TCM experienced greater reductions in facial pain, an effect that was sustained at 3 months.

CONCLUSION

Integrative medicine utilizes both complementary and conventional health approaches to optimize care of the whole person. In the case of Ms. S, several geriatric syndromes or issues were identified: gait disorder and falls, functional dependence, mild cognitive impairment, polypharmacy, multicomplexity, frailty, depression, and limited social support. **Figure 24-3** summarizes the approach to management by the interdisciplinary geriatrics team where each of the eight recommended management approaches is linked via the colored dots to the syndrome it addresses. A mind-body movement-based practice could be considered. In this case, the integrative modality tai chi was recommended given potential benefits for multiple geriatric syndromes, including gait disorder and falls, functional dependence, mild cognitive impairment, frailty, depression, and social support. In addition, the evidence regarding vitamin E was discussed and the patient decided to discontinue her supplement. Omega-3 fatty acid supplements were discussed as an option, but since the patient met criteria for polypharmacy, she elected not to start taking them at this time. By incorporating multimodal and noninvasive approaches, integrative medicine is poised to play a major role in the promotion of healthy aging and prevention and management of geriatric syndromes.

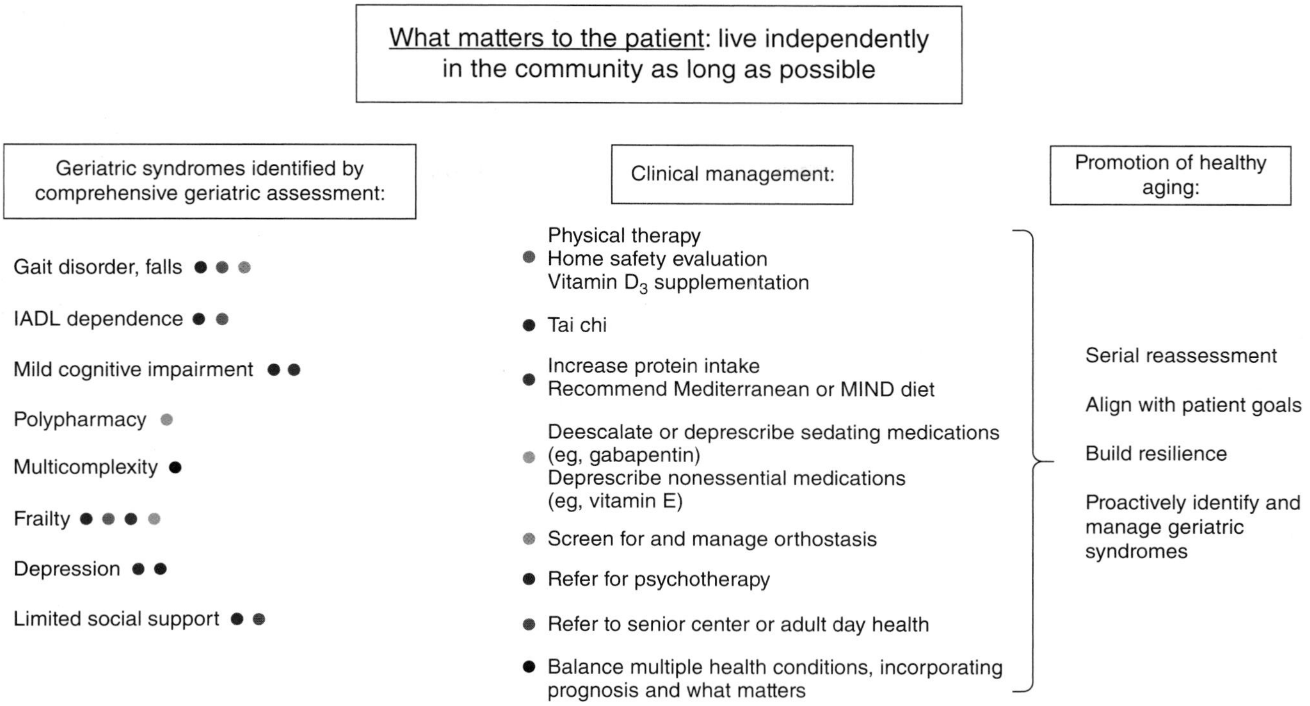

FIGURE 24-3. Geriatric syndromes and clinical management for patient case.

FURTHER READING

Abdelhamid AS, Brown TJ, Brainard JS, et al. Omega-3 fatty acids for the primary and secondary prevention of cardiovascular disease. *Cochrane Database Syst Rev.* 2020;3(2):CD003177.

Clarke TC, Barnes PM, Black LI, Stussman BJ, Nahin RL. Use of yoga, meditation, and chiropractors among U.S. adults aged 18 and over. NCHS Data Brief, no 325. Hyattsville, MD: National Center for Health Statistics. 2018.

Clarke TC, Black LI, Stussman BJ, Barnes PM, Nahin RL. Trends in the use of complementary health approaches among adults: United States, 2002–2012. *National Health Stat Report*; no 79. Hyattsville, MD: National Center for Health Statistics. 2015.

Food and Drug Administration. Dietary supplements, overview of dietary supplements and FDA's role in regulating them. 2019. Available at: https://www.fda.gov/food/dietary-supplements. Accessed April 7, 2021.

Frank J, Kisters K, Stirban OA, et al. The role of biofactors in the prevention and treatment of age-related diseases. *BioFactors* (Oxford, England). 2021;47(4):522–550.

Gahche JJ, Bailey RL, Potischman N, Dwyer JT. Dietary supplement use was very high among older adults in the United States in 2011–2014. *J Nutr.* 2017;147(10): 1968–1976.

George M, Avila M, Speranger T, Bailey HK, Silvers WS. AAAAI Work Group Report: Conducting an Integrative Health Interview. *J Allergy Clin Immunol Pract.* 2018;6(2): 436–439.e3.

Jou J, Johnson PJ. Nondisclosure of complementary and alternative medicine use to primary care physicians: findings from the 2012 National Health Interview Survey. *JAMA Intern Med.* 2016;176(4):545–546.

Khalsa SBS, Cohen L, McCall T, Telles S. *The Principles and Practice of Yoga in Healthcare.* New York, NY: Sage. 2016.

Kolasinski SL, Neogi T, Hochberg MC, et al. 2019 American College of Rheumatology/Arthritis Foundation Guideline for the Management of Osteoarthritis of the Hand, Hip, and Knee. *Arthritis Care Res.* 2020;72(2):149–162.

Li F, Harmer P, Fitzgerald K, et al. Effectiveness of a therapeutic tai ji quan intervention vs a multimodal exercise intervention to prevent falls among older adults at high risk of falling: a randomized clinical trial. *JAMA Intern Med.* 2018;178(10):1301–1310.

Liu H, Ye M, Guo H. An updated review of randomized clinical trials testing the improvement of cognitive function of ginkgo biloba extract in healthy people and Alzheimer's patients. *Front Pharmacol.* 2020;10: 1688.

344 Maiers M, Bronfort G, Evans R, et al. Spinal manipulative therapy and exercise for seniors with chronic neck pain. *Spine J.* 2014;14(9):1879–1889.

Mortensen SA, Rosenfeldt F, Kumar A, et al. The effect of coenzyme Q10 on morbidity and mortality in chronic heart failure: results from Q-SYMBIO: a randomized double-blind trial. *JACC Heart Fail.* 2014;2(6):641–649.

Okereke OI, Reynolds CF, Mischoulon D, et al. The VITamin D and OmegA-3 TriaL-Depression Endpoint Prevention (VITAL-DEP): Rationale and design of a large-scale ancillary study evaluating vitamin D and marine omega-3 fatty acid supplements for prevention of late-life depression. *Contemp Clin Trials.* 2018;68:133–145.

Quandt SA, Verhoef MJ, Arcury TA, et al. Development of an international questionnaire to measure use of complementary and alternative medicine (I-CAM-Q). *J Altern Complement Med.* 2009;15:331–339.

Rutjes AWS, Nüesch E, Reichenbach S, Jüni P. S-Adenosylmethionine for osteoarthritis of the knee or hip. *Cochrane Database Syst Rev.* 2009;2009(4):CD007321.

Scott IA, Hilmer SN, Reeve E, et al. Reducing inappropriate polypharmacy: the process of deprescribing. *JAMA Intern Med.* 2015;175(5):827–834.

Sherrington C, Fairhall NJ, Wallbank GK, et al. Exercise for preventing falls in older people living in the community. *Cochrane Database Syst Rev.* 2019;1(1):CD012424.

Vancampfort D, Stubbs B, Damme TV, et al. The efficacy of meditation-based mind-body interventions for mental disorders: A meta-review of 17 meta-analyses of randomized controlled trials. *J Psychiatr Res.* 2021;134:181–191.

Vickers AJ, Cronin AM, Maschino AC, et al. Acupuncture for chronic pain: Individual patient data meta-analysis. *Arch Intern Med.* 2012;172:1444–1453.

Wieland LS, Skoetz N, Pilkington K, et al. Yoga treatment for chronic non-specific low back pain. *Cochrane Database Syst Rev.* 2017;1(1):CD010671.

Witt CM, Chiaramonte D, Berman S, et al. Defining health in a comprehensive context: a new definition of integrative health. *Am J Prev Med.* 2017;53(1):134–137.

Chapter 25

Patient-Centered Management of Chronic Diseases

Caroline S. Blaum, Aanand D. Naik

INTRODUCTION

Chronic conditions are the major causes of morbidity and mortality among adults in developed countries, as well as the major drivers of health care utilization and cost. In 2020, COVID-19 for a short time was the third leading cause of death in the United States. It affected all-cause death rates and lowered life expectancy. A major risk for severe COVID-19 disease and death, along with advanced age, was the presence of chronic conditions. The management of chronic conditions has been the major focus of health care in the United States for decades, with the goals of preventing the worsening of a chronic disease, decreasing development of related chronic diseases, mitigating associated functional impairment and disability, and decreasing health care utilization and costs. As people age, they confront an increasing number and complexity of chronic conditions and disabilities. Nearly two-thirds (65%) of adults older than age 65 live with MCC, and an estimated 171 million Americans will have MCC by 2030.

For people with chronic conditions, the vast majority of their health care management is done by them in their homes. Even when people have MCC and see many clinicians sometimes many times a month, they still spend the vast majority of their time at home, and are implementing recommended clinical interventions by themselves, or with a family member or care partner, in their homes. Clinicians, researchers, and policy makers have long recognized that patients should not be left alone in their self-management efforts. Self-management support is now understood to be an important component of ongoing clinical care and that achieving good outcomes of chronic disease management depends on patients' engagement and partnership in their care. Clinicians, practices, and the health system have roles in assuring that patients and their care partners can self-manage chronic diseases. Because self-management support was not historically considered clinical care, it is only beginning to be reimbursed by payers. Now because it is understood to be central to the management of chronic diseases care, it is often a component of value-based payment models and some self-management support interventions (eg, diabetes education) are reimbursed.

The basic premise of patient self-management and self-management support is that self-management

Learning Objectives

■ Understand the heterogeneity of older adults and how chronic disease self-management and self-management support approaches differ depending on patients' health status and clinical complexity, and why self-management and self-management support based on single-disease clinical practice guidelines have limitations in people with multiple chronic conditions (MCC) and complex health status.

■ Acquire a basic foundation in (1) behavioral concepts underlying patient self-management and self-management support interventions; (2) types of self-management support interventions, including newer technology-based strategies; and (3) the evidence base for different models of self-management support.

■ Recognize the paradigm shift in the concepts of self-management of multimorbidity for people with MCCs and/or complex health status that involves patients/care partners engaging and partnering in their care and articulating their health outcomes goals and preferences, and clinicians aligning clinical decision making with patients' goals and preferences.

Key Clinical Points

1. People living with chronic diseases must "self-manage" these diseases every day. Self-management support for these patients is a key component of clinical chronic disease management.

2. Behavioral health theories and chronic disease management models are the basis of many self-management support interventions. Much research has investigated self-management support for chronic diseases, especially diabetes, hypertension, COPD, and heart diseases, and there are many high-quality systematic reviews in the literature that demonstrate improvements

(Continued)

(Cont.)

in outcomes related to self-management support.

3. However, there is minimal evidence upon which to base chronic disease management among people who have MCC and therefore self-management. People with MCC are not generally included in the studies that provided the evidence. Adherence to disease-specific guidelines may not improve care for patients with MCC and may sometimes cause harm.

4. Self-management support for patients with MCC must be part of a comprehensive approach involving identification of care that matters to these patients and clinical decision making and care plans that provide such care.

5. Patient Priorities Care (PPC) and VA Whole Health are examples of care approaches for older adults with MCC that base care on what matters to patients, and incorporate self-management support within a comprehensive, team-based, whole person approach to care.

is guided by disease-specific guidelines, often based on treatment randomized controlled trials (RCTs) that most often did not include older adults, people with multimorbidity, or people with complex health status. Therefore, clinical management based on these guidelines may not apply to the many older adults with MCC, frailty, or serious, life-limiting conditions. This chapter will explore the complex landscape of chronic disease self-management and self-management support in older adults through the lens of the heterogeneity of the older population. Many older adults are healthy and functional, while some are experiencing severe, life-limiting conditions. There is a big middle group who are accumulating or already have MCC and functional or cognitive impairments and disabilities. Self-management and self-management support interventions, and the clinical paradigms behind them, differ with health status complexity.

This chapter will review foundational behavioral concepts related to self-management of chronic diseases, and how both behavioral theory, and system-based concepts of chronic disease management, have been used to develop, implement, and evaluate disease-specific self-management support interventions.

Finally, it has long been recognized that establishment of a collaborative relationship between clinicians and patients is critical to successful health care. Collaborative and trusting relationships are assuming an even more

central place in clinical care as shared decision making and goal-directed care become more prominent ways to sort out the complexity of clinical decision making in patients with multimorbidity. Longstanding health care disparities and inequities in access and quality of health care, broader social determinants of health, and increasing social isolation of many older people can complicate trusting relationships between clinicians and patients, further impeding chronic disease self-management. This chapter will explore what is known about disparities in self-management and self-management support.

Self-Management and Self-Management Support—Definitions and Key Concepts

Many definitions of self-management of chronic diseases can be found in the literature. It can be defined as patients having the knowledge and skills to accomplish needed tasks to manage their chronic disease on an ongoing, day to day basis; "day to day management of chronic conditions by individuals over the course of an illness"; or "the practice of activities that individuals initiate and perform on their own behalf in maintaining life, health, and well-being, developing the skills needed to decide, implement, evaluate, and revise an individualized plan for lifestyle change." Lorig and Holman have described self-management as including six key competencies: (1) problem solving; (2) decision making; (3) resource utilization; (4) development of a patient/provider relationship; (5) self-tailoring; and (6) taking action. In this theoretical model, they described three self-management tasks: medical management, emotional management, and role management. Through competencies in these tasks, patients can address aspects of chronic disease management that require self-care, such as attention to appropriate diet and exercise, monitoring and taking medications, doing physiological and clinical activities to monitor effectiveness of management and progress of disease (eg, self-monitoring of weight or blood pressure), getting laboratory, imaging, or other clinical tests, going to their physician or other clinical appointments, and communicating with family, caregivers, and clinicians. Competency in these tasks can improve self-efficacy, or the confidence a patient has in managing a chronic disease and dealing with any problem or barriers that arise. Embedded in these ideas of self-management and self-management support is a collaborative relationship between clinicians and patients. Old "top down" ideas such as compliance with treatment imply that the patient is a passive participant in their health care. Patients need to be partners in their care for effective chronic disease self-management.

Self-management of chronic diseases is generally distinguished from related concepts that are also quite relevant to the older population such as wellness and self-care. "Wellness" is when a person engages in activities that promote general health such as exercise and healthy nutrition, not necessarily in response to a chronic illness or an identified personal risk of a chronic illness. Self-care is a term for activities that improve quality of life and well-being, such as taking a vacation, meditating, or seeking social engagement. One way to conceptualize how people's behaviors interact with health and disease is to use the public health framework of primary, secondary, and tertiary prevention. This framework is well-established, although its relationship to management of chronic conditions can sometimes be interpreted in different ways. A common interpretation is that primary prevention occurs before there are any risks or symptoms and signs of disease. Wellness and self-care behaviors would fit into this category. Secondary prevention addresses risks for chronic diseases, such as smoking cessation, or weight loss to prevent diabetes. Because some conditions (ie, hypertension) can be risks for other diseases, secondary prevention is sometimes invoked in management of these conditions, and patient behaviors addressing secondary prevention are also often termed "self-management." There are many interventions designed to support people in these activities. Some of the behavioral theories discussed below are also relevant to secondary prevention behaviors. However, this chapter concerns self-management of chronic diseases and will not review the extensive literature related to secondary prevention activities. Self-management of chronic disease(s) generally fits into tertiary prevention, defined as management to alleviate symptoms and prevent complications and/or worsening of chronic diseases that already are clinically evident.

Improving patients' competencies in chronic disease self-management through self-management support is an important strategy to improve patient outcomes related to chronic diseases, such as improved symptoms, quality of life, and prevention of complications. Self-management support can be considered as a group of tools and techniques that the clinician and/or the health care system can use to support patient self-management. These tools are more than just didactics and education about chronic disease; these tools help patients acquire the competencies and the confidence to handle their condition. Self-management support is sometimes applied to supportive interventions for lifestyle change, such as smoking cessation, weight loss, or increasing physical activity/exercise. The extensive literature on such interventions is beyond the scope of this chapter. Self-management support approaches for substance use are also important interventions and highly relevant to the older population. These are covered in Chapter 23.

Theoretical Frameworks for Self-Management and Self-Management Support

Ideas around self-management and self-management support interventions are grounded in two major theoretical frameworks, health behavior theories and models, and models for improving chronic disease management quality and outcomes. Self-management of disease is health behavior, and many clinicians and scholars have considered why people may or may not engage in chronic disease self-management, and how behavioral theory can be applied to enhance patient self-management through self-management support interventions. It is known that self-management of disease is more successful if related to a patient's goals while it may be less successful if self-management activities are bothersome to the patient and don't appear to help reach a goal. Patients may also need to cope with barriers (can't afford medication) or the excessive complexity of some self-management activities. Information and education are needed but not sufficient, and feedback is considered to be helpful.

Behind these familiar ideas are four major theories of health behavior that most often appear in the literature, although there are several others that have been described. The Health Belief Model has been discussed since the 1950s. It is most often discussed in the context of primary prevention. It has four major tenants as shown in **Table 25-1**, including perceived benefits and barriers related to health behaviors. The model does not account for some key areas of behavior but it has several useful validated components.

The transtheoretical stages of change model, described by Prochaska and DiClemente in 1982, may be the most familiar model. It is often discussed in relationship to smoking cessation interventions, or invoked in exercise program designs. People pass through the "stages of change," pre-contemplative to maintenance, as they make a change in their behavior. The stages, shown in **Table 25-1**, are not necessarily linear, and people can go back and forth between stages. The social cognitive theory, is probably the most widely used as the basis for self-management support interventions. It is a complex and comprehensive behavioral theory that stresses the importance of self-efficacy (a person's confidence in accomplishing and maintaining a change in behavior despite challenges) and reciprocal determinism (a person is both an agent for change and a responder to change). It connects behaviors to personal factors and environmental factors, and emphasizes the importance of observational learning and self-regulatory behavior. The social-ecological model is consistent with social cognitive theory and stresses the importance of the external environment in behavioral change, and that behaviors can also affect the external environment. It considers multiple external levels—interpersonal, organization, community, and public policy—and postulates that creating an environment conducive to behavior change will help such change occur.

Self-management support interventions are recognized as an integral component of chronic disease management, and they are often designed, implemented, and studied in the context of multicomponent interventions designed to improve the quality of chronic disease management. Several models are commonly used to guide such interventions (**Table 25-2**), which are generally implemented and studied in primary care or ambulatory care practices (pulmonary, diabetes, or cardiology).

TABLE 25-1 ■ KEY CHARACTERISTICS OF FOUR HEALTH BEHAVIOR THEORIES AND MODELS THAT ARE THE THEORETICAL BASIS OF MANY PATIENT-FACING AND COMMUNITY-BASED SELF-MANAGEMENT SUPPORT INTERVENTIONS

THEORIES/MODELS OF HEALTH BEHAVIOR	KEY ELEMENTS	OTHER ATTRIBUTES
Health Belief Model	Perceived susceptibility and perceived severity Perceived benefits and perceived barriers Cues to action Self-efficacy (recent addition)	Often used to describe prevention behaviors (secondary prevention)
The Transtheoretical Model and Stages of Change	• Precontemplation • Contemplation • Preparation • Action • Maintenance	Considered most often in health behavior change, such as smoking cessation
Social Cognitive Theory	• Observational learning • Reinforcement • Self-control • Self-efficacy	Postulates that personal, environmental, and behavioral factors interact An important component is "reciprocal determination"—a person can be both an agent for change and a responder to change The major current theory behind self-management support interventions
Social Ecological Model	• Multiple levels of influence: individual, interpersonal, organization, community and public policy • Behaviors both shape and are shaped by the social environment	Sometimes considered an extension of the social cognitive theory Provides framework for some current self-management support interventions

TABLE 25-2 ■ KEY CHARACTERISTICS OF THREE COMMON FRAMEWORKS FOR CHRONIC DISEASE MANAGEMENT

CHRONIC CARE MODEL	PATIENT-CENTERED MEDICAL HOME	PRINCIPLES OF EFFECTIVE PRIMARY CARE
• Community • Healthcare system • Practice setting • Patients • Delivery system design • Self-management support • Decision support • Clinical information systems • Engaged patients • Proactive practice team	• Continuity and accessibility of care • Team-based care • Trained and prepared staff • Efficient clinical operations • Patient engagement and whole-patient approach • Care coordination and integration • Clinical information systems • Ongoing quality improvement	• Engaged leadership • Data-driven improvement • Responsible for patient panels • Team-based care • Patient-team partnership • Population management • Continuity of care • Prompt access to care • Comprehensive and coordinated care • "Template of the future"

The chronic care model was developed as a framework to describe the effective delivery of care for chronic diseases. It considers how the community, health care system, practice setting, and patients interact through six components of chronic care delivery: delivery system design, self-management support, decision support, clinical information systems, leading to a proactive practice team and informed, engaged patients.

The Patient-Centered Medical Home was developed over 15 years ago by the major primary care professional organizations: the American Academy of Pediatrics, the American Academy of Family Physicians, the American College of Physicians, and the American Osteopathic Association. Although it has evolved over the years, it is based on several key principles including continuity and accessibility of care, team-based care, trained and prepared staff and efficient clinical operation, patient engagement, care coordination and integration, effective health information, and ongoing quality improvement. Similarly, the 10 principles of effective primary care were articulated in 2014 by Bodenheimer as including "4 foundational elements—engaged leadership, data-driven improvement, empanelment, and team-based care—that assist the implementation of the other 6 building blocks—patient-team partnership, population management, continuity of care, prompt access to care, comprehensiveness and care coordination, and a template of the future." These models are completely consistent with ambulatory geriatric practice and have in common team-based and coordinated care, "whole-patient" orientation, access and continuity of care, and recognition of the importance of ongoing quality improvement. Geriatrics care, however, also explicitly recognizes the challenges of multimorbidity, functional impairment, frailty, and serious illness among older adult patients, which adds even more complexity to chronic care delivery for these patients.

The self-management support interventions that have been implemented and evaluated in the past 15 years are generally based on components of both behavioral change theories and chronic disease management models. Some are more purely behavioral and "patient facing," while some feature substantial health system redesign; many are multicomponent. Evidence suggests that self-management support interventions are more successful if connected to the health care delivery system rather than only being community based.

Heterogeneity of Older Adults

Supporting patients in self-management of chronic disease is foundational to improving outcomes of chronic disease management. However, the biggest problem faced by a large minority of older adults, about 40% of Medicare patients, is multimorbidity, and self-management strategies for these patients are much less developed. In older adults, MCC are highly prevalent, produce significant morbidity, and contribute to high illness burden. Among the over 5 million active users of the Veterans Health Administration, nearly 1.5 million (29%) have three or more chronic conditions and about 370,000 have five or more chronic conditions. Half of patients with MCC are 65 years or older. The effect of MCC on important and well-studied health and health care utilization outcomes, including decreased quality of life, higher mortality, and increased health care costs are a result of the intrinsically poorer health of persons with MCC.

The premise of self-management and self-management support is different in these multimorbid patients, because most evidence for clinical management is incomplete or absent. A paradigm shift in clinical decision making and chronic disease management is occurring with the recognition that care delivery should be based on the patients' goals and preferences. Emerging evidence is showing that care that matters to people with complex health care needs is associated with decreased care burden and improved patient satisfaction.

The Limitations of Clinical Practice Guidelines in Older Adults With Multimorbidity

Figure 25-1 illustrates a framework for understanding self-management approaches and challenges across the heterogeneous older adult population. In the idealized world of evidence-based medicine, clinical decision making for patients that leads to clinical interventions and patients' self-management, is based on evidence from single-disease clinical practice guidelines. Practice guidelines are typically developed from the best available evidence drawn from narrowly constructed randomized clinical trials. These studies typically focus on a single chronic condition and a target population with tight eligibility criteria. Therefore, most clinical practice guidelines are single-disease guidelines that typically reflect the care of a middle-aged and/or healthy older adult population without significant comorbidities. When understood from this framework (see Figure 25-1, left side), it becomes clear that guidelines optimize outcomes best when applied to functional adults with few chronic conditions who resemble people in the RCTs and other studies that established the guidelines. For this group, interventions typically prevent disease-specific negative outcomes and promote longevity without substantial trade-offs. The implicit goal of health care within the framework of single-disease guidelines is life prolongation through the elimination of disease. It is for this group, and those guidelines, that self-management is defined and self-management support has been developed and investigated. However elegant this perspective appears, it falters

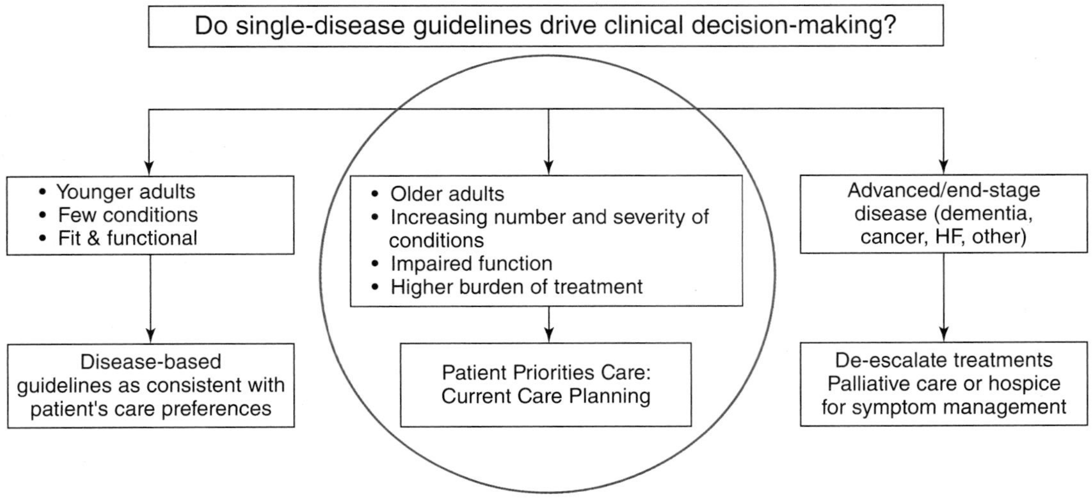

FIGURE 25-1. Heterogeneity of patients drives appropriate use of guidelines. The heterogeneity among older adults and how health status, including multimorbidity and function, determine the appropriateness of chronic disease guidelines for clinical decision making. HF, heart failure. (Adapted with permission from Blaum CS, Rosen J, Naik AD, et al. Feasibility of implementing patient priorities care for older adults with multiple chronic conditions. *J Am Geriatr Soc.* 2018;66[10]:2009–2016.)

as persons age and acquire additional chronic conditions. Many trials and studies exclude people with MCC, or with cognitive impairment, or people of advanced age, or with serious illness, or with disability, that is, people with complex health status. For such people the results of the studies cannot be extrapolated.

An alternative approach (see **Figure 25-1**, right side), focused on symptom management rather than single-disease guidelines, works well in palliative care. Some older people have severe illness, often in the context of multimorbidity, and may be in the last 1 to 2 years of life. For these patients the primary goal is to control urgent symptoms from a serious illness. For these people and their families and care partners, self-management by either the patient or a caregiver must be individualized. There is strong evidence that advance care planning, attention to symptom management, and a palliative care approach are appropriate for this group. However, there is also complexity and heterogeneity among this group. Many people may have advanced cancer or advanced heart failure, where there can be tension between disease-specific management interventions and a palliative approach. The implicit goal of health care shifts in this context to short-term quality of life rather than quantity of life. Guidelines exist for palliative care in people with advanced illness, but they are distinctly different from single-disease guidelines.

Neither of these approaches addresses the decisions faced in the management of older adults with MCC (see **Figure 25-1**, middle), often with functional impairments, who are not experiencing an imminent, life-limiting illness. Older adults with MCC often describe a broad array of short- and intermediate-term outcome goals. Decision making for their health care often involves trade-offs among conditions and dealing with burdens from managing MCC. Clinical practice guidelines designed for single diseases are simply inadequate in their design and application to be useful for older adults with MCC. These practice guidelines are not adjusted for older adults with MCC, do not consider burden of treatment, and do not factor potential harms from drug-drug, drug-disease, and disease-disease interactions. Furthermore, single-disease guidelines often focus on process measures that are very clinician-centered (eg, lipid screening and HDL control) and often do not target outcomes that matter most (eg, improving mobility and social engagement) to older adults who are self-managing their MCC. While for healthier and highly functional people there are few trade-offs in pursuing disease-specific guidelines, many older adults favor less treatment burden due to possible tradeoffs of harms versus benefits, and risks of treatment impacting competing, personally meaningful outcomes. We cannot rely on health care decisions made on single-disease guidelines applied to older adults with MCC that may create a risk of leading to increased harms and potential injuries.

Disease-Specific Self-Management and Self-Management Support Interventions

In middle-aged and healthy older adults who remain functional with few chronic conditions, however, disease-specific self-management and self-management support interventions are relevant. Important and high-quality clinical and health services research has addressed how to translate evidence-based/guideline-based management of chronic disease into practice and investigated whether this improves important outcomes such as decreased symptoms and complications, prevention of disability, decreased health care utilization, and better health-related quality of life. Patient self-management and self-management support interventions have been described and studied as part of the effort to optimize management of chronic diseases, and many self-management support interventions, as discussed below, have been shown to improve selected patient outcomes and have become an important part of the delivery of care to people who are beginning to develop chronic disease (**Table 25-3**). Some of the interventions that have been implemented and studied are likely to be applicable as the development and evaluation of self-management support for people with MCC increases. Self-management support interventions for patients with diabetes, hypertension, heart failure, asthma and COPD, and arthritis predominate, but interventions have also addressed stroke, CVD, bipolar disease, depression, rheumatoid arthritis, chronic low back pain, cancer-related fatigue, and use of oral anticoagulants, and many other chronic conditions.

The published literature is extensive and the behavioral and health services information is well established, with best practices available for implementation. There are multiple scoping reviews, systematic reviews, and meta-analyses that summarize evidence for disease-specific self-management support programs and related models of care.

Many of these interventions have been developed for primary care, although for some conditions they could be

TABLE 25-3 ■ SELF-MANAGEMENT SUPPORT TARGETS, TYPES, AND STRATEGIES		
DISEASES MOST OFTEN TARGETED FOR SELF-MANAGEMENT SUPPORT	**TYPE OF SELF-MANAGEMENT SUPPORT INTERVENTIONS**	**SELF-MANAGEMENT SUPPORT INTERVENTION STRATEGIES**
• Diabetes • Hypertension • COPD • Cardiovascular disease • Multiple others	• Patient education • Community-based, behavioral • Component of chronic disease management program in delivery system • Mixed	• Nurse/team member led • Group visits • Peer support • Technology enabled: telephonic, apps, remote monitoring, patient portal • Mixed

implemented in specialty clinics. Some have been implemented in community settings or use technology, and have variable links to the delivery system. Delivery system interventions are common and include care team member assistance, often a nurse, trained medical assistant, social worker, or pharmacist. Self-management support can occur telephonically, in the clinic, or sometimes in the home. Group visits in the clinical setting especially in diabetes are common self-management support interventions. Other common clinical models use nurse-based interventions, either telephonic/telehealth or in the home (see **Table 25-3**).

Community-based self-management support programs are common and have been investigated extensively. These are often purely patient facing and may or may not link to the clinical delivery system; multiple intervention types are represented in the literature. These can feature group visits (common in exercise or physical activity programs and weight loss), classes, peer counseling, use of technology such as automatic phone calls, websites or smart phone/tablet apps, videos, or intermittent mailings.

Technology and health IT-based interventions are becoming increasingly used and tested for self-management support and directed toward patients (although they can also be directed toward clinician behavior). Besides those mentioned, increased patient use of the EHR with increasingly interactive patient input, may influence patient self-management through better communication with clinicians. Patient portals are widely available with increasing patient uptake and patients can now read and add to clinical notes. Smart phone or tablet apps have become widely used for self-management support and have been evaluated in multiple systematic reviews and meta-analyses. In some early adopter systems, phone or tablet apps used by both patients and providers can seamlessly connect to EHR workflow and these types of connections will become much more widespread as digital interoperability among different platforms for health data, particularly patient generated data, improves.

Other types of chronic disease management interventions are less commonly used in self-management support interventions, although financial incentives for patients have been implemented and studied (eg, gift cards or money for hypertension control).

Specific Self-Management Interventions for Single Chronic Diseases

Below is a brief overview of some of the more common self-management interventions that have been tried in specific chronic diseases. There are many more examples in the literature but those below represent self-management support interventions that can often be found now in primary care or other ambulatory practices.

Diabetes Diabetes is the target of many existing self-management support programs and the disease most often targeted in published self-management support interventions. Multiple types of interventions have been studied and many are effective on some relevant outcomes. Diabetes

Self-Management Support (SMS) can be community based, educational, connected to the primary care or diabetes clinic, use technology, or be a combination of methods. Mobile phone and tablet apps are commonly used in diabetes with many descriptions of such programs and reviews in the literature. Diabetes self-management education has been shown to improve outcomes and Certified Diabetes Educators are reimbursed for this activity. Community-based educational and task competency interventions have been shown to improve patient level outcomes. There has been some attention to self-management support for diverse populations and the CDC has reported that diabetes self-management support is effective in Hispanic patients. Multiple diabetes self-management apps are available for mobile phones, some of which are sponsored by the American Diabetes Association.

Arthritis The first major SMS program based in behavioral theory was the Arthritis Self-Management Program (ASMP) developed by Lorig in 1979. The behavioral foundation of ASMP is social cognitive theory and the development of patient self-efficacy. The program consists of several sessions with trained facilitators and teaches medication management, communication with health care providers, strategies to cope with pain, nutrition, and exercise. It has been evaluated for decades and has been shown to improve patient self-efficacy, self-management behaviors, and possibly general health status, and it has been reported to be associated with cost savings.

The Chronic Disease Self-Management Program (CDSMP) Based on the success of the ASMP, Lorig and colleagues at Stanford applied similar behavioral concepts to self-management support for several diseases, including diabetes, cardiovascular disease, pulmonary diseases, cancer, pain, and HIV, because the skills taught can apply generally to chronic diseases. The different self-management support programs maintain the same format of several sessions with two facilitators and teach similar skills. After many years as part of Stanford University, the Chronic Disease Self-Management Program is now a non-profit called the Self-Management Resource Center (SMRC) that licenses and trains facilitators to implement the program throughout the country. It has relatively broad dissemination.

Hypertension and cardiovascular disease (CVD) CVD continues to be the major cause of death and a significant contributor to morbidity and mortality, and as such has been a major target of SMS interventions. Hypertension is highly prevalent with substantial benefit of treatment. Multiple intervention methods have been used in both, including nurse telephonic support, group visits, and the CDSMP behavioral approach. Mobile apps are thought to be an important tool for hypertension self-management and multiple studies evaluating their use are available. A brief scan of mobile device app stores demonstrates multiple self-management apps for hypertension and CVD.

Heart failure (HF) HF is generally a disease of older adults, whether associated with reduced or preserved ejection fractions. The morbidity, utilization, and mortality associated with heart failure have been a target of disease management programs, self-management support interventions, care delivery redesign, and much clinical and health services research for decades. Despite all this focus, outcomes for HF patients have improved only slightly, and reviews of disease management programs show small to moderate effects on some outcomes. Patients' self-management in HF is complex, and patients must recognize symptoms, manage diet, physical activity and complex medical regimens, recognize and react to physiological changes, and interact with caregivers and clinicians. SMS has generally been included within a multifaceted disease management program that is connected to clinical care, remote monitoring, telephonic/telehealth support, and sometimes home visits. A 2017 Cochrane review cataloged a wide variety of HF disease management programs that included self-management support, and reviewed multiple outcomes where some successes were noted. Now, however, it is widely recognized that fewer than 5% of HF patients only have HF and most patients have five to six comorbidities, often including cognitive impairment, complex health status, and limited life expectancy. Many of these HF patients may fit into a different paradigm of self-management related to their multimorbidity, with attention to goals and preferences.

COPD Self-management support interventions for COPD also feature several models. Similar to other chronic diseases, the CDSMP approach, patient education, and telephonic support are used. Patient action plans and technology approaches providing education and digital management support are also available.

Obesity While clinicians and experts in metabolism and nutrition can debate whether obesity is a disease, there are many self-management support interventions that target weight loss. However, the picture in older adults is not always clear and there is evidence that a body mass index (BMI) in the "overweight range" is protective for older adults. There is likely a U-shaped relationship of BMI index in older ages, where very low and very high BMIs are associated with poor outcomes. Body composition changes with age and loss of muscle appears to occur with aging leading to sarcopenia (discussed in Chapter 30). Weight loss can impact both fat and muscle; loss of muscle mass can exacerbate sarcopenia. Fat composition also changes with age, and even at a relatively low BMI an older adult may have excess fat relative to muscle mass. In obese older adults, sarcopenic obesity, where there is low muscle mass in the setting of obesity, and "fat frailty," where obese older adults meet various criteria defining frailty, have been described and are associated with poor outcomes. The picture may also be confused due to unintentional weight loss that is common in older adults either due to chronic diseases or unmet personal care needs. Studies that have combined weight loss with exercise, in diabetes interventions for example, have shown improved outcomes related to mobility and metabolic parameters. For the "young" old, where obesity is impacting chronic diseases such as diabetes and hypertension, weight loss programs similar to those for middle aged people are likely appropriate and there is an extensive literature in this area. However, it is incumbent upon the geriatrician and clinicians caring for older adults in general to understand when the picture becomes more complex as people age, accumulate MCC, and demonstrate changes in body composition.

Do Disease-Specific Self-Management Support Interventions Improve Outcomes?

Because self-management support is an integral component of the management of chronic diseases, major systematic reviews and meta-analyses often include self-management support within a suite of "disease management" interventions, which can be at the delivery system level, community level, clinician level (which can be multidisciplinary—physician, nurse, social worker, pharmacist, etc.), and patient level. There is debate over what outcomes should be considered in these evaluations, and different studies consider different outcomes. Outcomes that are evaluated are generally in three program categories: system level, provider level (such as provider behavior), and patient level. Patient level outcomes are the target of self-management support. Common patient level outcomes include: adherence to treatment, physiological markers of disease, risk behavior, quality of life, mental health status, satisfaction, function, knowledge, medication use, and health services use. Costs are also sometimes evaluated. Systematic and formal meta-analytic reviews usually tackle the entire disease management program, and use a variety of outcomes related to components of the chronic disease model, or Cochrane Organization's Effective Practice and Organization of Care (EPOC) taxonomy. The EPOC taxonomy considers outcomes related to multiple practice domains and sub-domains including care implementation strategies, service delivery interventions, and financial and governance arrangements. Some reviews, however, drill down to specific components of a self-management support program, evaluating interventions involving apps, telehealth, nurse led, peer led, community based, educational, group visits, home visits, and others.

A recent review of self-management support for chronic diseases, while not focused specifically on older adults, concerns behavioral self-management support, and provides an understandable guide through the evidence for the effectiveness of these interventions. It considers recent Cochrane reviews of self-management support interventions in diabetes, CVD, asthma, and arthritis and has a concise review of the behavioral foundations of self-management support interventions. It concludes that these interventions have a low to moderate effect on important outcomes on health behavior, health status, and health care utilization for selected chronic conditions.

Several systematic reviews focus on self-management support interventions in primary care. One evaluated 58 studies of self-management support in primary care in order to identify effective strategies within the interventions, and the impact of the interventions on multiple patient outcomes. Self-management support was conceptualized as a "portfolio of techniques and tools" that patients and care partners can use as they self-manage chronic disease, as well as a realignment of the patient/clinician relationship so that the patient is fully engaged and a true partner in disease management. The review assessed self-management support interventions that addressed many single conditions—diabetes, COPD, and depression were the most common. Several themes of successful self-management support interventions were identified that emphasize its multicomponent nature. Components of successful interventions include patient goal setting, personalized interventions tailored to patient needs, combinations of strategies to improve patient knowledge of the disease as well as techniques for monitoring symptoms and disease activity, coping and stress management strategies, problem-solving and decision-making skills. Eighteen outcomes were evaluated, and disease-specific and quality of life indicators were most often favorably affected.

Another review of chronic disease management interventions in primary care assessed self-management support as one of the several chronic disease management interventions. This review demonstrated that self-management support was among several interventions for chronic disease management; others include delivery system design changes and clinician decision support. Findings were that self-management support was both the most commonly studied intervention and had the most effect on patient outcomes, particularly for diabetes and hypertension. Self-management support interventions were found to improve patient level outcomes of physiological measures of diseases, risk behavior, satisfaction, and knowledge.

There are also multiple reviews of separate components of self-management support interventions such as nurse led interventions, peer support, and shared medical visits. One systematic review and meta-analysis of nurse led interventions reviewed 29 studies, most from the United States but some from the EU and Australia. It reviewed the effectiveness of a wide range of nurse led interventions including telephonic, in home, in clinic, and involvement by advanced practice nurses and RNs. Content included educational programs, problem solving, and self-management skills development. Most interventions involved hypertension and diabetes, and physiologic markers of disease were the outcomes most often improved (BP, HbA1c). Effects on quality of life and mortality were inconclusive. This review noted that self-management support programs that featured specially trained nurses were more effective. It also noted that nurse led self-management support was not effective in people with multimorbidity.

The literature has many studies and several reviews of peer support interventions. Peer support is generally used to support self-management of cardiovascular disease risk factors and diabetes. Although the evidence is mixed, peer support shows promise in these areas. Evidence suggests it improves glycemic self-management and systolic blood pressure in diabetes, and decreases cigarette smoking in people with cardiovascular risk factors.

Shared medical visits, often called group visits, are common in many current primary care settings. They have been used for over two decades for several conditions, but in middle aged and older adults they mainly focus on diabetes. A major review by Department of Veterans Affairs researchers in 2012, updated in 2014, found some evidence for effectiveness in glycemic control and diabetes knowledge. However, no evidence was found about subgroups who might benefit more, patient satisfaction was not different in those with shared medical appointments, and there was insufficient evidence to assess the relationship of the intensity of the intervention (length of time, group size, medication changes, follow-up visits) to outcomes. A general systematic review of shared medical visits again noted the predominance of such visits in diabetes and findings were consistent with the earlier VA evaluations.

Technology use is a big part of self-management support interventions in current clinical settings, and evaluations of its effectiveness are ubiquitous in the literature. A 2017 metareview (ie, a systematic review of systematic reviews) of telehealth interventions for diabetes, hypertension, heart failure, COPD, and asthma reviewed 56 systematic reviews and 256 studies. Findings were that the systematic reviews were inconsistent, and some but not all showed improved physiological markers of disease.

In the past few years, mobile phone and tablet apps have been used in and studied clinical settings. These technologies have been used most in diabetes, obesity, COPD, and hypertension. A brief scan of PubMed will yield many systematic reviews and meta-analyses from around the world. Most reviews show acceptability and feasibility, but the studies tend to be short-term and many do not use rigorous methodology. Despite some positive results in some reviews, the general consensus is that the effectiveness remains unclear. Regardless, in the current clinical environment, apps are often used by patients for self-management and, when connected with a clinical program providing feedback, for self-management support. The developing interoperability environment that will digitally connect data from mobile apps to the EHR could potentially improve mobile device supported self-management.

Self-Management Support for People With MCC

Clinicians and investigators have begun to consider the theoretical foundations and some interventions regarding self-management support for patients with MCC. There are several systematic reviews in the literature related to clinical and community interventions that attempted to improve outcomes for patients with multimorbidity. A broad range of diseases were considered part of multimorbidity interventions, but diabetes, hypertension, depression, CVD, and

COPD were most often included. An example of such reviews is a 2017 Cochrane review, updated in 2021, that considered interventions in primary care and in the community using the EPOC framework. It included both randomized and nonrandomized interventions reported from 1996 to 2015. The self-management support interventions evaluated were similar to those for single diseases. Most studies included either delivery system changes, such as case management by nurses or other care team members, or patient-oriented self-management support such as educational programs. The results of these self-management support interventions included: (1) no effect on clinical outcomes and utilization; (2) mixed effects on medication use, some patient reported outcomes such as quality of life, and health behaviors; and (3) improved mental health outcomes (when depression was one of the included diseases) and clinician behaviors. Confidence in the outcomes found was generally judged as low or moderate, although the impact on depression was high.

Given the modest to small impact of self-management support on improving care for people with multimorbidity, there is broad recognition that clinical management of people with MCC/complex health status, including self-management support, is inadequate and does not improve the quality of care for multimorbidity patients. A recent review presented a thematic analysis of observational and qualitative literature addressing self-management challenges for people with complex health status, defined broadly. Their screening process identified 22 articles from 980 papers screened, from which they identified six themes: need for prioritization; lack of motivation; risk for depression; risk of poor self-efficacy; increased risk of receiving conflicting information; and opportunity to use personal experience. A systematic review and expert consensus by an international and interdisciplinary group reviewed eight international guidelines of clinical principles for management of multimorbidity and polypharmacy and identified 246 recommendations. The consensus panel summarized all this information into four guiding principles, and each guiding principle was associated with a self-management approach. The self-management principles included: establishing the self-management burden in the context of the persons' capacity and need for support; encouraging patients to clarify goals, values, and priorities; considering use of individualized care plans and medication plans, telehealth use, and care coordinators; and assuring review and follow-up of self-management plans, particularly related to medication-related concerns.

HF, whether with preserved or reduced ejection fraction, is nearly always associated with multimorbidity. A recent systematic review evaluated 14 studies that assessed self-management of HF with reduced ejection fraction in people with cognitive impairment. The involvement of family and care partners was not emphasized. The review found that cognitive impairment predicted poor self-care ability, self-care maintenance, disease management, and self-confidence. Cognitive impairment contributed to poor engagement in self-care, worse health outcomes, and increased mortality.

The complexity of HF self-management, and the ubiquity of multimorbidity in HF, led leading HF clinical researchers to develop a "pragmatic framework to optimize health outcomes HF and multimorbidity." They noted that many HF self-management support interventions are directed only toward HF and fail to account for multimorbidity, and that multiple studies have shown disappointing outcomes from that approach. These investigators maintain that five steps to reorganize HF self-management support could potentially improve HF outcomes: "1) acknowledge multimorbidity; 2) profile hospitalized HF patients for multimorbidity; 3) identify priorities and patient-centered goals; 4) support individualized home-based case management to supplement standard HF management; and 5) evaluation of other health outcomes beyond hospitalization."

Self-Management and Self-Management Support in Diverse and Underserved Populations

As reviewed above, the effectiveness of self-management interventions for single chronic conditions is modest or, in the case of multimorbidity, generally small, although in some cases there are important favorable patient outcomes. Unfortunately, effectiveness is further diminished among racial and ethnic minorities, lower income groups, and those living in rural areas. Inadequate housing, food insecurity, and financial challenges make self-management of chronic conditions difficult, even assuming health care access. However, health care access is often inadequate in low-income areas, and mistrust of the health care system, and dysfunctional provider/patient relationships certainly complicate the ability of some Black, indigenous, and people of color and immigrant people with chronic diseases to self-manage chronic conditions, whether they have one or many.

Interventions featuring community support, perhaps designed for community health centers using culturally appropriate self-management support strategies, are needed to improve both access and effectiveness of self-management and self-management support in populations with health disparities. Strategies that use more common health information technology like mobile phones hold potential promise. Telemedicine and telehealth approaches that incorporate health educators and health professionals are more effective because they mirror the structure of other evidence-based management approaches while broadening access. Formal involvement of family and friends in self-management support is another strategy for improving the outcome of self-management among minority populations. An ecological approach that involves social networks and social support (especially group-based interventions) for self-management and health behaviors may improve the outcomes of chronic illnesses in minority populations. Augmentation with technology, such as proactive calls from a nurse educator, may further enhance reach and adoption given the difficulty of attending in-person group visits among all populations.

Evidence for self-management interventions targeting older adults with multiple morbidities from minority populations is minimal. However, a few insights drawn from other studies suggests that a focus on whole-person functional status and symptoms is important. An ecological approach that places a vulnerable older adult within the context of a family and community for self-management support is likely critical. Communities of color and other disadvantaged populations will benefit from the integration of community resources, such as community health centers, into the design and delivery of self-management interventions. The use of widely available technologies that augment reach, access, and adoption hold promise for improving the uptake and outcomes of self-management interventions, especially for older, multimorbid, and minority populations.

Deficiencies of Current Self-Management and Self-Management Support Interventions in People With MCC

Many clinicians, investigators, and experts, supported by the emerging literature, realize that the current approach to self-management and self-management support for patients with MCC, based on managing chronic conditions by adherence to single-disease clinical practice guidelines, is inadequate to improve outcomes for these patients. Among potential reasons why this may occur, three stand out. First, older adults with MCC are at increased risk of adverse outcomes from the application of multiple clinical practice guidelines, including drug-drug, disease-disease, and drug-disease interactions and the harms of polypharmacy. These adverse outcomes may be of greater importance than the disease-specific outcomes that guidelines often target. Self-management support for all of their conditions based on disease-specific guidelines could well increase adverse events. Second, clinical practice guidelines fail to focus on outcomes most important to older adults, including living independently in one's home, increasing physical function, and engaging in meaningful social relationships. People may not be engaged in self-management that does not help them achieve the outcomes they care about. Third, older adults, caregivers and clinicians are burdened by the workload of multiple disease-specific interventions, and may wish to decrease this burden, particularly when the workload is not aligned with the goals of the older adult and caregiver. Self-management support interventions may sometimes actually add to this burden.

The presence of MCC exposes an older adult to significant risk for adverse outcomes arising from acute exacerbations from a serious illness and interactions of one or more chronic illnesses. This burden of multimorbid illnesses is defined as the "cumulative impact on the older adult from numerous acute and chronic diseases and general impairments, affecting multiple domains rather than a single organ system or isolated impairment." High levels of illness burden significantly impact quality of life, daily

TABLE 25-4 ■ PATIENT SELF-MANAGEMENT ACTIVITIES

Self-management tasks: diet, exercise, monitor physical signs such as blood pressure, HbA1c, weight, edema
Medication management: monitor, maintain supply, identify adverse effects, deal with complexity of dosing and administration, report perceptions of effectiveness
Health care appointments: number of clinician visits, emergency department visits, hospitalizations, laboratory tests, imaging
Procedures: time, discomfort, anxiety, complications, time to recover

functioning, symptom burden, and carry a significant economic impact on personal finances.

In addition to the burden of illness, adults with MCC face an excessive burden of treatment that impacts their daily life, relationships, and well-being. Multimorbidity imposes burdens on older adults and their caregivers related to frequent health system interactions, demands for self-care activities, and medication burdens from polypharmacy and drug interactions (Table 25-4). Burden of treatment consists of the everyday demands arising from interacting with the health system and frequent clinician visits, negotiating conflicting information about symptoms and treatments, adapting recommendations into daily routines, managing medications, and relying on supportive services.

Patients with MCC and their family caregivers spend 2 hours a day on self-care plus an additional 2 hours for every visit to a health care facility (ie, travel time, wait time, and time receiving care). Patients with Medicare typically visit five or more specialists annually. Higher burden is associated with poor medication adherence and morbidity. For older adults with cognitive and functional impairment, the capacity to manage the complexities of treatment is often diminished. Over time, the persistent imbalances between complexity and capacity create stress, fatigue, and inability to perform necessary care tasks, which then results in poorer health outcomes. Burden of treatment for older adults with MCC is not only considered a harm in and of itself, but also impacts health care access, use, self-management, and health outcomes.

New Approaches to Care for People With MCC

A paradigm shift in clinical decision making that results in the provision of the appropriate amount of care is needed to achieve what matters most for older adults and their families. An approach that focuses care on what matters most for older adults rather than adherence to single-disease guidelines holds more promise for increasing quality of care for patients with multimorbidity, and is likely to increase engagement and partnership with clinicians and reduce self-management burden, allowing patients to achieve health outcomes that matter to them. Several approaches have been described and are diffusing throughout the delivery system where people with multimorbidity receive care. One is the Veterans Administration

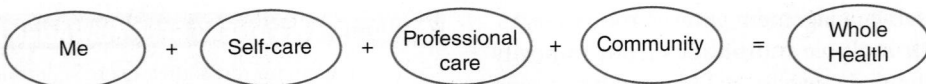

FIGURE 25-2. Veterans Administration Whole Health Program. The Veterans Administration's Whole Health Program provides a whole-person, patient-centered, comprehensive view of health, and its components are described within circles. For example, the "Me" component involves the patient's identification of 'what matters most to you' and working toward a personal health plan by identifying missions, aspirations, purpose, and shared goals. The next circle is your self-care. These are the circumstances and choices you make in your everyday life. The next circle represents professional care you receive. Professional care may include tests, medications, supplements, surgeries, examinations, treatments, and counseling. This also includes complementary approaches such as acupuncture and mind-body therapies. The fourth circle represents the people and groups with whom you are connected. (Data from US Department of Veterans Affairs Whole Health https://www.va.gov/WHOLEHEALTH/circle-of-health/index.asp.)

Whole Health Program (**Figure 25-2**), which focuses on the array of health, social, spiritual, and wellness needs of whole persons rather than a narrow focus on prolonging life and eliminating symptoms.

Investigators have demonstrated that older adults with MCC describe a consistent set of health-related priorities ("what matters most") that typically include: social and spiritual engagement; function and independence; life enjoyment activities and roles; and managing health that balances quality with quantity of life. Older adults with MCC report wanting their clinicians to know their priorities (and assume they do know them), but few patients describe having specific discussions about their priorities. Outcome goals that help older adults with MCC live according to what matters most to them, within the context of what treatments they are willing and able to engage in, should be the basis for guiding treatment decisions and subsequent patient self-management efforts. Such an approach is much more consistent with the foundational definition of patient-centered care.

Another prominent approach is Patient Priorities Care (PPC) (**Figure 25-3**), which also seeks to align clinical decision making for people with MCC with their health outcome goals and care preferences to deliver care that matters to people.

The key premise of such approaches is that people are much more likely to engage in their care, partner with clinicians to achieve the goals that matter to them, and self-manage care that respects and aligns with their preferences, when they are willing and able to achieve

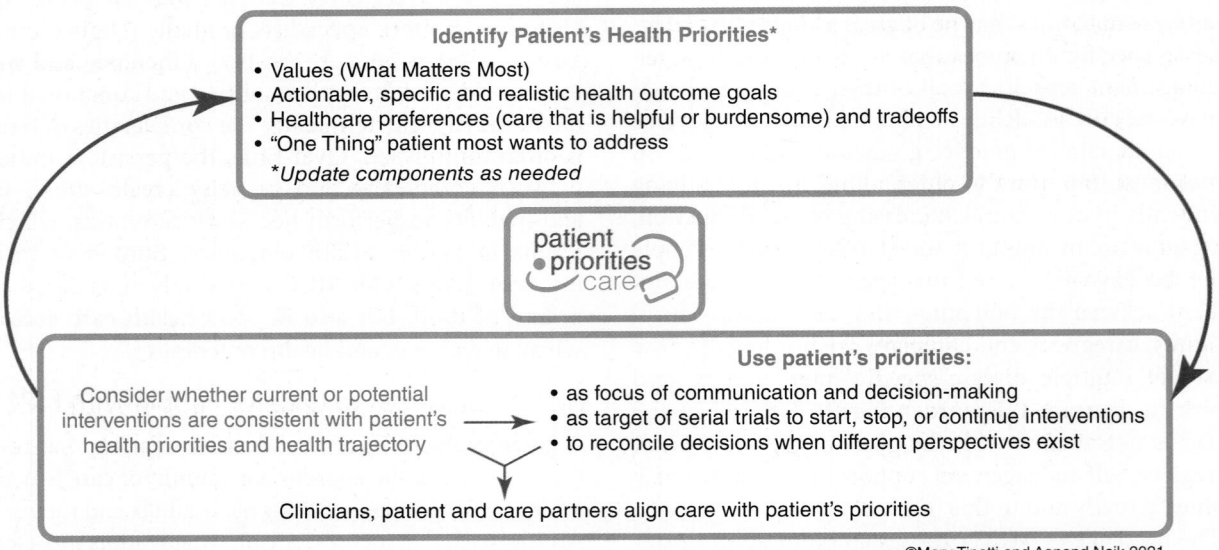

©Mary Tinetti and Aanand Naik 2021

FIGURE 25-3. The key steps involved in Patient Priorities Care are illustrated. Patient health priorities are identified either through a self-directed process (https://myhealthpriorities.org/) or with a health professional. The health priorities are transmitted to the patient's clinician who then considers whether current or potential interventions are consistent with patient's health priorities. Clinicians and patients align care with the identified health priorities by using the patient's priorities as a focus of communication and decision making, as a target of serial trails to start, stop, or continue care, and to reconcile decisions when different perspectives exist. Self-management support is provided to assist the patient if necessary to carry out the clinical interventions that will help the patient achieve or make progress on her/his priorities.(Reproduced with permission from Mary Tinetti and Aanand Naik 2021.)

their goals, that is, what matters to them. The PPC and the whole health approach are completely consistent with health behavioral theories for successful patient chronic care self-management: care that stresses goal setting, patient communication and engagement with clinicians, self-efficacy, and removing barriers to care.

The case scenario presented illustrates the problems a patient with MCC can face in self-management, and how a new approach to clinical decision making and care delivery can simplify his treatment burden, and direct self-management and self-management support toward his personal health outcome goals.

Case scenario: Older adult with MCC Mr. T is an 80-year-old man with type 2 diabetes, hypertension, and stable congestive heart failure (ejection fraction of 40%) who is presenting to his primary care physician today for follow-up. Additional comorbidities include osteoarthritis of his knees, benign prostatic hypertrophy, and age-related macular degeneration. His wife accompanies him to the visit. Mr. T is independent in all activities of daily living but has mobility impairment requiring a cane and has trouble with stairs. He needs assistance with some of his instrumental activities of daily living; his wife does the housekeeping, driving, shopping, and cooking. He manages his medications.

Over the past several months Mr. T's blood pressure has been at goal. His hemoglobin A1c values have been between 7.5% and 7.8%. He saw a podiatrist within 6 months, but he has missed two ophthalmology visits over the past year. He is taking two oral hypoglycemics as well as insulin, five evidence-based medications, and three medications for symptoms. He has six specialists.

Mr. T's primary complaint over the past few months is that he is weak and tired. He has been skipping church, where he was very active for years, because he can't climb up steps. A medical evaluation has ruled out acute illnesses or new conditions. Side effects of medications are being considered as contributing to some symptoms. Mr. T has been getting mixed messages from his health care team. His primary care clinician decreased his beta-blocker, but his cardiologist increased the dosage again. The primary care clinician then initiated a trial of decreasing Mr. T's insulin, but his endocrinologist increased the insulin at a later visit.

Mr. T and wife are frustrated with conflicting recommendations and he states that he does not feel any better. His wife is stressed and angry that his clinicians "can't get on the same page." Both Mr. T and his wife say that "we don't know who to listen to and it scares us—we don't know the right thing to do."

The primary care physician is also frustrated with the conflicting recommendations and concerned that the patient has missed several appointments and may start skipping some meds. What Mr. T wants from his health care is to have more energy, go to church, and have less "work of being a patient." Is this approach to managing Mr. T's chronic conditions, while guideline-driven and well-intentioned, helping Mr. T and his wife? How do Mr. T and his wife decide upon and implement self-management tasks, given conflicting recommendations, treatment burden, and their realization that the treatments for all his conditions are not helping him do what matters to him.

Management of MCC Including Self-Management Support for Mr. T

Management of Mr. T's multimorbidity would be based on delivering care that matters to Mr. T and helping him achieve his health outcome goals while respecting his care preferences. Such support would be connected to his primary care or geriatrics practice, or perhaps the practice where he receives most of his care (eg, cardiology,

MEDICAL CHART FOR MR. T		
Diagnoses	**Medications**	**Clinician Visit Schedules**
Diabetes mellitus, type 2	Metformin 500 mg twice daily	Primary care physician every 3 months
Congestive heart failure	Glyburide 10 mg twice daily	Cardiology every 6 months
Hypertension	Insulin glargine 15 units nightly	Endocrinology every 6 months
Hyperlipidemia	Aspirin 81 mg daily	Podiatry every 3 months
Osteoarthritis	Furosemide 40 mg twice daily	Ophthalmology every 6 months
Benign prostatic hyperplasia	Metoprolol XL 100 mg daily	Urology every year
Age-related macular degeneration	Lisinopril 10 mg twice daily	**Self-Management and Monitoring Tasks**
	Spironolactone 25 mg daily	**Daily medications as above**
	Atorvastatin 80 mg daily	Check blood sugar twice daily and as needed
	Tamsulosin 0.4 mg nightly	Check feet daily
	Acetaminophen 650 mg twice daily	Daily weight
		DASH diet daily
		Physician visits as above
		Hemoglobin A1c and basic metabolic panel quarterly
		Prostate-specific antigen and lipid panel annually
		Echocardiogram and electrocardiogram annually

endocrine). The practice would include team-based care and a member of the care team, perhaps a nurse, social worker, care management professional, or other team member, and would coordinate Mr. T's self-management. Self-management support activities would be incorporated into several care delivery components that could include:

1. Identifying What Matters to Mr. T (his goals and preferences): A trained member of the care team would work with Mr. T and his wife to find out what he wants from his health care, what matters to him—framed as specific outcome goals—and what he is able and willing to do to achieve his goals.

2. Coordinating with community resources so Mr. T can access those resources that will help him achieve his goals (physical therapy, fall prevention programs, and faith-based activities).

3. Using available evidence for targets of management for his chronic diseases. For example, evidence is available regarding HbA1c and BP targets, and DM management interventions appropriate for his age and health status.

4. Coordinating medications among different clinicians involved in Mr. T's care, using emerging evidence regarding regimen simplification and de-intensification of medication and other self-management activities, reducing Mr. T's self-management burden.

5. Using emerging telehealth standards to determine which clinical visits are appropriate for telehealth so Mr. T. can go in-person only to those visits that need to be in-person (ophthalmology). Innovative use of telehealth could allow two to three specialists on the same telehealth visit with patient to coordinate care. Fewer clinical visits would reduce self-management burden.

6. Using technology such as phone or tablet apps, the EHR patient portal, or physiological monitoring, to engage Mr. T in relevant self-management activities and maintain between-visit communication.

7. Communicating the patient's health outcomes goals and preferences through the EHR/HIE, fully visible to Mr. T and his wife, to drive care integration so his various specialists and community care (PT) clinician can align their clinical interventions to help him achieve the outcomes that matter to him (go to church, be less tired, have less work of being a patient) from his health care.

Patient Priorities Care

Care for chronically ill older adults would benefit from a personalized, person-centered approach whereby clinicians recommend primarily the care that achieves the outcomes that matter most to an older adult (ie, outcome goals) while being consistent with what the person is willing or able to do to achieve those outcomes (ie, care preferences). PPC is a clinical approach, developed and validated by a multidisciplinary clinical team that identifies the priorities of an older adult and then aligns treatment decisions to achieve those identified priorities. Patient priorities refer to the specific health outcome goals that individuals most desire from their health care given what they are willing and able to do to achieve these outcome goals within the context of their preferences. Patient priorities encompass: (1) health outcome goals—the health and life outcomes that people desire from their health care, and (2) health care preferences—health care activities (eg, medications, self-management tasks, health care visits, diagnostic testing, procedures) that people are willing and able (or not willing or able) to perform and the care they are willing (or not willing) to receive. To inform decision making, outcome goals should be specific, realistic, and timely and aligned with what matters most to the individual (health-related values).

PPC is a structured process (see **Figure 25-3**) whereby a health care professional *first* guides an older adult through a clinical encounter to *identify* her/his priorities. The health care professional documents the patient priorities within an electronic health record (EHR) and transmits them to the clinician. Second, clinicians review the priorities to *decide* which current therapies should be changed, enhanced, or stopped, and which new treatments or care options should be considered to better achieve the identified priorities, *aligning* health care to meet patient priorities rather than disease endpoints. In the third step, the clinical team *monitors* how management is working to help the patient achieve priorities, and *communicates* these priorities and the aligned clinical care to all people involved with the patient's care, including the patient and family/care partner.

The feasibility and effectiveness of the PPC approach has been demonstrated in a nonrandomized clinical trial within a large private practice with primary care providers and cardiologists. Compared to usual care (UC), patients in this study reported greater reductions in treatment burden ($\beta = -5.0$; $p = .01$) and more deprescribing (odds ratio = 2.05 [1.43 – 2.95]). A subsequent pilot study adapted PPC for a VA geriatrics clinic setting, and found similar results. These results suggest PPC is effective at reducing burdensome care (eg, inappropriate medications) and recommending a wider range of care (including home and community services and supports) that aligns with priorities. Furthermore, PPC is innovative by focusing on care that achieves patient priorities rather than clinical practice guidelines.

Whole Health Approach to Care Expands Care Options

Similar to the PPC approach, the Department of Veterans Affairs cultivated VA Whole Health—an innovative approach to care that supports the health and well-being of veterans. The VA Whole Health approach has gained traction and now exists at all VA facilities across the country. The VA Whole Health approach is not specific to the care of veterans; it is applicable to all patients who desire care that is focused on "what matters to you, not what is the matter with you." The VA Whole Health approach begins by guiding veterans through the process of developing a personalized health plan based on what matters most. The process is facilitated by a whole health coach who guides the veteran by first exploring the Circle of Health (https://www.va.gov/WHOLEHEALTH/images/components-of-whole-health.svg), which is a structured process for exploring health-related values. Using the circle of health, veterans can complete their personalized health plan which also includes shared goals and health care preferences. The personalized health plan encourages veterans to expand their health care options beyond traditional health care services including alternative and complementary care, yoga and acupuncture, multimodal pain management, exercise, and nutrition. The VA Whole Health program has made tremendous strides in impacting the care of younger and middle-aged veterans. The program is now working with the VA Geriatrics and Extended Care office to address the needs of older veterans, including a partnership with the PPC developers.

An expanded understanding of what older adults would like to achieve from their health care often involves more self-management support than the traditional medical system offers. Community-based self-management support can be provided by community-based services that support multimorbid patients and their families/care partners in self-management of chronic conditions including functional or cognitive impairment. For example, the VA implementation pilot for PPC noted increased use of home and community services and supports as complementary services to align with and achieve patient priorities, generally through supporting self-management of the wanted care. Home and community-based services and supports, including adult day services and home services (skilled nursing, physical therapy, homemaker) are increasingly recommended in VA to help older adults achieve outcomes that matter to them. Personal care support for instrumental and basic activities of daily living are important interventions for helping people achieve goals that matter and also provide self-management support of chronic diseases. Treatment recommendations that promote the use of home and community based long-term services and supports aligned with patient priorities are not only patient-centered but also beneficial to the health system.

PPC and the Whole Health approach to care provide a conceptual and empiric foundation for moving the focus of care away from strict adherence to clinical practice guidelines and inappropriate care delivery and self-management expectations. The alternative motivation for health care lies in an emphasis on the priorities of older adults, defined concretely as outcome goals and what patients are willing to do to achieve their goals (care preferences). Self-management and self-management support would be directed toward helping the patients achieve their goals, given their care preferences. Adherence to evidence and practice guidelines remains important but only as a means to achieving patient priorities rather than the primary measure of health care quality.

There remain other issues to face regarding how to support people with multimorbidity in their self-management of chronic diseases and conditions in order for them to achieve their goals. Important problems include: how to involve and support families and care partners in helping patients' goal achievement: how to disseminate new care approaches for multimorbidity management to different clinicians; how to incentivize providers to both deliver care that matters and follow up with clinical decision making and care plans that help patients achieve their goals; and how emerging technological capabilities, especially EHR communication between clinicians and patients, and interoperability among EHR systems and mobile technology, will impact self-management and health outcomes of patients with multimorbidity. Emerging approaches to care of patients with MCC, focused on patient-defined health outcomes, that support patients' self-management to achieve their own goals hold promise to improve chronic disease management and, most importantly, outcomes that matter to older people.

FURTHER READING

Allegrante JP, Wells MT, Peterson JC. Interventions to support behavioral self-management of chronic diseases. *Annu Rev Public Health*. 2019;40:127–146.

Bandura A. Health promotion by social cognitive means. *Health Educ Behav*. 2004;31(2):143–164.

Blaum C, Rosen J, Naik A, et al. Feasibility of implementing patient priorities care for older adults with MCC. *J Am Geriatr Soc*. 2018;66(10):2009.

Bodenheimer T, Ghorob A, Willard-Grace R, Grumbach K. The 10 building blocks of high-performing primary care. *Ann Fam Med*. 2014;12(2):166–171.

Bodenheimer T, Wagner EH, Grumbach K. Improving primary care for patients with chronic illness: the chronic care model, Part 2. *JAMA*. 2002;288(15):1909–1914.

Contant É, Loignon C, Bouhali T, Almirall J, Fortin M. A multidisciplinary self-management intervention among patients with multimorbidity and the impact of socioeconomic factors on results. *BMC Fam Pract*. 2019;20(1):1–8.

Dineen-Griffin S, Garcia-Cardenas V, Williams K, Benrimoj SI. Helping patients help themselves: a systematic review of self-management support strategies in primary health care practice. *PloS One*. 2019;14(8):e0220116.

Effective Practice and Organisation of Care (EPOC). EPOC Taxonomy; 2015. epoc.cochrane.org/epoc-taxonomy. Accessed July 6, 2021.

Fortin M, Chouinard MC, Dubois MF, et al. Integration of chronic disease prevention and management services into primary care: a pragmatic randomized controlled trial (PR1MaC). *CMAJ Open.* 2016;4(4):E588.

Gaudet T, Kligler B. Whole health in the whole system of the veterans administration: how will we know we have reached this future state? *J Altern Complement Med.* 2019;25(S1):S7–S11.

Gobeil-Lavoie A-P, Chouinard M-C, Danish A, Hudon C. Characteristics of self-management among patients with complex health needs: a thematic analysis review. *BMJ Open.* 2019;9(5):e028344.

Hanlon P, Daines L, Campbell C, McKinstry B, Weller D, Pinnock H. Telehealth interventions to support self-management of long-term conditions: a systematic metareview of diabetes, heart failure, asthma, chronic obstructive pulmonary disease, and cancer. *J Med Internet Res.* 2017;19(5):e172.

Hardman R, Begg S, Spelten E. What impact do chronic disease self-management support interventions have on health inequity gaps related to socioeconomic status: a systematic review. *BMC Health Serv Res.* 2020;20(1):150.

Heitkemper EM, Mamykina L, Travers J, Smaldone A. Do health information technology self-management interventions improve glycemic control in medically underserved adults with diabetes? A systematic review and meta-analysis. *J Am Med Inform Assoc.* 2017;24(5):1024–1035.

John JR, Jani H, Peters K, Agho K, Tannous WK. The effectiveness of patient-centered medical home-based models of care versus standard primary care in chronic disease management: a systematic review and meta-analysis of randomised and non-randomised controlled trials. *Int J Environ Res Public Health.* 2020;17(18):6886.

Kneipp SM, Horrell L, Gonzales C, et al. Participation of lower-to-middle wage workers in a study of Chronic Disease Self-Management Program (CDSMP) effectiveness: implications for reducing chronic disease burden among racial and ethnic minority populations. *Public Health Nurs Boston Mass.* 2019;36(5):591–602.

Lorig K, Holman H. Arthritis self-management studies: a twelve-year review. *Health Educ Q.* 1993;20:17–28.

Lorig KR, Holman HR. Self-management education: history, definition, outcomes, and mechanisms. *Ann Behav Med.* 2003;26(1):1–7.

Lovell J, Pham T, Noaman SQ, Davis M-C, Johnson M, Ibrahim JE. Self-management of heart failure in dementia and cognitive impairment: a systematic review. *BMC Cardiovasc Disord.* 2019;19(1):99.

McBrien KA, Ivers N, Barnieh L, et al. Patient navigators for people with chronic disease: a systematic review. *PloS One.* 2018;13(2):e0191980.

McCabe C, McCann M, Brady AM. Computer and mobile technology interventions for self-management in

chronic obstructive pulmonary disease. *Cochrane Database Syst Rev.* 2017;5:CD011425.

Muth C, Blom JW, Smith SM, et al. Evidence supporting the best clinical management of patients with multimorbidity and polypharmacy: a systematic guideline review and expert consensus. *J Intern Med.* 2019;285(3):272–288.

Naik AD, Dindo LN, Liew JR, et al. Development of a clinically feasible process for identifying individual health priorities. *J Am Geriatr Soc.* 2018;66(10):1872–1879.

Naik AD, Hundt NE, Vaughan EM, et al. Effect of telephone-delivered collaborative goal setting and behavioral activation vs enhanced usual care for depression among adults with uncontrolled diabetes: a randomized clinical trial. *JAMA Network Open.* 2019;2(8):e198634-e.

Reynolds R, Dennis S, Hasan I, et al. A systematic review of chronic disease management interventions in primary care. *BMC Fam Pract.* 2018;19(1):11.

Smith SM, Soubhi H, Fortin M, Hudon C, O'Dowd T. Managing patients with multimorbidity: systematic review of interventions in primary care and community settings. *BMJ.* 2012;345.

Smith SM, Wallace E, O'Dowd T, Fortin M. Interventions for improving outcomes in patients with multimorbidity in primary care and community settings. *Cochrane Database Syst Rev.* 2016;3:CD006560.

Stewart S, Riegel B, Boyd C, et al. Establishing a pragmatic framework to optimise health outcomes in heart failure and multimorbidity (ARISE-HF): a multidisciplinary position statement. *Int J Cardiol.* 2016;212:1–10.

Takeda A, Martin N, Taylor RS, Taylor SJ. Disease management interventions for heart failure. *Cochrane Database Syst Rev.* 2019;1:CD002752.

Tinetti ME, Esterson J, Ferris R, Posner P, Blaum CS. Patient priority–directed decision making and care for older adults with MCC. *Clin Geriatr Med.* 2016;32(2):261–275.

Tinetti ME, Naik AD, Dindo L, et al. Association of patient priorities–aligned decision-making with patient outcomes and ambulatory health care burden among older adults with MCC: a nonrandomized clinical trial. *JAMA Intern Med.* 2019;179(12):1688–1697.

Vaccaro JA, Exebio JC, Zarini GG, Huffman FG. The role of family/friend social support in diabetes self-management for minorities with type 2 diabetes. *J Nutr Health.* 2014;2(1):1–9.

Wadsworth KH, Archibald TG, Payne AE, Cleary AK, Haney BL, Hoverman AS. Shared medical appointments and patient-centered experience: a mixed-methods systematic review. *BMC Fam Pract.* 2019;20(1):97.

Whitehead L, Seaton P. The effectiveness of self-management mobile phone and tablet apps in long-term condition management: a systematic review. *J Med Internet Res.* 2016;18(5):e97.

Chapter 26

Legal Issues

Marshall B. Kapp

INTRODUCTION

The law regulates human relationships prospectively and retrospectively in a variety of ways. To a large extent, the legal implications of medical practice are generic, in the sense that they apply to patients of all ages. Rules developed to deal with the care of younger adults apply with full force to older persons, whose rights do not diminish just because of advanced chronological age. However, a patient's advanced years may raise issues demanding particular attention by involved participants in the professional/patient relationship. This chapter concentrates on selected aspects in which the law influences the delivery of geriatric services through its impact on the recognition and enforcement of respective rights and responsibilities of the parties, within the dynamics of an older patient/health care provider relationship.

OVERVIEW OF HEALTH CARE REGULATION

The U.S. Constitution establishes a federal system of government, under which health care delivery, financing, and other matters are regulated at the national (federal), state, and local levels. Under separation of powers principles, regulation takes the form of (1) constitutional (federal, state, and local) provisions, (2) statutes enacted by elected legislatures, (3) rules or regulations promulgated by executive branch administrative agencies such as health or social service departments on the basis of authority conferred on the agency by the legislature via statute, and (4) common law doctrines created by courts as a matter of public policy and prior case precedent. These various forms of regulation may impose specific or general duties on parties, may authorize but not require parties to act in specific ways, or may prohibit parties from engaging in particular conduct. Health care regulation may be directed at individual health professionals or at health care facilities, agencies, institutions, and other organizations.

Regulation of Health Professionals

One primary mechanism for regulating health professionals to assure adequate qualifications and acceptable conduct is licensure, which entails the requirement that an individual satisfy—on both an initial and continuing basis—certain enumerated standards to be permitted to

Learning Objectives

- Appreciate the general legal environment within which physicians and other health care professionals function when providing medical care to older patients.
- Understand the elements of a medical malpractice claim brought against a health care provider.
- Engage in the process of shared decision-making and informed consent with older patients in a legally appropriate manner.
- Advise patients and families about available tools to facilitate advance health care planning.
- Apply in clinical practice the legal requirements for confidentiality of patient information and permissible exceptions to those requirements.

Key Clinical Points

1. Maintain and apply in clinical practice an acceptable level of knowledge and skill for your specialty (ie, keep up with your field).
2. Engage in the process of informed and voluntary shared decision-making with your patients or their decision-making surrogates.
3. Discuss the topic of advance health care planning in a timely and supportive manner with patients, ascertaining the patient's relevant values and treatment preferences in various contingencies and documenting them in the medical record.
4. Respect and safeguard the confidentiality of patients' medical information, but understand the circumstances under which it is legally permissible or even mandatory to reveal what would otherwise be confidential information.

practice a particular profession. Professional licensure ordinarily occurs at the state level through statutes (such as state Medical Practice Acts or Nursing Practice Acts) and regulations promulgated by a state's licensing body (such as the Medical Board or Nursing Board) to implement the Practice Act. Licensure statutes and regulations limit certain activities to licensed professionals; engaging in those activities without prior state approval is practicing medicine or nursing without a valid license and subjects the wrongdoer to civil fines and potential criminal sanctions.

Many statutory and regulatory requirements or prohibitions imposed on health professionals occur as conditions attached to payment for professional services under government insurance programs, especially Medicare and Medicaid. Professionals who treat patients covered by these government programs must satisfy the positive (eg, "Thou shalt" maintain adequate patient records) or negative (eg, "Thou shalt not" engage in self-referral) strings placed on the payment of public dollars to receive compensation for services rendered.

Another manner of health professional regulation under the civil law is tort liability in private lawsuits claiming malpractice (discussed below). Particularly egregious, intentional misbehavior (such as patient abuse or billing fraud) may subject a health professional to criminal law punishments.

Significant regulatory sanctions imposed on certain health professionals, as well as any monies paid on behalf of a health professional as a result of a professional liability claim, must be reported to the federal Department of Health and Human Services' National Practitioner Data Bank (NPDB). An individual's NPDB file is confidential except in circumstances specified in federal regulation.

Regulation of Health Care Facilities and Agencies

Besides regulating individual health professionals, government regulates provider facilities and agencies through licensure requirements, conditions attached to compensation under public insurance programs including Medicare and Medicaid, criminal prohibitions on specific behaviors such as the filing of false claims, and civil liability for malpractice claims brought by or on behalf of individual patients. For example, Congress enacted the Nursing Home Quality Reform Act, 42 US Code §#1395i-3(a)-(h), as part of the Omnibus Budget Reconciliation Act (OBRA) of 1987, Public Law No. 100-203. This Act contains many of the recommendations proposed in a 1986 Institute of Medicine report that Congress had directed the Department of Health and Human Services to commission. OBRA 1987 amended the Social Security Act, Titles 18 (Medicare) and 19 (Medicaid), to require substantial upgrading in nursing home quality and enforcement. To implement this legislation, the Department of Health and Human Services (DHHS) published regulations in 1989, 42 Code of Federal Regulations Part 483. These regulations were substantially updated on October 4, 2016, at 81 Federal Register 68688-01.

Violation of these regulations subjects nursing homes to a range of sanctions, up to decertification from participation in the Medicare and Medicaid programs.

During the national Public Health Emergency declaration issued in 2020 in response to the COVID-19 pandemic, DHHS temporarily waived a number of regulatory requirements that otherwise would bind nursing homes.

STANDARDS OF CARE AND PROFESSIONAL LIABILITY

Overview of Malpractice Liability

In a private civil lawsuit predicated on a theory of professional negligence, the plaintiff is required to establish four distinct elements by a preponderance of the evidence (a more likely than not standard) (**Table 26-1**). First, the plaintiff has the burden of proving that the professional/provider defendant owed the patient an obligation defined by the appropriate standard of care. The existence of this duty ordinarily is established by showing that there existed, within the relevant timeframe, a professional relationship between the patient and provider; that is, the plaintiff was a patient of the provider for diagnostic and/or therapeutic purposes.

Second, the plaintiff must present sufficient evidence that the professional/provider breached or violated the appropriate standard of care within the professional relationship. The professional/provider does not guarantee particular results, let alone perfection. By the same token, it is not enough for professionals/providers to "do their best" if their conduct does not rise to the applicable level of care, even when the errors or omissions were unintentional (ie, negligent). How the law determines the applicable level of professional care is discussed below.

The third element a medical malpractice plaintiff is required to prove is the occurrence of some financially compensable injury or damage. Besides special or economic (pecuniary) damages that include such quantifiable items as lost income and past and future health care–related costs, plaintiffs may be awarded general or noneconomic (nonpecuniary) damages for such difficult to quantify things as pain and suffering, mental anguish, grief, and other emotional complaints. In the past few decades, some juries have become more willing to award substantial noneconomic damages to older patients claiming medical negligence that

TABLE 26-1 ■ ELEMENTS OF A PROFESSIONAL NEGLIGENCE CLAIM
1. Duty owed by professional/provider to the patient
2. Breach or violation of duty
3. Damage or injury to the patient
4. Causal (both general and proximate) link between the professional/provider breach of duty and the injury suffered by the patient

has caused, for example, loss of function such as the ability to ambulate, drive, or toilet independently, chronic physical pain, diminution in mental capacity, or loss of ability to engage in sexual relations. In very rare circumstances, punitive or exemplary damages may be awarded over and above compensatory damages, where the defendant's conduct has been not merely negligent, but reckless or malicious. For example, a jury might award punitive damages when it finds that a patient developed serious pressure ulcers because of a hospital's or nursing home's demonstrated ongoing pattern of neglect. Liability insurance policies purchased by health professionals (or purchased for them by their employers) ordinarily do not cover punitive damages.

The final component of proof in a professional malpractice lawsuit is the element of causation. To succeed, the plaintiff must persuade the jury, to a reasonable (not absolute) degree of medical certainty, that the injuries were the result of the defendant's negligence. The plaintiff must prove not only that the defendant's negligence was a "substantial factor" in bringing about the injury or that "but for" (*sine qua non*) the defendant's negligence the injury would not have happened, but further that there were no intervening, superceding (not reasonably foreseeable) forces that acted to break the chain of proximate or direct causation between the defendant's negligence and the patient's injury. For example, a physician might negligently fail to diagnose cancer in an older patient in a timely manner and the patient, on learning that cancer is at a stage that it cannot be treated effectively, commits suicide. Assuming the availability of effective treatment if the cancer had been properly diagnosed in a timely manner, representatives of the deceased patient may argue that "but for" the physician's negligence the death would not have taken place; however, the physician would respond that the patient's act of committing suicide was an intervening, superceding (not reasonably foreseeable) factor that disrupted the chain of proximate causation between the physician's negligence and the patient's injury.

Developing and Disseminating Standards of Care

Legal standards of care have been established mainly by the courts as a matter of common law on an incremental, case-by-case basis. State statutes, such as those containing professional licensure requirements, also help to define the required standards of care.

Under the traditional formulation, a professional who is accused of negligent acts or omissions in a medical malpractice claim is held to a standard requiring the professional to have and exercise that level of knowledge and skill ordinarily possessed and exercised by competent, reasonable professional peers (in most states, determined on a national rather than local basis) in similar circumstances. Put differently, under long-standing tort principles of negligence, professionals have been judged legally according to the prevalent practice or custom of peer professionals in clinical circumstances like the situation that

confronted the particular defendant in the case immediately before the court.

There is a significant trend in many states to evolve from the traditional customary professional standard of care in favor of imposing more objective, external standards of "reasonableness" against which the professional's behavior is to be evaluated by the jury. An objective, evidence-based standard of reasonableness may exceed (ie, require more knowledge and sophistication than) the prevailing customary practice within the professional community at the time in handling a specific clinical challenge presented by a patient. Thus, the state of the art in a particular area of care, required under a reasonableness standard, frequently might not be synonymous with and reflected in the current customary practice within the practitioner community. Courts adopting a reasonableness standard often recite the famous maxim of Judge Learned Hand: "Courts must in the end say what is required; there are precautions so imperative that even their universal disregard will not excuse their omission."

When a reasonableness standard is imposed on malpractice defendants, expert witnesses may be allowed to testify, and thereby educate the lay jurors, regarding the appropriate professional conduct under the circumstances. To establish reasonable conduct, the parties may also introduce other kinds of evidence to supplement the testimony of the expert witnesses (**Table 26-2**). Additional forms of evidence introduced for this purpose may include professional codes of ethics, medical journal literature, textbooks (learned treatises), the *Physician's Desk Reference* (PDR) and pharmaceutical package inserts (PPIs) pertaining to the correct use and dosage of prescription drugs, pertinent statutes or regulations, voluntary accreditation standards such as those of the Joint Commission, and, of increasing importance, pertinent clinical practice guidelines (CPGs) or parameters.

Leaders in health care delivery and financing acknowledge that a good deal of routine medical practice has long been predicated more on habit and inertia than on solid empirical evidence establishing clinical efficacy. Out of a concern about both wasteful resource usage and the quality of patient care, professional organizations and

TABLE 26-2 ■ PROOF OF THE STANDARD OF REASONABLE CARE UNDER THE CIRCUMSTANCES

1. Expert testimony about appropriate care
2. Professional codes of ethics
3. Medical journal literature
4. Textbooks (learned treatises)
5. *Physician's Desk Reference* (PDR) and pharmaceutical package inserts (PPIs)
6. Relevant statutes or regulations
7. Voluntary accreditation standards
8. Clinical practice guidelines or parameters

specialty societies, including the American Geriatrics Society and the Society for Post-Acute and Long-Term Care Medicine (AMDA), governmental agencies led by the federal Agency for Healthcare Research and Quality (AHRQ), and the Patient-Centered Outcomes Research Institute (PCORI), independent bodies such as the U.S. Preventive Services Task Force, and individual institutions and agencies in the United States and elsewhere have engaged in a concerted movement to develop, collect, and disseminate to practicing clinicians a variety of evidence-based CPGs or parameters to educate practitioners about whether particular diagnostic or therapeutic interventions have actually been demonstrated to produce desired health benefits for patients. The Institute of Medicine has defined CPGs as "systematically developed statements to assist practitioner and patient decisions about appropriate health care for specific clinical circumstances." Deviations from relevant CPGs may be permissible in the case of particular patients, but the health professional should document the justification for such deviation.

In a related vein, the American Board of Internal Medicine Foundation and Consumer Reports have partnered in a Choosing Wisely initiative designed to encourage and enable patients and physicians to share in making decisions about medical care that is supported by available evidence, not duplicative of other tests or procedures already received, and necessary for that particular patient. Numerous medical specialty organizations have joined in this initiative, identifying common practices in their respective specialties for which physicians and patients ought to ask questions about the value obtained from routine use.

The legal ramifications of CPGs or parameters continue to evolve. Nevertheless, there is a growing tendency for the courts to admit into evidence, on behalf of either side to a malpractice dispute (ie, for either inculpatory or exculpatory purposes), properly validated, scientifically supported contemporary practice parameters on the issue of the standard of care to be applied under any particular set of circumstances. This development already has consequences, in that informal surveys show that plaintiffs' attorneys consider health professionals' compliance with or deviation from relevant practice parameters in making decisions about whether to initiate malpractice litigation at all and how to conduct settlement negotiations for claims that are pursued.

Because of added strains and resource limitations experienced by health care providers due to the COVID-19 pandemic, at least a dozen states enacted legislation providing immunity for providers shielding them against certain kinds of COVID-19-related liability claims. Congress has considered but not passed national legislation in this area.

INFORMED CONSENT

Basics of Informed Consent

Informed consent is the legal component of a broad modern shared decision-making approach that puts health care professionals in the role of decision facilitators or guiders rather than decision makers. The informed consent doctrine originates with the ethical principle of autonomy or self-determination, especially regarding the physical integrity and dignity of one's own body.

A health professional/provider may be held civilly liable, usually under a negligence theory but in rare cases under a battery or intentional tort theory, for subjecting a person to any diagnostic, therapeutic, or research-related intervention without that person's effective consent. In their legal formulation, the substantive parts of the informed consent rule have evolved over time as a function of state common (judge-made) law. Moreover, the majority of states have enacted statutes and regulations spelling out a jurisdiction's specific details regarding informed consent, for clinical care generally and/or within particular settings such as nursing homes or public mental institutions.

For a patient's decision about whether to accept or reject a suggested medical intervention to be considered legally valid, three separate but interrelated elements must be present (**Table 26-3**).

First, the patient's participation in the decision-making process and final decision(s) regarding intervention must be voluntary, not unduly dictated by force, fraud, duress, or any other actual or perceived ulterior form of constraint or coercion. Second, the patient's agreement or disagreement with recommended interventions must be properly informed. The professional is obligated to disclose sufficient information about the proposed intervention to empower the patient to make a knowledgeable, intelligent consent or refusal. The third essential element of legally effective medical decision-making is adequate capacity on the part of the patient to cognitively and emotionally understand and manipulate pertinent information about medical matters.

In terms of the informed component of informed consent, there are two competing standards for determining how much information about a proposed medical intervention must be shared with the patient in advance. The medical custom or reasonable professional standard

---

TABLE 26-3 ■ ELEMENTS OF LEGALLY VALID MEDICAL DECISION-MAKING

1. Voluntary
2. Informed
   a. Diagnosis or nature of the problem
   b. Expected benefits
   c. Risks
   d. Alternatives, including complementary and alternative interventions
   e. Risks and benefits of refusal
   f. Cost implications
   g. Level of uncertainty
3. Competent/capable decision maker

requires the disclosure of information that an objective reasonable, prudent professional would disclose under similar circumstances. By comparison, the materiality or patient orientation standard compels the sharing of information that might make a difference or be material in the decision-making process of a reasonable patient in similar circumstances. The states are approximately evenly split between these two competing standards of information disclosure.

Under either, the materiality or the reasonable professional standard, the basic components of information disclosure implicated by the professional's fiduciary or trust obligations include the following: diagnosis or nature of the patient's medical problem; nature and purposes (expected benefits) of the proposed interventions; reasonably foreseeable risks associated with the intervention, specifically, the likelihood of a risk materializing and the severity if it does occur; reasonable alternative interventions and their anticipated risks and benefits; and the reasonably foreseeable risks and benefits of not undergoing the proposed intervention. Other informational items that a health professional should seriously consider disclosing to the patient are complementary medicine alternatives, which are increasingly popular with older individuals; cost ramifications to the patient of proposed alternatives; professional-specific information pertinent to the particular intervention (eg, the professional's own track record with the particular intervention or financial incentives the professional has regarding the patient's course of care); and the level of uncertainty within the medical community concerning the particular intervention.

Informed consent to a medical intervention may be implied or expressed. There are many situations in which a patient's permission to proceed with a medical intervention does not need to be put into words but, instead, may be implied from the context. This happens when, through demonstrative actions, the patient indicates a wish (or at least willingness) to undergo a specific intervention by voluntarily submitting to it in a manner that the health professional can reasonably rely on to conclude that the intervention has been authorized. Implied consent is appropriate for most routine, noninvasive, non-risky kinds of medical interventions such as taking a patient's blood pressure or listening to the heart. Implied consent is not an exception to the informed consent requirement, but just a different (created by behavior instead of words) form of permission.

Express consent (put into spoken or written words), by contrast, is more appropriate when the proposed medical intervention is intrusive and/or significantly more risky than ordinary, everyday life. With a small number of exceptions created by particular state statutes for designated kinds of interventions (such as testing for the HIV virus), express consent in the form of spoken rather than written patient words is legally adequate, as long as the consent is voluntarily and competently given on the basis of sufficient information being disclosed. However, for particularly intrusive or risky interventions, the professional/provider

should consider documenting the patient's decision to consent or refuse by asking the patient to sign a separate written form, in addition to the professional making a progress note in the patient's medical record. Also, voluntary accreditation standards with which the provider purports to comply, such as those of the Joint Commission, may require the use of separate written consent forms for particular sorts of medical interventions.

Decisional Capacity Issues

Sometimes, a patient is not cognitively and/or emotionally capable of assimilating pertinent information and engaging in a rational, voluntary decision-making process about proposed and alternative medical interventions. Some older persons with dementia, depression, or other age-related mental disorders are so impaired that they fall into this category. When the patient personally lacks adequate decisional capacity, the health professional is not relieved of the duty to obtain informed consent but, instead, must work with someone else who is willing to act as a surrogate on the patient's behalf.

Assessing decisional capacity entails a functional inquiry. Among the basic questions to be posed are (**Table 26-4**): (1) Can the person make and communicate in an understandable form any decisions at all? (2) Is the person able to offer reasons for the choices made, indicating some degree of reflection and consideration? (3) Are the reasons given based on logical reasoning proceeding from factually accurate suppositions? (4) Can the patient appreciate the ramifications (ie, likely risks and benefits) of the options outlined and choices expressed, and the reality that these ramifications apply to that patient? (5) Does the individual comprehend the practical implications of different choices?

A patient's present cognitive and emotional capacity should be evaluated on a decision-specific, rather than a global or all-or-nothing, basis. A patient may be capable of making some kinds of decisions, but not others; partial or limited capacity, especially with adequate assistance and support by family or friends, is possible even when total capacity is not. Moreover, capacity may fluctuate within a specific patient according to variables such as time of day, day of the week, physical location, acute and transient physical problems, other persons available to support or coerce the patient's choice, and medication reactions. Older individuals may be especially vulnerable to fluctuations in capacity induced by these factors. Some of these factors

TABLE 26-4 ■ COMPONENTS OF FUNCTIONAL ASSESSMENT OF DECISIONAL CAPACITY
1. Ability to communicate decisions
2. Ability to give reasons for decisions
3. Reasons given are logical and factually accurate
4. Appreciation of ramifications
5. Comprehension of ramifications

may be susceptible to manipulation by caregivers (eg, by changing timing of drug administration) so that discussions with the patient (rather than or in addition to the surrogate) about the care plan can take place under the most lucid circumstances possible.

Advance Health Care Planning as Prospective Decision-Making

There are several legal mechanisms available to maximize a patient's medical autonomy prospectively. An older person may, while still capable of making health care decisions, execute certain legal instruments to anticipate and prepare for eventual incapacity by voluntarily delegating or directing the exercise of future medical decision-making power. Although oral advance medical directives are theoretically legally valid, patients should be encouraged to execute written versions to maximize the likelihood that the directive ultimately will be respected by family members and health professionals. Organizational providers are required by the federal Patient Self-Determination Act to initiate discussions with competent patients about the availability of advance medical directive opportunities.

The **durable power of attorney (DPA)** consists of a written document in which an individual (the principal) appoints an agent, or attorney-in-fact, to make various kinds of decisions for the principal. Each state has enacted statutes that explicitly authorize the use of a **DPA for health care (DPAHC)** to empower an agent (including a nonfamily member) to make medical choices on a patient's behalf, should the patient later lose decision-making capacity. Examples of DPAHC templates for individual states are available on the internet. A DPAHC may be immediate, meaning that it comes into effect as soon as the agent is named. In a springing DPAHC, on the other hand, the legal authority transfers (springs) from the patient to the agent only on the occurrence of some specified future event, like a declaration of the principal's incapacity by a designated number of examining physicians. The patient should be informed by attending health professionals when they have decided to act as though decision-making authority has sprung to the designated agent, so that the patient can utter a protest, if desired, to the agent's exercise of power.

The DPAHC is a proxy directive, and hence distinguishable from a **living will** or instruction-type directive. In an instruction directive, a competent patient documents his or her wishes regarding future medical treatment (eg, "no extraordinary measures" or "keep me alive forever no matter what pain or expense") rather than naming an agent to make future treatment decisions in the case of eventual incapacity. The two kinds of legal devices are not mutually exclusive; indeed, patients may be encouraged to execute them in tandem because the living will can help an agent named under a DPAHC to exercise the patient's substituted judgment (defined below) more accurately.

When a patient is incapable of making their own health care decisions but has not previously executed an instruction or proxy directive, in most states health professionals may rely on legislation empowering family members and enumerated other persons to make medical decisions for incapacitated persons. In states with such family consent statutes, the approved procedure usually consists of documenting unanimous agreement among the attending physician, specified relatives or others (listed in a stated preference order), and sometimes consultant physicians as well.

When there is no valid proxy or instruction directive, family consent statute, or judicial precedent in one's jurisdiction authorizing the family to act as patient surrogate, or in those relatively uncommon situations in which family members strongly and irreconcilably disagree about the best course of care for their relative, judicial creation of a **guardianship or conservatorship** (nomenclature varies by jurisdiction) may be advisable to transfer decision-making power formally from an incapacitated patient to a single, specific surrogate. However, the official legal process (ordinarily entailing significant financial, time consumption, and emotional costs) should not be initiated unless and until less formal approaches, such as mediation or consultation with an **institutional ethics committee** or ethics consultation service, have been exhausted in an effort to reach a sufficient level of agreement among the interested stakeholders. In a guardianship/conservatorship case, professionals who have evaluated and/or treated the alleged incompetent person usually are called to provide evidence to the court in the form of a written affidavit and/or live sworn testimony. Many jurisdictions have public or volunteer guardianship programs that operate to provide surrogate decision makers for individuals with substantially impaired cognitive and/or emotional capacity who have no suitable family members or other private parties who can serve as guardians for them.

In the past, a surrogate was expected to make decisions consistent with the guardian's view, as a trust agent, of the patient's best interests. The modern approach, however, is toward a substituted judgment standard of proxy decision-making, whenever it is realistically feasible. Under this latter approach, the surrogate is obligated to make those decisions that the patient would make, according to the patient's own preferences and values to the extent these can be accurately ascertained, if the patient were presently able to make and express decisions competently.

Another innovation in advance health care planning is the **Physician Orders for Life-Sustaining Treatment (POLST)** paradigm (also known as Portable Medical Orders; see https://polst.org/). The precise title for this concept varies among jurisdictions. In some states, it is named Medical Orders for Life-Sustaining Treatment (MOLST; see https://molst.org/) and has also been named Physician Orders for Scope of Treatment (POST; see https://www.indianapost.org/). POLST is a mechanism to convert a patient's treatment wishes into the tangible form of a written physician's order. Because health professionals are accustomed to carrying out medical orders, there is evidence that when treatment instructions are expressed in the form of a POLST they are substantially more likely to be honored in practice than are wishes expressed only in the form of a patient's prior expression or a surrogate's current representation of the patient's inferred preferences. Unlike an advance directive, a POLST is appropriate only for a patient who is so seriously ill that a physician exercising sound judgment would not be surprised if that patient died within the next year or two. Individual states are at different points concerning the degree of POLST penetration in medical practice and statutory and/or regulatory codification. There are no laws in the United States that prohibit either physicians from writing a POLST today for an appropriate patient or emergency medical services (EMS) or other health professionals from following a POLST.

CONFIDENTIALITY

While providing care, health professionals routinely are exposed to private information about patients and their families. Professionals owe patients a fiduciary responsibility to hold in confidence all sensitive patient information entrusted to them as a consequence of the professional/patient relationship. This ethical obligation, predicated on the patient's important interest in protecting personal privacy and avoiding the social stigma and potential discrimination that breach of one's medical privacy might entail, is enforceable legally under both state and federal law.

State Law

Every state, both within its state professional Practice Acts and in separate statutes pertaining to particular health care delivery settings, has enacted provisions pertaining to the confidentiality duties of health care professionals, institutions, and agencies. Often, state agencies publish accompanying regulations to implement these statutes. Moreover, a strong common law health care confidentiality doctrine has been forged by state court decisions rendered over time. Violation of state common law or the relevant statutory or regulatory requirements regarding confidentiality of patient information may subject erring health professionals/providers to civil damage suits, brought by or on behalf of the patient whose privacy was improperly infringed; additionally, violation of state Practice Act provisions may subject the violator to administrative sanctions, including license suspension or even revocation.

However, numerous exceptions to the general confidentiality rule have been recognized by the courts as part of the common law or embedded in state legislation or regulation (**Table 26-5**). First, the most prominent exception occurs when a patient, expressly or impliedly, voluntarily and knowingly waives, or gives up, the right to assert the confidentiality of particular information. These waivers take place daily to make information available to third-party payers (for instance, Medicare claims processors and

TABLE 26-5 ■ EXCEPTIONS TO THE DUTY OF CONFIDENTIALITY
1. Patient permission (waiver)
2. Danger to others
3. Mandatory or permissive reporting statutes
4. Legal process (court order)
5. "Treatment, payment, and health care operations" (HIPAA)

private health insurers), quality of care auditors (such as Joint Commission surveyors), and other public and private entities like health care surrogates authorized to make medical decisions on behalf of a patient who is not capable of making their own decisions. Because the modern delivery of health care is a team endeavor, each patient implicitly gives permission for the sharing of certain otherwise private pieces of information among the members of the treatment team. Internal information sharing of this nature is essential to optimal care, especially for accomplishing coordination and continuity of long-term care for older patients with disabilities. Indeed, failures in communication among the multiple providers involved in the care of a patient needing such coordination and continuity may form the basis for negligence liability claims when harm results.

Second, the usual confidentiality duty may be outweighed in situations of jeopardy to innocent, at-risk third parties, such as happens when a patient with serious sensory or cognitive impairments insists on continuing to drive an automobile or maintain loaded firearms in the home for protection against intruders. Particular details regarding methods for the health professional to discharge the responsibility to report a credible threat of harm to public health or law enforcement authorities vary on the basis of state statutory and case law.

Third, the patient's reasonable expectation of privacy must give way when the health professional is mandated by state statute to report to enumerated public health or law enforcement authorities (eg, Adult Protective Services [APS]) the professional's reasonable suspicion that certain conditions or activities have occurred or are occurring. Such reportable conditions or activities may include elder mistreatment or neglect (in many states including cases of self-neglect is also within that definition), domestic violence, infectious diseases, and births and deaths. Some states that have declined to mandate the reporting of particular situations to public authorities nonetheless encourage voluntary reporting; a few states have pursued this approach regarding cases of suspected elder abuse or neglect. Those states supply an incentive for voluntary reporting by expressly providing legal immunity against civil or administrative liability for covered persons making good faith reports to public authorities. Mandatory and voluntary reporting statutes embody the state's exercise of either its inherent police power to protect and promote the general health, safety, welfare, and morals of the community or its *parens patriae* power to step up and safeguard individuals (such as persons with serious cognitive or emotional disabilities) who are not capable of protecting themselves. Further, a health professional may be compelled to reveal otherwise confidential information about particular patients by the force of legal process, namely, by a judge's issuance of a court order requiring such release. This is a possibility in any civil or criminal lawsuit involving a factual dispute about a patient's physical or mental condition. A court order (as opposed to a subpoena or subpoena *duces tecum*, which is issued simply as an administrative, nondiscretionary matter by the court clerk rather than by a judge) requiring one to produce personally identifiable patient information may override the state's provider/patient testimonial privilege statute that ordinarily prohibits the provider from testifying in a legal proceeding regarding private patient information. Every state testimonial privilege statute provides for judicially compelled testimony on the part of the health professional when, for example, the patient has placed his or her own health condition and medical treatment in issue in a lawsuit. This could occur when, for instance, the individual challenges the allegations propounded by others about one's mental impairments made in a guardianship/conservatorship petition.

Federal Law

Particular health care settings There are a variety of federal statutes and regulations imposing on health providers particular confidentiality obligations when care is provided within specific types of health care settings, including federal penal institutions, Veterans Affairs facilities, military institutions, federal community health centers, and facilities specializing in the treatment of persons having drug and alcohol addiction. Violation of these laws may result in substantial civil fines. Statutes and regulations setting the conditions for receipt of Medicare and Medicaid payments contain confidentiality provisions, set within general patients' rights standards, applicable specifically to nursing homes and home health agencies. Noncompliance with those provisions could trigger a range of regulatory sanctions, at the extreme including decertification of the facility or agency from participation in federal health care financing programs.

Health Insurance Portability and Accountability Act Federal regulations at 45 Code of Federal Regulations Parts 160 and 164 implement the Health Insurance Portability and Accountability Act (HIPAA) of 1996 (Public Law No. 104-191, title XI, Part C). These regulations, published as a Privacy Rule and a Security Rule, impose on covered health care entities (defined in part as health providers who transmit identifiable patient information electronically) an extensive set of requirements regarding the handling of personally identifiable medical information contained in patient records. These regulations impose severe criminal and civil sanctions for unauthorized disclosures of personal health information. Substantively, HIPAA and its implementing regulations in essence codify preexisting state statutory and common law protections for patients, with the addition of provisions making it clear that patients have the right to access the information contained in their own medical records. (Previously, state law varied or was unclear regarding the issue of patient access to records.) Patient access to their own electronic medical records was expanded further in 2020, through the 21st Century Cures Act, to include clinical notes.

HIPAA contains provisions authorizing covered entities to transmit personal health information to certain others for purposes of "treatment, payment, and health care operations" such as quality assurance or marketing. These and other exceptions explicitly contained in HIPAA basically track the preexisting state statutory and common law exceptions discussed in the previous section.

SUMMARY

Individual health professionals and organizational providers serving older patients inevitably and continuously interact with laws and the legal system. This chapter has outlined a handful of the arenas in which this interaction is likely to occur. For advice in particular circumstances, especially pertaining to relevant state law, specialized legal consultation should be sought from knowledgeable attorneys in private practice, counsel and/or risk managers employed or retained by the health provider, the professional's or provider's liability insurance carrier, or an institutional ethics committee.

FURTHER READING

Baker T, Silver C. How liability insurers protect patients and improve safety. *DePaul Law Rev.* 2019;68(2):209–237.

Blease C, Walker J, DesRoches CM, Delbanco T. New U.S. law mandates access to clinical notes: implications for patients and clinicians. *Ann Intern Med.* 2021;174(1):101–102.

Bookman K, Zane RD. Surviving a medical malpractice lawsuit. *Emerg Med Clin N Am.* 2020;38(2):539–548.

Cohen AB, Costello DM, O'Leary JR, Fried RT. Older adults without desired surrogates in a nationally representative sample. *J Am Geriatr Soc.* 2021;69(1):114–121.

Comer AR, Slaven JE, Montz A, et al. Nontraditional surrogate decisionmakers for hospitalized older adults. *Med Care.* 2018;56(4):337–340.

Cooke BK, Worsham E, Reisfield GM. The elusive standard of care. *J Am Acad Psychiatry Law.* 2017;45(3):358–364.

Dillon E, Chuang J, Gupta A, et al. Provider perspectives on advance care planning documentation in the electronic health record: the experience of primary care providers and specialists using advance health-care directives and physician orders for life-sustaining treatment. *Am J Hosp Palliat Care*. 2017;34(10):918–924.

Frolik LA, Kaplan RL. *Elder Law in a Nutshell*. 7th ed. St. Paul, MN: West Academic Publishing; 2019.

Glaser J, Nouri S, Fernandez A, et al. Interventions to improve patient comprehension in informed consent for medical and surgical procedures: an updated systematic review. *Med Decision Making*. 2020;40(2):119–143.

Grosso S. What is reasonable and what can be proved as reasonable: reflections on the role of evidence-based medicine and clinical practice guidelines in medical negligence claims. *Ann Health Law*. 2018;27(1):74–100.

Hooper S, Sabatino CP, Sudore RL. Improving medical-legal advance care planning. *J Pain Symptom Manage*. 2020;60(2):487–494.

Jacobsen J, Blinderman D, Cole CA, Jackson V. "I'd recommend…"—How to incorporate your recommendation into shared decision making for patients with serious illness. *J Pain Symptom Manage*. 2018;55(4):1224–1230.

Jain N, Bernacki RE. Goals of care conversations in critical illness: a practical guide. *Med Clin N Am*. 2020;104(3):375–389.

Lee RY, Modes ME, Sathitratanacheewin S, et al. Conflicting orders in physician orders for life-sustaining treatment forms. *J Am Geriatr Soc*. 2020;68(12):2903–2908.

Mack DS, Dosa D. Improving advanced care planning through physician orders for life-sustaining treatment (POLST) expansion across the United States: lessons learned from state-based developments. *Am J Hosp Palliat Care*. 2020;37(1):19–26.

Oza VM, El-Dika S, Adams MA. Reaching safe harbor: legal implications of clinical practice guidelines. *Clin Gastroenterol Hepatol*. 2016;14(2):172–174.

Pope TM, Bennett J, Carson SS, et al., on behalf of the American Thoracic Society and American Geriatrics Society. Making medical treatment decisions for unrepresented patients in the ICU. *Am J Respir Crit Care Med*. 2020;201(10):1182–1192.

Schoenfeld EM, Mader S, Houghton C, et al. The effect of shared decision-making on patients' likelihood of filing a complaint or lawsuit: a simulation study. *Ann Emerg Med*. 2019;74(1):126–136.

Shen MJ, Manna R, Banerjee SC, et al. Incorporating shared decision making into communication with older adults with cancer and their caregivers: development and evaluation of a geriatric shared decision-making communication skills training module. *Patient Educ Couns*. 2020;103(11):2328–2334.

Sulmasy LS, Bledsoe TA, for the ACP Ethics, Professionalism and Human Rights Committee. American College of Physicians Ethics Manual, 7th ed. *Ann Intern Med*. 2019;170 (Suppl.):S1–S32.

U.S. Department of Health and Human Services, Health Resources and Services Administration. *NPDB Guidebook*. Rockville, MD: U.S. Department of Health and Human Services; 2018. Available at https://www.npdb.hrsa.gov/resources/aboutGuidebooks.jsp. Accessed February 2, 2021.

Chapter 27

Perioperative Care: Evaluation and Management

Shelley R. McDonald

INCREASED RISK IN THE OLDER SURGICAL PATIENT

Inherent Vulnerabilities with Aging

Surgery in the older adult is different because of the increased risks of poor outcomes with seemingly simple or "routine" procedures but also because it can be challenging to identify those risks. Older adults preparing for surgery represent an incredibly diverse group of individuals not only because of the many available types and approaches to delivering surgical therapy but also because of the underlying vulnerabilities. Even though it is widely acknowledged that older adults are a heterogeneous group of patients they are also a distinctly vulnerable group of surgical patients who overall, experience disproportionately higher rates of postoperative complications, morbidity, and mortality. Thus, it is imperative to fully weigh the anticipated benefits of surgical interventions to the risks and explore whether this aligns with each patient's preferences, their goals for the surgery, and overall health goals.

Identifying a person's true baseline before surgery in terms of functional status as well as cognitive abilities can help more accurately assess an older individual's tolerance of surgical stressors, which in turn allows for more realistic goal setting, permits sufficient time for presurgical optimization and prehabilitation, and enables planning for recovery if additional resources need to be lined up. Examples of this frequently include friends or family traveling from out of town or requesting leave from work, an older adult temporarily moving to a friend or child's home, or being a participant in choosing a postacute care facility that would be potentially acceptable if they needed more assistance and therapy during recovery.

Learning Objectives

- Understand how to identify older adults who are at increased risk of poor surgical outcomes and implement strategies to modify patient-factor vulnerabilities to mitigate risk.
- Describe evidence-based perioperative practices that improve surgical outcomes for older adults that utilize interprofessional teamwork.

Key Clinical Points

1. Older adults are a distinctly vulnerable group of surgical patients and need to be evaluated for high-risk characteristics including, advanced age, impaired cognition, dependency in functioning, impaired mobility, malnutrition, dysphagia, and discordance of goals for surgical outcomes.

2. Thoughtful use of screening tools increases discrimination for assessing surgical risk in older adults, but the use can be challenging because predictive validity and feasibility is widely varied with different instruments.

3. Person-centered care for older adults delivered using evidence-based interventions is done more efficiently and effectively using structured processes that include interdisciplinary teams engaged throughout the continuum of surgical care.

Over 16% of the US population is older than 65 years and roughly 10,000 adults turn 65 years of age each day. Longitudinal studies show as aging continues so do increases in chronic medical conditions, mobility limitations, widowhood, loneliness, and institutionalization. Older adults are at increased risk of cognitive and functional decline. Those older than 85 years are even more likely to have accumulated age-related physiologic declines, leading to increased comorbidity, decreased functional abilities, decreased cognition, and malnutrition. These conditions create an increased vulnerability or frailty, which is an important predictor of adverse surgical outcomes. The cohort of high-risk older adults being considered for surgical therapy is going to be a sizable because by 2050, 20 million Americans will be 85 years or older. Despite increased physiological vulnerabilities, the demand for surgery will likely remain strong because subjective well-being remains positive over the course of old age and often surgeons use a communication strategy in which the surgical intervention is presented as restoring normalcy known as the "fix-it" model that may not fully explain the value of a planned surgical intervention and how it may impact someone's lifestyle.

Prevalence of Surgery in Older Adults

Nearly 40% of all surgical procedures are performed on older adults. Major surgery is a very common occurrence in the lives of adults older than 65 years. The 5-year cumulative risk for those in the United States is 14% (95% confidence interval [CI], 12.2%–15.5%) and remains relatively high even for those 90 years or older, 12% (95% CI, 9.9%–14.4%). **Table 27-1** (data in bold) shows that half of

TABLE 27-1 ■ TOP 10 OPERATING ROOM PROCEDURES IN THE US

RANK	PROCEDURE IN US	PER 100,000 POP
1	**Arthroplasty knee**	**223**
2	Percutaneous coronary angioplasty (PTCA)	170
3	**Laminectomy, excision intervertebral disc**	**149**
4	**Hip replacement, total and partial**	**149**
5	**Spinal fusion**	**144**
6	Cholecystectomy and common duct exploration	129
7	**Partial excision bone**	**108**
8	Hysterectomy, abdominal and vaginal	99
9	Colorectal resection	97
10	Excision, lysis peritoneal adhesions	97

Note: This table shows that over half of the top 10 procedures performed in the United States are to address musculoskeletal issues, which are frequently related to degenerative changes related to aging.

Data from Fingar KR, Stocks C, Weiss AJ, et al. Most Frequent Operating Room Procedures Performed in U.S. Hospitals, 2003–2012. HCUP Statistical Brief #186. December 2014. Agency for Healthcare Research and Quality, Rockville, MD.

the top 10 procedures performed in the United States are to address musculoskeletal disorders, which are frequently related to degenerative changes of aging. More importantly the deconditioning and decreased mobility from degenerative musculoskeletal disorders and potentially inappropriate medications to treat symptoms are directly related to increased risk of poor postsurgical outcomes, increased postoperative complications, and prolonged recovery after surgery.

ASSESSING SURGICAL RISK IN COMPLEX OLDER PATIENTS

There are many individual markers or observable characteristics that can be used when assessing an older adult's fitness for surgery either as discrete or composite measures. Recognizing these as **geriatric-specific** risk factors for poor surgical outcomes is important so that the risks can be anticipated and thus a plan put into place for appropriate shared decision making and risk mitigation.

Age over 80 years: How do we prognosticate? Advanced age should not be considered as the primary risk factor for predicting poor surgical outcomes because cognitive and physical abilities do not uniformly decline as we age. Physiologic reserve also differs significantly between older adults as well as between major organ systems within individuals. Thus, age alone cannot be used to estimate surgical risk because of the increasing heterogeneity in older age. Despite this variance, older age is associated with a greater burden of chronic diseases and when we assess outcomes for the older cohorts of older adults there is a greater risk for adverse outcomes. When the outcomes for major noncardiac surgery are examined in patients older than 80 years for morbidity and mortality, those with who experienced any postoperative complication had a higher 30-day all-cause mortality than those who did not have any complications (26% vs 4%, p < 0.001). Thirty-day all-cause mortality has also shown to be higher in those older than 80 years after cardiac surgery. Age is the bluntest tool we have for assessing risk in older adults and it can remind us to be more aware of screening for a true baseline in physical and cognitive functioning, but it should not be the sole factor in the decision to proceed or not with surgical therapy.

Frailty: The oldest of old patients are more likely to be frail, which is a clinical syndrome characterized by low physiological reserve leading to increased vulnerability. Frailty can be a thought of as a general descriptive term or a defined geriatric syndrome with measurable traits with many different instruments to assess this in a clinical setting. The features observed with Fried's phenotypic frailty are unintentional weight loss, weakness, exhaustion, low physical activity, and slow walking speed. Preoperative frailty in older adults is known to be associated with increased incidence of adverse postoperative outcomes, including more postoperative complications, increased length of hospital stay, and greater likelihood of being discharged to a skilled nursing or assisted-living facility. Because of the many available frailty scales, it is important to understand the strengths and weaknesses of the differing scales used. The phenotypic frailty scale is more often used for research and strongly associated with the development of postoperative delirium, whereas the Edmonton Frail Scale was a better predictor of complications, and the Clinical Frailty Scale tends to be more strongly associated with mortality and for discharge locations other than directly back to home. Acceptability, implementation, and feasibility are potential barriers to the use of frailty scales but selected use of these instruments can improve risk assessment particularly when used in combination with other risk-assessment tools. **Table 27-2** reviews

TABLE 27-2 ■ SELECTED FRAILTY SCALES USED IN SURGICAL RISK ESTIMATION

SCALE	DOMAINS	ASSOCIATED POST-SURGICAL OUTCOMES
Frailty phenotype	5 domains: Exhaustion, weakness, low physical activity, slow walking speed, and unintentional weight loss	• Postoperative delirium
FRAIL Scale	5 domains: Fatigue, resistance, ambulation, illnesses, loss of weight	• Postoperative delirium • Predictive for mortality and complications in emergency surgery
Edmonton Frail Scale	17 deficits: Cognition, general health status, functional independence, social support, medication use, nutrition, mood, continence, and functional performance	• Postoperative complications • Weakly to moderately discriminative for mortality
Clinical Frailty Scale	9-point scale: Judgment-based tool to broadly stratify the degrees of fitness/frailty	• Mortality • Discharge not to home
Risk Analysis Index	14-item questionnaire including: gender, age, cancer, comorbidity, residence, and ADLs	• Weakly to moderately discriminative for mortality • Prediction of longer-term outcomes up to 1 year
The Frailty Index	At least 30 health variables	• Moderate to strong discrimination for mortality • More sensitive to health change

ADLs: activities of daily living.
Note: This table shows the domains that make up the more commonly used frailty assessment instruments and associated postoperative outcomes.

some of the more common scales mainly used during assessments preceding elective surgery unless otherwise noted. See Chapter 42 for more discussion of frailty.

Gait speed: Gait speed is a direct or indirect component of many frailty scales, and slower gait speeds are associated with poor health and reduced ability to function. This single measure used during preoperative evaluation before cardiac surgeries is an independent predictor for increased in-hospital mortality, major complications, and discharge to a health care facility. As there are multiple factors that impact walking abilities, gait speed should be used to refine estimates of surgical risk and to identify those who may need more in-depth presurgical evaluation.

Weight and muscle mass: Weight loss is reflective of poor nutrition and/or poor utilization of nutrition, and in older adults is associated with many negative outcomes including loss of lean body and bone mass, development of pressure sores, slow wound healing, increased risk of infection, longer length of hospitalization, greater likelihood of hospital readmission after discharge, and increased mortality. Significant age- and disease-related reductions in skeletal muscle mass (sarcopenia) decrease the capacity of the older patient to make a functional recovery, possibly resulting in a discharge to a subacute or long-term care facility. Furthermore, weight loss preceding surgery increases the likelihood of delirium and postoperative pulmonary complications. All older adults need to be screened for nutritional risk before surgery because approximately one-third of older adults living in the community are at risk of being malnourished or are malnourished. This prevalence increases to a staggering 86% for those hospitalized. When an older adult has lost more than 10% of their body weight in the 6 months leading up to surgery or more than 5% in 1 month prior, further nutritional screening and assessment should be done to develop a nutritional support plan based on the nature, extent, and underlying causes of the malnourishment. The Mini Nutritional Assessment (MNA) is one well-established and validated nutritional screening tool in older persons. Obese older adults should also be screened because they are more likely to experience postsurgical complications. Furthermore, the comorbidities most related to obesity such as diabetes, coronary heart disease (CHD), congestive heart failure (CHF), atrial fibrillation (A-fib), stroke, cancer, and arthritis also increase the risks of postsurgical complications and can contribute to slower recoveries after surgical therapy. See Chapter 49 for more discussion of sarcopenia.

Functional status and falls: Accurate assessment of functional abilities for managing day-to-day affairs of maintaining a household (IADLs) and performing self-care (ADLs) as adults age into advanced age provides important information about cognitive and physical limitations, available social supports, need for adaptive interventions, and the impact of their illness and risks for postoperative complications. Dependency in just one ADL (toileting, feeding, dressing, grooming, transferring, or bathing) prior to surgery has been shown to be associated with 75% greater odds of postoperative death compared to a matched cohort of functionally independent older adults. When examined in older adults undergoing elective colorectal or cardiac surgery, falling only one time in the 6-month period before surgery is another discrete factor associated with having at least one postoperative complication, an increased 30-day readmission rate, and higher risk of being discharged to an institution. A positive inquiry about falling should trigger further assessment for high-risk medication use, sensory impairments, neuromuscular limitations, cognitive deficits, mood disturbances, or environmental barriers. The ACS NSQIP©/AGS Best Practice Guidelines recommends evaluating function using the four-question Short Simple Screening Test for Functional Assessment:

1. Can you get out of bed or chair yourself?
2. Can you dress and bathe yourself?
3. Can you make your own meals?
4. Can you do your own shopping?

If an older adult being considered for surgery cannot perform any of these activities, then a full inquiry should be performed about ADLs and IADLs to identify areas that need to be addressed both before and after surgery. Please see Chapter 43 for more about falls.

Cognition: Cognitive impairment, dementia, or history of prior delirium are significant risk factors for developing delirium following surgery. When dementia-level cognitive impairment is present before surgery as measured by the Mini-Cog screening tool, older adults are more likely to have increased complications, longer length of stay, higher discharge rates to institutional facilities, and long-term mortality as measured up to 4.5 years after a major elective surgery. Too often patients with cognitive impairment and dementia are excluded from clinical trials, thus there is limited literature on cognitive impairment as an independent risk factor for other postoperative complications. Nevertheless, delirium is the most common postsurgical complications for older adults and results in a sequalae of events that lead to increased likelihood of other complications including falls, aspiration, prolonged hospital stay, functional and cognitive decline, institutionalization, and death. Furthermore, postsurgical outcomes in older adults are worse when delirium occurs compared to postsurgical outcomes without delirium. This leads to an enormous loss of personal independence and financial burden with the 1-year direct cost of delirium in the United States estimated to be $33 billion. Therefore, it is critical to have a screening protocol in place to have a better understanding of an older adult's cognitive abilities prior to surgery with more in-depth assessment for those who do not do as well as expected on the cognitive screening or for those with previously unrecognized cognitive impairment. When neurocognitive deficits are recognized, it then

becomes important to allow for anticipated surgical risks and benefits to be presented in the most meaningful way for the patient and discussed in context of what is that person's overall health goals and with the input of any surrogate decision makers. Please see Chapter 9 for more on cognitive assessment.

Depression and mood: Identification of mental health disorders including depression, anxiety, posttraumatic stress disorder (PTSD), and substance abuse disorders should be deliberately explored as part of preoperative geriatric risk screening. Older patients who present with depressive symptoms before surgery have a greater risk of experiencing postoperative delirium and longer postoperative hospital lengths of stay. Anxiety is also associated with increased lengths of stay, and PTSD is associated with risk for emergence delirium (ED), which is defined as fearful, aggressive, and agitated behaviors that occur immediately following surgery upon awakening from anesthetic agents. Alcohol dependence may be overlooked in older adults but should also be screened for because it is associated with increased risk of postoperative complications.

The recognition of any mental health disorder should trigger scrutiny for actual use of prescribed medications including benzodiazepines, opioids, alcohol, illicit substances, and over-the-counter medications. Anticipatory guidance should include education/reassurance for the surgical procedure and plans for anesthesia and hospital and posthospital management of pain. Nonpharmacologic management should include exercise as tolerated, deep breathing, cognitive behavioral techniques for stress reduction, or integrated approaches such as music, aromatherapy, or massage. See Chapter 65 for more on depression and mood disorders.

Cardiopulmonary fitness: Poor cardiorespiratory fitness is the most significant independent predictor for postoperative mortality and length of hospital stay over age alone. Age-associated changes in cardiac physiology illustrate how age increases operative risk. This is primarily a result of a loss of vascular compliance, the left ventricle demonstrates an increase in stiffness, impaired diastolic relaxation, and an increase in filling pressures. These changes subsequently make the ventricle less tolerant of shifts in intravascular volume. An acute increase in volume (eg, from intravenous fluids administered during surgery) leads to a further increase in left ventricular filling pressures and could result in pulmonary congestion as a consequence of the age-related increase in diastolic stiffness. Conversely, an acute loss of intravascular volume, such as the third spacing of fluid or intraoperative blood loss, reduces preload to the stiffened ventricle and could produce a marked reduction in systolic blood pressure. Coronary artery disease (CAD), a common comorbidity, also increases risk; adding the intraoperative burden of myocardial ischemia to the already impaired diastolic relaxation leads to a further worsening of ventricular filling pressures and increases the risk of pulmonary edema.

When cardiac risk measures such as the Society of Thoracic Surgery and EuroScore II cardiac surgery risk models are added to frailty measures, the results are better model discrimination for postoperative outcomes.

Cardiac complications: CAD and heart failure (HF) are highly prevalent in older populations and remain the primary cause of death for the older patient. An estimated 25% to 30% of all perioperative deaths are attributed to cardiac causes. Because older adults are more likely to have significant CAD and HF, patients should be carefully screened for signs and symptoms of occult or overt disease. The left ventricular ejection fraction (LVEF) is an independent risk factor for major adverse cardiac events (MACE) with an increased risk of death when the LVEF falls below 40%. The risk of MACE is also higher among patients with HF with preserved LVEF than those without HF. Two-thirds of older adults with HF have normal left ventricular systolic function, and as previously noted the age-associated increases in vascular and left ventricular stiffness result in a greater sensitivity to volume shifts. Age-related declines in the electrical conduction system place the older patient at a greater risk of drug-induced bradycardia or high-grade atrioventricular blocks. A history of prior myocardial infarction or a low LVEF is associated with a greater risk of ventricular tachycardia. Older age (> 65 years) is also an independent risk factor for perioperative stroke and a history of stroke is a predictor of perioperative MACE.

Review **Table 27-3** for age-related physiological changes by organ system and the relationship to postoperative outcomes.

In summary, because normal aging does not account for the bulk of operative risk, the clinician's task is to identify underlying illnesses in older patients and assess its impact on perioperative risk.

SPECIFIC CONSIDERATIONS IN OLDER ADULTS

Pulmonary Complications

Postoperative pulmonary complications are another important cause of postoperative morbidity and mortality. Besides patient-related risk factors such as cigarette smoking and history of chronic lung disease, advanced age is an important predictor of adverse postoperative pulmonary complications. With increasing age, the respiratory system demonstrates several changes in function, which may include a loss of pulmonary elastic recoil, decreased diffusion capacity, and reduced cough and gag reflexes, as a consequence of either neurologic injury or respiratory muscle weakness. Postoperatively, it is common for older patients to experience atelectasis or aspiration. An estimated 14% of older patients will have a major pulmonary perioperative complication (atelectasis, pneumonia, respiratory failure, exacerbation of chronic lung disease, bronchospasm,

TABLE 27-3 ■ PHYSIOLOGIC CHANGES OF AGING AND EFFECTS ON PERIOPERATIVE CARE

SYSTEM	CHANGE	SIGNIFICANCE
General	↓ Skeletal muscle mass ↓ Thermoregulation	Altered volume of distribution Potential drug toxicity Greater frailty ↓ Functional recovery
Skin	↓ Re-epithelialization ↓ Dermal blood vessels	↓ Rate of wound healing
Cardiac	↑ Vascular stiffness ↑ Ventricular stiffness Conduction system degeneration Valvular degeneration ↓ Maximal heart rate Cardiopulmonary deconditioning ↑ Prevalence of coronary artery disease	↑ Blood pressure and ventricular vascular load Hypertension Ventricular hypertrophy ↑ Sensitivity to volume shifts ↓ Heart rate response ↑ Risk of high-grade arteriovenous blocks ↑ Risk of myocardial ischemia
Pulmonary	↓ Elastic recoil ↑ Chest wall stiffness ↑ V/Q mismatch ↓ Airway protections	↑ Potential for respiratory failure (eg, sedative drugs) ↑ Risk of aspiration and infections
Renal	↓ Number of nephrons ↓ Decreased sodium and water excretion Prostatic hypertrophy	↓ Half-life of drugs cleared by the kidney ↑ Risk for fluid overload ↑ Urinary retention and infection risk
Immune	↓ Immune function	↑ Risk of infections
Hepatic	↓ Blood flow ↓ Microsomal oxidation	↑ Half-life for drugs cleared by the liver
Endocrine	Insulin resistance Impaired insulin secretion	Hyperglycemia

Note: This table details the age-related physiological changes by organ system and the relationship to postoperative outcomes.

pleural effusion, pneumothorax, and airway obstruction), particularly after an abdominal or a cardiothoracic procedure. Postoperative pneumonia in older patients is associated with a 15% to 20% mortality rate. A detailed pulmonary and occupational exposure history prior to surgery can help predict impaired respiratory function. Because neurologic events that may impair airway protection are occasionally subtle, obtaining a history of swallowing difficulties or prior aspiration may prompt postoperative interventions aimed at reducing aspiration risk.

Renal Complications

Renal function is reduced as a result of glomerular and tubular senescence. The progressive sclerosis of glomeruli that occurs with increasing age is hastened by comorbid conditions such as hypertension, diabetes mellitus, and CAD. In the older patient, the serum creatinine often does not fully reflect the reduction in renal function. The age-associated reduction in skeletal muscle reduces creatinine production, so a reduced creatinine clearance is not always as apparent, even in the setting of diminished filtration. Baseline renal insufficiency results in greater risk for volume and acid-base disturbances in the perioperative period. Older adults are more susceptible to preoperative dehydration, intraoperative fluid shifts, hypotension, and hypovolemia, factors associated with the development of acute tubular necrosis, the most frequent cause of postoperative renal dysfunction. Certain medications and use of contrast dye can also contribute to renal toxicity. Also, alterations in renal (and hepatic) metabolism place the older patient at a greater risk of perioperative drug toxicities.

Infectious Complications

Postoperative infectious complications represent a major source of morbidity and mortality for older adults. In addition, the development of a surgical site infection or other health care–acquired infection can substantially increase length of stay and associated health care costs. The extended use of indwelling devices, prolonged ventilation, and length of stay are important risk factors for postoperative infections. Infections associated with devices and prosthetic material can present unique treatment challenges. The treatment of significant infections often requires extended courses of parenteral and/or oral antimicrobial therapy, which can raise issues related to safety and tolerability of antimicrobial agents, including nephrotoxicity. Prolonged need for antimicrobials can also increase the risk of *Clostridium difficile* infection. Prevention strategies are evolving and include targeted preoperative decolonization for *Staphylococcus aureus.*

Emergency Surgeries

While emergency surgeries are associated with a higher overall death rate in all age groups, this finding is most apparent among older patients who have the highest mortality rates as a consequence of a greater number of complications. The causes for the increased risk are multifactorial. The identical surgical disease in the older adult may present later in its course, and diagnosis can be delayed because of an atypical presentation. Also, the older patient may undergo surgery later due to efforts to "optimize" comorbidities prior to surgery. In the older patient, a delay in a needed nonemergent surgery may have a greater risk if the delay could result in an emergent procedure. Therefore, clinicians should be aware that if the time needed to optimize the patient for surgery is extended, an anticipated elective procedure could become a higher-risk emergent procedure.

Other Concerns

A neurologic event, such as a stroke, may increase the risk of aspiration by impairing the ability to swallow, to move food through the esophagus, and to control respiratory secretions. Advancing age is also associated with a decrease in esophageal peristaltic wave amplitude, reduced tone of the lower esophageal sphincter, a greater incidence of hiatal hernias, delayed gastric emptying, and increased gastroesophageal reflux, all of which are factors that may increase the perioperative aspiration risk. Impaired glucose regulation and risk for stress hyperglycemia are common in this age group and may increase infection risks. Thus, careful monitoring to control blood sugars perioperatively may have important benefits. Pressure injuries are another important postoperative complication (see Chapter 46 "Pressure Injuries"). Age-related changes in mobility and sensation can contribute to breakdown of skin integrity. Aggressive preventative measures including frequent assessment and pressure unloading are essential aspects of postoperative management.

Taking the time to thoroughly discuss what is involved with a particular surgery with older patients and their families can help promote a clearer understanding of risk and benefits and reduce false expectations. Incorporating regular patient and family conferences can be helpful. In such discussions, it is often apparent that an older patient has a different outlook and acceptance of a specific level of care. Shorter-term goals, such as the quality, not quantity, of life may be most important. Additionally, the overall tolerance of surgery may be different than that of a younger person. The understanding that a longer time to recover may be necessary is often best communicated in this forum. It is also important to inform the patient and family that an intermediate-care program may be needed, such as a subacute care center, a rehabilitation unit, as well as the extended use of home care services.

Period of Risk

Anesthesia is generally considered a safe procedure in older patients, with a progressive decline in complication rates being observed in recent years. Preoperative risk factors are a better predictor of 7-day mortality than is the duration of anesthesia or the experience of the anesthesiologist. Once the preoperative risk factors are controlled for, the type of anesthesia (eg, spinal vs general) fails to predict outcomes. The greatest period of risk for complications remains the time immediately after surgery, with half of adverse events occurring within 3 weeks of surgery.

Limited social support is also a risk factor. Among orthopedic patients, those with adequate social support are doing better 6 months after surgery.

Cancer adds a unique challenge for older adults going for surgery because they may require chemotherapy or radiation therapy before their surgical intervention; they may go into surgery with worse health status compared to prior to cancer diagnosis. Cancer also adds psychological stressors because uncertainties related to their condition add anxiety, increasing the risk for delirium and poor outcomes.

APPROACHES TO PREOPERATIVE ASSESSMENT AND PLANNING

A systematic way to organize the complex factors that older adult bring to surgical decision making and planning is essential in order to provide care that aligns both with the technical capabilities of the surgery and the goals for the patient in pursing surgical therapy.

Older adults may have very different goals for their surgery, so it is very important to have a shared decision-making process during the perioperative assessment and planning for older adults. All available data should be gathered, including clear direction from the surgeon about surgical goals and outcomes, as well as risk related to differing surgical techniques. Planning for a potential ostomy is an example where sometimes patients may not fully understand the chances of this outcome or the required lifestyle modifications unless it is explicitly addressed. It is also recommended to have someone accompany the patient during their clinic visits because their friends and family may want to discuss the surgical goals, overall health goals, preoperative preparation, and planning for recovery in more detail after the clinic visit.

Preoperative clinics should leverage community resources, family members, and an interdisciplinary team to address and optimize perioperative risk factors unique to older adults, in accordance with best practices.

The older patient may be unable to adequately communicate concerns or clinical history to a health care provider. Therefore, maximizing the communication and exchange of data between the surgical team and the medical providers can help ensure the best possible outcome for the older patient. Clinical programs that foster close communication among surgeons and consulting internists or geriatricians have demonstrated improved surgical outcomes and greater functional recoveries. Teamwork and communication between the various services are critical to promoting the best possible understanding of the patient's clinical situation, helping to mitigate surgical risk.

ACS NSQIP©/AGS Best Practice Guidelines: The American College of Surgeons (ACS) with the American Geriatrics Society (AGS) provided evidence-based guides for best practices approach to identify risk and focus on prevention in preoperative assessment of older adults undergoing surgery (**Table 27-4**). These best practices create a framework for engaging older patients and their caregivers to create a patient-centered approach that guides every member of the interdisciplinary and interprofessional team caring for the older adult. The integration and coordination of care in the older surgical patient undergoing elective surgery begins when the surgery is scheduled. When this framework is used, patient-centered and collaborative

TABLE 27-4 ■ ACS NSQIP ®/AGS BEST PRACTICE GUIDELINES FOR OPTIMAL PERIOPERATIVE MANAGEMENT OF THE GERIATRIC SURGICAL PATIENT	
RECOMMENDED PREOPERATIVE ASSESSMENTS	**ASSESSMENT AND MANAGEMENT STRATEGIES**
What Matters Most	• Determine the patient's treatment goals and expectations in the context of the possible treatment outcomes
Mentation	• Assess the patient's cognitive ability and capacity to understand the anticipated surgery • Screen for depression • Identify risk factors for developing postoperative delirium
Mobility	• Determine baseline frailty score • Document functional status and history of falls
Medication	• Take accurate/detailed medication history and consider appropriate perioperative adjustments. Monitor for polypharmacy • Screen for alcohol and other substance abuse/dependence
Multimorbidity/Multicomplexity	• Perform a preoperative cardiac evaluation according to the American College of Cardiology/American Heart Association (ACC/AHA) • Identify risk factors for postoperative pulmonary complications and implement appropriate strategies for prevention • Assess nutritional status and consider preoperative interventions if the patient is at severe nutritional risk • Determine family and social support system • Order appropriate preoperative diagnostic tests focused on older adults

(Continued)

TABLE 27-4 ■ ACS NSQIP ®/AGS BEST PRACTICE GUIDELINES FOR OPTIMAL PERIOPERATIVE MANAGEMENT OF THE GERIATRIC SURGICAL PATIENT (CONTINUED)

RECOMMENDED DAILY POSTOP ASSESSMENTS	ASSESSMENT AND MANAGEMENT STRATEGIES
Delirium/cognitive impairment	• Pain control • Optimize physical environment (eg, sleep hygiene, sleep protocol, minimize tethers, encourage family at bedside) • Vision and hearing aids accessible • Remove catheters • Monitor for substance withdrawal syndromes • Minimize psychoactive medications • Avoid potentially inappropriate medications
Perioperative acute pain	• Ongoing education regarding safe and effective use of institutional treatment options • Directed pain history • Multimodal, individualized pain control • Vigilant dose titration
Pulmonary complications	• Chest physiotherapy and incentive spirometry • Early mobilization/ambulation • Aspiration precautions
Fall risk	• Universal fall precautions • Vision and hearing aids accessible • Appropriate treatment of delirium • Early mobilization/ambulation • Early physical/occupational therapy if indicated • Assistive walking devices
Ability to maintain adequate nutrition	• Resume diet as early as feasible • Dentures made available • Supplementation if indicated
Urinary tract infection (UTI) prevention	• Daily documentation of Foley catheter indication • Catheter care bundles, hand hygiene, barrier precautions
Functional decline	• Care models and pathways • Structural: uncluttered hallways, large clocks and calendars • Multidisciplinary rounds • Early mobilization and/or PT/OT • Family participation • Nutritional support • Minimize patient tethers
Pressure ulcers	• Reduce/minimize pressure, friction, humidity, shear force • Maintain adequate nutrition • Wound care

PT/OT, physical therapy/occupational therapy.
Note: This table shows adapted checklist evaluations from the ACS NSQIP ®/AGS Best Practice Guidelines for both optimal preoperative assessment and optimal perioperative management of the geriatric surgical patient.

patient care is delivered, representing the best chance to improve surgical care for an aging population. Structured perioperative care around evidence-based best practices improves the quality of care, reduces unnecessary hospital admissions, reduces hospital acquired complications, while providing a patient-centered approach by eliciting individual goals and preferences for each patient. If the decision is to pursue surgery, this approach creates the opportunity for collaboration across different settings of health care delivery during the entire continuum of surgical need, until full recovery.

Geriatric 5 Ms: Age-friendly health systems are recognizing four or five evidence-based elements of high-quality care that organize the complexities of assessing the surgical risks and surgical planning for an older adult into a framework organized by: What Matters Most, Mentation, Mobility, Medication, and Multimorbidity/Multicomplexity.

Interdisciplinary teams: Preoperative clinics should leverage community resources, family members, and an interdisciplinary team to address and optimize perioperative risk factors unique to older adults, in accordance with best practices. Many of the clinical care points in recognizing and mitigating surgical risk can be acted upon by many members from a variety of professions. Interestingly, the Clinical Frailty Scale is valid for use by health care professionals with a license or registration for example MD, RN, LPN, OT, PT, SW, or psychologist.

Comprehensive geriatric assessment: This would be the "gold standard" means to use multidimensional, interdisciplinary, interprofessional process and teams to fully assess in a complete manner an older adult's medical, psychological, and functional status within their social and environmental circumstances. This information allows for a patient-centered plan to manage and treat their surgical needs beginning with optimizing targeted areas before surgery and creating an integrated plan for treatment during hospitalization and throughout recovery.

POSTOPERATIVE MANAGEMENT

Postoperative management includes the appropriate use of medications for pain, increasing mobilization, proper use of urinary catheters, the treatment and prevention of delirium, and anticoagulation use.

Pain control: Pain is often undertreated in older patients because of the concern of using potent analgesics in older patients and a misconception that pain sensations are diminished in such patients. Postoperative patients should be regularly asked about the severity of their discomfort using analog scales, and analgesics should be given according to anticipated needs rather than "as needed." Simply scheduling pain medications is another useful approach. Comments on the management of persistent pain, medication dosing, and metabolism, as well as associated toxicities, are well summarized by the AGS comprehensive review of this topic. See Chapter 68 for more detail about pain management.

Early mobilization: Prolonged bed rest can adversely affect the older patient. Changes noted with prolonged immobility include a decrease in cardiac output and aerobic capacity, baroreceptor desensitization and orthostatic hypotension, skeletal muscle deconditioning, bone loss, hypercalcemia, joint contractures, constipation, incontinence, pressure sores, sensory deprivation, an increased risk for deep vein thrombosis (DVT), atelectasis, hypoxemia, and pneumonia. Early mobilization from bed is vital, helping to reduce the risk for complications. If the recovery process prevents full mobilization, then a physical therapy referral for range-of-motion exercises and the maintenance of an upright posture (chair) may reduce the frequency and severity of these complications.

Catheters: Postoperative urinary drainage is often managed by an indwelling catheter but this predisposes to urinary tract infection and associated complications. Catheter use should be short, with a goal of prompt removal by the morning after surgery. If there is a concern for urinary retention or bladder distension, then intermittent catheterization should be considered. The use of a urinary catheter beyond 48 hours should be avoided, except when retention cannot be managed by other means. Patients requiring long-term use of a urinary catheter should not be given prophylactic antimicrobials.

Postoperative delirium: An acute confusional state occurs in 10% to 15% of older patients undergoing general surgery, 30% of cardiac surgery patients, and, in one study, up to 50% of hip fracture repairs. Delirium is also a marker for worse functional recovery, and older patients with in-hospital delirium are at risk of significant long-term reduction in cognitive function (see Chapter 58 on delirium).

Delirium is often subtle and can easily be missed. Clinical factors key to the diagnosis are a rapid onset, a disturbed level of consciousness, decreased attention and environmental awareness, memory deficits, disorientation, perceptual disturbances, and evidence of a condition that contributes to its development. A history of dementia as well as prior delirium, advanced age, and a prior decline in cognitive function are risk factors for perioperative delirium. As a rule, delirium fluctuates and may not be evident during all visits. Nursing staff and family members are often the most reliable source for the serial assessments of an at-risk patient.

Delirium often compromises postoperative care and extends the length of stay. Behaviors can often be controlled with environmental measures, such as a bedside sitter, increased visitations by family, frequent orientation, minimizing abrupt relocations, and permitting patients to return to a more normal day-night cycle. If medically appropriate, the use of a sleep protocol is often helpful. Symptomatic control of agitation to prevent harm is occasionally needed. Unfortunately, no single drug has an accomplished record. High-potency antipsychotics such as risperidone, haloperidol, olanzapine, and quetiapine should be cautiously titrated to improve symptoms. Lower-potency drugs such as chlorpromazine and thioridazine should be avoided because of their associated anticholinergic and arrhythmogenic effects. If delirium is secondary to alcohol withdrawal, short-acting benzodiazepines can be used with close monitoring for excessive sedation. Formal delirium prevention protocols can be helpful, especially in the intensive care unit setting.

Other complications: Postoperative surveillance for myocardial ischemia, infarction, arrhythmias, and DVT should ideally lead to a reduction in mortality. Postoperative myocardial ischemia is the strongest predictor of cardiac morbidity. Anginal pain may be masked by narcotics or may be difficult to verbalize during recovery. Postoperative ST-segment changes on electrocardiogram (ECG) are indicative of myocardial ischemia and are an independent predictor of events. Such changes are associated with a worse long-term survival. The optimal surveillance strategy for the diagnosis of postoperative ischemia or infarction has not been defined. In patients without documented CAD, surveillance should be restricted to patients who develop signs or symptoms of cardiovascular dysfunction. Cardiac troponin measurements should be part of the diagnostic plan for myocardial infarction detection, but additional research is needed to correlate outcomes to the magnitude of an isolated cardiac troponin elevation. As a rule, postoperative myocardial infarctions have a similar pathology to infarction occurring in a nonsurgical patient, the spontaneous thrombosis of the coronary artery. Therefore, when this complication occurs, appropriate medical management as well as an aggressive attempt at opening the infarct-related artery should be considered in the appropriate postoperative patient.

Postoperative arrhythmias are often caused by correctable noncardiac problems such as infection, hypotension, metabolic abnormalities (hypokalemia and hypomagnesemia), and hypoxia. Ventricular arrhythmias (frequent ventricular ectopic beats or nonsustained ventricular tachycardia) may occur in more than one-third of high-risk patients. Prophylactic use of antiarrhythmics other than β-blockers is not recommended. Sustained ventricular tachycardia with or without hemodynamic complications requires consultation with a cardiologist. Postoperative A-fib is common. Approximately 25% of older patients develop this rhythm. Age and the type of surgery are strong predictors for the development of A-fib. The prophylactic use of a β-blocker and amiodarone has shown some benefit by reducing the frequency of this rhythm, but is not routinely recommended.

Hemoglobin levels often fall after major surgery. Transfusions should be reserved for patients with symptoms and possibly those with levels below 7 g/dL. Small trials have demonstrated that administering intravenous iron infusions in anemic patients prior to hip and knee replacement surgery reduced the need for postoperative blood product transfusions.

Cognitive decline has been noted following a variety of surgeries. The International Study of Postoperative Cognitive Dysfunction found that 26% of patients older than 60 years who had either intra-abdominal or orthopedic procedures had a significant decline in cognitive function 1 week after surgery. Risk factors included older age, greater use of anesthetics, and postoperative respiratory and infectious complications. In coronary artery bypass surgery, where the aorta is often cross-clamped and a bypass pump is used, embolization of both gas and particulates occurs. As a result, central nervous system ischemic damage is often noted after these procedures. Postoperative cerebral infarcts (many subclinical) are the likely cause of cognitive decline noted with cardiac surgery. Off-pump coronary artery bypass surgery seems to have a lower rate of short-term decline in cognitive function (21% vs 29%), but

similar decline is noted at 6 months (31% vs 38%). The risk of further decline in cognitive function should be incorporated into the decision process for patients with underlying dementia who are not undergoing emergent or lifesaving surgery. Finally, postoperative critical pathways involving regimens, including low-dose opiates, early extubation, and an emphasis on accelerated functional recovery, can be safely applied to older patients.

The management of anticoagulants prior to surgery is briefly summarized. For patients on chronic warfarin with an international normalized ratio (INR) goal of 2.0 to 3.0, four scheduled doses should be withheld to allow the INR to normalize to less than 1.5 before surgery. If the INR is typically kept above 3.0, then longer periods without a warfarin dose may be required. The INR should be measured on the day of surgery to ensure that it has reached an acceptable range. If the INR is excessive, a small dose of vitamin K (eg, 1 mg intravenously or 2.5 mg orally) may be given, which will further reverse the INR within 24 hours. If rapid reversal of the INR is required, fresh frozen plasma can be administered. When the INR is less than 2.0, other prophylactic antithrombotic interventions should be considered.

Elective surgery is best avoided for at least 3 months following a DVT or pulmonary embolism (PE) event to ensure adequate duration of anticoagulation treatment. If this is not possible, then anticoagulation bridging with low-molecular-weight heparin (LMWH) should be given before and after the procedure for patients on warfarin while the INR is less than 2.0. LMWH should be stopped 24 hours before surgery; restarting LMWH can be considered 24 to 48 hours after surgery, depending on the type of surgery, bleeding risk, and thrombotic risk of the patient. Patients receiving one of the newer oral anticoagulants (eg, dabigatran, rivaroxaban, or apixaban) do not require perioperative bridging therapy given the relatively short half-life of these agents. These medications can be discontinued 1 to 4 days prior to surgery depending on the patient's risk of thrombosis, surgical bleeding risk, and renal function.

SUMMARY

As our society ages, the need for surgical procedures will continue to increase among older adults. Age alone is not a reliable predictor of operative risk and should not be the sole criteria for deciding who should and who should not have surgery. However, age is associated with a higher prevalence of chronic diseases, which, in turn, are strong predictors of operative risk and help determine who might benefit from surgery and preoperative testing. The AHA and ACC have published updated guidelines, which help guide preoperative cardiac risk assessment. Perioperative care requires a careful medical evaluation and comprehensive postoperative observation that anticipates potential complications. Newer techniques related to minimally invasive surgery appear promising. Besides decreasing recovery time and postoperative pain, there is some suggestion that overall operative risk may be decreased. Future studies examining clinical outcomes of interest in older adults will be an essential component of evaluating the relative risks and benefits of new interventions.

ACKNOWLEDGMENT

Many thanks to Satyen S. Nichani, Paul J. Grant, and Preeti N. Malani for their contributions to the Perioperative Evaluation and Management components of this chapter in earlier editions of this book.

FURTHER READING

Afilalo J, Kim S, O'Brien S, et al. Gait speed and operative mortality in older adults following cardiac surgery. *JAMA Cardiol.* 2016;1(3):314–321.

Arteaga AS, Aguilar LT, González JT, et al. Impact of frailty in surgical emergencies. A comparison of four frailty scales. *Eur J Trauma Emerg Surg.* 2021;47(5):1613–1619.

Aucoin SD, Hao M, Sohi R, et al. Accuracy and feasibility of clinically applied frailty instruments before surgery: a systematic review and meta-analysis. *Anesthesiology.* 2020;133(1):78–95.

Becher RD, Vander Wyk B, Leo-Summers L, Desai MM, Gill TM. The incidence and cumulative risk of major surgery in older persons in the United States. *Ann Surg.* 2021; Epub ahead of print.

Centers for Disease Control and Prevention. National Hospital Discharge Survey. Atlanta, GA; 2010.

Chow WB, Rosenthal RA, Merkow RP, Ko CY, Esnaola NF. Optimal preoperative assessment of the geriatric surgical patient: a best practices guideline from the American College of Surgeons National Surgical Quality Improvement Program and the American Geriatrics Society. *J Am Coll Surg.* 2012;215(4):453–466.

Gou RY, Hshieh TT, Marcantonio ER, et al. One-year Medicare costs associated with delirium in older patients undergoing major elective surgery. *JAMA Surg.* 2021;156(5):430–442.

Hamel MB, Henderson WG, Khuri SF, Daley J. Surgical outcomes for patients aged 80 and older: morbidity and mortality from major noncardiac surgery. *J Am Geriatr Soc.* 2005;53(3):424–429.

Inouye SK, Westendorp RGJ, Saczynski JS. Delirium in elderly people. *Lancet.* 2014;383(9920):911–922.

Kaiser MJ, Bauer JM, Ramsch C, et al. Frequency of malnutrition in older adults: a multinational perspective using the mini nutritional assessment. *J Am Geriatr Soc.* 2010;58(9):1734–1738.

Katlic MR, Robinson TN. The costs of postoperative delirium. *JAMA Surg.* 2021;156(5):470–471.

Kruser JM, Pecanac KE, Brasel KJ, et al. "And I think that we can fix it": mental models used in high-risk surgical decision making. *Ann Surg.* 2015;261(4):678.

Makary MA, Segev DL, Pronovost PJ, et al. Frailty as a predictor of surgical outcomes in older patients. *J Am Coll Surg.* 2010;210(6):901–908.

Mohanty S, Rosenthal RA, Russell MM, Neuman MD, Ko CY, Esnaola NF. Optimal perioperative management of the geriatric patient: a best practices guideline from the American College of Surgeons NSQIP and the American Geriatrics Society. *J Am Coll Surg.* 2016;222(5): 930–947.

Passel JS, D'Vera Cohn D. US population projections, 2005–2050. Pew Research Center Washington, DC; 2008.

Robinson TN, Wu DS, Pointer L, Dunn CL, Cleveland JC Jr, Moss M. Simple frailty score predicts postoperative complications across surgical specialties. *Am J Surg.* 2013;206(4):544–550.

Robinson TN, Wu DS, Pointer LF, Dunn CL, Moss M. Preoperative cognitive dysfunction is related to adverse postoperative outcomes in the elderly. *J Am Coll Surg.* 2012;215(1):12–17; discussion 17–18.

Scarborough JE, Bennett KM, Englum BR, Pappas TN, Lagoo-Deenadayalan SA. The impact of functional dependency on outcomes after complex general and vascular surgery. *Ann Surg.* 2015;261(3):432–437.

Chapter 28

Anesthesia

Leanne Groban, Chandrika Garner

INTRODUCTION

By the year 2024, people 65 years and older will represent over a quarter of the global population. Soon, there will be more older people than children and more people at the extremes of old age than ever before. This trend in population aging will undoubtedly translate into increasing numbers of older adults in developed countries requiring invasive and minimally invasive procedures for revascularization (joint repair and replacement), urologic, and gynecologic-, gastrointestinal-, and ophthalmologic-related surgeries, and more. In the United States, for example, older adults already account for approximately 40% of all in-patient operations and about one-third of outpatient procedures performed annually. One of the major challenges of treating older patients is the heterogeneity of the geriatric population—and the need to individualize care for each patient to provide the best outcome. As the incidence of comorbidity increases with age, so does the risk for postoperative complications and longer hospital stays which underscores the collaborative roles that geriatricians, anesthesiologists, and surgeons are certain to play, moving forward in the care of the older surgical patient. Indeed, high quality care for older adults undergoing major and even minor surgical procedures requires a well thought-out and all-inclusive approach to risk stratification, communication, and coordination. Accordingly, in July 2019, the American College of Surgeons initiated the Geriatric Surgery Verification (GSV) Program that provides hospitals with a validated list of 30 evidence-based and patient-centered standards for geriatric surgery, which hospitals can implement to continuously optimize surgical care for this vulnerable population. These standards define the resources and processes that hospitals need to have in place to perform operations effectively, efficiently, and safely in older adults (defined by 75 years and older), while also always prioritizing what matters most to individual patients with regard to their needs and treatment goals. At the time of composing this chapter, one hospital had achieved Level 1 verification of being a Geriatric Surgery Hospital, and 11 other institutions, among seven states, were at the "Commitment Level" of the verification process. Given the aging demographics and expected uptick in the need for surgical services in those 75 years and older, it is likely that all major

Learning Objectives

- Recognize the various types of anesthesia and associated drugs used in the intraoperative management of the older surgical patient.

- Review the impact of, and controversy around anesthesia and surgery as a cause of postoperative cognitive morbidity.

- Give general descriptions of the types of surgical approaches and associated anesthetic and monitoring techniques used in the older cardiac patient for treatment of coronary artery disease, aortic valve stenosis, and atrial fibrillation.

- Summarize the plan for the older patient who requires anesthesia for a procedure near the end of life who has an "Allow Natural Death" order in place and/or an implantable cardiac defibrillator.

Key Clinical Points

1. To date, there is no conclusive evidence that suggests one anesthetic technique is superior to others in the older surgical patient in terms of limiting postoperative dysfunction, for example, delirium and cognitive dysfunction, the most common postoperative complications in older persons.

2. As older adults are more sensitive to intravenous anesthetics, volatile agents, and opiates due to age-related changes in pharmacokinetics and pharmacodynamics, anesthetic dosing is age-adjusted and anesthetic depth continuously monitored by end-tidal anesthetic concentrations and physical signs. Because many of the assumptions about anesthetic depth might not be as reliable in older patients as they are in younger patients, brain function monitoring with processed electroencephalography (pEEG) or a bispectral index (BIS) monitor is often used.

(Continued)

3. While there is no recommended pharmaceutical for preventing postoperative delirium, best practice consensus guidelines advocate nonpharmaceutical interventions (eg, staff education, early mobilization, adequate pain control and assessments, frequent orientation, sleep-wake cycle preservation, early postoperative use of hearing and visual aids, etc) and avoidance of high-risk medications.

4. Limiting excessive anesthetic depth while avoiding awareness and recall after surgery in older patients is important for mitigating neurotoxicity and the potential for perioperative neurocognitive dysfunction, but it also reduces the risk of acute kidney injury, adverse cardiac events (eg, myocardial infarction [MI] or injury), and central nervous system ischemic events as a result of anesthetic-induced intraoperative hypotension.

5. The benefit of off-pump coronary artery bypass (OPCAB), regardless of the surgical approach, is the avoidance of manipulation of the aorta and need for a cardiopulmonary bypass (CPB) circuit and its associated risks. While no evidence supports OPCAB over CABG for reducing all-cause mortality, cardiac complications, or success of revascularization in the general population, subgroup analyses suggest improved outcomes in the geriatric cardiac surgery population.

6. Aortic stenosis is the most common single valve disease, with prevalence between 2% and 10% in patients over age 75. While there may be a benefit to avoiding CPB in the geriatric population, overall complication rates for transcatheter aortic valve replacement (TAVR) are as high as 20%, which includes a stroke rate of 2%.

7. Surgical procedures are common at the end of life. Conversations with the patient and/or decision maker regarding the perioperative course of action are necessary and should involve both the surgeon and anesthesiologist. Automatic suspension of Allow Natural Death (AND) is not acceptable and any modifications must be discussed with the patient and documented, including verification of the "time" the modification is in place.

medical centers will move in the direction of GSV certification. It is nearly certain that geriatricians will play key roles in the shared decision-making process and interdisciplinary approach to continuously optimize surgical care for older adults. In view of this, this chapter will provide the reader with a general understanding of: (1) intraoperative management strategies (eg, regional vs general anesthesia [GA] vs sedation) aimed to minimize risk of some of the common complications of older patients (eg, postoperative delirium [POD] and cognitive dysfunction); (2) special concerns attached to geriatric cardiac procedures performed within and outside the operating room (eg, hybrid cardiovascular and electrophysiology suites); and (3) perioperative issues that relate to Allow Natural Death (AND) orders.

TYPES OF INTRAOPERATIVE ANESTHESIA

The decision as to which kind of anesthesia that will be used is dependent on several factors including the patient's medical history, the surgical procedure that is to be performed, the preference of the surgeon and anesthesiologist, and the patient's first choice. As the primary goal is to provide the safest anesthetic with the best outcome possible, the anesthesiologist, who is the perioperative medicine expert, will thoroughly explain the options to the patient and surrogate while also discussing the rationale for recommending one over another method. The types of anesthesia that might be used include general anesthesia, regional (peripheral nerve blocks) or neuraxial anesthesia (eg, spinal or epidural), combined general and regional anesthesia, and conscious sedation (**Figure 28-1**). When either general or neuraxial anesthesia is deemed appropriate for an older adult, for instance in the case of hip fracture repair, neuraxial is often the preferred choice. With all anesthesia modalities, the patient's breathing, oxygenation, heart rate, blood pressure (BP), and body temperature are closely monitored intraoperatively and in the postanesthesia care unit. To appreciate the latest medical literature on how anesthetic type might influence the most common postoperative complications among older adults undergoing surgery and anesthesia, a basic understanding of the different techniques available and the anesthetic agents used to ensure safe outcomes is warranted.

To begin with, **GA** is the state produced when a patient receives medications for amnesia, analgesia, muscle relaxation, and sedation. An anesthetized patient is considered being in a state of controlled, reversible unconsciousness. General anesthetics, in the form of inhalational (eg, isoflurane, sevoflurane, desflurane, nitrous oxide, and xenon) and/or intravenous agents (eg, propofol, ketamine, and etomidate) depress the central nervous system to a sufficient degree to permit the performance of surgery and other noxious or unpleasant procedures. To control breathing, the anesthesia care provider inserts either an endotracheal tube or a laryngeal mask airway into the trachea or pharynx,

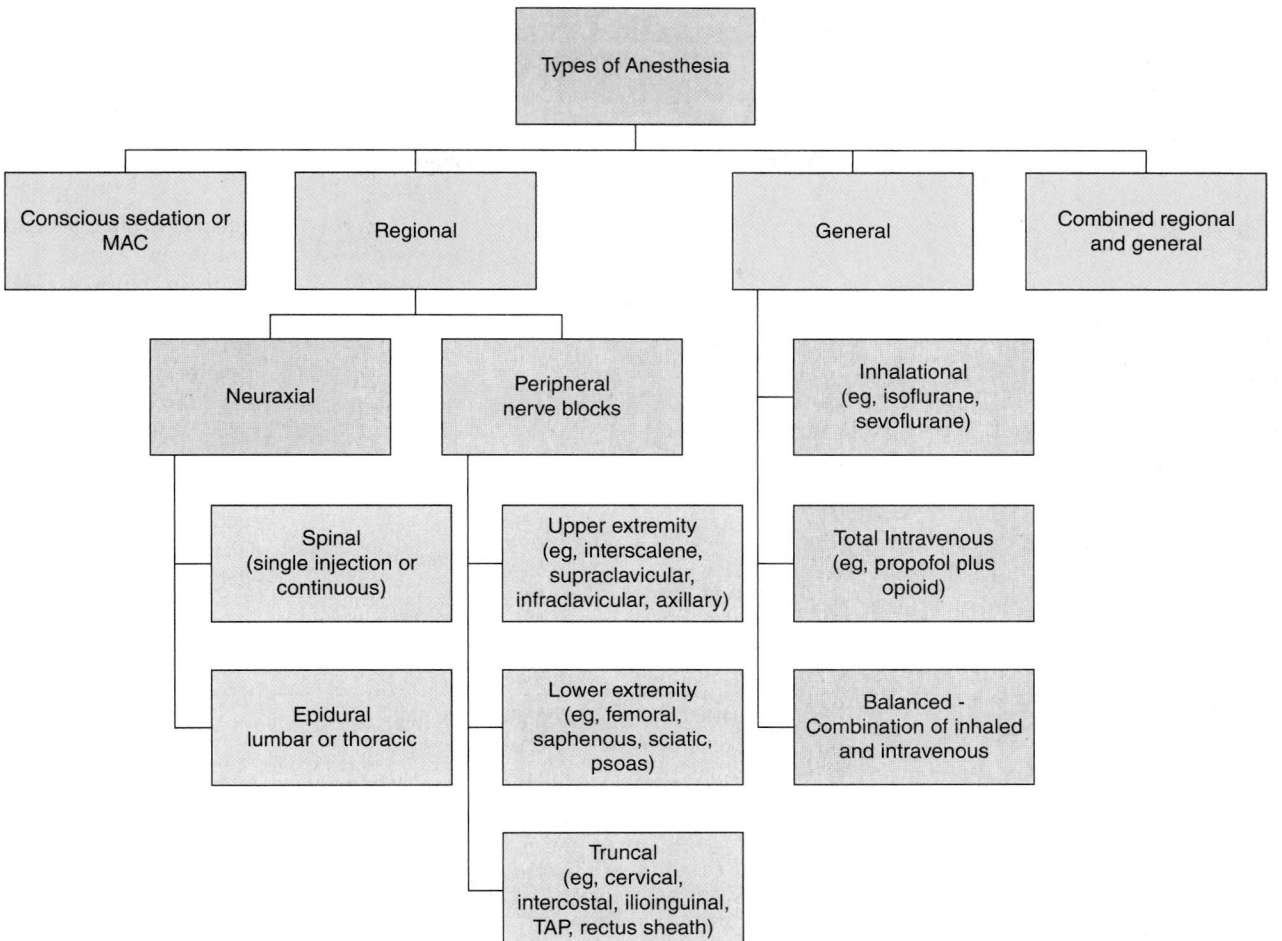

FIGURE 28-1 Schematic displaying the types of anesthetic techniques for older patients requiring surgery and minimally invasive procedures in and outside the operating room. MAC, monitored anesthesia care; TAP, transverse abdominal plane.

respectively, after the patient is rendered unconscious following induction of anesthesia. Maintenance anesthesia is commonly provided with volatile or inhalational anesthetics, which offer reliable control over the depth of anesthesia. Short-acting opioids (eg, fentanyl, sufentanil, or alfentanil) are used for analgesia along with the inhalational agent, because the latter has only weak analgesic properties. To facilitate endotracheal intubation and minimize the need for high-dose volatile anesthetics, neuromuscular blocking agents (eg, succinylcholine, rocuronium, vecuronium, or cisatracurium) are often used. **Table 28-1** shows the commonly used intravenous drugs, their side effects/contraindications, and dosing concerns/recommendations for the older patient. Standard monitoring, including pulse oximetry, electrocardiogram (ECG), noninvasive BP device, temperature monitor, measurement of end-tidal carbon dioxide, inspired oxygen concentration, and low oxygen concentration and ventilator disconnect alarms are employed in all older adults undergoing a general anesthetic. A peripheral nerve stimulator is also used to guide dosing of short-acting neuromuscular

blocking agents and to ensure complete reversal of neuromuscular blockade, if extubation is planned at the end of the surgical procedure. Indeed, even a small amount of leftover neuromuscular blockade can have profound effects on pharyngeal muscle function, predisposing the older patient to aspiration pneumonia. As older adults are more sensitive to intravenous anesthetics, volatile agents, and opiates due to age-related changes in pharmacokinetics and pharmacodynamics, anesthetic dosing is age-adjusted and anesthetic depth continuously monitored by end-tidal anesthetic concentrations and physical signs. Because many of the assumptions about anesthetic depth might not be as reliable in the older adult as they are in younger patients, brain function monitoring with processed electroencephalography (pEEG) or a bispectral index (BIS) monitor is often used. Limiting excessive anesthetic depth while avoiding awareness and recall after surgery in older patients, is a key tenet of the American Society of Anesthesiologist's Brain Health Initiative. Not only is this important for mitigating neurotoxicity and the potential for perioperative neurocognitive dysfunction, but it also reduces the risk of

385

PART II PRINCIPLES OF GERIATRICS

TABLE 28-1 ■ COMMONLY USED INTRAVENOUS ANESTHETIC-RELATED DRUGS

CLASS	AGENT	INDICATION	SIDE EFFECTS/ CONTRAINDICATIONS	AGING-RELATED CONCERNS/ DOSING RECOMMENDATIONS
SEDATIVE HYPNOTICS				
Barbiturate	Thiopental	Induction (fast onset)	Involuntary movements, cough, laryngospasm, hypersensitivity reaction	Initial distribution of all hypnotic drugs is often impaired in older patients contributing to their "increased sensitivity." Liver blood flow declines with age, reducing clearance of hepatically extracted drugs. Induction doses should be reduced and dosed incrementally and slowly due to altered initial distribution and heightened and often delayed hemodynamic effects.
Barbiturate	Methohexital	Induction (fast onset) (ECT therapy)	Pain on injection, marked excitatory phenomenon, induce seizure in epileptics	
Phenol derivative	Propofol	Induction (fast onset)/ maintenance/antiemetic	Hypotension, pain on injection	
Imidazole group	Etomidate	Induction (fast onset) particularly in patients with dilated cardiomyopathy/low ejection fraction	Inhibits cortisol production (not ideal in septic patient), involuntary movements, nausea and vomiting, pain on injection	
Phencyclidine derivative; NMDA antagonist	Ketamine	Induction (hypotensive cases); analgesic for dressing changes	Dissociative anesthesia, hallucinations on emergence (less if premedicated with BDZ), excessive salivary and bronchial secretions; SNS activation; avoid in increased intracranial pressure	
Benzodiazepine	Midazolam	Induction (slow onset); premedication for anxiolysis, antegrade amnesia	Avoid in older patients— contributes to postoperative delirium; reversal— flumazenil (short-acting)	
ANALGESICS				
Opioid, naturally occurring (opium)	Morphine	Used intravenously, intramuscularly, subcutaneously, orally, intra-articular, intrathecal, epidural, and occasionally nebulized	Respiratory depression; may precipitate histamine release and bronchospasm; contraction of sphincter of Oddi, constipation; pruritus; muscle rigidity (eg, chest wall) urinary retention. Metabolite morphine-6-glucuronide elimination is impaired in renal failure patients. Reversal: naloxone	Increased central nervous system sensitivity to all opioids in older patients; reduce dosing by 50% in patients ≥ 80 y; titrate to effect; consider short-acting agent (eg, remifentanil) via controlled delivery system.

(Continued)

TABLE 28-1 ■ COMMONLY USED INTRAVENOUS ANESTHETIC-RELATED DRUGS (CONTINUED)

CLASS	AGENT	INDICATION	SIDE EFFECTS/ CONTRAINDICATIONS	AGING-RELATED CONCERNS/ DOSING RECOMMENDATIONS
ANALGESICS (Cont.)				
Synthetic opioid	Fentanyl (100× more potent than morphine)	Used intravenously (fast onset due to high lipid solubility), intrathecally, epidurally, orally, and transdermally	Respiratory depression; chest wall rigidity at high doses	
Synthetic opioid	Sufentanil	Used intravenously	Respiratory depression Reversal: naloxone	
Ultra-short-acting opioid	Remifentanil	Target-controlled intravenous; infusion/ titratable	Respiratory depression Reversal: naloxone	
Synthetic opioid: short-acting	Alfentanil	Intravenous short-acting (often used to blunt airway reflexes upon intubation without muscle relaxation)	Clearance reduced upon coadministration of erythromycin	
NEUROMUSCULAR BLOCKING AGENTS (NMBAs)				
Nondepolarizing	Pancuronium (long-acting)	Facilitate endotracheal intubation and improve surgical conditions	30%–70% excreted unchanged in urine, prolonged action if reduced GFR—avoid in renal disease; may cause transient increase in heart rate	Muscle relaxant action is slow in onset and usually longer duration of action in older patients, except for cisatracurium—recovery not modified. Because older patients are prone to silent aspiration in the recovery room, use of NMBA with minimal or no organ elimination (eg, cisatracurium) is favored. Carefully monitor and completely reverse neuromuscular blockade in older patients. Neostigmine or sugammadex is used to reverse vecuronium and rocuronium.
Nondepolarizing	Rocuronium (intermediate-acting)		Avoid nondepolarizing NMBA in patients with neuromuscular diseases, eg, myasthenia gravis (prolonged effects)	
Nondepolarizing	Vecuronium (intermediate-acting)			
Nondepolarizing; benzylisoquinolinium	Cisatracurium (intermediate-acting)			
Depolarizing	Succinylcholine (short-acting)	Intravenous, intramuscular; rapid sequence induction; ECT treatment; breaking laryngospasm		

acute kidney injury, adverse cardiac events (eg, myocardial infarction [MI] or injury), and central nervous system ischemic events as a result of anesthetic-induced intraoperative hypotension. In general, BP is maintained within 20% of the patient's baseline and mean arterial pressure (MAP) is kept at 65 mm Hg or above (and systolic BP $\geq$ 100 mm Hg). However, in older patients and particularly those with preexisting hypertension, target mean BPs are best kept well above 65 mm Hg. Indeed, increasing evidence in the anesthesia literature shows that even brief periods (eg, $\geq$ 10 minutes) of perioperative hypotension (defined as systolic BP < 100 mm Hg or MAP < 60–70 mm Hg) associate with adverse cardiac events.

Regional or neuraxial anesthesia is the injection of a local anesthetic around major nerves (eg, axillary, femoral, interscalene, and intercostal nerve blocks) or in the subarachnoid (spinal anesthesia) or epidural spaces (epidural anesthesia), to block a limb and/or a large region of the body (eg, hip fracture repair). Regional anesthesia (RA) provides excellent muscle relaxation in addition to intraoperative and postoperative pain control, given that local anesthesia-induced blockade of sodium channels can last 8 to 12 hours, depending upon the dose, or employment of a catheter for continuous local anesthetic delivery for analgesia (eg, epidural catheter). Upon placement of the regional or neuraxial block, small, incremental doses of intravenous fentanyl or remifentanil might be given to help position the patient. Intraoperatively, low-dose propofol, or dexmedetomidine infusions, is oftentimes administered to provide conscious sedation, as needed. As RA has been linked to improved postoperative pain scores and patient satisfaction, reduced opioid consumption, and opioid-related side effects (eg, nausea, ileus, respiratory depression), it should be considered part of a multimodal pain-reducing approach (eg, surgical field infiltration with local anesthetics, utilization of peripheral nerve blocks, nonsteroidal anti-inflammatory agents, clonidine, and dexmedetomidine) whenever possible in older patients prone to developing postoperative respiratory depression.

It might seem intuitive to care providers that the procedure becomes "less intrusive" by choosing RA, and accordingly, leads to better outcomes. Indeed, seeing patients back in their respective rooms, awake, oriented, eating, and conversing with family members after an orthopedic procedure implies a speedy and favorable recovery. However, the controversy persists as to whether RA is better than GA with respect to patient mortality and morbidity. For hip fracture repair, for example, the International Fragility Fracture Network recently shared no preference for or against general or neuraxial anesthesia, but rather stated that hospitals should follow their own local guidelines. In a 2018 systematic review and meta-analysis, no differences in 30-day mortality or serious events (eg, pneumonia, acute MI, renal failure, or delirium) were found for RA compared to GA for patients undergoing hip fracture surgery. Moreover, a retrospective cohort study by Neuman and colleagues

published in 2014, involving over 56,000 patients 50 years or above undergoing hip repair surgery could not find a difference in 30-day mortality when RA was compared to GA, but did show that RA led to a modestly shorter length of hospital stay. Until the completion of two large-scale, multicenter, randomized controlled trials that are examining the efficacy of RA versus GA for hip fracture surgery in older individuals—the REGAIN trial with a primary endpoint of walking after 60 days and other patients-centered outcomes up to 1 year postop, and the iHOPE trial with an endpoint of all-cause mortality or cardiac or pulmonary events within 30 days postoperatively—anesthesiologists base anesthetic modality choice on patient's preferences, and the patient's comorbid conditions and potential for postoperative complications.

Because many older adults are taking anticoagulant and antiplatelet medications for the prevention of stroke and thromboembolism, these patients are at a heightened risk for neuraxial bleeding and the development of an epidural hematoma. While this does not necessarily preclude the use of neuraxial techniques (eg, spinal or epidural), or paravertebral blocks, deep plexus blocks, and deep peripheral nerve blocks (eg, in anatomic locations not amenable to the application of pressure to control hemorrhage), it does require careful planning and communication among members of the patient's perioperative care team, the patient's primary physician, and the patient. The American Society of Regional Anesthesia and Pain Medicine 2018 consensus guidelines for patients receiving hemostatic altering medications provide anesthesiologists with information on timing of drug cessation prior to neuraxial techniques, bridging therapy in cases of warfarin usage, maintenance of neuraxial catheters, and timing for starting medications after a neuraxial technique or removal of the neuraxial catheter. For many of the newer medications, recommendations are based on elimination half-lives. The mechanism of drug elimination and clearance is also taken into consideration as many of the antiplatelet drugs are renally metabolized and have prolonged action in those older patients with reduced renal function.

Monitored anesthesia care is the intravenous administration of short-acting sedatives, analgesics, and anxiolytics to help a patient relax during minor procedures (eg, colonoscopy, transesophageal echocardiogram, and interventional radiologic procedures) that do not require GA. This is sometimes referred to as conscious sedation. Because of the increased risk for postoperative neurocognitive dysfunction among older patients, benzodiazepine administration should be avoided and sedation and analgesia be achieved with propofol, ketamine, or dexmedetomidine. Because of the "fine line" between light and deep sedation in older individuals, all dosing of sedatives and analgesics are reduced, and the spontaneously breathing patient receiving supplemental oxygen is continuously monitored for respiratory rate, oxygen saturation, end-tidal carbon dioxide, in addition to all other standard

ASA (American Society of Anesthesiologists) monitoring. Changes in capnography values and waveforms often help clinicians understand a patient's level of comfort, sedation, and respiratory function during procedural sedation. Indeed, if the patient is not communicative or unable to cooperate, reluctant to be awake, and/or if the procedure length is deemed to be longer than usual, GA might be a better choice to achieve the goal of a rapid recovery.

POSTOPERATIVE COMPLICATIONS IN OLDER ADULTS

It is well accepted that older age is a risk factor for perioperative mortality and morbidity, including cardiovascular, pulmonary, renal, and neurocognitive complications. Of the postoperative complications, cognitive morbidity in the form of POD and persistent cognitive decline are significantly more prevalent when compared to any of the other complications (**Table 28-2**). Accordingly, this section will provide insight on the impact that anesthesia and surgery might have on the development of perioperative neurocognitive disorders (PND) and strategies that are used to help mitigate its occurrence. See Chapter 27, Perioperative Care: Evaluation and Management, for specifics on risk factor assessment for PND.

In order to unify the neurocognitive disorders seen by anesthesiologists with the cognitive classifications observed in the general population based on the *Diagnostic and Statistical Manual for Mental Disorders,* fifth edition (DSM-5), the term "perioperative neurocognitive disorders" was established in 2018. This term encompasses patients presenting for surgery with preexisting neurocognitive disorders (eg, mild cognitive impairment and Alzheimer disease), and those with POD, delayed neurocognitive recovery (cognitive decline up to 30 days after surgery), and postoperative neurocognitive disorder (defined as a decline in cognition that persists or is diagnosed up to 12 months after the procedure). Delayed neurocognitive recovery and postoperative neurocognitive disorder align with mild cognitive impairment and dementia. In this chapter,

TABLE 28-2 ■ POSTOPERATIVE COMPLICATIONS IN OLDER SURGICAL PATIENTS

COMPLICATION	INCIDENCE
Pulmonary embolism	0.2%–0.5%
Acute renal failure	0.4%–0.6%
Stroke	0.3%–1%
Myocardial infarction	0.4%–2%
Pneumonia	2%–4%
Death	2%–5%
Heart failure	0.6%–6%
Cognitive dysfunction	10%–16%
Delirium	12%–24%

postoperative cognitive dysfunction (POCD) and postoperative neurocognitive disorder are used interchangeably given that much of the literature to date has used the former term.

Postoperative Delirium: Impact of Anesthesia

POD is a common and serious complication of anesthesia and surgical care. Unlike emergence delirium, which occurs immediately after emergence from anesthesia and resolves quickly, POD may show up a week after the procedure or even at the time of hospital discharge. It has severe consequences to the patient including increased risk of mortality, need for discharge to an institution, accelerated cognitive and functional decline, and an increased risk of falls. At the medical center level, POD associates with increased length of stay and higher readmission rates—both leading to increased costs. POD not only affects perioperative care, it takes a tremendous psychological toll on caregivers and the patient. While the surgical procedure might have gone flawlessly, the older patient might be referred to by his or her family as "just not the same." For the patient, this can also be very isolating and contribute to posttraumatic stress disorder.

The occurrence of POD in older patients after noncardiac surgery in past studies has ranged between 5% and 52%. In a 2020 systemic review and meta-analysis involving 17,241 patients (35 studies) undergoing GA for noncardiac surgery, and 15,090 patients (19 studies) for cardiac surgery the pooled incidence of POD was 17% (95% confidence interval [CI]: 14%–9.2%) and 15% (95% CI: 13%–18%), respectively. In another recent study involving over 20,000 surgical inpatients, people 65 years or older, the unadjusted average rate of delirium occurrence across 30 institutions was 12%. By specialty, the highest rates of POD occurred for cardiothoracic (14%), orthopedic (13.0%), and general surgery (13.0%), and the lowest rates were associated with urologic (6.6%) and gynecologic procedures (4.7%). Multivariate analyses further indicate that patients at highest risk of POD are older, have more comorbidities (eg, higher ASA classification), more likely to have undergone emergent surgery, and more likely to have preexisting cognitive impairment. Indeed, many of the same patients who develop POD are also those who are frail. Frailty is common in older elective surgical populations; 38% to 54% of those greater than or equal to age 70 in one study scored as prefrail and 35% to 41% as frail on comprehensive frailty measures. Screening for frailty and cognitive impairment preoperatively using the FRAIL scale and the Animal Verbal Fluency test in older elective spine surgery patients identified those at high risk for the development of postoperative delirium. Accordingly, it is important to inform older patients who screen positively for preoperative frailty or cognitive impairment that their risk for developing POD is increased and their anesthesia care team will take a proactive approach to minimize this risk. Furthermore, educating family and caregivers as to what to look for postoperatively will help identify POD early, if it occurs.

Currently, there is limited evidence in support of one anesthetic modality over another to reduce POD. In a 2018 Cochrane database review, no differences with regard to safety and postoperative delirious symptoms were shown between total intravenous anesthesia (eg, propofol) versus use of volatile agents, including Xenon, in older patients undergoing noncardiac surgery. The effect of RA versus GA on delirium in hip fracture repair patients also remains inconclusive, in part because rigorous and adequately powered studies, to date, are lacking.

Adjunctive pharmacologic therapies have been examined for their benefit in reducing the occurrence of POD. The selective alpha-2 adrenergic receptor agonist dexmedetomidine is one such drug that has shown promise in reducing the risk of POD. In three meta-analyses conducted over the past several years, intraoperative infusions of dexmedetomidine were found to lower the incidence of POD in older non cardiac surgical patients, albeit with a potential increase in bradycardia. Unfortunately, there remains insufficient evidence for dexmedetomidine administration to have the same POD-reducing benefit in older cardiac surgery patients. Other adjuvants have been tested with the goal of improving pain control without excessive need for opioids. Both gabapentin and ketamine have been studied in randomized controlled trials, but no role for these adjuvants in reducing the incidence of POD was reported.

Guiding anesthetic depth with pEEG monitoring has been considered in the armamentarium of anesthesiologists to help limit the risk of delirium in some older patients. As the BIS monitor produces a single number between 0 and 100, it is assumed that the lower the number, the deeper the anesthesia. Titrating the dose of volatile or intravenous anesthesia to a BIS of 40 to 60 or 50 to 60 versus standard monitoring with end-tidal anesthetic concentration has been shown to reduce the rate of POD in four trials involving general anesthesia and in one study that randomized patients into receiving BIS target values of at least 80 (intervention) versus 50 (control) during sedation with propofol in spinal anesthesia. However, a large prospective trial entitled Electroencephalography Guidance of Anesthesia (ENGAGES) that randomized GA in adults (age > 60 years) undergoing major surgery (including cardiac, gastrointestinal, thoracic, gynecologic, hepatobiliary-pancreatic, urologic, and vascular procedures) to pEEG-guided or routine care found no difference in the incidence of delirium between groups (26% in the EEG group and 23% in usual care). Even so, favorable findings for brain depth monitoring for POD reduction in the ADAPT-2 trial (Anesthetic Depth and Postoperative Delirium Trial-2) suggests that cognitively vulnerable older patients may actually benefit from reducing time in burst suppression during the surgical procedure. While the existing data do not support routine use of pEEG monitoring for the prevention of POD in older patients, it remains a practical monitor to consider for those older adults who have preexisting PND, and when the goal is to facilitate rapid emergence and recovery.

In summary, except for possibly dexmedetomidine administration, none of the approaches (eg, intravenous vs inhalational anesthesia, regional vs general anesthesia, incorporation of processed EEG monitoring, use of adjuvants such a gabapentin or ketamine) have sufficient evidence to support their use in the reduction of POD in older patients. What we do have available are "best practice" consensus guidelines from various professional societies and working groups, including the American Geriatric Society (AGS), the American College of Surgeons (ACS) in conjunction with NSQIP, the European Society of Anesthesiology, the International Society Perioperative Neurotoxicity working group, and the American Society for Enhanced Recovery and Perioperative Quality Initiative Joint Consensus. A summary of the recommendations by these expert panels is presented in **Table 28-3**. Notably, multicomponent, nonpharmaceutical interventions (eg, frequent orientation, reinstitution of dentures, hearing and vision aids, early mobilization, preservation of day/sleep cycles, staff education, adequate and frequent pain assessment, early removal of indwelling catheters, adequate hydration, and early reinstitution of nutrition) and avoidance of high-risk POD medications (eg, Beers Criteria) are recommended by nearly all groups in the management of modifiable risk factors for delirium.

Postoperative Cognitive Dysfunction: Impact of Anesthesia

Two questions may surface among older patients slated for a surgical procedure—"does POD lead to dementia?" and/or "will anesthesia and surgery provoke dementia?"—for which geriatricians should have some knowledge. With respect to the first question, findings from several earlier studies (2008–2017) suggest that POD may be a predictor of progression to dementia and cognitive decline years after surgery. For example, Inouye and colleagues in 2016 found nondelirious patients crossing the trajectory of cognitive decline at 36 months when compared to their baseline cognitive status, whereas patients with POD crossed the trajectory to POCD at 12 months after surgery. However, more recent work suggests that delirium and cognitive dysfunction after surgery are independent and distinct entities. In a retrospective cohort study of 560 older noncardiac surgery patients, fewer than half of those who developed delirium (134 of 560 or 24%) went on to develop POCD at 1 month (47%), but this proportion dissipated after 2 (23%) and 6 months (16%), implying that POD and long-term POCD might be different disorders. The second question, "will cognitive function decline after surgery?" is justifiable. The association between exposure to anesthesia and surgery to long-term cognitive trajectory continues to be a topic of debate. Longitudinal data from a cohort of older adults (n = 1819) in the Mayo Clinic Study of Aging demonstrated a small decline in cognition in those who had undergone surgery versus those who had no exposure to anesthesia and surgery in the 20 years prior to their enrollment. Using participants from the Whitnall II cohort study, Krause

	YEAR PUBLISHED	PREOPERATIVE COGNITIVE SCREEN	DEPTH OF ANESTHESIA (pEEG MONITOR)	REGIONAL ANESTHESIA	MAINTENANCE OF CEREBRAL PERFUSION	MULTI-COMPONENT INTERVENTION	MEDICATION MANAGEMENT
American Geriatric Society	2015	Recommended	Recommended	Consider	N/A	Recommended	Avoid Beers medications
American College of Surgeons/ National Surgical Quality Improvement Practice	2012	Recommended	N/A	Consider	N/A	Recommended	Avoid Beers medications
European Society of Anesthesiologists	2017	Recommended	Recommended	N/A	Recommended	Recommended	Judicious benzodiazepine use
American Society of Anesthesiologists Brain Health Initiative	2018	Recommended	Recommended	Unable to Recommend	Recommended	N/A	N/A
Sixth Perioperative Quality Initiative	2020	Recommended	Unable to Recommend	Unable to Recommend	N/A	Recommended	Avoid Beers medications

pEEG, processed EEG.

et al reported *modest* reductions in cognition coincident with those who were admitted for major surgery, whereas a *strong* association with cognitive decline was found for those hospital admissions that were for medical only reasons. In a nationwide population-based cohort study from Korea involving nearly 45,000 patients (50 years and older) who required surgery, the hazard ratio for developing dementia over the 12-year study period was 1.28 after adjusting for covariates when compared to 175,000 age-matched controls. Taken together, POD is likely not part of a continuum to POCD or long-term dementia, but rather a separate entity. People who experience POCD do not necessarily have POD first. Also, hospital stays for surgery are not linked to higher risks for PND than admissions for medical only reasons.

To ascertain whether the brain is "injured" by anesthesia, the association between exposure to GA versus RA and the risk of developing dementia has been considered. In a population-based propensity study involving 41,700 community-dwelling individuals 66 years or older who underwent one of five elective surgeries by GA or RA, Velkers and colleagues found, after matching 7500 patients in each group, no difference in the onset of dementia up to 5 years after surgery. Going one step further, the effects of sevoflurane GA *without* surgery, in 59 healthy volunteers between 40 and 80 years, was reported to have no adverse influence on plasma biomarkers of neurological injury or systemic inflammation. In fact, a minimum alveolar concentration (MAC) of sevoflurane actually reduced plasma tau, neurofilament light (NF-L), and glial fibrillary acidic protein (GFAP) 5 hours after anesthesia when compared to respective baseline values.

As anesthesia alone does not appear to be a significant harbinger to the onset of dementia, others found that the extent of surgery has an impact on the development of neurocognitive decline. In a large data set from the Korean National Health Insurance Services, Choi et al identified nearly 64,000 patients with a diagnosis of gastric cancer who underwent curative gastrectomy surgery and compared them to 203,000 age-matched controls for onset of dementia. Interestingly, these investigators found no differences in dementia after surgery in the *partial* gastrectomy group but a 1.3-fold higher risk of dementia development in the *total* gastrectomy group when compared to controls. This finding points to the potential for a "dose response" effect of surgery on postoperative neurocognitive disorders, which should be considered when planning surgery in older patients.

Taken together, PNDs are common complications in older adults undergoing anesthesia and surgery which have serious consequences. The etiology underlying postoperative delirium, delayed cognitive recovery and/or postoperative cognitive decline remains poorly understood, and is unlikely a distinctive cause. In those who are at an increased risk for PND, for example, preexisting dementia, minimally invasive or less extensive procedures, or a surgery that might be linked to functional improvement (eg, cataract surgery), or one that associates with dementia risk reduction (eg, carotid endarterectomy, abdominal aortic aneurysm repair) should be considered. To date, no recommended intraoperative anesthetic technique or pharmaceutical PND prevention exists, but rather standardized therapeutic concepts in the perioperative period (eg, staff and patient education, early mobilization, good

TABLE 28-4 ■ PERIOPERATIVE MEDICAL MANAGEMENT AND PRECAUTIONS

CLASS	EXAMPLES	ADVERSE EFFECTS/PRECAUTIONS/AVOIDANCE
Antiemetics (postoperative nausea and vomiting [PONV] management)	Propofol infusion; aprepitant (for very high-risk PONV); ondansetron (4 mg IV q6h); haloperidol (0.5–1 mg q6h); metoclopramide (5 mg IV once)	Avoid dexamethasone (especially doses > 4 mg); avoid when possible: diphenhydramine (Benadryl); hydroxyzine (Vistaril); lorazepam (Ativan); prochlorperazine (Compazine); scopolamine
Nonsteroidal anti-inflammatory drugs (NSAIDs)	Diclofenac, ibuprofen, etodolac, meloxicam, naproxen	Increased risk of GI bleeding or PUD in high-risk patients, including those 75 years and older and/or those taking corticosteroids, anticoagulants, or antiplatelet agents
	Ketorolac	Increased risk of GI bleeding, PUD, or acute renal injury in the older patient—avoid
	Indomethacin	CNS adverse effects more likely than other NSAIDs
Sedative hypnotics	Benzodiazepines	Avoid (except for specific indications such as seizure)
	Gabapentin	Reduce dose when GFR < 60; avoid in patients with ESRD
	Meperidine	Avoid, especially in patients with chronic kidney disease (renally cleared metabolite)
Anticholinergics	Scopolamine; promethazine (Phenergan); prochlorperazine (Compazine); diphenhydramine (Benadryl); hydroxyzine (Vistaril); tricyclic antidepressants	Avoid; all contribute to increased risk of oversedation, central anticholinergic side effects (including delirium)
Other psychoactive medications	Steroids (dexamethasone); antipsychotics	Avoid or use cautiously—all associated with an increased risk of delirium

ESRD, end-stage renal disease; GFR, glomerular filtration rate; GI, gastrointestinal; PUD, peptic ulcer disease.

pain control and adequate pain assessments, maintenance of normothermia, avoiding excessive BP fluctuations, and avoiding benzodiazepines and anticholinergic medications) are being incorporated into hospital practice bundles and electronic medical record alert systems to help ensure safe and optimal outcomes in the geriatric surgical population. **Table 28-4** lists recommendations for the prevention and management of postoperative nausea and commonly used classes of other perioperative drugs that require caution with use or avoidance in older patients.

CARDIAC PROCEDURES COMMON TO OLDER ADULTS: ANESTHETIC IMPLICATIONS

Both structural and electrical cardiac diseases are common in patients over the age of 75. Structural cardiac disease includes coronary artery disease (CAD) and valvular pathology—particularly aortic stenosis and mitral regurgitation (MR). Among the electrical cardiac diseases regularly diagnosed in the older adult are atrial fibrillation (AF) and sinus node dysfunction. Procedures to treat these diseases are routinely performed in patients over the age of 75 years. While there is a tendency to prefer less invasive procedures in this patient population, correction of certain cardiac lesions requires GA with endotracheal intubation, invasive arterial pressure monitoring, and central venous access. The standard anesthetic for cardiac surgery in the older adult provides hemodynamic stability, amnesia, analgesia, end-organ protection, and the ability for rapid emergence postoperatively. Numerous studies have attempted to show advantages of specific anesthetic drugs and adjuvants over others to achieve these goals but results remain equivocal.

Patients with significant cardiac disease, whether or not they are undergoing procedures to address their cardiac disease, often require specific monitoring beyond typical GA monitors described earlier in this chapter. In patients with reduced ventricular function or severe valvular disease, an arterial pressure monitor called an arterial line is often placed in one of the radial arteries prior to, or immediately after, induction of GA. Preinduction placement of an arterial line allows for the anesthesiologist to measure beat-to-beat arterial BP variations during anesthetic induction. As discussed earlier, induction of GA can lead to changes in BP because many of the agents used to induce and maintain GA cause peripheral vasodilation and hypotension. Patients with severe cardiac disease may not tolerate long periods of hypotension; while invasive pressure monitoring will not prevent or treat hypotension, it will allow the anesthesiologist to closely monitor BP and treat small changes more quickly than would be possible with a noninvasive BP monitoring system that measures only every few minutes. Transesophageal echocardiography (TEE) allows for real-time monitoring of cardiac ventricular and valvular function. TEE is commonly performed after induction of GA and endotracheal intubation in patients undergoing cardiac surgery and sometimes in those with reduced systolic function or "tight" aortic stenosis who require noncardiac surgery. TEE is more invasive than transthoracic echocardiography (TTE), but TEE has the advantages of being performed by an anesthesiologist at the head of the bed without interfering with a sterile surgical field, and it provides significantly better image quality than TTE for most patients. Central venous access is typically obtained via the right internal jugular vein. An introducer placed in this vein can allow the anesthesiologist to place a pulmonary artery catheter in selected patients having cardiac surgery with cardiopulmonary bypass. Postprocedure, patients are typically transferred to the intensive care unit (ICU) for continued monitoring and mechanical ventilation. Specific considerations for selected cardiac diseases and associated interventions that require anesthesia are discussed further.

Anesthesia for Coronary Artery Bypass Grafting and Percutaneous Interventions

As patients age, the incidence of CAD increases. An estimated 30% of patients over the age of 75 have clinically significant coronary disease, compared with 8% of patients younger than 65 years. While many of these patients can be treated by a percutaneous intervention (PCI), certain lesions are best repaired surgically. Benefits of coronary artery bypass graft (CABG) surgery over PCI are less well-defined in patients 75 years and older than in those younger than 75 or middle-aged. Standard CABG surgery is performed under GA with invasive arterial pressure monitoring, endotracheal intubation, central venous line placement with or without a pulmonary arterial catheter. Adverse outcomes associated with CABG surgery include stroke, renal injury, and postoperative neurologic dysfunction. Studies show that older patients are more likely to have more severe disease, such as left main or multivessel CAD with concomitant left ventricular dysfunction. In combination with enhanced cardiac disease severity, decreased functional capacity, frailty, and cognitive impairment may lead to worse outcomes in this patient population when compared to their younger counterparts. Other risk factors widespread in this population, including smoking, obesity, diabetes, and hypertension, further contribute to less favorable outcomes than in younger cardiac surgical patients.

As an alternative to traditional CABG with cardiopulmonary bypass (CPB), certain surgeons will offer off-pump coronary artery bypass (OPCAB) surgery to patients with select lesions. OPCAB can be performed via a conventional sternotomy or a minimally invasive approach via a left thoracotomy. The minimally invasive approach may include a robotic surgical technique. The incision for minimally invasive OPCAB is smaller than a traditional sternotomy, but the pain score associated with the thoracotomy is often higher than that of a sternotomy. Surgery performed via a thoracotomy requires lung deflation on the surgical side. To achieve this, the anesthesiologist must selectively ventilate one lung while the surgeon is working. This approach may not be appropriate for patients with significant lung disease, as they may not tolerate one-lung ventilation. The benefit of OPCAB, regardless of the surgical approach, is the avoidance of CPB and its associated risks. OPCAB versus CABG has been extensively studied; however, no clear data, to date, demonstrate a significant advantage of one over the other in all-cause mortality, cardiac outcomes, or success of revascularization in the general population. Interestingly, some subgrouping analyses suggest improved outcomes of OPCAB over CABG in the geriatric population. Indeed, OPCAB that avoids manipulation of the ascending aorta (eg, which is usually cross-clamped prior to the initiation of CPB in CABG surgery) may lead to improved neurologic outcomes. Some patients are best served by a hybrid approach that typically combines off-pump surgical revascularization for the left anterior descending artery with a PCI to repair other high-grade lesions. This staged approach allows for complete revascularization while limiting the time under GA.

Anesthesia for Aortic Valve Replacement

Aortic stenosis is the most common single valve disease, with a prevalence between 2% and 10% in patients over age 75. Because senile calcific aortic stenosis increases with aging, procedures that replace the aortic valve are offered to patients in this age group. Indications for aortic valve replacement include severe aortic stenosis and symptomatic moderate aortic stenosis. Aortic valve replacement can be performed in a variety of ways. The standard approach is via a midline sternotomy with CBP. Minimally invasive aortic valve replacement can be performed on CPB via an upper hemi-sternotomy or anterior thoracotomy. All three surgical approaches have a clinically equivalent 1.2% risk of stroke. As with OPCAB, thoracotomy approaches require lung isolation. An alternative to surgical valve replacement is a transcatheter aortic valve replacement (TAVR). While TAVR tends to be more commonly performed in the "middle- and oldest-old" (mean age of 83 years) age groups, improvements in technology and reductions in associated complication rates have expanded its potential to the "youngest-old" (65–74 years) and to those considered to be at low-risk. TAVR is typically performed in a percutaneous manner via the femoral artery. The valve is delivered retrograde up the descending aorta and deployed without removing the patient's native aortic valve. At some centers, TAVR is performed with GA and endotracheal intubation; at others, it is performed with a local anesthetic at the femoral puncture site along with varying levels of conscious sedation. Even for cases where sedation is planned, conversion to GA is not uncommon. Reasons for conversion to GA include the patient's inability to cooperate by remaining motionless and/or inability to breathe comfortably while lying flat, or the proceduralist has a need for better imaging of the aortic valve—thereby necessitating placement of a transesophageal probe for TEE, or because of a procedural complication. TAVR often is typically performed with invasive BP monitoring and robust intravenous access. In patients who have significant distal aortic, iliac, or femoral arterial disease, transfemoral placement of the valve may not be possible. For these patients, surgical cutdown to one of the major arteries (femoral, axillary, carotid, or aortic) may be required for TAVR placement. Due to the discomfort associated with surgical cutdown, GA with endotracheal intubation is required. Patients who require intubation during the procedure are typically extubated at the end of the procedure, although due to the femoral vessel access, they must remain supine for several hours in order to reduce bleeding risk. Post TAVR, patients may not require ICU admission and are able to leave the hospital after 1 or 2 days, representing a lower level of required postoperative care compared with surgical aortic valve replacement. Even so, overall complication rates for TAVR are still as high as 20%; with stroke rates, significant postprocedure paravalvular leaks, and major bleeding accounting for 2%, 3.6%, and 6%, respectively.

Anesthesia for Mitral Valve Repair/Replacement

MR is the most frequently acquired valvular heart disease in the United States; this may be due to the many underlying causes of MR. Up to 50% of patients with left ventricular dysfunction have some MR. The mitral valve can be repaired or replaced surgically utilizing CBP with GA, endotracheal intubation, invasive BP monitoring, and TEE. After addressing MR, the left ventricular afterload can be dramatically increased; patient selection for mitral valve intervention is important because some patients will not be able to tolerate this increased afterload. In the hands of an experienced surgeon, operative risks and recurrence of MR are low. Overall, surgical mortality is estimated at less than 2% in patients with an average age of 60 years. Newer technology for addressing MR is constantly being developed. There are several methods for decreasing MR including edge to edge repair techniques, annuloplasty bands to decrease the size of the valve, neochords, and percutaneous mitral valve replacement. The nonsurgical techniques for mitral valve repair are not as well established as those for treating aortic stenosis, and thus are reserved for patients who are a prohibitive surgical risk. As of 2020, only the MitraClip (Abbott) is Food and Drug Administration (FDA) approved in the United States. The MitraClip clasps the edges of the two leaflets together in both phases of the cardiac cycle to decrease regurgitation. This procedure requires GA, invasive arterial pressure monitoring, and TEE guidance. Patients are typically extubated at the end of the procedure, although due to the large caliber venipuncture,

they must remain supine for several hours in order to reduce bleeding risk. Patients who cannot tolerate the flat time, due to dyspnea or poor cooperation, may need to remain intubated with sedation during this recovery period.

Atrial Fibrillation and Anesthesia for Cardiac Ablation Procedures

AF is a common comorbidity in the geriatric population; the median age of patients with AF is 75 years. Incidence of AF increases with age and is 2.3% in people older than 40 years, 5.9% in those older than 65 years, and 10% in those older than 80. Patients with AF are anticoagulated to decrease the risk of stroke from embolization of left atrial clot; the proportion of strokes due to AF is likely greater than 20%. Due to the high prevalence of AF in this patient population and the increased risk of anticoagulation in older patients who are at increased risk of falls, AF ablation procedures are frequently performed in this group. Recurrence in AF is less than 50% after catheter-based ablation compared with 80% for those treated with antiarrhythmic medicines alone. AF ablation is typically a catheter-based procedure with access via the femoral vein. Anesthetic management includes GA with endotracheal intubation, possible TEE to assess for cardiac muscle paralysis, and arterial access. Arterial access is generally placed after anesthetic induction for monitoring of BP and heparinization. The patient must be heparinized during the procedure because the catheter crosses the interatrial septum into the left atrium to gain access to the pulmonary veins for ablation. As long as the catheter is in the left atrium, the patient must be anticoagulated to an activated clotting time (ACT) of 250 seconds in order to decrease risk of generation of thrombus that can cause harmful emboli. Patients are typically extubated at the end of the procedure, although due to the large caliber venipuncture, they must remain supine for several hours in order to reduce bleeding risk. In patients for whom rhythm control cannot be achieved and anticoagulation is not tolerated, left atrial appendage occluder devices can be placed. Because 90% of left atrial thrombi are located in the left atrial appendage, these devices may decrease stroke risk in patients with AF who cannot tolerate anticoagulation. There are several commercially available devices, with both percutaneous and surgical techniques as options. The anesthetic requirement for these devices is similar to that of AF ablation, including GA, TEE, and often invasive arterial pressure monitoring for frequent blood draws to monitor the level of anticoagulation.

Anesthesia for Cardiac Implantable Electrical Devices

Implantation of cardiac rhythm devices is another frequently performed procedure in the geriatric population, since the largest risk factor for sinus node dysfunction is aging. Sinus node dysfunction is the most common indication for pacemaker placement, accounting for 50% of all implants in the United States. Anesthetic management is similar for all device placements. In many cases, device placement can be performed with sedation. In order for this to be successful, the patient must be able to cooperate and there must be adequate pain control. To ensure patient comfort during the procedure, the electrophysiologist performing the procedure must be able to give adequate local anesthetic to numb the insertion site and the pocket where the generator will be implanted. The patient must be able to stay still for the procedure and respond to directions in order to prevent vascular injury associated with patient movement. Some electrophysiologists prefer to perform the procedure under GA in order to avoid the potential discomfort of a sedated patient, both for the patient and the proceduralist. In addition to preference of the proceduralist, some patients may require GA with or without endotracheal intubation due to their inability to tolerate the procedure with sedation. This may be due to patient anxiety, airway obstruction due to sedation (ie, obstructive sleep apnea), or an inability of the patient to tolerate lying still due to pain or dyspnea.

As anesthesia for cardiac procedures and cardiac surgery require that the anesthesiologist possess much of the knowledge typically within the jurisdiction of the cardiologist and cardiac surgeon, in addition to having a proficient skillset in performing and interpreting TEE examinations, a fellowship-trained cardiac anesthesiologist will be leading the intraoperative management, in parallel with the surgical/proceduralist team and perfusionist, particularly when a CPB circuit is needed. There is no doubt that older adults with cardiac disease, and the various clinicians caring for them, are faced with difficult and often multiple reasonable options. Shared decision-making enables both the patient and clinician the ability to contribute their differing but equally important areas of expertise to find the best path toward the patient's personal care goals. Having general knowledge of the anesthetic techniques involved in many of the more common cardiac surgery procedures will provide the geriatrician with a foundation of information that can aid in their contribution to the shared decision-making process.

Goals of Care: "Allow Natural Death" and Anesthesia

Given that many people at the end of life have surgical procedures, the impact of Do Not Resuscitate and Allow Natural Death (AND) orders should not be ignored. In a medical beneficiary study from 2008 involving over 1.8 million older individuals, 32% underwent an inpatient surgical procedure during their last year before death, 18% underwent a procedure in their last month of life, and 8% underwent a surgery in their last week of life. In part because of these data, and the fact that it is becoming more common to encounter an older patient scheduled for surgery who has an AND in place, hospitals accredited by The Joint Commission are required to have an AND policy. Indeed, procedures requiring anesthesia can create an ethical dilemma when AND/Do Not Intubate/Limited Resuscitation orders are in place prior to a surgery because "resuscitation" is nearly always ongoing to some degree in

the operating room while a patient is undergoing surgery with anesthesia. In the case of a patient with a documented AND, the four main tenets of health care ethics come to the forefront. First, the patient has the right to be informed and to make decisions regarding his/her care, particularly at the end of life. Automatic suspension of an AND constitutes betrayal of autonomy. Second, the procedure being offered must be of some benefit to the patient in either quantity or quality of life. Also, with respect to beneficence, patients do not have a right to a treatment that is not deemed to have a benefit. Certainly, nonmaleficence or "do no harm" underscores all aspects of medicine. Lastly, the principle of justice comes to play when health care providers offer resources (eg, surgical procedures) that are limited to those who will best benefit from them.

The American Society of Anesthesiologists state that physicians must communicate and document any modifications that are made to the patient's wishes and advanced directives prior to surgery. This should be done with the patient while in the presence of both the surgeon and anesthesiologist. Most often the patient's wishes to hold the AND can be met under one of the following three categories: (1) full attempt at resuscitation within the perioperative period, (2) limited attempt at resuscitation defined in regard to specific procedures (eg, chest compression, intubation), and (3) limited attempt at resuscitation defined with respect to the patient's goals and values. Importantly, automatic suspension of the AND is not acceptable and any modifications must be discussed with the patient and documented. These discussions require time and should be conducted well before the surgical procedure and then readdressed immediately prior to surgery, with the patient and the lead perioperative team members present so that everyone is aligned with the plan and the patient's wishes. Under the best circumstances these discussions should also include the primary care provider, nursing staff in the operating room/recovery room, and possibly a chaplain. It is important to reassure the patient and his/her family that having an AND order does not mean "do not treat." In a retrospective analysis using the American College of Surgeons NSQIP database 2007–2013, 5000 patients with AND orders in place had, as expected, an increased incidence of mortality, however, there was no difference in morbidity at 30 days when compared to non-AND matched patients by procedure, and after adjusting for preoperative factors. This tells us that patients received routine treatment for complications after surgery such as wound infection, renal failure, stroke, deep venous thrombosis, and pulmonary embolism but did not necessarily receive advanced cardiac life support. In summary, older patients are having procedures at the end of life. Conversations with the patient and/or decision maker regarding the perioperative course of action are needed. If an AND is modified, it must be documented along with verifying the "time" the modification is in place. Because many geriatricians initiate advanced directives and code status discussions with their patients independent of surgery, their presence and input are critical in this shared decision-making.

Many older patients with implantable cardioverter defibrillators (ICDs) undergo surgical and minimally invasive procedures. Studies show that 30% to 40% of patients with ICDs might experience depressive and posttraumatic stress symptoms related to their need for the device. It is the role of the anesthesiologist to take these symptom burdens into account when these patients present to the perioperative area and to allay any anxiety by letting them know how their heart function will be continuously monitored (eg, continuous ECG, pulse oximetry, and arterial pressure monitoring to provide beat-to-beat display, if indicated). Other nuances specific to the intraoperative management of ICDs include readily available urgent transcutaneous pacing, defibrillation or cardioversion, careful cautery pad placement so that the current from the electrocautery unit does not interfere with the ICD generator or leads, and the surgeon's use of bipolar as opposed to monopolar cautery. Importantly, all anesthesiologists, irrespective of their subspeciality, are expected to understand equipment characteristics, troubleshooting, and rescue strategies when patients with ICDs are under their care.

The geriatrician can aid in preoperative assessment of such patients by communicating with the anesthesiologist and/or preoperative physician as to the reason for the pacemaker or an ICD placement as well as whether or not the patient is dependent on the pacemaker function. Patients with severe atrial-ventricular (AV) nodal dysfunction or AV nodal ablation will be pacemaker-dependent. Patients who have biventricular pacemakers, 100% ventricular pacing is a sign of a properly functioning device and is not necessarily indicative of pacemaker dependency. For patients who have ICDs, it is important for the anesthesiologist to know if the device was placed for primary prevention in a patient with risk factors for lethal arrhythmias due to decreased ejection fraction or for secondary prevention in a patient who has a history of lethal arrhythmias. Taken together, it is important for the geriatrician to communicate with the anesthesiologist as to any information they might have regarding the patient's ICD, and to also help allay any anxiety relating to the planned procedure, device function, and/or dependency.

SUMMARY

Based on the current literature, there is unconvincing evidence that one anesthetic technique or cardiac surgical approach is superior to others in the older surgical patient in terms of limiting postoperative dysfunction, for example, delirium and cognitive dysfunction, the most common postoperative complications in the older adult. As older adults are more sensitive to intravenous anesthetics, volatile agents, and opiates due to age-related changes in pharmacokinetics and pharmacodynamics, anesthetic dosing is age-adjusted and anesthetic depth continuously monitored by end-tidal anesthetic concentrations, physical signs and often brain function monitoring with processed EEG. While there is no recommended pharmaceutical for preventing POD after noncardiac and cardiac surgery, best practice consensus guidelines advocate nonpharmaceutical interventions (eg, staff education, early mobilization, adequate multimodal pain control and assessments, frequent orientation, sleep-wake cycle preservation, early postoperative use of hearing and visual aids, etc) and avoidance of high-risk medications such as benzodiazepines. As a member of the interdisciplinary care team, anesthesiologist's role extends from focusing on comorbidities and initiating preoperative optimization to intra- and postoperative care strategies aimed at analgesia, while maintaining homeostasis and minimizing the risk of PNDs. Given that surgical procedures are common at the end of life, preoperative and then immediately presurgical conversations with the patient and/or decision maker regarding the perioperative course of action should involve the surgeon, anesthesiologist, and the patient's primary care physician to ensure that the patient's wishes and goals of care are understood and documented.

FURTHER READING

Arnold SV, Manandhar P, Vemulapalli S, et al. Impact of short-term complications of TAVR on longer-term outcomes: Results from the STS/ACC transcatheter valve therapy registry. *Eur Heart J Qual Care Clin Outcomes.* 2021;7(2):208–213.

Berian JR, Zhou L, Russell MM, et al. Postoperative delirium as a target for surgical quality improvement. *Ann Surg.* 2018;268:93–99.

Brignole M. Sick sinus syndrome. *Clin Geriatr Med.* 2002;18:211–227.

Choi YJ, Shin DW, Jang W, et al. Risk of dementia in gastric cancer survivors who underwent gastrectomy: a Nationwide Study in Korea. *Ann Surg Oncol.* 2019;26(13):4229–4237.

Daiello LA, Racine AM, Yun Gou R, et al. Postoperative delirium and postoperative cognitive dysfunction: overlap and divergence. *Anesthesiology.* 2019;131:477–491.

Evered L, Silbert B, Knopman DS, et al. Recommendations for the nomenclature of cognitive change associated with anaesthesia and surgery-2018. *Br J Anaesth.* 2018;121:1005–1012.

Ghoreishi M, Thourani VH, Badhwar V, et al. Less-invasive aortic valve replacement: trends and outcomes from the STS database. *Ann Thorac Surg.* 2021;111(4):1216–1223.

Hamel MB, Henderson WG, Khuri SF, Daley J. Surgical outcomes for patients aged 80 and older: morbidity and mortality from major noncardiac surgery. *J Am Geriatr Soc*. 2005;53:424–429.

Krause BM, Sabia S, Manning HJ, Sing Manoux A, Sanders RD. Association between major surgical admissions and the cognitive trajectory: 19 year follow-up of Whitehall II cohort study. *BMJ*. 2019;366:l4466.

Liu LL, Leung JM. Predicting adverse postoperative outcomes in patients aged 80 years or older. *J Am Geriatr Soc*. 2000;48:405–412.

O'Donnell CM, Black N, McCourt KC, et al. Development of a core outcome set for studies evaluating the effects of anaesthesia on perioperative morbidity and mortality following hip fracture surgery. *Br J Anaesth*. 2019;122:120–130.

Schulte PJ, Roberts RO, Knopman DS, et al. Association between exposure to anaesthesia and surgery and long-term cognitive trajectories in older adults: report from the Mayo Clinic Study of Aging. *Br J Anaesth*. 2018;121:398–405.

Sessler DI, Bloomstone JA, Aronson S, et al. Perioperative Quality Initiative consensus statement on intraoperative blood pressure, risk and outcomes for elective surgery. *Br J Anaesth*. 2019;122:563–574.

Shaefi S, Mittel A, Loberman D, Ramakrishna H. Off-pump versus on-pump coronary artery bypass grafting—a systematic review and analysis of clinical outcomes. *J Cardiothorac Vasc Anesth*. 2019;33:232–244.

Susano MJ, Grasfield RH, Friese M, et al. Brief preoperative screening for frailty and cognitive impairment predicts delirium after spine surgery. *Anesthesiology*. 2020;133:1184–1191.

Tang CJ, Jin Z, Sands LP, et al. ADAPT-2: a randomized clinical trial to reduce intraoperative EEG suppression in older surgical patients undergoing major noncardiac surgery. *Anesth Analg*. 2020;131:1228–1236.

Velkers C, Berger M, Gill SS, et al. Association between exposure to general versus regional anesthesia and risk of dementia in older adults. *J Am Geriatr Soc*. 2021;69:58–67.

Vizzardi E, Curnis A, Latini MG, et al. Risk factors for atrial fibrillation recurrence: a literature review. *J Cardiovasc Med (Hagerstown)*. 2014;15:235–253.

Wenk M, Frey S. Elderly hip fracture patients: surgical timing and factors to consider. *Curr Opin Anaesthesiol*. 2021;34:33–39.

Wildes TS, Mickle AM, Ben Abdallah A, et al. Effect of electroencephalography-guided anesthetic administration on postoperative delirium among older adults undergoing major surgery: the ENGAGES Randomized Clinical Trial. *JAMA*. 2019;321:473–483.

Surgical Quality and Outcomes

Hiroko Kunitake

INTRODUCTION

The US population is aging and increasing numbers of older adults are undergoing surgery. Adults 65 and older account for more than 40% of all inpatient operations and 33% of outpatient operations performed annually in the United States. With advances in care and surgical technique, it is not uncommon to have surgical patients in their 80s and 90s and beyond. However, operations in older adults are associated with a high risk of prolonged hospitalization, surgical complications, and functional decline. As we place increasing focus on improving these outcomes, we have found that chronological age is not sufficient for predicting surgical risk. Frailty has been shown to be a stronger predictor of perioperative morbidity and mortality than age alone, and we are now working to refine how we assess frailty in surgical patients so that we can have meaningful discussions with patients and their families about the impact and possible outcomes of surgery.

In contrast to younger patients, many older surgical patients value maintenance of functional independence and quality of life (QOL) as much as or even more than quantity of life. In this context, the long-standing traditional measures of surgical quality and a successful surgical outcome—short hospital stay, few postoperative complications, and avoidance of 30-day readmission must be reconsidered. Functional recovery following surgery is now perhaps the most important measure of surgical success in this older patient population and globally encompasses physical well-being as well as cognitive, psychological, emotional, social, and even economic recovery over a period of a year or more.

This chapter will review traditional surgical outcomes as well as patient-centered outcomes of functional and cognitive recovery and QOL for older patients undergoing surgery.

TRADITIONAL SURGICAL OUTCOMES

Older patients have more comorbidities, less physiologic reserve, and often a less robust social support network to withstand the physical insult of surgery as well as the stress put on their nutritional, psychological, and emotional well-being. Several studies using the American College of Surgeons National Surgical Quality Improvement Program

Learning Objectives

- To understand what older patients undergoing surgery consider a successful outcome in contrast to the traditional surgical outcomes of length of stay, postoperative complications, and readmission.

- To understand the long-term effects of surgery including associated complications and readmissions on the ability of patients to achieve functional recovery (physical, cognitive, psychological, emotional, social, and economic recovery) after surgery.

- To review the effect of delirium and postoperative cognitive dysfunction on postoperative recovery.

Key Clinical Points

1. Many older surgical patients value maintenance of functional independence and quality of life (QOL) as much as or even more than quantity of life and make decisions regarding their surgical care based on these values.

2. Frailty is a stronger predictor of perioperative morbidity and mortality than chronological age alone. A comprehensive and efficient frailty assessment for patients in the preoperative period should be standardized.

3. Hospitalized older adults undergoing surgery are at risk for geriatric events (delirium, dehydration, falls or fractures, failure to thrive, and pressure ulcers), which can contribute to worse outcomes.

4. Geriatric co-management of patients has been associated with improved outcomes including shorter length of stay and lower rates of complications and mortality for older patients.

(ACS NSQIP) database, which includes patients having a wide range of surgical procedures at academic and community hospitals across the country, showed that older patients, as a group, had significantly higher morbidity (1.2–2 times higher) and 30-day mortality (2.9–6.7 times higher) than younger patients. Additionally, patients older than 75 years were significantly more likely to have a prolonged hospital stay. Approximately 60% of patients older than 75 years remained in the hospital longer than 7 days after a major gastrointestinal tract operation.

In the past, we used patient's age to guide expectations on postoperative recovery and even to decide whether we would offer surgery to a patient. However, if selected appropriately, older patients undergoing even very high-risk procedures can have good outcomes and benefit from surgery. Frailty, or physiological decline and increased vulnerability to stressors, is a key factor in determining an older patient's ability to withstand and recover from surgery. Frailty does not correlate with chronological age and may not correlate with the American Society of Anesthesiologists physical status classification score. There are many methods to try to determine frailty in surgical patients but regardless of how frailty is measured, frail patients have been shown in multiple studies to have increased in-hospital, 30-day, 90-day, and 1-year mortality, increased rates of postoperative complications, longer lengths of stay, and increased need for institutionalization at discharge compared to nonfrail geriatric surgery patients.

A 2014 study of 180 patients who underwent surgical treatment for gastric cancer reported that postoperative mortality was 23% among patients who were frail, compared with 5% among patients who were fit. A 2016 systematic review including 23 studies of patients with mean age of 75–87 years undergoing a wide variety of oncologic or nononcologic surgery and using 21 different instruments to measure frailty found that frail patients had increased 30-day mortality (odds ratio [OR] 1.4–8.33), 1-year morality (OR 1.1–4.97), 2-year mortality (OR 4.01), and 5-year mortality (OR 3.6) compared with nonfrail patients. Finally, in a large study of over 14,000 inpatient and outpatient operations, increasing frailty correlated with increased rates of major morbidity, readmission, mortality, and discharge to facility for inpatient procedures as well as increased unplanned admission for outpatient procedures. Not surprisingly, direct costs per patient also increased with increasing frailty in the inpatient cohort (Modified Hopkins Frailty Score: low, $7045; intermediate, $7995; high, $8599).

In addition to postsurgical complications, hospitalized older adults undergoing surgery are at risk for geriatric events (delirium, dehydration, falls or fractures, failure to thrive, and pressure ulcers), which can contribute to worse outcomes. A large study using the National Inpatient Sample including over 800,000 patients undergoing one of the five most common elective procedures in adults 65 years or older (total knee arthroplasty, right hemicolectomy, carotid endarterectomy, aortic valve replacement, and radical prostatectomy) analyzed the rates of perioperative geriatric events. Among admissions for adults 65 years or older,

2.4% experienced a geriatric event. Rates of geriatric events increased with age and varied by procedure, ranging from 1.0% in admissions for radical prostatectomy to 10.3% in admissions for aortic valve replacement. The most common geriatric event in adults 65 years or older was dehydration (1.1%). Among patients 75 years or older, the most common geriatric event was delirium (1.7%).

Looking more specifically at high-risk geriatric surgery (operations associated with a > 1% inpatient mortality in patients ≥ 65 years old), a study including over 500,000 geriatric patients found that the overall inpatient mortality rate was 4.6%. The median postoperative length of stay was 5.4 days and rate of discharge to nursing facility was 28.8%. In this study, mortality, postoperative length of stay, and rate of discharge to nursing facility were influenced by the volume of high-risk geriatric operations performed at the hospital and the proportion of high-risk operations at that center which were performed on geriatric patients. Higher proportion was associated with decreased mortality and shorter length of stay suggesting that these centers may be better equipped to manage the unique health care needs of these older adults undergoing high-risk surgery and provide high-quality geriatric-focused care.

Geriatric-Focused Care and Co-management to Improve Surgical Outcomes

Surgical outcomes in older patients are improved when these patients are treated in a geriatric-focused health system and several organizations are prioritizing the improvement of geriatric patient care. Some physicians may be fortunate to work in an Age-Friendly Health System, which strives to provide evidence-based high-quality care based on the geriatric 4Ms—What Matters Most, Medication, Mentation, and Mobility—to all adults in their system (Multicomplexity being implicit in this patient population and not a separate M). The Age-Friendly Health System movement began in 2017 and now comprises several hundred hospitals, practices, and postacute long-term care communities who are focused on caring for older adults. Another entity striving to improve the care of older surgical patients is the American College of Surgeons Geriatric Surgery Verification Program, which includes 32 surgical standards designed to systematically improve surgical care and outcomes for this patient population. These standards overlap with the framework of the Age-Friendly Health System and bridge preoperative, postoperative, and transitions of care periods for the patient, but also include recommendations on improving facilities, equipment, data surveillance, and community outreach to build an infrastructure that is focused on the surgical care of older adults.

Geriatric co-management of patients has been associated with improved outcomes including shorter length of stay and lower rates of complications and mortality for older patients. Currently, the most common co-management model is the orthogeriatric care model for the management of hip fractures in older patients. Each hospital has developed their own unique co-management model and these fall into three categories: Routine Geriatric Consultation (routine geriatrician consultation on older patients in an orthopedic ward); Geriatric Ward (care within a geriatric ward with the orthopedic surgeon acting as consultant); and Shared Care (integrated care model with both orthopedic surgeon and geriatrician sharing responsibility for the care of the patient). Routine Geriatric Consultation is the most common orthogeriatric model. Most studies of this model show that orthopedic geriatric collaboration improves outcomes versus standard of care for older patients although the types of outcomes differ in various studies.

In another retrospective study of over 1800 patients (≥ 75 years old) who underwent elective cancer-related surgery, patients who received geriatric co-managed care were compared with those who did not. Although adverse surgical events were not significantly different, the probability of death within 90 days was 4.3% for the geriatric co-management group versus 8.9% for the surgical service group. Patients in the geriatric co-management group also received more inpatient physical and occupational therapy, speech and swallow rehabilitation, and nutrition services than patients managed by the surgical service alone and this geriatric-focused multidisciplinary care may have contributed to their improved outcomes. Most hospitals now use standardized enhanced recovery after surgery (ERAS) pathways tailored to specific operations that span the preoperative, intraoperative, and postoperative periods. These ERAS pathways have been very successful in decreasing complications and length of stay, but the same pathway is used for young and old surgical patients and patients who are frail or fit. One current area of innovation is in tailoring the ERAS pathway to address the unique needs of older surgical patients and in many cases, this includes automated consults to inpatient support services such as physical therapy and nutrition services based on certain screening criteria.

PATIENT-CENTERED SURGICAL OUTCOMES

Functional Recovery

In a 2002 seminal paper exploring the treatment preferences of older adult patients with serious illnesses, patients were more likely to be willing to undergo a treatment if the possible outcome was death than undergo the same treatment if the possible outcome was severe cognitive or functional impairment. This study and many subsequent studies pushed us to realize that our traditional surgical outcomes measures were not appropriate for the unique older surgical patient population. Older patients wanted to know about their expected cognitive and functional recovery after surgery and their ability to remain independent before making a decision about whether to proceed with the surgery. Until recently we did not measure these outcomes, which were difficult to quantify and required a much longer follow-up period of up to a year or longer, compared with traditional outcomes. Several prospective longitudinal cohort studies of older adults have contributed to our understanding of functional recovery after surgery. In most studies, majority

of patients had an initial functional decline, but were able to recover to close to their presurgery level of function over a period of 6 months to a year.

The Precipitating Events Project is a longitudinal study of 754 community-dwelling persons 70 years or older who were initially nondisabled in four basic activities of daily living: bathing, dressing, walking, and transferring. These participants were queried using monthly interviews to evaluate functional status (whether they need assistance for four essential activities [bathing, dressing, walking, and transferring], five instrumental activities [shopping, housework, meal preparation, taking medications, and managing finances], three mobility activities [walk ¼ mile, climb flight of 7 stairs, and lift/carry 10 pounds], and whether they had driven a car in the past month) in addition to comprehensive assessments every 18 months. From 350 admission for major surgery, 69 admissions had no change or improved disability at the first follow-up. The remaining 216 participants undergoing 266 major surgeries had initial increased postoperative disability but by their 6 month follow-up, 174 (65.4%) had recovered to their presurgery level of function, 76 (28.6%) had not reached their presurgery level of function but were alive, and 16 (6%) had died. Two factors significantly associated with an increased likelihood of functional recovery were having an elective operation (hazards ration [HR] 1.72) and being nonfrail (HR 1.60). Additionally, in this cohort, intervening illnesses and injuries leading to hospitalization, emergency department (ED) visit, or restricted activity were common in the year after major surgery and were more closely associated with functional decline than were traditional risk factors such as chronic conditions, obesity, depressive symptoms, or hearing impairment. Ultimately, a quarter of patients did not recover to their premorbid level of function in the year following surgery and the vast majority of patients experienced at least one episode of functional decline during the study period.

In addition to the impact of major surgery, subsequent hospitalizations are also associated with functional decline. The Successful Aging after Elective Surgery (SAGES) study, an ongoing prospective cohort study of 566 adults aged 70 and older undergoing major scheduled noncardiac surgery, showed that readmissions, whether associated with the index surgery or not, were associated with delays in functional recovery. Over an 18-month period, 253 participants (45%) had 503 readmissions (143 patients had one, and 112 had two or more, with a maximum of 12); 203 (36%) participants reported 345 readmissions that were unrelated to the index hospitalization. The degree of functional impairment increased progressively with the number of readmissions, potentially due to the harmful effects of delirium, immobilization, sleep deprivation, malnutrition, and psychological stress experienced during each hospital admission.

Another measurement of functional decline, loss of independence (LOI), is now gaining attention. The definition of LOI varies across studies, but it encompasses a decline in functional status or increased care needs. In a study of patients undergoing inpatient surgery at a hospital participating in the ACS NSQIP Geriatric Surgery Pilot Project, LOI was measured at discharge and was characterized by one of three changes: a decline in function according to activities of daily living (ADLs), a decline in mobility requiring a new mobility aid, or an increase in care needs, such as a need for new home-care services or discharge to a nonhome destination. At the time of discharge, 26% of patients experienced a decline in functional status and 30% had a decline in mobility. Forty-six percent of patients had increased care needs (27.8% required additional supportive services at home, 18.2% required discharge to a nonhome destination). Overall, 60% of patients experienced at least some degree of LOI. LOI increased significantly with age: 50% of patients between 65 and 74 years, 67% of patients between 75 and 84 years, and 84% of patients 85 years and older.

Delirium and Postoperative Cognitive Dysfunction

Delirium is the most common surgical complication in older adults, affecting up to half of patients postoperatively, and it is closely linked to poor patient outcomes. Postoperative delirium is associated with a two- to fivefold increased risk of major postoperative complications, a threefold increased risk of institutional placement at discharge, longer hospital stays, and increased rates of readmission and mortality. In addition, Medicare cumulative costs attributable to delirium in older surgical patients were found to be $44,291 per patient over 1 year following surgery and $56,474 per patient with severe delirium over the year following surgery. Despite these significant adverse results, postoperative delirium is significantly underrecognized and therefore undertreated. It is equally important to note that delirium is preventable in up to 40% of patients with relatively simple adjustments in perioperative care. The prevention and management of delirium in surgical patients need as much targeted emphasis in surgical education as other more traditional complications.

An episode of postoperative delirium has as significant an impact on patient outcomes as a major postoperative complication. In a large cohort of patients 70 years or older undergoing major orthopedic, vascular, or abdominal surgery, 8.3% developed a major postoperative complication and 24% developed delirium. Patients who had a major complication such as unstable arrhythmia, respiratory failure, or stroke, but did not have delirium had increased length of stay (relative risk [RR], 2.8; 95% confidence interval [CI] 1.9–4.0). However, patients with delirium but no major complication had prolonged length of stay (RR 1.9; 95% CI 1.4–2.7) as well as increased institutional discharge (RR 1.5; 95% CI 1.3–1.7) and increased 30-day readmission (RR 2.3; 95% CI 1.4–3.7). Patients who had both a major complication and delirium had the highest rates of adverse outcomes with a mean length of stay of 13 (SD 11) days and increased institutional discharge (RR 1.8; 95% CI 1.4–2.5) and 30-day readmission (RR 3.0; 95% CI 1.3–6.8).

A number of studies have looked at the relationship between postoperative delirium and postoperative cognitive dysfunction. Postoperative delirium and postoperative cognitive dysfunction share risk factors and may co-occur, but their relationship over the postoperative period is unclear. A study looking at the association between postoperative delirium and the risk of postoperative cognitive dysfunction at 1 month, 2 months, and 6 months after major noncardiac surgery showed that postoperative delirium increased the risk of postoperative cognitive dysfunction at 1 month postoperatively, but there was no association between postoperative delirium and cognitive dysfunction at 2 and 6 months after major noncardiac surgery.

The Postoperative Cognitive Dysfunction in Elderly Cancer patients (PICNIC) study was a prospective observational study of patients aged 65 or older who underwent oncologic surgery. Three cognitive domains (memory, executive function, and information processing speed) were evaluated at baseline (approximately 2 weeks before surgery) and 3 months postoperatively. Of the 219 patients included in the analysis, 26 (12%) had cognitive decline 3 months postoperatively, whereas 117 (53%) patients had improved cognitive scores. Advanced age (> 75 years old), lower preoperative Mini-Mental State Examination (MMSE) score, and major surgery (surgery with anesthesia lasting > 210 minutes) were risk factors for cognitive decline at 3 months postoperatively. In patients with advanced age (> 75 years) or those undergoing major surgery, 18% showed cognitive decline and in patients who additionally had a lower preoperative MMSE score, the incidence was 37%. During the study, 10% of patients were diagnosed and treated for postoperative delirium.

Quality of Life

Quality of life (QOL) is tightly intertwined with functional and cognitive recovery, but studies show that postoperative QOL can exceed the preoperative level even for patients who have postoperative functional decline or suffer a complication. A study of patients age 75 and older undergoing surgery for colorectal or gastric cancer measured activities of daily living (ADLs) and QOL at baseline and then at 1 month, 3 months, and 6 months postoperatively. Twenty-four percent of patients showed a decrease in ADL at 1 month postoperatively, but most patients recovered with only 3% showing a decline at the sixth postoperative month. QOL of the patients similarly fell immediately after surgery but then rapidly recovered to equal or better than their preoperative level, 3 to 6 months after surgery. In another study of patients 70 years or older undergoing elective resection for colon or rectal cancer evaluated with the EORTC-QLQ-C30, emotional function and QOL improved for both frail and nonfrail patients at 3 months. At long-term follow-up (median time 22 months after the operation), emotional function and QOL scores had decreased from the postoperative peak but still remained above baseline.

Another measure of QOL or independence is the amount of time spent at home following oncologic surgery. In a study of over 80,000 people undergoing oncologic surgery, older adults spent more than 98% of their time at home over the 5 years following surgery. The amount of time at home varied with the type of oncologic surgery. Breast surgery had the highest likelihood of spending time at home and gastrointestinal surgery had the lowest likelihood of spending time at home over the 5 years following surgery. The amount of institutionalized time increased over time. Most patients who survived the surgery were likely to have 14 or less institution days per year for the first four postoperative years. However, in the fifth year, 50% of patients who were still alive were likely to experience more than 14 institution days per year. Advancing age, preoperative frailty, lower socioeconomic standing, rural residency, high-intensity surgical procedure, and gastrointestinal, gynecologic, or oropharyngeal cancers were associated with less time at home.

Minimally invasive surgery is now expected by most patients but the benefits in older patients are not always as clear. QOL was compared between patients undergoing laparoscopic versus open pancreatic resection to determine if minimally invasive surgery improved QOL. In both the minimally invasive and open surgery groups, physical, functional, and QOL scores decreased in the immediate postoperative period but returned to baseline by 6 months postoperatively. Patients who experienced a severe complication had greater declines in QOL than patients who did not have a complication regardless of the surgical approach, emphasizing that a safe operation is the best approach to optimize patient QOL.

Future Directions

In order to give older patients the best understanding of their anticipated surgical outcomes, we can no longer rely simply on estimates of traditional outcome measures such as morbidity and mortality but must find a way to incorporate geriatric patient-centered outcomes as well. This is a complex and multidimensional risk calculation that is unique to each patient and yet must be determined in a timely manner so that surgical decisions can be made. The ACS NSQIP Surgical Risk Calculator is a decision support tool that provides estimates of risk for 12 30-day outcomes using 21 preoperative risk predictors. Using data collected from 21 ACS NSQIP Geriatric Surgery Pilot Project hospitals, six new geriatric risk factors (living situation, fall history, mobility aid use, cognitive impairment, surrogate-signed consent, and palliative care on admission) were added in order to predict four postoperative geriatric outcomes (pressure ulcer, delirium, new mobility aid use, and functional decline). Using a geriatric-enhanced surgical risk calculator like this is critical to enabling clinicians to better guide patients and their families as they make decisions about their health care and ultimately to improving surgical outcomes for these patients.

Additionally, older patients can benefit from a personalized care plan that incorporates their complex needs and personal goals. At our institution, we are striving to develop and improve this model, which will span the preoperative, intraoperative, and postoperative segments of a patient's experience and will provide the foundation for improving surgical quality and outcomes for our older patients (**Figure 29-1**).

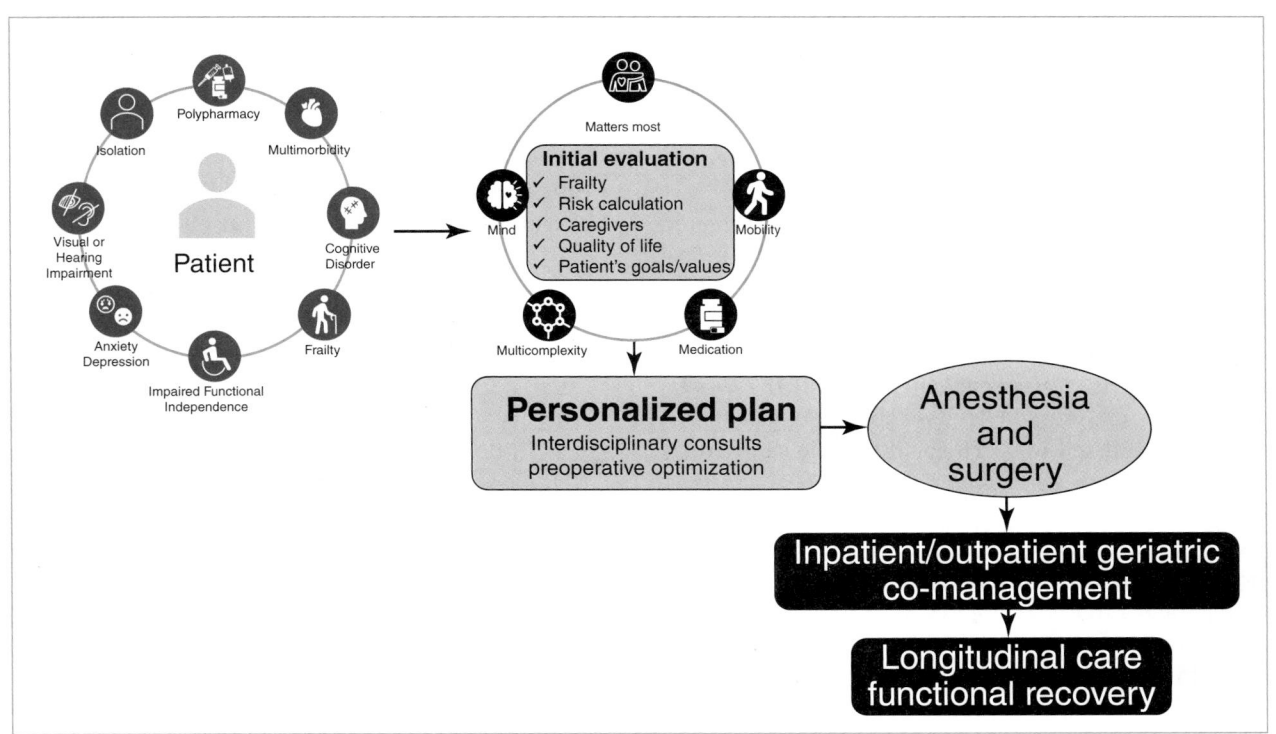

FIGURE 29-1. The future: personalized surgical care for older adults.

CONCLUSIONS

Older adults as a group become more diverse in their health care conditions and their personal goals as they age. The definition of surgical quality and a good outcome is unique to each patient. As surgeons, perhaps the most important thing we can do is to ask patients: What matters most to you? For some patients, this may be resecting their tumor, regardless of the risks. For others, it may be living independently for as long as possible. And for others, the best outcome may be focused on symptom relief and palliative care. As surgeons, we are in a unique position to have informed discussions about surgery in the framework of what matters most to the patient and their loved ones and to put patients on the trajectory toward their goals, even if surgery is not desired. In this way, we will be able to help older patients achieve the best outcomes possible.

FURTHER READING

Amemiya T, Oda K, Ando M, et al. Activities of daily living and quality of life of elderly patients after elective surgery for gastric and colorectal cancers. *Ann Surg.* 2007;246(2):222–228.

Becher RD, Murphy TE, Gahbauer EA, Leo-Summers L, Stabenau HF, Gill TM. Factors associated with functional recovery among older survivors of major surgery. *Ann Surg.* 2020;272(1):92–98.

Bentrem DJ, Cohen ME, Hynes DM, Ko CY, Bilimoria KY. Identification of specific quality improvement opportunities for the elderly undergoing gastrointestinal surgery. *Arch Surg.* 2009;144(11):1013–1020. Erratum in: *Arch Surg.* 2010;145(3):225.

Berian JR, Mohanty S, Ko CY, Rosenthal RA, Robinson TN. Association of loss of independence with readmission and death after discharge in older patients after surgical procedures. *JAMA Surg.* 2016;151(9):e161689.

Centers for Disease Control and Prevention. National Center for Health Statistics: Number of Discharges from Short-stay Hospitals, by First-listed Diagnosis and Age: United States, 2010. www.cdc.gov/nchs/data/nhds/4procedures/2010pro4_numberprocedureage.pdf. Accessed February 28, 2021.

Chesney TR, Haas B, Coburn NG, et al. Patient-centered time-at-home outcomes in older adults after surgical cancer treatment. *JAMA Surg.* 2020;155(11):e203754.

Daiello LA, Racine AM, Yun Gou R, et al. Postoperative delirium and postoperative cognitive dysfunction: overlap and divergence. *Anesthesiology.* 2019;131(3):477–491.

Dworsky JQ, Childers CP, Gornbein J, Maggard-Gibbons M, Russell MM. Hospital experience predicts outcomes after high-risk geriatric surgery. *Surgery.* 2020;167(2):468–474.

Dworsky JQ, Shellito AD, Childers CP, et al. Association of geriatric events with perioperative outcomes after elective inpatient surgery. *J Surg Res.* 2021;259:192–199.

Fried TR, Bradley EH, Towle VR, Allore H. Understanding the treatment preferences of seriously ill patients. *N Engl J Med.* 2002;346(14):1061–1066.

Gill TM, Han L, Gahbauer EA, Leo-Summers L, Murphy TE, Becher RD. Functional effects of intervening illnesses and injuries after hospitalization for major surgery in community-living older persons. *Ann Surg.* 2021;273(5):834–841.

Gou RY, Hshieh TT, Marcantonio ER, et al. One-year Medicare costs associated with delirium in older patients undergoing major elective surgery. *JAMA Surg.* 2021;156(5):430–442.

Hall MJ, Schwartzman A, Zhang J, Liu X. Ambulatory surgery data from hospitals and ambulatory surgery centers: United States, 2010. *Natl Health Stat Report.* 2017;(102):1–15.

Hornor MA, Ma M, Zhou L, et al. Enhancing the American College of Surgeons NSQIP Surgical Risk Calculator to Predict Geriatric Outcomes. *J Am Coll Surg.* 2020;230(1):88–100.e1.

Lawrence VA, Hazuda HP, Cornell JE, et al. Functional independence after major abdominal surgery in the elderly. *J Am Coll Surg.* 2004;199(5):762–772.

Lin HS, Watts JN, Peel NM, Hubbard RE. Frailty and postoperative outcomes in older surgical patients: a systematic review. *BMC Geriatr.* 2016;16(1):157.

Marcantonio ER. Delirium in hospitalized older adults. *N Engl J Med.* 2017;377(15):1456–1466.

Pisani MA, Albuquerque A, Marcantonio ER, et al. Association between hospital readmission and acute and sustained delays in functional recovery during 18 months after elective surgery: the successful aging after elective surgery study. *J Am Geriatr Soc.* 2017;65(1):51–58.

Tegels JJ, de Maat MF, Hulsewé KW, Hoofwijk AG, Stoot JH. Value of geriatric frailty and nutritional status assessment in predicting postoperative mortality in gastric cancer surgery. *J Gastrointest Surg.* 2014;18(3):439–445; discussion 445–446.

Turrentine FE, Wang H, Simpson VB, Jones RS. Surgical risk factors, morbidity, and mortality in elderly patients. *J Am Coll Surg.* 2006;203(6):865–877.

Chapter 30

Nutrition Disorders, Obesity, and Enteral/Parenteral Alimentation

Dennis H. Sullivan, Larry E. Johnson, Jeffrey I. Wallace

INTRODUCTION

Throughout life, nutrition is an important determinant of health, physical and cognitive function, vitality, overall quality of life, and longevity. The quantity and variety of available foods, as well as the meaningfulness of the social interactions provided by meals, are important to psychological well-being. The composition of the diet and the amount that is consumed are strongly linked to physiologic function. When a well-balanced diet adequate to meet the body's metabolic demands is not maintained, malnutrition may develop with consequent detrimental effects on health and well-being.

Malnutrition can have many manifestations. As outlined below, a diet that is deficient in one or more required nutrients (eg, calories, protein, minerals, fiber, or vitamins) can lead to a state of nutritional deficiency. The greater the magnitude and duration of the nutritional deprivation and the more fragile the individual, the more likely nutritional deficits will produce noticeable body compositional changes, functional impairments, or overt disease. Even borderline dietary deficiencies can have important health consequences such as producing subtle organ system impairments, diminished vitality, or increasing the individual's susceptibility to disease. Protein and protein-energy undernutrition are two of the most common, frequently unrecognized, and potentially serious forms of nutritional deficiency. The prevalence of these conditions is particularly high among chronically ill older individuals and those in hospitals, nursing homes, and other institutional settings. Although there is a complex interrelationship between nutrition, disease, and clinical outcomes, protein and protein-energy undernutrition appear to be significant contributors to disease-related morbidity and mortality in these populations.

Learning Objectives

- Describe the important interrelationship between diet and physical activity in maintaining or restoring lean body mass (LBM) and the resulting effects this interaction has on total body mass in older adults.
- Describe the changes in body composition that occur over the adult life span and what physiologic, dietary, lifestyle, and disease factors are responsible for these changes.
- Describe the changing prevalence of obesity among older adults and be able to assess the impact of excess weight on the health status of older patients.
- Advise older adults about what constitutes an optimal diet and the advisability of using nutrient supplements given their health status.
- Describe common factors contributing to undernutrition in older adults.
- Identify the three most common causes of weight loss in older adults.
- Determine appropriate nutritional support interventions for persons with protein-energy malnutrition (PEM).

Key Clinical Points

1. With advancing age, the ratio of fat to total body mass increases regardless of whether total body weight increases or remains constant.

2. Although skeletal muscle mass generally declines with advancing age, the rate of decline in healthy individuals is highly dependent on the individual's habitual level

(Continued)

(Cont.)

of physical activity and the quality of his/her diet.

3. Although the impact of excess weight (ie, body mass index [BMI] > 25 kg/m²) on long-term survival is highly controversial, there is a strong direct relationship between the level of obesity and the risk of developing disabling chronic diseases such as severe osteoarthritis, type 2 diabetes, and heart disease.

4. There is no evidence of benefit for any micronutrient supplement in healthy older adults who do not have a documented deficiency of the given nutrient or a condition that places them at high risk for the development of such a deficiency. Supplements of vitamins and minerals do not prevent or treat cardiovascular disease (CVD), cancer, or dementia.

5. Vitamin and mineral supplements, above the recommended upper limit (UL), increase adverse health outcomes. The National Academy of Medicine provides evidence-based guidelines for Recommended Dietary Allowances of vitamins and minerals for most individuals.

6. Laboratory blood tests of serum proteins (such as albumin and prealbumin) are indicators of inflammatory status, disease severity, and morbidity risk, rather than nutritional status.

7. Weight loss of 5% or more of baseline body weight over 6 to 12 months is associated with increased morbidity and mortality and should prompt clinical investigation.

8. When malignancy is the cause of weight loss, the diagnosis is usually readily made with standard evaluations that include a careful history, physical examination, and basic laboratory tests.

9. High-protein, high-calorie oral nutritional supplements may reduce morbidity and mortality when provided to hospitalized malnourished patients age 75 or older.

10. Enteral nutrition (EN) is preferred over parenteral nutrition (PN) for patients who are in need of nutritional support and have a functional gastrointestinal (GI) tract.

At the other end of the spectrum, the persistent consumption of excess quantities of one or more nutrients can have similar untoward consequences. Forms of malnutrition that result from excess consumption include hypercholesterolemia, hypervitaminosis, and obesity. Obesity is the most common nutritional disorder of advanced age in western societies, with a high prevalence among noninstitutionalized free-living older adults. Many obese older individuals have other nutritional disorders. Among chronically ill or functionally debilitated obese older individuals, protein undernutrition is a common, serious, and frequently unrecognized problem that can develop for many reasons including an imbalanced diet, disease, and inactivity.

Recognizing and maintaining an optimally balanced diet is an important challenge, particularly when individuals age. The challenge is particularly great for older people who already are malnourished, especially if they have nutritional disorders that developed earlier in life, such as obesity, osteoporosis, or protein undernutrition. Even healthy individuals often fail to maintain an optimal diet due to lack of knowledge, resources, or willpower. Age-related acute and chronic diseases, physical disabilities, social isolation, use of multiple medications, depression, impaired cognitive ability, and dysregulation of appetite control may contribute further to poor eating habits and the development or exacerbation of nutritional disorders. In turn, inappropriate dietary intake and poor nutritional status can impact the progression of many acute and chronic diseases such as coronary heart disease (CHD), cancer, stroke, diabetes, and osteoporosis, which are among the 10 leading causes of death in the United States. Approximately two-thirds of all deaths within the United States are due to diseases associated with poor diets and dietary habits.

Assessing diet quality of the older people is critical to addressing issues relevant to their health and nutritional status. Such an assessment must be based on knowledge of what constitutes a balanced diet for a given individual. The goal of this chapter is to identify an approach to nutrition evaluation and management that takes into account the unique needs, limitations, and desires of each older individual. The chapter examines the interrelationship between nutrition, activity, disease burden, and health outcomes and then focuses on age-related changes in body composition and appetite regulation that affect nutritional status and nutrient requirements. The chapter includes discussion of both undernutrition and obesity as well as specific dietary considerations for optimal health.

THE INTERRELATIONSHIP BETWEEN NUTRITION, ACTIVITY, AND DISEASE

Although nutrition is a vital component of good health, it cannot be evaluated in isolation. The relationship between nutrient intake and health is influenced by other factors, most notably activity level, disease burden, and advancing age. A basic understanding of these interrelationships is essential in order to assess the potential benefits and limitations of nutritional interventions.

Nutrition-Activity Interrelationship

Nutrition and physical activity are closely linked, each having vitally important and interacting effects on body composition, functional ability, and well-being. The balance between nutrient intake and physical activity is particularly important in determining muscle mass and strength, body fat content and distribution, and bone density and resilience. A detailed description of the importance of physical activity in these relationships is provided in Chapter 54.

To preserve existing muscle mass and strength, it is necessary to maintain both an adequate level of physical activity and a balanced diet that includes sufficient protein, energy, vitamins, and minerals to meet metabolic demands and prevent negative nitrogen balance (as discussed in detail further). It is not known precisely what level of physical activity is needed to prevent loss of existing muscle mass and strength in older adults. However, even a week or two of bed rest or similar degrees of activity restriction can result in noticeable loss of muscle mass, strength, and function even when the diet is adequate, and the individual is otherwise healthy. When an inadequate diet and inflammation are combined with inactivity, as occurs with serious illness, muscle loss can be even more rapid and profound. Overfeeding does not prevent muscle atrophy associated with inactivity and may exacerbate the functional consequences since the excess nutrients are converted to fat.

Consumption of a protein meal stimulates muscle protein synthesis. However, nutrition alone has never been demonstrated to be an effective method of repleting muscle mass, improving strength, or increasing endurance in frail older individuals who have experienced a recent loss of weight. Efforts at repletion should focus on both increasing nutrient intake and exercise. Based on studies of healthy older men, the combination of progressive resistance muscle strength training and a high protein diet (containing up to 1.6 g of protein/kg body weight/day) may be the most effective method of improving muscle mass. The role of special formula amino acid supplements has yet to be determined.

Exercise and nutrition also play a critical role in maintenance of optimal bone density and strength. As discussed in Chapter 51, the nutrient needs of bone include the correct balance of protein and energy and adequate intake of vitamins and minerals, especially vitamin D and calcium. The importance of exercise for optimal bone health is also described in Chapter 54. Osteopenia can develop despite an optimal diet if exercise or other weight-bearing activities are not adequate. Because of its apparent beneficial effects on bone mineral density (BMD), exercise should be combined with an appropriate diet for both prevention and treatment of osteoporosis and fracture-related disability.

Having both direct and indirect effects on numerous metabolic processes within muscle, bone, and adipose tissues, exercise has a major impact on how nutrients are utilized by the body during health and illness. By inducing an increase in the mass and metabolic capacity of muscle, exercise effects energy expenditure, glucose metabolism, and size of protein reserves in a manner that counteracts some of the effects of aging and thus has important nutritional implications for individuals as they grow older. Total energy expenditure (TEE) represents the sum of basal energy expenditure, post-prandial thermogenesis, and the energy expenditure of activity. Muscle represents not only the primary source of energy expenditure during physical activity, it is also the primary contributor to basal energy expenditure, which may represent 50% to 80% of TEE. With advancing age, there is a parallel decline in muscle mass and both basal and total daily energy expenditure that may be partially or fully accounted for by the fact that people tend to become more sedentary as they grow older.

Exercise-induced increases in muscle size or protein content result in greater body protein reserves that can be critical to survival during episodes of nutritional deprivation that usually accompany profound physiologic stress such as trauma, sepsis, or other acute disease. Such physiologic insults trigger an acute inflammatory response that causes ketogenesis to be suppressed, leaving glucose as the primary energy source available to the body. The problem is invariably compounded by reduced nutrient intake that results as a consequence of the anorexia and gastrointestinal tract dysfunction induced by the inflammatory response. With nutrient intake suppressed, gluconeogenesis becomes the predominant source of glucose. Since the substrate for gluconeogenesis is provided by catabolism of skeletal muscle, LBM becomes an important determinant of survival. Once LBM falls below a critical level, the chance of surviving a serious acute illness diminishes dramatically. Studies conducted within the Warsaw Ghetto, hospital intensive care units, and other settings suggest that a loss of more than 40% of baseline lean mass is incompatible with life. Indeed, very few healthy people have a LBM that is less than 70% of the mean for that of adults between 20 and 30 years.

In addition to inducing muscle hypertrophy, exercise also affects insulin sensitivity and glucose disposal directly and plays a synergistic role with diet in maintaining a healthy weight and a sense of well-being. These effects of exercise can be important adjuncts to good nutrition in the prevention and treatment of hypertension, diabetes, and osteoporosis.

Nutrition-Disease Interrelationship

There is a complex interrelationship between nutrition, health status, and clinical outcomes. Although a full discussion of this topic is beyond the scope of this chapter, it is important to emphasize several key points. First, nutrient requirements and the ability to metabolize select nutrients are influenced by many disease states. In addition, many diseases compromise the older individual's ability to consume adequate amounts of all nutrients. This can occur through a number of mechanisms including disease-induced suppression of appetite, alteration of the normal swallowing mechanism, maldigestion or absorption, or loss of self-feeding ability.

The detrimental effects of disease on nutrient metabolism often become more pronounced with advancing age. This is particularly true of the many acute and chronic diseases that induce an inflammatory response, including acute and chronic infections, congestive heart failure, chronic pulmonary disease, cancer, end-stage renal disease, and rheumatoid arthritis. As described in detail in Chapter 3, with advancing age, the inflammatory response often becomes dysregulated as indicated by persistently elevated serum concentrations of proinflammatory cytokines and other inflammatory mediators including interleukin (IL)-6, IL-1(beta), tumor necrosis factor (TNF)-alpha, and possibly IL-8 and others. IL-1, IL-6, and TNF-alpha all contribute to the loss of skeletal muscle, fat tissue, and bone mass that characterizes inflammation-associated cachexia. Although anorexia is almost always a contributing factor, the inflammation-induced loss of fat and lean mass is often refractory to nutrition support. Through a number of different mechanisms, proinflammatory cytokines create a state of muscle hypercatabolism by suppressing muscle protein synthesis and/or accelerating muscle protein breakdown independent of dietary factors.

Since these potentially deleterious effects of disease can be difficult to predict, older individuals with one or more acute or chronic health problems should have frequent reassessments of their nutritional status and their nutritional care plan revised as necessary. Although nutrient intake may not be adequate to completely reverse inflammation-induced catabolism, a low nutrient intake will accelerate the development of cachexia. Optimally, good nutritional care should be part of the overall plan of medical intervention aimed at treating the underlying pathology as well as addressing protein and energy deficits. Although a number of specific nutrients are being studied to determine their value in counteracting inflammation-induced loss of LBM, there is not yet adequate evidence that any given dietary supplement is more effective than current standard dietary or nutrition support practices.

AGE-RELATED CHANGES THAT AFFECT NUTRITION

Changes in Body Composition

With advancing age, there are significant changes in body composition that affect the nutritional needs of the individual. Weight increases steadily on average from age 30 to 60 years primarily due to an increase in total body fat. After age 60, weight usually stabilizes, and then begins to decline.

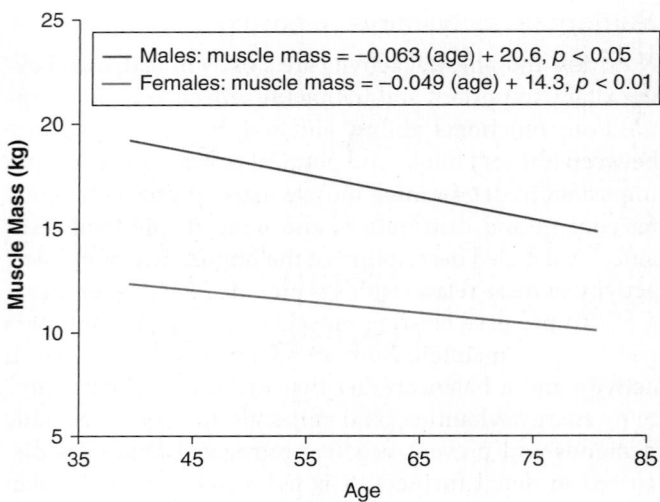

FIGURE 30-1. Declining muscle mass with increasing age. (Data from Janssen I, Heymsfield SB, Wang ZM, et al. Skeletal muscle mass and distribution in 468 men and women aged 18-88 yr. *J Appl Physiol* (1985). 2000;89[1]:81–88.)

The incidence as well as the potential causes of weight loss increase with age, particularly beyond age 75.

Regardless of whether or not weight changes, advancing age is characterized by a progressive loss in LBM, a relative increase in fat mass, and a redistribution of fat from peripheral to central locations within the body. These changes generally begin in the third decade and increase at an accelerated rate after age 65. This late acceleration may be due to loss of LBM plus the increased prevalence of chronic diseases in old age. The loss of LBM consists predominantly of skeletal muscle, particularly type II or fast twitch fibers. Central LBM, such as the liver and other splanchnic organs, is relatively preserved. As reviewed in detail in Chapter 49, muscle mass may decline by up to 45% between the third and eighth decade of life (see **Figures 30-1** and **30-2**). The quality of muscle may also change. With advancing age, there is a gradual infiltration or replacement of muscle by fat, as has been documented by computed tomography. Even accounting for body size, height, and other aspects of body composition, fatty infiltration into muscle is associated with symptomatic functional decline, poorer physical function, and change in strength.

The loss of muscle mass with age appears to be the result of multiple interrelated factors including age-related changes in metabolism, function, or structure of organ tissues, disease, medical therapeutics, heritability, and behavior and lifestyle choices of the individual (Chapter 49). The declines in nutrient consumption and activity level that often accompany older age are possibly modifiable contributors to the loss of muscle mass. An accelerated loss of muscle mass can occur when a serious illness requires treatment with steroids or other antianabolic drugs or is accompanied by low nutrient intake and the need for prolonged bed rest.

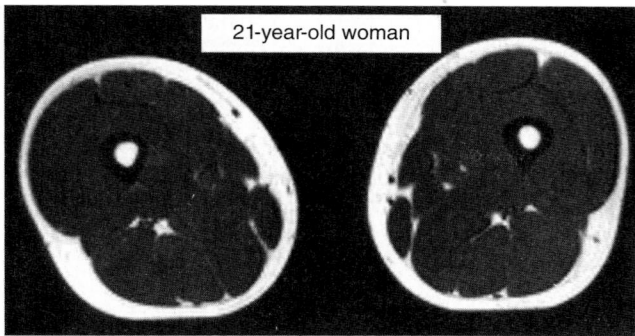

21-year-old woman

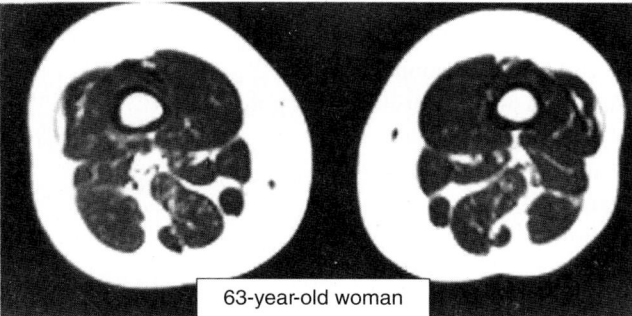

63-year-old woman

FIGURE 30-2. Cross-sectional computed tomography images of the midthighs of a younger and an older woman demonstrating the decline in muscle mass and relative increase in fat mass with age.

TABLE 30-1 ■ FACTORS CONTRIBUTING TO INADEQUATE NUTRITION IN OLDER ADULTS	
SOCIOECONOMIC	**PHYSIOLOGIC**
Fixed income	Impaired strength/aerobic capacity
Reduced access to food	
Social isolation	Impaired mobility/dexterity (arthritis, stroke)
Inadequate storage facilities	Impaired sensory input (smell, taste, sight)
Inadequate cooking facilities	Poor dentition/oral health
Poor knowledge of nutrition	Malabsorption
Dependence on others	Chronic illness (via anorexia, altered metabolism)
Caretakers	Alcohol
Institutions	Drugs (**Table 30-2**)
PSYCHOLOGICAL	**ACUTE ILLNESS/ HOSPITALIZATION**
Depression	Failure to monitor dietary intake and record weights
Bereavement	Failure to consider increased metabolic requirements
Anxiety, fear, paranoia	
Dementia	Iatrogenic starvation (eg, NPO[a] for diagnostic tests)
	Delay in instituting nutritional support

[a]Nothing by mouth.

The loss of muscle mass with age is closely linked with a reduction in muscle strength and exercise capacity, which contribute to functional impairments and disability as well as to the development of CHD, diabetes mellitus, and other diseases that can contribute to further decline in a vicious cycle leading to frailty (see Chapter 42).

In parallel with the loss of LBM, there is an increase in the relative amount and the distribution of body fat with advancing age. Between the second and ninth decades of life, the percentage of body weight that is fat increases by 35% to 50% in women and to an even greater extent in men. Whether or not total body weight changes, intra-abdominal (visceral) fat increases quantitatively and proportionally more than peripheral fat mass. In females, the accumulation of intra-abdominal fat accelerates at menopause and represents primarily a shift from peripheral sites. In males, the increase in intra-abdominal fat with age represents primarily an increase in total body fat mass. For a given waist circumference, older adults have greater visceral fat than young adults, and men have greater visceral and less subcutaneous fat than women.

Changes in Appetite and Energy Intake Regulation

Maintenance of a stable weight requires a steady balance between nutrient intake and energy expenditure. With advancing age, the metabolic, neural, and humoral pathways that normally maintain this delicate balance by regulating appetite and hunger begin to lose their compensatory responsiveness to changes in energy demands. Psychological, socioeconomic, and cultural influences and numerous disease processes further contribute to the dysregulation (**Table 30-1**). From the third to seventh decade of life, these factors integrate to create an imbalance usually favoring a tendency toward weight gain and increased fat deposition, at least in societies where food is plentiful and the physical demands of life are light. However, after age 70, the risk of losing weight increases steadily with each year of survival. Loss of body weight correlates with low dietary energy intake, which is common among both healthy and frail older adults. The late-life weight decline is associated with many chronic conditions that increase risk of death in old age, including Alzheimer disease.

Pathophysiologic Changes that Lead to Loss of Taste, Smell, and Appetite with Advancing Age

Numerous pathologic and age-related physiologic changes can have a deleterious effect on eating habits and the likelihood of maintaining an adequate diet (see **Table 30-1**). This can include deterioration in sight, olfactory function, taste sensation, or ability to feel the temperature and texture of food in the mouth, all of which can contribute to a diminished appetite. Even healthy older individuals experience

TABLE 30-2 ■ CLASSES OF MEDICATIONS THAT CAN SUPPRESS APPETITE AND ALTER OLFACTORY FUNCTION[a]

Antidepressants

Antiinflammatories

Antihypertensives and other cardiac medications

Lipid-lowering drugs

Antihistamines

Antimicrobials

Antineoplastics

Bronchodilators and other asthma medications

Muscle relaxants

Drugs for the treatment of parkinsonism

Anticonvulsants

Vasodilators

[a]Numerous drugs in each category can alter appetite and olfactory function.

TABLE 30-3 ■ HORMONES AND CHEMICALS THAT MAY PLAY A ROLE IN APPETITE AND OBESITY

Adiponectin

Amylin

Cholecystokinin (CCK)

Cholesterol and other lipid fractions

Estrogen

Gastrin

Gastrin-releasing peptide (GRP)

Ghrelin

Glucagon

Glucagon-like peptide 1 (GLP-1)

Glucocorticoid hormones

Glucose-dependent insulinotropic polypeptide (GIP)

Growth hormone

Guanylin

Insulin

Leptin

Motilin

Neurotensin

Nonesterified fatty acids (NEFAs)

Oxyntomodulin

Pancreatic polypeptide

Peptide YY

Proopiomelanocortin

Secretin

Serotonin

Sex hormone–binding globulin (SHBG)

Somatostatin

Substance P

Testosterone

Thyroid hormones

Triacylglycerol

Vasoactive intestinal polypeptide (VIP)

such changes. Much greater losses in taste and smell occur in association with medication usage and other health-related concerns. **Table 30-2** contains a representative listing of medications that can cause appetite suppression and losses of olfactory function and taste sensation. Poor oral health (Chapter 32) and many diseases that decrease mastication, salivary flow, or ability to swallow (Chapter 31) can also lead to deterioration in taste and smell to adversely affect appetite.

In addition to the special senses, there are various neural and humoral pathways within the gut that may change with advanced age and possibly contribute to the inability of many older individuals to adequately regulate food intake. There are also large numbers of hormones and other gut-derived substances that are thought to influence appetite and food metabolism, as shown in **Table 30-3**. It is theorized that age-related changes in some or all of these substances may adversely affect food intake in older adults.

Psychological, Socioeconomic, and Cultural Influences on Appetite

After the seventh decade of life, psychological, socioeconomic, and cultural factors are increasingly important for an adequate diet (see **Table 30-1**). Depression is a highly prevalent, frequently unrecognized, and potentially treatable cause of a poor appetite and weight loss. Similarly, bereavement is associated with a lack of appetite. Eating alone may be associated with a lower energy intake, and the presence of family and close friends leads to greater nutrient intake. Within institutional settings, particularly nursing homes, physical environment and ambience within the dining areas are known to affect appetite and can often be improved. Elimination of therapeutic diets (eg, low salt or low cholesterol) may also be of benefit. Such restricted diets often make meals much less appetizing for the older residents and may add little to disease management. For these reasons, the American Dietetic Association in collaboration with the Centers for Medicare and Medicaid Services, Pioneer Network, and others published a position statement suggesting that use of therapeutic diets in nursing homes be restricted.

OBESITY

Definition and Prevalence

Obesity is defined as an unhealthy accumulation of body fat, which leads to a higher risk of medical illness and premature death. Although not ideal, body mass index (BMI) and waist circumference are the most widely utilized metrics for classifying overweight and obesity. Both are easily obtained and highly validated measures. BMI is calculated as body weight in kilograms divided by height in meters squared (kg/m^2), while waist circumference is a direct measure obtained halfway between the iliac crest and the lower anterior ribs, with the individual standing, and at the end of expiration.

The definition of body weight categories does not currently vary by age or race. Normal weight is considered to be a BMI between 19 and 25; overweight, a BMI of 25 to less than 30; and obesity, a BMI of 30 or more. Waist circumference is used as an index of central/abdominal adiposity and is clinically useful in further categorizing an individual based on cardiometabolic risk. Traditionally, abdominal obesity is defined as a waist circumference 89 cm (35 inches) or more for women and 102 cm (40 inches) or more for men. A waist-to-hip ratio greater than 1.0 in men and 0.8 in women is another indicator of central obesity. As with BMI, there is controversy as to whether different reference ranges should be used depending on age and ethnicity. While overweight consistently increases morbidity risk in old age, the data on mortality are less consistent, suggesting that guidelines for both BMI and waist circumference should be liberalized for older individuals.

Based on National Health and Nutrition Examination Survey (NHANES) data and current definitions, obesity is highly prevalent among older adults, especially the young old (ie, individuals between the ages of 65 and 80 years). The variability in rates of obesity by race, gender, and age is shown in **Figure 30-3**. In all race-by-gender groups, the prevalence declines steadily with each decade of life after age 70. In part, this may be a cohort effect. Reflecting trends for the nation as a whole, prevalence rates of obesity in older adults increased significantly between 1999 and 2010, especially among men (see **Figure 30-4**). It was only among the oldest-old, those older than 80 years, that the prevalence remained stable during this time.

Potential Benefits and Adverse Consequences of Obesity

There is controversy regarding the potential benefits and adverse consequences of being overweight or obese after age 65. Potential benefits include protection against bone fractures and a possible survival advantage, at least for select populations of older adults. The lower fracture risk is related to increased fat mass: obese older adults place more stress on their bones and convert more androstenedione to estrone than do slimmer individuals of similar age. Both of these factors contribute to increased BMD. Fat also can also serve as a cushion to protect against the impact of a fall, creating further protection against bone fractures.

Assessing the impact of weight on survival in old age is more complex. Overweight and obese older adults may have a survival advantage during periods of protracted illness, an effect thought to be the result of their greater energy and protein reserves. In general, obesity is associated with greater lean mass; during periods of catabolic stress, the fat and lean mass serve as a functional nutritional reserve.

The impact of obesity on survival in the general population of community-residing older adults usually shows a "J-shaped" relationship (**Figure 30-5**). There is a consistent higher mortality with a BMI less than 19. However, this does not necessarily indicate that older

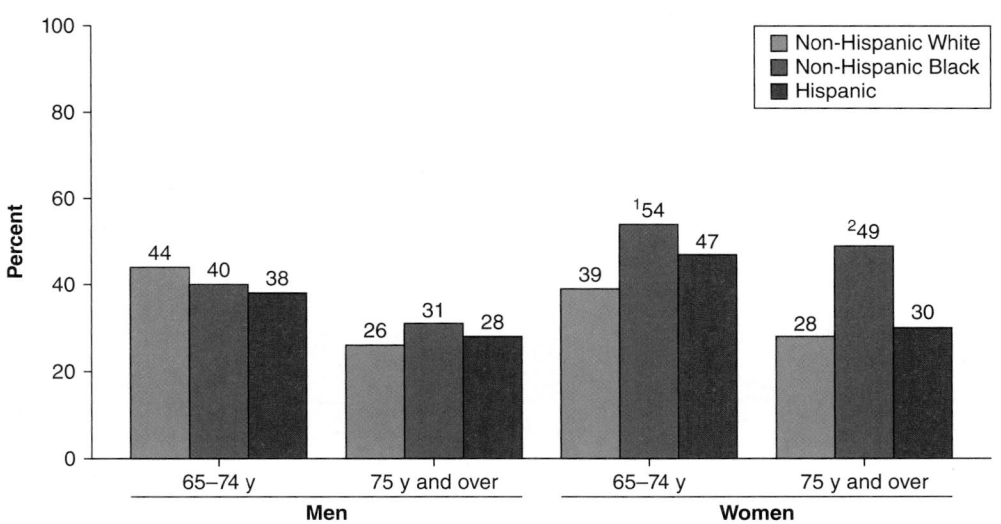

[1]Significantly different from non-Hispanic White.
[2]Significantly different from non-Hispanic White and Hispanic.

FIGURE 30-3. Prevalence of obesity among adults age 65 and over by sex and race/ethnicity: United States, 2007–2010. (Reproduced with permission from the National Center for Health Statistics Data Brief No. 106, September 2012, Centers for Disease Control and Prevention, U.S. Department of Health and Human Services.)

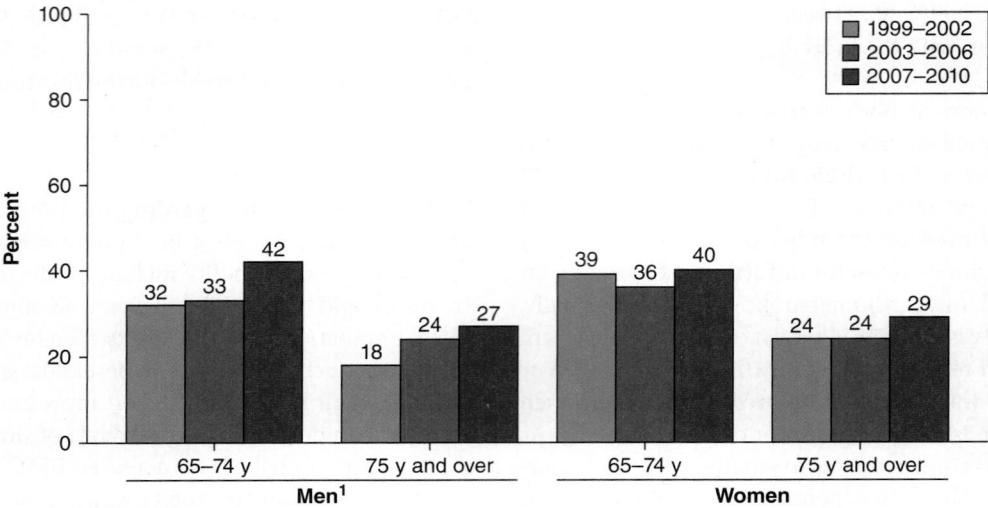

¹Significantly linear trend.

FIGURE 30-4. Trends in the prevalence of obesity among adults age 65 and over by sex: United States, 1999–2010. (Reproduced with permission from the National Center for Health Statistics Data Brief No. 106, September 2012, Centers for Disease Control and Prevention, U.S. Department of Health and Human Services.)

adults who have been slender all of their lives are at increased risk of mortality. Rather, the higher mortality probably reflects recently lost weight due to disease in many older adults with a low BMI. However, low protein reserves, whether the result of weight loss or a thinner body habitus, may be the critical factor that is contributing to risk of death in older adults with a low BMI.

Due to the heterogeneity of various study results, it is unclear what range of BMI is optimal for survival and at what level of obesity all-cause mortality risk begins to increase. However, when different methodologic approaches are used, which in some cases include controlling for cohort mortality and age-related survey selection bias, all-cause mortality appears to increase in direct relationship with BMI in the

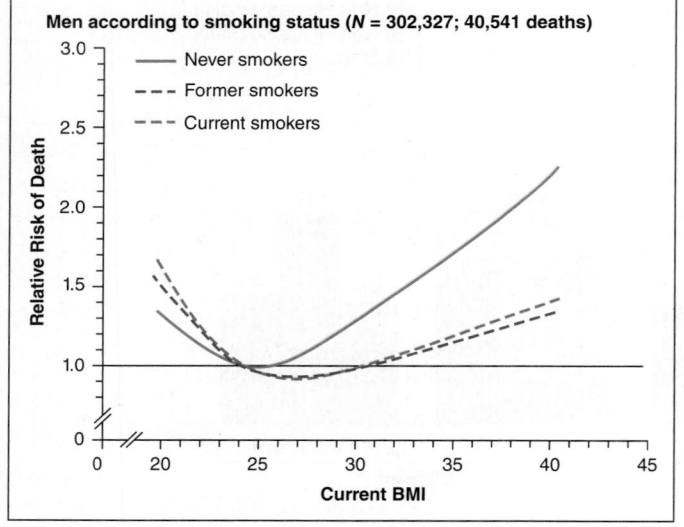
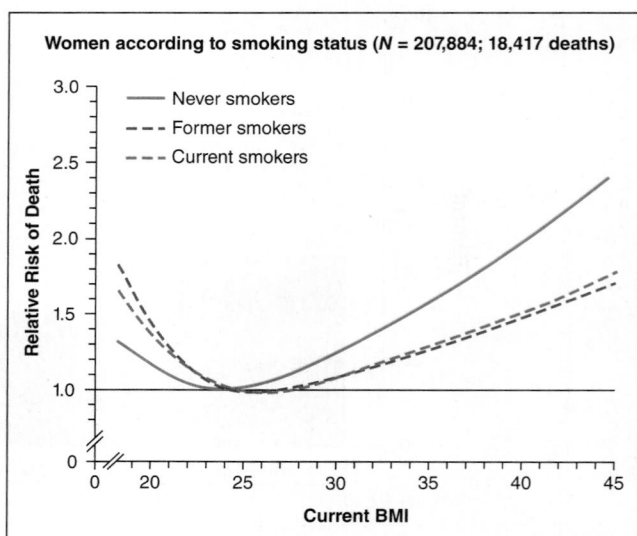

FIGURE 30-5. Data from the National Institutes of Health-AARP cohort age 50 to 71 years and followed for a maximum of 10 years. Men (left) and women (right) shown by smoking status in relation to their current BMI. Risks for never smokers are thought to most accurately estimate risk because they remove the effect of smoking on body weight and risk of death. Data adjusted for age, race or ethnic group, level of education, alcohol consumption, and physical activity.

range of 25 to more than 40. Further complicating the issue, mortality risk in old age may relate to fat distribution as well as total body mass. For any given body weight, mortality risk increases with increasing waist circumference, or more specifically, increasing intra-abdominal or visceral fat mass as measured by modern imaging modalities. Although waist circumference is strongly correlated with intra-abdominal fat mass, the two metrics are not the same, and direct measures of intra-abdominal fat are more powerful indictors of cardiovascular (CV) risk. However, the mortality risk associated with obesity after controlling for intra-abdominal fat mass is also controversial. Given the many uncertainties about the impact of obesity on overall survival, it is important to consider what other effects excess weight has on the health of older adults.

Weight-Associated Morbidity

The impact of obesity on overall health, functional status, and quality of life in older adults is more certain. Overweight in old age is associated with the same risks for disease as in younger populations, and it also exacerbates many age-associated diseases (**Table 30-4**). In addition to the detrimental metabolic effects of excess body fat, there are adverse mechanical consequences. For example, a relative excess in total body weight to muscle mass leads to osteoarthritis and other disabling conditions while increasing the work required to perform many activities of daily living. The result is a lower functional reserve, chronic

TABLE 30-4 ■ DISORDERS DIRECTLY CAUSED OR EXACERBATED BY OBESITY

Atherosclerotic cerebrovascular disease and stroke
Depression
Hypoventilation/obstructive sleep apnea
Pulmonary hypertension
Heart failure
Coronary heart disease
Peripheral vascular disease
Metabolic syndrome
Varicose veins/venous insufficiency
Hypertension
Dyslipidemia
Type 2 diabetes
Fatty liver diseases
Cholelithiasis
Various forms of cancer
Skin problems
Degenerative disease of large joints
Back pain
Degenerative disc disease
Urinary incontinence
Postoperative complications

pain, and an increased risk of disability. Some heavier individuals have relatively less muscle mass than expected on the basis of size, a situation described as sarcopenic obesity (see Chapter 49); for these individuals, the risk of disability is especially high.

Because of its contribution to many age-related diseases that lead to deterioration in central or peripheral nervous system, cardiopulmonary, or musculoskeletal function, obesity is a major risk factor for functional disability with advancing age. As a result of both these diseases and the treatments required for their control, obese older adults are far more likely to develop physical impairments or disabilities than are other older adults. Obesity also makes it more challenging to obtain the needed level of care when disabled, all of which can lead to a deterioration in quality of life.

Interventions Targeting Obesity

Given the increased risk of disability associated with obesity, controlled weight loss may be an appropriate therapeutic option for selected older adults. Short-term clinical trials in older people show that appropriate interventions can lead to moderate weight loss, resulting in improvements in CV risk factors (such as hypertension, insulin resistance, and metabolic syndrome) and other clinical outcomes. However, weight loss could produce more long-term adverse than beneficial results in some older adults. In fact, there is a strong association between weight loss in older adults and an increased risk of subsequent adverse clinical outcomes such as hospitalization and death. Even when trying to control for voluntary versus involuntary weight loss, there have been conflicting findings. Furthermore, when dietary restriction is the primary mechanism for weight loss, the loss of fat is accompanied by loss of both LBM (particularly skeletal muscle mass) and BMD. Although the percentage loss from each of these tissue compartments with dieting is the same in old and young adults, the adverse consequences could be much greater in older people who have lower functional reserves and higher fracture risk. This is particularly true for older people with sarcopenic obesity, as even a small further loss of muscle mass might cause significant functional impairment.

Thus, a primary focus of any weight loss intervention in older adults should be on preserving or improving LBM and BMD. The only approach to date that has proven successful in accomplishing this dual-purpose goal is the combination of an energy-restricted, normal to high-protein diet with moderate-to-intense exercise (also see Chapter 54). In obese older adults, diet and exercise together can lead to clinically meaningful improvements in key metabolic parameters, physical performance, self-reported physical function, and quality of life; the beneficial effects are greater and the loss of both BMD and LBM less than with either intervention alone. To attain these benefits, only moderate weight loss (in the range of 10%) is required. The target of the weight loss should be improvement in the target weight-related health conditions.

Although randomized, controlled trials provide strong evidence of benefit, little is known about how best to achieve these results with obese older adults in routine clinical settings. Efforts to increase physical activity and to decrease caloric intake are the best options for older adults, as surgical and pharmacological options are limited, usually untested in this population, and generally much riskier. Selective glucagon-like peptide (GLP)-1 receptor agonists such as semaglutide (approved for weight loss by the Food and Drug Administration [FDA] in 2021) and most recently a dual GLP-1 receptor and glucose-dependent insulinotropic peptide agonist have been used effectively to promote weight loss in overweight adults both with and without type 2 diabetes. However, the safety and effectiveness of these agents to promote weight loss while preserving LBM, bone mass, and physical function in specific subpopulations of older adults remain to be determined. In the absence of relevant long-term clinical trial data on outcomes with weight reduction, advice on weight loss should be guided by symptoms related to obesity and its associated diseases, anticipated short-term health benefits, and the general level of health status of the patient.

To be considered a candidate for a weight loss program, an obese older adult needs to have a weight-related problem that is likely amenable to weight loss plus the motivation to commit to the necessary lifestyle changes that are required to meet program goals. In order to have any lasting benefits, changes in dietary habits and level of physical activity need to be maintained long-term. Such a vigorous program would likely require the individual patient to be relatively healthy.

Components of a Weight Loss Program for Older Adults

Upon committing to a weight loss program, an older adult should undergo a careful medical evaluation, which should include a detailed history and physical examination as well as a very careful assessment of the potential risks and benefits of both exercise and diet. American College of Sports Medicine guidelines (see Chapter 54) should be used to assess the risks of exercise and need for more detailed diagnostic testing such as cardiac stress tests. Successful programs generally include an assessment of the individual's insight, motivation, and readiness to make the necessary lifestyle changes. Using motivational interviewing or other techniques, the individual's personal goals should be illuminated, and a personalized intervention strategy devised that includes short- and long-term goals and timelines. Support from or coparticipation by family and significant others can be critical to success.

Ideally, both the dietary and exercise interventions need to be consistent with the individual's lifestyle, abilities, interests, and personal goals. When an established program is not available to which the individual can be referred, input and support from a multidisciplinary team of professionals is crucial. Such a team may include a dietitian/nutritionist, physical therapist, nurse, physician, social worker, or other health professionals. The diet should include at least 1.0 g/kg/day of high quality protein, adequate micronutrients, and only moderate energy restriction (eg, 1100–1300 kcal/day) with the goal of 1 to 2 pounds of weight loss or less in a week. The exercise intervention should include a combination of endurance and progressive-resistance muscle strength training and be tailored to the individual (see Chapter 54 for details).

Once an obese older adult starts an exercise/weight loss program, the quality and frequency of follow-up support become crucial. Early in the intervention, frequent follow-up is often needed, but the intervals between contacts can be gradually extended once the individual demonstrates an acceptable trajectory of success. Follow-up can be accomplished by recurring clinic visits, phone calls, or any of a variety of electronic means. These follow-up visits can be used to monitor progress (eg, checking exercise and weight logs), provide ongoing support and assistance to deal with setbacks and barriers to success, and provide guidance in advancing exercise intensity or setting new goals. The level of involvement of a nurse or other appropriately trained health professional in the follow-up assessments needs to be determined based on the medical complexity of the participant.

NUTRIENT REQUIREMENTS TO MAINTAIN HEALTH

Energy

Daily energy requirements per kilogram of body weight generally decline with age, dropping as much as 33% between the third and ninth decade of life. Male gender and chronic disease are associated with a greater rate of decline. However, a decrease in energy requirements with age occurs even among those who remain healthy, in part because of the age-related loss of muscle mass described above. Muscle is much more metabolically active than adipose tissue. As muscle mass decrease the ratio of fat to lean mass increases, leading to a greater drop in the basal or resting metabolic rate (RMR) than predicted by the decrease in total body mass. Since RMR generally accounts for 60% to 75% of TEE, the end result of the muscle loss is a significant decline in TEE, and thus energy requirements.

A second mechanism accounting for the decline in energy requirements with age is a decrease in physical activity. Energy expenditure of physical activity (EEA) generally declines with age to the same extent as RMR, accounting for about 15% to 35% of TEE in the majority of older adults. However, EEA can range from 5% in those who are bedridden to 50% in highly active, physically fit older adults. Lifestyle plays a big role in determining EEA of older people, just as it does in those who are younger. Although the increased prevalence of chronic disabling diseases accounts for some of the decline in physical activity with advancing age, even healthy older adults tend to be more sedentary than younger individuals.

Some chronic conditions may result in an increased TEE, although this remains controversial. Examples include individuals with Alzheimer disease who constantly pace and individuals with a constant tremor. Even when an individual appears to be rather sedentary, their EEA may be greater than expected. For example, a patient with hemiparesis or amputation likely requires high levels of energy expenditure to complete basic activities of daily living due to low neuromuscular energy efficiency.

The usual decline in energy requirements with advancing age means that many older persons need to consume less food in order to maintain their weight and customary activity level. This places the older individual at risk of developing protein and micronutrient deficiencies, since requirements for other nutrients may not decrease as much as energy. Consequently, it is important that older individuals increase their activity level and change their diet to protein- and micronutrient-rich foods.

Protein

Because of the paucity of high-quality nutrition studies with adequate representation from older age groups, current recommendations for protein intake do not differentiate adults over the age of 65 from those who are younger. The latest (2005) version of the Recommended Dietary Allowance (RDA) for protein, released by the Food and Nutrition Board and the National Academy of Medicine, is 0.8 g/kg body weight/day for both men and women over age 19. However, some contend that the recommended protein intake for older adults should be 1.0 to 1.25 g/kg/day. Given the variability in estimates of protein requirements in older adults, it may not be possible to resolve this controversy until better measurement techniques become available.

Factors That Influence the Protein Requirements of Older Individuals

The protein requirements of an individual can change with time, being influenced by age, nonprotein content of the diet, activity level, medications, and health status. The energy content of the diet is particularly important. The protein intake required to maintain nitrogen balance increases the further total energy intake falls below 126 kJ/kg (30 kcal/kg). A negative energy balance usually precipitates a negative nitrogen balance, especially in individuals who are ill or who have a low level of activity. As a general rule, protein requirements increase with high levels of activity such as sustained high-intensity exercise. Thus, the role of a high protein diet, perhaps combined with resistance training, to prevent loss of LBM in older obese individuals during voluntary caloric restriction and increased physical activity to achieve weight loss (as described above) merits further study.

Many disease states and medications can induce a catabolic state for protein by altering the normal balance between protein synthesis and degradation. Older individuals who are both confined to bed and have an injury, infection, or another acute inflammatory condition are at particularly high risk of developing a profoundly negative nitrogen balance that can lead to a rapid loss of LBM, particularly skeletal muscle mass. High doses of corticosteroids can have a similar effect. The amount of protein that needs to be consumed in order to minimize loss of LBM and optimize recovery from such disease states is often difficult to determine. In general, older hospitalized patients who are acutely ill or recovering from major surgery or trauma warrant a protein intake of 1.5 g/kg of body weight/day or higher (also see discussion of Malnutrition below and **Table 30-9**) unless they have a condition that necessitates protein restriction such as renal or hepatic insufficiency. Whether one source of protein is better than another in meeting the nutrient needs of older adults is controversial. Although it is generally recognized that all older adults should consume a diet that provides adequate quantities of all essential amino acids, there is otherwise little consensus as to the importance of the dietary protein source.

Fat and Cholesterol

Fat serves as a key source of energy and essential fatty acids as well as a vehicle for transporting fat-soluble vitamins. Even when obesity and elevated cholesterol or triglycerides are a concern, fat intake should not fall below 10% of total energy requirements in order to allow for adequate absorption of fat soluble vitamins (A, D, E, K), and to ensure that the requirements for the essential fatty acids are met. There are two main types of essential fatty acids, the omega-6 series, derived from linoleic acid (eg, arachidonic acid and gamma-linoleic acid), and the omega-3 series, which could be derived from alpha-linolenic acid (from plant sources) or contained in krill oils or certain cold water fish (eg, eicosapentaenoic acid [EPA] and docosahexaenoic acid [DHA]); the omega-3 fatty acids obtained from fish are synthesized by microalgae, which the fish consume. The essential fatty acids are required for the synthesis of cell membrane phospholipids and eicosanoids, which include prostaglandins, leukotrienes, and hydroxy acids. Cell membrane phospholipids influence the biomechanical properties of the membranes and their membrane-bound receptors. The eicosanoids, derived predominantly from arachidonic acid and EPA, serve many functions including modulation of inflammation and host defenses. The eicosanoids made from omega-6s are generally more potent mediators of inflammation, vasoconstriction, and platelet aggregation.

Clinical deficiency of the essential fatty acids is rarely seen in adults since western diets generally include adequate amounts of these nutrients, and adipose tissue provides an additional reserve of 0.5 to 1 kg. When a deficiency does develop, it is usually a result of profound cachexia or extensive small bowel disease or necrosis and the inadequate provision of nutrition support. This is particularly true of the omega-6 fatty acids, which are abundant in many of the foods common to the average American diet including most vegetable oils, nuts, cereals, seeds, and legumes.

In contrast, the average American diet may provide suboptimal amounts of omega-3 fatty acids. Although current recommendations call for the omega-3 derivatives of alpha-linolenic acid to be at least 0.2 % of total food energy, many nutritionists suggest higher intakes due to their purported beneficial effects on metabolism. Oils from a variety of cold water fish species including halibut, mackerel, herring, and salmon are potentially high in the omega-3 fatty acids. Currently, nutritional labeling does not indicate the amount of omega-3 fatty acids that is contained in fresh fish; farm-raised fish may have more or less omega-3 fatty acids than wild caught fish, depending on the food they are fed. Many omega-3 fatty acid supplements are available commercially, but these provide varying amounts of marine-based EPA and DHA. There is inadequate evidence that these supplements provide the same benefits as consuming fish. Alpha-linolenic acid, a precursor of EPA, is found primarily in plant products such as soybeans, canola oil, flaxseed oil, and walnut oil. However, humans may be able to convert as little as 10% of alpha-linolenic acid to EPA.

The optimal fat intake for older adults needs to be determined on an individual basis. For example, reduced fat intake may be considered for a patient with CHD. However, the importance of dietary fat as a contributor to CHD risk after the age of 65 remains controversial. It is not known whether fat- and cholesterol-restricted diets have any beneficial effects in reducing CHD mortality in this age group. In fact, such diets may have detrimental consequences, especially in those who are having problems maintaining their weight. Therefore, it seems prudent to limit fat intake only in older individuals with CHD who otherwise would not be adversely affected by such dietary restrictions.

Increasing the ratio of monounsaturated and polyunsaturated fat to saturated fat, without changing total fat intake, may be beneficial in some situations. For this reason, some experts support the use of the Mediterranean-style diet, which promotes the use of olive oil, tree nuts, peanuts, fatty fish and other seafood, and white meat, and discourages intake of red and processed meats. Concern has also been raised about the use of partially hydrogenated fats rich in trans fatty acids, as these products may have an adverse effect on lipid metabolism. Although more study is needed, it is probably prudent to emphasize the use of natural fats derived from vegetable oils (predominantly monounsaturated), nuts, and fish while reducing those from animal products and avoiding foods containing trans fatty acids. However, this approach may not be applicable to frail older individuals, especially those who are losing weight involuntarily, have a BMI less than 20, or have diseases limiting their nutrient intake. Since fats have twice the energy content per gram as carbohydrates and protein, a diet high in fat may be necessary for such frail older individuals in order to meet their maintenance energy requirements or to replete deficits. Thus, restricting the types of foods these individuals consume may have detrimental consequences.

Carbohydrates

Recommendations for carbohydrate content of the diet are generally based on two considerations, the source of the carbohydrates and the energy requirements of the individual. Ideally, food sources should be rich in fiber (see section on fiber content of diet below) and provide primarily complex carbohydrates rather than simple sugars. The amount of carbohydrates that should be included in the diet is usually determined by default. The energy, protein, and fat requirements of the individual are determined first. Carbohydrate requirements are then determined by subtracting the amount of energy supplied by protein and fat from the total energy requirements. Since protein requirements represent approximately 15% of the total energy content of the diet and fat ideally should be less than 30%, carbohydrates usually represent 55% to 70% of the total. When carbohydrates are totally excluded from the diet, energy requirements of the body are partially met by the incomplete oxidation of fatty acids, which leads to ketosis and may cause lethargy and depression. Ketosis can also contribute to anorexia, which is part of the appeal of high-fat, low-carbohydrate weight loss diets. To prevent ketosis, at least 50 to 100 g of carbohydrates should be consumed each day.

Water

Although fluid requirements do not change appreciably with age in adults, people over the age of 65 have a reduced ability to regulate their fluid intake and to limit urinary water losses. Thus, they are much more likely than young adults to become dehydrated (and hypernatremic) when their health status or environment changes. Regulation of water and sodium balance in older people, and recognition and management of dehydration/hypernatremia are reviewed in Chapter 39. Chronic disease and injuries that cause a deterioration of cognitive or physical function increase the risk of dehydration further by altering the perception of thirst, reducing the ability to express the desire for water, or diminishing the capability to access and drink adequate amounts of fluids. When an acute febrile illness occurs in an older individual who is already physically or cognitively impaired, life-threatening dehydration can develop rapidly. This scenario occurs with alarming frequency in nursing homes. The failure of many health care providers, family members, and personal aid assistants to recognize the risk factors and early warning signs of dehydration contributes to the danger that a frail older individual will become severely dehydrated. Many older adults themselves do not recognize their risks and may inappropriately restrict their fluid intake, sometimes as a method of controlling incontinence.

Care must be taken to prevent dehydration by recognizing those at highest risk, especially older individuals with cognitive and physical deficits, swallowing problems, ongoing weight loss, diarrhea, fever, or poorly controlled diabetes, or receiving enteral feeding, diuretics, or laxatives. The minimum daily intake for inactive adults in moderate climates is estimated to be between 1 and 3 L/day; a reasonable target is roughly 30 mL/kg/day for most healthy older adults. Requirements increase with fever, activity, or prolonged exposure to an elevated environmental temperature (also see Chapter 39). Patients, family, and all health care staff, especially in nursing homes, need to be trained to recognize the importance of maintaining an adequate fluid intake at all times, and to carefully monitor intake if there is a change in mental status, activity level, or health status, or if fluid requirements increase, as may occur during heat waves.

Fiber

Dietary fiber is derived from structural components of plant cell walls and consists of plant polysaccharides and lignin, which are resistant to digestion by intestinal enzymes. Many professional health organizations recommend a diet containing 20 to 35 grams of fiber a day or 10 to 13 grams dietary fiber per 1000 kcal consumed. Although dietary fiber may be associated with health benefits including a decreased rate of certain forms of cancer, diabetes, heart disease, and obesity, the average American diet is very low in fiber with consumption usually in the range of only 10 to 15 grams daily.

There are two general categories of dietary fiber: water-insoluble fibers, such as cellulose, hemicellulose, and lignin; and water-soluble fibers, such as gum and pectin. Each category of fiber has a somewhat different spectrum of beneficial effects. Both types lower the energy density of the diet. The added bulk also has a short-term satiety effect that helps control appetite and prevent overconsumption. Water-insoluble fiber has the further effect of holding water within the intestinal contents, which results in an increased fecal bulk, a decreased gut transit time, and a lower intraluminal pressure within the colon. These properties of water-insoluble fiber make it an important dietary component since it reduces constipation and may help prevent the formation of colonic diverticula. Sources of insoluble fiber include fruits, vegetables, dried beans, wheat bran, seeds, popcorn, brown rice, and whole grain products such as breads, cereals, and pasta. About two-thirds to three-fourths of the dietary fiber in typical mixed-food diets is water-insoluble. There are many excellent web sites that provide tables listing the soluble and insoluble fiber content of foods (eg, https://www.helpguide.org/articles/healthy-eating/high-fiber-foods.htm; https://www.medicalnewstoday.com/articles/146935#recommended-intake; https://www.northottawawellnessfoundation.org/wp-content/uploads/2017/11/NOWF-Fiber-Content-of-Foods.pdf).

Water-soluble fiber increases the viscosity of intestinal contents, prolongs gut transit time, and decreases the rate of small intestinal absorption of carbohydrates and bile acids. These effects may have important physiologic implications that can be used to advantage clinically. By slowing the rate of carbohydrate absorption, a very high soluble-fiber diet can be effective in reducing the postprandial surge in the serum glucose, which may be beneficial in the treatment and prevention of diabetes. Through its effects on bile acid absorption, soluble fibers can lower total cholesterol and low-density lipoprotein (LDL) cholesterol by 3% to 10%. There is an inverse association between the total dietary fiber intake and the rate of fatal and nonfatal myocardial infarctions; several meta-analyses demonstrate that higher intake is also associated with decreased all-cause mortality. Most of these effects of soluble fibers were demonstrated using fiber concentrates. Comparable amounts of fiber can be obtained from food sources, such as apples, oranges, pears, peaches, grapes, vegetables, seeds, oat and rice bran, dried beans, oatmeal, barley, and rye. Diets that are high in fiber from food sources also provide essential micronutrients and nonnutritive compounds such as xenobiotics, antioxidants, and phytoestrogens that may have important health-promoting consequences.

As a general rule, a diet rich in fresh fruits, vegetables, legumes, and whole grain products is recommended. As portrayed in the USDA Choosemyplate.gov, this should include two cups of fruit, 2 1/2 cups of vegetables, and 6 ounces of grains each day (**Figure 30-6**). Since most fruits and vegetables contain less than 2 grams/serving total fiber and most refined grain products contain less than 1 gram/serving, legumes, whole grains, and cereal brans should be substituted for other foods whenever possible in order to increase the amount of both kinds of fiber. Supplementing the diet with any of the commercially available concentrated fiber sources may be necessary, especially in frail older people. Concentrated sources of dietary fiber may also be helpful in the treatment of chronic constipation when a limited variety of food is available or the amount of food consumed

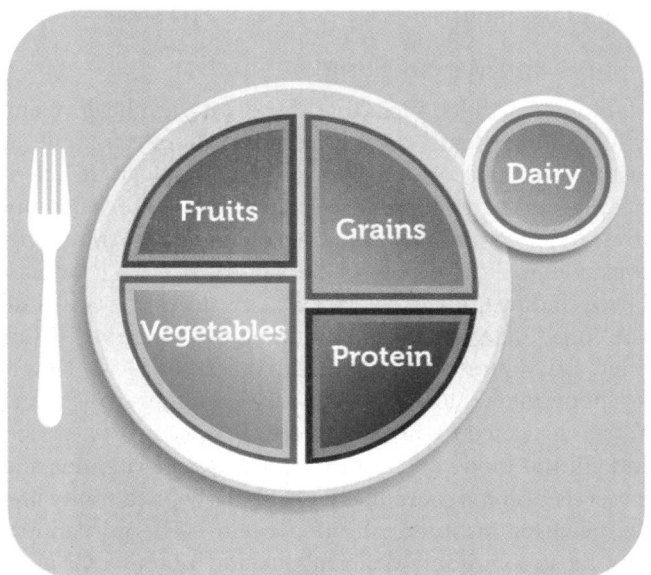

FIGURE 30-6. ChooseMyPlate.gov, U.S. Department of Agriculture, Center for Nutrition Policy and Promotion, June 2, 2011, USDA Center for Nutrition Policy & Promotion (CNPP). (Reproduced with permission from http://choosemyplate.gov/.)

is inadequate. A large increase in fiber over a short period of time may result in bloating, diarrhea, gas, and general discomfort. It is important to add fiber gradually over a period of several weeks to avoid abdominal problems. Fiber supplements should always be taken with adequate fluid in order to avoid worsening constipation.

VITAMINS AND MINERALS

Recommended Intakes

The Food and Nutrition Board of the US National Research Council developed the dietary reference intakes (DRIs), which updated the earlier RDAs for vitamins and minerals. The DRIs include separate intake recommendations for adults from age 51 through 70, and for adults older than 70 years. There are not enough scientific data to calculate requirements for all micronutrients, and any person with a medical disorder may need more or less than the DRI for some nutrients. **Table 30-5** lists the recommended intakes for various vitamins, as well as the recommended tolerable upper limits (ULs) intake. Intakes of micronutrients that are lower than the UL usually pose little risk for toxic side effects in healthy people. The UL allows patients and health care workers to understand possible risks if large amounts of vitamins and minerals are consumed. Understanding and consuming the DRI for vitamins and minerals reduces the risk for classic deficiency disorders (eg, scurvy, pellagra, beriberi, etc), but the ideal intake of vitamins and minerals needed for optimum health, which may be higher than the DRIs or ULs, remains controversial. Changes to the DRIs are often contentious, and they can have major medicolegal and financial implications for fortified foods and the supplement/ health food industry.

Vitamin and Mineral Supplementation

Many older adults, including those who are healthy and living independently as well as those who are frail, ill, or institutionalized, are at risk for micronutrient deficiencies. Several population-based nutritional surveys demonstrate that community-dwelling older adults commonly consume as little as 50% of the DRIs for many vitamins. These findings reflect the fact that even healthy adults do not consistently consume recommended amounts of fortified dairy products, fruits, and vegetables. Risk factors for poor intake, adverse drug-nutrient interactions, and nutrition-related diseases all increase as a function of age, and clinical (and subclinical) deficiencies of vitamins and minerals become more likely, particularly once frailty and the need for institutionalization occurs. The micronutrients most commonly deficient include vitamins C, D, E, B_{12}, thiamine (B_1), and folic acid, and the minerals calcium, magnesium, and zinc. Because of this, many nutritionists recommend that older adults add a daily, iron-free, general vitamin and mineral supplement supplying the DRI for

most micronutrients, although evidence in support of benefit from this recommendation is lacking. Studies of multivitamin supplementation in noninstitutionalized people have found no benefit in reducing CV or cancer risk. It also remains unclear as to whether intakes of individual micronutrients above the DRI in selected populations are beneficial. High intakes of some micronutrients (such as vitamins A, D, and pyridoxine) are well known to cause toxicity, which may be so subtle and nonspecific that the harmful effects may not be easily diagnosed. High supplemental intakes of other vitamins or provitamins (such as vitamin E and β-carotene) that had been thought to be risk-free have now been associated with adverse health consequences. Thus, older adults should be counseled not to exceed the tolerable ULs (see **Table 30-5**) for vitamin intake and to

TABLE 30-5 ■ ADULT DIETARY REFERENCE INTAKES AND TOLERABLE UPPER LIMITS FOR SELECTED VITAMINS AND MINERALS

VITAMIN OR MINERAL	RECOMMENDED DAILY INTAKE[a]	TOLERABLE UPPER LIMIT
Vitamin A (retinol)	900 µg (males) 700 µg (females)	3000 µg
Vitamin D	600 IU (age 9–70) 800 IU (age > 70)	4000 IU
Vitamin E	15 mg 22 IU (natural vitamin E) 33 IU (synthetic vitamin E)	1000 mg 1500 IU
Vitamin K	120 µg (males) 90 µg (females)	[b]
Vitamin B_1 (thiamin)	1.2 mg (males) 1.1 mg (females)	[b]
Vitamin B_2 (riboflavin)	1.3 mg (males) 1.1 mg (females)	[b]
Niacin (nicotinamide)	16 mg (males) 14 mg (females)	[b]
Vitamin B_6 (pyridoxine)	1.7 mg (males) 1.5 mg (females)	100 mg
Vitamin B_{12} (cobalamin)	2.4 µg	[b]
Folic acid (folate)	400 µg	1000 µg
Vitamin C (ascorbic acid)	90 mg (males) 75 mg (females) (increase by 35 mg for smokers)	2000 mg
Calcium	1000–1200 mg	2500 mg
Selenium	55 µg	400 µg

[a]The recommended daily intake is the daily intake that will fulfill the nutritional needs of most healthy adults. The tolerable upper limit (UL) is the highest level of daily nutrient intake that is likely to pose no adverse health risk in most people. As intake above the UL occurs, there is an increasing risk of adverse effects.
[b]Tolerable upper limit not yet determined.

disclose all vitamin and mineral supplement use whenever medications are reviewed by health professionals. Vitamin and mineral supplementation should not substitute for an overall program of healthy nutrition (eg, high fruit, vegetable, and whole grain intake and reduced simple sugar and saturated and trans-fat intake).

Vitamin B$_{12}$ (Cobalamin)

Low serum vitamin B$_{12}$ levels become more common with aging, and about 10% to 15% of older adults have vitamin B$_{12}$ deficiency. Pernicious anemia, an autoimmune disorder causing decreased gastric intrinsic factor production, is a rare cause of deficiency in an older adult. Cobalamin deficiency in older adults is more commonly due to malabsorption of cobalamin in foods; usually due to atrophic gastritis and hypochlorhydria (**Table 30-6** lists multiple other causes). Supplemental B$_{12}$ in crystalline form is not affected by atrophic gastritis and continues to be well absorbed. Stomach acid helps remove the vitamin from food and make it bioavailable. Disorders that interfere with enterohepatic absorption (such as ileal disease or surgery) will lead to deficiency more rapidly than low intake because the high efficiency of enterohepatic vitamin B$_{12}$ reabsorption will be impaired, and the vitamin lost in the stool.

Vitamin B$_{12}$ deficiency can present clinically with two relatively independent disorders. There is a hematologic disorder that causes macrocytosis and anemia. And there is a neurologic disorder that can cause a peripheral neuropathy, including paresthesias and numbness; spinal column lesions, including loss of vibration and position sense, sensory ataxia, limb weakness, orthostatic hypotension, and plantar extensor responses; and neuropsychiatric symptoms. These signs and symptoms of vitamin B$_{12}$ deficiency are nonspecific and common in many older adults with comorbid disorders. When there are several possible causes for the neurologic signs and symptoms, vitamin B$_{12}$ supplementation is usually accompanied by disappointing, small measurable neurologic or behavioral improvement. The older the patient is and the more profound the signs and symptoms are, the less likely is the recovery. However, some patients may respond, especially if deficiency is relatively recent. Since patients with more severe hematologic signs often have less neurologic impairment, and vice versa, it is important to consider vitamin B$_{12}$ deficiency even if the patient lacks macrocytosis and anemia. Thus, screening older adults for vitamin B$_{12}$ deficiency should be considered, and supplementation of all deficient patients is recommended.

Many patients with "low normal" vitamin B$_{12}$ serum levels (< 350 pg/mL) have measurable biochemical abnormalities, including elevated methylmalonic acid (MMA) (> 270 nmol/L) levels, which improve with supplementation. Although these patients often appear to be asymptomatic, it is probable that borderline serum vitamin B$_{12}$ levels represent an early preclinical deficiency state. If this is the case, current laboratory norms for vitamin B$_{12}$ are too low, since they may not identify patients with early deficiency. Secondary tests for low B$_{12}$ status are also nonspecific and rarely useful; for example, MMA may also be elevated with renal failure, and homocysteine levels are also affected by folate and vitamin B$_6$ status.

An approach to screening for vitamin B$_{12}$ deficiency and treatment guidelines are presented in **Table 30-7**. Intramuscular or oral replacement is most common; alternative formulations (such as nasal gels) are more costly and have not been rigorously tested. There is no scientific basis for prescribing vitamin B$_{12}$ supplementation as a general tonic, and it is not recommended. Oversupplementation of vitamin B$_{12}$ is not recommended and may be associated with increased mortality.

Folate (Folic Acid)

Folate deficiency is associated with general malnutrition (particularly that accompanying alcohol abuse) or with specific folate antagonists, such as methotrexate, phenytoin, sulfasalazine, primidone, phenobarbital, and triamterene. Like vitamin B$_{12}$ deficiency, it can present as a megaloblastic macrocytic anemia. Although measures of both vitamin B$_{12}$ and folate status are often included in the evaluation of macrocytosis, low folate is a rare cause of this disorder. Folate supplementation alone may improve the macrocytosis and anemia in vitamin B$_{12}$ deficiency, without correcting the ongoing neurologic disorder of vitamin B$_{12}$ deficiency, and may even cause a more rapid neurologic/cognitive deterioration. However, in B$_{12}$-deficient patients with restored normal B$_{12}$ status, high folate intake is associated with protection from cognitive impairment. There are very rare case reports of neuropathy associated with folate deficiency. Slowed mental processing, including

TABLE 30-6 ■ CAUSES OF VITAMIN B$_{12}$ DEFICIENCY

Atrophic gastritis and hypochlorhydria

Chronic antacid use (histamine-2 blockers, proton pump inhibitors)

Gastric surgery

Ileal surgery

Diseases of the small intestine and terminal ileum: Crohn disease, sprue, malabsorption syndromes

Helicobacter pylori infection

Pancreatic insufficiency

Parasitic infections of the small bowel (eg, fish tapeworm)

Bacterial overgrowth syndromes

Strict vegetarianism

Acquired immune deficiency syndrome (AIDS) and AIDS treatment (eg, zidovudine)

Pernicious anemia

Metformin

TABLE 30-7 ■ EVALUATION AND TREATMENT OF VITAMIN B₁₂ DEFICIENCY IN OLDER ADULTS

1. **Screening**: Obtain a serum vitamin B_{12} level in any older adult with
   - Frailty
   - Macrocytosis or neutrophil hypersegmentation with or without anemia
   - Peripheral neuropathy
   - Gait disorder
   - Unexplained neuropsychiatric symptoms
2. **Interpretation:**
   - Vitamin B_{12} deficiency: level < 200 pg/mL (150 pmol/L)
   - Vitamin B_{12} borderline deficiency: level 200–350 pg/mL (150–260 pmol/L)
3. **Management**
   - B_{12} deficiency can be treated with B_{12} supplementation, usually without further investigation
   - In rare cases, it is essential to evaluate for pernicious anemia
   - For an otherwise healthy patient whose deficiency is found incidentally and who is otherwise asymptomatic:
     - A trial of oral supplementation with 1 mg daily
     - Serum vitamin B_{12} level in 1 month to verify GI absorption
     - Periodic (once or twice yearly) serum vitamin B_{12} thereafter
   - For patients with possible symptoms of vitamin B_{12} deficiency:
     - Parenteral supplementation with intramuscular B_{12} (1000 μg) several times within days to weeks, then monthly injections indefinitely

GI, gastrointestinal.

poorer performance on mental status testing, and depressive symptoms (particularly impaired motivation and social withdrawal) have been described in patients with folic acid deficiency. It is uncertain if folate deficiency has an association with major depression, and whether genotype testing for mutations in the MTHFR (5,10-methylenetetrahydrofolate reductase) gene or supplementation with the more expensive L-methylfolate (which crosses the blood–brain barrier more easily) improves response to treatment-resistant depression. Fortification of grains with folic acid began in the United States in 1998 (to reduce the incidence of neural tube defects in developing fetuses). Consumption of a diet rich in fruits and vegetables, along with fortified grains, continues to be recommended as the best source for folic acid, but folate in supplements is more bioavailable.

Folate status may be assessed by measuring serum folate if dietary intake (diet or vitamin supplementation) has not been recently changed or with erythrocyte (red blood cell [RBC]) folate levels if there has been a recent change in diet (as after hospital admission). Homocysteine levels can be elevated in folic acid deficiency, but may also be increased with renal insufficiency, and with vitamin B_{12} or B_6 deficiency.

Vitamin D

Vitamin D plays a critical role in maintenance of normal bone health (see Chapter 51). The complex physiology of vitamin D, its relationship to calcium and bone metabolism, nutritional and other causes of vitamin D deficiency, and the clinical features and treatment of vitamin D deficiency are all covered in Chapter 97, so are not addressed here. While vitamin D has been postulated to have multiple physiologic functions beyond those related to bone and calcium metabolism, these effects are controversial.

Routine screening of healthy older adults with 25(OH) D levels is controversial and expensive. The Choosing Wisely initiative does not recommend routine vitamin D screening, and the US Preventive Services Task Force (USPSTF, 2021) reports that there are no studies directly evaluating benefits or harms of screening. Vitamin D supplementation does not prevent or improve nonskeletal conditions, including mood disorders, cognitive decline, diabetes mellitus, adiposity, fatigue, osteoarthritis, chronic pain, cardiovascular disease (CVD) (including atrial fibrillation), strength, or colorectal adenomas. There is weak evidence that supplementation may prevent viral illnesses and asthma exacerbations. High-dose vitamin D does not benefit BMD, muscle function, muscle mass, or falls, and may increase harms (falls, death, and hospitalization). Based on multiple studies, the USPSTF (2018) recommends against D supplementation to prevent falls in community-dwelling older adults. It also found Insufficient Evidence to recommend vitamin D and calcium supplementation to prevent fractures in community-dwelling postmenopausal women and asymptomatic men without osteoporosis or vitamin D deficiency.

Calcium

From adolescence onwards, both men and women should consume between 1000 and 1200 mg of elemental calcium daily, unless there are unique nutrition requirements. Many older adults consume far less than this amount. In addition, calcium absorption declines with age and varies depending on dietary source. The UL for calcium intake is 2000 mg/day for people over age 50. The important role of calcium intake in management of osteoporosis is covered in Chapter 51.

A cup of milk or yogurt contains about 300 mg of calcium. Green vegetables contain some calcium, but they also contain other phytochemicals that interfere with calcium absorption. Therefore, calcium bioavailability from vegetables may be limited. Because of dietary limitations or other factors, many older adults are unable to consistently obtain the recommended intake of calcium from natural sources and may need to take calcium supplements. Some brands of orange juice and candy now contain added calcium, which can add to dietary sources of this element. Calcium is also available in pill form. Calcium carbonate is least expensive but should be consumed with food (although high-fiber foods may reduce absorption somewhat). Some other formulations, such as calcium citrate, are better absorbed but may cost more, or have less calcium per pill. Calcium supplements can increase constipation in some individuals. Persons who develop calcium oxalate kidney stones should not drastically limit their calcium intake from foods, as dietary calcium can bind with and reduce food oxalate absorption and decrease risk of stone formation. Observational studies have identified a possible association between calcium supplementation and increased risk for CVD. Until this issue is clarified, emphasis should be placed on maximizing calcium intake from food sources.

SPECIFIC DIETARY CONSIDERATIONS FOR OPTIMAL HEALTH

Vitamins and Cognition

Although numerous vitamins have been linked to cognitive decline with advancing age and to the pathogenesis of Alzheimer disease, most of this evidence is from observational studies. For example, there are associations between dietary intake of foods high in carotenoids and a diminished risk of cognitive impairment. These findings highlight the potential importance of maintaining a well-balanced diet, but do not provide evidence of cognitive benefit of using supplements containing any vitamin.

Nutrition, Cardiovascular Disease, and Cancer

There is a growing body of evidence that nutrition plays an important role in CVD prevention. Diets that are lower in saturated fat, contain poly- and monounsaturated fatty acids, and include an abundance of fruits and vegetables are associated with a reduced risk of CVD events. A number of dietary regimens fall into this category including the Mediterranean-style diet (described in the Fat and Cholesterol section), which reduced major CVD events in persons at high risk.

Antioxidants have also been promoted as protective for CVD and cancer. The rate of cardiac death may be lower in people who consume a diet rich in the antioxidant vitamins and minerals, particularly vitamins E and C, and carotenoids. These findings are difficult to interpret as diets rich in antioxidants are also higher in fiber and lower in cholesterol and saturated fat; and people who consume large amounts of fruits and vegetables, or who take vitamin supplements, often have healthier lifestyles. Meta-analyses of randomized clinical trials for primary prevention of CVD have not confirmed a beneficial effect of any vitamin, antioxidant, or fish oil supplement. In fact, increased morbidity or mortality was found with the use of supplemental β-carotene, vitamin E, and selenium; high supplemental vitamin E may increase risk for hemorrhagic stroke and all-cause mortality. High-dose omega-3 fatty acid supplementation, including mixed EPA-DHA, carboxylic acid formulations, and icosapent ethyl (IPE) formulations, have produced mixed but generally negative results on improving CVD, bone health, falls risk, nonvertebral fractures, and infection rates, and are not yet recommended. However, possible benefit for certain subgroups continues to be investigated.

There is currently no convincing evidence that any vitamin, mineral, or antioxidant supplementation prevents cancer. It is very likely that people with cancer or other serious illnesses will try alternative therapies, including megavitamin and mineral supplements, and herbal or folk remedies. Although it is generally thought that the toxicity of antioxidant vitamins and most B vitamins is low for intakes below the UL, there is increasing evidence of potential harms. Some of this evidence has come from intervention trials which have reported an increased incidence of lung cancer in high-risk patients treated with β-carotene supplements, an association between selenium supplementation and skin cancer, and an increased incidence of prostate cancer in men who took vitamin E. These risks should be discussed proactively with patients so that they can have the best information available to make their decisions and toxic side effects can be prevented. Tolerable ULs should not be exceeded.

Nutrition and Age-Related Eye Diseases

Evidence to support a protective effect of individual vitamin and mineral supplements on age-related eye diseases is conflicting. The Age-Related Eye Disease Study (AREDS) found a slight reduction in progression (not prevention) of age-related macular degeneration (AMD) using a combination of higher-dose vitamins C and E, β-carotene, zinc, and cupric oxide. In the AREDS2 study, the addition of omega-3 fatty acids (DHA and EPA) and/or lutein and zeaxanthin (macular xanthophylls) and removal of β-carotene did not decrease AMD progression. The AREDS2 supplementation also did not reduce CVD risk in the older adult participants. Observational studies have identified an association between dietary antioxidant content and a lower risk of age-related cataracts. However, there is also no evidence that regular high doses of antioxidant vitamin and mineral supplements are effective in preventing cataracts.

ASSESSMENT OF NUTRITIONAL STATUS

Initial Screening Assessment

The risk of developing one or more nutritional disorders increases with age. Prevention and early intervention are the best approaches to keeping older individuals optimally nourished because many forms of malnutrition, particularly protein and energy undernutrition, are very difficult to reverse. Providers should routinely screen their older patients to determine if they have or are at risk of developing nutritional problems, at least annually and whenever there is a change in the patient's health. Like other screening instruments, the nutritional screen should use simple criteria, be relatively easy to complete, have relatively low attendant costs, and provide a valid assessment of nutritional risk with a reasonable degree of sensitivity and specificity. Examples of screening instruments include the Malnutrition Screening Tool (MST), Malnutrition Universal Screening Tool (MUST), and the Mini-Nutrition Assessment (MNA). Individuals identified by the screen to be at risk of having or developing nutritional disorders should be scheduled for a more in-depth assessment.

For the initial screening assessment, older individuals who have experienced a recent deterioration in their socioeconomic or health status should be considered at high risk. Since many older individuals facing financial hardship do not volunteer this information, it is important to assess whether financial resources are inadequate to meet living expenses, including the purchase and preparation of an appropriate variety and quantity of foods. Food insecurity is an important issue for some older adults (see Chapter 21). When the older person is dependent on others for meal preparation or feeding assistance, caregiver neglect and other forms of abuse can pose serious threats and often require careful vigilance to identify. The nutritional screen should also assess psychological stressors, particularly the loss of a spouse or other family members. Older individuals should always be evaluated for depression. Alcohol and drug abuse are serious but frequently unrecognized problems that can cause a variety of nutritional disorders; screening tools include the CAGE Alcohol Questionnaire and Alcohol Use Disorders Identification Test (AUDIT).

The list of medications that can adversely affect nutrient intake is very long (see **Table 30-2**). Any drug that is being taken, including over the counter (OTC), herbals, and folk medications, should be considered suspect when anorexia or weight loss occur. Many drugs produce subtle side effects that older individuals may tolerate when feeling well. However, these same side effects, which may include alterations in appetite, taste sensation or salivary secretion, nausea, constipation, diarrhea, or a depressed sensorium, can contribute to the development of anorexia during periods of ill health. Swallowing problems can also adversely affect nutrient intake (see Chapter 31). Besides choking or coughing while eating or drinking liquids, the signs and symptoms may be far more subtle and can include only food avoidance. Older patients who are hospitalized are at very high risk of developing nutritional deficits prior to discharge. Prolonged bed rest, acute inflammation, and inadequate nutrient intake, which are common during hospitalization, rapidly lead to the depletion of both lean and total body mass, placing the older patient at high risk for subsequent mortality. For this reason, any acute hospitalization should be recognized as a nutritional risk factor.

A careful weight history, possibly the most important component of the nutrition screen, should be obtained from all older patients. Since patients often provide inaccurate accounts of their weight history, prior weights from the medical record may be useful. A weight loss of 5% or more within the prior 3 months or 10% or more within the

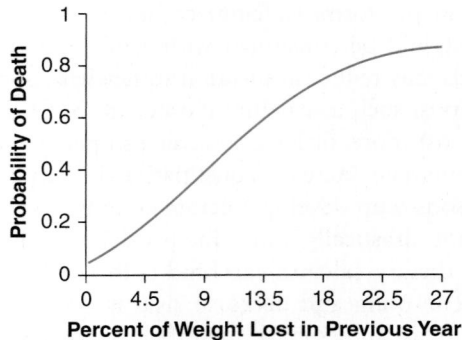

FIGURE 30-7. The relationship between the amount of weight that was lost in the prior year and the estimated risk of mortality within the subsequent year. Based on a study of 750 patients age 65 and older discharged from an acute care hospital.

prior 6 months to 3 years should be considered indicative of a potentially serious nutritional problem unless the weight fluctuation can be ascribed with certainty to alterations in fluid balance, such as those with heart failure or on hemodialysis. There is a clear and direct correlation between the amount of weight that is lost and increased risk of subsequent mortality (**Figure 30-7**), even if older individuals state that they voluntarily lost the weight. Voluntary weight loss in frail older adults has the same adverse implications as involuntary weight loss, likely because few older individuals successfully lose weight volitionally and keep it off while healthy. Thus, "voluntary" weight loss is the result of underlying pathology in many older individuals.

As part of the general physical examination, a weight and height should be obtained. If significant kyphosis or scoliosis is present, the patient's estimate of peak adult height can be utilized for current height. From the weight and height measurements, the patient's BMI and weight as a percentage of usual weight can be calculated. Since poor oral health may contribute to the development of nutritional problems, a careful oral examination is indicated.

Comprehensive Nutritional Assessment

Anthropometrics Neither BMI nor the skinfold measurements are good measures of total body fat mass if there is significant intra-abdominal fat accumulation, as often occurs with advanced age. Waist circumference and the waist-to-hip ratio are reasonably useful indicators of abdominal fatness, as defined earlier.

Laboratory assessment

Albumin A random serum albumin, interpreted without regard to clinical context, has low sensitivity and specificity and only limited clinical utility as a nutritional indicator. While albumin synthesis decreases by 30% to 50% after only 24 to 48 hours of protein and energy deprivation, there may be little change in the serum albumin concentration even after a much more prolonged period of fasting in an otherwise healthy individual. During periods of inadequate nutrient intake, a decreased rate of albumin degradation and mobilization of albumin from the extravascular space may contribute to the maintenance of a normal serum albumin concentration. For these reasons, albumin is not a very sensitive screening test for early stages of nutritional deterioration. Conversely, a low albumin concentration has low specificity as an indicator of protein-energy undernutrition. Acute and even chronic subclinical inflammation and other disease conditions are usually the primary contributors to the development and maintenance of a low serum albumin. Although in healthy individuals serum albumin has a half-life of approximately 20 days, during periods of acute physiologic stress (such as major surgery or sepsis), the serum concentration can decline by up to 30 g/L within a few days. This effect on the albumin concentration is probably mediated by cytokines that are believed to increase vascular permeability to albumin. The concentration of albumin is normally much greater within the intravascular compared to the extravascular space (35–50 g/L compared to ~ 10 g/L). With inflammation-induced changes in vascular permeability, there is a rapid loss of the normal concentration gradient between the intra- and extravascular space and an apparent sequestration of albumin in extravascular sites. These same cytokines also suppress albumin synthesis and may trigger an increased rate of albumin degradation with a resultant drop in the serum concentration to 25 g/L or less. Prolonged hypoalbuminemia can also develop in association with advanced liver disease (cirrhosis), severe congestive heart failure, nephrotic syndrome, and protein-losing enteropathies. When these conditions are not present, a persistently low serum albumin probably represents ongoing inflammation and is associated with a high risk of adverse outcomes, including death. The independent effect of nutritional deprivation on low albumin is unclear. Since it is not currently possible to differentiate the effects of inflammation from those of nutritional deprivation, a low albumin indicates only that the patient is at risk for being undernourished, and for increased morbidity and mortality. Serum albumin does not increase rapidly with refeeding and should not be utilized as an indicator of the adequacy of nutritional support.

Prealbumin Although it has limited specificity as a nutritional indicator, serum prealbumin may respond to changes in nutrient intake if there is no persistent inflammation or other active disease processes that are keeping the serum levels suppressed. Despite its name, prealbumin is not a precursor to albumin. Its more descriptive name is transthyretin because it transports both thyroxine and retinol (vitamin A). In health, prealbumin has a half-life of 2 to 3 days and a much smaller volume of distribution compared to albumin. Like albumin, prealbumin is a negative acute-phase reactant. In response to systemic inflammation, liver production declines and the serum concentration drops rapidly. Low levels are also found in association with end-stage liver disease, iron deficiency, and nutrient deprivation. Renal failure and high-dose steroid therapy are associated with elevated prealbumin concentrations.

Because of its relative short half-life, prealbumin is more sensitive to changes in nutrient intake and disease activity than is albumin. The serum concentration begins to drop after 3 to 5 days of very low nutrient intake in an otherwise healthy individual and can decline by 50% or more after a major physiologic insult. In the latter case, the nadir value is usually reached within 3 to 5 days and corresponds to the period of maximal negative nitrogen balance. With resolution of the inflammatory process, the serum concentration will climb rapidly to the normal range if nutrient intake is adequate. A rising prealbumin correlates with positive nitrogen balance. This fact may be used to advantage to assess the adequacy of nutrition support. Failure of the serum concentration to increase by at least 20 mg/L in 1 week is considered an indication of inadequate nutrient intake and/or ongoing inflammation and should prompt a careful assessment of the patient and the nutrient regimen being employed.

Assessment of Nutrient Intake

Although frequently difficult to obtain, a detailed nutrient and caloric intake assessment is often the most critically needed part of the nutritional assessment. In the outpatient setting where both over- and undernutrition may be a concern, a 24-hour recall or a 3-day food intake diary can be effective tools for estimating nutrient intake and identifying where dietary modifications need to be made, especially if a dietitian or comparably skilled health care provider gives the patient and the family adequate instructions on how to collect the needed data. The employment of more accurate methods of measuring nutrient intake is often especially necessary within hospitals and nursing homes.

Unfortunately, many older patients are maintained throughout their hospitalization on nutrient intakes that are far less than their estimated maintenance energy requirements. Contributing to the problem, the attending health care team often overestimates how much food the older patient is consuming. In one study, over 20% of non-terminally ill older hospitalized patients had an average daily nutrient intake while hospitalized that was less than 50% of their maintenance energy requirements. This lack of adequate nutrient intake was associated with a significant deterioration in protein-energy nutritional status by discharge and a sevenfold increased risk of mortality. Low nutrient intake may be an even more widespread problem within nursing homes. Only by carefully monitoring each older individual's nutrient intake during their institutional stay can this problem be recognized. However, resources are often not available to support monitoring efforts. Within the hospital setting, older patients who are not recovering as rapidly as expected, have been placed on clear liquids or nothing by mouth for more than 24 hours, have a persistently low serum prealbumin, or are unexpectedly losing weight, should have their nutrient intake measured each day until they resume an adequate diet. A dedicated team of appropriately trained staff members may be needed to perform this daily nutrient intake assessment, since accuracy often suffers when the regular nursing and dietary staff performs this function. Within nursing homes, any resident experiencing an acute illness, change in mental status, loss of weight, or decline in functional status should have their nutrient intake monitored in a similar fashion.

MALNUTRITION

Definition

Protein-energy malnutrition (PEM) is present when insufficient energy and/or protein is available to meet metabolic demands. PEM may develop because of poor dietary protein or caloric intake, increased metabolic demands, or increased nutrient losses. Proposed clinical criteria from the Academy of Nutrition and Dietetics and the American Society for Parenteral and Enteral Nutrition to diagnose adult malnutrition are listed in **Table 30-8**.

Epidemiology

Prevalence data, relying on a variety of measures of nutritional adequacy, suggest that deficiencies in macronutrients (protein energy) and micronutrients (vitamins and minerals) are very common among older adults. National survey data indicate that 40% to 50% of noninstitutionalized older adults are at moderate to high risk for nutritional problems, and up to 40% have diets deficient in three or more nutrients. Prevalence estimates in selected populations over age 65 indicate that 6% to 15% of older persons seen in outpatient clinics, 12% to 50% of hospitalized older persons, and 25% to 60% of older persons residing in institutional settings have one or more nutritional inadequacies—with PEM being the most common. Physical and psychosocial factors that may lead to inadequate nutrition were discussed earlier and are listed in **Table 30-1**.

As discussed earlier in this chapter, energy intake declines with age, attributable in part to decrements in LBM and physical activity that often accompany aging. A still greater reduction in caloric intake to levels that may be below daily requirements has been a consistent finding of nutritional surveys conducted among community-dwelling older adults. The National Health and Nutrition Examination Survey (NHANES III) found that the mean daily energy intake of persons age 70 and older was approximately 1800 kcal/day for men and 1400 kcal/day for women, and more than 10% of older adults reported consuming less than 1000 kcal/day. Even if this limited energy intake met the caloric needs of less-active older adults, it is unlikely that all noncaloric nutrient needs (vitamins and minerals) would be met unless the diet was extremely diverse and rich in nutrients. Although micronutrient deficiencies are common when PEM is moderate to severe, it is the PEM that tends to have the greater clinical impact. Poor nutritional status and PEM are associated with altered immunity, impaired wound healing, reduced functional status, increased health care use, and increased mortality. Despite the confounding effect of coexisting nonnutritional factors, poor nutrition remains an independent source of increased morbidity and mortality after adjustment for nonnutritional factors.

Pathophysiology

PEM may occur as a consequence of inadequate intake alone (eg, starvation) or in association with disease-activated physiological mechanisms that affect body metabolism, composition, and appetite (ie, cachexia). In the former (primary caloric deficiency state) the body adapts by using fat stores while conserving protein and muscle, and the resulting physiologic changes are often reversible with resumption of usual intake and activity. Cachexia is a complex metabolic syndrome that is associated with elevated inflammatory cytokines (eg, TNF-α and IL-6) and increased protein and muscle degradation that may not be mitigated or reversed by refeeding. Although cachexia is usually associated with specific chronic disease conditions (eg, cancer, renal failure, chronic obstructive pulmonary disease [COPD]), this state may develop in older persons without obvious underlying disease.

Presentation and Evaluation

Despite its clinical importance, malnutrition is often missed clinically. Effective management of frail or ill older adults mandates an evaluation of nutritional status to better allow for early recognition of PEM and consideration of appropriate interventions. Assessment of nutritional status by standard anthropometric, biochemical, and immunologic measures can be complex, as both nutrient intake and non-nutrition-related factors can affect these parameters (see preceding section on Assessment of Nutritional Status). The close monitoring of body weight, a readily obtainable measure that reflects imbalance between caloric intake and energy requirements, is a simple and reliable way to screen for malnutrition, particularly in the outpatient setting. Weight loss of 5% or more of usual body weight over 6 to 12 months is associated with increased morbidity and mortality in the outpatient setting, and so is the degree of weight loss that should prompt investigation.

TABLE 30-8 ■ CLINICAL CHARACTERISTICS RECOMMENDED FOR THE DIAGNOSIS OF ADULT MALNUTRITION[a]

Insufficient energy intake

Weight loss

Loss of muscle mass (eg, temporal wasting, reduced pectoralis, deltoid, quadriceps, other muscle)

Loss of subcutaneous fat (eg, orbital, triceps, fat overlying ribs)

Localized or generalized fluid accumulation (eg extremity or genital edema, ascites)

Decreased functional status as measured by reduced handgrip strength

[a]A minimum of two or more characteristics is recommended to diagnose malnutrition.

TABLE 30-9 ■ ESTIMATION OF DAILY ENERGY AND PROTEIN NEEDS

I. Daily energy requirements (kcal/d)

  A. Quick estimate: maintenance 25–30 kcal/kg; stress 30–40 kcal/kg; sepsis 40–50 kcal/kg (tends to overestimate requirements for older and obese patients)

  B. Estimates based on resting metabolic rate (RMR, kcal/d):

    1. First estimate RMR (using either equation below)

      a. Harris-Benedict:

$$RMR_{women} = 655 + [9.5 \times wt\ (kg)] + [1.8 \times ht\ (cm)] - (4.7 \times age)$$

$$RMR_{men} = 66 + [13.7 \times wt\ (kg) + [5 \times ht\ (cm)] - (6.8 \times age)$$

      b. Schofield

$$RMR_{women} = [wt\ (kg) \times 9.1] + 659$$

$$RMR_{men} = [wt\ (kg) \times 11.7] + 588$$

    2. Then multiply RMR by adjustment factor to estimate total energy requirement:

Total daily energy requirement = RMR × 1.3 for mild illness/injury

= RMR × 1.5 moderate illness/injury

= RMR × 1.7–1.8 severe illness/injury

II. Daily protein requirements (g/d) (may overestimate if patient obese)

RDA healthy nonpregnant adults	0.8 g/kg
Minimally stressed patients	1.0 g/kg
Injury/illness	1.2–1.4 g/kg
Severe stress/sepsis	1.4–1.8 g/kg

In the hospital setting, where acute illness or injury often coexists with inadequate intake, alterations in nutritional parameters associated with PEM may develop rapidly. Elevated levels of inflammatory mediators appear to be responsible for the greater losses in LBM and the rapid declines in albumin that often accompany PEM in physiologically stressed patients. While serial weight measures remain clinically relevant, early detection and correction of PEM in acutely ill hospitalized patients is enhanced by determination of dietary intake relative to metabolic requirements. Although registered dietitians often provide this information, all members of the clinical care team should be aware of dietary intake and can readily estimate caloric and protein requirements using formulas presented in **Table 30-9**. Biochemical and immunologic measures (eg, albumin, prealbumin, transferrin, and lymphocyte counts) can provide prognostic information, but their lack of specificity limits their utility as markers of PEM. An effective assessment of nutritional status requires synthesis of information provided from the dietary history, physical examination, and biochemical data. There are no definitive criteria for classifying degrees of PEM. However, when weight loss exceeds 20% of premorbid weight, serum albumin is less than 21 g/L, transferrin is less than 1 g/L, and total lymphocyte count is less than 800/µL, PEM is generally considered to be severe.

Assessment for Causes of Weight Loss

Initial management of patients with PEM and/or weight loss should include a thorough evaluation to identify underlying causes, and if found, to aggressively attempt to correct potentially remediable factors. In the acute care setting the cause(s) of malnutrition are often readily evident, although depression may be a contributing factor that is frequently overlooked. In contrast, reasons for poor nutrition and weight loss among community-dwelling older persons may be multiple and not as readily discernible. Depression, gastrointestinal (GI) maladies (eg, peptic ulcer, motility, or malabsorption disorders), and cancer are the three most common causes of involuntary weight loss in older adults when a single predominant cause is present (**Table 30-10**). When cancer is the cause of weight loss, the diagnosis is rarely obscure. Most diagnoses are readily made after standard evaluations that include a careful history and physical examination and basic screening tests, with additional tests only as directed by signs and symptoms. If the initial basic evaluation is unrevealing, as will occur in roughly 25% of cases, it is best to enter a period of "active surveillance" rather than pursue more extensive undirected testing. A diagnostic algorithm (**Figure 30-8**) focusing first on verifying actual weight loss (patients may inaccurately report a history of weight loss) and then on whether caloric intake is adequate can help guide an appropriate work-up.

Management

General considerations Older persons who are not meeting their protein and caloric requirements through oral intake should be considered for nutritional support. **Table 30-11** outlines approaches to nutritional support and factors to consider in deciding whether to pursue specific interventions. The urgency for nutritional interventions relates to the degree of protein-calorie depletion at the time of diagnosis coupled with the expected magnitude and duration of inadequate nutrition. In the hospital setting, clinicians must consider that patients may have been suffering from PEM for some time prior to admission. Therefore, delay in instituting nutritional support while waiting for improved intake should be avoided. One approach is to intervene if a patient has a 5- to 7-day period of severely limited intake or for weight loss more than 10% of preillness weight in a hospitalized patient. However, attempts should be made to prevent PEM rather than wait for this degree of PEM to develop because weight loss and undernutrition are associated with worse clinical outcomes, and recovery of lost LBM is often difficult. This is particularly important in severe stress states (eg, sepsis, major injury) where protein catabolism can lead to LBM losses that approach 0.6 kg/day. In support of early intervention when the development of PEM is likely, a trial of enteral nutrition among patients with major injury found that early (within 24 hours) enteral feeding had clinical benefits over tube feeding started later in the course of hospitalization.

Patient preference The effect of the planned intervention on the patient's quality and/or quantity of life should be addressed before proceeding with nutritional support.

TABLE 30-10 ■ DIAGNOSTIC SPECTRUM OF INVOLUNTARY WEIGHT LOSS

	STUDY (STUDY SIZE)									
	MARTON (N=91)	RABINOVITZ (N=154)	HUERTA (N=50)	LANKISCH (N=158)	LEVINE (N=107)	THOMPSON (N=45)	METALIDIS (N=101)	BILBAO-GARAY (N=78)	WU (N=136)	BOSCH (N=2677)
Study population	70% Inpt 30% Outpt	Inpatient	Inpatient	Inpatient	Outpatient	Outpatient	57% Inpt 43% Outpt	Outpatient	Inpatient	Outpatient
Weight loss definition[a]	≥ 5%/6 mo	≥ 5%/not stated	≥ 10%/6 mo	≥ 5%/6 mo	≥ 5%/6 mo	≥ 7.5%/6 mo	≥ 5%/6–12 mo	≥ 5%/3 mo or ≥ 10%/6 mo	≥ 5%/6–12 mo	> 5%/6–12 mo
Mean age	59	64	59	68	62	72	64	59	80	64
Gender (% male)	100%	45%	64%	44%	53%	33%	46%	49%	81%	51%
Diagnosis %										
Neoplasm	19	36	10	24	6	16	22	23	17	33
Gastrointestinal	14	17	18	19	6	11	15	6		17
Psychiatric	9	10	42	11	22	18	16	33	24	14
Endocrine	4	4	10	11	5	9	2	6		5
Cardiopulmonary	14		2	10	9		5	3		1
Other medical diagnoses[b]	18	9	8	8	16	22	13	17	34	14
Unknown	26	23	10	16	36	24	28	11	26	14

[a]Weight loss study definition: percent body weight lost per time interval in months.

[b]Neurologic, infectious, alcohol, medication, renal, inflammatory disease, multifactorial. Wu study did not report specific medical diagnoses separately.

Data from Bilbao-Garay J, et al. Assessing clinical probability of organic disease in patients with involuntary weight loss. Eur J Intern Med 2002;13:24. Bosch X, et al. Unintentional weight loss. PLOS ONE 2017 12(4):e0175125. Huerta G, Viniegra L. Involuntary weight loss as a clinical problem. Rev Invest Clin (Spanish). 1989;41(1):5. Lankisch PG, et al. Unintentional weight loss: diagnosis and prognosis. J Intern Med. 2001;249:41. Levine MA. Unintentional weight loss in the ambulatory setting: etiologies and outcomes. [Personal communication and abstract]. Clin Res 1991;39(2):580A. Marton KI, et al. Involuntary weight loss: diagnostic and prognostic significance. Ann Intern Med. 1981;95:568. Metalidis C, et al. Involuntary weight loss. Does a negative baseline evaluation provide adequate reassurance? Eur J Intern Med 2008;19:345. Rabinowitz M, et al. Unintentional weight loss. Arch Int Med. 1986;146:186. Thompson MP, Morris LK. Unexplained weight loss in the ambulatory elderly. J Am Geriatr Soc. 1991;39:497. Wu JM, et al. Evaluating diagnostic strategy of older patients with unexplained unintentional body weight loss. Arch Gerontol Geriatr 2011;53:e51.

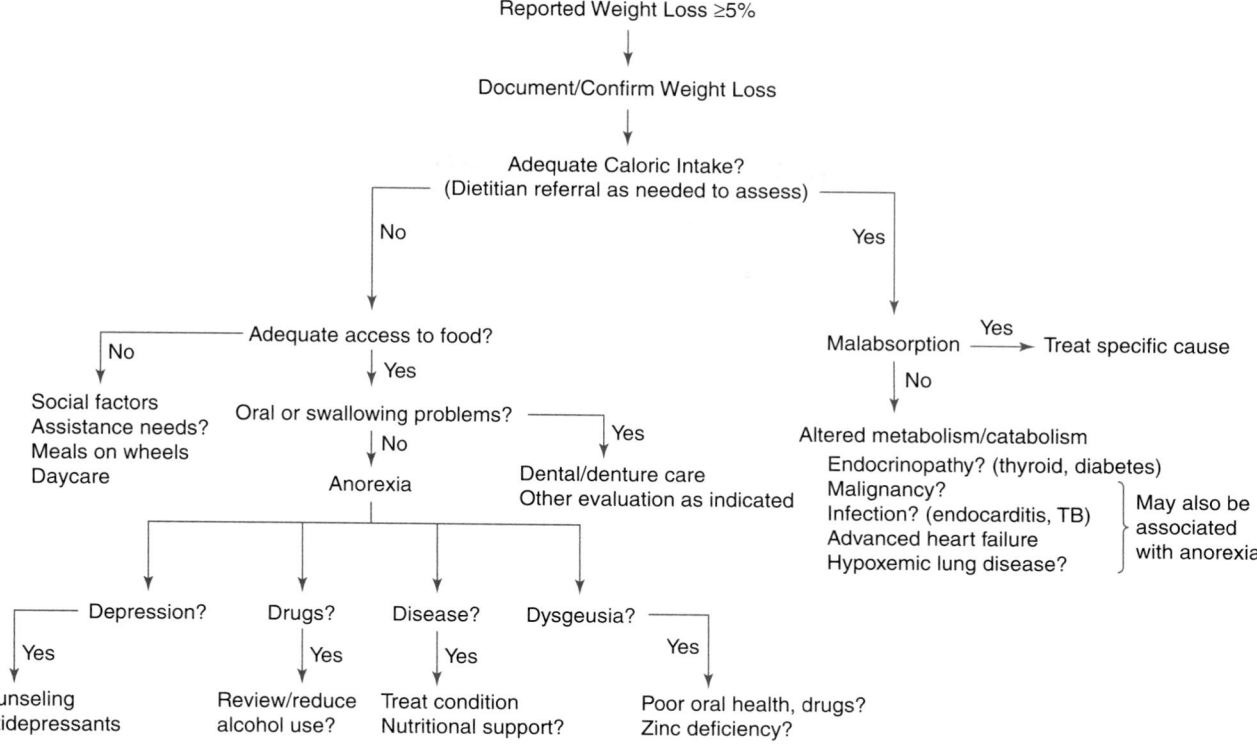

FIGURE 30-8. Weight loss evaluation algorithm.

Although nutritional support interventions may improve weight and other nutritional parameters, evidence demonstrating their ability to improve clinical outcomes is still limited, particularly when PEM is associated with serious (eg, critically ill intensive care unit [ICU] patients) or irreversible underlying disease (eg, cancer). While efforts to improve nutrition, even in patients with serious underlying disease, are often warranted, late in the course of disease appropriate palliative care may include, if not mandate, discontinuing such efforts. Determination of the care preferences of the patient is a critical component of the decision-making process. Patient and family counseling prior to implementing nutritional support should include a review of the interventions being considered and their potential for adverse, as well as beneficial, effects. **Figure 30-9** provides an algorithm to help guide nutritional support decisions.

Enhancing oral intake

Nonpharmacologic approaches Although it is uncommon for hospitalized older persons with PEM to be able to increase their food consumption sufficiently to correct their nutritional deficits, trials of strategies to improve voluntary intake are reasonable for stable patients with mild PEM (no definitive criteria exist, but parameters consistent with mild-moderate PEM include weight 85%–90% of premorbid weight, albumin 25–30 g/L, transferrin 1.5–2.0 g/L, total lymphocyte count 800–1200/μL). As previously outlined, underlying causative or contributing condition(s) to PEM should be sought, identified, and addressed. Strategies to help overcome anorexia and improve oral intake include assessing and meeting food preferences, providing frequent small meals and snacks, use of fortified and flavor-enhanced foods, providing company at meals and feeding assistance as needed, and minimizing dietary restrictions. A dietitian may aid greatly in these efforts.

TABLE 30-11 ■ APPROACHES TO IMPLEMENTING NUTRITIONAL SUPPORT	
AVAILABLE INTERVENTIONS	**FACTORS TO CONSIDER**
Enhance oral intake	Degree of baseline protein-calorie depletion
Frequent meals, snacks	
Provide favorite foods, fortified foods, minimize/remove dietary restrictions	Current intake relative to requirements
	Expected duration of inadequate nutrition
Feeding assistance, company at meals	Effect of intervention on clinical outcomes
Protein-calorie supplements	
Multivitamins	Potential benefits
	Potential adverse effects
Appetite stimulants?	Burden of intervention
Anabolic agents	Potential for reversibility
Enteral nutrition	Quality of life
Parenteral nutrition	Patient care preferences

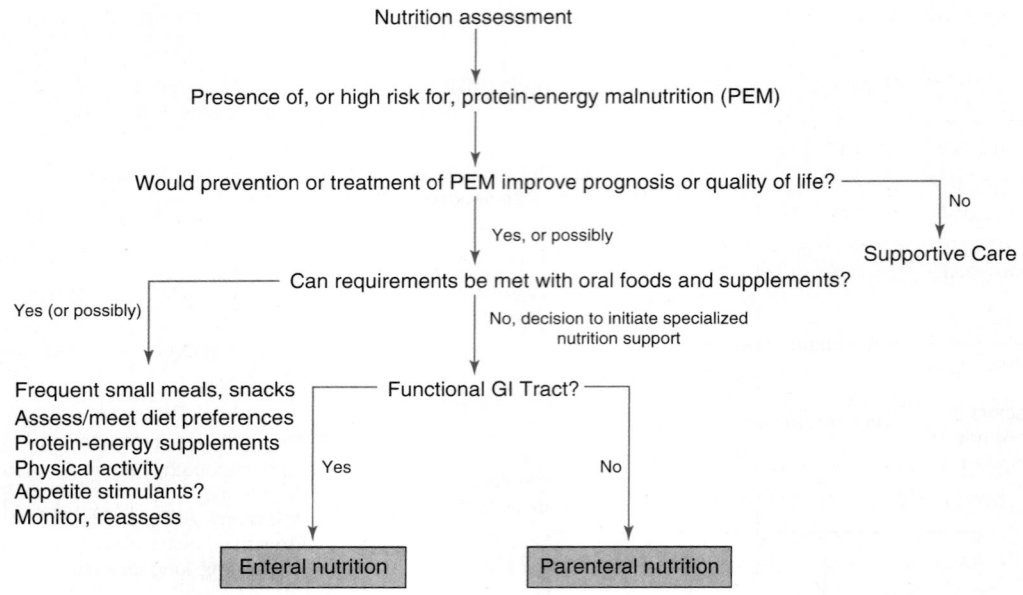

FIGURE 30-9. An algorithmic approach to nutritional support.

The role for high-protein, high-calorie oral nutritional supplements is not clear. While meaningful clinical benefits may occur in malnourished older adults, the effects are less clear in persons with dementia or other progressive illnesses, particularly in the outpatient setting. A Cochrane Library review concluded that oral nutritional supplements produce modest (2% on average) weight gain, may reduce mortality in undernourished individuals, and may reduce hospital complications, but evidence for functional benefits or reduced length of hospital stay is lacking. As the greatest mortality impact was found in hospitalized malnourished patients age 75 or older who received high-calorie supplements, it seems reasonable to recommend such supplements in older hospitalized patients with, or at high risk for, PEM. Higher-calorie "plus" variety nutritional supplements (1.5–2.0 kcal/mL) are preferred over standard (1 kcal/mL) formulas, as costs are only slightly higher. Furthermore, because they deliver higher calorie content per milliliter ingested, patients do not need to drink as much volume to improve caloric intake. Supplements should be provided between, rather than with, meals as this appears to result in less compensatory decreases in food intake at mealtime, thereby more effectively increasing total daily caloric intake. However, even if total caloric intake is only marginally improved, the provision of energy from nutritionally dense supplement sources may be beneficial due to improved protein and micronutrient intake.

A standard multivitamin supplement should also be considered for all older adults with PEM. Although study results are not consistent, some have demonstrated that improving micronutrition with multivitamins, particularly in malnourished or at-risk persons, may improve clinical outcomes (eg. infection rates). Increased physical activity

is an important adjunct that can help maintain LBM and improve appetite, thereby leading to improved caloric intake and functional status.

Drugs Pharmacologic approaches to stimulate appetite and promote weight gain can be considered on an individual basis with the knowledge that the few agents (megestrol acetate [MA], dronabinol, cyproheptadine) that may improve intake in some patient populations (eg, cancer, human immunodeficiency virus, anorexia nervosa) have not been shown to be effective in older adults and may cause serious side effects. Further, the weight gain that has been observed with these agents has usually been small, disproportionately fat mass, and not associated with improved function, quality of life, or decreased morbidity and mortality. MA increases risks of thrombotic events, fluid retention, and mortality. The American Geriatrics Society Beers Criteria lists both MA and cyproheptadine as medications to be avoided in older adults. Dronabinol has not been carefully studied in older adults and at best has shown limited promise in small nonrandomized trials conducted in nursing home patients. If initiated, MA may not have a demonstrable effect on appetite for several weeks, but if no effect is seen by the eighth week, MA should be discontinued. If positive effects are demonstrated without significant side effects, MA may be continued for up to 12 weeks. Treatment for more than 8 to 12 weeks can suppress the adrenal–pituitary axis, resulting in adrenal insufficiency and insufficient response to acute stressors. MA also appears to blunt the beneficial effects of progressive resistance exercise, consistent with an undesirable glucocorticoid-like catabolic effect.

If depression is felt to be a contributing factor to poor intake, a trial of therapy is usually warranted. Selective serotonin reuptake inhibitors (SSRIs) are first-line anti-depressant agents that may improve appetite by improving depression. Mirtazapine leads to more weight gain than SSRIs, but it is not clear that mirtazapine has a significant advantage over other antidepressants when weight loss is a predominant presenting sign in a depressed older adult. There is no high-quality evidence to support the use of mirtazapine for weight gain in the absence of depression.

Maintaining Lean Body Mass and Functional Status

Anabolic agents Anabolic hormones (eg, growth hormone [GH], testosterone, oxandrolone) have received considerable attention in the search to find strategies to help preserve or increase LBM in patients with malnutrition and weight loss. Although adequate nutrition is essential for patients with weight loss, a physiologically stressed catabolic patient may lose significant LBM despite aggressive nutritional support (and the weight gain that does occur with nutritional support and appetite stimulants may be primarily fat and water). GH has generally failed to demonstrate benefits on muscle mass or muscle strength in older adults, even in association with resistance training. The use of GH in intensive care and congestive heart failure patients has also yielded disappointing results with evidence of increased mortality. The cost, need for injection, and potential side effects of GH (eg, arthralgias, edema, insulin resistance, tumor growth) further limits its clinical role. Testosterone increases muscle protein synthesis mass and strength, and improvements in functional outcomes have been observed in small, controlled trials in selected male populations (eg, older men after knee replacement surgery, deconditioned older men on a Geriatric Evaluation and Management unit). Although testosterone might be considered in men with documented clinical hypogonadism (see Chapter 97), its role in the setting of malnutrition and/or cachexia remains to be clarified, especially in light of known safety concerns (in particular CV). Oxandrolone, a synthetic testosterone derivative with an increased anabolic to androgenic effect ratio, has shown some utility for patients with weight loss in association with AIDS/HIV or burns, and preliminary data also suggest benefit in patients with COPD. This agent can cause hepatitis, hirsutism, and fluid retention, and is contraindicated in patients with breast or prostate cancer. Selective androgen receptor modulators (SARMs), for example enobosarm, have the potential to provide desirable anabolic effects on muscle and bone without androgenic effects elsewhere, but these agents are still under study and not yet available clinically. Other anabolic agents that are under study include myostatin inhibitors and ghrelin analogues. Myostatin is expressed in skeletal muscle and inhibits muscle protein synthesis and promotes fibrosis. Blocking these effects may provide a novel approach to prevent muscle loss and promote muscle growth. Ghrelin is an endogenous GH secretagogue that increases appetite and has anabolic properties that can lead to increases in LBM. Anamorelin is an oral ghrelin analogue that has shown promise in patients with cancer-associated anorexia/cachexia. It remains under study and is not commercially available.

Physical activity Efforts to increase physical activity are an important adjunct to any nutritional intervention as positive effects of exercise include enhanced appetite and improved functional status. The benefits (and safety) of exercise in older populations are reviewed in Chapter 54.

NUTRITIONAL SUPPORT

Enteral Nutrition

Enteral nutrition (EN) is defined as the nonvolitional delivery of nutrients by tube into the GI tract. EN should be considered for patients with PEM, or at high risk for it, who cannot meet their nutritional requirements through oral intake. However, specific indications regarding if and when to provide EN are not clearly established, and patient prognosis and preference are critical factors that must be taken into account. EN requires a functional GI tract and is contraindicated in patients with bowel obstruction, inadequate bowel surface area, major upper GI bleeding, GI ischemia, or intractable vomiting or diarrhea. Purported benefits of enteral tube feedings relative to parenteral nutrition (PN) include the maintenance of GI structure and function, more physiological delivery of nutrients, less risk of overfeeding and hyperglycemia, and lower costs. Although some of these advantages may be more theoretical than actual, EN is preferred when GI function is adequate. EN and PN should not be considered mutually exclusive. For patients unable to fully meet their nutritional requirements through EN, a mixture of PN and EN is preferable to PN alone.

Efficacy EN can improve prognostically important intermediate nutritional parameters but the effects of EN on clinical outcomes (eg, functional status, medical complications, mortality) are unclear owing to limited and/or mixed data. EN is often not initiated until advanced PEM is present, which is a clear impediment to the potential positive effects of nutritional therapy. There is prospective clinical trial evidence that EN can improve both nutritional parameters and clinical outcomes (eg, length of stay, infectious complications, and mortality) in older undernourished hip fracture patients. Further study is needed to determine which older hospitalized patients might benefit most from aggressive nutritional support. In the interim, sufficient rationale exists to consider EN for patients who are undernourished or at high risk for undernutrition and cannot meet their nutritional needs with oral intake.

Tube placement The route selected for tube feeding depends on the anticipated duration of feeding, the potential for aspiration, and the condition of the gastrointestinal tract (eg, esophageal or gastric obstruction). Nasogastric (NG) or nasointestinal tubes provide the simplest approach for patients requiring relatively short-term EN (< 30 days). Patient comfort is often problematic, and tolerance is best when a small-diameter, soft feeding tube is used rather than a standard large-bore NG tube. The use of longer specialized feeding tubes also allows the tube to reach beyond the pylorus into the distal duodenum or jejunum (ie, beyond the ligament of Treitz), which is the preferred site of placement for patients who have delayed gastric emptying or are at high risk for aspiration. Methods to promote passage of the tube past the pylorus when postpyloric feeding is desired include ensuring adequate tube length, having the patient lie on their right side, prescribing erythromycin or metoclopramide, or using endoscopic or fluoroscopic guidance to position the tube. However, postpyloric feeding can be a challenge to maintain as even endoscopically placed tubes may migrate back into the stomach. After placement, the desired tube position should be verified radiologically before starting feedings and the tube should be marked at its exit point to help identify if subsequent movement occurs.

Percutaneous tube placement (gastrostomy, gastrojejunostomy, jejunostomy) is indicated when long-term tube feeding is anticipated (> 4 weeks). Percutaneous placement of gastrostomy tubes (G-tubes) can be performed either endoscopically or under radiographic guidance. The risks of major complications with either procedure are generally low, but infection, hemorrhage, and peritonitis have each been reported at rates of 1% to 3%. Placement of feeding tubes directly into the jejunum may be required for patients with abnormal or inaccessible stomachs (eg, gastrectomy, duodenal obstruction). Although direct jejunostomy tube (J-tube) placement can be accomplished using percutaneous methods, a J-tube traditionally requires an open surgical procedure and is often placed at the time of laparotomy when the need for prolonged nutritional support is anticipated.

Tube feeding is associated with an increased incidence of aspiration. However, most aspiration pneumonias are the result of difficulty handling endogenous (oropharyngeal or gastric) secretions rather than aspiration of material introduced through the tube. Thus, it is not entirely surprising that although postpyloric feeding tube placement is generally advised in older and sicker patients, the reduction in the incidence of pneumonia is small.

Formula selection Adult enteral formulas fall into one of the following categories: standard, concentrated, predigested (previously called elemental or semi-elemental), and disease-specific. All consist of varying mixtures of protein (often casein), carbohydrate (often cornstarch), and fat (usually vegetable oils), and most do not contain lactose. Formula variability includes nutrient composition, nutrient density, osmolarity, fiber content, and cost (cost tends to be substantially higher for disease-specific specialty formulas, and up to 10-fold higher for critical care and predigested specialty formulas). Isotonic standard formulas with caloric densities of 1.0 to 1.2 kcal/mL are usually the initial products of choice. Higher caloric density formulas (1.5–2.0 kcal/mL) may be useful when volume

restriction is paramount (eg, in patients with renal failure) but their higher viscosity increases the risk of tube clogging and their higher osmolarity may be less well tolerated if delivered rapidly via tubes placed beyond the pylorus. There is no evidence that routine supplementation of EN with fiber prevents diarrhea, but supplemental fiber may be tried if patients receiving EN are having problems with diarrhea or constipation. Predigested formulas differ from standard EN because their carbohydrates are less complex and proteins have been hydrolyzed to short-chain peptides. Although they are promoted for patients with diminished ability to digest nutrients, it is uncommon for patients to be incapable of digesting and absorbing standard formulas unless they have significantly impaired gastrointestinal function (assuming appropriate adjustments are made in rates of feedings, osmolality, and fiber content).

Disease-specific/specialty formulas are available for patients with renal failure, liver failure, diabetes mellitus, pulmonary disease, gastrointestinal dysfunction, and critical illness. However, as costs are usually substantially higher and no clear clinical benefits have been consistently demonstrated, disease-specific formulations are not routinely recommended. Renal formulas, which are low in electrolytes and dense in calories, do have a place in renal failure patients who have need for fluid and/or electrolyte restrictions. These formulas may be useful before dialysis but are not necessary for most patients once on dialysis. Formulas have been developed for diabetic patients but use of cheaper standard formulas with adjustments in glucose control regimens as necessary is adequate for most diabetic patients. Formulas for pulmonary patients have higher fat and lower carbohydrate content based on the now known erroneous rationale that this alteration in fuel source reduces carbon dioxide production. Clinical studies have failed to show any benefit to support the use of pulmonary EN formulations. Hepatic formulas have specific amino acid mixtures (high in branched chain, low in aromatic amino acids) that are less likely to cause or exacerbate hepatic encephalopathy. They are only indicated when, despite appropriate medical therapy, hepatic encephalopathy limits the delivery of adequate protein to a patient with liver disease.

A number of specialty formulations have been designed for critically ill patients. Some of these products are enriched with glutamine (an amino acid associated with improved nitrogen balance and gut barrier function as well as immune-modulating effects when delivered parenterally), arginine (a conditionally essential amino acid associated with improved nitrogen balance and immune function), and/or other immune modulators (eg, antioxidants, selenium, omega-3 fatty acids). However, meta-analyses have not shown convincing clinical benefits and a large trial of "immunonutrition" in an ICU population found that early provision of glutamine or antioxidants did not improve clinical outcomes, and glutamine was associated with increased mortality. Pending further study, use of these products in EN formulas is not recommended.

Administration guidelines After desired tube placement location is confirmed, tube feeds (TFs) can be started at a rate of 10 to 30 mL/hour. Two basic approaches to advancing TF flow rates are: (1) maintain a lower "trophic" feeding goal of 25% to 30% of estimated needs for 6 days before increasing to target rate; versus (2) advance TF rate to goal as quickly as tolerated over 24 to 48 hours. The American Society for Parenteral and Enteral Nutrition favors the latter for patients who are severely malnourished or at high nutritional risk while noting that EN was better tolerated in mechanically ventilated ICU patients (eg, less vomiting, reduced use of prokinetic agents) and clinical outcomes were similar when feeding rates were kept low (10–30 mL/hour, roughly 30% of target rate) for 6 days before increasing by 25 mL/hour every 6 hours as tolerated to target rate. In non-ICU settings feeding rates can be advanced 25 mL/hour every 6 to 12 hours based on individual tolerance, until target rate is reached. Routine checking of gastric residual volume (GRV) lacks benefit and is no longer recommended unless abdominal distension, abdominal pain, nausea, or change in clinical status occur. An evaluation for remediable factors (eg, medications, high fat-content formulas) should be conducted if GRV exceeds 250 mL, and feedings should be held if GRV exceeds 500 mL. Once daily requirements are reached, further adjustments to deliver nutrients primarily at night can allow more freedom of movement during the day. Nocturnal feeds probably offer little benefit in terms of decreased satiety and improved intake during the day relative to continuous feeds. Intermittent bolus gastric feedings without a pump offers convenience advantages but generally should be avoided in persons with delayed gastric emptying and those at high risk for aspiration.

As all feeding products consist of no more than 70% to 80% water, they are unable to meet basal free-water requirements of roughly 30 mL/kg per day. Most patients require additional water beyond the routine water flushes that occur with medication and TF administration to avoid tube clogging. Attention must also be paid to water and electrolyte requirements as they will need to be increased with excess losses due to diarrhea, high urinary output, or increased insensible losses. For patients with fever, an additional 300 to 400 mL of water is needed for each degree centigrade of temperature elevation. Monitoring of weight and electrolytes can help detect any necessary adjustments, with additional free-water needs given in divided boluses three or four times a day.

Risks and complications Proper consideration of whether to proceed with EN entails an understanding of common adverse effects (**Table 30-12**). NG tubes are often not well tolerated, with agitation and self-extubation being particularly common among patients with cognitive impairment or delirium. Self-extubation may lead to consideration of physical or chemical restraints, but such restraints are not justified to prevent NG tube self-extubation alone. Also, EN in actual practice often involves delayed and inadequate

TABLE 30-12 ■ ADVERSE EFFECTS OF ENTERAL NUTRITION AND MANAGEMENT APPROACHES

ADVERSE EFFECTS	MANAGEMENT

Poor tolerance
  Frequent self-extubation
  Agitation
	Consider
	  Parenteral nutrition
	  Percutaneous gastrostomy tubes

Pulmonary Aspiration	Elevate head of bed $\geq 30°$ (ideally 45°) Good oral hygiene Postpyloric feeding

Gastrointestinal
  Gastric retention
  Nausea/vomiting
  Diarrhea
	
	Low-fat formula, metaclopramide
	Postpyloric feeding
	↓Delivery rate, ↑fiber, antidiarrheals

Metabolic complications
  Hyperglycemia
 	
  Fluid and electrolytes
 	
  Refeeding syndrome
	
	Routine monitoring glucose, electrolytes
	Monitor weight, volume status, free water
	Monitor phosphate, magnesium, potassium

Mechanical problems
  Insertion site irritation/infection
  Tube plugging
 	
  G-tube, J-tube extubation
  Nasopharyngitis, sinusitis, local pain, epistaxis
	
	Local skin care
	
	Warm water or pancreatic enzyme flushes
	See text
	Use small-bore flexible tube and avoid prolonged nasal intubation (> 4–6 wks)

Drug interaction considerations	
Tube feeds ↓ bioavailability (eg, ciprofloxacin, azithromycin)	Hold feedings 15 min before and after medications
Frequent medications interrupt nutrition	Alternate medication routes (IV, IM, rectally, transdermal)

nutritional support because of frequent problems with tubes (eg, self-extubation, plugging) or GI intolerance (eg, high residuals, bloating, diarrhea). These factors may explain why attempts to provide EN to older persons are often abandoned after only a short course of therapy. Some have advocated for an early switch to PN, or starting with PN, particularly if patients are confused or delirious and the expected duration of therapy is short (1–2 weeks). If longer-term support is likely, early use of percutaneous gastrostomy tubes, which tend to be better tolerated by uncooperative or confused patients, may be considered (along with a reevaluation of overall patient care preferences and intervention goals before proceeding with this more invasive approach).

Pulmonary aspiration is a relatively common complication of EN, but unless aspiration causes an overt clinical event (eg, aspiration of a large volume), it is not clear that aspiration causes untoward clinical outcomes such as higher rates of pneumonia. Nonetheless, strategies to reduce aspiration are generally advised. Patients with gastric retention, decreased gag reflex, and altered levels of consciousness are at increased risk for aspiration, and mechanically ventilated patients should not be considered protected by the presence of an endotracheal cuff. The risk of aspiration can be reduced as outlined in **Table 30-12**. EN-related GI issues and their management are also presented in **Table 30-12**. When significant diarrhea occurs, infectious causes (particularly *Clostridium difficile*) must first be excluded. Metabolic abnormalities related to tube feedings include high potassium and phosphorous requirements in the first few days after nutritional support is started because of extracellular to intracellular shifts that accompany nutrient utilization, particularly among very malnourished patients ("refeeding syndrome"). Fluid retention can occur in older adults with impaired renal or cardiac function. To minimize these problems, monitoring protocols should include frequent evaluation of GI tolerance, daily weights, and daily monitoring of glucose and electrolytes until stable.

Increased problems with tube clogging often occur when more viscous higher-calorie formulas and medications (especially fiber and calcium supplements) are passed via small-bore (smaller than no. 10 French) catheters. Tube maintenance with regular water flushing every 4 to 8 hours for patients on continuous feeds, and before and after the delivery of intermittent TFs or medications (with 30 mL warm water) can reduce clogging problems. When possible, medications should be given by mouth rather than by feeding tube. If clogging occurs flush with 30 to 60 mL warm water, or a solution containing pancreatic enzymes. Cola or cranberry juice flushes have not been shown to be any more effective than water for resolving occlusions, and when used their dried residuals can narrow the lumen of the tube and contribute to clogging. Another common mechanical problem is the replacement of a gastrostomy or jejunostomy tube that has fallen out. Feeding tube fistula tracts are generally not well established for at least 1 to 2 weeks after placement (and often substantially longer given malnutrition's adverse effect on wound healing). Tubes that come out early (in the first 2–3 weeks after placement) require replacement by the original specialist. If the fistula tract is well established, patients or care providers should be able to gently replace tubes that have fallen out. Delay in doing so for more than 6 to 12 hours risks spontaneous closure of the tract. However, feeding should not be resumed until proper tube placement is radiologically confirmed.

Parenteral Nutrition

PN, the delivery of nutrients by vein, should be considered to prevent the adverse effects of malnutrition in patients who are unable to obtain adequate nutrients by oral or enteric routes (ie, EN is not possible or effective). However, specific indications regarding if and when to institute PN, as well as the utility of PN once instituted, have not been clearly delineated. In general, the decision to institute PN depends on the severity and expected course of the underlying disease(s) and the severity of preexisting and anticipated undernutrition. For critically ill patients who are adequately nourished on admission and have contraindications to EN, guidelines from the Society of Critical Care Medicine and American Society for Parental and Enteral Nutrition recommend against PN during the first week as early PN likely increases the risk of infections and other complications without conferring benefit. Conversely, in the situation where EN is not possible and the patient is severely malnourished or at high nutrition risk on admission, these same guidelines recommend consideration of PN as soon as possible after ICU admission. They also advise supplemental PN be considered after 7 to 10 days (but not before) for patients unable to meet more than 60% of energy and protein requirements by the enteral route alone. Decisions to institute PN require careful consideration of the patient's clinical condition and prognosis, clinical judgment about the patient's ability to tolerate undernutrition, and insight regarding patient care needs and preferences.

Efficacy The European Society for Clinical Nutrition and Metabolism concluded that PN can reduce morbidity and mortality in geriatric patients, but the evidence that PN improves clinical outcomes in older adults is not robust. There are limited data on beneficial effects of PN in the following settings: perioperatively in patients with GI cancers; in patients undergoing major elective surgery who are severely malnourished (generally when weight loss exceeds 10%–15% and serum albumin level is < 33 g/L, or, in the absence of weight loss, if albumin is < 28 g/L); and in bone marrow transplant recipients, malnourished critically ill patients, and patients with short bowel syndrome. Overall, there is still a paucity of studies and many unanswered questions about the efficacy and safety of PN in older adults.

Administration guidelines

Intravenous access Total parenteral nutrition (TPN), the delivery of all required nutrients by vein, requires the use of hypertonic solutions that can only be tolerated when delivered into large venous vessels, preferably into the superior vena cava. Because peripheral veins are limited to solutions containing lower concentrations of amino acids and dextrose (< 10% dextrose), peripheral parenteral nutrition (PPN) alone usually cannot deliver nutrients in sufficient quantity to meet all requirements. Although the infusion of lipids can improve energy delivery and vessel tolerance to PPN, its role in PN is extremely limited given the uncertain clinical benefits of short-term PPN and the ease of obtaining central venous access for TPN. Short-term TPN in the hospital setting is preferably delivered via a peripherally inserted central catheter (PICC). PICC lines offer reduced risks of central placement complications (eg, pneumothorax, inadvertent arterial puncture, and hemorrhage) and may have a reduced risk of infectious complications compared to subclavian or internal jugular venous catheters. Tunneled central venous catheters (eg, Hickman or Groshong catheter) are generally preferred over PICCs for long-term TPN (eg, home TPN) owing to lower infection rates. Regardless of the placement method used, proper line position needs to be confirmed by x-ray before initiating TPN.

TPN composition Standard TPN solutions contain carbohydrate (dextrose), protein (amino acids), electrolytes, vitamins, minerals, and trace elements. Lipid emulsions (traditionally soybean or safflower oil with egg phospholipids) may be infused separately or added to the mixture. Although clinicians should have a basic knowledge of usual TPN formula composition (**Table 30-13**), PN should be initiated and monitored by a team (usually physicians, nutrition specialists, and pharmacists) with an advanced understanding of factors such as nutrient metabolism and solute compatibility. Clinicians should also be aware that electrolyte requirements are highly variable and often require adjustments as they are influenced by the patient's underlying diseases (eg, heart failure, renal dysfunction) and factors such as renal or GI fluid losses.

The optimal proportions of fat and carbohydrate to meet energy needs are controversial. All standard formulas contain hypertonic glucose (10%–70% dextrose before mixing), but because diabetes and glucose intolerance are so common in older people, slow upward titration in delivery rates is necessary. Aggressive glucose monitoring and treatment is important, as hyperglycemia is associated with increased infection risk and worse clinical outcomes in critically ill patients. Glucose infusion rates should not exceed 5 mg/kg/min (about 500 g/day for a 70-kg person on continuous TPN) because the rate at which stressed patients can metabolize glucose as energy is limited. Overfeeding with glucose can lead to not only hyperglycemia, but also increased carbon dioxide production and the conversion of excess glucose calories into fat (which requires energy and contributes to fatty liver changes).

Lipids in the form of 10% to 20% fat emulsions are added to TPN as a source of concentrated energy and to supply essential fatty acids. Delivery of fat emulsions two to three times a week is usually sufficient to prevent essential fatty acid deficiency. Fat emulsions are isotonic and are generally well tolerated, but patients occasionally develop hyperlipidemia and, less frequently, have allergic reactions (usually to the egg phospholipid component). Increasing the proportion of energy supplied by fat can reduce hyperglycemia and carbon dioxide production, but fat delivery should not exceed 2.5 g/kg/day (or 50%–60% of nonprotein calories) to avoid possible adverse

TABLE 30-13 ■ "AVERAGE" TPN FORMULA COMPOSITION AND PARAMETERS FOR DAILY VITAMIN, MINERAL, AND ELECTROLYTE REQUIREMENTS

MACRONUTRIENTS[a]	
Protein	15%
Carbohydrate	55%–65%
Fat	20%–30%

MICRONUTRIENTS	
Vitamins	
Vitamin A	3300 IU
Vitamin D	200 IU
Vitamin E	10 IU
Thiamine (B-1)	6 mg
Riboflavin (B-2)	3.6 mg
Niacin (B-3)	40 mg
Pantothenic acid (B-5)	15 mg
Pyridoxine (B-6)	4 mg
Biotin (B-7)	60 µg
Folic acid (B-9)	600 µg
Cobalamin (B-12)	5 µg
Vitamin C	200 mg
Trace Elements	
Zinc	5 mg
Copper	1 mg
Chromium	10 µg
Manganese	0.5 µg
Selenium	60 µg
Electrolytes	
Sodium	60–150 mEq
Potassium	40–100 mEq
Chloride	Equal to sodium
Magnesium	16 mEq
Phosphorus	10–30 mmol
Calcium	10 mEq

[a]Percent of total calories.

consequences associated with fat overload. The fat overload syndrome is characterized by hyperlipidemia with diffuse fat deposition that can cause organ and reticuloendothelial system dysfunction and increased risk of sepsis. Newer lipid emulsions that contain omega-3 fatty acids (eg, mixtures that include fish oil as well as olive oil) may have anti-inflammatory properties that could be beneficial during critical illness, but to date evidence is inadequate to recommend their routine use.

Formula delivery Infusion rates usually start at 25 to 50 mL/h and are increased every 8 to 12 hours as metabolic status allows until fluid and nutrition goals are met. At some institutions, carbohydrate, fat, and protein TPN components are mixed together into a single bag (total nutrient admixture or 3-in-1 formula), which may have cost and convenience benefits compared to traditional TPN

TABLE 30-14 ■ GUIDELINES FOR MONITORING PATIENTS ON TPN

CLINICAL DATA	LABORATORY DATA
Vital signs three times per day until stable	Glucose chemsticks qid until stable
Daily weights	Daily: Electrolytes, glucose, creatinine, blood urea nitrogen, calcium, phosphorus, magnesium until stable, then twice weekly
Daily fluid input and output	
Daily line and skin inspection	
Efficacy of nutritional support	
	Weekly: LFTs, albumin, CBC, PT, triglyceride

CBC, complete blood count; LFTs, liver function tests (alanine and aspartate aminotransferase, alkaline phosphatase, bilirubin); PT, prothrombin time.

TABLE 30-15 ■ TPN COMPLICATIONS AND POTENTIAL CORRECTIVE MEASURES

CONDITION	PREVENTION/MANAGEMENT
Metabolic	
Fluid overload	Restrict fluid by ↑ macronutrient concentrations
Hyperglycemia	↓ Carbohydrate delivery (rate, concentration), insulin IV; consider ↑ proportion energy from fat
Hypoglycemia	Avoid sudden cessation/interruption of TPN
Refeeding syndrome	Start/titrate TPN slowly, avoid overfeeding
Hypertriglyceridemia	↓ Fat infusion rates and/or frequency of lipids
Hyperchloremic metabolic acidosis	↑ Acetate/↓ chloride; consider renal/gastrointestinal causes
Metabolic alkalosis	Consider renal/gastrointestinal causes; replete K+; ↓ acetate
Respiratory (hypercarbia)	↓ Total calories, ↑ proportion energy from fat
Nonmetabolic	
Line infection	Hand hygiene and maximal barrier precautions during insertion, single-lumen catheter; dedicated TPN line; aseptic line
Catheter occlusion	Regular flushes; no line blood draws; urokinase
Hepatic	
Steatosis/↑ liver function tests	Avoid carbohydrate overfeeding; rule out other causes
Biliary (cholestasis)	Enteral feed if possible; rule out other causes

administration of dextrose and amino acids (2-in-1) with separate intravenous (IV) fat emulsion infusions. In most circumstances, daily TPN volumes are infused continuously over the full 24 hours. This allows slower delivery of carbohydrate (which can help reduce hyperglycemia), and the continuous flow may decrease the risk of catheter occlusion while avoiding interruptions that might lead to hypoglycemia. Shorter infusion schedules with brief periods off TPN (cyclic TPN) are occasionally desirable, but this is more of an issue for long-term TPN in the home care setting. Because TPN formulas (especially the lipid component) can suppress appetite, it may be desirable to reduce or hold lipid emulsions for a few days to help improve oral intake prior to planned discontinuation of TPN.

Patient monitoring and complications Older persons receiving TPN should be monitored closely (**Table 30-14**), with adjustments made in frequency of monitoring depending on the patient's acuity and stability. **Table 30-15** details common complications and their prevention and/or treatment. Correction of dehydration and volume depletion can most readily be accomplished with standard IV fluids, which can be infused separately or added to TPN bags for convenience. Fluid overload can be managed by using higher concentrations of macronutrients to limit total volumes infused, with diuretics added as needed. Although insulin can be added directly to TPN solutions to help control hyperglycemia, it is best to give insulin separately until caloric delivery and glucose control are stabilized. IV insulin is preferred over subcutaneous insulin owing to the latter's potential for erratic absorption in malnourished patients. Infection and volume depletion need to be considered if hyperglycemia is a persistent problem. As with EN, potassium and phosphate must be monitored closely because they may drop precipitously after initiating TPN in malnourished patients. In most cases, electrolyte requirements stabilize within 1 week. The relative amounts of chloride (which can lead to metabolic acidosis) and acetate (which can be metabolized to bicarbonate and lead to metabolic alkalosis) can be adjusted as needed depending on the patient's acid–base balance.

Infection of the access line is uncommon in the first 72 hours, so early fevers are usually a result of other causes. The risk of infection can be reduced by following optimal insertion techniques and providing aseptic vigilant catheter care. The line site should be monitored daily for erythema, tenderness, or discharge. The increased rates of sepsis that have been observed in some trials of TPN (and which possibly diminished the potential for TPN trials to demonstrate improved clinical outcomes) may have been related to overfeeding and hyperglycemia. Avoidance of hyperglycemia (in particular glucose levels > 200 mg/dL) may decrease the risk of TPN-associated infections. Liver abnormalities that can occur with TPN include fatty liver with elevated liver function tests (often occurs early, likely related to carbohydrate overfeeding, generally benign/reversible) and cholestasis (tends to occur later, after 3+ weeks). EN, even in small amounts, may reduce problems with cholestasis.

Efforts should be made to transition to EN or oral intake as soon as feasible. As tolerance to EN improves, the amount of PN energy should be reduced and PN should be discontinued when EN or oral intake is providing more than 60% of energy requirements.

Special Issues

Comorbidity Responses to nutritional support may vary substantially owing to heterogeneity in underlying disease states associated with PEM (particularly the presence and severity of inflammatory/catabolic states). Limited data on the interaction between nutritional support and specific comorbid conditions and care settings include the following:

Hip fracture As many as half of all older patients who present with hip fractures are malnourished. Undernutrition may directly contribute to hip fracture events via increased presence of osteoporosis, increased risk of falls due to reduced LBM and strength, and reduced fat to "cushion" a fall. Nutritional intervention, primarily with oral nutritional supplements, improves energy balance and reduces complications and hospital length of stay following hip fracture. Accordingly, attention to nutrition is an important aspect of post hip fracture care, particularly in undernourished patients. As nasogastric feedings are not well tolerated after hip fracture and do not improve mortality, EN should be reserved for patients with more severe levels of malnutrition with poor intakes not responsive to oral supplementation.

Chronic obstructive pulmonary disease Prevalence estimates of malnutrition in patients with COPD range from 20% to 70%. Causes are likely multifactorial and include increased inflammatory activity, higher metabolic rate due to work of breathing and diminished intake due to dyspnea, chronic sputum (can alter taste), flattened diaphragm (may contribute to early satiety), and medication side effects (eg, adverse GI effects). Nutritional support (most often with oral supplements) has beneficial effects on a wide range of COPD outcome measures that include anthropometrics, immune function, muscle strength, respiratory function, and quality of life. Given their relative low cost and potential for benefit, nutritional support should be considered for all patients with COPD and evidence of PEM.

Nursing home Very high prevalence rates of PEM and weight loss have been documented in nursing home patients, likely because conditions associated with reduced intake are so common (see earlier discussion and **Table 30-1**), In this setting, simple interventions such as fortified foods, high-calorie snacks, nutritional supplements, and assisted feeding, can improve nutritional parameters and help stabilize weight. Although it is not clear that improvements in nutritional parameters translate to improved clinical outcomes, such interventions may enhance quality of life and are reasonable and appropriate for most nursing home residents.

Dementia Use of TFs in patients with advanced dementia is not advised. Tube feeding patients with advanced dementia does not improve nutritional status, decrease pressure sores or infections, reduce aspiration problems, or improve functional status or survival. Potential adverse effects of TFs in these patients include increased risk of aspiration, discomfort and complications from tube placement, agitation driving increased use of physical and chemical restraints, worsening pressure ulcers from increased urine and fecal output, and diminished quality of life from decreased interaction at mealtime and loss of gustatory pleasure from food intake. The lack of demonstrable benefits combined with considerable potential for harm led the American Geriatrics Society to advise clinicians not to recommend percutaneous feeding tubes in patients with advanced dementia and instead focus on oral-assisted feeding with food as the preferred nutrient.

FURTHER READING

Baldwin C, Smith R, Gibbs M, Weekes CE, Emery PW. Quality of the evidence supporting the role of oral nutritional supplements in the management of malnutrition: an overview of systematic reviews and meta-analyses. *Adv Nutr.* 2021;12(2):503–522.

Beavers KM, Nesbit BA, Kiel J, et al. Effect of an energy-restricted, nutritionally complete, higher protein meal plan on body composition and mobility in older adults with obesity: a randomized controlled trial. *J Gerontol A Biol Sci Med Sci.* 2019;74(6):929–935.

Cetin DC, Nasr G. Obesity in the elderly: more complicated than you think. *Cleve Clin J Med.* 2014;81:51–61.

Despres JP. Body fat distribution and risk of cardiovascular disease: an update. *Circulation.* 2012;126:1301–1313.

Fakhouri TH, Ogden CL, Carroll MD, Kit BK, Flegal KM. Prevalence of obesity among older adults in the United States, 2007-2010. *NCHS Data Brief.* 2012;106:1–8.

Gingrich A, Volkert D, Kiesswetter E, et al. Prevalence and overlap of sarcopenia, frailty, cachexia and malnutrition in older medical inpatients. *BMC Geriatrics.* 2019;19(1):120.

Jenkins DJA, et al. Supplemental vitamins and minerals for cardiovascular disease prevention and treatment. *J Am Coll Cardiol.* 2021;77:423–436.

Jensen GL, Compher C, Sullivan DH, et al. Recognizing malnutrition in adults: definitions and characteristics, screening, assessment, and team approach. *JPEN J Parenter Enteral Nutr.* 2013;37:802–807.

436 Kim Y, et al. Dietary fiber intake and total mortality: a meta-analysis of prospective cohort studies. *Am J Epidemiol.* 2014;180:565.

Manson J, et al. Vitamin D supplements and prevention of cancer and cardiovascular disease. *N Engl J Med.* 2019;380:33–44.

Michos Erin D, et al. Vitamin D, calcium supplements, and implications for cardiovascular health. *J Am Coll Cardiol.* 2021;77:437–449.

Miller J, Wells L, Nwulu U, Currow D, Johnson MJ, Skipworth RJE. Validated screening tools for the assessment of cachexia, sarcopenia, and malnutrition: a systematic review. *Am J Clin Nutr.* 2018;108(6):1196–1208.

Milne AC, Potter J, Vivanti A, Avenell A. Protein and energy supplementation in elderly people at risk from malnutrition. *Cochrane Database Syst Rev.* 2009;(2):CD003288.

Morton RW, Murphy KT, McKellar SR, et al. A systematic review, meta-analysis and meta-regression of the effect of protein supplementation on resistance training-induced gains in muscle mass and strength in healthy adults. *Br J Sports Med.* 2018;52:376–84.

Nicholls SJ, et al. Effect of high-dose omega-3 fatty acids vs corn oil on major adverse cardiovascular events in patients at high cardiovascular risk: the STRENGTH randomized clinical trial. *JAMA.* 2020;324:2268–2280.

Otten JJ, et al (eds). *Dietary Reference Intakes: The Essential Guide to Nutrient Requirements.* Washington, DC: The National Academies Press; 2006.

Perera L, Chopra A, Shaw A. Approach to patients with unintentional weight loss. *Med Clin North Am.* 2021; 105:175–186.

Protein and amino acid requirements in human nutrition. WHO Technical Report Series No. 935:2007. https://apps.who.int/iris/handle/10665/43411. Accessed December 15, 2021.

Reedy J, Krebs-Smith SM, Miller PE, et al. Higher diet quality is associated with decreased risk of all-cause, cardiovascular disease, and cancer mortality among older adults. *J Nutr.* 2014;144:881–889.

Reinders I, Volkert D, de Groot LCPGM, et al. Effectiveness of nutritional interventions in older adults at risk of malnutrition across different health care settings: pooled analyses of individual participant data from nine randomized controlled trials. *Clin Nutr.* 2019;38(4): 1797–1806.

Sobotka L, Schneider SM, Berner YN, et al. ESPEN guidelines of parenteral nutrition: geriatrics. *Clin Nutr.* 2009;28(4):461–466.

Struijk EA, Beulens JW, May AM, et al. Dietary patterns in relation to disease burden expressed in disability-adjusted life years. *Am J Clin Nutr.* 2014;100:1158–1165.

Taylor B, McClave S, Martindale R, et al. Guidelines for the provision and assessment of nutrition support therapy in the adult critically ill patient: Society of Critical Care Medicine and American Society for Parenteral and Enteral Nutrition. *Crit Care Med.* 2016;44(2):390–438.

Ukleja A, Gilbert K, Mogensen K, et al. Standards for nutrition support: adult hospitalized patients. *Nutr Clin Pract.* 2018;33(6):907–920.

US Department of Agriculture, Center for Nutrition Policy and Promotion. ChooseMyPlate.gov. USDA Center for Nutrition Policy & Promotion (CNPP). June 2, 2011. Available at http://choosemyplate.gov/. Accessed December 15, 2021.

Volkert D, Beck AM, Cederholm T, et al. ESPEN guideline on clinical nutrition and hydration in geriatrics. *Clin Nutr.* 2019;38(1):10–47.

Wilding JPH, Batterham RL, Calanna S, et al. Once-weekly semaglutide in adults with overweight or obesity. *N Engl J Med.* 2021;384(11):989.

Yang Y, et al. Association between dietary fiber and lower risk of all-cause mortality: a meta-analysis of cohort studies. *Am J Epidemiol.* 2015;181:83.

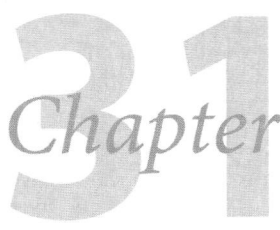

Chapter 31

Disorders of Swallowing

Nicole Rogus-Pulia, Steven Barczi, JoAnne Robbins

INTRODUCTION

Demographic changes related to aging necessitate that clinicians have the resources to address eating and swallowing difficulties present in older adults. The capacity to effectively and safely eat or swallow is one of the most basic human needs and also can be a great pleasure. Therefore the loss of this capacity can have far-reaching implications. Many would argue that swallowing is one of the cardinal behaviors needed to sustain life. The process of swallowing requires orchestration of a complex series of psychological, sensory, and motor behaviors that are both voluntary and involuntary. Dysphagia refers to difficulty swallowing that may include oropharyngeal or esophageal problems. More specifically, there may be difficulty in oral preparation for swallowing and/or moving material from the mouth to the esophagus and from the esophagus to the stomach.

Although age-related changes and comorbidities place older adults at risk for dysphagia, an older adult's swallow is not inherently impaired. *Presbyphagia* refers to characteristic changes in the mechanism of swallowing of otherwise healthy older adults. Clinicians need to be able to distinguish among *dysphagia*, presbyphagia, and other related diagnoses such as globus to avoid misdiagnosis and overtreatment of dysphagia. Older adults can be more vulnerable and, with additional stressors such as acute illness and certain medications, they can cross over from having a healthy older swallow (*presby*phagia) to experiencing *dys*phagia. This chapter reviews the normal swallowing process and presbyphagia, as a healthy aging evolution, dysphagia outcomes, multidisciplinary approaches to diagnosing and managing dysphagia, and rehabilitation strategies for dysphagia care.

Learning Objectives

- To understand the anatomy and physiology of the normal swallowing process.
- To distinguish between presbyphagia (healthy age-associated changes in swallowing) and dysphagia.
- To identify age-related diseases and conditions most commonly associated with the development of dysphagia.
- To describe screening and assessment techniques, instrumental and noninstrumental, for identifying and characterizing dysphagia.
- To summarize options available for treatment of dysphagia, including compensatory and rehabilitative approaches.

Key Clinical Points

1. Changes in swallowing that occur with healthy aging, termed presbyphagia, combined with age-associated diseases and conditions place older adults at risk for the development of dysphagia.
2. Swallowing is a complex patterned response that involves coordination of 30 oral and pharyngeal muscle pairs across both the cranial and spinal nerve systems.
3. An interdisciplinary team approach to early identification and comprehensive assessment of dysphagia will allow for effective treatment through both compensatory and rehabilitative techniques.

IMPACT OF DYSPHAGIA

Dysphagia prevalence depends on the specific population sampled, with community-dwelling and more independent individuals having rates near 15%. Upward of 40% of people living in institutional settings, such as assisted living and nursing homes, are dysphagic. Given the projected increases in the geriatric population over the next several decades, the prevalence of dysphagia is expected to increase substantially. With a greater number of individuals in assisted-living facilities and nursing homes, there is a compelling need to address dysphagia not only in ambulatory and acute care settings but also in long-term care settings.

The consequences of dysphagia vary from social isolation because of the embarrassment associated with choking or coughing at mealtime to physical discomfort (eg, food sticking in the throat) to potentially life-threatening conditions. The more serious sequelae include dehydration, malnutrition, and both overt and silent aspiration, precipitating pulmonary complications. For the purposes of this chapter, aspiration is defined as the entry of material into the airway *below* the level of the true vocal folds. Silent aspiration refers to the circumstance in which a bolus comprising saliva, food, liquid, medication, or any foreign material enters the airway below the vocal folds *without* triggering overt symptoms such as coughing or throat clearing. Both overt and silent aspiration occur more frequently in older adults and may lead to pneumonitis, pneumonia, exacerbation of chronic lung disease, or even asphyxiation and death.

Dysphagia is an independent risk factor for the development of aspiration pneumonia. The reported prevalence of dysphagia in older patients hospitalized for pneumonia ranges from 55% to 86%. Dysphagia is also an independent risk factor for hospital readmission due to aspiration and nonaspiration pneumonia in patients 70 or older discharged from an acute geriatric unit. Dysphagia is an independent risk factor for malnutrition as well.

Signs of bolus flow abnormality in dysphagia, using instrumental assessments (videofluoroscopy and fiberoptic endoscopic evaluation of swallowing [FEES]), include (1) the duration, direction, and completeness of bolus flow; (2) the duration and extent (range) of anatomic structural movements; and (3) the relationship between bolus flow and structural movements as well as between physiologic and anatomic parameters such as pressure generation and muscle/fat structure. Bulbar innervated swallowing mechanisms may provide targets specific for novel treatment paradigms aimed at improving swallowing function. Other clinical outcomes of dysphagia have become important end points in assessing interventions that aim to make it possible for patients to eat and drink adequately and safely. Key outcome measures are summarized in **Table 31-1**. Additionally, pneumonitis, overt aspiration pneumonia, and other forms of pulmonary damage are monitored. Nonetheless, it has been difficult to attribute mortality directly to dysphagia because it is often a secondary rather than a primary diagnosis.

Dysphagia profoundly influences quality of life (QOL). Patients with swallowing difficulties, especially those who relinquish oral eating, manifest significant changes in psychosocial status, functional status, and emotional well-being. Eating and drinking are social events that relate to friendship, acceptance, entertainment, and communication. As such, major adjustments in the process of feeding and eating can lead to distressing responses such as shame, anxiety, depression, and isolation. Practical dysphagia-specific, comprehensive, QOL measures are available. By monitoring functional outcomes in clinical practice, physicians and other health care providers may be able to better assess and adjust their treatment of dysphagia.

SWALLOWING PROCESS

Swallowing is an orchestrated activity that balances the competing behaviors of ingestion, speaking, and breathing. Approximately 30 oral and pharyngeal muscle pairs and multiple nerves must perform precisely on cue so that the upper aerodigestive tract is reconfigured from a mechanism that channels air for breathing and speaking (**Figure 31-1**) to a food-propelling mechanism that accomplishes ingestion (**Figure 31-2**). The four morphologic regions serving these purposes are the oral cavity, pharynx, larynx, and esophagus. Of these, the first three collectively are termed the upper aerodigestive tract because they also serve the airway-dependent functions of respiration and speech production. In humans, with our upright posture, it is the adjacent position of the anatomy for breathing to the anatomy for food passage that facilitates gravitational influences on food to flow into an unprotected airway. Such anatomy and physiology require precision to satisfy the delicate balance between swallowing physiology and breathing—each a life-sustaining function that must occur during cessation of its counterpart. Thus, a basic understanding of the relationship between the anatomic components and the functional interaction of this mechanism is essential to an understanding of normal swallowing and the effects of age and age-related diseases on it.

Normal Swallowing

Swallowing is an integrated neuromuscular process consisting of a combination of volitional and relatively automatic movements. Although normal swallowing is usually conceptualized as a continuous sequence of events, the process of deglutition has been conveniently described as occurring in two, three, or four phases or stages. Moreover, the system engaged in swallowing can be divided into two basic structural subsystems, horizontal and vertical (**Figure 31-3**), that mirror the direction of bolus flow and the potential for gravitational influence on it.

Horizontal subsystem The oral cavity components comprise the horizontal subsystem, which handles the initial, largely volitional, processing and transport phases of swallowing—the swallow preparatory phase and the oral transport phase. The *swallow preparatory phase* is characterized by food acceptance, containment, and manipulation. The lips and the buccal musculature act in complex patterns, varying the size and shape of the oral opening to allow acceptance and/or containment of food within the oral cavity. The process of chemically changing the material requires that numerous labial and lingual glands secrete into the oral cavity an enzyme-rich fluid that maintains and lubricates the mucosa and is directly incorporated into the food. Textural manipulation of food and the mechanical formation of a bolus once it is modified by saliva are accomplished largely by the tongue. The tongue positions the bolus between the teeth and moves in a complex three-dimensional chewing pattern if the bolus requires mastication. The moistening of the food in the oral cavity is essential for normal bolus transit

TABLE 31-1 ■ SUMMARY DESCRIPTIONS OF SELECTED TOOLS FOR ASSESSING OUTCOMES RELATED TO EATING AND SWALLOWING

DOMAIN	TOOL	SHORT DESCRIPTION
Nutrition/Dietary Intake	Functional Oral Intake Scale (FOIS)	Describes the functional level of oral intake of food and liquid (1 = tube dependent; 7 = unrestricted oral intake).
	International Dysphagia Diet Standardization Initiative-Functional Diet Scale (IDDSI-FDS)	Captures the nature and degree of diet texture modification using the IDDSI framework.
Patient-Reported Outcomes	Eating Assessment Tool (EAT-10)	10-item questionnaire focused on self-perceived oropharyngeal dysphagia.
	Swallowing Quality of Life (Swal-QOL)	Questionnaire designed to measure quality of life related to oropharyngeal dysphagia.
	Sydney Swallow Questionnaire (SSQ)	17-question self-report inventory developed to measure symptomatic severity of oropharyngeal dysphagia.
	MD Anderson Dysphagia Inventory (MDADI)	Self-administered questionnaire designed specifically for evaluating the impact of dysphagia on quality of life of patients with head and neck cancer.
Clinical Assessment of Swallowing Function	3-ounce water swallow test (WST)	Screening technique for aspiration risk. Involves administering 3 ounces of water to the individual and monitoring for signs of aspiration before, during, and after administration.
	Yale Swallow Protocol	Screening protocol designed to identify patients at high risk for aspiration. Incorporates assessment of cognition, oral motor function, and the 3-ounce water swallow test.
	Toronto Bedside Swallow Screening Test (TOR-BSST)	Screening tool administered at the bedside by trained screeners that identifies patients at risk for dysphagia following stroke.
	Timed Water Swallowing Test (TWST)	Timed test of swallowing capacity with water designed for use in patients with neurogenic dysphagia.
	Test of Mastication and Swallowing Solids (TOMASS)	Quantitative clinical assessment of solid bolus ingestion.
Instrumental Assessment of Swallowing Function	Penetration-Aspiration Scale (PAS)	Scale designed to capture multidimensional depth of airway invasion during the modified barium swallow assessment.
	Modified Barium Swallow Impairment Profile (MBSImP)	Standardized assessment of swallowing impairment on the MBS study through examination of 17 physiologic components and associated standardized impairment scores.
	Dynamic Imaging Grade of Swallowing Toxicity (DIGEST)	Grading scale for use with MBS studies that reflects the interaction between safety (airway invasion) and efficiency (pharyngeal residue) to yield a global grade of pharyngeal dysphagia.
	Yale Pharyngeal Residue Severity Rating Scale	Anatomically defined and image-based tool to determine residue location and severity based on Fiberoptic Endoscopic Evaluation of Swallowing (FEES).
Global Functional Scales	American Speech-Language-Hearing Association (ASHA) National Outcomes Measurement System (NOMS) Functional Communication Measure (FCM) for Swallowing	Assessment of overall swallowing function on a 7-point scale based on level of oral intake/method of feeding, need for compensatory strategies, and level of cueing.
	Dysphagia Outcome and Severity Scale (DOSS)	7-point scale developed to systematically rate the functional severity of dysphagia based on instrumental assessment (MBS or FEES) and recommendations for diet level, independence level, and type of nutrition.

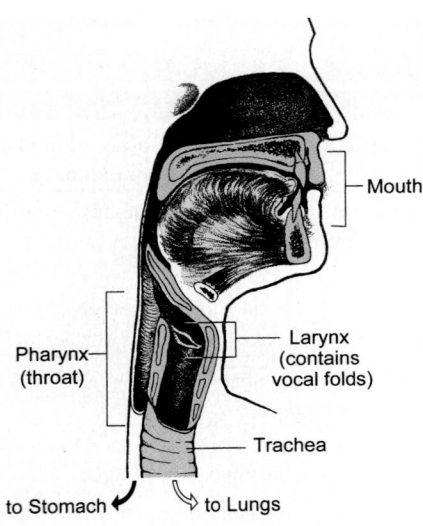

FIGURE 31-1. Aerodigestive tract channeling air for breathing from the nose and mouth through the open larynx into the lungs and back up and out. For speaking, air is channeled similarly, but the vocal folds vibrate to produce voice. (Modified with permission from Weihofen D, Robbins J, Sullivan PA. *The Easy to Swallow, Easy to Chew Cookbook.* New York, NY: John Wiley and Sons; 2002. Illustration ©2002 by Kathryn M. Kleckner.)

and/or flow and clearance, particularly because gravity provides no assistance until the vertical phases of swallowing.

The *oral transport phase* comprises movement of the cohesive bolus (masticated if necessary) posteriorly (and horizontally when the subject is in a normal upright seated posture) to the inlet of the superior aspect of the vertical subsystem, the pharynx (**Figure 31-4**). The intrinsic tongue muscles change the shape and position of the tongue,

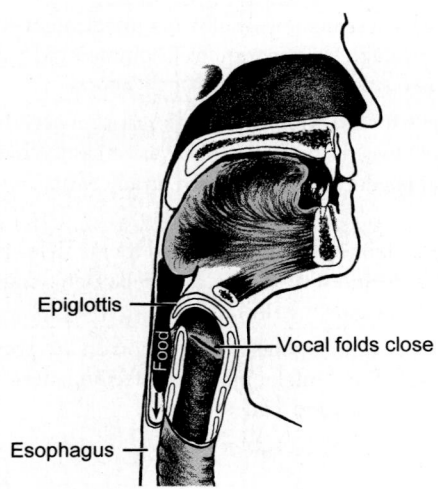

FIGURE 31-2. Aerodigestive tract reconfigured from an air channel to a food-propelling mechanism during swallowing. The tongue propels food into the throat; the epiglottis covers the larynx, which is the airway entrance; and the vocal folds close to protect the trachea and lungs from foreign material. (Modified with permission from Weihofen D, Robbins J, Sullivan PA. *The Easy to Swallow, Easy to Chew Cookbook.* New York, NY: John Wiley and Sons; 2002. Illustration ©2002 by Kathryn M. Kleckner.)

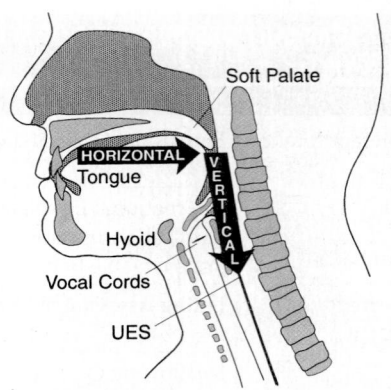

FIGURE 31-3. The oropharyngeal swallowing mechanism can be divided into two basic structural subsystems, horizontal and vertical, that mirror the direction of bolus flow. UES, upper esophageal sphincter. (Adapted with permission from Robbins J. Normal swallowing and aging. *Semin Neurol.* 1996;16[4]:309–317.)

forming grooves along its body and anterior and lateral seals to facilitate containment (**Figure 31-4A**), and then progressively arching the tongue posteriorly to transport the bolus to the vertical subsystem (**Figures 31-4B and C**).

Vertical subsystem The pharyngeal and laryngeal components, in conjunction with the tongue dorsum, comprise the superior aspect of the vertical subsystem, where gravity begins to assist in the transport of the bolus. The anatomic juxtaposition of the entrance to the airway (laryngeal vestibule) and the pharyngeal aspect of the upper digestive tract demand biomechanical precision to ensure simultaneous airway protection and bolus transfer or propulsion through the pharynx. To this end, the pharyngeal transport phase is characterized by a sequence of rapid, highly coordinated neuromuscular events that cause pressure changes critical to bolus transport or transit in a safe, timely, efficient manner.

Linguapalatal contact sequentially moves the bolus against the posterior pharyngeal wall, contributing to the positive pressures imparted to the bolus and propelling it downward. Simultaneously, the pharyngeal constrictors begin to contract in a descending sequence, first elevating and widening the entire pharynx to engulf the bolus (**Figures 31-4D and E**), and clean up residue after swallowing is completed. Tight closure of the velopharynx during the pharyngeal transport phase provides a seal at the superior aspect of the vertical system, preventing nasal leakage of the bolus and contributing to the generation of high positive pressures, which are applied to the bolus.

Several mechanisms ensure the redundancy by which airway protection is accomplished. Three levels of sphincteric closure include (1) the aryepiglottic folds, (2) the false vocal folds, and (3) the true vocal folds, with closure of the true vocal folds (the lowest of the three sphincters) providing "the last line of defense" to prevent aspiration of invasive material. The hyolaryngeal complex is lifted upward and forward by the combined contraction of the suprahyoid muscles, thyrohyoid muscles, and pharyngeal elevators.

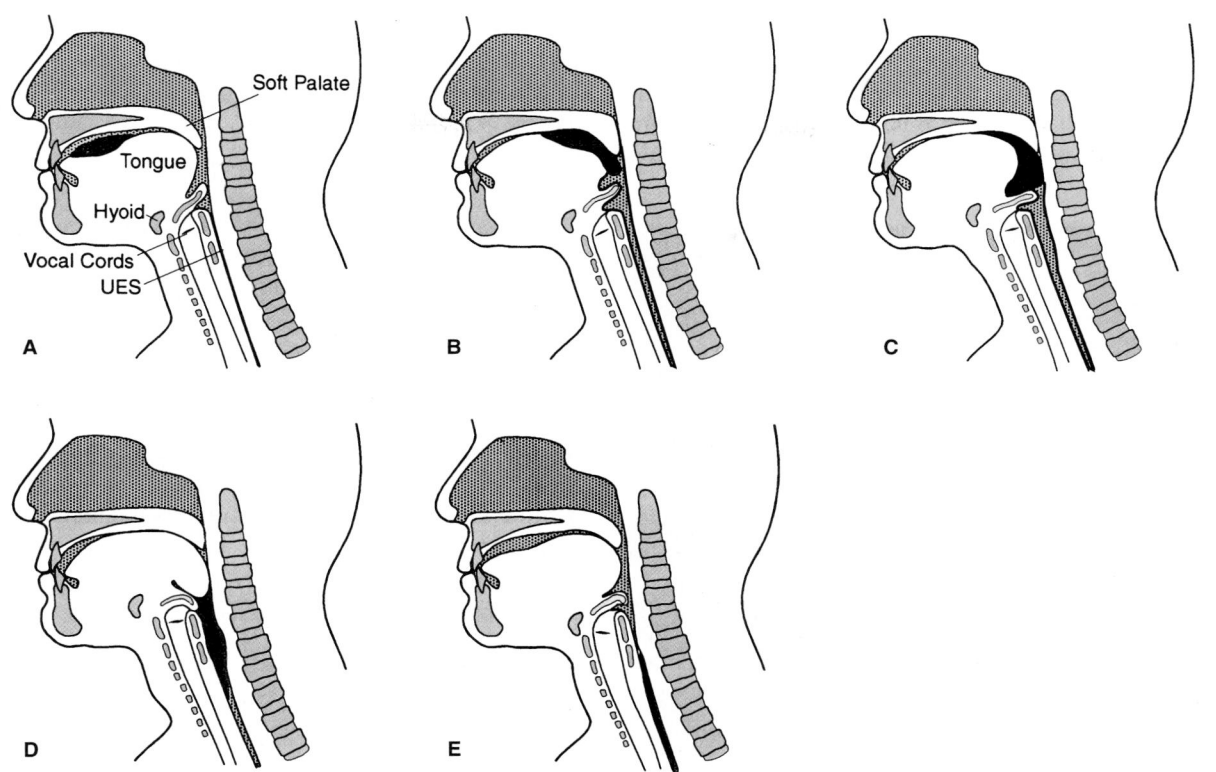

FIGURE 31-4. Lateral view of bolus propulsion during swallowing. **A.** Voluntary initiation of the swallow by tongue "loading." **B.** Bolus propulsion by tongue dorsum and upper esophageal sphincter (UES) opening anticipating bolus arrival. **C.** Bolus entry into pharynx associated with epiglottal downward tilt, hyolaryngeal excursion, and UES opening. **D.** Linguapharyngeal contact facilitating bolus passage through the pharynx. **E.** UES closing and completion of oropharyngeal swallowing; then the entire bolus is in the esophagus. (Adapted with permission from Robbins J. Normal swallowing and aging. *Semin Neurol.* 1996;16[4]:309–317.)

This hyolaryngeal elevation and anterior movement, coupled with retraction of the tongue base, covers the laryngeal vestibule and diverts the bolus laterally around the airway. Timely relaxation and opening of the upper esophageal sphincter (UES) permits continuous vertical passage of the bolus into the esophagus. The UES functions as a mechanical valve. For it to open normally, four criteria must be met: (1) relaxation of muscle tone, (2) compliant tissue, (3) traction force provided by sufficient hyolaryngeal excursion, and (4) pulsion force imparted by the bolus. In normal swallowing, UES relaxation and opening occur prior to bolus arrival at the hypopharynx.

Neurophysiology of Oropharyngeal Swallowing

Historically, swallowing was largely viewed as a sequence of pharyngeal and esophageal events and was defined as reflexive. However, it is now clear that normal swallowing is a patterned response rather than a traditional reflex.

Sensorimotor control of swallowing requires the coordinated activity to be distributed across both the cranial and spinal nerve systems, including the peripheral nerves, their central nuclei, and their neural centers, as summarized in **Table 31-2**. This neural network spans all levels of the neuraxis from the cerebrum superiorly to the brain stem and spinal nerves inferiorly and muscles and

end organs at the periphery. This relatively diffuse network is designed to integrate and sequence both the volitional and automatic actions of swallowing.

Healthy persons depend on a highly automated neuromuscular sensorimotor process that intricately coordinates the activities of chewing, swallowing, and airway protection. To accomplish a normal swallow, which occurs

TABLE 31-2 ■ NEUROMUSCULAR CONTROL OF SWALLOWING

NEURAL CONTROL

- Afferent sensory fibers contained in cranial nerves
- Cerebral and midbrain fibers that synapse with brainstem swallowing centers
- Paired swallowing centers in the brain stem
- Efferent motor fibers contained in cranial nerves and the ansa cervicalis

MUSCLE CONTROL

- The masseters, temporalis, and pterygoids (innervated by cranial nerve V)
- The lip and buccal musculature, the orbicularis oris, and the buccinator (innervated by cranial nerve VII)
- The intrinsic and extrinsic lingual muscles (innervated by cranial nerve XII).

in 2 seconds or less, the muscles of chewing interact with 26 pairs of striated pharyngeal and laryngeal muscles (see **Table 31-2**). Optimal structural integrity and precise neural mediation result in continuous, rapid bolus flow from the mouth to the esophagus (**Figures 31-5A, B, and C**) that

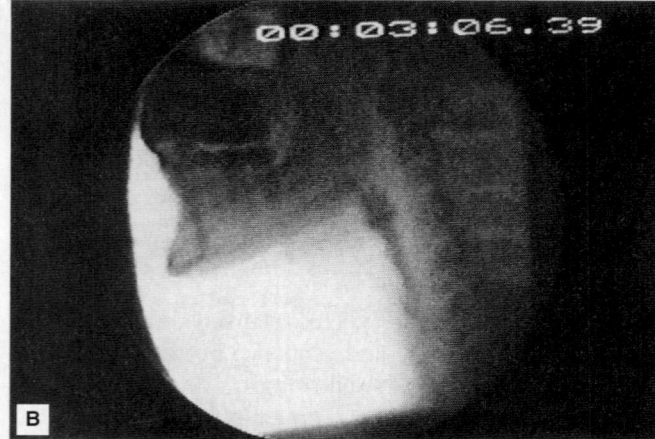

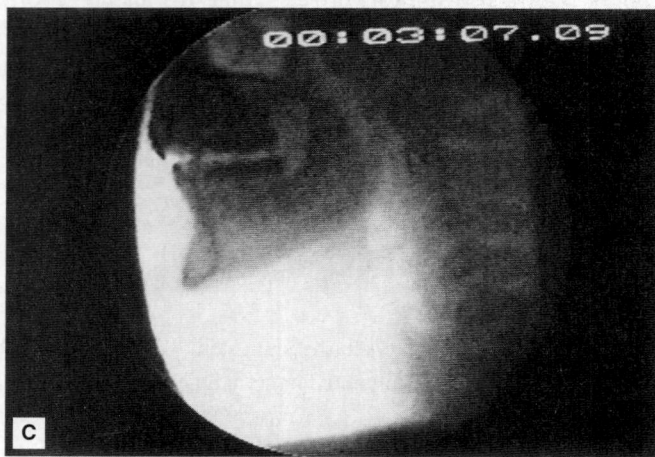

FIGURE 31-5. Healthy young swallowing documented with video-fluoroscopy. **A.** Bolus in oral cavity, ready to be swallowed. **B.** Bolus appears as a "column" of material swiftly moving through the pharynx. **C.** Oropharynx cleared of material when the swallow is completed. (Adapted with permission from Robbins J. Normal swallowing and aging. *Semin Neurol.* 1996;16[4]:309–317.)

accommodates variations in bolus size, texture, and temperature and the individual's intent to swallow, chew, or just hold the bolus in the mouth.

SENESCENT SWALLOWING

Traditional thinking suggests that the causes of dysphagia are always disease-related, with direct or indirect damage to effector end-organ systems of swallowing. However, the swallowing changes with healthy aging, progressive changes of the anatomy, and physiology of the oropharyngeal swallowing mechanism put the older population at increased risk for dysphagia (**Figure 31-6**). Dysphagia occurs when an older healthy adult with diminished functional reserve is faced with increased stressors that elicit dysphagia only in a vulnerable individual. Such stressors include central nervous system (CNS)-altering medications, mechanical perturbations (eg, a nasogastric [NG] tube or a tracheostomy), or medical conditions (eg, frailty).

Age-Associated Changes in Swallowing

The swallow of an older healthy adult is relatively slow. In people older than 65, the initiation of laryngeal and pharyngeal events, including laryngeal vestibule closure, maximal hyolaryngeal excursion, and upper UES opening, takes longer than in adults younger than 45. Although the specific neural underpinnings have not been confirmed, oral events may become uncoupled from the pharyngeal response. Thus, in older healthy adults, the bolus may remain adjacent to an open airway by pooling or pocketing in the pharyngeal recesses longer than in younger adults (**Figure 31-7**).

Aspiration and airway penetration are the most significant adverse clinical outcomes of misdirected bolus flow, as reflected in the high rates of pneumonia with increasing age and disease. While airway invasion is generally believed to be absent in healthy adults, under demanding conditions (eg, endurance = demanding), older individuals are less able to compensate and are more at risk for aspiration than younger people. Findings such as these differentiate presbyphagia from clinically abnormal swallowing.

Age-related changes in the generation of lingual pressure also define presbyphagia. Healthy older individuals have reduced isometric tongue pressures compared with younger individuals. In contrast, the generation of maximal lingual pressure during swallowing (which requires submaximal pressures) remains "young" in magnitude but slows in the time necessary to achieve those "young" swallowing pressures. The relationship between maximum isometric pressure and peak swallowing pressures can be considered an indication of the functional reserve available for swallowing. As people get older, slower swallowing may allow time to recruit the necessary number of motor units required for pressures critical for adequate bolus propulsion through the oropharynx. However, fluids

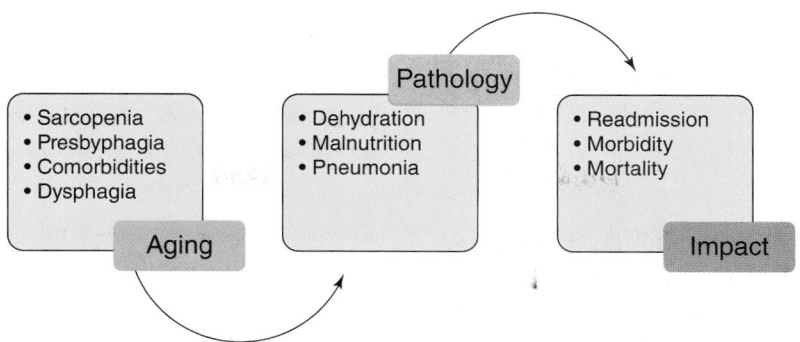

FIGURE 31-6. Model for interactions of aging effects leading to clinical outcomes of dysphagia. The onset of sarcopenia along with other factors leads to *presby*phagia, or age-associated changes in swallowing, in healthy older adults. When older adults experience comorbid age-related disease or conditions, such as stroke or dementia, they are at increased risk for the development of *dys*phagia. Dysphagia is associated with a variety of negative health outcomes, including dehydration, malnutrition, and pneumonia, that increase the risk for hospital readmissions, morbidity, and even death.

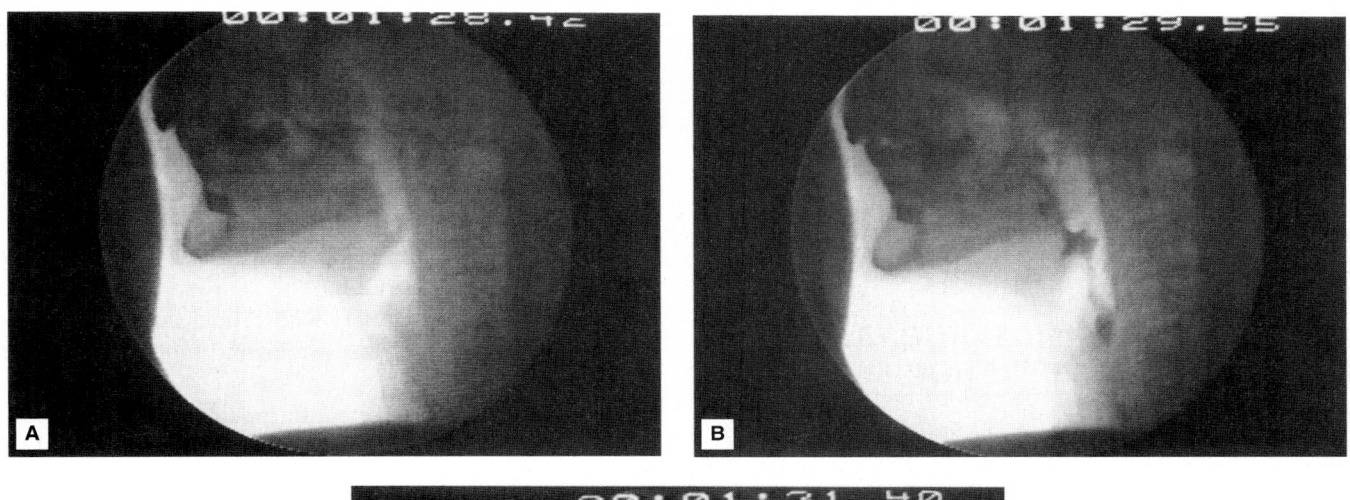

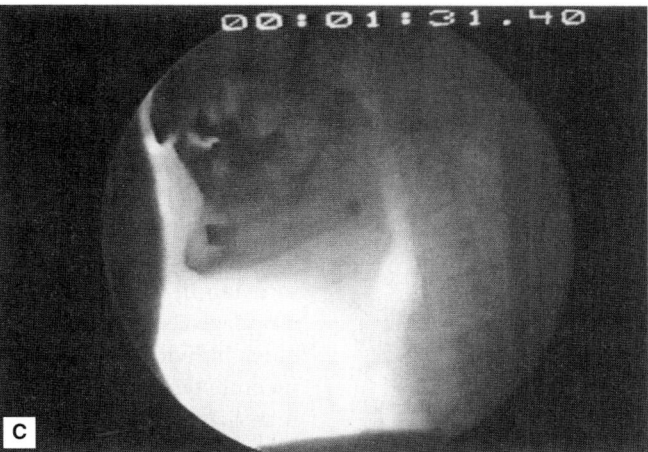

FIGURE 31-7. Healthy old swallowing documented with videofluoroscopy. **A.** Bolus in mouth ready for swallowing. **B.** Bolus pooled in vallecula and pyriform sinus during delayed onset of pharyngeal response. **C.** Bolus cleared of material when the swallow is completed. (Adapted with permission from Robbins J. Normal swallowing and aging. *Semin Neurol.* 1996;16[4]:309–317.)

of low viscosity (eg, water, tea), by their composition, are likely to move more quickly than the physiology to handle them safely and thus put older people at increased risk for aspiration.

Neurophysiologic Correlates of Senescent Swallowing

The relationship between slower swallowing and increased number and severity of periventricular white-matter hyperintensities (PVHs) in the brain suggests that voluntary control of swallowing is mediated by corticobulbar pathways traveling within the periventricular white matter. These PVHs may explain, at least in part, the relatively asymptomatic decline in oropharyngeal motor performance observed in older people. Cerebral atrophy, a common finding in asymptomatic older individuals, may be another contributing factor to presbyphagia.

Changes in the periphery with age may be a function of changes in various sensory mechanisms or caused by muscle atrophy. Similar to the age-related loss of limb skeletal muscle, there are changes with age in muscle composition, muscle tension, muscle strength, and muscle contraction in facial, masticatory, and lingual musculature. Rather than reflecting CNS deterioration, slowed swallowing that remains coordinated and effective, as found in most healthy old people, may represent a compensatory strategy for achieving pressure-generation values that may be critical to successful bolus propulsion.

DIFFERENTIAL CONSIDERATIONS FOR DYSPHAGIA AND ASPIRATION

Etiologies

Older adults are at increased risk for developing dysphagia because of a number of age-associated phenomena, comorbid conditions, and medications. By targeting high-risk groups and intervening with acceptable compensatory and rehabilitative approaches, it is hoped that the ultimate burden of dysphagia on the geriatric population will decline.

As illustrated in **Figure 31-6**, decreased physiologic reserve can combine with a number of age-related, disease-related, or iatrogenic changes to transform an at-risk individual into an older adult with dysphagia. Sarcopenia, described in detail in Chapter 49, affects the head and neck musculature involved in swallowing. In fact, anterior and posterior isometric tongue pressure positively correlates with hand grip strength and with jump height and power. Furthermore, sarcopenia and worsening frailty status predict dysphagia prevalence in older adults.

Several anatomic or pathologic perturbations occurring throughout the orobuccal cavity, the laryngopharyngeal region, and the esophagus are also important cofactors in the onset of dysphagia. Additionally, age-related alterations

in the neural coupling between respiration and swallowing result in more frequent occurrences of swallowing during the inspiratory phase in older adults. When the inspiratory phase is interrupted for swallowing rather than the expiratory phase, there is an increased risk for entry of material into the airway once inhalation is resumed.

Age-related conditions Age-related changes throughout the upper aerodigestive tract can influence swallowing integrity. Oral risks are also discussed in Chapter 32. During the oral phase, the food bolus may be inadequately prepared because of poor or absent dentition, periodontal disease, ill-fitting dentures, or inappropriate salivation caused by xerostomia. Salivary flow rate declines with advancing age and is exacerbated by xerostomia-inducing medications often prescribed to older adults. Certain organic components within whole saliva, including secretory immunoglobulin A and mucoglycoproteins, also are reduced in older adults thereby altering the compositional makeup of saliva and affecting oral health. This decline in mucous properties can change the viscoelastic properties of saliva that may be important for bolus formation.

Musculoskeletal factors such as weakness of the muscles of mastication, arthritis of the temporomandibular joint or larynx, osteoporosis of the jaw, or changes in tongue strength and coordination of the oropharyngeal events can deter efficient swallowing. Sensory input for taste, temperature, and tactile sensation changes in many older adults. This disruption of sensory-cortical-motor feedback loops may interfere with proper bolus formation and timely response of the swallowing motoric sequence and detract from the pleasure of eating.

Material can penetrate into the upper airway in normal individuals if the bolus is not properly prepared, if the timing of the swallow is delayed, or if the intake is too rapid. Important risk factors for aspiration include altered level of attention during feeding (eg, delirium), altered sensory discrimination in the oropharynx, feeding problems, mechanical ventilation, and feeding tube placement. In the latter circumstance, the rate of tube feeding, the position of the patient, altered intestinal transit times, and the ability of the patient to protect their airway all influence the occurrence of reflux and aspiration and are discussed in detail in Chapter 30. There are subtle changes in lower esophageal sphincter (LES) function even in asymptomatic older individuals. Gastroesophageal reflux caused by LES incompetence as well as intraesophageal reflux (defined as material moving proximally within the esophagus prior to crossing the LES) also predispose individuals to micro- or macroaspiration.

Age-related disease Neurologic and neuromuscular disorders are principal risks for dysphagia (**Table 31-3**). Stroke, brain injury, Alzheimer disease, other dementia syndromes, and parkinsonism all place older adults at increased risk for dysphagia with its incipient consequences.

TABLE 31-3 ■ NEUROLOGIC DISORDERS CAUSING DYSPHAGIA

Stroke

Head trauma

Parkinsonism and other movement and neurodegenerative disorders

Progressive supranuclear palsy
  Olivopontocerebellar atrophy
  Huntington disease
  Wilson disease

Torticollis
  Tardive dyskinesia

Alzheimer disease and other dementias

Motor neuron disease (amyotrophic lateral sclerosis)

Guillain-Barré syndrome and other polyneuropathies

Neoplasms and other structural disorders
  Primary brain tumors
  Intrinsic and extrinsic brainstem tumors
  Base of skull tumors
  Syringobulbia
  Arnold-Chiari malformation
  Neoplastic meningitis

Multiple sclerosis

Postpolio myelitis syndrome

Infectious disorders
  Chronic infectious meningitis
  Syphilis and Lyme disease
  Diphtheria
  Botulism
  Viral encephalitis, including rabies

Myasthenia gravis

Myopathy
  Polymyositis, dermatomyositis, inclusion body myositis, and sarcoidosis
  Myotonic and oculopharyngeal muscular dystrophy
  Hyper- and hypothyroidism
  Cushing syndrome

Iatrogenic conditions
  Medication side effects
  Postsurgical neurogenic dysphagia
    Neck surgery
    Posterior fossa surgery
    Irradiation of the head and neck

TABLE 31-4 ■ WARNING SIGNS ASSOCIATED WITH DYSPHAGIA AND ASPIRATION RISK

Decreased alertness or cognitive dysfunction
  Stupor, coma, heavy sedation, delirium, "sundowning," dementia, agitation
  Playing with food, inappropriate size of bites, talking or emotional lability during attempts to swallow

Changes in approach to food
  Avoidance of eating in company
  Increase in amount of food remaining on plate
  Special physical preparation of food or avoidance of foods of specific consistency
  Prolonged mealtime, intermittent cessation of intake, frequent "wash downs"
  Compensatory measures (head and neck movements)
  Laborious chewing, repetitive swallowing
  Coughing and choking on swallowing, increased need to clear throat

Manifestations of impaired oropharyngeal functions
  Dysarthria
  Wet, hoarse voice and other voice changes
  Dysfunction of focal musculature (facial asymmetries, abnormal reflexes or dystonia, dyskinesias or fasciculations)
  Drooling or oral spillage, pooling and pocketing of food
  Frequent throat clearing

Patient complaints or observations of
  Difficulty initiating a swallow
  Sensation of obstruction of bolus in the throat or chest
  Regurgitation of food or acid
  Inability to handle secretions
  Unexplained weight loss
  Impaired breathing during meals or immediately after eating
  Pain on swallowing
  Leakage of food or saliva from a tracheostomy site

with dementia. The inability to eat safely is one of the most life-threatening impairments for these patients frequently leading to pneumonia onset. Between 50% and 75% of patients who have had a recent acute stroke develop eating and swallowing problems, with ensuing complications of malnutrition and pneumonia. Brainstem or bilateral hemispheric strokes predictably produce dysphagia, but unilateral lesions also can contribute to dysphagia.

A host of common problems involving the head and neck can directly damage the effector muscles of swallowing and increase the risk for dysphagia. Head and neck injury, carcinoma, complex infections, thyroid conditions, and diabetes are associated with age-related dysphagia. Although vertebral osteophytes are common, these bony growths alone rarely cause dysphagia. Dysphagia more commonly results from the presence of osteophytes in conjunction with neuromuscular weakness or discoordination.

Because cognitive function and/or communication may be impaired, it is important for the practitioner to note the warning signs associated with dysphagia and risk of aspiration (**Table 31-4**). The entire eating process, which includes self-feeding (transferring food from the table to the mouth) in addition to swallowing, is affected in patients

This can be caused by combinations of several underlying conditions or comorbidities such as diabetes, chronic obstructive pulmonary disease, congestive heart failure, renal failure, an immunocompromised status, and/or cachexia for which an individual no longer can sustain adequate reserve to effectively compensate.

Sometimes dysphagia can be a direct consequence of a treatment provided for another disease process. Health care interventions can result in drug-induced delirium, protracted hospital stays, and ultimately malnutrition. Indwelling NG tubes, prolonged airway intubation resulting in laryngeal injury, and medication effects may all predispose a frail older adult with borderline airway protection to develop frank aspiration.

Older adults are much more likely to be taking medications for multiple medical conditions. These medications can influence salivary flow, intestinal peristalsis, cognition, or psychomotor status, thereby interfering with normal oropharyngoesophageal function or altering airway protection. More than 2000 drugs can cause xerostomia or reduced salivary flow via anticholinergic mechanisms. The list is extensive and can include common antidepressants, antihistamines, antipsychotics, and antihypertensive agents. Likewise, delirium-promoting drugs can produce adverse consequences through either anticholinergic or other central mind-altering effects. Certain agents can directly relax the LES and increase acid reflux and esophageal problems. Finally several psychotropic drugs can produce delayed neuromuscular responses or extrapyramidal effects, thereby influencing the tongue and bulbar musculature. **Table 31-5** provides a partial list of these agents and how they can contribute to dysphagia.

An altered level of attention and cognition may also produce special concerns with regard to safe eating and swallowing. Delirium is frequently underrecognized and undertreated in both hospital and institutional settings. In general, testing an inattentive adult for dysphagia results in the poorest evaluation. If swallowing is assessed during one of these episodes, aspiration is likely to occur. If a staff member at a hospital or nursing home feeds a patient during one of these intervals, the outcome may be disastrous.

Several different treatments can either directly or indirectly damage swallowing effector organs as described previously. Head and neck cancer surgeries, some spinal cord surgeries, thyroid surgeries, and any intervention that can jeopardize the recurrent laryngeal nerve may result in dysphagia. A number of chemotherapy and radiotherapy regimes can cause oropharyngeal injury. The prospective outcome of dysphagia should be incorporated into the risk-benefit discussions of these procedures.

Symptoms

Medical history plays a critical role in establishing a diagnosis of dysphagia (**Table 31-6**). A detailed history can elucidate the proper diagnosis in some dysphagic adults and is

TABLE 31-5 ■ MECHANISMS BY WHICH COMMON MEDICATIONS CONTRIBUTE TO DYSPHAGIA

Xerostomia
Anticholinergic effects
  Tricyclic antidepressants
  Antipsychotic agents
  Antihistamine drugs
  Antispasmodic drugs
  Anti-parkinsonism drugs
  Antiemetic drugs
Other mechanisms
  Antihypertensives (eg, diuretics, calcium channel blockers)

Reduction in esophageal and/or laryngeal peristalsis
Antihypertensive drugs (eg, dihydropyridine calcium channel blockers)
Antianginal drugs (eg, nitrates)

Delayed neuromuscular responses
Drugs that promote delirium (eg, anticholinergic agents, opiates, benzodiazepines)
Drugs that have extrapyramidal side effects (eg, antipsychotic drugs)

Esophageal injury and/or inflammation
Drugs that relax the lower esophageal sphincter (eg, calcium channel blockers, nitrates)
Large pills that have incomplete esophageal transit

an important first step in the evaluation process. Dysphagia may present in a more subtle fashion, without symptoms, but with recurring exacerbations of an underlying disease such as chronic obstructive pulmonary disease.

Patients may initially complain of difficulty swallowing liquids, solid food, or pills. Caregivers or nursing personnel may note such difficulties experienced by the patient including "pocketing" of pills within the oral cavity. The patient may report more effort needed while eating. The patient or the patient's observant family members may complain of the increased time needed to complete a meal. The patient or the practitioner may identify weight loss without any other localizing explanation. However, clinicians must distinguish these dysphagia or aspiration symptoms from a myriad of other common health problems that may mimic dysphagia in older adults. For example, in frail individuals, depression or early Parkinsonism may be manifested solely by weight loss and slowed eating. Without a complete history, these patients may be sent for a dysphagia work-up before an attempt is made to manage their "root problem."

Symptoms of esophageal dysphagia include food "hanging up" behind the sternum, neck pain, chest pain, and heartburn. A specific problem with solid food dysphagia suggests a mechanical obstruction. If the symptoms are intermittent, a lower esophageal ring may be present. If the symptoms are progressive, a peptic stricture or carcinoma

TABLE 31-6 ■ HISTORICAL DATA USED FOR CLINICAL DIAGNOSIS OF DYSPHAGIA

Site or timing of impairment
  Oral (problems with chewing, bolus gathering, initiation of swallow)
  Pharyngeal (problem immediately on swallowing, choking after a long delay, suggestive of passage of residue from the pharynx into the larynx)
  Esophageal (seconds after swallow, behind chest bone)

Onset, frequency, and progression
  Duration, sudden onset related to a specific event (stroke, pill impaction, etc), or gradual
  Frequency (constant, intermittent)
  Progression and severity (including more and more foods and impairing nutrition and hydration)

Aggravating factors and compensatory mechanisms
  Food consistency (solids and/or liquids)
  Temperature
  Usefulness of sucking, turning, and tilting of head, and so on
  Intermittent, constant, or fatiguing symptoms

Associated symptoms
  Change in speech or voice
  Weakness; lack of control of musculature, particularly of the head and neck
  Choking or coughing
  Repetitive swallows or increased need to clear the throat
  Regurgitation (pharyngeal and nasal, or esophageal and gastric; immediately on swallow, or long delay, undigested food, putrefied or secretions?)
  Fullness/tightness in the throat (globus sensation)
  Pain, localized or radiating
  Odynophagia (pain on passage of bolus)

Ancillary symptoms and evidence of complications
  Loss of weight or loss of energy (including from dehydration)
  Change in appetite; attitude toward food, toward eating in company; preparation of foods
  Respiratory problems (cough, increased sputum production, shortness of breath, pneumonias and other respiratory infections)
  Sleep disturbances (secondary to secretion management or regurgitation)
  Changes in salivation (water brash or dry mouth)

is more likely. If there are difficulties in ingesting solids and liquids, a neuromuscular or dysmotility etiology must be considered.

SCREENING ACROSS A CONTINUUM OF CARE SETTINGS

Dysphagia evaluation varies depending on the clinical setting. The comprehensive diagnostic approaches available for hospitalized older patients with dysphagia may not be logistically feasible for bedbound nursing home residents. Likewise, interdisciplinary dysphagia teams are frequently available in academic settings or in larger hospital systems and less common in other settings. When such a team is not available, the responsibility for screening for swallowing problems falls on the primary provider or the hospital staff. Speech language pathologists, who are usually the swallowing therapists, are well trained to conduct bedside (also referred to as noninstrumental) examinations that include history taking, oral motor assessment, voice evaluation, and assessment of trial swallows. Prior to this referral though, clinicians can provide a focused secondary screening during their encounter with the patient. A number of attempts have been made to identify a simple screening tool for use in ambulatory clinics or at the patient's bedside. A systematic review focused on dysphagia screening techniques for inpatients 65 years or older without stroke or Parkinson disease concluded that existing evidence is not sufficient to recommend the use of bedside tests in a general older population. While none of these approaches has proven altogether effective, certain approaches warrant mention (see **Table 31-1** for an overview of selected available tools). However, along with the risk of false negatives, bedside screening provides no information about the underlying pathophysiology of the swallow or for selecting specific interventions.

Despite these issues, owing to the high prevalence of swallowing difficulties in geriatric patients, some mechanism of primary screening needs to take place within a primary care clinic setting. Several validated screening tools are listed in **Table 31-1**. Because swallowing is not something a patient usually mentions, it may be necessary to ask related questions until a particular word or phrase triggers an association with the patient's experience (eg, swallowing, chewing, moving food to the throat, coughing, choking). Nonetheless, once dysphagia is suspected, a more complete assessment is necessary not only to validate its presence but also to define and construct a treatment plan that modifies the underlying sensorimotor pathophysiology.

TEAM APPROACH TO DYSPHAGIA

An interdisciplinary team approach offers the stated advantage of a more efficient comprehensive assessment with shared responsibility for interventions and often makes timely consultation possible. The responsibilities of team members are often divided among disciplines and can include reviewing health issues, obtaining pertinent swallowing history, and an examination (which may include instrumental studies), providing education and counseling to the patient and to the family or the care provider, conducting psychosocial screening, and reviewing advance directives. Core teams frequently include a speech language pathologist, a dietitian, a social worker, and either a physician or a nurse practitioner.

A major function of the swallowing team is to perform a thorough assessment of the swallowing mechanism and its function. Most commonly, the speech language pathologist plays a major role, performing a two-part examination consisting first of a clinical (bedside) noninstrumental evaluation often followed by an instrumental assessment of swallowing.

Noninstrumental Swallowing Assessment

The clinical evaluation is noninstrumental and although often referred to as a "bedside" procedure can be performed in a variety of environmental settings including an outpatient office. It usually involves four types of assessment: (1) history taking; (2) speech and voice assessment; (3) oropharyngeal sensorimotor assessment; and (4) performance on trial swallows. The specific methods and measures preferred and most frequently used by clinicians when working with dysphagia of neurogenic origin, which is frequently the case in older patients, are shown in **Table 31-7**.

Although a noninstrumental assessment provides a breadth of information, it can only increase the suspicion of aspiration through findings such as increased secretions or a wet and/or gurgly voice quality. Given the possibility of silent aspiration as a result of decreased cognition or diminished sensation in older people, coughing and throat clearing, which are the characteristic signs of aspiration, may be absent. To rule out aspiration with an acceptable level of confidence, an instrumental assessment is often necessary. Moreover, effective dysphagia intervention relies on an accurate diagnosis of the specific pathophysiology. That is, the underlying movement disorder that results in disordered bolus flow in terms of direction, duration, and clearance, must be defined and remediated in order to eliminate or minimize the dysphagia. Most frequently, instrumental methods are necessary to clarify the aspects of the swallowing sequence that must be modified to effect safe and efficient bolus flow. Although clinicians must pursue a complete oropharyngeal and esophageal assessment of many dysphagic patients, this section focuses on oropharyngeal dysphagia, and the reader is referred to Chapter 85 for a discussion of esophageal disorder.

Instrumental Examination

Oropharyngeal videofluoroscopic swallowing evaluation An oropharyngeal videofluoroscopic swallowing evaluation, or Modified Barium Swallow (MBS) study, is most commonly used to assess the integrity of the oropharyngeal anatomy, swallowing physiology, and bolus flow. Structural abnormalities and mucosal lesions are identified by the barium that is swallowed and used to outline the soft tissue structures it passes. Perhaps the two greatest strengths of the videofluoroscopic swallow evaluation are that the swallow is recorded in motion and preserved digitally or on videotape for replay. This method permits viewing of the dynamic swallow. All oropharyngeal

TABLE 31-7 ■ CLINICAL AND BEDSIDE SWALLOWING METHODS AND MEASURES

History	Oral motor
Patient report of problem	Tongue strength/range of motion
Family report of problem	Lip seal/pucker
History of pneumonia	Jaw strength/lateralization
Type of neurologic insult	Soft palate movement/symmetry
Nutritional status	Dysarthria
Gastrointestinal anomaly	Speech intelligibility
Structural abnormality	Oral apraxia
Previous surgery	Volitional cough
Other disease	Ability to follow directions
Medications	Management of secretions
Voice	**Trial swallows**
Breathiness	*Bolus type:*
Harshness	Thin liquid
Wet/gurgly	Thick liquid
Strained/strangled	Puree
Overall dysphonia/aphonia	Solid
Resonance	*Swallowing-related events:*
	Oral transit estimate
	Estimate swallow duration
	Laryngeal elevation
	Voice quality after swallow
	Ability to feed self
	Swallows per bolus
	Spontaneous cough
	Estimate of penetration/aspiration
	Estimate of oral stasis
	Observation of meal

Reproduced with permission from McCullough GH, Wertz RT, Rosenbek JC, et al. Clinicians' preferences and practices in conducting clinical/bedside and videofluoroscopic swallowing examination in an adult/neurogenic population. Am J Speech Lang Pathol. 1999;8(2):149–163.

structures can be examined with regard to their contribution to the coordinated (or uncoordinated) swallow in terms of timing and range of motion. Their impact on bolus flow is made apparent. Therefore, the specific pathophysiology and its impact on bolus flow are clarified and can be targeted for treatment.

An oropharyngeal videofluoroscopic swallow study is not designed simply to determine if a patient is aspirating or even why a patient is aspirating or retaining residue. It is designed also to assist a clinician in determining if a patient can safely receive oral nourishment and allows for trials of proposed interventions to maximize efficacy and safety. During the study, the clinician often varies bolus characteristics sufficiently to be able to offer a diet recommendation (such as thickened liquid or semisolid). Additional recommendations may be simple postural adjustments, such as tucking the chin, which are shown under fluoroscopy to improve direction or efficiency of bolus flow.

Although videofluoroscopy is the instrumental method most commonly used to assess swallowing, it is limited in the following ways:

1. The amount of information obtained is restricted to a few minutes in an effort to limit radiation exposure.
2. The environment can be distracting for patients with cognitive deficits.
3. The material ingested is barium, not food, and may not simulate the swallow evoked when real food is used as a stimulus (taste, smell).

Despite these limitations and exposure to a small amount of radiation (equivalent to 2 years of natural background radiation or a set of dental x-rays), videofluoroscopy is preferred for the breadth of information it provides with regard to anatomy, physiology, bolus flow, and assessment of trial intervention.

In addition, a fluoroscopic examination can easily be extended to the esophagus when indicated. Merging of the videofluoroscopic swallow study directly into esophagraphy, which results in a distinct third test referred to as an oropharyngeal esophagram, may reveal anatomic or physiologic findings for the referred sensation. Findings may include a Schatzki ring, an esophagus-narrowing web or stricture, a delay in LES opening or esophageal stasis, or other esophageal etiologies for the dysphagia. Thus, an oropharyngeal esophagram permits a more organized, efficient, cost-effective process for professional personnel and for the patient. Most importantly, it optimizes the potential for comprehensive findings and facilitates immediate intervention.

Fiberoptic endoscopic evaluation of swallowing Fiberoptic endoscopic evaluation of swallowing (FEES) is second to videofluoroscopy in frequency of instrumental approaches used with older patients. It combines the traditional endoscopic examination, in which the flexible scope allows direct visualization of the nasal cavity, the entire nasopharynx, the oropharynx, the larynx, and the hypopharynx, with dynamic recording of swallowing. Although FEES permits only limited observation of the pharyngeal swallow because it is "whited out" or visually obliterated during swallowing caused by constriction of the anatomy, the method provides a valuable alternative to a noninstrumental clinical assessment. It is being used with increased frequency in long-term care facilities where videofluoroscopy is unavailable and also with bariatric patients or those who cannot be moved to radiology because of medical instability. Other advantages are its repeatability, the use of real food and fluid during the assessment, and its potential as a biofeedback tool.

In addition to limited visualization of the dynamic oropharyngeal swallow, the limitations of FEES involve risks related to endoscopy, which include nosebleed, mucosal injury, gagging, allergic reaction to the topical anesthesia, laryngospasm, and vasovagal response. The unlikely possibility of encountering an adverse reaction during a flexible endoscope examination must be balanced against the daily risks faced by patients with dysphagia.

DYSPHAGIA INTERVENTION

Adherence to dysphagia-related recommendations, whether thickened liquids or an exercise regimen, is known to be problematic. Reasons include not aligning therapy with the patient's goals, poor insight into the extent of swallowing-related deficits, a lack of understanding regarding the importance of treatment for dysphagia, and inadequate patient education on the part of the clinician. A variety of patient-reported outcome measures, including the SWAL-QOL, Eating Assessment Tool (EAT-10), Sydney Swallow Questionnaire (SSQ), and the MD Anderson Dysphagia Inventory, allow clinicians to gauge the patient's perspective of his or her swallowing impairment in order to tailor treatment to the needs of the patient, thereby supporting improved adherence.

Treatment for dysphagia is usually compensatory, rehabilitative, or a combination of the two approaches. Compensatory interventions avoid or reduce the effects of impaired structures or neuropathology and resultant disordered physiology and biomechanics on bolus flow. Rehabilitative interventions have the capacity to directly improve dysphagia at the biological level. That is, the targets of therapy are aspects of anatomic structures (eg, muscle) or neural circuitry that may have a direct influence on physiology, biomechanics, and bolus flow.

Compensatory Dysphagia Interventions

Traditionally, interventions for dysphagia in older patients are compensatory in nature and are directed at modifying bolus flow by targeting neuromuscularly induced pathobiomechanics or by adapting the environment.

Postural adjustments Postural adjustments are relatively simple to teach to a patient, require little effort to employ, and can eliminate misdirection of bolus flow through biomechanical adjustment. A general postural rule for facilitating safe swallowing is to eat in an upright posture so that the vertical phase of the oropharyngeal swallow capitalizes on gravitational forces at work. For patients with hemiparesis, a common strategy is a head turn toward the hemiparetic side, effectively closing off that side to bolus entry and facilitating bolus transit through the nonparetic pharyngeal channel. If the pathophysiologic condition is the uncoupling of the oral from the pharyngeal phase of the swallow, a simple chin tuck (45 degrees) reduces the speed of bolus passage, thereby giving the neural system time to initiate the pharyngeal and airway protection events prior to bolus entry.

Food and liquid rate and amounts Although we live in a "fast food" society, older individuals and especially those with dysphagia take longer to eat. Eating an adequate amount of food becomes a challenge not only because of the increased time required to do so but also because fatigue frequently becomes an issue. Typically, smaller amounts per swallow are less likely to enter or block the airway, but in individuals who experience a sensory loss in the mouth or throat, larger amounts of food or liquid may be necessary to trigger a swallow. To promote a safe, efficient swallow in most individuals with swallowing and chewing difficulties, the following recommendations are useful:

- Eat slowly and allow enough time for a meal.
- Do not eat or drink when rushed or tired.
- Take small amounts of food or liquid into the mouth—use a teaspoon rather than a tablespoon.
- Concentrate on swallowing—eliminate distractions like television.
- Avoid mixing solid food and liquid in the same mouthful.
- Place the food on the stronger side of the mouth if there is unilateral weakness.
- Alternate between liquids and solids.
- Use sauces, condiments, and gravies to facilitate cohesive bolus formation and prevent pocketing or small food particles from entering the airway.

Adaptive equipment Eating and drinking aids can assist in placing, directing, and controlling the bolus of food or liquid and in maintaining proper head posture while eating. For example, modified cups with cutout rims (placed over the bridge of the nose) or straws prevent a backward head tilt when drinking to the bottom of a cup. A backward head tilt, which results in neck extension, should be avoided in most cases because when the head is tilted back, food and liquid are more likely to be misdirected into the airway. A speech pathologist or swallowing clinician can make suggestions regarding appropriate aids for optimizing swallowing safety and satisfaction. Occupational therapists are experts in the area of adaptive equipment and can be helpful in obtaining products that are often available only commercially.

Diet modification The most common compensatory intervention is diet modification, a totally passive environmental adaptation. Withholding thin liquids such as water, tea, or coffee, which are most easily aspirated by older adults, and restricting liquid intake to thickened liquids is almost routine in nursing homes in an attempt to minimize or eliminate thin-liquid aspiration, presumably the precedent to the long-term related outcome, which is pneumonia. Despite the huge impact these seemingly unappealing practices may have on patient QOL, they have been commonly implemented in the absence of efficacy data.

Both chin-down posture and thickened liquids (nectar and honey viscosity) have been shown to be effective for patients with Parkinson disease and/or dementia. In the short term, aspiration is reduced with honey-thick liquids as compared with both nectar-thick and chin-down posture interventions. Both chin-down posture and thickened liquids were equally effective in pneumonia prevention over 3 months.

Additional diet modifications include a pureed diet and a soft food diet in which the bolus maintains itself in a cohesive mass during transit but has more texture than the pureed diet. The use of sauces and gravies to minimize the formation of dry particles that may easily be misdirected into the airway is a common practice. Other strategies are also available, so the dietitian should work closely with the team to ensure that the safest diet is provided and that it is effective in maintaining adequate nutrition and hydration, while also acceptable to patients in order to enhance compliance.

Free water protocols Approaches have been developed to encourage intake of water to avoid dehydration in those patients with dysphagia who require thickened liquids. These "free water" protocols involve intensive oral care followed by ingestion of thin liquids between meals but thickened liquids during meals. While initial studies have shown no increased risk for lung complications in patients following these protocols, the findings are limited by small sample sizes and strict exclusion criteria that focus only on patients who are ambulatory, acute rehabilitation inpatients, and cognitively intact. More research is needed to examine the safety and outcomes of these protocols in various older adult populations prior to clinical implementation.

Rehabilitative Dysphagia Interventions

Rehabilitative exercises are, by nature, more active and rigorous. Often a rehabilitative approach to dysphagia intervention is withheld from older patients because such a demanding activity is assumed to deplete any limited remaining swallowing reserve, thus potentially exacerbating dysphagia symptoms. Sufficient treatment efficacy data are unavailable, and so assumption-based patterns of practice prevail.

Given that progressive resistance training appears to be safe and effective for limb musculature in older adults, such training has been systematically applied to the muscles of swallowing. Several exercise regimens with efficacy data have been utilized with older adult populations including systematic tongue strengthening over 8 weeks, expiratory muscle strength training over 5 weeks, and a simple isotonic/isometric neck exercise (lying flat on back while lifting head with shoulders flat) over 6 weeks. Additionally, preventative approaches that incorporate swallowing-related exercise regimens have begun to be implemented with older adults with the goal of minimizing the effects of presbyphagia and increasing swallowing functional reserve.

OPTIMIZING SWALLOWING AND RELATED HEALTH THROUGH PREVENTION

Medications

Minimizing medications that may put a patient at risk for dysphagia is an important goal. Furthermore, pills are often described by patients as being difficult to swallow. Patients should be informed about medications that can be crushed, can be mixed with foods, or are available in liquid form. Pill-induced damage to the esophagus can occur if pills are taken when lying down or with inadequate amounts of liquid.

Oral Hygiene

Poor oral hygiene is a risk factor for pneumonia, and aspiration of saliva, whether or not it is combined with food or fluid, can increase the likelihood of infection. The risk for periodontal disease as well as dental caries increases with age. Therefore, patients should be encouraged to perform oral hygiene several times a day and undergo periodic dental examinations. Furthermore, products to relieve oral dryness in the form of saliva substitutes, as well as alcohol-free mouth care products, can be recommended.

TuBe or Not TuBe—Oral Versus Nonoral Intake

Oropharyngeal dysphagia is potentially life threatening. In the older population, critical decisions often must be made that impact on the patient's safety, health, and QOL. Among these perplexing issues is the question of continuing oral intake or providing nonoral enteral or parenteral nutrition. This dilemma is also reviewed in Chapter 30.

Enteral nutrition, the delivery of nutritive products to the digestive system through nonoral means, is often selected for the temporary prevention of aspiration in acutely ill patients. It also is chosen for permanent replacement in patients whose disease process results in confirmed or suspected swallowing-related aspiration or malnutrition and dehydration. In the case of longer-term or permanent nutritive supplementation, the clinician's impressions often direct decisions relating to tube feeding for weeks, months, or even years in older patients whose chronic disease processes are overlaid on reduced functional reserve for safe, sufficient swallowing. However, it would clearly be narrow and short-sighted to make decisions with such an impact solely on the basis of empirical swallowing abilities or even instrumental physiologic and bolus flow test results. For an issue that may be a critical source of a patient's sense of autonomy, self-respect, dignity, and QOL, swallowing ability is merely one factor in a decision-making formula. It is also important to consider that feeding tubes are associated with their own risks and poor long-term outcomes. NG tubes can result in agitation, nasal irritation, and sinus infection while gastrostomy tubes may lead to cellulitis, fasciitis, and bacteremia. Both types of feeding tubes increase the risk of diarrhea as well as pressure ulcers with slower healing of existing sores. There is currently no evidence to support that feeding tubes prolong survival in patients with dementia and dysphagia or that early placement improves recovery of function or length of stay in patients with post-stroke dysphagia. In fact, the Ethics and Clinical Practice Committees of the American Geriatrics Society published a comprehensive review of the evidence about feeding tubes and dementia in 2014 and issued position statements that suggest placement of feeding tubes in patients with dementia should be seriously reconsidered. Other approaches, such as hand feeding, are preferred for this population.

In summary, while oropharyngeal dysphagia may be life threatening, so are the alternatives, particularly for frail older patients. Therefore, contributions by all team members are valuable in this challenging decision-making process. The patient's family or care provider's point of view is also critical but second, of course, to that of the competent patient, himself. The state of the evidence calls for more research, including randomized controlled trials (RCTs) in this area. Until then, the many behavioral, dietary, and environmental modifications described in this chapter and being further refined are compassionate and, in many cases, preferred alternatives to the always present option of tube feeding.

FURTHER READING

American Geriatrics Society Ethics Committee and Clinical Practice and Models of Care Committee. American Geriatrics Society feeding tubes in advanced dementia position statement. *J Am Geriatr Soc (JAGS)*. 2014;62(8): 1590–1593.

Barczi SR, Sullivan P, Robbins J. How should dysphagia care of older adults differ? Establishing optimal practice patterns. *Semin Speech Lang*. 2000;21(4):347–361.

Buehring B, Hind J, Fidler E, Krueger D, Binkley N, Robbins J. Tongue strength is associated with jumping mechanography performance and handgrip strength but not with classic functional tests in older adults. *J Am Geriatr Soc*. 2013;61(3):418–422.

Cabre M, Serra-Prat M, Force L, Almirall J, Palomera E, Clave P. Oropharyngeal dysphagia is a risk factor for readmission for pneumonia in the very elderly persons: observational prospective study. *J Gerontol A Biol Sci Med Sci*. 2014;69(3):330–337.

Christmas C, Rogus-Pulia N. Swallowing disorders in the older population. *J Am Geriatr Soc*. 2019;67(12):2643–2649.

Gillman A, Winkler R, Taylor NF. Implementing the Free Water Protocol does not result in aspiration pneumonia in carefully selected patients with dysphagia: a systematic review. *Dysphagia*. 2017;32(3):345–361.

Huckabee ML, McIntosh T, Fuller L, et al. The Test of Masticating and Swallowing Solids (TOMASS): reliability, validity, and international normative data. *Int J Lang Commun Disord*. 2018;53(1):144–156.

Jardine M, Miles A, Allen JE. Swallowing function in advanced age. *Curr Opin Otolaryngol Head Neck Surg*. 2018;26(6):367–374.

Logemann J, Gensler G, Robbins J, et al. A randomized study of three interventions for aspiration of thin liquids in patients with dementia or Parkinson's disease. *J Speech Lang Hear Res*. 2008;51:173–183.

Malandraki GA, Johnson S, Robbins, J. Functional MRI of swallowing: from neurophysiology to neuroplasticity. *Head Neck*. 2011;33 Suppl 1(0 1):S14–S20.

Malandraki GA, Perlman AL, Karampinos DC, et al. Reduced somatosensory activations in swallowing with age. *Hum Brain Mapp*. 2011;32(5):730–743.

Martin-Harris B, Brodsky MB, Michel Y, et al. MBS measurement tool for swallowing impairment- MBSImp: establishing a standard. *Dysphagia*. 2008;23(4):392–405.

Newman R, Vilardell N, Clave P, et al. Effect of bolus viscosity on the safety and efficacy of swallowing and the kinematics of the swallow response in patients with oropharyngeal dysphagia: white paper by the European Society for Swallowing Disorders (ESSD). *Dysphagia*. 2016;31(2):232–249.

Nicosia MA, Hind JA, Roecker EB, et al. Age effects on the temporal evolution of isometric and swallowing pressure. *J Gerontol A Biol Sci Med Sci*. 2000;55(11):M634–640.

Raphael C. Oral health and aging. *Am J Public Health*. 2017;107(S1):S44-S45.

Robbins J, Coyle J, Rosenbek J, et al. Differentiation of normal and abnormal airway protection during swallowing using a penetration-aspiration scale. *Dysphagia*. 1999;14(4):228–232.

Robbins J, Gensler G, Hind J, et al. Comparison of 2 interventions of liquid aspiration on pneumonia incidence: a randomized trial. *Ann Intern Med*. 2008;148:509–518.

Rogus-Pulia NM, Rusche N, Hind J, et al. Effects of device-facilitated (D-F) isometric progressive resistance oropharyngeal (I-PRO) therapy on swallowing and health-related outcomes in older adults with dysphagia. *J Am Geriatr Soc*. 2016;64(2):417–424.

Suiter DM, Leder SB. Clinical utility of the 3-ounce water swallow test. *Dysphagia*. 2008;23(3):244–250.

Teno JM, Gozalo PL, Mitchell SL, et al. Does feeding tube insertion and its timing improve survival? *J Am Geriatr Soc*. 2012;60(10):1918–1921.

CHAPTER 31 DISORDERS OF SWALLOWING

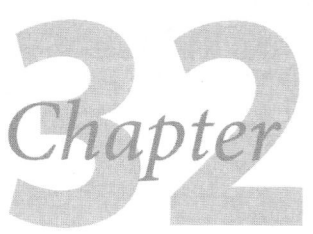

Chapter 32

Oral Health

Joseph M. Calabrese, Judith A. Jones

INTRODUCTION

The centrality of the mouth to human health, function, and behavior is clear. The abilities to eat, smile, speak, and interact with others are essential functions. This chapter presents the contributions of the mouth to health and function in an older person's life. The components of the oral cavity are described along with age-related and disease-related changes, how to evaluate geriatric patients' oral conditions, and when to refer. The impacts of oral conditions on quality of life are described, as are disparities in access to and outcomes of oral health care and the importance of prevention in health status. Finally, goals of long-term oral health care are described, along with options for long-term oral health care.

ESSENTIAL FUNCTIONS OF THE ORAL CAVITY

Specialized tissues have evolved in the orofacial region that allow us to speak, process food, and protect us from pathogens and trauma (**Table 32-1**). The teeth, the periodontium, and the muscles of mastication prepare food for swallowing. The tongue plays a central role in communication and is a key participant in food bolus preparation and translocation. Salivary glands provide secretions with multiple functions; saliva lubricates oral mucosal tissues keeping them intact and pliable, and moistens the food bolus into a swallow-acceptable form. These activities are finely coordinated; a disturbance in any one function can compromise speech, alimentation, and the quality of a patient's life (**Table 32-2**).

The oral cavity is exposed to the external world and is vulnerable to infectious, traumatic, and environmental insults. Mechanisms have evolved to protect the mouth and permit normal oral function. Local infections that can affect the oral cavity are summarized in **Table 32-3**.

The oral cavity is richly endowed with sensory systems that contribute to the enjoyment of food and alert an individual to potential problems. These systems include taste (and its inextricable relationship with smell); thermal, textural, and tactile sensation; and pain discrimination. Saliva plays an important protective role and contains a broad spectrum of antiviral, antibacterial, and antifungal proteins

Learning Objectives

- Describe normal healthy tissue, abnormal tissue (hard and soft) and lesions in the oral cavity.
- List the primary barriers to professional oral health care: finances, perceived need, access to care, and the clinician's inability to care for the challenges that face this population.
- Identify patient limitations that decrease their ability to perform daily oral hygiene care.
- Recognize why being part of an interprofessional health care team along with oral health care providers (dentists, hygienists, dental assistants, caregivers) ensures good oral health in long-term care facilities.
- Identify the oral health challenges that frail homebound patients will face.
- Recognize when to refer and what criteria are most important when referring an older adult patient to an oral health professional.

Key Clinical Points

1. Oral health screening should be part of the patient's initial history and physical examination.
2. A preventive model of oral health care for all older adult patients includes fluoride-containing gels, varnishes, rinses and pastes, antibacterial rinses, electric toothbrushes, floss threaders, and other adaptive methods.
3. Many common medications have adverse effects on the oral cavity and oral health.
4. Disease in the oral cavity can diminish a patient's overall health and quality of life.
5. Common systemic medical conditions may affect oral health and vice versa, and may affect dental treatment.

TABLE 32-1 ■ ORAL TISSUES AND THEIR FUNCTIONS

ORAL TISSUE	FUNCTION
Teeth	Mastication, bone regeneration
Periodontium	Mastication, bone regeneration, host defense
Salivary glands	Lubrication, buffering acids, antimicrobial activity, mechanical cleansing, mediation of taste, remineralization of teeth, oral mucosal repair
Taste buds	Taste, host defense
Oral mucosa	Host defense, mastication, swallowing, speech
Muscles of mastication and facial expression	Mastication, swallowing, speech, posture

that modulate oral microbial colonization. Biomarkers of systemic (eg, C-reactive protein [CRP], interleukin [IL]-6) and oral inflammation are present in saliva. Other proteins maintain the functional integrity of teeth by keeping saliva supersaturated with respect to calcium and phosphate salts and provide the first role in repairing early dental caries (tooth decay) via a remineralization process.

TOOTH LOSS AND DENTAL CARIES

The loss of teeth has long been associated with aging. However, older adults lose teeth not because of age per se, but because of dental diseases. National surveys in the United States (NHES, NHANES) demonstrate that each successive age cohort has less tooth loss than the prior one. Thus, the percent of 65- to 74-year-olds who had lost all their teeth decreased from 55% in 1958 to 1959 to 29% in 1988 to 1994, to 24% in 1999 to 2004, and 13% in 2011 to 2016.

Tooth loss has two major causes: dental caries (discussed later) and periodontal diseases (discussed in the next section). Dental caries mostly affect exposed tooth surfaces, and periodontal diseases affect the supporting bony and ligamentous dental structures. With the current trends toward increasing tooth retention in aging populations,

TABLE 32-2 ■ ORAL-PHARYNGEAL PROCESSES IN OLDER ADULTS

PROCESS	HEALTHY OLDER ADULTS	MEDICALLY COMPLEX OLDER ADULTS
Taste	Unaffected	Diminished
Smell	Diminished	Diminished
Food enjoyment	Unaffected	Diminished
Salivary output	Unaffected	Diminished
Chewing efficiency	Slightly diminished	Diminished
Swallowing	Slightly diminished	Diminished

TABLE 32-3 ■ CLINICAL MANIFESTATIONS OF ORAL INFECTIONS

DISEASE	ORAL MANIFESTATIONS
Dental and periodontal infections	
Dental caries	Soft to hard discolored defect on tooth surface
Gingivitis and periodontitis	Erythematous, edematous, and hemorrhagic gingiva, which may be accompanied by gingival recession and tooth mobility
Viral infections	
Primary herpes simplex infection	Clear to yellow vesicles that rupture and form shallow, painful ulcers on all mucosal surfaces; gingival tissues inflamed, edematous, and painful
Recurrent herpes simplex infection	Burning or tingling prodrome in lesion sites (lip, hard palate, attached gingiva); whitish-gray vesicles rupture to form painful ulcers, which then develop a crust
Herpes zoster	Unilateral vesicular eruptions in areas following the distribution of ophthalmic, maxillary, or mandibular divisions of trigeminal sensory nerves
Cytomegalovirus	Mononucleosis-like symptoms, petechial hemorrhages, enlarged salivary glands, pharyngotonsillitis
Fungal infections	
Pseudomembranous candidiasis	Soft, white or yellow plaques that can be wiped off to expose an underlying erythematous mucosa
Hyperplastic candidiasis	Leukoplakic or keratotic lesions that cannot be removed by scraping
Erythemic or atrophic candidiasis	Painful erythematous oral mucosal lesions; tongue appears "bald"; diffuse inflammation of denture-bearing areas
Angular cheilitis	Erythematous cracked or fissured lesions at the lip commissures
Salivary gland infections	
Acute sialoadenitis	Tender salivary gland swelling with purulent discharge on palpation of the gland duct
Chronic sialoadenitis	Recurrent, tender swellings of salivary gland progressing to a firm and atrophic gland

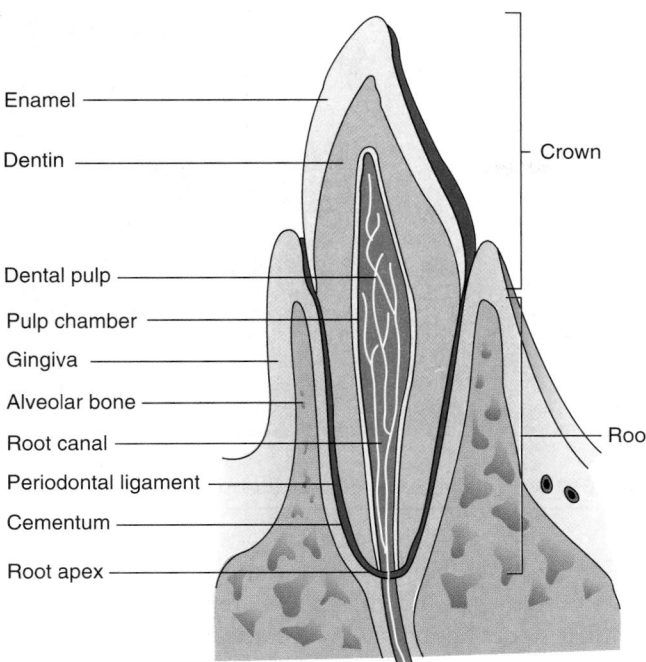

FIGURE 32-1. Cross-section of tooth.

Enamel
Dentin
Crown
Dental pulp
Pulp chamber
Gingiva
Alveolar bone
Root canal
Root
Periodontal ligament
Cementum
Root apex

Acid production by plaque bacteria dissolves the mineral content of the enamel, dentin, or cementum. The exposed proteins are destroyed by hydrolytic enzymes, resulting in early dental caries. Dental plaque is considered a primary etiologic factor in dental caries, as well as a principal source of pathogenic organisms in periodontal diseases.

As older adults live longer and maintain their permanent dentition, there is susceptibility to coronal caries due to recurrent decay bordering existing fillings and the increased prevalence of root surface caries. There are many risk indicators for root surface caries: increased age, decreased exposure to fluoride, coronal caries, periodontal attachment loss, diminished oral-motor skills required for oral hygiene, and additional medical, behavioral, and social factors.

For an older adult with teeth, dental caries is a significant concern and may be a source of pain, infection, and difficulty chewing or swallowing, resulting in a compromised diet or malnutrition. Dental caries will appear as orange to dark brown lesions that frequently are associated with dental plaque (**Figure 32-2A and B**). Long-standing dental caries ultimately result in the destruction of the tooth with the possibility of local or disseminated infection in the maxillofacial tissues, space infections in the head

there is a correspondingly greater risk for the development of both of these disease entities.

A tooth consists of several mineralized and non-mineralized components supported by the periodontal ligament and the alveolar bone (**Figure 32-1**). The outer dental structure (enamel) is the hardest mineralized component, approximately 95% hydroxyapatite. Enamel covers the coronal portion of the tooth and is the first hard tissue exposed to caries-causing bacteria. Dentin, approximately 72% mineralized, constitutes the main portion of the tooth structure, extending almost the entire length of a tooth. It is covered by enamel on the crown and by cementum on the root. Cementum is the least mineralized of the three components (~ 50%) and is the component most susceptible to caries-causing bacteria. The central, nonmineralized portion is the dental pulp, which houses the vascular, lymphatic, and neuronal supply to the tooth. Stem cells are present in pulpal tissues.

There are two classifications of dental caries, depending on the tooth surface affected. Coronal caries occurs when the enamel and dentin of the crown portion of the tooth (usually above the gums) are affected. In older adults, if gingival (gum) recession or periodontal disease causes the root surfaces of the tooth to become exposed to the oral environment, root surface caries may occur.

The primary caries-causing microorganisms are *Streptococcus mutans*; oral streptococci, *Actinomyces*, and lactobacilli are also associated with coronal and root surface lesions. These bacteria reside on the tooth surface in dental plaque, a soft, firmly adherent mass that contains bacteria, food debris, desquamated cells, and bacterial products.

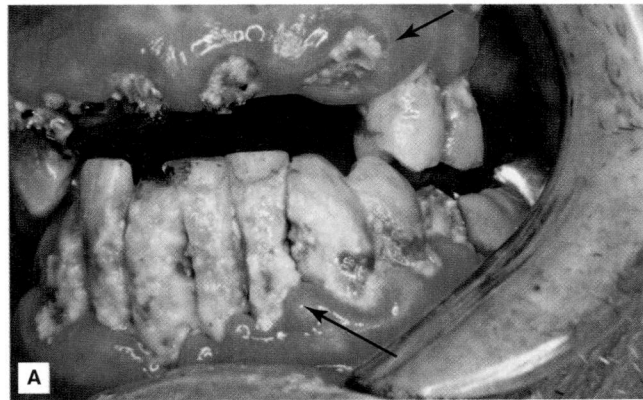

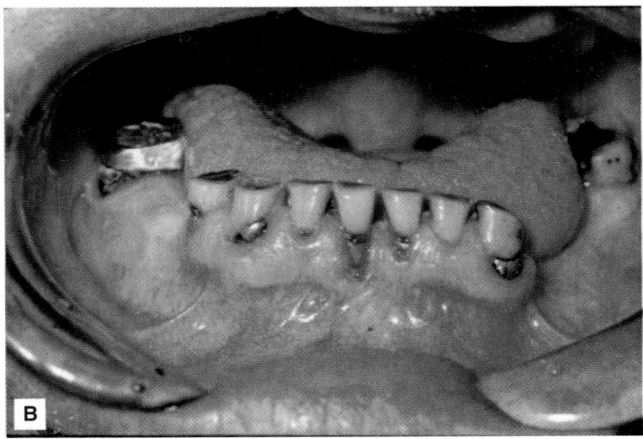

FIGURE 32-2. A. Dental caries, dental plaque, and **B.** gingival recession in two patients with dementia.

and neck, and infection in the systemic circulation (septicemia). Once teeth have been destroyed from dental caries or periodontal disease, mastication, phonation, and swallowing are perturbed. Finally, social contact and nutritional status may be affected in an edentulous aging individual.

The prevention of dental caries in an older adult includes use of fluoride in many forms, daily effective oral hygiene, and regular visits to dental professionals. Tooth surfaces can become resistant to decalcification and decay through repeated exposure to fluoride in water supplies, toothpaste, rinses, high-strength prescription gels, and varnishes. However, even resistant tooth surfaces can decay when oral hygiene is poor and the mouth is dry and/or exposed repeatedly to fermentable carbohydrates. When detected early, dental caries can be debrided from a tooth, and the missing tooth structure can be restored with a wear-resistant, insoluble restorative material (eg, amalgam or composite resin). Some restorative materials contain fluoride (glass ionomers) and can help reduce caries risk. Replacements for lost teeth are available with complete or partial dentures, crowns, bridges, or implants.

PERIODONTIUM AND PERIODONTAL DISEASES

The periodontium consists of the tissues that invest and support the teeth. It is divided into the gingival unit (gums) and the attachment apparatus (cementum, periodontal ligament, and alveolar bony process) (see **Figure 32-1**). Gingivitis occurs when the gingival unit alone is inflamed. Periodontitis (periodontal disease) exists when there is inflammation, infection, and an appreciable loss of the attachment apparatus as a result of the presence of pathogenic microorganisms. Microbial species (eg, *Porphyromonas gingivalis*, *Bacteroides*, *Fusobacterium*, *Prevotella*, *Actinobacillus*, *Actinomyces*, *Capnocytophaga*, and others) cross through the gingival epithelium and enter subepithelial tissues, where they activate host defense mechanisms. Eventually, this causes tissue destruction, including bone loss, mobility, pain on eating, and tooth loss.

Periodontal diseases are more prevalent in the aging population than with younger adults. Sixty-four percent of persons in the United States age 65 and older have moderate or severe periodontal diseases. Older persons experience greater gingival recession and loss of periodontal attachment (see **Figure 32-3**). Periodontal disease proceeds through a series of episodic attacks rather than occurring as a slowly progressing continuous process. Bone destruction results from an overly aggressive local immune reaction to the pathogenic organisms, triggering a cascade of cytokine and immunologic events that can produce irreversible loss of alveolar bone. Among healthy adults, periodontal attachment loss occurs at small increments in all age cohorts and does not occur in

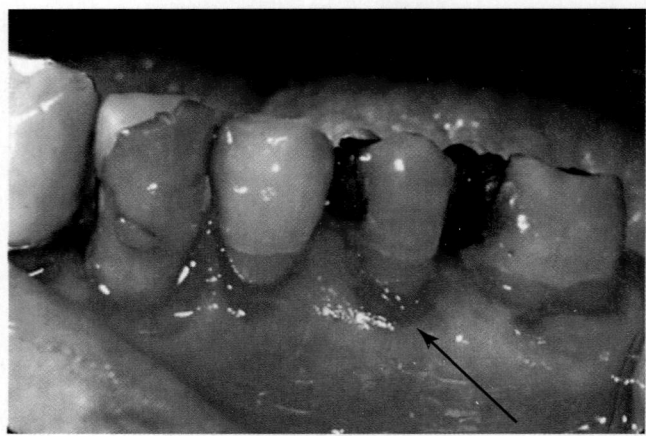

FIGURE 32-3. Periodontal and gingival disease.

greater amounts in older healthy adults. However, many systemic diseases and therapeutic regimens commonly found in older individuals adversely affect periodontal health. Therefore, older, medically compromised adults and smokers are especially susceptible to developing periodontal diseases and at risk for associated dental-alveolar infections, pain, and tooth loss.

Medication-induced changes: Several classes of medications commonly prescribed for older people are associated with gingival enlargement and hyperplasia, a condition that if left untreated, predisposes people to both dental caries and destructive periodontitis. Some calcium channel blockers (eg, nifedipine), phenytoin, and cyclosporine can cause this unwanted drug side effect, which may require periodontal surgery.

Periodontal-systemic connections: Periodontal diseases have oral and systemic effects on health. They are directly associated with halitosis, gingival bleeding, tooth mobility, and tooth loss. Untreated periodontitis has been reported to interfere with blood glucose control in patients with diabetes; and cardiovascular disease is associated with periodontitis after controlling for traditional risk factors such as body mass index (BMI), gender, tobacco use, age, and blood lipid levels. Gram-negative bacteria are implicated in the pathogenesis of periodontal disease, and colonization of the oropharynx with gram-negative bacilli predisposes a patient to pneumonia. Aspiration pneumonia can occur when oropharyngeal secretions are aspirated into the lungs, causing infection. Bacteria from the gingival sulcus in persons with periodontitis have been isolated from patients with pneumonia. Risk factors for aspiration pneumonia include older age, immunocompromised state, mechanical ventilation, feeding problems and/or feeding tubes, deteriorating health status, and wearing dentures during sleep. Importantly, debilitated older patients who do not have adequate oral hygiene care are highly susceptible to aspiration pneumonia.

Treatment of gingivitis and periodontitis starts with good oral hygiene in the form of tooth brushing for

2 minutes twice daily and flossing daily. Electric tooth-brushes can assist older patients who have arthritis, motor, and/or cognitive disorders. Periodontal therapy ranges from local (dental prophylaxis, local debridement, scaling, and root planing) to pharmacologic (intrasulcular anti-microbial solutions, systemic low-dose doxycycline as an immunomodulator) to surgical techniques (debridement, excision of hyperplastic tissue), depending on the extent of periodontal infection and bony destruction. Several anti-microbial and anticollagenase drugs have been approved for treatment: oral rinses (chlorhexidine 0.12%), subgin-gival antimicrobials (minocycline hydrochloride 1-mg microspheres), short-term antimicrobials (clindamycin 300 mg QID or metronidazole 400 mg TID for 7–10 days), or anticollagenases (doxycycline 20 mg). While periodon-tal healing after surgery tends to be slower even in healthy older persons, the long-term results of periodontal therapy are indistinguishable from those in younger adults. The decision either to save the dentition and restore periodontal health or to extract teeth with moderate periodontal dis-ease should be determined after all oral and systemic fac-tors have been evaluated. The health and functional status of a person, rather than age per se, should determine the extent of periodontal treatment.

SALIVARY GLANDS, HYPOFUNCTION, AND XEROSTOMIA

There are three major pairs of salivary glands (parotid, sub-mandibular, and sublingual) and numerous minor glands (labial, palatal, and buccal); their principal function is the exocrine production of saliva. Each gland type makes a unique secretion derived from either mucous or serous cell types, forming the fluid in the mouth termed *whole saliva*. Saliva includes many constituents that are critical to the maintenance of oral health. Saliva lubricates the oral mucosa, promotes remineralization of teeth, and protects against microbial infections. Saliva helps prepare the food bolus for deglutition, dissolves foods, and delivers tastants to the taste buds.

Salivary output does not appreciably diminish with increasing age. Nevertheless, there is a common clinical observation that older individuals have xerostomia (dry mouth) and voice concern of said condition. Further, there appear to be no significant alterations in the composition of saliva in older, healthy persons.

The physiologic findings contrast with the morpho-logic changes seen in aging salivary glands. Major salivary glands lose approximately 30% of their parenchymal tis-sue over the adult life span. The loss primarily involves acinar or fluid-producing components, while propor-tional increases are seen in ductal cells and in fat, vascu-lar and connective tissues. Because acinar components are primarily responsible for the secretion of saliva, it is not known why, in the presence of a significant reduction in the gland acinar volume, total fluid production does

TABLE 32-4 ■ CAUSES OF SALIVARY HYPOFUNCTION IN OLDER ADULTS

CATEGORY	EXAMPLES
Medications	Anticholinergics
	Antidepressants
	Antihistamines
	Antihypertensives
	Anti-Parkinson disease
	Anxiolytics
	Diuretics
Oncologic therapy	Cytotoxic chemotherapy
	Head and neck radiotherapy
Oral conditions	Bacterial and viral infections
	Salivary gland obstructions
	Traumatic lesions
	Neoplasms
Other conditions	Alzheimer disease
	Cerebrovascular accidents
	Dehydration
	Diabetes mellitus
	Late-stage liver disease
	Sjögren syndrome
	Systemic lupus erythematosus
	Thyroid disorders (hyper and hypo)

not diminish with increasing age. Current thinking is that salivary glands possess a functional reserve capacity that enables them to maintain fluid output throughout the human adult life span. There is evidence that with a reduced reserve capacity, additional burdens placed on aging salivary glands (eg, anticholinergic medications) increase vulnerability to functional decline. Therefore, salivary hypofunction (the objective finding) and com-plaints of xerostomia (the subjective finding) should not be considered normal sequelae of aging but instead are indicative of a variety of diseases and their treatments (**Table 32-4**). Many medications taken by older adults reduce or alter salivary gland performance, as can dehy-dration. In addition, radiation for head and neck neo-plasms and cytotoxic chemotherapy have direct and dramatic deleterious effects on salivary glands.

The most common disease affecting salivary glands is Sjögren syndrome, an autoimmune exocrinopathy that occurs predominantly in postmenopausal women. Alz-heimer disease, diabetes, dehydration, rheumatoid arthri-tis, and cerebrovascular accidents may also affect salivary output. Several oral inflammatory and obstructive salivary gland disorders (eg, bacterial infections, sialoliths, trauma, neoplasms) result in salivary dysfunction, as well as benign and malignant salivary tumors.

A clinician is likely to encounter many older patients with oral complaints related to salivary gland hypofunc-tion. Clinical examination includes palpation of all major

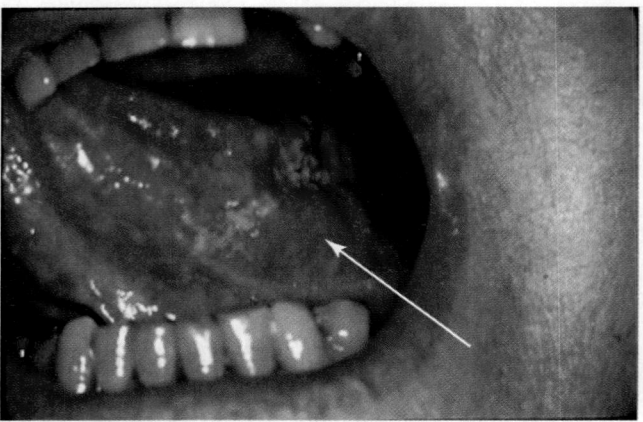

FIGURE 32-4. Candidiasis of lateral border of tongue.

glands and inspection of the duct orifices while milking the glands to ensure gland patency. The application of a mild solution of citric acid or lemon juice to the tongue can help determine whether a patient's salivary glands will respond to a gustatory stimulus. Regardless of etiology, any of the major oral physiologic roles influenced by saliva (see **Table 32-1**) may be affected adversely. With impaired glandular output, dental caries will increase, increasing the possibility of tooth loss. The oral mucosa becomes desiccated and cracked, leaving the host more susceptible to microbial infection (**Figure 32-4**). Older adults with salivary gland hypofunction may experience difficulty swallowing or speaking at length, pain (which may arise from either the teeth or the oral soft tissues), impaired denture use, altered taste, and diminished food enjoyment.

Treatment of salivary dysfunction starts with identification of the etiology. Medication-induced salivary problems can be eliminated by stopping unnecessary medicines, modifying drug use and dose, or substituting one drug with another drug that has fewer anticholinergic side effects. Even when no reduction in the daily dose is recommended, the splitting of a dose into several smaller and more frequently taken doses may alleviate or diminish the sensation of oral dryness. To enhance salivary production, gustatory (*sugar-free* mints, candies), masticatory (*sugar-free* gums), and pharmacologic (pilocarpine 5 mg TID and qhs, cevimeline 30 mg TID) stimulants can be useful in a patient who has remaining salivary function. Salivary substitutes, rinses, and moisturizing gels can assist a patient who has little or no remaining salivary function. Prevention of xerostomia is essential and can be achieved with the frequent use of noncarbonated, caffeine- and sugar-free beverages, topical fluoride, and routine oral hygiene no less than twice daily. Full (complete) and partial removable prostheses (dentures) must be kept clean and out of the mouth during sleeping hours. Frequent lubrication of the lips will help prevent lip cracking, trauma, and infections.

SENSORY FUNCTIONS

When food enjoyment, recognition, and sensory function decline in an older person, significant nutritional deficits can result. The question of whether there is a true anorexia (loss of appetite) associated with aging is confounded by many comorbidities, common in older people, that may cause anorexia, and social and psychological factors that may reduce oral food and fluid intake. Perturbations in taste, smell, and other oral sensory modalities can occur with age and with dental/periodontal problems, thereby reducing the rewards of eating and contributing to a diminished interest in food by some older persons.

The taste receptors of the human gustatory system are distributed throughout the oropharynx and are innervated by three cranial nerves: VII, IX, and X. The number of lingual taste buds does not diminish with age. The registration of a taste phenomenon is complex, because multiple factors are involved: gustation, olfaction, and central nervous system function. The ability to taste is often evaluated at two levels: (1) *threshold*, the most common measure, a "molecular-level" event, which reflects the lowest concentrations of a tastant that an individual can recognize as being different from water, and (2) *suprathreshold*, a measure that is reflective of the ability to taste the intensity of substances at functional concentrations encountered in daily life. In addition to detection, recognition, and intensity, the normal sensation of taste involves a hedonic component: the degree of pleasantness.

Taste function among healthy, community-dwelling individuals changes modestly with increased age. In contrast, a threefold increase in the frequency of subjective taste complaints has been observed among older persons who take prescription medications. Objective threshold and suprathreshold evaluations of gustatory function in healthy older adults have been reported for all four taste qualities (sweet, sour, salty, and bitter). In general, the changes detected with increased age are modest and taste-quality-specific. For example, the ability of older adults to detect salt decreases slightly with age, while no changes in the detection threshold for sucrose (sweet) are noted. The importance of medication usage and place of residence in the evaluation of taste dysfunction has been confirmed in clinical studies in which institutionalized persons and those using more prescription medications had elevated taste thresholds.

Older adults perform less well in the more complicated problems of flavor perception, food recognition, and food preference. This is probably a result of diminished olfactory performance rather than the modest changes that accompany taste function with aging. Olfactory performance data show declines in thresholds, suprathreshold intensity judgments, and odor recognition in both men and women with increasing age. Among older adults, average thresholds are higher, the ability to perceive suprathreshold intensities is blunted, odor recognition is impaired, and the judgment of pleasantness is reduced compared with younger subjects. Moreover, longitudinal studies demonstrate that as people get older, recognition decrements become even more severe.

Normal chemosensory function does not operate independently of good oral health. Numerous oral conditions can directly or indirectly affect smell and taste by altering the underlying biology of the taste or smell system or by introducing exogenous stimuli into the mouth or nose. Fungal/bacterial/viral infections, vesiculobullous diseases, salivary gland hypofunction, poorly fitting prostheses, and oral manifestations of systemic diseases can cause chemosensory dysfunction. Inadequate removal of food particles allows their breakdown or by oral microorganisms to noxious, unpleasant substances. Periodontal diseases can result in accumulations of putrefied materials that may leak into the oral cavity and alter taste sensation. Similarly, dental-alveolar bacterial infections with subsequent fistula formation may contribute continuously low levels of purulent matter in the mouth.

The complaint of a smell or taste problem may be indicative of a chemosensory disorder or could be the manifestation of an oral and/or systemic medical problem. For example, the sudden loss of either smell or taste may be a sign of brain tumor or COVID-19. Alternatively, gradual diminishment in food enjoyment may be related to multiple sources. Examples include a poorly fitting removable prosthesis (**Figure 32-5**), an oral fungal infection (see **Figure 32-4**), decreased smell identification, or use of a new drug. A patient should be asked if he or she can specifically identify the four basic tastants and distinguish between different odorants; such patients could be given the University of Pennsylvania Smell Identification Test. A thorough multidisciplinary approach is required for a patient presenting with chemosensory complaints because of the wide range of potential oral, systemic, physiologic, cognitive, and pathologic factors that are involved in oral sensory functioning.

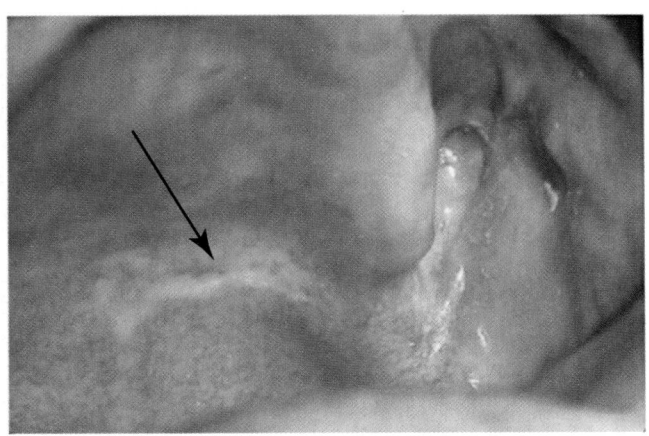

FIGURE 32-5. Denture scar on palate in patient with xerostomia (dry mouth). Arrow highlights the denture scar on palate.

Three general types of soft tissue line the mouth: (1) well-keratinized tissue with a dense layer of connective tissue and firmly attached to underlying bone (marginal gingiva, palatal mucosa), (2) slightly keratinized and freely movable tissue (labial and buccal mucosa, floor of the mouth), and (3) specialized mucosa (dorsum of the tongue). The primary function of the oral mucosa is to act as a barrier to protect the underlying structures from desiccation, noxious chemicals, trauma, thermal stress, and infection. The oral mucosa plays a key role in the defense of the oral cavity.

Aging can be associated with changes in the oral mucosa similar to those in the skin, with the epithelium becoming thinner, less hydrated, and more susceptible to injury. The reasons for these changes are complex and include alterations in protein synthesis and responsiveness to growth factors and other regulatory mediators. Cell renewal (ie, mitotic rates) and the synthesis of proteins associated with oral mucosal keratinization occur at a slower rate in aging individuals. Normal tissue architecture and patterns of histodifferentiation, which probably are dependent on complex interactions with the underlying connective tissue, do not display any changes with age. Overall, changes in the vascularity of oral mucosa likely contribute to alterations in mucosal integrity because of reductions in cellular access to nutrients and oxygenation. Mucosal, alveolar, and gingival arteries can be affected by arteriosclerosis. Varicosities on the floor of the mouth and the lateral and ventral surfaces of the tongue (comparable to varicosities in the lower extremities) are also observable in some geriatric patients.

The maintenance of mucosal integrity depends on the ability of the oral epithelium to respond to insults caused by physical factors (trauma), exposure to chemical or microbiological toxins, microbial infections, and oral and/or systemic conditions. Although the immune system generally declines with age (see Chapter 3), it is unknown whether this decline extends to mucosal immunity. If so, the oral mucosa and gingival tissues may be more susceptible to transmission of infectious diseases as well as delayed wound healing.

Although age has no effect on the clinical appearance of the oral mucosa, the use of removable prostheses has a potentially adverse effect on the health of the oral mucosa. The denture-bearing mucosa of aged maxillary and mandibular ridges shows morphologic changes. Ill-fitting dentures can produce mechanical trauma to the oral tissues (see **Figure 32-5**) and cause mucosal hyperplasia. Oral candidiasis can frequently be found on denture-bearing areas in an edentulous individual, often occurring with angular cheilitis (deep fissuring and ulceration of the epithelium at the commissures of the mouth). The clinician should ask the patient to remove all removable dentures before conducting an oral screening.

Oral mucosal alterations in an older person are often a result of multiple oral and systemic factors (**Table 32-5**). Many medications have been associated with oral mucosal changes, and long-term use of antibiotics frequently results in oral candidal infections, while drugs with xerostomic side effects (see earlier) increase the potential for mucosal injury. Bisphosphonate drugs used for cancer metastasis and osteoporosis (especially those administered intravenously) are associated with increased risk for osteonecrosis, a severe destruction of oral mucosa and bone. However, risk for the rare event of osteonecrosis must be balanced against the benefit of bisphosphonate drugs for common osteoporosis-related fractures. Drugs used in older patients for arthritic conditions, hypertension, cardiac arrhythmias, seizures, and dementia are associated with lichenoid-like reactions. The withdrawal of a causative drug usually results in complete resolution of the lesion within 2 to 3 weeks, but if there is no clinical improvement, a definitive diagnosis should be obtained with a biopsy specimen.

Many oral mucosal disorders can affect older people, ranging from benign (eg, recurrent aphthous ulcers and traumatic lesions) to malignant (eg, squamous cell carcinomas) (**Figure 32-6A and B**). The diagnosis of mucosal diseases requires a detailed history and a thorough head and neck and oral examination, including all mucosal tissues. For vesiculobullous and erosive diseases, a simple three-item classification is helpful: (1) acute multiple lesions (eg, erythema multiforme, herpes simplex, herpes zoster, allergic reaction), (2) recurring oral ulcers (eg, recurrent aphthous stomatitis, traumatic ulcer), and (3) chronic multiple lesions (eg, pemphigus vulgaris, mucous membrane pemphigoid, lupus erythematosus, lichen planus, dysplasia, squamous cell carcinoma). If a lesion does not resolve after 2 to 3 weeks, a tissue biopsy is required. For lesions that are suspected to be oral manifestations of autoimmune connective tissue disorders (eg, pemphigus, pemphigoid,

TABLE 32-5 ■ CONDITIONS ASSOCIATED WITH ORAL MUCOSAL CHANGES

CLASSIFICATION	DISEASE/DISORDER	EXAMPLES
Oral conditions	Infections	Candidiasis, herpes simplex, herpes zoster
	Ulcerative conditions	Recurrent aphthous stomatitis
	Cancer	Oral squamous cell carcinoma
	Periodontal diseases	Gingivitis, periodontitis
	Prosthodontic problems	Poorly fitting dentures, denture stomatitis
	Salivary gland hypofunction	Desiccated oral tissues
	Food allergies	Lichenoid changes
	Trauma	Traumatic fibroma, mucocele
Systemic diseases	Dermatologic disorders	Systemic lupus erythematosus, lichen planus, pemphigus vulgaris, cicatricial pemphigoid, erythema multiforme
	Endocrine disorders	Diabetes mellitus
	Neurologic disorders	Alzheimer, Parkinson, CVA
	Immunocompromising disorders	HIV, AIDS, rheumatoid arthritis
Medical therapies	Medications	Diuretics, calcium channel blockers, antibiotics, antiseizures, immunomodulating drugs, bisphosphonates
	Radiotherapy	Head and neck radiotherapy
	Cytotoxic chemotherapy	Methotrexate, 5-FU, cyclosporine

5-FU, 5-fluorouracil; AIDS, acquired immunodeficiency syndrome; CVA, cerebrovascular accident; HIV, human immunodeficiency virus.

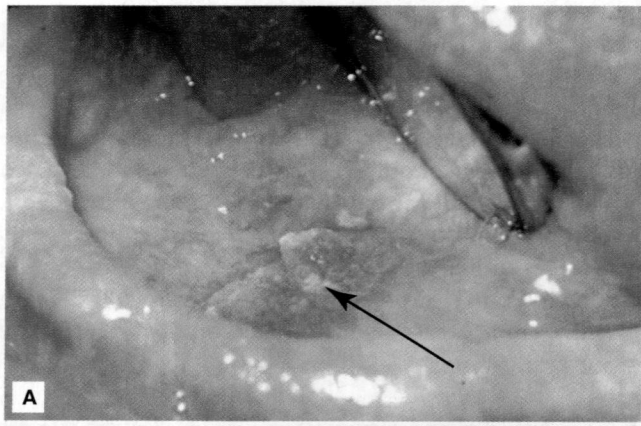

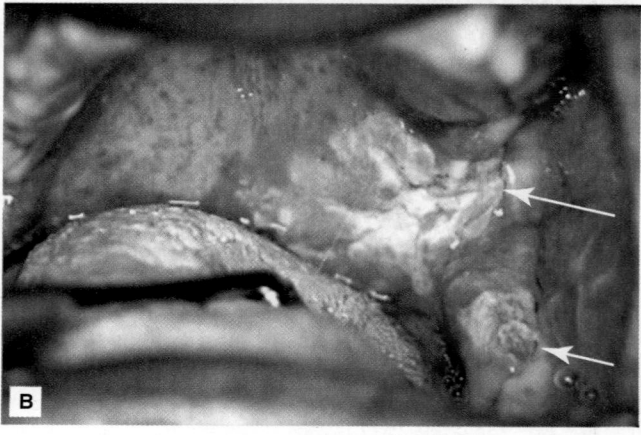

FIGURE 32-6. A. Squamous cell carcinoma, floor of the mouth. **B.** Squamous cell carcinoma, soft palate, retromolar pad.

TABLE 32-6 ■ TREATMENT OF COMMON VESICULOBULLOUS AND EROSIVE DISEASES IN OLDER ADULTS

MEDICATION	REGIMEN
Topical treatments[a–d] Fluocinonide gel 0.05% Triamcinolone acetonide in gel base 0.1% Clobetasol propionate gel 0.05%	Apply to affected regions TID and QHS
Oral rinses[b,c,e] Dexamethasone elixir 0.5 mg/5 mL Diphenhydramine elixir 12.5 mg/5 mL	Rinse and spit 10 mL QID for 5 min
Systemic medications[b,f,g] Prednisone 5 mg	12 tabs QOD × 2 d, decreasing by 2 tabs every other day
Azathioprine 50 mg	1 tab BID

[a]If extensive gingival lesions are present, use with a custom-fabricated tray.
[b]Oral candidiasis may result, and concomitant antifungal therapy may be necessary.
[c]Taper as indicated by clinical response.
[d]Can be combined in a 1:1 mixture with orabase.
[e]Can be combined in a 1:1 mixture with sucralfate, Kaopectate, or Maalox.
[f]Dose and duration depend on severity of disease and concomitant systemic diseases.
[g]Azathioprine in combination with prednisone permits use of lower doses of prednisone.

lichen planus), biopsies should also include specimens for direct immunofluorescence. If trauma from an injury or an ill-fitting denture is suspected, removal of the etiology should allow the lesion to heal. Many of these conditions have an immunologic etiology, and therefore management strategies involve topical and/or systemic immunomodulating agents (**Table 32-6**).

ORAL CANCER

The oral mucosal disease with the greatest potential morbidity and mortality is cancer (see **Figure 32-6A and B**). Oral cancers represent 2.9% of all cancers. There were an estimated 53,260 new oral and pharyngeal cancers in the United States in 2020 and 10,750 cancer deaths. The 5-year survival rate is 66%. Median age at diagnosis is 63; 80% of new cancers occur after age 55; and median age at death is 68. Five-year survival for localized cancers (29% of oral and pharyngeal cancers) is 85%, for cancers that spread to regional nodes (48%) is 67%, and for metastatic oral and pharyngeal cancers (19%) is 40%. The greatest risk factors for developing oral cancer are age, tobacco, heavy alcohol use, and human papillomavirus (HPV). Males are more than twice as likely to develop oral cancer as females.

Carcinoma should be considered part of the differential diagnosis of any oral lesion. Any oral lesion that does not heal *completely* in 2 to 3 weeks after removal of suspected etiologies (eg, ill-fitting denture, change in medication) should undergo a diagnostic biopsy procedure.

The treatment of oral cancers involves head and neck surgery, radiotherapy, chemotherapy, or a combination of any of these three modalities, depending on the tumor's histopathology and stage. Before receiving definitive therapy, the patient should have a comprehensive oral examination so that focal areas of infection or potential infection (dental caries, periodontal disease, dental-alveolar infections, soft and hard tissues lesions) can be treated *before* surgery, radiotherapy, or chemotherapy. The patient must be educated about many potential risks: surgery-related sensory, esthetic, and functional problems; radiotherapy-induced mucositis, salivary gland hypofunction, and osteoradionecrosis; and chemotherapy-induced mucositis and immunosuppression.

MOTOR FUNCTION

The oral motor apparatus is involved in routine yet intricate functions (speech, posture, mastication, and swallowing). Regulation of these activities may occur at three levels: the local neuromuscular unit, central neuronal pathways, and systemic influences. While aging is associated with changes in neuromuscular systems, animal studies suggest that age-associated deficiencies in motor function are unrelated to the composition and contractile function of skeletal muscles. Rather, these changes probably are related to other factors such as neuromuscular transmission and propagation of nerve impulses.

Dentition status (the number of teeth), and not age, influences mastication. While older adults with an intact dentition prepare food more slowly for swallowing than do younger individuals, and minor alterations in performance (mastication, swallowing, oral muscular posture, and tone) can be expected with increased age, changes are more common among completely or partially edentulous persons rather than among persons with a natural dentition. Any diminution in masticatory efficiency can be exacerbated in individuals with a compromised dentition (persons with dental caries, periodontitis, missing teeth, and removable dentures).

Swallowing changes in older persons are usually caused by sensory, muscular, and neurologic deterioration. A thorough review of swallowing problems in older people is provided in Chapter 31, Disorders of Swallowing. Normal aging has minor adverse effects on swallowing, although in a healthy older person, even advanced age does not appear to cause any clinically important dysfunction. However, a host of conditions common in the older adult population can cause clinically significant swallowing deficiencies. Salivary hypofunction (described earlier) impairs swallowing times and under severe conditions increases the likelihood of aspiration. Patients with neuropathies have been reported to have oral swallow times four- to sixfold longer than those in healthy controls; these persons may not even be able to produce the recognizable characteristics of an oral swallow. Neurovascular conditions (eg, cerebrovascular accidents, dementia, motor neuron disease) and Parkinson disease are likely to cause dysphagia and predispose a person to the danger of aspiration.

The temporomandibular joint (TMJ) is located between the glenoid fossa and the condylar process of the mandible, and exhibits a functionally unique gliding and hinge movement. It is of particular interest to clinicians, for it is the focus of several craniofacial pain disorders. Radiographic and postmortem evaluations suggest that the components of this joint undergo degenerative alterations with increasing age. However, TMJ functional impairment is not a "normal" age-associated event. Rather, temporomandibular disorders (TMD) in older adults are linked with many common oral and systemic conditions. Orofacial pain in an older patient may be a result of a variety of problems of the craniomandibular complex and other extraoral diseases, making diagnosis and treatment challenging and frequently requiring a multidisciplinary approach.

In general, two types of pathology are associated with the TMJ: *articular*, related to the joint itself, and *nonarticular*, pathology occurring in structures unrelated to the joint but causing similar or referred symptomatology. Articular abnormalities common to all joints may also affect the TMJ: for example, trauma, ankylosis, dislocation, and arthritis. Nonarticular disorders may result from trigeminal neuralgia, headache, migraine, otitis, dentoalveolar pain/infection, and masticatory myalgia. Orofacial habits (eg, jaw clenching and tooth grinding) and poor head and neck posture can produce muscle fatigue and spasm. Psychological conditions (stress and depression) can exacerbate underlying articular and nonarticular disorders. Clinically, the patient will present with pain in many regions: TMJ, temporal, neck, masticatory muscles, and the oral cavity. Diagnosis is challenging because symptoms primarily occur in any of these sites with regular, irregular, or no pain referred to the TMJ region. Limited jaw opening (< 40 mm from the maxillary central incisor to the mandibular central incisor edges) and pain on mastication or during jaw movements may be indicative of TMD. Treatment, as with other arthritic or muscular disorders, requires an appropriate diagnosis and ranges from conservative and reversible regimens (anti-inflammatories, analgesics, muscle relaxants, physical therapy, oral bite splints) to more invasive procedures for unresolved painful conditions (eg, TMJ surgery). Pain in the jaws and/or face is present in 3% to 6% of persons age 65 and older.

Speech is another function of the oral structures; speech undergoes changes with increasing age, including shape of the tongue and its function during sound production and frequency variability. Among healthy older persons, these changes do not compromise or alter speech in any perceptible way. Tongue strength decreases with age, even among healthy adults, yet tongue endurance is similar between younger and older persons. There are also age-associated alterations in intraoral and maxillofacial posture. Drooping of the lower face and lips in the older adult results from the loss of supporting hard tissues and diminished tone of the circumoral muscles. The latter changes may elicit esthetic concerns and can lead to embarrassment from drooling or food spills caused by the inability of an older individual to close the lips competently while eating or speaking. Often, drooling caused by reduced circumoral muscle tone can result in complaints of excess salivation. Finally, oral motor disorders also may result from therapeutic drug regimens, such as the frequent association of tardive dyskinesia with phenothiazine therapy. These dyskinesias may include diminished performance and speech pathologies as well as alteration in movement (eg, chorea).

ORAL CONDITIONS AND QUALITY OF LIFE IN OLDER ADULTS

Poor oral health diminishes the quality of life among persons with poor general health. There is a strong association between poor general health and poor oral health (**Figure 32-7A and B**). Persons who report poor general health are more likely to have complete tooth loss compared to older people reporting good or better general health. Older adults with teeth reporting poor general health also have two to four fewer teeth than persons reporting good or better general health. Further, the mean number of teeth in persons 50 years and older reporting poor general health is below the threshold for a functional dentition (20 teeth are considered the minimum for a functional dentition). Persons reporting poor general health are also more likely to report painful aching in their mouth. Conditions that increase the likelihood of reporting pain include arthritis, chronic obstructive pulmonary disease (COPD), cardiovascular disease (CVD), diabetes, and low/no vision. One in five adults between age 65 and 74 who report poor general health also report avoiding particular foods because of poor oral health (problems with their teeth, dentures, or mouth).

DISPARITIES IN ACCESS TO AND OUTCOMES OF CARE

Nearly 73 million baby boomers will turn 65 by 2030. Most will lose dental insurance upon retirement. **Medicare** does not cover dental care except in very narrowly prescribed circumstances. **Medicaid** coverage varies by state; in 2011, 22 states provided "comprehensive," 7 provided limited, 14 provided emergency, and 7 provided no dental coverage for adults. However, Medicaid is only for people at or below the poverty level. Thus, a large "middle" group of older people are on a fixed income with limited access to sponsored dental care coverage. Such people need private dental coverage and/or effective, community-based prevention programs.

There are important disparities in access to dental care, tooth loss, unfilled caries, periodontal diseases, and

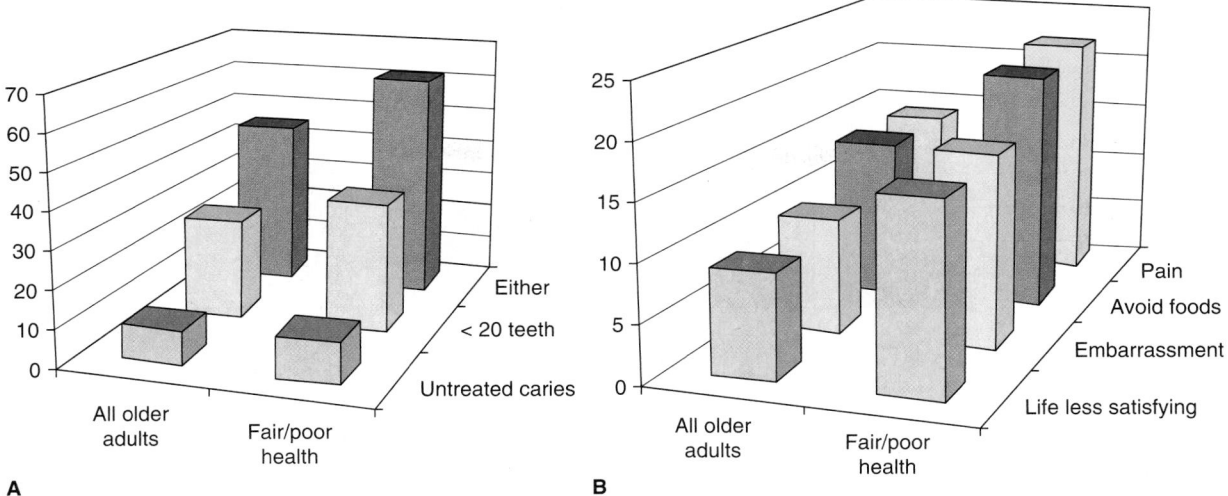

FIGURE 32-7. A. Tooth loss and caries are more prevalent in older adults with fair/poor health. **B.** Oral quality of life by self-reported health. The Y axis in both A and B is percent prevalence. (Data from Griffin SO, Jones JA, Brunson D, et al. Burden of oral disease among older adults and implications for public health priorities. *Am J Public Health.* 2012;102[3]:411-418.)

oral cancers among the poor, near poor, and racial and ethnic minorities. Insurance affects access for persons age 65 and older : "54% of adults with private health care coverage had visited dental professional within the past 6 months, compared with 41% of adults who had only Medicare and 25% who had Medicare plus Medicaid" (CDC, 2014). Thus, the so-called dual eligibles are the most likely group of older persons to not have access to dental care. In addition, while past dental care use has improved slightly among persons age 65 and older since 1999 to 2004 for persons above 200% of the federal poverty level (FPL), it is lower among persons below 200% of this level (**Figure 32-8A**).

Baby boomers will be keeping their teeth longer and in greater numbers than ever before; however, dental decay (caries) is now as much of a problem in older adults as in children. NHANES caries data from 1999 to 2004 and 2011–2016 (**Figure 32-8B**) showed that among persons age 65 and older, prevalence of unfilled caries was higher among persons below 200% of the FPL (18% vs 25%) in contrast with persons 200% or more of the FPL, where unfilled caries rates were lower in 2011 to 2016 (16% vs 14%). NHANES data from 2011 to 2016 show that unfilled decay was highest among Mexican Americans, non-Hispanic Blacks and the poor, while complete tooth loss (edentulism) is lowest among Whites and highest among the poor and African-Americans (**Figure 32-8C**). Disparities in access and dental conditions are the starkest in nursing homes and senior centers. In nine Basic Screening Surveys across the United States, edentulism ranged from 25% to 43% (median 33%) and unfilled caries from 25% to 53% (median 40%). National SEER data show that new oral and pharyngeal cancer rates are highest among male Whites, yet death rates are highest among African-American men (**Figure 32-9**).

COMPREHENSIVE ORAL EXAMINATIONS AND EVALUATIONS

The initial examination and radiographic series by an oral health professional can yield the greatest diagnostic value. This information will not only serve as a diagnostic tool for the immediate treatment needs but also as a baseline that can be used to map the progression of disease or a decline in the patient's oral health. For frail medically compromised (homebound or institutionalized) older adults, subsequent visits can be more challenging when there has been an overall decline in the patient's medical and physical condition or psychological state.

For nondental health professionals on the interdisciplinary geriatrics team, it is important to take a couple of minutes to complete an intraoral evaluation. Any clinical findings that differ from the routine normal color and structure are indications for referral to a dental health professional. Along with the clinical intraoral evaluation, it can be very helpful for the nondental health professional to ask two simple questions:

"Do you have any pain or discomfort in your mouth?"
"Do you have any trouble biting or chewing your food?"

A positive response to one or both predicts the need for treatment. Any combination of positive responses to these questions should also trigger a referral for consultation to an oral health care provider with formal training or experience with special needs adults or geriatric dental medicine. Often the most important step is the early identification of the clinical problem, and referral to the appropriate provider. Lack of an early referral may result in a missed opportunity to aid the patient with their oral health needs. The interdisciplinary team working together can ensure

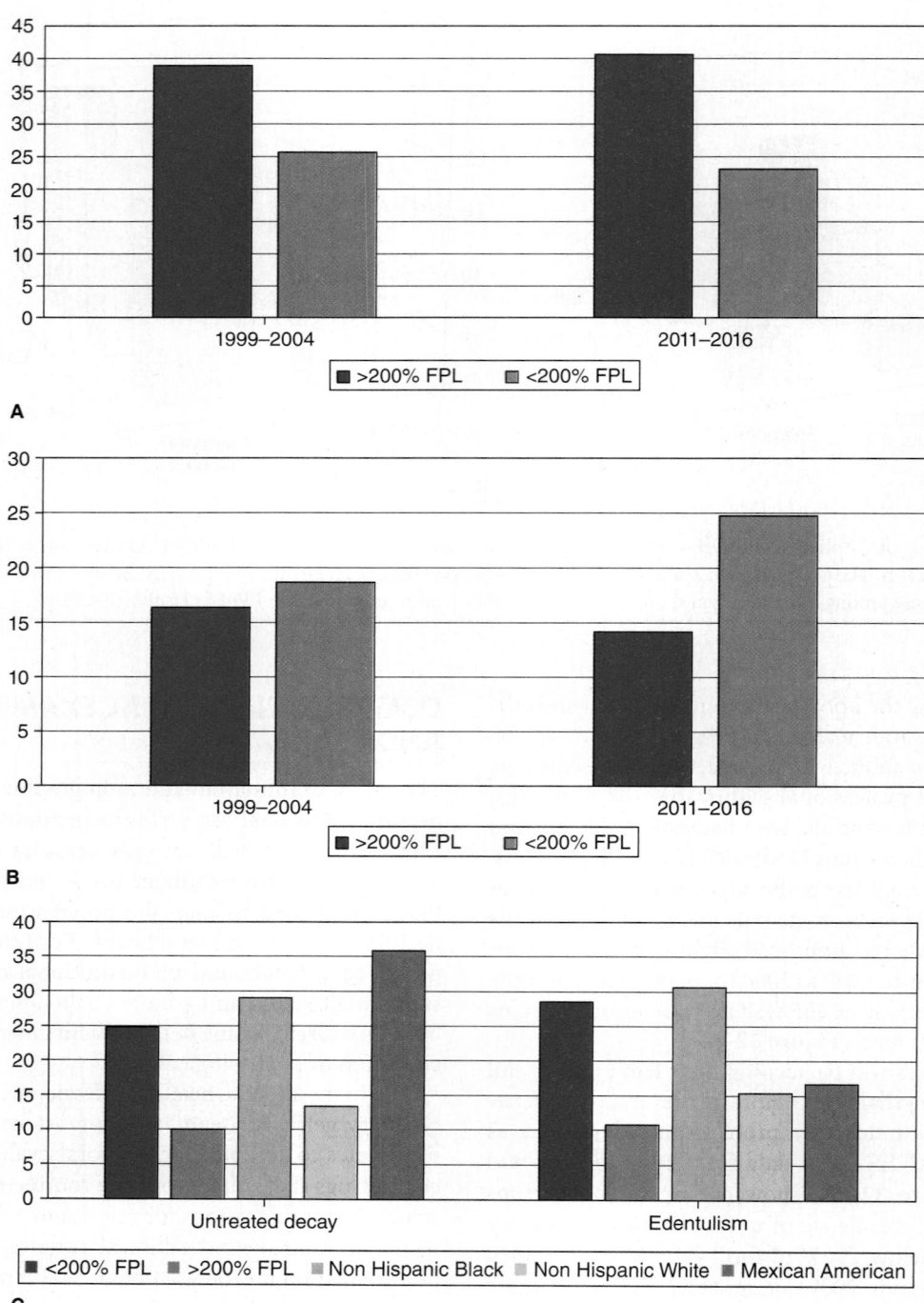

FIGURE 32-8. A. Percent with past year dental care use among 65+ year olds, USA, 1999-2004 and 2011-2016. **B.** Percent with untreated dental caries among 65+ year olds, USA, 1999-2004 and 2011-2016. **C.** Percent with edentulism and untreated dental caries among 65+ year olds by income, race and ethnicity, USA, 2011. Federal poverty level (FPL) is a measure of income issued every year by the Department of Health and Human Services (HHS). (A & B, Data from Griffin SO, Thornton-Evans G, Wei L, et al. Disparities in dental use and untreated caries prevalence by income. *JDR Clin Trans Res.* 2021;6[2]:234–241. C, Data from Griffin SO, Griffin PM, Li CH, et al. Changes in older adults' oral health and disparities: 1999 to 2004 and 2011 to 2016. *J Am Geriatr Soc.* 2019;67[6]:1152–1157.)

that the needs of the patient are addressed in a timely and thorough manner. Important interactions may involve the primary care physician, specialist physician, nurse, nurse practitioner, physician assistant, dentist, dental specialist, dental hygienist, dental assistant, and health aides. One key goal is to determine the need for antibiotic premedication prior to dental treatment. Premedication is often considered for patients with risk for endocarditis, autoimmune

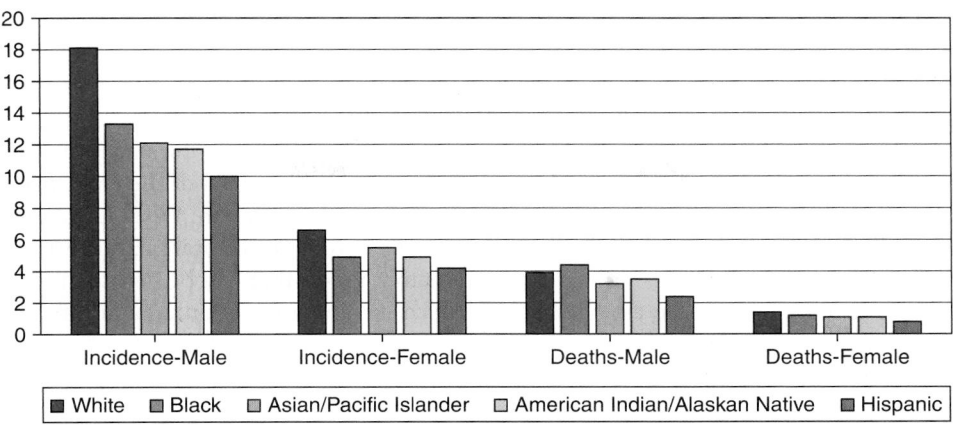

FIGURE 32-9. Oral and pharyngeal cancer incidence and deaths by race and ethnicity, sex, per 100,000, USA, 2013-2018. (Data from SEER: https://seer.cancer.gov/statfacts/html/oralcav.html.)

disease, chemotherapy, joint replacement, or heart murmurs. Another goal is to establish appropriate antianxiety premedication regimes for patients with psychiatric, social, and medical conditions to ensure that optimal dental treatment can be rendered efficiently.

KEY FEATURES OF AN ORAL EXAMINATION FOR NONDENTAL CLINICIANS

When performing an intraoral assessment, the clinician should use a strong light source and take the time to systematically review all anatomic landmarks in the oral cavity. An instrument such as a dental mirror or tongue blade plus use of fingers with a dry gauze can be used to isolate and retract tissues within the oral cavity to properly access and evaluate each structure. For example, it is impossible to evaluate the floor of the mouth without physically retracting the tongue and gaining direct vision. At a minimum, an oral health screening should include the hard palate, soft palate, uvula, tongue, cheek, lips, floor of the mouth, gingiva/gums, and teeth. It is important to document and report any findings in a referral for dental treatment. This report should include any mobile, decayed, missing, or fractured teeth along with any structure that is loose or does not follow normal size, color, or texture. Any sign or symptom of an abscess or infection in the oral cavity should be reported immediately. If a physician starts the patient on a course of antibiotic for a dental infection, that should also be noted to avoid repetition of the antibiotic.

ORAL HEALTH IN LONG-TERM CARE

By the time of transition to a nursing home for long-term care, many frail older adults already need dental care. There is a clear need for community-based prevention *before* older people require long-term care. Prior to embarking

on programs to prevent caries and other oral diseases in older people using, for example, fluoride varnish, patient navigation, and patient-centered counseling, it is important to take a community-based participatory approach to find out what older people want, and what would be acceptable options for preventive care.

As the end of life draws near either in the long-term care setting or at home, goals of dental care may shift from aggressive treatment to a focus on comfort, safety, dignity, and preservation of function. In a Delphi study of the goals of oral health in long-term care, the 10 most important goals are shown in **Table 32-7**.

The overall goal in these special populations is to be proactive as opposed to waiting for problems to arise. Prevention and early detection are paramount to avoid more complex problems that may require a more invasive treatment plan for the patient. In many cases, this increases the financial burden for the patient, the family, or the facility.

First, it is important to identify any limitations the patient may have. Oral health care should ideally be

---

TABLE 32-7 ■ TOP 10 ORAL HEALTH OUTCOMES IN LONG-TERM CARE

Patient will be free from oral pain.

Patient will not be at risk for aspiration of teeth, crowns, dentures, and dental material.

Emergency dental treatment will be available when needed.

Prevent mouth infections.

Daily mouth care is as much a part of daily care as shaving or brushing hair.

Prevent discomfort from loose teeth or sore gums.

Teeth will be brushed thoroughly once a day.

Staff will be able to provide oral hygiene care as needed.

Provide dental care to prevent problems eating.

Recognize oral problems early.

practiced in the morning when the patient wakes up, after each meal, and at their hour of sleep. In some cases, patients are not able to gain access to care at each of these points in a day due to the lack of available assistance. When assistance is available, the oral hygiene should be practiced as often as possible, but *no less than twice daily*.

When obstacles are introduced, such as a patient with arthritis who is unable to hold the small handle of a toothbrush, the plan needs to be modified so it is doable. The solution to this example could be as simple as creating a larger handle by wrapping a sponge around the brush and securing it with medical tape, placing two small slits in a tennis or racquet ball and sliding the brush into the slits, securing the brush in a bicycle handle or purchasing an electric toothbrush with a larger handle. In most cases, the action of the electric brush can take the place of the movements that once were accomplished by the patient.

It is also important for patients to continue to see the oral health team on a regular basis. The number of visits needed for older adults could range from quarterly to semi-annual or an annual evaluation for the edentulous patient. These routine visits along with a strong care plan for twice-daily oral hygiene will greatly decrease the risk of complex problems arising in the oral cavity. The patient's physician should communicate any major health changes to the oral health team, who will be able to assist in finding solutions for new barriers. When delivering oral health care within a long-term facility it is important to consider the cooperation and participation of the staff, patients, their families, and the administration. Without the support of the administration, delivery of oral health care is difficult. There are many models that can be designed to best fit the needs of each specific population. At a minimum, the facility should provide the space and time required to properly treat each patient and allow staff access for in-service training as required by the facility.

ACKNOWLEDGMENTS

The late Dr. Jonathan Ship wrote this chapter in the 6th edition. While we are not able to include him as an author in this chapter, much of the material from that chapter has been retained in this edition. The authors are grateful for Dr. Ship's enduring leadership and lifetime contributions to the field of geriatric dental medicine and oral health in the older adult population.

FURTHER READING

Atkinson JC, Grisius M, Massey W. Salivary hypofunction and xerostomia: diagnosis and treatment. *Dent Clin North Am*. 2005;49(2):309–326.

Bernabé E, Sheiham A. Age, period and cohort trends in caries of permanent teeth in four developed countries. *Am J Public Health*. 2014;104(7):e115–e121.

Calabrese J, Friedman P, Rose L, Jones J. *Using the GOHAI to Assess Oral Health Status of Frail Homebound Elders: Reliability, Sensitivity & Specificity*. Special Care in Dentistry, October 1999.

Chalmers JM, Carter KD, Spencer AJ. Caries incidence and increments in community-living older adults with and without dementia. *Gerodontology*. 2002;19(2):80–94.

Dye BA, Li X, Beltrán-Aguilar ED. Selected oral health indicators in the United States, 2005–2008. *NCHS Data Brief, No 96*. Hyattsville, MD: National Center for Health Statistics; 2012.

Dye BA, Li X, Thornton-Evans G. Oral health disparities as determined by selected Healthy People 2020 oral health objectives for the United States, 2009–2010. *NCHS Data Brief, No 104*. Hyattsville, MD: National Center for Health Statistics; 2012.

Eke PI, Dye BA, Wei L, et al. Prevalence of periodontitis in adults in the United States: 2009 and 2010. *J Dent Res*. 2012;91(10):914–920.

Gibson G, Jurasic M, Wehler C, Jones JA. Supplemental fluoride use for moderate and high caries risk adults: a systematic review. *J Pub Health Dent*. 2011;71:171–184.

Greenberg MS, Glick M, Ship JA. *Burket's Oral Medicine: Diagnosis and Treatment*. 11th ed. Hamilton, OH: BC Decker; 2007.

Griffin SO, Griffin P, Li CH, Bailey WD, Brunson D, Jones JA. Changes in older adults' oral health and disparities: 1999 to 2004 and 2011 to 2016. *J Am Geriatr Soc*. 2019;67(6):1152–1157.

Griffin SO, Jones JA, Brunson D, Griffin P, Bailey WD. Burden of oral disease among older adults and implications for public health priorities. *Am J Public Health*. 2012;102(3):411–418.

Griffin SO, Regnier E, Griffin PM, et al. Effectiveness of fluoride in preventing caries in adults. *J Dent Res*. 2007;86(5):410–415.

Jones JA, Brown EJ. Target outcomes for long-term oral health care: a Delphi approach. *J Public Health Dent*. 2000;60(4):330–334.

Jones JA, Spiro A III, Miller DR, Garcia RI, Kressin NR. Need for dental care in older veterans: assessment of patient-based measures. *J Am Geriatr Soc*. 2002;50:163–168.

Migliorati CA, Siegel MA, Elting LS. Bisphosphonate-associated osteonecrosis: a long-term complication of bisphosphonate treatment. *Lancet Oncol*. 2006;7(6):508–514.

Musacchio E, Perissinotto E, Binotto P, et al. Tooth loss in the elderly and its association with nutritional status, socio-economic and lifestyle factors. *Acta Odontol Scand*. 2007;65(2):78–86.

National Cancer Institute. SEER Stat Fact Sheets: Oral Cavity and Pharynx Cancer. Available at https://seer.cancer.gov/statfacts/html/oralcav.html. Accessed October 26, 2020.

Pretty IA, Ellwood RP, Lo EC, et al. The Seattle Care Pathway for securing oral health in older patients. *Gerodontology*. 2014;31(suppl 1):77–87.

Slade GD, Akinkugbe AA, Sanders AE. Projections of U.S. edentulism prevalence following 5 decades of decline. *J Dent Res*. 2014;93(10):959–965.

Spielman AI, Ship JA. Taste and smell. In: Miles TS, Nauntofte B, Svensson P, eds. *Clinical Oral Physiology*. Copenhagen: Quintessence Publishing Co. Ltd; 2004: 53–70.

Terpenning M. Geriatric oral health and pneumonia risk. *Clin Infect Dis*. 2005;40(12):1807–1810.

Yoshikawa M, Yoshida M, Nagasaki T, et al. Aspects of swallowing in healthy dentate elderly persons older than 80 years. *J Gerontol A Biol Sci Med Sci*. 2005;60(4): 506–509.

Chapter 33

Low Vision: Assessment and Rehabilitation

Gale R. Watson, Katharina V. Echt

DEMOGRAPHICS AND ECONOMICS

Population Studies

Many large, population-based, cross-sectional studies have documented the increase in prevalence of eye disease and visual impairment with increasing age, particularly in people older than 75 years. Greater prevalence of vision loss in the population with advancing age is a common feature across available data reports, despite a fair degree of variability in estimates and projections as a function of data type, source, definitions, and approach. Year 2020 prevalence estimates for vision loss in the United States, for instance, are 4.8% (16 million) of the population and 10% of those age 50 and older (12 million; International Agency for Prevention of Blindness *Vision Atlas*, https://www.iapb.org/learn/vision-atlas). The Centers for Disease Control and Prevention (CDC) and the National Centers for Health Statistics (NCHS) estimate the prevalence of significant visual impairment among Americans age 18 to 44 is 5.5%; the prevalence in those age 45 to 74 is approximately 12% and is rising to more than 15% for those age 75 and older. Indeed, according to a 2016 National Academies of Sciences, Engineering, and Medicine Report, of all adults with vision impairment or blindness who were 40 years and older in 2015, nearly half (48% or 2 million) were at least age 80. Projections for the year 2050 indicate the proportion of US adults age 80 and older will expand to account for 63% (5.6 million) of adults age 40 and older with vision impairment or blindness. After age 85, one in four older people are vision-impaired—unable to read, drive, recognize faces, and perform everyday activities without assistive devices and rehabilitation training. The prevalence of all forms of vision loss are projected to increase. Higher numbers of visually impaired older adults are non-Hispanic White women.

Learning Objectives

- Understand the prevalence of vision impairment among older adults, its functional implications, as well as the costs to the older adult who develops it, to the family, and to society.

- Understand the normal age-related vision changes, and recognize functional indications and losses of the most prevalent age-related eye diseases.

- Care for older adults who have vision loss with evaluations, recommendations, supportive education, and appropriate referrals to eye care and rehabilitation providers.

- Assure that older adults with low vision who are in long-term and palliative care have their specific visual needs addressed.

Key Clinical Points

1. Visual impairment among older adults is treated through examination, prescription, and recommendation of assistive devices and interventions, rehabilitation training, and education of family and other health professionals.

2. Vision loss among older adults is associated with depression, comorbid health problems, and other disabilities. Treatment and rehabilitation for vision loss increase independence and mental health.

(Continued)

3. Geriatricians can play an important role in assuring that older adults receive low-vision rehabilitation and supporting the full range of services that can be provided.

4. Addressing visual impairment and assuring that older adults maintain their visual abilities and strategies can be included as a part of long-term and palliative care plans.

Cost of Age-Related Vision Loss

Age-related visual impairment is not only challenging to the person who develops it, but also affects society as a whole. The total economic burden of eye disorders and vision loss in the United States has been estimated at $139 billion for the year 2013. More than half of these costs ($77 billion) were incurred by Americans age 65 and older, with $30 billion direct medical expenditures for eye disorders and low vision care, vision aids, adaptations, devices and assistance.

Medicare beneficiaries with coded diagnoses of vision loss incurred yearly eye-related costs ranging from $237 to $407 per patient depending on severity of loss. Beneficiaries with vision loss were also shown to incur an additional $2.1 billion in non–eye-related medical costs. Additional non–eye-related costs per patient yearly were $2193, $3301, and $4443, respectively. Health utility (distress, pain, depression, lack of mobility, social limitations) was converted into quality-adjusted life years, and the total lost value for this factor was $11 billion. Significantly higher overall health care utilization and expenditures among patients with vision loss relative to patients without vision loss is a persistent issue consistent with comparatively higher prevalence of chronic comorbidities in this population. Vision loss may in fact amplify mortality and morbidity risk associated with this greater chronic comorbidity burden.

Patients with vision loss experience a number of health care access barriers. Gaining physical access to providers and other health professionals and health facilities as well as difficulties with patient–provider communication and limited availability of accessible health education and information to support adherence to recommendations and self-care following health care visits and stays elucidate some of the ways in which vision loss can limit effective patient-centered care. Having vision impairment was associated with lower patient satisfaction with care ratings among Medicare beneficiaries in 2017.

Recent analytic population health reports describing specific health care utilization disparities among older adults with vision loss affirm prior reports regarding the economic impact of eye disorders and vision loss in the United States. Older adults with vision loss were less likely to complete recommended preventive health screenings,

had longer average length of hospital stay, higher readmission rates, and higher incurred hospitalization and post-discharge costs relative to comparisons without vision loss. While more remains to be understood, it is clear that prevention of vision loss in the first place, or early detection and timely referral for low vision assessment and rehabilitation are key to minimizing the significant health, disability, and economic burdens exacted by vision loss in aging.

Related Impairments

Vision loss is reason enough for a decline in function among older people, but vision loss has also been associated with declines in cognition, hearing, mobility, well-being, and overall quality of life. Older visually impaired people are twice as likely to have difficulty walking as do sighted peers, three times more likely to have difficulty getting outside, more than twice as likely to have difficulty getting in and out of a bed/chair, and three times more likely to have difficulty preparing a meal.

The most prevalent age-related causes of visual impairment in the United States are macular degeneration, diabetic retinopathy, glaucoma, and cataract. Approximately 60% of people with visual impairments who are not institutionalized have one or more additional impairments. These include the loss of hearing, impaired mobility and greater falls risk, decreased energy and stamina from respiratory and heart disease, and cognitive changes resulting from stroke or dementia. Vision loss has been ranked third, behind arthritis and heart disease, among the most common chronic conditions causing older people to require assistance with activities of daily living (ADLs). Because the majority of people with visual impairments have useful vision, rehabilitation services and vision-enhancing techniques and devices offer opportunities to increase their visual and general functional capacity.

AGING AND LOSS OF VISION

Normal Age-Related Changes in Vision

Every older person experiences age-related changes in vision. The majority of these age-related changes are not amenable to correction with spectacles. **Table 33-1** summarizes the age-related changes that cause functional declines for older people. Decreased transmission of the ocular media, increased scatter in the cornea, lens, vitreous body, and retina as well as decreased pupil size are related to anatomic changes in the aging eye. The age-related changes discussed here are those that have the greatest impact on function in daily life. The importance of accommodating these typical, age-related changes in visual function cannot be overstated. Age-related changes in vision affect nearly all older adults and manifest in the absence of eye pathology. Their impacts on aspects of health self-management and cognitive function, for instance, are only beginning to be appreciated. Age-related changes in vision must be taken in account when considering the daily living, quality of life, and the design of facilities for all older people.

TABLE 33-1 ■ NORMAL AGE-RELATED CHANGES IN VISION

CHANGES	REASON	IMPLICATIONS FOR DAILY LIFE
Loss of accommodation	• Crystalline lenses lose flexibility • Ciliary muscles lose tone	• Increasing inability to focus on close targets beginning around age 45. • Plus lenses prescribed in a bifocal, reading glasses, or contact lenses; required to compensate for loss of accommodative ability.
Loss of low-contrast acuity	• Decreased transmission of ocular media • Decreased pupil size	• Functional loss of acuity under glare or low lighting may cause small targets to be missed, bumping or tripping into low-lying objects.
Increased sensitivity to glare	• Increased light scatter in cornea, lenses, vitreous body, and retina	• Discomfort even in low glare conditions such as cloudy days. High glare causes decreased acuity and difficulty in seeing targets in the environment. • Sun lenses, hats, visors, and umbrellas provide more comfort outdoors; tinted lenses may be prescribed for indoors.
Increased difficulty with light and dark adaptation	• Losses in ocular transmittance and pupillary miosis	• Require longer to adjust to sudden or extreme shifts in lighting conditions, such as when moving bright to dim environments or vice versa. Risk for stumbling or falling is greater under these circumstances. Fear of balance problems or falling may cause compensatory behaviors such as shuffling, reaching for hand-holds, etc. Change environmental lighting to avoid light/dim areas. If not possible, wear sunglasses outdoors and remove coming indoors. When emerging into disabling light, wait before ambulating.
Loss of color discrimination	• Smaller pupil diameter, reduced light transmission through the lens, changes in photoreceptors and neural pathways	• Difficulty detecting differences in dark colors and pastels and distinguishing hues of blues/greens/violet; adding directional lamps with daylight bulbs or matching colors near a sunny window helps.
Loss of attentional visual field	• Decline of higher-order visual processes such as selective and divided attention and rapid processing speed	• Risk factor for balance and mobility problems and vehicle crashes in driving. Training improves performance.
Increased difficulty with visual reading ability	• Related to attentional visual field, low-contrast acuity and slower, less accurate eye movement performance	• Reading speed of older readers reduced by one-third that of younger readers; text navigation skills decline with age. Training improves performance as does attention to typographical design (font, size, contrast, spacing, etc.).

Accommodation The ability to accommodate for focus on visual targets from distance to near, which is dependent on a flexible crystalline lens and the ciliary muscle, is altered with age, beginning around age 45. During this change, an increasing amount of plus in a concave lens (usually prescribed in bifocal lenses or reading glasses) is required to boost the focusing power of the eye to compensate for the loss in refracting ability of the lens for near tasks.

Visual acuity The visual acuity of nonvisually impaired older people shows only a modest decrease under high-contrast conditions, but reducing the illumination of an acuity chart, reducing the contrast of the acuity chart, and/or adding surrounding glare, produces drastic age-related acuity losses, as compared to young observers. For example, in a sample of 900 older observers, for those at age 82, the median high-contrast visual acuity was 20/30, low-contrast high-luminance acuity was 20/55, low-contrast low-luminance acuity was 20/120, and low-contrast acuity in glare conditions was 20/160. The added challenge of less than optimal lighting and/or contrast between the letters and their

background means that older adults have difficulty resolving detailed visual information at the same distance as younger observers. The combined challenge of low contrast stimuli *and* less than optimal illumination significantly reduces visual acuity relative to young comparisons. A young observer loses only about one line of acuity under similar conditions. Thus, older adults' visual acuity is dramatically reduced under less than optimal viewing conditions. Older people need higher contrast and two to three times more light to see than a younger person. Low contrast and low lighting adversely impact the visual function of older people, and modification of visual materials and environmental lighting are helpful.

Adaptation to changing lighting conditions Because of anatomic changes in the eye and media, older people require more light to support adequate vision; however, they are also more sensitive to glare, such as very bright direct light or reflected bright light in the environment. As a result, older adults are more likely to experience momentary glare disability and take longer to recover from glare exposure (eg, camera flash, bright headlights) relative to younger persons. The adverse effects of glare may have the most impact on activities such as walking outdoors or driving, but may affect indoor activities as well. Because adaptation to changing levels of light is slowed in aging, the momentary vision loss and visual discomfort experienced when moving between dim and very bright environments (eg, from a dim restaurant, or theater, into a sunny day) may limit how well important targets that must be viewed for the sake of safety are seen. Glare sensitivity has been associated with motor vehicle accidents for older drivers.

Attentional visual field Attentional visual field, the visual field area over which one can detect and process rapidly presented visual information, declines with age. Unlike conventional measures of visual field that assess visual sensory sensitivity (such as static flashing lights), attentional visual field relies on higher-order processing skills such as selective and divided attention and rapid processing speed. Decreased attentional visual field has been correlated to a greater incidence of driving accidents and is related to a greater risk for balance and mobility problems for nonvisually impaired older people. Attentional visual field can be improved with training, but such training is not widely available.

Reading rate Visual reading ability decreases with age as well. The reading rate of older people who do not have a vision loss and have good high-contrast visual acuity still decreases by as much as a third of that of young readers. Accuracy of reading, however, can remain comparable to that of younger readers. Reading performance among older people with good acuity (20/30) is highly correlated with attentional visual field; those with good reading performance into very old age also retain good attentional fields as well. Low-contrast visual acuity is also correlated with reading performance for this population; older people with poor low-contrast acuity tend to read more slowly. Even when high-contrast acuity is good, older people, especially the oldest old, are at risk for reading difficulties that may arise from a combination of reduced attentional visual field, reduced accuracy and efficiency of eye movements, and poor low-contrast visual acuity. Reading ability can be supported by optimizing lighting, contrast and typography (font size and type, spacing, leading, kerning, line length) of text materials. Moreover, reading rate for nonvisually impaired older adults with good high-contrast acuity and good comprehension skills can be improved with training. Training in reading efficiency that emphasizes improvements in eye movements for reading similar to those exercises used to improve reading for school children has given good results for this population. Such training, however, is not widely available.

Color discrimination Color discrimination is another aspect of vision that declines with advancing age. People who are older have greater difficulty detecting differences between very dark colors (eg, brown, black, or navy). Particularly challenging are tasks that involve green-blue-violet color discriminations, or distinguishing between very light, pastel colors (eg, light yellow, peach, light green, light blue—common medication pill colors). Loss of color vision in old age is related to smaller pupil diameter (miosis), reduced light transmission through the lens which yellows and thickens with age, and changes in photoreceptors and neural pathways.

Dark adaptation Dark adaptation ability and speed decline as a result of losses in ocular transmittance and pupillary miosis resulting from the aging process. Difficulty with slowed dark adaptation can be limiting to older adults moving from light to dim environments and vice versa. The risk for stumbling or falling may be greater under these circumstances (eg, exiting a theater into a bright, sunny day). During the protracted adaptation period the nonvisually impaired older person may function as if severely visually impaired when required to transition quickly between environments with drastically different levels of illumination.

Spectacles and falls risk Although not related to a change in vision per se, care must be taken in providing refractive correction in spectacle form for geriatric patients. Multifocal spectacle lenses either in the form of bifocals or varifocals are commonly prescribed but are associated with a higher risk of "edge of step" accidents, and multifocal lens wearers are twice as likely to fall as single-focus lens wearers. A large percentage of these falls are reported to occur outside the home, perhaps as a result of tripping or stumbling resulting from obstacles not seen in the near-vision correction of the lower visual field. The bifocal portion of a spectacle correction provides additional dioptric power to provide vision at near distance for reading, etc. This means that objects outside this near-focal range, such as steps, curbs, stairs, pets, etc., are blurred and indistinct. This effect is greatest in older patients, as the need for extra dioptric power for near vision increases with age. Patients with multifocal correction are encouraged to tuck their chins and look over the top of the bifocal correction when moving so that they can look through the distance correction in the upper portion of the lenses, but head flexion significantly increases postural instability. Encouraging those who are at risk for falling to explore these issues with their eye care specialists, who may recommend separate "near" and "distance" spectacles or other solutions, can be an important aspect of falls prevention.

The changes in healthy aging vision described above are common and experienced by nearly all people as they grow older. This does not minimize the importance of using, and recommending, the strategies described above to minimize the impacts of age-related changes in visual function on daily life. The impacts of the aging visual system described are evident in the absence of eye conditions or disease and amplify functional impairments if pathology does develop. The most prevalent age-related causes of *visual impairment* are described next.

Prevalent Age-Related Causes of Visual Impairment

Age-related macular degeneration Functional vision loss due to age-related macular degeneration may include metamorphopsia (visual images appear distorted and wavy), relative scotomas, as well as dense central scotomas for those whose pathology progresses to visual impairment. Individuals with central scotomas in both eyes usually develop a strongly preferred retinal locus or loci (PRL) that performs as the primary fixation reference, although the patient may not always be aware that there is a scotoma present. The loss of central visual field results in loss of visual acuity and contrast sensitivity. The ability to use the PRL that develops for fixation may be difficult for many people. The effects of macular degeneration on daily life include difficulty with reading print, inability to recognize faces (that can lead to reluctance to participate in social activities), difficulty with distance and depth cues (that adversely affect safe mobility), and loss of color and contrast sensitivity (that interferes with a variety of household and work/leisure tasks) (**Table 33-2**).

Diabetic retinopathy The progression of diabetic retinopathy includes macular edema that may cause blurred vision if the fovea is involved, retinal hemorrhages (and/or laser treatments), which may result in scattered central, peripheral, and/or midperipheral scotomas, and retinal detachment, which can cause larger areas of field loss if not reattached. Diabetic retinopathy can progress to total blindness. Loss of function can include decreased visual acuity, scattered field loss over the retina, metamorphopsia across the retina, increased sensitivity to glare, and loss of color and contrast sensitivity. If the fovea is lost to scotoma, then a PRL or multiple PRLs will likely develop. Vision fluctuations can be manifested over time as macular swelling increases or subsides, and can also be related to hemorrhage. Sudden vision loss is common following hemorrhage, with the patient describing episodes of smoky vision, a dropped veil over the eye(s), or seeing black or red strings across the field of view. Treatment and absorption of blood can improve acuity, though not usually to normal levels. The effects on daily life include difficulty reading print materials, difficulty recognizing faces, increased sensitivity to glare and light/dark adaptation, difficulty with distance and depth cues, loss of color and contrast sensitivity, and fluctuating vision.

TABLE 33-2 ■ AGE-RELATED CAUSES OF VISUAL IMPAIRMENT

CONDITION	COMMON CLINICAL PRESENTATION	IMPLICATIONS FOR REHABILITATION
Macular degeneration	• Reduced visual acuity • Loss of central visual field and contrast sensitivity	Difficulty with tasks requiring fine detail vision such as reading, inability to recognize faces, distortion or disappearance of the visual field straight ahead, loss of color and contrast perception, mobility difficulties related to loss of depth and contrast cues.
Diabetic retinopathy	• Reduced visual acuity • Scattered central scotomas • Peripheral and midperipheral scotomas • Macular edema	Difficulty with tasks requiring fine detail vision such as reading, distorted central vision, fluctuating vision, loss of color perception, mobility problems because of loss of depth and contrast cues.
Cataract	• Reduced visual acuity • Light scatter • Sensitivity to glare • Altered color perception • Loss of contrast sensitivity • Image distortion • Possible myopia	Usually remedied by lens extraction and implant, except in extreme cases. If not managed by implant, difficulty with detail vision, difficulty with bright and changing light, color perception, decreased contrast perception, some mobility problems caused by loss of perception of depth and distance, sensitivity to glare, and loss of contrast.
Glaucoma	• Degeneration of optic disk • Loss of peripheral visual fields	If not managed by medication or surgery, reduced peripheral fields result. Reading and mobility problems because of restricted visual fields. People suddenly appearing in the small visual field seen as "jack in the box."
Traumatic brain injury and stroke	• Loss of hemi/quadrant visual field, or paracentral scotoma • Possible visual neglect • Visual perceptual difficulties • Visual agnosia	Mobility and reading problems due to visual field loss and spatial perceptual difficulties that reduce ability to drive, reach accurately, and execute eye movements related to reading; difficulty with visual and cognitive processing. Visual neglect may include inability to complete shaving and/or dressing. Difficulty completing other rehabilitation assessments and interventions because visual impairment may not be recognized as disabling.

Cataract Age-related cataract is manifested by gradual opacity of the lens, which interferes with the passage of light, causing reduced visual acuity, light scatter, sensitivity to glare, altered color perception, and image distortion (straight lines appear wavy). People with cataracts may experience trouble with glare and loss of contrast, may have decreased acuity, and report areas of metamorphopsia or small scotomas in the visual field. When the cataract has begun to interfere with lifestyle, surgery may be performed to remove either the entire lens or the posterior portion. Correction for the removal of the lens is provided primarily through intraocular lens implants, but occasionally eyeglasses or contact lens are used instead. Cataract surgery is the most common major surgical procedure done for people older than age 65 who are receiving Medicare funding. Cataract surgery with lens implantation is associated with improved objective and subjective measures of function in ADLs, as well as improved levels of vision to normal acuity in most cases.

Glaucoma Glaucoma is an increase in intraocular pressure caused by an abnormality in flow of aqueous fluid from the anterior chamber. It can cause a degeneration of the optic disk, loss of visual fields, and severe visual impairment. When left untreated, or if treatment is not successful, glaucoma results in a loss of peripheral fields and can lead to blindness. The effect of peripheral field loss on daily life is most problematic in safe ambulation. Because of field restrictions, the patients may not see objects in their path and may bump into objects that fall outside the field of view in any direction (street signs, tree branches, other people, etc). In addition, a person outside the patient's field of view may suddenly be seen as a "jack-in-the-box" and create a startle effect. Peripheral field loss may also create problems in reading and writing as only a small portion of the page can be seen at once.

Traumatic brain injury and stroke Head injury to older adults from falls or automobile accidents resulting in traumatic brain injury (TBI), as well as brain injury due to strokes, can lead to visual impairment. Between 20% and 40% of strokes result in visual disorder that can inhibit cognitive functioning and may reduce the effectiveness of rehabilitation of the TBI. Visual field disorders can result from injury to the visual pathway anyway between the retina and the striate cortex. The optic chiasm is an anatomic landmark that differentiates the peripheral (prechiasmatic) and the central (postchiasmatic) visual pathway. Unilateral injury to the prechiasmatic pathway affects the ipsilesional field only, but postchiasmatic injury causes visual deficits in both monocular hemifields that are referred to as homonymous. Visual field disorders must be discerned by visual field measurement techniques called perimetry. Patients are often unaware of field loss and may not report the lost visual field/s, but they may suffer from their effects, for example, bumping into objects, tripping, falling, being unable to read, etc. Vision can be completely lost in the missing field, or some vision function (eg, light detection) may remain. The most common visual field losses are hemianopsia (loss of half the visual field), followed by quadranopsia (loss of one quadrant) and paracentral scotoma (island of vision loss in the parafoveal region). Recovery of some visual field following injury may be spontaneous, and some patients learn spontaneously to adapt to visual field loss by oculomotor strategies; shifting gaze may reveal what is missing in the field of view of a street scene (such as an oncoming car) or the missing portion of a line of text. Systematic training in oculomotor adaptation and visual perceptual training can improve vision function and has the ability to improve the perceived visual field. Visual field loss may also be accompanied by visual neglect. Older adults with neglect may not spontaneously be able to attend to the neglected side. TBI may also result in disorders of visual space perception, which affect reach (over- or underreaching for objects, knocking objects over), driving (accidents resulting from inability to judge distance and depth), and reading (inability to plan and execute accurate eye movements). Visuospatial localization and orientation may be improved through training, but may not reach pre-TBI thresholds. Visual agnosia, a failure to visually recognize an object because of "mistaken identity," is a disorder that is based in both visual-perceptual and visual-cognitive functions. Typically, misidentifications result from the incomplete or inappropriate use of object features such as size, shape, or color. Older adults with TBI may be unaware that they are ignoring other features that might assist with correct identification. Cognitive and/or communication disorders can make visual impairment more difficult to detect following TBI. Undetected or untreated visual impairment in TBI can limit the effectiveness of other TBI rehabilitation. For example, many cognitive and functional assessments use visual items that cannot be appropriately identified by older people with vision loss; visual motor assessments require eye-hand coordination. If TBI vision loss is not detected and treated to the extent possible, the examiner or therapist may get a false-negative impression of the level of TBI disability. In addition, the TBI patient will be frustrated and troubled unduly by participating in rehabilitation that does not simultaneously address the vision deficit. Integrated, interdisciplinary team-based care is key.

ROLE OF THE GERIATRICIAN IN VISION REHABILITATION

After diagnosis and medical management of the patient's vision loss, the geriatrician can play an important role in assuring that visually impaired people receive rehabilitation services that are of high quality, are sought in a timely manner, and provide all the benefit that the patients might be able to derive from them.

A geriatrician can provide the following services for their patients related to vision rehabilitation:

1. A visual acuity evaluation. Current best practice includes the use of a logarithmic visual acuity chart.

2. A contrast sensitivity function evaluation. The Pelli-Robson chart is recommended for its ease of use and reliability.

3. A referral to a low-vision eye care specialist (ophthalmologist or optometrist) for the appropriate clinical low-vision evaluation and prescription of optical low-vision devices for tasks the older person can no longer perform, such as reading, writing, watching television, and recognizing street signs.

4. A referral to certified vision rehabilitation professionals for assessment and instruction of vision, and assistive devices for literacy, ADLs, safe travel, hobbies, etc. These therapists can also provide environmental analyses and teach the use of environmental cues.

5. Assistance to patients in preparing for rehabilitation by providing information and encouraging them to consider the goals they would like to achieve. **Table 33-3** provides the questions and rating scale for the VA Low-Vision

Visual Functioning Questionnaire-20 (VFQ-20). The VA VFQ-20 is a modified 20-item questionnaire that is effective in assessing the impact of vision impairment on quality of life and is helpful in assisting patients in setting goals for rehabilitation.

6. Counseling or referral for coping with psychosocial issues related to visual impairment. Patients may not be forthcoming about these issues, so the physician must ask. Adjustment disorder and depression are associated with visual impairment for older people. When patients are dealing with loss of independence and control, lowered self-esteem, and strained social relations, counseling and/or psychotherapy may be recommended for both patients and family members.

7. Reinforcement of simple strategies to improve abilities, such as the use of saturated colors and contrast in the home environment, and the use of simple devices, such as sun lenses outdoors and brighter indoor environments.

8. Providing information to the patient and family about the variable nature of low vision, its effect on daily life tasks, and the variable nature of visual abilities according to fluctuations of light and contrast.

9. Sponsorship of, or referral to, support groups where older people with vision loss and their families can discuss problems, coping, and rehabilitation strategies they have learned with other patients.

10. Assistance in community awareness about the prevalence, treatment, and rehabilitation of visual impairment among older people.

Patients likely to benefit from vision rehabilitation include those with reduced acuity of less than 20/50 in the better-seeing eye, central or peripheral field loss with intact visual acuity, reduced contrast sensitivity, glare sensitivity, and/or light/dark adaptation difficulties as well as those with TBI. Candidates for cataract surgery with macular disease might also benefit from preoperative low-vision assessment and coincident rehabilitation training that enhances postoperative visual performance and satisfaction with a cataract procedure.

ADAPTATIONS OF CLINICAL AND FUNCTIONAL EVALUATIONS FOR OLDER ADULTS

The clinical and functional low-vision examinations for older people should distinguish aging from treatable disease processes; focus holistically; incorporate family and caregiver support; identify what matters most to the patient; and set realistic patient-centered goals as part of interdisciplinary team-based plans of care to improve functional status and quality of life.

In health care service delivery to older adults with low vision, certain aspects of the examination sequence are adapted to accommodate these principles.

TABLE 33-3 ■ VA LOW-VISION VISUAL FUNCTIONING QUESTIONNAIRE-20 (WITHOUT OVERALL SCORING)

Directions: Select one of the responses listed below to indicate the level of difficulty for each activity which pertains to the following question: "Is it difficult to_____?"

1. Not difficult
2. Slightly/moderately difficult
3. Extremely difficult
4. Impossible
5. Unscored/don't do because of *nonvisual* reasons

Note: *If you use a low-vision device, adaptive device, or an adaptive technique to assist with the activity, respond as though you were using the device or technique.*

ACTIVITY	LEVEL OF DIFFICULTY
1. Read newspaper or magazine articles	
2. Read mail	
3. Read menus	
4. Read small print on package label	
5. Keep your place while reading	
6. Read street signs and store names	
7. Read print on TV	
8. See photos	
9. Find something on a crowded shelf	
10. Identify medicine	
11. Tell time	
12. Watch TV	
13. Handle finances	
14. Get around outdoors in places you know	
15. Adjust to bright light	
16. Take a message	
17. Prepare meals	
18. Use appliance dials	
19. Groom yourself	
20. Eat and drink neatly	

Because most age-related visual impairments result in a central scotoma, most patient complaints will be related to the loss of acuity, loss of central visual field, and resultant decrease in contrast sensitivity and color sensitivity. Patient goals for rehabilitation will usually include reading, writing, independence in ADLs such as meal preparation and household maintenance, management of glare and other illumination concerns, leisure activities, and safe independent movement and travel. Older people may also have specific health-related activities that require the use of vision (eg, loading a syringe with insulin, changing an ostomy bag); these will be goals as well.

This information may be taken by a pre-examination telephone interview to lessen the amount of time the first examination visit might require. Because low-vision rehabilitation requires a great deal of energy and motivation from the patient, it will be guided by their personal goals for rehabilitation and by those tasks that are difficult or impossible to perform because of low vision. In this regard, the intake interviewer may find that some education is necessary in order to set reasonable goals for low-vision treatment. Because most low-vision interventions and assistive devices are "task specific," it is important to state treatment goals as specifically as possible.

Because of the nature of the older person's vision loss, professionals should become familiar with some key accommodations that assist in providing quality health care, such as the following:

- Always face, make eye contact, and speak directly to the older adult with visual impairment.
- Allow the older adult to take your arm when moving from place to place in the environment, and use appropriate sighted guide techniques. If you are guiding a person with visual impairment by having the person take your arm, you are responsible for assuring that the path you are taking is wide enough to accommodate both of you. If the path is not wide enough (eg, a crowded hallway), ask the person to step behind you, while still holding your arm when walking.
- Say your name when first coming into the room, and tell the older adult when you are leaving the room.
- Do not leave the older adult with low vision standing alone in a hallway or room without a wall or furniture near to touch for orientation and balance.
- Avoid using directional cues that are visual in nature such as pointing or giving directional references that are unclear to those with low vision. For example, instead of saying, "take that chair over there" say, "take the red chair against the white wall to your immediate right."

Clinical Low-Vision Evaluation

The low-vision eye care specialist (who may be an ophthalmologist or an optometrist) must be flexible and adaptable to a variety of different environments, schedules, and communication styles. The conventional pattern of the low-vision examination will be followed including distance and near acuities; internal and external ocular health examination; retinoscopy; tonometry and slit-lamp biomicroscopy; ophthalmoscopy; ophthalmometry; determination of central and peripheral fields; color vision and contrast-sensitivity testing; glare testing; and near and distance testing of vision-enhancing devices, including optical, electronic, and nonoptical devices. For many older adults, especially those in long-term care facilities, a careful refraction and update of conventional spectacles may provide significant improvement in vision. **Table 33-4** summarizes the aspects of the clinical low-vision examination.

Because of the nature of medical and long-term care service delivery to older adults, the low-vision examination and therapeutic intervention is often taken out of the office or clinical setting. There is a growing trend of providing low-vision services as a part of outpatient hospital care, comprehensive outpatient rehabilitation facilities, and long-term care facilities, such as nursing homes and private homes of older adults.

Long-Term Care Facilities

Despite the fact as many as half the people in nursing homes have visual impairment, few nursing home residents receive low-vision care. For example, one study estimated only 25% of visually impaired patients at a long-term care facility who could potentially benefit from vision rehabilitation were referred for these services. Another study found that there was no difference in the referral rate for vision services for nursing home residents between those who complained about their vision and those who did not. Another study found that only 11% of all residents in 19 nursing homes had

TABLE 33-4 ■ CLINICAL LOW-VISION EXAMINATION	
Settings for the examination	• Long-term care facilities • Individual's home • Community service agency • Rehabilitation center
Aspects of the examination	• Distance/near acuities • Internal/external health examination • Retinoscopy • Tonometry • Slit-lamp biomicroscopy • Ophthalmoscopy • Ophthalmometry • Central/peripheral field measurement • Color vision testing • Contrast-sensitivity testing • Evaluation of low-vision devices (optical, nonoptical, and electronic)

received eye examinations in the last 2 years. Providing information about vision and vision impairment to the nursing home staff is important for assisting residents in using their remaining vision effectively. Because stroke is another common medical condition requiring rehabilitation for older adults, it is important that the low-vision team work closely with those professionals who diagnose, treat, and rehabilitate older adults who have experienced cerebrovascular accident. Currently, Hadley School for the Blind provides an online curriculum in visual impairment for in-service training for people with visual impairment and their family members as well as professionals and technicians who work with them (www.Hadley.edu). The use of curricular materials by long-term care staff has proven effective in increasing staff knowledge and positive outcomes for patients.

Hospital Settings

Low-vision care is routinely provided to older veterans in the hospital system of the Veterans Health Administration (VHA). In the inpatient Blind Rehabilitation Centers, a veteran who is severely disabled is seen for up to 10 weeks of rehabilitation, including low-vision rehabilitation. Results from a national outcomes study indicate positive outcomes and veteran satisfaction from these programs that exceed the outcomes of rehabilitation in the private sector. The VHA also provides low-vision rehabilitation for veterans who are visually impaired but have remaining vision. In 2009, the VHA expanded low-vision services at medical facilities and in patients' homes providing $40 million in funding for a continuum of care closer to veterans' homes. Outcome studies of all VA vision rehabilitation services indicate that veterans who are provided low-vision services regain their ability to perform independent activities of daily living (IADLs) independently and become active community participants. VHA is the only national medical system that completely integrates vision and blind rehabilitation into the system of care. In fiscal year 2014, VHA provided inpatient, outpatient, and home-based vision and blind rehabilitation to approximately 29,000 unique patients. Further, there are approximately 50,000 severely disabled blind veterans on the rosters of VHA case managers, who assure that this vulnerable population receive all the VA benefits that should accrue to them. Hospitals in the private sector are increasingly providing services to older people as a part of outpatient services, and low-vision rehabilitation is often provided.

Community Service Agency Settings

The Older Americans Act (OAA) is a major source for the organization and delivery of social and nutrition services for older adults as well as their caregivers. The OAA authorizes many services through a national network of 56 state agencies on aging, 629 area agencies on aging, 244 tribal organizations, and 2 native Hawaiian organizations representing 400 tribes. The OAA programs include community service employment for low-income older Americans; training, research, and demonstration activities in the field of aging; and vulnerable elder rights protection activities. The Administration on Aging (AoA) oversees these OAA programs and services and maintains an online National Eldercare Locator searchable for local agencies and resources. Low-vision services or vision rehabilitation agencies in your area can be located by searching your state's rehabilitation agency website or searching the American Printing House for the Blind's Directory of Services (VisionAware: https://visionaware.org/), which includes directories of state agencies, independent service providers, and organizations that provide vision rehabilitation services.

Private Home Settings

Pew Research Center estimates that 4 in 10 adults in the United States are caring for a sick or older family member at home. The number of caregivers increased 10% between 2010 and 2013; most caregivers surveyed were between 30 and 64 years. Approximately 70% of the older population requiring long-term care resides in the community. Senior residential retirement centers have increased in number. Most frail older people requiring care are living at home with family members and not in long-term care facilities. It is crucial that family members and caregivers understand the sometimes contradictory nature of visual impairment; for example, visual performance varies widely under different levels of illumination and can decline if the older person is fatigued. Comorbid conditions such as dementia, mobility impairment, and depression can affect how the older person uses vision and interprets visual images. Understanding the interaction of these factors will help family members in supporting the older adult achieve their goals for vision rehabilitation.

Functional Visual Assessment

Whenever possible, a functional assessment should take place in the older adult's daily environment. Specific goals for using vision independently stated by the older adult will guide the functional assessment to discover what visual target size, target distance, and visual skills are required to achieve that goal. For example, if the patient's goal is to read the newspaper again, the target size requires approximately 20/40 or better visual acuity with spectacles and magnification, the target distance will be determined by the magnification device, and the visual skills required are precise visual fixation and saccades while maintaining the focal distance of the magnification device. The older adult must learn not only new visual strategies, but also new cognitive strategies to aid comprehension, even with a slower rate of reading. The functional assessment can also uncover the need to address other goals, the need for environmental assessment and modification, and to provide ongoing opportunities to educate the older adult and family about vision and rehabilitation. **Table 33-5** presents the key aspects of the functional vision assessment.

TABLE 33-5 ■ KEY ASPECTS OF THE FUNCTIONAL VISUAL ASSESSMENT

Functional visual acuities	Distance and lighting required for discriminating detail of objects in the environment
Functional visual fields	Ability to perceive objects in the environment in central and peripheral quadrants of the visual field at near and distance
Color/contrast discrimination	Ability to detect objects, their color, and contrast with the varying light/dark backgrounds at varying distances
Ocular motor skills	Ability to maintain fixation and move the eyes/head/body to fixate, scan, track, and localize targets in the environment
Visual perceptual skills	Ability to make sense of what is seen; recognize critical features, perceive part-to-whole relationships, identify figure-ground, etc
Lighting	Analysis of the usefulness of environmental lighting; need for greater/less illumination and controls such as filters, sun lenses, etc.
Use of visual and non-visual cues	Availability and use of visual and nonvisual cues in the environment that enhance task performance
Performance of activities of daily living and instrumental activities of daily living that are affected by vision	Observe for ability to perform, ease and speed of performance, comfort and stress level, safety

The functional low-vision assessment may be completed by a wide variety of rehabilitation professionals. Traditionally, the functional low-vision assessment of older people has been provided by a low-vision therapist, a rehabilitation teacher for the visually impaired, an orientation and mobility specialist, or some other professional from the field of visual impairment, such as an eye care technician or technologist. Now, as vision rehabilitation is increasingly a part of hospital services and comprehensive outpatient rehabilitation facilities, the functional assessment may be provided by a rehabilitation nurse, an occupational therapist, or some other rehabilitation professional who has received specialized training in low vision.

Regardless of the background of vision rehabilitation professionals, they should be well versed and experienced in basic optics of the eye, lenses, and low-vision devices; methods of observation and evaluation of visual skills for all daily tasks; the causes and functional implications of visual impairments; basic techniques of sighted guide and basic orientation and mobility; assessment of safety (falls, medication access, sharps, burns, etc); assessment

of literacy (reading, numeracy); assessment of the visual aspects of environment; and basic techniques of assessing and using technology such as optical devices (eg, magnifiers, spectacles, monoculars) and electronic devices (eg, Braille writer, smartphones, tablets, computers, and closed-circuit television [CCTV] system). The rehabilitation professional providing the evaluation may also be the rehabilitation therapist, in which case they must be familiar with techniques of instructing visual-motor skills for all daily, vocational and avocational tasks (with and without optical devices and access technology), task analyses, organization and time management, basic orientation and mobility, basic techniques of literacy, and safety in the home. The professional must also be familiar with tools and techniques that do not require the use of vision. There are situations in which using vision is not the safest or most efficient way to complete a task. In that case, other nonvisual strategies such as voice-over, use of Braille tags, use of a long cane on a dark street, etc, are more helpful. The rehabilitation professional will work closely with the eye care specialist providing the clinical low-vision examination, and the low-vision team may also include a counseling professional and any other professionals who are providing care associated with vision impairment or comorbid disabilities. Because many older people are at risk for multiple impairments, this team may also include other physicians, such as a geriatrician or physiatrist, orthopedist, speech, physical, respiratory, and recreational therapists, nurses, and technicians.

MANAGEMENT OF LOW VISION

Developing a Vision Rehabilitation Plan

The clinical low-vision examination and functional visual assessment culminate in a vision *rehabilitation plan* that summarizes the information obtained in the evaluations into clearly stated goals and objectives. If Medicare is funding the low-vision services, the plan will follow that format and requirements. In many cases, family members also may be involved. The implementation of the vision rehabilitation plan should emphasize a process using the principles of andragogy, or adult learning, that incorporate the older person's values, beliefs, attitudes, and life experiences.

Following the clinical examination and functional assessment, the low-vision team will recommend low-vision devices (including optical, electronic, nonoptical, and environmental modifications) that will be evaluated to assess their usefulness by the older adult. There should be additional focus on the rehabilitation program and its adaptation for older individuals. Successful use of low-vision devices is related to the intensity of the instructional program. Research shows that specialized therapy in the use of visual skills and low-vision devices improve the abilities of low-vision individuals who are older to a greater extent than do the services provided by eye care specialists alone.

Low-Vision Therapy

Low-vision therapy is a crucial aspect of providing care. Therapy is dependent on the goals of the older adult and might include the following:

- Visual skills rehabilitation training including fixation, PRL ability for reading, and visual scanning for other visual tasks such as locating a traffic light or street sign.
- Literacy assessment and training to improve reading accuracy, speed, comprehension, and duration.
- Legible handwriting and written expression (including being able to read one's own handwriting).
- Use of low-vision devices for daily tasks.
- Modification of the environment to enhance safety and ability to complete activities including lighting, contrast, organization, labeling, glare control, removal of hazards, and other safety measures.
- Use of access technology such as computers, smartphones, tablets, global positioning devices, etc.
- Guidance on safe functional movement within the known environment.
- ADLs such as home maintenance, meal preparation and cleanup, clothing care, grooming, etc.
- Strategies for self-management of health such as organizing and accessing medications, blood pressure check, diabetic management, ostomy care, etc.
- Assessment and modification of work stations at home or away.
- Information and education of caregivers such as understanding the functional implications of low vision and their effect on daily life, understanding the use of assistive devices.
- Visual strategies for safe driving, or managing daily routines without driving.
- Use of community resources for people who are visually impaired such as support groups, free services such as *Library for the Blind* talking books, Treasury Department's free money identifier, low or no cost transportation, etc.
- Referral to other practitioners in a broader low-vision team, for example, referrals for assessment and training in the use of long white cane for mobility, guide dog, Braille training, diabetic education, etc.
- Emerging technology for adults with vision impairment has reduced much of the frustration of literacy and recognition of friends and family due to new technology.

Instruction and Guided Practice Using Remaining Vision and Low-Vision Devices

Working with a low-vision therapist will provide an opportunity for the older adult to develop the appropriate visual skills; use optical devices and access technology; and learn to apply principles of color, illumination, and contrast that make the environment as conducive as possible to the use of remaining vision. It is important to assist caregivers in understanding how rehabilitation interventions aid the older adult in accomplishing visual tasks. Family members and caregivers can provide important social support in this regard, but must understand the process in order to be most helpful. In a study of visually impaired older veterans, a supportive caregiver was the most strongly correlated variable to continued use of low-vision devices 1 to 2 years after they were prescribed. If at all possible, devices should be loaned for use in the daily environment before they are prescribed to assure that they are useful.

Some aspects of instructing the use of vision, prescribed devices, and access technology are particularly important when working with older people with low vision. Because of the potentially devastating consequences of falling, the low-vision therapist must be certain to address safety issues related to using low-vision devices that will prevent falls. Nausea, dizziness, and other aspects of motion sickness can be side effects of using magnification, and reducing them is an important aspect of instruction. Monoculars and binoculars should be used as spotting devices only, and older adults must never attempt to walk while viewing through them. If the older person's goal is watching television or spectator sports, binoculars that are spectacle-mounted may be provided and the older person will use them only while seated.

Another factor to be explored in the use of low-vision devices for older adults is hand tremor. Hand tremor may be severe enough that handheld magnifiers or telescopes are not useful. The low-vision team may want to explore spectacle-mounted devices to avoid the difficulty of maintaining focus, if hand tremor is problematic.

Postural support and ergonomic considerations are important to using devices for people who are older. Because of the prevalence of back and neck pain, as well as limited stamina, it is important that the therapist assure the older person to be as comfortable as possible. The low-vision therapist will evaluate and demonstrate the use of appropriate ergonomic devices such as the appropriate chair and table, lumbar and cervical support, footstool, lamps, and reading stands. One study demonstrated that older adults who were supported according to ergonomic standards achieved significantly better reading performance.

Cognitive decline may limit the usefulness of low-vision devices for independent functioning; however, an additional goal can be added for rehabilitation—reducing caregiver burden. Vision rehabilitation for older adults with cognitive decline may include ergonomic solutions for comfort, increasing safety by providing good lighting for ambulation and other visual tasks, judiciously adding bold color and contrast for cuing activity and movement, and using simple assistive devices for common activities (eg, watching television on a larger screen, reading large-print books, getting a bright-colored snack from the refrigerator).

Finally, illumination is an important aspect of the instruction. Most older people need more light, but some may be extremely sensitive to light. An evaluation of a variety of lamps and overhead lighting situations is necessary, with the use of illumination controls that are individually recommended such as filters, absorptive lenses, hats with brims, and pinhole glasses.

Low-Vision Devices

Low-vision devices are optical devices, electronic devices, lighting devices, ergonomic devices, access technology such as global positioning devices, accessible smartphones and tablets, and other tools that enhance the use of vision. Some devices, such as those optical devices that incorporate refractive correction, require special prescription. Others are simpler, such as lamps, reading stands, or large-print books. During the clinical evaluation and functional assessment, the low-vision team will discover whether magnification, minification, voice-over, or other nonoptical devices (such as large-print books, lamps, reading stands, etc.) will be useful for enhancing the vision. **Table 33-6** summarizes the types of devices available and their uses. Devices are prescribed/recommended based on the goals of the older person and most people require instruction and practice in their use.

Magnification devices may be categorized as four types: relative distance, relative size, angular, and electronic. Relative distance magnification is provided by bringing the device to be viewed closer to the eyes. Often older adults who want to recognize someone will move more closely to the face they want to see, exhibiting this type of magnification. Spectacle-mounted magnifiers focus the target image, such as print for reading, at ranges closer than the older eye can accommodate, and allow very close distances to be maintained. These lenses must be prescribed by an eye care specialist experienced in low vision in order to incorporate the refractive correction of the older person when required. Typically, these devices require a close focal distance and have a short depth of focus. Depending on the power and focal distance, they can be used for near tasks such as reading, writing, and viewing photographs.

Magnification may also be provided by stand or handheld magnifiers, which are often more familiar to older adults who may have used them previously for maps

TABLE 33-6 ■ LOW-VISION AND SPEECH-OUTPUT DEVICES

OPTICAL/ELECTRONIC DEVICES	TYPICAL USE
Stand or handheld magnifiers (both optical and electronic, eg, smartphones with universal design)	Short-term reading or writing tasks such as checking a price tag or recipe, signing a check
Spectacle-mounted magnifiers	Long-term reading such as newspaper; used for writing in low powers
Handheld monoculars or binoculars	Traffic or street signs, spectator events
Spectacle-mounted monocular or binocular telescope	Television viewing, spectator events, possible driving Short-focus telescope can be used for cards, reading music, games, woodworking, etc
Closed-circuit television system (may be free-standing or incorporated into computer)	Reading, writing, independent activities of daily living, with distance camera, can be used like a telescope with very wide field of view
Field-expansion devices: • Reverse telescope • Field-expansion prisms • Hemianopic mirrors	Field expansion for ambulating or obstacle detection, identification, and/or avoidance Best with normal or near-normal acuity
NONOPTICAL DEVICES	**TYPICAL USE**
Lamps	Provide brighter illumination, primarily used as task lighting
Illumination control devices	Control glare, may increase contrast: sun lenses, hats, visors, colored filters
Handwriting implements	Felt-tip pens, bold-line paper, check- and letter-writing stencils, allow user to stay on line and write legibly
Posture and focal distance support	Upright reading stand, footstool, chair with arms and high back Cervical and lumbar support: provide comfort and allow user to read or write for a longer period
Large print	Large-print books and news, large phone dials, etc, to enhance visibility
Color/contrast aids	Brightly colored tape/paint for marking dials, edge of steps, etc, to enhance visibility and safety
Speech-output (aka voice-over) devices	Software, hardware, or applications that provide salient electronic information in spoken format. Spoken format reduces reading fatigue for long-term reading tasks or mobile tasks, such as electronic global positioning systems with spoken format.

or coins. These devices do not require a close eye-to-lens distance, but the closer to the eye the lens is held, the wider the field of view. Some are available with built-in illumination, which overcomes the problem of illuminating the target the older adult is viewing. Handheld magnifiers require a steady hand to maintain focus and may be fatiguing to use for long periods. Older adults who use stand magnifiers must wear their bifocal correction for visual accommodation, as the lens is set slightly inside the true focal distance of the lens in order to provide a better optical image at the periphery of the lens.

Relative size magnification is used whenever a target to be viewed is made physically larger. Examples of this are magazines and books that are printed larger than normal. Environments such as older adult high-rise apartments or condominiums and planned communities may also use enlarged signage, another example of relative size magnification.

Telescopic devices provide angular magnification by the use of a positive and negative lens in housing (galilean) or by the use of two positive lenses with an erecting prism (keplerian). Older adults may have used monoculars or binoculars in the past for sporting or other events and may have developed basic skills in their use. Older adults may use telescopic devices for identifying targets that are further away, such as street signs, sporting events, or television. The telescope may be handheld or may be mounted into spectacles for hands-free viewing. Mounted short-focus telescopes may be used for tasks that are closer, such as reading music from a stand or identifying cards on a table. Some older adults with visual impairment who meet visual and driving requirements may use miniature mounted telescopes (called bioptics) for driving.

The CCTV system, used by people who are visually impaired, is an example of electronic magnification. The CCTV provides a camera to focus on the visual task and the older adult sees the image projected onto an enlarged screened monitor or his television set. The visual task may be reading and writing from a desktop or the camera may be positioned for visual tasks at a greater distance such as seeing the minister and choir at church. The advantages of the CCTV include more magnification than any other device, a wider field of view, and color and contrast enhancement capability. CCTV offers a mechanism for the development of new technologies such as miniaturization, head-worn devices, and contrast enhancement.

Computer configuration with the CCTV can use multiple cameras to provide split-screen images for designing a workstation that simultaneously accesses computer, print viewing, word processing, and distance viewing.

Expanded field devices are helpful to older adults who maintain normal or near-normal acuity while experiencing decreased field of view, such as that caused by glaucoma or hemianopsias. Expanded field devices provide the ability to find targets by increasing the perceived view of a scene. For example, an older adult with restricted fields wishes to find the arriving and departing flight monitors in an airport. By using a field-expansion device, these monitors can be more easily located and the user then moves closer to them in order to read the information without the device if central vision is intact. A reverse telescope functions similar to a peephole in a door, but with better optics. Another type of field-expanding device minifies in the horizontal meridian only. The visual field may also be expanded by the use of base-out prisms incorporated into spectacles. The base-out prism shifts the image in, allowing a small eye movement to see the expanded field. Small mirrors attached to spectacles may also be used for field expansion.

Universal design in small portable electronic devices such as smartphones and tablets has revolutionized the field of vision rehabilitation. These devices are manufactured with sensory access (both vision and hearing enhancements) included in each one manufactured. The visually impaired user merely accesses the settings to turn on magnification or voice-over controls in the device, and then downloads a myriad of applications that provide the ability to ask the current location; use navigation systems; read; capture spoken commands, notes and documents; turn on a flashlight in the device; take a picture and ask what the picture depicts; use a wireless keyboard to use the device as a computer and other activities too numerous to mention. Universal design for access is becoming a marketing strategy for companies; one large cable company recently announced voice-over for navigating channels and finding desired programming. For older adults who are technologically adept, accessible smartphones and tablets are quickly learned and highly used. For older adults who have struggled with computers and other technology such as "smart" microwave ovens, these access devices may be very frustrating. However, even very old adults who are cognitively intact can master these intricate but powerful devices with good rehabilitation techniques.

If a smartphone, tablet, computer, CCTV, or other electronic device is to be used visually, the eye care specialist will assure that the older adult's vision is best corrected for the viewing distance of the screen. A pair of reading spectacles may be prescribed.

Instruction in the Use of Devices That Enhance Remaining Vision

A sequence of instructional procedures covers several areas:

- Use of visual skills without low-vision devices
- Use of visual skills with low-vision devices
- Use of vision and low-vision devices for individualized functional tasks that lead to the accomplishment of defined goals

Instruction in the use of visual skills without devices covers fixation, spotting, localization, scanning, tracing, and tracking. Individuals with maculopathy (such as age-related macular degeneration or diabetic retinopathy) may require additional instruction in the development and maintenance of visual skills using the PRL.

Instruction in the use of visual skills with low-vision devices includes integrating unaided visual abilities with the unique demands of a low-vision device such as maintaining the focal distance or focusing the device, and adjusting eye and head movements to compensate for a restricted field of view through the lens. If the individual is using eccentric viewing (the use of a PRL other than the fovea), the instructor assures that the device selected allows the opportunity to maximize field and acuity in the eccentric position.

Reading and Writing with Low-Vision Devices

Reading is a task that is so fundamental to our society and so disrupted by age-related visual impairment that it is the primary goal for vision rehabilitation among older adults. Readers with low vision can develop visual skills that are well-adapted to reading if they receive appropriate intervention. Most readers develop a strong PRL following the onset of central scotoma. The PRL is an area that will take over the function of fixation in an eccentric, nondamaged area of the retina. The reader may require instruction and practice in using the PRL for reading, especially because of the demands of using magnification to compensate for acuity loss. A Swedish study found that 71% of older adults with low vision could read the newspaper following rehabilitation, although at a 3-year follow-up that number had dropped to 48%. However, the number of fluent readers (70 words per minute or better) had increased from 41% to 48% over the 3-year period. These results indicate that those older adults with vision loss who persevere with rehabilitation strategies are able to continue improving their skills over time. In another study, people with macular loss who had a PRL below the scotoma exhibited faster reading rates, and the size of the atrophic area in the macula was the predominant limiting factor in reading; the larger the atrophy, the lower the reading rate. Reading rate is also related to visual span (number of characters available in the field of view) and the reserves of acuity and contrast sensitivity provided by the visual system and low-vision device. Accuracy of word identification and comprehension of reading, however, can remain near normal for readers with macular loss despite their slow rates. Readers with low vision often supplement visual reading with speech output devices such as spoken computer programs and books on audiotape.

Older adults with low vision can write effectively using a combination of magnification devices, lighting devices, stencils (templates for checks, envelopes, letters, etc. that assure that writing is spatially correct), and pens that provide more visibility.

Older adults who have good computer skills can substitute desktop computer, laptop, or smart phone for most low-vision devices and use the universally designed magnification, voice-over, and/or both to achieve reading and writing goals.

ENVIRONMENTS FOR OLDER PEOPLE

The onset of visual impairment for older adults can make even the most familiar environment seem strange and hazardous. It is important that older adults be oriented to familiar and unfamiliar environments, and that the environment be as "user-friendly" as possible to increase independence and safety. There are a variety of rehabilitation techniques that assist in accomplishing this task. **Table 33-7** presents the basic strategies.

Improving the Lighting

Most older people require two to three times more light than do younger people for the same tasks, but those with cloudy media (cataract, keratoconus, vitreous floaters, etc) are more sensitive to glare. The challenge is to get enough light without creating glare, which can be disabling. For example, the glare from a sunny window onto a waxed

TABLE 33-7 ■ WAYS TO MAKE AN ENVIRONMENT MORE VISUALLY ACCESSIBLE	
Change the real or perceived size of objects to be viewed	For loss of detailed vision: • Increase size (large print) • Move closer (move chair closer to the television) • Use magnification For loss of peripheral fields with normal acuity: • Minify image (reverse telescope) • Move further away • Use field-enhancement devices such as mirrors
Improve lighting	Use appropriate environmental lighting to decrease glare and increase overall light level; use illumination controls such as sun lenses, hats with brims, visors, colored filters; use task lighting such as flex-arm lamps
Increase contrast between objects and background	Eliminate busy background patterns, mark down steps with contrasting color on risers; increase contrast between furniture, eating utensils, etc, and their background
Use bright, clear colors	Mark light switches, dials, etc, with colored tape; use large areas of bright color for discrimination of objects
Organize the environment for ease and safety	Doors completely open or closed, chairs under table when not in use, furniture against the wall, organize clothing for color and function, organize and mark food stuff, etc
Consider alternative strategies that do not use vision	Use of other senses for task performance, such as voice-output for reading materials, use of long white cane for safe travel, olfactory cues for doneness of food, etc

floor, tabletops, and glass could cause objects in the dining room of a senior community to be obscured. An older person with low vision might function as if blind in that environment and be unable to find a chair, recognize his friends, serve his plate, or identify the food in a buffet line.

In an environment that is conducive for the function of older people, it is important to manage not only light, but also shadow, which can be conducive to function, for example, a triangular shadow at the end of a step indicates the height and depth of the step as well as how many steps are there. But shadow can also be hazardous, such as the shadow of a garden wall that obscures a sidewalk curb, causing a person to trip or fall.

Lighting is best if controllable, no matter what type it is. Many older people with low vision will require task lighting that can be positioned closer to reading/writing material or craft activity. Because the intensity of light is inversely related to the square of distance from its source, adding light at ceiling height will not provide adequate task illumination for older viewers. Task lights must be used that can be positioned closely, and therefore flex-armed lamps are best in this regard.

There are a variety of different types of bulbs that are useful and recommended for older viewers with low vision.

- Fluorescent lighting spreads evenly, is inexpensive and energy efficient, but provides less contrast because of that evenness and produces less shadow. It is a harsh light and flickers and may be bothersome to some viewers, causing headache and eye strain. Covering or shading fluorescent bulbs or bouncing the light from the ceiling to the eye may be helpful.
- Incandescent light is easily directed and provides more contrast and shadow. But the light can pool, especially if provided by one bulb suspended from the ceiling, causing pinpoint glare or pools of light within relative darkness. Using multiple incandescent fixtures can eliminate this problem. Incandescent lamps are good for task lighting such as reading, sewing, or hobbies.
- Halogen light uses the glow of halogen gas, as well as the incandescent filament to create a brighter light. The light is more blue and therefore may require filtering. Ultraviolet or blue light may generate superoxide and hydroxide free radicals that may be related to damage in the eye. Although controlled clinical studies have not been done, blue light has been suggested as increasing risk of cataract and macular degeneration. Subsequent studies have not shown a correlation to visible light exposure and risk, but many rehabilitation services are cautious about "blue light hazard." An Australian study suggests that people with less melanin (ie, light-colored iris, fair skin) are at more risk from light.
- Neodymium oxide and incandescent bulbs are currently touted as "full-spectrum lighting." These bulbs emit fewer ultraviolet and infrared rays and provide a sharp drop in the emission of yellow light. The effect is a more vivid "true" color, similar to sunlight, so contrast is increased.

These types of lighting can be mixed to achieve effects that are most pleasing and comfortable for older people with low vision. A study exploring these types of lighting in reading lamps found strong preferences among older readers with low vision, but no differences in objective measures of reading performance based on the type of light. Thus, informed reader choice should guide the selection of the type of light for older readers.

Light/dark adaptation is another aspect of environmental lighting that must be considered. Most older people have difficulty traveling from bright areas to dim ones because their dark adaptation is not as efficient as in young adults. People with severely restricted field loss (eg, advanced glaucoma) become functionally blind in dim lighting. Avoiding light/dark areas in the environment such as a bright dining room and dim hallway is helpful. When these areas are unavoidable, the older person could use illumination controls such as sunglasses or brimmed hats to assist with light/dark adaptation. People with severely restricted visual fields who are at risk for falling when ambulating at night may use lightweight, very bright, portable lamps with long battery life that have been designed for night hunters.

Increasing Contrast

Light/dark contrast is produced by the amount of light that is reflected from different surfaces (a light object is brighter than a dark one). A greater contrast between objects and their backgrounds make them easier to see. Therefore, providing an area of dark background and an area of light background in the bathroom, kitchen, and bedroom can help a person more easily identify possessions. For example, if a comb and brush are of light color, they may be kept on a dark tray. Most TV remotes are black, so they should be placed on a very light background. Similarly, marking the edge of stairs with contrasting colored tape makes each step more visible.

Using Color

The ability to identify colors, especially darks and pastels, diminishes with age. Certain visual impairments, especially those that affect the cones, such as macular degeneration, also reduce color vision. However, bright, clear colors can be seen by most older people with low vision. For example, yellow against navy blue is very visible, because it combines both color and contrast cues.

Using Organizational Strategies

Organization can be extremely helpful for the person with low vision. For example, always making sure that doors are completely open or completely closed, and placing chairs under the table when not used increases the safety of the environment. Organizing and labeling clothing by color and function in closets and drawers and organizing the kitchen can assist an older person in continuing to live independently. Learning new ways of performing daily tasks can make the loss of vision less of a problem in independent living. For example, retrieving a pair of spectacles that have fallen onto a light carpet might be difficult for some older adults. Learning a visual scanning pattern that begins at the site where the spectacles seem to have fallen and then continues in a circular pattern outward until they are found will assist in retrieving them.

Using color coding can be helpful as well. For example, chicken soup cans could be marked with wide yellow rubber bands, and tomato soup cans could be marked with wide red rubber bands. These markers could be quickly identified, avoiding the necessity for identifying the soup with a magnifier each time a can is retrieved from the cabinet. Brightly colored and nubby stick-on "dots" may be provided that provide both contrast and tactual cues for marking dials, buttons, and controls of appliances.

Using Alternative Strategies

Even when an older adult with low vision retains useful vision for a wide variety of tasks, it is sometimes helpful to use alternative techniques that do not require the use of vision because vision may not be the most efficient or safest way of accomplishing some tasks. For example, even though an older adult may have useful vision for walking, he may find it best to use a long white mobility cane in order to detect drop-offs, so that vision can be used to seek landmarks for orientation. An older adult with low vision may use speech output (a program that speaks symbols or words) for most computer word processing so that limited stamina for reading and writing may be used for reading mail, which must be done visually. A metal plate called a "flame-tamer" may be placed on the eyes of a gas stove in order to avoid burns in the kitchen. Knowledge of a wide variety of rehabilitation strategies and tools will assist older adults with low vision in developing a repertoire of techniques and devices that allows them to complete tasks safely, efficiently, and effectively.

Orientation to a new setting requires some basic alternative techniques that can be used anywhere. Some older adults may be able to use all of the techniques; some may only need one or two. It is important to remember not to rush the older adult in orientation, whether it is a long-term care facility or physician's office. These exercises may be repeated as often as necessary. Teaching family members these techniques may be helpful when new environments come up in the future. **Table 33-8** presents an overview of these techniques.

PSYCHOSOCIAL CONSIDERATIONS

Adaptation to Vision Loss

Anxiety and depression are common reactions to loss, and age-related visual impairment is complicated by the other losses associated with aging. There are two schools

TABLE 33-8 ■ ORIENTATION TO A NEW SETTING FOR OLDER ADULTS WITH VISION LOSS	
Using a starting/ending point	Begin at one starting/ending place in the room, such as the door. While leading an older adult via human guide, have the older adult reach out and feel both sides of the doorway, then describe the contents of the room. While leading him, allow him to trail his hand against the wall and furniture to feel their features. Give simple names to the walls using some feature of the wall (eg, the wall to the right is the bed wall, the wall opposite is the window wall).
Using compass directions or clock face	Some older adults will be more familiar with compass directions. Using the same starting point of the doorway, proceed as the older adult's human guide and use north wall, south wall, east wall, and west wall to name the four sides of the room. Use compass directions as the way of finding and naming locations in the room. Use clock face numbers in a similar manner for those who can more easily understand them.
Using landmarks and cues	Use familiar landmarks for orientation to a new environment, for example, the smell of food is a landmark for the dining room. The audible hum and red glow of a soft-drink machine may be another landmark.

of thought on the timing of rehabilitation related to adaptation. Some rehabilitation professionals subscribe to a "loss theory" of psychological adjustment. This theory proposes that the person must "die" as a sighted person, and be "reborn" as a visually impaired person, incorporating the visual impairment into the sense of self. According to this theory, attempting rehabilitation would be fruitless until the process is complete. Others subscribe to the theory that anxiety and depression are related to a person's negative stereotypes about visual impairment and a lack of confidence and motivation to attempt rehabilitation, but that if rehabilitation is successful, depression and anxiety should be reduced.

Older adults may hold many negative stereotypes associated with visual impairment: increased helplessness, inhabiting a world of darkness, increased vulnerability to crime, and the perception that use of devices marks them as different or to be pitied. Older adults with low vision may attempt to pass as fully sighted in order to avoid having others project these negative stereotypes onto them. But attempting to pass as fully sighted may cause other difficulties. For example, older adults with low vision do not recognize faces well, and the lack of a friendly hello when passing acquaintances may be interpreted as unfriendliness. Failure to use alternative techniques for identifying targets and moving in the environment may lead to falls, burns, or other safety hazards.

Support groups and peer counseling for older adults with low vision can be extremely helpful in coping with vision loss. Support groups may be found through local multiservice agencies for people who are visually impaired or may be started by senior citizen's centers or other groups. Short-term professional counseling in conjunction with rehabilitation may be very helpful.

Family and Social Support

In a recent study of low-vision device use among veterans, most of whom were older males with macular degeneration, family support was the most powerful predictor of continued use of devices up to 2 years following their prescription. Providing information and support to family members who are experiencing the impact of an older member's vision loss can be powerful. Visual impairment is experienced by the entire family or caregiving system, not just by the older person, and both social and psychological concerns must be addressed. The loss of vision by one family member can disrupt roles in the family, create economic demands, and add stress when tasks previously performed by the older adult must be performed by someone else.

For family members who understand the functional implications of visual impairment, understanding the behavior of their older adult with low vision is easier. For example, understanding the effect of changing lighting conditions, the effects of glare, and the adaptation times when traveling from dim light to bright and vice versa, can help explain behaviors like shielding the eyes, shuffling the feet, hesitation, fear of falling, and ceasing previously enjoyed activities. The fact that an older adult with restricted visual fields may pick up a dime from the floor, then bump into a partially open door seems contradictory, but is perfectly explained by the functioning field of view.

Assisting older adults with low vision in continuing social activities, such as hobbies, crafts, games, and traveling can aid them in maintaining important contacts with family and peers. Social support and contact are associated with less depression in older adults with low vision. Support groups can assist older adults with low vision in completing and using their rehabilitation, as well as facilitating adaptation to vision loss. Peer support or mutual aid groups who meet regularly to share their concerns may be especially beneficial for older adults who may be overprotected, abused, or treated paternalistically by those who do not understand visual impairment or aging. Facilitating assertiveness for older adults with low vision is recommended because it is linked to less depression and more social support. Social skill training in assertiveness for older adults with low vision has been shown effective in decreasing depression, and in deriving greater satisfaction in life.

FUNDING FOR LOW-VISION REHABILITATION

Rehabilitation Services Administration

Vision rehabilitation services have been funded through private pay, or through vocational rehabilitation services for individuals who were preparing for the work force. Funding for services to older adults with vision impairment has been a critical health care issue in the United States. Public funding through Rehabilitation Administration Service for the *Independent Living Services for Older Individuals Who Are Blind* program under the Rehabilitation Act is minimal, with approximately $495 million allocated nationally in fiscal year 2014. These funds provide services in the traditional "blindness" system—state services or private agencies for the blind. State governments may also allocate funding for low-income older people to receive vision and blind rehabilitation as well.

Veterans Health Administration

Prior to 2002, only older veterans with legal blindness who served in the US military and whose disability is service-connected had full access to comprehensive blindness and services through the Department of Veterans Affairs Medical Centers. However, most visually impaired veterans have age-related vision loss and their income is such that a copayment is required from them or from their private insurance carrier. Vision rehabilitation services were developed initially to meet the needs of blinded veterans returning from World War II. Young war-blinded men had few other medical problems, so efforts to rehabilitate them for the work force spawned the professions of orientation and mobility instructors, rehabilitation teachers for the blind, and low-vision therapists in order to meet their unique needs. Services for veterans who are visually impaired but not legally blind were provided nationally beginning in 2008. This specialized "blindness and low-vision" rehabilitation was not considered part of the broader medical rehabilitation. Credentialing of vision-rehabilitation professionals developed separately from occupational or physical therapists, and their practice was autonomous, requiring neither medical referral nor physician supervision. As a result, many medical professionals are unaware of their services and do not understand the "blindness" rehabilitation system in which their practice began. The Department of Veterans Affairs model of service delivery in vision rehabilitation continues today in the same vein. Services are provided nationally by teams of professionals. Ophthalmologists or optometrists provide the medical eye care services, and the vision and blind rehabilitation professionals are orientation and mobility specialists, rehabilitation teachers, and low-vision therapists. Recently the Department of Veterans Affairs appropriated $40 million to provide vision rehabilitation services in a continuum of care for patients who have low vision as well as those who are blind, in recognition that veterans are aging in place and require services close to home. The vision/blind rehabilitation service in this milieu is also unique in that prosthetic devices are provided. Devices such as magnifiers, telescopes, binoculars, CCTV system, computer equipment, accessible smartphones, and tablets are dispensed according to Veterans Affairs (VA) policy at no cost to veterans as a part of the VA's commitment to vision/blind rehabilitation services.

Medicare Funding for Vision Rehabilitation

The rise in older adults with low vision has spurred Medicare to produce a national policy of reimbursement as well. In 2002, the Centers for Medicare and Medicaid Services (CMS) released a national program memorandum to alert the provider community that Medicare beneficiaries who are blind or visually impaired are eligible for physician-prescribed rehabilitation services from approved health care professionals on the same basis as beneficiaries with other medical conditions that result in reduced physical functioning. This memorandum was issued in response to the committee report accompanying the FY 2002 Labor/Health and Human Services/Education appropriations bill.

The memorandum further directed that the patient receiving services must have a potential for restoration or improvement of lost functions and must be expected to improve significantly within a reasonable and generally predictable amount of time. The rehabilitation that is covered is to be short term and intense; maintenance therapy is not covered. Applicable Health Care Common Procedural Coding System therapeutic procedures are outlined in the memorandum, as are applicable International Classification of Diseases (ICD)-9 codes that support medical necessity.

The effect of the program memorandum has been to increase the visibility of Medicare provisions for vision rehabilitation, but it is not a national coverage decision. Medicare carriers are not compelled by the memorandum to develop a Local Medical Review Policy as a result, and are still able to deny all claims that the local carrier does not deem medically reasonable or necessary.

In 2003, Congress authorized the Secretary of Health and Human Services to carry out a nationwide outpatient vision rehabilitation services demonstration project. The purpose of the project was to examine the impact of standardized national coverage for vision rehabilitation services in the home by physicians, occupational therapists, and certified vision/blind rehabilitation professionals. The 2003 Demonstration Project did not provide coverage for adaptive equipment (low-vision and blindness devices). The project proceeded for 2 years without clear results. The outcome of the project was status quo, with no new practitioners added to Medicare for reimbursement in providing care for older people with low vision.

To date, the national funding sources for providing vision and blind rehabilitation care continue to be CMS, Department of Veterans Affairs, and Rehabilitation Services Administration.

PALLIATIVE CARE FOR OLDER ADULTS WHO ARE VISUALLY IMPAIRED

Palliative care for older adults with visual impairment may focus on assuring that patients are able to see as well as participate in activities that mean the most to them; continue hobbies and other desired activities that relieve stress and help them to feel that life is as normal as it can be; participate in diversions that may assist in managing pain; participate in spiritual activities such as reading or listening to devotional materials that strengthen faith and may reduce anxiety and depression; and reduce caregiver burden.

In addition to the suggested strategies in the section of this chapter titled "Environments for Older People," the following considerations may assist patients with visual impairment in palliative care.

- Assure that spectacle correction in eyeglasses is up-to-date. Assure that spectacles, magnifiers, and other useful devices are within patient's reach, and are kept in the same known place, so that they may be used whenever desired.
- Assure that patient's autonomy is respected in long-term care. When entering the patient's room, knock on the door and ask to enter the room; address the patient by name and identify yourself.
- If the patient is not in their home environment, ask the patient how he or she performs ADL such as bathing, eating, and dressing, and how you can help. Include the patient, family, and palliative team in the plan.
- Talk in a normal, natural tone of voice, face the patient directly, and if possible, make eye contact and explain what you're going to do in detail before you do it (eg, taking blood or vital signs); ask permission or notify the patient before you touch him or her.
- Always address the patient directly, even if family members are present. Don't worry about saying the words "look," "see," or "blind."
- If the patient is in palliative care in a facility, describe the room layout including dimensions. Use compass directions to describe the location of objects in relation to the bed (eg, "you are facing north in the bed," "the door is to the west").
- Place the phone, call bell, and bedside table within the patient's reach in a known location, and let the patient know where they are. Do not move them.
- Place the item in the patient's hand, or the patient's hand on the item, if needed.
- Once you've oriented the patient to the room, alert staff to leave things in position. Notify the patient before you move, take, or add any objects (eg, furniture, trash can, grooming aids).

- If the patient is mobile, use the "Human Guide" technique to assist the patient with ambulating:
  - Ask the patient from which side he or she would prefer to be approached and guided.
  - Extend your arm so that it touches the patient's; he or she can grasp and follow your elbow.
  - While the patient is holding your arm, walk to his or her side, one step ahead, at a pace that is comfortable for him or her.
- Use clock coordinates to describe the location of food on the plate and all items on his food tray. Ask the patient what assistance is needed.

- Indicate to the patient when you are leaving the room so she will know you are leaving.
- Encourage the patient to use assistive devices (eg, talking clocks/watches, radios, speech-output reading devices, etc.).
- Encourage the patient to use reading technology for pleasure reading, devotionals, etc. If the patient does not have the stamina for reading, experiment with talking books or voice-over devices. Reading to the patient with visual impairment may be a bonding experience for family members and friends.
- Craft activities and games are available that are enlarged and use bright saturated colors and good contrast.

FURTHER READING

American Academy of Ophthalmology. *Preferred Practice Pattern: Age-Related Macular Degeneration.* San Francisco, CA: American Academy of Ophthalmology; 2019.

American Academy of Ophthalmology. *Preferred Practice Pattern: Diabetic Retinopathy.* San Francisco, CA: American Academy of Ophthalmology; 2019.

American Academy of Ophthalmology. *Preferred Practice Pattern: Primary Angle Closure Disease.* San Francisco, CA: American Academy of Ophthalmology; 2020.

American Academy of Ophthalmology. *Preferred Practice Pattern: Primary Open-Angle Glaucoma.* San Francisco, CA: American Academy of Ophthalmology; 2020.

American Academy of Ophthalmology. *Preferred Practice Pattern: Vision Rehabilitation.* San Francisco, CA: American Academy of Ophthalmology; 2017.

Casten R, Rovner B. Depression in age-related macular degeneration. *J Vis Impair Blind.* 2008;102:591–599.

Echt KV. Designing web-based health information for older adults: Visual considerations and design directives. In: RW Morrell (ed). *Older Adults, Health Information, and the World Wide Web.* Mahwah, NJ: Erlbaum; 2002:61–87.

Echt KV, Saunders GH. Accommodating dual sensory loss in everyday practice. *Perspectives on Gerontology.* 2014;19:4–16.

Haegerstrom-Portnoy G. Vision in elders—summary of findings of the SKI study. *Optom Vis Sci.* 2005;82:87.

National Eye Institute. Prevalence of adult vision impairment and age-related eye diseases in America. https://www.nei.nih.gov/eyedata/adultvision_usa. Accessed February 16, 2022.

Schuchard RA, Fletcher DC. Preferred retinal locus: a review with applications in low-vision rehabilitation. *Ophthalmol Clin North Am.* 1994;7:243–256.

Silverstone B, Lang MA, Rosenthal B, et al. (eds). *The Lighthouse Handbook on Vision Impairment and Vision Rehabilitation.* New York, NY: Oxford University Press; 2000.

Stelmack J, Massof B. Using the VA LV VFQ-48 and LV VFQ-20 in low vision rehabilitation. *Optom Vis Sci.* 2007;30:705–709.

Stelmack J, Tang XC, Reda DJ, et al. Outcomes of the Veterans Affairs Low Vision Intervention Trial (LOVIT). *Arch Ophthalmol.* 2008;5:608–617.

Watson GR. Low vision in the geriatric population: rehabilitation and management. *J Am Geriatr Soc.* 2001;49:317–330.

Watson GR, Echt KV. Aging and vision loss. In: AL Corn, AJ Koenig (eds). *Foundations of Low Vision: Clinical and Functional Perspectives.* New York, NY: AFB Press; 2010:871–916.

Chapter 34

Hearing Loss: Assessment and Management

Su-Hua Sha, Kara C. Schvartz-Leyzac, Jochen Schacht

INTRODUCTION

The sense of hearing is unequalled by our other sensory modalities in terms of its sensitivity, dynamic range, and discrimination of the finest nuances in stimuli. It does serve us well through a part of our lifetime, but beginning in our 40s (slightly earlier for men and later for women) our inner ears suffer the influence of aging in a very subtle yet progressive manner. Age-related hearing loss (ARHL) affects most people aged 65 and older and represents the predominant neurodegenerative disease of aging.

(The terms "age-related hearing impairment" and "age-related hearing loss" are interchangeably used in the literature whereby "loss" does not imply a complete loss of hearing but may signify any degree of auditory dysfunction. Individuals with hearing loss are generally referred to as "hard-of-hearing.")

Hippocrates had already noted deafness to be more prevalent among his older patients and in *The Comedy of Errors*, Shakespeare's older merchant, Aegeon, complains of his own "dull deaf ears." Thus, ARHL or presbycusis is not a disease of modern societies but has been accepted for centuries as one of Lord Byron's inevitable "woes that wait on age" that it still appears to be today. It was the New York otologist St. John Roosa who first drew the attention of his colleagues to hearing loss of older adults as a medical condition. In 1885 he proposed the name presbycusis that he had coined from the Greek πρέσβυς, old man, and ακούειν, to hear. Systematic studies of the anatomical pathology began in the late nineteenth century, leading by the 1930s to the realization that the decreased auditory acuity could be attributed to deterioration of the auditory sensory cells and the auditory nerve. These changes frequently affect the perception of the upper frequencies first, resulting in high-frequency (high "pitch") hearing loss as a hallmark of presbycusis. However, ARHL is not a uniform condition, but a multifactorial one combining genetic predispositions with a plethora of lifetime insults to the hearing organ because, in all its versatility and efficacy, our sense of hearing is also uniquely vulnerable to environmental influences. These may include noise, chemicals, and solvents at the workplace, lifestyle (eg, smoking), and leisure activities (from iPods to rock concerts and target shooting), diseases (eg, diabetes, respiratory disorders), viral or bacterial infections, and

Learning Objectives

- Learn the epidemiology, pathophysiology, diagnosis, clinical features, risk factors, and treatment of hearing impairments in older adults.

- Understand the interplay between common medical comorbidities, medications, genetics, and hearing disorders in older patients.

- Gain a clear understanding of tests used to distinguish various kinds of hearing impairments.

- Learn about recent technological advances involving hearing aids and cochlear implants, as well as emerging therapies targeting hair cell regeneration.

Key Clinical Points

1. Age-related hearing loss (ARHL) is the most common sensory impairment in older adults, and its prevalence increases steadily with age.

2. Men develop ARHL earlier than women. Family history and specific genes increase risk for presbycusis. Over 55% of ARHL in older patients can be attributed to heritability.

3. Diabetes mellitus and cardiovascular disease, two of the most common comorbidities seen in older adults, promote hearing loss and cochlear pathology.

4. Pure tone audiometry, tympanometry, acoustic reflex measurements, and word recognition scores are the most common methods for hearing assessment.

5. Older patients often present with difficulties in speech recognition rather than inability to hear sound.

even the adverse effects of the very medications (aminoglycosides, cisplatin) designed to cure diseases and infections. This spectrum of potential abuse of our auditory organ yields an exceedingly intricate etiology and pathology of hearing loss in older adults. Age-related pathology of the central auditory system adds to the complexity of the problem. Consequently, presbycusis has been defined as hearing loss associated with various types of auditory dysfunction, peripheral or central, that accompany aging and that cannot be accounted for by extraordinary ototraumatic, genetic, or pathologic conditions.

Animal models provide hope to resolve some of the basic mechanisms that underlie the deterioration of hearing and point to ways and means to delay or prevent presbycusis. By virtue of the availability of molecular and genetic information and of transgenic and knock-out animals, mice have become one of the preferred model animals although, as we shall point out later, caveats do apply here too. This review will illustrate the features of human presbycusis and draw on animal models to discuss its potential molecular basis.

EPIDEMIOLOGY OF AGE-RELATED HEARING LOSS

ARHL is the most frequent sensory loss in older adults and the prevalence of the disorder increases with age. In humans, as in most other species, ARHL mostly begins at the high frequencies and progresses gradually into the lower speech range. Males experience ARHL earlier than females, beginning in the late 30s to early 40s while women will match the men's deficits in the later decades of their lives. Approximately 44% of people suffer from a significant hearing loss in their 60s; this number rises to 66% between the ages of 70 and 79 years, and skyrockets to 90% after age 80. With an increased life span of the population worldwide, especially in developed countries, the impact of ARHL will continue to increase in the future.

The individual rate of decline in hearing, however, is exceptionally variable and some people may maintain excellent hearing with "golden ears" late into life as a result of genetic traits that have yet to be elucidated. Superimposed on the gender differences, race apparently also plays a role, although whether this role is causative or correlative is unknown. One study of over 2000 older Americans aged 73 to 84 found the incidence of high-frequency hearing loss to be 92% in Caucasian American men, 76% in African-American men, 74% in Caucasian American women, and 59% in African-American women.

RISK FACTORS MODULATING AGE-RELATED HEARING LOSS

The large variability in the age of onset, rate of progression, and the nature and severity of the hearing loss suggests that ARHL is a complex genetic disorder with superimposed environmental and health-related risk factors.

Genetics

Family history plays a role in predisposition to presbycusis. An analysis of hearing thresholds in sibling or parent/child pairs versus spousal pairs (controls) in Framingham Heart Study patients found that the inherited genetic effects were significant. The predictive power of family history appeared stronger for females than males and stronger for a "flat" rather than sensorineural high-frequency type hearing loss (see the classification of age-related hearing loss in the section on "Peripheral Pathology of Age-Related Hearing Loss in Humans"). Overall, the study suggested that about 55% of ARHL in older adults can be ascribed to heritability.

Further studies detailing genes that contribute to ARHL in humans have pointed largely those involved in detoxification of reactive oxygen species (ROS) and include glutathione S-transferase polymorphisms (in the *GSTM1* and *GSTT1* genes), an *N*-acetyltransferase 2 gene polymorphism, and superoxide dismutase 2 promoter variants. A genome-wide association study (GWAS) of presbycusic subjects at the Audiological Center of the Antwerp University Hospital found no variants with genome-wide significance. Previously reported genes for ARHL could not be confirmed, indicating that ARHL is highly polygenic in nature, with probably no major determining genes involved.

Gender and Hormonal Factors

The fact that ARHL sets in earlier in males than in females is seen both in the human population and in experimental animals. Differences between males and females diminish in the later decades of life, suggesting a modulation of ARHL by the hormonal status of an individual. In support of this notion, receptors for steroid hormones have indeed been located in the cochlea. In further support of a link between ARHL and hormonal levels, fluctuations in hearing thresholds have been observed during the menstrual cycle; estrogen therapy slowed the development of ARHL in postmenopausal women. Furthermore, in patients (and mouse models) with Turner syndrome who synthesize inadequate levels of estrogen, ARHL sets in early and sensorineural hearing loss often presents in childhood. While estrogen seems to be protective of hearing, progesterone replacement is detrimental in postmenopausal women, negatively affecting the auditory nerve pathway and neurotransmitters. Generally, sex-hormone replacement therapy in premenopausal, perimenopausal, and postmenopausal women has revealed a number of serious side effects in addition to hearing loss, including strokes, breast and ovarian cancer, and cardiovascular problems.

Another class of steroid hormones, mineralocorticoids, may also influence ARHL. A correlative study in human subjects showed a protective effect of elevated serum levels of aldosterone on auditory thresholds and an improvement of speech perception ("hearing-in-noise") in older individuals. Although aldosterone primarily acts on water and ion resorption in the kidney, aldosterone receptors have also been localized to the inner ear. They are hypothesized to influence the ionic composition of inner ear fluids, which is essential for cochlear homeostasis and the transduction of sound (see section on "Anatomy of the Auditory Periphery").

Diseases

A contribution of specific diseases to the rate and severity of hearing loss has long been speculated but firm evidence is challenging to ascertain. The complex etiology of ARHL and the multitude of potential noxious influences renders it difficult to account for all potentially confounding factors in human population studies. Nevertheless, good evidence exists for diabetes and cardiovascular disease as risk factors in ARHL.

Diabetes mellitus Both type 1 and type 2 diabetes promote hearing loss and cochlear pathology in humans and in animals. Deficits in several aspects of auditory function were significantly more pronounced in a group of people with type 2 diabetes aged 60 or older compared with a group of age- and sex-matched controls and excluding those with other significant health issues or a history of hearing problems. Furthermore, plasma concentrations of glycosylated hemoglobin (HbA_{1c}), an indicator of potentially elevated glucose levels, have been found to correlate with ARHL in a cohort aged 65 or older, even in those without levels high enough to be diagnosed with diabetes.

Diabetes mellitus and associated deregulated blood glucose levels exact a multitude of stresses on a cellular level, which could lead to loss of function in the delicately balanced hearing organ with time and age. Fundamentally, increased blood glucose levels lead to cellular hypoxia and a build-up of ROS and lipid metabolic byproducts, as well as changes in the collagen and microtubule structure of the cells. In addition, diabetes has profound effects on the vasculature, including atherosclerosis and vessel wall dystrophy. In the inner ear, which depends on the highly vascularized stria vascularis to maintain the endocochlear potential, this could result in impaired sensory function. Patients with diabetes mellitus also demonstrate abnormal processing of auditory signals at the level of the brain stem and cortex.

Cardiovascular disease All conditions that affect the function of blood vessels such as hyperlipidemia, hypercholesterolemia, hypertension, hyperlipoproteinemia, and cardiovascular disease have been implicated in ARHL. Specifically, a flat ARHL (see next section) appears to be associated with those conditions because the maintenance of the endolymphatic potential and driving force for the transduction process is most vulnerable to any restriction of blood flow. Just as in diabetes, any disease leading to vascular compromise will impair these processes and diminish the sensitivity of the cochlear organ to sound.

Lifestyle and Environmental Factors

Poor health habits with regard to exercise, smoking, and diet are also considered risk factors for ARHL based on data from population studies. Since some of these habits influence cardiovascular function and other potential risk factors for ARHL, it remains open to what extent lifestyle directly influences the auditory organ or whether the resulting effects are secondary to general health. Additional major environmental risk factors include exposure to excessive or even moderate noise, ototoxic medications (primarily aminoglycoside antibiotics and anticancer agents of the cisplatin class), and several industrial solvents.

Even at levels that do not necessarily inflict acute damage by themselves, these environmental factors appear to sensitize the auditory system to subsequent loss and aggravate any age-related changes. This notion was borne out in experiments in which mice at a young age (1–3 months) received a moderate noise exposure that resulted in temporary hearing loss only. Although their hearing recovered to normal baseline levels within a few days or a week after the noise exposure, these mice developed a significantly greater hearing loss with progressing age than control animals. Therefore, the initial recovery might not have been a return to normal but to a "hidden hearing loss." The implication of this finding is that occupational or recreational noise exposure, even if no deficit is noted at the time, will take its toll in later years.

Psychology

Interestingly, adherence to negative stereotypes about older adults, that is, the concept in many societies that aging is met with an inevitable decline in function of all faculties, demonstrates as a predicting risk factor for ARHL. External stereotyping (the prevalence of stigmata with aging in the individual's culture) and negative internal perception (extent of internalization of these stigmata) acted as independent risk factors on hearing loss with age, and had a stronger impact than gender or race. This predicts an observable phenomenon wherein cultures with positive concepts of aging do not expect their elders' hearing to become enfeebled and, in fact, the incidence of ARHL is then lower. Here again, an influence on the auditory system maybe secondary to the effect of stigmata on general well-being and levels of stress hormones in particular. Furthermore, a stimulating social engagement in a positive environment might delay not only cognitive decline but also an associated hearing loss.

BASICS OF HEARING AND HEARING LOSS

In order to understand the different forms of presbycusis and their underlying mechanisms, some knowledge of auditory anatomy and physiology is required. The following sections briefly summarize the essentials.

Anatomy of the Auditory Periphery

Not only is ARHL shaped by many influences, it also shows a variety of morphological manifestations. An early framework for classifying ARHL was proposed by Schuknecht in 1964 based on the histopathology of human temporal bones, and has since been modified on the basis of further human and animal studies. The mammalian auditory organ, the cochlea (**Figure 34-1**), is encased in bone, and its tissues

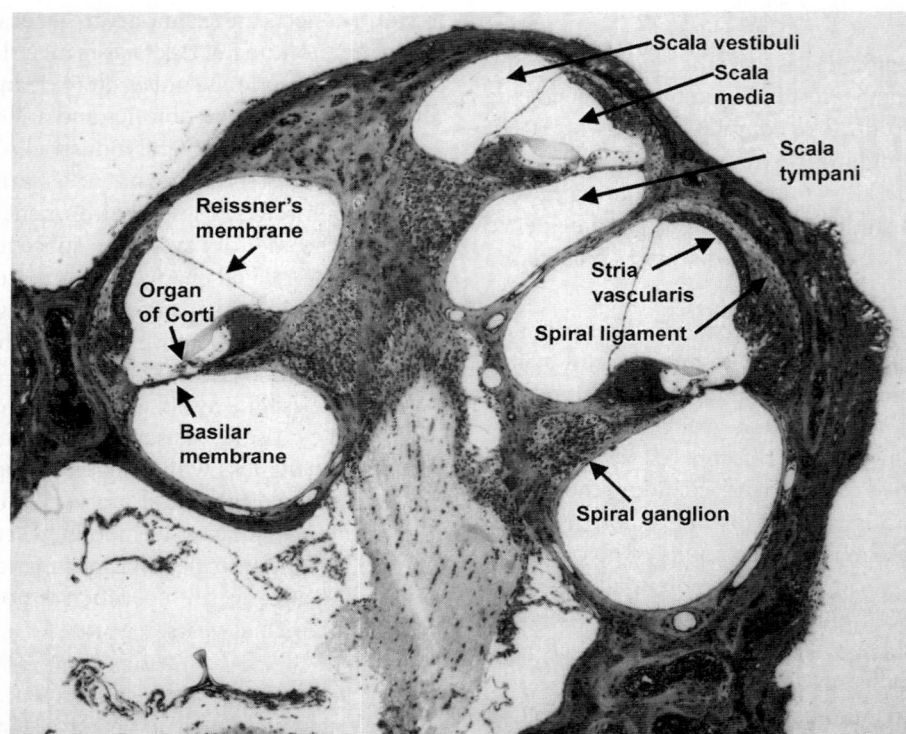

FIGURE 34-1. Anatomy of the cochlea. A low-magnification light micrograph of a near midmodiolar cross section illustrates the tissues and fluid-filled spaces of the 2½ turns of the mouse cochlea. As indicated in the upper turn, the fluid spaces are the scala tympani and scala vestibuli filled with perilymph, and scala media filled with endolymph. They are separated by the thin Reissner membrane and by the basilar membrane upon which the organ of Corti is located. When sound reaches the ear, the vibrations of the tympanic membrane (ear drum) are passed along the middle ear ossicles to the cochlea where they initiate a traveling wave in the fluids which, in turn, move the basilar membrane. The tectorial membrane, an acellular structure, rests on the stereocilia of the hair cells. Spiral ganglion neurons run from the organ of Corti where they contact the hair cells through the modiolus to the central auditory system. The stria vascularis and spiral ligament, tissues involved in setting up the ionic composition and high (+70 to +100 mV) potential of the endolymph, lie along the lateral wall of the cochlea.

and fluids coil "snail-like" for 2½ to 4½ turns (depending an species) and a total length of a few centimeters without any relationship to body size. A human cochlea, for example, on average extends for 33 mm in 2½ turns while the dimensions in the guinea pig are 20 mm and 4½ turns. In all species, however, the cochlea is tonotopically organized, meaning that high frequencies are processed in its basal part, low frequencies in the apex.

Several structures with distinctly different functions and susceptibility to environment and age-related insults can be discerned within this membranous labyrinth and are best seen in a midmodiolar section that transverses the length of the cochlea. The lumen of the cochlea is separated into three fluid-filled compartments by the basilar membrane and Reissner membrane. Scala vestibuli and scala tympani contain perilymph, similar in composition to extracellular fluids. Scala media contains endolymph, unique among body fluids by its high concentration of K^+ and low Na^+, creating a large positive endolymphatic potential (also referred to as endocochlear potential) as a driving force for the transduction current, which is used by

the sensory cells. Scala media is bounded laterally by spiral ligament and stria vascularis, the tissues that are responsible for maintaining the ionic composition and hence the potential of endolymph. These tissues are also highly vascularized and provide most of the oxygen and nutrient supply to the cochlea.

The organ of Corti (**Figure 34-2**), located on the basilar membrane, is the auditory end organ containing sensory cells and supporting cells. Sensory cells include one row of inner hair cells (IHCs) and three rows of outer hair cells, numbering several thousand in all species. The name "hair cell" is derived from the stereocilia that protrude from the apical end of the cells (**Figure 34-3**) and contain the mechano-transduction channels. IHCs are the primary sensory cells that convert the mechanical acoustic input into receptor potentials and release of neurotransmitter, triggering action potentials that are carried to the brain by the spiral ganglion neurons (SGNs). Most of the afferent innervation by this auditory nerve converges on the IHCs. The major function of outer hair cells, which receive mostly efferent innervation from auditory centers in the brain, is

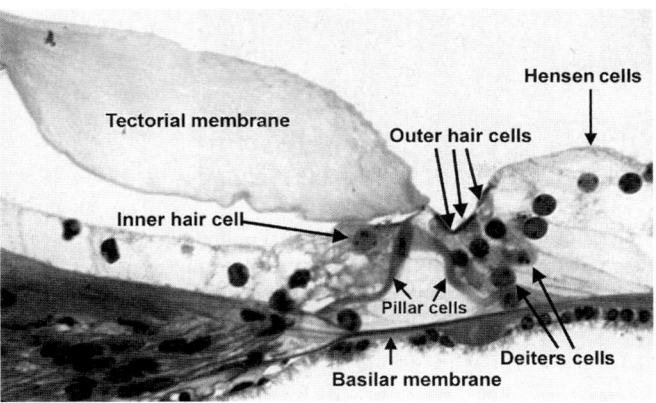

FIGURE 34-2. The organ of Corti. A cross section shows details of the mouse organ of Corti located on the basilar membrane. The sensory cells are arranged in one row of inner hair cells and three rows of outer hair cells. Inner hair cells are the primary transducers of sound and receive most of the afferent innervation of the spiral ganglion nerve. Outer hair cells amplify transduction and receive most of the efferent innervation. Supporting cells include Deiters', Hensen's, and pillar cells. The tectorial membrane does not extend to its full length because of preparation artifacts.

to enhance the performance of the cochlea, particularly at low intensities of sound. Supporting cells include the inner pillar, outer pillar, Deiters', Hensen's, and Claudius' cells, about whose function we know less.

The cells in the sensory epithelium are highly differentiated. Hair cells, once lost, are not regenerated by

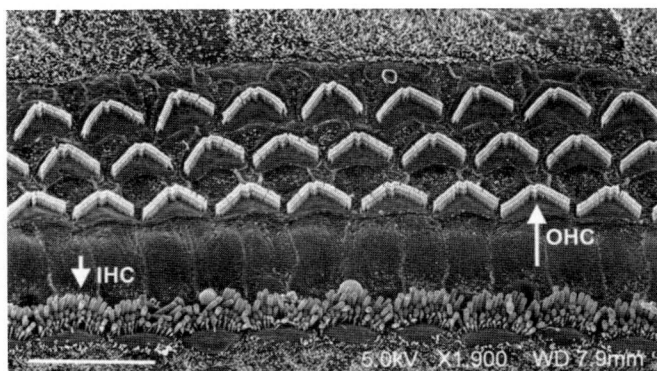

FIGURE 34-3. Hair cells and their stereocilia. A scanning electron micrograph of a "surface preparation" gives a top view of the organ of Corti, presenting the apical aspects of hair cells and supporting cells. The hair cells are distinguished by their stereocilia, the white tufts arranged in linear (inner hair cells, IHC) and W-like (outer hair cells, OHC) form. During sound transduction, the stereocilia are deflected by a shearing motion generated between the basilar membrane and the tectorial membrane, causing transduction channels to open for influx of potassium from the endolymph. This influx triggers a receptor potential and release of neurotransmitter (glutamate) at the synapse between the inner hair cell and the spiral ganglion nerve. Scale bar: 20 μm. (Scanning electron micro-graph from mouse cochlea kindly provided by Dr. Andrew Forge, Institute of Laryngology and Otology, University College London, UK.)

other cell types in the mammal but are replaced by permanent "scars" (**Figure 34-4**). Consequently, any damage to these cells leads to irreversible hearing loss. Considerable research effort is currently expended on determining any factors that might regenerate hair cells from supporting cells or enable the differentiation of putative stem cells into hair cells.

Functional Assessment of Hearing

From a clinical functional aspect, pure tone audiometry, tympanometry, acoustic reflex measurements, and word recognition scores with behavioral tests are the most common and important methods for hearing assessment. Tympanometry and acoustic reflex (stapedius reflex) test the integrity of the middle ear while audiometry yields information about acoustic thresholds at distinct frequencies. Word recognition tests, in contrast, explore more complex tasks that involve both the auditory periphery and central processing of the information. Auditory brain stem response (ABR) and otoacoustic emission measurements provide information on the integrity of the auditory pathway and outer hair cells, respectively. They are passive sound-evoked responses and therefore suitable for testing infants or incapacitated individuals and most easily adapted to routine testing in animals. Some invasive methods, essentially limited to animal experimentation, such as recordings of cochlear microphonic potential (largely derived from outer hair cells), cochlear whole nerve action potential, and single unit recordings, can be used to assess hair cell transduction and synaptic activity, the function of auditory afferent nerves, and individual neurons of the cochlear and vestibular nerves.

Frequencies and Sound Intensity: What Constitutes Hearing Loss?

A significant hearing loss of any origin will eventually lead to difficulties in communication and a decreased awareness of the environment. In addition to the social isolation, individuals with early-onset presbycusis may suffer economic consequences from difficulties in employment or professional advancement. The question of what constitutes a significant hearing loss is complex as it involves consideration of both the magnitude of sensitivity loss and the frequencies at which the loss occurs. Although the most convenient assessment criterion for ARHL is a subjective one—that is, posing the question, "Do you have a hearing problem?" or answering a more elaborate questionnaire like the Hearing Handicap Inventory for the Elderly-Short (HHIE-S)—a more quantitative evaluation can be obtained by an audiogram. While there is not one set paradigm for classification of audiograms into handicapping and non-handicapping hearing thresholds, the American Speech-Language-Hearing Association and the American Academy of Audiology set the bar at a threshold shift (hearing loss) of 25 dB or above at any frequency between 250 Hz and 8000 Hz.

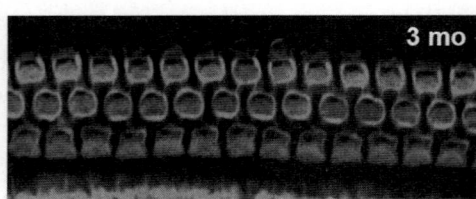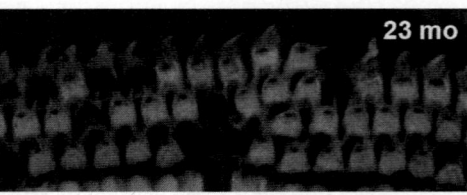

FIGURE 34-4. Loss of hair cells with age. Surface preparations of the mouse cochlea are stained with phalloidin to visualize F-actin, a major component of stereocilia and hair cells. Three rows of outer hair cells are complete and arranged in an orderly fashion in an animal of 3 months of age. At 23 months, the structure is disturbed and some cells are missing.

What does a loss of 25-dB hearing acuity mean in everyday terms? The bel or decibel (dB) scale of sound pressure ("intensity") is logarithmic, such that an increase in 3 dB represents approximately a doubling of the sound intensity. Therefore, a reduction of sensitivity of 25 dB is considerable. In rough terms, a difference of 25 dB in threshold makes normal conversation equivalent to a whisper, and a whisper equivalent to silence (**Table 34-1**). The affected person will still hear the crying baby—albeit subdued—but not the leaves rustling in the forest or the crickets in summer.

There is one caveat. Defining hearing loss as beginning at a threshold shift of 25 dB in one ear is clinically useful but does not necessarily mean that an afflicted person even notices the deficit. Auditory impairment may be asymmetrical, affecting primarily one ear only (recreational shooters or combatants are good examples). Such a unilateral impairment might remain unnoticed since the better ear will provide a "normal" hearing in most situations.

ARHL poses a specific problem as the hearing loss progresses slowly and mostly sets in at the high frequencies. The frequency spectrum of human hearing, at its best, ranges from about 60 Hz to 16 kHz but speech frequencies and hence, basic hearing needs, mostly center on the 1000 Hz to 2000 Hz range (**Table 34-2**). A hearing loss at the very high frequencies may therefore not produce any communicative disadvantages particularly when conversations occur in a quiet environment; even musical instruments have a limited range in their fundamental frequencies.

Since the progression of ARHL is also slow, the individual maybe unaware of the gradual loss of overtones in speech or instrumental music (which can extend two or three octaves higher than the fundamentals) for a long time.

TABLE 34-1 ■ TYPICAL SOUND LEVELS

DB	SOUND
15	Pin drop at close range
15–20	Rustling leaves, dripping faucet
35	Whisper
50–60	Normal conversation
60–70	Vacuum cleaner
70–90	Screaming child
85	*Safety limit for an 8-h workday*
100	*Safe for 15 min or less*
105–110	Gas engine mower, chain saw
110	Car stereo at maximum volume
110	*Safe for 1 min 29 s*
115	Maximum volume from an iPod
116	*Human body perceives low frequency*
120	Front row at a rock concert
120–130	Jet plane taking off
127	*High risk of tinnitus*
130–140	Gun shot from a hunting rifle
140	*Hearing deficit at exposures < 1 s*

Intensity levels of some familiar sounds can provide a guide to understanding the impact of hearing loss as discussed in the text. The comparison of these levels to safety standards also illustrates the potential impact of environmental noise exposure on the complex manifestations of presbycusis.
Data from DHHS (NIOSH) Publication No. 98–126 on Occupational Noise Exposure. US Department of Health and Human Services. Public Health Service Centers for Disease Control and Prevention. National Institute for Occupational Safety and Health. Cincinnati, Ohio. June 1998.

TABLE 34-2 ■ FREQUENCY RANGES OF COMMON SOUNDS

SOUND	APPROXIMATE FUNDAMENTAL FREQUENCY RANGE (HZ)
Guitar	82–1175
Truck engine	125–250
Dog's bark	200–300
Violin	196–4400
Soprano singer	200–1400
Most spoken consonants	250–500
Middle C of the musical scale	264
Spoken vowels	500–750
Crying baby	750–1000
Consonants: c, p, ch, g, h, sh	1000–2000
Telephone ring	3000–4000
Consonants: f, k, s, t, th	3000–8000
Birds chirping	4000–8000

In addition to these fundamental frequencies, most sources of sounds and musical instruments, in particular, produce overtones that add to the richness of the sound. These overtones reach two to three times the fundamental frequencies. Comparison of the frequencies to the classical pattern of high-frequency age-related hearing impairment illustrates the early impact on specific speech features and the quality of music appreciation.

However, losses at higher frequencies like those in ARHL cost the ability to discriminate between many words with f, p, k, s, t, th sounds (see **Table 34-2**). For example, to a person with high-frequency hearing loss, "sick" and "thick" may be difficult to differentiate, and "three socks" may sound like "free fox" unless the listener has developed the ability to read the speakers lips for supplementary information or can interpret them in context. Such communication errors may seem trivial, but can cause enormous social disability when they happen in work situations or become cumulative.

Audiological examinations routinely include frequencies up to 8000 Hz and could reveal the presbycusic changes although the individual may still be told by the audiologist that their hearing is "normal for the age." Such a statement should not be taken to mean that a hearing aid is not necessary or not useful. Quite frequently, an individual with a reasonably reliable pure-tone audiogram and good one-on-one communication skills may experience difficulties in speech perception in a noisy environment such as a restaurant, a party, or a conference because high frequencies are essential for auditory discrimination in the presence of background noise. This "party effect" is often the first signal indicative of presbycusis, and such individuals may greatly benefit in their enjoyment of conversation and music by modern hearing aids fitted to their particular needs.

PERIPHERAL PATHOLOGY OF AGE-RELATED HEARING LOSS IN HUMANS

A classification of the various forms of presbycusis has limitations because of the complexity of functional deficits and pathologic changes. However, broad categories of ARHL are as follows: (1) *Sensorineural* ARHL refers to a primary degeneration of hair cells ("sensory ARHL") of the organ of Corti that begins in the base, yielding an audiogram that is abnormal only at the high frequencies (**Figure 34-5A**). Current data suggest that ARHL in humans largely follows such a pattern of a high-frequency hearing loss. A *neural* component of ARHL mainly reflects loss of afferent neurons while cochlear structures remain relatively normal, leading to a loss of word discrimination ability. In general, aging people lose afferent neurons only slowly and significant changes in the audiogram may require a loss of up to 90% of neurons. The incidence of purely neural ARHL is therefore controversial. As hair cells degenerate, secondary neuronal degeneration follows, so that the term "sensorineural" ARHL is favored over a separation of sensory and neural ARHL. (2) A *"flat configuration" (or metabolic)* ARHL shows an audiogram that is significantly depressed at all measured frequencies. It is thought to be caused primarily by a dysfunction of the supporting structures in the cochlea that maintain the endocochlear potential, the driving force for auditory transduction. A decrease of the endocochlear potential will affect the entire cochlea and hence all frequencies (**Figure 34-5B**). Human and animal studies have connected a metabolic ARHL to pathology of the stria vascularis and the adjacent spiral ligament but a lack of such correlation has been noted in some human temporal bones and points to a potentially more complex etiology. (3) *Cochlear conductive* ARHL *or mechanical* ARHL is caused by changes in the stiffness of the basilar membrane. An audiogram of this type shows a linear decline of over 50 dB at all frequencies without degeneration of any cochlear cells or structures. Only a small portion of ARHL is estimated to fall into this category. (4) Mixed ARHL is the overlap of multiple pathologies. About 25% of cases may be of mixed pathology.

In evaluating ARHL, it is oftentimes difficult to determine the individual contributions of environmental influences that might damage the hair cells in the organ of Corti, such as exposure to noise, industrial solvents, or ototoxic medications. Aminoglycoside antibiotics (exemplified by streptomycin, gentamicin, kanamycin, and related drugs), in particular, destroy hair cells in a base-to-apex progression, causing an initial high-frequency hearing loss reminiscent of sensorineural presbycusis. Noise-induced hearing loss usually differs in its pattern as the site of cochlear damage relates to the frequency of the exposure, creating a "notch" in the audiogram. A fingerprint of noise trauma in hunters and shooters, for example, is a unilateral hearing deficit in the 4-kHz region (**Figure 34-5C**). Damage from industrial noise would be expected to be bilateral and create a broader area of hearing loss.

The recent discovery of a "hidden hearing loss" has spurred an interest in more subtle cochlear morphological changes than overt hair cell loss, in particular the integrity of synaptic connections. SGNs, bipolar cochlear neurons that conduct auditory information to the brain, transmit sound information from hair cells to the central auditory system via two type synapses: cochlear synapses and auditory nerve synapses. The pathophysiology of cochlear synapses at peripheral terminals of the SGNs has been well characterized in animal models: moderate noise exposure can induce loss of IHC synapses as a consequence of excessive glutamate release from overstimulated IHCs (excitotoxicity). This concept is further supported by the protection of cochlear synapses from noise exposure via a blockade of calcium-permeable AMPA receptors that are thought to mediate excitotoxicity. Such damages of cochlear synapses lead to loss of SGNs with aging and accelerate ARHL. This "cochlear synaptopathy" may also occur in humans, as recently revealed in human temporal bones. However, the prevalence of cochlear synaptopathy is clinically unknown because it is difficult to assess cochlear synaptopathy in patients.

CENTRAL AUDITORY ASPECT OF AGE-RELATED HEARING LOSS

In addition to deficiencies in peripheral auditory processing, advanced age can lead to changes in the central auditory system, which can essentially be classified into two

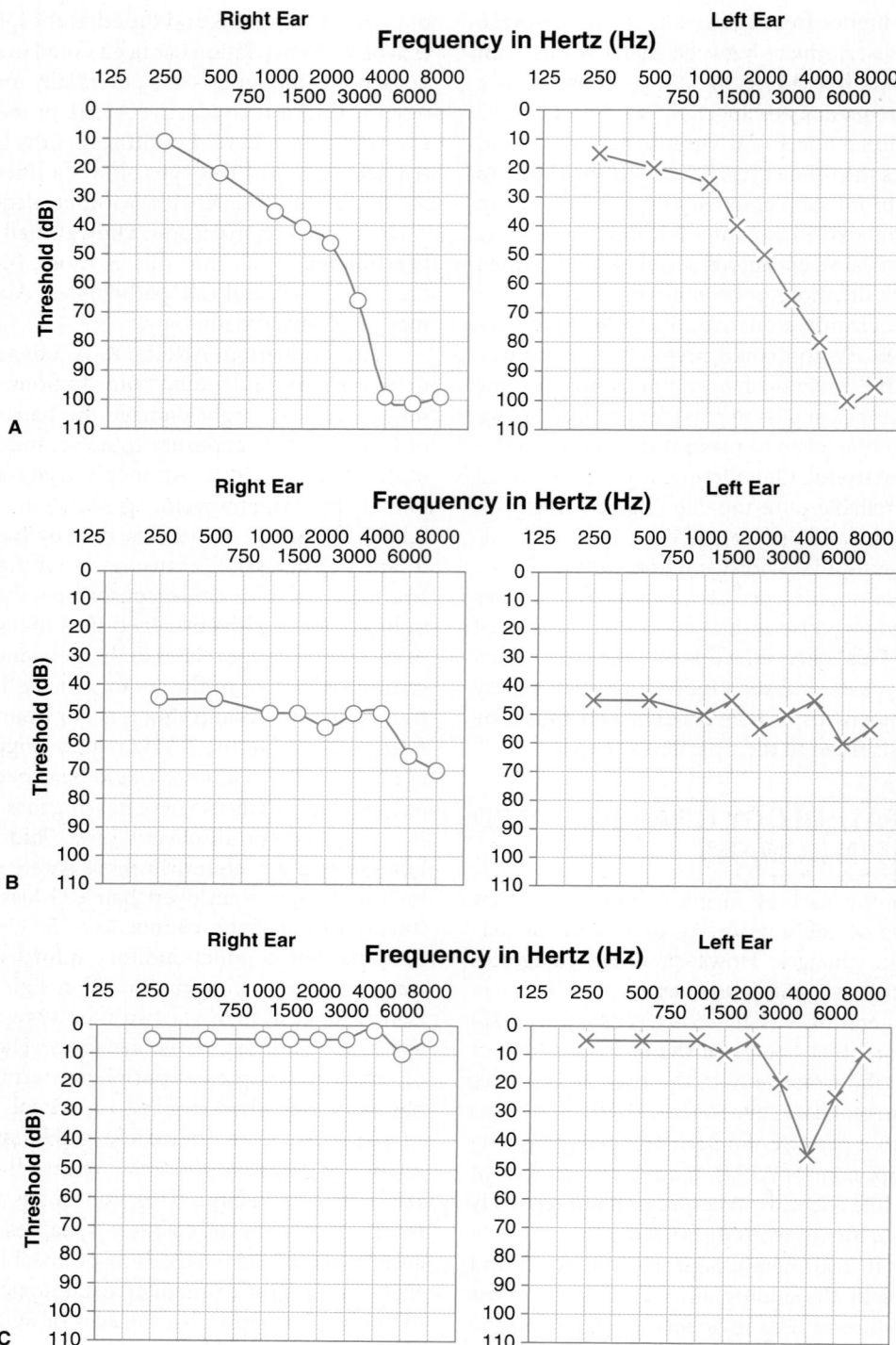

FIGURE 34-5. Audiograms of different degrees and configurations of hearing loss. Pure tone audiograms record the auditory thresholds, that is, the minimal sound level necessary to elicit a response in the listener at specific frequencies. Typical audiograms cover the range from 250 to 8000 Hz and the increasing intensity of the sound is plotted downward on the y-axis. A normal ear (**Figure 34-5C**, right) would yield an audiogram with flat responses around 0 to 25 dB; if the threshold is increased in an individual, the curve drops lower. Thresholds of 25 to 30 dB suggest a mild hearing loss, while thresholds of 70 dB and above would make average speech inaudible without hearing aids or a cochlear implant. **A.** The sloping audiogram from a 62-year-old man shows progressive high-frequency hearing loss in both ears. Lower speech frequencies are within normal limits or moderately affected but thresholds in the higher frequencies are sufficiently poor to cause difficulty with speech understanding in background noise **B.** The flat audiogram from a 64-year-old man shifted to higher thresholds is indicative of a "metabolic" presbycusis. **C.** The audiogram from a 32-year-old man shows a sharply defined hearing loss of 45 dB only at 4 kHz in the left ear. Such a "notch" in the audiogram is typical for noise damage, here from target shooting or hunting.

major types. The first is referred to as "peripherally induced central effects," which presents with changes in the cochlear nucleus driven by the decline of peripheral cochlear inputs that occur with age, typically starting with hearing loss at high frequencies. The other is referred to as "true aging" neurodegenerative changes in the brain. In this case, ARHL shares similarities or common mechanisms with other central nervous system conditions of the aged such as Alzheimer and Parkinson diseases. Age-dependent changes in auditory structures include declines in the number of ventral cochlear nucleus and lemniscal nerve fibers.

Indicative of deficits in sound processing in the higher auditory or cognitive centers, older adults often present with difficulties in speech recognition, rather than an inability to hear sound. Despite audiograms within the normal range, such patients might still require a stronger speech-to-noise signal or might experience better comprehension when speech is slowed down. Specific comprehension tests, for example, of speech perception in noise (QuickSIN test) can be used to better define such a condition, and can often identify difficulties understanding speech in noise independent of degree of hearing loss. Additionally, measures of complex auditory function (eg, speech in noise, comprehension of temporally compressed ["rapid"] speech) have been shown to relate to cognitive measures of working memory in adults. Cognitive screening examinations, such as the Hearing-Impaired Montreal Cognitive Assessment (HI-MoCA) are sometimes used in patients with ARHL in order to parse out contributions of peripheral and central factors to communication difficulties.

Animal models have helped to illuminate some central consequences of degeneration of the auditory periphery. However, the interrelationship of the pathophysiology of the auditory nerve and how it may contribute to central processing deficits in the cochlear nucleus needs further study. With age, synaptic connections may also change in number, spontaneous activity, or in their inhibitory or excitatory properties. It is possible, although yet unknown, if these changes directly affect speech understanding in humans. For patients with cochlear implants, who often have degeneration of the auditory nerve due to auditory deprivation, we know that the integrity of the auditory nerve matters to optimize speech understanding. Nevertheless, cochlear implants can still be very successful in older patients with a long duration of hearing loss (and loss of peripheral nerve connections) suggesting that the success of cochlear implants and hearing aids is at least partially dependent upon more central factors.

LESSONS FROM ANIMAL MODELS

Suitability of Different Species

A large variety of species has been studied for age-related auditory pathology, including chinchillas, guinea pigs, primates, dogs, and rodents. These species cover the range of cochlear pathologies, including organ of Corti, neural,

and strial degeneration, and the majority of animals show a complex mix. Mongolian gerbils are considered a model for metabolic (strial) presbycusis, presenting with strial atrophy, decreased endocochlear potential, and decreased cochlear blood flow. Degeneration of spiral ganglion cells, vacuolization of fibrocytes, and interstitial edema in the spiral ligament are also observed. In cats and rats, the underlying pathology has been linked to a combination of hair cell and spiral ganglion cell loss. Recently, a metabolic-type of hearing loss was also observed in the rat underscoring the fact that a singular "pure" type of hearing loss maybe rare in any species.

Mice have become favored for study of ARHL, because of availability of molecular and genetic information and of transgenic and knock-out animals. A caveat, however, is that each mouse strain differs significantly in its rate of hearing loss, ranging from those such as CBA and CAST, which exhibit minimal hearing loss by 18 months of age, to those such as C57BL/6 and DBA, which exhibit significantly accelerated hearing loss by approximately 8 and 3 months of age, respectively. The accelerated loss of hair cells and hearing found in C57BL/6 and BALB/cJ mice correlates with the presence of a recessive locus on proximal mouse Chr 10, the age-related hearing loss (Ahl) gene. The Cdh23^{ahl} allele (cadherin 23 or otocadherin) promotes degeneration of the organ of Corti in the cochlear base and high-frequency hearing loss beginning after 1 year of age as shown in congenic B-6.CAST-Cdh23^{ahl}. Furthermore, Cdh23^{ahl} also promotes noise-induced hearing loss, suggesting a connection between noise and ARHL. Since BALB/cJ and C57/BL mice are genetic mutations, they may not reflect a normal biological aging process. In fact, one genetic analysis of human presbycusis found no evidence for the presence of a mutation in cadherin 23.

The CBA/J mouse is among the strains in which the progression of ARHL more closely approximates human presbycusis. CBA/J mice lose hearing sensitivity late in their life span, advancing from high to low frequencies. ARHL begins around 12 months of age—here again the onset is earlier in males than in females—and progresses slowly until 18 months, after which point a more rapid rate of hearing loss is seen. The hearing loss at high frequencies is accompanied by loss of outer hair cells and a moderate degeneration of spiral ganglion cells. Since the CBA/J strain maintains normal morphology of the stria vascularis and normal endocochlear potential in aging, a sensorineural origin of the observed auditory deficits can be inferred.

Molecular Mechanisms

Significant progress has been made in our understanding of the pathologic and functional changes that occur in the inner ear with age using animal models. However, less is known about the specific molecular and genetic mechanisms contributing to ARHL. Recent work suggests to place "auditory aging" in animals—at least for sensorineural presbycusis—into the category of oxidant-stress related events. Oxidant stress is caused by the metabolic overproduction of ROS or reactive nitrogen species (RNS), including singlet oxygen, superoxides, peroxides, hydroxyl radicals, and hypochlorous acid or nitric oxide-derived compounds such as nitroxyl anion, nitrosonium cation, higher oxides of nitrogen, S-nitrosothiols, and dinitrosyl iron complexes. Maintaining cellular redox homeostasis depends on the rate of production of ROS and their removal by cellular antioxidants. If such homeostasis is disrupted, cell death is a potential consequence. Markers of oxidative stress are indeed elevated in the cochlea of the aging CBA/J mouse while antioxidant defense systems decrease. Other suggestive evidence for an involvement of oxidative stress comes from heterozygous mice lacking superoxide dismutase; ARHL developed earlier and with greater severity, as evidenced by an increased hair cell loss following the canonical base-to-apex progression. Consistent with oxidative stress is also the observation that the severity of ARHL in humans correlates with plasma levels of hydroxyl radicals and hydrogen peroxide, although a causal relationship cannot be inferred. While oxidative stress may be a contributing factor, failed attempts to slow the progression of cochlear degeneration and hearing loss with antioxidants point to a more complex picture (see section on "Prevention of Age-Related Hearing Loss"). Recent studies in lower organisms suggest that low levels of mitochondrial ROS (mROS) regulate immunity and autophagy, which positively affects aging. The dual function of ROS to both promote cell damage and promote cell adaptation to stress responses makes them challenging as potentially therapeutic targets.

Deletions in mitochondrial DNA are also an established indicator of cumulative oxidative damage to a tissue and have been observed in the aging—including human—cochlea. DNA in mitochondria, in contrast to nuclear DNA, is particularly vulnerable because these organelles possess less efficient machinery to repair DNA damage, leaving mutations uncorrected and prone to adversely affect mitochondrial function. A mtDNA[4977] deletion is the most common mutation found in human temporal bones and significantly correlated with individual audiometric thresholds and the severity of presbycusis.

Vascular abnormalities are another pathologic change with aging potentially affecting supply of nutrients and oxygen as well as mitochondrial respiration, thus adding to oxidant stress in the inner ear. As a case in point, suppression of cochlear blood flow promotes mitochondrial DNA mutations and may impact hearing loss. In addition, and as already mentioned, reduction of cochlear blood flow from age-related degeneration could lead to a compromised function of the stria vascularis and an inability to maintain cochlear homeostasis for the maintenance of transduction currents and tissue integrity. The sum of these considerations supports the general concept that ARHL is a consequence of accumulated environmental injuries to the cochlea along with the intrinsic genetically controlled aging process.

Genetic Contributions

The majority of so-called mouse models of genetic hearing loss exhibit sensory dysfunction soon after birth; in other words, these are models of accelerated hearing loss not necessarily reflecting human pathology. Hence, the utility of these models for understanding presbycusis-type later-onset hearing loss is unclear. In contrast, a genetically heterogeneous population of four-way cross mice at the age of 8, 18, and 22 months was tested for auditory hearing function by auditory brain stem response (ABR), and genotyped at 128 markers to identify loci that modulate late-life hearing loss. Polymorphisms significantly affecting hearing at 18 or 22 months of age were noted on several chromosomes. Such phenotypic variability strongly suggests that ARHL is a complex polygenetic disorder possibly involving numerous alleles on multiple genes. These conclusions from an animal model fit well with the previously mentioned GWAS study in humans.

PREVENTION OF AGE-RELATED HEARING LOSS

Avoiding noise, ototoxins, and smoking, but engaging in regular exercising and maintaining a healthy diet may aid in slowing progressive hearing loss as it will contribute to general health. The question as to what extent interventive strategies can specifically delay ARHL cannot yet be conclusively answered but some data from animal experimentation point to the general concept that the rate of ARHL can be influenced.

"Augmented acoustic environment" is a concept to influence the progression of presbycusis by exposure to controlled stimuli. This environment could be created by an enhanced ambient acoustic background or by delivery of specific stimuli through hearing aids. Studies in mice, although mostly on inbred strains with accelerated hearing loss, confirm that the auditory system responds to such treatment but not necessarily in predictable ways. While amelioration of some forms of age-related changes was found, other effects were detrimental, leaving final judgment to future experimentation.

Dietary restriction has been widely used in aging studies and can slow certain age-related physiological declines and extend longevity. For the auditory system, results of such studies are inconclusive and emphasize the point that organ-specific effects of a generalized treatment are impossible to predict. Caloric restriction had positive effects on the progression and magnitude of ARHL in rats but was ineffective in rhesus monkeys. A comprehensive study of 15 mouse strains brought every conceivable result from an apparent amelioration of the rate or severity of presbycusis to no effects and to an acceleration of hearing loss. Such results indicate a major influence of genotype on the outcome, cautioning that similar problems might be encountered in presbycusis therapy in humans.

Antioxidant therapy in animal models, based on the premise that oxidant stress is a contributor to ARHL, has shown inconsistent results. Rats that were placed on vitamin supplementation (vitamins C and E) shortly after birth outperformed their placebo controls in hearing tests at old age but the number of animals in this study was exceedingly low and the results might have been skewed by a more robust health of the surviving small cohort. When the supplementation with antioxidants (acetyl carnitine and lipoic acid) in rats was started later in life and upheld for 6 weeks, results were less convincing. Dogs, on the other hand, fed an antioxidant diet for the final 3 years of their life had better preserved auditory neurons; a confounding factor, however, might have been the high noise level in the kennels which can contribute to noise-induced hearing loss which may be attenuated by antioxidants. In a long-term longitudinal study, 10-month-old female CBA/J mice were maintained on either a control or antioxidant-enriched diet and monitored through 24 months of age; ARHL showed no difference between the two groups. The simple approach to attenuate ROS generation may therefore be an inadequate therapy, perhaps due to the dual role of ROS in adaptation to stress and promotion of cell damage.

Nevertheless, human studies suggest the hypothesis that ARHL can, to some extent, be influenced by dietary or therapeutic intervention. Daily supplementation of folic acid for 3 years positively affected the hearing of older participants in a study in the Netherlands. The effect was significant but very small on low-frequency hearing while age-related changes in high-frequency hearing, the area normally most afflicted by presbycusis, proceeded unaffected. Since low-frequency hearing is important for speech, the result can be considered encouraging. The underlying mechanism of this protection has yet to be established but the effect goes hand-in-hand with controversial observations that patients with higher erythrocyte and serum concentrations of folate maintain lower hearing thresholds. It should be noted however that routine folic acid supplementation of foods is not permitted in the Netherlands but is common in other industrialized countries. Results therefore may differ in countries where basic folate levels in the population can be expected to be higher. Finally and quite intriguingly, several surveys indicate alcohol consumption as a possible modulator of ARHL. Moderate use of alcohol was associated with better hearing in older individuals in three independent studies, an effect in line with—somewhat controversial—observations that low alcohol intake can be beneficial for general health. Heavy drinkers, in contrast, had a tendency toward more pronounced high-frequency hearing loss.

MANAGEMENT OF AGE-RELATED HEARING LOSS

Restoration of normal hearing is currently not possible since lost hair cells, a major cause of ARH, cannot regenerate. The current choice for rehabilitation of ARHL, therefore,

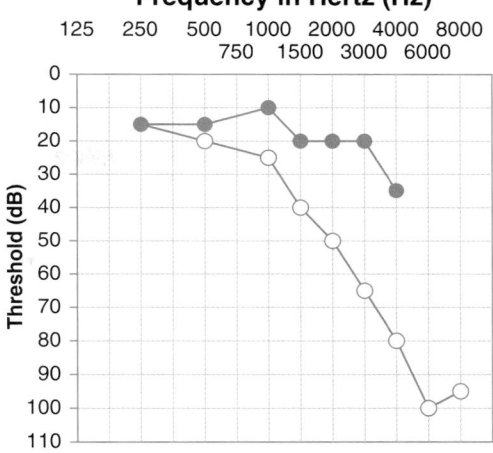

FIGURE 34-6. Typical effects of a hearing aid. The unaided audiogram (open circles) shows presbycusic high-frequency hearing loss. With hearing aids in place (closed circles), acuity is improved to near-normal levels for frequencies up to 3000 Hz. Note that low frequencies deliberately are not boosted and that rescue of the elevated thresholds at high frequencies is not possible.

is hearing aids. Digital hearing aids present a wide range of user options and have advanced technologically in all aspects including the tolerance of a noisy environment and improved cosmetology. Hearing aids, individually tailored to a user's audiogram, provide clearly increased hearing ability and speech discrimination (**Figure 34-6**). However, knowledge about the benefits and acceptance of hearing aids is low. About one-half of older people who could benefit from a hearing aid never try; others are dissatisfied after short use and only 10% to 30% continue to wear hearing aids. Rejection to a large extent depends on personal idiosyncrasies, education, and cultural aspects. Health care costs do not appear to be a decisive factor. The compliance rate is the same in the United States (where patients pay or co-pay for the hearing aid) and the United Kingdom (where they are free), around 15%. In some instances the pathophysiological basis may lie beyond the cochlea. "I can hear but I can't understand" may point to a central auditory deficit that cannot be easily corrected by enhancing the peripheral stimulus.

If the magnitude of the hearing loss exceeds the corrective capability of hearing aids, cochlear implants (CI) are recommended with increasing frequency to older patients. Cochlear implant candidacy is quickly expanding and is beneficial in patients who score at less than 60% on sentences, in quiet or in noise, in the poorer hearing ear. While a hearing aid essentially amplifies sound to the cochlea and therefore depends on remaining sensory cells, the cochlear implant bypasses the sensory cells and directly stimulates the auditory nerve electrically. To achieve an effective transformation to an electrical stimulus, the acoustic information needs to be preprocessed and delivered to the nerve via an electrode implanted into the cochlea. The success depends on appropriate coding paradigms and a healthy complement of cochlear nerve innervation. Since the degeneration of the cochlear nerve is slow in humans, much of the aging population presenting with presbycusis should be good candidates. The outcome of implantation is variable but almost all of the patients greatly improve speech perception and most even acquire the ability to carry on telephone conversations. Challenges that remain are speech recognition in unfamiliar contexts and the enjoyment of music. In older patients, cognitive status will also affect cochlear implant outcomes. Unlike acoustic hearing aids, cochlear implants are typically covered by medical insurance (including Medicare) and age is not a contraindication to success. There is some evidence that older patients perform slightly poorer overall with a CI compared to their younger counterparts, but in these patients, it is difficult to parse out effects of chronological age and duration of hearing loss/neural degeneration. Importantly, CIs are successful and beneficial in the overwhelming number of older recipients.

ASSOCIATION BETWEEN HEARING LOSS AND COGNITIVE DECLINE

More recently, there has been a shift in focus and awareness of potential effects of hearing loss on cognitive decline in the aging population. It has long been recognized that even in the absence of significant measurable hearing loss, older individuals demonstrate slowed auditory processing when compared to younger peers. Even older patients with relatively normal hearing can have difficulty understanding speech in the presence of background noise or when the speaker talks at rapid pace; for older individuals with hearing loss, these effects are even more pronounced, and studies have pointed to underlying differences in cognitive processing to help account for senescent declines in speech understanding.

Several studies have identified a potential link between untreated hearing loss and a higher prevalence of cognitive decline in older adults; however, the precise nature or direction of this relationship is yet unknown. Epidemiologic studies suggest that hearing loss is independently associated with more rapid cognitive decline in older patients, and a single study from Johns Hopkins University (JHU) reported a 24% increased risk for cognitive loss among those with ARHL. Additional studies reveal that the severity of hearing loss also plays a role; among 1103 participants, only those with moderate to severe hearing loss showed an increased risk of cognitive dysfunction compared to normal hearing controls. A radiologic study conducted at JHU reported that even among patients without cognitive loss observed on behavioral screenings, those with hearing loss show changes in microstructural integrity of the temporal lobe and reduced grey matter in the hippocampus.

It is not yet understood whether hearing aids and/or CIs can be used to help slow the onset of cognitive decline associated with untreated hearing loss. However, a retrospective study at the University of Michigan including 114,862 adults aged 66 or older suggests that the use of hearing aids can delay the diagnosis of Alzheimer and dementia, and also results in lower incidences of anxiety and falls. Additional studies in older patients who use CIs have reported improved performance on behavioral measures of cognitive function, when preoperative and postoperative scores are compared. While studies are underway, there is currently insufficient data using prospective, randomized controls to help determine if hearing aids and CIs can help to prevent early-onset cognitive changes in these populations.

OUTLOOK

ARHL is an exceedingly complex disease besetting an organ of even greater complexity. It appears to be a sequel to numerous morphological and molecular changes that befall the auditory system as we age and that are being characterized with increasing acuity by basic and clinical research. One of the major reasons for the lack of treatment of ARHL is the extensive phenotypic variability in hearing loss among human subjects. Our understanding and ability to design interventive and curative therapies will much depend on advances into the molecular and cellular mechanisms of auditory pathologies and identification of genetic variants associated with ARHL. Recent new technologies such as next-generation sequencing including DNA-Seq, RNA-Seq, ChIP-Seq, Methyl-Seq, targeted sequencing utilizing Illumina HiScanSQ, and Ion Torrent instrumentation will provide the platform to perform a large-scale genome-wide phenotype association studies with ARHL.

Given the partial success of pharmacological protection, this approach should yield the first practical results. Appropriate agents for and timing of interventions will be explored in animal models, both independent of and tied into interventions in extending life span and general health. Gene therapy also shows promise as a possible strategy to protect hair cells. To date, research has successfully focused on prevention of hearing loss caused by acute traumata like drugs and noise. Such model systems might be modified to serve hearing loss from aging as the etiology of these insults shows similarities to age-related sensorineural hearing loss. As a major caveat, any intervention into ARHL would necessitate lengthy trials that may prevent the implementation of prospective solutions in the near future.

In the area of rehabilitation, technological advances of hearing aids and cochlear implants will improve not only speech recognition but also music appreciation, an area currently of difficult rehabilitation. A direct nerve implant, already successfully tested in an animal model, may replace the cochlear implant for better efficacy of stimulation and a wider range of frequency and intensity perception. The following generation of prostheses will bypass the cochlea and its nerve and stimulate higher auditory centers. Although clinical application of auditory midbrain implants is less common, a handful of patients have already been treated albeit with more limited success compared to hearing aids or cochlear implants. Such prosthetic therapy could prove advantageous for patients with massive degeneration of the auditory periphery and/or degeneration of the auditory nerve as in a severe neural type of ARHL.

Lastly, functional hair cell regeneration is the final frontier in the field. Recent studies have shown that cells in the organ of Corti, such as supporting cells, may mitose or transdifferentiate into hair cells if appropriately stimulated. The challenges, however, are highly complex: not only hair cells need to be (re)generated, they also have to be incorporated into the intricate cytoarchitecture of the cochlea and find their appropriate connections to the central auditory structures. Stem cell research may likewise provide new insights for replacement of hair cells and the regeneration of the auditory nerve.

Although presbycusis is not yet preventable or treatable, progress in basic and clinical research promises hope for the future. Most realistic in the near term seem protective pharmacological strategies to delay or attenuate ARHL and improved rehabilitation through next-generation hearing aids and implants. A plausible clinical therapy for the regeneration of new and functional hair cells may, despite recent encouraging advance, still be decades away.

ACKNOWLEDGMENT

The authors wish to thank Andra E. Talaska for her contributions to the previous versions of this chapter. Dr. Schacht's and Sha's research on age-related hearing loss was supported by program project grant AG-025164 from the National Institute on Aging, NIH. Dr. Sha's research is supported by R01 grant DC009222 from the National Institute on Deadness and Other Communication Disorders.

FURTHER READING

Durga J, Verhoef P, Anteunis LJ, Schouten E, Kok FJ. Effects of folic acid supplementation on hearing in older adults: a randomized, controlled trial. *Ann Intern Med.* 2007;146:1–9.

Fransen E, Bonneux S, Corneveaux JJ, et al. Genome-wide association analysis demonstrates the highly polygenic character of age-related hearing impairment. *Eur J Hum Genet.* 2015;23(1):110–115.

Frisina RD, Walton JP. Age-related structural and functional changes in the cochlear nucleus. *Hear Res.* 2006;216–217:216–223.

Gates GA, Cooper JC Jr, Kannel WB, Miller NJ. Hearing in the elderly: the Framingham cohort, 1983–1985. Part I. Basic audiometric test results. *Ear Hear.* 1990;11:247–256.

Helzner EP, Cauley JA, Pratt SR, et al. Race and sex differences in age-related hearing loss: the Health, Aging and Body Composition Study. *J Am Geriatr Soc.* 2005;53:2119–2127.

Jiang H, Talaska AE, Schacht J, Sha S-H. Oxidative imbalance in the aging inner ear. *Neurobiol Aging.* 2007;28:1605–1612.

Johnsson LG, Hawkins JE. Sensory and neural degeneration with aging, as seen in microdissections of the human inner ear. *Ann Otol Rhinol Laryngol.* 1972;81:179–192.

Kujawa SG, Liberman MC. Acceleration of age-related hearing loss by early noise exposure: evidence of a misspent youth. *J Neurosci.* 2006;26:2115–2123.

Levy BR, Slade MD, Gill TM. Hearing decline predicted by elders' stereotypes. *J Gerontol B Psychol Sci Soc Sci.* 2006;61:P82–P87.

McFadden SL, Ding D, Salvi R. Anatomical, metabolic and genetic aspects of age-related hearing loss in mice. *Audiology.* 2001;40:313–321.

National Institute on Deafness and Other Communication Disorders. Presbycusis. https://www.nidcd.nih.gov/health/age-related-hearing-loss.

Ohlemiller KK. Contributions of mouse models to understanding of age- and noise-related hearing loss. *Brain Res.* 2006;1091:89–102.

Pickles JO. Mutation in mitochondrial DNA as a cause of presbyacusis. *Audiol Neurootol.* 2004;9:23–33.

Rosenhall U, Karlsson Espmark AK. Hearing aid rehabilitation: what do older people want, and what does the audiogram tell? *Int J Audiol.* 2003;42(Suppl 2):2S53–2S57.

Schacht J, Altschuler RA, Burke DT, et al. Alleles that modulate late life hearing in genetically heterogeneous mice. *Neurobiol Aging.* 2012;33:1842.e15–1842.e29.

Schacht J, Hawkins JE. Sketches of otohistory. Part 9: presby[a]cusis. *Audiol Neurootol.* 2005;10:243–247.

Schuknecht HF. Further observations on the pathology of presbycusis. *Arch Otolaryngol.* 1964;80:369–382.

Sha S-H, Kanicki A, Halsey K, Wearne KA, Schacht J. Antioxidant-enriched diet does not delay the progression of age-related hearing loss. *Neurobiol Aging.* 2012;33:1010.e15–1010.e16.

Van Eyken E, Van Camp G, Van Laer L. The complexity of age-related hearing impairment: contributing environmental and genetic factors. *Audiol Neurootol.* 2007;12:345–358.

Willott JF, Chisolm TH, Lister JL. Modulation of presbycusis: current status and future directions. *Audiol Neurootol.* 2001;6:231–249.

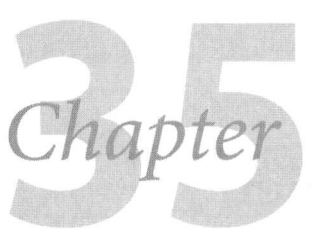

Chapter 35

Sexuality, Sexual Function, and the Aging Woman

Monica Christmas, Kaitlyn Fruin, Stacy Tessler Lindau

INTRODUCTION

Sociological evidence about sexuality of women in middle and later life has increased substantially over the last decade, but sexual function and outcomes among middle age and older women are still largely overlooked in the context of medical care. Negative societal attitudes about aging, sexuality among older people, and women's sexuality, in particular, present a significant barrier to scientific inquiry and medical attention to older women's health concerns. Proven interventions for promoting female sexual well-being or treating women's sexual problems are limited. Although older women experience high rates of sexual problems and the majority of partnered older women are sexually active, physicians infrequently discuss sexual health with older women. Public health attention to older women's sexuality remains sparse.

The 2005–2006 National Social Life, Health and Aging Project (NSHAP), funded by the National Institutes of Health, provided the first comprehensive, population-representative biosocial data on sexuality among middle age and older women and men in the United States, and it informs many of the insights presented in this chapter (https://www.norc.org/Research/Projects/Pages/national-social-life-health-and-aging-project.aspx). In 2010 and 2011 (NSHAP Wave II), 75% of participants in the baseline NSHAP study (Wave I) participated in follow-up interviews. Between 2015 and 2016, 2409 surviving Wave I respondents and an additional new cohort of respondents born between 1948 and 1965 participated in Wave III (accessed at https://www.icpsr.umich.edu/web/NACDA/studies/36873). This chapter first locates older women's sexuality in a sociodemographic context, then describes sexual activity, behaviors, and problems experienced by women in later life; reviews physiologic changes that affect

Learning Objectives

- Understand a biopsychosocial model for research, diagnosis, and care of sexual concerns among aging women.
- Integrate into clinical practice knowledge of population norms of sexual activity, behaviors, and problems among aging women.
- Use knowledge of sexual physiology in aging to inform sexual history-taking, diagnosis, and treatment of sexual problems in older women.

Key Clinical Points

1. Older women, including those without a partner, value their sexual function and expect physicians to counsel them about sexual side effects or expected outcomes of medical conditions and treatments.

2. An older woman with sexual dysfunction is likely to be bothered or distressed by the sexual problems, and this distress can have deleterious effects on her overall physical and mental health and intimate relationships.

3. Older women who identify as members of a sexual minority group are marginalized and stigmatized in medical care generally, and they are particularly vulnerable with respect to receiving appropriate medical attention for their sexual concerns.

sexual functioning as women age; and recommends a clinical approach to evaluation, prevention, and treatment of sexual problems common among older women. Older women, and their sexual relationships, are very heterogeneous. Generalizations made in this chapter, based on population data from the NSHAP study and findings from other sources, are rooted in statistical norms but should not be interpreted as a normative prescription for older women's sexuality.

Interactive Biopsychosocial Model

The interactive biopsychosocial model (IBM) provides a conceptual framework for understanding the bidirectional relationship between sexuality and health throughout the life course (**Figure 35-1**). To the degree that medicine attends to matters of sexuality, the orientation is largely negative. The medical model approach to understanding sexuality focuses on sexual dysfunction as a problematic consequence of aging, disease, or treatment.

Sexual behavior can result in health problems, such as sexually transmitted infection and victimization. Aging, physical and mental health problems, surgeries, medications, and other medical treatments can cause sexual dysfunction. The IBM acknowledges this reciprocal relationship between sexuality and health but incorporates the possibilities that sexuality may also be health promoting and that aging, or even illness, may confer advantages for sexual life.

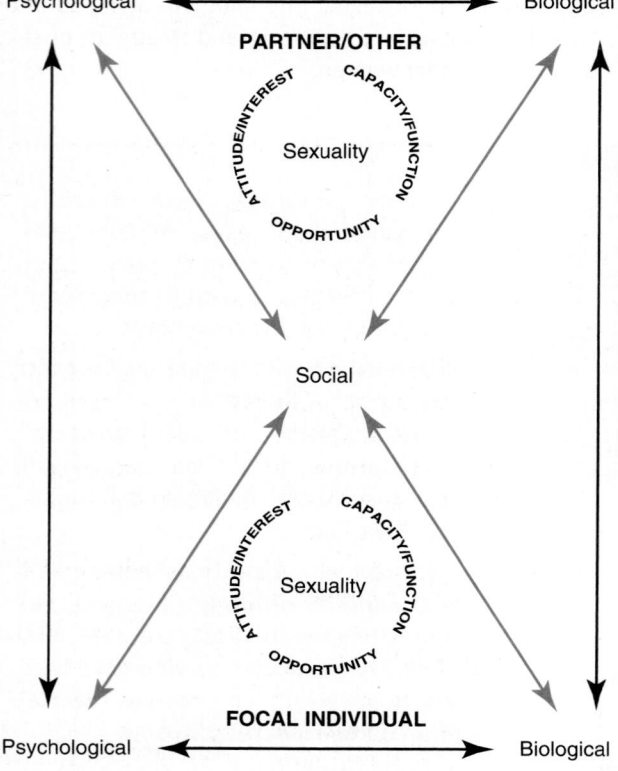

FIGURE 35-1. The interactive biopsychosocial model.

In this model, health comprises biological, psychological, and social components and is conceptualized as jointly produced by a woman in conjunction with her spouse or other intimate partner(s). Joint production of health means that partners contribute assets (or liabilities) to the "health endowment," and these assets and liabilities impact the health of the other(s). The hourglass shape symbolizes the dynamic nature of both health and intimate relationships over time. Clinically, this model can be used as a mnemonic for the broad domains of inquiry pertinent to assessing a patient's sexual history and reminds the clinician of the importance of ascertaining the presence, and health, of the patient's intimate partner(s).

SOCIODEMOGRAPHIC CONTEXT OF OLDER WOMEN'S SEXUALITY

Sexuality in later life commonly occurs in the context of a long-term marital relationship. Men are significantly more likely than women to have a spouse or other romantic partner in later life and to be engaging in a satisfying sexual relationship, despite a high prevalence of erectile difficulties. As a result of greater longevity, women, in contrast, are much more likely to experience aging, illness, and death without a partner (**Figure 35-2**).

Still, many older women regard sexuality as important for health and relationships and, among those with a spousal or other intimate relationship, many engage in regular sexual activity. Women tend to be less satisfied with sex in later life than men, and they also report a high frequency of sexual problems including low desire, vaginal dryness, and difficulty experiencing orgasm. An older married woman is often healthier and more vital than her spouse and commonly assumes a caregiver role, which can interfere with the romantic dynamic of the relationship. Physical health problems, medications, and medical treatments affect the sexual lives of older couples; older heterosexual adults with a spouse or other intimate partner who are not sexually active most commonly attribute this to the male partner's health problems. Although some aspects of aging are regarded as detrimental to sexual life, older women also identify ways in which aging is beneficial for sexuality (**Table 35-1**).

Lack of formal sexuality education combined with widely restrictive social, religious, and cultural practices around female sexuality during much of the twentieth century have influenced the current generation of older women's sexual expectations throughout their lives. As a result, many report that they have never discussed nor would they initiate discussion of sexual matters with anyone, including their spouses. Most older women report that they have never spoken of sexual matters with a physician, yet feel that sexuality is an appropriate issue for physicians to address and that the physician, rather than the patient, should initiate the discussion (**Table 35-2**). Gender and age differences between women and their physicians can also

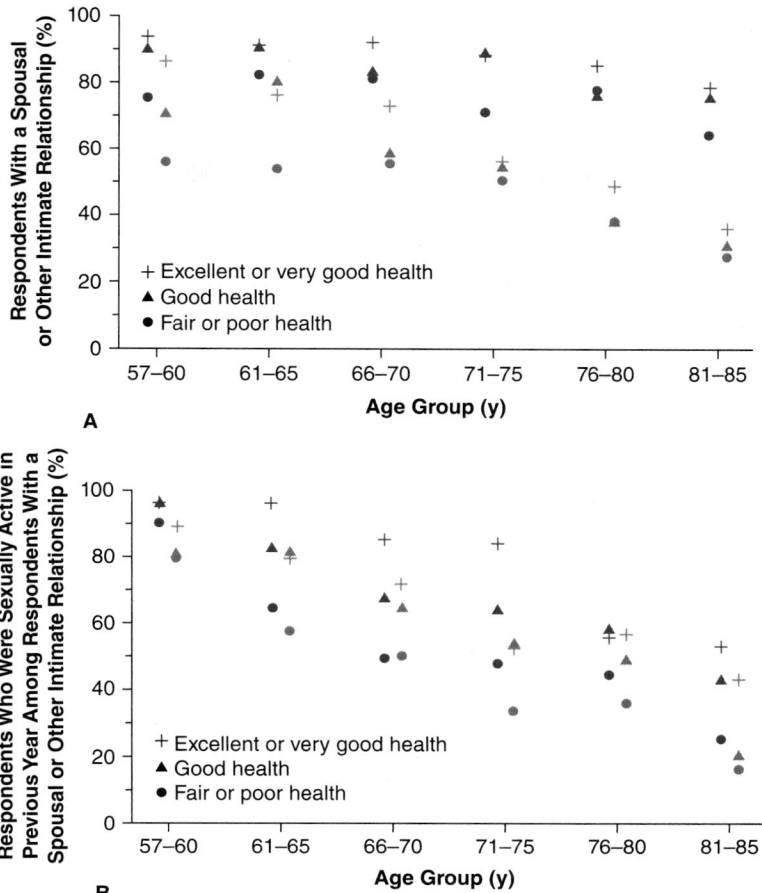

FIGURE 35-2. Prevalence of relationships and sexual activity by age and health status. *Note: Red symbols denote men; yellow symbols denote women.* (Reproduced with permission from Lindau ST, Schumm LP, Laumann EO, et al. A study of sexuality and health among older adults in the United States. *N Engl J Med.* 2007;357[8]:762–774.)

present barriers to communication about sexual matters. In addition, older women perceive physicians to be poorly trained to deal with patients' sexual concerns and that physicians presume older women to be asexual or disinterested (see **Table 35-2**).

Aging of the baby boomers, the generation of the sexual revolution, is increasing demand for medical attention to sexual matters. Although male longevity is expected to increase, older women will continue to outnumber older men through 2050; this presents a significant gender disparity in the opportunity for formation of new sexual relationships in later life and, in some cases, results in multiple women sharing a single male partner. Little is known about the health implications of emerging trends among older adults including nonmonogamy, rising rates of divorce, unmarried cohabitation, same-sex marriages, and later life dating.

Sexuality and Cognitive Function

Until recently, most of what was known about sexuality in the context of cognitive dysfunction derived from studies of sexual behavior among people with dementia living in nursing home settings. NSHAP Wave II included the first nationally representative study of sexuality among community-dwelling people with cognitive impairment and dementia. This study found that cognitively impaired men were much more likely than women to be partnered (83% vs 57%), about half of all partnered women and men with cognitive impairment, including 40% of those aged 80 to 91, were sexually active. Sexual problems, including a lack of interest in sex, were reported by a quarter of men and one in ten women with cognitive impairment. Yet, very few cognitively impaired people had addressed sexual function concerns with their partner or a physician. Because cognitive impairment can impede consent for sexual activity, and an individual's understanding of sex or ability to express their desire for sex can wax and wane in the course of dementia, it makes sense to include an individual's wishes for sexual activity in their documentation of advance directives. NSHAP, in fact, reported that 14% of women and 17% of men with cognitive impairment engaged in obligatory sex or sex without feeling aroused. Currently, an estimated 3 million older people with cognitive impairment or dementia are both community-dwelling

TABLE 35-1 ■ OLDER WOMEN'S VIEWS ON SEXUALITY AND AGING

	EFFECTS OF AGING ON SEXUALITY	EFFECTS OF SEXUALITY ON AGING
Beneficial	• Partners know each other better • Decreased sexual inhibition • More time • Fewer distractions • Know own body	• Better circulation • Form of exercise • Feeling of youthfulness or completeness • Security of not being alone • Pride in body • Optimistic outlook on life • Indicative of general good health • Happiness/ endorphins • Physical release, outlet • Alleviates arthritic pain
Detrimental	• Less intense physical sexual response • Increased inhibition due to poor body image • Societal prejudice • Need for secrecy	• Worry about transmitting or contracting infection • Loss of status as respected elder

Data from ST Lindau funded by the John A. Hartford Foundation, 1993.

TABLE 35-2 ■ OLDER WOMEN'S PERCEPTIONS ABOUT BARRIERS TO DISCUSSING SEX WITH A PHYSICIAN

WHY PATIENTS DON'T DISCUSS SEX	WHY DOCTORS DON'T DISCUSS SEX
• Patients "don't know what we don't know" • Feel intimidated • Feel it might be disrespectful to physician • Feel uncomfortable discussing sex with male physician • Feel uncomfortable discussing sex with younger physician • Fear that a physical examination may be embarrassing, uncomfortable, or painful • Worry that difference in sexual orientation between patient and physician will threaten relationship • Think physicians not capable of or interested in discussing sex, so no value in raising the issue • Feel the physician would raise the topic if relevant	• Doctors assume older people are not interested in talking about sex or having sex • "Look upon us as their parents" • Don't know enough to feel qualified to talk about sex • Assume someone else is dealing with these issues • Focused on treating older people for illness rather than maintaining health and quality of life • Don't have time • Have their own hang-ups about sex • Embarrassed to talk about sex with older female patients • Religious beliefs interfere

Data from ST Lindau funded by the John A. Hartford Foundation, 1993 and the University of Chicago Program in Integrative Sexual Medicine Registry (2008–2014).

and sexually active. This number is expected to double by 2050. Best practice for care of older adults with cognitive impairment should include early and ongoing discussion about the effects of impairment on sexual function, sexual behavior (which can include an increase or change in sexual behavior in some cases), and decision making about engaging in partnered sexual activity.

Sexuality in Long-Term Care Institutions and Palliative Care

The early literature on sexuality and aging in the nursing home or long-term care setting focused on strategies for staff to restrict this behavior. Residents of long-term care institutions are less likely to be sexually active than community-residing older adults, and they cite lack of partners, lack of privacy, lack of interest, sexual dysfunction, and negative attitudes of staff as limiting sexual expression. Older lesbian, bisexual, and transgender individuals are at increased risk of stigma and discrimination, especially in settings where the right to privacy is limited.

Increasingly, as a human rights matter, long-term care institutions provide private rooms for residents and have trained their providers to understand and accept sexuality in a respectful manner. Sometimes,

sexual relationships form among people with dementia who have, but may not remember, a community-residing spouse. Likewise, community-residing spouses may initiate new intimate relationships while maintaining involvement with and commitment to their institutionalized spouse. The implications of these relationships for health and integrity in later life are a growing reality, but poorly understood and often a cause of distress for families. Sexual exploitation and abuse of older women living in residential facilities (and in the community) are poorly documented, but vulnerability is heightened by cognitive impairment, which can interfere with a woman's ability to consent to sexual relations.

Palliative care, whether provided in an institutional or community setting, presents another opportunity to address a patient's capacity for sexual function and fulfillment. Palliation for sexual function could entail providing sex hormone therapy to a patient even if she has a history of an estrogen-sensitive cancer. It could also involve treatment aimed specifically at alleviating nonhormonal causes of dyspareunia, such as timing breakthrough pain medications prior to sexual activity. While some patients bring closure to their sexual lives before entering palliative care, other patients may wish to remain intimate with their partners as long as possible. Optimization of sexual function for older women in palliative care is understudied and often overlooked, but is an area of increasing attention.

SEXUAL ACTIVITY, BEHAVIOR, AND PROBLEMS

Sexual Partnership

Population-based normative data for older women show that sexual activity is largely determined by availability of a sexual partner. Among women aged 57 to 64 in the 2005–2006 NSHAP study, about 85% had a current spouse or other romantic or intimate partner. Nearly all of these relationships were reported as heterosexual, monogamous, and involving sexual activity. The proportion of women with a partner declined with age, because of earlier male mortality. By age 85, only about 40% of women had a partner, and fewer than 20% of all women engaged in sexual activity.

As compared with findings for younger women, women 57 years and older reported fewer total sexual partners over the lifetime. Most sexually active older women reported that their current relationship was monogamous. In the NSHAP baseline study, nearly 1 in 10 married women and twice as many nonmarried women with a sexual partner believed that their current partner had other sexual partners during the relationship.

In the NSHAP baseline study, 5% of women reported ever having a female sexual partner and only five women (0.3%) reported currently being in a relationship with another woman. Although population data on lesbian relationships at older ages are only just beginning to emerge, estimates from the younger population suggest that women in this study may have underreported same-sex relationships. Qualitative research and clinical experience reveals cases of older women choosing or demonstrating receptivity to intimacy with female partners for the first time in later life. Some women explain this as a choice caused by the scarcity of males in later life, while others are fulfilling, for the first time, a lifelong interest. The Caring and Aging with Pride study (2010), a national community-based survey of lesbian, gay, bisexual, transsexual (LGBT) aging, found that among individuals 50 years and older, lesbian and bisexual adults were less likely to have a partner or be married than people identifying as heterosexual.

The low representation of sexual minorities in studies of older adults, the frequent exclusion of older adults in studies of sexual minorities, and the lack of inclusion of questions ascertaining sexual orientation in routine research practice render older LGBT adults largely invisible in most research. This invisibility is perpetuated in clinical settings when providers do not ask about sexual orientation and when patients feel unsafe disclosing their sexual orientation. Further research is necessary to understand the barriers to accessing care and the health needs of aging sexual minorities so that culturally competent care and targeted interventions can be delivered. With marriage equality declared a constitutional right, older adults who identify as members of a sexual minority group will be more likely to disclose their status in research, clinical, and institutional living settings.

Sexual Activity

Among those who are sexually active (defined in the NSHAP study as engaging in "any mutually voluntary activity with another person that involves sexual contact, whether or not intercourse or orgasm occurs" during the prior 12 months), the kinds and frequency of sexual activity in which women engage are similar to those observed among younger women. Most commonly, sexual activity involves vaginal intercourse, hugging, kissing, or other forms of sexual touching, and about 45% of sexually active women engaged in oral sex. On average, the frequency of sexual activity for those with a sexual partner ranges from one to three times per month, similar to that observed among younger sexually active adults. About a quarter of women aged 57 to 85 reported masturbating in the previous year. The prevalence of masturbation among women without a partner is the same as among women with a partner. This is also true for older men (50% report masturbating) and suggests that older adults maintain an individual desire for sexual activity, even in the absence of a sexual partner.

Sexually Active Life Expectancy

Sexually active life expectancy projects population patterns of sexual activity to estimate the number of years, for any given age, of expected future sexual activity. As calculated based on 1995–1996 and 2005–2006 data, at age 55, sexually active life expectancy is about 16 years for women with a spouse or other intimate partner (**Figure 35-3**). Among sexually active women, good health was associated with a gain of 3 to 6 years of expected future sexually active life. Communication of normative expectations to

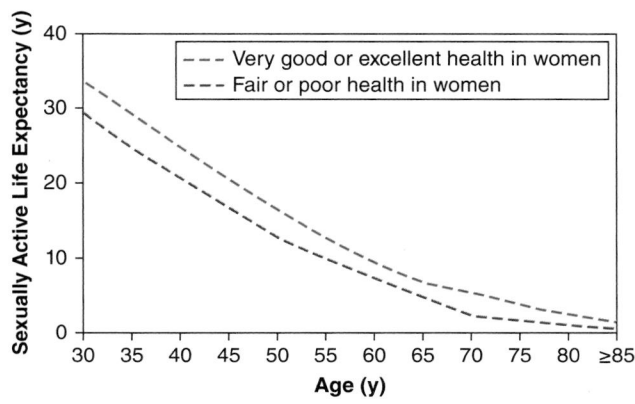

FIGURE 35-3. Sexually active life expectancy. (Adapted with permission from Lindau ST, Gavrilova N. Sex, health, and years of sexually active life gained due to good health: evidence from two US population based cross sectional surveys of ageing. *BMJ*. 2010;340:c810.)

patients about the longevity and quality of their sexually active lives assuming good health could motivate patients to stop smoking, adhere to medication regimens, exercise regularly, or engage in other health-promoting behaviors. Further research is needed to evaluate the potential impact of sexually active life expectancy projections on individual health behavior. The sexually active life expectancy measure also quantifies years of sexually active life lost in the absence of knowledge and treatments to preserve sexual function as people age.

Sexual Problems

Among sexually active women, approximately half reported having one bothersome sexual problem; almost one-third reported having two. The most common sexual problems experienced by older women are summarized in **Table 35-3**. Lack of interest in sex, pain with intercourse, unpleasurable sex, and inability to experience orgasm are much more common among older women as compared to men and somewhat more common compared to younger women. Because some sexually inactive women discontinued sexual activity as a result of bothersome sexual problems, the NSHAP baseline study underestimates the prevalence of problems in the whole population. On the other hand, many women engage in sex despite bothersome problems. The rewards or gains of sexual engagement may outweigh the experience of sexual pain or lack of physical pleasure; some women may obligatorily participate in sex to satisfy their partner while others may lack agency to refuse.

Problems related to sexuality in later life can result from sexually transmitted infection, trauma, and sexual violence or abuse. These topics are discussed below. Sexual dysfunction, including clinical diagnosis and treatment, is discussed later in this chapter.

Sexually Transmitted Infections (STIs)

Data from the NHANES and the baseline NSHAP study provide the population prevalence of STIs among older women. Overall, the prevalence of most STIs in the general older adult population is very low (< 1% for *Chlamydia trachomatis*, *Neisseria gonorrhea*, and syphilis), although rates of some infections may be higher in residential communities or geographic regions with high concentrations of sexually active older adults (eg, Florida and Hawaii in the United States), or in other subpopulations. A prevalence estimate for *Trichomonas vaginalis* among older US women is not available; late twentieth-century data from Danish and Chinese epidemiologic studies indicate that very few cases occur among women 60 years and older. Changes in the cervical epithelium caused by loss of estrogen in older women may account for reduced susceptibility to these infections. Although there is no evidence for an epidemic, STI prevalence among older adults is likely underestimated because of lack of uniform tracking systems and under-identification in the clinical setting. One study showed that physicians were likely to counsel older African-American and married women about human immunodeficiency virus (HIV) and other STIs, but the majority of older women reported that a physician has never initiated such discussion.

Viral infections, including genital herpes simplex virus (HSV) and human papillomavirus (HPV), are the

TABLE 35-3 ■ MOST COMMON SEXUAL PROBLEMS AMONG A POPULATION-BASED SAMPLE OF OLDER WOMEN IN THE UNITED STATES (*N* = 1550)			
	PERCENTAGE BY AGE GROUP (95% CONFIDENCE INTERVAL)		
	57–64	65–74	75–85
Lack of interest in sex (*n* = 504)	44 (37–52)	38 (30–47)	49 (37–62)
Difficulty with lubrication (*n* = 495)	36 (30–42)	43 (35–52)	44 (27–60)
Inability to climax (*n* = 479)	34 (28–40)	33 (25–41)	38 (24–53)
Pain during intercourse (*n* = 506)	18 (13–22)	19 (11–26)	12 (4.3–19)
Sex not pleasurable (*n* = 498)	24 (18–30)	22 (15–29)	25 (15–35)
Anxiety with performance (*n* = 500)	10 (6.3–15)	13 (6.1–19)	9.9 (1.7–18)
Avoided sex because of problems (*n* = 357)	34 (25–44)	31 (22–39)	23 (9.4–36)

Note: Estimates are weighted to account for differential probabilities of selection and differential nonresponse. Data in this table reflect prevalence among those of 1550 women surveyed in the National Social Life, Health and Aging Project who reported having sex in the last 12 months and having at least one sexual problem.
Data from Lindau ST, Schumm LP, Laumann EO, et al. A study of sexuality and health among older adults in the United States. N Engl J Med. 2007;357(8):762–774.

more prevalent STIs among older women. HSV-2 sero-prevalence among men and women 70 years and older based on NHANES III data (1988–1994) was 28%, but women had a higher overall prevalence than men and rates were much higher among African-Americans (74%) and Mexican Americans (45%). High-risk, or oncogenic, HPV (HR-HPV) prevalence among women aged 57 to 85, based on 2005–2006 NSHAP data, was 6% and did not vary significantly across age or racial/ethnic groups. The prevalence of HR-HPV among older women is similar to that documented by NHANES for women aged 50 to 59. HR-HPV is an important factor in both cervical dysplasia and cervical cancer, a leading cause of female cancer death in the world. In the United States, about 20% of cervical cancer cases, but more than a third of cervical cancer deaths, occur in women aged 65 and older. Most screening and prevention strategies, including HPV vaccine, use age-based eligibility criteria that exclude older women.

The rate of new HIV infection among older women in the United States, particularly those of minority racial and ethnic groups, has been increasing over the last several years, due mostly to transmission by heterosexual sex. Mucosal atrophy (vaginal, rectal) related to menopausal estrogen depletion increases an older woman's susceptibility to mucosal tears and abrasions that can facilitate HIV transmission. In 2010, 27% of Americans diagnosed with HIV/AIDS after age 50 were women. Public health messages regarding HIV/AIDS prevention and detection do not target older women, and physicians rarely offer HIV counseling or testing to this group. The effects of HIV/AIDS and treatments on sexual function among older women have been minimally investigated. Please see Chapter 107 for further discussion of HIV in later life.

STI prevention strategies for older adults have not been well-tested. Counseling women with new or multiple sexual partners warrants discussion of STI prevention, including education about barrier methods such as male and female condoms and dental dams (for oral sex) (**Figure 35-4**). Few older adults, including those in nonmarital sexual relationships, report using condoms. Condom use by older couples to prevent STIs may be compromised by the belief that condoms are not necessary if there is no risk of pregnancy; by changes in male and female physiology that occur with age;

and by knowledge, communication, and cultural barriers as seen in younger age groups. A male condom is best applied when the penis is fully erect, but for some older men, full erection may not occur until after coitus is initiated. Female condom use does not require a fully erect penis and may be preferable for some couples.

For women, increased susceptibility to condom-induced vaginal irritation or abrasion may result from vaginal dryness and/or atrophy caused by estrogen depletion. Foreplay is encouraged to stimulate full penile erection and maximal female arousal before attempting vaginal or other penetration. Use of water or silicone type lubricants is recommended to reduce vaginal and vulvar friction in couples using condoms (oil-based lubricants can reduce condom effectiveness). Because they dry quickly, water-based lubricants may actually increase vaginal friction. Condoms with spermicide are not necessary for post-reproductive age women and should be avoided because they have a shorter shelf-life and have been associated with urinary tract infection in younger women. Nonlatex male and female condoms and dental dams are available for individuals with latex sensitivities and allergies, and they have physical and performance properties that some individuals may prefer. Male and female condoms and dental dams are for one-time use only.

Medicare annual wellness visits are an ideal opportunity for physicians to assess their patients' sexual history, although sexual history-taking is not included in the CMS quick reference document for the annual wellness visit. Medicare does cover HIV testing, and, for at-risk individuals, chlamydia, gonorrhea, syphilis, and hepatitis B tests. People at increased risk of STIs can receive up to two individual 20- to 30-minute, intensive in-person behavioral counseling sessions each year. These counseling sessions can include education, skills training, and guidance on safe sexual behavior and may help mitigate the competing clinical issues that prevent discussion of safer-sex practices during routine visits.

Sexual Trauma, Violence, and Abuse

Early life events, including sexual trauma in the form of abuse, exploitation, genital injury, and rape, can have lasting effects on sexuality and health that persist into later life.

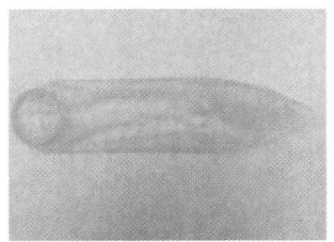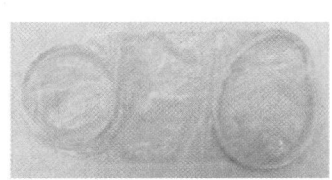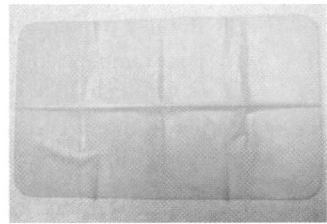

FIGURE 35-4. Barrier methods of sexual protection. Latex male condom *(left)*, nitrile female condom *(middle)*, dental dam *(right)*.

Lifetime estimates among older women indicate that 20% to 26% of women experience intimate partner violence; nearly 40% in one study reported that this was severe, including forced sex or sexual contact. In the NSHAP baseline study, 9% of women aged 57 to 85 reported a lifetime history of forced sex (which may or may not have been with an intimate partner); of these, nearly 40% reported that the most recent event occurred at or younger than age 19 and 16% reported that the most recent event occurred after age 40. Sexual dysfunction, particularly conditions such as vaginismus, dyspareunia, inability to experience orgasm, lack of pleasure with sex, and disturbing fantasies are more common among women with a history of sexual trauma, violence, or abuse. In conjunction with medical treatment and/or physical therapy, psychotherapy can be effective in helping women cope with sexual violence and experience positive sexual relationships.

Elder mistreatment, or abuse, discussed in Chapter 48, is defined by the US CDC to include sexual abuse or abusive sexual contact but is not limited to an intimate partner. In fact, lack of a spouse or other partner, cognitive impairment, and institutionalization are risk factors for female sexual abuse and rape in later life. Very little is known about how commonly older women experience sexual violence or abuse; 3% of women aged 60 and older in one study reported having been pressured to have sex in a way they did not like or want since age 55. Few older women report that a physician has ever asked questions to ascertain sexual victimization. There is not sufficient evidence to support the accuracy of existing screening tools to identify abuse in older adults, and studies of interventions to address sexual trauma focus almost exclusively on younger women, perhaps explaining why physicians may feel ill-prepared to screen for victimization among older women. Screening questions for identifying intimate partner violence in the clinical setting are summarized in **Table 35-4** and should be part of routine assessment of the older woman.

In acute or emergency care settings, intimate partner violence and sexual abuse should be considered when a woman presents with physical injury, vague symptoms (especially in recurrent visits), acute mental status changes,

TABLE 35-4 ■ SAMPLE INTIMATE PARTNER VIOLENCE SCREENING QUESTIONS

When to ask	**In private settings** **During new patient visits and annual examinations**
How to frame	**Normalize topic** For example, "We've started talking to all of our patients about safe and healthy relationships because it can have such a large impact on your health."
How to ensure confidentiality	**Explain confidentiality** For example, "Before we get started, I want you to know that everything here is confidential, meaning that I won't talk to anyone else about what is said…" **Note disclosure laws** For example, "…unless you tell me that [insert the laws in your state about what is necessary to disclose]"[a]
Sample questions	**"Does your partner threaten you or make you feel afraid?"** For example, threatened to hurt you if you did not do something, controlled who you talked to or where you went, went into rages **"Has your partner ever hit, choked, or physically hurt you?"** For example, hit, slapped, licked, bitten, pushed, shoved you **"Has your partner forced you to do something sexual that you did not want to do?"**
For women with disabilities:	**"Has your partner prevented you from using a wheelchair, cane, respirator, or other assistive device?"** **"Has your partner refused to help you with an important personal need, or threatened not to help you with these personal needs?"** For example, taking your medicine, getting to the bathroom, getting out of bed, bathing, getting dressed, or getting food or drink
For older women[b]:	**"Has anyone prevented you from getting food, clothes, medication, glasses, hearing aids, or medical care, or from being with people you wanted to be with?"**[b] **"Has anyone made you afraid, touched you in ways that you did not want, or hurt you physically?"**[b]

[a]For more information on mandatory reporting policies in your state, refer to Mandatory Reporting of Domestic Violence by Health Care Providers, available for free download from Futures without Violence http://www.futureswithoutviolence.org/mandatory-reporting-of-domestic-violence-by-healthcare-providers/.

[b]Items are from the Elder Abuse Suspicion Index (Yaffe MJ, Tazkarji B. Understanding elder abuse in family practice. *Can Fam Physician*. 2012;58:1336–1340). Please see Chapter 48 for complete screening tool for elder abuse.

Adapted with permission from ACOG Committee Opinion No. 518. Intimate partner violence. Obstet Gynecol. 2012;119(2 Pt 1):412–417.

and/or is accompanied by a partner or other individual who interferes with the patient's interaction with health care providers.

FEMALE SEXUAL RESPONSE CYCLE

The Masters and Johnson model of the female sexual response cycle (**Figure 35-5A**), based on physiologic research initiated in the 1960s with a convenience sample of local sex workers, other volunteers, and patients presenting for treatment of sexual problems or contraception, remains the most widely represented model in medical textbooks and historically was the foundation for the Diagnostic and Statistical Manual definitions for sexual dysfunction. This traditional, linear model describes four phases of human sexual response: excitement, plateau, orgasm, and resolution (sex therapist Helen Singer Kaplan modified this model in 1979 to include orgasm, excitement, and desire) and illustrates notable differences in female as compared with male sexual physiology.

According to Masters and Johnson, the female sexual response is more variable than that of males, and female orgasm may be single and peak-like similar to male orgasm, more gradual or undulating, and/or repetitive during a single sexual encounter. The typical male sexual response is described as much more uniform, peaking in a single orgasm, and includes a latency period during which a subsequent orgasm cannot occur. Arousal for women tends to require direct clitoral or periclitoral stimulation and, for many women, nipple areolar complex stimulation, before, during, and/or after intercourse (which may involve penile-vaginal, penile-anal, oral, or manual penetration) in order to experience orgasm. Sufficient arousal with vaginal lubrication (physiologic or with a lubricant) before vaginal penetration may be particularly important for the older woman engaging in vaginal intercourse with a male sex partner because of reduction in the firmness and fullness of the male erection in later life.

The pattern of female sexual response may vary across time and relationships, although little is known empirically about the physiology of the female sexual response cycle in later life or in the context of very long-term (several decades or more) relationships. Psycho-emotional changes, and changes in physical appearance with age, can negatively or positively affect an older woman's feeling of attractiveness, and can influence her interest in sex. Some women indicate decreased psychological inhibition about physical appearance or improved self-image with age, both of which can be sexually liberating.

As men age, the sexual response becomes more similar to that of women (a phenomenon some refer to as "feminization of the male sexual response cycle"). Tactile stimulation and foreplay are increasingly important for older male arousal, the time to erection and orgasm is longer, and latency between orgasms (the refractory period) is increased. Because few older men or women are aware of these phenomena, these changes often cause unnecessary anxiety and shame, leading some couples to cease sexual activity as a consequence. The changes to sexual physiology that occur with age may be beneficial to some couples, as the mutual need for foreplay and the longer arousal phase in men makes it easier for some couples to experience simultaneous orgasm. Older couples should be provided basic information about the normative changes to sexual function that occur with aging. The National Institute on Aging offers an "AgePage" on this topic (http://www.nia.nih.gov/health/publication/sexuality-later-life); the American Association of Retired Persons (AARP) also offers accessible, consumer-focused information about sexuality and intimacy in its publications. WomanLab.org, a resource from the University of Chicago Program in Integrative Sexual Medicine, was codeveloped with aging women to fill gaps in public and clinician understanding of female sexuality in the context of aging and illness.

Building on the pioneering work of Masters and Johnson, Basson proposed a widely referenced intimacy-based, cyclical model of the female sexual response that incorporates the quality and duration of the relationship as well as the psycho-emotional component of female sexuality (**Figure 35-5B**). In women, sexual desire may occur before or following sexual arousal. This model emphasizes the role of intimacy in generating female sexual desire and suggests that lack of intimacy and unsatisfying sexual encounters can raise the threshold for interest and arousal in a subsequent sexual encounter. Rather than linear and discrete, the phases of the female sexual response are described by Basson as variably overlapping in a way that "blends mind and body."

Further empirical characterization of the physiology and psychosocial aspects of the female sexual response cycle in later life, including how it might fluctuate within relationships over long durations of time, across relationships, and with aging, is needed both to inform women's expectations and the clinical approach to older women's sexuality.

FEMALE SEXUAL PHYSIOLOGY IN LATER LIFE

Effects of senescence on the endocrine, neurovascular, musculoskeletal, genitourinary, and gastrointestinal systems are particularly salient to sexual function in later life. Global changes in physical appearance, sensory function (hearing, vision, olfaction, taste, and tactile sensation), cognitive function and memory, and body aromas such as scent, breath, and genital odor can also affect sexual engagement and enjoyment. The female sexual response involves a complex and highly interconnected series of physiologic events connecting mind and body. Disruptions in these physiologic systems caused by age-related changes, physical or mental illness, or medical procedures and medication use can alter the sexual response and the ability of a

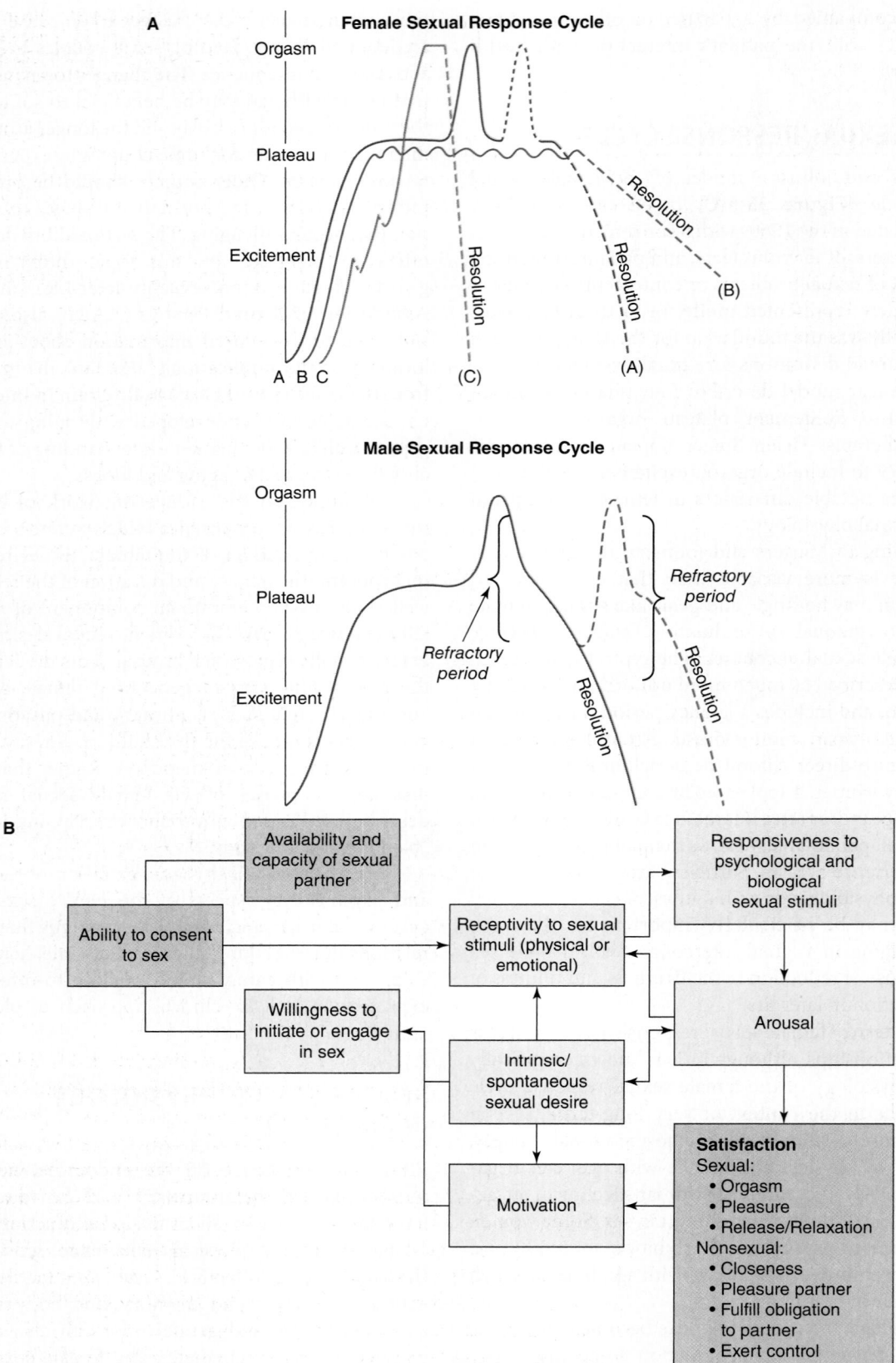

FIGURE 35-5. A. Masters' and Johnson's models of sexual response cycles for females and males. *Note: In female sexual response cycle, A, B, and C refer to three different sexual response patterns found in females.* **B.** Adaptation (blue) of Basson's model (pink) of the partnered female sexual response cycle highlighting features pertinent to older women (blue). (A, Reproduced with permission from Masters W, Johnson V. *Human Sexual Response.* Boston, MA: Little, Brown and Company; 1966. B, Adapted with permission from Basson R. The female sexual response: a different model. *J Sex Marital Ther.* 2000;26[1]:51–65.)

woman to derive pleasure and satisfaction from her sexual encounters.

Endocrine System, Menopause, and the Genitourinary System

Loss of estrogen due to menopause is a dominant physiologic event that can affect many aspects of older women's sexual function. Women can live a third or more of life in menopause: the median age of natural menopause in the United States is 51 and average female lifespan is 81 years. Surgical menopause occurs when a woman undergoes bilateral oophorectomy (or loses ovarian function as a result of other interventions such as chemotherapy or radiation) prior to natural menopause. In the NSHAP study, about one in five US women aged 57 to 85 reported a history of surgical menopause. Women who have undergone bilateral oophorectomy, pre- or postmenopause, also experience an abrupt and irreversible loss of androgen production.

Estrogen is important for maintaining skin, subcutaneous, mucosal (vaginal, bladder, and rectal) and musculoskeletal integrity, the vaginal microenvironment (pH balance and microflora), vascular flow to the vagina and clitoris via regulation of nitric oxide synthase expression, and sensory perception. Over time, low estrogen results in vaginal dryness, loss of epithelial cell glycogen, shortening of the vagina, narrowing of the introitus, thinning of the labia, and diminution of the fat pad underlying the mons pubis. Loss of vaginal acidity results from glycogen depletion and can increase propensity for bacterial vaginitis. Urinary and fecal incontinence can be exacerbated by estrogen depletion and inhibit social and sexual relationships as well as sexual function. The term genitourinary syndrome of menopause (GSM) was adopted in 2014 to encompass the constellation of genital and urinary signs and symptoms attributed to the absence of estrogen and aging (**Table 35-5**). Maintenance of sexual activity in later life appears to offset some of these local genital changes, in part by maintaining elasticity of the vulvovaginal tissues, pelvic floor musculature, and pelvic joints. Additionally, sexual activity and other forms of physical contact may mitigate estrogen-related decline in sensory perception and function with age and may play a role in female attractiveness. Exogenous estrogen is approved by the US Food and Drug Administration (FDA) for treatment of moderate to severe dyspareunia in women. Details of estrogen treatment, including a table of available preparations, and treatment of other genitourinary disorders affecting sexual function are provided in Chapter 36.

Testosterone, along with dehydroepiandrosterone (DHEA), plays an important role in female libido, arousal, genital sensation, and orgasm. Loss of testosterone can exacerbate vaginal mucosal atrophy, thinning of pubic hair, and may compromise an older woman's sense of general well-being. Female androgen insufficiency as a treatable condition is controversial. While levels of endogenous androgens have not been found to be predictive of sexual function, a large meta-analysis confirmed that testosterone

TABLE 35-5 ■ AGE-ASSOCIATED GENITOURINARY CHANGES & SYMPTOMS

ANATOMIC CHANGES
Narrowing and shortening of vaginal barrel
Decreased elasticity of vaginal mucosa
Atrophy of vaginal mucosa
Hypopigmentation of vaginal mucosa and erythema
Loss of vaginal folds
Increased vaginal fragility/friability/fissures/petechiae
Loss of labia minora
Uterine/vaginal prolapse
Urethral eversion, prolapse, or atrophy

PHYSIOLOGIC CHANGES
Decreased lubrication
Reduced vaginal blood flow
Increased vaginal pH
Decreased epithelial glycogen content and lactobacilli

SYMPTOMS
Vulvovaginal dryness/irritation/burning/tenderness
Vulvovaginal itching
Recurrent urinary tract infections
Dysuria/pain or discomfort with urination
Increased urinary frequency/urgency
Bleeding associated with intercourse
Dyspareunia/pain or discomfort with intercourse
Decreased arousal/libido
Difficulty achieving orgasm

Note: Although these are common symptoms associated with age, they do warrant medical evaluation for treatment and to rule out other causes like contact irritant dermatitis, vulvar dermatoses, infections, and dysplasia or cancer of the urogenital tract. *Data from Portman DJ, Gass ML; Vulvovaginal Atrophy Terminology Consensus Conference Panel. Genitourinary syndrome of menopause: new terminology for vulvovaginal atrophy from the International Society for the Study of Women's Sexual Health and the North American Menopause Society. Maturitas. 2014;79(3):349–354.*

therapy for low libido was effective in clinical trials involving women with bilateral oophorectomy or total loss of ovarian function, as well as postmenopausal women with or without use of estrogen therapy (estrogen reduces bioavailable testosterone by increasing sex hormone–binding globulin production). However, the FDA has not approved testosterone for this indication. Use of testosterone or DHEA to treat female sexual dysfunction is currently off-label in the United States and most countries, and requires close monitoring for side effects. Although rare, irreversible deepening of the voice and growth of facial hair may occur with testosterone use. In the 2019 Global Consensus Position Statement, an international task force found physiologic dosing of testosterone was not associated with severe side effects; however, long-term safety and efficacy have not been established in postmenopausal women.

CHAPTER 35
SEXUALITY, SEXUAL FUNCTION, AND THE AGING WOMAN

Central Effects on Sexual Function

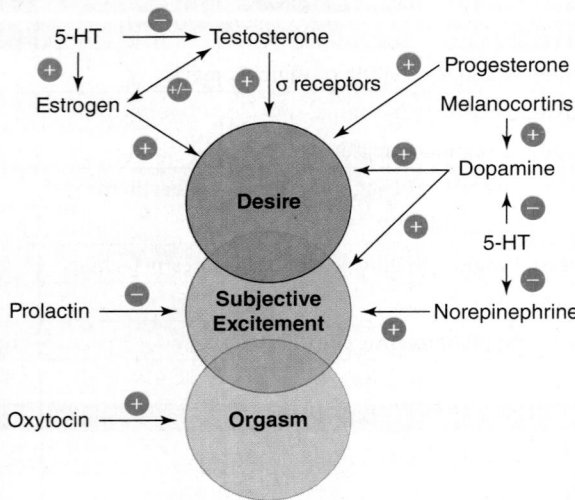

Peripheral Effects on Sexual Function

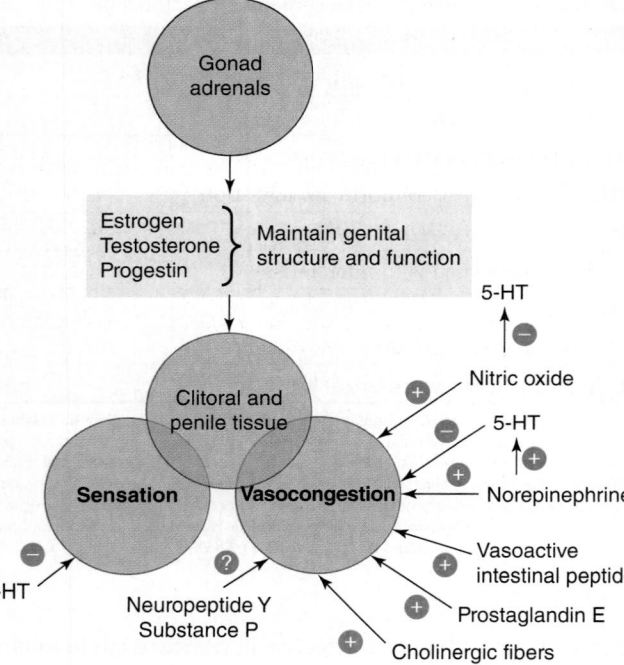

FIGURE 35-6. Central and peripheral effects on sexual function. *Note: + indicates a positive effect, – indicates a negative effect, ? indicates the effect is unknown; 5-HT: 5-hydroxytryptamine (serotonin). (Adapted with permission from Clayton AH. Sexual function and dysfunction in women. Psychiatr Clin North Am. 2003;26[3]:673–682.)*

Figure 35-6 summarizes central and peripheral hormonal mediators of sexual function (see also Chapter 97). Understanding centrally mediated neuroendocrine changes that occur with senescence is an active area of discovery, focused heavily on understanding cognitive pathophysiology. In women and female animal studies, interest in the cascade of neuroendocrine events resulting in menopause has been similarly driven by an effort to understand the role of sex hormones and hormone therapy in neuroplasticity and degeneration, as well as by efforts to treat female infertility. Application of this knowledge to female sexual function in later life, particularly sex differences in endocrine regulation of the sexual response cycle, is nascent.

Aside from its peripheral effects, estrogen plays an important central role via direct membrane receptor activity and modulation of neurotransmitters. Estrogen appears to exert neurotrophic and neuroprotective activity in the brain that mitigates hypothalamic damage that occurs with age. Estrogen also interacts with serotonin and norepinephrine metabolism, which may explain the role of estrogen depletion in sleep, mood, memory, and, through these and no doubt other mechanisms, the female sexual response cycle in later life.

The hypothalamic-pituitary-adrenal (HPA) axis mediates the human physiologic stress response and, of course, is the pathway or pacemaker through which sex hormonal regulation occurs. The loss of temporality and pulsatility in HPA neural signaling is a key event in menopause; the dynamics of HPA function over the portion of the lifespan following menopause and the implications for female sexual functioning in later life are much less well-defined. Vasoactive intestinal peptide (VIP), now recognized to play a role in female sexual arousal via vasocongestion of the clitoral tissue, also signals time of day information for central gonadotropin-releasing hormone (GnRH) regulation. Rhythmic synthesis of VIP in the brain appears to wane by middle age in women and may be an important triggering event in the loss of hypothalamic-pituitary-ovarian access coordination required for ovulation and menstruation. The peripheral effects of changes in central VIP metabolism for later life sexual arousal in women are unknown.

Neurovascular System

Neurovascular physiology, mediated by the sympathetic and parasympathetic nervous systems and a growing list of nonadrenergic/noncholinergic neurotransmitters (eg, nitric oxide and VIP), is particularly important for the arousal and orgasm phases of the female sexual response cycle. Arousal involves vascular engorgement of the genitopelvic organs, including the labia, vagina, and clitoris; lengthening, dilation, and lubrication of the vagina; retraction of the clitoral hood; and tumescence of the clitoris. Microvascular integrity is important for genital sensation and orgasm. Clitoral sensation, in particular, can be compromised by microvascular disease as seen in chronic smokers and women with hypercholesterolemia or diabetes. Although clinical guidelines for diabetes care in men advise assessment and treatment of erectile problems, clinical guidelines for women do not go beyond screening for sexual dysfunction. Research on effective treatment options for sexual dysfunction among older women with diabetes is needed to inform clinical guidelines. Women with diagnosed diabetes are less likely than men to have discussed sexual problems with a physician and more likely to cease all sexual activity.

Cardiovascular disease can impair women's sexual function in later life both through psychological and physiologic mechanisms. Although practice guidelines recommend that physicians communicate with patients about the sexual implications of heart disease and potential sexual side effects of treatment, these issues are commonly omitted from counseling, and men are significantly more likely than women to receive such counsel.

Treated and untreated hypertension are both associated with lower rates of sexual activity among older women. However, among sexually active older women, the rate of sexual problems is similar among women with treated hypertension, untreated hypertension, and no hypertension. No one class of antihypertensives has been consistently associated with female sexual dysfunction, particularly in older women. Based on expert opinion, older women with hypertension should be counseled that treatment of hypertension is likely to improve overall sexual function and longevity.

Acute myocardial infarction (AMI) is an important health problem in older women. United States and European practice guidelines state that patients with uncomplicated AMI can resume sexual activity within a week of AMI. Based on the largest study to date of sexual outcomes in AMI among older women, the majority of those who were sexually active before their AMI resume sexual activity within 1 year following AMI. Receipt of counseling by a physician about resuming sex is the single most important predictor of whether a woman resumes sexual activity after AMI.

Phosphodiesterase inhibitors are used in men to treat neurovascular causes of erectile dysfunction; similar effectiveness has not been found in women. The only FDA-approved device for treatment of female sexual dysfunction, the Eros Therapy (UroMetrics) clitoral pump, may assist some women with microvascular disease in experiencing improved clitoral sensation, vaginal lubrication, and orgasm.

Musculoskeletal System and Body Fat

Parity, childbirth-related injury, pelvic or lower extremity trauma, obesity, and sedentariness can compromise the integrity of the vulvar, pelvic floor, and lower extremity musculature, contributing to incontinence and pelvic organ prolapse. Effective contraction and relaxation of the peri-introital, perineal, and pelvic floor muscles are important for penetration, arousal, orgasm, and the relaxation phase following orgasm. Loss of flexibility of hip muscles and compromised stability and mobility of hip joints, commonly experienced by women with arthritis or hip fracture, can interfere with sexual functioning in later life. Skeletal changes in the hips and vertebrae caused by loss of bone density, osteoporosis, vertebral compression and fracture, and arthritis can make vaginal penetration, particularly using "missionary" (female supine with hips and knees flexed) position, difficult and may be accommodated by use of alternative sexual positioning such as side-lying or

sex without vaginal penetration. Prevention and treatment of these conditions with attention to maximizing musculoskeletal strength and flexibility can improve overall physical functioning and help preserve sexual capacity for aging women. Endorphin release associated with pleasurable sexual activity may help alleviate musculoskeletal pain.

Although more than a third of women age 65 and older are obese, little is known about the effect of obesity on older women's sexual function and satisfaction. Research is further complicated by women's varying self-appraisals of their body size and attractiveness, the frequent co-occurrence of obesity and chronic disease among older women, and the potentially different contributions of abdominal adiposity, generalized obesity, and relative weight gain postmenopause.

Gastrointestinal System

Gastrointestinal changes with aging that are most relevant to female sexual function include incontinence of stool and flatus, hemorrhoids, and borborygmi. Anal or stool incontinence typically results in cessation of sexual activity and can be socially isolating. Hemorrhoids can be exacerbated by sexual activity, particularly anal intercourse, and may result in bleeding during or following sex. Borborygmi can be controlled to some degree by timing of meals in relation to symptoms. Constipation can be a cause of dyspareunia; this can be overcome by treating the primary cause of constipation and educating the patient to time sexual activity after moving her bowels. Older women should be screened and evaluated for anal and urinary incontinence, especially those who have ceased and/or wish to resume sexual activity after a hiatus, as both are commonly overlooked as contributors to female sexual function. Treatment should be initiated in order to prevent embarrassing or painful sexual experiences that can be very detrimental to sexual self-image and function.

Cancer and Female Sexual Function

The vast majority of cancers affecting older women involve treatment with local or systemic therapies that impair or surgically remove the sexual organs. Most women who develop cancer value their sexual function and wish to preserve the possibility of future sexual activity. All women, regardless of age or current partner status, undergoing treatment for cancer should be counseled about the potential effects of cancer or its treatment on future sexual function, and baseline sexual activity and function (prior to cancer treatment) should be documented. Women undergoing pelvic radiation should be offered vaginal dilation therapy to preserve vaginal capacity for sexual activity and future gynecologic examinations. The most common sexual function problems in this patient population include dyspareunia, commonly resulting from or exacerbated by severe vulvovaginal atrophy (VVA), and diminished or no libido. Compromised sexual function and painful or unsatisfying sexual activity may strain intimate partnerships and provoke anxiety about cancer recurrence. Repeated studies show that women with cancer, including older women, believe that physicians should discuss sexual outcomes and side effects of treatment. As in cardiovascular disease, women who report discussing sex with a physician are significantly less likely to avoid sex because of a sexual problem or to exhibit complex sexual morbidity.

SEXUAL HISTORY-TAKING

There is ample evidence that older women, including those who are not currently sexually active, regard sexual function as an important aspect of health, believe it is appropriate for physicians to discuss sexual issues in the context of medical care, and want physicians to be proactive in counseling about sexual outcomes or side effects of treatment. Avoidance of these matters can be deleterious, particularly for women who identify as a member of a sexual minority group. Geriatricians can signal their openness to all patients by posting commonly recognized symbols such as a rainbow flag or an explicit statement of respect for all human rights (**Figure 35-7**).

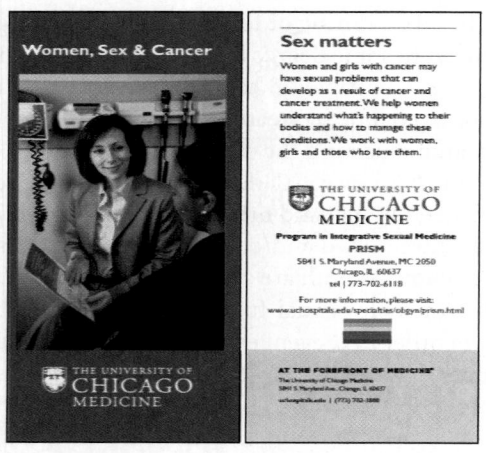

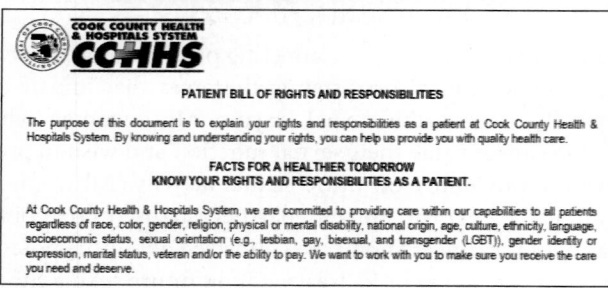

FIGURE 35-7. Examples of image and text indicating freedom from discrimination for lesbian, gay, bisexual, transsexual (LGBT) patients. Front (top left) and back (top right) of brochure for the Program in Integrative Sexual Medicine at the University of Chicago, showing rainbow flag icon indicating that LGBT patients are welcome; bottom: excerpt from patient bill of rights and responsibilities for the Cook County Health and Hospitals System indicating nondiscrimination policy. (Top, Reproduced with permission from anneryanphoto.com. Bottom, https://cookcountyhealth.org/wp-content/uploads/2014-03-27-Pt-Bill-of-Rights_2013-07-11-FINAL-English.pdf.)

Table 35-6 lists basic sexual history questions that can be incorporated into a routine geriatrics encounter and should be tailored to the individual's needs.

The geriatrician is also encouraged to include on patient self-report or review of system checklists a simple item such as, "Do you have any sexual problems or concerns?" The widely used PLISSIT model or the "therapeutic moment" approach described in **Tables 35-7A and B** can help guide a preliminary conversation about sexual concerns. When a patient presents with multiple concerns in addition to a sexual concern, the geriatrician should work with the patient to prioritize issues for the current visit, acknowledge the sexual concern, and suggest, if necessary, that the patient return for a visit focused specifically on that issue. The IBM (see **Figure 35-1**) provides a useful framework for more in-depth assessment of a patient's sexual concern. The geriatrician should inquire about the patient's biological or medical problems, psychological or emotional problems, and relational or social problems. If the patient is in a current relationship, the history should also inquire about the partner's health in these domains, whether there has been communication with the partner about the patient's sexual concerns, and whether the partner also has any sexual function difficulties.

FEMALE SEXUAL DYSFUNCTION

Use of terms like "dysfunction," "normal," and even "healthy" in relation to human sexuality requires caution and has been criticized, particularly in the feminist and psychology literatures. What is a normal level of sexual desire for older women? Is celibacy unhealthy? Few older women report same-sex partners, so is lesbianism abnormal? Is a distressing sexual difficulty a "dysfunction" or a "normal" response to unhappy circumstances in a relationship? Critiques are rooted in a painful history of sexual discrimination, particularly in the United States, and partially in medical history; as recently as the early 1990s, female sexual dysfunction could be diagnosed as a sexual problem experienced by a woman even if it was only troublesome to her partner. In addition, skeptics of the "medicalization" of female sexuality question how "normal" or "functional" sexuality can be defined as the absence of problems, given the high prevalence of sexual problems in the population.

Diagnostic Classification of Female Sexual Dysfunction

The *Diagnostic and Statistical Manual of Mental Disorders*, Fifth Edition (DSM-5) updates classification of female sexual dysfunction for clinical diagnosis (**Table 35-8**). The DSM-5 merges the conditions dyspareunia and vaginismus (classified separately in the DSM-IV) as genitopelvic pain/penetration disorder. Hypoactive sexual desire disorder and female arousal disorder are now defined as female sexual interest/arousal disorder.

TABLE 35-6 ■ SEXUAL HISTORY-TAKING AND SEXUAL EDUCATION IN THE ROUTINE GERIATRICS ENCOUNTER

Context	Ensure privacy Communicate comfort and matter-of-fact attitude If proxy required or requested, educate and engage that person	Educate patient about typical changes in sexuality that can occur with age and specific health conditions/treatments Educate about safety in sexual relationships
Transition	"To round out my understanding of your health/your health concerns today, may I ask you a couple of questions about your sexual life?"	Not always necessary, but can be useful if no other obvious transition Screening sexual history can easily come after questions ascertaining home setting, eg, "Who lives at home with you?" and "Are you safe in your home?"
Questions	"Do you currently have a spouse or other romantic, intimate, or sexual partner?" "How many partners have you had in the last year?" "Does your partner/partners have other sexual partners?" "Is your partner/partners male, female, or both?" "When is the last time you had sex?" *If no longer having sex:* "What are the reasons you stopped having sex?" "What type of sexual contact do you have: genital, anal, oral?" "Are you satisfied with your sexual life?" "Do you have any worries or difficulties with regard to your sexual life?" "How's your partner's health?" "Is your partner having any sexual problems?" "Has anyone ever forced you to have sex or sexual contact?" *If new partner or concern about risk factors:* "Have you and your partner been tested for sexually transmitted infections, including HIV/AIDS?" "Have you or your partner/partners tested positive for a STI?" "If so, which STI, how long ago, and were you both treated?" "Do you use condoms or other barrier methods to prevent sexually transmitted infection?" "If not, what is the reason?"	Opportunity to communicate awareness to the possibility of nonmonogamy Opportunity to communicate nonjudgment about same-sex relationships If patient responds yes, pursue questions summarized in **Table 35-10** or defer to a subsequent visit (see Conclusion) If patient responds yes or reveals risk factors, pursue questions summarized in **Table 35-4** Educate about testing, inform about confidential versus anonymous testing and meaning of test results Plan follow-up visit to provide posttest counseling Educate about barrier methods for sexually transmitted infection (STI) prevention
Conclusion	*If no problems identified or patient not sexually active:* "I want to encourage you to feel comfortable talking with me about any sexual concerns should they arise." *If problem(s) identified:* "I'm concerned about the problem you're having. Would you (and your partner) be willing to return (or be referred) to discuss this further?"	

Data from American College of Obstetricians and Gynecologist. Sexual Health. ACOG Committee Opinion No 706 Summary. Obstet Gynecol. 2017;130(1):25–252 and Simon JA, Davis SR et al. Sexual well-being after menopause: An International Menopause Society White Paper. Climacteric. 2018;21(5):415–427.

Population estimates of sexual problems from the cross-sectional NSHAP study (**Figure 35-8**) and other studies are useful for quantifying the baseline prevalence of sexual problems in later life, or even bothersome sexual problems, but should not be expected to translate precisely into population rates of female sexual dysfunction, clinically defined. Prevalence estimates for older women can be estimated from prior studies, but are needed for the newly

TABLE 35-7A ■ THE PLISSIT MODEL FOR ADDRESSING SEXUAL HEALTH NEEDS

P	Permission	Give the patient *permission* to raise concerns about her sexual health, legitimizing her concerns and acknowledging her sexuality	Ask, "Do you have any sexual problems or concerns?"
LI	Limited information	Give the patient *limited information* about the sexuality changes common to the patient's condition	General educational resources; eg, National Institute on Aging's "AgePage" on sexuality in later life Condition-specific resources; eg, American Cancer Society's patient information booklet on cancer
SS	Specific suggestions	Give the patient *specific suggestions* about sexual dysfunction and resumption of sexual activity	
IT	Intensive therapy	Give the patient more *intensive therapy* by connecting them with other professionals that can help with sexual concerns	The International Society for the Study of Women's Sexual Health (www.isswsh.org) Society for Sex Therapy and Research (www.sstarnet.org/) American Physical Therapy Association Section on Women's Health (www.womenshealthapta.org) International Organization of Physical Therapists in Women's Health (www.ioptwh.org)

Note: An extended version of the PLISSIT model (Ex-PLISSIT) was published by Davis and Taylor in 2006. The "extended" version includes permission-giving at each stage of interaction.
Adapted with permission from Annon J. The PLISSIT model: a proposed conceptual scheme for the behavioral treatment of sexual problems. J Sex Educ Ther. 1976;2(1):1–15.

defined classes of genitopelvic pain/penetration disorder and female sexual interest/arousal disorder.

Causes of Female Sexual Dysfunction

Sexual dysfunction in later life can be primary, such as a life-long history of bothersome low sexual desire, or secondary. Secondary causes include (1) interpersonal and personal psychological factors including depression and substance use, (2) biological factors including a wide spectrum of illnesses, injuries, physical disabilities, and their medical and surgical treatments (note that earlier life illness such as cancer and its treatment may have long-lasting effects on sexual function in survivors), and (3) social factors. The patient's psychosexual history and her current partner's physical and mental health, medications, substance use, and sexual function must also be investigated in order to gain a full picture of the patient's sexual functioning and to appropriately tailor therapeutic interventions. Common medications implicated among iatrogenic causes of sexual dysfunction are summarized in **Table 35-9**. Evidence for the effects of drugs on sexual dysfunction is mixed overall and very limited with respect to older females, specifically. Treatment of underlying disease and health concerns, including common problems like incontinence, vaginal atrophy, sleep dysfunction, and depression, is an essential first step to addressing sexual function problems. Sexual side effects of medications can be offset by improvement of disease-related symptoms and better overall health.

TABLE 35-7B ■ THERAPEUTIC MOMENT MODEL FOR ADDRESSING SEXUAL HEALTH NEEDS AS FOLLOWS:

	PROVIDER BEHAVIOR	EXAMPLE PROVIDER STATEMENT
Empathy	Acknowledge sexual health need and concerns	"I understand that this problem has been painful for you."
Validation	Share normative data and patient resources	"You are not alone. Other women experience this, but few talk about it."
Healing	Convey appropriateness of treating sexual health needs	"I would like to work with you to help solve this problem."
Expectations	Communicate that care may require multiple visits and limits of evidence in field	"More information is needed to fully understand and solve this problem."
Hope	Communicate positive outlook and realistic prognosis	"I am optimistic that we can make some changes to improve this problem."

TABLE 35-8 ■ DEFINITIONS OF FEMALE SEXUAL DYSFUNCTION FROM THE DSM-5

FEMALE SEXUAL INTEREST/AROUSAL DISORDER

Diagnostic Criteria

302.72 (F52.22)

A. Lack of, or significantly reduced, sexual interest/arousal, as manifested by at least three of the following:

1. Absent/reduced interest in sexual activity.
2. Absent/reduced sexual/erotic thoughts or fantasies.
3. No/reduced initiation of sexual activity, and typically unreceptive to a partner's attempts to initiate.
4. Absent/reduced sexual excitement/pleasure during sexual activity in almost all or all (approximately 75%–100%) sexual encounters (in identified situational contexts or, if generalized, in all contexts).
5. Absent/reduced sexual interest/arousal in response to any internal or external sexual/erotic cues (eg, written, verbal, visual).
6. Absent/reduced genital or nongenital sensations during sexual activity in almost all or all (approximately 75%– 100%) sexual encounters (in identified situational contexts or, if generalized, in all contexts).

B. The symptoms in Criterion A have persisted for a minimum duration of approximately 6 mo.

C. The symptoms in Criterion A cause clinically significant distress in the individual.

D. The sexual dysfunction is not better explained by a nonsexual mental disorder or as a consequence of severe relationship distress (eg, partner violence) or other significant stressors and is not attributable to the effects of a substance/medication or another medical condition.

Specify whether:

• **Lifelong:** The disturbance has been present since the individual became sexually active.

• **Acquired:** The disturbance began after a period of relatively normal sexual function.

Specify whether:

• **Generalized:** Not limited to certain types of stimulation, situations, or partners.

• **Situational:** Only occurs with certain types of stimulation, situations, or partners.

Specify current severity:

• **Mild:** Evidence of mild distress over the symptoms in Criterion A.

• **Moderate:** Evidence of moderate distress over the symptoms in Criterion A.

• **Severe:** Evidence of severe or extreme distress over the symptoms in Criterion A.

FEMALE ORGASMIC DISORDER

Diagnostic Criteria

302.73 (F52.31)

A. Presence of either of the following symptoms and experienced on almost all or all (approximately 75%–100%) occasions of sexual activity (in identified situational contexts or, if generalized, in all contexts):

1. Marked delay in, marked infrequency of, or absence of orgasm.
2. Markedly reduced intensity of orgasmic sensations.

B. The symptoms in Criterion A have persisted for a minimum duration of approximately 6 mo.

C. The symptoms in Criterion A cause clinically significant distress in the individual.

D. The sexual dysfunction is not better explained by a nonsexual mental disorder or as a consequence of severe relationship distress (eg, partner violence) or other significant stressors and is not attributable to the effects of a substance/medication or another medical condition.

Specify whether:

• **Lifelong:** The disturbance has been present since the individual became sexually active.

• **Acquired:** The disturbance began after a period of relatively normal sexual function.

Specify whether:

• **Generalized:** Not limited to certain types of stimulation, situations, or partners.

• **Situational:** Only occurs with certain types of stimulation, situations, or partners.

Specify if:

• **Never experienced an orgasm under any situation.**

(Continued)

TABLE 35-8 ■ DEFINITIONS OF FEMALE SEXUAL DYSFUNCTION FROM THE DSM-5 *(CONTINUED)*

FEMALE ORGASMIC DISORDER (Cont.)

Specify current severity:

- **Mild:** Evidence of mild distress over the symptoms in Criterion A.
- **Moderate:** Evidence of moderate distress over the symptoms in Criterion A.
- **Severe:** Evidence of severe or extreme distress over the symptoms in Criterion A.

GENITO-PELVIC PAIN/PENETRATION DISORDER

Diagnostic Criteria

302.76 (F52.6)

A. Persistent or recurrent difficulties with one (or more) of the following:

1. Vaginal penetration during intercourse.
2. Marked vulvovaginal or pelvic pain during vaginal intercourse or penetration attempts.
3. Marked fear or anxiety about vulvovaginal or pelvic pain in anticipation of, during, or as a result of vaginal penetration.
4. Marked tensing or tightening of the pelvic floor muscles during attempted vaginal penetration.

B. The symptoms in Criterion A have persisted for a minimum duration of approximately 6 mo.

C. The symptoms in Criterion A cause clinically significant distress in the individual.

D. The sexual dysfunction is not better explained by a nonsexual mental disorder or as a consequence of a severe relationship distress (eg, partner violence) or other significant stressors and is not attributable to the effects of a substance/medication or another medical condition.

Specify whether:

- **Lifelong:** The disturbance has been present since the individual became sexually active.
- **Acquired:** The disturbance began after a period of relatively normal sexual function.

Specify current severity:

- **Mild:** Evidence of mild distress over the symptoms in Criterion A.
- **Moderate:** Evidence of moderate distress over the symptoms in Criterion A.
- **Severe:** Evidence of severe or extreme distress over the symptoms in Criterion A.

Note: For more information on substance/medication-induced sexual dysfunction or other specified and unspecified sexual dysfunction refer to the DSM-5.
Reprinted with permission from the Diagnostic and Statistical Manual of Mental Disorders. 5th ed. (Copyright ©2013). American Psychiatric Association. All Rights Reserved.

CHAPTER 35   SEXUALITY, SEXUAL FUNCTION, AND THE AGING WOMAN

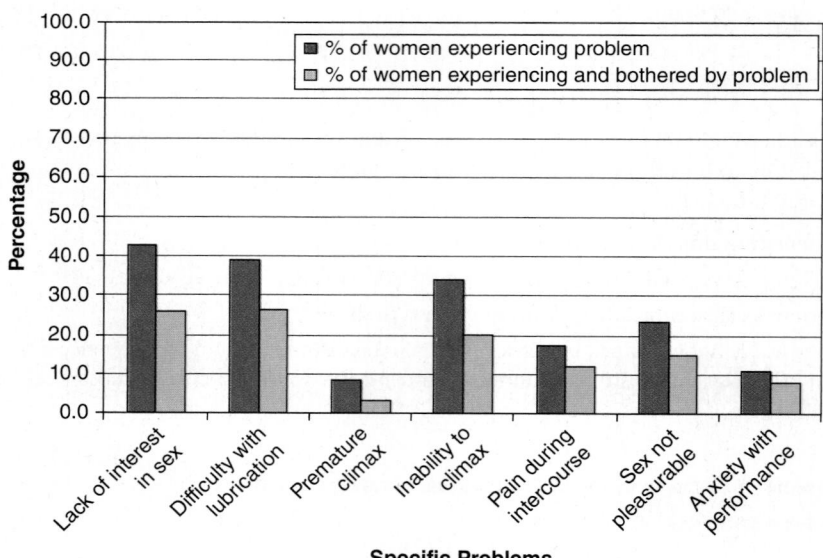

FIGURE 35-8. Prevalence of sexual problems and associated distress among a population-based sample of older women in the United States (*n* = 1550). *Note: Estimates are weighted to account for differential probabilities of selection and differential nonresponse. Data in this graph reflect prevalence among those of 1550 women surveyed in the National Social Life, Health and Aging Project who reported having sex in the last 12 months and having at least one sexual problem.* (Data from Lindau ST, Schumm LP, Laumann EO, et al. A study of sexuality and health among older adults in the United States. *N Engl J Med.* 2007;357[8]:762–774.)

TABLE 35-9 ■ DRUGS IMPLICATED IN SEXUAL DYSFUNCTION, ALTHOUGH RESEARCH IS NEEDED TO BUILD THE EVIDENCE BASE FOR THE EFFECTS OF MEDICATION ON FEMALE SEXUAL FUNCTION

Antiepileptics

Carbamazepine, phenobarbital, phenytoin, primidone

Cardiovascular and antihypertensive medications

Amiodarone, β-Adrenergic blockers,[a] calcium channel antagonists (diltiazem, nifedipine), clonidine, digoxin, diuretics (hydrochlorothiazide), lipid-lowering agents, methyldopa, prazosin, reserpine, spironolactone

Drugs affecting hormones

Aromatase inhibitors, cimetidine, raloxifene, spironolactone, tamoxifen

Histamine H$_2$ receptor blockers

Hormones

Estrogens, gonadotropin-releasing hormone agonist, progestins

Ketoconazole

Narcotic analgesics

Psychoactive/psychotropic medications

Amphetamines and related anorexic drugs, antipsychotics, barbiturates, benzodiazepines, lithium, monoamine oxidase inhibitors (MAOIs), opioids, selective serotonin reuptake inhibitors (SSRIs), serotonin-norepinephrine reuptake inhibitors (SNRIs), tricyclic antidepressants

Steroids

[a]No one class of antihypertensives has been consistently associated with female sexual dysfunction, particularly in older women.
Data from Phillips NA. Female sexual dysfunction: evaluation and treatment. Am Fam Physician. 2000;62(1):127–136; Drugs that cause sexual dysfunction: an update. Med Lett Drugs Ther. 1992;34:73–78; Kingsberg S. Taking a sexual history. Obstet Gynecol Clin North Am. 2006;33:535–547; Parish SJ, Hahn SR, et al. The International Society for the Study of Women's Sexual Health Process of Care for the Identification of Sexual Concerns and Problems in Women. 2019;94(5):842–856; Walsh KE, Berman JR. Sexual dysfunction in the older woman. Drugs Aging. 2004;21(10):655–675.

Clinical Evaluation of Sexual Dysfunction

Health care providers should routinely inquire about sexual function during visits to normalize the topic and establish a safe space to discuss concerns. Questions to assess sexual dysfunction are summarized in **Table 35-10**. Identification of the level of personal distress caused by each problem can be assessed informally by asking, "How much does this problem bother you?" and can be noted as a lot, somewhat, or not at all. Not uncommonly, an older woman will say she is not bothered by the problem, but is motivated to address it for relational purposes. The Derogatis Female Sexual Distress Scale (2002) and other research tools can be used to track change in distress over time, but have not been validated in geriatric-age women. We recommend the PROMIS sexual function measures (http://www.nih-promis.org/measures/availableinstruments).

Although many adult female sexual function problems have a psychosocial component, a thorough gynecologic physical examination by a skilled practitioner is needed to

TABLE 35-10 ■ QUESTIONS TO ASSESS SEXUAL DYSFUNCTION IN THE PRIMARY CARE SETTING

WHO	QUESTIONS
Individual *(Interview patient alone; interview partner alone if patient gives permission for partner to be interviewed)*	1. Clarify individual's view of the problem(s) and how s/he thinks s/he is coping 2. Review individual's sexual response to self-stimulation (see note in text regarding older women and masturbation) 3. Ask about individual's past partnered sexual experiences, including positive and negative aspects 4. Determine individual's developmental history: any losses or traumas, and how s/he coped 5. Inquire if individual ever experienced sexual, emotional, or physical abuse, whether as a child or as an adult

Couple	1. Ask couple to explain their sexual problem(s) in their own words
	2. Establish duration of problems, generalized or situational
	3. Determine context of sexual problems, including relationship quality
	4. Ask about the erotic context:
	  • What frequency of sex is expected or attempted?
	  • Are there concerns about safety from STIs or privacy?
	  • Adequacy of partner's sexual skills?
	  • Is there mutual communication about sexual needs?
	5. Determine the rest of the sexual response for each partner
	6. Inquire how each partner has reacted to the problem(s)
	7. Note any previous treatment(s), their compliance and benefit; clarify why couple is seeking help now and assess their motivation to make changes

Data from Basson R. Women's sexual dysfunction: revised and expanded definitions. CMAJ. 2005;172(10):1327–1333.

evaluate for underlying gynecologic pathologies that may be contributing to sexual function issues. Details of the routine gynecologic examination can be found in Chapter 36. A vulvar cotton swab test can be used to quantify and localize vulvar pain, although some have questioned specificity of this test. Graded vaginal dilators can be used to demonstrate to the patient her vaginal capacity and to educate her about dilation, a useful modality in women seeking to resume sexual intercourse after a long hiatus, in women with vaginal stenosis related to radiation or extreme atrophy, and in women with vaginismus. Using a hand mirror or diagram during the pelvic examination allows the patient to visualize genital findings and the depth of penetration with the examining finger, speculum, or a vaginal dilator. This information can be therapeutic and facilitate education about the patient's genital anatomy and any physical findings.

Clinical Management of Female Sexual Dysfunction

Although the evidence base for treatment of sexual problems in women is growing, few studies to date include women 65 years and older. Treatment of many sexual problems benefits from an interdisciplinary approach when possible, including thorough medical evaluation, and in some cases, physical and/or psychotherapy. Despite improved coverage of mental health services for Medicare beneficiaries, very few mental health professionals with expertise in geriatrics are also certified in sex therapy. The overview of clinical management presented here draws heavily on recommendations by the Female Sexual Dysfunction Practice Bulletin (Number 2013) updated in 2019 by the American College of Obstetricians and Gynecologists (ACOG), as well as the International Menopause Society White Paper

on sexual well-being after menopause, and uses DSM-5 classifications. It aims to give primary care providers initial treatment options. If available and affordable, referral to a specialist with experience in treatment of female sexual dysfunction may be optimal. Psychotherapy, including couples' and sex therapy, cognitive-behavioral approaches, mindfulness, and sensate focus techniques have been successfully implemented for treatment of female sexual dysfunction and can be adapted to the needs of older women and couples.

Genitopelvic Pain/Penetration Disorder

Genitopelvic pain/penetration disorder is more common during and after menopause, exacerbated by thinning of the vaginal mucosa, decreased vaginal lubrication, prolapse of the pelvic organs, and shortening of the vagina caused by natural or iatrogenic loss of estrogen. Pain, attributed to these physiologic changes, is a common reason for cessation of sexual activity among older women and couples. Management involves treatment of the underlying condition, as covered in Chapter 36. Lubricants are typically used to reduce friction during vaginal or anal penetration in women with dyspareunia and are also available in hundreds of variations over the counter (**Table 35-11**). Both moisturizers and lubricants may be used in conjunction with hormone therapy. Pelvic physical therapy is an

TABLE 35-11 ■ OVERVIEW OF VAGINAL LUBRICANTS AND MOISTURIZERS

	PROS	CONS
Lubricants (*Use immediately before or during intercourse to reduce friction*)		
Water-based	Inexpensive Compatible with latex and silicone Some varieties do not decrease sperm motility Best for women prone to yeast infections	Can dry out quickly Can feel tacky May contain glycerin and/or paraben[a]
Silicone-based	Does not dry easily Can be used in water Feels lush Compatible with latex	More expensive than water-based Difficult to wash off Incompatible with silicone and rubber Impairs sperm motility Not recommended for women prone to yeast infections
Oil-based	Stays slick longer Good for masturbation Natural Inexpensive Food-grade (eg, vegetable, olive, coconut, vitamin E oil)	Degrades condoms Impairs sperm motility
Moisturizers (*Use routinely, 2–3 times per week*)		
	Helps moisturize vaginal lining May make vaginal/surrounding tissue stronger and more pliable Works for several days Compatible with condoms	May contain glycerin[a]

[a]Glycerin has been suggested to increase the risk of yeast infection, although vaginal candidiasis is unlikely in a hypoestrogenic woman; paraben preservative is a common allergen.

effective modality for treating dyspareunia when there is a pelvic, abdominal, and/or low-back component to the dyspareunia and when vaginismus is present. Vaginal dilation with graded dilators or other devices and behavioral, sex, or couples' therapy are additional modalities that benefit many women with sexual pain disorders. Although, not FDA approved for treatment of VVA, energy-based laser devices, such as microablative fractional CO_2 and Erbium YAG lasers have shown promising short-term benefit in alleviation of symptoms due to VVA. It is important to note that in 2018 the US FDA issued warnings about injuries attributed to intravaginal lasers used as treatment for VVA.

Orgasm Disorder

Management depends heavily on whether the disorder is lifelong or acquired and situational or generalized. Acquired situational orgasmic disorder is most common and occurs in the setting of decreased libido and/or relational strain. Treatment primarily focuses on instruction in masturbation, also known as "sexual skills training." Because older women, particularly those 75 years and older, report less experience with masturbation (some report they have never masturbated), ability to assess orgasmic ability may be limited. Encouragement to self-stimulate either manually or with a vibrator must take into account the woman's experience with and attitudes about masturbation. Psychotherapy to assess psychological issues and attitudes regarding orgasm and to complement physical interventions may be necessary. Education about vulvar anatomy, the role of the clitoris in orgasm, and variations in female orgasm may be therapeutic for some women. Women with arousal disorders also commonly have difficulty experiencing orgasm, so evaluation of arousal should be included in women with this complaint. Sleep dysfunction is a common comorbidity in women with libido, arousal, and orgasm disorders.

Medical Therapy for Female Sexual Dysfunction

Currently there are three FDA-approved medical treatments for postmenopausal women experiencing sexual dysfunction: conjugated equine estrogen, ospemifene, and intravaginal prasterone, as discussed earlier. Other systemic and local exogenous estrogen products, especially local vulvovaginal estrogen cream and vaginal estrogen tablets and rings, are commonly used off-label to treat dyspareunia in menopausal women.

Hormone products have not been approved for use to treat female sexual interest/arousal disorder, but women treated with these products for VVA may experience improvement in desire and arousal that results from alleviation of dyspareunia. Two pharmaceuticals have been approved for treatment of "hypoactive sexual desire disorder," a term that was eliminated with the 2013 revisions to the DSM-5: flibanserin, a serotonin agonist/antagonist taken daily by mouth; and bremelanotide, a melanocortin-receptor-4 agonist given as a self-injection as needed before a sexual encounter. Neither drug has been approved for use in postmenopausal women

Androgen therapy, including testosterone and DHEA formulations, is being used off-label in some cases for treatment of sexual interest/arousal disorder. Systematic reviews have not shown efficacy with any of the DHEA formulations, but testosterone use has shown some benefit. However, side effects can be irreversible and safety is not established in older women. Tibolone, a synthetic steroid hormone, has been investigated for the treatment of sexual dysfunction in postmenopausal women but evidence of its benefits is limited and it is not approved by the FDA. Treatment of depression can improve sexual desire and interest, but some antidepressants, particularly selective serotonin reuptake inhibitors (SSRIs), can inhibit sexual interest. There is limited clinical data to inform treatment options for SSRI-induced sexual dysfunction, but decreasing or ceasing the SSRI dose, switching antidepressants, or using bupropion in combination with SSRIs to offset this side effect may be effective for some women.

Off-label use of phosphodiesterase inhibitors has also been tried for women with genital arousal disorder (a very small subset of women with sexual dysfunction); again, safety has not been established in older women and there is no convincing evidence that benefit outweighs risk. Tricyclic antidepressants and anticonvulsants are being used by some practitioners for treatment of vulvovestibulitis (a cause of dyspareunia), but these should be used with caution because of central nervous system side effects that may be exaggerated in older women, particularly those taking other medications.

Funding for intervention research in the area of female sexual dysfunction comes primarily from pharmaceutical sources supporting clinical trials of small numbers of young, healthy subjects followed for brief periods; even studies of postmenopausal women include only small numbers of older women. Building an evidence base is a necessary step to offering safe and effective medical, psychological, and other treatments for female sexual dysfunction in later life. Several drugs for treatment of female sexual dysfunction, particularly sexual interest/arousal disorder, are currently in preclinical and clinical trials. The FDA has held a patient-focused drug development public meeting and scientific workshop on female sexual dysfunction to learn from patients about their perspectives on female sexual dysfunction and the treatments currently available. As more treatment options for female sexual dysfunction become available, an increase in sexual activity among women in later life may occur.

CONCLUSION

Many aspects of older women's health have been neglected by researchers and clinicians, including sexuality. Sexual and intimate relationships in later life can promote health and well-being and sustain a basic human need.

Many older women engage in sexual relationships despite sexual problems and pain, while others discontinue sex caused by problems that could be treated. Physicians caring for older women can positively impact their patients' sexual functioning and overall well-being by initiating and fostering an open and ongoing dialogue about sexual matters in the context of healthy aging or in relation to medical conditions and their treatments. Public health messaging and medical education addressing the continued importance of sexual health discussions past reproductive age could help normalize late life female sexuality and validate older women's sexual health concerns. Research is needed to establish trajectories of older women's sexuality with aging especially among people identifying with racial, ethnic, and sexual minority groups, and to provide an evidence base for diagnosis and treatment of female sexual dysfunction in later life.

ACKNOWLEDGMENTS

We would like to acknowledge Amber Matthews, BA, and Isabella Joslin, BA, research assistants in the Lindau Laboratory at the University of Chicago, for their contribution to the review and synthesis of the literature. Additionally, we would like to acknowledge Amber Matthews for her work on data visualization, figures, and editing.

FURTHER READING

American College of Obstetricians and Gynecologists. Female sexual dysfunction. ACOG Practice Bulletin No. 213. *Obstet Gynecol.* 2019;134(1):203–205.

American College of Obstetricians and Gynecologist. Sexual Health. ACOG Committee Opinion No 706 Summary. *Obstet Gynecol.* 2017;130(1):251–252.

American Psychiatric Association. *Diagnostic and Statistical Manual of Mental Disorders: DSM-5.* Washington, DC: American Psychiatric Association; 2013.

Baron SR, Florendo J, Sandbo S, Mihai A, Lindau ST. Sexual pain disorders in women. *Clinician Reviews*; 2011. http://www.clinicianreviews.com/the-publication/past-issues-single-view/sexual-pain-disorders-in-women/59f19a0743f02eceb02c4bd7196c235c.html. Accessed March 24, 2016.

Basson R. The female sexual response: a different model. *J Sex Marital Ther.* 2000;26(1):51–65.

Basson R, Wierman ME, Van Lankveld J, Brotto L. Reports: summary of the recommendations on sexual dysfunctions in women. *J Sex Med.* 2010;7(1):314–326.

Davis SR, Baber R, Panay N, et al. Global consensus position statement on the use of testosterone therapy for women. *J Clin Endocrinol Metab.* 2019;104(10):4660–4666.

Fredriksen-Goldsen KI, Kim HJ, Emlet CA, et al. *The Aging and Health Report: Disparities and Resilience among Lesbian, Gay, Bisexual, and Transgender Older Adults.* Seattle, WA: Institute for Multigenerational Health; 2011.

Gaster B, Larson EB, Curtis JR. Advance directives for dementia: meeting a unique challenge. *JAMA.* 2017;318(22):2175–2176.

Hughes C. What you need to know about the Medicare preventive services expansion. *Family Pract Manag.* 2011;18(1):22–25.

Islam RM, Bell RJ, Green S, Page MJ, Davis SR. Safety and efficacy of testosterone for women: a systematic review and meta-analysis of randomized controlled trial data. *Lancet Diabetes Endocrinol.* 2019;79(10):754–766.

Joy M, Weiss KJ. Consent for intimacy among persons with neurocognitive impairment. *J Am Acad Psychiatry Law.* 2018;46(3):286–294.

Lindau ST, Dale W, Feldmeth G, et al. Sexuality and cognitive status: a U.S. nationally representative study of home-dwelling older adults. *J Am Geriatr Soc.* 2018; 66(10):1902–1910.

Lindau ST, Gavrilova N. Sex, health, and years of sexually active life gained due to good health: evidence from two US population based cross sectional surveys of ageing. *BMJ.* 2010;340:c810.

Lindau ST, Laumann EO, Levinson W, Waite LJ. Synthesis of scientific disciplines in pursuit of health: the Interactive Biopsychosocial Model. *Perspect Biol Med.* 2003; 46(suppl 3):S74–S86.

Lindau ST, Schumm P, Laumann, EO, Levinson W, O'Muircheartaigh C, Waite L. A national study of sexuality and health among older adults in the United States. *N Engl J Med.* 2007;357(8):762–774.

Lusti-Narasimhan M, Beard JR. Sexual health in older women. *Bull World Health Organ.* 2013;91(9):707–709.

Masters W, Johnson V. *Human Sexual Response.* Boston, MA: Little, Brown and Company; 1966.

Moyer VA. Screening for intimate partner violence and abuse of elderly and vulnerable adults: U.S. preventive services task force recommendation statement. *Ann Intern Med.* 2013;158(6):478–486.

National Institutes of Health. PROMIS: dynamic tools to measure health outcomes from the patient perspective. https://www.healthmeasures.net/explore-measurement-systems/promis. Accessed December 13, 2021.

National Institute on Aging. AgePage: sexuality in later life; Revised 2017. http://www.nia.nih.gov/sites/default/files/sexuality_in_later_life_0.pdf. Accessed December 14, 2020.

Parish SJ, Hahn SR, Goldstein SW, et al. The international society for the study of women's sexual health process of care for the identification of sexual concerns and problems in women. *Mayo Clin Proc.* 2019;94(5): 842–856.

Portman DJ, Gass ML. Vulvovaginal Atrophy Terminology Consensus Conference P. Genitourinary syndrome of menopause: new terminology for vulvovaginal atrophy from the International Society for the Study of Women's Sexual Health and the North American Menopause Society. *Maturitas.* 2014;79(3):349–354.

Russell BA, Bachmann GA, Chudnoff S, et al. Finding solutions for female sexual dysfunction. The American Congress of Obstetricians and Gynecologists; 2010. https://www.womentc.com/wp-content/uploads/2014/04/Finding-Solutions-for-FSD-ACOG.pdf. Accessed December 13, 2021.

Simon JA, Davis SR, Althof SE, et al. Sexual well-being after menopause: an International Menopause Society White Paper. *Climacteric.* 2018;21(5):415–427.

US Department of Health and Human Services, Centers for Medicare & Medicaid Services. Your guide to Medicare's preventive services; Revised 2018. https://www.medicare.gov/Pubs/pdf/10110-Medicare-Preventive-Services.pdf. Accessed December 13, 2021.

World Health Organization. *Defining Sexual Health: Report of Technical Consultation on Sexual Health.* Geneva: World Health Organization; 2002.

Gynecologic Disorders

Thomas Clark Powell, Russell Stanley, Holly E. Richter

INTRODUCTION

The population of older women, generally defined as those greater than 65 years of age, is the fastest growing segment of the US population and as such deserves exceptional medical care from all health care providers. Primary and high-quality preventative care are an important challenge and opportunity for the health care workforce for older women. When gynecologic care is provided by geriatric primary care practitioners, they must be more mindful than ever about risks, symptoms, and unspoken issues. Lifetime risk of a gynecologic cancer (excluding breast cancer) is over 5%, greater than a woman's lifetime colorectal cancer risk. Pelvic floor symptoms bother at least 40% of women age 70 to 79 and more than 50% of women greater than or equal to 80 years. Sexual problems are prevalent in half of older women who are still sexually active. This chapter seeks to address the most common and important gynecologic and urogynecologic issues encountered in a geriatrics practice, with practical tips and suggestions. Urinary incontinence (UI) is not included in this chapter but is covered in detail elsewhere (see Chapter 47). Topics are presented anatomically, in approximately the same order as a physical examination is approached, along with the major corresponding clinical issues.

GYNECOLOGIC WELL-WOMAN VISIT

Gynecologic history and review of systems and medication list are mainstays of the primary care approach to gynecologic care. This should be targeted to assess cancer and infectious disease risks, to anticipate and interpret problems, and to promote function and quality of life. If a new patient visit is focused on other concerns, an assessment of vaginal bleeding and pelvic or vulvovaginal pain should be obtained at a minimum, since these are most indicative of urgent issues.

Key points in the gynecologic history and physical examination are listed in **Table 36-1**. If gynecologic surgery was performed, note the indication. For pain, prolapse, and incontinence surgeries, determine whether symptoms are resolved. Lifetime hormonal status and exposure, family cancer history, and cancer screening since age 55 are important in assessing current cancer risks.

Learning Objectives

- Establish personal and familial risk factors for gynecologic cancer in female patients.
- Review criteria that should be met to discontinue screening for cervical cancer.
- Describe the approach to the initial evaluation of vulvovaginal complaints.
- List multiple options to treat atrophic vaginitis.
- Understand the indications for specialty referral versus reassurance in a woman with pelvic organ prolapse (POP).

Key Clinical Points

1. Primary care providers are increasingly responsible for routine gynecologic care of older women.

2. Cervical cancer has a higher case-fatality rate in older women, and if a cervix is in situ, screening should be discontinued only in low-risk women age 65+ after three negative cytologies or two negative HPV co-tests in the previous decade.

3. Endometrial cancer associated with a false-negative screening ultrasound is frequently of the more aggressive type.

4. Although ultrasound and serum (CA-125) screening for ovarian cancer is ineffective in a low-risk population, imaging should be considered in women with suspicious symptoms involving abdominal and pelvic pain/discomfort, bloating, gastrointestinal disturbances, and urinary complaints.

5. Pelvic pain is not commonly due to pathology of reproductive organs; the urinary tract, gastrointestinal (GI) tract, and musculoskeletal systems should be thoroughly

(Continued)

(Cont.)

investigated with history and physical examination.

6. Pessaries can successfully relieve symptoms for many types of POP and stress urinary incontinence and should be offered.

7. Genitourinary syndrome of menopause and atrophic vaginitis are results of hypoestrogenism and can be readily treated using vaginal estrogen without systemic effects.

Diethylstilbestrol (DES) is an often-forgotten cancer risk factor that should be assessed. It was synthesized in 1938 and prescribed to pregnant women until 1971 in the United States and the early 1980s in some European countries. An estimated 5 to 10 million women worldwide took DES during pregnancy. An increased breast cancer risk has been seen in both women who received DES and their female fetuses exposed in utero (DES daughters). The increased risk of vaginal clear cell adenocarcinoma and cervical neoplasia in DES daughters continues into the fifth decade, but little is known about epidemiology of these conditions in advanced age.

Physical Examination

The physical examination serves four main purposes: (1) to understand the patient's anatomic status, (2) to detect unrecognized problems at an early stage, (3) to detect significant current problems in the cognitively or neurologically impaired, and (4) to provide the patient an opportunity to discuss embarrassing and private issues. A surprising number of gynecologic and urologic symptoms are only voiced or discovered during the pelvic examination, despite a thorough history and review of systems. An annual pelvic examination helps the practitioner assess the condition of the vaginal tissue, the vulva and perineum for any abnormalities that may be present. Although

TABLE 36-1 ■ GYNECOLOGIC HISTORY AND EXAMINATION

	COGNITIVELY INTACT	COGNITIVELY IMPAIRED[a]
History	Hormones: menarche, menopause, past and current hormone use	Current hormone use
	Breast complaints: pain, lump, nipple discharge	Staining of brassiere or clothing, pain
	Vulvovaginal issues: bulge, bleeding, discharge, pain	Apparent discomfort in perineal area
	Urinary issues: incontinence, urinary frequency, urinary urgency, hesitancy, nocturia, dysuria, hematuria, infections	Toileting practices, pad use
	Defecation issues: constipation, fecal incontinence (gas, liquid, solid stool)	Defecation frequency, stool consistency
	Sexual health issues: sexual activity, contacts, satisfaction, potential sexual abuse	Sexual behaviors
	Family history of gynecologic, breast, intestinal, endocrine malignancies	
Physical examination	Breast examination (annually)	Breast examination if tolerated
	Pelvic examination • Upon assuming care for new patient • For symptoms • For vague concerns • To ensure optimal referral Routine examinations controversial, low yield	Annual inspection of the external genitalia is probably useful. Initial internal examination may also be worthwhile. Subsequent internal examinations are indicated for symptoms or to rule out fecal impaction.
	External genitalia and perineum: architecture and integument	
	Urethra: meatus, caruncle	
	Bladder: tenderness, fullness	
	Vagina: mucosal tissue quality, discharge, mass, prolapse	
	Cervix: lesions, mobility	
	Uterus: size and mobility	
	Adnexa: palpability or mass	
	Rectum: anal sphincter tone, mass, stool for occult blood	

[a]Suggestions for examination in the cognitively impaired older woman (moderate or severe impairment) are based on clinical experience (Level D evidence).

Normal Anatomy	Fecal Impaction
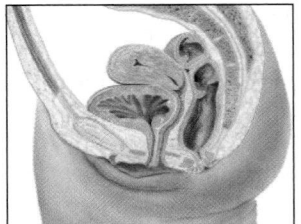	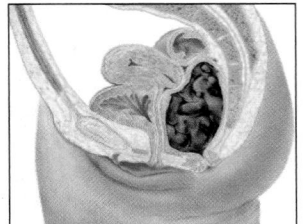
Mid-sagittal view–Female pelvis	Mid-sagittal view–Female pelvis
A	**B**

FIGURE 36-1. Sagittal view of normal pelvic anatomy (**A**) and fecal impaction (**B**). Note how a large impaction can compress the bladder, urethra, and surrounding innervation and other tissues.

there is some debate regarding the utility of this examination, assessing the health of the vulva and vagina remains important for primary care providers and gynecologists to provide complete care. Periodic examination of "asymptomatic" but concerned women is indicated. A patient may not be able to articulate the concerns she has. Appropriate speculum size, shape, and use is essential to perform a thorough but painless vaginal examination. Topical lidocaine at the posterior introitus as needed limits discomfort. This can also be applied liberally to the vulva and vagina to facilitate examination in cognitively impaired women. Fecal impaction should be ruled out in older women as a cause of a difficult vaginal examination. Fecal impaction can also compress the urethra and bladder and the surrounding innervation (**Figure 36-1**), cause urinary symptoms in addition to abdominal discomfort, and requires evaluation of underlying causes as well as treatment. (See Chapter 87, Constipation.)

The American College of Obstetricians and Gynecologists (ACOG) is unique in clearly recommending that "annual examination of the external genitalia should continue" beyond age 65. The utility of annual external genitalia examination may be most important in women who are cognitively impaired. Given the possible association with vaginal cancer, ACOG also recommends continuing annual internal pelvic examinations indefinitely in DES daughters, even those who have had a hysterectomy.

BENIGN BREAST DISEASE

While numerous studies address breast cancer, less is known about the epidemiology of benign breast disease in older women, but it may represent a significant number of primary care encounters. The breast is a complex structure subject to many pathologic conditions, both intrinsic and extrinsic. These may involve skin, connective tissue, ligaments, nerves, vasculature, lymphatics, and muscles in addition to mammary ducts and alveoli.

A clinical breast examination begins with inspection to evaluate overall symmetry and presence of skin changes such as erythema, swelling, and bulging or retraction of the nipple and areola. Palpation should include axillary, supraclavicular, and infraclavicular lymph nodes. Pertinent positive and negative findings should be documented, ideally in all patients, but especially if there is any breast complaint. Symptomatic problems can be categorized as a lump, pain, nipple discharge, or inflammation and should be evaluated and appropriately documented.

Breast Lump

It is important for the clinician to remember that it is not possible to distinguish between malignant from benign or solid from cystic masses by clinical examination alone. However, when combining findings from clinical examination, interpreted in combination with pathology and imaging, one can better evaluate and develop a treatment plan for breast lumps. Evaluation of a lump includes noting the size, position, consistency, and character. Location can be described referencing the areola as a clock face and measuring distance from the areolar border. While a myriad of pathologic entities could result in a breast lump, age is a consistent risk factor for malignancy. All discrete lumps should be evaluated by a breast specialist. The diagnostic mammogram and ultrasound may be performed before or after consultation, per consultant preference. If a lump found by the patient is not palpated by the physician, additional consultation is in order. If both the patient and physician agree that now there is no palpable abnormality, reassessment in 2 months to reconfirm is advisable.

Mastalgia

Mastalgia is common and rarely indicates pathology. The prevalence of breast pain is 66% and is higher for women nearing menopause than for premenopausal women. The precise etiology of mastalgia is currently unknown. Mastalgia is generally classified as either noncyclic or cyclic. Noncyclic mastalgia is often focal and does not have any relationship to the menstrual cycle. Focal mastalgia is frequently caused by a simple cyst, but breast cancer can occasionally present as localized breast pain. Thus, careful examination, imaging, and possible needle biopsy should be considered. Of note, cyclic mastalgia is usually bilateral, diffuse, and is most severe during the late luteal phase of the menstrual cycle and is most prevalent in the premenopausal population.

Symptoms may be unilateral or bilateral, intermittent, or persistent, sharp, or aching. Only half of women with significant breast pain seek medical attention. Cancer uncommonly presents with breast pain, and mastalgia is not an indication for a diagnostic mammogram. Focal persistent pain may be associated with cancer in 1% to 3% of patients, but primarily in younger women. If focal persistent pain is concerning, a diagnostic mammogram and ultrasound can adequately rule out cancer, or the patient may be referred.

Pain sources intrinsic to the breast include fibrocystic disease, duct ectasia, trauma, sclerosing adenosis, and stretching of Cooper ligaments. Conditions external to the breast but perceived as breast pain include costochondritis (Tietze syndrome), cervical radiculopathy, intercostal neuralgia, thrombophlebitis of the thoracoepigastric vein (Mondor disease), herpes zoster, angina, cholecystitis, and hiatal hernia. The affected breast(s) should be palpated to differentiate breast from chest wall pain. If findings are negative and mammographic screening is current, the patient can be offered reassurance and follow up. Interference with activities such as physical contact, sexual activity, exercising, and sleeping may indicate a need for more aggressive pain management, starting with a well-fitted brassiere with good support and nonsteroidal anti-inflammatory drugs or acetaminophen. Prescription pharmacologic agents for mastalgia have side effects and are supported by limited data. Danazol is the only FDA-approved medication for mastalgia. Tamoxifen has also shown efficacy. However, both of these medications come with significant side effects and are targeted for the treatment of cyclic breast pain, which should not be found in the older population.

Nipple Discharge

Breasts are secretory organs and discharge is a common symptom. Important nipple discharge characteristics are whether it is spontaneous or expressed, unilateral or bilateral, involving single or multiple ducts, and the color. The examiner should try to elicit discharge palpating each breast quadrant from the outside toward the areola, and then gently squeezing the areola. A patient may also demonstrate expressing the discharge. A mass should be ruled out, particularly under the areola. Whereas unilateral, single-duct, spontaneous, bloody, or watery discharge is more concerning for neoplasia, bilateral, expressed, non-bloody discharge from multiple ducts is not associated with cancer. Pathologic nipple discharge is defined as a spontaneous single-duct discharge that is either bloody or serous. The rate of underlying malignancy ranges from approximately 2% for young women with no associated clinical or imaging findings to approximately 20% for older women without associated findings. Most pathologic nipple discharges are caused by benign intraductal papillomas, which are simple milk duct polyps. Consultation should be obtained for all bloody or recurrent spontaneous discharge. A thick gray or green grumous or purulent discharge may indicate duct ectasia (dilated lactiferous ducts with inspissated secretions) or subareolar abscess. Duct ectasia is also the most common cause of blood-stained discharge from multiple ducts. Duct ectasia is benign but may be excised to rule out underlying cancer. Hyperprolactinemia is rare in older women. A serum prolactin is indicated if galactorrhea is observed or suspected. Eczematous and other skin conditions may imitate nipple discharge.

Breast Inflammation

Inflammatory conditions intrinsic to the breast include duct ectasia, fat necrosis, a ruptured inflammatory cyst, an inflammatory abscess due to obstructed ducts, idiopathic granulomatous mastitis, foreign body, radiation, and inflammatory carcinoma. Smoking, diabetes, and rheumatoid arthritis predispose to abscesses. The most common pathogen is *Staphylococcus aureus*. Risk factors for methicillin-resistant *S aureus* include diabetes and residence in long-term care. Most abscesses respond well to drainage and antibiotics. Consultation should be obtained for recurrent or persistent abscess. Conditions extrinsic to the breast that may present with inflammation include metastatic lung cancer, Wegener granulomatosis, sarcoidosis, and other skin diseases.

PELVIC PAIN

Perceived "pelvic" pain may arise from any component between the umbilicus and the upper thigh. Bladder pain syndrome, also known as interstitial cystitis (IC), is discussed later in this chapter. A strictly gynecologic cause of either acute or chronic pelvic pain is uncommon in older women except with advanced malignancy. Although many women fear that the pain indicates an ovarian problem, other causes are more likely. After menopause, the ovaries have decreased to about the size of an almond in its shell and are largely inactive, making painful cysts rare and torsion highly unlikely. Benign ovarian cysts and masses are usually asymptomatic until they are quite large. A complaint of "pain" is not likely to herald a gynecologic malignancy; nonspecific abdominal and pelvic fullness or discomfort are more common descriptions associated with cancer. Infection and neoplasm could be gynecologic causes of acute pain. But a non-gynecologic cause would be more likely, such as constipation, diverticulitis, herpes zoster, or pelvic insufficiency fracture.

Older women rarely experience the same type of chronic pelvic pain (≥ 6 months) that plagues women in their reproductive years, with "cross-talk" between pelvic organ structures, pelvic tension myalgia, and central sensitization. POP is a more common ailment in the geriatric population and may cause low back or pelvic pain. Pelvic floor repair with synthetic mesh may result in chronic pain. More likely etiologies of chronic pelvic pain involve the gastrointestinal and musculoskeletal systems. The abdomen, low back, and hips should be evaluated. Myofascial pain with trigger points in the lower abdomen is a particularly notorious pelvic pain impostor. This occurs in 30% of patients with chronic abdominal pain, frequently misrepresented as visceral or functional pain. A finding of myofascial trigger points with the Carnett test (increased point tenderness with partial sit-up tensing the abdominal muscles) does not completely rule out internal causes of pain, but initial treatment of this will clarify the etiology.

Following evaluation of the abdomen, back, bony pelvis, and hips, the pelvic examination should proceed slowly, assessing sensation and tenderness from external to internal. Urethra, bladder, and pelvic musculature can be sequentially palpated. If abdominal pain or tenderness is present, begin the "bimanual" examination of the uterus and ovaries using only the vaginal hand. After assessing cervical, uterine, and adnexal tenderness without abdominal palpation, proceed to bimanual evaluation. If the cause is unknown, repeating the examination at subsequent visits is valuable, as the findings typically vary somewhat. Vulvovaginal pain examination is addressed below.

VULVAR AND VAGINAL ISSUES

Examination of the Vulva

Normal vulvar architecture consists of labia minora, labia majora, clitoris, clitoral hood, and intact urethral meatus (**Figure 36-2**). Advanced age and estrogen deficiency

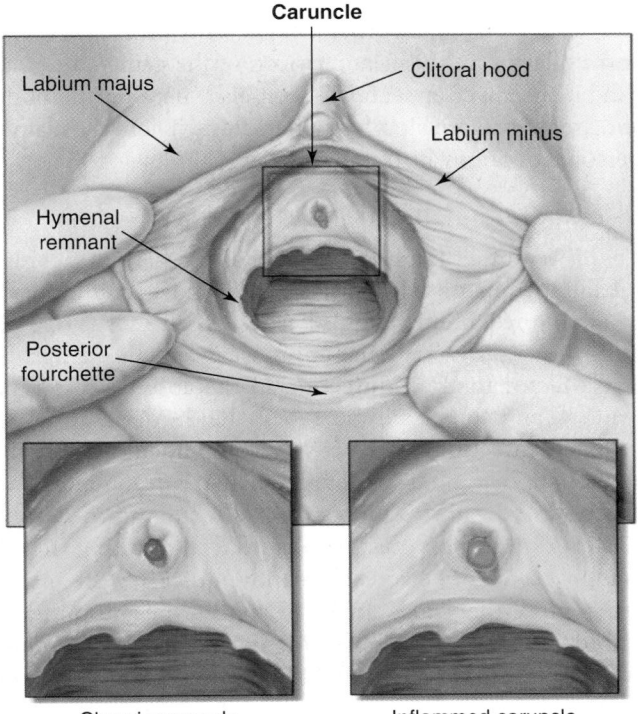

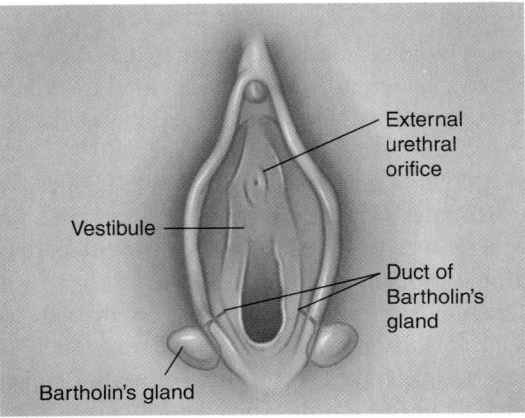

FIGURE 36-2. Illustration of pelvic examination landmarks and a urethral caruncle.

may lead to a loss of vulvar architecture, especially of the labia minora. Cherry angiomata and epithelial inclusion cysts on the labia majora are common and not concerning. Asymmetrical pigmented lesions should be noted and considered for either biopsy or follow-up examinations. Punch biopsies of the vulva are simple, rarely become infected, and can be performed in the office under local anesthesia. Bartholin glands are in the inferior (dorsal) aspect of each labium majus. An asymptomatic Bartholin cyst does not require referral if there is no detectable mass associated with the cyst, but rare Bartholin gland malignancies do occur. Thus, a symptomatic Bartholin cyst or abscess in the postmenopausal woman should be drained and biopsied and consideration given to full excision if symptoms persist.

Benign Conditions of the Vulva

The hundreds of benign vulvar disorders generally fall into categories of infection, neoplasia, and dermatosis, some of which may reflect systemic disorders. Inflammatory disorders may be difficult to recognize, even by dermatologists, because the warm, moist, frictional environment alters their otherwise typical appearance. Establishing a nomenclature that is both clinically useful and pathologically appropriate is challenging. The current International Society for the Study of Vulvar Diseases (ISSVD) classification relies primarily on histologic morphology (**Table 36-2**). Realizing its limitations, they have since formulated an approach that allows highly accurate diagnoses with just clinical observations. Estrogen deficiency may increase susceptibility to trauma, irritation, and secondary infection, but is not a primary cause of vulvar problems.

Lichen Simplex Chronicus

Lichen simplex chronicus is characterized as an eczematoid disease of hyperkeratotic, scaling plaques with varying pigmentation that is found to be associated with severe vulvar pruritis. This can be seen in conjunction with other vulvar skin disorders and is ultimately brought on by chronic scratching and subsequent irritation from dermatological and environmental processes. Lichen simplex chronicus is associated with patients who have a history of atopic disease in up to 75% of patients and typically presents later in adult life. The diagnosis of lichen simplex chronicus is based on history of pruritis, typical hyperkeratotic lesions on examination, and vulvar irritation. Biopsy may be done to identify underlying disease such as lichen sclerosus or cultures may be sent to identify yeast. First-line therapies involve treating the underlying conditions, utilization of topical corticosteroids, and even a combination of steroid and antifungal ointments if an underlying yeast infection is suspected. Hygiene measures such as controlling the amount of vulvar wetness and avoiding potential irritants (strong soaps, perfumes, or detergents) are key to cutting down on things that exacerbate and prolong the condition.

TABLE 36-2 ■ CLASSIFICATION OF VULVAR DERMATOSES: PATHOLOGIC SUBSETS AND CLINICAL CORRELATES (2006 INTERNATIONAL SOCIETY FOR THE STUDY OF VULVOVAGINAL DISEASE CLASSIFICATION)

Spongiotic pattern
  Atopic dermatitis
  Allergic contact dermatitis
  Irritant contact dermatitis

Acanthotic pattern (formerly squamous cell hyperplasia)
  Psoriasis
  Lichen simplex chronicus
    Primary (idiopathic)
    Secondary (superimposed on lichen sclerosus, lichen planus, or other)

Lichenoid pattern
  Lichen sclerosus
  Lichen planus

Dermal homogenization/sclerosus pattern
  Lichen sclerosus

Vesiculobullous pattern
  Pemphigoid, cicatricial type
  Linear IgA disease

Acantholytic pattern
  Hailey-Hailey disease
  Darier disease
  Papular genitocrural acantholysis

Granulomatous pattern
  Crohn disease
  Melkersson-Rosenthal syndrome

Vasculopathic pattern
  Aphthous ulcers
  Behçet disease
  Plasma cell vulvitis

Lichen Sclerosus

Lichen sclerosus is a chronic inflammatory disease that can occur at any age, its highest prevalence being after menopause. It may have an autoimmune etiology and is frequently associated with other autoimmune disorders. Pruritus is characteristic, but it may be asymptomatic. Typical lesions are porcelain white papules and plaques, often with areas of ecchymosis or purpura. Perianal involvement can create the classic "figure of eight" appearance. In more advanced cases, vulvar architecture is lost, with labial fusion, clitoral hood phimosis, and fissures. Scarring may lead to introital narrowing. The malignant potential of lichen sclerosus is debated but may be as high as 4% to 5%. Biopsy confirmation of the diagnosis and visual inspection at least annually are advisable. Treatment is necessary only to control symptoms. Typical regimens involve moderate strength topical glucocorticoids for at least 4 weeks, then tapering to a lower dosing frequency. A subsequent maintenance regimen of daily or twice-daily emollient may reduce the frequency of symptomatic flares. Estrogen has little or no effect on lichen sclerosus but can improve the resilience of unaffected areas, and estrogen cream can serve as an emollient.

Lichen Planus

Lichen planus exhibits a wide range of morphologies. Of women with oral lichen planus, approximately 20% to 25% have vulvovaginal lesions. The erosive form may cause pain and vaginal discharge, and lead to agglutination and resorption of labial architecture, rarely with complete obliteration of the vaginal orifice. As with lichen sclerosus, biopsy can be utilized for confirmation of diagnosis and to rule out malignancy. Treatment options include topical or systemic corticosteroids or immunomodulators. Other autoimmune disorders to consider are Zoon disorder (plasma cell vulvitis), Behçet disease, Crohn disease, aphthous ulcers, and Hailey-Hailey disorder (fragile and inflamed vulvar and axillary skin). Psoriatic lesions of the genitalia do not exhibit the silver appearance seen elsewhere on the body, and are more often simply erythematous. There is usually a personal or family history of psoriasis.

Ulcerations and Infections of the Vulva

The differential diagnosis of genital ulceration includes sexually transmitted diseases, the most common of which in the United States is herpes simplex virus (HSV). Immune suppression, including very advanced age, is a risk factor for HSV infection in the absence of sexual contact, and for herpes zoster of the S3 dermatome. A primary infection is usually accompanied by lymphadenopathy, vaginal discharge, urinary frequency and urgency, and painful ulcers on the labia and/or cervix. Zoster can inhibit detrusor function resulting in an inability to void. Lesions clear more quickly with antiviral agents. Other causes include syphilis, the autoimmune disorders listed above, blistering dermatologic disorders, and of particular concern in older women, excoriated or ulcerated neoplasia.

Vulvar Neoplasia

Vulvar carcinoma is a rare malignancy and represents less than 5% of all cancers in the female genital tract. However, even though vulvar carcinoma remains uncommon, the incidence is increasing with an estimated 6020 new cases of vulvar carcinoma diagnosed in the United States annually and an estimated 1150 deaths from the disease. The average age of diagnosis is 68.7 with 70% of vulvar cancer diagnoses occurring in women over the age of 60.

Squamous cell carcinomas (SCC) of the vulva are the most common histologic subtype, accounting for 90% of vulvar cancers. There are two distinct pathways involving the pathogenesis of SCC of the vulva and its precursor lesion, vulvar intraepithelial neoplasia (VIN). In the past, VIN included grades 1 to 3, but the nomenclature has recently changed, and VIN now refers only to high-grade lesions of the vulva. Human papillomavirus (HPV)-associated VIN, also referred to as usual type VIN, occurs more frequently in younger women and is mostly associated with the carcinogenic HPV genotypes, most commonly HPV 16. HPV-independent VIN, or differentiated VIN, occurs more frequently in older women and is associated with chronic inflammation that is secondary to underlying dermatologic conditions such as lichen sclerosus or lichen planus. The HPV-associated VIN develops slowly and then will spontaneously regress. On the other hand, the HPV-independent VIN is more likely to progress rapidly to invasive squamous cell cancer. Presentation is often with vulvar burning or pruritus.

Vulvar cancer is surgically staged. The presence or absence of lymph node metastasis is the most important prognostic factor for women with this disease. Five-year survival in the absence of nodal metastasis is 91% compared to only 57% for patients with node-positive disease.

Vulvar melanoma is the second most common type of malignancy of the vulva and makes up 5% to 10% of vulvar malignancies. Many vulvar melanomas occur in the older patient population and is more common in the Caucasian population. Compared to the cutaneous version of melanoma and other mucosal melanomas, the prognosis for women with vulvar melanoma is poor with a 5-year survival rate of less than 50%. Similar to cutaneous melanomas, an approach of wide local excision with sentinel lymph node biopsy has been adopted as the treatment of choice for patients.

Vulvar Pain, Vaginal Pain, and Dyspareunia

To evaluate vulvar or vaginal pain, the perineum from the mons pubis to the anus should be inspected for vulvar architectural changes, which may or may not be pathologic, including fissures, ulcers, erythema, and other signs of inflammation. Palpation of the vulva and around the vaginal introitus with a cotton swab will better establish the location and extent of tenderness than digital palpation. Areas to assess are the base of hymeneal remnants, posterior fourchette, and periurethral Skene glands.

Vulvodynia is chronic vulvar pain that persists for greater than 3 to 6 months in the absence of another clinically identifiable condition. In 2015, the ISSVD updated vulvar pain classifications into two categories: (1) vulvar pain caused by a specific disorder (infection, inflammation, neoplasm, trauma, hormonal deficiency, neurologic disease, or iatrogenic etiology) and (2) vulvodynia, defined as vulvar pain of at least 3 months' duration, without an identifiable cause. While the true prevalence of vulvodynia is unknown, estimated prevalence is between 10% and 16% over a woman's lifetime and tends to be more common in older patients. Women may have both a specific disorder and vulvodynia and may require concurrent or sequential management since vulvodynia is a diagnosis of exclusion.

Vulvodynia may be provoked, unprovoked, or both, and generalized or localized. "Localized provoked vulvodynia" denotes the condition formerly termed vulvar

vestibulitis. The suffix "itis" is technically inaccurate as inflammation is not usually present. Pain located specifically in the vestibule is referred to as vestibulodynia. This is not particularly associated with aging or atrophy. This condition is poorly understood and may be frustrating for patients and can be difficult to treat. After ruling out known causes of discomfort (infection, dermatitis, genitourinary syndrome, post herpetic neuralgia, etc.), the approach to continued vulvodynia generally must be multimodal and often interdisciplinary to address physical as well as psychosocial causes and effects. Pelvic floor physical therapy, cognitive behavioral therapy, couples' therapy, and/or sexual therapy all may be utilized depending on the specific attributes of a woman's pain and setting in which it occurs. Neuropathy is thought to be one of the many components and may be addressed using antidepressants that modulate serotonin and norepinephrine as well as low-dose tricyclic antidepressants; however, evidence for the most appropriate agent, dose, and duration are limited and often extrapolated from experience with other chronic pain syndromes. Similarly, other agents such as gabapentin, pregabalin, and carbamazepine may be used as adjunct treatment with physical and cognitive therapies. Topical estrogen is appropriate to ensure that tissue atrophy is not a contributing factor. Glucocorticoid or lidocaine topical preparations rarely improve symptoms for long duration but are reasonable to try both for the effect of their active ingredients and emollient properties. Persistent symptoms may require coordination of care with a pain management specialist.

Unlike the vulva, the vagina is rarely an isolated source of pain unless the patient is sexually active. Simple postmenopausal vaginal atrophy is usually asymptomatic, but dyspareunia is common. Dyspareunia evaluation is guided by historical factors such as past sexual experiences, exact symptoms during intercourse, and examination. The anterior, lateral, and posterior vaginal walls and apex should be inspected and palpated as separately as possible. Atrophic vaginitis considerations are presented below. Patients with presumed atrophic vaginitis that has not responded to estrogen frequently have an unrecognized vulvar condition. Isolated vaginal pain in the absence of intercourse should prompt consideration of surrounding organs and structures, including the pelvic floor musculature and urinary and gastrointestinal tracts.

Vaginitis, Vaginosis, and Vaginal Discharge

Symptoms of vaginitis, vaginosis, and vaginal discharge overlap with each other and with those of vulvar conditions. A true bacterial vaginitis is uncommon in the absence of an underlying epithelial disorder. Bacterial vaginosis incidence increases with age, but only requires treatment for bothersome symptoms or planned vaginal surgery. Yeast infection incidence declines with age, but antibiotics, diabetes, immune suppression, and estrogen therapy are risk factors. *Trichomonas* can be carried asymptomatically and occur recurrently without partner treatment. Coexistence with bacterial vaginosis is common. Either estrogen initiation or replacement of vaginal prolapse with a pessary may cause benign white discharge from an increase in epithelial turnover. Desquamative inflammatory vaginitis is an uncommon cause of discharge, burning, and dyspareunia, and may be a manifestation of erosive lichen planus. Rare causes of purulent malodorous discharge include an enterovaginal fistula secondary to diverticulitis, inflammatory bowel disease, or prior surgery.

Evaluation of vaginal discharge in younger and older women is largely the same except for vaginal bleeding. Any history of a brown or red discharge necessitates endometrial evaluation. Physical examination is essential to evaluate vaginal discharge as findings often differ from the presumption based on history. With aging and estrogen deficiency, vaginal pH rises, providing a less hospitable environment for both lactobacilli and yeast. However, vaginal candidiasis still occurs and stereotypically is accompanied by symptoms of odorless, thick, white discharge and pruritis. The vulva may be involved with erythema, excoriations, and satellite lesions. On microscopy, pseudohyphae are diagnostic. In contrast, bacterial vaginosis causes a thin, malodorous, gray discharge that on microscopy demonstrates clue cells, which are squamous epithelial cells surrounded by bacteria. If microscopy is not available, commercial tests are available for bacterial vaginosis and *Trichomonas vaginalis*, and yeast can be cultured. A trichomoniasis diagnosis should prompt sexually transmitted infection screening and treatment of partner(s). Current recommendations for detection and treatment of sexually transmitted diseases are maintained on the website of the Centers for Disease Control and Prevention (www.cdc.gov/std/default.htm).

Vaginal atrophy due to hypoestrogenism involves several changes including mucosal thinning; loss of rugae, elasticity, and distensibility; an increase in subepithelial connective tissue and vaginal pH (> 4.5); and reduced secretions which collectively contribute to genitourinary syndrome of menopause. Changes in the vaginal microbiome predispose to urinary tract infections (UTIs). Atrophic "vaginitis" is poorly defined apart from simple atrophy, but is usually diagnosed when symptoms (dryness, itching, irritation, burning, dyspareunia, irritative voiding) or signs (pale, thin, shiny vaginal mucosa, telangiectasias, petechiae, patches of inflammation, discharge) are present (**Figure 36-3**). A cytologic maturation index would reveal 60% to 100% parabasal cells but is not necessary for the diagnosis.

Low-dose topical estrogen remains the preferred treatment for atrophic vaginitis in most women. It is the most proven for symptom relief, and there are several delivery options, via ring, tablet, capsule, or cream. Examples of low- and moderate-dose vaginal estrogen therapies are listed in **Table 36-3**. The ring can remain in the vagina for 3 months, releasing 6 to 9 μg of estradiol daily. Tablets containing 10 μg of estradiol may be inserted nightly for 2 weeks, then twice a week indefinitely. Daily use is required initially to stimulate mucosal remodeling, because the very low maintenance dose alone is not sufficient. The dose and absorption of both the ring and the tablet are specific and well-studied. Serum estradiol rises briefly in the first 24 hours then remains within the postmenopausal range.

Exact low dosage is difficult to achieve with creams, but cream has other advantages. The vehicle soothes the mucosa. Creams are often the least costly approach. The amounts needed to treat atrophic vaginitis are smaller than the lowest measurements on the applicator; using an estimated 1/4 to 1/2 g twice weekly is reasonable. Some women find fingertip application of a pea- or chocolate chip–size amount placed into the vagina easier than inserting an applicator.

The lower urinary tract is also estrogen sensitive, as estrogen receptors are found in the bladder and urethra. The symptoms of dysuria, urethral discomfort, overactive bladder (OAB, consisting of urinary urgency, frequency, urgency urinary incontinence, nocturia), hematuria, UTIs, and UI are associated with aging. Estrogen has been a mainstay of treatment in urinary tract symptoms. There is a role for transvaginal estrogen in preventing recurrent UTIs.

Vaginal estrogen use in breast cancer survivors is controversial and best prescribed in consultation with an oncologist. Oral estrogen is contraindicated during breast cancer treatment, but no harm has been detected from use of low-dose intravaginal preparations with a history of breast cancer. Patients taking aromatase inhibitors may achieve undesirably high premenopausal serum estrogen levels, warranting extra precaution or consultation before and during any estrogen treatment. Concerns seem to only apply to hormone-sensitive cancers as no increased recurrence of hormone receptor–negative cancers has been found with any type of postmenopausal hormone therapy. Nonetheless, women with a history of breast cancer should try nonhormonal treatments first.

With these low doses, progestins to prevent endometrial hyperplasia or endometrial surveillance are not required. However, estrogen absorption varies considerably among individuals, and endometrial growth could possibly be stimulated. Any brown or red discharge necessitates evaluation of the endometrium as would be performed with any postmenopausal bleeding. Ospemifene is an oral estrogen agonist/antagonist, or selective estrogen receptor modulator (SERM), approved by the FDA for dyspareunia due to vaginal atrophy. It is effective for vulvovaginal atrophy and appears to have favorable effects on bone, neutral effects on the endometrium and the cardiovascular system, and no clinically significant estrogenic effect on the breast. Risks and contraindications are like those for estrogen, including venous thromboembolism. Vasomotor symptoms are bothersome in 10% of patients.

Other non-estrogen therapies are less reliable in reducing dyspareunia and irritative voiding symptoms, but often relieve mild symptoms. Vaginal moisturizers are used on a regular basis, daily to weekly, to maintain epithelial moisture and vaginal pH. In addition, vaginal lubricants may be used for intercourse. Frequent sexual activity helps maintain supple tissues. Alternative hormonal agents

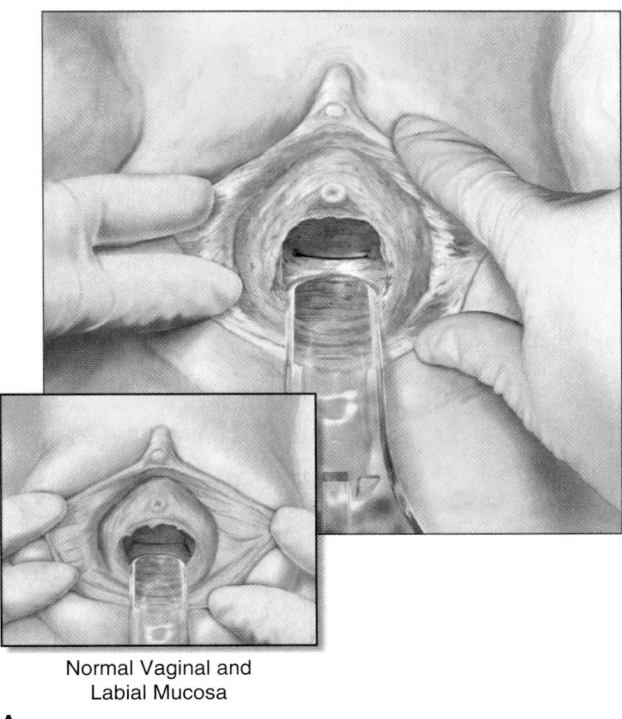

A

Normal Vaginal and
Labial Mucosa

B

FIGURE 36-3. (**A**) Illustration of atrophic vaginitis versus normal mucosa. Signs of atrophic vaginitis may include pale, smooth, shiny mucosa with patches of inflammation and petechiae. (**B**) Illustration of remodeling of vaginal mucosa in response to topical estrogen therapy. (B, Reproduced with permission from Reiter S. Barriers to effective treatment of vaginal atrophy with local estrogen therapy. *Int J Gen Med.* 2013;6:153–158.)

(dehydroepiandrosterone, other SERMs, testosterone) are promising but not yet sufficiently studied.

Vaginal Cancer

Vaginal cancer accounts for 1% or less of female genital tract cancers. Metastatic disease of the vagina is more common than primary vaginal cancer, notably from cancers of the endometrium, cervix, vulva, ovary, breast, rectum, and kidney. The most common primary vaginal cancer is SCC, but adenocarcinoma, sarcoma, melanoma, and others occur. Vaginal SCC is often preceded by vaginal intraepithelial neoplasia, which is associated with concomitant cervical or vulvar neoplasia in about 50% of cases. It is usually asymptomatic and not easily visible, but induration may be palpable. Two-thirds of cases occur in the upper vagina. Risk factors for primary vaginal cancer are the same as those for cervical cancer, including prior gynecologic cancer and radiation therapy. Bleeding, discharge, pain, and urinary or rectal complaints are presenting symptoms. Survival drops precipitously beyond stage II.

CERVIX UTERI

Examination of the Cervix

The location of the squamocolumnar junction, the border between squamous (ectocervical) and mucous (endocervical)

TABLE 36-3 ■ CHARACTERISTICS OF LOCAL VAGINAL HORMONAL TREATMENTS

FORMULATION	BRAND NAME	GENERIC AVAILABLE	USUAL CLINICAL DOSING	COMMENTS
LOW-DOSE VAGINAL ESTROGEN (SERUM ESTRADIOL < 20 pg/mL)				
4 µg estradiol insert	Imvexxy	No	1 insert daily for 2 wk, then 1 insert twice weekly	Formulated as a medium-chain triglyceride
7.5 µg estradiol ring	Estring	No	1 ring per vagina every 90 d	Should not be confused with Femring, which is a systemic vaginal estrogen ring
10 µg insert and tablet	Imvexxy and Vagifem	Yuvafem	1 insert daily for 2 wk, then 1 insert twice weekly	
MODERATE-DOSE VAGINAL ESTROGEN (SERUM ESTRADIOL > 20 pg/mL, INTERMITTENTLY)				
0.5 g (0.3 mg) CEE cream	Premarin vaginal cream (0.625 mg/g)	No	0.5–1 g 1–3 times/wk	FDA-approved frequency includes daily for 21 d then off 7 d, but may lead to higher systemic absorption
HIGHER-DOSE VAGINAL ESTROGEN (SERUM ESTRADIOL CAN INTERMITTENTLY REACH PREMENOPAUSAL LEVELS)				
≥ 1g (0.625 mg) CEE cream	Premarin vaginal cream (0.625 mg/g)	No	0.5–1 g 1–3 times/wk	FDA-approved dose is up to 2 g, which may lead to higher systemic absorption
≥ 0.5 gm (50 µg) estradiol cream	Estrace cream (100 µg/g)	Estradiol	0.5–1g daily for 2 wk, then twice/wk	FDA-approved dose: 2–4 g daily, then 1 g 1–3 times/wk, which may lead to higher systemic absorption
VAGINAL DHEA				
6.5 mg (0.5%) DHEA insert	Intrarosa, Prasterone	No	1 insert daily	

CEE, conjugated equine estrogen; FDA, Food and Drug Administration.

Modified with permission from Crean-Tate KK, Faubion SS, Pederson HJ, et al. Management of genitourinary syndrome of menopause in female cancer patients: a focus on vaginal hormonal therapy. Am J Obstet Gynecol. 2020;222(2):103–113.

epithelia, changes location over a lifespan. It is usually within the endocervical canal in older women and not visible. Its importance lies in the fact that it is the most common site of cervical neoplasia. Cystic structures near this border are almost invariably Nabothian cysts. These are not true cysts, but collections of mucus trapped during metaplastic transition, when squamous cells cover mucus-secreting crypts. They do not require biopsy. Any lesion whose benignity is uncertain should be biopsied or referred. Cytology is a screening test and alone is not an appropriate evaluation of a visible lesion.

Cervical Cancer

Worldwide, cervical cancer is the most common gynecologic cancer and the fourth most common cancer overall in women. Most incident cases and 87% of cervical cancer-related deaths occur in less-developed countries due to the lack of access to appropriate screening and treatment of preinvasive disease. In the United States, there are an estimated 12,820 cervical cancer diagnoses and 4210 deaths annually. The risk of cervical cancer increases with age, and the case-fatality rate is higher in older women. While women over age 65 years represent approximately 14% of the US female population, more than 20% of new cervical cancer cases and a disproportionate amount of

cervical cancer deaths are in this age group. Most of these are in unscreened or inadequately screened women. Three-fourths of cervical cancers are SCC; the remaining adeno-, adenosquamous, and clear cell carcinomas have higher mortality rates. In older women only half to two-thirds of cervical cancers are associated with HPV. Postcoital bleeding may occur at an early stage, but other symptoms (pain and bowel or bladder symptoms) are absent. Radical hysterectomy is the primary treatment for early-stage cervical cancer. Radiation therapy is used for locally advanced disease, as adjunctive treatment, when surgery is not an option, and along with chemotherapy for palliation.

Cervical Cancer Screening (Table 36-4)

The excess deaths from this mostly preventable malignancy are only avoided through screening, including "adequate" screening of older women. Screening older women provides equivalent benefit to screening younger women, that is, an equivalent reduction in severe cervical intraepithelial neoplasia (CIN) and, by inference, of cancer. However, due to low cancer incidence and long lead time, routine screening after age 65 provides little benefit *if women have been adequately screened prior to this.* The key to safe discontinuation is knowing the patient's screening and risk factor history. The three main issues in

TABLE 36-4 ■ CRITERIA (ALL OF WHICH SHOULD BE MET PRIOR TO DISCONTINUING CERVICAL CANCER SCREENING)

Age > 65 **OR** 25 years post hysterectomy if performed for CIN2 or greater dysplasia	
Low risk	No preceding CIN2 or 3 Not diagnosed with HIV or other immunosuppression
Adequate negative screening	3 consecutive negative cervical cytology tests OR 2 negative cytologic tests with negative HPV co-testing in the past 10 years, the most recent within the last 5 years

older women are (1) when to discontinue screening, (2) in whom to continue screening, and until what point, and (3) the best screening modalities.

Cervical cancer screening has evolved from microscopy of exfoliated cells in the vagina to detect current cancer, introduced by Georgios Papanikolaou in 1928, to prevention of cancer through HPV genotyping, with or without cervical cytology. Testing options, recommendations, and guidelines have changed several times in recent years, and will continue to evolve. Cervical cytology with HPV co-testing should be obtained every 5 years in women over age 30. Updated guidelines and algorithms are available from the American Society for Colposcopy and Cervical Pathology (www.asccp.org).

The ACOG, American Society for Colposcopy and Cervical Pathology (ASCCP), the United States Preventive Services Task Force (USPSTF), the American Cancer Society (ACS), and other organizations recommend discontinuing cervical screening after appropriate criteria are met. The criteria include that the patient should be age 65 or older, low risk, and have had adequate negative screening. Adequate is defined as three consecutive negative cervical cytology tests or two negative cytologic tests with negative HPV co-testing in the past 10 years, the most recent of which was within the past 5 years. Ideally the final test would include HPV genotyping. Women older than 65 should continue with screening until these criteria are met. Screening should continue for at least 25 years after documented regression or treatment of a precancerous lesion, even if this extends after age 65. Having a new sexual partner after age 65 does not necessitate additional screening.

Screening of women who have undergone a total hysterectomy (*corpus et cervix uteri*) is not recommended unless the hysterectomy was performed for dysplasia, for cancer or the woman is a DES daughter. The positive predictive value of vaginal cuff cytology after hysterectomy for benign disease is approximately zero. Many women do not know whether their hysterectomy was total or supracervical (*corpus* alone). This can be determined at the initial pelvic examination. If a cervix is unexpectedly discovered, adequate screening should be performed before discontinuation.

Risk factors for cervical cancer include an abnormal Pap smear within the past decade, a history of moderate or severe CIN (CIN 2 or 3) within the past 25 years; a history of cervical, vaginal, or vulvar cancer; immune suppression; and DES exposure in utero. These groups are excluded from major society guidelines for lengthening screening intervals and discontinuation, but without sufficient alternative recommendations. As mentioned earlier, screening should continue for at least 25 years following successful treatment for CIN 2+. Women infected with human immunodeficiency virus (HIV) should continue annual screening indefinitely. Other causes of immune suppression including solid organ transplant, autoimmune disorders, treatment with glucocorticoids, and chronic antineoplastic therapies are not addressed. The relevance of DES exposure in utero to cervical or vaginal cancer risk in advanced age is uncertain. Although ACOG recommends continuing annual internal pelvic examinations indefinitely in DES daughters, it does not specifically address cervical or vaginal cytology.

CORPUS UTERI AND VAGINAL BLEEDING

Benign Conditions of the Uterus

Both the uterus and leiomyomata (fibroids) typically decrease in size after menopause. Therefore, a palpably large uterus (navel orange or grapefruit sized) is unusual. Previous medical records would probably clarify whether this is a new finding. If unclear, sonographic evaluation would inform the need for further evaluation or referral to a gynecologic specialist. Uterine tenderness is also unusual. Bacterial endometritis is uncommon, but can occur even in the absence of uterine manipulation. It is usually associated with a purulent, odorous discharge and/or bleeding.

Uterine Cancer

Endometrial cancer is the most common gynecologic malignancy in developed countries and the second most common in developing countries. The mortality rate has been declining slowly, but more than 10,000 women still die annually in the United States of this disease. An estimated 61,380 new cases of uterine cancer are diagnosed annually in the United States, and 10,920 women die per year because of this disease. Patients 65 and older account for 44.3% of new endometrial cancer diagnoses and 66.6% of endometrial cancer deaths. Incidence rates in Europe and North America have risen since the 1980s, possibly related to increases in obesity and life expectancy with a concomitant decrease in birth rates. Ninety percent of uterine cancers originate in the endometrium. Three-fourths are type I endometrioid adenocarcinoma. Type II is more aggressive and characterized by clear cell and papillary serous tumor histology. Papillary serous carcinoma accounts for only 10% of uterine cancers but 40% of uterine cancer deaths.

Type I endometrial cancer is associated with traditional risk factors related to estrogen abundance and inadequate progestin. It tends to present at an earlier stage and younger age than does type II. Risk factors include early menarche and late menopause, obesity, chronic anovulation, type 2 diabetes, hypertension, and nulliparity. Pregnancy, lactation, hormonal contraceptives (including a progesterone-releasing intrauterine device), and postmenopausal hormone therapy with continuous (not intermittent) progestins are protective historical factors. Pathogenesis and risk factors for type II endometrial cancer are less well understood. Although the effect size of risk and protective factors is stronger in most studies for type I cancer than for type II, the factors are surprisingly similar. Risk factors include body mass index, early menarche, and diabetes; protective factors are higher parity, oral contraceptive use, and cigarette smoking.

Endometrial cancer is the most common sentinel cancer in Lynch syndrome, an autosomal dominant condition caused by germline mutations in mismatch repair genes. Lynch syndrome accounts for 2% to 5% of endometrial cancers and is more associated with younger age and type I histomorphology. The question of universal versus selective genetic screening in endometrial cancer patients remains to be resolved. The 2014 Clinical Practice Statement from the Society for Gynecologic Oncology (SGO) recommends that "all women who are diagnosed with endometrial cancer should undergo systematic clinical screening for Lynch syndrome (review of personal and family history) and/or molecular screening. Molecular screening of endometrial cancers for Lynch syndrome is the preferred strategy when resources are available."

A hysterectomy with bilateral salpingo-oophorectomy, lymph node sampling, and tumor debulking is required for endometrial cancer staging and is the mainstay of treatment. Radiation and/or chemotherapy may be used adjunctively or in women who are too frail to undergo surgery. Overall, 5-year survival is estimated at 82% since bleeding usually leads to early diagnosis and treatment. Older age is associated with a worse prognosis because more aggressive tumors are relatively more common, as well as due to comorbidity, late diagnosis, and lack of aggressive treatment.

Malignant lesions of the myometrium include leiomyosarcoma and other sarcomatoid tumors. These are less likely to cause bleeding in early stages, and may only be detected by the presence of an enlarging uterus or pelvic mass, or be discovered after hysterectomy. Incidence of leiomyosarcoma peaks in the sixth and seventh decades. They are aggressive tumors with high metastatic potential. Treatment involves surgery, chemotherapy, and radiation. Extension of tumor beyond the confines of the uterus is associated with a poor prognosis.

Approach to Vaginal Bleeding

Abnormal vaginal bleeding occurs in up to 20% of postmenopausal women, 10% to 20% of the time due to endometrial hyperplasia or neoplasia. Studies invariably analyze "postmenopausal" as one group, so these statistics misrepresent the risks in older women. Older women bleed less often, but older age increases the risk of malignancy and of a higher-grade cancer. Although most women with postmenopausal bleeding will be referred to a gynecologist, a focused history and examination will ensure the best referral. A rectal polyp, urethral mucosal prolapse, vulvovaginal pathology, or neglected pessary may be discovered.

All pelvic bleeding sources should be investigated, including hematuria, hematochezia, vulvovaginal pathology, and trauma (**Table 36-5**). The external genitalia, vagina, and cervix are inspected for ulcerations, atrophy, abrasions, polyps, etc. If the cervix appears normal, screening with

TABLE 36-5 ■ DIFFERENTIAL DIAGNOSIS OF VAGINAL BLEEDING IN OLDER WOMEN

Uterus (corpus uteri)	Endometrial atrophy
	Endometrial proliferation from estrogen stimulation
	Endometrial polyp
	Endometrial hyperplasia
	Endometrial cancer
	Endometritis
	Myometrial cancer
Cervix (cervix uteri)	Cervical polyp
	Cervicitis
	Cancer
Vagina	Atrophy
	Infection
	Cancer
	Trauma
	Foreign body
	Prolapse with abrasion
Vulva	Ulcerations
	Excoriations
	Cancer trauma
Urinary tract	Urethral caruncle
	Urethral mucosal prolapse
	Hematuria
Gastrointestinal tract	Rectal polyp
	Rectal prolapse
	Hemorrhoids
	Hematochezia
Other (rare causes)	Oviduct cancer
	Ovarian cancer
	Metastatic nongynecologic cancer
	Endometriosis
Systemic illness	Coagulation disorder
	Hepatic cirrhosis
Iatrogenic	Anticoagulation
	Estrogen therapy

both cytology and HPV genotyping (co-testing) is advisable unless recently performed. An abnormal appearing cervix warrants biopsy. Bimanual and rectal examinations will help rule out pelvic masses, tissue induration, and rectal pathology.

Regardless of other findings, the endometrium must be evaluated with a biopsy or transvaginal ultrasound in the setting of postmenopausal bleeding. Office biopsy can have greater than 99% sensitivity, but not all devices achieve this. ACOG states that endometrial sampling may be deferred if the endometrial thickness is 4 mm or less. However, biopsy for tissue diagnosis is preferable to sonography to evaluate the endometrium in older women or in those with recurrent or persistent bleeding regardless of imaging.

No guidelines have been established for the evaluation of vaginal bleeding in frail, impaired older women. Even if aggressive treatments are not an option, palliative management improves when the disease process is understood. Evaluation of vaginal bleeding including biopsy can always be recommended, guided by clinical judgement and the patient's wishes.

OVARY AND ADNEXAL MASSES

Adnexal Mass

"Adnexa" is a plural word meaning "parts." *Adnexa uteri* refers to the fallopian tube and ovary. Adnexal masses can be, accordingly, of either the tube or ovary, but many other gynecologic and non-gynecologic pathologies masquerade as adnexal masses. Definitive diagnosis of an ovarian mass generally requires excisional surgery. However, imaging can obviate surgery in most patients. Although the chance of malignancy is increased after menopause, most adnexal masses are benign.

Menopause occurs when the ovary ceases its cyclic reproductive function and shrinks to an average volume of less than 4 cm^3. It continues to be an important source of androgen production, but not of estrogen. Functional cysts, normally associated with development of mature ova, still occur often after menopause. These generally resolve without intervention. Benign lesions are overwhelmingly epithelial tumors, usually cystadenomas. Tumors may also arise from stromal or germ cells, but most of these occur at younger ages. An endometrioma may persist indefinitely and is unlikely to grow or become newly symptomatic in older women.

Transvaginal ultrasound is the preferred imaging study for adnexal masses. Magnetic resonance imaging (MRI) is best suited to clarify the malignant potential if ultrasound is unreliable or cannot be performed transvaginally. When extraovarian disease is suspected or needs to be ruled out, computed tomography (CT) scan is the most reliable technique. Ultrasonography may be useful even when the adnexal mass was discovered on another imaging study, sometimes adding information that better characterizes the ovaries and uterus. For cysts that will be followed,

it is best to measure size over time with the same imaging modality, and ultrasound is less expensive.

Simple cysts less than 10-cm diameter will resolve spontaneously in half of older patients, indicating they were functional cysts. Most of the persistent ones eventually excised are benign epithelial tumors. Complex ovarian masses, with loculations or solid components, comprise 3% of postmenopausal adnexal masses. These are more concerning for neoplasia, but up to half may also resolve spontaneously. If an asymptomatic simple cyst is smaller than 10-cm diameter on transvaginal ultrasound and the serum CA-125 is not elevated, the usual plan is to repeat these studies in 3 to 6 months. Indications for urgent gynecologic consultation include size greater than or equal to 10 cm, complex components, or an elevated CA-125.

Ovarian Cancer

Ovarian cancer is the deadliest of the gynecologic cancers and is the fifth leading cause of cancer death in women in the United States. Approximately 1 in 70 women will be diagnosed with ovarian cancer in their lifetime. In 2020, an estimated 21,750 women were diagnosed with ovarian cancer in the United States, and 13,940 died from this disease. The median age at diagnosis is 63. The age-specific incidence peaks at age 80 to 84, and subsequently plateaus. Survival rates are poor primarily because of diagnosis at advanced stage. Initial symptoms are nonspecific, such as abdominal or pelvic pain, bloating, urinary complaints, and constipation. It is now appreciated that early-stage cancers are often symptomatic. In retrospect, most ovarian cancer patients have had symptoms for several months prior to diagnosis. While a transvaginal ultrasound and CA-125 blood test perform poorly as screening tests in low-risk women, they are useful to rule out ovarian cancer when abdominal, pelvic, gastrointestinal, or urinary symptoms are present. Early evaluation of symptoms has not been proven to improve survival, but some evidence suggests it identifies more women with completely resectable disease. Genetic testing is evolving rapidly. It is now thought that approximately 25% of ovarian cancers have a germline mutation.

Most ovarian malignancies in older women are epithelial. The paradigm of epithelial ovarian cancer pathogenesis has undergone radical changes in the past decade. Rather than arising from the ovarian cortex, most cancers are likely derived from the fallopian tube or the endometrium. Epithelial ovarian cancers are now divided into two broad categories. The relatively indolent type I tumors are comprised of low-grade serous, low-grade endometrioid, clear cell, and mucinous carcinomas, and Brenner tumors. Type II tumors are high-grade serous, high-grade endometrioid, and other aggressive carcinomas. While these new distinctions have few direct implications for geriatrics practice, they have expanded preventive surgical strategies. ACOG recommends performing incidental bilateral salpingectomy whenever possible. Older women already routinely undergo bilateral salpingo-oophorectomy incidental to abdominal hysterectomy, but not routinely during vaginal surgery. This should be considered in preoperative planning, but there are inadequate data to fully inform this decision.

Surgery is indicated for most women with ovarian cancer, even in advanced age, both for staging and improved survival with optimal tumor debulking. Treatment outcomes are better on average when the initial surgery is performed by a gynecologic oncologist rather than a general gynecologist, due to more complete staging and debulking. Having one surgery for diagnosis and partial treatment, then a subsequent one to finish the staging and treatment is associated with worse outcomes. This may have implications for referrals from a geriatrics practice.

HORMONES

Menopause

Menopause is defined as 12 months of amenorrhea secondary to cessation of ovulation. This can also be attained by surgical oophorectomy, chemotherapy, or radiation. The transition to menopause referred to as the perimenopause begins approximately 4 years prior to the last menstrual period and starts with irregular cycles during which time estrogen levels can be normal or elevated. Progesterone and estradiol levels decrease with an increase in follicle-stimulating hormone (FSH) levels. The postmenopausal estradiol levels are usually less than 20 pg/mL, while FSH is most often more than 70 mU/mL. Symptoms attributed to menopause include vasomotor (hot flushes and night sweats), vaginal atrophy (pruritis, dryness, and dyspareunia), UI, sleeping difficulty, depression, anxiety, mood changes, cognitive decline, and somatic complaints. Migraine prevalence may also increase in perimenopausal women due to estrogen fluctuations. Therefore, consideration of hormone therapy and the alternatives is important for symptom management and quality of life.

Hormone Therapy

Estrogen and estrogen plus progestin hormone therapy (HT) following menopause has a complex constellation of statistically small benefits and risks, and symptoms can often be managed with nonhormonal alternatives. Estrogen therapy is by far the most effective treatment for vasomotor symptoms of menopause. However, the use of systemic estrogen has been complicated by the results of the Women's Health Initiative (WHI), which found that the use of systemic estrogen alone increased the risk of stroke (relative risk 1.39), while the addition of progestin increased the risk of coronary events (relative risk 1.28), breast cancer (relative risk 1.26), and pulmonary embolism (relative risk 2.13). The absolute risk of these events is much lower in younger premenopausal women.

While initiation of HT after age 65 is contraindicated, continuation of HT taken since menopause should be decided on an individualized basis. The ACOG and the North American Menopause Society (NAMS) recommend that the lowest effective dose of systemic estrogen (plus progestin if uterus is present) should be used and estrogen replacement not be used for disease prevention. The marginal risk of continuation is very small. However, given the association with stroke and cardiovascular events, most women over age 65 will choose to discontinue HT. The issue then becomes how to discontinue without suffering excessive menopausal symptoms.

Four randomized trials studying fewer than 300 women have evaluated abrupt discontinuation versus tapering over 2 weeks, 4 weeks, 4 months, and 6 months. Overall successful discontinuation rates were similar, but symptoms were generally greater in the abrupt discontinuation groups. Roughly half of women tolerate sudden cessation but do better with ongoing clinical support for up to 3 years. Others experience unacceptable vasomotor symptoms, insomnia, irritability, short-term memory loss, or fatigue and resume HT. Anecdotally, tapering over an even longer time would yield greater success with fewer symptoms. Unless urgent, this can be done as slowly as necessary, reducing the dose every few months or annually. When the lowest commercially available dose has been reached, the taper can be continued dropping one weekly dose at a time once a month or as tolerated. Vasomotor symptoms can also be ameliorated with nonhormonal medications. Paroxetine, clonidine, and gabapentin have all shown efficacy in symptom management; however, paroxetine is the only nonhormonal agent with FDA approval for this indication. These may be trialed as initial therapy or as management after discontinuation of hormonal therapy. Each of these drugs have significant side effects in the older population.

Occasionally an older woman not taking estrogen experiences new-onset vasomotor symptoms. Pertinent history includes onset, frequency, duration, timing during the day or night, facial erythema, perspiration, flushed feelings, associated activities, and her symptoms at the time of menopause. Medications or supplements are often implicated in new symptoms; however, other etiologies should be evaluated including thyroid function. While hormone-related vasomotor symptoms do not suddenly arise years after a decline in estrogen, it is unclear in some cases whether hormones could be involved. A trial of estrogen therapy for 1 to 3 months can be informative or educational. Transdermal administration would minimize the risk of a vascular event as this avoids first-pass metabolism in the liver.

UROGYNECOLOGIC AND PELVIC FLOOR SUPPORT ISSUES

POP, UI, and UTI are very common gynecologic problems experienced by older women. Incontinence and infection are covered in more detail elsewhere. This section will focus on several specific conditions common in urogynecology and female urology including POP as well as bladder and urethral disorders such as IC, urethral caruncle, urethral cancer, urethral stricture, and urethral diverticulum. Urinary incontinence is discussed in Chapter 47.

Urethral Disorders

Several disorders of the female urethra occur with greater incidence and prevalence in older women compared to their younger counterparts. A urethral caruncle generally appears as a polypoid red mass protruding from the urethra at the 6 o'clock position. This is often asymptomatic and identified incidentally on physical examination (see **Figure 36-2**). Some patients may notice it and are often concerned for possible malignancy. Urethral caruncles are typically soft to palpation, although they may bleed due to irritation. They represent an incomplete prolapse of the urethral mucosa with possible loss of support of the periurethral muscular-connective tissue. Topical estrogen is generally effective and may lead to reduction in size or complete involution of the caruncle.

Urethral prolapse, in contrast to caruncles, is complete circumferential mucosal prolapse. It is managed similarly to a caruncle and, in most cases, resolves with topical estrogen. If there is persistent pain, bleeding, or other concerns, referral is warranted for further evaluation and consideration of surgical management.

In contrast, urethral cancers in women may present with bleeding and are typically hard or firm to palpation. The tumor can extend proximally toward the bladder neck, or into the vagina. Treatment is typically surgical, although radiation may also be used in select cases or for palliation.

Urethral strictures in women are uncommon. Surgical excision and reconstruction are the most effective form of therapy. Urethral dilation should be avoided in women and is not particularly effective for long-term therapy. There are no data to support routine urethral dilation for treatment of UTI or voiding dysfunction in most women.

Urethral diverticulum results from an outpouching of tissue in the urethra associated with a defect in the midline fusion of the urethral plate. Women often experience the "3-Ds" of dysuria, dyspareunia, and dribbling incontinence; they may also be associated with recurrent UTIs. Differential diagnosis for urethral diverticulum includes vaginal wall cysts from an embryologic remnant (Gartner's duct cyst) or local gland (Skene's duct cyst) and ectopic ureterocele. Surgical excision with urethral closure or reconstruction is typically indicated. Urethral malignancy has been found in approximately 6% to 9% of patients with a urethral diverticulum; the most common type of malignancy is adenocarcinoma. Magnetic resonance imaging is the imaging modality of choice prior to surgical management.

Interstitial Cystitis and Painful Bladder Syndrome

Interstitial cystitis (IC), also called painful bladder syndrome (PBS), is a chronic condition of the bladder typically associated with a constellation of symptoms including urinary urgency, frequency, and pelvic pain. It is generally diagnosed in women in their 30s or 40s but must

be chronically managed throughout a woman's lifetime as there is no cure. Patients generally experience worse pain with bladder filling, which is relieved at least temporarily by voiding. Pain is a hallmark symptom and helps to differentiate the condition from overactive bladder (OAB) and other forms of lower urinary tract dysfunction. The exact etiology of IC is unknown although theories include autoimmune components, direct chemical irritants in the urine, effects from inflammatory mediators, and defects in the bladder epithelial barrier layer. Other conditions that should be ruled out in cases of possible IC include bladder cancer, bladder carcinoma in situ, UTI, and bladder stones. Continued symptoms in the context of persistent negative urine cultures should prompt the clinician to consider IC.

Diagnosis can be made based on clinical symptoms and ruling out other etiologies. Cystoscopy with hydrodistension of the bladder under anesthesia is a useful diagnostic tool and may also be therapeutic for many patients. Reduced bladder capacity and mucosal changes including petechial hemorrhage are commonly seen in cases of IC. Ulcerations of the bladder mucosa occur less commonly but may represent more severe disease. Cystoscopy also offers the clinician the opportunity to visually examine the bladder to rule out other serious conditions such as bladder cancer, particularly in older women where the rates of bladder cancer increase compared to young women. Bladder wash cytology and biopsies may also be used to help aid in the diagnosis of bladder cancer. Patients may be treated for IC or PBS without cystoscopic confirmation of the condition, but in older patients it is wise to eliminate other potential pathologies. Referral to Urology is indicated if a patient has persistent or progressive symptoms not adequately managed with conservative therapy.

Pelvic Organ Prolapse

POP can be quite bothersome for older women. Incidence and prevalence rates of POP increase with advancing age. Risk factors include prior hysterectomy, obesity, smoking, parity, poor tissue quality, and connective tissue disease. Several different types of prolapse occur depending on the involved anatomy. Patients may experience a bulging sensation from the vagina or may complain of pressure or discomfort in the pelvis or lower back. Bleeding and discharge are common symptoms, particularly in women with large prolapse extending out of the vaginal canal, and may be associated with erosion, ulceration, or keratinization of the exposed vaginal mucosa.

Evaluation of Pelvic Organ Prolapse

Clinical evaluation includes careful history and physical examination (**Table 36-6**). Symptoms should be identified to help gauge the degree of bother experienced by the patient, which in turn can help determine the types of treatment that can be considered. In patients with little symptomatic bother and minimal other signs or symptoms,

TABLE 36-6 ■ EVALUATION AND MANAGEMENT OF PELVIC ORGAN PROLAPSE

History

Vaginal bulge, pressure or pain (often worse in late afternoon or evening)

Vaginal bleeding or discharge

Urinary frequency or incontinence

Difficulty initiating urinary stream

Sense of incomplete bladder emptying

Constipation

Fecal incontinence

Need to elevate the bladder to urinate or "splint" the perineum or rectum to defecate

Physical examination

Vaginal bulge

Mucosal abrasions or ulcerations

Degree of descent of prolapse

   Does prolapse extend beyond midpoint of vagina

   Does prolapse extend beyond the vaginal introitus/hymenal ring

   Does prolapse increase with maximal Valsalva or cough effort

Anterior vaginal wall, posterior vaginal wall, vaginal apex

Cervix and uterus—support and mobility

Urethra and bladder neck—support and mobility

Postvoid residual urine volume and urinalysis

Management

Nonsurgical

   Observation

   Pessary

   Estrogen cream—to prevent and treat ulcerations and improve mucosal quality

   Barrier creams or ointments to protect vaginal mucosa

   Truss-strong elastic support

Surgical-reconstructive

   Transvaginal

   Transabdominal

   Laparoscopic/robotic

   Uterosacral or sacrospinous ligament fixation of vaginal vault

Surgical-vaginal obliterative

   Colpocleisis

   Colpectomy

observation may be adequate. Careful pelvic examination is critical in making the correct diagnosis of POP. Prolapse of the anterior vaginal wall is a cystocele, and the posterior vaginal wall is typically a rectocele. Loss of support of the vaginal apex may include small bowel which is known as an enterocele. Uterine prolapse may also occur due to loss of support of the cardinal or uterosacral ligaments. Complete vaginal eversion may occur in women with a prior hysterectomy, or "procidentia" if the uterus is in situ.

Physical examination is important for complete assessment. On simple inspection, it can be difficult to differentiate the portion of the vagina involved in the prolapse. A single-blade speculum is useful for this purpose. The speculum is initially inserted to depress the posterior vaginal wall. The speculum is then reinserted in the reverse position to elevate the anterior vaginal wall allowing inspection of the posterior compartment for evidence of rectocele. Asking the patient to cough and Valsalva can help to demonstrate prolapse that may increase with abdominal straining. It can be useful to also examine the patient in the standing position if possible, as some prolapse may only be evident with standing.

A cystocele occurs because of a weakness of the anterior vaginal wall muscular-connective tissue. The bladder protrudes into the vaginal space, and in some cases may extend beyond the hymenal ring. Cystoceles may or may not be associated with stress UI. Some women with large cystoceles may have trouble voiding due to obstructive angulation of the urethra or poor bladder contractility (**Figure 36-4**). In some cases, women with large cystoceles may report having to put their fingers in the vagina to elevate the tissue to straighten out the urethra to urinate or to completely empty the bladder. Despite this, high-grade obstruction in women is rare, and development of upper tract deterioration with hydronephrosis and renal insufficiency is uncommon. Hydroureter and hydronephrosis can occur if there is substantial ureteral kinking at its insertion into the bladder in cases of complete vaginal vault prolapse. This is more likely if the uterus is present. Serum blood urea nitrogen and creatinine level and renal ultrasound are useful in determining the extent of renal impairment.

A rectocele is a protrusion of the rectum through the posterior wall of the vagina and is caused by weakness in the perirectal muscular-connective tissue (**Figure 36-5**). Some patients may describe difficulty with defecation, including an increased sense of pressure or need to strain. Some women describe needing to "splint" or press on the posterior vaginal wall or perineum to completely evacuate their stool.

An enterocele is a herniation of small bowel and peritoneum through the apical vagina or between the uterosacral ligaments and rectovaginal space (**Figure 36-6**). It is the only true hernia among the various forms of POP. It is more common in women who have undergone prior hysterectomy. However, it can be present in any posterior vaginal wall prolapse, and rarely in anterior compartment prolapse.

Rectal prolapse involves protrusion of the rectum through the anal sphincter with tissue extending beyond the anal verge. It may or may not be associated with hemorrhoids. Symptoms of rectal prolapse can include pain, bleeding, or defecatory dysfunction. Many patients experience both fecal incontinence and constipation. Careful examination is needed to determine if the rectal prolapse can be reduced. In cases where reduction is not possible,

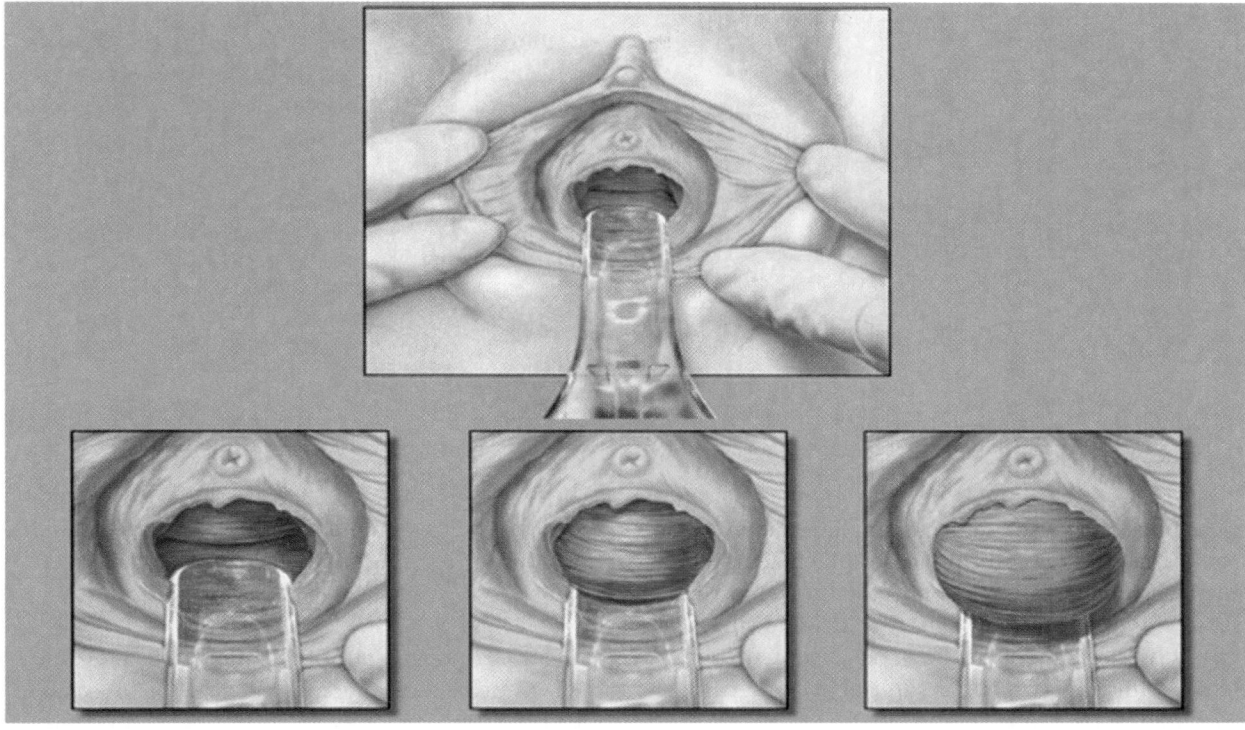

A

Cystocele

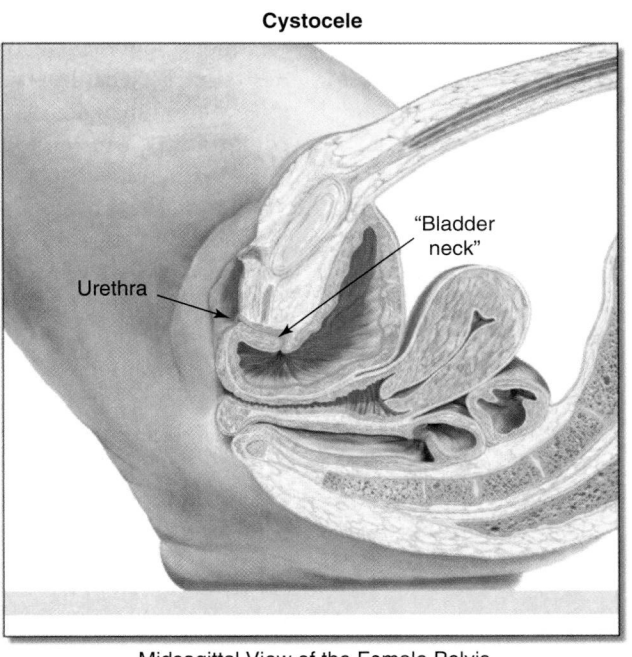

"Bladder neck"

Urethra

Midsagittal View of the Female Pelvis

B

FIGURE 36-4. Anterior and sagittal views of a cystocele. Note the increasing size of a cystocele (**A**) and that it can cause angulation of the urethra and contribute to symptoms of voiding difficulty and urinary retention (**B**).

tissue incarceration and necrosis may develop. Patients with rectal prolapse should be referred to a colorectal surgeon or gastroenterologist for additional evaluation and treatment.

Several different systems have been designed to grade the degree of POP based on anatomic changes. The

Baden-Walker system was commonly used in clinical practice, and classifies the degree of prolapse based on whether it extends beyond the midpoint of the vagina or beyond the vaginal introitus, when it is more likely to become symptomatic. The POP-Q system is more commonly used in

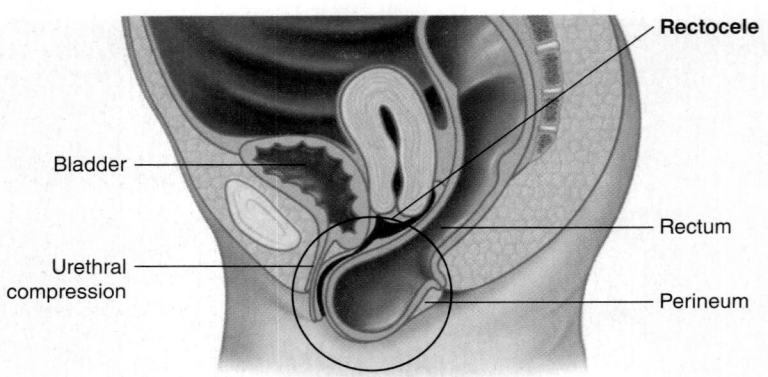

FIGURE 36-5. Sagittal view of a rectocele.

research settings but is also useful in a simplified approach in defining the leading edge of the prolapse. It includes multiple anatomic measurements in relation to the vaginal introitus. In most systems, the hymenal ring is used to define the vaginal introitus. A clear understanding and documentation of the extent of prolapse is useful for surgical planning and for following progress over time (**Figure 36-7**).

Treatment of Pelvic Organ Prolapse

Most treatments are aimed at reducing the prolapse back into the vaginal canal and correcting vaginal anatomy (see **Table 36-6**). Ulcerations of the vaginal epithelium may respond to topical estrogen therapy. Barrier compounds may also be helpful to reduce tissue irritation.

Treatment of POP may be surgical or nonsurgical and depends to some degree on the amount of bother experienced by the patient. It also depends on overall health status, and goals of therapy. The main conditions necessitating definitive treatment or specialist referral include nonhealing ulcerations, bleeding, elevated postvoid residual urine volume causing recurrent UTIs, and hydronephrosis. If none of these are present and the patient is not particularly bothered by her symptoms, then reassurance and observation are appropriate. Application of estrogen cream once or twice a week is advisable for preventive care and can help

reduce tissue irritation and ulceration. Some patients may find comfort in using supportive underwear.

Nonsurgical Treatment of POP and UI

Nonsurgical treatment of POP and UI includes such treatment as behavioral therapy (pelvic floor muscle exercises including stress and urgency incontinence strategies), medications, as well as the use of intravaginal support devices. One should consider first starting with a conservative treatment approach in older women who do not have a desire for surgical intervention or in cases where surgical intervention may not be an ideal choice due to the medical comorbidities causing the increased surgical risk.

With respect to pelvic floor muscle exercises, they may limit the progression of mild prolapse and related symptoms, but less response has been noted with prolapse beyond the vaginal introitus. Pelvic floor muscle exercises are usually employed to treat accompanying urinary and/or fecal incontinence. Results are generally dependent on patient motivation and the patient's willingness to comply with an exercise treatment program.

The use of a pessary has been considered an excellent option for nonsurgical management of POP and UI. Patient acceptance is relatively high when appropriately counseled. There are a number of different sizes and shapes

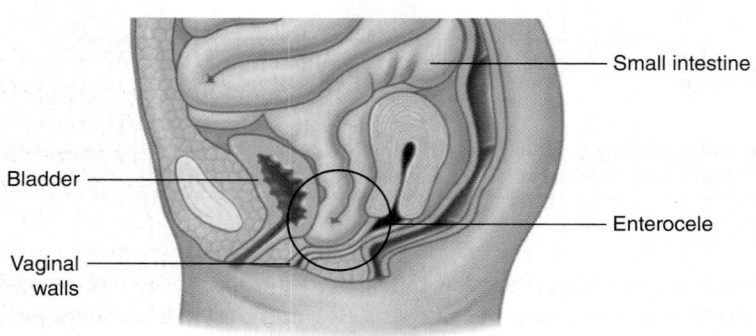

FIGURE 36-6. Sagittal view of an enterocele.

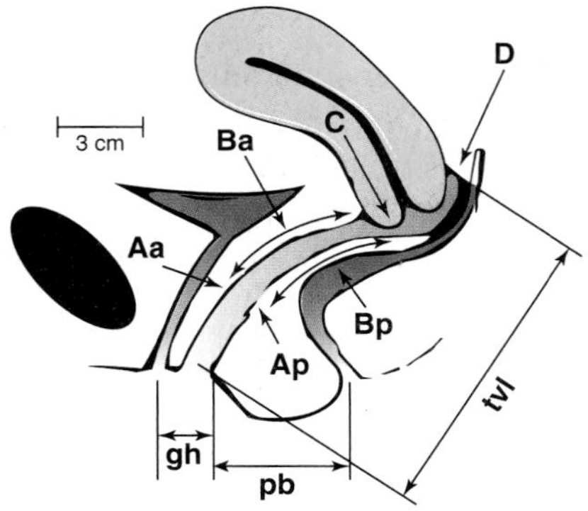

Anterior wall Aa	Anterior wall Ba	Cervix or cuff C
Genital hiatus gh	Perineal body pb	Total vaginal length tvl
Posterior wall Ap	Posterior wall Bp	Posterior fornix D

FIGURE 36-7. Treatment of pelvic organ prolapse. (Reproduced with permission from Bump RC, Mattiasson A, Bø K, et al. The standardization of terminology of female pelvic organ prolapse and pelvic floor dysfunction. *Am J Obstet Gynecol.* 1996;175[1]:10–17.)

for pessaries and most of them are made from silicone. The risk factors for a failed fitting include a large genital hiatus and a short vaginal length. Pessaries provide pelvic organ support within the vaginal vault. There are two categories of pessaries for POP: support pessaries and space-filling pessaries. The ring pessary (with a diaphragm) is one of the most used support pessaries while the Gellhorn pessary is a commonly used space-filling pessary. Most women who have a stage II or stage III prolapse are successfully fitted with ring pessaries while women with stage IV prolapse usually require a Gellhorn pessary.

Some of the possible complications from pessaries include odor and vaginal discharge. There may also be a failure to retain a pessary or the pessary may be too large, which could lead to excoriation or irritation. There may also be increased stress incontinence with reduction of the vaginal prolapse and in rare instances more severe complications such as fistula formation.

Ideal follow-up for pessaries should be tailored to the patient. Some patients can remove pessaries by themselves and clean them while other patients are less mobile and are cognitively impaired and may need very close follow up within 1 to 3 months. Each clinician should evaluate the tissue health of the patient, the cognitive and mobility status of the patient, type of pessary being utilized, and the patient's home/living situation and then assess the patient for the appropriate treatment plan for each patient depending on the aforementioned factors. Assessing tissue health and the use of vaginal estrogen cream accompanying the pessary are important aspects of managing pessary care.

Surgeries

Surgical management of POP includes either reconstructive or obliterative procedures. Reconstructive options aim to reduce the prolapse and reestablish normal vaginal anatomy. Examples include anterior and posterior colporrhaphy and enterocele repair. Prolapse of the vaginal apex may require more advanced repair techniques including vaginal, abdominal, laparoscopic, or robotic approaches to the vaginal apex. For example, one can perform a vaginal uterosacral or sacrospinous ligament fixation, in which the apex of the vagina is sutured to a fixed point in the pelvis. In some cases, mesh or other supporting material is needed to perform this type of repair such as sacrocolpopexy. Potential complications include mesh erosion through the vaginal wall or other surrounding structures. Colpocleisis is an obliterative procedure in which the prolapse is reduced and the vagina is essentially closed to prevent recurrence. For a specialist, it is technically straightforward and may offer an option for older women with substantial comorbidity who may not be good candidates for more involved reconstructive procedures. However, patients need to be carefully counseled that penetrative sexual activity will not be possible after colpocleisis. Studies have shown that in carefully selected patients, satisfaction rates are high with low rates of regret regarding the procedure. Rectal prolapse is typically treated surgically with either reduction, fixation, or excision of the prolapsed portion of the rectum. Treatments to prevent chronic constipation are indicated after all types of POP repair to avoid significant straining with bowel movements and prevent prolapse recurrence.

SUMMARY

Although gynecologic issues comprise a small part of geriatric care, large impacts can be made on function and quality of life. A thorough personal and family history will guide cancer prevention and detection. An initial pelvic examination will provide the basis for understanding symptoms and anticipating problems, potentially for years to come. Querying problems in a systematic fashion addressing all potential gynecologic concerns will encourage the patient to voice symptoms when they arise. Persistence in addressing incontinence and pelvic floor issues can help maintain physical activity and prevent isolation. Ensuring adequate cervical cancer screening, early recognition of endometrial and vulvar cancer, and early investigation of abdominopelvic complaints to rule out ovarian cancer will reduce disease burden. Proactive assessment of pelvic floor conditions may also impact quality of life.

ACKNOWLEDGMENT

Karen L. Miller and Tomas L. Griebling contributed to this chapter in the 7th edition and some material from that chapter has been retained here.

FURTHER READING

General

Meyer I, Howard TF, Smith HJ, Kim KH, Richter HE. Gynecologic disorders in the older woman. In: Rosenthal R, Zenilman M, Katlic M (eds). *Principles and Practice of Geriatric Surgery*. Cham: Springer; 2020.

The 2017 hormone therapy position statement of The North American Menopause Society. *Menopause*. 2017;24(7): 728–753.

Breast

ACOG Practice Bulletin No. 164. Diagnosis and Management of Benign Breast Disorders. *Obstet Gynecol*. 2016;127(6):e141–e56.

Pain

ACOG Practice Bulletin No. 218. Chronic pelvic pain. *Obstet Gynecol*. 2020;135(3):e98–e109.

Lindsetmo RO, Stulberg J. Chronic abdominal wall pain—a diagnostic challenge for the surgeon. *Am J Surg*. 2009;198(1):129–134.

Vulva

ACOG Practice Bulletin No. 224. Diagnosis and Management of Vulvar Skin Disorders. *Obstet Gynecol*. 2020;136(1):e1–e14.

The 2020 genitourinary syndrome of menopause position statement of the North American Menopause Society. *Menopause*. 2020;27(9):976–992.

Bornstein J, Bogliatto F, Haefner HK, et al. The 2015 International Society for the Study of Vulvovaginal Disease (ISSVD) terminology of vulvar squamous intraepithelial lesions. *J Low Genit Tract Dis*. 2016;20(1):11–14.

Gerfus KB, Lee AW, Baradaran N, et al. Pathophysiology, clinical manifestations, and treatment of lichen sclerosus: a systematic review. *Urology*. 2020;135:11–19.

Marnach ML, Torgerson RR. Vulvovaginal issues in mature women. *Mayo Clin Proc*.; 2017;92(3):449–454.

Vagina

ACOG Practice Bulletin No. 215. Vaginitis in nonpregnant patients. *Obstet Gynecol*. 2020;135(1):e1–e17.

Shifren JL. Genitourinary syndrome of menopause. *Clin Obstet Gynecol*. 2018;61(3):508–516.

Cervix

Malagon T, Kulasingam S, Mayrand MH, et al. Age at last screening and remaining lifetime risk of cervical cancer in older, unvaccinated, HPV-negative women: a modelling study. *Lancet Oncol*. 2018;19(12): 1569–1578.

Perkins RB, Guido RS, Castle PE, et al. 2019 ASCCP Risk-Based Management Consensus Guidelines for Abnormal Cervical Cancer Screening Tests and Cancer Precursors. *J Low Genit Tract Dis*. 2020;24(2):102–131.

Uterus/Bleeding

ACOG Practice Bulletin No. 149. Endometrial cancer. *Obstet Gynecol*. 2015;125(4):1006–1026.

SGO Clinical Practice Statement. Screening for Lynch syndrome in endometrial cancer. March 2014. https://www.sgo.org/clinical-practice/guidelines/screening-for-lynch-syndrome-in-endometrial-cancer/. Accessed December 12, 2020.

Ovary/Adnexal Mass

ACOG Practice Bulletin No. 174. Evaluation and management of adnexal masses. *Obstet Gynecol*. 2016;174: e1–e17.

ACOG Practice Bulletin No. 182. Hereditary breast and ovarian cancer. *Obstet Gynecol*. 2017;182:e1–e17.

Urogynecological Issues

ACOG Practice Bulletin No. 214. Pelvic organ prolapse. *Obstet Gynecol*. 2019;134(5):e126–e142.

Bump RC, Mattiasson A, Bø K, et al. The standardization of terminology of female pelvic organ prolapse and pelvic floor dysfunction. *Am J Obstet Gynecol*. 1996;175(1): 10–17.

De Albuquerque Coelho SC, de Castro EB, Juliato CR. Female pelvic organ prolapse using pessaries: systematic review. *Int Urogynecol J*. 2016;27(12):1797–1803.

Chapter 37

Sexuality, Sexual Function, and the Aging Man

J. Lisa Tenover, Alvin M. Matsumoto

Sexuality is a basic human need that exists throughout life and is a significant component to quality of life of many older individuals. Although 70% of adult patients in a large sample study considered sexual matters to be an appropriate topic for a general clinician or geriatrician to discuss, sexual problems are noted in fewer than 2% of primary care physicians' notes. Sexuality and sexual function in the aging female are addressed in Chapter 35. Sexuality, sexual function and dysfunction in the aging male, and the use of testosterone replacement therapy for male sexual dysfunction caused by male hypogonadism will be discussed in this chapter.

SEXUALITY AND SEXUAL FUNCTION IN OLDER MEN

Sexual Behaviors

Numerous cross-sectional and longitudinal epidemiologic studies of sexuality and aging report that, although sexual activity decreases with age, many older adults are sexually active. Sexual expression can encompass many forms, but most studies report data on sexual intercourse, oral sex, and masturbation.

Figure 37-1A depicts the age-related prevalence of male sexual activity from two large studies. Both studies defined sexual activity as activity with a partner and occurring within the 12 months prior to the data collection. In these studies, the likelihood of sexual activity with a partner did decline with age, but nearly 40% of men at age 75 to 80 reported some sexual activity, and 54% of these reported sex at least two to three times a month.

Reasons reported by older men for not engaging in sexual activity are varied, involving social factors as well as physical and psychological health. Partner availability (no partner, partner not interested, or partner with physical limitations) is a major factor. Psychological conditions, such as anxiety and depression, can affect libido and sexual function; and many medical problems are linked to sexual dysfunction.

Changes in Male Sexual Physiology With Age

Overall there is a gradual slowing of sexual physical response time as men age. It takes more time to achieve sexual arousal, complete the sexual act, and become rearoused

Learning Objectives

- Identify the factors affecting sexual function in the older man, including changes in sexual physiology, coexisting medical problems, and psychosocial issues.
- Describe the initial evaluation of erectile dysfunction (ED) in an older man, using knowledge of possible etiologies to guide evaluation and treatment recommendations.
- Identify older men with sexual dysfunction who might benefit from testosterone treatment.

Key Clinical Points

1. Male sexual activity declines with aging, due to social factors and changes in physical and psychological health; yet many older men are sexually active into late life.

2. The most common causes for ED in older men are vascular in origin, not hormonal, and thus current predominant therapies are phosphodiesterase-5 (PDE-5) inhibitors and vacuum devices.

3. Testosterone treatment improves libido, sexual activity, and erectile function in older men with hypogonadism (ie, men with symptoms and signs of testosterone deficiency and consistently low morning serum testosterone concentrations), but not in older men with normal testosterone concentrations.

for further sexual activity. **Table 37-1** lists the specific changes in the male sexual response cycle with age. Some of the changes have been shown to be impacted, at least in part, by low testosterone levels, while others are unaffected by hormone levels.

The Aging Gay, Bisexual, or Transgender (GBT) Male

As of 2017, somewhere between 1.4% and 2.4% of older men identified themselves as GBT. Older GBT men have similar sexual problems as older heterosexual men, but

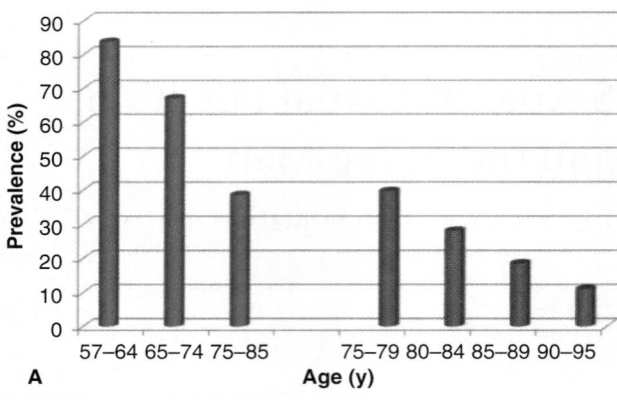

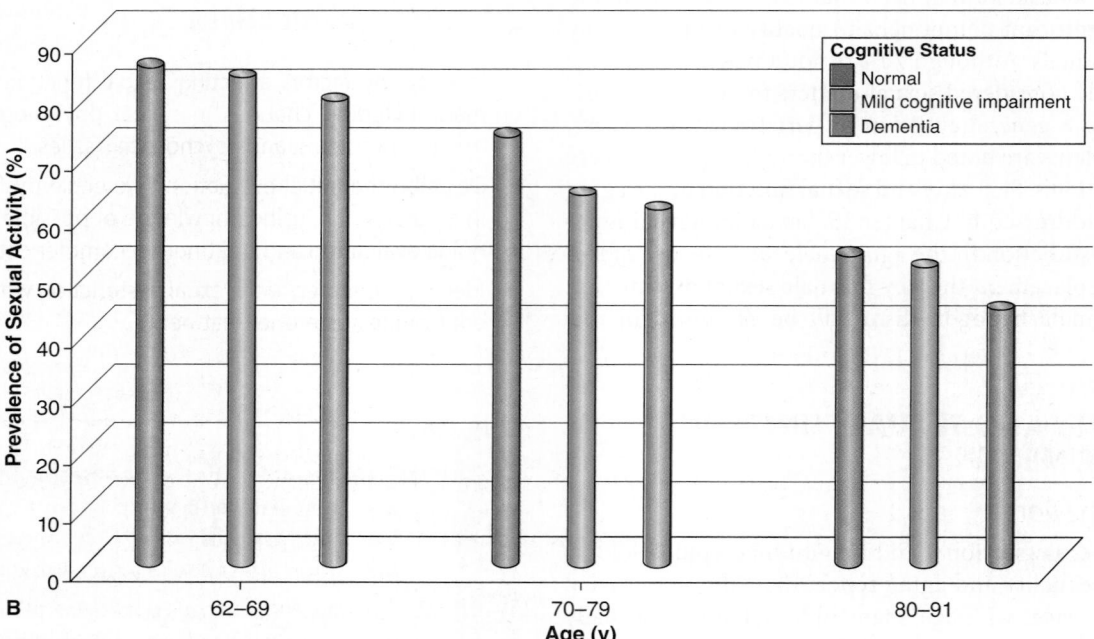

FIGURE 37-1. **A.** Prevalence, by age group, of male sexual activity with a partner in previous 12 months obtained from a survey of a probability sample of 3000 US adults age 57 to 85 and from a population-based cohort study of 3274 men age 75 to 95. **B.** Prevalence of male sexual activity with a partner in previous 12 months, by age group, and of cognitive status as determined by short cognitive assessment tool, obtained from a survey of a probability sample of community-dwelling men aged 62 to 91. (A, blue bars, Data from Lindau ST, Schumm LP, Laumann EO, Levinson W, O'Muircheartaigh CA, Waite LJ. A study of sexuality and health among older adults in the United States. *N Engl J Med.* 2007;357[8]:762–774. A, red bars, Data from Hyde Z, Flicker L, Hankey GJ, et al. Prevalence of sexual activity and associated factors in men aged 75 to 95 years: a cohort study. *Ann Intern Med.* 2010;153[11]:693–702. B, Data from Lindau ST, Dale W, Feldmeth G, et al. Sexuality and cognitive status: a U.S. nationally representative study of home-dwelling older adults. *J Am Geriatr Soc.* 2018;66[10]:1902–1910.)

may suffer additional problems. GBT older men can face discrimination when seeking health care, and many service providers are poorly prepared to work with them. Additionally, these older men are likely to suffer additional stress while trying to find a partner, especially if their living situation changes and they move into assisted-living facilities or nursing homes. While assisted living and long-term care facilities have been evolving to become more welcoming to the LGBT community, disparities in care still exist. Specific organizations that address issues of aging gay, bisexual, or transgender persons have formed across the country.

Unprotected sex occurs in approximately 10% of older gay men. Compared to younger gay men, however, older gay men get tested less often for sexually transmitted diseases, including testing for acquired immunodeficiency syndrome (AIDS). The incidence of AIDS is increasing in older men. Education about safe sex practices is important for the older population. Older males with a history of anal sex need to be regularly examined for anal cancer, as the prevalence increases in such persons.

Older GBT males should be encouraged to make advance directives for health and to specifically designate their durable power of attorney for health care in order to

TABLE 37-1 ■ CHANGES IN THE MALE SEXUAL RESPONSE CYCLE WITH AGE

Lengthening of the excitement (plateau)
Decreased penile rigidity[a]
Longer interval to ejaculation (plateau) phase
Fewer and less forceful contractions of the urethra
Lower ejaculatory volume
Less well-defined sense of impending orgasm[a]
Shortening of the ejaculatory event and orgasmic phase[a]
Increased occurrence of resolution without ejaculation[a]
More rapid detumescence
Lengthening of the refractory period

[a]Aspects that may be somewhat affected by testosterone levels.

facilitate the ability of their partners to make their health decisions.

Sex in Long-Term Care

While there is no reason to believe the desire for intimacy is lost on entering a residential long-term care facility, persons who live in nursing homes frequently have no opportunity for a private or sexual life; many couples are separated due to the residential care admission. Federal regulations provide some right to privacy, and nursing home staff are becoming more educated about resident sexuality and issues that may arise as a result, but barriers to sexual expression in long-term care often are significant. Issues surrounding romantic liaisons between two unmarried residents in a nursing home can be problematic. Ethical concerns can arise around the assessment of sexual behaviors and whether they are "sexually inappropriate" or not, and may involve balancing a resident's need for sexual expression against expectations and beliefs of caregivers and family members. If the sexual conduct involves one or both persons who are cognitively impaired, individual capacity to consent to sexual activity needs to be assessed. There is considerable variability by state in the definitions of capacity to consent to sexual activity and sexual consent is complicated, involving knowledge, capacity, and voluntariness. There are no surrogate decision makers for sexual relations. Psychological evaluation for capacity to consent to sexual activity may need to be sought. Also see Chapter 35, as similar challenges affect older women in these settings.

Sex and Cognitive Impairment/Dementia

Development of cognitive impairment does not equate with loss of sexuality or sexual function. Although age-adjusted rates of partnered sexual activity are lower in those with worse cognitive function, the majority of community dwelling partnered older men with dementia are sexually active. In one study (**Figure 37-1B**), more than 40% of partnered men, ages 80 to 91 and who screened positive for dementia, were sexually active, although compared to

the same age men with normal cognition, those men with dementia were more likely to report obligatory sex and sex without arousal. Issues of sexuality, however, can be especially complex for those individuals who have significant dementia and can include loss of partner recognition, loss of memory of past sexual activity, and role changes, where one's sexual partner now also is one's caregiver. Physicians of demented male patients need to ask the spouse or partner about sexual issues or conflicts. Placing the problems in the context of dementia can assist with discussion of coping strategies. Nonsexual ways of expressing one's intimacy, such as touching, holding hands, and massages, might be suggested.

Inappropriate sexual behavior (ISB) in individuals with dementia reportedly ranges from 7% to 25% with higher prevalence in men, in residents of nursing facilities, and in persons with more severe cognitive impairment. There is no universally accepted definition of ISB, but it has been described as sexually related activities or heightened sexual drive that interferes with function and is pursued at inappropriate times or with nonconsenting persons. Included in ISB are unwanted verbal remarks, unwanted touching, disrobing, public masturbation, unwanted sexual advances, and sexual aggression. ISB can cause conflict between a patient's autonomy and the prevention of psychological and physical trauma. It impacts families, care providers, and, especially in long-term care facilities, may threaten others who might be unable or unwilling to give informed consent.

There are no established treatment protocols for ISB. Some environmental and behavioral strategies that have been tried include redirection, distraction, clothing modification, avoidance of external cues, and in long-term care facilities, provision of single rooms. Supportive psychotherapy for spouses and families can be helpful. There are no controlled trials of pharmacologic therapies for ISB, but medications that have been reported to reduce ISB include the selective serotonin reuptake inhibitors (SSRIs), venlafaxine, both first-generation and atypical antipsychotics, medroxyprogesterone acetate, gonadotropin-releasing hormone (GnRH) analogues, cyproterone acetate, cholinesterase inhibitors, pindolol, and gabapentin.

SEXUAL DYSFUNCTION IN THE AGING MALE

Categories of Male Sexual Dysfunction

The major categories of sexual dysfunction in older men include erectile dysfunction (ED), lack of interest in sex (low libido), performance anxiety, and inability to climax. ED is by far the most prevalent. ED is defined as the inability to obtain and sustain a penile erection adequate for intercourse. Age alone is a major risk factor for ED, and its incidence, prevalence, and severity increase with age. In the Massachusetts Male Aging Study, a community-based

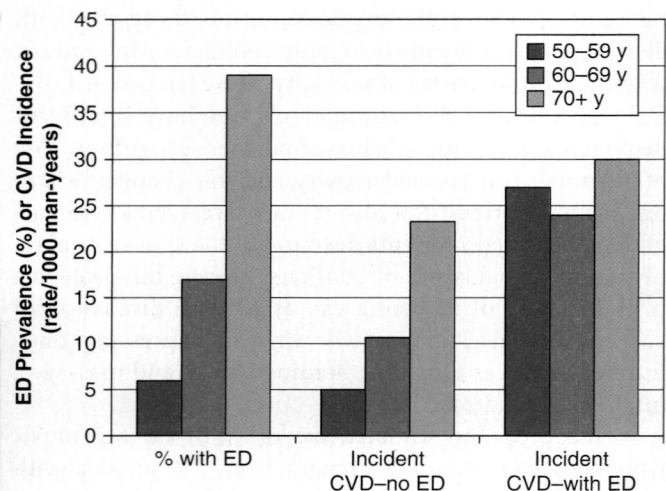

FIGURE 37-2. Prevalence, by age group, of erectile dysfunction (ED) from a longitudinal population-based study of community-dwelling men, and the 10-year follow-up incidence of cardiovascular events as a function of baseline presence or absence of ED. (Data from Inman BA, Sauver JL, Jacobson DJ, et al. A population-based, longitudinal study of erectile dysfunction and future coronary artery disease. *Mayo Clin Proc.* 2009;84[2]:108–113.)

study of middle-aged and older men, the reported incidence of some degree of ED was 55% for men at age 60, and 65% for men at 70 years; the prevalence of total ED was 15% at age 70. In a population-based prospective cohort study in Olmsted County, Minnesota, ED prevalence was 6% in men aged 50 to 59, 17% in men aged 60 to 69, and 39% in men aged 70 and older (**Figure 37-2**).

Libido is dependent on learned responses, general health-related quality of life, and, to some extent, serum testosterone levels. As will be discussed later in this chapter, testosterone levels decline in men with normal aging, and some men may reach levels that are low enough to affect libido. Similarly, treatment of prostate cancer with androgen deprivation therapy (ADT) resulting in severe testosterone deficiency can be associated with loss of libido.

Performance anxiety is common in older men and often a result of equating masculinity with speed and magnitude of sexual activity. A man may become so preoccupied by his performance that his confidence and sexual capacity lessen, leading to ED. Depression and psychosocial stresses also are prevalent in older men and contribute to sexual problems. "Widower's syndrome," where a man fails to achieve erection after the death of spouse, is a reported entity.

Inability to reach climax or resolution of climax without ejaculation can occur. In the University of Chicago study, this occurred in about 16% in the 57- to 64-year age range, but increased to 33% in the 75-year and older age group.

Erectile Dysfunction

Etiologies **Table 37-2** lists the major etiologies of ED. Vascular disease, which includes both atherosclerotic arterial

TABLE 37-2 ■ MAJOR ETIOLOGIES OF ERECTILE DYSFUNCTION

Vascular disease
   Atherosclerotic arterial occlusive disease, corpora venous leak
Neurologic disease
   Neuropathy, cord injury, stroke, multiple sclerosis, temporal lobe epilepsy, Parkinson disease
Diabetes mellitus
   Both vascular and neurologic effects
Other systemic diseases
   Renal failure, chronic obstructive pulmonary disease
Hormonal
   Hyper- and hypothyroidism, hypercortisolemia, severe hypogonadism
Urologic
   Lower urinary tract symptoms (LUTS) due to BPH
Surgery/radiation/trauma
   Prostate cancer surgery or radiation therapy, Peyronie disease
Lifestyle related
   Obesity, smoking, heavy alcohol use
Medications
Psychogenic
   Depression, anxiety

occlusive disease and corpora cavernosal venous leak, is the most common cause of ED. The likely mechanism is that penile hypoxia leads to replacement of corpora smooth muscle by connective tissue, which results in impaired cavernosal expandability and inability to compress subtunical venules.

Cardiovascular disease (CVD) and ED share etiologies. Diabetes mellitus, hypertension, hyperlipidemia, and smoking are major risk factors for both ED and CVD. The penis is a high blood flow system during erectile function, so ED may be an early sign of vascular inadequacy on the basis of atherosclerosis. Numerous studies suggest that ED is one of the sentinel symptoms of occult CVD, particularly in men under the age of 70 (see **Figure 37-2**). It is recommended that men under the age of 70 presenting with ED should be provided appropriate screening and treatment for CVD.

Diabetes mellitus is the most common single disease to cause ED. Although the severity of hyperglycemia has been suggested as a predictor of ED, age, duration of diabetes, autonomic neuropathy, and other diabetic complications appear to be better predictors. Sometimes ED is the first symptom of diabetes mellitus, so all men who present with newly diagnosed ED should be evaluated for possible diabetes.

Neurologic diseases, such as peripheral neuropathy, spinal cord injury, stroke, multiple sclerosis, temporal lobe epilepsy, and Parkinson disease all can cause ED. In men who develop multiple sclerosis, about half of them present initially with ED. In these men, ED may be present for a time, then resolve and recur at the next exacerbation. Men with stroke-related ED also tend to have ejaculatory problems.

Significant other systemic diseases that can cause ED are renal failure and chronic obstructive pulmonary disease (COPD). Chronic renal failure impacts erectile function through effects on the vascular system and via the development of autonomic neuropathy. In addition, many men with end-stage renal disease are severely hypogonadal. Neither hemodialysis nor testosterone replacement in men with renal failure has been shown to improve ED. Men with COPD and low PaO_2 have decreased cavernosal nitric oxide. Oxygen therapy may improve erectile function in some men with COPD.

Hypercortisolemia and hyper- and hypothyroidism have been associated with low libido and ED. Hypothyroidism also is associated with delayed ejaculation, while hyperthyroidism is associated with premature ejaculation. Normalization of thyroid function frequently leads to improvement in both ED and ejaculatory dysfunction, although it may take up to 6 months after achievement of a euthyroid state for these functions to normalize.

Serum testosterone levels in men decline with aging, but the amount of contribution of this testosterone decline to the development of ED is not clear. In the Massachusetts Male Aging Study, where serum testosterone levels were measured throughout the study duration, 16% of the men who had no ED at baseline developed erectile problems within the next 8 years. Of the men who developed ED, 22% were in the lowest tertile for serum testosterone levels, but 12% were in the highest tertile. In the Concord Health and Ageing in Men study, where men 70 years and older were followed for 2 years, no association of ED and testosterone levels was found. Conversely, in the European Male Ageing Study, where men 40 to 79 were followed for over 4 years, becoming hypogonadal (as defined by serum total testosterone < 10.5 nmol/L) was significantly associated with development of ED. Unlike ED, a number of studies have reported that in healthy older men, libido does tend to correlate with serum testosterone levels.

ED and lower urinary tract symptoms (LUTS), occurring as the result of benign prostatic hyperplasia (BPH), frequently coassociate. A study in older men who had both ED and LUTS and were treated with the PDE-5 inhibitor, sildenafil, reported that both ED and LUTS symptoms improved with the sildenafil treatment.

While transurethral resection of the prostate (TURP) for BPH seldom results in ED, surgery for prostate cancer is more extensive and results in some degree of ED in about 60% of men. Nerve-sparing surgery offers a greater chance of preserving sexual potency. In addition, penile rehabilitation with PDE-5 inhibitors immediately following surgery helps prevent complete ED. ED also has been reported to be associated with pelvic radiation in up to 36% of cases.

Peyronie disease, where fibrosis of the penile corpora cavernosa occurs, also can lead to erectile problems.

A number of lifestyle factors have been associated with the development of ED. Obesity alone is associated with a 20% increased risk of developing erectile problems. Weight loss may improve erectile function in obese patients. Smoking also can cause ED, both from direct effects of nicotine on penile smooth muscle and from longer-term effects on accelerating atherosclerosis. Heavy alcohol consumption (> 3 drinks/day) is associated with ED. Physical activity alone, regardless of weight, can improve or delay development of ED.

A large number of medications have produced adverse drug events reports involving male sexual dysfunction, usually ED. By and large, the effects on sexual function are medication class effects, based on mechanisms of action. The more common medications that have been reported to be associated with ED are beta blockers, diuretics, antiandrogens, opioids (chronic use), and antidepressents, particularly the SSRIs, venlafaxine, and the tricyclics. It is unlikely that medications would precipitate symptomatic ED in a man who had absolutely no erectile problems prior to initiating the medication, but for men with mild preexisting ED, these medications may precipitate clinically significant ED.

Evaluation of Sexual Dysfunction

The first step in evaluation of sexual dysfunction is often the most difficult: eliciting the information. Asking a brief question about sexual activity in all patients can legitimize the topic for conversation. Examples of possible screening questions include: "Are you satisfied with your sexual activity?"; "How has your illness affected your sex life?" if the patient has a chronic illness; or "Many of my male patients your age have noticed some change in their sexual function; how about you?"

If sexual dysfunction is discovered during screening, then a more extensive sexual and health history and physical examination are warranted. A careful history from the man's sexual partner also can be helpful. If psychological or couples' problems exist, or if the patient is depressed, these should be treated. As noted earlier, an evaluation for general vascular disease and for diabetes, as well as a medication evaluation, should be done.

Treatments for Erectile Dysfunction

After addressing lifestyle modifications, medications and reversible causes of ED, the next step is consideration of direct medical treatments. **Table 37-3** lists the current medical treatments for ED that are available in the United States.

The most common first-line therapy of ED is an oral phosphodiesterase type 5 (PDE-5) inhibitor because of their efficacy (from 45% to 90%), ease of use, and generally favorable side effect profiles. The PDE-5 inhibitors available currently in the United States are sildenafil, vardenafil, tadalafil, and avanafil. Systemic reviews and pooled data across trials support that all four PDE-5 inhibitors

TABLE 37-3 ■ CURRENT MEDICAL TREATMENT OPTIONS FOR ERECTILE DYSFUNCTION AVAILABLE IN THE UNITED STATES

Medications

Oral

PDE-5[a] inhibitor

Sildenafil, vardenafil, tadalafil, avanafil

α-Adrenergic blocker (rarely used)

Yohimbine, phentolamine

Intramuscular injection or transdermal patch

Testosterone (see Chapter 97)

Intracavernous injection

Alprostadil (PGE1)[b]

Papaverine (PDE inhibitor) ± phentolamine (α-adrenergic blocker)

Transurethral

Alprostadil (PGE1)

Vacuum erection devices

Penile prosthetic implants

[a]PDE-5: phosphodiesterase type 5.
[b]PGE1: prostaglandin E1.

have similar efficacy. Tadalafil has a longer duration of action and avanafil may have a more rapid onset of action compared to the others. Sildenafil and vardenafil must be taken on an empty stomach, as high-fat meals and/or alcohol delay their absorption, but food does not interfere significantly with the absorption of tadalafil or avanafil. They all require sexual stimulation to work effectively. Men with diabetes mellitus or after prostatectomy usually have more severe ED at baseline, so they often respond less well to PDE-5 inhibitors. Men who are hypogonadal may find PDE-5 inhibitors more effective if combined with testosterone therapy.

PDE-5 inhibitors have some vasodilatory activity and interact with nitrates. Therefore they are contraindicated in men taking nitrates. Men with LUTS/BPH who are taking α-adrenergic blockers, medications which also can lower blood pressure, should be cautioned when starting a PDE-5 inhibitor. Most common side effects of these agents are headaches, flushing, rhinitis, dyspepsia, myalgias, dizziness, back pain, and lowering of blood pressure. Sildenafil and vardenafil have some cross-reactivity with PDE-6, which may explain some reports of visual disturbances (usually a "blue haze") with use of these medications.

Intracavernous injections with prostaglandin E1 (PGE1) or a PDE-5 inhibitor, with or without intracavernosal co-injection of an α-adrenergic blocker, have efficacy of 65% to 90%. Side effects include mild local pain (10%–15%), penile fibrosis, prolonged erections, and rhinitis. PGE1 (Alprostadil) also can be delivered via urethral insertion, followed by vigorous penile massage to assist with medication delivery. Reported efficacy is between 45% and 65% and side effects include mild pain, minor urethral

bleeding, dizziness, and lowered blood pressure; there is a rare risk of anterior optic neuropathy.

Vacuum erection devices consist of a vacuum cylinder connected to a pump to create controlled negative pressure, and one or more constriction rings that go at the base of the penis after vacuum-induced engorgement has occurred. Intercourse occurs with rings in place, but the ring should not be left on for more than 30 minutes. Erection satisfactory for intercourse occurs in 75% to 90% of users. Overall satisfaction rate is 65% to 70% if the method is chosen and used, but only about 12% of men select the vacuum device as an initial choice of therapy. Side effects or reasons for dissatisfaction include pain, inconvenience, and premature loss of rigidity. There are few contraindications to its use, but if on anticoagulants, these devices should be used with care.

Penile prosthetic implants are either semirigid (noninflatable) or inflatable. Designs have improved over the last decades, and the 5-year failure rates for the inflatable prosthesis are low. Infection is the most significant complication and varies from less than 1% to 16%.

Oral α-adrenergic blockers, such as yohimbine or phentolamine, have been used to treat ED, but with low efficacy (10%–20%) and are rarely used. Testosterone replacement therapy, with or without concomitant PDE-5 inhibitor treatment, has been used successfully to treat ED in some hypogonadal men (see following section).

Testosterone and Male Sexual Function

Testosterone and its active metabolite, estradiol, play important roles in maintaining normal sexual function in men. Libido, sexual activity, and erectile function are reduced by severely low, castration-range, serum testosterone concentrations produced by ADT in older men with prostate cancer. In a recent study, healthy older men were treated with a gonadotropin-releasing hormone agonist (to induce experimental castration) and various dosages of testosterone (to produce very low to normal serum testosterone concentrations) for 16 weeks. In this study, sexual desire and erectile function were reduced slightly at serum testosterone concentrations less than 200 ng/dL; however, they were not reduced significantly relative to controls until serum testosterone levels were less than 100 ng/dL. These results suggest that the threshold of testosterone concentrations to maintain sexual function is relatively low and support results from previous observational studies.

Testosterone treatment is only indicated for men with hypogonadism (see Chapter 97). As per the Endocrine Society clinical practice guidelines, the diagnosis of hypogonadism requires clinical manifestations (ie, symptoms and signs) of testosterone deficiency and consistently low morning (preferably fasting) serum testosterone concentrations on at least two occasions. Sexual dysfunction symptoms (eg, low libido, loss of spontaneous erections, ED, and reduced sexual activity) are prominent manifestations of hypogonadism.

Meta-analyses have reported inconsistent effects of testosterone treatment on sexual function. Earlier meta-analyses utilized testosterone treatment trials in which men without symptoms or signs of testosterone deficiency or who had normal to low-normal testosterone levels were included. A more recent meta-analysis, however, included only the small number of randomized, placebo-controlled studies of 1779 men who had at least one symptom or sign of testosterone deficiency and morning testosterone concentration less than or equal to 300 ng/dL who received testosterone replacement therapy for more than or equal to 12 weeks. In this meta-analysis, compared to placebo, testosterone treatment of hypogonadal men was associated with a modest but significant improvement in libido, erectile function, and sexual satisfaction.

The results of the Testosterone Trials (T Trials) are worth noting. This was a large, multi-center, double-blind, placebo-controlled study in older men (average age 72 years) with unequivocal hypogonadism (symptoms and signs of testosterone deficiency and two morning total testosterone levels by mass spectrometry < 275 ng/dL) for no apparent reason other than age. More details of the T Trials are provided in Chapter 97. Of the 459 men with low sexual desire (low libido) enrolled in the Sexual Function Trial of the T Trials, testosterone versus placebo treatment for 1 year resulted in moderate and sustained improvements in sexual activity, libido, and erectile function in older men with age-associated hypogonadism. The effect of testosterone therapy on ED as assessed by the International Index of Erectile Function (IIEF) was clinically meaningful, but less than that reported for PDE-5 inhibitors. In contrast to improvements in libido and sexual activity in testosterone-treated men that correlated with incremental changes in serum total or free testosterone and estradiol levels, the improvement in ED did not correlate with sex steroid concentrations. Also, no threshold testosterone concentration was apparent for any of the sexual function outcomes.

In contrast to men with hypogonadism, testosterone treatment does not improve libido, sexual activity or erectile function in men with normal testosterone (ie, eugonadal men). Also, in men with ED who fail to respond to PDE-5 inhibitors, the addition of testosterone treatment may improve erectile function as well as libido and sexual activity in men who have severe hypogonadism, but not in eugonadal men.

FURTHER READING

Ahern T, Swiecicka A, Eendebak RJAH, et al. Natural history, risk factors, and clinical features of primary hypogonadism in ageing men: longitudinal data from the European Male Ageing Study. Clin Endocrinology. 2016;85:891–901.

American Geriatrics Society Ethics Committee. American Geriatrics Society care of lesbian, gay, bisexual and transgender older adults position statement. J Am Geriatr Soc. 2015;63:423–426.

Araujo AB, Mohr BA, McKinlay JB. Changes in sexual function in middle-aged and older men: longitudinal data from the Massachusetts Male Aging Study. J Am Geriatr Soc. 2004;52:1502–1509.

Cunningham GR, Stephens-Shields AJ, Rosen RC, et al. Testosterone treatment and sexual function in older men with low testosterone levels. J Clin Endocrinol Metab. 2016;101(8):3096–3104.

Finkelstein JS, Lee H, Burnett-Bowie SM, et al. Dose-response relationships between gonadal steroids and bone, body composition, and sexual function in aging men. J Clin Endocrinol Metab. 2020;105(8):2779–2788.

Hay B, Cumming RG, Blyth FM, et al. The longitudinal relationship of sexual function and androgen status in older men: the Concord health and ageing in men project. J Clin Endocrinol Metab. 2015;100:1350–1358.

Hyde Z, Flicker L, Hankey GJ, et al. Prevalence of sexual activity and associated factors in men aged 75 to 95 years. Ann Intern Med. 2010;153:693–702.

Inman BA, St. Sauver JL, Jacobson DJ, et al. A population-based, longitudinal study of erectile dysfunction and future coronary artery disease. Mayo Clin Proc. 2009;84:108–113.

Lindau ST, Dale W, Feldmeth G, et al. Sexuality and Cognitive Status: A U.S nationally representative study of home-dwelling older adults. J Am Geriatr Soc. 2018;66:1902–1910.

Lindau ST, Schumm LP, Laumann EO, et al. A study of sexuality and health among older adults in the United States. N Engl J Med. 2007;357:762–774.

Ponce OJ, Spencer-Bonilla G, Alvarez-Villalobos N, et al. The efficacy and adverse events of testosterone replacement therapy in hypogonadal men: A systematic review and meta-analysis of randomized, placebo-controlled trials. J Clin Endocrinol Metab. 2018;103(5):1745–1754.

Snyder PJ, Bhasin S, Cunningham GR, et al. Effects of testosterone treatment in older men. N Engl J Med. 2016;374(7):611–624.

PART II PRINCIPLES OF GERIATRICS

553

Chapter 38

Benign Prostate Disorders

Catherine E. DuBeau, Christopher D. Ortengren

DEFINITIONS

Many terms are used to describe benign prostate disease, often interchangeably. Precision is important, however, because the conditions overlap only partially (**Figure 38-1**). Benign prostate hyperplasia (BPH) is a histologic condition characterized by benign proliferation of stromal and/or epithelial prostate tissue. Its prevalence increases with age and is nearly universally present in men by the ninth decade. Benign prostate enlargement (BPE) occurs in about half of men with BPH, and is quantified by milliliters of prostate tissue (eg, as measured by ultrasound). Bladder outlet obstruction (BOO) occurs in only a subset of men with BPE.

Common voiding symptoms are urgency, frequency, nocturia, slow stream, hesitancy, incomplete emptying, postvoiding dribbling, and incontinence, which may be related to BPH, BPE, BOO, age-related physiologic changes in the lower urinary tract, and/or comorbid conditions and medications. However, women may experience these same symptoms. Therefore, voiding symptoms are best described by the nonspecific term lower urinary tract symptoms (LUTS).

EPIDEMIOLOGY AND NATURAL HISTORY

Early autopsy and epidemiologic studies demonstrated a marked rise in prevalence of BPH and BPE with age, especially during the sixth and seventh decades, and a similar relationship between age and "clinical BPH" (LUTS and BPE on examination) (**Figure 38-2**). In a racially, ethnically, and socioeconomically diverse population in the United States, the overall prevalence of LUTS was 19% and increased with age (11% at age 30–39 to 26% at age 70–79) but did not differ by sex or race/ethnicity. Other studies suggest that 28% to 35% of older men without previous prostate surgery have moderate to severe LUTS. More recent data from longitudinal epidemiologic studies and placebo arms of treatment trials confirm that the incidence of benign prostate disease gradually and variably increases with age until the ninth decade (**Figure 38-3**). Only weak correlations exist between BPE, BOO, and LUTS, suggesting that their relationships are nonlinear and complex.

Learning Objectives

- Understand the epidemiology and pathophysiology of benign prostate disease in older men.
- Perform an evaluation of older men with lower urinary tract symptoms (LUTS) that incorporates an understanding of the role of etiologic factors beyond benign prostate disease.
- Manage evidence-based stepped treatment of LUTS, including appropriate specialist referral.

Key Clinical Points

1. Benign prostate hyperplasia (BPH), prostate hypertrophy, and bladder outlet obstruction are related but not always coincident common conditions in older men.

2. The natural history of benign prostate disease and lower urinary symptoms is variable and includes symptom regression.

3. Multimorbidity, medications, and functional and cognitive impairment may be the predominant cause of LUTS even in men with benign prostate disease.

4. Many men with LUTS can be effectively managed with medical treatment.

Some data suggest that African-American men have a higher risk of benign prostate disease, urinary retention, and BPE/BOO surgery, possibly because they have higher levels of 5α-reductase and larger prostate transitional zone volume (see section "Pathophysiology"). The very limited available data suggest that Hispanic men have similar risk of BPH and characteristics of BPE as non-Hispanic White men. Asian men generally have lower rates of benign and malignant prostate disease, although this may differ by country of origin.

Progression of benign prostate disease is defined as worsening LUTS, acute urinary retention (AUR), and/or the need for surgical treatment. LUTS can vary significantly over time, and abate as well as progress. In a prospective

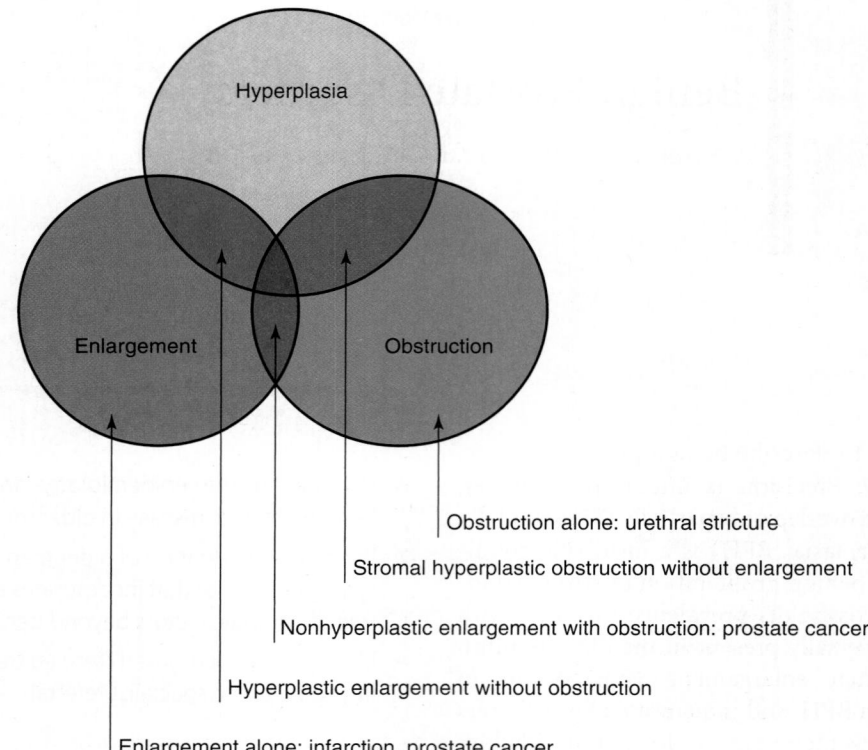

Obstruction alone: urethral stricture

Stromal hyperplastic obstruction without enlargement

Nonhyperplastic enlargement with obstruction: prostate cancer

Hyperplastic enlargement without obstruction

Enlargement alone: infarction, prostate cancer

FIGURE 38-1. Overlap between benign prostatic hyperplasia (BPH), benign prostatic enlargement (BPE), bladder outlet obstruction (BOO), and lower urinary tract symptoms (LUTS) in men.

cohort of men with moderate LUTS, by 1 year, symptoms had improved in 16% and worsened in only 24%, and at 4 years, symptoms were only mild in 13%, unchanged in 46%, and worse in 41%. The worsening of LUTS and the

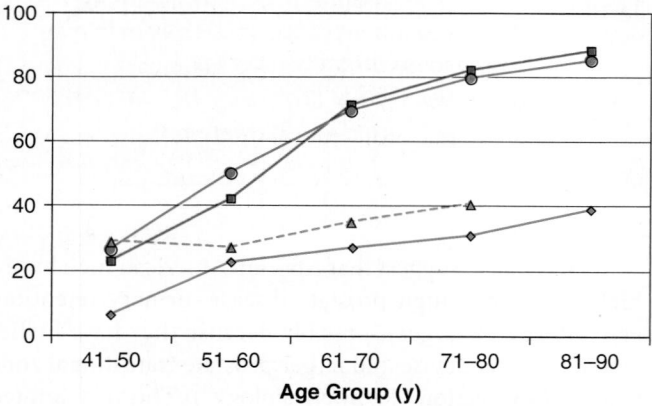

FIGURE 38-2. Autopsy evidence of prostate hyperplasia (percentage of prostates, solid line with ■), mean weight (mL) of all prostates (solid line with ◆), mean weight of prostates with hyperplasia (dashed line with ▲), and percentage of men with lower urinary tract symptoms (LUTS) (solid line with •). (Data from Berry SJ, Coffey DS, Walsh PC, et al. The development of human benign prostatic hyperplasia with age. *J Urol.* 1984;132:474–479 and Guess HA, Arrighi HM, Metter EJ, et al. Cumulative prevalence of prostatism matches the autopsy prevalence of benign prostatic hyperplasia. *Prostate.* 1990;17:214–216.)

need for medication and surgery differ by age, with the proportion developing severe LUTS and treatment increasing with age (**Figure 38-4**). The incidence of AUR in men with LUTS and benign prostate disease is low; in a meta-analysis including 6100 moderately symptomatic men, the incidence of AUR was 13.7 per 1000 patient-years in all men, and considerably higher in men aged 70 or older or taking anticholinergic agents (34.7 per 1000 patient-years). Higher baseline prostate-specific antigen (PSA) levels are associated with greater risk of AUR and surgery; 7.8% of men with PSA levels up to 1.3 ng/mL develop AUR and/or require surgery by the fourth year, compared with 13% of men with PSA levels 1.4 to 3.2 ng/mL, and 20% with PSA levels 3.3 to 12 ng/mL. Change in PSA over time (PSA velocity), however, is not associated with AUR or surgery. As PSA is strongly correlated with prostate volume, it is not surprising that higher volumes (> 30–40 mL by ultrasound) are associated with worsening LUTS and AUR. Other factors that increase AUR risk include previous episode(s) of retention, baseline postvoiding residual volume (PVR) greater than 100 mL, worsening LUTS, and failure to respond to α-blocker treatment. It is important to remember that not all men with BPE will have LUTS.

LUTS are strongly related to poorer health and decreased quality of life. Bother from urinary symptoms and poorer health status (self-reported health, SF-12 Physical Summary Scale, or difficulty with instrumental activities

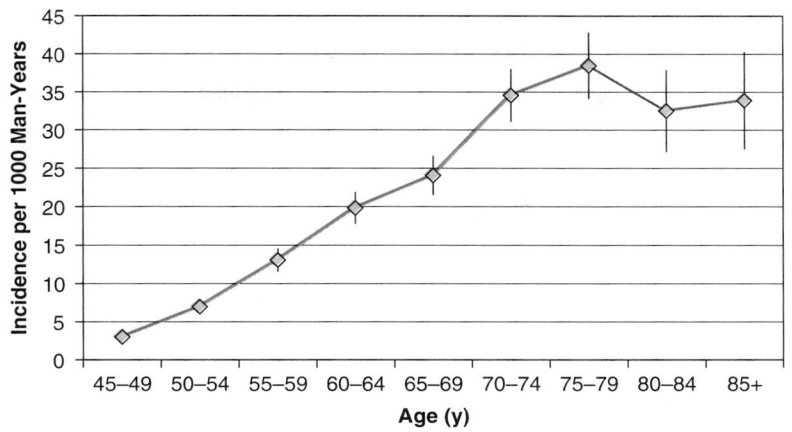

FIGURE 38-3. Incidence of benign prostatic hyperplasia (BPH) by age. (Data from Verhamme KM, Dieleman JP, Bleumink GS, et al. Incidence and prevalence of lower urinary tract symptoms suggestive of benign prostatic hyperplasia in primary care—the Triumph project. *Eur Urol.* 2002;42[4]:323–328.)

of daily living [IADLs]) are strongly associated with older age. Over half of men with severe LUTS report they would feel unsatisfied, unhappy, or terrible if they were to spend the rest of their life with their urinary condition.

PATHOPHYSIOLOGY

Hyperplasia

Prostate hyperplasia occurs when prostate cell proliferation exceeds programmed cell death (apoptosis) as a result of stimulated cell growth, inhibition of apoptosis, or both.

BPH occurs predominantly in the prostatic periurethral transitional zone, unlike prostate cancer, which tends to occur in more peripheral areas. BPH and prostate cancer are genetically distinct, and one is not a risk factor for the other.

The development of stromal and epithelial hyperplasia in BPH is androgen- and aging-dependent, and involves numerous paracrine and autocrine factors. The trophic androgen for prostate growth is dihydrotestosterone, produced from testosterone within the prostate by the enzyme 5α-reductase (thus the utility of 5α-reductase inhibitors

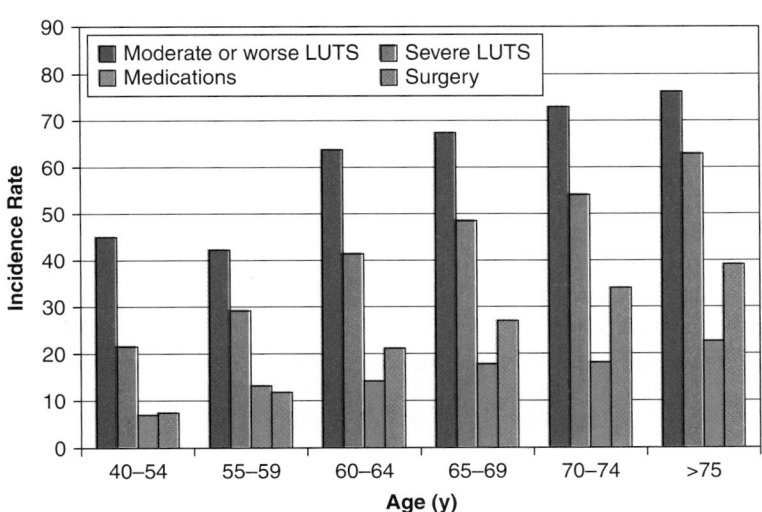

FIGURE 38-4. Progression of lower urinary tract symptoms (LUTS) over 18 years regarding worsening symptoms, need for medication, and need for surgery, by age group. Data are incidence rates per 1000 man-years over 18 years from the Physicians Health Study. At baseline, all men had International Prostate Symptom Score (IPSS) of < 7. Progression to "moderate or worse" LUTS was defined as IPSS of ≥ 15, surgery, or medication use. Progression to "severe" LUTS was defined as IPSS of ≥ 20, surgery, or medication use. (Data from Platz EA, Joshu CE, Mondul AM, et al. Incidence and progression of lower urinary tract symptoms in a large prospective cohort of United States men. *J Urol.* 2012;188[2]:496–501.)

[5αRIs] for treatment). In the absence of 5α-reductase, even high serum levels of testosterone will not cause BPH. Additional factors supporting prostate cell growth include inflammatory cytokines (eg, interleukin-8), autocrine cytokine growth factors, and neuroendocrine cell products. Stromal-epithelial interactions regulating proliferation also involve interactions between androgens, estrogens, and stimulatory and inhibitory peptide growth factors (eg, fibroblast growth factor-2, transforming growth factor-β). Other regulatory factors include nitric oxide (nitric oxide synthetase levels are low in BPH), vitamin D, and local autonomic innervation and activity. Thus, the development of BPH is the end result of numerous pathways involved in regulating sympathetic activity, androgen-estrogen balance, and smooth muscle proliferation.

The divergence in prevalence between BPH, BPE, BOO, and LUTS results from many lower urinary tract factors (**Table 38-1**). In addition, numerous medical conditions, medications, and functional impairment may cause or worsen LUTS independent of prostate disease (see Chapter 47 on incontinence).

Risk Factors

Factors associated with the development of benign prostate disease and LUTS include age, physical inactivity, high meat and fat intake (especially polyunsaturated fats), diabetes, high insulin levels, obesity, low high-density lipoprotein levels, and arteriovascular disease. Vasectomy is not a risk factor and the data on smoking are inconclusive. Potentially modifiable risk factors for BPH and/or LUTS are obesity, a diet high in meat and fat, medications (antidepressants), and physical inactivity.

EVALUATION

Benign prostate disease may be asymptomatic, but most commonly presents with LUTS; other symptoms include urinary retention, recurrent urinary tract infections (UTIs), or hematuria (from prostatic varices). **Figure 38-5** lists the recommended evaluation and management in men presenting with LUTS suggestive of benign prostate disease from the American Urological Association (AUA) 2021 guideline on the management of BPH. The sections below highlight aspects of the evaluation especially relevant to older men.

History

The evaluation of older men with LUTS closely parallels that of older persons with urinary incontinence (UI; see Chapter 47). The history should include the onset, progression, and associated factors for the common LUTS (slow stream, urgency, nocturia, etc), and quantification of LUTS using a symptom index (see below). Distinguishing between "irritative" and "obstructive" LUTS is not useful, because the terms are poorly specific and do not correlate with symptom bother, severity,

TABLE 38-1 ■ LOWER URINARY TRACT FACTORS UNDERLYING THE DIVERGENCE IN PREVALENCE BETWEEN BPH, BPE, BOO, AND LUTS

FACTOR	IMPACT
Ratio of stromal to epithelial hyperplasia (stromal proliferation predominates in 50%, glandular in 25%, and mixed in 25%)	Stromal glands tend to be smaller, more symptomatic, and have worse symptomatic outcomes to prostatectomy
Location of BPH nodules	Adenomas, which occur predominantly in central transitional and periurethral zones of the prostate, predispose to prostatic urethra compression. Adenomas in the median lobes may compress the bladder base without causing BOO.
Fibroelastic properties of prostate capsule	Altered compliance may increase urethral compression in the absence of mechanical BOO.
α-Adrenergic innervation of prostate	Increased number of α-adrenergic receptors promotes smooth muscle contraction.
Variability in detrusor muscle structure and function	Detrusor contractility can be affected by BPE/BOO-associated increased connective tissue infiltration; smooth muscle hypertrophy and disintegration; decreased autonomic neuronal number; and conversion from predominantly β-adrenergic (inhibitory) to α-adrenergic (stimulatory) responsiveness.
Detrusor overactivity	Detrusor overactivity (DO) is found in about two-thirds of men with BOO. Causality is unclear as DO occurs in normal asymptomatic older men and women. DO resolves in up to two-thirds of men after TURP, yet tends to persist in older adults.
Atherosclerotic disease	May cause detrusor ischemia leading to impaired contractility, and acute BOO from prostate infarction.
Neurologic disease	Depending on type and location of involvement, may cause DO, impaired contractility, and/or sphincter dysfunction including neurologically mediated BOO.

BPH, benign prostatic hyperplasia; BPE, benign prostatic enlargement; BOO, bladder outlet obstruction; LUTS, lower urinary tract symptoms; TURP, transurethral resection of the prostate.

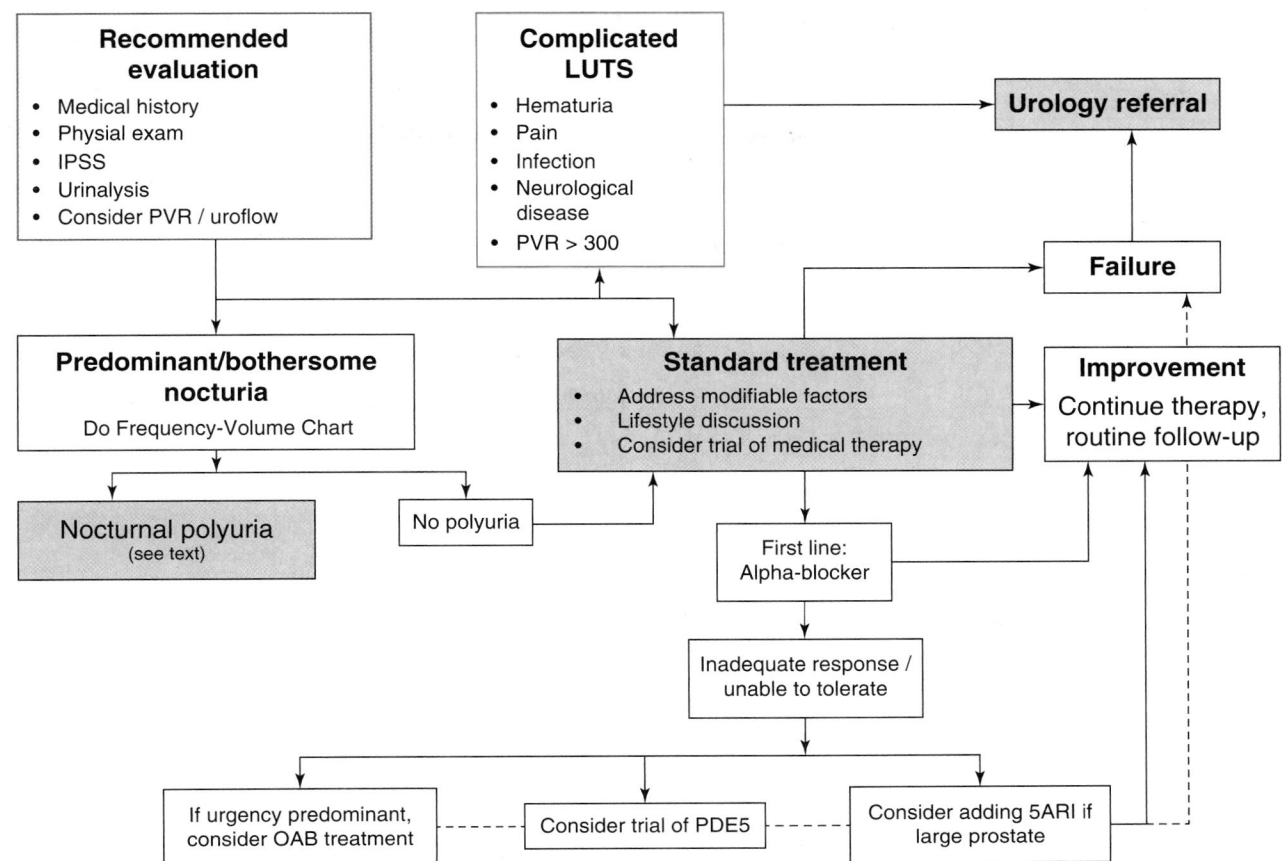

FIGURE 38-5. Algorithm for management of symptomatic benign prostatic hyperplasia (BPH). 5ARI, 5α-reductase inhibitor; OAB, overactive bladder; IPSS, International Prostate Symptom Score; LUTS, lower urinary tract symptoms; PDE5, phosphodiesterase 5; PVR, postvoiding residual volume; UTI, urinary tract infection. (Data from Parsons JK, Lerner LB, Barry MJ, et al. Management of Benign Prostatic Hyperplasia/ Lower Urinary Tract Symptoms: AUA Guideline 2021. American Urological Association.)

or physiologic measures. Older men always should be evaluated for causes of LUTS other than prostate disease. The history and review of systems should question patients about hematuria, dysuria, and pelvic pain (rare in benign prostate disease, more suggestive of infection, bladder stone, prostate or bladder cancers); episodes of urinary retention; cardiac symptoms (regarding possible congestive heart failure in patients with nocturia); bowel and sexual function; type and amount of fluid intake (in relationship to frequency and nocturia symptoms); and sleep disturbance. All medications (including nonprescription drugs) must be reviewed, with a focus on drugs that can decrease detrusor contractility (anticholinergics, calcium channel blockers), diuretics, drugs that can cause pedal edema and contribute to nocturia, and α-adrenergic agents.

Symptom Indices

The International Prostate Symptom Score (IPSS) and American Urological Association Symptom Index (AUASI) are identical indices that quantify the severity of BPH-associated LUTS on a scale 0 to 35; scores of 0 to 7 indicate mild symptoms, 8 to 19 moderate, and 20 to 35 severe (**Table 38-2**). An additional question, not tallied in the total score, assesses disease-specific quality-of-life impact. The IPSS is widely translated. A change in AUASI of ± 5 points has an 80% probability of indicating a true clinical change. The threshold for clinical change varies with symptoms severity (minimum perceptible difference is 2 points for AUASI < 20 and 6 points for AUASI ≥ 20). Any magnitude of change, however, may be caused by interval changes in comorbidity and medications and not prostate disease.

The Benign Prostatic Hyperplasia Impact Index (BII) measures the impact of BPH-associated LUTS on a scale 0 to 13 (**Table 38-3**). Results from randomized controlled treatment trials suggest that the minimal clinically perceptible difference for the BII is a mean decrease of 0.5 to 1.7 points. BII correlates well with the AUASI, but not with objective measures of BPH-associated LUTS severity (eg, urine flow rate or prostate size).

TABLE 38-2 ■ AMERICAN UROLOGICAL ASSOCIATION SYMPTOM INDEX

1. Incomplete emptying: Over the past month, how often have you had the sensation of not emptying your bladder completely after you finished urination?

Not at all	Less than 1 time in 5	Less than half of the time	About half of the time	More than half of the time	Almost always	Your score
0	1	2	3	4	5	

2. Frequency: Over the past month, how often have you had to urinate again less than 2 h after you finished urinating?

Not at all	Less than 1 time in 5	Less than half of the time	About half of the time	More than half of the time	Almost always	Your score
0	1	2	3	4	5	

3. Intermittency: Over the past month, how often have you found that you stopped and started again several times when you urinated?

Not at all	Less than 1 time in 5	Less than half of the time	About half of the time	More than half of the time	Almost always	Your score
0	1	2	3	4	5	

4. Urgency: Over the past month, how often have you found it difficult to postpone urination?

Not at all	Less than 1 time in 5	Less than half of the time	About half of the time	More than half of the time	Almost always	Your score
0	1	2	3	4	5	

5. Weak stream: Over the past month, how often have you had a weak stream?

Not at all	Less than 1 time in 5	Less than half of the time	About half of the time	More than half of the time	Almost always	Your score
0	1	2	3	4	5	

6. Straining: Over the past month, how often have you had to push or strain to begin urination?

Not at all	Less than 1 time in 5	Less than half of the time	About half of the time	More than half of the time	Almost always	Your score
0	1	2	3	4	5	

7. Nocturia: Over the past month or so, how many times did you get up to urinate from the time you went to bed until the time you got up in the morning?

None	1 time	2 times	3 times	4 times	5 times	Your score
0	1	2	3	4	5	

ADD UP THE SCORES FOR THE TOTAL AUA SCORE =

Quality of Life Due to Urinary Symptoms: If you were to spend the rest of your life with your urinary condition just the way it is now, how would you feel about that? (circle)

Delighted	Pleased	Mostly Satisfied	Mixed	Mostly Dissatisfied	Unhappy	Terrible

Adapted with permission from Barry MJ, Fowler FJ Jr, O'Leary MP, et al. The American Urological Association symptom index for benign prostatic hyperplasia. The Measurement Committee of the American Urological Association. J Urol. 1992;148(5):1549–1557.

OTHER MEASURES OF LUTS AND QUALITY OF LIFE

There is a variety of other measures of LUTS and their impact. Some of the more widely used are the International Consultation on Incontinence Questionnaire (ICIQ) male module (ICIQ-MLUTS). To assess sexual function, the Derogatis Interview for Sexual Functioning Self-Report and the International Index of Erectile Function can be used. Depending on the patient's symptoms, other potentially useful scales are the Incontinence Impact Questionnaire and ICIQ Urinary Incontinence Short Form, and UI-specific and general quality-of-life measures; for

example, ICIQ-LUTSqol, Urogenital Distress Inventory, Urge Impact Scale, and the SF-12.

The impact of LUTS on quality of life is critical to evaluate because it is the primary determinant of treatment. Quality-of-life impact may include interference with daily activities, work, sleep, and sexual function; worry, embarrassment, and impaired self-esteem; and physical discomfort. Patients' perception of bother may be independent of LUTS severity, and bother from an individual symptom may be more important than from all symptoms. Determining a patient's most bothersome symptom can help target evaluation and treatment; for example, nocturia is often extremely bothersome, yet

TABLE 38-3 ■ BENIGN PROSTATE HYPERPLASIA IMPACT INDEX

OVER THE PAST MONTH:	0	1	2	3		SCORE
1. How much physical discomfort did any urinary problems cause you?	None	Only a little	Some	A lot		
2. How much did you worry about your health because of any urinary problems?	None	Only a little	Some	A lot		
3. Overall, how bothersome has any trouble with urination been during the past month?	Not at all bothersome	Bothers me a little	Bothers me some	Bothers me a lot		
	0	**1**	**2**	**3**	**4**	
4. How much of the time has any urinary problem kept you from doing the kind of things you would usually do?	None of the time	A little of the time	Some of the time	Most of the time	All of the time	
					Total Score:	

Reproduced with permission from McVary K, Roehrborn C, Avins A, et al. American Urological Association Guideline: Management of Benign Prostatic Hyperplasia (BPH), Revised 2010. American Urological Association Education and Research, Inc.

many prostate-specific treatments are not very effective for it.

Nocturia

Nocturia is defined as voiding at least once during the normal hours of sleep. Almost 80% of older men have nocturia, which is the most bothersome of all of the LUTS associated with benign prostate disease. Moreover, nocturia 2 or more times a night is associated with hypertension, cardiovascular disease, and increased mortality. The three main causes of nocturia are LUT pathophysiology, nocturnal polyuria, and sleep disturbance (**Table 38-4**). The latter two causes are especially important in older men because of the many age-related changes, comorbid conditions, and medications that can cause them.

Nocturnal polyuria is defined as the excretion of one-third or greater of the daily (24-hour) urine output during normal sleeping hours. Older persons are prone to nocturnal polyuria, possibly due to higher nocturnal atrial natriuretic peptide levels and/or altered secretion of vasopressin. Some older persons may excrete 50% or more of their 24-hour urine output during the night. For this reason, one episode of nocturia is considered normal in older persons and even the best treatment may not be able to completely eliminate nocturia. Another cause of nocturnal polyuria is peripheral edema; because edema fluid mobilizes when the patient reclines, leading to increased urine output. Sleep apnea is an underappreciated cause of nocturnal polyuria; apnea should be suspected when the patient or his partner report loud snoring, apneic periods, excessive daytime sleepiness, and morning headaches, and in men who are obese and/or have hypertension. Tools such as the Epworth Sleepiness Scale or STOP-BANG can help assess apnea risk. Importantly, treatment of apnea with continuous positive airway pressure (CPAP) reduces nocturia. (See Chapter 44 on sleep disorders.)

When aroused owing to primary sleep disorders, patients may sense their bladder volume (which tends to be higher at night) and get up and void, and report these episodes as "nocturia." Common causes of sleep disturbance in older persons include age-related changes in sleep architecture (see Chapter 44), pain (eg, from arthritis), depression, restless leg syndrome, gastric reflux, pulmonary and cardiac diseases, dementia, Parkinson disease, and the effects of many medications (see **Table 38-4**).

Physical Examination

Given the many medical causes of LUTS in older men, a complete physical examination is required and should include evaluation of cognition, function, and mobility. In men with impaired emptying without other evident cause, a neurologic examination should include the bulbocavernosus reflex, anal wink, and perineal sensation to assess sacral nerve integrity. Digital rectal examination (DRE) should be done to assess prostate nodularity, rectal tone, masses, and stool impaction. DRE is not accurate for assessing prostate volume, even when performed by specialists, because BPH adenomas can occur in the anterior and median lobes that are inaccessible to rectal palpation. Prostate volume is not associated with BOO, and is important only for decisions regarding surgical approach for prostatectomy. Although higher volume is associated with disease progression and response to 5α-reductase inhibitor treatment, it should not be routinely assessed for this purpose because accurate measurement requires ultrasound.

Laboratory Tests

Only urinalysis is needed in routine assessment, primarily to check for microscopic hematuria. The decision of whether to do PSA testing in men with LUTS should follow the recommended guidelines for prostate cancer screening (see Chapter 90 on prostate cancer). Serum creatinine is not

TABLE 38-4 ■ CAUSES OF NOCTURIA

1. **Nocturnal polyuria**
   a. Age-related delay in urine excretion
   b. Fluid intake
      i. Late afternoon and evening intake
      ii. Caffeine
      iii. Alcohol
   c. Peripheral edema
      i. Venous insufficiency
      ii. Congestive heart failure
      iii. Medications
         1. Gabapentin
         2. Pregabalin
         3. Thiazolidinediones
         4. Nonsteroidal anti-inflammatory agents
         5. Pyridine calcium blockers (eg, nifedipine)
   d. Medical conditions
      i. Obstructive sleep apnea
      ii. Uncontrolled diabetes mellitus
2. **Sleep disturbance**
   a. Insomnia
   b. Depression
   c. Congestive heart failure
   d. Obstructive sleep apnea
   e. Pain (eg, arthritis)
   f. Restless leg syndrome
   g. Medications
      i. Stimulants
      ii. β-Blockers
      iii. Steroids
      iv. Thyroxine
      v. Selective serotonin reuptake inhibitors antidepressants
      vi. Withdrawal from alcohol, narcotics, benzodiazepines
3. **Lower urinary tract dysfunction**
   a. Decreased functional bladder capacity
      i. Detrusor overactivity
      ii. Increased postvoiding residual volume
         1. Impaired contractility
         2. Outlet obstruction

required because of the extremely low prevalence of renal insufficiency in men with LUTS. Vitamin B_{12} level may be considered in men with a high PVR or urinary retention.

Postvoiding Residual and Urine Flow Rate

PVR is not required in the initial evaluation, especially in men with mild-moderate LUTS who can be managed with watchful waiting or medical therapy. PVR is small in randomly selected community men (75th percentile, 35 mL). In a large trial of men with moderate LUTS, the baseline mean PVR was 110 ± 74 mL. PVR correlates modestly with prostate volume, but is not significantly associated with age, AUASI, quality-of-life indices, BOO, or the need for invasive therapy.

PVR should be considered in men with complex neurologic disease (eg, Parkinson disease, spinal cord injury), new impairment in renal function without other evident cause, medications that can decrease detrusor contractility (anticholinergics, opiates, calcium channel blockers), or who have failed empiric therapy. Inability to pass a urethral catheter for PVR measurement is more likely a result of sphincter spasm than BOO; this can be overcome using intraurethral lidocaine jelly and patient relaxation. Older men tend to have a larger PVR in the morning, which can increase within-patient PVR variability.

Urine peak flow rate measurement is commonly used in urologic practice. In the AUA BPH guideline, flow rate can be considered in the initial evaluation, and recommended in men who inadequately respond to medical therapy. Low urine flow rate is not specific for BOO, as it can also occur with impaired detrusor contractility (intrinsic or extrinsic [eg, from medications]) and/or a low bladder volume. A normal peak flow rate is very sensitive for BOO (peak flow > 12 mL/s with void $\geq$ 150 mL excludes BOO).

Frequency-Volume Charts (Bladder Diaries)

Frequency-volume charts are very helpful to determine if polyuria contributes to frequency and/or nocturia symptoms (**Table 38-5**). To complete the diary, the patient records the time and volume of all voids (continent and incontinent). Several studies (albeit primarily in women) confirm that bladder diaries are reliable and valid, especially when done for 3 days.

Specialized Testing

Urodynamic studies Urodynamic studies are not required in the initial evaluation of men with LUTS, especially in men with mild-moderate symptoms, The AUA guideline recommends urodynamics, along with PVR and frequency voiding charts, in men who have inadequate response to medical therapy. Urodynamics may also be considered in frail older men (especially those with Parkinson disease or spinal cord injury) who desire surgical treatment, in order to exclude conditions such as detrusor hyperactivity with impaired contractility. The urodynamic tests to evaluate LUTS are cystometry and pressure-flow study. Cystometry measures bladder pressure during filling to determine detrusor stability (vs overactivity), contractility, and compliance. The standard for diagnosing BOO is pressure-flow study, which simultaneously measures flow rate versus bladder pressure during voiding. A high bladder pressure combined with a low flow rate is indicative of BOO.

Other tests AUA guideline recommends cystoscopy in men who have inadequate response to medical therapy. Cystoscopy also is recommended for men with hematuria (especially those with risk factors for bladder carcinoma such as smoking), positive cytology, or pelvic pain. Cystoscopy should not be used to diagnose BOO. Renal ultrasound may be considered in men with new renal impairment, yet even

TABLE 38-5 ■ USE OF A FREQUENCY-VOIDING CHART IN THE EVALUATION OF LUTS AND NOCTURIA

DATE	TIME	VOIDED VOLUME (ML)	ARE YOU WET OR DRY?	ESTIMATED LEAKAGE	COMMENTS	
4/5	3:05 PM	240	Dry			
	6:10 PM	210	Dry		Beer with dinner	
	8:15 PM	150	Dry			
	10:20 PM	150	Dry			
	10:30 PM	45	Dry		Went to bed	
4/6	3:15 AM	270	Wet	Tablespoons		
	5:50 AM	300	Dry			
	7:40 AM	120	Dry		Coffee	Total nocturnal output = 690
	9:50 AM	60	Dry			
	11:20 AM	90	Dry			
	12:50 PM	120	Dry			
	1:40 PM	120	Dry			
	3:35 PM	90	Dry			
	6:00 PM	90	Dry			
	8:40 PM	215	Dry			
	10:25 PM	180	Dry		Went to bed	Total daytime output = 965
4/7	1:00 AM	240	Dry			
	3:50 AM	400	Dry		Almost didn't make it	
	5:20 AM	200	Dry			
	8:00 AM	180	Dry		Coffee	Total nocturnal output = 1020
	11:15 AM	90	Dry			
	4:00 PM	120	Dry			

Bladder diary of 75-year-old man with LUTS and bothersome nocturia. Shaded portions are the nighttime urine output (from time of sleep up to and including first morning void). The diary demonstrates nocturnal polyuria ranging from 690 to 1020 mL. On 4/6, nocturnal polyuria constituted ~ 50% of the 24-hour urine output (965/[1020 + 965]). The diary also demonstrates the common finding of lower voided volumes during the day compared to night (60–240 mL vs 45–400 mL). Even with the higher functional bladder volume at night, the volume of polyuria ensures that he would have to awaken to void almost three times (1020 mL/400 mL = 2.6 voids). Thus, the evaluation of this patient should first focus on possible non-LUT causes of nocturnal polyuria.

Adapted with permission from DuBeau CE, Resnick NM. Evaluation of the causes and severity of geriatric incontinence. A critical appraisal. Urol Clin North Am. 1991;18(2):243–256.

in this group, hydronephrosis is usually only found in men who also have PVR greater than 150 mL.

MANAGEMENT

Overview

For the majority of men, treatment of benign prostate disease will focus on management of LUTS. Generally, fewer than 10% will need upfront surgical intervention for severe obstruction, urinary retention, or gross hematuria. This section focuses on stepped, evidence-based management of LUTS based on the AUA BPH guideline (see **Figure 38-5** and **Table 38-6**), emphasizing shared decision making. The discussion assumes that contributory multimorbidity, medications, and impairments have been addressed and minimized to the extent possible.

Shared Decision Making

Treatment decisions must be patient-centered because benign prostate disease has variable impact on patients and only a small absolute risk of morbidity. No treatment prolongs life or guarantees durable cure, and watchful waiting and lifestyle changes provide relief with little risk for many men. Only the small minority of men with hematuria, significant renal impairment, hydronephrosis, recurrent UTIs, retention, and large PVR (eg, over 200 mL) require immediate referral to a urologist. Issues to discuss in making management decisions include symptom severity and quality-of-life impact, risk for disease progression, preferences for immediate versus delayed symptom improvement, likely treatment outcomes and adverse effects, short- and long-term costs, and ability to comply with long-term monitoring. Providers should offer guidance in tailoring treatment so that men are supported in—and not burdened by—decision making. There are video and print decision aids to help both patients and providers weigh treatment risks and benefits. Men with nocturia should be offered prostate-specific medical and invasive therapy *only* after treatment of any contributing polyuria and/or sleep disturbance.

TABLE 38-6 ■ MEDICAL TREATMENT OF LUTS/BPH

2021 AUA GUIDELINE STATEMENT	GERIATRIC CONSIDERATIONS
Management decisions Patients should be counseled on options for intervention, which can include behavioral/lifestyle modifications, medical therapy, and/or referral for discussion of procedural options. (Expert Opinion)	1. Treatment decisions in older men should consider preferences and goals of care for symptom management, and overall goals for quality of life. 2. Before initiating medical therapy, evaluate all patients for comorbid conditions, medications, and functional impairments that may be causing or worsening LUTS. 3. Before initiating medical therapy, consider existing burden of polypharmacy, potential drug-drug and drug-disease interactions, and costs of therapy.
α-Adrenergic blockers (α-blockers) 1. Clinicians should offer one of the following α-blockers as a treatment option for patients with bothersome, moderate to severe LUTS/BPH: alfuzosin, doxazosin, silodosin, tamsulosin, or terazosin. (Moderate Recommendation; Evidence Level: Grade A) 2. Choice of α-blocker should be based on patient age and comorbidities and different adverse event profiles (e.g., ejaculatory dysfunction, changes in blood pressure). (Moderate Recommendation; Evidence Level: Grade A) 3. When initiating α-blocker therapy, patients with planned cataract surgery should be informed of the risk of floppy iris and be advised to discuss these risks with their ophthalmologists. (Expert Opinion)	Choice of α-blocker should consider which ADE(s) is most important to avoid for a particular patient: 1. Tamsulosin may have slightly less effect on blood pressure than alfuzosin, and both have less blood effect than doxazosin and terazosin. 2. α-Blockers for BPH/LUTS should not be used as primary treatment for hypertension. 3. Tamsulosin and silodosin more likely to cause ejaculatory dysfunction. 4. The Beers Criteria list doxazosin and terazosin as Potentially Inappropriate Medications to avoid in older persons. They are especially inappropriate in men with orthostatic hypertension and diastolic dysfunction.
5α-Reductase inhibitors (5-ARIs) 1. 5-ARI monotherapy should be used as a treatment option in patients with LUTS/BPH with prostatic enlargement as judged by a prostate volume of > 30 cc on imaging, a prostate-specific antigen (PSA) > 1.5 ng/dL, or palpable prostate enlargement on digital rectal exam (DRE). (Moderate Recommendation; Evidence Level: Grade B) 2. 5-ARIs are recommended as a treatment option to prevent progression of LUTS/BPH and/or reduce the risks of urinary retention and need for future prostate-related surgery. (Strong Recommendation; Evidence Level: Grade A) 3. Before starting a 5-ARI, clinicians should inform patients of the risks of sexual side effects, certain uncommon physical side effects, and the low risk of prostate cancer. (Moderate Recommendation; Evidence Level: Grade C)	1. The delayed onset of symptom relief (up to 6 mo) with these drugs may not be consistent with a patient's goals of care. 2. Treatment decisions predicated on PSA and/or prostate volume are difficult to operationalize in many older men. PSA measurement may not be appropriate and digital rectal examination is neither sensitive nor specific for prostate size.
PDE5 inhibitors 1. For patients with LUTS/BPH irrespective of comorbid erectile dysfunction (ED), 5 mg daily tadalafil should be discussed as a treatment option. (Moderate Recommendation; Evidence Level: Grade B) 2. Do not combine low-dose daily 5 mg tadalafil with α-blockers for the treatment of LUTS/BPH as it offers no advantages in symptom improvement over either agent alone. (Moderate Recommendation; Evidence Level: Grade C)	Insurance coverage for daily tadalafil may be very limited.

(Continued)

TABLE 38-6 ■ MEDICAL TREATMENT OF LUTS/BPH (*CONTINUED*)

2021 AUA GUIDELINE STATEMENT	GERIATRIC CONSIDERATIONS
Antimuscarinic agents Antimuscarinic agents, alone or in combination with an α-blocker, may be offered as a treatment option to patients with moderate to severe predominant storage LUTS. (Conditional Recommendation; Evidence Level: Grade C)	1. All trials involving older men have used antimuscarinics only in combination with α-blockers. 2. The Beers Criteria list anticholinergic drugs as Potentially Inappropriate Medications to avoid in older persons. 3. There is increasing evidence for an association of anticholinergic medications with immediate and long-term cognitive impairment. 4. IPSS improvement with combined α-blocker and anticholinergic compared to α-blocker alone is variable and generally small, so risks of combination therapy are likely greater than additive benefit.
Beta-3-agonists Beta-3-agonists in combination with an α-blocker may be offered as a treatment option to patients with moderate to severe predominate storage LUTS. (Conditional Recommendation; Evidence Level: Grade C). Monotherapy with beta-3-agonists is not effective.	1. Beta-3-agonists may be poorly covered by insurance. 2. Blood pressure should be monitored in patients started on beta-3-agonists because of the risk of hypertension.

AUA, American Urological Association; BPH, benign prostatic hypertrophy; LUTS, lower urinary tract symptoms.
Data from Parsons JK, Lerner LB, Barry MJ, et al. Management of Benign Prostatic Hyperplasia/ Lower Urinary Tract Symptoms: AUA Guideline 2021. American Urological Association.

PART II PRINCIPLES OF GERIATRICS

Multiple medical problems, frailty, and short life expectancy need not preclude treatment of benign prostate disease. The broad range of available therapies permits tailoring to the desired immediacy of symptom relief, avoidance of specific adverse effects, and patient comorbidity. Noninvasive treatment is possible in care settings where adequate clinical monitoring and medication adjustment are possible. Assisted-living residents and other vulnerable men may require skilled nursing facility care after surgical interventions in order to monitor PVR and provide physical therapy for improved mobility. Across settings, surgery may not be desirable for men at high risk for in-hospital functional and cognitive decline.

Treatment decisions include the efficacy, durability, and associated adverse effects of therapy. **Table 38-6** summarizes 2021 AUA guideline statements on treatment along with associated geriatric considerations. **Figure 38-5** shows the suggested treatment algorithm modified from the 2021 AUA guideline.

General Geriatric Medicine Considerations in BPH/LUTS Treatment

Management of benign prostate disease and LUTS in older men should incorporate important principles central to the practice of geriatric medicine. These are as follows:

- *Goals of care*: Specific treatments may be effective for some, but not other individuals with LUTS, and have differing time to maximum effect. It is important to ask these questions: Which LUTS are the most bothersome or troubling to the patient and/or caregiver? How urgent is symptom relief? To what degree is the patient accepting of possible surgical treatment? How does the time course of treatment fit within the patient's remaining life expectancy?

- *Avoiding harms from treatment*. Several medications used to treat LUTS are included in the Beers Criteria of potentially inappropriate medications in older persons (see Chapter 22, Medication Prescribing and De-Prescribing). These include antimuscarinics and α-blockers (in patients with falls and previous fractures). LUTS management frequently involves medications or treatments that can cause or worsen erectile dysfunction (ED). The likely harm from a specific treatment in a particular patient must be carefully considered.

- *Appropriate prescribing*: These principles include starting at the lowest possible dose, and avoidance of drug-drug and drug-disease interactions. For example, all α-blockers can cause significant hypotension (especially in patients with hypertension), several interact with other drugs that induce or inhibit the P450 system, and doxazosin can exacerbate congestive heart failure. The half-lives of silodosin (34 hours) and tamsulosin (15 hours) may allow for off-label, less than daily dosing.

Indications for Urology Referral

Absolute indications for prompt urologic referral and intervention are urinary retention (> 250–300 mL—acute or chronic), recurrent UTIs, bladder stones, and hematuria (gross and microscopic). Urology referral should also be considered for men with LUTS and prior bladder or prostate cancer, history of urethral stricture, complicated neurologic disease (Parkinson disease, spinal cord injury), and those who fail noninvasive treatment.

Medical Therapy

Watchful waiting The natural history of benign prostate disease and LUTS and the large placebo effects seen in randomized controlled treatment trials support the use of watchful waiting as a specific intervention. Men most appropriate for watchful waiting have mild to moderate LUTS, are comfortable with this approach, and are amenable to regular follow-up. Clinicians should be "watchful" and not passive in monitoring these patients, with regular follow-up, and careful monitoring for men taking anticholinergics, opioids, or calcium channel blockers. Men should be counseled on general voiding hygiene and behavioral approaches to decrease LUTS (see Chapter 47 on incontinence), counseling to avoid medications that can cause retention (eg, over-the-counter "cold" tablets containing α-agonists and antihistamines), and instructions on the signs of symptoms of retention.

Self-management techniques can be effective. One such program, comprising education and reassurance, lifestyle modifications, and behavioral interventions (ie, adjustment in fluid intake), resulted in 30% to 50% less need for medication or surgery than standard care. In the largest randomized trial of watchful waiting versus transurethral resection of the prostate (TURP) (n = 556 men with moderate LUTS), TURP had significantly greater symptom improvement at 3 years, yet the watchful waiting results were not trivial (mean decrease in symptom score 66% and 38%, respectively). One-third of men on watchful waiting crossed over to TURP, but absolute failure rates with watchful waiting were low (urinary retention 2.9%, PVR > 350 mL 5.8%, worsening LUTS 4.3%). There were no significant differences in sexual function, general well-being, or social activities. The improvement in LUTS was less in men with the least symptom bother, especially after TURP. In the Medical Therapy of Prostatic Symptoms (MTOPS) trial, only 17% of men in the placebo (watchful waiting) arm had "clinical progression" at 4 years, of which 80% had progression solely by clinically significant increase in AUASI of 80% of greater than or equal to four points.

Medications (Table 38-7)

α-Adrenergic Blockers α-Adrenergic blockers are the mainstay of medical treatment for BPH-related LUTS. A recent network meta-analysis found α-blockers more effective than all other medications for BPH-related LUTS. They work by several mechanisms: decreased contractility of prostatic tissue, capsule, and urethra; increased apoptosis caused by higher levels of tumor growth factor-β; and improved vascular flow to the detrusor. The nonselective agents—terazosin and doxazosin—target α_{1B} and α_{1D} receptors, which are also found outside the LUT and can lead to adverse effects, especially cardiac. There are scant data on prazosin for treatment of BPH-associated LUTS. Selective agents target the α_{1A} receptors that are specific to the prostate, and include tamsulosin (0.4–0.8 mg daily), alfuzosin (10 mg daily), and silodosin (8 mg daily [4 mg with renal impairment]).

Time to onset of action for all α-blockers is 2 to 4 weeks. Randomized controlled trials (RCTs) show no significant differences in LUTS reduction between these

TABLE 38-7 ■ MEDICATIONS FOR TREATMENT OF LOWER URINARY TRACT SYMPTOMS IN MEN

α-Blockers	
Nonselective	Doxazosin 4–8 mg once daily
	Terazosin 2–10 mg once daily
Selective	Alfuzosin 10 mg once daily
	Silodosin 4–8 mg once daily
	Tamsulosin 0.4–0.8 mg once daily
5α-Reductase inhibitors	Dutasteride 0.5 mg once daily
	Finasteride 5 mg once daily
Antimuscarinic agents[a]	Darifenacin 7.5–15 mg once daily
	Fesoterodine 4–8 mg once daily
	Solifenacin 5–10 mg once daily
	Tolterodine ER 4 mg once daily
Beta-3-agonists	Merabegron 25–50 mg once daily
	Vibegron 75 mg once daily
Phosphodiesterase type 5 inhibitors[a]	Tadalafil 5 mg once daily

[a]Includes only those agents and doses with published evidence.

agents. Efficacy is greater in men with more severe LUTS, and appears durable, although most long-term data are from open-label trials. α-Blockers do not prevent urinary retention and are not very effective in reducing nocturia.

For all of these agents, withdrawal rates in published trials are 10% to 15%, and may be higher in clinical practice. All can cause asthenia, headache, dizziness, and hypotension, but dizziness and hypotension are less marked with the selective α_{1A} agents, making them preferred for use in older men. Slow titration from minimal starting doses and nighttime dosing help mitigate first-dose hypotension. Alfuzosin is taken within an hour of a meal to maximize bioavailability. Although seemingly parsimonious, α-blockers should be avoided as first-line antihypertensive agents in men with LUTS and hypertension.

Tamsulosin is associated with retrograde ejaculation and a high risk of floppy iris syndrome during cataract surgery. To prevent the latter complication, special surgical approaches are necessary and men taking tamsulosin should alert their ophthalmologist. The impact of stopping tamsulosin preoperatively is unclear, as some cases occurred months after discontinuation. Concomitant use of phosphodiesterase type 5 (PDE-5) inhibitors for ED can cause potentially dangerous hypotension with all α-blockers, although possibly less likely with tamsulosin.

5α-Reductase Inhibitors The 5αRIs finasteride and dutasteride decrease prostate size by blocking the 5α reduction of testosterone to dihydrotestosterone, the active androgen for prostate growth. 5αRIs decrease prostate volume over 6 months by a maximum of 30%. They have a slow onset of action, and improvement in LUTS may take 6 to 10 months; they will not help men who want rapid symptom improvement or have a short life expectancy. Lifetime use is necessary to prevent recurrent BPE and LUTS, raising the potential for higher lifetime treatment costs. In one study, finasteride was more cost-effective for men with moderate LUTS than watchful waiting (up to 3 years) and TURP (up to 14 years), but cost-effectiveness decreased over time. Unlike α-blockers, 5αRIs are considered "disease modifying" because they decrease the risk of BPE-related complications (ie, worsening symptoms, AUR, need for surgery), as first demonstrated in the PLESS trial (Proscar Long-term Efficacy and Safety Study) in men with moderate to severe LUTS and BPE. Finasteride decreased the incidence of AUR (absolute risk reduction [ARR] 5% [95% CI 10%–5%], number needed to treat [NNT] 26–49) and prostatectomy (ARR 4% [95% CI 7%–3%], NNT 18–31). Risk reduction was apparent by 1 year and was greatest in men with large glands (prostate volume > 58 mL and/or PSA ≥ 1.4 ng/mL). Similar results were seen with dutasteride in the Reduction by Dutasteride of Prostate Cancer Events (REDUCE) trial. At baseline, men had prostate size greater than 40 mL and AUASI less than 8. At 4 years, clinical progression occurred in 21% in men taking dutasteride versus 36% in men on placebo (NNT 7). Sexual dysfunction with finasteride was 8% greater than placebo (absolute difference).

Although 5αRIs maintain or even increase serum testosterone levels, they can cause adverse sexual effects including decreased libido (6%) and impotence (8%). There is conflicting data from cohort studies whether 5αRIs increase the risk of depression, primarily due to differences in pharmaco-epidemiology methods. Data from the prospective Prostate Cancer Prevention Trial did find evidence of a possible association. A sub-analysis of the PLESS trial and subsequent case-control and population-based studies found no association of finasteride or dutasteride with osteoporosis or hip fracture.

The relationship between 5αRIs and prostate cancer is complex. 5αRIs decrease PSA levels by 40% to 60% in the first year. PSA should be monitored and biopsy done if PSA remains stable or rises only in older men for whom prostate cancer screening is appropriate (which should be uncommon). Long-term use of 5αRIs may increase the risk of high-grade prostate cancer. In the initial report from the Prostate Cancer Prevention Trial (PCPT), finasteride lowered prostate cancer rates (18% vs 24% with placebo), but there was a statistically significant increase in high-grade cancer in the finasteride group (6.4% vs 5.1%). Results were very similar in the subsequent REDUCE trial with dutasteride: overall prostate cancer rates were lower with the 5αRI (23% relative reduction, absolute reduction 5%), but there were significantly more high-grade tumors. However, a higher rate of high-grade tumors was still present but no longer statistically significant in the 2013 PCPT analysis with an extra year of data. Furthermore, at 10-year analyses, there were no differences in overall or prostate cancer–specific mortality. However, the Food and Drug Administration (FDA) maintains a black box warning of risk of high-grade prostate cancer with these drugs.

Phosphodiesterase Type 5 Inhibitors Randomized trials demonstrate statistically significant but modest decreases in AUASI with daily doses of PDE-5 inhibitors used for ED. Trials have included tadalafil 5 mg daily, vardenafil 10 mg daily (only studied in men < 65 years), and sildenafil 25 mg daily, but only daily tadalafil is FDA-approved for treatment of male LUTS.

PDE-5 inhibitors may decrease BPH-associated LUTS by regulation of smooth muscle tone and tissue oxygenation. However, there is ongoing controversy about whether the observed efficacy of PDE-5 inhibitors for LUTS is a direct effect or secondary to subjects being "unblinded" to their randomization to drug by improvement in ED symptoms. A review of four randomized trials found no significant interaction of baseline ED severity and improvement in IPSS, and similarly no significant interaction between baseline IPSS severity and ED outcomes.

Combination Therapy

α-Adrenergic blockers and bladder relaxants. The most bothersome LUTS are typically urgency, frequency, and nocturia, which are less responsive to drug therapy than other LUTS. This led to interest in using antimuscarinic agents and the beta3 agonist mirabegron to treat male LUTS. The vast majority of trials studied these drugs in combination with α-blockers, due to concern about incomplete emptying and retention with monotherapy. In addition, most only included men with PVR less than 200 mL, and had a relatively short follow-up (12 weeks, maximum in one study for 4 months). The additive benefit from antimuscarinics or mirabegron is clinically modest at best, and mostly for reducing frequency but not urgency, nocturia, or incontinence. This modest benefit must be weighed against the risks of antimuscarinics and the potential blood pressure effects of mirabegron, as well as added cost. Because of their different mechanisms of action, combination treatment with α-blockers and 5αRIs has the potential for additive benefit. The pivotal Medical Therapy of Prostate Symptoms (MTOPS) study randomized nearly 3000 men with moderate LUTS to placebo, doxazosin, finasteride, or both drugs with a mean follow-up of 4.5 years. The primary outcome was "clinical progression," not LUTS reduction. At 1 year, only doxazosin (alone or in combination) was significantly more effective than placebo, but at 5 years, finasteride was more effective than doxazosin, and combination therapy more effective than either finasteride or doxazosin alone (albeit with high withdrawal rates and adverse effects). Men with baseline prostate volume greater than 40 mL and/or PSA greater than 4 ng/mL benefited the most from combination therapy. Disease progression was associated with rising PSA and prostate volume during the trial in men on placebo or doxazosin, but not finasteride or combination therapy. The Symptom Management After Reducing Therapy (SMART) trial evaluated whether the efficacy of short-term combination therapy is maintained with a 5αRI alone. After 24 weeks of dutasteride ± tamsulosin, stopping tamsulosin caused increased symptoms only for men with severe baseline LUTS. The CombAT trial (Combination of Advodart and Tamsulosin) randomized men with symptomatic LUTS to tamsulosin 0.4 mg, dutasteride 0.5 mg daily, or both. At 4 years, AUR or surgery occurred in 4.2% on combination therapy, versus 5.2% with dutasteride and 12% with tamsulosin. Symptom progression was less likely with combination (13%) than dutasteride (18%) or tamsulosin (22%).

α-ADRENERGIC BLOCKERS AND PDE-5 INHIBITORS. There is no clear benefit from adding PDE-5Is to α-blockers. A meta-analysis including 11 RCTs and a total of 855 patients found statistically but not clinically significant decrease in IPSS (pooled mean difference −1.66, 95% CI −3.03 to −0.29; minimum clinically significant difference is 3 or more). Tadalafil is approved as a single agent for treating LUTS and ED.

Phytotherapy Saw palmetto, β-sitosterols, and cernilton are some of the plant-derived compounds used to treat BPH-related LUTS, especially outside of the United States. Most phytotherapy trials suffer from short-term treatment (typically 4–24 weeks) and lack of standardized preparations. Although a Cochrane systematic review concluded that saw palmetto significantly improved LUTS and decreased nocturia, a subsequent RCT found no difference from placebo in men with moderate to severe LUTS. Cochrane meta-analyses also found that β-sitosterols and cernilton statistically significantly reduce LUTS, but the source trials were heterogeneous and small. Phytotherapeutic agents have few reported side effects in the data that exist, yet more rigorous and long-term data are lacking.

Emerging drug therapies Drugs under investigation for LUTS treatment include $α_{1D}$ antagonists and agents targeting novel therapeutic pathways (vitamin D_3 and calcitriol analogs; agonists/antagonists of endogenous peptides; intraprostatic botulinum toxin; intraprostatic fexapotide triflutate [which targets caspase, tumor necrosis factor and beta lymphoma pathways causing prostate epithelial involution]; and the gonadotropin-releasing hormone antagonist cetrorelix).

Surgery The role for surgical management of benign prostate disease is well established with Level 1 evidence of robust and durable symptom improvement. Surgery should be considered for patients with moderate to severe symptoms (AUASI > 8) who have failed appropriate medical management or wish to avoid daily medications. More stringent indications exist for conditions where medical therapy is often inappropriate such as patients with renal insufficiency due to BOO, bladder stones, gross hematuria related to BPH, recurrent urinary retention, or UTI.

For the past century, surgical treatment has involved removing obstructing adenomatous tissue from primarily the transition zone of the prostate with either a transurethral (TURP) or open surgical approach (simple prostatectomy). These procedures differ from a radical prostatectomy, preformed for prostate cancer, in that prostatic tissue and capsular structure are left in place obviating the need for an anastomosis between the bladder neck and urethra that is required when the entire gland is removed. The TURP has classically been performed utilizing a monopolar resectoscope, an instrument inserted into the urethra with a lens for visualization and an electrified wire loop to remove obstructing adenoma surrounding the urethra. Irrigation with a nonconductive fluid such as glycine or water is needed with monopolar TURP and prolonged operative time increases the risk for transurethral resection syndrome (dilutional hyponatremia and hypervolemia). Due to this risk, open surgical approaches (retropubic, suprapubic, perineal) are used to treat larger prostates. Both open simple prostatectomy and TURP require regional or general anesthesia, variable length of hospital admission, and have known complications such as blood loss requiring transfusion, urethral stricture, bladder neck contracture, stress urinary incontinence, ED, and retrograde ejaculation. More recently alternatives to classic monopolar TURP and open simple prostatectomy have been developed to mitigate need for general anesthesia, hospital admission, discontinuation of anticoagulation therapy, or open surgery, and surgical candidacy has been expanded to older and more comorbid individuals.

Transurethral Resection of Prostate TURP remains the gold standard for surgical treatment of LUTS attributed to BPH. TURP is highly effective, resulting in up to 90% decrease in LUTS and 10-point decrease in AUASI. Symptom decrease may be less in older men (< 80% decrease in symptoms). TURP is superior to watchful waiting in preventing worsening LUTS, elevated PVR, and AUR over 5 years (10% vs 21%, NNT 9). Urodynamic evaluation may be helpful in identifying men most likely to have the best symptomatic outcomes (BOO present without detrusor overactivity or underactivity). Efficacy declines over time, from 87% decrease in LUTS at 3 months to 75% at 7 years, and reoperation rates average 1% to 2% per year.

There are two types of TURP, the original monopolar resection (M-TURP) and the newer bipolar resection (B-TURP); the difference is that the electrical generator of B-TURP allows for isotonic irrigation fluid, eliminating the risk of TURP syndrome. A 2019 Cochrane systematic review, including more than 50 RCTs with overall moderate quality of evidence, suggests that 1-year (and likely longer) symptomatic and objective outcomes from M-TURP and B-TURP are similar, but B-TURP has less post-TURP syndrome, decreased need for postoperative blood transfusion, and reduced overall adverse events. In practice, B-TURP has become the new standard modality.

Perioperative complications of TURP have declined over time. Adverse effects of TURP include retrograde ejaculation (74%); immediate surgical complications (12%); UI (1%); bleeding requiring transfusion (3%); postoperative urinary retention (7%); and UTI (6%). There are conflicting data on erectile function after TURP with some studies finding improved function while others have rates of ED as high as 14 %. One study found no difference in ED and UI rates between TURP and watchful waiting and the percentage of men who were sexually active was unchanged before and after TURP. Men older than age 80 have higher rates of complications (early 30%–40%, late 13%–22%), reoperation (4% per year), and perioperative mortality (2%–3% vs 0.4%), but no change in long-term survival. Older men may be at higher risk of postoperative myocardial infarction, although the level of evidence is weak. Many of the studies in older men, however, did not adjust for increased comorbidity, and there is some evidence that higher Charlson scores are associated with increased morbidity post-TURP. There is significant risk associated with TURP in the anticoagulated patient with increased risk of hemorrhage needing transfusion, bladder clots, and thromboembolic events. Laser-based prostate procedures are generally preferable in patients who are unable to discontinue anticoagulation.

Laser Prostatectomy Laser technology is an increasingly used alternative to TURP. The main laser systems currently used are holmium or thulium lasers for enucleation of the prostate (HoLEP, ThuLEP) and the GreenLight laser for photovaporization of the prostate (PVP). Lasers are able to provide rapid vaporization and coagulation of prostatic tissue with minimal tissue depth penetration, providing better coagulative properties than either monopolar or bipolar TURP.

Laser enucleation of the prostate consists of transurethral en-bloc excision of the transitional zone of the prostate gland using a combination of mechanical dissection with a rigid cystoscope and laser energy to enucleate the prostatic adenoma and move it to the bladder where it is morcellated. This procedure has a significant learning curve and is disproportionally utilized by urologists who have exposure in fellowship training. It provided similar outcomes when compared to TURP as measured by IPSS (AUASI) and IPSS-Qol outcomes and lower likelihood for either peri- or postoperative blood transfusions. Laser enucleation is likely a more durable treatment as well. Laser enucleation can be completed on any sized prostate gland but is frequently utilized as an endoscopic option for the treatment of large prostate glands (> 80 mL) and provides similar outcomes to open prostatectomy for men with AUR with significant BPE.

GreenLight laser photovaporization of the prostate (PVP) utilizes a 532-nm wavelength laser that is preferentially absorbed by hemoglobin and provides targeted tissue vaporization and coagulation. The PVP, like a TURP, utilizes a cystoscope and gradual removal of prostatic adenoma starting from the lumen of the prostatic urethra and moving out to the surgical capsule of the prostate. Unlike TURP and laser enucleation procedures, there is no tissue for pathologic examination at the completion of PVP because all tissue is vaporized by laser energy. In a multicenter, industry-sponsored RCT in 269 patients, PVP was noninferior to TURP with 24 month follow-up data, including similar adverse events related to UI and overall need for reoperation. PVP patients had shorter catheterization times

and shorter hospital stay. A single center study comparing M-TURP, B-TURP, and 120W PVP through 36 months found similar change in IPSS and IPSS-QOL between PVP and the TURP cohorts. Per AUA guidelines, PVP should be considered for patients at higher risk for bleeding (eg, treated with heparin, warfarin, clopidogrel, or direct oral anticoagulant drugs) due to lower transfusion rates compared to TURP and good safety outcomes reported in this population.

Side effects of laser enucleation vary by technique, and can include impotence, retrograde ejaculation, increased urgency and frequency, UI, and bladder neck stricture.

Simple Prostatectomy Men with large prostate volume (> 60 mL) have traditionally required open prostatectomy (via an abdominal or perineal approach) because the operative time needed for TURP significantly increases perioperative complications. With the introduction of B-TURP, laser enucleation, laparoscopic, and robotic-assisted surgeries, open procedures have become less common and account for less than 5% of prostatectomies for benign indications, and some surgeons prefer to perform an "incomplete" TURP to avoid the morbidity of abdominal or perineal surgery. In the case of very large prostate glands, simple prostatectomy (open, laparoscopic, or robot-assisted) continues to be a reasonable option. In retrospective studies, open prostatectomy has lower reoperation rate and mortality than TURP, but these analyses did not adequately control for the higher age and comorbidity in TURP patients or the secular trend of decreasing TURP mortality. A more recent RCT evaluated laparoscopic simple prostatectomy compared to B-TURP and found similar risk of blood transfusions, need for reoperation, UI, and similar change in IPSS through 36 months,

Minimally Invasive Procedures

PROSTATIC URETHRAL LIFT. The prostatic urethral lift (PUL) alters prostate anatomy without removing tissue by utilizing transprostatic suture implants delivered through a cystoscope. The implants consist of two T-shaped bars attached to a length of suture that are deployed through the prostate with one bar located outside the prostate capsule and the other within the prostatic urethral lumen. The tension across the implant helps widen the prostatic urethra. A single RCT compared the PUL to TURP and found 73% of patients with PUL reported 30% or greater reduction in IPSS at 1 year compared to 91% who had TURP. At 2 years patients with TURP had an average 6 point greater reduction in IPSS and significantly better Qmax than those with PUL. PUL was found to have less likelihood of altering sexual function than TURP with no evidence of altered ejaculatory or erectile dysfunction, and ejaculatory bother improved by 40% at 1 year while intensity of ejaculation and amount of ejaculate improved by 23% and 22%, respectively. Another study compared PUL to sham and found modest improvements in IPSS (mean decrease −5.2; CI: −7.45, −2.95) at short-term follow-up and with both sham and PUL remaining significantly improved at 5 years. Rates of serious and non-serious harm are similar between TURP and PUL and reoperation rates at 2 years are similar. Long-term data are limited but this procedure has gained popularity over the past decade partly due to the ability to complete it in an office setting without the use of general anesthesia.

PROSTATE INCISION. Transurethral incision of the prostate (TUIP) is a technically simpler procedure used in men with small glands (< 30 mL). TUIP is done under local anesthesia with shorter operation time and less bleeding than TURP. TUIP has similar symptomatic efficacy to TURP at 1 year. In a select case series, at 2 years only 8% of TUIP patients had required a subsequent TURP. TUIP has the potential to be a safe and effective alternative for obstructed older men with smaller prostates who have high operative risk and have failed noninvasive treatment.

Transurethral needle ablation (TUNA) employs transurethrally placed radiofrequency needles to heat prostate tissue, causing coagulation necrosis and a tissue defect. Symptomatic efficacy is lower and less durable than with TURP, and no studies compare TUNA to other procedures, medical therapy, or watchful waiting. Transurethral microwave thermotherapy is a related outpatient procedure that requires repeated treatments. Symptomatic improvement is typically modest, and in short-term trials is inferior to TURP, sham procedures, and terazosin. The future of these procedures is uncertain.

Urethral stents to facilitate voiding should be reserved for high-risk patients with recurrent AUR who are unfit for surgery or for whom long-term indwelling catheterization is undesirable. Permanent absorbable stents are complicated by encrustation, pain, and infection, and failure rates range from 20% to 30%. Nonabsorbable temporary stents are complicated by migration, UTI, stricture, and encrustation. Due to lack of efficacy, thermotherapy and urethral stents are no longer recommended to treat BPH-related LUTS.

PREVENTION

Data on risk and protective factors suggest that increased physical activity, a diet low in meat and fat and high in vegetables and micronutrients, and moderate alcohol consumption may prevent or slow the progression of benign prostate disease. Weight loss for obese men, glycemic control in diabetes, and treatment of high cholesterol also may be important. However, there are no intervention trials to support these suggestions.

FURTHER READING

Alexander CE, Scullion MMF, Omar MI, et al. Bipolar versus monopolar transurethral resection of the prostate for lower urinary tract symptoms secondary to benign prostatic obstruction. *Cochrane Database Syst Rev.* 2019;12(12):CD009629.

American Urological Association (AUA) guidelines on the management of benign prostatic hyperplasia. https://www.auanet.org/guidelines/guidelines/benign-prostatic-hyperplasia-(bph)-guideline. Accessed August 29, 2021.

Bachmann A, Tubaro A, Barber N, et al. A European multicenter randomized noninferiority trial comparing 180 W GreenLight XPS laser vaporization and transurethral resection of the prostate for the treatment of benign prostatic obstruction: 12-month results of the GOLIATH study. *J Urol.* 2015;193(2):570–578.

Barry MJ, Link CL, McNaughton-Collins MF, McKinlay JB. Boston Area Community Health (BACH) Investigators. Overlap of different urological symptom complexes in a racially and ethnically diverse, community-based population of men and women. *BJU Int.* 2008;101:45–51.

Biester K, Skipka G, Jahn R, Buchberger B, Rohde V, Lange S. Systematic review of surgical treatments for benign prostatic hyperplasia and presentation of an approach to investigate therapeutic equivalence (noninferiority). *BJU Int.* 2012;109(5):722–730.

Crawford EF, Wilson SS, McConnell JD, et al. Baseline factors as predictors of clinical progression of benign prostatic hyperplasia in men treated with placebo. *J Urol.* 2006;175:1422–1427.

Füllhase C, Chapple C, Cornu J-N, et al. Systematic review of combination drug therapy for non-neurogenic male lower urinary tract symptoms. *Eur Urol.* 2013;64: 228–243.

Hollingsworth JM, Wilt TJ. Lower urinary tract symptoms in men. *BMJ.* 2014;349:g4474.

Kaplan SA, Herschorn S, McVary KT, et al. Efficacy and safety of mirabegron versus placebo add-on therapy in men with overactive bladder symptoms receiving tamsulosin for underlying benign prostatic hyperplasia: a randomized, phase 4 study (PLUS). *J Urol.* 2020;203(6)1163–1171.

Knapp GL, Chalasani V, Woo HH. Perioperative adverse events in patients on continued anticoagulation undergoing photoselective vaporisation of the prostate with the 180-W Greenlight lithium triborate laser. *BJU Int.* 2017;119(Suppl 5):33–38.

Kumar N, Vasudeva P, Kumar A, Singh H. Prospective randomized comparison of monopolar TURP, bipolar TURP and photoselective vaporization of the prostate in patients with benign prostatic obstruction: 36 months outcome. *Low Urin Tract Symptoms.* 2018;10(1):17–20.

Kupelian V, Wei JT, O'Leary MP, et al. Prevalence of lower urinary tract symptoms and effect on quality of life in a racially and ethnically diverse random sample: the Boston Area Community Health (BACH) Survey. *Arch Intern Med.* 2006;166(21):2381–2387.

Lerner LB, McVary, KT, Barry MJ, et al. Management of lower urinary tract symptoms attributed to benign prostatic hyperplasia: AUA Guideline part I, initial work-up and medical management. *J Urol.* 2021;206(4):806–817.

Lerner LB, McVary, KT, Barry MJ et al. Management of lower urinary tract symptoms attributed to benign prostatic hyperplasia: AUA Guideline part II, surgical evaluation and treatment. *J Urol.* 2021;206(4):818–826.

Lerner LB, McVary, KT, Barry MJ et al. Management of lower urinary tract symptoms attributed to benign prostatic hyperplasia: AUA Guideline part I, initial work-up and medical management. *J Urol.* 2021;206:806.

Platz EA, Joshu CE, Mondul AM, Peskoe SB, Willett WC, Giovannucci E. Incidence and progression of lower urinary tract symptoms in a large prospective cohort of US men. *J Urol.* 2012;188(2):496–501.

Sarma AV, Wei JT. Clinical practice. Benign prostatic hyperplasia and lower urinary tract symptoms. *N Engl J Med.* 2012;367:248–257.

Saigal CS. Quality indicators for benign prostatic hyperplasia in vulnerable elders. *J Am Geriatr Soc.* 2007;55(suppl 2):S253–S257.

Toren P, Margel D, Kulkarni G, Finelli A, Zlotta A, Fleshner N. Effect of dutasteride on clinical progression of benign prostatic hyperplasia in asymptomatic men with enlarged prostate: a post hoc analysis of the REDUCE study. *BMJ.* 2013;346:f2109.

Ückert S, Kedia GT, Tsikas D, Simon A, Bannowsky A, Kuczyk MA. Emerging drugs to target lower urinary tract symptomatology (LUTS)/benign prostatic hyperplasia (BPH): focus on the prostate. *World J Urol.* 2020;38(6):1423–1435.

Unger JM, Till C, Thompson IM Jr, et al. Long-term consequences of finasteride vs placebo in the Prostate Cancer Prevention Trial. *J Natl Cancer Inst.* 2016;108(12):djw168.

Walton A. Managing overactive bladder symptoms in a palliative care setting. *J Palliat Med.* 2014;17(1):118–121.

Weiss JP, Blaivas, JG, Blanker MH, et al. The New England Research Institutes, Inc. (NERI) Nocturia Advisory Conference 2012: focus on outcomes of therapy. *BJU Intl.* 2013;111(5):700–716.

Xie JB, Tan YA, Wang FL, et al. Extraperitoneal laparoscopic adenomectomy (Madigan) versus bipolar transurethral resection of the prostate for benign prostatic hyperplasia greater than 80 ml: complications and functional outcomes after 3-year follow-up. *J Endourol.* 2014;28(3):353–359.

Zhang J, Li X, Yang B, et al. Alpha-blockers with or without phosphodiesterase type 5 inhibitor for treatment of lower urinary tract symptoms secondary to benign prostatic hyperplasia: a systematic review and meta-analysis. *World J Urol.* 2019;37:143–153.

Geriatric Conditions

Chapter 39

Systems Physiology of Aging and Selected Disorders of Homeostasis

George A. Kuchel

"Besides more or less obvious physical changes in old age, physiological investigation may reveal increasing limitation of the effectiveness of homeostatic devices which keep the bodily conditions stable."

Walter Bradford Cannon (1871–1945)

OVERVIEW

All organ systems undergo physiological changes with aging. However, the rate and nature of such changes varies both among organ systems and across individuals. This book includes individual chapters that address physiological changes associated with aging within the context of specific organ systems or tissues (see Part V: Organ Systems and Diseases).

Nevertheless, approaches to the older patient, which do not consider the entire person and ignore considerations cutting across different organ systems or disciplinary perspectives often fail to produce clinically meaningful improvements in the health of older adults, especially in the context of multiple morbidity (see Chapter 41). This chapter discusses physiology of aging using an integrative systems-based approach designed to address these issues via several complementary perspectives. First, in order to fully understand aging it is essential to consider cross-cutting physiological patterns that are observed with aging across different organ systems. Second, efforts to improve the health and function of frail older adults with common geriatric syndromes and multiple morbidities require an understanding and appreciation of the impact of physiological changes in the context of these additional complexities. Finally, the full impact of aging on physiological responses can only be understood when considering the ability of older adults to respond to common stressors experienced in life ranging from changes in ambient temperature to fluctuations in fluid balance to ability to maintain an adequate blood pressure and brain perfusion when standing up, among many others. Given the importance of temperature and fluid/salt balance regulation, physiological principles and clinical approaches to these problems are discussed in additional detail in this chapter.

Learning Objectives

- Describe general features of physiological aging shared across tissues and organ systems including loss of complexity, increased heterogeneity, loss of resilience, homeostenosis, diminished physiological reserves, diminished end-organ responsiveness, loss of negative feedback, and allostatic load.

- Understand the concepts of homeostasis and homeostenosis.

- Describe the impact of aging on homeostatic mechanisms which help maintain a normal physiologic body temperature and fluid/salt balance in the face of lowered or increased ambient temperature, as well depletion or overload of fluids and sodium.

- Describe the clinical features—including epidemiology, symptoms, signs, results of diagnostic tests and treatment— of hypothermia, hyperthermia, and water and sodium excess or depletion.

- Describe the impact of aging on the ability to maintain a normal blood pressure in the face of orthostasis, meal ingestion, hypovolemia, and volume overload.

Key Clinical Points

1. In addition to tissue- and organ-specific changes, shared features of physiological aging include loss of complexity, increased heterogeneity, loss of resilience, homeostenosis, diminished physiological reserves, diminished end-organ responsiveness, loss of negative feedback, and allostatic load.

2. Homeostasis reflects the aggregate effect of varied mechanisms that maintain normal physiologic constancy in the face of different extrinsic challenges. Aging is associated with impaired homeostasis, or

(Continued)

(Cont.)

homeostenosis, in the form of diminished capacity to respond to varied challenges.

3. Aging is associated with a failure of several different homeostatic mechanisms that enhance the risk of hypothermia in the face of decreased ambient temperature.

4. Aging is associated with a failure of homeostatic mechanisms that enhance the risk of hyperthermia and heatstroke in the face of increased ambient temperature.

5. The clinical presentation of hypothermia and hyperthermia may be subtle in older adults, requiring a high index of suspicion and careful supportive management in order to avoid the high rate of mortality associated with these conditions in late life.

6. Aging is also associated with homeostatic deficits when confronted with the assumption of the upright posture, eating, hypovolemia or a fluid challenge, increased or decreased sodium level, increased or decreased glucose level, bladder filling or bladder outlet obstruction, major burns or trauma, bed rest, or exercise.

AN INTEGRATIVE APPROACH TO THE PHYSIOLOGY OF AGING

Cross-Cutting Physiological Changes of Aging

Loss of complexity Geriatricians are in many ways experts in clinical complexity and in dealing with complicated decisions that arise from multiple morbidity, the multifactorial nature of most geriatric conditions, and the complex multidimensional needs of many older adults. However, declines in complexity involving critical structural and functional components accompany and greatly contribute to these clinical manifestations. Selected examples include losses with aging in the complexity of dendritic arborizations (**Figure 39-1A**), neuronal circuits (Chapter 56), and bone architecture (Chapter 51). Further discussion is provided in the section on systemic patterns of change later in this chapter.

Increased heterogeneity Descriptions of aging often emphasize comparisons of means or medians. However, changes in variability with aging also need to be considered. Most, but not all, physiological parameters show evidence of increased heterogeneity in aged populations (**Figure 39-1B**) and also in older individuals examined repeatedly over time (**Figure 39-1C**). Such increases in heterogeneity are seen both for many physiological parameters

that on average decline with aging (eg, gait speed) and others that typically increase with aging (eg, systolic blood pressure).

Decreased resilience Resilience represents the ability of a physiological system or individual to maintain normal function (black line in **Figure 39-1D**) or to rapidly and completely regain normal function (blue line in **Figure 39-1D**) when exposed to a stressor. As discussed below, relevant stressors may be as varied as a stressful "fight or flight" response, exposure to a decreased or increased ambient temperature, orthostasis, meal ingestion, hypovolemia, hyperglycemia, hypoglycemia, fluid challenge, dehydration, bladder outlet obstruction, major burn, trauma, bed rest, exercise, medications interfering with signaling pathways (eg, anticholinergic, antidopaminergic), or neuronal degeneration. When a stressor or a combination of stressors overcome an individual's resilience mechanisms, delayed recovery (red line in **Figure 39-1D**), partial recovery with new disability (purple line in **Figure 39-1D**), or even death (stippled red line in **Figure 39-1D**) may result.

Homeostenosis reflects a narrowing of the capacity to maintain normal homeostasis which results in the aged system being overwhelmed by stressors (#2 and #3 in **Figure 39-1E**) that would normally not pose any difficulty (#1 in **Figure 39-1E**).

Diminished physiological reserve Physiological reserves (blue in **Figure 39-1F**) decline with aging and therefore may no longer be available (red in **Figure 39-1F**) to come into play when initial resilience mechanisms are overwhelmed, thus resulting in lost function and even system decompensation (red in **Figure 39-1E**). There may be decreased synthesis and release of specific neurotransmitters with aging, such as declining dopamine release in brain circuits involved in motor and behavioral control, or decreased levels of circulating hormones (eg, testosterone in men, 17β-estradiol in women).

Diminished end-organ responsiveness Many physiological systems demonstrate decreased responsiveness with aging (**Figure 39-1G**). There is often a decline of end-organ receptor numbers (eg, post-synaptic beta adrenergic receptors) or decreased responsiveness at the level of individual receptors (eg, functional uncoupling of the platelet alpha 2-adrenergic receptor-adenylate cyclase complex). Any of these individual or combined changes can result in delayed onset and diminished magnitude of end-organ functional responses.

Loss of negative feedback with basal activation and system sluggishness Declines with aging in the ability of systems to provide negative feedback have been described in the context of neural circuits, endocrine systems, and immune response loops (**Figure 39-1H**). These impair the ability of the aged sympathetic nervous system (SNS), hypothalamic-pituitary-adrenal (HPA) axis, and inflammatory mediators to dampen and downregulate the activation of these systems (**Figure 39-1H**). As a result, with aging, basal levels of

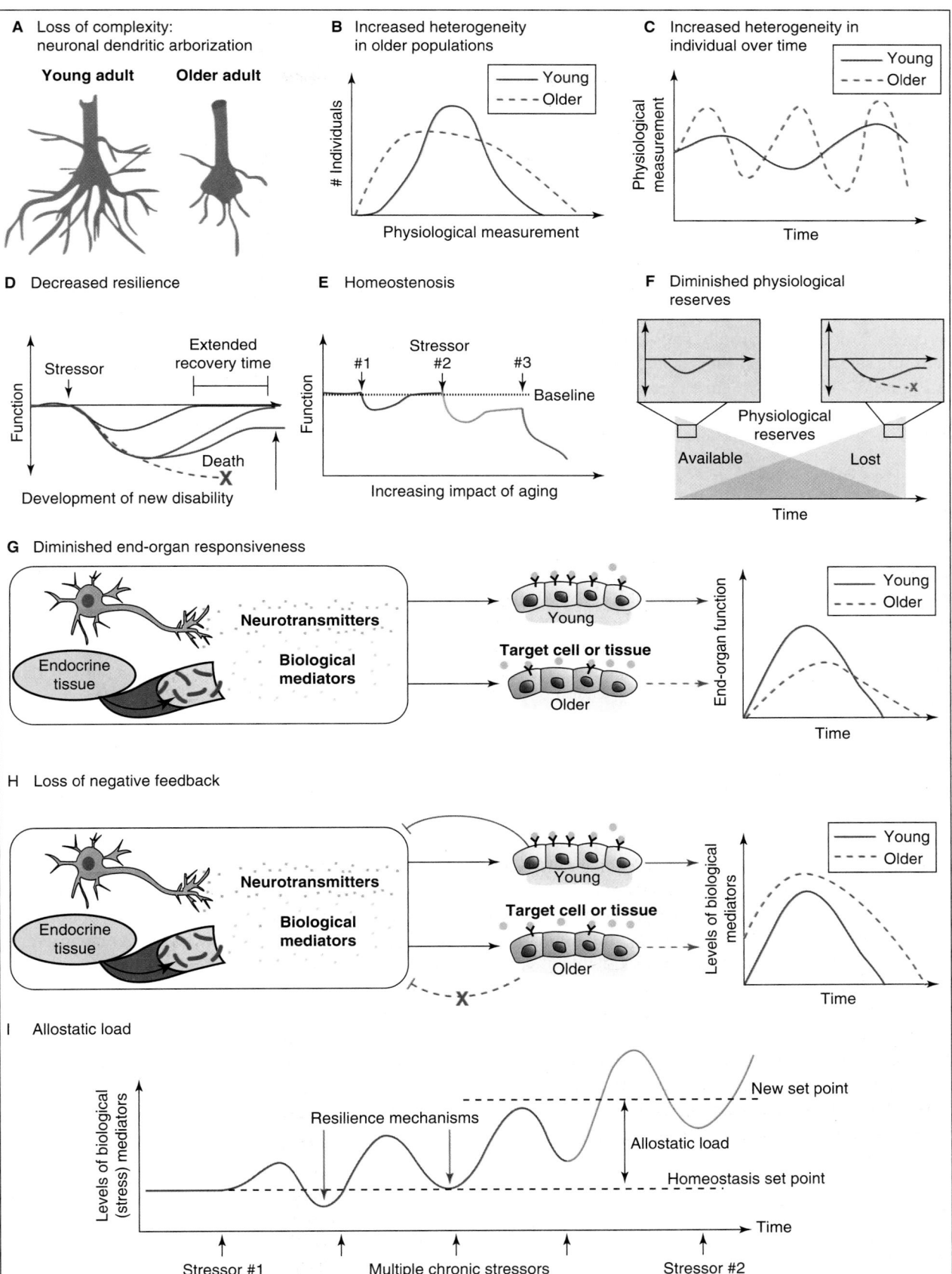

FIGURE 39-1. Cross-cutting physiological changes of aging.

mediators of SNS function (eg, norepinephrine), stress (eg, cortisol), and inflammation (eg, interleukin [IL]-6) are elevated with healthy aging and even more so in the context of frailty, multiple morbidity, and disability. Moreover, poststimulation increases in these mediators tend to be higher and remain for a longer period of time in older adults.

Allostatic load Individual physiological and behavioral stressors do not occur in isolation from the many other similar and different events that may have preceded these homeostatic challenges. To that end, the term allostatic load was coined to measure "the wear and tear on the body" that accumulates as an individual is exposed to repeated or chronic stress. From a resilience perspective this means that repeated multiple chronic stressors can reset the homeostatic set point so that subsequent stressors (stressor #2 in **Figure 39-1I**) result in enhanced levels of biological mediators of stress (red line in **Figure 39-1I**) together with increased likelihood of system decompensation.

Attributing Physiological Changes to Aging and/or Disease

Age-related physiological changes influence nearly all aspects of older patients' health status and functional independence. These include clinical symptoms, health trajectories, and responsiveness to therapies, as well as related conditions such as resilience and frailty. Physiological declines with geriatric syndromes and chronic diseases of aging often represent quantitatively augmented versions of otherwise similar physiological changes with typical healthy aging. Recognition of these common shared physiological motifs as well as their transition from "normative" to pathological aging requires sophisticated clinical expertise. In fact, one of the key features of comprehensive geriatric care is the ability of skilled experts such as geriatricians to take into consideration the nature of physiological changes attributable to aging and/or varied aging-related disease processes when making diagnostic and therapeutic decisions regarding individual patients.

A growing body of knowledge has highlighted the nature of many physiological changes attributable to aging in the absence of overt diseases, although interpretation of such work requires a clear understanding and definition of disease versus "normative" aging. Exclusion of older adults from research continues to represent a major problem. To that end, in 2017 the National Institutes of Health (NIH) established a policy whereby individuals of all ages, including children and older adults, must be included in all human research, conducted or supported by the NIH, unless there are scientific or ethical reasons not to include them. Nevertheless, two major problems remain. First, most studies still fail to recruit older adults whose health status in the form of multiple morbidity with presence of varied common chronic diseases (Chapter 41) reflects the types of real-world patients seen by most geriatricians. At the other extreme in terms of health status, there continues to be a great deal of confusion as to the selection and

recruitment of appropriate older "controls" when seeking to disentangle the role of aging versus diseases.

Furthermore, research that focuses on older adults who have no evidence of any chronic disease presents significant challenges since it excludes the vast majority of older adults, including many living healthy and independent lives in the community. Moreover, this approach to recruitment is more reflective of "exceptional" aging as opposed to usual or typical healthy aging. The latter construct is more broadly translatable to real-world clinical care since it reflects physiological aging in the context of far greater numbers of independent and generally healthy older adults with extremely common and well-controlled chronic conditions such as hypertension, hyperlipidemia, osteoarthritis, and others.

Nevertheless, and in spite of the above complexities and the fact that even healthy aging is associated with a great deal of interindividual heterogeneity, geriatricians must possess a deep understanding of the nature of physiological changes attributable to aging and other changes attributable to specific chronic diseases. While such a task might seem overwhelming and perhaps even insurmountable at first, two foundational principles of aging physiology greatly facilitate even a novice's approach to these otherwise challenging issues.

First, in the majority of cases, the physiological changes involving a specific organ or tissue that are attributable to aging do not differ qualitatively from those that are observed with individual chronic diseases or geriatric syndromes. Instead, these disease processes and geriatric syndromes for which aging represents a major risk factor generally reflect a quantitative amplification of individual and often multifaceted physiological changes described with aging.

Second, the otherwise highly disparate, distinct, and multifactorial chronic diseases, geriatric syndromes, and other common conditions that afflict older adults do share a common overarching feature—biological aging as a common and shared risk factor. As a consequence of these underlying biological mechanisms or drivers that are shared with aging, individual chronic diseases and geriatric syndromes also generally share common physiological patterns or motifs. Moreover, the shared biological drivers also represent opportunities for intervening in these physiological declines via geroscience-guided interventions (see Chapter 40).

Physiological Changes in the Context of Geriatric Syndromes

In addition to being highly prevalent in frail older people, geriatric syndromes also exert a substantial impact on quality of life and disability. Moreover, these are complex multifactorial conditions in which large numbers of underlying and provocative risk factors involving different organ systems interact in influencing ultimate clinical presentation, course, response to treatment, and outcome. These unusual features present important challenges for the clinician since the patient's chief complaint may point away from, rather than toward, the specific pathologic condition, which actually underlies the change in health status. At times, the two processes may involve distinct and distant organs with an apparent "disconnect" between the site of the underlying insult and the site involved in specific functional declines and/or clinical symptoms as reported by the patient. For example, an infection involving the urinary tract can precipitate delirium, and it is often the altered neural function in the form of cognitive and behavioral changes which are the patient's presenting symptoms. The underlying urinary tract infection may be missed unless carefully searched for.

Grouping distinct conditions together as geriatric syndromes also highlights those common features that may help in the development of innovative clinical and research strategies. One of the primary goals of geriatric medicine has been to maintain functional independence in frail older adults, addressing the very common scenario of an older patient who is able to maintain usual function under basal conditions, yet decompensates when exposed to seemingly common every day and even minor challenges. In fact, the clinical dilemma of a frail older adult who is at significant risk of delirium, falls, or incontinence can be restated within a homeostatic framework. Viewed in this manner, function is determined by a complex balance between underlying physiology and health; the nature, number, and intensity of the challenges being experienced; as well as overall physiological plasticity expressed as the effectiveness of relevant homeostatic mechanisms. This approach has several advantages, above all, permitting a clinical and research conceptualization of health and aging that moves beyond traditional paradigms and to an approach that is able to capture the highly dynamic and multifactorial reality of geriatric care.

However, some of the most complex, common, debilitating, and costly clinical problems seen in geriatrics are extremely challenging, precisely because they defy conventional medical wisdom by crossing traditional organ- and discipline-based boundaries. Termed "geriatric syndromes," they are discussed subsequently (Chapters 42–48). Nevertheless, given the central importance of these diverse conditions to the practice and science of geriatric medicine, it is also important to address their common features which range from their multifactorial etiology to their association across multiple different tissues of augmented versions of physiological motifs associated with aging (see **Figure 39-1**).

Physiological Changes in the Context of Multiple Morbidity

The coexistence of multiple chronic conditions and morbidities is common in older people, especially in patients typically seen by geriatricians (Chapter 41). Unfortunately, there is limited information regarding the likely impact on physiological parameters of the multiple morbidity state

or even more importantly the coexistence of specific pairs or clusters of chronic conditions. This lack of information exists because most physiological studies conducted in older adults focus on one single organ system at a time, not considering and often formally excluding the presence of other common chronic conditions.

One example of such a knowledge gap involves sarcopenia. Although there have been great advances in our understanding of muscle aging and sarcopenia (see Chapter 49), their interface with varied chronic conditions is much less well explored. For example, while aging, deconditioning, sepsis, congestive heart failure, cirrhosis, and cancer are all associated with significant declines in muscle mass and function, it remains unclear to what extent similar or distinct physiological changes or mechanisms are involved. These considerations have important clinical implications regarding the choice and responsiveness to varied existing and future interventions.

Conversely, different chronic conditions may have competing and at times even opposing effects on a shared physiological measure. For example, the coexistence of congestive heart failure with chronic kidney disease can result in conflicting care priorities with strategies focused on heart function emphasizing diuresis to reduce blood volume, while those focused on renal performance highlight the importance of maintaining sufficient renal perfusion by increasing blood volume via salt and water loading. As a result, patients with these conditions and their caregivers may sometimes receive conflicting guidance as to the use of diuretics and fluid restriction versus fluid increases from different providers.

HOMEOSTASIS IN A HISTORICAL CONTEXT

The term homeostasis was first coined by Claude Bernard in the mid-nineteenth century and is now extensively used to refer to the body's attempts at maintaining an internal constancy, which is required for optimal function. Far from reflecting physiologic "stasis," effective homeostasis actually requires that all relevant compensatory mechanisms remain suitably vibrant, responsive, and well calibrated. During the twentieth century, it became increasingly clear that overall health status, as well as many individual disease processes, may impair an individual's ability to appropriately respond to common homeostatic challenges. The recognition that aging can also exert a measurable impact on homeostatic mechanisms came later, but is not recent, as illustrated by the 1932 quote preceding this chapter from the great physiologist Walter Cannon. Finally, in the modern era, several events have greatly affected our understanding of homeostasis. In an extension of the concept of homeostasis, Yates introduced the term homeodynamics to emphasize that the resiliency of living organisms requires a dynamic interplay of multiple regulatory mechanisms rather than a constancy of the internal environment. Advances in basic research have also permitted investigators to explore homeostatic principles at the level of subcellular processes ranging from gene expression to protein turnover. Most recently, some of the limitations inherent in purely reductionist studies have led to a trend toward systems biology, emphasizing an integration of relevant homeostatic processes from the level of individual cells to tissues and organisms. Moreover, it is now possible to begin defining mechanisms in a manner which reflects the multifactorial and systemic nature of typical geriatric conditions or syndromes.

HOMEOSTATIC REGULATION IN OLD AGE

General Considerations

Physiologic systems responsible for maintaining homeostatic regulation may control variables as divergent as body temperature, blood pressure, intracellular calcium, or serum cortisol, among many others. At the same time, even among distinct systems, it is possible to observe shared common physiologic principles by which they all exert homeostatic control (**Table 39-1**). With these considerations in mind, efforts are being made to identify unifying and preferably specific "fingerprints" by which aging affects homeostatic control within different physiologic systems.

Systemic Patterns of Change

Homeostenosis of old age has been viewed as the diminished capacity to respond to various homeostatic challenges. Even healthy older adults may exhibit homeostenosis when exposed to a cold or hot environment, on rapidly assuming upright posture, and while responding to an acute fluid challenge or hypovolemia. Traditionally, these deficits were attributed to a loss of physiologic reserve, an appealing, yet somewhat ill-defined concept emphasizing static (eg, losses in neuronal numbers, declines in renal function) rather than dynamic explanations. A focus on physiologic categories of relevant complexity that decline with aging may provide a better basis for understanding the dynamic nature of stability in old age, disease, and frailty. For example, study of aged bone and brain demonstrates evidence of declining complexity in terms of trabecular or neuronal architecture. Other examples of declining complexity involve physiologic processes such as narrowing of auditory frequency responsiveness, declines in recognizable blood pressure patterns over time, and increased randomness or stochastic activity of cardiac intervals. It has been proposed that such alterations in dynamics of physiologic systems contribute to functional decline and frailty. Note that complexity and variability are different concepts, with aging often having distinct and at times directly opposite effects. For example, aging *increases* interindividual and intraindividual variability in blood pressure measurements, while observable patterns over time involving the complexity of these readings *decrease* with aging. Finally, proponents of the concept of allostatic load have used population-derived measurements (eg, blood pressure, waist-hip ratio, cholesterol, glycosylated hemoglobin, cortisol, catecholamines, and dehydroepiandrosterone sulfate [DHEA-S]) as an estimate of cumulative physiologic burden exacted on the body through attempts to adapt to life's demands.

Alterations in Specific Homeostatic Mechanisms

In addition to systemic perspectives of homeostasis, there has also been a growing interest in uncovering specific homeostatic mechanisms that are impaired in old age. For example, markers of SNS activity such as peripheral norepinephrine (NE) levels are elevated in older adults under basal conditions. At the same time, a variety of different stimuli result in an elevation in peripheral NE levels, which are both enhanced and prolonged in older adults. Another common feature is a decline in end-organ responsiveness of many, but not all, receptors to their relevant ligand in the form of a neurotransmitter or hormone. Finally, decreased tissue responsiveness translates in many cases to lessened effectiveness of negative feedback mechanisms as shown for a number of hormones, including corticosteroids.

Reconciling Different Views of Homeostatic Dysregulation

Although many different aspects of homeostatic dysregulation in old age have been described, common unifying principles can sometimes be identified. For example, in simple gene circuits negative feedback loops enhance the complexity and stability of such systems, permitting more precise and rapid responses to homeostatic challenges. Thus, declines in negative feedback demonstrated for many mammalian homeostatic systems could also contribute to some of the other commonly described features of homeostatic dysregulation in old age and frailty. Moreover, a marker of "allostatic load" such as peripheral cortisol is not only a predictor of future cognitive and functional impairment, but can also contribute to neuronal cell death involving hippocampal cells involved in cognition, while also contributing to a decline in the ability of cortisol to downregulate its own synthesis and release.

SPECIFIC HOMEOSTATIC CHALLENGES

General Considerations

As discussed earlier, under normal basal conditions, many older adults are able to maintain their usual level of function even in the presence of a large number of health problems. However, once exposed to additional challenges, the same individuals may experience rapid and at times even catastrophic declines in their health status and functional independence. **Figure 39-1** provides an overview of our current understanding of the impact of aging on the ability

TABLE 39-1 ■ IMPACT OF AGING ON PHYSIOLOGICAL RESPONSES TO SPECIFIC HOMEOSTATIC CHALLENGES

HOMEOSTATIC CHALLENGE	SELECTED BIOMARKERS UNDER BASAL CONDITIONS	IMPACT OF AGING ON RESPONSE TO SPECIFIC CHALLENGE
"Fight or flight" challenge or mental stress	↑ Norepinephrine ± Epinephrine ↑ Sympathetic neural recordings ± Cortisol levels	Prolonged ↑ in norepinephrine levels, sympathetic neural activity, and cortisol levels
Decreased ambient temperature	± Temperature ↓ Metabolic rate	↓ Sensation of cold ↓ Shivering intensity ↓ Thermogenesis ↓ Vasoconstriction
Elevated ambient temperature	± Temperature	↓ Sweating responses ↓ Vasodilatation ↓ Ability to raise cardiac output
Orthostasis, meals, and hypovolemia	± Blood pressure	Hypotension risk ↑ with frailty, polypharmacy, cardiovascular diseases and autonomic failure
Hyperglycemia and hypoglycemia	↑ Fasting glucose	↓ Glucose-insulin dynamics Response to hypoglycemia unaffected or small ↓
Fluid challenge and dehydration	± Serum sodium ± Osmolarity	↓ Plasma volume ↑ Impact of given amount of fluid depletion on osmolality ↓ Glomerular filtration rate generally ↓ Ability to concentrate urine and retain Na⁺ in salt depletion ↓ Ability to excrete Na⁺ in salt loading ↓ Ability to excrete free water ↓ Thirst perception ↑ Ability of hyperosmotic stimuli to raise AVP ↓ Ability of hypovolemic stimuli to raise AVP
Bladder outlet obstruction	↓ Detrusor contractility mildly	↓ Ability to raise detrusor pressure ↑ Likelihood of detrusor decompensation with muscle degeneration and fibrosis
Major burns and trauma		↓ With comorbidity favorable outcome
↓ Physical activity		↑ Extent and speed of deconditioning
Anticholinergic medications		↑ Xerostomia, cognitive problems, constipation, urinary retention
Antidopaminergic medications		↑ Rigidity, poverty of movement

AVP, arginine vasopressin.

to effectively respond to specific homeostatic challenges in terms of the most relevant biomarkers or physiologic measurements. However, it must also be noted that aging may influence some of these measurements under basal conditions. Note that some of these topics are discussed in greater detail in chapters addressing specific organ systems (see **Table 39-1**). Finally, when evaluating the information provided in **Table 39-1** and **Figure 39-1**, several overarching principles must be kept in mind. First, while animal studies largely support results of human research, occasional species-specific differences have been noted.

Thus, all summary findings in **Table 39-1** are based on human research. Second, most of the changes reported in **Table 39-1** can be attributed to normal or "usual" aging, with common geriatric illnesses often enhancing such vulnerabilities. In many cases, it remains unknown whether individuals who age particularly well or successfully also exhibit some or all of these changes.

"Fight or Flight Response"

When confronted with a stressful situation, animals and humans respond in a fairly predictable fashion involving a series of predetermined responses collectively referred to as the fight or flight response. Although thought to have evolved as a response to the risk of attack by a predator, in the context of our patients, such responses are more commonly activated during mental stress for any reason, while caring for an ill or disabled spouse or during bereavement. Stress results in the activation of hypothalamic and brainstem neurons, leading to increased stimulation of SNS preganglionic neurons, which regulate cardiac and adrenal medullary function, and activation of the HPA axis. These events result in both local and systemic release of corticosteroids and catecholamines, which are ultimately responsible for mediating most of the clinical features of the response to stress. The above sequence of reactions can ultimately influence a broad range of systemic functions including cardiac performance, energy metabolism, as well as immune and inflammatory responses.

Under basal conditions, overall SNS activity appears to be increased with aging. This basal activity increase is manifested in the form of increased SNS nerve activity on microneural recordings, elevated basal plasma NE, and less consistently epinephrine levels, while basal cortisol levels do not appear to be altered with aging. In contrast, both systems demonstrate somewhat similar patterns of dysregulation in old age with enhanced and prolonged responsiveness following exposure to varied challenges. For example, assuming the upright posture, an oral glucose meal, insulin infusion, isometric exercise, and mental stress all result in enhanced elevation of peripheral NE levels in older subjects, while cortisol responses to surgical stress are also increased. Moreover, demonstrated deficits in terms of decreased negative feedback have been proposed as being major contributors to exaggerated SNS and HPA axis activation with aging. For example, the ability of clonidine or elevated blood pressure to downregulate SNS activity via central nervous system (CNS) α_2-receptors or baroreceptor activation, respectively, is impaired in old age. This is in addition to well-described declines in the ability of peripheral catecholamines to increase heart rate via β-adrenergic receptors or to mediate arterial vasoconstriction via α-adrenergic receptors. Similarly, the ability of circulating corticosteroids to downregulate HPA activity via hypothalamic and hippocampal receptors is also diminished in old age.

Lowered Ambient Temperature

Epidemiology Older adults are less able to adjust to extremes of low temperature. For example, one report from the United Kingdom described hypothermia among 3.6% of individuals 65 years and older admitted to the hospital, with nearly 10% of community-dwelling older adults found to demonstrate evidence of borderline hypothermia. Hypothermia also occurs often in North America, including hypothermia-related deaths in sunbelt states with advanced age, chronic medical conditions, substance abuse, and homelessness as contributing risk factors. Moreover, a number of individual case series have highlighted the need to remain vigilant to the development of hypothermia among frail and immobile residents of air-conditioned long-term care facilities. Concerns have also been raised about the role played by medications, which may enhance the risk of hypothermia.

Pathophysiology While basal body temperature remains unaltered with aging, older adults are less able to sense and respond to cold challenges when exposed to lowered ambient temperatures. Relevant mechanisms include a decreased sensation of cold, as well as declines in shivering intensity, thermogenesis, and vasoconstriction. Such changes may be related to both physiologic declines associated with aging or with specific diseases. For clinical purposes, hypothermia is generally defined as a core body temperature of less than 35°C (95°F), obtained using tympanic, rectal, or esophageal probes. Nonetheless, significant clinical consequences may occur at slightly higher body temperatures. Moreover, the development of frank hypothermia depends on a balance between the severity and length of the cold exposure and an individual subject's ability to sense and mount an effective response to such a challenge. Ultimately, aging, frailty, comorbidity, and diseases may all contribute to determining an individual's specific vulnerability.

Normal body temperature is regulated by the hypothalamic thermoregulatory center, which controls heat loss and heat generation by regulating sweating, blood vessel tone, as well as shivering and nonshivering (chemical) thermogenesis. Older adults demonstrate evidence of deficits in both afferent and efferent thermoregulatory pathways (see **Table 39-1**). For example, a diminished sensitivity to changes in environmental temperature may have both physiologic and behavioral consequences. As a result, already compromised compensatory mechanisms may be overwhelmed if an older individual does not seek suitable shelter or clothing in the cold. Declines in shivering thermogenesis may be particularly catastrophic in older adults, given the importance of these mechanisms in normal responses to cold temperature. Other contributing physiologic risk factors for hypothermia include deficient autonomic mechanisms with a decreased vasoconstrictor response, which is more common among older adults with orthostatic hypotension, as well as decreased ability of β-adrenergic stimuli to effect thermogenesis. Decreases in lean body mass with a lower metabolic rate also enhance the vulnerability of older adults, and relatively low fat mass may provide frail older adults with less insulation against heat loss.

A large number of potentially reversible factors also need to be considered (**Table 39-2**). Thus, a clinician's approach to hypothermia requires a comprehensive assessment of medical, cognitive, social, and economic factors that may contribute.

Clinical presentation Early manifestations of hypothermia may be subtle and nonspecific. Moreover, older adults may

TABLE 39-2 ■ POTENTIALLY REVERSIBLE FACTORS CONTRIBUTING TO HYPOTHERMIA IN OLDER PEOPLE

- Malnutrition
- Hypothyroidism
- Hypoglycemia
- Immobility/decreased physical activity with low ambient temperature (eg, lack of heating in winter or excessive air conditioning in long-term care facilities)
- Severe sepsis
- Medications
  ○ Alcohol
  ○ Phenothiazines
  ○ Barbiturates
  ○ Benzodiazepines
  ○ Opioids
  ○ General anesthetics
  ○ Antidepressants
  ○ Neuroleptics
- Hypothalamic neural injury
  ○ Anoxia
  ○ Vascular event
  ○ Trauma
  ○ Malignancy
- Socioeconomic factors
  ○ Self-neglect
  ○ Poor judgment
  ○ Lack of financial resources for adequate heating

TABLE 39-3 ■ CLINICAL FEATURES OF HYPOTHERMIA

Early hypothermia (core temperature of 32°C–35°C/90°F–95°F)
- Fatigue
- Lethargy
- Apathy
- Slow gait
- Slurred speech
- Confusion
- Cool skin

Advanced hypothermia (core temperature 28°C–32°C/82°F–90°F)
- Skin cold and cyanotic
- Hypopnea
- Altered consciousness progressing to coma
- Slowing of neurologic reflexes
- Sluggishness of pupillary responses
- Bradycardia
- Atrial and ventricular arrhythmias
- Hypovolemia (cold-induced water and solute diuresis)
- Risk of hypotension and cardiovascular collapse

Near death (core temperatures below 28°C/82°F)
- Unresponsive
- Apneic
- Very cold skin
- Ventricular fibrillation
- Absent neurologic reflexes
- Fixed and dilated pupils

become hypothermic even without exposure to extremely cold temperatures. Thus, a high index of suspicion is essential, as is a thermometer capable of recording very low temperatures. Clinical features vary with the severity of hypothermia and are summarized in **Table 39-3**. Challenging the diagnosis is the nonspecific nature of these symptoms and signs, combined with the finding that some hypothermic older patients may not complain of feeling cold and may not shiver. Individuals who have survived early cardiovascular complications of severe hypothermia are at risk for pneumonia, aspiration, pulmonary edema, pancreatitis, gastrointestinal hemorrhage, acute renal failure, and intravascular thrombosis. Common electrocardiogram (ECG) changes with hypothermia are listed in **Table 39-4**. Abnormal J (Osborne) waves are relatively specific to hypothermia and disappear as temperature returns to normal. Finally, individuals who present with hypothermia may have underlying severe hypothyroidism (myxedema coma, see Chapter 98) as a cause of the hypothermia, so thyroid stimulating hormone (TSH) measurement is mandatory. A history of previous thyroid disease or a surgical scar in the thyroid region may provide the only clues.

Management

Emergency Care Severe hypothermia represents a medical emergency. If outdoors, such individuals need to be immediately moved away from severe cold, wet clothing must be removed, and warmed blankets applied. Early cardiac

monitoring is essential since even minor stimuli can trigger significant dysrhythmias. Procedures such as chest compression or pacemaker placement should be avoided as long as a heartbeat is detectable and the patient is breathing spontaneously. However, cardiopulmonary resuscitation may be required. Since a cold heart is relatively unresponsive to drugs or electrical stimulation, such efforts must be pursued aggressively and need to include warmed

TABLE 39-4 ■ ELECTROCARDIOGRAM CHANGES IN HYPOTHERMIA

Specific: Abnormal J (Osborne) waves following each QRS

Nonspecific
- Bradycardia
- Prolonged P-R interval
- Prolonged QRS complex
- Prolonged QT segment
- Atrial fibrillation
- Premature ventricular contractions
- Ventricular fibrillation
- Similarity to acute myocardial ischemia/infarction

intravenous fluids (eg, 5% dextrose normal saline without potassium).

General Support Severe hypothermia is associated with a mortality exceeding 50%. These figures worsen further with advanced age and with associated comorbidity. As a result, such patients require close supportive care in an intensive care unit. Such supportive care must include treatment of contributing conditions such as infection, hypoglycemia, and hypothyroidism. Clinicians need to have a high index of suspicion for infection in hypothermic older adults, administering broad-spectrum antibiotics without waiting for results of confirmatory cultures. When administering thyroid hormone for suspected hypothyroidism, corticosteroids may also be required in order to avoid inducing adrenal insufficiency. While ECG monitoring is necessary, central lines should be avoided, given cardiac irritability in these subjects. Pharmacodynamic and pharmacokinetic properties of many commonly used drugs may become dramatically altered in hypothermic patients, creating therapeutic challenges. Such drugs may accumulate as metabolism is delayed and as ever-increasing doses are administered because of a lack of response at lower temperatures, causing potential problems as responsiveness to accumulated doses of these medications increases during body warming. Insulin is ineffective at temperatures below 30°C (86°F), so should not be administered until some rewarming has occurred. Volume depletion as well as hypoxemia needs to be corrected. Intubation may be required, and blood gases should be monitored.

Rewarming strategies need to be undertaken immediately following stabilization, since cardiac arrhythmias, acidosis, fluid, and electrolyte disorders may be resistant to treatment until the core body temperature is raised. For patients who are only mildly hypothermic (core temperatures of 32°C–35°C or 90°F–95°F), passive rewarming techniques using insulating materials and transfer to a warm environment generally suffice. For such individuals, active external rewarming using electric blankets, warm mattresses, hot water bottles, or warm water baths are generally not necessary. Moreover, such treatment can be associated with significant risk as warmth-induced peripheral vasodilatation may precipitate hypovolemic shock in vulnerable individuals.

For individuals in more severe hypothermia (core temperatures under 32°C or 90°F), active core rewarming is necessary. A variety of techniques are available, with peritoneal dialysis rewarming by rapid instillation and removal of warm (40°C or 104°F) potassium-free dialysate representing the most practical solution in most institutions. It can provide safe core warming within six to eight fluid exchanges. Mediastinal lavage involves a major surgical procedure, while extracorporeal circulation requires special equipment and carries risks of hypotension and heparin-induced hemorrhage. Gastric lavage using balloons filled with warm fluid is simple, yet rate of warming may be slow and pharyngeal irritation may induce arrhythmias.

Raised Ambient Temperature

Epidemiology Heatstroke is a major public health problem with over 600 US deaths attributed to extreme heat each year, nearly 40% of which occurring in those older than 65 years. Heat waves in the United States (eg, Chicago) and abroad (eg, France) have graphically illustrated the vulnerability of older adults to excessively high temperatures. Given a growing awareness of the need to be vigilant for the development of hyperthermia in institutional settings, nursing home cases have fortunately become rarer. Nevertheless, older adults living in the community, especially those who are frail, suffer from disabilities, and live alone are at great risk. In addition to the risk of heatstroke, hyperthermia also contributes to excessive cardiac mortality and morbidity.

Pathophysiology As in the case of hypothermia, heatstroke represents an example of homeostatic decompensation in which older adults' deficient or sluggish compensatory mechanisms are unable to maintain normal body temperature in the face of increased environmental temperature. Excess mortality in older adults during heat waves may be attributed to heat-provoked cardiac events or to primary thermoregulatory failure. In recent years, there has been a growing awareness that heatstroke is a form of hyperthermia, which is associated with an excessive systemic inflammatory response contributing to multiorgan dysfunction. Impairments of thermoregulatory systems may occur at a number of different levels and, as in the case of hypothermia, may result from aging or from associated comorbidity and diseases. Sweating responses to thermal, pharmacologic, and chemical stimuli are reduced with aging, representing a significant contributor to homeostatic decompensation by older adults faced with significant heat challenges. Moreover, older adults require higher body core temperatures before compensatory sweating mechanisms are activated. During times of heat stress, younger individuals depend on being able to increase their skin heat loss by shunting blood flow from core toward peripheral blood vessels. In older individuals, the extent and speed of these important compensatory homeostatic mechanisms is impaired as a result of decreased cardiac output and a diminished vasodilatation of peripheral blood vessels. However, some of the above changes may also be the result of occult cardiac disease or physical deconditioning. For example, maximum oxygen uptake appears to be a much more important predictor of sweat rate and forearm flow during exercise than is chronological age. Moreover, with increased physical activity, older adults are able to improve some of these physiologic responses to heat challenge toward those seen in younger individuals. Finally, as for hypothermia, presence of significant comorbidity, medications, as well as social and environmental factors may further place older adults at risk of homeostatic decompensation during heat waves. For example, decreased mobility or impaired judgment caused by dementia or psychiatric illness may keep some older adults from seeking assistance and from taking sensible precautions such as removal of heavy clothing and increasing fluid intake. Moreover, air conditioning may not be an option for individuals living on a fixed income. Common chronic conditions such as congestive heart failure, diabetes mellitus, chronic obstructive pulmonary disease (COPD), and alcoholism further enhance the risk of heatstroke. Anticholinergic agents used for urge incontinence, depression, or behavioral problems may also contribute to hyperthermia by inhibiting normal sweating mechanisms, while diuretics may lead to hypovolemia. Finally, neuroleptic medications have been associated with an increased risk for hyperthermia in the rare but highly dangerous neuroleptic malignant syndrome.

Clinical presentation Earliest warnings of thermoregulatory failure or heat exhaustion may be subtle and nonspecific (**Table 39-5**). Frank heatstroke is defined clinically as a core body temperature above 40°C (105°F) that is accompanied by hot, dry skin, and major CNS abnormalities. Multiorgan dysfunctions are also common (see **Table 39-5**). Rhabdomyolysis, disseminated intravascular coagulation, and acute renal failure may occur in older adults, but are more common in exertional heatstroke typically seen in younger athletes.

Management Heatstroke is a medical emergency, requiring prompt and aggressive therapy. Rapid cooling is essential since its pathophysiology involves thermoregulatory failure rather than a reset thermostat point. Immediate on-site management must include removal of clothing, cooling the patient's skin with cold water or ice packs, and transfer to a cooler setting. Cool intravenous fluids should be considered, as oral hydration may lead to aspiration. Other effective cooling techniques include ice water baths, cold water gastrointestinal lavage, or the administration of cool water followed by warm air to promote evaporation. Irrespective of the technique chosen, speed is of the essence with careful continuous monitoring in order to prevent hypothermic overshoot. Careful fluid balance management and cardiovascular monitoring are also essential. However, given the high prevalence and mortality associated with heatstroke, preventive measures are extremely important. Above all, vulnerable older adults, as well as their families and neighbors, must be educated regarding both the seriousness of this problem and commonsense strategies, which can help reduce its toll.

Orthostasis, Meals, and Hypovolemia

An ability to appropriately respond to the challenge of assuming the upright posture is absolutely critical to remaining independent. Under normal conditions, significant or symptomatic orthostatic hypotension is rare among healthy older adults. However, aging does blunt the ability of older individuals to defend against more major hemodynamic challenges, especially among frail individuals, in the presence of significant comorbidity and following exposure to multiple provocative factors (**Table 39-6**). For example, while meal ingestion induces only negligible and asymptomatic blood pressure changes in most healthy older adults, frail older people may develop symptomatic postprandial hypotension, which may even contribute to altered mental status and syncope.

TABLE 39-5 ■ CLINICAL FEATURES OF HYPERTHERMIA

SYMPTOMS/EXAMINATION FINDINGS

- Core body temperature above 40°C (105°F)[a]
- Hot, dry skin[a]
- Feeling of warmth
- Lethargy/confusion
- Weakness
- Dizziness
- Anorexia
- Nausea/vomiting
- Headache
- Dyspnea

MULTIORGAN DYSFUNCTION

- Central nervous system[a]
  - Delirium
  - Convulsions
  - Coma
- Heart
  - Congestive heart failure
  - Arrhythmias
  - Hypovolemic shock
- Hepatic: necrosis
- Pulmonary/renal
  - Respiratory alkalosis
  - Metabolic acidosis
  - Hypokalemia

[a]Defining features of heat stroke.

TABLE 39-6 ■ RISK FACTORS FOR ORTHOSTATIC HYPOTENSION

Aging: Decreased baroreceptor sensitivity and ventricular compliance

AGE-RELATED DISEASES/CONDITIONS

- Frailty
- Hypertension
- Diabetes mellitus
- Aortic stenosis
- Parkinson disease
- Autonomic neuropathy

CONCURRENT CHALLENGES

- Meal ingestion
- Drugs/polypharmacy
  - Diuretic-induced sodium depletion
  - Other medications for hypertension
  - Antidepressants
  - Antipsychotics

Hyperglycemia and Hypoglycemia

Aging is associated with glucose intolerance (see Chapter 99). Even in healthy individuals who do not meet criteria for diabetes mellitus or for impaired glucose tolerance, aging is associated with a dramatic slowing in the return of glucose levels back to normal following glucose ingestion. In contrast, most healthy older adults are able to respond adequately to hypoglycemia. Nevertheless, diabetes, malnutrition, medications, as well as a number of comorbidities may significantly attenuate older adults' ability to recover from a hypoglycemic episode.

Fluid Challenge and Dehydration

Aging is accompanied by impairments in nearly all aspects of the regulation of water and salt balance. With aging, body fat increases with declines in total body water as well as blood and plasma volume. As a result of these declines in fluid compartments with aging, an equivalent acute loss or gain of body water will result in enhanced flux in osmolality with greater increases in osmolality in older adults as compared to younger individuals. At the same time, in most but not all older adults, glomerular filtration rate (GFR) declines with aging. This is accompanied by decreased capacity to excrete free water or to concentrate the urine and retain sodium when confronted by osmotic and volume stressors. Ability to perceive thirst and to then respond to such challenges is also impaired. While secretion of arginine vasopressin (AVP), the antidiuretic hormone (ADH), increases with aging both under basal conditions and in response to hyperosmotic stimuli, ability of hypovolemic stimuli to induce AVP secretion is impaired in many older adults. Moreover, renal responsiveness to AVP may be impaired with aging.

As a result of the above changes, older adults tend to have greater difficulty in appropriately diluting their urine when confronted with a major water challenge. While less well-studied, declines in GFR tend to compromise the ability of the aged kidney to deal effectively with a sodium load. Difficulties with water disposal can predispose older individuals to develop hyponatremia, while decreased capacity to adapt to increased salt load may contribute to dependent edema, nocturia, hypertension, and congestive heart failure. The aged body's capacity to prevent dehydration is also affected. Aging is associated with a decreased sensation of thirst even in the setting of significant dehydration. Moreover, aging is associated with a delay in the time required for the kidney to appropriately concentrate urine in response to sodium restriction. Large numbers of medications, as well as the presence of significant comorbidity, can further enhance the clinical impact of these aging-related changes.

Hyponatremia

Epidemiology Hyponatremia is the most common electrolyte abnormality in clinical medicine, resulting primarily from the inability to excrete a water load due to excessive ADH presence or due to lack of sufficient solute excretion. It affects approximately 10% of ambulatory older individuals and is even more common in hospitalized or institutionalized patients with estimates ranging from 25% to 50%. Hyponatremia frequently accompanies common medical conditions that affect older adults such as congestive heart failure, cirrhosis, many cancers, and chronic kidney disease. Hyponatremia is also seen with chronic CNS disorders and chronic pulmonary disease and is a side effect of a number of medications such as thiazide diuretics, chemotherapeutic agents, pain medications, and antipsychotics. The most common cause of hyponatremia in older individuals is the syndrome of inappropriate ADH secretion (SIADH). However, in spite of its frequency, hyponatremia is an independent predictor of mortality, as well as falls, osteoporosis, fractures, hospital readmissions, and need for long-term placement.

Clinical presentation Symptoms of hyponatremia vary depending on severity and underlying clinical conditions. Many may be completely asymptomatic, especially if the serum sodium is greater than 130 mEq/L, and the condition is discovered serendipitously on routine laboratory evaluation. However, even mild degrees of hyponatremia may produce symptoms—commonly fatigue, inanition, weakness, and nausea. As the hyponatremia worsens, more significant signs and symptoms become apparent including a clouded sensorium, inability to concentrate on tasks, falls, seizures, and coma. When evaluating symptomatic status, it is important to ascertain the individual's baseline mental function. As a general rule, the more chronically and gradually the hyponatremia has developed, the fewer the overt symptoms even with serum sodium concentrations as low as 120 to 125 mEq/L. However, serum sodium less than 115 mEq/L is virtually always accompanied by symptoms, even if chronic.

Pathophysiology

Pseudohyponatremia. In contrast to true hypo-osmolar hyponatremia, pseudohyponatremia can be seen with significant hyperglycemia, where the osmotically active glucose obligates egress of water from the intracellular space, thus diluting the serum sodium. In these cases, the serum osmolality will be high, while the serum sodium is low. A simple equation to estimate the "true" serum sodium in the setting of hyperglycemia is the following: ([Measured glucose – 100]/100) × 1.5 + measured serum Na = corrected serum Na. If the corrected serum sodium falls within the normal range, then the patient has pseudohyponatremia. Serum sodium may also be low with severe hyperlipidemia, particularly hypertriglyceridemia, or hyperproteinemia as may be seen with multiple myeloma or other paraproteinemias. In these instances, a measured serum osmolality will be normal. Further testing and therapy then should be directed toward diagnosis and management of these underlying conditions.

Renal Diluting Capacity Ability of the kidneys to appropriately respond to the hyponatremia by diluting the urine is best assessed by measuring urine osmolality or specific gravity. Ability to excrete excess water by diluting the urine declines with aging and in the context of hyponatremia it may suggest that excess ADH is present. The vast majority of cases of hyponatremia are associated with an inappropriately high urine osmolality, that is, an inability to excrete a free water load.

Role of Volume Status Managing hyponatremia in a physiologically guided manner requires assessment of fluid status (**Table 39-7**). Hypovolemia is suggested by a low blood pressure, orthostatic hypotension, weight loss, and a low urine sodium (< 20–40 mEq/L). Hypervolemic hyponatremia is suggested by the presence of hypertension and/or peripheral or pulmonary edema. All categories of hyponatremia are commonly seen in older adults given underlying physiological predispositions combined with increasing prevalence of the varied chronic conditions and multiple morbidities that may contribute to hyponatremia.

Management Although hyponatremia is defined by serum sodium levels, management of older adults with this problem must also encompass other closely inter-related physiological parameters and conditions. To that end, accompanying alterations in fluid volume must also be treated and underlying and precipitating diseases and geriatric syndromes that contributed to the hyponatremia must not be ignored.

Most instances of hyponatremia are mild and asymptomatic with serum sodium ranging between 130 and 135 mEq/L. The benefits of correcting such mild asymptomatic cases by stopping potentially offensive medications or use of mild fluid restriction remain unclear. Severe symptomatic hyponatremia is a medical emergency warranting immediate treatment, no matter what the underlying cause is. The goal for treatment is to raise the serum sodium to a level where life-threatening symptoms abate, generally aiming for an increase of no more than 8 mEq/L within the first 24 hours. The rate at which such an increase is most safely accomplished remains an area of intense study with some advocating a rapid increase followed by stabilization while others recommend a steady gradual increase over the 24-hour period. The mechanism for achieving this increase will very much depend on the underlying cause. Patients afflicted with SIADH, with a high urine osmolality, respond most effectively to hypertonic saline with or without the use of a loop diuretic to enhance free water excretion. Hypovolemic individuals will respond to 0.9% saline with correction of the hyponatremia. Hypervolemic individuals such as those with heart failure will respond to a combination of high-dose loop diuretic and water restriction. In contrast, individuals who are already excreting a dilute urine may be able to correct themselves without specific intervention. In all circumstances, frequent monitoring of serum sodium is critical to ensure adequate but not excessive correction of the serum sodium within the critical first 24-hour period.

Hypernatremia

Epidemiology Hypernatremia occurs far less frequently than hyponatremia but is especially common in the setting of heat waves and in frail older adults. For example, a prevalence of between 0.3% and 8.9% has been described in nursing home patients, while up to 30% of nursing home residents develop hypernatremia during admission to a hospital. Presence of hypernatremia is associated with enhanced risk of morbidity and mortality.

Clinical presentation Clinical features of acute hypernatremia may range from none to lethargy, weakness, irritability, and even seizures and comma. As with hyponatremia, the gradual onset of chronic hypernatremia may be associated with milder symptoms.

Pathophysiology This hyperosmolar condition generally results from a loss of water through renal or extrarenal mechanisms and/or inability to sense or respond to thirst by increasing fluid intake. Older individuals with reduced thirst sensation have lost a critical mechanism to prevent the development of hypernatremia. Moreover, such

TABLE 39-7 ■ APPROACH TO DIFFERENTIAL DIAGNOSIS OF HYPONATREMIA BY EVALUATION OF VOLUME STATUS		
HYPOVOLEMIC	**EUVOLEMIC**	**HYPERVOLEMIC**
GI losses; nausea, vomiting, diarrhea	Age-related excess release or lack of suppression of ADH causing idiopathic hyponatremia	Liver cirrhosis
Sweating	SIADH from pulmonary diseases, malignancies such as small cell cancer of the lung, lymphomas, strokes, head trauma, subdural hematoma, medications, HIV infection	Congestive heart failure
Diuretics, especially thiazides	Hypothyroidism	Nephrotic syndrome
Cerebral salt wasting	Primary adrenal insufficiency	
Salt-losing nephropathy	Drugs such as NSAIDs, haloperidol, SSRIs, antidepressants	
	Postoperative hyponatremia due to infusion of hypotonic solutions, anesthesia	

ADH, antidiuretic hormone; GI, gastrointestinal; NSAIDs, nonsteroidal anti-inflammatory drugs; SIADH, syndrome of inappropriate ADH secretion; SSRI, selective serotonin reuptake inhibitor.

individuals are frequently unable to concentrate the urine maximally, thus obligating more water losses through renal excretion. One common clinical scenario associated with the development of hypernatremia is an older individual debilitated by stroke or other major limitation to mobility rendering them unable to obtain fluids. Other situations include severe diarrhea leading to profound intestinal fluid losses, advanced chronic kidney disease, or uncontrolled diabetes mellitus with severe polyuria. More rarely, partial or complete central diabetes insipidus will develop in the setting of head trauma after a fall or surgery.

Renal Concentrating Capacity The renal response to hypernatremia is elaboration of a low-volume, highly concentrated urine, generally with a urine output of less than 20 mL/h and a urine osmolality of greater than 600 mOsm/kg. If the hypernatremic person exhibits this response, then the cause of the hypernatremia is extrarenal water losses such as diarrhea or inability to obtain water to drink due to immobility. Diagnostic and therapeutic efforts should be directed toward determination of the cause of the failure to obtain adequate fluid or the cause of the extrarenal fluid loss. If the hypernatremic person has polyuria with a urine output greater than 50 to 100 mL/h and/or a urine osmolality of 300 mOsm/kg or less, then the cause is likely renal loss of water due to an osmotic diuresis as is seen commonly with uncontrolled diabetes mellitus or insipidus.

Management Aside from treating any underlying cause of water loss or water deprivation, the cornerstone of therapy for hypernatremia is water replacement. As for hyponatremia, correction of hypernatremia should be judicious in rate, limiting the decrease of serum sodium to approximately 8 to 10 mEq/L/24 h, although some have suggested that 50% of the water deficit can be safely corrected in the first 24 hours. The water deficit can be estimated by the following equation:

$$\text{Water deficit (L)} = \frac{\text{Measured [Na] mEq/L} - 140 \text{ mEq/L}}{140 \text{ mEq}} \times (0.45 \times \text{body weight [kg]})$$

If the water deficit is less than 3 L and the patient is able to drink safely, then oral water repletion is reasonable. If not, then the deficit will need to be addressed with intravenous administration of 5% dextrose in water. Frequently, patients with hypernatremia are also intravascularly volume-depleted and may be frankly hypotensive. If the cardiovascular status is in jeopardy, then the initial fluid of choice is 0.9% saline to ensure adequate intravascular volume. Once the volume status is established, switching to more hypotonic fluid is reasonable. If the degree of volume depletion is felt to be moderate, then initial therapy with 5% dextrose in 0.45% saline is a reasonable choice, taking into account that twice as many liters would be required to deliver the volume of free water equivalent to that delivered using 5% dextrose in water. Serum sodium should be carefully monitored throughout the therapy as the above calculation is based on several assumptions that may not apply to the individual person, such as the estimated percentage of body weight that is comprised of body water, the projected volume of distribution of the fluid, and ongoing salt and water losses.

Physiologic Regulation of Sodium Balance

From a clinical standpoint, regulation of sodium balance may be considered as being equivalent to the regulation of extracellular fluid volume. Aging has several notable effects on cardiovascular, neural, and humoral factors involved in sodium balance. As noted, older individuals have more difficulty in excreting a sodium load due to the age-related decrease in GFR as well as concomitant medical conditions such as heart failure, and have more difficulty adjusting to an abrupt decrease in sodium ingestion or frank sodium loss. The former defect predisposes the older person to significant volume overload and exacerbation of hypertension, while the latter defect potentiates the development of volume depletion. Interestingly, despite the overall tendency for older individuals to retain sodium, atrial natriuretic peptide (ANP) levels are higher in older individuals and the ANP response to a sodium load is more pronounced, as is the renal natriuretic response to ANP. In contrast, the renin response to the upright position is dampened in older adults and the levels of aldosterone tend to be lower. These alterations in hormone balance would be predicted to result in renal salt wasting, yet older individuals are more likely to exhibit salt-sensitive hypertension, being either more susceptible to sodium retention or perhaps more sensitive to the effects of sodium on blood pressure. The explanation for these apparent discrepancies has not been fully established.

Sodium/Volume Depletion

Older individuals are more prone to extracellular fluid volume depletion—total body sodium depletion—than younger individuals. Volume depletion is a common reason for admission to the hospital for older patients. A major consequence of aging is a slowed ability of the kidney to increase sodium reabsorption in response to volume depletion, thus potentiating sodium losses. Furthermore, when faced with a salt-losing condition such as food deprivation, aged animals ingest less sodium than younger animals, suggesting age-related defects in the sensing mechanisms for sodium loss in addition to intrinsic defects in the renal response to volume depletion. The consequence is an increase in the susceptibility to volume depletion. Assessment of volume status relies heavily on physical examination and selected laboratory findings.

Clinical presentation Physical examination findings of volume depletion in older adults are similar to those in younger patients, but may not be as obvious. Also complicating the evaluation of volume status in older adults are the changes in body composition that occur with aging, including loss of muscle mass and increase in fat mass, resulting in an overall reduction in total body water. Hypotension with tachycardia and orthostatic hypotension are commonly used parameters to detect volume depletion. These findings may not be as reliable in older individuals due to peripheral neuropathy, medications, or deconditioning, all of which may result in orthostatic hypotension even in the absence of volume depletion. In addition, older women manifest a lesser increase in heart rate in response to volume depletion than do younger women.

Laboratory findings suggestive of volume depletion may also be less reliable in older adults than in younger people. A blood urea nitrogen (BUN)/creatinine ratio of greater than 20:1 is consistent with volume depletion, but in older adults could be due to a decrease in muscle mass and not volume depletion. Conversely, poor protein intake could result in a lower BUN/creatinine ratio, masking the presence of underlying volume depletion. A low urine sodium concentration of 20 mEq/L or less or a low fractional excretion of sodium less than 1% are commonly used parameters to help determine volume status; however, in older individuals, this valuable clue to volume depletion may be lost due to impaired renal sodium reabsorption. Additionally, measurement of A or B natriuretic peptide, cortisol, and aldosterone levels may have limited value due to aging effects on these hormones as well as the time required to obtain the results.

Management Treatment of volume depletion in older adults centers around the cause and the status of other underlying conditions. Common causes of volume depletion include gastrointestinal fluid losses, bleeding, anorexia associated with infection or chronic disease, diuretic use, and adrenal insufficiency. In particular, primary adrenal insufficiency or isolated aldosterone deficiency can present with repeated episodes of fatigue and hypotension that responds to parenteral saline administration. Frank hyperkalemia may be present, but often is not, and urine studies will show a relatively high urine sodium. Thus, the diagnosis of mineralocorticoid deficiency may not be initially suspected. The treatment of volume depletion is administration of sodium either orally, parenterally, or both. Diuretics should be discontinued and their ongoing use reevaluated once the sodium deficit is replenished. If the index of suspicion is sufficiently high, measurement of fasting morning cortisol, renin, and aldosterone may also be considered. If frank adrenal insufficiency is diagnosed, then treatment with both glucocorticoid and mineralocorticoid replacement is indicated. If isolated mineralocorticoid deficiency is diagnosed, then therapy with a mineralocorticoid-specific replacement such as fludrocortisone 0.1 mg daily should be initiated.

Sodium Excess

Peripheral and pulmonary edema are the hallmarks of volume overload or sodium excess. Lower extremity edema is common and can be attributed to local or systemic factors. It is important to determine if a patient has a systemic cause of edema, as treatment of the edema will center around the treatment of the systemic disorder. In contrast, local causes of edema such as venous insufficiency are addressed through local measures such as compression stockings. Systemic causes of edema, including congestive heart failure (Chapter 76), chronic kidney disease (Chapter 83), and liver failure (Chapter 86) are discussed elsewhere. Medications that may contribute to volume overload include nonsteroidal anti-inflammatory drugs, thiazolidinediones, direct vasodilators, calcineurin inhibitors, and steroid hormones that have mineralocorticoid effects such as prednisone. Even in the absence of heart failure, these drugs may cause sodium retention and subsequent edema.

Bladder Filling and Bladder Outlet Obstruction

The ability of older adults to sense and respond appropriately to bladder filling appears to be diminished. These sensory processing deficits may be contributing to a form of homeostatic dysregulation involving lower urinary tract mechanisms in response to bladder filling. It remains to be seen to what extent these changes contribute to common voiding disorders of late life involving urgency and/or impaired bladder emptying.

Bladder outlet obstruction is a relatively common complication of benign prostatic hyperplasia, and older men with this problem are much more likely to develop urinary retention with detrusor decompensation than are their younger counterparts. Normally, during a compensatory phase, bladder emptying is maintained with an increased bladder muscle mass, mostly caused by hypertrophy of individual muscle cells. During a subsequent decompensation phase, the bladder undergoes muscle loss, collagen infiltration, and axonal degeneration. Aging appears to increase the likelihood of detrusor decompensation, with its associated degenerative changes.

Major Burns and Trauma

For any given total percentage of body surface burned, advanced age contributes to a measurable decrease in survival. Such systemic vulnerability has been attributed to a combination of progressive reductions in the function of many organs, together with simultaneous reductions in varied homeostatic capabilities and functional impairments associated with specific disease states. In spite of remarkable improvements in the perioperative care of older adults, older individuals have significantly worse outcomes than their younger counterparts following burns, road traffic injuries, and head trauma. While more research is needed, this differential vulnerability may be related to the catastrophic nature of these events, as well as underlying vulnerabilities and presence of significant comorbidity.

Immobilization/Bed Rest

Older adults are particularly vulnerable to loss of function and the development of adverse events following bed rest. With immobilization, muscle mass can be lost at a rate of up to 5% a week, which together with disruptions in subcellular muscle structure, can result in losses in muscle strength, which may approach 40% by 6 weeks. When unloaded, aged muscle cells are more likely to atrophy or to degenerate via apoptotic mechanisms. Strategies, which can diminish the impact of bed rest, include opting for minimally invasive surgery whenever possible, rapid mobilization following surgery or injury, exercise, nutritional supplementation, as well as efforts to decrease offending medications and to address relevant comorbidity. Increased physical activity represents an extremely attractive option since contrary to conventional wisdom, even frail institutionalized older adults experience significant benefits from exercise in terms of muscle mass, muscle performance, and improvements in relevant homeostatic mechanisms.

Anticholinergic and Antidopaminergic Medications

Anticholinergic While systematic literature is lacking, older adults appear to be highly sensitive to anticholinergic effects of commonly used medications including altered cognitive function, dry mouth, constipation, and urinary retention. Some of this vulnerability can be attributed to the presence of underlying disease or preclinical pathology. For example, subjects with Alzheimer disease develop new learning deficits at lower scopolamine doses than do age-adjusted normal controls, while the presence of detrusor underactivity predisposes older adults to develop urinary retention when treated with anticholinergic agents. In addition, there is enhanced anticholinergic vulnerability with aging alone, as shown by an augmented and prolonged inhibition of stimulated parotid flow rate in healthy older adults following exposure to an intravenous anticholinergic drug (glycopyrrolate). Increased blood–brain permeability in old age and in the setting of specific diseases has been proposed as one mechanism that could mediate an augmented vulnerability to develop cognitive or other CNS problems with anticholinergic medications. Other relevant contributing mechanisms include a decreased homeostatic capacity with declines in both numbers and complexity of relevant cellular elements, as well as an aging-associated loss in the ability of muscarinic receptors to be upregulated when exposed to anticholinergic agents.

Antidopaminergic Older adults often develop extrapyramidal side effects when given neuroleptic agents with potent antidopaminergic properties. Interestingly, adverse events such as acute dystonia are relatively rare in old age, while others including rigidity, poverty of movement, and tardive dyskinesia appear to be more common in old age. In many cases, early or preclinical Parkinson disease may render individuals more vulnerable to pharmacologic disruption of relevant CNS dopaminergic circuits. Moreover, aging-associated declines in numbers and function of CNS dopaminergic neurons, as well as a decreased capacity to compensate for additional losses by upregulation of dopaminergic receptors or by neuronal plasticity involving surviving dopaminergic fibers, are also likely to contribute to the loss of such homeostatic mechanisms.

ACKNOWLEDGMENT

Many thanks to Eleanor Lederer and Vibha Nayak for their contributions to the Disorders of Fluid and Electrolyte Balance chapter in the 7th edition of this book, some components of which were used in this chapter.

FURTHER READING

Aalami OO, Fang TD, Song HM, Nacamuli RP. Physiological features of aging persons. *Arch Surg.* 2003;138(10):1068–1076.

Burke SN, Barnes CA. Neural plasticity in the ageing brain. *Nat Rev Neurosci.* 2006;7(1):30–40.

Carpenter RH. Homeostasis: a plea for a unified approach. *Adv Physiol Educ.* 2004;28(1–4):180–187.

Epstein Y, Yanovich R. Heatstroke. *N Engl J Med.* 2019; 380(25):2449–2459.

Ferrara N, Komici K, Corbi G, et al. Beta-adrenergic receptor responsiveness in aging heart and clinical implications. *Front Physiol.* 2014;4:396.

Ferrucci L, Kuchel GA. Heterogeneity of aging: individual risk factors, mechanisms, patient priorities, and outcomes. *J Am Geriatr Soc.* 2021;69(3):610–612.

Goldstein DS. How does homeostasis happen? Integrative physiological, systems biological, and evolutionary perspectives. *Am J Physiol Regul Integr Comp Physiol.* 2019;316(4):R301–R317.

Hadley EC, Kuchel GA, Newman AB, Workshop Speakers and Participants. Report: NIA Workshop on Measures of Physiologic Resiliencies in Human Aging. *J Gerontol A Biol Sci Med Sci.* 2017;72(7):980–990.

Hart EC, Charkoudian N. Sympathetic neural regulation of blood pressure: influences of sex and aging. *Physiology (Bethesda).* 2014;29(1):8–15.

Inouye SK, Studenski S, Tinetti ME, Kuchel GA. Geriatric syndromes: clinical, research, and policy implications of a core geriatric concept. *J Am Geriatr Soc.* 2007;55(5):780–791.

Kuchel GA, Hof PR. *Autonomic Nervous System in Old Age.* Basel: Karger Press; 2004.

Kuchel GA. Frailty and resilience as outcome measures in clinical trials and geriatric care: are we getting any closer? *J Am Geriatr Soc.* 2018;66(8):1451–1454.

Lee PG, Halter JB. The pathophysiology of hyperglycemia in older adults: clinical considerations. *Diabetes Care.* 2017;40(4):444–452.

Masoro EJ. *Handbook of Physiology: Section 11 Aging.* New York: Oxford University Press; 1995.

Morley JE. Dehydration, hypernatremia, and hyponatremia. *Clin Geriatr Med.* 2015;31:389–399.

Pignolo RJ. Physiology of human ageing. In: Heidt PJ, Bienenstock J, Bosch TCG, Zasloff M, Rusch V, eds. *Ageing and the Microbiome.* Herborn, Germany: Old Herborn University Foundation; 2018, pp. 5–23.

Reske-Nielsen C, Medzon R. Geriatric trauma. *Emerg Med Clin North Am.* 2016;34(3):483–500.

Schneider A, Ruckerl R, Breitner S, Wolf K, Peters A. Thermal control, weather, and aging. *Curr Environ Health Rep.* 2017;4(1):21–29.

Studenski S, Ferrucci L, Resnick NM. Geriatrics. In: Robertson D, Williams GH, eds. *Clinical and Translational Science. Principles of Human Research.* Amsterdam: Academic Press; 2009, pp. 477–495.

van Beek JH, Kirkwood TB, Bassingthwaighte JB. Understanding the physiology of the ageing individual: computational modelling of changes in metabolism and endurance. *Interface Focus.* 2016;6(2):20150079.

van den Beld AW, Kaufman JM, Zillikens MC, Lamberts SWJ, Egan JM, van der Lely AJ. The physiology of endocrine systems with ageing. *Lancet Diabetes Endocrinol.* 2018;6(8):647–658.

Applied Clinical Geroscience

Sara E. Espinoza, Jamie N. Justice, John C. Newman,
Robert J. Pignolo, George A. Kuchel

"There is nothing more deceptive than an obvious fact. Besides, we may chance to hit upon some other obvious facts which may have been by no means obvious."

Sherlock Holmes in *The Adventures of Sherlock Holmes.* Arthur Conan Doyle (1892)

WHAT IS THE GEROSCIENCE HYPOTHESIS?

Geroscience is a relatively new field in aging that focuses on understanding the relationships between biological aging and age-related diseases. Key terms and language in this new discipline are shown in **Table 40-1**. The **geroscience hypothesis** states that fundamental biological mechanisms of aging drive the susceptibility of aged individuals to not just one, but multiple chronic diseases, such as cardiovascular disease, type 2 diabetes, malignancy, and dementia.

Geroscience is based on evidence that a set of interrelated cellular biologic processes drive aging and the varied phenotypes observed with aging: macromolecular damage, metabolism, proteostasis, inflammation, adaptation to stress, epigenetics, cell senescence, and stem cells/regeneration. These processes have been coined the hallmarks or pillars of aging (**Figure 40-1**).

Hallmarks of Aging

Aging is no longer a mysterious "black box." It used to be common for a researcher studying a certain component of aging to argue that they were studying the single most important part of the aging process. Fortunately, such arguments and competing theories or visions of aging have been mostly superseded by a realization that there are several biological contributors to aging, and that the manipulation of one modulator of aging has implications for the entire system. Discovery of mutations in genes that radically alter lifespan and rates of aging in simple model organisms such as the nematode worm *Caenorhabditis elegans*, which have clear analogues to human biology, demonstrate that aging is a malleable biological process. Many fundamental discoveries in cell biology have shown that biological regulation is a normal part of aging in vivo. Finite cellular replicative lifespan is one such example. It is apparent that manipulating the rates of biological aging can be accomplished using genetic manipulations and drug-like molecules. Therefore,

Learning Objectives

- Understand how hallmarks of biological aging contribute to age-related diseases and conditions in older adults.

- Understand that since advances in aging research show that aging is modifiable, geroscience research focuses on preventing and delaying age-related diseases and conditions through interventions that target aging mechanisms.

- Discuss use of biomarkers of aging for clinical geroscience trials.

- Understand the principles of translational geroscience as they apply to clinical trials studying interventions in fundamental aging processes.

Key Clinical Points

1. Aging is a universal human experience that looms large in popular and commercial culture. Geroscience is a new field, and some of the early interventions being studied include repurposed drugs or over-the-counter agents that target aging mechanisms.

2. Common sense clinical judgment should prevail when providers are asked about using such substances ahead of rigorous clinical data and Food and Drug Administration (FDA) approvals. A plausible link to mechanisms of aging does not mean an intervention will be effective or risk-free. Unregulated clinics are not the same thing as carefully controlled and regulated clinical trials.

3. Attempting to reverse the many ways our bodies change as we age is not always appropriate or helpful, as some changes may be adaptive, or represent consequences rather than causes of aging.

(Continued)

(Cont.)

4. Providers and consumers should remember that most investigational drugs and therapies fail, and that typically older adults are at greater risk for harm by the misuse of medications or procedures.

5. Geriatricians will need to gain knowledge in geroscience so that they can function as content experts in geroscience-guided therapies as they are developed and approved for clinical use.

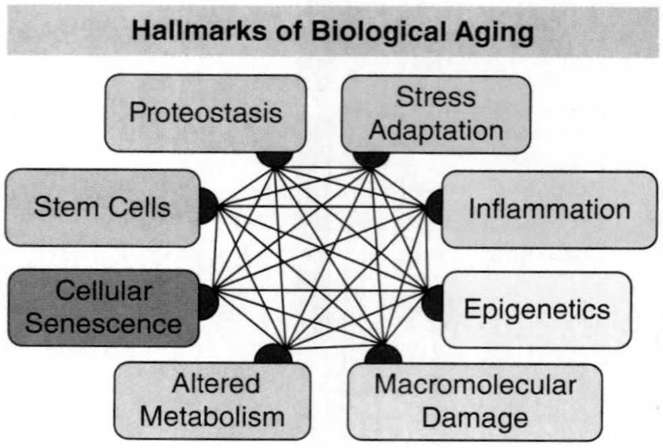

TABLE 40-1 ■ GEROSCIENCE GLOSSARY

- **Geroscience.** Posits that fundamental biological mechanisms play important roles in the susceptibility of aged individuals to multiple chronic diseases
- **Healthspan.** Duration of healthy, active life before the occurrence of functional limitation and dependence
- **Lifespan.** Normal duration of life of members of a given species, typically as median lifespan
- **Hallmarks or pillars of aging**: Interrelated cellular biologic processes that are manifest with aging and could be potential targets to extend healthspan
  - **Macromolecular damage.** Accumulation of damaged proteins, lipids, and DNA often attributed to oxidative damage
  - **Altered metabolism.** Processes of cellular biochemistry, signal transduction pathways, and energy homeostasis that lead to age-related changes in pathways that regulate growth, metabolism, and nutrient sensing
  - **Proteostasis.** Impaired folding during synthesis of protein and failure to renew or degrade misfolded proteins leading to damaged cellular components
  - **Inflammation.** Non-cell-autonomous processes leading to elevated levels of blood inflammatory markers that are both consequent of and causative to chronic disease
  - **Stress adaptation.** Continuum from psychological to molecular stresses that encompass both beneficial short-term stress and prolonged exposure to stress can overwhelm compensatory responses
  - **Epigenetics.** Changes in how genes are turned on or expressed, inclusive of DNA methylation, histone modification, chromatin remodeling, and enzymatic systems
  - **Cellular senescence.** Cell cycle arrest and a proinflammatory senescent cell phenotype triggered by molecular damage and metabolic stressors
  - **Stem cells / regeneration.** Loss of adult stem cells and ability of cells or tissues to regenerate
- **Multifactorial complexity.** Conditions caused by many contributing factors or do not stem from a single genetic cause
- **Geriatric syndrome.** Unifying features of multifactorial clinical conditions that involve multiple systems and do not fit into discrete disease categories (eg, frailty, falls, delirium, incontinence)

FIGURE 40-1. Hallmarks/pillars of aging.

a wealth of diverse research into the biology of aging has led to the identification of "clusters" of biological mechanisms, now referred to as hallmarks or pillars, that individually and collectively appear to "drive" aging (see **Figure 40-1**; **Table 40-2**).

These insightful discoveries suggest that aging processes can be modified to increase lifespan through more than one pathway intervention. Such an approach was first shown viable with laboratory-based genetic interventions that extended median lifespan, and this approach is further supported by decades of research demonstrating the aging-related benefits of dietary restriction (see Chapter 1, Biology of Aging and Longevity). It was first observed in the 1930s that restricting the food intake of laboratory rodents, without malnutrition, would extend their lifespan up to 40%. While there are important genetic and environmental variables, this basic effect has now been replicated in many species including non-human primates. Careful mechanistic studies in model organisms revealed that many of the biological effects of dietary restriction on conditions of aging are mediated by specific molecular signaling pathways that can be manipulated genetically or pharmacologically. We are now witnessing an emergence of pharmacological approaches that may extend median lifespan and healthspan in model organisms. First among these were studies conducted using worms (*C. elegans*), fruit flies (*Drosophila*), and rodents, demonstrating that targeting pathways such as mammalian target of rapamycin (mTOR) signaling with drugs or drug-like molecules could also extend lifespan and healthspan.

TABLE 40-2 ■ GEROSCIENCE HYPOTHESIS: SUPPORTING OBSERVATIONS AND DISCOVERIES

1. Biological aging involves categories of distinct processes referred to as the hallmarks or pillars of biological aging.
2. These processes can be manipulated in animal models using genetics and drugs.
3. Such manipulations can result in favorable changes to lifespan and/or healthspan.
4. Biological aging represents the greatest shared factor for multiple chronic diseases.

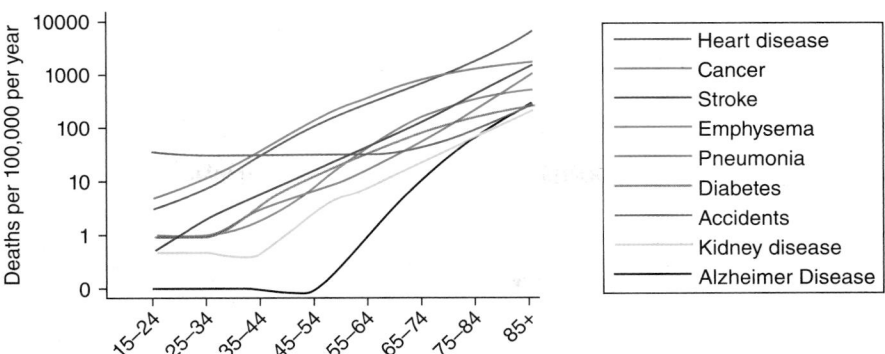

FIGURE 40-2. Age (y axis) represents the major shared risk factor of death from most chronic diseases.

Geroscience-Driven Interventions to Modulate Aging in Humans

Aging represents the major shared risk factor for death from most chronic diseases (**Figure 40-2**). The **promise of geroscience** is that interventions will be found that target aging processes, thereby simultaneously preventing, delaying the onset of, or slowing the progression of multiple chronic diseases. Supporting observations and discoveries are listed in **Table 40-2**. While grounded to a large extent in the biological sciences, the geroscience hypothesis is highly congruent with clinical observations that overlapping and interacting predisposing factors influence the risk of multiple different chronic diseases or geriatric syndromes, and that interventions designed to target such shared upstream or downstream risk factors may help improve highly diverse and varied clinical phenotypes and outcomes. Targeting the overlapping and interacting molecular and cellular mechanisms of aging via hallmarks or pillars that drive many chronic predisposing factors is the translational geroscience approach.

Multifactorial complexity

Some Challenges The term "geriatric syndrome" has been used to capture the unifying features of distinct and disparate clinical conditions that do not fit into discrete disease categories. Research into common geriatric syndromes has shown that no single risk factor typically determines their onset. Instead, in the case of conditions as varied and complex as delirium, falls, incontinence, and frailty, multiple coexisting risk factors need to be considered, with each individual risk factor contributing only modestly to the overall risk of such conditions. Given the nature of this type of multifactorial complexity, it has been difficult to envision a path from basic mechanistic studies to interventions with the potential to prevent or slow the progression of these complex conditions.

Early Insights The observation that multifactorial risk profiles often include both predisposing and precipitating risk factors has raised the possibility that some chronic factors may contribute as "drivers" throughout the entire disease process, while other more acute events may play a role as precipitating events in later stages. Similarly, four independent predisposing risk factors (slow-timed chair stands, decreased arm strength, decreased vision and hearing, and either a high anxiety or depression score) were associated with the risk of distinct and disparate outcomes raised for the first time the specter of shared risk factors for these geriatric syndromes (**Figures 40-3** and **40-4**).

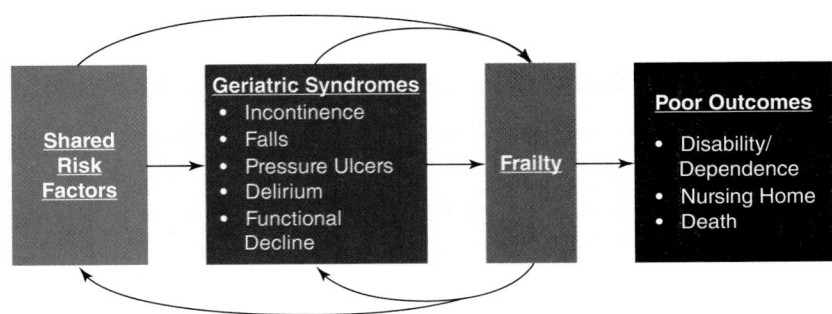

FIGURE 40-3. Shared risk factors may contribute to multiple different geriatric syndromes. (Reproduced with permission from Inouye SK, Studenski S, Tinetti ME, et al. Geriatric syndromes: clinical, research, and policy implications of a core geriatric concept. *J Am Geriatr Soc.* 2007;55[5]:780–791.)

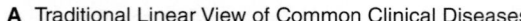

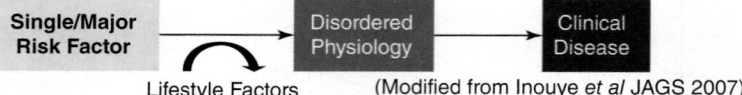

A Traditional Linear View of Common Clinical Diseases

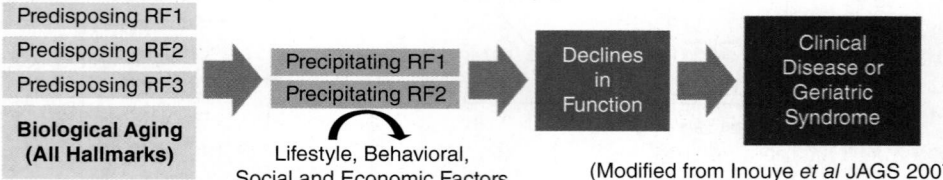

B Biological Aging as a Major Risk Factor (RF) for Clinical Diseases and Geriatric Syndromes

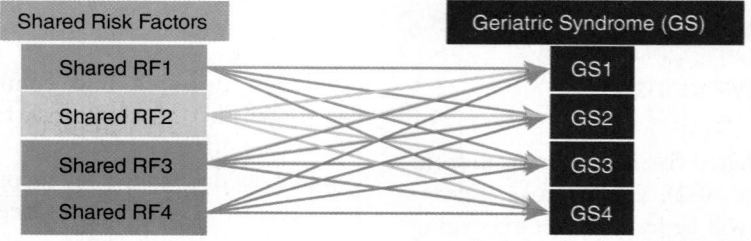

C Functional Domains as Shared Risk Factors (RF) for Common Geriatric Syndromes

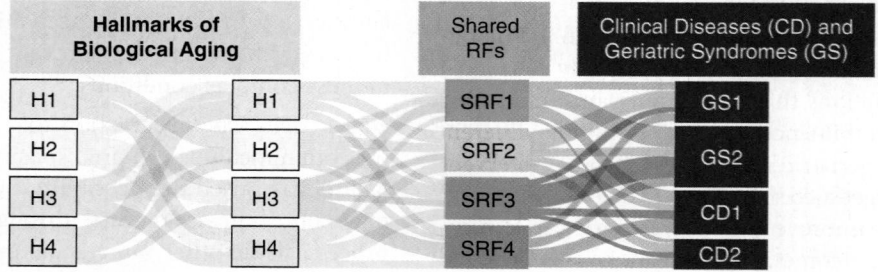

D Hallmarks of Aging as Shared and Modifiable Risk Factors for Clinical Disease and Geriatric Syndromes

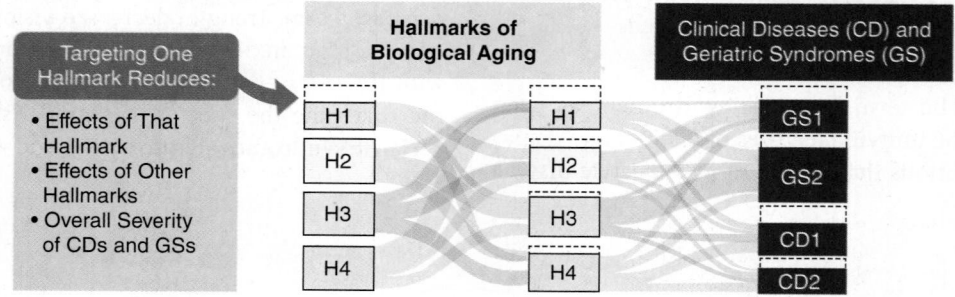

E Targeting Hallmark(s) of Aging Can Improve Functional Clinical Disease and Geriatric Syndromes

FIGURE 40-4. The evolving view of multifactorial complexity and hallmarks of biological aging in geriatric syndromes and clinical diseases.

Therefore, interventions such as exercise and physical activity may result in functional improvements across diverse outcomes because they target shared risk factors for different conditions or geriatric syndromes. Such approaches offer a path to treating individuals with multiple morbidities. Moreover, evidence that some combinations of risk factors may influence each other and mediate their downstream effects via common shared pathways opens the possibility of targeting such points of risk factor synergism.

The Path to Geroscience The pathophysiology of many conditions, particularly those that are inherited, can be viewed along a traditional linear model in which a single or one major predominant risk factor results in disordered physiology which then progresses to overt clinical disease

(**Figure 40-4A**). In the case of some inherited conditions, onset of disease is inevitable and independent of lifestyle factors with its full manifestations becoming evident at birth or even in utero. In the case of many other conditions, even those that are attributable to a single gene mutation, the onset and progression of physiological and clinical manifestations is highly sensitive to varied lifestyle factors. For example, while phenylketonuria (PKU), an inborn error of metabolism that results in decreased metabolism of the amino acid phenylalanine, is not currently treatable, if diagnosed early in life, functional declines and disease can be fully averted by controlling phenylalanine in the diet.

However, in spite of its simplicity and appeal, this linear model does not apply to most adult chronic diseases since the etiology of such conditions is typically multifactorial. Such multifactorial complexity is particularly important when seeking to understand and manage geriatric syndromes. While extremely heterogeneous, geriatric syndromes share a number of overarching features. First, these conditions are highly prevalent in frail older adults with a substantial impact on function, independence, and quality of life. Second, clinical features and functional effects of any given geriatric syndrome often involve multiple different and even distant organ systems, defying and challenging traditional organ and discipline-based boundaries. Third, the underlying etiology and pathophysiology of all geriatric syndromes is highly multifactorial with each single risk factor contributing only modestly to the overall risk of such conditions. Moreover, this multifactorial complexity is further enhanced by temporal factors whereby multiple different chronic predisposing risk factors collectively enhance the future risk of these conditions, while other more acute precipitating factors can subsequently induce declines in function and the emergence of a clinical diagnosis of a specific geriatric syndrome (see **Figure 40-4B**).

Functional domains as shared risk factors for common geriatric syndromes

In addition to a multifactorial pathogenesis involving each specific geriatric syndrome, many individual risk factors, especially those involving varied measures of function, are shared by different geriatric syndromes (**Figure 40-4C**). For example, it has been shown that declines in lower extremity function, declines in upper extremity function, and neurobehavioral changes in the form of anxiety or depression represent independent but shared risk factors for urinary incontinence, falls, and functional dependence. Although published nearly three decades ago, this description of shared functional risk factors for varied geriatric syndromes offers seminal insights into translational geroscience when examining the role of varied individual facets of biological aging as shared predictors and/or drivers of different geriatric syndromes (**Figures 40-4D and E**). Moreover, these considerations provide an explanation of why an intervention such as exercise can have benefits on conditions as diverse as urinary incontinence, falls, and functional dependence since it can positively influence each of the above risk factors (**Figure 40-4B**).

The much belated recognition that aging represents the single largest risk factor for most chronic diseases and geriatric syndromes represented one foundational element for the emergence of the geroscience hypothesis. Nevertheless, a need arose to reconcile these observations drawn mostly from the study of populations toward more mechanistic research. Most evidence suggest a role for biological aging exerting its predisposing effects over time while other more traditional risk factors also enhance the risk and progression of chronic diseases and geriatric syndromes (**Figure 40-4B**).

Varied biological hallmarks of aging as shared and modifiable risk factors for chronic diseases and geriatric syndromes

Since many diverse biological processes clearly contribute to the aging process, no one single molecule or biological pathway should be considered responsible. As in the case of shared functional predictors, such as lower extremity performance, a growing body of knowledge supports varied biological hallmarks of aging as shared risk factors or drivers for multiple different chronic conditions (**Figure 40-4D**). Moreover, evidence that modifying hallmarks of aging using genetic and pharmacological manipulations can slow biological aging provided additional support for the geroscience hypothesis. Finally, the ability of geroscience-guided interventions to target one or more biological hallmarks of aging, each representing a shared risk factor for different chronic diseases, offers insights into why interventions focused on a primary biological mechanism may offer such broad and pleiotropic beneficial effects (**Figure 40-4E**).

Impact of targeting upstream vs downstream hallmarks of aging

While hallmarks of aging generally have broad effects on aging-related conditions (including other hallmarks; **Figure 40-4E**), some appear to have more widespread effects because of the ability to target such hallmarks "upstream" of other hallmarks. This offers insight into why some geroscience-guided interventions focused on more downstream biological pathways (eg, inflammation) have at times shown lesser functional and clinical benefit compared to interventions targeting more upstream biological pathways (eg, cellular senescence) that have biological effects on multiple downstream pathways, including inflammation.

Basic and Preclinical Research in Support of Geroscience

A broad range of preclinical studies has established the feasibility of geroscience-guided treatments in animal models. For example, mouse studies have clearly established a role for low-dose rapamycin (mTOR inhibitor) in extending both lifespan and healthspan. In other studies, drugs with senolytic properties (such as dasatinib and quercetin, which kill potentially harmful senescent cells) also increase lifespan and improve a broad variety of physiological measures including mobility performance and cognitive

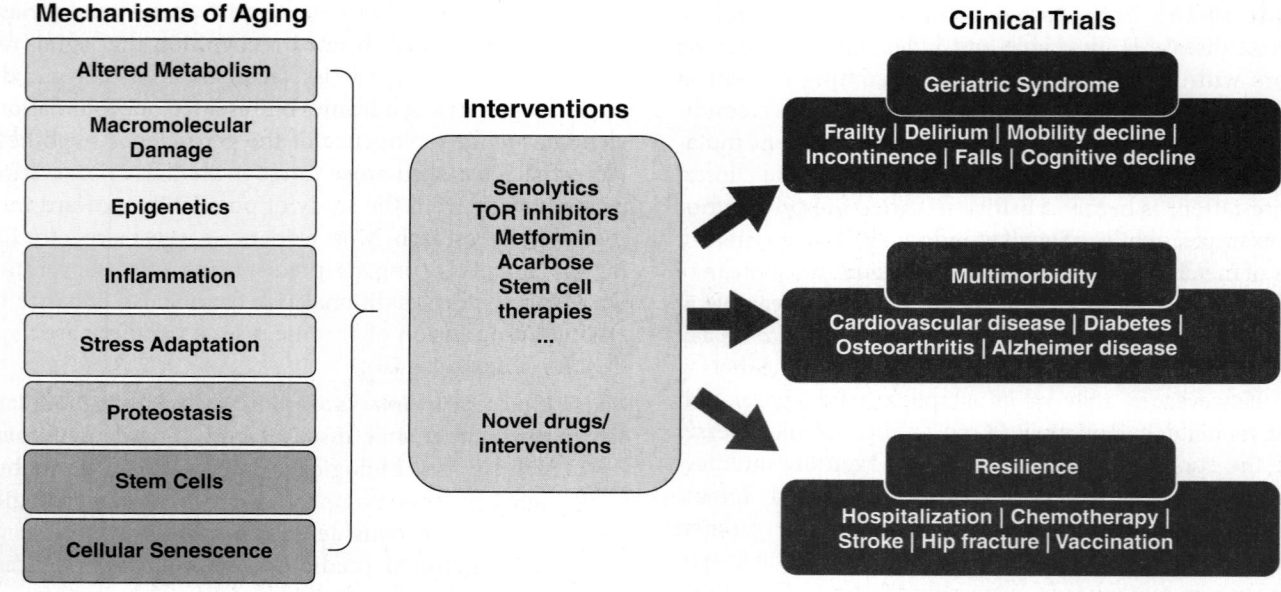

FIGURE 40-5. Categories of geroscience-guided interventions.

function, while also improving geriatric syndromes such as frailty, sarcopenia, and late-life osteoporosis (**Figure 40-5**).

Types of Geroscience Interventions Based on Preclinical Studies

One way to assess the likelihood of successful translation of a geroscience-based intervention into clinical trials is to weigh the evidence from preclinical studies. Thus, a major prediction of translational geroscience is that healthspan, and perhaps lifespan, would be extended in model organisms. The National Institute on Aging (NIA) Interventions Testing Program (ITP) tests drugs to determine if they prevent disease and extend lifespan in genetically heterogeneous (outbred) mice. The ITP has shown that of 26 drugs tested to date, 7 extended lifespan significantly: nor-dihydroguaiaretic acid, aspirin, acarbose*, protandim*, rapamycin, 17-α-estradiol*, glycine, and a synergistic combination of rapamycin + metformin (*indicates mainly effective in males). **Table 40-3** lists examples of interventions that successfully target primary aging processes to extend health- and lifespans, healthspan alone, or lifespan alone. Several interventions include currently available pharmacologic agents that have been repurposed for studying effects on human aging, such as rapamycin, angiotensin-converting enzyme (ACE) inhibitors/angiotensin II receptor blockers (ARBs), metformin, and so-called "senolytic" compounds.

Senotherapeutics as an Example of Geroscience Discovery-to-Translation

Progress has been made toward targeting fundamental aging processes, and multiple interventions are currently being explored, especially cellular senescence. Senolytic agents

TABLE 40-3 ■ PRECLINICAL EVIDENCE FOR GEROSCIENCE-BASED INTERVENTIONS

Extension of healthspan and lifespan
Caloric restriction/food-clocking/ketogenic diets
Exercise
Rapamycin
17-α-estradiol
Angiotensin-converting enzyme (ACE) inhibitor, angiotensin II receptor blockers (ARBs)
Metformin
Senolytics: dasatinib, quercetin, navitoclax, piperlongumine, fisetin, A1331852, A1155463, FOXO4-related peptide, others
Extension of healthspan[a]
Flavonoids/resveratrol/sirtuin activators
Senescence-associated secretory phenotype (SASP) inhibitors: ruxolitinib, rapamycin, metformin
Extension of lifespan[b]
Acarbose
Nordihydroguaiaretic acid (NDGA; median lifespan only)
Protandim
Methionine restriction
Aspirin (median lifespan only), salicylic acid
Other potential interventions
Anti-GDF8, GDF11, anti-activin A
CD38 inhibitors, NAD mimetics
Humanins
Protein aggregation inhibitors

[a]In some cases, information on lifespan extension is not available
[b]In some cases, information on healthspan extension is not available.

were first described on the basis of their inhibition of senescent cell apoptotic pathways. In preclinical models, clearance of senescent cells improves age-related phenotypes, such as chronic diseases, poor resilience, and geriatric syndromes including frailty. Interventions that genetically or pharmacologically remove senescent cells in animal models of aging offer proof-of-concept that they can be translated to human conditions associated with aging, especially those with heavy senescent cell burden. There are many potential interventions proposed to intervene in primary aging processes that may be distinct from cellular senescence; however, these processes are not necessarily mutually exclusive, and in fact may be interdependent. This suggests that any intervention that targets a single fundamental aging process could affect multiple processes that impact aging. Translation of promising pharmacologic senolytic agents has begun with assessments of safety and target engagement, and these early studies will provide lessons for future geroscience-based interventions.

Human studies using such approaches include evidence that a rapamycin analogue administered to community-dwelling older adults improves influenza vaccine responses, while also enhancing general immune responses and decreasing rate of reported infections. A randomized controlled trial of 25% calorie restriction in nonobese adults, CALERIE, showed that dietary restriction is safe and well tolerated, and can improve clinical measures of aging-related diseases as well as biomarkers of aging. Also, the intermittent use of a combination of two senolytics (dasatinib and quercetin) has been shown to be well-tolerated and safe in an open-label pilot study in individuals with idiopathic pulmonary fibrosis, a chronic, ultimately fatal, condition driven mostly by cellular senescence. As a result of these encouraging findings, examples of relevant clinical trials currently underway include studies testing dasatinib and quercetin for Alzheimer disease, while another senolytic called fisetin is being studied for frailty. Many other studies are about to begin recruitment.

Moreover, in the context of COVID-19, for which aging and chronic diseases jointly represent the greatest risk factor for severe illness and death, separate studies are underway testing the use of a rapamycin analogue, fisetin, or metformin in older adults residing in the community and nursing homes. Finally, the Targeting Aging with Metformin trial has been designed to forge a regulatory pathway for aging biology as a target for drug development (https://www.afar.org/tame-trial, accessed 02/14/2022).

TRANSLATIONAL GEROSCIENCE

Principles

Translation of therapies rooted in the basic concepts of the geroscience hypothesis includes the following general principles:

- Any pharmacological, dietary, or exercise-derived intervention that targets fundamental aging processes;

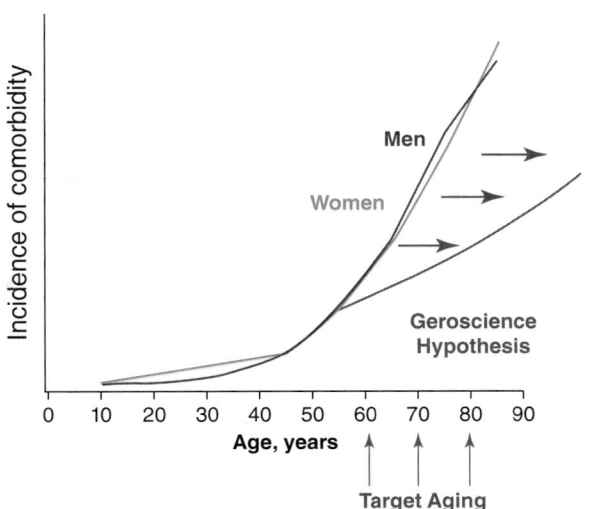

FIGURE 40-6. Targeting biological aging processes could delay the incidence of multiple age-related diseases. (Reproduced with permission from Justice JN, Niedernhofer L, Robbins PD, et al. Development of clinical trials to extend healthy lifespan. *Cardiovasc Endocrinol Metab.* 2018;7(4):80–83.)

- Geroscience-based clinical trials are built upon strong findings from preclinical studies utilizing relevant animal models and/or human studies demonstrating efficacy for single, chronic disease states with supporting evidence for age-related pleiotropic effects;
- The intervention ultimately works to prevent, delay, ameliorate, or reverse multiple chronic conditions or geriatric syndromes (**Figure 40-6**);
- Efficacy of geroscience interventions are based on clinically meaningful outcomes that will benefit healthspan, resiliency, and possibly lifespan;
- Pilot or proof-of-concept human studies provide early insight into safety and administration (dosing, etc), possible efficacy in terms of surrogate biological outcomes and aging mechanistic target engagement, as well as initial data on clinical outcomes that inform the design of larger clinical trials; and
- The successful intervention is generally applicable to older adults with multimorbidity, functional decline, and decreased resilience, and to those of racial, ethnic, and gender diversity who also live in diverse residential settings.

These general principles of translational geroscience serve to identify and target primary aging mechanisms in older adults; confirm efficacy through disease-based, functional, and other outcomes; "de-risk" interventions in a vulnerable population; and assure wide applicability in real-world settings.

Framework for Geroscience-Based Clinical Trials

Conceptually, two categories of clinical trial approaches for geroscience-based therapies have emerged—those aimed at prolonging healthspan and those focused on improving

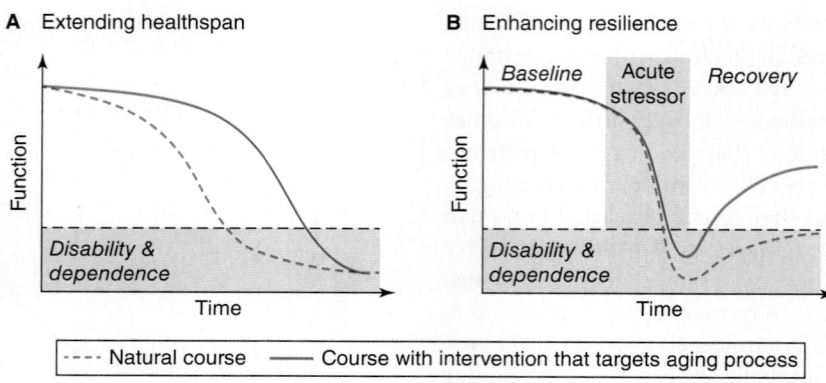

FIGURE 40-7. Extending healthspan and enhancing resilience with interventions that target aging. (Reproduced with permission from Newman JC, Milman S, Hashmi SK, et al. Strategies and challenges in clinical trials targeting human aging. *J Gerontol A Biol Sci Med Sci.* 2016;71(11):1424–1434.)

resilience (**Figure 40-7**). In the first approach, expected declines in healthspan due to progressive loss of physiological and physical function, as well as accumulation of multiple chronic diseases and geriatric syndromes, are targeted to avoid resultant disability and dependence. The advantages of this strategy are that, if successful, it would have high clinical impact on multimorbidity and quality of life, leverage known pathophysiology, and be suited to various interventions. Weaknesses include the difficulty in separating effects of an intervention on a single disease from an underlying effect on primary aging and the challenge of conducting mechanistic studies with multifactorial conditions.

In the second approach, the effects of an acute event that cause sudden, severe morbidity and functional dependence is targeted to optimize recovery to prior functioning and independence. Resiliency, or rebound after an acute event to prior baseline functional and health status, is difficult to achieve in older, frail individuals. In this approach, the goal would be to evaluate interventions that would minimize common physiological stressors such as surgery, trauma, or myocardial infarction. A successful intervention would reduce the severity of consequences in older individuals, including longer recovery times, higher risk of death, and lower likelihood of recovery to baseline function and independence. Strengths of this strategy include the focus on acute events that cause the most disability (eg, trauma) and the potential to evaluate short-term, high-impact outcomes for high-incident acutely deleterious events (eg, 30-day survival after myocardial infarction). Weaknesses are the likely heterogeneity of a specific stressor and the population or circumstances of the acute event as well as the greater possibly for harm associated with very serious stressors.

Outcome Measures

There are many potential outcome measures that capture aspects of fundamental aging processes and clinical measurements related to multimorbidity and physical function that would support the major predictions of the geroscience hypothesis. Several endorsements have been made for the following outcome measures in clinical trials of geroscience-based therapies: (1) mortality; (2) active life expectancy or expected disability-free survival; (3) markers of geriatric syndromes including gait speed, frailty indices, assessments of physical and cognitive functions, and activities of daily living; (4) accumulation of age-related diseases and co-occurrence with disabilities and geriatric syndromes; (5) composite outcomes from subsets of chronic diseases; and (6) other outcomes, including the rate of accumulation of new, age-related diseases, as well as indices of multimorbidity, such as the Charlson Comorbidity Index. Consideration for grouping chronic diseases with shared risk factors and underlying mechanisms into the same categories has been proposed in order to distinguish that an intervention is effective in slowing the aging process rather than having an effect related to a particular shared mechanistic pathway. Additional potential clinical outcome measures are listed in **Table 40-4**.

Outcome measures for geroscience clinical trials should be designed to evaluate time to onset of a new, age-related chronic disease as well as to assess major age-related functional outcomes (mobility, cognitive function, or activities of daily living limitation) and biomarkers of aging as secondary and tertiary outcomes (see biomarkers section on next page). Key features of this design are a primary clinical outcome that represents diverse disease families that are not expected to share etiologic mechanisms except as related to primary aging processes. The secondary outcome related to functional changes is only partially explained by multimorbidity and so key aspects of physical decline likely also reflect fundamental aging.

Populations

Geroscience-based clinical trials must adopt a geriatric-centric design so as to not arbitrarily exclude individuals with coexisting chronic diseases or those who reside in diverse settings, to assure appropriate functional outcome measures, and to avoid focusing on interventions that target only single disease states. These principles optimize

TABLE 40-4 ■ OUTCOME MEASURES FOR CLINICAL TRIALS ON TRANSLATIONAL GEROSCIENCE

All-cause mortality
Age-related diseases
Functional disability
Disease-free survival
Time to incidence of a second or third age-related disease
Composite outcomes (ie, from subsets of chronic diseases)
Time to incidence of impairment of a first activity of daily living (ADL)
Time between disability and death[a]
End-of-life functional trajectory[a]
Quality of death[a]
Length of stay after elective surgery[b]
Gait speed[c]
Grip strength[c]
Mobility stress test[c]
Basic and instrumental ADLs[c]
Number of chronic prescription medications
Cognitive tests (eg, digit symbol substitution test)
Surrogate endpoint biomarkers (see biomarker section)

[a]Could be included in longer clinical trials.
[b]For clinical trials on resilience.
[c]Quantitative intermediate or secondary outcome.

the generalizability of study findings for typical geriatric patients with multiple coexisting conditions, support patient preferences involving function and independence, acknowledge aging as a major risk factor for multimorbidity, and help to validate geroscience-guided therapies in multiple residential and other settings.

Aging studies centered on geroscience-based interventions must be broadly inclusive to capture the heterogeneity of the aging population with respect to gender, race and ethnicity, genetics, socioeconomic status, physical functioning, comorbidities, disabilities, and complex physiology. Exclusion based on very old age or multiple comorbidities would limit those who would most likely benefit from geroscience interventions. Design strategies that may increase statistical power and clinical benefit include stratification by function, comorbidities, or surrogate biomarkers, as well as targeting patients at higher risk for the primary outcome. These approaches may also decrease the time to carry out the study and increase the likelihood of detecting an effect of the intervention. Caveats must be considered for inclusion of individuals with many major morbidities and/or profound functional impairment with limited life expectancy to avoid futile intervention or possible harm. Conversely, recruitment of older individuals lacking any age-related conditions and disabilities could minimize detection of new onset disease or disability during the prescribed study period.

Lastly, standardization of geroscience-based clinical trial outcomes across interventional studies offers the advantages of comparing efficacy and safety findings, establishing benchmarks for assays of target engagement and changes in clinically meaningful endpoints, and assuring quality measures associated with reproducibility. Standardized outcome measures would necessarily apply to a common or core set of measurements and would vary slightly depending on target population (outpatient/community-dwelling, in-hospital, skilled nursing facility).

BIOMARKERS OF AGING FOR CLINICAL TRIALS IN GEROSCIENCE

As highlighted previously, there is no single accepted endpoint for clinical trials testing promising geroscience interventions. The clinical endpoints necessary to ascertain intervention efficacy would be impractical in many trials. Consequently, there is a great deal of activity in developing and validating biomarkers that might (1) change over a much shorter period of time, (2) serve to identify promising intervention candidates, and (3) inform mechanisms or change in the underlying aging biology.

Importantly, biomarkers for clinical trials must have a strong statistical link to the desired outcome. Though biomarkers might lie on the causal pathway, primary interest is identifying biomarkers that move in a direction after intervention to predict clinical outcomes. In other words, biomarkers for geroscience trials reflect the *interaction* between the *change in underlying biology* and the *change in clinical endpoint* (healthspan, lifespan). For example, dysregulated inflammatory signaling and chronic low-grade inflammation is a pillar of biological aging that is strongly associated with mortality and multiple age-related health events. Interventions targeting specific inflammatory pathways, such as anakinra (interleukin [IL]-1 receptor antagonist), canakinumab (human anti-IL-1β monoclonal antibody that neutralizes IL-1β signaling), and tocilizumab (monoclonal IL-6 receptor antibody), are successfully used in the treatment of inflammatory disease. Yet there is little evidence that specifically targeting these inflammatory signaling pathways confer direct benefit on lifespan or aging per se in the absence of underlying disease. This does not diminish the importance of chronic inflammation in aging biology or etiology of chronic disease, nor does this limit utility as a biomarker for intervention effect. Many geroscience-guided interventions that robustly extend lifespan and healthspan broadly affect sources of systemic chronic inflammation that precede and predict health indicators and mortality in model organisms and humans. Thus, inflammatory biomarkers reflect the interaction between a change in underlying aging biology and change in organismal health.

This concept is counter to biomarker development and validation in the context of specific disease. For example, serum high low-density lipoprotein cholesterol (LDL-C) is a biomarker for atherosclerotic heart disease. Elevated

TABLE 40-5 ■ CRITERIA FOR BIOMARKERS OF AGING IN CLINICAL TRIALS

1. Association with chronologic age
2. Association with long-term mortality
3. Association with multiple age-related conditions/outcomes
4. Sensitivity to change
5. Changes in the biomarker associated with change in risk of outcome
6. Evidence of mediation in the context of effective interventions

LDL-C is related to higher coronary heart disease risk, and interventions that lower LDL-C also lower the risk of heart disease. The link is so well established that new drugs can be approved on the basis of their cholesterol-lowering properties rather than proving a reduction in heart disease risk. The strength of LDL-C as a biomarker for heart disease is based on its causal role in the promotion of atherosclerosis.

The search for biomarkers of longevity or use in clinical trials in geroscience is complicated by the fact that no single pathway or mechanism that leads to long life has been identified. Nevertheless, it is possible to propose criteria for biomarkers such that if they were positively affected by a treatment, one would expect life or health extension with some confidence (**Table 40-5**).

Collaborative efforts to develop and validate biomarkers of aging for use in clinical research and practice are underway. Several candidate biomarkers outlined below reflect underlying cellular and molecular aging pathways, are associated with long-term mortality, and show association with multiple age-related conditions and outcomes other than mortality. The latter criteria are most difficult to meet. Longitudinal assessment of biomarkers not implicated in specific disease pathways are infrequently measured clinically or in large cohort studies; this greatly limits evaluation of sensitivity to change and association of change in biomarker with change in outcome risk. In order to meet the final criteria, "evidence of mediation in the context of effective intervention," there must first be: (1) an accepted outcome for a geroscience trial, and (2) an intervention that is proven effective at changing the risk of that outcome. The field is making strides to meet these challenges. Aging outcomes trials are in progress, and interventions are under investigation that could one day demonstrate efficacy. Such investigations will provide needed validation of biomarkers of aging for use in clinical trials targeting aging biology.

Importantly, use of a panel of biomarkers is considered collectively to examine an intervention's effects on multiple aging pathways. Many options are possible to construct a multivariable score of blood-based biomarkers of biological age: statistical modeling or principal component analyses, or a simple rank-based biomarker index. For example, in the Cardiovascular Health Study, an index of five circulating biomarkers was constructed; the hazard ratio for mortality per point of the biomarker index was 1.30 (95% confidence interval 1.25–1.34) and attenuated the association of age on mortality by 25%. Investigations testing the utility of biomarker indices in clinical trials and association with outcomes such as multimorbidity and physiologic function are underway.

Another class of biomarker strategy uses multisystem physiologic, phenotypic, and clinical measures to calculate a composite score representing biologic age that differs in older cohorts compared with a reference population. Examples include homeostatic dysregulation, phenotypic age, and Klemera-Doubal methods, which include measures that might not be associated with chronological age when considered independently, but considered collectively in each of these models, may represent a meaningful biomarker of biological age. For example, several groups have applied the Klemera-Doubal method that takes biochemical measures and uses a reference population to calculate what an individual's predicted chronologic age would be. This method was used in a post-hoc analysis of the CALERIE trial, which showed that caloric restriction for 2 years reduced the advancement of physiologic age compared to control participants.

Aging is associated with changes to DNA including distinct patterns of DNA methylation and telomere loss. The gradual erosion of telomeres limits the replicative capacity of a cell in vitro, known as the Hayflick limit, and so in vivo telomere length was an early focus of aging biomarkers efforts. In practice, telomere length in peripheral white blood cells has shown some association with aging and age-related conditions but with substantial variability that has limited clinical applications so far. Epigenetic biomarkers take advantage of observed chronologic changes in DNA methylation to calibrate "clocks" that can estimate age and aging-related risk. Many aging metrics based on patterns of DNA methylation have been developed, and each "clock" or DNA methylation biomarker is unique to its calibration method. For example, they may be calibrated to chronological age, multifactorial aging phenotypes, or aging-related biomarkers. These estimators can detect a myriad of age-related diseases, predict mortality and adverse health events, and reliably identify persons who appear physiologically older than their chronologic age. A few small studies suggest that methylomic patterns can change in response to an intervention, but much more work needs to be done.

COUNSELING PATIENTS ON "ANTI-AGING" THERAPIES

Aging is a uniquely universal human experience that looms large in popular and commercial culture. Geroscience is a new field, and some of the early interventions being studied include repurposed drugs or over-the-counter agents that may be implicated in aging mechanisms. Common sense clinical judgment should prevail when providers are asked about using such substances ahead of rigorous clinical data and FDA approvals. A plausible link to mechanisms of aging does not mean an intervention will be effective or risk-free. Unregulated clinics are not the same thing as carefully controlled and regulated clinical trials. Attempting to reverse the many ways our bodies change as we age is not always appropriate or helpful, as some changes may be adaptive, or represent consequences rather than causes of aging. Providers and consumers should remember that most investigational drugs and therapies fail, and that typically older adults are at greater risk for harm by the misuse of medications or procedures.

BARRIERS TO RAPID PROGRESS IN GEROSCIENCE AND A PATH FORWARD

Despite the rapidly growing scientific foundation of geroscience, and the promise for transforming the health and health care of older adults, translational progress has been slow. Many of these barriers are related to the newness of the field. Geroscience is a new branch of translational research requiring a unique combination of expertise in geriatric medicine, biology of aging, clinical research methods, and clinical research in older adults that few investigators possess. In spite of these challenges, the geroscience approach holds promise as a means of leveraging advances in the biology of aging to make tangible strides toward improving human health with aging. Geriatricians and other clinicians who are fully focused on the care of older adults will need to acquire and maintain content expertise in geroscience and in the use of geroscience-guided therapies in order to optimally function as specialists and providers.

FURTHER READING

Burch JB, Augustine AD, Frieden LA, et al. Advances in geroscience: impact on healthspan and chronic disease. *J Gerontol A Biol Sci Med Sci.* 2014;69 Suppl 1:S1–S3.

Campisi J, Kapahi P, Lithgow GJ, Melov S, Newman JC, Verdin E. From discoveries in ageing research to therapeutics for healthy ageing. *Nature.* 2019;571(7764): 183–192.

Hickson LJ, Langhi Prata LGP, Bobart SA, et al. Senolytics decrease senescent cells in humans: preliminary report from a clinical trial of dasatinib plus quercetin in individuals with diabetic kidney disease. *EBio Medicine.* 2019;47:446–456.

Inouye SK, Studenski S, Tinetti ME, Kuchel GA. Geriatric syndromes: clinical, research, and policy implications of a core geriatric concept. *J Am Geriatr Soc.* 2007; 55(5): 780–791.

Justice J, Miller JD, Newman JC, et al. Frameworks for proof-of-concept clinical trials of interventions that target fundamental aging processes. *J Gerontol A Biol Med Sci.* 2016;71(11):1415–1423.

Justice JN, Niedernhofer L, Robbins PD, et al. Development of clinical trials to extend healthy lifespan. *Cardiovasc Endocrinol Metab.* 2018a;7(4):80–83.

Justice JN, Ferrucci L, Newman AB, et al. A framework for selection of blood-based biomarkers for geroscience-guided clinical trials: report from the TAME Biomarkers Workgroup. *Geroscience.* 2018b;40(5-6): 419–436.

Justice JN, Nambiar AM, Tchkonia T, et al. Senolytics in idiopathic pulmonary fibrosis: results from a first-in-human, open-label, pilot study. *EBio Medicine.* 2019;40: 554–563.

Kennedy BK, Berger SL, Brunet A, et al. Geroscience: linking aging to chronic disease. *Cell.* 2014;159(4):709–713.

Kulkarni AS, Gubbi S, Barzilai N. Benefits of metformin in attenuating the hallmarks of aging. *Cell Metab.* 2020;32(1):15–30.

Lopez-Otin C, Blasco MA, Partridge L, Serrano M, Kroemer G. The hallmarks of aging. *Cell.* 2013;153(6): 1194–1217.

Mannick JB, Del Giudice G, Lattanzi M, et al. mTOR inhibition improves immune function in the elderly. *Sci Transl Med.* 2014;6(268):268ra179.

Mannick JB, Morris M, Hockey HP, et al. TORC1 inhibition enhances immune function and reduces infections in the elderly. *Sci Transl Med.* 2018;10(449):eaaq1564.

Miller RA. Extending life: scientific prospects and political obstacles. *Milbank Q.* 2002;80(1):155–174.

Newman JC, Milman S, Hashmi SK, et al. Strategies and challenges in clinical trials targeting human aging. *J Gerontol A Biol Sci Med Sci.* 2016;71(11):1424–1434.

Newman JC, Sokoloski JL, Robbins PD, et al. Creating the next generation of translational geroscientists. *J Am Geriatr Soc.* 2019;67(9):1934–1939.

Pignolo RJ, Passos JF, Khosla S, Tchkonia T, Kirkland JL. Reducing senescent cell burden in aging and disease. *Trends Mol Med.* 2020;26(7):630–638.

Sanders JL, Arnold AM, Boudreau RM, et al. Association of biomarker and physiologic indices with mortality in older adults: cardiovascular health study. *J Gerontol A Biol Sci Med Sci.* 2019;74(1):114–120.

Tinetti ME, Inouye SK, Gill TM, Doucette JT. Shared risk factors for falls, incontinence, and functional dependence. Unifying the approach to geriatric syndromes. *JAMA.* 1995;273(17):1348–1353.

Xu M, Pirtskhalava T, Farr JN, et al. Senolytics improve physical function and increase lifespan in old age. *Nat Med.* 2018;24(8):1246–1256.

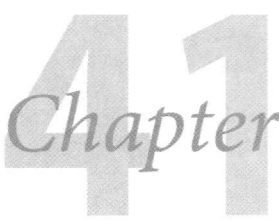

Managing the Care of Patients with Multiple Chronic Conditions

Stephanie Nothelle, Francesca Brancati, Cynthia Boyd

INTRODUCTION

Worldwide, one in three adults has more than one chronic condition, and in the United States, more than half of older adults have three or more chronic conditions. Multiple chronic conditions present unique challenges for older adults, their families, and clinicians. Older adults with multiple chronic conditions are at greater risk of death, functional decline, diminished quality of life, and long-term care placement. Clinicians who care for adults with multiple chronic conditions have limited evidence to draw upon and are often asked to follow disease-specific guidelines with conflicting and interacting treatment plans. Providing person- and family-centered care for older adults with multiple chronic conditions is a key skill of geriatric medicine.

This chapter will review the epidemiology and impact of multiple chronic conditions for individuals, clinicians, and society. We will also discuss common challenges that result when caring for someone with multiple chronic conditions and present a suggested approach to caring for older adults with multiple chronic conditions. We will also briefly review the evidence for interventions focused on older adults with multiple chronic conditions. Many chapters in this book focus on individual organ systems and common diseases. This introductory focus on multiple chronic conditions will provide an important context to be considered as each of the subsequent organ- and disease-specific chapters are read.

TERMINOLOGY

A challenge in addressing the topic of multiple chronic conditions is the lack of consensus around terminology and definitions of the terms used. Two of the most commonly used terms or phrases to describe this issue are "multiple chronic conditions" and "multimorbidity." While comorbidity is often used synonymously, comorbidity refers to the presence of a second condition in reference to an index condition. For example, a clinician focused on treating hypertension might consider a patient's comorbid chronic renal disease when choosing an appropriate therapy. When older adults have multiple chronic conditions, it is disjointed and disease-centric to consider each disease as being "index" in sequence, and many times to patients

Learning Objectives

- Discuss implications of multiple chronic conditions for older adults and their families, the health care system, and society.
- Describe one common clinical challenge in the care of a person with multiple chronic conditions.
- Explain suggested approaches to the care of an older adult with multiple chronic conditions.

Key Clinical Points

1. Having multiple chronic conditions is the most common condition—over 63% of Americans older than 65 years have at least two chronic medical conditions.

2. A challenge in providing care to older adults with multiple chronic conditions is reconciling their care with the specific clinical practice guidelines and recommendations for each of their conditions, given the increased likelihood for polypharmacy and treatment burden.

3. Focusing on older adults' goals and priorities for their health care, what matters most, is key to providing care in the context of multiple chronic conditions.

there is not one central or focal condition. Herein we will use the phrase "multiple chronic conditions."

In its simplest form, having multiple chronic conditions means having more than one chronic condition. A chronic condition, while also variably defined, is defined per the Centers for Disease Control and Prevention as a condition that lasts at least a year and requires ongoing medical attention and/or limits activities of daily living. However, simply counting chronic conditions fails to acknowledge that not all chronic conditions or combinations of chronic conditions are equal in terms of their effect on patients, their effects on other conditions, or their effect on outcomes such as function and quality of life. The approach to two

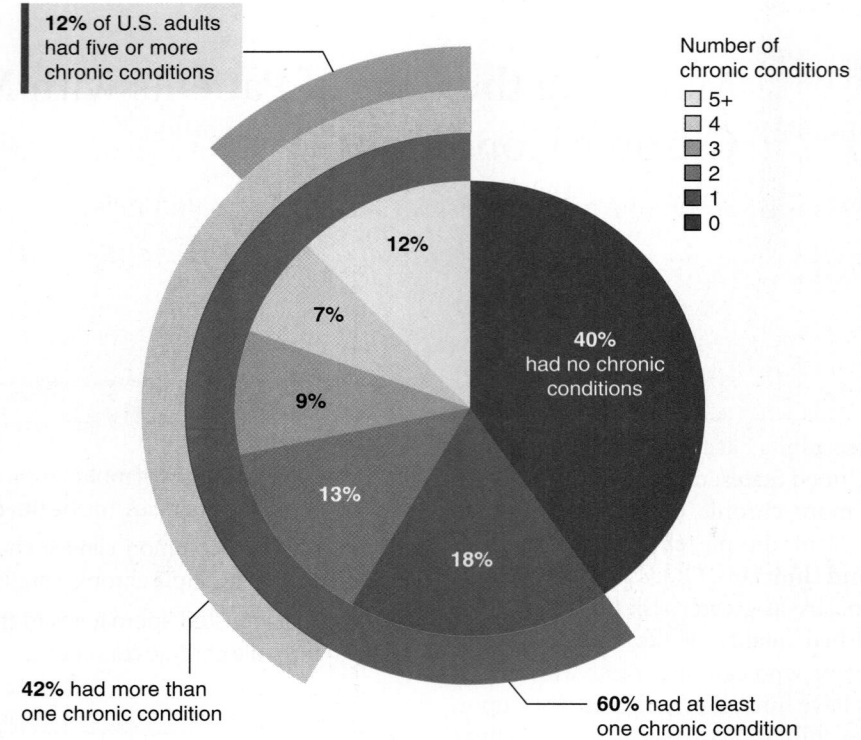

12% of U.S. adults had five or more chronic conditions

Number of chronic conditions
☐ 5+
☐ 4
☐ 3
☐ 2
☐ 1
☐ 0

12%

7%

9%

13%

40% had no chronic conditions

18%

42% had more than one chronic condition

60% had at least one chronic condition

FIGURE 41-1. Percentage of US adults with chronic conditions, by number of chronic conditions (2014). Note: Percentages may not total 100 because of rounding. (Reproduced with permission from Buttorff C, Ruder T, Bauman M. *Multiple Chronic Conditions in the United States*. Santa Monica, CA: RAND Corporation; 2017. https://www.rand.org/pubs/tools/TL221.html.)

disparate conditions, osteoarthritis and hypothyroidism, is different than the approach to two conditions such as congestive heart failure and chronic kidney disease, where the management of one is intricately tied to the other. Thus, determining which chronic conditions "count" in a definition of multimorbidity is another area of disagreement.

In this chapter we will use the National Quality Forum definition, which states, "Persons with multiple chronic conditions are defined as having two or more concurrent chronic conditions that collectively have an adverse effect on health status, function, or quality of life and that require complex healthcare management, decision-making or coordination."

EPIDEMIOLOGY

Due to the variability in definitions of multiple chronic conditions, statistics on multiple chronic conditions can vary dramatically depending on what conditions are being considered. These definitions may include just a handful of common chronic conditions, dozens of physical conditions, or any mental or physical health condition that persists for more than one year and requires ongoing medical attention or limits activities of daily living.

Recent estimates demonstrate that over 42% of American adults have at least two chronic conditions and up to 12% have five or more chronic conditions when including

any physical or mental chronic condition (**Figure 41-1**). When considered by age group, up to 50% of Americans between ages 45 and 65, and over 80% of Americans older than age 65, have multiple chronic conditions. Prevalence of multiple chronic conditions is highest in non-Hispanic White adults at 31% and lowest among Hispanic adults and non-Hispanic Asian adults, at 18% and 16%, respectively, when considering 10 common physical conditions. Men and women older than age 65 have an equal prevalence of multiple chronic conditions. Differences in multimorbidity prevalence by insurance status have also been demonstrated. In adults older than age 65, patients on both Medicare and Medicaid have the highest prevalence of multiple chronic conditions (77%), while patients on Medicare fee-for-service have the lowest prevalence of multiple chronic conditions (59%). Sixty-three percent of both Medicare with Medicare Advantage and private insurance holders have multiple chronic conditions, with similar or higher rates likely among the uninsured.

The most common chronic conditions in the United States are hypertension (27% of American adults aged 18 and older in 2014), high cholesterol (22%), and mood disorders (12%). Currently the chronic disease that is most associated with a second chronic condition is kidney disease, with 81% of chronic kidney disease patients on Medicare having at least one other chronic condition (usually diabetes or congestive heart failure) (**Figure 41-2**). Among American adults between 2008 and 2014, men saw the highest increase

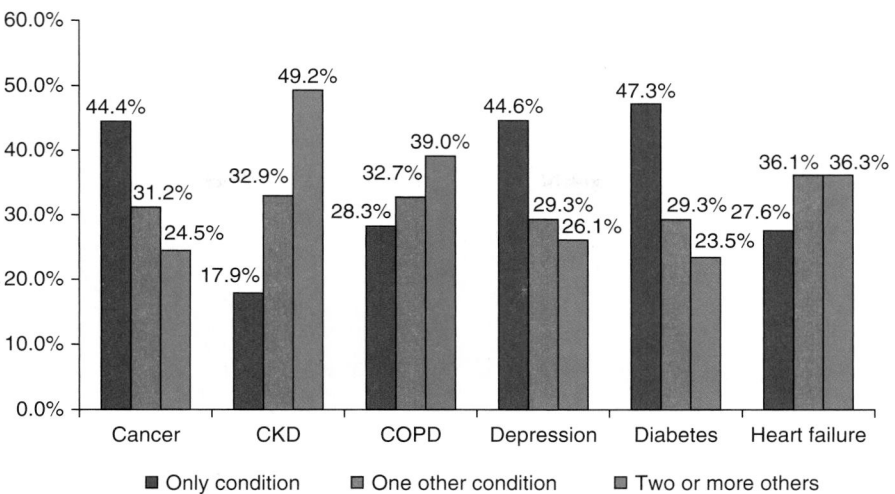

FIGURE 41-2. Proportion (%) of Medicare beneficiaries with multiple chronic conditions by select chronic condition (2005). (Reproduced with permission from Schneider KM, O'Donnell BE, Dean D. Prevalence of multiple chronic conditions in the United States' Medicare population. *Health Qual Life Outcomes.* 2009;7:82.)

in prevalence of hypertension (2.5% increase) while women saw the highest increase in mental health conditions (4% increase in anxiety disorder alone). Studies that include mental health in their definition of chronic conditions demonstrate a positive correlation between the number of chronic conditions and the onset of depression. Depression was found in 14% of adults between ages 50 and 74 with one physical chronic condition, 21% of people with two chronic conditions, 30% of people with three chronic conditions, and 37% of people with four chronic conditions. In 2014, mood and anxiety disorders were the third and fifth most prevalent chronic conditions in American adults.

In the United States, rural populations have a higher prevalence of multiple chronic conditions than urban populations (35% vs 26%). Socioeconomic status has also been found to impact the prevalence of chronic multimorbidity in high income countries. A 2012 study found that on average, populations living in the poorest areas of Scotland had a 10- to 15-year earlier onset of multimorbidity compared to their peers living in most affluent neighborhoods. The disparity in the prevalence of multiple chronic conditions by socioeconomic status begins in the second decade of life and disappears in the eighth decade, perhaps due to survival bias (**Figure 41-3**). All socioeconomic groups show a steep increase in the prevalence of multiple chronic conditions starting at age 50 (see **Figure 41-3**). This study also found that low socioeconomic status was found to be particularly linked to the presence of mental health disorders co-occurring with multiple chronic conditions. However, there is only a weak correlation between socioeconomic status and multiple chronic condition prevalence globally. This is potentially because many behaviors that confer risk for chronic conditions (smoking, physical inactivity, alcohol consumption, unhealthy diet, etc) are more common among people of low socioeconomic status in high-income countries but

are more common among those with higher socioeconomic status in low- and middle-income countries.

IMPACT

The impacts of multiple chronic conditions on older adults and their families/friends, the health care community, and society are extensive. Impacts include use of health care, complications from health care, and functional and quality of life outcomes relevant to the daily lives of older adults and their loved ones.

Patients with multiple chronic conditions require more health care resources. When taking all chronic conditions into account, Americans who have three or more chronic conditions make up 28% of the population but 67% of health care expenditures. The more concurrent chronic conditions a patient has, the greater health care expenditures they incur. In 2005, Medicare beneficiaries with no chronic conditions amassed health care costs of about $3000, while patients with two and three or more chronic conditions amassed costs of about $16,400 and $35,700, respectively. Further, patients with three or more chronic conditions spend 6.6 times as much on medications than their peers with no chronic conditions and 2.1 times more than their peers with one or two chronic conditions. Patients with multiple chronic conditions also use a greater proportion of the resources in the health care system, seeing both primary care and specialty physicians 2 to 5 times more often than their peers without chronic conditions. The number and duration of hospital stays also correlates with the presence of multiple chronic conditions; older adults with three or more chronic conditions have 14.6 times more hospital stays and spend 25 times more nights in a hospital than their peers without any chronic conditions. Further, older adults with four or more chronic conditions are 90 times as

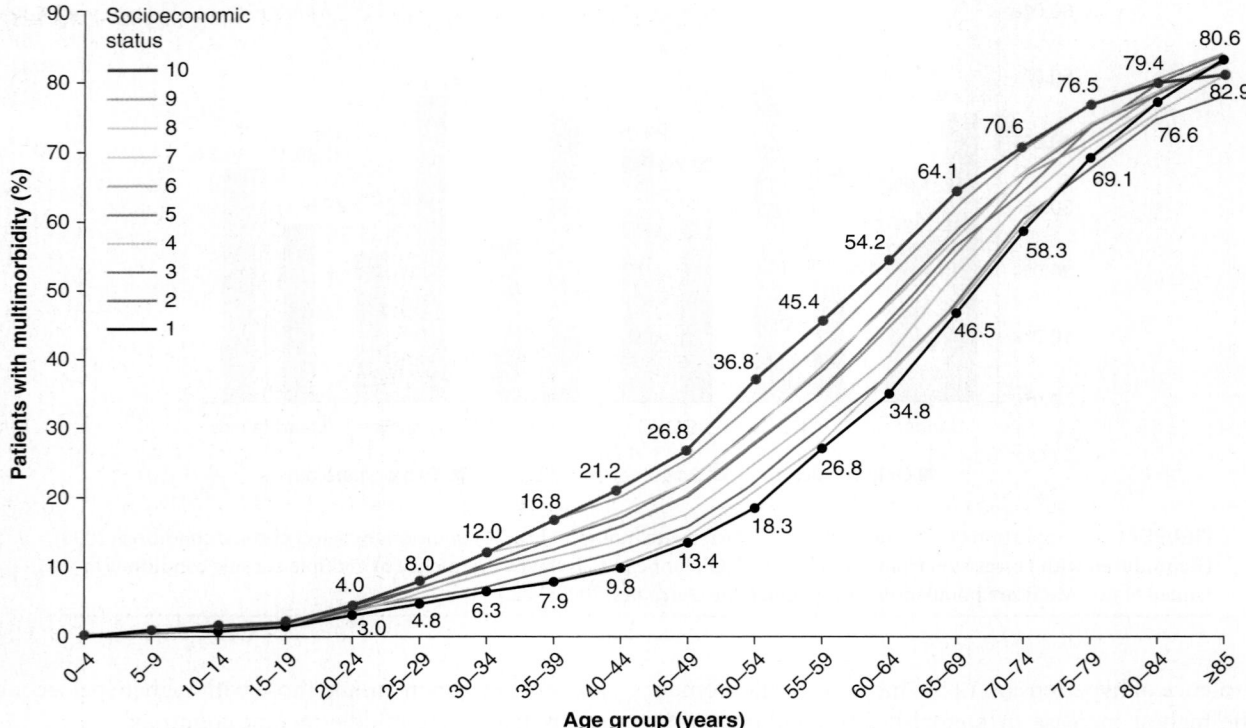

FIGURE 41-3. Prevalence of multiple chronic conditions as a function of age, stratifying on socioeconomic status. On socioeconomic status scale, 1 = most affluent and 10 = most "deprived." (Reproduced with permission from Barnett K, Mercer SW, Norbury M, et al. Epidemiology of multimorbidity and implications for health care, research, and medical education: a cross-sectional study. *Lancet.* 2012;380[9836]:37–43.)

likely to incur hospital admissions than someone without any chronic conditions.

In addition to increased cost of care, older adults with multiple chronic conditions also tend to experience a lower quality of care. Older adults with multiple chronic conditions are more likely to experience adverse drug effects, including drug-drug interactions, as well as experience greater difficulty in participating in their own care due to the complexity of their health conditions, when compared to adults without multiple chronic conditions. Additionally, different combinations of conditions are associated with receiving lower quality treatment. Adults with both psychoses and arthritis, for example, are less likely to receive treatment for arthritis than individuals with arthritis alone. For other combinations of conditions, however, the opposite trend is seen. For instance, older adults are more likely to be treated for psychiatric disorders if they have a concurrent somatic chronic condition, such as diabetes.

Older adults with multiple chronic conditions report experiencing a lower quality of life and greater functional disability than their peers, though some conditions have a larger impact on quality of life and disability than others. Adults with multiple chronic conditions require more help with activities of daily living and experience more social, home, work, physical, and cognitive limitations than their peers without chronic conditions—these limitations

increase with the number of chronic conditions a person has (**Figure 41-4**). Older adults in particular experience more limitations in daily activity and cognitive ability than younger adults with the same number of chronic conditions.

Out of 10 common chronic conditions, a 2014 cross-sectional study of Spanish adults older than 50 years found depression, anxiety, and stroke to have the greatest impact on quality of life and disability scores. Hypertension had the least impact on both quality of life and disability scores, as defined by the World Health Organization Quality of Life instrument and Disability Assessment Schedule. While an increasing number of chronic conditions generally correlated with worse quality of life and disability scores in both genders, women tended to report worse quality of life and disability scores than men for the same number of conditions. Women with two chronic conditions, for example, had an average disability score of 9.9, compared to 7.3 for men. Additionally, there was some variation in the impact of certain conditions on disability scores between the sexes. Women reported worse disability outcomes for anxiety and angina than men did, while men reported worse disability outcomes for edentulism and asthma than women. It should be noted that not all concurrent chronic conditions confer worse quality of life than having a single chronic condition. Chronic obstructive pulmonary disease (COPD) and asthma, for example, have overlapping symptoms and therefore have not been shown to

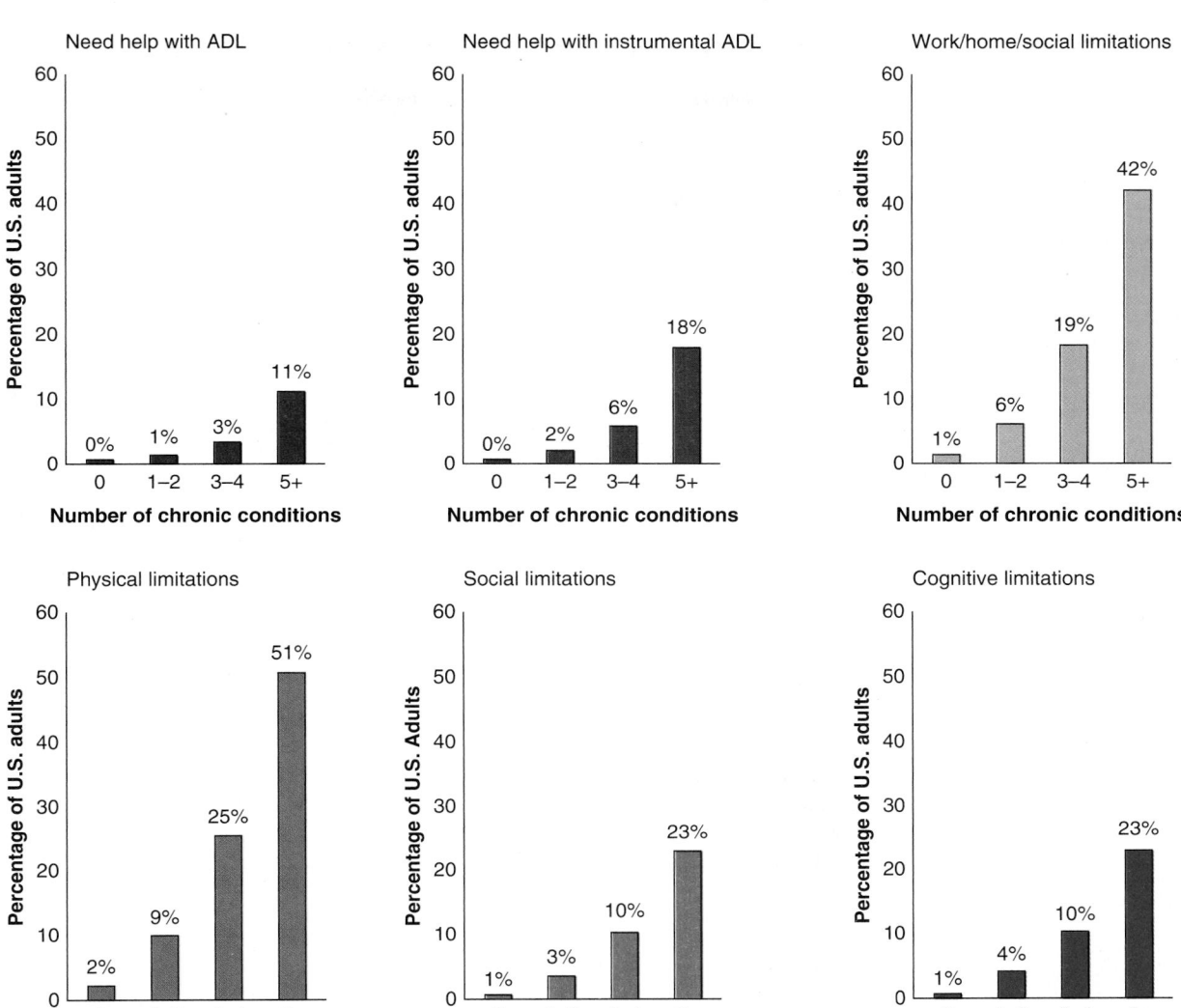

FIGURE 41-4. Functional, physical, social, and cognitive limitations, by number of chronic conditions (2014). (Notes: ADL include such basic functions as being able to bathe, dress, eat, go to the bathroom, or do light activity—for example, walking up a flight of stairs. Instrumental ADL include light housework, preparing meals, paying bills, and shopping. We used the composite variables constructed in MEPS for the ADL and IADL, which indicate whether a person reponed needing supervision to complete at least one ADL or instrumental ADL activity. A work/school/home limitation is defined as an impairment or a physical or mental health problem that limits a person's ability to work at a job, do housework, or go to school. A physical limitation is defined as having difficulties walking, climbing stairs, grasping objects, bending or standing for long periods of time. MEPS defines social limitations as whether a person has trouble participating in social or family activities because of a physical or cognitive impairment. A cognitive limitation exists if the person has trouble with memory is esaily confused, has trouble marking decisions, or needs to be supervised for his or her own safety.) (Reproduced with permission from Buttorff C, Ruder T, Bauman M. Multiple Chronic Conditions in the United States. Santa Monica, CA: RAND Corporation; 2017. https://www.rand.org/pubs/tools/TL221.html.)

worsen quality of life in patients with both conditions compared to patients with only one.

CHALLENGES AND POTENTIAL SOLUTIONS

There are numerous challenges for patients, their families, clinicians, and society as a result of multiple chronic conditions. In this section of the chapter, we will focus on a few of the most commonly encountered challenges in clinical practice.

Clinical Practice Guidelines

Many people with multiple chronic conditions experience disease-focused, not patient-centered care, in part due to the focus of clinical practice guidelines on specific diseases. Single disease-focused clinical practice guidelines are often applied in the care of people with multiple chronic conditions, despite the fact that there are limitations to the applicability of these guidelines to this population.

TABLE 41-1 ■ IT'S NOT EASY LIVING WITH MULTIPLE CHRONIC CONDITIONS

TIME	MEDICATIONS	NONPHARMACOLOGIC THERAPY	ALL DAY	PERIODIC
7 AM	Ipratropium MDI Alendronate 70 mg weekly	Check feet Sit upright 30 min Check blood sugar	Joint protection Energy conservation Exercise (non-weight-bearing if severe foot disease, weight-bearing for osteoporosis) Muscle strengthening exercises, aerobic exercises, ROM exercises Avoid environmental exposures that might exacerbate COPD Wear appropriate footwear Albuterol MDI PM Limit alcohol Maintain normal body weight	Pneumonia vaccine, yearly influenza vaccine All provider visits: Evaluate self-monitoring blood glucose, foot examination, and BP Quarterly HbA1c, biannual LFTs Yearly creatinine, electrolytes, microalbuminuria, cholesterol Referrals: Pulmonary rehabilitation Physical therapy DEXA scan every 2 y Yearly eye examination Medical nutrition therapy Patient education: High-risk foot conditions, foot care, footwear, Osteoarthritis COPD medication and delivery system training Diabetes mellitus
8 AM	HCTZ 12.5 mg Lisinopril 40 mg Glyburide 10 mg ASA 81 mg Metformin 850 mg Naproxen 250 mg Omeprazole 20 mg Calcium + vitamin D 500 mg	2.4 g Na, 90 mm K, adequate Mg, ↓ cholesterol and saturated fat, medical nutrition therapy for diabetes, DASH		
12 PM	Ipratropium MDI Calcium + vitamin D 500 mg	Diet as above		
5 PM	Eat dinner	Diet as above		
7 PM	Ipratropium MDI Metformin 850 mg Naproxen 250 mg Calcium + vitamin D 500 mg Lovastatin 40 mg			
11 PM	Ipratropium MDI			

Data from Boyd CM, Darer J, Boult C, et al. Clinical practice guidelines and quality of care for older patients with multiple comorbid diseases: implications for pay for performance. JAMA. 2005;294(6):716–724.

A study that delineated the treatment regimen that would arise from implementation of clinical practice guidelines for an older woman with five common chronic conditions (COPD, hypertension, diabetes, osteoarthritis, and hypertension) resulted in 12 different medicines, in 19 doses per day, with a high degree of medication regimen complexity (**Table 41-1**)

Many single disease guidelines only address people with multiple chronic conditions in a limited fashion, and many fail to incorporate many patient-centered topics, like how to incorporate patient preferences. Applying the guidelines to older adults with multiple chronic conditions thus takes interpretation on the part of the clinician. Suggestions for interpreting the evidence in the context of multiple chronic conditions and incorporating guideline-based recommendations into the overall care plan are outlined below.

Polypharmacy, Potentially Inappropriate Medications, and Deprescribing

As expected, having multiple chronic conditions is a strong risk factor for polypharmacy. Approximately 50% of people 65 years or older take more than five regular medications and up to 91% of people living in long-term care take five or more regular medications.

Polypharmacy has significant negative consequences for patients. Taking more than four medications is associated with a higher risk of injurious falls and the risk of having a fall further increases with each additional medication, regardless of the type of medication. Polypharmacy can be appropriate in some patients (referred to as "evidence-based polypharmacy"), but even when the medications are recommended for individual conditions (ie, in guidelines), they may not always be effective or safe in a person with multiple chronic conditions.

Frequently people with polypharmacy are taking potentially inappropriate medications, in which the risks of medication use may outweigh the benefit (eg, high risk and unnecessary medications). Twenty to seventy-nine percent of older adults are taking at least one potentially inappropriate medicine, which puts them at increased risk of adverse drug events and mortality.

Several assessment tools exist for potentially inappropriate medications including explicit tools such as the Beers Criteria, STOPP (Screening Tool of Older People's Prescriptions), and START (Screening Tool to Alert to the Right Treatment), and implicit criteria such as the Medication Appropriateness Index. The Beers Criteria are regularly updated by a panel through the American Geriatrics Society and contain a list of medications for which the risk of adverse effects may exceed the benefit of the medication. The STOPP and START criteria have clear standards to guide clinicians in decision making about stopping a potentially risky medication and starting a new, alternative medication. In contrast, the Medication Appropriateness Index relies on 10 questions to ask about each medication. This tool relies on physician judgment, which allows for a more patient-centered approach but is much more time consuming to apply than the explicit tools such as the Beers Criteria and STOPP and START.

Although there is considerable information to guide prescribers in the safe and effective initiation of new medications, there is a proportionate lack of guidance regarding how inappropriate medications should be safely and effectively discontinued. Stopping or decreasing medications is referred to as deprescribing. Patients are more likely to consider deprescribing if their physician recommends it. Reasons to consider deprescribing a medication include, but are not limited to, lack of a valid indication for the medication in the patient's medical history, duplicative therapy (eg, proton pump inhibitor and H_2-blocker), dose adjustment for hepatic or renal impairment, drug-drug/drug-food/drug-disease interactions, lack of time to benefit, low magnitude of effect, adverse drug events, and medication cost.

Patient and family preferences and goals of therapy need to be considered when selecting medications for deprescribing. Once a medication is selected for deprescribing, a plan should be made to taper or stop the medication and to monitor for effects of the change. Guidelines including algorithms to stop certain medications (eg, proton pump inhibitors, antihyperglycemics) as well as shared decision-making aids are available through the Canadian Deprescribing Network at www.deprescribing.org.

Limited Evidence

Older adults with multiple chronic conditions are often excluded from clinical trials that are focused on examining a single disease. The average clinical trial participant has half the number of chronic conditions as the average primary care patient. The lack of evidence on how to treat an older adult with multiple chronic conditions can be frustrating for clinicians who are forced to make assumptions about how other conditions and treatments may interact.

Enrolling large numbers of older adults with multiple chronic conditions for participation in clinical trials is challenging given typical exclusion criteria and study protocols. Once recruited, retention in studies requires specific protocols and resources that maximize the participation of older adults. Concerns about missing data can be addressed with proactive attention to retention and analytic approaches, as the NIH Inclusion Across the Life Span program advocates. Moreover, as noted above, multiple chronic conditions can be very heterogeneous, which presents challenges when trying to create counterfactual populations in clinical trials, but analyses based on multivariate risk prediction are

opportunities to avoid the challenges of multiple subgroup analyses. Innovative approaches to address the net balance of benefits and harms, across multiple dimensions of heterogeneity can help synthesize the evidence base in such a way that existing data can inform care for older adults with multiple chronic conditions. However, currently we have inadequate evidence to inform many decisions for older adults with multiple chronic conditions. The lack of evidence on how to treat an older adult with multiple chronic conditions can be challenging for clinicians who are forced to make assumptions about how other conditions and treatments may interact as they care for older adults.

To help clinicians address this challenge, the American Geriatrics Society Expert Panel on the Care of Older Adults with Multimorbidity has proposed several questions to consider when reviewing the literature for adults with multiple chronic conditions as part of a set of Guiding Principles, described further. First, the panel suggests considering whether older adults with multiple chronic conditions were included in the trial and if so whether specific chronic conditions modified the treatment effect; for example, whether chronic renal disease made a given treatment less effective or more likely to cause side effects.

The panel also suggests considering the strength or quality of the evidence and whether the outcome examined is one that is important to older adults with multiple chronic conditions. Clinical trials will often include endpoints that are markers of disease (eg, low-density lipoprotein level or change in forced expiratory volume in 1 second). Such an outcome is likely seen as less important to an older adult than whether or not they have a stroke that requires hospitalization or if the distance they can walk is limited by their shortness of breath.

Harms and benefits should also be weighed. In addition to considering whether a treatment effect was observed, a clinician might consider whether adverse effects were sufficiently explored and reported and how the proposed treatment might interact with an older adult's other treatments. Specifically, financial cost and treatment burden or complexity of the treatment should be considered as they are associated with adherence.

Finally, two concepts to consider when interpreting the results include absolute risk reduction (ARR) and time to benefit. Many studies report the relative risk reduction (RRR) rather than the ARR. The ARR is the difference in risk between the two groups being compared (eg, baseline risk compared to risk of an outcome with a treatment) while the RRR is the ARR divided by the baseline risk. As an example, if the risk of a negative outcome is 2% in the placebo group and 1% in the treatment group, this amounts to a 1% ARR and a 50% RRR. Presence of multiple chronic conditions can impact the baseline risk of a given outcome and may change the magnitude of the RRR, making interpretation of these values challenging. Focusing on the RRR promotes overestimation of the effect. Thus, focusing on the ARR can help ground the clinician's interpretation of effect. Lastly, time to benefit is the time it takes to achieve an observable and clinically meaningful change in a given outcome as a result of the treatment. Time to harm is a similar concept that examines the time it takes to observe an adverse effect. These values can help guide a clinician who is treating an older adult with multiple chronic conditions who may have limited life expectancy. If the time to benefit from a treatment is 5 years, but the older adult is unlikely to live that long, then it may not be helpful to start the treatment.

Coordination of Care

Older adults with multiple chronic conditions typically see many clinicians from many specialties, which require coordination of care. The number of different physicians seen each year by the average Medicare beneficiary ranges from 4 for those with just 1 condition to 14 for those with 5 or more chronic conditions. As the number of physicians seen increases, the need for coordination across providers increases in turn.

Coordination of care is important for older adults with multiple chronic conditions. Care that is scattered across providers increases risk of unnecessary tests and procedures, which exposes individuals to harm and adds burden to the patient and his/her caregivers who need to arrange for what is ordered. Much of this fragmentation reflects a health care system that was designed for single disease, episodic care, and has been slow to adapt to the care of older adults with multiple chronic conditions.

Historically, the primary care clinician has been seen as the physician responsible for coordinating care across providers, however, given time constraints and administrative burdens, it may be challenging for primary care clinicians to coordinate across all of the specialists involved in an older adult's care. To address the gap in coordination, health care entities are increasingly employing professionals in coordination roles. While the titles for these positions are varied, care manager or case manager is commonly used. Typically, these positions are filled by someone who is a nurse or social worker by training. The care manager is charged with helping a panel of complex older adults, usually with multiple chronic conditions, with coordination of care and disease self-management. While data on the success of these programs is mixed, some have showed the ability to improve outcomes and lower health care costs. Further discussion on interventions targeting older adults with multiple chronic conditions is below.

Including the Caregiver

Most of the care for older adults with multiple chronic conditions is provided by informal caregivers. Herein, we will use the term "caregiver" to refer to an unpaid family member or friend who assists the patient with their care and daily activities and "care recipient" to refer to the person with multiple chronic conditions who is receiving the care. In addition to helping with self-care, emotional support, and household activities, almost half of caregivers also help

with health care activities (eg, coordinating and attending health care visits, managing medications). Individuals who primarily help with health care activities may not view themselves as caregivers; the phrase "care partners" is increasingly used to recognize that care can be bidirectional or that the care recipient can still play an active role in their care. For example, among two spouses, each may help each other with different tasks. Caring for persons with multiple chronic conditions has been associated with increased caregiver burden and reduced health related quality of life for the caregiver; however, having a caregiver is associated with improved medication adherence, healthy lifestyle behavior promotion, and reduced emergency services utilization for the care recipient.

Despite the significant role caregivers play in delivering care to a person with multiple chronic conditions, caregivers are not routinely identified or supported in health care delivery, which is typically focused on the patient (the care recipient). Further, evidence from national studies suggest that almost one half of older adults' caregivers were not asked during routine health care encounters if they needed help managing older adults' care. Some of this may be a consequence of health care providers such as physicians and nurses feeling uncertain about how to interact with caregivers. It may be challenging to effectively partner with a caregiver while respecting patient privacy and autonomy and balancing differences in health care priorities and goals between the care recipient and caregiver. Although the evidence regarding how to be work with caregivers in the health care setting is still limited, some best practice suggestions have been put forth by the National Academies for Science, Engineering, and Medicine in their report "Families Caring for an Aging America" including routinely identifying caregivers who are involved in an older adult's care, assessing the caregiver's needs, and supporting identified needs through appropriate referrals and connections to services in the health care system and community.

APPROACH TO THE PATIENT WITH MULTIPLE CHRONIC CONDITIONS

Given the limited evidence surrounding care of older adults with multiple chronic conditions, many of the currently available recommendations are derived from expert opinion. The American Geriatrics Society convened two work groups to create five guiding principles for the management of multiple chronic conditions and a framework with Action Steps to translate the principles into patient care decisions. Below we provide some suggestions for approaching clinical care for adults with multiple chronic conditions based on the Action Steps proposed by the American Geriatrics Society.

Focus on Patient Goals and Priorities

Older adults with multiple chronic conditions are likely to vary significantly in their care preferences, medical condition, and life context. Thus, eliciting and communicating a patient's goals and priorities for their health care are vitally important in the care of older adults with multiple chronic conditions.

There are several validated tools to elicit a patient's health priorities. For all older adults with multiple chronic conditions the "Patient Priorities Identification" tool (available at: www.patientprioritiescare.org) and validated questions available through the American Geriatrics Society (GeriatricsCareOnline.org) can help guide a conversation. Others such as VITALtalk (www.vitaltalk.org) and Prepare for your Care (www.prepareforyourcare.org) are more appropriate in advanced illness. Priorities and goals can shift over time so reviewing and updating established goals and priorities, particularly after a major change in condition or life circumstances (eg, functional decline, loss of a spouse), is important. Finally, once the priorities and goals are identified, they should be clearly documented in the medical record and shared with all members of the care team.

Consider the Patient's Health Trajectory

Assessing and discussing a patient's health trajectory is also important in the overall care of older adults with multiple chronic conditions. Health trajectory refers to likely pathways or patterns of change in function, health status, or quality of life, including likelihood of death. While there are unfortunately few tools to estimate changes in function, health status, or risk of death, a discussion with the patient and family of general expectations for changes in quality of life or function may be just as helpful as a more precise prognosis. For example, framing a decision or discussion into time frames of 1–2, 2–5, 6–10, or 10+ years can be helpful. An online repository of calculators to estimate life expectancy is available at www.eprognosis.org. Other practical considerations for specific clinical care decisions include using the estimated "time to benefit" or lag time for an estimated intervention. For example, the time to benefit for many cancer screenings is estimated at 10 years while the time to the benefit from antihypertensive therapy is 2 to 3 years. Having this information in mind can help guide a patient to make a decision about what is best for them.

Prior to discussing health trajectory and life expectancy with a patient, it is wise to explore whether and how much the patient would like to discuss this topic and what information he or she is interested in knowing (eg, need for repeated hospitalizations or need to move to a more supportive living environment). Potential ways to bring up this conversation include asking "What is your understanding of how your illnesses will affect your day-to-day life and your health?" and following up with, "Would you like to talk more about this?" Some patients may have a hard time articulating what they do or do not want to know and providing options can be helpful. For example, "Some of my patients want a big picture view of what to expect; others want lots of details about what might happen; and some don't want to talk about this at all. What is best for you?"

Consider Treatment Complexity and Treatment Burden

Older adults with multiple chronic conditions are asked to take on a great number of health care and self-management tasks (also discussed in Chapter 25). The negative effect of managing health related treatments and tasks on quality of life is referred to as treatment burden. Approximately 40% of older adults report some degree of treatment burden. Older adults and their caregivers spend an average of 2 hours a day on health care related tasks (eg, measuring blood sugar) and 2 hours for each health care visit. Treatment burden increases the risk of nonadherence to effective treatments, which may lead to poor outcomes (eg, uncontrolled blood pressure) that in turn lead to health care professionals further intensifying the treatment. Minimizing treatment burden is thus not only important for patient and family quality of life but it also provides an opportunity to stop burdensome care and start more beneficial and goal concordant care. While tools to measure treatment burden exist, they are multiquestion surveys which in current form are likely more useful in the research than in the clinical setting.

Refine the Treatment Plan Based on Patient Priorities and Health Trajectory

Using the patient's care priorities as a guide, all health care activities (medications, visits, self-management tasks) should be reviewed and modified as appropriate from time to time. Care that is harmful, burdensome, or misaligned with patient care priorities should be stopped. Consider a patient's health trajectory and the time to benefit (lag time) for treatments such as cancer screening and each medication when deciding whether to start, continue, or stop a medication.

A key step in refining care for older adults with multiple chronic conditions is to align care decisions across all parties—patients, family, and other clinicians. Having all parties agree and focus on the patient's health priorities and health trajectory as guiding principles in care decisions can be helpful. Further, patients and family involved in care should be invited to be active participants in the decision-making process.

Aligning the perspectives of all parties can be challenging when individuals have different perspectives. For example, patients and clinicians may have different perspectives about starting or stopping a medication. Sometimes this is due to a disconnect between the patient's goals and their preferences (what they are willing to do) and discussing this discrepancy can help decision making. Other times, patients and clinicians may simply not agree and it is best to accept the patient's decision and move forward, revisiting the topic in the future if appropriate. When clinicians have different perspectives, it can help to focus on the patient's priorities instead of individual diseases using the principles of collaborative negotiation (eg, define the issue around a common goal, make sure all parties are using the same information, identify sources of differing recommendations, brainstorm therapeutic alternatives).

INTERVENTIONS TARGETING CARE OF PEOPLE WITH MULTIPLE CHRONIC CONDITIONS

A Cochrane review published in 2015 examined 17 interventions aimed at improving care for persons with multiple chronic conditions. Most of the studies (12 of 17) utilized an organizational or system level approach to improving care through utilization of a care or case manager to assist with coordination of care and self-management. The remaining five studies focused on patient education and engagement directly through chronic disease self-management and patient engagement workshops. The interventions resulted in modest improvements in mental health outcomes and possible improvements in functional outcomes, in the studies that reported these outcomes. However, there were no clear positive improvements in clinical outcomes (eg, blood pressure, symptom scores), health service use, medication adherence, patient-related health behaviors, health professional behaviors, or costs. The authors suggest that interventions are most successful when they are integrated into existing health care systems and when they focus on specific problems or outcomes experienced by people with multiple chronic conditions.

CONCLUSIONS

Effectively caring for the growing population of older adults with multiple chronic conditions is a key component of geriatric medicine. While there are several challenges to caring for this population such as limited evidence to guide care and disease-based clinical practice guidelines, focusing on patient and family preferences and considering the patient's overall health trajectory and burden of treatment can help a clinician effectively tailor care. In many chapters of this book, several common conditions and their treatments are reviewed in detail within the confines of each individual organ system. We encourage the reader to remember the key principles of this chapter when considering how to implement disease-specific recommendations in the care of an older adult who has multiple chronic conditions.

FURTHER READING

American Geriatrics Society Expert Panel on the Care of Older Adults with Multimorbidity. Patient-centered care for older adults with multiple chronic conditions: a stepwise approach from the American Geriatrics Society: American Geriatrics Society Expert Panel on the Care of Older Adults with Multimorbidity. *J Am Geriatr Soc.* 2012;60(10):1957–1968.

Barnett K, Mercer SW, Norbury M, Watt G, Wyke S, Guthrie B. Epidemiology of multimorbidity and implications for health care, research and medical education: a cross-sectional study. *Lancet.* 2012;380(9836):37–43.

Boersma P, Black LI, Ward BW. Prevalence of multiple chronic conditions among US adults, 2018. *Prev Chronic Dis.* 2020;17:200130.

Boyd CM, Darer J, Boult C, Fried LP, Boult L, Wu AW. Clinical practice guidelines and quality of care for older patients with multiple comorbid diseases: implications for pay for performance. *JAMA.* 2005;294(6):716–724.

Boyd C, Smith CD, Masoudi FA, et al. Decision making for older adults with multiple chronic conditions: executive summary for the American Geriatrics Society Guiding Principles on the Care of Older Adults with Multimorbidity. *J Am Geriatr Soc.* 2019;67(4):665–673.

Buttorff C, Ruder T, Bauman M. Multiple chronic conditions in the United States. Santa Monica, CA: RAND Corporation, 2017. Available at https://www.rand.org/pubs/tools/TL221.html. Accessed February 2, 2022.

Garin N, Olaya B, Moneta MV, et al. Impact of multimorbidity on disability and quality of life in the Spanish older population. *PLoS One.* 2014;9(11):e111498.

Goodman RA, Ling SM, Briss PA, Parrish RG, Salive ME, Finke BS. Multimorbidity patterns in the United States: implications for research and clinical practice. *J Gerontol A Biol Sci Med Sci.* 2016;71(2):215–220.

Guiding principles for the care of older adults with multimorbidity: an approach for clinicians. Guiding principles for the care of older adults with multimorbidity: an approach for clinicians: American Geriatrics Society Expert Panel on the Care of Older Adults with Multimorbidity. *J Am Geriatr Soc.* 2012;60(10):E1–E25.

Hajat C, Stein E. The global burden of multiple chronic conditions: a narrative review. *Prev Med Rep.* 2018;12:284–293.

Lehnart T, Heider D, Leicht H, et al. Review: health care utilization and costs of elderly persons with multiple chronic conditions. *Med Care Res Rev.* 2011;68(4):387–420.

Schneider KM, O'Donnell BE, Dean D. Prevalence of multiple chronic conditions in the United States' Medicare population. *Health Qual Life Outcomes.* 2009;7(1):82.

Vogeli C, Shields AE, Lee TA, et al. Multiple chronic conditions: prevalence, health consequences, and implications for quality, care management, and costs. *J Gen Intern Med.* 2007;22(Suppl 3):391–395.

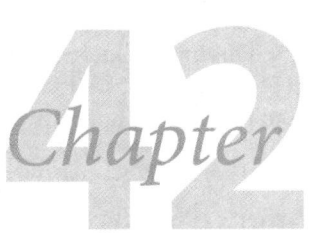

Chapter 42

Frailty

Luigi Ferrucci, Jeremy D. Walston

INTRODUCTION

Over the past century, the science of clinical medicine, the identification of risk factors for disease states, and the discovery of specific pathophysiologic mechanisms have greatly improved treatment and preventive strategies and increased longevity around the world. From 1900 to 2013, and in spite of the aging of the population, the percentage of the population who died every year fell from 2.5% to 0.7% and life expectancy at birth rose from 47 to 79 years. Death rates have been strongly affected by improvement in living conditions, availability of energy and clean water, and later on by smoking reduction, treatment of hyperlipidemia and hypertension, and to some extent progress in medicine. For example, heart disease death rates declined by almost two-thirds during the past 50 years, and stroke rates declined by more than three-quarters (http://www.cdc.gov). In spite of the relative success in the early detection of major diseases, the current approach remains "watch and wait" and then intervene to manage the symptoms of many chronic diseases. As a consequence, the mortality of chronic disease patients declined, and many older adults live into a period of life characterized by disease-related multimorbidity and disability (see Chapter 2).

Geriatrics is the medical specialty that first developed the concept that a specific disease diagnosis or an assemblage of diagnoses could not encompass the substantial heterogeneity and complexity of the health problems of many older patients. Knowing the diseases and their clinical stage is not enough to explain presence and severity of physical and cognitive limitations. Prompt diagnosis and optimal care of specific diseases remain an important goal, but the criteria for the definition of "optimal care" may change substantially. There is also evidence that older people respond differently to many treatments when they are affected

Learning Objectives

- Gain perspective about the general concept of frailty in older persons.
- Understand alternative operational definitions of frailty.
- Recognize frailty in older persons.
- Understand the etiologic contributions to frailty.
- Understand clinical conditions that may impact frailty in older adults.
- Understand frailty as the final stage of processes that start early in life and are due to the progressive imbalance between damage accumulation and resilience capacity.

Key Clinical Points

1. Frailty is a syndrome often observed in older persons. It is strongly associated with a broad range of adverse outcomes, including physical and cognitive disability, increased health care utilization, and early death.

2. Although there are many operational definitions of frailty, the most widely utilized in clinical and epidemiological studies is physical frailty, which includes measures of unintentional weight loss, weakness, slow gait, exhaustion, and low activity.

3. Aging phenotypes that are closely related to frailty and late-life decline include (1)

(Continued)

imbalance in the signaling networks that maintain homeostatic equilibrium and stress responses, (2) changes in body composition, (3) imbalance between energy availability and energy demand, and (4) neurodegeneration/neuroplasticity.

4. Frailty occurs when mechanisms of resilience that reduce damage accumulation are exhausted and the potential to recover from even subliminal stresses declines.

5. The failing of resilience and the accumulation of damage are associated with a chronic proinflammatory state.

6. Frailty can be conceptualized as a final common outcome of accelerated aging processes.

7. Frailty ascertainment is essential to optimize medical and surgical treatment of older persons who may be vulnerable to related adverse outcomes.

8. The paradigm of precision medicine provides an ideal entry point for frailty measurement into clinical medicine.

by multimorbidity, disability, and geriatric syndromes, although mechanisms for such differential response are still not understood. In other words, to understand and potentially improve the health of their patients, geriatricians should complement their knowledge of internal medicine with sound theory about how multimorbidity, frailty, and functional and cognitive impairment affect prognosis, response to treatments, care needs, and quality of life. As the recognition of rising burden that the aging of the population imposes on people, families, the health care system, and the society as a whole, we have started asking whether the burden imposed by aging was unavoidable or, at least to some extent, could be prevented or "compressed." In this chapter, we describe the concept of "frailty" as relevant both in the assessment and care of older patients as well as a "state of reference" in the science aimed at identifying individuals who are aging faster than others and at developing interventions that slow down aging and prevents its consequences.

FROM COMPREHENSIVE GERIATRIC ASSESSMENT TO FRAILTY

Historically, a major focus of geriatric medicine has been to conceptually capture the complexity of older patients and develop standard tools for measuring it. This effort has demonstrated unequivocally that health status in older

patients is best measured by the ability to function in the environment and that functional status provides powerful prognostic information on multiple adverse health outcomes independent of disease status. An array of large epidemiologic studies provided robust evidence that even minor declines in physical function are associated with substantial deterioration of quality of life, are good metrics of disease severity progression, are more accurate and predictive than traditional organ-specific measures, and provide prognostic information for multiple health-related outcomes, including health care resources utilization, progression of disability, and mortality. This bulk of knowledge created the premises for the conceptualization of frailty as a status of susceptibility that is related to diseases, but evolves independently.

FRAILTY CONCEPTUAL DEVELOPMENT AND THE "LAYERS" OF FRAILTY

Most health care professionals recognize that there are complexities that are unique to geriatric patients. Despite extensive research with a focus on the development of functional assessment tools and overall functional status, there is still a vacuum of knowledge about the complexity of aging and its relationship with diseases and disability. Understanding physical and cognitive function is clearly important, but this understanding often does not provide clear and specific paths to interventions. Furthermore, since addressing each single disease does not necessarily require information on functional status, ouside the world of geriatric assessment functional status has often been ignored.

Although there is a broad awareness that recognizing diseases is a necessary component of clinical care, there is also evidence that making a diagnosis is not enough to infer prognosis or expected response to treatments and to fully understand health and functional status of older patients. The conceptualization and operationalization of frailty is an attempt to capture the missing components of deteriorating health status that are often overlooked in the traditional medical approach based on disease diagnoses, in order to find the most vulnerable subset of older adults and ultimately develop treatment strategies that can improve their conditions.

It is often argued that clinicians can easily recognize frail older persons when they see and interact with them. This assumption was examined by a formal multistage Delphi process conducted between 2011 and 2012 that asked a large number of geriatricians, health care providers, and experts to identify the critical characteristics that define a frail older person. Not unexpectedly, results were mixed. The majority of participants agreed that frailty should be (1) considered a clinical syndrome that involves multiple physiologic systems, (2) characterized by decreased reserve and impaired ability to respond to stress, and (3) useful in different settings to identify individuals at high risk of developing adverse health outcomes. However, there was very little agreement on a specific set of clinical measurements and laboratory biomarkers useful for diagnosis. Because of the lack of clarity and the need to determine whether there was sufficient information available to justify systematic screening for frailty, a consensus conference was convened in December 2012. The project was endorsed by experts from six major international scientific societies and included the participation of other independent top experts in the field. Consistent with the previous experience, a construct of frailty emerged as a "medical syndrome with multiple causes and contributors characterized by diminished strength, endurance, and reduced physiologic function that increases an individual's vulnerability for developing increased dependency and/or death." There was consensus that because frailty screening is particularly important to identify individuals at risk of disability, the definitions of frailty and disability should not overlap and that frailty cannot be exhaustively defined by the presence of sarcopenia or multimorbidity. The published report from the conference supported screening for frailty in all individuals 70 and older using some of the operational criteria developed and validated. However, the rationale provided in support of population screening was less than robust as there are still no follow-up recommendations to be made to frail individuals. Indeed, at the current time, there is no strong evidence that frailty can be prevented, although observational studies have suggested that following a Mediterranean style diet and being physical active are associated with lower risk of developing frailty. Also, no randomized controlled trial has yet demonstrated that frailty and its consequences on health and function can be reversed. The lack of this information is likely the most important obstacle to the introduction of frailty in routine assessment of older persons.

Specific guidelines on how the presence of frailty should modify treatment strategies are now being published and endorsed by diverse medical societies: surgery, diabetes, pain management, renal and cardiac failure, oncology, pulmonary diseases, and many others. Almost surprisingly, the practice of frailty assessment is being incorporated into the clinical evaluation of these specialties more than in general geriatrics, perhaps because evidence-based general clinical guidelines of management and treatment of frailty have not yet appeared.

Starting from the consensus conclusions above, the complexity of typical frail patients can be conceptualized by considering their features in concentric layers, like the layers of an onion (**Figure 42-1**). The first layer is the clinical presentation characterized by *multimorbidity, impaired physical function* (including loss of mobility), *cognitive impairment,* and *mental health problems.*

These characteristics can be considered as the common beacon at the confluence of all frailty characteristics that contribute to the clinical syndrome. The clinical tools to evaluate this layer convey most of the demonstrated prognostic information for disability, mortality, and many

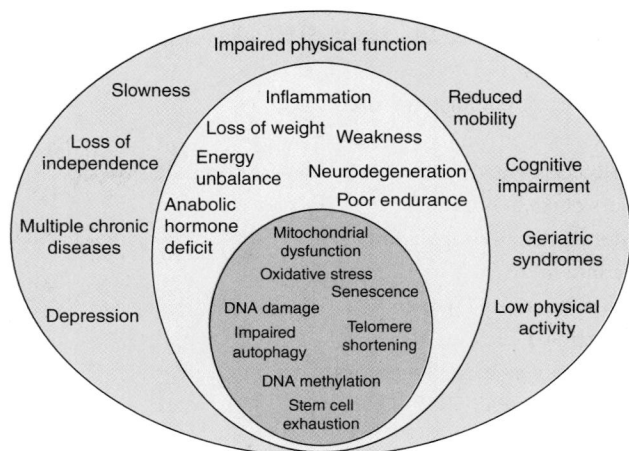

FIGURE 42-1. Frailty can be conceptualized as a construct with three overlaying dimensions, similar to layers of an onion. The clinical presentation, including cognitive and physical impairments, is in the first, most superficial layer. The second layer includes a number of hypothetical pathophysiologic mechanisms and can also be considered as the "area of biomarkers." The third, most inner layer includes the biological mechanisms that are hypothesized to be primary causes of frailty. (Reproduced with permission from Ferrucci and Fabbri, unpublished data.)

other adverse health outcomes. Examples are *walking speed, poor lower extremity performance, reduced physical activity, reduced muscle strength, poor memory, number of diseases, number of drug treatments,* and many others. Part of this first layer is also a dynamic dimension that is clinically observable, characterized by *reduced functional reserve, impaired resilience* to a number of stresses, and *delayed and incomplete recovery* after homeostatic perturbations, health instability, and impending deterioration of health and functional status.

Older patients who come to the observation of geriatricians often present these characteristics. In spite of medical treatment aimed at promoting recovery and stabilization, many patients show a spiral of progressive health deterioration with a wide range of clinical features, as listed in **Table 42-1**. Such patients may already have or soon develop one or more "geriatric syndromes" (see subsequent Chapters 43–48). It can be quite useful to consider the geriatric syndromes as an overt manifestation of different combinations of the aging phenotypes.

The next, second layer closer to the frailty core could be defined as the "area of biomarkers" and departs from a purely descriptive interpretation of frailty by providing some information on possible mechanisms. Frailty includes impairments across multiple physiologic systems and organs: (1) muscle mass and strength are reduced and fat mass increased beyond what is expected from aging alone, and these changes may be accompanied by extreme bone fragility; (2) level of fitness is poor and accompanied by altered resting metabolic rate due in part to change in body composition and in the most severe cases to impaired

TABLE 42-1 ■ CHARACTERISTICS OF FRAILTY

Increased vulnerability
Reduced physiologic reserves
Decreased resistance to stressors
Reduced capacity to maintain internal homeostasis
Loss of resilience
Multisystem dysregulation
Failure to thrive
Accumulation of deficits
Functional decline
Dependence in daily activities
Impaired mobility
Disability
Comorbidity
Cognitive impairment
Poor health function
Poor psychological functioning
Depression
Unintentional weight loss
Sarcopenia/muscle wasting
Weakness
Low strength
Slow motor performance
Slow walking speed
Decreased balance
Low energy expenditure
Low physical activity
Low fitness
Poor endurance
Exhaustion
Gait abnormality
Impaired vibration sense tremor
Vision and/or hearing deficits

oxidative capacity and reduced energetic efficiency, which likely contribute to fatigue and reduced mobility; and (3) some homeostatic mechanisms/stress response systems are impaired, show low reserve and reduced ability to respond to perturbation, and have reduced ability to recover a stable level of equilibrium (described in detail in Chapter 39). Perhaps the most pervasive homeostatic dysregulation feature is the development of a proinflammatory state, demonstrated by chronically elevated levels of cytokines and associated with blunted immune responses to vaccination and/or to infection, thereby predisposing to infections. The etiology of the age-related proinflammatory state is complex and not completely understood (see discussion later in this chapter). Kidney function in frailty is often substantially impaired beyond normal aging changes. Anemia and malnutrition are also prominent features. Broad involvement of the nervous system (including central, peripheral, and autonomic components) likely plays an important role in the physical and

cognitive manifestations of frailty. Frailty is associated with leukoaraiosis as well as micro- and macroischemic lesions in the white matter on brain imaging, longer reaction time, and reduced performance in dual tasks that involve both cognitive and physical challenges. There is motor neuron loss and fragmentation of the neuromuscular junction, which probably contributes to sarcopenia and poor mobility. Impaired orthostatic hemodynamics, heart rate control, and reduced intestinal peristalsis are signs of autonomic dysfunction. While many studies have considered relationships of frailty with single physiologic and pathologic features, the constant involvement of multiple physiologic systems in frailty suggests that most of them are driven by some unifying cause, perhaps an acceleration of the same mechanisms that at the molecular and cellular level account for the phenotypic manifestations of aging.

In parallel to the conceptual development of frailty as a clinical entity with profound functional consequences and poor prognosis, its biological basis is being investigated. The biological basis of frailty represents the deeper, third layer of the onion-like frailty syndrome model, which is mechanistic and still largely hypothetical. Attempts to understand the core mechanisms of frailty provide the basis for making a connection between the biology of aging and the experience of geriatric practice. As explained in Chapter 40, the geroscience hypothesis is that accelerated aging-related biological processes ("hallmarks of aging") drive the accumulation of tissue and organ damage across many physiologic systems that eventually leads the development of the aging-related phenotype including frailty and other geriatric syndromes. The identification of these mechanisms and the development of pathophysiological changes is at the front edge of the science of frailty and ultimately has strong potential for translation. Interestingly, most of the "hallmarks of aging" may trigger an inflammatory response. For example, senescent cells produce large quantities of proinflammatory cytokines and chemokines that appear in the circulation. Unrepaired DNA damage causes genomic instability that further precipitates cellular senescence. Damaged mitochondria not eliminated and recycled due to defective mitophagy can trigger both the production of interleukin 1 (IL-1) and IL-18 through the NLP3 inflammasome and type I interferons through the stimulator of interferon genes (STING) signaling pathway. Because of this connection, it has been proposed that "inflammaging" is a global biomarker of the mechanisms involved in the biology of aging.

FROM SPECULATION TO PRACTICE: OPERATIONAL DEFINITIONS OF FRAILTY

Functional assessment attempts to assess and track the consequences of physiologic declines that occur with aging and to characterize the consequences regardless of the causes and mostly for management purposes.

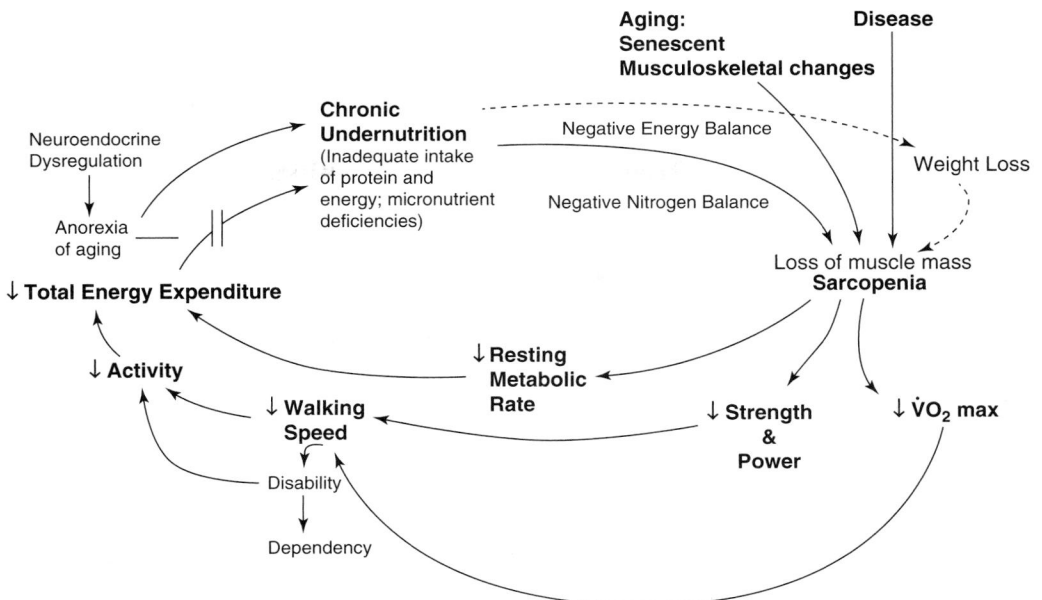

FIGURE 42-2. Schematic representation of the pathologic vicious cycle proposed to lead to a progressive decline in health and function according to the physical frailty model. (Reproduced with permission from Fried LP, Tangen CM, Walston J, et al. Frailty in older adults: evidence for a phenotype. *J Gerontol A Biol Sci Med Sci.* 2001;56[3]:M146–M156.)

In contrast, the concept of frailty implies the existence of underlying pathophysiologic mechanisms responsible for the phenotypical manifestations. Although different interpretative frameworks for frailty have been developed, with different operational criteria, most connect frailty directly or indirectly with the biology of aging. In summary, individuals become frail when their residual resilience capacity can no longer cope with the simple stress of being alive. This is the reason why frailty can rapidly progress and is associated with very high risk of disability and mortality.

FRAILTY AS A SYNDROME OR PHENOTYPE

The operational model of frailty developed by Linda Fried and others working in the Cardiovascular Health Study (CHS) hypothesized the existence of an identifiable phenotype of frailty and has been supported by a large body of strong methodological work. According to this model, frailty is the result of dysregulation of the stress response systems responsible for organismal resilience, leading to loss of homeostatic capabilities, increased susceptibility to stress, and the emergence of a distinct syndromic phenotype that is predictive of a range of adverse clinical outcomes. The syndromic attribution to frailty in CHS was later validated by the Women's Health and Aging Study, and implies that the criteria used for the clinical definition are not exhaustive of the syndrome but rather represent biomarkers that in the aggregate allow for the identification of a group of subjects likely to be affected by the intended condition with some level of sensitivity and specificity.

In describing their theoretical construct of frailty, the authors of the frailty index consider the diagnostic criteria as the milestones of a pathologic vicious cycle of declining energetics and reserve that leads to a progressive decline in health and function. The visual representation of this cycle has become part of the background culture in geriatrics and gerontology (**Figure 42-2**). The updated model has helped to facilitate the testing of biological hypotheses related to frailty and other adverse health outcomes often observed in older adults (**Figure 42-3**). This evolution toward a deeper biological and etiologic understanding remains key to progress in this field.

Thus, the defining elements of frailty represent both the diagnostic criteria for the syndrome and the core features of its pathophysiology. In particular, the phenotype of frailty was defined by five characteristics (**Table 42-2**): unintentional weight loss, weakness, exhaustion, slowness, and low activity.

Those individuals who meet at least three of the five criteria are considered frail, while those individuals who meet two criteria out of five are considered as prefrail. Of note, the presence of one criterion alone may constitute a risk factor but does not represent frailty itself, because frailty is considered a multisystemic syndrome. Using this operational definition, the severity of frailty is associated with risk for disability and loss of independence, even in the absence of an acute precipitant. In addition, frailty is associated with the presence of specific chronic diseases, particularly those with an inflammatory etiology, and patients with chronic multimorbidity are likely to be frail or have high risk of developing frailty. While frailty incidence

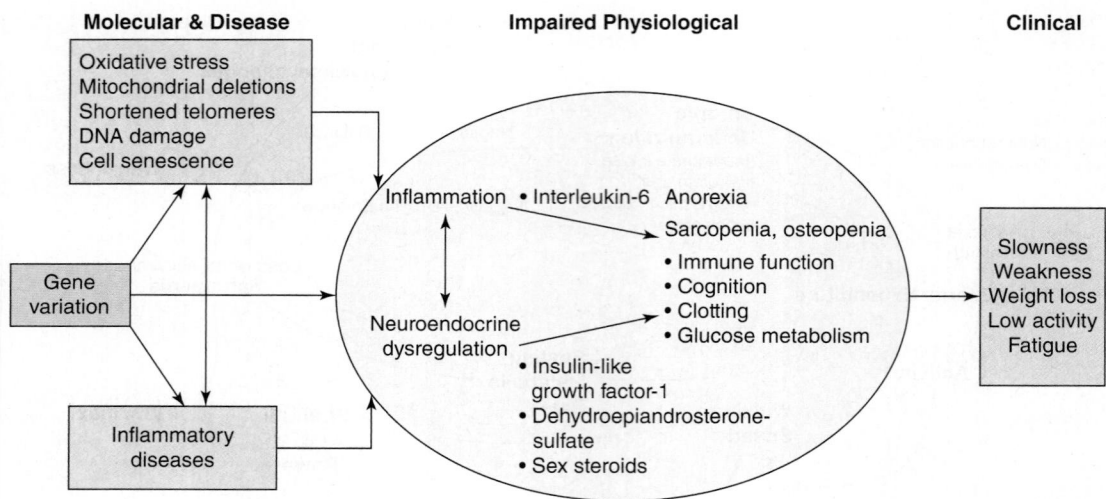

Molecular & Disease   **Impaired Physiological**   **Clinical**

FIGURE 42-3. A model pathway of physical frailty derived from the cycle presented in **Figure 42-2** that links biology and disease to physiology and signs and symptoms of physical frailty. (Reproduced with permission from Walston J, Hadley EC, Ferrucci L, et al. Research agenda for frailty in older adults: toward a better understanding of physiology and etiology: summary from the American Geriatrics Society/National Institute on Aging Research Conference on Frailty in Older Adults. *J Am Geriatr Soc.* 2006;54[6]:991–1001.)

rises with increasing age independent of chronic diseases, the association with such chronic diseases, including cardiovascular, kidney, and rheumatologic diseases, suggests that there may be both a primary, aging-related frailty and a phenotype of frailty that is secondary to chronic disease or jointly related to a shared etiology.

The phenotypic approach to frailty is appealing because it can be assessed easily and quickly using the Physical Frailty Phenotype, per **Table 42-3**, and also because it is based on a solid pathophysiologic model that highlights opportunities for interventions. However, this approach to frailty also has a few drawbacks. The first problem is the lack of a specific cognitive dimension, which is in contrast with the clinical experience that cognitive impairment often accompanies frailty. Indeed, the subgroup of older patients who experience "dual" decline of mobility and cognition appear to be at very high risk of developing functional decline and disability. A second problem is the inclusion of weight loss in the syndrome. Unexplained weight loss is a strong biomarker of health decline with aging. However, given the increasing prevalence of obesity, a sarcopenic-obesity variant of frailty is becoming more and more frequent, and this variant may be missed by the weight loss criterion. Third, the threshold selected for the definition of some of the criteria are based on distributions in the CHS population, which may not be fully representative of all clinical populations in the United States. Despite these limitations, this definition of frailty has proven to be a useful tool both for research and clinical applications, and it has been adapted for many studies and uses. Examples of the many successful applications are given later in this chapter.

FRAILTY AS A DEFICIT ACCUMULATION

Another major school of thought that has been a mainstream in frailty research is the approach developed by Ken Rockwood and colleagues. In this approach, frailty is considered an accumulation of illnesses, signs, symptoms, and laboratory abnormalities, based on the observation that "the more things individuals have wrong with them, the higher the likelihood that they will be frail." Using data from two population-based Canadian studies, Rockwood and his collaborators combined a series of 70 measurements (jointly referred to as "deficits") in order to generate a multisystem, broad, graded, and conceptually simple

TABLE 42-2 ■ CRITERIA FOR FRAILTY SYNDROME ACCORDING TO FRIED AND COLLEAGUES	
CHARACTERISTICS OF FRAILTY	**CARDIOVASCULAR HEALTH STUDY MEASURE**
1. Weight loss (unintentional)/sarcopenia (loss of muscle mass)	> 10 lb lost unintentionally in prior year
2. Weakness	Grip strength: lowest 20% (by gender, body mass index)
3. Exhaustion/poor endurance	"Exhaustion" (self-report)
4. Slowness	Walking time/15 ft: slowest 20% (by gender, height)
5. Low activity	kcal/wk: lowest 20% males: < 383 kcal/wk; females: < 270 kcal/wk

Adapted with permission from Fried LP, Tangen CM, Walston J, et al. Frailty in older adults: evidence for a phenotype. J Gerontol A Biol Sci Med Sci. 2001;56(3):M146–M156.

TABLE 42-3 ■ SUMMARY OF FRAILTY TOOLS

INSTRUMENT	PUBLICATION(S)	DOMAINS/ITEMS	SCORING
Physical Frailty Phenotype	Fried et al, *J Gerontol*, 2001	Physical function (gait speed, grip strength), physical activity, weight loss, and exhaustion	Score range: 0–5 Frail = ≥ 3 criteria present Intermediate/prefrail = 1–2 criteria present Robust/nonfrail = 0 criteria present
Deficit Accumulation Index or Frailty Index (FI)	Mitnitski et al, *The Scientific World*, 2001; Mitnitski et al, *J Gerontol Med Sci*, 2004; Rockwood et al, *J Am Geriatr Soc*, 2006; Rockwood et al, *J Gerontol Med Sci*, 2007a; Rockwood et al, *J Gerontol Med Sci*, 2007b	Diseases, activities of daily living (ADLs), health attitudes/values, and symptoms/signs from clinical and neurologic examinations	Number of deficits present and divided by the number of deficits taken into consideration Higher proportion equates to a higher level of frailty Number of deficits may vary
Gill Frailty Measure	Gill et al, *N Engl J Med*, 2002	Physical function (gait speed, chair stand)	Moderately frail if rapid gait speed back and forth over 10-ft course is > 10 s; or could not stand from the chair. Severely frail if meet both criteria
Edmonton Frail Scale (EFS)	Rolfson et al, *Age Ageing*, 2006	9 domains: cognition, general health status, functional independence, social support, medication use, nutrition, mood, continence, and functional performance	Score range: 0–17 (higher = more frail)
Clinical Frailty Scale (CFS)	Rockwood et al, *CMAJ*, 2005	Clinical judgment from very fit to severely frail: 1 = Very fit—robust, active, energetic, well motivated, and fit; these people commonly exercise regularly and are in the most fit group for their age; 2 = Well—without active disease, but less fit than people in category 1; 3 = Well, with treated comorbid disease—disease symptoms are well controlled compared with those in category 4; 4 = Apparently vulnerable—although not frankly dependent, these people commonly complain of being "slowed up" or have disease symptoms; 5 = Mildly frail—with limited dependence on others for instrumental activities of daily living; 6 = Moderately frail—help is needed with both instrumental and noninstrumental activities of daily living; 7 = Severely frail—completely dependent on others for the activities of daily living, or terminally ill	Physician assigns score of 1–7 based on clinical judgment Physicians making the initial assessment given access to diagnoses and assessments related to these variables and other measures of comorbidity, function, and associated features that inform clinical judgments about the severity of frailty A secondary review and scoring performed by a multidisciplinary team

(Continued)

PART III

GERIATRIC CONDITIONS

TABLE 42-3 ■ SUMMARY OF FRAILTY TOOLS (CONTINUED)

INSTRUMENT	PUBLICATION(S)	DOMAINS/ITEMS	SCORING
Brief Frailty Instrument	Rockwood et al, *Lancet*, 1999	Four levels of classification, representing fitness to frailty: 0 = Those who walk without help, perform basic activities of daily living (eating, dressing, bathing, bed transfers), are continent of bowel and bladder, and are not cognitively impaired 1 = Bladder incontinence only 2 = One (two if incontinent) or more of needing assistance with mobility or activities of daily living, has cognitive impairment with no dementia (CIND), or has bowel or bladder incontinence 3 = Two (three if incontinent) or more of totally dependent for transfers or one or more activities of daily life, incontinent of bowel and bladder, and diagnosis of dementia	Higher classification means higher grade of frailty
Vulnerable Elders Survey (VES-13)	Saliba et al, *J Am Geriatr Soc*, 2001	Age, self-rated health, physical function, and ADL/IADL disability	Score range: 0–10 Frail = score ≥ 3
FRAIL Scale	Abellan Van Kan, *J Nutr Health Aging*, 2008; Abellan Van Kan, *J Am Med Dir Assoc*, 2008	Fatigue, physical function (resistance: ability to climb a single flight of stairs; and ambulation: ability to walk one block), illnesses (more than 5), weight loss (more than 5%)	Score range 0–5 No frailty = 0 deficits Intermediate frailty = 1 or 2 deficits Frailty = 3 or more deficits

Adapted with permission from Buta BJ, Walston JD, Godino JG, et al. Frailty assessment instruments: systematic characterization of the uses and contexts of highly-cited instruments. Ageing Res Rev. 2016;26:53–61.

tool into the Deficit Accumulation Index, usually referred to as the Frailty Index (FI). This approach conceptualizes frailty as a stochastic accumulation of structural and functional deficits in almost any physiologic system or organ and operationalizes it as a simple unweighted count of the number of deficits. The FI, in particular, is the ratio of the deficits present in a person to the total number of deficits considered. Therefore, according to this definition, it is the proportion of all potential deficits considered for a given person rather than their specific nature or combination that best expresses the likelihood and the severity of frailty. The FI and multiple shorter versions of the original FI have most often been used as a means of assessing individual aging and risk of mortality as described below.

The FI has a strong face validity; it shows an age-specific, nonlinear increase (similar to Gompertz law), higher values in females, strong associations with adverse outcomes (eg, mortality), and a universal limit to its increase (at FI ~ 0.7). This approach is reproducible and highly correlates with mortality, but it is unwieldy for clinical use because of the large number of variables that need to be collected. Therefore, Rockwood and collaborators developed a much simpler approach, the seven-category Clinical Frailty Scale (CFS), based on the clinician's overall impression. The CFS has similar predictive power to FI for institutionalization and death. The seven CFS categories are described in **Table 42-3**. The CFS mixes items such as comorbidity, cognitive impairment, and disability that other groups separate in focusing on physical frailty.

The FI approach has several attractive features but some drawbacks as well. First, as a prognostic tool, the FI is a sensitive predictor of adverse health outcomes, in part because it includes multiple related factors known to share causal relationships with adverse outcomes. The clinical version of the FI is very direct and intuitive, and shorter versions of FI can be generated quickly from medical records. The stochastic approach of the FI approximates the idea of aging as a rise in entropy, which makes intuitive sense and is supported by a wealth of research data and solid mathematical models. Because of the flexibility of the criteria used for definition, the FI can be operationalized widely, which explains in part its increasing popularity. Indeed, the FI is one of the strongest predictors of dementia development and predicts the risk of COVID-19 infection and mortality, both in nursing homes as well as in patients admitted to intensive care units (ICUs).

However, the purely stochastic nature of the FI definition of frailty limits any link with biological mechanisms. This and the lack of a focused list of measures make the development of specific mechanistic, biological, and intervention development studies needed to move toward focused clinical strategies more challenging. Finally, the FI, even with multilevel variables, is still based on the assumption of equality of deficits, although that does not appear to limit its clinical value of predicting adverse outcomes.

The Edmonton Frail Scale (EFS) is a clinical tool for the assessment of frailty now used widely. The EFS was developed for clinicians who have limited time but want to evaluate frailty in their practice even though they may not have specialized geriatric training. The EFS assesses nine domains: cognition, general health status, functional independence, social support, medication use, nutrition, mood, continence, and functional performance. The EFS provides information on frailty and vulnerability that is organized into domains that are consistent with a comprehensive geriatric assessment. The EFS has been validated against many other screening tools, such as the Mini Mental State Examination and the Geriatric Depression Scale, in hospitalized older patients.

OTHER OPERATIONAL DEFINITIONS OF FRAILTY

There are many other operational definitions of frailty beyond the ones described above, although most of them arise from the already discussed concepts. The most relevant operational definitions are summarized in **Table 42-3**. The wide variety and number of published tools document the very lively discussion in the field about the definition and interpretation of frailty, which has occupied many hours in meetings, workshops, and roundtables.

A NOVEL APPROACH: FRAILTY AS AGE-RELATED BIOLOGICAL DECLINE

While agreement on an operational definition of frailty is very important for translational purpose, until the pathophysiology of frailty is fully understood, operational definitions of frailty should be considered temporary and amenable to change. Importantly, the theoretical discussion and research on the biological and mechanistic origin of frailty does not completely depend on a specific operational definition. We recently proposed an agnostic approach, which assumes that frailty is, in fact, a syndrome of accelerated aging and, therefore, phenotypes of aging as well as frailty can be identified as those physiologic dimensions that change with aging in all humans and, perhaps, in all living organisms. For example, the risk of developing a clinical disease such as coronary artery disease (CAD) increases with aging but not all individuals develop CAD. Therefore, CAD cannot be considered a phenotype of aging. On the other hand, percent body fat, especially visceral fat, increases with aging in all individuals and, therefore, increased visceral fat could be considered a phenotype of aging.

Based on these assumptions, we proposed that the phenotypes of aging can be clustered in discrete interactive domains, whose impairments are pervasive across body systems and, therefore, can serve as proxy measures of the rate of aging. In particular, we identified four main "aging phenotypes" that we hypothesize are closely related

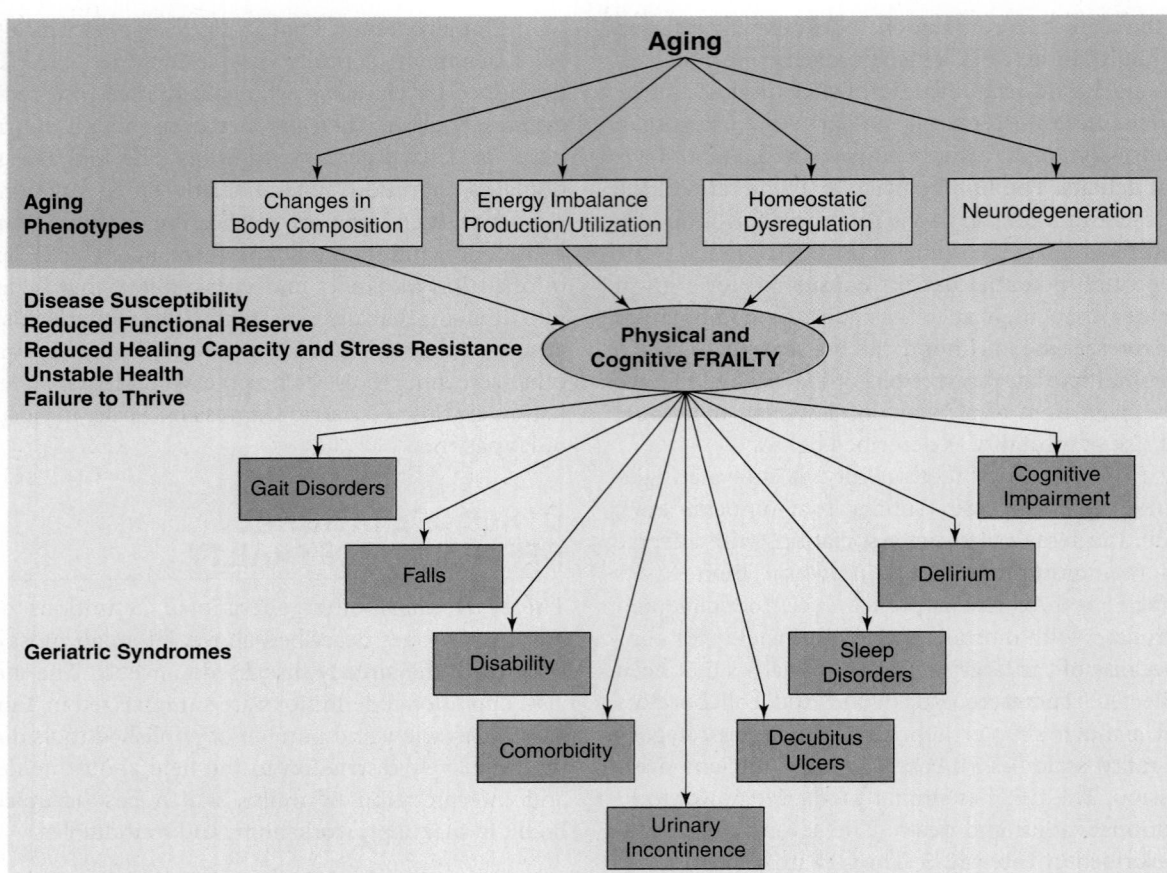

FIGURE 42-4. Schematic representation of the domains of the aging phenotype and their relationship with frailty and multiple downstream geriatric syndromes. (Reproduced with permission from Longo DL, Fauci AS, Kasper DL, et al. *Harrison's Principles of Internal Medicine.* 18th ed. New York, NY: McGraw Hill; 2012.)

to frailty and late-life decline: (1) signaling networks that maintain homeostasis; (2) body composition; (3) balance between energy availability and energy demand; and (4) neurodegeneration/neuroplasticity, whose changes occur in parallel in all aging individuals and are strongly intercorrelated (**Figure 42-4**). Extensive evidence, in fact, shows that physical frailty is associated with overt changes in these four main interacting domains regardless of its operational definition. Such conceptualization of frailty also recognizes the heterogeneity and dynamic nature of the aging process. Aging is a universal phenomenon, but the progressive multisystem instability and deterioration that characterize aging are very heterogeneous among different individuals. The conceptualization of frailty as a result of various levels of impairment in the "aging phenotypes" represents an interconnecting and dynamic interface between the clinical presentation of the syndrome (first layer of frailty in **Figure 42-1**) and its biological bases (the inner and deeper layer or biological core of frailty). This model also illustrates a causal link to the development of multiple geriatric syndromes as well as some chronic disease states, whose occurrence can be interpreted as clinical expression of alterations in specific combinations of aging phenotypes.

Signaling Networks That Maintain Homeostasis

A remarkable and pervasive biological feature of aging and frailty is the presence of a chronic and mild proinflammatory state, revealed by elevated levels of serum proinflammatory cytokines such as IL-6 and tumor necrosis factor α (TNF-α). Such a proinflammatory signature of aging, also called "inflammaging," has been described across different animal models and tissues, and is even present in individuals who are free of diseases, disabilities, and cardiovascular risk factors. Moreover, higher levels of proinflammatory biomarkers have been associated with loss of physiologic reserve and function across multiple organs and system in older adults. In addition, some of these inflammatory cytokines are known to damage tissues and organs and depress stem cell replenishment processes over time. These biomarkers are strong independent predictors of adverse health outcomes including multiple chronic diseases, disability, hospitalization, and mortality. More details on the proinflammatory state of aging are provided in Chapter 3.

Another important mechanism that connects the biology of aging with inflammation and frailty is cellular senescence. Cells that undergo different types of stress express mediators that cause arrest of replication, probably as a cancer avoidance mechanism, and secrete large amounts of immune modulators, growth factors, proteases, microRNA, DNA fragments, and other bioactive molecules, which are collectively named the senescence-associated secretory phenotype. Studies in animal models have demonstrated that the removal of senescent cells is allocated with the delayed phenotypic aging, and randomized controlled trials of senolytic drugs (drugs that selectively remove senescent cells) to prevent a number of geriatric conditions, including components of frailty, are now in the field. The accumulation of senescent cells in multiple tissues and the spilling of Senescence Associated Secretory Phenotype (SASP) molecules in the circulation may account, at least in part, for the high circulating levels of inflammatory markers in older persons. Indeed, recent studies that use assay methods that detect the concentrations of thousands of proteins in the circulation have found that many of the proteins whose concentration increases with aging are SASP proteins.

An additional and relevant characteristic of the aging process is the occurrence of complex and profound hormonal changes, including a decline in multiple anabolic hormone concentrations (dehydroepiandrosterone sulfate [DHEAS], testosterone, estrogens, growth hormone [GH]/insulin-like growth factor 1 [IGF-1], and vitamin D), with a relative preservation of catabolic hormones (thyroid hormones, cortisol). A single hormonal alteration, in fact, is unusual in older persons and usually is a sign of a specific impending disease. More often, aging individuals experience a complex "multiple hormonal dysregulation," characterized by simultaneous and synergistic mild multiple anabolic hormonal deficiencies, which may be an important contributor to progressive loss of resilience and high vulnerability in older adults. Multihormonal dysregulation has also been associated with the development of numerous geriatric conditions, including sarcopenia and cognitive decline as well as high risk of disability, comorbidity, and mortality.

Body Composition

Aging is also characterized by major changes in body composition that negatively affect metabolism and functional status. These changes contribute to impaired mobility, disability, and other adverse health outcomes in older adults. Details regarding the age-related decline of lean body (ie, muscle) mass and muscle strength and increase of fat mass, especially visceral and intermuscular fat, are provided in Chapter 30. After the age of 70, fat-free mass and fat mass tend to decrease in parallel, with consequent decreasing weight. The decrease in muscle strength exceeds what is expected on the basis of the decline in muscle mass alone, especially after the age of 60 to 70, suggesting that other factors related to muscle quality may play a major role in the decline in muscle strength and physical function in older adults. The causes of these changes are not completely known but several lines of evidence are emerging,

as described in detail in Chapter 49, Muscle Aging and Sarcopenia. There is evidence that volumetric changes in specific brain areas are associated with decline of muscle strength. Progressive muscle denervation secondary to progressive failure of the denervation/reinnervation cycle and to dysfunction of the neuromuscular junction is probably responsible for part of the decline of muscle mass and quality with aging. Furthermore, there is increased fat infiltration within the muscle, which probably results from age-related changes in body composition and includes storage of lipids in adipocytes located between the muscle fibers (also termed intramuscular fat) and between muscle groups (intermuscular fat) as well as lipids stored within the muscle cells themselves (intramyocellular lipids). This fat infiltration is thought to be largely responsible for the deterioration of muscle quality, impaired muscle force production, and mobility decline in older adults. Interestingly, visceral and intramuscular adipocytes are among the cell types most likely to become senescencent and produce proinflammatory moleculles that contribute to a proinflammatory phenotype local and systemic often seen in frail older adults. Another focus has been on energy availability. The muscle tissues are highly energetically demanding, with energy consumption raising as much as 100-fold between rest and contraction. There is strong evidence that mitochondrial mass and mitochondrial function decline with aging, and lower mitochondrial function has been associated with mobility loss through the mediation of its negative impact on muscle strength. The failure of mechanisms of the maintenance and repair of damaged muscle fibers, mainly due to the limited energy and reduced regenerative capacity of satellite cells (stem cells resident in muscle tissue) may be particularly important in late life when continued and intensive repair is require because of the rapid accumulation of damage. Again, chronic inflammation and specifically chronic elevations in the cytokine IL-6 may be driving some of these events. Overall, the decline in muscle mass and muscle strength with aging plays a critical role in the development of the frailty syndrome.

Balance Between Energy Availability and Energy Demand

Although the idea that longevity and health are linked to energy metabolism was introduced over a century ago, the role of energy metabolism in human aging and chronic diseases is still not fully understood. As described earlier, Fried and colleagues conceptualized frailty as a vicious cycle of declining energetics and reserves. Indeed, the integrity of energetic metabolism is a prerogative for successful aging because resilience strategies at the biological and phenotypic level require substantial amounts of energy to be effective. In fact, the degenerative processes that characterize aging occur when organisms lose the ability to produce the extra energy required for resilience. From this perspective, lack of energy could be the root causes of progressively higher morbidity and mortality with aging.

Resting metabolic rate (RMR) is the energy required to maintain structural and functional homeostasis at physical rest, in fasting and neutral conditions. RMR reflects, at least in part, the energy used continuously to cope with damage accumulation through repair, recycling, or novel biogenesis of molecules or organelles.

RMR accounts for 60% to 70% of the total daily energy expenditure and can be assessed by indirect calorimetry. RMR normalized by body size declines rapidly from birth up to the end of the third decade, and then continues to decline more slowly from adulthood until death, mostly but not completely, as a consequence of the age-related loss of lean body mass. Consistent with the idea that high RMR reflects in part higher need for compensation and repair, in older adults higher RMR is an independent risk factor for mortality and predicts future greater burden of chronic diseases; consequently it should be considered a marker of health deterioration. Studies conducted in large samples have shown a complex relationship between RMR rate and the presence of chronic diseases. In the initial phase, RMR may be higher than expected because of the high energetic cost of compensation; however, later on as frailty develops, the production of energy becomes the limiting factor and RMR declines. An interesting hypothesis is that when this shift in RMR occurs, there is accelerated and irreversible deterioration of health. Specifically, the initial increase of RMR is a resilience mechanism that copes efficiently and effectively with internal and environmental challenges to maintain homeostatic equilibrium; however, the later decline of RMR in spite of critical stresses indicates a failure of the resilience mechanism. The maximum energy that can be produced by an organism over extended time periods, or fitness, which can be estimated from the peak oxygen consumption during a maximal treadmill test, also declines with age, as described in detail in Chapter 54, Therapeutic Exercise.

Neurodegeneration

An important biomarker of aging and frailty is the age-related degeneration of the central and peripheral nervous system. As result of these changes, declining performance in specific cognitive abilities, such as memory, processing speed, executive function, reasoning, and multitasking, is commonly experienced with aging. All of these so-called "fluid" mental abilities are important for carrying out everyday activities, living independently, and leading a fulfilling life. Interestingly, it is becoming clear that individuals who experience "dual decline" of mobility and cognitive function are at particularly high risk of dementia and other health outcomes.

Age-related changes occur also at the level of the peripheral nervous system, especially after the age of 60, with a progressive degeneration in structure and function from the spinal cord motor neuron to the neuromuscular junction. The number of motor neurons declines with aging, likely contributing to the age-related loss of muscle strength and quality. Age-related motor unit remodeling

leads to changes in fiber-type composition because denervation occurs preferentially in the fast muscle fibers with reinnervation occurring by axonal sprouting from slow fibers. As a consequence, motor units decrease in number and become progressively larger but less functional with aging, leading to reductions in fine motor control. Furthermore, the efficiency of segmental demyelination-remyelination processes declines with aging, resulting in slower nerve conduction and consequent decreased sensation as well as slower reflexes.

THE EPIDEMIOLOGY OF FRAILTY

The prevalence of frailty varies enormously among studies according to different definitions, countries, and settings. Among community-dwelling adults aged 65 and older the average prevalence is 11% (but the reported range is 4.0%–59%). Use of a broader definition of frailty results in a higher prevalence than use of the Fried tool (14% vs 10%). Moreover, prevalence of frailty increases with age, reaching 16% in individuals aged 80 to 84 and 26% in those aged 85 or older. Independent of the type of definition, the prevalence is higher in women than men (Fried Scale: 9.6% vs 5.2%; FI: 39% vs 37%). The relationship between frailty and body mass index (BMI) is U-shaped, with higher rates of frailty in individuals at both low and very high BMI. The prevalence of frailty has varied from 27% to 80% in older hospitalized patients and from 30% to 70% in institutionalized older adults. Using the CHS definition, exhaustion seems to be the criterion that contributes most to frailty status and most likely to appear first, followed by the other criteria.

The clinical relevance of frailty is mainly due to its being an important predictor of serious adverse outcomes, such as disability, health care utilization, and death. A linear relationship between mortality rate and frailty as accumulation of deficits has also been demonstrated. In addition, physical frailty indicators are strong predictors of disability in activities of daily living in community-dwelling older people. Slow gait speed and low physical activity/exercise seem to be the most powerful predictors followed by weight loss, lower extremity function, balance, muscle strength, and other indicators. Moreover, increasing frailty is associated with increasing length of hospital stay, nursing home institutionalization, high health care utilization and costs, and mortality. Furthermore, frailty negatively impacts quality of life, directly or indirectly (through associated comorbidity), and prescribing drugs for these vulnerable individuals is difficult and frequently complicated by iatrogenesis.

Finally, using the Fried definition, nearly 60% of people older than age 70 have at least one transition between any two of the three frailty states over 4.5 years. Transitions to states of greater frailty are more common than to states of lesser frailty, and the probability of transitioning from being frail to nonfrail is very low. Although a person who has already entered the frail state is unlikely to transition back to no frailty, the evidence that frailty is a dynamic process in which older adults gradually progress through different frailty states suggests the opportunity for prevention.

COGNITION, DEMENTIA, AND FRAILTY

Traditionally, operationalization of frailty has been mostly focused on the physical aspects of the syndrome. However, the contribution of cognition to frailty and their complex interrelationship have been increasingly recognized. There is a higher prevalence of cognitive impairment and lower cognitive performance in frail older adults than in fit ones. Moreover, frailty increases the risk of future cognitive decline and incident dementia. As a consequence, the term "cognitive frailty" has been used to describe a clinical condition characterized by the simultaneous occurrence of both physical frailty and cognitive impairment, in the absence of a diagnosis of dementia or underlying neurologic conditions. In particular, the operational definition of cognitive frailty is based on the following criteria: (1) physical frailty; (2) mild cognitive impairment (MCI), according to the Clinical Dementia Rating (CDR, score equal to 0.5); and (3) exclusion of Alzheimer disease (AD) and other dementias. Moreover, it has been suggested that the occurrence of physical frailty should precede the onset of cognitive impairment, in order to differentiate between a physically driven cognitive decline versus a cognitive deterioration independent of physical conditions. Furthermore, frailty is a significant effect modifier in the pathway to dementia. In particular, the risk of dementia associated with accumulation of brain pathology as evidenced by neuroimaging is substantially higher in those who are frail compared to those who are not frail, although the mechanism of this synergic association is not clear. Future research in this field should better define the epidemiology and clinical presentation of this condition as well as the underlying biological and pathophysiologic pathways.

FRAILTY IN THE CONTEXT OF SPECIFIC MEDICAL CONDITIONS

The robust scientific progress generated in understanding functional status as a prognostic marker has induced other specialties to incorporate frailty into clinical decision making.

1. *Frailty to evaluate surgical risk.* Despite progress in medical and anesthesia support techniques, older surgical patients have an excess risk of postoperative adverse outcomes. The main reasons are the frequent presence of comorbid conditions and reduced functional reserve across multiple systems. In addition, surgical diseases and surgery itself are stressors that may alter physiologic homeostasis. Therefore, assessing frailty has a particular clinical relevance for older patients who are considered as candidates for surgery.

Frailty status identifies individuals who are far more likely to experience postoperative complications such as pneumonia, delirium, and urinary tract infections; have prolonged hospital stays; be discharged to nursing homes or long-term care facilities; and have higher mortality. Although surgical decision making is very challenging due to the heterogeneity of health status and level of fitness among older adults, frailty measurement tools are increasingly being applied to identify higher risk older adults. This is in part because traditional risk assessment measures have substantial limitations as they are mostly based on specific comorbid conditions or on single organ system, and they do not estimate individual physiologic reserve. "Alternative" tools, whose cornerstone is the assessment of frailty, are also emerging. One example is a multidimensional frailty score which was more useful than conventional methods for predicting outcomes in geriatric patients undergoing surgery. In addition, a modified FI strongly predicted the risk of postsurgical morbidity and mortality, suggesting that preoperative frailty assessment may improve surgical decision making.

2. *Frailty and cancer.* Emerging evidence suggests that the pathogenesis of age-related degenerative diseases and cancers may share many common denominators, in particular cellular senescence. One of the major issues facing physicians who deal with older adults with cancer is the heterogeneity of their physiologic reserve, including levels of physical and cognitive fitness. Consequently, it is difficult to predict their ability to tolerate aggressive surgical and nonsurgical treatments that may be necessary to improve their prognosis. Thus, as described in detail in Chapter 88, a comprehensive geriatric assessment is useful in the evaluation of older adults with cancer, with particular attention to functional status, presence of comorbidities, social support, cognitive status, and presence of geriatric syndromes. Even in very old patients with a diagnosis of cancer but who are apparently healthy, physically active, and cognitively intact, susceptibility to stress cannot be evaluated with traditional approaches. In these cases, the conceptual framework provided by the physical phenotype of frailty is particularly useful to estimate the risk of side effects of potentially harmful treatments and make the most appropriate choices among different treatment options. It now appears that the susceptibility to the side effects of cancer chemotherapic treatment can be estimated based on the percent of senescent cells in the circulation. This finding provides a conceptual bridge between the biology of aging and frailty.

3. *Frailty and chronic kidney disease (CKD).* Reduced renal function, even when still in the range considered "normal aging," is one of the main factors associated with unsuccessful aging. Older adults with the more severe stages of CKD are often frail individuals with reduced physiologic reserves, homeostatic

dysregulation, comorbid conditions, polypharmacy, geriatric syndromes, disability, need for institutional care, frequent hospitalization, and high mortality rate. CKD even at earlier stages has been associated with clinical manifestations of frailty. Individuals in the CHS population with CKD had a twofold risk of being frail and disabled because of disease-related conditions such as protein-energy wasting, anemia, inflammation, acidosis, and hormonal disturbances. Frailty is also extremely common among patients starting dialysis and is associated with adverse outcomes among incident dialysis patients, including higher risk of hospitalization and death. In these patients, frailty may be either a result of uremia or independent of CKD. Frail patients are started on dialysis earlier (at a higher estimated glomerular filtration rate) on average than nonfrail patients, although there are no data to suggest that frail patients derive any benefit from early initiation of dialysis either in the form of improved survival or functional status.

4. *Frailty and cardiovascular disease (CVD)*. Frailty has become a high priority in the management of CVD patients due to their increasing aging and complexity. Frailty is about three times more prevalent among persons with CVD than in those without CVD. In the CHS, frail subjects were more likely to have subclinical CVD, and subjects with subclinical CVD were more likely to have impaired physical or mental function during follow-up. Similarly, women with coronary artery disease (CAD) in the Women's Health Initiative Study were more likely to develop de novo frailty over 6 years (12% vs 5%), and the Health, Aging, and Body Composition study showed that older adults with objectively measured frailty were more likely to develop CAD events (3.6% vs 2.8% per year). **Table 42-4** lists CVD

TABLE 42-4 ■ CARDIOVASCULAR CONDITIONS WITH HIGH FRAILTY PREVALENCE AND POOR FRAILTY-RELATED OUTCOMES

- Coronary artery disease (CAD)
- Percutaneous coronary intervention (PCI)
- Aortic valve replacement (transcutaneous)
  - ↑ mortality
  - ↑ institutional care
- Heart failure
  - ↑ mortality
  - ↑ emergency department visits
  - ↑ hospitalizations
    - ↑ length of stay
    - ↓ activities of daily living
    - ↑ higher readmissions
    - ↑ mortality
- Cardiac surgery
  - ↑ postoperative mortality and morbidity
  - ↑ need for rehabilitation
  - ↑ institutional care

conditions with high frailty rates and adverse frailty-related outcomes. Thus, identifying frailty has important implications for clinical care of older patients with CVD. The assessment of frailty is particularly relevant when counseling older patients with CVD regarding their prognosis following a procedure in order to plan personalized management and treatment and increase their likelihood of positive outcomes.

5. *Frailty and diabetes*. In the CHS, both frail and prefrail subjects had higher rates of diabetes than nonfrail subjects. Furthermore, frail CHS participants were more likely to have higher glucose and insulin levels at baseline and on oral glucose tolerance testing than those who were not frail. Thus, there is no doubt that diabetes and frailty are closely interrelated, but what is uncertain is whether frailty leads to glucose disorders, glucose disorders lead to frailty, or both are casually related to other common factors. Insulin resistance predicts incident frailty, and diabetes accelerates the loss of skeletal muscle strength—an important component of frailty. Increased expression of inflammatory markers in frail older adults may negatively influence late-life glucose tolerance leading to the development of diabetes and may also have an adverse impact on the microvascular complications of diabetes.

6. *Frailty and HIV*. Patients with HIV experience accelerated aging and greater risk of frailty and difficulty with daily activities than HIV-negative people of the same age. Prevalence of frailty in younger HIV-infected individuals is similar to that in older adults, ranging from 5% to 20%. A decline in prevalence of frailty was observed with increased use of effective antiretroviral therapy. Duration of HIV infection and other markers of advanced HIV disease (CD4+ T-cell count < 350 cells/mm^3) are independently associated with the occurrence of a frailty-related phenotype. The presence of clinical AIDS, previous opportunistic illnesses, and CD4+ T-cell count less than 100 cells/mm^3 are further risk factors for HIV-related frailty. A low serum albumin, which may represent an end point of chronic low-grade inflammation from concomitant comorbidities, weight loss, and/or nutritional and metabolic disturbances, is also associated with HIV-related frailty and is an important independent predictor of death in untreated HIV-infected persons. Frail HIV-infected persons have greater comorbidities including CKD, cognitive impairment, and depression; higher rates of nonelective hospitalization; and longer inpatient admissions.

7. *Frailty and transplantation*. An increasing number of older adults are referred for and have access to organ transplantation and also are donating organs. Organ allocation systems vary by specific organ and by programmatic tendencies. For example, the lung allocation score, which includes age as a variable, grades disease severity and physiologic reserve. The Model

for End-Stage Liver Disease (MELD) predicts waitlist mortality but predicts posttransplant outcomes only at scores above 35. Although short-term outcomes are acceptable for older transplant recipients across organs, long-term outcomes differ by age. Older donor organs also have been associated with inferior long-term outcomes, for example, increased risk for graft loss. Transplant recipients are often selected based on the likelihood of successful outcomes, and age is often used as a determinant. However, comprehensive risk assessment, based on stronger predictors than age and accounting for end points such as independence and quality of life, is needed to evaluate risk versus benefit for older recipients. One prospective study of 487 patients with end-stage liver disease referred for liver transplant demonstrated that frailty, defined using the Fried criteria, is a better indicator of quality of life than severity of liver disease measured as MELD.

MULTIMORBIDITY, FRAILTY, AND OTHER GERIATRIC SYNDROMES ARE PARALLEL MANIFESTATION OF ACCELERATED AGING

As people age, they not only tend to lose their physical and cognitive integrity, but also become highly susceptible to many chronic diseases and geriatric syndromes. Indeed, the terms multimorbidity and multiple chronic conditions, the co-occurrence of at least two chronic diseases in the same person at the same time, are mainly used to refer to an age-related phenomenon, as described in detail in Chapter 41. Consistent with the ideas that aging is the root cause of chronic diseases and that the rate of biological aging is heterogeneous, in some individuals the number of chronic diseases is higher and in some others is lower than expected, which further supports the notion that aging is the main risk factor for most chronic diseases.

If frailty is the aggregation of subclinical losses of reserve across multiple physiologic systems, it is not surprising that it may present itself through different clinical manifestations such as multimorbidity, the geriatric syndromes, or the aging phenotypes that are considered part of the frailty syndrome. Attempts to operationalize frailty mainly focus on the identification of preclinical measures of high vulnerability to stressors with consequent increased risk to develop adverse outcomes, including disability, cognitive decline, multimorbidity, geriatric syndromes, and ultimately death.

Consistent with this idea, multimorbidity is strongly associated with the main clinical manifestations of frailty such as impaired physical function and cognitive decline. Multimorbidity is associated with reduced response to flu vaccination as well as with the risk of COVID-19 infection and COVID-19 mortality. In addition, multimorbidity is strongly associated with several aging phenotypes (second layer of frailty—see **Figure 42-1**). In the InCHIANTI study,

higher baseline levels and steeper increases over time of IL-6 strongly predicted accelerated longitudinal accumulation of chronic diseases in older adults. Moreover, multimorbidity was also related to higher RMR, and RMR higher than expected for a certain age, sex, and body composition predicted future greater development of chronic diseases. In addition, obesity is associated with greater burden of diseases compared to normal weight and overweight status. However, in older adults who are obese at baseline, loss of weight over time rather than gain of weight is associated with the most dramatic rise in number of chronic conditions. Thus, weight loss, which is also one of the diagnostic criteria for the physical phenotype of frailty, when it occurs in obese older adults, may represent a sign of ongoing health status deterioration and steeper accumulation of multimorbidity.

The relationship between multimorbidity and the basic biological mechanisms of frailty is still largely unexplored. Age-related pathologies once thought to be distinct from each other are now understood to share the same underlying molecular and cellular mechanisms, some of which are also the biological underpinnings of the aging process.

GEROSCIENCE AS A POSSIBLE INTERFACE BETWEEN FRAILTY AND PRECISION MEDICINE

The manifesto of geroscience (see Chapter 40) embraces the conceptual approach outlined in the onion frailty model. According to this view, slowing down aging would be considerably more effective to improve the health of older persons than addressing any disease or risk factor separately. Although biological mechanisms of aging are still poorly understood, research in animal models strongly suggests that the rate of aging can be modified and even reversed by several nonpharmacological and pharmacological interventions (see Chapter 1). Some of the hypothetical mechanisms of the biology of aging can now be tested in humans to verify whether one or more of them are related and change in parallel with frailty, thereby validating the hypothesis that they are true drivers of the aging process. While it would be difficult and prohibitively expensive to apply routinely sophisticated techniques of molecular biology to the evaluation of frail older patients, it may be possible to identify basic biomarkers that capture the biological nature of the processes at the core of frailty. These processes (illustrated in **Figure 42-5**) could be targeted for potential interventions.

High-throughput genetic and genomic biomarkers are increasingly employed to study aging and age-related medical conditions and may have value in understanding the core of frailty and translate this knowledge into clinical applications. Studies that combine measures of aging biology, such as high-throughput biomarkers and in-depth phenotyping, may create a convergence between geroscience

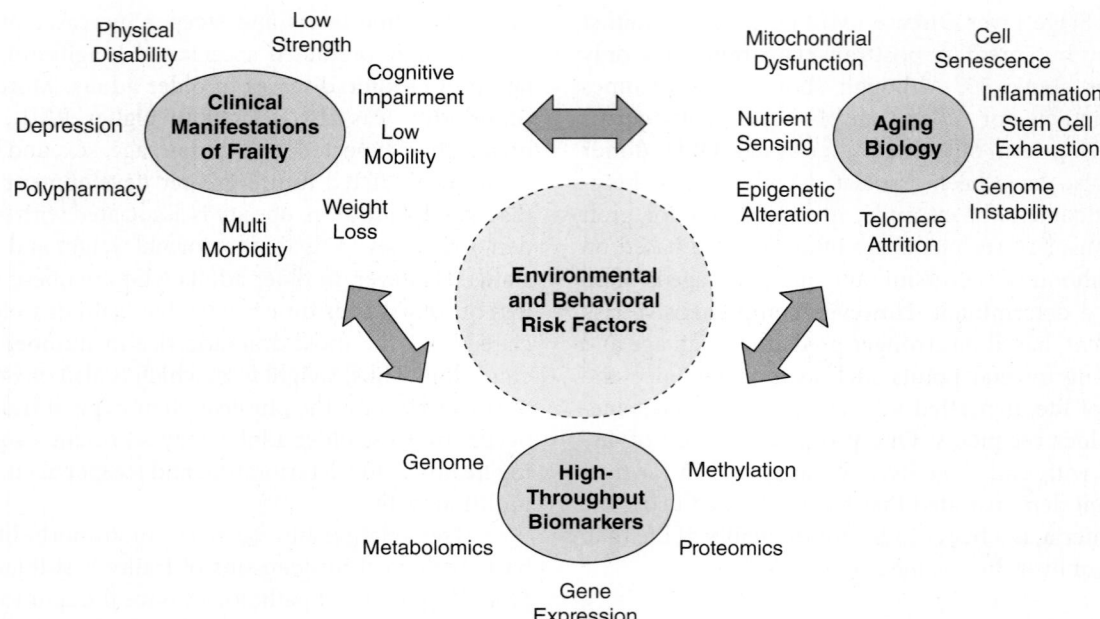

FIGURE 42-5. Potential targets of frailty-focused research aimed at understanding the relationship between accelerated aging and frailty. (Reproduced with permission from Ferrucci and Fabbri, unpublished data.)

and "precision medicine." Precision medicine assumes that individual patients can be classified into subpopulations that differ in some key biological characteristics that make them susceptible to specific medical conditions or outcomes. Preventive or therapeutic interventions could then be tailored to those patients with specific characteristics, thereby maximizing effectiveness and sparing expense and side effects. Frailty appears to result from perturbing and stressful events that act on a background predisposition leading to multisystem dysregulation. The biological mechanisms responsible for the frailty syndrome could be identified as those that are cross-sectionally and longitudinally correlated with some predefined phenotypes. The nature of these relationships might be further described by a signature biomarker set derived from genetic, gene expression, epigenetic, or proteomic biomarkers. Once these relationships have been robustly established, such methods could be used to classify patients to receive different targeted therapeutic interventions. In fact, a number of circulating proteins that are strongly associated with frailty and predict the development of frailty have been identified and replicated in separate populations. Some of these biomarkers are already proposed for clinical utilization.

The new paradigm of precision medicine provides an almost ideal entry for the frailty concept into the mainstream of modern medicine. Beyond the variety of operational

definitions, at the heart of precision medicine is the attempt to better understand the pathology in the context of the physiology of a specific individual, so that prevention and treatment strategies can be selected that account for variability across individuals. To accomplish this goal, precision medicine relies on state-of-the-art molecular profiling and the emerging ability of computational biology and systems biology to extract meaningful information from "big data." An attractive feature of precision medicine is the agnostic approach to patient subgroup classification that excludes preconceived assumptions about etiology and pathophysiology. Under the assumption that biological mechanisms underpinning the aging process are also involved in the pathophysiology of chronic diseases and frailty, namely that multimorbidity and frailty result from accelerated aging, the agnostic approach proposed by precision medicine may be able to capture their nature. Prevention and treatment strategies driven by precision medicine will have to take into account the core mechanisms of aging and, perhaps, will be able to distinguish pathologic conditions that have a unique, intrinsic pathophysiology from those that are mostly age related. To accomplish this goal, it is critical that the next-generation studies that derive the molecular signature of pathology include measures of multimorbidity and frailty and that geriatricians and gerontologists be involved in the development of these new tools.

FURTHER READING

Ferrucci L, Fabbri E. Inflammageing: chronic inflammation in ageing, cardiovascular disease, and frailty. *Nat Rev Cardiol.* 2018;15(9):505–522.

Ferrucci L, Studenski S. Clinical problems of aging. In: Longo DL, Fauci AS, Kasper DL, et al., eds. *Harrison's Principles of Internal Medicine.* 18th ed. New York, NY: McGraw Hill; 2012.

Kennedy BK, Berger SL, Brunet A, et al. Geroscience: linking aging to chronic disease. *Cell.* 2014;159(4): 709–713.

Morley JE, Vellas B, van Kan GA, et al. Frailty consensus: a call to action. *J Am Med Dir Assoc.* 2013;14(6):392–397.

Usher T, Buta B, Thorpe RJ, et al. Dissecting the racial/ethnic disparity in frailty in a nationally representative cohort study with respect to health, income, and measurement. *J Gerontol A Biol Sci Med Sci.* 2021;76(1):69–76.

Walston J, Bandeen-Roche K, Buta B, et al. Moving frailty toward clinical practice: NIA Intramural Frailty Science Symposium Summary. *J Am Geriatr Soc.* 2019; 67(8):1559–1564.

Chapter 43

Falls

Stephen R. Lord, Jasmine C. Menant

EPIDEMIOLOGY OF FALLS AND FALL-RELATED INJURIES IN OLDER PEOPLE

A fall is "an event which results in a person coming to rest inadvertently on the ground or floor or other lower level." Prospective studies undertaken in community settings have reported fall incidence rates of 32% to 40% in people aged 65 and older and fall rates of 40% to 50% in people beyond the age of 75. Prospective studies in residential aged care facilities (RACFs) report fall incidence rates between 30% and 56%. Falls also occur frequently when people are in hospital, with incidence rates ranging between 2% in general hospitals to 27% in acute hospital geriatric wards.

Fall-related injuries can be severe and lead to a decline in the quality of life of an older person. Around 37% to 56% of all falls lead to minor injuries, while 10% to 15% of falls cause major injuries. Falls are the leading cause of injury-related hospitalizations in people aged 65 and older, and account for 14% of emergency admissions and 4% of all hospital admissions in this age group. Falls that do not result in physical injuries can also have serious consequences including significant fear of falling, which can lead to reduced mobility and frailty through the avoidance of daily activities. Furthermore, falls constitute a key predisposing factor for older people requiring institutional care.

RISK FACTORS OF FALLS

Many sociodemographic, medical, neuropsychological, and sensorimotor factors are strongly related with falls. As a result of age-related changes, disease, or adverse medication effects, sensorimotor and balance systems can be impaired and predispose to falls (**Figure 43-1**). **Table 43-1** summarizes the findings of numerous prospective cohort studies and rates each risk factor according to the strength of published evidence.

Psychosocial and Demographic Risk Factors

Falls are associated with increased age and female gender in community-living older people. The difference in fall rates between men and women has been attributed to more women living alone, being underweight, using more psychotropic medications and having reduced muscle strength. Additionally, older women are also more likely

Learning Objectives

- To be aware of the extent of the problem and consequences of falls in older people.
- To appreciate the broad range of risk factors for falls, and in particular, the risk factors that are amenable to correction through fall prevention initiatives.
- To be aware of appropriate fall-risk screens and assessments for the community setting, and validated assessments for hospital and residential aged care settings.
- To have knowledge of effective single and multifaceted interventions for preventing falls and the populations for which appropriate interventions should be targeted.

Key Clinical Points

1. Falls are common in older people and frequently have serious consequences including fractures, significant fear of falling, reduced mobility, increased dependency, and need for institutional care.

2. A broad range of risk factors for falls have been documented. Key among these are factors directly or indirectly influencing balance control and gait stability.

3. Evidence-based assessments are available for community, hospital, and residential aged care settings.

4. Single intervention strategies shown to successfully prevent falls include exercise, enhanced podiatry, occupational therapy interventions, expedited cataract extraction, provision of single lens glasses for regular multifocal glasses wearers, cardiac pacing for carotid sinus hypersensitivity, and vitamin D supplementation in people with low levels of vitamin D living in RACFs.

5. Tailored multifaceted and multifactorial interventions are the most effective interventions for preventing falls in high-risk populations including RACF residents.

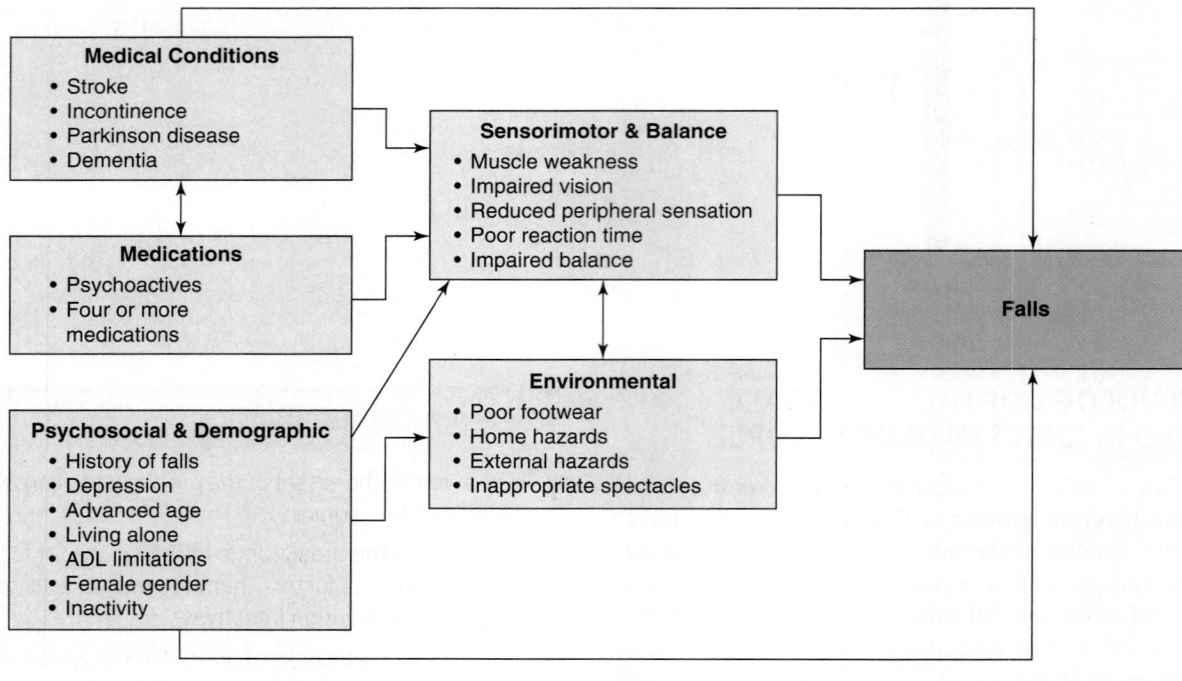

FIGURE 43-1. Risk factors for falls in older people.

to sustain fall-related fractures due to a higher prevalence of osteoporosis. However, in hospitals and institutions, fall incidence is similar for men and women, or even, higher in men. The finding that living alone is a risk factor for falls is most likely confounded by gender and increased age, in that women comprise most of the very old population.

As outlined in the intervention section later, physical activity can improve strength, balance, and functional abilities in older people. However, being more physically active does not always prevent falls, which likely reflects more physically active older people take part in activities which increase exposure to fall-risk situations. In addition, frail older adults taking up physical exercise training are likely to overestimate their balance abilities early in the program. Clearly, the risk related to increased exposure to falls should be balanced against other benefits of exercise including increased physical functioning and independence.

The most surprising finding regarding associations between sociodemographic factors and falls is that alcohol consumption has not been shown to be a fall-risk factor. Despite examining the issue, no significant associations have been found between alcohol use and falls in several large cohort studies. The lack of a positive association between alcohol use and falls may be due to response and selection biases, in that heavy alcohol consumers are likely to underreport their drinking levels or simply decline participation in research studies. There is strong evidence that long-term high alcohol intake can lead to multiple medical problems including osteoporosis, cerebellar atrophy, and peripheral neuropathy. Emergency department data for fall-related presentations also indicate that traumatic brain injuries are twice as prevalent among older people presenting with an indication of alcohol use prior to the fall.

Medical Factors

Many diseases and associated impairments have been identified as risk factors of falling, mainly through impairing neuropsychological function and balance control. Major conditions include stroke, Parkinson disease, multiple sclerosis, dementia, depression, dizziness, urinary incontinence, and arthritis. These conditions increase the risk of falls in both community and institutional settings, although the importance of some of these factors such as incontinence and impaired cognition are of greater importance in institutions. On the other hand, certain conditions commonly thought to be strong risk factors for falls, such as vestibular disorders and orthostatic hypotension, have not been found to be strong risk factors in community-based research studies but may be important in clinical populations, for example, orthostatic hypotension in Parkinson disease.

Medications

Both community and institutional studies have demonstrated consistent associations between medication use and falls in older people, particularly for psychoactive medication (benzodiazepine, antidepressant, and antipsychotic) and multiple medication use. These studies indicate that use of psychoactive medications leads to a two to threefold increased risk of falls and a twofold increased risk of experiencing a hip fracture. The association between the use of nonsteroidal anti-inflammatory drugs and falls is

TABLE 43-1 ■ RISK FACTORS FOR FALLS

DOMAIN	RISK FACTOR	ASSOCIATION
Psychosocial and demographic factors	Advanced age	***
	Female gender	**
	Living alone	**
	History of falls	***
	Inactivity	**
	ADL limitations	***
	Alcohol consumption	-
Medical factors	Stroke	***
	Parkinson disease	***
	Dementia	***
	Incontinence	**
	Acute illness	**
	Vestibular disorders	*
	Arthritis	**
	Foot problems	**
	Dizziness	**
	Orthostatic hypotension	*
Medication factors	Psychoactive medication use	***
	Antihypertensive use (acute effects)	**
	NSAIDs	-
	Use of 4+ medications	***
Balance and mobility factors	Impaired stability when standing	**
	Impaired stability when leaning and reaching	***
	Inadequate responses to external perturbations	***
	Slow voluntary stepping	***
	Impaired gait and mobility	***
	Impaired ability in standing up	***
	Impaired ability with transfers	***
Sensory and neuromuscular factors	Visual acuity	**
	Visual contrast sensitivity	***
	Visual field loss	**
	Reduced peripheral sensation	***
	Reduced vestibular function	*
	Muscle weakness	***
	Poor reaction time	***
Neuropsychological factors	Impaired cognition	***
	Depression	***
	Fear of falling	***
Environmental factors	Poor footwear	*
	Inappropriate spectacles	*
	Home hazards	*
	External hazards	-

***Strong evidence (consistently found in high-quality studies); **moderate evidence (usually but not always found); *weak evidence (occasionally but not usually found); and - little or no evidence (not found in published studies despite research to examine the issue).

PART III

GERIATRIC CONDITIONS

inconsistent across studies but the most recent and comprehensive systematic review found that these medications do not increase fall risk in an adjusted analysis. Results of studies into use of antihypertensive medications have been conflicting and have also highlighted the importance of examining drug classes rather than grouping all antihypertensive medications together. In fact, there is evidence that some classes of antihypertensive agents (ie, angiotensin system blocking medications) are protective against falls but the mechanisms underpinning this effect are unclear. These findings also need to be interpreted in the context of medication initiation and prescription changes as a time-risk analysis has shown the risk of falls is significantly increased within the 24-hour periods following the initiation of an antihypertensive or change in antihypertensive dose.

Balance, Mobility, and Gait Factors

The ability to rise from a chair, turn while walking, and ascend and descend stairs all require good balance control. Aging is associated with impairments in sensorimotor systems that contribute to balance, which in turn can impair ability to safely perform a range of functional tasks. Gait changes are also common with increasing age. Older adults tend to walk with slower speed, shorter step length, increased step time variability, wider step width, and a relatively increased proportion of time spent in the double-support phase. It is likely these changes are due to both physical limitations and adaptive strategies to improve safety; but nonetheless, these spatiotemporal gait patterns are predictive of falls. Older adults at risk of falls are also less able to adapt their gait on short notice to negotiate obstacles and recover from unexpected trips and slips. In addition, older people at high risk of falls have difficulty controlling the accelerations of their trunk and head while walking, which may impair their gaze stability.

Sensory and Neuromuscular Factors

Good balance requires the complex integration of sensory information regarding the position of the body relative to the surroundings and the ability to generate appropriate motor responses to control body movement. Reduced balance and mobility in older people can result from impairments in sensory, motor, and central processing systems. Impairments may result from a specific pathology affecting a particular system, or a progressive age-related loss of function. Visual input provides a continually updated reference frame regarding the position and motion of body segments in relation to each other and the environment. Impaired vision, particularly reduced contrast sensitivity and depth perception, is a risk factor for falls and fractures as it increases the likelihood of misjudging obstacles in the environment. In addition, sensory systems provide information about the nature of balance perturbations. Decreased lower limb muscle strength also has important ramifications for balance and falls in older people, and in large community-based studies, reduced knee extension

strength has been shown to increase fall risk. Similarly, in RACFs, knee extension and ankle dorsiflexor weakness have been found to be major risk factors for falls. Finally, adequate central processing and reaction time are necessary for voluntarily correcting balance perturbations.

Neuropsychological Factors

Several studies have shown that walking is not a fully automated process and that increased cognitive resources are required for balance control in older age. For example, a significant percentage of older people in residential aged care are unable to answer a simple question while maintaining walking, with such people at increased risk of falls. Older people who fall also do poorly in tests of executive functioning and attention. Recording of cortical activity using functional near-infrared spectroscopy while people step, walk, and negotiate obstacles has also confirmed the increased reliance on the prefrontal cortex with increasing task complexity, and that older people exhibit neural inefficiency (stagnation or decrease in behavioral performance with concurrent increases in cortical activity). Fear of falling and depression, both prevalent in older people, may have detrimental effects on several domains of life, including restricting activities of daily living and enjoyable pastimes, and in consequence lead to physical inactivity and social isolation. Older people with high levels of fear or generalized anxiety have also been shown to select inadequate postural control strategies, such as excessive stiffening in threatening conditions (such as when standing at height).

Environmental Factors

It has been estimated that extrinsic factors are involved in 35% to 45% of falls that result in injuries, and one prospective study with repeated assessments over the follow-up period found the presence of home hazards was a significant risk factor for falls in frail older people. The interaction between an older person's abilities and their exposure to environmental factors is particularly important. People with high physical abilities can withstand a bigger range of environmental challenges without falling, yet when faced with an extreme challenge, such as an icy footpath, may still fall. People with lower physical abilities can generally cope well in an environment that offers few challenges, such as in their own home, but in people with very poor abilities, falls may occur in relatively safe, hazard-free environments. In addition, the extent of a person's risk-taking behavior or exposure to fall-risk situations plays an important role in the interaction between an older person's abilities and their environment. There is evidence that environmental hazards play a greater role in falls that occur away from the home where, depending on the population studied, about one quarter to one half of falls occur. Falls occurring away from the home more frequently involve stairs or slipping and tripping hazards, or temporary hazards that cannot be anticipated. In addition, environmental factors can play a role in whether a fall will lead to a serious injury. For example, a fall on stairs is associated with a twofold increase in risk of injury.

FALL-RISK SCREENING AND ASSESSMENT

Several tools for screening fall risk have been validated for use in older people living in the community (**Table 43-2**). In this setting, fall-risk screening provides an efficient means of identifying those people at greatest risk of falling who should have a comprehensive fall-risk assessment performed. A simple, easy-to-administer screen is to ask older people about their history of falls in the past 12 months and assess their balance and mobility status. Several studies have identified previous falls as one of the strongest predictors for falling again in the following year. It has therefore been suggested that health care practitioners should ask all older people about any falls they have experienced.

Best practice guidelines recommend the Timed Up and Go (TUG) Test as a simple screening tool to identify people warranting an assessment of balance and gait. It involves measuring the time taken for a person to rise from a chair, walk 3 meters at normal pace and with usual assistive devices, turn, return to the chair, and sit down. However, a systematic review involving 25 studies found the predictive value of the TUG for falls in community-dwelling older adults was limited and no cut-point for impaired performance could be recommended. Alternatives

TABLE 43-2 ■ EXAMPLES OF VALIDATED FALL-RISK SCREENING TOOLS

The Timed Up and Go Test	The Timed Up and Go Test (TUG) measures the time taken for a person to rise from a chair, walk 3 meters at normal pace with their usual assistive device, turn, return to the chair, and sit down. Both quality of the walk and transfers and the time taken to complete the tests should be recorded.
The Alternate Step Test	The Alternate Step Test measures the ability of patients to alternatively place their left and right feet as fast as possible onto an 18-cm high step. A test time > 10 sec to complete eight alternating steps indicates an impaired performance.
The Sit to Stand Test	The Sit to Stand Test measures the ability of patients to complete five chair rises as fast as possible. A test time > 12 sec to complete the test indicates an impaired performance.
The Short Physical Performance Battery	The Short Physical Performance Battery comprises simple assessments of standing balance, chair rise ability, and gait. Each test is graded from 0–4 with a total test score of 12.

to the TUG that are simple to administer and have good predictive accuracy for falls include the Alternate Step Test, the Sit to Stand Test, and the Short Physical Performance Battery (**Table 43-2**).

Assessment – Community

Older people living in the community with a history of one or more falls in the past year who perform poorly on a simple test of balance or gait should be assessed further to develop an individualized fall prevention care plan. Assessment tools provide detailed information on the underlying deficits contributing to overall risk and should be used to guide interventions. Assessing fall risk typically involves either the use of multifactorial assessment tools that cover a wide range of fall-risk factors or individual functional mobility assessments that focus on the physiologic and functional domains of postural stability, including vision, strength, coordination, balance, and gait.

Assessment – Hospitals

The UK NICE guidelines recommend that hospital patients aged 65 and older or those aged 50 to 64 who have an underlying condition that places them at risk, such as a recent stroke, should be assumed to be at risk and automatically undergo multifactorial assessments and interventions. Such assessments should have good predictive accuracy, validation across multiple hospitals, and evaluate risk factors for falls that can be addressed or managed during the inpatient stay, such as postural instability, cognitive impairment, visual impairment, continence issues, and medication use. This information should then form the basis for an individualized fall prevention plan.

Assessment – Residential Aged Care

Some guidelines recommend that residents who score at risk of falls on a screening tool should undergo a comprehensive fall-risk assessment, as well as residents who experience a fall, or who move to or reside in a setting where most people are considered to have a high risk of falls (eg, high-care facilities, dementia units). In many residential care settings, however, most residents are at an increased risk of falls so it may be pragmatic to omit the screening process and implement regular fall-risk assessments of all residents.

The CaHFRiS Fall Screen comprises easily collectable measures and provides a simple way of quantifying the probability with which a care home resident will fall over a 6-month period. The CaHFRis items are: MMSE less than 17, presence of impulsivity, reduced standing balance, reliance on a walking frame, a fall in the previous year, and use of antidepressants and/or hypnotics/anxiolytics with the absolute risk of falling increasing from zero in those with no risk factors to 100% in those with six or more risk factors. While described as a fall risk screen, this tool assists in identifying important explanatory risk factors for falls that may be amenable to targeted interventions.

A range of comprehensive assessment tools have been developed for use in a range of settings—see https://fallsnetwork.neura.edu.au/resources/. The choice of tool depends on the time and equipment available and the level of ability of the older people being assessed.

FALL PREVENTION STRATEGIES

There is now a strong body of evidence to support interventions for preventing falls in older people. Single intervention strategies shown to successfully reduce falls in randomized controlled trials (RCTs) include exercise, enhanced podiatry, occupational therapy interventions, expedited cataract extraction, provision of single-lens glasses for regular multifocal glasses wearers, and cardiac pacing for carotid sinus hypersensitivity. Multifactorial interventions, which target risk factors identified in a fall-risk assessment, have also been shown to prevent falls in community, hospital, and residential aged care settings. For a full overview, please refer to systematic reviews from the Cochrane Collaboration and the "Further Reading" list.

Single Fall Prevention Strategies

Exercise Exercise has a major role to play in preventing falls among older people and is recommended in evidence-based guidelines for fall prevention. Overall systematic review findings from 64 RCTs indicate that community-dwelling older people allocated to well-designed exercise programs had 23% fewer falls than those allocated to control programs. Exercise, however, covers a wide range of physical tasks (balance, strength, flexibility, etc.) delivered in many formats, some of which result in bigger reductions in falls than others. A systematic review showed that greater effects are seen in programs that provide a high challenge to balance and three or more hours per week of prescribed exercise. This work also showed that exercise is effective in reducing falls even in the oldest subgroups (75 years and older), and regardless of whether it is delivered in a group or individual setting, by a health professional, or by a trained exercise leader. Four contrasting examples of effective exercise interventions for preventing falls that contain challenging balance and functional exercise training are outlined in **Table 43-3**. In addition to these more traditional exercise interventions, training programs aimed at improving rapid stepping, a key balance recovery response, have been shown to reduce falls by 52% in a meta-analysis of seven RCTs.

Most activities of daily life require concurrent motor execution together with attention and additional executive function skills, for example, inhibition and task switching. Crossing a busy road, walking while talking on a mobile phone, and walking through crowded malls are some examples. Several small trials have been conducted to investigate whether exercise training combined with cognitive function training can reduce falls in older adults. Some of these have examined the roles of exergames (performed on balance boards, step mats [see example in **Figure 43-2**] or using virtual reality technology). The findings from these studies indicate exergame training can improve physical and cognitive factors associated with falls in older people and are equivalent to traditional exercise interventions in their effect on fall-risk factors. Research is underway to determine whether such training can also prevent falls.

Exercise as a single intervention in certain high-risk populations, however, may not be an effective fall prevention strategy. Systematic review findings indicate that while exercise interventions are effective among

TABLE 43-3 ■ EXAMPLES OF EFFECTIVE EXERCISE FALL PREVENTION STRATEGIES

EXERCISE	DESCRIPTION
Individually prescribed home exercise	Individually prescribed home exercise programs to be undertaken three times per week. Exercises include: standing with one foot directly in front of the other; walking placing one foot directly in front of the other; walking on the toes and walking on the heels; walking backward, sideways, and turning around; stepping over an object; bending and picking up an object; stair climbing in the home; rising from a sitting position to a standing one; knee squats; moderate-intensity strengthening exercises with ankle cuff weights and a walking program.
LiFE program	Integration of balance and strength training into daily life activity. Rather than a prescribed set of exercises conducted several times a week, LiFE activities occur whenever the opportunity arises during the day. The strategies to improve balance include reducing base of support, moving to limits of sway, shifting weight from foot to foot, stepping over objects, and turning and changing direction.
Hybrid home-group program	Progressive group exercise programs with a supplementary home program. The exercise classes comprise balance-specific, individually tailored and targeted training for dynamic balance, strength, bone, endurance, flexibility, gait, and functional skills. The home exercises comprise strength and balance training to be undertaken twice a week.
Tai chi	Group exercise involving practiced controlled leaning movements, multidirectional weight shifting, awareness of body alignment, and multi-segmental (arms, legs, and trunk) movement coordination with synchronized breathing.

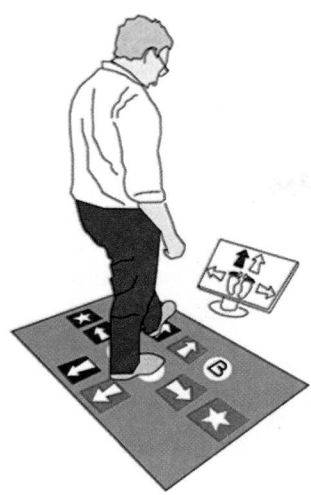

FIGURE 43-2. A step mat training intervention. The participant is undertaking a choice stepping reaction time task: one of four arrows on the screen changes color and the participant is asked to step as quickly as possible onto the same location of the pad.

people with Parkinson disease and those with cognitive impairment, they do not reduce fall rates among long-term stroke survivors or older people recently discharged from hospital. In fact, one home-based exercise program significantly *increased* falls in older people recently discharged from hospitals by 43%. This area requires further investigation, as it may be that to be effective; exercise needs to form part of multifactorial interventions or be supplemented with educational components in these frailer populations.

The effect of exercise alone as a fall prevention intervention in acute hospitals is not known, but in subacute hospital settings, three RCTs have shown that balance and mobility interventions can prevent falls. The evidence for exercise programs in RACFs as a single intervention is also mixed, but a recent trial of twice-weekly combined progressive resistance and balance training for 25 weeks improved physical performance and reduced falls by 55% in long-term aged-care residents. In addition, several multifaceted programs that have included exercise have shown positive effects in preventing falls. For example, an intervention program that involved staff training and feedback, information and education for residents, environmental adaptations, hip protectors, and twice-weekly exercise in groups of six to eight people delivered by exercise instructors reduced falls by 45%.

Visual interventions Two trials have examined the effects of expedited cataract surgery in reducing falls. The first examined the efficacy of cataract surgery in the first eye and showed that the fall rate in the operated group was significantly lower (a 34% reduction) than that observed in the control group. The second trial showed that cataract surgery for the second eye reduced falls by a similar amount (ie, 32%) in the operated group, but this reduction did not reach statistical significance. In addition, a recent prospective cohort study found that cataract surgery is associated with fewer falls in older adults, providing spectacle lens power updates of the operated eye are cautious (<±0.75 diopter change).

In contrast, the evidence for updating glasses to ensure the use of correct prescription glasses is less clear. One RCT evaluated a vision improvement intervention in people with impaired vision and found that this intervention strategy did not significantly reduce the rate of falls. A second RCT that assessed vision and provided vision-related treatments, if required, showed a significantly *increased* fall rate, by about 50%. A third RCT provided single lens distance glasses to community-dwelling older people at risk of falls who regularly used multifocal glasses outdoors. This visual intervention involved counseling as a core intervention component to demonstrate how multifocal glasses blur ground level hazards (**Figures 43-3** and **43-4**) and was effective in significantly reducing all falls (by 40%), outside falls, and injurious falls in the subgroup of people who regularly took part in outside activities.

Some older people have impaired vision that cannot be corrected. A targeted home safety assessment and modification program designed for older people with low vision has been shown to reduce the rate of falls by 41% in people with severe visual impairment.

Medication management Centrally acting medications have consistently been shown to increase fall risk. While initial trials found withdrawing centrally acting medications could significantly reduce falls in community and residential care settings, a more recent systematic review involving five trials and 1309 participants in clinical trials found fall-risk inducing drugs withdrawal strategies (mostly targeting centrally acting medications) did not significantly reduce fall rates (RaR: 0.98, 95% CI: 0.63, 1.51) in older people over a 6- to 12-month follow-up period. This suggests strategies to prevent the initial uptake of centrally acting medications are warranted. Furthermore, the prescription of benzodiazepines, z-drugs, or other psychotropic medication for the management of insomnia in older persons should be avoided, unless there is a clear pattern of addiction or inability to complete a withdrawal program. Nonpharmacological approaches to the management of insomnia should also be considered.

Current evidence from systematic reviews and mega-trials indicates vitamin D supplementation does not improve physical function or prevent falls in community-dwelling older adults, even in those with vitamin D deficiency, but may reduce falls in older adults living in RACFs.

Home safety interventions Home safety interventions are effective in high-risk groups and when delivered by an occupational therapist. A meta-analysis showed that intensive interventions carried out by occupational therapists

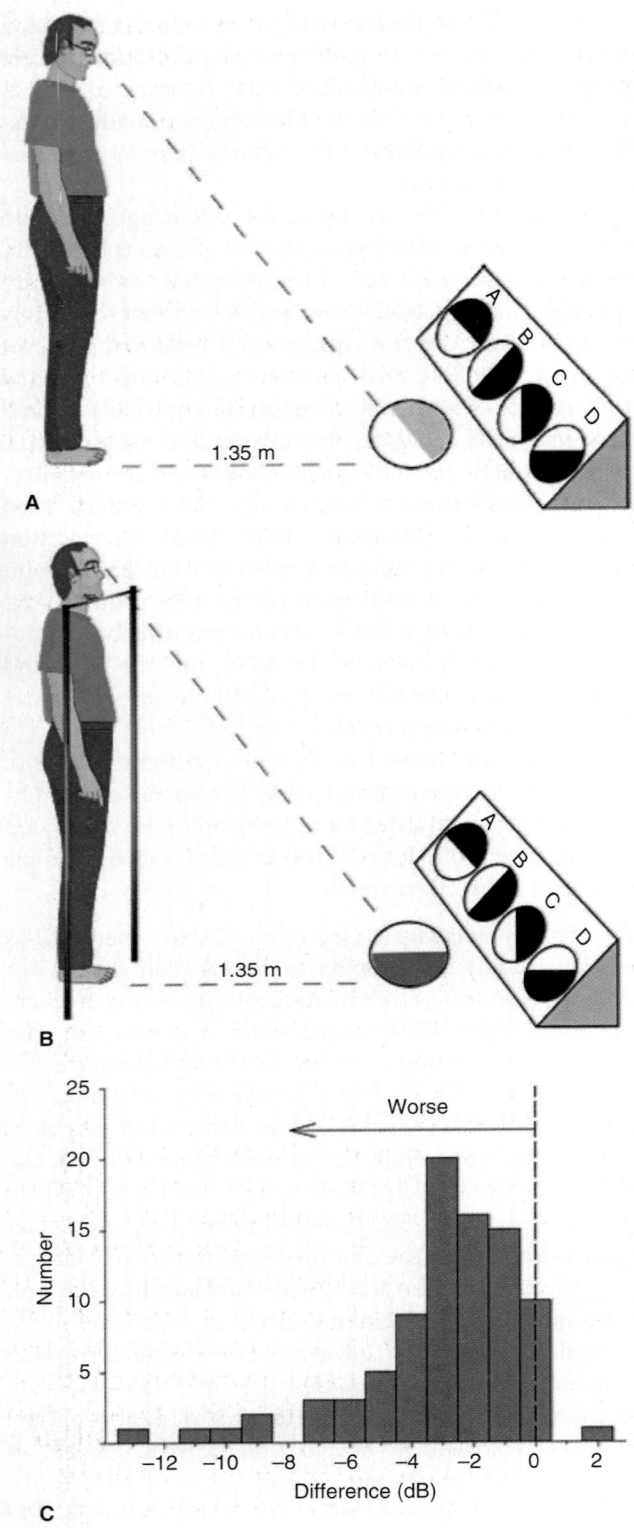

FIGURE 43-3. Contrast sensitivity assessments of edge stimuli (24 separate plates with reducing contrast edges) placed at floor level. In panel A the participant views the edge stimulus through the upper lens of bifocal spectacles. In panel B the participant is forced to view the edge stimulus through the lower lens. Participants are then shown the difference between their upper and lower lens contrast vision. For reference, panel C shows differences between upper and lower lens edge contrast sensitivity scores for 87 regular multifocal glasses wearers.

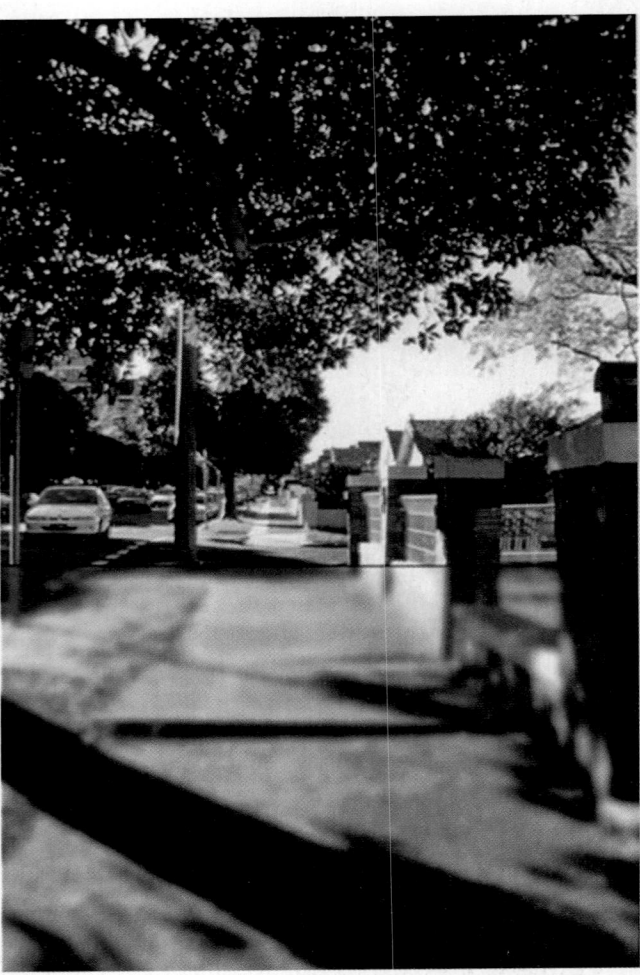

FIGURE 43-4. Simulated view of a street scene used in counseling to demonstrate how bifocal glasses blur ground level hazards such as pavement misalignments.

can reduce fall risk by 21% overall and by 39% for high-risk groups. These interventions included a comprehensive evaluation process of hazard identification and adequate follow up and support for adaptations and modifications, while involving the older person in priority setting.

The effectiveness of home safety interventions appears to depend on safe mobility advice and subsequent behavioral change rather than purely on environmental modification as successful interventions have had an impact on outdoor falls as well as indoor falls. Home-modification interventions can also reduce injuries from falls. In a cluster RCT of 842 households benefiting from government aids, home modifications reduced the rate of injuries from falls by 26% and injuries specific to the home-modification intervention by 39%.

Feet and footwear Multifaceted podiatry interventions and multifactorial interventions incorporating podiatry can reduce falls by 23% and 27%, respectively, in older people living in the community, according to a meta-analysis and systematic review. These interventions comprise the provision of foot orthoses and/or new safe footwear, advice on footwear, foot and ankle exercises, and routine podiatry. One pilot study has investigated the effect of a podiatry intervention in RACFs residents, showing small protective effect on falls directly after the intervention delivery (3 months), which disappeared at 6-month follow-up.

Psychological interventions There is limited evidence on psychological interventions in relation to fall prevention. Most cognitive behavioral programs when implemented as sole interventions have not prevented falls in people with fear of falling. However, the addition of cognitive behavioral therapy principles to multifactorial fall prevention interventions, especially in combination with exercise programs, may be more effective in reducing fall risk in people with fear of falling compared to exercise alone. Other psychological conditions, such as depression, anxiety, and sleep disorders, have been identified as risk factors for falls. There is a good evidence that cognitive behavioral therapy is an effective treatment of these conditions in older people, but this approach has not been investigated in relation to fall prevention.

Cardiovascular interventions Not all falls are caused directly by gait and balance problems. Individuals presenting with recurrent falls and no obvious balance or mobility impairment can benefit from a specialist assessment and specific diagnostic investigations. Three studies have evaluated the efficacy of implantation of pacemakers as a fall prevention strategy for people with cardioinhibitory carotid sinus hypersensitivity—an abnormal hemodynamic response to massage of the carotid sinus that is characterized clinically by unexplained dizziness and/or syncope. Overall, these studies indicate that pacemakers are effective in reducing drop attacks and syncope and reducing falls frequency.

Multifactorial Fall Prevention Strategies

Multifactorial interventions involve identifying a range of risk factors associated with falls and interventions based on the identified risk profile, and a recent Cochrane review of 43 trials conducted in community-dwellers found that multifactorial interventions reduced falls overall by 23%. Common strategies in multifactorial prevention programs are medication adjustment, home safety modifications, exercise programs, and education.

Residents of RACFs have a high prevalence of physical frailty and cognitive impairment, and in this setting, single approaches to intervention have generally not been shown to be effective. In contrast, multifactorial interventions provided by multidisciplinary teams with appropriate staff education have been shown to significantly reduce falls. Some of these trials have included comprehensive geriatric assessments of each patient whereas others have used specific fall-risk assessments. Multifactorial interventions

successful at reducing falls in hospital inpatients include combinations of supervised exercise and balance training, resident and staff education, medication review, vitamin D supplementation, environmental review, walking aids, and provision of hip protectors.

Impact of Multifactorial Interventions on Fall-Related Injuries

Two recent very large trials have tested the impact of multifactorial fall prevention interventions on fractures (n = 5451) and serious fall injuries (n = 9803), respectively. Both were undertaken in General Practice settings and sought to implement interventions within existing services primarily using existing resources and both found that their interventions did not significantly reduce falls or factures. These studies raise interesting questions about the challenge of funding and implementing fall prevention interventions as well as the ability of investigators to support and even measure uptake of intervention components in very large trials. Overall, it appears that multifactorial interventions are difficult to implement in practice and require greater commitment from participants and health care professionals than single component interventions. It also seems that multiple risk factor interventions are more effective in reducing falls if the interventions are provided directly, and less effective if the interventions rely on referral to routine service providers.

CONCLUSION

Many RCTs have shown interventions for preventing falls in older people. These have built on large epidemiological studies that have identified risk factors for falls amenable to intervention and validated assessments that can identify individuals at high risk of falls. A range of single intervention strategies have been shown to successfully reduce falls, including exercise containing medium-high intensity balance training, enhanced podiatry, home safety interventions, expedited cataract extraction, cardiac pacing for people with carotid sinus hypersensitivity, and vitamin D supplementation in people living in RACFs. Further research is required to clarify the roles medication reviews, visual interventions, and cognitive behavioral therapy can play in preventing falls. Tailored multifaceted and multifactorial interventions are particularly effective in preventing falls in high-risk populations including RACF residents. The translation of research findings into clinical practice remains a challenge. A combination of population health initiatives for lowering fall risk in the general population of older people combined with targeted interventions for those at increased risk is required to realize fall reductions at the population level.

Bhasin S, Gill TM, Reuben DB, et al. A randomized trial of a multifactorial strategy to prevent serious fall injuries. *N Engl J Med.* 2020;383:129.

Cameron ID, Dyer SM, Panagoda CE, et al. Interventions for preventing falls in older people in care facilities and hospitals. *Cochrane Database Syst Rev.* 2018;9:CD005465.

de Vries M, Seppala LJ, Daams JG, et al. EUGMS Task and Finish Group on Fall-Risk-Increasing Drugs. Fall-risk-increasing drugs: a systematic review and meta-analysis: I. Cardiovascular drugs. *J Am Med Dir Assoc.* 2018;19:371.e1.

E JY, Li T, McInally L, et al. Environmental and behavioural interventions for reducing physical activity limitation and preventing falls in older people with visual impairment. *Cochrane Database Syst Rev.* 2020;9:CD009233.

Gillespie LD, Robertson MC, Gillespie WJ, et al. Interventions for preventing falls in older people living in the community. *Cochrane Database Syst Rev.* 2012;9:CD007146.

Hewitt J, Goodall S, Clemson L, et al. Progressive resistance and balance training for falls prevention in long-term residential aged care: a cluster randomized trial of the Sunbeam program. *J Am Med Dir Assoc.* 2018;19:361.

Hopewell S, Copsey B, Nicolson P, et al. Multifactorial interventions for preventing falls in older people living in the community: a systematic review and meta-analysis of 41 trials and almost 20,000 participants. *Br J Sports Med.* 2020;54:1340.

Lamb SE, Bruce J, Hossain A, et al. Prevention of fall injury trial study group. Screening and intervention to prevent falls and fractures in older people. *N Engl J Med.* 2020;383:1848.

Lamb SE, Jorstad-Stein EC, Hauer K, et al. Development of a common outcome data set for fall injury prevention trials: the Prevention of Falls Network Europe consensus. *J Am Geriatr Soc.* 2005;53:1618.

Lee J, Negm A, Wong E, et al. Does deprescribing fall-associated drugs reduce falls and its complications? A systematic review. *Innov Aging.* 2017;1:268.

Mackenzie L, Beavis AM, Tan ACW, et al. Systematic review and meta-analysis of intervention studies with general practitioner involvement focused on falls prevention for community-dwelling older people. *J Aging Health.* 2020;32:1562.

Okubo Y, Schoene D, Lord SR. Step training improves reaction time, gait and balance and reduces falls in older people: a systematic review and meta-analysis. *Br J Sports Med.* 2017;51:586.

Oliver D, Papaioannou A, Giangregorio L, et al. A systematic review and meta-analysis of studies using the STRATIFY tool for prediction of falls in hospital patients: how well does it work? *Age Ageing.* 2008;37:621.

Schoene D, Wu SM, Mikolaizak AS, et al. Discriminative ability and predictive validity of the timed up and go test in identifying older people who fall: systematic review and meta-analysis. *J Am Geriatr Soc.* 2013;61:202.

Seppala LJ, Wermelink AMAT, de Vries M, et al. EUGMS task and Finish group on fall-risk-increasing drugs. Fall-risk-increasing drugs: a systematic review and meta-analysis: II. Psychotropics. *J Am Med Dir Assoc.* 2018;19:371.e11.

Sherrington C, Fairhall NJ, Wallbank GK, et al. Exercise for preventing falls in older people living in the community. *Cochrane Database Syst Rev.* 2019;1:CD012424.

Tiedemann A, Shimada H, Sherrington C, et al. The comparative ability of eight functional mobility tests for predicting falls in community-dwelling older people. *Age Ageing.* 2008;37:430.

Weber M, Belala N, Clemson L, et al. Feasibility and effectiveness of intervention programmes integrating functional exercise into daily life of older adults: a systematic review. *Gerontology.* 2018;64:172.

Whitney J, Close JCT, Lord SR, et al. Identification of high-risk fallers among older people living in residential care facilities: a simple screen based on easily collectable measures. *Arch Gerontol Geriatr.* 2012;55:690.

Wylie G, Torrens C, Campbell P, et al. Podiatry interventions to prevent falls in older people: a systematic review and meta-analysis. *Age Ageing.* 2019;48:327.

Chapter 44

Sleep Disorders

Armand Ryden, Cathy Alessi

INTRODUCTION

Problems with sleep are frequently encountered in older adults. More than two-thirds of older people with multiple comorbidities report sleep problems. These problems commonly include difficulty falling asleep, difficulty staying asleep, or sleepiness during the day. This chapter will explore the epidemiology, pathophysiology, clinical presentation, diagnosis, and management of sleep disorders commonly encountered in older adults.

SLEEP AND AGING

Sleep is a reversible behavioral state that is characterized by a decreased responsiveness to the environment and can be detected by observing stereotypical changes in the electroencephalogram (EEG). Each sleep period involves a progression of sleep stages that tend to cycle every 90 minutes. There are two major sleep states: rapid eye movement (REM) and nonrapid eye movement (NREM) sleep. REM sleep is characterized by having brain activity that is more similar to wake, rapid eye movements, and a complete loss of skeletal muscle tone. When people awaken from REM sleep they usually report vivid dreaming; hence REM sleep is often thought of as dreaming sleep. NREM sleep is divided into three stages: N1, N2, and N3. N3 sleep is also known as slow wave sleep. As sleep progresses from N1 through N3, people become more difficult to arouse; hence N1 sleep is considered light sleep, while N3 sleep is considered deep sleep. As people age there is a reduction in sleep efficiency, which is the amount of time actually asleep divided by time spent in bed (**Figure 44-1**). There are also significant changes to sleep architecture with aging. Longer time to initiate sleep and more fragmented sleep occur with aging. Furthermore, the amount of N3 sleep decreases with age starting in early adulthood. The reduction in N3 sleep with age is more prominent in men. Whether there are changes in REM sleep with aging is less clear. There is conflicting evidence regarding age as a risk factor for excessive daytime sleepiness. Objective measures of sleep have shown that healthy older adults have a lower propensity to fall asleep when given nap opportunities, suggesting a lower sleep drive. However, naps and unplanned naps are more common in older adults. These naps are associated

Learning Objectives

■ Recognize sleep disorders that are most common or particularly important in the care of older adults.

■ Understand that there may be a link between poor sleep and the development of Alzheimer dementia.

■ Identify key differences in the presentation and recognition of common sleep disorders in older compared to younger adults.

■ Describe evidence-based treatment for sleep disorders in older adults, including insomnia, obstructive sleep apnea (OSA), and other common conditions.

■ Summarize important issues in the management of sleep disturbance in special populations of older adults, such as those with dementia and those living in institutional settings.

Key Clinical Points

1. Poor sleep is common in older adults and is more closely associated with comorbidities than with chronological age.

2. Many important health outcomes are associated with poor sleep in older adults, including cognitive decline, increased medication use, and higher health care utilization.

3. Insomnia is common in older adults, and many of the pharmacologic therapies are relatively contraindicated in this population. Cognitive behavioral therapy for insomnia has a strong evidence base as a safe and effective treatment of insomnia in older adults.

4. In older adults, OSA is less likely to present with classic signs and symptoms and has been linked with important health outcomes including hypertension, cardiovascular disease, diabetes, and cognitive impairment. Continuous positive airway

(Continued)

(Cont.) pressure (CPAP) for the treatment of OSA can be successful in older adults, including those with mild to moderate dementia.

5. Rapid eye movement (REM) behavior disorder (RBD), which is characterized by dream enactment and lack of normal muscle atonia during REM sleep, can be comorbid with and even the precursor to neurodegenerative disorders such as Parkinson disease, multiple system atrophy, and Lewy body dementia.

6. Sleep-wake cycle disruption is common in nursing home patients and may be improved by behavioral interventions such as exposure to bright light, maintenance of a regular day-night cycle and melatonin.

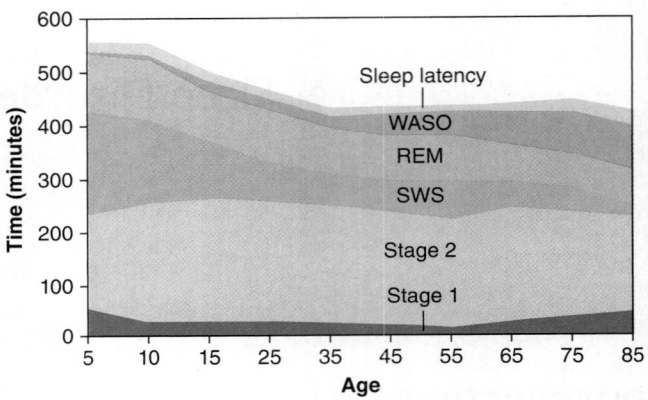

FIGURE 44-1. Change in sleep stages with age. Time spent in wake after sleep onset (WASO) increases significantly while time spent in slow wave sleep (SWS) decreases with age. REM, rapid eye movement. (Reproduced with permission from Krieger MH, Roth T, Dement WC. *Principles and Practices of Sleep Medicine*. 5th ed. St. Louis, MO: Elsevier Saunders; 2011.)

with comorbidities such as depression, pain, and nocturia. The changes in sleepiness with aging may reflect the accrual of comorbidities rather than being a product of the natural aging process.

Many experts believe that the age-related changes in sleep are due to a decreased ability to sleep rather than a decreased need to sleep. There is growing evidence that short and disturbed sleep are associated with poor cognitive and health outcomes. When older poor sleepers and good sleepers are compared, poor sleepers have worse health-related quality of life, increased medication use, and greater health care utilization. Having longer time awake after sleep onset has been associated with greater cognitive decline among older adults. One of the most active areas of research over the past several years has been in the potential relationship between sleep and dementia, particularly Alzheimer disease (AD). Sleep appears to be important in the clearance of beta-amyloid (Aβ) protein, the build-up of which is implicated in the pathogenesis of AD. Basic animal models have shown that Aβ is cleared through the glymphatic system during sleep. Excessive daytime sleepiness and napping have been associated with Aβ in the cerebral spinal fluid as well as being associated with the development of Aβ positivity on longitudinal assessments. There is also evidence that experimentally induced acute sleep deprivation can induce Aβ accumulation in healthy adults. It is hypothesized that sleep disruption with aging may lead to a decline in cognitive functioning because of the accumulation and deposition of these pathologic proteins. However, since these abnormal proteins may impact brain systems involved in sleep-wake homeostasis, excessive sleepiness and poor sleep may be an early symptom of a neurodegenerative condition. It would be reasonable to posit that there may be a bidirectional relationship between sleep symptoms and neurodegenerative diseases.

Many of the illnesses associated with aging can disrupt sleep, which may inhibit the normal progression through sleep stages. Thus, chronological age itself may not be the greatest predictor of sleep quality. Numerous epidemiologic studies have found a U- or J-shaped relationship between sleep time and subsequent mortality with both long and short sleep durations being associated with an increased risk of death. The cause of this relationship is still unknown given all of the potential confounders, despite controlling for known comorbidities. Changes in sleep architecture in aging may contribute to metabolic changes that occur in older adults. For instance, N3 sleep is associated with growth hormone secretion and the reduction in N3 sleep with aging may be partly responsible for the decrease in growth hormone in older men. Decreased sleep has also been linked to the metabolic conditions that impact healthy aging such as obesity and diabetes mellitus. Given the link between insufficient and fragmented sleep, quality of life, and health outcomes, there is a need for awareness, evaluation, and treatment of sleep disorders that commonly affect older adults.

SLEEP-DISORDERED BREATHING

Definition

Sleep-disordered breathing (SDB) is characterized by disturbed respiration during sleep arising from repetitive events of complete (ie, apnea) or partial (ie, hypopnea) cessation of airflow lasting at least 10 seconds. This is classified as obstructive sleep apnea (OSA) when the events are due to an obstructed airway, which is determined by the persistence of respiratory effort. On the other hand, if there is concomitant cessation of breathing effort, the disorder is classified as central sleep apnea (CSA) because there is a momentary defect in the central control of breathing

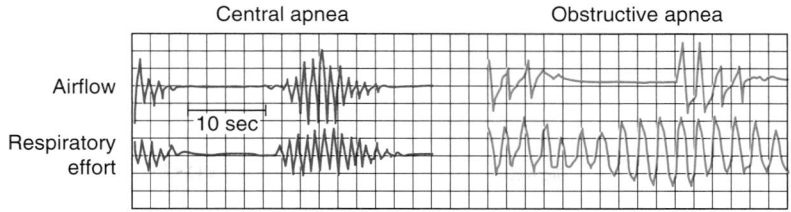

FIGURE 44-2. Obstructive versus central sleep apnea. (Reproduced with permission from Krieger MH, Roth T, Dement WC. *Principles and Practices of Sleep Medicine.* 5th ed. St. Louis, MO: Elsevier Saunders; 2011.)

(**Figure 44-2**). OSA is by far the most common sleep-related breathing disorder; however, there is often overlap between the two clinical syndromes. CSA can be associated with several different clinical conditions. Heart failure is the most commonly recognized cause of CSA and is often characterized by Cheyne-Stokes respiration, which is periodic cycling between hypoventilation and hyperventilation (**Figure 44-3**). Other common causes of CSA include stroke, opioid use, and hypoventilation syndromes. The severity of SDB is generally determined by the apnea hypopnea index (AHI), which is the number of apneas and hypopneas per hour of sleep. SDB can be diagnosed when the AHI is greater than 15, or when it is greater than 5 with significant symptoms or related comorbidities. An AHI greater than 30 is generally considered to indicate severe SDB.

The consequences of respiratory events during sleep include arousals from sleep, intrathoracic pressure swings, and cyclical drops in the blood oxygen level. This ultimately leads to sleep fragmentation and nocturnal hypoxemia, which may lead to significant health consequences.

Epidemiology

Many of the risk factors for OSA increase with age (**Table 44-1**). Estimates of the prevalence of OSA have

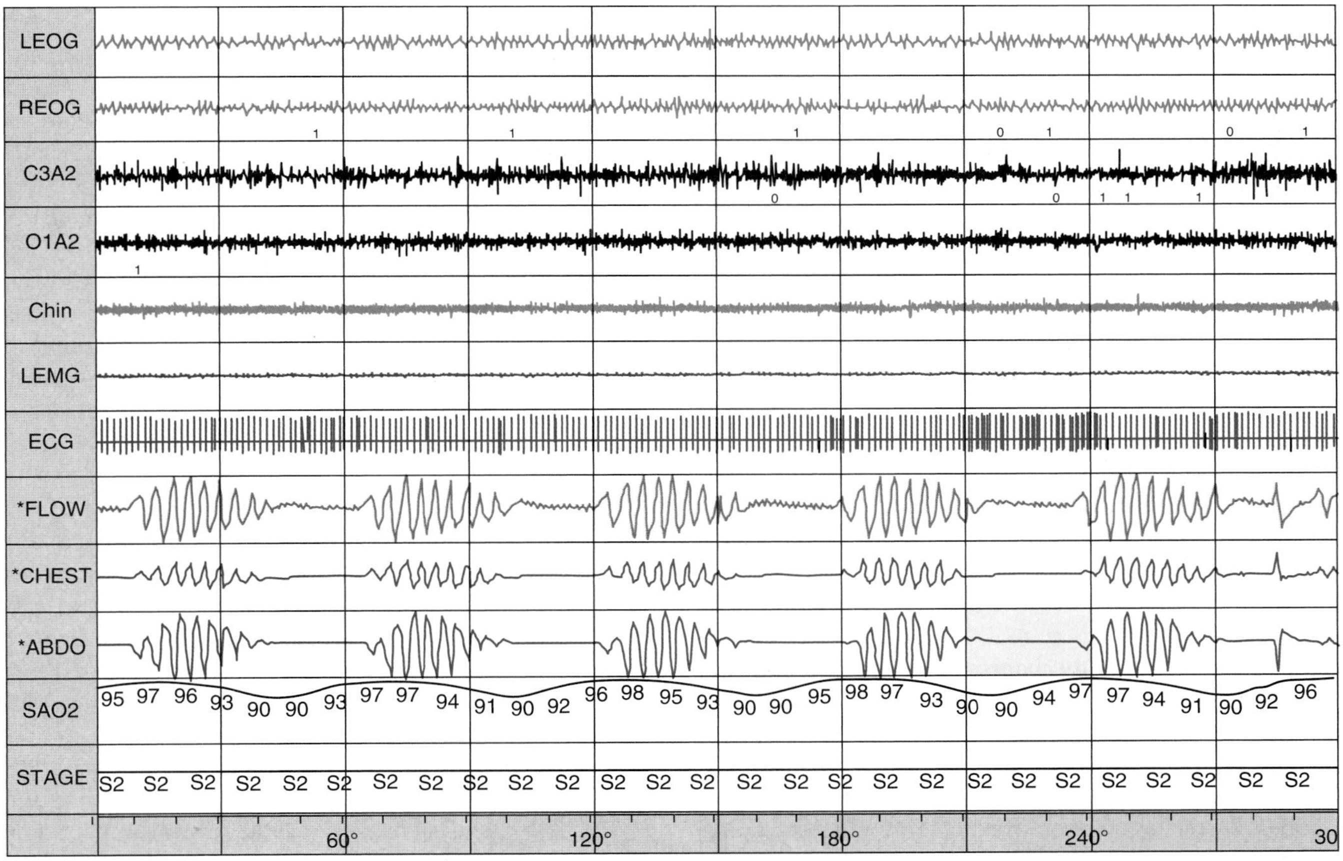

FIGURE 44-3. This figure represents central sleep apnea with a Cheyne-Stokes breathing pattern. During the periods of apnea there is no chest or abdominal effort. (Reproduced with permission from Javaheri S, Randernath WJ. Opioid-induced central sleep apnea: mechanisms and therapies. *Sleep Med Clin.* 2014;9[1]:49–56.)

TABLE 44-1 ■ POTENTIAL AGE-DEPENDENT RISK FACTORS IN SLEEP-DISORDERED BREATHING
Increased body mass index (central obesity)
Decreased muscle tension
Changes in airway anatomy
Increased airway collapsibility
Decreased thyroid function
Decreased lung volume

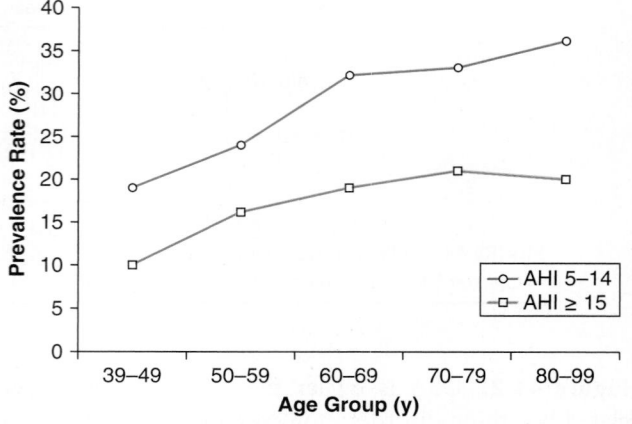

FIGURE 44-4. Association of obstructive sleep apnea (OSA) with age. Mild obstructive sleep apnea is shown in red while moderate to severe obstructive sleep apnea is shown in green. AHI, apnea hypopnea index. (Reproduced with permission from Norman D, Loredo JS. Obstructive sleep apnea in older adults. *Clin Geriatr Med.* 2008;24[1]:151–165.)

varied widely and are dependent on the populations studied. A cohort between 2007 and 2010 of middle-aged adults has estimated moderate to severe SDB to occur in 6% of women and 13% men. Evidence suggests that OSA is underdiagnosed in the general population, particularly in women. If the rate of obesity and overweight continues to increase, the rates of SDB will also increase. Less is known about the epidemiology of SDB in an older population; however, most studies have shown that the risk of OSA increases with increasing age until the age of 70 at which time there is a plateau (**Figure 44-4**). Furthermore, premenopausal status appears to protect against OSA meaning that the gender discrepancy between men and women narrows in the older population. OSA may be more severe in African-American and Asian populations compared to the Caucasian population.

The risk of CSA increases substantially with aging. CSA is two to three times more prevalent in those aged 65 to 90 than in those aged 39 to 64. Most likely this is due to the accrual of conditions that predispose to CSA such as congestive heart failure, atrial fibrillation, chronic kidney disease, and chronic pain conditions requiring opiates. It is estimated that upwards of 50% of patients with stable heart failure have some form of SDB. Many of these patients have a combination of CSA and OSA.

Pathophysiology

There are three types of SDB events: central, obstructive, and mixed. Central events result from a failure of the respiratory control center to send a signal to breathe. This often occurs because of an abnormal sensitivity of the respiratory controller, which can lead to oscillations between hyperventilation and hypoventilation. Obstructive events occur from anatomic obstruction of the upper airway despite respiratory effort. The major factor that governs the presence of obstructive events is an anatomically narrow airway; however, other mechanisms such as failure of adequate upper airway neuromuscular activation are thought to play a role. Features that govern the size of the upper airway include excess adiposity, craniofacial structure, excessive tonsillar and peritonsillar soft tissue, and lower lung volumes. Mixed events comprise central and obstructive components.

The most significant immediate consequence of OSA is excessive daytime sleepiness and the risk of motor vehicle accidents. Significant epidemiologic associations of OSA

with adverse cardiovascular and metabolic consequences have been reported. The association between SDB and these comorbidities is likely multifactorial. SDB results in sleep fragmentation, which has been shown to increase sympathetic nervous system activation, increase nocturnal cortisol levels, and interfere with insulin sensitivity. The potential downstream effects of these neurohumoral changes include the development of hypertension and diabetes. Increased intrathoracic pressure can occur and increase atrial natriuretic peptide levels potentially contributing to nocturia. Furthermore, the cyclic deoxygenation and reoxygenation that occurs with OSA leads to endothelial cell injury and inflammatory changes, which predispose to coronary and cerebral vascular disease (**Figure 44-5**). The intrathoracic pressure changes associated with increasing respiratory effort against a closed airway can lead to esophageal reflux as well as potentially deleterious hemodynamic effects in heart failure.

Clinical Presentation

The major symptoms of SDB include excessive daytime sleepiness and nocturnal snoring. The patient may present to the clinic complaining of sleepiness or at the request of a loved one with the complaint of snoring. The paradigmatic patient with SDB is an obese male with nocturnal snoring, witnessed apneas, frequent nocturnal awakenings, and excessive daytime sleepiness. However, these associations are less predictive in an older population. Other important symptoms of SDB include nocturia, insomnia, morning headaches, nocturnal confusion, and daytime impairments in mood and cognition. Sleepiness can be assessed with a standardized measure such as the Epworth Sleepiness Scale. It is often helpful to obtain corroborating information from a bed partner regarding snoring, witnessed apneas as well

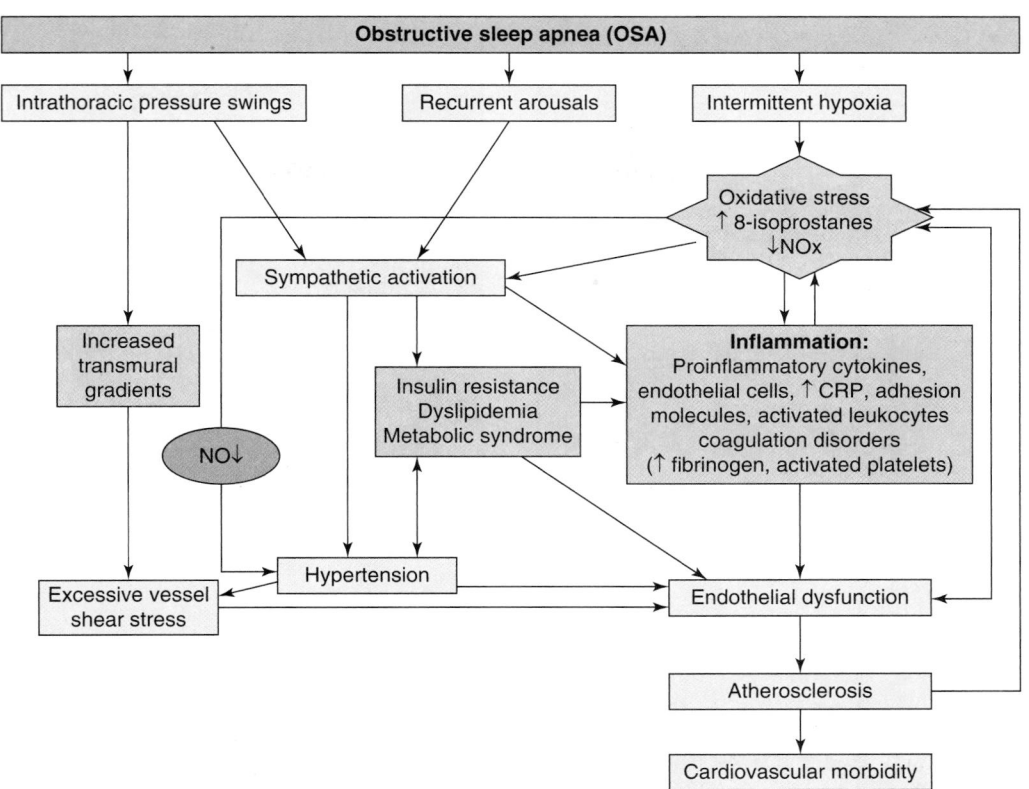

FIGURE 44-5. Model explaining why obstructive sleep apnea (OSA) might be associated with increased cardiovascular risk. NOx, nitrogen oxides; NO, nitrous oxide. (Reproduced with permission from Jullian-Desayes I, Joyeux-Faure M, et al. Impact of obstructive sleep apnea treatment by continuous positive airway pressure on cardiometabolic biomarkers: a systematic review from sham CPAP randomized controlled trials. *Sleep Med Rev.* 2015;21:23–38.)

as additional features that may point to a comorbid sleep disorder. Snoring is indicative of a partially collapsed airway and is a useful predictor of the presence of OSA or future development of the condition. The lack of classic symptoms and findings of OSA should not preclude further evaluation for SDB, particularly in older patients.

Physical features that predict increased risk of OSA include an elevated body mass index (BMI), a large neck circumference, and a crowded upper airway. In older adults, an elevated BMI has less predictive value of the likelihood of OSA. In clinic the airway can be assessed using a modified Mallampati score known as the Friedman classification, with positions III and IV conferring a high risk for OSA (**Figure 44-6**). In general, the less posterior oropharynx that can be visualized indicates a greater risk of SDB. Neck circumference greater than 17 inches in men and 16 inches in women is another predictor for SDB on physical examination. However, the predictive value of neck circumference is not as strong in older patients.

The presence of disturbed sleep in a patient with congestive heart failure may be indicative of SDB. As mentioned previously, a high percentage of patients with heart failure have OSA, CSA with Cheyne-Stokes respiration, or a combination of the two conditions. It can be difficult to

tease apart symptoms of heart failure such as orthopnea and paroxysmal nocturnal dyspnea (PND) from those of SDB. Opioid medication use is a risk factor for another form of CSA, which should be considered whenever patients on opioids present with sleep complaints.

Evaluation

Patients suspected of having SDB should be referred for sleep testing. An attended in-laboratory polysomnography (PSG) is considered the gold standard test for SDB. This involves traveling to a sleep laboratory to spend the night. The test involves the use of EEG, electromyogram (EMG), and electrooculogram (EOG) leads to determine presence and stage of sleep. There is measurement of airflow with a nasal pressure transducer as well as an oronasal thermistor. Respiratory effort is measured using chest and abdominal belts; and occasionally with an esophageal pressure monitor or accessory muscle EMG. An alternative approach to the diagnosis of SDB is the home sleep apnea test (HSAT). The patient takes the sleep testing equipment home and puts it on before bed. These tests are not generally able to measure sleep directly. Most of these tests measure airflow, effort, and pulse oximetry. Alternative testing includes the inference of respiratory events from peripheral

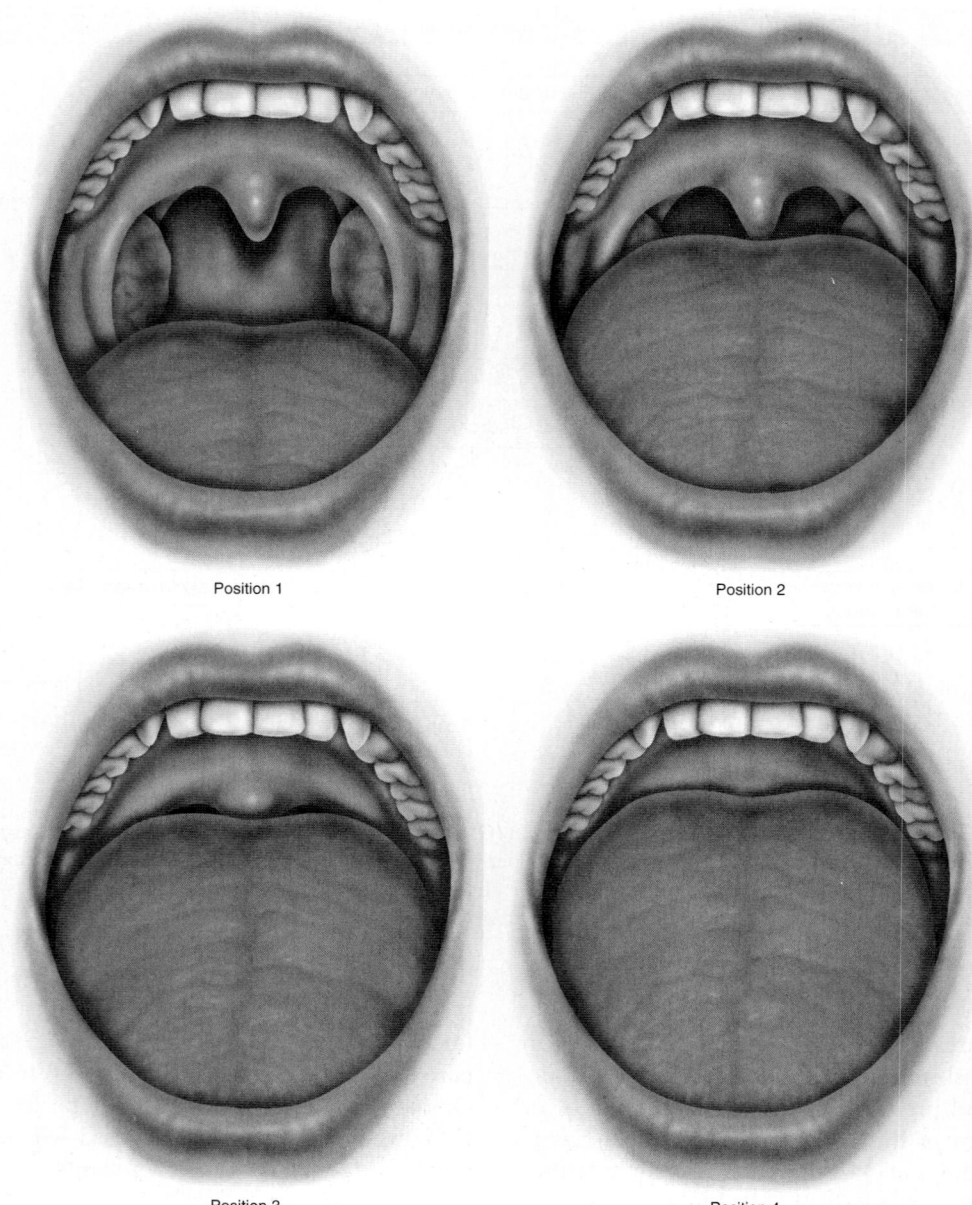

FIGURE 44-6. Friedman palate position. Positions 3 and 4 are associated with increased risk of obstructive sleep apnea (OSA). (Reproduced with permission from Friedman M, Ibrahim H, Bass L. Clinical staging for sleep-disordered breathing. *Otolaryngol Head Neck Surg.* 2002;127[1]:13–21.)

arterial tone changes due to changes in sympathetic activity resulting from the respiratory events that can be correlated with pulse oximetry. Such devices may be easier for some patients to self-administer, particularly those with cognitive or dexterity issues. However, these devices are not validated for the measurement of central apneas and should not be used in those taking alpha-adrenergic blocking medications or in those with atrial fibrillation. HSAT is only recommended for patients with a high pretest probability of having OSA who do not have significant cardiopulmonary comorbidities.

The advantages of an attended full-channel PSG include a higher reliability of the data, the ability to carefully define AHI by measuring sleep directly, and the simultaneous assessment for alternative sleep diagnoses to SDB. The advantages of HSAT include lower cost, the convenience for patients to sleep at home, and increased access to sleep testing. In populations at high risk for OSA, studies have shown that out-of-center sleep testing leads to similar patient outcomes compared to in-laboratory PSG. The limited studies in older patients have shown that HSATs can be used to accurately diagnose OSA. Due to cost issues third-party payers are increasingly pressuring practitioners to move toward HSAT. However, HSAT may be difficult for some older patients due to the need for the patient or caregiver to independently place the sensors. Another consideration is that older patients are more likely to have the comorbidities that preclude HSAT as modality due to the possibility of CSA. It must also be emphasized that a negative HSAT does not rule out OSA. An HSAT may be negative simply because the patient did not sleep during the test or due to technically inadequate data.

Management

The first-line treatment for SDB is positive airway pressure therapy. The most basic of these therapies is continuous positive airway pressure (CPAP), which has been available since the early 1980s. CPAP delivers a constant positive pressure in order to splint the airway open preventing collapse. To apply this pressure an airtight interface goes in the nose, over the nose, or over the nose and mouth, and then connects to a CPAP machine via a hose. Traditionally, the amount of air pressure (usually between 5 and 20 cm H_2O) is manually determined in the sleep laboratory with the sleep technologist adjusting the pressure to eliminate respiratory events and snoring. There is evidence that patients who have mild to moderate dementia are able to tolerate CPAP therapy and such a condition is not a contraindication to CPAP initiation.

Auto-titrating CPAP (APAP) is now available, in which the machine adjusts the pressure based on events and flow characteristics using internal algorithms that are proprietary to the device manufacturers. APAP can be used to determine a fixed CPAP pressure or can be used as the primary modality of therapy. APAP has been found to have a very small but statistically significant advantage in adherence over CPAP in randomized studies. Individual patients, however, particularly those with very different CPAP needs depending on body position or sleep stage, may find APAP to be more comfortable than fixed CPAP. The main advantage of APAP is the ability to determine, or provide, a therapeutic pressure without requiring a resource-intensive in-laboratory PSG.

CPAP is usually effective in eliminating obstructive apneas and hypopneas and has been found to substantially improve excessive daytime sleepiness and nocturnal sleep quality. CPAP has only recently been studied in older adult populations. Overall, these studies have found that CPAP improves sleepiness, quality of life, mood, and is cost effective in adults older than 65 years. There has been some suggestion that short-term memory and executive function can be improved with CPAP in those with severe OSA. Observational studies have found that CPAP is well tolerated and beneficial in older patients above the age of 80 and in those with mild to moderate dementia. The major downside to CPAP is that in general long-term adherence can be difficult to achieve. Estimates are that at the end of a year only 50% to 70% of all adult patients are adherent to CPAP

therapy. Factors that may improve CPAP adherence include early follow-up, education and setting of expectations, humidification, attention to interface comfort, expiratory pressure relief, possible early use of hypnotics, and desensitization to therapy. Each of these interventions has small but important impacts in individual patient acceptance to therapy. Studies on whether aging is a factor in nonadherence have been mixed. Any changes in CPAP adherence with age are most likely due to factors other than age itself.

Positive airway pressure therapy has to be individualized in patients who have CSA. Many patients who have Cheyne-Stokes respiration will respond to a combination of CPAP and/or supplemental oxygen. Likewise, the majority of patients with obesity-hypoventilation syndrome respond to CPAP alone. However, many patients require more advanced ventilatory modalities to eliminate CSA. Regardless of the particular mode, these advanced devices involve applying bilevel pressure with a back-up respiratory rate. The amount of pressure support given during a certain breath can be controlled by sophisticated proprietary algorithms in order to achieve specific desired clinical effects.

Adaptive servo-ventilation (ASV) is used for CSA syndromes that are not due to hypoventilation. Safety concerns of ASV in heart failure patients were raised with the SERVE-HF trial which found increased mortality in those who were randomized to ASV for CSA among in an ejection fraction (EF) less than 45%. Therefore, ASV is generally not recommended in those with an EF less than 45%. In older patients with preserved EF and central or combined central and OSA there is some evidence that ASV can improve sleep-related symptoms and daytime functional status.

Dental devices that move the jaw forward (mandibular advancement or mandibular repositioning devices) are a treatment alternative to positive airway pressure in OSA. The principle behind such therapy is that when the lower jaw moves forward the tongue is also pulled forward, thus opening up the airway. These devices are generally thought to be more effective in mild to moderate OSA rather than severe OSA. However, the severity of OSA may not necessarily predict response to mandibular advancement therapy in all patients. In general, mandibular advancement therapy does not reduce the residual AHI to as great of an extent as positive airway pressure therapy. However, comparative effectiveness studies suggest equivalence for major outcomes is likely due to the fact that adherence rates tend to be higher for mandibular advancement therapy. Side effects include temporomandibular joint pain and occlusion abnormalities. One of the major limiting factors to mandibular advancement therapy, particularly in older adults, is that teeth are generally required to anchor the device in place. Tongue repositioning/retaining devices can be used in patients who lack their native teeth. However, these devices have been less extensively studied and are less likely to be effective.

Other therapies have been utilized in OSA. One of these therapies is expiratory positive airway pressure

(EPAP) provided through nasal valves, which makes it more difficult to breathe out than breathe in. This causes pressure build up that helps stent the airway open, as well as causing an increase in lung volume that may prevent obstructive respiratory events. This therapy is less well validated but may be used as a salvage therapy or in mild cases.

One therapeutic modality that has recently been developed is hypoglossal nerve stimulation. This therapy involves an implanted lead that goes to the respiratory muscles to sense the onset of inspiration and a lead that goes to the hypoglossal nerve that causes tongue contraction to open the airway with inspiration through direct action as well as muscular coupling with the soft palate. Randomized trials found promising results in a highly selected group of patients with a BMI less than 32 kg/m^2 who could not tolerate CPAP therapy. Initial trials had limited numbers of older patients. A recent cohort study of 62 patients aged 65 to 80 found significant reductions in AHI and sleepiness scores in this population with hypoglossal nerve stimulator therapy.

Surgery is also an alternative therapy for SDB. There are multiple surgical techniques that are available to otolaryngologists for the treatment of SDB. The most common technique is the uvulo-palato-pharyngoplasty (UPPP). This procedure has variable success rates depending on anatomic factors and the degree of obesity. Furthermore, even after successful therapy SDB may reoccur due to growth of scar tissue.

A more aggressive surgical approach is a maxillary mandibular advancement. In this approach both the maxilla and mandible are cut and advanced forward. This surgery requires the patient's jaw to be wired shut for several weeks. Although this is the most effective surgery for SDB, many patients opt to not undergo such an extensive procedure.

Other behavioral changes that the patients with SDB can implement to help treat the syndrome include weight loss, sleeping on the side, and the avoidance of alcohol and other sedatives. In particular, positional techniques to encourage sleeping on the side may be beneficial when SDB occurs primarily in the supine position.

It is becoming increasingly recognized that while positive airway pressure therapy eliminates SDB more effectively than other interventions, it is essentially ineffective in a subset of patients who cannot tolerate its use. The use of multiple modalities of therapy, with each having a modest effect on AHI, may be able to achieve adequate control of SDB in those who cannot tolerate CPAP.

Pharmacologic Therapy

There are limited pharmacologic agents available for SDB and none that are approved for this indication. However, occasionally patients who are successfully treated for SDB with CPAP will have residual excessive daytime sleepiness. Modafinil and armodafinil, central nervous system stimulants, have Food and Drug Administration (FDA) approval for the treatment of residual excessive daytime sleepiness in treated OSA. Acetazolamide has an unclear role in some CSA syndromes. Ventilatory stimulants such as progesterone have been tried unsuccessfully in obesity hypoventilation syndrome.

Prevention

There is no specific disease prevention strategy for SDB. Addressing factors that contribute the subsequent development of SDB contributes to prevention. Since elevated BMI is the most potent risk factor for the development of OSA, weight loss and lack of weight gain are the most important preventative measures for OSA. Preventing decompensation of heart failure may be a way to prevent the development of heart failure–related CSA.

Patient Preference

Patient preference is clearly a key factor in determining the therapy of choice. CPAP and mandibular advancement devices can both be difficult to tolerate due to the need for equipment use and potential discomfort. The health benefit of treating minimally symptomatic SDB in older patients is unclear. Therefore, it is reasonable to withhold SDB treatment if the patient declines treatment and they have minimal symptoms. In patients who are sleepy and drive, it is more imperative to encourage SDB therapy. Also, in sleepy older patients with SDB, the treatment may have a greater beneficial impact on the prevention of SDB-related comorbidities and improvement in quality of life.

Comorbidity

SDB is associated with significant mental and physical comorbidities. Given the association between obesity and SDB, many of the comorbidities of obesity and SDB overlap. However, there are several lines of evidence suggesting an independent relationship between SDB and the development of hypertension, atrial arrhythmias, heart failure, coronary artery disease, cerebrovascular accidents, and diabetes mellitus. Most of these relationships have been elucidated from observational population studies and basic science investigations. Direct evidence that treatment of SDB can reverse some of these comorbidities is more limited. However, treatment of OSA does result in modest improvement in blood pressure among hypertensive patients. In addition, treatment of OSA after cardioversion for atrial arrhythmias such as atrial fibrillation has been found to increase the likelihood of staying in sinus rhythm. Large randomized controlled trials have failed to show that CPAP therapy leads to a reduction in cardiovascular events. The major limitation to these studies has poor adherence to CPAP. Due to ethical concerns those with excessive daytime sleepiness were excluded. Thus, it is unclear whether an individual who is adherent to CPAP therapy might gain cardiovascular benefit from therapy.

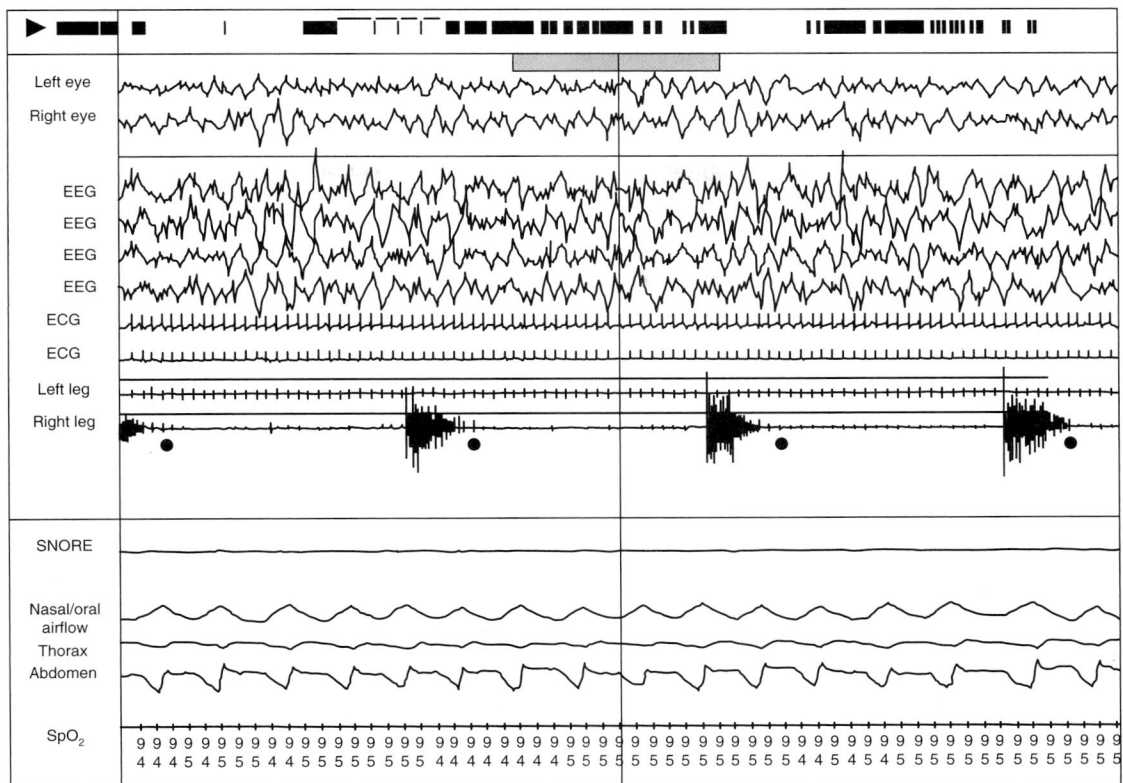

FIGURE 44-7. Periodic leg movements in sleep (PLMS) seen on polysomnography (PSG). (Reproduced with permission from Avidan AY. Sleep disorders in the older patient. *Prim Care.* 2005;32[2]:563–586.)

Insomnia is an important comorbidity of SDB. In fact, SDB itself may contribute to insomnia by disrupting sleep architecture and even preventing stable sleep onset due to OSA respiratory events. Sometimes insomnia improves with the treatment of SDB. However, insomnia may be exacerbated by the invasiveness of positive airway pressure or mandibular advancement. For a successful treatment outcome both disorders must be addressed. SDB and other mental illnesses such as anxiety, depression, and posttraumatic stress are frequently present in the same patient. Once again, the SDB may exacerbate some of the symptoms of these mental illnesses, and these illnesses may present barriers to acceptance of therapy.

RESTLESS LEGS SYNDROME AND PERIODIC LIMB MOVEMENT DISORDER

Definition

Restless legs syndrome (RLS), also known as Willis-Ekbom disease, is characterized by the urge to move one's legs. Most often patients with RLS have uncomfortable sensations in their legs, and sometimes arms, which lead to this urge. The other defining features of RLS are that the symptoms are improved with movement, worsen with relaxation, and occur later in the day. RLS can also affect and may even be limited to the arms. There is no objective test to diagnose RLS.

Periodic leg movements in sleep (PLMS) are characterized by cyclic movements of the lower limbs during sleep. These consist of stereotyped movements that typically involve the flexion of the big toe with partial flexion of the ankle, knee, and sometimes hip. PLMS last between 0.5 seconds and 10 seconds with a period between movements of 5 to 90 seconds (**Figure 44-7**). At least four movements in a row must occur to count as PLMS. Periodic limb movement disorder (PLMD) can be diagnosed if there are at least 15 PLMS per hour, the PLMS cause sleep disturbance and the symptoms are not better explained by another sleep disorder or a medical illness. Since PLMS are often seen in RLS (80%–90%), REM behavior disorder (70%), and narcolepsy (45%–65%), PLMD can only be diagnosed in the absence of these sleep disorders. A PSG is required to define PLMS and thus diagnose PLMD.

Epidemiology

The prevalence of RLS increases with age and is estimated to affect up to 8% of older adults, making it a very commonly encountered disorder in the outpatient setting. RLS is 1.5 to 2 times more common in women than in men. Iron deficiency and family history increase the odds of developing RLS. The prevalence of RLS is two to five times greater in patients with chronic renal failure. Taking antihistamines and most antidepressants are risk factors for the development of RLS. The development of comorbidities may partially explain why RLS is more common in older adults. RLS severity correlates with a reduced health-related quality of life when comorbid with other conditions. Large population studies have found associations between RLS and cardiovascular disease.

The exact prevalence of PLMD is not known. PLMS increases in frequency with age. PLMS are seen on PSG in up to 45% of older people. The presence of PLMS often does not impact individuals in a clinically meaningful way. The existence of comorbidities with aging makes a clear-cut diagnosis of PLMD difficult. Having a family history of RLS may make PLMD more likely.

Pathophysiology

RLS and PLMS are often thought of as sharing a similar pathophysiology, with RLS being a sensory manifestation and PLMS a motor manifestation. The exact mechanisms of RLS and PLMS are not exactly known. There appears to be a defect in the homeostatic regulation of iron that then leads to a dysfunction in the dopamine system.

Clinical Presentation

RLS may present with complaints of specific RLS symptoms or simply with a primary complaint of insomnia. The most classic presentation is of a creepy crawly sensation that is predominately in the lower calf and gets better with walking. It is worse at night and with rest. Sometimes RLS symptoms involve the upper extremities as well. By definition the symptoms occur while awake. Patients who are not able to describe symptoms due to significant dementia or aphasia may be seen rubbing or massaging the legs or may present with increased motor activity at night. Pacing, cycling movements, and foot tapping can also be signs that there may be RLS symptoms. Since 80% to 90% of patients with RLS have PLMS the observation of kicking during sleep makes the diagnosis of RLS more likely. It is often difficult to distinguish RLS symptoms from peripheral neuropathy. The nighttime onset of symptoms and relief of symptoms with movement help distinguish the two conditions. For patients with both conditions present, determining the contribution of RLS over neuropathy remains challenging.

PLMD may present with a patient or bed partner complaint of kicking at night. The patient may simply present with complaints of disturbed sleep, insomnia, and/or excessive daytime sleepiness. Since PLMS are so common in older adults, significant clinical sleep disturbance and/or daytime sleepiness are required to make the diagnosis. The symptom of waking up kicking has to be distinguished from hypnic jerks or sleep starts—total body jerking often with a sensation of falling that occurs at sleep onset. Hypnic jerks are very common and generally not pathologic.

Evaluation

The diagnosis of RLS can be based on clinical criteria alone. A PSG is sometimes helpful to rule out other sleep disorders, particularly SDB which may be a comorbid cause of sleep disturbance. Presence of PLMS on PSG is suggestive of RLS but neither rules in nor rules out RLS.

A sleep study with limb electrode measurement is required for the diagnosis of PLMD because this is the only way for PLMS to be accurately measured. Furthermore, since PLMD is a diagnosis of exclusion other sleep disorders must be ruled out at the same time. A diagnosis of PLMD requires at least 15 movements per hour of sleep. Some clinicians also count the PLMS that occur with arousal in making the diagnosis.

Patients with RLS or PLMD should have a serum ferritin measured to rule out any degree of iron deficiency contributing to these conditions.

Management

Pharmacologic management The treatment options for RLS and PLMD are similar. However, whether to initiate treatment for PLMD is more controversial. For either condition the decision to treat needs to be individualized, based on the severity of symptoms and the impact on quality of life.

Patients should receive iron supplementation if the serum ferritin is less than 75 mcg/L. This entails a much more aggressive iron replacement strategy than is typically used in patients without RLS. Newer evidence even suggests using IV iron in those with moderate to severe RLS and a ferritin less than 300 mcg/L, although IV iron is usually reserved for those with iron malabsorption.

There are two accepted classes of medications that can be used for first-line treatment of RLS. The long-established treatment of choice has been dopamine agonists. Recently more of a role has been established for α2δ calcium channel ligands, which include gabapentin, gabapentin enacarbil, and pregabalin. Recent guidelines on RLS therapy have suggested limiting the dosage of dopamine agonists and considering the use of α2δ calcium channel ligands as first-line agents (**Table 44-2**).

The primary long-acting dopamine agonists that are used for persistent RLS include ropinirole, pramipexole, and rotigotine transdermal. These agents should be taken approximately 2 hours before bedtime. Carbidopa-levodopa can be used in patients for as-needed dosing when symptoms are infrequent. The major drawback to the use of dopaminergic agents is a phenomenon called augmentation. Augmentation is a worsening of RLS manifested by: the onset of RLS symptoms earlier in the day, and/or increased intensity of RLS symptoms, and/or spread of symptoms to the upper extremities and trunk when these areas were previously unaffected. Augmentation is much more frequent with carbidopa-levodopa, which is why this agent is reserved for use when symptoms are infrequent. Estimates of augmentation on the long-acting dopamine agonists have ranged between 2% and 15% per year. The risk of augmentation is higher with higher doses and longer duration of therapy. Thus, it is recommended that maximal

TABLE 44-2 ■ PHARMACOLOGIC TREATMENT OF PLMS/RLS

CLASS	GENERIC	BRAND	DOSE
Dopaminergic agents	Ropinirole	Requip	0.25–4 mg
	Pramipexole	Mirapex	0.125–2 mg
	Carbidopa/levodopa[a]	Sinemet	25/100–25/200 mg
α2δ calcium channel ligands	Gabapentin encarbil	Horizant	600–1200 mg
	Gabapentin[a]	Neurontin	100–1800 mg
	Pregabalin[a]	Lyrica	300 mg
Benzodiazepines	Clonazepam[a]	Klonopin	0.25–2 mg
	Temazepam[a]	Restoril	15–30 mg
Opiate agents	Codeine[a]	Tylenol #3/#4	30–60 mg (codeine)
	Tramadol[a]	Ultram	50–100 mg
	Oxycodone[a]	Roxycodone	5–15 mg
	Hydrocodone[a]	Vicodin	5–15 mg
	Methadone[a]		5–10 mg

[a]Off-label.

doses recommended for RLS are not exceeded. Augmentation can sometimes be managed by giving an additional dose of dopamine agonist earlier in the day, switching to a different dopamine agonist, or preferably switching to a different class of medication. Other important side effects of dopamine agonists include daytime sleepiness, headaches, and nausea. Behavioral disinhibition is a potentially dangerous side effect that can threaten a patient's livelihood. There is no evidence that tolerability of these agents changes with ageing.

The other agents that have good evidence for RLS therapy are the α2δ calcium channel ligands. Only gabapentin enacarbil is FDA approved for RLS treatment. These agents may be particularly useful when the patient also has peripheral neuropathy. A recent randomized controlled trial showed that pregabalin was as efficacious as pramipexole, with a lower rate of augmentation. Major adverse effects from these medications can include drowsiness, dizziness, and suicidal ideation. There may be significant variability in the pharmacokinetics in these drugs with aging, particularly if there is a reduction in renal function. Careful monitoring is required.

Other medications that can be used for the treatment of RLS include benzodiazepines and opiates. Benzodiazepines have a long history of use for intermittent RLS; however, the evidence base for this practice is limited. Low-dose opiates including methadone can be used for treatment of refractory RLS. Clearly, benzodiazepines and opiates may have adverse cognitive effects in older patients and should be used with caution. The American Geriatric Society recommends avoiding opiates when combined with other central nervous system depressants.

Nonpharmacologic therapy Behavioral strategies that can be used for RLS include moderate exercise, pneumatic compression, massage, and yoga. There are novel devices available for the treatment of RLS; however, the data available

are extremely limited. Avoidance of possible triggers for RLS should also be recommended. These include sleep deprivation, caffeine, and alcohol use. Also, most antidepressants are known to elicit or provoke RLS symptoms. However, bupropion is less frequently associated with RLS, and therefore, a switch from a selective serotonin reuptake inhibitor (SSRI) or serotonin-norepinephrine reuptake inhibitor (SNRI) to bupropion when RLS symptoms are present could be considered.

Prevention

There is no specific prevention for RLS. Adherence to a healthy lifestyle may be beneficial. This includes moderate exercise, a regular sleep schedule, and limiting caffeine and alcohol intake.

Patient Preference

The focus of RLS management is symptom relief. The medications used for the treatment of RLS may have important side effects. Therefore, therapy is determined by the balance between symptom control and side effects, in addition to patient input and preferences.

Comorbidities

Frequently encountered comorbidities of RLS include Parkinson disease, chronic kidney disease, iron deficiency anemia, and peripheral neuropathy. It is essential to address both the underlying disease process and the RLS symptoms at the same time. There is some evidence that both RLS and PLMS are associated with cardiovascular disease.

REM SLEEP BEHAVIOR DISORDER

Definition

REM sleep behavior disorder (RBD) is defined as recurrent complex movements or vocalizations during sleep characterized by dream enactment. Normally during REM sleep there is complete loss of skeletal muscle tone (atonia). However, in RBD there is REM sleep without atonia, which is required for the diagnosis of RBD, in addition to dream enactment behavior.

Epidemiology

RBD is a male-predominant syndrome, which usually occurs after the age of 50. The prevalence of RBD has been estimated to be around 1% in those older than age 40 and around 2% in those older than age 60. Clinical series have shown that patients present for evaluation in their mid-60s. Thus, RBD can be considered to be a disease of aging. This is likely due to the fact that RBD is more common in certain neurologic disorders such as Parkinson disease, multiple system atrophy, and Lewy body dementia.

Pathophysiology

There is an association between neurodegenerative disorders and RBD, particularly synucleinopathies, which result from a pathologic lesion of aggregates of insoluble α-synuclein protein. These aggregates are linked to degradation of specific brain regions and clinical symptoms. The most important clinical diagnoses of synucleinopathies are Parkinson disease, dementia with Lewy bodies, and multiple system atrophy. The α-synuclein protein aggregates can be found in the brain areas responsible for producing active atonia during REM sleep. Up to 90% of patients who present with RBD develop another synucleinopathy disorder over the course of a 10- to 15-year follow-up (**Figure 44-8**).

RBD is also strongly linked with narcolepsy, which may be a different form of REM sleep motor-behavior dysregulation. The RBD may be worsened by the use of SSRIs to treat cataplexy. Other neurologic disorders have been associated with RBD including cerebrovascular disease, multiple sclerosis, Guillain-Barre syndrome, normal pressure hydrocephalus, Tourette syndrome, and autism.

Clinical Presentation

RBD will often present with sleep-related injury that results from the enactment of dreams that are often violent. It is rare for patients with RBD to calmly walk and carry out other complex tasks. Patients are usually not able to leave the room they are in because they are not attentive to their environment. Because RBD occurs during REM sleep, it usually appears at least 90 minutes after sleep onset and is more likely to occur later in the sleep period. Often RBD is the first manifestation of Parkinson disease or dementia with Lewy bodies, but may also present later in patients with these disorders.

Evaluation

The evaluation of RBD includes a neurologic and sleep history. The history should focus on common associated conditions such as Parkinson disease and associated dementia. Other early signs of an α-synucleinopathy include loss of smell and constipation. The presence of vivid dream enactment makes RBD more likely than an NREM sleep parasomnia. A predilection for events to occur later in the sleep period also makes RBD more likely. A detailed neurologic

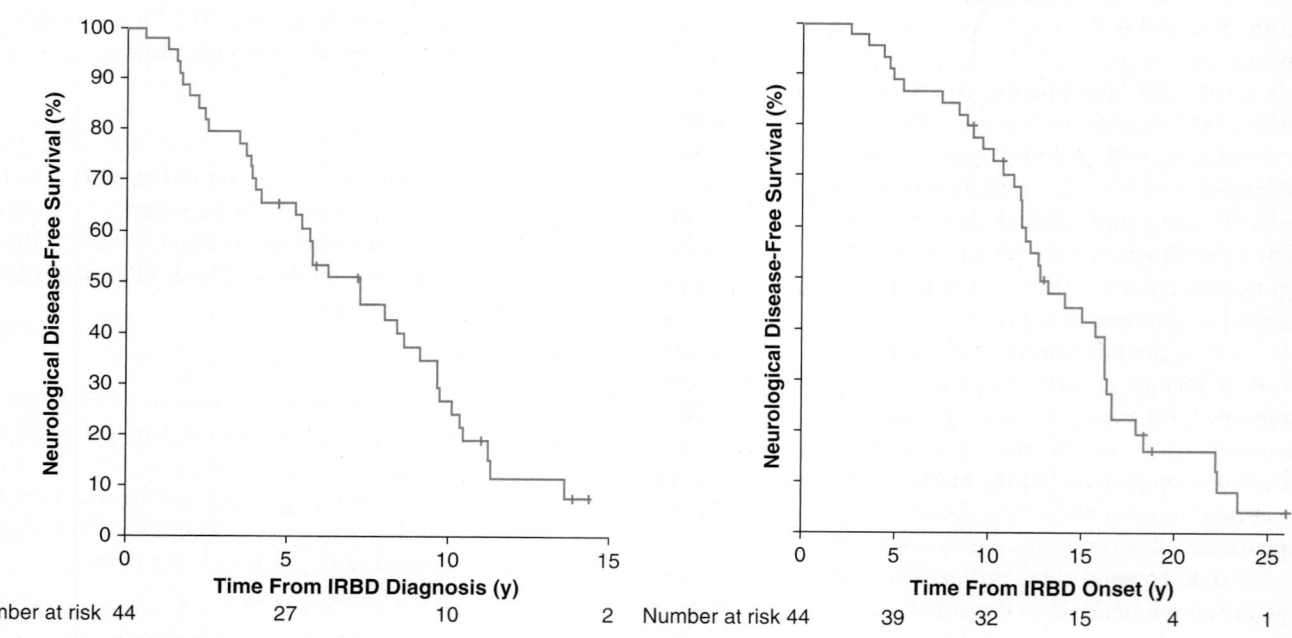

FIGURE 44-8. Relationship between the diagnosis of idiopathic REM behavior disorder (IRBD) and the development of a neurodegenerative disorder. (Reproduced with permission from Iranzo A, Tolosa E, Gelpi E, et al. Neurodegenerative disease status and post-mortem pathology in idiopathic rapid-eye-movement sleep behaviour disorder: an observational cohort study. *Lancet Neurol.* 2013;12[5]:443–453.)

examination can elucidate a comorbid neurodegenerative disorder. It may be difficult to distinguish RBD symptoms from those of other parasomnias, nocturnal seizures, and the nightmares of posttraumatic stress disorder (PTSD). SDB can cause RBD-like symptoms, which typically resolve with effective SDB therapy.

An attended in-laboratory PSG is the gold standard for diagnosing RBD. Acting out of dreams in REM sleep during the sleep study is typically sufficient for diagnosing RBD. However, often patients will not have RBD behavior events during PSG. In this case, finding substantial REM sleep with increased muscle tone with a history of dream enactment behaviors can support an RBD diagnosis. The diagnosis can be complicated in patients who have PTSD, as there is emerging evidence that PTSD may predispose to RBD and that PTSD may be associated with atonia in REM sleep independent of RBD.

Management

Pharmacologic management There are no currently FDA-approved therapies for RBD. The goal of treatment is to avoid injury and prevent sleep disruption. The two major pharmacologic treatments are melatonin and clonazepam. Avoiding benzodiazepines is generally preferable in older patients making melatonin the primary first choice for therapy in most circumstances. There is evidence from small trials that melatonin reduces the amount of REM sleep with excessive muscle tone as well as the clinical manifestations of RBD. The mechanism by which melatonin improves RBD is unknown. Often fairly high doses of melatonin can be used, however there is uncertainty as to how high the dosing should go. The major drawback to melatonin is that it is not an FDA-regulated pharmaceutical. Therefore, quality and strength may not be as tightly regulated. Clonazepam at low doses has been successfully used to treat RBD symptoms. A single-center retrospective study of RBD patients found that both melatonin and clonazepam improved RBD symptoms; however, only melatonin was associated with reduced injuries and falls. Moreover, melatonin had a better side effect profile than clonazepam.

Nonpharmacologic therapy The most important intervention in patients with RBD is ensuring the safety of both the patient and any bed partners. The patient should consider sleeping separately from their bed partner for that person's safety. Sharp furniture and other sharp objects should be removed from the patient's bedroom. Likewise, any weapons should not be freely accessible. If falling out of bed has been an issue, moving the mattress to the floor can be considered. Alarms have been developed to wake patients as they leave the bed. Some patients have gone so far as to sleep in sleeping bags to prevent injuring themselves.

Well-recognized precipitating factors for RBD symptoms include the use of SSRIs, venlafaxine, mirtazapine, and other antidepressants except for bupropion. Hence, tapering off these medications or switching to bupropion should be considered. Any sort of comorbid SDB disorder should be aggressively treated, which may help with RBD symptoms.

Prevention

There are no known preventative measures for RBD.

Patient Preference

Since the treatment of RBD is symptom based, patient preferences often dictate the intensity and type of therapy. Many patients may opt for melatonin therapy given that its side effect profile appears to be favorable to clonazepam. The desire for the patient to know the ramifications of an RBD diagnosis as a predictor of development of a future neurodegenerative disorder needs to be carefully elucidated.

Comorbidities

As discussed previously presence of RBD strongly predicts the subsequent development of an α-synucleinopathy such as Parkinson disease, multiple system atrophy, and dementia with Lewy bodies. Often RBD is the first manifestation of one of these disorders. Therefore, RBD will eventually coexist with one of these neurodegenerative disorders in most patients. RBD can also present in patients with narcolepsy. There are some cases in which RBD and NREM parasomnias coexist as well.

OTHER PARASOMNIAS

Other parasomnias occur in NREM sleep, which include sleep walking, confusional arousals, and sleep terrors. These disorders are much more common in children and young adults, and generally do not first present in old age. The distinguishing features of these conditions are that they predominantly occur in the first part of the night and the patients are difficult to arouse and do not have recollection of the event or associated dream imagery. One aspect of these NREM parasomnias relevant to older adults is that nonbenzodiazepine hypnotics (eg, zolpidem, zalepelon, eszpicolone) can be associated with very complex sleep behaviors such as sleep cooking, sleep eating, and sleep driving. This is a rare but possibly dangerous side effect of these medications.

CIRCADIAN RHYTHM DISORDERS

Definition

Circadian rhythms refer to the 24-hour biological rhythms that control functions such as hormone secretion, core body temperature, and the sleep-wake cycle. The endogenous circadian rhythms originate in the suprachiasmatic nucleus (SCN), which is the internal circadian pacemaker. The SCN synchronizes itself using other internal rhythms from hormone secretion patterns and external signals, the most potent of which is light. The sleep-wake cycle is driven by melatonin secretion and body temperature, which are both governed by the SCN. However, external light can disrupt this cycle.

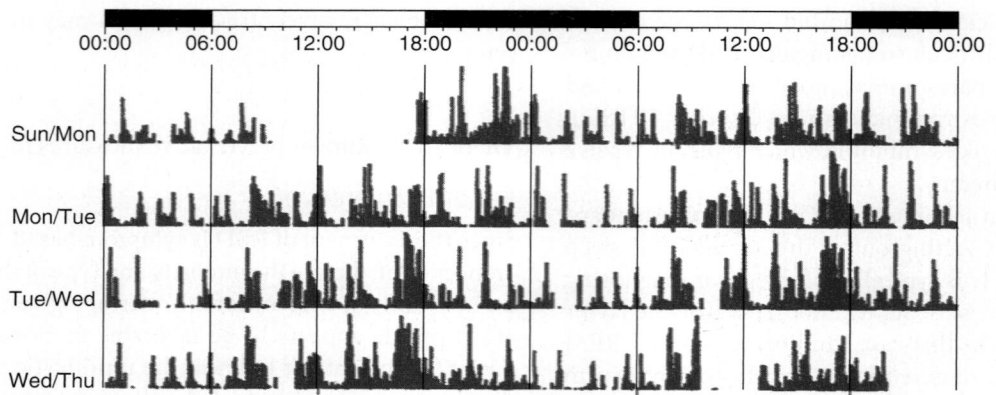

FIGURE 44-9. Actigraphy of a patient with irregular sleep-wake disorder. The red lines indicate bouts of movement and activity. In this patient there is not a set time when there is activity versus inactivity. (Reproduced with permission from Kryger MH, Avidan AY, Berry RB. *Atlas of Clinical Sleep Medicine.* 2nd ed. Philadelphia, PA: Elsevier; 2014.)

Circadian rhythm disorders are a chronic or recurrent pattern of sleep-wake rhythm disruption due to a misalignment between the patient's endogenous circadian rhythm and their desired or red sleep-wake cycle. For this to be considered a disorder it must cause bothersome insomnia symptoms and/or excessive sleepiness. For instance, a retired person who is not bothered by going to bed at 8 PM and waking up at 4 AM does not have a disorder.

Delayed sleep-wake phase disorder is a delay in the phase of the endogenous major sleep episode with respect to the desired major sleep episode such that the patient complains of an inability to fall asleep and difficulty waking up at the desired time.

Advanced sleep-wake phase disorder is an advance in the phase of the endogenous major sleep episode with respect to the desired major sleep episode such that the patient complains of difficulty staying awake until the desired bedtime, with an inability to remain asleep until the desired awakening time.

Irregular sleep-wake rhythm disorder is characterized by a lack of a clearly defined circadian rhythm resulting in insomnia at night and excessive sleep during the day (**Figure 44-9**). This disorder is often associated with neurodegenerative diseases and is likely common in the nursing home setting.

Non–24-hour sleep-wake rhythm disorder usually occurs from a patient's inability to entrain their circadian rhythm to light due to complete blindness. The natural circadian rhythm is typically longer than 24 hours. Thus, each subsequent day, the patient will go to bed and wake up a little later. This leads to episodes of insomnia and hypersomnia (**Figure 44-10**).

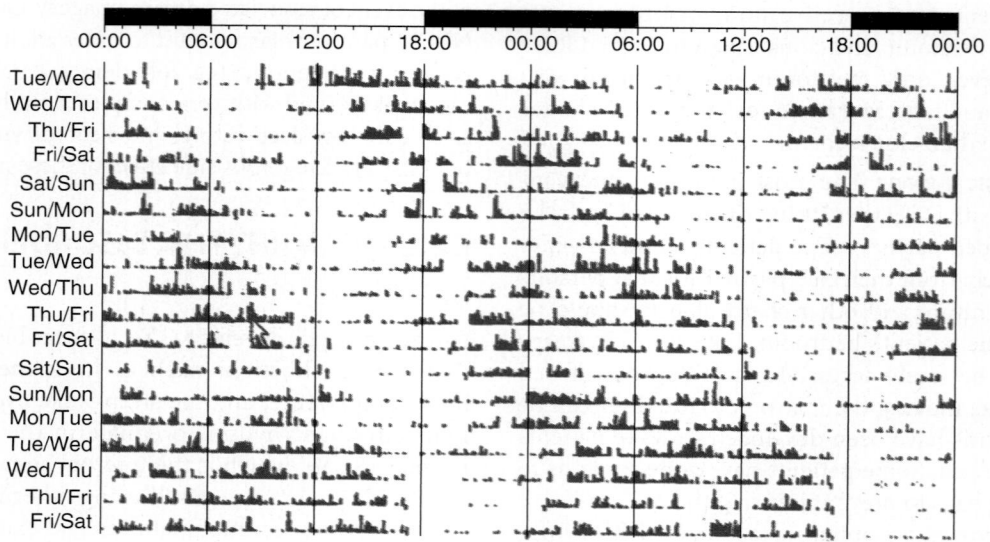

FIGURE 44-10. Actigraphy of a patient with non–24-hour sleep-wake rhythm disorder. Because the internal circadian rhythm is longer than 24 hours, each night the patient goes to bed later and wakes up later, causing a drift in the sleep period over time. (Reproduced with permission from Kryger MH, Avidan AY, Berry RB. *Atlas of Clinical Sleep Medicine.* 2nd ed. Philadelphia, PA: Elsevier; 2014.)

Epidemiology

Delayed sleep-wake phase disorder is more common among adolescents and young adults; however familial patterns and psychiatric disorders are risk factors for development of delayed sleep-wake phase disorder in later life.

The prevalence of advanced sleep-wake disorder is not fully known and is thought to comprise 1% of a middle-aged population. Advanced age appears to be a risk factor, given that aging is associated with the development of morning tendencies. However, older patients may be more tolerant of these changes in endogenous circadian rhythm.

Irregular sleep-wake rhythm disorder is commonly seen in older adults with neurodegenerative disorders such as AD, Parkinson disease, and Huntington disease.

Pathophysiology

Possible causes of advanced sleep-wake phase disorder include a loss of the ability for the circadian clock to phase delay, a tendency to abnormally phase advance to entraining stimuli or a shorter endogenous circadian pacemaker. The latter of these has been shown to underlie the pathophysiology in select familial patients with circadian clock gene mutations.

There are several factors that may cause irregular circadian rhythms with aging. These may include (1) degeneration of the SCN with age, (2) a blunting of melatonin secretion at night, (3) decreased sensitivity to entraining cues, and (4) less availability to cues such as bright light. Furthermore, neurodegenerative disorders may result in physical disruption of circadian rhythm pathways. Irregular sleep patterns prevent the normal sequence of progression through sleep stages.

Clinical Presentation

Patients with delayed sleep phase disorder present with sleepiness in the morning and an inability to sleep in the evening. Patients with advanced sleep phase disorder present with sleepiness in the evening, and an inability to sleep in the early morning. These patients will essentially present with insomnia complaints. However, an ability to sleep when the patient aligns their sleep-wake cycle with their endogenous circadian rhythm will be indicative of a circadian rhythm disorder rather than insomnia. Patients with advanced sleep phase syndrome may develop a self-imposed sleep deprivation from trying to adhere to a "normal schedule" but will wake up too early. A strong familial pattern may also suggest a circadian disorder.

Patients with irregular sleep-wake rhythm disorder will present with poorly consolidated sleep. Caregivers of patients with dementia who have this condition may notice nighttime wandering and agitation. In fact, sundowning may be a phenotype of a circadian rhythm disturbance. Patients will generally sleep for less than 4 hours at a time, and will have many short periods of sleep and wake throughout the day and night.

Evaluation

The key component in evaluating patients with suspected circadian rhythm disturbances is a comprehensive sleep history. Sleep logs for 1 to 2 weeks are helpful in establishing the diagnosis of a circadian disorder. Wrist actigraphy (a device with an accelerometer) can also be useful, particularly in patients who cannot fill out sleep logs, or for those in whom the accuracy of the sleep logs is doubtful. Newer actigraphy monitors that have a light sensor can also give the clinician a sense of the patient's light exposure. PSG is only indicated when other sleep disorders are suspected.

Management

The primary management for circadian rhythm disorders involves the use of appropriately timed bright light therapy. Appropriately timed melatonin can be used as an alternative to, or in conjunction with, bright light therapy. However, there is less evidence for this approach. There are commercially available light boxes, or where feasible, natural sunlight can be used. In general, exposure to bright light in the morning will advance the circadian rhythm, while exposure in the evening will cause a delay in rhythm. Patients with advanced sleep-wake phase disorder should wear sunglasses in the morning and spend late afternoons outdoors without sunglasses.

For irregular sleep-wake rhythm disorder a strong routine with natural light and increased activity during the day and darkness with decreased noise at night may be helpful. Tasimelteon is a melatonin agonist for the MT1 and MT2 receptors with greater affinity for the MT2 receptor. This agent is only approved in adults for non–24-hour sleep-wake rhythm disorder.

INSOMNIA

Definition

Insomnia is defined as the inability to fall asleep, the inability to stay asleep, or waking up earlier than desired. In order to have a clinical diagnosis of insomnia the patient must have an adequate sleep opportunity and adequate sleep environment. The sleep disturbance must also have an impact on their quality of life by causing any of the following: fatigue, impaired cognitive performance, mood disturbance, daytime sleepiness, behavioral problems, reduced motivation, proneness for errors, or worry about sleep. Insomnia is categorized as chronic if it persists more than 3 months and short term if it has lasted fewer than 3 months. The most recent International Classification of Sleep Disorders no longer emphasizes previously distinguished insomnia subtypes or insomnia comorbid with mental or medical disorders. Even when insomnia is related to another condition, treatment of the comorbid condition often does not cure the insomnia. Furthermore, individual patients often have an overlap across insomnia subtypes.

Epidemiology

Insomnia is a highly prevalent sleep disorder, affecting up to 10% of young adults and increases to about 30% to 48% in those older than 65 years. The prevalence of insomnia is higher in older adults, which is likely due to age-related reductions in sleep efficiency and the accrual of comorbidities that are associated with insomnia. However, among older adults the diagnosis of insomnia does not necessarily increase with increasing age. Insomnia is more prevalent in women than men even in older adults.

Comorbid psychiatric conditions increase the likelihood of developing chronic insomnia. Depression is perhaps the most common and strongly associated mental illness with insomnia. Anxiety is also a risk factor for developing insomnia; as is being a caregiver for an ill family member, with up to 40% of caregivers reporting taking sleep aids for insomnia.

A wide variety of medical problems are associated with insomnia. Many studies have linked sleep disturbances with worsened health-related quality of life, nursing home placement, and even death. Epidemiologic evidence shows a greater prevalence of insomnia in hypertension, heart disease, arthritis, lung disease, gastrointestinal reflux, stroke, and neurodegenerative disorders, to only name a few. Symptoms of medical illnesses that can disrupt sleep include pain, paresthesias, cough, dyspnea, reflux, and nocturia.

Many medications can impair sleep or change sleep architecture. If stimulating medications (eg, caffeine, sympathomimetics, bronchodilators, activating psychiatric medications) are taken too near to bedtime, sleep can be disturbed (**Table 44-3**). Furthermore, sedating medications can lead to daytime sleeping, which often decreases the ability to sleep at night.

Late-life insomnia is often a long-lasting problem. One study showed that a third of older patients had persistent severe insomnia symptoms at 4-year follow-up. Among women older than 85 years, more than 80% reported sleeping difficulties, with many using over-the-counter (OTC) sleeping medications. Lastly being a caregiver for others, which often occurs later in life, is a contributing factor to the development of insomnia.

TABLE 44-3 ■ EFFECT OF COMMON DRUGS TAKEN BY OLDER ADULTS

SEDATING	ALERTING
Hypnotics	Alcohol/nicotine
Antihypertensives	CNS stimulants
Antihistamines	Thyroid hormones
Antpsychotics	Bronchodilators
Antidepressants	Corticosteroids
	β-Blockers
	Calcium channel blockers

Pathophysiology

The causes of insomnia are often multifaceted. One popular theoretical model for insomnia posits that there are predisposing factors, precipitating factors, and perpetuating factors. Predisposing factors are a vulnerability to insomnia and may include anxiety, depression, or hyperarousal. Precipitating factors are triggers for insomnia such as loss of a spouse, retirement, moving to a new home, or any other sort of stressor. Perpetuating factors are maladaptive habits or beliefs that the patient has acquired to deal with the insomnia such as spending long periods in bed or taking naps.

As noted earlier, insomnia in older adults is often comorbid with medical or psychiatric illnesses. The symptoms such as pain, dyspnea, or nocturia may be so significant that these become the primary driving factors behind the sleep disturbance.

Clinical Presentation

Patients with insomnia may present to their primary care provider with specific complaints about either not being able to fall asleep or stay asleep. However, many patients do not talk to their doctors about their sleep complaints. Instead, the presence of insomnia may be revealed by eliciting self-medication with over-the-counter therapies or alternative sedatives.

A careful sleep history and evaluation should be conducted in patients with insomnia in order to assess whether there are comorbid sleep disorders, such as SDB, underlying the sleep disturbance. The presence of undiagnosed OSA is common in those with insomnia.

Evaluation

PSG and other sleep studies are not necessary in the evaluation of insomnia; however, they should be obtained if a comorbid sleep condition is suspected. Sleep diaries with daily entries over 1 to 2 weeks, with caffeine, alcohol, and medication use noted can be very helpful in determining the severity of the insomnia as well as identifying possible perpetuating factors such as irregular bedtimes or late-night caffeine (**Table 44-4**). This may help the patient gain more insight into their sleep problem. Wrist actigraphy in conjunction with a sleep diary can be used to obtain a more objective measure of the patient's overall sleep-wake pattern. This device is particularly helpful when accuracy of the sleep diary is questionable or when sleep-wake misperception is suspected. The accuracy of direct to consumer devices, such as fitbits, has not been rigorously tested, but they may be useful adjuncts in practice.

Management

Behavioral and nonpharmacologic interventions appear to have better long-term efficacy with fewer side effects than pharmacologic interventions. Therefore, behavioral interventions are preferred for the treatment of insomnia, particularly in older patients. However, access to highly skilled

TABLE 44-4 ■ SAMPLE SLEEP DIARY

NAME:	DATE:		TO				
	MONDAY	TUESDAY	WEDNESDAY	THURSDAY	FRIDAY	SATURDAY	SUNDAY
1. Bedtime							
2. Time taken to fall asleep (after lights off)							
3. Number of nighttime awakenings							
4. Wake-up time							
5. Time out of bed (morning)							
6. Total sleep time (night only)							
7. Total wake time (night only)							
8. Nap time (if any)							
9. Medication (time/dosage)							
10. Alcohol (time/dosage)							
11. How was your sleep last night?[a]							
12. How tired were you in the morning?[b]							

[a]1 = excellent to 5 = very poor; [b]1 = not tired to 5 = very tired.

professionals trained in such interventions may be limited in some health care systems. Cognitive behavioral therapy for insomnia (CBT-I) has been recommended as the first-line treatment for all insomnia in adults by multiple practice guidelines.

Pharmacologic management Most pharmacotherapy for insomnia is designed and approved for the treatment of transient sleep disturbances. Pharmacotherapy can be considered when insomnia is triggered by an acute event or when chronic insomnia persists despite behavioral insomnia treatment. Sedative-hypnotics have been associated with adverse side effects in older adults, such as falls, cognitive slowing, fractures, and even mortality. Therefore, if a sedative-hypnotic is used in older individuals, the smallest dose of an agent with the least risk of adverse events should be chosen for the shortest duration necessary. In general, short-acting drugs should be used for patients who have trouble falling asleep while intermediate-acting drugs should be used when patients have trouble staying asleep (**Table 44-5**).

Benzodiazepines have had a long history of being used for insomnia. These drugs bind nonselectively to the γ-aminobutyric acid benzodiazepine (GABA-A) receptor subunits. The overall effects of these drugs are to induce anxiolysis, sedation, and amnesia. Temazepam, lorazepam, triazolam, and estazolam are intermediate-acting agents that are most commonly used for insomnia, while triazolam is a shorter-acting agent that is also used for insomnia. Due to next-day effects, the longer-acting agents, flurazepam and quazepam, should not be used in older adults. Benzodiazepines do decrease the time to fall asleep by about 10 minutes on average and the number of awakenings, thereby increasing the total sleep time by 30 to 60 minutes during the nighttime. The side effects associated with this class of medications include confusion, falls, rebound insomnia, tolerance, and withdrawal symptoms on discontinuation. Benzodiazepines have been linked to increased pneumonia in those with AD. These agents are all listed as potentially inappropriate for use in geriatric patients in the Beers Criteria.

Nonbenzodiazepine-benzodiazepine receptor agonists (NBRAs [such as eszopiclone, zolpidem, and zaleplon]) are structurally unrelated to benzodiazepines but bind selectively to the GABA-A receptors. They generally produce sedation and amnestic effects without the anxiolytic properties. These agents likely have similar efficacy to benzodiazepines but with a somewhat better side effect profile, in part due to their relatively short duration of action. In healthy older adults without comorbidities, NBRAs are relatively well tolerated. Zolpidem and zaleplon should only be taken immediately before bed because of their rapid onset of action. Eszopiclone has a longer duration of action than the other NRBAs, and is better for sleep maintenance but may cause drowsiness in the morning. There is also an extended-release form of zolpidem that can be used for sleep maintenance insomnia. Guidelines only recommend these medications for use in short-term insomnia, however studies have shown efficacy in chronic insomnia. Concerns remain regarding the risks of falls, confusion, and fracture in older adults, particularly in those with frailty. The emergence of complex sleep-related behaviors such as sleep driving and sleep eating has been seen with zolpidem, which may be class side effect with these agents. NRBAs are also on the Beer's list of potentially inappropriate medications for older adults.

Melatonin receptor agonists (eg, ramelteon) are approved for insomnia. Rather than activating GABA receptors, ramelteon is selective for the MT1/MT2 melatonin receptors. Ramelteon has been shown to reduce total sleep latency and increase sleep time in older adults, with fewer

TABLE 44-5 ■ PRESCRIPTION MEDICATIONS COMMONLY USED FOR INSOMNIA IN OLDER ADULTS

CLASS, MEDICATION	STARTING DOSE (MG)	USUAL DOSE (MG)	HALF-LIFE (H)	COMMENTS
INTERMEDIATE-ACTING BENZODIAZEPINE				
Temazepam	7.5	7.5–30	8.8	Psychomotor impairment, increased risk of falls
SHORT-ACTING NONBENZODIAZEPINES				
Eszopiclone	1	1–2	6	Reportedly effective for long-term use in selected individuals; may be associated with unpleasant taste, headache; avoid administration with high-fat meal
Zaleplon	5	5–10	1 (reportedly unchanged in older adults)	Reportedly little daytime carryover, tolerance, or rebound insomnia
Zolpidem	5	5	1.5–4.5 (3 in older adults, 10 in hepatic cirrhosis)	Reportedly little daytime carryover, tolerance, or rebound insomnia
MELATONIN RECEPTOR AGONIST				
Ramelteon	8	8	1.5 (2.6 in older adults)	Dizziness, myalgia, headache, other adverse events reported; no significant rebound insomnia or withdrawal with discontinuation
SEDATING ANTIDEPRESSANTS				
Doxepin	3	3–6	15.3 (doxepin); 31 (metabolite)	Somnolence/sedation, nausea, and upper respiratory tract infection reported; antagonizes central H_1 receptors (antihistamine); active metabolite; should not be taken within 3 h of a meal
Mirtazapine	7.5	7.5–45	31–39 in older adults; 13–34 in younger adults; mean = 21	Increased appetite, weight gain, headache, dizziness, daytime carryover; used for insomnia with depression
Trazodone	25–50	25–150	Reportedly 6 ± 2; prolonged in older adults and obese individuals	Moderate orthostatic effects; administration after food minimizes sedation and postural hypotension; used for insomnia with depression
DUAL OREXIN RECEPTOR ANTAGONISTS				
Lemborexant	5	5–10	17–19	Next day drowsiness, complex sleep-related disorder, abnormal dreams, and sleep paralysis may occur. Metabolism through CYP3A4.
Suvorexant	5	10–20	12	Next day drowsiness, complex sleep-related disorder, abnormal dreams, and sleep paralysis may occur. Metabolism through CYP3A4.

side effects. However, somnolence, dizziness, headache, and fatigue can be side effects of this agent. Ramelteon does not seem to be associated with significant withdrawal or rebound insomnia effects. The major downside of ramelteon is that its lack of amnestic properties makes it somewhat less effective for subjective improvement in sleep.

Dual orexin receptor agonists (DORAs). There are two new agents for insomnia that target the orexin (also known as hypocretin) system, suvorexant and lemborexant. Damage to the orexin-secreting neurons of the hypothalamus were discovered to be the principle cause of narcolepsy with cataplexy. It was found that this system stabilizes wakefulness. DORAs decrease sleep drive by blocking the effects of both orexin receptors. DORAs have been shown to increase subjective sleep time and quality to a modest degree. The most common side effect is somnolence as well as possible impairment in driving. The half-lives of these medications, particularly lemborexant, are fairly long. Also, REM instability such as mild cataplexy, sleep paralysis, and sleep onset/offset hallucinations have also been reported. DORAs are metabolized by the CYP3A system leading to potential drug-drug interactions. Of note, suvorexant is the only medication specifically approved for insomnia among those with Alzheimer dementia. This was based on a relatively small trial of 277 participants with mild to moderate AD and insomnia. There was increased sleep time of around half an hour after 2 weeks and few adverse effects.

Other agents are available for treatment of insomnia. The tricyclic antidepressant doxepin has recently been developed for insomnia in a low-dose formulation (3–6 mg). For comparison, the usual antidepressant dose of doxepin is 100 to 300 mg per day. At these low dosages doxepin selectively antagonizes H1 receptors, which is believed to have sleep-promoting effects. Data suggests that low-dose doxepin does not have more anticholinergic effects than placebo. The duration of action for doxepin makes it more attractive for problems with sleep maintenance rather than sleep onset. The use of low doses of other sedating antidepressants such as trazodone and mirtazapine at bedtime is common. However, there is limited evidence to support this practice. In fact, a study in the use of trazodone for nondepressed patients showed that there was short-term benefit, which dissipated after 2 weeks. Thus, the benefits may be very small compared to the potential for side effects. However, if there is comorbid depression it should be treated, and sedating antidepressants may be a good choice as primary or adjunctive therapy. Trazadone has been associated with daytime sleepiness, headache, and orthostatic hypotension as well as priapism.

Although sedating antipsychotics are sometimes used to treat insomnia, there is scant evidence demonstrating their efficacy, and these medications can have significant adverse events, including increased mortality particularly in older adults with dementia. Guidelines suggest that sedating antipsychotics should not routinely be used in the management of insomnia in older adults without coexisting serious psychiatric conditions that warrant use of these agents.

Almost half of all older adults report the use of non-prescription over-the-counter (OTC) sleeping agents. Common nonprescription agents include sedating antihistamines, acetaminophen, alcohol, melatonin, and herbal products. The sedating antihistamines (eg, diphenhydramine) are the most common ingredients in these OTC drugs marketed for sleep. Diphenhydramine is sedating through its potent antihistaminergic effects, and tolerance to its sedating effect develops rapidly. The long half-life of diphenhydramine may result in next-day sedation. Patients may also experience dry mouth, urinary retention, delirium, decreased cognition, constipation, and increased ocular pressure. For these reasons, diphenhydramine should not be used as a primary treatment for insomnia in older patients. Many patients may use alcohol to self-medicate for insomnia; however, it can interfere with sleep in the later evening and worsen sleep difficulties.

Other supplements are available OTC, such as melatonin and valerian. One drawback of these supplements is the lack of standardization and oversight of traditional pharmaceuticals. Due to lack of solid evidence recent AASM guidelines do not recommend their use. There is evidence that melatonin improves time to fall asleep and sleep efficiency in older adults. However, the results of studies have been mixed. Valerian is a herbal product marketed for insomnia due to its mild sedative properties. Some valerian preparations contain multiple botanicals, which may increase the chance of side effects. Kava, another herbal product marketed for insomnia, has a significant risk of adverse events, including hepatotoxicity, and is not recommended.

Behavioral and other nonpharmacologic interventions
Behavioral treatment of insomnia is the safest, and perhaps, the most effective therapy for insomnia in older adults. It is the recommended first-line treatment for insomnia in all adults. Effective behavioral interventions for insomnia go beyond sleep hygiene, which is not generally effective when used alone for chronic insomnia. Several randomized trials and systematic reviews provide strong evidence for cognitive behavioral therapy for insomnia (CBT-I). CBT-I usually combines sleep hygiene, stimulus control, sleep restriction, and cognitive therapy, each of which will be discussed in greater detail below. CBT-I has reliably been shown to produce improved sleep efficiency, decreased nighttime wakefulness, and greater satisfaction with sleep. In at least two randomized trials with older adults comparing CBT-I with a prescription sedative-hypnotic agent, participants reported better improvement in sleep and more satisfaction with CBT-I therapy. One consistent finding of studies comparing CBT-I to pharmacologic therapy is that the improvements with CBT-I are more sustained. One of the major downsides to CBT-I is the limited access to practitioners who are trained in this specific therapy, but efforts are underway in some health care systems to increase access. Also, CBT-I requires significant buy-in from the patient. New delivery models that involve the use of the internet, nonspecialist providers, and telehealth-based CBT-I have yielded promising results.

Sleep hygiene is education on general practices to maintain a healthy sleep-wake routine. When a sleep history is performed behaviors that contribute to disruptive sleep should be ascertained. Examples of these behaviors include sleeping with the television on, or excessive caffeine consumption. Patients should be educated about behaviors that may contribute to poor sleep and insomnia (**Table 44-6**).

Stimulus-control therapy is designed to break the negative associations patients have with their sleep

TABLE 44-6 ■ SLEEP HYGIENE RULES FOR OLDER ADULTS

Check effect of medication on sleep and wakefulness.
Avoid caffeine, alcohol, and cigarettes after lunch.
Limit liquids in the evening.
Keep a regular bedtime-waketime schedule.
Avoid naps or limit to 1 nap a day, no longer than 30 min.
Spend time outdoors (without sunglasses), particularly in the late afternoon or early evening.
Exercise—but limit exercise immediately before bedtime.

662

CHAPTER 44 SLEEP DISORDERS

TABLE 44-7 ■ INSTRUCTIONS FOR STIMULUS-CONTROL THERAPY FOR OLDER ADULTS
1. Patient should only go to bed when tired or sleepy.
2. If unable to fall asleep within 20 min, patient should get out of bed (and bedroom if possible). While out of bed, do something quiet and relaxing.
3. Patient should only return to bed when sleepy.
4. If unable to fall asleep within 20 min, patient should again get out of bed.
5. Behavior is repeated until patient can fall asleep within a few minutes.
6. Patient should get up at the same time each morning (even if only a few hours of sleep).
7. Naps should be avoided.

TABLE 44-8 ■ INSTRUCTIONS FOR SLEEP RESTRICTION THERAPY FOR OLDER ADULTS
1. Calculate the average amount of time asleep per night reported by patient.
2. Patient is only allowed to stay in bed for this amount of time plus 15 min.
3. Patient must get up at the same time each day.
4. Daytime napping should be strictly avoided.
5. When sleep efficiency has reached 80%–85%, patient can go to bed 15 min earlier.
6. This procedure should be repeated until patient can sleep for 8 h (or period needed for a good night's sleep).

environment, which have come about from maladaptive behaviors. Patients are instructed to not have any other in-bed activities aside from sleep or sex, and to only go to bed when tired enough to fall asleep. They should unwind prior to going to bed and should not watch an alarm clock. If the patient cannot fall asleep within approximately 20 minutes they should get out of bed and do a relaxing activity and only return to bed when able to fall asleep. For a regular pattern to develop the patient needs to avoid napping and should get out of bed the same time each day. Daytime sleepiness may increase early in this therapy particularly when paired with sleep restriction (**Table 44-7**).

Sleep-restriction therapy was developed from the observation that many patients with insomnia spend a large amount of time in bed unsuccessfully attempting to sleep. Sleep-restriction therapy is guided by the patient's sleep diary. The amount of time the patient actually sleeps is calculated and the patient is only allowed to spend that amount of time plus around 15 minutes in bed each night for the following week. Since the amount of sleep will be less, this will lead to sleep deprivation and an increased sleep drive. The increased sleepiness makes it easier for the patient to subsequently fall asleep more quickly and have more consolidated sleep. Once the patient has significantly consolidated, time in bed is increased gradually until the patient is getting adequate sleep (**Table 44-8**).

Cognitive therapy in CBT-I addresses the maladaptive thoughts or dysfunctional beliefs patients have about their sleep. This is essential to be addressed to ensure adherence to the behavioral aspects of the therapy. Other components of CBT-I may include various relaxation techniques and scheduled worry time. Image rehearsal therapy may be helpful with patients who have trouble sleeping from nightmares related to PTSD. Mindfulness and other relaxation techniques can be strong adjuncts to the behavioral and cognitive components of CBTI.

There are several small studies that have found a beneficial effect of bright light, either from natural sunlight or light boxes, on the sleep of older adults. The reported effects of light on insomnia are more variable than those reported for circadian rhythm disorders. Evening light exposure may be useful for those who go to sleep and wake up too early (ie, advanced sleep phase), while morning exposure may be useful in patients who stay up and sleep in late (ie, delayed sleep phase).

There is less evidence to support other behavioral interventions, but individual patients may find them useful. For example, bathing before sleep can enhance sleep quality in some older individuals, which is likely related to changes in body temperature. A moderate exercise program can improve sleep in healthy sedentary older adults. However, strenuous exercise should not be done close to bedtime because this may interfere with sleep. Studies have shown a beneficial effect of Tai chi on symptoms of insomnia.

SLEEP IN INSTITUTIONALIZED OLDER ADULTS AND NEURODEGENERATIVE DISORDERS

Sleep in older adults living in nursing homes is well known to be disturbed, particularly in patients with neurodegenerative disorders. The prevalence of disturbed sleep in neurodegenerative disorders may be due to damaged brain structures responsible for regulation of sleep and circadian rhythms. Furthermore, a lack of exposure to light and alerting activities during the day can contribute to poor sleep at night. At the extremes, some patients may not spend a full hour fully awake or fully asleep in a 24-hour period. This lack of consolidated sleep prevents the normal sequence through various sleep stages and results in light nonrestorative sleep. In noninstitutionalized patients with significant dementia, progressive disturbances in the sleep-wake cycle often reach a point where nighttime behaviors become a significant stressor for caregivers. In fact, frequent nocturnal wandering and confusion is a leading cause of institutionalization.

The presence of dementia and other neurodegenerative disorders may impact therapy for sleep disorders. Severe dementia may impair the ability of patients to use CPAP for SDB; however, studies have shown that CPAP can be successfully used in mild to moderate dementia. Treatment of SDB in these patients can actually improve cognitive function. Furthermore, dementia can impact appropriateness of CBT for insomnia, where patients may not be able to participate. Behavioral treatment programs for insomnia that involve the caregiver have been used in patients with dementia. Most pharmacologic therapies for insomnia are relatively contraindicated in those with significant dementia. However, there are behavioral interventions that may be helpful in nursing home patients (**Table 44-9**). Recent data suggest that the most promising approaches are increased daytime light exposure, nighttime use of melatonin, and acupressure.

TABLE 44-9 ■ SLEEP HYGIENE RULES FOR NURSING HOME PATIENTS

Limit the amount of time in bed, particularly during the day.

Limit naps to 1 hour once a day, early in the afternoon.

Keep regular sleep-wake schedule (if possible similar to prior home routine).

Keep regular meal schedule (if possible, patients should not eat in bed).

Avoid caffeinated beverages and food.

Limit nighttime noise.

Ensure that patient rooms are as dark as possible during the night.

Ensure that patient environment is brightly lit during the day.

Encourage exercise appropriate for each patient.

Match roommates on sleep-wake behavior.

Assess patients for possible sleep problems and initiate specific treatment.

Check medications for sedating/alerting effects.

FURTHER READING

Allen RP, Chen C, Garcia-Borreguero D, et al. Comparison of pregabalin with pramipexole for restless legs syndrome. *N Engl J Med.* 2014;370(7):621–631.

American Academy of Sleep Medicine. *International Classification of Sleep Disorders.* 3rd ed. Darien, IL: American Academy of Sleep Medicine; 2014.

American Geriatrics Society 2019 Updated AGS Beers Criteria® for Potentially Inappropriate Medication Use in Older Adults. *J Am Geriatr Soc.* 2019;67(4):674–694.

Auger RR, Burgess HJ, Emens JS, Deriy LV, Thomas SM, Sharkey KM. Clinical Practice Guideline for the Treatment of Intrinsic Circadian Rhythm Sleep-Wake Disorders: Advanced Sleep-Wake Phase Disorder (ASWPD), Delayed Sleep-Wake Phase Disorder (DSWPD), Non-24-Hour Sleep-Wake Rhythm Disorder (N24SWD), and Irregular Sleep-Wake Rhythm Disorder (ISWRD). An Update for 2015: An American Academy of Sleep Medicine Clinical Practice Guideline. *J Clin Sleep Med.* 2015; 11(10):1199–1236.

Aurora RN, Kristo DA, Bista SR, et al. The treatment of restless legs syndrome and periodic limb movement disorder in adults—an update for 2012: practice parameters with an evidence-based systematic review and meta-analyses. *Sleep.* 2012;35(8):1039–1062.

Aurora RN, Zak RS, Maganti RK, et al. Best practice guide for the treatment of REM sleep behavior disorder (RBD). *J Clin Sleep Med.* 2010;6(1):85–95.

Bloom HG, Ahmed I, Alessi CA, et al. Evidence-based recommendations for the assessment and management of sleep disorders in older persons. *J Am Geriatr Soc.* 2009;57(5):761–789.

Cowie MR, Woehrle H, Wegscheider K, et al. Adaptive servo-ventilation for central sleep apnea in systolic heart failure. *N Engl J Med.* 2015;373(12):1095–1105.

Donovan LM, Kapur VK. Prevalence and characteristics of central compared to obstructive sleep apnea: analyses from the sleep heart health study cohort. *Sleep.* 2016;39(7):1353–1359.

Epstein LJ, Kristo D, Strollo PJ Jr, et al. Clinical guideline for the evaluation, management and long-term care of obstructive sleep apnea in adults. *J Clin Sleep Med.* 2009;5(3):263–276.

Espie CA, MacMahon KM, Kelly HL, et al. Randomized clinical effectiveness trial of nurse-administered small-group cognitive behavior therapy for persistent insomnia in general practice. *Sleep.* 2007;30(5):574–584.

Kapur VK, Auckley DH, Chowdhuri S, et al. Clinical practice guideline for diagnostic testing for adult obstructive sleep apnea: an American Academy of Sleep Medicine Clinical Practice Guideline. *J Clin Sleep Med.* 2017;13(3): 479–504.

Kripke DF, Langer RD, Elliott JA, Klauber MR, Rex KM. Mortality related to actigraphic long and short sleep. *Sleep Med.* 2011;12(1):28–33.

Mander BA, Winer JR, Walker MP. Sleep and human aging. *Neuron.* 2017;94(1):19–36.

Martínez-García M, Chiner E, Hernández L, et al. Obstructive sleep apnoea in the elderly: role of

PART III

GERIATRIC CONDITIONS

continuous positive airway pressure treatment. *Eur Respir J.* 2015;46(1):142–151.

McCurry SM, Pike KC, Vitiello MV, et al. Increasing walking and bright light exposure to improve sleep in community-dwelling persons with Alzheimer's disease: results of a randomized, controlled trial. *J Am Geriatr Soc.* 2011;59(8):1393–1402.

McMillan A, Bratton DJ, Faria R, et al. Continuous positive airway pressure in older people with obstructive sleep apnoea syndrome (PREDICT): a 12-month, multicentre, randomised trial. *Lancet Respir Med.* 2014;2(10): 804–812.

Posadas T, Oscullo G, Zaldívar E, et al. Treatment with CPAP in elderly patients with obstructive sleep apnoea. *J Clin Med.* 2020;9(2):546.

Qaseem A, Kansagara D, Forciea MA, Cooke M, Denberg TD. Clinical Guidelines Committee of the American College of Physicians. Management of Chronic Insomnia Disorder in Adults: A Clinical Practice Guideline From the American College of Physicians. *Ann Intern Med.* 2016;165(2):125-133.

Raggi A, Ferri R. Sleep disorders in neurodegenerative diseases. *Eur J Neurol.* 2010;17:1326–1338.

Ramar K, Dort LC, Katz SG, et al. Clinical practice guideline for the treatment of obstructive sleep apnea and snoring with oral appliance therapy: an update for 2015. *J Clin Sleep Med.* 2015;11(7):773–827.

Richards KC, Lambert C, Beck CK, et al. Strength training, walking, and social activity improve sleep in nursing home and assisted living residents: randomized controlled trial. *J Am Geriatr Soc.* 2011;59(2):214–223.

Sateia MJ, Buysse DJ, Krystal AD, Neubauer DN, Heald JL. Clinical Practice Guideline for the Pharmacologic Treatment of Chronic Insomnia in Adults: An American Academy of Sleep Medicine Clinical Practice Guideline. *J Clin Sleep Med.* 2017;13(2):307–349.

Spira AP, Covinsky K, Rebok GW, et al. Objectively measured sleep quality and nursing home placement in older women. *J Am Geriatr Soc.* 2012;60(7):1237–1243.

Stone KL, Blackwell TL, Ancoli-Israel S, et al. Sleep disturbances and risk of falls in older community-dwelling men: the outcomes of Sleep Disorders in Older Men (MrOS Sleep) study. *J Am Geriatr Soc.* 2014;62(2):299–305.

Webster L, Costafreda Gonzalez S, Stringer A, et al. Measuring the prevalence of sleep disturbances in people with dementia living in care homes: a systematic review and meta-analysis. *Sleep.* 2020;43(4):zsz251.

Xie L, Kang H, Xu Q, et al. Sleep drives metabolite clearance from the adult brain. *Science.* 2013;342(6156):373–377.

Yu J, Zhou Z, McEvoy RD, et al. Association of positive airway pressure with cardiovascular events and death in adults with sleep apnea: a systematic review and meta-analysis. *JAMA.* 2017;318(2):156–166.

Chapter 45

Syncope and Dizziness

Ria Roberts, Lewis A. Lipsitz

DEFINITIONS

Syncope

Syncope is defined as a transient loss of consciousness secondary to cerebral hypoperfusion, characterized by unresponsiveness and loss of postural tone, with spontaneous, complete recovery. It is often a cause of otherwise unexplained falls in older adults. Syncope can result from one or more underlying processes that temporarily impair consciousness. Transient ischemia of the vertebrobasilar circulation, hypoxemia, and hypoglycemia are examples of other transient causes of loss of consciousness, but according to the definition above, they are technically not syncope if they are associated with focal neurologic abnormalities or do not recover spontaneously without intervention (eg, oxygen or glucose administration). Seizures may occur during a syncopal event as a consequence of cerebral hypoperfusion, but are rarely a cause of syncope.

Dizziness

Dizziness is an abnormal perception of the body's relationship to space, which is often described as postural instability or imbalance. Patients frequently complain of dizziness alone or as a prodrome to syncope or falls. Dizzy symptoms can be classified into four subtypes, which present with distinct temporal patterns: vertigo and presyncope are acute and often episodic, while disequilibrium and other types are usually chronic and sustained. Dizziness can also be attributable to a cardiovascular diagnosis especially if associated with pallor, syncope, prolonged standing, palpitations, or improvement when lying down or sitting.

EPIDEMIOLOGY

Syncope

Syncope has a lifetime prevalence of up to 47% in healthy adults, and accounts for 3% of emergency department (ED) visits. The incidence is 0.6% per year, increasing to 2% to 6 % in older adults. The outcome of ED visits for syncope, based on a 1-year meta-analysis, showed a 7% mortality, 16% recurrence rate requiring hospitalization, and 6.0% incidence of device insertion, demonstrating that syncopal patients suffer long-term morbidity and mortality. Syncope is the seventh most common reason for emergency

Learning Objectives

- Define and understand the typical presentations of syncope and dizziness.
- Outline the common causes of syncope and dizziness.
- Discuss age-related physiologic changes that predispose older adults to syncope and dizziness.
- Detail pathophysiology and etiology of syncope and dizziness.
- Discuss management and prevention of syncope and dizziness.

Key Clinical Points

Syncope:

1. Syncope is a common symptom throughout life; however, its presentation is often atypical in older adults who are less likely to have a warning or prodrome prior to syncope, and often have amnesia for loss of consciousness. Syncope is also one of many causes of falls in the older adult.

2. The etiology of syncope in older adults is typically multifactorial and often medication related. Modification or cessation of cardiovascular, psychotropic, and other medications is often needed to prevent syncope in older adults.

3. Causes of syncope can be cardiac or noncardiac. Cardiac causes are most prevalent in older adults and are associated with increased morbidity and mortality.

4. Age-related physiologic changes that predispose older adults to syncope include baroreflex impairment, decreased cerebral blood flow, reduced renal salt and water conservation, decreased thirst, impaired early diastolic ventricular filling, and an age-related decrease in vascular response to sympathetic activity.

(Continued)

5. Monitoring blood pressure during common daily activities is a useful tool to identify causes of syncope; and implantable loop recorders are recommended as an early diagnostic tool in the evaluation of unexplained syncope given the relatively high diagnostic yield.

Dizziness:

1. Dizziness is an abnormal perception of the body's relationship to space, which is often described as postural instability or imbalance. In older adults, it is often associated with fear of falling, mood disorders, polypharmacy, and functional disability.

2. Dizzy symptoms can be classified into four subtypes, which present with different temporal patterns: vertigo, presyncope, disequilibrium, and other.

3. Patients frequently complain of dizziness alone or as a prodrome to syncope or falls.

4. Several age-related changes increasing older adults' susceptibility to dizziness include reduction in sensory receptors of the vestibular system, decreased vision and visual-vestibular reflexes, and decreased proprioceptive sense.

5. Visual, proprioception and balance exams, with and without eyes closed, as well as hearing assessment are all important elements of the dizziness work-up. Neuroimaging and specialized vestibular testing should be reserved for patients with chronic dizziness, vertigo, and/or focal neurologic findings.

6. Patients with chronic vestibular diseases (Meniere disease, labyrinthitis, vestibular neuritis, and ototoxicity) may benefit from vestibular desensitization exercises.

7. In the absence of a single etiology, treatment of each contributing factor can reduce dizzy symptoms.

admission of patients older than 65 years, and accounts for 1% of all hospital admissions. Syncope-related hospitalizations have been estimated to cost the US $2.4 billion annually, and up to 40% of cases remain unexplained despite extensive inpatient evaluations. In the young, the peak incidence of syncope occurs between 10 and 30 years of age and is mostly neurally mediated (vasovagal). Older adults on the other hand are more likely to have cardiovascular causes of syncope.

Dizziness

The prevalence of dizziness ranges from 4% to 30% in persons aged 65 or older, with a higher prevalence in females. In older adults, comorbid conditions associated with chronic dizziness include falls, functional disability, orthostatic hypotension (OH), syncope, and stroke. Chronic dizziness is also associated with worsening depressive symptoms, self-isolation, and decreased participation in social activities.

PATHOPHYSIOLOGY, ETIOLOGY, AND PRESENTATION OF SYNCOPE

Pathophysiology of Syncope

A syncopal episode results from temporary hypoperfusion of the brain, including the brain stem reticular activating system, which is responsible for consciousness. Standing in an upright posture results in the pooling of 500 to 1000 cc of blood in the lower extremities and splanchnic circulation, resulting in a decrease in venous return to the heart, reduced ventricular filling, decreased cardiac output, and a fall in blood pressure. The decrease in blood pressure reduces the stretch of baroreceptors in the carotid sinus and aortic arch, resulting in a baroreflex response to hypotension, which plays an important role in preventing syncope. The baroreflex response includes an increase in sympathetic outflow and a decrease in vagal activity from the central nervous system. This in turn increases heart rate, peripheral vascular resistance, venous return, and cardiac output, limiting the fall in blood pressure. Disruption in the baroreflex response is a cause of OH and resultant cerebral hypoperfusion.

Aging is commonly associated with a decline in baroreflex sensitivity and predisposes older adults to syncope during preload reduction. Due to a defect in beta-adrenergic receptor signal transduction, the older heart does not respond as well to sympathetic activation, as is evident in the diminished heart rate response to exercise or posture change in an older person. Although sympathetic outflow is greater with aging, several studies show a diminished cardioaccelerary and vasoconstrictor response. These changes can result in hypotension during common daily activities that reduce venous return to the heart, such as standing up, eating a meal, or taking medications that reduce cardiac preload such as diuretics or nitrates.

Older adults are also prone to reduced blood volume due to excessive salt wasting by the kidneys as a result of a decline in plasma renin and aldosterone, a rise in atrial natriuretic peptide, a reduced thirst response to hyperosmolality, and, often concurrent diuretic therapy. Low blood volume, together with age-related diastolic dysfunction and a blunted heart rate response to hypovolemic stress can lead to low cardiac output and an increased susceptibility to OH. Cerebral autoregulation, which maintains a relatively constant cerebral circulation over a wide range of blood pressures, is altered in the presence of hypertension and possibly by aging—the latter is still controversial. In general, it is agreed that sudden declines in blood pressure can markedly affect cerebral blood flow and render an older person particularly susceptible to presyncope and syncope. Syncope may thus result either from a single process that abruptly decreases cerebral blood flow and oxygen delivery to the brain, or from the cumulative effect of multiple processes, each of which contributes to reduced cerebral oxygen delivery.

Etiology of Syncope

The etiology of syncope can be cardiac or noncardiac, as shown in **Table 45-1**. Cardiac causes can be divided into structural heart disease, myocardial dysfunction, and arrhythmias, and are associated with higher mortality rates irrespective of age. Noncardiac causes include: respiratory causes (acute respiratory failure, pulmonary hypertension), vascular causes (hemorrhage, aortic dissection, pulmonary embolism, and cervical spondylosis that compresses vertebral arteries), neurologic conditions (seizure disorder, stroke, transient ischemic attack), neurally mediated syncope (vasovagal syncope, situational syncope, reflex syncope), and unexplained causes. Examples of situational syncope include: drug-induced hypotension, postprandial hypotension, OH, and dehydration. Examples of reflex syncope include: cough syncope, swallow syncope, post-micturition syncope, defecation syncope, and carotid sinus hypersensitivity.

Cardiac Syncope

Cardiac syncope may be secondary to structural heart disease, myocardial dysfunction and/or arrythmia (bradyarrhythmia and tachyarrhythmia). Specific etiologies are listed in **Table 45-1**. The prevalence of cardiac disease, including structural heart disease and arrhythmias, rises dramatically with age and is responsible for about one-third of cases of syncope in older patients. Cardiac syncope is associated with higher morbidity and mortality rates, and may be preceded by dyspnea, chest pain, palpitations, and/or cyanosis during unconsciousness. Persistent cardiac symptoms, elevated serum troponin and B-type natriuretic peptide levels, and an abnormal electrocardiogram (ECG) may persist after a cardiac syncopal event. Myocardial infarction (MI) can also present atypically as syncope. The older patient may not recall cardiac symptoms that may have preceded the event, making it more challenging when evaluating causes of syncope.

Noncardiac Causes of Syncope

Noncardiac causes of syncope are listed in **Table 45-1**. Below, we discuss some of the most common noncardiac causes.

Orthostatic hypotension Orthostatic hypotension (OH) is defined as a 20 mm Hg or greater decline in systolic BP and/or 10 mm Hg or greater decline in diastolic BP when changing from a supine or sitting to standing position, usually measured immediately and after a short delay upon standing (eg, at 1 and 3 minutes). Characteristic symptoms of OH include falls, dizziness, weakness, nausea, palpitations, tremulousness, headache, presyncope, fatigue, and weakness.

OH can be caused by volume depletion, medications, adrenal insufficiency, and/or autonomic failure. Paradoxically, older patients with hypertension are more prone to OH due to the combination of age and hypertension-related impairments in blood pressure regulatory mechanisms.

TABLE 45-1 ■ CARDIAC AND NONCARDIAC CAUSES OF SYNCOPE

CARDIAC CAUSES			NONCARDIAC CAUSES			
STRUCTURAL HEART DISEASE	MYOCARDIAL DYSFUNCTION	ARRHYTHMIA	NEUROLOGIC CONDITIONS	NEURALLY MEDIATED SYNCOPE	RESPIRATORY CAUSES	VASCULAR CAUSES
Severe aortic stenosis	Dilated cardiomyopathy	**Bradyarrhythmias** Atrioventricular block	Seizure disorder	Vasovagal syncope	Acute respiratory failure	Hemorrhage
Hypertrophic cardiomyopathy	Myocarditis	Sinus node dysfunction	Stroke	Situational syncope	Pulmonary hypertension	Aortic dissection
Valvular disease			Transient ischemic attacks	Reflex syncope		Pulmonary embolism
Prosthetic valve dysfunction		**Tachyarrhythmias** Supraventricular tachycardia				Cervical spondylosis that compresses vertebral arteries
Coronary artery anomalies		Ventricular tachycardia				
Cardiac masses		Long QT syndrome				
Myocardial infarction/ ischemia		Wolff-Parkinson-White syndrome				
Pericardial disease						

668 Volume depletion for any reason is often a common sole or contributing cause of OH and, in turn, syncope. Of note, in the older adult, a postural increase in heart rate is not a reliable indicator of hypovolemia because of baroreflex impairment.

Medications found to be contributory to OH include: antipsychotics (particularly MAO inhibitors and tricyclic antidepressants), diuretics, beta-blockers, and vasodilators, particularly nitrates and alpha blockers. The combination of alpha- and beta-blockade is especially dangerous. Since older adults are effectively partially beta-blocked due to age-related baroreflex impairment, the addition of an alpha blocker, like terazosin or tamsulosin for urinary frequency, can precipitate OH and syncope.

Dysautonomia can also result in OH and syncope through impaired cardioacceleratory and vasoconstrictor mechanisms that would normally compensate for reduced venous return to the heart during upright posture. In addition to OH and syncope, other symptoms of dysautonomia include defective sweating, erectile dysfunction, urinary incontinence, and bowel disturbances (diarrhea or constipation). The etiology includes both central nervous system neurodegenerative conditions and peripheral autonomic neuropathies. Neurodegenerative diseases that impair the autonomic nervous system include: multiple systems atrophy, Parkinson disease, Lewy body dementia, multiple strokes, myelopathy, and brain stem lesions. Causes of peripheral autonomic neuropathies include diabetes, amyloidosis, paraneoplastic syndromes, autoimmune diseases, pure autonomic failure, and less commonly, infections (botulism, HIV, syphilis, Chagas disease, leprosy, diphtheria), nutritional deficiencies (vitamin B_{12}), and various neurotoxins (alcohol, dioxin, heavy metals, and chemotherapeutic agents).

Multiple systems atrophy (MSA) is a multisystem neurodegenerative disease due to striatonigral degeneration, cerebellar atrophy, or pyramidal lesions that is characterized by dysautonomia and motor disturbances. Clinical manifestations of MSA include muscle atrophy, distal sensorimotor neuropathy, pupillary abnormalities, restriction of ocular movements, life-threatening laryngeal stridor and respiratory insufficiency, dysphagia, constipation, bladder disturbances, and OH. Resting plasma norepinephrine levels are usually within the normal range but fail to rise on standing or tilting. The parkinsonian manifestations of MSA can be distinguished from Parkinson disease and Lewy body dementia by the absence of hallucinations and cognitive defects. Also, unlike Parkinson disease, MSA does not respond to dopamine, and there is poor or absent response to an adequate trial of levodopa.

OH is also a common clinical manifestation of Parkinson disease and the side effect of dopaminergic medications used to treat it. Cognitive impairment, in particular, abnormal attention and executive function, is more common in Parkinson disease with OH. This may be due to the effects of hypotension on the brain, including watershed hypoperfusion and cerebral infarction in executive and attention control regions.

Other non-neurogenic mediated conditions associated with OH include myocarditis, atrial myxoma, aortic stenosis, constrictive pericarditis, hemorrhage, prolonged diarrhea or vomiting, ileostomy fluid loss, burns, hemodialysis, salt-losing nephropathy, diabetes insipidus, adrenal insufficiency, fever, extensive varicose veins, deconditioning, dehydration, and hypertension. As noted above, hypertension increases the risk of hypotension by impairing baroreflex sensitivity and reducing ventricular compliance.

Older persons with hypertension are more vulnerable to cerebral ischemic symptoms even with modest OH because the threshold for cerebral autoregulation is shifted to higher blood pressures. This may result in decreased cerebral blood flow at higher blood pressure values, thereby increasing the risk of cerebral ischemia from sudden declines in blood pressure, even within "normal" ranges. Additionally, the acute administration of antihypertensive agents when blood pressure regulatory mechanisms and cerebral autoregulation are impaired may further increase the risk of OH and syncope. However, paradoxically, the chronic treatment of hypertension may improve blood pressure regulation, reduce the risk of OH, and increase cerebral blood flow in older adults.

Postprandial hypotension (PPH) PPH, an often overlooked cause of syncope in older adults, is defined as a 20 mm Hg or greater decline in systolic BP within 2 hours of the start of a meal. Postprandial physiologic changes that predispose to PPH include pooling of blood in the splanchnic circulation, a decrease in venous return to the heart, and failure to increase sympathetic nervous system activity, heart rate, and vascular resistance. The vasodilatory effects of insulin and other gut peptides released after a meal, including neurotensin and vasoactive intestinal peptide (VIP), may contribute to the hypotension. PPH has a prevalence of 24% to 36% of nursing home residents, and 23% of older adults admitted to a geriatric hospital with syncope or falls. It has also been found in 50% of older adults with unexplained syncope. Like OH, PPH is associated with hypertension, autonomic insufficiency, Parkinson disease, diabetes, renal failure, angina, transient ischemic attack, lacunar infarcts, and leukoaraiosis, alcohol use disorder, and polypharmacy. PPH may or may not coexist with OH in older patients. PPH is causally related to recurrent syncope and falls in many older persons, but the clinical significance of a fall in blood pressure after meals is difficult to quantify.

Vasovagal syncope The hallmark of vasovagal syncope is transient hypotension and/or bradycardia sufficiently profound to produce cerebral ischemia and transient loss of neural function. The possible mechanism involves a sudden fall in venous return to the heart, rapid fall in ventricular volume, and partial collapse of the ventricle in combination with vigorous ventricular contraction. The net result of these events is stimulation of ventricular mechanoreceptors and activation of the Bezold-Jarisch reflex leading to peripheral vasodilatation (hypotension) and bradycardia. Several neurotransmitters, including serotonin, endorphins, and vasopressin may play an important role in the pathogenesis of vasovagal syncope possibly by central sympathetic inhibition, although their exact role is not yet well understood.

Vasovagal syncope has been classified into cardioinhibitory (bradycardia), vasodepressor (hypotension), and mixed (both) subtypes depending on the blood pressure and heart rate response. In most patients, the manifestations occur in three distinct phases: a prodrome or aura, loss of consciousness, and postsyncopal phase. Many older adults do not experience a prodrome or aura, making vasovagal syncope hard to diagnose. A precipitating factor or stressful situation is identifiable in many patients. Common precipitating factors include extreme emotional stress, anxiety, mental anguish, trauma, a warm environment, air travel, prolonged standing, physical pain or anticipation of physical pain (eg, anticipation of phlebotomy). Some patients experience vagal responses to specific situations such as micturition, defecation, and coughing. Thus, situational and vasovagal syncope may overlap. Prodromal symptoms include extreme fatigue, weakness, diaphoresis, nausea, visual defects, visual and auditory hallucinations, dizziness, vertigo, headache, abdominal discomfort, dysarthria, and paresthesias. The duration of the prodrome varies greatly from seconds to several minutes, during which time some patients are able to take actions such as lying down to avoid an episode. The syncopal period is usually brief during which some patients develop involuntary movements—usually myoclonic jerks, but tonic-clonic movements may occur. Thus, vasovagal syncope may masquerade as a seizure. Recovery is usually rapid but older patients can experience protracted symptoms such as confusion, disorientation, nausea, headache, dizziness, and a general sense of ill health. Avoidance of precipitating factors and preventative actions such as lying down during prodromal symptoms have great value in preventing episodes of vasovagal syncope. Of note, healthy older persons are not as prone to vasovagal syncope as younger adults.

Carotid sinus hypersensitivity and carotid sinus syndrome

The carotid sinus is a dilated area in the carotid bifurcation where the internal and external carotid arteries meet to make the common carotid artery. This neurovascular structure contains baroreceptors, which, when stretched, activate the parasympathetic nervous system and suppress the sympathetic nervous system, resulting in vasodilation, bradycardia, and hypotension. In some patients, hypersensitive receptors in the carotid sinus cause an exaggerated response called carotid sinus hypersensitivity (CSH). The incidence of CSH increases with age and predominantly affects males with atherosclerotic vascular disease. It is diagnosed by carotid sinus massage sequentially on each side of the neck while blood pressure and heart rate are being monitored. This maneuver should not be performed in people who have any history or evidence

of carotid occlusion or heart block, in those with carotid bruits, or those who have had a recent cerebrovascular event or MI. The recommended duration of carotid sinus massage is from 5 to 10 seconds. The maximum fall in heart rate usually occurs within 5 seconds of the onset of massage. Complications resulting from carotid sinus massage are uncommon but may include sinus arrest, cardiac arrhythmias, and neurologic sequelae. Fatal arrhythmias are extremely uncommon and have generally only occurred in patients with underlying heart disease undergoing therapeutic rather than diagnostic massage. Neurologic complications result from either occlusion of, or embolization from, the carotid artery.

CSH is objectively defined as asystole of 3 seconds or longer (cardioinhibitory), and/or a fall in systolic BP exceeding 50 mm Hg (vasodepressor), or a combination of the two (mixed) while a carotid sinus massage is performed, with or without symptoms. When carotid sinus stimulation results in syncope, this condition is called "carotid sinus syndrome (CSS)." Other hypotensive disorders such as vasovagal syncope and OH may coexist in one-third of patients with CSH. Patients with a history of coronary artery disease or hypertension, or those taking digoxin, β-blockers, or α-methyldopa are most susceptible. Syncope may be precipitated by mechanical pressure on the carotid sinus due to head turning, tight neckwear, or neck pathology such as fibrosis from prior thyroid or head and neck cancer radiotherapy. In a significant number of patients, no triggering event can be identified. CSS is associated with appreciable morbidity. Approximately half of patients sustain an injury, including a fracture, during symptomatic episodes.

Unexplained Causes of Syncope

Despite the multitude of diagnostic tests, expensive technologies, and medical services that are used to evaluate syncope, approximately 40% of cases remain unexplained at end of the evaluation. Orthostatic, postprandial, and drug-induced hypotension, as well as structural heart disease and occult cardiac arrhythmias, are common causes of otherwise unexplained syncope.

PRESENTATION OF SYNCOPE

The presentation of syncope is often atypical in older adults as they are less likely to have a warning or prodrome prior to syncope and often have amnesia for loss of consciousness. Since syncope may be unwitnessed, it is often mistaken for a fall. Therefore, history alone cannot be relied upon when assessing an older patient who is found on the ground. Injurious events such as fractures and head injuries are more common in syncope, because the victim lacks protective reflex responses when they lose consciousness. In some forms of syncope, particularly during hypotensive or vasovagal events, there may be a premonitory period in which various symptoms (eg, light-headedness, nausea, sweating, weakness, visual disturbances) offer warning of an impending syncopal event. Often, however, loss of consciousness occurs without warning or recall of warning. Recovery from syncope is usually accompanied by almost immediate restoration of appropriate behavior and orientation. The post-recovery period may be associated with fatigue of varying duration, which can lead to misdiagnosis as a seizure.

SYMPTOMS AND PRESENTATION, PATHOPHYSIOLOGY, AND ETIOLOGY OF DIZZINESS

Symptoms and Presentation of Dizziness

Dizzy symptoms can be classified into four subtypes, which can present with acute, episodic, or chronic temporal patterns. The dizzy symptom subtypes are: vertigo, presyncope, disequilibrium, and other.

Vertigo is defined as a sensation of spinning or motion due to an imbalance of tonic vestibular signals arising from the inner ear, brain stem, or cerebellum. Common causes of vertigo in older persons include benign paroxysmal positional vertigo (BPPV), cerebrovascular disease, acute labyrinthitis, and vestibular neuronitis. Acute labyrinthitis refers to the swelling and inflammation of the labyrinth of the inner ear whereas vestibular neuronitis refers to inflammation of the vestibular nerve located in the inner ear. Acute labyrinthitis and vestibular neuronitis commonly occur after viral infections, with the main presenting symptom being vertigo.

Presyncope is a sensation of impending loss of consciousness due to diffuse cerebral ischemia that typically arises from vascular or cardiac causes, as described for syncope above.

Disequilibrium is a sensation of unsteadiness and of being off-balance, which can result from disturbances of visual, vestibulospinal, proprioceptive, somatosensory, cerebellar, and/or motor functions. The feelings of unsteadiness or imbalance primarily involves the lower extremities or trunk rather than the head. In older adults, disequilibrium can be secondary to strokes, peripheral neuropathy, vestibular deficits, multiple neurosensory deficits, musculoskeletal weakness/physical deconditioning, neuromuscular disease, and cerebellar disease. Symptoms suggestive of cerebellar disease include double vision, limb ataxia, and numbness.

Other subtypes of dizziness are often associated with vague symptoms that are difficult for patients to describe, and may be associated with anxiety disorders and other psychological diagnoses. Although dizziness may be a symptom of one or more discrete diseases, multifactorial etiologies of dizziness are common in older persons.

Temporal Pattern of Dizzy Symptoms

As previously noted, dizzy symptoms may present in episodic or continuous patterns. Hence, the frequency and duration of dizzy symptoms should always be assessed.

Meniere disease, transient ischemic attack (TIA), migraine, and BPPV present with episodic dizziness, the latter precipitated by specific movements. Episodic dizziness less than 1 minute suggests BPPV, episodes lasting 20 to 120 minutes suggest (TIA) or migraine, and episodes more than 120 minutes to 2 days suggest Meniere disease or recurrent vestibulopathy. With continuous dizziness, symptoms are present daily. Common causes of continuous dizziness include multisensory impairments, psychogenic dizziness, stroke, cerebellar atrophy, peripheral neuropathy, unresolved labyrinthitis, medications such as aminoglycosides resulting in bilateral vestibular damage, and deconditioning.

PATHOPHYSIOLOGY OF DIZZINESS

Maintenance of balance and equilibrium requires a complex integration multisensory information from the vestibular, proprioceptive, visual, and auditory systems in the cerebral cortex and cerebellum which allows appropriate balance-maintaining responses. Abnormalities in one or more of these systems results in multisensory impairment, which precipitates imbalance and the sensation of dizziness.

Dizziness may be difficult to diagnose, specifically in older persons, as it often represents multisystem dysfunction. Several age-related changes increasing older adults' susceptibility to dizziness include: reduction in sensory receptors of the semicircular canals, utricle and saccule of the inner ear, proprioceptive nerve and retina; diminished synapses; vascular disease affecting the microenvironment surrounding neurons; decreased vision and visual-vestibular reflexes; and decreased proprioceptive sense.

The vestibular system maintains spatial orientation at rest and during acceleration. Elements of the vestibular system and its connecting pathways include the semicircular canals, utricle, saccule, vestibular nerve, vestibular nuclei, vestibulospinal tracts, and vestibulocerebellar pathways. Diseases affecting the vestibular system that result in dizziness include Meniere disease, BPPV, labyrinthitis, vestibular neuronitis, acoustic neuroma, and drug toxicity (especially aminoglycosides and loop diuretics).

Proprioception contributes to equilibrium by providing information about changes in body position and mediates the body's response to positional change. Mechanoreceptors in the large joints of the body, including ankles, knees, hips, and spine provide information to the brain about how the body is oriented in space. Therefore, degenerative arthritis of these joints can disrupt the acquisition of proprioceptive information and results in a sense of disequilibrium. Other common disorders of proprioception include peripheral neuropathy secondary to diabetes, vitamin B_{12} deficiency, and cervical spondylosis or stenosis.

Vision provides important information on spatial orientation and is particularly important when vestibular and/or proprioceptive function is impaired. Common ocular diseases include cataracts, macular degeneration, and glaucoma. Age-related visual changes include a decrease in visual acuity, dark adaptation, contrast sensitivity, and accommodation.

Hearing also provides spatial clues, but to a lesser extent than vision. Impairment in hearing, common in older persons, may be secondary to age-related changes previously discussed, or to disease processes.

The cerebral cortex and cerebellum, along with their synaptic networks, integrate information and supply the musculoskeletal system with information for appropriate postural responses. Because of multiple and complex connections, essentially any central nervous system disorder can lead to imbalance, which may manifest as dizziness.

ETIOLOGY OF DIZZINESS

Key causes of dizziness syndromes in older adults include postural dizziness with and without OH, positional vertigo, acute labyrinthitis, vestibular neuronitis, recurrent vestibulopathy, Meniere disease, vertebrobasilar transient ischemic attacks, stroke, cervical dizziness, physical deconditioning, psychologic factors, and drug-induced dizziness.

Strokes that typically present with dizziness include: vertebrobasilar stroke syndrome, cerebellar infarction, anterior inferior cerebellar artery infarction, and lacunar strokes. Cervical dizziness can be classified into vascular cervical dizziness and proprioceptive cervical dizziness. Vascular cervical dizziness is caused by disruption in blood flow through vertebral arteries, commonly from an osteoarthritic spur; proprioceptive cervical dizziness results from overstimulation of the proprioceptive receptors of the facet joints of the neck. Physical deconditioning, likely due to limited exercise, typically results in muscle weakness, reduced coordination, and dizziness. Psychologic factors such as anxiety disorder, adjustment disorder, depressive disorder, and conversion disorder also commonly cause dizziness.

Many classes of drugs can cause or contribute to dizziness, resulting in drug-induced dizziness. Common examples include antihypertensives, antiarrhythmic agents, anticonvulsants, antidepressants, anxiolytics, antibiotics (aminoglycosides, macrolides, and vancomycin analogs), antihistamines, nonsteroidal anti-inflammatory agents, and over-the-counter cold and sleep preparations. These agents cause dizziness through different mechanisms. Antihypertensive agents, particularly calcium channel blockers, nitrates, and hydralazine, can cause dizziness simply by lowering blood pressure to a level at which symptoms occur. Loop diuretics, such as furosemide can cause dizziness by ototoxicity and/or volume depletion. Antiarrhythmics, anticonvulsants, and anxiolytics are responsible for dizziness through their direct effects on the central nervous system. Tricyclic antidepressants, antihistamines, and cold preparations cause dizziness via their sedating and anticholinergic properties. Antibiotics (eg, aminoglycosides, macrolides, and vancomycin analogs), nonsteroidal anti-inflammatory agents, and loop diuretics cause dizziness through ototoxicity, especially in the presence of impaired renal function, which decreases their clearance. The aminoglycosides are especially hazardous because of their toxicity to both the kidney and the vestibular system.

EVALUATION OF SYNCOPE AND DIZZINESS

Evaluation of Syncope

The initial step in the evaluation of syncope is to obtain a careful history of the event, going back 1 to 2 hours in time and asking the patient or proxy about activities that may have precipitated syncope. Did the patient take hypotensive or sedating medications, eat a meal, exercise, stand up, or perform a valsalva maneuver while straining, defecating, or urinating? One should also assess for pertinent past medical history and medications. History of heart disease, neurologic deficits, and risk factors for acute GI bleeding are all important. The presence of heart disease is an independent predictor of a cardiac cause of syncope, with a sensitivity of 95% and a specificity of 45%. Blood pressure should also be assessed during activities that may have precipitated syncope such as posture change, meals, and medications to assess for situational hypotension. To facilitate this, patients can be asked to bring a meal or their medications to an office visit, and a medical assistant can take blood pressure measurements before and at 30 and 60 minutes after consuming them.

For syncopal patients, a baseline ECG should be obtained. Blood studies can be helpful to identify conditions such as dehydration, hemorrhage/anemia, adrenal insufficiency, MI, hypoxia, pulmonary embolism, and causes of autonomic failure such as diabetes. If patients have cardiac symptoms, MI must be ruled out with cardiac enzymes (troponin) and serial ECGs. Based on a systemic review, an abnormal troponin level, B-type natriuretic peptide (BNP) greater than or equal to 300 pg/mL and NT-proBNP greater than 156 pg/mL have all been found to be independently associated with major adverse cardiovascular events (MACE) after an ED evaluation for syncope.

Cardiac Syncope

The gold standard for the diagnosis of cardiac syncope is symptom-rhythm correlation—that is, contemporaneous **heart rate and rhythm recording** during syncope. Cardiac monitoring may identify diagnostic abnormalities, such as asystole in excess of 3 seconds and rapid supraventricular (SVT) or ventricular tachycardia (VT). The absence of an arrhythmia during a recorded syncopal event excludes arrhythmia as a cause. Since cardiac arrhythmias are evident in up to 50% of patients with an ejection fraction of less than 40%, and atrial fibrillation occurs in one in five men older than age 80, an evaluation for arrhythmias is an important component of the syncopal workup. However, the commonly used **24-hour ambulatory ECG or Holter monitor** has limitations. It has low diagnostic yield, only

1% to 2% in unselected populations, and in the absence of symptoms it does not exclude a causal arrhythmia. Furthermore, some older adults may have difficulty operating it. Implantable loop recorders (ILRs) are quickly replacing ambulatory ECG monitors. These small devices are implanted or injected subcutaneously in the left side of the chest under local anesthesia and continuously record patients' ECG during spontaneous symptoms. Given their higher diagnostic yield, ILRs are now recommended as an early diagnostic tool in the evaluation of unexplained syncope, especially in older patients. Difficulties with ILRs include inability to activate the device, particularly if patients have cognitive impairment; however, automated recordings and remote monitoring have much improved their operability and diagnostic yield.

Echocardiography (echo) should be performed in syncope patients with known heart disease and in whom a structural cardiac abnormality is suspected. The prevalence of structural cardiac abnormalities increases with age. The test is of most benefit in older patients with aortic stenosis or mitral regurgitation, and to evaluate ejection fraction.

Exercise stress testing is indicated in patients who present with exercise-induced syncope. It is not always possible in older patients who may be unable to exercise, so pharmacologic stress tests or angiography may be necessary.

Electrophysiologic study is indicated in the older patient with syncope when a cardiac arrhythmia is suspected but not evident on prolonged cardiac monitoring. Diagnosis is based on confirmation of an inducible arrhythmia or conduction disturbance. The benefit is dependent on pretest probability based on the presence of organic heart disease or an abnormal ECG. Electrophysiologic study has the advantage of providing both diagnosis and treatment in the same session (transcatheter ablation). It is most effective for the identification of sinus node dysfunction in the presence of significant sinus bradycardia of 50 beats/min or less, impending high-degree atrioventricular block in patients with bi-fascicular block, inducible monomorphic VT in patients with previous MI, and inducible SVT with hypotension in patients with palpitations.

Noncardiac Syncope

Carotid sinus massage, previously described, is used to evaluate for CSH. It should be done in patients with no evidence of cerebrovascular disease or cardiac conduction disease, if there is no other identifiable cause of syncope.

Neurologic imaging studies have been found to have low diagnostic utility, especially in the absence of any focal neurologic findings. The American Academy of Neurology discourages the use of carotid artery imaging for syncope and the American College of Physicians and American College of Emergency Physicians discourages the use of CT scans and MRIs for syncope in the absence of focal neurologic signs. Neurologic evaluation is indicated when syncope is suspected to be epilepsy or due to autonomic failure.

In patients with possible situational syncope, **ambulatory BP monitoring** should be included in the initial work-up. They should have orthostatic vital signs measured, preferably with 2 values over 5 minutes during supine rest to obtain a baseline average, then at 1 and 3 minutes of standing to detect immediate and delayed OH. If a suspicious murmur is auscultated, an echocardiogram is warranted. If the patient presents with focal neurologic findings or seizures, an EEG or brain CT scan may be helpful, but these are rarely useful in the absence of neurologic signs.

Tilt tests and **autonomic function tests** may be useful to help diagnose autonomic failure. However, OH can usually be detected during a physical examination and tilt studies have many false positives. Therefore, tilt studies should be reserved for patients with unexplained syncope, the evaluation of neurohumoral responses to posture change, or to assess the effect of therapeutic interventions.

Unexplained Syncope

While evaluating unexplained syncope, orthostatic, postprandial, and drug-induced hypotension should be ruled out as they are common causes of otherwise unexplained syncope. It is important to recognize that syncope occurs when there is inadequate delivery of oxygen and metabolic substrate to the brain, which almost invariably is due to hypotension. Unfortunately, when a patient is first evaluated in the ED, orthostatic blood pressures are rarely measured, often due to fear that the patient may have injured themselves and cannot safely stand up. Sometimes, intravenous fluids are given before orthostatic blood pressures are taken, thus obviating the value of the test. Although patients often spend several days in the hospital to evaluate syncope, it is rare that blood pressures are examined before and after a meal or in response to medications they were taking at the time of an event. In one review of 2106 patients 65 years and older admitted to the hospital following a syncopal episode, postural blood pressure measurements, while performed in only 38% of episodes, had the highest yield of all diagnostic tests with respect to affecting diagnosis (18%–26%) or management (25%–30%) and determining etiology of the syncopal episode (15%–21%). Therefore, the presence of hypotension must be carefully sought during the same activities that were associated with the syncopal event.

Another cause of unexplained syncope is occult cardiac arrhythmias and the presence of structural heart disease. In these patients, cardiac evaluation consisting of echocardiography, stress testing, and prolonged electrocardiographic monitoring or an electrophysiologic study are recommended. Of note, although cardiac arrhythmias are commonly sought during hospitalizations, monitoring is usually done while patients are at rest in bed, rather than engaging in activities that may have precipitated syncope. Therefore, ambulatory cardiac monitoring with an external or implantable continuous monitor is ideal. Electrophysiologic studies may be necessary in some patients with suspicion of heart block or inducible arrhythmias.

TO HOSPITALIZE OR NOT

Approximately 10% of patients with syncope who present to the ED will suffer from a serious outcome within 7 to 30 days of their visit; hence, it is important to note the characteristics of syncopal patients who should be considered candidates for hospital admission. These include patients with persistently abnormal vital signs in the emergency room, signs and symptoms of volume depletion/inability to maintain a normal volume status, gastrointestinal bleed or acute change in hematocrit to less than 30, acute coronary syndrome, dysfunction of an implantable cardiac device, valvular heart disease, the presence of a previously undiagnosed cardiac murmur, family history of sudden death, and new-onset dyspnea or features of congestive heart failure. Additionally, those with evidence of conduction disease including prolonged QT, fascicular block, repetitive sinoatrial block or sinus pauses, slow atrial fibrillation (< 40 bpm), ventricular arrhythmias, persistent bradycardia (< 40 bpm), or Brugada pattern on ECG (incomplete right bundle branch block and ST elevations in the anterior precordial leads) are also considered high risk for hospitalization. Lastly, those with syncope during exertion, when supine or in a sitting position, as well as those with immediate onset of palpitations following the syncopal event warrant hospitalization.

According to the 2018 European Society of Cardiology guidelines for the diagnosis and management of syncope, patients with high-risk features are more likely to have cardiac syncope and are at increased risk for sudden cardiac death (SCD) and increased overall mortality. Hence, it is crucial to identify such patients to ensure early, rapid, and intensive investigation, and those with cardiac devices should undergo prompt device interrogation. Additionally, patients with recurrent symptoms, those without anyone to observe them, and those unable to seek help if needed should be hospitalized for at least 24 hours for observation. On the other hand, patients with reflex or situational syncope, including syncope due to OH, can be discharged from the ED if they can be observed, maintain adequate hydration, and be kept safe at home.

EVALUATION OF DIZZINESS

A stepwise approach is recommended for the evaluation of dizziness, proceeding from a careful history and physical examination, medication history, and screening laboratory tests. Providers should inquire about the precipitating factors of dizziness if any, such as missing a meal, drinking alcohol, taking medications, standing from a lying position, rolling over in bed, changing head or neck position, urinating, or defecating. Frequency and duration of dizzy symptoms should be queried to determine whether they are intermittent or continuous. If vestibular causes of dizziness are suspected, it should be determined if it is central or peripheral.

A focused physical examination is an essential component of the work up. Orthostatic blood pressure and heart rate should be assessed as described for syncope above. The examiner should look for spontaneous nystagmus on cranial nerve testing. In central lesions, nystagmus is vertical and non-suppressible by visual fixation. In peripheral lesions, nystagmus is horizontal or rotatory, and can be suppressed by visual fixation. An ocular examination for near and distant vision should be performed, as well as a hearing test (whisper test or audioscope) and an otoscopic examination to rule out cerumen impaction or structural abnormalities. Palpation and assessment of range of motion of the neck is also important to assess for cervical arthritis and vestibular dysfunction. Of note, patients may voluntarily restrict the range of neck movement in order to minimize dizziness secondary to vestibular causes, and such patients may respond well to vestibular rehabilitation.

A neurologic examination should include cranial nerves, the motor and sensory systems, and gait and balance. In the cranial nerve examination, one should look for diplopia, dysarthria, or facial paresthesia to rule out vertebrobasilar involvement. The absence of a corneal reflex suggests acoustic neuroma, especially if accompanied by unilateral hearing loss, tinnitus, and cerebellar signs. The presence of cogwheel rigidity and bradykinesia is suggestive of Parkinson disease. Although most of the abnormalities detected in the balance examination are not specific, the presence of a positive Romberg sign with the eyes closed is suggestive of an abnormality of proprioception and/or of the vestibular system. It also suggests that vision is needed to maintain balance. This should lead to interventions that maximize vision and ambient lighting in order to improve postural control. A wide-based stance and an improvement in gait with minimal handheld assistance of the examiner suggest a proprioceptive deficit or peripheral neuropathy.

In addition to the history and physical examination, clinicians should also perform certain provocative tests, such as the Dix-Hallpike maneuver (**Figure 45-1**), which establishes the diagnosis of BPPV. In this test, the patient is asked to sit on an examination table with the head rotated 45 degrees to one side. The patient is then asked to fix his/her vision upon the examiner's forehead. The examiner, while holding the patient's head firmly in the same position, moves the patient from a seated to a supine position with the head hanging below the edge of the table. If the ipsilateral ear is affected, then this maneuver will result in vertigo and nystagmus. If present, the direction, latency, duration of nystagmus, and duration of vertigo should be noted. The diagnostic criteria for BPPV are (1) vertigo accompanied by a rotatory nystagmus; (2) a latency of 1 to 5 seconds between the completion of the maneuver and the onset of vertigo and nystagmus; (3) paroxysmal nature

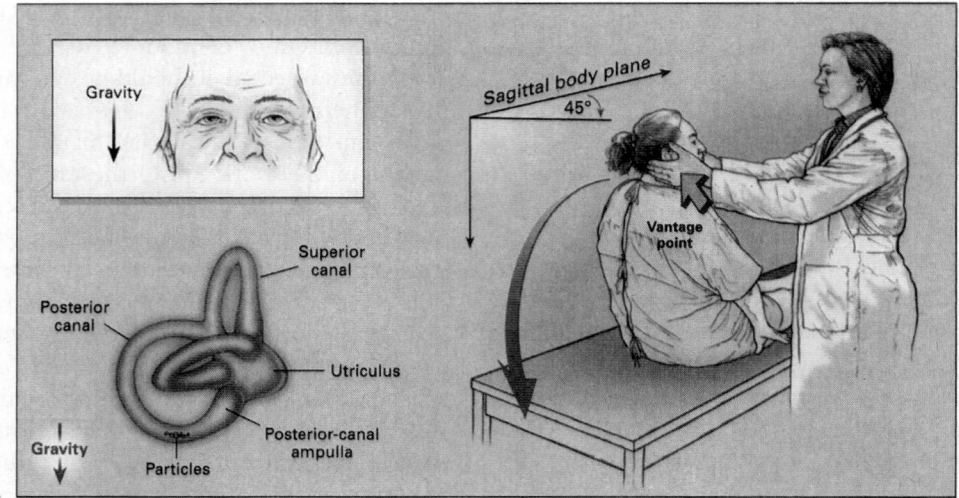

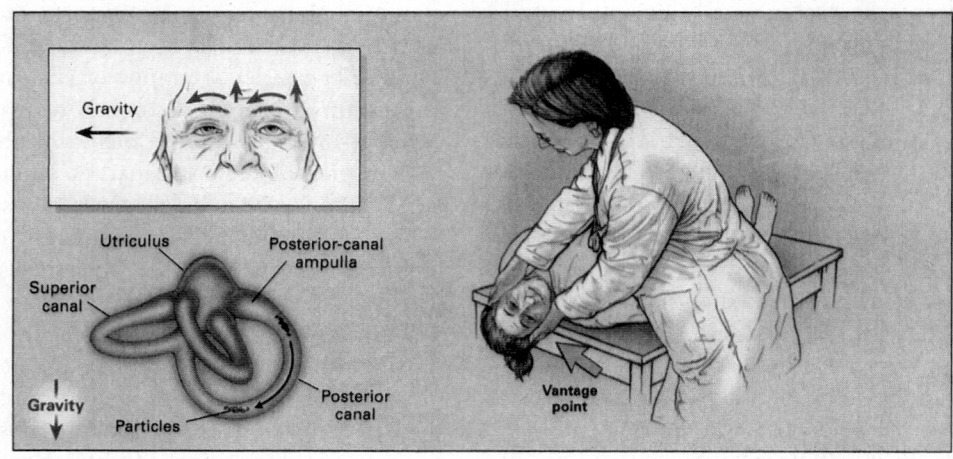

FIGURE 45-1. The Dix-Hallpike maneuver. (Reproduced with permission from Furman JM, Cass SP. Benign paroxysmal positional vertigo. *N Engl J Med.* 1999;341(21):1590–1596.)

of the vertigo and nystagmus (lasting for 10–20 seconds); and (4) fatigability, that is, a decrease in the intensity of the vertigo and nystagmus with repeated testing.

Baseline laboratory tests, including hematocrit, hemoglobin A1c, metabolic panel, thyroid function tests, and vitamin B$_{12}$ levels, should be done to rule out common modifiable contributors to dizziness such as anemia, diabetes, azotemia, hypothyroidism, and vitamin B$_{12}$ deficiency.

If the dizziness is presyncopal or associated with syncopal episodes, the above work-up for syncope should be initiated, including a careful search for cardiac arrhythmias using long-term continuous ambulatory cardiac monitoring.

Audiometry should be done in patients with a history of fluctuating or gradual hearing loss. An audiogram will reveal sensorineural loss in both Meniere disease and acoustic neuroma; the hearing loss will be greater in lower frequencies in Meniere disease and in higher frequencies in acoustic neuroma, often unilaterally.

Furthermore, in patients with a suspicion of cervical osteoarthritis, imaging of the cervical spine can be considered, but the frequency of false positives is great. Neuroimaging is needed when a stroke or cerebellopontine tumor is suspected. Magnetic resonance imaging (MRI) is preferred over computed tomography (CT) scans because of its greater sensitivity, particularly for lesions in the brain stem. Routine MRI is unlikely to reveal specific causes of dizziness. Transcranial Doppler studies or a magnetic resonance angiogram (MRA) may be needed to detect vertebrobasilar insufficiency if there is high suspicion.

Abnormalities of the peripheral vestibular system can be evaluated by performing special tests, such as electronystagmography (ENG) with caloric testing, a rotational chair test, and computerized posturography. These tests are performed by consultants in otorhinolaryngology. However, one must keep in mind that abnormalities are common in older persons without dizziness, so a positive test is neither sensitive nor specific.

A targeted battery of more elaborate and expensive tests is indicated only when routine evaluation suggests a specific disease entity and the results of these tests are likely to influence management. Neuroimaging and specialized vestibular testing should be reserved for patients with chronic dizziness, vertigo, and/or focal neurologic findings. When the etiology is multifactorial, identifying and treating the contributing sensory deficits may improve, if not eliminate the dizziness.

GENERAL PRINCIPLES FOR THE MANAGEMENT OF SYNCOPE AND DIZZINESS

Management of Syncope

Avoidance of precipitating factors and correction of the underlying cause, whether cardiac or noncardiac in origin, is paramount. Withdrawal or modification of culprit medications is often the only necessary intervention in older persons. Many patients experience symptoms without warning, necessitating drug therapy. A number of drugs are reported to be useful in alleviating symptoms and are discussed below.

The treatment of OH and postprandial hypotension (PPH) starts with nonpharmacologic treatment and progresses to pharmacologic interventions, if necessary. For OH, any offending medication should be withdrawn, substituted, or reduced in dose, and warm environments and straining activity should be avoided. Squatting and leg crossing when symptoms develop can help increase blood pressure. Adequate hydration, increasing salt intake, wearing pressure-graded support stockings—preferably waist-high—abdominal binders, and sleeping in a 30 to 45 degree head-up position can be helpful. For PPH, antihypertensive medications should be given between, rather than with, meals. It is also important to avoid preload reduction (diuretics or prolonged sitting) and maintain adequate intravascular volume. Avoiding alcohol use, eating multiple small frequent meals high in protein and fat, walking after meals, and eating cold rather than warm meals may also be therapeutic.

Pharmacologic treatment for severe forms of OH and PPH includes caffeine consumption, 250 mg (2 cups brewed) in the morning, fludrocortisone 0.1 to 0.5 mg po daily, midodrine 2.5 to 10 mg po TID, and octreotide 50 mg subQ, 30 minutes pre-meal.

For patients with symptomatic cardioinhibitory CSS, atrioventricular sequential (dual chamber) cardiac pacing is the treatment of choice. With appropriate pacing, syncope is abolished in 85% to 90% of patients. For vasodepressor CSS, a recent small randomized controlled trial showed benefit from the alpha-agonist midodrine. Surgical denervation of the carotid sinus may be a treatment option in refractory situations.

Cardiac syncope treatment options are summarized as followed: For cardiac syncope caused by symptomatic atrioventricular (AV) conduction disease/AV block and sick

sinus syndrome, cardiac pacing is the treatment of choice. In syncope due to intrinsic cardiac tachyarrhythmias, SVT and VT, antiarrhythmic drug therapy or catheter ablation is recommended in order to prevent syncope recurrence. An implantable cardiac defibrillator (ICD) is indicated in patients with syncope due to VT and an ejection fraction (EF) less than 35%, in patients with syncope and previous MI, and in patients who have VT induced during electro-physiologic studies. ICD should be considered in patients with an EF greater than 35% with recurrent syncope due to VT when catheter ablation and pharmacological therapy have failed or could not be performed. Of note, older patients with unexplained syncope, who have bi-fascicular bundle branch block and have undergone a reasonable workup, might benefit from empirical pacemaker implantation, especially if syncope is unpredictable (with no or short prodromes) or has occurred in the supine position or during effort.

In older adults, a multifactorial approach is recommended as there is likely more than one cause for syncope. Additionally, it may be appropriate to place pacemakers in frail older adults if the pacemaker can improve their quality of life and prevent falls or syncope.

MANAGEMENT OF DIZZINESS

The goal of treatment for dizziness is to identify and treat modifiable factors and to decrease associated disability. Systemic disorders such as anemia, metabolic derangements, vitamin B_{12} deficiency, and thyroid abnormalities, as well as vision and hearing deficits should be corrected. Visual correction with bifocal lenses can increase, rather than decrease dizziness if the lenses are worn while walking and looking down, because the short-distance correction in the lower part of the lens may distort the longer-distance view of the ground. Separate glasses may be needed for short and long-distance vision. Anxiety and depression should be treated, recognizing the dilemma that most antidepressants can also cause dizziness. Identify and minimize the impact of multiple contributors, particularly drugs. Stopping potentially offending medications is preferable to adding new ones.

Although recommendations for the pharmacologic treatment of dizziness include vestibular suppressants such as antihistamines (eg, meclizine), anticholinergic agents (eg, scopolamine), and benzodiazepines (eg, diazepam), these are dangerous medications in older adults, often responsible for falls, confusion, and other adverse events. Therefore, if medications are needed, these should be used in low doses and for acute episodes of dizziness. Their prolonged use may compromise central and peripheral adaptation, and thus, paradoxically, prolong the dizziness. Benzodiazepines may at times be indicated as a long-term vestibular suppressant in persons with severe unilateral lesions who are not surgical candidates. In one study, selective serotonin reuptake inhibitors were found to be effective in treating chronic dizziness associated with anxiety.

Vestibular rehabilitation has been shown to improve symptoms, postural instability, and dizziness-related handicap in patients with chronic dizziness. Vestibular rehabilitation consists of exercises combining movements of eyes, head, and body designed to stimulate the vestibular system. At first, these exercises may worsen the dizziness, but with continued practice and gradual increase in frequency, these exercises can improve dizziness, probably through central adaptation and habituation. These exercises also may help patients alleviate anxiety and fears in performing various activities. Improvement is usually seen after 6 to 8 weeks of vestibular rehabilitation. Patients should perform these exercises initially under the supervision of a trained specialist, such as a physical therapist, and later independently at home. In patients with cervical dizziness, physical therapy can substantially decrease the frequency and severity of dizziness and neck pain and can improve postural stability. Some patients may also benefit from cervical collars or cervical traction.

Patients diagnosed with BPPV can be treated by performing the Epley canalith repositioning procedure (**Figure 45-2**), which moves free-floating particles from the posterior semicircular canal into the utricle of the labyrinth by the effects of gravity, thereby eliminating turbulence and fluctuation of the endolymphatic pressure in the semicircular canals. In this five-position procedure, the patient is asked to sit on a table and a vibrator is applied to the ipsilateral mastoid process. Next, the patient is made to lie down supine on the examining table with the head rotated 45 degrees toward the affected ear and hanging below the edge of the table, similar to the Dix-Hallpike test. This position will induce vertigo. Once the vertigo subsides, the head is rotated 45 degrees to the opposite side, which may induce vertigo again. Then the head and body are rotated further in the same direction until the head is facing downward. Subsequently, while holding the head in the same position, the patient sits up. Finally, the head is turned forward with the chin down by about 20 degrees. The examiner holds the head in each of these positions for approximately 10 to 15 seconds or until the vertigo subsides. The patient should be told not to lie flat for the next 24 to 48 hours. Alternatively, a cervical collar can be used to prevent loose particles from sliding back to the posterior semicircular canals. These maneuvers can be performed without using the vibrator, although the results are said to be not as good. This maneuver can be repeated at weekly intervals until vertigo ceases and the Dix-Hallpike test is negative.

Surgery is reserved for a small group of patients who fail pharmacologic or vestibular rehabilitation, or who have cerebellopontine angle tumors. Patients with uncontrolled Meniere disease can have a transmastoid labyrinthectomy, partial vestibular neurectomy, or endolymphatic sac decompression. Very rarely, patients with BPPV who do not respond to repeated canalith repositioning procedures may benefit from disabling of the semicircular canal either by singular neurectomy or by occluding the posterior semicircular canal.

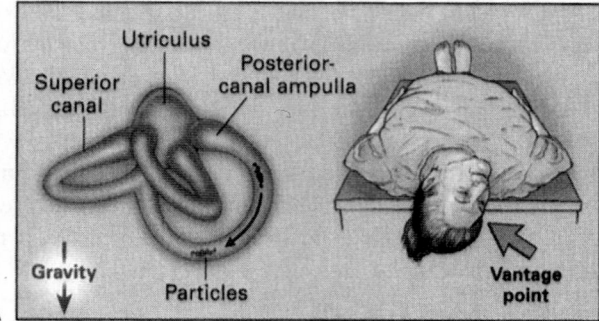

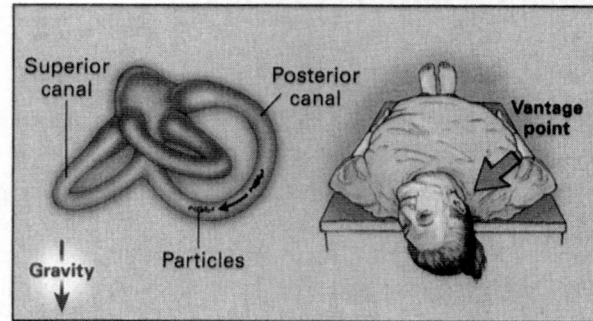

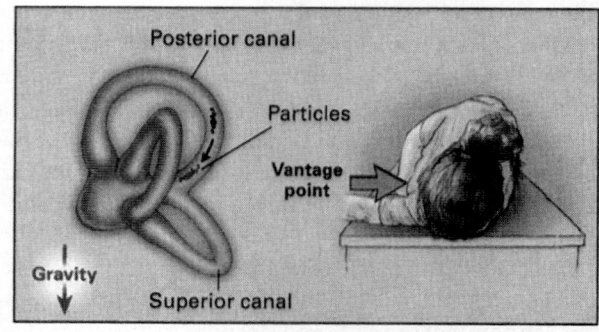

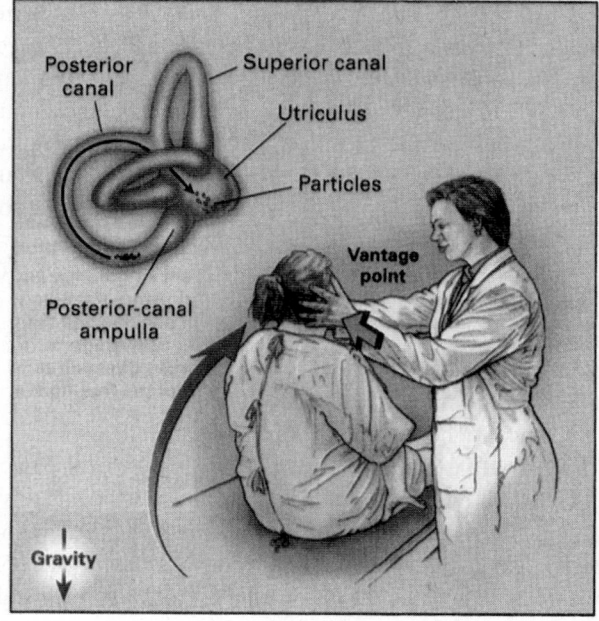

FIGURE 45-2. The Epley Canalith repositioning procedure. (Reproduced with permission from Furman JM, Cass SP. Benign paroxysmal positional vertigo. *N Engl J Med.* 1999;341(21):1590–1596.)

FURTHER READING

Albassam OT, Redelmeier RJ, Shadowitz S, Husain AM, Simel D, Etchells EE. Did this patient have cardiac syncope? The rational clinical examination systematic review. *JAMA*. 2019;321(24):2448–2457.

Brignole M, Moya A, de Lange FJ, et al. 2018 ESC Guidelines for the diagnosis and management of syncope. *Eur Heart J*. 2018;39(21):1883–1948.

Grossman SA, Bar J, Fischer C, et al. Reducing admissions utilizing Boston Syncope Criteria. *J Emerg Med*. 2012;42(3):345–352.

Jansen S, Bhangu J, de Rooij S, Daams J, Kenny RA, van der Velde N. The association of cardiovascular disorders and falls: a systematic review. *J Am Med Dir Assoc*. 2016;17(3):193–199.

Kharsa A, Wadhwa R. Carotid Sinus Hypersensitivity. [Updated 2020 Nov 7]. In: StatPearls [Internet]. Treasure Island (FL): StatPearls Publishing; 2020 Jan. Available from: https://www.ncbi.nlm.nih.gov/books/NBK559059/.

Leafloor CW, Hong PJ, Mukarram M, Sikora L, Elliott J, Thiruganasambandamoorthy V. Long-term outcomes in syncope patients presenting to the emergency department: a systematic review. *Can J Emerg Med*. 2020;22(1):45–55.

Lipsitz LA. Syncope in the elderly. *Ann Intern Med*. 1983;99(1):92–105.

Lipsitz LA, Nyquist RP Jr, Wei JY, Rowe JW. Postprandial reduction in blood pressure in the elderly. *N Engl J Med*. 1983;309(2):81–83.

Mendu ML, McAvay G, Lampert R, Stoehr J, Tinetti ME. Yield of diagnostic tests in evaluating syncopal episodes in older patients. *Arch Intern Med*. 2009;169(14):1299–1305.

Pournazari P, Oqab Z, Sheldon R. Diagnostic value of neurological studies in diagnosing syncope: a systematic review. *Can J Cardiol*. 2017;33(12):1604–1610.

Sloane PD. Evaluation and management of dizziness in the older patient. *Clin Geriatr Med*. 1996;12(4):785–801.

Solbiati M, Casazza G, Dipaola F, Sheldon RS, Costantino G. Cochrane corner: implantable loop recorder versus conventional workup for unexplained recurrent syncope. *Heart (British Cardiac Society)*. 2016;102(23):1862–1863.

Thiruganasambandamoorthy V, Ramaekers R, Rahman MO, et al. Prognostic value of cardiac biomarkers in the risk stratification of syncope: a systematic review. *Intern Emerg Med*. 2015;10:1003–1014.

Viau JA, Chaudry H, Hannigan A, Boutet M, Mukarram M, Thiruganasambandamoorthy V. The yield of computed tomography of the head among patients presenting with syncope: a systematic review. *Acad Emerg Med*. 2019;26(5):479–490.

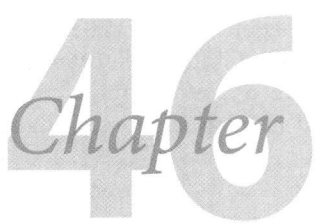

46 Chapter

Pressure Injuries

Joyce M. Black

As recently as 2014, pressure injury (PI) among older adults has been called a global "public health problem." This conclusion was reached based on the high rates of PI among nursing home residents as well as hospitalized patients.

DEFINITION

A PI is localized damage to the skin and underlying soft tissue usually over a bony prominence or related to a medical or other device. The injury can present as intact skin or an open injury and may be painful. The injury occurs because of intense and/or prolonged pressure or pressure in combination with shear. According to the National Pressure Injury Advisory Panel (NPIAP), the tolerance of soft tissue for pressure and shear may also be affected by microclimate, nutrition, perfusion, comorbidities, and condition of the soft tissue. The most common bony prominences are sacrum, heels, ischial tuberosities, trochanters, lateral malleoli, and heels. PI on the sacrum and heels are most common. However, PI can occur on any soft tissue exposed to pressure, so the clinician should not be guided only by the location of the wound to determine its etiology. Other terms for PI include pressure ulcer, bedsore or decubitus ulcer. The later terms imply development only in those confined to bed. Since the major causative factor is pressure, and because PI occurs in positions other than just lying down, PI is the preferred term.

EPIDEMIOLOGY

Pressure injuries occur in all health care settings. About 70% of PIs occur in people older than age 65, and they are seen in 9% to 22% of nursing home (NH) residents and 5% to 32% of patients in hospitals. Among minority NH residents in the United States, the prevalence of PI is nearly twice that of Whites. The prevalence of PI in American hospitals is often reported through the National Database of Nursing Quality Indicators (NDNQI). More than 2000 US hospitals and 98% of Magnet recognized facilities participate in the NDNQI program to measure nursing quality and improve their outcomes; those outcomes include PI rates. NDNQI directs participating institutions to conduct a quarterly survey of all patients to determine the prevalence of PI. Participating hospitals receive data on PI rates

Learning Objectives

- Identify the four pathophysiologic factors of pressure injury (PI) development.
- Describe the six PI classifications according to the National Pressure Injury Advisory Panel's (NPIAP's) guidelines.
- Outline the process for PI risk screening and risk assessment.
- Describe the essential strategies for a successful PI prevention program.
- Describe the standard of care for treatment of full-thickness PI.

Key Clinical Points

1. Pressure injuries are caused by mechanical force compressing tissues between the bony skeleton and external surfaces directly damaging the cell wall leading to cellular death. Ischemia from occluded capillaries and lymphatics and release of oxygen free radicals from reperfusion injury contribute to the extent of the injury.

2. Prevention includes screening for risk followed by risk assessment using standardized risk assessment tools to determine individual-specific risk and implementing targeted prevention interventions based on identified risk factors.

3. Scheduled repositioning programs, use of reactive and active support surfaces, assessment and management of nutrition, and use of prophylactic dressings are key prevention strategies.

4. Adequate, timely, and complete debridement of necrotic tissue, identification and treatment of infection and management of

(Continued)

> **(Cont.)** biofilm development, and providing a moist wound environment are the key tenets of appropriate pressure injury care.
>
> 5. Medical record documentation must include pressure injury risk status, prevention strategies, pressure injury assessment (size, stage, location, and description of wound bed minimally), treatment plan, and evaluation of treatment success.
>
> 6. Partial-thickness pressure injuries (stage 2) should heal within 60 days maximum; full-thickness pressure injuries (stage 3/4/unstageable) should demonstrate improvement in overall injury status every 2 to 4 weeks.

and can evaluate their PI programs against hospitals of like size and complexity.

PIs are a quality issue for all areas of health care. PI incidence and severity are used as markers of quality care by regulators in long-term care facilities, home care agencies, and acute care hospitals. The Joint Commission estimates that 2.5 million patients in acute care hospitals are treated for PI each year and this number is likely to increase as the population ages. Unlike facility-specific conditions (such as surgical site infection or ventilator-associated pneumonia), PI present across all care settings and patients, especially among geriatric populations.

MORBIDITY AND MORTALITY ASSOCIATED WITH PRESSURE INJURY

PI can lead to pain and disfigurement. Of those persons with PI who are able to report pain, 87% report pain with dressing changes, 84% report pain at rest, and 42% report pain at rest and during dressing changes. Further, 18% of those persons reporting dressing change-related wound pain report pain at the highest level (eg, "excruciating"). Yet, only 6% of those persons reporting PI pain receive any medication for pain. There is some evidence that a higher proportion of persons with stage 3 or 4 injuries report injury pain compared to those with stage 2 injury and they report more severe pain than those with stage 2 PI.

PIs also reduce the quality of life when they are located on visible body areas, have odorous drainage, and require the patient to limit time up in a chair in order to reduce pressure on the wound.

Septicemia is the most severe complication from PI. The incidence of bacteremia from PI is approximately 1.7 per 10,000 hospital discharges. When the PI is the source of bacteremia, overall mortality is 48%. Further, septicemia is reported in 40% of PI-associated deaths. Clinicians should be aware that transient bacteremia occurs after PI debridement in as many as 50% of patients. Other infectious complications of PI include wound infection, cellulitis, and osteomyelitis. Infected PI are one of the most common infections found in skilled nursing facilities and are reported in 6% of residents.

Prolonged hospitalization, slow recovery from comorbid conditions, and increased death rates are consistently observed in older individuals who develop PI in both hospitals and nursing homes. Hospital-acquired PI development is associated with higher in-hospital mortality (11%), mortality 30 days after discharge (15%), and longer hospital stays (11.6 ± 10.1 days for those with hospital acquired PI vs 4.9 ± 5.2 days for those without).

In addition, failure of a PI to heal or improve has been associated with a higher rate of death in nursing home residents. Nursing home residents whose PI healed within 6 months show a lower mortality rate (11% vs 64%) than residents with injuries that did not heal within 6 months. The link between PI and mortality may be related to an unidentified causal pathway, to PI as a marker for coexisting morbidity in frail, sick patients, or to the association between fatal sepsis and PI as cause of death. Whatever the link, PIs are reported as a cause of death among 114,000 persons per year (age-adjusted mortality rate of 3.8 per 100,000 population).

PIs are costly. Annual costs were estimated at $27 billion for 2016 and this figure does not include other costs of care which are not reimbursable. The cost for managing a single full-thickness PI is as much as $70,000 to $130,000. The Centers for Medicare and Medicaid Services (CMS) reports the cost of treating a PI in acute care (as a secondary diagnosis) is just over $43,000 per hospital stay. Contributing cost factors include increased length of stay due to PI complications such as pain, infection, high-tech support surfaces, and decreased functional ability. The Agency for Healthcare Research and Quality (AHRQ) reported that PI-related hospitalizations ranged from 13 to 14 days and cost $16,755 to $20,430 compared to the average stay of 5 days and costs approximately $10,000. As a result, PI remain on the national agenda for improving quality. This emphasis on PI across the spectrum of health care settings highlights the importance of the condition for clinicians. PIs have also received attention in the courtroom. Organizations have been prosecuted for negligence related to PI care and development, and, in a landmark case, one health care facility operator was found guilty of manslaughter for a resident's death related to improper care for her PI.

PATHOPHYSIOLOGY

PI forms from external or extrinsic causes (pressure and shear) in tissue with diminished tolerance or intrinsic causes (protein–calorie malnutrition, incontinence).

Pressure Pressure is the perpendicular force or load exerted on a specific area. The gravitational pull on the skeleton causes loading and deformation of the soft tissue between the bony prominence and external support surface. PIs are the result of mechanical injury to the cell membrane of the muscle. The membrane is directly deformed or destroyed by pressure of a high magnitude, such as a person lying on the floor after a fractured hip. As the amount of soft tissue available for compression decreases, the pressure gradient increases; thus, most PIs occur over bony prominences where there is less tissue for compression and the pressure gradient within the vascular network is altered. Deformation of tissues is a key factor in the damage seen in deep tissue pressure injury (DTPI) and full-thickness PI (stages 3 and 4) and may be the force that initiates cell death. The degree of tissue deformation depends on the tissues (ie, size and shape of the different tissue layers), the mechanical properties of the involved tissues (eg, stiffness, strength, shape of the bone), and the magnitude and distribution of the external mechanical force applied to the tissues. The tissues' ability to withstand deformation can change with time due to aging, lifestyle changes, injury, or disease. High-pressure body areas in the semi-reclined position are the occiput, sacrum, and heels. In the erect sitting position, the ischial tuberosities exert the highest pressure, and the trochanters are affected in the side-lying position.

Several investigators have examined the reaction of cells to deformation. Observing single muscle cells has demonstrated that deformations exceeding 80% have consistently ruptured cell membranes, causing immediate and irreversible damage. Observations of an entire muscle have demonstrated similar findings; 2 hours of sustained deformation at strains higher than 50% inflicted irreversible damage to muscle tissue. Muscle tissue is metabolically active and when ischemic it is more sensitive to deformation forces, and irreversible damage may be present at the muscle layer without such damage occurring in the skin or subcutaneous layers. The cell death and local tissue necrosis change the geometry and characteristics of the tissues, which further increases the deformation force exacerbating the PI. Heat accumulation or increased skin temperature intensifies the effects of ischemia and hypoxia on tissues. Increased skin temperature causes an increase in metabolic rate, which increases the need for oxygen in the tissues.

Inflammation in the injured tissue increases interstitial fluid pressure which further impedes arteriolar circulation. The capillary vessels collapse, and thrombosis occurs. Lymphatic flow is decreased, allowing further tissue edema, and contributing to the tissue necrosis.

Less intense pressure, over time, occludes blood and lymphatic circulation, causing deficient tissue nutrition and accumulation of cellular waste products. If pressure is relieved before a critical time is reached, a normal compensatory mechanism, reactive hyperemia, restores tissue nutrition and compensates for compromised circulation. If pressure is not relieved, the blood vessels collapse and thrombose. The tissues are deprived of oxygen, nutrients, and waste removal. In the absence of oxygen, cells use anaerobic pathways for metabolism and produce toxic by-products. The toxic by-products lead to tissue acidosis, increased cell membrane permeability, edema, and eventual cell death.

These cellular changes result in inflammation and edema locally at the site of injury. The inflammatory changes exist in the tissues before any damage is fully visible on the skin surface. This is the nonvisible spectrum of pressure-induced tissue damage, the preclinical stage of disease in the physiology cascade leading to frank ulceration. These inflammatory changes with tissue edema can occur from 2 to 7 days before visible skin breakdown.

When prolonged pressure is finally relieved, the damage does not end. As the vascular network is relieved of pressure, the tissues are re-perfused and re-oxygenated. The sudden entry of oxygen into previously ischemic tissues releases oxygen-free radicals known as superoxide anions, hydroxyl radicals, and hydrogen peroxide, all of which induce new endothelial damage and decrease microvascular integrity causing postischemic or reperfusion injury.

Shear Shear stress is a parallel force applied to an area of the body, in contrast to pressure which is a perpendicular force. Shear stress leads to tissue deformation or distortion, which is called shear strain. Clinically, the term "shear" encompasses both ideas, a force and the resultant injury or strain on tissues. Shear also deforms the cell membrane. The mechanical physical forces of shear which is the force applied against a surface as it moves or slides in an opposite but parallel direction stretching tissues and displacing blood vessels laterally and deformation which stretches and pulls cells are also key factors in PI development.

Friction Friction is a superficial force applied to the skin and not considered a true cause of PI. However, friction damages the upper layers of skin and makes it less tolerant of the other forces. Chronic friction injuries can develop and are seen in patients who slide out of chairs to stand or move between one surface and another (bed to chair). The tissue becomes hyperkeratotic and often hyperpigmented. These tissue changes are not classified as PI.

Tolerance for pressure Comorbid conditions of the body also change the tolerance of soft tissue for pressure. Protein calorie malnutrition, in which the patient has a low body mass index, reduces the padding provided by adipose tissue over the bony prominences. Further, undernourished patients are often hospitalized for a longer stay in intensive care units, with a reduced functional status, and an increased acuity of illness, higher comorbidities, and higher mortality. However, obesity also creates risk for PI. The soft tissue of the severely obese patient is difficult to offload creating tissue-on-tissue pressure. For example, the abdominal pannus is often resting on the thighs or the pubis creating PI.

Impaired arterial flow, either from peripheral vascular disease or the use of vasopressors, decreases the body's ability to reperfuse tissue that has been exposed to pressure and shear. Impairment of arterial inflow leads to local ischemia, delayed reperfusion of ischemic tissue, and impaired lymphatic drainage, all reducing tissue tolerance and the threshold to develop PI. When ischemia is present, the time to develop PI of the heel is shortened. Anemia is often suggested as a risk factor for PI development, but data remain inconclusive.

Lack of sensation, from neurologic disease or injury, diabetic neuropathy, or medication-inducted sedation (anesthesia, sedation for mechanical ventilation), increases risk for PI because the patient lacks the normal protective sensation to move to restore blood flow. Lack of sensory perception from diabetic neuropathy is a major risk factor to heel PI development. Stroke, degenerative neurologic disease, and spinal cord injury are major factors for development of ischial PI that form when the patient is sitting for prolonged periods of time in a chair, recliner, or wheelchair. Distinguishing between PI and diabetic and ischemic ulcers can be difficult and there are overlapping signs.

Exposure to moisture weakens the bonds in the epidermis and decreases tolerance for pressure and shear. Urinary incontinence leads to moisture-associated skin damage; this is not a PI, but often leads to many small open wounds that do not tolerate pressure. Diarrhea also damages the skin, but the wounds are more severe, a form of chemical burn.

Previous full-thickness injury that has closed with scar tissue is also at higher risk for future damage from pressure and shear. Scar tissue does not ever acquire the strength of the native tissue. Scar tissue has a tensile strength of 40% that of native tissue. So, if a patient had a prior stage 4 PI on the sacrum, that scar tissue will be at increased risk for future PI.

Four hypotheses for the pathophysiology behind PI development include the following:

1. High-magnitude pressure leading to direct deformation of tissue cells
2. Ischemia caused by capillary occlusion
3. Shear leading to ischemia of tissues
4. Reduced tolerance for pressure from comorbid conditions such as malnutrition, arterial disease, neuropathic conditions, exposure to moisture, or previous full-thickness injury to the skin

ASSESSMENT

Multiple factors act together synergistically to cause PI in the functionally impaired frail older population. A comprehensive approach is required for these patients with multiple comorbidities to prevent development of PI. Assessment involves screening for risk of developing PI, assessment of the severity of the tissue damage (staging), and evaluation of injury healing over the course of treatment.

Risk Screening and Risk Assessment

Screening is particularly useful for acute care hospitals and specific populations. Given that PI forms from exposure to pressure, the insensate, immobile patient is at highest risk. Severely restricted mobility is the most important risk factor for all populations and a necessary condition for the development of PI. A study of geriatric patients, who were monitored for movements using devices on the bed, showed that none of the individuals with more than 50 movements a night developed PI, whereas 90% of individuals with 20 or fewer spontaneous body movements at night developed a PI. Therefore, the simplest screening tool for PI development is "Does the patient move his body? His leg?" If the answer is no, or not without help, the patient is at risk for PI development.

Screening can be expanded to include those patients who were exposed to intense or prolonged pressure prior to admission. The advantage of a second screen to determine risk is that it allows practitioners to procure support surfaces, turning sheets or overlays or wedges in advance of the patient's arrival on the unit. High-risk patients include:

- Demographic characteristics: African-American race and advanced age (older than 75 years).
- Persons with limited mobility or for whom movement is not possible without staff or caregiver assistance including persons who are unable to move due to sedation.
- Persons admitted to the hospital from a nursing home. These individuals are already frail as they require nursing home care and are now acutely ill.
- Persons admitted to the critical care unit from the emergency department.
- Persons older than 65 years admitted to the acute care hospital who are scheduled for a surgical procedure anticipated to be 3 hours or longer.
- Patients who experienced intraoperative hypotensive episodes.
- Persons admitted to the hospital who were found down for a prolonged time.
- Patients undergoing special therapy, for example, oncology patients admitted for bone marrow transplant or with graft-versus-host disease.
- Patients with hospital transport times more than 1 hour.
- Patients readmitted to a nursing home from the hospital.
- All persons who have had a previous PI and especially persons with spinal cord injury or neurologic dysfunction with prior PI.
- Patients admitted with any diagnosis reducing the tolerance of skin for pressure and shear including nutritional deficiencies, vascular disease, diabetes, and anemia.
- Patients admitted with conditions that will require a long time for recovery including paralysis, senility, respiratory failure, acute kidney injury, stroke, and heart failure.

- Patients admitted with infection: sepsis, osteomyelitis, pneumonia, bacterial infections, and urinary tract infections.
- Intensive care unit patients with sepsis, surgery times more than or equal to 8 hours, or long-term vasopressor therapy (consider at high risk).

Risk assessment tools Early intervention based on screening is an excellent means to reduce risk for PI. A more specific risk assessment tool focused on PI risk factors should follow. Risk assessment is recommended in all clinical practice guidelines for PI. The purpose in identifying patients at risk for PI development is to allow for appropriate use of resources for prevention.

Nurses often use a formal risk assessment tool, such as the Braden Pressure Sore Risk Assessment. This tool is scored in six areas of risk and provides direction to target interventions to those specific risk factors. There is, however, limited evidence to support a direct link between use of risk assessment tools and decreased incidence of PI in part because once risk is identified, interventions to reduce risk are provided. Use of risk assessment tools is linked to increased documentation of prevention interventions and is better than use of clinical judgment alone, particularly for those patients at moderate risk.

PI risk assessment should be performed on admission to the health care setting and at periodic intervals thereafter. The frequency of reassessment is based on the likelihood of the condition of the patient changing. In acute care hospitals, risk assessment should be repeated every shift. In home health settings, risk assessment should be conducted weekly for the first 4 weeks with every other week reassessments thereafter depending on patient condition and frequency of home visits. Nursing home residents should be reassessed for PI risk status weekly for the first 4 weeks

following admission followed by quarterly assessments. Whenever the patient's condition changes in that he is more immobile or eating less, PI risk should be recognized.

PREVENTION

PI prevention involves scheduled turning and repositioning programs, use of support surfaces to reduce/relieve pressure, nutritional support, and general skin care. Prevention interventions should be implemented for persons at risk for PI development and those with existing PI as part of the treatment plan. **Table 46-1** presents general prevention interventions directed at risk factors for PI development.

Turning and Repositioning

Patients at risk for PI who are unable to move independently should be placed on scheduled repositioning programs. The recommended time interval for full change of position or turning while in bed is every 2 to 3 hours, depending on the individual patient profile and the use of support surfaces. An old practice of turning patients every 2 hours has long lacked data to support this intervention. Some patients turn themselves relatively frequently, and turning and repositioning may be an unnecessary use of staff time and sleep disruptive at night. Turning activity can be detected by bed sensors, actigraphy, and other pressure mapping strategies (see below). And with the use of improved pressure-reducing support surfaces (eg, foam, air, gel-filled mattress overlays, low-air-loss therapy devices), frequency often need not be every 2 hours. A randomized clinical trial of PI incidence and turning schedules was conducted on 942 nursing home residents at moderate or high risk for PI development. Residents were placed on high-density foam mattresses and randomly assigned to turning schedules of every 2, 3, or 4 hours. There was no significant difference

TABLE 46-1 ■ PRESSURE INJURY PREVENTION INTERVENTIONS	
RISK FACTOR	**PREVENTION INTERVENTONS**
Immobility	Scheduled repositioning programs, use of pressure reduction/relief surfaces in bed and chairs.
Inactivity, limited mobility	Use of trapeze bars for self-movement in bed, encourage ambulation, rehabilitation as appropriate.
Decreased sensory perception	Scheduled repositioning programs, verbal reminders to move/reposition, use of pressure reduction/relief surfaces in bed and chairs.
Malnutrition	Nutritional assessment to determine deficits, nutritional supplementation (high protein), and daily multivitamin if indicated and appropriate to goals.
Excess moisture and incontinence	Scheduled toileting or prompted voiding programs if responsive, routine check and change programs with pads and adult briefs for persons who do not respond to scheduled toileting or prompted voiding, use of skin creams and ointments for protection from moisture.
Friction and shearing	Use of trapeze bars for those with upper body strength, turn sheets and draw sheets for moving in bed, use of corn starch or lubricants to limit friction between surfaces, thin film or dressings, and pads over bony prominences subject to friction, use of footboards to help prevent sliding while in bed.
Dry skin	Use warm water, gentle cleansers, and limited force for cleansing when soiled and for routine bathing, lubricate and moisturize dry skin, inspect skin daily paying particular attention to bony prominences, avoid massage of reddened areas.

in PI incidence between the turning groups; 2.5% of those turned every 2 hours, 0.6% of those turned every 3 hours, and 3.1% of those patients turned every 4 hours developed PI. There also was no difference in PI rates between the high- and moderate-risk groups of residents.

The patient should be positioned to avoid direct pressure on the sacrum and heels. Position the patient at a 30-degree side-lying position (eg, 30-degree angle to the support surface) with the upper leg forward of the lower leg to reduce the tendency of the patient to fall back onto the sacrum. The legs should be separated with a pillow to reduce pressure. Maintain the head of the bed at the lowest degree of elevation consistent with medical conditions and limit the amount of time the head of the bed is elevated. This position will decrease exposure of the sacral area to shear forces that may predispose to PI in general and especially DTPI. Patients with arterial disease should have their heels off the bed. If the patient will remain positioned on a pillow that "floats the heel", that is all that is needed. However, many patients kick the pillows away or are at extremely high risk—for those patient heel offloading boots or "donuts" made of foam placed above the ankles that elevate the heel are used.

There are techniques to make turning patients easier and less time consuming. Turning sheets, draw sheets, and pillows are essential for passive movement of patients in bed. Turning sheets and overlays are useful in repositioning the patient to a side-lying position, and for pulling the patient up in bed and help to prevent dragging the patient's skin over the bed surface.

Use of real-time pressure mapping systems has been used to improve frequency of repositioning activities by caregivers. Pressure mapping systems may have a positive impact on PI development because the duration and amount of pressure over specific bony prominences are displayed for caregivers allowing for more accurate offloading of bony prominences.

Similar approaches are useful for patients in chairs. Individuals at risk for PI development should avoid uninterrupted sitting in chairs and should be repositioned every hour. The rationale behind the shorter time is the extremely high pressure generated on the ischial tuberosities when sitting erect in the chair and sacrum when reclined or slouched in the seated position. When possible, individuals who are able should be taught to shift weight every 15 minutes while seated. Full-body change of position involves standing the patient and reseating them in the chair. This process can be labeled "Stand and March in Place" and reduces the usual process of manually pulling patients up in the chair, a process which greatly increases back and shoulder injury to staff and shear for the patient. Use of footstools and the foot pedals on wheelchairs and appropriate 90-degree flexion of the hip (may be achieved with pillows, special seat cushions, or orthotic devices) can help prevent chair sliding. Attention to proper alignment and posture is essential. Patients who mobilize by

wheelchair benefit from "tilt-in-space" chairs that recline the patient by tilting the backrest back.

Repositioning for preventing PI at the heel location involves completely offloading the heel using suspension devices, foam donuts (mentioned above), or pillows. The goal is to keep the heels free of all pressure or "float" the heels. Elevating the lower leg and calf with pillows or suspension devices spreads the pressure to the lower legs and the heel is no longer subjected to pressure. Heel suspension devices are preferable for long-term use over pillows as it can be difficult for patients to keep their legs on pillows over longer time frames.

Support Surfaces

Most institutions that care for patients or residents use a 4-inch viscoelastic foam mattress on the beds. This mattress is adequate for the patient or resident who can self-turn and move the legs. For patients at higher risk, reactive or active support surfaces should be used. Some mattresses are replaced, sometimes an overlay can be placed on the usual mattress, and sometimes the entire bed system is replaced. These decisions stem from the relative risk for PI development. The higher the risk, the more aggressive the support surface needs to be. How frequently a patient needs to be repositioned by the staff when lying on a specialty support surface has not been fully studied.

The definitions of types of support surfaces stem from the support surface initiative by the National Pressure Injury Advisory Panel. The premise of a support surface is that if pressure can be redistributed over a larger body area, the relative pressure at any one area will be less. Think of the analogy of pushing your hand onto a surface of many nails versus one nail. Reactive support surfaces are powered or nonpowered surfaces with the ability to only change load distribution properties in response to an applied load. Reactive surfaces reduce pressure by immersion and envelopment of the body into the surface to reduce the deformation of tissue caused by pressure over the bony prominence. A foam mattress is an example of a nonpowered reactive surface. Active support surfaces are powered surfaces that inflate and deflate cells of air to change pressure over a body area. Active surfaces reduce pressure by periodically shifting the areas of support on anatomic locations so that deformation is not sustained over one area. In general, active support surfaces are recommended for persons at higher risk for PI development when frequent repositioning is not possible. An alternating air mattress is an example of an active powered support surface.

Additionally, clinicians should advocate for use of support surfaces in the operating room to reduce intraoperative acquired PI. High-risk patients for PI development during surgery are those whose operation will exceed 3 hours, those with American Society of Anesthesiologists (ASA) scores of 3 or higher, and those who are prone for surgery. The areas of the body exposed to pressure during surgery vary by the position used for the operation. Staff familiar with the position required should place prophylactic dressings on areas of high risk or pad the table to protect those body areas.

Providing topical preparations or fabrics/linens (silk or noncotton blends) to eliminate or reduce the surface tension between the skin and the bed linen or support surface will assist in reducing friction-related injury. Use of appropriate techniques when moving patients so that skin is not dragged across linens will lessen friction-induced skin breakdown. Patients who exhibit voluntary or involuntary repetitive body movements (particularly of the heels or elbows) require stronger interventions. Use of a protective film, such as a transparent film dressing or a skin sealant; a protective dressing, such as a thin hydrocolloid; or protective padding will help to eliminate the surface contact of the area and decrease the friction between the skin and the linens. Even though heel, ankle, and elbow protectors do nothing to reduce or relieve pressure, they can be effective aids against friction. Hip fracture patients are especially vulnerable to heel injuries. Elevation of the heel off the bed surface is a useful preventive measure.

Use of prophylactic silicone foam dressings over bony prominences has demonstrated significantly decreased heel (3% vs 12% favoring dressing) and sacral (1% vs 5% favoring dressing) PI among critical care patients with the number needed to treat of 10 to prevent any injury. Similar outcomes exist in long-term care residents showing reduction in PI rates even in the incontinent resident. Use of prophylactic silicone foam, hydrocolloid, foam, or silicone gel dressings around medical devices has also been shown to decrease PI development related to medical devices including tracheostomy tubes, nasal intubation tubes, and nasal continuous positive airway pressure (CPAP) devices.

General skin care should include routine skin inspection, incontinence assessment and management, and skin hygiene interventions to maintain skin health. Routine skin inspection should occur daily with particular attention to bony prominences. Reddened areas should not be massaged. Massage can further impair the perfusion to the tissues. The skin should be evaluated for dryness and cracking and use of moisturizers can be helpful. Attention should also be focused on gentle handling to prevent skin tears. Incontinence assessment and management with scheduled toileting or prompted voiding programs and for those unresponsive to these programs check and change schedules are important. Prompt cleansing after incontinent episodes with warm water and gentle cleansers and use of protective ointments and creams help maintain perineal skin health.

Nutrition

Malnutrition and/or weight loss has been associated with fourfold higher risk of PI development. Other studies have demonstrated that the severity of the PI is associated with the severity of the malnutrition. Although it seems intuitive, it has proven difficult to define a specific causal relationship between malnutrition and PI development. Multiple studies have demonstrated a relationship between different markers of malnutrition (eg, dietary protein intake, inability to feed self, and weight loss) and PI formation. Modest evidence exists to support providing oral nutritional supplements to persons at risk for PI with relative reduction in PI incidence of 25%.

Nutritionists should routinely assess patients and residents at risk for PI. A comprehensive nutritional assessment should be completed to provide information on adequacy of nutritional intake, anthropometric measures of current and usual body weight, height and body mass index (BMI), physical examination findings that highlight nutritional issues such as muscle wasting, edema, micronutrient deficiencies, and functional status. Nutritionists also consider the patient/resident's ability to eat independently. For many years, serum albumin and prealbumin were considered biochemical markers of malnutrition. However, these laboratory values should not be the sole basis of a malnutrition or failure to thrive diagnosis because serum protein levels reflect severity of inflammatory response rather than nutritional status. Both intake of calories and protein often need to be optimized in patients at risk for PI. There are no studies that show PI rates to be lower in those persons given nutritional supplementation, but providing supplements represents good clinical practice. When dietary intake is inadequate, or deficiencies are suspected or confirmed, provide a vitamin and mineral supplement. Dietary restrictions should be revised or modified/liberalized when limitations result in decreased food and water/fluid intake. These adjustments should be managed by a registered dietitian whenever possible.

DIAGNOSIS OF PRESSURE INJURY

The diagnosis of a PI begins with a history of the patient's exposure to pressure. Consider the events that preceded the onset of the wound, such as supine with the head of the bed elevated, sitting in a bedside chair or wheelchair, being unable to move the legs as the likely precipitant events to PI. Conditions that reduce the tolerance of skin and soft tissue for pressure and shear include reduced arterial perfusion, exposure to moisture, and protein calorie malnutrition. Differential diagnoses include arterial ulcers, diabetic foot ulcers, skin tears, and moisture-associated skin damage. Deep tissue PI is almost always preceded by exposure to intense pressure in the prior 48 to 72 hours. Differential diagnoses of deep tissue PI include traumatic injury, such as pelvic hematoma and embolic disease.

Detection of Early Pressure Injury

Detection of early pressure-induced tissue damage is important because early intervention may prevent evolution into more severe pressure damage. There are several nonvisual methods of detecting pressure damage currently being explored for use in clinical practice by wound care specialists: ultrasound, thermography, spectroscopy, and surface electrical capacitance. Of these, ultrasound, thermography, and surface electrical capacitance show promise for use clinically.

High-resolution ultrasound is one of the earliest noninvasive methods to visualizing skin and soft tissues that provides echogenic images of skin and deeper tissues. Early work showed tissue edema in nursing home residents at risk for PI. Nearly 80% of those with abnormal ultrasound images did not have documentation of erythema suggesting that ultrasound technology can detect tissue damage before clinical signs occur. Despite the advantages to ultrasound the equipment is large and expensive, requires skilled technicians to obtain useful images, and requires trained providers to interpret images.

Thermography, the measurement of skin surface temperature and temperatures of tissues below the skin surface, may provide a method for detecting nonvisual pressure damage and resultant ischemia or inflammation. Both increased and decreased skin temperature (compared to adjacent normal tissue) are associated with stage 1 PI in rehabilitation patients with pressure-induced erythema. Skin temperature variability also differentiates between nursing home residents at high and low risk for PI development and between those residents who do and do not develop PI. A study of nursing home residents using a thermographic camera found that areas of blanchable erythema with cooler skin temperatures were more likely to develop necrotic ulcers in 7 days.

Measurement of the subepidermal water content of the skin and underlying tissue can be accomplished using surface electrical capacitance devices. These devices detect and measure water or edema as the initial inflammatory response of injured tissues below the stratum corneum. When cells are injured, such as occurs with early pressure-induced tissue damage, cellular permeability increases and the action potential across the cell membrane is decreased allowing quick, high electrical charges to pass through the tissues. Devices to measure these charges are small, portable, handheld dermal phase meters, which require light skin touch with readings available within 3 to 8 seconds. In nursing home residents, critical care patients, veterans with spinal cord injury, and persons with dark skin tones, this technique has detected inflammatory changes in the tissues, identifying pre-stage 1, stage 1, and deep tissue PI on the sacrum and heels.

Early Presentation

PIs are labeled using a staging system: stages 1 to 4, unstageable, and deep tissue PI (see **Figure 46-1**).

While there is no label for preclinical or pre-stage 1 PI, there are often signs of reperfusion of tissue after pressure is relieved. Blanchable erythema presents as discoloration of a patch or flat, nonraised area of the skin larger than 1 cm.

Assessment of Pressure Injury Stage

PIs are commonly classified using a staging or categorical system based on the observable depth of tissue loss. The stage is determined on initial assessment by noting the deepest layer of tissue involved. The injury is not restaged unless deeper layers of tissue become exposed. The numeric classification system suggested an orderly evolution of PI; however, PI do not progress, heal, or deteriorate in a linear fashion.

The most used staging system is the National Pressure Injury Advisory Panel's (NPIAP) system describing six classifications of PI. The NPIAP staging system was updated in 2016. **Figure 46-1** presents the definitions for PI stages. When more than one tissue type is present in a wound, stage the wound to the highest level of damage because this will dictate the treatment needed.

Stage 1 Intact skin with nonblanchable erythema involves more severe damage to underlying tissues including lymphatic and capillary occlusion. Skin temperature is cool compared with healthy tissues, and the area may feel indurated. This stage of tissue injury is also reversible, although tissues may take 1 to 3 weeks to return to normal.

Stage 2 An open wound with exposure of the dermis. The wound is superficial, with indistinct margins. Fluid-filled blisters (open or closed) may be seen. If properly treated, these wounds should heal in 2 to 4 weeks. Stage 2 PI often develops as a result of friction (rubbing heels on the bed) or chronic exposure to moisture, which reduces the tolerance of skin for pressure.

The remaining four stages of PI are full-thickness wounds; that is, exposure of body structures beneath the skin. These wounds are often the outcome of deep tissue PI.

Deep tissue PI Initially appears as purple or maroon intact skin over an area of the body exposed to intense pressure about 48 hours prior. The initial injury was deformation and destruction of muscle cells, but due to the low metabolic demand of skin the skin stays alive for a time after the muscle beneath it is destroyed. The skin lyses off, creating a blistered look to the wound and then the damage becomes apparent. Eschar usually forms and surgical debridement is often needed.

Stage 3 Full-thickness loss of skin with exposure of adipose tissue. Because of the location of PI over bony prominences, this stage is not common. However, as wounds heal they appear to be stage 3 PI because they are filled with granulation tissue.

Stage 4 Full-thickness loss of skin with exposure of bone, muscle, tendon, ligament, or cartilage. Osteomyelitis is a common outcome when there is exposure of bone and should be considered the cause of nonhealing in any stage 4 PI.

Unstageable A PI that is most likely a full-thickness PI, but it cannot be determined if the ulcer is a stage 3 or 4 because the extent of the damage cannot be visualized due to slough or eschar in the wound bed.

Mucous membrane PI Medical devices lead to many PI. They tend to be made of hard plastic and often rest on muscle membrane (endotracheal tubes, nasogastric tubes, catheters). These PI cannot be staged using the PI staging system because the anatomy of mucous membrane is not the same as skin.

Skin failure/terminal ulcers Clinicians have long reported change in skin color usually on the sacrum near the time of death. At times, these changes are labeled skin failure to parallel the failure of other body organs, citing the idea that the skin is the largest organ of the body and therefore can also fail. However, the wounds are not large enough to lead to death on their own, such as would be seen with epidermolysis bullosa or Steven-Johnson syndrome. The condition needs a different name; the reader may see changes in the terminology in the future.

PRESSURE INJURY STAGE	DEFINITION AND CLINICAL DESCRIPTION	PHOTOGRAPH
Stage 1	Intact skin with a localized area of non-blanchable erythema, which may appear differently in darkly pigmented skin. Presence of blanchable erythema or changes in sensation, temperature, or firmness may precede visual changes. Color changes do not include purple or maroon discoloration; these may indicate deep tissue pressure injury.	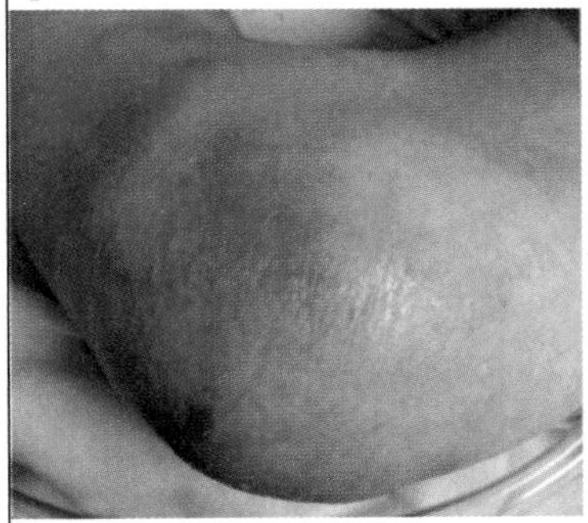 *Left medial knee*
Stage 2	Partial-thickness loss of skin with exposed dermis. The wound bed is viable, pink or red, moist, and may also present as an intact or ruptured serum-filled blister. Adipose (fat) is not visible and deeper tissues are not visible. Granulation tissue, slough, and eschar are not present. These injuries commonly result from adverse microclimate and shear in the skin over the pelvis and shear in the heel. This stage should not be used to describe moisture-associated skin damage (MASD) including incontinence-associated dermatitis (IAD), intertriginous dermatitis (ITD), medical adhesive–related skin injury (MARSI), or traumatic wounds (skin tears, burns, abrasions).	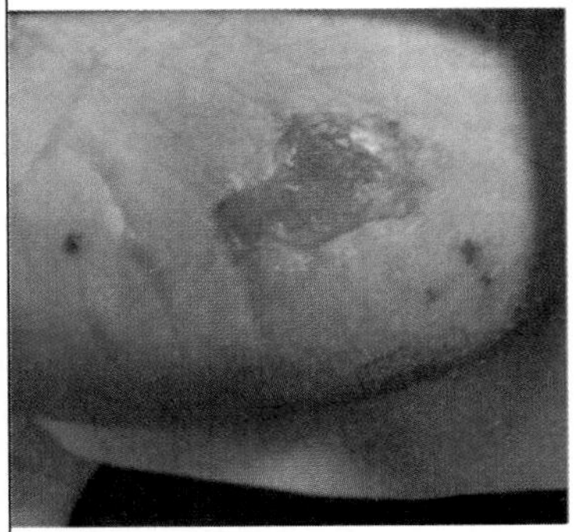 *Left lateral heel*
Stage 3	Full-thickness loss of skin, in which adipose (fat) is visible in the ulcer and granulation tissue and epibole (rolled wound edges) are often present. Slough and/or eschar may be visible. The depth of tissue damage varies by anatomical location; areas of significant adiposity can develop deep wounds. Undermining and tunneling may occur. Fascia, muscle, tendon, ligament, cartilage, and/or bone are not exposed. If slough or eschar obscures the extent of tissue loss this is an unstageable pressure injury.	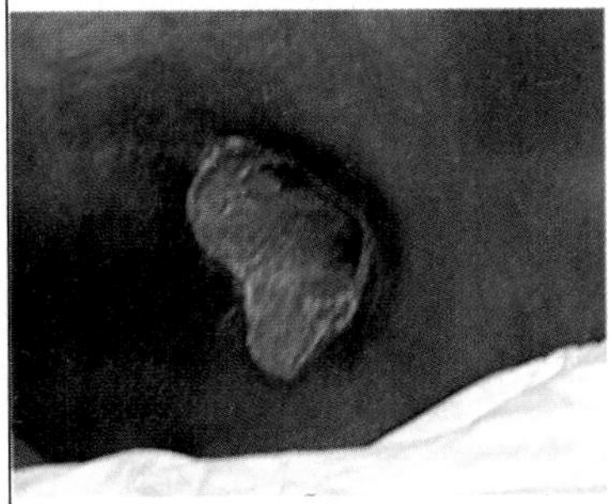 *Sacrum*

FIGURE 46-1. Stages of pressure injury.

Stage 4	Full-thickness skin and tissue loss with exposed or directly palpable fascia, muscle, tendon, ligament, cartilage, or bone in the ulcer. Slough and/or eschar may be visible. Epibole (rolled edges), undermining, and/or tunneling often occur. Depth varies by anatomical location. If slough or eschar obscures the extent of tissue loss, this is an unstageable pressure injury.	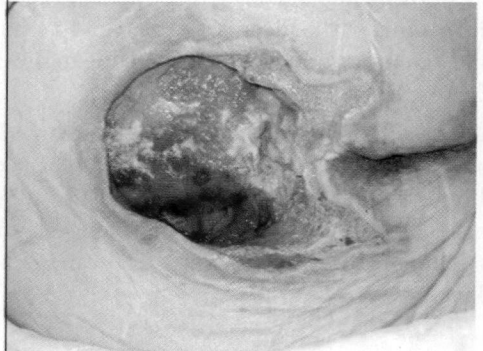 *Sacrum*
Unstageable	Full-thickness skin and tissue loss in which the extent of tissue damage within the ulcer cannot be confirmed because it is obscured by slough or eschar. If slough or eschar is removed, a stage 3 or stage 4 pressure injury will be revealed. Stable eschar (ie, dry, adherent, intact without erythema or fluctuance) on an ischemic limb or the heel(s) should not be removed.	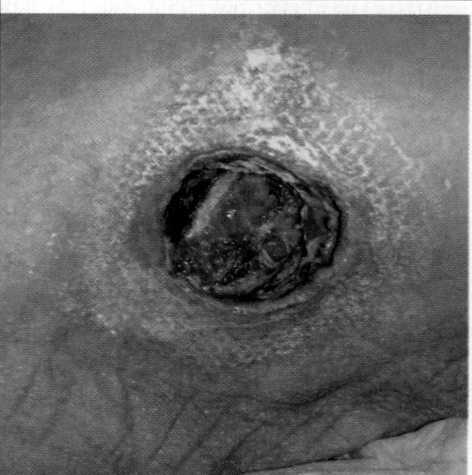 *Right greater trochanter*
Deep tissue pressure injury	Intact or nonintact skin with localized area of persistent nonblanchable deep red, maroon, purple discoloration or epidermal separation revealing a dark wound bed or blood-filled blister. Pain and temperature change often precede skin color changes. Discoloration may appear differently in darkly pigmented skin. This injury results from intense and/or prolonged pressure and shear forces at the bone-muscle interface. The wound may evolve rapidly to reveal the actual extent of tissue injury or may resolve without tissue loss. If necrotic tissue, subcutaneous tissue, granulation tissue, fascia, muscle, or other underlying structures are visible, this indicates a full-thickness pressure injury (unstageable, stage 3 or stage 4). Do not use DTPI to describe vascular, traumatic, neuropathic, or dermatologic conditions.	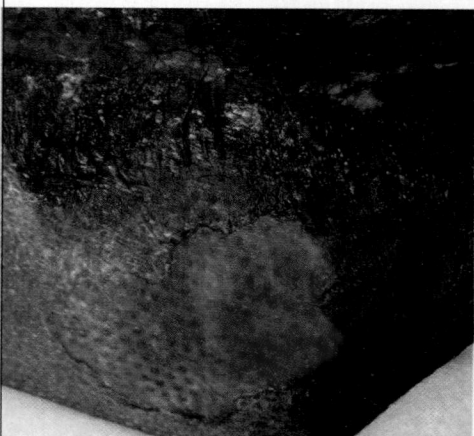 *Right lateral buttock*

FIGURE 46-1. (Continued)

MANAGEMENT OF PRESSURE INJURY

Pressure Injury Assessment

The healing of a PI is routinely assessed, usually weekly, by measuring the size of the wound, the type of tissue in the wound, the condition of the periwound, and the type of drainage and signs of infection. Nurses usually complete this activity, and the direction of the wound indicates if the current treatment needs changing. A good practice method is to reconsider the treatments in place

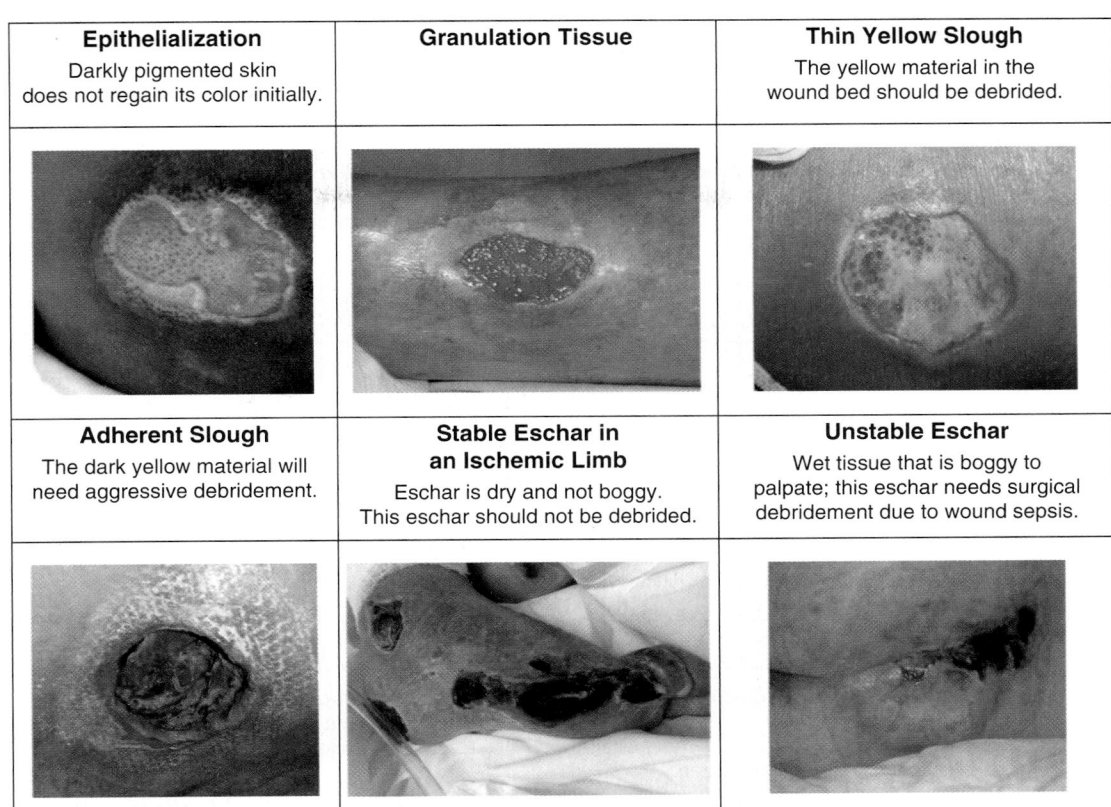

Epithelialization	Granulation Tissue	Thin Yellow Slough
Darkly pigmented skin does not regain its color initially.		The yellow material in the wound bed should be debrided.

Adherent Slough	Stable Eschar in an Ischemic Limb	Unstable Eschar
The dark yellow material will need aggressive debridement.	Eschar is dry and not boggy. This eschar should not be debrided.	Wet tissue that is boggy to palpate; this eschar needs surgical debridement due to wound sepsis.

FIGURE 46-2. Tissue types in pressure injuries.

if the wound does not show signs of healing in 2 weeks. Of course, if the wound is deteriorating, there is no benefit to waiting 2 weeks to change treatments. Signs of healing include the wound size decreasing, the exudate (drainage) from the wound decreasing, no signs of infection, and the reduction in the amount of necrotic or nonviable tissue with the development of granulation tissue. Final wound closure is measured by the presence of epithelium covering the wound. Improvement rates for stage 3 and 4 injuries are slower than stage 2 injuries with 75% of stage 2 wounds healing in 60 days, while only 17% of stage 3 or 4 injuries heal in the same time period. Tissue types seen in wounds are shown in **Figure 46-2**.

There are two research-based PI assessment tools for evaluating wound status and healing, NPIAP's Pressure Ulcer Scale for Healing tool (PUSH) (**Figure 46-3**) and the Bates-Jensen Wound Assessment Tool (BWAT) (**Figure 46-4**). Clinical practice guidelines, expert panels, and federal nursing home guidelines recommend standardized assessment of PI, and many groups recommend use of a standardized tool for ongoing PI assessment.

The PUSH tool incorporates surface area measurements, exudate amount, and surface appearance. The clinician measures the size of the wound, using length and width to calculate surface area and chooses the appropriate size category of 10 categories. Exudate is evaluated as none

(0), light (1), moderate (2), and heavy (3). Tissue type is rated as closed (0), epithelial tissue (1), granulation tissue (2), slough (3), and necrotic tissue (4). Each of the three items is scored, then the three sub-scores can be summed for a total score. The PUSH tool offers a quick assessment to predict healing outcomes, but assessment of additional wound characteristics may still be needed in order to develop a treatment plan for the PI.

The BWAT evaluates 13 wound characteristics using a five-point numerical rating scale and rates them from best (scored as 1) to worst (scored as 5) possible (see **Figure 46-4**). Characteristics include size, depth, edges, undermining or pockets, necrotic tissue type and amount, exudate type and amount, surrounding skin color, peripheral tissue edema and induration, granulation tissue, and epithelialization. Similar to the PUSH tool, once characteristics have been scored, they can be summed for a total score (range 13–65).

Redistribution of Pressure and Reduction in Shear

PIs occur due to exposure to pressure and shear; therefore, pressure must be reduced for the wound to heal. In general, the patient should not be positioned on the PI, but this is easy to say and sometimes difficult to do. If the patient can tolerate or is unaware of being positioned off the wound, the plan of care should indicate which positions are to be

PUSH Tool 3.0

Patient Name:_____   Patient ID#:_____

Ulcer Location: _____   Date:_____

DIRECTIONS:
Observe and measure the pressure ulcer. Categorize the ulcer with respect to surface area, exudate, and type of wound tissue. Record a subscore for each of these ulcer characteristics. Add the subscores to obtain the total score. A comparison of total scores measured over time provides an indication of the improvement or deterioration in pressure ulcer healing.

Length	0	1	2	3	4	5	
	0 cm²	< 0.3 cm²	0.3–0.6 cm²	0.7–1.0 cm²	1.1–2.0 cm²	2.1–3.0 cm²	
× Width		6	7	8	9	10	**Subscore**
		3.1–4.0 cm²	4.1–8.0 cm²	8.1–12.0 cm²	12.1–24.0 cm²	> 24 cm²	
Exudate Amount	0	1	2	3			**Subscore**
	None	Light	Moderate	Heavy			
Tissue Type	0	1	2	3	4		**Subscore**
	Closed	Epithelial Tissue	Granulation Tissue	Slough	Necrotic Tissue		
							Total Score

Length × Width: Measure the greatest length (head to toe) and the greatest width (side to side) using a centimeter ruler. Multiply these two measurements (length × width) to obtain an estimate of surface area in square centimeters (cm²). Caveat: Do not guess! Always use a centimeter ruler and always use the same method each time the ulcer is measured.

Exudate Amount: Estimate the amount of exudate (drainage) present after removal of the dressing and before applying any topical agent to the ulcer. Estimate the exudate (drainage) as none, light, moderate, or heavy.

Tissue Type: This refers to the types of tissue that are present in the wound (ulcer) bed. Score as a "4" if there is any necrotic tissue present. Score as a "3" if there is any amount of slough present and necrotic tissue is absent. Score as a "2" if the wound is clean and contains granulation tissue. A superficial wound that is reepithelializing is scored as a "1." When the wound is closed, score as a "0."

4 - Necrotic Tissue (Eschar): black, brown, or tan tissue that adheres firmly to the wound bed or ulcer edges and may be either firmer or softer than surrounding skin.
3 - Slough: yellow or white tissue that adheres to the ulcer bed in strings or thick clumps, or is mucinous.
2 - Granulation Tissue: pink or beefy red tissue with a shiny, moist, granular appearance.
1 - Epithelial Tissue: for superficial ulcers, new pink or shiny tissue (skin) that grows in from the edges or as islands on the ulcer surface.
0 - Closed/Resurfaced: the wound is completely covered with epithelium (new skin).

Version 3.0: 9/15/98
©National Pressure Ulcer Advisory Panel

FIGURE 46-3. National Pressure Injury Advisory Panel Pressure Ulcer Scale for Healing Tool. (© National Pressure Injury Advisory Panel.)

used (eg, side to side positioning). However, the more common issue is that patients often developed a PI by lying or sitting in a preferred position and it will be difficult to convince them to change. If the PI is on the sacrum, side to side turning, with confirmation that the sacrum is free from pressure, is the ideal practice. If the patient refuses to stay off the wound, consider upscaling the mattress or adding an overlay for additional immersion into the bed. These devices do not replace turning, but the increased immersion reduces pressure on soft tissue.

When PI occurs on the ischium in chairbound patients, a specialized chair cushion with high immersion is needed. Again, time spent lying on the sides will reduce

pressure on the ischium. However, ischial wounds are very slow to heal, and it is difficult to convince a patient to lie in bed for months. Usually a compromise is best, for example, being up a few hours at a time in the chair and then back to bed on the left or right side.

PI on the heel should be managed with a heel off-loading device (HOLD); pillows should not be used. Pillows are unreliable, often collapse under the weight of the leg, or get kicked off the bed. If the leg cannot be placed in a HOLD, apply a pressure redistribution foam dressing to the heel.

Trochanteric PI occurs in patients with contractures, who lie on their sides. Pressure redistribution in these patients is difficult because the PI are often bilateral, and

BATES-JENSEN WOUND ASSESSMENT TOOL

NAME

Complete the rating sheet to assess wound status. Evaluate each item by picking the response that best describes the wound and entering the score in the item score column for the appropriate date. If the wound has healed/resolved, score items 1, 2, 3, & 4 as = 0.

Location: Anatomic site. Circle, identify right **(R)** or left **(L)** and use **"X"** to mark site on body diagrams:

____ Sacrum & coccyx	____ Lateral ankle	
____ Trochanter	____ Medial ankle	Other Site
____ Ischial tuberosity	____ Heel	

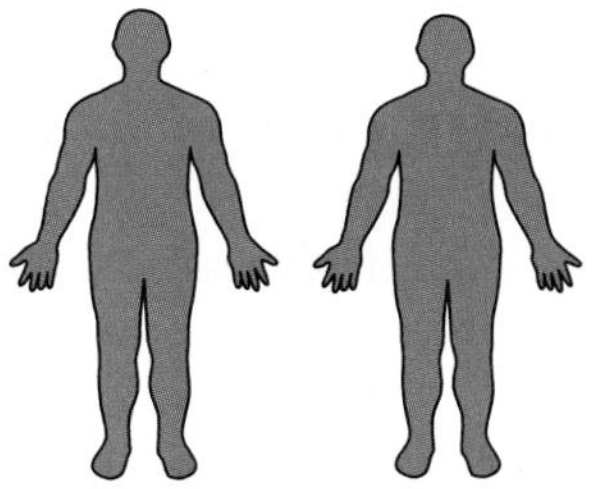

Shape: Overall wound pattern; assess by observing perimeter and depth.
Circle and <u>date</u> appropriate description:

____ Irregular	____ Linear or elongated	
____ Round/oval	____ Bowl/boat	Other Shape
____ Square/rectangle	____ Butterfly	

Item	Assessment	Date Score	Date Score	Date Score
1. Size*	*0 = Healed, resolved wound 1 = Length × width < 4 sq cm 2 = Length × width 4–< 16 sq cm 3 =Length × width 16.1–< 36 sq cm 4 = Length × width 36.1–< 80 sq cm 5 = Length × width > 80 sq cm			
2. Depth*	*0 = Healed, resolved wound 1 = Nonblanchable erythema on intact skin 2 = Partial thickness skin loss involving epidermis &/or dermis 3 = Full thickness skin loss involving damage or necrosis of subcutaneous tissue; may extend down to but not through underlying fascia; &/or mixed partial & full thickness &/or tissue layers obscured by granulation tissue 4 = Obscured by necrosis 5 = Full-thickness skin loss with extensive destruction, tissue necrosis or damage to muscle, bone or supporting structures			
3. Edges*	*0 = Healed, resolved wound 1 = Indistinct, diffuse, none clearly visible 2 = Distinct, outline clearly visible, attached, even with wound base 3 = Well-defined, not attached to wound base 4 = Well-defined, not attached to base, rolled under, thickened 5 = Well-defined, fibrotic, scarred, or hyperkeratotic			
4. Under-mining*	*0 = Healed, resolved wound 1 = None present 2 = Undermining < 2 cm in any area 3 = Undermining 2–4 cm involving < 50% wound margins 4 = Undermining 2–4 cm involving > 50% wound margins 5 = Undermining > 4 cm or tunneling in any area			
5. Necrotic Tissue Type	1 = None visible 2 = White/grey nonviable tissue &/or nonadherent yellow slough 3 = Loosely adherent yellow slough 4 = Adherent, soft, black eschar 5 = Firmly adherent, hard, black eschar			
6. Necrotic Tissue Amount	1 = None visible 2 = < 25% of wound bed covered 3 = 25% to 50% of wound covered 4 = > 50% and < 75% of wound covered 5 = 75% to 100% of wound covered			
7. Exudate Type	1 = None 2 = Bloody 3 = Serosanguineous: thin, watery, pale red/pink 4 = Serous: thin, watery, clear 5 = Purulent: thin or thick, opaque, tan/yellow, with or without odor			

FIGURE 46-4. Bates-Jensen Wound Assessment Tool.

PART III

GERIATRIC CONDITIONS

the patient cannot be positioned supine as the weight of the flexed legs pulls them back onto their sides. These patients require upscaled beds, side lying positioning at less than 90 degrees with wedges, and protection of the ankles and knees from the contracted legs.

Use of reactive support surfaces such as mattress overlays or active surfaces such as low-air-loss therapy for patients with stage 1 or 2 PI who cannot be positioned off the wound.

Healing full-thickness injury is aided by air-fluidized therapy beds or low-air-loss beds. One retrospective, multisite, comparison study showed faster healing of existing PI with air-fluidized therapy compared to both pressure reduction support surfaces and low-air-loss therapy (mean healing rate of 5.2 cm²/wk for the air-fluidized surface group compared to 1.5 cm²/wk for pressure reduction support surface group and 1.8 cm²/wk for low-air-loss therapy group).

Nutrition

Inadequate nutritional intake and undernutrition have been linked to the severity of PI and protracted healing. Providing 30 to 35 kcal/kg of calories and 1.3 to 1.5 g/kg of protein daily has been shown to significantly improve PI healing. The preferred method of feeding is orally and if nutritional requirements cannot be met orally, any dietary restrictions should be revised or modified/liberalized when they result in decreased food and water/fluid intake. Evidence on the efficacy of extra protein and energy via oral supplements is substantial. High energy, high protein supplements are beneficial, especially those with arginine, zinc, antioxidants, and micronutrients when provided for more than 4 weeks. However, providing tube feeding to persons with PI has not consistently achieved positive results. Individuals receiving enteral nutrition via a percutaneous endoscopic gastrostomy (PEG) or nasogastric tube often have significantly more major complications (eg, weight loss, aspiration pneumonia, recurrent tube displacement, and death) that were deemed to be related to the intervention compared to individuals receiving an oral diet. Tube feeding formulas also contribute to diarrhea, often contaminating open wounds. Free water will need to be added to the intake of patients on supplemental feeding. Additional fluids may be needed for fever, prolonged vomiting, profuse sweating, diarrhea, and/or heavily exuding wounds.

No evidence exists for use of supplemental vitamins or minerals (eg, vitamin A, E, C, iron) in persons with PI with no coexisting specific vitamin/mineral deficiency to improve PI healing. A daily multivitamin and mineral supplement that provides recommended daily allowances of vitamins and minerals is recommended for persons with suspected nutritional deficiencies.

Clinically, one of the most challenging aspects of nutrition is helping the anorexic elder eat. Many elders struggle with poorly fitted dentures or missing teeth, comorbid conditions or medications that reduce appetite, depression, and lack of usual social environments for eating, and lack of preferred foods when institutionalized but the most common complaint is "I'm just not hungry!" Family bringing in favorite foods can sometimes help. The use of appetite stimulants may be helpful in some people. Megestrol acetate (Megace) has never been shown to be effective in older patients or nursing home residents and has steroidal side effects. With increasing availability of medical marijuana some clinicians and patients are using it as a potential appetite stimulant. A nutritionist will be helpful to fully investigate the issues surrounding not eating.

When the patient is in palliative care or end of life/hospice care, the goals are to provide comfort and minimize symptoms. If providing supplemental nutrition assists in providing comfort to the individual and is mutually agreed upon by the individual, family caregivers, and health professional, then supplemental nutrition (in any form) is very appropriate for palliative or end of life/hospice wound care. If the individual's condition is such that to provide supplemental nutrition increases discomfort and the prognosis is expected to be poor, then providing supplemental nutrition should not be a concern and is not appropriate for palliative or end of life/hospice wound care.

Local Treatment

PI management includes cleaning the open wound, debriding necrotic tissue, reducing risk of infection and biofilms, and using appropriate topical therapy. As PIs are healing, dressings with nonstick surfaces should be used when dressing changes are required frequently; using typical gauze dressings can interfere with healing by removing healed tissue when they are changed.

Cleansing Solutions

PI cleansing at each dressing change is recommended in clinical practice guidelines. Cleansing removes surface contaminants, remnants of previous dressings, and microorganisms on the wound surface. Saline and water have no antiseptic properties and should seldom be used on PI because these wounds are colonized with bacteria. Antiseptic cleansing solutions include hypochlorous acid, dilute sodium hypochlorite (0.25% "half strength" Dakin's solution), and dilute povidone iodine (10% povidone with 1% free iodine [Betadine]). Hydrogen peroxide should not be used on open wounds. Some wound cleansers are cytotoxic to fibroblasts if used in high concentrations and should not be used for long periods of time. The general time frame is to apply the cleanser to the open wound for 10 to 15 minutes and then apply the new dressing. Surfactant antimicrobial cleansing solutions for use on the wound bed include polyhexamethylene biguanide and octenidine dihydrochloride. These solutions help to loosen slough in the wound bed.

Cleansing Lavage

The use of low-pressure lavage (4–15 lb per square inch [psi]) to mechanically lift fibrin and slough from PI has been recommended for many years. Several methods can be used to achieve this pressure, from items as simple as a needle and syringe to noncontact, low-hertz frequency ultrasonic mist to pulsed lavage systems. To remove the debris in the wound bed, the force of the irrigation stream must be greater than the adhesion forces holding the debris to the wound surface. Using wound cleanser as the lavage fluid provides additional benefits.

In general, if a PI contains necrotic debris or is infected, then reducing antimicrobial activity is more important than preventing cellular toxicity. The chemical and mechanical trauma of wound cleansing should be balanced by the dirtiness of the wound. For wounds with large amounts of debris, more vigorous mechanical force and stronger solutions may be used, while for clean wounds, less force and physiologic solutions such as normal saline can be used.

Dressings

Topical therapy for PI should be provided using moist wound healing dressings. Randomized controlled trials as well as several comparative studies provide compelling support for use of moist wound healing dressings instead of any form of dry gauze dressings for PI. Moist wound healing allows wounds to re-epithelialize up to 40% faster than wounds left open to air. Controlled trials suggest that the use of semi-occlusive dressings such as hydrocolloid dressings and foam dressings improve healing of stage 2 PI. These dressings are changed every 3 to 5 days, which allows wound fluid to gather underneath the dressing, facilitating epithelial migration. As noted above, regular gauze should not be used when dressing changes are more frequent; only dressings with nonstick surfaces should be used. **Table 46-2** presents general characteristics of moisture retentive dressing categories.

Biofilm Formation

PIs are colonized with bacteria and the longer the wound is open and not healed, the greater the risk for biofilm formation. PIs are typically colonized with greater than or equal to 10^5 organisms/mL of normal skin flora. Although greater than or equal to 10^5 organisms/mL of normal skin

PART III

GERIATRIC CONDITIONS

TABLE 46-2 ■ GENERAL CHARACTERISTICS OF MOISTURE RETENTIVE DRESSING CATEGORIES

DRESSING CATEGORY	DEFINITION	USES	NOTES
Composite Dressings	Combine one dressing group with another to address wound characteristics. For example, gauze/foam and transparent film dressing properties, hydrocolloid and alginates, etc.	Absorbent (depends on combination of dressings used in the composite) Wicks away excess moisture Nonadherent to wound bed Use depends on the combination of dressings used in the composite	• Some may be difficult to apply • If nonadherent to wound bed then requires secondary dressing to hold in place • Can be confusing to caregivers as combines various dressing category properties
Transparent Film Dressings	Polyurethane and polyethylene membrane film coated with a layer of acrylic hypoallergenic adhesive. Moisture vapor transmission rates (MVTR) vary	Appropriate for partial-thickness wounds Promotes epithelialization Semipermeable Bacterial barrier Autolysis Wound visible Protects against friction Self-adhesive	• May reinjure area on removal • Nonabsorbent so can lead to wound edge maceration • Tendency to remove prematurely • Indicated for minimal exudate, does not absorb drainage • Not indicated for moderate to heavy exudate
Hydrocolloids Regular or thin wafers, paste, granules	Gelatin, pectin, carboxymethylcellulose in a polyisobutylene adhesive base with a polyurethane or film backing	Absorbs low to moderate wound fluid Autolysis Thermal insulation Bacterial barrier Reduces pain Translucent to opaque Easy to apply Controls odor until dressing removed Impermeable to semi-permeable	• Not indicated for heavy exudate, limited absorbent abilities when used alone • Use with other products increases absorbent abilities • Odor on removal • Regular wafers are opaque, thin wafers allow some wound visualization • Edges may melt down and stick to linens • Some difficult to remove • Possible sensitivity to adhesive backing • Use with close supervision on immunosuppressed and diabetic patients, extensive burns, infected lesions

(Continued)

TABLE 46-2 ■ GENERAL CHARACTERISTICS OF MOISTURE RETENTIVE DRESSING CATEGORIES (CONTINUED)

DRESSING CATEGORY	DEFINITION	USES	NOTES
Hydrogels Sheets, wafers Amorphous gels Impregnated gauze	May or may not be supported by a fabric net, high water content, varying amounts of gel-forming material (glycerine, copolymer, water, propylene glycol, humectant)	Absorbs low to moderate drainage Autolysis Nonadhesive, may have adhesive borders Semipermeable or impermeable depending on backing Thermal insulation Reduces pain Conformable Carrier for topical medication	• Can dry out • May macerate surrounding tissues • Requires secondary dressing or tape to keep in place • Does not cause reinjury upon removal • Cooling effect can help relieve wound pain • Candidiasis may present from inappropriate usage
Wound Fillers (Exudate absorbers) Beads, flakes Pastes, powders	Consists of copolymer starch, dextranomer beads, or hydrocolloid paste that swell on contact with wound fluid to form gel, dextranomers, polysaccharides, starch, natural polymers, and colloidal particles	Moisture retentive Absorptive (moderate to large) Useful to fill cavities, pockets, undermining Can be used with topical medications	• Nonadhesive • Requires a secondary dressing to hold in place • May have burning sensation on application • May have odor • Some require mixing • Some require wound irrigation for nontraumatic removal
Alginates Ropes, pads, wafers	Calcium–sodium salts of alginic acid (naturally occurring polymer in seaweed)	Absorptive (moderate to large) Useful to fill cavities, pockets, undermining Moisture retentive Can use with topical medications or on infected wounds Reduces pain Thermal insulation	• Nonadherent, requires secondary dressing to hold in place • Hemostatic properties • May require wound irrigation for removal • No reinjury on removal • May dry out, should not be used on wounds with low exudate
Foams Wafers (thick or thin), pillows, composite dressings with thin film covers, available with surfactant impregnated or charcoal layer	Inert material that is hydrophilic and nonadherent, modified polyurethane foam	Absorptive (moderate to large) Autolysis Can be used with topical medications and on infected wounds Conformable Thermal insulation	• Nonadhesive unless used with composite dressing • Requires tape or secondary dressing to hold in place • Nontraumatic removal • Opaque • Waterproof, inert
Hydrofibers Pads, wafers, ropes	Soft nonwoven pad or ribbon dressings made from sodium carboxymethyl-cellulose fibers, similar absorbent material used in hydrocolloid dressings	Absorptive (moderate to large) Autolysis Thermal insulation Reduces pain	• Nonadherent, requires secondary dressing to hold in place • Hemostatic properties • May require wound irrigation for removal • No reinjury on removal

flora can cause local infection in intact skin and impair wound healing in surgical wounds, chronic wounds such as PI may bear microbial growth at this level for prolonged periods without noticeable clinical manifestations of infection and with evidence of some healing. While not healing, the wound stays inflamed. Chronic inflammation impairs healing because the proinflammatory cytokines (interleukin 1 and tumor necrosis factor) increase the level of matrix metalloproteinases (MMPs). The MMP family is a group of calcium-dependent zinc-containing enzymes that are involved in the degradation of extracellular matrix. MMPs play a crucial role in all stages of wound healing by modifying the wound matrix, allowing for cell migration and tissue remodeling. However, in chronic wounds, there is excessive expression of MMPs, which retards healing while promoting ongoing inflammation.

Biofilms are microbial communities in which the bacteria are encased in exopolysaccharide (EPS) and are less metabolically active than their free-living counterparts. Clinical studies show 60% of chronic wounds contain a biofilm. Biofilms also promote chronic inflammation. The nature of the EPS makes biofilms very resistant to endogenous antibodies and phagocytic cells and exogenous antibiotics and antimicrobial solutions. Bacterial biofilms may be the underlying pathology preventing PIs from healing. Biofilm is not visible to the naked eye, but it should be suspected in all chronic wounds. The best method of preventing biofilm development is adequate, timely, and complete debridement of necrotic tissue followed by appropriate topical therapy. Cadexomer iodine, medical-grade honey, silver, and polyhexamethylene biguanide (PHMB) dressings retard the development of new biofilm. Regardless of the type of topical treatment, the biofilm will reform, and maintenance debridement is required.

Pressure Injury Infection

Infection is a common cause of nonhealing or worsening PI. PIs are chronic, ischemic wounds and as such, they are more susceptible to infection and they occur in malnourished or poorly perfused patients who cannot mount a full immune response. The most common organisms identified in pressure ulcers are *Staphylococcus aureus*, *Proteus mirabilis*, *Pseudomonas aeruginosa*, and *Enterococcus faecalis*. Infected PI also can serve as reservoirs for infections with antibiotic-resistant bacteria. Methicillin-resistant *Staphylococcus aureus* (MRSA) colonization in infected PI is now reported commonly.

Stage 3, 4, and unstageable PI should be evaluated for acute and chronic infection. Tissue biopsy or quantitative swab technique to determine wound "tissue" bioburden is the preferred method to diagnose infection. Do not rely on cultures of the wound surface or wound drainage; they will present only the surface contamination. Tissue biopsy is the gold standard, but is not always feasible. Levine's technique uses light pressure on the wound bed to draw wound fluid for culture.

Osteomyelitis has been reported in 32% of patients with stage 4 PI. The strongest clinical indicator of osteomyelitis is palpable soft or rough bone or visible bone. Most infections are polymicrobial, with a predominance of *S aureus*, *Enterobacteriaceae* spp., and anaerobes. Plain film x-ray is useful in identifying probable osteomyelitis, but the final diagnosis is best made from MRI and bone biopsy with cultures. Management of osteomyelitis includes surgical debridement of infected bone and antibiotics. Infectious diseases specialists vary in their prescribed duration of antibiotics based in part on the level of infection (eg, infection limited to cortical bone may not require a full 6 weeks of therapy). Antibiotics are not risk free and often lead to diarrhea further contaminating the wound bed. When exposure to fecal matter cannot be controlled and the PI is contaminated from it, fecal diversion with catheters and diverting colostomy should be considered.

In patients with large, infected PI, or patients who cannot improve perfusion to a limb, more aggressive procedures such as amputation and hemicorporectomy are sometimes required. Surgical complication rates (including dehiscence, infection, necrosis, and hematoma) for both younger paraplegic patients and nonparaplegic older patients are as high as 50%, and PI recurrence at the same site has been reported ranging from 30% to 70%. Thus, the long-term outcomes have not been ideal even though 70% to 80% of surgically treated PI are healed upon discharge from the hospital. Further, while recurrence of PI at the same site is lower for older patients (40%) compared to younger paraplegic patients (more than 70%), 30% of older patients develop new injury sites, and mortality in older patients ranges from nearly 50% to 68%.

Hyperbaric oxygen therapy (HBOT), delivered within a hyperbaric chamber, can be a useful adjunct in the nonoperative management of chronic refractory osteomyelitis. Chronic refractory osteomyelitis is loosely defined as osteomyelitis that persists despite appropriate medical and/or surgical management. Unfortunately, in PI associated with chronic refractory osteomyelitis, the soft tissue and bony involvement tends to be quite advanced, so that outcomes with HBOT are suboptimal. HBOT can also be utilized to improve perfusion in failing or threatened soft tissue flaps following surgical reconstruction of advanced PI. Overall benefits of HBOT include:

- Enhanced osteoclast function
- Improved leukocyte bacterial killing
- Stimulation of vascular endothelial growth factor and platelet-derived growth factor
- Enhanced angiogenesis

Debridement

Wound debridement is recognized as an important component of wound bed management. It reduces devitalized or necrotic tissue, decreases risk for infection, and promotes granulation tissue formation. Benefits of debridement also may include removal of senescent fibroblasts and nonmigratory hyperproliferative epithelium, and stimulation of blood-borne growth factors. Maintenance debridement is a common phrase used to describe repeated, sometimes weekly, debridement of wound beds. Today, there are clinicians who examine and debride wounds in long-term care settings, reducing the need of the resident to leave the facility. In hospital settings, more aggressive surgical debridement can be performed under anesthesia.

Five methods of debridement (eg, surgical or sharp, mechanical, autolytic, enzymatic, bio-surgical) are available. Choice of debridement method is based on clinician preference and availability rather than specific evidence. Clinical practice guidelines on PI treatment recommend wound debridement with surgical or sharp debridement for extensive necrosis or when obtaining a clean wound bed quickly is important, and more conservative methods are recommended (autolytic and enzymatic) for wounds that are not acutely infected but rather stagnant in healing. Those patients tend to be in long-term care or home care environments. Debridement should only be performed when there is adequate perfusion to the wound. A vascular assessment prior to debridement of lower extremity PI should be performed to determine whether arterial supply is sufficient to support healing of the debrided wound. For this reason, stable eschar on ischemic limbs is not debrided, without arterial supply, the wound cannot heal. Patients with significant comorbid burden or who are at the end of life should not be repeatedly debrided when healing is not possible. Debridement of wounds may be done for control of odor or to unroof the wound and drain pockets of purulence.

Surgical debridement involves use of a scalpel, scissors, or other sharp instruments to widely excise the nonviable tissue. It is the most rapid form of debridement. A PI should be surgically debrided when there is a clinical need for extensive debridement; the degree of undermining and sinus tract or tunneling cannot be determined; there is advancing cellulitis; bone and infected hardware must be removed; and/or the individual is septic from the PI. Relative contraindications include anticoagulant therapy and bleeding disorders. Surgical debridement extends into viable tissue, and the resultant bleeding stimulates the production of bloodborne endogenous growth factors acting as chemoattractants for inflammatory cells and mitogens for both fibroblasts and epithelial cells. Health care professionals who use sharp debridement must demonstrate their competency in sharp wound debridement skills and meet licensing requirements. One multicenter, randomized, controlled trial comparing the effects of topical growth factor versus placebo on healing noted that independent of treatment effects, centers that used sharp debridement more frequently experienced better healing rates than those that used sharp debridement less frequently.

Sharp debridement can be performed with a scalpel, curette, scissors, or rongeurs. This form of debridement is done outside of the operating room but should be a sterile procedure. It is vital that health professionals who perform conservative sharp debridement possess knowledge of anatomy and adequate training and experience. Maintenance debridement is generally done using these methods.

Mechanical debridement involves the use of wet-to-dry dressings, wet-to-moist dressings, monofilament/microfiber debridement pads, and hydro-surgery. Wet-to-dry and wet-to-moist gauze dressings continue to be used for debridement, despite the significant disadvantages of increased labor time for application and removal of the dressings, removing viable tissue as well as nonviable tissue, and pain. This method of debridement should be used cautiously, as it can traumatize new granulation tissue and epithelial tissue, and adequate analgesia should be administered when this method is employed. It is not recommended in clinical practice guidelines. A monofilament/microfiber debridement pad removes slough and devitalized tissue, and potentially disrupts biofilm within the wound bed. The hydro-surgical water knife is an alternative tool to achieve surgical-type debridement. Little evidence on its use exists in PI wound management. Clinical evidence in wounds of different etiology indicates that hydro-surgery can achieve faster debridement than other nonsurgical methods. Grossly infected PI can be surgically debrided and then continually lavaged with antiseptic instillations using negative pressure wound systems to draw the fluid from the wound.

Enzymatic debridement involves applying a concentrated, commercially prepared proteolytic or fibrinolytic enzyme to the surface of the necrotic tissue, in the expectation that it will aggressively degrade necrosis by digesting devitalized tissue. The main enzymatic ointment available in the United States is collagenase. A common practice is to use enzymatic debridement following sharp debridement. Enzymatic ointments have yielded consistently positive results for their efficacy in wound debridement. Debridement with enzymatic ointments is faster than with autolysis, and more conservative than sharp debridement. Nanocrystalline silver can be inhibited when used in combination with collagenase, whereas iodine inhibits the activity of collagenase. Consult package inserts for details on which dressing materials are safely combined with collagenase.

Autolytic debridement is the process of using the body's macrophages and proteolytic enzymes to remove nonviable tissue. Use of occlusive dressings maintains a moist wound environment that allows enzymes within the wound fluid to digest necrotic tissue. Autolytic debridement will be slower to achieve a clean wound bed than other methods. Autolytic debridement is contraindicated in the presence of untreated infection or extensive necrotic tissue, in large PI with undermining and sinus tracts, and in individuals with compromised immunity or severe malnutrition.

Biosurgery is the fifth method of debridement. Biosurgery is the application of maggots (disinfected fly larvae, *Phaenicia sericata*) to the wound typically at a density of 5 to 8/cm^2. Comparative controlled studies evaluating the use of maggot therapy for PI debridement have shown a higher proportion of complete debridement in maggot-treated wounds versus standard debridement therapy (80% vs 48%, respectively). Biosurgery may not be acceptable to all patients and may not be available in all areas.

Advanced Wound Therapy

Evidence supporting use of advanced wound therapy in PI is building. Collagen dressings are mostly derived from bovine, porcine, or avian skin made into sheets and pads, as particles, and as gels. In chronic wounds such as PI, collagen lowers the elastase level, altering the chronicity of the wound and enhancing the healing process through dermal fibroblast proliferation, migration of the cells, and development of the capillary bed. Growth factors commonly stimulate the proliferation of neutrophils, macrophages, and keratinocytes, all of which are active in different stages of wound healing. Exogenous growth factors, platelet-risk plasma, and recombinant human platelet-derived growth factor have also been shown to improve healing of PI. These fairly novel approaches to PI healing should be used when the wound bed is clean and free of infection and the patient's ability to heal is enhanced with adequate nutrition and control of comorbid conditions that delay healing.

Compelling evidence exists for the use of electrical stimulation to treat stage 2 through 4 PI. Electrical stimulation has been strongly recommended in many guidelines with A level evidence from randomized clinical trials, yet the implementation of this treatment lags. Physical therapists often use electrical stimulation for this purpose.

Ultrasound is an acoustic therapy in which mechanical vibration is transmitted in a wave formation at frequencies beyond the upper limit of human hearing. Noncontact low frequency ultrasound therapy (NCLFUS) has been used for the resolution of deep tissue PI, but the quality of the evidence is modest. NCLFUS must begin while the deep tissue PI is still evolving, which is often an issue in using the therapy.

Negative pressure wound therapy (NPWT) applies vacuum to the wound to remove third space edema, thereby enhancing nutrient and oxygen delivery. It has its greatest efficacy in reducing wound volume, and therefore it can serve as an adjuvant therapy when combined with debridement and other treatments that promote healing, such as nutritional support and pressure redistribution. NPWT is intended for use in PI free of necrotic tissue. Therefore, NPWT therapy should begin after debridement. PI that has failed to improve with standard care with moist wound healing and has poor granulation tissue or excess exudate can also benefit from NPWT.

Surgical Reconstruction

Surgical reconstruction of PI most often uses myocutaneous and fasciectomies flaps to close wounds. Flap surgery is considered when patients have been unable to heal a full-thickness wound, despite adequate nutrition, control of risk factors (such as smoking), and adherence to offloading. Patients with nonhealing severe PI should be referred to an experienced surgeon to evaluate the eligibility for surgical repair of the PI. Expectations of the operation and the ability of the individual to tolerate surgery and surgical recovery should be discussed and understood.

Drugs

Pharmacologic interventions for PI include antibiotics and analgesics. Antibiotics may be systemic or local. Clinicians should institute systemic antibiotics for patients exhibiting signs and symptoms of systemic infection such as sepsis or cellulitis with associated fever and an elevated white blood cell count. Systemic antibiotics should be initiated for osteomyelitis or for the prevention of bacterial endocarditis in persons with valvular heart disease and who require debridement of a PI. Because of the high mortality of sepsis associated with PI despite appropriate antibiotics, broad-spectrum coverage for aerobic gram-negative rods, gram-positive cocci, and anaerobes is indicated in pending culture results in patients with suspected bacteremia. For oral therapy for methicillin-sensitive *Streptococcus* and methicillin-sensitive *Staphylococcus*, cephalexin, cefadroxil, dicloxacillin, and clindamycin are recommended. For suspected MRSA, clindamycin, amoxicillin with doxycycline, or trimethoprim-sulfamethoxazole can be used. When parenteral therapy is indicated, many drugs can be used but cefazolin, ceftriaxone, and clindamycin are generally used for empiric therapy. Vancomycin may be required for MRSA. If anaerobic infection is suspected, metronidazole, a carbapenem, or a beta lactamase inhibitor should be used. PI with odorous drainage in patients who are not able to undergo debridement can be managed by applying ground metronidazole to the wound bed.

Antiseptics should be used in full-thickness PI. Topical cadexomer iodine, silver, honey, or PHMB dressings are the preferred antiseptics because they reduce the bioburden in the wound bed. Mupirocin is effective against MRSA. On the other hand, clinicians should not use povidone-iodine, iodophor, sodium hypochlorite, hydrogen peroxide, or acetic acid as topical therapies on clean and healing PI. These antiseptic agents have been shown to be toxic to fibroblasts and to impair wound healing in in vitro laboratory studies, and how these solutions affect human wounds is unclear.

Using nonpharmacologic pain management strategies to reduce pain associated with PI reflects good practice. There is no direct evidence from the literature search on the effectiveness of nonpharmacologic pain management strategies for treating pain associated with PI; however, nonpharmacologic pain management strategies are well-acknowledged as being useful in pain management.

PI-related pain can be minimized by keeping the wound bed moist and covered. Use of hydrogels, hydrocolloids, alginates, polymeric membrane foams, and soft silicone dressings allows for less frequent dressing changes, and less trauma and pain on removal as they are nonadherent to the wound bed.

Pharmacologic strategies for severe wound pain include providing opioids and/or nonsteroidal anti-inflammatory drugs (NSAIDs) 30 minutes prior to the procedure and afterward and administering topical anesthetics or topical opioids using hydrogels as a transport media. Two options have been successful for use in chronic wound pain, EMLA cream (eutectic mixture of lidocaine 2.5% and prilocaine 2.5%) and diamorphine gel. EMLA cream reduces debridement pain scores in chronic venous injuries and may have a cutaneous vasoactive effect. Use of EMLA cream in venous injuries has been associated with a reduction in pain scores (measured on a 100-mm scale) of 21 mm. Low-dose topical morphine (diamorphine) has been used in several small, randomized, placebo-controlled studies to successfully control PI-related pain.

PALLIATIVE PRESSURE INJURY TREATMENT

Not all PI can be healed. Palliative PI care means that the goals are comfort and limiting the extent or impact of the PI but without the intent of healing. Palliative care may be indicated for terminally ill patients such as those with end-stage cancer or in the terminal stages of other diseases. Institutionalized older adults with multiple comorbidities or older adults with severe functional decline may also benefit from palliative care. Palliative PI care may include adequate debridement of necrotic tissue and identification and treatment of infection. PI should be dressed with highly absorptive dressings to reduce the frequency of dressing changes. Odorous drainage should be treated with metronidazole placed into the wound. The odor can be concealed with room deodorizers. Pain management should be a priority. Prevention should still consist of use of reactive or active support surfaces and attention to scheduled repositioning, although time frames may be adjusted or lengthened to ease the burden on the patient. Providing pain medication 30 to 40 minutes prior to repositioning activity and use of positioning devices may help those with pain on movement.

SUMMARY

PIs are chronic wounds and, as such, require patience and diligence by clinicians. Some PI never heal, and most require long periods of treatment with slow progress. Thus, identification of persons at risk for developing PI and aggressive prevention interventions to actively avoid PI

from starting are essential. Prevention includes screening for risk followed by risk assessment using standardized risk assessment tools to determine individual specific risk and implementing targeted prevention interventions based on identified risk factors. Scheduled repositioning programs, use of reactive and active support surfaces, assessment and management of nutrition, and use of prophylactic dressings are key prevention strategies. More research is needed to define optimal turning intervals for various support surfaces, to better elucidate the effect of nutrition interventions on both preventing PI and healing PI.

For those persons who do develop PI, clinicians should provide appropriate treatment during early injury stages to capitalize on healing progress in the initial 3 months. Offloading and nutrition are imperative. Adequate, timely, and complete debridement of necrotic tissue, identification and treatment of infection and management of biofilm development, and providing a moist wound environment are the key tenets of appropriate PI care. All preventive and therapeutic interventions, and progress of the injury, should be carefully documented in the medical record. Unfortunately, no intervention or combination of interventions has demonstrated the ability to completely eliminate PI. Thus, even as we develop more refined and specific screening, detection, and preventive interventions, it is likely we will continue to see PI in all health care settings. The information presented in this chapter should provide a foundation for developing a successful approach to both those at risk for PI development and those with existing PI.

ACKNOWLEDGMENT

This chapter is updated from the previous editions written by Barbara M. Bates-Jensen, PhD, RN, FAAN, and Anabel Patlan, BS.

FURTHER READING

National Pressure Ulcer Advisory Panel, European Pressure Ulcer Advisory Panel and Pan Pacific Pressure Injury Alliance. In: Haesler E, ed. *Prevention and Treatment of Pressure Ulcers: Clinical Practice Guideline.* Perth, Australia: Cambridge Media; 2019.

Padula WV, Delarmente BA. The national cost of hospital acquired pressure injuries in the United States. *Int Wound J.* 2019;16(3):634–640.

Schultz G. Bjarnsholt T, James GA, et al. Consensus guidelines for the identification and treatment of biofilms in chronic nonhealing wounds. *Wound Repair Regen.* 2017;25(5):744–757.

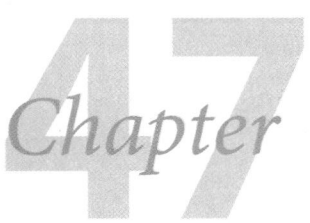

Chapter 47

Incontinence

Camille P. Vaughan, Theodore M. Johnson, II

DEFINITION AND EPIDEMIOLOGY

Defined as the complaint of any involuntary leakage of urine, urinary incontinence is a common and bothersome condition in older adults. Incontinence prevalence increases with age and with increasing frailty, and is 1.3 to 2.0 times greater in older women than older men. Among community-dwelling older women, the prevalence of any urinary incontinence is approximately 35%; among older men, it is approximately 22%. The prevalence of daily urinary incontinence in older community-dwelling persons is approximately 12% for women and 5% for men. The prevalence is higher among nursing home residents approaching 60%. Incontinence ranges in severity from rare episodes of dribbling small amounts of urine to continuous urine leakage with concomitant fecal incontinence. In addition, many older people who do not "leak urine" may have bothersome lower urinary tract symptoms such as urgency, frequency, and nocturia (waking from sleep at night to void) impacting their lives.

Physical health, psychological well-being, social status, and the costs of health care can all be adversely affected by incontinence. Urinary incontinence can be cured or greatly improved, especially in those who have adequate mobility and mental function. Even when not curable, incontinence can always be managed to improve comfort, reduce caregiver burden, and minimize costs of caring for the condition. Because many older patients are embarrassed to discuss their incontinence unaware that treatment is available, it is essential for providers to periodically ask about incontinence and to note this concern as a problem (**Table 47-1**). This chapter covers the basic pathophysiology of urinary incontinence in older persons, provides detailed information on the evaluation and management, and briefly addresses fecal incontinence.

PATHOPHYSIOLOGY AND CLASSIFICATION

Continence requires effective functioning of the lower urinary tract, adequate cognitive and physical functioning, motivation, and an appropriate environment (**Table 47-2**). Normal urination is a complex process and the neurophysiology of urination remains incompletely understood. Proper bladder filling and emptying are influenced by

Learning Objectives

- Identify different types of urinary incontinence based on clinical assessment.
- Describe initial management strategies for incontinence in the older adult, which involve soliciting patient preferences and goals for care.
- Determine when referral to a urologic or gynecologic specialist is indicated.

Key Clinical Points

1. Incontinence in the older adult is often the result of potentially reversible and modifiable conditions.
2. Multicomponent interventions, including lifestyle and behavioral therapies, are effective first-line treatments for incontinence in the older adult.
3. Treatment of incontinence in the older adult, particularly drug therapy, should involve consideration of patient preferences and comorbid conditions.

higher centers in the brain stem, cerebral cortex, and cerebellum. The brain stem facilitates urination and the cerebral cortex exerts a predominantly inhibitory influence. Additionally, the loss of the suprapontine inhibitory influences over the sacral micturition center from diseases such as stroke and Parkinson disease can produce incontinence in older patients. Even in the absence of specific, overt neurologic lesions, poor bladder control is associated with inadequate activation of the orbitofrontal cortex and white matter hyperintensities (evidence of white matter wasting) in the right inferior frontal cortex. Disorders of the brain stem and lesions rostral to the lumbosacral spinal cord can interfere with the coordination of bladder contraction and urethral relaxation leading to detrusor-sphincter dyssynergia. Interruptions of the sacral innervation can

TABLE 47-1 ■ ASKING ABOUT URINARY INCONTINENCE

Questions about incontinence should be open-ended and phrased in language easily understood by the patient:

"Tell me about any problems you are having with your bladder?"

"Tell me about any trouble you are having holding your urine (water)?"

If the responses to the above questions are negative, following up with questions may be helpful:

"How often do you lose urine when you don't want to?"

"How often do you wear a pad or other protective device to prevent urinary accidents?"

Adapted with permission from Fantyl JA, Newman DK, Colling J, et al. Urinary Incontinence in Adults: Acute and Chronic Management. Clinical Practice Guideline No. 2, 1996 Update. Rockville, MD: U.S. Dept of Health and Human Services, Public Health Service, Agency for Health Care Policy and Research; 1996. AHCPR publication 96–0682.

TABLE 47-2 ■ REQUIREMENTS FOR CONTINENCE

Effective lower urinary tract function

Storage

Bladder accommodation with increasing urine volumes while maintaining low pressure

Closed bladder outlet

Appropriate sensation of bladder fullness

Absence of involuntary bladder contractions

Emptying

Bladder capable of contraction

Lack of anatomic obstruction to urine flow

Coordinated lowering of outlet resistance with bladder contractions

Adequate mobility and dexterity to use toilet

Adequate cognitive function to recognize toileting needs

Motivation to be continent

Absence of environmental and iatrogenic barriers

Reproduced with permission from Kane RL, Ouslander JG, Resnick B, et al. Essentials of Clinical Geriatrics. 8th ed. New York, NY: McGraw Hill; 2018.

cause impaired bladder contraction and problems with continence.

At the most basic level, urination is governed by a reflex in the sacral spinal cord. During normal bladder filling, afferent pathways (via somatic and autonomic nerves) carry information regarding bladder volume to the spinal cord. Motor output is adjusted accordingly (**Figure 47-1**). Sympathetic tone closes the bladder neck and inhibits parasympathetic tone (thus relaxing the dome of the bladder); somatic innervation maintains tone in the pelvic floor musculature (including striated muscle around the urethra). Voluntary pelvic floor muscle contracture also leads to inhibition of parasympathetic tone. For bladder emptying, sympathetic and somatic tones diminish, and parasympathetic, cholinergic-mediated impulses cause

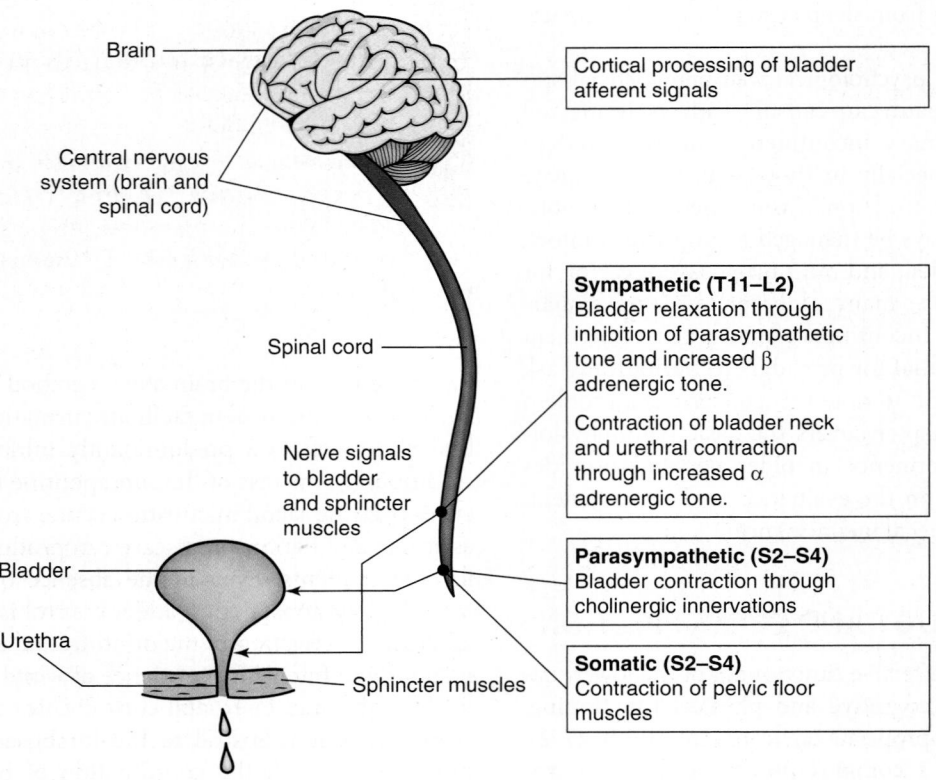

FIGURE 47-1. Central and peripheral nervous system involvement in micturition.

the bladder to contract. Normal urination is a dynamic process, requiring the coordination of several physiologic processes. Under normal circumstances, as the bladder fills, bladder pressure remains low (≤ 15 cm H_2O). The bladder volume at first urge to void is variable, but generally occurs at between 150 and 350 mL; normal bladder capacity is 300 to 600 mL. When normal urination is initiated (usually every 3 to 4 hours during wakefulness), the detrusor contracts and detrusor pressure increases until it exceeds urethral resistance (which lowers immediately prior to bladder contraction). Urine flow occurs typically over less than 2 minutes. If at any time during bladder filling, total bladder pressure exceeds outlet resistance, urinary leakage occurs. Transmitted intra-abdominal pressure alone by coughing or sneezing may cause leakage in someone with low outlet resistance pressure or urethral sphincter weakness. Alternatively, the bladder can contract involuntarily and cause urinary leakage.

Risk Factors

As is the case for a number of other common geriatric problems, multiple disorders often interact to cause urinary incontinence. Determining the cause or causes facilitates proper management.

Several age-related changes can contribute to the development of urinary incontinence. In general, postvoid residual (PVR) urine volume is greater with increasing age. Reduced functional bladder capacity has been associated with advanced age, yet this may be due to the higher prevalence of involuntary bladder contractions and detrusor overactivity in older persons. Involuntary bladder contractions are found in 40% to 75% of older incontinent patients, but also in 5% to 10% of older continent women and in up to one-third of older men with no or minimal urinary symptoms. Detrusor overactivity has been associated with specific anatomical findings (protrusion junctions and ultra-close abutment of detrusor muscle cells) on bladder biopsy and with evidence of cortical changes, which suggests impaired integration of bladder afferent signals. While involuntary bladder contractions do not always result in urinary incontinence, when combined with impaired mobility, these contractions likely account for a substantial proportion of incontinence in older functionally disabled patients. Aging in women is also associated with a decline in bladder outlet and urethral resistance pressure. While prior childbirths (either via vaginal deliveries or Caesarean section) are associated with a greater risk of future incontinence, this association is weaker for women older than 65 years. Additionally, in older populations, poor vaginal support is more closely associated with obstructive urinary symptoms than with urinary leakage and urgency. Obesity, deconditioned muscles, and hysterectomy predispose women to future development of incontinence. White women are more likely, as a group, to have stress urinary incontinence than women of other racial or ethnic groups. Oral estrogen therapy has also been identified as a risk factor for subsequent development of urinary incontinence in women.

Older men with prostatic enlargement may have decreased urine flow rates and detrusor muscle instability. Aging is also associated with more frequent nocturia, which may in part be related to higher urine production at night. Many older men and women have detrusor hyperactivity combined with poor bladder contractility (which has been termed "*detrusor hyperactivity with impaired contractility*"). These individuals have evidence of widespread muscle degeneration on detrusor muscle biopsy.

Acute or Reversible Causes

The difference between acute (or reversible) forms of incontinence and persistent (or established) incontinence is clinically meaningful although not always distinct. *Acute incontinence* refers to those situations where the incontinence is of sudden onset, usually linked to an acute illness or an iatrogenic problem, and subsides once the illness or problem has been resolved. *Persistent incontinence* refers to incontinence that is not precipitated by an acute illness and endures over time. Reversible factors related to acute incontinence may also contribute to persistent incontinence.

The potentially reversible causes of urinary incontinence are outlined in **Table 47-3**. These causes include impaired ability (or reduced willingness) to reach a toilet, conditions that affect the lower urinary tract, such as an infection, atrophic vaginitis, or surgical procedure, conditions that cause or contribute to polyuria, and iatrogenic factors. Because of urinary frequency and urgency, many older persons, especially those limited in mobility, carefully arrange their schedules (and may even limit social activities) in order to be close to a toilet. Thus, an acute illness can precipitate incontinence by disrupting this delicate balance. Hospitalization, with its attendant environmental barriers (such as catheters, tubes, lines, and bedside rails), and the delirium and immobility that often accompany acute illnesses in older patients can contribute to acute incontinence. Acute incontinence in these situations is likely to resolve with resolution of the underlying acute illness. In a substantial proportion of patients, incontinence may persist for several weeks after hospitalization and should be further evaluated.

Constipation and resultant fecal impaction are common in both acutely and chronically ill older patients. Impaction may cause mechanical distension of the bladder and outlet impingement that can interfere with adequate bladder emptying and cause reflex bladder contractions. Relief of a fecal impaction and effective treatment of constipation can lead to resolution of urinary, as well as fecal, incontinence (see Chapter 87, Constipation).

An elevated PVR should be considered in any older patient who suddenly develops urinary incontinence. In addition to fecal impaction, causes of incontinence with a high PVR in an older patient include immobility; anticholinergic, narcotic, calcium channel blocking, and

TABLE 47-3 ■ REVERSIBLE CONDITIONS THAT CAUSE OR CONTRIBUTE TO URINARY INCONTINENCE IN OLDER PERSONS

CONDITION	MANAGEMENT
Conditions affecting the lower urinary tract	
Urinary tract infection (symptomatic with frequency, urgency, dysuria, etc.)	Antimicrobial therapy (not for asymptomatic bacteriuria)
Atrophic vaginitis/urethritis	Topical estrogen
Postprostatectomy (incontinence will often resolve during first year)	Exercise-based behavioral interventions; avoid further surgical therapy during first year until it is clear condition will not resolve
Stool impaction	Disimpaction; appropriate use of bulk-forming agents and laxatives if necessary; implement high fiber intake, adequate mobility, and fluid intake
Drug side effects (see **Table 47-4**)	Discontinue or change therapy if clinically appropriate. Dosage reduction or modification (eg, flexible scheduling of rapid-acting diuretics) may also help
Increased urine production	
Metabolic (hyperglycemia, hypercalcemia)	Better control of diabetes mellitus; therapy for hypercalcemia depends on underlying cause
Excess fluid intake	Reduction in intake of total fluids or diuretic fluids (eg, caffeinated or alcoholic beverages)
Volume overload	Diuretic therapy (may also increase risk of incontinence)
Venous insufficiency with edema	Peripheral compression stocking
	Leg elevation
	Sodium restriction
	Diuretic therapy (may also increase risk of incontinence)
Congestive heart failure	Medical therapy
Impaired ability or willingness to reach a toilet	Assistance and/or environmental modifications; prompted voiding, as appropriate
Delirium	Diagnosis and treatment of underlying cause(s) delirium (see Chapter 58)
Chronic illness, injury, or restraint that interferes with mobility	Regular toileting
	Use of toilet substitutes
	Environmental alterations (eg, bedside commode, urinal)
Psychological	Remove restraints if possible
	Appropriate pharmacologic and/or nonpharmacologic treatment

Reproduced with permission from Kane RL, Ouslander JG, Resnick B, et al. Essentials of Clinical Geriatrics, 8th ed. New York, NY: McGraw Hill; 2018.

beta-adrenergic medications (**Table 47-4**). In addition, urinary retention may be an acute manifestation of an underlying CNS process (eg, spinal cord compression or stroke).

Inflammation of the lower urinary tract may precipitate or exacerbate incontinence. Atrophic vaginitis and urethritis are common among older women (part of genitourinary syndrome of menopause), which can result in dysuria, urgency, frequency, and even incontinence (see Chapter 36, Gynecologic Disorders). Physical signs include patchy erythema and increased vascularity of the labia minora and vaginal epithelium, petechiae and friability, and urethral erythema often with an inflamed caruncle (dark or bright red epithelium usually at the inferior aspect of the urethra). Topical estrogen therapy may be helpful in older women with these findings (discussed further later in chapter). Acute urinary tract infection can precipitate or exacerbate incontinence. However, urine loss among older patients with *chronic* incontinence, especially frail nursing home residents, with otherwise asymptomatic bacteriuria (with or without pyuria) does not appear to improve with bacteriuria treatment. These patients, therefore, should not be treated with antibiotics because of the costs and risks unless the incontinence is new or acutely worsened.

Diuretics (especially rapid-acting loop diuretics) and conditions that cause polyuria, including hyperglycemia and hypercalcemia, can precipitate acute incontinence. Patients with volume-expanded states, such as those with congestive heart failure and lower extremity venous insufficiency, may have polyuria at night, which can contribute to nocturia and nocturnal incontinence. As is the case in many other conditions in geriatric patients, a wide variety of medications can play a role in the development of incontinence in older adults (see **Table 47-4**). When feasible, stopping the medication, switching to an alternative, or modifying the dosage schedule can be beneficial and may be the only necessary treatment for incontinence. In addition

TABLE 47-4 ■ MEDICATIONS THAT CAN POTENTIALLY AFFECT CONTINENCE

TYPE OF MEDICATION	POTENTIAL EFFECTS ON CONTINENCE
Diuretics	Polyuria, frequency, urgency
Anticholinergics	Urinary retention, overflow incontinence, stool impaction
Psychotropics	
Antidepressants	Anticholinergic actions, sedation
Antipsychotics	Anticholinergic actions, sedation, immobility
Sedative–hypnotics	Sedation, delirium, immobility, urethral relaxation
Narcotic analgesics	Urinary retention, fecal impaction, sedation, delirium
Alpha adrenergic blockers	Urethral relaxation
Alpha adrenergic agonists	Urinary retention
Cholinesterase inhibitors	Urinary frequency, urgency
Angiotensin-converting enzyme inhibitors	Cough precipitating stress incontinence
Beta adrenergic agonists	Rarely may contribute to urinary retention
Calcium channel blockers	May contribute to urinary retention, edema (nocturia)
Gabapentin, pregabalin, glitazones	Edema (nocturia)
Alcohol	Polyuria, frequency, urgency, sedation, delirium, immobility
Caffeine	Polyuria, bladder irritation

Reproduced with permission from Kane RL, Ouslander JG, Resnick B, et al. *Essentials of Clinical Geriatrics. 8th ed.* New York, NY: McGraw Hill; 2018.

to medications, drinking multiple caffeinated or alcoholic beverages can cause urinary frequency and urgency, which may precipitate incontinence.

Persistent Incontinence

Table 47-5 lists the clinical definitions and common causes of persistent urinary incontinence. These types can overlap with each other, and an individual patient may have more than one type simultaneously. Incontinence results from one or a combination of two basic abnormalities:

1. Failure to properly store urine, caused by a hyperactive or poorly compliant bladder or by diminished outflow resistance; and/or
2. Failure to properly empty the bladder, caused by a poorly contractile bladder or by increased outflow resistance.

Stress incontinence is common in older women, especially in ambulatory clinic settings. The symptoms of stress incontinence are very specific: leakage coincident with increases in intra-abdominal pressure caused by coughing, sneezing, laughing, or exercising. Stress incontinence may be infrequent and involve very small amounts of urine. It may need no specific treatment in women who are not bothered by it; on the other hand, it may be so severe and/or bothersome that it renders the person housebound. Among women, it is most often associated with weakened supporting tissues, resulting in hypermobility of the bladder outlet and urethra and caused by lack of estrogen, obesity, previous vaginal deliveries, and/or surgery. Some women, generally those who have had previous lower urinary tract surgery, have intrinsic urethral weakness with failure of the urethra to fully close and prevent urine loss. These patients tend to have severe incontinence and occasionally have constant wetting. Stress incontinence is unusual in men, and it mainly occurs following transurethral interventions for benign prostatic conditions or after surgical or radiation therapy for lower urinary tract malignancy when the anatomic sphincters are damaged.

Urgency incontinence can be caused by a variety of lower genitourinary and neurologic disorders (see **Table 47-5**). This type of incontinence is characterized by a sudden strong desire to void, accompanied by a fear of leakage, and followed by urine loss. The amount of urine lost can be large but varies depending on sphincter function and the ability of the patient to abort a bladder contraction. Urgency incontinence, when it occurs along with urinary urgency, daytime urinary frequency, and nocturia, has been called "*wet overactive bladder.*" Urgency incontinence is most often, but not always, associated with involuntary bladder contractions. Some patients have a poorly compliant bladder without involuntary contractions (eg, interstitial cystitis or following irradiation). A subgroup of older incontinent patients with detrusor hyperactivity also have impaired bladder contractility, emptying less than one-third of their bladder volume with involuntary contractions on urodynamic testing. These patients may be predisposed to significant urinary retention and may require training to learn to completely empty their bladder with voiding.

The use of the term "overflow incontinence" has come in and out of favor, but related terms such as *acute* or *chronic urinary retention* and (either stress or urge) *incontinence with a high PVR* are also common. *Acute retention of urine* is "a painful, palpable or percussable bladder, when the patient is unable to pass any urine"; and *chronic retention of urine* is where the patient has a "non-painful bladder, which remains palpable or percussable after the patient has passed urine. . . (and) the patient may be incontinent." A high PVR can result from anatomic or neurogenic obstruction to urinary outflow, a hypotonic or acontractile bladder, or both. Prostatic enlargement, diabetic neuropathic bladder, and urethral stricture commonly cause urinary symptoms and may occasionally cause incontinence. Low spinal cord injury and anatomic obstruction in women (caused by pelvic prolapse and urethral distortion) are less common causes of overflow incontinence in older patients. Several types of drugs also can contribute to this type of persistent incontinence (see **Table 47-4**). Some patients with lesions

TABLE 47-5 ■ BASIC TYPES AND CAUSES OF PERSISTENT URINARY INCONTINENCE

TYPE	DEFINITION	COMMON CAUSES
Stress	Involuntary loss of urine (usually small amounts) with increases in intra-abdominal pressure (eg, cough, laugh, exercise)	Weakness of pelvic floor musculature and urethral hypermobility Bladder outlet or urethral sphincter weakness Postprostatectomy sphincter weakness
Urgency	Leakage of urine (variable but often larger volumes) because of inability to delay voiding after sensation of bladder fullness is perceived	Detrusor hyperactivity, isolated or associated with one or more of the following: Local genitourinary condition such as tumors, stones, diverticuli, or outflow obstruction Central nervous system disorders such as stroke, dementia, parkinsonism, spinal cord injury, multiple sclerosis
Mixed (stress and urgency)	Combination of above	
Functional	Urinary accidents associated with inability to toilet because of impairment of cognitive and/or physical functioning, psychological unwillingness, or environmental barriers	Severe dementia and other neurological disorders Psychological factors such as depression and hostility
High postvoid residual (formerly referred to as "overflow")	Leakage of urine (usually small amounts) resulting from either mechanical forces on an overdistended bladder resulting in stress leakage or from other effects of urinary retention on bladder and sphincter function contributing to urge leakage	Anatomic obstruction by prostate, urethral stricture, severe cystocele Acontractile bladder associated with diabetes mellitus or spinal cord injury Neurogenic (detrusor–sphincter dyssynergy), associated with multiple sclerosis and other suprasacral spinal cord lesions Medication effect (see **Table 47-4**)

Reproduced with permission from Kane RL, Ouslander JG, Resnick B, et al. Essentials of Clinical Geriatrics. 8th ed. New York, NY: McGraw Hill; 2018.

rostral to the lumbosacral spinal cord lesions (such as multiple sclerosis) develop detrusor–sphincter dyssynergia and consequent urinary retention, which must be treated similarly to overflow incontinence; in some instances, a sphincterotomy is necessary.

Functional incontinence results when an older person is unable to reach a toilet on time due to impaired cognitive function and/or mobility. Recognizing and removing barriers to continence, such as inaccessible toilets and psychological disorders, is critical. These factors also exacerbate other types of persistent incontinence. Patients with functional factors contributing to incontinence also may have abnormalities of the lower genitourinary tract, most commonly detrusor overactivity. In some patients, it can be very difficult to determine whether the functional factors or the genitourinary factors predominate without a trial of specific types of treatment.

Many older patients have more than one type of incontinence. Most common are the combination of urgency and stress incontinence (often called *mixed incontinence*) among older women as well as the combination of urge and functional incontinence among nursing home residents.

In addition, many older patients have a syndrome of "*overactive bladder*," where urinary urgency is present sometimes with urinary symptoms such as frequency, and nocturia, and may or may not be continent. These patients

should be assessed and treated similar to patients with symptoms of urgency incontinence.

EVALUATION

Guidelines recommend a basic diagnostic evaluation, which includes a history (which can be enhanced by a bladder diary record), a physical examination, and a urinalysis. A PVR may not be needed in all older patients with incontinence, but reasonably should be done for patients at risk for urinary retention (see below). Other diagnostic studies may be indicated in selected patients (**Table 47-6**). **Figure 47-2** summarizes the recommended diagnostic evaluation of incontinent older patients.

The objectives of the basic evaluation are threefold:

1. To identify potentially reversible conditions potentially contributing to incontinence (see **Table 47-3**).
2. To identify conditions requiring further diagnostic tests and/or gynecologic or urologic referral.
3. To develop a management plan, which may include referral for further evaluation or a therapeutic trial of behavioral and/or pharmacologic therapy.

In patients with recent or sudden onset of incontinence (especially when following an acute medical

TABLE 47-6 ■ COMPONENTS OF THE DIAGNOSTIC EVALUATION OF PERSISTENT URINARY INCONTINENCE[a]

All Patients

Focused history (a bladder diary record may be helpful in some patients)

Targeted physical examination

Urinalysis

Postvoid residual determination[b]

Selected Patients

Laboratory studies

    Urine culture

    Urine cytology

    Blood glucose, calcium

    Renal function tests

Renal and/or bladder ultrasound

Gynecologic evaluation

Urologic evaluation

Cystourethroscopy

Urodynamic tests

    Simple

        Observation of voiding

        Standing cough test for stress incontinence

        Simple (single channel) cystometry

        Urine flowmetry (for men)

    Complex

        Multichannel cystometrogram

        Pressure-flow study

        Leak point pressure

        Urethral pressure profilometry

        Sphincter electromyography

        Videourodynamics

[a]See also Table 47-7.
[b]The recommendation for a postvoid residual determination in all incontinent elderly patients is controversial (see text).
Reproduced with permission from Kane RL, Ouslander JG, Resnick B, et al. Essentials of Clinical Geriatrics. 8th ed. New York, NY: McGraw Hill; 2018.

condition and/or hospitalization), the potentially reversible causes of acute incontinence (see **Table 47-3**) should be ruled out by a brief history, a physical examination, and basic laboratory studies including urinalysis, culture, and tests for serum glucose or calcium, if indicated.

The history should focus on characteristics of the incontinence, including current problems and medications, and on the impact of the incontinence on the patient and caregivers. The incontinence should be characterized in terms of frequency, amount, and timing of leakage; and symptoms of voiding difficulty including hesitancy, intermittent stream, and straining to void. Symptoms of urgency versus stress incontinence should be sought, recognizing that symptom history does not perfectly predict subtype of urinary incontinence. For those with nocturia, or nocturnal incontinence, questions regarding sedating medications and/or sleep dysfunction are indicated. Bladder

diary records, such as the one shown in **Figure 47-3**, can be helpful in characterizing symptoms, as well as in following the response to treatment. The physical examination includes abdominal, rectal, and genital examinations, as well as an evaluation of lumbosacral innervation. The abdominal examination is insensitive for an elevated PVR or chronic urinary retention, but gross bladder distention (eg, ≥ 500 mL) should be easily detected. In acute urinary retention, the distended bladder is a firm, midline mass that emanates from the pelvis and is dull to percussion. In gross distention with either acute or chronic retention, the superior margin of the bladder is often identifiable by either palpation or percussion.

The pelvic examination in women includes inspection for significant prolapse, signs of vaginal tissue inflammation, and a cough test to detect stress incontinence. The *cough stress test* can corroborate stress urinary incontinence (UI) symptoms and can be performed with the patient standing or in the lithotomy position. Sensitivity is highest when the patient is standing. The patient should have a comfortably full bladder at approximately half-capacity (200 mL) and is instructed to cough vigorously once (followed by three additional coughs, if negative). It is insensitive if the patient cannot cooperate, is inhibited, or the bladder volume is low. Leakage simultaneously with coughing documents stress incontinence; delayed leakage (eg, after 3 seconds) or the initiation of voiding generally indicates a cough-induced bladder contraction.

Special attention should be given to assessing mobility and mental status, because impairments may be either causing the incontinence or interacting with urologic and neurologic disorders to worsen the condition. Patients with nocturia or nocturnal incontinence should be examined for signs of congestive heart failure or venous insufficiency with edema.

Urinalysis should be performed to look for evidence of infection, hematuria, and glucosuria. Clean urine specimens are often difficult to obtain from frail incontinent patients, but can be performed reliably without first resorting to in-and-out catheterization. For men who cannot void spontaneously, a condom-type catheter can be used after cleaning the penis to collect a specimen that accurately reflects bladder urine. While there is a clear relationship between acute symptomatic urinary tract infection and incontinence, the relationship between asymptomatic bacteriuria and incontinence is controversial. In nursing home populations, there is no benefit to treating bacteriuria in patients with chronic, stable incontinence. For patients in other settings, it is difficult to make clear recommendations. For the initial evaluation of incontinence among noninstitutionalized incontinent patients, it is reasonable to initially eradicate the bacteriuria to observe the effect on the incontinence.

A determination of PVR should be performed in patients at risk for retention, including those with diabetes with neuropathy, neurologic disorders, symptoms of

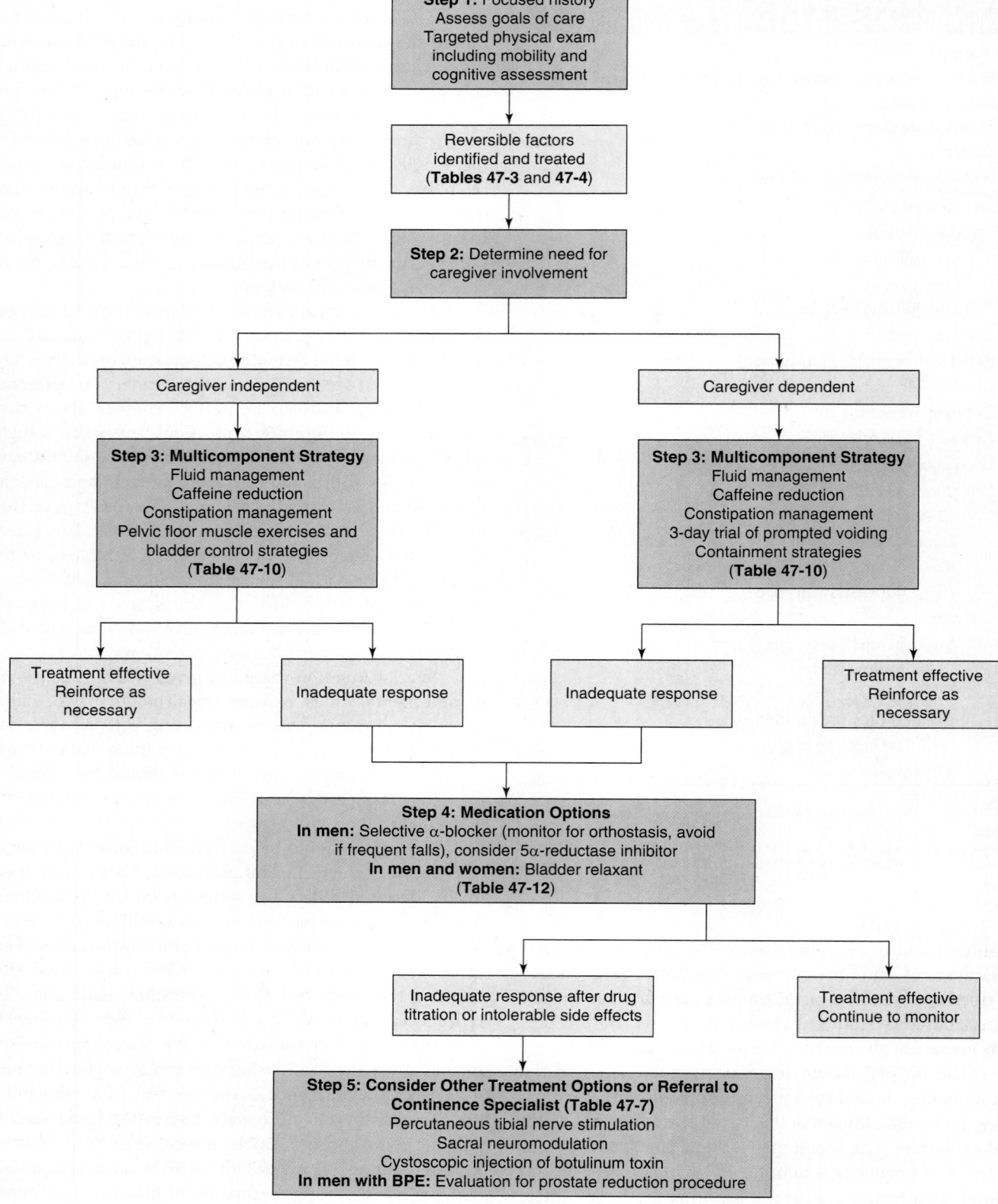

FIGURE 47-2. Summary of assessment and initial management of geriatric urinary incontinence. (See referenced tables and text for details.)

Your Daily Bladder Diary

This diary will help you and your health care team figure out the causes of your bladder control trouble. The "sample" line shows you how to use the diary.

Your name: _____

Date: _____

Time	Drinks		Trips to the Bathroom		Accidental Leaks	Did you feel a strong urge to go?	What were you doing at the time?
		What kind? How much?	*How many times?*	*How much urine? (circle one)*	*How much? (circle one)*	*Circle one*	*Sneezing, exercising having sex, lifting, etc*
Sample	Coffee	2 cups	✓✓	⊙ ○ ● sm med lg	○ ⊙ ● sm med lg	Yes (No)	Running
6-7 A.M.				○ ○ ●	○ ○ ●	Yes No	
7-8 A.M.				○ ○ ●	○ ○ ●	Yes No	
8-9 A.M.				○ ○ ●	○ ○ ●	Yes No	
9-10 A.M.				○ ○ ●	○ ○ ●	Yes No	
10-11 A.M.				○ ○ ●	○ ○ ●	Yes No	
11-12 noon				○ ○ ●	○ ○ ●	Yes No	

FIGURE 47-3. Example of a bladder record for ambulatory care settings. (Adapted with permission from Diagnosis of Bladder Control Problems (Urinary Incontinence). How do doctors find the cause of a bladder control problem? National Institute of Diabetes and Digestive and Kidney Diseases (NIDDK). National Institutes of Health.)

PART III

GERIATRIC CONDITIONS

voiding difficulty, or a history of urinary retention, and those taking medications with significant anticholinergic effects. Neither the history nor the physical examination is sensitive or specific enough for this purpose in geriatric patients. In these patients the PVR determination can be done by portable ultrasonography if equipment is available. To be accurate, the PVR determination should be done within a few minutes of a spontaneous continent or incontinent void. PVR values of less than 100 mL in the absence of straining to void generally reflect adequate bladder emptying in geriatric patients, whereas PVR values greater than 200 mL are abnormal. Values between 100 mL and 200 mL must be interpreted in the context of other patient symptoms. Noninvasive measurement of urinary flow rate in men may be helpful in identifying obstruction and/or bladder contractility problems.

Clinical practice guidelines do not recommend a complex urologic, gynecologic, or urodynamic evaluation for all incontinent older patients. Many patients can be treated with a trial of behavioral and/or drug therapy after a basic evaluation is completed and potentially reversible factors are addressed. **Table 47-7** lists examples of criteria for referring incontinent geriatric patients for further urologic, gynecologic, and/or urodynamic evaluations.

MANAGEMENT

Several therapeutic modalities are used in managing incontinent patients (**Table 47-8**). Special attention should be paid to the management of acute incontinence, which is common in older patients in acute care hospitals or nursing homes. Unfortunately, older incontinent patients may be managed in the acute hospital setting with indwelling catheterization. Rarely, this is justified by hemodynamic instability and the hourly need to assess urine output during the acute phase of an illness, yet often it is unnecessary. This practice poses a substantial and unwarranted risk of catheter-induced infection and interferes with mobility. Widespread use of quality indicators may reduce the frequency of these practices. Although time-consuming and more difficult, making toilets and toilet substitutes accessible and combining this accessibility with some form of scheduled toileting is a more appropriate approach. Indwelling catheters may be appropriate in the palliative setting at end of life. All the factors that can cause or contribute to a reversible form of incontinence (see **Table 47-3**) should be attended to in order to maximize the potential for regaining continence.

Management should be guided by the type of incontinence, and more importantly by patient and/or family

TABLE 47-7 ■ EXAMPLES OF CRITERIA FOR REFERRAL OF INCONTINENT GERIATRIC PATIENTS FOR FURTHER UROLOGIC, GYNECOLOGIC, OR URODYNAMIC EVALUATION

CRITERIA	DEFINITION	RATIONALE
History		
Recent history of lower urinary tract or pelvic surgery or irradiation	Surgery or irradiation involving the pelvic area or lower urinary tract within the past 6–12 months	A structural abnormality relating to the recent procedure should be sought
Recurrent symptomatic urinary tract infections	Two or more symptomatic episodes in a 12-month period	A structural abnormality or pathologic condition in the urinary tract predisposing to infection should be excluded
Physical Examination		
Marked pelvic prolapse	A prominent cystocele that descends the entire height of the vaginal vault with coughing during speculum examination	Anatomic abnormality may underlie the pathophysiology of the incontinence, and selected patients may benefit from surgical repair
Marked prostatic enlargement and/or suspicion of cancer	Gross enlargement of the prostate on digital examination; prominent induration or asymmetry of the lobes	An evaluation to exclude prostate cancer may be appropriate
Postvoid Residual		
Difficulty passing a 14-French straight catheter	Impossible catheter passage, or passage requiring considerable force or a large, rigid catheter	Anatomic blockage of the urethra or bladder neck may be present
Postvoid residual volume ≥ 200 mL	Volume of urine remaining in the bladder within a few minutes after the patient voids spontaneously in as normal a fashion as possible	Anatomic or neurogenic obstruction or poor bladder contractility may be present
Urinalysis		
Hematuria	Greater than or equal to 3 red blood cells per high-power field on microscopic examination in the absence of infection	A pathologic condition in the upper urinary tract, bladder, or urethra should be excluded
Therapeutic Trial		
Failure to respond to adequate trials of behavioral and/or pharmacologic therapy	Persistent symptoms that are bothersome to the patient after adequate trials of behavioral and/or drug therapy	Urodynamic evaluation may help guide specific therapy

Reproduced with permission from Kane RL, Ouslander JG, Resnick B, et al. Essentials of Clinical Geriatrics. 8th ed. New York, NY: McGraw Hill; 2018.

preferences. Patients should be carefully questioned about the degree of bother the incontinence is causing and how much risk and cost they are willing to undertake to address it. Supportive measures are critical in managing all forms of incontinence and should be used in conjunction with other, more specific treatment modalities. Education, environmental manipulations, appropriate use of toilet substitutes, avoidance of iatrogenic contributions to incontinence, modifications of diuretic and fluid intake patterns (especially caffeine), treatment of constipation, and good skin care are all important. Additionally, in women there is evidence that modest weight loss (approximately 5%–10% of body weight) leads to reduction in urinary incontinence episodes.

Specially designed incontinence undergarments and pads can be very helpful in many patients, but they must be used appropriately. Although they can be effective, several caveats should be raised:

1. Garments, external devices, and pads are a nonspecific treatment.

2. Many patients are curable if treated with specific therapies, and some have potentially serious factors underlying their incontinence that must be diagnosed and treated.

3. Patients often prefer more specific incontinence therapy designed to restore a normal pattern of voiding and continence.

4. Incontinence devices, garments, and pads are expensive and rarely covered by third-party payers.

To a large extent, the optimal treatment of persistent incontinence depends on identifying the type or types. **Table 47-9** outlines the primary treatments for the basic types of persistent incontinence in the geriatric population. Each treatment modality is briefly discussed below.

Behavioral Interventions

Many types of behavioral interventions are available for the management of urinary incontinence. These may be categorized as **patient dependent** (ie, require adequate

TABLE 47-8 ■ TREATMENT OPTIONS FOR URINARY INCONTINENCE IN OLDER ADULTS

Behavioral Interventions (see **Table 47-10**)

Patient-dependent
    Pelvic muscle exercises
    Bladder training
    Bladder retraining
    Adjunctive techniques
        Biofeedback
        Electrical stimulation
    Weight loss
Caregiver-dependent
    Scheduled toileting
    Habit training
    Prompted voiding

Drugs (see **Table 47-12**)

Bladder relaxants
Alpha agonists
Alpha antagonists
Topical estrogen

Surgery or Procedure Based

Bladder neck suspension (retropubic suspension or sling procedure)
Removal of obstruction or pathologic lesion
Sacral neuromodulation
Percutaneous tibial nerve stimulation
Periurethral injections
Botulinumtoxin A cystoscopic injections

Mechanical Devices

Urethral plugs (female only)
Artificial sphincters
External penile clamps

Nonspecific Supportive Measures

Education
Modifications of medication intake
Avoid caffeine and alcohol
Use of toilet substitutes
Environmental manipulations
Garments and pads

Catheters

External
Intermittent
Indwelling

Adapted with permission from Kane RL, Ouslander JG, Resnick B, et al. Essentials of Clinical Geriatrics. 8th ed. New York, NY: McGraw Hill; 2018.

TABLE 47-9 ■ PRIMARY TREATMENTS FOR DIFFERENT TYPES OF GERIATRIC URINARY INCONTINENCE

TYPE OF INCONTINENCE	PRIMARY TREATMENTS
Stress	Pelvic muscle (Kegel) exercises Other behavioral interventions Alpha adrenergic agonists (none are FDA indicated for such use in the United States) Periurethral injections Surgical bladder neck suspension
Urgency	Bladder training Bladder relaxants Topical estrogen (if atrophic vaginitis present) In men: Alpha antagonists
Functional	Behavioral interventions (caregiver dependent) Environmental manipulations Incontinence undergarments and pads
High postvoid residual	Surgical removal of obstruction Intermittent catheterization (if practical) Indwelling catheterization

Reproduced with permission from Kane RL, Ouslander JG, Resnick B, et al. Essentials of Clinical Geriatrics. 8th ed. New York, NY: McGraw Hill; 2018.

generally involve the patient's continuous, self-monitoring use of a bladder diary record such as the one depicted in **Figure 47-3**. In several studies, behavioral therapies are equivalent to drug therapy, with approximately three-fourths of patients reporting improvement. Frequently, these behavioral interventions are the preferred treatment modality by patients.

To be successful, patient-dependent interventions require a functional, motivated patient capable of learning and practice. These interventions also require a skilled, enthusiastic trainer and frequent patient contact, though positive results can be achieved by motivated patients who are self-directing their behavioral treatment following brief consultation with a provider or through assistance of a pamphlet or book. Pelvic floor muscle (Kegel) exercises are effective in men and women for the treatment of urge, stress, mixed stress–urge incontinence, and incontinence following prostatectomy. These exercises consist of repetitive contractions of the pelvic floor muscles. These exercises can be taught by brief verbal or written instructions, or instruction provided by having a patient squeeze the examiner's inserted finger during a vaginal or rectal examination (without doing a Valsalva maneuver, which is opposite of the intended effect). Once learned, the exercises should be practiced many times throughout the day (eg, three sets daily of 15 contractions building up from 3 seconds to 10 seconds in duration). Computer-assisted or manual biofeedback can be especially helpful for teaching patients who bear down (increasing intra-abdominal pressure) when attempting to contract pelvic floor muscles.

function and motivation of the patient), in which the goal is to restore a normal pattern of voiding and continence, or **caregiver dependent**, which can be used for functionally disabled patients, in which the goal is to keep the patient and the environment dry. **Table 47-10** summarizes these interventions. The patient-dependent interventions

TABLE 47-10 ■ EXAMPLES OF BEHAVIORAL INTERVENTIONS FOR URINARY INCONTINENCE

PROCEDURE	DEFINITION	TYPES OF INCONTINENCE	COMMENTS
Patient-Dependent			
Pelvic floor muscle (Kegel) exercises	Repetitive contraction and relaxation of pelvic floor muscles with use in everyday situations that precipitate leakage	Stress and urgency	Requires adequate function and motivation; biofeedback often helpful for teaching
Bladder training	Use of education, bladder records, pelvic muscle, and other behavioral techniques	Stress and urgency	Requires trained therapist, adequate cognitive and physical functioning, and motivation
Bladder retraining	Progressive lengthening or shortening of intervoiding interval, with intermittent catheterization used in patients recovering from overdistension injuries with persistent retention	Acute (eg, post-catheterization with urge or overflow, poststroke)	Goal is to restore normal pattern of voiding and continence; requires adequate cognitive and physical function and motivation
Caregiver-Dependent			
Scheduled toileting	Routine toileting at regular intervals (scheduled toileting)	Urgency and functional	Goal is to prevent wetting episodes; can be used in patients with impaired cognitive or physical functioning; requires staff or caregiver availability and motivation
Habit training	Variable toileting schedule based on patient's voiding patterns	Urgency and functional	Goal is to prevent wetting episodes; can be used in patients with impaired cognitive or physical functioning; requires staff or caregiver availability and motivation
Prompted voiding	Offer opportunity to toilet every 2 h during the day; toilet only on request; social reinforcement; routine offering of fluids	Urgency, stress, mixed, functional	Same as above; 25%–40% of nursing home residents respond well during the day and can be identified during a 3-d trial

Reproduced with permission from Kane RL, Ouslander JG, Resnick B, et al. Essentials of Clinical Geriatrics. 8th ed. New York, NY: McGraw Hill; 2018.

Biofeedback involves the use of bladder, rectal, or vaginal pressure or electrical activity recordings, or the examiner's finger in the vagina or rectum with a hand placed on the abdomen, to train patients to contract pelvic floor muscles while leaving the abdominal muscles relaxed. Electrical stimulation, introduced either vaginally or rectally, and magnetic stimulation have also been used to help identify and train muscles in the management of stress incontinence and inhibit involuntary bladder contractions in patients with urgency incontinence. The applicability of pelvic floor electrical or magnetic stimulation is limited because of equipment needs and that it may not be acceptable to many older patients in the United States.

Once these muscles are strengthened, and better muscle control is achieved, the patient must be taught to use the exercises in everyday life under circumstances that precipitate the incontinence in order to be effective. With practice, a pelvic floor muscle contraction can be done immediately prior to a cough, laugh, or sneeze to assist with stress incontinence; and used in rapid serial contractions to abort detrusor contractions associated with urinary

urgency. Pelvic floor muscle exercises are also effective in certain situations to prevent urinary incontinence and, if done preoperatively, allows a more rapid return to continence in the postoperative period.

Other forms of patient-dependent interventions include bladder training and bladder retraining. Bladder training involves the educational components taught during biofeedback, without the use of biofeedback equipment. Patients are taught pelvic muscle exercises and urge suppression strategies to manage urgency and are taught to use bladder diary records regularly. There is some evidence that these techniques are as effective as drug therapy in cognitively intact, motivated older adults. Bladder retraining as described here is used primarily after a period of temporary bladder catheterization. **Table 47-11** is an example of a bladder-retraining protocol. This protocol is applicable to patients who have had an indwelling catheter for monitoring of urinary output during a period of acute illness or for the treatment of urinary retention with overflow incontinence. Such catheters always should be removed as soon as possible, and this type of bladder-retraining

TABLE 47-11 ■ EXAMPLE OF A BLADDER-RETRAINING PROTOCOL

Objective: To restore a normal pattern of voiding and continence after the removal of an indwelling catheter.

1. Remove the indwelling catheter (clamping the catheter before removal is not necessary)
2. Treat urinary tract infection if present
3. Initiate a toileting schedule. Begin by toileting the patient:
   a. Upon awakening
   b. Every 2 h during the day and evening
   c. Before getting into bed
   d. Every 4 h at night
4. Monitor the patient's voiding and continence pattern with a record that allows for the recording of:
   a. Frequency, timing, and amount of continent voids
   b. Frequency, timing, and amount of incontinence episodes
   c. Fluid intake pattern
   d. Postvoid catheter volume
5. If the patient is having difficulty voiding (complete urinary retention or very low urine outputs, eg, ≤ 240 mL in an 8-h period while fluid intake is adequate):
   a. Perform bladder ultrasonography or in-and-out catheterization, recording volume obtained, every 6 to 8 h until residual values are ≤ 200 mL
   b. If the postvoid residual is > 300–400 mL, then catheterize with a Foley catheter and plan another voiding trial in a few days.
   c. Instruct the patient on techniques to trigger voiding (eg, running water, stroking inner thigh, suprapubic tapping) and to help completely empty the bladder (eg, bending forward, suprapubic pressure, double voiding).
   d. If the patient continues to have high residual volumes after 3 to 4 wk, consider urodynamic evaluation.
6. If the patient is voiding frequently (ie, more often than every 2 h):
   a. Perform postvoid residual determination to ensure the patient is completely emptying the bladder.
   b. Encourage the patient to delay voiding as long as possible and instruct the patient to use techniques to help completely empty bladder.
   c. If the patient continues to have frequency and nocturia, with or without urgency and incontinence:
      (1) Rule out other reversible causes (eg, urinary tract infection medication effects, hyperglycemia, and congestive heart failure).
      (2) Consider trial of bladder relaxant if postvoid residuals are low.

Reproduced with permission from Kane RL, Ouslander JG, Resnick B, et al. Essentials of Clinical Geriatrics. 8th ed. New York, NY: McGraw Hill; 2018.

protocol should enable most indwelling catheters to be removed from patients in acute care hospitals as well as some residents in long-term care settings. A patient who continues to have difficulty voiding after 1 to 2 weeks of such a bladder-retraining protocol should be examined for other potentially reversible causes of voiding difficulties. When difficulties persist, a urologic referral should be considered.

The goal of caregiver-dependent interventions such as scheduled toileting, habit training, and prompted voiding is to prevent incontinence episodes rather than to restore a normal pattern of voiding and complete continence. Highly motivated caregivers and cooperative patients are essential for these interventions to be successful. Scheduled toileting involves assisting the patient to the toilet at regular intervals, usually every 2 to 3 hours during the day regardless of the presence or absence of the patient's expressed desire to void. Habit training involves a schedule of toileting that is individually modified according to the patient's pattern of continent voids and incontinence episodes. *Prompted voiding* is a behavioral protocol that involves focusing the patient's attention on his or her bladder by asking if the patient is wet or dry, asking (prompting) the patient to attempt to void (up to three times) every 2 hours during the day, toileting the patient if he or she responds positively, giving praise as a social reward for attempting to toilet and maintaining continence, and offering fluids routinely. Between 25% and 40% of nursing home residents respond very well to daytime prompted voiding, and these responders can be identified by carrying out a 3-day trial of the intervention. Care for incontinence at night should be individualized. Routine incontinence care can be very disruptive to sleep. Because older people tend to awaken frequently at night, one way to individualize toileting in a long-term care setting is to check on the patient every hour or two, and only prompt to toilet when the patient is found awake.

Drug Treatment

Table 47-12 lists the drugs used to treat incontinence. In general, carefully selected older research participants have been able to achieve roughly equivalent efficacy from drug treatment compared to their younger counterparts. Drug treatment should generally be prescribed in conjunction with one or more behavioral interventions.

For urgency incontinence, drugs with bladder smooth-muscle relaxant properties are used and are available in two different classes: antimuscarinic (anticholinergic) and beta-3-agonist (noradrenergic). Antimuscarinic drugs are available in immediate release, controlled release, and topical preparations, while beta-3-agonist therapy is available in a once daily formulation. Most studies suggest a reduction of 60% to 70% in the frequency of incontinence episodes with drug therapy in selected older adults. While different drugs are likely equivalent on average, a particular patient who does not respond to one drug (either because of lack of efficacy or presence of adverse effects) may benefit from a trial on a different agent. Some patients may not respond for 2 weeks or even longer, so a 2- to 4-week trial should be undertaken when a new drug is prescribed.

TABLE 47-12 ■ DRUGS COMMONLY USED IN THE UNITED STATES TO TREAT URINARY INCONTINENCE

DRUGS	DOSAGES	MECHANISMS OF ACTION	POTENTIAL ADVERSE EFFECTS
Bladder Relaxants for Urgency Incontinence	In general, reduced dosages for renal and hepatic impairment		
Antimuscarinic		Increase bladder capacity; diminish involuntary bladder contractions	
Darifenacin (Enablex)	7.5–15 mg qd		Anticholinergic, lower dose if reduced hepatic function
Fesoterodine (Toviaz)	4–8 mg qd		Anticholinergic
Oxybutynin (Ditropan, immediate release, available as generic)	2.5–5.0 mg tid		Anticholinergic (dry mouth, blurry vision, elevated intraocular pressure, delirium, constipation)
Patch (Oxytrol)	3.9 mg qd Patch applied twice weekly		Above, but with less dry mouth, available over-the-counter
Oxybutynin gel (Gelnique)	3% pump or 10% gel packet One application daily		Above, but with less dry mouth
Solifenancin (Vesicare)	5–10 mg qd		Anticholinergic, lower for severe renal impairment or reduced hepatic function
Tolterodine (Detrol)	1–2 mg bid		Anticholinergic, lower dose for severe renal impairment or reduced hepatic function
Tolterodine (Detrol LA)	4 mg qd		Above, but with less dry mouth
Trospium chloride (Sanctura)	20 mg bid 20 mg once daily qhs with CrCl < 30 or in patients > 75 yo Give on an empty stomach > 1 h before a meal		Anticholinergic
Trospium chloride (Sanctura XR)	60 mg q am Give on an empty stomach > 1 h before a meal		Avoid in severe renal impairment or reduced hepatic function
Beta-3-agonist		Inhibits bladder contraction	
Mirabegron (Myrbetriq)	25–50 mg qd		Beta-3-agonist, max 25 mg/d with CrCl 15–20, reduced hepatic function (hypertension, tachycardia)
Vibegron (Gemtesa)	75 mg qd		Beta-3-agonist, avoid in severe renal or hepatic impairment; headache
Vaginal Estrogen[a]		Strengthen periurethral tissues and reduces inflammation from atrophic vaginitis	Contraindicated in women with a personal history of gynecologic cancer, relative contraindication in women with a personal history breast cancer
Topical	0.5–1.0 g per application		
Vaginal ring (Estring) (estradiol acetate)	One ring every 3 mo		
Drugs for Stress Incontinence[b]		Increase urethral smooth-muscle contraction	

(Continued)

TABLE 47-12 ■ DRUGS COMMONLY USED IN THE UNITED STATES TO TREAT URINARY INCONTINENCE (*CONTINUED*)

DRUGS	DOSAGES	MECHANISMS OF ACTION	POTENTIAL ADVERSE EFFECTS
Pseudoephedrine[c] (Sudafed)	30–60 mg tid		Headache, tachycardia, elevation of blood pressure
Duloxetine (Cymbalta)	30–60 mg daily		Nausea, xerostomia, headache
Drugs for Overactive Bladder Symptoms including Urgency UI in Men[d]		Relax smooth muscle of urethra and prostatic capsule	
Alpha adrenergic antagonist			
Doxazosin (available as generic, or Cardura)	1–8 mg qhs		Postural hypotension, dizziness, lowers blood pressure
Terazosin (available as generic, or Hytrin)	1–10 mg qhs		Same as above
Prazosin (Minipress)	1–2 mg tid		Same as above
Alfuzosin (Uroxatral)	10 mg qhs		Less effects on blood pressure
Silodosin (Rapaflo)	4–8 mg qd		Less effects on blood pressure; CrCl 30–50 use 4 mg qd
Tamsulosin (Flomax)	0.4–0.8 mg qd		Less effects on blood pressure (when used at 0.8 mg dose, greater blood pressure effects)
Phosphodiesterase Inhibitors		Inhibits PDE type 5, enhancing effects of nitric oxide–activated increases in cGMP	
Tadalafil	5 mg daily		Orthostatic hypotension, flushing, headache (contraindicated with terazosin/doxazosin/prazosin)
Other phosphodiesterase inhibitors given daily may be effective			
5-Alpha Reductase Inhibitor		Inhibits type II 5-alpha reductase, interfering with conversion of testosterone to 5-alpha-dihydrotestosterone	
Finasteride	5 mg daily		Sexual dysfunction, gynecomastia, decreased overall risk of prostate cancer with increased risk of high-grade prostate cancer
Dutasteride	0.5 mg daily	Inhibits type I and II 5-alpha reductase, inhibiting conversion of testosterone to dihydrotestosterone	Sexual dysfunction, decreased overall risk of prostate cancer with increased risk of high-grade prostate cancer

[a]For urgency UI associated with atrophic vaginitis.
[b]The primary initial treatment for stress UI is behavioral, with consideration of surgery for severe stress UI; there are no FDA-approved medications for stress UI.
[c]Contraindicated in patients with hypertension and cardiovascular disease.
[d]Can be used in combination with bladder relaxants.
Adapted with permission from Kane RL, Ouslander JG, Resnick B, et al. Essentials of Clinical Geriatrics. 8th ed. New York, NY: McGraw Hill; 2018.

Antimuscarinic drugs may have recognizable, bothersome systemic anticholinergic side effects such as dry mouth and constipation, which are most common with immediate-release formulations. They should be used carefully in patients with glaucoma and severe gastroesophageal reflux. Patients with Alzheimer disease and other forms of dementia must be followed for the development of drug-induced delirium when placed on antimuscarinic medications because of their anticholinergic effects. While the short-term cognitive effects of these agents are well understood, multiple epidemiologic studies suggest bladder antimuscarinic drug therapy (dose intensity, duration) is associated with a 50% relative increase in the odds of developing dementia. The results of these studies do not, however, preclude a treatment trial in the older adult population in the context of shared decision making. Beta-3-agonists could potentially lead to elevated blood pressure and should be not be used in persons with uncontrolled hypertension. Bladder relaxants may rarely precipitate urinary retention in some patients; men with some degree of outflow obstruction, diabetic patients, and patients with impaired bladder contractility are at the highest risk and should be followed carefully.

For older men with overactive bladder symptoms (with or without urinary incontinence), alpha adrenergic antagonists may be a better choice for first-line drug therapy. Bladder relaxants may also be used as single drug therapy in men, and the combination of a bladder relaxant and an alpha antagonist combined with pelvic floor muscle exercise-based behavioral therapy may be more effective in many older men.

Drug treatment for stress incontinence is less efficacious than is drug treatment for urgency incontinence, and no drug is approved for this indication in the United States. Duloxetine, a drug approved for depression in the United States, also has alpha adrenergic effects on the lower urinary tract through a spinal cord mechanism, and is recommended in other countries only as second-line therapy for the treatment of stress incontinence for those who prefer medication to surgical treatment. More recent studies have shown, for either opposed or unopposed oral conjugated estrogen therapy, an increased risk of developing or worsening of incontinence. Topical estrogen either chronically or on an intermittent basis (ie, 1- to 2-month course) may be effective for the treatment of irritative voiding symptoms and urgency incontinence in women with atrophic vaginitis and urethritis. Although no specific topical treatment regimen has been shown to be more effective than others, therapy usually involves 0.5 to 1 g of vaginal cream nightly for 1 to 2 weeks and then a maintenance dose two or three times per week or a controlled, slow-release vaginal ring. Several months of therapy are often necessary to observe therapeutic benefit.

Many older women have a combination of both urgency and stress incontinence or mixed incontinence. Treatment of mixed incontinence should initially target the symptoms the individual finds most bothersome.

Drug treatment in the setting of chronic urinary retention or urinary incontinence with high PVR, with either a cholinergic agonist or an alpha-adrenergic antagonist, is usually not efficacious. Although alpha-adrenergic blockers and 5-alpha reductase inhibitors are useful for treatment of symptoms suggestive of benign prostatic hyperplasia, they may not obviate the need for surgical intervention or requirement for catheter drainage in patients with bladder outlet obstruction who have chronic urinary retention or urinary incontinence with high PVRs (ie, residuals consistently greater than 200–300 mL).

Surgical Approaches

Surgery is a well-established treatment for stress urinary incontinence. Surgery should be considered for older women with stress incontinence and for women with a significant degree of pelvic prolapse associated with stress incontinence or incontinence with urinary retention who are unresponsive to nonsurgical treatment. As with many other surgical procedures, patient selection and the experience of the surgeon are critical to success. Any woman being considered for surgical therapy should have a thorough evaluation, before undergoing the procedure. Urodynamics are not necessarily required for stress incontinence or stress-predominant mixed incontinence without voiding difficulties. In general, surgical treatment is designed to correct urethral closure problems and to remedy defects in support of the urethra–vesicular angle. Mid-urethral slings with a synthetic mesh or the use of periurethral collagen injections are outpatient procedures. A pubovaginal sling using autologous fascia and bladder neck suspension using the Burch culposuspension procedure also have high rates of initial success, although subjective treatment outcomes are strongest with the mid-urethral sling. Additional long-term studies are needed.

Men with stress urinary incontinence (and usually with continuous urinary leakage) can be treated with the implantation of an artificial urinary sphincter (or other similar mechanical device designed to reversibly block urine outflow in the penile urethra). Newer "sling" procedures have been used in men, also.

While procedural approaches have previously been considered only for stress incontinence, there are also approaches for the treatment of refractory urgency incontinence. Approaches include neuromodulation and botulinum toxin A injection. Percutaneous tibial nerve stimulation (PTNS) is a minimally invasive procedure, which provides electrical stimulation using a small needle electrode placed in proximity to the posterior tibial nerve as it travels near the medial malleolus of the tibia. Patients undergo weekly 30-minute stimulation sessions in an outpatient clinical setting for up to 12 weeks. PTNS is generally well tolerated with minimal discomfort and has demonstrated effectiveness in adults without underlying neurogenic bladder. Sacral neuromodulation involves a two-stage operation with general anaesthesia and implantation of a pacemaker-like generator near the hip and sacral leads to stimulate the pudendal and sacral nerves. The procedure can be a safe, effective, and durable treatment, though cure rates for older adults and those with multiple medical comorbidities have been lower than in younger, healthier populations. The use of botulinum toxin A for refractory urgency incontinence has proven effective in several randomized, double-blinded, controlled studies, and is approved by the US Food and Drug Administration. Botulinum toxin A is accomplished via cystoscopy under direct visualization with injections into multiple bladder sites. Benefit is believed to be because of an effect on both efferent and afferent pathways, and early trial results suggest that the therapy lasts 6 months and is equally effective in older and younger age groups.

Surgery may be indicated in men in whom incontinence is associated with outflow obstruction. Men may have either chronic urinary retention, or acute urinary retention that is *precipitated* (use of an anticholinergic drug, recent instrumentation, or alpha agonist drug) or *spontaneous*. Those who have had complete acute urinary retention requiring mechanical drainage, and particularly those with *spontaneous* retention, are likely to have another episode within a short period of time and should be evaluated for a prostatic resection, as should men with incontinence associated with enough residual urine to be causing recurrent symptomatic infections or hydronephrosis. In men who do not meet these criteria, the decision should be based on weighing carefully the degree to which the symptoms bother the patient, the potential benefits of surgery (obstructive symptoms often respond better than irritative symptoms), and the risks of surgery (which may be minimal with newer prostate resection techniques).

MECHANICAL DEVICES, UNDERGARMENTS, CATHETERS, AND OTHER SUPPORTS

Three basic types of catheters and catheterization procedures are used for the management of urinary incontinence: external catheters, intermittent straight ("in-and-out") catheterization, and chronic indwelling catheterization. External catheters for men generally consist of some type of condom or adhesive connecting the penis to a drainage system. Improvements in design and observance of proper procedure and skin care when applying the catheter decrease the risk of skin irritation, as well as the frequency with which the catheter falls off. Existing data suggest that patients with condom catheters are at increased risk of developing symptomatic infection compared to incontinent adults depending upon absorbent pads or diapers. External catheters should be used only to manage intractable incontinence in male patients who do not have urinary retention and who are extremely physically dependent or pursuing a palliative approach to care. An external catheter that fits over the urethra for use in female patients is available commercially, but presently is not widely used.

Intermittent catheterization can help in the management of patients with urinary retention and overflow incontinence. The procedure can be carried out by either the patient or a caregiver and involves straight catheterization two to four or more times daily, depending on residual urine volumes. The goal is to keep residual urine volume generally less than approximately 300 to 400 mL. In the home setting, the catheter should be kept clean (but not necessarily sterile). Studies conducted largely among younger paraplegic patients show that this technique is practical and reduces the risk of symptomatic infection compared with the risk associated with chronic catheterization. The technique may be especially useful following removal of an indwelling catheter in a bladder-retraining protocol (see **Table 47-11**). However, older nursing home residents, especially men, may be difficult to catheterize. Anatomic abnormalities commonly found in the lower urinary tracts of older adults may increase the risk of infection because of repeated straight catheterizations. In addition, using this technique in an institutional setting, which may have an abundance of organisms relatively resistant to many commonly used antimicrobial agents, may yield an unacceptable risk of nosocomial infections. Using sterile catheter trays for these procedures would be very expensive. Thus, it may be extremely difficult to implement such a program in a typical nursing home setting.

Chronic indwelling bladder catheterization has higher risks than other forms of management, and should be sparingly used and only as indicated. On occasion, experts may recommend suprapubic catheters over urethral catheters for chronic use. Chronic bladder catheterization over months to years, has been shown to increase the incidence of chronic bacteriuria, bladder stones, periurethral abscesses (urethral catheters), urethral injury including penile erosion (urethral catheters), and even bladder cancer. Older nursing home residents managed with chronic indwelling bladder catheters frequently are at a higher risk of developing symptomatic infections. The limited evidence available to date does not suggest that routine changing of indwelling bladder catheters is warranted, though this is a common practice. Given these risks, it seems appropriate to recommend that the use of chronic indwelling bladder catheters be limited to certain specific situations (**Table 47-13**). When indwelling catheterization is used, certain principles of catheter care should be observed in an attempt to minimize complications (**Table 47-14**). In situations where there is reduced urinary output, increased leakage around

TABLE 47-13 ■ INDICATIONS FOR CHRONIC INDWELLING CATHETER USE

Urinary retention that
    Is causing persistent overflow incontinence, symptomatic infections, or renal dysfunction
    Cannot be corrected surgically or medically
    Cannot be managed practically with intermittent catheterization

Skin wounds, pressure sores, or irritations where incontinent urine contributes to excessive moisture and results in poor healing.

Care of terminally ill or severely impaired for whom bed and clothing changes are uncomfortable or disruptive

Patient preference

TABLE 47-14 ■ KEY PRINCIPLES OF CHRONIC INDWELLING CATHETER CARE

SUMMARY OF MAJOR RECOMMENDATIONS

Category I. Strongly Recommended for Adoption

Educate personnel in correct techniques of catheter insertion and care

Catheterize only when necessary

Emphasize hand washing

Insert catheter using clean technique is an acceptable and more practical alternative to sterile technique

Secure catheter properly

Maintain closed sterile drainage

Obtain urine samples aseptically

Maintain unobstructed urine flow

Category II. Moderately Recommended for Adoption

Periodically re-educate personnel in catheter care

Avoid irrigation unless needed to prevent or relieve obstruction

Refrain from daily meatal care with povidone–iodine solution as this may result in an increased infection rate

Replace the catheter and collecting system using aseptic technique and sterile equipment when the sterile closed drainage has been violated

Category III. Weakly Recommended for Adoption

Consider alternative techniques of urinary drainage before using an indwelling urethral catheter

Use smallest suitable bore catheter

Do not change catheters at arbitrary fixed intervals

Data from Gould CV, Umscheid CA, Agarwal RK, et al. Guideline for prevention of catheter-associated urinary tract infections 2009. Infect Control Hosp Epidemiol. 2010;31(4):319–326.

the catheter, or increased pain, it is important to perform an abdominal and genital examination to make certain the catheter is in the bladder and not obstructed. In these situations, it is often necessary to replace the catheter.

In men with post-prostatectomy urinary incontinence who are not a candidate for or do not desire surgical therapy, an external penile clamp for compression of the urethra may be a useful adjunctive therapy. Patients must be able to remember, monitor, and physically be able to remove the clamp every 2 hours. Some women with urinary incontinence and pelvic prolapse may respond well to use of a vaginal pessary, which is a device to slow the progression of prolapse by adding support to the vagina and increasing tightness of the tissues and muscles of the pelvis. Pessaries are made of rubber, plastic, or silicone, and come in a variety of types. Often patients need to be individually fitted with the device.

There are a variety of available absorbent products and undergarments that can help patients contain leakage, including disposable inserts, reusable and single-use adult diapers, and disposable underwear. Additionally, there are pads that can protect beds and/or chairs. Criteria for success of these devices revolve around fit, odor control, cost, and ability to hold urine. More frequent changing of pads

is expensive and inconvenient, but frequently helps control odor. Less frequent changing leaves skin wetter and likely more vulnerable to friction and abrasion.

In general, older adults want general information on urinary incontinence and sources of help. There are multiple consumer advocacy groups for those with incontinence that are dedicated to improving the lives of patients with urinary incontinence, for example, the National Association for Continence (www.nafc.org), and the Simon Foundation (www.simonfoundation.org) in the United States, that provide educational materials, reviews of available products, and links to researchers and manufacturers who provide incontinence materials.

FECAL INCONTINENCE

Fecal incontinence is less common than urinary incontinence. Its occurrence is relatively unusual in older patients who are continent of urine. Thirty to fifty percent of older patients in institutional settings with frequent urinary incontinence, however, also have episodes of fecal incontinence. This coexistence suggests common pathophysiologic mechanisms.

Defecation, like urination, is a physiologic process that involves smooth and striated muscles, central and peripheral innervation, coordination of reflex responses, mental awareness, and physical ability to get to a toilet. Disruption of any of these factors can lead to fecal incontinence.

The most common causes of fecal incontinence are problems with constipation and laxative use, neurologic disorders, and colorectal disorders (**Table 47-15**). In patients who are fed by enteral tubes, hyperosmotic feedings can precipitate diarrhea and fecal incontinence. Diluting the feedings or using slow continuous infusion is sometimes helpful. Constipation is extremely common in older persons and, when chronic, can lead to fecal impaction and incontinence. Hard stool in a fecal impaction irritates the rectum and results in the production of mucus and fluid.

TABLE 47-15 ■ CAUSES OF FECAL INCONTINENCE

Fecal impaction

Constipation

Laxative overuse or abuse

Hyperosmotic enteral feedings

Neurologic disorders
  Dementia
  Stroke
  Spinal cord disease

Colorectal disorders
  Diarrheal illnesses
  Diabetic autonomic neuropathy
  Rectal sphincter damage

Reproduced with permission from Kane RL, Ouslander JG, Resnick B, et al. Essentials of Clinical Geriatrics. 8th ed. New York, NY: McGraw Hill; 2018.

This fluid leaks around the mass of impacted stool and precipitates incontinence. Constipation is difficult to define; technically, it indicates fewer than three bowel movements per week, although many patients use the term to describe difficult passage of hard stools or a feeling of incomplete evacuation. Poor dietary and toilet habits, immobility, and chronic laxative abuse are the most common causes of constipation in older persons. Appropriate management of constipation prevents fecal impaction and resulting fecal incontinence. The management of constipation is discussed thoroughly in Chapter 87.

Fecal incontinence is sometimes amenable to biofeedback therapy. For those patients with end-stage dementia, a program of alternating constipating agents (if necessary) and laxatives in a routine schedule (such as giving regular osmotic laxatives as weekly enemas) may be effective in controlling defecation in many patients with fecal incontinence. Functionally dependent patients should be toileted regularly after a meal to take advantage of, or possibly regain, the gastrocolic reflex. Experience suggests that these measures should permit management of even severely cognitively impaired patients. As a last resort, specially designed incontinence undergarments are sometimes helpful in managing fecal incontinence and preventing skin irritation and other complications.

FURTHER READING

Brown JS, Vittinghoff E, Wyman JF, et al. Urinary incontinence: does it increase risk for falls and fractures? Study of Osteoporotic Fractures Research Group. *J Am Geriatr Soc.* 2000;48:721–725.

Burgio KL, Kraus SR, Johnson TM II, et al. Combined behavioral and two-drug therapy for lower urinary tract symptoms in men: the COBALT randomized clinical trial. *JAMA Intern Med.* 2020;180:411–419.

Burgio KL, Locher JL, Goode PS, et al. Behavioral versus drug treatment for urge urinary incontinence in older women: a randomized controlled trial. *JAMA.* 1998;280: 1995–2000.

Coupland CAC, Hill T, Dening T, et al. Anticholinergic drug exposure and the risk of dementia: a nested case-control study. *JAMA Intern Med.* 2019; 179: 1084–1093.

Fowler CJ, Griffiths DJ. A decade of functional brain imaging applied to bladder control. *Neurourol Urodyn.* 2010;29:49–55.

Gibson W, Johnson T II, Kirschner-Hermanns R, et al. Incontinence in frail elderly persons: report from the 6th International Consultation on Incontinence. *Neurourol Urodyn.* 2021;40(1):38–54.

Goode PS, Burgio KL, Locher JL, et al. Effect of behavioral training with or without pelvic floor electrical stimulation on stress incontinence in women: a randomized controlled trial. *JAMA.* 2003;290:345–352.

Guralnick ML, Fritel X, Tarcan T, et al. ICS Educational Module: Cough stress test in the evaluation of female urinary incontinence: introducing the ICS-Uniform Cough Stress Test. *Neurourol Urodyn.* 2018;37:1849–1855.

Hendrix SL, Cochrane BB, Nygaard IE, et al. Effects of estrogen with and without progestin on urinary incontinence. *JAMA.* 2005;293:935–948.

Kane RL, Ouslander JG, Resnick B, Malone ML. *Essentials of Clinical Geriatrics.* 8th ed. New York, NY: McGraw-Hill; 2018.

Lightner DJ, Gomelsky A, Souter L, Vasavada SP. Diagnosis and treatment of overactive bladder (non-neurogenic) in adults: AUA/SUFU Guideline. *J Urol.* 2019;202:558–563.

McVary KT, Roehrborn CG, Avins AL, et al. Update on AUA guideline on the management of benign prostatic hyperplasia. *J Urol.* 2011;185(5):1793–1803.

NICE treatment guidelines (NG 123) for Urinary Incontinence and pelvic organ prolapse in women. www.nice. org.uk/guidance/ng123. Last updated 24 June 2019. Accessed January 31, 2021.

Ouslander JG. Management of overactive bladder. *N Engl J Med.* 2004;350:786–799.

Subak LL, Wing R, West DS, et al. Weight loss to treat urinary incontinence in overweight and obese women. *N Engl J Med.* 2009;360:481–490.

Thom DH. Variation in estimates of urinary incontinence prevalence in the community: effects of differences in definition, population characteristics, and study type. *J Am Geriatr Soc.* 1998;46:473–480.

Vaughan CP, Markland AD. Urinary incontinence in women. *Ann Intern Med.* 2020;172:ITC17–ITC32.

Elder Mistreatment

Mark S. Lachs, Tony Rosen

DEFINITIONS

In the broadest context, *elder mistreatment* subsumes a variety of activities perpetrated upon an older person by others. There is as yet no universally agreed definition or classification of elder mistreatment. Proposed strategies for defining or classifying elder mistreatment have included using the type of abuse (eg, physical vs verbal abuse), motive (eg, intentional vs unintentional neglect), perpetrator relationship (eg, family vs paid caregiver), and setting (eg, community vs nursing home). Nonetheless, the clinician attempting to care for a victimized older person or to understand the spectrum of elder mistreatment will encounter several thematically similar definitions. For example, the Older Americans Act of 1975 defines elder abuse as "the willful infliction of pain, injury, or mental anguish." This definition has been adopted, and/or modified, by many state protective service agencies that investigate cases of abuse. An encompassing definition created by a 2002 expert panel convened by the National Academy of Sciences added the concept that elder mistreatment involves *a trusting relationship between an older person and another individual in which that trust is violated in some way*. The definition that likely best captures current understanding of elder mistreatment is that developed for the 2014 Elder Justice Roadmap, a report prepared by a large, multidisciplinary team of stakeholders inside and outside the US government:

- Physical, sexual, or psychological abuse, as well as neglect, abandonment, and financial exploitation of an older person by another person or entity
- That occurs in any setting (eg, home, community, or facility)
- Either in a relationship where there is an expectation of trust and/or when an older person is targeted based on age or disability

Table 48-1 lists representative examples of types of elder mistreatment. Whatever definition is employed, a consistent and important feature of elder mistreatment, and other forms of family violence, is that multiple types of mistreatment, such as physical and verbal abuse, neglect, and financial exploitation frequently coexist in the same abuser-victim dyad.

Learning Objectives

- Elder mistreatment, including physical abuse, sexual abuse, neglect, financial exploitation, psychological abuse, and abandonment, is common and may have serious medical and social consequences.
- Elder mistreatment is significantly underrecognized by clinicians and underreported to the authorities.

Key Clinical Point

1. Though researchers have described potential risk factors and are working to identify forensic markers associated with elder mistreatment, a high index of clinical suspicion in all encounters with geriatric patients and routine screening are currently the best tools physicians have to identify this often subtle geriatric syndrome.

Virtually all experts, clinicians, and reasonable laypersons will agree that egregious instances of physical violence such as punching, hitting, slapping, or assaulting an older person with a gun or other weapon are elder abuse. The most contentious definitional (and clinical) area relates to elder neglect, because the term neglect immediately implies that a caregiving obligation—such as providing food, medicines, or care—has not been met. This, in turn, raises difficult questions that must, with clinical judgment and experience, be considered in the context of the older adult's environment. For example, what are reasonable community standards for the frequency of bathing an assaultive spouse with Alzheimer disease? Does that standard change if the designated caregiver also suffers from chronic diseases that preclude perfect hygiene for their impaired family member? What if this inadequate care enables the "victim" to live at home long after other families would have considered nursing home placement?

TABLE 48-1 ■ REPRESENTATIVE DEFINITIONS OF ELDER MISTREATMENT

MISTREATMENT CATEGORY	DEFINITION	EXAMPLES
Physical abuse	Acts of violence that may result in pain, injury, impairment, or disease	• Pushing, striking, slapping, force-feeding • Incorrect positioning • Improper use of restraints or medications • Sexual coercion or assault
Neglect	The failure to provide the goods or services necessary for optimal functioning or to avoid harm	• Withholding of health maintenance care • Failure to provide physical aids such as eyeglasses, hearing aids, false teeth • Failure to provide safety precautions
Financial or material abuse	The misuse of the older person's income or resources for the financial or personal gain of a caretaker or advisor	• Denying the older person a home • Stealing money or possessions • Coercing the older person into signing contracts
Psychological, emotional, or verbal abuse	Conduct that causes mental anguish	• Verbal berating, harassment, or intimidation • Threats of punishment or deprivation • Treating the older person like an infant • Isolating the older person from others
Abandonment	The desertion of an older person by an individual who has assumed responsibility for providing care for the older adult or by a person with physical custody	
Violation of a trusting relationship	Meant to encompass all forms of abuse in that all forms involve the older person relying on and trusting another party, who through acts of omission or commission, violates that trust, without regard to intent	

Data from Aravanis SC, Adelman RD, Breckman R, et al. Diagnostic and treatment guidelines on elder abuse and neglect. Arch Fam Med. 1993;2(4):371–388.

Who exactly is the responsible caretaker, especially when multiple adult children are available to assume that role, but only one has "stepped up" because of birth order or some other arbitrary circumstance? And is it fair to label that adult child an "elder neglector" when caregiving becomes physically or psychologically impossible?

These difficult questions also highlight the fact that clinicians caring for elder abuse victims often find themselves working closely with alleged perpetrators of abuse and neglect, as these individuals are often the primary caregivers.

Another challenge in conceptualizing and defining elder mistreatment is how to include adults who have been victims of family violence chronically during their adult lives. Do these victims become elder mistreatment sufferers after they reach an arbitrary age cutoff or if they become functionally dependent or suffer cognitive decline?

EPIDEMIOLOGY

However it is defined, elder mistreatment is common. Recent prevalence studies, conducted in different countries, suggest that as many as 10% of community-dwelling older adults suffer from abuse, neglect, or exploitation each year. Multiple smaller studies suggest that nearly 50% of dementia sufferers are victims of mistreatment by caregivers. Psychological/emotional abuse (4.6%–13%), financial mistreatment (3.5%–6.6%), and neglect (5.1%–5.4%) are most commonly reported, with physical mistreatment (0.2%–2.1%) and sexual abuse (0.3%–0.6%) reported less frequently.

Unfortunately, despite its frequency, research suggests that as few as 1 in 24 cases of elder mistreatment is identified by the authorities. Victims may be unable to report abuse due to isolation, severe illness, or dementia, or may be reluctant to report due to fear of reprisal, guilt, desire to protect the abuser, cultural beliefs, or fear of institutionalization. Many older adults who suffer from abuse endure it for years before having it discovered. For others, it may not be until after they have died that their morbidity and early death are considered to be due to abuse. Both of these scenarios lead to delays in identification and intervention.

Much research has focused on identifying risk factors for elder mistreatment perpetrators and victims, with inconsistent results (**Table 48-2**). The most consistent findings relate to the relationship of the abuser to victim; most studies report that spouses and adult children are the most common perpetrators. Studies also show that when adult children are the abusers, sons and daughters are often equally implicated. At least one study found daughters to be the more common abuser. These findings must be viewed cautiously in that women are far more likely to be the de

TABLE 48-2 ■ POSSIBLE RISK FACTORS FOR ELDER MISTREATMENT

FACTOR	MECHANISM
Victim's poor health and functional disability	Disability reduces the older person's ability to seek help and/or defend self.
Cognitive impairment	Aggression toward caregiver and disruptive behaviors resulting from dementia precipitate abuse. Higher rates of abuse have been found among patients with dementia.
Abuser deviance	Abusers are likely to abuse alcohol or drugs and to have serious mental illness, which, in turn, leads to abusive behavior.
Abuser dependency	Abusers are very likely to depend on the victim financially, for housing, and in other areas. Abuse results from relative's (especially adult children's) attempts to obtain resources from the older person.
Living arrangement	Abuse is much less likely among older persons living alone. A shared living situation provides greater opportunities for tension and conflict that generally precede abusive incidents.
External stress	Stressful life events and chronic financial strain decrease the family's resistance and increase likelihood of abuse.
Social isolation	Older adults with fewer social contacts are more likely to be victims. Isolation reduces the likelihood that abuse will be detected and stopped. In addition, social support can buffer against the impact of stress.
History of violence	Particularly among spouses, prior history of violence in the relationship may be predictive of elder abuse in later life.

Reproduced with permission from Lachs MS, Pillemer K. Abuse and neglect of elderly persons. N Engl J Med. 1995;332(7):437–443.

facto or designated care providers to frail older adults and are, therefore, more "at risk" for being accused of mistreatment should caregiving fall short of any arbitrary standard.

Studies suggest that women represent two-thirds of elder mistreatment victims. Also, in cultures where women have inferior social status, older women are at high risk of neglect through abandonment when they are widowed, and their property is seized. While current research suggests that older adults with lower socioeconomic status are at greater risk for mistreatment, studies evaluating race and ethnicity have been contradictory. A particularly contentious area has been spawned by the "dependency theory" of mistreatment, which holds that mistreatment occurs when the victim becomes inordinately dependent on the caregiver for a variety of medical and nonmedical needs. Again, studies show an inconsistent relationship between functional disability in an older adult and elder mistreatment. In fact, a more consistent finding in the literature is the converse—the perpetrator is often dependent on the older adult victim for financial support and housing. Characteristically, an adult child unable to achieve independence is reliant on the older person for these needs.

Inconsistencies in findings from risk factor research may be related to the heterogeneous nature of elder mistreatment cases. Older adult protective services workers and clinicians experienced in elder mistreatment know that the term elder mistreatment subsumes many situations—abusive spousal relationships that have "aged," caregivers to dementia patients who lash out in frustration, and physically abusive adult children with poorly managed mental health or substance abuse problems are but a few examples. Epidemiologic studies that attempt to discern risk factors without acknowledging this reality probably are measuring an "average" effect, thus possibly missing important sets of risk factors among subgroups of abused or neglected older populations.

Whatever risk factors are identified in previous and future research should not foster a complacency wherein an absence or paucity of such factors causes the clinician to lower his or her guard. Elder mistreatment crosses all ethnic and socioeconomic boundaries. A high index of clinical suspicion is critical for identification.

PATHOPHYSIOLOGY

Theories of elder mistreatment abound; three deserve detailed discussion here, because they may have clinical relevance with regard to the types of interventions contemplated in confirmed cases of mistreatment. The most commonly cited theory contends that family violence is a learned behavior; abused children grow up to potentially abuse not only their children, but also perhaps spouses and their parents. This is sometimes referred to as the transgenerational violence theory of mistreatment.

The dependency theory of mistreatment holds that abuse is fostered by situations in which victims have a degree of functional and/or cognitive disability that results in activities of daily living impairment and overwhelming care needs. Closely associated with this paradigm is another theory—that of the "stressed caregiver."

The psychopathology of the abuser theory shifts focus away from the victim and argues that elder mistreatment is firmly rooted in mental health problems of the abuser. Examples include personality disorders, poorly or undertreated schizophrenia, alcoholism, and other substance abuse problems.

Discerning the underlying causes of elder mistreatment is essential in fashioning an intervention plan (see "Management" later in this chapter).

PRESENTATION

For a variety of reasons, the identification of elder mistreatment is one of the most difficult clinical challenges in geriatric medicine. First, many highly prevalent chronic diseases in older adults may have clinical manifestations that mimic abuse. If elder abuse is present, the clinician may ascribe those findings to chronic disease rather than family violence. Conversely, the clinician may erroneously attribute findings from another disease to elder mistreatment. Second, the setting in which an elder mistreatment evaluation occurs is often quite challenging. The assessment may be hurried (eg, the emergency department is the often-chaotic environment where acute injuries are evaluated). The presence of the suspected abuser only adds pressure to what is already likely to be a stressful encounter. The perpetrator, and also the victim, may have incentives to actively conceal the mistreatment from the clinician. Lastly, the competent identification and management of mistreatment may create significant additional work and propel the clinician into a world that he or she is likely to be unfamiliar with—a world that includes mandatory reporting statutes, adult protective service workers, and a criminal justice system with a vocabulary that is foreign to many medical professionals. Given these educational, emotional, and systemic obstacles, it is not surprising that elder mistreatment often is missed or unreported in the context of "customary care." In fact, research suggests that only 1.4% of cases reported to Adult Protective Services (APS) come from physicians, and, in a survey of APS workers, of 17 occupational groups, physicians were among the least helpful in reporting abuse.

Elder abuse forensics is a recent area of intense and growing focus. Of particular interest has been whether there are diagnostic and/or clinical signs and symptoms of abuse presentations, either during life or at autopsy, that are highly specific for elder mistreatment, as have been identified in child abuse (eg, shaken baby syndrome and bucket-handle metaphyseal fracture). Researchers have begun to search for physical injury patterns associated with abuse. Research has shown that physical abuse and assault-related injuries most commonly occur on the head/face, neck, and upper extremities. One study showed that, in comparison to other older adults, victims of physical abuse have bruises that are more often large (> 5 cm) and more commonly on the face, lateral right arm, or posterior torso. Physical abuse victims are much more likely than older adults presenting to the emergency department after a fall to have injuries to the left cheek/zygoma, neck, or ears. Additionally, physical elder abuse victims are more likely to have maxillofacial/dental/neck injuries combined with no injuries or their upper or lower extremity injuries. Medical and laboratory markers potentially suggestive of elder mistreatment have been suggested by experts, including malnutrition, dehydration, alterations in status of chronic illness, hypothermia/hyperthermia, rhabdomyolysis, and toxicologic findings, but these have not yet been systematically evaluated.

Until rigorous research identifies reliable forensic markers, clinicians need to consider elder mistreatment in the differential diagnosis of many or most of the clinical presentations they encounter. Fractures may result from osteoporosis or force or both. Depression may be related to neurotransmitter imbalances or a hopeless abusive environment. Malnutrition may be the result of any number of chronic illnesses inexorably worsening, or from the withholding of sustenance.

Dramatic injuries or neglect pose no particular diagnostic challenge. Fractures, burns, contusions, and lacerations, in concert with a credible history, immediately lead to the diagnosis. At the other extreme, subtle presentations that mimic chronic disease are highly challenging. Examples include chronic diseases that frequently decompensate despite a care plan and adequate resources (eg, repeated emergency department visits for congestive heart failure or chronic obstructive pulmonary disease exacerbation). Indeed, because elder mistreatment can be defined so broadly, there are very few presenting signs or symptoms in the geriatric patient for which elder mistreatment is not in the differential diagnosis.

Many instruments have been devised for the screening or evaluation of elder mistreatment, but they are not applicable to all settings. The Elder Abuse Suspicion Index (EASI) is a short screening instrument that has been validated for cognitively intact patients in a primary setting with a sensitivity of 0.47 and a specificity of 0.75. The EASI (**Figure 48-1**) is a tool to identify older adults at risk of mistreatment and includes five questions for the patient and one for the physician, with more than or equal to one "yes" response suggesting further assessment is needed.

All screening instruments may assist the clinician by serving as "checklists" to ensure a thorough evaluation. **Table 48-3** suggests a system-by-system approach. The importance of heightened awareness cannot be overemphasized in considering the diagnosis. Frequently, clues about potential mistreatment come from ancillary staff members (eg, office reception staff) or home care nurses who observe the abuser-victim dyad away from the health care provider. A general sense that something is amiss in the patient's environment such as caustic interaction between parties, poor hygiene or dress, frequently missed medical appointments, or failure to adhere with a clearly designated treatment strategy can all be important clues.

The patient and the alleged perpetrator should be interviewed separately and alone. Although there is an

Questions 1 through 5 are answered by the patient. Question 6 is answered by the physician.

1. Have you relied on people for any of the following: bathing, dressing, shopping, banking, or meals?

2. Has anyone prevented you from getting food, clothes, medication, glasses, hearing aids, or medical care or from being with people you wanted to be with?

3. Have you been upset because someone talked to you in a way that made you feel shamed or threatened?

4. Has anyone tried to force you to sign papers or to use your money against your will?

5. Has anyone made you afraid, touched you in ways that you did not want, or hurt you physically?

6. Doctor: Elder abuse may be associated with findings such as poor eye contact, withdrawn nature, malnourishment, hygiene issues, cuts, bruises, inappropriate clothing, or medication compliance issues. Did you notice any of these today or in the last 12 months?

The patient can answer "yes," "no," or "unsure." A response of "yes" on one or more of questions 2 through 6 should prompt concern for abuse or neglect.

FIGURE 48-1. Elder Abuse Suspicion Index (EASI). (Reproduced with permission from Yaffe MJ, Wolfson C, Lithwick M, et al. Development and validation of a tool to improve physician identification of elder abuse: the Elder Abuse Suspicion Index (EASI). *J Elder Abuse Negl.* 2008;20[3]:276–300.)

emerging consensus that patients of all ages should be routinely screened for family violence, an optimal strategy or instrument has not emerged. Patients should be asked candidly and calmly about the etiology of any unexplained injuries or other findings. Often patients are at first unwilling to speak candidly about being an elder abuse victim for reasons of embarrassment, shame, or fear of retribution from the perpetrator who is frequently a caregiver.

Interview of the suspected abuser is a tricky and potentially dangerous undertaking. On the one extreme, elder abusers who are presented with an empathetic, nonjudgmental ear to describe their stresses and actions will sometimes describe their situations at great length and in great detail. On the other hand, all forms of domestic abuse share a pattern wherein abusers gain and control access to their victims. An elder abuser graphically confronted with allegations of mistreatment may move to sequester a frail victim in such a way that a frail isolated older adult loses access to critically needed medical and social services. Whenever possible, assistance from providers skilled in elder abuse evaluation and management should be enlisted to assist in such undertakings.

MANAGEMENT

Elder abuse and neglect are morbid and mortal. Mistreatment is associated with adverse health outcomes for victims, including significant increases in emergency department usage, hospitalization, dementia, depression, and nursing home placement. Also, research has shown that mistreatment victims have a threefold risk of death compared to nonabused controls. Thus, intervention is critical.

Unfortunately, there are no randomized trials of reasonable quality addressing interventions for elder mistreatment. The clinician confronted with a confirmed case of elder abuse is best served by a resourceful approach that combines experience, clinical judgment, and local resources. One developing trend is large interdisciplinary groups who convene regularly to discuss cases of mistreatment, not only for the purpose of planning intervention, but also to consider case-by-case forensics, cross train disciplines, and provide general support to one another in this difficult field. However, there is no evidence-based evaluation of this strategy.

Whatever the approach to intervention, a dogmatic or algorithmic strategy to address all elder mistreatment cases is likely misguided. A rigid, inflexible approach ignores the enormous heterogeneity of the entity, including the type(s) of mistreatment being concurrently perpetrated, the underlying mechanisms, patient comorbidities, caregiver burden issues, and the available resources (both familial and community) that can be brought to bear on the issue. A more sensible approach may be the multipronged strategy increasingly used to treat other geriatric syndromes that have multifactorial etiologies. The paradigm may be a useful one in that elder mistreatment can be likened to geriatric syndromes. That is, there may be multiple "host" and environmental contributors; decompensation may be accelerated by other medical and social problems; and some of the contributors may be more remediable than others. The elder physical abuse victim with severe chronic obstructive pulmonary disease and an abusive schizophrenic child-caregiver will need an entirely different series of interventions than the spouse with progressive dementia who has suffered lifelong domestic violence that is now worsening.

The first step in confronting any confirmed case of family violence is ensuring the safety of the victim. First, the immediate threat of danger to the victim should be ascertained. Even if there is no immediate threat, a *safety plan* is critical in the management of all forms of family

TABLE 48-3 ■ CLINICAL MANIFESTATIONS OF POTENTIAL MISTREATMENT WITH RECOMMENDED ASSESSMENT

TARGET	ASSESSMENT
History from older adult	Interview patient alone; directly inquire regarding physical violence, restraint use, or neglect; ascertain precise details about nature, frequency, and severity of events
	Assess functional status (amount of dependence with activities of daily living [ADLs])
	Determine who the designated caregiver is if ADLs disability is present
History from abuser	Potential abuser should also be interviewed alone; this interview is best done by professionals with experience in this area; avoid confrontation in the information-gathering phase; interview other sources if possible
	Assess recent psychosocial factors (eg, bereavement, financial stresses)
	Ascertain caregiver understanding of patient's illness (eg, care needs, prognosis, etc)
	Elicit caregiver's explanations for injuries or physical findings
Behavioral observation	Withdrawal
	Infantalizing of patient by caregiver
	Caregiver who insists on providing the history
General appearance	Hygiene
	Cleanliness and appropriateness of dress
Skin/mucous membranes	Skin turgor, other signs of dehydration; multiple skin lesions in various stages of evolution
	Bruises, decubiti; evidence of care for established skin lesions
Head and neck	Traumatic alopecia (distinguishable from male pattern alopecia on the basis of distribution)
	Scalp hematomas
	Lacerations, abrasions
Trunk	Bruises, welts; shape may suggest implement (eg, iron/belt)
Genitourinary	Rectal bleeding
	Vaginal bleeding
	Decubiti, infestations
Extremities	Wrists or ankle lesions suggest restraint use or immersion burn (stocking/glove distribution)
Musculoskeletal	Examine for occult fracture, pain; observe gait
Neurologic/psychiatric	Thorough evaluation to assess focality of neurologic deficits
	Depressive symptoms, anxiety
Mental status	Formal mental status testing (eg, Mini Mental State Examination); cognitive impairment suggests delirium or dementia and plays a role in assessing decision-making capacity
	Psychiatric symptoms including delusions and hallucinations
Imaging	As indicated from the clinical evaluation
Laboratory	As indicated from the clinical evaluation (drug levels)
	Albumin, blood urea nitrogen, and creatinine toxicology
Social and financial resources	Determine whether there are other members of social network available to assist the older person with financial resources
	These resources are crucial in considering interventions that include alternate-living arrangements and home services

Reproduced with permission from Lachs MS, Pillemer K. Abuse and neglect of elderly persons. N Engl J Med. 1995;332(7):437–443.

violence (**Table 48-4**). What are the specific steps the victim should take if the perpetrator of mistreatment becomes acutely violent? Options include calling the local police department, accessing shelters, emergency department use/hospital admission, or respite care in some evolved systems of long-term care. Additionally, in most states, cases of elder abuse must be reported to adult protective services agencies. This typically results in a home visit to adjudicate the veracity of such a report. State protective service agencies vary widely with respect to their caseloads and

available resources; ideally a coordinated approach that brings to bear their expertise and resources in collaboration with the physician and multidisciplinary team produces the best response.

The safety plan paradigm will have limited utility in many cases of elder mistreatment, however, because of victim frailty and/or cognitive impairment that limits the use of self-protective behaviors. Frequently, clinicians find themselves in the predicament of caring for an elder mistreatment victim who lacks capacity. In these cases, the

TABLE 48-4 ■ SAFETY PLAN FOR VICTIMS OF ELDER MISTREATMENT OR OTHER VICTIMS OF FAMILY VIOLENCE WITH CAPACITY WHO INSIST ON REMAINING IN AN ABUSIVE ENVIRONMENT

TIME FRAME	ACTIVITY
Prior to violent or abusive episode	Recognize patterns that lead to abusive behavior (eg, abuser alcohol use).
	Determine who in the social network is available to assist when such an episode occurs through explicit conversations with neighbors, friends, other relatives.
	Be aware of elder domestic violence programs, shelters, and other resources in the local community available to assist; know their contact numbers.
	Have essential resources readily available if the patient needs to leave quickly (eg, money, ATM cards, credit cards, driver's license, keys, identification, Social Security card, other important documents).
	Practice implementing safety plan (eg, mock 911 call). Consider creating a "code" with a friend or neighbor so that the patient can communicate danger in the presence of the abuser.
During violent or abusive episode	Implement safety plan quickly and with discretion.
	Consider appeasing abuser briefly (if this does not cause a danger) so that safety plan may be implemented.
	Use of self-protective behaviors such as a weapon should be considered with utmost caution.
After violent or abusive episode	Recognize that family violence is a chronic problem that usually recurs and escalates.
	Change locks as soon as possible.
	Strongly consider order of protection.
	Let neighbors and landlord know that abusive individual no longer lives in the home.

likely intervention will involve the appointment of a guardian in collaboration with adult protective service agencies or other elder social service programs in the community that serve such functions. In such a proceeding, the clinician's role is to provide objective evidence that documents the lack of decision-making capacity. The clinician may also have a role in ensuring the alleged perpetrator of mistreatment does not become the guardian.

One of the most frustrating situations for professionals working with victims of family violence is the individual who retains decision-making capacity and insists on remaining in an abusive environment. Here the clinician's role is to educate the patient about the tendency of family violence to escalate and to review the safety plan created. The clinician should also explain to the patient that even if services are refused, the physician remains an important and available resource, should the situation change.

In general, the physician who suspects elder abuse would do well to employ the same creative strategies he or she uses to manage a variety of clinical problems in older adults. There may be local social services agencies in the community who provide an array of services such as meals on wheels or friendly visit. These services could represent a new resource for the patient, but also additional "eyes and ears" to ascertain what the home situation is like. A local adult day care referral might also enable a more detailed ongoing evaluation of a client while decompressing a stressful caregiving situation. A financial management program for the patient with cognitive impairment can shed light on the possibility of financial exploitation. The physician need not diagnose elder abuse while these useful services are being proffered.

Physicians should strive to provide trauma-informed care to potential elder abuse and neglect victims. This involves recognizing and being sensitive to the deep impact of stressful and traumatic experiences on a patient's physical and mental health. Elder abuse or neglect, which may occur every day for years, may cause depression, anxiety, or post-traumatic stress disorder, as may other life experiences. Practicing trauma-informed care involves maximizing a victim's choice and control and trying to minimize re-traumatization through treatment. Delivering trauma-informed care includes specific strategies: emphasizing the intention to maintain a patient's privacy and confidentiality, asking permission before touching a potential victim, limiting how much a victim has to talk about the mistreatment, and avoiding words such as violence/abuse/neglect/mistreatment/criminal behavior if the victim does not initially conceive of what has occurred in this way. Physicians should also use a trauma-informed approach when treating cognitively impaired patients, as they may also be profoundly impacted by current or previous traumatic exposures.

SPECIAL SITUATIONS

Elder mistreatment may also occur in institutional settings. The physician and nurse have roles in detecting these cases as well. Substantial regulatory safeguards have been progressively enacted since the 1970s to protect residents of long-term care facilities. These safeguards include mandatory criminal background checks of all employees, ombudsman programs to adjudicate complaints of mistreatment, and components of the Omnibus Budget Reconciliation Act of 1987, which includes residents' rights provisions (eg, minimization of restraints). In some contexts, the failure to create or follow a reasonable plan of care for the long-term care residents may be viewed as abusive or neglectful.

While the focus of elder abuse in long-term care has been on staff abuse of residents, this is probably far less common than previously when regulatory scrutiny was lacking. Recently, resident on resident abuse has been identified as a far more common and pervasive problem among nursing home residents. This includes verbal, physical, and sexual mistreatment. Although there are no prevalence data on the phenomenon, preliminary and indirect evidence suggests that it is highly prevalent. For example, more than 50% of nursing aides in long-term care report the personal experience of being physically hit by a resident in the previous year, typically in the course of providing direct care. Given that the prevalence of dementia and associated behavioral disturbance in long-term care facilities is high, it stands to reason that behavior of this type occurs frequently between residents.

Another recent area of interest has been abuse and neglect that occurs in long-term care environments other than nursing homes (eg, assisted living and board and care environments), because these facilities generally are under considerably less regulation. Interest in mistreatment in assisted-living facilities has also grown in recent years as much sicker patients begin to inhabit these institutions; many believe the higher acuity and generally lower levels of staff and supervision are a dangerous admixture in which abuse and neglect are more likely to occur. Data are lacking on the prevalence of abuse, or on the type of abusers, in these settings.

Physicians and other care providers have an important role in the detection of these institutional cases, because they may see potential manifestations of nursing home elder mistreatment in facilities or emergency departments as part of providing customary care. Physicians who suspect institutional abuse have an obligation to immediately report their suspicions to the long-term care ombudsman in their state.

SUMMARY

Elder mistreatment is a prevalent problem with many potential manifestations. The epidemiology of injuries and other clinical findings is not completely understood, but this does not preclude the clinician from taking an active role in its detection and management. Studies show elder mistreatment victims to be at substantial independent risk of death and quality-of-life decline. The syndrome should be afforded the same vigilance that health care providers devote to other "traditional" medical problems in geriatrics.

FURTHER READING

Acierno R, Hernandez MA, Amstadter AB, et al. Prevalence and correlates of emotional, physical, sexual, and financial abuse and potential neglect in the United States: the National Elder Mistreatment Study. *Am J Public Health.* 2010;100:292–297.

Bonnie J, Wallace RB, eds. *Elder Mistreatment: Abuse, Neglect, and Exploitation in an Aging America.* Washington, DC: National Academy of Sciences Press; 2003.

Dong XQ. Elder abuse: systematic review and implications for practice. *J Am Geriatr Soc.* 2015;63(6):1214–1238.

Lachs MS, Pillemer KA. Elder abuse. *Lancet.* 2004;304: 1236–1272.

Lachs MS, Pillemer KA. Elder abuse. *N Engl J Med.* 2015; 373(20):1947–1956.

Lachs MS, Teresi JA, Ramirez M, et al. The prevalence of resident-to-resident elder mistreatment in nursing homes. *Ann Intern Med.* 2016;165(4):229–236.

Lachs MS, Williams C, O'Brien S, et al. Risk factors for reported elder abuse and neglect: a nine-year observational study. *Gerontologist.* 1997;37:469–474.

Lachs MS, Williams CS, O'Brien S, et al. The mortality of elder mistreatment. *JAMA.* 1998;280:428–432.

Laumann EO, Leitsch SA, Waite LJ. Elder mistreatment in the United States: prevalence estimates from a nationally representative study. *J Gerontol B Psychol Sci Soc Sci.* 2008;63(4):S248–S250.

Mosqueda L, Burnight K, Gironda MW, Moore AA, Robinson J, Olsen B. The abuse intervention model: a pragmatic approach to intervention for elder mistreatment. *J Am Geriatr Soc.* 2016;64(9):1879–1883.

National Center for Elder Abuse. *The Elder Justice Roadmap: A Stakeholder Initiative to Respond to an Emerging Health, Justice, Financial, and Social Crisis.* https://www.justice.gov/file/852856/download. Accessed June 3, 2021.

Pillemer K, Burnes D, Riffin C, Lachs MS. Elder abuse: global situation, risk factors, and prevention strategies. *Gerontologist.* 2016;56(Suppl 2):S194–205.

Pillemer K, Finkelhor D. The prevalence of elder abuse: a random sample survey. *Gerontologist.* 1988;28:51–57.

Rosen T, LoFaso VM, Bloemen EM, et al. Identifying injury patterns associated with physical elder abuse: analysis of legally adjudicated cases. *Ann Emerg Med.* 2020;76(3):266–276.

Rosen T, Pillemer K, Lachs M. Resident-to-resident aggression in long-term care facilities: an understudied problem. *Aggress Violent Behav.* 2008;13(2):77–87.

Under the Radar: New York State Elder Abuse Prevalence Study: Self-Reported Prevalence and Documented Case Surveys 2012. https://ocfs.ny.gov/main/reports/Under%20the%20Radar%2005%2012%2011%20final%20report.pdf. Accessed June 3, 2021.

Wiglesworth A, Austin R, Corona M, et al. Bruising as a marker of physical elder abuse. *J Am Geriatr Soc.* 2009; 57(7):1191–1196.

Wiglesworth A, Mosqueda L, Burnight K, et al. Findings from an elder abuse forensic center. *Gerontologist.* 2006; 46:277–283.

Yaffe MJ, Wolfson C, Lithwick M, Weiss D. Development and validation of a tool to improve physician identification of elder abuse: the Elder Abuse Suspicion Index (EASI). *J Elder Abuse Negl.* 2008;20:276–300.

Chapter 49

Muscle Aging and Sarcopenia

Alfonso J. Cruz-Jentoft

INTRODUCTION

Age-related losses of muscle mass and strength are common and can lead to sarcopenia, a condition typically consisting of a combination of loss of strength, physical function, and muscle mass. This chapter will cover concepts related to the process of muscle aging as well as the current status of sarcopenia detection, evaluation, and management.

The human body is made up of more than 600 skeletal muscles, accounting for around 40% of the total body mass. Excluding water, muscles are composed of about 80% protein, or about 50% of total body protein. The main functions of skeletal muscle are mobility and regulation of proteins. Adults tend to lose muscle mass at a rate of about 8% per decade after age 40. At age 70, an adult will have lost a mean of 24% of the muscle mass present at age 30. The rate of muscle mass loss accelerates and almost doubles after age 70. It is essential to note that adults lose muscle strength much faster; about 3% to 4% per year after age 50. Strength loss renders older persons vulnerable to physical disability.

MOTOR UNITS AND THEIR REGULATION

The basic functional unit of skeletal muscles is the motor unit. Each motor unit consists of a neuron, its axon, and the muscle fibers innervated by that neuron. The neuron terminal is connected to the muscle fiber through the neuromuscular junction, where neurons release neurotransmitters that bind to muscle cells receptors. A single motor neuron may innervate from a few to thousands of muscle fibers, depending on the muscle, with neurons responsible for higher force production innervating a higher number of fibers. Human muscles harbor three types of muscle fibers: type I, type IIa, and type IIx (formerly named IIb). Type I

Learning Objectives

- Summarize age-related changes in the skeletal muscle and motor units.
- Appraise the evolving concept of sarcopenia and the characteristics of the different definitions proposed in the past two decades.
- Use muscle mass and function to diagnose sarcopenia in clinical practice.
- Develop a treatment plan for sarcopenic patients.

Key Clinical Points

1. Muscle aging involves anatomical and physiological changes in motor units and their regulation.
2. Sarcopenia is a progressive and generalized disease involving the accelerated loss of muscle mass and function. The concept of sarcopenia has evolved from low muscle mass alone to include muscle function.
3. Around 10% of the older persons living in the community suffer from sarcopenia, with a higher prevalence in other clinical settings.
4. Measures of muscle mass, muscle strength, and physical performance are used to diagnose sarcopenia in clinical practice.
5. Treatment of sarcopenia requires resistance exercise. Nutrition may have a role. No drugs are yet available for this condition.

TABLE 49-1 ■ CHARACTERISTICS OF MUSCLE FIBERS

	TYPE I	TYPE IIA	TYPE IIX
Contraction speed	Slow	Fast	Very fast
Diameter	Small	Intermediate	Large
Fatigue resistance	High	Intermediate	Slow
Contractile force	Low	High	Very high
ATP activity	Low	High	High
Energy	Aerobic	Combined	Anaerobic

fibers (slow-twitch) are well adapted to perform aerobic exercise and are highly resistant to fatigue, having high oxidative capacity and a low capacity to generate adenosine triphosphate (ATP). Type IIx fibers (fast-twitch) contract several times faster but fatigue rapidly, adapted to brief, intense contractions (as in weight lifting) and have a high ATP-generating capacity and low glycolytic capacity. Type IIa fibers (also fast-twitch) are also fast but are fatigue-resistant (**Table 49-1**). Muscle myofibrils are made of two main contractile proteins actin and myosin, with a double helix structure, regulated by troponin and tropomyosin.

The nervous system regulates recruitment of motor units to carry out movements by generating action potentials in the motor cortex of the brain, that propagate down to the neuromuscular junction, triggering contraction of muscle fibers in a highly energy dependent process. The motor cortex is regulated by many other brain regions.

MUSCLE AGING

Age-related changes have been described at all levels of the motor unit. With increasing age the number of muscle fibers is reduced, reflected in a loss of almost one-third of muscle mass in late life. This loss seems to be faster in type II than in type I muscle fibers. Compared to younger adults, more than one-third of motor neurons are typically lost in older adults. By age 70, the number of motor units is reduced about 40% compared with the number found in 25-year-olds. Continued loss with age after age 70 can lead to nonagenarians having only one-third of the number of motor units of young persons, even in apparently healthy aging. Apoptosis of motor neurons with denervation of the innervated muscle fibers leads to muscle weakness. This process has been associated with sarcopenia. An adaptive response to motor neuron loss is motor unit remodeling in a denervation-innervation cycle, where the same nerve fiber reinnervates larger bundles of muscle fibers to counteract neuron loss (**Figure 49-1**). This process preferentially involves fast fibers, which may gradually become slower and thus reduce muscle force and muscle power (the ability to use full force in a given period of time).

The firing capacity of motor units is also reduced with age during submaximal and maximal intensity contractions, a phenomenon that has been linked to motor unit remodeling, by shifting the fastest firing fibers to a slower phenotype. The consequence is that older persons need to increase the number of activated fibers and come closer to maximal effort to perform usual tasks such as climbing stairs or rising from a chair. The control of muscle contraction and movement also depends on other integrative neural mechanisms that show age-related changes, including neural excitability and brain connectivity.

The magnitude of change in muscle size and function is strongly associated with long-term lifestyle, especially with the degree of physical activity and the amount of endurance exercise. This was first demonstrated in animal models, where long-term exercise is associated with reduced loss of motor neurons and muscle fibers compared to sedentary animals. Studies in runners have shown that at least part of the age-related motor unit loss may be prevented or retarded by usual physical exercise, perhaps via an increase of the reinnervation capacity of denervated units. A low protein intake over long periods of time is also associated with reduced muscle mass loss and may help upregulate the balance between muscle protein anabolism and catabolism. Other genetic and molecular changes involved in age-related changes of the skeletal muscle and the motor unit are still largely the focus of research.

SARCOPENIA: CHANGING DEFINITIONS ALONG TIME

Sarcopenia is the most frequent age-associated disease of the skeletal muscle. It is defined as a progressive and generalized disease involving the accelerated loss of muscle mass and function that is associated with increased likelihood of adverse outcomes including falls, frailty, physical disability, and mortality. It may be considered "skeletal muscle insufficiency," similar to cardiac or renal insufficiency as a useful clinical construct.

The term "sarcopenia" is derived from the Greek words for "poverty of flesh." It was first described in the 1980s as an age-related decline in lean body mass affecting mobility, nutritional status, and independence. Initial studies of sarcopenia focused mostly on body composition (for some, sarcopenia is still a synonym of low skeletal muscle mass). However, over the years it has become clear that muscle mass measures or estimations with any available method are poor predictors of clinical outcomes, including physical disability. On the other hand, functional measures (muscle strength and some measures of physical performance, especially gait speed) were confirmed to be good predictors of disability and other relevant outcomes. Such evidence radically changed the concept of sarcopenia in recent years. This is not surprising; cardiac muscle function

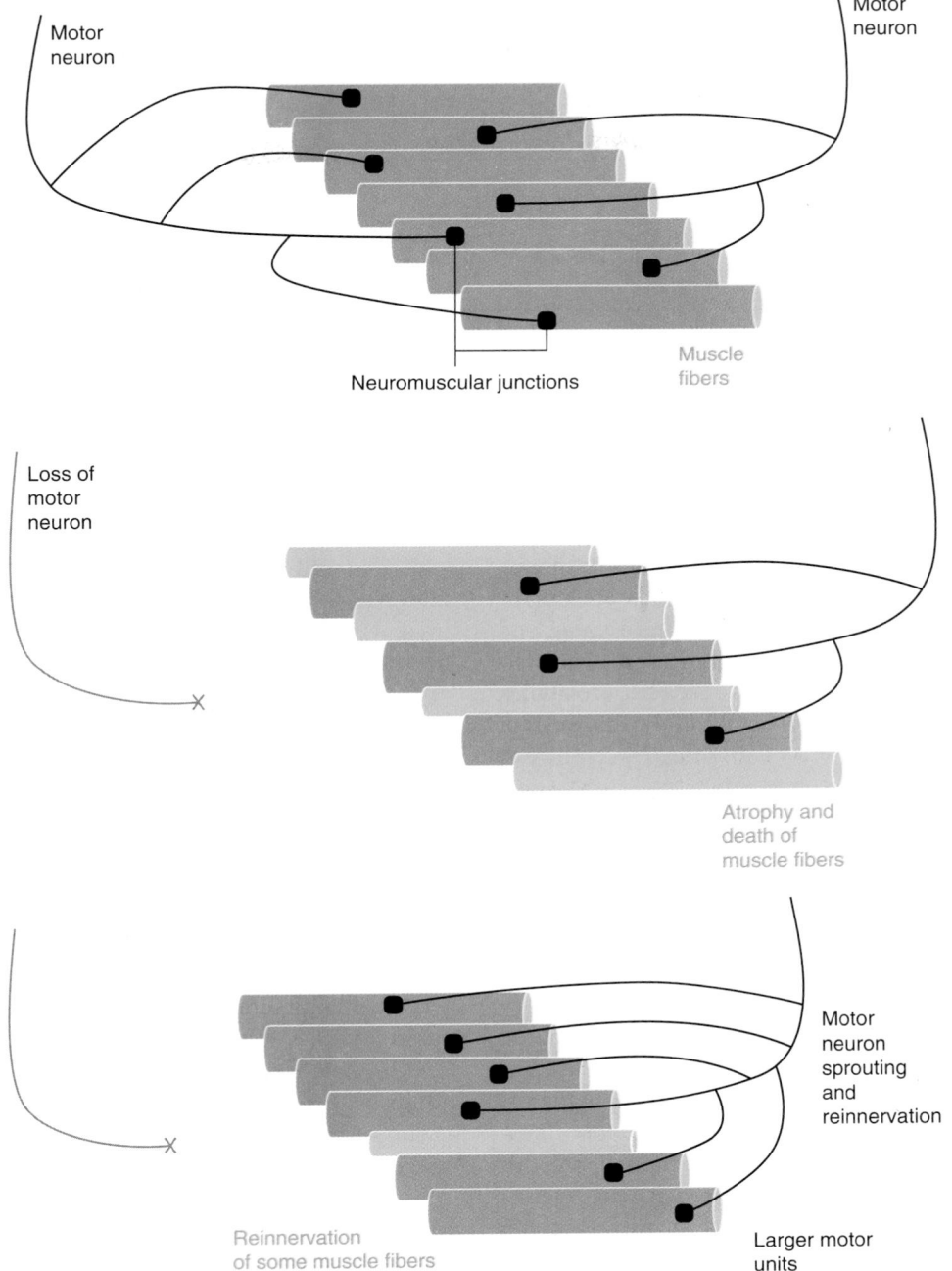

FIGURE 49-1. Motor unit remodeling in a denervation-innervation cycle.

is also more relevant than mass, except for diseases linked to reduced distensibility, a property that is not relevant for most skeletal muscles.

Building on this evidence, six expert consensus definitions were published from 2010 to 2014 by different groups and organizations: some working groups of the European Society for Clinical Nutrition (ESPEN), the European Working Group on Sarcopenia in Older People (EWGSOP, nurtured by the European Geriatric Medicine Society and ESPEN), an International Working Group on Sarcopenia (IWGS), a group around the Society on Sarcopenia, Cachexia and Wasting Disorders (SSCWD), the Asian Working Group for Sarcopenia (AWGS), and the US Foundation of the National Institutes of Health (FNIH) (**Table 49-2**). Although not equivalent, all definitions added functional measures to muscle mass estimates, were widely accepted by the scientific community, and triggered an increase in research that confirmed that defining

TABLE 49-2 ■ PARAMETERS INCLUDED IN DEFINITIONS OF SARCOPENIA AROUND 2010

DEFINITION	MUSCLE MASS	MUSCLE STRENGTH	PHYSICAL PERFORMANCE	CUTOFFS DEFINED	TIMES CITED*
ESPEN (2010)	▪		▪	▪	967
EWGSOP (2010)	▪	▪	▪		6368
IWGS (2011)	▪		▪	▪	1727
SSCWD (2011)	▪		▪	▪	613
AWGS (2014)	▪	▪	▪	▪	2036
FNIH (2014)	▪	▪		▪	1005

*Web of Science. https://www.webofscience.com/wos/alldb/basic-search. Accessed mid-December 2021.

sarcopenia as low muscle mass plus low muscle function was a relevant clinical construct that predicted outcomes and was potentially amenable to improve with interventions. These advances led to the recognition of sarcopenia as a disease with an ICD-10-CM code in 2016.

In recent years, measures and estimations of muscle mass have gradually lost credibility. Methods are unreliable, clear cutoff points could never be agreed upon, and the lack of correlation of muscle mass measures with relevant outcomes was confirmed. This reduced credibility, among other factors, led to a low uptake of the diagnosis of sarcopenia in clinical practice, missing the opportunity to prevent or reverse some outcomes. Therefore, some working groups decided to update their definitions, highlighting the importance of low muscle function and reducing the role of muscle mass in the diagnosis of sarcopenia, with the declared aim to make the diagnosis more friendly to practitioners.

The first update came from the EWGSOP (EWGSOP2) in 2019. This advanced definition opted to move muscle strength to the first parameter to be measured when sarcopenia is suspected, with muscle mass used as confirmation of the involvement of muscle in strength loss. In fact, the EWGSOP2 proposes the use of the term "suspected sarcopenia" for patients with low muscle strength when muscle mass has not been measured. It also suggests alternative use of measures of muscle quality (both in terms of muscle composition and in the ability of muscle mass volume to deliver strength) to replace muscle mass. For the EWGSOP2, low physical performance (defined as the full body ability to move or endure, as measured with walking or chair standing tests) is a marker of severity of sarcopenia that increases the risk of adverse outcomes. There is some evidence than mild or moderate sarcopenia may respond to some treatments that could be insufficient to tackle severe sarcopenia. This group also includes the concept of case finding (already suggested by the SSCWD group) by clinical symptoms or questionnaires with the aim to improve the detection of sarcopenia in clinical settings.

The AWGS (whose first definition was identical to the EWGSOP with distinct cutoff points for Asian populations) also published an updated version in 2020, where case-finding is also the first diagnostic step, albeit the algorithm, instruments or suspicion depend on the clinical setting (community vs other care settings). In specialized settings, muscle strength would be the first measure, followed by physical performance and muscle mass. However, this definition still requires impairments in either muscle mass and function to define sarcopenia, and in both to consider it severe.

Finally, the FNIH group, now named Sarcopenia Definition and Outcomes Consortium (SDOC), recently published an international expert panel position on 13 statements on the putative components of a sarcopenia definition. They confirmed by new analyses of available epidemiologic databases that low muscle strength is associated with physical performance (slowness) and that both low grip strength and low gait speed independently predict falls, self-reported mobility limitation, hip fractures, and mortality in community-dwelling older adults. On the other hand, they found again that lean mass measured by DXA was not associated with incident adverse health-related outcomes in community-dwelling older adults with or without adjustment for body size. This group recommends that low grip strength and usual gait speed should be included in the definition of sarcopenia, while low muscle mass (measured by DXA) should not be included. The evolution of definitions of sarcopenia is depicted in **Figure 49-2**.

EPIDEMIOLOGY

Sarcopenia is a relatively common condition in old age with adverse effects on current as well as future health. Estimates of disease prevalence and incidence are changing with the availability of more accurate definitions. The prevalence of sarcopenia using definitions that only consider low muscle mass can be as high as 40% in community dwelling older persons. However, when muscle function is also included, estimates of the prevalence of sarcopenia in the community are around 10% to 15%. The incidence of new cases of sarcopenia in older adults may be higher than 3% per year, although this has been less studied. There are no clear

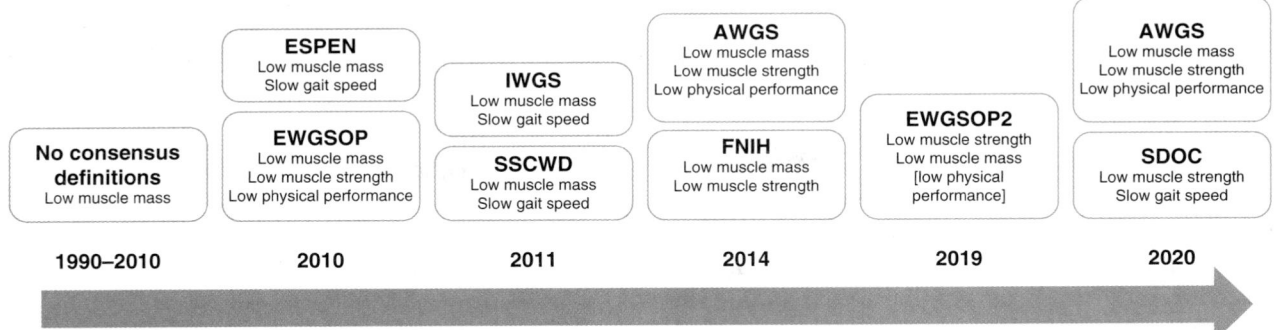

FIGURE 49-2. Guide to the evolution of the definition of sarcopenia.

differences in the prevalence of sarcopenia in males and females. However, the prevalence may be higher in acutely ill hospitalized patients (especially those with severe chronic diseases, present in > 20% of hospitalized older patients), in post-acute and rehabilitation settings (where prevalence may be > 50%), and in nursing homes (> 40% of residents will be sarcopenic).

Many risk factors for sarcopenia have been described. The association with age is probably related to long-term lifestyle. Protein intake has been shown to be related to muscle mass and function in epidemiological studies. People in the lowest quartile of protein intake show a higher age-related loss of muscle mass that those in the upper quartile. A slight deficit in protein intake, when sustained for many years, may have a strong impact on muscle mass and function in old age. Low levels of vitamin D, omega 3 fatty acids, and some micronutrients (magnesium, selenium) may also be associated with impaired muscle function, although evidence is still weak. Dietary patterns are also important to muscle health. Good adherence to a Mediterranean diet or having high scores in other measures of healthy eating (usually involving higher intake of fruits, vegetables, fatty fish, or whole grains) are also related to better muscle function and reduced disability than less healthy diets.

Low physical activity and sedentariness are usually considered risk factors for sarcopenia, but evidence is weak, as no robust long-term studies have shown an association between lifetime physical activity and exercise and muscle health. Chronic diseases may also be a risk factor for sarcopenia, especially when they limit mobility or appropriate nutrition in old age. Low-grade inflammation has been shown to be associated with sarcopenia. When inflammation is severe, sarcopenia blends into cachexia. Diabetes mellitus is also an established risk factor of sarcopenia; sarcopenia is more common in persons with diabetes compared to those without. On the other hand, sarcopenia may contribute to the development and progression of diabetes through altered glucose disposal due to low muscle mass and intramuscular adipose tissue accumulation.

Obesity and sarcopenia are also related, in a construct named sarcopenic obesity. Patients with sarcopenic obesity have high adiposity and low lean mass. However, this condition is still ill defined, as some patients may have adequate muscle mass (compared with standard population measures) but have muscle strength that is unable to move an increased total body mass. There is an initiative under the auspice of ESPEN to propose a definition of sarcopenic obesity that may advance the field, expected to be released in 2022.

Sarcopenia is associated with many adverse health consequences. Many studies have confirmed that mortality is 3 to 4 times higher in sarcopenic compared with non-sarcopenic persons with otherwise similar health conditions, and the impact of sarcopenia on mortality may be even higher in persons older than 80 years. Sarcopenia is also associated with a much higher risk of physical and cognitive frailty, functional decline, and disability. The risk of falls and fractures is also slightly increased in sarcopenia, although evidence about this association is not yet unequivocal. Sarcopenia also seems to increase the risk of hospitalization, readmission, and impaired health-related quality of life, whether assessed by general instruments or disease-specific instruments. Whether sarcopenia increases the risk of nursing home admission or global health care costs remains to be elucidated.

PATHOPHYSIOLOGY

Processes leading to sarcopenia are complex and interacting. They include anatomical and functional changes imposed on an aging skeletal muscle and nervous system, and also changes in hormonal regulatory mechanisms. Research is continuing, but it may well be that the phenotype of sarcopenia is produced through different mechanisms in different individuals, which could be relevant when tailoring interventions to individual patients.

Aging disturbs skeletal muscle homeostasis, which requires balance between hypertrophy and regeneration through complex and not yet fully understood mechanisms and pathways. Aging modifies the balance between muscle protein anabolic and catabolic pathways, with reduced protein uptake and probably increased catabolism, leading to an overall loss of skeletal muscle mass. As mentioned above, cellular changes include a reduction in the size and number of myofibers, particularly affecting type II fibers, with a partial transition of muscle fibers from type II to type I. Satellite cells (muscle progenitor cells) decrease, especially those associated with type II fibers. Extracellular fat increases with aging, as do intra- and intermuscular fat, infiltrating muscles in a process named myosteatosis. The metabolic and hormonal interrelations between adipose and muscle tissue seem to be important in the pathogenesis of sarcopenia. This may help to explain the still confusing relation between sarcopenia and obesity. Mitochondrial integrity in myocytes is altered, with an impairment in intracellular energy processes. Other intracellular signaling pathways, including insulin-like growth factor 1 (IGF-1), mTOR, and FoxO transcription factors, have also been shown to be altered in sarcopenic muscles. Changes in muscle gene expression, probably mediated through epigenetic changes, have also been described.

Age-related changes in neurologic signaling and central nervous system control mechanisms, as described above, also have a role in the pathogenesis of sarcopenia. However, it is unknown to what degree, as research in this area is still limited. Untangling the role of muscle and nervous changes is urgent, as it has a direct impact on therapeutic approaches. For example, the fact that nutritional interventions to promote increasing muscle show mixed results may be due to the fact that such interventions would not improve neural mechanisms. Also, innovative treatments aiming to improve cortical and associative brain areas may well be useful, at least in some instances. Physical exercise, the best-established treatment for sarcopenia, has been shown to act through both muscular and neural pathways.

Finally, the relation between bones and muscles is currently being explored. Both are key to mobility and they are anatomically and physically related. Osteoporosis and sarcopenia frequently coexist and, when present together, exponentially increase the risk of some adverse outcomes, so the term "osteosarcopenia" is gaining momentum. Research has found evidence of cross-talk between muscle and bone through endocrine factors such as myostatin, irisin, osteocalcin, and many other substances, although the relevance of this communication in the pathogenesis of sarcopenia has not been established.

DIAGNOSIS OF SARCOPENIA IN CLINICAL PRACTICE

Awaiting a global consensus on the definition of sarcopenia, clinicians will probably opt to choose one of the most recent definitions and use it in their practice. The diagnosis

TABLE 49-3 ■ COMPONENTS OF THE SARC-F SCREENING TEST
AREAS ADDRESSED BY THE QUESTIONS OF THE SARC-F:
• Perceived muscle strength
• Assistance in walking
• Rising from a chair
• Climbing stairs
• Falls

of sarcopenia using any modern definition is relatively straightforward and requires measurement of a combination of muscle mass, muscle strength, and physical performance. All definitions use at least two of these three, suggesting different cutoff points depending on the measure used and the population.

Screening

At this time, screening for sarcopenia has not been proved to be cost-effective, either universally or in defined care settings or populations. A screening instrument, the SARC-F questionnaire, which explores five items and can be self-administered, has the strongest evidence, with high sensitivity with low cutoffs (> 1 point) and a good specificity when using high cutoffs (> 4) (**Table 49-3**). This instrument can be used in clinical scenarios with a high expected prevalence of sarcopenia, including geriatric outpatient clinics, hospitalized older patients, rehabilitation settings, or nursing homes. Some modified versions have been proposed, including other elements such as muscle calf circumference.

Also, the diagnosis of sarcopenia may be triggered by the presence of signs and symptoms associated with this condition, including complaints of weakness, slowness, muscle wasting, falls, difficulties carrying out activities of daily living, or problems in rising from a chair or bed.

Muscle Strength

Because it is the most widely used definition worldwide, here we follow the suggestions of the updated EWGSOP2 that proposes a stepwise approach to the diagnosis of sarcopenia. The AWGS suggests a similar—but not identical—approach that differs in primary care or specialized settings. The SDOC has not provided recommendations for clinical practice.

The recommended first parameter to be measured when sarcopenia is suspected clinically or by a positive SARC-F is muscle strength, usually through handgrip strength. Although measuring leg strength would seem to be more intuitive, it requires expensive equipment, cutoffs have not been defined for populations, and the link between leg strength and grip strength is consistent enough to use the latter as a proxy. Most evidence from grip strength comes from studies that use a hydraulic (Jamar) dynamometer, but other models are being progressively incorporated into clinical practice. Grip strength measures need to be standardized by using a validated protocol (as is true for blood pressure

TABLE 49-4 ■ CUTOFF POINTS TO DEFINE LOW GRIP STRENGTH AND REDUCED GAIT SPEED

DEFINITION	GS MALES	GS FEMALES	GAIT SPEED
EWGSOP2	< 27 kg	< 16 kg	≤ 0.8 m/s
AWGS	< 28 kg	< 18 kg	< 1.0 m/s
SDOC	< 35.5 kg	< 20 kg	≤ 0.8 m/s*

*SDOC does not propose a precise cutoff; this is based on the 2014 FNIH consensus.

or other physical measures). If grip strength is below the reference values for gender and population (**Table 49-4**), sarcopenia should be suspected, as it is the most frequent reason of muscle weakness. However, the differential diagnosis is wide and other potential causes for low muscle strength should be considered—for example hand osteoarthritis, low motivation, or neurological disorders. Low grip strength is highly predictive of a range of adverse outcomes, disregarding its cause, and merits the launch of therapeutic interventions even when no further diagnostic tests are available.

Muscle Mass and Quality

The second step may be measuring muscle mass, although all experts do not agree on the need of having a muscle mass measure to diagnose sarcopenia. As mentioned, this is because all available measures are in fact estimations of muscle mass based on a number of presumptions that depend on the technique, results have a high inter- and intra-rater variability, cutoff points are inconsistent and a low muscle mass has not been consistently shown to be linked to adverse outcomes. Also, a low muscle mass may be due to malnutrition or cachexia and thus not directly caused by sarcopenia. Being said, an estimation of muscle mass would help linking low muscle strength to a muscle problem. More accurate techniques, such as the creatine dilution test are in development to measure active muscle mass. If more consistent links with outcomes are shown, they may help solve the limitations of available methods in the near future.

The most widely used methods to estimate muscle mass in practice at present are dual energy X-ray absorptiometry (DXA) and bioimpedance absorptiometry (BIA). The first has the widest evidence and definitions usually refer to it when defining cutoff points. It has the advantage that bone mineral density can be measured simultaneously. Usually, appendicular lean mass (skeletal muscle in the extremities) is measured, and in most cases adjustment for height is added to define cutoff values. BIA is useful as a bedside test; but as BIA equations and cut points are population- and device-specific, there is a lack of standardization that limits its accuracy. CT and MRI can also estimate muscle mass, usually by a cross-sectional image of the psoas muscle or the thigh. As such images are obtained routinely in some conditions and disciplines (surgery, oncology), they may be helpful in these settings, although

the link to outcomes is still to be defined in larger populations. Ultrasound has also been proposed as a simple alternative to measure muscle mass in clinical practice, and a standardization of measures (the SARCUS project) has been proposed by a European Geriatric Medicine Society working group, but it still lacks validated cutoff points for major muscles. Finding a very low muscle mass with any of these techniques, together with a low grip strength, would make sarcopenia very likely, while measures closer to the cutoff points used (that depend on gender, population, and method) may be more equivocal.

Muscle quality is a widely used term for an ill-defined concept. It may refer at least to two different concepts: (1) the relation between muscle strength and muscle mass (ie, the amount of strength delivered by each muscle mass unit) or (2) some observable characteristics of the muscle, either macroscopically or microscopically (such as inter- or intramuscular adiposity, or the rates between different muscle fiber types). Quality may prove to be a relevant concept, but as yet is not sufficiently defined for use in clinical practice. An estimation of fat infiltration or muscle heterogeneity in imaging (CT, MRI, or ultrasounds), if shown to be relevant to outcomes, would be a simple and useful approach to define a muscle problem as the cause of low muscle strength.

Physical Performance

Physical performance has been defined as the ability to carry out physical tasks in order to function independently in daily life. It measures composite functions of the whole body as opposed to the function of a single organ and depends on an intact musculoskeletal system integrated with the central and peripheral nervous systems, with significant involvement of a range of other body systems (cardiovascular, vision, balance, and other). Measures of physical performance usually involve standing or walking, and may include measures of mobility, strength, power, balance, and endurance. The most commonly used test in geriatric practice is gait speed in a 4- to 6-m track, again using standardized protocols. Gait speed has been shown to be related to functional outcomes and mortality along the whole spectrum of results, and even small losses (0.1 m/s) are predictive of impaired outcomes. Cutoffs have been proposed (**Table 49-4**). There is no agreement yet on the exact position of gait speed in the definition of sarcopenia: as an outcome (FNIH), as part of the core definition (EWGSOP, AWGS) or as a measure of severity of sarcopenia that shows the impact of a reduced muscle function in body function (EWGSOP2, AWGS). Nevertheless, gait speed is probably a basic vital sign in geriatric practice.

Other measures of physical performance that are not unusual in geriatric practice are used as well to define sarcopenia or its severity. The Short Physical Performance Battery (SPPB) adds a measure of balance and of muscle strength/power/endurance (sit to stand test) to gait speed. It has been validated in many clinical settings and is associated with frailty. The sit-to-stand test has also been proposed as a proxy for muscle strength when a dynamometer is not available (EWGSOP2 and AWGS). The Timed Up and Go (TUG) test is a widely used and useful measure of physical performance. Other walking tests (6 minutes, 400 m) may be chosen in some clinical and research settings.

Biomarkers

Most of the proposed diagnostic measures are (physical) biomarkers of sarcopenia. However, clinicians are used to including blood biomarkers in the diagnostic scheme of most diseases, so a search for such blood (or other tissues) biomarkers of sarcopenia is underway. Many of the elements that are known to be altered in sarcopenia, including the neuromuscular junction, inflammation, micro-RNAs, hormones, metabolic by-products, and others, have been proposed as potential biomarkers. Research in this area is complex and to date results are inconclusive. It may well be that composite panels including several biomarkers, rather than individual biomarkers, are needed.

Underlying Causes

Once sarcopenia has been confirmed, a systematic approach that includes a comprehensive geriatric assessment is recommended to search for potential underlying causes. Frequent causes of sarcopenia are described in **Table 49-5**. Most older patients will have more than one associated condition, and not all may be treatable. However, understanding the full picture of the individual patient will be

TABLE 49-5 ■ FREQUENT UNDERLYING CAUSES OF SARCOPENIA

TYPE	SOME EXAMPLES
Diseases that may cause sarcopenia	Bone and joint diseases (eg, arthritis, osteoporosis)
	Cancer (with or without cachexia)
	Cardiorespiratory (eg, heart failure, chronic obstructive pulmonary disease)
	Endocrine and metabolic disorders (eg, diabetes mellitus, hypoandrogenism)
	Liver and kidney chronic disorders
	Neurological diseases
Activity	Low level of physical activity, sedentary
	Prolonged bed rest, immobility
Nutritional	Anorexia (aging, oral problems)
	Low food intake (especially low protein intake)
	Micronutrient deficiencies
	Malabsorption and other gastrointestinal conditions
Iatrogenic	Drugs (eg, corticosteroids)
	Hospital admission
	Medical recommendation to limit mobility or activities

helpful when deciding a therapeutic approach. When no evident cause of a gradual-onset chronic sarcopenia is present in an older person, age-associated (primary) sarcopenia is diagnosed, and further exploration of long-term habits that may have led to sarcopenia is appropriate.

DIFFERENTIAL DIAGNOSIS WITH CACHEXIA, MALNUTRITION, AND FRAILTY

The recent global definition of malnutrition, the Global Leadership Initiative on Malnutrition (GLIM), includes low muscle mass as one of the three phenotypic criteria that are part of the five criteria that define malnutrition (the three phenotypic criteria are nonvolitional weight loss, low body mass index, and reduced muscle mass, and the two etiologic criteria are reduced food intake or assimilation and inflammation or disease burden). Thus, when low muscle mass is found in a given patient, checking if any of the other four proposed GLIM criteria are present can help determine if malnutrition is present, since the coexistence of sarcopenia and malnutrition is not infrequent. When low muscle mass is not associated with low muscle function, malnutrition will probably be present and will be the main diagnosis of that patient. When both low muscle mass and low muscle function are present in a malnourished patient, the most usual scenario will be that malnutrition has caused sarcopenia.

"Cachexia" is a term used to describe severe weight loss and muscle wasting associated with cancer, HIV infection, or end-stage organ failure. The most common definitions of cachexia include the presence of a low muscle mass as well. In fact, cachexia and sarcopenia may coexist. Cachexia has a complex pathophysiology including excess catabolism and inflammation, and endocrine and neurological changes that are different from those described in sarcopenia. Conceptually, cachexia may be the end result of some disease-related cases of sarcopenia. International consensus definitions of cachexia may guide clinical judgment to decide if sarcopenia or cachexia predominate; this is relevant for the choice of treatment, as cachexia would not respond to sarcopenia treatment.

Frailty, addressed in Chapter 42, has a physical aspect that is closely related to sarcopenia. In fact, the three elements that define sarcopenia are embedded in the Fried physical frailty phenotype: unintentional weight loss—that usually involves muscle mass loss, weakness (low grip strength), and slow walking speed. Sarcopenia is a major determinant of physical frailty, as it impairs the main mobility-related organ. Of course, physical frailty can be caused by nonmuscular diseases, and mild sarcopenia may not lead to frailty. Thus, they are distinct but overlapping constructs.

TREATMENT

Because sarcopenia is a complex condition—and a quite recently defined one—evidence about treatment is still limited. Understanding the pathophysiology of sarcopenia is key to developing effective new interventions and translational research in this area is needed. Of course, addressing the causes and risk factors that are found in the comprehensive geriatric assessment may be useful in treating sarcopenia and preventing relapses, but to date no trials have been carried out with a multimodal approach. The first available evidence-based clinical practice guideline only places a strong recommendation on physical activity as the cornerstone for treatment of sarcopenia.

Physical Exercise

There is compelling evidence that supports the benefits of resistance exercise in improving skeletal muscle function and mass both in younger and older persons, and this evidence extends to patients with sarcopenia. However, the optimal mode, duration, and intensity of exercise are still ill-defined. Resistance exercise uses weights or elastic bands in repetitive movements to improve strength and power of groups of muscles. To treat sarcopenia, both lower and upper extremities should be exercised, at least twice a week. The minimum expected time to obtain an objective improvement seems to be close to 3 months. Ideally, exercises should be started under the advice and vigilance of an expert exercise or physical therapist, in order to teach the correct way to perform each exercise and avoid injuries. Gradually the patient will be able to start unsupervised exercise. Compliance is key to obtain results; it may be improved with supervision or peer support in an exercise group.

Many trials have shown that resistance exercise can be embedded in a multifaceted exercise program that includes aerobic (cardiovascular) and balance training, and possibly stretching and joint range-of-motion movements. However, patients should be aware that the usual cardiovascular exercise that physicians recommend widely to improve aging and well-being (walking, swimming, dancing, bicycling) will not have an impact on sarcopenia. Including resistance exercise is key to improve muscle function.

A recommendation to increase physical activity and reduce sedentariness in usual life is common sense; it is perceived to help in the prevention and treatment of sarcopenia and other conditions. However, this has not been tested as a treatment for sarcopenia and should not replace a formal exercise program as the cornerstone of treatment.

Nutrition

The evidence about nutrition interventions in treating sarcopenia is less consistent, with only conditional or weak recommendations in the clinical practice guideline. However, some recommendations can be made. Protein intake is key to muscle health, and the recommendations for protein intake in older people have recently been raised from the former 0.8 g per kg of body weight per day to 1–1.2 g in healthy older adults, and up to 1.5 g in disease. Most older persons do not reach these targets, so a careful review of patient food intake by an expert nutritionist is needed

to consistently increase protein intake. This approach has been shown to be feasible and effective in a large multicenter randomized controlled trial. When the required levels of protein intake cannot be reached with usual food, the use of high protein nutritional supplements may be considered (usually in the form of oral nutritional supplements rather than protein-only supplements).

Some individual nutrients may also be useful to improve muscle mass and function. The essential amino acid leucine and its metabolite beta-hydroxy beta-methylbutyric acid (HMB) have shown some effects in improving muscle mass and function in randomized controlled trials, although it is not yet clear which individuals benefit most. Mild sarcopenia seems to respond better. Trials have usually included leucine and HMB in full oral supplements, so the effect of leucine and HMB in isolated forms in older people is unknown. There is also some evidence supporting the use of fish oil–derived n-3 (omega-3) polyunsaturated fatty acids (PUFA) and creatine. Vitamin D has not been shown to improve muscle function in sarcopenic patients. It may be useful in improving muscle function in persons with severe vitamin D deficiency.

Some trials have explored nutrition interventions in combination with physical exercise in the treatment of sarcopenia, with mixed results; only a few trials show some synergistic effects. Since physical exercise increases energy needs, energy intake (carbohydrates and fat) should be adjusted to the new requirements to increase the caloric content of the diet. Supplements may be occasionally needed. Also, incorporation of proteins into muscles seems to be limited in terms of time in older people and has a higher threshold in older compared to younger adults. Therefore, a timed boost of proteins seems to be better than increasing protein content over the day. Basic research has shown that aged muscle will most avidly take up proteins immediately after exercise.

Pharmacologic Treatments

At this time, there are no drugs approved for sarcopenia, nor are any expected in the short term. There are many reasons for this situation, including the lack of guidance from drug approval agencies on what would be acceptable clinical trial outcome measures for drug approval, uncertainty about which particular groups of patients with sarcopenia would benefit more, issues about the optimal trial design and timing, lack of strong basic science research to support most drugs, and the multifaceted pathophysiology of the condition.

Trials to date have been performed mostly with hormones. Combined estrogen–progesterone, dehydroepiandrosterone (DHEA), growth hormone, growth hormone-releasing hormone, combined testosterone-growth hormone, and insulin-like growth factor-1 have all shown negative results, but many studies have not included well-defined sarcopenic patients. Testosterone may increase muscle mass in men with low serum testosterone levels

(< 200–300 ng/dL), but physical function does not seem to improve, and this drug is not devoid of side effects. In more recent trials, the initial interest in selective androgen receptor modulators (SARMs, which may be used in women as well as men) from small phase I and II trials has not been followed by convincing results from larger studies. Pioglitazone and angiotensin-converting enzyme inhibitors have also been explored with negative results.

Myostatin is a myokine, a growth factor that inhibits muscle cell growth. There is evidence that myostatin inhibition may be able to increase muscle mass, consistent with the recognition that myostatin acts as a brake on muscle differentiation, hypertrophy, and protein synthesis. A phase II proof of concept trial reported that a myostatin antibody was associated with increased muscle mass and improvement in some measures of physical performance in older, weak patients with a history of falling (but not diagnosed sarcopenia). Bimagrumab has been shown to increase muscle mass and reduce adiposity in diabetic patients, but again the effects on muscle function and physical performance seem to be limited. Myostatin inhibitor research seems to be evolving to explore changes in body composition and moving away from muscle function.

ASSESSING THE EFFECT OF TREATMENTS

There is still no agreement on what intermediate and final outcomes should be expected to improve with an intervention for sarcopenia. In clinical practice, the simplest approach is to assess changes in the parameters used for the diagnosis. Gains in muscle mass are usually difficult to assess (due to the mentioned technical issues of available instruments) and do not seem to be relevant for most older patients. Gains in muscle strength may be easier to assess but more difficult to obtain with available treatments. The minimum clinically significant difference for muscle strength is not yet defined in older patients with sarcopenia. At present, there is a case for using physical performance measures to assess improvement in clinical practice. Improvements gait speed over 0.1 m/s or over 1 point in the SPPB are accepted as being clinically relevant. Improvement in final outcomes including activities of daily living, the number of falls, or quality of life are even more relevant but not as straightforward to determine. Patients rate improved mobility as the most desired outcome of treatment, followed by the ability to manage domestic activities, a lower risk of falls, reduced fatigue, and a better quality of life.

FURTHER READING

Beaudart C, Zaaria M, Pasleau F, Reginster J-Y, Bruyère O. Health outcomes of sarcopenia: a systematic review and meta-analysis. *PloS One.* 2017;12:e0169548.

Bhasin S, Travison TG, Manini TM, et al. Sarcopenia definition: the position statements of the sarcopenia definition and outcomes consortium. *J Am Geriatr Soc.* 2020;68:1410–1418.

Bruyère O, Beaudart C, Ethgen O, Reginster J-Y, Locquet M. The health economics burden of sarcopenia: a systematic review. *Maturitas.* 2019;119:61–69.

Buckinx F, Landi F, Cesari M, et al. Pitfalls in the measurement of muscle mass: a need for a reference standard. *J Cachexia Sarcopenia Muscle.* 2018;9:269–278.

Calvani R, Picca A, Cesari M, et al. Biomarkers for sarcopenia: reductionism vs. complexity. *Curr Protein Pept Sci.* 2018;19:639–642.

Chen LK, Woo J, Assantachai P, et al. Asian Working Group for Sarcopenia: 2019 consensus update on sarcopenia diagnosis and treatment. *J Am Med Dir Assoc.* 2020;21:300–307.e2.

Cruz-Jentoft AJ, Bahat G, Bauer J, et al. Sarcopenia: revised European consensus on definition and diagnosis. *Age Ageing.* 2019;48:16–31.

De Spiegeleer A, Beckwee D, Bautmans I, Petrovic M. Pharmacological interventions to improve muscle mass, muscle strength and physical performance in older people: an umbrella review of systematic reviews and meta-analyses. *Drugs Aging.* 2018;35:719–734.

Dent E, Morley JE, Cruz-Jentoft AJ, et al. International clinical practice guidelines for sarcopenia (ICFSR): screening, diagnosis and management. *J Nutr Health Aging.* 2018;22:1148–1161.

Dodds RM, Syddall HE, Cooper R, et al. Grip strength across the life course: normative data from twelve British studies. *PloS One.* 2014;9:e113637.

Evans WJ, Hellerstein M, Orwoll E, Cummings S, Cawthon PM. D3-creatine dilution and the importance of accuracy in the assessment of skeletal muscle mass. *J Cachexia Sarcopenia Muscle.* 2019;10:14–21.

Frontera WR, Zayas AR, Rodriguez N. Aging of human muscle: understanding sarcopenia at the single muscle cell level. *Phys Med Rehabil Clin N Am.* 2012;23:201–207, xiii.

Ida S, Kaneko R, Murata K. SARC-F for screening of sarcopenia among older adults: a meta-analysis of screening test accuracy. *J Am Med Dir Assoc.* 2018;19:685–689.

Manini TM, Clark BC. Dynapenia and aging: an update. *J Gerontol A Biol Sci Med Sci.* 2012;67:28–40.

Pavasini R, Guralnik J, Brown JC, et al. Short physical performance battery and all-cause mortality: systematic review and meta-analysis. *BMC Med.* 2016;14:215.

Perkisas S, Baudry S, Bauer J, et al. Application of ultrasound for muscle assessment in sarcopenia: towards standardized measurements. *Eur Geriatr Med.* 2018;9:739–757.

Roberts HC, Denison HJ, Martin HJ, et al. A review of the measurement of grip strength in clinical and epidemiological studies: towards a standardised approach. *Age Ageing.* 2011;40:423–429.

Rosenberg IH. Sarcopenia: origins and clinical relevance. *J Nutr.* 1997;127:990S–991S.

Sayer AA, Syddall H, Martin H, Patel H, Baylis D, Cooper C. The developmental origins of sarcopenia. *J Nutr Health Aging.* 2008;12:427–432.

Yoshimura Y, Wakabayashi H, Yamada M, Kim H, Harada A, Arai H. Interventions for treating sarcopenia: a systematic review and meta-analysis of randomized controlled studies. *J Am Med Dir Assoc.* 2017;18: 553.e1–553.e16.

Chapter 50

Mobility Assessment and Management

Valerie Shuman, Caterina Rosano, Jennifer S. Brach

INTRODUCTION

Mobility problems are pervasive in older adults. Mobility limitations affect personal independence, need for human help, and quality of life. Limited mobility predicts future health, function, and survival. Like other geriatric syndromes, mobility disorders are often caused by diseases and impairments across many organ systems; so evaluation and management require multiple perspectives and disciplines. Health care providers should be able to assess and treat mobility problems. They should be able to measure and interpret clinical indicators of mobility such as gait speed and the short physical performance battery. They should know the physiologic and biomechanical mechanisms underlying normal and abnormal mobility, the differential diagnosis of the causes of mobility disorders, and the approaches to management of mobility problems. With rapid technological advancements in the measurements of mobility, geriatricians should be aware of novel assessments that could be used in the clinic.

DEFINITIONS AND METHODS OF CLASSIFICATION

Defining Mobility

Mobility is the ability to move one's own body through space. Mobility requires force production and feedback control systems to navigate the mass of the body through a three-dimensional environment. Walking is the fundamental mobility task for human life. Mobility also includes a wide range of other important activities that require moving one's body, from turning over in bed to climbing stairs. Mobility tasks have an inherent hierarchical order based on the biomechanical and physiologic demands made on the body. This orderedness is apparent in the developmental tasks of infancy and childhood when mobility independence is first achieved. The simplest and first mobility task is turning over in bed, followed by sitting upright, transferring from lying to sitting and from sitting to standing. From there, individuals progress to locomotion with an increased base of support (like crawling or using a walker), independent two-legged walking, and finally to more challenging tasks like ascending and descending stairs, running, climbing ladders, and playing sports.

Learning Objectives

- Describe the prevalence and consequences of mobility disorders in older people.
- Identify strategies to detect and evaluate mobility disorders.
- Characterize approaches to the management of mobility disorders.

Key Clinical Points

1. Loss of mobility is a major cause of disability in older people but is rarely assessed in typical clinical practice.
2. The assessment of mobility involves taking a history and performing a physical examination that identifies cardiopulmonary, musculoskeletal, psychological, and neurologic contributors.
3. Mobility can be assessed by a number of simple performance tests including gait speed, the short physical performance battery, and the Timed Up and Go test.
4. Interventions to promote mobility include addressing underlying impairments, therapeutic exercise, assistive devices, home adaptations, and caregiver training.

Mobility disability is best defined within a conceptual framework such as that of the World Health Organization's International Classification of Functioning, Disability and Health (ICF) (**Table 50-1**). The concept of disability in general has transitioned from being considered a biological consequence of pathologic processes to a social construct influenced by personal and environmental factors. For example, the inability to climb 12 stairs may be considered a disability in a region with primarily two-story homes but not in an area largely made of ranch-style homes. Mobility disability occurs at the level of the whole person and can be manifested by difficulty in carrying out basic hygiene activities such as bathing or by limitations in participating

TABLE 50-1 ■ MOBILITY DISABILITY AND THE DISABLEMENT PROCESS

INTERNATIONAL CLASSIFICATION OF FUNCTIONING, DISABILITY, AND HEALTH COMPONENT	FACTORS RELATED TO MOBILITY DISABILITY
Health condition	Mobility limitations
Body functions and structures	Structures: losses of strength, endurance, coordination, balance, and range of motion Functions: problems with transfers, walking, and climbing stairs
Activities	Difficulty bathing, toileting, dressing, cooking, driving, or dancing
Participation	Loss of capacity to work, attend spiritual gatherings, volunteer
Personal factors	Decreased motivation, fear of falling, limited resiliency, negative self-perception of physical limitations
Environmental factors	Limited social support, few community or institutional resources for exercise or transportation, low neighborhood walkability, high general environmental demands

in life roles, such as shopping for family members. Mobility disability is often defined by functional limitations in walking, transferring, or climbing stairs, which are caused by problems with strength, endurance, coordination, balance, and range of motion. Impaired dual-task capacity, such as attending to cognitive tasks while walking, is another clinical manifestation of mobility disability. These functional limitations can be caused by numerous pathologic processes at the body structure level. Mobility disability can precipitate a cycle of negative consequences because it often leads to decreased activity, which in turn worsens functional limitations and causes organ system deconditioning, including muscle weakness, loss of joint range of motion, and poor cardiovascular endurance. Whether or not an individual is classified as having mobility disability can be modified by psychological, social, and environmental factors.

Classification Methods for Mobility

Mobility classification is often driven by a tacit assumption of orderedness. Few single current instruments assess the full range of mobility from the lowest levels of rolling over in bed to the highest levels of endurance and coordination required for athletics or dance. The Patient-Reported Outcomes Measurement Information System (PROMIS®) measures, an NIH-funded initiative, include both computer-adaptive tests and fixed short forms that are highly comprehensive assessments of domains, such as mobility. These batteries are used in both research

and clinical practice. Mobility assessment tools for older adults generally address one or more of the following three mobility levels: nonambulatory, ambulatory, and vigorous, corresponding broadly to Tinetti's levels of frail, transitional, and vigorous mobility status. Mobility levels are surprisingly stable. While day-to-day variability does occur, people in general tend to remain in one level or decline very gradually unless a major event has occurred. Within the nonambulatory level, there are important mobility skills that affect independence in personal care activities, care needs, and demand for human help; these activities include bed mobility, self-transfer skills, and wheelchair mobility. Within the vigorous mobility level, the degree of fitness, as represented by the ability to perform demanding or challenging mobility activities, may be a useful indicator of the extent of physiologic reserve. As an indicator of the extent of physiologic reserve, vigorous mobility status may be a marker of ability to tolerate physiologic stressors such as acute illness, surgery, or periods of reduced activity.

Mobility can be assessed by self-report, professional observation, or performance-based measures. Instruments to assess mobility from all three perspectives have been developed. We selected instruments with established reliability and validity for use with older adults (**Table 50-2**). Each has advantages and disadvantages, including floor or ceiling effects. These tools have been used to estimate the population incidence and prevalence of mobility disorders, predict the consequences of mobility problems, screen patient populations, determine care needs, and determine reimbursement of services in rehabilitation settings. More detailed instruments have been developed specifically for sorting out causes and mechanisms. Detailed instruments for diagnosing the etiology of mobility limitations will be discussed separately in the section on causes of mobility limitations. Mobility measures have varying strengths and limitations, depending on characteristics such as reliability and validity, respondent burden, feasibility and convenience of use, and assessor skill required.

Self-report measures are the easiest type of measure to obtain when gathering data from large populations. Self-report measures have high face validity in that they reflect the opinion of the person themselves. Various self-reported walking measures predict performance of functional mobility in older adults. Since self-report measures usually ask about a period of time, such as recent weeks or months, they can identify fluctuating ability over time. Self-report measures can be limited by problems with reliability, accuracy, and nonresponse. Because these are usually ordinal scales, they lack ability to discriminate small but important differences.

Professional observation measures reflect the opinion of an experienced assessor and may be more feasible when an individual is considered an unreliable informant or is unable to cooperate with testing (eg, individuals with severe cognitive decline). Professional report is limited by

TABLE 50-2 ■ INSTRUMENTS USED TO SCREEN AND CLASSIFY MOBILITY

INSTRUMENT NAME	RANGE	ITEMS	SCORING	MEANINGFUL VALUES/COMMENTS
SELF-REPORT MEASURES				
Patient-Reported Outcomes Measurement Information System (PROMIS®) mobility domain	Nonambulatory, ambulatory, and vigorous	Items vary from low-demand mobility tasks, such as standing, to high-demand tasks like dancing energetically or running 10 miles	Items scored based on Likert scale of ability to complete tasks. Scoring varies per format, but higher scores indicate better function	Administered as a short, fixed form or with computer-adaptive testing
Avlund mobility; Mob-T and Mob-H	Nonambulatory, ambulatory, and vigorous	Report of fatigue (Mob-T) and need for help (Mob-H) in six activities, from transfers to stairs and walking outside	Score of 1 given for each item subject can complete without help/fatigue; range 0–6 with 6 indicating independence in all tasks	
Mobility modifications	Ambulatory	Report of changing the way one walks ½ mile or climbs stairs	Not applicable	Identifies preclinical mobility limitations
Rosow-Breslau	Ambulatory to vigorous	Complete heavy household work, walk ½ mile, climb 12 stairs	Score of "1" given for each item reported unable to be done	Can be used as single items
Short Form 36 (SF-36), physical function subscale	Ambulatory to vigorous	Ten items, many directly related to mobility, from walk across a room to walk 1 mile	Weighted Likert scale transformed from 0 (negative health) to 100 (positive health)	Insensitive at lower levels of mobility
PERFORMANCE-BASED MEASURES				
Long-term care survey	Nonambulatory to ambulatory	Walking inside and bed/chair transfers	Not applicable	Can be used as single items
Barthel mobility items	Nonambulatory to ambulatory	Walking (or wheeling), transfers, and stairs	10 items scored 0/5/10/15 for total potential score of 100, 100 indicating independence in all tasks	Minimal clinically important difference 9.8 points
Functional independence measure (FIM)	Nonambulatory to ambulatory	Mobility-related items include transfers, locomotion (walk or wheelchair use, stairs), and activities of daily living	Each item scored from 0 (unable to perform) to 7 (performs independently)	Mandated for use for reporting and reimbursement in inpatient rehabilitation facilities until 2019
Minimum data set (MDS)	Nonambulatory to ambulatory	Bed mobility, transfers, locomotion (walking or wheelchair)	Each item scored from 0 (requires helper for full task) to 6 (requires no help)	Mandated for use for reporting and reimbursement in Medicare/Medicaid-certified skilled nursing facilities. Used as single items
Short Physical Performance Battery (SPPB)	Ambulatory	Timed 4-m walk, 5 chair rises, and 3 standing balance challenges	Walking and chair items scored 0–4 (4 being best) and balance items scored 0–1 or 2 (higher being better)	Substantial meaningful change is 1.0 point. Less than 10 points indicates risk of disability

(Continued)

TABLE 50-2 ■ INSTRUMENTS USED TO SCREEN AND CLASSIFY MOBILITY (CONTINUED)

INSTRUMENT NAME	RANGE	ITEMS	SCORING	MEANINGFUL VALUES/COMMENTS
Gait speed	Ambulatory	Timed walk	Varying distances, instructions, and procedures, like rolling vs standing start	Desired older adult speed > 1.2 m/s Slow walking < 0.6 m/s, very slow < 0.4 m/s Gait speed < 1.0 m/s indicates risk of future disability Small meaningful change in gait speed is 0.05 m/s, substantial meaningful change is 0.10 m/s
Timed Up and Go (TUG)	Ambulatory	Time to rise from chair, walk 10 feet, turn around, walk back, and sit down	Number of seconds to complete task once rater says "Go"	Other formats include TUG-cog to challenge dual tasking < 10 s normal < 20 s able to move in community > 30 s needs assistance for mobility
6-min walk test	Ambulatory to vigorous	Distance covered in 6 min	Completed in defined, uninterrupted area	Community ambulators should walk at least 300 m Small meaningful change is 20 m, substantial meaningful change is 50 m
Long distance corridor walk	Ambulatory to vigorous	Distance covered in 2 min, followed by time to complete 400 m walk	Completed in 20-m-long course	Each minute increase in time to complete test associated with 52% higher rate of mobility disability

the need for assessor experience and training and can be vulnerable to problems with inter-assessor reliability unless extensive efforts to standardize assessment are made. Since professional reports are usually based on ordinal scales, ability to discriminate small but important differences might be limited.

Performance-based measures are independent of assessor opinion. Most performance measures produce continuous quantitative results, which allow for discrimination of small but important or subclinical differences. Performance-based measures are limited in that they require direct observation, subject understanding and cooperation, and standardization of instructions and procedures. These tools measure capability rather than actual daily mobility activities (ie, the assessment of gait speed in a clinician's office is not a valid assessment of a person's gait speed at home). The need for subject cooperation can lead to problems with nonresponse. Performance-based measures do not account well for short-term fluctuations over hours to weeks. Despite these limitations, performance-based testing may have direct application in clinical settings because it is brief and can provide useful information.

Psychological aspects of fear, attention, mobility confidence, and activity avoidance can have great effect on mobility disability, separately or in combination with observable mobility limitations. Several instruments to assess psychological factors related to mobility disability have been developed (**Table 50-3**). Items from these scales might have use in the clinical setting.

EPIDEMIOLOGY

Prevalence

The epidemiology of mobility disability can be considered from the perspective of basic or higher-level mobility. Basic mobility problems map to the nonambulatory to ambulatory range; higher-level mobility problems map to the ambulatory to vigorous range.

Mobility disability increases dramatically with age; dependence in getting around inside increases from 5% of persons aged 65 to 74 years to 30% of persons aged 85 or older. Women tend to have higher rates of mobility disability than men, 30% compared to 23% of those 65 years and older. Racial differences exist in older adults as well; 34% of Blacks/African Americans, 23% of Asian Americans, 35% of other/multiracial background, and 25% of White people self-report experiencing mobility disability. Those with higher levels of depression report greater prevalence of mobility limitations.

Basic mobility problems include tasks such as getting around inside the house and transferring from bed or chair. Examples of higher-level mobility problems are getting around outside the house, ability to walk one-quarter or one-half mile, and ability to climb stairs. Basic mobility problems are uncommon in community-dwelling older persons but are very frequent in institutionalized older people. Among community-dwelling persons aged 65 and older, approximately 5% are dependent in getting in and out of a chair or bed and 7.5% are dependent in getting around inside. Among institutionalized persons older than

TABLE 50-3 ■ INSTRUMENTS TO ASSESS PSYCHOLOGICAL FACTORS RELATED TO MOBILITY		
INSTRUMENT NAME	**SCORING**	**COMMENTS**
FEAR		
"Are you afraid of falling?"	Yes/no	Community-dwelling older adults and those in long-term care
"How would you rate your fear of falling?"	Five-point numerical rating 0–4	Helps to provide further discrimination than dichotomous question
SELF-EFFICACY/CONFIDENCE		
Falls Efficacy Scale (FES)	Ten items, rated 1–10 with 1 very confident and 10 not confident at all	Community-dwelling older adults, those in inpatient rehabilitation, and those in long-term care > 80 increased risk of falling
Activities-Specific Balance and Confidence Scale (ABC)	Sixteen items rating confidence in doing multiple activities, scale 0–100 with 100 representing complete confidence	
Modified Gait Efficacy Scale (mGES)	Seven-item scale rated 1 (no confidence) to 10 (complete confidence) for walking activities	Spans walking on level surfaces to outdoor surfaces and long distances
AVOIDANCE		
"Has fear of falling made you avoid activities?"	Yes/no	
ATTENTION		
Digit Symbol Substitution Test	Scores range from 0 to 100, with higher scores indicating higher cognitive function	

65 years, approximately 80% are dependent in getting in and out of a chair or bed and getting around inside.

In the past decade, basic mobility problems have decreased in prevalence for those older than 85 years, while remaining stable for those aged 65 to 84 years old. The decline in prevalence observed in the oldest old may be due to decreasing rates of disability in some chronic diseases in late life; for example, arthritis and heart disease, the two diseases that have been most associated with increased disability, have become less disabling. With advances in the management of these conditions, progression is delayed; consequently, the disabling effect on mobility is reduced. At the same time, there has been an increase in the incidence of obesity and sedentary lifestyle in middle age and among young old: these are also major contributing factors to disability, and these trends may explain why there is not a reduction in disability among the younger old.

Higher-level mobility problems, defined as difficulty walking a quarter mile or climbing stairs, increase with age, are more common in women than in men, and appear to be decreasing. Approximately 13% of Americans older than 60 years report higher-level mobility problems in that they have difficulty going outside the home alone. There is a marked increase with age. There is also geographic variation; self-reported difficulty going outside the home alone is more common among older adults in the southern United States.

Risk of Adverse Consequences Associated with Mobility Status

Mobility problems have serious consequences. Mobility status predicts mortality. Older people with difficulty walking 2 km or climbing one flight of stairs are twice as likely to die during the next 8 years compared to those with no difficulty. Mortality risk is even higher among those who have mobility difficulty and are also physically inactive. Poor mobility performance, even in the absence of self-reported mobility limitations, is an independent predictor of death. Among persons who report no mobility problems, gait speed less than 1.0 m/s is associated with an increased risk of death. Older persons who have a 0.1 m/s decline in gait speed over 1 year have a double risk of dying during the subsequent 5 years, whereas older persons who have a 0.1 m/s improvement in gait speed over 1 year have a 40% decreased risk of dying in the following 8 years. Improving mobility through exercise is associated with reduced risk of future falls. In a pooled analysis of over 30,000 community-dwelling older adults, each 0.1 m/s faster gait speed was associated with a 13% reduction in risk of mortality.

Poor mobility performance is an independent predictor of future self-care difficulty and mobility disability. Among community-dwelling persons older than 70 years without disability, baseline physical performance score was a powerful predictor of incident disability in both activities of daily living and in higher-level mobility disability. Mobility self-report and performance have been shown to predict disability in older populations from numerous countries and cultures, including Mexican American, British, Italian, French, Dutch, Spanish, Scandinavian, Australian, Japanese, and Chinese.

Poor mobility performance is also an independent predictor of hospitalization and nursing home placement. In a population-based study of nondisabled older adults, poor baseline physical performance score was associated with a twofold increased risk of hospitalization and more days in the hospital over the following 4 years, independent of baseline health status. The risk was mostly associated with hospitalization for dementia, pressure ulcer, hip fractures, other fracture, pneumonia, and dehydration.

Mobility may be part of an underlying constellation of core factors that link multiple outcomes associated with aging. Poor mobility, as measured by timed chair stands, is one of four factors proposed to be common risk factors for geriatric syndromes (the others are incontinence, falls, and functional decline). Conversely, good mobility, along with good cognition and nutritional status, is an independent predictor of recovery of functional independence after a period of disability. Abnormalities of gait and slow gait speed have been found to precede the onset of cognitive decline and dementia, especially vascular dementia. Among older adults, simultaneous abnormalities of mobility, cognition, and mood are more common than would be expected by chance, perhaps implying potential common underlying causes.

Severe mobility disability, sometimes called immobility, has widespread and devastating consequences. It accelerates impairments in multiple organ systems, including bone, muscle, heart, circulation, lung, skin, blood, bowel, kidney, nutrition, and metabolism. Loss of organ system function can be rapid and severe; muscle strength can decline by 1% to 5% per day of enforced bed rest. Skin breakdown and pressure ulcers start to occur after only hours of persistent and unrelieved pressure. Major consequences of clinical significance include decreased plasma volume, orthostatic hypotension, accelerated loss of bone density, muscle weakness, decreased pulmonary ventilation, and constipation leading to fecal impaction. When even temporary bed rest is combined with the increased vulnerability of aging and acute illness, there is a marked increased risk of death, disability, and institutionalization.

PATHOPHYSIOLOGY

The causes of mobility problems are complex. Unique and complementary etiologic perspectives can all contribute to a better understanding of mobility. Three perspectives are described here: biomechanical, biomedical, and biopsychosocial. Each has advantages and disadvantages when used as frameworks to understand mobility problems.

Biomechanical Perspective: Direct Assessment of the Body in Motion

Age affects the biomechanics of walking. Normal gait can be defined in terms of the gait cycle with two main phases:

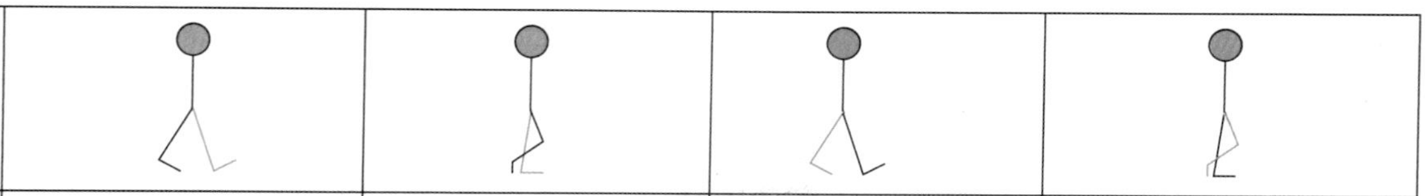

Right Lower Extremity (LE)	Heel strike	Stance	Toe off	Swing
Ankle Joint:	Neutral position (90°)	Neutral position (90°)	Plantar flexion for push off	Dorsiflexion for foot clearance
Muscles:	Ankle dorsiflexors active to support position of ankle	Plantar flexor torque drives foot into floor, ankle dorsiflexors eccentrically active to slow foot	Plantar flexors active	
	Weight rolls from heel to toe			
Knee Joint:	Extended to prepare for weight bearing	Slight knee flexion (shock absorbing) progressing to full extension for stable weight bearing	Extension progressing to passive knee flexion to prepare for swing	Knee flexion for foot clearance progressing to passive extension for limb advancement
Muscles:	Initially, knee extensors (quadriceps) active then both quadriceps and hamstrings active for knee stabilization	Quadriceps eccentrically active to decelerate knee flexion		Hamstrings and gastrocnemius active for knee flexion, relax for knee extension
Hip Joint:	Hip flexed ~30°	Progressive hip extension	Hyperextension of the hip progressing to hip flexion	Hip flexing to advance limb
Muscles:	Hip extensors active for stability	Hip extensors active initially; hip abductors active to keep pelvis neutral	Hip flexion initiated by hip abductors and hip flexors	Hip adductors and flexors active for swing, hamstrings active to terminate swing
Left LE*	Toe off	Swing	Heel strike	Stance
SUPPORT	Double support	Single support (right)	Double support	Single support (left)

*Note: When the right LE is at heel strike, the left LE is approaching toe off and vice versa. When the right LE is in stance the left LE is in swing and vice versa.

FIGURE 50-1. Human walking.

PART III

GERIATRIC CONDITIONS

stance and swing (**Figure 50-1**). A normal cycle begins with a push off from the forefoot, then a swing through and heel strike, timed tightly to be followed by the push off of the other leg; normal gait initiates at the ankle, not the hip. Normal gait has highly characteristic patterns of foot, ankle, knee, hip, pelvis, trunk, and arm motion. Gait biomechanics can also be viewed from the perspective of the pattern of steps (footprints) (**Figure 50-2**). Step length is the forward distance between two foot falls. Stride length is the distance covered by one foot until it falls again. Stride length is, therefore, twice the step length, assuming the step lengths are the same on both sides. Step width is the lateral distance between two foot falls. With age, gait speed slows, step length decreases, and the proportion of the gait cycle when both feet are in contact with the ground (double support time) increases. During gait, older people compared to young adults tend to have more thoracic kyphosis, more posterior pelvic tilt, decreased hip extension, and greater external rotation of the foot. Older people tend to generate less power from the ankle and use hip flexion to compensate more than young adults. Normal gait has a very regular spatial and temporal pattern. An irregular gait can be either regularly irregular, like a limp, or irregularly irregular, with no pattern at all (**Figure 50-3**). Irregularly irregular gait, often called gait variability, predicts falls and mobility disability.

Normal walking maximizes energy efficiency. When walking changes owing to biomechanical alterations caused by disease or aging, walking becomes more energy demanding. Normal walking also requires excellent control of balance and timing. When problems develop with balance and timing, the priority for safe walking may be to increase stability and support at the expense of losses of energy efficiency. Thus, many changes with aging increase the energy cost of walking and decrease gait efficiency.

A biomechanical perspective can be applied broadly to mobility and balance, based on the increasing biomechanical demand placed on the body in motion. Typically, tasks are considered more challenging as the base of support narrows and transfers of mass over the base become more demanding. Thus, difficulty increases from sitting to standing to walking, to climbing stairs, walking a line, or running. A biomechanical approach to postural alterations and body-segment movement abnormalities can be useful

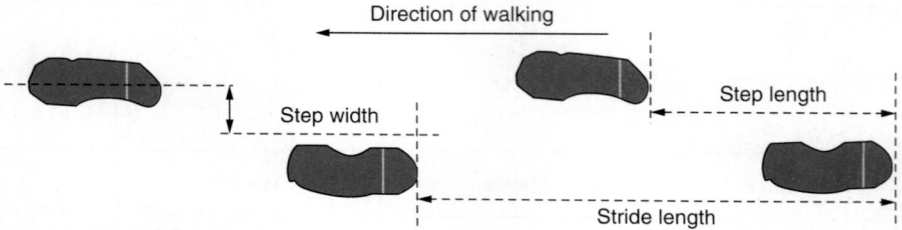

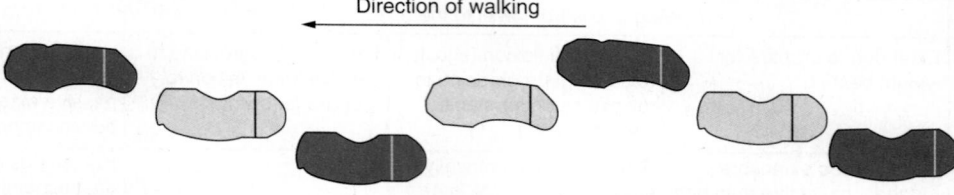

Step length = the distance between two consecutive footprints on opposite sides of the body.
Stride length = the distance between two consecutive footprints on the same side of the body.
Step width = the distance between the inner most borders of two consecutive footprints.

Dark-colored footprints represent foot placement during walking.
Quick clinical inspection for approximation of normal gait:
Step length = 1 step length between right and left steps (light-colored footprint).
Step width = 1 foot width (light-colored footprint) between right and left steps

FIGURE 50-2. Step patterns in human walking.

for identifying causes of, and solutions to, mobility problems. Specific abnormalities can be addressed by targeting rehabilitative programs or the type of assistive devices. Limitations to the biomechanical framework include lack of consideration of how various physiologic or external factors impact mobility problems.

A. Usual gait: right and left step lengths approximately equal.

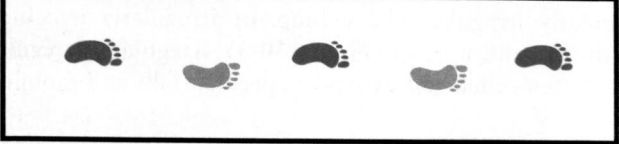

B. Asymmetric gait (limp): right step length consistently shorter than left step length. All left step lengths approximately equal and all right step length approximately equal.

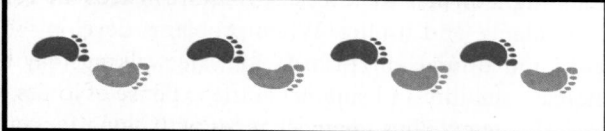

C. Variable gait: inconsistent right and left step lengths.

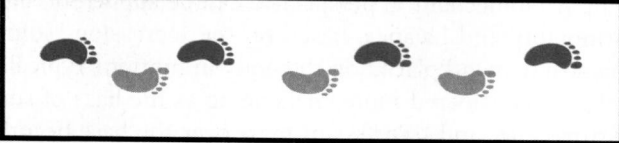

Blue = left foot prints, Grey = right foot prints

FIGURE 50-3. Gait patterns.

Biomedical Perspective: Using Organ System Impairment to Link Function and Disease

The causes of mobility limitation can be assessed from a physiologic standpoint. There are three main physiologic components of mobility: balance control (neurologic system), force production (cardiopulmonary and muscular systems), and structural support (skeletal system—bone and joints). Ferrucci created a framework that identifies six main physiologic subsystems that influence walking ability: central nervous system, perceptual system, peripheral nervous system, muscles, bones and joints, and energy production. Another way of organizing the systems that affect walking is to consider inputs and outputs. In this approach, the physiologic elements of mobility can be assigned to three main components based on a sequence of information from (1) sensory inputs to (2) central processing to (3) effector factors that carry out instructions from the brain. Sensory inputs include vision, vestibular function, and peripheral sensation. Central processing includes level of attention, rapid integration of sensory inputs, coordinated timing of multiple segmental body motions, and postural reflexes. Effector-related factors include generation of muscle strength and power, endurance, pain, speed of reaction, and flexibility. There are several important emerging areas of knowledge related to our understanding of the physiologic contributors to walking. Brain abnormalities found on magnetic resonance imaging (MRI) are associated with alterations in attention, rapid processing and integration of multiple sensorimotor inputs, and abnormal gait. Small vessel cerebrovascular disease in the absence of stroke and MRI findings of "white matter disease" or focal grey matter atrophy are associated with slower gait speed, even among high-functioning older adults. These MRI findings predict the onset of mobility disability. Such brain abnormalities appear to be most pronounced in the frontal areas and basal ganglia, regions that are most vulnerable to changes in cerebral perfusion with older age. These areas have been found to concurrently affect mobility, cognition, and mood and may suggest a shared underlying cerebrovascular process. Another emerging area of knowledge is related to subclinical losses of dopaminergic transmission in the brain in the aged. These losses of dopaminergic function also contribute to altered mobility and may present clinically in patterns that differ from traditional Parkinson disease. Dopamine deficiency in the aged may be related to cerebrovascular disease. Loss of oxygen-carrying capacity because of anemia has been recognized as a potential contributor to mobility limitations, especially in Caucasians, perhaps owing to decreased endurance but also possibly because of chronic subclinical ischemic effects on the brain. Disorders of glucose regulation, including poorly controlled diabetes, may also affect the integrity of brain motor areas and compromise mobility control. Research on the links among cardiovascular risk factors, brain structural abnormalities, mobility, cognition, and mood is developing rapidly. In the future, it may be possible to refine these observations into diagnosable and possibly treatable disorders. It is possible that attention to cardiovascular and metabolic risk factors might reduce the risk of developing some of these brain abnormalities and thus potentially reduce the incidence of mobility problems.

A physiologic perspective on mobility helps define organ system impairments, which can be linked to treatable diseases, conditions, and pathologic processes, as described by the disablement process in **Table 50-1**. A physiologic perspective is also helpful when accounting for the multiple interacting health problems of many older adults. When more than one organ system that is important for mobility is impaired, the risk of mobility problems increases. Thus, mobility can be affected when one system is severely disrupted, when several are modestly disrupted or when many are mildly disrupted. A physiologic perspective also helps account for the phenomenon of stress-induced disability. Organ systems have excess capacity, called physiologic reserve. Losses of organ system function can be clinically unapparent because these are losses of unused reserve or because one system is compensating for another. Many subclinical physiologic losses may not be recognized until stress is placed on the system by further physiologic decline or by an unexpected high demand on the system. When sufficient reserve is lost or a compensating organ system fails, mobility disability becomes overt. For example, when persons with many subclinical physiologic losses face an unexpected mobility demand, such as walking on ice at night, they may face a demand that is greater than their mobility capacity. Mobility reserve can now be assessed. One way to challenge reserve is to perform simultaneous physical and cognitive tasks. Described as "dual tasks," older individuals may deteriorate significantly when asked to walk and talk or walk and perform a mental calculation. Mobility tests that incorporate obstacles also assess reserve. Tests of gait variability may be another way to detect subclinical change in mobility.

A physiologic perspective can help define interventions, based on the disablement structure described in **Table 50-1**. Treatments could be aimed at managing the underlying pathologic conditions that are causing the impairment (eg, improving cardiac ejection fraction through treatment of congestive heart failure), treating the impairments themselves (eg, strength training), or creating compensations and adaptations at the level of functional limitations (such as using a cane). A physiologic approach offers a constructive way to connect biomechanical and clinical mobility assessment to a biomedical model of diagnosis and treatment. The individual is the focus of the biomedical model, however, and addressing biomechanical and clinical factors may improve the physiologic impairments of mobility problems but not address mobility disability.

Biopsychosocial Perspective: Addressing Personal, Social, and Environmental Contributions

The experience of mobility disability can be viewed as mismatched personal capacities (physiologic and psychologic) and social and environmental demands. Psychological factors that influence mobility include negative attitudes toward aging, fear of falling, and poor attention and emotional vitality. Self-reported conditions associated with increased risk of new higher-level mobility disability include baseline and incident heart attack and stroke, baseline hypertension, diabetes, angina, dyspnea, exertional leg pain and incident cancer, and hip fracture. Epidemiologic risk factors for the onset of higher-level mobility disability include demographics, diseases, and health behaviors. Among the demographic factors associated with increased risk, advancing age has the strongest effect, with lower income, and lower educational level also playing a role. Behavior-related risk factors include current smoking, alcohol abstention, low physical activity, high body mass index, and high waist circumference. Exposure to some of these factors as early as in mid-life can influence development of disability later in life. Physical activity, a health behavior that is a key to mobility, is influenced by multiple psychological, social, and environmental factors. Common reasons given by older adults for limiting or avoiding physical activity include lack of an exercise companion, lack of interest, fatigue, fear of falling, weather, and safety. Self-reported conditions identified as major barriers to physical activity by older adults include arthritis and past injury.

Environmental demands can exacerbate mobility limitations or reinforce positive behaviors. The experience of disability is lessened when older adults' physical capacities match the challenges present. An overly challenging environment reduces access, for example, an ambulatory older adult who struggles with stairs cannot enter a restaurant which lacks a ramp. Alternatively, inappropriate simplification of environments reinforces maladaptive behaviors with negative health consequences, for example, use of a power lift chair by an individual with intact lower extremity strength reduces use of leg muscles, potentially initiating muscle mass loss and resulting in difficulty standing from chairs without assistance. Social support follows a similar pattern. Too little social support increases mobility disability, whereas inappropriately high support diminishes opportunities to reduce development of mobility limitations.

Advantages of the biopsychosocial model include a holistic view of all influencing factors related to mobility disability. Disadvantages are the complexity in identifying, evaluating, and intervening on disposing factors.

Gait Speed as an Integrator of Multiple Approaches

Walking is the foundation of mobility, is influenced by biomechanical and physiologic processes and environmental factors and is a major driver of disability. Walking speed is considered a "vital sign" in older adults. While there are several influences on measures of gait speed such as leg length, gender, or periods of acceleration and deceleration, in general, gait speed can be interpreted clinically. Normal usual walking speed in the older adult should be at least 1 m/s. When measuring a fixed walk distance, this means that the time should be less than the distance in meters. For example, a 4-m walk time should be less than 4 seconds. When measuring a fixed time, this means that the distance should be more than the time in seconds. For example, the distance walked in a 6-minute walk (360 seconds) should be more than 360 m. The normal step frequency of walking (called the cadence) is a little more than two steps per second or somewhat more than 120 steps per minute. With approximately two steps per second at a normal pace of 1 m/s, there is approximately 0.5 m or 20 in. in a step. Clinically, this translates into approximately two shoe-lengths per step, or an imaginary "shoe" in between each step (see **Figure 50-2**).

As a general rule, there are links among walking speed, energy expenditure, and disability. Energy expenditure can be measured in metabolic equivalents (METs). One MET is the energy requirement for lying in bed. Two METs is twice the energy requirement for lying in bed and is approximately the energy requirement for self-care activities. The usual energy cost in METs of walking at various speeds has been reported in relationship to miles per hour, and walking speed can be translated directly between meters per second and miles per hour. Therefore, the energy requirements in METs and the expected activity level can be associated with gait speed, as described in **Table 50-4**. This conversion table allows clinicians and researchers to approximate the functional status of individuals or populations based

TABLE 50-4 ■ TRANSLATING WALKING SPEED: WALKING SPEED, METS, AND FUNCTION

WALKING SPEED				
M/S	MPH	6-MIN WALK DISTANCE (M)	METS	FUNCTION
0.67	1.5	240	< 2	Self-care
0.89	2.0	320	2.5	Household activities
1.0	2.2	360	2.7	
1.1	2.5	400	3.0	Carry groceries and light yard work
1.3	3.0	480	3.5	Climb several flights of stairs

METs, metabolic equivalents.

on any measure of gait speed. Using METs as a basis for function, a sequence of mobility capacities is described in **Table 50-5**.

EVALUATION

Strategy for the Clinical Encounter

There are no established standards for the overall evaluation and treatment of mobility problems in older adults. Currently, the most common approach is similar to the ones used for other geriatric syndromes. These approaches are all based on a biopsychosocial model that incorporates

TABLE 50-5 ■ EXAMPLE OF A SEVEN-LEVEL CLASSIFICATION OF MOBILITY BASED ON ENERGY EXPENDITURE

Level 1	Able to perform sustained physical activity for at least 30 min at a vigorous pace like running, jogging, and tennis. Greater than 4 METs, sustained activity
Level 2	Able to perform sustained physical activity for at least 60 min at a usual pace like walking 1 or more miles. 3.5–4 METs, sustained activity
Level 3	Able to perform physical activity at a usual pace for at least 15 min like walking 1/2 mile. 2.5–3.5 METs, limited duration of activity
Level 4	Physical activity limited. Able to walk one block. May have slowed gait speed. May use an assistive device like a cane to walk. 2.0–2.5 METs
Level 5	Physical activity limited. May have difficulty walking one block but able to walk across a room. May use assistive device like a cane or a walker. < 2 METs
Level 6	Mobility severely limited. Requires wheelchair for indoor mobility. Transfers independently. 1.5 METs
Level 7	Mobility profoundly limited; requires assistance with transfers from chair or bed. 1 MET

METs, metabolic equivalents.

biomedical, rehabilitative, and psychosocial elements and a multidisciplinary team. The initial goal of assessment is to classify the mobility problem into one of three large groups: **nonambulatory, ambulatory, or vigorous**. For the person who presents in a wheelchair or bed, one can screen for ability to stand or walk with assistance. For ambulatory individuals, a quick sorting strategy is to observe gait. Since most gait parameters are highly interrelated, abnormal gait can be grossly distinguished from normal by a few simple characteristics like use of a gait aid, gait speed less than 1 m/s (or step length less than twice foot length), or step asymmetry. Persons with normal gait can be assessed for higher level fitness by use of one or more screening tests for higher level abilities such as single foot stand for 30 seconds, ability to tandem walk or ability to walk more than 450 to 500 m in 6 minutes. Persons with normal walking but inability to perform higher level tasks might be good candidates for exercise programs for well elders or for further evaluation if the mobility change is recent or causing problems.

Further assessment of the nonambulatory or for those with abnormal gait depends in part on the treatment goals. The team can select a basic strategy; either to try to improve mobility or to compensate for irreversible mobility loss (**Figure 50-4**). This decision is based on patient preferences, the time course of the mobility loss, the potential to reverse impairments, and the ability of the patient to participate in treatment. For example, a person with severe cognitive deficits or severe irreversible motor paralysis might be considered more appropriate for compensation than for interventions to improve mobility. Planning for compensation might target mobility care needs and resources. For the person considered to have potential for improving mobility, the major decisions are the timing and value of interventions directly on mobility (usually through exercise and rehabilitation) and on underlying physiologic impairments (usually through medical team care). In primary care, the provider can screen and triage function by recognizing mobility disorders, assessing potential for intervention, and referring to other providers as appropriate.

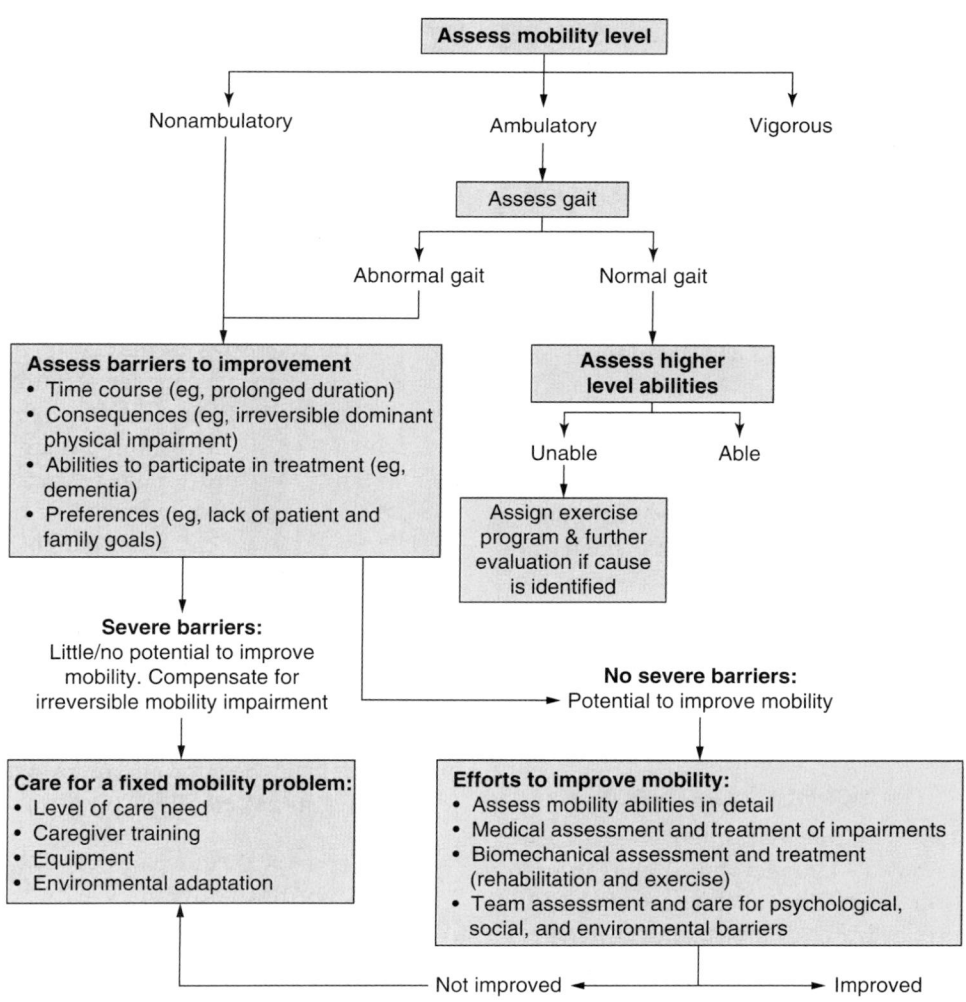

FIGURE 50-4. A clinical strategy for assessment and management of mobility problems.

TABLE 50-6 ■ BRIEF EVALUATION OF MOBILITY PROBLEMS FOR USE IN PRIMARY CARE

SYSTEM	SYMPTOMS LIMITING WALKING	CLINICAL FINDINGS
Cardiopulmonary (lung, heart, and blood)	Dyspnea and fatigue	FEV_1, O_2 saturation with activity, hemoglobin, and ejection fraction
Neurologic (frontal, motor, extrapyramidal, and peripheral)	Unsteady and hesitant	Tone, timed tapping, executive cognitive function, and peripheral sensation
Musculoskeletal (bones and joints, muscles)	Pain and stiffness	Knee, hip, low back range of motion, and pain. Manual muscle tests and chair rise

Table 50-6 gives examples of a quick system of assessment for symptoms and clinical findings based on the three main involved organ systems. The primary provider can identify and treat overt clinical impairments that can be detected quickly in the clinic, like weight-bearing pain caused by osteoarthritis, or dyspnea caused by congestive heart failure. When the cause of the mobility problem is less obvious, a referral to multidisciplinary team for comprehensive mobility assessment should be considered. Since the potential causes range across many organ systems, this strategy might be more efficient than referral to several organ system–based specialists. Research into mobility problems is an active and high-priority area in aging; in the future, efficient clinical practice and referral may be better informed by evidence.

The comprehensive approach to the clinical assessment of treatable causes of mobility is currently a specialized referral function that is resource intensive. Evaluation starts with the clinical assessment of the severity, course and consequences of mobility limitation, and the determination of potential to improve mobility. Mobility performance is assessed in more detail, including biomechanical aspects of functional limitations during movement. Potential contributing factors are identified based on physiologic impairments, and evidence is sought for psychosocial and environmental influences.

Clinical Assessment of Mobility Performance

In ambulatory patients, simple assessment of gait speed is a useful place to start. The gait speed can be used to estimate function as described above. Gait can be assessed in more detail from a biomechanical perspective (**Table 50-7**). Gait can be examined for general characteristics like path deviations, irregular or variable stepping, or a widened base of support and for altered motion of the component parts: trunk, arms, hip, knee,

ankle, and foot. Mobility tasks can be examined for performance difficulty or altered movement patterns as task demands increase. Sometimes, the finding of an abnormal body-segment movement or gait characteristic suggests a specific impairment or disease. More often, the abnormality is nonspecific but is amenable to direct intervention in rehabilitation. Clinical gait assessments that capture many of these biomechanical elements (eg, variable stepping, path deviation, hip range of motion, arm swing) are the modified Gait Abnormality Rating Scale and the Tinetti Performance Oriented Mobility Assessment.

Mobility assessment scales usually have a functional rather than a biomedical perspective and are not designed to detect specific impairments. These scales can be used to identify areas for task practice or adaptation in rehabilitation and to assess the effects of treatment. When selecting an assessment tool, level of mobility of the patient should be considered. For nonambulatory patients, assessments should focus on bed mobility and transfers. The Hierarchical Assessment of Balance and Mobility assesses mobility, transfers, and balance and detects multiple levels within the bed and chair. For ambulatory patients, assessments should focus on walking including unchallenged (straight path walking) and some challenged walking. For patients with vigorous mobility, assessments should focus on more challenging walking tasks such as uneven surfaces, obstacles, curved paths, dual task, and walking for longer distances. Some clinical measures focus on one mobility group (ie, nonambulatory) but many clinical assessments of mobility are based on a hierarchy of task difficulty and will span the various mobility groups. One such measure, the Berg Balance Scale, assesses 14 tasks of progressive difficulty from sitting balance to one leg standing and rising onto a step. The Physical Disability Index has eight mobility tasks including six items for nonambulatory persons. The Activity Measure for Post-Acute Care (AM-PAC) was developed specifically for use across post-acute care settings (from inpatient to outpatient settings) and can also capture a range of mobility. The AM-PAC is based on patient responses and clinician observation, and captures three domains: basic mobility, daily activities, and applied cognitive. The Dynamic Gait Index, which includes eight challenging gait items such as changing gait speed, walking with head turns, and stepping over an obstacle, may be appropriate for patients with higher level (ie, vigorous) mobility.

Differential Diagnosis Based on a Physiologic Perspective

A clinical schema for the comprehensive evaluation of mobility that is derived from Ferrucci, Tinetti, and the authors' own work is proposed in **Table 50-8**. Many impairments are detectable through the usual geriatric clinical history and physical examination. Some sensory

TABLE 50-7 ■ EXAMPLES OF A BIOMECHANICAL ASSESSMENT OF COMMON GAIT ABNORMALITIES AND POSSIBLE CAUSES

GAIT ELEMENT	GAIT ABNORMALITY	POSSIBLE CAUSES
BODY SEGMENTS		
Ankle and foot	Forefoot strikes floor simultaneously with initial heel contact (foot slap)	Weak ankle dorsiflexors and decreased proprioception
	Initial contact is by forefoot	Leg length discrepancy, plantar flexion contracture, and painful heel
	Heel and toe leave floor together during push off	Fixed ankle, weak plantar flexors, and painful forefoot
	Forefoot drags during swing (foot drop)	Weak ankle dorsiflexors
	Tendency to roll from plantar to medial surface of the foot while walking	Weak lateral ankle stabilizers and varus knee deformity
Knee	Knee flexed at initial contact	Painful knee, weak knee extensors, leg length discrepancy, and knee flexion contracture
	Decreased knee extension during swing	Knee pain or decreased range
	Hyperextension of the knee in stance	Weak knee extensors
Hip	Decreased hip flexion at initial contact	Weak hip flexors and decreased range of motion
	Increased hip flexion during swing (steppage gait)	Compensation for foot drop
	Decreased hip extension during late stance	Hip flexion contracture
	Hip circumduction with lateral movement of entire limb	Weak hip flexors and inability to flex leg
	Pelvis drops on one side, lateral instability when walking	Contralateral hip abductor or gluteus weakness
	Excessive elevation of the ipsilateral side of the pelvis during swing (hip/pelvic hiking)	Inadequate hip or knee flexion or excessive plantar flexion
GAIT PATTERN		
Gait initiation	Hesitation	Parkinson disease, frontal lobe disorders, and normal pressure hydrocephalus
Stance width	Increased	Cerebellar disorders and peripheral neuropathy
Path	Weaving	Vestibular disorders
	Scissoring (steps cross over laterally)	CNS disorders
	Increased variability	CNS disorders (eg, white matter hyperdensities and lacunar infarcts)

PART III

GERIATRIC CONDITIONS

systems are amenable to clinical evaluation. Some impairments are hard to detect in the clinic and require further testing. Vestibular testing may be helpful when there is unsteadiness that is not well explained by other impairments or when specific vestibular symptoms are present. Electrodiagnostic testing of nerve conduction velocity or abnormal muscle activity may be indicated when neurologic findings are suspicious. Exertional chest pain or dyspnea requires appropriate cardiac and pulmonary testing and a screen for anemia. Leg pain on exertion suggests testing for peripheral vascular disease or lumbar stenosis.

Psychosocial and Environmental Assessment

Mobility limitations are influenced by psychological, social, and environmental factors (**Table 50-9**). Depression can have a powerful effect on the desire to be mobile. Fear of falling, lack of confidence, lower attention, and low self-efficacy can also adversely influence a person's mobility. Screens for these conditions can include a single question or multiple questions

(see **Table 50-3**) and should be part of a comprehensive mobility assessment. Apathy and lack of motivation are a common concern in geriatric rehabilitation. Formal and informal social support resources can be critical for the person with mobility limitations. Cultural and financial factors can influence attitudes toward disability and resources for addressing the problem. The safety and accessibility of the living environment can be a barrier or facilitator for persons with mobility problems. Self-report measures, such as the life-space mobility questionnaire, quantify how often and with what level of difficulty older adults engage with progressively wider environments (eg, leaving bedroom, going outside, traveling beyond neighborhood, etc.). A home visit for assessment can offer many opportunities for creative problem solving.

In recent years, mobile health technologies, such as wearable devices and smartphones, have become widely used to monitor physical activity in the person's own environment. These devices could also be used to gain insights into spatiotemporal parameters of gait.

TABLE 50-8 ■ ASSESSMENT AND TREATMENT OF ORGAN OR SYSTEM IMPAIRMENTS THAT CAUSE MOBILITY PROBLEMS

FUNCTIONAL DOMAIN	ORGAN SYSTEM	IMPAIRMENT	ASSESSMENT	RELATED CAUSES	TREATMENT
Sensory	Eye	Acuity	Near and far by Snellen chart	Presbyopia and cataracts	Lenses and surgery
	Eye	Peripheral vision	Confrontation	Glaucoma and stroke	Prisms
	Eye	Depth	Depth testing	Monocular	Lighting, contrast, and avoid multifocal lens while walking
	Eye	Dark adaptation	Self-report	Miotic agents for glaucoma	Change medications and lighting
	Vestibular	Otoliths	Self-report of inappropriate spinning sensation, generally lasting 1–2 minutes	Benign positional vertigo	Canalith repositioning maneuver (formerly Eppley maneuver) and vestibular rehabilitation
	Vestibular	Semicircular canals	Ability to perceive rotation and acceleration	Ménière disease	Medications and vestibular rehabilitation
	Peripheral nerve	Neuropathy	Filaments and vibratory sense	Diabetes and peripheral vascular disease	Haptic enhancement (see text) and footwear
Central	Circulation	Decreased brain perfusion	Hypotension and orthostasis	Medications, arrythmias, postprandial hypotension, and dehydration	Change medications, anti-arrythmics, or pacemaker; increase fluid intake
	Brain	Processing speed	Level of attention, Digit Symbol Substitution Test, and Trail Making B Test	Medications and CNS disorders (white matter hyperdensities, focal atrophy, and brain infarcts)	Change medication, exercise, and blood pressure control
	Brain	Postural reflexes	Righting reflexes	Parkinson disease and other CNS disorders diseases	Trial of anti-Parkinson medications
Effector	Muscle	Strength	Manual muscle tests and strength-based motions (chair rise and squat)	Multiple neurologic conditions and inactivity	Exercise, bracing, and medication adjustment
	Musculoskeletal	Flexibility	Contractures and range of motion (ROM)	Injury, arthritis, and inactivity	Active and passive ROM and orthotics
	Heart endurance	Cardiomyopathy	Dyspnea at rest or on exertion, fluid retention, and echocardiogram	Systolic or diastolic dysfunction	Standard care for systolic and diastolic dysfunction
	Lung endurance	Hypoxia or reduced air flow	Dyspnea rest or on exertion, hypoxia, and decreased peak flow	Chronic obstructive pulmonary disease, asthma, and other lung	Standard pulmonary care and oxygen
	Circulation endurance	Peripheral vasculature	Leg pain on exertion, decreased pulses, and bruits	Arteriosclerosis and venous insufficiency	Medical and surgical, and exercise
	Hematologic endurance	Anemia	Dyspnea or fatigue on exertion	Multiple causes	Treat based on cause and transfusion for severe
	Muscle endurance	Sarcopenia	Leg fatigue on exertion	Inactivity	Exercise and possibly trophic agents in the future
	Musculoskeletal pain	Bone and joint deficits	Weight-bearing pain	Osteoarthritis, osteoporotic fractures, periarticular conditions, and foot problems	Pain medications, injections, assistive devices, and orthoses
	Neurologic pain	Spinal cord, roots, and nerves	Leg and back pain with activity	Spinal stenosis, radiculopathies, peripheral neuropathies, and CNS disorders	Injections, surgery, and medications

TABLE 50-9 ■ PSYCHOSOCIAL AND ENVIRONMENTAL ASSESSMENT AND MANAGEMENT OF MOBILITY

AREA	TYPE	ASSESSMENT	MANAGEMENT
Psychological	Depression	Standard screen (see Chapter 65)	Antidepressants and counseling
	Self-efficacy	Interview	Counseling
	Motivation	Interview and observation	Stimulants and social therapies
	Attention	Standard test	Counseling, social therapies
Social	Emotional and instrumental supports	Interview	Community programs and family engagement
	Culture	Interview	Cultural consultation
	Finances	Interview	Community resources
Environment	Physical barriers	Home visit	Environmental adaptations
	Access	Interview and home visit	Community programs

MANAGEMENT

Intervening Directly on Mobility

Interventions directed at functional limitations are often rehabilitative in nature and involve exercise, adaptive equipment, and environmental modifications. Mobility limitations can be addressed through mobility task practice and exercise to improve specific impairments in strength, balance, endurance, and/or flexibility. Deconditioning is almost always present as a direct consequence of reduced mobility and inactivity, and deconditioning has been found to be treatable in many older adults who are sick or frail. General conditioning programs of exercise are frequently indicated. Task-specific exercises and assistive and orthotic devices can improve stability and reduce weight-bearing pain. The evidence for the effectiveness of rehabilitation and exercise interventions is growing and has been examined in older adults with varying levels of mobility limitations. In general, increasing the amount of time spent walking, even at moderate pace and in the absence of direct cardiovascular beneficial effects, can improve mobility and reduce disability. Recent studies suggest that a focus on neural control of walking through the development of progressively more complex motor skills may be especially effective in improving walking speed and the energy efficiency of walking. Chapter 55 on rehabilitation and Chapter 54 on exercise present these interventions in more detail.

Treating Impairments

Some impairments can be linked to diseases and pathologic processes that are amenable to medical treatment, and some impairments can be improved directly regardless of pathologic cause (see **Table 50-8**). Peripheral sensory disorders are often not correctable, but compensation can be achieved with lighting to improve visual information and increasing haptic feedback (for example, through use of a cane). Haptic perception is demonstrated by the remarkable decrease in sway with eyes closed, seen in persons with peripheral sensory or vestibular disorders,

when they are allowed even minimal, nonsupporting contact with a stable surface such as a table, wall, or assistive device. Shoe inserts that increase sensory feedback are in development.

Progress in rehabilitation technology demonstrates some beneficial effects on recovery of mobility after a stroke or other injuries. For example, individuals with unilateral cerebral lesions after stroke may improve symmetric stepping in walking following split-belt treadmill training, in which the legs move at different speeds to encourage post-training even stepping. Other technologies include body weight–supported treadmill training, although evidence indicates that robust physical therapy leads to similar benefits. These technological advancements can potentially revolutionize the approach to physical therapy for older adults.

The slowed gait of Parkinson disease can be responsive to medication although the balance disorder is not. Parkinson patients may move faster when medications are initiated and thus increase their risk of fall injury unless appropriate rehabilitative measures are coordinated. Likewise, current evidence indicates individuals with BPV benefit from a combination of the canalith repositioning maneuver and balance rehabilitation more than from the repositioning maneuver alone. From the lens of improving mobility limitations, most pharmacologic interventions work best in concert with rehabilitation.

Attention to Factors That Modify Behavior and Environment

The modifiable psychosocial factors that influence physical activity may offer opportunities to intervene (see **Table 50-9**). Depression can be managed medically or with psychotherapy. Social support and encouragement can be promoted through group activities. Exercise (ie, balance, strength training, Tai chi/dance) may reduce fear of falling without increasing the risk or frequency of falls. The beneficial effects of physical activity on mobility could also be indirect, for example because it promotes attention, alertness, mood, as well as increasing one's motivation to move better and more. Physical environmental adaptations in the home include ramps and railings, bathroom modifications, proper lighting, and strategic placement of stable furniture items. Further modifications are often indicated in institutional settings.

Care for the Immobile Person

Interventions to reduce the consequences of immobility include determining the level of care need and living setting, training others to properly position and move the patient, implementing a mobilization plan, use of pressure-reducing devices to prevent pressure ulcer, and, sometimes, using equipment to aid in transfers (see Chapter 46). Persons who are responsible for carrying out transfers of immobile patients, including health aides and family caregivers, need training in proper techniques that reduce injury to the patient and the assistant. Appropriate assistive devices, such as wheelchairs or powerchairs should be considered to increase environmental accessibility.

Absolute bed rest is almost never indicated and should be discouraged in all settings. Mobility-related activities such as scooting in bed, sitting up, and standing can promote improved physiologic function when walking is not feasible. Mobilization, including walking, has been shown to be feasible even in the intensive care setting and is associated with reduced intensive care unit delirium. An exception to routine mobilization might be for humanitarian reasons when an individual is actively dying, where routine mobilization might cause suffering without associated benefit. Mobilization, rather than bed rest, during hospitalization for acute illness has been one of the most consistently efficacious interventions in geriatric care units.

SUMMARY

Mobility disorders are widespread in older adults. Mobility limitations constrain many functions required for independent living and are powerful indicators of future problems. Mobility can be classified using simple screening. Evaluation starts with a triage function or simple measures like gait speed. Many common contributors to mobility limitations can be managed in the primary care setting. A comprehensive mobility evaluation is resource intensive and requires a multidisciplinary team. Evaluation and management include a biomechanical approach to function, a biomedical approach to the physiologic components of mobility, and a biopsychosocial and environmental approach to modifying factors.

FURTHER READING

Bevilacqua R, Maranesi E, Riccardi GR, et al. Non-immersive virtual reality for rehabilitation of the older people: a systematic review into efficacy and effectiveness. *J Clin Med.* 2019;8(11):1882.

Brach JS, VanSwearingen JM. Interventions to improve walking in older adults. *Curr Transl Geriatr Exp Gerontol Rep.* 2013;2(4).

Cohen JA, Verghese J. Gait and dementia. *Handb Clin Neurol.* 2019;167:419–427.

Ferrucci L, Bandinelli S, Benvenuti E, et al. Subsystems contributing to the decline in ability to walk: bridging the gap between epidemiology and geriatric practice in the InCHIANTI study. *J Am Geriatr Soc.* 2000;48:1618–1625.

Freedman VA, Spillman BC, Andreski PM, et al. Trends in late-life activity limitations in the United States: an update from five national surveys. *Demography.* 2013;50:661–671.

Fried LP, Bandeen-Roche K, Chaves PH, Johnson BA. Preclinical mobility disability predicts incident mobility disability in older women. *J Gerontol Med Sci.* 2000;55A: M43–52.

Guralnik JM, Ferrucci L, Simonsick EM, et al. Lower-extremity function in persons over the age of 70 years as a predictor of subsequent disability. *N Engl J Med.* 1995;332:556–561.

Jorstad EC, Hauer K, Becker C, et al. Measuring the psychological outcomes of falling: a systematic review. *J Am Geriatr Soc.* 2005;53:501–510.

Kendrick D, Kumar A, Carpenter H, et al. Exercise for reducing fear of falling in older people living in the community. *Cochrane Database Syst Rev.* 2014;11:CD009848.

Li KZH, Bherer L, Mirelman A, et al. Cognitive involvement in balance, gait and dual-tasking in aging: a focused review from a neuroscience of aging perspective. *Front Neurol.* 2018;9:913.

Moskowitz S, Russ DW, Clark LA, et al. Is impaired dopaminergic function associated with mobility capacity in older adults?. *Geroscience.* 2021;43(3):1383–1404.

Pahor M, Guralnik JM, Ambrosius WT, et al. Effect of structured physical activity on prevention of major mobility disability in older adults: the LIFE study randomized clinical trial. *JAMA.* 2014;311(23):2387–2396.

Peel NM, Kuys SS, Klein K. Gait speed as a measure in geriatric assessment in clinical settings: a systematic review. *J Gerontol A Biol Sci Med Sci.* 2013;68(1):39–46.

Perera S, Mody SH, Woodman RC, et al. Meaningful change and responsiveness in common physical performance measures in older adults. *J Am Geriatr Soc.* 2006; 54:743–749.

Rosano C, Rosso AL, Studenski SA. Aging, brain, and mobility: progresses and opportunities. *J Gerontol A Biol Sci Med Sci.* 2014;69(11):1373–1374.

Schaap LE, Koster A, Visser M. Adiposity, muscle mass, and muscle strength in relation to functional decline in older persons. *Epidemiol Rev.* 2013;35:51–65.

Studenski S, Perera S, Patel K, et al. Gait speed and survival in older adults. *JAMA.* 2011;305(1):50–58.

VanSwearingen JM, Studenski SA. Aging, motor skill, and the energy cost of walking: implications for the prevention and treatment of mobility decline in older persons. *J Gerontol A Biol Sci Med Sci.* 2014;69(11):1429–1436.

Warmerdam E, Hausdorff JM, Atrsaei A, et al. Long-term unsupervised mobility assessment in movement disorders. *Lancet Neurol.* 2020;19(5):462–470.

Wennberg AM, Savica R, Mielke MM. Association between various brain pathologies and gait disturbance. *Dement Geriatr Cogn Disord.* 2017;43(3–4):128–143.

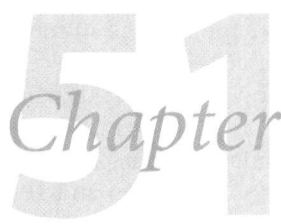

Chapter 51

Osteoporosis

Gustavo Duque, Mizhgan Fatima, Jesse Zanker, Bruce R. Troen

DEFINITION OF OSTEOPOROSIS

The term osteoporosis was first introduced in the nineteenth century based on histologic diagnosis ("porous bone"). Osteoporosis is a "disease characterized by low bone mass and microarchitectural deterioration of bone tissue leading to enhanced bone fragility and a consequent increase in fracture incidence." Osteoporosis may also be defined either by the presence of a fragility fracture (a fracture resulting from a fall from standing height or less) or by bone mineral density (BMD) measurement. In defining BMD criteria for osteoporosis, the World Health Organization (WHO) used as the standard the BMD of young adult women who were at the age of peak bone mass. For each standard deviation below peak bone mass (or 1 unit decrease in T-score), a woman's fracture risk approximately doubles. As seen in **Table 51-1**, a T-score less than −2.5 defines osteoporosis; osteopenia (low bone mass) and normal bone mass are also defined.

A BMD measurement may confirm the diagnosis of osteoporosis and indicates that interventions are needed prior to fracture in older adults. In addition, individuals with osteopenia could be still at risk of fractures. They, therefore, should be followed carefully for further bone loss while also promoting nonpharmacologic interventions that maintain bone health. Although the original standards for definitions of osteoporosis were determined in White women, the standards for men and Hispanic women are similar to those of White and African-American women. However, defining osteoporosis solely by T-score does not effectively capture all patients at risk of a fracture. Greater than 50% of all hip fractures occur in those with T-scores that are better than −2.5. Failure to evaluate and treat such patients adds to the individual and societal cost and consequences of osteoporosis. Therefore, we are still faced with the challenge of improving the identification of the individual patient at risk of fracture and subsequently optimizing both prevention and treatment for older adults.

Primary or idiopathic osteoporosis has been historically classified as postmenopausal or senile osteoporosis. Postmenopausal osteoporosis occurs in women between 51 and 75 years. It is related to estrogen deficiency seen with the menopausal transition, which associates with very high levels of bone resorption. In contrast, senile osteoporosis typically occurs in persons older than 60 years. It affects both men and women and has different pathophysiology, which involves reduced levels of bone turnover due to a reduction in the numbers of bone-forming cells (osteoblasts). Increasing evidence points to a progressive age-related alteration in stem cell physiology that favors adipogenesis and thereby reduces osteoblastogenesis and bone formation. Nevertheless, estrogen probably plays a role in the pathophysiology of senile osteoporosis as well. Secondary osteoporosis is the result of underlying conditions or medications that adversely affect bone. This chapter will focus on the typical characteristics of senile osteoporosis from its pathophysiology to therapeutic approaches.

Learning Objectives

- To understand the features of osteoporosis in older persons
- To identify fracture risk in older persons
- To learn fracture prevention strategies in older persons

Key Clinical Points

1. Both older men and women are at risk of osteoporotic fractures.
2. Fracture risk assessment, including clinical factors, should be performed in every person older than 65.
3. Calcium and vitamin D should be an essential component of any osteoporosis treatment.
4. Antiresorptives (bisphosphonates and denosumab) and anabolics (teriparatide and romosozumab) are effective and safe treatments for osteoporosis in older persons.

TABLE 51-1 ■ WORLD HEALTH ORGANIZATION CRITERIA FOR OSTEOPOROSIS	
WHO CLASSIFICATION	BMD T-SCORE
Normal	> −1
Osteopenia	≤ 1 but > −2.5
Osteoporosis	≤ −2.5
Severe osteoporosis	≤ −2.5 + fragility fracture

EPIDEMIOLOGY

Due to the increasing osteoporosis prevalence with age, the worldwide aging of the population and the changing lifestyle habits, the prevalence of osteoporosis has risen significantly and will continue to in the future. In 2018, the National Osteoporosis Foundation (NOF) announced that 54 million Americans, half of all adults age 50 and older, are at risk of breaking a bone and should be concerned about bone health; this means that approximately 10 million adults in the United States have osteoporosis, with an additional 43 million having low bone mass. In addition, women have more than 250,000 and 500,000 hip and spine fractures per year, respectively. Men account for an additional 250,000 fractures per year, of which 75,000 are hip fractures.

On reaching the age of 90, one-third of women and one-sixth of men will suffer a hip fracture. Both women and men have a similar lifetime vertebral fracture risk of 12%. The consequences of osteoporotic fracture include diminished quality of life (QoL), decreased functional independence, and increased morbidity and mortality. Pain and kyphosis, height loss, and other changes in body habitus resulting from vertebral compression fractures diminish the QoL in women and men. These changes lead to declines in functional status, such as the inability to bathe, dress, or ambulate independently and decrease pulmonary and gastrointestinal function. Approximately 50% of women do not fully recover prior function after hip fracture; older adults have 20% to 25% mortality in the year following hip fracture. Indeed, men are at a higher risk of dying after a hip fracture than women. Osteoporosis-related bone breaks cost patients, their families, and the health care system. The estimated annual cost of osteoporotic fractures in the United States is more than $22 billion, and by 2025 the NOF predicts that osteoporosis will be responsible for 3 million fractures costing $25 billion annually, which is higher than the money spent treating cardiovascular disease. Therefore, prevention and early diagnosis and treatment of osteoporosis are vital to improving the health of older adults.

PATHOPHYSIOLOGY

New advances in understanding bone physiology have elucidated an active interaction among bone and bone marrow cells, growth factors, and hormones responsible for maintaining calcium levels, skeletal structure, and resistance to trauma. Bone is not simply a mineralized structure but a complex system of cell–cell, cell–matrix, and cell–hormone interactions influenced by genetic background, lifestyle, and diet.

Bone is composed of inorganic (calcium phosphate crystals) and organic compounds (90% collagen and 10% noncollagenous proteins). Noncollagenous proteins include albumin, osteopontin, osteocalcin, α2-HS-glycoprotein, and growth factors, constituting the so-called bone matrix. The bone matrix is produced by osteoblasts and is the environment in which bone and external factors interact in a well-coordinated manner. There are two types of bone: cortical and trabecular. Cortical bone predominates in the long bones of the extremities, while trabecular bone predominates in the vertebrae and pelvis and makes up 80% of skeletal mass. While both types of bone have an active remodeling process, trabecular bone is metabolically more active than cortical bone and more acutely responsive to alterations in sex steroid hormone status. The bone marrow is also a complex environment in which bone cells interact with hematopoietic and marrow adipose tissues (**Figure 51-1**), playing an essential role in regulating bone turnover.

During childhood and adolescence, skeletal growth occurs at growth plates, areas in which cartilage proliferates and gradually undergoes calcification, resulting in new bone formation. However, bone remodeling is a lifelong process that maintains bone to harbor bone marrow, support the body, protect vital organs, and provide a source of minerals. Remodeling replaces older, frailer bone with newer, more resilient bone in an organized manner. The end product of remodeling is the maintenance of skeletal homeostasis and the preservation of anatomical integrity. With aging or with menopausal transition, the once-coordinated mechanism of bone remodeling with balanced formation and resorption becomes uncoupled, leading to bone loss and increased risk of fracture.

BONE CELLS

The cells involved in bone turnover are osteoclasts, osteoblasts, and osteocytes (**Figure 51-2**). Osteoclasts are macrophage-like cells that secrete proteolytic enzymes and hydrogen ions required to remove the deposited bone matrix. The remodeling cycle begins when osteoclast precursors interact with other marrow cells and are activated, becoming multinucleated osteoclasts, which initiates resorption. Bone resorption occurs within the resorption lacuna, a tightly sealed zone beneath the ruffled border of the osteoclast where it has attached to the bone surface. Resorption depends on acidification of this extracellular compartment leading to demineralization. Subsequently, the organic matrix is degraded by cysteine proteases, chief of which is cathepsin K. Osteoclasts consequently create a functional extracellular lysosome, containing both an acidic environment and specific lysosomal enzymes.

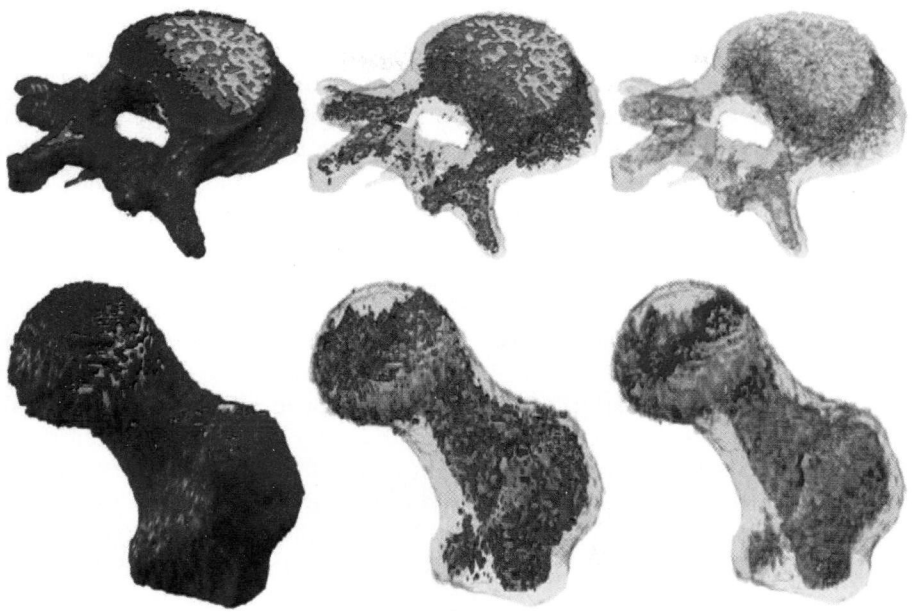

FIGURE 51-1. Components of bone structure. Computed tomography (CT) images of osteoporotic bone (vertebrae and proximal femur) from a 70-year-old woman analyzed using a specialized image analysis software (Tissue Compass™) that depicts bone toward marrow, left to right. Cortical and trabecular bone is illustrated in blue. Note that the marrow is occupied mainly by fat (yellow) at the expense of hematopoietic (red) marrow.

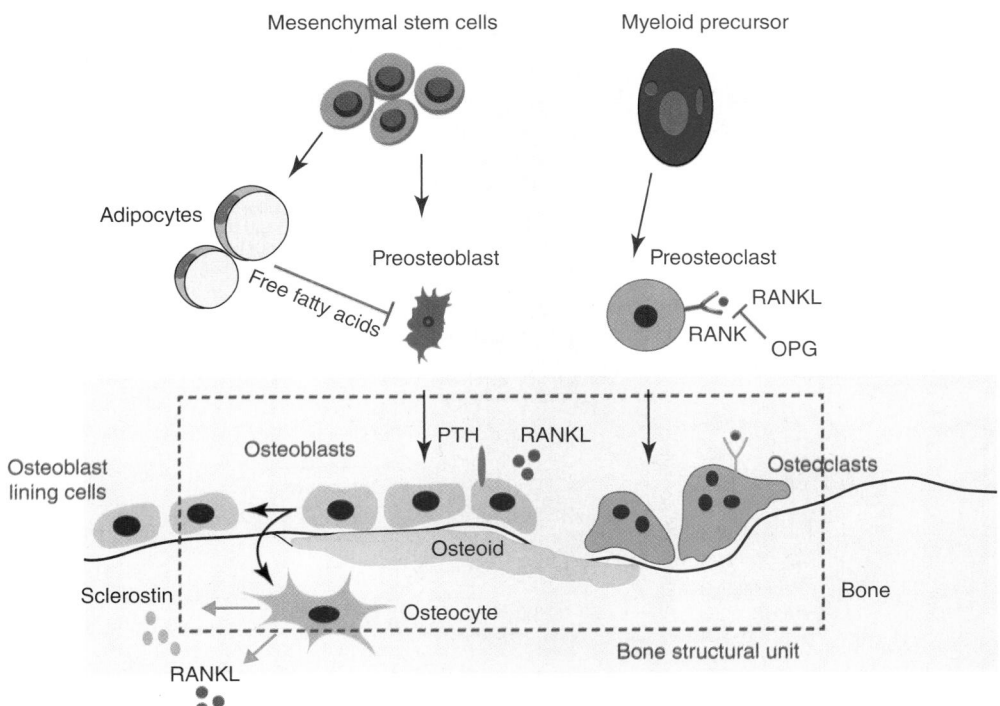

FIGURE 51-2. The cellular components of bone turnover. After the expression of specific transcription factors, mesenchymal precursors differentiate into osteoblasts. In contrast, osteoclasts differentiate from mononuclear precursors and act as bone-resorbing cells in the bone multicellular unit. After the completion of bone resorption, osteoclasts undergo apoptosis and are replaced by active osteoblasts responsible for forming new bone. Osteoblasts finally end as lining cells, as osteocytes embedded into the osteoid, or undergo apoptosis. Osteocytes are neuron-like cells representing end-stage osteoblast that have become embedded in the bone matrix (osteoid). (Reproduced with permission from Al Saedi A, Stupka N, Duque G. Pathogenesis of Osteoporosis. *Handb Exp Pharmacol.* 2020;262:353–367.)

In cortical bone, the resorption period lasts approximately 30 days; the final result is a resorption tunnel that osteoblasts will later fill in in a haversian manner, in which plates of bone are laid down in layers of concentric rings around a central channel. The apposition of these haversian canals takes the shape of a "cut onion," which gives the cortical bone its typical morphology. In trabecular bone, the erosion period lasts approximately 43 days, resulting in a trench between the trabeculae. The life span of osteoclasts is around 2 weeks; once these cells complete their role as bone-resorbing cells, they undergo apoptosis or programmed cell death.

Osteoblasts are fibroblast-like cells derived from pluripotent mesenchymal cells that localize on periosteal surfaces (**Figure 51-2**). Such pluripotent stromal cells can be induced to differentiate along the osteoblastic, adipocytic, fibroblastic, or chondrocytic lineages when required. When bone integrity has to be conserved, mesenchymal stromal cells are committed toward the osteoblastic lineage. Many factors are involved in the process of osteoblastogenesis (**Figure 51-3**), including the bone morphogenic protein family; bone morphogenic proteins 2, 4, and 7 are potent inducers of osteoblast differentiation. A transcription factor called Runx2/Cbfa1 plays a crucial role in osteoblast differentiation; mice lacking Runx2/Cbfa1 do not form bone. A mature osteoblast is a cuboidal cell with a large nucleus and enlarged Golgi highly enriched in alkaline phosphatase. It produces type I collagen and specialized bone-matrix proteins such as osteoid, the primary protein for further bone formation and mineralization. Osteoblasts produce alkaline phosphatase, the specific function of which has yet to be determined. Nevertheless, it is used as a marker of osteoblast differentiation and activity and indirectly as a marker of subsequent osteoclast resorption. Mice lacking functional alkaline phosphatase suffer from hypophosphatasia characterized by impaired mineralization of cartilage and bone matrix. After osteoblasts complete their bone-forming function, they face one of three fates: (1) they become embedded in the newly formed matrix, becoming osteocytes; (2) they remain on the surface of the newly formed bone and become lining cells; or (3) they undergo apoptosis. Hormonal changes, the presence or absence of growth factors, inflammatory conditions, and the aging process in bone determine the ultimate fate of the osteoblast.

In contrast, osteoclasts belong to the macrophage lineage and express multiple very potent degradative enzymes.

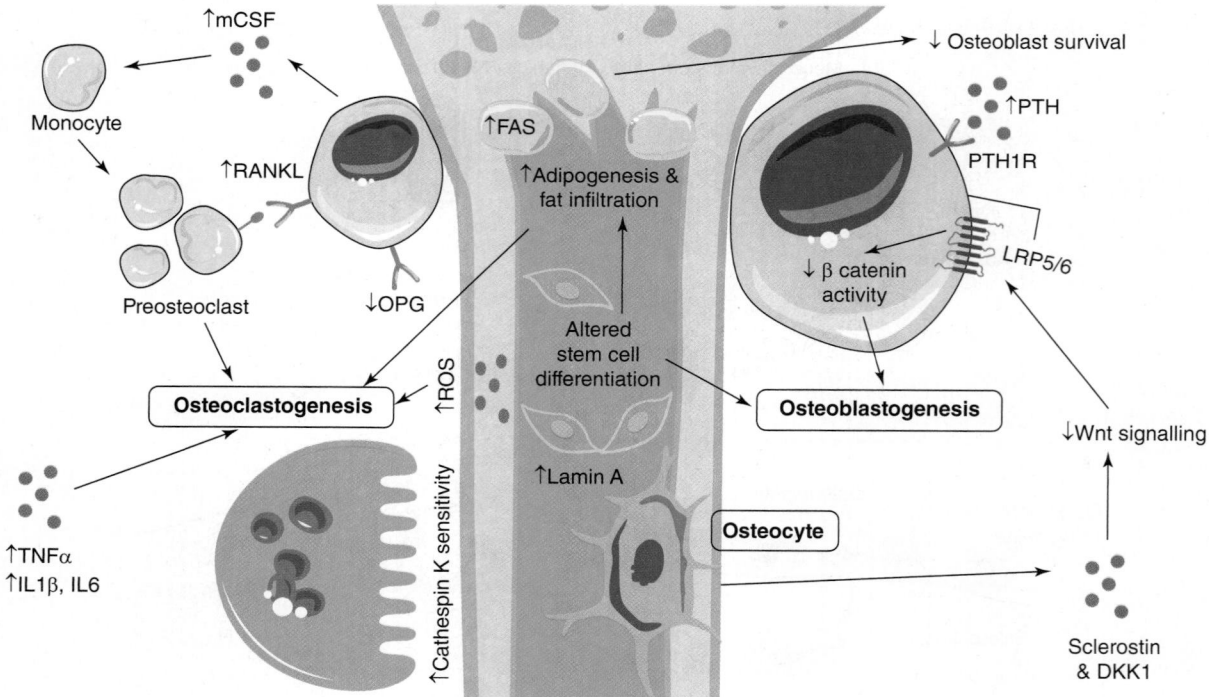

FIGURE 51-3. Factors that regulate bone cell differentiation and bone turnover. The Wnt signaling pathway is the most critical stimulator of osteoblastogenesis. Wnts activate β catenin, which translocates to the nucleus and stimulates the expression of osteogenic transcription factors such as RUNX2. Intermittent exposure to parathyroid hormone also has an osteogenic effect. Osteocytes regulate osteoblastogenesis via two major inhibitory factors, sclerostin and DKK1. Osteoclastogenesis is stimulated by the receptor activator of nuclear factor kappa-B ligand (RANKL), which is secreted by stromal cells and mature osteoblasts. Inflammatory factors such as TNFα and interleukins induce RANKL expression. In addition, adipocytes secrete adipokines and fatty acids that cause osteoblast and osteocyte apoptosis and induce osteoclast differentiation and activity. (Reproduced with permission from Feehan J, Al Saedi A, Duque G. Targeting fundamental aging mechanisms to treat osteoporosis. *Expert Opin Ther Targets.* 2019;23[12]:1031–1039.)

Osteoclast differentiation, formation, and, to a lesser degree, activation depend upon the proximity and products of the osteoblast (**Figure 51-3**). Without exception, the fate of the osteoclasts is to die by apoptosis.

Osteocytes constitute the third group of bone cells that are involved in bone metabolism. These cells are the most abundant cell type in bone and are the focus of intense research. Osteocytes are postmitotic terminally differentiated osteoblasts that are entrapped within the new bone matrix. Once considered inert, these cells are now recognized as key regulators of skeletal metabolism, mineral homeostasis, and hematopoiesis. Osteocytes are the critical responders to mechanical forces and orchestrators of bone remodeling and mineral homeostasis (**Figure 51-3**). Although osteocytes are entombed within their hosting lacunae, they are not isolated and instead maintain close communication with other cells and micro environments through a complex network of channels (canaliculi) in which osteocyte projections (cilia) are in close contact with blood vessels. Several functions attributed to osteocytes include the synthesis of matrix molecules such as osteocalcin and an essential role in direct communication with surface osteoblasts through molecules known as connexins. Two of those connexins, sclerostin and DKK1, are potent inhibitors of osteoblast differentiation and function and play an important role in the activation and regulation of bone metabolism in response to physiologic and mechanical stimuli. These modulate the response of bone during functional adaptation of the skeleton to mechanical forces and the need for repair of microdamage. Any mechanical force applied on the bone (ie, exercise) will have an inhibitory effect on sclerostin and DKK1, thus facilitating osteoblast differentiation and function. Osteocytes are very long-lived cells with a half-life of 25 years, after which most undergo apoptosis.

BONE TURNOVER

Bone homeostasis depends on the intimate coupling of bone formation and bone resorption. After osteoclasts resorb bone, preosteoblasts differentiate into osteoblasts and migrate to the area of excavated bone and begin to deposit osteoid, which is eventually mineralized into new bone. Osteoclasts and osteoblasts belong to a temporary structure known as a basic multicellular unit (see **Figure 51-2**). The coordinated process of bone resorption and formation by the basic multicellular unit lasts 6 to 9 months and results in newly mineralized bone. Osteoblasts are not only active as bone-forming cells, but these also play an important role in the regulation of osteoclast activity. The interaction between osteoblasts and osteoclasts requires a complex system of factors facilitated by integrins and cadherins (see **Figure 51-4**). Briefly, the primary

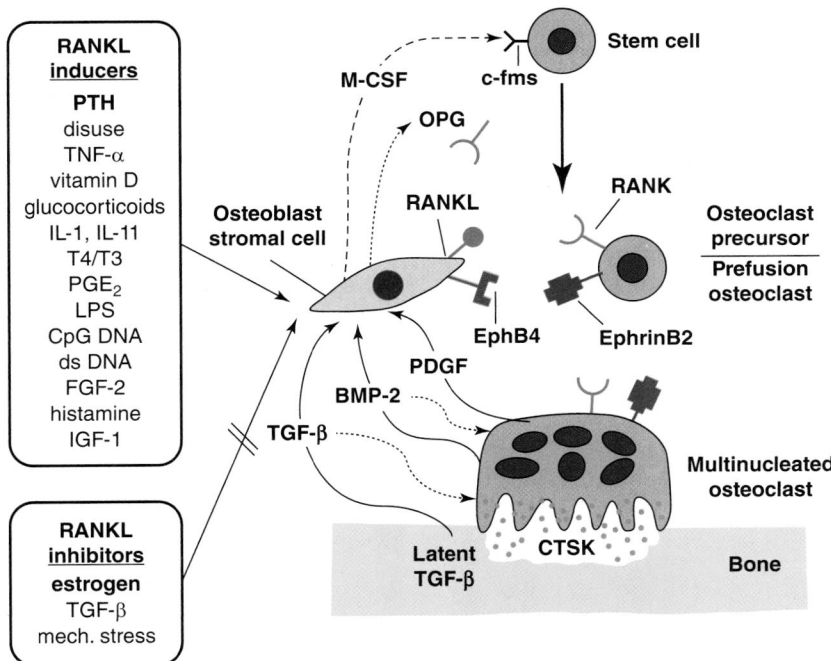

FIGURE 51-4. Osteoblast–osteoclast coupling and the regulation of RANK ligand expression. Osteoblast production of M-CSF and RANKL play critical roles in the differentiation and activation of osteoclasts. M-CSF acts to maintain monocytic stem cell survival, and subsequently, RANKL acts to commit the cell toward osteoclast differentiation, fusion, polarization, and activation. EphB4 and ephrinB2 interact both to limit osteoclast activity and stimulate osteoblast differentiation. TGF-β acts only upon release from the extracellular matrix after osteoclastic resorption, which is mainly mediated by the excretion of CTSK. BMP-2, bone morphogenetic protein-2; CTSK, cathepsin K; M-CSF, macrophage colony-stimulating factor; PDGF, platelet-derived growth factor; RANKL, RANK ligand; TGF-β, transforming growth factor-β.

osteoclast/osteoblast interaction depends on the expression by osteoclast precursors and mature osteoclasts of a membrane receptor known as receptor activator of nuclear factor-κ B (RANK), which belongs to the family of tumor necrosis factor (TNF) receptors. Osteoclast differentiation, maturation, and survival depend on RANK activation by its cognate ligand (RANK ligand—RANKL), which is produced by osteocytes, osteoblasts, and osteoblast precursors after exposure to different stimuli such as hormones and cytokines (**Figure 51-4**). Multiple other factors also act to either enhance or suppress osteoclast formation and activation and subsequent bone resorption (see **Table 51-2**).

RANKL is mainly a cytoplasmic membrane-bound molecule; to a lesser extent, it is secreted. Mature osteoblasts and osteocytes also produce a decoy receptor for RANKL called osteoprotegerin (OPG). OPG competitively binds to RANKL and prevents the interaction between RANK and RANKL, thus decreasing osteoclastogenesis and osteoclastic bone resorption and increasing osteoclast apoptosis. More recently, a group of molecules known as ephrins has been identified as key players in regulating osteoblast/osteoclast interaction. This cellular communication is bidirectional and involves a trans-membrane ligand known as ephrinB2, expressed by osteoclasts, and its receptor EphB4 expressed by osteoblasts (see **Figure 51-4**). This signaling seems to limit osteoclast activity while enhancing osteoblast differentiation. Consequently, osteoblastogenesis and osteoclastogenesis, along with corresponding bone formation and resorption, are tightly and ineluctably coupled. The differentiation and activation of both osteoblasts and osteoclasts depend critically on each other; however, recent evidence indicates that osteocytes also play an essential role in bone turnover by regulating osteoblast function and survival as well as osteoclast function; all modulated by hormones, growth factors, and mechanical forces.

GENETICS

Genetics plays a role in the determination of peak bone mass. Racial differences in the incidence of osteoporosis have been reported, including a lower relative risk of fractures and higher peak bone mass in African-American women compared with White women. No single gene, gene product, or polymorphism has yet been credibly identified to account for the variance seen in BMD in specific geographic areas. Several environmental factors, such as diet, topography, and yearly sunlight exposure, almost certainly interact with a genetic predisposition to explain the variance seen in periosteal expansion before puberty and trabecular number and thickness and periosteal-endosteal remodeling during aging. Candidate genes for determining peak bone mass are the vitamin D receptor, vitamin D binding protein, the peroxisome proliferator activator gamma, the Jagged 1 gene, and the low-density lipoprotein receptor-related protein 5. All these polymorphisms have been associated with different levels of peak of bone mass and predisposition to fractures in adulthood. However, multiple studies have shown that BMD and fracture predisposition are complex traits controlled by multiple genetic loci. More generally, there does appear to be a familial predisposition to osteoporotic fracture. Therefore, the fracture risk increases if an immediate family member (most typically a mother or sister) has experienced an osteoporotic fracture.

MECHANICAL FACTORS

Approximately 95% of peak adult bone mass is gained by the end of puberty. The level of peak bone mass attained and the subsequent rate of bone loss are the primary factors that determine an individual's bone mass in early and late adulthood. Initial bone formation does not require a mechanical stimulus, but further appositional and endochondral growth is dependent on the mechanical forces generated by the muscles. The magnitude of this loading is directly related to body mass and physical activity. There is some evidence that after mechanical load, microfractures may occur in bone, with subsequent activation of interleukins (ILs) and growth factors, thereby regulating bone turnover and formation. In addition, osteocytes play an important role in the response to mechanical stress by stimulating bone turnover and facilitating bone formation

TABLE 51-2 ■ LOCAL FACTORS REGULATING BONE CELL INTERACTION AND ACTIVITY

STIMULATORS OF BONE RESORPTION	STIMULATORS OF BONE FORMATION
RANK ligand	Vitamin D
Interleukins-1, -6, -8, -11	Estrogen
Macrophage colony-stimulating factor	Androgen
Vitamin D	Insulin-like growth factors
Glucocorticoids	Transforming growth factor
Parathyroid hormone	Mechanical force
Tumor necrosis factor	Fibroblast growth factors
Reduced mechanical force/low gravity	Platelet-derived growth factor
Epidermal growth factor	Bone morphogenetic proteins
Platelet-derived growth factor	
Fibroblast growth factors	
Leukemia inhibitory factor	
Prostaglandins	
Thyroid hormone	

INHIBITORS OF BONE RESORPTION	INHIBITORS OF BONE FORMATION
Estrogen	Sclerostin
Androgen	Dickkopf
Osteoprotegerin	
Interferon-γ	
Interleukin-4	
Calcitonin	

through the release of RANKL and the inhibition of sclerostin and DKK1.

LOCAL FACTORS

Local factors are important in regulating bone turnover and in the interaction between bone matrix and systemic factors and hormones (see **Table 51-2** and **Figures 51-2 to 51-4**). The skeleton responds to mechanical forces by several regulatory mechanisms, including the release of cytokines, such as macrophage colony-stimulating factor (M-CSF) and granulocyte colony-stimulating factor regulating cell differentiation. Mediators and regulators of cell–cell interaction include insulin-like growth factor (IGF)-1 and IGF-2, parathyroid hormone (PTH)-related peptide, IL-1, IL-6, and TNF-α. In addition, TNF-α, IL-6, IL-1, and prostaglandins largely mediate the response to sex-steroid hormones. Although high levels of these factors are necessary for osteoblast–osteoclast regulation and pathogenesis of osteoporosis–their usually stable systemic levels suggest that alterations in local secretion and concentration are critical to bone physiology. These local factors largely determine the activation or inhibition of bone cells, cell recruitment, cell differentiation, and life span.

SYSTEMIC HORMONES

A number of systemic hormones affect bone metabolism, including vitamin D, PTH, calcitonin, and sex-steroid hormones (estrogens and androgens) (see **Table 51-2**). The major effect of vitamin D is to maintain calcium homeostasis by increasing the efficiency of the small intestine in absorbing dietary calcium. Vitamin D also plays a role in bone resorption by inducing RANKL expression by osteoblasts, thereby inducing osteoclast differentiation and activation and subsequent bone formation by stimulating osteoblastogenesis and inhibiting apoptosis of mature osteoblasts. Hypovitaminosis D, widespread in older adults, is associated with lower BMD, frequent falls, and more osteoporotic fractures.

The parathyroid glands secrete PTH through a calcium sensor mechanism. When calcium levels decrease, PTH is released and exerts its function on two primary target tissues: kidney and bone. In the kidney, PTH acts on the proximal tubule to reduce PO_4 resorption and to increase the activity of 1-α-hydroxylase, the enzyme that converts 25(OH)-vitamin D to 1,25(OH)2-vitamin D_3, the active form of vitamin D. In bone, PTH increases osteoclast-induced bone resorption by inducing RANKL expression and subsequent signaling via RANK. Hypovitaminosis D is often, but not always, accompanied by elevated PTH—secondary hyperparathyroidism. Acute and cyclical exposure to PTH in bone has an antiapoptotic as well as an anabolic effect on osteoblasts. This is the basis for using PTH to treat severe osteoporosis (see further discussion below). Calcitonin is a hormone secreted by thyroidal C cells in mammals. Its main biologic effect is the inhibition of osteoclastic bone resorption. In vitro and in vivo studies in animals demonstrate that calcitonin causes the osteoclast to shrink and retract from the bone surface, decreasing its bone-resorbing activity and enhancing bone-forming osteoblasts.

Sex-steroid hormones play a variety of roles in bone turnover. Although some aspects of its effects remain unclear, estrogen increases the level of OPG, inhibiting osteoclastogenesis. Estrogen also induces osteoclast apoptosis and regulates the action of IL-1, IL-1 receptor antagonist (IL-1Ra), IL-6, and TNF-α, and their binding proteins and receptors. Declining estrogen levels lead to increased expression of IL-1, IL-6, and TNF-α, all of which enhance bone resorption. In response to diminished estrogen, osteoblasts produce more RANKL and less OPG, which induces RANKL–RANK interaction and signaling, further stimulating osteoclast differentiation and activation. Since estrogen increases osteoblast differentiation and decreases osteoblast apoptosis, bone formation declines at the time of menopause. Overall, there is a high turnover state with predominant bone resorption, which results in bone loss and susceptibility to fractures.

Androgens play an important role in the formation of adolescent bone by regulating cytokines in the bone matrix. The effect of progesterone on bone seems to be indirect and limited through its regulation of calcitonin secretion and thus bone resorption.

Women are at higher risk of osteoporosis because they have lower peak bone mass than men and experience accelerated bone loss during menopause, as described above. Histomorphometric data on the skeletal changes associated with postmenopausal bone loss show increased bone turnover in both cancellous and cortical bones. Biochemical markers also reflect high bone resorption after menopause. These markers return to normal with estrogen replacement. Trabecular bone is affected earlier in menopause than cortical bone because it is more metabolically active. Thus, rapid bone loss is seen primarily in the spine (3% per year) for approximately 5 years after menopause. Subsequently, there is a slower rate of bone loss that is more generalized (> 0.5% per year at many sites). A consistent finding in untreated postmenopausal women is a reduction in wall width of bone, indicating decreased osteoblast activity. Although this could be related to the loss of the antiapoptotic effect of estrogen on osteoblasts, studies are inconclusive.

AGE-RELATED MECHANISMS OF OSTEOPOROSIS

Age-related bone loss is a complex phenomenon, with many factors involved in its pathogenesis (see **Figures 51-4 and 51-5**). As individuals age, distinct changes occur in trabecular bone, cortical bone, and bone marrow. The onset and triggers of age-related bone loss are still not fully defined. However, densitometric studies show a slow

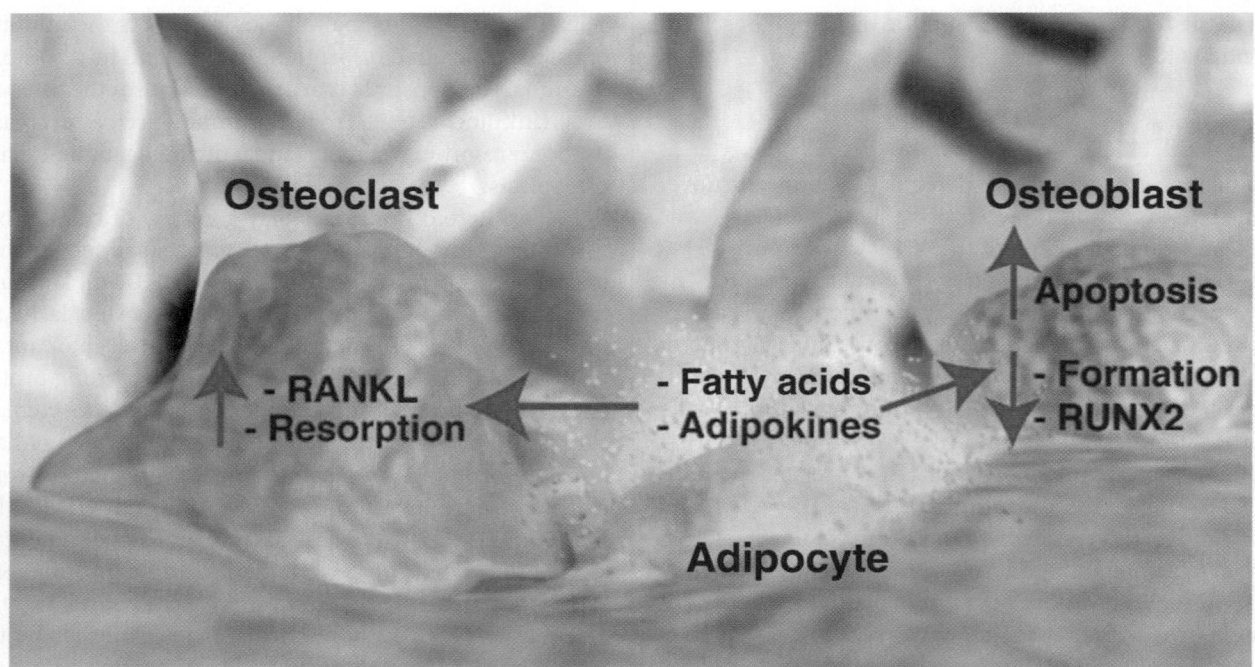

FIGURE 51-5. The role of fat in aging bone. Increasing bone marrow fat levels observed in aging bone are associated with the local secretion of lipotoxic factors (fatty acids and adipokines), reducing osteoblast differentiation and inducing apoptosis in osteoblasts and osteocytes. At the same time, they also stimulate osteoclast differentiation and activity.

and progressive decline in BMD after the third decade of approximately 0.5% per year, even though serum levels of estrogens are still within the normal range. With aging, osteoblastogenesis decreases, resulting in lower numbers of osteoblast precursors and increasing bone marrow adiposity (see **Figures 51-1** and **51-4**). The bone marrow of a young individual is virtually devoid of adipocytes. However, in older adults, adipose deposits may occupy up to 90% of the bone marrow cavity.

Pluripotent mesenchymal cells within the bone marrow stroma are, by default, programmed to differentiate into adipocytes, but the presence of specific osteogenic factors in the bone marrow induces osteoblastic differentiation. With aging, those osteogenic factors are decreased, generating a predominant adipocyte differentiation of those precursors. In addition, osteoblast and osteocyte apoptosis increase with aging. Histomorphometric data demonstrate that 50% to 70% of the osteoblasts present at the remodeling site cannot be accounted for after the enumeration of lining cells and osteocytes. The discrepancy in osteoblast numbers is believed to be a consequence of osteoblast apoptosis. This phenomenon may account for the significant reduction in bone formation associated with aging, which is added to high levels of marrow adipogenesis.

In addition, increasing marrow fat levels directly negatively affects bone metabolism by regulating the function and survival of bone cells. By secreting fatty acids and adipokines, marrow adipocytes inhibit osteoblast differentiation, function, and survival and osteocyte survival. This effect has been described as lipotoxicity, defined as the

ectopic accumulation of lipid and lipid products in nonadipose tissues leading to cellular dysfunction, cell death (lipoapoptosis) and disease. Additionally, adipocyte-secreted factors (primarily fatty acids) affect autophagy, defined as the conserved process whereby aggregated proteins, intracellular pathogens, and damaged organelles are degraded and recycled. Autophagy appears to play a significant role in skeletal maintenance after recent reports reveal that suppression of autophagy in osteocytes mimics skeletal aging. Furthermore, marrow adipocytes induce osteoclastic activity by facilitating the release of RANKL into the bone marrow milieu, thus stimulating bone resorption in addition to decreasing bone formation (**Figure 51-5**).

The early changes associated with age-related bone loss are similar in men and women, as described above. However, women also experience accelerated bone loss of approximately 3% to 5% per year during menopause. In men, the decline in bone mass is gradual until very late in life, when the risk for fractures increases rapidly. Concurrent with osteoblast and adipocyte formation changes, multiple factors enhance osteoclastogenesis and bone resorption (see **Figure 51-4**). In particular, the interactions between osteoblasts, osteocytes, and osteoclasts, crucial to the dynamic equilibrium that maintains healthy bone, are altered. Consequently, the combination of decreased bone formation and increased bone resorption leads to diminished BMD, more flawed bone structure and quality, and, ultimately, enhanced fragility and fractures.

Muscle-secreted factors could also explain the cellular changes observed in aging bone. There is growing evidence

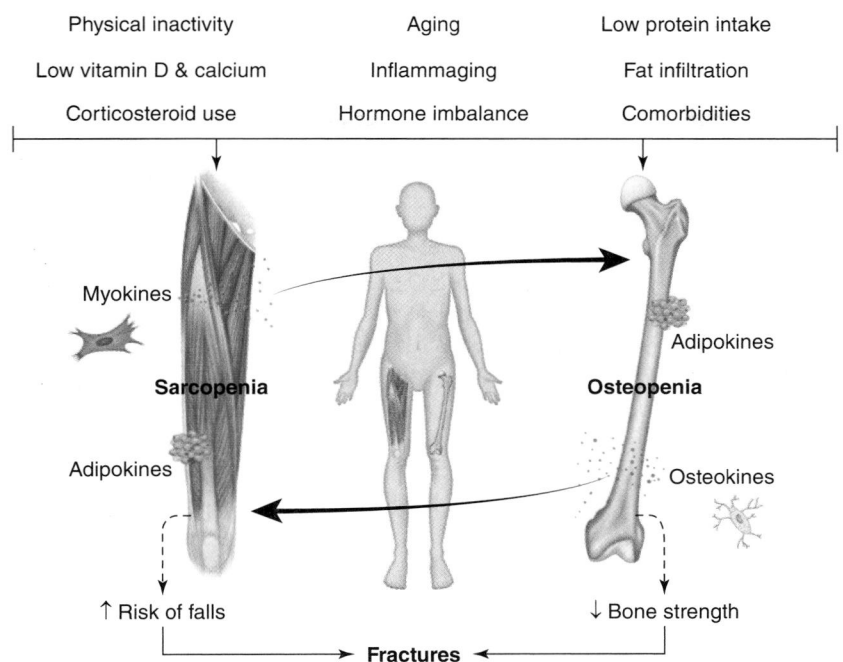

FIGURE 51-6. Muscle-bone cross-talk (myokines, osteokines, adipokines) and the pathophysiology of osteosarcopenia. (Reproduced with permission from Kirk B, Zanker J, Duque G. Osteosarcopenia: epidemiology, diagnosis, and treatment-facts and numbers. *J Cachexia Sarcopenia Muscle.* 2020;11[3]:609–618.)

that a complex bone/muscle cross-talk system exerted via osteokines and adipokines plays a critical regulatory role in bone metabolism (**Figure 51-6**). This cross-talk is affected by aging and other factors such as hormones and inactivity, associated with reduced osteogenic myokines levels. In addition, adipokines and fatty acids are also involved in this cross-talk by affecting bone and muscle structure and function. Overall, this growing evidence on the communication and close interaction between muscle and bone allowed us to propose the term osteosarcopenia as a new geriatric condition in which both osteopenia/osteoporosis and sarcopenia (loss of muscle mass, function, and strength) simultaneously occur in the same subject, increasing their risk of falls and fractures.

In addition to cellular changes, there are two major changes in calciotropic hormones that impact aging bone. Vitamin D levels decrease with age and reduce calcium absorption. Changes in the aging skin lessen the amount of 7-dehydrocholesterol, the precursor of cholecalciferol (vitamin D_3), and its conversion rate. Furthermore, declining renal function leads to a reduction in the production and activity of 1-α-hydroxylase, the enzyme responsible for the activation of vitamin D_3. Consequently, a negative calcium balance ensues, which activates the calcium sensor receptor in parathyroid glands. PTH is secreted as a physiologic response, stimulating osteoclast activity, maintaining normal serum calcium levels at the expense of bone mineralization. This theory of secondary hyperparathyroidism was once the definitive explanation for age-related bone loss. However, not all individuals with hypovitaminosis

D exhibit secondary hyperparathyroidism. Therefore, it is just one of the elements of a syndrome that results in osteoporosis in older adults. However, this mechanism has been recently associated with additional important risk factors for fractures: sarcopenia and falls. Vitamin D and PTH appear to modulate neuromuscular function, particularly in frail older adults. Serum levels of 25(OH)-vitamin D lower than 35 nmol/L increase the risk of falls by 30%, which highly predisposes to fractures. Patients with serum levels between 35 and 80 nmol/L, which were considered normal in the past, are still at risk of falls, suggesting that the therapeutic goal should be to obtain serum levels greater than 80 nmol/L.

In summary, age-related bone loss results from changes at the cellular level, including decreased osteoblastogenesis, shortened osteoblast and osteocyte life span, increased adipogenesis and lipotoxicity, simultaneous occurrence of sarcopenia, and hormonal changes, including decreased levels and activity of sex-steroid hormones and vitamin D, and increased levels and activity of PTH.

OSTEOPOROSIS IN MEN

Although the pathophysiology of osteoporosis in men has been a subject of active research in recent years, the relative contribution of hormones and aging, per se, remains to be elucidated. It is well established that androgen levels decrease with aging. Testosterone levels decrease by approximately 1.2% per year, and the binding protein levels increase with aging, resulting in lower bioavailable testosterone. There is evidence that androgens exert their effect on bone through the action of IGF-1. IGF-1 levels are increased during puberty and are closely related to sex-steroid levels.

With aging, lower levels of sex-steroid hormones result in decreased levels of IGF-1, with a reduction in bone formation and bone mass. Dehydroepiandrosterone, another androgen, declines slightly in the sixth decade without significant changes after that. Contradictory evidence is available about the importance of this decline in dehydroepiandrosterone and its administration in treating male osteoporosis. Thus, osteoporosis in men appears to result from cellular and hormonal changes, including lower levels of testosterone, dehydroepiandrosterone, and IGF-1 with subsequent lower osteoblast activity and higher osteoblast apoptosis. However, further study is necessary to delineate the specific roles of these factors in the decline of BMD and the high rate of fractures in men after the seventh decade of life.

Case reports of low bone mass and increased bone turnover in men with estrogen deficiency—either from an estrogen receptor abnormality or an absence of aromatase, the enzyme responsible for converting testosterone to estrogen—suggest that estrogen is required for normal bone homeostasis in men. Serum estrogen levels better predict BMD in men than do serum testosterone levels. In older men in whom both gonadotropin secretion and aromatase conversion are suppressed, estrogen acts as the principal sex-steroid-regulating bone resorption. Blocking the conversion of testosterone to estrogen using an aromatase inhibitor has been shown to increase bone resorption in a short-term study conducted in healthy older men, further supporting a role for estrogen in bone metabolism. Some of the effects of testosterone on bone may be mediated through aromatization of testosterone to estrogen, a possibility that warrants further study.

PRESENTATION

Osteoporosis is frequently underdiagnosed and undertreated by medical professionals. Osteoporosis is a silent disease, and symptoms may not appear until an incident fracture. Both men and women can have osteoporosis (as characterized by low BMD according to the WHO criteria) prior to a fracture, which is why it is so important to consider clinical risk factors, use risk identification tools (see further), and perform BMD measurement in those at risk of osteoporosis. Osteoporosis may be detected on plain x-rays (usually a chest x-ray) either by the presence of vertebral fractures or by "osteopenia" in the x-ray report. As many as a third or more of those with "osteopenia" on an x-ray may have T-scores worse than −2.5, and as many as half will have T-scores in the −2.5 to −1.0 range. Therefore, persons who are diagnosed with "osteopenia" by plain x-ray are candidates for BMD measurement. Osteoporosis may also present as an acute fracture. Most fractures that occur

in old age are caused, at least in part, by osteoporosis, and it is crucial to initiate a therapeutic regimen in these adults.

Even after a minimal trauma fracture, the diagnosis is often not considered. Three-quarters of postmenopausal women with a distal radius fracture were either undiagnosed or not treated in one study. As many as 50% of women with a hip fracture leave the hospital without treatment. The overall risk of repeat fracture within the first year is 20%. Fractures that are likely related to osteoporosis and thus should trigger therapy with an approved agent include wrist, vertebral, and hip fractures. Frequently, these fractures are classified as fragility fractures because there is often little or no trauma associated with the event. Those with such fractures do not require BMD testing, although a baseline BMD is usually helpful to assure treatment adherence and response.

In older persons, several clinical findings could indicate the presence of vertebral fractures. This includes height loss and progressive kyphosis. It is recommended that older persons be assessed routinely and that simple measurements such as occiput/wall distance be performed to identify those patients with asymptomatic vertebral fractures.

SECONDARY CAUSES OF OSTEOPOROSIS

The diagnosis of primary osteoporosis is made by BMD measurement before fracture or by incident fracture. Secondary osteoporosis is the consequence of diseases or drugs affecting bone directly (involving changes in bone cells or bone matrix composition) or indirectly (by increasing endogenous or ectopic hormonal production). It is important to exclude diseases that may present as a fracture or low BMD in evaluating women and men with osteoporosis. **Table 51-3** lists the major secondary causes of osteoporosis along with laboratory tests used to exclude each disease. These laboratory tests should be considered in persons who present with acute compression fracture or who present with a diagnosis of osteoporosis by BMD measurement, particularly in those with Z scores below 2 SD. Men are more likely to have a secondary cause of osteoporosis than are women. The most commonly reported secondary causes of osteoporosis in men include hypogonadism and malabsorption syndromes. An additional secondary cause of osteoporosis in men relates to using luteinizing hormone-releasing hormone agonists in prostate cancer. Luteinizing hormone-releasing hormone agonists suppress the pituitary gland, decrease testosterone and estrogen to castrate levels, and render men at increased risk of osteoporosis. Several retrospective studies have found increased fracture rates in this population of men. Many studies demonstrate rates of bone loss that are up to three- to four-fold higher in men treated with luteinizing hormone releasing hormone agonists, compared with annual rates of bone loss in normal aging men.

Medications also may have a detrimental effect on bone. Consideration should be given to dose adjustment,

TABLE 51-3 ■ RECOMMENDATIONS FOR EVALUATION OF SECONDARY CAUSES OF OSTEOPOROSIS

DISEASE	EVALUATION
ENDOCRINE ABNORMALITIES	
Primary hyperparathyroidism	Ionized calcium, PTH
Paget disease	Alkaline phosphatase
Osteomalacia	Serum + urine Ca, PO_4, alkaline phosphatase, 25(OH)D
Hyperthyroidism	T_4, thyroid-stimulating hormone
Hypogonadism (men only)	Bioavailable testosterone, prolactin
Cushing syndrome	Urinary free cortisol
NEOPLASTIC CONDITIONS	
Multiple myeloma	Complete blood count, serum, and urine protein electrophoresis
Bone metastases	Serum calcium, bone scan
OTHER CONDITIONS	
Alcoholism	Medical history
Malabsorption syndromes	Medical history, antigliadin and antiendomysial antibodies
MEDICATIONS	
Glucocorticoids	Medical history
Anticonvulsants	25(OH)D, alkaline phosphatase
Heparin (long term)	Medical history
Excess thyroid hormone replacement	Thyroid-stimulating hormone

discontinuation of the drugs, or preventive treatment. Medications that adversely affect BMD include glucocorticoids, proton pump inhibitors (PPIs), excess thyroid supplementation, anticonvulsants, methotrexate, cyclosporine, and heparin. In older adults, glucocorticoids, PPIs, and thyroid hormone are used quite commonly; accordingly, clinicians should consider the effects of these medications on the already increased fracture risk when prescribing these to older adults.

The prevalence of osteoporosis in adults taking glucocorticoids is approximately 30%. Bone loss typically occurs in the first 6 months of therapy, usually associated with doses of ≥7.5 mg/d administered for longer than 3 months. The risk also increases with increasing glucocorticoid dose. Glucocorticoids both suppress bone formation through direct effects on osteoblasts and increase resorption through indirect effects on osteoclasts. Glucocorticoid-induced osteoporosis is preventable if treatment is considered when therapy with corticosteroids is initiated. Replacement of gonadal hormones and treatment with anti-resorptives (bisphosphonates and denosumab) or intermittent PTH has been shown to prevent bone loss in patients taking glucocorticoids. Other measures for preventing bone loss are calcium and vitamin D supplementation and reduction of glucocorticoid dose to the lowest effective dose for the underlying disease.

In most cases, secondary osteoporosis can be either prevented or treated if suspected by the clinician. Immobilization predisposes to bone mineral loss and osteosarcopenia; thus, a program of early mobilization of hospitalized older patients is essential. Mild-to-moderate vitamin D deficiency may give rise to osteoporosis rather than osteomalacia; oral replacement may prevent its occurrence. Finally, a comprehensive medication review could also identify those medications placing the patient at risk of osteoporosis; thus, adjusting their doses or reevaluating their indications constitutes the most appropriate approach.

EVALUATION

Risk Identification

While approaches to the patient with osteoporosis have often based treatment on T-scores, assessing clinical risk factors can facilitate early identification of individual patients who are more likely to suffer from vertebral and nonvertebral fractures. This is particularly important, since most fractures occur in postmenopausal women with T-scores that are better than −2.5. The age of the patient is the most critical contributor to fracture risk. Additional important factors include a previous fracture history as an adult, history of fracture risk in a first-degree relative, body weight less than 127 lb, current history of smoking, and corticosteroid use for more than 3 months (**Table 51-4**). Impaired vision, early estrogen deficiency, dementia, frailty, recent falls, low calcium and vitamin D intake, low physical activity, and alcohol consumption of more than two drinks per day are additional clinical risk factors. Prior recent fracture is a robust predictor of future fracture. The increased risk is similar in both men and women and is

TABLE 51-4 ■ RISK FACTORS FOR OSTEOPOROTIC FRACTURE

POTENTIALLY MODIFIABLE	NONMODIFIABLE
Current cigarette smoking	Personal history of fracture
Low body weight (< 127 lb)	History of fracture in a first-degree relative
Estrogen deficiency	Advanced age
Early menopause (< 45 years of age)	Female sex
Prolonged premenopausal amenorrhea (> 1 year)	White or Asian race
Low calcium intake (lifelong)	Dementia
Alcoholism	History of corticosteroid medication
Taking sedative medication	Taking seizure medication
Impaired eyesight	Poor health/frailty
Recurrent falls	
Inadequate physical activity	
Arms usually required to stand	
Poor health/frailty	

PART III

GERIATRIC CONDITIONS

the same as the risk of the first fracture in a woman who is 10 years older. Half of the patients will refracture within 10 years, and half of those will occur within 2 years of the first fracture. Therefore, most older patients with a prior fracture are candidates for treatment.

Identifying patients at risk of osteoporosis and osteoporotic fractures should be routine practice in geriatric medicine. The presence of risk factors (see **Table 51-4**) has a very high predictive value for osteoporotic fractures, especially in older persons. However, except for age, which has the highest predictive value, these risk factors have a different weight in predicting the absolute risk of future fractures. Therefore, to help the clinician accurately calculate a patient's risk of suffering a fracture within 5 or 10 years, two online assessment tools have been widely validated.

The FRAX index (http://www.shef.ac.uk/FRAX) estimates the absolute risk of suffering a fracture in 10 years. This calculator has been demonstrated to be extremely useful since it includes specific data obtained from large cohorts worldwide. However, a major limitation of this tool is that falls are not included in the algorithm. Considering that falls are an important risk factor for fractures, the FRAX tool could be underestimating the level of risk in frequent fallers, particularly in frail older adults. In contrast

to the FRAX tool, the Garvan tool (http://www.garvan.org.au/bone-fracture-risk) includes a history of previous falls in its algorithm. Although it has been recently tested in non-Australian populations, this tool was initially developed and validated using the Dubbo Osteoporosis Study database. Another major advantage of this tool is that it calculates fracture risk at 5 and 10 years, providing valuable information that could be easily shared with the patient.

Since many osteoporotic fractures result from falls (Chapter 43) or the simultaneous presence of sarcopenia (Chapter 49), it is essential to assess patients for fall risk and sarcopenia and institute preventive measures where appropriate. **Figure 51-7** proposes a practical diagnostic algorithm to identify osteoporosis and sarcopenia in clinical practice. The risk factors for osteoporosis and sarcopenia are almost identical; thus, identification of secondary causes of osteoporosis should trigger the assessment for the presence of sarcopenia. The causes of falls are often multifactorial and include medications, poor vision, impaired cognition, maladaptive devices, alcohol, orthostatic hypotension, impaired balance and gait, environmental hazards, and lower extremity weakness. Recent studies suggest that specific performance measures can help to identify those at greater risk of falling. Individuals who

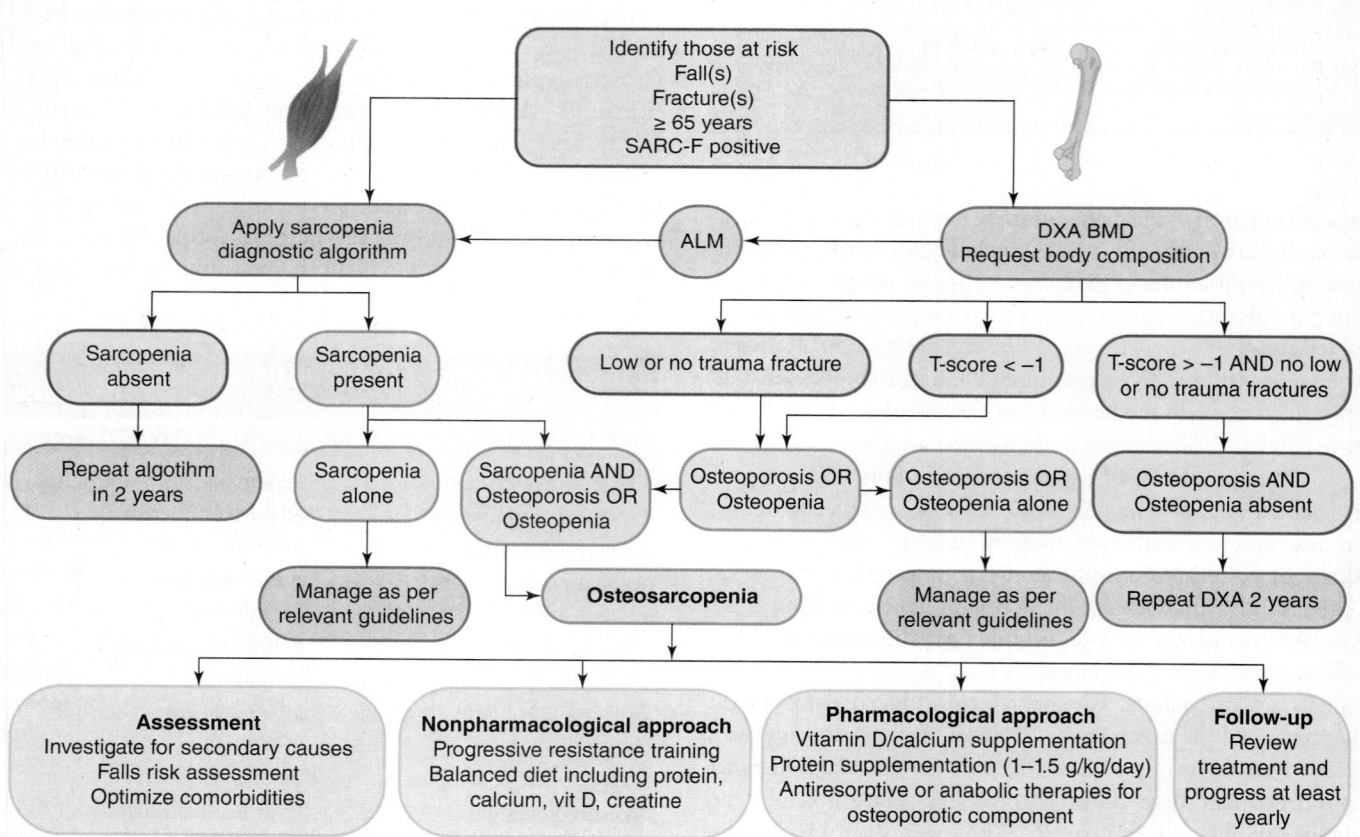

FIGURE 51-7. Clinical algorithm for the combined assessment and management of osteoporosis and sarcopenia in older persons. (Reproduced with permission from Kirk B, Zanker J, Duque G. Osteosarcopenia: epidemiology, diagnosis, and treatment-facts and numbers. *J Cachexia Sarcopenia Muscle.* 2020;11[3]:609–618.)

cannot maintain a semi tandem stand for 10 seconds with their eyes open are at increased risk. A gait velocity of less than 0.8 m/s also predicts a greater propensity to fall. Additional office-based screening tests that identify potential fallers include the inability to complete the timed up and go test in 14 seconds, the inability to maintain a one-leg stand for at least 5 seconds, and a score of less than 19 in the performance-oriented mobility assessment. Finally, the SARC-F questionnaire (Strength, Assistance with walking, Rising from a chair, Climbing stairs, and Falls) has a high specificity (~95%) to detect sarcopenia. The criteria are: (1) difficulty lifting and carrying 10 pounds, (2) difficulty walking across a room, (3) difficulty transferring from a chair or bed, (4) difficulty climbing a flight of 10 steps, and (5) falls in the past year. The first four criteria are scored as none = 0, some = 1, and a lot = 2. The last criterion is none = 0, 1 to 3 falls = 1, and ≥ 3 falls = 2. A score of 4 or greater is predictive of clinically important sarcopenia and is associated with adverse outcomes.

Bone Mineral Density (BMD) Assessment

BMD measurement has historically been considered the gold standard for the diagnosis of osteoporosis in the clinical setting. Various techniques could be used to measure BMD of the hip, spine, wrist, or calcaneus. The preferred method of BMD measurement is dual-energy x-ray absorptiometry (DXA). BMD of the hip, anteroposterior spine, lateral spine, and wrist can be measured using this technology. Quantitative computerized tomography is also used to measure BMD of the spine. Specific software can adapt computerized tomography scanners for BMD measurement. The advantages of DXA over quantitative computerized tomography include lower cost, lower radiation exposure, and better reproducibility over time. Peripheral DXA (measures wrist BMD) or ultrasonography of the calcaneus may be helpful for general osteoporosis screening, and these have the advantage of reduced cost and portability. Peripheral bone densitometry (performed at the heel, finger, or forearm) is highly predictive of hip, spine, wrist, rib, and forearm fractures for the subsequent 12 months.

Assessment of BMD should be considered for (1) postmenopausal women younger than 65 years with one or more additional risk factors (other than menopause); (2) all women older than 65 years, regardless of additional risk factors; and (3) patients with a history of minimal trauma fracture in which osteoporosis treatment is being started (as a baseline BMD assessment and to evaluate future therapeutic response). A study of more than 200,000 postmenopausal women from more than 4000 primary care practices in 34 states reported that approximately 50% of this population had low BMD previously undetected, including 7% of women with osteoporosis. An additional study found that screening postmenopausal women with BMD reduced the incidence of hip fracture by 36%. These studies suggest that efforts should be made to increase BMD measurements in postmenopausal women.

Postmenopausal women with significant kyphosis and clinical risk factors also do not require BMD testing to confirm the diagnosis of osteoporosis. Instead, both of these subsets of patients deserve treatment. In a cohort of over 8000 women participating in the Study of Osteoporotic Fractures, of the 243 that suffered a hip fracture, 54% had a total hip BMD T-score better than −2.5 at the start of the study. Similarly, in a study of 257 men aged 70 and older, although those with lower T-scores had a higher fracture rate, the majority of fractures occurred in men with T-scores better than −2.5. These studies emphasize that BMD is not the fundamental determinant of fracture risk; the microarchitecture and quality of bone are also important, which is not directly assessed with densitometry, as is the propensity to fall.

As noted above, clinical risk factors need to be assessed. Furthermore, it is imperative to recognize that age is a much more significant factor than BMD in determining fracture risk. The 10-year probability of a fracture in an 80-year-old is more than twice as great as the probability of fracture in a 50-year-old with the same BMD T-score. BMD may also be used to establish the diagnosis and severity of osteoporosis in men and should be considered in men with low-trauma fracture, radiographic changes consistent with low bone mass, or diseases known to place an individual at risk of osteoporosis. Data relating BMD to fracture risk were initially derived from studies completed in women, but recent data suggest that similar associations may be valid in men as well. Assessment of BMD should also be strongly considered in both perimenopausal women and older men who are about to undergo long-term treatment with corticosteroids. Bone densitometry can be used to assess response to therapy. However, usually 2 years between tests are necessary to obtain accurate and valuable information. Biochemical markers of bone turnover yield much quicker details about compliance and success of therapy.

Biochemical Markers of Bone Turnover

Serum and urine biochemical markers that reflect collagen breakdown (or bone resorption) and bone formation help monitor osteoporosis treatment. Higher levels of resorption markers have been associated with increased hip fracture risk, decreased BMD, and increased bone loss in older adults in some studies. However, biochemical markers in many patients with osteoporosis will lie within the normal range. In addition, there is often a substantial overlap of marker values in women with high and low bone density or rate of bone loss. Therefore, at this time, markers are not recommended for screening or diagnosis of osteoporosis. In addition, few studies have compared the response of a particular marker (or combination of markers) and BMD to therapy in order to determine the magnitude of decrease of a biochemical marker necessary to prevent bone loss or, more importantly, fracture. Markers are most useful in assessing the response of an individual patient to treatment.

Markers of bone resorption and formation decrease in response to antiresorptive therapy and increase in response to PTH, treatment with anabolic properties. The advantage of the serum versus urinary markers is that the intra-patient variability tends to be lower with serum markers, thus reducing error. Many of the osteoclast-specific markers can then be rechecked as early as 6 weeks after beginning therapy. Successful antiresorptive therapy, which also means compliance, will reduce serum levels of markers of both resorption and formation, since these processes are tightly coupled. However, changes in bone formation markers will lag several months behind changes in bone resorption markers.

MANAGEMENT

Osteoporosis develops in older adults when the normal processes of bone formation and resorption become uncoupled or unbalanced, resulting in bone loss. Osteoporosis prevention and treatment programs, then, should focus on strategies that minimize bone resorption and maximize bone formation, as well as strategies that reduce falls. Several nonpharmacologic and pharmacologic options are available to health care providers. Importantly, modifying risk factors (see **Table 51-4**) should be the first step in preventing osteoporotic fractures in older adults.

Nonpharmacologic Interventions

Exercise Exercise is an essential component of osteoporosis treatment and prevention programs. Data in older men and women suggest a positive association between current exercise and hip BMD. Among regular exercisers, those who reported strenuous or moderate exercise had higher BMD at the hip than those who reported mild or less-than-mild exercise. Similar associations were seen for lifelong regular exercisers and hip BMD. In a randomized study of women at least 10 years past menopause, the group receiving calcium supplementation plus exercise had less bone loss at the hip than those assigned to calcium alone. Furthermore, high-intensity strength training effectively maintains femoral neck BMD and improves muscle mass, strength, and balance in postmenopausal women compared to nonexercising controls, suggesting that resistance training would be helpful to maintain BMD and to reduce the risk of falls in older adults.

A marked decrease in physical activity or immobilization results in a decline in bone mass; accordingly, it is essential to encourage older adults to be as active as possible. However, not all types of exercises have proved to be beneficial. Progressive resistance strength training of the lower limb improved BMD at the neck of the femur in postmenopausal women. In contrast, aerobic exercises and low impact activities like brisk walking and cycling have failed to increase BMD at any site. Whole-body vibration (WBV) has been shown to increase BMD in some studies; however, some trials have also reported no effect. Evidence regarding the role of exercise in preventing fracture is limited as no randomized controlled trial (RCT) has so far evaluated the role of exercise as a single intervention to prevent fractures. However, exercise and focused physical therapy can prevent falls, which are significant contributors to increased fracture risk. Concerning exercise, an important consideration in older people is configuring a program according to comorbidities and functional status, as adherence may vary depending upon underlying conditions, particularly osteoarthritis and/or cardiopulmonary disease.

Physical therapy is an integral part of osteoporosis treatment programs, especially after an acute vertebral compression or hip fracture. The physical therapist can provide postural exercises, alternative modalities for pain reduction, and suggest changes in body mechanics that may help prevent future falls and fractures. Gait training or balance training and muscle strengthening can help prevent falls, even for relatively frail older persons. A meta-analysis of randomized clinical trial interventions to reduce falls concluded that all types of exercises achieved similar benefits in balance, endurance, flexibility, and strength. The key message is to prescribe a program for those patients who are mobile and functional enough, in addition to cognitively capable, to participate.

Nutrition (calcium and vitamin D) Calcium and vitamin D are required for bone health at all ages. Elemental calcium, 1200 to 1500 mg/day, for postmenopausal women and men older than 65 is needed to maintain a positive calcium balance. The amount of vitamin D required is at least 800 IU/day, although evidence suggests that as much as 2000 IU of cholecalciferol per day and more are necessary to achieve serum levels (25[OH] vitamin D $\geq$ 75 nmol/L) that are optimally effective for fall and fracture prevention.

Overall, adequate calcium and vitamin D should be recommended for all older adults, regardless of BMD, to maximize bone health. In osteoporotic patients who require pharmacologic treatment, administration of calcium and vitamin D alone is not recommended. Indeed, supplementation with vitamin D enhances the BMD response to osteoporosis treatment. It is also worth noting that all pivotal trials of anti-osteoporotic agents (antiresorptive, anabolic, or dual-action agents) have included supplementation with calcium and vitamin D.

Despite our understanding of the role of calcium and vitamin D in bone physiology, recent analyses have raised some controversies about their role in increasing BMD and fracture prevention. Several recent meta-analyses showed that calcium intake from diet or supplements produced only a small increase in BMD. Notably, the increase was considered unlikely to decrease fracture risk. There is also controversy regarding supplementation with a high dose of calcium, as some reports have suggested an increased risk of cardiovascular disease. However, a recent systematic review and dose-response meta-analysis of prospective cohort studies found that total calcium intake was associated with lower cardiovascular mortality in post-menopausal women. Dietary calcium was associated with all-cause mortality, and supplemental intake was not associated with the risk of all-cause, cancer, or cardiovascular mortality.

Like calcium, the role of vitamin D supplements in improving BMD and decreasing fracture risk is debated as the latest meta-analyses have failed to show any benefit in improving BMD or reducing fracture risk. This is despite earlier analyses conclusively stating the positive role of vitamin D supplements in osteoporosis management by decreasing the risk of nonvertebral fractures. This lack of apparent benefit could be due to the inclusion of a significant number of healthy people with no risk factors for osteoporosis, with normal serum levels of vitamin D, or with different doses of vitamin D supplements in RCTs. To add to the controversy surrounding its use, high doses of vitamin D by bolus administration (500,000 IU/year or 60,000 IU/monthly) have consistently been shown to increase the risk of falls and trends to increased fractures. Despite these controversies, it is accepted that vitamin D has a role in osteoporosis (and sarcopenia) management, particularly in those with vitamin D deficiency. While frank vitamin D deficiency ($\leq$ 30 nmol/L) should be treated with a loading dose of 50,000 IU cholecalciferol or ergocalciferol, it is recommended that all others be treated with an appropriate daily dose of 1000 to 4000 IU cholecalciferol.

Nutrition (additional factors) Two prospective studies examined the effect of additional nutritional factors on bone loss and fracture risk in older adults. The Framingham Osteoporosis Study found that higher baseline magnesium, potassium, and fruit and vegetable intakes were associated with higher baseline BMD. In men, increased potassium and magnesium intakes were associated with lower bone loss at the femoral neck. Additionally, this study showed a correlation of hip fractures with higher serum levels of homocysteine. Although homocysteine levels are associated with vitamin B_{12}, serum levels of this vitamin have not been associated with lower BMD, suggesting that the role homocysteine plays in bone biology remains to be elucidated. However, other studies have not found a clear association between homocysteine levels and fracture. In addition, lower baseline protein intake or percent of total energy from animal protein has been associated with more significant bone loss at the femoral neck and lumbar spine. In another prospective cohort study, the Study of Osteoporotic Fractures, BMD was not related to the ratio of animal to vegetable protein intake. Still, a higher proportion of animal to vegetable protein intake was associated with more significant femoral neck bone loss and an increased risk of hip fracture. These studies suggest that nutritional factors other than calcium and vitamin D are essential for bone health in older adults. Prospective randomized studies are indicated to elucidate further the role of nutrition in preventing and treating osteoporosis in older adults.

PHARMACOLOGIC TREATMENT (TABLE 51-5)

Estrogen Replacement Therapy

Multiple studies demonstrate that postmenopausal estrogen use will prevent bone loss at the hip and spine when initiated within 10 years of menopause. However, there have been few prospective studies of estrogen replacement therapy and fracture prevention. One small study demonstrated a reduction in vertebral fractures in postmenopausal women with transdermal estradiol compared to placebo. The Women's Health Initiative study showed a 24% reduction in all fractures and a 33% reduction in hip fractures in women taking estrogen plus progestin. However, the Women's Health Initiative study also concluded that the overall risks of estrogen plus progestin outweighed the benefits, including those associated with reducing fractures. Few studies have evaluated the use of estrogen in women older than 70 years. Observational data, however, from the Study of Osteoporotic Fractures support a protective effect of current estrogen use against hip fracture, even in the oldest women.

Lower doses of estrogen also effectively reduce bone resorption and bone loss in older women; the lower doses also result in fewer side effects than the usual replacement doses typically used by clinicians. 17β-estradiol 0.25 mg/day was as effective as 0.5 and 1.0 mg/day in reducing biochemical markers of bone turnover in 75-year-old women compared to placebo. The side-effect profile of 0.25 mg/day was similar to placebo and significantly different from the two higher doses. In a longer-term study, 0.3 mg/day of conjugated equine estrogen plus 2.5 mg/day of medroxyprogesterone acetate increased bone density of the hip and spine in older women who were vitamin D replete. While a recent report from the Women's Health Initiative study demonstrates cardiovascular benefit in women aged 50 to 59 who took estrogen, at this time, better alternatives to the treatment of osteoporosis in older patients exist. Therefore, in older patients, particularly those at least 5 to 10 years postmenopausal, estrogen is not recommended.

Bisphosphonates

Bisphosphonates decrease bone resorption by inhibiting osteoclast action and survival while promoting secondary mineralization. They are structurally similar to pyrophosphates, which bind to hydroxyapatite on the bone surface and inhibit osteoclast activity.

Alendronate The efficacy of alendronate has been well established in increasing BMD at all sites and reducing the risk of vertebral fracture in older persons. However, evidence regarding its effectiveness for nonvertebral or hip fracture is less robust. Alendronate treatment for 3 years in postmenopausal women (mean age 71) with existing vertebral fracture and low femoral neck BMD decreased the risk of new morphological and clinical vertebral fractures. For postmenopausal women (mean age 68) with no preexisting

TABLE 51-5 ■ PHARMACOLOGIC AGENTS FOR THE TREATMENT OF OSTEOPOROSIS

CLASS	DRUG NAME	MECHANISM OF ACTION	FORMULATION (TREATMENT DOSAGE)	PATIENTS STUDIED	EFFICACY	KEY SIDE EFFECTS/ PRECAUTIONS
Bisphosphonate	Alendronate (Fosamax®, Binosto®, generic)	Inhibition of osteoclast activity	70 mg weekly orally	Men and post-menopausal women with osteoporosis	Reduced hip and vertebral fractures by approx. 50% over 3 years	Contraindicated eGFR < 35 mL/min
	Ibandronate (Boniva®, generic)		150 mg monthly tablet or 3 mg intravenously 3-monthly	Corticosteroid-induced osteoporosis	Reduced vertebral fractures by approx. 50% over 3 years	Common–gastrointestinal
	Risedronate (Actonel®, Altevia®, generic)		35 mg weekly, 75 mg on 2 consecutive days monthly, or 150 mg monthly orally		Reduce vertebral fractures by 41% to 49% and nonvertebral fractures by 36% over 3 years. Approved for use in patients on glucocorticoid therapy	Uncommon–eye inflammation
	Zoledronic acid (Reclast®, Aclasta®)		5 mg intravenous infusion yearly × 3		Reduced vertebral fractures by 70%, hip fractures by 41%, and nonvertebral fractures by 25% over 3 years	Rare–ONJ (highest risk in patients with cancer), atypical femoral fracture (> 5 years use)
Synthetic parathyroid hormone	Teriparatide (Forteo®)	Anabolic activity resulting in new bone formation	20 mcg daily subcutaneous injection for a maximum of 24 months	Men and women with osteoporosis Corticosteroid-induced osteoporosis	Reduced risk of vertebral fractures by 65% and non-vertebral fractures by 53% after 18 months	Caution or avoidance in those at increased risk of osteosarcoma; Paget disease, previous radiation therapy, hypercalcemia, skeletal metastases; or those with a history of prostate cancer or lymphoma. Common–leg cramps, nausea, and dizziness Increased risk of osteosarcoma shown in rats
Parathyroid hormone-related protein (PTHrP) analog	Abaloparatide (Tymlos®) [Approved in some locations]		80 mcg daily subcutaneous injection for a maximum of 24 months	Postmenopausal women with osteoporosis	Reduced risk of vertebral fractures by approx. 57%	
Biologic— RANK-ligand inhibitor	Denosumab (Prolia®)	Inhibits coupling of osteoclasts and reduces bone resorption	60 mg 6-monthly subcutaneous injection	Men with low bone mass and postmenopausal women Corticosteroid-induced osteoporosis	Reduced vertebral fractures by 68%, hip fractures by 40%, and nonvertebral fractures by 20% over 3 years	Rapid bone loss after cessation Uncommon–hypocalcemia, cellulitis, skin rash Rare–weak immunosuppressant with increased risk bacterial infections, ONJ, atypical femoral fracture

(Continued)

TABLE 51-5 ■ PHARMACOLOGIC AGENTS FOR THE TREATMENT OF OSTEOPOROSIS *(CONTINUED)*

CLASS	DRUG NAME	MECHANISM OF ACTION	FORMULATION (TREATMENT DOSAGE)	PATIENTS STUDIED	EFFICACY	KEY SIDE EFFECTS/ PRECAUTIONS
Hormone replacement therapy (HRT)	Various	Maintenance estrogen levels Prevents bone resorption	Oral or transdermal in a wide variety of formulations	Postmenopausal women or women with hysterectomy	WHI study–5 years HRT reduced vertebral fractures by 34% and other fractures by 23%	Increased risk of myocardial infarction, breast cancer, pulmonary emboli, deep vein thrombosis No increase in cardiovascular disease if starting within 10 years of menopause
Selective estrogen receptor modulators (SERMs)	Raloxifene (*Evista®*)	Estrogen agonist in bone preventing resorption	60 mg daily orally	Postmenopausal women	Reduced risk vertebral fractures by approx. 30% in patients with prior vertebral fracture, and 55% in those without a previous vertebral fracture over 3 years	Uncommon–leg cramps, deep vein thrombosis
	Bazedoxifene (*Duavee®*)		0.45 mg/20 mg daily orally		Reduced incidence of vertebral fracture by approx. 30% at 3 years	Uncommon–muscle spasms, gastrointestinal complaints, dizziness, neck pain Uncommon–deep vein thrombosis

eGFR, estimated glomerular filtration rate; HRT, hormone replacement therapy; ONJ, osteonecrosis of the jaw; WHI, Women's Health Initiative.
Reproduced with permission from Zanker J, Duque G. Osteoporosis in Older Persons: old and New Players. J Am Geriatr Soc. 2019;67(4):831–840.

PART III

GERIATRIC CONDITIONS

fracture, alendronate was only effective in reducing the risk of clinical fracture in those with femoral neck BMD ≤ −2.5. Additionally, a subanalysis showed a decrease in the risk of nonvertebral fractures in those with femoral neck BMD ≤ −2.5. Alendronate treatment was equally effective in those ≤ 75 and those > 75 and reduced the risk of vertebral fracture by 51% and 38%, respectively after 12 months. There was not enough power to conduct subgroup analyses to determine if alendronate prevented hip fracture in older people (aged ≥ 75). The time to therapeutic benefit for alendronate in individuals ≥ 70 was calculated to be 8 months. Therefore, limited life expectancy in older and frail people should not delay the clinical decision to commence treatment. Furthermore, in a study of older women with osteoporosis living in residential aged care, alendronate treatment for 2 years was well tolerated and increased BMD at all sites.

Risedronate Risedronate has reduced the cumulative incidence of new vertebral fracture over 3 years by 41% in postmenopausal women (mean age 69) with established osteoporosis. Risedronate also has reduced the incidence of hip fracture in postmenopausal women (mean age 74) and an older group with osteoporosis (aged ≥ 80, mean age 83). However, the risk of hip fracture in the older cohort with nonskeletal risk factors (such as propensity for falls) remained unaffected. The lack of efficacy may be explained by the fact that bone density was not measured in those > 80, so that group would have likely included women who did not have osteoporosis as measured by BMD. A pooled analysis of multiple trials found that risedronate treatment for 3 years in women > 80 reduced the risk of vertebral fracture by 44%. As the risk and prevalence of vertebral fractures increase with age, older people are more likely to benefit from risedronate, evidenced by a higher absolute risk reduction—similar to that seen with alendronate. For nonvertebral fractures, the reduction in the cumulative incidence over 3 years was not statistically different between the risedronate group and placebo in the same cohort. The lack of apparent benefit for nonvertebral fracture in older adults could be due to nonskeletal risk factors for fragility fracture in this age group (age ≥ 80); however, further analysis is required to confirm this.

Zoledronic acid In postmenopausal women (mean age 73) with osteoporosis (BMD ≤ −2.5 or radiological evidence of at least one vertebral fracture), intravenous infusion of zoledronic acid yearly for 3 years reduced the risk of vertebral fracture by 70%, nonvertebral fracture by 25%, and hip fracture by 41%. In postmenopausal women with a previous hip fracture (mean age 74), zoledronic acid reduced the risk of any new clinical fracture by 35%. Moreover, zoledronic acid treatment had an additional benefit for all-cause mortality, with fewer deaths in the subjects receiving zoledronic acid (9.6%) than the placebo (13%). Zoledronic acid also significantly reduced the incidence of clinical vertebral, nonvertebral, or any clinical fracture in adults aged 75 or older.

Zoledronic acid was shown to be safe and well-tolerated by older adults in the trial at the once-a-year dose (5 mg IV). The most common adverse effects were postinfusion influenza-like symptoms that include fever, arthralgia, myalgia, and headache; however, these symptoms decreased with subsequent infusions. Although bisphosphonate therapy in frequent and high doses in cancer patients is associated with osteonecrosis of the jaw (ONJ), when used to treat osteoporosis in the recommended dose, ONJ is very rare (estimated incidence 0.001%–0.01%). The antifracture effectiveness of bisphosphonates persists even after discontinuation. This, together with recommended yearly infusion doses, improves compliance and efficacy in older adults who often struggle with compliance due to pill burden. Intravenous zoledronic acid also avoids gastrointestinal side effects commonly encountered with oral preparations of bisphosphonates, particularly frequent in older adults. Prolonged use of bisphosphonates is associated with an increased risk of atypical femoral fracture (AFF). However, absolute numbers are small, and the relative risk is much smaller than the risk of osteoporotic hip fracture and its significant adverse consequences and the significant reductions in the risk of hip and other fractures. The risk of AFF increases with more prolonged treatment of any bisphosphonate and should be investigated with x-ray in patients complaining of groin or thigh pain, as fracture precedes pain in most cases. Further investigations with a bone scan or MRI may be required. The risk of AFF rapidly diminishes after the termination of bisphosphonate treatment.

Denosumab

Denosumab is a humanized monoclonal antibody that binds to RANKL and inhibits osteoclast activation and activity. Denosumab (60 μg) given subcutaneously every 6 months to postmenopausal women (age 60–90; mean 72) over 3 years reduced hip fracture by 40%. Denosumab also decreased the risk of new radiological vertebral fracture by 68% and nonvertebral fracture by 20%. Denosumab was very effective in individuals aged 75 or older and significantly decreased the risk of hip fractures. Very interestingly, the denosumab group experienced fewer falls compared to the placebo group. However, preliminary analyses conducted by comparing a strength-related questionnaire did not reveal any difference between the treatment and placebo groups. Prospective clinical studies are needed to investigate the effects of denosumab on muscle function. However, decreasing the risk of falls by improving muscle function would reduce the risk of fragility fracture in older adults. Denosumab was well-tolerated, and the ease of administration by subcutaneous route every 6 months

makes it a preferred choice in many older adults. However, unlike bisphosphonates, denosumab is not incorporated into bones. Therefore, its effect diminishes when treatment is ceased. The antifracture effect declines to pretreatment levels 12 months after discontinuing therapy, and the risk of fracture increases markedly in those with prior vertebral fracture. The risk of atypical fractures increases with prolonged treatment; however, the risk to benefit ratio is small and should not preclude denosumab use. Indeed, denosumab treatment in long-term care residents may be preferred over other osteoporosis treatment modalities given the route of administration, the paucity of side effects, and the certainty of compliance.

Teriparatide

Teriparatide is a synthetic analogue of PTH and promotes both bone resorption and synthesis. Intermittent doses of teriparatide (20 mcg/d subcutaneously) exert an anabolic effect on bone, whereas continuous infusion promotes catabolic action. Treatment with teriparatide in postmenopausal women (mean age 71) over 18 months increased BMD at all sites. It also decreased the risk of vertebral fracture by 65% and nonvertebral fracture by 53%. Teriparatide was as effective in individuals 75 years or older as in a younger cohort younger than 75 years. In adults 75 years or older, after a median treatment period of 19 months, teriparatide reduced new vertebral fractures by 65%; the number needed to treat was 11. The risk of hip fracture was not investigated as a primary endpoint in this trial. In a head-to-head comparison of teriparatide with risedronate in postmenopausal women (mean age 72), the teriparatide treatment group had a 56% less cumulative incidence of new vertebral fracture over 24 months.

Indications for teriparatide include a T-score worse than −3.5 or prevalent fractures in the setting of a T-score worse than −2.5. In addition, patients who continue to fracture or lose BMD after 2 years of bisphosphonate treatment are also candidates for teriparatide. The major limitations to the use of teriparatide in older adults are its significant cost and the mode of administration, since subcutaneous dosages require an appropriate cognitive status, a high degree of motivation, and a considerable level of functional independence. At present, studies suggest that teriparatide should not be combined with bisphosphonate therapy since concurrent bisphosphonate treatment appears to blunt the BMD response to teriparatide. Due to concerns regarding osteosarcoma in animal studies, teriparatide therapy should continue no longer than 2 years. It is also contraindicated in Paget disease and those at risk of osteosarcoma or unexplained alkaline phosphatase elevation. However, it is imperative to treat with an antiresorptive after discontinuation of teriparatide to maintain gains in BMD.

Abaloparatide

Abaloparatide is a synthetic analogue of PTH-related peptide (PTHrP) and, due to preferential binding with PTH receptor, differs from teriparatide with predominantly anabolic action on bones. In a phase 3 trial, abaloparatide (80 mcg/d subcutaneously) given for 18 months to postmenopausal women (mean age 69) improved total hip BMD and reduced the risk of new vertebral fractures by 86% and nonvertebral fracture by 43%. A subgroup analysis in participants 80 years or older demonstrated that abaloparatide effectively increased BMD in both the hip and the spine. However, while there were numerical reductions in vertebral and nonvertebral fracture risk, they were not significantly different from placebo. Like teriparatide, the use of abaloparatide is restricted to a maximum of 2 years, based on the results of nonclinical studies on teriparatide, where it was associated with an increased risk of cancer. In general, as anabolic agents, both abaloparatide and teriparatide should be considered as starting therapy for patients with very high fracture risk and/or history of multiple fractures.

Romosozumab

Romosozumab is a humanized monoclonal antibody to sclerostin and thereby antagonizes its inhibitory impacts on osteoblasts. Romosozumab differs from other antiosteoporosis agents as it has dual effects on bone by decreasing bone resorption and increasing bone formation. Romosozumab administered for 12 months, followed by 12 months of denosumab treatment. lowers the risk of vertebral fracture by 75%. Romosozumab was compared with alendronate in postmenopausal women (mean age 74) and, after 2 years, was associated with 48% lower risk of vertebral fracture, 19% lower risk of nonvertebral fracture, and 38% lower risk of hip fracture versus alendronate. When compared with the anabolic agent teriparatide, romosozumab treatment significantly increased spine BMD and trabecular hip BMD. Romosozumab treatment was also very effective in men with osteoporosis (mean age 72) and after 1 year markedly increased BMD at the lumbar spine and the hip.

Romosozumab, due to its anabolic effect on bone and ease of administration (210 mg monthly SC), when compared to teriparatide (20 mcg daily SC), has the potential to be the preferred agent to treat osteoporosis and therefore decrease the risk of fractures. Its use is currently restricted to a maximum of 12 months due to concerns regarding increased risk of cardiovascular events as observed in one phase 3 clinical trial and the potential for oncogenesis due to previous known association of teriparatide with cancer in rodents. The subanalysis of the antifracture efficacy of romosozumab in old and very old adults is still awaited.

OSTEONECROSIS OF THE JAW AND ATYPICAL FEMORAL FRACTURES

Longer-term administration of antiresorptives has been associated with two major complications: ONJ and AFFs. ONJ is defined as the presence of exposed and necrotic bone in the maxillofacial region that does not heal within 8 weeks. The risk of ONJ may be increased in those undergoing invasive dental procedures, such as tooth extractions. The risk of ONJ in patients with postmenopausal osteoporosis taking oral bisphosphonates is proportional to the duration and cumulative dose of antiresorptive agents and is exceedingly low with an estimated incidence of 0.02% to 0.06%. Therefore, in general, the minimal risk of ONJ associated with bisphosphonate use appears to be significantly outweighed by the potential benefit of fracture risk reduction and the reduction in subsequent morbidity due to fractures. Overall, a professional dental checkup should *not* delay osteoporosis treatment initiation in older persons, particularly those at a very high fracture risk.

AFFs are stress or insufficiency fractures located in the subtrochanteric region and diaphysis of the femur. Radiographically, AFFs are located in the lateral cortex and with a transverse short oblique configuration, and are associated with cortical thickening (periosteal stress reaction). They have been reported in patients taking bisphosphonates and patients treated with denosumab, but they also occur in patients with no exposure to these drugs. The absolute risk of AFFs in patients on bisphosphonates is very low, ranging from 3.2 to 50 cases per 100,000 person-years. However, long-term use may be associated with a higher risk (> 100 per 100,000 person-years). More importantly, however, the number of fragility fractures prevented by bisphosphonate therapy far outweighs the number of AFFs that occur. To enable early detection, intervention, and prevention of AFF, clinicians should be vigilant and obtain imaging studies when patients on an antiresorptive present with thigh pain, as this may be an early sign of an AFF.

DRUG HOLIDAYS IN OSTEOPOROSIS TREATMENT

All long-term trials with bisphosphonates and denosumab have demonstrated sustained therapeutic efficacy and a very low incidence of side effects. Findings from pooled analyses of three long-term extension trials involving bisphosphonates reveal that patients who received 6 years or more of bisphosphonates had fracture rates of 9.3% to 11%, whereas the fracture rate for patients switched to placebo was 8.0% to 8.8%. Consequently, it is reasonable to evaluate whether continued therapy imparts additional benefit. However, it is still crucial to evaluate future fracture risk when considering patients who may benefit from a drug holiday. A drug holiday may be considered after 3 to 5 years of antiresorptive therapy in patients with moderate or low risk of fracture because stopping these medications for a short period of time poses minimal risk to the patient. In high-risk patients, careful consideration for a drug holiday's timing and/or duration is needed, as these patients may derive benefit from treatment beyond 5 years.

There is increasing concern about the underdiagnosis and undertreatment of patients with osteoporosis in particular settings, such as long-term care institutions. Institutionalized patients, whether mobile or immobile, are at high risk of osteoporosis. Residents should be assessed upon admission and multifactorial prevention measures implemented. All should be treated with a combination of vitamin D (minimal dose of 800 IU/day) plus calcium (1200 mg/day). Because frail older adults may be markedly hypovitaminotic D or exhibit an unpredictable response to supplementation, the serum level of 25(OH) vitamin D should be obtained before beginning supplementation. Between 1500 and as much as 4000 IU/day may be needed. If the 25(OH) vitamin D level is less than or equal to 50 nmol/L, patients should be started on 2000 IU/day of cholecalciferol. Individuals with levels ≤ 30 nmol/L should be started on a loading dose of 50,000 IU and then continued with a dose of 3000 to 4000 IU/day. Additionally, the presence of risk factors and/or previous fractures strongly supports the use of pharmacologic treatment with either antiresorptives or anabolic agents. Since osteosarcopenia is highly prevalent in this population, a combined diagnostic and therapeutic approach for osteoporosis and sarcopenia should be implemented. The clinician should consider the patient's level of functionality, QoL, and life expectancy before starting pharmacologic treatment for osteoporosis in a long-term care setting. However, since hip fractures lead to a decline in QoL and life expectancy, and fracture risk reduction can be achieved as quickly as 6 months of treatment, pharmacologic approaches are justified in institutionalized patients who are at risk. Bisphosphonates are the first-line choice, and intravenous administration is likely to achieve better adherence. Denosumab appears to offer equal protection and may enhance adherence because of its subcutaneous administration. Anabolic agents such as teriparatide, abaloparatide, and romosozumab are not first-line agents and should only be used in those with severe osteoporosis and repeated fractures in the setting of antiresorptive treatment.

FURTHER READING

Cauley JA, Giangregorio L. Physical activity and skeletal health in adults. *Lancet Diabetes Endocrinol.* 2020;8(2):150–162.

Chiodini I, Merlotti D, Falchetti A, Gennari L. Treatment options for glucocorticoid-induced osteoporosis. *Expert Opin Pharmacother.* 2020;21(6):721–732.

Coll PP, Phu S, Hajjar SH, Kirk B, Duque G, Taxel P. The prevention of osteoporosis and sarcopenia in older adults. *J Am Geriatr Soc.* 2021;69(5):1388–1398.

Colón-Emeric C, Whitson HE, Berry SD, et al. AGS and NIA Bench-to Bedside Conference summary: osteoporosis and soft tissue (muscle and fat) disorders. *J Am Geriatr Soc.* 2020;68(1):31–38.

Cosman F, Dempster DW. Anabolic agents for postmenopausal osteoporosis: how do you choose? *Curr Osteoporos Rep.* 2021;19(2):189–205.

Devlin MJ, Rosen CJ. The bone-fat interface: basic and clinical implications of marrow adiposity. *Lancet Diabetes Endocrinol.* 2015;3(2):141–147.

Diab DL, Watts NB. Updates on osteoporosis in men. *Endocrinol Metab Clin North Am.* 2021;50(2):239–249.

Dominguez LJ, Farruggia M, Veronese N, Barbagallo M. Vitamin D sources, metabolism, and deficiency: available compounds and guidelines for its treatment. *Metabolites.* 2021;11(4):255.

Farr JN, Khosla S. Cellular senescence in bone. *Bone.* 2019;121:121–133.

Feehan J, Al Saedi A, Duque G. Targeting fundamental aging mechanisms to treat osteoporosis. *Expert Opin Ther Targets.* 2019;23(12):1031–1039.

Fink HA, MacDonald R, Forte ML, et al. Long-term drug therapy and drug discontinuations and holidays for osteoporosis fracture prevention: a systematic review. *Ann Intern Med.* 2019;171(1):37–50.

Jain S. Role of bone turnover markers in osteoporosis therapy. *Endocrinol Metab Clin North Am.* 2021;50(2):223–237.

Kanis JA, Harvey NC, Johansson H, Odén A, McCloskey EV, Leslie WD. Overview of fracture prediction tools. *J Clin Densitom.* 2017;20(3):444–450.

Kennedy CC, Ioannidis G, Thabane L, et al. Successful knowledge translation intervention in long-term care: final results from the vitamin D and osteoporosis study (ViDOS) pilot cluster randomized controlled trial. *Trials.* 2015;16:214.

Khosla S, Hofbauer LC. Osteoporosis treatment: recent developments and ongoing challenges. *Lancet Diabetes Endocrinol.* 2017;5(11):898–907.

Kirk B, Feehan J, Lombardi G, Duque G. Muscle, bone, and fat crosstalk: the biological role of myokines, osteokines, and adipokines. *Curr Osteoporos Rep.* 2020;18(4):388–400.

Liu J, Curtis EM, Cooper C, Harvey NC. State of the art in osteoporosis risk assessment and treatment. *J Endocrinol Invest.* 2019;42(10):1149–1164.

Troen BR. Falls: to D or not to D-that is not the (only) question! *Ann Intern Med.* 2021;174(2):261–262.

Zanker J, Duque G. Osteoporosis in older persons: old and new players. *J Am Geriatr Soc.* 2019;67(4):831–840.

Osteoarthritis

Michele R. Obert, Ernest R. Vina, Jawad Bilal, C. Kent Kwoh

INTRODUCTION

Osteoarthritis (OA) is a highly prevalent and disabling disease and has been designated as a serious disease by the US Food and Drug Administration (FDA). Approximately 240 million people worldwide are affected by symptomatic OA, including at least 32 million in the United States. This number is expected to rise with longer life expectancies and the worsening obesity epidemic. OA is the third leading cause of years lived with a disability in the United States and is the most common cause of mobility limitation among older adults. Overall, there is a 1 in 2 lifetime risk of developing symptomatic knee OA. In addition, OA is associated with an increased risk of dying prematurely and with increased prevalence of comorbid conditions such as cardiovascular disease, diabetes mellitus, and depression. Those with hip or knee OA have a 20% excess mortality compared to those without it, partly due to limitation in their physical activity levels. Finally, OA-associated economic burden is highly significant due to direct medical costs and indirect costs (eg, lost wages, home care, hospital expenditures). It is estimated that wages lost due to OA approximate $65 billion, and medical costs can exceed $100 billion annually in the United States.

EPIDEMIOLOGY, CAUSES, AND PREDISPOSING FACTORS

Age, Sex, and Race

Age is the strongest risk factor for developing OA. The prevalence of the disease increases with increasing age. Among adults older than age 60 in North America, approximately 20% to 40% have radiographic evidence of hand OA while 30% to 40% have radiographic evidence of knee OA. Symptomatic OA is less prevalent, with 13% to 26% of all adults having symptomatic hand OA and 10% to 14% having symptomatic knee OA. At age 50, the pooled radiographic prevalence of thumb base OA is 5.8% for men and 7.3% for women; whereas at age 80, the pooled radiographic prevalence of thumb base OA for men and women are 33% and 39%, respectively. Among adults 45 years or older, the prevalence of symptomatic hip OA is about 10%. In one study, symptomatic foot OA was present in 17% of adults older than 50 years, with disabling symptoms presenting in 9.5%.

Women are more likely than men to be affected by hand OA, hip OA, and knee OA, especially after menopause. The prevalence of OA may also vary by race and ethnicity. OA of the knee is more common in African Americans than in non-Hispanic Whites or Mexican Americans. OA of the hip is more common in people of European descent compared to those of Asian or African descent. Compared to older Whites in the United States, older Chinese subjects in China have higher prevalence of knee OA but lower prevalence of hip and hand OA. Increasing evidence shows that the prevalence of arthritis-attributable activity and work limitation and severe joint pain is significantly higher among Hispanics compared to non-Hispanic Whites.

Obesity

Obesity is the strongest modifiable risk factor for the development of OA. It is estimated that the reduction of body weight from obese to normal weight would reduce knee OA incidence by 21% in men and 33% in women. Obesity is also associated with having an increased risk of developing hand and foot OA. However, there is less consistent data supporting the relationship between hip OA and obesity.

Occupation, Sports, and Joint Trauma

OA has also been linked to certain occupations. Working as a farmer or a construction worker/laborer increases the risk of developing knee and hip OA, especially among those who are overweight. Specific occupational activities such as more than 30 minutes of squatting, more than 30 minutes of kneeling, and climbing more than 10 flights of stairs per day increase the risk of developing radiographic knee OA. Among older adults, recreational walking, jogging, and other recreational activities do not seem to increase the risk of developing knee OA. However, high-impact sports are associated with increased risk of OA in certain joints: American football (knees, feet, ankles); baseball (shoulders, elbows); soccer (knees, hips, ankles); ice hockey (knee); and boxing (carpometacarpal). These often account for the development of OA at joints that are not usually affected by OA.

The increased risk of OA from occupational and sports activities is likely due to injury rather than participation in these activities. Hip dislocation and femoral acetabular impingement are associated with the development of hip OA. Ligamentous or meniscal damage in the knee and/or surgical meniscectomy increases the risk of knee OA. In parallel, quadriceps muscle weakness is linked to tibiofemoral and patellofemoral knee OA. Prior foot or ankle injuries have also been linked to the development of foot OA.

Malalignment and Physical Abnormalities

Joint malalignment may also increase the risk of developing OA. Varus alignment or knee extensor muscle weakness increases the risk of knee OA development and progression. This increased risk is most prominent in overweight and obese persons. Similarly, congenital hip dysplasia or cam deformity increases the risk of hip OA, especially in middle-aged (55–65 years) and younger (< 50 years) individuals. Specific physical attributes, such as leg length inequality, having a higher knee height and having an index finger shorter than the ring finger have all been associated with an increased risk of developing radiographic knee OA.

Genetics

The number of OA genetic risk loci has recently increased significantly through genome-wide association studies and now includes 90 genome-wide significant loci for OA. The effect size associated with these genes is small, however. Genes that code for structural proteins of the cartilage's extracellular matrix seem to have a role, especially those that code for collagen type II (COL2A1). Genes that code for different interleukins (eg, IL-1A, IL-1B, IL-1RN, IL-4R, IL-17A, IL-17F, and IL-6) may also affect genetic susceptibility to OA. Other genes that have been implicated in the development of OA include the estrogen receptor α gene, vitamin D receptor gene, frizzled related protein gene, asporin, and proteins related to cartilage and bone development and bone homeostasis. In addition, genes related to height, hip shape, bone area, and developmental hip dysplasia may also play a role.

CLASSIFICATION AND PATHOPHYSIOLOGY

Classification

OA has traditionally been classified as either primary (idiopathic) or secondary to known causes (Table 52-1). Primary OA most commonly affects the joints of the hands, knees, hips, spine, and feet. Nodal generalized OA is characterized by polyarticular finger involvement (distal interphalangeal [DIP], proximal interphalangeal [PIP], first carpometacarpal [CMC] joints) and a predisposition to OA of the knee, hip, and spine. It commonly affects middle-aged women with a strong family history of OA. Inflammation is being increasingly recognized as having a role in the pathophysiology of OA. Only a minority of OA patients have inflammatory symptoms, such as swelling and redness of the joints, however, and often these symptoms are mild and intermittent. Erosive OA is a variant that occurs when there is an additional erosive/inflammatory component, often involving the DIP and PIP joints of the hands. Other individuals may have a phenotype that indicates a larger role for mechanical factors in the pathophysiology. Secondary OA occurs when another disease or condition causes OA. Conditions that can lead to secondary OA include trauma; inflammatory arthritis (eg, septic arthritis, rheumatoid arthritis, seronegative

TABLE 52-1 ■ SECONDARY CAUSES OF OSTEOARTHRITIS	
Anatomical abnormalities	Bone dysplasia, congenital hip dislocation
Metabolic/endocrine	Diabetes mellitus, hemochromatosis, acromegaly, hyperparathyroidism, ochronosis
Crystal deposition disease	Gout, pseudogout
Inflammatory arthritis	Rheumatoid arthritis, systemic lupus erythematosus, seronegative spondyloarthropathy, juvenile idiopathic arthritis
Trauma	Fracture, surgery, infection
Others	Avascular necrosis, neuropathic charcot joints

spondyloarthropathy, gout); metabolic/endocrine disorders (eg, hemochromatosis, hyperparathyroidism); neuropathic disorders; and anatomical abnormalities.

The American College of Rheumatology (ACR) has proposed specific criteria to standardize the classification of OA of the knee, hip, and hands for clinical and epidemiologic studies. These criteria are based on a combination of features such as patient age (> 50 years), clinical symptoms (ie, pain, < 30 minutes of morning stiffness), physical examination (ie, presence of crepitus, bony enlargement/tenderness), laboratory findings (ie, normal inflammatory parameters, synovial fluid consistent with OA and negative rheumatoid factor), and radiographic findings (ie, presence of osteophytes). These criteria only apply to patients with symptomatic disease, exclude patients with secondary OA, and are intended to classify and not diagnose OA.

Pathophysiology

OA can be thought of as a failed repair of joint damage due to abnormal intra- and extra-articular processes involving a combination of biomechanical, biochemical, and genetic factors. A single or a combination of insults to the joints, including biomechanical trauma, chronic inflammation, genetic and metabolic factors, oxidative damage, and chondrocyte senescence, can trigger or contribute to the cascade of events that leads to OA. In the earliest stage of OA, fibrillation of the superficial layer of the articular cartilage may be observed with loss of glycosaminoglycan content in those areas. Eventually, the fibrillation extends to the subchondral bone, the cartilage fragments into the joint, the matrix degrades, and the cartilage is completely lost, leaving a denuded bone.

Chondrocytes in the articular cartilage react to insults in the joint, leading to changes in cellular function and matrix elements. Chondrocytes and synovial cells release matrix metalloproteinase (MMP) enzymes, such as collagenases, stromelysins, and gelatinases responsible for cartilage degradation. While these MMPs may be susceptible to MMP inhibitors, synthesis of MMPs is enhanced and the inhibitors are overwhelmed in OA. Cytokines have been implicated in the regulation of this process. Interleukin-1 (IL-1), a catabolic cytokine, is known to suppress type 2 cartilage synthesis and to induce proteases. IL-1 level and cell sensitivity are increased in OA. Anabolic cytokines, such as insulin-like growth factor-1 and transforming growth factor β, on the other hand, are found in decreased levels in the serum and synovial fluid of OA patients. Besides cartilage degradation, subchondral bone may also increase in density, potentially reflective of healing response to microfractures that have occurred. Cyst-like bone cavities may form, in addition to synovial inflammation and hypertrophy, which is not seen in normal aging joints. Osteophytes, or bony projections that form along joint margins, are often considered a hallmark of OA.

Several other factors have also been implicated in the development of OA. Crystals, including calcium pyrophosphate dihydrate and basic calcium phosphate crystals, have been identified in the synovial fluid of OA joints. Other than their ability to induce inflammation, their role in the pathogenesis of OA remains unclear. Protein levels of nuclear receptor erythroid 2-related factors 1 and 2 (NRF1 and NRF2), which regulate antioxidant gene expression for cellular protection, are present in lower levels in chondrocytes of persons with OA. An imbalance in antioxidant production by the chondrocyte compared to reactive oxygen species production has been found to damage lipids, protein, DNA, and normal cell signaling, contributing to the development of OA. In addition, the complement system may stimulate inflammatory mediators and enzymes that can contribute to the pathogenesis of inflammatory OA, while nitric oxide, known to activate MMPs in articular cartilage, may also mediate the osteoarthritic development process. Supported by epidemiologic studies, sex-related hormones have also been considered to play a role in the development of OA, especially in women.

PRESENTATION

Symptoms

Patients with symptomatic OA most commonly present with pain in the joint. Pain tends to worsen with increased activity or weight-bearing and to improve with rest. Early in the disease, patients may complain of pain that is sharp, intermittent, and unpredictable. These features may often lead patients to limit their activity to avoid pain. As the disease progresses, the pain becomes more constant and aching in nature. Late in the disease, pain may be noted with progressively less activity, possibly occurring even at rest and at night. Patients may also complain of morning stiffness that typically resolves within 30 minutes or less. Joint stiffness may also occur after periods of prolonged inactivity, also known as the "gelling" phenomenon. Other patients may report joint locking or joint instability. In contrast, joint stiffness lasting more than an hour, joint pain and stiffness that improve with activity, and persistent joint swelling all suggest an inflammatory type of arthritis, such as rheumatoid arthritis, instead of OA.

Knee OA patients may complain of localized pain, often in the medial and lateral joint lines, or diffuse knee pain. They may have difficulty climbing the stairs or walking for even short periods of time. With laxity in the knee joint, patients may have feelings of knee instability, which may lead to falls. Hip OA patients may complain of pain in the anterior hip or inguinal area. Less commonly, their pain may also be felt laterally (ie, in the trochanter) or referred to the knee. They may have difficulty crossing their legs or putting on a pair of shoes.

Hand OA patients may report pain involving the DIP, PIP, and first CMC joints. Gripping, pinching, holding, or lifting objects may be particularly challenging in patients with symptomatic hand OA. Foot OA can cause such disabling foot pain with ambulation that can lead to significant functional limitations and increased risk of falls.

OA most commonly affects the cervical and lumbar spine areas. Cervical spine OA typically causes neck pain but can also cause occipital headaches, upper extremity radicular pain, shoulder pain, and loss of dexterity of the hands. Rarely, large osteophytes may compromise the spinal canal, causing lower-extremity spasticity and gait disturbance. Lumbar spine OA can often cause lower back pain that may radiate into the lower extremities and worsen with bending ipsilateral to the involved joint. Lumbar facet joint osteophytes can lead to lumbar canal stenosis with symptoms of claudication and/or pain at night; symptoms of spinal stenosis are often relieved by bending slightly forward (eg, walking uphill, upstairs or leaning forward on a shopping cart) and worsened by bending backward (eg, walking downhill or downstairs). Other symptoms of spinal stenosis include pain, tingling, numbness, and weakness,

Physical Examination

OA patients may have a completely normal physical examination. Typically, they have joint-line tenderness, crepitus (ie, a peculiar crackling, crinkly, or grating feeling on palpation, which may also be audible) and bony enlargement. There may be joint swelling that tends to be intermittent and without palpable warmth. Synovitis can also be noted in OA, and some patients may have prominent joint effusions. With disease progression, the joint's range of motion may decrease. Joint deformity, contractures, and/or laxity may also develop later in the disease.

In hand OA, there may be tenderness of the affected finger joints and/or tenderness of the first CMC joint. Enlargement of the first CMC joint can result in a squared appearance of the hand. Prominent bony enlargements of the DIP and PIP joints are known as Heberden and Bouchard nodes, respectively.

In knee OA, there is often crepitus on active knee motion and bony tenderness. There may also be effusion (without warmth) and a limited range of motion. The joint fluid may migrate into the semimembranosus bursa posteriorly, causing swelling along the posterior knee known as a popliteal or "Baker's" cyst. Knee varus ("bow-legged") or valgus ("knock-kneed") deformities may be observed later in the disease. Medial/lateral knee joint laxity may be evident on examination and lead to joint instability.

In hip OA there may be reproducible pain along the anterior hip or the inguinal area with passive or active range of motion, particularly with extension and internal rotation. The range of motion in the hip joint may also be affected; limited internal rotation and/or extension may be an early indication of hip OA. Hip OA patients may also develop an antalgic gait in which the stance phase of the gait is abnormally shortened on the affected hip joint.

In foot OA, the first metatarsophalangeal (MTP) joint is most commonly affected, followed by the second cuneometatarsal (CMT) and talonavicular (TN) joints.

There are limited agreed upon guidelines for the clinical assessment of foot OA. For first MTP joint OA specifically, the patient may exhibit pain in that joint upon walking, limited dorsiflexion in the first MTP joint and pain on direct palpation of the joint. Other exam findings that may be present include hallux valgus, first interphalangeal joint hyperextension, and decrease in ankle joint dorsiflexion range of motion.

EVALUATION

Diagnostic Imaging

OA can usually be diagnosed clinically based on history and physical examination alone. Although conventional radiography can demonstrate the severity of damage and may be used to confirm the diagnosis with an atypical presentation, radiographs are not necessary to make a diagnosis. Before making a clinical diagnosis of OA, however, other diseases should be excluded. At the very least, OA should be distinguished from referred pain, inflammatory arthritis conditions (eg, rheumatoid arthritis, gout, pseudogout) and periarticular bursitis (eg, trochanteric bursitis of the hip, pes anserine bursitis of the knee). Radiographic findings suggestive of OA are very common in older adults, yet many of these patients have minimal to no OA-related symptoms. Radiographic features of OA include joint space narrowing, osteophytes, subchondral sclerosis, subchondral cysts, and/or altered bone contours. X-rays may also show calcification of cartilage or other structures and soft-tissue swelling.

Radiographic findings specific to knee OA patients include medial tibiofemoral and/or patellofemoral joint space narrowing, along with osteophyte formation. Lateral joint space narrowing may also be seen but is less common (**Figure 52-1**). Osteophytes may be seen anteriorly and medially at the distal femur and proximal tibia and posteriorly at the patella and tibia. Radiographic changes seen in hip OA include joint space narrowing (superior, axial, or medial), osteophyte (femoral or acetabular) formation, and subchondral sclerosis.

With hand OA, the first CMC, the DIP, and the PIP joints are most commonly involved. Joint space loss is typically nonuniform and asymmetric. Involvement of more than two metacarpophalangeal joints suggests different type of arthritis other than OA. Hand x-rays of those with erosive OA will reveal erosions and the "gull-wing" deformity (**Figure 52-2**). X-rays of patients with lumbar or cervical OA will reveal intervertebral disc narrowing and osteophytes arising from the vertebral body margins (**Figure 52-3**). Sclerosis and cyst formation may also be seen. Neural foraminal narrowing may result from osteophyte formation, but this is best seen using a computed tomographic (CT) scan.

With foot OA, a foot-specific atlas that grades osteophytes and joint space narrowing can be used to classify radiographic OA in the commonly affected areas, although

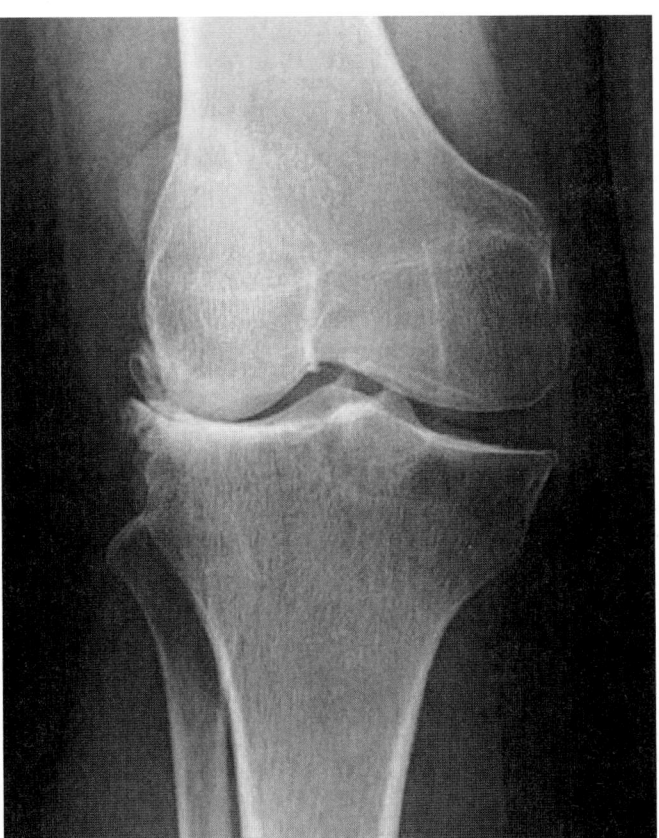

FIGURE 52-1. Knee x-ray anteroposterior view showing severe joint space narrowing within the lateral compartment, genu valgus, and joint effusion.

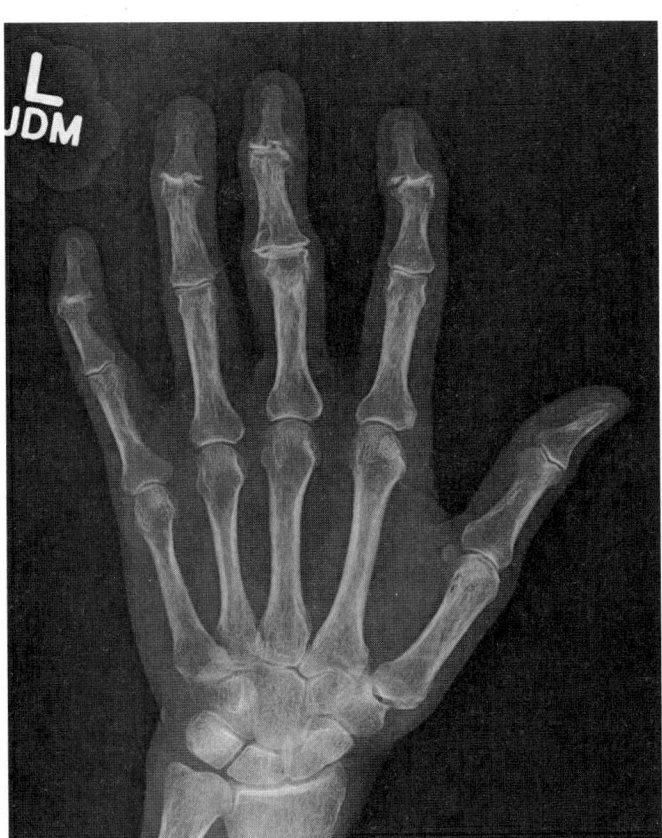

FIGURE 52-2. Hand x-ray showing joint space narrowing of the index, middle, ring, and small finger DIP joints and middle finger PIP joint. There are possible central erosions of the index and ring finger DIP joints, suggestive of erosive osteoarthropathy.

this requires both dorsoplantar and lateral views to be taken while standing.

It is important to remember that conventional radiographs have limited resolution and cannot detect early OA. They also only provide images of bony structure and are two-dimensional projections of three-dimensional joints, meaning multiple views are necessary to visualize the joint and detect possible OA involvement properly.

As a research tool, MRI has allowed the detection of preradiographic OA. It offers greater resolution than an x-ray, provides depiction in three dimensions, and allows visualization of bone and soft tissue structures. MRI allows visualization of subchondral cyst-like lesions, subchondral bone attrition, joint effusion, synovitis and meniscal damage. The integrity of ligaments, periarticular cysts and bursae, and osteophytes may also be assessed through MRI. It is important to remember that although research with MRI has contributed to understanding the relevance of these structures in explaining pain and structural progression in OA, MRI is not necessary to diagnose OA.

Laboratory Studies

Laboratory tests are unhelpful in diagnosing OA but are helpful in excluding other causes of arthritis such as

rheumatoid arthritis, gout, or infectious arthritis. Inflammatory markers, such as erythrocyte sedimentation rate and C-reactive protein level, and immunologic tests, such as antinuclear antibodies and rheumatoid factor, should not be routinely ordered unless there are signs or symptoms suggestive of inflammatory arthritis or autoimmune disease. Uric acid level may be ordered if gout is suspected.

Performing an arthrocentesis may be valuable in evaluating patients with presumptive OA. Synovial fluid findings in OA often show a white blood cell count of less than 2000 cells/mm^3. Counts that are greater than 2000 cells/mm^3 suggest an inflammatory or infectious arthritis etiology. Under polarized microscopy, there should be no visible crystals. The presence of gout or pseudogout crystals suggests crystalline arthritis as the underlying cause of joint pain.

A variety of OA-related biomarkers have been identified and validated for several OA outcomes. They are products of cartilage and bone turnover (eg, urine/serum carboxy-telopeptide of type II collagen, serum hyaluronan). However, their utility in diagnosing OA, determining the risk of disease progression, and assessing the response to OA therapies is unclear and currently under investigation.

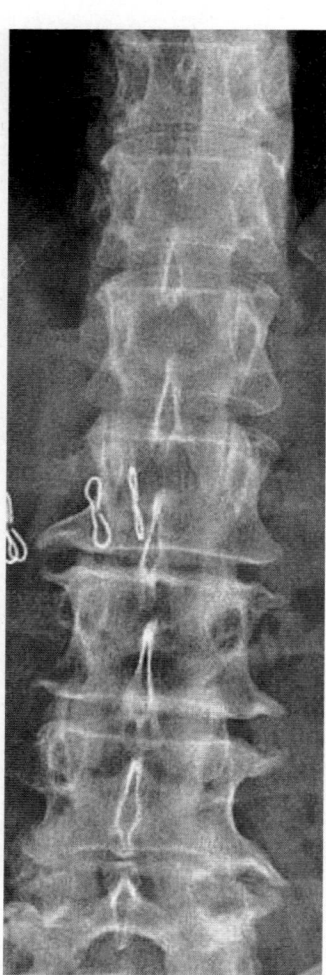

FIGURE 52-3. Lumbar spine x-ray showing extensive osteophyte formation.

MANAGEMENT

The ACR/Arthritis Foundation (AF) and the Osteoarthritis Research Society International (OARSI) have published updated recommendations for management of OA. The main goals of management are to minimize OA-related pain, improve physical functioning and optimize the quality of life of patients with OA. There are nonpharmacologic, pharmacologic, and surgical treatment options for the management of OA (**Figures 52-4** and **52-5**). OA management should be tailored to the individual patient, and optimal management likely includes a combination of these treatment modalities. For example, evidence suggests that patient education, exercise programs, weight reduction, and wedge insoles all offer additional benefit in combination with an analgesic or nonsteroidal anti-inflammatory drug (NSAID).

Physical, Psychosocial, and Mind-Body Approaches

Self-efficacy and self-management OA patients should be taught the goals of OA treatment, the importance of changes in lifestyle, exercise, pacing of activities and weight loss, and various ways to minimize joint loading. The educational focus should be on initiating self-help and patient-driven treatments that reflect the nature and course of the disease rather than simply accepting therapies delivered by providers. Thereafter, the emphasis should be on maintaining adherence to nonpharmacologic and pharmacologic therapies. Such information may be taught through group courses, individual consultations, and regular telephone calls. Participants in these programs report reduction in pain, improvement in function, and weight loss. These programs may also increase patient self-efficacy and physical activity, and decrease the number of OA-related physician visits.

Exercise Aerobic exercise and muscle strengthening can significantly improve the physical health and symptoms of patients with OA. Regular aerobic activities that older adults can engage in include walking, bicycling, swimming, and tai chi. Quadriceps muscle strengthening can be particularly helpful for a patient with knee OA. In general, there is no significant difference in reducing arthritis-related symptoms and disability in knee and hip OA patients between aerobic and resistance training. In addition, balance exercises may be beneficial by improving a person's ability to control and stabilize their body position.

For patients with advanced OA, mobilization exercises (ie, stretching and flexibility training) and isometric strengthening exercises can initially be prescribed. Mobilization exercises increase length and elasticity in muscles and periarticular tissues. Mobilization of the sesamoid apparatus and strengthening of hallux plantar flexors is beneficial for first MTP joint OA. During isometric exercises, muscle length does not noticeably change and the affected joint does not move. Isometric exercises for older adults include chair leg extensions, wall sits, and hip extensions. The exercise regimen may then progress toward isotonic strengthening and aerobic exercises. During isotonic exercise, muscle tension remains unchanged but muscle length changes. Beneficial isotonic exercises include squats, wall slides, and leg presses. Finally, water-based exercise is a low-impact activity that takes the pressure off joints, muscles, and bones. It is particularly beneficial for those with severe OA and marked deconditioning.

Physical therapists are valuable for providing instructions and appropriate exercises. They are essential for outlining individualized treatment and a progressive home exercise program. Indeed, a physical therapy regimen that includes strengthening and neuromuscular training can improve symptoms in two-thirds of patients with advanced knee OA. Physical therapy evaluation may also result in provision of assistive devices, such as canes and walkers, as necessary.

In summary, exercise can be a joint-specific range of motion and/or strengthening program or a general aerobic conditioning regimen. Exercise may be supervised on land, in water or in a self-directed home-based program. Regardless of the type of exercise regimen, extra attention

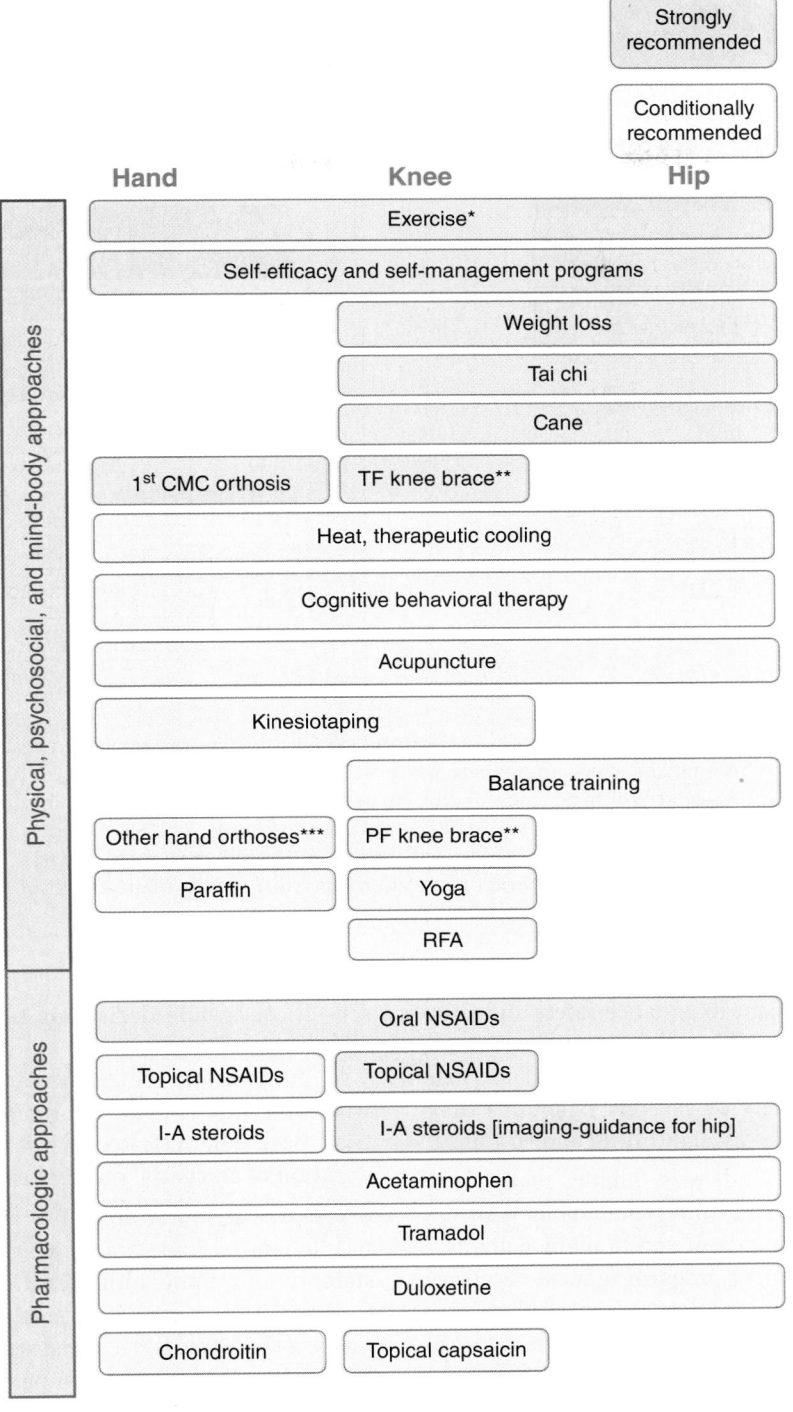

FIGURE 52-4. Nonpharmacologic and pharmacologic treatment options that are recommended for the management of OA. Recommended therapies for the management of osteoarthritis (OA). Strongly and conditionally recommended approaches to management of hand, knee, and/or hip OA are shown. No hierarchy within categories is implied in the figure, with the recognition that the various options may be used (and reused) at various times during the course of a particular patient's disease. * = Exercise for knee and hip OA could include walking, strengthening, neuromuscular training, and aquatic exercise, with no hierarchy of one over another. Exercise is associated with better outcomes when supervised. ** = Knee brace recommendations: tibiofemoral (TF) brace for TF OA (strongly recommended), patellofemoral (PF) brace for PF OA (conditionally recommended). *** = Hand orthosis recommendations: first carpometacarpal (CMC) joint neoprene or rigid orthoses for first CMC joint OA (strongly recommended), orthoses for joints of the hand other than the first CMC joint (conditionally recommended). IA = intraarticular; NSAIDs = nonsteroidal anti-inflammatory drugs; RFA = radiofrequency ablation. (Reproduced with permission from Kolasinski SL, Neogi T, Hochberg MC, et al. 2019 American College of Rheumatology/Arthritis Foundation Guideline for the Management of Osteoarthritis of the Hand, Hip, and Knee. *Arthritis Care Res (Hoboken)*. 2020;72[2]:149–162.)

A

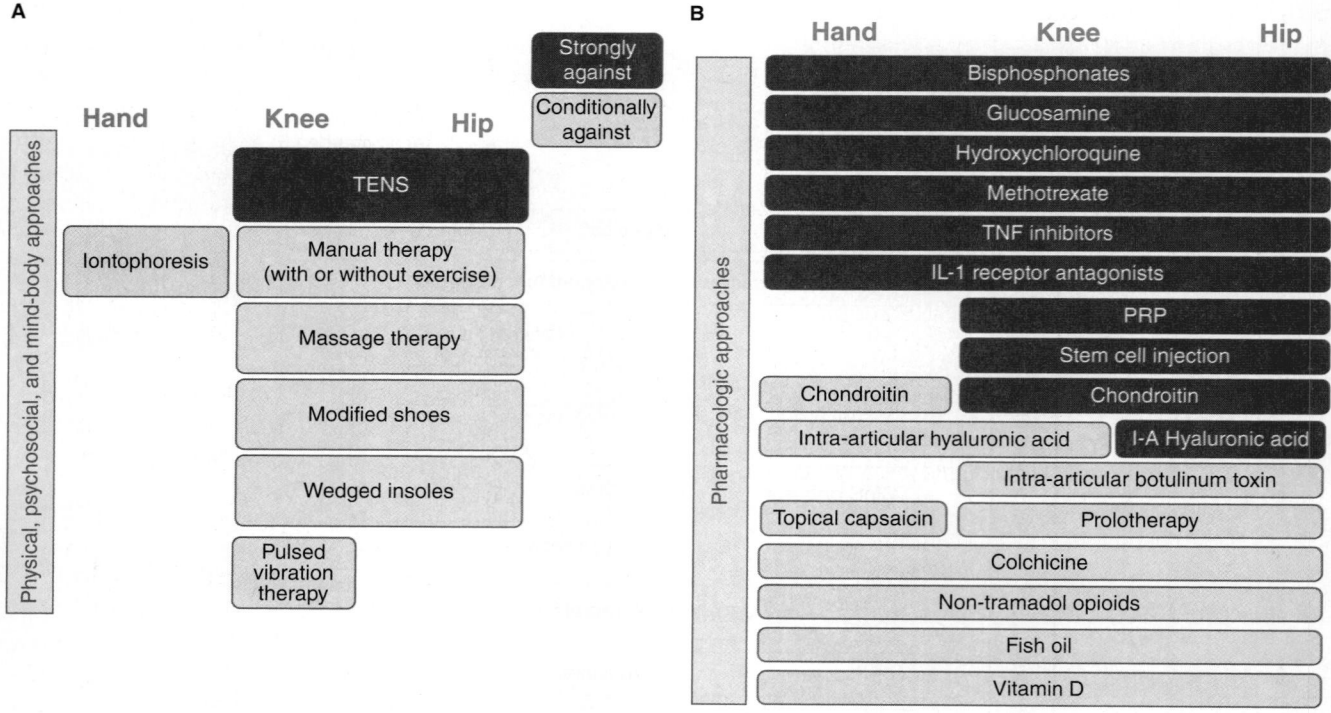

B

FIGURE 52-5 Nonpharmacologic and pharmacologic treatment options that are recommended against for the management of OA. Therapies recommended *against* physical, psychosocial, and mind-body approaches (**A**) and pharmacologic approaches (**B**) in the management of hand, knee, and/or hip osteoarthritis. No hierarchy within categories is implied in the figure. I-A = intraarticular; IL-1 = interleukin-1; PRP = platelet-rich plasma; TENS = transcutaneous electrical nerve stimulation; TNF = tumor necrosis factor. (Reproduced with permission from Kolasinski SL, Neogi T, Hochberg MC, et al. 2019 American College of Rheumatology/Arthritis Foundation Guideline for the Management of Osteoarthritis of the Hand, Hip, and Knee. *Arthritis Care Res (Hoboken).* 2020;72[2]:149–162.)

is needed for the older patient to enhance safety and compliance with the program, taking into account potential comorbidities. Those with knee or hip OA should also cautiously engage in moderately or severely strenuous exercises (eg, stair climbing, heavy weightlifting and running).

Weight loss All existing guidelines highly recommend weight loss in overweight and obese individuals with OA of the hip or knee for OA management. In many patients, a structured weight management program may be necessary. An effective program focuses on developing healthy eating and physical activity habits. It should include a plan for the individual to lose weight slowly and steadily to maintain weight loss over the long run. Patients should avoid fad diets, which often result in rapid weight loss in the short term, but weight gain over the longer term. A realistic goal is weight loss of more than 5% to be achieved within a 20-week period. The program may include ongoing feedback, monitoring, and support. Weight reduction has been shown to improve knee and hip OA-related pain, stiffness and disability.

Tai chi and acupuncture Tai chi, a practice that originated in China, is referred to as "moving meditation." Practitioners move their bodies slowly, gently, and with awareness while incorporating deep breathing, meditation, and relaxation. It may be beneficial in improving strength, balance, and self-efficacy while decreasing the risk of falls in patients with lower extremity OA.

In contrast, the efficacy of acupuncture in patients with knee, hip, or hand OA remains controversial. Clinical trials have demonstrated that it may provide a short-lived duration of analgesia, mostly for those with knee OA.

Braces and taping A tibiofemoral knee brace, and at times patellofemoral knee braces, can reduce pain and improve stability and ambulation, leading to lower risk of falling for knee OA patients with varus or valgus instability. Separately, a brace and a neoprene sleeve offer additional beneficial effects for knee OA compared with medical treatment alone. A brace tends to be more effective than a neoprene sleeve, however. Medially directed patellar taping may also benefit patients with knee OA.

Orthoses All patients with knee, hip, or foot OA should receive advice regarding appropriate footwear. However, laterally and medially wedged insoles have not demonstrated clear efficacy or benefit. Hand orthoses may benefit patients with first digit CMC joint OA of the hand, although evidence supporting hand orthoses for OA in other joints of the hand has not yet been established. With foot OA, footwear known as a "rockersole," where the sole of the shoe is curved, reduces the need for first MTP joint dorsiflexion and has been shown to reduce the pressure under the first MTP joint. Foot orthoses include shoe-stiffening inserts and contoured orthoses that may reduce foot pain.

Assistive devices Walking aids can reduce OA-related pain in patients with knee and hip OA. A cane can significantly reduce joint loading and pain. In addition, it can provide additional stability in a patient where joint disease affects ambulation. It should be properly fitted to approximately the level of the greater trochanter of the hip. Patients should be instructed to use the cane with the hand opposite the affected knee or hip. The final bend to the elbow when walking with the cane should be approximately 15 to 20 degrees. When disability is more severe or when OA is bilateral, a walker may be a better option. Assistive devices, such as zipper pulls, built-up handles on pencils/pens, cushioned carrying tools, and meal preparation devices, can be very beneficial for patients with hand OA. Occupational therapists are likely to be helpful in recommending lifestyle modifications and assistive devices to patients with arthritis symptoms.

Heat and cold therapy Thermal modalities may be effective for relieving OA symptoms, but the benefits may be temporary. All patients with hand, knee, and hip OA should be instructed in the use of thermal agents. Heat can be administered by various techniques, including the application of heat packs, ultrasound, electrically delivered heat, immersion in warm water, and paraffin baths. There are also store-bought heat patches, belts, packs, and wraps. Patients should be instructed that heat therapies should be limited to 20-minute intervals to reduce the risk of burns. Cold (or cryotherapy) can be administered by application of ice packs or massage with ice. It can decrease inflammation, minimize muscle spasms, and reduce pain. Patients should also be instructed to limit the use of ice or cold packs to 20 minutes. The choice of heat or cold is often based on patient preference.

Topical Agents

Capsaicin and rubefacients Topical capsaicin creams contain a lipophilic alkaloid extracted from chili peppers, which activates and sensitizes peripheral c-nociceptors. Both 0.03% and 0.08% topical capsaicin have been shown to reduce pain in knee OA, although a dose of 0.03% topical Capsaicin is better tolerated than a dose of 0.08%. At this time, efficacy in treating hand OA has not been well demonstrated, and the risk of contaminating the eyes is high. Capsaicin has also not demonstrated any benefit in treating hip OA, likely due to the depth of the joint under the skin. Topical capsaicin can be considered as an adjunct therapy or used instead of topical NSAIDs for foot OA as studies have shown similar improvement in pain. Rubefacients containing salicylates (eg, trolamine salicylate, hydroxyethyl salicylate, diethylamine salicylate) may also be used as adjunctive agents, albeit supportive data is scant. Skin burning, stinging and erythema are potential side effects.

Topical NSAIDs Topical NSAIDs, such as diclofenac sodium gel, are recommended as first-line pharmacological therapy to treat hand and knee OA prior to starting oral NSAIDs, given their favorable side effect profile and efficacy of pain relief. They are also recommended as first-line pharmacologic therapy for the treatment of symptomatic foot OA. In February 2020, the FDA approved Voltaren gel (diclofenac sodium topical gel 1%) for sale over the counter. Topical NSAIDs have a high safety margin and are not associated with acute renal failure or gastrointestinal adverse events when used as instructed. Thus, they may be particularly useful in patients with cardiac, renal, or gastrointestinal comorbidities. They may be less ideal for those with a large number of affected joints, in which case systemic therapy would be preferred. Similar to capsaicin, topical NSAIDs are not recommended for treating hip OA due to the depth of the joint under the skin precluding their efficacy.

Oral Pharmacologic Therapies

Acetaminophen Acetaminophen has traditionally been used as a first-line agent in treating mild-moderate OA. However, some meta-analyses have shown that acetaminophen was no better than placebo for symptom control. Other studies showed its use was associated with minimal improvement in pain control, which may be outweighed by the side effect profile of the medication. Acetaminophen use may still play a role in the treatment of knee, hip, hand, or foot OA for short treatment durations, or in patients who have contraindications precluding the use of oral or topical NSAIDs. The FDA has reduced the maximum daily dose of acetaminophen to 3 g/day. Regular monitoring for hepatotoxicity is recommended in those with prolonged use, especially for those taking the maximum recommended daily dose.

Oral NSAIDs NSAIDs inhibit the activity of cyclooxygenase (COX)-1 and -2 enzymes, providing analgesic and anti-inflammatory effects. They are recommended as first-line oral pharmacotherapy over all other oral medications and can be very helpful for OA patients who do not respond to topical NSAIDs, have multiple joint involvement, or suffer from moderate-to-severe levels of pain. There is no strong evidence that a particular NSAID is more effective than other NSAIDs, but the side effect profiles make some safer than others for specific patients. Some patients may prefer specific NSAIDs (eg, meloxicam, naproxen) based on the frequency of dosing for convenience.

Patients may be started on a low-cost NSAID with a short half-life, such as ibuprofen. Initially, the medication should be started on the lowest possible dose, and if the response is not satisfactory after a few weeks, then the medication dosage may be slowly increased up to the maximum recommended dose. Switching to a different NSAID is another OA treatment management option.

While efficacious, NSAIDs should be prescribed with caution, particularly in patients with comorbidities that may increase NSAID toxicity. Gastrointestinal complications such as peptic ulcers and bleeding are potential side effects. This risk increases with older age, concurrent use of other medications (eg, glucocorticoids, anticoagulants), and longer therapy duration. Using either a COX-2 selective inhibitor or a nonselective NSAID in combination with a proton-pump inhibitor reduces this risk. Nephrotoxicity is another potential toxicity. Patients with chronic kidney disease (CKD) stage IV or V (estimated glomerular filtration rate < 30 cc/min) should avoid NSAIDs. Nonacetylated salicylates, sulindac, and nabumetone may be less nephrotoxic than other NSAIDs.

Patients with cardiovascular disease are also at increased risk for cardiovascular adverse events (eg, myocardial infarct or stroke) associated with NSAIDs, particularly with the use of diclofenac. Patients should be made aware of such risks and monitored closely during treatment. Finally, concomitant use of low-dose aspirin and nonselective NSAIDs (eg, ibuprofen) may also render aspirin less effective when used for cardioprotection and stroke prevention.

COX-2 selective inhibitors A COX-2 inhibitor (ie, celecoxib) or a COX-2 selective NSAID (eg, meloxicam) can be a better treatment option for a subset of OA patients. They can effectively relieve painful OA symptoms with significantly less risk of GI side effects as compared to nonselective NSAIDs. Prescribing these medications to patients with cardiovascular risk factors should be done with caution however, as they may increase the risk of myocardial infarct, stroke, and other related conditions.

Narcotic analgesics Tramadol is a weak μ-opioid receptor inhibitor that inhibits the reuptake of serotonin and norepinephrine. It can relieve pain in patients with hand, knee, or hip OA, but should only be used when they have contraindications to NSAIDs, inadequate response to other pharmacologic and nonpharmacologic treatment modalities, or are not a good surgical candidate. Tramadol should be trialed prior to any nontramadol opioids. Like other narcotic agents, it can also cause nausea, dizziness, somnolence, vomiting, and increased mortality risk. Long-term use may also lead to physical dependence. However, respiratory depression and constipation are considered less of a problem with tramadol.

More potent narcotic medicines, such as oxycodone, hydrocodone, or morphine sulfate, may be considered in some OA patients only after failure of all other treatments. Patients who continue to have severe OA-related pain and disability despite trying other pharmacologic and nonpharmacologic OA treatments may be good candidates. Those who are unwilling or unable to undergo joint replacement surgery due to comorbid conditions (eg, significant cardiac or pulmonary disease) may also be reasonable candidates.

Narcotic agents are poorly tolerated in older people due to increased sensitivity to certain side effects, including constipation, urinary retention, confusion, and sedation. The risk of falls may also be increased in a population already vulnerable to falls due to joint disease and other risk factors. If narcotic medicines are to be started in older people, then the lowest dose should be prescribed for the

shortest possible length of time. Adjuvant therapies with nonnarcotic pain relievers should also be considered.

Nutraceuticals Glucosamine and chondroitin sulfate are naturally occurring constituents of cartilage proteoglycans. They are popular "nutritional supplements" used by many OA patients, but their use is highly controversial. Although several clinical trials showed their efficacy in improving pain and function, these trials were primarily industry-sponsored and utilized a pharmaceutical grade of glucosamine sulfate, which is not available in the United States. The best available data with the lowest risk of bias indicate that these supplements were no more effective than placebo. The ACR/AF and OARSI recommend against the use of either glucosamine or chondroitin sulfate to treat knee or hip OA.

Other nutraceuticals have been investigated for their potential benefits in the treatment of OA. A number of nutraceuticals have reported a short-term reduction of pain, but most of the current studies on nutraceuticals are small, exhibit various forms of bias, and have short follow-up times.

Other options The use of serotonin and norepinephrine reuptake inhibitors, such as duloxetine, seems promising in the treatment of OA. It has shown moderate efficacy in treating symptoms for knee OA when used alone or when combined with NSAIDs, and its effects are likely to be similar in the treatment of hip and hand OA. The tolerability of the medication may be a limiting factor, however.

Disease-modifying osteoarthritis drugs (DMOADs) can potentially inhibit the structural disease progression of OA and improve OA-related symptoms. At present, there are no DMOAD therapies available on the market. However, several research studies are being conducted to determine DMOAD efficacy and safety. Many studies have focused primarily on preventing hyaline cartilage loss. Because the pathogenesis of OA involves multiple tissues, more recent studies are also targeting other tissues, including the subchondral bone. Most DMOADs under investigation have an anti-catabolic effect on cartilage and may also structurally modify subchondral bone. Studies of bisphosphonates showed no efficacy in the control of OA pain or improvement in function. Similarly, tumor necrosis factor inhibitors and IL-1 receptor antagonists administered subcutaneously or intra-articularly did not prove to be efficacious for treating erosive OA and are not recommended for use. Other options under investigation include inducible nitric oxide synthase inhibitors, MMP inhibitors, aggrecanase inhibitors, doxycycline, Wnt inhibition, intra-articular injection of an anabolic growth factor, fibroblast growth factor 18, and a cathepsin K inhibitor.

Intra-Articular Therapies

Glucocorticoid agents Intra-articular glucocorticoid (eg, methylprednisolone, triamcinolone) injections can significantly relieve pain due to OA. They can be most beneficial to OA patients with one or a few joints that continue to be bothersome despite oral pharmacologic therapies. They are particularly efficacious in patients with knee or hip OA. Knee joint injection can be administered in an ambulatory care setting. Hip joint injection, though, is often done with ultrasonographic or fluoroscopic guidance. When proper technique is used, complications from intra-articular injections such as bleeding and infection are rare. Benefits may be short-lived, however, and pain relief typically lasts for up to 2 months. More than three injections within a 6-month period are not recommended, and the long-term effects these steroids have on the cartilage are still controversial.

Viscosupplementation Viscosupplementation, the intra-articular injection of hyaluronic acid, has been used for symptomatic knee OA. Hyaluronic acid is a large molecular weight glycosaminoglycan, which is a constituent of synovial fluid. Hyaluronic acid in OA joints is often of low molecular weight, losing its biomechanical and anti-inflammatory properties. Recent meta-analyses demonstrated no clear benefit of intra-articular hyaluronic acid injection for the treatment of OA symptoms after addressing the component of bias from studies, especially in hip OA. Although the ACR/AF and OARSI OA management guidelines do not recommend using viscosupplementation based on the lack of evidence for treatment benefit, there may be individual patients who would benefit from a trial after the failure of all other treatment options.

Platelet-rich plasma and mesenchymal stem cell therapy Platelet-rich plasma (PRP) and mesenchymal stem cell (MSC) therapy are heavily marketed for many conditions including OA. These therapies are still experimental, have not been approved by the FDA, and should not be administered or obtained except in the case of an FDA-approved clinical trial. They may be marketed as "FDA-approved," but only the equipment used to obtain and administer the PRP or MSC therapy has been FDA-approved.

Surgical Interventions

Surgical intervention should be considered in OA patients who continue to have significant pain and disability despite maximal use of nonpharmacologic and pharmacologic therapies. Patients must also be healthy enough to withstand surgery. Shared decision making has been shown to be beneficial for patients and surgeons with regards to expectations, satisfaction, and outcomes.

Arthroscopic debridement and joint lavage Arthroscopic debridement is the removal of loose bodies, debris, mobile fragments of articular cartilage, unstable torn menisci, and impinging osteophytes. The procedure invariably also includes joint lavage. While it is a relatively common procedure, its practice is highly controversial. While a few uncontrolled studies have demonstrated short-term efficacy, most studies have shown that this procedure is no better than placebo in providing symptomatic relief for knee OA. Arthroscopic debridement or joint lavage alone is not recommended as treatment options in the OARSI OA management guidelines.

Osteotomy Osteotomy is a surgical procedure in which the bone is cut to shorten, lengthen, or change bone alignment. High tibial osteotomy is a potential surgical treatment for knee OA. It is appropriate for unilateral knee OA with varus malalignment. Realignment of the varus deformity would reduce stress on the medial compartment of the knee by redistributing the weight of the body from the arthritic medial compartment to the healthier lateral compartment. Although the overall failure rate at 10 years is approximately 25%, the procedure can reduce pain, improve function, and delay the need for joint replacement.

Intertrochanteric varus or valgus osteotomy has been used for hip OA treatment for nearly a century. Pelvic or femoral osteotomies have also been used to correct the biomechanics and joint congruency in young patients with hip dysplasia to prevent the development of hip OA. Evidence in the efficacy of these procedures, however, is limited.

Joint replacement Joint replacement surgery is an irreversible procedure used in those with severe OA who have failed conservative treatment modalities, have persistent pain, and have had associated loss of function secondary to their symptoms. The average age at the time of knee replacement is the mid-sixties, although this procedure is being done more and more often in younger patients. Patients who undergo surgery often attain substantial improvements in pain, quality of life, and physical functioning; however, between 20% and 30% of patients have reported not being satisfied with surgery outcomes after total joint replacement. Maximal improvements are usually observed in the first 3 to 6 months with long-term benefit plateauing after 9 to 12 months. Quality of life indicators following joint replacement also improve approximately a year after surgery and only decline gradually over time. Certain patient characteristics such as advanced age, obesity, and comorbidities may limit improvement in patient-reported outcomes after surgery and increase rates of complications, but the presence of these characteristics should not prevent patients from being offered surgery; rather, these factors should inform the shared decision-making process. With current advances, implants typically last 15 years or more. The risk of revision is higher in patients with diabetes, obesity, and those who received surgery before 65 years compared to those aged 65 or older.

Unicompartmental knee arthroplasty involves replacement of a part or section of the knee that is arthritic. It may be considered in patients with discrete knee pain and disease localized to the medial compartment. Compared to total knee arthroplasty, it may also improve knee pain and function and requires a smaller surgical incision. Consequently, there is less postoperative pain, and hospital stays are shorter. The rehabilitation process also tends to be more rapid. Postsurgical complications, such as deep vein thrombosis and infection, are also fewer with unicompartmental than total knee replacement surgery. However, unicompartmental knee arthroplasty may make subsequent total knee replacement surgery more complex and has a shorter lifespan than a total knee arthroplasty joint, making rates of revision higher.

Joint fusion Joint fusion surgery, also known as arthrodesis, may be selected in patients with severe OA of the wrist, ankle, or first MTP joint. It may also be used as a salvage procedure when knee joint replacement has failed. During the procedure, two bones on each end of a joint are fused, eliminating the joint itself. While a fused joint loses flexibility, it can bear weight better and may leave the patient completely pain-free.

Hand surgeries Surgery is considered when nonsurgical treatment options have not significantly helped patients with OA of the thumb base or OA of the interphalangeal joints. In the case of the first CMC joint OA, trapeziectomy is the procedure of choice. More complicated surgical techniques have not proven to be more effective and are linked to increased rates of adverse events such as pain, instability, nerve dysfunction, chronic regional pain syndrome, and infections. The procedure of choice for OA in the PIP joint is arthroplasty with a silicone implant, except for the second PIP joint, for which arthrodesis is the preferred surgical method. Similarly, arthrodesis is the best approach for the DIP joints.

PREVENTION

There are currently no therapies known to prevent the progression of joint damage due to OA. However, current research efforts are trying to identify preclinical biochemical and imaging biomarkers that will provide opportunities to diagnose and treat OA earlier in the disease course. Hence, we may eventually be able to prevent the development and further progression of the disease.

There are also known potential theoretical targets for primary and secondary prevention of OA. A person's weight is the largest identified modifiable risk factor for the development and progression of OA. The risk of knee OA has been shown to increase along with an increase in BMI. Therefore, weight loss for those who fall into the obese and overweight categories is important in primary prevention. Patients need to be educated on the benefits of weight loss and the need to achieve a normal body weight.

The *Physical Activity Guidelines for Americans* recommend at least 150 minutes of moderate-intensity aerobic physical activity or 75 minutes of vigorous-intensity physical activity per week; walking is a great way to accomplish this. Repetitive use due to a job, hobby, or sport and joint-related injuries have also been linked to OA. Therefore, avoidance of repetitive movements and education on joint protection techniques (eg, using good body mechanics) to reduce joint injury while working or playing sports are important. Finally, joint malalignment is one of the strongest predictors for progressive OA. Nonsurgical and surgical strategies may be considered to correct anatomical abnormalities.

CONCLUSIONS

OA is a highly prevalent disease among older adults worldwide. Older age, obesity, structural abnormalities, and previous injury are among the known risk factors for disease development. Patients often present with chronic pain, stiffness, and functional disabilities. Diagnosis is based on history and physical examination, and can be supported by characteristic radiographic findings. Management of OA should be tailored to the individual patient. Treatment may include a combination of nonpharmacologic, pharmacologic, and surgical approaches, with different approaches being used at appropriate timepoints throughout the natural history of the disease.

FURTHER READING

Bannuru RR, Osani MC, Vaysbrot EE, et al. OARSI guidelines for the non-surgical management of knee, hip, and polyarticular osteoarthritis. *Osteoarthritis Cartilage.* 2019; 27(11):1578–1589.

Ferguson RJ, Palmer AJ, Taylor A, Porter ML, Malchau H, Glyn-Jones S. Hip replacement. *Lancet.* 2018;392(10158): 1662–1671.

Fernandes L, Hagen KB, Bijlsma JW, et al.; European League Against Rheumatism (EULAR). EULAR recommendations for the non-pharmacological core management of hip and knee osteoarthritis. *Ann Rheum Dis.* 2013;72(7):1125–1135.

Hunter DJ, Bierma-Zeinstra S. Osteoarthritis. *Lancet.* 2019;393:1745–1759. doi:10.1016/S0140-6736(19) 30417-9.

Katz JN, Arant KR, Loeser RF. Diagnosis and treatment of hip and knee osteoarthritis. *JAMA.* 2021;325(6):568. doi:10.1001/jama.2020.22171.

Kloppenburg M, Kroon FPB, Blanco FJ, et al. 2018 update of the EULAR recommendations for the management of hand osteoarthritis. *Ann Rheum Dis.* 2019;78:16–24. doi:10.1136/annrheumdis-2018-213826.

Kolasinski SL, Neogi T, Hochberg M, et al. 2019 American College of Rheumatology/Arthritis Foundation Guideline for the Management of Osteoarthritis of the Hand, Hip, and Knee. *Arthritis Rheumatol.* 2020;72(2): 220–233.

Liu X, Machado GC, Eyles JP, Ravi V, Hunter DJ. Dietary supplements for treating osteoarthritis: a systematic review and meta-analysis. *Br J Sports Med.* 2018;52(3):167–175.

Loeser RF, Collins JA, Diekman BO. Ageing and the pathogenesis of osteoarthritis. *Nat Rev Rheumatol.* 2016;12(7): 412–420.

Paterson KL, Gates L. Clinical assessment and management of foot and ankle osteoarthritis: a review of current evidence and focus on pharmacological treatment. *Drugs Aging.* 2019;36(3):203–211.

Price AJ, Alvand A, Troelsen A, et al. Knee replacement. *Lancet.* 2018;392(10158):1672–1682.

Reynard LN, Barter MJ. Osteoarthritis year in review 2019: genetics, genomics and epigenetics. *Osteoarthritis Cartilage.* 2020;28(3):275–284.

Roddy E, Menz HB. Foot osteoarthritis: latest evidence and developments. *Ther Adv Musculoskelet Dis.* 2018; 10(4):91–103.

van der Oest M, Duraku L, Andinopoulou E, et al. The prevalence of radiographic thumb base osteoarthritis: a meta-analysis. *Osteoarthritis Cartilage.* 2021;29(6): 785–792. https://doi.org/10.1016/j.joca.2021.03.004.

Vina ER, Kwoh CK. Epidemiology of osteoarthritis: literature update. *Curr Opin Rheumatol.* 2018;30(2):160–167.

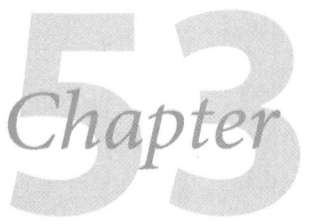

Chapter 53

Hip Fractures

Ellen F. Binder, Simon Mears

INTRODUCTION

Hip fracture is a major public health problem with significant consequences for older patients, their families, and the health care system. In 2010, there were approximately 260,000 adults aged 65 and older hospitalized for a hip fracture in the United States and this number is expected to increase to 289,000 by 2030 due to the aging of the population and people living longer. Recent worldwide estimates are in the order of 1.7 million hip fractures annually, and are expected to surpass 6 million by the middle of this century. As seen in **Figure 53-1**, hip fracture incidence increases exponentially in both men and women with advancing age. The average age of a patient with hip fracture is 82 years. Among those who reach age 85, approximately 19% of women and 12% of men will experience a hip fracture and, of those who reach 90 years, 30% of women and 20% of men will sustain a hip fracture. Although the majority of hip fractures occur in older White women, 25% to 30% of hip fractures occur in men and, in the United States, 8% occur in non-Whites. Prominent risk factors for hip fracture are osteoporosis and propensity to fall. Underlying these essential conditions for having a hip fracture are the reduced bone strength and quality that are characteristic of osteoporosis and the multiplicity of medical, psychosocial, and environmental factors that lead to falls.

The direct medical and indirect nonreimbursed costs (eg, unpaid caregiving services and lost wages of patients and caregivers) of hip fracture have been estimated to be as high as $20 billion annually in the United States. Over the past few years, measures have been taken in an attempt to reduce costs of care for hip fractures. This approach, called bundling, gives a single standardized payment that includes the total cost for all care for the patient for 90 days after surgery. Hospitals with high costs are at risk to lose money with bundled care. The largest costs are typically postacute care and readmissions. The switch to bundled care forces hospitals to work to reduce readmissions and complications when possible, and attempt to send patients home rather than to subacute care. Bundling also promotes interaction between surgeons, geriatricians, and postacute care centers to try to focus rehabilitation goals and reduce length of stay in the postacute center.

Learning Objectives

- To be able to describe the surgical and medical issues commonly experienced by older hip fracture patients.
- To be able to describe the physiological and functional changes and psychosocial issues commonly experienced by older hip fracture patients during the year after the fracture event.
- To be able to understand the impact of bundled care on hip fracture management.
- To understand the role of the geriatrician in providing care to older hip fracture patients during the perioperative and recovery periods.

Key Clinical Points

1. Hip fracture in older adults is associated with significant morbidity and mortality.
2. Complications of hip fracture can be prevented or mitigated, through careful perioperative screening and intervention strategies initiated during the acute hospitalization, during a period of formal rehabilitation services, and over the course of the year after the fracture event.
3. Geriatricians can play a critical role in coordinating care for hip fracture patients, initiating appropriate state-of-the-art interventions, and optimizing communication between the patient, family members, and the health care team.

Among those who have experienced a hip fracture, approximately 18% of women and 36% of men are expected to die within the first year of their fracture. The highest mortality rates occur within the first few months after a fracture among those who are in the poorest health. In addition, comparison of survival rates of female hip fracture patients to similarly impaired women without fractures indicates that

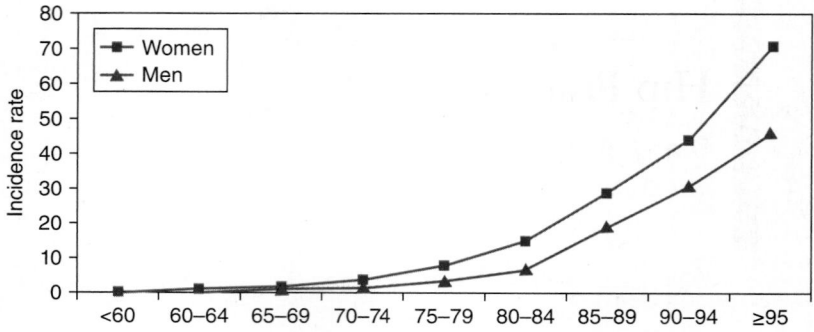

FIGURE 53-1. Age-specific incidence rates of hip fracture (per 1000 person-years): the Framingham study. (Reproduced with permission from Samelson EJ, Zhang Y, Kiel DP, et al. Effect of birth cohort on risk of hip fracture: age-specific incidence rates in the Framingham Study. *Am J Public Health.* 2002;92[5]:858–862.)

the fracture itself is responsible for nine extra deaths per 100 patients during the first 4 years following the fracture. Epidemiological data from studies of women indicate that even in those with the lowest number of medical comorbidities and best functioning at the time of fracture, the mortality attributable to hip fracture continues to increase well beyond the first year post fracture. Causes of death in women and men are similar and approximately four times greater than their nonfracture counterparts for heart disease, three times greater for cerebrovascular disease, and three times greater for chronic obstructive pulmonary disease. Interestingly, one study showed that men are far more likely than their nonfracture counterparts to die from infectious causes such as septicemia and pneumonia, in the first 2 years following hip fracture.

The intent of this chapter is to provide information about the medical and psychosocial status of the older patient who presents with a hip fracture and to discuss strategies for care and the role of the geriatrician in providing care during the acute hospital stay and the subsequent year or more of follow-up care.

WHAT TO EXPECT WHEN SEEING PATIENTS IN HOSPITAL

Medical Presentation and Fracture Characteristics

Classically, a patient with a hip fracture presents with a painful, shortened, and externally rotated lower extremity after a fall and landing on the affected hip. Most patients are unable to weight bear on the extremity. A small percentage of fractures are nondisplaced or "hairline" fractures and the patient may be able to bear weight and ambulate with pain. Nondisplaced fracture may progress to displaced fractures if not recognized. Patients having pain with gentle rolling of the lower extremity and a history of trauma should be evaluated for fracture. If plain radiographs are negative, magnetic resonance imaging (MRI) should be performed to look for bone marrow edema and fracture. MRI is more sensitive than computed tomography. If a nondisplaced fracture is found, treatment is either with non–weight bearing or in situ fixation to prevent propagation.

Approximately half of all hip fractures occur in the area of the femoral neck (or "intracapsular fractures"), and the other half occur in the area between the greater and lesser trochanters ("intertrochanteric fractures" or "extracapsular fractures"). Less common are fractures that occur within 5 cm below the lesser trochanter; these are called "subtrochanteric fractures." Patients with intertrochanteric fractures tend to be older than those with femoral neck fractures and are more likely to have multiple medical comorbidities. A schematic of the hip anatomy is shown in **Figure 53-2**, which indicates the anatomy of the vascular supply to the hip region. This schematic is useful to understand the various surgical approaches to hip fracture care and the potential for blood loss at each site. As demonstrated in the schematic, the regions of the femoral neck and the femoral head derive their main blood supply from fine retinacular arteries that stem from the medial circumflex femoral artery. These delicate vessels are closely apposed to the femoral neck in this region. A fracture in the femoral neck is more likely to disrupt the vascular supply to the femoral neck and head, which can result in longer-term nonunion and osteonecrosis. Thus, fractures in the femoral neck region, particularly displaced fractures, are usually managed with joint replacement or arthroplasty rather than internal fixation. Arthroplasty may be partial or total replacement. Total hip replacement is thought to give better long-term results and less pain for patients who are active. In contrast, the blood supply to the intertrochanteric area is plentiful and redundant, such that nonunion and osteonecrosis are less common in this region, and fractures can heal well after internal fixation procedures. Internal fixation is most commonly performed with a hip plate and screw or with an intramedullary hip screw. All of these procedures allow the patient to bear weight as tolerated after hip fracture repair.

Impact of Age-Associated Physiological Changes and Comorbidities

The cumulative effect of environmental exposures, lifestyle, and genetic factors results in a remarkably heterogeneous

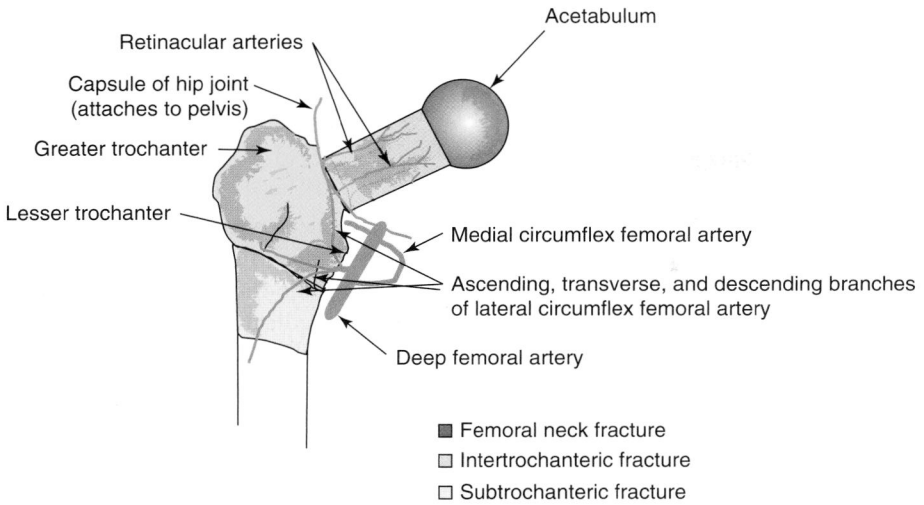

Retinacular arteries

Capsule of hip joint
(attaches to pelvis)

Greater trochanter

Lesser trochanter

Acetabulum

Medial circumflex femoral artery

Ascending, transverse, and descending branches
of lateral circumflex femoral artery

Deep femoral artery

■ Femoral neck fracture
☐ Intertrochanteric fracture
☐ Subtrochanteric fracture

FIGURE 53-2. A schematic diagram of the anatomy of the hip.

geriatric population. Aging impacts most organ systems, although the degree to which organs are impaired from aging varies from individual to individual. In addition, several chronic medical conditions may also exist in a given individual. Medical care of the patient with hip fracture must, therefore, be adapted to the individual patient's needs. This requirement for a tailored approach to care provides opportunities for challenges and satisfaction from the practice of geriatric medicine.

The changes that occur with aging physiology result in decreased resilience to stress, or the so-called "homeostenosis" in most organs. For example, older individuals may have lung volumes and decreased mucociliary clearance of their lungs, resulting in an increased propensity for postoperative atelectasis and pneumonia. Because of decreased physiological reserve, older individuals are at particular risk for a wider range of iatrogenic complications and do not recover as well when complications and adverse events occur. Older individuals are more susceptible to delirium during the pre- and postoperative period. This complication not only increases the patient's risk of dying in the subsequent year, but also can impair an individual's ability to participate in rehabilitation. Many of these complications are predictable and the geriatrician plays a critical role in team coordination and preventing complications. Hip fracture brings all of these known and unknown challenges together with the psychological insult of an acute fracture and need for surgical repair. The geriatrician must work with the surgical team to rapidly get the patient to surgery and progress the patient thought rehabilitation to hopefully bring them back to their baseline function.

Cognitive Status

Dementia is a prominent risk factor for falls and fractures and, not surprisingly, a significant number of patients with hip fracture have underlying cognitive impairment.

Delirium is a common occurrence both at time of presentation to the emergency department and postoperatively, occurring in up to 60% of patients after hip fracture repair. Underlying dementia is a major risk factor for the development of delirium. The presence of delirium and cognitive impairment portend a worse functional recovery for patients with hip fracture. Identification of underlying dementia and risk factors for delirium is important for both prognostication, and so that modifiable risk factors can be avoided or minimized. Given the high risk of delirium in this patient population, it is particularly important to prepare the patient and family emotionally for this potential complication as it can be quite frightening to unprepared family members.

Risk factors for delirium in hospitalized patients have been well described. Some of the most consistently reported risk factors include advanced age, chronic cognitive impairment or dementia, sensory impairment, male sex, presence of comorbid psychiatric disease, polypharmacy and use of psychoactive and narcotic medications, infection, use of restraints, sleep deprivation, and undertreatment of pain. Among hip fracture patients, admission from an institutional setting and congestive heart failure (CHF) are important risk factors for delirium. Multi-component and nonpharmacologic interventions, preferably implemented by an interdisciplinary team, can prevent delirium and are cost-effective. Studies of proactive geriatric consultation with targeted recommendations, such as oxygen delivery, fluid balance, analgesia, elimination of unnecessary medications, regulation of bowel and bladder function, nutritional intake, mobilization, prevention of postoperative complications, assessment of environmental stimuli, and treatment of agitated delirium, have shown reductions in the incidence of delirium overall by a third, and in one study, a reduction in the incidence of severe delirium by half.

Nutritional Status and Physiologic Changes after Hip Fracture

Due to a number of factors, including pain and medications, reduced appetite is common during the acute hospital and rehabilitation period, and a significant number of patients will have difficulty meeting their caloric needs. Many hip fracture patients are undernourished prior to the fracture and therefore at high risk for malnutrition during their recovery.

Changes in body composition also are notable after a hip fracture. The average woman who fractures a hip can expect to lose 3% to 6% of her muscle mass within 2 months of the hip fracture and to have an increase in fat mass of 3% to 4% during the post fracture year. Losses of bone mineral density also are profound in this already osteoporotic group of older women. Older women lose nearly 3% of their total hip bone mineral density and more than 4.5% of their bone mineral density in the contralateral femoral neck during the year following a hip fracture. This is 12.5 times more than the loss of 0.5% that would have been expected in a group of women of the same age, comorbid disease status, and starting level of bone mineral density (**Figure 53-3**). Older men with hip fracture also show accelerated loss of bone mineral density in the contralateral hip that are greater than that expected from aging. Pharmacologic interventions to prevent secondary fractures should be considered for both women and men after hip fracture.

In addition, the prevalence of vitamin D deficiency among hip fracture patients is very high, and contributes to the observed losses in bone density and muscle strength, and fall and fracture risk.

The Geriatrician's Role in Preoperative Care

The geriatrician can serve a central role in caring for patients upon admission to the acute care hospital by evaluating the medical and perioperative issues, ensuring maximal medical stabilization prior to surgery, and providing early detection and ongoing vigilance regarding risks for and development of, postoperative medical complications. The geriatrician is well positioned to discuss with the patient and family the anticipated hospital and postacute care procedures and transitions, thereby reducing uncertainty and alleviating anxiety at this unanticipated and challenging time.

Studies indicate that a multidisciplinary approach to acute care for hip fracture can improve clinical outcomes. Several models of orthogeriatrics comanagement have been developed. Models vary from geriatric consultation or liaison services, management on a geriatric ward with orthopedic consultation, and integrated inpatient orthogeriatric units. A systematic review and meta-analysis of 18 studies found that orthogeriatric collaboration was associated with reduced in-hospital mortality, reduced long-term mortality, and reduced length of stay. A randomized trial of orthogeriatric care provided on a geriatrics ward (vs an

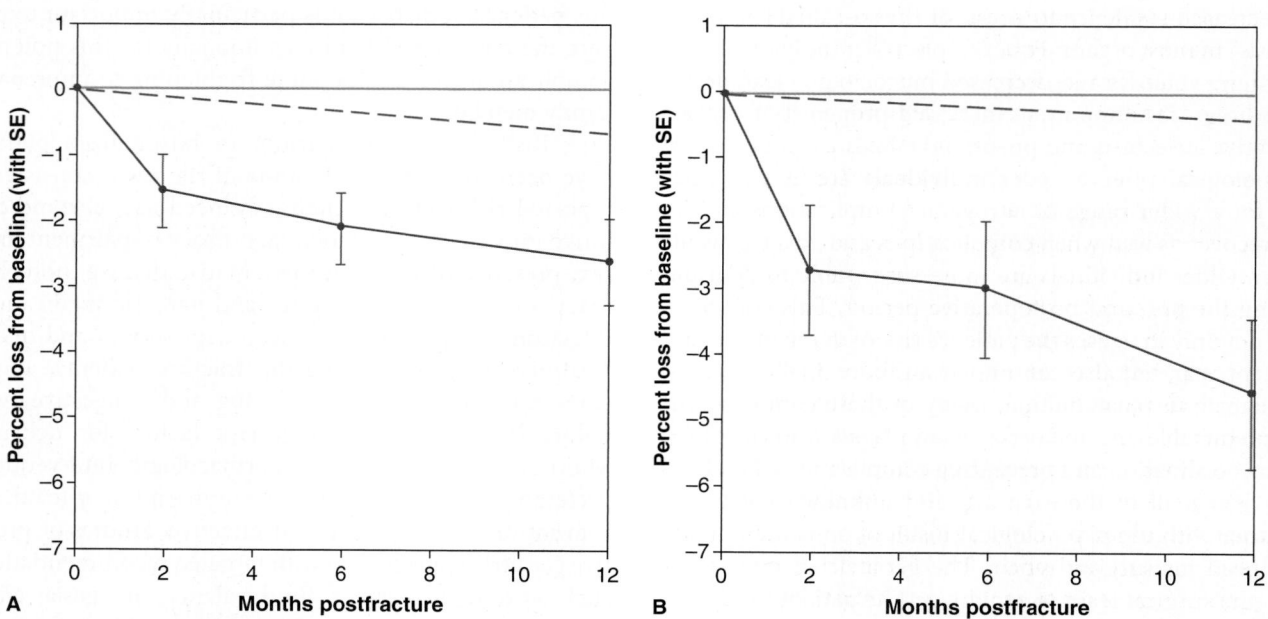

FIGURE 53-3. Expected and observed change in total hip bone mineral density (**A**) and femoral neck bone mineral density (**B**) during the 12 months following fracture. Legend for both panels: solid line, hip fracture (observed mean and standard error); broken line, Study of Osteoporotic Fractures (SOF; expected mean based on interpolated data obtained for a 42.3-month period). (Reproduced with permission from Magaziner J, Wehren L, Hawkes WG, et al. Women with hip fracture have a greater rate of decline in bone mineral density than expected: another significant consequence of a common geriatric problem. *Osteoporos Int.* 2006;17[7]:971–977.)

orthopedic ward without geriatrics consultation) did not reduce the rate of in-hospital delirium, but did improve mobility at 4 months after surgery.

The majority of patients with a hip fracture will undergo surgical repair. The types of surgical approach and anesthesia employed are largely the purview of the surgeon and the anesthesiologist and often depend on local practice patterns and physician training. No differences have been found in mortality between general and spinal anesthetic. Preoperative regional anesthetic with a nerve block has been shown to decrease pain in hip fracture patients. The nerve block can be done by an anesthesiologist or a trained emergency room physician. The pain relief from the nerve block may make the use of a Foley catheter unnecessary. The geriatrician should help to limit the use of catheters to those who can't roll or get on a bed pan because of pain.

To prepare the patient for hip fracture surgery, the attending physician should determine the risks of cardiovascular, pulmonary, and other complications and strive to reduce those risks. (Refer to Chapter 27, Perioperative Care: Evaluation and Management, for more details on the use of preoperative testing for risk stratification, preoperative pulmonary treatments, and the use of β-blockers and other medications to reduce the risk of perioperative adverse cardiac events in high-risk patients.) Medication reconciliation is particularly important. The patient may not have an accurate medicine list upon presentation to the emergency department, and calls to the pharmacy and/or primary care physician may be necessary to obtain correct information or clarify questions.

While surgical approaches usually offer more benefits than nonsurgical approaches, nonsurgical approaches should be considered for some selected patients. The clearest benefit of surgery over the nonsurgical approach is that surgery results in better anatomic alignment and better likelihood of ambulation. Nonsurgical approaches may be considered in patients who are unable to ambulate prior to the fracture, those with advanced dementia and contractures, those with little pain from the fracture, and those in whom surgical risks are very high or life expectancy is very short. The geriatrician can help by providing a "big picture" view of whether or not the patient will benefit from surgical repair of the hip or whether palliative care should be considered. The determination of what may be most appropriate for a patient requires a thorough understanding of the patient's pre-fracture functional and cognitive status, comorbidities, psychosocial factors, and the patient's prior goals, values, and priorities. If it is determined that the patient is not a good surgical candidate, the geriatrician should be prepared to discuss the patient's care goals and priorities and the palliative care management strategies and resources and to refer to palliative care and hospice colleagues and providers, as appropriate. Discussion of options for those not considered good candidates for surgery, including palliative and hospice care, also can be initiated and led by the geriatrician.

The Geriatrician's Role in Postoperative Care

In the United States, a patient will usually remain in the acute hospital setting for 1 to 5 days after surgery for hip fracture. Patients should be mobilized the day of surgery if possible and certainly by postoperative day number 1. Early mobilization has been shown to be safe and effective for minimizing deconditioning and reducing the risk of complications such as delirium, constipation, pneumonia, thromboembolism, and pressure ulcer formation. If a catheter was placed, this should be removed the morning after surgery. Adequate treatment of postoperative pain is important for maximizing participation in physical therapy and increasing mobility. The optimal pain medication regimen has not been determined. The preoperative nerve block often helps postoperative pain considerably and intravenous pain medicine is not required after surgery. Care should be taken to prescribe a customized regimen that provides sustained pain relief early in the postoperative period, minimizes sedation, and also anticipates episodic increases in pain associated with activities such as therapy sessions.

The geriatrician must monitor the patient closely for the development of postoperative complications and is in a key position to detect subtle delirium that could be a harbinger of an ominous underlying complication, such as pulmonary embolus, urinary tract infection, and pneumonia. Postoperative pulmonary complications are among the most lethal complications in this population. Deep breathing exercises with or without an incentive spirometer, early mobility, and use of physical and/or pharmacologic approaches to reduce the risk of deep venous thrombosis should all be instituted. Other important postoperative medical considerations the geriatrician may be particularly adept at managing are reducing polypharmacy, pressure ulcer detection and management, maximizing sensory input, explaining the treatments and progression of care to patients and family, and communicating across the transitions of care to reduce errors during this vulnerable time. Atrial fibrillation and CHF are other typical postoperative complications. Worsening of CHF often happens after hospital discharge and this should be taken in account if the patient is transferred to a subacute nursing facility.

The geriatrician should also determine the patient's risk for subsequent falls and fractures. A falls history should be obtained, including a complete description of the fall that led to the fracture as well as any previous falls, with particular attention to remediable risk factors to be addressed prior to discharge back to home (see Chapter 43, Falls). The geriatrician should discuss with the patient, family, and other providers the issue of osteoporosis treatment (see Chapter 51, Osteoporosis). To facilitate optimal secondary fracture prevention measures, many hospitals have enrolled in the International Osteoporosis Foundation "Capture the Fracture" program (www.capturethefracture.org) to implement a postfracture care coordination program. Such programs bring together and coordinate a multidisciplinary team of providers who can assess and manage osteoporosis and fall prevention.

If antiresorptive therapy is being considered for treatment of osteoporosis, the vitamin D level should be repleted prior to starting a bisphosphonate. Therefore, if not performed recently, a serum vitamin D level should be checked during the acute hospital admission.

Discharge Planning

Prior to discharge from the in-patient setting, a multidisciplinary assessment involving the geriatrician, the orthopedic surgeon, nursing, social work, physical therapy, and occupational therapy should be performed. The goal of this assessment is to decide on discharge plans and rehabilitation needs and goals. The following considerations should be taken into account: the patient's current level of mobility, the patient's postoperative medical and skilled nursing needs, the home environment, social support and economic resources available, self-care skills, and requirements for activities of daily living (ADL). The geriatrician plays a key role in coordinating the patient's care and communicating with patients and families as they transition through the health care system. A critical role for the geriatrician is to ensure continuity of care. Recent studies have shown that, with each transition to a different site of care, there is the potential for an adverse effect on the care of patients with hip fracture, and physicians must, therefore, be vigilant to ensure adequate communication and good continuity of care to minimize this risk.

While a patient's medical diagnoses and baseline functional status are important considerations for maximal functional recovery, his or her social support network and home environment are equally important. Social support will often dictate how long a patient needs to stay in in-patient rehabilitation before safe to discharge to home or the appropriate level of care. For example, if a patient had been previously living independently in a multistory home where the bathroom and bedroom are on the second floor and the kitchen on the first floor, one of three things would need to occur prior to discharge home: (1) the patient would need to be able to negotiate a full flight of stairs independently and safely; (2) the patient would need to rearrange the home to live on the ground floor and be able to transfer and ambulate short distances on a level surface independently and safely; (3) the patient would need a responsible caregiver to assist with daily tasks; or (4) the patient would need to stay with a family member on one floor. Not all patients have access to, or resources for, assistance in their homes, but some have families or friends who are able to provide this support, which is usually unreimbursed. This can also be a major stressor when the caregiver has to take time off from work and/or travel long distances to provide assistance. In collaboration with the interdisciplinary team, the geriatrician can assist family members and caregivers to anticipate and prepare for the patient's upcoming needs. An assessment of the home environment by an occupational and/or physical therapist provides essential information for home discharge planning.

Transitions of Care

After the acute hospital stay, the hip fracture patient may be discharged home or to a postacute setting. This is typically an acute rehabilitation center or a subacute nursing facility. Very functional patients with capable families and good social support should be discharged home if possible. Those who cannot return home upon hospital discharge will require a short-term stay in an acute inpatient rehabilitation facility or a subacute skilled nursing facility (SNF). Transitions of care to these facilities are difficult and fraught with potential for medical errors. The accepting physician may rarely see the patient in the facility and the amount of rehabilitation services provided can vary. In the best situation, a trained geriatrician will continue care for the patient at the site of rehabilitation, and a handoff can be performed prior to transfer. A detailed consultation note immediately prior to the date of transfer, which details the comorbidities that are being managed by the geriatrician and the plan of care, can be extremely helpful to the accepting physician and rehabilitation team.

Changes in Hip Fracture Care: Bundled Care for Hip Fracture and COVID-19

Bundled care means that one payment is given to the hospital for the entirety of care of a patient for 90 days after surgery. This rate is set by Medicare. Hip fractures are part of several voluntary bundles which are radically changing the way care is delivered. If a hip fracture is treated with arthroplasty, the patient may be part of the arthroplasty bundle. This includes mostly elective patients with osteoarthritis. Another bundle includes care of other procedures of the entire femur bone which include hip fractures. This bundle also includes periprosthetic fracture treated with plates and patients with fixation of the mid or lower portion of the femur. Bundled care is different, because any complication requiring hospital readmissions is included within the single payment given for the bundle. The payment also includes the cost of any postdischarge care, including inpatient or outpatient services. The most expensive portion of care for the hip fracture patient is generally the postacute care and readmission and not the initial hospital stay. Participation in a bundle requires active involvement of the entire care team to minimize postsurgical complications, facilitate communication and continuity across transitions of care, shorten postacute stays without reducing quality of care, and avoid readmissions. This can involve follow-up via telemedicine, and close monitoring of patients while in a subacute facility. Utilizing rehabilitation facilities or programs with a relationship to the acute care hospital or medical center can be helpful to try to ensure that clearly articulated rehabilitation goals are set and achieved to get the patient home earlier.

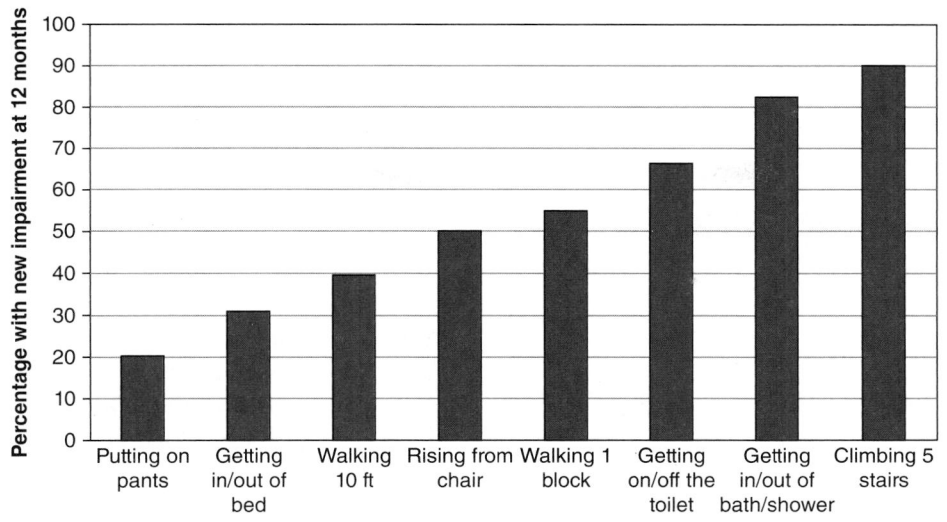

FIGURE 53-4. Lower extremity activities of daily living—percentage of those unimpaired before fracture with impairment at 12 months after fracture. (Data from Magaziner J, Hawkes W, Hebel JR, et al. Recovery from hip fracture in eight areas of function. *J Gerontol A Biol Sci Med Sci.* 2000;55[9]:M498–M507.)

The COVID-19 virus changed hip fracture care. The treatment of patients with active COVID-19 and hip fracture depends upon the severity of the COVID-19 infection. Those who have respiratory symptoms and fracture seem to have poor outcomes. Those who are asymptomatic should probably have early surgery as is usually performed. Postoperative visits are often curtailed if patients are COVID-19-positive and telemedicine visits must be used. The COVID-19 epidemic also made patients fearful of being in the hospital or of being in a nursing home, and this further stressed the importance of home discharge when possible.

POSTFRACTURE CHANGES IN PHYSICAL AND PSYCHOSOCIAL FUNCTION AND IMPLICATIONS FOR CARE

Physical Function

Hip fractures have significant effects on functioning and body composition. **Figure 53-4** shows the proportion of patients with hip fracture who, prior to their fracture, were able to perform routine tasks involving lower extremities but were not able to perform them a year later. Twenty percent of those who could put on their own pants without assistance prior to their fracture required assistance to do so 1 year later. More striking is the proportion of patients who needed assistance from another person or required the use of equipment to walk across a small room (40%), use the toilet (66%), or climb five stairs (90%). Instrumental tasks also are affected, with 62%, 53%, and 42% who could do their own housecleaning, get to places out of walking distance independently, and shop without assistance, respectively, prior to their fracture, requiring

assistance to perform these tasks a year later. Other functional consequences of hip fracture include increases in cognitive impairment and depressive symptoms, as well as increases in problems with gait and balance. Despite advances in surgical procedures, postoperative care, and long-term rehabilitation, hip fractures rank in the top 10 of all impairments worldwide in terms of causing disability and functional decline.

Psychological Status

The diagnosis of hip fracture conveys to patients and families a significant degree of psychological stress. Most lay persons are quite aware of the risk of mortality and poor recovery of function after a hip fracture, the high rate of nursing home use and long-term placement and, for those who do return home, the high rates of dependency on others for care. Although not the case for most patients, many patients and families believe that having a hip fracture signifies the "beginning of the end." These psychological stressors may contribute to the high rates of postoperative depression that have been described. Patients may endorse depressive symptoms during their hospital stay and for up to 6 months after fracture; those who report symptoms of depression even transiently tend to recover less well than those who do not endorse depressive symptoms at all.

FUNCTIONAL RECOVERY POSTHIP FRACTURE

Recovery in function following a hip fracture can be anticipated in most patients, although many will fail to reach their prefracture functional levels. This recovery appears to follow a sequence that may be instructive for management

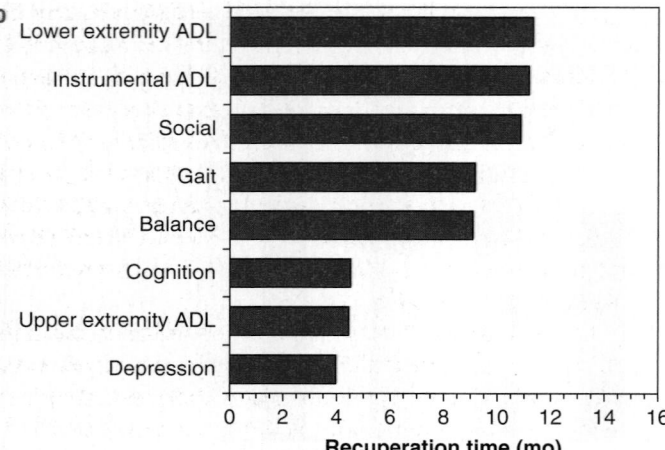

FIGURE 53-5. Time to recuperation following hip fracture in eight areas of function. ADL, activities of daily living. (Reproduced with permission from Magaziner J, Hawkes W, Hebel JR, et al. Recovery from hip fracture in eight areas of function. *J Gerontol A Biol Sci Med Sci.* 2000;55[9]:M498–M507.)

during the initial year after the fracture. Depression, upper extremity ADL, and cognitive function reach their peak level of recovery by approximately 4 months postfracture, while tasks associated with mobility, such as balance and gait, reach a plateau at approximately 9 months postfracture. Interestingly, the more complex tasks that are indicative of disability, such as performing lower extremity activities and instrumental tasks, recover by approximately a year (**Figure 53-5**).

Patients who recover more slowly than anticipated should have an assessment of factors that may be contributing, such as persistent delirium, depression, polypharmacy, vitamin D and other nutritional deficiencies, and social isolation, so that a targeted multidisciplinary plan can be developed to address the issues of concern.

POSTFRACTURE REHABILITATION

Rehabilitation Services

The majority of patients with hip fracture will undergo a period of rehabilitation therapy after the fracture repair (see Chapter 55, Rehabilitation). Rehabilitation services are provided only if both of the following requirements are fulfilled: (1) the patient has a functional loss and (2) is able to participate in rehabilitation efforts. Individuals with severe cognitive impairment or those with unresolved delirium that interferes with participation in standard rehabilitation, those with severe prefracture disability (eg, bed-bound), and those with terminal illness, may not qualify for standard rehabilitation services. Alternative approaches may be required. The geriatrician can judge potential benefits and work with the multidisciplinary rehabilitation team to recommend the most appropriate rehabilitative care.

Rehabilitation services can be provided in one or more of the following settings: an inpatient acute rehabilitation unit, a subacute rehabilitation unit in a SNF, or on an outpatient basis, either at home or in a clinic. The location of postdischarge rehabilitation is determined by a number of factors, including the patient's functional impairments, comorbidities, ability to participate in skilled therapy sessions, social support, and personal preferences. In the United States, rehabilitation is typically limited by Medicare reimbursement and rarely goes beyond 30 days. In one study, approximately 50% of hip fracture patients were discharged to a SNF subacute unit, 20% were discharged to an acute inpatient rehabilitation unit, 15% were discharged to home, and 14% were discharged directly to a long-term care facility. The COVID-19 pandemic shifted services more toward home care, when feasible.

Inpatient acute rehabilitation units are usually located in specialized units of an acute care hospital, or in a dedicated rehabilitation hospital. Patients with complex medical or rehabilitation needs and with good endurance may receive their rehabilitation in the acute setting. The requirements for acute rehabilitation are that the individual must be able to participate in therapy for at least 3 hours/day, and at least two rehabilitation therapeutic disciplines be involved (eg, physical therapy and occupational therapy).

Patients with less complex medical or rehabilitation needs, who are not able to participate in 3 hours/day of rehabilitation but who otherwise have a functional decline that would benefit from rehabilitation and are unable to be discharged to home, can receive rehabilitation in the subacute SNF setting. These patients typically receive interventions from a licensed professional 5 days a week, however, on a less intense basis than in the acute rehabilitation setting.

Patients with more mild functional and mobility impairments or with good support at home may receive their rehabilitation on an outpatient basis, either at home or at an outpatient facility. In order to qualify for home rehabilitation, patients must have a functional decline that would benefit from rehabilitation, have sufficient caregiver support to enable them to be cared for at home, and be homebound and therefore unable to attend rehabilitation at an outpatient clinic. Since rehabilitation will be delivered by homecare professionals in the patient's home, heavy equipment must not be required.

For individuals with less complex rehabilitation needs, services may be delivered in an outpatient clinic. Outpatient rehabilitation may also continue after acute, subacute, and homecare services, to facilitate attainment of rehabilitation goals.

The Role of the Geriatrician in the Rehabilitation Setting

The geriatrician can also play a key role in medical management at rehabilitation settings, especially at SNFs.

Regardless of the rehabilitation setting, medical care should focus on the following principles: treatment of chronic medical conditions, continued postoperative hip fracture care, prevention of complications from the associated functional decline and immobility, and prevention of future falls and fractures.

Despite ongoing therapy by rehabilitation professionals, increased risk for complications related to immobility, such as DVT, pressure ulcers, and constipation, persist at the rehabilitation setting. Thus, continued vigilance to their prevention and detection must be exercised. Based on current recommendations, DVT prophylaxis should be continued for 21 to 31 days after hip fracture surgery. Pressure ulcers are common after hip fracture surgery, with reports of an incidence rate of stage II or greater ulcers within 21 days of fracture of approximately 5%. Given the decreased mobility and frequency of use of narcotic analgesics for postoperative pain, constipation is a common occurrence and efforts should be made to prevent this with an adequate bowel regimen. Continued monitoring by the geriatrician of the patient's weight, nutritional status, symptoms of depression and cognitive impairment, and the success of related interventions is very important for ensuring optimal recovery.

Many patients with hip fracture in the acute and subacute rehabilitation settings receive their medical care from a physician who was not their primary care provider prefracture and may not be familiar with their history or support system. Care for these patients represents a challenge for the attending physician, as these patients are typically older and with significant and complicated comorbid disease. More than 75% of patients with hip fracture have at least four comorbid medical conditions prior to their fracture. In addition to supervising the care of the hip fracture and any sequelae, the attending physician must ensure that these chronic medical conditions continue to be addressed.

What to Tell the Patient and Family to Expect With Regard to Function

Because hip fracture may result in persistent functional limitations and disability, patients with hip fracture may anticipate significant changes in their lifestyle. The geriatrician needs to provide support and encouragement during the initial recovery period following hip fracture surgery when pain and disability are greatest. Patients and their families can be reassured that significant improvements in lower extremity function during the first few months postfracture are likely to occur, while at the same time cautioned that lower extremity limitations can be prolonged. Up to 50% of older adults who had previously been independent may be dependent on mobility aids, such as a cane or a walker, for ambulation at 1 year postfracture. These limitations and fear of recurrent falls may result in self-limitation of daily activities.

These declines in function may result in loss of independence in the older patient, and, as a result, the older patient with hip fracture may be facing the prospect of moving from their independent residence to a higher level of care for the first time. Individuals who have an injury as a result of a fall, such as a hip fracture, are 10 times more likely to be admitted to a SNF. This may be one of the most frightening aspects of the postfracture recovery period, and helping patients to understand that this is an expected reaction to having a hip fracture may enable them to overcome this fear and resume their activities more quickly.

Older patients and those with multiple health conditions may need to be told that their recovery may be slower than for others. Compared to younger patients, those who are older than 85 years have been found to require longer rehabilitation stays, have worse recovery of lower extremity function, are more likely to be discharged to long-term care, and are more likely to have persistent pain, which may be accompanied by ADL limitations and reduced quality of life. Depression and cognitive limitations should also be discussed with patients and families. It is important for them to understand that depressive symptoms and cognitive limitations are common after a hip fracture. They should also be informed that these changes are not always persistent, as depressive symptoms and cognitive limitations will frequently resolve with limited intervention within 2 months, and that treatment for mild depression is often useful to avoid any lingering anxiety or depression that accompanies the hip fracture.

The Geriatrician's Role after Formal Rehabilitation for the Hip Fracture

After the patient has returned home, the focus of follow-up care should be to monitor whether the patient is making expected gains in recovery, evaluate barriers if expected gains are not achieved, and prevent subsequent falls and injury. Most hip fracture patients plateau in their functional level by 6 months after fracture event. The occurrence of complications may alter that course and many will continue to realize gains with longer amounts of time. Geriatricians are well trained to identify barriers to recovery after a hip fracture and initiate interventions that can further enhance recovery and reduce fall risk. Optimally, the patient should be reevaluated at the time of discharge from the acute rehabilitation setting, and again upon discharge from home physical therapy, to assess the patient's recovery level, physical impairments, and need for outpatient services. Multidisciplinary fall risk assessment (eg, home environment assessment, medication review, vision testing, postural blood pressure measurement, gait and balance testing, and targeted neurological, musculoskeletal, and cardiac examinations) followed by interventions directed at these risks can reduce fall risk and are cost-effective in older adults at risk of recurrent falls.

Continuation of an exercise program after formal rehabilitation services have ended has been shown to

TABLE 53-1 ■ FOCUS OF THE GERIATRICIAN AT VARIOUS STAGES OF CARE FOR PATIENTS WITH HIP FRACTURE

SETTING OF CARE	WHAT THE GERIATRICIAN IS FOCUSED ON
Acute hospital—preoperative	1. Do surgery or nonoperative approaches best meet this patient's goals? 2. What are the preoperative cardiac, pulmonary, cognitive, and other risks for this patient and what can be done to reduce these? 3. What must be done to prevent postoperative complications, especially pressure ulcers, delirium, anemia, DVT, CHF, and pneumonia? 4. Why did this person fall and how can this information be used to ensure that medical status is optimized for surgery or nonoperative management?
Acute hospital—postoperative	1. What can be done to prevent postoperative complications, such as pressure ulcers, delirium, anemia, DVT, CHF, and pneumonia? 2. Is pain adequately treated? 3. Is there delirium and how can it be addressed? 4. Has serum vitamin D level been measured recently? 5. What is the next appropriate level of care and when is the patient ready to go there? 6. Who will provide medical care after discharge and how can continuity of care be ensured? 7. What are the plans for osteoporosis management?
Subacute setting—rehab	1. Is pain adequately treated? 2. Are there any complications requiring treatment, such as constipation, delirium, pneumonia, venous thrombosis, deconditioning, weight loss or poor nutrition, and pressure ulcers? 3. Are there signs of active depression limiting participation in rehabilitation and what can be done to address this during rehabilitation and after discharge? 4. Why did this person fall and what can be done to reduce the chances of future fractures? 5. Is the patient on vitamin D supplementation? Is follow-up scheduled for osteoporosis management? 6. What does this person need to do to be able to go home safely? 7. Who will next provide medical care and how can continuity of care be ensured?
Outpatient setting—primary care	1. Is this person receiving appropriate interventions to prevent falls and fractures and increase activity level and reengagement into community life? 2. Is this person safe in the current living arrangement? 3. Is recovery occurring in the expected sequence and in the expected time frame? 4. Has pain resolved? 5. Is the patient participating in outpatient therapy and/or an exercise program?

improve physical function during the year following surgical repair of the fracture. Exercise programs that include progressive-resistance training appear to be most effective at improving measures of physical function and quality of life. However, home-based exercise programs for hip fracture patients have also shown modest improvement in physical function. The physician should discuss with patients their options for continued outpatient therapy and/or exercise, determine their preferences, and provide appropriate referrals and prescriptions.

Although hip protectors have received attention for their potential to reduce hip fractures, meta-analyses suggest that these offer little or no benefit for patients in randomized studies. As a result, these devices should not be considered as alternatives to the other fall reduction and bone-strengthening interventions discussed above.

CONCLUSION

Care for older patients with hip fracture represents one of the greatest challenges for the geriatrician because of the multiplicity of medical and psychosocial factors involved in postfracture care. A summary of some of the key issues a geriatrician should focus on at various stages of hip fracture care appears in **Table 53-1**. Answering these questions requires vigilant attention preoperatively, postoperatively, in the rehabilitation setting, and after rehabilitation efforts have terminated. Although a hip fracture event has significant consequences for patients and their families, through this attention and communication with patients, families, and the other clinicians involved in the care of patients as they transition through the various sites of care, it is the goal of the geriatrician to minimize long-term adverse effects and to ensure that the overall well-being of the patient is maximized.

FURTHER READING

Dyer SM, Crotty M, Fairhall N, et al. A critical review of the long-term disability outcomes following hip fracture. *BMC Geriatr.* 2016;16(1):158.

Falaschi P, March DR (eds). *Orthogeriatrics: The Management of Older Patients With Fragility Fractures* [Internet]. Cham (CH): Springer; 2021.

Grigoryan KV, Javedan H, Rudolph JL. Orthogeriatric care models and outcomes in hip fracture patients: a systematic review and meta-analysis. *J Orthop Trauma.* 2014;28:e49–e55.

HEALTH Investigators, Bhandari M, Einhorn TA, et al. Total hip arthroplasty or hemiarthroplasty for hip fracture. *N Engl J Med.* 2019;381(23):2199–2208.

Malik AT, Khan SN, Ly TV, Phieffer L, Quatman CE. The "hip fracture bundle"—experiences, challenges and opportunities. *Geriatr Orthop Surg Rehabil.* 2020;11: 2151459320910846.

Perracini MR, Kristensen MT, Cunningham C, Sherrington C. Physiotherapy following fragility fractures. *Injury.* 2018; 49(8):1413–1417.

Reyes BJ, Mendelson DA, Mujahi N, et al. Postacute management of older adults suffering an osteoporotic hip fracture: a consensus statement from the International Geriatric Fracture Society. *Geriatr Orthop Surg Rehabil.* 2020;11:2151459320935100.

Sieber FE, Neufeld KJ, Gottschalk A, et al. Effect of depth of sedation in older patients undergoing hip fracture repair on postoperative delirium: the STRIDE randomized clinical trial. *JAMA Surg.* 2018;153(11):987–995.

Smith T, Pelpola K, Ball M, Ong A, Myint PK. Pre-operative indicators for mortality following hip fracture surgery: a systematic review and meta-analysis. *Age Ageing.* 2014; 43:464–471.

Chapter 54

Therapeutic Exercise

Kerry L. Hildreth, Kathleen M. Gavin, Christine M. Swanson,
Sarah J. Wherry, Kerrie L. Moreau

AGING AND BENEFITS OF EXERCISE

A common belief among the lay public, as well as among many health care professionals, is that much of the disease and functional decline that accompanies aging is inevitable, a result of the "aging process" itself. However, much of the physical decline and reduced physiologic reserve attributed to aging is, in fact, caused by complex interactions of disuse, environmental and lifestyle factors, disease, and genetics.

Physical activity level and fitness are associated with a greater average lifespan and inversely related to the risk of mortality. Among adults older than 60 years, engaging in at least 150 minutes per week of moderate to vigorous physical activity is associated with a 28% reduction in all-cause mortality. Even a modest dose of moderate to vigorous physical activity confers a mortality benefit compared to no activity. Higher cardiorespiratory fitness is associated with lower mortality, with a striking 80% reduction in mortality risk between elite performers (those > 2 standard deviations above the mean for age and sex) and the lowest performers.

With respect to resistance exercise, older adults performing guideline-concordant strength training had 46% lower odds of all-cause mortality than those who did not. A recent meta-analysis of more than 1400 studies reported that compared to no exercise, any resistance training was associated with 21% reduction in all-cause mortality. Combining resistance and aerobic exercise appears to confer even greater benefit than either alone. In the above meta-analysis, resistance exercise plus aerobic exercise was associated with a 40% reduction in all-cause mortality. Among older women, those who participated in both strength training and greater than or equal to 150 minutes per week of aerobic activity had a 46% lower risk of all-cause mortality.

An inverse dose–response relationship has also been noted between physical activity and the risk of developing many chronic diseases, as discussed later in this chapter. Despite the overwhelming benefits of physical activity, only 35% of persons older than 60 years meet current recommendations for physical activity (these recommendations are included in **Table 54-3**, discussed later in this chapter); this percentage drops significantly in older age groups.

Learning Objectives

■ Describe the changes in aerobic exercise capacity and in skeletal muscle strength and power that occur with aging.

■ Describe the effects of aerobic and resistance exercise training on aerobic exercise capacity, skeletal muscle strength and power, and physical function in older adults.

■ Describe the role of exercise in the prevention and treatment of common geriatric disorders.

Key Clinical Points

1. **The physiologic responses to aerobic and resistance training on aerobic exercise capacity and muscle strength and power are preserved in older adults.**

2. **Because the relation between physiologic impairment and functional limitations is nonlinear, older adults with little or no physiologic reserve may realize large functional improvements with exercise.**

3. **Older adults can safely engage in even high-intensity exercise; exercise and physical activity recommendations should be specific and tailored to the individual to enhance long-term adherence.**

It is increasingly clear that many of the health benefits of exercise can be accrued simply through a more active (nonsedentary) lifestyle. This concept may be especially helpful in trying to encourage older individuals who feel they are unable or unwilling to engage in formal exercise training.

Sedentary behavior includes activities that require an energy expenditure of more than or equal to 1.5 times resting energy expenditure, and encompasses activities such as sitting, watching TV, using a computer, reclining, or lying down during waking hours. Objective measurements of sedentary time in the National Health and Nutrition Examination Survey (NHANES) indicate that adults aged 60 or older spend more time engaged in sedentary behaviors (8–9 hours per day, or 60% of their waking time) than any other segment of the population. In older adults, sedentary behavior is associated with an increased risk of sarcopenia and functional limitations, and inversely associated with physical function. Prolonged periods of sedentary behavior appear particularly deleterious, particularly for metabolic health. In older adults, the number of breaks in sedentary time is associated with higher levels of physical function, independent of moderate to vigorous physical activity. Changing sedentary behavior may have an immediate impact on the health of older adults. In one study, older adults who reduced their sedentary time over a 2-year period had a lower risk of all-cause mortality compared to those who either increased or did not change their sedentary time.

AGING AND EXERCISE

Aerobic Exercise Capacity

One of the key physiologic changes that occurs with aging and contributes to the decline in physical function is a decline in aerobic exercise capacity, best measured by the amount of oxygen consumed at maximal or peak exercise (maximal or peak aerobic power; VO_{2max} or VO_{2peak}). Longitudinal data indicate that the rate of decline in VO_{2peak} accelerates markedly with each successive decade, reaching more than 20% per decade from the 1970s onward (**Figure 54-1**).

Age-associated declines in VO_{2max} can be attributed to alterations in both central and peripheral determinants of exercise capacity. Reductions in maximal heart rate and in the maximal ability of muscle to extract oxygen from the blood, driven in large part by the age-associated loss of muscle mass, appear to contribute to declines in VO_2 max in older adults (also see Chapter 73, The Aging Cardiovascular System). In all age groups, endurance-trained adults have a higher VO_2 max than their age-matched sedentary peers, suggesting that participation in habitual aerobic exercise may attenuate the age-related decline in VO_2 max.

Despite declines in VO_{2max} with aging, the response to an aerobic exercise training program in previously sedentary, healthy older adults is comparable to that observed in younger subjects, with improvements mediated by both central and peripheral adaptations (also see Chapter 73). Improvement in VO_{2max} has been reported to be between 6% and 30%, with significant improvements observed in as little as 3 weeks.

Skeletal Muscle Strength and Power

Aging is associated with a significant loss in skeletal muscle mass, and consequently in muscle strength (maximum force exerted) and power (rate of force development) in men and women, independent of physical activity status. The loss in muscle strength also accelerates with advancing age; by age 80, strength is approximately 30% to 40% of peak. The rate of decline in muscle power, which is a stronger determinant of physical function in older age than muscle strength, appears to be even greater than the decline in strength. The loss of muscle strength and power is associated with both mortality and physical disability in older adults; however, both can be increased by improving muscular function (eg, muscle cell hypertrophy) or by improving neurological function (eg, learning).

To a large extent, the age-associated loss of muscle strength and power reflects loss of muscle mass. However, other factors are clearly involved. In the Health, Aging and Body Composition (Health ABC) Study, for example, the decline in muscle strength over 3 years was three times greater than the parallel rate of decline in muscle mass. Regular physical activity may prevent or attenuate some of the age-related loss in strength. Importantly, vigorous strengthening exercise can produce substantial gains in strength in older adults.

A primary mechanism for the effects of resistance exercise is muscle hypertrophy, and older adults appear to achieve increases in muscle fiber size and cross-sectional area comparable to those in younger adults. However, even modest increases in muscle fiber size or cross-sectional area are accompanied by proportionally greater increases in strength, again suggesting involvement of other mechanisms. Proposed mechanisms include learning effects from improvements in motor skill coordination, and neural adaptations such as increased voluntary muscle activation, reflecting recruitment, firing and synchronization of motor units, and better coordination of synergistic and antagonist muscle cocontraction.

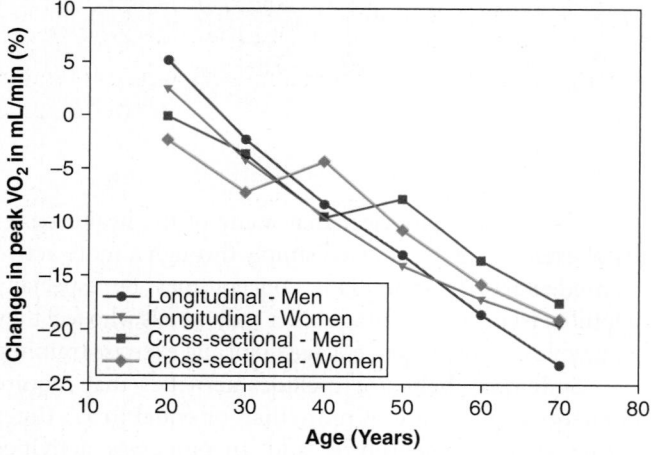

FIGURE 54-1. Per-decade percent cross-sectional and longitudinal changes in peak VO_2 by gender and age decade. (Reproduced with permission from Fleg JL, Morrell CH, Bos AG, et al. Accelerated longitudinal decline of aerobic capacity in healthy older adults. *Circulation.* 2005;112[5]:674–682.)

Nonlinear Relationship Between Physiologic Impairment and Functional Limitation

Healthy humans have excess physiologic capacity not tapped during most daily activities and can thus lose a fair amount of physiologic reserve before functional limitations occur.

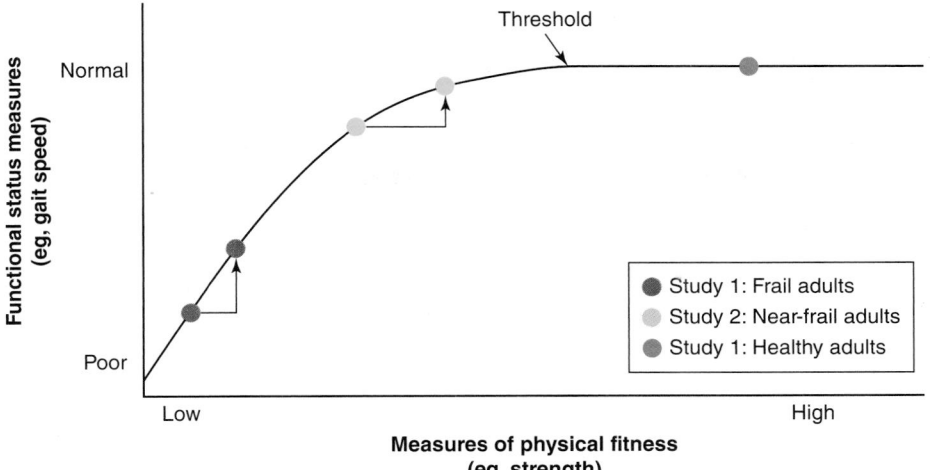

FIGURE 54-2. Theoretical relationship between physical fitness and functional status. The curvilinear relationship shows a threshold effect: above the threshold level of fitness, functional status is normal; below it, function is impaired. A curvilinear relationship implies that the benefit from exercise depends on the target group. Three hypothetical exercise studies are shown. Each study produces the same absolute improvement in fitness. In the frail adults of study 1, exercise produces a large improvement in functional status. In the healthy adults of study 3, no benefit on functional status is seen. Study 2 shows intermediate benefits. (Data from Buchner DM, Larson EB, Wagner EH, et al. Evidence for a non-linear relationship between leg strength and gait speed. *Age Ageing.* 1996;25[5]:386–391.)

Indeed, the relationship between leg strength and walking speed is nonlinear. This nonlinear relationship is intuitive: if strength was linearly related to walking speed, highly trained weightlifters would walk ridiculously fast (16–30 km/h) because they are several times as strong as normal adults, who walk at around 5–8 km/h. That is, above a certain threshold level of adequate physiologic reserve, function is normal; below the threshold, function is impaired (**Figure 54-2**). The exact shape of the curve depends on the task and the physiologic capacity of interest. **Figure 54-2** may oversimplify the situation because most tasks have multiple physiologic determinants that may interact to affect behavioral ability.

To illustrate the concept of thresholds, consider that in steady-state measures of oxygen consumption, walking on a level grade at 5 km/h requires 3.2 METs (1 MET = 3.5 mL O_2/kg/min). With illness or inactivity, aerobic capacity may fall below the 3.2 METs required for walking. Because exercise can increase aerobic capacity, it should improve walking in this situation. However, aerobic exercise would not affect ability to walk at 5 km/h in adults whose aerobic capacity already exceeds 3.2 METs.

Thus, exercise may produce a large improvement in function in frail adults with little or no physiologic reserve. Indeed, well-designed studies of exercise in frail adults report improvements in functional limitations with exercise. For example, the Lifestyle Interventions and Independence for Elders (LIFE) study of frail older adults (70–89 years) demonstrated that a structured, moderate-intensity physical activity intervention reduced the risk of mobility disability compared to a control health education program. The greatest risk reduction (HR = 0.75) was observed in older adults

with lower physical function at baseline, compared to those with moderate functional impairments at baseline (HR = 0.95). In contrast, exercise would be expected to have much smaller effects on functional limitations in healthy older adults, at least in basic activities of daily life.

EXERCISE AND COMMON GERIATRIC DISORDERS

A number of common geriatric disorders can be improved with exercise, although many questions remain about the type and intensity of exercise, sex differences in response to exercise, and mechanisms underlying the benefits. **Table 54-1** summarizes the current knowledge of the effects of different exercise modalities on several common geriatric disorders.

Cardiovascular Diseases

Although the mortality rates attributable to cardiovascular diseases (CVD) have declined, CVD burden in older adults remains high. There is a consistent, independent inverse relationship between aerobic fitness and physical activity levels and CVD mortality. Both short bouts and longer continuous sessions of physical activity are equally effective for reducing coronary heart disease (CHD) risk, provided the total energy expended is similar. Although a dose response has been demonstrated in some studies, even low to moderate physical activity can reduce risk for CVD mortality, with no additional protection from participating in more vigorous activities.

In contrast to the overwhelming evidence of the benefit of aerobic exercise to reduce CVD risk, few data exist

TABLE 54-1 ■ EXERCISE EFFECTS IN COMMON GERIATRIC DISORDERS

DISORDER	AEROBIC EXERCISE	RESISTANCE EXERCISE	COMBINED EXERCISE	ALSO SEE CHAPTER #
Coronary heart disease	+	+	+	Chapter 74
Heart failure	+	+	+	Chapter 76
Peripheral artery disease	+	?	?	Chapter 78
Stroke	+	+	+	Chapter 62
Hypertension	+	?	?	Chapter 79
Diabetes mellitus	+	+	+	Chapter 99
Obesity	+	?	+	Chapter 30
Osteoporosis	+	+	+	Chapter 52
Falls	+	?	?	Chapter 43
Arthritis	+	?	+	Chapters 52, 102, and 103
Cancer	+	+	+	Chapter 88
Depressed mood	+	+	+	Chapter 65
Impaired cognition	+	+	+	Chapter 59
Sleep disorders	+	?	?	Chapter 44
Parkinson disease	+	+	?	Chapter 61

+ = benefit; ? = unknown benefit.

on the association between strength training and CVD risk. Strength training is generally associated with reduced CVD mortality; however, the relationship may be J-shaped, with low to moderate levels (1–50 minutes per week) associated with the lowest risk of CVD mortality.

Similar to physical activity, fitness has been reported as being at least as good a predictor of both overall and CVD-related death as blood pressure, obesity, smoking, or diabetes. Because of the reported benefit of increasing physical activity and fitness levels on CVD risk, aerobic exercise and strength training are typically prescribed for older adults with CVD as part of a comprehensive cardiac rehabilitation program to increase aerobic capacity, improve CVD risk factors, prevent disease progression, and reduce the risk for future cardiovascular events and death. In fact, individuals with stable coronary artery disease randomized to exercise training improved their aerobic capacity and had a higher event-free survival (reduced repeat revascularization and hospitalizations) than those receiving percutaneous coronary intervention.

Both aerobic exercise and strength training improve aerobic exercise capacity to a similar degree in patients with CHD, and the improvements are enhanced when the two exercise modalities are combined. Aerobic exercise and strength training are also beneficial in improving exercise tolerance and quality of life in other CVD patient populations including heart failure (see Chapter 76) and peripheral arterial disease (PAD, see Chapter 78). Supervised aerobic exercise training is associated with reduced mortality (35%) and hospital readmission (28%) in patients with chronic heart failure. In patients with PAD, any physical activity greater than light intensity is associated with reduced mortality compared to no physical activity or only light-intensity activities. Because walking is effective in improving absolute claudication distance (ACD), guidelines recommend that individuals with PAD participate in a supervised walking program that gradually increases speed and distance as an initial noninvasive approach, using walking claudication pain—either onset of pain, or mild to moderate or maximal level tolerable—for prescribing exercise intensity. Other modes of exercise also improve ACD. However, the data are insufficient, particularly with regard to resistance training, to make any clinical recommendations. Thus, there is a need for further definitive, large clinical trials of alternative or complementary exercise interventions for PAD in older adults.

Exercise training programs in CVD patients have numerous physiologic effects on the cardiovascular system and CVD risk factors (**Table 54-2**). Improvements in VO_{2max} of 15% to 25% are driven by either central

TABLE 54-2 ■ EFFECTS OF EXERCISE TRAINING ON THE CARDIOVASCULAR SYSTEM AND CARDIOVASCULAR RISK FACTORS

- Improved maximal oxygen uptake (VO_{2max})
- Improved insulin sensitivity
- Improved glucose homeostasis
- Reduced arterial stiffness
- Improved endothelial function
- Improved blood lipid profile
  - Increased high-density lipoprotein (HDL)-C and HDL2-C
  - Reduced triglycerides
  - Reduced very-low-density lipoprotein (VLDL)
  - Reduced apolipoprotein A-I

(ie, improved myocardial oxygenation, enhanced left ventricular function) and/or peripheral adaptations, depending on the population. For example, in coronary artery disease (CAD) and heart failure patients, those with depressed left ventricular function may not show cardiac adaptations, but rather, the improvements in VO_{2max} are largely attributed to improvements in maximal arteriovenous oxygen difference due to improved mitochondrial oxidative enzymatic capacity.

In addition to improving multiple CVD risk factors, exercise training programs reduce arterial stiffness and improve vascular endothelial function in patients with CVD, measures that are important for overall vascular homeostasis. In general, aerobic exercise training programs improve vascular function in older adults independent of disease state. However, there are noted sex differences between the magnitude of improvement with exercise training, with near restoration of endothelial function to youthful levels in healthy older men, but attenuated or minimal improvements in postmenopausal women not on estrogen-based hormone therapy. Exercise training may also increase circulating bone marrow derived endothelial progenitor cells (EPCs) and improve EPC function. EPCs facilitate vascular repair and vasculogenesis, and are reduced in CVD patients. Other potential mechanisms of exercise training on CVD could be related to regression of coronary artery stenosis and formation of collateral vessels, resulting in enhanced myocardial perfusion.

The benefits of exercise on CVD risk are thought to be due at least in part to improvements in lipid profiles. Higher levels of physical activity are associated with less atherogenic lipoprotein profiles in young and middle-aged individuals, although data in older adults are lacking. There is no consistent effect of resistance training on lipoproteins.

Although exercise training is beneficial overall for CVD patients, there are a few conditions in which exercise may not be as beneficial and actually contraindicated. These conditions include unstable angina, uncontrolled hypertension, uncontrolled cardiac arrhythmias, recent myocardial infarction, severe aortic stenosis and other valvular diseases, acute pericarditis, and decompensated heart failure.

Hypertension

Hypertension is covered in Chapter 79. Over 80% of adults age 60 or older with hypertension are treated with antihypertensive therapies, and more than 30% of hypertensive adults age 80 or older are taking three or more classes of antihypertensive medications. Although antihypertensive medications produce long-term benefit, these medications can have numerous side effects, especially in older patients. Thus, using nonpharmacologic treatments (eg, weight loss, low-sodium diet, and exercise) is appealing, especially in older adults with mild to moderate hypertension.

Both leisure-time activity and aerobic exercise capacity (ie, VO_{2max}) are inversely related to risk for hypertension, with the lowest risk for hypertension in the most active and fit people. Hypertensive older Swedish men (born in 1914) who regularly exercised vigorously had an adjusted relative risk of 0.43 for total mortality and 0.33 for cardiovascular mortality. Given the apparent benefits of increased physical activity on aerobic exercise capacity and reduced hypertension risk, the Eighth Report of the Joint National Committee on Prevention, Detection, Evaluation, and Treatment of High Blood Pressure (JNC 8) recommends increased physical activity designed to enhance aerobic exercise capacity as initial therapy to prevent, treat, and control hypertension.

Aerobic exercise training programs effectively lower blood pressure in older adults with mild to moderate hypertension. Overall, aerobic exercise training programs or increasing physical activity of moderate intensity and of adequate volume result in a 4 to 10 mm Hg decline in systolic blood pressure and a 3 to 8 mm Hg decline in diastolic blood pressure in individuals with stage 1 hypertension, regardless of age or sex. The effects of aerobic exercise training in older adults with stage 2 hypertension, or those with resistant hypertension are less clear. In resistant hypertension, moderate-intensity exercise training reduced 24-hour ambulatory blood pressure similarly to that reported for mild to moderate hypertensives. Although there are limited data comparing different exercise intensities, low- to moderate-intensity exercise may be more effective at lowering blood pressure than more vigorous exercise. Indeed, even light Tai chi exercise or increasing daily walking can reduce and even normalize blood pressure in sedentary older hypertensive patients.

There is limited and inconsistent data on the effect of strength training on blood pressure in older hypertensive adults. Excessive blood pressure elevations can occur during high-intensity resistance training, especially if associated with Valsalva. However, with low- to moderate-intensity strength training and proper breathing techniques, this is not a concern. Overall, progressive resistance training results in a 3 mm Hg decrease in both systolic and diastolic blood pressure. However, the effect of resistance training on systolic blood pressure in adults older than 50 years and on systolic and diastolic blood pressures in hypertensives is less and not significant. Given the small number of studies available in hypertensive older adults, additional research is warranted to provide recommendations on the effect of resistance training for blood pressure reduction in hypertensive older adults.

The mechanisms underlying the blood pressure lowering effects of exercise in hypertensive adults are not completely understood, although changes in body composition, sympathetic nervous system activity, peripheral vascular resistance, and insulin levels have all been postulated. For example, weight loss alone or combined with exercise provides a greater blood pressure lowering effect than exercise alone. Aerobic exercise training decreases arterial stiffness and improves endothelial function in hypertensive adults. However, whether the decreases in blood pressure with exercise are due to improvements in arterial stiffness and endothelial function, or vice versa, are unclear.

Obesity

As described in Chapter 30, obesity is associated with increased morbidity and mortality from multiple medical complications, and has been consistently correlated with mobility impairment and poor physical function, especially in older adults. While weight loss alone can improve cardiometabolic risk factors, fitness, function, and quality of life in obese older adults, it is also associated with loss of fat-free mass (FFM) and decreases in bone mineral density (BMD). Given these potential harms, there is general agreement that exercise should be a component of any weight loss intervention, in order to minimize loss of muscle and bone with weight loss in older obese adults.

Diet plus exercise interventions improve multiple cardiometabolic and functional outcomes in older adults, although effects on cardiovascular events or mortality have not been demonstrated yet. For example, the Diabetes Prevention Program (DPP) lifestyle intervention of moderate-intensity exercise and modest weight loss (7%) was very effective in preventing progression to diabetes in older (60–85 years) participants. Compared to younger people in the DPP, older participants had greater reductions in waist circumference, lost more weight, and were more likely to achieve the goal of at least 150 minutes of exercise per week.

A randomized, controlled trial by Villareal et al. provides the most compelling evidence for including exercise in any weight loss intervention in older obese adults. They compared 52 weeks of weight loss diet, exercise (aerobic and strength training), or both in more than 100 older obese adults with mild to moderate functional impairment. Participants receiving the diet intervention lost weight, whereas weight remained stable in the exercise only group. Physical and metabolic function improved in all groups, but was greatest in the diet plus exercise group. The expected decreases in FFM and BMD with weight loss were attenuated in the diet plus exercise group, but not completely reversed. Because the negative effects of weight loss on body composition and BMD in older obese adults are not fully offset by exercise, an important question is whether weight loss per se is necessary, or whether exercise alone can confer most of the benefits without the associated risks of weight loss in this population.

Osteoporosis

The decline in BMD with age is well recognized (see Chapter 51), and there is an epidemic of osteoporotic fractures that affects women more than men and that primarily involves hip, vertebral, and wrist fractures. Mechanical loads are critical to skeletal integrity. Animal studies confirm the importance of mechanical strain to bone modeling and remodeling. They have also identified that (1) the osteogenic response to mechanical loading is optimized with relatively few repetitions of high-magnitude forces; (2) the

application of force must be in a dynamic, rather than static, fashion; and (3) fast strain rates are more osteogenic than slow strain rates. Furthermore, the osteogenic response to mechanical loading is mediated locally in skeletal regions subjected to the strain, highlighting the need for exercises to specifically target regions of the skeleton at risk of fracture. It appears that bone cells lose sensitivity to mechanical loading after relatively few loading cycles. For example, four sets of 90 load applications per day were more osteogenic than one set of 360 loading cycles, and interposing an 8-hour recovery period between loading sessions resulted in a greater osteogenic response than when the recovery period was 0.5 hour. These concepts have not been rigorously evaluated in humans, but they suggest that multiple short bouts of exercise per day may be more effective in preserving bone health than a single, longer daily session. The concept of allowing bone to "rest" between loading cycles may also have implications for resistance training. For example, if the intent is to perform three sets of eight repetitions of several exercises, it might be of greater benefit to bone to perform one set of each exercise and then cycle back through for the second and third sets, rather than doing three consecutive sets of each exercise.

The effects of exercise on bone mass have been estimated by comparing athletes who participate in different sports or physically active versus sedentary people. For example, the humerus in the dominant arm of tennis players had approximately 30% greater cortical bone thickness when compared to the nondominant arm. Athletes who participate in muscle-building activities (eg, weight lifting and body building) and in activities that involve jumping or vaulting (eg, volleyball and gymnastics) also tend to have elevated BMD. These data suggest that exercise in younger individuals may increase peak bone mass—an important protective factor for reducing osteopenia later in life. In contrast, the primary benefit of physical activity in older adults may be to preserve, rather than increase, bone mass.

Although both weight-bearing aerobic exercise and resistance exercise can increase bone mass in older women and men, increases in BMD appear to require a vigorous level of exercise, which supports the contention that the osteogenic response to exercise is attenuated with aging. In postmenopausal women, exercise may increase BMD by up to 5%, as compared to no-exercise controls, but average increases generally are only 1% to 3%. These modest increases may reflect difficulty reaching the strain threshold needed for bone remodeling to occur due to decreased muscle mass and strength, declines in hormones and growth factors that affect the sensitivity of bone to strain, and/or insufficient calcium and vitamin D.

There is also evidence that exercise can prevent fractures. Results from prospective cohort studies, such as the Nurses' Health Study and the Study of Osteoporotic Fractures, suggest that the risk for hip fracture is reduced by approximately 50% in the most physically active quintile of the population. In evaluating the potential benefit of simple walking activity, the Nurses' Health Study found a dose-response benefit for both duration and speed of walking, such that more hours per week spent walking and fast walking speed conferred reduced fracture risk. Even hours per week spent standing was inversely related to hip fracture incidence. Perhaps most importantly, changes in physical activity for several years were related to hip fracture incidence in the expected manner: decreases in physical activity were associated increased risk and vice versa. Such findings suggest that any type of ambulatory physical activity may confer skeletal benefits and that increased physical activity should be advocated at any age as a strategy to reduce fracture risk.

The low frequency of fractures makes well-designed, adequately powered randomized controlled trials extremely expensive. Very few exercise trials have included fractures as an outcome, or reported fractures as an observation. Analysis of 11 exercise intervention studies that reported fractures found that exercise reduced the risk of overall fracture by approximately 50% and vertebral fracture by approximately 40% compared to controls, although the authors urged caution due to the strong likelihood of publication bias. The Erlangen Fitness and Osteoporosis Prevention Study compared fracture incidence among 137 postmenopausal osteopenic women either participating in a supervised exercise intervention (two group and two home sessions per week), or a sedentary control group for 12 years. Although fewer fractures occurred in the exercise group, the difference between groups did not reach statistical significance.

Important areas for future research include determining the effects of age and sex in the response of bone to exercise. In addition, new methods such as peripheral quantitative computed tomography may provide important information on bone quality (eg, strength and geometry) in response to exercise.

Cancer

Cohort and case control studies consistently support an inverse relation between physical activity and overall cancer incidence and mortality. The effects appear to be stronger in men than in women, but many studies excluded women. Overall, occupational and leisure physical activities were associated with a 30% independent protective effect on overall cancer risk in men, and men who engaged in regular vigorous activities had a 20% reduction in cancer risk compared to sedentary men. Analysis of more than 15,000 cancer deaths over 12 years in the NIH-AARP Diet and Health Study found that compared to those who reported rarely or never engaging in moderate to vigorous physical activity, those who reported more than 7 hours/week had a lower risk of cancer mortality (HR = 0.89).

In persons diagnosed with cancer, exercise is associated with improved surgical outcomes, decreased symptoms and side effects of treatment, and improved physical function and psychological health. Participation in exercise post cancer diagnosis has been estimated to increase cancer survivorship by 50% to 60%.

To date, the most compelling data involve the relationship between activity and risk of colon or breast cancer. A reduced risk of colon cancer (relative risk, 0.4–0.9) has been found in groups with high physical activity levels compared to those with low levels. In general, controlling for other cancer risks including tobacco, alcohol, age, obesity, and diet does not diminish the relationships, and this finding has been demonstrated in men and women of different racial and ethnic groups. Among patients with colon cancer, any prediagnosis physical activity was associated with a 25% reduction in colon-cancer mortality, and a 26% reduction in all-cause mortality compared to patients who reported no physical activity prior to diagnosis. Moderate to high levels of postdiagnosis physical activity were also associated with reductions in all-cause mortality ranging from 24% to 39%.

Physical activity reduces the risk of breast cancer overall by 15% to 20%. The strongest effect appears to be in postmenopausal breast cancer, where the risk reduction ranges from 20% to 80% when comparing the most active to the least active groups. These associations remain even after adjusting for potential confounding factors such as age, body mass index (BMI), reproductive history, tobacco use, and diet. There appears to be a dose response, with higher levels of activity associated with greater risk reduction. As with colon cancer, exercise in breast cancer patients is associated with better physical function and fewer treatment-related side effects.

Depressed Mood

Subjects who exercise regularly consistently report an improved sense of well-being and reduced tension and anxiety. Large epidemiological studies have demonstrated an association between low levels of physical activity and depressive symptoms. These studies have also shown physical activity to be an independent predictor of the development of depressive symptoms. In the National Health and Nutrition Education Survey I Epidemiologic Follow-Up Study, low levels of physical activity predicted depressive symptoms 8 years later in White women, with those reporting little to no physical activity twice as likely to develop depressive symptoms as those reporting moderate to high levels.

As for treatment for clinical depression, structured, mixed exercise programs result in a modest reduction in symptom severity. The effects of exercise appear to be comparable to those of behavioral or pharmacologic therapy. Proposed mechanisms for the effects of exercise on mood include increases in endorphin and monoamine levels, as well as social engagement and improvements in self-efficacy and self-esteem.

Impaired Cognition

There may be a positive effect of exercise on cognition. Numerous cross-sectional and longitudinal studies including the Nurse's Health Study and the Mayo Clinic Study on Aging have found an association between higher levels of physical activity and both better cognitive test scores and reduced risk of cognitive impairment and dementia. Among 1200 older adults in the Framingham Study, a hazard ratio of 0.55 was found for incident all-cause dementia after 10 years of follow-up in participants reporting moderate to heavy physical activity compared to less active participants. Among those in the lowest quintile of physical activity, the hazard ratio for incident dementia was 1.45.

Results from exercise intervention studies have been mixed, although the balance of evidence supports moderate positive effects of exercise training on cognition in both cognitively normal and cognitively impaired individuals. In older adults without known cognitive impairment, 8 of 11 studies using aerobic exercise interventions found positive effects on cognitive function that coincided with improvements in maximal oxygen uptake (VO_{2max}). A meta-analysis of 16 trials in older patients with dementia found a significant positive effect on cognitive function with exercise training, although the authors emphasized caution given the substantial heterogeneity between trials.

Some studies have also reported cognitive benefits with resistance training alone, but the greatest cognitive effects were observed with mixed training paradigms. Exercise appears to improve function in multiple cognitive domains, with the strongest effects in executive control functions. Important areas for further study include determining the duration and intensity of exercise needed to realize cognitive benefits, and potential sex differences in the cognitive responses to exercise.

The bases for the exercise-associated improvements in cognition are presently an active area of investigation. Animal studies support a neuroprotective effect of exercise through promotion of neuroplasticity, increases in brain-derived neurotrophic factor and enhanced neurogenesis.

Sleep Disorders

Age effects on sleep and sleep disorders are covered in Chapter 44. Physical activity and regular exercise are beneficial for sleep in older adults. Higher levels of cardiorespiratory fitness and physical activity in older adults are associated with better self-reported sleep quality. For instance, objectively measured indices of sleep quality (eg, sleep onset latency, wake time after sleep onset, sleep efficiency) are better in physically fit older men compared to sedentary controls, and higher levels of physical activity are protective against insomnia in older adults. Although few longitudinal exercise studies have specifically focused on older adults, a systematic review and meta-analysis of six studies in adults older than 40 years demonstrated that 10 to 16 weeks of aerobic exercise has positive effects on self-reported sleep quality measured using the Pittsburgh Sleep Quality Index.

It appears that slow wave sleep (SWS), which plays a role in the restorative functions of sleep, is particularly sensitive to exercise training. Older physically fit men have more SWS than sedentary older men, and exercise training increases SWS in older men and women. One longer-term study (12 months) demonstrated that in older adults with mild to moderate sleep problems, exercise was associated with decreases in stage 1 sleep, increases in stage 2 sleep, and fewer awakenings.

There remain many questions regarding the effects of exercise on sleep in older adults. For example, most studies in older adults have examined the effects of aerobic training, but at least one study has shown that progressive resistance training can improve subjective measures of sleep quality. It is not known if aerobic, resistance, or a combination is most effective for improving sleep. The effects of exercise intensity have not been established, but lower intensity activities such as yoga and Tai chi also improve self-reported measures of sleep quality. Similarly, lower-intensity exercise (eg, stretching and flexibility) was associated with greater improvements in self-reported sleep quality than higher-intensity exercise performed at 60% to 75% of maximal heart rate. The effects of frequency of exercise have also not been defined, but a study in older men (~64 years) showed that after a 16-week exercise training period, SWS increased on a day when exercise was performed, but not on a sedentary day. These findings suggest that physical activity should be done on most days of the week to maximize the benefits on sleep. Whether exercise has different effects in men and women is not known.

It should also be recognized that there may be a reciprocal relationship: poor sleep is associated with lower levels of physical activity. For example, in sample of subjects from the Healthy Women Study (~73 years), greater self-reported sleep efficiency and less sleep fragmentation were associated with higher physical activity levels the following day. Thus, there appears to be a circular association whereby increased physical activity improves sleep, and improved sleep facilitates greater physical activity levels.

Parkinson Disease

Exercise is associated with reduced mortality rate and with improvements in functional mobility and activities of daily living in individuals with Parkinson disease (see Chapter 61). Though data are limited, controlled trials of both resistance and aerobic training in individuals with Parkinson disease have demonstrated improvements in mobility, gait, and quality of life. The intensity of exercise required to realize benefits in Parkinson disease is an area of active investigation, as some studies have found greater improvements with a higher dose of exercise, while others have not.

Despite impaired force production and increased fatigability, individuals with Parkinson disease are able to participate safely and effectively in high-intensity resistance exercise, and appear to derive benefits similar to those in neurologically healthy adults. In one study, 12 weeks of high-force eccentric resistance training in adults with Parkinson disease was associated with a 6% increase in muscle hypertrophy, a 24% increase in torque, and an 18% improvement in 6-minute walk time compared to a standard exercise program. Aerobic exercise interventions—mainly treadmill exercise—consistently improve gait, mobility, and quality of life.

Stroke

Stroke is a leading cause of disability in older adults, with 20% to 25% of stroke survivors requiring at least some assistance with activities of daily living (see Chapter 62). These functional deficits predispose patients to a sedentary lifestyle, further increasing the risk of stroke and CVD, the leading causes of death among stroke survivors. Physical rehabilitation in stroke patients has traditionally focused on the first few months after the event, as prevailing wisdom held that further functional improvements were unlikely after this time. However, improvements in aerobic capacity and sensorimotor function can be achieved with continued rehabilitation. Physical activity and exercise recommendations for stroke survivors from the American Heart Association identify three primary goals: (1) preventing complications from prolonged inactivity; (2) decreasing the risk of recurrent stroke and cardiovascular events; and (3) increasing aerobic fitness. Specific recommendations for aerobic exercise and strength training are similar to those recommended for all adults. In addition, incorporation of stretching and balance/coordination activities is recommended to prevent muscle contractures, and to improve the ability to safely perform activities of daily living.

RISKS ASSOCIATED WITH EXERCISE

Despite the overwhelming evidence that exercise confers multiple benefits and can be performed safely even in frail older adults, concerns about potential injury and other adverse events are common among patients and health care providers. These fears may prevent patients from engaging in the amount and intensity of exercise needed to realize health benefits, thus presenting a potential barrier to increasing physical activity levels.

"Overuse" injuries involving soft tissues are by far the most common and are likely to increase with advancing age. Eccentric exercise (eg, lowering a weight that has been lifted) may predispose to excess muscle injury. Appropriate warm-up and cool-down periods, as well as emphasis on stretching and flexibility, are likely to be especially important in reducing soft-tissue injury in an older population.

The prevalence of asymptomatic coronary artery disease is higher in older compared to younger adults, and there is a transient increase in the risk of sudden death occurring during a bout of vigorous exercise, especially in previously sedentary individuals. However, the small increased risk of a cardiovascular event with exercise is clearly outweighed by the reduction in risk during the nonexercising period of the day. Thus, the overall risk of sudden death in active men is only 30% of that in sedentary men. Furthermore, there is lower cardiovascular-related and overall mortality in active individuals.

In older patients with diabetes mellitus, careful attention to the possibility of exercise-induced hypoglycemia is critical because of the sustained improvement in insulin sensitivity for 24 to 48 hours following vigorous exercise. Meticulous foot care and supportive, well-fitted shoes are also important for the exercising diabetic patient. Patients with proliferative retinopathy should avoid anaerobic (specifically isometric) exercise, such as power lifting, because of the increased ocular and systemic pressure occurring with the Valsalva maneuver.

In the past, a pre-exercise assessment, including a complete history and physical examination, and an exercise stress test were recommended for adults older than 60 before vigorous exercise. Such an evaluation is expensive and could present a significant barrier to exercise. Furthermore, there are little data to substantiate this recommendation. Current recommendations suggest that asymptomatic individuals who plan to exercise at moderate intensity do

TABLE 54-3 ■ SUMMARY OF PHYSICAL ACTIVITY RECOMMENDATIONS FOR OLDER ADULTS

- Perform (1) moderate-intensity endurance activities at least 30 min/d in bouts of at least 10 min each to total 150–300 min/wk; (2) at least 20–30 min/d or more of vigorous-intensity endurance activities to total 75–150 min/wk; or (3) an equivalent combination of moderate and vigorous activity.
- Perform 8–10 strengthening activities involving the major muscle groups between moderate and vigorous intensity (8–12 repetitions) at least 2 d/wk.
- Perform flexibility exercises that use sustained stretches involving the major muscle groups with static movements at moderate intensity at least 2 d/wk.
- For frequent fallers or individuals with mobility problems, perform balance exercises including (1) progressively difficult postures that gradually reduce the base of support (eg, two-legged stand, semitandem stand, tandem stand, one-legged stand), (2) dynamic movements that perturb the center of gravity (eg, tandem walk, circle turns); (3) stressing postural muscle groups (eg, heel stands, toe stands); or (4) reducing sensory input (eg, standing with eyes closed).
- The intensity and duration of physical activity should be low at the outset for older adults who are highly deconditioned, functionally limited, or have chronic conditions that affect their ability to perform physical tasks. The progression of activities should be individual and tailored to tolerance and preference. Muscle-strengthening activities and/or balance training may need to precede aerobic training activities among very frail individuals. Older adults should exceed the recommended minimum amounts of physical activity if they desire to improve their fitness. If chronic conditions preclude activity at the recommended minimum amount, older adults should perform physical activities as tolerated so as to avoid being sedentary.

Data from American College of Sports Medicine, Chodzko-Zajko WJ, Proctor DN, et al. American College of Sports Medicine position stand. Exercise and physical activity for older adults. Med Sci Sports Exerc. 2009;41(7):1510–1530.

not need screening before initiating an activity program. The geriatric medicine axiom of "start low and go slow" should be applied to beginning a safe physical activity program. It is appropriate for patients to notify their health care providers of their intent to begin an exercise program, because adjustments in medications or dosages may be necessary. The health care provider can also work with the individual to tailor the exercise program to the individual's abilities and be a source of ongoing support and encouragement.

RECOMMENDATIONS

There is now ample evidence that older adults can safely engage in both aerobic and resistance exercise training, and that exercise has beneficial effects on numerous important health-related end points in this population. Despite these acknowledged benefits, older adults are the least physically active age group. Potential barriers to exercise in older adults include perceptions of safety, chronic conditions and physical limitations, and access to exercise programs or facilities.

Consensus recommendations for physical activity in older adults are summarized in **Table 54-3** and were updated in 2018 by the Department of Health and Human Services (DHHS) in the Physical Activity Guidelines for Americans, 2nd edition. The DHHS guidelines stress the importance of avoiding sedentary behavior, and that any amount of physical activity provides some health benefits. The specific modifications for older adults include: (1) being as physically active as their conditions allow if the target of 150 min/week is not possible because of chronic conditions; (2) engaging in balance exercises for individuals at risk of falling; (3) determining the level of effort for physical activity relative to level of fitness; and (4) understanding how chronic conditions may affect the ability to safely engage in regular physical activity. Key to recommendations for exercise in older adults is the need to individualize the program of physical activity. While there is a dose-response relationship between the intensity of exercise and the improvement in most outcome measures, significant cardiovascular and metabolic improvements can be obtained when less intense exercise is maintained over sufficiently long periods of time. Less intense exercise regimens may be more acceptable to some older individuals and appear to make long-term compliance more likely. Low-intensity programs may be necessary in frail populations, such as those with stroke, heart failure, and chronic lung disease, in which more intensive exercise is not tolerated. While multiple short bouts of exercise (at least 10 minutes each) may be effective in improving certain outcome measures, longer sessions remain preferable if these can be tolerated.

Because the physical activity goals may seem daunting, especially for inactive older adults, specific instructions are more helpful than general advice to "increase physical activity." Provision of written exercise prescriptions from health care providers increases activity levels among previously sedentary adults. In addition, an increasing array of technologies allows individuals to set activity goals and to monitor and track activity in real time.

Changes in lifestyle are difficult to maintain at any age, and recidivism rates for exercise programs are high. This problem may be reduced by: (1) careful attention to warm-up periods and slow progression in an effort to reduce early injuries; (2) enthusiastic leadership; (3) regular assessment of improvement with personalized feedback and praise; (4) spousal and family support for participation; (5) flexible goals (time rather than distance) set by the participant; and (6) use of distraction techniques such as music.

ACKNOWLEDGMENTS

Dr. Robert Schwartz and Dr. Wendy Kohrt wrote this chapter in the 6th edition, and Dr. Edward Melanson contributed to the 7th edition chapter. Some material from the previous versions has been retained in this edition. The authors also gratefully acknowledge the advice and encouragement of Drs. Schwartz and Kohrt in the preparation of this chapter.

FURTHER READING

Billinger S, Arena R, Bernhardt J, et al. Physical activity and exercise recommendations for stroke survivors. A statement for healthcare professionals from the American Heart Association/American Stroke Association. *Stroke.* 2014;45(8):2532–2553.

Bottaro M, Machado SN, Nogueira W, Scales R, Veloso J. Effect of high versus low-velocity resistance training on muscular fitness and functional performance in older men. *Eur J Appl Physiol.* 2007;99:257–264.

Chodzko-Zajko WJ, Proctor DN, Fiatarone Singh MA, et al. Exercise and physical activity for older adults. *Med Sci Sports Exerc.* 2009;41(7):1510–1530.

Diabetes Prevention Program Group. Reduction in the incidence of type 2 diabetes with lifestyle intervention or metformin. *N Engl J Med.* 2002;346:393–403.

Feskanich D, Willett W, Colditz G. Walking and leisure-time activity and risk of hip fracture in postmenopausal women. *JAMA.* 2002;288:2300–2306.

Hollings M, Mavros Y, Freeston J, Singh MF. The effect of progressive resistance training on aerobic fitness and strength in adults with coronary heart disease: a systematic review and meta-analysis of randomised controlled trials. *Eur J Prev Cardiol.* 2017;24(12):1242–1259.

Hupin D, Roche F, Gremeaux V, et al. Even a low-dose of moderate-to-vigorous physical activity reduces mortality by 22% in adults aged ≥60 years: a systematic review and meta-analysis. *Br J Sports Med.* 2015;49:1262–1267.

Kesaniemi YK, Danforth E Jr, Jensen MD, Kopelman PG, Lefebvre P, Reeder BA. Dose-response issues concerning physical activity and health: and evidence-based symposium. *Med Sci Sports Exerc.* 2001;33:S351–S358.

Kohrt WM, Bloomfield SA, Little KD, Nelson ME, Yingling VR. American College of Sports Medicine Position Stand: physical activity and bone health. *Med Sci Sports Exerc.* 2004;36:1985–1996.

Kramer AF, Erickson KI, Colcombe SJ. Exercise, cognition, and the aging brain. *J Appl Physiol.* 2006;101:1237–1242.

Kraschnewski JL, Sciamanna CN, Poger JM, et al. Is strength training associated with mortality benefits? A 15 year cohort study of US older adults. *Prev Med.* 2016:87;121–127.

Latham NK, Bennett DA, Stretton CM, Anderson CS. Systematic review of progressive resistance strength training in older adults. *J Gerontol A Biol Sci Med Sci.* 2004;59A:48–61.

Orchard TJ, Temprosa M, Goldberg R, et al. The effect of metformin and intensive lifestyle intervention on metabolic syndrome: the Diabetes Prevention Program randomized trial. *Ann Intern Med.* 2005;142:611–619.

Pahor M, Guralnik JM, Ambrosius WT, et al. Effect of structured physical activity on prevention of major mobility disability in older adults: the LIFE study randomized clinical trial. *JAMA.* 2014;311:2387–2396.

Rejeski WJ, Bray GA, Chen SH, et al. Aging and physical function in type 2 diabetes: 8 years of an intensive lifestyle intervention. *J Gerontol A Biol Sci Med Sci.* 2015;70(3):345–353.

Tanaka H, Seals DR. Endurance exercise performance in masters athletes: age-associated changes and underlying physiologic mechanisms. *J Physiol.* 2008;586(1):55–63.

US Department of Health and Human Services. *Physical Activity Guidelines for Americans*, 2nd edition. Washington, DC: US Department of Health and Human Services; 2018.

Villareal DT, Chode S, Parimi N, et al. Weight loss, exercise, or both and physical function in obese older adults. *N Engl J Med.* 2011;364:1218–1229.

von Stengel S, Kemmler W, Kalender WA, Engelke K, Lauber D. Differential effects of strength versus power training on bone mineral density in postmenopausal women: a two year longitudinal study. *Br J Sports Med.* 2007;41:649–655.

Williams MA, Haskell WL, Ades PA, et al. Resistance exercise in individuals with and without cardiovascular disease: 2007 update. *Circulation.* 2007;116:572–584.

Zoico E, Di Francesco V, Guralnik JM, et al. Physical disability and muscular strength in relation to obesity and different body composition indexes in a sample of healthy elderly women. *Int J Obes Relat Metab Disord.* 2004;28:234–241.

Rehabilitation

Cynthia J. Brown

DEFINING REHABILITATION

The purpose of rehabilitation is to restore some or all of a person's physical and mental capabilities that have been lost as a result of disease, injury, or illness and to help achieve the highest possible level of function, independence, and quality of life. The techniques and modalities used to achieve these goals are numerous and typically do not differ for younger versus older persons. However, rehabilitation outcomes and approaches are frequently different for the older adult. For example, most young adults experience a single acute event that results in disability. Older adults are more likely to have multiple comorbid conditions that, over time, result in disability. Even if the older persons have acute events, like a hip fracture or a stroke, their underlying comorbid conditions may impact on the outcomes of rehabilitation. Older patients may also have subclinical physical or cognitive comorbidities, which become evident when challenged by a new disability. For example, mild cognitive impairment may be first recognized during rehabilitation after a hip fracture, when the patient has difficulty learning how to use a new assistive device.

Goals of rehabilitation for older adults usually focus on recovery of self-care ability and mobility, while for younger persons reentering the workforce or returning to school may be the goal. In general, recovery for older adults requires a longer period of time to achieve, and functional outcomes are usually worse when compared with younger adults. It is important to discuss rehabilitation goals with all patients and focus therapy toward achieving those goals. For example, older persons may have been avid golfers or fishermen, and return to this activity may be important for their quality of life. Rehabilitation efforts and goals of care may also be impacted by a person's values and beliefs about exercise and social roles. For example, if a patient has never cooked and does not believe that this is an important task to learn, taking the patient to the kitchen to learn how to prepare a meal may be viewed as a useless task. Participation by the patient and family in the development of the goals of rehabilitation is critical to achieve a successful outcome.

Disability is common in older persons and can have a significant impact on function and quality of life. In order to better understand the process of disablement, a variety

Learning Objectives

- Name and describe the conceptual models used as the framework for rehabilitation.
- Explain the advantages and disadvantages of each site of care for rehabilitation.
- List providers who are commonly members of the interprofessional rehabilitation team.
- Identify common rehabilitation interventions, in addition to exercise.
- Name at least two types of adaptive aids and how they are used.

Key Clinical Points

1. In addition to the history and physical examination, an evaluation should include assessments of cognition, motivation, depression, social support, and financial resources, as these factors can have a significant impact on rehabilitation outcomes.

2. It is important for the provider to understand the range of available rehabilitation settings, both inpatient and community based, and the advantages and disadvantages of each setting.

3. An interdisciplinary team is often required to meet the complex rehabilitation needs of older patients, and while team members have defined roles and functions, there is considerable overlap in the services provided.

4. Exercise is the cornerstone of physical rehabilitation, with each prescribed exercise being related to achievement of a goal and ultimately to an improvement in function.

5. Adaptive aids include devices that allow persons with physical limitations to

(Continued)

(Cont.) participate in activities, such as basic and instrumental activities of daily living, with greater ease and/or less pain. Categories of adaptive aids include mobility aids to assist people to move around within their home and community, bathroom aids to assist with bathing and toileting, and self-care aids that assist with dressing, personal hygiene, cooking, and other activities.

of theoretical models have been explored and are presented below.

History of the Disability Framework

In an attempt to provide a framework for the discussion of the consequences of disease and injury, Nagi developed the first disablement model in the 1960s (**Figure 55-1**). The model uses four related yet distinct phenomena considered by Nagi to be the basis of rehabilitation and include active pathology, impairment, functional limitation, and disability. Active pathology was described as a disruption in the normal cellular function and the body's efforts to regain a normal state. Impairment, which usually results from active pathology, referred to an abnormality or loss at the tissue or organ level. Functional limitation described restrictions at the individual level, while disability described a physical or mental limitation in a social context. Nagi's view of disability was a product of the interaction between individuals and their environment. Importantly, individuals could have similar functional impairments that result in different patterns of disability, depending on the environment in which they function.

In 1980, the World Health Organization's (WHO) *International Classification of Impairments, Disabilities, and Handicaps* (ICIDH) was developed in Europe. Like Nagi's disablement model, the ICIDH characterized three distinct concepts related to disease and health conditions: impairments, disabilities, and handicaps. While the ICIDH was developed to classify function and disability, it failed to receive endorsement by the World Health Assembly.

A major criticism of these early disablement models was that these presented the response to disease or illness as a static process with a linear progression through the disablement process. It was recognized that the interaction between disease and disability is more complex, particularly for older persons. Recognition of this complexity led to significant dialogue within the rehabilitation community and to a major revision of the ICIDH.

In 2001, the WHO released the *International Classification of Functioning, Disability, and Health* (ICF) (**Figure 55-2**), which attempted to incorporate, from a biological, personal, and social perspective, a biopsychosocial view of health. The ICF characterizes decreases in function as the consequence of a dynamic interaction between various health conditions and contextual factors. Health conditions are described as diseases, disorders, injuries, or aging. Contextual factors are divided into two categories: environmental factors and personal factors. Environmental factors include the physical, social, and attitudinal environment in which people live. These might include individual environment like furniture placement in the home or societal environment like policies regarding access to buildings. Personal factors are characteristics of the individual, which are not part of the health condition or illness. These might include gender, fitness, or coping styles. Listed across the center of the model are the three domains of human function: body functions and structures, activities, and participation. Body functions and structures are the physiologic functions and the anatomic parts of the body. The execution of a task or action by a person is an activity, while participation is the application to a real-life activity. For each of these three domains of human function, there are several levels on which the function can be experienced. These include functioning at the level of the body or body parts and the level of the whole person and the whole person in their environment. Disability is defined as any decline at any of these levels.

Using the ICF model, we could describe an older woman, who has a history of osteoarthritis of the knees and hypertension, who presents to rehabilitation after a hip fracture. She lives alone in a second-floor apartment and has a daughter who lives at a distance 6 hours away. The patient has a large circle of friends and regularly attends social gatherings at the local senior center. **Figure 55-3**

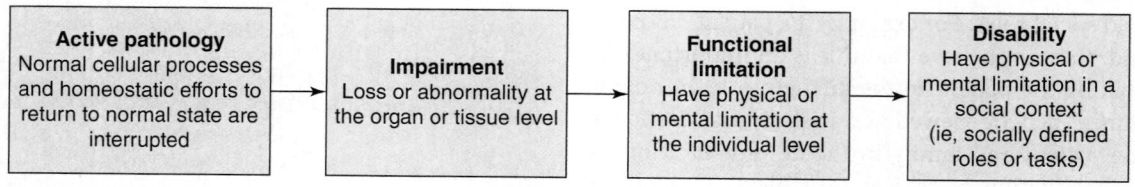

FIGURE 55-1. Schematic of the Nagi disablement model with definitions. The first disablement model was described by Nagi in the early 1960s. The initial disablement model focused on a linear progression to disability and has been replaced over time with new models such as the International Classification of Functioning, Disability, and Health (ICF). Importantly, the Nagi model was the first attempt to describe the process of disability.

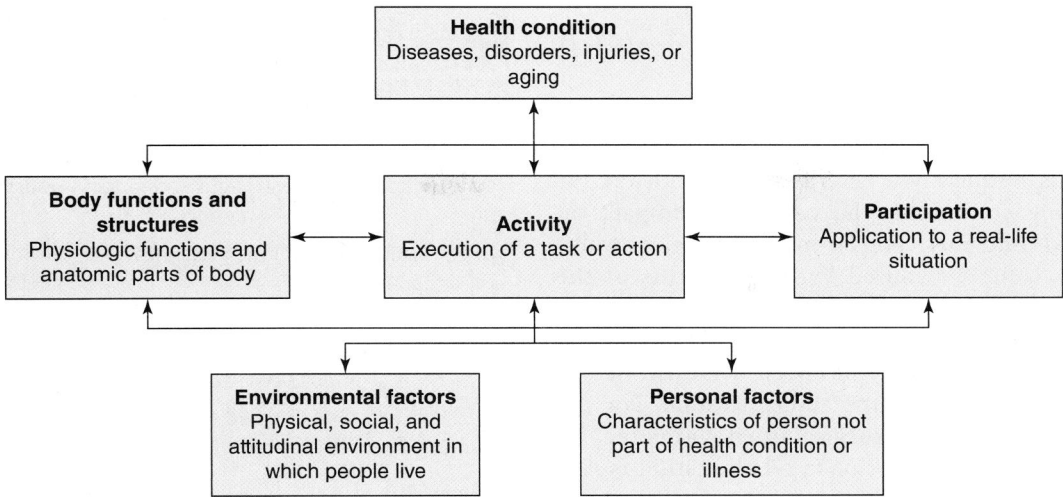

FIGURE 55-2. International Classification of Functioning, Disability, and Health (ICF). The latest version of the ICF focuses on the interaction between various factors and the impact these factors have on health and functioning. Prior models focused on disability and portrayed the path to disability as a linear process. This model attempts to incorporate, from a biological, personal, and social perspective, a biopsychosocial view of health. (Reproduced with permission from World Health Organization. *Towards a Common Language for Functioning, Disability and Health.* Geneva, Switzerland: ICF; 2002.)

demonstrates how this patient's problems might be placed in the ICF model, with the goal of generating hypotheses about the best treatment options. Important issues include not only improving the patient's strength and walking ability but also addressing where she will live after discharge and how to keep her active in her community. Understanding the relationships between the different components and addressing them is the key to a successful rehabilitation.

It is believed by many that the ICF framework has the potential to provide a standard disablement language, which could facilitate dialogue across disciplines. The ICF model attempts to reflect the interactions between different components of health and avoids the linear view of previous models. This framework also looks beyond disease and mortality to focus on how people live with their disabling conditions.

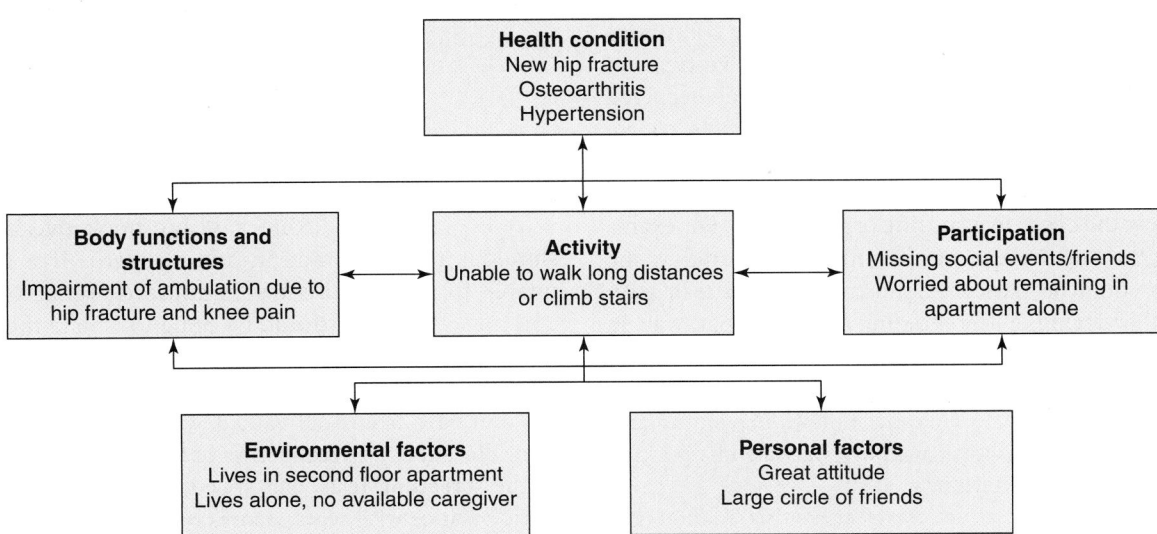

FIGURE 55-3. Using the ICF model to describe patient function. This figure demonstrates how a patient's problems might be placed in the ICF model with the goal of generating hypotheses about the best treatment options. In the case of this patient with osteoarthritis and new hip fracture, the ICF model illustrates how addressing where the patient will live after discharge and how to keep the patient active in the community are as important as improving the patient's strength and walking ability. Understanding the relationships between the different components and addressing them is the key to successful rehabilitation. (Data from WHO ICF model.)

Goals of Evaluation

An important goal of evaluation is to identify the cause of the disability for which rehabilitation is required. While there is frequently a final common pathway for many disabling conditions, the cause may impact on treatment and outcomes. For example, a person's walking difficulty could be caused by osteoarthritis of the knee or a meniscal tear. For the patient with osteoarthritis, an exercise program focused on strengthening the musculature around the knee has been demonstrated to decrease pain and improve the ability to walk. For the patient with a meniscal tear, surgical intervention may be a better option. Evaluation prior to rehabilitation is also important to identify comorbidities that may directly or indirectly affect rehabilitation outcomes. While the older person may have osteoarthritis causing limited walking ability, they may also have poor cardiac or pulmonary function that further limit walking ability. Another goal of evaluation is to determine the best site for rehabilitation to occur. Several settings are available, including an inpatient rehabilitation facility, a subacute nursing home, or a home. The appropriate setting is usually determined through evaluation of the disability and comorbid conditions that may affect rehabilitation. The next section outlines the evaluation process and focuses on creation of an individual treatment plan that addresses the patient's unique disabling conditions.

Function-Oriented History and Physical Examination

During the initial evaluation, the history and physical examination can help characterize the disabling conditions and lead the clinician toward the most effective types of treatment. Determining if the functional decline occurred suddenly or has taken a more slowly progressive course may be very helpful in determining the cause of the disability. Symptoms associated with a given activity may also help narrow the cause to a specific organ system. For example, while the impairment may be difficulty in walking, the limitation could be caused by shortness of breath or pain with weight bearing. Differentiating the causal pathway, in this case cardiopulmonary versus musculoskeletal, helps to refine the work-up required and assists the provider in targeting the appropriate therapy. Functional status and residence prior to the illness or injury may also help guide expectations of rehabilitation.

Table 55-1 lists several brief screening maneuvers, which can be done in the physician's office when evaluating a patient for disability. These assessment tools can be used to quickly assess baseline functional status as well as monitor progress during rehabilitation. If these screening tests are positive, additional testing should be performed, as the screening tests are often not as accurate as more detailed maneuvers. A variety of standardized measures are

TABLE 55-1 ■ PHYSICAL PERFORMANCE TESTS USED TO ASSESS FUNCTION

SCREENING ACTIVITY	ATTRIBUTE ADDRESSED	FUNCTIONAL IMPLICATION
Put a heavy book on an overhead shelf	Upper extremity strength and range of motion	Ability to perform housework
Grasp a piece of paper and resist its removal	Pinch strength	Grooming and feeding self
Write a sentence	Fine motor coordination	Feeding self
Timed rise to standing five times[a]	Lower extremity strength	Ambulation and stair climbing
Gait speed[a]	Dynamic balance, predicts falls, and morbidity and mortality	Ambulation and general function with ADLs
Standing balance[a]; feet side by side, semitandem and tandem	Static balance	Balance with progressively smaller base of support
Life space assessment[b]	Mobility within the home and community in the 4 weeks prior to assessment	Addresses factors in addition to physical function that might impair mobility
Rhomberg; standing with eyes closed and assess sway or loss of balance	Proprioception	Ability to balance without visual input

Data from [a]Studenski SA, Perera S, Wallace D, et al. Physical performance measures in the clinical setting. J Am Geriatr Soc. 2003;51(3):314; [b]Peel C, Sawyer-Baker P, Roth DL, et al. Assessing mobility in older adults: the UAB Study of Aging Life-Space Assessment. Phys Ther. 2005;85:1008–1019.

available to further test function during basic and instrumental activities of daily living (IADLs).

For example, lifting a heavy book overhead tests shoulder range of motion and strength. If a person is unable to achieve this task, additional range of motion and muscle testing should be done to isolate the cause of the difficulty.

Many of the screening tests listed have normative values and have been well validated for the geriatric population. The short physical performance battery includes three of the screening tests, gait speed, timed chair stands, and static balance with worse scores being associated with falls, nursing home placement, and mortality. The University of Alabama at Birmingham (UAB) Study of Aging Life-Space Assessment is a validated instrument that measures a person's mobility in the home and community during the month preceding the assessment. Importantly, the Study of Aging Life-Space Assessment goes beyond measuring the individual's ability to perform specific tasks by assessing the person's actual pattern of mobility, which may help identify factors other than physical impairment, such as emotional or socioeconomic factors, which might be limiting mobility.

In addition to the history and physical examination, an evaluation should include assessments of cognition, motivation, depression, social support, and financial resources, as these factors can have a significant impact on rehabilitation outcomes. A variety of validated assessment tools can be used to screen for cognition and depression, such as the Montreal Cognitive Assessment (MoCA) and the Geriatric Depression Scale, respectively. Assessment of current methods utilized by the patient for coping with disability, including use of ambulatory or assistive devices, level of assistance needed, and any limitation of activities, should also be explored.

Determining Rehabilitation Potential

Many factors influence the choice of who would benefit from rehabilitation and the success of those rehabilitation efforts. Assessment for rehabilitation potential needs to be done when the acute medical illness has resolved. A patient with a hip fracture and concurrent delirium may do poorly on initial assessment but, once the delirium clears, may progress nicely with rehabilitation. At times, the medical condition will need to be treated concurrently with rehabilitation efforts. After a prolonged intensive care unit (ICU) stay, a patient may have significant orthostatic hypotension, which will resolve as they regain the upright position during rehabilitation. **Table 55-2** lists a variety of acute medical illnesses that might delay referral to rehabilitation until these are resolved.

Other determinants of rehabilitation benefit include motivation, cognition, and prior functional status. Comorbid illness may have a significant effect on rehabilitation efforts and may even cause a change in rehabilitation approaches. For example, a patient with chronic obstructive pulmonary disease (COPD) on home oxygen who falls and fractures a hip may not be able to tolerate more than 5 minutes of therapy at one time. The rehabilitation approach might be changed to include frequent walks of short duration by therapy and nursing, as opposed to an hour-long therapy session twice a day. **Table 55-3** lists a variety of factors that might influence either the use of rehabilitation or the goals of the rehabilitation. In some cases, like terminal illness with a short life expectancy, the goals of care may need to be addressed with the patient and family, and palliative care may be a more appropriate option. For other factors, like lack of motivation, well-defined patient-centered goals that are easily measured may help overcome this potential obstacle.

After careful evaluation, including a function-oriented history and physical examination, assessment of factors that may impact on rehabilitation outcomes, and the development of goals with the team, including the patient and

TABLE 55-2 ■ FACTORS FOR WHICH REHABILITATION MAY NEED TO BE DELAYED UNTIL RESOLVED

FACTOR OF INTEREST	REASON FOR POSSIBLE DELAY IN REHABILITATION
Delirium or altered level of consciousness	Unable to cooperate or learn
Hemodynamic instability	May make it unsafe to carry out certain types of exercise
Occult fracture and bony metastasis	Weightbearing or resistance exercise could worsen fracture or cause fracture
Acute infections (eg, bladder infection and pneumonia)	May cause confusion, fatigue, and/or hypotension
Acute skin or joint infection	May cause fatigue, pain, and/or muscle splinting
Acute inflammatory disease (eg, certain rheumatologic and neuromuscular conditions)	Resistive exercises may impair recovery
Acute orthopedic conditions	Joint instability may preclude use of certain exercises, and functional goals may be limited

TABLE 55-3 ■ FACTORS THAT MAY INFLUENCE THE SUCCESS OF REHABILITATION INTERVENTIONS

Cognitive impairment	Goals may be more limited. Take advantage of skills patient already has, use interventions that do not require carryover.
Disability has been present for many years	Goals may be more limited and directed to compensatory strategies or treatment of deconditioning.
Motivation is limited	Goals need to be well defined and reached in measurable steps.
Patient had prior rehabilitation for the same problem	Rehabilitation may be limited unless new functional decline has occurred.
Terminal illness	Intervention is directed toward reducing caregiver burden and patient discomfort.
Severity of disability	Extremely mild disability may not require intervention. Extremely severe disability may have very limited potential for benefit.
Social and cultural circumstances	Absence of a caregiver, financial limitations, and cultural beliefs may preclude use of certain techniques or technologies.
Malnutrition	Unable to build muscle; rehabilitative interventions may be limited unless nutritional status is improved.

the family, we are ready for the final step prior to initiation of rehabilitation, choosing the site for rehabilitation. Determining the optimal setting in which rehabilitation should occur is based on many of the factors previously evaluated, as well as patient preference.

COMPONENTS OF REHABILITATION

The Organization of Rehabilitation

Settings for care A variety of settings are available, both inpatient and community based, in which to receive rehabilitation services. It is important for the provider to understand the range of available settings and the advantages and disadvantages of each setting. While the provider may be responsible for helping match the patient to the optimal setting, insurance and cost also play a role. Rehabilitation services are available through Medicare Part A on a time-limited basis. Patients must demonstrate that they are making progress with rehabilitation goals in order to qualify for services.

Inpatient rehabilitation is offered in rehabilitation centers and Medicare-skilled nursing facilities. In order to qualify as a Medicare-certified inpatient rehabilitation hospital, a certain percentage of all admitted patients must have at least one of 13 conditions, which include diagnoses like stroke, burns, and neurologic disorders. Patients must be managed by an interdisciplinary team of skilled nurses and therapists, be seen daily by a physician, and require 24-hour rehabilitation nursing care. Rehabilitation is intensive with patients receiving a minimum of 3 hours of therapy daily. As the rehabilitation center offers 24-hour-a-day medical care, patients in need of close medical supervision during therapy can receive it. However, the patient must be able to tolerate the intensity of therapy provided, which may be difficult for the older patient.

Like the rehabilitation center, Medicare-approved skilled nursing facilities must provide 24-hour nursing care. While physicians must be available 24 hours a day, they supervise care and can visit the patients less frequently. Interdisciplinary care may not occur, although therapy services, dietary, pharmacy, and social services are available. There are no requirements for intensity or duration of therapy sessions, or any required case mix. This setting allows for a slower rehabilitation pace, which may be necessary for some older patients with multiple comorbid diseases. The availability of 24-hour nursing care is also a benefit for persons who are unable to care for themselves or who do not have caregivers at home.

Home health benefits for rehabilitation, including part-time nursing and therapy services, are also available through Medicare to patients who are defined as "homebound." This includes patients for whom leaving the home is difficult or who require help of another person to get out of the home. A physician or allowed practitioner (advanced practice providers or clinical nurse specialists) must order Medicare home health services, certify a patient's eligibility for the benefit, and a face-to-face encounter must occur within the 90 days prior to the start of home health care, or within the 30 days after the start of care. These services must be recertified every 60 days. While the intensity of the rehabilitation is less and the nursing services are part time, many patients prefer rehabilitating in their own home. If the patient has the necessary support system, this can be an excellent option.

While a number of studies have examined the effect of the rehabilitation setting on outcomes, the results remain unclear. For patients with hip fracture, the setting of care does not appear to have an impact on outcomes. After a stroke, patients who are treated in inpatient rehabilitation hospitals or special stroke units are more likely to be discharged to home and with improved function. Ultimately, factors such as patient prognosis, level of medical and nursing care needed, and intensity of therapy the patient can tolerate will help determine the optimal setting for rehabilitation.

Rehabilitation Team Members

An interdisciplinary team is often required to meet the complex rehabilitation needs of older patients. While team members have defined roles and functions, there is considerable overlap in the services provided. For example, while the physical therapist may focus on transfer and gait training, the occupational therapist may also encourage practice of transfers while performing self-care skills. In addition, there are different levels of education and licensure required for different providers. **Table 55-4** outlines the types of rehabilitation team members and their usual roles, methods of evaluation, and treatment.

Key members of this interdisciplinary team are the patient and the family. Indeed, the patient and family are at the center of the interprofessional team. An important component of chronic disease management is patient self-management, and patients must be active participants in the decision-making process. The team is responsible for establishing goals, in collaboration with the patient and the family, and developing a treatment plan to achieve those goals. In addition to teaching the patient, a key component of rehabilitation is training the caregiver or the family. Specifically, caregivers must be taught how to assist with exercise programs, ambulation, and activities of daily living (ADLs). The caregiver may need to know how to use adaptive equipment or even how to transfer the patient safely, if the patient is not independent with this task. Communication among all team members, including the patient and their family, is critical for success.

Process of Care: Rehabilitation Interventions

A variety of interventions are available to treat physical impairments and disability. The selection of intervention strategy is determined by the results of the assessment. All interventions should either directly or indirectly lead to an improvement in activity and/or participation. Major categories of interventions include (1) exercise/physical

TABLE 55-4 ■ REHABILITATION TEAM MEMBERS, TYPICAL ROLES, AND METHODS USED FOR EVALUATION AND TREATMENT

TEAM MEMBER	PRIMARY METHODS OF EVALUATION AND TREATMENT
Chaplain or spiritual care provider	• Provides spiritual support to patient and family
Dietician	• Assess nutritional status • Alter diet to maximize nutrition
Nurse	• Evaluation of self-care skills • Evaluation of family and home care factors • Self-care training • Patient and family education • Liaison with community
Occupational therapist	• Evaluate self-care skills and other activities of daily living • Home assessment • Self-care skills training; recommendations and training in use of assistive technology • Fabrication of splints
Pharmacist	• Collaborate with providers to determine most appropriate medication regimen and dosage • Identify potential interactions between medications
Physical therapist	• Assessment of motor control and impairments such as joint range of motion, muscle strength, and balance • Assessment of gait and mobility • Provision of appropriate assistive devices • Exercise training to increase range of motion, strength, endurance, balance, coordination, and gait • Treatment with physical modalities (heat, cold, ultrasound, and electrical stimulation), soft tissue and manual therapy techniques
Physician/advanced practice provider	• Manage complex medical conditions • Coordinate patient care services of the interprofessional team
Prosthetist orthotist	• Makes and fits prosthetic limbs • Makes a variety of orthotics including braces, ankle-foot orthoses, splints, and shoe inserts • Assesses fit of orthotics
Psychologist/neuropsychologist	• Assessment of brain function through testing • Counseling
Recreation therapist	• Assess leisure skills and interests • Involve patients in recreational activities to maintain social roles
Social worker	• Evaluation of family and home care factors • Assessment of psychosocial factors • Counseling
Speech therapist	• Assessment of all aspects of communication • Assessment of swallowing disorders • Treatment of communication deficits • Recommendations for alterations of diet and positioning to treat dysphagia

activity; (2) modalities including thermal agents and electrotherapy; (3) adaptive aids such as walkers, canes, and devices to improve ADLs; and (4) orthotics (splints and braces) and prosthetics (artificial limbs).

Exercise/physical activity

General Principles of Exercise Exercise is the cornerstone of physical rehabilitation. Each exercise prescribed for a patient should be related to achievement of a goal, and all goals should lead to improvement in function. For example, a common exercise for patients is elbow and shoulder flexion. Typical goals related to these exercises are feeding one's self, dressing one's self, or reaching overhead to retrieve an item from a shelf. The expected functional outcome for each exercise should be shared with the patient and his/her family. The involvement of the patient and the family is important to maximize adherence.

In setting goals for exercise programs, it is important to consider any pathology that is present. If there is irreversible damage to the neuromuscular system, then the potential for improvement in muscle function is limited. Amyotrophic lateral sclerosis is an example of a pathology in which improvement in muscle function is limited. However, in most cases, decline in muscle strength results from a combination of pathology and deconditioning occurring secondary to inactivity. The deconditioning component is reversible, and therefore some improvement in muscle strength is possible.

A common question often asked is whether exercise is safe for older adults. The number of adverse events reported as a result of exercise in adults is relatively low, with adverse events being more common with vigorous exertion and in persons with atherosclerotic heart disease. To facilitate a safe response, close monitoring before exercise, during exercise, immediately after exercise, and 24 hours after exercise is important. In addition, prior to the initiation of an exercise program, it is important for medical conditions such as congestive heart failure and diabetes to be stable and under optimal medical management. Exercise should be supervised initially to assure appropriate changes in heart rate and blood pressure. There is an expectation that minor muscle soreness will occur with most types of exercise, and patients should be counseled to expect some discomfort. Some patients with osteoarthritis may actually experience a decrease in joint discomfort with exercise. Because increased activity typically has a positive effect on insulin resistance, patients with diabetes may experience a need for less medication to control blood glucose levels.

For exercise to cause a change in physical function, the body must be stressed greater than the usual stress of everyday life. Therefore, it is important that patients are challenged in their exercise programs. For example, when a patient achieves a specific goal, such as walking 30 m at 0.5 m/s, the goal needs to be increased to a greater distance and/or speed. In comparison to younger adults, older adults need a longer recovery time both during an exercise session (between bouts) and between sessions. Improvement may also take longer for older versus younger adults, which should be considered when setting time frames for the achievement of goals.

There are many classification systems for types of exercise. In the following discussion, we will describe exercise types based on the anticipated outcome, including exercise to increase muscle strength, aerobic capacity, balance, flexibility, and motor control.

Exercise to Increase Muscle Strength

A typical exercise program to increase muscle strength involves movements performed against resistance. The resistance can be weights, rubber tubing or bands, or the person's own body weight. To achieve optimal results, the resistance should be 60% to 80% of the person's maximal lifting ability. For the majority of older adults who are starting an exercise program, it is wise to begin at a lower level (~ 40%–50% of maximal capacity) until the person has mastered the movement patterns.

Bone density can be positively affected by exercises designed to increase muscle strength. Prior to initiating a program to increase muscle strength, it is important to know the individual's bone status, or the extent and location of osteoporosis and/or osteopenia. In persons with osteoporosis, the amount of resistance may need to be modified to avoid overstressing bones and causing a fracture.

Exercise to Increase Aerobic Capacity

Exercise programs designed to increase aerobic capacity involve continuous activity (such as walking, cycling, and stair stepping), usually performed for at least 20 minutes at an intensity that is 50% to 80% of one's maximal oxygen consumption. Older adults who are beginning a program may need to start with 5 to 10 minutes of continuous activity at a lower intensity. In fact, several sessions of shorter duration (ie, 10 minutes) per day have shown similar benefits as one session of 30 minutes. To achieve benefits, endurance training needs to be performed three to five times per week. For older persons in rehabilitation programs who have physical limitations, the specific activities may need to be modified. For example, cycling may not be possible for a person who has significant hemiparesis after a stroke. Adaptations, such as securing the person's foot to the pedal, may allow the individual to exercise. Moving to another venue, such as a therapeutic pool, may be another option.

A benefit of aerobic capacity training is an increase in maximal oxygen consumption, which is defined as the amount of oxygen consumed while performing the maximal workload that one can perform for 2 to 3 minutes. Improving the maximal amount of work that a person can perform is not necessarily a direct benefit because daily activities are performed at submaximal, rather than maximal, levels of exertion. However, with an increase in maximal oxygen consumption, a given amount of submaximal work is performed at a lower percent of maximal oxygen consumption. Consequently, as a result of aerobic capacity training, submaximal work expressed as a percentage of maximal oxygen consumption is lower. From a functional perspective, activities such as dressing, bathing, and performing housework can be performed with less fatigue and for longer time periods.

Aerobic exercise has positive benefits for persons with hypertension, hypercholesterolemia, and obesity. Regular aerobic exercise has been shown to decrease resting blood pressure, resulting in either a decrease in the amount of or a need for medications. Although aerobic exercise often does not decrease total cholesterol, many studies have shown positive benefits for high-density lipoprotein cholesterol and triglyceride levels. For both treatment and prevention of obesity, aerobic exercise is a key component of a successful program.

Aerobic exercise also has benefits for cardiovascular and pulmonary diseases. For persons with angina, participation in a regular endurance exercise program produces an increase in the "anginal threshold," allowing persons to exercise at higher levels prior to the onset of angina. Persons with chronic pulmonary disease typically experience less breathlessness with activities, as a result of a regular exercise program. One of the most effective treatments for claudication is walking to the onset of pain, which ultimately produces an increase in the distance walked prior to the onset of claudication.

Exercise to Improve Balance Balance, defined as the ability to remain upright as the body's center of gravity shifts relative to the base of support, declines as people age. The somatosensory, visual, and vestibular systems contribute to our ability to maintain balance. Balance is an essential component to walking because walking involves a continuous shift of the body's center of gravity relative to the base of support.

Balance exercises are important for persons who have fallen or who are at high risk of falls. Exercises are prescribed that are appropriate for the individual's current level of function. For example, low-level exercises may involve standing and shifting one's center of gravity. As the person progresses, he/she may practice standing on one extremity or walking on a balance beam. Exercises performed with eyes closed force the use of the vestibular and somatosensory systems. Exercises performed on altered surfaces, such as foam or carpet, force the use of the visual and vestibular systems. For persons with a specific abnormality of the vestibular system, such as benign positional vertigo, there are specific exercises that often are helpful.

Flexibility Exercises The goal of flexibility exercises is to increase range of motion of a body part by increasing muscle length and/or joint motion. The most effective and safe approach is a prolonged, low-intensity stretch of the muscle/joint with limited motion. Having a sufficient amount of motion is important for many functional activities. For example, going up and down stairs using a reciprocal gait pattern requires at least 90 degrees of knee flexion. Reaching overhead requires 120 to 150 degrees of shoulder flexion and abduction. In addition, sufficient range of motion at the hip and ankle is important for maintaining standing balance. Excessive range of motion, however, decreases stability and can lead to pain, decreased mobility, and falls.

Parkinson disease is an example of a common condition in older adults in which flexibility exercises are important. Persons with Parkinson disease assume a flexed posture, resulting in loss of cervical and thoracic extension. Prescribing exercises early in the course of the disease may prevent the severity of the postural abnormalities. Maintaining spinal extension is important to prevent compromise of respiratory capacity and to minimize gait and balance disorders.

Task-Oriented Exercises to Improve Motor Control Older persons may lose their ability to perform tasks because of abnormal tone (spasticity) and/or muscle weakness. Task-oriented exercises are used to improve coordination and motor performance. Constraint-induced movement therapy (CIMT) is one method used to improve motor function. With CIMT, the stronger, less affected extremity is "constrained" using a cast or mitt. The person is forced to use the affected extremity and practice tasks needed for daily living. This method typically involves participation in therapy for 4 to 6 hours per day. The approach is based on learning theory and assumes plasticity of the central nervous system with reforming of neural connections after injury. A Cochrane review reported greater improvements in upper extremity motor function in persons poststroke with CIMT compared to conventional treatment. These differences were not significant at 6 months.

A second method used to improve walking performance and balance is treadmill training with partial body support. A harness is connected to an overhead system, which is mounted on a treadmill. By providing partial weight support in combination with a speed-controlled treadmill, patients can perform a greater amount of task-specific practice compared to traditional methods of gait training. A Cochrane review of treadmill training with and without body weight support after stroke concluded that persons who are able to walk appear to benefit the most from this intervention. Potential benefits include an increase in walking speed and walking endurance.

Designing Exercise Prescriptions Exercise should be prescribed in an individualized manner similar to prescriptions for medications. The components of an exercise prescription include mode (type of activity), frequency (number of times per day or week), intensity (level of exertion), and duration (length of time of each individual session). Sufficient research is not available to determine the ideal exercise prescription for older adults with the variety of comorbidities that are typically present. However, for some types of exercise, such as moderate- to high-intensity strength training, there is evidence that exercising every other day or every third day is optimal because of the need for recovery time. Because specific guidelines for persons with pathology are not available, pre- and postexercise monitoring is essential. Vital signs and blood glucose levels (if diabetes is present) need to be checked prior to and after exercise. Persons who are beginning an exercise program or increasing their current exercise level need to be asked how they are feeling 24 hours after exercise. Severe muscle soreness and general body fatigue are signs that the exercise stress was excessive.

Physical modalities Physical modalities that are often used with older adults include heat and cold agents, aquatic or pool therapy, electrotherapy, and phototherapy (monochromatic infrared energy—MIRE). For most of these agents, there is limited evidence of effectiveness as a sole intervention. However, when used in combination with other therapies, especially exercise therapy, these modalities can enhance the effectiveness of the overall intervention. The most common indication for use of physical modalities is pain management. Because older adults may have reduced mental status, or impaired circulation and sensation, using modalities in older adults requires caution. Educating patients and their families on the rationale for use of modalities is essential, especially if these are to be used in the home environment.

Thermal Agents (Including Aquatic Therapy) Thermal agents include superficial and deep heating modalities and cryotherapy. Physiologic effects of heat include increased blood flow and edema, increased extensibility of connective tissue structures, and decreased pain. Superficial modalities primarily increase the temperature of the skin and underlying subcutaneous tissue and include hot packs, heating pads, and paraffin. Superficial heat is beneficial for persons with osteoarthritis, rheumatoid arthritis, and conditions resulting in cervical and low-back pain. The most popular deep heating modality is ultrasound, a form of acoustic energy, which when absorbed by tissues is converted into heat. Ultrasound is often used for tissue contractures, tendonitis, and pain resulting from musculoskeletal disorders. Ultrasound should not be administered close to the brain, eyes, reproductive organs, pacemakers, or arthroplasties.

Cryotherapy includes cold packs, ice massage, cold water immersion, and vapocoolant sprays. Physiologic effects of cold include cutaneous vasoconstriction, decreased nerve conduction velocity, decreased spasticity, and increased joint stiffness. Cold therapy provides short-term analgesia and often allows patients to move when movement otherwise would be too painful. Cold therapy should be avoided in persons with arterial insufficiency, impaired sensation, cold hypersensitivity, and Raynaud disease.

Aquatic or pool therapy is an alternative to physical modalities and/or exercise on land. A therapeutic pool provides a combination of heat and buoyancy for support of upright activities. Patients with muscle weakness and pain often can walk and exercise in a therapeutic pool when movement on land is limited. Because total body heating produces significant vasodilation, patients with cardiac insufficiency may experience chest pain. All patients need to be careful exiting the pool because of the possibility of postural hypotension. Persons with heat intolerance, such as those with multiple sclerosis, may require a "cool" pool with temperatures below 90°F.

Electrotherapy Electrotherapy can be used as an intervention for pain management, muscle activation, wound healing, and urinary incontinence. Transcutaneous electrical nerve stimulation (TENS), a popular treatment for pain, involves placing electrodes over peripheral nerves, nerve roots, or painful areas. The mechanism of action is unclear but probably involves the release of endogenous endorphins in the cerebrospinal fluid, which block pain by binding to opiate receptors. Adverse effects of TENS are minor and typically involve skin irritation secondary to sensitivity to the electrodes or gel. Contraindications to the use of TENS include persons with impaired sensation and/or cognition and persons with either a pacemaker or an implanted cardiac defibrillator. A recent Cochrane review was unable to conclude that, in people with chronic pain, TENS is beneficial for pain control, disability, health-related quality of life, or use of pain relieving medicines.

Neuromuscular stimulation is used to activate muscles addressing treatment goals in persons after stroke, spinal injury, or knee surgery. For persons poststroke, electrical stimulation can be used to enhance functional movement patterns, such as contraction of the anterior tibialis muscle to prevent foot drop during the swing phase of gait or contraction of the quadriceps at heel strike during gait. After knee surgery or injury, persons often "forget" how to contract the quadriceps muscle as a result of pain and/or joint effusion. Neuromuscular simulation can be used to "retrain" the quadriceps muscle countering atrophy that occurs with immobilization.

An important difference between normal muscle contraction and electrically induced muscle contraction is the order of recruitment of motor units. With normal muscle contraction, the smaller fatigue-resistant motor units are recruited first, followed by larger, fatigable motor units. With electrical stimulation, the larger-diameter fatigable fibers are recruited first. The consequence is that fatigue occurs fairly quickly with neuromuscular stimulation. Providing adequate rest periods and limiting the duration and frequency of contractions are strategies to lessen fatigue.

Electrotherapy used for wound healing involves application of electric current either directly to a wound or to the skin surrounding the wound. Electrical stimulation is approved for Medicare coverage for the treatment of stasis, arterial pressure, and diabetic ulcers that have not responded to conventional therapy. Animal and human studies have shown that electrical stimulation increases both DNA and collagen synthesis; directs epithelial, fibroblast, and endothelial cell migration into wound sites; inhibits the growth of some wound pathogens; and increases the strength of scar tissue. The effectiveness of electrical stimulation is demonstrated in randomized controlled trials, with the strongest evidence being demonstrated in the treatment of pressure ulcers.

Phototherapy (MIRE) Devices that deliver MIRE were approved by the Food and Drug Administration (FDA) in 1994 to increase circulation and decrease pain. This treatment involves placing pads over the lower leg and foot. The pads contain diodes that emit light energy in the near-infrared spectrum (890-nm wave length). The typical treatment protocol involves 30-minute treatments, three times a week, for a total of 12 treatments. The infrared photo energy is thought to release nitric oxide from hemoglobin. Nitric oxide relaxes smooth muscle cells, dilating blood vessels and improving circulation. MIRE has been used for the treatment of peripheral neuropathy, with the goal to improve sensation and decrease neuropathic pain. Research studies are conflicting; however, the majority of them have shown that MIRE was no more effective than placebo in improving sensation.

Adaptive aids Adaptive aids include devices that allow persons with physical limitations to participate in activities, such as basic and IADLs, with greater ease and/or less pain. Categories of adaptive aids include mobility aids to assist people to move around within their home and community, bathroom aids to assist with bathing and toileting, and self-care aids that assist with dressing, personal hygiene, cooking, and other activities. It is not unusual for older persons to have devices that they do not need, often as a gift from a friend or relative. The opposite also occurs when older persons need devices that are not prescribed. The devices described below need to be prescribed by a professional, and the patient or family or caregiver needs to be instructed in their use. Devices that are used incorrectly can lead to falls and other adverse events. It can be helpful for the professional (typically a physical or occupational therapist) to make a home visit to assess whether the prescribed adaptive devices can be used safely in the patient's home.

Mobility Aids Canes are the most popular mobility aid for older adults because they are lightweight and easy to use when space is limited. Canes are used to decrease weight bearing (and pain) in an extremity with an arthritic joint and to improve balance by increasing the base of support. When adjusted to the proper height, the handle of the cane is at the level of the wrist when the arm is fully extended. Canes should be used in the hand on the side opposite of the involved extremity. Many people will incorrectly use the cane in the hand on the side of the involved extremity. The cane then acts as a brace for the involved extremity, producing an abnormal gait pattern and limiting range of motion of both the hip and the knee of the involved side. To achieve a normal gait pattern, patients are instructed to hold the cane in the hand opposite the involved extremity and advance the cane and the involved extremity simultaneously. Patients then swing through with the uninvolved extremity while bearing weight on the cane and, to a lesser degree, the involved extremity. For stairs, patients are taught to go "up with the good and down with the bad." To ascend the stairs, the uninvolved extremity is advanced up the stairs first, while the involved extremity and the cane remain on the lower step. To descend the stairs, the involved extremity and the cane are lowered first and then the uninvolved extremity descends to the same step. For persons with decreased sensation in the lower extremities, a cane can also provide proprioceptive input to the brain by transmitting information from intact proprioceptors in the hand.

Two major types of canes are straight and quad canes. Straight canes are usually made of aluminum or wood, with a variety of handles available. Quad canes are aluminum canes with a four-legged base. One advantage of a quad cane is that the cane does not fall if the person releases the handle. A disadvantage of some quad canes is that their base is too large to place on stairs, making stair climbing difficult.

Crutches are usually not used with older adults because a higher level of coordination and skill is required.

The two major types of crutches are axillary and forearm crutches. If axillary crutches are used incorrectly, shoulder injury and/or axillary nerve damage can occur. Forearm crutches are more functional because a cuff secures the crutch on the patient's arm allowing use of the hand to manipulate objects. Crutches are usually used to provide bilateral support. However, a single crutch can be used instead of a cane if additional unilateral support is needed.

A walker usually is prescribed when a cane does not provide sufficient support. Walkers provide bilateral support and are easier to use than crutches. Walkers should be adjusted so that the user maintains an erect posture and is not required to lean forward to reach the walker. There are several types of walkers that vary in stability and function. The standard four-point or "pick-up" walker requires that the person pick it up with each step, requiring arm strength and endurance, and producing a slow walking speed. With a two-wheeled rolling walker, the person can use a more normal gait pattern and speed. Having two rather than three or four wheels provides more stability. A four-wheeled walker, called a "rollator," has hand brakes so that it can be locked when the user is standing up and sitting down. This type also has a platform seat for resting and a basket for carrying objects. The rollator requires greater skill because of the use of the hand brakes. It is preferred for outdoor use because the wheels are larger and move easier over sidewalks and slightly rough terrain. A final option is the Merry Walker, which provides the maximal amount of support. This type of walker includes front, side, and back bars, and a seat for resting. Merry Walkers are larger and more difficult to manipulate in homes. They are often used in institutional settings for persons with severe balance and coordination deficits.

A wheelchair should be prescribed for a person who can no longer walk safely or when walking endurance is low. The wheelchair allows the person to continue to do activities such as shopping that require extended periods of standing and walking. Quality of life is maintained and social isolation is avoided. Two main types of wheelchairs are manual and power chairs. There are many options available for customizing a chair for individual needs. In considering the optimal chair, both stability and mobility need to be considered. For example, a back height that is too high makes propelling the chair independently difficult thus impairing mobility, whereas a back height that is too low may not provide adequate trunk support. There are a variety of manual wheelchairs available with many different features. The width of the seat can range from narrow to wide to accommodate larger persons. Removable arm rests and foot rests are available and make transfers easier and safer. Fixed foot rests are not recommended because they can contribute to falls. Consultation with the occupational therapist or physical therapist is recommended, as the therapist would know best how to order appropriate parts to maximize function.

Manual wheelchairs are lighter in weight than power chairs and are fairly easy to fold and load into a car for travel. Power chairs and scooters provide enhanced mobility outdoors and in the community. Most power chairs are difficult to maneuver in homes. In addition, a car carrier is needed for travel.

Prescribing a wheelchair for use is an important decision, and the advantages and disadvantages for each patient need to be considered. For patients who are able to walk, having a wheelchair may discourage walking, leading to decreased muscle strength and endurance and increasing the probability of falling. However, not prescribing a wheelchair as walking ability declines can negatively affect quality of life. Patients and families need to be counseled on appropriate use of a wheelchair based on their unique needs.

Table 55-5 illustrates some of the commonly prescribed types of canes, walkers, and power chairs and describes some of the benefits and drawbacks of using the different mobility aids as well as clinical situations in which the device might be useful.

TABLE 55-5 ■ KEY FEATURES AND CLINICAL SITUATIONS WHERE AMBULATORY DEVICES MIGHT BE BENEFICIAL

AMBULATORY DEVICE	SUPPORT PROVIDED	DEVICE BENEFITS	DEVICE DRAWBACKS	CLINICAL SITUATIONS WHERE DEVICE MIGHT BE BENEFICIAL
Straight cane	Unilateral	Assists with balance and proprioception Reduced weight bearing on opposite side	May not provide enough support Doesn't stand up on its own, making it difficult to carry objects and open doors	Osteoarthritis of knee or hip Peripheral neuropathy
Quad or 4-point cane	Unilateral	More stable than straight cane Allows greater weight bearing on device	Heavier than single-point cane Increased base of support may increase risk of tripping over device	Stroke with hemiparesis
Standard "pick-up" walker	Bilateral	Very stable and allows non-weight-bearing movement	Must be lifted and advanced requiring strength and coordination Gait pattern and turns not smooth due to lack of wheels	Hip fracture where non-weight-bearing needed Unilateral amputation, prior to prosthesis
Two-wheeled rolling walker	Bilateral	Easier to advance than standard walker Allows smoother, faster gait pattern than standard walker	Less stable than standard walker Turns less smooth than rollator due to fixed wheels	Deconditioning Parkinson disease
Rollator or 4-wheeled walker	Bilateral	Allows for smoother, faster gait than standard walker Turns easily due to front rotating wheels Good for outside walking because of large wheels Has seat for resting	Less stable than standard or rolling walker Requires increased coordination due to brakes More expensive than rolling or standard walkers	Cardiopulmonary disease Peripheral neuropathy with balance difficulty
Manual wheelchair	Full body	Often used by caregivers and in nursing homes for ease of patient mobility	Requires use of arms and some cardiopulmonary endurance or someone to push the chair	Nonambulatory patients with cognitive impairment Low-level spinal cord injury patients with good endurance
Power wheelchair	Full body	Allows community mobility for those with limited ambulatory ability Controls do not require intact UEs	Need cognitive ability to operate safely May need home modifications	Neurologic diseases (eg, high-level spinal cord injury, MS, ALS) Multiple limb amputations
Scooter	Full body	Similar benefits to power wheelchair, but may be more acceptable to patient than power wheelchair	Need to be able to operate controls with UEs	Significant cardiopulmonary disease

ALS, amyotrophic lateral sclerosis; MS, multiple sclerosis; UEs, upper extremities.

Bathroom and Self-Care Aids For many older adults with physical disabilities, the bathroom is a challenging and unsafe place. Devices are available for use in a typical home bathroom to make activities easier and safer. Grab bars located close to the toilet and shower or tub should be considered for all older adults. Many older adults have difficulty rising from a regular toilet seat because of the low height. A raised toilet seat can be secured to a regular toilet. For persons who need more assistance, bedside commode chairs are available. Some bedside commode chairs have wheels, and can be rolled over a regular toilet. Tub benches are available for individuals who have difficulty getting out of a regular tub, and shower chairs are available for persons who cannot stand independently to take a shower.

Devices are also available to assist patients with ADLs. Occupational therapists can assist with identifying the most appropriate adaptive aids. Some examples for dressing include aids to assist with manipulating buttons, securing pants, and putting on/off shoes and socks. For eating, enlarged handles on utensils and modified plates are available. Having an appropriate aid often results in independence in performing a task versus needing to ask for assistance.

Electronic Devices (Environmental Control Units/Augmentative Communication Aids) Devices are available that use more sophisticated technologies to allow patients a greater degree of independence and enhanced communication. Environmental control units typically are used for patients with severe disabilities to allow turning on/off lights and controlling other electronic devices. Whatever voluntary motion is available is used to control the unit, usually through a joystick, mouth stick, or eye motion. Devices used to enhance communication include communication boards, voice amplifiers, and telephone adaptations. For strategies to enhance communication, consultation with a speech and language pathologist is recommended.

Orthotics and prosthetics Orthotics and prosthetics are external devices used to enhance function. Orthoses typically are used to either restrict or assist motion and are named according to the joints or body parts that are affected. For example, ankle-foot orthoses (AFOs) include the foot and ankle, and knee-ankle-foot orthoses extend from the thigh to the foot.

The most commonly used orthoses for older adults are foot orthoses and AFOs. Foot orthoses include shoe inserts and other devices placed inside the shoe. Inserts can be used to relieve pain or to protect insensitive feet. Examples of commonly used foot orthoses include heel spur cushions, scaphoid pads to correct flattening of the arches, and metatarsal pads to transfer weight from the metatarsal heads to the metatarsal shafts. AFOs are used for patients with either weakness or paresis of dorsiflexors to prevent foot drop during gait. These orthoses can be made of plastic or metal. Plastic orthoses can be interchanged between shoes but do not provide as much support as metal orthoses.

Appropriate use of foot and ankle orthoses can improve function by providing a safe, more comfortable gait.

For individuals with diabetes and severe diabetic foot disease, Medicare will cover one pair of therapeutic shoes and inserts or shoe modifications each year. Physicians must provide a pedorthist or podiatrist with certification that the person has diabetes.

Many older adults require prostheses because of amputation resulting from vascular disease. In prescribing prostheses for older adults, important considerations include ease of donning and doffing, stability during activities, and overall function. In persons with severe dementia or advanced cardiopulmonary disease, wearing a prosthesis may not be practical. Persons who are not independent in basic ADLs skills, such as transferring and dressing, typically are not good candidates for prosthetic use. To achieve the optimal outcome, the patient should be involved in a preprosthetic training program to improve strength and endurance. The physician should work closely with the physical therapist and prosthetist to assure that the prosthesis is evaluated for correct fit and that the patient receives training on use of the prosthesis.

SPECIFIC CONDITIONS TREATED WITH REHABILITATION

Pulmonary Rehabilitation

Patients with chronic respiratory diseases frequently experience disability owing to decreased exercise tolerance and symptoms like dyspnea and anxiety. The established benefits of pulmonary rehabilitation (PR) include improved exercise capacity, a decreased sensation of dyspnea, and overall improvement in quality of life. The cornerstone of most PR programs is exercise, although other components may include education and behavioral modifications like energy-conservation techniques. As with other rehabilitation programs, PR can occur in inpatient, outpatient, and home settings with equal success. Exercise programs are individually tailored to meet the patients' needs, and patients are usually encouraged to exercise three times a week or more to a level where they experience moderate dyspnea. Training regimens vary, depending on the goal of the rehabilitation. For example, many patients with COPD experience dyspnea with upper body activity, like bathing or grooming. An exercise program that targets strengthening of the arms with elastic bands or light weights helps decrease the dyspnea and work effort required for these tasks. Treadmill or track training will improve walking endurance but not strength, so a variety of training exercises are usually utilized.

A Cochrane review concluded that PR showed both statistical and clinical improvements in dyspnea and disease-specific quality-of-life-measures and current guidelines recommend PR for all patients with COPD who experience ongoing symptoms despite optimal pharmacologic therapy. Supervised programs offered greater benefit than unsupervised ones, and patients with severe disease appeared to benefit the most when compared to those with mild-to-moderate COPD. However, many questions still remain about what components are essential and how to best assess outcomes after rehabilitation.

Cardiac Rehabilitation

Cardiac rehabilitation (CR) is increasingly recognized as an important component of an interdisciplinary treatment strategy for patients with a history of myocardial infarction (MI) and stable angina and patients after coronary artery bypass graft (CABG) surgery. Many of the benefits of CR occur through the exercise component of these programs. Exercise training has been found to decrease coagulability, increase fibrinolysis, improve endothelial function by moderating inflammation, and improve endothelium-dependent vasodilation. These beneficial effects can be demonstrated by the reduction in C-reactive protein seen with exercise and the improvement in hyperemic myocardial flow after CR. Disability or functional decline is often associated with a variety of cardiac conditions, and participation in CR can improve fitness and reduce the signs and symptoms of exercise intolerance. This can lead to improved functional independence. In addition to exercise training, CR provides a structured environment for risk factor management through patient monitoring plus support of compliance and adherence. However, despite evidence of the beneficial effects, CR remains underutilized, with approximately one-third of eligible patients receiving CR.

In low-risk individuals with heart failure and after MI or stenting, exercise-based CR has been found to be safe with no increase in short-term mortality and effective with demonstrated reductions in risk of hospital admission and improvements in patient's health-related quality of life compared with control. Studies have also demonstrated equal effectiveness of home-based and center-based programs in improving outcomes of exercise-based CR. In a study of more than 600,000 Medicare patients hospitalized for acute coronary syndrome, percutaneous coronary intervention, or CABG, the 12% who participated in CR had a lower rate of mortality compared to nonparticipants (2.3% vs 5.3%). This benefit was sustained at 5 years with a mortality rate of 16% for participants versus 25% for nonparticipants. In addition, there was a dose-response relationship with participants who attended 25 or more sessions having a 20% lower 5-year mortality rate compared to those who attended fewer than 25 sessions.

For patients with congestive heart failure, randomized clinical trials conducted during the last decade have demonstrated that CR can improve exercise tolerance, quality of life, and disease-related symptoms, without adversely affecting left ventricular function. While there is no consensus regarding the optimal exercise program, guidelines support the use of regular aerobic and/or strengthening exercises. Exercise training induces peripheral and central adaptations, including improvement in vasodilation among active muscle, decreased sympathetic nervous system activation, and increases in peak cardiac output, heart rate, and stroke volume. These adaptations lead to a reduction in the commonly observed exercise intolerance because of fatigue and dyspnea. Using peak oxygen consumption (VO_2) to measure exercise capacity, improvements have ranged from 15% to 30%. Other common symptoms associated with heart failure such as shortness of breath, ability to perform ADLs, anxiety, depression, and general well-being have all been improved with CR. The magnitude of improvement has ranged from 15% to 50% for each of these variables, and improvements in quality of life can be seen as early as 2 months after initiation of the exercise program. In addition to improvements in symptoms and quality of life, reduction in mortality has also been demonstrated. Increased sympathetic nervous system activity and higher plasma and tissue cytokine concentrations are associated with worsening disease and poorer prognosis in patients with heart failure. Exercise training causes a downregulation of these systems, with a resultant 28% reduction in total mortality and hospitalization and a 29% reduction in death rate. Prior to initiation of an exercise program, patients must be clinically stable with controlled fluid status for at least 3 to 4 weeks.

The literature demonstrates a beneficial effect of CR for a variety of cardiac diagnoses, including acute MI, congestive heart failure, and after CABG surgery. Exercise training positively affects both the basic pathophysiology of coronary artery disease and the underlying disease process. This, in turn, minimizes the impact of disability, improves quality of life, and reduces mortality. Referral to CR increases the likelihood of participation and long-term compliance, which can have significant beneficial effects for the patient.

Peripheral Arterial Disease

Studies have demonstrated that the optimal exercise rehabilitation program for improving the distance walked prior to the onset of claudication uses intermittent walking to the onset of pain. The increased distance achieved occurs through improvements in cardiopulmonary function, peripheral circulation, and walking economy. Improvements require an exercise program of at least 6 months duration to be effective. Treadmill walking has been shown to be more effective than strength training in achieving these results.

Amputation

During the initial postoperative period, goals include relieving pain, preventing medical complications, and preventing mobility problems, particularly muscle atrophy and contractures. Between 60% and 80% of persons undergoing a lower extremity amputation experience phantom limb pain. Approximately 10% of those who experience phantom pain rate the pain as severe enough to be disabling. Conflicting evidence exists regarding the success of adequate pain control preoperatively or perioperatively on the incidence of phantom pain. However, there is little controversy regarding the importance of adequate pain control for persons undergoing amputation.

Common medical problems after amputation include poor wound healing, skin breakdown, and falls. Early mobilization with or without a prosthesis is critical for recovery of function. Older persons who already have decreased lean muscle mass are at risk of additional muscle atrophy. Joint contractures occur when patients spend significant periods of time sitting in a chair or a wheelchair and can have a negative impact on their ability to ambulate with prosthesis. Initially after amputation, older persons are instructed in the basics of self-care and mobility and then discharged to home. Rehabilitation occurs later after healing of the amputation site and can occur in a rehabilitation facility, in the home, or as an outpatient.

For the older adult, comorbid conditions and premorbid functional status impact the success of the surgery and subsequent rehabilitation. Prior to surgery, the older person should be medically stable, with special attention being paid to cardiopulmonary status. Level of amputation should also be considered. The energy expenditure required for a transtibial amputee is much less than for a transfemoral amputee and may predict a person's ability to regain ambulatory ability. However, while preserving the knee joint may be beneficial, preoperative evaluation should carefully assess the risk and benefit of knee preservation to avoid surgical revisions and longer lengths of stay in the hospital.

Prosthesis use can decrease energy expenditure with transfers and ambulation and should at least be considered, irrespective of age. While firm criteria for prosthetic prescription do not exist, Medicare has developed a guide for selection of prosthetic knee and ankle components. Indications for prosthesis are based on the likelihood that a person will reach or maintain a defined functional state within a reasonable time and that the person is motivated to ambulate. For example, an individual with the potential to be ambulatory at a household level may qualify for a lower performance prosthetic knee than someone with the potential to be active in the community and/or pursue athletic activities.

Considerations in determining the potential functional status of someone after an amputation may include prior ability to walk, medical status as it relates to the person's ability to meet the physiologic demands associated with prosthetic use, and ability to learn new skills. These measures would certainly be useful when developing goals for the patient after amputation. A variety of lower limb prosthetic devices are available. To date, studies have not included a large enough sample of older persons to determine the optimal socket or foot design for this population. This determination should be made with the input of the patient, physician, prosthetist, therapists, and insurance company.

Stroke Rehabilitation

Rehabilitation after stroke can begin as early as 24 to 48 hours poststroke once the patient is medically stable and focuses on return to previous mobility and self-care activities, as well as the prevention of medical complications like pressure ulcers or deep vein thrombosis, and minimization of spasticity. Provision of emotional support to the patient and family is essential. There appears to be a statistically significant and clinically important benefit from organized inpatient interdisciplinary rehabilitation in the postacute period. In several randomized controlled trials, either organized inpatient interdisciplinary rehabilitation or stroke unit care demonstrated improved outcomes, including reduced odds of death. Guidelines for the management of stroke were developed by Veterans Affairs and the Department of Defense and rate the quality of available evidence. The guidelines present algorithms for initial assessment as well as management after rehabilitation referral.

Techniques used during stroke rehabilitation vary and are tailored to the needs and deficits of an individual patient. Strengthening, facilitation techniques that progress movement and task-oriented approaches, like constraint-induced therapy, are common. The goal of therapy, no matter the approach, is improvement of function and quality of life.

After a stroke, patients may have a variety of impairments in addition to muscle weakness. Dysphagia places patients at risk of aspiration and can be silent in up to one-third of patients with dysphagia. Communication disorders including aphasia also occur in one-third of patients, with prognosis being worse for patients of advanced age, or with delayed treatment. During the first month after a stroke, the incidence of bladder incontinence is 50% to 70%, although it returns to levels seen in the general population by 6 months. Treatment can include timed voiding schedules and monitoring of postvoid residuals. Hemiplegic shoulder pain is also a common occurrence, affecting 34% to 84% of patients poststroke. Major risk factors include advanced age and changes in muscle tone, which occur after the stroke. Treatment involves proper positioning to avoid joint subluxation and early range-of-motion exercises to prevent contractures and spasticity. There is some evidence that electric stimulation can improve hemiplegic shoulder pain for up to 6 months after treatment. Depression is another frequent complication after stroke, one that can have a significant negative effect on rehabilitation. Incidence ranges from 15% to 70% depending on the study, and several antidepressant medications have been associated with improvement. An organized, interdisciplinary team approach helps to address these common sequelae after stroke.

Parkinsonism

At this time, there are no guidelines or generally accepted rehabilitation techniques for persons with Parkinson disease. Traditionally, therapy has focused on improving posture, range of motion, exercise capacity, and gait. There is evidence that exercise programs including resistive and flexibility exercises can improve physical function. One review demonstrated improvements in gait speed, balance and freezing episodes with exercise. Another commonly used technique is an external cueing strategy where auditory pacing, use of a walking stick, or visual cues can help improve gait and decrease episodes of freezing for some patients. Because of the success of rhythmic cueing, studies are being done to explore the use of treadmill training as a method to improve the gait pattern of patients with parkinsonism. Results from a systematic review are promising, with improvements in gait speed, stride length, and walking distance being seen. The "Training Big" program is being used increasingly frequently to improve motor performance through the use of repetitive high-amplitude movements. Originally used to amplify voice, studies are reporting significant improvements in gait speed and other functional measures. The long-term benefits of all the exercise interventions are still unknown.

Osteoarthritis and Total Joint Replacement

Several randomized trials have demonstrated the efficacy of strengthening exercises to lessen pain and improve function. Weight loss combined with strengthening exercises was shown to be more effective than weight loss alone for improving function and reducing pain. If pain occurs with an exercise, that exercise should be avoided, and monitoring by a physical therapist during the initial rehabilitation period is reasonable. Osteoarthritis of the hip is less amenable to exercise, probably because improving strength in the ball and socket hip joint does not provide the same support as strengthening the hinged knee joint. Efforts to relieve pain will help the person with arthritis maintain physical activity levels and minimize the effects of deconditioning and muscle weakness.

Total joint arthroplasty is the most common elective surgical procedure done in the United States. The primary indications for arthroplasty are mobility limitation and progressive pain, despite conservative treatments like exercise and use of mobility aids. After total joint replacement, the principal goal is to attain the highest level of functional independence possible. Rehabilitation after a total hip replacement focuses on strengthening exercises and gait training. Precautions to reduce the risk of hip dislocation may be required during the initial months of post hip replacement. For example, in the early stages of recovery from the traditional posterolateral approach, patients may need to avoid crossing their legs, flexing their hips more than 90 degrees and rolling their legs in and out to decrease the risk of hip dislocation. Raised toilet seats are also recommended to prevent excessive hip flexion during the first few months after surgery. After total knee replacement, rehabilitation is focused on pain control, reduction of swelling, improving range of motion, and strengthening the muscles around the knee. Recovery from total knee replacement requires the patient work hard to attain and maintain range of motion during the first few months after surgery, which is distinct from hip replacement surgery.

Hip Fracture

The initial rehabilitation efforts are focused on early mobilization to prevent complications of bed rest, like deconditioning and deep vein thrombosis. Post repair, decreased weight bearing on the fractured limb is standard and patients are taught to walk with an appropriate assistive device. The amount of weight that can be placed on the repaired limb depends on fracture stability. If possible, patients should be allowed to bear weight as tolerated as opposed to "touchdown" weight bearing, which is often difficult for older patients to achieve. There is mounting evidence that exercise following hip fracture is beneficial with higher-intensity/duration programs showing more promising outcomes, although the optimal exercise program to maximize function after hip fracture has not been determined.

Sarcopenia and Deconditioning

While no consensus exists regarding the optimal training program, numerous studies have demonstrated resistance exercises to be very beneficial in the treatment of sarcopenia and deconditioning. Increased muscle mass and strength occur with loading the muscle at 60% to 80% of one-repetition maximum (1RM), two to three times a week. (Some researchers also recommend that at least once a week low-intensity, high-velocity resistance training should be done to address the loss of power that occurs with sarcopenia.)

Improvement in muscle strength and power through endurance exercise can reduce the difficulty older adults may experience in performing daily functional activities and may promote spontaneous additional physical activity. While sarcopenia owing to aging may not be reversible, other components of the observed decline in physical activity can be ameliorated with exercise.

PHYSICAL ACTIVITY AND EXERCISE POSTREHABILITATION

Many people complete rehabilitative episodes of care with persistent impairments and loss of function. These individuals are at higher risk for the development of secondary and tertiary complications due to lack of physical activity and exercise. Facilitating the transition of individuals with disability from rehabilitation to community-based physical activity and exercise programs is one strategy that is proving to be successful in increasing activity. Physicians and other professionals should be aware of the importance of promoting healthy lifestyles in individuals postrehabilitation.

CONCLUSION

Because disability is common among older persons, rehabilitation is an important component of geriatric health care. Defining the cause or causes of disability will allow the rehabilitation team to provide treatment in the optimal setting for the individual patient. Much remains unknown about the most effective rehabilitation techniques for patients with multiple comorbidities; however, available literature supports the continued use of rehabilitation to improve function, independence, and quality of life for older persons.

FURTHER READING

Anderson L, Sharp GA, Norton RJ, et al. Home-based versus centre-based cardiac rehabilitation. *Cochrane Database Syst Rev.* 2017;6(6):CD007130.

Bourbeau J, Gagnon S, Ross B. Pulmonary rehabilitation. *Clin Chest Med.* 2020;41:513–528.

Gerhard-Herman MD, Gornik HL, Barrett C, et al. 2016 AHA/ACC guideline on the management of patients with lower extremity peripheral artery disease: a report of the American College of Cardiology/American Heart Association Task Force on Clinical Practice Guidelines. *Circulation* 2017;135(12):e686–e725.

Jette AM. Toward a common language for function, disability, and health. *Phys Ther.* 2006;86(5):726–734.

Kumar KR, Pina IL. Cardiac rehabilitation in older adults: new options. *Clin Cardiol.* 2020;43:163–170.

Lee DJ, Costello MC. The effect of cognitive impairment on prosthesis use in older adults who underwent amputation due to vascular-related etiology: a systematic review of the literature. *Prosthet Orthot Int.* 2018;42(2):144–152.

Lee KJ, Um SH, Kim YH. Postoperative rehabilitation after hip fracture: a literature review. *Hip Pelvis.* 2020;32(3):125–131.

Lindsay LR, Thompson DA, O'Dell MW. Updated approach to stroke rehabilitation. *Med Clin N Am.* 2020;104:199–211.

Marzetti E, Calvani R, Tosato M, et al. Physical activity and exercise as countermeasures to physical frailty and sarcopenia. *Aging Clin Exp Res.* 2017;29(1):35–42.

McDonnell MN, Rischbieth B, Schammer TT, Seaforth C, Shaw AJ, Phillips AC. Lee Silverman Voice Treatment (LSVT)-BIG to improve motor function in people with Parkinson's disease: a systematic review and meta-analysis. *Clin Rehab.* 2018;32(5):607–618.

Mehrholz J, Thomas S, Elsner B. Treadmill training and body weight support for walking after stroke (Review). *Cochrane Database Syst Rev.* 2017;8(8):CD002840.

Mora JC, Valencia WM. Exercise and older adults. *Clin Geriatr Med.* 2018;34(1):145–162.

Peel C, Sawyer-Baker P, Roth DL, et al. Assessing mobility in older adults: the UAB Study of Aging Life-Space Assessment. *Phys Ther.* 2005;85:1008–1019.

Pereira AP, Marinho V, Gupta D, Magalhaes F, Ayres C, Teixeira S. Music therapy and dance as gait rehabilitation in patients with Parkinson disease: a review of evidence. *J Geriatr Psychiatry Neurol.* 2019;32(1):49–56.

Rutherford RW, Jennings JM, Dennis DA. Enhancing recovery after total knee arthroplasty. *Orthop Clin N Am.* 2017;48:391–400.

Smith TO, Jepson P, Beswick A, et al. Assistive devices, hip precautions, environmental modifications and training to prevent dislocation and improve function after hip arthroplasty. *Cochrane Database Syst Rev.* 2016;7(7):CD010815.

Stinear CM, Lang CE, Zeiler S, Byblow WD. Advances and challenges in stroke rehabilitation. *Lancet Neurol.* 2020;19:348–360.

Studenski SA, Perera S, Wallace D, et al. Physical performance measures in the clinical setting. *J Am Geriatr Soc.* 2003;51(3):314.

Treat-Jacobson D, McDermott MM, Bronas UG, et al. Optimal exercise programs for patients with peripheral artery disease. A scientific statement from the American Heart Association. *Circulation.* 2019;139:e10–e33.

Urits I, Seifert D, Seats A, et al. Treatment strategies and effective management of phantom limb-associated pain. *Curr Pain Headache Rep.* 2019;23:64.

Winstein CJ, Stein J, Arena R, et al. Guidelines for adult stroke rehabilitation and recovery. *Stroke.* 2016;47:e98–e169.

The Aging Brain

Luigi Puglielli

The success of modern medicine during the last century has been followed by a sharp increase in the average lifespan of the world population. As a result, we have transitioned to a society where problems linked to age-associated disabilities and diseases are highly prevalent. These disabilities and diseases currently absorb a growing fraction of the costs associated with health care management. Importantly, within the next decade, the disability caused by cognitive decline and dementia combined is expected to become the most expensive. Therefore, efforts to study how aging affects brain functioning and why these changes predispose us to cognitive decline and/or dementia have become a priority for our society. Many cellular and molecular aspects of brain aging are shared with other organ systems, including defective autophagy, reduced efficiency in maintaining protein homeostasis, accumulation of intracellular and extracellular protein aggregates, increased oxidative damage to proteins, nucleic acids and membrane lipids, and impaired energy metabolism. However, given the molecular and structural complexity of neural cells, which express approximately 50 to 100 times more genes than cells in other tissues, there are age-related changes that are unique to the nervous system. For example, complex cellular signal transduction pathways involving neurotransmitters, trophic factors, and cytokines that are involved in regulating neuronal excitability and plasticity are subject to modification by aging. These events are immediately reflected by changes in synaptic plasticity, functional connectivity, and global cognitive adaptability. This chapter describes cellular and molecular changes that occur in the brain during aging and how such changes may predispose to neurodegenerative diseases.

Learning Objectives

- Understand how aging affects the brain at the histologic, cellular, and molecular levels, and how these changes are linked to cognitive decline and common neurodegenerative diseases.
- Gain a clear understanding of the most prominent biochemical and molecular aspects of the aging brain.
- Learn about the effects of aging on cognition and neurodegenerative diseases.
- Recognize novel active areas of research in the field of cognitive neuroscience.
- Learn how environmental factors influence normal brain aging.

Key Clinical Points

1. Given the steady increase in average human lifespan, the number of individuals who will experience some degree of cognitive decline is rising.
2. Healthy aging is associated with atrophy of the gray matter; however, it is not indicative of presence of a disease.
3. Comprehensive clinical evaluation is necessary to differentiate mild cognitive impairment and dementia from normal aging-associated cognitive decline.
4. Specific aging-associated histologic, cellular, and molecular changes can predispose to neurodegenerative diseases.
5. Environmental factors can be modified to mitigate potential effects of aging on brain functions.

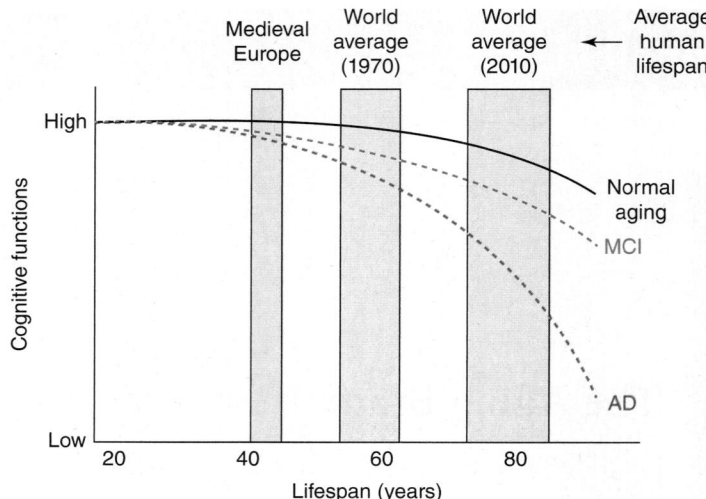

FIGURE 56-1. Cognitive changes as a result of aging. Trends of normal aging, mild cognitive impairment (MCI), and dementia due to Alzheimer disease (AD) are shown. Due to the progressive increase in lifespan, a higher number of individuals can now reach the age where specific cognitive changes (as a result of normal aging, MCI, or AD) are observed.

AGING AND COGNITION

A large segment of the world population will experience some degree of cognitive decline during aging (**Figure 56-1**). This decline most typically affects working memory as well as short-term and delayed memory recall; however, a smaller group of individuals will also experience reduced information processing speed and spatial memory. Most of the decline appears to occur after the age of 60 with minimal or nonexistent changes occurring between the age of 20 and 60. Functional magnetic resonance imaging and positron emission tomography studies suggest that the cognitive decline might be linked to the progressive reduction in the volume of specialized memory-forming and processing brain areas (**Figure 56-2**). Similar age-associated changes have been observed in nonhuman primates, dogs, rats, and mice, suggesting intrinsic age-associated events. Nonmedical interventions, such as physical exercise, cognitive stimulation, and diet together with treatment of common medical comorbidities, such as obesity, hypertension, hypercholesterolemia, diabetes, and metabolic/hormonal imbalances, might help mitigate age-associated declines.

It is widely projected that an exponentially increasing number of individuals will suffer from dementia and other cognitive disorders that will affect their daily function and increase mortality (see **Figure 56-1**). In 2000, the number of patients with dementia worldwide was estimated to be over 20 million. This number is projected to exceed 100 million by 2040, with an average of 5 million new cases every year. Rates of increase are not uniform. Developed countries initially shared most of the "dementia burden"; however, as a result of significant improvement in economic and social conditions, developing countries are now experiencing a larger disease burden. Consequently, the rate of increase

in the number of patients with dementia is projected to be almost 100% in developed countries and over 300% in developing countries. Major attention is now being given to the diagnosis of mild cognitive impairment (MCI), a transitional stage between normal aging and dementia. Patients with MCI display more severe cognitive deficits and more evident brain structural changes. In general, when diagnosed, they retain independence and are able to function normally within the society. However, they are at high risk to develop dementia, most typically Alzheimer disease, with an annual rate of conversion between 10% and 15%. Careful memory evaluation, lifestyle changes, and medical correction of existing risk factors might help delay conversion into clinical dementia.

The ability of the brain to reorganize, develop, and prune neural pathways is called synaptic plasticity. There are two components of synaptic plasticity that are thought to be important for learning and memory formation: long-term potentiation (LTP) and long-term depression (LTD). LTP involves a rapid influx of calcium into the neuronal cell, leading to the enhancement of cell excitability by the activation of intracellular signaling cascades that increase protein transcription, translation, and the insertion of new receptors into the cell membrane. LTD has the opposite effect, modulating transcription, translation, and the induction of receptors back into the cell that leads to decreased cell excitability. It is commonly believed that LTP and LTD are the cellular correlates of learning and memory and, therefore, great attention has been devoted to understanding how they are influenced by aging. In general, aged rodents show consistent deficits in induction and maintenance of LTP in the cornu ammonis area 1 (CA1) and in the dentate gyrus, two essential memory-forming areas of the brain.

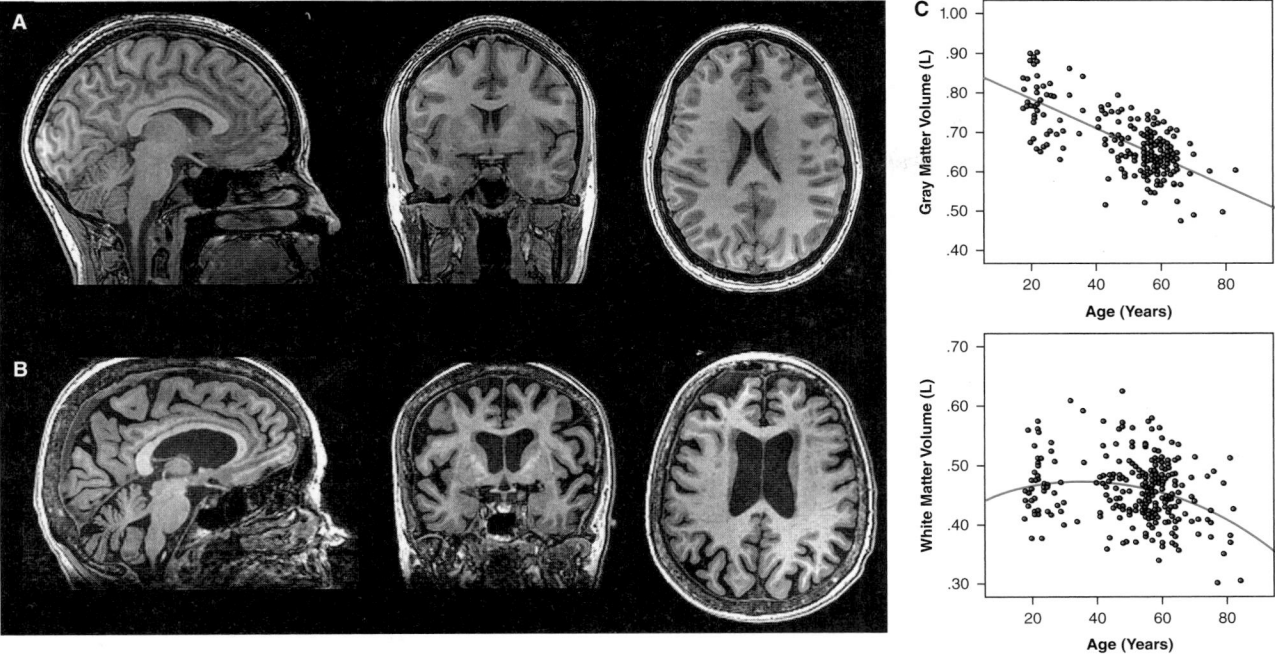

FIGURE 56-2. Volumetric changes in the human brain as a function of age. **A.** Magnetic resonance imaging (MRI) sections from a 24-year-old healthy woman; **B**. MRI sections from an 80-year-old healthy woman (nondemented, Mini Mental State Examination = 30, *APOE* ε3/ε3). The older brain has more atrophy, larger sulci, larger ventricles, and different shape of ventricles due to loss of tissue. Atrophied cerebellum is also noticeable. **C.** Scatter plots of total gray matter volume (*upper panel*) and white matter volume (*lower panel*) derived from healthy volunteers who underwent T_1-weighted MRI. Gray matter shows a linear decline with age, whereas white matter (largely myelin) shows a nonlinear decline. (Reproduced with permission from Dr. Barbara Bendlin, Department of Medicine, University of Wisconsin-Madison.)

These deficits correlate with performance in hippocampal-dependent memory tasks. Furthermore, LTP is reduced in the hippocampus of aged rats that demonstrate cognitive impairments relative to aged unimpaired (*resilient*) rats. Studies have also demonstrated that aged impaired rats are more susceptible to LTD. Specifically, the stimulus threshold for the induction of LTD is lower in aged rats, perhaps making it easier to erase memories. Finally, mouse models of accelerated aging display early and evident deficits in both LTP and LTD that correlate with memory impairment on behavioral tests.

In conclusion, the normal aging process is accompanied by specific changes in neuronal activities that are related to the formation and consolidation of memory, thus leading to a decline in cognitive functions. Given the significant increase in average lifespan that we are experiencing, the cognitive decline is becoming more evident forcing us to devote significant efforts in understanding the genetic, molecular, and biochemical changes that characterize the aging brain.

A similar important target of research is trying to understand why a subset of the aging population retains sufficient cognitive functions to remain fully functioning and independent throughout most of their life while others do not. This *resistance* or *resilience* to age-associated cognitive

decline or to age-associated dementia is observed even in the face of similar post-mortem brain alterations. Indeed, brain abnormalities that are typical of the aging brain (as well as the diseased brain), such as amyloid plaques, neurofibrillary tangles (NFTs), Lewy bodies, vascular changes, cortical atrophy, and hippocampal sclerosis, can be equally observed in brain autopsy among individuals that displayed age-associated cognitive decline or age-associated dementia and those that were able to maintain their cognitive functions. Therefore, dissection of the genetic, molecular, and biochemical events that underlie this evident resistance and resilience to aging itself or to age-associated dementia might help us understand how the brain adapts to age and disease, and identify appropriate preventive/therapeutic strategies.

STRUCTURAL CHANGES IN THE AGING BRAIN

Aging is characterized by significant molecular, structural, cytoskeletal, neurochemical, and vascular changes (see **Figure 56-2**) in the brain. Structural changes (**Figure 56-3**) are diffuse and affect the cerebellum as well. Gray matter volumes show a linear decline, while white matter volumes show a nonlinear decline. At the cellular level, all major cell

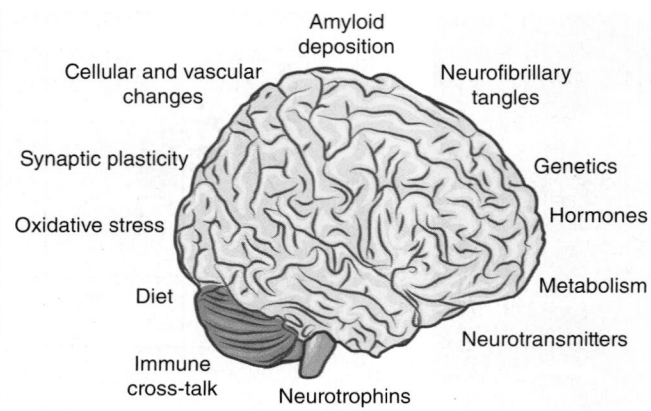

FIGURE 56-3. Simplified view of changes affecting the brain as a function of age.

types in the brain undergo structural changes as a function of age. These changes include nerve cell death, dendritic retraction and expansion, synaptic loss and remodeling, and glial cell (specifically, astrocytes and microglia) reactivity. Such structural changes may result from alterations in cytoskeletal proteins and the deposition of insoluble proteins such as tau and α-synuclein inside neuronal cells and amyloid in the extracellular space. Finally, alterations in cellular signaling pathways that control cell growth and motility may contribute to both adaptive and pathologic structural changes in the aging brain. **Table 56-1** provides a brief summary of the most prominent changes.

Functional Connectivity Changes

MRI-based analysis of structural and functional connectivity has revealed that the brain has highly connected regions, such as the hippocampal formation, cingulate gyrus, cuneus, precuneus, and superior frontal and parietal regions. These regions have a high density of intra- as

---

TABLE 56-1 ■ MOST PROMINENT STRUCTURAL CHANGES OF THE AGING BRAIN

- **Amyloid plaques**—accumulate in the parenchyma; main component: β amyloid
- **Astrocytes**—increased number of activated astrocytes
- **Microglia**—increased number of activated microglia
- **Mitochondria**—changes in morphology
- **Neurofibrillary tangles**—accumulate within neurons; main component: phospho-tau
- **Neuronal loss**
- **Neuronal morphology**—reduced dendritic branches and spines; cell body overall unchanged
- **Synapses**—reduction in number and changes in morphology
- **Vascular**—increase in atherosclerosis and arteriosclerosis
- **Volume**—reduction in gray matter volumes

---

well as inter-connectivity. Several cross-sectional studies support the conclusion that old age is associated with lower "within-network" and higher "between-network" connectivity. This shift is associated with reduced performance on memory- and executive-based tasks. The between network connectivity might reflect a compensatory attempt to maintain functional regional activity. Interestingly, there is also evidence that older adults display increased bilateral brain activation, while younger adults display preferential unilateral activation to achieve the same task-based performance. A major caveat of these studies is that they are almost exclusively cross-sectional; indeed, the few longitudinal studies performed so far have generated inconclusive results.

Vascular Changes

As in other organ systems, vessels that supply blood to the brain are vulnerable to age-related atherosclerosis and arteriosclerosis, which render the vessels susceptible to occlusion or rupture (stroke), a major cause of disability and death in the older population. Reduced brain perfusion in the absence of overt stroke may play a role in age-related cognitive dysfunction. Decreased cerebral blood flow occurs with advancing age and is accompanied by declines in cerebral metabolic rate for oxygen and glucose use. Age-related changes in cerebral vasculature are generally similar to those that occur in vessels elsewhere in the body and are therefore likely to result from common cellular and molecular changes, including accumulation of atherosclerotic plaques, oxidative damage to vascular endothelial cells, and an inflammatory response in which macrophages may penetrate the blood-brain barrier.

Age-dependent cerebral vascular changes are strongly linked to heart disease and hypertension. Interestingly, apolipoprotein E polymorphisms are linked to increased risk of both atherosclerosis and Alzheimer disease, with the apolipoprotein E4 increasing the risk. This association suggests that age-related vascular changes may make an important contribution to the neurodegenerative process in Alzheimer disease. Finally, important transport functions of cells (endothelial cells and astrocytes) that comprise the blood-brain barrier may also be impaired in the aging brain and more so in Alzheimer disease. Many of the same medical, behavioral, and dietary approaches now recognized to forestall cardiovascular disease may also forestall cerebrovascular disease; these approaches include correcting existing risk factors such as hypertension and hypercholesterolemia, engaging in physical and mental activities, preventing and/or correcting obesity, and taking a low-calorie and a high antioxidant diet.

Synaptic Changes

Synapses are dynamic structural specializations where neurotransmission and other intercellular signaling events occur. There is considerable evidence for synaptic "remodeling" in the brain as we age. Most studies using nonbiased methods indicate that aging does not induce a substantial loss of total neurons in memory-forming and processing areas of the brain. However, several studies in rodents and nonhuman primates indicate that neurogenesis decreases in the aging brain, with the greatest decline occurring in middle-age groups. In addition to decreased neurogenesis, evidence suggests that aging is accompanied by loss of synapses. As an example, the extent of synaptic loss in the hippocampus has been correlated to the severity of learning impairment observed in aged rodents, supporting the notion that the loss of hippocampal synapses directly contributes to the cognitive impairment. The synaptic loss observed in the hippocampus of aged rats may be due to the loss of both presynaptic and postsynaptic terminals. Ultrastructural studies using electron microscopy have also revealed age-related changes in the type of terminals formed. For example, aged female monkeys with memory impairment have fewer multiple-synapse boutons and twice as many nonsynaptic boutons in the dentate gyrus. Furthermore, aged rodents and monkeys display significant loss of postsynaptic spines in the hippocampus and cortex associated with reduced cognitive performance.

Synapse loss occurs in neurodegenerative disorders and strongly correlates with clinical symptoms. Accumulating data suggest that synaptic degeneration, resulting from excitotoxic events localized to synapses, may initiate the neuronal death process in Alzheimer disease, Parkinson disease, Huntington disease, and stroke. Glutamate receptors are highly concentrated in postsynaptic dendritic spines, which represent sites of massive calcium influx during normal physiologic synaptic transmission. Age-related decreases in energy availability and increases in oxidative stress, and disease-specific alterations, such as amyloid β-peptide (Aβ) accumulation in Alzheimer disease and trinucleotide expansions of the huntingtin protein, may render synapses vulnerable to excitotoxic injury.

Cytoskeletal Changes

The cell cytoskeleton consists of polymers of different sizes and protein compositions. The three major types of polymers are actin microfilaments (6 nm in diameter), microtubules (25 nm in diameter), which are composed of tubulin, and intermediate filaments (10–15 nm in diameter), which are made of specific intermediate filament proteins that differ in different cell types (eg, neurofilament proteins in neurons and glial fibrillary acidic protein in astrocytes). To regulate the processes of filament assembly and depolymerization, and to link the cytoskeleton to membranes and other cell structures, neurons and glial cells employ an array of cytoskeleton-associated proteins. For example, neurons express several microtubule-associated proteins (MAPs) that are differentially distributed within the complex architecture of the cells; MAP-2 is present in dendrites but not in the axon, whereas tau is present in axons but not in dendrites. While there are no major changes in the levels of the most abundant cytoskeletal proteins with aging, there are changes in the cytoskeletal organization and in posttranslational modifications (PTMs) of cytoskeletal proteins.

For example, increased amounts of phosphorylated tau occur in some brain regions, particularly those involved in learning and memory (eg, hippocampus and basal forebrain). In addition, there is evidence that calcium-mediated proteolysis of MAP-2 and spectrin (a protein that links actin filaments to membranes) is increased in some neurons during aging. Oxidation of certain cytoskeletal proteins is suggested by studies demonstrating their modification by glycation and covalent binding of the lipid peroxidation product 4-hydroxynonenal. A consistent feature of brain aging in humans and laboratory animals is an increase in levels of glial fibrillary acidic protein, a marker of astrocyte activation, which may represent a reaction to subtle neurodegenerative changes.

Tau proteins are perhaps the most studied MAPs in neurobiology. They consist of a group of alternatively spliced proteins that ensure microtubule-dependent neuronal functions by binding and stabilizing the microtubules. In general, the degree of phosphorylation inversely correlates with binding. As a result, hyperphosphorylated tau proteins dissociate from microtubules and aggregate to form cytosolic filaments, which ultimately result in NFTs, pathogenic aggregates that characterize different forms of age-associated frontotemporal dementias (globally referred to as tauopathies) as well as Alzheimer disease. The number and distribution of NFT also increase as a function of age. In addition to the phosphorylation status, the pro-aggregating properties of tau depend on the differential splicing of the *MAPT* gene, which results in the different tau isoforms. The pattern of phosphorylation and splicing of tau differs in the fetal and adult brain and in the central and peripheral nervous system. It also differs among mammals, probably explaining why only humans and nonhuman primates develop classical NFT. Work in multiple mouse models has shown that abnormal tau metabolism can cause memory deficits. Furthermore, genetic disruption of tau in mouse models of Alzheimer disease can rescue the cognitive deficits associated with the disease phenotype. Finally, mutations in the gene encoding tau proteins (*MAPT*) have been associated with hereditary forms of frontotemporal dementias, whereas polymorphisms in the same gene appear to act as genetic risk factors for sporadic progressive supranuclear palsy and corticobasal degeneration.

Intraneuronal pathogenic aggregates are also observed in other neurodegenerative diseases, underscoring common features. In Parkinson disease, degenerating neurons of the central nervous system accumulate Lewy bodies, which are composed of α-synuclein, ubiquitin, and neurofilament protein, with associated MAPs (particularly MAP-1b) and actin-related proteins such as gelsolin. In amyotrophic lateral sclerosis, lower motor neurons are filled with aggregates made of superoxide dismutase 1 (SOD1), TDP-43, and neurofilaments, which concentrate in proximal regions of the axon. The specific molecular events involved in the formation of cytoskeletal alterations in different neurodegenerative disorders have not been clearly and definitively established. More information on specific pathogenic aggregates that characterize different neurodegenerative diseases can be found in Chapters 59, 61, and 63.

Amyloid Accumulation

The amyloid β-peptide (Aβ) is a 38- to 49-amino acid peptide that arises from a much larger membrane-spanning precursor, the amyloid precursor protein (APP). During normal aging, and to a much greater extent in Alzheimer disease, Aβ forms insoluble aggregates in the brain parenchyma and vasculature. Of the above different Aβ species, the 40- and 42-aa long peptides are by far the most abundant; Aβ40 preferentially accumulates in the vasculature, while Aβ42 preferentially accumulates in the parenchyma. Small Aβ aggregates (oligomers) can be neurotoxic and can increase neuronal vulnerability to metabolic, excitotoxic, and oxidative insults. Aβ aggregates are organized as fibrils of approximately 7 to 10 nm in the amyloid plaques (also referred to as senile plaques), which accumulate in the brain parenchyma and are intermixed with nonfibrillary forms of the peptide and often surrounded by dystrophic neurites.

In addition to Alzheimer disease brains, amyloid/senile plaques are also present in the hippocampus and neocortex of cognitively normal aged individuals and tend to increase in an age-dependent fashion. Although still under debate, it is now becoming apparent that the number and/or distribution of amyloid plaques does not immediately correlate with cognitive decline. The synaptic loss and the number/distribution of NFTs appear to be better predictors of memory deficits. Indeed, the neuronal/synaptic loss of the hippocampal formation, entorhinal cortex, and entorhinal-hippocampal association system appears to be the only feature able to distinguish normal aging from MCI and the early stages of Alzheimer disease. Although amyloid plaques do not closely correlate with memory deficits, a high plaque load is rarely observed in the absence of cognitive impairment.

Aβ originates from proteolytic cleavage of a much larger precursor, the APP, a type I membrane protein that inserts in the endoplasmic reticulum (ER) before being transported to the neuronal surface. Proteolysis of APP can occur within the secretory pathway while transiting to the cell surface or on the cell surface itself. Substantial evidence indicates that intracellular Aβ aggregates are more pathogenic than amyloid plaques and strongly associate with neuronal and synaptic loss.

Detailed information on the mechanisms that lead to the generation and accumulation of Aβ in the brain as well as Alzheimer disease–relevant pathogenic features can be found elsewhere in this book (see Chapter 59).

Inflammatory Microglia

Microglia are different for other brain-resident cells in the sense that they do not originate from the neural tube. They derive from the yolk sac and invade the central nervous system at approximately the same time neurons are formed. As the brain develops, microglia establish close connections with neurons and participate in many important developmental functions such as neurogenesis, synapse pruning, and modeling of synaptic networks. In the adult brain, microglia maintain strong connections with mature neurons and continue participating in essential neuronal functions. They respond to neuronal activity but are also capable of triggering neuronal responses. An essential aspect of microglia biology is their ability to respond to a variety of *noxae* and transition from a quiescent to an immune-active state. The quiescent state is recognized by a ramified morphology and is mostly maintained through soluble molecules that are secreted by healthy neurons. In the presence of neuronal damage, microglia assume phagocytic features and become ameboid-like. When activated, microglia can migrate to the site of injury and secrete proinflammatory cytokines that are essential during the acute phases of injury. Fundamental functions of activated microglia include elimination of damaged/dystrophic neurites, phagocytosis of cellular debris and toxic protein aggregates, promotion of neuronal repair, and neurotrophism.

Compelling evidence indicates that microglia can undergo a process of cellular aging that significantly alters their functions. "Senescent" microglia have dystrophic morphology with process abnormalities such as shortening, deramification, and swelling, as well as cytoplasmic fragmentation and cytorrhexis. They also display reduced motility and phagocytic abilities. The most consistent cellular features of senescent microglia include ER stress, reduced autophagy, accumulation of iron, and secretion of many proinflammatory molecules. This altered proinflammatory signature appears to be a fundamental aspect the aging brain. Importantly, the transcriptome of activated, senescent microglia differs significantly from the transcriptome of normal activated microglia supporting the concept that indeed these are two different cellular states. Such a profile is also observed during age-associated neurodegenerative diseases including Alzheimer disease, Parkinson disease, and tauopathies. Dystrophic "senescent-like" microglia are found in close proximity of amyloid plaques, NFTs, and Lewy bodies. They also appear to react to protein aggregates such as Aβ, NFTs, or α-synuclein. Finally, mutations and genetic variants in genes related to microglia functions have been linked to different late-onset/sporadic forms of neurodegenerative diseases. Examples are TREM2 and CD33 in Alzheimer disease, TLR2 and LRRK2 in Parkinson disease, and CSF1R in dementia with parkinsonism.

ALTERATIONS IN ENERGY METABOLISM AND MITOCHONDRIAL FUNCTION IN THE AGING BRAIN

During the aging process, changes that occur in cerebral blood vessels, as well as in the neural cells themselves, appear to result in reduced energy availability to neurons. These age-related changes may be accelerated in several different neurodegenerative disorders including Alzheimer disease and Parkinson disease.

Cerebral Metabolism

Reduced glucose use, and changes in enzymes involved in energy metabolism, may occur during normal aging, but are not dramatic. Studies of aging rodents document decreases in glucose and ketone body oxidation, oxygen consumption, local cerebral glucose use, and glycolytic compounds (eg, fructose-1,6-diphosphate). Additional studies show that brain cells in older animals exhibit increased vulnerability to metabolic stresses. Incorporation of glucose into amino acids declines in the brain of aging mice, and older people are much more vulnerable to metabolic encephalopathy than young people. In contrast to normal aging, activities of several enzymes involved in energy metabolism are severely reduced in Alzheimer disease brain tissue. Three such enzymes, which are involved in mitochondrial oxidative metabolism, are the pyruvate dehydrogenase complex, the α-ketoglutarate dehydrogenase complex, and cytochrome c oxidase. These defects may result from age-associated oxidative damage to the DNA encoding these enzyme systems and/or reduced activity of the proteins in these systems.

Another factor that may contribute to reduced neuronal energy metabolism is impairment of the function of glucose transporter proteins in neuronal membranes. Studies of postmortem brain tissue of Alzheimer disease patients document reduced levels of glucose transporters, and experimental studies of cultured hippocampal neurons and synaptosomes show that insults relevant to the pathogenesis of Alzheimer disease (exposure to Aβ and oxyradical-generating agents) can impair glucose transport. Impairment of glucose transport and mitochondrial dysfunction would be expected to lead to ATP depletion and render neurons vulnerable to excitotoxicity.

Mitochondrial Function

Age-related structural changes in synaptic mitochondria have been reported and include a decrease in numbers and increase in size. During normal aging, levels of mitochondrial protein synthesis are unchanged. However, decreases in synthesis of specific mitochondrial proteins that are components of the electron transport chain occur in aging rodents. Damage to mitochondrial DNA progressively increases in somatic cells during the aging process, with the most pronounced damage occurring in postmitotic cells such as neurons. Mitochondrial dysfunction has been linked to several neurodegenerative disorders. In Parkinson disease, there are marked decreases in complex I and α-ketoglutarate dehydrogenase activities. Exposure of cultured dopaminergic neurons to insults relevant to the pathogenesis of Parkinson disease (eg, MPTP and Fe^{2+}) causes mitochondrial dysfunction. In Alzheimer disease, cytochrome c oxidase and α-ketoglutarate dehydrogenase activity levels are markedly reduced in vulnerable

brain regions. Interestingly, mitochondrial deficits are also observed in nonneuronal cells, including platelets and fibroblasts, of Alzheimer disease patients. When mitochondria from platelets of Alzheimer disease patients are introduced into cultured neuroblastoma cells, levels of oxidative stress are increased, suggesting an important contribution of mitochondrial alterations to the increased oxidative stress present in neurons of Alzheimer disease brain. Mitochondrial alterations in neurons have been documented in studies of mouse models of Alzheimer disease (APP and presenilin mutant mice), Parkinson disease (α-synuclein mutant mice), Huntington disease (huntingtin mutant mice), and stroke (middle cerebral artery occlusion).

NEURONAL ION HOMEOSTASIS IN THE AGING BRAIN

Among the properties of neurons that set them apart from many other cell types is their excitability, which is regulated by a complex array of neurotransmitters and ion channels. Neurons express voltage-dependent sodium channels, as well as multiple types of calcium and potassium channels that are differentially expressed among neuronal populations, and are segregated in different cellular compartments (eg, L-type calcium channels in the cell body, N-type calcium channels in the dendrites, and T-type calcium channels in presynaptic terminals). In addition, neurons possess ion-motive ATPases that play critical roles in reestablishing ion gradients following neuronal stimulation. A variety of age-related alterations in electrophysiologic parameters of neurons have been described in rodents (described earlier in this chapter) and, in some cases, in humans, including increased thresholds for induction of action potentials in cranial nerves, increased after hyperpolarizations in hippocampal neurons, and impaired LTP/LTD of synaptic transmission in the hippocampus. Moreover, a generalized decrease in neuronal inhibition appears to occur during the aging process.

The calcium ion plays fundamental roles in regulating neuronal survival and plasticity in both the developing and adult nervous system. Calcium mediates some of the effects induced by neurotransmitters and neurotrophic factors on neurite outgrowth, synaptogenesis, and cell survival in many different regions of the developing nervous system. Furthermore, in the adult nervous system, calcium regulates neurotransmitter release from presynaptic terminals and influences postsynaptic changes associated with learning and memory processes. Aging may result in decreases in the activity of the plasma membrane calcium ATPase and in levels of calcium-binding proteins, while increasing calcium influx through voltage-dependent channels and increasing the activation of calcium-dependent proteases.

Several studies have measured and determined changes in calcium transmission across the neuronal membrane in aged rodents. The final step in synaptic transmission that triggers LTP or LTD is dependent on the amount of calcium entering the cell. Therefore, changes in calcium conductance across the cell membrane could have significant effects on synaptic plasticity in aged animals. Studies have revealed that aged rats display an increased density of L-type Ca^{++} channels in CA1 pyramidal cells, leading to increased L-type Ca^{++} currents. In addition, CA1 pyramidal cells from aged rodents also show an increased duration of calcium-mediated action potentials. The inward flux of calcium in response to an action potential activates a calcium-mediated inward potassium current. These potassium channels are slower to open and close than calcium channels, which leads to a temporary after-hyperpolarization of the cell following an action potential. Studies have revealed that this phenomenon is increased in aged rodents and rabbits, leading to less frequent firing of action potentials in response to a prolonged depolarizing current. Taken together, these data demonstrate that age-related changes in calcium transmission underlie detrimental changes in synaptic plasticity and may partially explain the deficits in plasticity seen over the course of aging.

NEUROTRANSMITTER SIGNALING IN THE AGING BRAIN

A number of alterations in different neurotransmitter systems have been documented in studies of aging rodents and in analyses of brain tissues from humans with age-related neurodegenerative disorders. While some of these alterations likely result from neuronal degeneration, others appear to occur in the absence of cell injury.

Cholinergic Systems

Acetylcholine is employed as a neurotransmitter in select populations of neurons in the brain, prominent among which are basal forebrain neurons that innervate widespread regions of the neocortex and hippocampus; these cholinergic neurons are known to play key roles in learning and memory processes in humans and rodents. Deficits in one or more aspects of cholinergic signal transduction may occur with aging including choline transport, acetylcholine synthesis, acetylcholine release, and coupling of muscarinic receptors to their GTP-binding effector proteins. Cholinergic deficits are much more severe in Alzheimer disease patients and differ qualitatively from the changes observed during normal aging. Particularly striking is a reduced ability of muscarinic agonists to activate GTP-binding proteins in cortical neurons. Increased levels of membrane lipid peroxidation in neurons may contribute to impaired cholinergic signaling; for example, Aβ, Fe^{2+}, and the lipid peroxidation product 4-hydroxynonenal can impair coupling of muscarinic receptors to the GTP-binding protein G_{q11}.

Dopaminergic Systems

Prominent reductions in both pre- and postsynaptic aspects of dopaminergic neurotransmission occur during brain aging. Decreases in dopamine levels and dopamine transporter levels in the striatum occur with advancing age, and there is an age-related decrease in levels of D_2 receptor-binding sites in striatum. As with cholinergic signal transduction, there also appears to be an age-related impairment of coupling of dopamine receptors to their GTP-binding effector proteins. The contribution of oxidative stress to changes in dopaminergic signaling has not been established, although the prominent role of oxyradicals in the pathogenesis of Parkinson disease argues that similar oxidative processes contribute to dopaminergic dysfunction during normal aging. These changes in dopaminergic signaling likely play a role in age-related deficits in motor control and may explain the fact that the older adults are susceptible to extrapyramidal effects of dopamine receptor antagonist drugs.

Monoaminergic Systems

Norepinephrine and serotonin are the major monoamine neurotransmitters in the brain. Noradrenergic neurons are located primarily in the locus caeruleus and serotonergic neurons in the raphe nucleus; both types of neurons project to widespread regions of cerebral cortex. There are several subtypes of receptors for norepinephrine, some of which couple to GTP-binding proteins. There are also several subtypes of serotonin receptors; some couple to GTP-binding proteins while others are ligand-gated ion channels. There appears to be increased levels of norepinephrine with aging in some brain regions, while levels of α_2-adrenergic receptors may decrease in cerebral cortex with advancing age. Levels of serotonin may decrease in the striatum, hippocampus, and cerebral cortex. Age-related decreases in levels of evoked serotonin release and of serotonin-binding sites have been reported and may contribute to affective disorders such as depression.

Amino Acid Transmitter Systems

The amino acid glutamate is the major excitatory neurotransmitter in the human brain. Glutamate stimulates ionotropic receptors that flux calcium and sodium; excessive activation of ionotropic glutamate receptors may play a role in the degeneration of neurons in several age-related disorders including stroke, Alzheimer disease, Parkinson disease, and Huntington disease. Levels of ionotropic glutamate receptors were reported to decrease with aging, but these decreases may be the result of degeneration of the neurons expressing the receptors. The contribution of dysfunction of glutamatergic transmission, in the absence of neuronal death, to age- and disease-related deficits in brain function is unknown. The major inhibitory neurotransmitter in the human brain is γ-aminobutyric acid (GABA). Relatively little information is available concerning the impact of aging on GABAergic systems, although levels of glutamate decarboxylase and GABA-A binding sites may be decreased. Interestingly, GABAergic interneurons are typically spared in various neurodegenerative disorders including Alzheimer disease.

NEUROENDOCRINE CHANGES IN THE AGING BRAIN

A variety of age-related alterations in neuroendocrine systems have been documented. Of particular importance for human brain aging and neurodegenerative disorders are changes in levels of steroid hormones, particularly glucocorticoids and estrogens. There is considerable evidence for age-related alterations in the diurnal regulation of circulating glucocorticoid levels and an increase in the mean level. Moreover, regulation of the hypothalamic-pituitary-adrenal axis is altered in Alzheimer disease patients, such that plasma levels of glucocorticoids are increased. Increased levels of glucocorticoids, including those induced by physiologic or psychological stress, can increase the vulnerability of hippocampal neurons to injury and death caused by ischemic and excitotoxic insults, suggesting that glucocorticoids may have a negative impact on the outcome of both acute (eg, stroke) and chronic (eg, Alzheimer disease) age-related neurologic disorders. Estrogen (17β-estradiol) may have a beneficial effect on brain aging. Epidemiologic studies suggest a reduced risk of Alzheimer disease in postmenopausal women who take estrogen replacement therapy, and older women who take estrogens perform better on cognitive tasks. Surgical ovariectomy in rodents causes changes in neurotrophin receptor signaling, promotes the generation and accumulation of Aβ, and is associated with memory deficits. These effects are abrogated by exogenous estrogens. Finally, animal and cell culture studies have shown that 17β-estradiol can protect neurons from being damaged and killed by insults relevant to ischemia and Alzheimer disease, including glucose deprivation, exposure to Aβ, and expression of Alzheimer disease–linked presenilin mutations. Results of clinical findings, however, have not provided convincing evidence that estrogen treatment either reduces risk for Alzheimer disease or related illnesses or enhances cognition.

IMMUNOLOGIC FACTORS IN THE AGING BRAIN

While the blood-brain barrier limits access of circulating lymphocytes to neurons in the brain, it is becoming increasingly evident that the brain is by no means devoid of immune responses. The brain possesses resident immune effector cells called microglia (described earlier in this chapter) that may respond to age- and disease-related neurodegenerative processes. Some data suggest that a decline in peripheral immune function during aging may lead to an autoimmune-like phenomenon in the brain wherein microglia is activated. Inflammatory processes are associated with, and contribute to, the neurodegenerative process in Alzheimer disease and other age-related neurodegenerative disorders; these include activation of microglia in the affected brain regions, increased local cytokine production in association with the neuropathologic changes,

and activation of components of the complement cascade system. Collectively, the emerging data suggest a role for chronic inflammatory reactions in the pathogenesis of at least some neurodegenerative disorders. Recent studies have revealed that the choroid plexus, an epithelial monolayer that produces cerebrospinal fluid (CSF) and maintains a dynamic interface between the CSF and the blood, undergoes age-associated changes that are consistent with a type I interferon effect. Importantly, blocking type I interferon activity in aged mice is sufficient to reestablish a "young" choroid plexus activity and improve memory functions. Also intriguing is the fact that these changes appear to be driven by inflammatory changes that originate from both the brain parenchyma and the systemic circulation. Together, these results suggest that changes in inflammatory markers in the brain or in the periphery can influence (positively or negatively) memory functions; they also suggest that the choroid plexus plays an important role in the age-associated cognitive decline.

NEUROTROPHIC FACTORS IN THE AGING BRAIN

Cells in the nervous system produce a variety of proteins that serve the function of promoting neuronal survival and growth, and protecting the neurons against injury and death. Examples of such "neurotrophic factors" (also referred to as neurotrophins) include nerve growth factor (NGF), brain-derived neurotrophic factor (BDNF), neurotrophin-3, neurotrophin-4, basic fibroblast growth factor (bFGF), and insulin-like growth factor (IGF). Neurotrophic factors are remarkable in that they can protect neurons against a variety of insults relevant to the pathogenesis of age-related neurodegenerative conditions. For example, bFGF can protect hippocampal and cortical neurons against metabolic, oxidative, and excitotoxic insults, and can greatly reduce brain damage in rodent models of stroke. One or more neurotrophic factors have also been shown to protect neuronal populations against neurodegenerative disorder-specific insults. Examples are the ability of BDNF to protect dopaminergic neurons against MPTP toxicity (Parkinson disease model) and hippocampal neurons against Aβ-mediated toxicity (Alzheimer disease model). The precise mechanism(s) whereby neurotrophic factors can rescue or prevent neuronal degeneration are unclear and might be different in different neuronal populations. In addition to preserving existing neurons, neurotrophic factors may stimulate the production of new neurons from neuronal stem cells. Such neural stem cells may be able to replace lost or damaged neurons and are therefore receiving considerable attention for their potential use in the treatment of neurodegenerative disorders. An intriguing feature of neurotrophic factors is that their expression is increased by activity in neuronal circuits. Experimental studies in cell culture and in vivo show that such activity-dependent production of neurotrophic factors plays a major role in promoting neuronal survival and neurite outgrowth. Rearing of rodents in an "intellectually enriched" environment results in expansion of dendritic arbors and increased numbers of synapses in hippocampus and certain regions of cerebral cortex.

The activity and the specificity of neurotrophic factors depend on specific cell-surface receptors. Examples are the tyrosine-kinase family of receptors, TrkA, TrkB, and TrkC, and the p75 neurotrophin receptor (p75^{NTR}). These receptors can assemble as homo- and heterodimers, which display different affinity to specific neurotrophic factors and provide signaling specificity. For example, TrkA:p75^{NTR} heterodimers have higher affinity to NGF than TrkA:TrkA and p75^{NTR}:p75^{NTR} homodimers. Therefore, depending on how these receptors assemble on the neuronal surface, they can transduce slightly different or completely different signals. During aging the levels of TrkA decrease while those of p75^{NTR} increase, thus an expression pattern that favors the formation of TrkA:TrkA homodimers will switch toward an expression pattern that favors the formation of TrkA:p75^{NTR} heterodimers and p75^{NTR}:p75^{NTR} homodimers. While this switch occurs, the levels of NGF remain overall unchanged. However, since the affinity of the above receptor complexes for NGF is different, the signaling cascade will change as a result of aging. As an example, the above TrkA-to-p75^{NTR} switch has been linked to cognitive decline and increased risk of Alzheimer disease in rodents. A TrkA-to-p75^{NTR} switch has also been observed following surgical menopause in rodents, suggesting a possible impact in postmenopausal women.

The above competing activity of neurotrophin receptors is further complicated by the competing activity of neurotrophins. An example is BDNF competing with NGF for binding on TrkA:TrkA homodimers and pro-NGF competing with NGF for binding on p75^{NTR}:p75^{NTR} homodimers and TrkA:p75^{NTR} heterodimers. Importantly, levels of pro-NGF increase as a function of age while those of NGF remain unchanged. Mice with increased levels of pro-NGF develop a brain phenotype that resembles Alzheimer disease, and postmortem Alzheimer disease brain tissues express more pro-NGF than age-matched controls. In conclusion, complex scenarios can result as a function of aging leading to different neurotrophin-receptor interactions and, ultimately, to different biological effects. Since some of these changes are brain areas specific, we can expect different physiologic/pathologic outcomes.

AUTOPHAGY AND THE AGING BRAIN

Autophagy is an evolutionary conserved catabolic process that enables the cell to respond to both extracellular and intracellular stress signals in order to maintain cellular homeostasis. It helps dispose of large toxic protein aggregates that form within the cell, digest sick/damaged organelles, respond to pathogenic infections, and manage a plethora of metabolic challenges. The basic process of autophagy requires "sequestration" of unwanted material (ie, toxic protein aggregates or damaged organelles) into a double-membrane vesicular structure called autophagosome, which then will fuse with lysosomes where enzymatic digestion of the entire autophagosome occurs. This process is tightly regulated and involves more than 40 different proteins collectively referred to as the "autophagy machinery." To ensure correct activation and recruitment of this machinery, the cell has devised a series of organelle- and compartment-specific receptors that allow autophagy to be activated in a very specific and targeted fashion. Words like reticulophagy/ER-phagy, mitophagy, and nucleophagy are examples of commonly used expressions to indicate ER-specific autophagy, mitochondria-specific autophagy, and nucleus-specific autophagy, respectively.

Malfunction of autophagy contributes to the progression of many diseases across lifespan, including sporadic and hereditary forms of neurodegeneration, cancer, inflammation, and many age-associated diseases. Reduced or malfunction of autophagy is also considered a hallmark of cellular aging. Many progressive forms of neurodegenerative diseases, including Alzheimer disease, Parkinson disease, and taupoathies are characterized by the aberrant accumulation of toxic protein aggregates. Compelling data indicate that increased levels of autophagy can be beneficial in mouse models of diseases characterized by increased accumulation of toxic protein aggregates. As such, improving normal proteostatic mechanisms is an active target for biomedical research, thus explaining the large number of ongoing clinical trials exploring the therapeutic potential of stimulating autophagy.

Genetic or pharmacological stimulation of autophagy in *Caenorhabditis elegans*, *Drosophila Melanogaster*, and mammals improves metabolic health and proteostasis (protein homeostasis), and extends lifespan. The lifespan extension can go from as low as 20% to as high as 80% indicating a rather robust effect. Conversely, genetic manipulations that reduce or block the autophagic response lead to reduced lifespan and a plethora of phenotypic manifestations that are consistent with accelerated forms of pathogenic aging. An example of this complexity is the ER acetylation machinery, which is responsible for the disposal of toxic protein aggregates that form within the ER and secretory pathway. ER acetylation is ensured by a membrane transporter, AT-1, which translocates acetyl-CoA from the cytosol into the ER lumen. In the ER lumen, acetyl-CoA is used by two ER-based acetyltransferases, ATase1 and ATase2, which acetylate ER resident- and transiting-nascent glycoproteins. Genetic manipulations that lead to increased influx of acetyl-CoA into the ER and increased ER acetylation in the mouse (AT-1 sTg mice) cause a segmental form of progeria. The phenotype is reminiscent of the progeria-like manifestations of patients with gene duplications of AT-1, and includes alopecia, skin lesions, rectal prolapse, osteoporosis, cardiomegaly, muscle atrophy, cognitive impairment, systemic inflammation, and accumulation of senescent cells. Biochemical inhibition of the ATases, downstream of AT-1 can restore the proteostatic function of the ER and rescue the progeria phenotype of AT-1 sTg mice. Furthermore, genetic or biochemical inhibition of the ATases can significantly delay the progression of Alzheimer disease in the mouse.

A major caveat of the translational approaches aimed at stimulating autophagy and improving the proteostatic capacity of the cell is the fact that—as mentioned above—autophagy itself is highly selective and can be triggered to dispose of toxic protein aggregates in different places (ie, ER and secretory pathway, cytosol, mitochondria). Therefore, a "one-approach strategy" that fits all neurodegenerative diseases will not be viable, and different autophagy-stimulating compounds will have high degree of disease specificity.

GENETIC FACTORS IN BRAIN AGING AND NEURODEGENERATIVE DISORDERS

Several microarray studies have now been performed in mice, rats, nonhuman primates, and humans to analyze the genetic profile of the aging brain. They all indicate that normal aging is not accompanied by a genome-wide dysregulation of transcription but rather by specific changes that affect only a small subset of genes, which accounts for about 3% to 5% of all the genes expressed in the brain. These changes (**Table 56-2**) will not be discussed here as their overall biological significance is still uncertain. Of note, a similar expression profile was also found in patients with

TABLE 56-2 ■ GENETIC PATHWAYS OF THE BRAIN THAT ARE AFFECTED BY AGING

Glucose metabolism	Some up, some down
Fatty acid metabolism and transport	Overall down
Mitochondria β-oxidation	Overall down
Protein synthesis and modification	Some up, some down
Protein turnover	Overall down
Vesicular/protein transport	Overall down
Stress response (antioxidant, DNA repair, metal ion homeostasis, etc)	Overall up
Inflammatory molecules	Overall up
Microglia activation	Overall up
Neurogenesis	Overall down
Growth factors	Overall down
Myelination	Overall up
Synaptic turnover and activity	Overall down
Synaptic plasticity	Overall down
Ca++ homeostasis	Overall down
Intraneuronal signaling (kinases, G proteins, etc)	Overall down
Hormonal regulation	Some up, some down

Alzheimer disease supporting the view that a *continuum* might exist between normal aging and Alzheimer disease.

Longevity Genes

It is now evident that specific genetic, biochemical, and molecular pathways are intrinsically related to aging. Some of these pathways were initially identified in lower organisms and then later confirmed in higher organisms, while others were immediately identified in higher organisms. These include the insulin-like growth factor 1 receptor (IGF-1R), Delta40p53, and Klotho.

Among them, IGF-1R has probably received more attention. The first evidence that IGF-1R signaling can regulate the progression of aging came from *C elegans*, where mutations that reduce IGF-1R activity were able to increase the lifespan of the animal. Similar results were then obtained in *D melanogaster* and, later on, in mammals. Importantly, mutations that act on IGF-1R downstream targets were also able to modify the lifespan of the animals providing robust and definitive connection between IGF-1R and aging. Overall, reduced IGF-1R activity extends lifespan and delays age-associated events, while increased IGF-1R activity achieves the opposite effects. A partial block of IGF-1R signaling is also achieved by caloric restriction, which extends the maximum lifespan and delays many biological changes that are associated with aging. In humans, genetic variations that reduce IGF-1R signaling appear to be beneficial for old age survival and preservation of cognitive functions, suggesting that the mechanisms regulating lifespan and aging via this pathway are evolutionary conserved. Finally, reduced IGF-1R signaling can rescue Alzheimer disease in mouse models.

Delta40p53 is a short N-terminal truncated isoform of the tumor suppressor gene *TP53*. The common *TP53* gene generates at least 12 different proteins through a combination of alternative promoter usage, alternative splicing, and alternative initiation of translation. Of them, p53 is the most "famous" and most studied due to its pathogenic role in many forms of cancer. Delta40p53 (also referred to as p44 or p47) lacks the first N-terminal 39 amino acids of full-length p53 but retains the DNA-binding domain as well as one of the two transactivation domains. Delta40p53 retains some of p53 functions but lacks others; it retains some of the regulatory elements but lacks others. Mice overexpressing full-length p53 ("Super p53" mice) are resistant to cancer development but have normal maximum lifespan. In contrast, mice overexpressing Delta40p53 (p44$^{+/+}$ mice) display a segmental progeria phenotype that mimics an accelerated form of pathogenic aging. The phenotype includes early onset of diabetes, osteoporosis, memory impairment, and reduced lifespan. To date at least five additional mouse models with altered p53 activity have been shown to develop an accelerated aging phenotype providing robust and definitive connection between *TP53* and aging. Recent studies have also shown that Delta40p53 regulates the generation of Aβ as well as the phosphorylation status of tau, suggesting a possible connection with the accumulation of amyloid plaques and NFTs that characterizes the aging as well as the Alzheimer disease brain (discussed earlier in this chapter). Interestingly, mice engineered to overexpress p44 develop an accelerated form of Alzheimer disease neuropathology.

Klotho is a cell-surface membrane protein that can also be released in the circulation. Klotho has glycosidase-like activity. Its levels and enzymatic activity decline during aging. Genetic variants of *KLOTHO* are associated with human aging and klotho-deficient mice display a progeroid phenotype that resembles aging. The phenotype includes atherosclerosis, skin atrophy, osteoporosis, reduced fertility, emphysema, memory defects, and reduced lifespan. In contrast, mice overexpressing klotho display increased lifespan and increased resistance to several age-associated features. A possible connection between klotho and IGF-1R has also been delineated. Human variations that lead to increased circulating levels of klotho are associated with greater cortical volumes in the brain. Finally, overexpression of klotho in the mouse enhances cognition and rescues some of the deficits that characterize Alzheimer disease.

In addition to the above, polymorphisms that are associated with longevity and preserved physiologic functions have also been identified in two cholesterol-related genes, apolipoprotein E (*APOE*) and cholesteryl ester transfer protein (*CETP*). *APOE* carries cholesterol in the circulation, while *CETP* facilitates the transfer of cholesteryl esters and triglycerides between circulating lipoproteins. Individuals normally inherit two APOE alleles, of which there are three isoforms (E2, E3, and E4). The E2 allele has been linked to longevity and reduced incidence of Alzheimer disease. In contrast, the E4 allele has been linked to increased risk for Alzheimer disease. Certain *CETP* variants have been linked to increased levels of high-density lipoproteins (HDLs), reduced progression of atherosclerosis, and longevity. The "longevity effect" of *APOE* and *CETP* might be explained, at least in part, by their ability to reduce the progression of atherosclerosis in the vasculature.

Another possible longevity gene is that encoding an isoform of angiotensin-converting enzyme, although its mechanistic links to aging are unclear. Finally, the multigene major histocompatibility system appears to influence lifespan and may act by sustaining functions of the immune system. Additional information on longevity genes and their impact in age-associated events can be found in Chapter 1.

Disorder-Specific Genes

Considerable progress has been made in studying human genetic disorders that cause progeroid syndromes, which are characterized by a disease phenotype mimicking an "accelerated" form of aging. Although progeroid syndromes can be classified as *unimodal* (affecting one tissue/organ) and *segmental* (affecting multiple tissues/organs), the term progeroid syndrome is usually limited to the segmental forms of the disease (**Table 56-3**). Examples

TABLE 56-3 ■ SEGMENTAL PROGEROID SYNDROMES WITH COGNITIVE CHANGES

SYNDROME	INHERITANCE	MEAN LIFESPAN (Y)
Ataxia-telangiectasia	Autosomal recessive	~ 45–50
Berardinelli–Seip syndrome	Autosomal recessive	~ 40
Bloom syndrome	Autosomal recessive	Unclear
Cokayne syndrome	Autosomal recessive	~ 20
Down syndrome	Trisomy 21	~ 60
Hutchinson–Gilford progeria	Autosomal dominant	~ 10–15
Rothmund–Thompson syndrome	Autosomal recessive	Unclear
Trichothiodystrophy	Autosomal recessive	~ 10
Werner syndrome	Autosomal recessive	~ 45–50

include Werner syndrome, Bloom syndrome, Rothmund–Thomson syndrome, Hutchinson–Gilford progeria syndrome, and Cokayne syndrome. Patients affected by these disorders have limited lifespan and develop a complex array of disease manifestations, including type 2 diabetes, osteoporosis, hair loss, skin atrophy, atherosclerosis, cardiomyopathy, heart failure, chronic obstructive pulmonary disease, renal insufficiency, and neurologic abnormalities. The neurologic defects are often subtle and difficult to diagnose; when evident, they include bulbar, extrapyramidal and cerebellar symptoms, deafness, retinopathy, cognitive deficits, corticospinal symptoms, and peripheral neuropathy. Brain imaging shows diffused white matter pathology as well as different degrees of gray matter pathology in memory-forming and processing areas. The genetic defect has been mapped in most classical forms of progeroid syndromes. Specifically, Werner syndrome has been associated with mutations in *WRN*; Bloom syndrome has been associated with mutations in *BLM*; Rothmund–Thomson syndrome has been associated with mutations in *RECQL4*; Hutchinson–Gilford progeria syndrome has been associated with mutations on *LMNA*; and Cokayne syndrome has been associated with mutations in *ERCC8* and *ERCC6*. All the above genes encode proteins that are involved in different aspects of DNA transcription, repair, or recombination underscoring common pathogenic elements.

Although progeroid syndromes manifest with symptoms and physical features that are—at least in part—reminiscent of an accelerated form of aging, they must be viewed as diseases rather than true forms of accelerated aging. It is plausible to assume that the dissection of the molecular phenotype of these diseases will inform us about aging. However, it is also plausible to expect that the underlying defects of human progerias are substantially different from those of normal aging. Additional discussion of human progerias can be found in Chapter 1.

Considerable progress has also been made in identifying genetic factors that play pathogenic roles in Alzheimer disease, the most common form of dementia associated with aging. Specifically, disease-causing mutations in APP, PSEN1, and PSEN2 have been identified in familial (early-onset) forms of Alzheimer disease. In addition, several "predisposition" genes have been identified in which polymorphisms increase the risk for developing sporadic (late-onset) Alzheimer disease. Description of the most important polymorphisms identified to date as well as pathogenic roles of APP, PSEN1, and PSEN2 can be found in Chapter 59.

The Brain as a Regulator of Lifespan

Among the very first mouse models of extended lifespan were the Ames and the Snell dwarf mice. Both models had a selective defect in the secretion of key hormones from the pituitary gland, specifically, growth hormone (GH), prolactin, and thyroid-stimulating hormone. The 40% to 60% extension of lifespan was also accompanied by evidence of delayed aging. The increased lifespan of the Ames and Snell mice was primarily linked to the deficiency of the GH-IGF1 axis. GH is released in the circulation by the pituitary gland; upon binding to its own receptor in the liver, it causes secretion of IGF1, which then binds to IGF-1R and stimulates IGF-1R signaling. Mice with isolated deficiency in growth hormone secretion (Little mice) or lacking the growth hormone receptor (GHR-KO mice) also displayed longevity. The lifespan extension in the Little and GHR-KO mice was in the 25% to 55% range. Finally, mice with reduced secretion of IGF1 or reduced levels of IGF-1R also displayed different levels of increased lifespan. In essence, the Ames and Snell mice represent the very first evidence that the brain itself (or specialized sets of neurons in the brain) could influence the lifespan of the animals. Following studies in lower organisms (C elegans and D melanogaster) clearly confirmed this conclusion. More recently, genetic disruption of IRS2, an adaptor protein that acts downstream of IGF-1R and the insulin receptor, in the mouse brain ($bIrs^{-/+}$ and $bIrs^{-/-}$) also caused a significant increase in the lifespan of the animals. Regardless of the specific mechanism(s) involved in the phenotype of the above genetic models, it is now well accepted that in addition to being affected by aging, the brain (or the nervous system) itself can affect aging.

EMERGING AREAS OF STUDY

Epigenetics

A series of transcriptome-based studies across different species indicate that the aging brain is characterized by global changes within different genetic pathways. In general, genes involved in vesicular transport, synaptic turnover, and plasticity appear to be reduced, while genes involved with neuroinflammation and stress response appear to be upregulated. These changes are likely the result of alterations in the normal mechanisms of epigenetic regulation of gene expression, which include DNA methylation, histone PTMs, and small noncoding microRNA (miRNA).

DNA methylation of the pyrimidine ring of cytosine within CpG and non-CpG sites is associated with repression of transcription. Studies in aged cognitively animals have reported hypermethylation among synapse-related genes and hypomethylation among neuroinflammatory genes. However, these findings have not been consistently replicated across laboratories and animal species. This inconsistency might—at least in part—be explained by the different behavior of CpG and non-CpG sites with the former remaining unchanged and the latter becoming hypermethylated as a function of age. However, to date, the effect of age on DNA methylation in the brain remains unclear.

Histone PTMs include acetylation, methylation, phosphorylation, ubiquitination, and sumoylation. The effect of these modifications remains to be fully understood as it might depend on the specific modification, the extent of modification, and the location of the histone tag. As with DNA methylation, no general conclusions can be drawn on the effect of age on histone PTMs. Furthermore, the PTM profile of histone proteins does not appear to highlight specific changes in memory functions among young or old animals or to distinguish cognitively normal and impaired aged humans.

miRNAs are small (18–25 nucleotide long) noncoding RNAs that can pair with complementary sequences within coding mRNAs and inhibit translation. An intriguing aspect of miRNAs is that they can be found packed into small single-membrane circulating vesicles referred to as exosomes. Exosomes appear to originate from different cells and tissues and can cross biological membranes. As such, they might function as a general communication system connecting different cells, tissues, and organs by delivering cargo molecules. No study has reported consistent changes in either levels or types of miRNAs as a function of brain aging. However, the fact that miRNAs are present within exosomes has spurred great interest. So far, differences in experimental approaches as well as inconsistent characterization of exosomal preparations have limited the study outcomes. Furthermore, it is still unclear whether they can enter the brain or can interact with neurons (or other cell types) to deliver miRNA with high specificity.

The Glymphatic System

The glymphatic system serves as a "waste drainage" system for the brain. It includes a perivascular network for the flux of the CSF connected to the lymphatic system that is associated with meninges, cranial nerves, and large vessels exiting the skull. The flux of CSF is achieved by convection through the astrocyte end-processes and toward the perivenous space to ultimately reach the lymphatic system. CSF transport across the astrocyte network requires aquaporin 4 (AQP4), a member of the AQP family of water channels. Animal studies suggest reduced efficiency of glymphatic-mediated transport of cargo material as a function of age. A similar decline has been documented in mouse models of Alzheimer disease, stroke, and traumatic brain injury. Aging, stroke, and traumatic brain injury are the strongest risk factors for Alzheimer disease. Although it is still unclear how important the glymphatic system is for the removal of macromolecules from the brain, there are sufficient data indicating that both Aβ and tau oligomers use—at least in part—this route. Consistently, genetic knockout of AQP4 in the mouse appears to impair Aβ removal. A major area of concern is the fact that the glymphatic system has been almost entirely characterized in the rodent brain and it is unknown whether an identical system is in place in humans and whether it is efficient enough to play a fundamental role in the removal of macromolecules.

DIETARY FACTORS IN BRAIN AGING AND NEURODEGENERATIVE DISORDERS

It is now evident that the diet can affect one's risk of age-related neurodegenerative disorders. In particular, emerging findings indicate that several dietary risk factors for prominent age-related diseases including cardiovascular disease, cancer, and diabetes are also risk factors for Alzheimer disease, Parkinson disease, and stroke. A summary of possible preventive measures to improve brain health can be found in **Table 56-4**.

Calorie Intake

Apart from genetic manipulation, the only known means of increasing the lifespan of rodents and nonhuman primates is by decreasing their calorie intake; both maximum and mean lifespan can be increased by up to 40%. The average lifespan of humans is certainly decreased by overeating,

---

TABLE 56-4 ■ PREVENTIVE MEASURES TO PROTECT THE AGING BRAIN

- **Physical exercise.** Improves cardiovascular functions; reduces volume loss; stimulates neurogenesis.
- **Intellectual and outdoor activities.** Stimulate neurogenesis; stimulate synaptic plasticity; increase brain capacity.
- **Diet.** Improved brain health has been associated with diets that include a modest decrease in total calories and high consumption of fruits and vegetables. Antiaging effects have been associated with intake of poly- and monounsaturated fatty acids, vitamins, phytochemicals, polyphenols, and antioxidants.
- **Correction of existing medical conditions.** Examples include hypercholesterolemia, dyslipidemias, diabetes, and hypertension.
- **Minimize environmental stressors.** Disposition to stress is associated with poor brain health.

---

although it remains to be determined whether maximum lifespan can be increased through calorie restriction. Epidemiologic data suggest that individuals with a low-calorie intake are at a reduced risk for Alzheimer disease and Parkinson disease. Biochemical markers of aging, and deficits in learning and memory and motor function, are retarded in rodents maintained on dietary restriction. Neurons in the brains of rats and mice maintained on dietary restriction are more resistant to dysfunction and death in experimental models of Alzheimer disease, Parkinson disease, Huntington disease, and stroke. A 20-year longitudinal study in Rhesus macaques showed that a 30% reduction in daily calorie intake reduced the rate of age-related deaths as well as the incidence of typical age-associated diseases, such as diabetes, cancer, cardiovascular disease, and brain atrophy. The ability of calorie restriction to prevent brain atrophy was observed across several gray matter areas involved in both motor and executive functions. Magnetic resonance imaging also showed preserved volumes and insulin sensitivity in memory-forming and processing areas, while postmortem histology showed reduced astrogliosis. Therefore, a large body of evidence from lower organisms to nonhuman primates delineates a relationship between calorie intake and progression of aging and/or incidence of age-associated events. The mechanism whereby caloric restriction increases the resistance of neurons to the adverse effects of aging is not entirely known. Studies in yeast, worms, flies, rodents, and monkeys suggest that the reduced calorie intake causes a comprehensive metabolic reprogramming that involves key nutrient-responsive signaling pathways.

Folic Acid (Homocysteine)

It was recognized long ago that folic acid deficiency can cause abnormalities in the developing nervous system. Subsequently, it was shown that people with low levels of folic acid tend to have elevated levels of homocysteine and that this condition is associated with increased risk of cardiovascular disease and stroke. Homocysteine is produced during metabolism of methionine, and folic acid plays an important role in removing homocysteine via remethylation. Epidemiologic findings suggest that people with elevated homocysteine levels may be at increased risk of Alzheimer disease and Parkinson disease. Animal studies support a cause-effect relationship between elevated homocysteine levels and neuronal vulnerability to neurodegenerative disorders. For example, hippocampal neurons of APP mutant mice (Alzheimer disease model) and substantia nigra dopaminergic neurons in MPTP-treated mice (Parkinson disease model) exhibit increased vulnerability to degeneration when maintained on a folic acid–deficient diet. By increasing homocysteine levels, folic acid deficiency may promote accumulation of DNA damage by inhibiting DNA repair. In neurons, the increased DNA damage can trigger apoptosis, particularly under conditions of increased oxidative or metabolic stress. Of note, results of clinical studies to date have failed to provide any convincing evidence that folic acid supplementation either reduces risk for dementia or vascular diseases.

Stimulatory Phytochemicals and Antioxidants

Epidemiologic findings suggest that individuals who regularly consume vegetables and fruits have a lower risk of developing age-related neurodegenerative disorders compared to those who eat few such plant products. Several phytochemicals have been reported to enhance neuronal plasticity and survival in studies of animal models of neurodegenerative disorders. Examples include sulforaphane, curcumin, allicin, resveratrol, and other grape-derived polyphenols. Instead of functioning as direct antioxidants, many of these beneficial phytochemicals may stimulate mild adaptive stress responses that result in increased production of antioxidant enzymes, neurotrophic factors, and other protective proteins in neurons. The possible therapeutic benefits of several such stimulatory phytochemicals are currently being tested in human subjects with age-related neurologic disorders.

Epidemiologic findings also support a protective effect of antioxidants found in fruits and vegetables against stroke, and possibly Alzheimer disease. Studies in animal models of Alzheimer disease, Parkinson disease, Huntington disease, stroke, and amyotrophic lateral sclerosis have documented beneficial effects of some antioxidants. Positive effects have been reported for several commonly used dietary supplements, including vitamin E, creatine, and ginkgo biloba. However, the effects of such antioxidants are relatively subtle compared to the quite striking neuroprotective effects of dietary restriction.

PHYSICAL VERSUS COGNITIVE TRAINING AND THE AGING BRAIN

Several studies have revealed that both cognitive and physical training of older adults can cause changes in brain connectivity that is reflected in improved cognitive functions. Proposed mechanisms responsible for the positive changes imparted upon by physical training include angiogenesis and improved vascular functions, synaptogenesis, and neurotrophin-mediated signaling. Comparison of cognitive and physical training shows almost similar positive effects with the exception of the hippocampus and frontal brain regions, where physical training appears to induce effects that are more robust. When studying changes within specific cognitive domains, both trainings positively affect executive functions, as well as working-, short- and long-term memory. However, physical training appears to be more effective with spatial and speed memory, while cognitive training appears to be more effective with problem solving and multitasking. Whether physical and cognitive training can complement each other is currently unclear, although some studies do report complementary improvement of structural and functional connectivity.

BIOMARKERS OF AGING, BRAIN AGING, AND ALZHEIMER DISEASE

Given the steady increase in average human lifespan, there is a substantial need to identify old individuals that are at higher risk for morbidity or mortality. Several studies have tried to address this need by identifying "static" and/or "dynamic" biomarkers of aging that could predict the future onset of age-associated diseases. Ideally, such an instantaneous and unbiased profile would provide valuable information about the "biological age" of the body and the overall vulnerability to diseases and death. Such a "snapshot" would also provide opportunities to investigate how different variables, such as socioeconomic status, demographic distribution, and behavior, can interact with biological and genetic factors to influence rates of aging and disease vulnerability in individuals. The list of potential biomarkers differs among the different studies and can encompass more than 40 different variables (selected markers are listed in **Table 56-5**). In general, markers of cognitive performance, systemic inflammation, cardiovascular disease/failure, and metabolic imbalance appear to be strong predictors. However, there is discussion on whether static or dynamic profiles are more informative. For example, visit-to-visit variability of blood pressure appears to be a stronger predictor of cardiovascular risk and all-cause mortality among the 70 to 75 age group than stable moderate hypertension. In the case of Alzheimer disease, longitudinal changes in CSF- and MRI-based biomarkers and in cognitive test scores are stronger predictors. In essence, there is consensus that maintaining stable trajectory of certain "biomarkers" or risk factors for major age-associated diseases may be more beneficial to reduce both morbidity and mortality. The identification of a biomarker profile is complicated by the genetic profile and the socioeconomic makeup of the individual (and population). This is particularly evident when trying to assess cognitive abilities and functional independence, which are heavily influenced by intrinsic individual- and race-based differences.

The steady increase in average human lifespan has also been accompanied by a steady increase in both prevalence and incidence of Alzheimer disease. As discussed in Chapter 59, clinical diagnostic criteria for Alzheimer disease have limited accuracy, do not specifically separate Alzheimer disease from other neurodegenerative diseases, and do not correlate strongly with the severity of the neuropathology as assessed at autopsy. Therefore, there has been great effort to identify biomarkers of Alzheimer disease with the purpose of differentiating Alzheimer disease from other neurodegenerative diseases and from "normal" brain aging. In general, CSF-based biomarkers have shown much higher predicting power than peripheral blood-based biomarkers (see **Table 56-5**). Due to their central pathogenic role, it is not surprising that Aβ and tau have emerged as the strongest predictors. In the case of Aβ, the progressive decrease in CSF $A\beta_{42}$ differentiates Alzheimer

TABLE 56-5 ■ BIOMARKERS OF AGING AND ALZHEIMER DISEASE

CONDITION	TESTED	PREDICTING POWER
Age-associated vulnerability	Body mass index; blood pressure; hematocrit; red blood cell counts; white blood cell counts; cholesterol (total, HDL, LDL); triglycerides; glucose; insulin; albumin; bilirubin; hemoglobin; glycosylated hemoglobin; osteocalcin; calcium; sodium; potassium; chloride; iron; zinc; BUN-creatinine ratio; creatinine; vitamin D; alkaline phosphatase; ferritin; transferrin; α2-macroglobulin; ceruloplasmin; transaminases; testosterone; dehydroepiandrosterone; cortisol; epi/norepinephrine; C-reactive protein; interleukin 6; natriuretic peptide; homocysteine; uric acid; fibrinogen; amyloid A and P; pentraxin 3; adiponectin; malondialdehyde; carbonylated/nitrated proteins; nitric oxide products; sRAGE	Low
Alzheimer disease	PET amyloid imaging	High
	PET tau imaging	Uncertain
	CSF $A\beta_{42}$	High
	CSF $A\beta_{42}/A\beta_{40}$ ratio	High
	CSF tau	High
	CSF phospho-tau	High
	CSF neurogranin	Moderate
	CSF neurofilament light chain	Moderate
	Blood $A\beta_{42}$	Low
	Blood $A\beta_{42}/A\beta_{40}$ ratio	Low
	Blood tau	Low
	Blood neurofilament light chain	Low

disease patients from cognitively normal/stable individuals and correlates with the severity of the pathological changes observed at autopsy. Although there is no experimentally proven explanation for the association between reduced CSF $A\beta_{42}$ measured in living patients and the amyloid plaque load observed at the autopsy, the fact that they correlate has been consistently documented. The predicting power of measuring CSF $A\beta$ improves when both the 42 and 40 amino acid-long forms of the peptide are measured. Indeed, the $A\beta_{42}/A\beta_{40}$ ratio shows higher concordance with amyloid PET imaging. Again, although there is no experimentally proven explanation for the increased predicting value of the $A\beta_{42}/A\beta_{40}$ ratio, the association with the severity of the disease shows a mean sensitivity and specificity around 85% to 90%. Furthermore, the CSF $A\beta_{42}/A\beta_{40}$ ratio appears to resolve nonspecific features of $A\beta_{42}$ measures alone. Indeed, decreased CSF $A\beta_{42}$ levels are also observed in other forms of dementia, such as frontotemporal dementia and Lewy body dementia, while changes in CSF $A\beta_{42}/A\beta_{40}$ ratio are not. CSF levels of total tau appear to correlate very strongly with the severity of AD patients. Tau is a cytosolic protein and its release to the extracellular space can only occur as a result of neurodegeneration. As such, it is not surprising that levels of tau reflect the severity of the neurodegenerative damage. Although CSF levels of total tau do not differentiate Alzheimer disease from other neurodegenerative diseases, levels of phosphorylated (phospho)-tau appear to be quite specific for Alzheimer disease. Currently, different biochemical assays are available for the analysis of phospho-tau species. Combining $A\beta$ and tau

measures in the CSF offers improved diagnostic potential even in prodromal stages of the disease. The combination of these biomarkers with amyloid-based PET imaging seems to offer a very consistent and reliable way to follow the progression of the Alzheimer form of dementia in an unbiased fashion.

Among emerging CSF biomarkers of brain aging and neurodegeneration, neurogranin and the neurofilament light chain appear to hold the strongest potential. Both are cytosolic proteins and, therefore, as with tau, they reflect neurodegenerative events rather than early forms of neuronal toxicity. When looking at "naturally secreted" CSF biomarkers, the BDNF and the pro-nerve growth factor (pro-NGF) appear to be among the strongest predictors. Indeed, several studies have reported decreased CSF levels of BDNF and increased levels of pro-NGF as part of aging. Both BDNF and pro-NGF are members of the large family of neurotrophins and play fundamental biological functions for brain physiology. As such, they are particularly attractive. Neurotrophins and their receptors have been discussed earlier in this chapter.

CONCLUSION

Structural changes occur in the brain during aging and appear to be compensatory responses to adverse changes in cellular metabolism that accompany the aging process. There are several biochemical processes that may predispose neurons to dysfunction and death in aging and neurodegenerative disorders. The discovery that the lifespan of an organism can be regulated by specific genetic, molecular, and biochemical pathways has changed our view of aging itself and has spurred active interest in studying the basic biology of aging to understand diseases. At the same time, disease-driven research has helped discover pathways that are relevant for aging.

Convergence between age- and disease-related research has yielded an unprecedented body of information that will help us understand how the brain evolves and adapts to aging and how we can modulate these changes to improve the quality of life of a growing segment of our population.

FURTHER READING

Bishop NA, Lu T, Yankner BA. Neural mechanisms of ageing and cognitive decline. *Nature*. 2010;464:529.

Blennow K, Zetterberg H. Biomarkers for Alzheimer's disease: current status and prospects for the future. *J Intern Med*. 2018;284:643.

Bonafe M, Barbieri M, Marchegiani F, et al. Polymorphic variants of insulin-like growth factor I (IGF-I) receptor and phosphoinositide 3-kinase genes affect IGF-I plasma levels and human longevity: cues for an evolutionarily conserved mechanism of life span control. *J Clin Endocrinol Metab*. 2003;88:3299.

Cohen E, Paulsson JF, Blinder P, et al. Reduced IGF-1 signaling delays age-associated proteotoxicity in mice. *Cell*. 2009;139:1157.

Colman RJ, Anderson RM, Johnson SC, et al. Caloric restriction delays onset and mortality in rhesus monkeys. *Science*. 2009;325:201.

Costantini C, Scrable H, Puglielli, L. An aging pathway controls the TrkA to p75NTR receptor switch and amyloid β-peptide generation. *EMBO J*. 2006;25:1997.

de Cabo R, Carmona-Gutierrez D, Bernier M, Hall MN, Madeo F. The search for antiaging interventions: from elixirs to fasting regimens. *Cell*. 2014;157:1515.

Dubal DB, Yokoyama JS, Zhu L, et al. Life extension factor Klotho enhances cognition. *Cell Rep*. 2014;7:1065.

Frake RA, Ricketts T, Menzies FM, et al. Autophagy and neurodegeneration. *J Clin Invest*. 2015;125:65.

Freude S, Hettich MM, Schumann C, et al. Neuronal IGF-1 resistance reduces Aβ accumulation and protects against premature death in a model of Alzheimer's disease. *FASEB J*. 2009;23:3315.

Kapogiannis D, Mattson MP. Disrupted energy metabolism and neuronal circuit dysfunction in cognitive impairment and Alzheimer's disease. *Lancet Neurol*. 2011;10:187.

Madeo F, Zimmermann A, Maiuri MC, et al. Essential role for autophagy in life span extension *J Clin Invest*. 2015;125:85.

Mattson MP. Energy intake and exercise as determinants of brain health and vulnerability to injury and disease. *Cell Metab*. 2012;16:706.

Pehar M, O'Riordan KJ, Burns-Cusato M, et al. Altered longevity-assurance activity of p53:p44 in the mouse causes memory loss, neurodegeneration and premature death. *Aging Cell*. 2010;9:174.

Pehar M, Puglielli, L. Molecular and cellular mechanisms linking aging to cognitive decline and Alzheimer's disease. In: Perloft JW, Wong AH, eds. *Cell Aging*. New York: Nova Science Publishers Inc; 2012:153.

Peng Y, Shapiro SL, Banduseela VC, et al. Increased transport of acetyl-CoA into the endoplasmic reticulum causes a progeria-like phenotype. *Aging Cell*. 2018;17:e12820.

Puglielli L. Aging of the brain, neurotrophin signaling, and Alzheimer's disease: is IGF1-R the common culprit? *Neurobiol Aging*. 2008;29:795.

Chapter 57

Cognitive Changes in Normal and Pathologic Aging

Bonnie C. Sachs, Brenna Cholerton, Suzanne Craft

"Age does not depend upon years, but upon temperament and health. Some men are born old, and some never grow so."

Tyron Edwards

"A man is as old as his arteries."

Thomas Sydenham

The dogma that aging brings inevitable cognitive decline is being challenged by studies of the rapidly expanding oldest segment of our society, adults older than 60 years. Although some aspects of cognition are affected by aging, many changes in cognition previously considered the unavoidable consequence of brain senescence may instead result from incremental insults on brain function associated with aging-related medical conditions. The detection of such changes, which may stabilize or even reverse with appropriate intervention, and their differentiation from the cognitive changes associated with neurodegenerative disease or other neurologic disorders is a critical task. The primary goal of this chapter is to describe changes in various cognitive abilities that occur with normal aging and with common age-related medical and neurologic conditions.

THE EFFECTS OF NORMAL AGING ON COGNITIVE FUNCTION

General Intellectual Functioning

Age-related changes in intelligence are extremely variable, with notable interindividual differences. Overall, studies of aging have consistently shown that crystallized abilities (acquired knowledge and skills gained from experience) remain relatively intact with aging, while fluid intelligence, which involves flexible reasoning and problem-solving approaches, declines. This general pattern has been documented in both cross-sectional and longitudinal research designs. More specifically, it has been theorized that reductions in speed of information processing may account for many of the age-related changes noted in fluid intelligence. Below, we review the literature on the effects of normal aging on specific cognitive functions, summarized in **Table 57-1**.

Attention

Attention involves the ability to attend to, or focus on, one or more pieces of information long enough to register and make meaningful use of the data. Attention requires both

Learning Objectives

■ Describe the expected effects of aging on a variety of cognitive functions.

■ Identify age-related medical conditions that can negatively impact cognition.

■ Describe the key clinical features of Alzheimer disease (AD) dementia, as well as current primary tools used for diagnosis.

■ Describe the differences and similarities between AD dementia and other neurodegenerative diseases.

Key Clinical Points

1. Normal aging is associated with mild changes in circumscribed aspects of cognition; these changes are much less significant than cognitive effects associated with age-related medical conditions and neurodegenerative disease.

2. Physical disease is often linked with adverse cognitive consequences and increased risk for neurodegenerative disease; effective management of common age-related conditions may thus reduce the negative impact on cognition that is often considered an unavoidable outcome of aging.

3. Late-onset depression in older adults may be a symptom of prodromal neurodegenerative disease.

4. Certain medications can lead to adverse cognitive effects and even increased risk for dementia in older adults.

5. Alzheimer disease dementia is the eventual clinical manifestation of underlying pathology that is often present for years or decades before symptoms are noticed; thus,

(Continued)

(Cont.)

careful history-taking and new clinical and research tools may aid in early diagnosis.

6. Non-Alzheimer neurodegenerative diseases typically manifest with distinct cognitive and behavioral symptoms early in the disease process, although differentiation becomes more difficult with advancing dementia.

simple and complex immediate processing and provides a foundation for working memory and other cognitive functions. Sustained attention, or vigilance, entails attending to one type of information over a period of time. After controlling for reaction time and sensory changes, sustained attention and strategies for maintaining vigilance do not appear to change significantly with age. Divided attention, or the ability to concentrate on more than one piece of information at a time, may decline with age, although research in this area has produced mixed results. Increased distractibility (difficulty blocking out irrelevant stimuli), decreased use of effective strategies, and reduced processing speed may be responsible for some of the noted declines in divided attention. Pronounced impairment of attention is not typical of normal aging, however, and a complete evaluation of medical and psychosocial issues is warranted for individuals who demonstrate such changes. Attention can be negatively impacted by perceptual or sensory changes, illness, chronic pain, certain medications, and psychological disturbance (in particular, depression and anxiety), all of which are common in an older population. As the ability to effectively attend is a requisite for nearly all other cognitive functions, it is important to identify the cause/s of attentional impairment whenever possible and to implement any changes in medications or treatment that may help to resolve these problems.

Executive Functions

Executive functions include the ability to control, inhibit, and direct behavior, make meaningful inferences and appropriate judgments, plan and carry out tasks, manipulate multiple pieces of information at one time (working memory), complete complex motor sequences, and solve abstract and complex problems. Neuropsychological test performance on executive tasks declines slightly with age, and several current theories posit that deficits in working memory and executive function underlie many age-related changes in cognition. Neurocognitive tasks that require response inhibition, such as the Wisconsin Card Sort Test, Stroop Color Word Test, the Go-No-Go Task, and Brown–Peterson Distractor Test, may be affected.

Alternatively, many have suggested that a reduction in cognitive processing speed rather than executive function per se may be at least in part responsible for decreased performance on executive tasks. It should be noted that changes in the executive system that occur with normal aging are much less severe than the deficits associated with dysexecutive syndromes, including those caused by stroke, heavy and prolonged alcohol use, head injury, and some neurodegenerative diseases. In fact, successful aging appears to produce little impact on "real-world" executive functions requiring planning and executing multiple tasks. Thus, it is important to assess an individual's actual functional abilities in addition to performance on neuropsychological tests of executive function.

Memory

Memory changes are perhaps the most common cognitive complaints reported by older adults; reports of occasionally "walking into a room and forgetting why" are almost ubiquitous. Patients often wonder if their subjective concerns reflect normal age-related changes or some pathologic condition. For patients with a family history of Alzheimer disease (AD) or other forms of dementia, even minor memory failings can cause significant anxiety. One of the difficulties in answering such questions lies in the complex nature of the memory process. Different processes are invoked when learning new information (declarative memory), recalling prior life events (remote memory), recalling general knowledge not tied to a specific event (semantic memory), and remembering procedures for performing tasks such as riding a bicycle (procedural memory). In addition, some

TABLE 57-1 ■ COGNITIVE EFFECTS OF NORMAL AGING		
	PRESERVED COGNITION FUNCTIONS	**COGNITIVE FUNCTIONS SHOWING DECLINE**
General intellectual functioning	Crystallized, verbal intelligence	Fluid, nonverbal intelligence, speed of information processing
Attention	Sustained attention, primary attention span	Divided attention (possibly)
Executive function	"Real-world" executive functions	Novel executive tasks
Memory	Remote memory, procedural memory, semantic recall	Learning and recall of new information
Language	Comprehension, vocabulary, syntactic abilities	Spontaneous word finding, verbal fluency
Visuospatial	Construction, simple copy	Mental rotation, complex copy, mental assembly
Psychomotor functions		Reaction time

conditions result in modality-specific deficits, differentially affecting verbal or visual memory.

A number of models describe the different stages or processes involved in forming and recalling memories. One example, the modal model, describes memory processes in terms of sensory memory, short-term (working) memory, and long-term memory. First, when a patient senses and attends to a given stimulus, a large amount of information is briefly held in sensory memory. Information is then rehearsed or manipulated in short-term or working memory. Although many factors are involved in determining what information is transferred to long-term storage, sufficient rehearsal is a common requirement for successful transfer. Thus, it is clear that when a patient complains of memory changes, additional information is required to make sense of the problem.

Although it is true that some older adults continue to demonstrate memory performances comparable to young adults, on average even healthy older adults do show changes in some aspects of memory. For example, when a large group of healthy, nondemented older subjects were followed over a 7-year period, a general memory factor showed significant decline with time. Other studies have attempted to describe which aspects of memory change with healthy aging. In general, older adults without significant illness demonstrate increased difficulty learning new information compared to younger cohorts. When older adults are given repeated chances to practice learning new information, they demonstrate a slower learning curve and a lower total amount learned.

Although healthy older adults may retain slightly less information over time than younger adults, this effect is less pronounced than the slowed learning rate. For delayed memory tests, patients are generally asked to recall information 15 to 30 minutes after the initial presentation of the material. Although patients recall less information at the delay with age, the proportion of the information that they initially learned generally remains stable. In general, longitudinal studies of aging show only small declines in delayed memory with age, particularly on tests of visual memory. Some older adults also appear less likely to use cognitive strategies (eg, clustering information by category) to aid memory recall than younger subjects. This may be due to generational differences in learning style. However, it may be significant because the use of memory strategies reduces the age effect observed on free recall tests.

A number of memory processes do not appear to change with the typical aging process. Remote memory, or recall of events that occurred in the distant past, remains relatively intact, as does sensory memory. In addition, while older patients often have medical problems that limit physical movement, procedural memory appears to be unaffected by healthy aging. Lastly, semantic memory, such as vocabulary knowledge and general information about the world, remains largely unchanged by aging until very late in life.

Longitudinal studies have consistently shown that as groups age, the variability in cognitive performance increases. Overall, studies of healthy aging suggest that there are some statistically significant declines in memory in late life. However, the memory functions of patients who age successfully are typically adequate for the demands of independent living.

Language

Language abilities incorporate multiple levels of processing, and general language functions tend to remain relatively stable with increasing age. Some linguistic abilities, however, particularly those involving language output, show reliable declines in older adults. As with other cognitive functions, there are multiple potential intervening factors, including trauma, illness, and sensory disruption, that may lead to more severe changes in the language functions.

Language comprehension involves discerning the simple and complex rules of language and incorporating both visual and auditory information into a meaningful concept, and is generally associated with few age-related impairments. While hearing loss, which is common in older adults, does not affect language per se, it can impact the ability to successfully perceive spoken language and can mimic difficulties with true language comprehension. Therefore, this should be assessed and ruled out as a contributing factor in older adults complaining of comprehension difficulties.

The ability to recognize basic word structure and word representation is typically measured using "lexical-decision" tasks (in which letters are rapidly presented and the person is asked to identify whether or not it is a word) and simple word reading tasks. While some studies have suggested an inverse relationship between performance on these tasks and age, it is generally believed that such changes are the result of decreased reaction time and processing speed rather than the ability to comprehend word structure and meaning. In addition, there is some indication that the level of lexical processing changes slightly with age, in that older adults tend to rely more on word recognition than do younger adults, while ignoring other factors such as word length. Phonological understanding of language does not appear to change significantly with age, although hearing loss may appear to reduce auditory comprehension. Overall, it is generally accepted that language comprehension remains relatively intact throughout the lifespan.

Basic syntactic abilities also do not appear to change significantly with advancing age, although minor repetitions, longer pauses, and an increased use of pronouns and other vague words while speaking have been noted. Additionally, a recent longitudinal study suggests a decline in spoken grammatical complexity during the eighth decade of life. The authors note, however, that there is high interindividual variability throughout the lifespan in terms of syntactic aptitude.

Semantic abilities require aptitude with naming and retrieval of long-stored information. There is a steady increase in vocabulary knowledge throughout middle-adulthood, and such knowledge typically remains stable in the later years. A frequent complaint from older adults, however, involves the "tip-of-the-tongue" phenomenon, in which there is a notable struggle with spontaneous word finding. In contrast to the dysnomia that often accompanies dementia, however, such changes appear to result primarily from difficulties retrieving rather than storing information, and thus there is usually a marked improvement when cues are given. Tasks of verbal fluency, which are most akin to demands required in fluid, conversational speech, also appear to change somewhat with age. Multiple research findings support a decrease in semantic fluency ("name all the animals you can"), while phonemic fluency ("tell me as many words as you can that begin with the letter F") generally remains stable. Younger adults tend to produce more words and change categories more frequently than do older adults on semantic fluency tasks, while older adults may generate the same amount of words but more "clusters" on tasks of phonemic fluency. Thus, older adults likely rely more on structural word knowledge than on word meaning.

Visuospatial Skills

Visuospatial skills are commonly tested by constructional tasks in which patients are asked to draw figures or assemble objects. In general, as patients age, they become slower at completing visuospatial tasks. However, as noted previously, one of the more consistent findings in the field is that normal aging is associated with general slowing of psychomotor and cognitive speed. Therefore, performance on tests of visuospatial functioning is often confounded by generalized slowing. Some studies have attempted to separate the effects of the two domains. For instance, after controlling for processing speed and executive functioning, the effects of age on the commonly used Wechsler Block Design test were dramatically reduced. Similarly, an 11-year follow-up of older adult subjects analyzed both speed and quality of performance (errors) on a parallelogram test. As expected, speed declined with age, but the quality of the performance actually improved significantly. This body of literature suggests that declining speed contributes to some of the findings that report visuospatial processing deficits in normal aging.

Speed does not appear to account for all of the visuospatial changes observed in healthy aging, however. Mental rotations of objects or spatial coordinates, accurate copy of complex geometric designs, and mental assembly of objects typically worsen with age even when unlimited time is allowed to perform such tasks. Furthermore, when speed is included in scoring, some studies have reported disproportionate slowing on visuospatial tasks compared to verbal tasks. Overall, some studies may exaggerate the visuospatial decline observed in normal aging because of the role speed plays in many tasks used to assess visuospatial function. However, abstract spatial abilities may decline with age, even when speed is controlled.

Psychomotor Functions

Age-associated slowing in reaction time, related to both a general reduction in the speed of cognitive processing and to changes in peripheral motor skills, has been consistently reported. Age-related declines in brain dopamine activity and periventricular white matter changes may be associated with reduced cognitive speed and basic motor functions. As a result, performance on tests requiring speed and quick reaction to stimuli are likely to decline. As previously noted, increased psychomotor speed and reaction time are believed to underlie many of the age-related changes noted on neurocognitive testing, particularly tasks involving perceptual speed, attention, and working memory. In addition, changes in psychomotor functions can be associated with changes in real-world tasks, such as driving. As a result, it is important to monitor the manner in which physical changes are impacting an individual's level of safety in performing daily activities.

COGNITIVE EFFECTS OF COMMON AGE-RELATED MEDICAL CONDITIONS

In the following section, cognitive symptoms associated with common diseases affecting older adults are reviewed. Prevalence of common medical conditions that may impact cognition in older adults are presented in **Figure 57-1**. A summary of cognitive symptoms associated with common medical conditions is presented in **Table 57-2**.

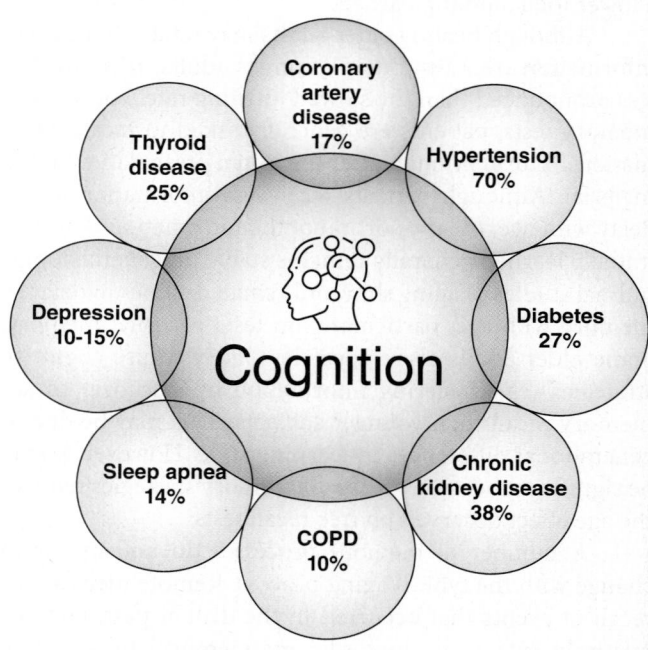

FIGURE 57-1. Prevalence of common medical conditions associated with cognitive impairment among US adults aged 65 and older. Data for most diseases obtained from cdc.gov. (Data from Diab N, Daya NR, Juraschek SP, et al. Prevalence and risk factors of thyroid dysfunction in older adults in the community. *Sci Rep.* 2019;9[1]:13156.)

TABLE 57-2 ■ POSSIBLE COGNITIVE EFFECTS OF COMMON AGE-RELATED MEDICAL CONDITIONS

	SYMPTOM COURSE	INCREASED RISK FOR DEVELOPING NEURODEGENERATIVE DISEASE?	MEMORY	ATTENTION	EXECUTIVE FUNCTIONS	LANGUAGE	VISUOSPATIAL FUNCTION	PSYCHOMOTOR FUNCTION	BEHAVIOR
Coronary artery disease	Can begin with subtle symptoms even early in the disease. Decline is variable depending upon cognitive domain. Limited evidence for improvement with cardiac rehabilitation, including exercise	AD, VaD, PD	Verbal memory deficits possible	Reduced attention occurs early	Variable, reduced reasoning and other executive deficits	Reduced verbal fluency and vocabulary	Visuospatial function may show greater longitudinal decline than other domains	Reduced psychomotor function occurs early	Associated with depression, anxiety
Cardiac surgery	Symptom onset immediate after surgery, often with improvement during the first year postsurgery. Risk for additional decline in some patients	AD, VaD	Verbal and visual memory deficits possible several years after surgery	Reduced attention	Variable	No significant changes noted	May lead to impaired visual organization and construction	Reduced reaction time, general slowing	Depression common after surgery
Hypertension	May improve with antihypertensive treatment and/or lifestyle changes	AD, VaD	Verbal and visual recall and recognition deficits in some patients	Reduced attention and vigilance	Impairment in working memory and other executive function	Reduced verbal fluency	May lead to impaired visual organization and construction; more likely with comorbid diabetes	Reduced reaction time, general slowing	Variable
Type 2 diabetes mellitus	Slow progression. May improve with oral antidiabetic agents and/or lifestyle changes	AD, VaD, PD	Verbal memory impairment related to deficits in encoding new information	Reduced complex attention, simple attention variable	Impairments in abstract reasoning and concept formation	No significant changes noted	Variable, more likely with comorbid hypertension	Reduced reaction time, general slowing	Depression common

(Continued)

TABLE 57-2 ■ POSSIBLE COGNITIVE EFFECTS OF COMMON AGE-RELATED MEDICAL CONDITIONS (CONTINUED)

	SYMPTOM COURSE	INCREASED RISK FOR DEVELOPING NEURODEGENERATIVE DISEASE?	MEMORY	ATTENTION	EXECUTIVE FUNCTIONS	LANGUAGE	VISUOSPATIAL FUNCTION	PSYCHOMOTOR FUNCTION	BEHAVIOR
Chronic kidney disease	Often improves with renal transplantation or dialysis	VaD, AD, PD	Immediate and delayed memory impaired in moderate and end stages of disease	Reduced attention in early stage of disease	Reduced reasoning, concept formation, and other executive functions in moderate stage of disease	Language may decline throughout the disease	Visuospatial impairment in end stage of disease	Processing speed declines in early stage of disease	Associated with depression, anxiety
Chronic obstructive pulmonary disease	May improve with oxygen therapy	AD, VaD	Verbal and visual memory deficits	Reduced attention	Impairment in general executive function	May have impaired verbal fluency, naming	May have impaired general visuospatial/construction	Reduced reaction time, general slowing	Depression common
Sleep apnea	Stronger association in younger and middle-aged adults. May improve with continuous positive airway pressure	AD, VaD	Verbal and visual memory deficits	Reduced attention	Impairment in general executive function	May have impaired verbal fluency, naming	May have impaired general visuospatial/construction	Reduced reaction time, general slowing	Depression and irritability related to sleep disruption and hypoxia
Nutritional deficiency	Mixed reports with supplementation; effects of low vitamin B$_{12}$ and vitamin D deficiency may persist	AD, Wernicke-Korsakoff syndrome	Variable depending upon nutrient deficit	Variable depending upon nutrient deficit	Variable depending upon nutrient deficit	Variable depending upon nutrient deficit	Variable depending upon nutrient deficit	Variable depending upon nutrient deficit	Variable
Thyroid disease	May improve with thyroid treatment, although some patients do not return to baseline	AD	Recall deficits, intact recognition	Variable.	Variable	No significant changes noted	Reduced visuospatial function	Reduced reaction time, general slowing	Depression

AD, Alzheimer disease; PD, Parkinson disease; VaD, vascular dementia.

Cardiovascular Disease

Cardiovascular disease increases risk for developing both debilitating cognitive decline due to large vessel stroke and/or vascular dementia (VaD) and milder cognitive deficits. While much of the cognitive dysfunction associated with cardiovascular disease can be discussed in terms of its effects on the cerebrovasculature and resulting vascular cognitive impairment (VCI), here we focus on independent cardiovascular disease–associated risk factors for cognitive decline in older adults, including the effects of coronary artery disease, cardiac surgery, and hypertension.

Coronary artery disease Subtle impairments in cognition can be seen early in the disease, including among patients diagnosed at midlife. Specific impairments have been reported across measures of reasoning and other executive deficits, verbal memory, vocabulary, semantic and phonemic fluency, visuospatial function, and global cognition. Increased length and greater severity of coronary artery disease are consistently associated with reduced cognitive performance even in the absence of strokes or obvious cerebrovascular disease. Indeed, among older adults without a history of stroke enrolled in the Cardiovascular Health Study, there was a greater than 60% prevalence of cognitive impairment. Factors associated with cognitive impairment among patients with coronary artery disease include cardiac surgery, presence of an apolipoprotein E (*APOE*) ε4 allele, presence and degree of heart failure, use of concurrent anticholinergic medications, hormone disruptions (eg, thyroid), and elevated inflammatory biomarkers (eg, interleukin-6, C-reactive protein, brain-derived neurotrophic factor).

Cardiac surgery In addition to the risk of immediate postoperative delirium following cardiac surgery, postoperative cognitive decline (POCD) after cardiac surgery is reported in 30% to 70% of patients at the time of hospital discharge. Factors that increase the risk of POCD include older age, cerebrovascular disease, underlying neurodegenerative disease, cardiopulmonary bypass time, manipulation of the ascending aorta, and cerebral hyperthermia. A wide range of cognitive deficits, including problems with attention and concentration, processing speed, memory, and visuospatial function, have been noted in patients immediately following surgery. Several reports suggest that postoperative cognitive function stabilizes or even improves after a period of approximately 12 months in those patients who demonstrate initial decline. However, the prevalence of cognitive dysfunction remains relatively high at 12-month follow-up (15–25%), and longitudinal data suggest that these patients are at higher risk for continued cognitive deterioration and multiple dementia types (including AD, VaD, and mixed dementias). Post-CABG neurocognitive status is related to overall quality of life, and current recommendations underscore the importance of closely monitoring cognitive status in the years following cardiac surgery.

Hypertension Essential hypertension is associated with risk of cognitive impairment independent of secondary disease or organ damage. Uncontrolled hypertension may impact cognition and increase dementia risk via several mechanisms, including arterial stiffening, inflammation in the blood vessels, disruption of the blood–brain barrier, development of subcortical white matter lesions, adverse impacts on cerebral blood flow, and disrupted energy substrate delivery. Potential cognitive effects of primary hypertension include reductions in mental status, slowed reaction time, reduced attention and vigilance, weakened executive function, poor verbal fluency, and impaired visual organization and construction. Memory functions, including spatial recall, verbal recall, and word recognition, may also be affected in some hypertensive patients. Beyond effects on specific cognitive functions, hypertension, particularly at mid-life, is a significant risk factor for later dementia. Thus hypertension has been identified as one of the major modifiable risk factors for dementia. Treating hypertension with medication and/or lifestyle changes may reduce dementia risk, although evidence regarding the use of specific antihypertensives to prevent later cognitive impairment is mixed. Interestingly, blood pressure often *declines* in the period immediately preceding the onset of AD, and it has been suggested that low blood pressure in older adults may compromise brain function as a result of hypoperfusion. In addition, sudden aggressive lowering of blood pressure in older adults with long-term hypertension may interact with their chronically upregulated cerebral vascular resistance and induce cerebral hypoperfusion. Thus careful monitoring of blood pressure and gradual titration of medication regimens is of particular importance. Additional interest has been focused on the question of whether particular treatment methods may confer particular protective effects on cognition. Additional controlled randomized trials are needed to answer this question.

Type 2 Diabetes Mellitus

Much attention has been given to the rampant epidemic of type 2 diabetes mellitus (T2DM) in older adults, a trend thought to be largely attributable to obesity and physical inactivity. Current prevalence estimates in the United States suggest that between 20% and 30% of adults older than 65 years are afflicted with T2DM. The negative impact of T2DM on multiple medical systems is well known. The clear impact of T2DM on cognitive function in older adults is less-widely known, but accruing evidence demonstrates that these patients show pronounced impairment in attention and verbal memory when compared to healthy age-matched adults and accelerated cognitive decline over time. Complex attentional impairment is most common, involving the inability to handle multiple streams of information or attend to information in the face of competing stimuli. Verbal memory deficits typically affect the ability to encode new verbal information. The magnitude of such impairment may vary from subtle subjective complaints to pronounced impairment that interferes with daily activities and may interfere with the patient's ability to adhere to complex treatment regimens. The mechanisms causing attentional and memory impairments are likely multifactorial and include vascular factors, as described earlier, in addition to the potential negative effects of hyperglycemia and glucose toxicity thought to cause oxidative injury. Notably, successful treatment of T2DM has been shown to improve cognitive function. Recent work also suggests that insulin resistance, independent of hyperglycemia, may have negative consequences on brain systems mediating memory and attention, suggesting that therapeutic strategies focused on improving insulin sensitivity may be preferable to those focused on augmenting insulin levels. The importance of treating and preferably preventing T2DM has been underscored by its associated risk for various forms of neurodegenerative disease, including AD, VaD, and Parkinson disease (PD).

Chronic Kidney Disease

Cognitive impairment among patients with chronic kidney disease (CKD) is quite common, with prevalence estimates ranging from 10% to 40% depending upon length and severity of disease. CKD patients perform more poorly than controls on tests of orientation, attention, abstract reasoning and concept formation, executive function, memory, language, and global cognition. Such changes can occur early in the disease, but progress at different rates depending on the domain assessed. For example, language may continue to decline, while other domains remain stable for long periods of time. The underlying cause of cognitive impairments in CKD patients is not entirely understood currently. Cerebrovascular disease is a common comorbidity of CKD and thus likely to underlie some of the cognitive impairments associated with the disease. However, as cognition often improves or stabilizes following dialysis and/or renal transplantation, underlying vascular disease is most likely not the sole culprit. Rather, it has been suggested that dialysis-related factors (hemodynamic instability, cerebromicrobleeds), uremic metabolites, anemia, and depression may all potentially impact cognitive function among those with CKD.

Chronic Obstructive Pulmonary Disease

Emphysema and chronic bronchitis obstruct airflow, resulting in hypoxemia and hypercapnia. Cognitive dysfunction is commonly observed in chronic obstructive pulmonary disease (COPD), although the specific skills affected appear to be broad and diffuse. Deficits in verbal and visual memory, attention, abstraction, psychomotor speed, information processing speed, and global cognition have all been reported. These changes in cognition appear to be due to hypoxemia. The decrease in arterial oxygen partial pressure correlates with neuropsychological impairments, and most studies indicate that oxygen therapy results in modest improvements in cognition. However, a diagnosis

of COPD, especially at midlife, does increase risk for later life mild cognitive impairment (MCI) and dementia.

Obstructive Sleep Apnea

The prevalence of obstructive sleep apnea (OSA) increases in geriatric populations. Cognitive changes in OSA can be diverse but may include reduced performance on measures of global cognition, attention, concentration, processing speed, working memory, executive functioning, and verbal and visual learning and memory. Interestingly, the association between cognitive impairment and OSA is stronger in younger and middle-aged adults. In older adults, OSA may have weaker or no association with specific cognitive impairments; however, there is increased risk over time for MCI, AD, and VaD. Cognitive deficits may be related to severity of hypoxia, hypersomnolence, or comorbid conditions. In addition, recent evidence suggests a possible association between OSA and presence of AD biomarkers. Continuous positive airway pressure treatment may improve aspects of cognitive functioning in some patients.

Nutritional Deficiency

Older adults are at considerable risk for nutritional deficiencies as a consequence of poor diet and malabsorption syndromes. Much research in this area has focused on deficiencies of B vitamins, antioxidants, and vitamin D.

Lower B_{12} levels and folate are associated with reduced cognition and increased risk of AD, although the evidence is mixed. B vitamins play an important role in homocysteine metabolism. Homocysteine is an independent risk factor for cerebrovascular and cardiovascular disease. In patients with both AD and VaD, elevated plasma homocysteine levels have been reported, and recent studies suggest that homocysteine levels are related to cognitive function in normal aging. Reduced performance on tests of mental status, nonverbal pattern abstraction, construction, and processing speed are reported in patients with high plasma homocysteine. Given that plasma homocysteine and folate levels are inversely related, it is conceivable that such cognitive deficits are related to reduced folate rather than to increased homocysteine per se. Recent data suggest, however, that homocysteine increases the risk for cognitive decline independent of both folate levels and other vascular risk factors. In addition, although supplementation of vitamin B is shown to reduce homocysteine levels in older adults, concurrent benefits on cognition have not been widely reported. Nonetheless, among older adults with cognitive deficits, routine laboratories and repletion of B vitamins are recommended when applicable.

There has been much debate about the potential protective effects of antioxidants in dementia. For example, both deleterious and protective effects of vitamin E have been reported. Overall there is little evidence that vitamin E supplementation reduces risk for cognitive decline. A large-scale clinical trial, however, showed reduced functional decline with high-dose vitamin E supplementation (2000

IU per day) for mild-to-moderate AD. Although these results appear promising, additional work is needed to clarify the risk-to-benefit ratio for vitamin E supplementation.

More recently, concerns about vitamin D deficiency have been raised in relation to increased risk for a number of negative health outcomes, including cognitive decline and dementia. Meta-analyses indicate associations between vitamin D deficiency and worse performance on tests measuring global cognition, visuospatial abilities, processing speed, and attention, while memory skills appear to be less affected. Unfortunately, vitamin D supplementation has not been strongly associated with improved cognition in older adults to date.

Thyroid Disease

Both hypo- and hyperthyroidism are associated with potential adverse cognitive changes, particularly in younger and middle-aged adults. Hypothyroidism may increase risk for dementia, as well as result in specific deficits in visuospatial skills, psychomotor speed, and memory. There is some evidence that the memory deficits associated with hypothyroid conditions are related to retrieval rather than immediate recall or learning; thus, disproportionately better performance may be observed on tests of cued or recognition memory than on free recall tests. Thyroid replacement therapy frequently improves cognitive functioning, although skills may not return to baseline levels in some patients. Hyperthyroid may also increase dementia risk, and related cognitive symptoms may include deficits in attention, executive functioning, and memory. Interestingly, dementia risk from hyper- and hypothyroid conditions does not appear to extend to adults in the older age ranges (eg, 75 and older). There is also some evidence for sex differences, such that a stronger relationship between thyroid disease and dementia risk in women as compared to men has been reported. Overall, however, thyroid hormone abnormalities occur in a large proportion of patients with dementia and thus should be routinely monitored as a treatable contributor to cognitive decline.

Depression

Depression is an increasingly common problem in older adults, with prevalence estimates ranging from 11% to 30%. Situational risk factors for depression in older age include the loss of social support, death of family members and close friends, changing social roles, illness, and physical limitations. Depressive symptoms, including lack of initiation, impaired executive function, cognitive slowing, poor attention and concentration, and mild memory impairment, can mimic early signs of dementia and may potentially lead to misdiagnosis and/or lack of appropriate medical intervention. As depression is a potentially reversible cause of cognitive impairment, the differential diagnosis between depression and dementia is vital when evaluating older patients. Factors that are useful in discriminating between depression and dementia include the clinical course of symptoms, relationship to a specific crisis or stressful event, history of previous psychiatric problems, quality of effort, and level of impaired processing on cognitive evaluation.

Late-onset depression is also an independent risk factor for the development of neurodegenerative diseases, including AD, VaD, and Lewy body disease (LBD). Depressive symptoms may thus represent a preclinical phase of progressive dementia in some patients. In patients with early cognitive loss, depressive symptoms may represent realistic self-evaluation of such decline and/or may coincide with actual changes in neuroendocrinologic status. In the absence of predisposing situational factors, late-onset affective disorders are quite rare. Thus, cognitive ability and independent functional status must be carefully evaluated in older patients, and an in-depth qualitative analysis of depressive symptoms may be useful. For example, major depressive disorder is associated with a range of affective, cognitive, and vegetative symptoms, while depressive symptoms in early dementia are more likely to include cognitive and motivational symptoms (eg, poor concentration, lack of initiation) in the relative absence of central affective disturbance. Continued monitoring of the cognitive status of depressed older patients is essential in order to rule out progressive cognitive decline.

Medications

A number of medications have the potential to cause both subtle cognitive changes and alterations in overall mental status, particularly in older adults. Medications known to adversely affect cognitive status include opiates and opioid-like analgesics, benzodiazepines, anticonvulsants, antipsychotic and antidepressant medications, antiparkinsonian agents, central nervous system stimulants, antihistamines and decongestants, and certain cardiovascular medications. Anticholinergic medications, used to treat a variety of conditions including insomnia, bladder spasms, gastrointestinal disorders, dizziness, and others, have been linked to an increased risk for dementia in older adults in a large-scale prospective community-based study. Despite this finding, these drugs are widely prescribed in older adult populations. A variety of other medications, particularly those that readily cross the blood–brain barrier, may impact cognitive function in certain individuals. In addition, drug interactions in older adults can lead to more serious physiologic and cognitive consequences than those observed in younger adults, and adverse medication interactions are more likely to occur in an older population. As a result, changes in cognitive status must be carefully evaluated in light of a patient's current medication profile.

Delirium

Older adults are at a significantly increased risk for developing delirium, particularly following surgery or in response to medication changes or interactions. Delirium is a reversible condition that can be distinguished from most neurodegenerative diseases by a rapid onset of symptoms that include significant disorientation and disturbance in consciousness, reduced awareness of the environment, and attention deficits. While recent memory is generally impaired, altered consciousness is the primary indicator of delirium. Hallucinations, delusional thinking, and other disturbed thought processes may also be present. Delirium usually resolves quickly, but may persist for several weeks. It should also be noted that postoperative delirium may signify the presence of a beginning dementia. A primary concern is to identify and treat the underlying cause while providing a supportive and nonthreatening environment for the patient.

NEURODEGENERATIVE DISEASE

The following section reviews the cognitive and behavioral profiles associated with common neurodegenerative disorders (**Table 57-3**). Early identification of such disorders, many of which are diagnosed solely on these parameters, has become increasingly important due to potential therapies that may delay disease progression.

Dementia Due to Alzheimer Disease

AD dementia, the most prevalent of the primary neurodegenerative disorders, is the clinical manifestation of underlying AD neuropathology, primarily the accumulation of β-amyloid protein and neurofibrillary tangles leading to neuronal loss and synaptic degeneration. Diagnostic criteria by the National Institutes on Aging and the Alzheimer's Association (NIA/AA) initially put forth in 2011 and updated in 2018 recognize AD as a continuum, with underlying neuropathologic processes often beginning 20 years or more before the onset of clinical dementia symptoms. These criteria allow use of biomarkers that reflect these processes, alongside supporting clinical information, for use in early differential diagnosis. Currently, cerebrospinal fluid (CSF), β-amyloid and phosphorylated tau, and imaging studies (amyloid or tau positron emission tomography [PET]) may be used to determine the presence of β-amyloid deposition and/or aggregated tau to provide diagnostic evidence for or against AD as the underlying pathology, and anatomic magnetic resonance imaging (MRI), fluorodeoxyglucose (FDG)-PET, and CSF total tau may be incorporated as markers of severity of neurodegeneration. Currently in development, several blood-based biomarkers may serve as useful diagnostic tools in the future, the most promising of which is plasma phosphorylated tau181, which is closely associated with CSF phosphorylated tau and tau PET, and may be useful in both staging of AD and in differentiating between AD and non-AD dementia types. In the absence of current availability of such tools, however, conventional diagnostic criteria are considered to be reasonably accurate, particularly when the evaluation is comprehensive and includes a complete medical and psychosocial history, medical evaluation, and neurocognitive testing.

The NIA/AA criteria for AD dementia require (1) that the patient meets criteria for dementia (cognitive symptoms that interfere with independently completing daily activities [managing medications or finances, driving, cooking, etc] that occur within at least two cognitive domains, represent a decline from previous function, and are not better explained by delirium or psychiatric disturbance), (2) evidence/report of an insidious onset, and (3) worsening cognition by report or observation of the patient, informant, or clinician. The initial cognitive symptoms may be amnestic or nonamnestic to account for variants that present with deficits in cognitive domains other than memory, such as posterior cortical atrophy (which presents with initial visuospatial deficits) or language-predominant forms, though amnestic presentations are by far the most common. The term "probable AD" should not be used if another medical/neurologic disease could account for the symptoms. "Possible" AD dementia may be diagnosed if the symptom history is atypical or unclear or if there is a mixed dementia picture.

Patient history A complete medical and psychosocial history is a vital component of any dementia assessment. Such a history should be obtained both from the patient and a reliable informant, preferably someone who has regular contact with the patient and who has an adequate opportunity to observe their daily functional abilities. Typically, a patient in the earliest stages of AD will not exhibit deficits in basic self-care activities, such as feeding or bathing. However, more complex daily tasks, including driving, managing finances, shopping, and other chores and activities, are likely to be affected. A gradually progressive course and insidious onset of cognitive symptoms is a hallmark of AD, and thus a careful history regarding the nature and timing of symptom onset and progression must be obtained. An inventory of all current medical and psychiatric concerns, family history, past major medical and mental health problems, and medications must be evaluated in order to rule out conditions that may be either causing cognitive problems or exacerbating their expression.

Medical examination An important goal of the medical evaluation is to exclude the presence of medical conditions that may be responsible for the observed cognitive deficits. It is critical to investigate potentially reversible causes of dementia such as uncontrolled liver or kidney disease, adverse reactions to medications, and delirium. Laboratory blood tests, such as complete blood count, complete metabolic panel, and B_{12} levels, can aid in ruling out systemic illnesses, vitamin deficiency, or organ malfunction. Structural brain scans, such as CT or MRI, are used to evaluate major cerebrovascular events, tumors, normal pressure hydrocephalus (NPH), and other neurologic conditions, while functional brain scans (eg, PET) can identify patterns of activity that may be useful in classifying dementia type. As noted, ruling out the possible contribution of psychiatric conditions, such as major depression, is also a critical piece of this examination.

TABLE 57-3 ■ EARLY COGNITIVE SYMPTOMS ASSOCIATED WITH DIFFERENT DEMENTIA TYPES

| | SYMPTOM ONSET | PROGRESSION RATE | MEMORY | | | | ATTENTION | EXECUTIVE FUNCTIONS | LANGUAGE | VISUOSPATIAL FUNCTION | PSYCHOMOTOR FUNCTION | BEHAVIOR |
			RECENT	RECOGNITION INTACT?	REMOTE INTACT?	PROCEDURAL INTACT?						
ALZHEIMER DISEASE (AD)												
	Insidious	Steady, gradual	Significantly impaired declarative recall	N	Y	Y	Intact primary span; impaired selective/divided attention	Mildly impaired working memory, response inhibition, general problem solving	Semantic organizational abilities significantly impaired, mild anomia	Simple construction intact, complex visual reasoning impaired	If present, symptoms are mild	Depression common
LEWY BODY DISEASES												
PD/PDD	Insidious	Varied	Possible deficits	Variable	Y	May be deficits due to impaired automation	Intact primary attention span, impaired selective/divided attention; fluctuations	Difficulty planning/shifting set	Verbal fluency, mechanical aspects of speech impaired	May be impaired	Resting tremor, bradykinesia, rigidity, postural instability, shuffling gait, impaired processing speed	Depression common, may exhibit hallucinations/delusions, less common than DLB
DLB	Insidious	Steady, gradual	Usually less impaired than AD	Variable	Y	Y	Significant fluctuations in attention	Variable	Variable; fluency may be impaired	Impaired construction, copy, visuospatial planning and problem solving	May exhibit a range of parkinsonian symptoms	Hallucinations, delusions, depression
VASCULAR DEMENTIA (VaD)												
	May be insidious or acute	Stepwise or gradual	Possible deficits	Varies	Y	Y	Intact primary span; impaired selective/divided attention	Significantly more impaired than AD and relative to performance on verbal memory tasks	Verbal fluency impaired	Relatively preserved, although may be affected by executive impairments	Slowing, possible discrete motor problems depending on distribution of vascular changes	Depression common

(*Continued*)

PART III

GERIATRIC CONDITIONS

TABLE 57-3 ■ EARLY COGNITIVE SYMPTOMS ASSOCIATED WITH DIFFERENT DEMENTIA TYPES (CONTINUED)

| | SYMPTOM ONSET | PROGRESSION RATE | MEMORY | | | | | ATTENTION | EXECUTIVE FUNCTIONS | LANGUAGE | VISUOSPATIAL FUNCTION | PSYCHOMOTOR FUNCTION | BEHAVIOR |
			RECENT	RECOGNITION INTACT?	REMOTE INTACT?	PROCEDURAL INTACT?						
FRONTOTEMPORAL LOBAR DEGENERATION (FTLD)													
Behavioral variant FTLD (FTLDbv)	Insidious	Steady, rapid	Relatively preserved	Y	Y	Y	Intact primary span; impaired selective/ divided attention	Impaired across a range of executive functions	Verbal fluency impaired	Relatively preserved, although may be affected by executive impairments	May exhibit ideational apraxia	Significant behavioral changes, may include behavioral disinhibition, apathy, loss of empathy/ sympathy, hyperorality
Primary progressive aphasia (PPA)	Insidious	Steady, varied	Preserved recall, may score poorly on verbal memory tests	Y	Y	Y	Preserved	Preserved	*Nonfluent:* poor articulation, dysarthria, relatively preserved comprehension; *Logopenic:* anomia, impaired repetition; *Semantic:* impaired comprehension, anomia, intact speech rate & prosody	In semantic dementia, may have visual agnosia	*Nonfluent PPA:* buccofacial apraxia	Changes unlikely

Progressive supranuclear palsy (PSP)	Insidious	Steady, gradual	Mild impairment, less than AD	Variable	Y	Y	Impaired selective/divided attention	Impaired across a range of executive functions	Verbal fluency impaired	May be impaired	Vertical supranuclear gaze palsy, postural instability	Apathy, disinhibition
Cortico-basal degeneration syndrome (CBS)	Insidious	Steady, gradual	Variable, may be severe	Variable	Y	Possible impairment	Impaired selective/divided attention	Impaired across a range of executive functions	May have a variety of language disturbances	Possible	Asymmetric motor symptoms, alien limb syndrome	A variety of neuropsychiatric disturbances possible
ALCOHOL-RELATED DEMENTIAS												
Persistent alcohol dementia	Deficits persist after d/c alcohol use	May worsen over time	Impairment on recall, not more than other functions	Variable	Y	Y	Impaired sustained attention	Abstraction, mental flexibility, perseveration, confabulation, impaired judgment, reduced ability to care for self	Preserved	Visual scanning, visuospatial organization impaired	May exhibit cerebellar tremor, impaired gait	Apathy, depression
Wernicke-Korsakoff syndrome	Acute (initial phase)	Steady, gradual (chronic phase)	Significant impairment on declarative recall relative to other deficits (semantic memory spared)	N	N	Variable	Impaired across all attentional functions	Similar profile to persistent alcohol dementia	Preserved	Visual scanning, visuospatial organization impaired	Impaired gait, abnormal reflexes, other movement abnormalities	Personality change prominent feature, inappropriate behavior
PRION DISEASE												
	Insidious	Steady, rapid	Nonspecific impairments reported	Y	Y	Y	Non-specific impairments reported	Reduced problem-solving ability	Generally preserved	Generally intact	May exhibit impaired reflexes and coordination	Apathy, emotional lability, impaired sleep, appetite loss

(Continued)

TABLE 57-3 ■ EARLY COGNITIVE SYMPTOMS ASSOCIATED WITH DIFFERENT DEMENTIA TYPES (*CONTINUED*)

| | SYMPTOM ONSET | PROGRESSION RATE | MEMORY | | | | ATTENTION | EXECUTIVE FUNCTIONS | LANGUAGE | VISUOSPATIAL FUNCTION | PSYCHOMOTOR FUNCTION | BEHAVIOR |
			RECENT	RECOGNITION INTACT?	REMOTE INTACT?	PROCEDURAL INTACT?						
NORMAL PRESSURE HYDROCEPHALUS (NPH)												
	Insidious	Varied, potentially reversible	Not prominently impaired	Y	Y	Y	Primary deficits in attention	Nonspecific impairments in executive function reported	Generally preserved	Generally intact	Wide-based gait or other balance disturbance, urinary incontinence	May present with a confusional state
HIV-ASSOCIATED NEUROCOGNITIVE DISORDER (HAND)												
	May occur at any time; severe dementia rare with antiretroviral drugs	Varied	Variable	Variable	Y	Y	Nonspecific impairments reported	Nonspecific impairments in executive function reported	Generally preserved	Generally intact	Slow, loss of coordination	Depression common
NEUROSYPHILIS												
	May occur at any time; severe dementia only with advanced disease	Varied, potentially reversible	Variable	Variable	Y	Y	Variable	Variable	Generally preserved	Generally intact	May be ataxic	Hallucinations, delusions, personality change, mood disturbance

DLB, dementia with Lewy bodies; PD, Parkinson disease; PDD, Parkinson disease with dementia.

Neuropsychological assessment Neuropsychological assessment of cognitive function not only provides confirmatory evidence for cognitive impairment but may also aid in disease staging and clarification of dementia type. Given the extensive variation in rate of AD progression between patients, successive neuropsychological examinations early in the disease can also provide information regarding an individual's rate of progression and remaining cognitive strengths, which is essential for advising patients and family about possible safety issues that arise. Perhaps one of the most valuable assets of neuropsychological evaluation is the sensitivity of the tests to detect early cognitive decline. While there has been debate regarding the usefulness of providing an early AD diagnosis, it is generally accepted that such a diagnosis will allow the patient to avail themselves of current and emerging therapies, as well as to make decisions regarding health care, finances, and legal issues while they still have the capacity to do so. In a typical neuropsychological evaluation, patients are given tests that sample a variety of domains of cognitive function. Results are compared to normative data based on age, and often education, and also to an individual's estimated premorbid abilities (based on educational and occupational background and performance on tests that tend to remain stable over time). Pattern analysis of test results, in combination with data from the patient history and medical evaluation, is then used to generate diagnostic possibilities. The following sections discuss cognitive impairment patterns typical in patients with AD.

Memory The hallmark of AD, and most often the first cognitive symptom of the disorder, is anterograde amnesia, evidenced by difficulty with learning and retaining new information, which is often described as "rapid forgetting." Deficits are noted in declarative memory as a result of prominent impairment in information encoding, retrieval, and in particular, storage of new material. Patients are likely to exhibit deficits in recent episodic recall, and they or their caregivers often report they misplace items, forget recent events or conversations, and frequently repeat questions or statements. In contrast to impaired episodic recall and difficulty learning new information, procedural memory is rarely impaired, and remote memory remains relatively intact until later stages of the disease.

In order to adequately evaluate short-term memory loss and establish a pattern of impaired learning and memory storage or retention, neuropsychological evaluations include tests of both immediate and delayed verbal and visual recall. While cognitive screeners such as the Folstein Mini-Mental State Examination (MMSE) and Montreal Cognitive Assessment (MoCA) assess general mental status and orientation, they are not adequate for a comprehensive understanding of memory impairment. To satisfactorily assess a person's true memory ability, tasks that are high in cognitive demand, that exceed the primary memory span (such as story recall and list learning tasks that include at least 10 items), and that have a recognition component are recommended. On neuropsychological examination, verbal and visual free immediate and delayed recall and recognition are significantly impaired in patients with AD relative to same-age peers, and patients typically exhibit a high number of intrusion errors and repetitions. Semantic recall is generally the most predominantly impaired, and thus verbal recall tasks are often the most sensitive to early memory loss.

Attention and Executive Function Certain aspects of attention and concentration are often impaired early in the disease process, and recent research has supported that it may in fact be one of the earliest abilities affected in AD. While patients with AD are likely to have relatively intact simple attention (eg, primary memory span), tests requiring selective, divided, and complex aspects of attention are likely to be impaired, particularly as task demands increase. This pattern of performance strongly supports the presence of a deficit in working memory (the ability to simultaneously attend, process, and respond to multiple pieces of information) early in the disease process, and a converging body of evidence supports a primary executive component in AD.

In addition to problems on tasks of complex attention and working memory, patients are likely to exhibit mild deficits in response inhibition, evidenced by intrusion errors and perseverative responses, on neuropsychological testing. Deficits in abstract reasoning, general problem-solving ability, and making appropriate judgments are also commonly noted. In assessing for judgment and abstraction, patients may be asked the meaning of proverbs (eg, "you can lead a horse to water but you can't make it drink") and are often given hypothetical situations in which they must decide an appropriate course of action (eg, "What would you do if you were in a crowded shopping mall and saw smoke and fire?"). On these tasks, even early AD patients may provide incorrect, concrete, or inappropriate responses.

Language Semantic processing is considered the primary language deficit in AD and is present in more than half of all AD patients at the time of diagnosis. Word finding problems are commonly reported in both AD and normal aging, but patients with AD have more severe deficits and are more likely to produce a significantly higher number of semantic paraphasias and circumlocutions. Patients are generally impaired on tasks of confrontational naming (eg, naming a visually presented item), and, unlike changes that occur with normal aging, are not likely to be assisted by phonemic cues (eg, providing the sound the word starts with). Syntactic processing, in contrast to semantic processing, is typically unaffected in mild AD. For example, patients with early AD can typically process even complex sentences at the same level as their healthy counterparts, and generally remain unimpaired on repetition and fluent speech. Verbal fluency tasks are particularly useful in evaluating both semantic and syntactic processing. Semantic, or category, fluency (eg, "Tell me as many animals as you can") is generally impaired disproportionately to syntactic, or phonemic, fluency (eg, "Tell me as many words that begin with the letter ___") in AD. While decreased information processing and working memory may impair an AD patient's responses on certain syntactic processing tasks, and comprehension and intelligible speech are likely to decline slowly as the disease advances, patients who present first with nonfluent aphasia or impaired comprehension should be carefully evaluated for conditions other than AD.

Visuospatial Function Deficits in visuospatial abilities are frequently seen in patients with AD, although they generally appear later than memory deficits. Patients may become lost while driving, or even in familiar places (eg, grocery store). Eventually, disorientation may lead to confusion in one's own home and subsequent wandering behavior. Early deficits, however, are more likely to involve visuospatial problem solving. Neuropsychological tests commonly used involve comparing simple construction or copying, typically not impaired early in the disease, to complex visual reasoning. The presence of constructional apraxia early in the disease may indicate greater pathology in visual processing areas of the brain and has been associated with more rapid symptom progression. In general, more complex drawing tasks, such as three-dimensional figure copy, may be more precise measures of the most common early visual spatial deficits in AD than simple copying tasks.

Motor Function While motor dysfunction has not been typically considered to be a defining symptom of AD, recent research suggests that AD patients may display impairments in gait, motor speed, and general level of activity, and these changes may even be evident during the prodromal phase of the disease. In addition, converging evidence provides support for greater neuropathologic overlap between AD and other conditions, such as dementia with Lewy bodies (DLB), making motor changes such as tremor or gait disturbance more likely in these patients. Importantly, there have been reports of gait disturbance in patients taking cholinesterase inhibitors, a factor that should be carefully monitored when prescribing these medications.

Patients with AD may also exhibit mild ideomotor and ideational apraxia (deficits in skilled movements) due to concrete responses, lack of sufficient external cues, or a disruption in conceptualization ability. However, moderate-to-severe apraxia is not generally present until later stages of the disease. Incorporating an apraxia assessment into a dementia evaluation is useful, particularly for excluding other disorders that may initially present with more severe skilled movement disorders.

Behavioral changes Mood disturbance is common in patients with AD and has even been recognized more recently as a possible prodrome to the development of dementia in older adults. Depression in AD may manifest as apathy, indifference, poor initiation, or emotional lability. Irritability, agitation, and paranoid ideation can also

occur in AD, and may worsen with disease progression, prompting wandering behavior and aggressive outbursts. Repetitive and aimless behavior may also increase as the disease progresses. More severe psychotic symptoms, such as hallucinations and severe delusions, are typically rare in earlier stages of AD in the absence of coexisting disorders. Given the wide range of behaviors that may be exhibited in AD, it is imperative that the patient's family be provided with ample dementia education, that they have access to social support, and that they possess the coping skills necessary to provide adequate care.

Awareness of deficits Patients in the early stages of AD typically vary in their level of deficit awareness. Whatever the starting point, deficit awareness declines with disease progression. Even when patients do acknowledge their cognitive decline, such awareness may not be "complete" as a result of deficits in executive function. For example, patients may be unable to translate cognitive problems into everyday functional difficulties, and as a result may not understand how their deficits affect certain activities, such as driving, cooking, and managing finances. Again, providing the patient's caregivers with ample education can increase the likelihood that patients and family will comply with physician recommendations to limit certain unsafe behaviors.

Variant AD presentations While most often the primary early deficit in AD involves recent memory, there are several, less common variant forms of AD that involve primary deficits in executive functioning, language (logopenic aphasia [LPA]) or visuospatial function (posterior cortical atrophy). In such cases, differential diagnoses, including frontotemporal lobar dementia (FTLD), primary progressive aphasia (PPA), Lewy body disease (LBD), and others, must be carefully considered prior to assigning a diagnosis of AD.

Mild Cognitive Impairment Due to AD

"Mild cognitive impairment" describes age-atypical levels of cognitive impairment that do not meet the criteria for dementia and that are not the result of a known medical condition or neurodevelopmental disorder. MCI and AD are not fully distinct entities and can be considered as existing on a cognitive and functional continuum. In its most common usage, the term MCI is assigned to cognitive impairments thought to be related to underlying AD pathology, although criteria for prodromes of other neurodegenerative dementias (eg, Parkinson disease dementia [PDD], FTLD) have been proposed. The clinical conceptualization of MCI relies largely on characteristic cognitive and functional symptoms. Current NIA/AA criteria for MCI due to AD include the following: (1) concerns regarding a change in cognition by either the patient, informant, or a skilled clinician, (2) objective impairment in one or more cognitive domains compared to the patient's estimated premorbid level of functioning based on age and education, (3) preserved independence in functional abilities, although patients may require some assistance or have mild impairments on more complex tasks such as financial management, navigation to unfamiliar places, etc, and (4) absence of dementia. Other causes, such as traumatic brain injury, cerebrovascular disease, and medical or metabolic abnormalities, should be ruled out as the primary etiology, though they may still play a smaller, contributing role.

While cognitive screeners can detect certain levels of cognitive impairment, they are not all equally sensitive to MCI, especially in persons with higher levels of educational attainment. Further, they may incorrectly identify cognitive impairment in individuals from diverse racial and ethnic backgrounds and those with lower levels of education. In contrast, a comprehensive neuropsychological evaluation is particularly useful in distinguishing normal age-related changes in cognition from MCI, as this type of testing can help ascertain subtle decrements in performance compared to an individual's estimated baseline level of functioning. Serial neuropsychological assessments are also helpful for monitoring subsequent change in cognition. On these types of assessments, scores that fall 1 to 1.5 standard deviations below the mean for age and education matched peers are typically considered "abnormal," though no formal cutoff thresholds exist. As is the pattern with AD, MCI typically, though not always, presents with early episodic memory impairment on cognitive testing.

Longitudinal research suggests that 80% of those diagnosed with MCI will go on to develop AD within 5 to 8 years, and will convert at a rate of approximately 10% to 15% per year compared to general population conversion rates of 1% to 2%. Amnestic forms of MCI are more likely to progress to AD than nonamnestic (eg, executive or language forms). However, the current criteria acknowledge that even initial nonamnestic presentations may also progress to AD. Progression to AD is also thought to be more likely when multiple cognitive domains are affected (amnestic-multi-domain MCI). In addition to converting to AD, both single-domain and multi-domain MCI may further progress to other forms of dementia such as vascular or Lewy body dementia. Because of the heterogeneity inherent to the construct of MCI, as many as 15% to 40% of those diagnosed with MCI may subsequently perform in the normal ranges on neuropsychological assessments or "revert" to normal. The exact reason that individuals with MCI may subsequently revert is multifactorial and incompletely understood. Studies have found that those from community- or population-based versus clinic-based samples are more likely to revert, as are those without positive biomarkers, those who are younger and have fewer medical conditions, and those with higher levels of education (**Figure 57-2**).

Biomarkers, while not yet commonplace in the clinical diagnosis of MCI, are playing an increasingly important role in understanding the pathophysiology of MCI and AD. Further, they can provide some support when deciding

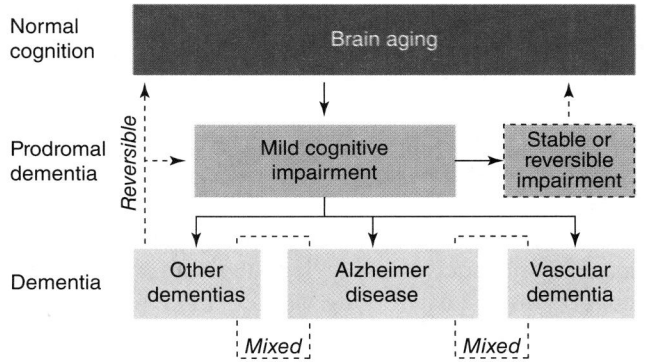

FIGURE 57-2. A conceptual model of mild cognitive impairment (MCI) as prodromal dementia. A minority of persons diagnosed with MCI may remain stable or even improve over time. Although individuals with MCI may decline to vascular or other forms of dementia, the majority of declining MCI patients evaluated in research clinics receive a diagnosis of AD (either in pure form or mixed with other dementia subtypes). (Reproduced with permission from Golomb J, Kluger A, Garrard P, et al. *Clinician's Manual on Mild Cognitive Impairment*. London, UK: Science Press; 2001.)

whether a particular clinical phenotype may be due to AD and in estimating likelihood of progression to dementia. For instance, one set of proposed criteria grade the likelihood of progression to AD on the basis of biomarker outcomes: MCI due to AD-high likelihood is assigned when there are positive biomarkers for both β-amyloid accumulation and neuronal injury on the basis of imaging and/or lumbar puncture, while the absence of positive biomarkers indicates a process that is unlikely to be related to AD. A more recent set of biomarker-based research criteria for MCI and AD incorporates measures of amyloid, tau, and neurodegeneration. However, these criteria are not yet recommended, nor widely used, in clinical diagnosis. In the future, these biomarkers as well as less invasive and less costly blood-based biomarkers currently in development (eg, plasma phosphorylated tau181) may eventually be widely used in both clinical and research settings to differentiate between MCI due to AD and other dementia types.

Palliative care concerns specific to AD Patients with AD generally have a gradual progression of cognitive and functional impairment, though the absolute course and trajectory is slightly different for each person. Education about the expected course of illness and potential safety concerns is useful, as it allows patients and families to prepare advance directives and durable powers of attorney. Some may also make other lifestyle changes, like moving to a single level house or considering a move to a continuing care retirement community. Addressing driving safety is important in AD and all varieties of dementia, as patients with dementia will ultimately need to refrain from driving. Behavioral or lifestyle interventions, such as increasing exercise, healthful eating behaviors, and engagement in cognitive and social activities, are also useful at this stage and help maintain physical health and quality of life. There are several pharmacological interventions that are approved by the US Food and Drug Administration for memory loss in AD, including donepezil, galantamine, rivastigmine (early-to-moderate stage), and memantine (moderate-to-severe-stage), that can be considered by the patient's treating physician. In moderate-to-later stages of the disease course, patients will become dependent for basic daily activities such as eating, bathing, and grooming, and may also display challenging behaviors like wandering or agitation. Maintaining a regular, predictable schedule that includes some form of activity, ensuring good nighttime sleep, and assessing for other causes of agitation (eg, infection; pain) can be helpful in these situations. Occasionally, medications can be prescribed to combat agitation or aggression, though certain types of medications (eg, antipsychotics, sedatives) often have unwanted side effects in older adults or those with dementia, so these decisions need to be made judiciously. Patients with late-stage disease often experience difficulties with swallowing, communication, and/or bladder and bowel control and need round-the-clock-care. In moderate to late stage disease, many families find they need to rely on hired caregivers or consider an assisted living facility for assistance in managing their loved ones' needs. Caregiver support and education is essential at all stages of the disease.

Lewy Body Disorders

Lewy body dementia (LBD) encompasses both DLB and PDD. The primary neuropathologic feature in both diseases is the accumulation of cortical Lewy bodies, resulting from abnormal aggregation of α-synuclein. However, additional pathologic features, including accumulation of tau protein, concurrent vascular and/or AD pathology, neurotransmitter abnormalities, and frontostriatal projections that have been disrupted by loss of dopaminergic neurons, can all contribute to the cognitive decline associated with these diseases.

Although PD and DLB have historically been considered related but separate clinical entities, many of the neuropathologic, clinical, cognitive, and psychiatric characteristics of the two diseases have considerable overlap. Both are associated with cognitive fluctuations, visual hallucinations, psychiatric symptoms, and REM sleep behavior disorder in the context of PD motor symptoms, and thus recent debates have examined whether PD, PDD, and DLB should be placed along a clinical continuum representing the same underlying pathology. Currently, the differential diagnosis is based on the timing of the onset of the cognitive symptoms. A patient with PD who develops dementia after 1 year of well-established motor symptoms is classified as "PDD," while a patient with motor symptoms occurring after the onset of dementia (or within one year of motor symptom onset) is classified as "DLB."

Parkinson disease Diagnosis of PD according to the United Kingdom Parkinson Disease Society Brain Bank clinical diagnostic criteria requires specific motor symptoms,

including bradykinesia and at least one of the following: muscular rigidity, rest tremor, and/or postural instability. Although motor symptoms have long been considered the defining feature of PD, a wide range of associated nonmotor symptoms, such as impaired sleep patterns, psychiatric symptoms, gastrointestinal dysfunction, and cognitive impairment, are increasingly recognized as having substantial impact on functional abilities and quality of life for these patients. Of these nonmotor symptoms, cognitive dysfunction is a substantial concern, with upwards of 80% of patients who live for 20 years or more with PD expected to develop PDD over the course of the disease. Current Movement Disorder Society task force recommended consensus diagnostic criteria for PDD include (1) a diagnosis of PD, (2) PD symptoms developed prior to the onset of dementia, (3) impaired global cognition (eg, on MMSE or MoCA), (4) cognitive impairment severe enough to impair activities of daily living, and (5) impairments in more than one cognitive domain on detailed neurocognitive testing. Additional supportive symptoms may include psychiatric symptoms (eg, depression, apathy, delusions) or impaired sleep. Even among patients without dementia, however, the rate of concurrent cognitive impairment can be quite high. PD-mild cognitive impairment (PD-MCI), similar to MCI due to AD, is characterized by subjective cognitive decline (noted by the patient, collateral, or clinician), objective impairments on neuropsychological assessment, and absence of functional impairment sufficient to significantly interfere with functional independence in the presence of clinically verified PD. PD-MCI is common, with overall prevalence estimates approximately 30% to 40%. Cognitive deficits often emerge early during the course of the disease, with 10% to 30% of newly diagnosed patients with PD identified with cognitive impairment. However, there is substantial variability in the nature and course of cognitive symptoms in PD, with many patients maintaining a stable or fluctuating course and others demonstrating more rapid decline (**Figure 57-3**). Several variables associated with more rapid cognitive decline have been identified, including age, disease duration, sex, and specific genetic mutations.

Most patients with PD exhibit at least some decline in attention, working memory, processing speed, or other executive functions, although the nature and degree of impairments across other domains are variable. PDD is often characterized by worsening visuospatial deficits, impaired verbal fluency, difficulty planning or shifting to a new stimulus, slowed information processing speed, and impaired memory. Memory impairment is most frequently attributable to a retrieval deficit since recognition is often intact. Procedural learning may be impaired, a pattern atypical in normal aging or in AD. Some language skills are intact, such as vocabulary, while others that tap additional cognitive domains, such as verbal fluency, may be impaired. Mechanical aspects of speech are often impaired as well. Although PDD has been previously characterized as a "subcortical" dementia to distinguish it from cortical dementias

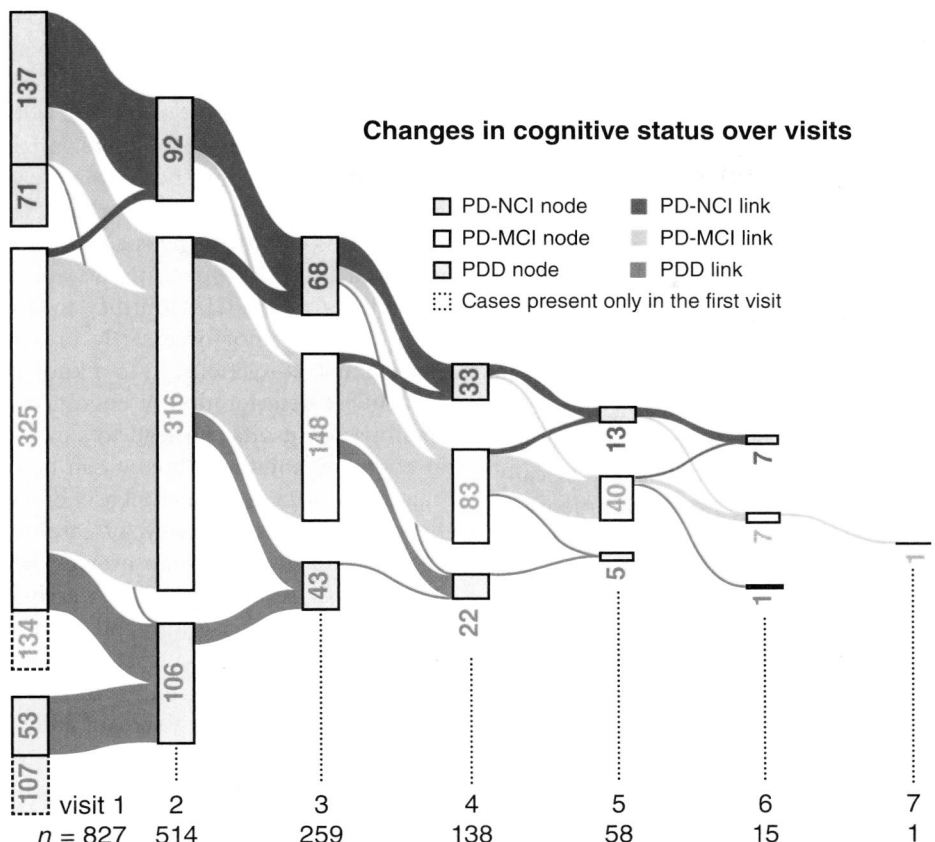

FIGURE 57-3. Change in cognitive diagnostic status over time in a multi-site Parkinson disease (PD) cohort. The number inside each node represents the number of people with the corresponding cognitive status indicated by its color. The nodes with dashed lines represent people with only data from the first visit. The links represent the group participants who continued to the next visit. PDD, PD with dementia; PD-MCI, PD with mild cognitive impairment; PD-NCI, PD with no cognitive impairment. (Reproduced with permission from Phongpreecha T, Cholerton B, Mata IF, et al. Multivariate prediction of dementia in Parkinson's disease. *NPJ Parkinsons Dis.* 2020;6:20.)

such as AD, this characterization has been criticized more recently and may serve simply as a gross depiction of the cognitive profile. Indeed, recent research suggests that while initial mild cognitive deficits in PD likely result from depleted dopamine in the midbrain and resulting defects in the frontostriatal loop, cortical pathology is required for progression to dementia.

Dementia with Lewy bodies Current consensus criteria for probable DLB include (1) a diagnosis of dementia (defined as cognitive impairment sufficient to impair functional abilities) and (2) two or more core clinical features (fluctuating cognition, well-formed visual hallucinations, rapid eye movement [REM] sleep behavior disorder, and/or one or more cardinal motor symptoms of PD), or one core clinical features in the presence of one or more indicative biomarkers (eg, reduced dopamine uptake on SPECT or PET scan, REM sleep disorder diagnosed by polysomnography). As discussed above, DLB and PDD share many of the same features, including cognitive fluctuations, neuropsychiatric features, and motor symptoms. However, the timing and severity of these symptoms may differ. Visual

hallucinations often occur earlier in DLB, delusions may be more common, and a differential response to antiparkinsonian medications has been reported. In terms of cognition, prominent visuospatial and executive impairments are noted, similar to PDD. Memory impairments, although not necessary for diagnosis, tend to be more prominent in DLB. It is thus unsurprising that among patients with DLB, there tends to be a likelihood of concurrent AD pathology.

Given the overlap in symptoms and pathology, differential diagnosis between DLB and AD can thus also be difficult. The presence of visual hallucinations in patients with MMSE scores greater than 20 is highly suggestive of DLB. Neuropsychological studies have identified typical cognitive profiles that may aid in diagnosis. In DLB, patients have more difficulty than AD patients in copying complex designs, assembling pieces of an object, or completing other tasks requiring visuospatial skills. In contrast, AD subjects generally show significantly more impairment on delayed recall tasks than patients with DLB. DLB patients have attentional skills that are generally equivalent to those of AD patients; however, patients with DLB exhibit significant attentional fluctuations. As a result, evaluating attention over time is more helpful than the overall severity of attention problems in the differential diagnosis. Finally, these cognitive profiles are most evident early in the course of the diseases. As the diseases progress, all cognitive functions become impaired and neuropsychological testing is less helpful for diagnosis.

Palliative care concerns specific to PD and DLB There is increasing recognition that appropriate palliative care that addresses cognitive changes in PD and DLB is both vital and underutilized. Given the range of symptoms in PD and associated caregiver and patient burden, an early focus on nonmotor symptom control, adjustment to cognitive changes, and advance care planning is strongly recommended in addition to routine care that has historically focused nearly solely on motor symptom management. To address the problems associated with increasing cognitive decline, occupational therapy, integrated care models, and psychoeducational programs for patients and family members may be helpful tools. In general, however, both patients and caregivers report that they are not provided with enough information about the nature and prognosis of the diagnosis, and thus lack the tools necessary to address end-of-life care issues and mitigate problems associated with advancing cognitive disease, such as medication reconciliation and home safety issues. DLB is associated with specific difficulties in accessing palliative care, largely due to lack of knowledge about the diagnosis in the general medical community and related difficulty in adequately diagnosing DLB. Further, patients with DLB often present with behavioral problems that may result in difficulty accessing resources. As a result, patients are often not appropriately medicated and physicians rarely discuss what to expect as the disease progresses. Assessment resources such as the Palliative Care Outcome Scale or the Edmonton Symptom Assessment System may be helpful to identify care needs in patients. However, provider education is a vital initial step to providing adequate community palliative care for PD/DLB.

Vascular Cognitive Impairment

VCI is an umbrella term that includes both mild VCI and major VCI (VaD) in the context of imaging evidence for cerebrovascular disease. A diagnosis of mild VCI requires impairment in at least one cognitive domain with mild or no impairment in activities of daily living that are independent from any motor or sensory impairments caused by the vascular event. A diagnosis of major VCI (or VaD) requires significant deficits in at least one cognitive domain along with correlated impairment in daily functional activities (again that are independent of any motor or sensory sequelae associated with the vascular event). VaD subtypes include poststroke dementia (the only subtype that requires a clear temporal relationship between vascular event and cognitive decline), subcortical ischemic VaD, multi-infarct dementia, or mixed dementia (representing combined suspected vascular disease and other neurodegenerative diseases including AD and LBD).

Cognitive profiles of patients with VCI, especially in mild or early forms, can be quite variable given the underlying neuropathologic heterogeneity associated with the diagnosis. Executive function deficits, reduced verbal fluency, and slow processing speed are common. Depression, irritability, and lack of initiative are also frequently seen in patients with VCI. Contrary to long-standing clinical lore, VCI does not necessarily present primarily with a clear temporal relationship to a known vascular event nor to stepwise deterioration in cognition. Rather, continuous small vessel insults can lead to slowly progressive decline in cognitive abilities. Thus, it can be difficult to differentiate VaD from AD on the basis of the clinical course of symptoms. Detailed review of cardiovascular risk factors and cognitive profile may provide better differentiation. A review of studies examining early-stage AD and VaD found that the latter group had more pronounced deficits in executive function on tests such as the Wisconsin Card Sorting Test and the executive function scale of the Mattis Dementia Rating Scale than did adults with AD. Interestingly, performance between the two groups was similar on tests of selective attention and working memory such as the Trail-Making Test and Stroop Color Word Interference Test. In contrast, VaD patients had better performance than AD patients on tests of verbal learning and story recall, such as the California Verbal Learning Test and the Logical Memory subtest of the Wechsler Memory Scale-Revised (WMS-R), with fewer intrusions. However, VCI can impact the structure and function of the hippocampus, thus leading to more notable memory deficits in some patients, although these impairments may not occur until later in the disease process. Because memory impairment is most often the reason patients seek evaluation, adults with VaD may have more progressed dementia and greater cognitive impairment at the time of diagnosis. It is important to note that as both VaD and AD progress, the cognitive profiles become more similar, so that differentiating mid-stage disease is very difficult. In addition, neuropathologic studies have shown that many patients previously diagnosed with VaD due to presence of vascular risk factors such as diabetes, hypertension, and radiologic evidence of ischemia have prominent AD pathology as well. Prevalence estimates of the co-occurrence of AD and VaD range from 20% to 40% of patients with dementia. Few studies have attempted to differentiate between mixed AD/VaD and either form of dementia on a neuropsychological basis, although it has been suggested that mixed dementia most closely resembles VaD from a cognitive perspective. Vascular pathology increases the likelihood that patients with neuropathologic AD will show significant cognitive impairment.

Palliative care concerns specific to VCI Given the variable (and often unknown) progression of cognitive symptoms in

VCI, palliative care concerns are likely to be patient-specific, and may include lifestyle interventions aimed at maximizing retained cognitive abilities, quality of life, and overall physical health. Occupational therapy, psychoeducation, managing comorbid depression, and training and support for caregivers may all be helpful interventions. In advanced major VCI, palliative care interventions and end-of-life planning and preparation similar to those used most frequently in AD are recommended.

Frontotemporal Lobar Degeneration

Frontotemporal lobar degeneration (FTLD) is caused by a range of underlying neuropathologic conditions (including intracellular inclusions of tau or transactive response DNA-binding protein [TDP-43], among others). FTLD onset occurs at slightly younger ages than other conditions such as AD, with onset occurring most commonly in the late 50s-to-early 60s. It is thought to be the second most common form of dementia in individuals under the age of 65. Roughly 30% to 40% of FTLD cases are linked to genetic mutations, including granulin (GRN) and microtubule-associated protein tau (MAPT) mutations, and patients with some types of genetic mutations may develop symptoms at even earlier ages. As with AD, FTLD patients show insidious onset of symptoms with a gradual progression. Various clinical presentations can be caused by FTLD, primarily resulting in gradually progressive disturbances in language and/or behavior. Although comparisons of AD and FTLD groups do not always reveal significantly different cognitive profiles, in general, FTLD patients show relatively spared memory performance in comparison to their executive and language functioning, especially when memory cues are provided. Apraxia is also more common in FTLD than in AD. Often a multidisciplinary approach may be most helpful in the differential diagnosis since studies indicate that up to 75% of pathologically confirmed FTLD patients also appear to meet clinical criteria for probable AD, and certain subtypes of FTLD are often misdiagnosed as a primary psychiatric disorder early on. The following diagnostic variants are currently recognized as most likely resulting from FTLD, although the extent to which these conditions may have shared pathology with other diseases, and the likelihood that these represent distinct disorders is not currently well defined.

Behavioral variant FTLD This diagnostic category (bvFTD) accounts for nearly 50% to 60% of all FTLD diagnoses. This variant most often presents initially with a prominent decline in social cognition and behavior and/or executive dysfunction, with relative sparing of other cognitive functions, and includes at least three of the following: (a) disinhibition, (b) apathy, (c) diminished empathy/sympathy, (d) perseverative, stereotyped, or compulsive behaviors, and/or (e) hyperorality/dietary changes. These behavioral and/or executive symptoms are the source of impairment in daily activities. While these criteria are sufficient for a

diagnosis of "possible" bvFTD, a diagnosis of "probable" bvFTD requires neuroimaging findings of disproportionate frontal or temporal lobe involvement, or a pathogenic mutation. Early in the disease process, performances on formal neuropsychological testing may be remarkably well preserved, underscoring the importance of a thorough diagnostic interview and history with the patient and an informant; however, many individuals do display impaired selective and divided attention, difficulty shifting mental set, poor abstraction and reasoning, impaired verbal fluency, and perseverations. Unfortunately, cognitive screeners such as the MMSE are not very helpful in screening for early bvFTD since many patients score within normal limits early in the disease.

Primary progressive aphasia PPA typically occurs in the fifth or sixth decade of life, and its rate of progression varies greatly. The diagnosis of PPA requires initial prominent language dysfunction with relative sparing of other cognitive domains early on, and the absence of radiologic evidence of cerebrovascular or other neurologic injury that would account for the aphasia. Because anomia and other language deficits may occur in a number of neurodegenerative conditions, the differential diagnosis of PPA rests on the clear demonstration that nonlinguistic cognitive and behavioral functions are intact during the initial stages of the disease. The clinician must carefully determine whether poor performance on memory and other nonlanguage tests is due to language deficits such as impaired comprehension of instructions. Differential diagnosis is also complicated by the heterogenous etiologies of PPA demonstrated by the different subtypes. Although not consistent across all cases, agrammatic PPA is often associated with tau pathology, logopenic PPA with AD pathology (although not always in brain regions typically associated with AD), and semantic PPA with TDP-43 pathology. PPA variants include (1) agrammatic/nonfluent aphasia and (2) semantic variant PPA (sometimes called semantic dementia [SD]). As noted, a third variant, LPA, is often included under the larger umbrella of PPA; however, neuropathologically, LPA is primarily attributed to AD-type pathology, so it is often considered a language-variant of AD.

Progressive Nonfluent/Agrammatic Aphasia Progressive nonfluent/agrammatic aphasia (PNFA) is characterized by labored articulation and/or agrammatism, frequently occurring alongside apraxia of speech. Patients with PNFA also typically have intact comprehension for simple speech and phrases but impaired comprehension for complex or syntactically irregular phrases. Semantic knowledge is also well preserved.

Semantic Dementia SD, on the other hand, involves a loss of ability to understand words (semantic knowledge of words and objects), which is accompanied by marked deficits in confrontational naming. Other deficits include difficulty with visual recognition of objects, dyslexia, and dysgraphia.

Patients with semantic dementia may display prominent visual agnosias and may not be able to demonstrate object use accurately. In contrast to PNFA, speech production remains intact in early disease as does repetition.

Logopenic Aphasia LPA is the most recently characterized PPA variant. LPA presents with impaired word retrieval in spontaneous speech and difficulty with naming, in addition to impaired sentence repetition, and in some instances, sentence comprehension. The hypothesized mechanism behind some of the language deficits in LPA, especially impaired sentence repetition, is a deficiency in short-term working memory, and hence, single-word repetition, which requires minimal working memory, is well preserved. The naming deficit in LPA is not as dramatic as in SD, and these patients also have preserved object knowledge. While patients with LPA demonstrate effortful word retrieval, this again is less severe than in PNFA and their speech is usually grammatically accurate and free from motor speech abnormalities, which marks another useful distinction between LPA and other PPA subtypes.

FTLD movement disorders Certain movement disorders, which may also include behavioral and/or language disturbance, may be caused by or associated with FTLD.

FTLD-Motor Neuron Disease Frontotemporal dementia with motor neuron disease (FTD-MND) tends to be a rapidly progressive condition, with death typically occurring 3 to 5 years after symptom onset. Age of onset is more variable and can range from 35 to 75, on average. The FTD-MND syndrome is typically characterized by gradual onset of both cognitive and psychiatric symptoms, in addition to, though not necessarily simultaneously to, development of classic upper and/or lower motor neuron dysfunction, such as muscle wasting, paraparesis, fasciculations, or abnormal reflexes. Early bulbar involvement can also lead to symptoms of dysphagia and pseudobulbar affect, or uncontrollable episodes of laughing or tearfulness. Behaviorally, these patients may display similar symptoms to patients with bvFTD. Cognitive symptoms can include variable language and executive dysfunction.

Progressive Supranuclear Palsy Although Lewy bodies are found in only the minority of progressive supranuclear palsy (PSP) cases, PSP is frequently misdiagnosed as PD. A core feature of the disorder is vertical supranuclear gaze palsy, although this symptom may not present early in the course of the disease. Patients also present with postural instability, and falls are often seen shortly after onset. Cognition is characterized by mental and psychomotor slowing and notable executive dysfunction, often fairly early in the disease course. Memory impairments are observed, but they are not as severe as in AD. Language functions resemble those seen in PD. Visual spatial deficits and increased apathy are also observed.

Corticobasal Syndrome Corticobasal syndrome (CBS) is the primary clinical phenotype of corticobasal degeneration, which is characterized by abnormal tau deposition, and relatively focal and asymmetric cortical atrophy in frontal and parietal brain regions on imaging. The mean age of onset for CBS is in the early 60s. CBS is characterized by progressive, asymmetric motor symptoms such as tremor, loss of coordination, rigidity, and myoclonus, and a higher prevalence of alien limb syndrome. Unilateral apraxia (most commonly ideomotor) is common. A range of language abnormalities including slowed verbal fluency, and/or executive dysfunction may also be seen in CBS. In contrast to AD, memory is typically well preserved early on, but may worsen with disease progression and may even become prominent in some patients. Neuropsychiatric and behavioral symptoms are common and can include apathy, personality change, disinhibition, and irritability.

Palliative care concerns specific to FTLD Given the heterogeneity in FTLD phenotypes, care recommendations vary by subtype. Many of the core symptoms of bvFTD and related subtypes, including impulsivity, poor judgment, and disinhibition, can be distressing for family members, so education about bvFTD and early support for family and caregivers is essential. Education about possible environment and behavioral modifications is recommended and typically focuses on mitigating safety risks (eg, driving impulsively, poor management of money, falling victim to scams, etc) given reductions in insight and self-awareness are quite common in bvFTD. Early consultation with a psychiatrist is often helpful as well; there is some evidence that treatment with selective serotonin reuptake inhibitors may be helpful in managing unwanted behavioral symptoms. Patients with either primary (PPA subtypes) or secondary language dysfunction (PSP; CBS; FTD-MND) may benefit from consultation with a speech-language pathologist (SLP) early on in the course of their disease, who may be able to provide useful strategies. Augmentative and alternative communication devices can also be employed as the condition progresses. SLPs may also be of benefit as part of a multidisciplinary team as some of these patients may have, or go on to develop, dysarthria and/or dysphagia. Physical therapy can also be a valuable tool to assist with early motor dysfunction in FTD-MND, PSP, and CBS. Like most neurodegenerative conditions, motor and/or sensory dysfunction can occur in other FTLD subtypes as well as the disease progresses to moderate or severe stages.

Dementia Due to Suspected Non-Alzheimer Disease Pathophysiology

Dementia due to suspected non-Alzheimer disease pathophysiology (SNAP) is a relatively new biomarker-based term that is used to describe individuals who have evidence of neurodegeneration on neuroimaging, but who lack biomarkers classic to AD—specifically, amyloid. SNAP is more prevalent with increasing age. While there is little evidence of SNAP in persons younger than 50, prevalence increases with increasing age after the age of 60. Most commonly, the term SNAP has been used to describe individuals with either normal cognition or MCI who lack evidence of clinically significant amyloid but have evidence of neurodegenerative changes in the brain. Neurodegeneration characteristic of SNAP is also observed in individuals with clinical dementia; however, these individuals' condition is usually attributed to a non-AD etiology based on clinical presentation (eg PPA, DLB), and it is hypothesized that TDP-43, hippocampal sclerosis, vascular disease, and/or other pathophysiological processes may be the causative factor. No definitive cognitive phenotype has been identified in individuals with SNAP who are deemed clinically normal, though SNAP does appear to confer risk for subsequent cognitive decline. Not surprisingly, those with SNAP and MCI have greater likelihood of progression to dementia than those with SNAP and no evidence of MCI. Further, those with SNAP, regardless of cognitive status, have a greater risk of decline compared to those without SNAP. The data is mixed on the risk of decline in SNAP compared to those without SNAP but who are amyloid and/or tau positive, though it is generally accepted that the presence of neurodegeneration, amyloid, and tau combined confers the greatest risk for accelerated cognitive decline.

Limbic-Predominant Age-Related TDP-43 Encephalopathy

Limbic-predominant age-related TDP-43 encephalopathy (LATE) is a common, but relatively recently described finding in those in their eighth or ninth decade of life. Estimates vary, but recent autopsy studies of individuals aged 80 and older have identified evidence of LATE in 5% to 50% of their samples. This proteinopathy was first discovered in autopsies of individuals with cognitive impairment that mimicked AD; that is, these individuals had an amnestic cognitive syndrome similar to AD. Like AD, LATE can also evolve to include multiple cognitive domains but the clinical presentation remains distinct from other TDP-related conditions such as FTLD-TDP. Given the occurrence in very late life, it is unsurprising that the pathological changes of LATE often co-occur with those of AD, LBD, and/or VCI. While data on this entity is still in its infancy, there is some indication cognitive changes progress more slowly in those who only have evidence of LATE compared to those with evidence of multiple pathologies.

Alcohol-Related Dementia

Contradictory evidence exists as to the role of mild-to-moderate alcohol and risk for developing certain dementias, including AD and VaD. Chronic and profound alcohol use, however, can have a negative effect on cognition and may exacerbate the cognitive symptoms of other dementias and brain injuries. Poor nutrition (thiamine

deficiency in particular) resulting from alcohol abuse is a primary contributor to the onset of cognitive problems. In addition, liver disease can interfere with thiamine regulation in the brain and may be a factor in the multiple cognitive and motor impairments associated with long-term alcohol use.

Persistent alcohol dementia Alcohol dementia involves impairment in more than one area of cognitive function that persists after the patient stops drinking for a period of time. Visuospatial problem-solving deficits and executive problems, including apathy, decreased judgment, and reduced interest in self-care, are prominent in these patients. Memory problems, in particular anterograde amnesia, are also common, but are generally not more impaired than other cognitive domains, and recognition is often intact. Typical neuropsychological sequelae include impairments on tasks requiring visual scanning, visuospatial organization, perceptual-motor speed, sustained attention, abstraction, and mental flexibility, while language functions are generally preserved. Perseveration and confabulation are common indicators of impaired executive function in the responses of patients with chronic alcohol use. It is also noteworthy that chronic alcohol use may potentiate the onset of AD, and produce a clinical picture of conjoint cognitive deficits.

Wernicke–Korsakoff syndrome The most severe neurologic outcome of heavy and prolonged alcohol use, and the result of critical malnutrition, is Wernicke–Korsakoff syndrome. In contrast to patients with persistent alcohol dementia, Wernicke–Korsakoff patients exhibit an acute symptom onset, often beginning with a grave confusional state, nystagmus, and significant ataxia. During this phase, symptoms progressively and rapidly worsen if treatment (immediate thiamine replacement) is not applied. This phase is almost always followed by a chronic and progressive stage that is associated primarily with impaired frontal and cerebellar functions. Unlike persistent alcohol dementia, Korsakoff patients have significant impairments in memory relative to other cognitive effects, and memory impairment includes both retrograde and anterograde amnesia for episodic events, frequently with prominent confabulation. In contrast to AD, semantic memory is relatively spared in the Korsakoff patient. Patients show a characteristic gradient of remote memory impairment, with better recall for remote events and progressively reduced recall of recent events. As with persistent alcohol dementia, executive dysfunction and visuospatial impairments are also significant symptoms of the syndrome. Cerebellar atrophy and peripheral nerve damage lead to impaired gait, decreased or abnormal reflexes, and other movement abnormalities in these patients.

Palliative care concerns specific to alcohol-related dementias Alcohol-related dementias, unlike progressive dementias such as AD and DLB, may be amenable to interventions if made in a timely manner (such as drinking cessation and nutritional supplementation), which may improve cognitive symptoms or stall further cognitive decline. Once these important interventions have been put in place, encouraging skill maintenance, providing adequate scaffolding for cognitive skills, maintaining daily structure and routine, and help with general self-care may be useful for maintaining maximal cognitive function.

Prion Diseases

The prion diseases are a group of rare fatal spongiform encephalopathies that result from mutations and polymorphisms in the prion protein gene (PrP), causing rapid neurodegeneration. These diseases, of which Creutzfeldt–Jakob is the most well-known, produce a profound and quickly progressive dementia, and may be sporadic, familial, or infectious. Sporadic cases are the most common, and are generally diagnosed in people in their 60s, with a typical age range between 40 and 80. Early cognitive signs of the prion diseases are usually vague and nonspecific, such as poor memory, concentration, and problem solving. Initially, there are also often psychiatric symptoms, including apathy, emotional lability, impaired sleep, and appetite loss. Early frank neurologic symptoms are not common, but as the disease progresses, hyperreflexia, impaired coordination, changes in saccadic eye movements, and incontinence may occur. Given the early vague symptoms and dearth of neurologic symptoms, patients are not likely to present for evaluation until they are in the more moderate-to-advanced stages, which can occur in a matter of months. Diagnosis typically involves measuring electroencephalographic changes, hyperintensities on MRI, and abnormal 14-3-3 protein deposits in the CSF. The most common differential diagnoses include depression, AD, and LBD. Given the generally rapid course of disease in combination with diagnosis that typically occurs in the later stages of disease, palliative care often consists largely of hospice care, social work interventions to address disability and making end-of-life decisions, and bereavement resources and interventions for caregivers.

Normal Pressure Hydrocephalus

NPH is a potentially reversible dementia that makes up about 6% of dementia cases. Abnormalities in the production, absorption, or flow of CSF result in ventricular dilatation. Patients may present with a triad of clinical symptoms that include gait or balance disturbance, urinary incontinence, and cognitive deficits. Unlike most other dementias, cognitive symptoms often present later in the course. This can make early clinical diagnosis difficult since gait abnormalities and incontinence have a variety of etiologies in geriatric populations. Radiographic evidence and intraventricular pressure measurement aid in the diagnosis. When cognitive deficits are present, they are most frequently observed in executive functioning. Although many subjects may have subjective memory complaints, memory deficits are not a prominent early symptom, and some memory declines are attributable to attention problems, which are more common. However, many of these patients may have concurrent underlying neurodegenerative disease, and thus may present with varied cognitive profiles.

When treated, a ventriculoperitoneal shunt is usually used to divert CSF for better absorption. However, surgery in geriatric populations always involves added risks, and the benefits of shunt surgery remain unclear. A wide variety of success rates have been reported, with better outcomes often reported after shorter follow-up periods. Patients with the full triad of symptoms appear to respond best to shunt surgery. Gait problems show the most frequent improvement, while cognitive function improves in the fewest patients. Recently, findings from a 5-year follow-up of NPH patients with and without shunt surgery showed that at the 6-month assessment, 83% of the shunt cases improved in gait and 46% improved in memory. Of surviving shunt cases 5 years after surgery, 39% remained improved in gait, and fewer than 10% continued to show improvements on cognitive tests. Results suggested that outcomes may be improved in younger patients. Palliative care may involve inpatient and outpatient rehabilitation, physical therapy, occupational therapy, and other interventions aimed at maximizing retained cognitive functions.

HIV-Associated Neurocognitive Disorder

Although there is often the perception that geriatric patients are not at risk for human immunodeficiency virus (HIV) infection, the Centers for Disease Control and Prevention reported that 10% of all HIV cases in the United States are in patients of 50 years or older, and these numbers are expected to grow. With the use of combination antiretroviral therapies, progression to HIV-associated dementia is rare (2–3%). However, the prevalence of milder cognitive deficits is more frequent, with prevalence estimates ranging from 50% to 60%. Commonly affected areas of cognition are speed of information processing, attention, and motor speed, although it is increasingly recognized that impairments in broader executive functions, learning, and prospective memory are prevalent. As a result, differentiating these symptoms from early AD can be difficult clinically and may require more careful evaluation of both AD- and HIV-related CSF and imaging biomarkers. Palliative care depends upon severity of disease but should focus on managing potential multiple medical and psychosocial comorbidities and end-of-life planning as appropriate.

Neurosyphilis

Despite successes in treatment and education, syphilis cases have continually increased since 2000. Neurosyphilis can occur any time during the disease; however, syphilitic dementia may occur as the disease advances (generally 5–25 years after initial infection) that may present with hallucinations, delusions, mood disturbance, personality change, strokes, ataxia, or cognitive decline. Deficits are observed in short-term memory and mental status with progressive cognitive decline in all areas of functioning. Although neurosyphilis is often classified as a reversible dementia, there is only limited evidence to support cognitive benefits with penicillin treatment. Thus, following treatment with penicillin, palliative care may include occupational therapy or cognitive rehabilitation to help maximize remaining cognitive function. Neurosyphilis is more likely to occur in patients with comorbid HIV, and thus both should be considered during differential diagnosis. Neurosyphilis should further be considered in a differential diagnosis of dementia of unclear etiology in geriatric patients.

CONCLUSION

We have greatly furthered our understanding that age-related medical conditions not considered classically neurologic in nature can nevertheless impact the central nervous system and thereby affect cognition. This knowledge has led to the realization that many of the changes in cognition previously thought to be unavoidable concomitants of normal aging are in fact preventable and in some cases even reversible. The deleterious consequences of not treating such disorders have become evident, given that many common diseases such as T2DM and hypertension appear to be risk factors for dementia. In turn, early identification of dementia or the prodromal condition MCI will become critical as therapeutic options for delaying disease progression proliferate. Careful characterization of cognitive status through neuropsychological assessment can provide the clinician with essential information to determine whether the patient is experiencing symptoms that warrant concern or further treatment. As the field of geriatrics approaches the goal of controlling or even preventing endemic late-life chronic diseases, it will become increasingly clear that deleterious cognitive changes that occur with healthy aging are fewer and more subtle than we thought, and that they are accompanied by age-related strengths in experience and knowledge that will enable us to lead vital, productive lives well into our 80s and beyond.

FURTHER READING

Albert MS, DeKosky ST, Dickson D, et al. The diagnosis of mild cognitive impairment due to Alzheimer's disease: recommendations from the National Institute on Aging-Alzheimer's Association workgroups on diagnostic guidelines for Alzheimer's disease. *Alzheimers Dement.* 2011;7(3):270–279.

Bennett S, Thomas AJ. Depression and dementia: cause, consequence or coincidence? *Maturitas.* 2014;79(2):184–189.

Berger I, Wu S, Masson P, et al. Cognition in chronic kidney disease: a systematic review and meta-analysis. *BMC Med.* 2016;14(1):206.

Biessels GJ, Despa F. Cognitive decline and dementia in diabetes mellitus: mechanisms and clinical implications. *Nat Rev Endocrinol.* 2018;14(10):591–604.

Burkauskas J, Lang P, Bunevicius A, et al. Cognitive function in patients with coronary artery disease: a literature review. *J Int Med Res.* 2018;46(10):4019–4031.

Cairns NJ, Bigio EH, Mackenzie IR, et al. Neuropathologic diagnostic and nosologic criteria for frontotemporal lobar degeneration: consensus of the Consortium for Frontotemporal Lobar Degeneration. *Neuropathol.* 2007;114(1):5–22.

Cheng C, Huang CL, Tsai CJ, et al. Alcohol-related dementia: a systematic review of epidemiological studies. *Psychosomatics.* 2017;58(4):331–342.

Emre M, Aarsland D, Brown R, Clinical diagnostic criteria for dementia associated with Parkinson's disease. *Mov Disord.* 2007;22(12):1689–1707.

Inouye SK, Westendorp RG, Saczynski JS. Delirium in elderly people. *Lancet.* 2014;383(9920):911–922.

Iwasaki Y. Creutzfeldt-Jakob disease. *Neuropathology.* 2017;37(2):174–188.

Krause D, Roupas P. Effect of vitamin intake on cognitive decline in older adults: evaluation of the evidence. *J Nutr Health Aging.* 2015;19(7):745–753.

Laursen P. The impact of aging on cognitive function: an 11-year follow-up study of four age cohorts. *Acta Neurol Scand Suppl.* 1997;172:7–86.

Litvan I, Goldman JG, Tröster AI, et al. Diagnostic criteria for mild cognitive impairment in Parkinson's disease: Movement Disorder Society Task Force guidelines. *Mov Disord.* 2012;27(3):349–356.

Loggia G, Attoh-Mensah E, Pothier K, et al. Psychotropic polypharmacy in adults 55 years or older: a risk for impaired global cognition, executive function, and mobility. *Front Pharmacol.* 2020;10:1659.

McKeith IG, Boeve BF, Dickson DW. Diagnosis and management of dementia with Lewy bodies: fourth consensus report of the DLB consortium. *Neurology.* 2017;89(1):88–100.

McKhann GM, Knopman DS, Chertkow H, et al. The diagnosis of dementia due to Alzheimer's disease: recommendations from the National Institute on Aging-Alzheimer's Association workgroups on diagnostic guidelines for Alzheimer's disease. *Alzheimers Dement.* 2011;7(3):263–269.

Olaithe M, Bucks RS, Hillman DR, et al. Cognitive deficits in obstructive sleep apnea: insights from a meta-review and comparison with deficits observed in COPD, insomnia, and sleep deprivation. *Sleep Med Rev.* 2018;38:39–49.

Oliveira LM, Nitrini R, Román GC. Normal-pressure hydrocephalus: a critical review. *Dement Neuropsychol.* 2019;13(2):133–143.

Skrobot OA, Black SE, Chen C, et al. Progress toward standardized diagnosis of vascular cognitive impairment: Guidelines from the Vascular Impairment of Cognition Classification Consensus Study. *Alzheimers Dement.* 2018;14(3):280–292.

Smail RC, Brew BJ. HIV-associated neurocognitive disorder. *Handb Clin Neurol.* 2018;152:75–97.

Chapter 58

Delirium

Matthew E. Growdon, Tanya Mailhot, Jane S. Saczynski, Tamara G. Fong, Sharon K. Inouye

Delirium, an acute disorder of attention and global cognitive function, is a common, serious, and potentially preventable source of morbidity and mortality for hospitalized older persons. Delirium affects as many as half of all people age 65 and older who are hospitalized. With the aging of the US population, delirium has assumed heightened importance because persons aged 65 and older presently account for nearly 40% of all days of hospital care. Total costs attributable to delirium spanning the hospital and posthospital period exceed $60,000 per patient; annually over $183 billion (in 2018 US dollars) of US health care costs are attributable to delirium. Importantly, delirium is preventable in up to 50% of cases. Substantial additional costs linked to delirium accrue after hospital discharge because of the increased need for institutionalization, rehabilitation services, closer medical follow-up, and home health care. Delirium often initiates a cascade of events in older persons, leading to a downward spiral of functional and cognitive decline, loss of independence, institutionalization, and ultimately, death. Delirium is a critical risk marker to identify patients at high risk for poor outcomes. Recently, this fact has been underscored in the care of patients affected by severe acute respiratory syndrome coronavirus 2 (SARS-CoV-2) during the COVID-19 pandemic, as those who present with delirium experience worse hospital outcomes compared to those who do not. With its common occurrence, its frequently iatrogenic nature, and its close linkage to the processes of care, incident delirium can serve as a marker for the quality of hospital care and provides an important opportunity for quality improvement.

DEFINITION

The definition of and diagnostic criteria for delirium continue to evolve. Standardized criteria for delirium in the American Psychiatric Association's *Diagnostic and Statistical Manual of Mental Disorders, Fifth Edition* (DSM-5, 2013) represent the current diagnostic standard. These criteria are based on (A) a disturbance in attention and awareness; (B) an acute onset and fluctuating course; (C) an additional deficit in cognition (such as memory, orientation, language, or visuoperceptual ability); (D) impairments not better explained by dementia and do not occur in context of severely impaired level of consciousness

Learning Objectives

- Learn the epidemiology, pathophysiology, clinical presentations, evaluation, and management of delirium in older adults.
- Understand the role of various predisposing and precipitating factors in increasing risk of older persons to delirium and associated prognosis and mortality.
- Learn the special relationship between dementia and delirium and the role of certain medications in predisposing older adults to delirium.
- Recognize that delirium is preventable in up to 50% of cases with proven effective nonpharmacologic approaches.
- Gain a clear understanding of the specific indications and efficacy of various treatments, including pharmacologic and nonpharmacologic strategies commonly used to manage delirium.
- Understand the latest concepts about special issues related to delirium, including the COVID-19 pandemic, patient preferences and decision making, nursing home care, and palliative and end-of-life care.

Key Clinical Points

1. Delirium is commonly encountered in older adults in various clinical settings and associated with significant morbidity and mortality, especially in intensive care units, inpatient settings, nursing homes, and following major medical illnesses or surgery.
2. Delirium is unrecognized in up to 70% of older patients and can lead to long-term functional and cognitive deficits.
3. The pathophysiology of delirium is currently unclear but posited to be the end result of multiple pathogenic pathways eventually culminating in the dysfunction of various neurotransmitters and major brain networks.

(Continued)

(Cont.)

4. Delirium is commonly due to multiple causes and is preventable in up to 50% of cases through addressing as many predisposing and precipitating factors as possible.

5. Among the precipitating factors, decreased mobility is strongly associated with delirium, and medical equipment and devices may further contribute to immobilization.

6. Dementia is the underlying risk factor in up to two-thirds of cases of delirium and must be suspected in patients with slowly progressive cognitive and functional deficits.

7. Acute onset, varying levels of alertness, and inattention are cardinal features of delirium, and obtaining historical details from a close family member or friend is critical in making a correct diagnosis of delirium.

8. Nonpharmacologic strategies are the preferred treatment for delirium in older patients, and medications are reserved for more severe symptoms that affect either medical management or patient safety.

or coma; and (E) evidence of an underlying medical etiology or multiple etiologies. Expert consensus was used to develop these criteria, however, and performance characteristics such as diagnostic sensitivity and specificity have not yet been reported for DSM-5 criteria. A standardized tool, the Confusion Assessment Method (CAM), provides a brief, validated diagnostic algorithm that is currently in widespread use for identification of delirium. The CAM algorithm relies on the presence of acute onset and fluctuating course, inattention, and either disorganized thinking or altered level of consciousness. The algorithm has a sensitivity of 94% to 100%, specificity of 90% to 95%, and high interrater reliability. Given the uncertainty of diagnostic criteria for delirium, a critical area for future investigation is to establish more definitive criteria, including epidemiologic and phenomenologic evaluations assisted by advances in neuroimaging and other potential diagnostic marker tests.

EPIDEMIOLOGY

Most of the epidemiologic studies of delirium involve hospitalized older patients, in whom the highest rates of delirium occur. Reported rates vary based on the subgroup of patients studied and the setting of care. Previous studies estimated the prevalence of delirium (present at the time of hospital admission) at 7% to 80% and the incidence of delirium (new cases arising during hospitalization) at 8% to 82%. The highest prevalence and incidence rates occur

among ventilated intensive care unit patients. The incidence rates of delirium in high-risk hospital venues, such as the intensive care unit and surgical settings, range from 16% to 82% and 8% to 58%, respectively. Delirium occurs in up to 48% of patients in nursing homes or postacute settings, and in up to 83% of all patients at the end of life. The rates of delirium in all older persons presenting to the emergency department in several studies have ranged from 8% to 27%. While less frequent in the community setting, delirium is an important presenting symptom to outpatient clinics and often heralds serious underlying disease. Delirium is often unrecognized. Previous studies have documented that clinicians fail to detect up to 70% to 85% of affected patients across all of these settings. Furthermore, the presence of delirium portends a potentially poor prognosis. Delirium in the intensive care unit is associated with a fourfold increased risk of in-hospital mortality and a sixfold increased risk of mortality at 6 months. In the emergency department, delirium is associated with a sevenfold increased risk of mortality at 6 months. Longer lengths of stay, cognitive and functional sequelae lasting up to 1 year postoperatively, and institutionalization are also consequences of delirium.

PATHOPHYSIOLOGY

The fundamental pathophysiologic mechanisms of delirium remain unclear. Delirium is thought to represent a functional rather than structural lesion. The characteristic electroencephalographic (EEG) findings demonstrate global functional derangements and generalized slowing of cortical background (alpha) activity. It has been hypothesized that delirium is mediated via a final common pathway of different but interacting pathogenic mechanisms leading to dysfunction of multiple brain regions and neurotransmitter systems and culminating in disruption of large-scale networks. Evidence for a single pathway is lacking, and it remains difficult to ascribe delirium to a distinct neurobiological mechanism. Another hypothesis which has gained favor is that delirium occurs in the setting of an acute stressor, such as surgery or sepsis, superimposed on an underlying brain vulnerability, such as cognitive impairment or frailty. This model suggests that as vulnerability increases, delirium can be triggered by relatively minor acute stressors. Numerous contributions to brain vulnerability have been suggested, such as structural lesions, vascular changes, alterations in brain connectivity, neuroinflammation, or neurodegeneration, and other age-related changes. Evidence from EEG, evoked-potential studies, and neuroimaging studies in delirium suggest focal dysfunction localized to the prefrontal cortex, thalamus, basal ganglia, temporoparietal cortex, fusiform, and lingual gyri of the nondominant cortex. Studies using computed tomography (CT) or magnetic resonance imaging (MRI) have found lesions or structural abnormalities in the brains of patients with delirium. Single-photon emission computed tomography (SPECT) studies have shown that delirium is mostly associated with decreased cerebral blood flow, but these results have been variable.

Associated neurotransmitter abnormalities involve elevated brain dopaminergic function, reduced cholinergic function, or a relative imbalance of these systems. Serotonergic activity may interact to regulate or alter activity of these other two systems, and serotonin levels may be either increased or decreased. Extensive evidence supports the role of cholinergic deficiency. Acetylcholine plays a key role in consciousness and attentional processes. Given that delirium manifests as an acute confusional state often with alterations of consciousness, it is likely to have a cholinergic basis. Anticholinergic drugs can induce delirium in humans and animals, and serum anticholinergic activity is increased in patients with delirium. Physostigmine can reverse delirium associated with anticholinergic drugs, and cholinesterase inhibitors appear to have some benefit even in cases of delirium that are not induced by drugs. Neurotransmitter systems can also be affected indirectly. For instance, in sepsis, the systemic inflammatory response triggers a cascade of local (brain) neuroinflammation, leading to endothelial activation, impaired blood flow, neuronal apoptosis, and neurotransmitter dysfunction. Neuroinflammation can lead to microglial overactivation, resulting in a neurotoxic response with further neuronal injury. Animal studies have found that neurodegeneration causes priming of astrocytes and microglia, resulting in a greater neuroinflammatory response, as well as alterations in vasculature, including the blood-brain barrier, which may render the brain more vulnerable to circulating inflammatory molecules. The stress response associated with severe medical illness or surgery involves sympathetic and immune system activation, including increased activity of the hypothalamic-pituitary-adrenal axis with hypercortisolism, and release of cerebral cytokines that alter neurotransmitter systems, the thyroid axis, and modification of blood-brain barrier permeability. Age-related changes in central neurotransmission, stress management, hormonal regulation, and immune response may contribute to the increased vulnerability of older persons to delirium. The description of delirium as "acute brain failure"—involving multiple neural circuits, neurotransmitters, and brain regions—suggests that understanding delirium may help to elucidate the underlying mechanisms of brain functioning.

ETIOLOGY

The etiology of delirium is usually multifactorial. Among older persons, delirium results from the interrelationship between patient vulnerability (ie, predisposing factors) and the occurrence of noxious insults (ie, precipitating factors). For example, patients who are highly vulnerable to delirium at baseline (eg, such as patients with dementia or serious illness) can experience delirium after exposure to otherwise mild insults, such as a single dose of a

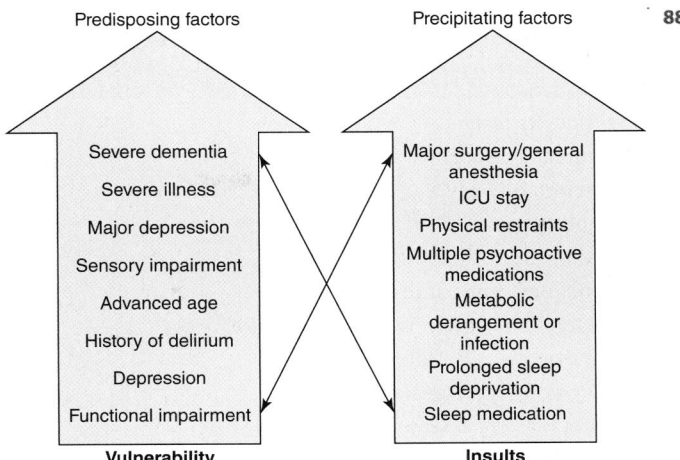

FIGURE 58-1. Multifactorial model for delirium. The etiology of delirium involves a complex interrelationship between the patient's underlying vulnerability or predisposing factors (*left axis*) and precipitating factors or noxious insults (*right axis*). For example, a patient with high vulnerability, such as with severe dementia, underlying severe illness, or hearing or vision impairment, might develop delirium with exposure to only one dose of a sleeping medication. Conversely, a patient with low vulnerability would develop delirium only with exposure to many noxious insults, such as general anesthesia and major surgery, intensive care unit (ICU) stay, multiple psychoactive medications, and prolonged sleep deprivation.

sedative medication. Older patients with few predisposing factors (low baseline vulnerability) are relatively resistant, with precipitation of delirium only after exposure to multiple potentially noxious insults, such as general anesthesia, major surgery, multiple psychoactive medications, immobilization, and infection (**Figure 58-1**). Based on validated predictive models for delirium, the effects of multiple risk factors appear to be cumulative. Clinically, the importance of the multifactorial nature of delirium is that removal or treatment of one risk factor alone often fails to resolve delirium. Instead, addressing many or all of the predisposing and precipitating factors for delirium is often required before the delirium symptoms will improve.

Predisposing Factors

Predisposing factors for delirium include preexisting cognitive impairment or dementia, a history of delirium, advanced age (> 70 years), severe underlying illness and multimorbidity, functional impairment, depression, alcohol abuse, a history of stroke, hypertension or transient ischemic attack, carotid artery disease and sensory impairments (vision or hearing) (**Table 58-1**). Preexisting cognitive impairment, including dementia, is one of the most powerful and consistent risk factors for delirium demonstrated across multiple studies in various settings, with patients with dementia having a two- to fivefold increased risk for delirium. Up to two thirds of delirious patients have underlying dementia. Nearly any chronic medical condition can predispose a patient to delirium, ranging from

TABLE 58-1 ■ PREDISPOSING AND PRECIPITATING FACTORS FOR DELIRIUM FROM VALIDATED PREDICTIVE MODELS

Predisposing factors

- Dementia or cognitive impairment
- Comorbidity/severity of illness
- Depression
- Vision and/or hearing impairment
- Functional impairment
- History of transient ischemia or stroke
- History of alcohol abuse
- History of hypertension
- Carotid artery disease
- History of delirium
- Age > 70

Precipitating factors

- Drugs (polypharmacy, psychoactive medications, sedatives, hypnotics)
- Use of physical restraints
- Indwelling bladder catheter
- Physiologic
  - Elevated BUN/creatinine ratio
  - Elevated serum urea
  - Abnormal serum albumin
  - Abnormal sodium, glucose or potassium
  - Metabolic acidosis
- Infection
- Iatrogenic complications
- Major surgical procedure (eg, aortic aneurysm repair, noncardiac thoracic surgery, and neurosurgery)
- Trauma admission
- Urgent admission
- Coma
- ICU stay > 10 days

diseases involving the central nervous system to diseases outside the central nervous system, including infectious, metabolic, cardiac, pulmonary, endocrine, or neoplastic etiologies. Predictive risk models that identify predisposing factors in populations, such as general medicine, intensive care, surgical patients (cardiac and noncardiac), cancer patients, and nursing home residents, can help identify patients at an increased risk of delirium.

Precipitating Factors

Major precipitating factors identified in validated predictive models include medication use (see section on "Drug Use and Delirium"), which are associated with up to a fivefold increased risk of delirium, use of indwelling bladder catheters, use of physical restraints, dehydration, malnutrition, iatrogenic events, infections, metabolic and electrolyte derangements, surgery, admissions that are urgent or involve trauma, extended ICU stays (> 10 days), and coma (see **Table 58-1**). Decreased mobility is strongly associated with delirium and concomitant functional decline. The use of medical equipment and devices (eg, indwelling bladder catheters and physical restraints) may further contribute to immobilization. Major iatrogenic events occur in up to 40% of older hospitalized adults (three to five times the risk when compared with adults younger than 65 years) and double the risk for development of delirium. Examples include complications related to diagnostic or therapeutic procedures, allergic reactions, and bleeding caused by over-anticoagulation. Disorders of any major organ system, particularly renal or hepatic failure, can precipitate delirium. Occult respiratory failure has emerged as an increasing problem in older patients, who often lack the typical signs and symptoms of dyspnea and tachypnea. In older adults, acute myocardial infarction and congestive heart failure may present with delirium or "failure to thrive" as the cardinal feature, and minimal symptoms of angina or dyspnea. Occult infection is a particularly noteworthy cause of delirium because older patients may not present with leukocytosis or a typical febrile response. Metabolic and endocrinologic disorders, such as hyper- or hyponatremia, hypercalcemia, acid-base disorders, hypo- and hyperglycemia, and thyroid or adrenal disorders, may also contribute to delirium. Precipitating factors for delirium in hospitalized older patients that have been validated include use of physical restraints, malnutrition, more than three medications added during the previous day (> 70% of these were psychoactive drugs), indwelling bladder catheter, and any iatrogenic event. The presence of each of these independent factors confers a two- to fourfold increased risk of delirium. The presence of multiple factors has a cumulative effect, yet each risk factor is potentially modifiable.

Drug Use and Delirium

In 30% or more of delirium cases, use of one or more specific medications contributes to its development. While medications often incite delirium, they are also the most common remediable cause of delirium. The most common culprit medications have psychoactive effects, such as sedative hypnotics, anxiolytics, narcotics, and medications with anticholinergic activity (**Table 58-2**). In previous studies, use of any psychoactive medication was associated with a fourfold increased risk of delirium; use of two or more psychoactive medications was associated with a fivefold increased risk. Sedative-hypnotic drugs are associated with a 3- to 12-fold increased risk of delirium; narcotics with a threefold risk; and anticholinergic drugs with a 5- to 12-fold risk. The incidence of delirium, similar to other adverse drug events, increases in direct proportion to the number of medications prescribed because of the effects of the medications themselves and the increased risk of drug–drug and drug–disease interactions. Suboptimal medication management, ranging from inappropriate use to overuse of psychoactive medications, occurs commonly in older adults, suggesting that many

TABLE 58-2 ■ MEDICATIONS ASSOCIATED WITH INDUCING OR WORSENING OF DELIRIUM (AMERICAN GERIATRICS SOCIETY BEERS CRITERIA, 2019)

- Anticholinergics (including antihistamines, antiparkinsonian agents, skeletal muscle relaxants, tricyclic antidepressants and paroxetine, antimuscarinics, antispasmodics, antiemetics including prochlorperazine and promethazine)
- Antipsychotics (chronic and as-needed use)
- Benzodiazepines
- Corticosteroids (oral and parenteral)
- H2-receptor antagonists (cimetidine, famotidine, nizatidine, and ranitidine)
- Meperidine
- Nonbenzodiazepine benzodiazepine receptor agonist hypnotics, including zolpidem, eszopiclone, and zaleplon
- Tricyclic antidepressants

Data from 2019 American Geriatrics Society Beers Criteria® Update Expert Panel. American Geriatrics Society 2019 Updated AGS Beers Criteria® for Potentially Inappropriate Medication Use in Older Adults, J Am Geriatr Soc. 2019;67(4):674–694.

cases of delirium and related adverse drug events may be preventable.

Relationship Between Delirium and Dementia

Delirium and dementia frequently coexist, with dementia being a leading risk factor for delirium and delirium resulting in worsened cognitive functioning. The contribution of delirium to permanent cognitive impairment or dementia is an area of active research, given the fact that after delirium, some patients never recover to their baseline level of cognitive function. Delirium and dementia may represent two ends along a spectrum of cognitive impairment with "chronic delirium" and "reversible dementia" falling along a continuum. Dementia is the leading risk factor for delirium, and fully two-thirds of cases of delirium occur in patients with dementia. Studies have shown that delirium and dementia are both associated with decreased cerebral metabolism, cholinergic deficiency, inflammation and abnormal glucose metabolism, reflecting their overlapping clinical, metabolic, and cellular mechanisms. Delirium can alter the course of underlying dementia, with dramatic worsening of the trajectory of cognitive decline, resulting in more rapid progression of functional losses and worsened long-term outcomes including hospitalization and mortality. Additionally, postoperative cognitive decline is accelerated among patients with delirium.

PRESENTATION

Cardinal Features

Acute onset and inattention are the central features of delirium. Determining the acuity of onset requires accurate knowledge of the patient's prior cognitive status and often entails obtaining historical information from another close observer, such as a family member, caregiver, or nurse. With delirium, the mental status changes typically occur over hours to days, in contrast to the changes that occur with dementia, which present insidiously over weeks to months. Another key feature is the fluctuating course of delirium; symptoms tend to wax and wane in severity over a 24-hour period. Lucid intervals are characteristic, and the reversibility of symptoms within a short time can deceive even an experienced clinician. Inattention is manifested as difficulty focusing, maintaining, and shifting attention or concentration. With simple cognitive assessment, patients may display difficulty with straightforward repetition tasks, digit spans, or recitation of the months of the year backward. Delirious patients appear easily distracted, experience difficulty with multistep commands, cannot follow the flow of a conversation, and often perseverate with an answer to a previous question. Additional major features include a disorganization of thought and altered level of consciousness. Disorganized thoughts are a manifestation of underlying cognitive or perceptual disturbances and can be recognized by disjointed and incoherent speech or an unclear or illogical flow of ideas. Clouding of consciousness is typically manifested by lethargy, with a reduced awareness of the environment that may show diurnal variation. Although not cardinal elements, other frequently associated features include disorientation (more commonly to time and place than to self), cognitive impairments (eg, memory and problem-solving deficits, dysnomia), psychomotor agitation or retardation, perceptual disturbances (eg, hallucinations, misperceptions, illusions), paranoid delusions, emotional lability, and sleep-wake cycle disruption.

Classification of Delirium

The clinical presentation of delirium can take three main forms: hypoactive, hyperactive, or mixed. The hypoactive form of delirium is characterized by lethargy and reduced psychomotor functioning and is the more common form in older patients. Hypoactive delirium often goes unrecognized and carries an overall poorer prognosis. The reduced level of patient activity associated with hypoactive delirium, often attributed to low mood or fatigue, may contribute to its misdiagnosis or underrecognition. By contrast, the hyperactive form of delirium presents with symptoms of agitation, increased vigilance, and often concomitant hallucinations; its presentation rarely remains unnoticed by caregivers or clinicians. Patients can fluctuate between the hypoactive and hyperactive forms—the mixed type of delirium—presenting a challenge in distinguishing the presentation from other psychotic or mood disorders. Recognition of partial or subsyndromal forms of delirium has brought attention to the persistence of symptoms among older patients, particularly during the resolution stages of delirium. Partial forms of delirium also adversely influence long-term clinical outcomes.

Delirium is an important independent determinant of prolonged length of hospital stay, increased mortality, increased rates of nursing home placement, and functional and cognitive decline. Delirium has long been thought to be a reversible, transient condition; however, accumulating evidence brings this into question. Delirium symptoms generally persist for a month or more; as few as 20% of patients attain complete symptom resolution at 6-month follow-up. Cognitive function is impacted for up to a year following delirium, and patients who develop delirium are at increased risk for development of dementia. The chronic detrimental effects are likely related to the duration, severity, and underlying cause(s) of the delirium in addition to the baseline vulnerability of the patient.

EVALUATION

There are numerous instruments for the identification of delirium. Each delirium instrument has strengths and limitations, and the choice among them depends on the goals for use. The most widely used is the CAM, of which the four-item short form has been applied in over 10,000 studies to date and translated into over 19 languages. The CAM has been adapted for use in other settings, including the intensive care unit (CAM-ICU), nursing home (NH-CAM), and emergency department (CAM-ED and B-CAM). The CAM-S derived from the CAM can be used to rate delirium severity and has demonstrated predictive validity for relevant clinical outcomes. Designed for clinicians with minimal training, several brief screening tools have been validated in postsurgical, medical, emergency department, and postacute care settings. For example, the Ultra-Brief CAM (UB-CAM) requires just 1 minute to complete and can identify delirium with high sensitivity and specificity. Selected screening tools are presented in **Table 58-3**. These can be used as an initial step in delirium detection and should be followed by a comprehensive assessment. Additionally, family-informed tools can be completed by health care professionals and/or families, yielding sensitivities ranging from 67% to 90% and specificities ranging from 56% to 90% in diverse populations.

The acute evaluation of suspected or confirmed delirium centers on three main tasks that occur simultaneously: (1) establishing the diagnosis of delirium; (2) determining the potential cause(s) and ruling out life-threatening

TABLE 58-3 ■ SELECTED DELIRIUM SCREENING TESTS

BRIEF SCREENING TEST	BRIEF DESCRIPTION
Confusion Assessment Method (CAM) Short Form	Widely adopted 5-min instrument to score 4-item algorithm based on 9 operationalized DSM-IIIR criteria for delirium; involves cognitive assessment; interviewer training recommended for optimal use
Ultra-Brief CAM (UB-CAM)	2-step protocol: The UB-2 (below) is performed first and, when positive, followed by a short interview (3D-CAM) and rating of the CAM diagnostic algorithm. Ultra-Brief 2-Item Screener (UB-2): 2 items. Question 1: "*Please tell me the day of the week.*" Question 2: "*Please tell me the months of the year backwards, say December as your first month.*" Positive screen if one or both is incorrect, followed by a more thorough diagnostic interview such as the 3D-CAM. 3-Minute Diagnostic Confusion Assessment Method (3D-CAM): 3-min version of CAM requiring minimal training; algorithm probes 4 cardinal features of delirium, with 2 essential features and at least 1 of 2 secondary features indicating delirium. Skip patterns can shorten administration.
Confusion Assessment Method—ICU version (CAM-ICU)	Modification of CAM 4-feature algorithm with nonverbal tasks that can be used in the ICU setting
Delirium Triage Screen (DTS), combined with Brief Confusion Assessment Method (bCAM)	DTS: 2 items. Assesses 2 features of delirium: altered level of consciousness (feature 1); attention (feature 2). Attention is assessed using the "LUNCH" backwards spelling test. Validated among emergency department patients. If positive, follow with bCAM. bCAM: 7 items. Like the CAM algorithm, a score is considered positive for delirium if 3 out of 4 features are present (features 1 and 2, and either 3 or 4). Validated in emergency department and palliative care settings.
Nursing Delirium Screening Scale (Nu-DESC)	5-item, 1-min screening scale designed for use by nurses and used during routine care on the hospital floor, scores range from 0 to 10 with higher scores indicating delirium
Recognizing Acute Delirium as part of Routine (RADAR)	3 observational items. Assesses 3 features of delirium: consciousness; attention/hyperactivity; psychomotor retardation. Validated in nursing home and emergency department patients.
4AT	2-min instrument for general practice includes 4 items; scores range from 0 to 12, with a score ≥ 4 suggesting possible delirium.

A complete listing of information about delirium tools, along with critical performance characteristics, can be found online from the Network for Investigation of Delirium: Unifying Scientists at https://deliriumnetwork.org/measurement/adult-delirium-info-cards/.

contributors; and (3) managing the symptoms while assuring patient safety. Delirium is a clinical diagnosis, relying on astute observation at the bedside, careful cognitive assessment, and history-taking from a knowledgeable informant to establish a change from the patient's baseline functioning. Identifying the potentially multifactorial contributors to the delirium is of paramount importance. Many of these factors are treatable, and if left untreated, may result in substantial morbidity and mortality. Because the potential contributors are myriad, the search requires a thorough medical evaluation guided by clinical judgment. The challenge is enhanced by the frequently nonspecific or atypical presentation of the underlying illness in older persons. In fact, delirium is often the *only* sign of life-threatening illness, such as sepsis, pneumonia, or myocardial infarction in older persons.

History and Physical Examination

A thorough history and physical examination constitute the foundation of the medical evaluation of suspected delirium. The first step in evaluation should be to establish the diagnosis of delirium through careful cognitive assessment and to determine the acuity of change from the patient's baseline cognitive state. Because cognitive impairment may easily be missed during routine conversation, brief cognitive screening tests, such as the Mini-Cog test or the UB-CAM assessment, should be used to rate the CAM. The degree of attention should be further assessed with simple tests such as a digit span (inattention indicated by an inability to repeat five digits forward or three digits backward) or recitation of the months of the year backward. A targeted history, focusing on baseline cognitive status and chronology of recent mental status changes, should be elicited from a reliable informant. Historical data including intercurrent illnesses, recent adjustments in medications, the possibility of withdrawal from alcohol, other substances, or medications, and pertinent environmental changes may elucidate precipitating factors of delirium.

The physical examination should comprise detailed review focusing on potential etiologic clues to an underlying or inciting disease process. Vital sign assessment is important to identify fever, tachycardia, or decreased oxygen saturation, each of which may point to specific disease processes. Auscultatory examination may suggest pneumonia or pulmonary effusion. A new cardiac murmur or dysrhythmia may suggest ischemia or congestive heart failure. Gastrointestinal examination should focus on evidence of an acute abdominal process, such as occult bleeding, perforated viscus, or infection. Patients with delirium may also demonstrate nonspecific focal findings on neurologic examination, such as asterixis or tremor. New focal neurologic deficits should raise suspicion of an acute cerebrovascular event or subdural hematoma. In many older patients and especially those with cognitive impairment, delirium may be the initial manifestation of a serious new disease process. Attention to early localizing signs on serial physical examinations is paramount.

A complete medication review, including over-the-counter medications, is critical. Any medications with known psychoactive effects should be discontinued or minimized whenever possible. Medications with potential for withdrawal should be tapered carefully. Because of pharmacodynamic and pharmacokinetic changes in aging adults, these medications may cause deleterious psychoactive effects even when prescribed at customary doses and with serum drug levels that are within the "therapeutic range."

Laboratory Tests and Imaging

Laboratory evaluation should be guided by clinical judgment and take into account specific patient characteristics and historical data. A thorough history and physical examination, medication review, focused laboratory testing (eg, complete blood count, chemistries, glucose, renal and liver function tests, urinalysis), and search for occult infection should help to identify the majority of potential contributors to the delirium. Additional laboratory testing such as thyroid function tests, B_{12} level, cortisol level, drug levels or toxicology screen, syphilis serologies, and ammonia level should be based on the specific clinical presentation. Further diagnostic work-up with an electrocardiogram, chest radiograph, and/or arterial blood gas test may be appropriate for patients with pulmonary or cardiac conditions. The indications for cerebrospinal fluid examination, brain imaging, or EEG remain controversial. Their overall diagnostic yield is low, and these procedures are probably indicated in fewer than 5% to 10% of delirium cases. Lumbar puncture with cerebrospinal fluid examination is indicated for the febrile delirious patient when meningitis or encephalitis is suspected. Brain imaging (such as CT or MRI) should be reserved for cases with new focal neurologic signs, with history or signs of head trauma, or without another identifiable cause of the delirium. Of note, some neurologic symptoms are associated with delirium, including tremor and asterixis. EEG, which has a false-negative rate of 17% and a false-positive rate of 22% for distinguishing between delirious and nondelirious patients, plays a limited role and is most commonly employed to detect subclinical seizure disorders and to differentiate delirium from nonorganic psychiatric conditions.

Differential Diagnosis

Distinguishing a long-standing confusional state (dementia) from delirium alone, or from delirium superimposed on dementia, is an important, but often difficult, diagnostic step. These two conditions can be differentiated by the acute onset of symptoms in delirium, with dementia presenting much more insidiously and by the impaired attention and altered level of consciousness associated with delirium.

The differential diagnosis of delirium can be extensive and includes other psychiatric conditions such as depression and nonorganic psychiatric disorders (**Table 58-4**).

TABLE 58-4 ■ DIFFERENTIAL DIAGNOSIS OF ALTERED MENTAL STATUS

CHARACTERISTIC	DELIRIUM	DEMENTIA	DEPRESSION	ACUTE PSYCHOSIS
Onset	Acute (hours to days)	Progressive, insidious (weeks to months)	Either acute or insidious	Acute
Course over time	Waxing and waning	Unrelenting	Variable	Episodic
Attention	Impaired, a hallmark of delirium	Usually intact, until end-stage disease	Decreased concentration and attention to detail	Variable
Level of consciousness	Altered, from lethargic to hyperalert	Normal, until end-stage disease	Normal	Normal
Memory	Impaired commonly	Prominent short- and/or long-term memory impairment	Normal, some short-term forgetfulness	Usually normal
Orientation	Disoriented	Normal, until end-stage disease	Usually normal	Usually normal
Speech	Disorganized, incoherent, illogical	Notable for parsimony, aphasia, anomia	Normal, but often slowing of speech (psychomotor retardation)	Variable, often disorganized
Delusions	Common	Common	Uncommon	Common, often complex
Hallucinations	Usually visual	Sometimes	Rare	Usually auditory and more complex
Organic etiology	Yes	Yes	No	No

Although perceptual disturbances, such as illusions and hallucinations, can occur with delirium in about 15% of cases, recognition of the key features of acute onset, inattention, altered level of consciousness, and global cognitive impairment will enhance the identification of delirium. Differentiating among diagnoses is critical because delirium carries a more serious prognosis without proper evaluation and management. Treatment for certain conditions such as depression or affective disorders may involve use of drugs with anticholinergic activity, which could exacerbate an unrecognized case of delirium. At times, working through the differential diagnosis can be challenging, and the diagnosis of delirium may remain uncertain. Because of the potentially life-threatening nature of delirium, however, it is prudent to manage the patient as having delirium and search for underlying precipitants until further information can be obtained.

Algorithm for the Evaluation of Altered Mental Status

Figure 58-2 presents an algorithm for the evaluation of altered mental status in the older patient. The initial steps center on establishing the patient's baseline cognitive functioning and the onset and timing of any cognitive changes. Chronic impairments, representing changes that occur over months to years, are most likely attributable to dementia, which should be evaluated accordingly (see Chapter 59). Acute alterations, representing abrupt deteriorations in mental status, occur over hours to weeks and may be superimposed on underlying dementia. They should be further evaluated with cognitive testing to establish the presence

of delirium. In the absence of notable delirium features (see "Presentation" earlier in this chapter), subsequent evaluation should focus on the possibility of major depression, acute psychotic disorder, or other psychiatric disorders (see Chapters 65, 60, and 66).

PREVENTION

Primary prevention—preventing delirium before it develops—is the most effective strategy for reducing delirium and its associated adverse outcomes. **Table 58-5** describes well-documented delirium risk factors and preventive interventions to address each risk factor. A controlled clinical trial demonstrated the effectiveness of a delirium prevention strategy targeted toward these risk factors, which were selected based on their clinical relevance and the degree to which they could be modified by employing practical and feasible interventions. Compared with standard care, implementation of these preventive interventions resulted in a 40% risk reduction for delirium in hospitalized older patients.

The Hospital Elder Life Program (HELP; now AGS CoCare HELP at https://help.agscocare.org/) represents an innovative strategy of hospital care for older patients, designed to incorporate the tested delirium prevention strategies and to improve overall quality of hospital care. Programs such as HELP underscore the importance of an interdisciplinary team's contributions to the prevention of delirium. For example, trained volunteers and family members can play roles in daily orientation, therapeutic recreation activities, and feeding assistance. Physical rehabilitation experts and nurses can assist with mobilization

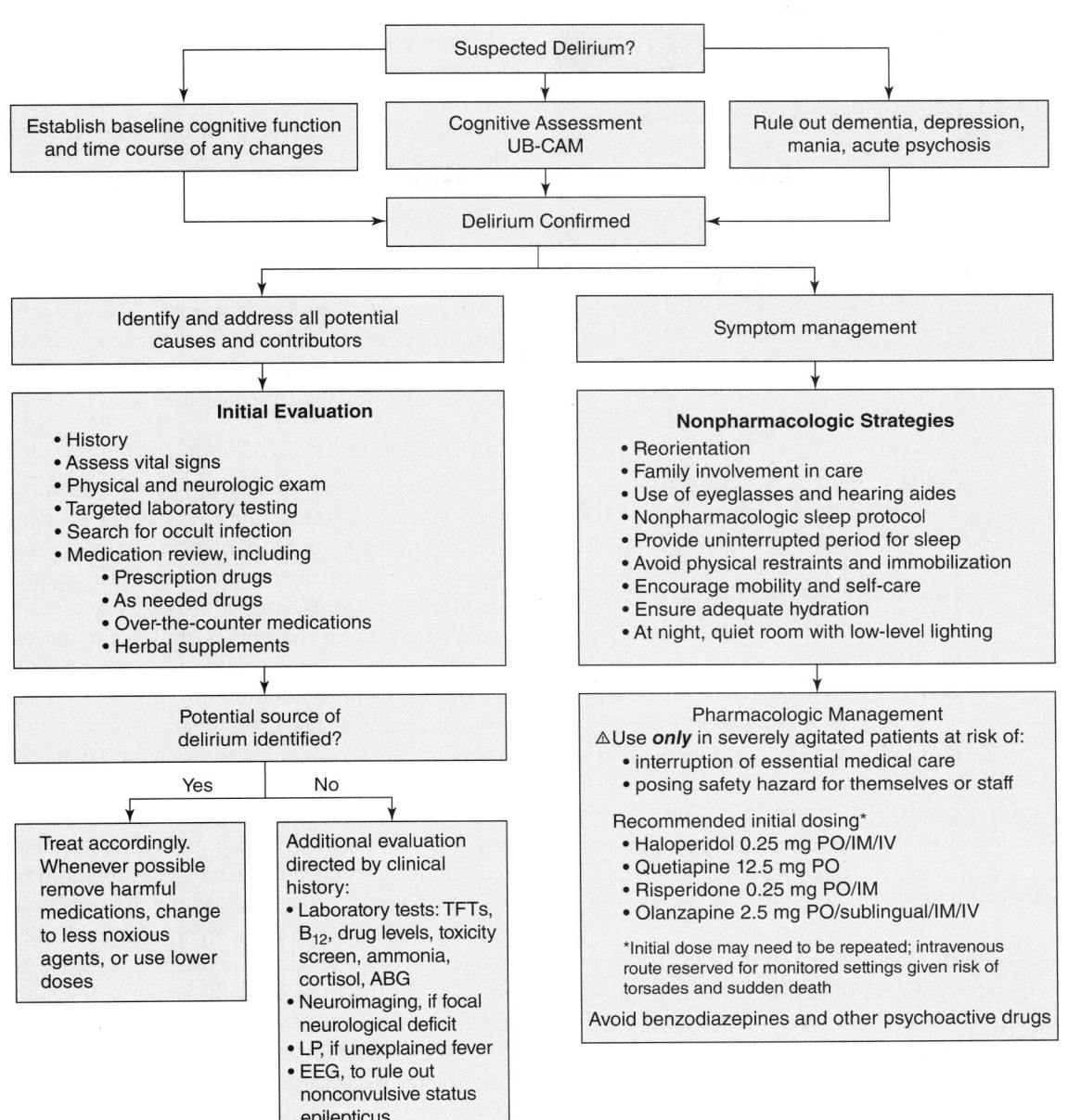

FIGURE 58-2. Flowchart for evaluation of suspected delirium in an older person. ABG, arterial blood gas; B_{12}, cyanocobalamin or vitamin B_{12} level; EEG, electroencephalography; IM, intramuscular; LP, lumbar puncture; PO, by mouth; TFTs, thyroid function tests (eg, T4, thyroid index, thyroid-stimulating hormone); UB-CAM, Ultra Brief Confusion Assessment Method.

and the incorporation of daily exercises to prevent functional decline. Dietitians can help to maximize appropriate caloric intake and oral hydration in acutely ill patients. Consultant pharmacists, chaplains, and social workers also may provide specialized expertise to address issues pertinent to individuals at risk for delirium.

At least 14 studies have examined primary prevention with nonpharmacologic multicomponent approaches to delirium in controlled trials with prospective sampling frameworks and validated delirium assessments. These studies applied multifactorial interventions or educational strategies targeted toward health care professionals, staff,

and families, and demonstrated significant reductions in delirium rates, in-hospital falls, health care–associated costs, and/or duration of delirium. Proactive geriatric consultation has been demonstrated to reduce the risk of delirium post hip fracture by 40% in a randomized controlled trial. Another trial found that home rehabilitation after acute hospitalization of older adults was associated with lower risk of delirium and greater patient satisfaction, when compared with an institutional setting. In all, trials suggest that up to 50% of cases of delirium may be preventable and that prevention strategies should begin early during hospitalization.

TABLE 58-5 ■ DELIRIUM RISK FACTORS AND TESTED PREVENTATIVE INTERVENTIONS

RISK FACTOR	INTERVENTION PROTOCOL
Cognitive impairment	• Orienting communication, including orientation board • Therapeutic activities program
Immobilization	• Early mobilization (eg, ambulation or bedside exercises) • Minimizing immobilizing equipment (eg, restraints, bladder catheters)
Psychoactive medications	• Restricted use of PRN sleep and psychoactive medications (eg, sedative-hypnotics, narcotics, anticholinergic drugs) • Nonpharmacologic protocols for management of sleep and anxiety
Sleep deprivation	• Noise-reduction strategies • Scheduling of nighttime medications, procedures, and nursing activities to allow uninterrupted period of sleep
Vision impairment	• Provision of vision aids (eg, magnifiers, special lighting) • Provision of adaptive equipment (eg, illuminated phone dials, large-print books)
Hearing impairment	• Provision of amplifying devices; repair hearing aids • Instruct staff in communication methods
Dehydration	• Early recognition and volume repletion

Data from Inouye SK, Bogardus ST Jr, Charpentier PA, et al. A multicomponent intervention to prevent delirium in hospitalized older patients. N Engl J Med. 1999;340(9): 669–676.

Preventive efforts for delirium will require system-wide changes and large-scale shifts in local and national policies and approaches to care. Recommended changes include routine cognitive and functional assessments on admission of all older patients, beginning in the emergency department setting; monitoring mental status as a "vital sign"; education of physicians and nurses to improve recognition and heighten awareness of the clinical implications; enhanced geriatric physician and nursing expertise; incentives to change practice patterns that lead to delirium (eg, immobilization, use of deliriogenic medications, bladder catheters, and physical restraints); and creation of systems that enhance high-quality geriatric care (eg, geriatric expertise, medication review, family involvement, case management, clinical pathways, and quality monitoring for delirium).

MANAGEMENT

Overview

The recommended management approach for all delirious patients begins with nonpharmacologic strategies, which usually result in successful symptom amelioration. In selected cases, such strategies must be supplemented with a pharmacologic approach, reserved for patients in whom delirium symptoms would result in interruption of needed medical therapies (eg, mechanical ventilation, central lines) or may endanger the safety of the patient or other persons. However, prescribing any drug requires balancing the benefits of delirium management against the potential for adverse medication effects because sedative drugs may prolong delirium and worsen clinical outcomes. The clinical team, family, and caregivers should understand that the choice of almost any medication may further cloud the patient's mental status, prolong delirium symptoms, and obscure efforts to monitor the course of the mental status change. Any drug should be initiated at the lowest starting dose for the shortest time possible.

Nonpharmacologic Management

Nonpharmacologic approaches are the mainstays of prevention and treatment for every delirious patient. These include strategies for reorientation and behavioral intervention, such as ensuring the presence of family members, use of sitters, and transferring a disruptive patient to a private room or closer to the nurse's station for increased supervision. Orienting influences such as calendars, clocks, and the day's schedule should be prominently displayed, along with familiar personal objects from the patient's home environment (eg, photographs and religious artifacts). Personal contact and communication are critical to reinforce patient awareness and encourage patient participation as much as possible. Communication should incorporate repeated reorientation strategies, clear instructions, and frequent eye contact. Correction of sensory impairments (ie, vision and hearing) should be maximized as applicable for individual patients by encouraging the use of eyeglasses and hearing aids during the hospital stay. Mobility and independence should be promoted; physical restraints should be avoided because they lead to decreased mobility, increased agitation, and greater risk of injury and worsening delirium. Patient involvement in self-care and decision making should also be encouraged. Other environmental interventions include limiting room and staff changes and providing a quiet patient care setting with low-level lighting at night. An environment with decreased noise allowing for an uninterrupted period for sleep at night is of crucial importance in the management of delirium. This may require unit-wide changes in the coordination of nursing and medical procedures, including medication dispensing, vital sign recording, and administration of intravenous medications and other treatments. Hospital-wide changes may be needed to ensure a low level of noise at night, including minimizing hallway noise, overhead paging, and staff conversations. Family involvement in nonpharmacologic management of delirium is critical and has been shown to reduce length of stay and ameliorate anxiety in family members.

Nonpharmacologic Sleep Protocol

Nonpharmacologic approaches for relaxation and sleep can be effective for management of agitation in delirious patients and for prevention of delirium through minimization of psychoactive medications. The nonpharmacologic sleep protocol includes three components: (1) a glass of warm milk or herbal tea, (2) relaxation music or tapes, and (3) back massage. This protocol was demonstrated to be feasible and effective, reducing use of sleeping medications from 54% to 31% in a hospital environment.

Antipsychotics

As a last resort, antipsychotics are the preferred agents for pharmacologic treatment of delirium. Haloperidol is the agent with the longest track record, although its use may be complicated by extrapyramidal side effects and acute dystonias. Many trials examining the efficacy of haloperidol and the atypical antipsychotics (such as quetiapine, risperidone, and olanzapine) have been low quality and/or inconclusive, with no effect on delirium duration, severity, relief of symptoms, length of stay or mortality. A recent placebo-controlled, randomized trial of haloperidol and ziprasidone in the intensive care setting similarly failed to show a benefit for these medications. Comparisons across antipsychotics have not found superior efficacy of any one agent. Additionally, there is evidence that antipsychotic drugs may prolong delirium and result in poor clinical outcomes. Moreover, official warnings have been issued regarding the increased mortality associated with the use of haloperidol and atypical antipsychotics in patients with dementia. Use of antipsychotics should be avoided in patients with Parkinson disease and Lewy body dementia.

If proceeding with antipsychotic administration, the intravenous route should be reserved for monitored settings due to the risk of torsades and sudden death. Parenteral administration is required in cases where rapid onset of action is required with short duration of action, whereas oral or intramuscular use is associated with a more optimal duration of action. The recommended starting dose is 0.25 mg of haloperidol orally or parenterally. The dose may be repeated every 30 minutes after vital signs have been rechecked. The clinical end point should be an awake but manageable patient, a goal that can be achieved by following the geriatric prescribing principle, "start low and go slow." Most older patients naïve to prior treatment with an antipsychotic should require a total loading dose of no more than 2.5 mg of haloperidol. A subsequent maintenance dose consisting of one-half of the loading dose should be administered in divided doses over the next 24 hours, with doses tapered over the ensuing 48 hours as the agitation resolves. Alternatively, an atypical antipsychotic may be considered at a low starting dose: quetiapine (starting dose, 12.5 mg; 24-h maximum, 25 mg), olanzapine (starting dose, 2.5 mg; 24-h maximum, 10 mg), or risperidone (0.25–0.5 mg; 24-h maximum, 1.5 mg). Patients should be reevaluated continually to assess for ongoing need and tapered off as soon as possible.

Other Pharmacologic Approaches

Benzodiazepines (eg, lorazepam) are not recommended as first-line agents in the treatment of delirium because of their propensity to cause oversedation and to exacerbate acute mental status changes. However, they remain the treatment of choice for delirium caused by seizures and alcohol- and medication-related withdrawal syndromes. While other drugs have been advocated for use in treatment of delirium, evaluation of their use has resulted in discrepant findings, and there is no consensus recommendation for their general use. Trials of the sedative dexmedetomidine in ventilated ICU patients found a reduction in delirium duration and length of ICU stay as well as better effectiveness and safety in haloperidol-resistant patients. Clonidine, an α2-agonist, has been shown to be safe, though no effect was detected on delirium. In randomized trials of melatonin and the melatonin receptor agonist ramelteon, the results have been mixed to date. Overall, data does not support the use of pharmacologic management of delirium, although the consensus in the field is for a limited role of medications for the treatment of intractable distress and agitation in which nonpharmacologic strategies have failed.

SPECIAL ISSUES

COVID-19

The arrival of the SARS-CoV-2 virus and associated COVID-19 in early 2020 has culminated in a global health crisis. Although COVID-19 typically manifests as an influenza-like respiratory illness, early reports of neurologic symptoms included altered mental status. In one study of older adults presenting to the emergency department with COVID-19, delirium was the sixth most common presenting symptom, and in some cases occurred without the typical symptoms of COVID-19. Rates of delirium during hospitalization with COVID-19 range from 25% to 84%. Delirium may be more severe or prolonged due to social isolation and use of personal protective equipment, resulting in poor communication, reduced social interactions, limited reorienting of patients, and prolonged need for mechanical ventilation, with increased immobilization, depth of sedation, or use of second-line medications due to drug shortages. Nonpharmacologic interventions for delirium prevention have been adapted for COVID-19 and are available online at https://help.agscocare.org/chapter-abstract/chapter/H00107/H00107_PART001_002.

Patient Preference and Decision Making

Given acute fluctuations in attention and decision-making capacity, delirium presents formidable challenges to the ethical care of affected patients (see Chapters 7 and 26). Cognitive assessments in patients with suspected delirium help to ensure that patients can be involved in decision making whenever possible and that appropriate surrogate decision makers are involved in representing a patient's wishes and understanding the risks and benefits of procedures and treatments. Because the patient may exhibit periods of lucidity in delirium, there may be times during which the decision-making and informed consent process can and must involve the patient. The clinician should be cognizant of ongoing subclinical manifestations of delirium, which may be important for both the long-term management and decision-making capacity of the patient.

Nursing Home Setting

For the postacute population receiving short-term rehabilitative care, persistent delirium after an acute hospitalization is a major concern. Prior studies demonstrated that 16% of admissions to postacute care met full CAM criteria for delirium, while another 50% demonstrated signs of subsyndromal delirium. Patients with delirium on admission to postacute care experience more complications such as falls, higher rehospitalization rates, and higher mortality. Of those admitted to postacute care with delirium, over 50% are still delirious 1 month later. Persistence of delirium prevents functional recovery in the postacute setting; only those patients whose delirium cleared within 2 weeks of admission recovered to their prehospitalization functional status. Persistent delirium is also associated with higher mortality.

The long-term care population represents a high-risk group for delirium, with a high prevalence of dementia and functional impairments. Incident delirium is common in this population, frequently heralding the onset of an acute illness that results in hospitalization and/or death. Nursing staffing ratios, high turnover, competing concerns, and the high prevalence of dementia make identification and prevention of delirium challenging in this setting. Nonetheless, these patients represent among the most vulnerable of older adults, and further attention to delirium in this setting is warranted. Research in long-term care settings is challenging, and results are mixed in this area. A recent trial involving nonpharmacologic delirium prevention strategies in the nursing home setting did not prevent delirium or reduce delirium symptoms, with greater than expected improvement in both intervention and usual care groups. This finding underscores the need for further research into effective delirium prevention strategies in this setting.

Palliative and End-of-Life Care

Because delirium occurs in more than 80% of patients at the end of life, it is considered nearly inevitable in the terminal stages by most hospice care providers and may serve as a marker of approaching death. Establishing goals of care with the patient and family is a crucial step, including discussions about the potential causes of the delirium, intensity of medical evaluations considered appropriate, and the potential trade-off between alertness and adequate control of pain and agitation. Some patients may wish to preserve their ability to communicate as long as possible, while others may focus on comfort perhaps at the expense of alertness. Physicians must be cognizant that even in the terminal phase, many causes of delirium are potentially reversible, and may be amenable to interventions (eg, medication adjustments, treatment of dehydration, hypoglycemia, or hypoxia) that may improve comfort and quality of life. However, the burdens of evaluation or treatment (eg, reduction in narcotic dose) may not be consistent with the goals for care. In all cases, symptom management should begin immediately, while evaluation is underway. Nonpharmacologic approaches should be instituted in all patients, with pharmacologic approaches for selected cases. Haloperidol remains the first-line therapy for delirium in terminally ill patients, although a recent randomized controlled trial did not support its use. In end-of-life care, sedation may be indicated as an additional therapy for management of severe agitated delirium in the terminally ill patient, which can cause considerable distress for the patient and family. Because sedation poses the risks of decreased meaningful interaction with family, increased confusion, and respiratory depression, this choice should be made in conjunction with the family according to the goals of care. If sedation is indicated, an agent that is short acting and easily titrated to effect is recommended. Lorazepam (starting dose 0.5–1.0 mg PO, IV, or SQ) is the recommended agent of choice.

FURTHER READING

American Geriatrics Society 2019 Beers Criteria Update Expert Panel. American Geriatrics Society 2019 updated Beers criteria for potentially inappropriate medication use in older adults. *J Am Geriatr Soc.* 2019;67:674–694.

American Psychiatric Association. *Diagnostic and Statistical Manual of Mental Disorders.* 5th ed. Washington, DC: American Psychiatric Association; 2013.

Fong TG, Davis D, Growdon ME, et al. The interface of delirium and dementia in older persons. *Lancet Neurol.* 2015;14:823–832.

Fong TG, Jones RN, Marcantonio ER, et al. Adverse outcomes after hospitalization and delirium in persons with Alzheimer disease. *Ann Intern Med.* 2012;156:848–856.

Girard TD, Exline MC, Carson SS, et al. Haloperidol and ziprasidone for treatment of delirium in critical illness. *N Engl J Med.* 2018;379:2506–2516.

Hshieh TT, Yue J, Oh E, et al. Effectiveness of multicomponent non-pharmacologic delirium interventions: a systematic review and meta-analysis. *JAMA Intern Med.* 2015;175:512–520.

Inouye SK, Bogardus ST Jr, Charpentier PA, et al. A clinical trial of a multicomponent intervention to prevent delirium in hospitalized older patients. *N Engl J Med.* 1999;340:669–676.

Inouye SK, Charpentier PA. Precipitating factors for delirium in hospitalized elderly persons: predictive model and inter-relationship with baseline vulnerability. *JAMA*. 1996;275:852–857.

Inouye SK, Marcantonio ER, Kosar CM, et al. The short- and long-term relationship between delirium and cognitive trajectory in older surgical patients. *Alzheimers Dement J Alzheimers Assoc*. 2016;12:766–775.

Inouye SK, van Dyck CH, Alessi CA, et al. Clarifying confusion: the confusion assessment method. A new method for detection of delirium. *Ann Intern Med*. 1990;113: 941–948.

Inouye SK, Westendorp RGJ, Saczynski J. Delirium in elderly people. *Lancet*. 2014;383:911–922.

Leslie DL, Marcantonio ER, Zhang Y, et al. One-year health care costs associated with delirium in the elderly population. *Arch Intern Med*. 2008;168:27–32.

Marcantonio ER. Delirium in hospitalized older adults. *N Engl J Med*. 2017;377:1456–1466.

Marcantonio ER, Flacker JM, Wright RJ, et al. Reducing delirium after hip fracture: a randomized trial. *J Am Geriatr Soc*. 2001;49:516–522.

Marcantonio ER, Goldman L, Mangione CM, et al. A clinical prediction rule for delirium after elective non-cardiac surgery. *JAMA*. 1994;271:134–139.

Motyl CM, Ngo L, Zhou W, et al. Comparative accuracy and efficiency of four delirium screening protocols. *J Am Geriatr Soc*. 2020;68:2572–2578.

Oh ES, Fong TG, Hshieh TT, Inouye SK. Delirium in older persons: advances in diagnosis and treatment (systematic review). *JAMA*. 2017;318:1161–1174.

Oh ES, Needham DM, Nikooie R, et al. Antipsychotics for preventing delirium in hospitalized adults: a systematic review. *Ann Intern Med*. 2019;171:474–484.

O'Mahony R, Murthy L, Akunne A, Young J. Synopsis of the National Institute for Health and Clinical Excellence guideline for prevention of delirium. *Ann Intern Med*. 2011;154:746–751.

Saczynski JS, Marcantonio ER, Quach L, et al. Cognitive trajectories after post-operative delirium. *N Engl J Med*. 2012;367:30–39.

Wilson JE, Mart MF, Cunningham C, et al. Delirium. *Nat Rev Dis Primer*. 2020;6:1–26.

Chapter 59

Dementia Including Alzheimer Disease

Cynthia M. Carlsson, Nathaniel A. Chin, Carey E. Gleason, Luigi Puglielli, Sanjay Asthana

Alzheimer disease (AD) is the most common neurodegenerative disorder affecting older adults, projected to affect more than 13 million Americans and 115 million individuals worldwide by 2050. Compared to projections in high-income countries, the number of individuals with AD in low- and middle-income nations is increasing at an even greater rate. The disease is characterized by diffuse functional and structural abnormalities in the brain that lead to progressive cognitive and behavioral deficits and functional decline. AD is associated with significant morbidity and mortality and is currently the sixth most common cause of death in the United States. The physical, psychological, functional, and socioeconomic impact of AD substantially affects the well-being and quality of life of patients and their caregivers. Caring for patients with AD places heavy financial burden on patients, families, communities, and the health care system at large. In the United States in 2020, the average lifetime cost of caring for a person with AD exceeded $350,000. The total cost of caring for Americans with AD exceeds $355 billion annually. Evidence is beginning to emerge on the economic impact of dementia care in low- and middle-income countries as most of the costs in these nations are related to informal care.

Recognizing the enormity of the burden of AD, international collaborations between clinicians, researchers, policy makers, patient advocacy groups, the media, and many others have increased public awareness of the global impact of the disease and have laid the foundation for the development of effective preventive and therapeutic strategies as well as improvements in care management for patients with AD. An example of such a coordinated effort is the 2011 United States National Alzheimer's Project Act (NAPA), a law designed to create and maintain an integrated national plan to address AD. The plan encompasses federal coordination of AD research and services and aims to improve early diagnosis and coordination of care, accelerate development of effective treatments, promote health equity in AD care among ethnic and racial minority populations, and stimulate coordination with international groups to address AD globally. Such national and international collaborations will help accelerate optimal diagnosis and care of patients at risk for AD and related dementias. Another example is the public health prevention effort underway to address 12 recognized modifiable risk factors that

Learning Objectives

- Describe the current diagnostic criteria for dementia, Alzheimer disease (AD), and mild cognitive impairment (MCI), and how these conditions differ from normal cognitive aging.
- Understand the effects of age and other genetic and nongenetic risk factors on risk of developing AD.
- Identify key neuropathologic features and mechanistic pathways associated with AD.
- Recognize common reversible causes of cognitive dysfunction.
- Describe an effective dementia care management plan across care settings and stages of disease, integrating use of pharmacologic and nonpharmacologic interventions, education, and community resources.

Key Clinical Points

1. AD is the most common neurodegenerative disorder affecting older adults with prevalence rates increasing with advancing age.
2. While aging is the most established risk factor for late-onset AD, various other genetic, lifestyle, and environmental factors also influence dementia risk.
3. The diagnostic evaluation for dementia, AD, and MCI depends heavily on a careful assessment of an individual's change in functional status, a structured cognitive assessment, a thorough clinical examination, and exclusion of other competing causes of cognitive decline.
4. There are currently no proven preventive or disease-modifying therapies for AD; however, aducanumab is the first FDA-approved medication that reduces amyloid burden in the brain, but without significant improvement in cognition. The current standard-of-care management plans integrate use of

(Continued)

(Cont.)

pharmacologic therapies to delay symptom progression; nonpharmacologic strategies to optimize function, behavior, and safety; and education and support for patients and their care partners.

5. Advanced care planning prior to loss of decisional capacity is of critical importance in developing patient-centered goals of care in persons with cognitive impairment.

contribute to dementia and recommend policy interventions to mitigate these risks. In the United States, this is the focus of the Alzheimer's Association's Centers for Disease Control and Prevention: Building Our Largest Dementia (BOLD) Public Health Center of Excellence on Dementia Risk Reduction supported by the BOLD Infrastructure for Alzheimer's Act—PL115-406.

DEFINITION

In defining AD features, it is widely recognized that the clinical cognitive and behavioral signs and symptoms do not always correlate with the degree of AD neuropathologic changes noted in the brain. The discrepancy between the neuropathologic changes and the individual clinical expression of disease is likely related to additional unidentified physiologic, metabolic, or genetic factors that either accelerate or slow cognitive decline. For example, some older adults with normal cognitive function just prior to death have been found to have significant AD neuropathology on autopsy. These individuals may have unrecognized neuroprotective factors that help preserve cognitive function despite notable neuropathologic changes. Thus, in order to disentangle the clinical syndrome from the neuropathologic changes, the current AD core clinical criteria are distinct from the AD neuropathologic guidelines, yet encourage clinicians and researchers to postulate the most likely neuropathology underlying the clinical presentation of disease.

In 2011, the National Institute on Aging and the Alzheimer's Association (NIA-AA) released cosponsored revised clinical diagnostic guidelines for dementia, dementia due to AD, MCI, and a theoretical framework for defining the preclinical stages of AD. Core clinical diagnostic criteria for dementia, AD, and MCI were designed for use in all clinical settings and are summarized in **Tables 59-1** and **59-2**. In 2013, the American Psychiatric Association published the *Diagnostic and Statistical Manual of Mental Disorders, Fifth Edition* (DSM-5). Within this edition, the term "dementia" was replaced with "major neurocognitive disorder" and the term "mild cognitive impairment" with "mild neurocognitive disorder." While the DSM-5

and NIA-AA terminologies differ, the diagnostic criteria for major neurocognitive disorder and dementia as well as those for mild neurocognitive disorder and MCI are nearly identical (see **Tables 59-1** and **59-2**) and, thus, in most circumstances are interchangeable. For simplicity, this chapter uses the terms "dementia" and "MCI."

EPIDEMIOLOGY

AD is the most common cause of dementia in older adults, currently affecting more than 6 million Americans. Worldwide more than 44 million individuals currently have AD or a related dementia. Unless effective preventive strategies are identified, it is anticipated that the prevalence of AD will double every 20 years. The United Nations predicts that the major rate of increase in the prevalence of AD will likely occur in developing countries that may not possess the essential resources, public health support system, or medical expertise to care for patients with AD. There is clear evidence that a number of risk factors significantly enhance the overall risk for developing AD. These risk factors relate to both genetic and nongenetic markers and are discussed below.

Aging

Age is the single most important and validated risk factor for AD. Epidemiologic studies indicate that the incidence and prevalence of AD both increase with age. Based on data from the 2010 US Census, the prevalence of AD was approximately 3% among adults between the ages of 65 to 74, 17% in persons aged 75 to 84, and 32% in individuals age 85 and older. With the average human lifespan increasing, the prevalence of AD is expected to accelerate at an even greater rate in coming decades. Although not clearly understood, converging research findings provide clues concerning the potential molecular pathway(s) underlying the association between aging and AD. Increases in the pathologic hallmarks of AD, notably amyloid plaques and neurofibrillary tangles, have been noted in the brains of older adults.

Age-related changes in molecular pathways involving insulin-like growth factor 1 receptor (IGF1-R), neurotrophin signaling, β-site amyloid precursor protein cleaving enzyme 1 (BACE1), and amyloid precursor protein (APP) metabolism may account for some of the increase in incidence and prevalence of AD with aging. Additionally, aging and IGF1-R signaling are both associated with cerebrovascular dysfunction, which may play a key role in the development of AD. An increased exposure time to age-dependent vascular risk factors or an interaction between aging and vascular risk factors may in part account for the effects of aging on the pathobiology of AD.

Apolipoprotein E Genotype

Late-onset AD is the most common form of the disorder, accounting for greater than 95% of all AD cases.

TABLE 59-1 ■ NIA-AA CORE CLINICAL DIAGNOSTIC CRITERIA FOR ALL-CAUSE DEMENTIA AND DEMENTIA DUE TO ALZHEIMER DISEASE

DEMENTIA

The patient has cognitive or behavioral symptoms that:

- Interfere with the ability to function at work or at usual activities
- Represent a decline from previous levels of functioning and performing
- Are not explained by delirium or major psychiatric disorder

Cognitive impairment is detected and diagnosed through a combination of:

- History-taking from the patient and a knowledgeable informant
- An objective cognitive assessment, either a "bedside" mental status examination or neuropsychological testing

The cognitive or behavioral impairment involves a minimum of two of the following domains[a]:

- Impaired ability to acquire and remember new information
- Impaired reasoning, judgment, and handling of complex tasks
- Impaired visuospatial abilities
- Impaired language functions
- Changes in personality, behavior, or comportment

PROBABLE DEMENTIA DUE TO ALZHEIMER DISEASE[b]

The patient meets criteria for dementia *and* has the following characteristics:

- Insidious onset over months to years, not sudden over hours or days
- Clear-cut history of worsening cognition by report or observation
- Initial and most prominent cognitive deficits are evident on history and examination in one of the following categories:
  - *Amnestic presentation* (most common presentation)—Deficits should include impairment in learning and recall of recently learned information, plus cognitive dysfunction in at least one other cognitive domain.
  - *Nonamnestic presentations*[c]:
    - *Language presentation*—The most prominent deficits are in word finding, but deficits in other cognitive domains should be present.
    - *Visuospatial presentation*—The most prominent deficits are in spatial cognition, but deficits in other cognitive domains should be present.
    - *Executive dysfunction*—The most prominent deficits are impaired reasoning, judgment, and problem solving, but deficits in other cognitive domains should be present.

The diagnosis of probable AD dementia *should not* be applied when there is evidence of:

- Substantial concomitant cerebrovascular disease (defined by a history of a stroke temporally related to onset or worsening of cognitive impairment or presence of multiple or extensive infarcts or severe white matter hyperintensity burden)
- Core features of dementia with Lewy bodies
- Prominent features of behavioral variant frontotemporal dementia
- Prominent features of primary progressive aphasia
- Active neurologic disease or a medical comorbidity or use of medication that could have a substantial effect on cognition

[a]Diagnostic criteria for DSM-5 "major neurocognitive disorder" require a significant cognitive decline in one or more cognitive domains (complex attention, executive function, learning and memory, language, perceptual-motor, or social cognition).

[b]The diagnosis of "probable AD dementia with increased level of certainty" is made when there is a documented cognitive decline and/or evidence of a causative genetic mutation (APP, PSEN1, or PSEN2, not APOE4) in addition to the above diagnostic criteria.

[c]Diagnostic criteria for DSM-5 "major neurocognitive disorder due to Alzheimer disease" require that one of the affected cognitive domains be memory and learning.

Data from McKhann GM, Knopman DS, Chertkow H, et al. The diagnosis of dementia due to Alzheimer's disease: recommendations from the National Institute on Aging-Alzheimer's Association workgroups on diagnostic guidelines for Alzheimer's disease, Alzheimers Dement. 2011;7(3):263–269.

Although some cases of younger-onset AD have strong links to the genes coding for *APP* and presenilin 1 (*PSEN1*) and 2 (*PSEN2*) proteins, many cases of late-onset AD are seen in individuals without any clear genetic predisposition. A common polymorphism in the apolipoprotein E (*APOE*) gene is the major determinant of risk in families with late-onset AD. Of the three allelic forms ($\varepsilon2$, $\varepsilon3$, and $\varepsilon4$), AD risk is increased fourfold in individuals with at least one $\varepsilon4$ allele and 12-fold in persons with two copies of the $\varepsilon4$ allele. While $\varepsilon4$ genotype modifies an individual's risk of the disease, by itself it is neither necessary nor sufficient for the development of AD.

In the Framingham study, 55% of $\varepsilon4$ homozygote carriers, 27% of $\varepsilon4$ heterozygote carriers, and 9% of noncarriers developed AD by age 85. *APOE* $\varepsilon4$ genotype may contribute to AD by influencing processes related to the development of AD, including altering the rate of production, clearance, or aggregation of amyloid β-peptide and/or influencing cerebral cholesterol metabolism and inflammation.

Vascular Risk Factors

Midlife vascular risk factors, including hypercholesterolemia, hypertension, diabetes mellitus, metabolic

TABLE 59-2 ■ NIA-AA CORE CLINICAL DIAGNOSTIC CRITERIA FOR MILD COGNITIVE IMPAIRMENT

MILD COGNITIVE IMPAIRMENT[a]
The patient, an informant who knows the patient well, or a clinician observing the patient notes a concern regarding a change in cognition in comparison to the patient's previous level.
There is evidence of lower performance in one or more cognitive domains (memory, executive function, attention, language, and/or visuospatial skills) that is greater than would be expected for the patient's age and educational background.
The patient maintains preserved independence in functional abilities, although they may take more time, be less efficient, and make more errors at performing such activities than in the past.
The patient does ***not*** meet criteria for dementia.

[a]DSM-5 "mild neurocognitive disorder" criteria also state that these deficits do not occur exclusively in the context of a delirium or other mental disorder (eg, major depressive disorder, schizophrenia). Identification and exclusion of other neurologic, psychiatric, and medical disorders is implied in the text of the NIA-AA MCI diagnostic criteria.

Modified with permission from Albert MS, DeKosky ST, Dickson D, et al. The diagnosis of mild cognitive impairment due to Alzheimer's disease: recommendations from the National Institute on Aging-Alzheimer's Association workgroups on diagnostic guidelines for Alzheimer's disease, Alzheimers Dement. 2011;7(3):270–279.

syndrome, obesity, and physical inactivity, have all been associated with a greater risk of developing AD in later life. High midlife total cholesterol and blood pressure levels are associated with a two- to nearly threefold increased risk of developing AD decades later and may convey an even greater risk than that caused by *APOE ε4* allele. Abnormal cholesterol metabolism is related to *APOE ε4* allele, suggesting that some of the adverse effects of this genotype on AD risk may be partially mediated through lipoprotein dysregulation. In a community-based cohort study, higher glucose levels were associated with an increased risk of dementia in populations both with and without diabetes mellitus. Metabolic syndrome is also associated with increased risk for AD, although this cluster of risk factors is more consistently related to greater risk of vascular dementia. Midlife obesity (RR 1.60, 95% CI 1.34–1.92) and physical inactivity (RR 1.82, 95% CI 1.19–2.78) are interrelated and both independently increase the risk for developing AD in late life. With more than 35% of current US adults meeting criteria for obesity, there is concern that this risk factor could further accelerate projected increases in AD incidence rates over the coming decades.

Studies support that vascular factors exert an independent additive effect on AD risk. The presence of multiple cardiovascular risk factors at midlife substantially increases the risk of late-life dementia in a dose-dependent manner. The positive corollary to these findings is that about a third of AD cases worldwide might be attributable to potentially modifiable risk factors, thus, providing a target for preventive strategies. Vascular risk factors exert their adverse effects on AD pathology through a variety of mechanisms, including modulation of β-amyloid (Aβ) metabolism, effects on insulin receptors, blood-brain barrier (BBB) integrity, endothelial dysfunction, and cerebral blood flow. These vascular-mediated changes subsequently lead to tissue hypoxia, increased oxidative stress, inflammation, and cognitive decline.

Traumatic Brain Injury

There is increasing epidemiologic evidence that moderate or severe traumatic brain injury (TBI) is a risk factor for AD in late life and may precipitate earlier onset of the disease. In longitudinal studies, the magnitude of AD risk increases with TBI severity. Compared to controls, World War II veterans with moderate TBI were twice as likely to develop AD, whereas the risk was fourfold in veterans with severe TBI with loss of consciousness. Neuropathologic examination of brains from patients with a history of head trauma generally reveals changes of diffuse amyloid plaques together with tau pathology, inflammatory response, and loss of cholinergic neurons. These pathologic changes may be related to transient upregulation of BACE1 together with increased generation of Aβ. These features are accompanied by tau hyperphosphorylation and increased caspase-mediated cleavage of APP. Thus, head trauma may lead to AD by triggering accelerated neurodegeneration.

Newer evidence demonstrates that recurrent mild TBI, including both concussive and subconcussive injuries, may also contribute to future risk of cognitive decline. However, it has been difficult to establish risk estimates of the impact of repetitive mild TBI on risk for AD due to a variety of methodologic challenges. The high frequency of concussive and subconcussive injuries, the variability in definitions and measurements of mild TBI, the heterogeneity of injuries among various cohorts (ie, military combat veterans vs contact sport athletes), and selection and recall biases have complicated research of this area. Repetitive concussive injuries may also lead to chronic traumatic encephalopathy (CTE), a condition that is neuropathologically distinct from AD. Symptoms of CTE frequently include headaches and disturbances in attention or concentration and depression—Chapter 64 provides additional details on CTE. Research is underway to clarify the varying types and severity of TBI and the effects of such injuries on risk for posttraumatic neurodegeneration.

Depression

More than 30% of patients with AD develop depression during the course of their illness, and some may present with depressive symptoms as their first clinical manifestation of underlying AD. While depression has long been recognized as a common psychiatric condition in older adults that may mimic dementia, depression is likely also a risk factor for AD. Findings of a meta-analysis involving over 20 population-based prospective studies supported an increased risk of AD in patients with a history of late-life depression (pooled risk OR [95% CI] 1.65 [1.42–1.92]). To date, the precise mechanisms underlying the association between depression and enhanced AD risk are unknown. Several potential mechanisms have been proposed that are common to both AD and depression, including elevated levels of cytokines, increased vascular risk factors, and the potential role of *APOE4* allele. More research is needed to better understand the biological basis of increased risk of AD in patients with a history of depression.

Race and Ethnicity

The assessment of differences in AD prevalence rates across geographic regions worldwide and among various racial and ethnic groups has proven to be challenging. Differences in education, literacy, life expectancy, access to health care, nutrition, social stressors, vascular risk factors, and cultural beliefs in what is considered normal aging can all influence AD prevalence estimates. In the Indianapolis/ Ibadan studies, the incidence and prevalence of AD were significantly lower among Africans in Ibadan, Nigeria, than among age-matched African Americans in Indianapolis, suggesting that differences in environmental factors may play a larger role than race in influencing the development of AD. The significant influence of environmental factors on AD risk is also supported by data showing that migrant populations tend to have dementia rates that fall between those seen in their homeland and adopted countries. Standardized approaches to case ascertainment of dementia and statistical comparisons across nations have been implemented to better assess variations in prevalence rates among low-, middle-, and high-income countries. These approaches have produced age-adjusted dementia prevalence estimates of approximately 5% to 9% in people older than age 60 across global regions.

Studies assessing ethnic and racial variations in dementia rates within countries have identified some group differences in AD incidence and prevalence. In a population-based study in the Washington Heights and Inwood communities of New York City, the cumulative incidence of AD was increased twofold among individuals of African-American and Caribbean Hispanic origin. The group differences in AD incidence did not change following corrections for differences in years of education or history of vascular risk factors. In a study in Houston, Texas, both the incidence and prevalence of AD were higher among older African-American and Hispanic individuals compared to non-Hispanic White adults. In Singapore, ethnic Malays and Indians had higher rates of dementia compared to ethnic Chinese, independent of vascular risk factors. While some research suggests there may be biological or genetic differences driving variations in AD risk, other studies support that these racial and ethnic group differences will not persist after rigorously accounting for important social, cultural, and environmental factors influencing risk of dementia.

Education

Low educational attainment, poor educational quality, and illiteracy have been shown to be associated with increased risk for AD. In a meta-analysis of 13 cohort and six case-control studies, low education had a pooled relative risk (RR) estimate for AD of 1.80 (95% CI 1.45–2.27) compared to high education, although the estimate from cohort studies (RR 1.59 [95% CI 1.35–1.86]) was significantly lower than the estimate based on case-control studies (2.40, [1.32–4.38]). Prospective cohort studies likely provide a more accurate assessment of the association between education and dementia since they allow for documentation of a decline from a previous level of cognitive performance. Some studies have found that education may be a marker of cognitive reserve as it modifies the association between AD neuropathology and level of cognitive function. For the same degree of brain pathology, persons with higher education demonstrate less cognitive impairment. In addition, higher levels of education may help individuals cope more effectively with cognitive changes. Access to higher levels of education may also be a marker of socioeconomic status, coexisting chronic diseases, access to health care resources, and premorbid intellectual abilities. Thus, while low educational attainment is associated with increased AD risk, it is not clear to what extent low education contributes to AD or whether early educational interventions will protect against the development of dementia.

Gender

There is some evidence that AD is more common among women, although study results are conflicting. In population-based studies, more than half reported a greater risk of AD in women, while the others found no difference. Some data support that estrogen deficiency following menopause may contribute to the development of AD; however, the effect of hormone replacement therapy on cognition remains controversial. The discrepant findings between studies assessing sex-based variations in dementia risk are likely due to methodologic differences in accounting for potential gender-related variability in life-expectancy, education, occupation, and lifestyle factors that can directly affect AD risk.

PATHOPHYSIOLOGY

Genetics of Alzheimer Disease

Based on the onset of symptoms, AD is normally divided into two groups: younger-onset (< 65 years) and late-onset (> 65 years) disease. Younger-onset patients include individuals with familial AD which accounts for between 1% and 5% of all AD cases and to date has been linked to mutations in the genes for the APP (gene name *APP*) on chromosome 21, presenilin 1 (PS1; gene name *PSEN1*) on chromosome 14, and presenilin 2 (PS2; gene name *PSEN2*) on chromosome 1. Among these genes, more than 250 different mutations have so far been identified, accounting for approximately 40% of all cases of familial AD, yet only 0.5% of AD cases overall. Most of the mutations (~ 200) are found in the *PSEN1* gene and account for 78% of the familial AD mutations. *APP* mutations (~ 33) account for about 18% of younger-onset autosomal dominant cases and *PSEN2* (~ 22 mutations) for about 4%. Familial AD is characterized by younger onset of cognitive symptoms (typically in the late 40s or early 50s), but is clinically indistinguishable from late-onset AD.

Late-onset AD, also called sporadic AD, accounts for greater than 95% of all cases of the disease. *APOE* is the only established susceptibility gene consistently found associated with late-onset AD in both case-control and genetic studies. *APOE* maps to chromosome 19 in a cluster with the genes encoding translocase of outer mitochondrial membrane 40 (*TOMM40*), apolipoprotein C1, and apolipoprotein C2. The *APOE* gene exists as three major alleles (ε2, ε3, and ε4) that encode three different ApoE isoforms: ApoE2, ApoE3, and ApoE4. Interestingly, these isoforms only differ in amino acid sequences at either position 112 or 158 of the protein. The inheritance of the ε4 allele confers an increased risk for developing AD, while the ε2 allele confers protection. For example, presence of one copy of the ε4 allele increases risk of AD fourfold, whereas inheritance of two copies enhances the risk by 12-fold. However, unlike genetic mutations associated with familial AD, the presence of *APOE* ε4 alone is insufficient to cause AD without additional factors. Even though the first report of an association between *APOE* ε4 and AD was published decades ago, the precise molecular mechanisms underlying this association still remain elusive. It is currently unknown if the *APOE4* allele influences the rate of production, clearance, or aggregation of Aβ peptide or whether it influences cholesterol metabolism and inflammation that reportedly play a major role in the pathobiology of AD.

With the advent of genome-wide association studies (GWASs), a number of new genetic loci with genome-wide significance have been identified. In addition to *APOE4*, more than 40 other polymorphisms have been associated with increased risk for late-onset AD. However, none of these associations has been uniformly confirmed in every population group studied to date. Over 20 genetic loci have been associated with late-onset AD, leading to four main mechanisms: Aβ metabolism, lipid metabolism, immune response, and cell signaling. Further research is needed to clarify the impact of other genetic changes on AD risk, genetic-environmental interactions, and the impact of such genetic factors on mechanisms of neurodegeneration and neuroprotection.

Neuropathology of Alzheimer Disease

The neuropathologic hallmarks of AD include amyloid plaques, neurofibrillary tangles, and neuritic plaques (**Figure 59-1**). The latter are a subset of amyloid plaques that are closely associated with neuronal injury and occur with dystrophic neurites. Cerebral amyloid angiopathy (CAA) frequently co-occurs with amyloid plaques, resulting from deposition of Aβ into cerebral vessels. Sporadic CAA is observed in 80% to 90% of AD patients and may cause lobar intracerebral hemorrhages and microbleeds. Together these processes contribute to loss of neurons and

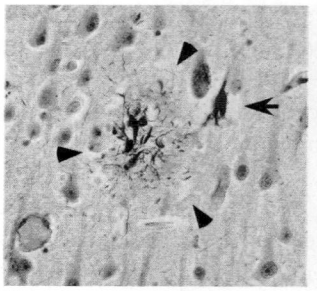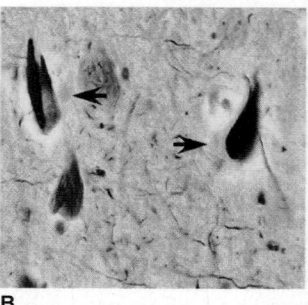

A   **B**

FIGURE 59-1. Small section of the neocortex from a patient with Alzheimer disease showing two classical neuropathologic lesions of the disease. **A.** The modified silver staining shows one dense senile (amyloid) plaque indicated by three arrowheads. The plaque consists of aggregated extracellular deposits of amyloid β-peptide (Aβ) fragments surrounded by silver-positive dystrophic neurites. The arrow indicates a neuron containing neurofibrillary tangles, which appear as dark masses of abnormal filaments occupying most of the cytoplasm. **B.** The image shows higher magnification of two neurons containing neurofibrillary tangles (*indicated by arrows*). (Reproduced with permission from Shahriar Salamat, MD, PhD, University of Wisconsin School of Medicine and Public Health, Department of Pathology and Laboratory Medicine.)

synapses in the neocortex, hippocampus, and other subcortical regions of the brain. The predominance of amyloid plaques versus neurofibrillary tangles or amyloid angiopathy can differ from one patient to another. However, neuronal/synaptic loss is a constant feature and eventually the direct cause of dementia. The distribution of the disease pathology seems to follow a region-specific pattern with amyloid plaques being more prevalent in the neocortex and neuronal/synaptic loss being more prevalent in the hippocampus, posterior cingulate, and corpus callosum—areas of the brain closely involved with memory formation and higher cortical activities. Finally, brains of persons with AD are also characterized by a diffuse and widespread invasion of reactive astrocytes, mostly concentrated in the hippocampus and around areas of neuronal loss. These astrocytic changes are not specific to AD and can be observed in other neurodegenerative disorders associated with inflammation and neurotoxic insults.

The dominant component of the amyloid plaque core is Aβ organized in fibrils of approximately 7 to 10 nm intermixed with nonfibrillar forms of the peptide. Neuritic plaques are characterized by a dense core of aggregated fibrillar Aβ, surrounded by dystrophic dendrites and axons, activated microglia, and reactive astrocytes. In addition, diffuse deposits of Aβ, likely representing a prefibrillary form of the aggregated peptide, are found without any surrounding dystrophic neurites, astrocytes, or microglia. These diffuse plaques can be found in limbic and association cortices, as well as in the cerebellum.

The other neuropathologic hallmark of AD is the presence of neurofibrillary tangles found exclusively in the cytoplasm of neurons (see **Figure 59-1**). The tangles appear as paired, helically twisted protein filaments composed of highly stable polymers of cytoplasmic proteins called tau. Tau comprises a group of alternatively spliced proteins found in the cytoplasm that possess either three or four microtubule-binding domains and can assemble with tubulin, thus helping the formation of cross bridges between adjacent microtubules. Tau proteins can be phosphorylated in multiple sites, and the degree of phosphorylation is inversely correlated with binding to microtubules. As a result, highly phosphorylated tau proteins dissociate from microtubules and polymerize into filaments forming neurofibrillary tangles. In addition to AD, the abnormal accumulation of filamentous tau is observed in frontotemporal forms of dementia, progressive supranuclear palsy, corticobasal degeneration, and Pick disease. Contrary to prior belief, tau proteins themselves can cause dementia, and multiple mutations in the *tau* gene have been found in frontotemporal dementia (FTD) with parkinsonism. The precise role of tau proteins in the pathogenesis of AD and their potential interaction with Aβ are still unclear.

In 2012, NIA and the Alzheimer's Association published revised criteria for AD neuropathologic change. These criteria recommended reporting on the presence and extent of hallmark lesions for AD observed at autopsy independent of the individual's cognitive state. These new guidelines took into account several well-established neuropathologic scoring criteria and integrated them into an "ABC score" based on three parameters (*Amyloid, Braak, CERAD*): criterion "A" ranks the Aβ plaque score (based on criteria from Thal et al.), criterion "B" measures the neurofibrillary tangle stage (modified from Braak criteria), and criterion "C" assesses the neuritic plaque score (modified from the Consortium to Establish a Registry for Alzheimer Disease [CERAD]). For reporting, these ABC scores are then transformed into one of four levels of neuropathic change: none, low, intermediate, or high. While CAA is not considered in the "ABC" score, the guidelines recognize that these changes frequently co-occur with parenchymal Aβ plaques and recommend neuropathologists comment on such changes separately within the neuropathology report.

Amyloid Precursor Protein Processing and Generation of Aβ

Aβ is a 39 to 43 amino acid hydrophobic peptide proteolytically released from a much larger precursor, APP. Although APP is the major source of toxic Aβ, it also exerts several important functions in the nervous system, including serving as a cell-surface receptor, growth factor, protease inhibitor, cell–cell interaction molecule, coreceptor/partner in the endocytic/lysosomal network, coagulation inhibitor factor, cell-surface scaffold protein, kinesin-interacting molecule for axonal transport, and transcription factor. The generation of Aβ from APP (**Figure 59-2**) requires the sequential recruitment of two enzymatic activities: β-secretase, also called BACE1, and γ-secretase, a multimeric protein

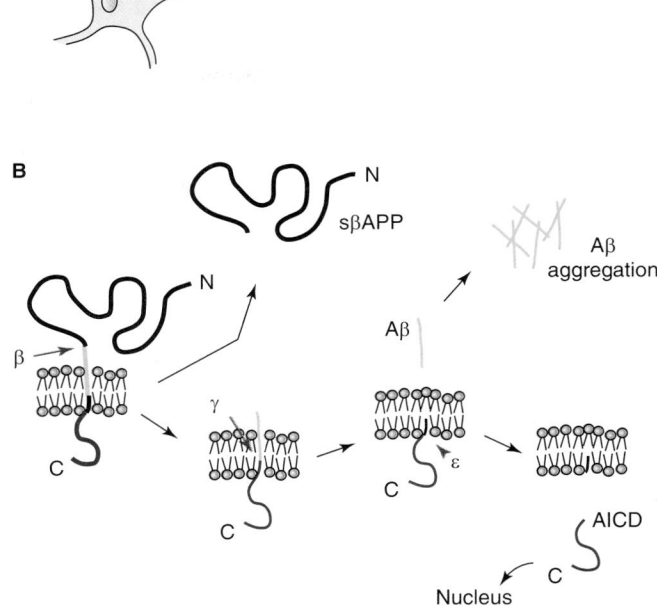

FIGURE 59-2. Generation of amyloid β-peptide (Aβ) from amyloid precursor protein (APP). APP is a type 1 membrane protein with a large extracellular domain, a single membrane-spanning domain, and a short cytoplasmic tail. The Aβ region of APP (*in yellow*) includes the first 12 to 14 amino acids of the membrane domain. **(A)** Shows a schematic image of APP on the cell surface of a neuron, whereas **(B)** provides a closer view of APP processing. The initial enzymatic step for the generation of Aβ requires proteolysis of APP at β-site (amino acid 1 of the Aβ region). This event liberates a large N-terminal fragment (sβAPP) that is rapidly secreted into the extracellular milieu and a small C-terminal fragment (β-APP-CTF) of 99 amino acids (also called C99). The removal of sβAPP most likely induces a conformational change that allows subsequent cleavage by γ-secretase. Once generated, the Aβ peptides aggregate in the brain in the form of plaques. Further cleavage of β-APP-CTF at the site liberates the signaling active APP intracellular domain (AICD). In addition to the above β/γ pathway, APP can also be cleaved at the α-site (between amino acids 16 and 17 of the Aβ region) precluding the generation of Aβ.

complex containing presenilin, nicastrin, Aph-1, Pen-2, and CD147. The β-cleavage is the rate-limiting step and occurs before the γ-cleavage. It liberates a large N-terminal fragment of the protein (sβAPP) that is released in the extracellular milieu and a small (~12 kDa) membrane-anchored fragment called β-APP-CTF (or C99). The release of the large N-terminal domain allows subsequent γ-cleavage, and liberation of Aβ and the signaling of active intracellular domain (AICD) of APP (see **Figure 59-2**). Generation of Aβ40 and Aβ42 results from γ-cleavage of Aβ at positions 40 and 42, respectively. The release of Aβ in the extracellular milieu is followed by oligomerization and aggregation in the form of fibrils and amyloid plaques. Additionally, small Aβ aggregates are also found in the soma of the neurons suggesting that the Aβ fragments can escape secretion and aggregate in the intracellular environment. The molecular mechanisms underlying the toxicity of Aβ are still being investigated and currently incompletely understood. However, research seems to indicate that small Aβ aggregates (oligomers), which represent the "preplaque" neurotoxic species of Aβ, act as the proximate cause of neuronal injury and synaptic loss associated with AD. Additionally, the C-terminal tail of APP can undergo further processing at amino acid 664 of APP695 liberating two small cytosolic fragments, Jcasp and C31. Both of these fragments are generated only after γ-cleavage, require caspase-mediated processing of APP, and can activate proapoptotic pathways in a variety of cellular systems.

The most critical clinical link between Aβ and AD came from the observation that patients with Down syndrome (trisomy 21) had a higher propensity for developing a clinical and pathologic phenotype resembling AD, thereby suggesting a potential association between AD and chromosome 21. This observation was further strengthened by the fact that Aβ was the major component in plaques from both patients with Down syndrome and AD, and that its genesis was related to a gene (*APP*) located on chromosome 21, close to the obligate Down syndrome region. Following the identification of APP, several groups found mutations in the *APP* gene that were linked to familial forms of AD. Given that the duplication of the *APP* locus could result in early AD and that Down syndrome patients with partial trisomy 21 developed AD only when the trisomy was proximal to the *APP* locus, the potential direct relationship between APP metabolism and AD seems strong. Furthermore, causative mutations in the genes that encode for PS1 and PS2, which are also implicated in the metabolism of APP, have been found and are associated with familial forms of AD, thereby conferring additional strength to the linkage between APP/Aβ metabolism and AD.

Although the generation of Aβ from APP seems to be a pivotal step in the pathobiology of AD, it does not explain all the neuropathologic changes observed in patients with AD. For example, examination of the brain of transgenic mice expressing human APP harboring one or more familial AD-associated mutations reveals the presence of amyloid plaques and some synaptic loss and cognitive deficits, but absence of tau pathology and astrocytosis. This suggests that additional biochemical/molecular events are required to develop the full pathologic spectrum of AD. To circumvent this issue, several new animal models have been generated where human APP is accompanied by additional genes. These genes include the *presenilins* (harboring familial AD-associated mutations), *tau*, and *APOE*. Recently, several transgenic mice models harboring three or five familial AD-associated mutations (respectively called 3X and 5X mice) in two or more genes have been generated. All of these models demonstrate that Aβ is an essential element for the development of AD-like neuropathology and revealed a close relationship between Aβ and the phosphorylation/aggregation state of tau. However, none of the mouse models fully reproduce the classical AD phenotype, thereby again suggesting that Aβ seems to be necessary but not sufficient to produce the entire spectrum of AD neuropathology. Transgenic mice expressing the human microtubule-associated protein tau develop the typical tau-related pathology found in individuals suffering from FTD with parkinsonism; however, they do not develop amyloid plaques, suggesting that tau is not required for the formation of plaques. Crossing these mice with APP transgenic mice potentiates tau-related pathology and neuronal loss but does not aggravate plaque pathology, suggesting that Aβ acts upstream of tau in the classical AD phenotype. However, studies from patients with AD, mouse models, and ex vivo cellular systems indicate that Aβ and tau can interact synergistically, thereby fostering their respective aggregation and neuronal loss. Thus, the true relationship between Aβ and tau is more complex than previously thought and likely involves additional molecular and biochemical pathways acting upstream of both Aβ and tau production in the AD brain.

CLINICAL PRESENTATION

The most common clinical onset of AD is an amnestic presentation, characterized by slowly progressive memory loss for recent events. Patients with AD frequently have problems remembering recent conversations, dates, appointments, and may misplace items. Many patients are not aware of these deficits and are brought to medical attention by their family members or friends. For some patients, memory loss symptoms are first noted by others during a stressful life event, such as the patient's hospitalization or the death of a spouse; however, a thorough interview frequently reveals that the cognitive deficits preceded such an event by months to years. The memory deficits of AD are generally differentiated from those caused by normal aging by the fact that AD-related deficits are progressive and interfere with the individual's usual daily activities. Memory loss leading to a change in functional status is not a part of normal aging and warrants further evaluation.

Nonamnestic presentations of AD are also common and may include prominent initial impairments in language abilities, visuospatial skills, and executive function. As these presentations are less commonly recognized by patients, families, and clinicians alike as being early symptoms related to AD, individuals with nonamnestic presentations are frequently misdiagnosed or experience a delay in diagnosis. In addition to the more common amnestic presentation, nonamnestic presentations are specifically identified in the NIA-AA diagnostic criteria for AD (see **Table 59-1**). Patients who initially present with language impairment frequently will complain of marked word-finding problems with subsequent progression to paraphasic errors and circumlocution. AD patients with a visuospatial presentation may have prominent deficits in spatial cognition, including poor object and face recognition, an inability to perceive multiple visual elements simultaneously, and difficulty understanding written language. Executive dysfunction is another common initial presenting symptom of AD, leading to impairments in reasoning, judgment, problem solving, and an inability to complete complex demanding tasks. Deficits in concentration and attention frequently occur in patients with AD, but these changes may also be notable in persons with depression, attention deficit disorder, sleep disorders, or adverse medication effects.

As the disease progresses, changes in personality are commonly seen in patients with AD and may include increased passivity, lack of interest, agitation, restlessness, and/or overactivity. AD patients may exhibit increased irritability when confronted with memory loss symptoms, such as when struggling to find a word, being reminded of a prior conversation or event, or searching for a misplaced item. More than 30% of persons with AD develop symptoms of depression, which may be the first clinical presentation of the disease. Early signs of depression in patients with AD include increased irritability, alterations in appetite or sleep, trouble concentrating or making decisions, low energy, social withdrawal, and a decline in physical function. Worsening of behavior and cognitive symptoms in the evening is also common in patients with AD and may be related to changes in circadian rhythm from loss of sunlight.

In the later stages of the disease, individuals may have increased confusion, dysphagia, impaired gait, and repeated falls. In some patients with AD, disruptive behaviors may increase with aggression, agitation, and physical or verbal hostility; in others, these behavioral symptoms lessen with disease progression. The majority of patients become increasingly frail and dependent for self-care and activities of daily living with many patients developing bowel and bladder incontinence. Persons in the late stages of AD may become immobile and bed-bound, which increases their risk of developing pressure sores, malnutrition, and dehydration. The most common causes of death in patients with AD include pneumonia, urinary sepsis, dehydration, pressure sores, fractures, and malnutrition. The median survival period from the time of diagnosis to death generally ranges from 7 to 10 years, although some patients, especially those with familial AD, die earlier.

EVALUATION

For many older patients with cognitive complaints, their evaluation, diagnosis, and management may be effectively completed within a primary care setting. If available, utilization of multidisciplinary team members from nursing, social work, psychology, and/or pharmacy can greatly aid a primary care physician in the diagnosis and management of patients with cognitive concerns. A smaller subset of patients will need more in-depth neuropsychological assessment and clinical evaluation from a dementia specialist.

The NIA-AA clinical diagnostic criteria for dementia, AD and MCI (see **Tables 59-1** and **59-2**) were designed to be used across all clinical settings, including primary care, specialty clinics, and long-term care. The clinical diagnoses of MCI and dementia are primarily ascertained through completion of a focused interview with the patient and an informant who knows the patient well, a thorough review of the patient's medical history and medication use, a comprehensive physical examination, a formal assessment of cognitive function, basic laboratory tests, and neuroimaging (**Table 59-3**). While the differential diagnosis for AD is extensive (**Table 59-4**), a systematic approach to dementia diagnosis can help primary care clinicians identify common confounding medical and psychiatric conditions and medications that can adversely affect cognition. In addition, a structured evaluation may facilitate accurate diagnosis of the most common causes of dementia—AD and AD mixed with vascular dementia as well as predementia syndromes such as MCI. Integrating various established diagnostic criteria, **Figure 59-3** shows a primary care diagnostic algorithm developed to guide clinicians in their assessment of patients with cognitive complaints.

Identification of a cognitive concern is the first step in the evaluation. While early cognitive changes in some patients may be readily identified by the individuals themselves, their families, and/or their clinicians, such symptoms may not be as apparent in other patients due to a variety of factors, including poor insight, attribution of such changes to normal aging, cultural views of dementia, or lack of corroborative history from others. Whether all older adults should undergo routine screening for dementia remains controversial. The US Preventive Services Task Force recommends against routine screening for dementia in asymptomatic older adults based on insufficient evidence that such widespread screening impacts individual or societal outcomes. However, the US Medicare Annual Wellness Visit requires that clinicians assess cognitive function by "direct observation," although no cognitive screening tool is endorsed. In an effort to operationalize the Medicare Annual Wellness Visit requirements, the Alzheimer's Association recommends using self-reported memory concerns, clinician observations, or concerns from a person who knows the patient well to trigger a formal memory assessment. Screening questions such as "Does your memory bother you?" or "Do you think your memory is worse than others of your age?" also may be used to determine which older patients need a formal evaluation of cognitive performance. Identifying memory concerns through self-report or screening questions may reduce the number of unnecessary formal cognitive screening tests administered to asymptomatic adults at low risk for dementia. However, individuals without a close informant may need structured cognitive tests to identify memory concerns. When a cognitive concern is identified, a separate clinic visit should be arranged to investigate the underlying cause (see **Figure 59-3** and **Table 59-3**).

TABLE 59-3 ■ EVALUATION OF THE PATIENT WITH COGNITIVE CONCERNS

History of cognitive changes

Primary symptom(s) at onset (memory loss, language/spelling errors, impaired reasoning, difficulties in multitasking, personality changes, etc)

Date of onset and time course of cognitive decline (gradually progressive, stepwise, fluctuating, abrupt, rapidly progressive, etc) and whether or not it was associated with delirium

Past and present function at higher level tasks (including tasks at work, hobbies, daily household chores including instrumental activities of daily living [IADLs])

Safety concerns (medication management, driving, kitchen safety, use of firearms or heavy equipment, wandering, financial scams, etc)

Other associated symptoms (depression, tremor, frequent falls, visual hallucinations, stroke and/or transient ischemic attack symptoms, ataxia, urinary incontinence, agitation, personality changes, etc)

Past medical and psychiatric history

Vascular risk factors (including how well they have been controlled over time)

Strokes and/or transient ischemic attacks (assess whether cerebrovascular event was associated with onset of cognitive symptoms)

Atrial fibrillation, carotid artery disease, patent foramen ovale, and/or other risk factors for stroke

Coronary artery bypass surgery (assess whether surgery was associated with onset of cognitive symptoms)

Other major central nervous system (CNS) event (traumatic brain injury with loss of consciousness, anoxic brain injury, postoperative cognitive dysfunction, etc)

Hearing and/or vision loss

Obstructive sleep apnea (including how well it is treated with continuous positive airway pressure [CPAP] or other modalities)

Alcohol or other substance abuse

Depression, anxiety, posttraumatic stress disorder, or other psychiatric illness

Parkinson disease, parkinsonism, amyotrophic lateral sclerosis, or multiple sclerosis

Seizure disorder

History of malignancy with or without prior treatment with chemotherapy

Medication review

Prescription and nonprescription medications and supplements (especially those with anticholinergic or sedating side effects)

Timing of onset of cognitive symptoms with medication/supplement initiation or dose change

Social history

Family, friends, and other social support

Use of community resources (including home aides, senior centers, meal services, etc)

Educational history (including formal years of education and/or technical training, any interruption in schooling or repeated grades, any suspected or diagnosed learning disabilities or attention deficit disorder, etc)

Work history (including types of responsibilities associated with occupation)

Military history (including exposure to combat or blast injuries)

Hobbies and other daily activities

Substance use history (including any prior history of heavy alcohol use)

Family history

History of AD or other dementias (including age of onset of symptoms in affected family members)

History of other neurodegenerative disorders, strokes, psychiatric illnesses, etc

Physical examination

General appearance (attention, comprehension, cooperation, personal hygiene and grooming, social appropriateness, psychomotor slowing, word-finding difficulties)

Mental status (behavior, attitude, mood, affect, insight, judgment, thought content, thought process, speech, language)

Cranial nerves (facial symmetry, visual acuity, pupillary responses, eye movements, visual fields, hearing impairment)

Motor function and integration (strength, tone, cogwheeling, simulation of motor actions to test for apraxia)

Sensory function and integration (sensation to light touch, identification by touch of an object placed in the hand or a number written on the hand, ability to perceive simultaneous bilateral tactile stimuli)

Coordination (rapid alternating movements, finger-to-nose testing, heel-shin testing)

Deep tendon reflexes

Gait

(Continued)

TABLE 59-3 ■ EVALUATION OF THE PATIENT WITH COGNITIVE CONCERNS (*CONTINUED*)

Screening cognitive tests (time to administer)
Mini Mental State Examination (MMSE) (5–10 min)
Montreal Cognitive Assessment (MoCA) (10 min)
Saint Louis University Mental Status (SLUMS) Examination (5–10 min)
Mini-Cog (3 min)
Memory Impairment Screen (MIS) (3–4 min)
General Practitioner Assessment of Cognition (GPCOG) (4 min)

Depression screen
Geriatric Depression Scale—Short Form (GDS-SF) (5–7 min—may be self-administered)

Informant assessment
Eight-Item Interview to Differentiate Aging and Dementia (AD8) (3 min)
GPCOG Informant Questionnaire (2 min)
Informant Questionnaire on Cognitive Decline in the Elderly (IQCODE) (10–15 min)

Laboratory evaluation
Vitamin B_{12}, thyroid-stimulating hormone (TSH), 25-OH vitamin D, complete blood count, glucose, blood urea nitrogen and creatinine, basic metabolic profile, liver enzymes

Neuroimaging
Noncontrast head CT
MRI

TABLE 59-4 ■ DIFFERENTIAL DIAGNOSIS FOR ALZHEIMER DISEASE

DEPRESSION	LEWY BODY DEMENTIA
Adverse medication effects	Vascular dementia/vascular cognitive impairment
Delirium	Frontotemporal dementia
Acute alcohol intoxication	Parkinson disease dementia
Substance use disorders	Progressive supranuclear palsy
Obstructive sleep apnea	Corticobasal degeneration
Other sleep disorders	Prion-related diseases (Creutzfeldt–Jakob, bovine spongiform encephalopathy)
Chronic hypoxia and/or hypercapnia	Normal pressure hydrocephalus (NPH)
Recurrent hypoglycemia	Huntington disease
Thyroid diseases	Alcohol-related dementia
Other metabolic-endocrine disorders	Wernicke–Korsakoff syndrome
Vitamins B_1 (thiamine), B_{12}, and/or D deficiencies	Traumatic brain injury
Uremia	Chronic traumatic encephalopathy (CTE)
Hepatic encephalopathy	Mass lesions (neoplasms, benign tumors, hematomas)
Environmental toxicity (lead, mercury, polychlorinated biphenyls [PCBs], dioxins, etc)	Central nervous system rheumatologic/autoimmune disorders (systemic lupus erythematosus, sarcoidosis, vasculitis, multiple sclerosis, etc)
Lyme disease	Paraneoplastic syndromes
HIV-associated neurocognitive disorders (HAND)	Cerebral autosomal dominant arteriopathy with subcortical infarcts and leukoencephalopathy (CADASIL)
Progressive multifocal leukoencephalopathy (PML)	Carotid artery disease
Chronic meningitis/encephalitis	Postoperative cognitive dysfunction
Neurosyphilis	Seizure disorder

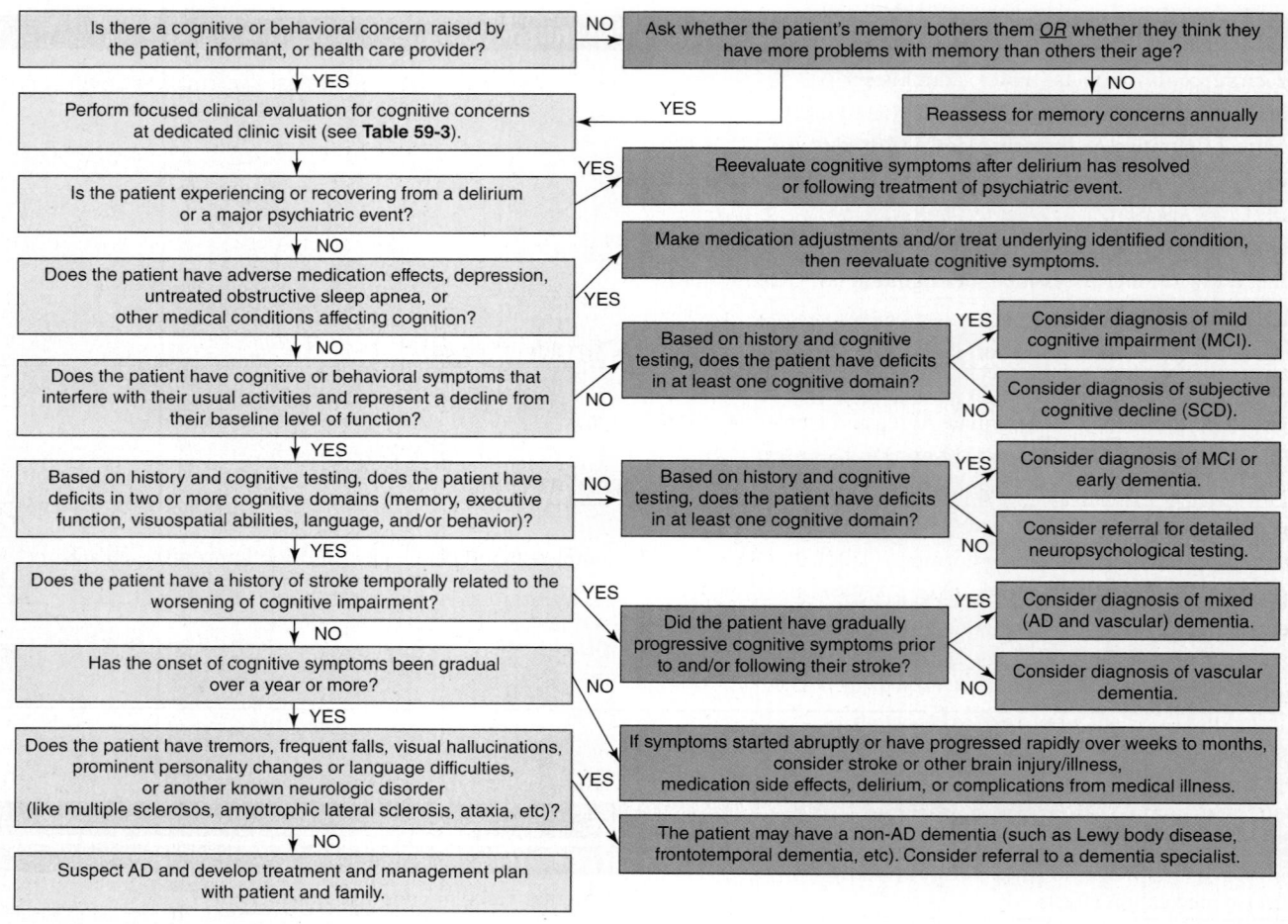

FIGURE 59-3. Algorithm for the clinical diagnosis of Alzheimer disease.

Within a dedicated primary care clinic visit, an optimal cognitive assessment includes gathering information not only from the patient's perspective, but also independently in a separate interview from an informant who knows the patient well. Depending on available time and resources, an independent informant interview may be accomplished through utilizing a variety of health care team members, such as social workers, medical assistants, nurses, or psychologists to conduct a brief structured informant interview or a full detailed assessment. Important historical elements include establishing when the cognitive symptoms began and the very first symptoms noted (such as problems with memory, language, executive function, apraxia, or personality changes). A careful delineation of the time course of progression will narrow the differential diagnosis and will help identify whether there are multiple contributing factors or one underlying process. Frequently, an inciting event that disrupts coping skills, such as a hospitalization or the death of a spouse, will draw the attention of family members to a patient's memory problems. The family may give a history of an acute onset of memory impairment following the inciting event, but careful questioning may identify cognitive

problems preceding that time period and point to a gradually progressive course.

A key component to the interview is establishing the patient's baseline cognitive and functional performance, taking into account past educational opportunities, estimated baseline intellectual function, occupational history, and prior established skills and abilities. Understanding the patient's baseline function will put neuropsychological test results into context in order to prevent over- or underdiagnosing dementia in patients who present with cognitive concerns. Changes in the person's ability to carry out tasks related to their occupation, hobbies, household management, and other volunteer activities should then be ascertained.

There are common reversible causes of cognitive dysfunction that next should be addressed. One of the first steps should be a careful review of prescription and nonprescription medications. Drugs with known anticholinergic properties (such as antihistamines, tricyclic antidepressants, bladder antispasmodic agents, etc) or sedating side effects (such as high-dose gabapentin, other antiepileptic medications, narcotic analgesics, benzodiazepines, sleeping aids, etc) should be carefully reviewed to see if the benefit of the offending medication outweighs the adverse cognitive effects. Patients should be included in shared decision-making with any medication adjustments as the value placed on various symptoms is likely to differ between individuals.

Clinicians should carefully evaluate their older patients for depression, anxiety, or other mood disorders that can affect cognitive performance. Depression may be a prodromal syndrome prior to dementia onset, but also commonly co-occurs with this syndrome. Pointed questions assessing for changes in sleep duration and/or quality, interest in activities, feelings of guilt, loss of energy, impaired concentration, changes in appetite, psychomotor slowing, and suicidal thoughts should be assessed. A brief screening tool such as the Geriatric Depression Scale (GDS) can be administered by a health care team member or self-administered while the patient is waiting for the clinician. Older patients with depression frequently complain of problems with poor concentration and forgetfulness and may perform poorly on tests of attention, speed of processing, and memory. In such patients, it is important to differentiate a loss of interest related to depression from a lack of initiative due to a neurodegenerative disorder. Treating depression and anxiety may lead to improvements in cognitive performance as well as mood.

Hearing loss may mimic cognitive dysfunction as patients who cannot hear well may not be able to properly encode new information from conversations or other auditory-received information. Questions on hearing loss symptoms and use and fit of any prescribed hearing aids can alert the provider as to whether hearing loss is contributing to cognitive symptoms or if further hearing evaluation is needed (see Chapter 34 for approach to screening for hearing loss).

A careful assessment of alcohol use should be completed in all patients, especially if cognitive performance varies widely from visit to visit or if the patient lives alone. Risk for obstructive sleep apnea should be assessed with several screening questions assessing the patient's snoring, witnessed apneic episodes, excessive daytime sleepiness, or nonrestorative sleep. In patients with diagnosed sleep apnea, their ability to effectively and regularly use their continuous positive airway pressure (CPAP) device should be assessed and any difficulties should be reported to the sleep medicine and/or respiratory therapy team to seek out other mask options for better fit and tolerance. Obstructive sleep apnea with its related hypoxia can cause profound effects on cognition.

Vascular disease may contribute to cognitive impairment through a variety of mechanisms. In addition to stroke causing acute cognitive decline, chronic low cerebral blood flow leading to subclinical hypoperfusion may also contribute to cognitive impairment and AD. Thus, a careful assessment of vascular risk factors should be completed to make sure they are well treated. Carotid bruits or a history of sudden cognitive changes should prompt work-up

for cerebrovascular disease with neuroimaging (computed tomography [CT] or preferably magnetic resonance imaging [MRI]) and either carotid ultrasound or magnetic resonance angiogram (MRA).

Delirium is associated with an acute or subacute onset of fluctuating cognitive dysfunction and may be caused by a wide variety of medical conditions and medications. In patients with delirium, a careful history frequently can tease out the temporal relationship between the onset of potentially reversible cognitive symptoms and contributing underlying medical problems or medications. Patients who have had a significant medial illness may exhibit signs of delirium for weeks to months following the inciting illness. Care should be made to avoid making a diagnosis of dementia in the presence of a resolving delirium. Since dementia is a risk factor for delirium, however, the presence of a delirium may suggest an underlying neurodegenerative disorder.

Additional information on safety should be obtained, including inquiries on medication management, driving, kitchen safety, use of firearms or heavy equipment or power tools, wandering, and susceptibility to financial scams. A review of systems should include questions on depression, tremors, falls, visual hallucinations, symptoms of stroke or transient ischemic attack, ataxia, dysphagia, urinary incontinence, waxing and waning level of consciousness, agitation, and personality changes.

The patient's past medical history should be reviewed for medical and psychiatric conditions affecting cognition, including cardiovascular and cerebrovascular disease and associated risk factors, surgical procedures including coronary artery bypass surgery, significant hearing loss, depression, Parkinson disease, TBI, seizures, and/or heavy alcohol use. A thorough medication review should be conducted to assess all prescription and nonprescription medications and the association of any medication initiation and/or dose adjustment with changes in cognitive symptoms. Patients should be encouraged to bring in all pill bottles to the clinic visit. The social history should assess the patient's education and occupational baseline, their social support network, and their use of community resources. An accurate assessment of prior or current alcohol or illicit drug use and a sexual history with special attention to sexually transmitted disease (notably syphilis and HIV) risk factors are critical to a correct diagnosis. An assessment of family history of dementia should include age of onset and time course of any symptoms of family members with memory loss.

The physical examination should include assessment of general appearance and a mental status examination (see **Table 59-3**). Careful observation upon interviewing a patient can provide rich information as to their ability to care for themselves, their organizational ability, their ability to provide detail within their conversation, and their comprehension of posed questions and the appropriateness of their response. Ears should be checked for any cerumen accumulation and/or hearing loss. A neurologic examination should screen for focal deficits, gaze palsies, increased muscle tone, cogwheeling, tremors, and ataxia. A detailed review of a comprehensive mental status and neurologic examination in older adults is described in Chapter 9. Cardiac arrhythmias, carotid bruits, or abdominal or femoral bruits may suggest a vascular contribution. The remainder of the physical examination should focus on ascertaining any major medical conditions that could have significant cognitive effects, such as hypoxia or significant active infection.

While there is no consensus as to which is the best cognitive screening tool, there are a variety of cognitive screening tests that have been validated in a primary care setting. Clinicians should identify several with which they are comfortable so that they can be used consistently over time with their patient population. The Mini-Mental State Examination (MMSE), the Montreal Cognitive Assessment (MoCA), and the Saint Louis University Mental Status Examination (SLUMS) have been widely used in primary care settings. The Alzheimer's Association recommends use of the General Practitioner Assessment of Cognition (GPCOG), the Mini-Cog, or the Memory Impairment Screen (MIS) for cognitive screening related to the Medicare Annual Wellness Visit, as these tests take less than 5 minutes to administer, have good psychometric properties, and can be administered by a variety of health care team members. Informant assessment of changes in patient performance may include the GPCOG informant questionnaire, the Eight-Item Interview to Differentiate Aging and Dementia (AD8), or the Informant Questionnaire on Cognitive Decline in the Elderly (IQCODE) (see **Table 59-3**). If time and resources allow, additional interview time with an informant may identify specific areas of safety concerns and help tailor the management plan.

In adults with high baseline cognitive functions, these screening tests may be normal in the presence of obvious functional impairment necessitating referral to a neuropsychologist for more detailed cognitive testing. In individuals with lower educational levels or learning disabilities, cognitive screening tests may suggest impairment, but the history may not suggest any changes in functional status. Thus, it is critical to use age- and education-adjusted norms, and integrate historical information on baseline function to decide if further neuropsychological testing is warranted or if abnormal testing actually reflects the patient's baseline cognitive performance.

Laboratory data can assist in identifying factors that may be contributing to cognitive decline. Rarely do these factors alone account for the overall cognitive changes that lead to the presentation of a patient with significant memory loss. Nevertheless, treating such factors may improve cognitive symptoms in patients with pronounced laboratory abnormalities, numerous comorbid illnesses, or an underlying neurodegenerative process. Recommended laboratory tests include vitamin B_{12}, folate, thyroid-stimulating

hormone (TSH), electrolytes, complete blood count, liver enzymes, and 25-OH vitamin D. If symptoms are atypical or if there are specific risk factors, then an HIV test or serologic test for syphilis may be performed. In patients with assumed heavy alcohol use, thiamine (vitamin B_1) levels should be checked. In some European countries, routine assessment of cerebrospinal fluid (CSF) for β-amyloid and tau levels is done as part of the clinical evaluation. While CSF β-amyloid and tau levels may increase diagnostic accuracy of MCI and dementia due to AD, in general they are not recommended for widespread clinical practice as in most cases they do not change a patient's management plan. CSF collection may be used in memory specialty clinics, though, to differentiate between different dementias, including Creutzfeldt–Jakob disease, normal pressure hydrocephalus (NPH), or other less-common causes of neurodegeneration (see **Table 59-4**). Genetic testing for *APOE ε4* genotype is not recommended in routine clinical practice. Testing for *PSEN1*, *PSEN2*, or *APP* genes should be reserved for specialists evaluating cases in which there is a suspicion for familial AD.

In patients with documented cognitive impairment, it is recommended that either a CT or MRI scan of the brain be obtained. If neuroimaging was obtained for another indication prior to the onset of cognitive symptoms, in most cases the patient should be reimaged. Typical findings for AD on neuroimaging can range from a fairly normal scan to focal or diffuse cerebral atrophy. A CT of the head without contrast is usually sufficient to screen for significant cerebrovascular disease, brain tumors, subdural hematoma, or NPH. MRI can provide more information if lacunar infarcts are suspected. MRA may be helpful in identifying significant stenosis that could cause hypoperfusion. In persons with suspected seizure disorder or Creutzfeldt–Jakob disease, an electroencephalogram (EEG) may be considered. Use of fluorodeoxyglucose (FDG) positron emission tomography (PET) and amyloid PET imaging to differentiate FTD from AD should be reserved for specialty clinic use. Tau PET imaging is a novel research tool that is not yet approved for clinical practice.

Formulating a Diagnosis

Once a cognitive concern is recognized and delirium is ruled out, the clinician should identify and document any impaired cognitive domains (such as memory, executive function, language, or visuospatial skills) on cognitive testing and any functional loss in the individual's daily activities. Each potentially reversible cause of cognitive impairment should be outlined (ie, medication side effects, alcohol, sleep apnea, depression, or other medical comorbidities) and a plan to address these conditions should be developed. Objective cognitive impairment in the context of a supportive clinical history plus a decline in the individual's daily functional abilities are key elements necessary to differentiate normal cognitive aging and subjective cognitive decline (SCD) from MCI and dementia. With normal aging, individuals may experience a decline in mental processing speed and may have more difficulty learning new material, but these cognitive changes should not affect their usual function within their daily activities. For example, a healthy older adult may have more difficulty recalling an acquaintance's name or learning a new computer program, but their cognitive testing should be normal and daily functional activities should remain intact. SCD is a term used primarily in research settings to broadly describe symptoms within a pre-MCI stage of neurodegeneration. SCD is currently defined as a self-identified persistent decline in cognitive capacity compared with the individual's previous normal status in a person who still performs in the normal range on standardized cognitive tests. An example would be a business manager with normal performance on cognitive testing, who has noticed a subjective decline in her efficiency in managing numerous projects simultaneously despite maintaining a similar work load for many years. It is not yet known what percentage of patients presenting with SCD progress on to MCI and eventually AD; however, there is converging evidence that risk for progression to MCI and dementia increases in persons with SCD. Identification of patients with SCD allows clinicians to complete a thorough evaluation for other medical, psychological, and medication factors that could contribute to cognitive decline. Patients with SCD should be screened for cognitive dysfunction annually to evaluate for objective evidence of a decline in cognitive performance.

Once a person with SCD develops deficits in at least one cognitive domain, they may meet criteria for MCI (see **Table 59-2**), a symptomatic predementia syndrome noted in up to 15% to 20% of older adults. Individuals with MCI may present with cognitive complaints and describe a variety of methods they use to compensate for these cognitive changes, such as increasing use of lists, calendars, alarms, and other reminders. They maintain their level of function, but are less efficient in doing so. For example, a cabinetmaker who demonstrates impairment in executive function on testing may complain that in order to complete a cabinet work order with his same level of quality workmanship, it now takes him 2 to 3 weeks, whereas a few years ago he could complete such an order in 1 week. Once an individual's cognitive impairment progresses to the point that they can no longer maintain their baseline level of function, they may meet criteria for dementia. In the previous example, as the cabinetmaker's cognition declines he may no longer be able complete a cabinet order at all or may finish it with poorer-quality workmanship. At that point he may have progressed to a dementia.

Approximately 12% to 15% of persons with MCI will progress each year to AD or other forms of dementia. MCI patients who have impairment in memory performance (single-domain amnestic MCI) or in memory plus another cognitive area (multidomain amnestic MCI) are more likely to progress to AD. Older individuals with nonamnestic MCI may be more likely to progress to other forms of

dementia, such as FTD, dementia with Lewy bodies, or vascular dementia. Once a diagnosis of dementia is suspected, the clinician must differentiate between various causes of dementia. AD is the most common form of dementia in the United States, accounting for 50% to 90% of all dementia cases. Dementia with Lewy bodies, vascular dementia, and FTD are other common forms of dementia (**Table 59-5**). Details of the clinical and pathologic features of these dementias are covered in Chapter 63. Differentiating AD from other causes of memory loss can help clinicians choose effective therapies, anticipate behavior changes and other potential complications, and provide patients and caregivers information on prognosis.

If a patient does not meet the criteria for AD yet clinical suspicion remains, the clinician may consider obtaining more detailed neuropsychological testing or repeating screening cognitive testing in 6 to 12 months to clarify the diagnosis as the symptoms become more apparent. Persons with suspected MCI should be reassessed on an annual basis to evaluate for progression to dementia. If the symptoms or course of the disease are atypical for AD, the level of functional decline is out of proportion to neuropsychological testing results, or if there are significant behavioral issues that need to be addressed, then referral to a geriatrician, neurologist, or psychiatrist with expertise in dementia is recommended.

Future Diagnostic Tools

Novel biomarkers are continually being investigated for use in the diagnosis of AD and other types of dementia, as well as in identifying predementia syndromes. Many of these tools are still used chiefly in research settings, but are being studied to evaluate their potential role in clinical practice. Current investigations are focusing on specific neuroimaging modalities and biomarkers (including blood and CSF) with strong relationships to clinically relevant outcomes that could be used not only for diagnosis of dementia, but also for identifying asymptomatic persons at risk for cognitive decline. Neuroimaging modalities have shown great promise in documenting not only the late effects of neuronal damage in AD (regional and global cerebral atrophy), but also in identifying preclinical pathology (such as in vivo amyloid and tau imaging on PET) and the functional consequences of such pathology (such as changes in activation patterns on functional MRI or glucose uptake on FDG-PET). CSF levels of Aβ and tau have been shown to predict risk for progression to AD in older adults and persons with MCI. With the recent advances in the safety and acceptability of lumbar punctures, CSF markers may eventually find their way into the widespread clinical diagnostic work-up of preclinical AD. Identification of reliable blood biomarkers is a rapidly expanding field with significant clinical applications. Future research is focusing on how novel biomarkers may be used in combination with cognitive tests to identify which individuals are at greatest risk for AD, who would benefit most from preventive therapies, and how effective

TABLE 59-5 ■ CLINICAL FEATURES OF COMMON DEMENTIAS

TYPE OF DEMENTIA	ALZHEIMER DISEASE	VASCULAR DEMENTIA	DEMENTIA WITH LEWY BODIES	FRONTOTEMPORAL DEMENTIA
MUST FIRST MEET DIAGNOSTIC CRITERIA FOR DEMENTIA (SEE TABLE 59-1)				
Typical Course	Insidious onset and gradually progressive	Acute onset of cognitive impairment with some stabilization (if only one vascular event) and/or stepwise deterioration (if multiple infarcts)	Progressive cognitive decline with fluctuating cognition, attention, and alertness	Insidious onset and gradually progressive
Cognitive Symptoms	Memory is the most commonly affected cognitive domain May also have impairments in executive function, language, and/or visuospatial skills	Various cognitive domains may be affected depending on the location of the clinical stroke(s) and/or severe subcortical cerebrovascular disease	Cognitive symptoms may fluctuate May have prominent impairment in visuospatial ability, attention, and/or executive function	Will have early behavioral disinhibition and apathy (frontal lobe predominance) or early prominent language abnormalities (temporal lobe predominance) Deficits are chiefly noted in executive tasks with relative sparing of memory and visuospatial skills
Other Associated Symptoms/ Signs	Some patients may have agitation and/or behavioral changes	May or may not have focal neurologic signs on examination Should have evidence of relevant cerebrovascular disease by brain imaging	May have recurrent well-formed visual hallucinations (usually people or animals), parkinsonism (including tremor, rigidity, and postural instability), recurrent falls and syncope, rapid eye movement (REM) sleep behavior disorder, neuroleptic sensitivity, and/or delusions	In behavioral variant frontotemporal dementia, may have early behavioral disinhibition, apathy, loss of empathy, perseverative behaviors, and hyperorality

these therapies are in modifying the underlying disease process in asymptomatic and symptomatic individuals.

Updated NIA-AA Research Framework

As noted earlier, the NIA-AA criteria for AD diagnosis were created in 2011. In April 2018, the NIA-AA released a report proposing a new research framework for studying AD that served to update the 2011 guidelines with subsequent scientific progress. The most important, paradigm-shifting change in the 2018 report was redefining AD by its biological changes in the brain rather than the clinical phenotype. By moving away from the prior definition based on clinical-pathological presentation to biological characterization, the NIA-AA framework aimed to create a common language in research studies, allow for more aligned comparison of research findings, and facilitate future clinical trials.

The current clinical framework for diagnosing AD is based on symptoms reported by the patient and corroborated by a collateral historian, together with an objective assessment of cognitive decline. The level of confidence in this diagnosis ranges from possible to probable, depending on the presence of typical symptoms, as well as the absence of alternative causes of cognitive decline. A biological diagnosis of AD, which is considered the only definitive

diagnosis, presently relies on autopsy findings of amyloid plaques and tau neurofibrillary tangles. Numerous studies have found discordant findings between clinical diagnoses and neuropathological outcomes. It is reported that 10% to 30% of clinically diagnosed persons with AD dementia do not display the neuropathological hallmarks of amyloid plaques and tau neurofibrillary tangles on autopsy. Differentiating the clinical syndrome, composed of symptoms not necessarily specific to AD, from the biological changes seen on neuropathology would allow discovery of novel mechanisms underlying AD neurobiology. Furthermore, enrollment of participants with biologically confirmed AD diagnosis will be critical in evaluating efficacy of disease-modifying therapies as they become available in the future.

The 2018 updated research framework proposed a biomarker classification system called AT(N). The framework categorizes individuals based on the presence or absence of the following core AD pathological features: aggregated amyloid beta protein (A), aggregated tau protein (T), and neurodegeneration or neuronal injury (N). The biomarkers for amyloid and tau were selected for their high specificity to AD-related changes found in autopsy studies. In the AT(N) framework, AD is defined by the presence of both amyloid (A) and tau (T). Since neurodegeneration is not a feature used in the neuropathological diagnosis of AD

TABLE 59-6 ■ CSF BIOMARKERS OF ALZHEIMER DISEASE

AD PATHOLOGY-RELATED MECHANISM	CSF MEASURE
Amyloid deposition	Aβ40, Aβ42, sAPPα, sAPPβ, Aβ oligomers, BACE1 levels/activity, ratios, eg, Aβ42/p-tau, Aβ40/Aβ42, N-terminal truncated Aβ42 APLP-1
Neurodegeneration	Total tau, p-tau, oligomeric forms of tau
Neuronal/axonal damage and white matter integrity	Neurofilament L (NFL)
Synaptic function/damage	Neurogranin, SNAP25, visinin-like-protein 1 (VLP1)
Neuroinflammation	YKL-40, MCP1, soluble form of TERM2, cytokines, chemokines, com3, S-100

and is seen in other neurodegenerative disorders as well, it is in parentheses in the proposed research framework. However, its inclusion in the framework was necessary to reflect disease severity. **Table 59-6** provides a list of validated biomarkers used to identify each component of the AT(N) framework.

The AT(N) framework has accelerated discovery of novel CSF and more recently blood-based biomarkers of amyloid, tau, neurodegeneration, neuroinflammation, and other pathological changes seen in AD. Many of these biomarkers, especially the core AD biomarkers including Aβ-42, total tau (t-tau), and phosphorylated tau-181 (p-tau-181), can now be reliably measured in CSF and correlate well with PET brain imaging and neuropathological findings. Although validation of various AD biomarkers in CSF, blood, and autopsy brain studies is ongoing, they are being actively used to enroll participants in treatment trials and clinical and translational studies. Based on data emerging from longitudinal cohort studies and randomized clinical trials, the reported accumulation of AD biomarkers over time points to a continuum of disease progression, as opposed to the older clinical conceptualization of distinct levels of disease staging.

There is converging evidence that amyloid deposition in the brain is the first neuropathological change seen in persons with AD. This conclusion is based on studies of people with early-onset AD due to an autosomal dominant mutation, those living with Down syndrome, and findings from transgenic animal models of AD. However, the presence of amyloid alone is viewed as only an early stage within the Alzheimer continuum and is necessary, but not sufficient, for the biological diagnosis of AD. While the amyloid cascade hypothesis suggests amyloid accumulation causes changes leading to tau accumulation and eventually neurodegeneration, it is also accepted that, unlike tau, amyloid is not strongly linked to cognitive function. Amyloid

may have downstream effects on tau and neurodegeneration, but the AT(N) framework does not assume an order of causality.

One of the most notable contributions of the AT(N) framework is to effectively screen and identify participants for enrollment in clinical trials based on their biomarker profile rather than nonspecific clinical presentations. The framework also provides validated and uniform biological outcome measures to assess the efficacy of disease modifying therapies, and determine dose-response relationships. Given AD is a chronic and slowly progressive condition, trials to find effective treatments are challenged with finding reliable surrogate outcomes that could change quickly, rather than wait for alterations in clinical or behavioral phenotype that would require longer and costly trials. The AT(N) framework would enrich treatment trials with biologically confirmed AD participants at higher risk of decline, as well as serve as a surrogate end-point in disease modifying therapy trials. Additionally, it could serve as a marker of treatment response.

The AT(N) framework is not meant to be comprehensive and exclusive, but rather adaptive to newer scientific discoveries. A new evolution in the framework is ATX(N), with "X" representing novel candidate biomarkers to help expand and explain underlying mechanisms in AD. Examples of potential mechanisms include neuroinflammation, synaptic dysfunction, microvascular changes, mitochondrial oxidative damage, glial activation, neurochemical deficits, and BBB dysfunction. The ATX(N) framework would help expand the scientific understanding of AD as well as investigate the heterogeneity of the disease.

AD Biomarkers

Cerebrospinal fluid AD biomarkers Amyloid and tau biomarkers are central in identifying AD pathology and will help explore disease heterogeneity. They will likely play critical roles in AD, including early diagnosis, disease progression, screening, risk prediction, target engagement, treatment monitoring, and validation of novel biomarkers. The core AD biomarkers, namely amyloid Aβ-42, t-tau, and p-tau181, have been validated through multiple CSF, PET brain imaging, and neuropathological studies. Given their proven reliability, amyloid and tau biomarkers will serve as a framework for identification of novel biomarkers to address contributions from potential coexisting pathologies, such as vascular insults, Lewy body dementia, Parkinson disease, and TDP (TAR DNA-binding protein)-43 that likely contribute to clinical symptoms and cognitive decline.

In the past decade, new CSF biomarkers have been identified representing multiple mechanisms active in AD. These mechanisms include glial activation, neuroinflammation, synaptic degeneration, and neuronal/axonal death. Importantly, many AD biomarkers can now be measured in CSF and several in blood as well. Although the validation of CSF biomarkers is currently ongoing, once approved, they will have major clinical applications in the diagnosis, progression, and treatment of AD and related disorders. **Table 59-6** summarizes CSF biomarkers representing various molecular pathways active in AD. While some of the CSF biomarkers, such as t-tau, NfL, YKL-40, and interleukins, may not be specific to AD, they elucidate disease progression and are related to symptoms. Measures of neurodegeneration may be particularly important, given clinical features of AD tend to track closely with synaptic dysfunction, and eventually neuronal death. Synaptic loss is an early pathological change in AD and closely associated with cognitive impairment.

Neuroimaging AD biomarkers The multimodal neuroimaging AD biomarkers, including CAT, MRI, amyloid PET, and tau PET brain scans, have been examined over years and validated as effective measures to help in the diagnosis and progression of AD, and exclusion of other treatable causes of dementia, such as stroke, tumor, or NPH. Recent advances in neuroimaging include novel PET radiotracers to image neuroinflammation and translocator protein (TSPO) PET and synaptic vesicle protein 2A (SV2A) PET, respectively, to study synaptic dysfunction and loss. Clinically, [18F] FDG PET is available to visualize synaptic dysfunction, neuronal cell loss, and metabolic dysfunction to help differentiate AD from non-AD dementias such as FTD and Lewy body disease. Additionally, amyloid PET and tau PET are available in research settings, but not yet approved for clinical use or reimbursement. Once approved, amyloid and tau PET scans will become important for biological diagnosis of AD.

Blood-based AD biomarkers Although highly informative, the utility of CSF and PET biomarkers is limited by their cost, logistical matters and practical barriers related to the lumbar puncture procedure. These limitations make CSF measures unlikely to become widely used in the clinical setting. Consequently, the pursuit of blood-based AD biomarkers has intensified. Several AD biomarkers can now be measured in blood through emerging analytical techniques. However, a major limitation in broad utility of these biomarkers is significant heterogeneity in results due to multiple factors, including variance in sample collection, storage, preanalytical processing, assays, and data analysis. Among the AD biomarkers that can be measured in plasma include Aβ42, Aβ40, total tau, p-tau181, p-tau217, p-tau231, neurofilament light (NfL), interleukins, and YKL-40. Highly sensitive mass spectrometry assays are used to measure plasma levels of Aβ42, Aβ40, and their ratios, while single molecule array (SIMOA) technology is used to assay NfL, interleukins, and p-tau and its analogues in plasma. Phosphorylation of tau occurs at multiple sites and certain isoforms, such as threonine 231 (p-tau231) and threonine 217 (p-tau217) change early in AD pathobiology and have been shown to accurately identify amyloid positivity along the AD biomarker continuum and clinical spectrum.

Plasma neurofilament light (NfL), a promising biomarker of neurodegeneration, albeit not specific to AD, has been shown to increase in persons with cognitive impairment due to many neurodegenerative disorders, including AD, Parkinson disease, FTD, and cerebral vascular disease. Elevated plasma NfL is a sign of early neuronal death and can increase during preclinical stages of AD. The field of plasma AD biomarkers is advancing rapidly and new biomarkers that change during early stages of AD will become invaluable for early diagnosis, progression from preclinical to symptomatic stages of AD, and treatment monitoring and response. However, these biomarkers are not yet ready for clinical applications, given that larger studies are necessary to validate, examine the relationship with clinical phenotype, and harmonize their measurement in plasma.

MANAGEMENT

Managing patients with AD involves presentation of the diagnosis, initiation of medical therapy, assessment and treatment of concomitant depression and/or behavioral concerns, identification of a social support network, education of patients and caregivers, provision of caregiver support, and initiation of appropriate safety measures.

Presenting the Diagnosis

Presenting the diagnosis of AD to a patient is difficult, as it may generate significant emotional responses from the patient and their family and trigger fear of future demise. Frequently, patients and family members suspect the diagnosis before it is presented, but how they respond to the news depends on personal coping mechanisms, cultural influences, family dynamics, and their preconceived understanding of AD. Clinicians may help patients and families adjust to this diagnosis by using an empathetic, yet honest approach and by providing them with educational and support resources, including those provided by agencies such as the Alzheimer's Association and the National Institute on Aging Alzheimer's Disease Education and Referral (ADEAR) Center. In addition, the clinician should emphasize the goals of diagnosing AD in order to take steps to protect the patient's memory, delay the progression of the disease, and maintain the person's safety. It is widely recommended to tell both the patient and family the diagnosis using the term "Alzheimer disease," thus, providing patients and families with a starting point for education. Encouraging both persons with the disorder and caregivers to utilize resources such as local support groups, community resources, and national Alzheimer organizations is an important part of the patient management plan.

Drug Therapy and Nonpharmacologic Therapy

Acetylcholinesterase inhibitors (AChEIs) are the mainstay of therapy for AD. AChEIs increase the levels of the neurotransmitter acetylcholine in neuronal synapses, thereby enhancing cholinergic activity in the affected brain regions. Although 18% to 48% of persons may experience improvements in cognition after taking these medications, the majority of patients do not have any noticeable improvement, but instead experience a plateau or slowing of their rate of cognitive decline. While prior studies raised questions as to the cost-effectiveness of treating AD patients with AChEIs, newer studies integrating generic drug cost estimates have demonstrated that these drugs are cost-effective. Delaying the progression of cognitive decline may lead to improvements in quality of life, reduced caregiver burden, and decreased economic cost associated with long-term care. AChEIs have not been shown to be effective in delaying progression from MCI to AD and, thus, are chiefly recommended for use in patients who already have a diagnosis of dementia.

Three FDA-approved AChEIs are actively prescribed in the United States: **donepezil (Aricept), galantamine (Razadyne), and rivastigmine (Exelon) (Table 59-7)**. While all three of these compounds are available as generic medications, some specific long-acting formulations and solutions of these drugs are still under patent (see **Table 59-7**) and, thus, are not yet available in generic form. In general, the most common adverse effects associated with AChEI use are nausea, anorexia, and diarrhea. Bradycardia, atrioventricular (AV) nodal block, and syncope and unintentional weight loss are additional potentially serious adverse side effects that would trigger deprescribing. It is recommended that patients are started on a low dose of the medication with dose increases approximately every 2 months until a therapeutic dose is achieved (see **Table 59-7**). Gastrointestinal side effects may be alleviated by taking the medications with food. Sleep disturbances are also common and may improve with altering the dosing schedule.

Memantine (Namenda) is an FDA-approved medication for use in moderate-to-severe AD. Memantine is an uncompetitive N-methyl-D-aspartate (NMDA) receptor antagonist. At high concentrations, memantine can inhibit mechanisms related to learning and memory, but at lower concentrations, it can preserve or enhance memory in animal models of AD. Memantine can protect against the excitotoxic destruction of cholinergic neurons and may inhibit β-amyloid production. In persons with moderate-to-severe AD, memantine may slow the progression of cognitive decline. In addition, studies support that use of memantine was well tolerated and led to better outcomes on measures of cognition, activities of daily living, and behavior. Additional studies are needed before memantine can be recommended for earlier stages of AD. In patients with moderate-to-severe AD, combined treatment with a cholinesterase inhibitor and memantine has not been shown to be superior to treatment with either agent alone with regards to cognitive, functional, and behavioral outcomes. In patients who do not tolerate cholinesterase inhibitors due to gastrointestinal side effects or bradycardia, memantine may be used as first-line therapy. With use of either AChEIs or memantine, clinicians should educate families on what to expect with use of the medications, namely that they work to delay the progression of symptoms and not to significantly improve cognition. Consideration should be given to the modest expected benefit and monthly cost of both types of medications.

In June 2021, the US FDA approved **aducanumab** under accelerated approval based on the reduction in brain amyloid demonstrated in its clinical trials in patients with MCI and early stage AD. Aducanumab is a human monoclonal antibody targeting aggregated amyloid and amyloid oligomers. It is designed to enter the brain through the BBB, bind to amyloid plaques and oligomers, and stimulate microglia to clear the amyloid protein. In two clinical trials leading to the FDA approval, aducanumab was shown to significantly lower amyloid burden in the brain assessed by amyloid PET scans, in some study participants to near normal levels. In one of the two trials, treatment resulted in a 22% reduced rate of cognitive decline in the primary outcome measure (the Clinical Dementia Rating—Sum of Boxes) over an 18-month period; however, no statistically significant benefit was seen in the other study. Importantly, the aducanumab studies were initially halted based on futility analyses; however, reanalysis of datasets including newly collected data revealed statistically significant reduction in the rate of cognitive decline in only the high-dose group. Importantly, administration of aducanumab was associated with adverse effects on MRI imaging. These side effects called amyloid-related imaging abnormalities-effusion (ARIA-E) and -hemorrhage (ARIA-H) were seen in 34% to 36% of participants receiving the high dose. Approximately 80% of those with ARIA did not have symptoms; however, those with symptoms experienced headache, dizziness, visual disturbances, and nausea.

Controversy has arisen over how the study data were analyzed, the true clinical benefit to an individual as measured by the study outcomes, and the social and political pressure on the FDA approval process. Despite these concerns, the FDA approval of aducanumab has ushered in a new research-clinical paradigm that, for the first time, utilized amyloid clearance as a surrogate measure in the approval of a disease-modifying therapy. It is projected that approval of aducanumab will lead to the discovery of newer analogues of antiamyloid monoclonal antibodies with more favorable adverse effect profiles and demonstration of clinical efficacy.

Additionally, there are no clear guidelines on several issues directly relevant to aducanumab treatment, including patient selection, inclusion/exclusion criteria, payment for amyloid PET scan and MRIs necessary to monitor presence and progression of ARIA, and duration of treatment.

In addition to targeting β-amyloid pathways, novel research is focusing on the effects of inhibitors of tau phosphorylation and aggregation and the stabilization

TABLE 59-7 ■ FDA-APPROVED MEDICATIONS FOR THE TREATMENT OF ALZHEIMER DISEASE[a]

MEDICATION	INDICATION	AVAILABLE FORMULATIONS	DOSE RANGE AND TITRATION	ADVERSE EFFECTS
ACETYLCHOLINESTERASE INHIBITORS				
Donepezil (available as generic donepezil or Aricept)	Mild-to-moderate AD	• 5- and 10-mg tablets • 5- and 10-mg oral disintegrating tablets	• 5–10 mg once daily at bedtime • May be taken with or without food • Oral disintegrating tablets should be dissolved on tongue and followed with water • Begin at 5 mg once daily for 4–6 weeks, then increase to 10 mg daily as tolerated • Effective dose: 5–10 mg daily	• Bradycardia or heart block, syncope, nausea, diarrhea, insomnia, vomiting, muscle cramps, fatigue, anorexia
Donepezil (available as generic donepezil in 10-mg tablets or Aricept in 10- or 23-mg tablets)	Moderate-to-severe AD	• 10- and 23-mg tablets • 10-mg oral disintegrating tablets	• 10 mg once daily at bedtime • If the clinician thinks there is a strong indication for increased dosing, a patient who has been on 10 mg for 3 mo may increase to the 23-mg tablet daily • 23-mg tablets should not be split, crushed, or chewed • Effective dose: 10 or 23 mg daily	• Bradycardia or heart block, nausea, diarrhea, insomnia, vomiting, muscle cramps, fatigue, anorexia
Galantamine (available as generic galantamine, galantamine ER, Razadyne, or Razadyne ER)	Mild-to-moderate AD	• 4-, 8-, and 12-mg immediate-release tablets • 4 mg/mL immediate-release oral solution • 8-, 16-, and 24-mg extended-release capsules	**Immediate-Release Tablets or Oral Solution:** • 4–12 mg twice daily • Should be taken with meals • Begin at 4 mg twice daily for at least 4 wk then increase to 8 mg twice daily for at least 4 wk then 12 mg twice daily as tolerated • For patients with moderate hepatic or renal impairment (creatinine clearance 9–59 mL/min), dose should not exceed 16 mg/d • Should not be used in patients with severe hepatic or renal impairment (creatinine clearance < 9 mL/min) **Extended-Release Capsules:** • 8–24 mg once daily • Should be taken in the morning with food • Begin at 8 mg once daily in the morning for at least 4 wk then increase to 16 mg once daily in the morning for at least 4 wk then 24 mg once daily as tolerated • Conversion from tablets (or oral solution) to extended release should occur at the same daily dosage with the last dose of the tablets (or oral solution) occurring in the evening and the extended-release formulation starting the next morning • Effective dose: 16–24 mg daily	• Nausea, vomiting, diarrhea, dizziness, headache, decreased appetite, weight loss

ACETYLCHOLINESTERASE INHIBITORS

Rivastigmine (available as generic rivastigmine capsules or Exelon capsules, oral solution, or transdermal patch)	Mild-to-moderate AD	• 1.5-, 3-, 4.5-, and 6-mg capsules • 2 mg/mL oral solution • 4.6 mg/24 h and 9.5 mg/24 h patches	**Capsules or Oral Solution:** • 1.5–6 mg twice daily • Should be taken with meals • Oral solution may be taken directly or mixed with beverage • Begin at 1.5 mg twice daily for minimum of 2 wk then increase to 3 mg twice daily for minimum of 2 wk then 4.5 mg twice daily for minimum of 2 wk then 6 mg twice daily as tolerated • Patients with mild or moderate hepatic impairment or moderate-to-severe renal impairment may be able to only tolerate lower doses • Effective dose: 6–12 mg daily **Patch:** • Begin at 4.6 mg/24 h patch daily for 4–6 wk then increase to 9.5 mg/24 h patch daily as tolerated • Apply patch on intact skin for 24-h period; replace with a new patch every 24 h • Effective dose: 9.5 mg/24 h	• Nausea, vomiting, anorexia, dyspepsia, weakness
Rivastigmine patch (available as Exelon transdermal patch)	Mild, moderate, and severe AD	• 4.6 mg/24 h, 9.5 mg/24 h, and 13.3 mg/24 h patches	**Patch:** • Begin at 4.6 mg/24 h patch daily for a minimum of 4 weeks then increase to 9.5 mg/24 h patch daily as tolerated; may increase to maximum of 13.3 mg/24 h after minimum of 4 wk • Apply patch on intact skin for 24-h period; replace with a new patch every 24 h • Consider dose adjustments in mild-to-moderate hepatic impairment and low (<50 kg) body weight • If switching to an Exelon patch from rivastigmine capsules (or oral solution), a patient on a total daily dose of <6 mg of oral rivastigmine can be switched to the 4.6 mg/24 h patch while a patient on a total daily dose of 6–12 mg can be switched to the 9.5 mg/24 h patch • If switching, apply the first patch on the day following the last oral dose • Effective dose: 9.5 mg/24 h or 13.3 mg/24 h	• Nausea, vomiting, diarrhea

N-METHYL-D-ASPARTATE (NMDA) RECEPTOR ANTAGONIST

Memantine (available as generic memantine tablets or Namenda tablets or oral solution)	Moderate-to-severe AD	• 5- and 10-mg tablets • 2 mg/mL oral solution	**Tablets or Oral Solution:** • 10 mg twice daily • May be taken with or without food • Begin at 5 mg once daily for 1 wk then increase to 5 mg twice daily for 1 wk then 10 mg in the morning and 5 mg in the evening for 1 wk then 10 mg twice daily as tolerated • In patients with severe renal impairment (creatinine clearance 5–29 mL/min) target dose is 5 mg twice daily • Effective dose: 20 mg daily	• Dizziness, headache, confusion, constipation

913

(Continued)

PART III

GERIATRIC CONDITIONS

TABLE 59-7 ■ FDA-APPROVED MEDICATIONS FOR THE TREATMENT OF ALZHEIMER DISEASE[a] (CONTINUED)

MEDICATION	INDICATION	AVAILABLE FORMULATIONS	DOSE RANGE AND TITRATION	ADVERSE EFFECTS
N-METHYL-D-ASPARTATE (NMDA) RECEPTOR ANTAGONIST (Cont.)				
Memantine extended release (available as Namenda XR)	Moderate-to-severe AD	• 7-, 14-, 21-, or 28-mg capsules	• Patients on memantine 10 mg twice daily may be switched to Namenda XR 28 mg daily the day following the last dose of 10-mg memantine • Patients with severe renal impairment (creatinine clearance of 5–29 mL/min) may be switched from memantine 5 mg twice daily to Namenda XR 14 mg once daily • May be taken with or without food • Capsules can be taken intact or may be opened and sprinkled on applesauce • Effective dose: 28 mg daily	• Headache, diarrhea, dizziness
COMBINATION THERAPY (ACETYLCHOLINESTERASE INHIBITORS AND NMDA RECEPTOR ANTAGONIST)				
Namzaric (memantine HCl ER and donepezil HCl) capsules	Moderate-to-severe AD	• 14-mg memantine HCl ER/10-mg donepezil HCl or 28-/10-mg capsules	• Once patient stabilized on a daily dose of memantine ER (10 mg twice daily or 28 mg ER once daily) and donepezil 10 mg daily may switch to Namzaric 28-/10-mg capsule once a day in the evening • Patients with severe renal impairment on memantine HCl (5 mg twice daily or 14 mg ER once daily) and donepezil HCl 10 mg daily may be switched to Namzaric 14-/10-mg capsule once a day in the evening • May be taken with or without food • Capsules can be taken intact or may be opened and sprinkled on applesauce • Capsules should not be divided, chewed, or crushed	• Headache, diarrhea, dizziness, anorexia, vomiting, nausea, ecchymosis
MONOCLONAL ANTIBODIES DIRECTED AGAINST AMYLOID				
Aducanumab (available as Aduhelm infusion)	MCI due to AD and mild AD	• Supplied in vials of 170 mg/1.7 mL or 300 mg/3 mL • Monthly IV infusion	• The first and second infusion doses are 1 mg/kg; the third and fourth infusion doses are 3 mg/kg; the fifth and sixth infusion doses are 6 mg/kg; the seventh infusion and beyond doses are 10 mg/kg	• Amyloid-related imaging abnormalities (ARIA) with brain effusion or hemorrhage • Headache, falls, and diarrhea

[a]Information obtained from prescribing information documents.

of microtubules. Other potential therapeutic agents are directed toward inflammation and oxidation, insulin signaling, mitochondrial function, and nerve growth factor signaling.

Clinical trials have not conclusively shown that treating vascular risk factors delays the development or progression of AD. However, aggressive treatment of vascular risk factors in many patients with memory complaints, including those associated with AD, may be warranted. Vascular risk factor modification has known cardiovascular benefits that may lead to reduction in cerebrovascular disease, stroke, myocardial infarction, and coronary artery bypass grafting—factors strongly linked to cognitive decline. Trials are under way to clarify if vascular risk factor reduction and improved cerebral perfusion modify the course of AD. Until the completion of such trials, clinicians should follow established cardiovascular prevention guidelines for patients presenting with memory complaints, taking into account the patient's comorbid illnesses, quality of life, treatment costs, and life expectancy.

Evidence also supports that encouraging AD patients to engage in nonpharmacologic interventions, including physical activity and exercise, mentally stimulating activities, and social activities, may lead to cognitive benefits. Depending on an individual's physical abilities, comorbid illness, social situation, and interests, clinicians should encourage AD patients and persons with cognitive impairment to seek out opportunities for exercise and activities that promote use of their intact areas of cognitive function. For example, an AD patient with prominent language deficits but intact visuospatial skills may find crosswords or word search puzzles very frustrating, but may enjoy playing checkers or painting birdhouses. Such activities may need to be adjusted over time to account for progressive cognitive changes.

Behavioral Management

Noncognitive neuropsychiatric symptoms of dementia include aggression, agitation, depression, anxiety, delusions, hallucinations, apathy, and disinhibition. Such behaviors may be more distressing to family and caregivers than the actual memory decline. Neuropsychiatric symptoms may be managed by nonpharmacologic as well as pharmacologic interventions. Nonpharmacologic therapies should in general be explored prior to using pharmacologic therapy, unless the person's agitation threatens his or her safety or living situation. Chapter 60 includes detailed information on pharmacological and nonpharmacological management of behavioral symptoms of dementia.

Safety Management

Reviewing common safety concerns in persons with dementia may help identify significant risks and provide an opportunity for educating family members and caregivers on what areas to monitor closely and what safeguards to take to protect the person with AD. Some patients may require further evaluation to assess driving safety, which can be done through some occupational therapy departments, local driving schools, state Department of Motor Vehicles, or other similar agencies. Pill boxes, electronic reminders, or other similar medication planners may facilitate correct administration of medications and allow family or caregivers to help in setting up the medications properly. Other safety concerns, such as proper use of the stove, woodworking equipment, and access to firearms, should be discussed and appropriate supervision and/or limitations be arranged.

Caregiver Support

There is convincing evidence that the effects of AD are felt not only by the patient but also by the caregivers. Caregivers have increased depression, work absence, and health problems compared to those not caring for a family member with dementia. Clinicians and health care team members should direct caregivers toward educational resources on the disease, practical tips on helping someone with AD optimize their function, effective communication strategies, legal and financial planning, and the importance of caregiver health and social support. Use of respite services from family, friends, neighbors, home health agencies, and local adult day centers may allow for caregivers to take the appropriate time needed to maintain their own health and social connections. Local support groups allow for caregivers to share ideas and experiences. Other initiatives such as memory cafés, dementia-friendly communities, and online resources may provide caregivers important support and interaction.

PREVENTION

The Systolic Blood Pressure Intervention Trial Memory and Cognition in Decreased Hypertension (SPRINT-MIND) randomized trial has shown that targeting a systolic blood pressure goal of 120 mm Hg relative to what was at the time standard, 140 mm Hg, led to a statistically significant, 19% reduction in the incidence of MCI (see Chapter 79 for details). Currently, there are no established preventive therapies for AD and no approved medications to treat MCI. Evidence supports that therapies that either delay or prevent the onset of AD may need to be started in midlife in high-risk populations in order to significantly influence the onset and course of the disease. As the underlying pathologic changes that eventually lead to clinical AD begin decades before the onset of symptoms, primary prevention trials with conversion to AD as their primary outcome will be costly and time consuming. Integrating biomarkers with strong relationships to clinically relevant outcomes into such primary prevention trials may allow for earlier identification of disease-modifying effects of potential preventive therapies. Given the multifactorial nature of AD, future preventive strategies will most likely target a variety of mechanisms related to disease progression, similar to those used in cardiovascular disease prevention. Some potential prevention therapies currently under investigation include antiamyloid therapies, vascular risk factor modification, anti-inflammatory medications, antioxidants, and lifestyle interventions such as exercise, social engagement, and cognitive stimulation.

SPECIAL ISSUES

Comorbidity

Managing comorbid illnesses in a person with AD can be challenging. Patients may forget to take important medications for comorbid conditions which, in turn, may exacerbate confusion. Persons with AD may not be able to remember symptoms related to other comorbid illnesses, such as recent episodes of chest pain, shortness of breath, or localization of arthritis pain. Thus, it is important to educate families and caregivers on how they can best assist their loved one in managing their comorbid illnesses. For example, a caregiver of an AD patient with diabetes may need to directly observe insulin administration and meal intake to maintain good glucose control. An AD patient with significant chronic pain may need their caregiver to write down the time of day that they become more agitated with the goal of optimizing the timing of their pain medications. Each management plan will need to be tailored to the AD patient's comorbid illnesses and social situation, utilizing community resources as available.

Persons with dementia are more likely to experience delirium in response to medical illness or surgery. Thus, educating families that acute episodes of confusion may suggest a harboring infection or other illness may help families seek out appropriate medical care when watching for behavioral changes. Caregivers should be forewarned that an AD patient is at increased risk for delirium following surgical procedures and that interventions such as avoiding anticholinergic and sedative hypnotic medications, maintaining good sleep-wake cycles, optimizing pain control, using hearing aids and glasses as appropriate, and establishing daytime activities may help reduce risk of escalating postoperative delirium (see also Chapter 58).

Care Settings

Ensuring a safe living environment is a high priority for patients with any form of dementia including AD. Patients living in their own house or independent apartment may need additional safety measures implemented around their home, such as by posting emergency numbers on the wall, using timers to remind them to turn the stove off, using medical alert systems, and optimizing use of home care services to assist with tasks such as bathing, cleaning, meal preparation, transportation, and medication administration. Once patients can no longer identify what to do in an emergency situation, then 24-hour supervision is recommended. Through partnering with family and friends and use of community resources, some individuals with

AD are able to stay in their own home their entire lives. However, a variety of social circumstances, medical or behavioral issues, or economic limitations may necessitate that a person with AD move to a more structured, supervised setting. The choice of setting (eg, assisted living facility, skilled nursing facility, or locked dementia unit) varies from patient to patient and depends on the degree of cognitive impairment, cultural preferences, comorbid illnesses, economic resources, and behavioral and safety concerns.

Palliative and End-of-Life Care

Upon diagnosis of AD, many patients and families have questions as to what to expect in the years ahead. Since the course of AD progression may depend not only on genetic and environmental factors but also comorbid medical conditions, the rate of decline is difficult to predict. Once an AD patient is medically treated and after all potentially reversible contributing factors have been addressed, obtaining repeat cognitive testing may give the clinician an idea of the trajectory of the individual's decline and help inform the family on what to expect in the years ahead. Providing information to family and caregivers early in the disease course on end-of-life planning may help smooth this difficult transition later in the illness. Use of respite services, home health aides or family members, or palliative care may help the person with AD stay in the home longer. If their social network cannot support the patient as care needs increase, then nursing home placement or hospice care may be necessary. Caregivers of AD patients may go through feelings of guilt when a loved one is moved from home to a facility, so appropriate support should be provided. Capacity for decision making should be assessed regularly throughout the course of the illness with appropriate activation of advanced care planning when the patient is no longer able to make their own health care decisions.

Advanced dementia is associated with poor nutritional intake, urinary incontinence, skin breakdown, and infections such as pneumonia. Palliative and end-of-life care services are increasingly being used for patients with end stages of AD and other forms of dementia. As the disease progresses, patients may reach a point when they are no longer able to express their needs. When patients are at a stage of disease where they no longer are able to engage meaningfully in social interactions or participate in self-care, then consideration should be given to discontinuing cholinesterase inhibitors and/or memantine therapy. At that point, medication regimens may be simplified to focus on therapies that optimize patient comfort. As swallowing difficulties develop, modified diets and one-on-one feeding may be needed to maintain a patient's nutritional status. Feeding tubes are not recommended in end-of-life for patients with advanced AD as they do not prolong survival or increase comfort and have not been shown to reduce the risk of pressure sores, infection, or aspiration.

Hospice care can help with symptom management late in the course of the illness. Caregiver involvement in Alzheimer support groups can provide comfort during the unique grieving process related to dementia, as family and caregivers watch the cognitive and personality transformations in their family member with AD.

SUMMARY

AD is the leading cause of dementia with 44 million individuals currently affected worldwide. Unless effective preventive strategies are identified, it is anticipated that the prevalence of AD will double every 20 years. Given the widespread prevalence of AD and its impact on the well-being and quality of life of patients and their caregivers, it is critical for clinicians to be well-trained in identifying early cognitive changes, differentiating AD from other common medical and psychiatric conditions, diagnosing the disorder, and developing an effective management plan with their patients and families. Knowledge and use of educational and community resources can provide additional culturally tailored support to AD patients and their caregivers. In most situations, AD can be effectively diagnosed and managed within a primary care setting, through careful history-taking, a physical examination, and brief cognitive testing. Ancillary laboratory tests and neuroimaging can help differentiate between various causes of memory loss and different types of dementia. AD treatment involves not only pharmacologic therapy—with cholinesterase inhibitors, NMDA receptor antagonists, and soon aducanumab and potentially other monoclonal antibodies directed against amyloid—but also careful assessment of safety, behavioral concerns, and education for the patient, family, and other caregivers. While preventive therapies have not yet been established, novel therapies are under investigation to delay or preferably arrest the development and progression of AD. Clinicians are encouraged to be active champions of educational and research efforts to improve early diagnosis, treatment, and prevention of AD by promoting clinical research participation among willing patients and families. Annual updates on large-scale initiatives such as the United States National Alzheimer's Project Act (NAPA), Alzheimer's Disease International's World Alzheimer Report, the Alzheimer's Association's Facts and Figures, and other international collaborations and publications will keep clinicians informed on global efforts to optimize early diagnosis and effective care of patients at risk for AD and related dementias.

FURTHER READING

Albert MS, DeKosky ST, Dickson D, et al. The diagnosis of mild cognitive impairment due to Alzheimer's disease: recommendations from the National Institute on Aging-Alzheimer's Association workgroups on diagnostic guidelines for Alzheimer's disease. *Alzheimers Dement.* 2011;7(3):270–279.

Callahan CM, Boustani MA, Unverzagt FW, et al. Effectiveness of collaborative care for older adults with Alzheimer disease in primary care: a randomized controlled trial. *JAMA.* 2006;295(18):2148–2157.

Cordell CB, Borson S, Boustani M, et al; Medicare Detection of Cognitive Impairment Workgroup. Alzheimer's Association recommendations for operationalizing the detection of cognitive impairment during the Medicare Annual Wellness Visit in a primary care setting. *Alzheimers Dement.* 2013;9(2):141–150.

Hyman BT, Phelps CH, Beach TG, et al. National Institute on Aging-Alzheimer's Association guidelines for the neuropathologic assessment of Alzheimer's disease. *Alzheimers Dement.* 2012;8(1):1–13.

Jack CR Jr, Bennett DA, Blennow K, et al. NIA-AA Research Framework: Toward a biological definition of Alzheimer's disease. *Alzheimers Dement.* 2018; 14(4):535–562.

Kales HC, Gitlin LN, Lyketsos CG; Detroit Expert Panel on Assessment and Management of Neuropsychiatric Symptoms of Dementia. Management of neuropsychiatric symptoms of dementia in clinical settings: recommendations from a multidisciplinary expert panel. *J Am Geriatr Soc.* 2014;62(4):762–769.

Livingston G, Huntley J, Sommerlad A, et al. Dementia prevention, intervention, and care: 2020 report of the Lancet Commission. *The Lancet.* 2020;396:413–446.

McKhann GM, Knopman DS, Chertkow H, et al. The diagnosis of dementia due to Alzheimer's disease: recommendations from the National Institute on Aging-Alzheimer's Association workgroups on diagnostic guidelines for Alzheimer's disease. *Alzheimers Dement.* 2011;7(3):263–269.

Norton S, Matthews FE, Barnes DE, Yaffe K, Brayne C. Potential for primary prevention of Alzheimer's disease: an analysis of population-based data. *Lancet Neurol.* 2014;13(8):788–794.

Sachdev PS, Blacker D, Blazer DG, et al. Classifying neurocognitive disorders: the DSM-5 approach. *Nat Rev Neurol.* 2014;10(11):634–642.

Sperling RA, Aisen PS, Beckett LA, et al. Toward defining the preclinical stages of Alzheimer's disease: recommendations from the National Institute on Aging-Alzheimer's Association workgroups on diagnostic guidelines for Alzheimer's disease. *Alzheimers Dement.* 2011;7(3):280–292.

US Department of Health and Human Services National Alzheimer's Project Act. http://aspe.hhs.gov/national-alzheimers-project-act. Accessed September 10, 2015.

US Food and Drug Administration Postmarket Drug Safety Information for Patients and Providers: Aducanumab (marketed as Aduhelm) Information. https://www.fda.gov/drugs/postmarket-drug-safety-information-patients-and-providers/aducanumab-marketed-aduhelm-information

Zetterberg H, Bendlin BB. Biomarkers for Alzheimer's disease—preparing for a new era of disease-modifying therapies. *Molecular Psychiatry*. 2021;26:296–308.

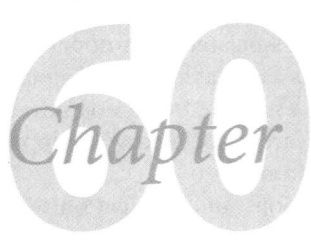

Chapter 60

Behavioral Symptoms of Dementia and Psychoactive Drug Therapy

Carol K. Chan, Constantine G. Lyketsos

EPIDEMIOLOGY

It is estimated that 5.3 million Americans live with Alzheimer disease (AD), the most common cause of dementia, and that 13.8 million people older than 65 years will be diagnosed in the United States by 2050. In the United States, annual health care costs for persons with AD are more than $172 billion, including $123 billion in costs to Medicaid and Medicare alone.

Neuropsychiatric symptoms (NPS) affect almost all persons with dementia over the course of illness. Although cognitive deficits are the hallmark of dementia, almost 98% of patients with AD experience depression, agitation, anxiety, psychosis, hallucinations, apathy, eating disorders, disinhibition, and/or sleep disturbances. Depression, apathy, and anxiety are the most common NPS in dementia. NPS are also present in the prodromal or mild cognitive impairment (MCI) stages of dementia. Depression and irritability are common even prior to the onset of MCI and dementia and appear to be the first symptoms of well over half of people who later develop dementia. Late-life onset of NPS of any severity in individuals without dementia, lasting for over 6 months, that are not attributable to another concurrent psychiatric disorder (such as major depressive disorder) are now referred to as mild behavioral impairment (MBI). While NPS are seen at all stages of dementia, including prior to cognitive decline, the severity of NPS increases with progressive cognitive decline both in community and nursing home populations.

The impacts of NPS on both patients and caregivers are significant: They are associated with worse quality of life, increased mortality, accelerated disease progression, and increased cost of care and caregiver burden/stress. Difficult behaviors and psychotic symptoms are among the highest determinants of institutionalization.

NPS are broadly categorized into four groups: (1) affective and motivational symptoms, such as depression; (2) psychotic symptoms, such as delusions or perceptual disturbances; (3) disturbances of basic drives, including feeding and sleeping; and (4) disinhibited and other socially inappropriate behaviors. Examples of symptoms in each category of NPS are in **Table 60-1**.

LEARNING OBJECTIVES

■ Learn the presentation, epidemiology, and pathophysiology of common neuropsychiatric symptoms (NPS), including behavioral disturbances, seen in patients with dementia.

■ Understand the best approach to evaluate NPS in patients with dementia and effective strategies to manage such symptoms.

■ Learn about the significance and efficacy of nonpharmacologic interventions.

■ Understand the appropriate indications, limitations, and adverse effects of pharmacologic interventions.

Key Clinical Points

1. NPS are seen in up to 98% of patients with dementia and are the result of high-order loss of behavioral control due to disease involvement of major brain networks and neurotransmitters.

2. Patients with NPS have higher mortality and progress more rapidly from mild to severe dementia.

3. Careful history-taking is essential and exclusion of delirium is paramount for proper diagnosis and management of NPS associated with dementia.

4. Onset of new NPS in patients with dementia, especially systematized delusions, can be mistaken for another psychiatric disorder, such as a major depressive disorder with psychotic features or schizophrenia.

5. Nonpharmacologic interventions should be the first-line treatment and antipsychotics should be avoided as much as possible, given their lack of efficacy in randomized trials and higher incidence of adverse treatment effects.

(Continued)

6. Appropriate indications for medications include failure of nonpharmacologic therapies and presence of NPS severe enough to interfere with the patient's overall quality of life and function.

7. If medications are started, use slow titration, use the lowest effective dose, and reassess its risk/benefit ratio on a regular basis.

PATHOPHYSIOLOGY OF NEUROPSYCHIATRIC SYMPTOMS

The underlying cause of NPS is multifactorial. Causal contributors include a combination of underlying brain circuitry disruptions, preexisting risk factors, and precipitating stressors. Disruptions in white matter and its associated cortices in sensory and limbic brain areas are thought to be involved in NPS in the context of dementia. In particular, disruptions to the corticocortical and frontal-subcortical circuits, key to regulating emotions and behaviors, have been implicated in the pathogenesis of NPS. AD pathologies, such as neuronal loss and neurofibrillary tangles, are abundant in the limbic system, which include the amygdala, basal forebrain, brainstem, and hypothalamus. The hypothalamus, among other things, is important for the regulation of appetite, circadian rhythms, and regulating emotional responses. Though these areas have been implicated in NPS, the degree to which pathologic involvement of these structures correlate with specific NPS has not been well studied.

Dysfunction in the projections of excitatory and inhibitory neurons from the brain stem to cortical regions modulating monoamines (dopamine, serotonin, and norepinephrine), glutamate, and acetylcholine, may also contribute to NPS. For instance, agitation and aggression have been associated with cortical dysfunction in the insula, amygdala, anterior cingulate gyrus, hippocampus, middle frontal gyrus, lateral frontal gyrus, and lateral temporal gyrus; these behaviors may be related to deficits in acetylcholine neurotransmission. Similarly, prominent aggressive behavior in patients with AD has been associated with loss of serotonin in the inferior frontal cortex. Psychosis is most prominently associated with functional deficits in the anterior cingulate cortex and frontal cortex, both of which receive dopaminergic innervation. Depressive symptoms have been related in part to disturbances in serotonin, norepinephrine, and dopamine, and have been associated with loss of serotonergic receptors in the hippocampus, noradrenergic neurons in the locus coeruleus, and serotonergic neurons in the raphe nucleus. The resulting imbalances of dopamine, noradrenaline, and serotonin neurotransmitters lead to NPS. Apathy is associated with dopamine and noradrenaline; depression is associated with serotonin and noradrenaline, psychosis is associated with dopamine, while agitation and aggression are associated with dopamine, noradrenaline, and serotonin.

These neurological disruptions, in combination with other underlying risk factors (such as personality factors, resilience, and psychiatric comorbidities), increase an individual's vulnerability to stressors or "triggers." Categories of stressors include patient factors (eg, physical discomfort, unmet needs, medical illness), environmental changes (eg, overstimulation or understimulation), and interpersonal stressors (eg, unrealistic caregiver expectations, negative communications). Thus, responses to these stressors in individuals with disruptions in brain circuitry due dementia may manifest as NPS.

DIAGNOSTIC APPROACH

History Taking

Due to the nature of cognitive impairment, a patient with dementia may not be able to provide an accurate history because of lack of insight, memory loss, and/or language problems. It is therefore critical to involve a reliable and knowledgeable informant during history taking. This helps elucidate a clear timeline of symptoms—whether the onset was insidious versus abrupt, the frequency if symptoms are episodic, and whether there have been precipitating events. Common stressors or "triggers" associated with NPS are in **Table 60-2** and should be considered during the history taking process. The severity of symptoms and associated distress (of both the patient and their caregiver) should be assessed. A thorough psychiatric and medical history is essential in considering differential diagnoses, which is discussed in greater detail below. An important part of history taking is asking caregivers how the behaviors are currently being managed and how the patient is responding to these interventions. Lastly, a careful history of physical symptoms should also be taken to determine whether medical causes and delirium may be contributing to the behavioral disturbance.

Physical Examination

Physical and neurological examination should be completed as part of the assessment to identify factors that may contribute to or worsen NPS, such as physical discomfort or delirium. Physical findings such as signs of infection, shortness of breath, pain, fluid overload or new neurological deficits may point to delirium due to an acute medical condition.

Clinical Measurements

The Neuropsychiatric Inventory (NPI) and its variations can be a useful tool in quantifying NPS. The NPI is the most widely used instrument for measuring NPS

TABLE 60-1 ■ NEUROPSYCHIATRIC SYMPTOMS

DOMAIN	EXAMPLES OF SYMPTOMS
Depression/dysphoria	Low mood Tearfulness Changes in sleep, appetite, energy Negative thoughts about him/herself (eg, putting him/herself down, feeling like a failure, feeling like he/she deserves to be punished, feeling like the family would be better off without him/her)
Anxiety	Frequently asking for reassurance Easily becoming upset when separated from caregiver Worry about planned events Periods of feeling shaky, unable to relax, feeling excessively tense Avoidance of certain places or situations that cause nervousness
Apathy/indifference	Indifference Disinterest in activities Poor motivation Less spontaneous (eg, less likely to initiate conversation)
Irritability/lability	Easily upset or frustrated Rapid changes in mood (eg, sudden flashes of anger over small things) Impatience (eg, having difficulty coping with small delays)
Agitation/aggression	Arguing Pacing Disruptive vocalizations Physical aggression (eg, throwing things, attempting to hit others) Rejection of care (eg, bathing, changing clothes) Repetitive questions
Disinhibition	Making socially inappropriate comments Talking openly about very personal or private matters Overfamiliarity with strangers Impulsive behaviors Overeating Overspending
Nighttime behaviors	Difficulty falling asleep Early awakening Excessive nighttime awakening (more than getting up once or twice to use the bathroom and falling back asleep immediately) Excessive napping during the day
Appetite/eating	Weight changes Loss of appetite or increase in appetite Change in types of food he/she likes (eg, eating too many sweets)
Motor disturbance	Wandering Rummaging Pacing Doing things repeatedly (eg, picking at things) Excessive fidgetting
Hallucinations	Hallucinations can occur in any sensory modality, but visual and auditory hallucinations (ie, seeing or hearing things that are not present) are most common
Delusions	False beliefs (eg, that others are stealing from him/her or planning to harm him/her, that their spouse is having an affair, that family members plan on abandoning them)
Elation/euphoria	Appearing excessively happy Laughing inappropriately Childish sense of humor Inflated sense of self (eg, claiming to have more abilities or wealth than is true)

TABLE 60-2 ■ COMMON CONTRIBUTING CAUSES OF NEUROPSYCHIATRIC SYMPTOMS

- A biological stress or delirium due to a recurrent or new medical condition
- A psychiatric syndrome that is either recurrent or associated with the dementia
- Reaction to cognitive disturbance (eg, reaction due to inability to express oneself)
- An environmental stressor (eg, excessive stimulation, unfamiliar surroundings)
- Unmet needs (eg, hunger, thirst, pain, constipation)
- Sensory deficit (eg, unable to see or hear properly without the use of eyeglasses or hearing aids)
- Unsophisticated caregiving (eg, poor communication, rushing patient)
- Medication side effects

in clinical research. It includes questions pertaining to changes in the patient's behavior with screening for the presence of NPS, in addition to ratings of their frequency and severity. The Neuropsychiatric Inventory-Questionnaire (NPI-Q) is a brief version suitable for use in clinical settings. It is a self-administered informant-based instrument that measures the presence and severity of 12 NPS, as well as informant distress. The Neuropsychiatric Inventory-Clinician Rating (NPI-C) is a clinician version that includes expanded domains and items.

Medication Review

A careful review of medications, including the time course of symptoms in relation to recent medication changes, is needed. Certain classes and combinations of medications may contribute to NPS. Classes of medications most likely to be associated with delirium, largely due to anticholinergic effects, include opiates, anticholinergics, benzodiazepines, antihistamines, tricyclic antidepressants (TCAs), muscle relaxants, and antiepileptic medications. Common examples of anticholinergic medications are in **Table 60-3**. Behavioral changes associated with these medications may include sedation, changes in sleep-wake cycle, and worse confusion or agitation. Medications used to treat Parkinson disease, such as dopaminergic agents, can precipitate impulsive behaviors. Anticholinergics, amantadine, dopaminergic agents, and catechol-O-methyl transferase (COMT) inhibitors, often used in Parkinson disease, can exacerbate psychotic symptoms, such as hallucinations and delusions.

Diagnostic Testing

For acute, new-onset NPS in dementia, work-up with a physical examination and laboratory studies is needed in many cases to evaluate for an underlying general medical cause. Laboratory testing typically consists of complete blood count, metabolic panel, liver function tests, and urinalysis/urine culture. Thyroid function tests, folate,

TABLE 60-3 ■ MEDICATIONS WITH ANTICHOLINERGIC ACTIVITY, WHICH HAVE INCREASED RISK OF CAUSING DELIRIUM

Amantadine (Symadine)
Benztropine (Cogentin)
Cyproheptadine (Periactin)
Digoxin (Lanoxin)
Diphenhydramine (Benadryl)
Dipyridamole (Persantine)
Doxylamine (Aldex, Doxytex, Nitetime Sleep-Aid, Sleep Aid, Unisom)
Furosemide (Lasix)
Hydroxyzine (Vistaril, Atarax)
Low-potency antipsychotics
Meclizine (Dramamine)
Metoclopramide (Reglan)
Oxybutynin (Ditropan)
Prochlorperazine (Compazine)
Promethazine (Phenergan)
Ranitidine (Zantac)
Scopolamine (Transderm-V)
Theophylline (Aerolate)
Tricyclic antidepressants

vitamin B_{12}, levels, toxicology, and electrocardiogram may be considered as additional tests if indicated based on history and physical examination. If there are signs and symptoms of a respiratory infection, chest radiography is indicated. Brain imaging, such as computed tomography (CT) or magnetic resonance imaging (MRI) may be indicated particularly if focal neurologic findings are present. Electroencephalogram (EEG) is indicated if seizures are suspected. Cerebrospinal fluid analysis is rarely needed but indicated if meningitis or encephalitis is suspected.

DIFFERENTIAL DIAGNOSIS

Differential diagnosis for NPS includes: medical conditions, delirium and primary psychiatric disorders such as major depression, bipolar disorder schizophrenia, etc. Presentation with acute changes in cognition and behavior should raise suspicion for delirium, and the underlying medical cause for delirium should be investigated accordingly.

In formulating a differential diagnosis, one should keep in mind that there may be more than one cause. Older individuals with primary psychiatric disorders such as major depressive disorder, bipolar disorder, anxiety disorders, and schizophrenia can develop dementia or delirium superimposed on their psychiatric illnesses. There are also late-onset forms of these disorders. Late-onset depression and anxiety are common among older adults (and among individuals with dementia), while late-onset bipolar disorder and schizophrenia are rare. However, if new psychiatric symptoms emerge in the setting of dementia, the underlying etiology is likely dementia as opposed to a separate, concurrent psychiatric disorder.

Delirium

If a patient exhibits a sudden drop or fluctuation of cognition, delirium should be considered in the differential diagnosis. Delirium is characterized by acute onset over hours or days with a fluctuating course. Cognitive deficits in delirium typically include inattention, disorganized thinking, or an altered level of consciousness. Delirium has a wide range of presentations, including hyperactive (eg, psychosis and agitation), hypoactive (eg, severe apathy, lethargy, and withdrawal), and mixed presentations where features of both hyperactive and hypoactive delirium are present. It is a syndrome with multiple potential etiologies. Providers should rule out delirium first in the setting of any acute change in cognition and/or consciousness, and assess for potential etiologies such as medication withdrawal, metabolic imbalance, infection, and intoxication.

Once the underlying cause is corrected, a patients' mental status and behavior should improve, though it commonly persists well beyond correction of the underlying cause—in some cases weeks to months. Some patients take a "cognitive hit" and may not fully return to their prior baseline. Short-term, low-dose use of oral or intravenous haloperidol or atypical antipsychotics can be considered for management of significant agitation in the context of delirium. Commonly used medications and starting doses include the following:

- Haloperidol (0.25–0.5 mg oral or intravenous every 6 hours as needed for agitation)
- Quetiapine (12.5–25 mg oral every 6 hours as needed for agitation)
- Olanzapine (2.5 mg oral or 1.25–2.5 mg intramuscular every 6 hours as needed for agitation)
- Risperidone (0.25–0.5 mg oral or intravenous every 6 hours as needed for agitation)

Depressive Symptoms

Major depressive disorder is a heterogeneous syndrome with a wide severity range. Symptoms include sleep disturbance, reduced energy, anhedonia, guilt, and suicidal ideation. It may include psychotic symptoms such as delusions and hallucinations. In individuals with dementia who experience new symptoms of depression, it can generally be presumed that the depressive symptoms are due to underlying neurodegeneration. Depressive symptoms of poor concentration, memory deficits, and anhedonia may be confused for cognitive deficits and apathy that are common to dementia.

Up to 50% of individuals with dementia will suffer from depression over the course of their illness, and it is one of the most common psychiatric symptoms in early dementia. Depression in dementia is associated with increased health care utilization, greater severity and acceleration of cognitive impairment, decreased quality of life for the affected individual and caregiver, and increased risk of suicide.

Among individuals with AD, risk factors for depression include older age, female gender, personal history of depression, and less education. Depression in individuals with dementia may go undetected because the symptoms they experience as part of a major depressive disorder can differ considerably from older individuals with normal cognition. For example, depression in dementia is more likely to present with agitation, irritability, and anxiety. Validated scales such as the Cornell Scale for Depression in Dementia and Geriatric Depression Scale (GDS) may be helpful as measures of depression.

Anxiety Symptoms

Symptoms of anxiety are relatively common in older adults and may be accompanied by agitation. They are often associated with comorbid depression and tend to go unrecognized. Similar to depression in dementia, new anxiety syndromes observed in dementia are most likely related to the underlying dementia as opposed to a separate anxiety disorder. The most common anxiety syndromes include generalized anxiety disorder, panic disorder, and phobias. Patients with posttraumatic stress disorder may become agitated when reexperiencing traumatic and painful memories ("flashbacks"). These episodes may become difficult for patients with dementia to distinguish from reality due to cognitive impairment (eg, short-term memory loss and disorientation) and because remote memory tends to be preserved until late in the course of many dementias. Clinicians should routinely inquire about a history of trauma when evaluating patients with dementia who are agitated.

Psychotic Symptoms

Psychotic symptoms, such as delusions and hallucinations, occur in 20% to 30% of patients with AD and in over 50% of patients with dementia with Lewy bodies (DLB) or Parkinson disease dementia. They may cause distress for the patient (and caregiver), and often contribute to the development of agitation.

Delusions are more common than hallucinations in dementia and can stem from cognitive impairment. For example, memory deficits may lead to the fixed and false belief that a misplaced item was stolen. Individuals with agnosia may misidentify formerly familiar individuals or objects. Less common delusions include delusions that they are being poisoned or that their partner has been unfaithful.

In AD, hallucinations are more likely to be visual than auditory, and tend to occur in the moderate to severe stages of dementia. In many circumstances, auditory hallucinations do not cause distress to the patient and as such, do not need to be treated pharmacologically. Visual hallucinations are more common in DLB than AD and may be the most clinically useful feature to distinguish DLB from AD. In DLB, hallucinations tend to be well-formed images of people, animals, or objects, but can also appear as simple shapes in the corner of one's eyes. Hallucinations are typically not distressing in DLB unless they are accompanied by delusions or occur in severely demented individuals.

Of note, many medications used to treat Parkinson disease, such as anticholinergic agents, amantadine, dopaminergic agents, and COMT inhibitors, can exacerbate visual hallucinations and delusions.

GENERAL MANAGEMENT

Dementia Care Models

The "DICE" (Describe, Investigate, Create, and Evaluate) approach (**Table 60-4**) provides a useful mnemonic for a methodic approach to the management of NPS.

TABLE 60-4 ■ DESCRIBE, INVESTIGATE, CREATE, AND EVALUATE (DICE) APPROACH

Describe	Caregiver describes problematic behavior
	Context of behavior
	Social and physical environment
	Patient perspective
	Degree of distress to patient and caregiver
Investigate	Provider investigates possible causes of problem behavior
	Undiagnosed medical conditions
	Underlying psychiatric comorbidity
	Limitations in functional ability
	Poor sleep hygiene
	Boredom, fear, sense of loss of control
	Medication side effects
	Sensory impairment
	Environmental factors
	Unmet needs
Create	Provider, caregiver, and team collaborate to create and implement treatment plan
	Respond to medical problems
	Strategize behavioral interventions
	Provide caregiver education and support
	Create meaningful activities for the patient
	Simplifying tasks
	Ensuring the environment is safe
	Enhancing communication with the patient
	Increasing or decreasing stimulation in the environment
Evaluate	Provider evaluates whether the interventions have been implemented by caregiver and whether they are effective

Data from Kales HC, Gitlin LN, Lyketsos CG, et al. Management of neuropsychiatric symptoms of dementia in clinical settings: recommendations from a multidisciplinary expert panel. J Am Geriatr Soc. 2014;62(4):762–769.

The "describe" phase involves characterization of the NPS, enabling the provider to identify underlying patterns or contributory factors to the behavior and establish treatment goals. In the "investigate" phase, the provider examines the patient and identifies potential underlying and modifiable causes. Behavioral disturbances are often multifactorial. As described in the previous section, common contributing factors may include delirium, pain, undiagnosed medical conditions (eg, dehydration, infection, constipation), medication side effects, underlying psychiatric comorbidity, sensory impairment, and environmental factors. In the "create" phase, the patient, caregiver, and treatment team collaborates to design and implement a treatment plan. This may involve both pharmacologic and nonpharmacologic interventions. The final step of the "DICE" approach is for the provider to "evaluate" whether recommended strategies were attempted and effective. If the caregiver did not implement the intervention, the provider should attempt to understand the barriers and brainstorm solutions with the caregiver. If interventions include a psychotropic medication, the provider and caregiver should monitor for changes in behaviors and potential side effects and evaluate the need for continued medication use on an ongoing basis.

Support for Patients and Caregivers

The Alzheimer's Association estimates that 60% to 70% of older adults with AD and other dementias live in the community and are cared for by family and friends. Nearly all have unmet needs regarding care, services, and support. The Maximizing Independence at Home (MIND at Home) Study found that 99% of patients had unmet needs. The most common domains with unmet needs included: safety (personal and home), general health and medical care, meaningful activities, legal issues, and advanced care planning. Higher unmet needs were reported in individuals who were minorities, had lower income, had fewer impairments in activities of daily living (ADLs), and more symptoms of depression. Caregivers, too, reported unmet needs. Ninety-seven percent reported having one or more unmet needs, with the most common domains being resource referrals, caregiver dementia education, mental health care, and general medical health care.

These findings highlight some of the areas that a dementia care team should address for every patient (**Table 60-5**). The care team should work with the patient and caregiver to maintain the patient's optimal physical and mental health, provide a safe environment that maximizes the patient's physical and cognitive abilities, and preserve the patient's dignity. Ideally, such an environment would allow patients to receive support for their ADLs and instrumental activities of daily living (IADLs), be well-nourished, maintain good sleep hygiene, and engage in activities and socialization. In-home activities tailored to the interests and capabilities of patients with dementia have been demonstrated to significantly increase the patient's engagement, reduce NPS, and reduce caregiver

TABLE 60-5 ■ SUPPORTIVE CARE FOR THE PATIENT WITH DEMENTIA

- Carefully evaluate the patient's dementia-related needs.
- Provide education about the diagnosis and trajectory of dementia to the patient (if appropriate) and caregiver.
- Manage medical comorbidities: Encourage routine follow-up with primary care, dental, vision, and hearing specialists. Assist with medical decision making.
- Address safety needs, particularly regarding falls, wandering, driving, ability to live alone, environmental hazards (eg, access to weapons, removing items patients may stumble upon), and medication management. Consider obtaining a home safety evaluation and driving evaluation. Encourage the use of monitoring devices.
- Provide comfort and emotional support.
- Provide meaningful activities, stimulation, and socialization. This may be achieved through adult day care, senior centers, and in-home activities.
- Maintain and document wishes for end-of-life care and distribution of finances after death. These should be addressed while individuals still have decision-making capacity.
- Provide quality nursing care in advanced stages.

burden. In-home occupational therapy assessments, using a functional assessment method such as the Assessment of Motor and Process Skills (AMPS), can provide useful data about a patient's care needs as well as assess the safety of the home environment. For more information about providing supportive care for patients, we refer you to the book *The 36-Hour Day* by Mace and Rabins (2017) and the Alzheimer's Association website (www.alz.org).

For caregivers, providing education about the disease and skills training in communication for dementia can significantly improve the quality of life for patients and increase positive interactions. A recent meta-analysis examining different caregiver interventions found that the most beneficial interventions address caregiving competency initially, then gradually addressing the care needs of the patient. In the United States, about 25% of people with dementia receive care from nonfamily caregivers, such as home health aids or nursing assistants hired directly by the family to care for a patient in the home setting. These caregivers may not always receive the necessary training to provide dementia care and face a challenging work environment. For nonfamily caregivers, interventions focused on facility staff training programs have been associated with reduction of NPS in patients and staff wellbeing. Some caregivers may benefit from encouragement to attend to their own emotional and personal needs. They should be encouraged to maintain their own medical appointments, hobbies, and social network. Utilization of respite from caregiving as needed, which can provide temporary relief for caregivers through provision of substitute care, should also be encouraged. Support groups can provide caregivers with the opportunity to share concerns, personal feelings, and seek support from peers. Psychological interventions, such as counseling and supportive therapy, have also been associated with positive impacts on psychosocial outcomes between patients and their informal caregivers.

NONPHARMACOLOGIC MANAGEMENT

Nonpharmacologic interventions are first-line in the management of NPS in dementia patients to avoid the risks and side effects associated with medications. An exception is emergency situations in which the safety of the patient or others is compromised, for example due to severe agitation.

Multiple small studies report modest improvement in quality of life and NPS with reminiscence therapy, music therapy, bright light therapy, aromatherapy, pet therapy, physical therapy, occupational therapy, exercise training, speech therapy, and multisensory stimulation. However, most studies of nonpharmacologic interventions included patients with mild to moderate NPS and few controlled data suggest that these nonpharmacologic interventions provide longer-term benefits, outside of the treatment session. Psychotherapy can be useful, particularly for patients in the early stages of dementia who are demoralized, depressed, or anxious.

Nonpharmacologic interventions that can be implemented by caregivers for common NPS are summarized in **Table 60-6**. Unfortunately, some of these can be difficult to implement in real-world settings or may not provide sufficient control of disruptive NPS. There is preliminary evidence that family caregiver interventions, such as promoting helpful coping, effective communication and scheduling of pleasant activities, and tailored activities for persons with dementia and their caregivers may improve quality of life in people with dementia living in the community.

PHARMACOLOGIC MANAGEMENT

Some patients who do not respond to nonpharmacologic approaches may require targeted medication therapy. It should be noted that while psychotropics are frequently prescribed for NPS in dementia, there are currently no pharmacotherapies with US Food and Drug Administration (FDA) approval for this purpose. Several classes of "psychiatric" medications have been studied specifically for NPS in dementia, but treatment response has been disappointing, with few randomized clinical trials (RCTs) showing clear efficacy of antipsychotics, antidepressants, or anticonvulsants. Risks and benefits of each class of medication are discussed in detail below.

Due to the inherent risks of using medications to treat NPS in dementia, nonpharmacologic approaches should be first-line therapy. Psychotropics should be used only after other efforts have been made to mitigate NPS, with three exceptions: (1) clear-cut major depression; (2) psychosis causing harm or with significant potential of harm to self or others; and (3) aggression causing harm or risk of harm to self or other.

TABLE 60-6 ■ GENERAL BEHAVIORAL STRATEGIES FOR COMMON NEUROPSYCHIATRIC SYMPTOMS

BEHAVIORS/SYMPTOMS	KEY STRATEGIES
Disorientation or confusion with person/object recognition	Provide reminders, cues, or prompts Identify individuals if patient does not remember names or has aphasia Use environmental cues (eg, calendars, keeping blinds raised during the day, keeping lights off at night) Keep objects for individual tasks in separate, labeled containers Use simple visual reminders (eg, pictures, arrows pointing to the bathroom)
Confusion/overwhelmed with tasks and environment	Eliminate noise and distractions while patient is engaged in an activity Break each task into very simple steps Offer simple choices (no more than two at a time) Provide simple verbal commands, using only one or two steps at a time Remove unnecessary items from the room while patients is engaged in a task Provide daily, structured, and predictable routines
Wandering or inability to respond appropriately to an emergency	Provide 24-hour supervision for the patient Place locks on all exits Develop an emergency plan. Inform neighbors, fire department, and police of the patient's condition Provide patient with medical alert and safe return ID bracelets
Nighttime wakefulness	Encourage good sleep hygiene (avoid stimulating activity, reduce caffeinated and alcoholic beverages that may affect sleep, limit daytime napping) Create a quiet routine for bedtime Evaluate environment for modifiable elements, such as temperature, noise level, light, shadows, and bed comfort
Anxiety, irritability, repetitive questioning, frustration	Use a relaxed and reassuring voice and light touch to help calm or redirect Avoid negative words and tone Allow patient sufficient time to respond to questions Help patient with aphasia find the words to express him/herself Allow extra time for tasks and activities Distract the patient as necessary Understand that behaviors are not always intentional
Boredom and restlessness	Create a structured, daily schedule that includes entertainment and exercise Provide meaningful activities that draw on preserved capabilities and interests Engage patients in activities involving repetitive motion (eg, folding towels, putting items in containers)
Delusions and hallucinations	Go along with patient's point of view of what is true. Avoid arguing or trying to reason as this can make the situation worse Ignore symptoms that are not distressing the person Distract the patient as necessary
Apathy	Give the patient a job at home, such as folding laundry Focus on the process of doing things rather than the results
Disinhibition	Distract from an inappropriate topic by calmly and firmly changing the subject Avoid television shows with violence or sexual content

Clinicians should obtain informed consent for medication use from the patient or their legal representatives after discussing potential risks (including so-called "black box warnings" of mortality in the case of antipsychotics) and benefits. Medications should be slowly titrated using starting doses appropriate for older individuals. Although a slow titration schedule is recommended for older adults, medications should still be increased as tolerated to produce an improvement in target symptoms. Behavior logs kept by the caregiver, documenting the timing and pattern of behaviors, may help identify optimal times for medication administration (eg, timing doses of medication to target difficult behaviors such as prior to bathing or dressing).

Clinicians should pay close attention to side effects and educate the caregiver about what to look out for. It is important to keep in mind that older individuals are at higher risk of adverse effects to medications due to (1) decreased renal clearance and slowed hepatic metabolism, (2) medical comorbidities, (3) potential for drug–drug interactions due to being on multiple medications, (4) increased risk of orthostatic hypotension and falls due to decreased autonomic regulation, and (5) elevated risk of delirium. The American Geriatrics Society Beers Criteria for Potentially Inappropriate Medication Use in Older Adults provides an overview of medications and guidelines on when they should potentially be avoided older adults.

In prescribing psychotropic medications for NPS, clinicians should keep potential pitfalls in mind. Though there are no FDA-approved medications for NPS in dementia, clinicians routinely prescribe psychotropics despite safety and efficacy concerns. In a study of newly admitted nursing home residents, only 12% received nonpharmacologic interventions within the first 3 months of admission, while 71% received at least one psychotropic medication. Moreover, more than 15% were taking four or more psychotropics. 64% and 71% of residents treated with psychotropics had not received psychopharmacologic treatment or a psychiatric diagnosis, respectively, for the 6 months preceding admission. Medications are widely used empirically based on similarities to other psychiatric conditions, such as depression, anxiety, or psychosis. Furthermore, psychotropics may be used without systematic identification of potential underlying causes of behaviors. NPS in dementia are the result of responses to stressors in individuals with increased vulnerability due to brain circuitry disruptions. Nonpharmacologic strategies targeted at mitigating or eliminating these triggers should be used and evaluated for effect first. Most dementias are progressive in nature and NPS can fluctuate over time. Thus, clinicians and caregivers may find themselves trying to manage several evolving behaviors simultaneously, often with multiple medications, leading to increased risks of adverse effects from medications and unpredictable results. Further complicating this matter is that psychotropics can cause side effects that exacerbate other domains of NPS. For example, antipsychotic medications may contribute to sedation, reversal in sleep-wake cycle, and delirium. If medications are indicated, it is important to follow several guidelines as listed in **Table 60-7**.

Antipsychotics

Antipsychotics provide (at times considerable) benefit to some patients with psychosis and agitation in dementia but have been associated with higher risk of death, cardiovascular disease, and cerebrovascular disease in this population. The use of antipsychotics in patients with dementia remains controversial because their efficacy is modest and they have been associated with adverse effects, including weight gain, parkinsonism, rapid cognitive decline, a higher risk of cerebrovascular or cardiovascular events, QTc prolongation, and mortality. The DART-AD trial reported an increased long-term risk of mortality in patients with AD prescribed antipsychotics. As a result, the FDA issued a "black box warning" for the use of atypical and conventional antipsychotics in treating patients with dementia-related psychosis. Retrospective cohort studies evaluating all-cause mortality in older individuals have found higher mortality risk with haloperidol than with risperidone,

TABLE 60-7 ■ GENERAL GUIDELINES FOR STARTING PSYCHOTROPIC MEDICATIONS FOR NEUROPSYCHIATRIC SYMPTOMS

- Explore potential contributing factors for neuropsychiatric symptoms. Consider the need for a medical work-up.
- Define specific targets for intervention
- Implement nonpharmacologic interventions concomitantly
- Be mindful that isolated neuropsychiatric disturbances are unlikely to respond to medications
- Use medications sparingly, starting at a low dose, monitoring for adverse effects (particularly delirium, sedation, orthostasis, falls), and using the lowest effective dose
- Change one medication at a time to allow for a clearer picture of how it affects target symptoms and to minimize adverse effects
- Be aware of potential drug–drug interactions
- Consider timing doses around difficult behaviors (eg, administering a dose half an hour prior to morning care)
- Psychotropic use (particularly antipsychotics) should be time-limited, as symptoms may resolve
- Obtain informed consent prior to starting medications. Routinely review the risk–benefit ratio of treatment with patients and caregivers
- Have a plan in place to manage after-hours crisis

olanzapine, aripiprazole, ziprasidone, or quetiapine. The highest risk of mortality occurs soon after therapy is initiated, and there appears to be a dose-dependent relationship to mortality. Given these risks, the American Psychiatric Association (APA) has published practice guidelines on the use of antipsychotics to treat agitation or psychosis in patients with dementia, emphasizing judicious use and reserving antipsychotics for when nonpharmacologic approaches have been tried, and when symptoms are severe and dangerous. They also recommend that if there is no significant response after a 4-week period, the medication should be tapered and withdrawn. In patients whose antipsychotic medications are being tapered, symptoms should be assessed at least every month during tapering and for at least 4 months after the medication is discontinued. Long-acting injectable antipsychotics should not be used unless administered for a co-occurring chronic psychotic disorder.

If a risk/benefit assessment favors the use of an antipsychotic for NPS in patients with dementia, treatment should be initiated at a low dose and titrated to the minimum effective dose as tolerated. The choice of antipsychotic should be guided by the target symptoms, side-effect profile, and formulation (eg, consider using medications that have solution or dissolving forms). The recommended dosing in patients with dementia and side effects of atypical antipsychotics discussed in this section are summarized in **Table 60-8**.

The Clinical Antipsychotic Trial of International Effectiveness—Alzheimer's Disease (CATIE-AD) was

TABLE 60-8 ■ SELECT ANTIPSYCHOTIC DOSAGES AND SIDE EFFECTS

MEDICATION	FORMULATIONS[a]	RECOMMENDED DAILY DOSE FOR TREATING NPS IN DEMENTIA	SIDE EFFECTS[b]
Risperidone	Oral tablet Oral solution Oral disintegrating tablets	0.25–1 mg	Orthostatic hypotension, dose-dependent EPS, tardive dyskinesia, hyperprolactinemia, risk of cerebrovascular events, weight gain, moderate risk of diabetes mellitus and dyslipidemia, sedation, cognitive effects
Olanzapine	Tablet Disintegrating tablets IM	2.5–10 mg	Sedation, anticholinergic effects at higher doses, gait disturbance, orthostatic hypotension, high risk of weight gain, hyperglycemia, diabetes mellitus, risk of cerebrovascular events, dose-dependent EPS
Quetiapine	Tablet	12.5–150 mg	Sedation, orthostatic hypotension, moderate risk of weight gain, diabetes mellitus, and dyslipidemia, anticholinergic effects at higher doses
Aripiprazole	Oral tablet Oral solution Oral disintegrating tablets	5–10 mg	Sedation, nausea, lower risk of EPS, weight gain
Haloperidol	Oral tablet Oral solution IM IV	0.5–5	High risk of EPS, sedation, orthostatic hypotension, seizure
Clozapine	Oral tablet	6.25–75 mg	Excessive sedation, sialorrhea, seizure, anticholinergic effects, agranulocytosis, orthostatic hypotension, sustained tachycardia, weight gain, diabetes mellitus, dyslipidemia. Requires weekly blood draws to monitor for agranulocytosis in the first 6 months of treatment.
Pimavanserin	Oral tablet	34 mg	Confusion, peripheral edema, GI distress, hypotension, weight gain

[a]Only short-acting formulations are listed. Long-acting injectable formulations are available for some antipsychotics, but are not recommended for use of neuropsychiatric symptoms in dementia.
[b]All antipsychotics have a black-box warning for increased mortality in individuals with dementia and can cause QT prolongation.
EPS, extrapyramidal symptoms; IM, intramuscular injection; IV, intravenous.

designed to compare the efficacy of antipsychotics to placebo in reducing psychotic symptoms or behaviors of agitation/aggression in outpatients with AD. Olanzapine and risperidone showed the most benefit in NPS reduction. However, the magnitude of improvement was modest, and use of atypical antipsychotics over 36 weeks was associated with worsening cognitive function at a magnitude consistent with 1 year's cognitive deterioration on placebo, and there were no observable improvements in functional measures. Similarly, an Agency for Healthcare Research and Quality (AHRQ) Comparative Effectiveness Review found that the most effective antipsychotics include risperidone (for psychosis and agitation), olanzapine (for agitation), and aripiprazole (for overall NPS). A meta-analysis of studies examining antipsychotic discontinuation in patients with dementia found that although the proportion of patients with NPS severity worsening was higher than those who continued on antipsychotics, no statistically significant difference in NPS severity was observed.

Due to the elevated risk of extrapyramidal side effects, typical antipsychotics, such as haloperidol, should not be used as a first-line neuroleptic in nonemergent situations. Extrapyramidal symptoms (EPS) include parkinsonism,

tardive dyskinesia, akathisia, and dystonias. Particular care should be taken when considering the use of antipsychotics in patients with DLB and Parkinson disease, as they are extremely sensitive to extrapyramidal side effects, with the exception of clozapine. Extrapyramidal side effects can include parkinsonian symptoms, acute dystonia, and neuroleptic malignant syndrome. Due to its low risk for causing EPS, clozapine is a good option for psychotic symptoms in DLB. However, the potential for serious adverse effects, particularly neutropenia, and the need for close laboratory monitoring makes it more challenging to use in routine clinical practice. Pimavanserin was approved by the FDA in 2016 for treatment of hallucinations and delusions associated with Parkinson disease psychosis. Clozapine and quetiapine, though not specifically approved for use in Parkinson disease, are less likely than other antipsychotics to worsen parkinsonian symptoms.

Antidepressants

Aside from depression, antidepressants are also used to treat other NPS, including anxiety, agitation, and apathy. Up to 50% of community dwelling older adults with dementia in the United States are prescribed antidepressants. Although systematic reviews of the literature have found limited evidence to support the efficacy of antidepressants in the treatment of depression, anxiety, and apathy in dementia, there is emerging evidence for their use in agitation. A summary of dosing and side effects of antidepressants is in **Table 60-9**.

Selective serotonin reuptake inhibitors Selective serotonin reuptake inhibitors (SSRIs) act on the serotonergic system by blocking its presynaptic reuptake. They are considered first-line therapy for late-life depression and are generally well tolerated compared to other classes of antidepressants such as TCAs. In the context of dementia, however, systematic reviews and meta-analysis have found little or no difference between groups treated with SSRIs and placebo in depressive symptoms. Fluoxetine has not been associated

with improvements in NPS. Though initial findings for sertraline reported promising effects for depression, subsequent larger studies have not found evidence that sertraline is superior to placebo in the treatment of depression in dementia. There is growing evidence, though, for a role of SSRIs in the management of agitation in dementia. The Citalopram for Agitation in Alzheimer's Disease (CitAD) study, a randomized placebo-controlled trial, found that participants in the citalopram group had significant improvement in agitation, measures of caregiver stress, improved performance on ADLs, and reduced use of emergency medications for agitation (lorazepam) compared to placebo. However, citalopram was associated with side effects including QT prolongation and worsened cognition, which may limit its use. Further analysis found that cognitive and cardiac changes were primarily associated with

TABLE 60-9 ■ ANTIDEPRESSANT ORAL DOSAGES AND SIDE EFFECTS

	INITIAL DAILY DOSE (mg)	MAX DAILY DOSE (mg)	SIDE EFFECTS
SELECTIVE SEROTONIN REUPTAKE INHIBITORS			
Citalopram	5–10	20	GI distress, sexual dysfunction, slight weight gain, QTc prolongation at doses > 20 mg, hyponatremia, SIADH
Escitalopram	5	10	GI distress, sexual dysfunction, slight weight gain, hyponatremia, SIADH, insomnia, fatigue
Fluoxetine	10	80	GI distress, sexual dysfunction, slight weight gain, abnormal dreams, hyponatremia, SIADH, insomnia, fatigue
Sertraline	25	200	GI distress, sexual dysfunction, slight weight gain, hyponatremia, SIADH, headache
Paroxetine Paroxetine CR	10 12.5	40 50	Anticholinergic effects may increase risk of delirium, may cause withdrawal effects due to short half life, GI distress, hyponatremia, SIADH
SEROTONIN NOREPINEPHRINE REUPTAKE INHIBITORS			
Duloxetine	30	120	GI distress, dry mouth, urinary hesitancy, headaches, fatigue, sedation, hyponatremia, hepatitis
Venlafaxine XR Venlafaxine IR	37.5 25–50	225 375	GI distress, minimal sedation, headaches, sexual dysfunction, weight loss, withdrawal symptoms, anxiety, dose-dependent hypertension, hyponatremia, mild anticholinergic effects
Desvenlafaxine	50	100	Dizziness, dry mouth, insomnia, decreased appetite, GI distress, dose-dependent hypertension, elevated cholesterol and triglycerides, hyponatremia
OTHER			
Mirtazapine	7.5	30–45	Dry mouth, GI distress, dizziness, QT prolongation, elevated cholesterol and triglycerides, weight gain, increased appetite, sedation
Bupropion XL Bupropion SR Bupropion IR	150 100 75	450 150 BID 150 TID	Mild anticholinergic effects, hypotension, high sedation, slight sexual dysfunction, serotonin syndrome, increased appetite, dry mouth
PREFERRED TRICYCLIC ANTIDEPRESSANTS			
Nortriptyline	10–25	75–150	Therapeutic window 50–150 ng/mL; anticholinergic effects, hypotension, sedation, sexual dysfunction, slight weight gain
Desipramine	10–25	50–150	Therapeutic window 150–300 ng/mL; mild anticholinergic effects, hypotension, slight GI distress, sedation, sexual dysfunction, slight weight gain

Maximum recommended dosage for patients greater than 60 years of age. BID, twice daily; CR, controlled release; GI distress, gastrointestinal distress (eg, nausea, vomiting, diarrhea, constipation); IR, immediate release; SIADH, syndrome of inappropriate secretion of antidiuretic hormone; TID, three times a day.

the R-enantiomer, whereas clinical improvements were primarily associated with the S-enantiomer, escitalopram. The effectiveness of escitalopram for agitation in AD is now being studied in the Escitalopram for agitation in Alzheimer's disease (S-CitAD) trial.

Though SSRIs are generally well tolerated, common side effects include nausea, diarrhea, anorexia, drowsiness, lethargy, sleep disturbance, tremor, and anxiety. These side effects usually improve after 1 to 2 weeks. Hyponatremia may occur with SSRI treatment and should be assessed particularly in older adults. Some SSRIs, such as paroxetine, have anticholinergic properties and should be avoided in older adults.

Serotonin norepinephrine reuptake inhibitors Serotonin norepinephrine reuptake inhibitors (SNRIs) include duloxetine, venlafaxine, and desvenlafaxine. While they are used in late-life depression, evidence for their efficacy in NPS in dementia is limited. A small 6-week randomized placebo-controlled trial of venlafaxine (14 in venlafaxine group, 17 placebo) did not find a significant difference in depressive symptoms between groups. A longer 12-week randomized double blind trial of 20 patients with moderate AD did not find any benefit in venlafaxine for symptoms of depression compared to baseline, though statistically significant change in cognitive and functioning scales were observed. Common side effects of SNRIs include gastrointestinal (GI) distress, headaches, sexual dysfunction, and hyponatremia.

Mirtazapine Mirtazapine is a nonadrenergic and specific serotonergic antidepressant. In the Health Technology Assessment Study of the Use of Antidepressants for Depression in Dementia (HTA-SADD) trial, there was no difference between mirtazapine and placebo, or mirtazapine and sertraline on depressive symptoms. Subsequent subgroup analysis found that mirtazapine reduced depressive symptoms over placebo in participants with primarily affective symptoms and severe endorsement of psychological symptoms, and an absence of sleep problems. A small, open-label study with 16 patients found a significant reduction of agitation. Mirtazapine can be sedating at lower doses and is sometimes used as a sleep aid. However, a more recent randomized placebo-controlled trial of mirtazapine in patients with dementia and sleep disturbances (24 in mirtazapine group vs 16 placebo) found no benefit over placebo in improving sleep duration of efficiency. The group receiving mirtazapine experienced increased daytime sleepiness, limiting its use.

Bupropion Bupropion is a dual inhibitor of norepinephrine and dopamine reuptake. Though it has been shown to be effective in depressed older adults, its use specifically for NPS has not been extensively studied. One RCT reported it was ineffective for the treatment of apathy in Huntington disease. Buproprion should be avoided in individuals with a history of seizures or psychotic symptoms.

Tricyclic antidepressants A number of older and smaller studies have investigated the use of TCAs in dementia. Two RCTs explored the effects of imipramine on depression in dementia reported no benefit over placebo. A RCT of clomipramine reported that participants receiving the treatment of significantly improved depressive symptoms on the Hamilton Depression Scale and rate of remission. A small RCT of desipramine in individuals with moderate AD found improvement in measures of function in the treatment group, but no differences in symptoms of depression. The use of TCAs is limited by their high risk of adverse events, relative to previously discussed classes of antidepressants.

Monoamine oxidase inhibitors The monoamine oxidase inhibitor (MAOI) moclobemide was found to be superior to placebo for depressive symptoms in one multisite, double-blinded, placebo-controlled trial of 649 older adults with symptoms of depression and cognitive decline. However, this antidepressant is not marketed in the United States. The use of MAOIs is limited by the required adherence to a low-tyramine diet and the risk of serotonin syndrome with concomitant use of other serotonergic antidepressants.

Anticonvulsants and "mood stabilizers" Many anticonvulsants are approved for used as so-called mood stabilizers in bipolar disorder. However, there is limited evidence for efficacy in treating NPS in dementia, with more evidence that their use can be harmful. Though initial case studies of valproic acid suggested possible efficacy for treatment of agitation in dementia, recent trials and a recent Cochrane meta-analysis suggested that valproate, when used solely for "organic brain disorders," is ineffective for treating agitation in people with dementia. Furthermore, valproic acid is poorly tolerated with numerous adverse effects such as sedation, diarrhea, ataxia, and thrombocytopenia.

Carbamezapine has been shown to improve NPS in one small (n=51), randomized trial in patients who were resistant to treatment with antipsychotics. Other trials have reported no benefit over placebo, but increased adverse effects including sedation, disorientation, confusion, and ataxia. Further limiting its use in older adults, carbamazepine is a potent hepatic enzyme inducer, with high potential for drug–drug interactions, is an auto-inducer (making its titration challenging), and is also associated with bone marrow toxicity and hyponatremia.

Studies examining the use of oxcarbazepine and topiramate for behavioral disturbances in dementia are limited. There has only been one randomized controlled study of oxcarbazepine in this context, where no difference was observed compared to placebo for aggression or agitation, while adverse events such as sedation, fainting, and ataxia occurred more frequently in the treatment group. No placebo-controlled trials involving topiramate for NPS in dementia have been conducted. One randomized study found it to have superior efficacy compared to risperidone.

The efficacy of gabapentin in treating NPS has been described in several case reports and open-label trials, including for treating behaviors of sexual inappropriateness.

However, despite its frequent off-label use, there are no current randomized controlled trials evaluating the use of gabapentin.

Case reports, retrospective chart reviews, and one open-label trial (which allowed for concomitant use of other psychotropic drugs) have reported modest clinical improvement in NPS using lamotrigine. No randomized-controlled trials have been conducted to date. The need for a slow titration schedule due to the risk of Stevens-Johnson syndrome may limit its use in the acute setting.

Lithium The use of lithium, an established treatment for bipolar and other mood disorders with symptoms of agitation, has been limited in dementia by its narrow therapeutic window, leading to adverse effects including toxicity, increased falls, and confusion in prior case reports and trials. There are currently no randomized controlled trials evaluating the use of lithium. However, the Lithium Treatment for Agitation in Alzheimer's disease (Lit-AD) clinical trial, which uses low-dose lithium, has recently completed recruitment. Though study results are not yet published, this study will serve as the first randomized, double-blind, placebo-controlled trial to assess the efficacy of lithium for symptoms of agitation and aggression, with or without psychosis, in older adults with AD.

Cholinesterase inhibitors and memantine Cholinesterase inhibitors (AChI), such as donepezil, galantamine, and rivastigmine, and memantine, a noncompetitive N-methyl-aspartate (NMDA) antagonist, are symptomatic therapies for cognitive symptoms in Alzheimer dementia. They are approved for treatment of mild to moderate AD, while memantine is approved for treatment of moderate to severe AD. Evidence for their efficacy in treating NPS is limited. Meta-analyses of randomized controlled trials have found that donepezil, galantamine, and memantine are superior to placebo in reducing emergence of NPS, though the effects are modest compared to that of neuroleptics. Combination therapy of AChI and memantine, which is sometimes used in moderate to severe AD, has been shown in meta-analysis to have superior outcomes in reducing NPS compared to monotherapy and placebo. In general, AChI and memantine should not be considered first-line pharmacologic agents in the management of acute NPS of moderate or greater severity. Given their potential benefit in delaying cognitive symptom progression and modest improvement of NPS, however, they remain reasonable options for treating chronic NPS in dementia.

Both AChI and memantine are generally well tolerated. Common side effects of AChIs include vomiting, diarrhea, dyspepsia, anorexia, eight loss, dyspepsia, headache, dizziness, insomnia, and vagotonic effects leading to bradycardia and heart block. Common side effects of memantine include dizziness, headache, confusion, constipation, and fatigue.

Stimulants Modafinil, a wakefulness-promoting medication, and methylphenidate, a stimulant, have both been evaluated as possible treatments for apathy associated with AD. Modafinil is FDA-approved to treat narcolepsy, shift work sleep disorder, and obstructive sleep apnea. One small randomized controlled trial in people with mild to moderate AD and clinically significant apathy at baseline did not observe statistically significant benefit over placebo for improving apathy or caregiver burden. Common side effects include headaches, nausea, diarrhea, anxiety, dyspepsia, and insomnia.

Methylphenidate is a dopamine reuptake inhibitor which is FDA-approved for treatment of attention deficit/hyperactivity disorder. Methylphenidate has been associated with significant reductions in apathy symptoms in AD in a 6-week and 12-week randomized, double-blind, placebo-controlled trial. Though generally well tolerated, side effects of methylphedniate include cardiovascular effects, insomnia, headaches, and decreased appetite. Psychiatric side effects may include increased impulsivity, hallucinations, and affect lability. As a result, methylphenidate and other stimulants should be avoided in individuals with a history of schizophrenia, bipolar disease, or impulse control disorders.

Benzodiazepines Benzodiazepines are used in 8.5% to 20% of patients with AD, despite limited evidence for their efficacy in reducing agitation or improving sleep quality. A systematic review reported few randomized-controlled trials comparing benzodiazepines to other medications in managing NPS in dementia, and that of the few that are available none have found evidence benzodiazepines are more effective in reducing NPS than antipsychotics. They should be avoided due to their cognitive and deliriogenic effects increasing the likelihood of falls and fractures. The exception is use in emergency situations in which severely agitated patients are at risk of harming themselves or others, or in situations where patients have not responded to alternative pharmacologic interventions. If used, benzodiazepines should be utilized sparingly, with short-acting preparations preferred as they do not accumulate with repeated dosing compared to long-acting. Many benzodiazepines are metabolized through the liver, and benzodiazepines metabolized through glucuronidation (eg, oxazepam, temazepam, or lorazepam) are preferable in individuals with complex medical comorbidities. They have no active metabolites and are less susceptible to drug–drug interactions.

Melatonin Circadian rhythm disturbances such as sleep disturbances and sundowning are common in dementia. Due to its role in maintaining the circadian rhythm, melatonin has been of interest as a pharmacologic therapy for NPS in dementia. A 2020 Cochrane review of pharmacotherapies for sleep disturbance in dementia reported five randomized controlled trials that examined the use of melatonin for sleep disturbances in dementia and found that there was low-certainty evidence that melatonin doses up to 10 mg may have little or no effect on sleep efficacy, time awake after sleep onset, number of nighttime awakenings, or mean duration of sleep. Of studies that have examined melatonin versus placebo in the context of agitation or sundowning behaviors, one RCT of 20 patients treated for 4 weeks with melatonin 3 mg reported benefits over placebo. One randomized controlled trial of ramelteon, a melatonin-receptor agonist, did not find any evidence of effect on sleep outcomes.

Newer medications Pimavanserin, an atypical antipsychotic with a novel mechanism of action as a selective inverse agonist at the serotonin receptor, was approved in 2016 by the US FDA for treatment of Parkinson disease psychosis. Although it has low risk of EPS due to its lack of dopamine blockade, it carries a similar side effect profile to other atypical antipsychotics, including QT prolongation and the black box warning for increased mortality in patients with dementia. There has been one phase 2, single-center study of nursing home residents using pimavanserin in the treatment of behavioral disturbances in AD. Participants treated with pimavanserin had reduced NPI scores at 6 weeks, but improvements were not sustained at 12 weeks compared to placebo.

Dextromethorphan-quinidine was approved by the US FDA in 2010 for the treatment of pseudobulbar affect. Dextromethorphan is a low-affinity, uncompetitive N-methyl-D-aspartate receptor antagonist, σ_1 receptor agonist, serotonin and norepinephrine reuptake inhibitor, and neuronal nicotinic $\alpha_3\beta_4$ receptor antagonist. Off-label use in AD for agitation has been examined in one phase 2 randomized, multicenter, double-blind, placebo-controlled study, which reported a significant reduction in symptoms, though significant adverse events were observed in the treatment group, including falls, diarrhea, and urinary tract infection.

Evidence for the effectiveness and safety of psychoactive cannabinoids, such as dronabinol and tetrahydrocannabinol (THC), has been varied. While some studies have reported significant improvements of NPS, two recent systematic reviews found a high risk of bias in studies with considerable variability with respect to study design, and that higher quality trials did not find evidence of improvement in NPS. Most adverse drug events reported were mild, and the most common adverse drug event was sedation. Further large, randomized controlled trials are needed.

CONCLUSION

NPS are common throughout the range of dementia severity. They can be disabling to the patient, onerous to the caregiver, and at times dangerous. The differential diagnosis of NPSs in dementia is wide, including underlying medical causes, delirium, medication effect, and primary psychiatric disorders. These differentials should be considered prior to implementing a treatment plan. A multidisciplinary dementia care team can be invaluable to delivering effective, personalized care to patients with dementia. Nonpharmacologic interventions should be considered first-line therapy, prior to implementing medications. Pharmacotherapy is appropriate when nonpharmacologic approaches have been unsuccessful, when symptoms are distressing or disruptive to the patient or caregiver, and in emergent situations. All psychotropic medications for behavioral symptoms are associated with adverse effects. Individuals with dementia and multiple medical comorbidities requiring many medications are at elevated risk of adverse effects and drug–drug interactions. When starting new medications, it is best to "start low and go slow," use the lowest possible dose, and frequently reassess the risk/benefit ratio of the medication.

FURTHER READING

2019 American Geriatrics Society Beers Criteria® Update Expert Panel, Fick DM, Semla TP, et al. American Geriatrics Society 2019 updated AGS Beers Criteria® for potentially inappropriate medication use in older adults. *J Am Geriatr Soc.* 2019;67(4):674–694.

Black BS, Johnston D, Rabins PV, et al. Unmet needs of community-residing persons with dementia and their informal caregivers: Findings from the maximizing independence at home study. *J Am Geriatr Soc.* 2013;61(12):2087–2095.

Canevelli M, Adali N, Voisin T, et al. Behavioral and psychological subsyndromes in Alzheimer's disease using the Neuropsychiatric Inventory. *Int J Geriatr Psychiatry.* 2013;28(8):795–803.

Cooper C, Mukadam N, Katona C, et al. Systematic review of the effectiveness of non-pharmacological interventions to improve quality of life of people with dementia. *Int Psychogeriatr.* 2012;24(6):856-870.

Gitlin LN, Kales HC, Lyketsos CG. Nonpharmacologic management of behavioral symptoms in dementia. *JAMA.* 2012;308(19):2020-2029.

Hane FT, Lee BY, Leonenko Z. Recent progress in Alzheimer's disease research, part 1: pathology. *J Alzheimers Dis.* 2017;57(1):1-28.

Hane FT, Robinson M, Lee BY, et al. Recent progress in Alzheimer's disease research, part 3: diagnosis and treatment. *J Alzheimers Dis.* 2017;57(3):645-665.

Kales HC, Gitlin LN, Lyketsos CG, Detroit Expert Panel on the Assessment and Management of the Neuropsychiatric Symptoms of Dementia. Management of neuropsychiatric symptoms of dementia in clinical settings: recommendations from a multidisciplinary expert panel. *J Am Geriatr Soc.* 2014;62(4): 762–769.

Lanctôt KL, Amatniek J, Ancoli-Israel S, et al. Neuropsychiatric signs and symptoms of Alzheimer's disease: new treatment paradigms. *Alzheimers Dement (N Y).* 2017; 3(3):440–449.

Mace NL, Rabins PV. *The 36-Hour Day: A Family Guide to Caring for People Who Have Alzheimer Disease, Other Dementias, and Memory Loss.* Baltimore, MD: JHU Press; 2017.

Porsteinsson AP, Drye LT, Pollock BG, et al. Effect of citalopram on agitation in Alzheimer disease: the CitAD randomized clinical trial. *JAMA.* 2014;19;311(7): 682–691.

Robinson M, Lee BY, Hane FT. Recent progress in Alzheimer's disease research, part 2: genetics and epidemiology. *J Alzheimers Dis.* 2017;57(2):317–330.

Schneider LS, Dagerman KS, Insel P. Risk of death with atypical antipsychotic drug treatment for dementia: meta-analysis of randomized placebo-controlled trials. *JAMA.* 2005;294:1934–1943.

Seitz DP, Gill SS, Herrmann N, et al. Pharmacological treatments for neuropsychiatric symptoms of dementia in long-term care: a systematic review. *Int Psychogeriatr.* 2013;25(2):185–203.

Sink KM, Holden KF, Yaffe K. Pharmacological treatment of neuropsychiatric symptoms of dementia: a review of the evidence. *JAMA.* 2005;293:596–608.

Chapter 61

Parkinson Disease and Related Disorders

Vikas Kotagal, Nicolaas I. Bohnen

DEFINITION AND TERMINOLOGY

Parkinsonism is the unifying term that describes a constellation of motor and nonmotor neurologic features. Parkinsonism can be defined as a variable combination of six specific, independent motor features: bradykinesia (slowness of movement), tremor at rest, rigidity, loss of postural reflexes, flexed posture, and freezing of gait (where the feet are transiently "glued" to the ground). Of these features, bradykinesia—either affecting the arms or legs ("appendicular bradykinesia") or midline structures including the trunk, head and neck, oropharynx, or eyes ("axial bradykinesia")—is the most central element of parkinsonism and is caused by loss of dopaminergic neurons in a midbrain structure called the substantia nigra pars compacta (SNpc) responsible for innervating a group of critical motor nuclei within the deep portions of the brain collectively labeled the basal ganglia.

There are multiple causes of parkinsonism. The most common and extensively studied is idiopathic Parkinson disease (PD), which is estimated to affect approximately 1% to 2% of people older than age 60. PD is a complex disorder with a wide variety of clinical presentations whose exact pathogenesis is incompletely understood. The eponymous name "Parkinson disease" was coined following the publication of "An Essay on the Shaking Palsy" by the British surgeon James Parkinson in 1817. In more recent years, the term "Parkinson disease" has been favored over "Parkinson's disease" given that Dr. Parkinson neither personally contracted nor "owned" the disease that over time has been associated with his surname.

There are numerous causes of parkinsonism, almost all of which becoming increasingly common with advancing age. These include (a) secondary parkinsonism caused by toxins, medications, or structural lesions in the brain; (b) atypical parkinsonian conditions including progressive supranuclear palsy (PSP), multiple system atrophy (MSA), corticobasal syndrome (CBS), and dementia with Lewy bodies (DLB); and (c) more rare neurodegenerative conditions with heterogeneous manifestations that can include parkinsonism such as juvenile Huntington disease, spinocerebellar ataxia type 3, and Wilson disease (**Table 61-1**).

Learning Objectives

- Learn the epidemiology, pathobiology, clinical manifestations, and genetics of Parkinson disease (PD).

- Understand the latest terminology and major clinical differences between parkinsonism and PD.

- Learn the common presenting features of diseases, such as progressive supranuclear palsy (PSP), corticobasal degeneration (CBD), and MSA that mimic and require differentiation from PD.

- Acquire new knowledge about the latest tests to diagnose PD and indications and adverse effects of cutting-edge therapies, including dopaminergic and nondopaminergic agents and surgical treatments for PD.

- Understand the significance of exercise, physical activity, and supportive care for management of patients with PD.

(Continued)

(Cont.)

5. Besides symptoms, dopamine transporter single-photon emission computed tomography (SPECT) imaging helps to diagnose PD and differentiate it from essential tremor.

6. Deep brain stimulation (DBS) surgery is typically indicated for patients with difficult motor complications and medication-refractory tremors.

It should be noted that there are a variety of overlapping and often outdated names frequently used to describe certain parkinsonian conditions that can be confusing to the nonspecialist. For example, the term olivopontocerebellar atrophy was formerly used to describe a collection of neurodegenerative conditions including MSA and some other progressive neurodegenerative cerebellar disorders. Similarly, the terms Lewy body dementia (LBD) and DLB are used interchangeably to refer to the same disorder. Finally, the term "diffuse Lewy body disease" is also used loosely by both clinicians and pathologists to describe the

TABLE 61-1 ■ CLASSIFICATION OF THE PARKINSONIAN STATES

Primary parkinsonism (Parkinson disease)

Sporadic

Known genetic etiology (see **Table 61-2**)

Secondary parkinsonism (environmental etiology)

  Drugs

    Dopamine receptor blockers (most commonly antipsychotic medications)

    Dopamine storage depletors (reserpine)

  Postencephalitic

  Toxins—Mn, CO, MPTP, cyanide

  Vascular

  Brain tumors

  Head trauma

  Normal pressure hydrocephalus

Parkinsonism-plus syndromes

  Progressive supranuclear palsy (PSP)

  Multiple system atrophy (MSA)

  Corticobasal syndrome (CBS)

  Dementia with Lewy bodies (DLB)

Heterodegenerative disorders

  Alzheimer disease

  Wilson disease

  Huntington disease

  Frontotemporal dementia on chromosome 17

  X-linked dystonia parkinsonism

topographical distribution of postmortem findings that can be seen in DLB.

EPIDEMIOLOGY

Like other insidiously developing progressive disorders of aging, there are inherent challenges in identifying the true prevalence of PD. The diagnosis of PD is typically made on the basis of clinical examination. There are numerous adjunctive clinical diagnostic measures, including a documented favorable response to a trial of dopaminergic medications, that can enhance certainty in the diagnosis of PD but these may not be used in large epidemiologic studies. The gold standard for making the diagnosis of PD remains autopsy where characteristic intracellular cytoplasmic inclusions of α-synuclein called Lewy bodies are seen in the SNpc and other brain and nervous system regions. Longitudinal clinical postmortem studies suggest that 10% to 20% of patients thought to have PD in life will have alternative diagnoses on autopsy. Interestingly, midbrain Lewy bodies are also seen on autopsy in about 20% of older individuals without a known history of parkinsonism suggesting that PD may be either underdiagnosed or not yet have manifested the typical motor features of the disease during life. Alternatively, these individuals may have so-called prodromal DLB.

Many epidemiologic studies of PD identify cases through medical records rather than through door-to-door examinations of well-defined populations. Incidence rates of PD vary not only by age but also by gender. Estimates across all possible ages and genders tend to range from 4.5 to 19/100,000 person-years reflecting differences in ascertainment methods and biological susceptibility. Among individuals older than age 60, incidence rates range from 27.2 to 107.2 cases/100,000 person-years. The median age of onset is in the early sixties and there is increasing risk for PD seen with each successive decade of life.

Since most people with PD live many years before death, prevalence rates of PD are higher than the incidence rates. Across all age ranges and genders, PD is thought to affect between 100 and 200 out of every 100,000 people. For people older than age 60, PD is thought to affect slightly more than 1 out of every 100 individuals. Parkinson disease is about 1.5 times more common in men than in women for reasons that may reflect differences in underlying biological susceptibility.

In most cases, PD is not a direct cause of death and frequently goes unmentioned on death certificates. Death in individuals with PD is occasionally due to secondary acute comorbidities seen in patients with mobility restrictions including aspiration pneumonia, traumatic falls, deep vein thrombosis, and pulmonary embolus. Mortality rates in PD are slightly higher in comparison to age- and gender-matched populations, although differences in life expectancy are most profound in individuals with early-onset PD. Individuals with PD and dementia also have a higher risk of death. PD patients who follow with a neurologist have a lower likelihood of death compared to those whose PD is managed exclusively by primary care physicians.

PD is caused by a complex interaction between genetic and environmental risk factors. Nevertheless, to date, relatively few environmental risk factors for sporadic PD have been identified. Exposure to pesticides containing the pyridine compound 1-methyl-4-phenyl-1,2,3,6-tetrahydropyradine (MPTP), industrial solvents, and heavy metals including manganese have all been suggested to associate with a higher risk of incident PD. Higher incidence in rural areas has been associated with farming-related exposures to pesticides and/or drinking from well water. There are several factors that have been consistently demonstrated to have an inverse relationship with PD risk including cigarette smoking, caffeinated coffee consumption, high plasma levels of uric acid, and endogenous estrogen exposure. The biological principles that mediate these associations are incompletely understood.

Although over 90% of cases of PD are considered sporadic, there is a growing understanding of the influence of primary monogenetic genetic causes of PD. Mendelian inheritance is implicated in several PD risk factor genes, all of which share a common naming schema as *PARK* genetic loci. To date, there are 20 *PARK* genes (**Table 61-2**). The most notable of these include *PARK1* or α-synuclein mutations, which were the first genetic variant identified to cause familial parkinsonism. There are now several identified autosomal-dominant and autosomal-recessive causes of PD some of which show variable penetrance depending on the underlying mutation. More recently, common haplotypes of genes known to play a role in other neurodegenerative conditions have been recognized as incremental risk factors for PD. These include the *MAPT* gene encoding the tau protein implicated in neurofibrillary tangles of Alzheimer disease (AD). Allelic variations including point mutations and deletions in the *GBA* gene, whose loss of function is implicated in causing impaired lysosomal activity in Gaucher's disease, have also been linked to cases of

TABLE 61-2 ■ GENETIC FORMS OF PRIMARY PARKINSONISM

NAME	GENE SYMBOL	PROTEIN	CHROMOSOME
AUTOSOMAL DOMINANT TRANSMISSION			
PARK1/PARK4	SNCA	α-Synuclein	4q21.3
PARK3	Unknown	Unknown	2p13
PARK5	UCH-L1	Ubiquitin C-terminal hydrolase-L1	4p14
PARK8	LRRK2	Leucine-rich repeat kinase 2	12p12
Dopa-responsive dystonia		GTP cyclohydrolase 1	14q22.1–q22.2
PARK13	HTRA2	High-temperature requirement protein	2p13
PARK17	VPS35	Vacuolar protein sorting 35	16q11
PARK18	EIF4G1	Eukaryotic translation initiating factor 4 gamma	3q27
AUTOSOMAL RECESSIVE TRANSMISSION			
PARK2	PRKN	Parkin (ubiquitin ligase)	6q25
PARK6	PINK1	PTEN-induced kinase 1 (PINK1)	1p36
PARK7	DJ-1	DJ-1	1p36
PARK9	ATP13A2	ATPase	1p36
PARK10			1p32
PARK14	PLA2G6	Phospholipase A2, group 6	22q13
PARK15	FBX07	F-box protein 7	22q12
PARK19	DNAJC6	DNAJC6	1p32
PARK20	SYNJ1	Synaptojanin 1	21q22
OTHER PD-ASSOCIATED GENES			
GBA	GBA1	β-Glucocerebrosidase	1q21
VPS35	VPS35	Vacuolar protein sorting 35	16p12.1-q12.1
PARK10	Unknown	Unknown	1p32
PARK11	GIGYF2	Unknown	2q36
PARK12	Unknown	Unknown	Xq21
PARK16	Unknown	Unknown	1p32

early-onset PD, particularly among individuals of Ashkenazi Jewish ancestry.

Understanding the pathobiology of these genetic PD subtypes has advanced the field's understanding of causative factors leading to the majority of "idiopathic" PD as well. PD is now thought to occur because of the confluence of several interrelated neurobiological risk states that each grow more problematic in the setting of aging. These include (1) autophagy-lysosomal dysfunction (ALD), (2) oxidative stress and dopamine toxicity, (3) selective neuronal vulnerability, and (4) network frailty and the prion-like spread of toxic alpha-synuclein pathology. First, ALD is implicated in PD with GBA1 and LRRK2 mutations and may play a bidirectional causative role in propagating toxic alpha-synuclein aggregation, which in turn may deleteriously affect autophagy-lysosomal function. Second, the generation of toxic oxidative species by neuronal dopamine metabolism may impair mitochondrial function, which may in turn lead to secondary ALD related to the turnover of dysfunctional mitochondria. Third, ALD and oxidative stressors may make certain projection neurons with unusually large axonal arborization characteristics particularly vulnerable to the effects of inefficient cellular metabolism. Certain neuronal groups affected by alpha-synuclein pathology show extensively branched axonal trees, perhaps making them particularly vulnerable. In some cases, this vulnerability can be accelerated by local neuroinflammation at the site of nascent neurodegeneration accelerated by adjacent glial cell populations. Finally, toxic alpha-synuclein appears to spread from one cell to the next in "prion-like" fashion where a misfolded peptide aggregate can seed a connected neuron in its functional network, thereby causing it to develop alpha-synuclein pathology as well. These findings have collectively set the stage for new disease-modifying approaches currently being tested in PD clinical trials.

Atypical parkinsonian conditions including PSP, MSA, and CBS manifest with a prevalence rate that is roughly 5% to 10% of PD prevalence. DLB is more common than the other atypical parkinsonisms, although prevalence estimates of DLB are confounded by its significant clinical and pathologic overlap with other common neurodegenerative conditions including PD and AD. Risks for developing PSP and CBS have been linked to allelic variation in the MAPT gene, and mutations in the GBA gene are seen with increased frequency in both PD and DLB.

PATHOPHYSIOLOGY

PD is most strongly associated with two specific postmortem hallmarks: (a) the development of cytoplasmic, eosinophilic inclusions of the misfolded synaptic protein α-synuclein called Lewy bodies and (b) the loss of SNpc dopaminergic neurons innervating the striatum.

Nigrostriatal dopaminergic denervation is seen as part of the spectrum of normal aging, albeit to a milder degree than is seen in PD. It is estimated that with every year of life after the third decade, we lose 0.5% to 1% of nigrostriatal nerve terminals, including the dorsal putamen a structure charged with mediating speed and precision of motor movements. By the time motor symptoms of PD are present, however, the posterior putamen has undergone profound denervation equating to the loss of over 60% to 80% of dopaminergic terminals. Although in this way, PD could be conceptualized as an accelerated form of nigrostriatal aging, the nerve terminal loss in PD has a particular predilection for the posterior and dorsal putamen compared to more anterior and ventral striatal regions. In contrast, normal aging is associated with more mild and diffuse striatal losses of nerve terminals.

Within the striatum, dopaminergic innervation is organized into two broad conceptual pathways: the direct pathway and the indirect pathway. Although this model is continually updated, it has formed the scientific basis accounting for a number of advances in neurobiology including the development of DBS. In this conceptual model, the striatum is viewed as a series of interconnected relay nuclei that upregulate or downregulate inputs from both the cortex and deep nuclei of the brain stem and spinal cord, yielding a well-regulated motor output to the cortex, thalamus, and brainstem pedunculopontine nucleus, which is part of the mesencephalic locomotor center.

The "direct pathway" is a monosynaptic, D1 receptor–mediated excitatory connection between the striatum and the globus pallidus pars interna (GPi) and substantia nigra pars reticulata (SNpr). When stimulated, these latter two nuclei lead to an increase in motor output via thalamocortical afferents. The "indirect pathway" is a polysynaptic pathway that depends on inhibitory D2 receptors affecting the globus pallidus pars externa (GPe) and the subthalamic nucleus (STN), which then innervate the GPi/SNpr. The net effect of the indirect pathway is to suppress motor output via thalamocortical afferents. Like many models of complex biological phenomena, the direct and indirect pathway model is an oversimplification of more nuanced network and has been challenged and revised over time. It nevertheless provides a useful conceptual framework to think about the pathologic changes in PD. Since D1 receptors are excitatory and D2 receptors are inhibitory, loss of dopamine in PD has the net effect of reducing transmission through the direct pathway (less stimulation of voluntary motor activity) and increasing transmission via the indirect pathway (more inhibition of motor activity) leading to an output that is characterized by a paucity of movement.

Significant advances in neurobiology over the last 20 years have improved our understanding of cellular pathology in PD. Abnormal processing of misfolded α-synuclein is now thought to occupy a central role in PD pathogenesis. α-Synuclein itself is an endogenously produced neuronal protein involved in synaptic vesicle trafficking. The breadth of mendelian genetic mutations linked to inherited forms of PD has given rise to several theories about the pathogenesis of sporadic PD, many of which coexist and contribute in additive fashion toward cell death in at-risk neuronal populations including the SNpc. These possibilities include (1) damage to the protein degradation properties of lysosomes leading to α-synuclein accumulation and aggregation; (2) effects from oxidative stress, such as the reaction of oxyradicals with nitric oxide; (3) impaired mitochondrial function leading to both reduced ATP production and accumulation of electrons that aggravate oxidative stress, with the final outcome being apoptosis and cell death; and (4) inflammatory changes in the nigra producing cytokines that augment apoptosis.

A description of contemporary models of PD pathogenesis would be incomplete without discussing the developing hypothesis that pathogenesis and disease progression of PD may be mediated through a prion-like cell-to-cell spread of misfolded α-synuclein. Prion proteins whose unusual morphology allows the induction of pathologic changes in adjacent cells by promoting misfolding of endogenous proteins, thereby transmitting cell death to adjacent neurons in an infectious-like fashion. In vitro and in vivo experiments in preclinical models of PD have shown the ability of misfolded α-synuclein to induce similar changes in adjacent neurons leading to neurodegeneration.

The "Braak model" of PD pathogenesis is a temporal and topographic schema of Lewy body or Lewy neurite deposition based on findings in a cohort of older individuals with Lewy bodies found on autopsy. In the originally proposed model, Lewy body formation begins in the medulla oblongata and then progresses in a rostral fashion to involve the upper brain stem followed by the diencephalon and cortex. Coincidentally, with the brainstem medulla deposition, this model posits also early deposition in the olfactory tubercle, which then may progress to adjacent regions. Lewy body deposition in the original Braak stage 3 (of total six stages) involves the nigra and is thought to correspond with the onset of motor features of PD. Braak stages 1 and 2 correspond with premotor features of PD, including olfactory, sleep, and autonomic symptoms that can often predate the diagnosis of PD by several years. Similarly, cortical Lewy body formation seen in Braak stages 5 and 6 correspond with cognitive impairment and dementia seen later in the disease course in PD. More recent revisions of this model suggest even earlier involvement of Lewy body deposition in peripheral autonomic nerve terminals, including the intestines, stomach, and myocardium antedating the motor symptoms of PD decades before.

Unlike PD, both PSP and CBS are not thought to be disorders of α-synuclein but instead are attributable to misfolded tau. The parkinsonism seen in these disorders is attributable to tau-based neurodegeneration of the SNpc and basal ganglia. MSA is characterized by the development of argyrophilic cytoplasmic inclusion bodies that are positive for α-synuclein in glial cells rather than typical neuronal Lewy bodies. DLB has neuropathological overlap with PD with dementia (PDD) in that both disorders are characterized by Lewy body formation in the cortex.

PDD is clinically defined by the so-called 1-year rule where motor symptoms antedate cognitive symptoms for over 1 year, whereas motor and cognitive symptoms coincide within a year in DLB. Although different in the temporal profile of the emergence of cognitive and neurobehavioral symptoms, typical features of DLB and/or PDD include hallucinations, especially visual, fluctuations in cognition and dream enactment behavior. DLB, however, also features significant cerebral amyloidopathy more characteristic of AD. Although DLB is often characterized as representing an overlap between PD and AD neuropathology, neurofibrillary tangles are less common in DLB compared to prototypical AD.

PRESENTATION AND EVALUATION

The diagnosis of PD is of prognostic importance, as well as of therapeutic significance, because PD almost always responds somewhat to dopaminergic medications whereas the atypical parkinsonian conditions often do not. In general, the features of PD that tend to improve the most with levodopa or dopamine agonists include bradykinesia, especially fine motor distal motor dexterity, and rigidity in the arms and legs. In some individuals, features of rest tremor can improve significantly with levodopa, especially in the presence of more prominent bradykinesia. Axial motor features including hypophonia, dysphagia, and postural instability are often medication refractory and signify the influence of nondopaminergic changes superimposed on top of nigrostriatal dopaminergic denervation.

While it may be difficult to distinguish between PD and Parkinson-plus syndromes in the early stages of the illness, with disease progression over time, the clinical distinctions of the Parkinson-plus disorders become more apparent with the development of other neurologic findings, such as loss of downward ocular movements in PSP or cerebellar ataxia and autonomic dysfunction (eg, postural hypotension, loss of bladder control, and impotence), which can be seen to a mild-moderate degree in PD but are often very prominent in MSA.

PD begins insidiously and gradually progresses. Three of the most helpful clues that one is likely dealing with an alternative cause of parkinsonism other than idiopathic PD are (1) a symmetrical onset of symptoms (PD often begins asymmetrically on one side of the body), (2) a lack of a substantial clinical response to adequate levodopa therapy, and (3) the absence of rest tremor—though this latter feature is less specific and is present to variable degrees in PD. There are three commonly cited clinical criteria for diagnosing PD: the UK Brain Bank Clinical Diagnostic criteria, the Gelb criteria, and the 2015 Movement Disorders Society (MDS) Criteria. Each criterion emphasizes that bradykinesia, the most prevalent motor feature of PD, must be present and that other causes of parkinsonism should preferably be excluded. The UK Brain Bank criteria use the presence of postural instability as an

TABLE 61-3 ■ CRITERIA TO EXCLUDE THE DIAGNOSIS OF PARKINSON DISEASE IN FAVOR OF ANOTHER CAUSE OF PARKINSONISM

	LIKELY DIAGNOSIS
History of:	
Encephalitis	Postencephalitic
Exposure to carbon monoxide, manganese, or other toxins	Toxin induced
Recent exposure to neuroleptic medications or metoclopramide	Drug induced
Onset of parkinsonian symptoms following:	
Head trauma	Posttraumatic
Stroke	Vascular
Presence on examination of:	
Cerebellar ataxia	MSA, primary ataxic disorders
Loss of downward ocular movements	PSP
Pronounced postural hypotension not because of concurrent medication	MSA
Pronounced unilateral rigidity with or without dystonia, apraxia, cortical sensory loss, alien limb	CBS
Myoclonus	CBS, MSA
Falling or freezing of gait early in the course of the disease	PSP
Autonomic dysfunction not because of medications	MSA
Excessive drooling of saliva	MSA
Early dementia or hallucinations from medications	DLB
Dystonia induced with low-dose levodopa	MSA
Neuroimaging (MRI or CT scan) revealing:	
Lacunar infarcts	Vascular parkinsonism
Capacious cerebral ventricles	Normal pressure hydrocephalus
Cerebellar atrophy	MSA, primary ataxic disorders
Atrophy of the midbrain or other parts of the brain stem	PSP, MSA
Effect of medication:	
Poor response to levodopa	PSP, MSA, CBS, vascular, NPH
No dyskinesias despite high-dose levodopa	Same as above

CBS, corticobasal syndrome; CT, computed tomography; DLB, dementia with Lewy bodies; MRI, magnetic resonance imaging; MSA, multiple system atrophy; NPH, normal pressure hydrocephalus; PSP, progressive supranuclear palsy.

inclusion criterion for PD, whereas the Gelb criteria deemphasize this feature—given that it can also be seen in atypical parkinsonian conditions—and suggest that asymmetry of motor presentation should be the key inclusion criteria for PD. The MDS criteria for "clinically established" PD require, the absence of exclusionary criteria, the presence of bradykinesia, and at least 2 of 4 supportive criteria: (1) a levodopa treatment response, (2) levodopa-induced dyskinesias, (3) rest tremor, and (4) either olfactory loss and/or cardiac sympathetic denervation. Clinical features suggesting an alternative parkinsonian diagnosis, so-called "red flags," are listed in **Table 61-3** and a comparison of diagnostic features for PD and atypical parkinsonian conditions is presented in **Table 61-4**. One common misdiagnosis is tremor due to essential tremor, which can even be unilateral, although it more commonly is bilateral. Helpful in the diagnosis is that the tremor caused by PD is a predominant rest tremor, whereas essential tremor is not typically present at rest, but appears with holding the arms in front of the body (postural tremor) and increases in amplitude with activity of the arm (kinetic or action tremor), such as with

handwriting or performing the finger-to-nose maneuver. The presence of mixed and asymmetric tremor syndromes can be particularly challenging as sometimes PD and essential tremor may coexist in the same patients.

Although the diagnosis of PD rests largely on the clinical history and examination, there are adjunctive diagnostic measures that can be useful in making the proper diagnosis. A history of a positive response to levodopa or other dopaminergic medications, for example, is seen in almost all patients with PD. That having been said, many patients with atypical parkinsonian conditions—in particular MSA and DLB—will also describe a generally milder improvement in certain motor features from dopaminergic medications. Dopamine transporter imaging through SPECT (I-123 ioflupane SPECT or DaTscan) scan provides molecular imaging evidence to confirm the loss of nigrostriatal dopaminergic nerve terminals, consistent with parkinsonism (**Figure 61-1**). It cannot, however, differentiate between PD and other causes of neurodegenerative parkinsonism, such as DLB, PSP, or MSA; all of these conditions will have evidence of nigrostriatal losses

TABLE 61-4 ■ COMPARISON OF DIAGNOSTIC FEATURES FOR PD AND OTHER ATYPICAL PARKINSONIAN CONDITIONS

DISEASE	RELATIVE INCLUSION CRITERIA	CRITERIA SUPPORTIVE OF THE DIAGNOSIS	RELATIVE EXCLUSION CRITERIA
PD	• Bradykinesia • Rigidity • Rest tremor • Asymmetric onset (++)	• Gradually progressive course • Good response to dopaminergic therapies (++) • Motor fluctuations (+++) • Dyskinesias (+++) • Motor symptom duration > 5 y • Olfactory impairment • Rapid eye movement (REM) sleep behavior disorder • Cardiac sympathetic denervation	• Focal brain lesions within the basal ganglia • Recent history of neuroleptic medication use • Severe dysautonomia unrelated to medications • Supranuclear gaze palsy • Prominent postural instability at initial presentation (−) • Prominent cerebellar atrophy on MRI (−) • Freezing of gait developing within 3 y of motor symptom onset (−)
PSP	• Supranuclear gaze palsy (+++) • Slowing of vertical eye movements/saccades (+++) • Tendency to fall in the first year following the onset of motor symptoms (++)	• Gradually progressive course • Symmetric parkinsonism • Increased neck tone and axial rigidity (++) • Early dysphagia • Early cognitive features including apathy, decreased verbal fluency, and pseudobulbar effect • Early frontal release signs on neurologic examination • "Hummingbird sign" on sagittal brain MRI (++)	• Alien limb syndrome • Hallucinations • Early cerebellar signs • Early dysautonomia
CBS	• Asymmetric motor findings at presentation (+) • Limb dystonia at presentation (+) • Limb myoclonus (++) • Alien-limb phenomenon (+++)	• Cortical sensory deficit (++) • Frontal lobe cognitive symptoms including executive dysfunction, behavioral/personality changes, aphasia (++) • Focal cortical parietofrontal atrophy on brain MRI	• Rest tremor • Good response to dopaminergic medications • Hallucinations • Cerebellar signs • Prominent dysautonomia
MSA	• Cerebellar features on examination (++) • Prominent dysautonomia (+++) • Hyperreflexia and other pyramidal tract findings (+)	• Relatively few cognitive features • Respiratory stridor (++) • Orofacial dyskinesias • "Hot cross bun" sign on axial brainstem MRI	• Dysautonomia only in relation to medications • Hallucinations
DLB	• Hallucinations (+++) • Fluctuations in level of alertness (++) • Dementia within 1 y of the onset of motor features of parkinsonism	• REM sleep behavior disorder (+) • Sensitivity to medications, especially neuroleptics (++)	• Active delirium explained by concurrent medications or an alternative process • Supranuclear gaze palsy

+/− denotes strength of association between a particular feature and a specific disorder. CBS, corticobasal syndrome; DLB, dementia with Lewy bodies; MSA, multiple system atrophy; PD, Parkinson disease; PSP, progressive supranuclear palsy; REM, rapid eye movement.
The above table presents a summary of published diagnostic criteria. The lists of inclusion and exclusion criteria for any given disorders are not exclusive/exhaustive of all possibilities. For any given disease, not all inclusion criteria are required to make an affirmative diagnosis. Similarly, the presence of a single exclusion criterion does not represent an absolute contraindication to diagnosing a specific disorder.

PART III

GERIATRIC CONDITIONS

on dopamine transporter imaging. Dopamine transporter SPECT imaging has been approved to distinguish essential tremor from PD in patients with atypical tremor manifestation. This imaging modality can also be helpful to distinguish PD from drug-induced parkinsonism. Impaired performance on olfactory identification testing has also shown good correlation with postmortem findings of PD in patients presenting for suspected parkinsonism but can also be seen in other neurodegenerative conditions, such as AD or DLB. Scratch-and-sniff tests for odor identification are available commercially and can be completed and scored in the clinic relatively quickly.

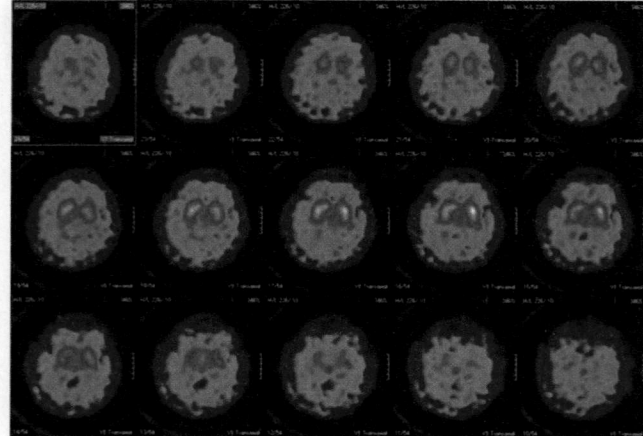

A   **Normal DaTscan: Essential tremor**

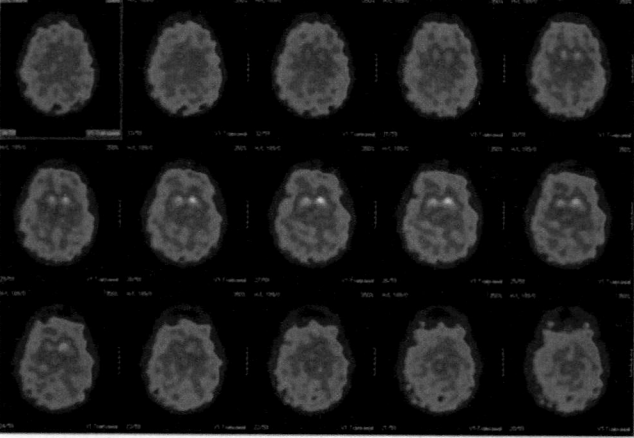

B   **Abnormal DaTscan: Primary parkinsonism**

FIGURE 61-1. A. Normal dopamine transporter imaging through single-photon emission computed tomography (DaT SPECT scan) in a patient with essential tremor. **B.** Asymmetric loss of putaminal dopaminergic nerve terminals affecting the right striatum more than the left consistent with a primary neurodegenerative parkinsonian condition.

Updated diagnostic criteria for DLB were published in 2017. Individuals meet the threshold for "probable DLB" if they show findings of a progressive dementia and have at least two of core features of DLB: (1) parkinsonism, (2) cognitive fluctuations, (3) rapid eye movement (REM) sleep behavior disorder (RBD), and (4) recurrent visual hallucinations. A positive biomarker test—including an abnormal striatal DaT SPECT, polysomnography findings consistent with RBD, or sympathetic denervation on myocardial scintigraphy—can also be substituted for one of these four core criteria in order to meet the "probable DLB" diagnostic threshold. The US Food and Drug Administration (FDA) has approved PET radiopharmaceuticals to detect the presence of amyloid plaques (eg, florbetapir) and neurofibrillary tangles (flortaucipir) and may be useful for diagnostic purposes if diagnostic uncertainty remains. The FDA is expected to review applications shortly for diagnostic

amyloid-beta blood tests that would allow the detection of cerebral amyloid disorders, including AD, in relevant clinical contexts. Whether these tests may be employed to distinguish different prognostic trajectories in individuals with common early synucleinopathies is a topic worth monitoring—this is especially true given that manifest DLB is characterized by higher cortical amyloid-beta plaque levels than idiopathic PD.

A recent proposal to distinguish the so-called body-first versus brain-first subtypes of PD may blur the line between PD and DLB diagnoses. The proposed subtyping is based on the temporal relationship between the onset of RBD and motor diagnosis of PD. A gut-first subtype would be defined when RBD precedes the motor diagnosis with at least 1 year compared to post-motor symptom emergence of this parasomnia or its absence. This subtyping may have an advantage of early stage prognostication but its utility in more advanced disease is questionable.

Although there are many motor features seen in early PD, the scope of nonmotor features associated with early PD is even larger. These can include (but are not limited to) olfactory impairment, sleep difficulties, depression, anxiety, chronic constipation, limb pain, apathy, erectile dysfunction, cognitive impairment, drooling, rhinorrhea, and other autonomic features. Although some of these features can be a secondary development due to disability accrued from PD, almost all of them are aggravated by primary Lewy body–related neuronal changes seen in various areas of the nervous system ranging from the enteric nerves of the gastrointestinal tract to the cholinergic nerves arising from the basal forebrain, which innervate the cerebral cortex. Although many of these features become increasingly common with age, the concomitant development of three or more of these features in an older individual without a clear alternate explanation should prompt a work-up for a parkinsonian condition.

Early cognitive changes seen in PD include difficulty with memory, attention, and executive dysfunction, the latter of which refers to planning, multitasking, and decision-making capacity. In some patients, these cognitive features may be stable for many years, whereas in others they may progress to dementia. It is estimated that about 50% of individuals with PD will develop dementia (PDD) within 10 years of their initial diagnosis.

MSA is a parkinsonian disorder characterized by aggressive α-synuclein–related cellular loss in the brain stem, cerebellum, and basal ganglia. The median age of onset is in the sixth decade of life with a mean time to severe disability of approximately 5 years from the time of diagnosis. Progressive cell death occurs not only in dopaminergic cells but in many different neuronal systems including the basal ganglia, substantia nigra, locus coeruleus, pontine nuclei, cerebellar Purkinje cells, and the intermediolateral cell column of the spinal cord. MSA is typically grouped into two clinical categories: MSA-P, where parkinsonism is seen, and MSA-C, where cerebellar features including ataxic gait, dystaxic limb movements, and ataxic speech predominate. Other characteristic features of both MSA-P and MSA-C that differ from PD include severe autonomic symptoms including orthostatic light-headedness, blood pressure fluctuations, and urinary dysfunction. Patients with MSA can also experience nocturnal stridor characterized by laryngeal obstruction secondary to vocal fold hypokinesia, which manifests with a high-pitched inspiratory noise. Unlike obstructive sleep apnea, nocturnal stridor can be acutely life threatening. While emergency tracheostomies have been performed in MSA for life-threatening stridor, this may be inconsistent with overall goals of care for such patients. Following with an otolaryngologist on an annual basis can be an effective method for monitoring this symptom overtime and some patients may benefit from nasal continuous positive airway pressure (CPAP). Unlike other atypical parkinsonian conditions, cognitive impairment is not a typical feature of MSA but may be present in a small subset.

PSP and CBS are both tauopathies associated with parkinsonism. PSP tends to present in the sixth and seventh decades of life with early oculomotor findings including downgaze impairment, axial rigidity, and postural instability. Patients with PSP also develop a frontal-predominant cognitive syndrome characterized by apathy, executive dysfunction, and pseudobulbar effect. CBS is the clinical diagnosis given for patients with suspected CBD, the latter of which refers specifically to neuropathologic findings. Clinically defined CBS is associated with several distinct postmortem histopathologies, including CBD, other forms of tau-related frontotemporal lobar degeneration, such as PSP, and AD. Motor manifestations of CBS also tend to occur in the sixth or seventh decade of life and are characterized by progressive asymmetric rigidity, myoclonus, parkinsonism, and an unusual motor phenomenon termed "alien limb" during which patients experience adventitious semipurposeful movements of one limb. CBS is one of the exceptions to the general rule that asymmetric limb motor involvement favors a diagnosis of PD. Early cognitive changes include praxis difficulties and language impairment. Cortical sensory loss can also be seen. The variable presence of these clinical features and their overlap with features seen in PSP, PD, and frontotemporal dementia (FTD) has led clinicians to use the term CBS to describe clinically probable, though not pathologically confirmed, CBD.

MANAGEMENT

Treatment of patients with PD can be divided into three major categories: medications, physical (and mental health) therapy, and surgery. Although the pharmacologic strategies described below apply primarily to PD, they can also be tried in atypical parkinsonian conditions. MSA, PSP, and CBD, however, are typically associated with a more limited response to medications, underscoring their overall worse prognosis.

TABLE 61-5 ■ DOPAMINERGIC AGENTS
Dopamine precursor: levodopa
Peripheral decarboxylase inhibitors: carbidopa, benserazide
Dopamine agonists: pramipexole, ropinirole, rotigotine, apomorphine
Catechol-O-methyltransferase inhibitors: entacapone, opicapone
Dopamine releaser: amantadine
Peripheral dopamine receptor blocker: domperidone
MAO type B inhibitor: selegiline, selegiline, rasagiline, safinamide
A2A antagonist: istradefylline

MAO, monoamine oxidase.

Dopaminergic Therapies

Dopamine replacement therapy is the primary medical approach to treating PD, and a variety of dopaminergic agents are available (**Table 61-5**). The most powerful oral drug is levodopa, the immediate precursor of dopamine. Levodopa, an amino acid precursor molecule of dopamine, can enter the brain, whereas dopamine is blocked by the blood-brain barrier. Levodopa is usually administered combined with a peripheral decarboxylase inhibitor (carbidopa or benserazide) to prevent formation of dopamine in the peripheral tissues, thereby increasing levodopa's bioavailability and also markedly reducing gastrointestinal side effects. The brand name Sinemet is a combination of carbidopa and levodopa; the brand name Madopar is a combination of benserazide and levodopa. Such combination drugs are available in standard (ie, immediate-release) and extended-release formulations. The former allows a more rapid and predictable "on," and the latter allows for a slightly longer plasma half-life, but with a slower and less predictable "on." The combination of the two release formulations can be administered in an attempt to smooth out and extend plasma levels of levodopa. A version of carbidopa/levodopa that dissolves under the tongue (Parcopa) and enters the stomach via swallowing saliva is also available. This orally dissolving formulation has particular usefulness for patients who have swallowing difficulties.

Although levodopa is the most effective drug to treat the symptoms of PD, over half of patients develop troublesome complications of disabling response fluctuations ("wearing-off") and/or dyskinesias after 5 years of levodopa therapy. Besides being metabolized by aromatic amino acid decarboxylase (commonly known as dopa decarboxylase), levodopa is also metabolized by catechol-O-methyltransferase (COMT) to form 3-O-methyldopa. Entacapone is a currently available COMT inhibitor. This agent extends the plasma half-life of levodopa with and also increases its peak plasma concentration, and thereby prolongs the duration of action of each dose of levodopa. Its clinical indication is to help reduce motor fluctuations, that is, increase "on" time and reduce "off" time. Because entacapone enhances levodopa's efficacy, it can increase dyskinesias and the dosage of levodopa may need to be lowered. Entacapone is very short acting, and each 200-mg tablet is taken simultaneously with levodopa. Entacapone is also available in a combination pill with carbidopa/levodopa (Stalevo). Tolcapone (100- and 200-mg tablets) is more potent and has a longer duration of action, but it is encumbered by a greater risk of diarrhea and hepatotoxicity, the latter of which has led to its removal from the market in the United States. After levodopa, the next most powerful oral drugs in treating PD symptoms are the dopamine agonists. Several of these are available. The ergot compounds of pergolide, bromocriptine, and cabergoline have the potential to induce fibrosis (cardiac valvulopathy and retroperitoneal, pleuropulmonary, and pericardial fibrosis), so these agents are not recommended; indeed, pergolide has been withdrawn from the US market. Pramipexole and ropinirole appear to be equally effective at therapeutic levels. Dopamine agonists are more likely than levodopa to cause hallucinations, confusion, and psychosis, especially in the older adults. Thus, it is safer to utilize levodopa in patients older than 70 years. On the other hand, clinical trials have shown that dopamine agonists are less likely to produce dyskinesias and the wearing-off phenomenon than levodopa. These differences are most likely due to the relatively lower potency/efficacy and longer half-life of dopamine agonists compared to levodopa. Slow-release preparations of ropinirole and pramipexole are also available. Other problems more likely to occur with dopamine agonists than levodopa are sudden sleep attacks, including falling asleep at the wheel, daytime drowsiness, ankle edema, and impulse control problems such as hypersexuality and compulsive gambling, shopping, and binge eating. The newest dopamine agonist is rotigotine which is applied via a dermal patch to the upper torso or arms. It is useful for those with swallowing difficulties and may help smooth out motor fluctuations and nocturnal akinesia when the last prebedtime dose of levodopa does not last throughout the night. Rotigotine is a high-potency agonist at human dopamine D1, D2, and D3 receptors with a lower potency at D4 and D5 receptors. Therefore, rotigotine differs from conventional dopamine D2 agonists used in the treatment of PD, such as ropinirole and pramipexole, which lack activity at the D1 and D5 receptors, but resembles that of apomorphine, which has greater efficacy in PD than other dopamine agonists. The preferential D1 receptor agonism may explain rotigotine's higher efficacy in treating freezing of gait in PD compared to pramipexole and ropinirole. Another advantage of rotigotine is the transdermal delivery facilitating more steady drug delivery throughout the day.

Apomorphine may be the most powerful dopamine agonist, but can cause intense nausea and historically has needed to be injected subcutaneously. It is used to provide faster relief to overcome a disabling "off" state. A newly developed formulation of Apomorphine is now available in a sublingual film (Kynmobi) and may be useful for treating patients with precipitous motor fluctuations (see Treatment of "Wearing Off").

Amantadine is adjunctive antiparkinsonian drug with several pharmacologic actions; it has mild antimuscarinic effects, but more importantly, it can activate release of dopamine from nerve terminals, block dopamine uptake into the nerve terminals, and block glutamate N-methyl-D-aspartate (NMDA) receptors. Its dopaminergic actions make it a useful drug to relieve symptoms in approximately two-thirds of patients, but it can induce livedo reticularis, ankle edema, visual hallucinations, and confusion. Its antiglutamatergic action is useful in reducing the severity of levodopa-induced dyskinesias, and in fact, is the only established effective antidyskinetic agent. The dose of amantadine for its anti-PD effect is usually 100 mg twice daily, but its antidyskinetic effect requires higher dosages, usually 300 to 400 mg/day. Unfortunately, the antidyskinetic effect tends to lessen over time. Older individuals often do not tolerate amantadine well because of mental adverse effects of confusion and hallucinations.

Domperidone is a peripherally active dopamine receptor blocker and is useful in preventing gastrointestinal upset from levodopa and the dopamine agonists. It is not available in the United States but is available in other countries including Canada. Monoamine oxidase type B (MAO-B) inhibitors (selegiline, rasagiline) offer mildly effective symptomatic benefit and are without significant hypertensive diet-linked side effects seen with MAO-A inhibitors, and therefore can be used in the presence of levodopa therapy. Although there has been considerable debate about possible protective or disease-modifying benefit of MAO-B inhibitors, numerous well-powered trials have failed to convincingly demonstrate a neuroprotective benefit. The results of these trials have been interpreted variably, however, given that selegiline and rasagiline appear to have a symptomatic benefit, which has contributed to some methodological concerns regarding specific trial designs. Selegiline, but not rasagiline, is metabolized to L-amphetamine and methamphetamine. Both of these drugs can reduce the severity of motor fluctuations with levodopa. The newly developed drug safinamide is thought to offer greater specificity for MAO-B, which in theory may reduce off target side effects related to diet.

Motor Complications of Dopaminergic Therapies

Many patients on levodopa therapy develop motor complications (**Table 61-6**). These motor complications, also referred to as "motor fluctuations," usually begin as mild wearing-off, which can be defined as when an adequate dose of levodopa does not last at least 6 hours and motor symptoms of bradykinesia, rigidity, or tremor emerge or worsen. Typically, in the first couple of years of treatment, there is a long-duration response so that the timing of doses of levodopa is not important. Over time, the long-duration response becomes lost, and only a short-duration response occurs; patients then develop the wearing-off phenomenon.

TABLE 61-6 ■ PATTERN OF DEVELOPMENT OF RESPONSE FLUCTUATIONS, DYSKINESIAS, AND OTHER COMPLICATIONS

Dyskinesias (chorea and dystonia)
- Peak-dose dyskinesias
- Diphasic dyskinesias (beginning and end of dose dyskinesias)

Fluctuations
- Wearing-off
- Delayed "ons"
- Dose failures
- Sudden, unpredictable "offs" (on-offs)
- Early morning "off" dystonia
- "Off" dystonia during day
- Nonmotor "offs" (eg, exacerbated fatigue, word-finding difficulty, restlessness, etc.)

Alertness
- Drowsy from a dose of levodopa
- Reverse sleep-wake cycle

Behavioral and cognitive
- Vivid dreams
- Mild hallucinations
- Severe hallucinations
- Delusions
- Punding
- Apathy
- Paranoia
- Delirium
- Dementia

The "off" episodes tend to be mild at first, but over time become more frequent or severe with more severe parkinsonism. Simultaneously, the duration of the "on" response becomes shorter. Eventually, some patients develop random, sudden "offs" in which the deep state of parkinsonism develops over minutes rather than tens of minutes, and they are less predictable in terms of synchrony with the dosing of levodopa. Many patients who develop response fluctuations also develop abnormal involuntary movements, that is, dyskinesias.

Treatment of "wearing-off"

The wearing-off phenomenon, when mild, may be ameliorated slightly with the addition of selegiline, rasagiline, or safinamide. Each MAO-B inhibitor potentiates the action of levodopa. A higher dose of levodopa may be necessary but more frequent dosing of levodopa may be the simplest approach to manage this motor complication. Many patients can require six or more doses of levodopa per day, and then, eventually, can develop dose failures owing to poor gastric emptying. These patients are often considered for duodenal infusion of levodopa or DBS (see Surgical Therapy later).

Continuous-release carbidopa/levodopa (Sinemet CR) can also be effective in patients with mild wearing-off in some patients or use the combination of both immediate- and extended-release formulations. Newer formulations of carbidopa/levodopa have attempted to address the clinical need for more uniform levodopa dosing throughout the day. These include Rytary—a capsule that contains immediate and extended release levodopa with carbidopa. Rytary and Sinemet make use of slightly different doses that may merit close monitoring when transition from one drug to the other. Optimally, Rytary may be a useful Sinemet substitution in patients who depend on levodopa administration every 2 to 4 hours throughout the day, hopefully allowing for less frequent dosing. A short-acting formulation of levodopa delivered in an inhaler (Inbrija) may be useful in the setting of precipitous motor "offs." It may start working within 10 to 30 minutes though—much like inhalers for pulmonary conditions—its efficacy can be altered by the technique of inhaler utilization. Dopamine agonists, which have a longer biological half-life than levodopa, can also be used in combination with immediate-release or continuous-release versions of carbidopa/levodopa. The addition of a dopamine agonist tends to make the "off" state less severe when used in combination with carbidopa/levodopa. COMT inhibitors have been found useful for treating wearing-off. Because of the short half-life of entacapone, it is given with each dose of carbidopa/levodopa and is about as equally effective as rasagiline in reducing the amount of daily "off" time. For those patients who have "offs" at a specific time of day, entacapone can be strategically given just with the dosage of carbidopa/levodopa that precedes this "off" period. Once daily dosing is now possible with a newly developed COMT inhibitor, opicapone. Adenosine A2A receptors are expressed in the striatum and a newly approved A2A-receptor antagonist (istradefylline) may serve to reduce activity of the basal ganglia's indirect pathway, thereby relieving parkinsonian hypokinesia. Istradefylline is a once-daily medication used to reduce off-time when used in conjunction with carbidopa/levodopa in PD patients with motor fluctuations.

Behavioral or sensory "offs" can also occur as do motor "offs," often in the absence of any motor "off," which means a return of parkinsonism. Behavioral and sensory "offs," tend not to be easily recognized, because visibly the treating physician sees no motor changes. Behavioral/sensory "offs" can consist of pain, akathisia, depression, anxiety, dysphoria, or panic, and usually a combination of more than one of these. Sensory "offs," like dystonic "offs," are very disabling. It is often the presence of one of these sensory and behavioral phenomena, more so than motoric parkinsonian or dystonic "offs," that drives the patient to take more and more levodopa, leading a few patients to develop an addictive relationship with dopaminergic medications, so-called dopamine dysregulation syndrome.

Dyskinesias are involuntary movements and occur in two major forms—chorea and dystonia. Choreiform movements are irregular, nonrhythmic, unsustained dance-like movements that seem to flow from one body part to another and can appear like benign fidgeting. Dystonic movements are more sustained, twisting contractions. Many patients have a combination of choreiform and dystonic dyskinesias.

Peak-dose dyskinesias occur when the plasma concentrations of levodopa or dopamine agonists are at their peak, and the synaptic brain concentration of dopamine is too high. Reducing the individual dosage can resolve this problem of peak-dose dyskinesias. However, the patient may need to take more frequent doses at this lower amount. An alternative approach is to add amantadine, which suppresses the severity of dyskinesias, possibly because of its antiglutamatergic action. Start with a dose of 100 mg BID and increase up to 200 mg BID if necessary. Buspirone in dose up to 20 mg/day may also of benefit in treating dyskinesias in some patients.

Some patients may develop "off" dyskinesias. In the absence of so-called early morning "off" dystonia, which responds well to dopaminergic therapies, such patients are encouraged to consider DBS (see later under Surgical Therapy). Depending on their distribution within the body and the disability associated with them, dystonic dyskinesias can also be treated with local injections of a chemodenervation agent such as botulinum toxin. This treatment can be associated with a significant improvement in quality of life but will also weaken a muscle group and thereby can impact a patient's function, particularly if the dystonic movements are occurring in the hands.

Diphasic dyskinesias are dyskinesias that occur at the beginning and end of dose, not during the time of peak plasma and brain levels of dopaminergic medications. They tend to particularly affect the legs with a mixture of chorea and dystonia.

Dopamine Medication–Related Nonmotor Complications

In addition to motor features, a number of nonmotor problems can also occur as complications from dopaminergic therapy. Mental changes of psychosis, confusion, agitation, hallucinations, paranoid delusions, punding, impulse control disorders, and excessive sleeping are probably related to activation of dopamine receptors in anteroventral striatal regions, or nonstriatal regions, particularly the cortical and limbic structures.

Drug-induced hallucinations tend to be mild, visual in nature rather than auditory, and not frightening. Consideration should be given to reducing the total dose of dopaminergic medication to whatever degree is tolerable for the patient. A complete review of medications is indicated as well to identify any other symptomatic treatments that might be worsening encephalopathy, including benzodiazepines, anticholinergics, and opioids. Adjunctive treatment can begin with the addition of either quetiapine, starting with 25 mg at bedtime or pimavanserin (17 mg 1–2 times daily, although dosing may need to be reduced in patients taking CYP3A4 inhibitors). Pimavanserin is a newer drug that targets serotoninergic neurotransmission through its action as an inverse agonist and antagonist at 5HT-2A receptors. Unlike quetiapine, pimavanserin has prospective clinical trial data supporting its efficacy for treating psychosis in PD. Even so, the relative safety and easy dosing of quetiapine have led to its continued use as symptomatic treatment. Currently, a head-to-head trial is underway aimed at comparing the safety and efficacy of these two drugs in PD with psychosis. The dose should be increased steadily until the hallucinations are brought under control. If quetiapine or pimavanserin are ineffective or if the hallucinations are frightening, clozapine, a stronger antipsychotic that will not worsen motor features of PD, should be considered. As mentioned previously, the reason clozapine is not the first drug of choice in dopaminergic-induced hallucinations is because clozapine causes agranulocytosis in approximately 1% to 2% of patients. Patients must have their blood counts monitored weekly for this potential complication, and then discontinue the drug if leukopenia develops. Both quetiapine and clozapine often cause drowsiness, so bedtime dosing is recommended.

If the psychosis is severe or if the patient is in an acute delirious state, hospitalization may be necessary, with immediate initiation of antipsychotic medications, and some reduction in anti-PD medication. These medications could even be withdrawn temporarily to overcome the psychosis, but this should be done stepwise over a 3-day period to avoid the neuroleptic malignant-like syndrome that could occur with sudden withdrawal of levodopa.

Dopamine agonist medications are associated with sleep attacks and impulse control disorders. Both of these issues can also be seen with levodopa but are much less common and less severe. Sleep attacks often manifest with a sudden wave of sleepiness that comes on with little warning and can be particularly dangerous for patients who are driving at the time. Impulse control disorders consist of behavioral changes such as compulsive gambling, shopping, and eating, and hypersexual behaviors. Not surprisingly, these changes can often have significant detrimental effects on family relationships. Both of these side effects are, to some degree, dose-dependent and typically necessitate reducing the dose of the dopamine agonists or stopping them altogether. Memantine, an NMDA receptor antagonist, has shown to be of benefit in some patients with dopamine agonist–induced impulse control disorders in PD.

Nondopaminergic Therapies

Nondopaminergic agents (**Table 61-7**) are useful to treat both motor and nonmotor symptoms of PD. Antimuscarinic drugs have been used since the 1950s to treat parkinsonian tremor but have limited efficacy and

TABLE 61-7 ■ NONDOPAMINERGIC AGENTS

Parkinsonian motor symptoms:

Antimuscarinics (for tremor): trihexyphenidyl, benztropine

Antiglutamatergics (to reduce dyskinesia): amantadine

Muscle relaxants: cyclobenzaprine, diazepam, baclofen

Nonmotor symptom control:

Depression: selective and nonselective serotonin reuptake inhibitors, tricyclics, electroconvulsive therapy

Psychosis (hallucinations, paranoia): clozapine, quetiapine

Insomnia: mirtazapine, trazodone, quetiapine, zolpidem

REM sleep behavior disorder: clonazepam, melatonin

Excessive daytime sleepiness: modafinil

Dementia: donepezil, rivastigmine

Orthostasis: fludrocortisone, midodrine, droxidopa

Restless legs: dopamine agonists, levodopa, gabapentin, opioids

frequently lead to cognitive impairment and hallucinations in the elderly population. For this reason, antimuscarinics should be avoided in patients older than 70 years. Furthermore, exposure to antimuscarinic drugs has been linked to a higher risk of developing freezing of gait in PD.

Depression is common in patients with PD, and often precedes the motor symptoms of PD. Selective serotonin reuptake inhibitors (SSRIs), serotonin-norepinephrine reuptake inhibitors (SNRIs), and other antidepressants including bupropion and tricyclic antidepressants are useful antidepressants. If insomnia is a problem for the patient, using an antidepressant that is also a soporific can be doubly advantageous: medications such as the tricyclic nortriptyline (which has fewer anticholinergic effects than amitriptyline) or an SNRI, such as low-dose mirtazapine, are good options. Recent data also suggest cognitive behavioral therapy (CBT) may improve PD depression more than existing medication-based approaches and can be delivered through telephone/virtual appointments.

Benzodiazepines including clonazepam are effective in reducing symptoms of dream enactment behavior attributable to rapid eye movement (REM) sleep behavior disorder (RBD). Nevertheless, they should be used with caution given their potential for cognitive side effects, increased risk of falls, rebound anxiety, and addictive potential.

Psychosis induced by levodopa and the dopamine agonists can usually be controlled by quetiapine and clozapine without worsening the parkinsonism. Other antipsychotic agents—be they typical or atypical neuroleptic mediations—are more likely to worsen the parkinsonism; therefore, they should be avoided. Clozapine is more effective than quetiapine, but because clozapine treatment requires weekly blood cell counts due to risk of agranulocytosis, low-dose quetiapine should be tried first.

Insomnia in PD requires a detailed history to distinguish specific causes of impaired sleep that may require different management approaches. Common causes of insomnia in PD include restless legs, persistent tremor, nocturnal akinesia, dream enactment behavior, bladder dysfunction, and early morning motor "off" symptoms or dystonia. Both sleep-onset insomnia and sleep-maintenance insomnia occur in PD, though sleep-maintenance insomnia may be more common and troublesome. Sleep-onset insomnia is treated conventionally with low doses of hypnotics and sedating antidepressants such as low-dose mirtazapine or trazodone. In demented patients, low nighttime doses of the atypical antipsychotic quetiapine may be useful if neurobehavioral disturbances occur at night. Sleep maintenance insomnia is due often to motor dysfunction. Bradykinesia with difficulty moving in bed or adjusting bedclothes is a common cause of sleep maintenance insomnia in PD. Levodopa has a relatively short serum half-life and a common experience is loss of levodopa effect in the middle of the night with worsening bradykinesia and nocturnal arousals. Medication schedule manipulations such as instituting or increasing a bedtime dose of levodopa may be useful. Similarly, use at bedtime of extended-release levodopa preparations, adjunctive agents that lengthen the levodopa half-life, or dopamine agonists that possess relatively long half-lives may ameliorate this form of sleep-maintenance insomnia. An additional common source of sleep-maintenance insomnia in more advanced PD is bladder dysfunction, which in men with PD may coexist with prostate enlargement. Specifically, autonomic dysfunction leading to urinary frequency, urgency, and incontinence is common in more advanced PD. Conventional approaches to treating bladder dysfunction may be useful. Nocturnal use of gabapentin can also be of benefit in some patients.

RBD is common in patients with PD, DLB, and MSA and often precedes the appearance of these disorders. RBD manifests with complex, nonstereotyped dream-enactment behavior and is usually associated with vivid or frightening dream content. Normally, dreaming in REM sleep is associated with muscle paralysis to all skeletal muscles outside of the eyes and diaphragm. This normal REM-associated muscle paralysis is reduced in RBD. RBD in PD, as in other settings, does not seem to cause daytime sleepiness but can result in injuries or disrupt bed partner rest. Infrequent and mild episodes of RBD probably do not require treatment but more severe episodes can be of dangerous to the bed partner or patient. Withdrawal of antidepressants that can precipitate or exacerbate RBD may be worthwhile. Safety measures within the sleeping room may be necessary. These can include use of separate beds, placement of mattresses on the floor, efforts to sleep on the first floor, and removing dangerous objects from the bedroom. The mainstay of medical treatment is use of hour-of-bedtime clonazepam (0.5–2 mg), which appears to be effective and is tolerated well by the majority of patients. Melatonin—though less effective—may be tried first and can be combined with clonazepam. In some patients, cholinesterase inhibitors may also help RBD symptoms. Dopaminergic therapy probably has little or no effect on RBD.

Periodic leg movements of sleep (PLMS) and restless legs syndrome (RLS) are estimated to be twice as common in PD as in matched populations. Despite this association, the relationship between PD and RLS is complex. While both RLS and PLMS may contribute to insomnia in PD, one study has shown no significant worsening in daytime sleepiness seen in PD patients with RLS compared to those without. No evidence exists that RLS predisposes patients to develop PD later in life. Though dopaminergic dysfunction may play a role in both PD and RLS, imaging studies of subjects with RLS without PD have not shown convincing evidence of a nigrostriatal dopaminergic deficit. These findings suggest that RLS may not in fact be a precursor to the cardinal motor symptoms of PD and may not be a "secondary" symptom of PD, but rather a separate disease entity that can be exacerbated by PD. Assessment and management of RLS in PD involve an evaluation for iron deficiency and iron supplementation when appropriate and use of low doses of dopaminergic agents such as long-acting dopamine agonists or L-dopa. In patients with poor or complicated responses to dopaminergic agents, gabapentin, clonazepam, or low-dose opiates may be useful.

Fatigue is an increasingly noted nonmotor symptom in PD of unclear etiology but has shown to be correlated with poor sleep and depression. Clinicians should attempt to differentiate fatigue from excessive daytime sleepiness, the latter of which is often due to poor quality of sleep at night or adverse effects associated with excess dopaminergic medications, necessitating a different approach to diagnostic work-up and management. Many patients describe fatigue as their first presenting symptom. Management should be aimed at underlying causes, such as depression. If needed, medications such as modafinil or nonprescription therapies such as liberalizing caffeine consumption can provide some benefit.

Mild cognitive symptoms can be seen in some PD patients with early disease and worsen with increasing disease duration. Early features typically include impaired attention, verbal memory, and executive dysfunction summarized as a subcortical-frontal syndrome. Dementia in PD is often associated with the development of significant visuospatial impairments, memory difficulties, and hallucinations—the latter of which may also be seen in response to dopaminergic or anticholinergic drugs. PDD and DLB patients are at a particularly high risk for developing delirium, either in association with new medications or because of underlying acute medical illnesses. Symptoms of delirium often involve profound disorientation and psychosis that can sometimes take weeks to resolve. Cholinergic deficits affecting subcortical and cortical structures are thought to play a significant role in PD cognitive impairment. Cholinesterase inhibitors, including donepezil and rivastigmine, are useful therapies for improving cognitive symptoms at all stages of PD. They are, however, limited in their efficacy due to limited central nervous system (CNS) bioavailability.

Orthostatic hypotension is common in PD and can be due to the disease itself or to dopaminergic medications, the latter of which lower blood pressure. It can also represent an early manifestation of an atypical parkinsonian condition, namely MSA. Fludrocortisone, midodrine, or droxidopa can overcome this symptom to some extent.

Constipation is common in PD. It may be further aggravated by anticholinergic medications. Besides changing dietary habits by increasing intake of more fiber and dried fruits, polypropylene glycol, or lubiprostone can be effective. For those who have bloating because of suppression of peristalsis when they are "off," keeping them "on" with levodopa can be beneficial.

Diet

There is emerging evidence that dietary pattern may modulate the course of PD, including at the prodromal level. A recent analysis of the Nurses' Health Study found that adherence to a Mediterranean diet was inversely associated with the presence of prodromal PD features, including constipation, excessive daytime sleepiness, and depression. Adherence to the Mediterranean diet is also associated with lower risk of PD. These studies are consistent with clinical research models highlighting the relevance of gut-brain axis functions in PD.

Exercise and Physical Activity

An active exercise program encourages patients to have ownership over their own care, allows muscle stretching and full range of joint mobility, increases aerobic capacity, muscle strength, motor skills, and improves a patient's mental attitude toward fighting the disease. Preclinical studies have shown that exercise slows the degeneration of dopamine neurons following local toxin, theoretically because exercise leads to an increase in brain neurotropic factors. There is also increasing evidence to suggest that sedentary behaviors, irrespective of the amount of formal exercise one performs, may have a deleterious impact on not only physical condition but also metabolic functions. These changes increase the risk for frailty among patients with PD subjects leading a decline in health. Encouraging patients to reduce the amount of time they spend seated each day is a good way to empower patients to regulate their own PD prognosis.

A regular routine of physical exercise, be it cardiovascular training or weight-based exercises, should be implemented as soon as the diagnosis is made, but is useful in all stages of disease. Stretching exercises may help to compensate for the tendency of patients to have a reduced range of motion. In moderate-to-advanced stages of PD, formal physical therapy is more valuable by keeping the joints from becoming frozen, and by providing guidance how best to remain independent in mobility, particularly with gait training and prevent injurious falls. One of the nonmotor symptoms of PD is the tendency toward apathy and conservative decision making with decreased motivation. Encouraging activity may help fight these symptoms.

Surgical Therapy

DBS surgery for PD was approved by the US FDA in 2002 and is associated with significant gains in quality of life for PD patients who are good surgical candidates. DBS surgery is typically indicated for PD patients with difficult-to-manage motor complications (fluctuations and/or dyskinesias) or with medication-refractory parkinsonian tremor. DBS involves placement of an impulse pulse generator (IPG) in the chest that looks much like a pacemaker. A lead from the IPG is tunneled under the skin surface to a specific region of the brain, either the STN or the GPi.

When stimulation is optimized, patients will experience an "on" state without disabling "off" features. Patients are also able to reduce their dose of dopaminergic medications, and in this way, are able to reduce dyskinesias as well. With the exception of tremor, motor features that generally do not improve with dopaminergic medications (eg, postural instability, other axial motor features, some gait freezing) also do not improve with DBS. DBS typically has little effect on the nonmotor features of PD unless they are directly related to on-off fluctuations seen with dopaminergic medications. Currently, DBS for PD is delivered in an "open loop" context, meaning that the type and intensity of stimulation delivered to each electrode is programmed and occurs constitutively once a stimulation paradigm is turned on in the IPG. The next important advance in DBS care will be the testing and validation of "closed loop" systems that can tailor stimulatory inputs to the brain based on DBS-detection of local neurophysiologic biomarkers that fluctuate in real-time depending on the neural correlates of relevant volitional movements.

Patients with significant speech, gait, depression with suicidal ideation or cognitive difficulties are usually not good candidates for DBS, not only because these symptoms do not respond to stimulation, but also because in some patients, these features may become notably worse after DBS, including the risk of suicide. The selection of appropriate candidates for DBS is often best done under the guidance of an experienced movement disorder neurologist. DBS is not suggested for patients with atypical parkinsonian conditions since the majority of these motor features do not respond to dopaminergic medications.

Focused ultrasound (FUS) was FDA-approved in 2018 for the treatment of parkinsonian tremor; it delivers a radiofrequency ablation to the STN and can be directed to other structures as well. FUS does not involve anesthesia and may be an appropriate therapy for those surgical candidates who cannot or do not wish to undergo conventional DBS surgery. One relative advantage is that unlike DBS, FUS does not necessitate future IPG replacements or frequent outpatient programming sessions. A disadvantage though is that FUS is permanent and nonprogrammable; compared to DBS, this limits FUS's ability to be titrated

to an individual's most disabling symptoms as the disease advances.

CARE CONSIDERATIONS

No two patients with PD are alike in their clinical presentation or their rate of disease progression. In addition, not all motor features of PD have the same clinical or prognostic significance. Gait and cognitive difficulties, for example, play a more significant role in patient autonomy, disease staging, and overall disability. Different motor phenotypes in PD have been distinguished, such as tremor-predominant or imbalance-predominant (so-called postural instability and gait difficulties [PIGD]) subtypes. PIGD features, however, tend to be less responsive to common medication strategies including dopaminergic therapies and can worsen at variable rates for reasons that appear to have little to do with dopaminergic neurotransmission.

There is an increasing body of literature implicating nondopaminergic or extranigral brain changes seen with aging as a mediator of disease progression in PD. Cerebral amyloid deposition and a decline in cerebrovascular integrity occur as part of brain aging. In individuals without PD, when these progressive changes exceed a critical threshold, patients who develop clinical symptoms are diagnosed with specific disorders including AD and vascular dementia. When these changes are milder, however, most people are able to use existing neuronal reserve to compensate and prevent the development of clinically significant disability. In PD, where the severe loss of striatal dopaminergic neurons is seen from the earliest stage of diagnosis, neuronal compensation mechanisms are relatively impaired, leading to the development of clinically significant disease features in the presence of even low levels of age-related comorbid brain pathologies (**Figure 61-2**). Longitudinal studies of PD have suggested that the severity of medical comorbidities is a chief determinant of progression to a disability, dementia, and death. For this reason, we recommend that all patients with PD attend carefully to common chronic medical conditions including cardiovascular risk factor reduction through physical exercise, appropriate diet, and medication management of comorbidities like hypertension and diabetes mellitus. The longitudinal role of a geriatrician or primary care doctor is hence indispensible for individuals with PD.

Recent data suggest that specialist care through a neurologist specifically is associated with reduced mortality in PD. Neurologists who are familiar with PD can be instrumental in making medication adjustments over time and can serve as an access point for newly approved medications and for DBS once patients have progressed from early-stage to mid-stage PD characterized by motor fluctuations. Multidisciplinary care models for delivering rehabilitative services have been trialed against standard physical therapy in carefully controlled settings and have been shown to improve quality of life. Home-based exercise programs have also been shown to improve off-state motor function

Pathologic stages of Parkinson disease

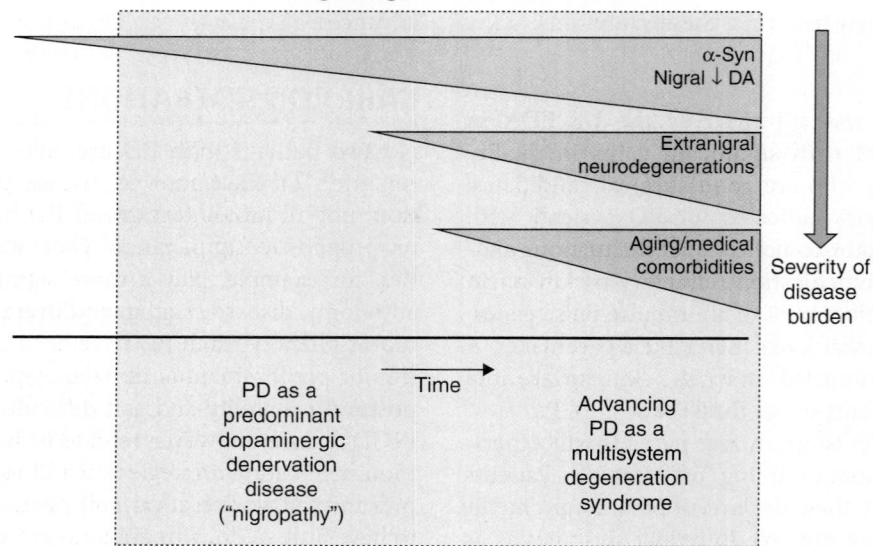

FIGURE 61-2. Schematic diagram depicting the natural history of progressive changes in Parkinson disease (PD) attributable to both dopaminergic and nondopaminergic ("extranigral") pathologies. With advancing disease duration, medical comorbidities and other neuropathologies exert additive/synergistic effects on overall motor and nonmotor disease burden in PD.

in PD in recent randomized trials. Developing reimbursement models to initiate, sustain, and broaden the impact of these clinical trial findings is an important priority for PD patients, advocates, and clinicians. Patients with late-stage PD or with significant disability from atypical parkinsonian conditions often benefit from consultations with palliative care physicians. This is particularly helpful for later-stage patients who are either confined to a wheelchair or who are considering nursing home placement because of inability to perform activities of daily living. Progressive dysphagia can be seen in some patients with advanced PD or atypical parkinsonian conditions and may necessitate a discussion about feeding tube placement. Discussing goals of care with patients at risk for loss of autonomy can empower patients to have control over a difficult disease.

CONCLUSION

Parkinsonian conditions including PD are common sources of disability in older individuals and are typically responsive to a wide variety of treatments. Longitudinal care with skilled geriatric and neurology providers is perhaps the most important step to ensure an individualized medical approach that prioritizes quality of life.

ACKNOWLEDGMENTS

We wish to thank Dr. Stanley Fahn, the previous author of this chapter.

FURTHER READING

Braak H, Ghebremedhin E, Rub U, Bratzke H, Del Tredici K. Stages in the development of Parkinson's disease-related pathology. *Cell Tissue Res*. 2004;318(1):121–134.

Chaudhuri KR, Healy DG, Schapira AH. Non-motor symptoms of Parkinsons disease: diagnosis and management. *Lancet Neurol*. 2006;5(3):235–245.

Cheng EM, Tonn S, Swain-Eng R, Factor SA, Weiner WJ, Bever CT Jr. Quality improvement in neurology: AAN Parkinson disease quality measures: report of the Quality Measurement and Reporting Subcommittee of the American Academy of Neurology. *Neurology*. 2010;75(22):2021–2027.

Dauer W, Przedborski S. Parkinson's disease: mechanisms and models. *Neuron*. 2003;39(6):889–909.

Deuschl G, Schade-Brittinger C, Krack P, et al. A randomized trial of deep-brain stimulation for Parkinson's disease. *N Engl J Med*. 2006;355(9):896–908.

Glimcher PW. Understanding dopamine and reinforcement learning: the dopamine reward prediction error hypothesis. *Proc Natl Acad Sci U S A*. 2011;108(suppl 3): 15647–15654.

Klein C, Schlossmacher MG. Parkinson disease, 10 years after its genetic revolution: multiple clues to a complex disorder. *Neurology*. 2007;69(22):2093–2104.

Krack P, Batir A, Van Blercom N, et al. Five-year follow-up of bilateral stimulation of the subthalamic nucleus in advanced Parkinson's disease. *N Engl J Med*. 2003; 349(20):1925–1934.

Langston JW. The Parkinson's complex: parkinsonism is just the tip of the iceberg. *Ann Neurol*. 2006;59(4):591–596.

Marras C, Lang A. Invited article: changing concepts in Parkinson disease: moving beyond the decade of the brain. *Neurology*. 2008;70(21):1996–2003.

Martínez-Fernández R, Máñez-Miró JU, Rodríguez-Rojas R, et al. Randomized trial of focused ultrasound subthalamotomy for Parkinson's disease. *N Engl J Med*. 2020;383:2501–2513.

Miyasaki JM, Shannon K, Voon V, et al. Practice parameter: evaluation and treatment of depression, psychosis, and dementia in Parkinson disease (an evidence-based review): report of the Quality Standards Subcommittee of the American Academy of Neurology. *Neurology*. 2006;66(7):996–1002.

Pahwa R, Factor SA, Lyons KE, et al. Practice parameter: treatment of Parkinson disease with motor fluctuations and dyskinesia (an evidence-based review): report of the Quality Standards Subcommittee of the American Academy of Neurology. *Neurology*. 2006;66(7):983–995.

Postuma RB, Gagnon JF, Montplaisir JY. REM sleep behavior disorder: from dreams to neurodegeneration. *Neurobiol Dis*. 2012;46(3):553–558.

Trinh J, Farrer M. Advances in the genetics of Parkinson disease. *Nat Rev Neurol*. 2013;9(8):445–454.

Williams-Gray CH, Mason SL, Evans JR, et al. The CamPaIGN study of Parkinson's disease: 10-year outlook in an incident population-based cohort. *J Neurol Neurosurg Psychiatry*. 2013;84(11):1258–1264.

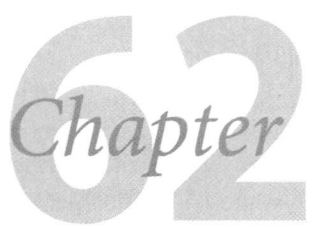

Chapter 62

Cerebrovascular Disease

Nirav R. Bhatt, Bernardo Liberato

Although stroke is the fifth leading cause of death in the United States, it remains the single most important cause of disability. Ischemic stroke and transient ischemic attack (TIA) are parts of the same spectrum, and their diagnosis usually implies inadequate blood flow to variable areas in the brain, brain stem, or cerebellum. Many varied pathologic processes lead to either occlusion of an extra- or intracranial artery or vein causing ischemic stroke or TIA, or rupture of an intracranial artery causing hemorrhagic stroke. A precise clinical diagnosis with appropriate localization strategies and determination of likely etiology are key to establishing appropriate treatment in the acute phase as well as planning the most adequate secondary prevention according to best practice and evidence available (**Figures 62-1** and **62-2**). This chapter focuses on identifying the pathology, clinical features, and treatment strategies that allow for the proper care of stroke victims, with a particular emphasis in the older population.

Learning Objectives

- Understand the pathophysiology and clinical presentations of different types of strokes, and specific symptoms and signs associated with the involvement of each major cerebral artery and location of infarction.

- Learn about the state-of-the-art neuroimaging techniques and other tests available to evaluate and diagnose stroke.

- Acquire latest information about the pharmacology, specific indications, and adverse effects of various drugs and surgical interventions available to treat different stages and types of strokes.

- Learn about the results of pivotal clinical trials forming the basis for latest guidelines to treat different types of strokes.

- Understand the rationale for various preventive strategies commonly used for different types of strokes.

EPIDEMIOLOGY

Stroke is a leading cause of mortality and morbidity in the United States. In 2018, according to statistics from the Centers for Disease Control and Prevention (CDC) and American Heart Association (AHA), one in every six deaths from cardiovascular disease (CVD) was due to stroke. In the United States, someone has a stroke every 40 seconds and every 4 minutes one death is due to a stroke. That burden is greater in the older population since stroke incidence and mortality increase with age which is reflected in the fact that approximately 66% of people hospitalized for a stroke will be 65 years or older. Stroke incidence becomes more evident in the aging population and its impact on greater longevity is demonstrated by the fact that 17% of all strokes will occur in patients 85 years and older. According to the AHA, stroke incidence is expected to more than double by 2050 with the greater increase in the population 75 years and older, underscoring the need for greater awareness and knowledge about stroke among those health professionals involved in the care of that group of patients. As in CVD in general, incidence by gender shows a predominance in men in the 60- to 79-year-old age group while women are slightly more affected in the 80 years and older age group.

Key Clinical Points

1. It is important to identify the pathophysiology in each stroke patient, as it drives selection of the best treatment choice.

2. Magnetic resonance imaging (MRI) brain scans with diffusion-weighted imaging (DWI) are the best way of identifying cerebral infarcts acutely and accurately. While computed tomography (CT) scan is less sensitive to detect recent infarcts of less than 12 hours, it is the initial method of choice in the hyperacute setting since most acute treatment decisions can be made based on its results.

3. Imaging of the cervical and cerebral large arterial system with CT angiography (CTA) or MR angiography (MRA) should be urgently performed to assess the arterial system. CTA offers the best resolution and suffices for acute decision making.

(Continued)

(Cont.)

4. Recombinant tissue plasminogen activator (rt-PA) initiated within 4.5 hours of symptom onset has been shown to reduce stroke-related disability. In general, benefits of rt-PA in older adults with stroke outweigh risks.

5. Mechanical thrombectomy for selected patients with large vessel occlusion is highly effective in reducing morbidity and mortality and is supported by Level Ia evidence.

6. Stroke carries a worse prognosis in older individuals overall; however, both intravenous rt-PA and mechanical thrombectomy have been found effective in this population and should be strongly considered when clinically appropriate.

7. Efficacy of carotid endarterectomy and carotid stenting for symptomatic disease with more than 70% stenosis is high and should be performed when clinically indicated. Clinical, demographic, and technical aspects should be considered when choosing the best method.

8. Oral anticoagulation is highly effective in preventing stroke in the setting of atrial fibrillation (AF) especially in the older population. Direct oral anticoagulants (DOACs) are used increasingly and present a better safety profile compared to warfarin.

9. Antiplatelet monotherapy continues to be the cornerstone for secondary prevention of noncardioembolic strokes, with dual antiplatelet therapy reserved for a short course in high-risk TIA/minor stroke. Dual antiplatelet therapy can also be considered in cases of strokes secondary to moderate to severe stenosis seen in intracranial atherosclerotic disease (ICAD).

Overall, prognosis is worse following a stroke in the older adults, and is associated with a higher risk-adjusted mortality, greater disability, longer hospitalization, and reduced chances of being discharged home after an admission to a hospital. However, despite an overall worse prognosis in older adults compared to younger age groups, more aggressive therapeutic and multitargeted secondary prevention strategies have resulted in more favorable stroke outcomes in the older population, including a decline in the crude stroke death rate. Importantly, these promising outcomes are seen across all older age groups including those 85 years and older.

ISCHEMIC STROKE OR TIA SUBTYPE

Pathophysiology and Clinical Presentation

It is important to recognize that ischemic stroke and TIA share the same pathological causation, such that efforts to define the underlying arterial pathophysiology of the ischemic stroke or TIA should be the focus of a treatment strategy. The term "cerebral vascular accident" or "CVA" should be discarded, and the terms "TIA" and "ischemic stroke" should be used with further characterization of the subtype of stroke according to its likely etiology, a definition that goes beyond nomenclature and carries implication when choosing the most appropriate therapeutic and prevention strategies. Despite more recent challenges to the classic etiologic categorization, in clinical practice, ischemic stroke/TIA can still be conveniently divided into five subtypes: (1) large artery atherosclerosis, including intra- and extracranial (25%); (2) small-vessel lacunar (25%); (3) cardioembolic (20%); (4) cryptogenic (25%); and (5) other (5%), such as arterial dissection, venous sinus occlusion, and arteritis. The prevalence of various ischemic strokes or TIA subtypes vary across different ethnic population groups. Specifically, African-Americans are at a relatively higher risk of having a lacunar stroke and atherothrombotic stroke, particularly that portion of atherothrombotic stroke caused by intracranial arterial atherosclerosis. Likewise, Asians have a higher frequency of intracranial arterial atherosclerotic disease. Conversely, extracranial atherosclerotic disease shows a predilection for Caucasians.

When transient or sustained focal neurologic symptoms or signs develop in a patient, history, general physical examination, and neurologic examination are important to diagnose stroke, localize the affected territory of the brain or spinal cord and the corresponding vascular distribution, and even suggest the pathophysiologic subtype. Strokes and TIAs require not only immediate imaging of the brain parenchyma but also noninvasive assessment of the extra- and intracranial arterial vasculature focusing on the arteries supplying the suspected symptomatic arterial territory. CT scan of the head is the neuroimaging modality of choice for the hyperacute evaluation of a suspected stroke, mostly to rule out other pathologies that could mimic an ischemic stroke, particularly hemorrhagic stroke. CT has nearly perfect sensitivity for acute intracerebral hemorrhage (ICH) (approaching 100%) and good sensitivity for acute subarachnoid hemorrhage (SAH) (~ 90%). Sensitivity for ischemic infarction in the acute setting is, however, much lower. Ischemic infarction may not be demonstrable by noncontrast CT for 12 to 14 hours after symptom onset. In addition, infarction involving only the cortical surface supratentorially, or infarction in the posterior fossa, can often be obscured by bone artifact. Therefore, the main reason for obtaining a head CT scan in the acute phase is to exclude intracranial hemorrhage and detect early signs of ischemia as well as define the extent of early ischemic changes. In the acute phase, vascular imaging, usually

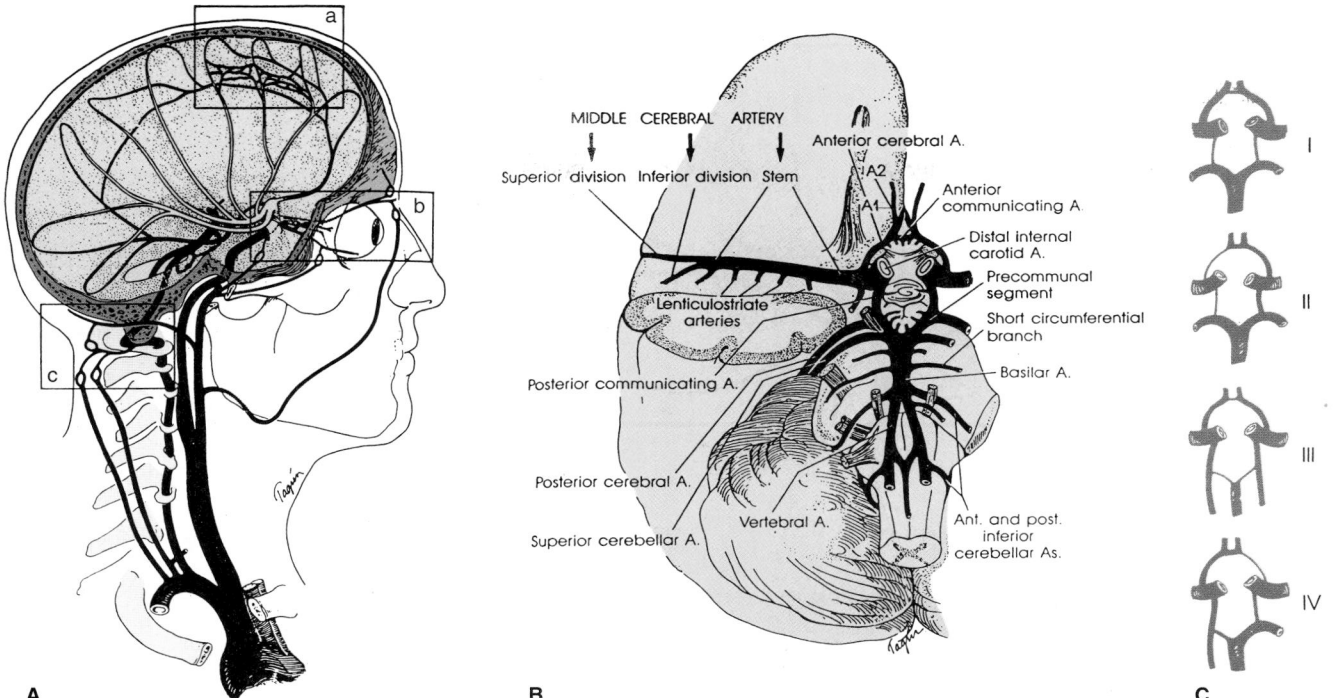

FIGURE 62-1. **A.** Arrangement of the major arteries of the right side carrying blood from the heart to the brain. Also shown are vessels of collateral circulation that may modify the effects of cerebral ischemia (a, b, and c). Not shown is the circle of Willis, which also provides a source for collateral circulation. *a.* The anastomotic channels between the distal branches of the anterior and middle cerebral artery, termed borderzone or watershed anastomotic channels. Note that they also occur between the posterior and middle cerebral arteries and the anterior and posterior cerebral arteries. *b.* The anastomotic channels occurring through the orbit between branches of the external carotid artery and ophthalmic branch of the ICA. *c.* Wholly extracranial anastomotic channels between the muscular branches of the ascending cervical arteries and muscular branches of the occipital artery that anastomose with the distal VA. Note that the occipital artery arises from the external carotid artery, thereby allowing reconstitution of flow in the vertebral from the carotid circulation. **B.** Diagram of the brain stem, cerebellum, inferior right frontal lobe, and temporal lobe transected. Principal branches of the vertebral basilar arterial system are pictured. Small branches of the vertebral and basilar artery that penetrate the medulla and pons are not pictured. The stem of the middle cerebral artery with its small, deep-penetrating lenticulostriate arteries and the circle of Willis with its small, deep-penetrating branches, are shown. **C.** Roman numerals I, II, III, and IV represent some of the possible variations of the circle of Willis caused by atresia of one or more of its arterial components. (A, Reproduced with permission from CM Fisher, MD.)

with CTA of head and neck, is mandatory to look for vessel pathology that could be responsible for the ischemic changes suggested by the neurological examination. Only with the precise knowledge of parent vessel pathology, or its absence, can therapy be properly considered. Also, given the well-defined role for mechanical thrombectomy (MT) in select patients with a large vessel occlusion (LVO) demonstrated on CTA, such imaging modality is essential part of the acute stroke evaluation. Even though MRI is the gold standard for identification of an ischemic stroke, its role in the hyperacute evaluation is limited given the longer examination time. Brain MRI, however, is indicated for most ischemic stroke patients early on after hospital admission, and other vascular imaging modalities that can be considered include a combination of MRA, carotid duplex ultrasound, and transcranial Doppler (TCD) (see **Figure 62-2**). A combination

of these imaging modalities is often necessary before a definite etiology can be determined and an appropriate preventive strategy can be devised. The following sections outline each of the four ischemic stroke and TIA subtypes, and intracerebral and SAH, in terms of their pathophysiologic process and clinical presentation. A discussion of a focused diagnostic approach to confirm that clinically presumed diagnosis follows. Based on the particular TIA or stroke subtype and its causative pathologic process, acute, subacute, and preventive management strategies can then be addressed.

Definition

The classical definition of a TIA is that of sudden focal neurological symptoms lasting less than 24 hours. This definition is purely a clinical one and does not take into consideration neuroimaging findings on MRI after an

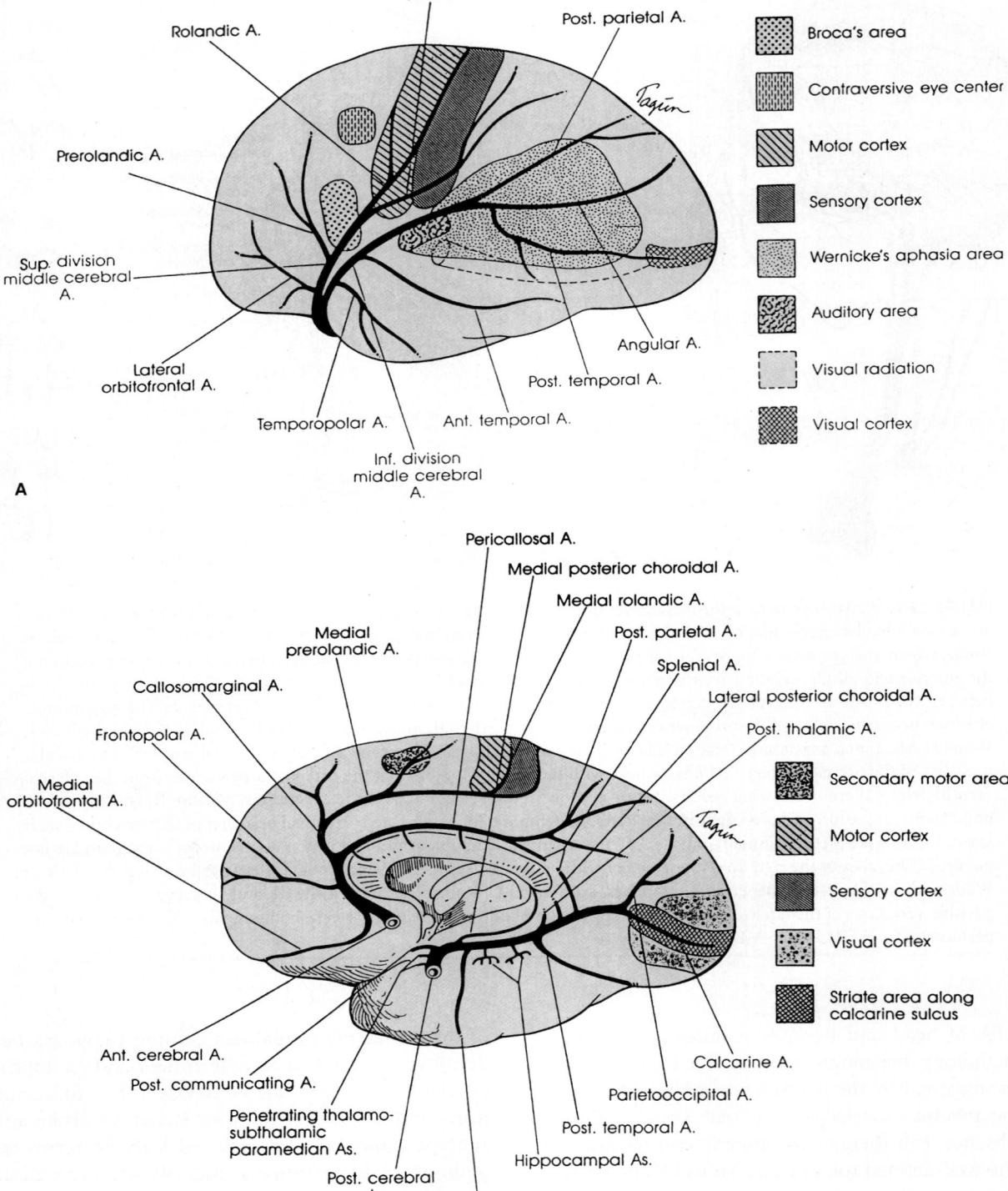

FIGURE 62-2. A. Diagram of a cerebral hemisphere, lateral aspect, showing the branches and distribution of the middle cerebral artery and the principal regions of cerebral localization. Note the bifurcation of the middle cerebral artery into a superior and inferior division. **B.** Diagram of a cerebral hemisphere, medial aspect, showing the branches and distribution of the anterior cerebral artery and the principal regions of cerebral localization. (Reproduced with permission from CM Fisher, MD.)

acute ischemic episode. The more complete definition establishes that if an acute focal neurological dysfunction shows an imaging correlate (DWI positivity on MRI) it is considered a stroke regardless of the persistence or not of the initial focal symptoms. In that case, it is called a minor stroke. For the majority of patients with persistent focal deficits beyond 24 hours (clinical stroke), neuroimaging will show a correlated lesion on MRI. The semantics do not carry great relevance for the diagnostic work-up for these patients since both a TIA and a stroke demand urgent and complete investigation. Its major importance lies in the fact that TIA or minor strokes carry an overall risk of about 10% for recurrent stroke in the following 90 days, the greatest risk being in the first 48 hours after its occurrence. This risk varies with the type of underlying vessel pathology, neuroimaging, and clinical features of the event. Based on clinical features, scales have been created to help stratify the short-term risk of recurrence of a TIA. The most commonly used scale is the ABCD2 scale where clinical features, when present, receive points and the sum of them will translate into higher risk of recurrence. The clinical features and the points assigned to each are as follows:

1. **A**ge > 60 years – 1 point
2. **B**lood pressure on presentation > 140/90 – 1 point
3. **C**linical features of the TIA—isolated speech (1 point), unilateral weakness (2 points)
4. **D**uration—< 10 min – 0 points; 10–59 min – 1 point; ≥ 60 min – 2 points
5. History of **D**iabetes—1 point

The sum of the points yields the final score and a score ≥ 4 represents an elevated risk for recurrence. This score was used in many acute prevention trials as criteria for enrolling patients (see below). The early time frame for highest recurrence risk underscores the need for urgent evaluation and implementation of therapeutic and preventive strategies after a TIA or minor stroke.

STROKE SUBTYPES

Large-vessel, atherothrombotic stroke/TIA subtype Atherothrombotic cerebral vascular disease accounts for approximately 25% of all ischemic strokes. To determine that a stroke is secondary to large-vessel atherosclerotic disease, it is required that the artery supplying the ischemic territory (extra- or intracranial) reveals a degree of vessel lumen stenosis > 50% of the normal lumen. It is divided into two categories according to the site of atherothrombotic involvement:

1. Extracranial atherosclerotic disease (ECAD)
2. Intracranial atherosclerotic disease (ICAD)

When considered as a group, atheromatous process commonly has a predilection for four extra- and

intracranial arterial locations (see **Figure 62-2**): (1) the internal carotid artery (ICA) origin, (2) the carotid siphon portion, (3) the middle cerebral artery stem, and (4) the vertebrobasilar junction. Although the origins of the common carotid and vertebral arteries (VA) also are sites of atheromatous disease, they are less often the cause of stroke or TIA. Atherosclerotic narrowing can also involve the proximal intracranial VA and origins of the posterior cerebral arteries (PCAs), but rarely involve the more distal branches of the cerebral and cerebellar arteries. At each of the sites of predilection, several mechanisms are possible and responsible for causing the stroke or TIA: (1) Embolism: thrombus forms on an atherothrombotic plaque and a piece of clot travels distally to occlude a more distal vessel. This is called an "artery-to-artery" embolus. (2) Thrombus propagation: this is less common, but if the thrombus propagates to occlude a distal vessel off the circle of Willis, large strokes can occur. (3) Hypoperfusion: the atherothrombotic process might occlude or narrow the vessel to such a degree that distal flow is diminished and not compensated via collateral flow through the circle of Willis. This low-flow state may result in border-zone infarctions where an area between the middle cerebral artery-anterior cerebral artery (MCA-ACA) or MCA-PCA territories is affected cortically or in the distal field of the lenticulostriate penetrating arteries, affecting the deep white matter.

In general, both artery-to-artery embolism and low-flow strokes occur when the vessel is narrowed to a degree that decreases pressure across the arterial segment. Low-flow stroke or TIA occurs less often from a cervical lesion because the circle of Willis can usually provide needed distal collateral circulation when a proximal stenosis becomes hemodynamically significant. Low-flow stroke or TIA occurs more often with atheromatous disease in the intracranial vasculature as this compromises the ability of the circle of Willis to provide sufficient collateral flow. In 70% of the population, the circle of Willis is incompetent, with one or more of the connecting arteries atretic or functionally inadequate (see **Figure 62-2**). In this circumstance, low-flow TIA or stroke may arise from atherothrombosis at the ICA origin or in its petrous or siphon portions.

a. ***Atherothrombotic disease of the anterior cerebral circulation (origin of the ICA, its major branches, and the common carotid artery)*** In the anterior circulation, atheroma occurs most often at the bifurcation of the common carotid artery (CCA), and usually begins on the posterior wall of the ICA origin.

- *Internal carotid artery*: Most often, atheroma at the origin of the ICA becomes symptomatic after it has narrowed the lumen to the point where the pressure begins to drop across the stenosis, allowing both embolic or low-flow ischemic TIA and stroke to occur. Embolism from thrombus forming in an ulcerated plaque may occur at 50% to 70% stenosis, but it is less common, and rarely occurs with lesser degrees of stenosis. Artery-to-artery embolism can also occur if the atheromatous process occludes the ICA origin forming a thrombus at the site. At times, the occluding thrombus may also propagate without embolization, reaching the ophthalmic artery origin and producing monocular blindness, or extending even more distally to the MCA origin and producing a devastating, full-territory stroke.

Low-flow symptoms caused by ICA origin stenosis are less common than artery-to-artery embolism, and occur only if two conditions exist: (1) the lesion has to be hemodynamically significant, that is, severe enough to provoke a drop in pressure across the lesion, (2) recruitment of the main collateral channels (circle of Willis and anastomotic connections between the external carotid artery and ophthalmic artery) is inadequate, leading to a low-pressure state either in the MCA or in one or both of the anterior cerebral arteries. If there is ICA occlusion and little distal collateral flow, then a complete middle cerebral syndrome may result. The PCA territory may also be vulnerable to low flow in the setting of carotid disease when this artery arises directly from the ICA, a variant called "fetal PCA" that is estimated to occur in up to 30% of the population. If the circle of Willis is complete, then occlusion of the ICA can be asymptomatic if it does not have an associated embolic or propagated thrombotic component.

The signs and symptoms of artery-to-artery embolism from the ICA are variable and depend on which intracranial branches are affected. The MCA, receiving majority of the blood flow originating from the ICA will be the most often affected but different symptoms can be the presentation of distal embolization, including from small emboli to the ipsilateral ophthalmic artery. In that case the symptom is called amaurosis fugax, in which a descending shade affecting the ipsilateral eye is usually described by the patient as a brief, usually self-limited phenomenon. In more extreme cases complete and persistent visual loss can occur, usually secondary to a central retinal artery occlusion (CRAO). This constitutes a neuro-ophthalmological emergency and should prompt emergent evaluation for the possibilities of an ipsilateral carotid disease either of atherosclerotic or inflammatory origin (giant cell arteritis [GCA]).

Atheromatous disease in the ICA siphon occurs less often but shares the same type of physiologic mechanisms for TIA and stroke as seen with atheromatous disease of the ICA origin. More proximal involvement, with CCA stenosis or occlusion, is much less common than ICA involvement and can present with similar symptoms.

- *MCA*: MCA territory symptoms can be divided into those involving the stem territory (M1 segment; see **Figure 62-2**) and those involving the superior or inferior territory divisions (M2 segments) or one of their cortical surface branches (see **Figures 62-1 and 62-2**). When the stem of the MCA is occluded (M1 occlusion), a complete MCA syndrome may occur. It produces a complete contralateral hemiplegia and sensory loss involving the face, arm, hand, leg, and foot. Gaze deviation toward the ischemic hemisphere occurs due to involvement of the frontal eye fields. Ischemia in the dominant hemisphere causes global or partial aphasia and ischemia of the nondominant hemisphere results in neglect (visuospatial and tactile) and anosognosia. The degree of cortical involvement, usually evident clinically by the presence of gaze deviation, aphasia, or neglect, depends on the level of occlusion and the degree of cortical surface collateral flow (see **Figure 62-1**). Smaller emboli cause single superior or inferior branch of the MCA syndromes, or partial branch syndromes. Superior division infarcts, typically present with either isolated contralateral weakness or isolated expressive aphasia or a combination of the two. Inferior division syndromes include difficulty with reading, writing, auditory comprehension of language, or fluent aphasic speech with no limb weakness. Paraphasic errors are common. Neglect of the left visual hemifield and extinction to double tactile stimulation are signs of cortical involvement seen most often in nondominant hemispheric syndromes but may also occur on the right with dominant syndromes.

- *Anterior cerebral artery (ACA)*: ACAs divide into two segments: A1 or stem, a part of the circle of Willis and A2 segment, distal to the anterior communicating artery (see **Figure 62-1**). The A1 segment gives rise to several deep penetrating arteries that supply the anterior limb of the internal capsule, the anterior perforated substance, portions of the anterior hypothalamus, and the posterior part of the head of the caudate nucleus. Infarction in these territories is more often caused by an embolus than by local atheromatous disease. ACA infarcts result predominantly in contralateral leg weakness with varying degrees of contralateral shoulder weakness. If the right and left A2 segments arise from a single anterior cerebral artery A1 segment due to contralateral hypoplastic A1 segment, a normal anatomic variant, an occlusion of this single A1 segment causes bilateral frontal lobe infarction resulting in bilateral leg weakness. Other symptoms of ACA infarcts include urinary incontinence, abulia, gait apraxia, and forced grasping of the hand.

- *Anterior choroidal artery (AChA)*: This artery arises from the ICA and supplies the posterior limb of the internal capsule and its adjacent white matter and medial temporal lobe, also supplying some geniculo-calcarine fibers. The complete clinical syndrome consists of contralateral hemiparesis, hemianesthesia, and hemianopia. However, because this territory is also supplied by penetrating vessels of the MCA stem and the posterior communicating and the posterior choroidal arteries, syndromes with minimal deficits can occur.

b. **Atherothrombotic disease of the posterior cerebral circulation: vertebrobasilar and posterior cerebral arteries and their branches** As seen in the anterior circulation, atherosclerosis has a predilection for certain parts of the posterior circulation—namely the proximal origins of the VA, which falls under the category of ECAD, the distal (intracranial) VA, the proximal to mid-basilar artery, and the proximal PCA, which fall under the category of ICAD (see **Figure 62-1**).

- *Vertebral and posterior inferior cerebellar artery*: An occlusion of the distal vertebral or its major branch, the posterior inferior cerebellar artery (PICA), may be caused by either atherothrombosis or by embolism from a proximal arterial source or the heart. VA dissection is another possibility. Atherothrombotic VA stroke is often heralded by TIA or minor stroke. Occlusion of either the VA or the PICA produces infarction in the lateral medulla, resulting in the lateral medullary (Wallenberg) syndrome. The symptoms and signs vary, but more commonly include vertigo, nausea and vomiting, hoarseness, dysphagia, ipsilateral facial numbness associated with impaired sensation of pain and temperature over the ipsilateral face and contralateral arm and leg, ipsilateral Horner syndrome, and ipsilateral limb ataxia. The PICA also supplies the posteroinferior cerebellum that may become infarcted if collateral circulation from the superior cerebellar artery (SCA) is inadequate. The infarct resulting from vertebral occlusion does not differ anatomically from that produced by PICA occlusion, except for a greater involvement of the restiform body (inferior cerebellar peduncle) in the latter. With moderate to large areas of cerebellar infarction, edema might occur and be fatal if not detected early and suboccipital craniectomy performed to relieve the mass effect on the brain stem.

- *Basilar artery*: TIA usually precedes atherothrombotic basilar artery occlusion and the consequent accompanying devastating brain stem infarction. The symptoms of a TIA in the territory of the distal vertebral and the basilar artery are more varied than in the carotid–middle cerebral territory because of the many different anatomic structures involved. Moreover, brain stem TIAs may be caused by disease of either of the small penetrating branches of the basilar or VA or disease of the basilar or VA

themselves. Penetrating branch disease may be due to atherothrombosis, involving the proximal origins of these small branch vessels, or lipohyalinosis, involving the small vessels deeper in the brain stem (see "Lacunar stroke/TIA subtype" later in this chapter). Therefore, when brain stem TIA or acute stroke occurs, it is extremely important to determine whether the problem lies in the basilar artery or in one of its smaller branches. Disease of a basilar branch produces unilateral infarction, whereas disease of the basilar artery itself usually causes bilateral infarction. Transient dizziness associated with diplopia, dysarthria, and numbness around the mouth strongly indicates the presence of basilar insufficiency. Other important symptoms occurring less often include a general profound feeling of weakness of the entire body, staggering, and/or a feeling of propulsion. Bilateral signs such as gaze paresis or internuclear ophthalmoplegia (INO) associated with ipsilateral sensory loss or weakness signify ischemic infarction in both sides of the pons, and therefore exclude single penetrating branch disease as the culprit.

Syndromes of unilateral brain stem infarction typically involve some combination of ipsilateral signs of the head and face, from involvement of cranial nerve nuclei or their fascicles, and contralateral motor and sensory signs in the limbs, from involvement of ipsilateral crossed long tracts, such as the corticospinal tract or spinothalamic tract respectively.

- *Major basilar branches—anterior inferior cerebellar artery (AICA), SCA, PCA*: These major branches of the basilar artery produce their own distinct pathophysiologic syndromes. They are most often caused by artery-to-artery embolism from an atherothrombotic source within the proximal basilar artery or the VA. An aortic or cardiogenic embolic source can be found, especially when the SCA is involved. Rarely, primary atherothrombotic stenosis or occlusion at their origins is the cause of the stroke or TIA.

- *SCA*: Occlusion of the SCA results in one or more of the following symptoms: ipsilateral cerebellar ataxia (caused by ischemia of the middle and/or superior cerebellar peduncle, or dentate nucleus); nausea and vomiting; dysarthria and contralateral loss of pain and temperature sensation over the extremities, body, and face (caused by ischemia of the spinal and trigeminal thalamic tract); and ataxic tremor or choreiform movements of the ipsilateral upper extremity. Ipsilateral Horner syndrome can be present. Partial syndromes occur frequently. Due to involvement of the cerebellar vermis, a pronounced truncal ataxia and gait impairment can be seen.

SCA territory infarction should prompt a thorough investigation for a potential embolic source.

- *Anterior inferior cerebellar artery (AICA)*: The territory it supplies usually includes the lateral midpons, middle cerebellar peduncle, cerebellum, and the labyrinth and cochlea. The principal symptoms may include ipsilateral deafness, facial weakness, vertigo, nausea, vomiting, nystagmus, tinnitus, cerebellar ataxia, Horner syndrome, and paresis of conjugate lateral gaze. Contralateral loss of pain and temperature sensation is also seen.

- *Paramedian and short circumferential branches of the basilar artery*: Occlusion of one of short circumferential branches of the basilar artery affects the lateral two-thirds of the pons and/or middle or superior cerebellar peduncle, whereas occlusion of one of the paramedian branches of the basilar artery affects a wedge-shaped area on either side of the medial pons. Many brain stem syndromes with cranial nerve abnormalities and crossed hemiplegia have been described.

- *PCA*: Arising from the bifurcation at the top of the basilar artery, each PCA divides into two segments: (1) P1 (proximal) segment, beginning at the top of the basilar artery and extending to the posterior communicating artery takeoff, with penetrating branches to the subthalamus, thalamus, and midbrain, (2) P2 segment, beginning at the posterior communicating artery takeoff, supplies the medial inferior temporal lobe and the medial occipital lobe. Twenty percent of the time, one or both of the right or left P1 segments are atretic and the P2 segment is supplied by the ICA via the posterior communicating artery. As discussed previously, this is referred to as a "fetal" PCA origin. The majority of ischemic syndromes result from embolism (artery-to-artery or cardiac) and less commonly atherothrombotic disease of the PCA.

- *P1 segment*: Syndromes are related to midbrain, subthalamic, and thalamic signs that vary depending on whether the embolus occludes the top of the basilar area, the right or left PCA proximal segment, or the penetrating artery branches that emerge from the proximal PCA. Top of the basilar artery occlusion results in the devastating syndrome of coma and quadriplegia, resulting from infarction of the reticular activating system and bilateral corticospinal tracts within the midbrain. Branch occlusions cause third nerve palsy and contralateral motor or sensory findings by involvement of the midbrain. The artery of Percheron is a normal anatomic variant in which a single large medial mesencephalic artery supplies both sides of the subthalamus and thalamus and part of the midbrain. Occlusion of this artery results in bilateral ptosis, paralysis of upgaze, and decreased consciousness, caused by involvement of both thalami and bilateral midbrain. When only a single penetrating artery territory is involved,

small-vessel lacunar disease results (see "Lacunar or Small-Vessel Disease" later in this chapter).

- *P2 segment*: Syndromes result from involvement of cortical branches to the medial inferior temporal lobe, giving rise to memory loss and delirium, and branches to the medial occipital lobe, giving rise to contralateral homonymous visual field defects. Distal field border zone ischemia of the PCAs and MCAs gives rise to visual impairment syndromes that include inability to recognize faces or pictures or to put items in a picture together to form an object (Balint syndrome).

Small-vessel, lacunar stroke/TIA subtype A lacunar infarct results from an occlusion of a small single penetrating artery arising from the circle of Willis, the middle cerebral stem, the basilar artery, or PCA and is defined as a small noncortical lesion measuring up to 1.5 to 2 cm in diameter. The cause is lipohyalinotic narrowing or occlusion in the mid- or distal part of the artery or atherothrombotic lesion at its origin; embolism is less often the cause. Lacunar strokes account for 25% of all ischemic strokes. These strokes cause recognizable clinical syndromes that evolve over hours to days, and may be preceded by transient symptoms (lacunar TIAs). The location of the ischemia determines the nature and severity of the symptoms. Recovery occurs often within days, but in some with especially strategically placed infarcts, significant disability is persistent and increasing age is associated with worse prognosis. Lacunar strokes are often asymptomatic but when multiple and recurrent are associated with more widespread white matter disease and an increased risk for cognitive decline and dementia.

The most common lacunar syndromes are the following:

- *Pure motor hemiparesis* is the most common lacunar stroke syndrome. It is usually from an infarct in the posterior limb of the internal capsule, corona radiata, or basis pontis. Less commonly, cerebral peduncle in the midbrain can be involved. The face, arm, leg, foot, and toes are equally paretic or plegic, but with no sensory deficit. The weakness may be intermittent (TIA), progress in a stepwise manner, or appear abruptly.

- *Pure sensory stroke* from an infarct in the ventrolateral thalamus. This type of infarct produces face, arm, and leg sensory involvement with numbness, tingling, and loss of pain and temperature. The patient generally recovers but often is left with an abnormal sensation. On rare occasions, an intolerable pain syndrome with dysesthesia occurs in the involved extremities some months afterward (Dejerine-Roussy syndrome).

- *Sensorimotor stroke* usually results from infarction between the thalamus and internal capsule and presents with contralateral weakness of face, arm, and leg as well as decreased sensation on the same side.

- *Ataxic hemiparesis* from an infarct usually in the basis pontis or the internal capsule. This results in contralateral weakness and ataxia.
- *Dysarthria—clumsy hand syndrome* caused by lacunar infarction of the genu of the internal capsule or, less frequently, the corona radiata or the paramedian rostral pons, with resulting mild contralateral arm ataxia or arm weakness, and dysarthric speech.

Cardioembolic stroke/TIA subtype Cardiomebolic strokes account for approximately 20% of all stroke subtypes and can reach twice this number in the older population. Despite the downtrend in stroke incidence worldwide, cardioembolic stroke incidence has tripled in the last few decades and is estimated to triple again in the next 30 years, possibly due to more extensive diagnostic evaluation. Many cardiac conditions predispose to stroke occurrence (**Table 62-1**).

On clinical grounds, it is usually diagnosed when a sudden deficit, reaching a peak soon after its onset, appears in the territory of a large intracranial artery or in one of its major branches, and the extra- or intracranial arterial supply to this ischemic territory zone does not have a significant stenotic or thrombotic occlusive lesion. In some cases, the embolic fragment may be seen, on imaging, to occlude the vessel or a distal branch. In other cases, the suspected embolic material is not visualized because it has already been dissolved by the endogenous fibrinolytic system, but not before significant ischemia has occurred.

The clinical presentations of embolism in the anterior and posterior cerebral circulation are similar to that of artery-to-artery embolism. The nature and severity of the symptoms depend entirely on the location of the embolic fragment occluding the artery and the spared collateral circulation to its cerebral territory. Which intracranial artery or arteries that get occluded will depend on the size of the embolic fragment and the extracranial artery it enters.

The radiological characteristics of an embolic infarction differ according to the size of the embolic material as well as the diameter of the artery affected. When a more proximal large artery is involved (such as the distal ICA or proximal MCA) a large area of ischemia, involving both deep and cortical structures, occurs. When the embolic material is smaller, it lodges in more distal branches and gives rise to the more typical embolic pattern of a cortically based, wedge-shaped ischemic lesion. The clinical suspicion together with the radiological appearance of a distal cortical-subcortical lesion should prompt a more aggressive investigation for a cardioembolic source such as a structural heart or aortic lesion or an atrial arrhythmia, even if clinically occult.

Many different heart conditions predispose to cardioembolic strokes (see **Table 62-1**), but AF is not only the most prevalent of these conditions but also the one with the best evidence-based treatment strategies. Estimated to affect more than 30 million people worldwide, it is associated with a three- to fivefold risk of stroke. Particularly relevant is its occurrence in the older population where, for individuals older than 65 years, its prevalence increases by 5% per year. Not only is it more prevalent with aging but the risk of stroke associated with it also increases in older adults, a notion emphasized by the fact that the proportion of ischemic strokes attributable to AF increases with age and can be as high as 40% in the oldest old age groups. The statistics of AF prevalence and stroke risk in the geriatric population should stress the importance of exhaustive search for AF in this age group, sometimes utilizing long-term rhythm monitoring strategies such as prolonged Holter monitoring or implantable rhythm monitoring device. In practical terms, the absence of an obvious etiology for an ischemic stroke, such as a lacunar or large vessel pattern, demands prolonged rhythm monitoring in the older population. With more studies demonstrating the effectiveness of prolonged rhythm monitoring strategies in detecting AF in stroke patients, it is also reasonable to consider such monitoring strategies in the older population, even when an alternative etiology is more immediately apparent.

Other conditions, even though less prevalent than AF, can represent high-risk conditions for embolic strokes and include congestive heart failure, recent myocardial infarction (MI) (both associated with left ventricular [LV] thrombus formation), complex aortic arch atheromas, valvular heart disease, and infective endocarditis.

TABLE 62-1 ■ EMBOLIC STROKE CLASSIFICATION

Cardiac source is definite: anticoagulant therapy generally considered standard of practice.
  Left ventricular thrombi
  Left atrial thrombi
  Rheumatic valvular disease
  Mechanical prosthetic valves
  Atrial fibrillation
  Nonbacterial thrombotic endocarditis

Cardiac source is definite: anticoagulation considered hazardous.
  Bacterial endocarditis
  Atrial myxoma

Cardiac source is possible: synonyms in the literature include "unknown source," "cryptogenic stroke"—these diagnoses are made by transthoracic or transesophageal echocardiogram.
  Mitral annular calcification
  Left ventricular dysfunction and dilated cardiomyopathy
  Postmyocardial infarction with or without left ventricular aneurysm or thrombi
  Left atrial spontaneous echo contrast
  Patent foramen ovale
  Atrioseptal aneurysm
  Valvular strands

Ascending aortic atheromatous disease: mobile plaque 4 mm or greater

Truly unknown-source embolic stroke.

Patent foramen ovale (PFO) is the consequence of failure of complete closure of the atrial septum primum and septum secundum immediately following birth, thereby leaving a communication between the right atrium and left atrium. PFO has been associated with stroke in epidemiologic studies, which indicate it is present in as many as 50% of patients with cryptogenic embolic stroke. Stroke may be more common in those with PFO because the atrial communication provides a channel by which a venous embolism can pass from the right to left side of the heart with the potential for subsequent cerebral embolism (so-called "paradoxical embolism"). Alternately, the PFO may itself be the source of thrombus formation with subsequent embolism. The PFO may be identified by transthoracic echocardiography with injection of agitated saline. Transesophageal echocardiography offers increased sensitivity. TCD ultrasound can also be used to detect the presence of right-to-left shunting by documenting the passage of agitated microbubbles into the cerebral circulation following a peripheral venous injection. It has equal or greater sensitivity than transthoracic echocardiography and can be used to guide the cardiac evaluation.

There is considerable controversy regarding the significance and therapeutic implications of PFO in stroke. PFOs are common and present in approximately 15% to 35% of the general population. After a thorough diagnostic work-up for stroke etiology, it is often difficult to determine if a PFO is related to the stroke or an "innocent bystander." If a PFO is identified, the patient should be screened for the presence of deep venous thrombosis (DVT), which would itself be an indication for a period of anticoagulation. PFO is likely more relevant in younger patients with few or no risk factors for stroke than in the older population, where other traditional cardiovascular risk factors make other stroke etiologies more likely.

Cryptogenic stroke In up to 30% of stroke patients, despite an extensive work-up, a causative etiology cannot be found, and the stroke is classified as cryptogenic. A minimally complete etiological work-up should include neuroimaging with CT or MRI, cervical and intracranial vessel imaging, and 24-hour heart rhythm monitoring. The absence of a clear etiology is more frequently seen in younger patients but can be seen in older individuals, even when multiple cardiovascular risk factors are present. Since a large-vessel stenotic atherosclerotic lesion and a lacunar pattern must be excluded, the majority of cryptogenic strokes will fall under the category of embolic stroke of undetermined source (ESUS). This most recent stroke subclassification acknowledges that many times cryptogenic strokes will appear indistinguishable from strokes from a known embolic source. Its radiological and clinical characteristics will be of an embolic looking stroke (above) with no obvious cardiac source of embolism. This entity is important not only because it is relatively frequent but because an even more extensive work-up in this group of patients often reveals an underlying cardioembolic source, namely atrial fibrillation. Studies have shown that in this group, after more prolonged heart rhythm monitoring (at least 6 months) with implantable monitoring devices, the prevalence of paroxysmal AF can be as high as 30%. Such results have obvious clinical significance given the superior protection that long-term oral anticoagulation offers for secondary prevention, when compared to antiplatelet therapy.

For the ESUS patients with no AF detected after months of continuous rhythm monitoring, the possibility that long-term anticoagulation might be more effective than antiplatelet therapy is being investigated by current studies where structural and electrical abnormalities of the left atrium (atrial cardiomyopathy) are considered as potential markers of increased embolic risk. Like AF, such a condition is more prevalent in older adults and likely predisposes to strokes. Results from such studies will help determine the best secondary prevention strategies for this group.

Other causes of cerebral infarction Although other causes of cerebral infarction account for only 5% of all ischemic strokes, they are extremely important because their precise pathophysiologic diagnosis can lead to effective treatment.

Dissection of the cervical cerebral arteries is the most common cause of stroke in this category subtype. A dissection is a tear in the arterial wall leading to intramural hematoma formation. A subintimal dissection occurs when an intramural hematoma is between the intima and the media layers and may lead to arterial narrowing and thrombus formation. A subadventitial dissection occurs when an intramural hematoma is between the media and the adventitia layers, and may lead to the formation of a dissecting aneurysm (sometimes referred to as pseudoaneurysm).

ICA dissections usually occur 2 cm distal to the carotid bifurcation near the base of the skull. VA dissections occur in the cervical transverse foramen but more commonly at the base of the skull, at the V3-V4 segments. Intracranial dissections are less common than cervical dissections and can lead to ischemic stroke and bleeding in the subarachnoid space. Trauma, either severe or trivial, are common causes of dissection, but Valsalva maneuvers associated with coughing and vomiting, weightlifting, contact sports, or chiropractic manipulations are other recognized associations. Spontaneous dissections, without a clear antecedent cause, are not uncommon. Dissections occur at all ages but tend to be less frequent in older individuals.

The most common symptom of arterial dissection is headache or neck pain. The clinical hallmark of carotid dissection is an ipsilateral Horner syndrome usually with unilateral cervical pain. Artery-to-artery embolism or low-flow syndromes occur, just as they do for atherothrombotic disease of the ICA. Similar pathophysiologic circumstances exist for VA dissections; with them, cervical spine pain and occipital headache are the suggestive symptoms. The most common site of infarction in vertebral dissection is the lateral medulla, with or without concomitant involvement of the PICA territory in the cerebellum. Dizziness, ataxia of gait, hiccups, nausea and vomiting with a unilateral Horner syndrome, and ipsilateral face numbness with contralateral body numbness are the hallmark symptoms (Wallenberg syndrome). Occasionally, diplopia and a hoarse voice are evident. Artery-to-artery emboli arising from a thrombus at the site of dissection in the VA may migrate to distal branches of the basilar artery, producing brain stem, cerebellar, or thalamic infarction. Sometimes spontaneous dissection can be seen in the context of underlying *fibromuscular dysplasia* (FMD), a noninflammatory, nonatherosclerotic vascular disease that can result in arterial stenosis, occlusion, aneurysm, or dissection. FMD most frequently involves the renal artery but can also involve the extracranial carotid and VA. It is usually seen in younger patients.

Vasculitis is inflammation of the blood vessels. There are numerous causes such as infection, malignancy, immune diseases, and drugs. Infectious vasculitis from bacterial or syphilitic infections is no longer a common cause of cerebral thrombosis. Infectious arteritis may rarely follow infection with varicella zoster virus (VZV), particularly if the ophthalmic division is involved, and is usually associated with involvement of larger caliber vessels. Cerebral arteritis may rarely accompany certain systemic vasculitides, including polyarteritis nodosa or Wegener granulomatosis. Necrotizing granulomatous arteritis, or primary angiitis of the central nervous system, involves the distal small branches (< 2 mm diameter) of the main intracranial arteries and produces small ischemic infarcts in the brain, optic nerve, and spinal cord. By definition, there is no systemic involvement. This rare disease is often relentlessly progressive. Presenting symptoms are varied and nonspecific, but headache is the most frequent complaint. MRI is frequently abnormal, but the findings are nonspecific. Findings include cortical and subcortical infarcts, parenchymal and leptomeningeal enhancement, subarachnoid and intraparenchymal hemorrhage, or mass lesions. Angiography can demonstrate areas of stenosis alternating with normal or dilated segments but both sensitivity and specificity are not ideal. Diagnosis of primary angiitis of the central nervous system can be difficult and typically requires either angiographic criteria be met or a tissue diagnosis.

Giant cell arteritis is a relatively common affliction of older persons, in which the external carotid system—particularly the temporal arteries—is the site of a subacute granulomatous infiltration with an exudate of lymphocytes, monocytes, neutrophilic leukocytes, and giant cells. The etiology of giant cell arteritis is not entirely clear, but it is likely secondary to multiple genetic and environmental factors with numerous infectious etiologies having been suspected in the past, including VZV. The pathogenesis is believed to involve an initial antigen-driven event that leads to the recruitment of T cells with subsequent inflammation potentially causing vascular damage and intimal hyperplasia, the result of which can cause stenosis or occlusion.

Clinically, the chief complaint is headache or jaw claudication. Systemic manifestations, through the release of inflammatory cytokines, can include fever, loss of weight, malaise, and polymyalgia rheumatica. Blindness of one or both eyes results from occlusion of the branches of the ophthalmic artery. Occasionally, an ophthalmoplegia caused by involvement of extrinsic ocular muscles occurs. In some cases, an arteritis of the aorta and its major branches, including the carotids, subclavian, coronary, and femoral arteries, has been found at postmortem examination. Significant inflammatory involvement of the intracranial arteries is rare, but strokes occur occasionally due to occlusion of the internal carotid, middle cerebral, or vertebral-basilar system with a predilection for affecting the latter.

Per the American College of Rheumatology, the diagnosis is made if three of the five following criteria are met: (1) age of onset is greater than 50, (2) new headache, (3) temporal artery abnormality (tenderness to palpation or decreased pulsation unrelated to arteriosclerosis of the cervical arteries), (4) elevated erythrocyte sedimentation rate (ESR) ($\geq$ 50 mm/h), and (5) abnormal findings on temporal artery biopsy. The hallmark neurologic symptom is transient monocular blindness, but ischemic stroke can rarely be the presenting feature. In older patients with new-onset headaches, especially if associated with visual complaints and/or ischemic stroke, high clinical suspicion warrants obtaining urgent ESR and C-reactive protein (CRP) levels.

Moyamoya disease is a poorly understood nonatherosclerotic occlusive disorder involving the progressive stenosis of large intracranial arteries, especially the distal ICA, the stem of the MCA, and the ACA. Even though being a disease predominantly seen in children and young adults, it can rarely be seen in adults older than 60 years.

Reversible cerebral vasoconstriction syndrome (RCVS) is a reversible angiopathy that presents with severe "thunderclap" headache, often recurrent, and fluctuating neurologic symptoms and signs as well as angiographic findings of alternating areas of constriction and dilation. It affects predominantly women in the fourth and fifth decades but has been reported in patients in their sixties and seventies. Brain imaging can be normal or show cerebral infarction, hemorrhage, or transient cerebral edema. The etiology is unknown. Eclampsia, the postpartum period, head injury, migraine, and sympathomimetic and SSRIs have all been associated with this entity. Conventional angiography is the gold standard for establishing the diagnosis although newer imaging techniques such as CTA and MRA are proving useful. Cerebrospinal fluid (CSF) is normal in most cases and this is one of the characteristics that helps distinguish this entity from primary angiitis of the central nervous system. The disease is self-limited, and, with adequate supportive care and withdrawal of the offending agent, partial or complete recovery occurs in most cases. The headaches and arterial vasoconstriction usually resolve within a few weeks.

Cerebral autosomal dominant arteriopathy with subcortical infarcts and leukoencephalopathy (CADASIL) is a rare primary arteriolopathy affecting small penetrating vessels to the basal ganglia, thalamus, and cerebral white matter. The disease is caused by a variety of mutations in the *Notch3* gene. The clinical presentation is varied, but there are five primary symptoms including late-onset migraine headaches with aura, subcortical ischemic strokes, mood disturbances, cognitive impairment, and apathy. It is part of the differential diagnosis of progressive cognitive impairment and diffuse matter after disease but is rarely seen in older adults.

Binswanger subcortical leukoencephalopathy, a rare cause of dementia, is a syndrome seen with advanced small-vessel hypertensive disease. Diffuse vascular lesions are seen in the subcortical layers of the cerebral hemispheres and there is widespread white matter demyelination. It usually affects individuals around 50 years and is characterized by fluctuations in mood and consciousness and perhaps even seizures. Dementia may be an early and prominent symptom preceded or accompanied by symptoms and signs of one or more small-vessel infarctions. Confusional states, memory difficulties, and abulia are prominent, and are sometimes accompanied by focal cortical-subcortical deficits such as aphasia, apraxia, or neglect. Focal neurologic deficits or uni- or bilateral limb signs may lead to a pseudobulbar state and gait difficulties are prominent. There is often evidence of vascular compromise in other body districts. Binswanger disease must be differentiated from disorders with prominent subcortical white matter involvement on CT or MRI such as hypertensive encephalopathy, cerebral amyloid angiopathy (CAA), and CADASIL.

Hematologic diseases such as acute and chronic leukemia, essential and secondary thrombocytosis, thrombocytopenia, and sickle cell disease can be complicated by ischemic or hemorrhagic stroke. Acquired hypercoagulable states, mainly with the detection of antiphospholipid antibodies can be part of the investigation of cryptogenic stroke in older patients while other hereditary conditions are more relevant in the investigation of stroke in the young. Cancer also increases the risk of hypercoagulability and hence ischemic stroke, and should be considered in older patients, especially when traditional stroke risk factors are absent.

Stroke can also occur during the course of a severe attack of migraine, especially migraine with aura ("migraine-induced stroke"). It is less often seen in the older population and is usually a diagnosis of exclusion, since other more common etiologies in that age group have to be considered and ruled out first.

EVALUATION

History, Physical Examination, and Initial Imaging Evaluation

The initial history and physical examination are the hallmark of the evaluation to obtain the pathophysiologic stroke or TIA subtype diagnosis. Urgent brain and vascular imaging must be performed in all patients. Noncontrast head CT, for most centers, is the initial imaging evaluation as it allows rapid exclusion of hemorrhage. While not sensitive enough to detect acute ischemic changes, especially small areas of infarction, in the first 12 hours after stroke, a head CT scan can answer the main questions in the acute setting such as:

1. Is there hemorrhage?
2. Is there an alternative diagnosis evident on initial imaging (tumor, abscess)?
3. Is the stroke already evident on initial imaging, and if so, how extensive is it?

Regarding the last question, part of the evaluation of the stroke characteristics on initial CT include estimating the extent of ischemic involvement mostly by determining areas of hypoattenuation and loss of gray-white matter differentiation. The ASPECTS scale (Alberta Stroke Program Early CT Score) is used to estimate extent of early ischemic changes and has been strongly related with prognosis. It divides the MCA-distribution territory in 10 different areas and subtracts 1 point for each area affected. A score < 6 is generally associated with a worse prognosis and is often used as a cutoff for guiding acute interventional therapies. However, it is not a strict rule and individual case-by-case decisions are still warranted when considering acute revascularization strategies in daily practice. Besides analysis of parenchymal involvement on noncontrast CT, acute vessel imaging with CT angiogram of the head and neck should be part of the acute stroke evaluation. Knowing the anatomy of intra- and extracranial vessels as well as presence and location of a LVO is critical information in the acute decision-making process. CT Perfusion (CTP) is also part of the same radiological armamentarium, and many times provides key information on tissue viability, especially in patients who present in an extended time window from stroke onset and might still be candidates for acute intervention (MT). Details of this modality can be found elsewhere but it consists of a CT scan modality in which a contrast bolus is tracked, by serial scanning, as it passes through the tissue and the results deconvoluted into a map of perfusion times. In practical terms, the critical information one looks for when obtaining a CTP in an acute stroke is whether there is still viable tissue (ischemic penumbra) that can potentially be saved by recanalization strategies (see below). For the reasons above, the information provided by CT or CTA (and in some cases CTP) is usually fast and reliable and in most cases will suffice to help determine eligibility for acute treatment, either intravenous thrombolysis (IVT) or MT (see below).

Despite a greater accuracy for detecting acute ischemic stroke changes, MRI of the head is less practical in the hyperacute setting and is usually reserved for completion of stroke evaluation at a later time or when a challenging case demands more information for the acute decision-making process. In patients who are not candidates for acute intervention, a more complete diagnostic work-up should be initiated. MRI of the brain with diffusion-weighted imaging (DWI) is the best way of identifying cerebral infarcts acutely and accurately. Susceptibility sequences identify subacute hemorrhagic infarcts and small areas of chronic hemorrhage (microbleeds) that might be associated with small-vessel diseases such as amyloid angiopathy or hypertensive vasculopathy. MRI is far more sensitive than CT scan not only for detecting infarction at different stages but also for identifying other pathologies that can mimic an acute stroke clinically such as brain tumor, abscess, and demyelinating/inflammatory lesions. MRI also has a high sensitivity and specificity for the detection of hemorrhage. Determining the location and pattern of ischemia on MRI is the first step in determining the most likely stroke etiology.

Imaging of the cervical and cerebral large arterial system with CTA, MRA, or carotid duplex and TCD ultrasound are modalities used for determining the vessel anatomy and its associated pathology. If done in the acute setting, CTA of the head and neck is usually sufficient and other modalities can be reserved for inconclusive studies or when administration of intravenous iodinated contrast is to be avoided. MRA of the head and neck does not offer the same anatomical resolution of the arterial system as conventional transfemoral angiography or CT angiography. MR perfusion-weighted imaging can, in an analogous way to CT perfusion imaging, identify areas of perfusion delay that indicate tissue at risk of progression to infarction.

Neurosonology tests include carotid duplex ultrasound and TCD assessment of the extra- and intracranial arterial system, respectively. Carotid duplex Doppler assesses flow in the CCA, its bifurcation, and the internal and external carotid arteries. In addition, flow in the middle portion of the VA is typically assessed to identify more proximal or distal obstructive lesions. TCD allows assessment of flow in the intracranial carotid artery and the ophthalmic artery through the transorbital approach. The transtemporal approach permits assessment of flow in the middle, anterior, and PCA stems. The occipital foramen magnum approach allows determination of flow in the distal VA and in the proximal and mid sections of the basilar artery. These tests have the advantage of being simple, noninvasive, and portable. Neurosonology tests can be used to follow the progression of the arterial pathology subacutely and chronically. Detection of microbubbles after injection of agitated saline is also helpful in detecting evidence of right to left shunt as seen in the presence of PFO. Prolonged monitoring with emboli detection and study of cerebral vasoreactivity are examples of the clinical utility of TCD in the etiological evaluation of ischemic strokes. The quantification of carotid artery atheromatous disease and its progression is an especially important use of carotid duplex combined with TCD.

Laboratory Evaluation

After completion of all acute neuroimaging modalities, the initial blood work should include the standard complete blood count, basic coagulation studies, and general chemistry examination. Checking a fasting lipid panel and screening for diabetes with hemoglobin A_{1c} should also be performed for stroke risk factor modification. Special clotting studies are not essential, but are often useful when a hypercoagulable state is suspected, mostly in younger patients. In the majority of older patients an extensive hypercoagulable panel is usually not warranted. The screen of thyroid function with a thyroid-stimulating hormone has helped us in identifying clinically inapparent hyperthyroidism, a condition that may be associated with AF or hyperlipidemia. ESR should be considered in the older population, especially when other risk factors are missing and there is suspicion of GCA or endocarditis as the cause of the stroke.

Cardiac evaluation In addition to obtaining a baseline electrocardiogram, cardiac echocardiography and cardiac rhythm monitoring should be performed, especially when a cardiac embolism is considered in the differential diagnosis. In practical terms, unless there is an obvious causative etiology identified (lacunar or large artery atherosclerosis), given the high prevalence of AF in the older population, cardiac rhythm monitoring should always be considered in this patient population. Outpatient prolonged cardiac rhythm monitoring, ideally with an implantable loop recorder device, is very helpful if AF or other cardiogenic arrhythmias are considered and is now standard of care to look for AF in cases of suspected cardiac embolism. The suggested duration of monitoring is usually for 6 months at least, or until paroxysmal AF is identified.

Therapeutic Strategies for Acute Ischemic Stroke

With the acute onset of neurologic deficits secondary to cerebral ischemia, the goal is to facilitate or reestablish blood flow to the ischemic zone. The therapeutic strategy should always be guided by the ischemic stroke pathophysiology and mechanism, whether presumed (history and physical examination) or confirmed (history, physical examination, and diagnostic data including neuroimaging, echocardiography, heart rhythm monitoring, and laboratory testing). The diagnosis should include not only the ischemic stroke or TIA subtypes noted earlier, but also the presence or absence of pathology in the parent vessel supplying the ischemic zone and the extent of the spared collateral flow to it. The time of onset to treatment determines the therapeutic options available, which typically include (1) acute reperfusion therapies, (2) early stroke prevention strategies, and (3) long-term stroke prevention strategies.

After the pathophysiologic diagnosis has been determined and the patient has been evaluated for therapies designed to facilitate or reestablish cerebral perfusion and prevent subsequent strokes, further management efforts

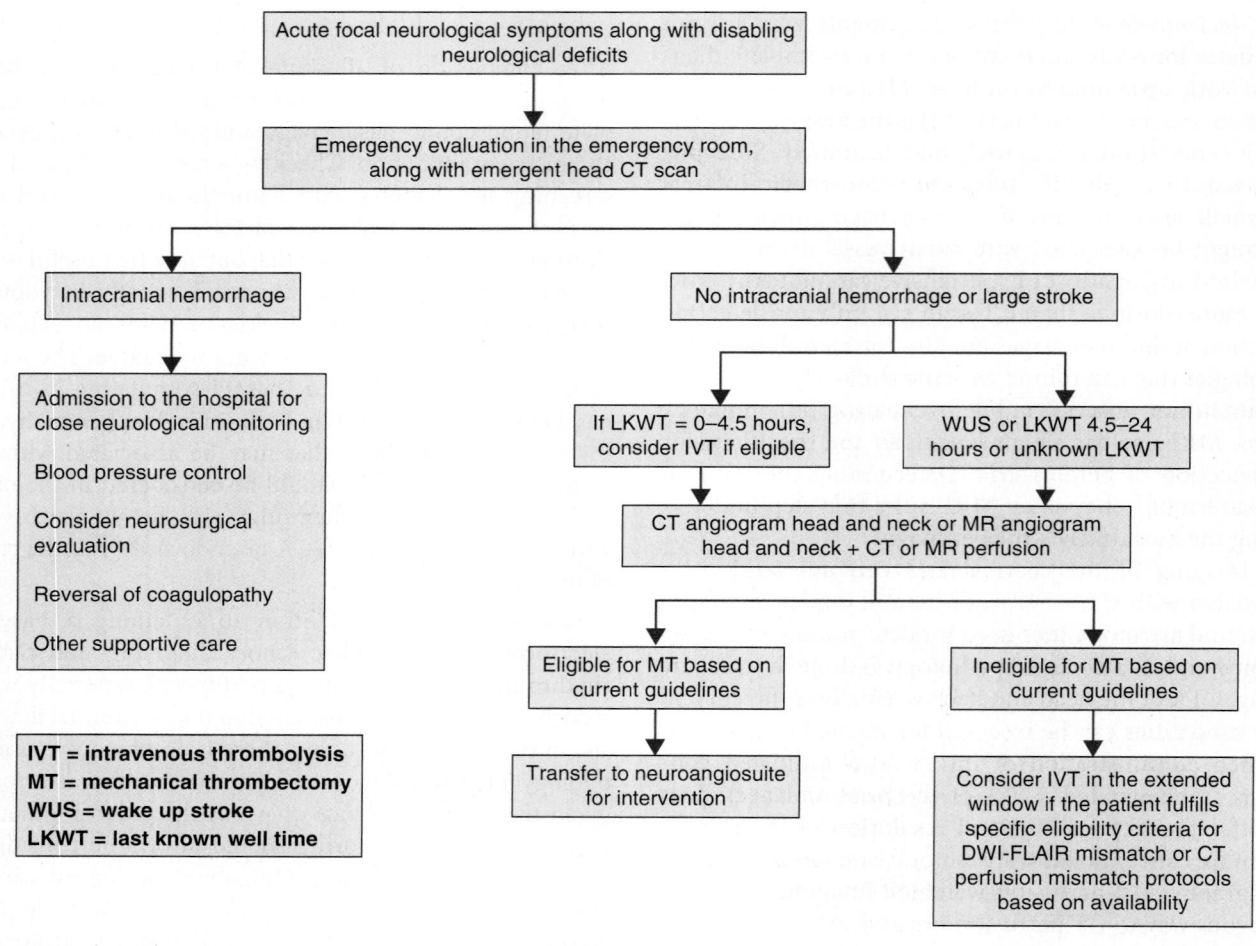

FIGURE 62-3. Algorithm for acute stroke treatment strategies.

are directed at preventing common complications, such as DVT and aspiration pneumonia, and assisting with neurologic recovery through rehabilitation.

Acute reperfusion therapies Within the first few hours of cerebral ischemia, rapid restoration of blood flow to the affected area is the cornerstone of acute stroke treatment, and this goal is achieved by either pharmacological treatment with IVT or mechanical clot removal via endovascular thrombectomy (EVT) or MT (see **Figure 62-3**).

Intravenous Thrombolysis For patients in whom treatment can be initiated within 3 hours of symptom onset, IVT with alteplase, at a dose of 0.9 mg/kg with 10% given as an immediate bolus and the remainder infused over 1 hour, has been shown to reduce stroke-related disability. In the pivotal National Institute of Neurological Disorders and Stroke (NINDS) rt-PA Stroke trial, patients treated with IVT had a 12% greater absolute chance of a good outcome, defined as minimal or no stroke-related disability. This benefit was present despite a 6% risk of symptomatic intracranial hemorrhage (sICH) in the IVT group, of which more than half were fatal. Posthoc analysis of the trial did

not show statistical evidence that the treatment effect varied by presumed stroke subtype, although the power to detect differences was modest. Subsequently, a trial of IVT given to patients with acute ischemic stroke within 3 to 4.5 hours showed a significant benefit of IVT as compared to placebo. In this study, the European Cooperative Acute Stroke Study (ECASS) III, the mean time to administration of rt-PA was 3 hours 59 minutes. Patients receiving IVT had a 7.2% absolute chance of a better outcome, defined as a modified Rankin score of 0 or 1 at 90 days. Mortality did not differ between the two groups. The rate of any intracranial hemorrhage was, as expected, higher in the IVT group (27% vs 17.6%) as was the rate of sICH (2.4% vs 0.3%), though lower than in the NINDS rt-PA trial. It is important to note that in ECASS III patients were excluded if older than age 80, if they had a severe stroke, or if they had a history of previous stroke and diabetes mellitus. However, updated AHA/ASA guidelines for acute stroke treatment cite a careful assessment of the published evidence to indicate that these exclusion criteria may not always be justified in clinical practice and recommend a detailed evaluation of individual risks versus benefits of IVT among patients presenting in the 3- to 4.5-hour time window. Further, both in NINDS and in ECASS III, the earlier the patients received IVT, the better were their outcomes. Therefore, it is of utmost importance to initiate thrombolytic therapy in patients with acute ischemic stroke as soon as possible, that is, aiming for shorter "door-to-needle" times.

Extended-window IVT: About 20% strokes occur during sleep, but a witnessed last-known-well (LKW) time of > 4.5 hours in these patients would disqualify them from receiving IVT due to the uncertainty regarding the true onset of stroke symptoms. Several studies have shown that a significant proportion of these patients suffer stroke symptoms in the early morning hours just before waking up because of the circadian fluctuations in blood pressure, heart rate, hemostatic processes, and occurrence of AF. Various neuroimaging modalities such as MRI (DWI-FLAIR Mismatch), CT perfusion, and MRI perfusion studies have been recently shown to reliably identify patients who may benefit from acute reperfusion therapies. The concept of DWI-FLAIR mismatch, that is, presence of an acute ischemic lesion on DWI in the absence of a hyperintense lesion on FLAIR serving as a surrogate marker of time elapsed since the actual onset of stroke symptoms has been recently evaluated in a randomized trial of MRI-guided intravenous thrombolysis in stroke patients with unknown time of symptom onset (WAKE-UP). The basis of this clinical trial was a proposition supported by previous studies that DWI-FLAIR mismatch on an MRI was reliably able to identify a majority of the patients whose stroke symptoms started within the preceding 4.5 hours. The trial included patients who presented with a new stroke, were LKW more than 4.5 hours earlier, had no thrombectomy planned, fulfilled the prespecified imaging criteria (DWI-FLAIR mismatch), and in whom treatment with IV alteplase could be initiated within 4.5 hours of symptom recognition. The trial was terminated prematurely owing to cessation of funding after the enrolment of 503 out of 800 patients and showed an excellent outcome in 53.3% patients receiving MRI-guided thrombolysis versus 41.8% in the control arm ($p = 0.02$). Alteplase was associated with a nonsignificantly higher risk of sICH (2% vs 0.4%, $p = 0.15$) and a nonsignificantly higher mortality at 90 days (4.1% vs 1.2%). Of note, the majority of the patients treated had mild to moderately disabling stroke with a median NIHSS of 6.

In acute ischemic stroke, there is a core of irreversibly damaged tissue surrounded by an ischemic penumbra representing potentially salvageable tissue, provided normal blood circulation within that tissue is rapidly restored (discussed later in this section). Studies have shown that a CT-perfusion or an MRI-perfusion study is able to identify the core and penumbra to a reliable extent, often represented as core/perfusion mismatch. The Thrombolysis Guided by Perfusion Imaging up to 9 Hours after Onset of Stroke (EXTEND) trial compared alteplase with placebo in patients presenting between 4.5 and 9 hours after stroke onset, or after awakening with stroke (if within 9 hours

from the midpoint of sleep), using predetermined CT or MRI core/perfusion mismatch criteria to select patients. After 225 of a planned 310 patients had been enrolled, the study was terminated because of a loss of equipoise after the publication of the WAKE-UP trial. This trial showed that alteplase was associated with an excellent 90-day outcome in 35.4% patients as compared to 29.5% patients receiving placebo (adjusted odds ratio 1.44, 95% CI 1.01–2.06, $p = 0.04$). The risk of sICH was higher in the alteplase group, 6.2% versus 0.9% (adjusted risk ratio 7.22, 95% CI 0.97–53.53, $p = 0.053$). The 90-day mortality was similar between the alteplase (11.7%) and placebo (8.9%) groups (adjusted risk ratio 1.17; 95% CI 0.57–2.40; $p = 0.67$). The publication of these trials among other studies has contributed to the expansion of IVT eligibility in a subset of acute stroke patients in whom the time they were LKW was either unknown or more than 4.5 hours prior to waking up with stroke symptoms, depending upon the center they are treated at and the resources available at that center. One limitation of the MRI-based approach is that it requires immediate access to an MRI scanner and collateral information from the patient/family members to establish MRI safety (absence of ICD/pacemakers or metallic prosthesis in the patient's body). On the other hand, a CT-perfusion-based approach requires access to an automated software that enables rapid calculation of ischemic core and penumbra estimates. Moreover, in both these trials, there were a substantial proportion of patients with a LVO who may have qualified for MT based on the updates from two novel endovascular trials that were subsequently published (discussed later in this section). These limitations have restricted the widespread adoption of these approaches depending upon the region, access to care, and resources available, but they may remain reasonable options for a select subgroup of acute stroke patients. The 2019 updates for the early management of acute ischemic stroke published by the AHA/ASA suggest the MRI-based approach (DWI-FLAIR mismatch) for IVT as a reasonable choice for a carefully selected group of acute ischemic stroke patients in the extended time window.

Because of the risks of hemorrhage, the decision to administer IVT should be based on an individual assessment of the benefits and risks for the specific individual, with careful attention to the treatment inclusion and exclusion criteria. Patients with acute disabling neurological deficits without hemorrhage or established infarct on initial head CT should be considered for IVT. Exclusion criteria must be reviewed carefully prior to IV rt-PA administration. An important concept to understand is the disabling nature of the neurological symptoms at presentation. A phase IIIb, double-blind, multicenter study to evaluate the efficacy and safety of alteplase in patients with mild stroke, rapidly improving symptoms, and minor neurologic deficits (the PRISMS trial) tested the efficacy of IV alteplase versus aspirin for emergent stroke with presenting symptoms that were deemed to be nondisabling in nature by the treating physician. Of a planned 948 patients, the trial was able to recruit 313 patients and failed to show a benefit of IV alteplase over aspirin, and consequently the current AHA/ASA guidelines recommend against IVT administration among patients who do not have presenting neurological deficits that would interfere with their daily lives. There has been concern about treatment of older adults because age may be a risk factor for IVT-related hemorrhage; however, the NINDS trial data show that this increased risk does not outweigh the potential benefit in older persons.

Although the rate of sICH after IVT is relatively low, it remains the most feared and sometimes fatal complication of this treatment. Rapid identification and administration of procoagulant factors such as cryoprecipitate or prothrombin complex concentrates (PCC) or tranexamic acid (or a combination of these aforementioned options) along with the provision of neurosurgical and hematological consultations under the care of experienced neurocritical care teams form the mainstay of management of sICH after IVT administration.

More recently, tenecteplase (TNK) instead of alteplase as the thrombolytic agent in acute ischemic stroke has been gaining some traction among the vascular neurology community. TNK is a recombinant tissue plasminogen activator like alteplase but exhibits a higher degree of fibrin specificity and a longer half-life that allows for a single bolus dose administration. Preliminary studies have shown that it is at least comparable, and in some situations, could be more effective than alteplase for acute ischemic stroke. Consequently, many centers worldwide are beginning to offer TNK as an alternative to alteplase as more evidence is awaited.

Mechanical thrombectomy EVT with thrombolytics/thrombus retrieval devices had been studied over the past two decades over many studies without much success in clinical outcomes. But, in 2015, several pivotal randomized clinical trials established an overwhelming benefit of EVT/MT in treatment of patients with acute ischemic stroke and a LVO who fulfilled certain criteria, establishing this treatment as a standard-of-care for this patient population. The reasons for such tremendous success of the newer trials were thought to be related to their better patient selection criteria and utilization of more effective reperfusion devices. The exact details differ among these trials, but overall, there were many common features that contributed to the success of these studies and EVT/MT, in general. First, all these trials required the presence of a LVO defined as an occlusion of the intracranial segment of the ICA or proximal segment of the middle cerebral artery (MCA), denoted by M1. The more distal blood vessels are denoted by M2, M3, and so on. Very few patients harbored an occlusion of M2 in these trials and none had more distal occlusions. Second, all trials except MR CLEAN (Multicenter Randomized Clinical trial of Endovascular treatment for Acute ischemic stroke in the Netherlands) required evidence of

absence of severe ischemic changes in the affected brain tissue on a noncontrast CT scan represented by an Alberta Stroke Program Early CT Score (ASPECTS), and although MR CLEAN did not have these requirements in the study entry criteria, it recruited very few patients who had evidence of advanced ischemic changes. Third, all trials encouraged rapid attempt at recanalization, and while most of the trials implemented 0- to 6-hour time window since LKW for study entry, ESCAPE (endovascular treatment for small core and anterior circulation proximal occlusion with emphasis on minimizing CT to recanalization times) and REVASCAT (randomized trial of revascularization with Solitaire FR device versus best medical therapy in the treatment of acute stroke due to anterior circulation LVO presenting within 8 hours of symptom onset) proved the benefit of MT in patients up to 8 hours from symptom onset. Fourth, for the majority of the patients, MT was carried out using the second-generation stent retriever devices. In this procedure, a catheter is advanced into an artery, and using fluoroscopic guidance, a stent retriever is inserted into the catheter. The stent reaches past the clot, expands to stretch the walls of the artery, and is retrieved, removing the clot. Finally, these trials required the patients to have decent baseline level of functioning for them to be able to participate. This allowed for adequate participation in the rehabilitation therapies following the thrombectomy procedure and promoted neurological recovery among the treated patients. A meta-analysis combining data from 1287 patients from five of these pivotal trials showed that the rate of successful recanalization among patients undergoing MT was 71%. Patients who underwent MT had a higher likelihood of achieving good 90-day clinical outcome with return to functional independence, 46% versus only 26.5% in the control group. Finally, the number needed to treat for one patient to have reduced disability was found to be 2.6, thus confirming the highly effective nature of MT as a treatment for anterior circulation LVO among acute ischemic stroke patients with disabling symptoms and who were LKW within 8 hours. Moreover, this benefit persisted across all age groups, even octogenarians, and although the overall mortality remained lower in the intervention group (15.3% versus 18.9% in the control group), this difference was not shown to be statistically significant.

The penumbra concept for patient selection: An intracranial occlusion causing complete cessation of blood flow to brain tissue it supplies renders that tissue at risk of irreversible damage. The larger the area supplied by this occluded vessel, the larger the tissue is at risk and while intracranial and extracranial collateral circulation may help compensate for some of the lack of blood flow, as time passes, even the collateral circulation runs the risk of failing, thereby causing irreversible tissue injury. Moreover, the normal average blood flow is about 50 mL/100 g/min. When this flow drops to 20 to 30 mL/100 g/min, there is a selective loss of neuronal functions with electrical

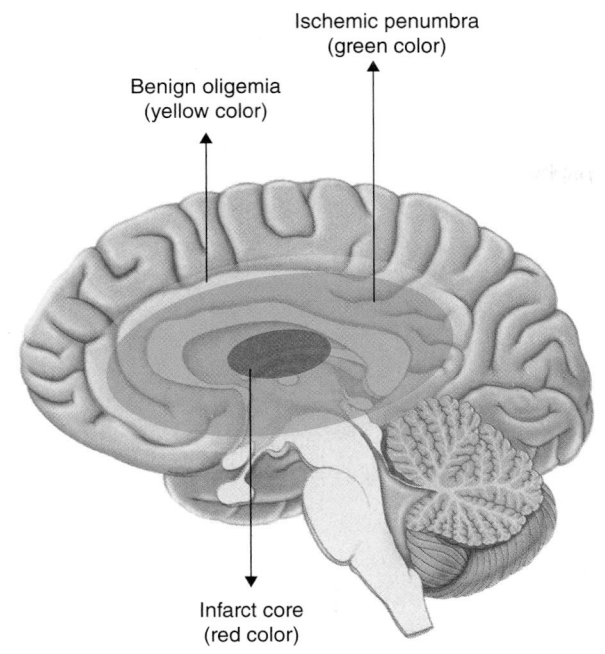

Benign oligemia
(yellow color)

Ischemic penumbra
(green color)

Infarct core
(red color)

FIGURE 62-4. Diagram of a cerebral hemisphere, lateral aspect, indicating the zones of ischemia (red), penumbra (green), and benign oligemia (yellow) that form in an acute ischemic stroke due to an intracranial LVO.

failure and inability to conduct the electrical impulses, but the cell structure is still intact. However, when this flow reduces below a critical level between 10 and 20 mL/100 g/min, there is loss of ATP function of the cell resulting in cell membrane damage, swelling, and subsequent cell death. Because of a close interplay of these phenomena, an intracranial occlusion leads to the formation of three zones of brain injury (see **Figure 62-4**): the ischemic core (tissue irreversibly injured), the ischemic penumbra (tissue with very slow blood flow, with cessation of neuronal functions but intact cell structure allowing for slow functional recovery if adequate blood flow is rapidly restored), and the zone of benign oligemia (tissue with milder reduction in the blood flow that does not lead to tissue at risk). Over the last few years, neuroimaging techniques with CT perfusion and MRI perfusion have been developed that can rapidly provide a reliable estimate of these zones of ischemia, penumbra, and benign oligemia. Although both the modalities have their pros and cons, they have been increasingly used in acute stroke imaging and form the basis of DAWN (DWI or CTP assessment with clinical mismatch in the triage of wake-up and late presenting strokes undergoing neurointervention) and DEFUSE 3 (endovascular therapy following imaging evaluation for ischemic stroke 3) trials published in 2018, which allowed for expansion of MT in patients who presented with acute disabling stroke symptoms beyond 6 hours of LKW time and had a salvageable penumbra measured by the automated quantitative

perfusion on CT perfusion or an MR perfusion study (see **Figure 62-5**). There were some differences in the clinical and imaging selection between the two trials, but essentially DAWN enrolled patients between 6 and 24 hours of their LKW time and DEFUSE 3 enrolled patients within 6 to 16 hours of their LKW time. DAWN enrolled 207 patients and showed the largest treatment effect size in terms of functional outcome with 49% of the patients undergoing MT achieving functional independence at 3 months versus only 13% patients in the medical management arm. Similarly, in DEFUSE, enrollment was terminated early for efficacy after 182 patients were randomized and showed the rate of return to functional independence in 41% patients undergoing MT versus only 15% in the medical management arm. The findings from these trials have shifted the paradigm of stroke treatment from being a strictly time-based approach toward a more inclusive salvageable tissue-based approach and expanded its eligibility to a much broader population. Like in the early time window, the efficacy for MT has been unequivocally accepted for all adult age groups, including octogenarians. Although these trials established the benefit of MT among patients in the extended time window, it is very important to understand that the patients who fulfill these criteria are relatively few and the survivability of the brain tissue depends upon the collateral circulation status of a patient. With time, this collateral circulation may fail, although definite timepoints at which this may happen are almost impossible to predict. Thus, even when dealing with a patient with favorable core/perfusion mismatch showing salvageable penumbra, it is crucial that these patients receive MT without any additional delay to harness the maximal benefit from reperfusion.

Post-reperfusion management: After the completion of the acute reperfusion therapies, patients should be admitted to a dedicated neurological care unit to monitor for neurological deterioration and cardiovascular or systemic complications and to complete investigations to determine the ischemic stroke mechanism. Upon successful reperfusion, the goal is to maintain hemodynamic stability, targeting gradual normotension. Severe resistant hypertension has been shown to increase the risk of ICH and so, after IVT, the widely accepted routine practice is to maintain blood pressure ranges < 180/105 mm Hg for at least 24 hours while avoiding rapid fluctuations, followed by a 24-hour CT scan or an MRI of the brain to rule out intracranial hemorrhage. To achieve this goal, intravenous antihypertensive medications such as labetalol, as needed, or continuous infusions of medications such as nicardipine are generally used. Typically, until the 24-hour CT/MRI scan rules out an ICH, pharmacological DVT prophylaxis and antithrombotic agents are avoided unless there is a strong indication to do so. There are no clear guidelines regarding optimal blood pressure goals after successful MT but depending on the degree of reperfusion, targeting normotension is a widely accepted routine practice until there

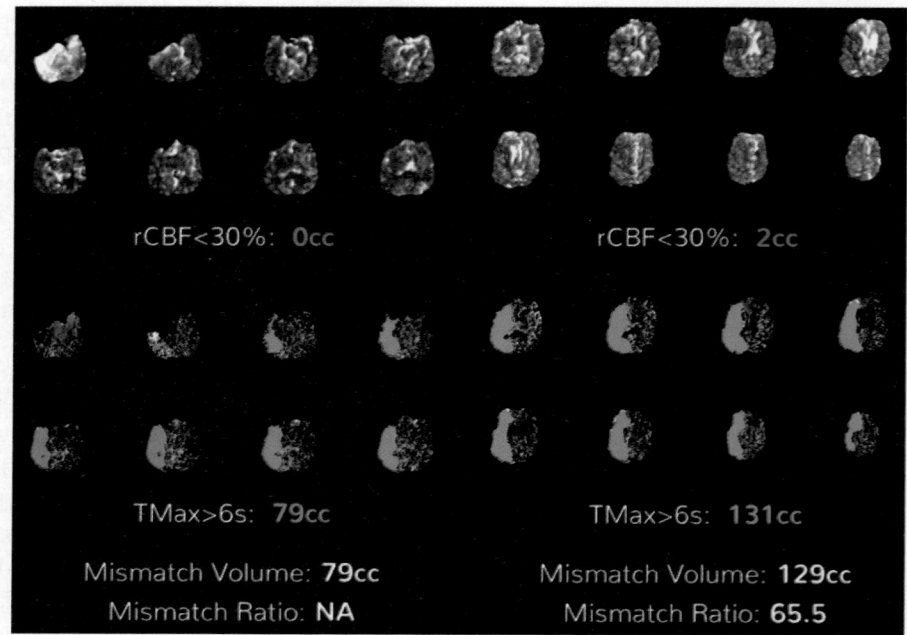

rCBF<30%: 0cc   rCBF<30%: 2cc

TMax>6s: 79cc   TMax>6s: 131cc

Mismatch Volume: **79cc**   Mismatch Volume: **129cc**

Mismatch Ratio: **NA**   Mismatch Ratio: **65.5**

FIGURE 62-5. An example of a CT perfusion obtained on a 73-year-old man who went to bed at 11 pm and woke up at 7 am with left-sided weakness, right gaze deviation, and left-sided homonymous hemianopia and neglect. His signs and symptoms were consistent with right MCA syndrome. The CTP shows an area of critically reduced cerebral blood flow (marked in red color) that represents possible core ischemic infarct surrounded by an area of hypoperfused tissue (marked in green color) that represents possible ischemic penumbra. The CT angiogram showed an intracranial M1 segment occlusion, which qualified the patient for MT. The patient was immediately taken to a neuroangiosuite, and an MT with stent-retriever device was performed. The patient's symptoms significantly improved on day 3 of his admission. His only neurological deficit was a mild left-sided facial droop.

is more robust data available. Similarly, hyperglycemia has been shown to be associated with poor stroke outcomes, and the patients admitted to the hospital who have severe hyperglycemia should be on standardized insulin protocols to treat and closely monitor their regular blood sugars. The Stroke Hyperglycemia Insulin Network Effort (SHINE) randomized controlled trial enrolled 1151 acute ischemic stroke patients and randomized nearly half of them to an interventional protocol with IV insulin to maintain blood sugar between 80 and 130 mg/dL and did not find any benefit in this group of patients when compared to the other half of the patients in the group that received standard care with subcutaneous insulin to maintain blood glucose between 80 and 179 mg/dL. Subsequently, intensive lowering of blood sugar is not currently recommended in routine practice caring for acute stroke patients. For patients who do not receive acute reperfusion therapies, maintaining cerebral perfusion pressures is critical, and the blood pressure is allowed to autoregulate with permissible systolic blood pressure (SBP) up to 220 mm Hg in the first 24 to 48 hours, subsequently aiming to gently lower blood pressure (with SBP goals of 160–180 mm Hg) within 24 to 72 hours of ischemic stroke onset. Close attention must be paid to the neurologic examination, as abrupt blood pressure drops may lead to hypoperfusion of an arterial territory at risk of infarction.

Common medical complications of stroke include aspiration pneumonia, DVT, and pulmonary embolism. When indwelling bladder catheters are used, urinary tract infection is an additional concern. All stroke patients with evidence of dysarthria, aphasia, cough, or aspiration should have a formal swallowing evaluation before being allowed to take food, liquid, or medicines by mouth. Some patients may require placement of a percutaneous endoscopic gastrostomy (PEG) feeding tube, which, in most cases, can be removed in several months when the ability to swallow improves. DVT can be prevented by the administration of subcutaneous heparin or the use of pneumatic compression boots, followed by ambulation as soon as possible. Attention should be made to avoid hyperthermia, which may lead to poorer stroke outcomes.

Early stroke prevention strategies Aspirin is the most common antithrombotic agent used for secondary stroke prevention after a stroke or a TIA. Typically, unless there are contraindications or excessive risks of bleeding, aspirin 50 to 325 mg/day is initiated as soon as possible after an ischemic stroke or a TIA. The risk of recurrent stroke after an ischemic stroke or a TIA is the highest in the first few days/weeks after the index event, thought to be as high as 10% within a week after a TIA or minor stroke, depending on the underlying stroke etiology. Although aspirin has been shown to be beneficial for long-term secondary stroke prevention, the most benefit is obtained in the first few days after the index TIA/stroke. Caution should be exercised when prescribing aspirin to patients who have known history of gastrointestinal ulceration/bleeding, although aspirin in 50 to 325 mg/day doses has been shown to be tolerated well in general. Clopidogrel is also used as a first-line agent for secondary stroke prevention. In a randomized, blinded trial of clopidogrel versus aspirin in patients at risk of ischemic events (CAPRIE) that randomized patients with a recent stroke, MI, or peripheral arterial disease to daily treatment with clopidogrel or aspirin, clopidogrel was associated with a modest reduction in overall primary outcome of stroke, MI, or vascular death, but in subgroup analysis, the outcomes between the two groups did not differ among patients who had a recent MI or a stroke. Some patients exhibit nonresponsiveness to clopidogrel, and although ticagrelor has been considered an effective substitute, it was not shown to be superior to aspirin alone for secondary prevention of stroke, MI, or death at 90 days in the Acute Stroke or Transient Ischemic Attack Treated with Aspirin or Ticagrelor and Patient Outcomes (SOCRATES) trial. The choice of antiplatelet therapy is dependent mainly on patient tolerance, contraindications, availability, and cost, and while the combination of aspirin plus extended-release dipyridamole has shown modest benefit over aspirin, its side effect profile with headache and gastrointestinal symptoms has limited its use. There is some data on the use of cilostazol as a second-line agent for patients with aspirin allergy in Asian patients, but high-quality data supporting the use of cilostazol in non-Asian ethnic groups is lacking and has limited its use.

Due to the high stroke recurrence rate in the early period after the index stroke/TIA, there has been an ongoing interest to find optimal treatment strategies to minimize this risk. The Clopidogrel in High-Risk Patients with Acute Nondisabling Cerebrovascular Events (CHANCE) trial randomized patients with acute high-risk TIA or a minor stroke to an interventional arm consisting of treatment with aspirin and clopidogrel for 3 weeks post the index event followed by placebo until 90 days and a control arm consisting of daily aspirin-treated patients and compared the primary outcome of recurrent stroke among these patients in 114 clinical centers in China. A total of 5170 patients were enrolled, and recurrent strokes occurred more frequently in the control arm at 11.7% versus the interventional arm at 8.2%, showing that addition of clopidogrel within first 24 hours after the index high-risk TIA or minor stroke for a total of 21 days resulted in 32% risk reduction for recurrent stroke, without increasing the bleeding risks significantly. Recently, a multicenter, multinational, randomized clinical trial, titled Platelet-Oriented Inhibition in New TIA and minor stroke (POINT), tested the efficacy of a combination of dual antiplatelet therapy (DAPT) in the intervention arm against single antiplatelet therapy in the control arm for a total of 90 days after the index high-risk TIA or

minor stroke and enrolled 4881 patients in North America, Europe, Australia, and New Zealand. The primary efficacy outcome for recurrent ischemic stroke, MI, or death from ischemic vascular causes was significantly lower in the intervention arm (5%) versus control arm (6.5%); however, the risk of major hemorrhage in the intervention arm (0.9%) was also higher as compared to the control arm (0.4%). The reason for higher risk of major hemorrhage was thought to be possibly related to the higher loading dose of clopidogrel, and a longer duration of treatment with DAPT in the POINT trial (3 months) as compared to CHANCE trial (3 weeks). Moreover, the benefit of DAPT in recurrent ischemic stroke reduction was shown to be maximum in the first 30 days after the index event, whereas the bleeding risk built up after a week of initiating the DAPT. Combining the findings of these two studies, the current AHA/ASA guidelines on early management of acute ischemic stroke strongly recommend considering a short course of DAPT with aspirin and clopidogrel initiated within 24 hours from symptom onset after a high-risk TIA or a minor ischemic stroke (provided the patient did not receive IVT) for a total of 21 days. This benefit of DAPT was mirrored in another randomized clinical trial, Acute Stroke or Transient Ischemic Attack Treated with Ticagrelor and ASA for Prevention of Stroke and Death (THALES), that utilized ticagrelor as the second antiplatelet agent substituting clopidogrel. However, the risk of major hemorrhage, including fatal and intracranial hemorrhage, was elevated among patients randomized to the intervention arm receiving aspirin plus ticagrelor for a total of 30 days.

Acute cerebral venous sinus thrombosis (CVST) may have varied presentations including ischemic stroke, ICH, headache, seizures, etc. It is routine practice to consider early anticoagulation with either unfractionated heparin (UFH) or low-molecular-weight heparin (LMWH) for the treatment of this condition, oftentimes even if the patient presents with baseline ICH. Following a period of neurological stabilization, the mode of anticoagulation is switched to oral anticoagulants, such as warfarin for a period of 3 to 6 months, or until resolution of CVST on follow-up imaging depending on the risks versus benefits. In a recent study, dabigatran was found to have similar efficacy in patients with mild to moderate CVST in preventing recurrent sinus thrombosis.

Extracranial cervical artery dissection is another established etiology of acute ischemic stroke, which is more common in young adults as opposed to the geriatric population. It may present with headache, Horner syndrome, cranial neuropathies, or ischemic stroke/TIA. Although evidence in support of optimal treatment is limited, it suggests that the either aspirin/dual antiplatelet therapy or anticoagulation for short term may be reasonable choices for secondary stroke prevention. The choice of antithrombotic regimen should be based on the treating physician's experience, radiological findings including size of stroke, if any, patient comorbidities after a detailed discussion of risks versus benefits with the patient, and consideration of patient preference for subsequent therapy.

Early recurrent stroke prevention management is dependent on the presumed stroke mechanism, as explored below.

Extracranial Large-Artery Atherosclerosis Surgical therapeutic options can be considered in this subacute phase. Carotid revascularization procedures may be applied in two distinct clinical settings: (1) symptomatic disease and (2) asymptomatic disease. The efficacy of carotid endarterectomy for symptomatic disease is high when there is a 70% to 99% stenosis, but modest when there is a 50% to 69% stenosis. Carotid endarterectomy for mild-to-moderate stroke or TIA in the territory of the ICA has been proven effective by the North American Symptomatic Carotid Endarterectomy Trial (NASCET) study, for patients with both 70% to 99% and 50% to 69% stenosis. Patients with severe stroke in the middle cerebral artery territory are not appropriate for carotid endarterectomy in the subacute phase. If the patient with severe stroke improves in rehabilitation to the point where worsening of the deficit would be problematic from recurrent stroke, then endarterectomy can be reconsidered. The surgical benefit for patients with symptomatic moderate stenosis was statistically significant but small, with only 1.5% absolute risk reduction per year, and therefore surgery should only be considered in centers with low perioperative rates of surgical morbidity. The decision to perform carotid endarterectomy for symptomatic moderate carotid stenosis should be made on an individual basis, considering the patient's surgical risk, center-specific perioperative complication rate, and the patient's life expectancy. Because the surgical risk occurs upfront during the perioperative period, the benefit from surgery accrues with increased years of life. For the older adults, the risks and benefits must be carefully weighed, and surgery should be withheld for patients with life expectancy fewer than 5 years. When there is symptomatic severe stenosis (70%–99% luminal narrowing), the surgical benefit is, by contrast, quite high, and most patients will benefit from surgical rather than medical management.

Carotid artery stenting (CAS) with angioplasty and stenting of the ICA plaque has gained ground as an alternative to carotid endarterectomy. Advantages include shorter hospital stay, lack of a neck incision, avoidance of general anesthesia, and a lower incidence of cranial neuropathy as a complication. A significant concern, however, is the risk of distal embolization of thrombus or fragments of atheroma dislodged during arterial access, balloon inflation, or stent deployment. An evolving array of embolization protection devices, deployed distal to the stent, are designed to limit this risk. Stenting is still an option for patients at high risk for complications from endarterectomy, including those with medical comorbidities, unfavorable neck anatomy, contralateral carotid occlusion, and restenosis at previous endarterectomy site. Randomized trials have addressed whether stenting can produce results as good as endarterectomy. Two trials, Endarterectomy versus Angioplasty in Patients with Symptomatic Severe Carotid Stenosis (EVA-3S) and Stent-Supported Percutaneous Angioplasty of the Carotid Artery versus Endarterectomy (SPACE), showed that, in symptomatic patients with greater than 60% ICA stenosis, carotid endarterectomy was associated with lower 30-day rates of major complications such as stroke and MI when compared to carotid stenting. By contrast, the Stenting and Angioplasty with Protection in Patients at High Risk for Endarterectomy (SAPPHIRE) trial, which included only patients who were deemed poor operative candidates for endarterectomy, showed equivalency between stenting and endarterectomy, with slightly lower complication rates in the stenting group. The Carotid Revascularization Endarterectomy versus Stent Trial (CREST) randomized patients with recent hemispheric TIA, ocular TIA, or minor stroke, with at least 50% to 70% carotid stenosis. There were no significant differences between endarterectomy and stenting for the composite outcome of stroke, MI, or death over a 4-year follow-up period. However, during the 30-day periprocedural period there were significantly higher risks of stroke in patients undergoing stenting, and of MI in patients undergoing endarterectomy. Of interest, an interaction between age and treatment efficacy was detected ($p = 0.02$), with a crossover at an age of approximately 70 such that CAS tended to show greater efficacy at younger ages, and carotid endarterectomy at older ages. Thus, the treatment choice for carotid revascularization in symptomatic carotid artery stenosis is dependent on multiple factors and is usually decided after a multidisciplinary discussion with the neurologists, neurointerventionalists, and specialists performing carotid endarterectomy with shared decision-making involving the patient/family members considering the risks/benefits and patient preference for each of these procedures.

The timing of carotid revascularization for ischemic stroke is of major importance. If the ischemic stroke is small, then early intervention, up to 2 weeks poststroke, is preferable. In more extensive strokes, however, the risk of cerebral reperfusion injury after a revascularization procedure is high, especially in severe or critical intracranial carotid stenosis. In this circumstance, carotid revascularization procedures should be deferred to a later date to allow the infarcted territory to heal and to allow normalization of the local cerebral blood volume. Precise assessment of the degree of severity of the stenosis and its effect intracranially is extremely helpful when determining the urgency of timing of surgery. In addition, an image through CTA or MRA is also helpful in identifying the pathology not only in the ICA origin, but also in the arteries distally and in those arteries providing collateral flow. On the other hand, the benefit of carotid revascularization procedures for asymptomatic carotid artery stenosis (lack of ipsilateral stroke or TIA in the past 6 months) is currently not well established.

Although earlier clinical trials provided some evidence of a modest benefit in this population, it is important to note that at the time of those trials, the medical management strategies were not as advanced as they are today and were not able to successfully achieve the currently accepted goals of lipid lowering, blood pressure reduction, and platelet inhibition. Moreover, with a strong emphasis on healthy lifestyle changes in addition to the medical management strategies, it is currently unclear whether carotid revascularization among patients with asymptomatic carotid stenosis is truly superior to conservative management with a combination of medical management and lifestyle changes for the goal of stroke prevention. As we eagerly await the results of CREST-2, carotid revascularization for asymptomatic carotid stenosis is not offered to patients routinely but considered on a case-by-case basis.

Cardioembolic Stroke For patients with nonvalvular AF, anticoagulant therapy with warfarin has been proven by randomized clinical trials to reduce the risk of recurrent cerebral or systemic embolism by close to 70%, as compared to aspirin. The international normalized ratio (INR) goal is 2 to 3. Novel oral anticoagulants (NOACs) such as the direct thrombin inhibitor dabigatran, and direct factor Xa inhibitors rivaroxaban, apixaban, and edoxaban have been shown to be noninferior to warfarin in prevention of cerebral or systemic embolism in nonvalvular AF. Further, NOACs as a group have a significantly lower risk of intracranial hemorrhage as compared to warfarin, despite a significantly higher risk of major systemic bleeding, mainly gastrointestinal. Despite this, there appears to be a net therapeutic benefit of NOACs over warfarin therapy. An additional advantage to these novel anticoagulants is that they do not require routine hematologic monitoring. Their current major disadvantage, however, is the limited availability of specific antidotes to counter bleeding from these medications. Anticoagulation is relatively contraindicated in infective endocarditis and in left atrial myxomatous syndromes because of associated cortical surface mycotic and myxomatous aneurysm with the risk of hemorrhage in the early phases of these diseases.

In advanced congestive heart failure, the risk of ischemic stroke or systemic embolism may be elevated due to the formation of intracardiac clots, especially in extensive anterior wall MI with an apical aneurysm. Anticoagulation may be recommended early on in this setting to prevent initial or recurrent embolism. The Warfarin versus Aspirin in Reduced Cardiac Ejection Fraction (WARCEF) study enrolled patients with left ventricular ejection fraction less than 35% and who were in sinus rhythm. Patients were randomized to aspirin 325 mg daily or warfarin with goal INR 2 to 3, and were followed up to 6 years, with mean follow-up of 3.5 years. There was no significant overall difference in the risk of ischemic stroke, hemorrhagic stroke, or death between treatment with warfarin and treatment with aspirin. A reduced risk of ischemic stroke with warfarin

was seen, but this was offset by an increased risk of major systemic hemorrhage. Thus, there is currently no clear evidence for anticoagulation of patients with congestive heart failure past the acute to subacute phases of ischemic stroke. A PFO as a source of paradoxical embolism (thromboembolism from the veins into the arteries) causing a stroke has attracted a lot of interest over the last several decades. Earlier clinical trials showed no benefit of endovascular PFO closure over medical management with antiplatelet therapy, but recently several trials have shown a modest reduction in the risk of secondary stroke in carefully selected patients that underwent endovascular PFO closure. It is important to note that all these trials enrolled patients between 18 and 60 years, who were thought to be higher risk of paradoxical embolism and majority of the patients had high-risk PFO morphology that rendered them at a higher risk of secondary stroke due to the PFO. It is currently unclear whether endovascular PFO closure among these patients is superior to therapeutic anticoagulation.

Lacunar Infarction The mainstay of early therapy in lacunar infarctions, in patients who do not receive IVT, is mostly supportive, aiming to avoid clinical decompensation, which can occur in the form of a stuttering lacunar syndrome in up to 30% of patients. Antiplatelet therapy should be instituted early on, blood pressure allowed to autoregulate, and glucose closely monitored. The choice of antiplatelet is mainly individual as all are equally effective for secondary ischemic stroke prevention, as discussed later in this section. Longer-term DAPT with aspirin 325 mg and clopidogrel 75 mg daily was not superior to aspirin therapy alone for reduction of recurrent lacunar stroke risk in the Secondary Prevention of Small Subcortical Strokes (SPS3) trial. Further, this combination promoted harm, leading to a significantly higher risk of bleeding and death. There is also no clear evidence that anticoagulation can improve clinical outcomes in lacunar stroke. Therefore, dual antiplatelet therapy and anticoagulation are not recommended for patients with lacunar stroke.

Intracranial Atherosclerosis For patients with symptomatic severe intracranial stenosis, warfarin was also shown in a randomized trial to be no more effective than aspirin in preventing recurrent stroke. A more recent trial, the Stenting and Aggressive Medical Management for Preventing Recurrent Stroke in Intracranial Stenosis (SAMMPRIS) trial, randomized patients with severe (> 70%) symptomatic intracranial stenosis to intensive medical therapy alone versus intensive medical therapy and intracranial stenting with the Wingspan device. All patients received aspirin 325 mg daily and clopidogrel 75 mg daily for 90 days. Intensive medical therapy consisted of management of primary and secondary risk factors, aggressive blood pressure control, and intensive lipid lowering (target LCL-C < 70 mg/dL). The trial was stopped prematurely as the rate of stroke or death was significantly higher in the stenting group as compared to the patients receiving medical management only.

This has led to widespread adoption of the medical management practices implemented in SAMMPRIS (DAPT, high-dose statins, tight blood pressure control, and healthy lifestyle and dietary habits for secondary stroke prevention in patients with symptomatic ICAD).

Cryptogenic Embolism In cryptogenic embolism, debate exists as to the efficacy of anticoagulant therapy. Aspirin or other antiplatelet agents have been prescribed in lieu of anticoagulant therapy, but their efficacy also has not been proven by randomized clinical trials. Stroke and TIA subtypes were not identified in those studies in which aspirin was compared to placebo or to another antiplatelet agent for the secondary prevention of recurrent stroke or TIA after a previous minor primary stroke or TIA. One study in which the primary and secondary stroke subtypes were accurately identified was WARSS, which compared the efficacy of warfarin to aspirin in secondary stroke prevention. When all the stroke subtypes were combined, there was no difference in the risk of stroke with warfarin compared to aspirin. When the data for primary individual stroke subtypes were analyzed in terms of secondary stroke prevention, there was a trend in favor of anticoagulant therapy for patients with cryptogenic embolism. More recently, ESUS has become a popular term denoting patients in whom there is a strong suspicion for an underlying embolic source, but without a definite diagnosis after a standard stroke work-up. Two large-scale randomized clinical trials investigated the benefits of utilizing anticoagulation with NOACs versus standard antiplatelet management among ESUS patients. The Rivaroxaban Versus Aspirin in Secondary Prevention of Stroke and Prevention of Systemic Embolism in Patients with Recent Embolic Stroke of Undetermined Source (NAVIGATE ESUS) enrolled 7213 participants and randomized half of them to receive the intervention with rivaroxaban 15 mg PO daily and the other half to standard of care aspirin daily. While rivaroxaban was not associated with any benefit in the rate of occurrence of primary outcome (recurrent ischemic or hemorrhagic stroke or systemic embolism), the rate of major bleeding, life-threatening bleeding, and hemorrhagic stroke was higher among patients receiving the study medication versus the standard of care. Similarly, another trial compared the efficacy of dabigatran against aspirin in patients with ESUS and found no benefit in reduction in the rate of recurrent stroke (ischemic or hemorrhagic), while increasing the risk of bleeding complications. Because of these two trials, routine anticoagulation among patients with ESUS is not recommended.

Giant Cell Arteritis (GCA) and Vasculitis Immunosuppression is the mainstay treatment for patients with tissue diagnosis of GCA or vasculitis. Maintaining a high index of suspicion is critical in the diagnosis of GCA, as early institution of glucocorticoids has been shown to minimize disability and to reduce the recurrence of flare ups in this condition. Long-term steroid therapy is usually pursued, with the introduction or other immunomodulatory medications such as tocilizumab, an IL-6 inhibitor to minimize recurrence of neurological and/or ophthalmological symptoms. The duration of immunosuppression is usually determined in a multidisciplinary setting with consensus from the treating neurologists, rheumatologists, and ophthalmologists in the context of patient's comorbidities that influence the risks versus benefits of such long-term immunosuppression. The role of antiplatelet therapy is not well studied and again is usually determined based on individual risks versus benefits of such therapy.

Management of malignant cerebral infarction Hemicraniectomy may be considered when progressive cerebral edema in the nondominant hemisphere becomes severe enough to compromise cerebral perfusion or cause brain herniation. This operation can prevent herniation and death by relieving intracranial pressure (ICP) but is unlikely to restore significant neurologic function because it is typically performed in the setting of extensive brain infarction. A pooled analysis of three small trials confirms that hemicraniectomy prevents severe dependency or death in patients younger than 60 years. Among patients 61 years or older with a malignant middle cerebral artery infarction, hemicraniectomy increased survival without severe disability. However, most survivors required assistance with most bodily needs.

In cerebellar ischemic strokes larger than 2 to 3 cm in diameter, decompressive posterior fossa craniectomy may also be performed if the patient shows signs of clinical deterioration, to avoid brain stem compression and upward herniation.

Long-term Preventive Strategies

Preventive strategies for controlling primary risk factors Treatment of hypertension is, by far, the most important aspect of risk factor control. Achieving and maintaining blood pressure treatment targets are probably more important than class effects of the drugs. Among other recommendations for a healthy cardiovascular health, AHA/ASA strongly encourages people to aim achieving optimal targets in seven metrics that compose Life's Simple 7 as follows: (1) no smoking or quitting smoking for > 12 months; (2) BMI < 25 kg/m^2; (3) physical activity of at least 150 min/week of moderate activity or at least 75 min/week of vigorous activity or at least 150 min/week of moderate and vigorous activity; (4) diet that includes (a) more than 4.5 cups/day of fruits and vegetables, (b) more than 2 servings/week of fish, (c) more than 3 servings/day or whole grains, (d) no more than 36 oz/week of sugar-sweetened beverages, and (e) 1500 mg/day of sodium; (5) blood pressure < 120/80 mm Hg, (6) total cholesterol < 200 mg/dL; and (7) fasting plasma glucose < 100 mg/dL. Following the Third Report of the National Cholesterol Education Program Expert Panel on Detection, Evaluation, and Treatment of High Blood Cholesterol in Adults (ATP III) guidelines for prevention of MI, the primary goal is lowering the low-density lipoprotein (LDL). Risk factor adjustments including diet, exercise, weight reduction, cessation of smoking, and diabetes management are all important first steps. Hydroxymethylglutaryl coenzyme A (HMG-CoA) reductase inhibitors ("statins") are associated with reduction in the risk of stroke, as well as reduction in the risk of MI. The Stroke Prevention with Atorvastatin to Reduce Cholesterol Levels (SPARCL) trial showed that, among patients with large-vessel atherothrombotic or lacunar stroke subtypes and LDL greater than 100 mg/dL, high-dose atorvastatin (80 mg every day) was superior to placebo in reducing subsequent stroke. Recently, the Treat Stroke to Target (TST) trial established the benefit of intensive treatment to achieve serum LDL < 70 mg/dL among patients who have had a recent stroke or a TIA and also have evidence of atherosclerotic disease (intracranial/extracranial atherosclerotic stenosis, history of coronary artery disease, or aortic arch atheroma) in preventing a composite primary outcome consisting of recurrent ischemic stroke, MI, new symptoms leading to urgent coronary or carotid revascularization, or death from cardiovascular causes.

Stroke recovery Patients with stroke-related disability should be evaluated by specialists in physical therapy, occupational therapy, or speech therapy as appropriate. A substantial number of patients may benefit from inpatient rehabilitation following their acute hospital stay. There is evidence from observational studies that patients treated in dedicated stroke units, with experienced physician, nursing and rehabilitation staff, have better outcomes than those treated in general medical or surgical wards.

Stroke recovery may require 6 months to a year, or even longer, because of the slow nature of neuroplastic changes following brain injury. Late complications of stroke include spasticity, contracture, pressure ulcers, shoulder joint dislocation, and depression. The injection of botulinum toxin in affected muscles has been shown to improve symptoms of stroke-related spasticity. Earlier, a recovery trial had shown that early use of fluoxetine with physical therapy enhanced motor recovery in stroke patients with moderate-to-severe deficits, independent of the drug's effect on mood; however, three recently concluded trials did not show the benefit of oral fluoxetine on functional outcome after stroke. However, it did show an increased risk of bone fractures among patients receiving fluoxetine and is as such not recommended routinely for indications other than mood disorders among stroke survivors.

INTRACRANIAL HEMORRHAGE

Intracranial hemorrhages are classified according to the site of origin. The diagnosis, treatment, and secondary prevention of intracranial hemorrhage depend on the assessment of the underlying specific pathophysiology, analogous to the way in which ischemic stroke diagnosis and treatment depend on identifying the ischemic stroke subtype. There are four locations of origin: intracerebral, subarachnoid, subdural, and epidural. Subdural and epidural hemorrhages

are predominantly traumatic and are not considered a form of hemorrhagic stroke. This section will therefore be concerned with ICH and SAH. Hemorrhagic stroke accounts for approximately 15% of all strokes. ICH may be further divided by location into deep ICH (arising in the deep hemispheric portions of the brain, including the basal ganglia, thalamus, brain stem, and cerebellum) and lobar ICH (arising in the cortex or at the junction of the cortex and the white matter). Hypertension is the most common cause of spontaneous ICH, while CAA is the most common cause of spontaneous lobar ICH in the older adults.

Intracerebral Hemorrhage

Deep hemispheric hemorrhage Hypertension is by far the major cause of hemorrhage in deep brain locations. The most common sites are the putamen, thalamus, pons, and cerebellum. A penetrating artery arising from one of the major intracranial arteries (middle cerebral stem or M1 segment, basilar artery, or PCA) is generally the source of the hemorrhage. These same vessels are also frequently affected by lipohyalinosis, and when occlusion occurs rather than rupture, lacunar infarction is the outcome.

Clinical Presentation

Each of the four sites of deep ICH produces a characteristic clinical syndrome. In *putaminal hemorrhage*, there is contralateral hemiplegia and conjugate deviation of the eyes toward the hemorrhage side. Stupor is evident at the onset in most cases. *Thalamic hemorrhage* typically presents with contralateral sensory loss and gaze abnormalities. Involvement of the internal capsule results in contralateral hemiparesis. Aphasia can occur in left thalamic ICH and visuospatial abnormalities can occur in right thalamic ICH. Involvement of the reticular activating system results in reduced consciousness and sleepiness. *Pontine hemorrhage* produces coma, quadriplegia, decerebrate rigidity, impairment of horizontal eye movements, and pinpoint pupils. *Cerebellar hemorrhage* typically presents with headache, vertigo, nausea, vomiting, and instability of gait. Facial weakness and gaze palsies can also occur. Coma may result from brain stem compression or upward or downward herniation of cerebellar structures.

Lobar hemorrhage Lobar hemorrhages occur spontaneously in the supratentorial white matter and cerebral cortex of all lobes of the brain. The manifestations are dependent on the area involved. Frontal hemorrhages may present with contralateral hemiparesis, expressive aphasia, and gaze deviation toward the hemorrhage. Parietal hemorrhages may result in contralateral neglect and sensory loss, while occipital hemorrhages could present with contralateral homonymous hemianopia. Temporal hemorrhages of the dominant hemisphere may present with receptive aphasia. Headache is sometimes present and may be most severe near the location of the hemorrhage. If the hemorrhage is large, then depressed consciousness may be present. The symptoms usually evolve over minutes or hours, in contrast to embolic ischemic stroke where the onset of symptoms is abrupt. A precise cause of lobar ICH is found in a significant number of cases: CAA and vascular malformations are the most common; metastatic disease is less frequent, but well known. A proportion of lobar ICH is likely caused by hypertension. Lobar ICH is more readily accessible for surgical evacuation because of its superficial location. A subgroup analysis of the Surgical Trial for Intracerebral Hemorrhage (STICH) showed a benefit for surgery, compared to initial conservative management, for ICH less than 1 cm from the cortical surface.

CAA is a common cause of both single and recurrent lobar hemorrhages in the older population and is diagnosed conclusively only by postmortem demonstration of amyloid in the media of cortical and leptomeningeal arterioles and capillaries. Sporadic amyloid angiopathy is caused by the deposition of β-amyloid only in the cerebral arteries, without systemic amyloidosis. But the clinical history of repeated supratentorial lobar hemorrhages and the demonstration of small, 1- to 2-mm areas of hypointensity on MRI susceptibility-weighted sequences, indicative of prior small asymptomatic hemorrhages (cerebral microbleeds), strongly suggest the diagnosis. These small, silent hemorrhages may be the cause of recurrent focal symptoms sometimes seen in these patients. A clinical-pathologic correlation study suggests that CAA is the cause of approximately 70% of primary lobar ICH in persons older than 55 years. Other than avoidance of antithrombotic medications, treatment options remain elusive. There is a high recurrence rate of 10% to 14% per year in sporadic lobar ICH, mostly caused by CAA, which is significantly higher than the recurrence rate of 2% to 4% per year observed in survivors of deep ICH. Careful control of associated hypertension, if present, seems prudent.

A small number of cases are associated with vascular or perivascular inflammation that frequently responds to a pulse of steroids, although late relapses may occur. Inflammatory CAA typically presents with cognitive impairment, seizure, or focal neurologic signs rather than hemorrhagic stroke. Asymmetric white and gray matter hyperintensities, often with small silent hemorrhages on susceptibility sequence, are observed on MRI. Biopsy is usually indicated to exclude other causes of vasculitis.

Lobar Hemorrhages Caused by Metastatic Disease Cerebral metastases, particularly malignant melanoma, may give rise to cerebral hemorrhage. Usually, the metastases are multiple and can easily be demonstrated by contrast MRI or CT scans.

Evaluation of ICH: Noncontrast head CT scan has excellent sensitivity for ICH and is the initial modality of choice in ICH diagnosis. There are no clinical signs or symptoms specific for ischemic stroke compared to hemorrhagic stroke, making CT mandatory in all patients presenting with potential stroke. Vessel imaging with CTA or MRA should be performed for the diagnosis of cerebral aneurysm or vascular malformation. Venous imaging with CT venography (CTV) or MR venography (MRV) should be performed if concern for venous sinus thrombosis exists. Catheter angiography should be performed if suspicion remains high for vascular abnormality despite negative CTA or MRA. Contrast-enhanced CT or MRI should be performed when suspicion of underlying mass lesion exists. A "spot sign" on CTA is the finding of contrast extravasation into a hematoma and is associated with hemorrhage expansion and poor outcome. MRI also has excellent sensitivity for detecting ICH. Hemorrhage on special T2-weighted sequences such as gradient recalled echo (GRE) or susceptibility-weighted imaging (SWI) appears as hypointensity or low signal compared to surrounding brain. Cerebral microbleeds are small areas of hypointensity that represent chronic small hemorrhage. Their location often points to an underlying etiology with deep microbleeds mainly due to hypertension and lobar microbleeds due to CAA. Older patients with a history of hypertension and hemorrhage in a typical location do not need angiographic assessment. In contrast, younger patients and those with an atypical-appearing hemorrhage should have angiography. When hemorrhages occur in atypical locations or in the absence of a history of hypertension, a follow-up MRI brain scan with and without contrast is performed in up to 3 months, following ICH resorption, to screen for an underlying lesion such as a vascular malformation or tumor. Acute laboratory assessment should include platelet count, prothrombin time, partial thromboplastin time, and INR to exclude bleeding diathesis. An ESR, CRP, and blood cultures should be considered in patients at risk for septic embolism from bacterial endocarditis. The history, physical examination, and imaging should exclude secondary causes of hemorrhage such as coagulopathy, brain tumor, aneurysm rupture, and hemorrhagic transformation of ischemic infarction.

The size and location of the hematoma determine the treatment and prognosis. Supratentorial hematomas greater than 5 cm in diameter have a poor prognosis. Infratentorial hematomas greater than 3 cm in size are generally fatal if they are in the pons. Other factors associated with poor prognosis are the presence of intraventricular blood and worse level of consciousness at presentation.

Treatment of ICH: All patients with ICH should be initially managed in an intensive care unit. General supportive care should be provided. Eunatremia, normoglycemia, and normothermia are mainstays of treatment. Seizures may occur and should be treated with anticonvulsant medications when they occur. Seizure prophylaxis is generally not recommended. Patients taking warfarin at the time of ICH must have the INR aggressively corrected emergently with vitamin K and vitamin K–dependent factors and the warfarin discontinued. Patients with ICH on antiplatelet medications should have these antiplatelet medications discontinued. A randomized clinical trial evaluated the utility of platelet transfusion in patients with spontaneous intracranial hemorrhage and found empiric platelet transfusion to be associated with a higher rate of death or dependence at 3 months as compared to standard of care and is currently not recommended routinely unless there is a neurosurgical procedure planned. Prompt anticoagulation reversal may be useful in reducing hematoma expansion and subsequent morbidity/mortality but this often comes at a cost of inadvertent procoagulant effects of the anticoagulant reversal agent that may contribute to thrombotic complications. For warfarin, IV vitamin K is used along with fresh frozen plasma/cryoprecipitate or prothrombin complex concentrate (PCC). NOAC-specific reversal agents (idarucizumab for dabigatran and andexanet alpha for direct thrombin inhibitors) are currently not widely available on a routine basis; therefore, PCC is often used in that scenario. The relationship between blood pressure and outcomes after ICH is complex. Although blood pressure reduction is crucial in prevention of hematoma expansion, the exact levels of blood pressure reduction have yet to be defined. Current guidelines state that it is likely safe to reduce SBP to 140 mm Hg acutely when the presenting SBP is between 150 and 220 mm Hg. For patients presenting with SBP > 220 mm Hg, aggressive reduction of blood pressure with continuous intravenous infusion of antihypertensive medication and frequent blood pressure monitoring to maintain SBP around 140 mm Hg to 160 mm Hg is recommended. In clinical trials, a more sudden reduction of blood pressure to achieve SBP < 140 mm Hg was associated with increased renal complications and was not clearly associated with any benefit in overall outcomes. Elevated ICP can result either from hematoma or associated cerebral edema. Patients with Glasgow Coma Scale (GCS) less than or equal to 8, evidence of transtentorial herniation or hydrocephalus, or significant intraventricular hemorrhage should have ICP monitoring and treatment. Osmotic agents such as mannitol or hypertonic saline are frequently used to lower ICP. Ventriculostomy with an external ventricular drain is often used in obstructive or communicating hydrocephalus.

The surgical indications for ICH depend mainly on the location of the ICH. Patients with cerebellar hemorrhages greater than 3 cm and neurologic deterioration or brain stem compression and/or hydrocephalus should have early hematoma evacuation. For other locations, surgical evacuation is controversial. The STICH trial failed to find a benefit for surgical evacuation over medical management. In STICH, patients with ICH less than 1 cm from the cortical surface had a trend toward favorable outcome with early surgery. Surgical evacuation for deep ICH accompanied by decreasing level of consciousness caused by increasing mass effect is also considered. Less invasive surgical methods are currently being developed and could be used widely in the future.

Vascular malformations Increasingly recognized with advances in neuroimaging techniques, vascular malformations are classified into four types: venous malformations, capillary telangiectasias, arteriovenous malformations (AVMs), and cavernous malformations or angioma. Vascular malformations may cause hemorrhage in either deep or lobar locations.

The management of patients with vascular malformations is best accomplished by an experienced team comprised of neurosurgeons and physicians who can consider both surgical and endovascular approaches, sometimes in combination. Radiosurgical obliteration may also be an option in some cases (ie, deep, inaccessible lesions associated with repeated hemorrhages or progressive neurologic deficits). Each case requires a unique approach that takes into account the extent and location of the vascular malformation, and the feasibility and safety of the various therapeutic approaches.

Subarachnoid Hemorrhage

The most common cause of atraumatic SAH is rupture of an aneurysm. Other less-common causes include blood dyscrasia or leukemia, tumors (such as ependymoma or meningioma, glioblastoma, renal cell, or metastasis), vascular malformation, or, rarely, venous sinus disease or meningitis.

Ruptured aneurysms occur at the branch points of arteries at the base of the brain and following rupture, give rise to SAH, or sometimes ICH. Histologic examination shows interruption of the internal elastic lamina with an aneurysmal outpouching that appears like a berry. Although usually single, aneurysms can be multiple in 15% to 20% of cases. The most common sites are the anterior communicating artery, junction of the posterior communicating artery with the ICA, middle cerebral stem bifurcation, top of the basilar artery, origin of the major branches of the basilar artery, and at the origin of PICA. Intracranial aneurysms can be associated with coarctation of the aorta and are more common in autosomal domination polycystic kidney disease.

Prodromal symptoms and signs, prior to rupture occur in as many as a third of cases. These symptoms may include headache, diplopia, or blurred vision. Pinpoint pain behind the eye with or without a third nerve palsy is the most common and indicates the presence of an aneurysm at the posterior communicating artery–ICA junction. It represents a medical emergency. Juxtaclinoid aneurysms compress the optic nerve, leading to amblyopia. Supraclinoid aneurysms can be confused with suprasellar tumors, sometimes producing a hypothalamic syndrome. Aneurysms in the vertebrobasilar system can produce occipital headaches and cerebellar or long-tract signs as well as cranial nerve deficits.

The most common symptom of aneurysmal rupture is a sudden, severe headache, often characterized as the "worst headache of life." Other symptoms may include loss of consciousness, nausea and vomiting, and meningismus. Focal neurologic signs occur infrequently. Focal signs occur when the hemorrhage ruptures into the brain parenchyma and help in localization of the rupture site. For example, anterior communicating artery aneurysmal rupture produces a slowed or abulic state with contralateral weakness of the leg while middle cerebral artery aneurysm rupture produces contralateral hemiparesis and aphasia if the dominant hemisphere is involved.

Evaluation of SAH: A noncontrast head CT is the initial modality of choice and has excellent sensitivity for SAH. At our institution a CTA of the head, to look for a cerebral aneurysm, is also performed at the time of the noncontrast head CT. If the head CT is negative for SAH, but high suspicion remains, a lumbar puncture (LP) must be performed. The main findings consistent with SAH on the LP are elevated red blood cell count, xanthochromia, and elevated opening pressure.

Delayed clinical syndromes mainly consist of re-rupture syndromes, hydrocephalus, and the syndromes resulting from cerebral vasospasm. *Re-rupture* is most frequent during the first 72 hours after the initial rupture. Early surgical or endovascular intervention now precludes many re-ruptures. *Fever* (≥ 38°C) in the absence of a discernible infective etiology is common in SAH, and in some instances, may be confused with florid meningitis. *Hydrocephalus* may be acute in the first day or two after the SAH and requires ventricular drainage. Delayed hydrocephalus presents several days to weeks after the SAH and may require ventriculoperitoneal shunting. Worsening stupor is a sign of both early and delayed hydrocephalus. *Cerebral vasospasm* usually develops between days 4 and 14 following the SAH. Its location and severity have been related to the extent and location of the subarachnoid blood, with thick clot typically present around the artery developing spasm. In 30% of cases, the spasm is severe enough to give rise to ischemic symptoms and infarction may ensue. In middle cerebral artery stem vasospasm, the resulting infarction may cause devastating cerebral edema. The extent and location of blood in the basal cisterns postoperatively may represent patients likely to have severe vasospasm to develop signs of ischemia or infarction.

Management of the patient with SAH from a ruptured berry aneurysm should focus on (1) medical stabilization, with aggressive treatment of elevated blood pressure and good supportive neurocritical care, (2) early surgical clipping or endovascular coiling in non-moribund patients to prevent re-re-rupture, and (3) prevention and treatment of delayed ischemia caused by vasospasm. The International Subarachnoid Aneurysm Trial (ISAT) showed that, for aneurysms equally accessible for surgical clipping or endovascular treatment with detachable coils, the endovascular strategy was associated with less death or dependency at 1 year. Volume expansion and blood pressure elevation together with calcium channel blockers are often used to prevent symptomatic ischemia from vasospasm. Oral nimodipine, 60 mg given every 4 hours, has been shown in multiple clinical trials to reduce mortality and the incidence of delayed ischemia. For refractory cases local intra-arterial infusion of vasodilators such as nicardipine, or angioplasty of the affected arteries, may alleviate arterial stenosis caused by vasospasm.

Given the above complications and expertise necessary to perform highly technical neurosurgical and endovascular approaches to obliterate aneurysms, the patient should be managed at a center capable of carrying out these maneuvers.

PALLIATIVE CARE

Palliative care is an approach that optimizes quality of life, comfort, and family-centered care by anticipating, preventing, and treating suffering. It involves addressing physical, intellectual, emotional, social, and spiritual needs of the patients and their loved ones. Stroke is associated with significant morbidity and mortality, especially in older adults. Large ischemic strokes, catastrophic ICHs and SAHs carry a significant mortality and disability in older patients and almost half of the deaths occur in an inpatient setting (acute care hospital or rehabilitation facilities). Primary palliative care is administered by the patient's primary treatment team that may consist of neurologists, hospital medicine specialists, physical and rehabilitation medicine specialists, speech therapists, etc. Pain is a significant symptom among poststroke patients and should be adequately addressed to enhance patients' well-being and neurological recovery. Some of the common pain syndromes include central poststroke pain, hemiplegic shoulder pain, and painful spasticity. While amitriptyline for relief of pain is often the drug-of-choice in younger patients, caution should be exercised when prescribing this medication to older adults because of its side effects, and often nortriptyline is the preferred treatment. For patients with hemiplegic shoulder pain, heat, ice, soft tissue massage, or intra-articular steroid injections, intramuscular botox injections, etc. are considered reasonable treatment choices. Other comorbidities such as fatigue, urinary incontinence, sleep-disordered breathing, depression, and anxiety should be promptly identified and addressed.

An essential part of establishing goals of care for a stroke patient is to obtain a thorough understanding of the aspects of functional recovery that are crucial to the individual patient—for example, ability to ambulate, ability to communicate, etc. A lot of patients express their strong desire to refrain from pursuing any lifesaving treatments if their current medical condition severely limits the likelihood of returning to their functional baseline in some of these aspects. Ideally, these goals of care discussions especially in the elderly should begin at the planning stage of administering acute stroke treatments, as often these treatments necessitate coadministration of other life-sustaining strategies such as mechanical ventilation, further requiring a variable amount of stay in a critical care unit as patients recover from their acute illness. As such, the discussions around risks versus benefits of acute stroke treatments should include a clear explanation of risks versus benefits of these additional life-sustaining measures that are necessary to obtain the maximum benefit from stroke treatment. While accurate prognostication regarding stroke recovery is prone to several uncertainties, a careful assessment of individual patient's comorbidities, size of stroke, and eloquence of the affected brain tissue may allow for a more informed shared decision-making between the patients/ families and the clinical teams. A sizable proportion of stroke patients suffer from dysphagia requiring artificial nutrition and hydration (ANH) through a nasogastric tube or PEG. In patients who cannot swallow safely, it is reasonable to offer a trial of a nasogastric tube for up to 2 to 3 weeks before considering a PEG. During this trial period, aggressive speech therapy making every effort at establishing the true extent of patients' swallowing capabilities should be made and reviewed with the patient/their family members. Finally, in patients who have suffered a severe degree of illness limiting their ability to achieve their desired outcome and wishing to pursue end-of-life or comfort measures, a multidisciplinary team approach in consultation with palliative care expertise should be promptly offered. Patients with a life expectancy of 6 months or less may be appropriate candidates for hospice. Depending on their health care needs, hospice care can be instituted in an inpatient setting or in appropriate context, even at home. Hospice care does not necessarily mean cessation of all medical treatments, but rather aims to offer comfort to the patient, prevent suffering, and focuses on the quality of life at the patient's terminal stage of illness.

ACKNOWLEDGMENT

The authors utilized information contained in a similar chapter in the 7th edition of this textbook and wish to thank Erica Camargo, MD, PhD, MSC, Ming-Chieh Ding, MD, PhD, Eli Zimmerman, MD, and Scott Silverman, MD, for their contributions to that chapter.

FURTHER READING

Albers GW, Marks MP, Kemp S, et al. Thrombectomy for stroke at 6 to 16 hours with selection by perfusion imaging. *N Engl J Med.* 2018;378(8):708–718.

Berkhemer OA, Fransen PSS, Beumer D, et al. A randomized trial of intraarterial treatment for acute ischemic stroke. *N Engl J Med.* 2015;372:11–20.

Brott T, Bogousslavsky J. Treatment of acute ischemic stroke. *N Engl J Med.* 2000;343(10):710–722.

Brott TG, Brown RD Jr, Meyer FB, Miller DA, Cloft HJ, Sullivan TM. Carotid revascularization for prevention of stroke: carotid endarterectomy and carotid artery stenting. *Mayo Clin Proc.* 2004;79:1197–1208.

Connolly ES, Rabinstein AA, Carhuapoma JR, et al. Guidelines for the management of aneurysmal subarachnoid hemorrhage: a guideline for healthcare professionals from the American Heart Association/American Stroke Association. *Stroke.* 2012;43(6):1711–1737.

Goyal M, Demchuk AM, Menon BK, et al. Randomized assessment of rapid endovascular treatment of ischemic stroke. *N Engl J Med.* 2015;372:1019–1030.

Goyal M, Menon BK, van Zwam WH, et al. Endovascular thrombectomy after large-vessel ischaemic stroke: a meta-analysis of individual patient data from five randomised trials. *Lancet.* 2016;387(10029):1723–1731.

Hemphill JC 3rd, Greenberg SM, Anderson CS, et al. Guidelines for the Management of Spontaneous Intracerebral Hemorrhage: A Guideline for Healthcare Professionals From the American Heart Association/American Stroke Association. *Stroke.* 2015;46(7):2032–2060.

Kern R, Ringleb PA, Hacke W, Mas JL, Hennerici MG. Stenting for carotid artery stenosis. *Nat Clin Pract Neurol.* 2007;3:212–220.

Kleindorfer DO, Towfighi A, Chaturvedi S, et al. 2021 Guideline for the Prevention of Stroke in Patients With Stroke and Transient Ischemic Attack: A Guideline From the American Heart Association/American Stroke Association. *Stroke.* 2021;52(7):e364–e467.

Nogueira RG, Jadhav AP, Haussen DC, et al. Thrombectomy 6 to 24 hours after stroke with a mismatch between deficit and infarct. *N Engl J Med.* 2018;378(1):11–21.

Powers WJ, Rabinstein AA, Ackerson T, et al. Guidelines for the Early Management of Patients With Acute Ischemic Stroke: 2019 Update to the 2018 Guidelines for the Early Management of Acute Ischemic Stroke: A Guideline for Healthcare Professionals From the American Heart Association/American Stroke Association. *Stroke.* 2019;50(12):e344–e418.

Chapter 63

Other Neurodegenerative Disorders

John Best, Howie Rosen, Victor Valcour, Bruce Miller

Alzheimer disease (AD) is the most common neurodegenerative disorder encountered by the practicing geriatrician; however, a sizable number of other neurodegenerative diseases will be seen in a typical practice, rendering a working knowledge of these disorders critical for clinicians. Furthermore, there is increasing evidence that with greater age, many individuals die with mixed pathology—with AD, vascular changes, frontotemporal lobar degeneration (FTLD), and Lewy body changes often seen in a single brain. This chapter provides an overview of the more common neurodegenerative disorders with emphasis on those that influence behavior and cognition early in the course. We begin by reviewing the clinical approach to neurodegenerative cognitive disorders and then review the clinical presentation, epidemiology, and examination findings of the more common neurodegenerative syndromes. We attempt to link clinical presentation to anatomy and neuropathology whenever possible.

APPROACH TO THE EVALUATION OF COGNITIVE AND BEHAVIORAL DISORDERS IN ADULTS

The evaluation of neurodegenerative disorders is multifaceted, requiring careful attention to the cognitive, behavioral, and motor history combined with a comprehensive neurologic examination aiming to identify the brain regions involved. Isolating anatomy in patients who present with slowly progressive neurodegenerative disorders greatly facilitates the determination of the correct diagnosis.

Emphasis should be placed on the earliest presenting symptoms, whether cognitive, behavioral, or motor in origin. These early features may be critical to the identification of the pathologic substrate. As diseases progress, signs and symptoms merge between the different disorders, making diagnosis more difficult. An early history of repeated falls, for example, should warrant concern for progressive supranuclear palsy (PSP), vascular dementia, or Parkinson disease. This finding is valuable when it is present early in the illness, although most dementias are associated with basal ganglia involvement later in their disease course, diminishing the value of falls for diagnosis in the later stages. Likewise, inappropriate behavior and disinhibition

Learning Objectives

- Learn about the epidemiology, common clinical presentations, diagnosis, and treatment of non-Alzheimer type of neurodegenerative diseases.

- Gain new knowledge about recent discoveries related to the genetics, pathology, and pathobiology of common tau- and α-synucleopathies in older adults.

- Learn about the specific behavioral and nonbehavioral symptoms, clinical signs, diagnostic criteria, and common neuroimaging, genetic, and laboratory tests used to diagnose non-Alzheimer types of dementia.

- Understand the scientific rationale, indications, and limitations of currently available and emerging therapies for common non-Alzheimer type neurodegenerative diseases.

Key Clinical Points

1. The evaluation of neurodegenerative disorders includes careful attention to the cognitive, behavioral, and motor symptoms along with a thorough neurologic examination.

2. In older age, it becomes increasingly common for there to be more than one type of pathology causing a dementia syndrome.

3. The characteristic features of Lewy body dementia include cognitive impairments with profound fluctuation, spontaneous parkinsonism, rapid eye movement (REM) behavior sleep disorder, and visual hallucinations.

4. About 30% of patients with Parkinson disease develop dementia. In these patients, unlike Alzheimer disease (AD), the motor and other symptoms of Parkinson disease generally predate dementia by many years.

5. The dominance of behavioral and personality changes in the absence of memory and

(Continued)

(Cont.)

perceptual symptoms is highly suggestive of the behavioral variant of frontotemporal dementia (FTD).

6. History of falls and dysphagia with abnormalities in vertical gaze and preserved oculocephalic reflex is suggestive of a diagnosis of progressive supranuclear palsy (PSP).

are commonly seen in patients with advanced dementia syndromes, regardless of disease etiology; however, when these findings are a prominent presenting feature in the relative absence of amnestic symptoms, frontotemporal dementia (FTD) should be considered more likely.

Cognitive histories should be comprehensive and must include evaluation of memory, language, visuospatial function, executive functioning, behavior, and attention (**Table 63-1**). The comprehensive history should probe for autonomic symptoms and sleep patterns, with emphasis on symptoms associated with disorders of REM sleep behavior and sleep apneas.

The assessment of behavioral symptoms can be particularly helpful and sometimes critical in non-Alzheimer neurodegenerative disorders. Behavioral variant frontotemporal dementia (bvFTD) is the most common cause of dementia in patients younger than age 60. Behavioral symptoms or personality change are commonly the presenting symptoms of this disorder (see discussion later in this chapter). Recent research criteria for bvFTD require three of the following six symptoms to meet "possible" criteria: early disinhibition, early apathy, early loss of sympathy or empathy for others, early repetitive motor behaviors, early hyperorality, and deficits in frontal

executive function with relative sparing of visuospatial abilities. For probable bvFTD, in addition to meeting the "possible" criteria just listed, frontotemporal atrophy or the presence of a known causative mutation is required. The emergence of predominant behavior and personality changes in the absence of episodic memory and perceptual complaints localizes disease to the frontal or anterior temporal lobes, although presence of memory loss does not rule out bvFTD.

The neurologic examination is a critical component to the assessment of neurodegenerative disorders and typically confirms the clinical impression obtained from the history. The motor examination identifies both pyramidal and extrapyramidal signs as well as features characteristic of FTD, dementia with Lewy bodies (DLB), corticobasal degeneration (CBD), and PSP. Examination of cranial nerves includes an assessment of eye movements and range of gaze. Abnormalities in vertical gaze, either reduced amplitude or complete palsy, with a preserved oculocephalic reflex are a characteristic finding in PSP. Horizontal gaze abnormalities are more typical of CBD. Abnormalities in saccadic eye movements can be seen in several neurodegenerative disorders ranging from AD to PSP. Saccadic movements are tested by asking the patient to focus on an object in front of them (such as a pen tip held by the examiner) then to quickly refocus on an item in their peripheral field (such as the examiner's finger) while the examiner watches carefully for saccadic latency (delay in initiation of movement), incomplete saccades (gaze palsy), and interrupted or jerky saccadic movement. Saccades should be tested in all four directions. The examiner should test ocular pursuit by having the patient track an object, such as the examiner's finger, in both horizontal and vertical directions.

The examination should probe for changes in cognition, behavior, and movement with emphasis upon the earliest abnormalities. It is important to realize that early symptoms reflect where the illness began, and this is usually helpful in the determination of disease etiology. Confirmatory imaging and laboratory work and standard laboratory tests to exclude treatable etiologies of cognitive impairment can then be completed (**Table 63-2**).

TABLE 63-1 ■ ASSESSMENT OF MAJOR COGNITIVE DOMAINS IN NEURODEGENERATIVE DISORDERS

Memory: repetitive statements, misplacing items, missed appointment or medications, recalling recent/remote events

Language: speech fluency, comprehension, reading, writing, articulation, word-finding, content of speech, output, spelling

Visuospatial: getting lost, driving, object perception, completing household repairs, parking

Executive: planning, flexibility/rigidity in thinking, organization, multistep tasks

Motor: gait, falls, tremor, dysphagia, weakness, handwriting, coordination

Autonomic: light-headedness, bowel/bladder function, impotence, hypotension

TABLE 63-2 ■ SOME LABORATORY TESTS COMMONLY USED IN THE EVALUATION OF COGNITIVE DISORDERS

Chemistries, including liver function tests and renal function tests

Complete blood count

Vitamin B_{12}

Homocysteine

Methylmalonic acid

Syphilis serology

HIV

Thyroid function

DISORDERS ASSOCIATED WITH α-SYNUCLEIN DEPOSITION

Dementia With Lewy Bodies

The precise role of α-synuclein in health and disease is not fully understood. High concentrations of α-synuclein in synaptic regions suggest a role in synaptic plasticity. In DLB, α-synuclein accumulates with the brain stem, basal ganglia, and cortex, resulting in a progressive neurodegenerative cognitive, behavioral, and motor disorder. The prevalence of DLB is still uncertain, and the coassociation of Lewy body and AD pathology is extremely common in aging dementia populations. Indeed, even with classical AD associated with apolipoprotein E4 genotype, more than 50% of subjects show Lewy bodies, and genetic disorders that predispose to Lewy bodies often show the coassociation of Aβ-42. Based on autopsy studies, DLB, especially cooccurring DLB and AD, is often underdiagnosed during life.

The reported mean onset of disease is 75 years with a range from 50 to 80 years, and there is a slight predominance of DLB in men compared to women. The clinical and pathologic overlap between DLB and AD and with Parkinson disease dementia (PDD) is well recognized, resulting in some diagnostic challenges. Accurate diagnosis has clinical implications, as patients with DLB compared to AD tend to have a robust response to cholinesterase inhibitors, and patients with DLB often have sensitivity to neuroleptic medications.

The core features of DLB are cognitive impairment with profound fluctuations in attention and cognition, spontaneous parkinsonism, REM behavior sleep disorder (the physical enactment of dreams), and recurrent well-formed visual hallucinations. The typical neuropsychological profile differs somewhat from that of AD. DLB often involves early executive dysfunction and, when present, more severe visuospatial dysfunction. In DLB there is typically better performance on episodic memory tasks, and recognition memory when compared to AD patients. Invariably, memory becomes impaired over time in both disorders. Combined cortical and subcortical deficits are common, and deficits in attention are a core feature of the disease.

The degree of cognitive fluctuation can be so profound as to affect Mini Mental State Examination (MMSE) scores up to 50% from day-to-day, and many patients repeatedly move in and out of delirium. Unfortunately, eliciting a history of fluctuation can be difficult, and this symptom may not be well described by caregivers. Clinicians should consider several different approaches, including questions focused on marked alteration in attention, staring spells, daytime sleepiness, and episodes of incoherent speech. On occasion, the fluctuation can be so severe as to result in emergency room evaluation for a transient ischemic attack (TIA) or delirium. Several structured scales exist to assist in assessment of fluctuation, including the One Day Fluctuation Assessment Scale and the Clinical Assessment of Fluctuation.

A common feature of neurodegenerative disorders with α-synuclein pathology is REM sleep behavior disorder (RBD), defined as vivid and often frightening dreams that are frequently acted out verbally or motorically. RBD occurs in 85% of DLB cases, compared to 15% of Parkinson disease patients and 60% of patients with multiple system atrophy (MSA). It is uncommon in other forms of dementia where α-synuclein pathology is absent. In the DLB diagnostic criteria, RBD is considered a core feature. Autonomic dysfunction is also common and can be profound with repeat syncope and unexplained loss of consciousness. When REM behavior occurs in association with severe autonomic symptoms, MSA rather than DLB should also be considered. Significant depressive symptoms occur in up to 40% of cases and can often precede other symptoms by years.

About two-thirds of DLB cases will exhibit visual hallucinations, misperceptions or, less frequently, delusional misidentification. When delusional misidentification, such as mistaking the spouse, friend, or relative as an impostor, occurs as the first symptom of a dementia, DLB is highly likely. The visual hallucinations of DLB can be vivid with distinct colors and the inclusion of human figures and animals. In contrast to the hallucinations sometimes seen with more advanced AD, visual hallucinations occur early in DLB. In one pathology-based study, visual hallucinations corresponded to a greater number of Lewy bodies in the anterior/inferior temporal lobes and to larger deficits in acetylcholine. Visual hallucinations often respond to boosting brain acetylcholine with cholinesterase inhibitors.

Spontaneous parkinsonism is a hallmark feature of DLB, eventually occurring in up to 70% of cases. Common findings include bradykinesia, axial and appendicular rigidity, postural instability, slowed response times, and hypomimia. In contrast to Parkinson disease, the parkinsonism of DLB is more commonly bilateral and less frequently includes tremor. Parkinsonism rarely occurs in isolation as an early finding in DLB although early features of the cognitive syndrome are commonly overlooked. Response to levodopa treatment is less frequent than the response seen in Parkinson disease; however, efficacy data may be biased. Clinicians are more likely to avoid such drugs in DLB patients for fear of adverse effects such as orthostasis or aggravations of hallucinations.

Parkinsonism contributes substantially to the disability in DLB and alters the clinical course. Mean survival among postmortem confirmed cases of DLB is 10 years, with a rate of disability at approximately 10% per year, often exceeding that of Parkinson disease. Cases of rapid progression to death in 1 to 2 years have been described. Risk factors for higher mortality include older age, hallucinations, greater degrees of fluctuation, and neuroleptic sensitivity.

Diagnostic criteria for DLB assist in identification of disease and are particularly useful for research purposes

TABLE 63-3 ■ MCKEITH CRITERIA FOR DLB[a]

Central features

Progressive cognitive decline with functional impairment

Prominent memory impairment may not occur early but is usually evident with progression

Deficits in attention, executive functioning, and visuospatial ability may be prominent early

Core features

Fluctuating cognition with prominent variations in attention and alertness

Recurrent visual hallucinations

Spontaneous parkinsonism

Suggestive features

REM sleep behavior disorder

Neuroleptic sensitivity

Low dopamine transporter uptake in the basal ganglia (SPECT, PET)

Supportive features

Repeated falls

Transient, unexplained loss of consciousness

Severe autonomic dysfunction

Systematized delusions

Depression

Hallucinations in nonvisual modalities

Relative preservation of medial temporal lobe structures on CT/MRI

Generalized low uptake on SPECT/PET with reduced occipital activity

Abnormal MIBG scintigraphy

Prominent slow wave activity on EEG with temporal lobe transient sharp waves

[a]Probable DLB requires two core features or one core feature and at least one suggestive feature.

Possible DLB requires one or more suggestive features. Probable DLB should not be based on suggestive features alone.

CT, computed tomography; DLB, dementia with Lewy bodies; EEG, electroencephalogram; MIBG, metaiodobenzylguanidine scintigraphy; MRI, magnetic resonance imaging; PET, positron emission tomography; SPECT, single-photon emission computed tomography.

Data from McKeith IG, Dickson DW, Lowe J, et al. Diagnosis and management of dementia with Lewy bodies: third report of the DLB Consortium. Neurology. 2005;65(12):1863–1872.

(**Table 63-3**). In the revised schema, core features include prominent fluctuation, recurrent visual hallucinations, RBD, and spontaneous features of parkinsonism such as rigidity, bradykinesia, and hypomimia. Supportive and suggestive features are also defined. To meet diagnostic criteria for probable disease, two core features or the combination of one core feature and one supportive feature are required. If one core feature without any suggestive features, or suggestive features are present in the absence of any core features, the term "possible DLB" is used.

The pathologic hallmark of DLB is the presence of neuronal spherical intracytoplasmic inclusions of α-synuclein, termed Lewy bodies (**Figure 63-1**). The Lewy bodies seen in DLB are very similar in appearance to those that are seen in Parkinson disease; however, in DLB, the distribution extends beyond the substantia nigra and locus coeruleus to involve the neocortex and limbic system. Cortical Lewy bodies lack the typical dense core with pale halo appearance that is seen in Parkinson disease. Other intraneuronal aggregates of α-synuclein (Lewy neurites), cortical senile plaques, and sparse tau pathology are all described in DLB. As described above, AD copathology is frequently encountered.

Currently, imaging studies do not add substantially to differentiating DLB from other neurodegenerative disorders and are only included as supportive features in diagnostic criteria. Structural magnetic resonance imaging (MRI) often identifies less atrophy of the medial temporal lobes in cohorts of DLB compared to AD and variably identifies greater atrophy in the basal ganglia structures and the dorsal midbrain. In group studies, single-photon emission computed tomography (SPECT) with ^{99m}Tc-hexamethylpropyleneamine oxime (HMPAO) tends to show decreased regional cortical brain activity in parietal-occipital regions of DLB compared to AD patients. This is relative sparing of the posterior cingulate cortical perfusion in DLB compared to the occipital cortex, a highly specific finding called the cingulate island sign. DLB patients exhibit decreased dopamine transport in the putamen and caudate by dopaminergic SPECT and decreased postganglionic sympathetic cardiac innervation by I-metaiodobenzyl guanindine (MIBG) SPECT imaging. The modest performance characteristics of these tests limits their clinical utility.

The clinical course of DLB is often faster than that seen in AD and a drop of four to five points on MMSE per year is common (in contrast to three points per year, which is typical for AD). Patients with DLB should be tried on cholinesterase inhibitors. Often this results in responses that exceed those seen in AD, including frequent reduction or elimination of hallucinations. Social stimulation and physical exercise to maximize balance and strength should be recommended. Symptomatic treatment with levodopa can be used, if indicated, for parkinsonian symptoms once fluctuation and visual hallucinations are stabilized with a cholinesterase inhibitor. Patients should be advised to avoid anticholinergic medications, including many common over-the-counter cold remedies. RBD, if severe, can be treated with melatonin or clonazepam. Atypical neuroleptic medications should be cautiously considered only if intolerable behavioral disturbances emerge.

Parkinson Disease Dementia

The temporal relationship between the onset of dementia and the development of parkinsonism is the primary clinical feature distinguishing DLB from PDD. In PDD, cognitive deterioration occurs in well-established Parkinson disease, typically years to decades after motor systems are identified. In contrast, research criteria for DLB require cognitive symptoms that predate parkinsonism by 12 months; although this "1-year rule" is often difficult to

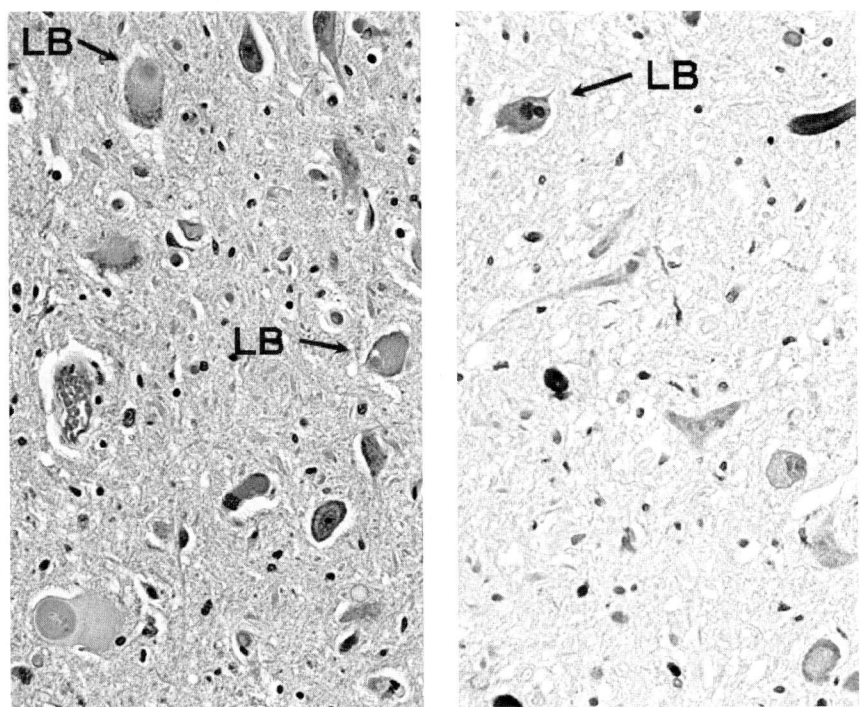

FIGURE 63-1. Lewy bodies (LB) seen with hematoxylin and eosin staining (*left*) and α-synuclein staining (*right*).

apply in the clinical setting. This temporal distinction is arbitrary, and many believe that the two disorders represent different points in the spectrum of the same disease, and abnormalities in α-synuclein accumulation underlie both disorders.

Approximately one-third of older Parkinson disease patients will develop sufficient cognitive symptoms during the course of their illness to impair function. Indeed, the diagnosis of Parkinson disease puts a patient at high risk for mild cognitive impairment (MCI) and then PDD following in many patients. In pure PDD, the prominent findings include motor and psychomotor slowing, decreased response times, and alterations in concentration and attention. The recognition that medications used to treat Parkinson disease can affect cognition and the understanding that, because of age, a substantial number of Parkinson patients will develop concurrent AD result in a scenario where cognitive symptoms in this population can be multifactorial. Possible predictors for dementia in Parkinson disease include older age at onset of motor symptoms, bradykinesia, nontremor prominent Parkinson disease, bilateral onset of motor signs, and declining response to levodopa. Depression and visual hallucinations may increase the risk as well. Patients with DLB typically exhibit a faster clinical decline than do patients with PDD.

Multiple System Atrophy

MSA is a sporadic disease marked by degeneration of multiple neurologic systems and resulting in relentlessly progressive clinical course. Death typically occurs within 6 to 10 years with an estimated 10-year survival of 40%. Relatively infrequent, the incidence is estimated to be 0.6/100,000 person-years or between 1.86 and 4.9/100,000 population. The incidence increases to 6/100,000 person-years among patients older than 50 years. The mean age of onset is 54. While currently speculated to have a combination of environmental and genetic predispositions, neither has been definitively established. Epidemiologic studies suggest a potential risk associated with exposure to pesticides. MSA is about three times more frequent in men than women and limited epidemiologic data suggest that it may be less frequent among smokers.

The term MSA was first used in 1969 and encompasses diseases previously labeled as striatonigral degeneration (now termed MSA-P for parkinsonism), Shy-Drager syndrome, and olivopontocerebellar degeneration (now termed MSA-C for cerebellar). The MSA subtypes are indicative of the predominant neurologic component involved. Patients with prominent orthostatic features tend to have decreased survival compared to other subtypes. Several derivations of diagnostic consensus statements exist with mixed sensitivity.

The presenting symptoms of MSA are variable and include cerebellar findings, autonomic failure, pyramidal findings, and parkinsonism. Parkinsonism (MSA-P) is prominent in most cases (80%) with cerebellar symptoms (MSA-C) more prominent in about 20% of cases. The more common presenting parkinsonian features are akinesia, rigidity, and postural (rather than resting) tremor. Autonomic symptoms precede motor symptoms in most cases. Gait instability is common but falls occur less frequently in early stages than in PSP. In early stages, MSA can mimic Parkinson disease but more symptoms evolve within 5 years. Gait ataxia, limb kinetic ataxia, and dysarthria are the more frequent presenting symptoms in patients with cerebellar-dominant MSA. The dysarthria caused by cerebellar dysfunction has a characteristic appearance of jerky, intermittently explosive, and slurred output often associated with poor separation of syllables.

Autonomic symptoms include orthostasis, erectile dysfunction, constipation, and urinary incontinence. While orthostasis is common, syncope occurs infrequently. Diagnostic criteria for the orthostatic component of MSA require a 30 mm Hg drop in systolic blood pressure; although in practice, a 20 mm Hg drop in systolic blood pressure or 10 mm Hg drop in diastolic blood pressure is thought to be significant in the absence of appropriate increased heart rate. Occurrence of symptoms suggestive of MSA in an individual younger than 30 years or in an individual with a family history of similar disease should raise suspicion for alternative diagnoses.

Most MSA patients complain of sleep problems, commonly sleep fragmentation (53%), early waking (33%), and insomnia (20%). As with other synucleinopathies, RBD is common, occurring in up to 60% of MSA patients. Nocturnal stridor and obstructive sleep apnea are also frequent in MSA. Stridor is associated with decreased survival and risk of sudden death.

Historically, MSA was characterized as a primary movement disorder without significant cognitive impairment. The current consensus criteria for MSA considered dementia as a nonsupporting feature. There is emerging evidence of higher prevalence of variable cognitive impairment, typically later in the clinical course. The pattern of cognitive impairment is most commonly frontal-executive dysfunction, likely secondary to deafferentation of frontostriatal neural pathways. Disruption of cerebellocortical circuitry in MSA-C can also lead to impaired attention, visuospatial function, and affect regulation.

Brain MRI changes occur in some patients but lack sensitivity and specificity for definitive diagnosis. These findings include hypointensity and atrophy of the putamen on T2-weighted images with a slit-like marginal hypointensity just lateral to the putamen on axial images. A characteristic "hot cross bun" sign has been described in the pons and middle cerebral peduncles thought to be caused by degenerative changes in pontocerebellar fibers. This finding lacks sensitivity and is sometimes seen in Parkinson disease, limiting specificity. Atrophy of the brain stem, middle cerebellar peduncles, and cerebellum may also be seen. Volumetric analyses of the striatum and brain stem, where atrophy is very severe in MSA but not in simple Parkinson disease, demonstrate some promise in discriminating these

two disorders. Electromyography (EMG) abnormalities at the anal sphincter can be seen in MSA, although the clinical utility for distinguishing MSA from Parkinson disease in early stages of disease has not been established.

The hallmark pathology of MSA is cell loss, gliosis, and glial inclusions in multiple neurologic systems including the spinal cord and cortex. Prominent abnormalities are also seen in the basal ganglia, substantia nigra, and olivopontocerebellar pathways, as suggested by the terminology, with anatomy reflecting symptoms. On gross inspection, the putamen is shrunken and displays a green-gray discoloration that can appear cribriform when disease is severe. As with DLB and Parkinson disease, there is an accumulation of α-synuclein as half-moon–, oval-, or conical-shaped argyrophilic glial cytoplasmic inclusions.

Treatment is generally symptomatic with about one-third of patients responding to levodopa in the early stages of the disease. Patients should be encouraged to sleep in a lateral decubitus rather than supine position to minimize airway obstruction. Use of positive airway pressure devices should be considered. Invasive means of controlling stridor and apneas have included tracheotomy but should be approached cautiously within the full context of ethical and quality-of-life considerations. RBD may respond to melatonin or low-dose clonazepam at night. Labile blood pressures may develop and should raise concern when symptomatic. Avoiding alcohol, heavy meals, or straining at micturition and defecation is recommended. Elastic stockings and elevating the head of the bed may provide some relief. Pharmacologic approaches designed to increase sympathetic tone (midodrine) or volume expansion (fludrocortisone) may be required. Patients with MSA-C tend to maintain function for a longer time than those with MSA-P.

NEURODEGENERATIVE DISORDERS ASSOCIATED WITH TAU, TDP-43, OR FUS PATHOLOGY

Frontotemporal Lobar Degeneration Syndromes

FTLD is the term used to capture a neuropathologically linked group of non-AD dementing conditions associated with frontotemporal and basal ganglia pathology. FTD subsumes three clinical syndromes, bvFTD, semantic variant primary progressive aphasia (svPPA), and nonfluent variant primary progressive aphasia (nfvPPA). Recent evidence indicates that FTLD is closely related to several other neurodegenerative disorders: CBD, PSP, and motor neuron disease (**Figure 63-2**).

The core anatomic feature of FTLD is the focal, often asymmetric cortical degeneration of frontal and anterior temporal regions with general sparing of posterior cortical structures. The resultant brain atrophy can be severe, sometimes described as "knife-edge," and the brain can weigh as little as 750 g at autopsy (**Figure 63-3**). Patients present

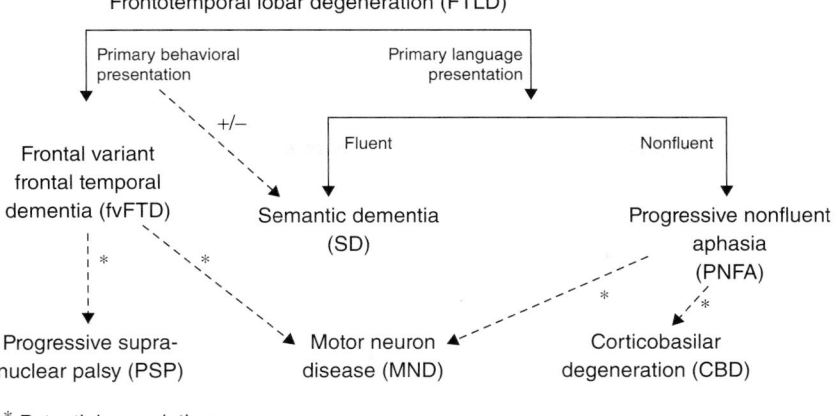

FIGURE 63-2. Frontotemporal lobar degeneration (FTLD) and potential associations to other neurodegenerative syndromes.

with a primary behavioral or language deficit that typically corresponds to the region of greatest brain atrophy and dysfunction. Patients presenting with primary behavioral deficits are classified as suffering with the behavioral variant of FTD (bvFTD). bvFTD overlaps considerably with the two syndromes that present with predominant language deficits: the semantic and nonfluent variants of primary progressive aphasia (svPPA and nfvPPA). In most centers bvFTD accounts for more than 50% of all cases with the others divided between svPPA and nfvPPA. The neuropathologic basis for nearly one-half of these diseases is the abnormal accumulation of tau protein with a similar percentage associated with abnormal aggregates of TDP-43. Less than 10% show aggregates of the fused in sarcoma (FUS) protein. Many FTD patients are misdiagnosed as having AD during life. In addition to changes in personality and behavior, features that should alert physicians to the possibility of FTD include early abnormalities in social conduct, loss of sympathy and empathy for others, repetitive motor behaviors, or hyperorality. When cognitive testing is completed, suspicion should be raised when abnormalities in executive functioning occur in the absence of prominent amnestic complaints or cognitive features localizing to posterior structures, such as problems with calculations and visuospatial tasks.

Patients who present with isolated language symptoms that exist for at least 2 years in the initial stages of cognitive decline are termed to have primary progressive aphasia (PPA). As a group, patients with PPA have greater atrophy on the left than the right of the perisylvian region, the anterior temporal lobes, and the basal ganglia. Inferior parietal lobule atrophy has also been described in PPA and is associated with predominantly word-finding deficits. Called logopenic aphasia by Gorno-Tempini and colleagues, this form of PPA is usually due to underlying AD pathology. As the syndrome progresses, patients presenting with nfvPPA go on to develop features of PSP or CBD or even amyotrophic lateral sclerosis (ALS). Thus, careful attention to the development of motor symptoms is necessary to help with the prediction of the underlying pathology. The emergence of artistic behavior has been described in some patients with primary language difficulty.

Efforts to distinguish the various PPA syndromes from each other may have clinical ramifications. Clinical, genetic, and imaging studies have indicated that the logopenic variety of PPA is usually a language presentation of AD. As the term implies, these patients have decreased speech output. They typically have slow speech with impaired syntactic comprehension and naming. lvPPA is associated with short-term phonologic memory deficits. These patients exhibit profound echoic memory deficits manifested as forgetting portions of longer phrases during repetition tasks and being able to partially paraphrase but not exactly repeat such phrases. If confirmed by imaging or other biomarkers to be AD in etiology, these patients may

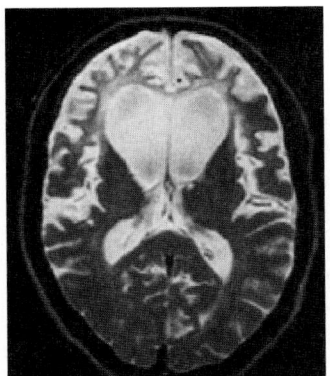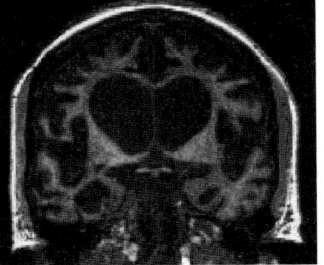

FIGURE 63-3. T2-weighted axial (*right*) and T1-weighted coronal (*left*) brain magnetic resonance imaging (MRI) in a 59-year-old woman with pathology-confirmed Pick disease.

be amenable to treatment with cholinesterase inhibitors or other emerging treatment strategies.

Nonfluent Variant Primary Progressive Aphasia

Patients with nfvPPA typically have apraxic, labored speech with errors in grammar, and difficulty with more complex syntax. Speech apraxia is the inability to produce speech caused by difficulty in programming the sensorimotor commands for the positioning and movement of muscles used to produce speech. This leads to difficulty with initiation of speech, sound substitutions, omissions, transpositions of syllables, and a slower rate of expressing sentences punctuated with inappropriate starts and stops. Patients may sound as if they are stuttering or having trouble enunciating, or otherwise mispronouncing words. The distortions can include sounds not present in their native language and the errors produced in apraxic speech are typically inconsistent. The problems are usually worse for multisyllabic words. Speech apraxia is localized to the left opercular and anterior insular region.

Anomia is variably present and phonemic paraphasias are frequently observed. Speech output is decreased and dropped words, often articles such as "the," occur. In patients with nfvPPA, sentences tend to have more nouns than verbs. In contrast to patients with svPPA, these patients maintain single word comprehension and semantic knowledge. Thus, nfvPPA is not likely in a patient who has preserved articulation, preserved grammar, and deficits in semantic knowledge. Insight into the condition can be exquisitely preserved with nfvPPA, and patients often develop depression. Other behavioral problems are uncommon in early stages of disease.

MRI studies of nfvPPA have revealed atrophy that is asymmetrically left-dominant with preferential involvement of the inferior frontal lobe, the insular region, and the caudate. Hypometabolism of the left frontal region can be observed on fluorodeoxyglucose positron emission tomography (FDG-PET). Most patients show tau pathology at autopsy with CBD being most common, followed by PSP and Pick changes. Approximately 20% show TDP pathology, usually TDP-43 type A.

Semantic Variant Primary Progressive Aphasia

In contrast to patients with nfvPPA, patients with svPPA have fluent speech that is grammatically accurate, but they exhibit the hallmark loss of semantic knowledge. Semantic memory is the encyclopedic knowledge of people, objects, facts, and words. Unlike episodic memories, individuals are not aware of where or when they learned these facts. Eventually individuals with svPPA lose all knowledge about the fact or word and exhibit features of a multimodality agnosia. Therefore, even when they are provided with the name of the object, the object is not recognized. Early in the disease, patients are often aware of word-finding difficulties and can also be aware of comprehension difficulties (eg, acknowledging that they don't recognize a word they

should know). Semantic paraphasias are frequent, with supraordinate substitutions of words and common use of nonspecific grouping words such as "stuff" and "things." Repetition and prosody are preserved, as are syntax and verb recognition.

Patients with svPPA display surface dyslexia manifest by difficulty pronouncing irregularly spelled words, such as "gnat," "heir," or "pint," when pronunciation does not follow standard phonologic rules. On neuropsychological testing, patients with svPPA have difficulty with category fluency and confrontational naming, particularly with low-frequency words. More recently, a right hemispheric variant of svPPA has been described. These patients have difficulty naming and recognizing famous people and develop a number of behavioral symptoms similar to bvFTD. In contrast to AD, many svPPA patients have greater deficits for remote compared to recent memory, when memory deficits become involved.

Of all the PPA syndromes, svPPA has the greatest propensity to include behavioral problems, which are included as supportive evidence in diagnostic criteria. As with FTD, the behavioral issues seen with svPPA often involve hyperorality, disinhibition, and aberrant motor behavior. Diagnostic criteria include behaviors such as loss of sympathy and empathy, narrowed preoccupations, and parsimony (excessive frugality, stinginess). Rigidity in thinking can be striking. svPPA patients can develop compulsions and have been described to have visual hypervigilance, such as recognizing that a hair is subtly out of place on an examiner or quickly seeing a coin on the street. They may exhibit difficulty in the interpretation of emotions, particularly negative emotions such as sadness, anger, and fear. Emergence of behavioral symptoms correlates with duration of illness but can also be an early finding. The presence of early behavioral issues in a patient with a PPA syndrome should alert to the possibility of svPPA.

Anatomic studies may explain why svPPA patients often exhibit behavioral abnormalities. The disorder begins in the amygdala and anterior temporal lobes. When it starts on the left side, language deficits predominate, while right-sided presentations are characterized by loss of empathy for others or deficits in the recognition of familiar people. These patients sometimes meet research criteria for bvFTD while others are more typical of svPPA. While svPPA begins in the anterior left temporal lobe, it typically spreads anteriorly to involve the frontal regions. Eventually it spreads to the right medial frontal lobe, the right orbitofrontal lobes, and the right insular region, areas associated with behaviors such as disinhibition and apathy. The absence of behavioral problems in the logopenic variety of PPA and in nfvPPA is likely due to the general sparing of these same structures in those diseases.

Patients with svPPA often have TDP-43 type C–positive, tau-negative inclusions at autopsy. The etiology for svPPA and for TDP type C aggregates is unknown. Rarely are these cases familial. Recent work suggests that a significant subset of these patients have a history of autoimmunity and increased levels of tumor necrosis factor (TNF) in the serum.

Behavioral Variant Frontotemporal Dementia

bvFTD presents with the insidious onset of change in personality and inappropriate behaviors. The mean age of onset is in the mid-fifties. Most commonly, symptoms include disinhibition, poor impulse control, loss of sympathy or empathy for others, overeating, compulsive behaviors, and deficits in executive control or multitasking (**Table 63-4**). Patients can develop stereotyped behaviors, defined as repetitive, invariant behaviors that lack purpose. Examples include counting, pacing, organizing, or the repetitive use of catch phrases. Socially inappropriate activities can include shoplifting and other criminal behavior, public urination, offensive speech, and public masturbation. Perseveration is common. Cravings for sweets are often observed. When associated with the decreased sense of satiety that can occur, large, unhealthy weight gain results. Hyperorality and oral exploratory behavior, similar to human Klüver-Bucy syndrome, can occur.

Patients with bvFTD are often misdiagnosed as having psychiatric illness. In other instances, any patient with an atypical dementia syndrome is considered to have bvFTD. Delusions can occur, often with bizarre or grandiose overtones. Patients exhibit lack of empathy and can have a cold, blunted effect. When the anterior cingulate and medial frontal lobes are involved, apathy can be particularly prominent, and some degree of apathy, especially in later stages, is almost universal. Some patients undergo large changes in their beliefs and attitudes, including religious sentiments. In contrast to AD, depression is uncommon in bvFTD.

TABLE 63-4 ■ SYMPTOMS IN BEHAVIORAL VARIANT OF FRONTOTEMPORAL DEMENTIA

Antisocial behavior

Apathy

Change in beliefs (hyperreligiosity, change in attitude)

Cravings (sweets, weight gain)

Criminal behavior (theft, assault, public urination)

Delusions

Disinhibition

Euphoria (inappropriate jocularity)

Hyperorality (oral exploratory behavior in late disease)

Hypersexuality (offensive statements, masturbation)

Impotence and decreased sexual drive

Impulsivity

Loss of empathy (coldness, self-centered)

Obsessive-compulsive behavior

Perseverative behavior

Poor insight

Stereotyped behavior (counting, pacing, repetitive use of catch phrases)

Neuropsychological testing demonstrates abnormalities in executive functioning, working memory, and social cognition with general sparing of visuospatial skills and verbal memory. Consequently, the MMSE score can be quite high even among patients with marked functional disability. BvFTD patients also display problems with set-shifting, concept formation, and abstract reasoning. They may demonstrate disinhibition, impulsivity, and poor judgment during testing. These behaviors can falsely lower verbal memory scores. When closely scrutinized, poor scores on such tests are accompanied by frequent intrusions of novel words and endorsement words that were not part of the original list learned (false positives on recognition testing). Although poor performance on executive function tasks is a feature bvFTD, it may not be present in early cases and can also be a feature of AD and other dementias, even early in the course. Thus, executive function tests should not be considered mandatory for a diagnosis of bvFTD, and when present it should not be the main reason for making a diagnosis of bvFTD. Rather, it should only be used to support a diagnosis when other, behavioral features of bvFTD are present.

Behavioral symptoms are a common late finding in most dementia syndromes. Thus, the emergence of behavior and personality symptoms in a patient with well-established dementia should be looked upon with caution when considering a change in diagnosis to bvFTD. The importance of the first symptom (often the presenting symptom) in the evaluation of patients with neurodegenerative disorders cannot be overstated.

Patients with bvFTD will typically have profound, usually bilateral, frontal, anterior insular, and anterior temporal lobe atrophy. Patients with greater atrophy on the right frontal lobe than left have more severe behavioral symptoms. Stages of atrophy have been described with the earliest stage involving only mild atrophy of the orbital and superior medial frontal lobes and hippocampus. As the disease progresses, the anterior frontal and temporal cortices and basal ganglia are increasingly involved. The severity of atrophy increases as disease advances. William Seeley has demonstrated that in many instances, the first neurons afflicted in bvFTD are von Economo neurons that sit in the anterior insular and cingulate cortex. These neurons are a unique feature in the brains of humans, other primates, and a few other species of mammals. SPECT and FDG-PET techniques have been used to differentiate FTD from AD with PET receiving Food and Drug Administration (FDA) approval for this indication. Both SPECT and FDG-PET demonstrate bilateral frontal hypometabolism/hypoperfusion in patients with FTD. Amyloid imaging is extremely valuable in separating AD from bvFTD, particularly in patients under the age 70 in whom the presence amyloid is not highly prevalent.

Pick Disease

Pick disease is a pathologic diagnosis and occurs in approximately 20% of clinical cases presenting with signs and symptoms of bvFTD. Less commonly it presents as nfvPPA. First described in 1892 by a German neurologist, Arnold Pick, the pathologic hallmark of Pick disease is argyrophilic cellular inclusions known as Pick bodies and swollen achromatic tau-positive neurons termed Pick cells. This is invariably associated with loss of large pyramidal neurons, resulting in a spongiform histologic appearance with selective atrophy of the frontal and anterior temporal lobes. Pick bodies are localized to the limbic cortex, paralimbic cortex, and predominantly the ventral aspect of the temporal lobe. The pre- and postcentral gyri are notably spared. The largest concentration of Pick bodies is found in the hippocampus and amygdala. Pick bodies are composed of randomly arranged tau filaments. In AD, tau pathology (neurofibrillary tangles) can spare the dentate gyrus; however, in Pick disease, this region is heavily involved.

Other FTLD Neuropathologies

FTLD is associated with tau pathology in about half of cases. The tau gene product has six isoforms, half of which result in three microtubule-binding repeats (3Rtau) and the other half result in four microtubule repeats (4Rtau). Pick disease is usually associated with 3Rtau. PSP and CBD, in contrast, are associated with 4Rtau. The clinical features and neuropathology of PSP and CBD are described later in this chapter.

Among FTLD cases that do not stain for tau protein, the histopathology will typically indicate a variable pattern of neuronal loss and gliosis with the presence of TAR DNA binding protein 43 (TDP-43) inclusions. TDP-43 neuropathology has been subdivided into four types, TDP-A to TDP-D, depending on the pattern of the TDP inclusions within the nucleus and cytoplasm. TDP type A is often associated with mutations in the progranulin gene, although sporadic cases have been seen. Type B is often associated with motor neuron disease, and the most common genetic mutation associated with familial FTD-ALS, C9orf72, often shows type B changes. TDP-C is the pattern associated with svPPA, while type D is seen with the rare FTD-causing mutation in valosin.

The Genetics of FTD

Our understanding of the genetics of FTLD is evolving. In 1998 it was discovered that a mutation in the microtubule-associated protein tau (MAPT) gene was responsible for a familial form of FTD associated with Parkinson disease (FTDP-17). This mutation appears to be more common in Southern Europe and France than in Northern Europe, and a few mutations have been reported in China and Japan. The disease onset with mutations is variable with several variants presenting in the third of fourth decade. Mean disease onset is approximately 52 years. The mechanism for disease pathogenesis with tau mutations appears to be variable. In some cases, a mutation in an intron adjacent to exon 10 leads to an excess of the 4R form of tau with abnormal aggregation of tau. In other mutations, abnormal microtubule-binding or excessive formation of oligomers appears to be the mechanism for neurodegeneration.

A mutation in the progranulin (GRN) gene (only 1.7 Mb away from the tau gene) was identified in 2006. This mutation appears to account for up to 11% of sporadic and 25% of familial FTD cases. Disease onset tends to be later than with tau, and approximately 10% of mutation carriers remain asymptomatic after age 70. There are mutations that modify progranulin expression that may be partially responsible for this clinical variability. The onset of disease can range from 35 to 80 years. The phenotype is more variable than with MAPT mutations, and syndromes vary from bvFTD, nfvPPA, CBD, and Parkinson disease to AD. Asymmetry is common, sometimes with one hemisphere being massively atrophic and the other relatively normal. The pathophysiologic mechanisms associated with GRN mutations are also debated; loss of neuronal growth attributed to low levels of the progranulin protein, excessive inflammation associated with low progranulin levels, and a relative increase in the granulin proteins cleaved from progranulin are all possible. All these hypothesized mechanisms probably contribute to illness. Autoimmunity is seen in more than 10% of mutation carriers and can precede neurologic disease.

In 2011 a mutation in the C9orf72 gene was discovered as the major cause for familial forms of FTD, ALS, and FTD-ALS. A large expansion of a hexanucleotide repeat in the intron of C9 leads to overproduction of RNA and the production of dipeptides generated from the RNA in a non-ATG manner. The clinical onset is typically in the sixth decade but patients in the fourth and eighth decades have been described. The illness can begin as a psychiatric illness with highly variable symptoms ranging from borderline personality disorder, bipolar illness, depression, and conversion disorder to drug addiction. Similarly, whether a mutation carrier is diagnosed with bvFTD or ALS is also variable, and in some instances, both syndromes emerge together. The mechanism for disease may reflect RNA-mediated neurodegeneration caused by large nuclear RNA aggregates that interfere with nuclear functions, the toxic effects of dipeptides, and possibly gene haploinsufficiency.

Other isolated cases of FTLD-related mutations have been described, including in the valosin-containing protein gene (VCP), and charged multivesicular body protein 2B (CHMP 2B) genes. Patients with the VCP mutation develop a rare disease with inclusion body myopathy, early Paget's disease of bone, and FTD (IBM-PDB-FTD). Additionally, predominantly ALS but sometimes bvFTD phenotypes can occur with mutations in the TDP-43 and FUS proteins. The list of mutations continues to grow, but thus far most of the more recently discovered mutations account for a small proportion of mutation related FTLD.

Treatment of FTLD

Treatment approaches for FTD and related disorders are generally aimed at symptom management, as there are not yet any effective disease-modifying therapies. Selective serotonin reuptake inhibitor (SSRI) medications may be beneficial for behavioral symptoms, including carbohydrate craving and compulsions. If delusions are problematic, atypical neuroleptics can be considered. There is no theoretical basis for the use of cholinesterase inhibitors, which can aggravate agitation. Attention to caregiver issues is important as the stressors often differ from those seen in typical AD and can be particularly burdensome. The different social and behavioral issues presented to FTLD compared to AD caregivers and the younger age of both patients and caregivers in FTLD can lead caregivers to feel isolated in support groups focused on typical AD.

Disease-modifying approaches are being investigated. Tau-lowering strategies are emerging for tau forms of FTD including tau mutations, Pick disease, PSP, and CBD. Monoclonal antibodies that target tau appear to show efficacy in animal models and have potential to diminish the brain's tau burden. Several other approaches are being investigated that could be effective for treatment of FTLD associated with TDP-43 inclusions, including sporadic and mutation-related disease.

AMYOTROPHIC LATERAL SCLEROSIS (LOU GEHRIG DISEASE)

ALS was first identified in 1869 by the French neurologist, Jean-Martin Charcot who described a progressive neurodegenerative disease with mixed upper and lower motor neuron signs. The disease's name is derived from myelin pallor identified in the lateral aspects of the spinal cord representing axonal degeneration from upper motor neurons as they descend to the limbs. In the United States, the disease is best known as Lou Gehrig disease, named after the famous baseball player who died of the disease in 1941. It occurs with an incidence of approximately 1 to 2/100,000 patients each year with a nearly 2:1 male-to-female predominance. About 5000 people develop ALS annually. As with FTLD, peak incidence occurs in midlife; however, disease can be seen in advancing ages.

Patients with ALS typically present with complaints of weakness in one or more limbs, resulting in unexplained tripping or dropping of items. Clumsy fine finger movements lead to difficulty with tasks such as buttoning clothes or writing. Patients often complain of cramping. Bulbar symptoms such as speech slurring, difficulties with swallowing, and hoarseness occur in many patients. Bulbar symptoms are presenting symptoms in about 25% of cases and more commonly occur in older patients. Patients may complain of difficulty chewing or swallowing. Up to 45% of patients will develop pseudobulbar effect characterized by episodes of uncontrolled laughter or crying, often in inappropriate settings. Many patients have symptoms of a slowly progressive behavioral syndrome including apathy, lack of insight, and loss of empathy.

The neurologic examination identifies both upper and lower motor neuron abnormalities. Muscle atrophy is seen, usually in the hands and often noted at the thenar or hypothenar eminence. Fasciculations and weakness are noted as lower motor neuron findings. Upper motor neuron findings include spasticity, hyperreflexia, and abnormal plantar responses. Much of the diagnostic work-up is aimed at ruling out alternative etiologies and EMG is diagnostic for ALS.

The clinical course is relentlessly progressive with only a 50% survival at 3 years, with aspiration or respiratory failure the most common cause of death. Mild muscle weakness progresses to inability to walk, difficulty with speaking, and dysphagia. The FDA has approved riluzole for treatment of ALS, which extends survival and delays the need for ventilation support. Treatment is otherwise directed at symptom control and quality of life. This is best achieved with a multidisciplinary approach, including ancillary services such as physical therapy, respiratory therapy, and social work.

The neuropathology of ALS includes neuronal cytoplasmic inclusions of a ubiquitinated protein, most commonly seen in lower motor neurons. These inclusions were shown to contain the 43-kDa TAR DNA-binding protein (TDP-43), the same protein that has been identified in FTLD-ALS or pure FTLD. This finding is consistent with previously recognized associations between ALS and FTD. The highly penetrant SOD1 mutation was previously thought to be the main cause of ALS prior to discovery of the *C9orf72* mutation. About 15% of patients with FTLD develop ALS. Similarly, about 50% of ALS patients develop cognitive and behavioral symptoms of FTLD, and a smaller percentage of these develop dementia.

CORTICOBASAL DEGENERATION

CBD is a tauopathy that was initially described in patients with dementia, apraxia, cortical sensory deficits, and asymmetric parkinsonism with a rigid akinetic arm. It is now recognized that the manifestations of CBD range from bvFTD, nfvPPA, executive and motor deficits to the asymmetric parkinsonian syndrome originally described. Often a bvFTD or nfvPPA syndrome is present for many years before the onset of motor symptoms. The mean age of disease onset for CBD is in the mid-sixties. A few series suggest that women may be more commonly affected than men. CBD is generally sporadic in occurrence, although familial cases have been described in association with both tau and progranulin mutations. Many cases are not correctly diagnosed during life.

When parkinsonian features emerge, they are often, but not always, asymmetric. Severe upper limb dystonia can result in internal contracture of the limb with the fingers clutching the thumb with flexion at the wrist. An alien limb phenomenon sometimes occurs with the limb not only levitating, but often hooking onto clothing or grabbing other body parts and behaving as if it were no longer under the control of the patient. On occasion, the alien limb will interfere with actions of the other hand. Simple levitation of the lower extremity is described as well but is less specific to CBD. Focal reflex myoclonus that is typically present first in the fingers, then in the hand, can be elicited with distal percussion.

Concurrent cortical sensory loss is seen without deficits to peripheral sensory modalities. This is identified by testing for agraphesthesia, agnosia, or problems with two-point discrimination. Bilateral limb apraxia is common, and apraxia of opening or closing the eyes can occur. Close evaluation of eye movements will often reveal saccadic latency with normal velocity, often in the horizontal plane. Supranuclear vertical gaze palsy can occur.

CBD shares many neuropathologic abnormalities with FTD and PSP, suggesting the possibility that they represent a spectrum of similar diseases linked by underlying tau pathology. Ballooned neurons throughout the neocortex associated with neuronal loss and astrocytic tau-staining plaques are the diagnostic histologic features of CBD. Unlike Pick disease, the distribution of ballooned neurons is extensive and involves both the primary sensory and motor regions. Pick bodies are absent. Commonly, the superior frontal lobes and the parietal lobes are most heavily affected and are reflected in patterns of neuropsychological testing. Secondary degeneration of the corticospinal tracts occurs. Grossly asymmetric atrophy of the parasagittal superior frontal gyrus and superior parietal lobule is common, with relative sparing of the temporal and occipital regions.

The treatment of CBD is symptomatic as disease-altering therapies are not known. Levodopa is beneficial in the minority of patients. Muscle relaxants and physical therapy with range-of-motion exercises can be useful, with occasional consideration of botulinum toxin therapy for dystonic limbs. Clonazepam may be instituted for myoclonus. There is no theoretical basis for the use of cholinesterase inhibitors in this disease.

PROGRESSIVE SUPRANUCLEAR PALSY

PSP, also referred to as Steele-Richardson-Olszewski syndrome, is a progressive neurodegenerative disease with prominent extrapyramidal motor findings and supranuclear ocular abnormalities. Patients with PSP present to both movement disorder clinics for motor abnormalities and behavioral clinics for cognitive or psychiatric complaints. The frequency of PSP in the general population is around 1 in 100,000, increasing to 7 in 100,000 among people older than 55 years. Diagnosis typically occurs in the sixth to seventh decade of life. There are only a few published reports of familial cases, suggesting that an autosomal-dominant mutation plays only a small role in the disease.

The initial descriptions of PSP emphasized abnormalities in movement with nearly all patients exhibiting early gait abnormalities, and 60% presenting with falls as the first manifestation of disease. Patients often pivot with turns and tend to fall backward. Increased tone (axial more than appendicular) and dysphagia (affecting 46% in the first 5 years) are other common motor findings while bradykinesia is seen in only about a quarter of autopsy-proven cases. Spastic dysarthria results in slurred speech. Ultimately patients become mute.

Eye movement abnormalities are the hallmark feature of the disease, with vertical supranuclear palsy a critical feature for diagnosis. While vertical gaze palsy can be upward or downward, downward gaze palsy has greater specificity for PSP because mild vertical gaze limitation is normal with aging. The oculocephalic reflex for vertical movement is preserved early in disease despite the vertical gaze palsy. Square wave jerks and both latency and hypometria of eye movements are often seen, typically greater with command (saccadic movements) rather than pursuit. A decreased blink rate and furrowed brow can be noticed when interviewing the patient.

Cognitive or psychiatric features are often present, even in the early stages of illness. The pattern of cognitive dysfunction is characterized by abnormalities localizing to the frontal and temporal lobes and subcortical structures. Thus, slowing of cognitive performance and below expectation performance in verbal fluency and executive functioning tasks are often documented, typically with retained verbal and visual memory performance. Behavioral symptoms of apathy, compulsions, perseveration, and utilization behavior are common. This pattern of neuropsychological and behavioral findings is similar to what is seen in FTD, consistent with the overlapping pathology of the two entities. Of note and differing from FTD, insomnia, depression and anxiety are often seen in PSP.

Treatment of PSP is focused on control of symptoms. Occupational therapy to address speech and visual limitations can be successful. Prevention of falls is critical but often challenging as impulsivity and lack of insight can limit the effectiveness of therapeutic interventions. Levodopa can be helpful in some patients with PSP, but eventually loses its efficacy. Survival is between 6 and 10 years at the time of diagnosis.

SPINOCEREBELLAR ATAXIA SYNDROMES

Spinocerebellar ataxias (SCAs) are a heterogeneous group of disorders with prominent, progressive cerebellar involvement. The current classification system corresponds to the order in which gene mutations have been identified. A comprehensive database, including scientific reviews and a listing of laboratories that will evaluate for mutations, is available at www.geneclinics.org.

Many of the SCA genetic mutations that have been identified to date are associated with expansion of repeated trinucleotides and are inherited in an autosomal-dominant manner. However, penetrance can vary greatly. The length of the polyglutamine repeat appears to be a major determinant

TABLE 63-5 ■ NEURODEGENERATIVE DISORDERS

SYNDROME	HISTORY "BUZZ" WORDS	UNDERLYING PATHOLOGY AND MORPHOLOGY	TYPICAL IMAGING FINDINGS
Alzheimer disease	Progressive episodic short-term memory loss	Amyloid β and tau	Hippocampal and precuneus atrophy
Dementia with Lewy bodies	Fluctuations, visual hallucinations, REM sleep disorder, parkinsonism	Alpha-synuclein	Minimal atrophy. ↓ parieto-occipital metabolism on FDG-PET with spared posterior cingulate
Parkinson disease dementia	Parkinsonism years/decades before cognitive changes	Alpha-synuclein	Decreased putamenal signal on DaTscan
Multiple system atrophy	Autonomic changes, cerebellar symptoms, postural tremor	Alpha-synuclein	T2 pontomedullary hyperintensity— "hot cross bun" sign
Behavioral variant frontotemporal dementia	Personality changes, loss of empathy/sympathy, stereotyped behaviors, hyperorality	Tau, TDP-43, less commonly	Frontal and/or anterior temporal lobe atrophy
Nonfluent variant primary progressive aphasia	Apraxic speech, agrammatism	Tau	Left inferior frontal gyrus atrophy
Semantic variant primary progressive aphasia	Loss of word meaning, multimodal agnosia, surface dyslexia	TDP-43	Left anterior temporal lobe atrophy
Logogenic variant primary progressive aphasia	Impaired word retrieval and repetition, phonologic errors, poor comprehension	Amyloid β and tau	Atrophy of left posterior superior temporal gyrus, middle temporal gyrus, inferior parietal lobule
Corticobasal syndrome (CBD)	Asymmetric parkinsonism, rigidity and dystonia, alien limb	Tau (CBD and PSP)	Perirolandic atrophy
Progressive supranuclear palsy (PSP)	Early falls, impaired vertical gaze, axial rigidity	Tau (PSP and CBD)	Dorsal midbrain atrophy with dilated third ventricle—"hummingbird sign"

PART III

GERIATRIC CONDITIONS

of age for disease onset in an inverse manner. Genetic analyses are estimated to identify only 40% to 60% of familial and less than 25% of sporadic cases. The likelihood that a gene mutation will be identified decreases with older age (> 40). The prevalence of SCAs is between 1 and 4/100,000 with variation by region caused by founder effects: SCA 2 (Cuba), SCA 3 (Azores), and SCA 10 (Mexico). These disorders most commonly present in the third decade of life with some presenting in youth; however, the range of age extends into older ages for many SCAs.

Phenotypic overlap is common in SCA syndromes, but progressive cerebellar disability often presenting early in disease is a common feature. SCA syndromes often affect the noncerebellar portions of the nervous system, particularly as the disease progresses, with neuropathology identified in the brain stem, basal ganglia, and cortex. Such clinical symptoms include oculomotor features (SCA 1, 2, 3), retinopathy (SCA 7), seizures (SCA 10, 17), peripheral neuropathy (SCA 1, 2, 3, 4, 8, 18, 25), or cognitive and behavioral deterioration (SCA 17, dentatorubral pallidoluysian atrophy).

Other neurodegenerative disorders should be considered in patients with progressive cerebellar dysfunction, including mitochondrial diseases, Huntington disease, leukodystrophies, Frederick ataxia, MSA, prion disease, and the premutation associated with fragile X syndrome. Paraneoplastic processes should be considered in patients presenting with subacute cerebellar dysfunction. Treatment for SCA is generally aimed at symptom management, physical and occupational therapy, and genetic counseling.

SUMMARY OF NEURODEGENERATIVE DISORDERS

Clinical diagnosis of neurodegenerative disorders can be difficult and requires a careful, comprehensive approach and evaluation to make the correct diagnosis. **Table 63-5** summarizes the distinctive features of common non-Alzheimer diseases that cause dementia.

EPILEPSY

Epilepsy in older adults can be caused by a variety of diseases, including ischemic and hemorrhagic strokes, mass lesions, infections, inflammatory etiologies, and neurodegenerative diseases. Cognitive comorbidities are frequently seen in people with epilepsy. There is a complicated interrelationship between cognitive dysfunction due to recurrent aberrant network activities during seizures, underlying degeneration or lesions, or antiepileptic medications themselves.

Acute and remote strokes are common causes of seizures in older adults. When a new seizure develops in the setting of a stroke, the cause is generally hemorrhagic, whereas both hemorrhagic and ischemic strokes can cause chronic seizures. A common causes of hemorrhagic stroke is hypertension; however, this generally causes hemorrhages in deep brain structures. Thus hypertension is not the most common cause of strokes associated with seizures. Cortical hemorrhages commonly occur in cerebral amyloid angiopathy (CAA). CAA is characterized by amyloid deposition in the small vessels of both the brain and leptomeninges. This is the same abnormal protein that accumulates in AD, with or without deposition of amyloid in the brain parenchyma. CAA predisposes to small microbleeds and larger intracerebral and subarachnoid hemorrhages.

Brain tumors are another common cause of epilepsy in older adults. Although primary brain tumors can cause seizures, metastatic lesions are the most common type of intracranial tumors that present with epilepsy in older persons. The tumors that most often metastasize to the brain originate from lung, breast, kidney, colon, rectum, and skin (melanoma).

Encephalitis due to underlying autoimmune or paraneoplastic diseases commonly presents with subacute cognitive or behavioral changes and seizures, and requires direct testing for antibodies for diagnosis. In addition to antiepileptic drugs, treatment of encephalitis requires immunosuppressive drugs, as well as identification and treatment of underlying malignancy. A wide variety of infections in the older adults can present with seizures. Given the higher prevalence of valvular heart diseases and cardiac surgeries, infections can present with septic emboli or even CNS abscesses from endocarditis and present with epilepsy.

Neurodegenerative disorders are another setting in which epilepsy can be a symptom. The rate of epilepsy in AD ranges from 10% to 22% across studies, and the prevalence of epilepsy in this disease is higher than that in other diseases causing dementia. The most common seizure type is complex partial seizures, often presenting with features that are typical of medial temporal lobe seizures, including auras such as deja-vu and olfactory hallucinations, and speech arrest in an unresponsive, awake state. Secondary generalization to tonic-clonic seizures also occurs commonly. Although these events were classically considered a feature of late stage AD, recent reports suggest they can develop when cognitive symptoms are mild or even in the asymptomatic stages of the disease. There are several proposed mechanisms for epileptogenesis in AD, including excessive presynaptic glutamate release as well as impaired GABAergic interneuron activity, especially in the dentate gyrus. Comorbid epilepsy and AD is associated with earlier onset of dementia and faster rate of decline; however, it is unclear if treatment of seizures can favorably alter the rate of disease progression.

A major factor in choosing epilepsy treatment in older adults is the potential for side effects, including cognitive dysfunction, reduction in bone mineral density and dizziness that may increase risk for falls. Choice of treatment should also include consideration of medical comorbidities, especially impaired hepatic or renal function and cardiac conduction abnormalities. These impairments together with other aging-associated changes in organ physiology may affect serum drug levels due to diminished adipose tissue mass, increased volume of distribution and differential liver or kidney function. In addition, polypharmacy and drug–drug interactions are a common concern in the older population. Given these concerns, ideal drugs should have minimal side effects and reduced chances for drug–drug interactions. Suitable agents for treatment of epilepsy in the older population include but are not limited to lamotrigine, levetiracetam, lacosamide, and oxcarbazepine.

ACUTE TRAUMATIC BRAIN INJURY

Traumatic brain injury (TBI) remains a common cause of neurologic dysfunction at all ages, including the older population. The impact of injury on neurological function depends on several factors, including the severity of injury, frequency of recurrence, and whether the injury is "penetrating" versus "nonpenetrating." There is converging evidence that repeated head blows that may cause only mild or no acute symptoms appear to increase risk of dementia. This entity, called chronic traumatic encephalopathy, is discussed in Chapter 64 in this textbook.

Penetrating traumatic brain injuries, also termed "open head injuries," are associated with the highest morbidity and mortality. A penetrating TBI is characterized by disruption of the dura mater, the outermost and thickest meningeal layer protecting and covering the brain. The typical mechanism of injury is a high velocity object such as a bullet or other fragments, as well as skull fractures with subsequent cavitation of bone into the cranial cavity. Due to the mechanism of injury, penetrating injuries are more common in younger people. Penetrating head injuries typically require intensive level care, especially for monitoring intracranial pressure and infections. Importantly, the risk of development of post-traumatic epilepsy is greater than 50% after a penetrating head injury.

Nonpenetrating (or closed) head injury is more typically seen in older people. Falls are the most common cause, with progressive visual and gait dysfunction, deconditioning, and use of sedating medications as important risk factors. Severity of head injury is defined by the Glasgow Coma Scale (GCS), with 13 to 15 being mild injury, 9 to 12 moderate injury, and < 9 defined as severe TBI. Subdural hematoma is a common complication of falls in older adults, and may be an explanation for subacute cognitive changes even after incidents that may have had minimal impact on the head. Notably, both head injury and subdural hematoma are risk factors for further cognitive decline and epilepsy.

Mild TBI, synonymous with "concussion" and defined as head injury with less than 30 minutes of loss of consciousness, less than 24 hours of posttraumatic amnesia and an initial GCS of 13 to 15, is frequently encountered in the older population following falls. Even after recovery from the acute trauma, people with mild TBI often report a constellation of symptoms termed "post-concussive syndrome," characterized by ongoing headaches, dizziness (especially vertigo), insomnia, or other sleep disturbances. There are also behavioral symptoms such as irritability, anxiety, and depression, and even subtle personality changes. Additionally, impaired memory and cognition, fatigue, and decreased cognitive stamina can occur. The prevalence of postconcussive syndrome following brain injury ranges from 30% to 80%; the severity of injury does not directly correlate with the development of postconcussive syndrome. Treatment is supportive and the symptoms generally resolve over time (sometimes many months); however, they may persist indefinitely.

CONCLUDING REMARKS ON NON-ALZHEIMER DISEASE NEURODEGENERATIVE DISORDERS

Scientific advances over the past decade have remarkably enhanced our understanding of non-AD neurodegenerative disorders. Yet, large knowledge gaps remain. In many cases, neuropathology can now be identified, facilitating the process of linking disease syndromes to pathologic substrate and supporting a deeper understanding of disease pathobiology. In such cases, clinical researchers can begin to accurately describe the clinical presentation of pathology-proven cases to provide clinicians with clues to neuropathology. When combined with emerging noninvasive diagnostic tools, we can achieve the ultimate goal of promoting pathology-driven treatment approaches, and one day a cure.

PART III

GERIATRIC CONDITIONS

FURTHER READING

Aarsland D, Creese B, Politis M, et al. Cognitive decline in Parkinson disease. *Nat. Rev Neurol.* 2017;13(4):217–231.

Fabbrini G, Fabbrini A, Suppa A. Progressive supranuclear palsy, multiple system atrophy and corticobasal degeneration. In: Reus VI, Lindqvist D, eds. *Handbook of Clinical Neurology* (3rd series, Vol. 165). Elsevier; 2019:155–177.

Lee SE, Khazenzon AM, Trujillo AJ, et al. Altered network connectivity in frontotemporal dementia with *C9orf72* hexanucleotide repeat expansion. *Brain.* 2014;137(pt 11): 3047–3060.

Manto MU. The wide spectrum of spinocerebellar ataxias (SCAs). *Cerebellum.* 2005;4(1):2–6.

McKeith IG, Boeve BF, Dickson DW, et al. Diagnosis and management of dementia with Lewy bodies. *Neurology.* 2017;89:88–100.

Miller B, Guerra JL. Frontotemporal dementia. In: Reus VI, Lindqvist D, eds. *Handbook of Clinical Neurology* (3rd series, Vol. 165). Elsevier; 2019:33–35.

Rascovsky K, Hodges JR, Knopman D, et al. Sensitivity of revised diagnostic criteria for the behavioural variant of frontotemporal dementia. *Brain.* 2011;134:2456–2477.

Vanes MA, Hardman O, Chio A, et al. Amyotrophic lateral sclerosis. *Lancet.* 2017;390:2084–2098.

Traumatic Brain Injury and Chronic Traumatic Encephalopathy

Ann C. McKee, Daniel Kirsch

TRAUMATIC BRAIN INJURY AND DEMENTIA

For decades, traumatic brain injury (TBI) has been considered a risk factor for Alzheimer disease (AD), yet recent large cohort studies indicate that TBIs of all severities (mild, moderate, severe) are a risk factor for dementia, but the neuropathology underlying this risk is largely unknown. Some of the difficulties in understanding the neuropathological consequences of TBI are that TBI is a heterogeneous condition, consisting of different grades of severity: mild, moderate, severe. The grade of severity is based on: the Glasgow Coma Scale; duration of loss of consciousness (LOC); development of posttraumatic amnesia; and frequency (single, multiple), types (focal, diffuse), nature (penetrating, blunt impact, blast), and presence or absence of skull fracture, hemorrhage, contusion, infarction, and/or other secondary processes. In a pooled analysis of 7130 participants from the Religious Orders Study, Memory and Aging Project (ROSMAP) and Adult Changes in Thought (ACT) cohorts, TBI with LOC was not associated with a clinical diagnosis of AD dementia or with AD neuropathological changes at autopsy. These findings were confirmed and extended by a recent study of more than 4000 autopsy participants from the National Alzheimer's Coordinating Center (NACC) that also found no association between TBI and AD neuropathological change or Alzheimer disease–related dementias (ADRDs) using Consortium to Establish a Registry for Alzheimer's Disease (CERAD) scores for neuritic plaques and Braak stage for neurofibrillary tangles (NFTs). There was also no association with cortical Lewy bodies (LBs), hippocampal sclerosis, infarcts, microinfarcts, or amyloid angiopathy. In contrast, exposure to repetitive mild TBI or repetitive head impacts (RHI) such as concussions and subconcussive impacts from contact sport participation, military service, or physical abuse, is associated with chronic traumatic encephalopathy (CTE), a distinctive hyperphosphorylated tau protein (p-tau)-based neurodegeneration. In CTE, the pathological diagnosis is based on its pathognomonic lesion consisting of a perivascular accumulation of p-tau in neurons and neurites in an irregular pattern at the depths of the cortical sulci (**Figure 64-1**). A supportive, yet nondiagnostic, feature of CTE is the preferential distribution of NFTs in the superficial regions of the cerebral cortex, quite

Learning Objectives

- Understand the epidemiology, pathophysiology, clinical manifestations, and adverse outcomes of traumatic brain injury (TBI) in older adults.

- Acquire cutting-edge knowledge about chronic traumatic encephalopathy (CTE) and the risk of developing dementia following repeated traumatic insults to the brain.

- Learn about the neuropathology, common clinical symptoms, diagnostic criteria, and progression of CTE over time.

- Recognize the various strategies and treatments used to address cognitive deficits associated with TBI and CTE.

Key Clinical Points

1. Chronic traumatic encephalopathy (CTE) is diagnosed neuropathologically and is a primary tauopathy with a distinct well-defined pattern of tau pathology.

2. The clinical presentations of CTE are nonspecific and can be grouped into behavioral, cognitive, dementia, and motor. Currently, there are no neuroimaging, laboratory, or cognitive tests that can definitively diagnose the disease during life.

3. The classic neuropathology of CTE includes a neurofibrillary tangle with "dot-like" neurites around a small arteriole in the brain.

4. In CTE, pathology becomes progressively worse over time with worsening of clinical presentations that are generally nonspecific.

5. CTE is associated with exposure to repetitive head impacts and pathology is increased with duration of exposure.

6. Over time, the CTE pathology progresses and involves other parts of the brain, including the hippocampus, entorhinal cortex, amygdala, brainstem, and cerebellum.

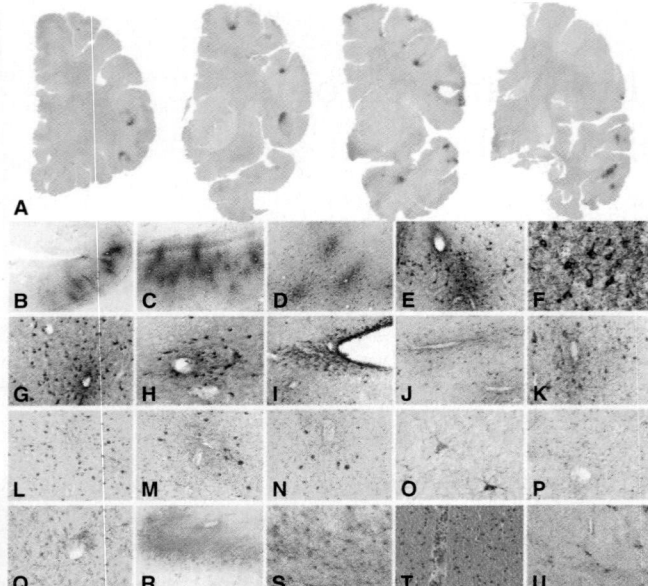

FIGURE 64-1. Histologic findings in stage II chronic traumatic encephalopathy (CTE). **A.** Whole mount coronal sections show multiple foci of p-tau pathology primarily located at the depths of the cortical sulci of the frontal and temporal lobes (free floating 50 μ sections, AT8 (p-tau) immunostain). **B–H.** Neuronal p-tau pathology consists of neurofibrillary tangles and dotlike and threadlike dystrophic neurites and is characteristically found around arterioles (**B–F**, free floating 50 μ sections, AT8 (p-tau) immunostain; **G, H**, 10 μ paraffin-embedded sections, AT8 (p-tau) immunostain). (**I**). Subpial astrocytic tangles (TSAs), which are nondiagnostic but supportive, can be found at the cortical depths (free floating 50 μ sections, AT8 (p-tau) immunostain). Other pathologies include pretangles (**J**), dystrophic neurites in the white matter (**K**), and occasional p-tau immunopositive astrocytes (**L**) (free floating 50 μ sections, AT8 (p-tau) immunostain). There may be marked astrocytosis of the white matter (**M, N**) (free floating 50 μ sections, glial fibrillary acidic protein immunostain). Hemosiderin-laden macrophages (**O**) (10 μ paraffin section, Luxol fast blue hematoxylin and eosin stain) and multiple perivascular foci of reactive microglia (**P**) are found around small vessels in the cerebral white matter (free floating 50 μ sections, LN3 immunostain).

unlike the laminar distribution of NFTs in cortical layers 3 and 5 found in AD. Because the criteria for the diagnosis of CTE were defined only recently and require the use of p-tau immunohistochemistry (IHC) beyond the standard silver staining recommended by CERAD, the prevalence of CTE in neurodegenerative disease brain banks is currently unknown. The few studies that have reexamined brain bank cohorts for CTE using newly defined National Institute of Neurological Disorders and Stroke (NINDS) criteria and p-tau IHC found CTE in 1% to 30% of cases, and some cases previously considered to be only AD have been rediagnosed comorbid AD and CTE.

There have been remarkably few detailed case studies of the neuropathology of remote moderate–severe TBI, although there are many speculative reviews. Several small neuropathologically focused studies support a relationship

between moderate–severe TBI and atypical AD neuropathological changes characterized by an unconventional distribution of p-tau and amyloid-beta (Aβ) pathology. Johnson et al. examined the brains of 39 individuals diagnosed with a single moderate–severe TBI after 1 to 47 years' survival and found that Aβ plaques were greater in density in the TBI group compared to controls. In addition, in subjects 60 years or younger at the time of death, NFTs were more frequent in the TBI group compared to age-matched controls and were distributed more commonly in the superficial layers of the cortex with clustering of NFTs among the depths of the sulci, an NFT distribution unlike AD and suggestive of CTE. Similarly, in a study of chronic severe TBI survivors without dementia, Scott et al. found increased Aβ accumulation by 11C-Pittsburgh compound positron emission tomography (PET) imaging in nine TBI subjects after severe TBI compared to age-matched controls and in a pattern distinct from the Aβ accumulation seen in AD patients. Clinical, neuroimaging, and neuropathological characteristics of two subjects who developed early onset dementia after sustaining a single moderate-severe TBI many years earlier have been described. One subject also had a history of RHI from military combat. Our study demonstrated the diversity and complexity of the neuropathology after remote TBI. In both cases, the pathologic findings included severe cerebral atrophy (brain weight < 930 g), white matter degeneration (which was particularly severe in the posterior corpus callosum), atypical AD, atypical CTE (with an unusual distribution of NFTs in the superficial layers of the cortex, but without the diagnostic pathognomonic perivascular lesion of CTE), widespread diffuse and sparse neuritic Aβ plaques, cerebral amyloid angiopathy (CAA), neuronal loss, and astrocytosis. Unusual α-synuclein and TAR DNA-binding protein 43 (TDP-43) proteinopathies were also found in one case. The size and distribution of the LBs and TDP-43 pathology were not characteristic of typical Lewy body disease (LBD) or frontotemporal lobar degeneration (FTLD). In a third recently reported case of a long-term survivor of moderate–severe TBI, there were widespread NFTs, α-synuclein positive LBs, diffuse Aβ plaques, and CAA. Other pathological changes reported in long-term survivors of TBI are axonal loss and disruption, reduced cortical thickness, blood-brain barrier dysintegrity, white matter degeneration, and chronic inflammation.

Axonal injury is one of the most common neuropathologies after TBI across all severities of injury. Hay et al. reported 47% of long-term individuals who experienced a single moderate–severe TBI who survived a year or more after injury had evidence of chronic blood-brain barrier disruption with multifocal abnormal fibrinogen and immunoglobulin G immunostaining in the cortex compared to limited localized immunostaining in controls. In this same group of long-term TBI survivors, Johnson et al. reported increased persistent neuroinflammation with significantly increased microglial density and reactive morphology, and reduced corpus callosum thickness compared to controls.

Findings in animal models of TBIs have also demonstrated axonal loss, myelin loss, white matter degeneration, astrocytosis, neuronal loss, and chronic inflammation.

These studies suggest that TBI is a heterogeneous entity that is influenced by the biomechanics of the acute traumatic event, secondary consequences of the acute injury, and chronic, poorly understood pathophysiological processes including deposition of multiple neurodegenerative disease proteins (p-tau, Aβ, TDP-43, α-synuclein), cerebral atrophy, white matter degeneration, axonal loss, blood-brain barrier disruption, and persistent neuroinflammation. Other factors that may exert substantial influence over the long-term outcome of TBI include the frequency and severity of the TBI (mild, moderate, or severe) as well as the underlying characteristics of the individual who experienced the TBI, including genetic factors, age, gender, cardiovascular health, and cognitive reserve, among others. Clearly, there is a fundamental need for rigorous clinicopathological case evaluations to determine the full spectrum of clinical features and neuropathological alterations that occur after remote TBI, much needed data that will advance the field and highlight pathways for successful intervention and treatment.

TRAUMATIC BRAIN INJURY AND PARKINSON DISEASE

Multiple studies have implicated any lifetime history of TBI as a risk factor for Parkinson disease (PD). Whether TBI sustained in older adulthood increases short-term risk of PD can be obscured by recall bias or reverse-causation. However, Gardner et al. found that among middle-aged and older patients, there is a 44% increased risk of being diagnosed with PD in those who experienced a TBI compared to those with nonbrain-related traumatic injury. Furthermore, the risk was significantly higher with more severe or more frequent TBI, providing additional support for a causal association. The Crane et al. study of ROSMAP and ACT participants also showed that TBI with LOC < 1 hour predicted increased risk for cortical LBs, and TBI with LOC > 1 hour predicted increased risk for cerebral microinfarcts. In addition, in the ACT cohort, TBI with LOC > 1 hour was associated with clinical diagnosis of PD. Contact sport athletes are also at increased risk of developing PD and parkinsonism. Adams et al. recently showed that the number of years an individual was exposed to RHI through contact sports was associated with the development of neocortical LBD, and LBD, in turn, was associated with parkinsonism and dementia. Furthermore, in the Framingham Heart Study (FHS) community cohort, years of contact sports play were associated with neocortical LBD (OR = 1.30 per year, p = 0.012), and in a pooled analysis, a threshold of more than 8 years of play best predicted neocortical LBD (ROC analysis, OR = 6.24, 95% CI = 1.5–25, p = 0.011), adjusting for age, sex, and APOE ε4 allele status.

CTE is a neurodegenerative tauopathy associated with repetitive mild head trauma, including concussion and asymptomatic subconcussive impacts. CTE has been identified in American football, ice hockey, soccer, baseball, and rugby players, professional wrestlers, a bull rider, military veterans exposed to blast, and victims of assault and domestic violence. In 2009, using 50 μm whole mount landscape slides and p-tau IHC, the distinctive regional pathology of CTE was described in two former boxers and one former National Football League (NFL) player. The findings were compared to the 48 cases of neuropathologically confirmed CTE previously reported. The pathology of CTE was distinctive from other tauopathies in that it was irregular, patchy, and perivascular, with a tendency to be most severe at the depths of the sulci in the frontal and temporal cortex (**Figure 64-2**). In addition, the p-tau neurites

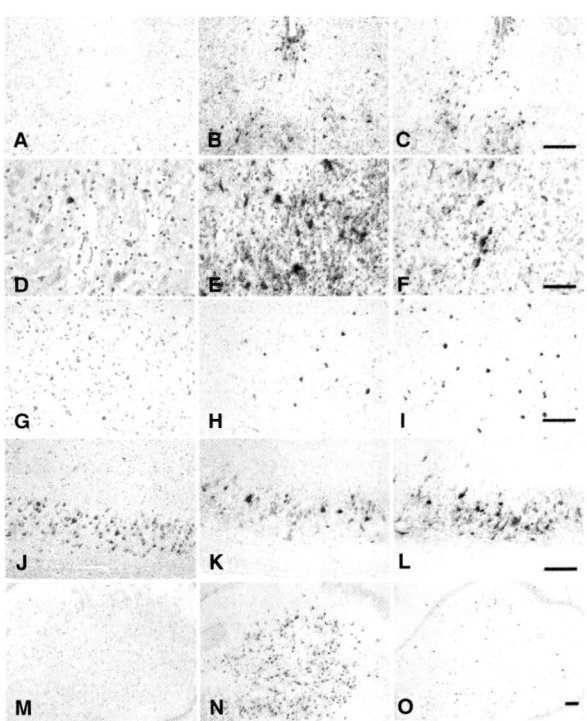

FIGURE 64-2. Patterns of p-tau isoforms 3R and 4R in chronic traumatic encephalopathy (CTE) in frontal and temporal lobes. **A, D.** 3R p-tau immunostaining shows scattered immunopositive neurons in the middle frontal cortex. **B, E.** 4R p-tau immunostaining shows many immunopositive neurons and astrocytic tangles in the subpial region of the middle frontal cortex and at the depth of the sulcus. **C, F.** AT8 (p-tau) immunostaining shows 3R and 4R p-tau immunopositive neurons and astrocytic tangles in the middle frontal cortex. **G, J, M.** 3R p-tau immunostaining shows scattered immunopositive neurons in CA1 (**G**), CA2 (**J**), and CA4 of the hippocampus (**M**). **H, K, N.** 4R p-tau immunostaining shows many immunopositive neurons in CA1 (**H**), CA2 (**K**), and CA4 hippocampus (**N**). **I, L, O.** AT8 (p-tau) immunostaining shows 3R and 4R p-tau immunopositive neurons in CA1 (**I**), CA2 (**L**), and CA4 hippocampus (**O**). All 10 μ paraffin-embedded sections, magnification bars 50 μm.

were dot-like, unlike the neuropil threads of AD, and there were p-tau immunoreactive astrocytes in the subpial and periventricular regions.

Clinical Symptoms and Diagnosis

The symptoms of CTE vary and generally include cognitive, behavioral, and motor symptoms that progress with the disease. The initial symptoms may include headache, loss of concentration, mood swings, short-term memory loss, and depression. With disease progression, these symptoms worsen and become associated with impairments in decision-making and judgment, explosive behavior, aggression, paranoia, parkinsonism, and gait abnormalities. Additional symptoms may include visuospatial abnormalities, verbal and physical violence, and suicidal ideation and attempts. In general, behavioral and mood symptoms are more common in younger patients, with motor and cognitive symptoms dominating in older adults.

Definitive diagnosis of CTE can only be made on autopsy; thus, patient evaluation should focus on characterizing the clinical phenotype and excluding other diseases that could account for the presenting symptoms. Clinical evaluation should focus on symptoms and history of exposure to contact sports, repeated head trauma, concussions, military employment with traumatic or blast injuries, and behavioral, cognitive, mood, or motor symptoms. Neurological examination should look for signs of LBD, muscle fasciculations, evidence of parkinsonism, language abnormalities, and motor neuron disease. Each patient should undergo neuropsychological testing to identify deficits in memory, attention, language, and visuospatial function. Routine labs and an MRI brain scan as well as amyloid and tau PET scans could be considered to confirm tau deposition in the brain. Alternatively, cerebrospinal fluid could be collected to assay amyloid, tau, and other analytes. Given the diagnosis of CTE can only be made on neuropathological examination of the brain, the remainder of this chapter is focused on the pathology of CTE.

Neuropathology of CTE

Preliminary criteria for the neuropathological diagnosis of CTE were presented in 2013 as part of a clinicopathological case series of 68 male subjects with CTE, ranging in age from 17 to 98 years (mean 59.5 years) and 18 age- and gender-matched controls without a history of brain trauma. The neuropathological criteria proposed by McKee et al. for CTE required the presence of focal epicenters of p-tau immunoreactive NFTs and abnormal neurites around a small vessel, distributed at the depths of the sulci in the cerebral cortex, NFTs distributed in the superficial layers of cortex, and p-tau immunoreactive astrocytes in the sub-pial layer at the depths of the sulcus most often found in the frontal and temporal cortices (**Figure 64-1**). Other frequent pathologies in CTE included axonal loss in the subcortical white matter and the cooccurrence of TDP-43 immunoreactive inclusions and neurites.

In addition, McKee and colleagues proposed a staging scheme for characterizing the progressive p-tau pathology in CTE (McKee CTE Staging Classification Scheme) (**Table 64-1**). The method of staging CTE p-tau pathology was based on the previous work of Braak and Braak in AD, who examined a series of 83 autopsy brains and found a characteristic distribution pattern of NFTs and neuropil threads (NTs) that permitted the differentiation of six pathological stages of AD. The Braak staging system for NFT forms the basis for the neuropathological diagnosis of AD used by the National Institute on Aging, and similar staging schemes are now available for Aβ plaques in AD and LBs in PD. Based on the 68 CTE cases, McKee and colleagues identified four pathological stages of CTE (I–IV), primarily using large hemispheric slides immunostained for p-tau (**Figure 64-3**). In the earliest stage of CTE, stage I, there are one or two isolated epicenters of NFTs and *dot-like* neurites (ie, "CTE lesions") arranged around small blood vessels at the depths of the sulci in the frontal, temporal, or parietal cortices. The small blood vessels at the center of the CTE lesions are usually small arterioles and may be associated with p-tau immunopositive thorn-shaped astrocytes (TSAs) in the subpial region. In stage II CTE, three or more CTE lesions are found in multiple cortical regions, the CTE lesions are larger, superficial NFTs are found along the sulcal wall and at gyral crests of the adjacent cortices, and there is more neurofibrillary pathology in the locus coeruleus and nucleus basalis of Meynert (**Figure 64-1**). In stage III CTE, confluent perivascular patches of p-tau mmunoreactive NFTs and dotlike- and threadlike-neurites are found at the sulcal depths, as well as NFTs in the superficial cortical laminae. Diffusely distributed NFTs are also found in medial temporal lobe structures, including the hippocampus, entorhinal cortex, perirhinal cortex, amygdala, as well as additional brainstem structures. Neurofibrillary degeneration in stage III CTE involves CA4 and CA2, as well as CA1 of the hippocampus (**Figure 64-4**). In CTE stage IV, CTE lesions and NFTs are densely distributed throughout the cerebral cortex, diencephalon, brain stem, cerebellar dentate nucleus, and spinal cord with neuronal loss and gliosis in the frontal and temporal cortices and astrocytic p-tau pathology (**Figure 64-5**). CTE pathology in stages I and II is considered to be mild and is considered to be severe in stages III and IV.

McKee and colleagues found a significant correlation between the stage of CTE pathology and duration of football career, supporting a dose-response relationship between cumulative head trauma exposure and CTE severity. They also found a significant association between CTE stage, number of years after retirement from football, and age at death, data supporting progression of p-tau pathological severity over time. By contrast, number of concussions, years of education, lifetime steroid use, and position played did not significantly relate to CTE stage.

Using the McKee criteria in 2015, the NINDS and National Institute of Biomedical Imaging and

TABLE 64-1 ■ CTE NEUROPATHOLOGICAL DIAGNOSTIC CRITERIA

Diagnostic lesion: p-tau aggregates in neurons, with or without thorn-shaped astrocytes, at the depth of a cortical sulcus around a small blood vessel, deep in the parenchyma, and not restricted to the subpial and superficial region of the sulcus.[a]

CTE SEVERITY[a]	LOW CTE	HIGH CTE
	< 5 of:	≥ 5 of:
	• NFT in gyral side adjacent to CTE lesion • NFT in gyral crest adjacent to CTE lesion • NFT in superficial cortical laminae (layer II) • NFT in CA4 of hippocampus (with dendritic swellings) • NFT in CA2 of hippocampus • NFT in entorhinal cortex • NFT in amygdala • NFT in thalamus • NFT in mamillary body • NFT in cerebellar dentate nucleus	

CTE STAGE[b,c]	MCKEE STAGE I	MCKEE STAGE II	MCKEE STAGE III	MCKEE STAGE IV
	• One or two cortical pathognomonic regions usually in frontal lobe • Pathognomonic lesions consist of foci of p-tau NFTs and thread and dotlike neurites • Sparse NFTs in locus coeruleus	• Three or more pathognomonic lesions affecting multiple cortical regions • Pathognomonic lesions consist of foci of p-tau NFTs and thread and dotlike neurites • Superficial NFTs in neocortex NFTs in locus coeruleus and nucleus basalis of Meynert	• Pathognomonic lesions in multiple cortical regions • Pathognomonic lesions consist of foci of p-tau NFTs, thread and dotlike neurites, and astrocytes • Clusters of p-tau at depth of sulcus may be larger • Superficial neocortical NFTs • NFTs in hippocampus, entorhinal and perirhinal cortices, and amygdala • NFTs in substantia nigra and locus coeruleus, thalamus, hypothalamus, and nucleus basalis of Meynert	• Pathognomonic lesions in multiple cortical regions • Pathognomonic lesions consist of foci of p-tau NFTs, thread and dotlike neurites, and astrocytes • NFTs distributed throughout the neocortex • Neocortical astrocytic p-tau pathology may be prominent • Neuronal loss and gliosis in the frontal and temporal cortices • Severe neurofibrillary degeneration of the medial temporal lobe • Neuronal loss and gliosis in medial temporal lobe • Severe neurofibrillary degeneration in diencephalon, including mammillary bodies, and brainstem • NFTs in cerebellar dentate, basis pontis, and spinal cord • Other pathologies, including myelin and axonal loss and TAR DNA-binding protein 43 (TDP-43) pathology

CTE, chronic traumatic encephalopathy; NFT, neurofibrillary tangles.
[a]Bieniek KF, Cairns NJ, Crary JF, et al. The Second NINDS/NIBIB Consensus Meeting to Define Neuropathological Criteria for the Diagnosis of Chronic Traumatic Encephalopathy. *J Neuropathol Exp Neurol.* 2021;80(3):210–219.
[b]Alosco ML, Cherry JD, Huber BR, et al. Characterizing tau deposition in chronic traumatic encephalopathy (CTE): utility of the McKee CTE staging scheme. *Acta Neuropathol.* 2020;140(4):495–512.
[c]McKee AC, Stein TD, Nowinski CJ, et al. The spectrum of disease in chronic traumatic encephalopathy. *Brain.* 2013;136(1):43–64.

Bioengineering (NIBIB) funded a consensus meeting of expert neuropathologists to evaluate 25 cases of various tauopathies blinded to all clinical, demographic, and gross neuropathological information. The tauopathies included CTE, AD, progressive supranuclear palsy (PSP), argyrophilic grain disease (AGD), corticobasal degeneration (CBD), primary age-related tauopathy (PART), and parkinsonism dementia complex of Guam (G-PDC). All cases were of moderate to severe pathological severity and without comorbid diseases. Unknown to the

PART III

GERIATRIC CONDITIONS

Stage I

Stage II

Stage III

Stage IV

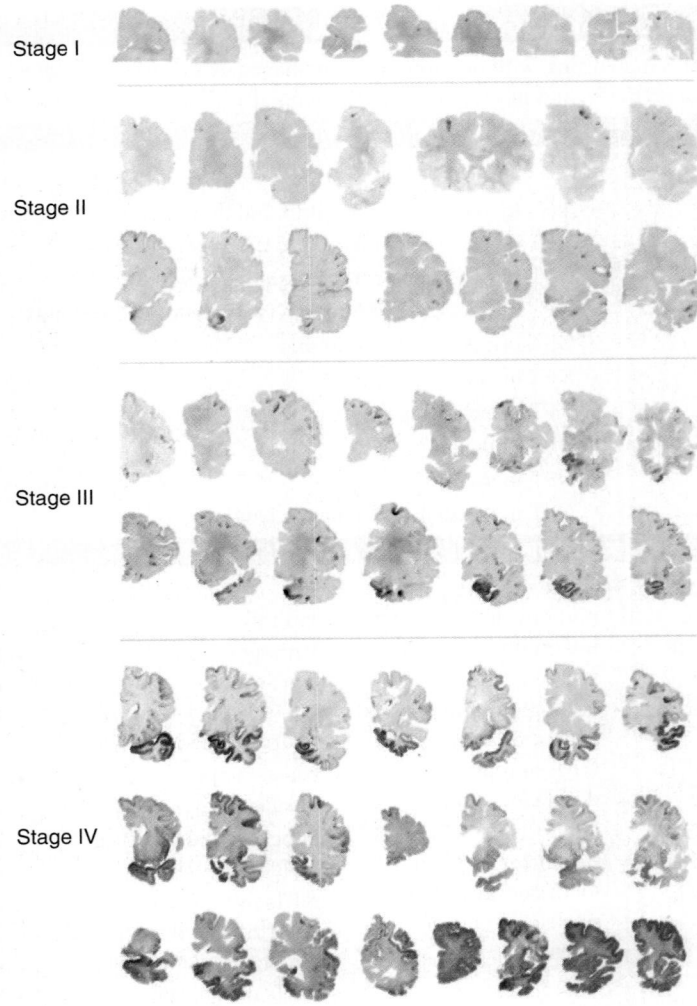

FIGURE 64-3. Coronal sections demonstrating stages of chronic traumatic encephalopathy (CTE). In stage I (top row) CTE, p-tau pathology is found in discrete foci in the cerebral cortex, most commonly in the superior or lateral frontal cortices, typically around small vessels at the depths of sulci. In stage II CTE (second row), there are multiple foci of p-tau at the depths of the cerebral sulci and localized spread of neurofibrillary pathology from these epicenters to the superficial layers of adjacent cortex. The medial temporal lobe is spared neurofibrillary p-tau pathology. In stage III CTE (third row), p-tau pathology is widespread; the frontal, insular, temporal, and parietal cortices show widespread neurofibrillary degeneration with greatest severity in the frontal and temporal lobes, and concentrated at the depths of the sulci. Also in stage III CTE, the amygdala, hippocampus, and entorhinal cortex show substantial neurofibrillary pathology that is not found in earlier stages. In stage IV CTE (fourth row), there is widespread and severe p-tau pathology affecting most regions of the cerebral cortex and the medial temporal lobe, sparing calcarine cortex in all but the most severe cases. All images, CP-13 (p-tau) immunostained 50 μ whole mount tissue sections.

neuropathologists before their analysis, the cases included 10 cases of suspected CTE that were part of the NINDS-funded Understanding Neurological Injury and Traumatic Encephalopathy (UNITE) or Veterans Affairs—Boston University—Concussion Legacy Foundation (VA-BU-CLF) brain bank at Boston University School of Medicine (BUSM), including seven cases of CTE with Aβ plaques and three cases without Aβ plaques. Five cases of AD with Braak stages V–VI, two cases of PSP, and two cases of CBD were also selected from the Alzheimer's Disease Center (ADC) brain bank at BUSM. Two cases of GPDC and two

cases of AGD were selected from the Alzheimer's Disease Research Center (ADRC) brain bank at Mayo Clinic-Jacksonville, and two cases of PART were selected from the ADRC brain bank at Columbia University. A single laboratory processed all the cases uniformly and the resulting slides were scanned into digital images that were provided to neuropathologists.

There was good agreement between the evaluating neuropathologists regarding the overall neuropathological diagnosis of all 25 cases (Cohen's kappa, 0.67), and even better agreement regarding the specific diagnosis of CTE

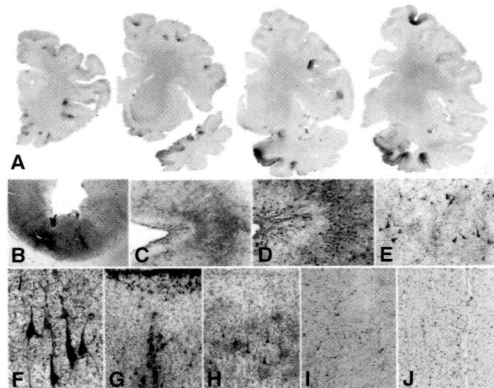

FIGURE 64-4. Histological findings in stage III chronic traumatic encephalopathy (CTE). (**A**) Whole mount coronal sections in stage III CTE that show multiple cortical foci of p-tau pathology throughout the frontal and temporal cortices. The cortical epicenters and depths of the sulci often consist of confluent masses of neurofibrillary tangles (NFT) and astrocytic tangles (ATs). (**B–D**) The p-tau pathology consists of NFTs, ATs, and dotlike and threadlike dystrophic neurites clustered around the penetrating cortical vessels, likely an arteriole. (**E**) Cortex adjacent to the cortical p-tau foci shows scattered NFTs. (**F**) The hippocampus shows dense neurofibrillary pathology. Subpial ATs (**G**) and p-tau immunopositive astrocytes may be prominent (**H**). There may be dystrophic neurites in the white matter (**I**). SMI-34 immunostaining shows reduction in axonal staining and numerous large, irregular axonal varicosities (**J**). (**A–I.** free floating 50 μ sections, AT8 (p-tau) immunostain; **J.** SMI-34 immunostain, 10-μ paraffin section.)

(Cohen's kappa, 0.78), using the proposed McKee criteria. Of the 10 cases submitted with the presumptive diagnosis of CTE, 64 of the 70 reviewer's responses (91.4%) indicated CTE as the diagnosis. There was a significant decrease of errors that paralleled the sequence of cases evaluated. The log of the expected errors significantly decreased by 0.43 for each case of CTE reviewed ($p = 0.024$). There were common additions to the CTE diagnosis, including "changes of Alzheimer's disease" (ADC) and AD in the cases with Aβ plaques. Other comorbid diagnoses included hippocampal sclerosis (HS), AGD, and PART. Of the 15 other tauopathy cases submitted for review with diagnoses other than CTE, the reviewers generally agreed with the submission diagnoses of AD (97.1% of responses), CBD (92.8%), and PART (78.5%); however, there were frequent discrepancies in cases with presumptive diagnoses of PSP, AGD, and GPDC.

The NINDS consensus group defined the single pathognomonic criterion for CTE as "an accumulation of abnormal p-tau in neurons, astrocytes, and cell processes around small vessels in an irregular pattern at the depths of the cortical sulci." They also concluded that the criteria reliably distinguished CTE from other tauopathies and made refinements of the original McKee criteria primarily in distinguishing CTE from age-related tau astrogliopathy (ARTAG).

The consensus panel defined supportive criteria for CTE as follows: "(1) abnormal p-tau-immunoreactive

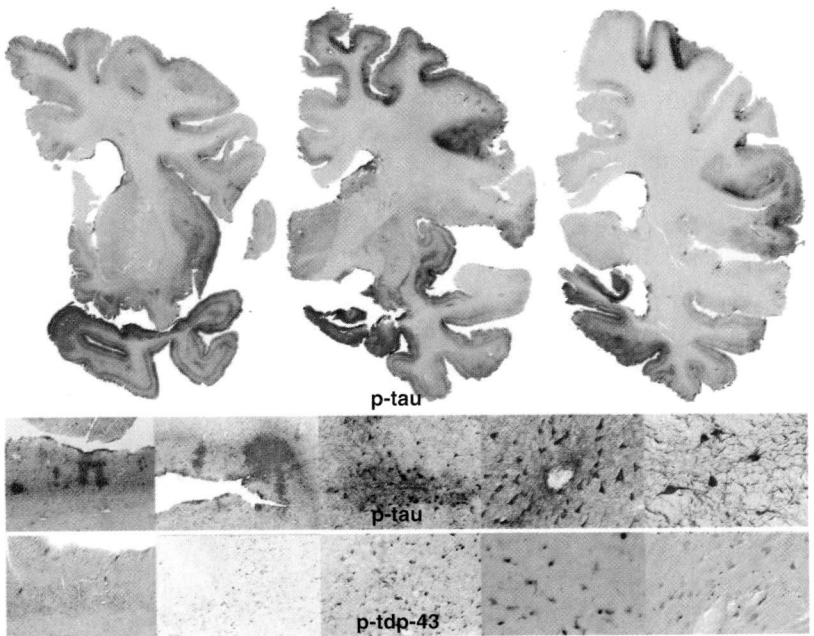

FIGURE 64-5. Histologic findings in stage IV chronic traumatic encephalopathy (CTE). **Top:** Whole mount coronal sections in immunostained for CP-13 (p-tau) show widespread p-tau pathology affecting most regions of the cerebral cortex and medial temporal lobe with characteristic concentration at the depths of the cortical sulci. **Middle:** In stage IV CTE, immunostainging for CP-13 (p-tau) shows prominent astrocytic tangles and marked neuronal loss in the cortex, amygdala, and hippocampus, in addition to dense neurofibrillary pathology. **Bottom:** Immunostaining for p-TDP-43 shows widespread pTDP-43 abnormalities in stage IV CTE. **All images:** 50 μ tissue sections.

pretangles and NFTs preferentially affecting superficial layers (layers II–III); (2) in the hippocampus, pretangles, NFTs or extracellular tangles preferentially affecting CA2 and pre-tangles and prominent proximal dendritic swellings in CA4; (3) abnormal p-tau-immunoreactive neuronal and astrocytic aggregates in subcortical nuclei, including the mammillary bodies and other hypothalamic nuclei, amygdala, nucleus accumbens, thalamus, midbrain tegmentum, and isodendritic core (nucleus basalis of Meynert, raphe nuclei, substantia nigra, and locus coeruleus); (4) p-tau-immunoreactive thorny astrocytes at the glial limitans most commonly found in the sub-pial and periventricular regions; and (5) p-tau-immunoreactive large grain-like and dot-like structures (in addition to some threadlike neurites)."

The panel noted that the diagnosis was often aided by inspection of the slide at low power inspection that revealed the distinctively irregular spatial pattern of p-tau in CTE. In addition, they observed that the pattern of superficial cortical involvement and hippocampal degeneration was unlike AD, the p-tau neurites were often dot-like, and that the TDP-43-immunoreactive inclusions in CTE were distinctive. They also made recommendations for the diagnosis and practical evaluation process of potential CTE cases.

The preliminary NINDS criteria for the pathological diagnosis of CTE were subsequently validated by Bieniek and colleagues in a study of participants from the Mayo Clinic Brain Bank in which the brains of 66 contact sport athletes and 198 controls without a history of brain trauma or contact sports were reanalyzed for p-tau pathology. Using the NINDS criteria, the authors found CTE in 21 of the 66 contact sport athletes (32%) and none of the 198 controls. Multiple international groups have used the NINDS criteria to evaluate and publish the neuropathological findings of CTE in various cohorts, including soccer players, American football players, a bull-rider, and rugby players.

In 2016, the consensus panel met again to validate and refine the preliminary pathological criteria for CTE, provided by the first NINDS consensus conference, using a second blinded sample of 27 cases of tauopathies (including 17 CTE cases representing all severities of disease) and blinded to clinical and demographic information to (1) develop the minimum threshold for diagnosis and (2) to determine whether the McKee CTE Staging Classification Scheme was reliable using a limited number of paraffin-embedded slides. Generalized estimating equation analyses showed a statistically significant association between the raters and CTE diagnosis for both the blinded (OR = 72.11, 95% CI = 19.5–267.0) and unblinded rounds (OR = 256.91, 95% CI = 63.6–1558.6).

In addition, the group discussed the minimum threshold for the diagnosis of CTE and the pathological features critical to a strict definition of "pathognomonic CTE lesion." The group endorsed a single pathognomonic lesion in the cortex as the minimum threshold for CTE. The group

also clarified that the pathognomonic lesion of CTE is a neuronal lesion characterized by NFTs and disordered neurites that may or may not contain p-tau immunoreactive astrocytes. The following features of the pathognomonic lesion were considered necessary: p-tau aggregates in neurons, with or without concomitant p-tau-immunoreactive TSAs, at the depth of the sulcus around small blood vessels, in deeper cortical layers not restricted to subpial and superficial regions. The panel unanimously confirmed that based on case material available, purely astrocytic perivascular p-tau lesions (including subpial ARTAG) did not meet criteria for CTE. Furthermore, clusters of p-tau immunoreactive astrocytes in the white matter of the frontal and temporal cortex, basal ganglia, or lateral or medial brain stem were considered consistent with ARTAG and not specific features of CTE.

Recognizing that the McKee criteria for staging CTE were based on a comprehensive panel of representative paraffin-embedded slides from multiple brain regions as well as hemispheric whole mount tissue sections, the panel suggested a simplified scheme to assess CTE severity using a restricted number of slides. The panel also proposed a working protocol for the diagnosis of CTE and assessment of CTE severity as "low CTE" or "high CTE," corresponding to CTE stages I–II and CTE stages III–IV, respectively (**Table 64-1, Figure 64-3**).

CTE Is a Primary Tauopathy

CTE is a primary tauopathy, and early stage CTE is characterized pathologically by a distinctive accumulation of p-tau in neurons as NFTs and dot-shaped NTs around small arterioles in the absence of any Aβ pathology. The arteriole at the center of the CTE lesion is often thickened and surrounded by a wide perivascular space containing occasional hemosiderin-laden macrophages. Subpial TSAs may be found in association with the CTE lesion, but in isolation, are not diagnostic for CTE. Moreover, Aβ deposition is not a feature of early CTE, but diffuse Aβ plaques commonly develop in CTE with aging and may occur in parallel with CTE p-tau pathology.

Astrocytes in CTE and Distinction from ARTAG

Age-related tau astrogliopathy (ARTAG) is a neuropathological entity often found as a comorbidity in older individuals. There are several publications in which ARTAG pathology is misclassified as mild CTE. These reports are accompanied by mistaken claims that CTE pathology is often found in normal controls. In contrast, a comprehensive study of p-tau pathology in 310 older Europeans showed no cases of CTE despite ARTAG presence in 38%.

Progression in CTE

P-tau pathology becomes progressively more severe in most subjects with CTE with age; this progressive pathology forms the basis of the McKee CTE Staging Classification

Scheme. Some individuals, however, show low levels of CTE pathology at an advanced age, supporting an indolent disease course. Nonetheless, for the majority of former American football players whose brains were donated to the UNITE brain bank, the McKee staging scheme correlates with duration of football career, number of years after retirement from football, and age at death, findings that support a progression of p-tau pathology severity with survival over time. Neuroinflammation, p-tau IHC staining density, and white matter rarefaction also increase in severity in association with the CTE stage and correlate with dementia. Among 177 American football players with CTE, semi-quantitative assessments of p-tau pathology showed a graded increase from stage I, where p-tau pathology was highest in frontal cortex and locus coeruleus; to stage II, where the p-tau pathology increased and was highest in the frontal, temporal parietal, septal, insular and entorhinal cortices, amygdala, thalamus, substantia innominata, substantia nigra, and locus coeruleus; to stage III, where there were further increases in p-tau pathology across all previous regions and hippocampus; to stage IV with still larger increases across all regions (**Figure 64-3**). The McKee CTE Staging Classification Scheme also correlates with quantitative regional assessments of p-tau pathology and dementia status. Other factors, such as the development of comorbidities with advancing age, may also drive progression of clinical symptoms in CTE in addition to increasing p-tau pathology.

SUMMARY

TBI is risk factor for dementia and parkinsonism, although the precise neuropathological underpinnings of these clinical conditions are unclear. TBI is a heterogeneous condition consisting of different grades of severity (mild, moderate, severe), frequency (single, multiple), types (focal, diffuse), nature (penetrating, blunt impact, blast), and presence or absence of skull fracture, hemorrhage, contusion, infarction, and/or other secondary processes. Neuropathological alterations after TBI include changes of AD, LBD, motor neuron disease, accumulation of p-tau or TDP-43, axonal disruption and loss, cerebral atrophy, blood-brain barrier dysintegrity, white matter degeneration, and chronic inflammation. Repetitive mild TBI or RHI, such as those typically experienced during contact sport participation, combat military service, and physical abuse, have been associated with CTE, a distinctive p-tau–based disorder. Histologically, CTE pathology is defined by irregular, patchy, and perivascular accumulation of p-tau NFTs and dotlike neurites, with a tendency to be most severe at the depths of the sulci in the frontal and temporal cortices. CTE is a progressive tauopathy that expands over time to involve deep brain structures such as the hippocampus, entorhinal cortex, amygdala, brainstem, and cerebellum. The pathological severity of CTE is divided into four (I–VI) stages using the McKee CTE Staging Classification Scheme that have been shown to correspond with quantitative regional assessments of p-tau pathology and significantly correlates with age at death and duration of football career. Recently, a NINDS consensus conference proposed an abbreviated scheme for classifying the pathology into low or high based on a limited number of paraffin-embedded blocks. At the current time, CTE can only be diagnosed by postmortem neuropathological evaluation; thus, there is an urgent need to develop diagnostic biomarkers to advance diagnosis during life and to evaluate potential therapeutic targets.

FURTHER READING

Barnes DE, Byers AL, Gardner RC, Seal KH, Boscardin WJ, Yaffe K. Association of mild traumatic brain injury with and without loss of consciousness with dementia in US military veterans. *JAMA Neurol.* 2018;75(9): 1055–1061.

Bieniek KF, Cairns NJ, Crary JF, et al. The Second NINDS/NIBIB Consensus Meeting to Define Neuropathological Criteria for the Diagnosis of Chronic Traumatic Encephalopathy. *J Neuropathol Exp Neurol.* 2021;80(3): 210–219.

Crane PK, Gibbons LE, Dams-O'Connor K, et al. Association of traumatic brain injury with late-life neurodegenerative conditions and neuropathologic findings. *JAMA Neurol.* 2016;73(9):1062–1069.

Dams-O'Connor K, Guetta G, Hahn-Ketter AE, Fedor A. Traumatic brain injury as a risk factor for Alzheimer's disease: current knowledge and future directions. *Neurodegener Dis Manag.* 2016;6(5):417–429.

Doherty C, O'Keeffe E, Keaney J, et al. Neuropolypathology as a result of severe traumatic brain injury? *Clin Neuropathol.* 2018;38:14–22.

Fann JR, Ribe AR, Pedersen HS, et al. Long-term risk of dementia among people with traumatic brain injury in Denmark: a population-based observational cohort study. *Lancet Psychiatry.* 2018;5(5):424–431.

Goldstein LE, Fisher AM, Tagge CA, et al. Chronic traumatic encephalopathy in blast-exposed military veterans and a blast neurotrauma mouse model. *Sci Transl Med.* 2012;4(134):134ra60–134ra60.

Jafari S, Etminan M, Aminzadeh F, Samii A. Head injury and risk of Parkinson disease: a systematic review and meta-analysis. *Mov Disord.* 2013;28(9): 1222–1229.

Johnson VE, Stewart W, Arena JD, Smith DH. Traumatic brain injury as a trigger of neurodegeneration. *Neurodegener Dis.* 2017;15:383–400.

1006 Kenney K, Iacono D, Edlow BL, et al. Dementia after moderate-severe traumatic brain injury: coexistence of multiple proteinopathies. *J Neuropathol Exp Neurol.* 2018;77(1):50–63.

Lee Y-K, Hou S-W, Lee C-C, Hsu C-Y, Huang Y-S, Su Y-C. Increased risk of dementia in patients with mild traumatic brain injury: a nationwide cohort study. *PloS One.* 2013;8(5):e62422.

Ling H, Morris HR, Neal JW, et al. Mixed pathologies including chronic traumatic encephalopathy account for dementia in retired association football (soccer) players. *Acta Neuropathol.* 2017;133(3):337–352.

Marras C, Hincapié CA, Kristman VL, et al. Systematic review of the risk of Parkinson's disease after mild traumatic brain injury: results of the international collaboration on mild traumatic brain injury prognosis. *Arch Phys Med Rehabil.* 2014;95(3, Supplement): S238–S244.

McKee AC, Cairns NJ, Dickson DW, et al. The first NINDS/NIBIB consensus meeting to define neuropathological criteria for the diagnosis of chronic traumatic encephalopathy. *Acta Neuropathol.* 2016;131:75–86.

McKee AC, Daneshvar DH, Alvarez VE, Stein TD. The neuropathology of sport. *Acta Neuropathol.* 2014;127(1): 29–51.

McKee AC, Stein TD, Nowinski CJ, et al. The spectrum of disease in chronic traumatic encephalopathy. *Brain.* 2013;136(1):43–64.

Mez J, Daneshvar DH, Abdolmohammadi B, et al. Duration of American football play and chronic traumatic encephalopathy. *Ann Neurol.* 2020;87(1):116–131.

Mez J, Daneshvar DH, Kiernan PT, et al. Clinicopathological evaluation of chronic traumatic encephalopathy in players of American football. *JAMA.* 2017;318(4): 360–370.

Nordström A, Nordström P. Traumatic brain injury and the risk of dementia diagnosis: a nationwide cohort study. *PLoS Med.* 2018;15(1):e1002496.

Ojo JO, Mouzon B, Algamal M, et al. Chronic repetitive mild traumatic brain injury results in reduced cerebral blood flow, axonal injury, gliosis, and increased T-tau and tau oligomers. *J Neuropathol Exp Neurol.* 2016;75(7):636–655.

Plassman BL, Grafman J. Traumatic brain injury and late-life dementia. *Handb Clin Neurol.* 2015;128:711–722.

Stewart W, McNamara PH, Lawlor B, Hutchinson S, Farrell M. Chronic traumatic encephalopathy: a potential late and under recognized consequence of rugby union? *QJM Int J Med.* 2016;109(1):11–15.

Wilson L, Stewart W, Dams-O'Connor K, et al. The chronic and evolving neurological consequences of traumatic brain injury. *Lancet Neurol.* 2017;16(10): 813–825.

Yaffe K, Lwi SJ, Hoang TD, et al. Military-related risk factors in female veterans and risk of dementia. *Neurology.* 2019;92(3):e205–e211.

Chapter 65

Major Depression

Whitney L. Carlson, William Bryson, Stephen Thielke

EPIDEMIOLOGY AND PATHOPHYSIOLOGY

Distinctive Features of Geriatric Depression

Various theories have tried to explain generally why people become depressed at different ages, but little fundamental understanding has developed around the causes of depression. Instead of sifting through theories and research, we summarize several generally accepted principles, which are usually taught as part of medical or psychology training, but which may be forgotten during a productive career. These, and the findings of research, form the groundwork for the recommendations we make about assessment and management.

Depression is not just part of getting older Although challenging life events, such as health problems and the loss of family and friends, may occur more often in later life, and although the prospect of one's own death may seem distressing, such cumulative negative events have not been shown to cause depression. In fact, aging generally involves resilience. Multiple studies demonstrate that around 5% of older adults meet criteria for major depression, which is lower than in other age groups. The likelihood of new-onset depression peaks in middle age. Among older adults, it appears that greater age involves a similar likelihood of becoming depressed, but a higher likelihood of remaining depressed. Therefore, it would be misguided and unproductive to normalize depression in older patients. Younger clinicians might learn from their older patients about how to navigate through the later stages of life.

Older age brings new challenges It is unlikely that any two people have ever experienced aging in exactly the same way, but certain generalizations hold. For our purposes, "older" means after the middle stage of life. Erik Erikson's theory of life stages conceives that mid-life (roughly age 40–65) involves a tension between generativity and stagnation. If individuals can continue to make progress in work, society, and family matters, they will feel comfortable, but if they lack direction or become stymied, they will experience distress. If navigated successfully, this stage builds the virtue which Erikson defined as "care." In later life (after age 65), the challenges shift to ego integrity versus despair: can individuals accept their lives in full, and conclude that they made some contribution to the world? Or do they feel

Learning Objectives

- Identify and characterize major depression; and understand how to recognize it within the context of common biological, psychological, social, and developmental challenges that older adults experience.

- Understand and select evidence-based treatment options for major depression in older adults, in light of their risks and limitations, and accounting for availability and patient preferences.

- Identify and be ready to apply practical strategies to support and develop therapeutic alliance with depressed older adults.

- Appreciate the importance of assessing suicide risk, and develop expertise in assessing suicidality in clinical encounters.

Key Clinical Points

1. Treating older adults with depression can challenge clinicians emotionally, and it is important to consider one's reactions to the experience. Clinicians interacting with depressed older adults can convey empathy and genuine human concern for their well-being.

2. Although aging is associated with new life challenges, depression is not a normal part of getting older. Depression should be identified and treated when present.

3. There is significant overlap between depression, social disconnection, and inability to meet basic human needs. The presence of anhedonia (lack of interest or pleasure) or hopelessness can indicate the presence of depression.

4. There are several evidence-based treatments for major depression in older adults, including medications, psychotherapy, and

(Continued)

(Cont.)

electroconvulsive therapy (ECT). Availability and patient preference are more important considerations than effectiveness.

5. In most cases, it is reasonable to consider tapering off an antidepressant after symptoms resolve or after an adequate trial produces no clear benefit. Exceptions would be a history of multiple depressive episodes or known decompensation with prior attempted dose taper.

6. All depressed older patients should be assessed for suicide risk. At minimum, this should entail evaluation of suicidal thoughts, intent to act on suicidal thoughts, suicidal plans, and access to lethal means.

guilty about their actions, and believe that everything was meaningless? If ego integrity is sustained through later life, people develop the virtue of wisdom. Although there is no necessary association with major depression and this theory, clinicians can remain attuned to this change in life tension and goals.

Depression is not just subjective distress Depression in later life has serious consequences for overall health and quality of life. It is associated with disability, cognitive impairment, perception of poorer health and quality of life, social disconnection, greater difficulty managing medical comorbidities and chronic pain, increased healthcare utilization, greater mortality, and higher costs. The relationship between depression and adverse health outcomes is likely bidirectional, with depression worsening health and function, and impaired health and function deepening

depression in return. Consequences of the relationship between depression and overall health and function include (a) the emergence of close connections between depression, social disconnection, and motivation to meet one's basic human needs, and (b) the potential for a downward spiral as depression and poor health exacerbate one another. We expand upon these consequences in the following section.

Interactions Between Geriatric Depression and Aspects of Health and Social Well-Being

Geriatric depression and basic human needs The relationship between depression and ability to meet one's basic needs is complex. Abraham Maslow's theory of human motivation, from which his hierarchy of needs derives, highlights clinical insights and potential pitfalls at the interface between depression and basic needs. Starting with basic physiological needs (eg, food, shelter, critical medicine) as the most fundamental source of motivation, the hierarchy progresses to basic physical and emotional safety, love and belonging, esteem, and, finally, self-actualization. Two core features of geriatric depression that distinguish it from other late-life mood disturbances are anhedonia (lack of interest or pleasure) and hopelessness. These, especially in combination, erode motivation to meet one's basic needs. It can be hard to identify depression as the underlying problem when other aspects of health and well-being are wanting, especially when deficits in basic needs are often more apparent than depressed mood. In these situations, anhedonia and hopelessness may be important clues to the presence of depression.

Life circumstances resulting in unmet basic needs can also precipitate depression in older adults. **Figure 65-1** illustrates this relationship. Deprivations in the higher levels of basic needs, self-actualization, and esteem tend to manifest as feelings of dissatisfaction and inadequacy, respectively, but not full-blown depression. Clinicians

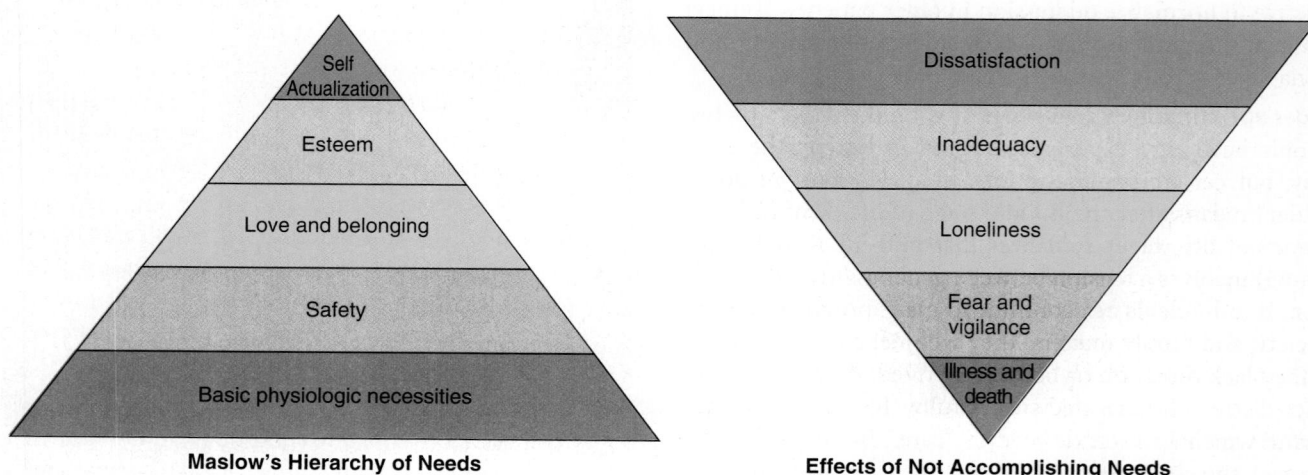

FIGURE 65-1. Depression erodes motivation to meet basic human needs (left), resulting in unmet needs and their associated consequences (right).

eager to diagnose and treat depression might overdiagnose it in these scenarios, by misinterpreting minor mood symptoms as a pathological condition. Depression tends to emerge when love and belonging needs are unmet. Abundant empirical evidence and theoretical frameworks, such as interpersonal theory, point to the critical importance of meaningful social connections in sustaining mood among older adults who experience changes in social roles (eg, retirement, grandparenthood), grief and loss, and, sometimes, functional and mobility limitations.

Although not inevitable or considered to be a part of normal aging, vulnerability to social disconnection can increase in these and other common scenarios, and such social deprivations are tightly linked to depression. Deficits in the most fundamental needs, including safety and basic physiological needs, are usually more urgent than love and belonging deficits and the depression that may accompany them. There is another potential pitfall here, as some clinicians will focus on treating depression as a more tractable issue than addressing safety and physiological needs (like housing and food insecurity), hoping that the patient will be able to find solutions to these more fundamental needs once depression is treated.

Social disconnection, loneliness, and depressed mood in older adults

The link between social disconnection and depression among older adults has become increasingly recognized as a general finding, a source of clinical concern, and an opportunity for intervention. Broadly, social disconnection is linked to physiologic and behavioral changes, such as chronic inflammation, changes in oxytocin and monoamine signaling, hypothalamic-pituitary-adrenal axis reactivity, unhealthy behaviors (eg, substance use, poor sleep hygiene, sedentary lifestyle), and challenges in coping and decision-making. The structural aspects of social connection include objective measures of network size (the number of contacts one has), frequency and duration of contacts, and living situation. Such connections sustain an individual's emotional well-being, and deprivation in structural connection is often termed *social isolation*. The term *loneliness* designates the perception that the function and/or quality of one's social connections are lacking. These distinct but closely related concepts offer another perspective from which to view geriatric depression, its health consequences, and treatment options.

Social isolation can develop in several common late-life scenarios, including retirement, widowhood, distance from adult children, sensory and mobility impairments, chronic medical comorbidities, and selective pruning of social contacts to the most meaningful few. Some forms of social isolation, such as living alone and selectivity, may reflect capability, independence, and preference, which are associated with positive health outcomes, so care must be taken not to assume that all social isolation signifies a problem.

Loneliness, however, is unlikely to be an adaptive coping mechanism. Someone can be surrounded by family and friends and still feel lonely if the quality of those

relationships is poor, or those people are offering kinds of support that the person does not want, but loneliness typically occurs in the context of some degree of social isolation. Loneliness is fundamentally related to the experience of depression, as the perceived lack of love and belonging overlap with depressed mood, negative self-appraisal, and feelings of worthlessness and being a burden. The opposite direction of causation, in which depression leads to loneliness, is also common, as depression inhibits motivation and ability to sustain relationships and feel good about them. The mutual reinforcement of social disconnection and depression can plunge older adults into a downward spiral that exacerbates morbidity and mortality. Treatment planning should consider the social factors that may either mitigate or compound it.

Practically addressing social disconnection in geriatric care

Psychosocial treatments have been developed to address the *social* aspects of depression, including interpersonal psychotherapy and behavioral activation. These are effective treatments for geriatric depression, but they require expertise that is not always available in geriatric medicine settings. An alternative, simpler model that was developed to support mental wellness at the population level and in clinical settings is **Act-Belong-Commit**. In basic terms, "Act" refers to doing something, which could include physical activity, reading, or hobbies. "Belong" refers to doing something with other people that fosters a sense of inclusion and community, like game nights or book clubs. "Commit" refers to doing something meaningful, like value-driven volunteer work. Act-Belong-Commit is straightforward and systematic enough to use in a busy geriatric medicine or primary care clinic, while also targeting depression through behavioral activation, love and belonging needs through social activity, and esteem and self-actualization needs through value-driven engagement. Prescriptions for specific kinds of desired social activity can help with credibility and accountability. While not a replacement for more traditional depression treatments, and not extensively studied in older adults, Act-Belong-Commit is a useful framework that geriatricians can incorporate into daily clinical practice.

Clinical symptoms and diagnosis of major depression

As a clinical phenomenon, depression deserves careful definition. Although people use the word "depressed" and "depression" in general speech to describe a low mood or feeling of distress, major depression involves specific hallmark findings. For the assessment of major depression in older adults, it is clinically useful and valid to use a brief, self-report rating scale such as the Patient Health Questionnaire-9 (PHQ-9) (**Figure 65–2**). The PHQ-9 is based on the *Diagnostic and Statistical Manual* (DSM)-5 of the American Psychiatric Association criteria for major depression. Note that symptom frequency is an important part of the assessment. Depression is thus quite different than having a bad day, or dealing with challenging circumstances. Scores of 0 to 4 indicate either no depression or

Patient Health Questionnaire-9 (PHQ-9)

ID #: ☐☐☐☐☐☐   Date: ☐☐ / ☐☐ / ☐☐☐☐

Timepoint: ☐☐

Over the *last 2 weeks*, how often have you been bothered by any of the following problems? (use "✓" to indicate your answer)

	Not at all	Several days	More than half the days	Nearly every day
1. Little interest or pleasure in doing things	0	1	2	3
2. Feeling down, depressed, or hopeless	0	1	2	3
3. Trouble falling or staying asleep, or sleeping too much	0	1	2	3
4. Feeling tired or having little energy	0	1	2	3
5. Poor appetite or overeating	0	1	2	3
6. Feeling bad about yourself—or that you are a failure or have let yourself or your family down	0	1	2	3
7. Trouble concentrating on things, such as reading the newspaper or watching television	0	1	2	3
8. Moving or speaking so slowly that other people could have noticed. Or the opposite—being so fidgety or restless that you have been moving around a lot more than usual	0	1	2	3
9. Thoughts that you would be better off dead, or of hurting yourself in some way	0	1	2	3
add columns:		+	+	+
(Healthcare professional: For interpretation of TOTAL, please refer to accompanying scoring.) **TOTAL:**				

10. If you checked off *any* problems, how *difficult* have these problems made it for you to do your work, take care of things at home, or get along with other people?	Not difficult at all (0) _____ Somewhat difficult (1) _____ Very difficult (2) _____ Extremely difficult (3) _____

FIGURE 65-2. Patient Health Questionnaire-9 (PHQ-9). (PHQ-9 is adapted from PRIME MD TODAY, developed by Drs. Robert L. Spitzer. Janet B.W. Williams, Kurt Kroenke, and colleagues, with an educational grant from Pfizer Inc. For research information. Contact Dr Spitzer at ris8@columbia edu. Use of the PHQ-9 may only be made in accordance with the Terms of Use available at *http://www.pfizer.com*, Copyright @1999 Pfizer Inc. All rights reserved. PRIME MD TODAY is a trademark of Pfizer Inc.)

Scoring of PHQ-9 Depression Assessment

Calculate the Total Number of Symptoms: Add the total number of symptoms in Questions 1-8 indicated by the patients as having experienced "more than half the days" or "nearly every day." Add an additional point if the patient answered question 9 [Suicidality Question] "several days, "more than half the days" or "nearly every day."

Total Number of Symptoms:

Calculate the Total (Severity) Score: Multiply the assigned point values by the number of responses given by the patient in each frequency column. Add these together to calculate the Total Score, which represents the severity of the symptoms:

"Several days"   _____ × 1 = _____ a
"More than half the days"   _____ × 2 = _____ b
"Nearly every day"   _____ × 3 = _____ c

    Total Score (a + b + c):   _____

Using the PHQ-9 for Diagnostic Assessment

Symptoms	Provisional Diagnosis	Treatment Recommendation*
1 to 4 symptoms (from gray areas on questions 1-9) plus functional impairment (#10)	Other	-Reassurance and/or supportive counseling -Education to call if deteriorates
2 to 4 symptoms (from gray areas on question 1-9), plus question 1 or 2, plus functional impairment (#10)	Minor depression	-Watchful waiting -Supportive counseling -If no improvement after one or more months use antidepressant or brief psychotherapy
3 to 4 symptoms (from gray areas on questions 1-9). plus question #2 (mood) with symptoms of 2 years, plus functional impairment (#10)	Chronic depression (probably) dysthymia	-Antidepressant and/or psychocherapy
5 symptoms (from gray areas on questions 1-9), plus questions 1 or 2, plus functional impairment (#10)	Major depression (severity score) **Moderate** (PHQ-9 score of 15 to 19) **Severe** (PHQ-9 score of 20)	**For moderate** -Patient preference for antidepressant and/or psychotherapy **For severe** -Antidepressants alone or in combination with psychotherapy

*Additional treatment considerations: Referral or comanagement with mental health specialty provider for patients with:

⊗ High suicide risk
⊗ Bipolar disorder
⊗ Inadequate treatment response
⊗ Complex psychosocial needs and/or
⊗ Other active mental disorders

FIGURE 65-2. (Continued)

clinically insignificant depressive symptoms. Scores of 5 to 9 indicate mild depression, generally subsyndromal, while scores of 10 or higher typically correlate with a diagnosis of clinical ("major") depression and warrant further evaluation and clinical intervention. The PHQ-9 is a good tool for measurement-based care to document the presence of symptoms and their change during treatment. Such instruments are also useful for educating patients and pinpointing which symptoms represent targets for intervention. Item 9 on the PHQ-9 asks the patient about death wishes or more intensive suicidal ideation; this is clearly an important part of the assessment. There is a broad range of risk and protective actors for suicide in older adults (**Figure 65–3**).

Although subsyndromal depression seems to have about the same effects on health and quality of life as major depression, antidepressant medications do not produce benefit in the treatment of subsyndromal depression. This creates a problem for clinicians. It is important to address patients' concerns, and the message, "You do not merit treatment" can seem discouraging or deflating. Instead of refusing to provide a treatment, we recommend using—and explaining—nonpharmacologic approaches. Subsyndromal depression might merit a "watch and wait" approach. And, as discussed below, major depression does not necessarily require treatment with an antidepressant medication, because other options exist, and patients prefer them to medications.

TREATMENT

Efficacy of Treatments in the Real World

Observational studies about real-world depression care paint a rather bleak picture. About 5% of older adults in primary care settings have clinically significant depression. Of these, about half are recognized and diagnosed. Of that group, about one in five receives guideline-concordant care. Therefore about 10% of depressed older adults are receiving what would be considered "adequate."

Unfortunately, such "adequate"—or guideline-concordant—care does not guarantee positive outcomes. Clinical research has identified a variety of treatments that show statistically better outcomes than either no treatment or placebo, but such findings do not translate well into real-world clinical practice. First, the clinical studies generally recruit a restricted group of patients who do not represent the real world, either because they do not have other problems or because researchers can recruit them easily. Second, the process of engaging in research entails additional attention, such as frequent check-ins, which does not happen in typical care. The "active" treatment arm receives more than just the treatment, as does the "control" arm. Third, most research studies last for weeks or months, and may produce short-lived outcomes. Finally, the benefits of treatment found in most clinical trials are relatively modest, often in the range of five or ten percentage points higher likelihood of a positive outcome.

The challenge of improving depression care in populations becomes evident in follow-up of collaborative care treatments for major depression. Collaborative care has, after extensive research and implementation, become recognized as the most effective structured approach for treating geriatric depression across primary care settings. Based on a large retrospective analysis of various clinic systems, patients in collaborative care had substantially greater likelihood of improvements in depression than those in usual care. Nevertheless, even in this "gold standard" approach, less than half of patients experienced a depression response (a ≥ 50% reduction in a symptom scale) at 6 months, and less than a third had remission of depression. Two-thirds of the patients in collaborative care thus remained effectively depressed. This "real-world" rate is considerably lower than in clinical trials of collaborative care. Tremendous heterogeneity in response was common: some clinics had less than 10% rates of depression response in patients who engaged in collaborative care, while others had over 80%.

This perspective may seem pessimistic, but it can be seen another way. By acknowledging that no single treatment will yield substantially better outcomes, clinicians can select from a variety of available options, and can engage with patients to identify approaches that will best suit patient preferences and resources. Despite the apparently low rates of response just mentioned, over time depression does and can improve. The challenge lies in finding ways to hasten response.

Selection of Best Treatment for the Patient

In busy clinical settings, medications have become the mainstay for treating depression. Most primary care providers have learned about depression and its management, and comfortably write prescriptions for antidepressant medications. Yet several other reasonable options exist, and the clinician will benefit from having considered them, both theoretically and with each patient. We propose several critical steps to increase the success of this process:

1. Elicit and discuss patient preferences for depression treatment.
2. Recognize that antidepressant medications involve risks, in particular falls, syndrome of inappropriate secretion of antidiuretic hormone, and mortality.
3. Address misconceptions about treatment options.
4. After selecting a treatment, ensure that it is (within bounds of safety) given a full trial.
5. Keep checking on symptoms during treatment.
6. If a treatment does not work, try another.

The core message for patients is, "We have a variety of treatments which might work for you. None is a guarantee, but let's try one that is safe and fits best with what you want. If that doesn't work, we'll try another."

The options that clinicians may want to consider are not all necessarily evidence-based, but some of them may

SUICIDE/SAFETY RISK FACTOR CHECKLIST

PHQ, Q9 ≥ 1
MADRS, Q10 ≥ 3
QIDS-SR Q12 ≥ 1

MR#: ____________
Subject Initials : ____________
Date: ____________

Suicidal Items

- Thoughts ____________
- Intent ____________
- Plan ____________
- Behavior ____________

Fill in all that apply:

Risk Factors

- o Hopelessness
- o Demographics, eg, male, Caucasian
- o Impulsivity/agitation/anxiety
- o Perceived burden to others
- o Chronic pain
- o Acute medical problems
- o NP status ____________
- o History of homicidal behavior
- o Aggressive behavior toward others
- o Available method(s) ____________
- o Refusal or inability to contract for safety
- o Significant recent loss
- o EtOH or substance use
- o Family Hx of attempts/completed suicide
- o Sexual orientation
- o Isolated
- o Hx of abuse ____________
- o Acute/chronic stressors, eg, caregiving, finances, grief

Risk Factors (cont.)

- o Insomnia, eg, hypnotics ____________
- o Suspicion of SI minimization
- o Unemployment
- o Previous suicide attempt
- o Discharge from psychiatric hospitalization
- o Homicidal ideation
- o Wish to join deceased
- o History of molestation

Protective Factors

- o Reasons for living ____________
- o Responsibility to others
- o Lives with others
- o Supports ____________
- o Fear of death or dying
- o Suicide is immoral
- o Cultural/spiritual beliefs
- o Engaged in work/school
- o Motivated to overreport SI
- o Ability to solve problem/make decisions

Firearm Form Status ____________

Action Plan ____________

Driving Precaution Documentation: Participant informed of possible risks associated with driving when starting a new medication. These include sedation and impaired decision making. He/she was advised to use extra caution when driving until any negative effects of the medication that MAY affect driving are known. Yes ☐ N/A ☐

AUDIT C completed: Yes ☐ No ☐ Reason why not ____________

____________ **Clinician Signature, No., & Date**

____________ **Supervisor Signature, No., & Date**

FIGURE 65-3. Suicide risk checklist. MADRS, Montgomery-Asberg Depression Rating Scale; QIDS-SR, Quick Inventory of Depressive Symptomatology-Self Scale.

resonate well with patients, and this gives a promising sign. Some modalities may not be available, especially in rural or underserved communities. The discussion below considers each option, and touches on some common preconceptions. Medications are treated separately.

Watch and wait Patients may recognize depression, but not want to take action. Especially if symptoms remain mild, it may be reasonable to continue to check in about them. This may seem antithetical to the mission of medicine, but it should be tempered by the discussion above about the effectiveness of treatments, and also by the recognition of low adherence. If the clinician has any concerns about safety or self-harm, this is obviously not a first choice.

Specialist referral In complex cases, such as the combination of depression with cognitive impairment or other forms of psychiatric illness, referral to a geriatric mental health specialist may provide the most benefit for the patient. Nevertheless, such management, even when available, does not provide any guarantees.

Electroconvulsive therapy (ECT) ECT has suffered from negative press and stereotypes. It remains by far the most effective treatment for depression, with response rates over 80%, and remission rates over 60%, in most studies. No trial has ever found medications to be more effective than ECT. Older patients seem to be even more responsive to ECT than younger adults. In its current form, ECT is a safe treatment with few side effects. Short-term memory loss almost always resolves within a few weeks after the course of treatment. The average initial course involves three to six treatments per week for 2 to 4 weeks.

Unfortunately, the beneficial effects tend to decay over time, even with medications, and "maintenance" ECT is sometimes required. ECT should be considered as an early option for patients with severe or psychotic depression, and for those who have had limited medication response.

Collaborative care As discussed above, collaborative care has the best record of success of any system-level intervention for geriatric depression. It involves coordination between the patient, a designated care manager (who checks in with the patient, develops plans, measures symptoms, and carries out brief interventions), the primary care provider (who prescribes medications), and a consulting psychiatrist (who monitors outcomes and communicates with the care manager). An information system tracks symptoms and treatments. Given the positive effects for patients and providers, systems that offer collaborative care can more efficiently and effectively manage geriatric depression. Yet also as discussed above, this approach does not guarantee remission of depression, and not all clinic systems have successfully applied the model.

Individual or group psychotherapy Various types of psychotherapy, such as cognitive behavioral therapy and interpersonal therapy, can produce lasting improvements in mood, and development of coping skills and insights. Group approaches, including reminiscence therapy, have been shown to yield significant effects. In the largest treatment trial of geriatric depression to date, 51% of participants preferred counseling or psychotherapy, and 38% preferred antidepressant medications. Research studies of psychotherapy have used structured, short-term interventions, lasting roughly 3 months at most. The treatments involve clear goals and processes, and they do not need to commit to "being analyzed." If no improvements have occurred after about 1 or 2 months, that particular psychotherapy modality may not be an effective strategy. Limited availability remains a key challenge.

Brief assessment of life stressors Depression, as a clinical syndrome, involves more than just a stressful situation or two. But sometimes patients can become so burdened by aspects of their lives that their ability to cope with or work through problems suffers. This may be especially true for individuals taking care of others, especially a spouse with dementia. The clinician can provide referrals for social support services, or respite care for the spouse of the patient. Sometimes caregivers require permission from an individual with expertise, such as a health care provider, that it is okay to take care of themselves instead of always providing care to others.

Physical activity Numerous studies have assessed the association between exercise and depression. Although it does not appear that exercise serves as a treatment for depression, people who exercised more often had lower rates of depression onset or recurrence. Because physical activity has other benefits, clinicians can sincerely recommend this as an approach to sustain mental and physical health.

Effective Use of Medications to Treat Depression

Antidepressant medications will likely remain the mainstay of treatment in most settings. Although research has identified some subtle differences between antidepressant classes and specific drugs, no single treatment has clear superiority. Because numerous sources, including electronic interaction checkers, address side effects, we will not discuss them here. Instead, we present several findings that clinicians may not recognize or remember. Chapter 60 contains detail about specific antidepressants and other psychotropics.

The placebo effect is powerful In quite a few studies, antidepressant medications have offered no statistically significant benefit over placebo, and response rates to placebo are often quite large. This appears especially so in less severe cases, and some meta-analyses have suggested that the actual effects of antidepressant medications (above and beyond the effects of placebo) occur only in more severe cases of depression. In all cases, the clinician can sincerely tell the patient that believing the medication will help increase the likelihood that it does help. Appreciating this point is especially important because most antidepressants take 6 to 8 weeks to have a measurable effect, and if a patient expects to feel better within a week or two, they may question whether the drug has any value.

Antidepressants treat major, not minor, depression Although antidepressant medications have a number of other indications, such as anxiety disorders, they do not show evidence of benefit for minor or subsyndromal depression. It may seem logically that "a little bit of antidepressant" will treat "a little depression," but this does not hold up under scrutiny. Starting an antidepressant for a condition that may resolve spontaneously runs the risk of assuming that the antidepressant produced the effect, thus committing the patient to continue the medication, or to face the problem of stopping it.

Antidepressants do not generally work in dementia Based on a large number of negative studies, there is general consensus that the usefulness of antidepressants in dementia is questionable. This creates a problem for patients with dementia, who are also unlikely to be able to engage in psychotherapy. Often other behavioral interventions, in particular related to caregiver support, can enhance mood. Insofar as polypharmacy is a significant problem in dementia care, it does not make sense to continue an antidepressant unless it yields a measurable benefit.

Slow up-titration may have benefits Older adults who were started on a lower dose of antidepressant, and then titrated up over multiple visits, had much better medication adherence than those who were started on a higher initial dose, even though they reached the same eventual dose. This is somewhat surprising, because one might expect that the sooner a target dosage is reached, the sooner a response would happen. More likely, the patient receives more personalized attention during dosage increases, and fewer side effects occur with titration.

There is no standard dosage for antidepressant effect Research about the dose-response curve for antidepressants does not support that there is a minimum effective dosage for each medication, or a narrow therapeutic window. For most antidepressants, there is only a small relationship between the dosage and the depression response, and the effect of zero dose (placebo) is substantial across all medications. Therefore, the best dosage is not a number fixed in stone, but rather the dosage that works for that individual patient. Safety, side effects, and interactions will dictate the maximum dosage.

Patients may not tell you about side effects Unless specifically asked, patients may be reluctant to report side effects, especially involving sexual dysfunction. They may choose instead simply to stop the medication. By presenting and normalizing the common side effects, including related to sexual issues, and by inquiring routinely about side effects of antidepressants, the clinician will enable patients to share concerns. If side effects are concerning enough, an antidepressant from another class could be tried, which is a better outcome than the patient deciding never to take an antidepressant again.

In an effort to improve adherence, patient satisfaction, and outcomes, astute clinicians will achieve better

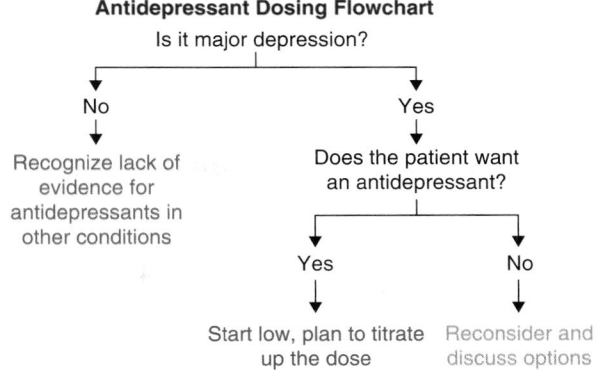

Antidepressant Dosing Flowchart

FIGURE 65-4. Antidepressant dosing flowchart.

responses by ensuring (1) that the condition is amenable to antidepressant treatment; (2) capitalizing on the placebo effect by increasing positive expectations; (3) planning to titrate up slowly rather than starting at a full dosage; (4) not assuming that each drug has a set therapeutic window that applies across patients; and (5) encouraging discussion of side effects. We propose the flowchart (see **Figure 65-4**) as a simple way to guide this decision.

Optimal Duration of Antidepressant Treatment

DSM-5 defines major depression as an "episode" for good reason: the symptoms typically will improve over time, even without treatment. Persistent depressive disorder (dysthymia) involves long-term, but less intense, symptoms, and is less common. This introduces a problem about ongoing medication use. If the depression remits, should the patient keep taking the medication to protect against future episodes? And if the depression does not improve, should the medication be kept simply because there is still a problem? Either case entails a sort of logical trap, which requires reasoning about what the condition would have been like, in an alternative world, if the antidepressant had not been started. This situation is impossible to resolve.

It is difficult to say how many older adults are prescribed antidepressants "unnecessarily," but it is likely a great many. In some populations, such as nursing home residents, almost half of individuals are prescribed an antidepressant, far higher than any estimates of depression prevalence. It is likewise difficult to quantify the harms and benefits that attend such a high level of prescription, except that polypharmacy in general, and some medications in particular, are consistently associated with negative consequences such as falls and hospitalizations. That especially becomes a problem if the medication is in fact providing no benefit.

Another important challenge is that cessation of many antidepressants, especially SSRIs and SNRIs, involves withdrawal effects. The typical effects include sweating, chills, dizziness, flu-like symptoms, GI upset, insomnia, vivid and excessive dreaming, depressed mood, vertigo, numbness,

PART III

GERIATRIC CONDITIONS

and shock-like sensations. These experiences can produce distress, and a sense that the mental health condition is worsening, or, in other words, a confusion of withdrawal with lack of efficacy. As a review by Shelton succinctly points out, "It is especially important to recognize the symptoms of discontinuation and to distinguish them from relapse and recurrence because a misdiagnosis may lead to unnecessary tests, useless treatments, and increased costs."

It is easy to be swayed by concerns about "doing no harm" into continuing medications that might provide no clear benefit, because (one reasons) they might also be preventing the return of a condition like depression. The safest defensive position would seem to involve a strong offense. Yet that metaphor does not apply well in this setting, and the potential benefits of treatment always come at a potential cost.

When studied scientifically, the risks of stopping antidepressant medications are surprisingly low. There have been few studies focusing on older adults, but, as Gueorguieva and colleagues indicate, across age groups, "the existence of similar relapse trajectories on active medication and on placebo suggests that there is no specific relapse signature associated with antidepressant discontinuation. Furthermore, continued treatment offers only modest protection against relapse." In other words, if a patient does well after an episode of depression, it may have nothing to do with the continued use of an antidepressant, and stopping the medication may be no different than continuing it.

Psychiatric research has shown that depression often relapses, even after complete remission, and that the likelihood of additional relapses increases with each additional episode. If someone has had a single episode of depression, she or he would have little need for a perpetual "maintenance" medication, but if the patient had had six or 10 such episodes, and did not relapse while taking a medication, she or he would most likely benefit from long-term use. The proof of the effect of medications ultimately lies in repeated experience, not in hypothesizing about potential effects. Also, medications do not provide a guarantee against relapse, and side effects may develop or worsen to a medication that was prescribed for years. All of this argues for thoughtful consideration, at every visit, of whether the antidepressant is providing a material benefit.

In this background, the only settings where antidepressants might reasonably be continued indefinitely and without reexamination are when depression has returned in relation to stopping the medication but not simply during withdrawal from it, or when multiple episodes of depression have occurred in the past (which is effectively the same situation, because presumably the medication was not in place at the time of the relapses). In other cases, it makes sense deliberately and slowly to consider discontinuing the medication, while monitoring symptoms. The time frames are not exact, but most SSRIs, SNRIs, and mirtazapine can be tapered over 2 to 4 weeks, and tricyclics require several months. Fluoxetine, which has a long half-life, does not require tapering, and can be used to smooth out the last stage of withdrawal (see below).

We propose this rough framework around stopping of antidepressants, which clinicians can tailor to their own practices:

1. Consider the end game when starting a medication. How long would you plan to use it, if there was a positive or a negative response?
2. At each appointment, reassess whether the antidepressant has benefit.
3. Allow time to taper off the medication. This will increase the likelihood that the patient does not experience distress, which will in turn increase the willingness to try medications again in the future if needed.
4. Continue to assess symptoms during withdrawal, and question whether symptoms can be attributed to withdrawal, lack of efficacy, or natural fluctuation.
5. If withdrawal symptoms happen even with a long taper, consider giving a single dose of fluoxetine 20 mg, which has a long half-life and tapers itself.

Practically, it is easier to start than to stop medications, and drug refills usually take but an instant. It may be expedient not to scrutinize the patient's medication regimen at each visit, but it ultimately undermines the goals of doing no harm and helping patients choose treatments that will work best for them.

APPROACH TO THE PATIENT

Challenges in Treating Older Adults With Depression

A common saying in geriatrics is that one of the best ways to care for the patient is to care for the caregiver. This applies to health care providers as well as to family, informal, and paid caregivers. Treating older adults who are experiencing symptoms of depression can challenge a clinician's patience and empathy. Even mental health providers who make it their life work often feel distress or frustration when interacting with people who have low mood, little energy, thoughts of death, and the other hallmark findings of depression. As is clear from the discussion above, patients with depression are almost never the "life of the party." We encourage providers to recognize and reflect on the feelings, both positive and negative, that develop when working with people faced with these problems. **Table 65-1** lists some of the challenges.

If clinicians start to feel especially negative emotions toward patients, or feel that they are emotionally exhausted by them, they might consider talking with a colleague, or taking a minute to reflect and recharge after an appointment that deals with mental health. It is especially important to remember that, despite our best efforts, we cannot

TABLE 65-1 ■ CHALLENGES WITH TREATING OLDER ADULTS WHO HAVE DEPRESSION

- People with depression are often slow to answer questions and do not offer straightforward or succinct replies. Talking with them can be like "pulling teeth."
- Hearing about and witnessing depressive symptoms can make the clinician feel emotionally drained, helpless, or depressed themselves.
- Older adults with depression may seem to have bottomless needs. They may report a variety of medical symptoms that require work-up, but that have no physiologic basis.
- Family members of people with depression are often concerned and want to explain at length what they have observed, and their wish to have their loved one "back to themselves." This is usually easier said than done.
- It requires emotional effort to cheer someone up, and people with depression often do not respond to attempts at cheering.
- The origins of the depression may seem easily fixable, but patients often seem unable or unwilling to do anything reasonable to solve their problems.
- Patients with depression may seem never to get better, and to be resistant to treatment. This tests the clinician's desire to heal and ease suffering, and may make the clinician feel like a failure.
- Treatments, when effective, usually take weeks or months to produce benefit.
- It is difficult to find providers willing and able to provide specialty care for older adults with depression, leaving the provider on their own.
- Suicidal thoughts may require time-consuming immediate action. A suicidal patient introduces medicolegal concerns about protecting the patient's safety and ensuring that the provider documents fully.
- If a patient does commit suicide, the provider often feels guilty that they could have done more, or that they will be in medicolegal jeopardy.

"fix" people's mental health problems for them. We can provide support, presence, and specific types of help, but ultimately individuals heal themselves (just as a wound heals itself, even if assisted by interventions). It can be frustrating to get the sense that one is doing nothing, but simply being emotionally present and listening to another person's distress is often enough.

Acknowledging Patients' Distress

Patients may express or demonstrate feeling sad, depressed, lonely, or ill, and this may or may not involve a clinical diagnosis of major depression. Some of the distress that older adults feel may relate to feeling a sense of disconnect from their medical providers and other people in their immediate circle. As the frequency of visits with primary care providers and specialty providers increases with new and chronic medical illnesses, the quality of these interactions will be important opportunities to help patients feel seen

and heard. Activities as basic as sitting down to talk to a patient, briefly touching them on the arm, and making regular eye contact instead of looking at notes, the computer, or phone can mean the difference between a meaningful interaction and one that does not result in a patient feeling understood. Asking a patient "Is there anything else I should know?" or "What other things are going on in your life?" also helps build genuine interactions and give a deeper context for a patient's presenting concerns. In other words, **simple human presence** is probably the most important way to ensure that older patients can express themselves.

How to Support Patients Between Appointments

It is difficult to ascertain what patients want. As Franz Kafka noted in a story, "To write prescriptions is easy, but to come to an understanding with people is hard." Some people might want a prescription, although research suggests that many do not. It is likely that what most people are truly seeking is genuine empathy and understanding and someone to help them navigate their circumstances and suffering. Therefore, regular contact with patients for check-ins when they are experiencing life stresses can make a significant difference. This is likely one of the reasons behind the relative success of collaborative care models. They have shown that the "person who cares" does not need to be a mental health professional. Staff in a busy primary care clinic such as nurses or care coordinators can play a role in checking in more informally with patients who need support in between visits. Helping patients identify helpful resources for connection and practical supports can also go a long way to helping to alleviate anxiety, frustration, and the overwhelm that older adults often experience trying to navigate our fast-paced and complex society.

Management of Suicidal Ideation

Suicidal ideation is sometimes the way a patient communicates the level of their suffering. It also may be a genuine wish to die. Suicidal thoughts are very difficult to understand. Some theories suggest that suicidality is mainly a problem-solving approach, in which the best course of action is not to be alive. Others have proposed that the suicidal condition represents a "negative quality of life," in which someone would take action to increase the quality of life to zero, that is, death. These theories may help a clinician to keep a balanced perspective, and to focus on effective problem-solving. In many instances, suicidal thoughts may help patients ensure they will receive support when they are feeling hopeless or overwhelmed with trying to navigate grief, social problems, or adjustments to the loss of function when they feel their needs are not being met or understood rather than a true desire to end their life.

Obviously, suicidal statements and expressions of hopelessness or a desire to die should always be taken seriously. Supporting a patient with such thoughts can come in many forms, often addressed by helping the patient have a way of talking about their suffering but also having readily at hand ways to connect them with mental health specialty and community support if that is needed. But there is no "one-size-fits-all" approach to addressing suicidality.

Several factors are associated with increased risk of suicide (see **Figure 65-3**), including male gender, social isolation, and substance abuse. Uncontrolled pain is one significant factor in expressions of suicidal ideation and a risk factor for completed suicide, particularly in older men. Those with more social connections and supports are often able to navigate difficult circumstances, particularly if they have been successful in attaining resolution of problems at other developmental life stages. However, the quality of their social supports is the most important factor in assessing whether others can be helpful when a patient expresses suicidal ideation.

It is most important to assess whether a patient expressing suicidal ideation has started to develop a plan or has one already formulated. If patients indicate that they have started rehearsing or gotten close to acting on a specified plan, this is an indication that the risk is especially high. Finding out if the patient has the means at hand, especially if their plan involves a firearm is especially important in these circumstances as removing the firearm or other means can decrease immediate risk. This may involve contacting someone in the patient's life about the situation, both to alert them of the concern as well as to assist in decreasing access to the means, especially where firearms are involved. Even when an expressed plan does not include the use of firearms, asking a patient if they own a gun is an important safety check.

Some patients may need to be considered for hospitalization, especially if they express that their plan is imminent and means are readily available. Hospitalization can provide a safe environment to better understand the circumstances that are contributing to the patient's feelings of hopelessness and assist in identifying supports and connections to community and mental health resources. Referral to a mental health professional for ongoing care can be an important step to help with ongoing assessment and care but may not be immediately available except in an emergency room setting. Patients with suicidal ideation who are expressing symptoms of psychosis are also at particular risk, particularly if their symptoms include command auditory hallucinations to harm themselves or others.

Quality of Life and Depression in Old Age

Older adults are often concerned about the quality of their life as they age, especially as they experience sensory deficits, loss of physical functioning, and pain. Goals of care should be discussed in depth and at frequent intervals. One of the benefits of the emergence of palliative care medicine is the identification of ways for such discussions to happen alongside primary care and specialty providers. One does not need to specialize in palliative care, however, in order to identify ways to alleviate suffering. Conversations about what a person sees as quality of life can often lead away from pursuing aggressive and potentially unsuccessful treatment. Alleviating suffering, including relieving pain, supporting practical needs, and identifying and providing meaningful emotional and spiritual supports are the cornerstones of palliative care medicine.

Palliative care should not be confused with end-of-life care or hospice as it applies to a much broader range of patients. Identifying ways to avoid unnecessary or unwanted treatments by discussing advanced care directives with patients is one important way of giving patients control over end of life situations. Primary care and specialty providers will also face situations where the family of a patient may not agree with choices their family member is expressing. Providing a place for difficult conversations to occur and supporting patient choices, options, and agency are some of the most important things providers can do to make patients feel supported.

Management of Depression in Long-Term Care Settings

Considering the setting of where there is a concern for a patient who might have depression also offers valuable opportunities for education of staff about ways to tailor a patient-centered care plan that can lead to alleviating patient and family concerns. Since antidepressants are commonly prescribed in nursing homes which then require consideration of gradual dose reduction, it is sometimes much easier to go about improving supports for patients in distress by identifying meaningful activities, social interactions and community supports as well as discussing issues in their environment and care delivery that are contributing to a less than satisfactory quality of life which often leads to feelings of helplessness and loss of control. Offering choices, managing environmental noise, reminding staff of important social interactions outside of care delivery, and identifying things a patient most values for comfort and peace are good places to start such conversations with the larger care network, including identifying caregiver stress that may be impacting those caring for patients either at home or in a long-term care setting. Reminiscence therapy has shown good benefits for improving depressive symptoms in long-term care settings.

Indications for Specialty Care Referrals

Not all patients with depression necessarily need to see a mental health specialist, though this is often part of the treatment plan when therapy is involved. If a patient with major depression is being treated and not improving, if their condition is worsening, or if ECT or complex augmentation strategies are being considered, this may be a time to consider a psychiatry consultation or referral. There are very few geriatric psychiatry specialists relative to the number of older adults needing care. Such subspecialty referral is not necessarily needed; most general psychiatrists should feel comfortable evaluating and treating older adults. Medically complex or cognitively impaired patients and those with a major depressive episode related to bipolar disorder or with psychotic features associated with their mood disorder may be best suited for geriatric subspecialty care given the risks of medications in this population.

Acknowledgment

Many thanks to Charles F. Reynolds, III, MD, for his contributions to the Depression chapter in the 7th Edition of this book. Material from that chapter on diagnosis of depression, including two figures, has been incorporated into this one.

FURTHER READING

Cameron IM, Reid IC, MacGillivray SA. Efficacy and tolerability of antidepressants for subthreshold depression and for mild major depressive disorder. *J Affect Disord.* 2014;166:48–58.

Carlson WL, Ong TD. Suicide in later life: failed treatment or rational choice? *Clin Geriatr Med.* 2014;533–576.

Casey DA. Depression in the elderly: a review and update. *Asia Pac Psychiatry.* 2012;4(3):160–167.

Donovan RJ, Anwar-McHenry J. Act-Belong-Commit: lifestyle medicine for keeping mentally healthy. *Am Lifestyle Med.* 2016;10:193–199.

Farina N, Morrell L, Banerjee S. What is the therapeutic value of antidepressants in dementia – a narrative review. *Geriatric Psychiatry.* 2017;32(1):32–49.

Gueorguieva R, Chekroud AM, Krystal JH. Trajectories of relapse in randomised, placebo-controlled trials of treatment discontinuation in major depressive disorder: an individual patient-level data meta-analysis. *Lancet Psychiatry.* 2017;4(3):230–237.

Hegerl U, Snhonknech P, Mergl R. Are antidepressants useful in the treatment of minor depression: a critical update of the current literature. *Curr Opin Psychiatry.* 2012;25(1):1–6.

Kobak KA, Taylor L, Katzelnick DJ, et al. Antidepressant medication management and Health Plan Employer Data Information Set (HEDIS) criteria: reasons for nonadherence. *J Clin Psychiatry.* 2002;63:727–732.

Lutz JL, Van Orden KA, Bruce ML, et al. Social disconnection in late life suicide: an NIMH workshop on state of the research in identifying mechanisms, treatment targets, and interventions. *Am J Geriatr Psychiatry.* 2021;29(8):731–744.

Maslow AH. A theory of human motivation. *Psychological Rev.* 1943;50:370–396.

National Academies of Sciences, Engineering, and Medicine. *Social Isolation and Loneliness in Older Adults: Opportunities for the Health Care System.* Washington, DC: The National Academies Press; 2019.

Ostrow L, Jessell L, Hurd M, Darrow SM, Cohen D. Discontinuing psychiatric medications: a survey of long-term users. *Psychiatr Serv.* 2017;68(12):1232–1238.

Park M, Unützer J. Geriatric depression in primary care. *Psychiatr Clin North Am.* 2011;34(2):469.

Phelps J. Tapering antidepressants: is 3 months slow enough? *Med Hypotheses.* 2011;77:1006–1008.

Santini ZI, Jose PE, Cornwell EY, et al. Social disconnectedness, perceived isolation, and symptoms of depression and anxiety among older Americans (NSHAP): a longitudinal mediation analysis. *Lancet Public Health.* 2020;5:e62-e70.

Schatzberg AF, Blier P, Delgado POL, et al. Antidepressant discontinuation syndrome: consensus panel recommendations for clinical management and additional research. *J Clin Psychiatry.* 2006;67(suppl 4):27–30.

Shelton RC. Steps following attainment of remission: discontinuation of antidepressant therapy. *Prim Care Companion J Clin Psychiatry.* 2001;3(4):168–174.

Thielke S, Diehr P, Unützer J. Prevalence, incidence, and persistence of major depressive symptoms in the Cardiovascular Health Study. *Aging and Mental Health.* 2010;14(2):168–186.

Tulner LR, Kuper IMJA, Frankfort SV, et al. Discrepancies in reported drug use in geriatric outpatients: relevance to adverse events and drug-drug interactions. *Am J Geriatr Pharmacother.* 2009;7(2):93–104.

Tveito M, Bramness JG, Engedal K. Psychotropic medication in geriatric psychiatry patients: use and unreported use in relation to serum concentrations. *Eur J Clin Pharmacol.* 2014;70:1139–1145.

Undurraga J, Baldessarini RJ. Randomized, placebo-controlled trials of antidepressants for acute major depression: thirty-year meta-analytic review. *Neuropsychopharmacology.* 2012;37:851–864.

Unützer J, Carlo AC, Arao, et al. Variation in the effectiveness of collaborative care for depression: does it matter where you get your care? *Health Aff.* 2020;39(11):1943–1950.

Unützer J, Katon W, Callahan CM, et al. Collaborative care management of late-life depression in the primary care setting: a randomized controlled trial. *JAMA.* 2002;288(22):2836–2845.

Wu C-H, Farley JF, Gaynes BN. The association between antidepressant dosage titration and medication adherence among patients with depression. *Depress Anxiety.* 2012;29:506–514.

General Topics in Geriatric Psychiatry

Ellen E. Lee, Jeffrey Lam, Dilip V. Jeste

MENTAL HEALTH ISSUES IN AGING

Relevant Population Demographic Information

The fact that the population in the United States will grow older in the coming decades is now widely recognized. Health care professionals continue to devote increasing time to the management of geriatric patients reflecting the dramatic growth in the old and very old adult populations. The overall structure of the population will also change. Projections by the United States Census Bureau estimate that by 2050, the number of individuals older than 65 years will increase from the 49 million in 2016 to 86 million. Those in the oldest age group, 85 years and older, will increase from 6.4 to 19 million individuals. **Figure 66-1** depicts the rapid growth in individuals 65 years or older between 1900 and 2060. Changes are also projected in racial and ethnic diversity with increases in both the older and the oldest old cohorts over the next four decades. By 2060, the self-reported racial distribution of those 65 and older will become more diverse, with White and non-Hispanic White groups decreasing, and all other groups increasing. Notably, from 2016 to the projections in 2060, Hispanic or Latino populations will increase their percent of resident population from 18% to 29%, Asians from 6.2% to 9.7%, and two or more races from 2.1% to 6.1%. While female life expectancy and proportion of older women are projected to continue to exceed those of men, this gap is narrowing, which could lead to secondary social and economic changes. Among the 65 years and older age group, the percentage of women will decrease from 56% in 2016 to 54% in 2060. Among those 85 years and older, the percentage of women will decrease from 65% to 61%.

The federal Administration on Aging data reveal the current living arrangements and incomes for older adults. In 2019, 57% of community-dwelling older adults lived with their spouse (72% of men and 49% of women) and 28% were living alone (19% of men and 35% of women). Over 2% of older adults lived in institutional settings, including nursing homes; however, this number increases substantially with increasing age and rises to 10% for those 85 years and older. **Figure 66-2** displays this information separately for men and women. Data from 2018 showed the median income of older persons was $26,000, $34,000 for men and $20,000 for women. These data varied by race

Learning Objectives

- Understand the prevalence of mental health and psychosocial problems associated with aging, and their adverse consequences on longevity and quality of life.

- Learn about the epidemiology, common clinical presentations, evaluation tools, and management of psychiatric conditions commonly seen in older adults.

- Acquire information necessary to recognize suicidal behavior in older adults, best ways to assess suicide risk, and effective strategies to manage suicidal patients.

- Understand the principles underlying use of antipsychotic medications in older adults, assessment of their risk-benefit ratio, clinical indications, side effect profile, and monitoring of clinical response.

- Learn about the prevalence, diagnosis, and treatment of substance use and personality disorders in older adults.

- Gain new knowledge about how "successful aging" can enhance emotional and psychological health in older adults, and promote longevity through salutary effects on cognition, physical function, and social interaction.

Key Clinical Points

1. The prevalence of psychiatric diseases increases with aging and exerts adverse effects on longevity, cognition, physical health, social interactions, and comorbid illnesses.

2. Mood disorders are common in older adults and associated with a high risk of suicide. It is important to recognize suicidal behavior and learn how to assess suicide risk and best ways to manage suicidal patients.

3. Use of antipsychotic medications in older adults is associated with serious adverse effects, including higher death rates in patients with dementia. None of these

(Continued)

(Cont.)

medications are Food and Drug Administration (FDA) approved for management of behavioral or psychological symptoms of dementia (BPSD), and there is no evidence from randomized trials that they are effective in managing psychotic symptoms.

4. Anxiety disorders are common in older adults and can present in many forms, including as generalized anxiety disorder (GAD), posttraumatic stress disorder (PTSD), obsessive-compulsive disorder (OCD), or panic disorder (PD). Additionally, anxiety symptoms are often associated with depression, dementia, medical comorbidities, and substance abuse. Psychotherapy and selective serotonin reuptake inhibitors (SSRIs) or serotonin-norepinephrine reuptake inhibitors (SNRIs) are the cornerstone of therapy for most anxiety disorders.

5. Promoting the principles of "successful aging" and positive psychological traits, such as optimism, resilience, and social engagement, enhances neuroplasticity and improves cognition, physical function, and overall quality of life.

with non-Hispanic Whites averaging a higher median income than Hispanics, African-Americans, and Asians.

Epidemiology of Psychiatric Disorders in Later Life

Mental well-being in older age is no less crucial than at any other stage of life. The Centers for Disease Control

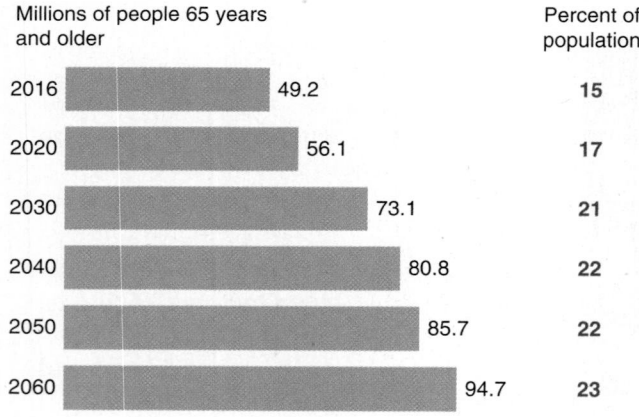

FIGURE 66-1 Number of persons in the United States, 65 years and older 1990 to 2060 (numbers in millions). This chart shows the large increases in the older population from 3.1 million people in 1900 to 43 million in 2012 and projected to 92 million in 2060. Note: Increments in years are uneven. (Reproduced with permission from U.S. Census Bureau, Population Estimates and Projections.)

and Prevention (CDC) estimates 20% of individuals older than 55 years suffer from a mental health disorder. In older adults, the burden from Alzheimer disease (AD) and other dementias increases, while the burden of other mental disorders, substance use disorders, and self-harm is reported to decrease over lifetime. However, this latter trend may be confounded by underreporting and underdiagnosis. The burden of mental health disorders among older adults is exacerbated by the stigma and lack of help-seeking. **Figure 66-3** presents additional information about the burden of mental disorders across the lifespan.

As the United States shifts from a youth-dependent population to an older-aged-dependent population and with the rise of the burden of neurocognitive disorders among older adults, the health care system must keep up with the growing demand for geriatric mental health care. The timely recognition, diagnosis, and treatment of neuropsychiatric illnesses are crucial to maintaining and bolstering the quality of life in older adults, but there is a substantial gap between the supply and demand of mental health care professionals for older adults, which is anticipated to only worsen over the coming years. As health care providers, it will be essential to prepare for these dramatic shifts in population demographics in order to ensure that a proportional growth in geriatric-specific mental health care occurs.

PSYCHOSOCIAL DEVELOPMENT ACROSS THE LIFESPAN

Health-defining, expected psychosocial developmental tasks or goals, sometimes referred to as psychological developmental milestones, vary according to age range. Psychologist Erik Erikson conceived of one of the most widely used and best-known models for human psychosocial development from infancy through old age and the end of life. Just like Sigmund Freud, Erikson believed that personality develops in a series of stages, however, Erikson's theory represented a marked a shift from Freud's psychosexual theory. While Freud's theory of psychosexual development essentially ended at early adulthood, Erikson's theory described development through the entire lifespan from birth until death and took into account the impact of social experience across the entire lifespan. The importance of Erikson's contribution to our modern understanding of psychosocial development cannot be overstated. For example, his efforts have inspired modern contemporaries such as George Valiant, author of a number of books in this area including the book *Aging Well*. In large part, because of the concepts and theories that Erikson espoused, it is now widely understood that adults of all ages, including the oldest old, may benefit from various forms of psychotherapy as long as these individuals have intact short-term memory and are motivated to make changes in their thoughts, beliefs, and behaviors.

In Erikson's model, the eighth and final stage of psychosocial development is characterized by the core conflict of

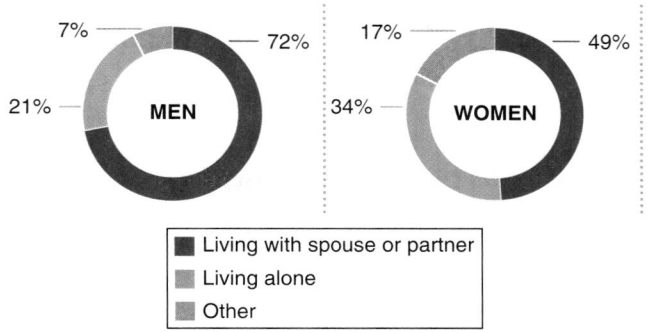

FIGURE 66-2. Living arrangements of men and women in the United States, 65 years or older, 2012. (Reproduced with permission from U.S. Census Bureau, Current Population Survey, Annual Social and Economic Supplement.)

integrity versus despair. This late adult stage includes those in the oldest age group 65 years and older. During this time, individuals grapple with answering deeper, existential questions such as, "Did I have a meaningful life?" and they reflect back on the life that they had. Wisdom is the "basic virtue" or resolution for this stage. Those who feel proud and satisfied with their accomplishments will master a sense of integrity. They have a sense of wisdom and acceptance when facing death and other end of life challenges. In contrast, someone who fails to master the developmental milestones of this stage may feel that his or her life has been wasted or lacked meaning and may experience feelings of regret, bitterness, and despair.

Ageism

In spite of the steadily growing interest among scientists, clinicians, and members of the general public, aging and later-life stages are often characterized by negative generalizations, myths, and stereotypes. While in the past, many scholars believed that aging was associated with increases in psychopathology, recent research demonstrates that older adults can be emotionally health, and on average may be

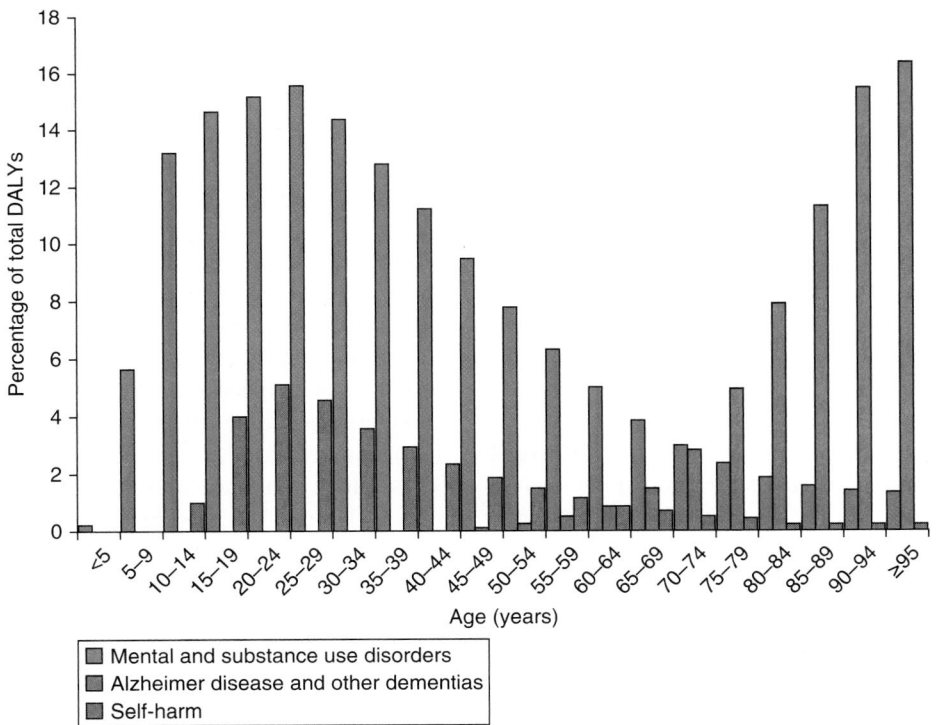

FIGURE 66-3. The global burden of mental and substance use disorders, Alzheimer disease and other dementias, and suicide (self-harm) in Disability-adjusted life years (DALYs) across the life course. (Reproduced with permission from Patel V, Saxena S, Lund C, et al. The Lancet Commission on global mental health and sustainable development. *Lancet*. 2018;392[10157]:1553–1598.)

PART III

GERIATRIC CONDITIONS

emotionally even healthier than younger and middle-aged adults. Depression and anxiety are not normal parts of growing older. The assumptions of inevitable decline in mental health with aging are often propagated by various forms of media and may even be perpetuated by health care professionals whose opinions are inaccurately biased by sampling error, for example, daily professional exposure to only those older individuals who are ill and in distress. In addition, the older individual may also adopt inaccurate understandings or expectations, when a pejorative view of later life obtained through media or some other type of exposure is internalized and enacted. In addition to stigmas associated with aging in general, an even greater stigma exits for people living with a diagnosis of neurocognitive impairment. Perceptions of the relationship between sexuality, aging, and dementia illustrate some of these misconceptions and stereotypes. While some studies have found sexual activity decreases in frequency with increasing age, there is no limit to sexual responsiveness, and many older people, including those with cognitive impairment, remain sexually active. Furthermore, sexuality has become increasingly important in successive groups of older cohorts. In professional training programs and in clinical care venues, there is a pressing need to challenge these biases and to correct these inaccurate views because of their potential to impact negatively the health and well-being of older adults. For example, because of the ageistic belief that older individuals do not engage in sexually intimate experiences, a clinician may omit questions about the older individual's recent and ongoing sexual experiences resulting in a missed opportunity to discuss how condom use is not only a form of contraception but also a good method to reduce the risk of sexually transmitted diseases. In addition, ageistic beliefs may be one reason that some clinicians are surprised to learn that many older adults living with dementia illness are leading meaningful, productive, and satisfying lives and may contribute to missed opportunities to help these older adults achieve the highest quality of life possible in spite of their dementia illness.

Common Emotional and Psychosocial Challenges Associated With Aging

With aging, certain mental health and psychosocial issues begin to emerge. Most notably, the later years of life may be characterized by various losses that for many may not have been present in earlier life stages. Some of these losses are specific to the individual such as loss of function, physical limitations, and decline in physical health and cognition. Medical comorbidities, injuries, or pain may limit mobility, while cognitive decline may jeopardize instrumental activities of daily living or other aspects of independence. As these new issues arise, aging adults may draw upon previous patterns of coping or discover opportunities for positive change and growth. Retirement is a common change and a potential challenge that arises later in life. Many look forward to retirement as the golden years of their life.

Although retirement may offer opportunities for traveling, spending time with family, nurturing old hobbies, and exploring new ones, it also marks a dramatic role transition and change in identity that may not measure up to idealized expectations and may contribute to social isolation. Many individuals also experience notable losses to their social support system including family members, friends, and peers during these years. In these settings, bereavement and grieving are normal responses to loss, but monitoring for an adjustment disorder, complicated grief, depression, or substance misuse may be warranted. Complex grief affects up to 7% of geriatric patients. It may present symptomatically like a major depressive disorder (MDD) triggered by a loss. An individual with complicated grief may meet criteria for MDD and may require treatment of the depression with pharmacotherapy, individual therapy, supportive counseling groups, referral to a specialist or some combination of these options. Feelings of self-worth are often preserved in normal grief reactions. Symptoms such as pervasive hopelessness, helplessness, guilt, diminished ability to experience pleasure, and suicidal ideation should raise concern for a major depressive episode. While a longing to be reunited with a deceased loved one or family member is often normal, careful screening and aggressive treatment may be indicated for more well-defined or active thoughts of suicide.

As physical and functional challenges arise in older patients, the need for a caregiver increases. The primary caregiver is often a spouse or adult child of the older patient. The role of a caregiver is wrought with physical, psychological, and emotional challenges when caring for someone with or without dementia. The caregiver may often suffer from significant morbidity and mortality, and new-onset mental health issues may arise in caregivers during this time. Screening for stressors, coping, and social support helps the clinician direct caregivers to helpful resources and information, which indirectly also helps support the patient and family or caregiving unit. Resources and support groups are often underutilized but effectively offer an opportunity for education, stress management, community, and solidarity. When resources are available, a hired caregiver may help ease the caregiving burden or may be necessary when support from family or close friends is not available.

Older adults are at a particularly high risk for loneliness, defined as the subjective distress arising from an imbalance between desired and perceived social relationships. Subjective loneliness differs from objective social isolation. Aging-related risk factors include widowhood, physical disability, poor health, and caregiving responsibilities. Several studies have found that loneliness increases with aging and that adults aged in the late 80s were more lonely than 60 to 80 year-old adults. Loneliness is associated with negative mental and physical health outcomes—including alcohol and drug abuse, poor nutrition, sedentary behaviors, poor physical functioning, as well as increased mortality. While the relationship is bidirectional, loneliness predicts development of depressive and anxiety symptoms. Nine longitudinal studies of nearly 41,000 older adults have reported loneliness to be a significant predictor of cognitive decline as well as development of mild cognitive impairment and dementia. Though the underlying biological processes have not been elucidated, increased amyloid-β and tau burden have been observed in cognitively normal older adults who are lonely.

Impact of COVID-19 Pandemic

The COVID-19 pandemic has disproportionately affected older adults. Older populations are at a higher risk of experiencing more severe complications and higher mortality when contracting SARS-CoV-2. Due to these heightened risks, older adults have been required to make important adjustments to their day-to-day lives, including stringent physical distancing measures to decrease the chances of exposure. Tragic cases of outbreaks in the nursing home settings and senior housing facilities have further restricted the everyday activities of these populations. As preventive social distancing measures have increased, social isolation has also proportionally increased. The COVID-19 pandemic has been particularly isolating to older adult populations given the lower familiarity levels with technologies to facilitate social interactions or virtual visits by family, friends, or even health professionals.

From a mental health perspective, the dynamic nature of the global COVID-19 pandemic has led to uncertainty, stress, and for some, bereavement. Preliminary evidence indicates that the combination of the challenges due to the pandemic has led to worsening mental health outcomes, including increased incidence of depression and anxiety among all age groups. However, contrary to expectations, preliminary evidence demonstrates that older adults have been more resilient, experiencing fewer negative mental health outcomes compared to other ages.

COMMON EVALUATION TOOLS

Cognitive Tests

Cognitive tests are effective tools for screening and diagnosis in ambulatory clinic and inpatient settings when patients are suspected to have cognitive impairment or a neurocognitive disorder. Several different tests are widely used, each with different strengths and weaknesses. Short questionnaires such as the Mental Test Score (MTS) or 6-Item Cognitive IT (6 CIT) are quick to administer but provide limited information. These are used most effectively as screening tools in a population with a high prevalence of cognitive impairment or deficits. The Clock Drawing Test, General Practitioner Assessment of Cognition (GPCOG), Mini-Cog, and Memory Impairment Screen have higher selectivity for neurodegenerative disease and are also quick to administer but similarly provide a limited amount of information. Multi-domain evaluation tools include the Mini-Mental State Examination (MMSE), Montreal

Cognitive Assessment (MoCA), St. Louis University Mental Status Examination (SLUMS), Addenbrooke's Cognitive Examination (ACE), and Test Your Memory (TYM). These tests provide broader and somewhat more comprehensive picture of the patient's cognitive abilities and may be best used to detect mild cognitive problems. Disadvantages of these tools include a longer time to administer with the exception of the TYM, which is a self-administered report. These tools are most helpful when assessing patients who are presenting with known memory problems. They help characterize the type and quantify the severity of cognitive deficits when they exist. While these tests are effective in identifying cognitive deficits, they are limited in their ability to diagnose or determine the etiology and type of a dementia.

The gold standard for diagnosing dementia and assessing neurodegenerative diseases and other cognitive deficits is a neuropsychological battery also called neuropsychiatric testing. This extensive and comprehensive assessment is performed by a specialist and may require at least 3 to 5 hours depending on the case. In addition to a full history and clinical interview, a complete neuropsychiatric battery often includes, but is not limited to, the following: California Verbal Learning Test (CVLT-2), Wechsler Adult Intelligence Scale (WAIS-4), subtests of the Wechsler Abbreviated Scale of Intelligence Second Edition (WASI-2), the Mattis Dementia Rating Scale (DRS), subtests of the Wechsler Memory Scale such as Visual Reproduction and Logical Memory, Test of Memory Malingering (TOMM), the Boston Naming Test (BNT), the Halstead-Reitan Battery, the Wide Range Achievement Test (WRAT-4), the Clock Drawing Test, the Trail Making Tests Part A and Part B, the Verbal Fluency tests from the Delis-Kaplan Executive Function Scale (D-KEFS), and the Wisconsin Card Sorting Test-64 (WCST-64). This type of testing also often includes screens for depression and anxiety symptoms which could be influencing cognitive performance such as the Geriatric Depression Scale (GDS) and Geriatric Anxiety Inventory (GAI), respectively. Other psychiatric screening tools which may be used in conjunction with, or in addition to, neuropsychiatric testing for clinical suspicion of other diagnoses or comorbidities include the PHQ-9 for depression, the Young Mania Rating Scale, GAD-7 for anxiety, PC-PTSD for PTSD, and Y-BOCS for OCD.

Other Evaluation Modalities

Other evaluation modalities, in addition to cognitive testing and screening, help determine the etiology of cognitive deficits or other psychiatric problems. For example, brain imaging, whether obtained from a computed tomography (CT) or magnetic resonance imaging (MRI), may help exclude a neurologic or general medical condition in the differential diagnosis. A brain CT or MRI may also help establish the etiology of dementia. Specifically, a brain CT or MRI assesses cerebral grey matter volume, cortical thickness, and vascular changes such as those that result from chronic untreated hypertension or atherosclerosis. Referrals to specialists in geriatric psychiatry and neurology may be warranted when considering or interpreting results of these tests. Other diagnostic tests and emerging methods specifically for making a diagnosis of Alzheimer dementia include cerebrospinal fluid (CSF) amyloid and tau, computer-assisted volumetric brain imaging, fluorodeoxyglucose positron emission tomography (FDG-PET), which measures cerebral glucose metabolism, and single-photon emission computed tomography (SPECT), a measure of cerebral perfusion. At present, Medicare will pay for an FDG-PET in cases when the clinician is not certain whether the patient has Alzheimer dementia or frontotemporal dementia. Future studies seek to identify reliable biomarkers or the combined use of several biomarkers for diagnosing dementia and its subtypes and engaging in prevention and treatment measures early in the course of the disease.

Evaluation for Delirium

Including delirium in the differential diagnosis is appropriate when assessing changes in mentation, confusion, notable behavioral changes from a previous baseline, and new or sudden onset of psychiatric symptoms. An evaluation for delirium involves a clinical interview and diagnostic evaluation of possible medical causes including medical conditions, medication side effects, or substance intoxication and withdrawal among others. The clinical hallmark of delirium is fluctuations in mental status, especially attention and alertness, and the symptoms are potentially reversible. Tools used in cognitive screening such as the MoCA or SLUMS and other cognitive exercises requiring sustained attention are especially helpful in making the diagnosis of delirium.

PSYCHOSIS IN OLDER PATIENTS

Introduction

Psychosis is a general term referring to a mental condition affecting thinking, perceptual experiences, and behaviors in a way that almost always impairs functioning. "Positive" psychotic symptoms include delusions, hallucinations, disorganized speech, and disorganized behavior. "Negative" psychotic symptoms may include reduced social interaction, reduced facial expressivity, reduced physical activity, reduced thought content, and reduced speech. Psychotic symptoms are common in older adults where they may be related to chronic psychotic disorders, mood disorders, neurocognitive disorders, or a symptom of delirium (ie, related to an underlying medical condition). Psychosis is almost always distressing for both patients and their families, and is associated with decreased quality of life and functioning, more caregiver distress, increased health care costs, and increased risk for placement in long-term care facilities. The most common primary psychotic disorders found in older adults are discussed here; mood disorders and delirium are discussed in detail elsewhere in the text.

Schizophrenia

Schizophrenia is a chronic psychotic disorder that causes significant social and occupational dysfunction. Symptoms of schizophrenia may include delusions, hallucinations, disorganized speech, disorganized or catatonic behavior, and negative symptoms. A diagnosis of schizophrenia requires at least two of these symptoms, one of which must be delusions, hallucinations, or disorganized speech. The symptoms must persist over at least a 6-month period of time and other conditions explaining the symptoms must be ruled out (eg, delirium, mood disorders). The prevalence of schizophrenia is estimated to be 0.6% among adults ages 45 to 64 and 0.1% to 0.5% in older populations. A minority of patients, approximately 20%, have onset of schizophrenia after age 40. Therefore, a majority of older adults with schizophrenia have had an earlier onset followed by a chronic course over many years. Studies suggest that schizophrenia with onset between the ages of 40 and 60, which is described as late-onset schizophrenia (LOS), differs from early-onset schizophrenia (EOS) in several important ways. Specifically, LOS is generally associated with a lower average severity of positive symptoms (ie, delusions, hallucinations, disorganized speech, or behavior), and lower average antipsychotic dose requirement. Further, the vast majority of patients with LOS are women. Accordingly, some have proposed that LOS is a distinct subtype of schizophrenia. At this time, it is not clear if LOS incidence in aging men will increase due to their gradually increasing life expectancy. However, the term LOS has not been incorporated into the *Diagnostic and Statistical Manual of Mental Disorders, Fifth Edition* (DSM-5), which states "late-onset cases can meet the diagnostic criteria for schizophrenia, but it is not yet clear whether this is the same condition as schizophrenia diagnosed prior to mid-life."

Delusional Disorder

Delusional disorder is characterized by the presence of delusions without other primary symptoms of schizophrenia (eg, hallucinations, disorganized speech or behavior, restricted affect). The disorder typically first appears in middle to late adulthood, with an average age at onset of 40 to 49 years for men and 60 to 69 years for women and is, therefore, more common in older adults than their younger counterparts. A diagnosis of delusional disorder can only be made when all other possible explanations for delusions have been ruled out (eg, delirium, neurocognitive disorders, mood disorders, and schizophrenia). According to DSM-5, the lifetime prevalence of delusional disorder is estimated to be 0.2%.

Psychosis in Neurocognitive Disorders

Psychotic symptoms are common in neurocognitive disorders. For example, it is estimated that 41% of patients with AD will experience psychotic symptoms at some point in the course of their illness. Some common psychotic symptoms in AD include misidentification of caregivers, suspiciousness, and delusions of theft. Hallucinations in AD are less common but may occur. Visual hallucinations are common in Lewy body disease and psychotic symptoms may also be associated with other neurocognitive disorders.

Evaluation

The evaluation of psychotic symptoms in older adults begins with a careful history, ideally by interview with both the patient and a reliable informant such as a family member. The time-course of symptoms can be particularly helpful as patients with chronic psychotic disorders (such as schizophrenia) and mood disorders, which are generally episodic, have a history of symptoms consistent with their diagnosis. Because psychosis is a common symptom of delirium, a medical evaluation should be performed to assess for any possible underlying medical condition. This evaluation may include a physical and neurological examination, laboratory tests, and brain imaging. A careful review of medications that could be contributing to the symptoms should also be done and substance use should be ruled out. The importance of a thorough medical evaluation cannot be over emphasized. Studies suggest that undetected contributing medical conditions may contribute to as many as 34% of hospital admissions for behavioral symptoms in older individuals. The possible explanations for this phenomenon have ranged from the influence of ageism (eg, the myth that paranoia is expected in older individuals), the extra time and effort required to obtain immediately useful historical information from older individuals due to normal age-associated changes in communication (eg, increasingly circumstantial speech, delayed retrieval of information stored in memory and slower speech production), discomfort associated with performing certain aspects of the physical examination in an older individual such as pelvic and rectal examinations, or the extra steps and staff needed to perform certain components of the physical examination in an older individual with a neurodegenerative illness, which has taken away the patient's ability to understand and cooperate with the examiner. In spite of these and other potential barriers to an optimal medical evaluation, accurately diagnosing and optimally treating medical conditions lead to more rapid restoration of the patient's health and avoid wasting increasingly precious resources. After assessment for contributing medical conditions and medication side effects referral to a geriatric psychiatrist may be helpful.

Management and Treatment

Antipsychotic and other medications Antipsychotic medications are commonly used to treat psychotic symptoms in older adults. Antipsychotic medications have been approved by the Food and Drug Administration (FDA) primarily for treatment of schizophrenia. In addition, some are FDA-approved for use in the treatment of bipolar disorder and for use in combination with antidepressants in the treatment of MDD. Antipsychotics are also widely used "off-label" in the treatment of psychosis related to neurocognitive disorders despite limited data to support the

long-term safety and effectiveness of these medications in this population. This widespread "off-label" use of antipsychotics reflects the lack of FDA-approved pharmacological alternatives for psychosis associated with neurocognitive disorders and the stress and suffering these symptoms cause for patients, their families, and others such as individuals living in the same residential care environment. In spite of what is known about the risks of prescribing antipsychotic medications to older individuals, it bears remembering that there are no FDA-approved medications from any class or category for the treatment of BPSD including psychosis nor have there been an adequate number and quality of head-to-head comparison studies of various antipsychotic medications versus medications from other classes or categories to determine if any of the other possibly helpful medications are better at reducing symptoms and/or less likely to cause serious side effects. The American Psychiatric Association Council on Geriatric Psychiatry recently published online a "Resource Document on the Use of Antipsychotic Medications to Treat Behavioral Disturbances in Persons with Dementia." This document is, perhaps, the most thoughtful, balanced, and helpful summary currently available to help guide clinicians and references recent longitudinal findings indicating that it may actually be the symptoms of psychosis and agitation that lead to increased rates of mortality and institutionalization rather than the antipsychotic medications themselves. In addition, this document emphasizes that nonpharmacological behavioral treatment strategies should be attempted as first-line approaches unless the behaviors are so severe that the patient or others are in imminent danger. Lastly, this document notes that the currently available evidence demonstrating that nonpharmacological approaches are safer or more effective than antipsychotics in the treatment of dementia-related psychosis or behavioral disturbance is limited.

Despite their widespread use, caution is warranted and the potential benefits and risks of antipsychotic use in each older individual patient must be carefully weighed. Pharmacokinetic and pharmacodynamic changes that occur with age lead to an increased sensitivity to antipsychotics in older individuals. Specifically, decreases in total body water and muscle mass combined with a relative increase in the proportion of adipose tissue result in an increased volume of distribution and slower elimination of antipsychotic medications, while decreased hepatic protein synthesis results in more "free" drug in the circulation. Further, increased permeability of the blood-brain barrier occurring with age can lead to higher concentrations of antipsychotic medications in the CNS. Aging is also associated with decreased synthesis and increased metabolism of dopamine, a decreased number of dopaminergic neurons, and decreased density of dopamine (D2) receptors in the brain. This age-related increase in sensitivity to antipsychotics often translates to lower antipsychotic dose requirements for treatment of psychotic symptoms in older adults and places older adults at greater risk for antipsychotic-induced side effects such as extrapyramidal symptoms (EPS, eg, parkinsonism). Also of concern in older adults is an increased risk of falls in those taking antipsychotics, likely due to a combination of the autonomic effects, EPS, and sedative properties of the medications.

Because second generation or "atypical" antipsychotics (eg, risperidone, olanzapine, quetiapine, ziprasidone, aripiprazole, paliperidone, iloperidone, asenapine, lurasidone) are generally associated with a lower risk for parkinsonism and tardive dyskinesia than first-generation antipsychotics, they have become popular for treatment of psychosis. Numerous studies, however, have now documented other liabilities associated with atypical antipsychotics including elevated risk of metabolic side effects and the FDA has issued a warning regarding increased risk for cerebrovascular adverse events and mortality in older patients with neurocognitive disorders treated with both atypical antipsychotics and, subsequently, for typical antipsychotics. One study evaluating the long-term safety and effectiveness of atypical antipsychotics in older adults compared four commonly prescribed atypical antipsychotics (aripiprazole, olanzapine, quetiapine, and risperidone) in 332 outpatients older than 40 years with psychotic symptoms related to a variety of psychiatric diagnoses over 2 years of treatment. Concerning findings included a high 1-year cumulative incidence of metabolic syndrome (36% in 1 year), high rates of both serious and nonserious (51%) adverse events, and no significant improvement in symptoms. Further, over half of the study participants discontinued their assigned medication within 6 months, most often due to side effects (52%) or lack of efficacy (26%). These findings suggest that the commonly used atypical antipsychotic medications may be helpful short-term but neither safe nor effective over longer periods of treatment in middle-aged and older adults.

The use of antipsychotic medications to treat schizophrenia in older adults is largely based on studies conducted on younger adults. Risperidone and olanzapine have been shown to be effective for treatment of psychotic symptoms in middle-aged and older adults with schizophrenia in short-term studies. Single short-term trials suggest that aripiprazole and paliperidone could also be beneficial. It is noteworthy that many older adults with early-onset schizophrenia have fewer and less severe delusions and hallucinations compared to their younger counterparts, and small minority of patients may experience sustained remission of illness. A reduction in dose or discontinuation of antipsychotic medication, therefore, may be possible in later years in some aging patients with schizophrenia. Their use for treatment of LOS has not been adequately studied. LOS is generally associated with a better prognosis and lower daily antipsychotic dose requirement than early-onset illness. Data regarding the pharmacological treatment of delusional disorder in older adults are limited in part because patients with delusional disorder tend to lack insight and

are difficult to enroll in randomized placebo-controlled trials. A survey of 48 experts in geriatric care in 2004 found antipsychotics to be the only recommended treatment for delusional disorder in older adults. Case studies and retrospective studies published since that time continue to support that view.

As noted above, there are currently no FDA-approved pharmacological treatments for psychosis related to neurocognitive disorders. However, given the lack of safe and effective evidence-supported alternatives, atypical antipsychotics continue to play a role in the treatment of some patients with memory illness, particularly when the symptoms are severe (with potential for harm to self or others) requiring aggressive treatment. The risk to benefit analysis in these situations is often complex. Potential benefits may include mitigation of agitation-associated injuries to patients (including falls), staff, and family members. Most dementia illnesses are progressive and the need for antipsychotic may recede as the patient's illness advances and associated additional brain injury has occurred. The only way to determine if antipsychotic medication is still required is to reduce the dose incrementally and observe whether problem symptoms reemerge on the lowered dose. Standardized measures of behavioral symptoms in neurocognitive disorders, such as the Pittsburgh Agitation Scale or the Cohen-Mansfield Agitation Inventory, can be useful to monitor the effects of treatment. Finally, it should be noted that patients with Lewy body disease are commonly sensitive to antipsychotic medications and particularly at risk for severe adverse reactions including parkinsonism, and anticholinergic and hypotensive effects. This sensitivity is most commonly associated with the antipsychotic medications, which are known to be potent dopamine receptor subtype 2 (D2) blockers, but it has also been observed and reported even with the very low-potency antipsychotics such as quetiapine.

Educating patients and their caregivers about possible risks and benefits associated with antipsychotic use in older adults and sharing the decision-making process are critical. Whatever treatment plan is implemented the prescribing clinician should carefully document in the patient's record the fact that informed consent was obtained from the patient or, when the patient lacks capacity for the decision, the appropriate proxy decision maker for the patient. If antipsychotic medications are used in older adults for any condition, we recommend starting with a low initial dose (25%–50% of that used in a younger patient) and titrating slowly. In patients who have been stably maintained on antipsychotic medications consideration should be given to incremental dose decreases in order to determine the lowest effective dose. Patients should be vigilantly monitored for side effects and to determine whether the prescribed medication is effectively treating their symptoms.

Non-Antipsychotic Medications In clinical practice, mood stabilizers, antidepressants, and sedative hypnotics are frequently used to treat psychosis and associated symptoms such as agitation and aggression, especially in persons with neurocognitive disorders. Yet, none of these medications have received FDA approval for those conditions. Moreover, they carry a clear risk of several major side effects. Therefore, considerable caution is warranted in using these medications in older patients.

Nonpharmacological interventions There are several nonpharmacological interventions which are beneficial for older adults with psychotic disorders. Cognitive Behavioral Social Skills Training (CBSST), a 36-session weekly group therapy program combining cognitive behavioral therapy (CBT), social skills training, and problem-solving training, resulted in improved functioning in of middle-aged and older patients with schizophrenia or schizoaffective disorder compared with a supportive therapy control. Helping Older People Experience Success (HOPES), a year-long program combining social skills training and preventive health care, was associated with improved community living skills and functioning, greater self-efficacy, and lower levels of negative symptoms in older adults with serious chronic mental illness, more than half of whom had schizophrenia or schizoaffective disorder. Functional Adaptation and Skills Training (FAST), a 24-week functional skills course, was also associated with improvement in functioning and decrease in utilization of emergency medical services in older adults with schizophrenia.

As noted above, data regarding psychosocial interventions for psychosis related to neurocognitive disorders are more limited. Small studies have reported benefit with interventions such as one-to-one social interaction, support groups, music therapy, dance therapy, aromatherapy, bed baths, person-centered bathing, and muscle relaxation therapy. Thus far studies testing these approaches, however, have been limited by small sample sizes, lack of appropriate control groups, and suboptimal outcome measures. More research is therefore needed in this area including better-powered, well-designed randomized controlled trials. Many studies of psychosocial interventions for behavioral symptoms in patients with neurocognitive disorders report a high placebo response rate suggesting that increased attention they receive as part of a research study is beneficial.

MOOD DISORDERS

Introduction and Suicidal Behavior

Given the preference of many older patients to seek mental health care from their primary care provider coupled with their reluctance to seek care from a mental health specialist, including psychiatrists, the primary care physician often is presented with the very challenging task of assessing and caring for older patients at risk for suicide. Although the emerging trend of "embedding" mental health providers within the primary care clinic environment seems to be an effective method of overcoming the resistance of older

individuals to receive care from psychiatrists and other mental health clinicians, for the time being most older individuals, including those at risk for suicide, will be evaluated and treated by primary care providers.

Chapter 65 of this text provides a very helpful summary of mood disorders in older individuals. This section of the current chapter provides additional information about three topics related to mood disorders: suicide, suicide risk assessment, and the treatment of suicidal ideation.

Older individuals account for a significant proportion of death by suicide in the United States. Statistics from the CDC in 2018 indicates that the rate of suicide among all older adults has increased in the last decade. In 2018, the most recent year for which data are available statistics show that those aged 55 to 64 have the highest suicide rates (20.20 per 100,000), with those aged 65 to 74, 75 to 84, and 85 and older also displaying relatively high numbers (16.31, 18.7, and 19.1 per 100,000, respectively). White males have the highest risk among all adult age groups. Moreover, older adults have the highest rate of completed suicides. With increasing age, the use of firearms as the method for completed suicide has become more common in the United States.

Suicide Risk Assessment

Establishing rapport is essential when caring for older patients. This is especially true when evaluating and assessing suicide. No matter how skilled the interviewers are, older patients are less likely to disclose thoughts about suicide and self-harm and yet the evaluation is an integral part of the treatment process because it opens up discussion between the patient and clinician, thereby allowing prevention through decreasing access to available means of suicide, building trust, facilitating a supportive therapeutic relationship, and tailoring treatment interventions.

Common barriers to open, effective communication about suicide with older patients include: (1) the belief that people should be able to deal with emotional problems without medical help; (2) the fear of being labeled "mentally ill"; and (3) the fear of being negatively judged by the clinician, fear of being referred to a psychiatrist, and the beliefs that primary care physicians do not understand and cannot help people suffering from depression. Using an empathic approach, the clinician should correct any misinformation. Educating patients and members of their social support system is essential. Tremendous benefits are usually obtained by sharing with the older patients that depressive illness is relatively common, that scientific research has begun to illuminate the underlying physiological basis for the illness and, therefore, views that depression is invariably a sign of character weakness or moral corruption are antiquated, and that scientifically proven, highly effective treatments are now available for depression and associated suicidal symptoms.

All patients with mood, substance use, and psychotic disorders should be assessed for suicide risk. This assessment need not be time consuming, especially when occurring in the context of an established therapeutic relationship. Simply asking questions pertaining to suicide can yield very helpful information. A suicide risk assessment requires the identification of suicidal ideation and intent, risk factors, and protective factors. The most important questions to ask concern present suicidal ideation. Contrary to the common belief, asking about suicidal ideation does not increase the likelihood of a patient subsequently developing suicidal ideation. Often using a "normalizing" statement as preface to questions about suicide is helpful. For example: "Sometimes individuals suffering from depression contemplate taking their lives. Have you had similar thoughts?" If a patient responds that he or she is having thoughts of suicide, the clinician should ask if any plans have been made. The lethality of plan should be weighed. For example, a plan to shoot oneself represents high lethality, whereas a plan to drink oneself to death represents lower lethality. If a plan has been made, the clinician should inquire if steps have already been made to carry out the plan such as buying ammunition for a firearm, purchasing rope, or stockpiling medications. Asking about a plan helps the clinician get a better sense of the patient's actual intent to act on the suicidal thoughts.

Another important part of the interview of a patient with depression is the identification of risk factors. A history of suicide attempts represents the most important risk factor for future attempts; however, most completed suicides are not preceded by unsuccessful attempts. Additional risk factors include hopelessness, including having no reason for living or no sense of purpose in life; feelings of helplessness; high levels of pessimism, rage, or anger; a desire for revenge; impulsiveness, increasing use of drugs or alcohol; withdrawal from friends and family; anxiety; agitation; insomnia; diminished "social connectedness" (eg, being single or living alone or living in a rural area); uncontrolled or chronic pain; male sex; and firearm access. Recent social losses also represent important risk factors, such as the death of a friend or family member, divorce, loss of employment, financial loss, and loss of housing. Worrisome activities include carrying out preparations for death, such as reassigning the responsibility of caring for dependents (children, pets, or a spouse), creating or updating wills, and giving away personal belongings.

Among psychiatric diagnoses, mood disorders carry the greatest risk. The majority of suicide occurs within the context of an active mood episode. The presence of an active substance use disorder along with a mood disorder leads to even greater risk. Physical illness, such as stroke, and disability are also important risk factors for suicide. Generally, the greater is the number of physical illnesses from which an individual suffers, the greater is the risk of suicide. Risk is also elevated the week following admission to, or discharge from, a psychiatric inpatient unit. The impact of neurocognitive disorder on suicide risk is difficult to establish; however, impairment in executive function has been found to be more prevalent in depressed older patients with a history of suicide attempts compared to those without a history of attempts.

Protective factors are also important to identify. High perceived social support, close interpersonal relationships, feelings of usefulness, perceived ability to achieve goals, a realistic and positive future outlook, and a successful adjustment to aging are examples of protective factors. The presence of these protective factors generally indicates a positive future orientation, meaning that the patient expects life to continue. Additional protective factors include religiousness and spirituality, being married, having children, and having a sense of responsibility to family. Using the above information, a general assessment of risk, should as low, moderate or high should be determined and should be documented in the patient's medical record. Determining the overall risk for suicide subsequently helps to determine the nature of the treatment that is required. **Table 65-1** in the Major Depression chapter (Chapter 65 of this text) outlines the risk factors for suicide as well as protective factors that may decrease the possibility of suicide.

To increase the reliability of the interview, structured suicidal assessment scales can be used. A commonly used suicide risk assessment tool is the Scale for Suicide Ideation, which is a 19-item clinician-rated measure that assess suicidal thoughts and behaviors during the preceding 7 days as well as for the worst moments in the patient's life as determined by the patient. The Scale for Suicide Ideation thoroughly measures many components of suicide, including suicidal plan, behavior, preparation for an attempt, and anticipation of an attempt. The Geriatric Suicide Ideation Scale is a recently developed, relatively easy to administer scale specifically developed for use with older individuals which has standardized administration and scoring procedures and is sensitive to suicide detection. This scale consists of 66 items and assesses four factors including suicidal ideation, death ideation, loss of personal and social worth, and perceived meaning of life. The SAFE-T is yet another recently developed structured suicide assessment. The SAFE-T reflects the American Psychiatric Association Practice Guidelines for the Assessment and Treatment of Patients with Suicidal Behaviors and consists of the following five steps: (1) eliciting any modifiable risk factors; (2) discovering protective factors that may help reduce suicide risk; (3) inquiring about current suicidal thoughts, behaviors, plans, and intent; (4) weighing factors 1 to 3 to calculate a level of risk and then identifying potential interventions to reduce risk; and (5) documenting risk, risk mitigation efforts and their respective rationales, and plans for follow-up. The well-written guidelines for use of the SAFE-T are available on the internet. In addition, a free pocket card of the SAFE-T is available on the Suicide Prevention Resource Center website (www.sprc.org).

Management and Treatment of Suicidal Patients

Any patient assessed to be at high, acute risk of suicide should receive an emergent mental health evaluation. If such services are not immediately available, most states have laws permitting emergency hospitalization for psychiatric evaluation of patients who, due to a mental illness, present an imminent risk of harming themselves. In general, various types of law enforcement officers are prepared to assist in securing and transporting patients for such an evaluation.

Managing and treating geriatric patients with suicidal tendencies initially involves three steps. The first is to diagnose and treat the current psychiatric disorder. The second step is to assess the suicidal intent and lethality with an emphasis on prevention. And the third is to construct a specific treatment plan tailored to the patient. Guidelines for managing suicide in adults were provided by the American Psychiatric Association's (APA) 2003 practice guidelines for the assessment and treatment of patients with suicidal behavior.

Major goals of treatment are to help the patient reduce modifiable risk factors while reinforcing protective factors. For example, prescribing no more than a 1-week supply of medication or less if the patient is taking multiple medications that, in combination in overdose, could be lethal. Enlisting the help of family members to remove firearms from the home is another valuable intervention especially given that removing the means of suicide is one of the most effective interventions in suicide prevention. Improving social support through increased supervision from family members and friends, as well as referrals as appropriate to home care and other supportive services, can also markedly diminish suicide risk. In any instance in which a clinician has significant concerns about suicide risk, a referral to a psychiatrist is highly recommended.

For older adults, specific guidelines for treating and managing suicide were provided from the Prevention of Suicide in Primary Care Elderly: Collaborative Trial (PROSPECT). **Table 66-1** shows the PROSPECT general recommendations for working with patients with suicide as well as management techniques for patients at high risk. In addition, guidelines for managing suicidal ideation in adults are provided by the American Psychiatric Association.

More recent reviews have identified collaborative primary-care-based depression screening and management as the intervention with the most evidence for preventing suicidal behavior. Other interventions include treatment with pharmacotherapy or psychotherapy, telephone counseling, and community-based prevention.

ANXIETY DISORDERS

Introduction

Anxiety disorders are the most common psychiatric disorders from which people suffer, and this remains true for individuals in later life. In fact, twice as many older individuals suffer from anxiety disorders as suffer from major neurocognitive disorders and anxiety disorders affect about five times more older individuals than do mood disorders. The nature of anxiety in older adults, however, does tend to differ in characteristic ways from that of their younger counterparts.

TABLE 66-1 ■ PROSPECT[a] RECOMMENDED GUIDELINES AND MANAGEMENT TECHNIQUES FOR WORKING WITH PATIENTS WITH SUICIDE

Guidelines while working with patients with suicidal ideation

- Be attentive
- Stay calm and nonthreatening
- Provide the patient with space and time to vent
- Be collaborative, use a team approach
- Be willing to say the word "suicide"

Management techniques for patients with high risk

- Directly assess the frequency and content of suicidal ideation and risk factors
- Explore the initial problem
- Have the patient describe reasons for and against suicide
- Assess the patient's access to means
  - Provide the patient with education regarding depression including its etiology, prognosis, and treatment
  - Decide how to manage an increase in suicidal ideation through either a formal contract or some other formality
  - Provide education regarding alcohol and illicit substances and encourage their discontinuation
- Meet with the patient weekly at minimum if suicidal ideation is present
- Write prescriptions for no more than 1 week until suicidal risk has decreased
  - Provide family education regarding suicide, including how to appropriately respond to the patient and assuring the living environment is safe (ie, remove firearms)
- Provide supportive and collaborative interaction with the patient

At each treatment assess hopelessness, suicidal ideation, and substance abuse

[a]PROSPECT, Prevention of Suicide in Primary Care Elderly: Collaborative Trial. *Data from Brown GK, Bruce ML, Pearson JL. High-risk management guidelines for elderly suicidal patients in primary care settings. Int J Geriatr Psychiatry. 2001;16(6):593–601.*

For example, in older individuals, somatic preoccupation is more common and more intense, and, due to a weakened autonomic response, the intensity of the physical symptoms associated with panic attacks is diminished. Fewer older patients meet full criteria for an anxiety diagnosis, though subthreshold anxiety affects a greater proportion of this population. Prevalence rates for full-criteria anxiety disorders among older adults have been estimated to range from about 5% to 15%, with a 2:1 female predominance.

Generalized anxiety disorder (GAD) represents approximately 50% of all anxiety disorders diagnosed in later life, and about half of all cases of GAD develop after an individual reaches 65 years of age. Specific phobia represents approximately 40% of anxiety disorders in older patients. The most common phobia in older adults is fear of falling. Approximately 60% of older adults with a history of falling and 30% of older individuals with no such history report this fear. PTSD, OCD, and PD represent almost all of the remaining 10% of anxiety diagnoses in older individuals.

Anxiety disorders often present atypically in older individuals including the reported frequency of certain symptoms of anxiety and the manner in which the anxiety symptoms are described. For example, shortness of breath or stomach discomfort may be the only way an older individual may be able to describe feelings of anxiety. In addition to differences in reporting, the diagnostic differential is far broader. A methodical approach to evaluation is recommended with the first step being to assess whether medical conditions and medications/substances might be mimicking, precipitating, or exacerbating the patient's anxiety symptoms. Medical conditions known to precipitate anxiety include delirium, chronic obstructive pulmonary disease (COPD), pulmonary embolism (PE), anemia, hypoglycemia, hyponatremia, hyperkalemia, angina, and arrhythmias. If the symptoms of anxiety are determined to indeed be the physiological consequence of a medical condition (such as panic attacks caused by a COPD exacerbation, or anxiety due to a seizure disorder), anxiety disorder due to another medical condition should be diagnosed.

Substance-induced anxiety disorder should be diagnosed if the anxiety symptoms are due to substance intoxication or withdrawal. The substance may or may not be a medication (eg, both cocaine and albuterol are "substances"). To accurately make this diagnosis (and, that is, to exclude a primary psychiatric or medical etiology of the anxiety), establishing timing of symptoms in relation to use of the substance(s) in question is crucial. Importantly, the anxiety symptoms should not have been experienced prior to use of the substance and the symptoms should not continue in the absence of continued use of the substance. Anxiogenic medications include anesthetics and analgesics, sympathomimetics and other bronchodilators, anticholinergics, insulin, thyroid preparations, oral contraceptives, antihistamines, antiparkinsonian medications, corticosteroids, antihypertensive and cardiovascular medications, anticonvulsants, lithium, antipsychotics, and antidepressants. In addition, alcohol or benzodiazepine withdrawal is commonly accompanied by intense anxiety, as is caffeine, cocaine, and amphetamine intoxication.

Primary psychiatric diagnoses should be considered after a medical etiology has been ruled out. The clinician should seek to ensure as much parsimony in diagnosis as possible. For example, might the pathology of an individual with three specific phobias be better explained by a diagnosis of GAD. The DSM-5 made few major changes to the diagnostic criteria for most anxiety disorders; perhaps the most substantial change was eliminating the requirement that a patient have insight that their anxiety is "excessive." Instead, the focus is placed on the frequency of the worry and degree of impairment it causes.

Specific Diagnoses

Neurocognitive disorder with features of anxiety Anxiety is common in the setting of neurocognitive disorder. In this clinical context, preexisting anxiety disorders may be altered in character or sometimes exacerbated and new-onset anxiety symptoms may arise. Degeneration in various brain regions has been implicated, including the dorsolateral prefrontal cortex, which is involved in modulating the anxious response. A bidirectional effect has been well established in this clinical setting: cognitive impairment tends to worsen anxiety symptoms and anxiety tends to worsen cognition. Just as neurocognitive disorder in the setting of a depressive episode is known to often portend the development of a neurocognitive disorder, so too can new-onset late-life anxiety be a prodrome of neurocognitive disorder. Parkinson disease, with its subcortical pattern of neurodegeneration and characteristic autonomic dysfunction, has been of particular interest because of its high association with not only anxiety but also depressive symptoms. Interestingly, PTSD has been shown to be a risk factor for neurocognitive disorder. Unfortunately, as a person's neurocognitive disorder progresses, the benefits of previous successful psychotherapeutic treatment may be lost and problematic symptoms may reemerge. Cognitive declines may result in loss of previously mastered coping strategies. For example, loss of inhibitory control in an individual suffering from PTSD can result in a return of anxious rumination about past traumas.

Depressive disorder with features of anxiety Approximately 25% of all older individuals with an anxiety disorder also suffer from MDD, while nearly 50% of older individuals with MDD also suffer from an anxiety disorder. In some individuals, anxiety may be of clinical significance only during depressive episodes, but in others the anxiety is chronic and seems to be an independent risk factor for developing late-life MDD. Those who suffer with both GAD and MDD may be more difficult to treat successfully. Fortunately, in many cases when depression is properly treated, patients will experience an improvement or even remission of anxiety.

Generalized anxiety disorder GAD represents the extreme on the continuum of human anxiety. The core feature is excessive, uncontrollable, an often irrational worry about a broad range of life circumstances. This clinical vignette highlights that in older individuals the focus of their anxiety is often related to their own health, including fears of memory loss and death. Worries also commonly include the health of loved ones, finances, falls, and loss of independence. The worries are also accompanied by physical symptoms such as muscle tension, insomnia, irritability, restlessness, being easily fatigued, and difficulty concentrating. The worries severely interfere with the patient's ability to function and, as a result, many people become more isolated and limit social and other activities.

When evaluating for GAD, it is important to ask about a broad array of age-appropriate topics that might be a source of anxiety, such as health and finances. With the patient's permission, interviewing friends and family may help to determine if the worry is substantially adversely affecting life quality and to obtain confirmation regarding the frequency and severity of symptoms. If new-onset GAD is suspected, it is recommended that the clinician also check closely for signs of a depressive disorder, as GAD-like anxiety can be a prominent feature of a major depressive episode. GAD is particularly important to diagnose and treat, as it is one of the least likely mental illnesses to spontaneously remit.

Panic disorder A panic attack is a brief, time-limited, well-circumscribed period of autonomic hyperarousal accompanied by physical symptoms (chest pain or palpitations, sweating, tremor) and cognitive symptoms (fear of imminent death or "losing control"). An individual who suffers repeat panic attacks and who develops a fear of future events as well as avoid situations which they associate with panic is said to suffer from PD. Fortunately, PD rarely develops after the age of 65, and, as previously noted panic attacks tend to be less severe. If an individual does develop panic attacks after the age of 65, there is a substantial chance the panic symptoms are related to a medical condition, such as Parkinson disease, exacerbations of asthma, COPD, or angina.

Agoraphobia Agoraphobia literally means "fear of the marketplace" and an individual suffering from this disorder tends to avoid public places because of fear they will be unable to escape should they develop a panic attack or other embarrassing symptoms (such as incontinence). The condition often develops after an event which the sufferer interprets as being traumatic, such as a myocardial infarction or fall-related injury. Stroke has been associated with late-life onset of agoraphobia. In DSM editions prior to the DSM-5, agoraphobia was linked with PD, but this is no longer the case. In DSM-5, the two are now recognized as distinct, but often overlapping, entities.

Posttraumatic stress disorder Following exposure to a traumatic (generally life threatening) stressor, the development of specific, characteristic symptoms defines PTSD. Briefly, the affected individual involuntarily reexperiences the event (via thoughts, flashbacks, or dreams), avoids situations that induce memories of the event (but may also experience generalized detachment from life), and develops abnormal symptoms of arousal/reactivity, such as an exaggerated startle response or irritability.

Compared to the general population, older adults are less likely to meet the full criteria for PTSD; in particular, fewer symptoms of hyperarousal and avoidance have been noted. Life events associated with aging, such as the death of a spouse, financial and physical decline, and chronic pain may cause reemergence of quiescent symptoms of PTSD (called "delayed PTSD").

Obsessive-compulsive disorder Unwanted, persistent obsessions and their repetitive, often ritualized compulsive responses, form the core of OCD. Most cases of geriatric OCD represent a continuation of an illness that most commonly has an onset in the teen years; in other words, new onset of OCD is quite rare in the geriatric population. Interestingly, brain lesions, especially in the basal ganglia, have been detected in those rare individuals who develop late-onset OCD, suggesting neurodegeneration and other brain injury as possible mechanisms.

Social anxiety disorder and illness anxiety disorder A fear of negative evaluation and the anxiety, avoidance, and other responses to social situations that follow characterize social anxiety disorder (SAD). SAD appears to decrease slightly in prevalence with age, as do the precipitating circumstances. Common concerns include incontinence, anxiety related to poor hearing or because of problems remembering people's names and embarrassment about personal appearance. Illness anxiety disorder, previously referred to as hypochondriasis, is characterized by worry about having a serious illness. One study has shown it to affect about 3% of the visitors to primary care settings. Individuals are often unconvinced by their physician's reassurances that, in fact, do not have such an illness.

Specific phobias and other specified anxiety disorder The essence of a specific phobia is fear or anxiety about circumscribed objects or situations that is out of proportion to the actual risk posed, coupled with avoidance behavior. Other specified anxiety disorder is diagnosed when the anxiety features do not meet full criteria for a specific anxiety disorder, such as panic attacks with less than four (of the possible 13) associated symptoms. Unspecified anxiety disorder (previously "anxiety disorder NOS") is most commonly given when an anxiety disorder is suspected, but further information and work-up would be needed to arrive at a more conclusive diagnosis (such as in emergency room settings). Adjustment disorder, with anxiety, should be diagnosed when the reaction to a stressor is out of proportion to reaction that would normally be expected.

Overview of Treatment

Psychotherapy is mentioned here first because, while it requires more time to administer and may present additional difficulties in the geriatric population, it is largely free of adverse side effects. The most rigorously studied modality is CBT. However, while the CBT literature consistently documents a positive response relative to no treatment, response rates in the older population, generally, are lower than for younger adults. Further, there is no consistent evidence that CBT provides greater benefit than other therapy modalities (eg, supportive therapy). Psychotherapy represents the prominent mode of treatment of agoraphobia, SAD, and illness anxiety disorder, and is used in conjunction with pharmacotherapy in the treatment of other anxiety disorders. Complementary therapy is also useful and largely without adverse side effect; examples include biofeedback, progressive relaxation, acupuncture, yoga, massage therapy, art, music, dance therapy, meditation, prayer, and spiritual counseling. A phobia of falling is first treated by accurately assessing the risk of falls and instituting fall-risk precautions, as well as vision optimization, weight-bearing exercise, and balance training such as Tai chi.

In terms of pharmacological management, the treating clinician should first consider which of the patient's medications might be removed. Older patients are particularly at risk for various forms of suboptimal prescribing, including unnecessary polypharmacy which, even in the absence of agents well-known to cause anxiety, may provoke subclinical delirium and associated anxiety symptoms. For example, a patient with overactive bladder suffering from anxiety might first be treated by testing the efficacy of a decreased dose of oxybutynin before prescribing an anxiolytic medication.

The cornerstone of pharmacological treatment is similar across anxiety disorders. Current evidence most strongly supports the use of an SSRI or SNRI at a dose higher than would be usually used to treat a depressive disorder. The recommended starting dose in geriatric individuals is generally half that recommended for a younger adult. The maximal antianxiety effect of an SSRI generally is achieved after 6 to 12 months of treatment with a therapeutic dose. In treating GAD, there is some evidence that buspirone is effective, but generally requires 2 to 4 weeks to reach maximal efficacy. Gabapentin and to a lesser extent pregabalin have also be studied and appear to be helpful. These medications can be given on a PRN basis, have little habit-forming potential and also possess analgesic properties. PD is typically treated with a high dose SSRI combined with psychotherapy (typically CBT and exposure therapy). Surprisingly few rigorous studies of pharmacologic treatment of PTSD have been conducted in older adults. Evidence of efficacy has been shown in individual studies of citalopram, mirtazapine and, for sleep-related PTSD problems only, prazosin. Caution is advised with the use of tricyclic antidepressants (TCAs), given their known cardiotoxicity and anticholinergic side effects (confusion, sedation). Benzodiazepines are also to be used with great caution in older patients, given their negative impact on cognition, tendency to cause physiologic dependence, increased risk of falls and risk of driving impairment. Prescribing benzodiazepines as a knee-jerk reaction to a complaint of anxiety also can reinforce a message to patients that anxiety must be immediately relieved. If benzodiazepines are used, there is only infrequently an indication to continue for more than 6 weeks. In addition to drug–drug interactions, SSRIs carry risks of hyponatremia, bleeding (particularly GI bleeding, and especially when used in conjunction with an NSAID), and may rarely cause parkinsonism and akathisia.

SLEEP DISORDERS

Introduction

The DSM-5 defines insomnia as "a predominant complaint of dissatisfaction with sleep quantity or quality," associated with at least one of the following: difficulty initiating sleep, maintaining sleep, and/or early morning wakening. The symptoms must cause "significant distress or impairment in functioning" and must occur at least 3 nights per week for at least 3 months.

In a survey of 9000 adults older than 65 years, more than 80% reported at least one problem with sleep, and more than half reported that at least one sleep complaint occurred nearly all the time. Poor sleep is distressing to patients and associated with poor outcomes including depression, anxiety, falls, mortality, long-term care placement, and decreased quality of life. Polysomnography (PSG) studies have confirmed age-related changes in sleep including increased fragmentation of sleep. The proportion of time spent in the lighter stages of sleep (stages 1 and 2) increases with age, especially between early adulthood and midlife, and there are reductions in both the amount of slow-wave (deep) sleep and rapid eye movement (REM) sleep. Most sleep disturbances in older adults, however, are not a normal part of aging. Sleep complaints are often comorbid with medical and psychiatric conditions, and a number of medications and substances are known to cause problems with sleep. Disturbed sleep is, therefore, often a multifactorial problem and careful assessment for all possibly contributing factors is required before concluding the patient's sleep complaints represent expected age-associated changes in sleep.

Older adults often have medical or psychiatric conditions that contribute to sleep problems. Conditions that cause pain or discomfort, respiratory symptoms, or nocturia are common causes of sleep disturbance. Gastroesophageal reflux disease, diabetes, cancer, neurodegenerative diseases, and mental illnesses are associated with high rates of sleep disturbance. It is also important to consider the effects of medications in older adults who are often taking multiple prescription and over-the-counter medications. Medications that may cause insomnia include stimulants, antihypertensives, bronchodilators, corticosteroids, decongestants, diuretics, and many antidepressants. In addition, sedating medications can cause daytime sleepiness and napping, disrupting nighttime sleep.

Sleep-Disordered Breathing

Breathing abnormalities occurring during sleep range from snoring to partial (hypopnea) or complete (apnea) cessation of airflow. These events may be caused by airway collapse during sleep or impaired central nervous system signaling and can lead to hypoxemia and repeated arousals throughout the night. A diagnosis of sleep-disordered breathing (SDB) is made when the total number of apneas plus hypopneas per hour is more than 5 to 10. Obstructive sleep apnea (OSA) syndrome is SDB with excessive daytime sleepiness. SDB is more common in older than younger adults. Young and colleagues reported the prevalence of SDB in 5615 adults older than 60 years to be 32% for those ages 60 to 69, 33% for ages 70 to 79, and 36% for ages 80 to 99.

Periodic Limb Movements in Sleep and Restless Legs Syndrome

Periodic limb movements in sleep (PLMS) are repetitive movements that can disrupt sleep usually by preventing the patient from falling asleep. The prevalence of PLMS may be up to 45% in adults older than 65 years. Restless legs syndrome (RLS) is a neurologic condition in which patients experience an urge to move the legs or arms, usually accompanied by a dysesthesia that is relieved or partially relieved by movement. The symptoms usually occur at rest or are worse during periods of rest and tend to be worse during the evening. RLS can be secondary to anemia or end-stage renal disease, and there is a growing body of evidence linking other chronic illnesses with RLS, including rheumatoid arthritis, chronic obstructive pulmonary disease, asthma, fibromyalgia, diabetes, Parkinson disease, and multiple sclerosis. The prevalence of RLS is between 8.7% and 19% in older adults and increases with age.

REM Sleep Behavior Disorder

REM sleep behavior disorder (RBD) is a condition in which the skeletal muscle atonia normally present in REM sleep is intermittently absent, resulting in movements such as punching, kicking, waving, or yelling during REM sleep. RBD typically affects older adults, mostly men. Associations between RBD and neurodegenerative diseases, including Parkinson disease, major neurocognitive disorder due to Lewy body disease, and multiple-system atrophy, have been established and RBD may precede the onset of the clinical neurologic symptoms by years.

Circadian Rhythm Disturbances

Ageing is associated with less robust circadian rhythms which can result in weaker sleep rhythms. Exposure to synchronizing cues changes with age. Older adults are exposed to less bright light, particularly those with neurocognitive disorders and those living in nursing homes. Less light exposure is associated with more awakenings. Nocturnal secretion of melatonin decreases with age. The timing of the sleep wake rhythm advances and sleep and wake times are routinely several hours earlier than conventional sleep and wake times. This phase shift causes problems if sleepiness in the early evening prevents individuals from engaging in activities they enjoy. Those who stay up may become tired when their wake time remains advanced. Falling asleep in the early evening, (napping) can lead to difficulty falling asleep at the desired and usual bedtime. In these cases, advanced sleep phase disorder is diagnosed. The prevalence of the disorder in older adults has not been established but age is a risk factor.

Evaluation

Because treatment strategies differ depending on the etiology of the sleep disturbance, a careful and systematic approach to diagnosis is recommended. Assessment of sleep disruption should begin with a detailed sleep history.

It can be helpful to have the patient complete a sleep diary and to get input from a caregiver who may be aware of symptoms (eg, snoring, gasping for air, limb movements) of which the patient is not aware. A medical history may reveal comorbid conditions. Both prescription and over-the-counter medications should be carefully reviewed. In addition, patients should be asked about caffeine, alcohol intake, and the use of recreational and illicit substances such as marijuana and methamphetamine. Primary insomnia is a diagnosis of exclusion when all other potential causes have been investigated and ruled out.

Older adults with SDB may present with symptoms similar to younger adults such as loud snoring, excessive daytime sleepiness, nonrestorative sleep, gasping arousals, witnessed apneas, dry mouth, or headaches upon awakening or may present with complaints of insomnia, nocturnal confusion, cognitive difficulties, enuresis, nocturia, or falls. Although body mass index is a risk factor, older adults with OSA may not be obese. Diagnosis is confirmed by PSG. Patients with PLMS may be unaware of them and may present with other complaints such as difficulty falling asleep, staying asleep, or excessive daytime sleepiness. The diagnosis of PLMS requires an overnight PSG. The diagnosis of RLS can be made on the basis of history. Patients can be asked about unpleasant, restless feelings in their legs, especially in the evening, that are relieved by walking or movement. In patients with significant cognitive impairment, signs of discomfort in the legs such as rubbing or kneading the legs and increased motor activity that are present or worse during inactivity and are lessened by activity may be observed. Exclusion of other conditions that may be mistaken for RLS, such as neuropathy, arthritis, akathisia, pruritus, vascular insufficiency, and anxiety, is important. The RBD screening questionnaire is a 10-item instrument asking questions about dreaming and movements which can be helpful in the assessment of RBD. The relationship between REM sleep and reported complex motor behaviors can be confirmed with PSG that includes video recording. In the assessment of circadian rhythm disturbances, examination of sleep patterns recorded in a sleep diary can be helpful. Objective assessment of sleep (eg, with actigraphy) can also be helpful but is not required.

Management and Treatment

Treatment of comorbid medical and psychiatric conditions should be optimized, medications that contribute to sleep disturbances avoided, and caffeine and alcohol consumption limited. Treatment of SDB begins with education. Weight loss, in appropriate patients, can yield a reduction in the severity of SDB. Continuous positive airway pressure (CPAP) is the gold-standard treatment. Respiratory depressants, which can increase the duration of apneas, should be avoided.

Treatment of secondary RLS necessitates treatment of the underlying disease. Otherwise treatment of RLS/PLMS in older patients involves the careful use of pharmacologic agents. Dopamine agonists (eg, ropinirole and pramipexole) have been shown to reduce the number of kicks and arousals and are the preferred therapy for RLS/PLMS in older patients. Treatment of RBD includes education of the patient and bed partner. Patients and their bed partners can consider taking measures to avoid being injured such as the use of bedrails or sleeping in separate beds. The long-acting benzodiazepine clonazepam is often used for treatment of RBD; however, older adults are more at risk for daytime sedation, falls, and cognitive symptoms with benzodiazepine use.

Evening light exposure has been found to delay circadian rhythms. Some, but not all, studies have shown improvements in objective sleep measures, while a subjective improvement in sleep is consistently observed. The optimal time for light exposure is between 7:00 PM and 9:00 PM, so light boxes are helpful, especially during the time of year when the length of daylight is the shortest. It can also be helpful to minimize morning light exposure by the use of sunglasses when outside in the first half of the day.

For primary insomnia, nonpharmacologic interventions, including education about sleep hygiene, are preferred in older adults. Cognitive behavioral therapy for insomnia (CBT-I) combines cognitive restructuring with one or more behavioral interventions (eg, stimulus control, sleep restriction, relaxation techniques). CBI-I is as effective as medications for short-term treatment of insomnia and is associated with better long-term outcomes in older adults.

In older adults it is especially important to consider potential side effects and medication interactions prior to considering pharmacological treatment. Long-acting hypnotics can cause excessive daytime sleepiness, impaired motor coordination, impaired cognition, respiratory depression and may be associated with tolerance and withdrawal symptoms upon discontinuation. There are data to support the short-term effectiveness of non-benzodiazepine receptor agonists (zolpidem, zolpidem MR, zaleplon, and eszopiclone) in older adults. Eszopiclone and zolpidem MR are FDA-approved for long-term use; however, safety concerns remain including increased risk for falls, cognitive symptoms, driving accidents, and psychiatric disturbances. Several studies support the effectiveness of ramelteon, a melatonin receptor agonist, in older adults with insomnia. Ramelteon is not extensively metabolized by the cytochrome P450 CYP3A4 isoenzyme, reducing the potential for drug–drug interactions but is metabolized by first-pass metabolism, which should be taken into account for patients with hepatic impairment. In practice, it is common to see medications from other classes prescribed for insomnia (eg, antihistamines, antidepressants, antipsychotics, anticonvulsants). There is no systematic evidence to support the effectiveness of these medications, while they are associated with risks in older adults.

SUBSTANCE USE DISORDERS

Introduction

According to the 2018–2019 National Survey on Drug Use and Health, estimates indicate about 62% use of alcohol, 21% use of tobacco products, 9.5% use of marijuana, and 0.6% use of cocaine in adults older than 50 years in the prior year. While other substances have not been examined closely in the older population, some estimates place hallucinogen use at 0.3%, inhalants at 0.2%, and methamphetamine at 0.4%. These studies also suggest a gradual increase in prevalence rates of drug misuse as younger cohorts age. Today an estimated 5.7 million older individuals need treatment for substance use disorders. According to this same survey, 3.4% and 1.1% of adults older than 50 years had alcohol use disorder and illicit drug use disorder, respectively. Unfortunately, substance misuse among older adults has not led to increasing emphasis on substance treatment for older adults. While these rates are lower than those in younger adult population, substance use disorders in older adults are often overlooked, understudied, underdiagnosed, and undertreated. Among the many suggested reasons for this is ageism and the associated inaccurate beliefs that the prevalence of substance use among the aging population is low and that the exploration of possible alcohol and substance misuse is not routinely indicated in older adults.

Alcohol Misuse

Alcohol is the most misused substance across the lifespan, the most well-studied substance and the substance most associated with an increased rate of other substance use in the older population. The National Institute on Alcohol Abuse and Alcoholism recommends no more than three servings of alcohol in 1 day and seven servings per week for older adults, both male and female. Approximately 16% of men and 11% of women older than 65 years meet this criterion for at-risk drinking. Research also indicates that these individuals are more likely to suffer from associated mental health issues such as depression and anxiety.

The impact of alcohol on the aging body should not be underestimated. Older adults experience significantly higher blood alcohol concentrations from a given quantity of alcohol as compared to younger adults; therefore, a safe amount of alcohol use significantly decreases with age. In addition to the normal age-associated physical and physiological changes, a higher rate of comorbid medical issues and the greater use of various medications in older adults also significantly increase the risk for serious adverse consequences from alcohol consumption in older individuals.

The best treatments for alcohol misuse are prevention, early screening, and early intervention. Screening for alcohol use should be routinely conducted in the context of a thorough medical and psychiatric history and physical. Special attention should be paid to the onset of use, the current and past use pattern, the frequency of use, the indications for tolerance, and any evidence of withdrawal symptoms.

Collateral information from family members or significant others is important as older adults may not report accurate alcohol use patterns due to impairment from use itself or from cognitive deficits. Physical signs of excessive alcohol such as an enlarged or tender liver, bilateral symmetric tremor of the hands, especially when the arms are extended, or changes in the skin such as red palms or acne rosacea, the latter of which is not caused by alcohol use but may be significantly worsened by alcohol. Helpful laboratory tests include elevated mean corpuscular volume, γ-glutamyl transpeptidase level, and aspartate aminotransferase levels. After chronic use, elevated carbohydrate-deficient transferase, serum uric acid, and decreased albumin levels are often seen. The CAGE questionnaire for alcohol use has variable sensitivity and specificity in older adults. Two 10-item questionnaires that have been specifically validated in older adult populations include the Short Michigan Alcohol Screening Test–Geriatric Version (SMAST-G) and the Alcohol Use Disorders Identification Test (AUDIT).

Alcohol contributes to significant morbidity in older adults. Isolated, often binge drinking episodes can lead to increased falls, confusion, poor executive functioning, and other traumatic events. Long-term, chronic use can lead to multiple organ system damage. Alcohol use in the older adult often accompanies depression and anxiety. In fact, often alcohol use treatment must take into account concurrent mental health disorder treatment. Notably, alcohol use is the second most common category of psychiatric risk for suicide attempts and completions. Additional consequences of alcohol use are sleep pattern changes and both short-term (black outs) and long-term (dementia) cognitive deficits.

If formal treatment is indicated, a combination of nonpharmacological and pharmacological treatment routes should be considered. Unfortunately, older-age-specific studies of nonpharmacological interventions for alcohol misuse have been characterized by small sample sizes and have yielded unclear outcomes. Pharmacological options for alcohol use are designed to either decrease craving or negatively reinforce use. Naltrexone is the most well-studied medication for alcohol use disorder in older adults and is an opioid-receptor antagonist that decreases craving by attenuating pleasure derived from alcohol use. Acamprosate is another drug with limited efficacy demonstrated in older adults that is believed to affect the reward pathway in the brain, also reducing craving. Disulfiram inhibits aldehyde dehydrogenase leading to uncomfortable accumulation of acetaldehyde, which results in flushing, sweating, nausea, and other uncomfortable symptoms. Disulfiram, however, is seldom used in older adults due to significant side effects such as changes in blood pressure and heart rhythm that can complicate heart disease and a number of significant drug–drug interactions due to inhibition of the metabolism of a number of medications including warfarin, phenytoin, isoniazid, and some benzodiazepines (eg, diazepam).

One of the most important aspects of alcohol misuse management in older adults is the accurate recognition and appropriate treatment of withdrawal. Alcohol withdrawal is especially dangerous in older patients due to the increased likelihood of seizures, irreversible damage to the brain, delirium, and other serious consequences. In the context of possible alcohol withdrawal, clinical assessment must be detailed and special attention must be paid to comorbid medical conditions and associated medication use. Supportive therapy must be initiated immediately to replace volume loss, correct electrolyte abnormalities, prevent falls, and correct vitamin deficiencies. The standard of care regarding medication to mitigate withdrawal symptoms and to prevent delirium tremens is a benzodiazepine. Unlike in younger adults, chlordiazepoxide is not the preferred or common choice of benzodiazepines. Lorazepam, oxazepam, or temazepam are preferred for older patients due to their intermediate half-life, relatively low lipid solubility, which minimizes undesirable accumulation in the lipid compartment, and their major biotransformation pathway of conjugation with glucuronic acid resulting in 70% to 75% of the administered dose being excreted as the glucuronide conjugate in the urine. This last characteristic allows for their use even in patients with severe hepatic dysfunction. Even with these advantages for the older patient, the use of one of these benzodiazepines must proceed with great care in order to avoid compounding the problems of withdrawal by increasing risks associated with excessive sedation and delirium including falls and respiratory sedation. The combined effect of the benzodiazepine with other medications being used by the older patient must be continuously assessed.

Benzodiazepine Misuse

While benzodiazepines are integral in treatment for alcohol withdrawal, they are also often misused in the older population. Commonly they are over prescribed and dosed above the amount required for the intended indication. Even when initially started at appropriate doses, benzodiazepines are continued without a definitive end point of use, which often leads to increased tolerance.

One of the most common reasons for benzodiazepine prescription is insomnia. As discussed in the section of this chapter devoted to sleep disorders, the causes and contributors to insomnia in older adults are various and include gender (higher risk for women), relationship status (single, widowed, or divorced), medical (multiple medical conditions), cognitive (dementia), polypharmacy, poor sleep hygiene, and mood disturbances. Despite these numerous possible etiologies of insomnia, benzodiazepines are often inappropriately used as the first-line agent for sleep complaints.

Another common reason for benzodiazepine prescription is for the treatment of anxiety. As with insomnia, causes of anxiety are often multifactorial and benzodiazepines are not be the ideal treatment in most instances.

Agarwal and Landon reported increasing rates of outpatient benzodiazepine prescribing over a 12-year period, yet Gerlach and colleagues found limited evidence of benefits from benzodiazepine usage in older adults. Over time many patients require increasing doses to achieve anxiety symptom abatement, which leads to complications, adverse events, and ultimately, the potential for dependence. As with alcohol, older adults have increased sensitivity to benzodiazepines, as metabolism is significantly slower in older adults. The risk for cognitive impairment, delirium, falls, sedation, and other unwanted effects are elevated. With physiological dependence setting in, benzodiazepine withdrawal mimics that of alcohol withdrawal and puts the older adult at similar risk as that of alcohol misuse. The evaluation and treatment of benzodiazepine withdrawal is virtually identical to that of alcohol withdrawal. To prevent benzodiazepine overuse, misuse, and complications, clinicians should carefully elicit the etiology of the sleep or anxiety complaints in order to find the optimal treatment and to minimize the use or benzodiazepines.

Opiate Misuse

Increased opioid misuse in older age cohorts has become an increasingly worrisome trend. Older adults are the most likely age group to be prescribed opioids long-term. A disturbing trend in the United States is opiate pain medication misuse. The most common rationale for opiate use is the treatment of chronic pain. Although the undertreatment of pain continues to be a problem for older adults, there is no evidence that sustained, long-term use of opiate-family pain medications leads to better outcomes. Opioids increase the risk of psychological and physiological tolerance. Furthermore, as older adults are more sensitive to medications, opiate misuse often causes sedation, constipation, cognitive impairment, and respiratory suppression, especially in context of polypharmacy and concurrent alcohol use.

Even with these unacceptable side effects, opioids remain one of the most potent pain-relieving medications. There is great controversy over appropriate guidelines on when and how to prescribe these medications. Many of the guidelines focus on curtailing long-term use, appropriate selection of drug and dose, and developing strategies for continual screening and monitoring.

Clinicians can prevent opiate misuse by maximizing the use for alternative treatments for pain in older adults. These other treatments can be tailored to each patient by examining the causes for the pain complaints and by not treating pain as a single entity unto itself. Even the medication alternatives to opiates for pain control also have potential serious adverse reactions and side effects. For example, overuse of NSAIDs can lead to gastropathies and TCAs are not well-tolerated in the older population. Considering acetaminophen as the first-line agent for pain control is recommended. Additionally, consideration should be given to SNRIs, gabapentin, and pregabalin as treatments for chronic pain. In context of opiate dependence, the clinician is advised to consider community substance use programs that include peer support and educational groups. The use of methadone, naltrexone as buprenorphine as treatments for opiate dependence has not been well studied in older populations.

Marijuana Misuse

Rates of marijuana use and misuse have increased substantially in the last few years. While marijuana use in adults older than 65 years in the United States was 0.4% in 2006, this rate has increased to 5.1% in 2019. The prevalence of marijuana use will likely continue to increase in older adults given marijuana use prevalence in younger cohorts and the growing movement toward marijuana legalization in the United States.

While there have been dramatic increases in marijuana use rates among older adults, scientists still know little about its effects on cognition, drug interactions, pharmacokinetics, and risk for adverse effects in this age cohort. In the older adult population, the full health impact of chronic marijuana use has yet to be determined, but recent studies indicate that marijuana negatively impacts cognitive function. Contrary to previous expectations, there is no adequate evidence to support the belief that marijuana can serve as an effective treatment for dementia or for symptoms of depression or anxiety. At this time, clinicians are recommended to screen for and provide counseling for possible marijuana misuse in older adults.

Misuse of Other Substances

Older adults also commonly misuse tobacco, with 8.2% of adults older than 65 years engaging in current cigarette smoking behavior. Despite widespread cigarette smoking prevention and cessation efforts, among older adults, misconceptions about nicotine use persist. For example, some continue to believe that in older adults, smoking cessation does not yield any benefit and that smoking can help with pain, mood, and cognition. None of these are validated nor should be reasons to omit screening for smoke cessation when caring for an older adult. Additionally, smoking is commonly related to comorbid anxiety and other substance misuse. Behavioral modifications can be very helpful for smoking cessation. Pharmacological methods for cessation include nicotine replacement therapy and medications designed to impact the reward pathway for smoking. Bupropion and varenicline have good evidence for smoking cessation in adults but evidence for their effectiveness in older adults is lacking. Bupropion is also potentially mood elevating and may lead to increased anxiety symptoms in some patients. For varenicline, there is a widely publicized negative effect on mood and potential to increase suicidal behavior. With a high prevalence rate of co-occurring anxiety and depression in older adults with substance use issues, it is important that varenicline's potential negative effect on mood and suicidal behavior is closely monitored by the clinician.

PERSONALITY DISORDERS

Research in personality and personality pathology in older cohorts is an emerging field primarily driven by the increasing number of older individuals, but already some patterns and key findings have emerged. Personality traits are enduring, consistent behaviors forming a unique profile that distinguishes individuals from each other and predicts an individual's response to experiences or stressors. These traits are apparent as older adults respond to normal milestones and pathology associated with aging. Because personalities are defined by long-standing patterns of behavior, global personality, and personality structure tend to remain stable with aging; however, neurologic or degenerative disease and brain injury in addition to positive changes associated with aging can lead to observed personality changes and shifts. For example, traits such as neuroticism, extraversion, and openness tend to decrease with age, while altruism and conscientiousness increase with age.

Personality disorders are organized into three groups or clusters in the DSM-5. Cluster A disorders include paranoid, schizoid, and schizotypal personality disorders. They are characterized by bizarre, eccentric behavior, and magical or delusional-type thinking. The cluster B disorders include antisocial, borderline, histrionic, and narcissistic personality disorders. Cluster B disorders are characterized by impulsive behaviors, interpersonal instability, and unstable or labile affect. The cluster C disorders are avoidant, dependent, and obsessive-compulsive personality disorders. Disorders in this cluster are driven by an anxious diathesis that leads to worry, fear, rigidity, and isolation.

The prevalence of personality disorders in the general adult population is about 12%. While personality disorders in older adults have not been well studied, large epidemiological surveys have found the prevalence of at least one personality disorder in older adults ranging from 11% to 15%. In certain geriatric subpopulations, however, the prevalence may be higher. For example, in geriatric patients with MDDs and dysthymia, up to a third also have a personality disorder, most commonly avoidant, dependent, or other cluster C disorders and traits. In older adults, the odd traits associated with cluster A personality disorder and the anxious behaviors of cluster C personality disorders are more common that the impulsive behaviors seen in cluster B personality disorders, which are more common in younger adults. Of those older adults in the psychiatric outpatient population, anywhere from 5% to 33% meet criteria for personality disorder. Rates increase in geriatric patients receiving inpatient mental health treatment with prevalence rates ranging from 7% to 80%. In some cases, the impact and severity of symptoms in those with a known diagnosis of a personality disorder may worsen later in life. For example, an exacerbation of symptoms and behaviors may occur in the setting of significant social stressors such as the loss of a supporting person or other stabilizing environmental factors such as a job. Currently, prevalence data

in older age groups are limited by the current methods and assessment tools used in epidemiologic studies directed at personality and personality disorders, which may inadequately correlate to the specific behaviors in older individuals. Further research and attention to this emerging field is needed to better understand the manifestation of traits and diagnosis of personality disorder in older adults. Additional disorders outside of this classification system include personality change due to another medical condition, other specified personality disorder and unspecified personality disorder.

In the DSM-5, personality disorders are defined as "an enduring pattern of inner experience and behavior that deviates markedly from the expectations of the individual's culture." This definition suggests a chronic course of long-standing, maladaptive coping behaviors with typical onset in adolescence or early adulthood that may persist into later life stages. The diagnosis of a personality disorder in an older adult requires integrating multiple sources of information such as patient information and medical history, self-reported autobiographical history, self-description, collateral from peers, family, supports or other informants, clinical observation of exhibited behaviors, and patterns of coping. Structured interviews or personality questionnaires may also aid in the diagnosis and synthesizing a formulation of personality and behavior patterns.

The diagnosis of a personality disorder can be challenging in the presence of an exacerbation of acute psychiatric symptoms, especially in the setting of limited history or collateral. For example, maladaptive coping behaviors and traits observed in an individual with a mood or anxiety disorder may be symptoms of the mental illness. In this case, further history or resolution of the behaviors or traits with treatment of the underlying mental illness may help clarify the diagnosis. Making a distinction between functional impairments due to psychological or environmental factors associated with aging and impairments resulting from personality pathology may further complicate assessment and diagnosis of a personality disorder.

Borderline personality disorder (BPD) is commonly encountered challenge in primary care and mental health settings with high comorbidity associated with other psychiatric disorders, chronic pain, fibromyalgia, and migraines. In addition, it is associated with worse outcomes in the treatment of other comorbid psychiatric illnesses. The disorder is characterized by interpersonal instability that is not only present in their personal life and support systems but may also play out in the doctor patient relationship through what is commonly referred to as transference and countertransference. Other traits include affective instability, emotional lability, impulsive behavior, identify disturbance, fear of abandonment, and feelings of emptiness or other dissociative symptoms. The etiology is often multifactorial including genetic vulnerability, brain abnormalities, developmental arrests, and experiences early in life especially with respect to trauma, abuse, abandonment, and absence of secure attachments. Remission rates are relatively high compared to other personality disorders; however, relapses can occur. In addition, remission of diagnostic criteria does not necessarily correlate with functional improvement. Up to 80% of patients with BPD exhibit suicidal behavior, and 60% to 70% make suicide attempts. Although this suicidal behavior does not necessarily lead to completed suicide, it remains a significant cause of death in this population. In addition, the severity or potential lethality of suicide attempts may increase or escalate with subsequent attempts or suicidal behaviors. Manualized, structured therapies such as dialectical behavior therapy (DBT), transference-focused psychotherapy, and mentalization-based therapy (MBT) are the mainstays of treatment. While symptom-focused psychopharmacology can be a helpful adjunctive treatment, polypharmacy should be avoided when possible.

Geriatric patients with personality disorders are at greater risk of depression, suicide, cognitive impairment, and social isolation. Developing a treatment plan that addresses the symptoms, behaviors, and associated functional impairments is an essential part of recovery and wellness in this population. There are several approaches to the treatment of personality disorder, and depending on the case, a multifactorial strategy may be warranted, especially in complicated or treatment-resistant cases.

In the evaluation and diagnostic period, the first step is to identify and treat any comorbid primary psychiatric illnesses. This will help clarify the target symptoms and clarify the nature of more long-standing maladaptive behaviors in contrast to symptoms of a mental illness. Common diagnoses or comorbidities to consider in the differential diagnosis include mood or depressive disorders, anxiety disorders, late-onset schizophrenia, delusional disorder, and delirium. Medical comorbidities should also be considered and ruled out. Somatization is a common symptom encountered in personality disorders where physical symptoms and perceptions may be psychologically driven. If somatic symptoms persist even after medical conditions have been ruled out, consideration of an underlying personality disorder, somatization disorder, or other commonly comorbid condition such as fibromyalgia and their respective treatments may be warranted.

Given the chronic and pervasive nature of personality disorders, full remission may be unrealistic, but evidence-based treatments have been characterized that improve the severity of symptoms, decrease impairment, and provide insight. Research in older adults with personality disorders demonstrates that DBT and schema therapy are effective treatment options. Other possible therapies include CBT, interpersonal therapy (ITP), and problem-solving therapy (PST). The efficacy of therapy may be more limited in the setting of significant neurocognitive disorders with associated memory and executive functioning impairments.

Other effective behavioral interventions include the implementation of structure and clear boundaries.

Clinicians can use aspects of the therapeutic treatment frame to set appropriate boundaries and limitations, schedule regular appointments to check in and prevent escalating crisis, and communicate with all providers to unify the treatment strategy and avoid common defenses such as splitting between members of the treatment team. Clear communication, minimizing polypharmacy, and learning how to respond to commonly encountered behaviors further enhances therapeutic rapport and positive treatment outcomes. The use of a behavior contract or treatment agreement is helpful, especially in cases problem behaviors persist despite the aforementioned measures. This is a document drafted in conjunction with the patient where boundaries, expectations, treatment goals, and consequences to nonadherence are agreed upon by the patient and the treatment team. Therapeutic power of a treatment agreement is increased if members of the patient's support system are allowed to read and then subsequently support its content. Signing such a document adds an additional level of clarity to boundary setting and commitment to the treatment.

Some studies also suggest improved outcomes with a combination of therapy and medications, which also speaks to the high rate of comorbidities between personality disorders and other psychiatric illness or diagnoses. When considering pharmacotherapy, strategies should consider targeting specific symptoms or the predominant presenting problems. Classes of medication to consider when targeting individual symptoms include second-generation antipsychotics, mood stabilizers, and serotonergic medications. Naltrexone and clonidine are used in the setting of self-mutilation and the associated impulsivity of this harmful, maladaptive behavior. Similar to treatment of any medical or psychiatric condition in a geriatric patient, safe and effective pharmacotherapy accounts for compliance and risk for noncompliance, abuse potential, pharmacokinetics, pharmacodynamics, interactions with other medications, and effect on other age-specific comorbidities.

SUCCESSFUL AGING

As part of the trend toward ever increasing life expectancy and the unprecedented increase in the proportion of the population which is older, a new focus has been placed on what is now called "successful aging." The concept of "successful aging" stands in stark contrast to the deep-rooted cultural and societal ageistic beliefs, which were discussed above and which affect our patients and how they may be perceived. The definition of "successful aging" and its determinants remains variable. The original model by Rowe and Kahn included three domains: absence of disease and disability, high cognitive and physical functioning, and active engagement with life. This model, however, has been criticized for its overemphasis on health and because it fails to account for many individuals who do not meet the Rowe and Kahn criteria for physical health and yet subjectively rate themselves as aging successfully and report a high degree of satisfaction in later life stages. Newer definitions of "successful aging" have been modified so that they apply to older individuals with and without medical and psychiatric morbidities. Qualitative studies of successful aging indicate that older adults consider the ability to adapt to circumstances and positive attitude toward the future as being more important than an absence of physical disease and disability. Investigations have revealed a paradox of aging: even as the physical health declines, self-rated successful aging and other indicators of psychosocial functioning improve in later life.

Neuroscience research during the past 15 years has demonstrated neuroplasticity of aging—that is, if there is optimal physical, cognitive, and social activity, development of new synapses, dendrites, blood vessels, and even neurons in specific regions such as dentate gyrus of the hippocampus can happen, in older animals and probably in humans. Clinical research supports a model in which positive psychological traits such as resilience, optimism, and social engagement interact with and feed into each individual's evaluation of the degree of well-being, and are a stronger predictor of outcomes such as self-rated successful aging than physical health. Moreover, several of these traits have been shown to have a positive effect on survival that rivals or exceeds that of well-established health risk factors such as smoking, hypertension, obesity, and sedentary lifestyle. One quality that has been reported to increase with age in some, but not all, studies is wisdom, conceptualized as a complex trait associated with advanced cognitive and emotional development, which is experience-driven. Research on wisdom has only recently gained some interest among scientists, although the concept of wisdom dates back to ancient times. Despite variability among the different published definitions of wisdom, there are several common elements, including prosocial attitudes and behaviors (eg, compassion, empathy), social decision making, insight,

decisiveness, acknowledgement of uncertainty, emotional regulation, openness to new experience, spirituality, and sense of humor. What unites these components is their utility for the self (eg, greater well-being) and for others (serving common good).

Successful aging is also seen in some people with serious mental illness. Studies have found that relative to their younger counterparts, middle-aged and older adults with schizophrenia tend to have better psychosocial functioning, including better adherence to medications and self-rated mental health, and lower prevalence of substance use and psychotic relapse. Survivor bias is not the primary explanation for this finding. A minority of older persons with schizophrenia experience sustained remission. Reported predictors of sustained remission include psychosocial support, early initiation of treatment, better premorbid functioning, and having been married.

Mental health and primary care providers have a unique opportunity to help promote "successful aging" by teaching patients and their family members the principles of health, nutrition, and wellness and by facilitating improved quality of life by treating symptoms, improving function, and developing psychosocial interventions. Ongoing studies of "successful aging" are continuing to clarify the definition and are focusing on findings that have clinical utility. Strategies to enhance successful aging include calorie restriction, physical exercise, stopping smoking and substance use, eating the so-called super foods (eg, broccoli, cabbage, cauliflower, spinach, vitamin E, curcumin) rich in antioxidants, and ensuring appropriate health care. Equally important are cognitive and psychological strategies such as developing positive attitudes and resilience, learning new skills, engaging in stimulating activities, and optimizing stress. An important principle to remember is that it is never too early nor too late to start on the path to successful cognitive and emotional aging.

FURTHER READING

Abrams RC, Bromberg CE. Personality disorders in the elderly: a flagging field of inquiry. *Int J Geriatr Psychiatry.* 2006;21:1013–1017.

American Psychiatric Association. *Diagnostic and Statistical Manual of Mental Disorders.* 5th ed. Washington, DC: American Psychiatric Association; 2013.

APA Council on Geriatric Psychiatry. Resource Document on the Use of Antipsychotic Medications to Treat Behavioral Disturbances in Persons with Dementia. Published online March 2014. http://www.psychiatry.org/practice/professional-interests/geriatric-psychiatry/geriatric. Accessed February 22, 2022.

Blazer DG, Wu LT. The epidemiology of substance use and disorders among middle aged and elderly community adults: National Survey on Drug Use and Health (NSDUH). *Am J Geriatr Psychiatry.* 2009;17(3):237–245.

Bostwick M, Rackley S. Addressing suicide in primary care settings. *Curr Psychiatry Rep* 2012;14:353–359.

Conwell Y, Van Orden K, Caine ED. Suicide in older adults. *Psychiatr Clin North Am.* 2011;34(2):451–468.

Granholm E, Holden J, Link PC, et al. Randomized controlled trial of cognitive behavioral social skills training for older consumers with schizophrenia: defeatist performance attitudes and functional outcome. *Am J Geriatr Psychiatry.* 2013;21:251–262.

Holt-Lunstad J, Smith TB, Baker M, Harris T, Stephenson D. Loneliness and social isolation as risk factors for mortality: a meta-analytic review. *Perspect Psychol Sci.* 2015;10(2):227–237.

Hornyak M, Trenkwalder C. Restless legs syndrome and periodic limb movement disorder in the elderly. *J Psychosom Res.* 2004;56(5):543–548.

Jeste DV, Savla GN, Thompson WK, et al. Association between older age and more successful aging: critical role of resilience and depression. *Am J Psychiatry.* 2013;170:188–196.

Jin H, Shih PA, Golshan S, et al. Comparison of longer-term safety and effectiveness of 4 atypical antipsychotics in patients over age 40: a trial using equipoise-stratified randomization. *J Clin Psychiatry.* 2013;74:10–18.

Kotwal AA, Holt-Lunstad J, Newmark RL, et al. Social isolation and loneliness among San Francisco Bay area older adults during the COVID-19 shelter-in-place orders. *J Am Geriatr Soc.* 2021;69(1):20–29.

Krendl AC, Perry BL. The impact of sheltering-in-place during the COVID-19 pandemic on older adults' social and mental well-being. *J Gerontol B Psychol Sci Soc Sci.* 2021;76(2):e53–e58.

Lee EE, Depp C, Palmer BW, et al. High prevalence and adverse health effects of loneliness in community-dwelling adults across the lifespan: role of wisdom as a protective factor. *Int Psychogeriatr* 2019;31(10):1447–1462.

Lenze EJ, Wetherell JL. Anxiety disorders. In: Blazer DG, Steffens DC, eds. *The American Psychiatric Publishing Textbook of Geriatric Psychiatry.* Arlington, VA: American Psychiatric Publishing, Inc; 2009:333–345.

Mohlman J, Bryant C, Lenze EJ, et al. Improving recognition of late life anxiety disorders in *Diagnostic and Statistical Manual of Mental Disorders*, Fifth Edition:

observations and recommendations of the Advisory Committee to the Lifespan Disorders Work Group. *Int J Geriatr Psychiatry.* 2012;27(6):549–556.

National Institute on Alcohol Abuse and Alcoholism. Alcohol and Aging. http://niaaa.nih.gov. Accessed February 22, 2022.

Neikrug A, Ancoli-Israel S. Sleep disorders in the older adult—a mini-review. *Gerontology.* 2010;56(2):181–189.

Norman D, Loredo JS. Obstructive sleep apnea in older adults. *Clin Geriatr Med.* 2008;24(1):151–165.

Okolie C, Dennis M, Simon Thomas E, John A. A systematic review of interventions to prevent suicidal behaviors and reduce suicidal ideation in older people. *Int Psychogeriatr.* 2017;29(11):1801–1824.

Penders KA, Peeters IG, Metsemakers JF, Van Alphen SP. Personality disorders in older adults: a review of epidemiology, assessment, and treatment. *Curr Psychiatry Rep.* 2020;22(3):1–14.

Stanley B, Brown G. Safety Plan Treatment Manual to Reduce Suicide Risk: Veteran Version. 2008. http://www.mentalhealth.va.gov/mentalhealth/suicide_prevention. Accessed February 22, 2022.

Uchida H, Mamo DC, Mulsant BH, et al. Increased antipsychotic sensitivity in elderly patients: evidence and mechanisms. *J Clin Psychiatry.* 2009;70(3):397–405.

Wenneberg AM, Canham SL, Smith MT, et al. Optimizing sleep in older adults: treating insomnia. *Maturitas.* 2013;76(3):247–252.

Woo BK, Daly JW, Allen EC, et al. Unrecognized medical disorders in older psychiatric inpatients in a senior behavioral health unit in a university hospital. *J Geriatr Psychiatry Neurol.* 2003;16(2):121–125.

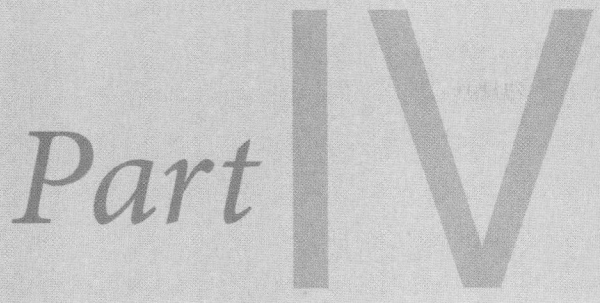

Part IV

Principles of Palliative Medicine and Ethics

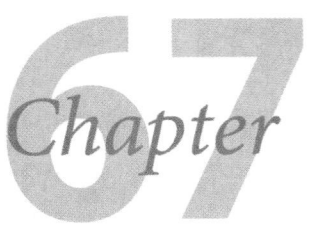

Chapter 67

Palliative Care and Special Management Issues

Paul Tatum, Shannon Devlin, Shaida Talebreza, Jeanette S. Ross, Eric Widera

INTRODUCTION

Palliative medicine is an essential skill set for health care professionals caring for older adults. Supporting the needs and goals of older adults as they age is a complex process that often involves balancing: goals of life prolongation, functional status preservation and restoration, risk and harm mitigation, and symptom relief. Palliative care aims to ensure that these goals match the individualized care plans through interprofessional care and careful communication and goal setting.

Palliative care for older adults poses distinct challenges. For older patients with diminished reserve to respond to stressors, the potential for harm of interventions can be substantially greater than younger populations. Cognitive impairment may limit the participation of patients at times when the most difficult decisions need to be made. The interaction of multiple illnesses in multimorbidity may reduce the potential benefit of interventions, which are otherwise therapeutic in single disease state.

DEFINING PALLIATIVE CARE

Palliative care aims to improve the quality of life for both the patient with serious illness and the family. Palliative care focuses on providing patients with relief from the symptoms, pain, and stress of a serious illness. It is appropriate for any type of diagnosis, any stage of a serious illness, and importantly, can be provided together with curative treatment.

Specialty palliative care consists of care by an interprofessional team of physicians, nurses, and social workers, chaplains and other individuals with expertise in palliative medicine, who work with patients' other health care professionals to provide care that matches patients' goals. In addition to palliative care specialists, the core principles of palliative care can be implemented by all health care professionals (often described as *primary palliative care*). The key components of primary palliative care include symptom management, coordination of care, communication about goals of care and advance care planning (ACP), caregiver support, and when needed, referral to specialist palliative care teams.

Hospice Care

Hospice care is a specialized form of palliative care for patients with limited life expectancy. Hospice care provides

Learning Objectives

- Identify the palliative needs of an aging population and recognize the potential benefits palliative care delivers in collaboration with or as part of geriatric medicine practice.

- Describe the unique palliative care needs of older adults including patients with dementia, frailty, or multimorbidity, as well as diverse populations.

- Distinguish the various advance care planning (ACP) formats and tools and adapt a three-step process to prognostication in older adults as part of ACP.

Key Clinical Points

1. Multiple randomized trials show palliative care improves outcomes including quality of life, satisfaction with care, reduced family distress, and increased hospice utilization.

2. For older adults with multiple chronic illness, a five-step approach to palliative care includes the following:
   a. Determine patient preferences.
   b. Interpret the evidence for treatment with recognition of the limitations applying it to an older adult population.
   c. Let prognosis frame clinical management decisions.
   d. Consider treatment complexity and feasibility as part of management decisions.
   e. Optimize therapies and care plans.

medical, psychosocial, and spiritual support to the patient. Hospice also supports family members coping with the complex consequences of illness, disability, and functional decline as death nears and includes bereavement support after death of the patient. Hospice care does not aim to shorten or prolong life, but rather provides comfort and support services to help people live out the time they have remaining to the fullest extent possible.

The Medicare hospice benefit employs an interdisciplinary team of professionals including doctors, nurses,

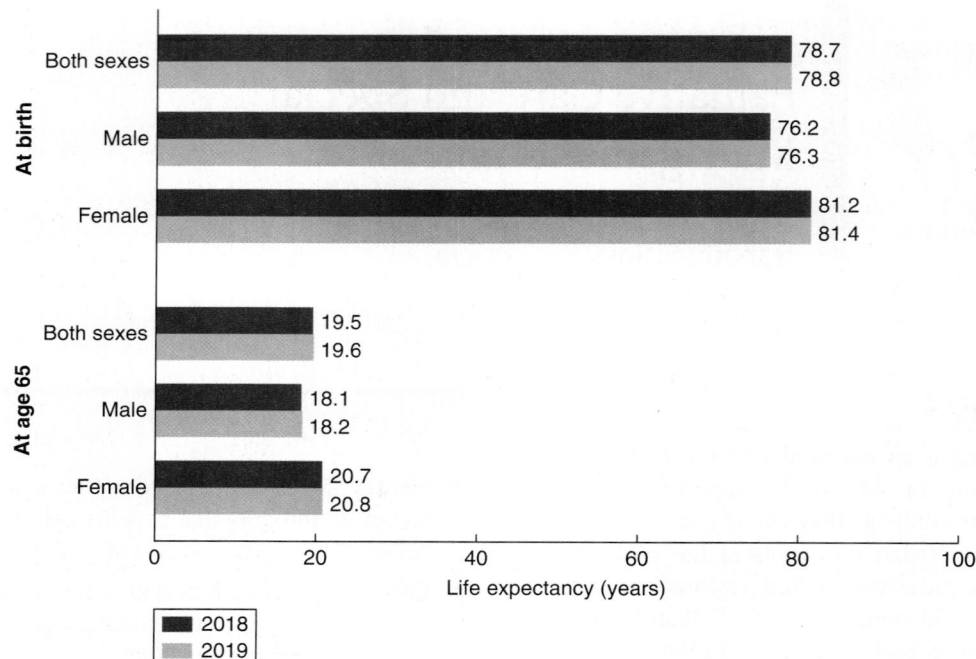

FIGURE 67-1. Life expectancy at birth and age 65, by sex: United States, 2018 and 2019. (Data from National Center for Health Statistics, National Vital Statistics System, Mortality.)

aides, social workers, and spiritual care coordinators to address the patient's physical, emotional, social, and spiritual needs. Under the Medicare hospice benefit, a patient is eligible for hospice care when the patient's attending physician and the hospice medical director certify that she or he is terminally ill with an expected prognosis of less than 6 months "if the disease runs its usual and expected course." The Centers for Medicare and Medicaid Services (CMS) has guidelines entitled local coverage determinations (LCDs) to help physicians determine a prognosis of 6 months or less. These LCDs are available on the CMS website and are *guidelines* to help determine prognosis, they *are not rules or requirements* for hospice admission. Once a patient is admitted, the hospice agency is required to provide services that are reasonable and necessary for the palliation and management of a patient's terminal illness and related conditions, including doctor and nursing visits, hospice aide and counseling services, medications, medical equipment and supplies, and short-term respite and inpatient stays to manage pain and symptoms.

PALLIATIVE CARE NEEDS OF AN AGING POPULATION

Health care in the United States has made tremendous advances which have allowed for an aging population. The typical death has been transformed from the nineteenth-century picture of an acute illness over a short time from infectious disease into a process of decline over years with increasing morbidity and functional dependency from chronic disease. The average age at the time of death in the United States per 2019 data is now 79 (81 years for females and 73 for males) and survivors to age 65 live on average another 20 years (**Figure 67-1**).

While chronic illness of older adults is increasingly complicated by multiple illnesses, in 2018 two major diseases, heart disease and cancer, still accounted for nearly half of all 2018 deaths. Apart from acute respiratory illness, accidents, and suicide, the majority of deaths of older adults are associated with a period of chronic disease. In 2018, two-thirds of people aged 65 and older had multiple chronic conditions per the Centers for Disease Control and Prevention (CDC).

The exponential increase in COVID-19 illness in the United States has led to a significant number of cases and mortality particularly in older adults in 2020 to 2021, becoming deadlier than heart disease and cancer. COVID-19's impact on older adults perfectly demonstrates the unique needs of the older adult population. Geriatric palliative care during the COVID-19 pandemic and future pandemics can work within systems to balance potentially burdensome interventions with complex goals and to deal with the common sequela of decline in performance status after infectious illness.

As the patient's number of comorbid conditions rises, the complexities of delivering care have had profound consequences. Patients with multimorbidity are at increased risk of disability and institutionalization, poorer quality of life, and higher risk of harm from medical treatments. Over time, the care that these patients get often becomes more fragmented. Among Medicare fee-for-service decedents in 2015, deaths in the home or community setting occurred in 40% and a change in the setting of care in the last 3 days of life occurred among 10% of decedents.

THE BENEFIT FOR PALLIATIVE MEDICINE

Palliative medicine is now well established as a discipline, and as the field matures, there is a growing body of literature showing its benefit.

The Evidence for Palliative Care Systems

The evidence for specialist palliative care interventions includes multiple randomized trials showing palliative care improves outcomes including quality of life, satisfaction with care, reduced family distress, and increased hospice utilization. The landmark Temel study demonstrated the value of concurrent care, that is, palliative care delivered early and simultaneously with curative, disease-focused care in advanced lung cancer patients. Early palliative care for newly diagnosed metastatic lung cell cancer patients was associated with higher quality of life, less depression, and a statistically significant longer median survival (12 months vs 8.9 months). Subsequent, larger cluster randomized trial of advance cancer patients with good performance status representing a wide variety of cancer types demonstrated improved quality of life with early palliative care. Notably, the statistical significance in many outcomes was not achieved until the fourth month of palliative care, emphasizing the importance of early referral to palliative care to impact quality of life measures beyond pain control. The ENABLE III study showed that initiating concurrent palliative care at the time of a cancer diagnosis had a significant impact on 1-year survival compared to initiating palliative care 3 months after initial cancer diagnosis (63% early vs 48% delayed) and involved multiple types of cancer not only lung cancer.

Extensive evidence is accumulating for palliative care delivery for noncancer diagnosis as well. A 2020 meta-analysis of 28 trials of palliative care in noncancer patients (13,664 patients, mean age 74) including patients with heart failure (10 studies), dementia (4 studies), chronic obstructive lung disease (3 studies), and multimorbidity (11 studies) showed that palliative care is associated with less emergency department use, less hospitalization, and lower symptom burden. Trials to date of palliative care have been least promising in dementia and highlight opportunities to better tailor palliative care to the special needs of persons living with dementia.

The Evidence for Hospice

Hospice has been shown in numerous studies to improve symptom control, increase patient satisfaction and quality of life, and help patients and families prepare for death. The highest-quality outcomes tend to occur for patients who were enrolled in hospice care for longer than 30 days. Since 2014 the CMS has collected quality data via the Hospice Item Set, which has seven key domains of patient quality.

A major benefit of hospice over usual care is that hospice allows patients to die in their own place of residence when that is the patient's wishes. Hospice care adds value by delivering high-quality care while reducing Medicare costs primarily through caring for patients in the home setting. Cost savings increase with greater time spent in hospice care. The maximum reduction in expenditures tends to occur when the hospice length of stay exceeded 50 days.

A specific concern of geriatricians and policy makers is whether hospice adds benefits for patients with dementia in long-term care. Nursing home residents with dementia and cancer who received hospice care in the last 30 days of life were less likely to die in a hospital than those who did not receive hospice, and hospice enrollment increases the likelihood that patients with dementia who have pain receive an opioid.

PALLIATIVE CARE IN SPECIAL POPULATIONS

Palliative care and geriatrics are both designed to serve the needs of the most vulnerable patients with a "common central philosophy of patient-centered commitment to holistic and humane care." Due to the growing geriatric population, there is an unprecedented need to provide excellent palliative care to older adults, especially those with dementia, frailty, and multimorbidity. Partnerships between geriatricians and palliative medicine specialists can be especially useful for management of patients with these conditions, with each specialty working together to ensure the highest level of evidenced-based compassionate care to older adults.

Dementia

Older adults with dementia have unique palliative medicine needs given the progressive nature of their illness with significant, prolonged disability and predictable increases in symptom burden as dementia advances. This population especially benefits from combined geriatric and palliative medicine approaches.

It is imperative that health care professionals provide appropriate management of behavioral and psychological symptoms of dementia. As discussed in detail in the management of agitation in Chapter 60, management should involve (1) identifying the specific problem behavior and its severity, (2) identifying potential triggers for the behavior, (3) removing underlying physiologic and environmental triggers whenever possible, (4) attempting nonpharmacologic interventions to improve behavior, and (5) as a final resort, using recommended targeted pharmacotherapy for behaviors that do not respond to attempts of nonpharmacologic management in situations that risk patient or caregiver safety. As part of the American Board of Internal Medicine (ABIM) "Choosing Wisely" initiative, the American Geriatrics Society (AGS) recommends against the use of antipsychotics as first-line treatment for behavioral and psychological symptoms of dementia. Notably, a cluster randomized trial of nursing home patients with behavioral problems using an empiric stepwise protocol to treat pain resulted in a decrease in the number of symptoms. Most patients were treated with the first step of the protocol, acetaminophen. Opioids may be tried for nonresponders. The Pain Assessment in Advanced Dementia (PAINAD) Scale may be a useful tool in this situation.

In advanced stages of dementia, weight loss and dysphagia are common with the latter putting patients at risk for aspiration pneumonia. Weight loss may be secondary to decreased appetite, depression, oral problems such as ulcers or ill-fitting dentures, increased wandering, or medication side effects. A reversible etiology for weight loss is not always present. The addition of nutritional supplements or appetite stimulants has not been shown to improve clinically important outcomes. For patients with dysphagia, several organizations, in the ABIM "Choosing Wisely" initiative, recommend *against percutaneous feeding tubes* and recommend *in favor of offering oral assisted feeding.* Studies have shown that feeding tubes in advanced dementia do not increase survival or quality of life, prevent aspiration pneumonia, or improve pressure ulcer healing or nutritional parameters (weight, albumin). In fact, feeding tube usage has been associated with the development of pressure ulcers and the use of pharmacologic and physical restraints. The majority of feeding tubes in patients with advanced dementia are inserted during an acute hospitalization.

Infections, specifically urinary tract infections and pneumonia, are frequently diagnosed in advanced dementia and commonly occur as patients near end of life. In nursing home residents with advanced dementia, observational data show suspected urinary tract infections rarely meet criteria for antibiotics; however, the majority are treated with them. Findings from a prospective cohort study suggest that the treatment of suspected urinary tract infections in this population does not prolong survival. Antibiotic therapy for aspiration pneumonia in advanced dementia has been associated with improved survival but not improved comfort. For aspiration pneumonia, the most aggressive treatment approaches with intravenous therapy and hospitalization have been associated with the greatest discomfort, and the survival benefit associated with antibiotic therapy was similar regardless of administration route. Interventions such as opioids, fans, and acetaminophen can increase comfort. In addition to using the minimal clinical criteria for the initiation of antibiotics, appropriate management of infections in advanced dementia requires an attention to a patient's primary goals (ie, life prolongation, comfort, safety) in order to avoid unnecessary or unwanted treatment burden.

Health care professionals caring for older adults with dementia should engage patients and their families in ACP early and include an assessment of understanding of diagnosis, prognosis, and disease trajectory. The hope is to align treatment preferences with patient values and decrease stress on future caregivers. ACP discussions may result in completion of an advance directive document in which the patient-specifies preferences for future care and/or designates an authorized surrogate decision maker to communicate their preferences in circumstances when they no longer possess medical decision-making capacity (see more details in Chapters 7 and 10). Dementia-specific advance directive documents are now available given dementia's distinct clinical course. While barriers to these conversations exist such as difficulty with prognostication, lack of decision-making capacity, and patient or family reluctance to engage, both geriatricians and palliative medicine specialists are well equipped to conduct these vital discussions. Online resources are available for assistance (**Table 67-1**).

ACP discussions with surrogate decision makers should continue as dementia progresses. Older adults with advanced dementia living in nursing homes who have proxies with an understanding of their terminal prognosis are less likely to receive burdensome interventions. Consideration for hospice care in end-stage dementia is also important as enrollment is associated with greater satisfaction in patient care. Determining a 6-month prognosis in advanced dementia can be challenging. Factors such as irreversible weight loss, low body mass index, functional dependence, and advanced age are associated with limited prognosis. Palliative medicine specialists can also help with prognostication.

Frailty

While the exact definition of frailty remains a subject of debate (see Chapter 42), frail patients are particularly vulnerable to adverse outcomes and have significant palliative care needs. For instance, severely frail older adults have shown poor response to treatment and may not benefit from intensive rehabilitation efforts. Attempting rehabilitation of the most frail may in fact cause harm. The key to

TABLE 67-1 ■ RESOURCES AVAILABLE FOR DEMENTIA-SPECIFIC ADVANCE CARE PLANNING
Dementia-Specific Advance Directive
https://dementia-directive.org
Communication Tools
https://www.capc.org/training/best-practices-in-dementia-care-and-caregiver-support/
For Caregivers and Surrogate Decision Makers
https://theconversationproject.org/wp-content/uploads/2020/12/DementiaGuide.pdf
https://www.alz.org
https://www.caregiver.org

managing the palliative needs of frailty is determining goals and recognizing the patient with poor potential to improve. When in doubt, a therapeutic trial of improving performance status is always appropriate, but if not achieved should prompt a repeat discussion of goals and prognosis.

Determining the severity of frailty and the potential for reversibility can help clinicians recommend appropriate treatment. Frailty definitions, staging, and recommended treatment options for each stage are described in **Table 67-2**.

Patients with frailty and multimorbidity may still be eligible for hospice even if they do not have a single terminal illness. While CMS has stated that frailty, debility, or adult failure to thrive are not accepted as the principal hospice diagnosis reported on the Medicare hospice claims form, this does not mean that frail patients are not eligible for the Medicare hospice benefit. A patient is considered hospice eligible if the attending physician and hospice medical director have certified the patient to be terminally ill with a prognosis of less than 6 months. This prognosis is determined based on the severity and irreversibility of the patient's frailty as well as their multimorbidity. The hospice Medical Director could utilize the hospice LCDs available on the CMS website to support their determination that the patient has a prognosis of less than 6 months.

Multimorbidity

Providing optimal care for older adults with multiple chronic conditions, or multimorbidity, presents one of the greatest challenges in geriatrics. Patients with multimorbidity have increased use of health care resources, poorer quality of life, higher rates of institutionalization, disability, and death. To address the challenge of providing patient-centered care to older adults with multimorbidity, a stepwise approach can integrate patient care with the key principles of geriatric and palliative medicine in five domains: (1) patient preferences, (2) interpreting the evidence, (3) prognosis, (4) clinical feasibility, and (5) optimizing therapies and care plans. The American Geriatrics Society's "Patient-Centered Care for Older Adults with Multiple Chronic Conditions: A Stepwise Approach: Expert Panel on the Care of Older Adults with Multimorbidity" is an excellent online resource: https://geriatricscareonline.org/ProductAbstract/Framework-for-Decision-making-for-Older-Adults/CL026 [geriatricscareonline.org].

Considerations for Providing Inclusive Care

The US population is ethnically diverse and there may be differences on perceptions and readiness for palliative care based on race and socioeconomic factors. Ornstein's 2020

TABLE 67-2 ■ A CLINICAL MANAGEMENT APPROACH TO FRAILTY

STAGE	CLINICAL	MANAGEMENT
Latent stage or "pre-frail" (1-2 frailty criteria met)	Not clinically apparent in the absence of stressors	Likely most responsive to **prevention**: • Minimize and/or treat precipitants. • Prevent and minimize immobility, and maintain physical activity. • Maintain muscle mass and strength through resistance exercises; this can be supplemented by aerobic and balance training. • Prevent nutritional inadequacy (including vitamin D deficiency). • Treat depression. • Reduce polypharmacy.
Early stage or "frail" (3 frailty criteria met)	Clinically apparent; earliest presentations tend to be weakness, slowed walking speed, and/or decreased physical activity	Likely most responsive to **intervention**: • Implement preventive measures (as above). • Encourage resistance and strength exercise. Evidence is substantial that resistance or strengthening exercise is effective in increasing muscle mass, strength, and walking speed in frail older adults. Other forms of exercise, including stretching, Tai chi, and aerobic exercise, are also helpful. • Prevent nutritional inadequacy; nutritional supplementation appears to be effective only when added to resistance exercise. • Offer "prehabilitation" before surgery.
End-stage or "severe frailty" (4-5 frailty criteria met and low cholestrol and albumin levels)	Severely frail older adults appear to be in an **irreversible**, pre-death phase with high mortality over 6-12 months; associated with high short-term mortality rates and suggest a poor response to treatment	Consider **palliative** approaches for these patients: • Focus on optimizing abilities needed to reach individual patient goals. • Compensate for diminished abilities by modification of living environment and/or increased support from caregivers.

Reproduced with permission of American Geriatrics Society. American Geriatrics Society and Talebreza S, ed. Frailty. In Geriatrics Evaluation & Management Tools. New York: American Geriatrics Society; 2021.

analysis of racial disparities in the use of hospice and end of life treatments found that Black individuals were significantly less likely to use hospice and more likely to have multiple emergency department visits and hospitalizations and undergo intensive treatment in the last 6 months of life compared with White individuals regardless of cause of death. Barzargan examined the awareness of palliative, hospice care and advance directives in a large sample of an ethnically diverse population. Hispanic and non-Hispanic Black participants are far less likely to report that they have heard about palliative and hospice care and advance directives than their non-Hispanic White counterparts. In this study, 75%, 74%, and 49% of Hispanics, non-Hispanic Blacks, and non-Hispanic White participants, respectively, claimed that they had never heard about palliative care.

Patients who are unable to speak the language of the care team are at risk of receiving care that may not match their wishes. Use of family members as interpreters risks information being withheld or incomplete translation. A trained medical interpreter at bedside or a telephone translator service is recommended.

The National Academy of Medicine (NAM) report on health care disparities and unequal treatment determined that patients' attitudes toward health care and treatment preferences were not the major source of disparities. At the level of clinical encounter, factors that lead to disparities include bias or prejudice, stereotypes (beliefs held by the provider about the behavior or health of minorities), and uncertainty about preferences. The key systems factors in disparities per the NAM study were factors such as cultural and linguistic barriers, fragmentation of health care systems, and the types of incentives in place.

While all persons with serious illness endure difficulties, those patients who are lesbian, gay, bisexual, and transgender/transsexual (LGBT) may face unique issues distinct from the heterosexual population. LGBT older adults have a history of having experienced stigmatization, discrimination, victimization, or violence during their lifespan by their families, school, workplaces, and even health care providers. LGBT persons may present at more advanced stages of illness because they are more reluctant to seek health care, or they lack health insurance. LGBT persons may need to rely on close friends rather than on family for caregiving. Nonfamily caregiving may be due to estrangement from the person's biological family or because LGBT persons are less likely to have children. Informal communities of support are also known as "lavender families" or "families of choice" and should be respected and included as family as identified by patients. The support from the "lavender family" may become essential in caring for an LGBT individual at the end of life. It may be challenging for LGBT persons who need custodial care to find a long-term care facility that is "LGBT friendly." LGBT patients may hide their sexual identities to be able to access a long-term care facility also known as "going back in the closet."

Transgender patients may face several unique stressors. Having a gender-variant body and requiring assistance for basic needs of daily living like bathing, dressing, or feeding puts the transgender individual in a vulnerable position and at risk of being physically abused.

It is of extreme importance that the LGBT person takes steps to legally document their preferences for health care and other legal matters. Individuals that may be closer to the LGBT person may not be identified as the default surrogate by law should the LGBT person no be able to make his or her own decision; and it is possible that the default decision maker may not be respectful of the individual's chosen gender identity.

LGBT patients should designate a Health Care Power of Attorney (HCPOA) and additionally explicitly give that person the power to direct health care professionals with the preferences of name, pronoun of choice, and appearance consistent with their gender identity. Given that the HCPOA and advance directives are no longer effective as soon as the person dies, it is important for LGBT persons to also put in place a Disposition of Bodily Human Remains (DBHR) document so that he or she can name who is the person to have authority over the remains of a person once deceased. For example, a same-sex partner who had HCPOA would not be able to claim the deceased body of his or her loved one unless he or she had been designated to do so in a DBHR document.

LGBT persons also may face challenges during the bereavement process, particularly if in the case of a same-sex relationship, the couple had not been openly acknowledged. The surviving individual may experience "silent mourning" and not have access to traditional grief support. **Table 67-3** offers open-ended inclusive questions to use to better understand patients' needs and to interact with them in a way that is aligned with their values and identity.

PROGNOSTICATION IN OLDER ADULTS

Prognostication is a vital aspect of decision making as it provides patients and families with information to determine realistic and achievable goals of care, is used in determining eligibility for benefits such as hospice, and helps in targeting interventions to those likely to live long enough to benefit from a proposed intervention. For example, it may take many years for the benefits to accrue for preventative interventions such as cancer screening and tight glycemic control. For frail older adults whose life expectancy is less than this time horizon to benefit, they are exposed to potential immediate harms of these preventative interventions without the possibility of receiving the benefits.

Prognostication can be broken into three general steps: (1) estimating the probability of an individual developing a particular outcome over a specific period of time, (2) the act of communicating the prognosis with the patient and/or family, and (3) the interpretation of the prognosis by the patient and/or family.

TABLE 67-3 ■ GETTING TO KNOW THE PATIENT IN AN INCLUSIVE WAY

QUESTION	RELEVANCE
What name do you use? How would you like me to address you?	• A person may have a legal name but may have a name of their choice they like to go by that may be different. • Listening to the patient pronounce their name gives you an opportunity to learn the pronunciation if it is a name you are not familiar with pronouncing.
What gender pronouns do you use?	• It can be awkward to ask a person their pronouns, and a way to achieve this is by introducing yourself and the pronouns you use. "My name is … and the pronouns I use are… [she/her, he/him, they/them]. What pronouns do you use?" • You don't have to assume based on the appearance of the person or their name what pronouns are preferred. • The person may not want to correct you.
To whom do you turn for support? Who are those you consider close to you that are either your family of origin or choice?	• Some persons may be estranged from the biological family and have informal communities of support. • Some patients may not be open about their sexual identity and may identify a significant other as a friend. • Asking broadly gives you the opportunity to gather information on who is important to the patient. • After a person dies, those important to the patient, whether they are the family of origin or choice or both, will benefit from bereavement care.
Do you have any groups or organizations that you belong to that are important to you?	• When asked broadly, this opens the opportunity for the patient to share what groups or organizations are meaningful to them. • The answers may be diverse and may include religious affiliation or groups like the Veterans of Foreign Wars (VFW) or the AA (Alcoholics Anonymous).
I'd like to learn about the things that give you meaning or strength. In times when you face challenges, what are some ways you cope and find strength?	• A question like this gives an opportunity for a wide range of answers to assess the spiritual or religious beliefs or existential concerns.
If you are unable to make your own decisions, who would make decisions for you? Have you formally named a medical decision maker?	• Do not assume that because a person refers to someone as their spouse that they are legally married. This is particularly relevant for unmarried LGBT couples, who may need to specify their preference in a formal document because the person the patient may choose may not be in the traditional surrogacy ranking. • Ask not only who their legal decision maker is (eg, the person they have appointed to serve as their durable power of attorney for health care or health care proxy) but also about who they would have included—and excluded—from discussions surrounding decisions about their care.

Step 1: Estimating Prognosis

Estimating prognosis in geriatric populations is more complicated than in younger populations, as older adults are more likely to have more than one chronic progressive illness that impacts life expectancy. Estimation of prognosis in multimorbid older adults requires clinicians to account for interaction of their medical problems, clinical and laboratory findings, and functional and cognitive status. While prognostication based on clinician judgment is correlated with actual survival, it is subject to numerous biases, most importantly that clinicians tend to overestimate patient survival by a factor of 3 to 5. Prognostic indices that incorporate age and clinical characteristics such as multimorbidity and functional status may improve the accuracy of prognostication compared to clinician judgment alone. A helpful repository of published geriatric prognostic indices can be found at www.ePrognosis.org.

Step 2: Communicating Prognosis

Numerous studies have shown that most individuals and their families want prognostic information, yet they are often not given the opportunity to discuss it with health care providers. This is despite evidence that effective communication around end-of-life issues can provide benefits to patients and families, without worsening of anxiety, hopelessness, or depression.

When delivering prognosis, it is first helpful to ask about the patient's understanding of their illness and perception of what the future may have in store for them. It is also helpful to assess the readiness of the patient and/or family member to have a discussion of prognosis by asking them permission to talk about it. Based on this information, the clinician should deliver prognostic information tailored to the patient's current desire and level of understanding.

When delivering prognostic estimates, clinicians should acknowledge the inherent uncertainty in most prognostic estimates. One way to do so is by giving ranges in prognostic estimates (ie, days to weeks, weeks to months, months to years to live) or by giving the best case, worst case, and most common scenarios. In addition, delivering information on prognosis is likely to bring emotional reactions in patients and their family members. Use of empathic statements, including naming the emotion, and the use of therapeutic silence can be helpful in supporting patients and their surrogate decision makers.

Step 3: Interpreting Prognosis

Patients' and surrogates' personal estimates of prognosis are often different, and generally more optimistic than what is communicated to them by health care providers. Furthermore, few surrogates solely rely on prognostication information delivered by physicians to determine their own prognostic estimates. Rather, their interpretation of prognosis is influenced by many factors, including perceptions of the patient's strength, will to live, unique history, individual observations of physical appearance, and the surrogate's presence, optimism, intuition, and faith. Given this information, it is helpful when delivering prognosis to include the factors that influence the clinician's prognostic estimate, as it may also influence the patient's or surrogate's interpretation of prognosis. It is also valuable to enquire how the clinician's prognostic estimate influenced how the patient or surrogate is currently thinking about the prognosis.

ADVANCE CARE PLANNING AND ADVANCE DIRECTIVES

ACP is a process that supports adults at any age or stage of health in understanding and sharing their personal values, life goals, and preferences regarding future medical care. ACP should be ongoing as the values or priorities of people may change as they go through life and should include continued support and preparation for future medical decision making. The focus of ACP is on meaningful conversations in order to create a care plan that aligns recommended treatments with patient preferences. There is evidence that ACP increases patient and surrogate satisfaction with both communication and medical care and decreases surrogate distress. ACP does not increase anxiety or lead to loss of hope. To effectively deliver ACP, health disparities, systemic racism, and cultural differences need to be addressed. These conversations are appropriate at any time in an older adult's life, but clinicians should especially consider initiating goals of care discussions if they answer "no" to the question "Would you be surprised if this patient dies in the next year?" Documentation of these discussions may include advance directives or physician orders further described in **Table 67-4**. **Advance directives** are written documents that state a patient's preferences for addressing *future* medical decisions. Advance directives can be

TABLE 67-4 ■ ADVANCE DIRECTIVES AND PHYSICIAN ORDERS

ADVANCE DIRECTIVES (FUTURE CARE)

Durable Power of Attorney for Health Care (DPOA-HC) or Health Care Proxy

1. Allows a patient to designate a person to make health care decisions on behalf of the patient should they lose decision-making capacity
2. Does not specify wishes for medical care
3. Ideal proxy is someone who the patient knows well, is a competent adult, and is willing/able to assist in health care decision making respecting the preferences of the patient should the need arise
4. Particularly important when the patient is estranged from their family or if the patient wants to name a friend who would not be in the hierarchy of surrogate decision makers

Living Will

1. Allows a patient to specify in writing wishes for future medical care in the hypothetical situation where they lose decision-making capacity
2. Difficult to cover all future possibilities making the health care proxy choice important

PHYSICIAN ORDERS (CURRENT CARE)

Physician Orders for Life-Sustaining Treatment (POLST)

1. Standing medical order specifying decisions regarding *current* medical care for patients with progressive chronic illnesses
2. Translates patient preferences for resuscitative efforts, artificial nutrition, and other life-sustaining treatment measures into an effective state-authorized medical order
3. Order accompanies patients in different settings (home, hospital, nursing home)

executed at any time by a competent adult person and go into effect when the person is no longer capable of making health care decisions.

Priorities in ACP discussions vary depending on the setting. In a *relatively healthy* person, the focus may be on making goals of care choices based on hypothetical situations or choosing a health care proxy. If a health care proxy is not chosen, the surrogate decision maker authorized to make health care decisions for an incapacitated patient is based on a hierarchy of closeness to the patient (eg, spouse, adult children, parents, etc), which may vary based on the state. In someone with a *predictable progressive condition* who is likely to lose functional or cognitive abilities, such as ALS or dementia, the conversation should include information on treatment options with significant long-term impact, such as tracheostomy or hemodialysis, as well as prognosis. In *a seriously ill* person, the choices are less hypothetical and an actual decision regarding treatment may be needed. In this circumstance, it is important to inform patients (or their proxies) of the risks, benefits, and alternative treatments available. Consideration should also be given to deactivating devices such as implantable cardioverter-defibrillators in patients close to death.

ACP is complex, and communication techniques differ based on the clinical situation. Chapter 71 expands on useful communication strategies. The Gerontological Society of America also has resources available to assist clinicians with communication with patients with cognitive and sensory impairments. A variety of resources to improve communication effectiveness in ACP are available online and include vitaltalk.org and capc.org. ICARE, a communication model used within the Veterans Health Administration, is provided as an example of discussing "Do not resuscitate orders" in **Table 67-5**. When having conversations about cardiopulmonary resuscitation (CPR), it is important to discuss the likelihood of this intervention meeting a patient's goals. A recommendation for or against CPR may differ, for example, for a patient who prioritizes maintaining independence and one who prioritizes living as long as possible. In adults older than 65 years, 17% of patients who undergo in hospital CPR survive to hospital discharge and 7% are discharged home. The presence of serious conditions such as metastatic cancer, sepsis, or multiple organ failure are associated with worse CPR outcomes.

In 2020 as the COVID-19 pandemic spread throughout the world, ACP required immediate attention and innovation. For older adults at high risk for serious disease, readdressing care plans and eliciting preferences specifically pertinent to COVID-19, such as hospitalization, intubation, and CPR, were urgently needed. Telehealth increased and remains a powerful tool for patient outreach. When using telemedicine for ACP, it is important to create a welcoming environment with the electronic device situated at eye level with adequate sound to promote patient engagement, to invite patients to include those they would want involved in the discussion, to provide an overview of a telehealth visit, and to monitor for nonverbal and environmental cues. Sending an electronic summary of the visit can also be helpful.

Addressing Spiritual Needs

Comprehensive palliative care attends to the whole needs of the patient. The founder of modern palliative care, Dr. Cicely Saunders, coined the term Total Pain, meaning that palliative care attended to the pain that was physical, psychological, social, and spiritual. An international consensus project defines spirituality as "a dynamic and intrinsic aspect of humanity through which persons seek ultimate meaning, purpose, and transcendence, and experience relationship to self, family, others, community, society, nature, and the significant or sacred. Spirituality is expressed through beliefs, values, traditions, and practices."

While patients with serious illness wish to have spiritual needs addressed as part of their care, most physicians report discomfort doing so. Screening for spiritual needs allows for referral for support, which can be in the form of pastoral support of a health care team or within the patient's own spiritual support network. A screening tool that has been well validated is FICA Spiritual History Tool. FICA asks questions about Faith, Importance, Community, and how to Address these issues. Additional questions for communication within the FICA framework can be found at https://smhs.gwu.edu/spirituality-health/.

TABLE 67-5 ■ ICARE GOALS OF CARE FOR CODE STATUS

Introduction	Orient patient or surrogate to the conversation	It is really important for us to honor our patient's choices. I'd like to spend a little time learning about things that are important to you and about the kind of medical treatments you would and would not want in an emergency. Does this sound OK to you?
Care goals	Patient's goals are the foundation of your recommendation	What matters most to you? What does a good day look like for you? As you think about your medical care, are there any medical treatments or procedures that aren't acceptable to you?
Alignment	Repeat what the patient said to ensure you got it right	As I listen, it sounds like what's most important to you is … [reflect back the patient's stated care goals].
Recommendation	Ask permission and make a recommendation aligned with the patient's goals	**If the outcomes of CPR do not align with the patient's goals:** Would it be OK if I offered a recommendation? Given what you have told me is most important, I'm concerned CPR won't help you live the life you want [repeat patient's goals]. For these reasons, I recommend we allow for a natural death instead of attempting CPR. **If the outcomes of CPR align with the patient's goals:** Would it be OK if I offered a recommendation? Given what you have told me is most important, it sounds like you would want to pursue any treatment that would give you a chance of living longer, even if that means your life might be supported by machines. For these reasons, I recommend we attempt CPR.
Exploration	Explore further if decision regarding code status seems inconsistent with stated goals	I worry that CPR won't help you reach your goals. Can you tell me more about what you are hoping for with CPR? Is there a situation you could imagine when you wouldn't want CPR?

CONCLUSION

An essential component of geriatric medicine is the routine delivery of effective primary palliative care that includes attention to symptom management, prognostication, communication, ACP, and individualized care plans. Appropriate referrals to specialty-level palliative care should also be considered when palliative needs are great, given the increasingly robust evidence base of benefit for both palliative care and hospice.

FURTHER READING

Acquaviva, KD. *LGBTQ-Inclusive Hospice and Palliative Care: A Practical Guide to Transforming Professional Practice.* New York, NY: Harrington Park Press; 2017.

American Geriatrics Society Expert Panel on the Care of Older Adults with Multimorbidity. Patient-centered care for older adults with multiple chronic conditions: a stepwise approach from the American Geriatrics Society: American Geriatrics Society Expert Panel on the Care of Older Adults with Multimorbidity. *J Am Geriatr Soc.* 2012;60:1957–1968.

American Geriatrics Society. Ten things physicians and patients should question, 2013. https://www.choosingwisely.org/societies/american-geriatrics-society/ [choosingwisely.org]. Accessed February 18, 2022.

Bakitas M, Tosteson T, Lyons K, et al. Early versus delayed initiation of concurrent palliative oncology care: patient outcomes in the ENABLE III randomized controlled trial. *J Clin Oncol.* 2015;33:1438–1445.

Bernacki RE, Block SD. American College of Physicians High Value Care Task Force. Communication about serious illness care goals: a review and synthesis of best practices. *JAMA Intern Med.* 2014;174:1994–2003.

Fried LP, Tangen CM, Walston J, et al. Frailty in older adults: evidence for a phenotype. *J Gerontol A Biol Sci Med Sci.* 2001;56:M146–M156.

Gerontological Society of America (GSA). *Communicating With Older Adults: An Evidence-Based Review of What Really Works.* Washington, DC: Gerontological Society of America. 2012.

Hanson LC, Ersek M, Gilliam R, Carey TS. Oral feeding options for people with dementia: a systematic review. *J Am Geriatr Soc.* 2011;59:463–472.

Husebo BS, Ballard C, Sandvik R, Nilsen OB, Aarsland D. Efficacy of treating pain to reduce behavioural disturbances in residents of nursing homes with dementia: cluster randomised clinical trial. *BMJ.* 2011;343:d4065.

IOM (Institute of Medicine). *Dying in America: Improving Quality and Honoring Individual Preferences Near the End of Life.* Washington, DC: The National Academies Press; 2014. https://www.nap.edu/catalog/18748/dying-in-america-improving-quality-and-honoring-individual-preferences-near [nap.edu]. Accessed February 18, 2022.

IOM (Institute of Medicine). *Unequal Treatment: Confronting Racial and Ethnic Disparities in Health Care,* 2002. http://nationalacademies.org/hmd/reports/2002/unequal-treatment-confronting-racial-and-ethnic-disparities-in-health-care.aspx. Accessed May 10, 2016.

IOM (Institute of Medicine). (US) Committee on Lesbian, Gay, Bisexual, and Transgender Health Issues and Research Gaps and Opportunities. *The Health of Lesbian, Gay, Bisexual, and Transgender People: Building a Foundation for Better Understanding.* Washington, DC: The National Academies Press; 2011. https://nationalacademies.org/hmd/reports/2011/the-health-of-lesbian-gay-bisexual-and-transgender-people.aspx. Accessed May 10, 2016.

Johnson KS. Racial and ethnic disparities in palliative care. *J Palliat Med.* 2013;16:1329–1334.

Mitchell SL, Teno JM, Kiely DK, et al. The clinical course of advanced dementia. *N Engl J Med.* 2009;361:1529–1538.

National Hospice and Palliative Care Organization. NHPCOs Facts and Figures. Hospice Care in America. http://www.nhpco.org/hospice-statistics-research-press-room/facts-hospice-and-palliative-care. Accessed May 10, 2021.

Quinn KL, Shurrab M, Gitau K, et al. Association of receipt of palliative care interventions with health care use, quality of life, and symptom burden among adults with chronic noncancer illness: a systematic review and meta-analysis. *JAMA.* 2020;324:1439–1450.

Sampson EL, Candy B, Jones L. Enteral tube feeding for older people with advanced dementia. *Cochrane Database Syst Rev.* 2009;2:CD007209.

Sidebottom AC, Jorgenson A, Richards H, Kirven J, Sillah A. Inpatient palliative care for patients with acute heart failure: outcomes from a randomized trial. *J Palliat Med.* 2015;18:134–142.

Singer AE, Meeker D, Teno JM, Lynn J, Lunney JR, Lorenz KA. Symptom trends in the last year of life from 1998 to 2010: a cohort study. *Ann Intern Med.* 2015;162:175–183.

Temel JS, Greer JA, Muzikansky A, et al. Early palliative care for patients with metastatic non-small-cell lung cancer. *N Engl J Med.* 2010;363:733–742.

Teno JM, Gozalo PL, Mor V, et al. Site of death, place of care, and health care transitions among US Medicare beneficiaries, 2000-2015. *JAMA.* 2018;320:264–271.

Zimmermann C, Swami N, Krzyzanowska M, et al. Early palliative care for patients with advanced cancer: a cluster-randomised controlled trial. *Lancet.* 2014;383:1721–1730.

Chapter 68

Pain Management

Roxanne Bavarian, Amber K. Brooks

OVERVIEW

Pain is one of the most common reasons adults seek medical care. Pain prevalence increases with age and is associated with wide-ranging adverse health outcomes including increased risk of falls, increased functional disability, declining mobility, cognitive decline, and decreased quality of life. The most common pain conditions in older adults include osteoarthritis, chronic neuropathic pain (eg, diabetes, herpes zoster), vertebral compression fractures (VCFs), pain associated with cancer and its treatments, and pain associated with other chronic illnesses. The prevalence of chronic (persistent) pain among older adults is estimated at 25% to 75% and higher in residential care settings. Chronic pain tends to be more complex in older adults with 60% to 70% of them describing multisite pain and more than 60% describing multiple types of pains. Diagnosing and treating chronic pain in older adults is further complicated by age-related changes in pathophysiology, such as cognitive impairment and organ system dysfunction; coexisting chronic medical conditions; and complex treatment considerations, such as polypharmacy and increased susceptibility to side effects, among other factors (**Table 68-1**).

CLASSIFICATION OF PAIN

Pain is defined as an unpleasant sensory and emotional experience associated with actual or potential tissue damage.

Acute Versus Chronic Pain

Acute pain is defined by its sudden onset, association with a noxious stimuli, and short duration of tissue healing (approximately ≤ 3 months). Examples of acute pain include trauma and postoperative pain. Poorly controlled acute postoperative pain is a particularly vulnerable period for older adults and is associated with increased stress response (ie, increased heart rate, blood pressure, and respiratory rate), limited mobility, prolonged hospital stays, and increased risk of developing chronic pain. Conversely, acute pain that is appropriately managed during the perioperative period may help prevent the development of chronic pain.

Learning Objectives

- Classify different types of pain.
- Describe pathophysiological findings in chronic pain.
- Review key aspects of pain evaluation and management.

Key Clinical Points

1. **Pain in older adults is often underdiagnosed and undertreated.**
2. **Careful evaluation of pain requires a thorough history, physical examination, and use of validated pain measures.**
3. **Comprehensive pain management in older adults requires a patient-centered, multidimensional pain management strategy that recognizes the biological and psychosocial complexities and utilizes a combination of medication and nonmedication therapies.**

Chronic Pain

Chronic (persistent) pain is defined as pain that persists or recurs for more than 3 months. In 2019, the International Association for the Study of Pain (IASP) updated its chronic pain classifications for the International Classifications of Diseases (ICD-11) (**Table 68-2**). Pain that is deemed a disease in its own right, such as fibromyalgia or nonspecific low back pain, is called "chronic primary pain." In the other six subgroups, pain is secondary to an underlying disease: chronic secondary musculoskeletal pain, chronic neuropathic pain, chronic secondary headache or orofacial pain, chronic secondary visceral pain, chronic cancer-related pain, and chronic postsurgical or posttraumatic pain.

High-impact chronic pain is defined as chronic pain that limits life or work activities on most days or every day during the past 6 months. In 2016, an estimated 8% of US adults (20 million) had high-impact pain, with higher

TABLE 68-1 ■ COMPLEXITIES OF PAIN AND AGING

Pathophysiology of Aging	Comorbidities
Cognitive impairment	Chronic complex medical conditions
Gastrointestinal system dysfunction	
Hepatic system dysfunction	
Renal system dysfunction	
Pulmonary system dysfunction	

Treatment Considerations	Diagnosis
Polypharmacy	Disparities in care (underdiagnosed, underreported, undertreated)
Side effects	
Caregivers	Multifactorial/multisite pain
Multiple specialists	Psychosocial considerations
Compliance	

prevalence among older adults (11% for 65 to 84-year-old adults and 16% for ≥85-year-old adults).

Pathophysiology of Chronic Pain

In a normal response to tissue injury with a noxious stimulus, the body will respond by activating immune cells, such as macrophages, leukocytes, and mast cells, that release proinflammatory mediators. These proinflammatory mediators include bradykinin, histamine, tumor necrosis factor, interleukin-1β, and interleukin-6, all of which promote the release of substance P and calcitonin gene-related peptide from nerve endings to ultimately activate spinal pathways that cause pain. These pain signals occur in response to the initial inflammation to help "teach" a person to avoid further injuring the damaged tissue during the healing process. In acute pain, healing occurs over the ensuing days to weeks, leading to resolution of inflammation and pain signals in the body. Contrarily, in patients with chronic pain, the nervous system will continue to send signals for pain even after the initial injury has subsided. The pathophysiology of chronic pain revolves around this concept of central plasticity of the brain ("neuroplasticity") in which neural connections are rewired and sensitivity to stimuli changes in response to an initial injury.

Neurological changes associated with chronic pain include hyperalgesia, allodynia, and the spread of pain. Hyperalgesia is defined as an increased sensitivity to painful stimuli, such as an exaggerated pain response to a gentle pinprick, scratch, or heat. Hyperalgesia occurs when the threshold of local nociceptors in the tissue is lowered, which increases the excitability of nociceptor neurons and pain pathways. Similarly, the receptive field of activation of these nociceptors can spread, leading to the spread of pain to adjacent, noninjured areas. Hyperalgesia and spread of pain is caused by a process known as peripheral sensitization, in which inflammation causes release of chemical mediators like histamine and bradykinin that influence the threshold and field of activation of nociceptors in the peripheral tissues. Central sensitization refers to the maladaptive plasticity within the central nervous system. This maladaptivity leads to an increase in the synaptic strength of pain pathways, with a reduction in pain inhibitory pathways, which ultimately lead to increased pain processing in the brain. Subsequently, allodynia may ensue: nonpainful touch stimuli activate mechanoreceptor neurons that have been rewired to stimulate pain pathways. Patients may also report their pain being triggered by a cool breeze against the painful area or the weight of their clothing or bedsheets brushing against the area.

Although the pathophysiological concepts behind chronic pain, such as hyperalgesia, allodynia, and spread of pain, have been verified in animal models of chronic pain, understanding why some patients develop chronic pain is a subject that warrants further research.

TABLE 68-2 ■ UPDATED CHRONIC PAIN CLASSIFICATIONS

CHRONIC PRIMARY PAIN	CHRONIC SECONDARY PAIN
MUSCULOSKELETAL PAIN	
Chronic primary musculoskeletal pain	Chronic secondary musculoskeletal pain
Chronic widespread pain	
NEUROPATHIC PAIN	
Complex regional pain syndrome	Chronic neuropathic pain
HEADACHE/FACIAL PAIN	
Chronic primary headache or orofacial pain	Chronic secondary headache or orofacial pain
VISCERAL PAIN	
Chronic primary visceral pain	Chronic secondary visceral pain
OTHER PAIN	
	Chronic cancer-related pain
	Chronic postsurgical or posttraumatic pain

Nociceptive Versus Neuropathic Pain

For treatment purposes, it is important to distinguish the underlying mechanism of pain in order to best tailor the treatment plan, particularly in regard to medications so as to minimize the risk of polypharmacy. Pain that results from the stimulation of pain receptors is called nociceptive pain. Nociceptive pain may arise from tissue injury, inflammation, or mechanical malformation. Examples include trauma, burns, infection, arthritis, ischemia, and tissue distortion. Pain from nociception usually responds well to analgesic medications.

Neuropathic pain, on the other hand, is caused by a lesion or disease of the somatosensory system, including peripheral nerves and central neurons, and affects 7% to 10% of the population. Neuropathic pain conditions commonly seen in older adults include diabetic peripheral neuropathy, postherpetic neuralgia, and posttraumatic neuralgia (postamputation or phantom limb pain). Neuropathic pain conditions are often persistent and difficult to treat in older adults, as they are more susceptible to the side effects of commonly used neuropathic pain medications such as oversedation and falls. However, it is important to begin treatment as early as possible with a regimen associated with the least amount of harm in order to prevent long-term complications of persistent pain such as physical and psychological disability.

Aging and Its Effect on Pain Perception

Age-related changes in the nervous system may alter pain perception. A decrease in the number of pain receptors in the skin and other organs, altered nerve conduction, and even central nervous system changes have been linked to altered sensory processing in older adults. Similarly, studies of experimental pain have also been linked to age-related changes in perception. These experimental pain studies used a heat probe, electrical stimulation, or other methods to induce pain in volunteers in an effort to identify a pain threshold or pain tolerance. These studies

reveal that aging may decrease sensitivity for pain of low intensity; reduced sensitivity is especially apparent for heat pain; and aging has no strong effect on pain tolerance. It is believed by most researchers that age-associated changes in pain perception are subtle, and their clinical relevance may be minimal. Conversely, older adults may have sensory impairments (visual or auditory), cognitive impairment, or sensory neuropathies that may interfere with the ability to appropriately communicate or even recognize pain symptoms.

Biopsychosocial Model for Older Adults With Pain

Chronic pain requires a multidimensional approach to treatment that incorporates the biological, psychological, and social factors that modulate a person's pain. The biopsychosocial model (BPS) of chronic (persistent) pain describes the intricate interplay between these factors. The original BPS model has since been adapted for older adults (**Figure 68-1**). A number of biological factors are associated with chronic pain in older adults, including age (usually described as ≥ 65 years of age), sex, multiple coexisting chronic medical conditions, genetic factors, common

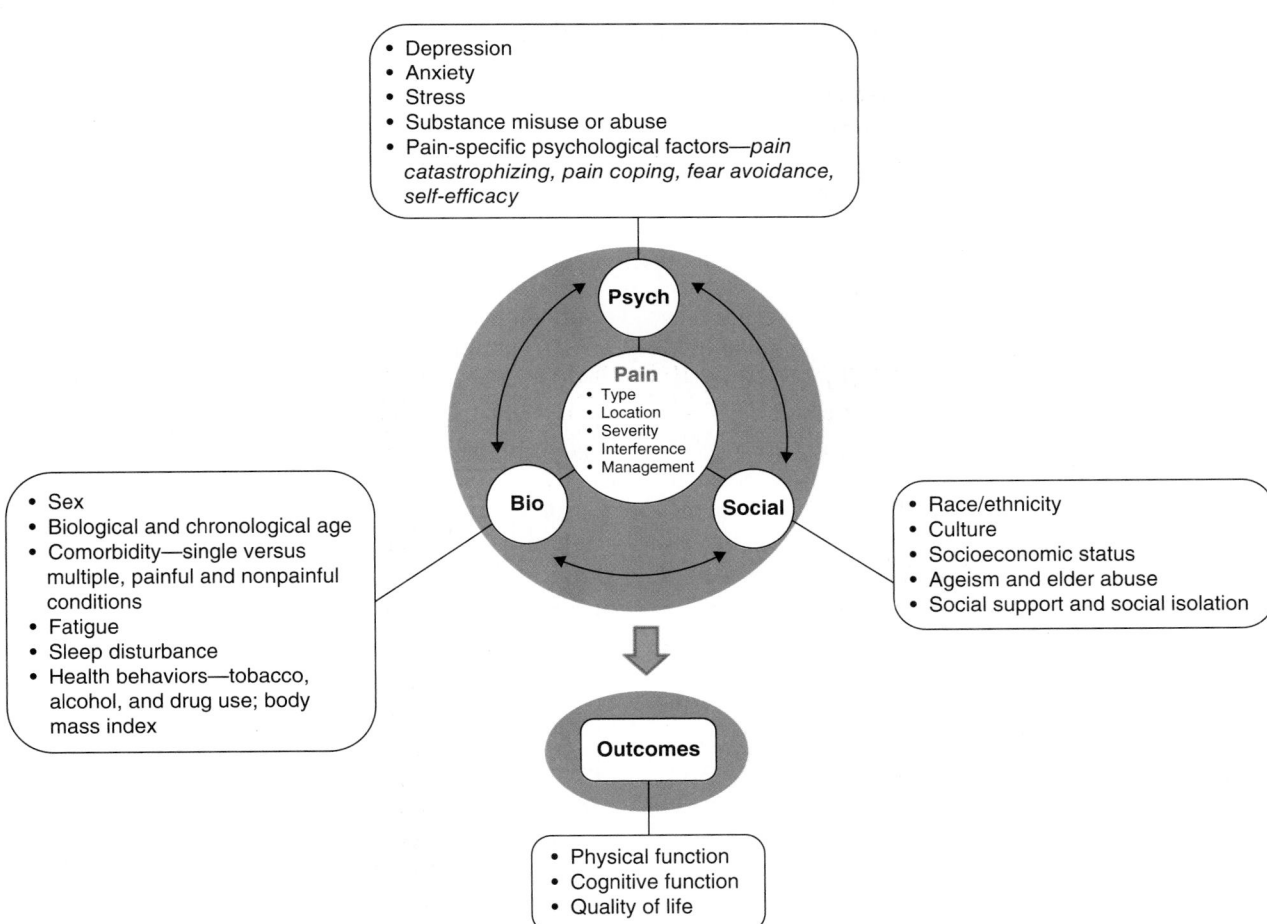

FIGURE 68-1. Biopsychosocial model of pain for older adults. (Reproduced with permission from Miaskowski C, Blyth F, Nicosia F, et al. A biopsychosocial model of chronic pain for older adults. *Pain Med.* 2020;21[9]:1793–1805.)

coexisting symptoms (fatigue and sleep disturbance), and a variety of health-related behaviors (smoking, alcohol use, and illicit drug use). Psychological considerations include depression, anxiety, stress, substance misuse or abuse, pain-specific psychological factors (pain catastrophizing, pain coping, fear avoidance, and self-efficacy). Social influences include race/ethnicity, culture, socioeconomic status, ageism and elder abuse, social support, and social isolation. Ultimately, it is the combination of these biopsychosocial factors that determine outcomes like physical function, cognitive function, and quality of life.

Diagnosis of Pain in Older Adults

The diagnosis of pain relies heavily on self-report from the patient, which is considered the gold standard in measuring pain in both clinical practice and research. A thorough assessment of pain should include a series of questions regarding the location of pain, along with its onset, frequency, intensity, quality of pain, and any modifying factors. When inquiring about pain intensity, it may be helpful to ask the patient about a range of their pain intensity over the past week, rather than solely in the present moment. The assessment of the pain characteristics should be done regularly, both at the initial visit to accurately diagnose a patient and the source of pain (ie, musculoskeletal, visceral, neuropathic, or a combination of the above) and also at follow-up visits to assess the benefit of any treatment rendered. As discussed in the previous sections, the longer pain goes untreated, the more likely for the pain to spread to neighboring areas of the body and become more difficult to diagnose.

Other pertinent questions in the assessment of pain include any history of trauma (eg, falls or injuries) or indirect trauma (eg, whiplash), especially given the risk for falls and occult fractures in older adults. Sleep quality should also be assessed for any indicators of poor sleep quality (eg, insomnia, frequent arousals, daytime hypersomnolence), which could impact the patient's perception of pain. With the patient's permission, a discussion of any recent personal stressors, such as the loss of a loved one, that may have contributed to the onset and/or intensity of pain may be relevant, particularly in neuropathic pain conditions where psychological stress is a known trigger.

In patients with pain, a review of systems should include whether the patient reports generalized muscle pain, generalized joint pain, swelling or erythema, or neurologic symptoms like numbness, tingling, or autonomic symptoms. The medical history should also be reviewed for any other chronic pain conditions and their history of management, which can help clinicians assess what treatment modalities have alleviated pain in the past. Other conditions associated with pain include psychiatric conditions, such as anxiety, depression, and posttraumatic stress disorder, which can potentially contribute or exacerbate symptoms of pain and may indicate a need for interdisciplinary treatment with a pain psychologist. Understanding the

patient's lifestyle and social history can also be informative, including their average daily activities, their stress levels, and their social support system. In addition, any history of drug addiction or alcoholism either in the patient or their family should be documented to assess their risk for opioid use disorder.

In older patients, obtaining an accurate history of their pain symptoms and review of systems may be difficult due to cognitive limitations and inability to respond to questions. In older adults, the line of questioning should be simple and transparent. For example, asking "Does this hurt?" may be more informative than "How are you doing?" For patients with difficulty responding to pain questions, a nonverbal observational pain scale may be indicated to better assess their pain. In patients with cognitive impairment or dementia, family or caregivers should also be asked to provide information regarding the patient's pain.

Various verbal and nonverbal pain assessment scales have been reviewed in the evaluation of pain in older patients. These scales are generally classified as unidimensional or multidimensional. A unidimensional pain scale focuses on a single factor, such as the severity of pain or impact of pain on function. In patients with chronic pain, the impact of the pain on physical and mental function, such as their mobility, mood, and fatigue, may be more meaningful than the pain intensity itself. **Table 68-3** provides a review of unidimensional pain scales. Multidimensional scales, on the other hand, include questions to assess pain intensity, interference with enjoyment of life, or history of pain treatments and relief. **Table 68-4** shows a review of multidimensional pain scales that can be useful in assessing pain in older adults.

Following the initial intake, a thorough physical examination should be completed. The affected location of pain should be evaluated for erythema or edema, which could be a marker of inflammation or infection. The musculoskeletal system can be evaluated by palpating for tender trigger points that duplicate the patient's chief complaint, as well as assessing range of motion, posture, and gait. A neurologic examination for signs of focal muscle weakness, atrophy, or sensory impairments such as numbness or tingling should also be performed to rule out any peripheral or central neuropathic condition.

TREATMENT

Physiologic Considerations and Medication Management in Older Adults

Age-related organ dysfunction poses significant challenges for nonopioid and opioid pain medication management in older adults. The gastrointestinal, hepatic, renal, and respiratory systems are particularly important to consider when initiating and dosing pain medications in this population. There is a plethora of age-related pharmacokinetic changes that clinicians should consider before prescribing pain medications (**Table 68-5**). Decreases in gastric secretion

TABLE 68-3 ■ UNIDIMENSIONAL SCALES FOR PAIN MEASUREMENT

SCALE	ORIENTATION OF SCALE	DESCRIPTION	RECOMMENDATIONS FOR OLDER ADULTS
Numeric Rating Scale (NRS)	Horizontal or vertical	Numeric range 0–5, 0–10, 0–20, or 0–100, where 0 represents no pain and 5, 10, 20, or 100 represent extreme pain	• May be difficult for older adults with cognitive impairment • Vertical orientation preferred over horizontal
Visual Analog Scale (VAS)	Horizontal or vertical	100 mm line, with one end representing no pain and the other end representing pain at its worst	• May be difficult for older adults to understand • High rates of failure and low reliability • Avoid in older adults
Colored Analog Scale (CAS)	Horizontal or vertical	Uses colors to represent increasing pain, with white representing no pain and increasing intensity of red representing extreme pain	• Can be used in older adults with and without cognitive impairment • May not be appropriate for all cultures • Requires visual acuity
Iowa Pain Thermometers (IPT)	Vertical	Utilizes a picture of a thermometer with use of colors to represent increasing pain, with verbal descriptors and numbers	• Allows for numeric rating of intensity and description of pain • Recommended in older adults, including those with cognitive impairment, as well as ethnic minorities • Requires visual acuity
Faces Pain Scale-revised (FPS-R)	Horizontal	Utilizes a series of faces expressing pain, where the first face (face 1) is zero pain and the last face (face 6) represents maximum pain	• Recommended in older adults and ethnic minorities • Requires visual acuity

and intestinal motility lead to altered absorption of certain medications. Aging is also associated with increased body fat and decreased lean body mass, total body water, and serum albumin—all of which affect the distribution of drugs throughout the body. Circulating albumin and other proteins bind analgesic medications, such as nonsteroidal anti-inflammatory drugs (NSAIDs) and tricyclic antidepressants (TCAs). More unbound drug can lead to increased toxicity and drug–drug interactions.

In addition, alterations in hepatic and renal function in older adults can affect drug metabolism and elimination.

Hepatic blood volume and blood flow decrease with age. Similarly, increasing age is associated with decreased renal blood flow and glomerular filtration rate, which may lead to increased serum concentrations of renally cleared medications and their metabolites. The resultant decline in hepatic and renal function may lead to increased risk for adverse medication events and drug–drug interactions secondary to elevated serum parent drug and metabolite concentrations.

Lastly, changes in the pulmonary systems such as decreased elasticity of the lung and increased chest wall

TABLE 68-4 ■ MULTIDIMENSIONAL PAIN SCALES FOR PAIN MEASUREMENT

SCALE	DESCRIPTION	COMMENTS
McGill Pain Questionnaire	78 words grouped into 20 categories that are related to pain	• Extensively studied; may discriminate between types of pain • Long, difficult to score
Brief Pain Inventory-Short Form (BPI-SF)	15 questions that assess pain intensity from 0 to 100, location, and interference with life, as well as any current treatments or medications	• Useful for gauging impact of pain on life, including activities of daily living • Helpful for assessing fall risk
Geriatric Pain Measure-Short Form	12 questions ask about pain intensity and interference with ambulation, social engagement, ability to accomplish tasks, and sleep	• Useful for gauging impact of pain on life, including activities of daily living • Involves more simple yes or no questions
Pain Intensity, Enjoyment in Life, and General Activity (PEG scale)	3 questions that assess pain intensity, interference on enjoyment in life, and general activity	• Can be given regularly to assess for benefits of treatment and level of pain control
Western Ontario and McMaster Universities Arthritis Index (WOMAC)	41 items in five domains: pain, stiffness, physical function, social function, and emotional function	• Specific for arthritis • Difficult to use

TABLE 68-5 ■ PHYSIOLOGICAL CHANGES ASSOCIATED WITH AGING

ORGAN SYSTEM	PHARMACOKINETIC CHANGES
Gastrointestinal system	Decreased gastric secretion
	Decreased intestinal motility
	Decreased absorption
Hepatic system	Decreased hepatic volume
	Decreased hepatic blood flow
Renal system	Decreased renal blood flow
	Decreased glomerular filtration rate
Pulmonary system	Decreased lung elasticity
	Increased chest wall rigidity

rigidity may lead to an increase in respiratory complications such as respiratory depression, which is of paramount importance when prescribing and dosing opioid medications.

Opioid Medication and Prescribing Practices for Older Adults

The first wave of the opioid epidemic began with the increased prescribing of opioids in the 1990s, with overdoses increasing since at least 1999. Furthermore, an analysis of Medicare beneficiaries' prescription opioid use in 2016 showed one in three Medicare Part D beneficiaries received a prescription for an opioid. Unfortunately, older adults are not immune from the detrimental consequences of opioid misuse disorder, including overdoses and deaths. The Centers for Disease Control and Prevention (CDC) reported an increase in drug overdoses and opioid deaths in the aging population, with a 7.7% increase in deaths related to opioid overdose in persons older than 65 years from 2013 to 2014. Older adults with opioid use disorder appear to be at higher risk of death compared to younger adults with the disorder. This disparity in death may be related to altered age-related organ function and accidental medication-related deaths.

In 2016, the CDC released its landmark guideline for prescribing opioids for chronic pain, which includes special considerations for prescribing practices in older adults. First, given reduced renal function and medication clearance even without renal disease, older adults may be more susceptible to the accumulation of opioids and, therefore, identifying the therapeutic window between safe dosages and higher dosages associated with respiratory depression and overdose may be extremely challenging. Cognitive impairment may increase the risk for medication-related errors and opioid-induced confusion. Prescribing providers should pay particular attention to prescribing immediate-release opioids (recommendation #4); prescribing the lowest effective dose possible (recommendation #5); and maintaining close follow-up within 1 to 4 weeks of starting opioid therapy, with subsequent follow-up at least every 3 months or more frequently

(recommendation #7). Clinicians should also consider instituting bowel regimens to prevent constipation, performing risk assessments for falls, monitoring for cognitive impairment, and performing random urine drug screen monitoring, especially when there are other caregivers involved in the patient's care. In response to the opioid epidemic in the United States, the CDC has also recommended that prescribers utilize state-wide prescription drug monitoring programs (PDMPs) prior to prescribing any opioid or other controlled substance to monitor a patient's use of controlled substances and minimize the risk for abuse, overdose, and diversion.

Commonly Used Opioid Medications

For patients with moderate acute or chronic pain that has failed to respond to conservative management with nonopioid medications or nonpharmacological therapies, weak opioids such as hydrocodone, codeine, and tramadol may be considered after a thorough discussion with the patient about potential risks versus benefit. In patients with severe acute or persistent pain, more potent opioids are available, including morphine, methadone, fentanyl, oxycodone, buprenorphine, hydromorphone, and oxymorphone. Of note, in opioids combined with nonopioid analgesics, the maximum dose is typically dictated by the maximum dose of acetaminophen, NSAID, or aspirin. A table of commonly used opioid medications with recommended starting doses is featured in **Table 68-6**.

Despite the number of different opioid medications, they generally possess similar mechanisms of action and pharmacokinetics. The mechanism of opioid medications in alleviating pain is mediated by their binding to opioid receptors in the central nervous system to inhibit the ascending pain pathway. In terms of pharmacokinetics, opioids are rapidly absorbed in the gut and then undergo a high rate of first pass metabolism in the liver, where they are conjugated and form metabolites. Opioids then vary in their distribution due to their differing protein affinity, and lastly are excreted via bile to feces or via the kidneys. As discussed above, older adults may be prone to side effects of opioids due to slower gastrointestinal transit time associated with aging and risk of increased gastric pH due to concurrent use of proton pump inhibitors or antacids. In addition, the increased adipose tissue and decreased lean body mass and total body water leads to changes in drug distribution and a longer time for elimination. Thus, with any opioid medication, older patients are at risk for side effects such as central nervous system depression, sedation, respiratory depression, and constipation. Because of the increased risk of side effects in older adults, it is recommended to start opioids at a lower dose, about 25% to 50% of the dose given to younger patients. The CDC recommends carefully evaluating a patient for benefits and risks of opioid doses beyond more than 50 morphine milligram equivalents per day (MME/day) and avoiding doses more than 90 MME/day.

TABLE 68-6 ■ COMMONLY PRESCRIBED ORAL OPIOID PAIN MEDICATIONS

DRUG	INITIAL DOSING	COMMENTS
Morphine, immediate release	10 mg every 4–6 hours	Titrate to comfort: continuous use for constant pain and intermittent use for episodic pain
Morphine, extended release	Tablet: 15 mg BID-TID Capsule: 30 mg QD vs 15 mg BID	Should be avoided in opioid-naive patients
Oxymorphone, immediate release (Opana)	5–10 mg every 4–6 hours	Titrate to comfort: continuous use for constant pain and intermittent use for episodic pain
Hydromorphone (Dilaudid, Exalgo)	1–2 mg every 3–4 hours	Titrate to comfort: continuous use for constant pain and intermittent use for episodic pain
Oxycodone, immediate release (Roxicodone)	5–10 mg every 4–6 hours	Titrate to comfort: continuous use for constant pain and intermittent use for episodic pain
Oxycodone, extended release (OxyContin)	Tablet: 10 mg BID Capsule: 9 mg BID	Should be avoided in opioid-naive patients
Hydrocodone-acetaminophen (Norco)	2.5–10 mg every 4–6 hours	Maximum dose dictated by acetaminophen 4 g total daily dose
Codeine (codeine, Tylenol 3)	15–60 mg every 4 hours as needed; maximum total daily dose: 360 mg/day	Variability in effectiveness between individuals due to drug metabolism into its seven active metabolites
Tramadol (Ultram)	25–50 mg every 4–6 hours; maximum total daily dose: 300 mg	• Acts both as an opioid receptor agonist and a serotonin-reuptake inhibitor • Avoid in patients with other serotonergic drugs or history of seizures
Methadone (Dolophine)	2.5–10 mg QD	Long half-life and risk of accumulation; difficult to titrate
Fentanyl, transdermal (Duragesic)	25-mcg patch (every-72-hour dosing)	• Should be avoided in opioid-naive patients • Dose dependent on previous 24-hour total morphine milligram equivalent dose
Tapentadol (Nucynta)	50 mg every q 4–6 hours moderate to severe pain	• Partial opioid and norepinephrine reuptake receptor activity • May be helpful in treating patients with neuropathic pain
Buprenorphine	Belbuca (SL): 75–150 mcg BID, max dose 900 mcg BID Butrans (transdermal): 5 mcg/h every 7 days, max dose 20 mcg/h Buprenex (IV/IM): 0.3 mg every 6 hours	• FDA-approved for the treatment of pain • Buprenorphine is a partial agonist at the mu opioid receptor with a high binding affinity to the mu receptor and slow dissociation from the receptor • May act as an antidepressant at the kappa receptor

A consideration in the use of opioids in managing chronic pain is the risk for development of opioid-induced hyperalgesia. Opioid-induced hyperalgesia refers to a state of nociceptive sensitization in which patients taking opioids for the treatment of pain develop hyperalgesia, or increased sensitivity to painful stimuli. The mechanism of opioid-induced hyperalgesia is not entirely clear, but is thought to be due to neuroplastic changes in the peripheral and central nervous system that lead to sensitization of pronociceptive pathways. While all patients receiving opioids are at risk for opioid-induced hyperalgesia, groups with increased risk include patients with a history of opioid use disorder, chronic pain patients receiving opioids, and patients on high doses of potent opioids. Clinical signs of opioid-induced hyperalgesia include lack of effectiveness of opioids in the absence of disease progression, which may be difficult to distinguish from opioid tolerance. However, in contrast to patients with opioid tolerance, patients with opioid-induced hyperalgesia will often show increased levels of pain with increased doses of opioids. Patients may also report symptoms such as diffuse allodynia beyond the region of the original pain. Management of patients with opioid-induced hyperalgesia includes attempting to gradually reduce or eliminate the opioid and evaluate symptoms. Combination therapy with nonopioid analgesics, opioids with unique properties such as buprenorphine, or NMDA receptor antagonists may prove to be more effective in patients with opioid-induced hyperalgesia.

Management of Acute and Postoperative Pain

Management of acute pain and pain around the time of surgery is challenging. Poorly controlled and undertreated pain is associated with prolonged hospitalization, delayed wound healing, increase in health care utilization and costs, poor patient satisfaction, and adverse psychological consequences. In addition, one of the most significant long-term consequences of poorly treated acute postsurgical pain is the development of chronic pain. However, advances in modern medicine offer promising new approaches for the management of acute pain, especially postoperative pain.

Enhanced Recovery after Surgery (ERAS) protocols have become more commonplace across the United States, especially in light of the opioid epidemic. The mainstay of ERAS protocols is the judicious use of multimodal analgesia. ERAS protocols attempt to minimize the use of opioids and offer opioid-sparing techniques such as intravenous or oral acetaminophen, intravenous or oral NSAIDs, intravenous lidocaine infusion, intravenous ketamine infusion, liposomal bupivacaine, neuraxial and peripheral regional anesthesia regional techniques for select surgeries, as well as patient-controlled modalities. Opioids still play an important role in the treatment of acute and postoperative pain, but are limited by their side effects and other sequelae, especially in older adults. If using opioid medications for acute pain in the inpatient setting, it is important to consider the following risk factors for opioid-related respiratory depression (and other adverse events), including a history of sleep apnea, obesity, concomitant administration of other respiratory depressant drugs such as benzodiazepines, opioid-naïve patients, opioid-tolerant patients, and chronic obstructive pulmonary disease. While supplemental oxygen is commonly used after surgery, it may produce acceptable oxygen saturation levels via pulse oximetry even with substantial hypoventilation. Thus, patients with risk factors for opioid-related respiratory depression should be considered for perioperative monitoring with continuous end-tidal carbon dioxide monitoring, especially during the first 24 hours after surgery.

Management of Chronic Pain

For patients with mild chronic pain, nonopioid analgesics, such as NSAIDs or acetaminophen, are recommended. These medications are available in tablet, capsule, topical, and injection form with many being available over the counter.

Acetaminophen Acetaminophen (Tylenol) is a widely available analgesic and antipyretic that can be used for mild-to-moderate pain of any etiology. While its mechanism of action is not yet fully understood, it is thought to activate descending serotonergic inhibitory pathways in the central nervous system to reduce pain perception. While acetaminophen is considered relatively safe in its side effect profile when compared to NSAIDs, the main adverse reaction is hepatotoxicity due to acetaminophen overdose. In older adults, initial dosing is recommended at 500 to 1000 mg every 6 hours. The maximum total daily dose of acetaminophen is 4000 mg. In patients with hepatic impairment or a history of alcohol use, a maximum daily dose of 2000 to 3000 mg is recommended. Given the availability of acetaminophen as an over-the-counter analgesic, prescribed medication, as well as combined with other medications,

such as opioids, it is important to review all of a patient's current medications to ensure the patient is not taking higher than the recommended dose.

Nonsteroidal anti-inflammatory drugs (NSAIDs) NSAIDs represent another class of widely available medications that has both anti-inflammatory and analgesic effects that alleviate mild-to-moderate pain, and in particular, pain of an inflammatory origin, such as osteoarthritis or rheumatoid arthritis. There are a variety of NSAIDs available either as a prescription or over the counter, each with different dosing regimens and tolerability profiles. Often, if one particular type of NSAID is not effective for a patient, it may be worthwhile trying a different NSAID. **Table 68-7** reviews the most common NSAID medications and their doses.

NSAIDs work to reduce pain by reversibly inhibiting the activity of cyclooxygenase enzymes, COX-1 and COX-2, and consequently preventing the synthesis of prostaglandins, which mediate inflammation as well as the transmission of pain. NSAIDs that act as nonselective COX inhibitors are not recommended for long-term use due to side effects associated with inhibition of COX-1. COX-1 is present throughout the body and plays a role in protecting the gastric mucosal lining and maintaining renal and hepatic function, among other functions. Inhibition of COX-1 is associated with increased risk for gastrointestinal ulcers and bleeding. Thus, patients on NSAIDs for any period of time should be monitored for any symptoms of gastrointestinal pain or bleeding. Caution should be given when prescribing either NSAIDs or aspirin to older adults who are on anticoagulant therapy due to increased risk of bleeding. Other complications of long-term NSAID use include increased risk for cardiovascular events and kidney disease.

COX-2, on the other hand, is present throughout the body in lower concentrations and is expressed in response to injury and inflammation. Utilization of NSAIDs that selectively target and inhibit COX-2 enzymes, such as celecoxib (Celebrex), can effectively reduce inflammation and pain, while sparing patients from the organ toxicity associated with other NSAIDs. However, COX-2-selective NSAIDs are not risk-free and, similar to nonselective COX-inhibiting NSAIDs are associated with increased risk for cardiovascular events.

For older adults at risk for adverse events associated with systemic NSAIDs, topical agents such as diclofenac 1% gel, represent a safe form of an anti-inflammatory treatment that can be massaged onto intact skin overlying painful areas, such as joints affected by osteoarthritis or other inflammatory conditions.

Other Adjunct Medications for Chronic Pain

In addition to opioids analgesics, a number of other medications may be helpful in the management of chronic pain depending on the diagnosis and etiology of the patient's pain. **Table 68-8** reviews common medications used in the

TABLE 68-7 ■ COMMONLY PRESCRIBED NONSTEROIDAL ANTI-INFLAMMATORY DRUGS (NSAIDs)

DRUG	DOSING	MECHANISM OF ACTION	COMMENTS
Celecoxib (Celebrex)	100–200 mg BID	Selective COX-2 inhibition	Reduced GI toxicity and platelet compared to other NSAIDs
Ibuprofen (Motrin, Advil)	2400 mg maximum total daily dose, dosed every 6–8 hours	Reversibly inhibits COX-1 and COX-2 to decrease formation of prostaglandin precursors	• High risk for side effects, particularly peptic ulcers, in older patients • Avoid long-term use due to GI, renal, cardiovascular toxicity • Older adults at risk for CNS side effects (confusion, agitation)
Naproxen (Aleve, Naprosyn)	1000 mg maximum total daily dose, dosed every 8–12 hours	Same as ibuprofen	Same as ibuprofen
Meloxicam (Mobic)	7.5–15 mg QD	Same as ibuprofen	Same as ibuprofen
Diclofenac (Cataflam)	150–200 mg maximum total daily dose, dosed every 6–12 hours	Same as ibuprofen	Same as ibuprofen
Indomethacin (Indocin)	25–50 mg, up to TID	Same as ibuprofen	Beers Criteria (AGS 2019): avoid use due to high risk for GI toxicity and acute kidney injury
Nabumetone (Relafen)	1,000 mg QD-BID	Same as ibuprofen	Same as ibuprofen
Ketorolac (Toradol)	**IM:** 120 per day, with 30–60 mg loading dose followed by half the loading dose **PO:** 60 mg per day, with 6-hour dosing	Same as ibuprofen	Beers Criteria (AGS 2019): avoid use due to high risk for GI toxicity and acute kidney injury
Diclofenac 1% topical gel (Voltaren gel)	2–4 g applied QID PRN	Same as ibuprofen	Topical gel to avoid systemic side effects, can be massaged onto intact skin

TABLE 68-8 ■ NONOPIOID COANALGESIC MEDICATIONS

DRUG	DOSING	MECHANISM OF ACTION	COMMENTS
Serotonin-norepinephrine reuptake inhibitors (SNRIs)			
• Venlafaxine (Effexor) • Duloxetine (Cymbalta)	37.5–75 mg QD 20–60 mg QD	Modulation of pain pathway via serotonin, norepinephrine	• Low sedation and anticholinergic effects compared to TCAs • Beers Criteria (AGS 2019): avoid SNRIs in patients with history of falls or fracture • Avoid abrupt discontinuation, slow taper over 4 weeks to avoid withdrawal symptoms
Tricyclic antidepressants (TCAs)			
• Amitriptyline (Elavil) • Nortriptyline (Pamelor)	10–50 mg QHS 10–50 mg QHS	Increases concentration of serotonin and/or norepinephrine to modulate pain pathways	• Beers Criteria (AGS 2019): avoid due to high anticholinergic activity; avoid in patients with history of falls or fracture • Avoid abrupt discontinuation, slow taper over 4 weeks to avoid withdrawal symptoms
Gabapentinoids			
• Gabapentin (Neurontin) • Pregabalin (Lyrica)	100 mg QHS, up to 900 mg TID PRN 25 mg QHS, up to 75 mg TID PRN	Block voltage-gated calcium channels to reduce neuronal hyperexcitability	• Initiate at lowest dose and gradually titrate • Contraindicated in those with renal impairment • Avoid in patients with concurrent opioid use
Sodium channel blockers			
• Carbamazepine (Tegretol) • Oxcarbazepine (Trileptal)	200–400 mg BID, maximum total daily dose of 1200 mg daily 150–300 mg BID, maximum total daily dose of 2400 mg daily	Block voltage-gated sodium channels to reduce neuronal hyperexcitability	• Consider testing for HLA-B*1502 allele • Risk for hyponatremia—monitor Na^+ and drug levels

PART IV PRINCIPLES OF PALLIATIVE MEDICINE AND ETHICS

(Continued)

TABLE 68-8 ■ NONOPIOID COANALGESIC MEDICATIONS (*CONTINUED*)

DRUG	DOSING	MECHANISM OF ACTION	COMMENTS
Benzodiazepines			
• Clonazepam (Klonopin) • Diazepam (Valium)	0.5 mg QHS 2–2.5 mg up to BID PRN	Increases activity of GABA to reduce neuronal excitability	• Initiate with low doses and monitor, particularly if any hepatic or renal impairment • Risk for sedation and falls—avoid in patients with concurrent opioid use
Muscle relaxers			
• Baclofen (Lioresal)	5–10 mg, up to TID	Muscle relaxer; inhibits transmission of monosynaptic and polysynaptic reflexes to reduce muscle spasticity	• Avoid if possible due to high risk of sedation and cholinergic effects • Gradual taper recommended if discontinuing
• Methocarbamol (Robaxin)	500 mg up to TID	Centrally acting skeletal muscle relaxer	Beers Criteria (AGS 2019): avoid use; limited efficacy at doses tolerated by older adults
• Tizanidine (Zanaflex)	2–4 mg up to QID	Alpha$_2$-adrenergic agonist, inhibits transmission of polysynaptic reflexes to reduce muscle spasticity	Caution in renally impaired patients
• Cyclobenzaprine (Flexeril)	5–10 mg up to TID	Centrally acting skeletal muscle relaxer	High risk of sedation and anticholinergic effects
• Metaxalone (Skelaxin)	800 mg up to QID	CNS depressant	Beers Criteria (AGS 2019): avoid use; limited efficacy at doses tolerated by older adults
Topical adjunct treatments			
• Topical lidocaine	Available as topical creams (3–5%), mucosal jelly 2%, mucosal solution 2%, and transdermal patches (1.8–5%)	Decreases neuronal membrane to sodium ions to reduce nerve initiation and	
• Capsaicin 0.075% cream	Apply thin film to affected area up to QID PRN	Binds TRPV-1 receptors on nociceptors, leading to increased pain followed by pain relief mediated by depletion of substance P	

management of chronic pain. These medications are often categorized as being "adjuvant" or "co-analgesics," as their initial indication was for conditions other than pain, such as depression or seizures; however, many of these medications can be used as a first-line treatment option for specific chronic pain conditions.

Tricyclic antidepressants (TCAs) and serotonin-norepinephrine reuptake inhibitors (SNRIs) can be used in the management of chronic pain. By increasing the activity of serotonin and norepinephrine, these medications modulate the pain pathway to inhibit ascending pain pathways and promote descending pain inhibitory pathways. These medications have been shown to be effective in treating neuropathic pain as well as musculoskeletal pain. Despite their efficacy at low doses, TCAs like amitriptyline and nortriptyline possess potent anticholinergic activity, which can lead to adverse effects, particularly in older individuals.

These adverse effects can include memory impairment, confusion, and hallucinations. Patients are also at risk for dry mouth, blurred vision, constipation, nausea, urinary retention, impaired sweating, and tachycardia. SNRIs should also be initiated with caution due to their serotonergic activity and risk for seizures. Additionally, Beers Criteria (American Geriatric Society, 2019) recommend avoidance of SNRIs in patients with a history of falls and fractures.

For patients with chronic neuropathic pain conditions, such as diabetic neuropathies, postherpetic neuralgia, and trigeminal neuralgia, medications in the category of anticonvulsants may be helpful. These include gabapentinoids, such as gabapentin and pregabalin, and sodium channel blockers, such as carbamazepine and oxcarbazepine. These medications have a high risk for side effects such as central nervous system depression, fatigue, dizziness, and disorientation. Such disorientation can cause patients to take the incorrect dosing or precipitate falls. Thus, dosing should always be initiated at a low dose with a gradual increase of the dose as needed to treat symptoms. Noteworthy, precautions include prescribing gabapentinoids with opioids due to the combined effects of central nervous system depression.

Clonazepam is a benzodiazepine that may be indicated for chronic neuropathic pain conditions, such as tinnitus or burning mouth syndrome, as well as movement disorders. However, benzodiazepines must be prescribed with caution in older adults because of the potential risk for sedation, confusion, and falls. For similar reasons, benzodiazepines and opioid medications should not be taken concomitantly. In addition, due to the risk for abuse and addiction, benzodiazepines such as clonazepam are included along with opioids in state-wide prescription drug monitoring programs and measured as lorazepam milligram equivalents (LMEs). Older adults taking daily benzodiazepines for more than 30 days may develop physiologic dependence and should be gradually tapered to avoid risk of withdrawal symptoms.

While sodium channel blockers like carbamazepine and oxcarbazepine represent highly efficacious frontline treatments for neuropathic pain such as trigeminal neuralgia, these medications require caution and close monitoring when prescribing. Due to the side effects of sedation, clinicians should consider advising the patient to have a family member or caregiver monitor the patient when first initiating carbamazepine or oxcarbazepine. Due to these drugs' effect on sodium levels and on the bone marrow, regular monitoring of sodium levels along with serum drug levels, a complete blood count with differential, and liver and renal function tests are recommended when initiating either of these medications. In addition, patients with either a HLA-B*1502 and HLA-A*3101 allele (most common in South Asian ancestry) are at risk for severe skin reactions, such as Stevens–Johnson syndrome, and thus, genotype screening may be indicated. Carbamazepine is also a potent cytochrome P 450 inducer that can interfere with the metabolism of other drugs, particularly those with narrow therapeutic indices like warfarin or lithium.

In patients with moderate-to-severe chronic musculoskeletal pain, muscle relaxants may be indicated to alleviate pain. A variety of muscle relaxants are available, including baclofen, methocarbamol, tizanidine, and cyclobenzaprine. While these medications are typically indicated on an as-needed basis to treat muscle spasm, patients with chronic musculoskeletal pain such as temporomandibular joint and muscle disorders caused by parafunctional habits (ie, jaw clenching and tooth grinding) may benefit from a nightly dose to reduce their pain. However, all muscle relaxants carry potential side effects of sedation and anticholinergic effects. The lowest possible dose is recommended when initiating therapy, with patients gradually increasing the dose either as needed or as tolerated.

Nonpharmacological Treatments

Chronic pain in older adults is often treated with a multimodal pain management approach: a combination of medications, physical therapy, psychological interventions, or interventional pain management. Interventional pain management is defined as the discipline of medicine devoted to the diagnosis and treatment of pain-related disorders, principally with the application of interventional techniques (commonly referred to as injection therapies), independently or in conjunction with other treatment modalities. Interventional pain procedures are performed by a myriad of providers, including, but not limited to, anesthesiologists, physiatrists, neurologists, neurosurgeons, orthopedic surgeons, rheumatologists, and radiologists. Interventional pain procedures have the added benefit of targeting specific nociceptive transmission sites with the goal of minimizing the intake of oral medications and their end organ effects. Thus, interventional pain management techniques offer older adults an alternative treatment pathway with potentially fewer side effects.

Low back pain *Lumbar epidural steroid injection* (ESI) is a commonly used procedure for treating lumbar spinal stenosis, lumbar disc herniation, lumbar degenerative disc disease, and lumbosacral radicular pain. Pertinent imaging such as plain films, magnetic resonance imaging (MRI), and computed tomography (CT) scans should be reviewed before performing an ESI, although physical examination findings and pain symptoms do not always correlate to image findings. ESIs are preferably performed with image guidance (CT or fluoroscopy) for increased accuracy using an interlaminar approach (midline or paramedian) or transforaminal approach. The transforaminal approach (placement of a needle within the neuroforamen) is preferentially used for patients with lumbosacral radicular pain who may also have low back pain. Contraindications to ESIs include coagulopathy, current anticoagulation use, infection (localized near injection site or systemic), uncontrolled diabetes, allergy to medication being injected (contrast, local anesthetic, steroid), anatomic changes that would prevent a safe procedure (congenital or surgical), or immunosuppression. Potential complications include bleeding, infection, neural injury, inadvertent injection of steroid or local anesthetic outside of the epidural space, and an allergic reaction to medications administered.

There is considerable controversy surrounding the efficacy of ESIs. The results of clinical trials are influenced by the type of interventional pain management specialist, injection approach (interlaminar vs transforaminal), pain type, and injectate. Nonetheless, there is general consensus that ESIs provide short-term relief (weeks to months) in well-selected patients. ESIs should be used in combination with other forms of pain management with the goal of reducing pain and improving function.

Lumbar Facet Injections Lumbar facet-mediated pain is a common cause of low back pain in older adults that is often associated with functional limitations. Lumbar facet joints, or zygapophyseal joints, are synovial joints in the lumbar region that are innervated by the medial branch (MB) nerves of the dorsal primary ramus. Lumbar facet-mediated pain may manifest in the low back and commonly refers pain to the groin, hip, or thighs, but rarely below the knee. Patients commonly report pain with bending over, twisting movements, lateral rotation, and prolonged sitting or standing. Typical examination findings include pain with direct palpation over the facet joints and pain with extension and lateral rotation, also known as facet loading. Diagnostic studies (plain films, CT, or MRI) can be helpful in characterizing the degree of lumbar facet arthropathy (mild, moderate, or severe). Lumbar facet mediated-pain injections can be performed by injecting directly into the joint space (intra-articular) or by aiming the injection at the junction of the superior articular process and transverse process where the MB nerves reside. Facet MB joint diagnostic nerve blocks are most commonly performed due to fair to good evidence regarding efficacy. In addition, an 80% reduction in pain after facet MB joint nerve blocks offers the added advantage of proceeding to MB nerve radiofrequency denervation in an attempt to provide longer lasting relief.

Sacroiliac Joint Injections The sacroiliac joints (SIJs) are small, diarthrodial joints located at the junction of the sacrum and ilium, whose primary purpose is to act as a shock absorber for the spine. The ability for the SIJ to absorb shock from the spine decreases with age and is associated with increased pain. SIJ degenerative changes may be seen on imaging studies (plain films, CT, or MRI). Physical examination findings may include tenderness to palpation directly over the joint space or positive provocative tests (ie, Faber, distraction, compression, Gaenslen's, or thigh thrust). The SIJ can refer pain to the hip, buttocks, sacrum, or thighs, but usually does not extend past the knee. It can be difficult to distinguish SIJ pain from other causes of low back pain like discogenic pain, lumbar myofascial pain, or lumbar facet-mediated pain. Like facet-mediated pain, intra-articular steroid injections or nerve blocks of the L5 dorsal primary rami and the lateral branch (LB) of the S1-3 dorsal rami may be performed. Evidence regarding the efficacy of intra-articular SIJ with steroids is limited. The best recommendation is to use these injections in combination with other multimodal pain management including physical therapy, medication management (muscle relaxants, anti-inflammatories), SIJ stretching exercises, heat, ice, or transcutaneous electrical nerve stimulation unit. If 80% relief from the nerve blocks is appreciated, the patient may proceed to radiofrequency denervation of the L5 dorsal primary rami and the lateral branch (LB) of the S1-3 dorsal rami for more prolonged relief.

Percutaneous Vertebral Augmentation for Compression Fractures VCFs are the most common fragility fracture reported in the literature. VCFs, by definition, compromise the anterior half of the vertebral body and the anterior longitudinal ligament leading to a characteristic wedge-shaped deformity. In older adults, the most common risk factor for VCFs is osteoporosis. The prevalence is highest among women older than 50 years, affecting an estimated 25% of postmenopausal women in the United States. An estimated 40% to 50% of people older than 80 years have sustained a VCF. Furthermore, people who have had one osteoporotic VCF are at five times the risk of sustaining a second VCF. Only a quarter of VCFs result from falls; most are precipitated by routine daily activities such as bending or lifting. VCFs most frequently occur at the thoracolumbar junction (ie, the segment from T12 to L3) and can be diagnosed with plain films, CT scan, or MRI. An MRI may provide more additional information regarding the acuity of the VCF, regarding whether it is, acute, subacute, or chronic. Patients afflicted with VCFs report wide-ranging symptoms including no pain, while others report severe pain. Symptomatic patients may benefit from conservative treatment including pain medications, immobilization via bracing, and physical therapy, while others fail to respond.

Two minimally invasive procedures, vertebroplasty (VP) and kyphoplasty (KP), are commonly used to treat persistent, acutely painful VCFs. In VP, cement is injected percutaneously into the fractured vertebral body via a cannula. KP is similarly performed percutaneously, but involves injection of the cement into an inflated balloon that creates a cavity that encapsulates the cement. Potential complications of both VP and KP include cement leakage into the spinal canal with resultant neurologic deficits and cement leakage into surrounding vascular structures with subsequent risk of pulmonary embolism. Contraindications to VP and KP include existing coagulopathy or use of blood thinners, burst fractures with retropulsed bone, and vertebral height loss greater than 66%.

Osteoarthritic joint pain and the use of interventional pain management Osteoarthritis (OA) is highly prevalent in older adults, with 60% of people 65 years and older diagnosed with arthritis or chronic joint pain. OA is a leading cause of disability, economic burden, and functional decline in older adults. OA is characterized by an active, dynamic process arising from an imbalance between the repair and destruction of joint tissues. Structural alterations in articular cartilage, adjacent bone, ligaments, synovium, and capsule have all been described in OA. Interventional pain management for knee and hip OA offers older adults nonsurgical and relatively low risk pain management therapy options. Interventional pain management for knee and hip OA is most often performed using fluoroscopy, MRI, CT scan, or ultrasonography (US) to help guide needle placement and increase accuracy of the procedure.

Intra-Articular Injections In general, three types of intra-articular injections may be performed including corticosteroid, hyaluronic acid (HA) also known as viscosupplementation, and platelet-rich plasma (PRP). These injections are commonly offered to patients with moderate-to-severe symptomatic OA that have responded unfavorably to physical therapy or nonsteroidal anti-inflammatory medications. Corticosteroid medications usually contain 40 to 80 mg of a depot steroid preparation such as triamcinolone acetate or methylprednisolone acetate in combination with a local anesthetic such as bupivacaine or lidocaine.

HA is naturally found in the knee and acts as a shock absorber and lubricant. Decreasing levels of HA are associated with OA. There are several commercially available HA preparations in the United States including Supartz, Synvisc, and Orthovisc. These formulations vary in origin (rooster combs vs bacterial), molecular weight, and the number of recommended injections (1–5).

PRP is the injection of autologous plasma with a high concentration of platelets into an affected joint or other area of interest. PRP injections are thought to relieve OA-related symptoms via the interaction of platelets, intrinsic joint tissues, and the release of growth factors and cytokines by activated platelets, which ultimately act to reduce inflammation and promote local healing.

In general, all three types of injections are safe and have relatively few side effects. Decisions about frequency, type, and imaging guidance for injection therapies are highly variable, but should be tailored to the patient.

Knee Pain Injection Treatments The knee is the largest joint in the body and the most common site of OA. Its prevalence is two times higher in men than women. Frequently reported symptoms are pain with ambulation, crepitus (cracking or popping sensation), warmth with palpation of the joint, or effusion (ie, swelling). Patients are good candidates for knee injections if they have radiographic evidence of moderate or severe OA. Corticosteroid, viscosupplementation, and PRP may be injected into the knee joint. In the short term (< 3 months), intra-articular steroid injections of corticosteroids and local anesthetic mixtures are more effective than placebo. However, long-term benefits are not well established. PRP injections for knee OA, especially end-stage OA, show promising efficacy (up to 12 months in some studies). However, there remains high variability in the administration of PRP including injection techniques, injection schedules, and number of centrifugations of autologous plasma, which can drastically alter the concentration of platelets injected.

Hip Pain Injection Treatments The hip joint is a ball and socket joint consisting of the articulation of the femoral head with the acetabulum. OA-related hip pain commonly travels to the groin but can also travel to the low back or buttock area. Patients report increased pain with standing and walking. Pain with internal rotation of the hip is a hallmark physical examination finding. Corticosteroid in combination with a local anesthetic is the most commonly performed intraarticular hip injection, which is done under the guidance of imaging (fluoroscopy, CT, or ultrasound). Additional clinical studies are needed to evaluate the short- and long-term efficacy of HA and PRP injections for hip pain.

Neuropathic pain conditions are more common in older adults, as the risk for conditions that cause neuropathic pain increase with age. For example, conditions like diabetes, herpes zoster, stroke, as well as cancer treatment can all result in neuropathic pain. While most patients respond to standard medications like anticonvulsants and gabapentinoids, older adults may not tolerate frontline treatment with anticonvulsants or gabapentinoids due to side effects of sedation and impaired cognition. Although relatively rare, neuropathic pain affecting the orofacial pain region, such as trigeminal neuralgia and postherpetic neuralgia, can be particularly difficult to manage due to its impact on speaking, chewing, and swallowing. Nerve blocks represent a safe, minimally invasive treatment option that can be both diagnostic, allowing clinicians to localize the source of pain, and therapeutic, in reducing the intensity or frequency of pain. For patients with suspected neuropathic pain of the facial region, an MRI of the brain with trigeminal protocol is recommended to rule out any mass lesion or vascular compression of the trigeminal nerve. Nerve blocks frequently performed in the orofacial region include inferior alveolar nerve blocks for trigeminal neuralgia of the V3 distribution, posterior superior alveolar nerve blocks for trigeminal neuralgia of the V2 distribution, occipital nerve blocks for occipital neuralgia and cervicogenic headaches, and sphenopalatine ganglion blocks for cluster headaches. While the duration of relief with a nerve block can be variable, for some patients, periodic nerve blocks can be helpful for treating flares of pain while avoiding polypharmacy with multiple analgesics and anticonvulsant medications. For older adults with persistent, refractory orofacial pain who cannot tolerate frontline treatments such as anticonvulsant medications, referral to neurosurgery is recommended for consideration of microvascular decompression of the trigeminal nerve, rhizotomy, or gamma knife radiosurgery targeting the trigeminal nerve.

Behavioral Therapies for the Treatment of Pain

In addition to the aforementioned pharmacological and nonpharmacological interventions, behavioral therapy plays a central role in the management of pain, particularly in older patients who are prone to the side effects of medications or may not be candidates for interventional treatment. Behavioral therapies represent safe and noninvasive techniques targeted to reduce pain, restore function and mobility, and improve overall physical and mental health. In fact, many patients themselves often directly state to their doctors that they are eager to try a more conservative treatment rather than initiate a new medication or undergo an invasive procedure.

For patients with chronic musculoskeletal pain, such as osteoarthritis or myofascial pain, physical therapy represents a noninvasive treatment to improve mobility, alleviate pain, and ultimately reduce disability and improve function for patients. For patients who do not have access to physical therapy, home care with stretching exercises and use of moist heat or ice as needed can help improve pain. In chronic pain conditions such as fibromyalgia, physical activity is recommended to reduce symptoms of pain and stiffness with the ultimate goal of improving daily function. While a combination of aerobic, resistance, and flexibility training is ideal, each regimen of exercise should be tailored to the individual and their functional goals. For example, in older patients with chronic pain and stiffness, a low impact alternative such as aquatic-based physical therapy or aquatic-based exercise may be indicated to maintain their mobility and reduce their pain.

Patients with chronic pain frequently experience significant emotional limitations due to their condition. In addition to their persistent, distressing pain, they may experience difficulties in obtaining a diagnosis and effective management, leading to feelings of discouragement and depressed mood. Some patients may develop disability due to their pain and isolate themselves from others. Psychological interventions have been well studied in the treatment of chronic pain conditions such as fibromyalgia, chronic low back pain, and rheumatoid arthritis. The goal of this treatment is to help patients cope with their pain and minimize any disability and distress. Evidence-based psychological interventions for patients with chronic pain

include both talk-based and behavioral therapy, such as cognitive behavioral therapy, acceptance and commitment therapy (ACT), and biofeedback. For patients who either lack access to a psychologist trained in cognitive behavioral therapy or are otherwise resistant to initiate treatment with a psychologist, mindfulness-based stress reduction techniques may be helpful as another mind-body approach to improve a patient's physical and mental health. Examples of stress reduction techniques include meditation, yoga, deep breathing exercises, and body scans. Such techniques are evidence-based to improve chronic pain such as low back pain, with the underlying goal of helping patients increase their awareness from moment to moment and allow them to accept any uncomfortable emotions and physical discomfort.

There are various complementary and alternative therapies that can potentially reduce pain, including acupuncture, massage therapy, Reiki healing, and dietary modifications or supplements, which many patients may seek out as an alternative to conventional Western medicine. As a clinician, it is important to support the patient as they develop their own approach to adapt to their chronic pain and maintain functionality and discuss these treatment options. Dietary modifications and supplements should also be reviewed with the patient to ensure no harmful side effects or interactions with their current medication regimen.

FURTHER READING

Booker SQ, Herr KA. Assessment and measurement of pain in adults in later life. *Clin Geriatr Med.* 2016; 32(4):677–692.

Brooks AK, Udoji MA. Interventional techniques for management of pain in older adults. *Clin Geriatr Med.* 2016;32(4):773–785.

By the 2019 American Geriatrics Society Beers Criteria® Update Expert Panel. American Geriatrics Society 2019 Updated AGS Beers Criteria® for potentially inappropriate medication use in older adults. *J Am Geriatr Soc.* 2019;67(4):674–694.

Centers for Disease Control and Prevention. (2016, January 1). Increases in drug and opioid overdose deaths—United States, 2000–2014. *Morbidity and Mortality Weekly Report.* https://www.cdc.gov/mmwr/preview/mmwrhtml/mm6450a3.htm?s_cid=mm6450a3_w. Accessed May 29, 2021.

Chau DL, Walker V, Pai L, Cho LM. Opiates and elderly: use and side effects. *Clin Interv Aging.* 2008;3(2):273–278.

Chiu IM, von Hehn CA, Woolf CJ. Neurogenic inflammation and the peripheral nervous system in host defense and immunopathology. *Nat Neurosci.* 2012;15(8):1063–1067.

Dahlhamer J, Lucas J, Zelaya, C, et al. Prevalence of Chronic Pain and High-Impact Chronic Pain Among

Adults — United States, 2016. *MMWR Morb Mortal Wkly Rep* 2018;67:1001–1006.

Department of Health and Human Services. (2016). Opioids in Medicare Part D: Concerns about extreme use and questionable prescribing. *Office of the Inspector General.* https://oig.hhs.gov/oei/reports/oei-02-17-00250.asp. Accessed May 29, 2021.

Dowell D, Haegerich TM, Chou R. CDC guideline for prescribing opioids for chronic pain—United States, 2016. *MMWR Recomm Rep.* 2016;65(No. RR-1):1–49.

Lautenbacher S, Peters JH, Heesen M, Scheel J, Kunz M. Age changes in pain perception: a systematic-review and meta-analysis of age effects on pain and tolerance thresholds. *Neurosci Biobehav Rev.* 2017;75:104–113.

Lee M, Silverman SM, Hansen H, Patel VB, Manchikanti L. A comprehensive review of opioid-induced hyperalgesia. *Pain Physician.* 2011;14(2):145–161.

Mitra S, Carlyle D, Kodumudi G, Kodumudi V, Vadivelu N. New advances in acute postoperative pain management. *Curr Pain Headache Rep.* 2018;22(5):35.

Pergolizzi J, Böger RH, Budd K, et al. Opioids and the management of chronic severe pain in the elderly: consensus statement of an International Expert Panel with focus on the six clinically most often used World Health Organization Step III opioids (buprenorphine, fentanyl, hydromorphone, methadone, morphine, oxycodone). *Pain Pract.* 2008;8(4):287–313.

Treede RD, Rief W, Barke A, et al. Chronic pain as a symptom or a disease: the IASP Classification of Chronic Pain for the International Classification of Diseases (ICD-11). *Pain.* 2019;160(1):19–27.

Williams ACC, Fisher E, Hearn L, Eccleston C. Psychological therapies for the management of chronic pain (excluding headache) in adults. *Cochrane Database Syst Rev.* 2020;8(8):CD007407.

Management of Common Nonpain Symptoms

Christine S. Ritchie, Alexander Smith, Christine Miaskowski

OVERVIEW: COMMON NONPAIN SYMPTOMS IN OLDER ADULTS

Advances in medicine have led to our ability to stave off many acute life-threatening events and have contributed to the development of numerous co-occurring chronic conditions defined as multimorbidity. The experience of multiple conditions is often characterized by an array of symptoms associated with these conditions and/or their treatments. The presence of bothersome symptoms in older adults may contribute to illness burden in ways that may not be predictable on the basis of any one diagnosed disorder. However, these symptoms have a negative influence on older adults' function and quality of life (QoL).

Many symptoms are addressed throughout this textbook: anorexia is covered in Chapter 30, sleep disorders in Chapter 44, dizziness in Chapter 45, pain in Chapter 68, depressed mood and anxiety in Chapters 65 and 66, and constipation in Chapter 87. The focus of this chapter is on overall symptom assessment, evaluation, and management of fatigue and shortness of breath, especially for those with advanced illness, and special considerations in the context of multimorbidity.

Multiple symptoms occur frequently in chronically ill older adults. Because many individual conditions, such as cancer, heart failure, and chronic obstructive pulmonary disease (COPD), are associated with high symptom burden, their accumulation contributes to a large and complex array of symptoms (**Figure 69-1**). In a nationally representative study of older adults that assessed for pain, fatigue, breathing difficulty, sleeping difficulty, depressed mood, and anxiety, 28% of the population had three or more symptoms. Of note, reduced physical function and falls were more common in those with higher symptom burden. In a population-based sample of older adults using a 10-item symptom tool, the average number of symptoms was 3.7 and one-third of the population had five or more. In this cohort, the most common nonpain symptoms were fatigue (48%), weakness (39%), constipation (36%), anxiety (36%), anhedonia or depression (37%), shortness of breath (35%), and poor appetite (17%). In a study of 318 adults followed by a housecalls program, 43% reported severe

Learning Objectives

- Review the prevalence of and assessment strategies used to evaluate common nonpain symptoms in older adults.
- Address the evaluation and management of fatigue and dyspnea.
- Describe symptom management considerations in the context of multimorbidity.

Key Clinical Points

1. Many older adults experience a higher symptom burden associated with multiple co-occurring conditions. Screening for common symptoms should be a routine component of a comprehensive geriatric assessment (CGA).

2. Multicomponent interventions that rely on nonpharmacologic treatments are most effective for the management of fatigue and breathlessness.

3. Because the evidence base for symptom management in older adults is sparse, especially for those with multiple chronic conditions, a thoughtful approach that is informed by patient preferences is necessary to optimize benefit and minimize adverse effects.

burden from one or more symptoms. The symptoms with the highest severity ratings were depression, pain, loss of appetite, and shortness of breath. Few longitudinal studies of the general older adult population have assessed changes in the symptom experience over time. Among 754 older adults in their last year of life, the monthly occurrence of one or more "restricting symptoms" was fairly constant in the first half of the year prior to death (20%). At approximately 5 months prior to death, the rate increased rapidly from 27% to 57% in the month prior to death.

	Cancer	CHF	COPD	CKD	Dementia	AIDS
1.	Pain (84%)	Breathlessness (88%)	Breathlessness (97%)	Fatigue (88%)	Breathlessness (46%)	Fatigue (73%)
2.	Fatigue (69%)	Fatigue (88%)	Fatigue (88%)	Sleep disturbance (82%)	Constipation (40%)	Pain (69%)
3.	Anorexia (66%)	Pain (75%)	Dry mouth (85%)	Anorexia (55%)	Pain (39%)	Dry mouth (54%)

FIGURE 69-1. Pain and nonpain symptoms in common chronic conditions. Top three most common (in rank order) symptoms by condition. AIDS, acquired immunodeficiency syndrome; CHF, congestive heart failure; CKD, chronic kidney disease; COPD, chronic obstructive pulmonary disease.

OVERALL EVALUATION OF SYMPTOMS

A CGA, historically did not include an assessment of pain or nonpain symptoms. More recent CGA versions have included systematic assessments of these symptoms.

Many symptom measures were developed initially for cancer patients and only evaluate symptoms over short time intervals. Other symptom measures focus on a particular disease without capturing the impact of nonindex conditions on symptoms. With few exceptions, nondisease-specific symptom inventories are not available for older adults with multiple conditions. One screening tool developed from a community-dwelling population of 1000 older adults, the Brief Symptom Inventory, assesses 10 common symptoms in older adults: shortness of breath, feeling tired or fatigued, problems with balance or dizziness, weakness, daily pain, stiffness, constipation, poor appetite, anxiety, and anhedonia. The tool shows discriminant and convergent validity. Another recently developed tool in Denmark captured 36 symptoms in a representative sample of 100,000 Danish people 20 years and older. The average number of symptoms reported by the population was 5.4. For each additional comorbid condition, one new symptom was added.

Many comprehensive symptom assessments were borrowed from oncology. The Memorial Symptom Assessment Scale (MSAS) measures the occurrence, severity, and distress of 32 symptoms and the Edmonton Symptom Assessment Scale measures 9 common symptoms on a 0 to 10 numerical rating scale. These instruments have been used to assess symptoms and multiple dimensions of the symptom experience in both geriatric and palliative care noncancer patients. The large number of items in the MSAS can be a practical barrier to its use in the clinical setting.

EVALUATION AND MANAGEMENT OF FATIGUE AND DYSPNEA

Evaluation of Fatigue

The prevalence of generalized fatigue in older adults varies from 5% to almost 70% depending on the measure used, the characteristics of the older adult population, the time of day fatigue is assessed, and the cut points used to determine fatigue. Regardless of the assessment tool, fatigue is associated with decreased function and increased mortality. In a study of 492 older primary care patients, the question "Do you feel tired most of the time?" identified older adults with a one and a half to almost twofold increased risk of mortality over 10 years. Other assessments for fatigue tend to be longer and assess multiple dimensions of fatigue, again, predominantly derived from oncology. The Brief Fatigue Inventory, a nine-item instrument that assesses severity of fatigue and the impact of fatigue on daily functioning in the past 24 hours, has good psychometric properties but has been predominantly used in cancer populations. More recently, the concept of fatigability developed as a complement to the symptom of fatigue. Fatigability measures how fatigued an individual feels in relation to defined activities (eg, how fatigued a person feels after a 5-minute treadmill test). It offers

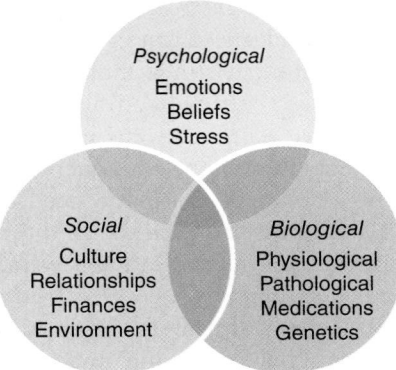

FIGURE 69-2. Biopsychosocial model.

a more standardized way to measure fatigue but is more difficult to integrate into standard practice.

A more comprehensive assessment of fatigue should address (1) when the fatigue began, whether the onset was sudden or more gradual; (2) the pattern of fatigue over the course of a day; (3) what exacerbates or improves the fatigue; and (4) the impact that fatigue has on daily function and relationships. Sleep characteristics and medications should be reviewed. Because psychological factors are often associated with fatigue, systematic assessment for depression is warranted.

The biopsychosocial model, commonly used to characterize pain, applies well to other symptoms, including fatigue. The biopsychosocial model posits that psychological, social, spiritual, and physical factors influence an individual's symptoms (**Figure 69-2**). In the case of fatigue, other factors such as obesity, depression, social isolation, loneliness, and spiritual distress may influence the experience of fatigue. A number of physical conditions are characterized by fatigue including electrolyte disturbances, occult malignancy, polymyalgia rheumatica, occult hepatitis, or HIV. Fatigue may be a silent harbinger of anemia or infection. In older adults, where atypical presentations of acute conditions are common, new-onset fatigue may indicate a recent myocardial infarction (MI) or heart failure. Hypogonadism is a less common cause of fatigue. Findings from the history and physical examination should dictate further diagnostic evaluation.

Management of Fatigue

Very few studies have addressed the management of fatigue in older adults; more trials have focused on chronic fatigue syndrome in younger adults. A few studies have evaluated fatiguability in context of frailty. Approaches that have not shown promise include protein supplementation, thyroid supplementation (in subclinical hypothyroidism), or testosterone (in men). Counseling, vitamin D3 (in those with vitamin D deficiency), and functional training have shown some promise. Improvement of older adults' sleep hygiene through both nonpharmacologic and pharmacologic

strategies (see Chapter 44) may reduce fatigue. While antidepressants may be beneficial, antidepressants with strong anticholinergic effects should be avoided (see Chapter 65). In the palliative care setting for older adults with advanced or life-limiting illnesses, psychostimulants such as methylphenidate or modafinil may be considered.

In a study of predominantly older prostate cancer patients (ages 52–94), methylphenidate reduced fatigue severity compared to control. However, a number of patients had to discontinue treatment due to increased blood pressure and tachycardia. A recent within-person crossover trial cast doubt on methylphenidate treatment of fatigue in advanced cancer. Among 43 participants who alternated between methylphenidate and placebo three times over a 9-day period, no improvement in fatigue during days with methylphenidate was observed. In older adults with known cardiovascular disease or arrhythmias, psychostimulants should not be used. While anecdotal reports touted the benefit of donepezil in treatment of opioid-induced fatigue in cancer patients, a subsequent clinical trial did not support these claims. In summary, fatigue is a common condition in older adults with likely multiple factors contributing to its prevalence.

Evaluation of Dyspnea (Breathlessness)

Due to the high rates of COPD and heart failure in older adults, along with an array of other comorbid conditions, shortness of breath (dyspnea) is very common in older adults. In an Australian primary care practice, over half of those who presented with shortness of breath were older than the age of 65. The prevalence of dyspnea in community-dwelling older adults ranges between 17% and 62%, depending on the population studied and cut point used to define "dyspnea." Dyspnea will likely occur at some point during a number of serious illnesses experienced by older adults (eg, cancer, heart failure, advanced lung disease), and at the end of life. The biopsychosocial model applies to dyspnea as well as it does to fatigue. Anxiety, disappointment, financial stressors, and questions about meaning often contribute significantly to the experience of dyspnea. Dyspnea, in turn, serves as a source of patient and caregiver distress and is associated with decreased QoL, decreased function, and increased health care utilization.

Physiologic mechanisms of dyspnea often fall under three categories: increased respiratory effort due to obstruction (eg, COPD, asthma, masses) or restriction (eg, obesity, pleural effusion); weakness (eg, multiple sclerosis, amyotrophic lateral sclerosis); or ventilation/perfusion mismatch (eg, anemia, pulmonary embolism, heart failure). More subtle systemic changes can contribute to the occurrence of dyspnea, especially at the end of life. For example, in the National Hospice Survey, 24% of patients with no known cardiopulmonary disease experienced dyspnea. The most appropriate measure of shortness of breath is the older adult's self-report. Dyspnea does not always correlate with hypoxia, hypercarbia, or the presence of tachypnea. Most self-report

GRADE	DEGREE OF BREATHLESSNESS
TABLE 69-1 ■ MEDICAL RESEARCH COUNCIL BREATHLESSNESS SCALE	
1	Not troubled by breathlessness except on strenuous exercise
2	Short of breath when hurrying on level ground or walking up a slight hill
3	Walks slower than most people on level ground, stops after a mile or so, or stops after 15 min walking at own pace
4	Stops for breath after walking about 100 yd or after a few minutes on level ground
5	Too breathless to leave the house, or breathless when undressing

tools to assess dyspnea come from the obstructive lung disease literature. One of the most common assessment tools is the Medical Research Council (MRC) breathlessness scale. First published in the 1950s, the MRC scale characterizes, through five statements, a range of disability caused by level of breathlessness (**Table 69-1**). It correlates well with other dyspnea scales and with other direct measures of function, such as walking speed.

Management of Shortness of Breath

Nonpharmacologic approaches to breathlessness have few side effects, unlike morphine for example, and avoid polypharmacy, a major concern in the older adults. They should be considered alongside pharmacologic approaches as first-line therapy. Nonpharmacologic approaches that can be helpful in the treatment of dyspnea include the use of a fan, breathing techniques, mindfulness and relaxation, anxiety management, and energy conservation. Breathing techniques that can reduce the sensation of dyspnea include pursed lip breathing, prolonged exhalation, and posture modification. In addition to mindfulness and relaxation, guided imagery and distraction strategies (eg, music, TV, reading by self or caregiver) were shown to reduce the sensation of breathlessness.

In patients with COPD and hypoxia, long-term oxygen therapy increases QoL and prolongs survival. Likewise, in a subset of patients with COPD, noninvasive ventilatory support such as with bilevel positive airway pressure (BiPaP) can improve QoL and prolong survival. In patients with advanced cancer and other nonpulmonary causes of dyspnea, the value of oxygen supplementation in improving outcomes is less clear. These results may be in part due to the fact that less than half of advanced cancer patients with dyspnea are hypoxic. In a study of nasal cannula–delivered air versus nasal cannula–delivered oxygen (median age 65), no difference was found in dyspnea relief between the two modalities when patients were not hypoxic; in two studies of hypoxic cancer patients, more

benefit from oxygen was noted. Recent studies of noninvasive ventilation in advanced cancer patients suggest that it may improve symptoms. In a multisite study of 200 predominantly older adults with advanced cancer (mean age 71), noninvasive ventilation was more effective than oxygen supplementation alone in reducing dyspnea and decreasing the amount of morphine needed to control symptoms. However, more patients in the noninvasive ventilation arm discontinued treatment primarily due to mask intolerance and anxiety.

Pharmacologic treatment for dyspnea should first and foremost be directed to the underlying cause of dyspnea, if known. Treatment may include a β-agonist for COPD or a diuretic in the case of heart failure. In a subset of patients, breathlessness persists at rest or on minimal exertion despite optimal treatment of the underlying chronic condition. These patients are described as having refractory dyspnea. In patients with refractory dyspnea, opioids may be beneficial. A number of studies of opioids for the treatment of refractory dyspnea in the setting of advanced illness demonstrate some benefit. However, the findings of reduced dyspnea (compared to control) are not consistent, and many studies remain underpowered to produce conclusive findings. Unfortunately, many of these studies use morphine, which has active metabolites (eg, morphine-6-glucornide, morphine-3-glucoronide). Morphine-3-glucoronide builds up in renal insufficiency, common in older adults and is responsible for symptoms of neurotoxicity (eg, hyperalgesia, allodynia, myoclonus). In older adults, opioids are associated with decreased mental functioning. For some patients, decreased mental functioning will not be acceptable despite its potentially positive impact on breathing.

IMPACT OF MULTIMORBIDITY ON SYMPTOM MANAGEMENT AND PATIENT DECISION MAKING

For older adults, multimorbidity is the norm not the exception. Over 90% of Americans age 65 and older have two or more chronic conditions. In older adults, symptom burden increases with increasing numbers of co-occurring conditions and is associated with doubled mortality rates and reduced QoL.

Symptom Management in Multimorbidity

Multimorbidity can constrain options for management of symptoms. Many pharmacologic treatments for symptoms have adverse effects that are magnified in patients with multimorbidity. For those with heart failure or hypertension, nonsteroidal anti-inflammatory agents often exacerbate these conditions. For those with cognitive impairment, opioids may make confusion more marked. Well known to those caring for older adults, initiation of one medication for one condition or symptom often leads to side effects that require use of a second medication to manage the side effects—the "prescribing cascade." Analgesics provide an apt illustration of this phenomenon. The use of a nonsteroidal anti-inflammatory drug (for those in whom it is not contraindicated) often requires additional medications to reduce the risk of potential negative gastrointestinal (GI) (eg, the addition of a proton pump inhibitor to reduce risk of GI bleeding) or cardiovascular (eg, the addition of aspirin to reduce the risk of MI or stroke) outcomes. In the case of opioids, patients must routinely be started on bowel stimulants or other laxatives to avoid the expected side effect of constipation.

Even without taking into account these challenges, many medications used to address symptoms have not been evaluated in older adults or in adults with multimorbidity. Among the symptom-focused studies done in older adults with advanced illness or multimorbidity, the most evidence exists for management of pain, and to a much lesser degree, dyspnea in cancer. There is a dearth of evidence for how to manage symptoms in noncancer illnesses, let alone in patients with several diseases. Therefore, the true benefits and the true risks are largely unknown. For this reason, pharmacologic management of symptoms warrants thoughtful discussions with the patient and/or family caregivers, as well as cautious initiation and careful monitoring of both the positive and negative effects of the treatment. For many older adults, symptom management involves both relief of discomfort and development of new drug-induced challenges. Anticipatory and ongoing discussion of the benefits and burdens of pharmacologic symptom management in the context of the patient's goals and preferences offers an ongoing person-centered approach to improving the older person's QoL.

The Role of Patient Preference in Symptom Management

Given the lack of evidence for optimal symptom management for older adults in general and in particular for older adults with multimorbidity, treatment strategies for symptom management are preference sensitive—that is there is often more than one reasonable treatment option, or a particular option offers uncertain benefit. For preference-sensitive decisions, the clinician must understand what is most important to the patient to determine what might be the best treatment option. A starting point may involve asking patients to prioritize a set of universal health outcomes that can be applied across individual diseases. Typical outcomes would include living as long as possible, maintaining function, staying cognitively intact, and alleviating pain and other symptoms. Other outcomes may include staying out of the hospital or dying at home. While not always mutually exclusive, understanding how patients prioritize these various outcomes can help guide decisions about symptom management. This broad-based approach provides a more

unified starting point, rather than asking patients or caregivers to make specific treatment decisions.

Optimal decisions regarding symptom management require that the patient is adequately informed about the expected benefits and harms of different treatment options for their symptoms, recognizing that in many instances optimal information is lacking. Actual decision-making preferences vary widely by patients and family caregivers. Some individuals prefer to make the decision themselves, while others prefer that the decision for a specific treatment be made by the clinician. In either instance, most individuals want their opinion used to guide the decision-making process. Then, the clinician can develop a management plan and evaluate at regular intervals whether the management plan remains concordant with patient's wishes. Reevaluation of treatment plans is critical as studies suggest that older adults with multimorbidity engage in dynamic reassessments of their conditions, as they shift between experiencing disruption from the condition and finding the ability to adapt to the condition's challenges.

The following case illustrates these decision-making issues. Consider an 86-year-old man with advanced COPD who presents to the emergency department acutely dyspneic. He wants to live a few more days to say goodbye to family members and friends, even if it means living in the hospital. He does not want to be intubated or sent to the intensive care unit (ICU). He agrees to try BiPAP while initiating diureses. He expresses immediate profound relief of dyspnea upon securing the mask. However, the next morning, he asks that the mask be removed as it seems suffocating. He has had the opportunity to talk to his family and the distress associated with the BiPAP mask no longer makes it worthwhile. The patient's clarity around what is important to him can guide the clinician in these preference-sensitive treatment decisions.

SUMMARY

Experiencing multiple symptoms is common in older adults and particularly common in older adults with multimorbidity. For most symptoms, pharmacologic and nonpharmacologic approaches have some evidence base. Unfortunately, the evidence base is very limited for older adults, especially for those with multiple chronic conditions. Because the evidence base for symptom management is so sparse, treatments are preference sensitive and should take into account the values and preferences of older patients and their caregivers. Universal outcomes around function, cognition, comfort, and survival may be good starting points regarding which treatment options make the most sense. Ultimately more research will be needed to ascertain which treatments are the most beneficial for older adults and those with multimorbidity.

FURTHER READING

Eldadah BA. Fatigue and fatigability in older adults. *PMR*. 2010;2(5):406–413.

Elnegaard S, Andersen RS, Pedersen AF, et al. Self-reported symptoms and healthcare seeking in the general population—exploring "The Symptom Iceberg". *BMC Public Health*. 2015;15:685.

Glynn NW, Santanasto AJ, Simonsick EM, et al. The Pittsburgh Fatigability Scale for older adults: development and validation. *J Am Geriatr Soc*. 2015;63(1):130–135.

Hardy SE, Studenski SA. Fatigue predicts mortality among older adults. *J Am Geriatr Soc*. 2008;56(10):1910–1914.

Jones PW, Harding G, Berry P, Wiklund I, Chen W-H, Leidy NK. Development and first validation of the COPD assessment test. *Eur Respir J*. 2009;34:648–654.

Jones PW, Quirk FH, Baveystock CM. The St George's respiratory questionnaire. *Respir Med*. 1991;85(suppl B): 25–31.

King DE, Xiang J, Pilkerton CS. Multimorbidity trends in United States adults, 1988-2014. *J Am Board Fam Med*. 2018;31(4):503–513

Lehti TE, Öhman H, Knuutila M, et al. Symptom burden is associated with psychological wellbeing and mortality in older adults. *J Nutr Health Aging*. 2021;25(3):330–334.

Mahmoud AM, Biello F, Maggiora PM, et al. A randomized clinical study on the impact of Comprehensive Geriatric Assessment (CGA) based interventions on the quality of life of elderly, frail, onco-hematologic patients candidate to anticancer therapy: protocol of the ONCO-Aging study. *BMC Geriatr*. 2021;21(1):320.

Martinez-Amezcua P, Simonsick EM, Wanigatunga AA, et al. Association between adiposity and perceived physical fatigability in mid- to late life. *Obesity (Silver Spring)*. 2019;27(7):1177–1183.

Mendoza TR, Wang XS, Cleeland CS, et al. The rapid assessment of fatigue severity in cancer patients—use of the Brief Fatigue Inventory. *Cancer*. 1999;85:1186–1196.

Mitchell GK, Hardy JR, Nikles CJ, et al. The effect of methylphenidate on fatigue in advanced cancer: an aggregated N-of-1 trial. *J Pain Symptom Manage*. 2015;50(3): 289–296.

Morris RL, Sanders C, Kennedy AP, Rogers A. Shifting priorities in multimorbidity: a longitudinal qualitative study of patient's prioritization of multiple conditions. *Chronic Illn*. 2011;7(2):147–161.

Nava S, Ferrer M, Esquinas A, et al. Palliative use of noninvasive ventilation in end-of-life patients with solid tumours: a randomised feasibility trial. *Lancet Oncol*. 2013;14(3):219–227.

Patel KV, Guralnik JM, Phelan EA, et al. Symptom burden among community-dwelling older adults in the United States. *J Am Geriatr Soc*. 2019;67(2):223–231.

Portenoy RK, Thaler HT, Kornblith AB, et al. The Memorial Symptom Assessment Scale: an instrument for the evaluation of symptom prevalence, characteristics and distress. *Eur J Cancer*. 1994;30A:1326–1336.

Ritchie CS, Hearld KR, Gross A, et al. Measuring symptoms in community-dwelling older adults: the psychometric properties of a brief symptom screen. *Med Care*. 2013;51(10):949–955.

Smith MEB, Nelson HD, Haney E, et al. *Diagnosis and Treatment of Myalgic Encephalomyelitis/Chronic Fatigue Syndrome. Evidence Report/Technology Assessment No. 219. AHRQ Publication No. 15-E001-EF*. Rockville, MD: Agency for Healthcare Research and Quality; December 2014. Addendum July 2016. www.effectivehealthcare.ahrq.gov/reports/final.cfm. Accessed January 3, 2022.

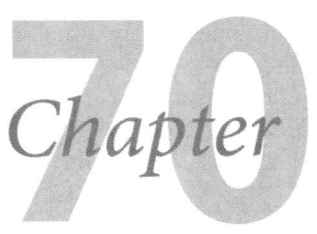

Chapter 70

Palliative Care Across Care Settings

Lisa Cooper, Laura Frain, Nelia Jain

INTRODUCTION

Consider Mrs. M, an 85-year old woman with congestive heart failure, mild cognitive impairment, and multijoint osteoarthritis, who lives alone in a second-floor, walk-up apartment. Mrs. M retired from her part-time secretarial work at the age of 70 to care for her husband with Lewy body dementia and has been widowed for the past 5 years. Mrs. M recently agreed to try ambulating with a walker after her third trip to the emergency room for falls but frequently forgets to use it. Her daughter, an only child, lives in the same city and helps her mother shop and clean. In the past, she accompanied her mother to medical appointments but has been unable to do so regularly in the past 2 years due to her work schedule and helping care for her grandchildren. Although Mrs. M never missed medical appointments in the past, she now has "no-showed" to most visits including for follow-up after being evaluated in the emergency room. Her daughter receives a call from a concerned neighbor who reports that her mother only rarely comes out of her apartment, and when she does, seems confused and unsteady. Her daughter has had similar concerns, and additionally worries that her mom appears to be in pain most days, depressed, and losing weight. She takes a day off from work to bring her mom to see her primary care doctor; but, prior to the appointment, she gets a call from the emergency room that her mother fell again resulting in a broken hip requiring surgery. Mrs. M's postoperative course is complicated by delirium and pain. She is transferred to a skilled nursing facility for rehabilitation where the team raises the concern that Mrs. M now has moderate dementia, frailty, and significant gait impairment. They recommend a more supportive living environment. Mrs. M moves in with her daughter and enrolls in a home-based primary care program. Initially, Mrs. M does well, with notable improvements in her mood, weight, walking, pain control, and cognitive health. However, over the next 2 years, her dementia progresses with increasingly severe behavioral and psychological symptoms and rising care needs. She becomes nearly wheelchair bound due to pain when walking. With limited support for her mom at home and now facing her own medical issues, her daughter admits Mrs. M to a nursing home. Mrs. M is hospitalized three times over the next year. She enrolls in hospice after the third hospitalization and survives another year.

Learning Objectives

- Conceptualize the ideal model of palliative care provision for the aging population facing multimorbidity and progressive functional impairment across care settings.
- Identify existing deficiencies and barriers to the adequate delivery of palliative care for older adults across the care continuum.
- Illustrate how effective collaboration between geriatrics and palliative care services with integration of palliative care interventions into existing models of care can help bridge these gaps.

Key Clinical Points

1. The palliative care needs of older adults differ from younger populations due to differences in illness trajectories, treatment preferences, and patterns of health care utilization.

2. Although the highest proportion of palliative care needs for older adults exists in the community setting, access to palliative care is concentrated in acute care settings and through hospice utilization.

3. Older adults often experience advancing frailty and multiple complex conditions, necessitating an integrated approach between geriatrics and palliative care specialties to meet the needs of this population across their trajectory of functional decline and increasing needs for care and support.

The case of Mrs M illustrates the need for a truly integrated system of palliative and geriatric care that meets the medical and social needs of older adults across the care continuum. Palliative care aims to improve the quality of life for persons with serious and advanced illness by decreasing symptom burden, addressing psychological and spiritual distress, and promoting well-being of patients and their families. The types of care that would help support Mrs. M's quality of life vary as her health circumstances and care settings change. These include, but are by no means limited to, (1) advance care planning conversations to delineate the patient's goals, values, and preferences and ensure goal-concordant care; (2) assessment and treatment of postoperative pain and delirium with heightened monitoring for postoperative cognitive and functional decline; (3) an interprofessional team that can provide longitudinal care for the patient across various settings; (4) caregiver training and support for the patient's daughter; and (5) functional assessment and home adjustments to address needs for adaptive devices and therapy services.

Unfortunately, in reality, our current health care system is fragmented with a disproportionate focus on acute care and immediate post-acute care, often leading to a lack of emphasis on matching treatments to patient goals. In this chapter, we will describe the ideal of a palliative care system for older adults that delivers integrated care across the care continuum, including hospice. We will contrast this ideal with the barriers to and lack of an integrated system for delivery of palliative care across the continuum. We will identify opportunities for improvement. We begin by discussing the tremendous overlap between the fields of geriatrics and palliative care.

GERIATRICS AND PALLIATIVE CARE ARE BETTER TOGETHER

The case of Mrs. M illustrates the blurred boundaries between geriatrics and palliative care (**Figure 70-1**). Geriatrics and palliative care both emphasize improving quality of life in late life. Both fields require excellence in management of persons with multimorbidity, dementia, and disability. Both fields emphasize attention not just to the patient, but also the patient's caregiver, and the situation of the patient within the context of family and community.

Both fields are directed primarily toward the sickest and most frail older adults, those that account for about half of health care spending in the United States.

By 2030, the number of Americans aged 65 or older is predicted to approach 73 million, representing 21% of the total US population. Eighty percent of all older adults have at least one chronic condition and 50% have a least two or more chronic conditions. Notably among these, the number of Americans living with Alzheimer disease is anticipated to double from 5.8 million, currently, to 13.8 million by 2050. It is also increasingly recognized that a substantial proportion of community-dwelling older adults are frail (~15%) and prefrail (45%). Like dementia, frailty is even more common at older ages, among women and racial and ethnic minorities, and with additional variability in prevalence based on geographic region, location of residence, and socioeconomic status.

In the setting of frailty and multiple chronic illnesses, older adults commonly experience long trajectories of functional decline and episodic fluctuations in health status. They frequently face repeated, nonlinear, and often difficult transitions across care settings, including the community, hospital, rehabilitation, and nursing facilities, and ultimately experience disjointed care. Older adults' family and physicians often have a poor understanding of their goals of care and have rarely engaged in discussions regarding treatment preferences.

Spurred by the needs of the aging population, there is increasing recognition that palliative care does not equate to "comfort care only" for the terminally ill. The recognition that geriatric palliative care approaches can have a major impact on symptom management, communication around goals of care, management of multiple chronic conditions, and caregiver support for all patients with advanced illness and frailty from the time of diagnosis is an invaluable step toward improving the quality of life for older adults.

The fields of geriatrics and palliative care have many common grounds, including providing goal-oriented care,

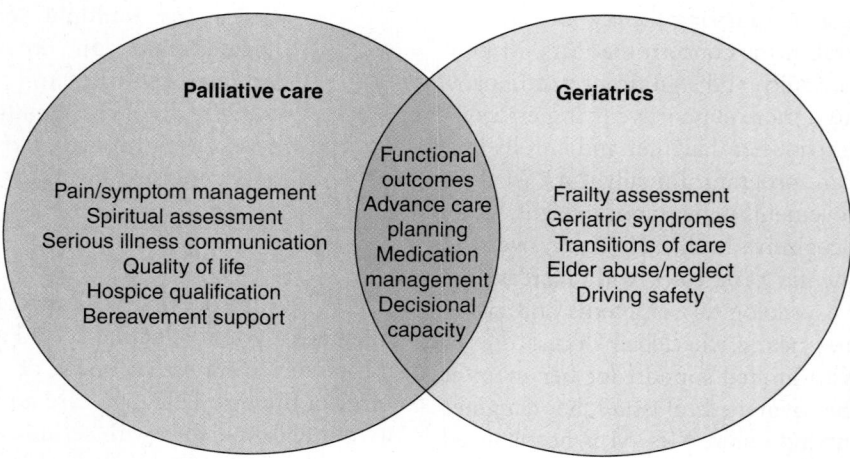

FIGURE 70-1. Intersection of palliative care and geriatrics.

working within an interprofessional team, using multidimensional assessments to identify unmet needs, attending to psychosocial factors, addressing caregivers' needs and including them in care planning and delivering, and adding valuable services to the most vulnerable and frail older adults. On the other hand, these intersections between geriatric medicine and palliative care give rise to unclear boundaries and limited understanding between the two professions. In addition, there are several gaps between the two fields. Palliative care contributes to patient care by offering intensive symptom management and psychosocial support; prognostication; alignment of goals and treatments between patients, families, and clinicians; and support in ethical decision making. Geriatric medicine offers a comprehensive geriatric assessment, including a better understanding of frailty and resilience, functional status, and expected trajectory. As such, the two specialties best serve patients when applied in a blended, interconnected way to deliver integrated patient care rather than in series (geriatrics, then palliative care). These care models can be implemented in different settings and best serve mutual patients as each specialty brings a unique and important aspect to the patient's care, with an ability to intensify or de-intensify a particular service's involvement depending on the patient's health state.

By simultaneously advocating for the holistic care of older adults, recognizing the specialized knowledge base and skills possessed by each discipline, and ensuring competency of future trainees in both geriatrics and palliative care, clinicians from both fields will be able to work together to target the sickest 5% of our population at highest risk, and match these patients with delivery models best suited to address their needs.

THE IDEAL OF A CARE CONTINUUM

The ideal of a continuum of care has been defined as, "a client-oriented system composed of both services and integrating mechanisms that guides and tracks clients over time through a comprehensive array of health, mental health, and social services spanning all levels of intensity of care." The introductory chapter in this section on palliative care introduced the concept that palliative care is appropriately initiated from the time of diagnosis with serious or advanced illness. For many, though not all, serious and advanced illnesses are diagnosed in the outpatient setting. The ideal care continuum would integrate palliative care into the settings where patients spend the most time after diagnosis, that is, in their homes. This would involve access to robust palliative care services along with integration of basic palliative care principles in ambulatory and home-based settings.

As patients develop more serious conditions, such as advancing frailty and dementia in the case of Mrs. M, they may require more care in acute institutional settings like skilled nursing facilities, hospitals, and nursing homes.

The ideal continuum of care would track patients as they move between settings, coordinate care across providers, and offer comprehensive services as people move between the community and the inpatient setting. As a patient's goals increasingly shift toward a focus on quality of life, high-quality palliative care services should take on a greater role in care, and be available in all settings.

THE REALITY OF PALLIATIVE CARE FOR OLDER ADULTS

Palliative care has been noted to improve quality of life and symptom management for patients, increase satisfaction of patients and their family members, and reduce health care costs. However, in the current health care system, palliative care is most readily made available to patients during times of crisis (acute inpatient hospitalization) or at the end of life (hospice). The majority of older adults' last months and years are still spent in the community, with institutionalization occurring only in the very late stages of life. There has been less progress noted in the area of nonhospice palliative care in nursing homes or the community setting, including assisted living and home-based programs, suggesting that the current level of palliative care services does not adequately address the needs of older adults.

Palliative care needs for older adults with advancing frailty differ from the needs of younger adults. Older adults tend to have prolonged illness duration with numerous chronic and complex medical conditions. Older patients experience greater functional and cognitive decline, and they also have increased caregiving needs for longer periods of time. Less is known about how older adults and their caregivers cope with the stressors of chronic illness compared to younger adults with sudden changes in health such as a new cancer diagnosis. Additionally, due to exclusion of older adults with multimorbidity from many research studies, there is a paucity of evidence to guide symptom management in this population. While older adults typically die of chronic, slowly progressive illnesses with multiple acute exacerbations, current Medicare coverage is targeted to the acute episodes of illness. This has resulted in palliative care that has been implemented in a reactionary fashion to these acute episodes. This approach insufficiently addresses patients' longer-term needs and creates missed opportunities for palliation along the disease trajectory (**Figure 70-2**).

In addition, frailty increases with age. While there are many different ways to define and capture frailty, they all are based on multidimensional vulnerabilities that cause susceptibility to stressors and reduced adaptive capacity and resilience to these acute events. Since increasing levels of frailty can present with gradual functional and cognitive decline, the trajectory might be less clear than single disease-based clinical evaluation. This also means that palliative care and supportive care might be needed for a longer period of time. Currently, there is no indicator of frailty in hospice-eligible criteria since the removal of

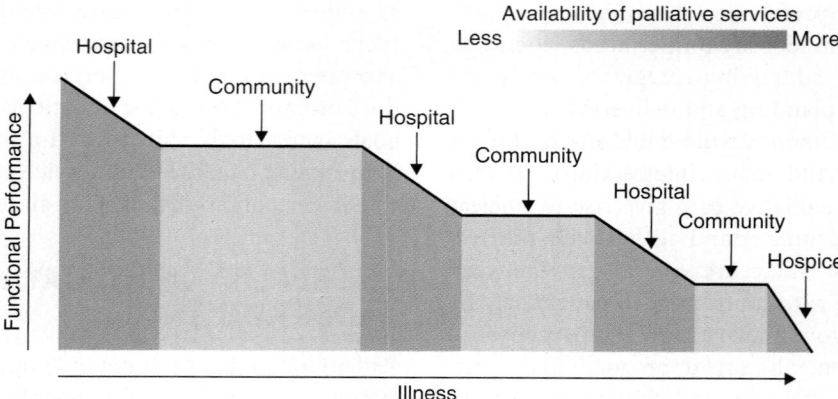

FIGURE 70-2. Gaps in palliative care services for older adults.

"adult failure to thrive" and "debility" as principle diagnoses for hospice eligibility in 2014 despite the Centers of Medicare and Medicaid Services 2009 report indicating a marked increase in the use of these diagnoses.

Better defining frailty and its expected trajectory, together with periodic measures and assessment of increasing health care needs, might assist in engaging palliative care approaches earlier and help in understanding poor outcomes from medical interventions. One area that can be addressed with increasing levels of frailty is polypharmacy and deprescribing, which has been shown to be beneficial in frail older adults, especially when the focus becomes more on quality of life and symptom control and avoiding side effects and medications that are unlikely to contribute any meaningful effect. Palliative care approaches are needed when patients and family are facing advancing frailty; however, due to the complexity of definition and wide range of presentation, these needs are often unmet. A true collaboration between geriatrics and palliative care experts can address this increasing gap.

In order to adequately address the needs of older adults, palliative care must be instituted in a timely manner, earlier in the course of a patient's illness. Upstream involvement of palliative care in the care of older adults, particularly while they are still residing in the community, allows for increased opportunities for shared decision making, constant evaluation of a patient's prognosis and symptom burden, and longitudinal care throughout different care settings. In addition to routine palliative care, clinicians have the opportunity to work with patients' primary care physicians, geriatricians, and specialists to emphasize function, financial planning, and maintenance of social roles within a community. This collaboration is even more integral when caring for older adults who often experience multiple concurrent progressive conditions that may challenge the formulation of prognostic estimates in terms of time and function. Effective palliative care for older adults will require moving away from a focus on single

disease trajectory toward understanding and assessment of patient's reserves and vulnerabilities in addition to their values and treatment preferences to guide medical decision making. This foundation will aid in easing transitions to higher levels of care and help patients avoid inappropriate or burdensome treatments.

PALLIATIVE CARE IN THE ACUTE CARE SETTING

Of all settings, palliative care services in the acute inpatient setting have enjoyed the most successful implementation and advancement in the last 20 years. In the inpatient setting, palliative care teams are interprofessional, comprised of a mix of physicians, social workers, nurses, and chaplains. These teams offer expertise in symptom management, support to medical teams as well as patients and families, knowledge about community-based palliative care services and hospice organizations, and assistance in prognostication over a variety of illnesses.

Given that the majority of patients with advanced or serious illness will spend some time in the hospital throughout the course of their illness, and that up to 50% of adult deaths occur in the hospital setting, ensuring adequate palliative care services in the inpatient setting is of particular importance. There is increasing evidence that inpatient palliative care interventions improve the quality of clinical care, increase patient and family satisfaction, improve transitions of patients out of the hospital, and reduce health care costs. Patients who receive inpatient palliative care consultations incur less laboratory and radiology costs, are less likely to be admitted to the intensive care unit (ICU), and spend less days in the ICU once admitted compared to patients receiving usual care, particularly among patients who die during hospitalization.

Older adults receiving palliative care consultation differ in characteristics and interventions compared to younger patients. Referral for palliative care consultation for older adults is more likely to be requested for disease processes other than cancer and for goals of care discussions rather than symptom management. Older adults tend to be referred to palliative care earlier in their hospital courses and have documented code statuses of "do-not-resuscitate" at time of consult. In the oldest subset of the population (80 and older), patients were more likely to be referred to palliative care for diagnosis of dementia, less likely to be included in discussions around goals of care due to lack of decisional capacity, and more likely to be discharged to nursing homes. In reviewing palliative care interventions offered by age, there are fewer interventions for pain or symptom management offered in older adults and an increased likelihood of limits placed on life-sustaining treatments after consultation. Given these differences, inpatient palliative care teams should be prepared to meet the unique palliative care needs of older adults.

Despite the advancements that have been made in inpatient palliative care, as well as the positive patient and family outcomes that have been observed, challenges remain in the delivery of palliative care in the inpatient setting. Inpatient palliative care teams continue to struggle with late requests for consultation. In addition, constant turnover of inpatient treatment teams, hesitation to move away from a curative focus, and varying levels of knowledge about and alignment with palliative care from referring clinicians pose ongoing barriers to optimal palliative care provision. Due to the acuity and complexity of medical issues present in the hospitalized patient population, it is often difficult for palliative care teams to address all of the needs of these patients during the acute hospitalization, particularly when caring for older adults with complex comorbidities and multifaceted care needs.

In order to address deficiencies that remain in the delivery of palliative care in the inpatient setting, there are opportunities to consider upstream involvement of palliative care as well as integration of palliative care services within existing models of care in the inpatient setting. Rates of presentation to the emergency department (ED) increase with age, and the percentages of patients requiring hospital admission are highest in older adults. As the population continues to age, there will be a rising number of seriously ill older adults who will present to the ED. These needs may be met by identification of ED palliative care "champions" such as nurse managers and care facilitators, routine use of screening tools to evaluate the need for palliative care assessment in this population, development of care pathways as a product of collaboration between ED and palliative care teams, availability of palliative care consultative services to the ED, and familiarity with community palliative care and hospice resources among ED teams.

An organized approach to the identification, assessment, and management of older adults' complex medical, social, psychological, and functional concerns and vulnerabilities is key. For patients admitted to inpatient hospital floors, utilization of such a systematic approach by an interprofessional team will ensure the needs of older adults are met. As previously discussed, older adults receiving palliative care consultation are more likely to have nononcologic diagnoses, which are associated with less predictable hospital courses and illness trajectories. As the hospital course unfolds, communication interventions should target the status of the patient's overall condition, estimated prognosis in terms of functional recovery and life expectancy, and available treatment options in the context of associated risks and likelihood of benefit. Clinicians with an understanding of basic palliative care assessment may be successful in appropriately identifying palliative care needs on day of admission, engaging palliative care teams upstream in the hospital stay of seriously ill older adults, monitoring progress on clinical improvement and achievement of patient's goals, and frequently reevaluating to identify new palliative care needs in the older adult population as they arise throughout the hospitalization (**Figure 70-3A and 3B**).

Emerging opportunities for early introduction of palliative care models include programs such as geriatric comanagement with orthopedic surgery and general surgery, with the geriatric-surgery verification program from the American College of Surgeons being adopted by an increasing numbers of medical centers, and with emerging geriatric-ED initiatives. Such programs advocate for early collaboration with geriatric medicine clinicians, who perform an early frailty, cognitive and functional assessment, and assist the team in tailoring treatment plans to specific characteristics and needs of the older patient. Within these models, comanagement with palliative care teams may be considered for patients in instances such as facilitation of complex communication and medical decision making, reevaluation of goals of care based on changes in the patient's clinical trajectory, or easing end of life transitions.

The ICU is another location in the inpatient setting with the most opportunities for successful delivery of palliative care to older adults. Older adults admitted to the ICU have high mortality rates during the course of their hospitalization, and older ICU survivors have elevated palliative care needs for ongoing physical and/or psychological distress. They also remain at increased risk for rehospitalization and 6-month mortality. Studies have demonstrated that patients, families, and clinicians may possess unrealistic expectations about prognosis and effectiveness of ICU interventions. Critically ill patients and their caregivers often seek more honest and open discussions regarding prognosis and appropriate therapies based on patients' values and goals. ICU clinicians should all receive training in core skills of primary palliative care, including serious-illness communication skills and symptom management. Palliative care "bundles" have been suggested to improve communication and promote the comfort of critically ill patients (IPAL-ICU). Key quality measures in these bundles include early identification and documentation of surrogate decision makers and advance directives, regular

1081

PART IV

PRINCIPLES OF PALLIATIVE MEDICINE AND ETHICS

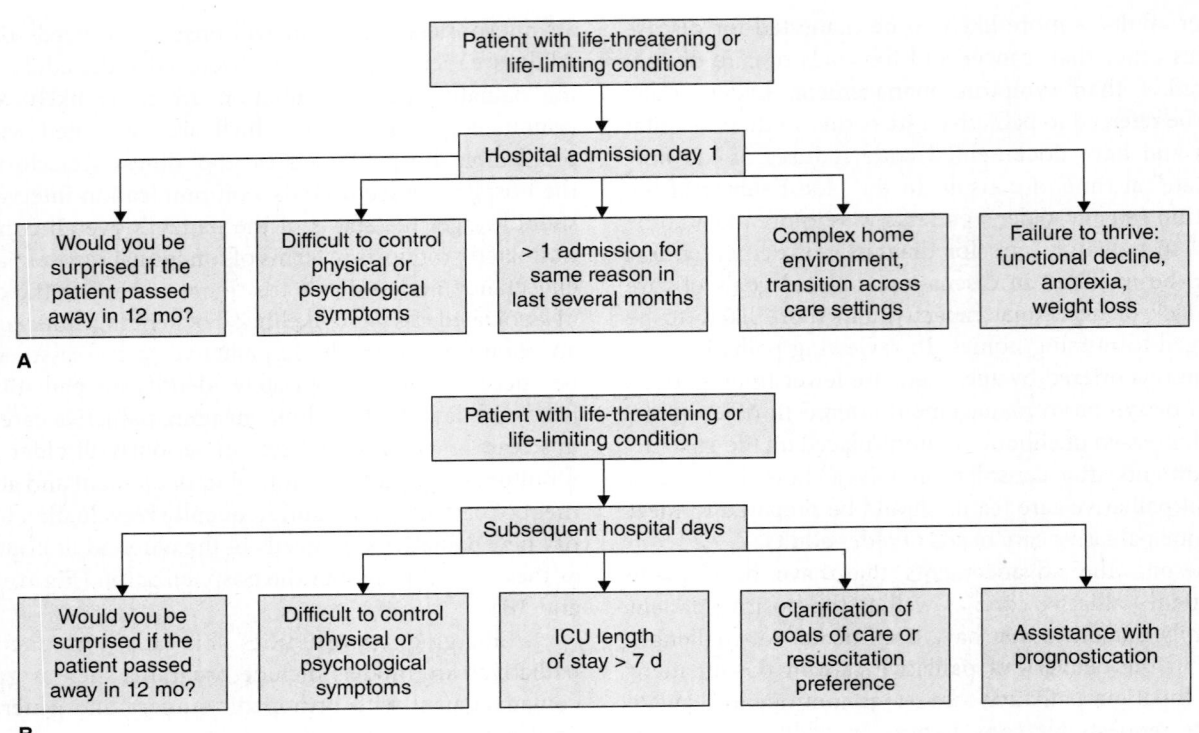

FIGURE 70-3 **A.** Inpatient criteria: guide for primary teams to prompt palliative care consultation on day of admission.
B. Inpatient criteria: guide for primary teams to prompt palliative care consultation on subsequent days of hospital admission.

symptom assessment, involvement of social work and spiritual care, and regular family meetings to update the patient and family on the status of the patient's illness. By emphasizing compassionate communication, symptom management, and shared decision making, palliative care can be successfully integrated for critically ill patients at all stages of illness.

Across the inpatient setting, collaboration between palliative care teams and patients' longitudinal outpatient clinicians, in particular geriatricians and/or primary care physicians, care managers or care transition specialists can bridge gaps in knowledge of patients' values and treatment preferences, communication, and appropriate identification of community resources to best meet the patients' needs for their current health state. Additionally, novel pathways to meet the unique hospital-based considerations of older adults offer further opportunity for palliative care integration and comanagement, particularly for patients experiencing high symptom burden or for those patients and families benefiting from ongoing goal clarification and assistance in complex medical decision making.

PALLIATIVE CARE IN POST-ACUTE CARE SETTINGS

Many older adults with complex care needs are living and now also dying in the community. Older individuals of advancing age often live alone, particularly women, with estimates of over 50% for women ages 85 and older in 2018. Approximately 21% of these community-dwelling older adults, totaling approximately 7.5 million individuals, are partly or completely homebound, and tend to be older, female, ethnic and cultural minorities, and have lower income. Despite a high burden of chronic conditions, especially dementia, and reports of lower health status, these older adults struggle or are not able to access the ambulatory care needed for their complex medical, psychosocial, and neurologic needs, and have high rates of hospitalization, leading to increased fragmentation of care. Despite the cycle of recurrent fluctuations in health and transitions in care, older adults' family (if present) and physicians often have limited understanding of their goals of care and care needs, prognosis, and have rarely engaged in discussions regarding treatment and care preferences. This is particularly problematic as family caregivers still provide the majority of direct care for US older adults with complex health conditions, and much of this care occurs in the community as opposed to nursing facilities. Additionally, growing evidence suggests that older adults living at home with dementia are more likely to have bothersome pain, dyspnea, and mood symptoms compared with people living in nursing or other residential facilities, with similar patterns seen among other vulnerable older adults in the community. Community-based palliative care services are currently available through both home-based and institutional-based models (**Figure 70-4**).

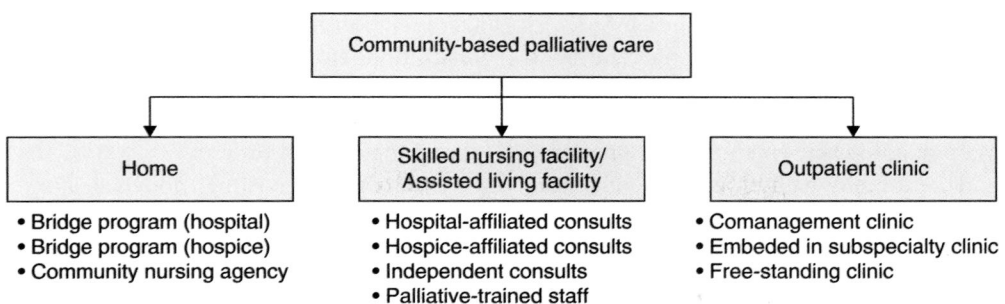

FIGURE 70-4. Palliative care delivery models in the community.

PALLIATIVE CARE IN THE CLINIC

For older adults whose functional status remains preserved or who have sufficient assistance to access care in the ambulatory setting, palliative care clinics facilitate the development of an early relationship between clinicians and patients, improve communication between primary care clinicians and other subspecialty clinicians, and increase satisfaction with care from the perspective of patients and their families. These clinics also serve as an appropriate setting for posthospital discharge follow-up for patients seen by inpatient palliative care teams.

There are a variety of existing models of palliative care clinics in our current health care system (Improving Outpatient Palliative Care [IPAL]). Some clinics are affiliated with particular specialties by which they generate all of their referrals. Other clinics are stand-alone clinics that function independently or share space and staffing with a primary care clinic or specialty clinic in a partially or completely embedded framework. Additionally, clinics vary in the focus of their care, ranging from providing task-specific to symptom-specific palliative care. Palliative care clinicians will often choose between providing care in a consultative or comanagement fashion for the majority of patients, while some patients will be taken care of entirely by the palliative care specialist. Finally, some clinics have the capability to extend their services beyond the clinic and into the community, providing visits to clinic patients who become homebound or transfer to a facility.

Outpatient palliative care services have been associated with improved patient outcomes, such as significant symptom improvement and high satisfaction with services. Care provided in palliative care clinics has also been associated with better maintenance of performance status, increased discussions about advance care planning and end-of-life care, and better long-term outcomes for caregivers. Patients receiving care in palliative care clinics in addition to usual care experience fewer hospital days and skilled nursing facility days, as well as increased hospice use. Clinicians also benefit, with increased rates of satisfaction observed in referring clinicians as well as palliative care clinicians.

Presently, the majority of outpatient palliative care clinics focus on care for patients with cancer diagnoses. As outpatient clinic services expand, particularly to nononcology populations, clinicians may face challenges, including the lack of standardization of the development process, need for adequate marketing, and insufficient staffing to accommodate anticipated growth of the clinics. Promising examples of outpatient palliative care for individuals with serious, life-limiting non–cancer-related diagnoses are emerging. A 2020 pragmatic trial of integrated palliative care at three academic tertiary centers for individuals with Parkinson disease and related disorders demonstrated better quality of life, improved symptom burden and motor symptoms, as well as higher rates and quality of advance care directives in the intervention group compared to those receiving standard of care. Additionally, the study was suggestive of a benefit on caregiver strain by 1 year. Although care at each site was provided in an ambulatory setting and by an interprofessional team using standardized checklists, the specific model of care varied by institution. Encouragingly, the impact on outcomes was equally effective across sites and suggests flexibility may exist in the design of integrated palliative care in the outpatient clinical setting if fidelity to key palliative care quality domains is maintained.

There are several limitations that impede the delivery of ideal palliative care in the clinic setting. Patients with severe and advanced illness, particularly those with chronic illnesses, are always at risk of declining to the point that they are unable to make their outpatient clinic appointments. Unless clinics are associated with bridge programs designed to extend palliative care services to homes and facilities until patients qualify for hospice, provided the latter is an acceptable option to them, chronically ill patients with progressive functional and cognitive decline often experience a gap in the continuation of their palliative care services. In addition, clinics are often limited by their hours of operation and staffing, particularly lacking coverage by a health care provider 24 hours a day to manage any acute crises that may arise. Finally, given the heavy reliance on referrals from the inpatient setting, primary care clinics, and subspecialty clinics, palliative care clinics require a certain amount of "buy-in" from other disciplines in order to continue to operate. As the population with chronic conditions continues to grow and age, increased attention to availability of palliative care clinics, reimbursement for palliative care services, and relationship building between hospitals, long-term care institutions, and community-based home care organizations is needed to ensure that this population of patients will be able to receive palliative care outside of the hospital setting.

PALLIATIVE CARE IN THE HOME

There are an increasing proportion of older adults living at home with chronic illness with intensive symptom management and advance care planning needs who do not qualify for hospice. As older adults become increasingly homebound, they are at increased risk for symptom and illness burden. Completely homebound patients have a 2-year mortality of approximately 40%, demonstrating a natural intersection of palliative care provision within home-based care. The ideal home-based palliative care model is comprised of an interdisciplinary team of physicians, nurses, social workers, chaplains, home health aides, and pharmacists (similar to the home hospice model) who are able to provide services in coordination with the primary care clinician and specialists. Services would include pain and nonpain management, medication management, discussions about health care decision making and goals of care, caregiver support, attention to spiritual concerns and quality of life, arrangement of respite care, and assistance with the transition to hospice if needed. Specifically tailored to the chronically ill, frail older adult, home-based palliative care would ideally integrate with home-based primary care or other community geriatric care models with an expanded focus that includes education and support for caregivers, timely access to medications, optimal use of applicable community resources, home safety and comfort, and 24/7 access to a health care clinician in order to ensure continuity of care and manage acute crises. A closely integrated model of home-based palliative care with home-based primary/geriatric care is especially beneficial for patients and families who are facing the strain of longer, often unpredictable, but ultimately terminal illness trajectories with challenging, day-to-day prognostication and frequent health exacerbations due to even minor physiologic stressors. This situation is commonly faced when caregivers and clinicians provide longitudinal care for patients with frailty, dementia, and complex multimorbidity. While highly integrated palliative and primary care models existed in limited, most often capitated, health care settings, the most notable and long-standing being the VA Home-Based Primary Care program, new partnerships are now arising between other home-based primary/geriatric and palliative care programs in the context of the United States' evolving alternative payment models and the growth of for-profit practices in home-based medical care. Home-based palliative care organizations would benefit from relationships with home-based primary care as well as institutions such as hospitals, primary care clinics, specialty clinics, nursing homes, and hospice agencies in order to increase the referral base and promote longitudinal care across the care continuum.

Studies on existing models of home-based palliative care have demonstrated beneficial outcomes. The patient populations receiving home-based palliative care include patients with both cancer and noncancer diagnoses (eg, dementia, cardiac disease, pulmonary disease, etc). Benefits noted include improved symptom scores in areas such as depression, dyspnea, and anxiety, decreased overall cost of care, increased completion of advance directives, and increased rates of dying at home. Fewer visits to the ED and lower rates of hospitalization have been observed, without a difference in overall survival. Rates of referral to hospice are higher than among control patients without home-based palliative care. Of the patients who do enroll in hospice, those who have received home-based palliative care prior to this transition are noted to have longer days of enrollment in hospice as compared to those with usual care.

Despite the positive impact home-based palliative care programs have on community dwelling patients with serious and advanced illnesses, the advancement of palliative care in the arena of home-based care has limitations. Home-based palliative care delivery is highly variable and delivered by diverse sources including hospitals and large health systems, community hospice and home health agencies, and individual practices or organizations. Programs face economic barriers such as insufficient reimbursement for services in proportion to time spent, particularly for professions other than physicians and nurses, and a lack of incentive to reduce costs. Organizational barriers exist as well, primarily driven by the lack of adequate staffing to meet the needs of homebound older adults, as well as the lack of recognition and training around quality standards and measurement. At present, there is no standardization of home-based palliative care practices or institutional support, leading to difficulty in translating the beneficial outcomes that have been noted in existing home-based palliative care models to the broader population. While progress has been made in developing a quality framework that adequately represents the needs of the homebound population, there are ongoing efforts to address implementation, measurement, and reimbursement challenges. These standardized quality metrics have the potential to ensure that frail, cognitively impaired and functionally limited people experience improved quality of life while potentially reducing burdensome hospital visits and health care costs.

PALLIATIVE CARE IN LONG-TERM CARE FACILITIES

In adults older than the age of 65, approximately 25% of all deaths will occur in a nursing home, with projections of an increase to up to 40% of deaths of older Americans occurring in nursing homes by 2030. The majority of residents in long-term care facilities are older adults, experience progressive frailty and functional impairment, and require increased assistance in activities of daily living. For older adults in long-term care facilities, life expectancies are typically shorter in the order of years. With projections suggesting that the number of frail older adults may triple or quadruple in the next 30 years, closer examination is needed on the state of palliative care services in long-term care facilities. For many long-term care residents, hospice is the only form of specialty palliative care available.

What is known about palliative care services in long-term care facilities at present is limited. There are several studies that demonstrate long-term care residents suffer from uncontrolled symptoms, depression, existential suffering, and difficulty adjusting to the long-term care facility as their permanent place of residence. Older adults who do receive palliative care consultation have lower rates of end-of-life hospitalizations, with those who receive consultation further upstream in their illness experiencing lower overall rates of hospitalization and an almost 50% reduction in potentially burdensome transitions such as an emergency room visit within 30 days of death or admission to hospice within 3 days of death.

A number of significant barriers to providing adequate palliative care in long-term care facilities exist. Demographics of patients in long-term care facilities, particularly nursing homes, are changing, with increased numbers of patients with chronic illness and multiple medical problems. A large percentage of these patients have noncancer diagnoses, leading to increased difficulty with prognostication and late referrals to hospice. Nursing home residents are often high utilizers of acute care settings, increasing the risk that patient's values and treatment preferences are unknown or have not sufficiently been elucidated. These issues are further complicated by the fact that there is often high staff turnover at long-term care facilities, making it difficult to sustain palliative care educational efforts and ensure palliative care competency among staff.

With current reimbursement policies focusing on rehabilitation needs and sustenance, a seemingly high proportion of patients undergo aggressive restorative treatment such as intravenous hydration or insertion of feeding tube placement instead of shifting to aggressive palliative care or hospice care. In addition, short-stay residents in nursing homes who are paid for under the Medicare skilled nursing facility benefit following a hospitalization are only able to access the Medicare Hospice benefit if they revoke the skilled nursing facility benefit and pay for room and board out of pocket. These out-of-pocket costs are a major financial disincentive to short-stay residents to exercise the Medicare hospice benefit.

Guidelines for quality palliative care in nursing homes emphasize that palliative care does not require patients to forgo curative treatments nor relinquish subacute rehabilitation or hospitalization (National Consensus Project Guidelines for Quality Palliative Care). Three different models of delivering palliative care services in nursing homes have been proposed: (1) hospice partnerships, (2) external palliative care consultation services, and (3) facility-based palliative care teams. Regardless of the approach taken, sustainability is key. Measures that are critical to sustainability of palliative care interventions in the long-term care facility setting include ongoing education efforts, "buy-in" of palliative care by nursing home staff and clinicians, increased availability of nurses and patient aides, and working relationships with hospitals and community organizations including hospice to ensure continuity of palliative care across all settings.

HOSPICE

Hospice care is the most well-known provider of palliative care services in the community. Hospice care is a philosophy of care in which patients facing a life-limiting illness are approached in a holistic manner, with a focus on medical care and symptom management, as well as an interest in the emotional, spiritual, and future planning needs of the patient and family. There are now more than 4600 hospice organizations nationally, and these organizations serve over 1.5 million people. Of Medicare beneficiaries receiving hospice care in 2018, greater than 60% were older adults aged 65 and older. The greatest increase in hospice utilization was observed in patients aged 85 and older. Research on hospice care has demonstrated increased survival compared to usual care, increased patient and family satisfaction with end-of-life care, increased rates of patients dying in their location of choice, and decreased inappropriate health care resource utilization. Despite tremendous growth in the use of hospice services over the last 30 years, hospice care is still underutilized. A substantial number of patients who would prefer to die at home still die in the hospital. At present, the majority of patients receive hospice care at home. Nationally, hospice is not available in all long-term care facilities, and only 6% of residents in nursing homes elect the hospice benefit annually, far lower than one would expect given the short lengths of stay prior to death for many long-term care facility residents.

The Medicare hospice benefit requires that patients have a life expectancy of 6 months or less. An unfortunate but common misconception is that palliative care and hospice care are equivalent. This leads to missed opportunities for palliative care involvement in patients independent of prognosis, as well as late referrals to hospice care until clinicians are confident the patient is dying. This has translated to a median length of service in a hospice organization of 18 days. Over half of patients are enrolled in hospice for 30 days or less, of which 28% of patients die in the first 7 days. The extent of comprehensive palliative care delivered by hospice organizations also varies, with larger hospice organizations having the ability to provide more intensive services such as 24-hour physician staffing, ethics committees, and regularly using standardized assessment tools for pain and symptom management.

Cancer remains the most frequent principal hospice diagnosis of beneficiaries of hospice care. As discussed previously, the diseases affecting older adults are largely chronic in nature, with fluctuating trajectories marked by acute exacerbations and difficulties in prognostication, which in turn may reflect the timing with which clinicians refer older adults for hospice. To avoid the continued pattern of late referrals of older adults to hospice until they are in an advanced terminal state, efforts will need to be shifted upstream, with increased emphasis on improved palliative care delivery across care settings, and increased communication and collaboration between primary care and/or specialty clinicians caring for older adults with specialists in palliative care and hospice. Access and utilization of hospice care by older adults will improve by expanding coverage of hospice services to patients with longer life expectancies and eliminating the need for patients to choose between hospice services and other home-care or institutional-level services. Newer programs such as the Medicare Care Choices Model are exploring opportunities to provide eligible beneficiaries access to hospice services while they continue to receive disease-modifying treatment. Thus far, participants in this program have demonstrated increased likelihood of hospice enrollment, decreased reliance on inpatient care, and positive caregiver experiences. By reconceptualizing the population for whom hospice care is offered away from eligibility based on prognosis, and instead, on patients and their caregivers with increasing vulnerabilities and need for care and in-home supports, older adults may be able to benefit from the supportive and holistic care provided by hospice agencies for longer periods of time.

CONCLUSION

The field of palliative care has enjoyed significant advancements over the years. Its rapid growth is evidenced by an increased number of clinicians choosing to train in the field and the increased availability of palliative care teams in a variety of care settings. The more widespread implementation of palliative care has led to improved quality of life and symptom management for patients; improved satisfaction among patients, families, and health care providers; and, decreased health care costs. However, the presence of adequate palliative care for older adults has lagged behind. Older adults have unique palliative care needs that are best met by providing longitudinal palliative care across the care continuum. Implementation of palliative care for older adults at the time of diagnosis of advanced or serious illness or at a time where they are noted to develop progressive frailty or cumulative burden from multiple comorbidities would be ideal. Increased involvement of palliative care with a focus on collaboration and comanagement with geriatricians and other longitudinal clinicians will help older adults reside longer in their communities, maintain their level of function, cope with care transitions, and participate in shared decision making regarding their treatment preferences. The health care system will also need to change in order to train clinicians in primary palliative care skills, expand access to specialty palliative care particularly in the community, and increase coordination of care among institutions and community organizations. Addressing these gaps in the current palliative care models will improve the quality of palliative care delivered to older adults across the care continuum.

FURTHER READING

Bandeen-Roche K, Seplaki CL, Huang J, et al. Frailty in older adults: a nationally representative profile in the United States. *J Gerontol A Biol Sci Med Sci.* 2015;70(11):1427–1434.

Bowman BA, Twohig JS, Meier DE. Overcoming barriers to growth in home-based palliative. *Care. J Palliat Med.* 2019;22(4):408–412.

Bryant EA, Tulebaev S, Castillo-Angeles M, et al. Frailty identification and care pathway: an interdisciplinary approach to care for older trauma patients. *J Am Coll Surg.* 2019;228(6):852–859.e1.

Chen CY, Thorsteinsdottir B, Cha SS, et al. Health care outcomes and advance care planning in older adults who receive home-based palliative care: a pilot cohort study. *J Palliat Med.* 2015;18(1):38–44.

Cooper L, Abbett SK, Feng A, et al. Launching a Geriatric Surgery Center: recommendations from the Society

for Perioperative Assessment and Quality Improvement. *J Am Geriatr Soc.* 2020;68(9):1941–1946.

Hamaker ME, van den Bos F, Rostoft S. Frailty and palliative care. *BMJ Support Palliat Care.* 2020;10(3):262–264.

Harrison KL, Ritchie CS, Patel K, et al. Care settings and clinical characteristics of older adults with moderately severe dementia. *J Am Geriatr Soc.* 2019;67:1907–1912.

Kamal AH, Currow DC, Ritchie CS, Bull J, Abernethy AP. Community-based palliative care: the natural evolution for palliative care delivery in the U.S. *J Pain Symptom Manage.* 2013;46(2):254–264.

Kluger BM, Miyaski J, Katz M, et al. Comparison of integrated outpatient palliative care with standard care in patients with Parkinson disease and related disorders: a randomized clinical trial. *JAMA Neurol.* 2020;77(5): 551–560.

Leff B, Carlson CM, Sailiba D, Ritchie C. The invisible homebound: setting quality-of-care standards for home-based primary and palliative care. *Health Affairs.* 2015;34(1):21–29.

Miller SC, Lima JC, Intrator O, Martin E, Bull J, Hanson LC. Palliative care consultations in nursing homes and reductions in acute care use and potentially burdensome end-of-life transitions. *J Am Geriatr Soc.* 2016;64(11):2280–2287.

Nelson JE, Curtis JR, Mulkerin C, et al. Choosing and using screening criteria for palliative care consultation in the ICU: a report from the Improving Palliative Care in the ICU (IPAL-ICU) Advisory Board. *Crit Care Med.* 2013;41(10):2318–2327.

Olden AM, Holloway R, Ladwig S, Quill TE, Van Wijngaarden E. Palliative care needs and symptom patterns of hospitalized elders referred for consultation. *J Pain Symptom Manage.* 2011;42(3):410–418.

Ornstein KA, Leff B, Covinsky KE, et al. Epidemiology of the homebound population in the United States. *JAMA Intern Med.* 2015;175(7):1180–1186.

Pacala JT. Is palliative care the "new" geriatrics? Wrong question—we're better together. *J Am Geriatr Soc.* 2014;62(10):1968–1970.

Ritchie CS, Leff B. Population health and tailored medical care in the home: the roles of home-based primary care and home-based palliative care. *J Pain Symptom Manage.* 2018;55(3):1041–1046.

Smith AK, Thai JN, Bakitas MA, et al. The diverse landscape of palliative care clinics. *J Palliat Med.* 2013;16(6):661–668.

Visser R, Borgstrom E, Holti R. The overlap between geriatric medicine and palliative care: a scoping literature review. *J Appl Gerontol.* 2021;40(4):355–364.

Voumard R, Rubli Truchard E, Benaroyo L, Borasio GD, Büla C, Jox RJ. Geriatric palliative care: a view of its concept, challenges and strategies. *BMC Geriatr.* 2018;18(1):220.

Zimbroff RM, Ritchie CS, Leff B, Sheehan OC. Home-based primary and palliative care in the Medicaid program: systematic review of the literature. *J Am Geriatr Soc.* 2021;69(1):245–254.

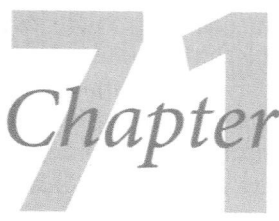

Chapter 71

Effective Communication Strategies For Patients with Serious Illness

Brook Calton, Matthew L. Russell

INTRODUCTION

Older adults are living longer, and with more chronic diseases, than ever before. The number of Americans ages 65 and older is projected to double from 52 million in 2018 to 95 million by 2060. The average US life expectancy increased from 68 years in 1950 to 79 years in 2017. Approximately 80% of older adults have at least one chronic medical condition; with 77% having at least two. In fact, the majority of hospice diagnoses are now noncancer related, such as congestive heart failure, chronic obstructive pulmonary failure, or dementia. Taken together, these data suggest effective communication around advanced illness is of ever-increasing importance for our older adults facing longer life trajectories, complex chronic illness, and debility and decline. Having achieved longevity, many older adults living with advanced illness prioritize goals such as function, comfort, and family support. Skillful communication is needed to ensure the treatments we offer align with these goals.

Effective communication with patients and families can have a number of benefits. It has been shown to improve diagnostic accuracy, health outcomes, treatment adherence, and patient satisfaction. In addition, effective end-of-life communication has been associated with decreased intensity of care, increased quality of life, and improved quality of dying for patients.

Studies consistently confirm the majority of patients facing advanced illness desire to have honest conversations about their goals, values, and end-of-life care with their providers. A recent systematic review of advance care planning in older adults found between 61% and 91% of older individuals wanted to discuss their end-of-life care with their providers. Benefits cited by patients included assurance their wishes would be respected, an opportunity to address important medical care and treatment issues before cognitive impairment or being physically unwell occurred, and to assist loved ones with decision making. They felt this responsibility to begin the discussion lies with physicians, they wanted to have the conversation in an open and honest manner, and preferred these conversations began early in their illness course.

However, despite the fact that communication around advanced illness is not only beneficial but also desired by

Learning Objectives

■ Describe a suggested six-step process for addressing goals of care and treatment preferences with patients who are seriously ill.

■ Identify unique challenges to communicating with seriously ill older adults and strategies to address them.

■ Summarize key communication techniques including ASK-TELL-ASK and SPIKES.

Key Clinical Points

1. **Data suggest patients and families generally desire to have open conversations with their medical providers around their goals of care, treatment preferences, and end-of-life wishes.**

2. **Conversations around goals, values, and treatment preferences should be held over time, as a patient's health status and/or perspectives evolve.**

3. **Clarifying patients, and families, understanding as well as effectively addressing emotions around serious illness can help make these conversations easier.**

most patients, this communication often remains inadequate. In studies, only an estimated 2% to 29% of frail older adults have discussed some form of end-of-life plans with a health care professional. In general, these discussions are often dominated by the clinician—in one study of 60 recorded patient-internist advance directive discussions, physicians spent 70% of the time talking and initiated more detailed discussions about patients values and goals less than 33% of the time. There are a number of challenges to effective communication that may contribute to the gaps described above. Potential barriers and suggested solutions are presented in **Table 71-1**.

In this chapter, we will provide an approach as well as key skills to prepare providers for having important

TABLE 71-1 ■ PROVIDER BARRIERS AND SUGGESTED SOLUTIONS TO ENHANCE COMMUNICATION AROUND ADVANCED ILLNESS

BARRIER	SUGGESTED SOLUTIONS
Provider time	• Reserve specific (and if possible, longer) visits for goals of care, advance care planning conversations • Have conversations over time, in small chunks, rather than in crisis only • Utilize resources (eg, prepareforyourcare.org) that help patients and family to reflect on their wishes before and after visits
Provider training	• Engage in standardized communication training during medical school and residency • Participate in continuing medical education (potential resources include Vital Talk and the American Academy of HealthCare Communication)
Prognostic uncertainty	• Acknowledge uncertainty upfront with patients • Frame discussions within best, worst, and most likely scenarios • Use prognostic calculators (eg, eprognosis.org)
Fear of offending patients	• Routinize goals of care and advance care planning conversations with all patients • Ask patient for permission to have conversation and how much information they want

conversations about goals of care and advance care planning with patients and families. We will also discuss unique challenges and situations specific to communication with older adults.

SUGGESTED APPROACH TO COMMUNICATING WITH PATIENTS WITH ADVANCED ILLNESS

Communication around advanced illness can take many forms. Potential conversations may include, but are not limited to, providing prognostic information, discussing treatment preferences, engaging in advance care planning, and transitioning to comfort care and/or hospice. It is important to remember, particularly in the outpatient setting, that any of these topics should be thought of as a process that occurs over time using open and honest communication that accounts for the patient's personal desire for information.

It is likely that patients' goals and preferences will shift over time as their illness progresses and/or what is important to them changes. Below we provide a suggested six-step approach that can be adapted to any of the conversations described above.

Step 1: Prepare

In the outpatient setting, if possible, it is optimal to ensure an adequate amount of protected clinic time to

have the conversation. Encourage the patient to bring family or caregivers with them that they would like to hear and/or participate in the conversation. Clarify medical treatment options and prognostic information with other providers engaged in the patient's care prior to the visit. In the inpatient setting, it is important to arrange for a private place to have the conversation and again, invite key family members, caregivers, and health care providers (eg, consulting MDs, bedside nurses, chaplains, etc) based on the patient's preferences. Prior to the conversation, meet briefly with the participating health care providers (premeeting) to agree upon an agenda, prognosis, suggested treatment course, etc.

Step 2: Clarify Patient's Understanding of Illness and Preferences for Information/Decision Making

Any conversation around advanced illness requires that the provider first assess the patient's understanding of their illness. If the patient is unable to participate in the conversation, the same process should be undertaken with the patient's family and/or designated medical decision maker, depending on the circumstances. This step, using open-ended questions, facilitates the provider's ability to successfully provide education around the patient's illness, discuss treatment options based on a shared understanding of the patient's condition, and avoid potential misunderstandings (**Table 71-2**).

Next, the patient's preferences for information and medical decision making should be clarified. This is critical because while most patients desire information about their illness and want to be involved in decision making, a significant minority do not. Asking these questions (and then proceeding accordingly) will build the patient's trust and empower them in these conversations (**Table 71-3**).

Step 3: Education and Exploration

Step 3 involves patient education and exploration of patients' hopes and values to facilitate medical decision making.

Once you have a sense of the amount of information the patient desires, the foundational communication skill ASK-TELL-ASK can be useful for providing patient education. You've already done the first "ASK" in step 2, by eliciting the patient's understanding of their illness. The provider should next "TELL" the patient in straightforward language the information they are hoping to

TABLE 71-2 ■ SUGGESTED LANGUAGE FOR ELICITING A PATIENT'S UNDERSTANDING OF THEIR ILLNESS

"Tell me how things are going for you."

"Just so we're on the same page, could you tell me what you have heard about your medical condition?"

"What do you understand about your current health situation?"

"What do you think is causing your illness?"

TABLE 71-3 ■ SUGGESTED LANGUAGE FOR ELICITING A PATIENT'S PREFERENCES FOR INFORMATION AND MEDICAL DECISION MAKING

Preferences for Information

"How much do you want to know about your illness?"

"I have information about your condition. Some patients want to know the details, other patients want me to talk to someone else. How do you feel?"

"Are you the type of person who wants detailed information about their health?"

Preferences for Medical Decision Making

"How involved would you like to be in medical decisions regarding your illness?"

"How do you like to make medical decisions with your doctors?"

"Some patients prefer to make medical decisions entirely on their own, others prefer to make the decision jointly with their doctor, and others prefer the doctor to decide for them. Where do you fall?"

convey (eg, help them better understand their illness, treatment preferences, difficult news, etc) in short, digestible chunks. The second "TELL" is an additional check for understanding or perspective. An easy way to ask is, *"To make sure I was explaining things clearly, can you summarize what I just said?"* This ASK-TELL-ASK cycle is often repeated several times during the same conversation, to ensure information is provided in a sensitive manner in digestible pieces.

Understanding a patient's hopes and values can help the provider provide sound medical advice in line with what is most important to the patient. A list of suggested questions is given in **Table 71-4**.

Step 4: Respond to Emotions

Providers often focus on the details of medical care and miss emotional cues. Responding to emotional cues is a key aspect of successful communication, building

TABLE 71-4 ■ SUGGESTED LANGUAGE FOR EXPLORING HOPES AND VALUES

Psychosocial Aspects of Illness

"What is the most difficult part of this illness for you and your family?"

What Gives Life Meaning

"As you think about what lies ahead, what is most important to you?"

"What do you enjoy?"

"How do you weigh quantity vs quality of life? What does quality of life mean to you?"

Hopes and Concerns

"When you think about the future, what do you hope for?"

"What do you fear about your illness?"

"When you think about getting very sick, what worries you the most?"

trust, and supporting patients. Clinicians can express empathy nonverbally and verbally. Eye contact, open body position, leaning in toward the patient, and when appropriate, light touch can be useful tools for showing nonverbal empathy. An invaluable tool for expressing verbal empathy employs the mnemonic "NURSE." Details of the mnemonic and sample language are provided in **Table 71-5**.

Step 5: Guide Decision Making

Every conversation is different and in many cases, exploring hopes, values, and emotions can be extremely beneficial, even without a specific medical decision to make. If there are decisions to make, the next step involves providing options to the patient that are consistent with what has been found out is important to them. Providers do not need to identify every possible option, particularly those that are inconsistent with the patient's expressed goals. Information should be given in small chunks and jargon should be avoided. Again, using Ask-Tell-Ask can allow for frequent stops to check for comprehension and provide clarifications or corrections if necessary. In many situations, based on what is understood about the patient's decision-making preferences from step 2, providers can ask for permission to provide a recommendation based on the patient's values and what is known about the medical circumstances. Many patients and families may need time and multiple discussions before they can make big changes in care or decisions, for example, to enroll in hospice or decide whether to go into a nursing home.

TABLE 71-5 ■ NURSE STATEMENTS AND SUGGESTED LANGUAGE

SKILL	TASK	SUGGESTED LANGUAGE
N: NAME	State the patient's emotion	*"It sounds like this experience has been frustrating."*
U: UNDERSTAND	Empathize with and legitimize the emotion	*"I can understand why you're nervous."*
R: RESPECT	Praise the patient for things they are proud of/have done well	*"You've taken incredible care of your mother."* *"I'm impressed by how thoughtfully you've approached this decision."*
S: SUPPORT	Show support	*"No matter what decision we make, I'll be here for you."*
E: EXPLORE	Ask the patient to elaborate on the emotion	*"Tell me more about how you're feeling."*

TABLE 71-6 ■ PROVIDING A RECOMMENDATION, SUGGESTED LANGUAGE

TASK	SUGGESTED LANGUAGE
Restate primary goal(s) and confirm understanding	*"Given what you have told me, it sounds like you want to continue treatments that may extend your life if your quality of life is similar to what it is now. Even if that means coming back to the hospital."* *"What I understand as most important to you is that you remain comfortable and we get you back home. Is that right?"*
Suggest possible plan(s) of care to meet goals	*"Have you heard of hospice? In my experience, it can be one of the best programs for achieving the goals you mentioned for symptom management and care in the home."* *"I'm hearing that you don't want a lot of medical interventions. Given that, I think we should consider focusing on symptom control as opposed to putting you on life support or doing CPR if your breathing gets worse. What do you think?"*

CPR, cardiopulmonary resuscitation.

In practice, this often means not expecting a decision to be made at the end of one discussion. Suggested language is in **Table 71-6.**

Step 6: Summarize and Plan

To close the conversation, the provider should summarize any decisions that were made during the discussion, offer to answer questions, and arrange a plan for follow-up. This is also an opportune time to reaffirm nonabandonment regardless of the outcome of the conversation and the goals of care. In both the outpatient and inpatient setting, this is also an opportune time to thank the patient for having this difficult conversation and remind them you are hoping this process of exploration and decision making will be an ongoing one, as time goes on and their health evolves.

STRATEGIES TO ADDRESS COMMUNICATION CHALLENGES WITH OLDER ADULTS

Communicating with older adults can come with a unique set of challenges. Specific age-related issues (eg, hearing and/or vision loss, decline in memory, slower processing of information) alongside psychosocial factors related to aging (eg, loss of identity, lessening of power/influence of one's life, and separation from family and friends) can impact communication. Studies have found in general, providers spend less time and take more of a paternal approach with older patients. Older patients may withhold information about symptoms or conditions the patient considers "normal for their age," such as pain—potentially hindering successful management of these important issues.

Hearing

Hearing loss is the third most common chronic condition reported by older adults.

Although older adults can compensate to a certain extent by devoting more cognitive effort to comprehension, this practice may limit the patient's ability to encode information into long-term memory, draw interferences, and follow complex conversations. Tips for communicating with patients with hearing loss include the following:

- Increase volume of speech slightly, speak a bit slower, and present information as clearly as possible.
- Avoid shouting as speaking loudly raises the pitch of the voice, making it difficult for patients with hearing impairment to understand.
- Keep good eye contact and sit directly facing the patient so the patient can supplement what they hear with lip reading. Keep lips at the patient's face level.
- Minimize use of the computer if possible.
- Make sure the meeting space is as quiet as possible. Close the door to noisy hallways. Turn off background music and TVs.
- Make use of pocket-talkers and encourage the patient to use their hearing aides, when available.

Memory Loss and Dementia

Working memory declines with age. Working memory is important for processing complex sentences (specifically, sentences with multiple imbedded clauses), which are common when discussing serious news, goals of care, and advance care planning with patients with advanced illness. To enhance comprehension, providers should attempt to break up individual pieces of information into separate sentences that could stand on their own. ASK-TELL-ASK (described earlier in this chapter) is a useful tool for confirming comprehension.

In cases where a patient suffers from dementia advanced enough to impair their ability to make their own medical decisions (or the patient lacks decision-making capacity for other reasons, such as delirium), effective communication with surrogate decision makers is critical. Important medical decisions by surrogates for patients with advanced dementia are common. In a study of 323 health care proxies for patients with advanced dementia, 40% recalled making at least one medical decision—the most common being around feeding (27%) and infections (21%). In a study of nursing home residents living with advanced dementia and in their last 3 months of life, surrogate decision makers who had an understanding of the patient's poor prognosis and the expected clinical complications in advanced dementia were much less likely to elect burdensome interventions than surrogates who lacked this understanding. This finding demonstrates the need for providers to, over time, educate the family for what to expect in the advance stages of dementia and to foreshadow what decisions may arise in the future.

In situations where a medical decision does need to be made by a surrogate decision maker for a patient with advanced dementia (or a patient who otherwise lacks capacity), the following communication approach is recommended. First, background information should be obtained, including reviewing the patient's advance directive with the surrogate decision maker, if available, and assessing what conversations the surrogate decision maker has had with the patient previously regarding their values and treatment preferences. This information may be sufficient to make some medical decisions, and in most situations, preferences on an advance directive should be honored.

When further discussion is needed, the next decision-making step relies on substituted judgment—asking what the patient would have wanted if he or she could tell us. Time spent with the surrogate decision maker reflecting on the patient's values (eg, what brought the patient pleasure of life, what did quality of life mean to them) can be invaluable in aiding with complex medical decisions. These include deceptively simple questions like, *Tell us about your mother.* We recommend, for this step, bringing the patient's "voice" into the decision-making process; for example, *"What would your mother choose if she could tell us?"* or *"Knowing your mother, what do you think would be most important to her right now?"* An appeal to substituted judgment may remove some of the burden, by framing the decision as the patient's own choice rather than the surrogate's.

When there is no reasonable basis on which to interpret how a patient would have made a medical decision, decisions should be made that are in the best interest of the patient. That is, the best path to promote the well-being of the patient as a unique person, in the context of their relationships, values, religion and spiritual beliefs, and culture. Providers should encourage surrogates to weigh the harms and benefit of various treatment options, including pain and suffering, the degree of and potential of benefit, and any impairments that will result from the treatment in question. Provider treatment recommendations, based on your understanding of the patient's values, can be very helpful here—and are encouraged. When best interest standards apply, the question becomes, *What do you think is best for your mother?* Occasionally, conflicts between what providers and surrogates feel is best to do arise, including questioning whether the surrogate is truly making decisions in the patient's best interest. Providers are encouraged to consult with their medical center's administration regarding next steps in these difficult, ethical situations.

Engaging the Supportive Network

Older patients may have formal or informal caregivers as well as family and friends who form a part of their support network. Engaging patient-identified supports is

key to promoting fruitful discussions. Family members and caregivers often accompany older adults to medical appointments. It is particularly important that caregivers (specifically, surrogate decision makers) be present for key conversations regarding an older adult's goals of care so they too can understand the patient's preferences. However, a common occurrence is that caregivers of older adults may unintentionally (or intentionally) fall into a pattern of "speaking for" the older patient. Sometimes, but not always, this is due to difficulties in communication including hearing or vision problems or memory impairment.

Although it is sometimes necessary for a caregiver to provide supplemental information, it should not serve as a substitute for direct communication between the older adult patient and provider. Maintain direct eye contact with the patient, allow extra time for the patient to answer questions, and avoid speaking in the third person about the patient. To help establish the patient's sense of autonomy and participation in their health care, continually attempt to redirect the conversation back to the patient if you find the caregiver is tending to talk over the patient.

Prognostic Uncertainty

As mentioned in the introduction, older adults are living longer, with more chronic conditions that affect their quality of life and prognosis. When it comes to prognosticating, this population can be more challenging to the provider than, for instance, patients with a more predictable, terminal illness such as metastatic cancer. Prognostic uncertainty may heighten providers' hesitancy to discuss prognosis with these complex patients. However we know these conversations are important, and desired by patients. In one study of frail older patients with a mean age of 73, a life-limiting illness, and a need for assistance in at least one instrumental activity of daily living, over half of the patients whose physician had never discussed prognosis reported wanting to discuss it. While providers often consider prognosis conversations as important to medical decision making (including, but not limited to, chronic disease management, cancer screening, initiation of dialysis, and advance care planning), many older adults find this information helpful in determining life choices (eg, financial decisions, long-term care and housing, and quality-of-life considerations like spending time with family). Using prognostic indexes, many of which can be found on the user-friendly E-Prognosis website (www.eprognosis.com), can help inform your estimates alongside the clinical picture for your individual patient. Additional techniques for approaching conversations where prognostic uncertainty is present are summarized in **Table 71-7.**

SPECIAL SITUATIONS
Discussing Difficult News

Difficult news is defined as any news that drastically and negatively alters the patient's view of his/her future. Although

TABLE 71-7 ■ ADDRESSING PROGNOSTIC UNCERTAINTY

TASK	SUGGESTED LANGUAGE
Acknowledge it is difficult to make a 100% certain prediction about the patient's prognosis	*"Like the weather, it is difficult for me to be 100% accurate regarding how long you have to live."*
Use NURSE statements to respond to the patient's emotion around uncertainty	*"I can imagine it's frustrating to not know exactly what will happen."*
Provide prognostic estimates using ranges, eg, days to weeks, weeks to months, months to years	*"My best estimate is that you have weeks to months to live."*
Provide estimates that relate to a population of patients, not just the patient in front of you	*"In patients with medical issues similar to yours, the data suggest patients live an additional 1–2 years."*
Ask open-ended questions that enhance understanding of what is important to your patient	*"How do you view your quality of life currently?"* *"How do you think about balancing quality of life with quantity?"* *"When you think about the future, what do you hope for?"* *"Would there be any circumstances under which you would find life not worth living?"*
After addressing emotion, gently encourage patients and families to refocus on the present, as opposed to fixating on uncertain future	*"What can we do now, given that we are unsure of exactly what the future will bring?"*

we often associate discussing difficult news with the practice of oncology, all providers, regardless of specialty, are called upon to discuss difficult news with patients. Difficult news may relate to a diagnosis (eg, terminal, chronic, cancer, etc), prognosis, test results significant for disease progression, a bad outcome, or even medical mistakes. For older adults, difficult news may come in the form of a loss of independence, such as being deemed unsafe to continue driving a car or, requiring a higher level of care that will force the patient to move from their home of many years. It is important to remember that (1) most patients want to know difficult news (in studies, 75–90%) and (2) how a patient responds to news is influenced by a patient's perspective, life experiences, occupation, personality and coping skills, religion, and social support. It is also important to recognize that a patient's desire for medical information and a family's desire to disclose such information (eg, the difficult news of a new cancer diagnosis) is influenced by a number of factors including, but not limited to, culture, ethnicity, religion, and past experiences with illness. Asking specifically about your patient's preferences regarding how much information they want to know about their health,

diagnosis, and treatment options and also how they prefer to make medical decisions is key to providing person-centered medical care.

When difficult news is communicated in an effective manner, it can have an important impact on patient satisfaction and decreasing patient anxiety and depression. Discussing difficult news poorly can not only negatively impact patient outcomes, but can also have short-term (eg, anxiety) and long-term (eg, feelings of failure, regret, identification, higher rate of "burn-out") effects on the provider. Challenges to discussing difficult news include providing information consistent with the patient's understanding of their disease, concerns about taking away patient hope, and addressing emotion. A useful roadmap for discussing difficult news uses the acronym SPIKES (**Table 71-8**). The GUIDE framework from VitalTalk (www.vitaltalk.org) can also be useful.

Tube Feeding in Advanced Dementia

Outcomes including death, aspiration pneumonia, functional status, and patient comfort are similar, if not better in some cases, for careful hand feeding compared to tube feeding in patients with advanced dementia (eg, bed-bound, unable to ambulate, and typically limited, if any, ability to communicate verbally alongside feeding difficulties, such as refusal of food, dysphagia, and/or recurrent aspiration). Additionally, the risk of hospitalization, ER visits, agitation, use of physical and chemical restraints, and incidence of pressure ulcers all appear to be higher with tube feeding as compared to careful hand feeding. Given this data, the American Geriatrics Society, in their "Choosing Wisely Campaign," does not recommend percutaneous feeding tubes in patients with advanced dementia and recommends oral assisted feeding instead.

Despite data that feeding tube placement in advanced dementia may not provide benefit, and may even cause harm, one of the most common communication challenges providers caring for older adults face revolves around these decisions. Insufficient education of patients and surrogates on the potential risks of tube feeding likely contributes to this challenge as does the important social and symbolic role food plays in many cultures and religions.

One of the best strategies for effectively addressing this issue is to start the conversation early. In most cases, outpatient providers will have an opportunity over months to years to observe their patient with advanced dementia's swallowing ability and progressively decreasing oral intake. After ruling out reversible causes, providers should continually educate patients (if able to engage), family members, caregivers, and surrogates that feeding difficulties are a sign of progressive, advanced dementia and you anticipate they will worsen over time. ASK-TELL-ASK, summarized earlier in *Step 3: Education and Exploration*, can be a particularly useful skill here to assess what a patient or family understands and provided targeted education around the natural history of dementia and feeding difficulties.

Discussions regarding preferences for feeding support should begin early in the course of dementia, ideally

TABLE 71-8 ▪ SPIKES FOR DISCUSSING DIFFICULT NEWS

S: Setup	• Ensure a private space where everyone can be seated • Obtain collateral information from other providers • Check in with yourself regarding your emotional status and worries regarding the conversation
P: Perception	• Use ASK-TELL-ASK to assess the patient's current understanding of their condition • Clarify misunderstandings
I: Invitation	• Find out how much information the patient wants to know (eg, *"How would you like me to talk with you about your test results?"* or *"I have some serious news about your health, would you like me to discuss with you or someone else?"*)
K: Knowledge	• Convey the difficult news in plain language without jargon (eg, *"The CT scan shows your cancer is not responding to the chemotherapy"* or *"Unfortunately, your vision has gotten worse to the point I think it is unsafe for you to be driving"*) • Pause for 10–15 seconds after you have delivered the difficult news to allow time for processing and emotion
E: Empathize	• Use empathetic statements to respond to patient emotions (draw upon the mnemonic NURSE found in **Table 71-5**) • Resist the temptation to make things better • Consider using "I wish" statements (eg, *"I wish I had better news"* or *"I wish things had turned out differently"*)
S: Summarize and Strategize	• Summarize the clinical information and plan next steps • Provide reassurance you will not abandon the patient • Ask patient to summarize information in his/her own words to check for understanding

when the patient's cognition is intact enough to express their own preferences. These discussions should not be delayed until a crisis develops. Any decisions made with the patient should be documented in the medical record and an advance directive. This decision-making process includes aligning what patients and families are hoping for, with the realistic expectations and potential outcomes of tube feeding. Questions that can be particularly helpful, both early in the patient's illness and in crisis situations (eg, recurrent hospitalizations for aspiration pneumonia in a patient with advanced dementia) include, *"What do you hope a feeding tube would do for you (or your loved one)?,"* *"What worries do you have about feeding tubes?,"* and *"Have you seen any other patients with severe dementia with a feeding tube? What do you think that experience was like for them?"*

End-of-Life Preferences

As older adults with advanced illness reach the end of their life it is important to be sure that the patients' wishes regarding resuscitation and ICU care are confirmed and documented. A recent study from Teno et al. found an evolving trend toward less in-hospital care, more deaths at home and in assisted living facilities, and fewer transitions of care among Medicare beneficiaries near the end of life. Equally if not more important is ensuring patients' wishes, including desire for hospitalization, hopes for what the end of their life would look like, and preferred place of death are discussed. Patient preferences should be revisited as their health status evolves as patient preferences for medical care change over time. When possible, it is critically important to ensure surrogate decision makers are present for

these important conversations so they are aware of the patient's wishes and appreciate nuisances of patient's preferences that may go uncaptured on advance care planning documents. Suggested language for exploring a patient's end-of-life preferences, beyond resuscitation, is given as following:

• *"If you were close to the end of your life, what would be most important to you?"*
• *"Do you have a sense of where you would prefer to be at the end of your life?"*
• *"Some patients feel strongly they'd like to die at home, while others don't have a preference. Do you?"*

CONCLUSION

Effective communication with older adults with advanced illness requires a diverse and flexible set of skills. Techniques including ASK-TELL-ASK, use of NURSE statements to address emotion, and the SPIKES model for delivering difficult news can be invaluable in overcoming some of the challenges to caring for older adults, including sensory deficits, memory problems, and prognostic uncertainty for patients facing multimorbidity and/or frailty. Despite the challenges, having these important conversations can be extremely rewarding. Most patients want to discuss these important issues with their providers. Furthermore, conversations around a patient's quality of life, goals of care, and advance care planning allow clinicians to match our treatment recommendations to patient's ultimate goals and values to provide them with the best care possible.

FURTHER READING

AGS Choosing Wisely Workgroup. American Geriatrics Society identifies five things that healthcare providers and patients should question. *J Am Geriatr Soc.* 2013; 61(4):622–631.

Back AL, Arnold RM, Baile WF, Tulsky JA, Fryer-Edwards K. Approaching difficult communication tasks in oncology. *CA Cancer J Clin.* 2005;55(3):164–177.

Back AL, Arnold RM, Tulsky JA. *Mastering Communication with Seriously Ill Patients: Balancing Honesty with Empathy and Hope.* Cambridge, MN: Cambridge University Press; 2009.

Clayton JM, Hancock KM, Butow PN, et al. Clinical practice guidelines for communicating prognosis and end-of-life issues with adults in the advanced stages of a life-limiting illness, and their caregivers. *Med J Aust* 2007;186:S77, S79, S83–108.

Fischer R, Ury W, Patton B. *Getting to Yes: Negotiating Agreement Without Giving In.* New York, NY: Penguin Books; 1981.

Mitchell SL, Teno JM, Kiely DK, et al. The clinical course of advanced dementia. *N Engl J Med.* 2009;361(16): 1529–1538.

Ritchie CS, Roth DL, Allman RM. Living with an aging parent: "It was a beautiful invitation." *JAMA.* 2011;306(7):746–753.

Smith AK, Williams BA, Lo B. Discussing overall prognosis with the very elderly. *N Engl J Med.* 2011;365(23): 2149–2151.

Sulmasy DP, Snyder L. Substituted interests and best judgments: an integrated model of surrogate decision making. *JAMA.* 2010 3;304(17):1946–1947.

Teno JM, Gozalo P, Trivedi AN, et al. Site of death, place of care, and health care transitions among US Medicare beneficiaries, 2000-2015. *JAMA.* 2018;320(3):264–271.

The Gerontological Society of America. *Communicating with Older Adults, An Evidence-Based Review of What Really Works.* Washington, DC; 2012.

van Vliet LM, Lindenberger E, van Weert JC. Communication with older, seriously ill patients. *Clin Geriatr Med.* 2015;31(2):219–230.

von Gunten CF, Ferris FD, Emanuel LL. The patient-physician relationship. Ensuring competency in end-of-life care: communication and relational skills. *JAMA.* 2000;284(23):3051–3057.

Widera EW, Rosenfeld KE, Fromme EK, Sulmasy DP, Arnold RM. Approaching patients and family members who hope for a miracle. *J Pain Symptom Manage.* 2011;42(1):119–125.

Chapter 72

Ethical Issues

Timothy W. Farrell, Caroline A. Vitale, Christina L. Bell, Elizabeth K. Vig

INTRODUCTION

Health care professionals who work with older individuals in diverse settings such as their homes, assisted living facilities, skilled nursing facilities, outpatient clinics, and hospitals may encounter ethical dilemmas in their work. Ethical dilemmas arise when there is uncertainty or disagreement between stakeholders about the right thing to do in a situation. Ethical dilemmas pertinent to older patients may include questions about the balance of patient privacy versus patient safety, patients' abilities to make their own medical decisions, decisions about preferred treatments at the end of life, and decisions made by surrogate decision-makers.

In this chapter, we will discuss a framework for approaching ethical dilemmas, and provide an overview of the ethics topics especially relevant to the care of older adults. Sections include: an approach to thinking about ethical dilemmas, moral distress in professional caregivers, breaking bad news, surrogate decision-making, ethical decisions at the end of life, dilemmas between honoring self-determination and individual/societal safety, ethical challenges in the nursing home setting, and resource allocation and ageism.

AN APPROACH TO THINKING ABOUT ETHICAL DILEMMAS

Case

Mrs. C is an 88-year-old woman with congestive heart failure, hypertension, atrial fibrillation, and chronic kidney disease. She lives alone in her own home. She was hospitalized last month for delirium secondary to a urinary tract infection. She is admitted again this month after a fall. While in the hospital, she is evaluated by physical therapy and occupational therapy who both recommend a short stay in a nursing home for rehabilitation. Mrs. C refuses to go to a nursing home and demands to return to her home. Her medical team insists that going directly home is not a safe discharge plan, and wants to require her to go to rehab.

Question: What is an ethically appropriate discharge plan for Mrs. C?

Health care professionals working with older patients may encounter ethical dilemmas, regardless of their discipline

Learning Objectives

- Discuss the steps in the CASES approach and how it is used to address ethical dilemmas.
- Define moral distress and identify risk factors for developing it.
- Explain the steps in the SPIKES approach to breaking bad news.
- Understand the need for surrogate decision-making to ensure appropriate care of many older adults.
- Explore the concepts of substituted judgment versus best interest.
- Gain insight into the experience of surrogate decision-makers and potential for surrogate distress after making difficult medical decisions.
- Describe the indications for palliative sedation.
- Recognize the barriers to cessation of driving.
- Discuss examples of ethical dilemmas that arise in nursing homes when the desire to maintain quality of care indicators is in conflict with promoting patient preferences and quality end of life care.
- Recognize ethical principles underlying health care resource allocation under conditions of resource scarcity, including arguments against excluding patients from healthcare resources based on age.

(Continued)

4. The majority of people want to be told if they have dementia.

5. Making medical decisions for loved ones can be very stressful for surrogate decision-makers.

6. Through a process of shared decision-making, patients or their surrogates share information about their goals and care preferences with clinicians, and their clinicians share pertinent medical information and make care recommendations based on the patient's values and goals.

7. Palliative sedation is a legal intervention of last resort to promote relief of intractable suffering for terminally ill patients who have comfort as their primary goal of care.

8. Physician aid in dying (PAD), also called physician-assisted suicide, is legal in some US states and countries. Euthanasia is not legal in the United States, but is legal in Belgium and the Netherlands.

9. Patients may raise the topic of PAD as a way to begin a conversation about the end of life. Clinicians should view this as an opportunity to talk about sources of intractable suffering and fears about dying regardless of whether or not they live in a state where the practice is legal.

10. Questions about whether or not to report concerns about an older individual's driving are answered by weighing the clinician's duty to protect the patient's safety, with the duty to maintain confidentiality, and the duty to protect the public. Some US states have mandatory reporting requirements.

11. Ethical issues prevalent in nursing homes include not only those in which the patient and family's care goals are in conflict, but also those in which regulations are in conflict with quality end of life care.

12. Triage committees, and not front-line health care providers, should make decisions about allocation of limited heath care resources under conditions of resource scarcity, and patient age should not factor into these decisions.

or work setting. Ethical dilemmas usually stem from a conflict in values between stakeholders. For example, an older patient with multiple comorbidities, who values being alive regardless of his condition, may disagree with his physician about the best way to manage his advanced kidney disease. To add complexity, older adults are a heterogeneous group with diverse values, preferences, and goals that may or may not be influenced by their race, ethnicity, or religious backgrounds. In terms of their beliefs about end-of-life care, for example, older patients may have more heterogeneous views than their clinicians. Because of this heterogeneity, clinicians should not assume that they know a patient's values and goals without engaging in a conversation with the patient.

Ethical dilemmas may be distressing to health care professionals. Although health care professionals learned about ethics in their training, many are not familiar with a standard approach to thinking about and responding to ethical dilemmas. Without knowledge of such an approach, ethical dilemmas encountered may lead to moral distress and burnout. Familiarity with a framework and using a standard approach to thinking about ethical dilemmas may help health care professionals to find ways to resolve them, while honoring patient preferences, and reducing their own stress.

Different frameworks for approaching ethical dilemmas exist. One approach is the four-box method from Jonsen et al., in which important information about the patient's medical condition, preferences, quality of life, and other contextual features of the case is collected. Another is the CASES approach to ethical dilemmas which has been developed and is used by ethics consultants throughout the Veterans Administration (VA) health care system (see **Table 72-1** and Further Reading). Although this approach was developed for use by ethics consultants, the approach also can be applied by others who are trying to better understand ethical dilemmas. Since the second step of the CASES approach is similar to the four-box method, let us apply the CASES approach to the case of Mrs. C above.

The first step of the CASES approach is to Clarify whether the dilemma is really about ethics or something else, such as a legal issue. This is done by identifying whether there is a conflict in values between two of the involved stakeholders about the right thing to do. To do this, we try to understand the perspectives and values of the involved stakeholders, and identify which values are in conflict. In the case of Mrs. C, the conflict in values is between Mrs. C, who doesn't want to go to a nursing home for rehab, but wants to go home, and her medical team that believes sending her home would be harmful to her. This dilemma also can be viewed as a conflict between ethical principles. In the case of Mrs. C, the conflict in principles is between honoring Mrs. C's autonomy/self-determination and promoting both beneficence and nonmaleficence.

In the second step of the CASES approach, information relevant to the case is Assembled. This information includes medical information, patient preferences, other parties' preferences, and ethics knowledge. In the case of Mrs. C, we already know that she has multiple medical problems, lives alone, is in her second hospitalization, and

TABLE 72-1 ■ THE CASES APPROACH

1. C—Clarify
   a. Does this case involve an ethics concern about the right thing to do?
   b. What is the conflict in values that is leading to the concern?
      i. Values are defined as strongly held beliefs, ideals, principles, or standards that inform ethical decisions or actions.
2. A—Assemble the relevant information
   a. What types of information is needed?
      i. Medical facts
      ii. Patients preferences and interests
      iii. Other parties' preferences and interests
      iv. Ethics knowledge
         1. Codes of ethics, ethics guidelines, and consensus statements
         2. Published literature
         3. Precedent cases
         4. Institutional policy and documents, and law
         5. Outside ethics experts
   b. Which stakeholders need to be interviewed?
3. S—Synthesize the information
   a. Analyze the information
      i. Review the range of ethically justifiable options
      ii. Weigh the different potential outcomes and the impact of these outcomes on the stakeholders
4. E—Explain the synthesis
   a. Communicate the ethically justifiable options to the key stakeholders
5. S—Support the consultation process
   a. Follow up with stakeholders

Data from Berkowitz KA, Chanko BL, Foglia MB, et al. Ethics Consultation: Responding to Ethics Questions in Health Care, 2nd ed. Washington, DC: U.S. Department of Veterans Affairs; 2015.

is staunch in her refusal to go to a nursing home for rehab. Knowing her reason for refusing this would be helpful. For example, she might tell us that her husband died in a nursing home after a prolonged decline from dementia, and that she gets flashbacks and panic attacks whenever she enters a nursing home. Or, she might tell us that she needs to get home to care for her frail neighbor. We would want to hear more from Mrs. C's medical team about their concerns, and what they believe they can and cannot allow their patients to do. In thinking about this case, it also might be helpful to look at the hospital's policies around informed consent and refusal of care, and to search for pertinent literature about this issue (see Further Reading).

Once we have gathered the relevant information about Mrs. C's case, including the stakeholders' perspectives, we would need to begin to consider the different possible options and the impacts of each option on the stakeholders. In the Synthesize step, we would weigh the potential risks and benefits to Mrs. C of honoring her preference and sending her home versus insisting that she be discharged to sub-acute rehab. An important aspect of the case is whether Mrs. C has decisional capacity

to make the "poor" decision to return to her home or not. (Decisional capacity is discussed in Chapter 10.) In assessing her capacity to make this specific decision, it would be important to find out if she understands the risks and benefits of going to a nursing home for rehab versus going directly home.

If Mrs. C has decisional capacity to make the decision to go home, her medical team cannot force her to go to a nursing home against her will. In light of this, her team should consider ways to promote her continued recovery and safety at home. This could include arranging for more resources in her home, such as a visiting nurse, physical therapist, occupational therapist, Meals on Wheels, and a product she could use to quickly call for help in the future. Or it might involve brainstorming about how to get help for her frail neighbor, so she would feel more comfortable going to the nursing home for rehab.

If Mrs. C lacks decisional capacity to make the decision to go home, then the medical team will need to involve her legal surrogate decision-maker to help make this decision. Since some states have laws forbidding placement of individuals in nursing homes against their will, finding a solution could prove to be difficult, and might involve substantial negotiating and developing creative solutions.

When the CASES approach is used by health care professionals to understand the nuances of ethical dilemmas in their work, the last two steps of the approach are less critical than they are for ethics consultants. These last two steps are included for ethics consultants to help ensure that their recommendations are shared with those involved with the case and that appropriate follow-up occurs. However, as a health care professional uses this approach and gains a deeper understanding of a case, he/she may want to share that information with others who are involved. It also may be helpful to identify recurrent ethical dilemmas within an organization, and determine if systems level interventions are needed.

ETHICAL DILEMMAS CAN LEAD TO MORAL DISTRESS IN PROFESSIONAL CAREGIVERS

Case

Mr. G is a 78-year-old skilled nursing facility resident with multiple medical problems, including mild dementia, who is admitted to the intensive care unit with pneumonia and possibly sepsis. He is intubated. Over the next 2 weeks, he develops acute respiratory distress syndrome (ARDS), *Clostridium difficile* colitis, and a pressure ulcer. His renal function is deteriorating. He remains delirious, and is therefore unable to participate in medical decision-making.

Mr. G's advance directive states that he wouldn't want life-prolonging measures for a terminal condition, and would want care focused on comfort. His wife, whom he designated as his health care agent through a Durable Power of Attorney for Health Care, insists that treatments with the goal of life prolongation be continued. His nurses are concerned that his prognosis is poor and his preferences aren't being honored. His physicians say he isn't "terminal" yet.

His nurses are concerned that he has pain. They note that he grimaces when they care for him. His wife refuses for him to have pain medications because of a fear that they will prevent him from waking up.

When the doctors, nurses, social workers, and the chaplain have tried to talk to Mrs. G about her husband's goals of care or his pain management, she becomes agitated and threatens lawsuits. Team members are frustrated. Rumors begin to circulate that Mrs. G is demented, in denial, revengeful, and wanting to keep him alive for his pension. Some have commented that scarce resources are being wasted in keeping him alive.

Question: In reading this case, can you sense the distress experienced by those caring for Mr. G?

Moral distress is a term that was coined by Jameton in 1984. Moral distress occurs when someone or something prevents you from doing what you believe is right, forcing you to act contrary to your core values. In other words, you believe you are providing care that is morally wrong. Although moral distress has been studied most in nursing, it has been documented in numerous health care professions, and even in health care leaders. Health care professionals who interact with older patients may personally experience moral distress, and also may interact with colleagues who are experiencing it.

There are numerous root causes of moral distress (see Table 72-2). These causes may be due to clinical factors of a case, but also may be due to individual characteristics of members of the care team, or to institutional factors. Multiple members of the care team may experience moral distress about a given case, but may experience this distress from different aspects of the case.

One theory of moral distress holds that one's level of distress does not return to baseline after experiencing an episode of moral distress, but that, with each case, one's "moral residue" increases to a new baseline. Thus, over time, there is a crescendo in a clinician's moral residue. This crescendo of moral residue and "untreated" moral distress can lead to burnout, to individuals leaving their positions, and even to individuals leaving their professions. This can be psychologically costly for individuals and financially costly for institutions (**Figure 72-1**).

After recognizing that a case is causing moral distress, what can health care professionals do about it? One helpful intervention is for the team to talk about the case and the aspects of the case that are giving each of them moral distress. Building one's moral resilience may be helpful (see Further Reading). Finally, if organizational factors are leading to moral distress in staff, these need to be brought to the attention of the organization's management.

TABLE 72-2 ■ SELECTED ROOT CAUSES OF MORAL DISTRESS

CLINICAL SITUATIONS

- Providing unnecessary/futile treatment
- Prolonging the dying process through aggressive treatment
- Inadequate informed consent
- Working with caregivers who are not as competent as care requires
- Lack of consensus regarding treatment plan
- Lack of continuity of care
- Conflicting duties
- Using resources inappropriately
- Providing care that is not in the best interest of the patient
- Providing inadequate pain relief
- Providing false hope to patients and families
- Hastening the dying process
- Lack of truth-telling
- Disregard for patient wishes

INTERNAL CONSTRAINTS

- Perceived powerlessness
- Inability to identify the ethical issues
- Lack of understanding the full situation
- Self-doubt
- Lack of knowledge of alternative treatment plans
- Increased moral sensitivity
- Lack of assertiveness
- Socialization to follow others

EXTERNAL CONSTRAINTS

- Inadequate communication among team members
- Differing inter- (eg, RN to MD) or intraprofessional (eg, RN to RN) perspectives
- Inadequate staffing and increased turnover
- Lack of administrative support
- Policies and priorities that conflict with care needs
- Following family wishes of patient care for fear of litigation
- Tolerance of disruptive and abusive behavior
- Compromising care due to pressures to reduce costs
- Hierarchies within healthcare system
- Lack of collegial relationships
- Nurses not involved in decision-making
- Compromised care due to insurance pressure or fear of litigation

Reproduced with permission from Hamric AB, Borchers CT, Epstein EG. Development and testing of an instrument to measure moral distress in healthcare professionals. Am J Bioeth Prim Res. 2012;3(2):1–9.

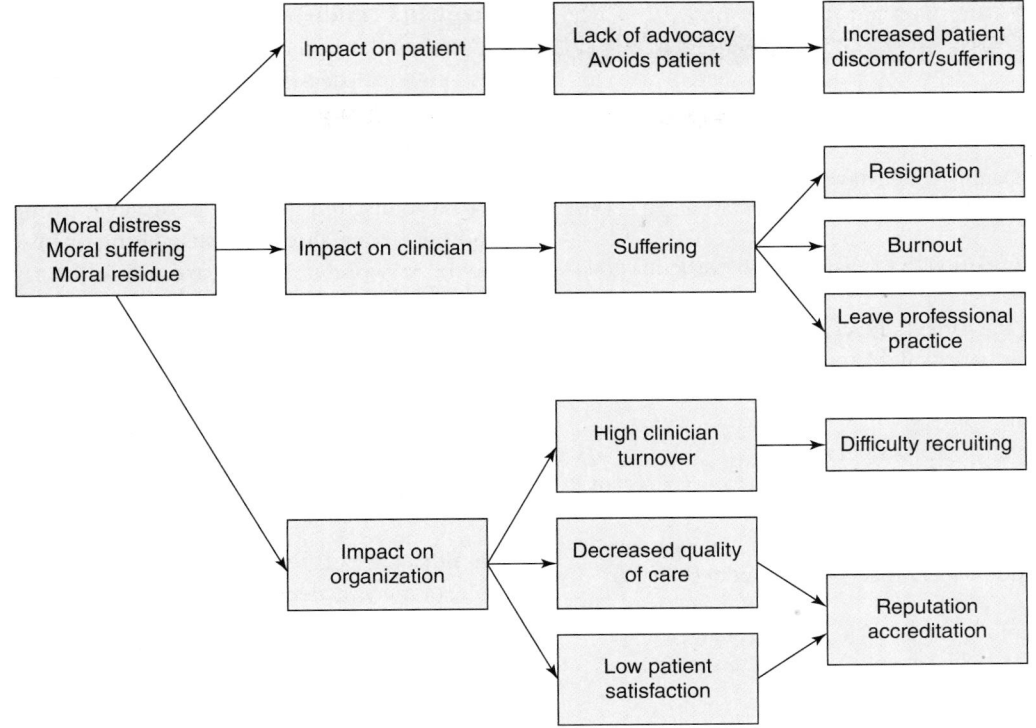

FIGURE 72-1. Impacts of moral distress on the patient, clinician, and organization. (Adapted with permission from Corley MC. Nurse moral distress: a proposed theory and research agenda. *Nurs Ethics.* 2002;9[6]:636–650.)

TRUTHFUL DISCLOSURE

Case

Mr. W is an 83-year-old man who is brought to see his primary care provider by his wife. She confronts the physician outside the examination room and expresses concern that her husband has become more forgetful and no longer is able to pay their bills. She remarks, "If he has Alzheimer's disease, please don't tell him."

Question: What is the ethically justifiable option for the clinician after he examines Mr. W?

In the past, when medicine was more paternalistic, physicians did not routinely inform patients of life-threatening diagnoses. The rationale for not sharing diagnoses, such as cancer, with patients was that this information would cause harm. However, most people want to know their diagnoses. A systematic review of 23 articles with over 9000 participants found that 91% of cognitively intact people and 85% of cognitively impaired people wanted to know if they had dementia. A second study found that there were no increases in rates of depression or anxiety after people learned of a dementia diagnosis.

As medicine has moved from being paternalistic to being patient-centered, the practice of withholding information from patients decreased. In this era of patient-centered care, patients should be offered the opportunity to learn about their medical conditions. Patients also have the right to decline to hear about their conditions. In certain cultures, it is still standard to not share information about serious illness with patients, but with their family members (ie, familismo). In some cultures, there is a belief that talking about bad things will make them happen. Thus if a patient doesn't want information, for any reason, giving this information without permission is not ethically justifiable, and could cause harm.

One method advocated for use when breaking bad news is the six-step SPIKES approach (see Further Reading). The steps of this approach are explained in **Table 72-3**.

In response to the case of Mr. W, it would be appropriate to understand Mrs. W's reasons for not wanting her husband to know his diagnosis. Perhaps he has asked her on multiple occasions not to ever tell him if he develops dementia, because of a previous experience with a family member who suffered from dementia. In this case, it might be appropriate not to share this information with Mr. W. Ultimately, however, he has a right to this information, if he wants it. After hearing her reasons, we could use the SPIKES approach to talk to Mr. W. We would ask about his understanding of his current situation and whether he would want information or not. In the case of dementia, it is appropriate to share information about the diagnosis with a patient with mild dementia who has decisional capacity to make the decision about whether or not to hear the cause of his memory loss. It might not be appropriate to repeat this information over and over to a patient with more advanced

TABLE 72-3 ■ THE SPIKES APPROACH TO BREAKING BAD NEWS

1. **S—Setting** up the interview
   a. Find a private, quiet room with room for all participants to sit down
   b. Encourage family and involved others to participate
   c. Minimize distractions—turn off sound from pagers and phones
   d. Establish rapport with the patient with eye contact and touch
2. **P**—Assessing the patient's **Perception**
   a. What do the patient and family understand about the patient's medical condition?
   b. Correct any misperceptions
3. **I**—Obtaining the patient's **Invitation**
   a. Ask the patient and family how much information and what kind of information they want or don't want
4. **K**—Giving **Knowledge** and information to the patient
   a. Start with a statement that you're about to share bad news
   b. Share the information succinctly in lay language
   c. Allow time for the patient and family to absorb this information
5. **E**—Addressing the patient's **Emotions** with empathic responses
   a. Acknowledge and validate the patient and family's emotional response
6. **S**—**Strategy and Summary**
   a. Summarize the conversation and answer questions
   b. Develop a clear plan for what comes next

Data from Baile WF, Buckman R, Lenzi R, et al. SPIKES-A six-step protocol for delivering bad news: application to the patient with cancer. Oncologist. 2000;5(4):302–311.

dementia, who might experience the emotional distress of receiving this diagnosis multiple times or might not be able to fully understand what this means.

DECISION-MAKING IN CHRONIC AND ADVANCED ILLNESS

Case

Mrs. S is an 82-year-old woman with mild dementia, coronary artery disease, hypertension, and peripheral vascular disease. She misses a meal in the dining room of her assisted living facility, and is found in her apartment lethargic and confused. She is sent to the hospital, admitted to the ICU, and diagnosed with urosepsis. She has a Physician Orders for Life-Sustaining Treatment (POLST) form, which accompanies her to the hospital, with preferences for Do Not Resuscitate status (DNR), Limited Additional Interventions, antibiotics to prolong life, and a trial of use of a feeding tube.

Despite aggressive care in the ICU, she remains delirious. Over the next 2 weeks in the ICU, she suffers a non-ST segment elevation MI, develops a pneumonia thought secondary to aspiration, and her kidney function worsens.

Her adult children, who are her legal decision-makers, are given regular updates, but are overwhelmed by the numerous medical decisions they are asked to make including: whether to insert a temporary feeding tube in her nose, followed later by whether to insert a more permanent tube in her stomach, and whether to start dialysis. Although they had initially told the ICU to do "everything" to make their mother better, short of resuscitating or intubating her, they begin to wonder if they are doing the right thing. They wonder how long their mother would want this level of care continued. During a routine meeting with the family, the ICU team uses the term "futile" and recommends that they change the goal of care to focus on maximizing their mother's comfort.

Question: What should the family and ICU team consider in deciding how to proceed?

In older patients with chronic medical conditions, a multitude of medical decisions may arise during acute illness, and in the course of worsening of the chronic conditions. When patients are unable to make their own decisions, surrogates are called on to make these decisions. Decision-making for others can be stressful for surrogates, while knowledge of a loved one's preferences can reduce the burden of decision-making for surrogates. In the case of Mrs. S, her children have attempted to implement her wishes, but her condition has worsened, and they are no longer sure of the right thing to do. In what follows, several decisions related to this case will be discussed.

We operate under the notion that the patient possesses a fundamental legal and moral right to have his or her care preferences respected. Understanding any prior conversations or specific directives (such as her POLST form), and knowing her overall values, hopefully Mrs. S's family would be able to speak on behalf of Mrs. S, as though they were relaying her explicit wishes, or "standing in her shoes." This concept illustrates the ethical principle of substituted judgment. When such patient preferences are known, it is expected that the patient's surrogate decision-maker would operate under this principle, communicating the patient's wishes, and choosing the option that would best fit her stated care preferences.

Often, the patient's explicit wishes regarding a specific clinical scenario are not known. It can be difficult to anticipate all of the different clinical scenarios and medical decisions that may need to be considered in one's future ahead of time. In this type of situation, surrogate decision-makers often need to rely on the principle of best interest. In deciding what satisfies a person's best interest, the surrogate decision-maker—ideally with guidance from the primary team of health care providers caring for the patient—is able to objectively weigh risks, potential benefits and treatment burdens to make an individualized decision for the patient. However, when evidence of the patient's wishes does exist, making decisions by substituted judgment should take precedence so that the patient's care preferences are honored.

At the beginning of her hospitalization, Mrs. S's children believed that they were doing what she would want in inserting a temporary nasogastric tube. When she didn't improve despite aggressive interventions and remained unable to swallow safely, her children were less sure if she would want a more permanent tube inserted. Although the literature, position statements from organizations such as the American Geriatrics Society, and the Choosing Wisely campaign have argued against the insertion of feeding tubes in patients with advanced dementia (which is discussed elsewhere), the appropriate use of feeding tubes in other situations is less clear. In Mrs. S's situation, the decision of whether or not to place a permanent feeding tube depends on her overall goals of care. It is not clearly right or wrong to place it.

Another decision that families often will make for their loved ones is whether to treat infections with antibiotics. Antibiotic therapy is thought to be beneficial and the usual standard of care in conditions such as pneumonia and urinary tract infections, which often arise among older adults. In some patients with advanced serious illness, however, antimicrobials can carry substantial risk and treatment burdens that need to be carefully weighed, especially among patients receiving end of life care. For example, patients receiving antimicrobials are at increased risk of acquiring infections with resistant organisms as well *C. difficile* infections. Some of the unintended consequences of antimicrobial therapy not only include burdens to the individual patient, but also extend to other patients, and to society through the possible selection of antimicrobial resistance. Studies are conflicting as to whether antimicrobial treatment of pneumonia may provide symptomatic benefit among patients with advanced dementia. A recent prospective study of patients with advanced dementia and pneumonia demonstrated an association between antimicrobials and increased discomfort. For patients receiving comfort-focused care near the end of life, the treatment of pain, fever, and dyspnea with opioids and antipyretics remains effective to provide symptomatic benefit. Whether a course of antibiotics is warranted will depend on the risks and benefits of the treatment and whether providing that course of treatment is consistent with the patient's goals of care.

In living with chronic conditions, older patients may have acute or chronic worsening of their kidney function. The number of older individuals who are beginning chronic dialysis is increasing. Many of these individuals start dialysis while in the hospital for an acute illness. Studies have shown that older people with poor functional status, multiple chronic conditions, and age over 85 when starting dialysis may not necessarily live longer with dialysis. Conservative management programs for older patients with advanced kidney disease who are forgoing dialysis are prevalent in the United Kingdom, but not elsewhere. In deciding about whether or not to begin dialysis, Mrs. S's children need to be fully informed about the risks and benefits of short- and long-term dialysis. As with other decisions, the decision to start dialysis depends on Mrs. S's goals of care.

After a trial of aggressive therapies aimed at life prolongation, Mrs. S's clinicians begin to talk about her situation being "futile." This term is used by health care professionals, but not by lay people, and therefore should not be used in routine conversations with patients or their loved ones. The term is also commonly used when clinicians don't believe that continuing on the current trajectory is "worth it." Different definitions of futility exist, including quantitative futility (very low probability of survival) and qualitative futility (patient's quality of life is below an acceptable standard). These definitions can be problematic because clinicians cannot accurately predict a patient's chances of survival and may not be able to separate their own views about acceptable quality of life from the patient's perceived quality of life. In the case of Mrs. S, decision-making might be easier if both the medical team and her family were clear about her goals of care; what makes life worth living for her (in keeping with the Institute for Healthcare Improvement and John A. Hartford Foundation's Age-Friendly Health Systems' 4Ms Framework in which eliciting what Matters to the patient is emphasized), and would she consider life to be acceptable if she lived in a nursing home, leaving three times a week for dialysis, and being fed through a tube.

When patients are very sick and care is focused on life prolongation, it can be hard for clinicians and family members to step back and examine the big picture. When the goal is to do "everything," medical teams may want to better understand what this means to a patient and family. They should not feel compelled to offer every intervention that is technically feasible. Instead, they should consider whether the intervention is clinically meaningful, and whether it will help to meet the patient's goals of care.

Mrs. S's medical team has recommended a change in the focus of her care from life prolongation to comfort care. Although this may be a clinically acceptable option, it is important that care recommendations be based on an understanding of the patient's values and preferences. Making recommendations tailored to patient preferences would be consistent with a shared decision-making approach. At the same time, it is important to acknowledge that although withholding and withdrawing care is ethically equivalent, withdrawing life prolonging measures may be more psychologically difficult for decision-makers.

In deciding how to proceed with Mrs. S's care, consulting a palliative care team may be helpful. The palliative care team could not only help the medical team develop a richer understanding of Mrs. S's values, care preferences, and goals of care by engaging in in-depth conversations with her children about her life, but also support her family during a stressful time.

MANAGING REFRACTORY SYMPTOMS CAUSING INTRACTABLE SUFFERING NEAR THE END OF LIFE

Case

Mr. P is a 90-year-old man with widely metastatic prostate cancer receiving hospice services in a nursing home. He continues to have severe bone pain from his metastatic disease despite the use of opioids, steroids, zolendronic acid injections, and a course of palliative radiation. As his opioid doses are increased, he develops myoclonus and confusion. Rotation to two different opioids over the next two weeks is minimally effective. His confusion worsens, becoming hyperactive delirium with bouts of yelling and attempting to climb out of bed. Addition of antipsychotic medications is only slightly effective.

His family and the nursing staff are distressed about his situation and their inability to ensure his comfort and safety.

Question: What are the ethically and legally appropriate options to reduce Mr. P's suffering?

In terminally ill patients such as Mr. P, questions may arise about ways to reduce his intractable suffering and promote his comfort at the very end of life, to ensure a peaceful death. His family may ask if there is something that could be done to end his suffering, such as euthanasia. Those taking care of him may wonder about the use of palliative sedation or physician aid in dying (PAD; also known as physician-assisted suicide) and whether alternative options exist. The differences between these entities can be confusing to families and clinicians, and are defined in **Table 72-4**.

TABLE 72-4 ■ KEY TERMS, DEFINITIONS, AND LEGAL STATUS OF INTERVENTIONS TO MANAGE INTRACTABLE SUFFERING AT THE END OF LIFE

TERM	DEFINITION	STATUS	SOURCE
Palliative sedation Also called terminal sedation, end-of-life sedation, total sedation, and proportional palliative sedation	Lowering of patient consciousness using medications for the express purpose of limiting patient awareness of suffering that is intractable and intolerable. Proportional palliative sedation is the process of reducing consciousness only as much as needed to reduce patient suffering. Patients may only be mildly sedated, not necessarily sedated to unconsciousness. Deep continuous sedation is used to describe the last step of a gradual process of palliative sedation in which the patient is sedated to deep unconsciousness.	Legal in the United States	Kirk et al. NHPCO Consensus JPSM 2010 AMA Code of Medical Ethics https://www.ama-assn.org/system/files/2019-06/code-of-medical-ethics-chapter-5.pdf AAHPM position statement 2014
Voluntary stopping of eating and drinking (VSED)	"An action of a competent, capacitated person who voluntarily and deliberately chooses to stop eating and drinking with the primary intention to hasten death because unacceptable suffering persists."	Legal in the United States	Wax JW, An AW, Kosier N, Quill TE. Voluntary stopping eating and drinking. *J Am Geriatr Soc.* 2018;66(3):441–445.
Physician aid in dying (PAD) Also called physician-assisted suicide (PAS) or physician-assisted death	A practice that "occurs when a physician facilitates a patient's death by providing the necessary means and/or information to enable the patient to perform the life-ending act." Medications are self-administered by the patient, thereby distinguishing it from euthanasia. Physician-assisted suicide is a term being used less often because of the impression that the patient commits suicide.	Legal in some US states, and in Canada, Belgium, the Netherlands, and Luxembourg	AMA Code of Medical Ethics https://www.ama-assn.org/system/files/2019-06/code-of-medical-ethics-chapter-5.pdf
Euthanasia	The administration of a lethal agent by another person, such as a clinician, to a patient for the purpose of relieving the patient's intolerable and incurable suffering by ending the patient's life. Intentionally ending the life of another person, usually with the goal of alleviating or avoiding suffering.	Not legal in the United States Legal in Belgium, the Netherlands, and Luxembourg under specific circumstances with procedures to guide use	AMA Code of Medical Ethics. https://www.ama-assn.org/system/files/2019-06/code-of-medical-ethics-chapter-5.pdf

Palliative sedation is legal in the United States. It is an intervention provided to relieve intractable and intolerable symptoms at the end of life, and is accomplished by intentionally lowering the patient's level of consciousness using sedating medications. Palliative sedation should be used as an intervention of last resort in the setting of a palliative care interdisciplinary team strategy to achieve symptom control within the spectrum of palliative care interventions. The American Medical Association, the American Academy of Hospice and Palliative Medicine, and guidelines from Europe, Canada, and Japan consider palliative sedation to unconsciousness to be appropriate as a last resort in terminally ill patients with goals for comfort and severe refractory distressing symptoms including agitated delirium, dyspnea, pain, nausea and vomiting, shortness of breath, urinary retention due to clot formation, gastrointestinal pain, uncontrolled bleeding, and myoclonus. Palliative sedation for suffering that does not result from physical symptoms, but from existential, psychological, or spiritual distress remains controversial.

The recommendations on palliative sedation from the American Academy of Hospice and Palliative Care in 2014 are summarized as follows: (1) it is ethically defensible if used after careful interdisciplinary evaluation and treatment of the patient; (2) it should be used when palliative treatments that are not intended to affect consciousness have failed or, in the judgment of the clinician, are very likely to fail; (3) it should be used where its use is not expected to shorten the patient's time to death; and (4) it should be used only for the actual or expected duration of symptoms. Ideally, the patient, family, and participating interdisciplinary health care professionals should be in agreement that this intervention is consistent with patient goals and is the right thing to do. Health care professionals who believe that participating in palliative sedation is morally wrong should not be forced to participate in the care of patients undergoing this intervention. Treatment of existential suffering should include the full interdisciplinary team including mental health and spiritual care experts. Respite sedation, or sedation for a limited time with subsequent removal of sedation to reassess the patient, may be an alternative approach.

An alternative to palliative sedation is the voluntary cessation of eating and drinking (also called voluntary stopping of eating and drinking or VSED). This practice is legal if chosen because of intractable suffering by a competent person with decisional capacity who is approaching the end of life. Many individuals who are approaching the end of life do not have an appetite, and thus do not experience discomfort from VSED. For others, symptoms resulting from voluntary cessation of eating and drinking may require intervention by a palliative care team. Individuals are encouraged to let their medical teams and families know if they decide to pursue VSED. However, there are cases in which older individuals who had decided to pursue this were evicted from long-term care facilities due to legal concerns.

VSED is a patient-initiated, voluntary process, which necessitates that the patient remains competent at least at the start of the process. The health care team may need to palliate symptoms of thirst and delirium, and sustain the continued withholding of food and fluids from some patients who pursue VSED. Due to the loss of decisional capacity inherent in the progression of dementia, VSED in the setting of dementia deserves further thoughtful consideration. While some dementia-specific directives allow for delineation of potential withholding or withdrawing of food and fluids (ie, stopping eating and drinking by advance directive, or SED by AD) when one's dementia progression reaches a certain point, implementation of these directives across varying state jurisdictions will need to be understood and studied further. While the concept of SED by AD has gained traction among some advocates for advance care planning, these directives have also been criticized for utilizing a potentially problematic ethical concept called "precedent autonomy" in which a fully cognizant and healthy patient directs their care preferences to be carried out after loss of decisional capacity, should their degree of functional incapacity and circumstance meet preset conditions, regardless of the clinical situation and social setting in which the patient might land. SED by AD is a process in which a surrogate decision-maker directs the withholding of food and fluids when a certain degree of cognitive and functional impairment is reached due to dementia progression. Advocates have focused on the ethical principle of patient autonomy to direct preferences for SED by AD, as is the case with more general advance directives. However, others, including a recent position statement put forth by the Ethics Subcommittee of AMDA—The Society for Post-Acute and Long-Term Care Medicine, argue that the principle of justice (the obligation to treat all individuals equally regardless of race, gender, cognitive or physical ability needs to be the overarching principle to guide these decisions), as well as the physician's obligations to beneficence and nonmaleficence, thereby advocating that comfort feeding should be implemented for those with advanced dementia. Some of the more detailed directives, that include specific preferences for SED by AD, are difficult to implement in care settings such as nursing homes and inpatient hospices. Specific instructions to discontinue hand feeding in advanced dementia or to instruct surrogates to not allow hand feeding if one loses the ability to feed oneself are potentially difficult to implement in care settings where the provision of oral food and fluids are considered basic and comfort-oriented care, especially if the patient appears to derive enjoyment comfort out of eating or tasting food. A policy of comfort feeding in advanced dementia, on the other hand, allows for continued assisted feeding for those who are accepting food and fluids as tolerated until their feeding behaviors indicate refusal or show signs of any distress with eating.

PAD, also called physician-assisted suicide or death with dignity, is legal in some US states and the

District of Columbia. The patient pursuing PAD intentionally self-administers lethal doses of medications with the intention of ending their suffering. The Death with Dignity laws in Oregon and Washington and similar laws in other states in the United States stipulate that only terminally ill patients who are decisionally intact and voluntarily making this request are eligible to use the law. Interested individuals are required to make two verbal and one written request, and must be adult residents of their state. Two attending physicians must verify that the patient is terminally ill with intact decisional capacity. The majority of people requesting this are already receiving hospice services, and often make the request because of concerns about loss of autonomy and control. Approximately one-third of individuals who obtain medications do not use them. Finally, patients may raise the subject of PAD with their clinicians as a way to begin a conversation about death and dying. Even if clinicians cannot or will not participate, they should still view this as an opportunity to talk about the patient's sources of unbearable suffering, and fears about dying.

Euthanasia is a process by which an individual, such as a clinician, intentionally administers a lethal dose of medication to a terminally ill patient, which directly ends their life. In contrast to PAD, euthanasia is not legal in the United States. Internationally, it is legal in Belgium and the Netherlands, which have widespread palliative care policies and availability of palliative care professionals. In these countries, the practice of euthanasia is considered one option to manage intractable suffering at the end of life, and is provided in conjunction with palliative care. Of note, a qualitative study characterizing the Dutch experience with euthanasia or physician-assisted suicide requests among older adults without terminal illness and with multiple geriatric conditions between 2013 and 2019 was recently published. These older adults attributed unbearable suffering to a combination of medical, social, and existential issues that include loss of mobility, fear of decline, social isolation, and loss of meaning. This study found that patients whose suffering was attributed to multiple geriatric conditions accounted for 4% of all cases of euthanasia or physician-assisted suicide in the Netherlands during this period, calling attention to the potential for a "slippery slope" of allowing the use of euthanasia or physician-assisted suicide for suffering due to nonterminal conditions that could instead be addressed with enhanced geriatric or palliative supportive efforts to enhance quality of life.

The ethical distinction between palliative sedation and euthanasia has been debated, hinging on three areas: intention, monitoring, and methods. Palliative sedation does not have the intention to hasten death, the patient is monitored to provide the minimum level of sedation required to provide symptom relief, and the medication is carefully titrated to achieve this minimum level of sedation required to provide symptom relief. The American Medical Association (AMA) asserts that the distinction between palliative sedation and euthanasia may be evident on examination of the medical record, as repeated doses and continuous infusions suggest palliative sedation, while one large dose or rapidly accelerating doses out of proportion to the level of immediate patient suffering may reflect an intention to hasten death. Other indications of inappropriate palliative sedation include inadequate communication and support between patients, relatives, and staff; inadequate evaluation of psychological distress and existential suffering; and inadequate monitoring. There are multiple published guidelines on appropriate indications, monitoring, and methods for palliative sedation, and most guidelines include the recommendation that cases in which this procedure is being considered should include a physician with expertise in palliative care.

BALANCING AUTONOMY AND SELF-DETERMINATION WITH INDIVIDUAL AND SOCIETAL SAFETY DRIVING

Case

Mr. J is an 89-year-old man living temporarily in a skilled nursing facility where he is receiving physical and occupational therapy after he fell and sustained a patellar fracture. He is doing well, and the interdisciplinary team informs you that he will be ready to discharge home soon. He lives in a one-story home with his wife. He drives to the neighborhood shopping center to meet his friends for lunch, buy groceries, and do other chores. During your assessment, you note that his memory is mildly impaired, with only one out of three items recalled after 5 minutes, and he has difficulty with attention. His clock-drawing test is markedly abnormal, with impaired spacing and numbering.

Questions for the interdisciplinary team: Should he still be driving? What do we do about it?

Decisions regarding older adults' driving ability can lead to ethical dilemmas for health care professionals, especially when the patient is upset at the loss of the independence and autonomy that driving provides. Common reasons for recommending driving cessation are epilepsy, stroke, dementia, visual impairment, and medication adverse effects. Strategies to employ when addressing driving decisions with patients are summarized in **Table 72-5**. Some key ethical considerations with regard to driving include protecting the patient's safety, the public's safety, and patient confidentiality. Protecting Mr. J would include counseling him about conditions or medications that may impair his ability to drive safely. Some states have mandatory reporting requirements for physicians regarding driving ability, and some states have found physicians liable for harm to others because their patients were not warned about conditions or medication side effects that could impair driving performance. Physicians must weigh the responsibility for ensuring patient confidentiality against the responsibility for the patient's safety and public safety. Involving patients and family, and carefully counseling patients,

TABLE 72-5 ■ STRATEGIES TO EMPLOY WHEN WORKING WITH OLDER ADULTS REGARDING DRIVING CESSATION

SITUATION	PROPOSED STRATEGIES
Patient threatens to sue physician if reported to Department of Motor Vehicles	• Clearly document how the patient was determined to be an unsafe driver (driving fitness evaluation, assessing driving-related skills [ADReS] battery, driving rehabilitation referral, medications, etc). • Advise patient that the state has the ultimate responsibility to determine licensing. • If physician is mandated to report in that state, physician must report. The physician should also advise the patient of this. • Check if the state has legislation protecting health professionals against liability for reporting unsafe drivers in good faith. • Consult malpractice insurance or legal counsel to determine degree of risk (physicians generally run little risk of liability for following mandatory reporting).
Physician identifies patient as an unsafe driver, state does not have mandatory reporting laws	• Attempt to counsel patient to stop driving voluntarily without revocation of license. • Explore ways to ensure that patient no longer drives. • If patient refuses to stop driving, physician must weigh breach of confidentiality vs potential injury to patient and others from a crash.
Patient had license suspended, but continues to drive	• Talk to the patient about why he or she continues to drive. • With the patient's permission, involve the patient's family or caregivers to identify transportation resources and alternative transportation. • Counsel patient that he or she is breaking the law, cite concerns about patient's safety, and discuss consequences of a crash (being injured, injuring others, financial and legal implications). • If the patient is cognitively impaired and lacks insight, counsel surrogate decision-makers regarding responsibility to prevent patient from driving. • Report patient as an unsafe driver again.
Patient threatens to find a new doctor if physician reports to Department of Motor Vehicles	• Diffuse the situation by reiterating how unsafe driving determination was made. • Convey concern for patient's safety, and safety of others who would be affected if patient crashed. • Remind patient that driving safety is part of good health care as much as other physician responsibilities. • Encourage patient to be evaluated by a driving rehabilitation specialist. • Emphasize that the state Department of Motor Vehicles makes the final determination of driving safety. • Maintain professional behavior by not expressing hostility even if he or she seeks a new physician.

Data from Clinician's Guide to Assessing and Counseling Older Drivers, 4th ed. New York, NY: American Geriatrics Society; 2019.

including providing a written letter of recommendations regarding driving cessation, can be helpful to navigate these challenging situations. Careful documentation of a patient's risks regarding driving and counseling provided, as well as additional referrals made to social workers, driving rehabilitation or other professionals, may reduce clinician liability. In addition, physicians must make sure they are in compliance with their own state reporting laws for physicians, available from each state's Department of Motor Vehicles (DMV). Six states have mandatory reporting requirements (California, Delaware, Nevada, New Jersey, Oregon, and Pennsylvania). In states without mandatory reporting laws, providers need to obtain release of information to report patients to the DMV, or they could be held liable for breach of confidentiality. Some states provide civil immunity if health care professionals report in good faith.

FIREARMS

The possession of firearms by people with dementia is another area in which the autonomy and self-determination of the individual needs to be weighed against the safety of the individual and of society. Of people with dementia, 60% have firearms in their homes and only 17% of families report storing these weapons unloaded and locked. Having firearms in the home increases the likelihood of suicide completion. Ten states and the District of Columbia require a permit to buy a firearm. Hawaii restricts persons with organic brain syndromes from possessing firearms, while Texas prohibits persons with dementia from obtaining a license to carry a handgun in public. There are "red flag laws" called extreme risk protection order (ERPO) laws in 17 states, which provide a means for court-ordered firearm removal based on reasonable or substantial threat. Strategies for assessing and counseling firearm safety in patients with dementia and their families are shown in **Table 72-6**. As dementia progresses, the recommendations become more focused on counseling families to restrict access to the firearm and remove the firearm from the home environment. A website has been developed to assist families and caregivers in discussing changes regarding safety in dementia, including firearms, driving and home safety (https://safetyindementia.org/).

TABLE 72-6 ■ RECOMMENDED STRATEGIES FOR COUNSELING PERSONS WITH DEMENTIA AND THEIR FAMILIES REGARDING FIREARMS

5 Ls (Loaded, Locked, Little Children, Low, and Learned)

Is it Loaded?

Is it Locked? (gun safe, trigger lock or cable lock in place, ammunition locked separate)

Are Little children present? (grandchildren at risk for injury)

Is the person feeling Low? (risk of suicide)

Is the person Learned? (knows how to use the weapon, or is the weapon inherited or not intentionally purchased, presence of dementia)

Firearm Safety Counseling Protocol Questions to Assess Access, Safety Profile, and Capacity

- Assess dementia severity:
  - Include person with dementia in assessment and counseling when dementia is mild.
  - As dementia severity increases, the protocol involves family members only.
- Risk assessment:
  - Firearm: type, number, status (locked, unloaded, with ammunition)
  - Patient: vision, neurological changes, PHQ-2
  - Environment: small children, teenagers
  - Behaviors: last time handled/disarmed firearm
- Counseling based on risk profile:
  - Safe storage (locked, unloaded, stored separate from ammunition, safety device)
  - Access for suicide and injury-related fatalities (Lethal Means Access)
  - Firearm sunset: ways to remove firearm from home, remove ammunition/ disable firearm (remove firing pins), red flag laws if family feels unsafe.

Data from Pinholt EM, Mitchell JD, Butler JH, et al. "Is there a gun in the home?" Assessing the risks of gun ownership in older adults. J Am Geriatr Soc. 2014;62(6):1142–1146 and Doucette ML, Dayton H, Lapidus G, et al. Firearms, dementia, and the clinician: development of a safety counseling protocol. J Am Geriatr Soc. 2020;68(9):2128–2133.

MANAGING SEXUAL INTIMACY AND OTHER ETHICAL ISSUES IN NURSING HOMES

Case

Mrs. N, an ambulatory 87-year-old nursing home resident with moderate dementia, is found by nursing staff in the room of Mr. O, an 85-year-old nursing home resident with COPD, Parkinson disease, and dementia. They are seated on Mr. O's bed, hugging. Mr. O is wearing his incontinence briefs, but no pants, and is audibly wheezing.

Question: What is the appropriate way to approach sexual intimacy in the long-term care setting?

Common ethical issues encountered in long-term care are summarized in **Table 72-7**. In general, ethical issues in the nursing home often involve tension between honoring resident autonomy and protecting their health and safety. During the COVID-19 pandemic, for example, many nursing homes prioritized beneficence and safety over resident

TABLE 72-7 ■ ETHICAL ISSUES IN LONG-TERM CARE FACILITIES

ETHICAL ISSUE	KEY CONSIDERATIONS
Conflict between resident autonomy and beneficence	Managing resident refusal of care, medications, bathing, or wanting to leave the facility. The facility staff and physician must communicate standards of care clearly with the patient and the surrogate decision-makers at the time of admission and at regular intervals.
Decision-making at the end of life	A facility ethics committee can assist with decisions regarding withholding, withdrawing, or otherwise limiting aggressive medical care.
Ethical issues in the care of LBGT persons in the long-term care setting	Adoption of congruent and appropriate wording on admission and procedure forms; nonrestriction of visitation and inclusion of partner in family meetings; create programs and staff education to facilitate respect; cultural competency and genuine inclusion; reducing isolation.
Role of ethics committees in nursing homes	Each nursing facility should have a mechanism to assist the facility, residents, physicians, leadership, and staff in managing ethical dilemmas, including policy development and review, quality assurance, education, monitoring judicial decisions and legislative action and consultation, and review of case-specific dilemmas.
Long-term care research	Autonomy and informed consent—residents may lack decision-making capacity necessitating consent by surrogate.

autonomy. This has resulted in isolation and cognitive decline.

Sexual intimacy in the long-term care setting requires a specific approach that is different from usual medical decision-making capacity evaluations. One recommended approach is summarized in **Table 72-8**.

In the case, the physician caring for Mrs. N and Mr. O must assess their capacity for sexual consent and the long-term care facility must develop a plan for sexual intimacy within the facility. Involving the residents' surrogate decision-makers is recommended for open communication and a coordinated approach that balances patient preference (if the patient is determined to have capacity for sexual consent) with safety and privacy.

RESOURCE ALLOCATION AND AGEISM

Case

A hospital system is approaching 100% ICU capacity due to the COVID-19 pandemic. This health system's crisis standards of care specify that adults older than age 85 should not enter the resource allocation algorithm, meaning that

TABLE 72-8 ■ COMPONENTS OF SEXUAL CONSENT IN THE NURSING HOME

COMPONENT OF DETERMINATION OF SEXUAL CONSENT	KEY CONSIDERATIONS
Is the person with dementia (PWD)...	
• Familiar with the sexual partner and the nature of that person's relationship to the PWD?	Can the PWD name the person who would be in sexual contact with them? Can the PWD accurately explain their relationship (ie, does the PWD mistake someone else for their spouse)?
• Able to describe or name the type of intimate sexual activity they are comfortable with?	Can the PWD state what kind of intimate sexual activity they would like to have with this person? (Note that the standard for capacity might be different, for example, for kissing their spouse versus sexual penetration.)
• Able to decline unwanted sexual activity?	Can the PWD say "no" to this person or to this activity? Can the PWD physically stop the person or the activity?
• Able to articulate what their reaction will be if sexual activity ends?	Can the PWD say how this activity will make them feel, react after it is over, or after the relationship ends?
Is this behavior consistent with previously expressed beliefs and preferences?	Observe the PWD in the long-term care setting: Are they acting in a manner that is consistent with how they would have acted prior to dementia?
Can the facility...	
• Enlist the PWD's proposed sexual partner in the assessment?	Observe partner for signs of cognitive impairment, awareness of the PWD's wishes, ability to assure their safety and privacy, and potential conflict of interest, coercion, or undue influence. Involve additional surrogate decision-makers if there are concerns.
• Address concerns of family or surrogate decision-makers?	Consider family members' personal, generational, and cultural background and acknowledge sensitive nature of the topic when discussing with family.
• Address concerns of staff members?	Elicit concerns from staff in a safe forum when developing plan regarding sexual intimacy and how to protect privacy and dignity of patients during sanctioned sexual activity.
• Address safety concerns?	Discuss with PWD, partner, and surrogate decision-maker the nature of the sexual activity and physical and other risks, including risk of falling, infection, or cardiovascular event. Develop plan for staff monitoring, if necessary.

Data from Metzger 2017 and American Medical Directors Association, 2008, White paper.

this group would be denied intensive care should crisis care standards need to be invoked.

Question: Which ethical principles should guide the fair allocation of health care resources under conditions of resources scarcity, especially when considering age?

The specter of denying health care resources to patients under conditions of resource scarcity is perhaps one of the starkest examples in which health care professionals rely on sound and transparent ethical principles for guidance. In usual conditions in Western societies, the principle of autonomy dominates health care decision-making, but under conditions of resource scarcity, the principle of justice has greater weight. During the 2009 H1N1 pandemic, many states began adopting crisis standards of care documents designed to provide guidance to hospitals faced with conditions of resource scarcity. More recently, the COVID-19 pandemic in 2020 brought renewed attention to these crisis standards of care as ICU capacity in terms of "space" (ie, ICU beds), "staff" (eg, intensivists, nurses, respiratory therapists), and "stuff" (eg, ventilators, remdesivir) was pushed to the brink, and many hospitals developed scarce resource allocation triage teams and revised relevant protocols.

A key ethical consideration with respect to allocating health care resources under conditions of resource scarcity

is that clinicians engaged in patient care on the "front line" should not be making decisions regarding resource allocation. Leaving resource allocation decisions to individual clinicians increases the chance that resources will be allocated in an ad hoc and not a systematic fashion, increases the risk of bias including the potential for decisions to disadvantage underrepresented groups (eg, a first-come, first-serve approach), and also burdens the clinician with moral distress. Each hospital should have an interdisciplinary triage committee that is removed from clinical care and that applies their state's crisis standards of care guidelines, with outcomes of these deliberations communicated to clinicians who apply the triage committee's recommendation. It is critically important that triage committees apply crisis standards of care fairly and that their decisions are subject to retrospective review. Otherwise, public confidence in the process by which limited resources are allocated may be undermined.

In early 2020, reports surfaced in Italy of rationing limited health care resources based on age. In the United States, some states' crisis standards of care included age-based cutoffs beyond which patients would not be eligible to receive limited health care resources. Additional age-related provisions include "tiebreaker" provisions in which older age counts against a patient if two patients have identical scores on measures of physiological function such as the MSOFA (Modified Sequential Organ Failure Assessment) score. Although the MSOFA is not based on age, other assessments used to distinguish between patients during times of crisis, such as the 4C mortality score, weight age heavily. While it is the case that older adults with COVID-19 have a higher overall mortality rate than younger adults with COVID-19, the use of age per se to ration health care resources has been criticized because the use of age alone does not consider individual differences that contribute to short-term prognosis. Other arguments to ration health care resources based on age include long-term predicted life expectancy and utilitarian frameworks such as maximizing "life-years saved." Long-term predicted life expectancy has been criticized in this context due to difficulty with prognosticating life expectancy and because, among underrepresented patients, it overlooks the fact that life expectancy may be shorter due to social determinants of health outside of patients' control. The "life-years saved" approach does not consider individual differences among patients and instead withholds resources based on membership in a class (ie, one's age group). Finally, the "fair innings" argument contends that older adults have a lesser claim on health care resources than younger adults since they have lived through more "innings." However, opponents of this argument argue that value judgments about which "innings" of life are more important than others cannot be made. Although situations in which patients are truly tied after an exhaustive consideration of individual characteristics such as physiological parameters should be rare, promising approaches to settling these ties using assessments that are not based on age, such as the Clinical Frailty Scale, are gaining acceptance.

Although the principle of justice outweighs the principle of autonomy under conditions of resource scarcity, autonomy should still be respected. It is critically important to consider the role of advance care planning in ensuring that older adults' preferences are honored even under these difficult conditions. Clinicians should engage in advance care planning conversations, but should be careful to avoid pressuring patients to make decisions for the sole purpose of conserving resources, regardless of whether the patient is healthy or ill at the time the advance care planning conversation occurs. Some have argued that adults should voluntarily relinquish their claim on health care resources to benefit younger generations, but this position is controversial and should not be assumed or imposed on older adults.

FURTHER READING

American Medical Directors Association, 2008, White paper, The role of a facility ethics committee in decision-making at the end of life. Available at https://paltc.org/amda-white-papers-and-resolution-position-statements/role-facility-ethics-committee-decision-making. Accessed February 22, 2021.

American Medical Association Code of Medical Ethics. Chapter 5: Opinions on caring for patients at the end of life. Available at https://www.ama-assn.org/system/files/2019-06/code-of-medical-ethics-chapter-5.pdf. Accessed February 7, 2021.

American Medical Directors Association. 2016, Capacity for sexual consent in dementia in long-term care. Available at https://paltc.org/amda-white-papers-and-resolution-position-statements/capacity-sexual-consent-dementia-long-term-care. Accessed January 10, 2021.

Baile W, Buckman R, Lenzi R, Glober G, Beale EA, Kudelka AP. SPIKES—a six-step protocol for delivering bad news: application to the patient with cancer. *Oncologist.* 2000;5:302–311.

Betz ME, McCourt AD, Vernick JS, Ranney ML, Maust DT, Wintemute GJ. Firearms and dementia: clinical considerations. *Ann Intern Med.* 2018;169(1):47–49.

Clinician's Guide to Assessing and Counseling Older Drivers. Fourth edition. American Geriatrics Society 2019. Available at https://geriatricscareonline.org/ProductAbstract/ clinicians-guide-to-assessing-and-counseling-older-drivers-4th-edition/B047. Accessed February 22, 2021.

Epstein, EG, Hamric AB. Moral distress, moral residue, and the crescendo effect. *J Clin Ethics.* 2009;20(4):330–342.

Farrell TW, Widera E, Rosenberg L, et al. AGS position statement: making medical treatment decisions for unbefriended older adults. *J Am Geriatr Soc.* 2017;65(1):14–15.

Farrell TW, Francis L, Brown T, et al. Rationing limited healthcare resources in the COVID-19 era and beyond: ethical considerations regarding older adults. *J Am Geriatr Soc.* 2020;68(6):1143–1149.

Fox E, Berkowitz KA, Chanko BL, Powell T. *Ethics Consultation: Responding to Ethics Questions in Health Care.* Second edition. Available at http://vaww.ethics.va.gov/docs/integratedethics/ec_primer.pdf. Accessed February 22, 2021.

Gruenewald DA. Voluntary stopping eating and drinking: a practical approach for long-term care facilities. *J Palliat Med.* 2018;21(9):1214–1220.

Metzer E. Ethics and intimate sexual activity in long-term care. *AMA J Ethics.* 2017;19(7):640–648.

Preshaw DHI, Brazil K, McLaughlin D, Frolic A. Ethical issues experienced by healthcare workers in nursing homes: literature review. *Nurs Ethics.* 2016;23(5):490–506.

Quill T, Arnold RM. Evaluating requests for hastened death #156. *J Palliat Med.* 2008;11:1151–1152.

Rushton, CH. Cultivating moral resilience. *Am J Nurs.* 2017;117(2 Suppl 1):S11–S15.

Wong SP, Sharda N, Zietlow KE, Heflin MT. Planning for a safe discharge: more than a capacity evaluation. *J Am Geriatr Soc.* 2020;68(4):859–866.

van den Berg V, van Thiel G, Zomers M, et al. Euthanasia and physician-assisted suicide in patients with multiple geriatric syndromes. *JAMA Intern Med.* 2021;181(2):245–250.

VHA National Center for Ethics in Health Care. Ethics guidance for pandemics 2020. Available at http://vaww .ethics.va.gov/ETHICS/activities/pandemic/Ethics_ Guidance_for_Pandemics_2020.pdf. Accessed February 22, 2021.

Wax JW, An AW, Kosier N, Quill TE. Voluntary stopping eating and drinking. *J Am Geriatr Soc.* 2018;66(3): 441–445.

Wright JL, Jaggard PM, Holahan T. Stopping eating and drinking by advance directives (SED by AD) in assisted living and nursing homes. *J Am Med Dir Assoc.* 2019;20(11):1362–1366.

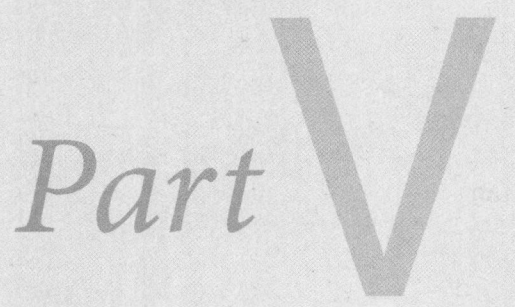

Organ Systems and Diseases

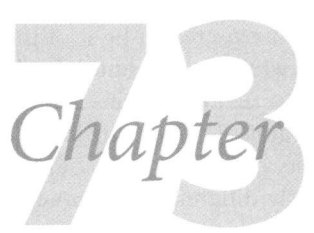

Chapter 73

The Aging Cardiovascular System

Ambarish Pandey, George E. Taffet,
Dalane W. Kitzman, Bharathi Upadhya

PRINCIPLES OF AGING BIOLOGY PERTINENT TO THE CARDIOVASCULAR SYSTEM

As the aging process begins after maturation, deteriorative, regenerative, and compensatory changes develop over time and result in diminished physiologic reserve capacity and an increased vulnerability to challenges, and, as a result, a decrease in the ability to fully recover from and survive challenges (resilience). Importantly, aging itself does not result in disease; however, it does lower the threshold for the development of disease and can intensify and accelerate the effects of the disease once initiated. The increased vulnerability with age to external or internal challenges is one of the tenets of geriatrics and gerontology.

These concepts are particularly relevant to the aging of the human cardiovascular system, especially older persons living in developed countries. When studying normal aging in these populations, it is essential to consider screening for clinical and subclinical disease, particularly atherosclerosis, and consider the impact of cultural and environmental factors and social determinants of health that are distinct from aging yet can mimic aging effects. These can manifest in human population studies as cohort and period effects, subtle or overt, and easily confused with aging. For example, numerous observational studies indicate that blood pressure increases with aging. However, recent studies comparing age–blood pressure associations over a lifetime (to age 60) in westernized versus non-westernized Amerindian communities, the Yanomami and the Yekwana, from remote rainforests in Venezuela, suggest the strong association between age and

Learning Objectives

- Understand the effects of normal aging on cardiac and vascular structure and function.
- Describe the effects of normal aging on the anatomy and physiology of the heart and vasculature.
- Understand the possible implications of the age-related changes in resting cardiovascular function.
- Understand the role of age-related changes on lowering the threshold for clinical disease.
- Describe the effect of age on the cardiovascular response during exercise.

Key Clinical Points

1. Normal aging is accompanied by substantial alterations in the anatomy and physiology of the heart and vasculature.

2. There are declines in most cardiovascular function aspects, which create significantly reduced reserve capacity, which becomes more apparent during exercise and stress.

3. Many of the age-related changes may lower the threshold for clinical disease and predispose to various cardiovascular disorders in older people.

(Continued)

(Cont.)

4. Awareness of the principles of aging biology, in general, will help clinicians tailor intelligent treatments to older patients.

5. Age-related declines in cardiovascular and exercise performance have been shown to be partially preventable and reversible with exercise training. Thus, maintaining regularly scheduled physical activity is an important strategy to mitigate the adverse effects of aging on cardiovascular function.

blood pressure may instead be due to diet and lifestyle. There is an age-associated increase in BP among individuals from the Yekwana community, who have been exposed to western lifestyle, but not in the Yanomami community, who are largely hunter-gatherers-gardeners and have remained isolated from western lifestyle influences. It has been proposed that a true age-related change should be absent in young persons, increase with age, be universally present in very old persons, and not be related to any known, definable disease.

In some early human aging studies, individuals with clinical and subclinical diseases were not excluded, leading to an overestimation of the effects of aging on the cardiovascular system. Coronary atherosclerosis is highly prevalent in western societies and is an important disorder that can be occult and can significantly affect cardiac function. Systemic arterial hypertension is even more common. Therefore, reasonable screening for these two most common disorders is prudent to separate aging from disease.

In addition to the effects of subclinical disease, there are additional effects of physical inactivity. Humans and many animals become increasingly sedentary as they age. For example, rats given free access to a running wheel will run 20 km/week when they are young, but this decreases to less than 7 km/week when approaching the age of 23 months. Many older people are even less active, with Americans older than 70 years on average engaging in less than 10 minutes per day of physical activity. Another increasingly important lifestyle-related factor relatively new to civilization is obesity. Adipose tissue owing to excess caloric intake has numerous adverse effects involving nearly all physiologic systems, including cardiovascular, and obesity increases substantially with age. Thus, the changes seen in an older population reflect the combination of all these factors, period, cohort, lifestyle, disease-related changes, and the biological effect of age itself. It is often challenging to precisely separate and discern, both qualitatively and quantitatively, the latter from the former. However, awareness of the important nuances of normal aging can help avoid most errors.

AGING CHANGES IN THE HEART

Substantial changes occur with aging in myocardial composition, cardiac structure, and cardiovascular function at rest and during exercise. The changes in anatomy are summarized in **Table 73-1**.

Cellular Changes of the Aging Heart

Myocyte hypertrophy and degeneration Cardiomyocyte hypertrophy has been recognized as part of the response to the arterial changes and increased afterload described below. However, this should be interpreted in light of the evidence that the heart is renewing itself, continuously repopulated from resident stem cell populations and/or those from the bone marrow. Age-associated cardiomyocyte hypertrophy may mark depletion of the process, as the youngest cells, those most recently differentiated into cardiomyocytes, are thought to be the smallest, and in mouse hearts, myocyte size heterogeneity increases dramatically with age. Interestingly, the largest cells are also the most vulnerable to stress.

The loss of myocytes with age is greater than the ability to repopulate the heart. This loss is due to aging-induced oxidative stress and mitochondrial damage that trigger cardiomyocyte death, including necrosis, apoptosis, and autophagy. The exact mechanisms of oxidative stress-induced aging are still not precisely known. Increased reactive oxygen species lead to cellular senescence, which may stop cellular proliferation in response to damage. The total number of cardiomyocytes may be reduced by 50% in healthy human and animal hearts across the lifespan. Those remaining cardiac myocytes are increased in size and are much more variable in size. Nearly universal findings in hearts from older individuals are focal basophilic degeneration resulting from abnormal glycogenolysis and lipofuscin, a "wear-and-tear" pigment, which results in a macroscopic darkened appearance of the aged myocardium. Lipofuscin occupies up to 10% of myocyte volume in very old hearts. Each mitochondrion has its own genome, with a relatively sparse ability to correct mutations. Several investigators find mitochondrial DNA deletions may increase with age. The implications of this finding remain

TABLE 73-1 ■ AGE-RELATED CHANGES IN THE ANATOMY OF THE HEART

- No significant change in left ventricular mass
- Fibrosis, collagen accumulation in the myocardium
- Left ventricular cavity size decreases, shortening of long axis, rightward shift and dilatation of the aorta, dilation of left atrium, senile septum
- Calcific and fatty degeneration of valve leaflets and annuli
- Coronary artery dilation and calcification
- Conduction system: fibrosis and loss of specialized cells and fibers: 75% of pacemaker cells in sinoatrial node lost; fibrosis of atrioventricular node and left anterior fascicle

uncertain since there are approximately 1000 mitochondria per myocyte, and there is evidence of active mitochondrial quality control mechanisms, which may also be altered with age.

Nowhere is cellular dropout more impressive than in the sinoatrial node, decreasing the sinoatrial node volume with age. The number of pacemaker cells is reduced (90% by the age of 70), with most volume replaced by fat. More modest cellular losses occur at the atrioventricular (AV) node, and minimal changes occur in the distal conduction system. The dropout of sinoatrial nodal cells is accompanied by a decrease in the slow, L-type calcium channel critical to the initiation of depolarization. Although the density of the L-type Ca^{2+} channels does not seem to be affected by age, the function seems to decline: a reduction in Ca^{2+} transient amplitude and slower channel inactivation has been associated with aging. The sensitivity of the older sinoatrial node to calcium channel blockers appears to increase, as assessed in the older guinea pig pacemaker.

Alterations in myocyte calcium homeostasis and active relaxation Older cardiomyocytes are intrinsically stiffer. In isolated papillary muscles from older rat hearts, a change in the pattern of contraction and relaxation is seen: slower force generation and slower relaxation with no change in peak force. The inotropic and lusitropic (facilitating relaxation) responses to sympathetic stimulation are also decreased with age. Calcium fluxes dictate cardiac contraction and relaxation. For contraction, a small amount of calcium enters the cells via the slow L-type calcium channels stimulating the release of 10- to 20-fold more calcium from the sarcoplasmic reticulum (SR), permitting actin and myosin to generate force. Active relaxation includes the calcium reuptake by the cardiac SR after contraction and extrusion from the cell by the Na-Ca exchanger and the SR Ca-ATPase (SERCA) pump. SERCA hydrolyzes ATP to translocate Ca^{2+} from the cytosol back into the SR, allowing relaxation of the cardiac muscle. In the young heart, 90% of calcium cycles in and out of SR. Aging reduces the capacity of SR to accumulate, retain Ca^{2+}, and inhibit excitation-contraction coupling in the cardiomyocytes by interfering with the calcium transient. Calcium reuptake into the SR is decreased by almost 50% in old hearts from rats and mice, and the content of SERCA is decreased in old human hearts as well. Concurrently, the old SR has enhanced calcium leak manifested by small spontaneous localized releases called calcium sparks. All these impede cardiac relaxation, perhaps increase diastolic calcium concentrations, and result in smaller Ca stores in the SR for release in the next contraction. To a small extent, compensation occurs in other calcium fluxes in that the SR Ca-ATPase activity is increased in old rat hearts. Gene therapy, increasing the SR Ca-ATPase, has improved the function of old rat hearts.

Connective tissue fibrosis and scarring Age-related cardiac fibrosis reflects the net result of multiple pathways modulated by natriuretic peptides, neurohormonal drive, endothelin (ET) effects, reactive oxidation species, inflammation, advanced glycosylation end products, hemodynamics, and other influences, many of which will be subject to polymorphic genetic variation. Diffuse foci of fibrosis are seen microscopically in the myocardium owing to an increase in interstitial collagen, a delicate pattern, unlike the patches of fibrosis seen after acute injuries, such as after myocardial infarction. Age-related fibrosis does not appear to require either ischemia or hypertension, although both disorders accelerate the process. Quantitatively, collagen content approximately doubles in the old heart as measured by magnetic resonance imaging (MRI). The collagenous weave is thicker and more cross-linked, conferring greater rigidity to the myocardium. Aging may produce a shift in the balance between matrix metalloproteinases (MMPs) and tissue inhibitors of MMPs that ultimately translates into increased matrix accumulation. Increased age-related fibrosis has been found in the cardiac conduction system (the SA node, the AV node, the His bundle, and the left bundle branch) and left ventricular (LV) tissue. These changes may partly underlie age-related alterations in diastolic filling. In addition, the proliferation of cardiac fibroblasts and collagen deposition in the atria with age will affect the myocardium's electrophysiological properties. Atrial fibrosis might lower the threshold for the development of atrial arrhythmias.

The association between healthy aging and myocardial fibrosis has been a matter of debate. In a small study, 32 healthy volunteers underwent cardiac MRI-based assessment of myocardial extracellular volume (ECV); older age was associated with greater myocardial fibrosis. These observations are consistent with animal studies by MRI and histological assessments. However, these findings have not been seen uniformly. In a subset of 314 healthy individuals from the Multiethnic Study of Atherosclerosis (MESA) cohort, the degree of myocardial fibrosis, as assessed by ECV, and myocardial scar burden, was not associated with aging.

Senile amyloid deposition Another histopathological change found in cardiac tissue of older adults is amyloid deposition. Senile cardiac amyloid deposition is seen to varying degrees in the majority of hearts from persons older than 90 years with a prevalence greater than 90% but is uncommon before age 60. It is easily recognized at autopsy, particularly along the left atrial (LA) endocardium. Its physiologic and clinical significance are incompletely understood, but it might contribute to LV diastolic stiffness. In some cases, amyloid deposition occurs at a level that leads to the progressive development of heart failure (HF). This infiltrative cardiomyopathy is defined as systemic senile amyloidosis (SSA). SSA is far less common than atrium-restricted amyloidosis.

Epicardial adiposity and intramyocardial fat deposition Aging affects all organ systems and alters body composition. Typically, fat mass increases with age and peaks at age 60 to 75 years. With aging, adipose deposits, particularly in the right ventricular (RV) epicardium and the AV groove. This is most pronounced in women and the obese. These observations at autopsy correlate with the increase in epicardial and pericardial fat stripes that superficially mimic pericardial effusion on echocardiography. In the Framingham Heart Study (FHS), the incidence and size of clear echocardiographic spaces (fat stripes) in the pericardium increased with age in both posterior and anterior regions. The increase in adipocytes may reflect a loss of control of differentiation of resident stem cells. Emerging data suggest that this adipose may impair cardiac function—the cells are metabolically and hormonally active and can generate various factors, including cytokines. Increased pericardial fat has been associated with atherosclerosis and coronary calcification, risk of atrial fibrillation (AF), and HF, particularly HF with preserved ejection fraction (HFpEF).

Besides epicardial fat deposition, myocardial triglyceride content increases with aging, which is further accentuated by comorbidities such as diabetes and obesity. Aging-associated increase in myocardial triglyceride content may be related to reduced fatty acid oxidation in the aging heart. As noted in older individuals, greater myocardial triglyceride content is associated with increased fatty acid intermediates in the myocytes that alter myocardial structure and function and lead to myocardial lipotoxicity and increased cardiomyocyte apoptosis. Clinically, this may manifest as impaired myocardial relaxation, reduced cardiac exercise reserve, and increased risk of HFpEF.

Neurohormonal signaling The two main pathways are the renin-angiotensin-aldosterone system (RAAS) and β-adrenergic signaling. RAAS plays an important role in regulating blood volume and systemic resistance. Several studies have revealed similarities between angiotensin II–treated heart and the aging heart, suggesting that angiotensin II may play a role in cardiac aging. These similarities consisted of the development of cardiac hypertrophy, fibrosis, and diastolic dysfunction. Neurohormonal signaling also involves β-adrenergic receptors. These receptors regulate heart rate, myocardial contractility, and ventricular structural remodeling after stimulation by catecholamines. With aging, circulating catecholamine levels increase, leading to uncoupling of β-adrenergic receptors from their effector, adenylyl cyclase. This explains the reduced β-adrenergic responsivity observed with age.

Changes in Cardiac Structure

Left ventricular mass Seminal autopsy studies from subjects aged 20 to 99 without a history of hypertension or coronary atherosclerosis demonstrated that mean heart weight indexed to body surface area was not associated with age in men but increased with age in women. The interaction between age and gender has also been confirmed in other autopsy studies using 2D-guided M-mode echocardiographic measurements of LV mass and in the Cardiovascular Health Study (CHS), an NHLBI-funded population-based, observational cohort study of 5000 older adults. Recent

studies evaluating cross-sectional and longitudinal associations between aging in healthy individuals (without cardiovascular disease [CVD] including hypertension, diabetes, smoking) and LV mass using echocardiographic and cardiac MRI examinations have demonstrated no significant changes in LV mass with aging in men and women, particularly after accounting for body size. Taken together, there are modest effects of age on LV mass, with no change to a slight reduction in LV mass noted with aging, particularly in middle-aged or older individuals.

Left ventricular and atrial size Changes in LV cavity size with aging have been a matter of debate, with some cross-sectional studies demonstrating a decrease in LV internal diameter in systole and diastole with aging while others showing no change to an increase. Cross-sectional analyses from the Baltimore Longitudinal Study of Aging (BLSA) using MUGA scan-based LV size assessment suggested increasing LV end-diastolic volume with aging in men but not women. However, these observations have not been confirmed in other studies, and a decline in the LV end-diastolic volume with aging has been demonstrated in a cohort of 104 healthy volunteers who were rigorously screened to exclude prevalent CVD. Larger cohort studies using cardiac MRI or echo-based assessment of LV parameters demonstrated a decline in LV end-diastolic volume with aging in cross-sectional as well as longitudinal analysis with repeated follow-up assessments.

Most echocardiographic and autopsy studies have found a significant age-related increase in LA size in subjects without apparent CVD, with an increase in LA dimension between ages 30 and 70. However, frankly increased LA volume before age 70 may reflect disease, whereas after age 70, increased LA volume can occur from aging alone. The mechanisms of this age-related increase in LA volume are unknown but may be related to the age-related alterations in diastolic LV function. Serial echocardiographic measurements of LA size in humans have indicated that age and disease have additive effects on increases in LA size over time. Some have suggested an assessment of LA size to evaluate the presence of HFpEF. However, this is likely confounded by the effects of aging alone. While LA size appears to reflect chronic elevations in LV end-diastolic pressures, it does not discriminate whether this is due to systolic or diastolic dysfunction or restriction from pericardial or infiltrative processes. Therefore, LA volume may not be helpful in discriminating between the types of cardiac dysfunction that cause the elevations in pressure or volume. However, age-related LA dilation likely has consequences for specific disorders common in older adults, such as AF. Further, in population-based cohorts, LA size is significantly associated with the age-adjusted risk for stroke and death in both sexes.

Left ventricular wall thickness and geometry In the large autopsy study described earlier, RV and LV free wall thicknesses remained relatively constant with age, while

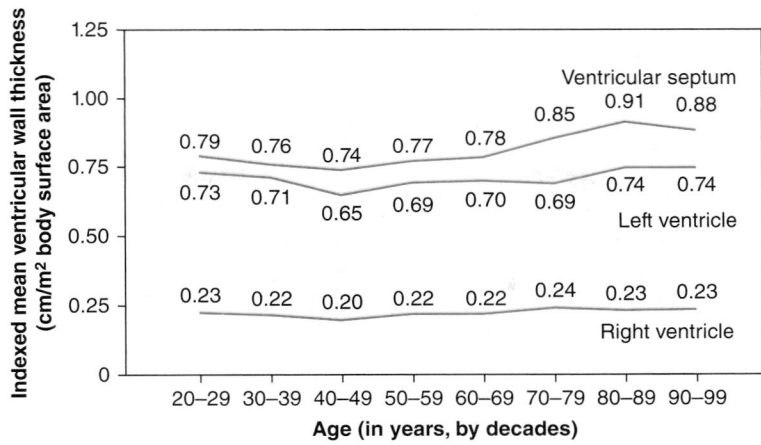

FIGURE 73-1. Ventricular wall thickness. Index mean ventricular wall thickness versus age in normal hearts from 765 adults. (Modified with permission from Kitzman DW, Edwards WD. Age-related changes in the anatomy of the normal human heart. *J Gerontol.* 1990;45[2]:M33–M39.)

ventricular septal thickness increased with age for both men and women, as shown in **Figure 73-1**. Wall thickness measurements at autopsy may not correlate well with those made in living individuals when measurements can be made in systole and diastole. However, most echocardiographic studies of healthy subjects confirmed autopsy-based findings showing mild age-related increases in ventricular septal and LV free wall thickness in women and men.

A frequent finding at autopsy and on echocardiograms of persons without apparent heart disease is the mild disproportionate thickening of the basal ventricular septum. This has been called sigmoid ventricular septum and senile septum and can confound to some degree the diagnosis of hypertrophic cardiomyopathy in older patients. The septal thickening may reflect hypertension rather than biological aging.

Due to increasing LV mass and free wall thickness and shrinking LV size, prior studies among healthy individuals demonstrated increasing relative wall thickness concentricity (mass/volume ratio) with aging. In more recent studies with MRI-based assessments, changes in relative wall thickness with aging have been less uniformly described. In a cross-sectional analysis from healthy individuals from MESA, the mass/volume ratio increased with aging in women but not men. In healthy individuals from the FHS, MRI-relative wall thickness did not increase with age in cross-sectional analysis. Among healthy Coronary Artery Risk Development in Young Adults (CARDIA) study participants, longitudinal echocardiographic assessment in young adulthood and middle age (20 years apart) did not show significant increases in relative wall thickness. These data suggest age-related changes relative to wall thickness are modest and may occur after middle age.

Valves The cardiac valves undergo several age-related changes. When measured at autopsy, the thicknesses of normal aortic and mitral leaflets increase, particularly along the closure margins. This is associated microscopically with collagen deposition and degeneration, lipid accumulation, and focal dystrophic calcification in the leaflets and annuli.

In those subjects most affected, this is recognized clinically and echocardiographically as aortic valve sclerosis, valve thickening without significant hemodynamic dysfunction. In the CHS, aortic sclerosis was found in 26% of participants, associated with male gender and hypertension. The relationship between age-related degenerative changes and the development of clinical aortic stenosis is incompletely defined, but aortic sclerosis is independently associated with a 1.5-fold increased risk of cardiovascular mortality, calling into serious question whether this should be considered a normal age-related change.

Age-related degenerative calcification of an otherwise normal-appearing tricuspid aortic valve may result in progressive aortic stenosis, the most common cause of aortic stenosis requiring valve replacement. The relationship between near-universal age-related thickening and mild calcification of the aortic valve leaflets and the development of degenerative calcific aortic stenosis is unclear, but the lack of efficacy of statins in modifying this natural history suggests that typical atherosclerosis is unlikely to be the driver.

The mitral annulus develops microscopic calcium deposits with aging, but gross mitral annular calcification is likely a disease process. Relatively little is known about the pathophysiology or natural history of mitral annular calcification. It is present in up to 40% of hearts from women older than 90 years with a large (4 to 1) female predominance. It is often associated with AV block and bundle branch block and modest mitral regurgitation but rarely with significant mitral stenosis.

The circumferences of all four cardiac valves, measured at autopsy, increase with age in normal hearts from

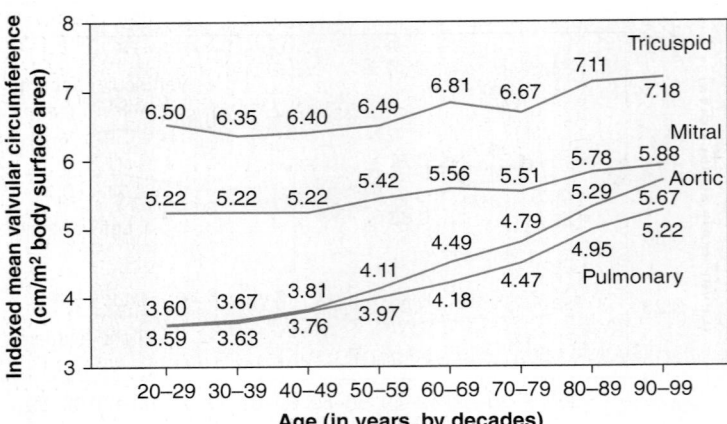

FIGURE 73-2. Normal indexed mean cardiac valve circumferences versus age. Results in 392 women. (Modified with permission from Kitzman DW, Edwards WD. Age-related changes in the anatomy of the normal human heart. *J Gerontol.* 1990;45[2]:M33–M39.)

women (**Figure 73-2**) and men and are associated with collagen degeneration and lipid accumulation in the valve annuli. This is most notable for the semilunar (aortic and pulmonary) valves than the AV (mitral and tricuspid) valves. In the case of the aortic annulus, this normal age-related dilatation has been confirmed in living subjects with echocardiography.

Annular dilatation likely contributes to the age-related increase in valvular regurgitation documented in healthy, normal, asymptomatic subjects. By the age of 80, 90% of apparently healthy subjects had multivalvular regurgitation; the aortic valve was affected earliest and to the greatest extent. The degree of valvular regurgitation caused by normal aging is always trivial or mild, central, and associated with normal (for age)-appearing leaflets. Age is the strongest risk factor for isolated severe aortic regurgitation. The idiopathic dilatation of the aortic annulus is the most common cause of aortic regurgitation in patients undergoing aortic valve surgery. This disease may exaggerate the age-related degenerative change with additional contributing factors as yet unidentified.

Pericardium Wavy bands of collagen bundles comprise the normal pericardium. The straightening of these wavy bands allows a degree of distensibility when pericardial pressure or volume increases acutely. With aging, these collagen bands become straighter, and the pericardium becomes thicker, and the pericardium of older subjects becomes stiffer. The significance of this is unknown, but it could impact diastolic compliance in older adults. As discussed earlier, the degree of epicardial and pericardial fat increases with age, particularly in women and obese persons.

Atrial septum The atrial septum thickens and becomes stiffer with age, probably owing to fatty infiltration and fibrosis. The atrial septum becomes less mobile with phasic respiration. If on echocardiography, a thin, hypermobile atrial septum is seen in an older person, then an atrial septal aneurysm (which often is accompanied by fenestrations),

patent foramen ovale, or atrial septal defect should be suspected and prompt further evaluation with color Doppler and peripheral venous injection of agitated saline contrast.

An exaggerated form of the age-related fatty infiltration of the atrial septum is found almost exclusively in older adults and is called lipomatous hypertrophy. It can mimic an intracardiac tumor but is recognizable by its characteristic dumbbell shape.

A patent foramen ovale is seen in approximately 35% of normal hearts younger than 30 years and in 20% at age 80. The lower prevalence of patent foramen ovale is accompanied by increased patent foramen ovale size in older individuals. While paradoxical embolism is usually considered when an atypical stroke occurs in a person younger than 55 years, it can contribute to strokes among older adults. Because of this, injection of venous-agitated saline contrast is often used as an adjunct to echocardiographic imaging even in older patients referred with atypical stroke.

Coronary arteries With aging, the coronary arteries become more dilated and tortuous, possibly because of hemodynamic drag. Coronary collaterals may increase in number and size with age, but this may reflect atherosclerosis. While atherosclerosis is a disease process, Mönckeberg medial calcification (arteriosclerosis) probably represents an age-related degenerative process. It is nearly universally found in the very old independent of gender. In the peripheral vasculature, it contributes to the age-related elevation in systolic blood pressure and arterial stiffening. Often seen in older patients and those with end-stage renal failure is the triad of cardiac calcifications (aortic cusps, mitral annulus, and coronary arteries), called the senile calcification syndrome. In these older persons, calcium metabolism is unaltered and, although a relationship with elevated serum cholesterol levels has been described, the etiology is unknown. These age-related changes could contribute to the loss of specificity of coronary calcium score in persons older than 75 years.

Overall Appearance

A characteristic geometric configuration is imparted to the older heart by these age-related changes, particularly those observed in the cardiac chambers: shortening of the long-axis dimension, a mild decrease in the internal systolic and diastolic LV cavity dimensions, dilatation, and rightward shifting of the aortic root, and dilatation of the left atrium as shown in **Figure 73-3**. These changes, plus mild regional calcification in the aortic and mitral valve annuli, are so characteristic that they serve as clues to help detect the age group of patients during blinded echocardiogram readings.

Changes in Cardiac Function with Age at Rest

Since there are significant changes in the anatomy of the cardiovascular system, one would expect alterations in cardiac physiology as well. Several important age-related

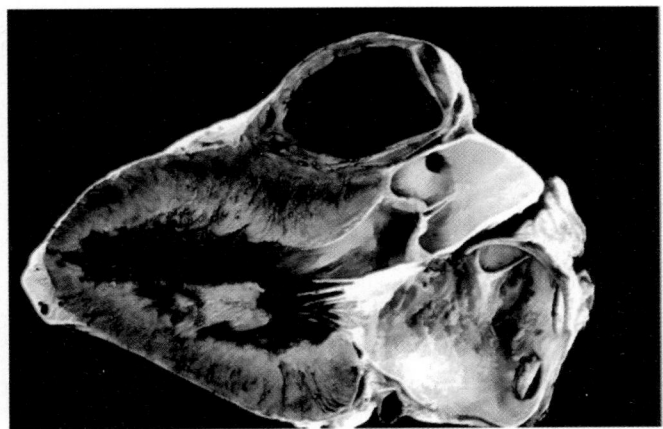

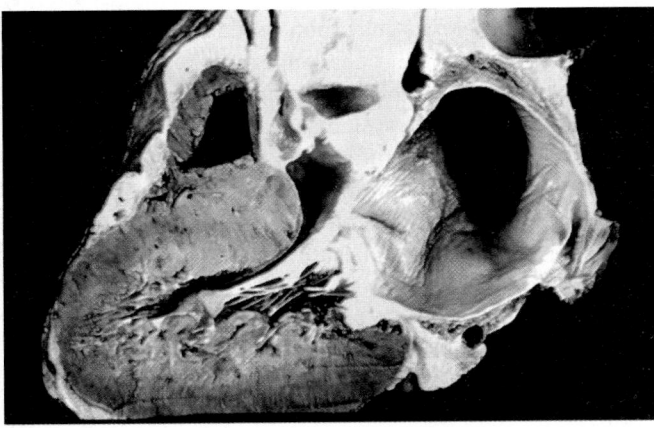

FIGURE 73-3. Age-related changes in the cardiac chambers. **A.** Normal heart from an 18-year-old for comparison (left ventricular long-axis views). **B.** Normal heart from an 84-year-old man demonstrates shortening of the base-to-apex (long-axis) dimension, decreased internal left ventricular dimension, aortic root dilatation with rightward shift, sigmoid-shaped septum, and left atrial dilatation. (Reproduced with permission from Bradenburg R, Fuster V, Giuliani ER, et al. *Cardiology Fundamentals and Practice.* Chicago, IL: Year Book Medical Publishers; 1987.)

TABLE 73-2 ■ AGE-RELATED CHANGES IN CARDIOVASCULAR PHYSIOLOGY
• Peak exercise capacity declines
• Peak cardiac output declines
• Peak heart rate declines
• Peak ejection fraction declines
• LV stiffness increases, diastolic relaxation decreases
• Valvular regurgitation develops
• Prolongation of PR, QRS, QT; left axis deviation
• Arteries stiffen, aortic impedance increases
• Peripheral oxygen extraction reserve declines

changes have already been discussed briefly earlier, including changes in valvular function and the potential anatomic substrates for impaired diastolic function. While the effect of age on cardiac function has long been a research topic, only recently have studies been performed using adequately robust techniques combined with appropriately screened reference populations. However, it is still true that little information is available regarding how these changes in function impact the epidemiology, presentation, diagnosis, prognosis, and therapy of CVD. Changes with age in cardiovascular function are summarized in **Table 73-2**.

Most earlier studies of cardiovascular function at rest show either no substantial change in cardiac output, stroke volume, heart rate, and ejection fraction with aging or mild-to-moderate and significant increases in systemic and pulmonary arterial blood pressure, with resultant increases in left and right ventricular afterload. However, in a cohort of healthy, well-screened individuals who underwent detailed resting and exercise hemodynamic and radionuclide assessment of LV volumes, there was a significant cross-sectional association between older age and smaller LV size, higher LV filling pressure, and lower stroke volume at rest, suggesting alterations in Frank-Starling mechanisms.

Heart rate and rhythm There is no change in resting heart rate with healthy adult aging (**Figure 73-4**). However, as will be discussed in the section on exercise, there is a clear and marked decrease in maximum heart rate in response to exercise that is highly predictable and can easily be estimated by a simple equation. For healthy adults, the equation (208 − [0.7 × age]) predicts the maximum heart rate for exercise testing.

The age-related change in maximum heart rate is perhaps the most substantial change in cardiac function, both in magnitude and in consequence. Although its mechanism(s) are not fully understood, several studies have been performed. In the presence of the β-adrenergic antagonist, propranolol, and the parasympathetic antagonist, atropine, ablating both sympathetic and parasympathetic input to the heart, the intrinsic heart rate is seen. Intrinsic heart rate decreases by 5 to 6 beats/min each decade of age so that the resting heart rate in an 80 years old is not much slower than the intrinsic heart rate. At rest, the parasympathetic

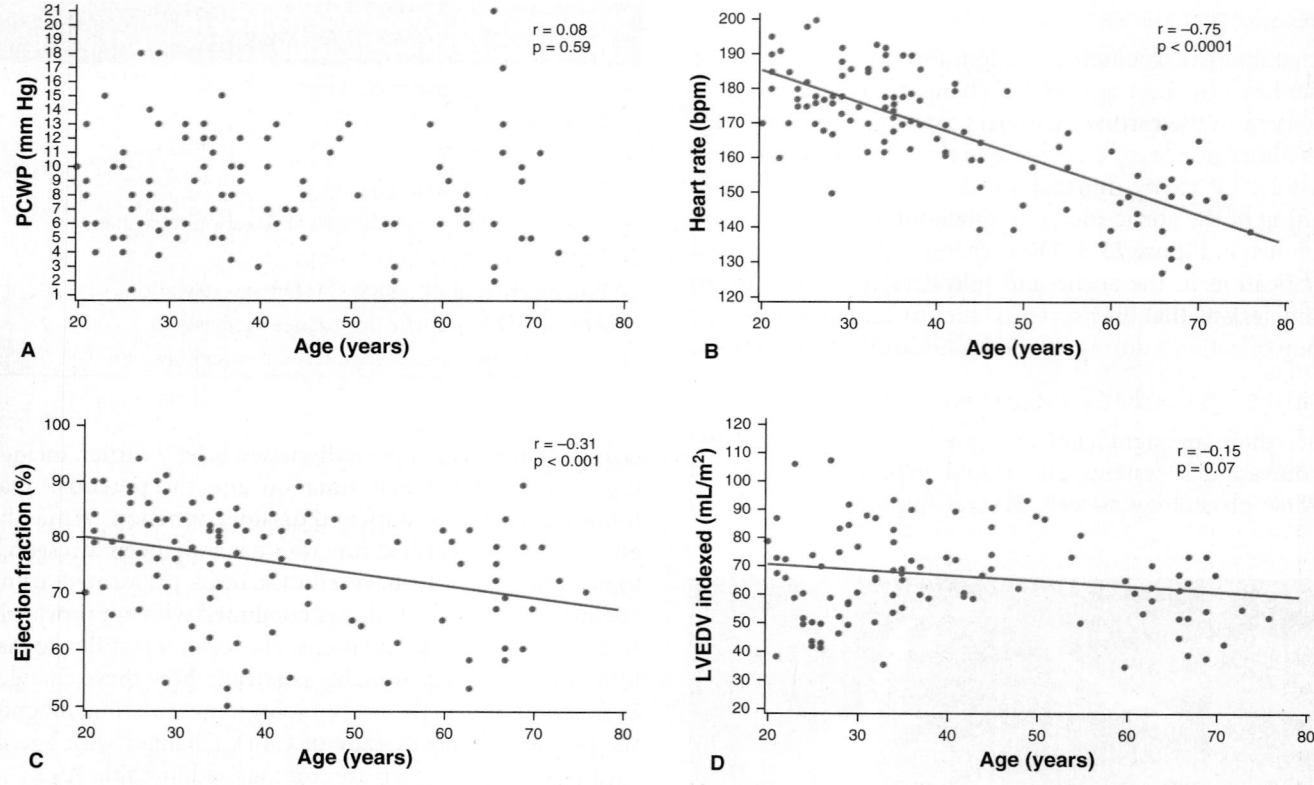

FIGURE 73-4. Correlation between age and resting measures of (**A**) diastolic function assessed invasively using pulmonary capillary wedge pressure, (**B**) heart rate, (**C**) systolic function assessed as ejection fraction, and (**D**) left ventricular end-diastolic volume among healthy, community-dwelling volunteers without cardiovascular disease. (Reproduced with permission from Pandey A, Kraus WE, Brubaker PH, et al. Healthy aging and cardiovascular function: invasive hemodynamics during rest and exercise in 104 healthy volunteers. *JACC Heart Fail.* 2020;8[2]:111–121.)

nervous system is minimally slowing the heart. As would be expected, the increase in heart rate after atropine is less in older adults than the young.

There is also decreased response to sympathetic agonists. Administration of sympathomimetic agents to healthy young and old adults demonstrated chronotropic effects were attenuated in the old. At doses that increased heart rate by 25 beats/min in young males, heart rate increased only 10 beats/min or less in older adults.

Supporting the decline in maximal heart rate as a primary age-related biological change is that it is not modified by vigorous exercise training; it is not a consequence of reduced physical activity. Also, it does not appear to reflect inadequate sympathetic stimulation, as plasma norepinephrine levels are increased, not decreased, at rest in normal older adults. Further, norepinephrine increases even more with exertion in older than in young persons under similar stress.

Perhaps as a direct reflection of the decreased parasympathetic nervous system input and decreased responsiveness to autonomic input, there is a significant decrease in heart rate variability. Heart rate variability measures the variations in instantaneous heart rate (or RR interval) over time. Loss of variability results in decreased complexity,

which correlates with the decrease in physiologic reserve. Any loss of complexity may then render the older individual less likely to tolerate challenges to their homeostasis. Furthermore, the loss of complexity with age occurs in a number of physiologic systems and is forestalled by interventions like exercise training.

In highly screened older adults, to exclude potential confounding effects of disease, the prevalence of atrial premature beats (APBs) reaches 88% on 24-hour ambulatory monitoring. Because there is no association with cardiac risk over the next decade with the presence of APBs, they are not thought to reflect subclinical coronary artery disease. At exercise testing, isolated ventricular ectopic beats occurred in more than half of highly screened adults older than 80 years. Therefore, the increases in ectopy of both atrial and ventricular origin are considered normal aging processes.

Diastolic function Increased LV stiffness associated with aging using invasive techniques was first described in young and old beagles. Ten years later, similar findings were identified by invasive techniques in humans. The advent of spectral Doppler echocardiography in between these two developments greatly expanded the ability for noninvasively assessing LV diastolic filling. All studies, including the large population-based databases from the FHS and the CHS, have uniformly found that diastolic LV filling is substantially altered in older normal adults. In addition, similar changes with aging are found in monkeys, rats, dogs, and mice.

The age-related changes in diastolic LV filling patterns—measured by reduction in early diastolic LA emptying, increased late diastolic emptying from atrial contraction, and increase in isovolumic relaxation time on pulsed Doppler echocardiography—have been confirmed in noninvasive human studies. The echocardiographic indexes of diastolic filling may be altered early in the course of various disorders that are common and sometimes unrecognized in older adults. A number of physiologic variables significantly influence them. Thus, it had been questioned whether the age-related alterations in Doppler diastolic filling indexes were simply secondary to these or whether they occurred independently of CVD and other confounding physiologic variables. However, physiologic studies with invasive and noninvasive hemodynamic assessments in old and young healthy volunteers rigorously screened for CVD have confirmed that an alteration in diastolic LV filling pattern is a primary, biologic effect of aging, intrinsic to the aged human heart, and not explicable by other physiologic and pathologic changes that frequently accompany the aging process.

Since normal healthy older individuals are expected to have an altered Doppler LV filling pattern, what should be considered abnormal? Data from echocardiographic assessments in older healthy adults without CVD included in large community-based cohort studies such as the CHS and FHS have yielded important data informing the normative range for diastolic function parameters in older men and women. Thus, Doppler diastolic filling patterns within this range should be considered normal in patients in this age range. Accordingly, it is preferable to use the term "delayed relaxation" or "normal for age" in clinical descriptions of this finding, rather than the terms "impaired relaxation" or "abnormal relaxation," which denote abnormality and are inconsistent with aging principles. In addition, findings obtained in older patients during basal conditions that fall outside these ranges should be considered abnormal, regardless of age. Second, the pattern of LV filling is helpful. Certain patterns, such as the pseudonormalized and restrictive patterns can be more easily discerned from normal and can be more specific for disease when found in older than in younger patients because these differ more from the expected pattern. Mitral annulus tissue Doppler has significantly boosted the ability to assess LV diastolic function noninvasively because the annular velocity measures are relatively load-dependent. As would be expected, based on the above study, age alters the tissue Doppler velocities as well. Unfortunately, age-related normative reference data are relatively sparse.

The age-related differences in LV diastolic function and LV compliance have also been assessed by invasive hemodynamic studies. Among healthy, community-dwelling individuals age 20 to 76 well-screened for CVD, a cross-sectional assessment demonstrated higher pulmonary capillary wedge pressure and smaller LV size with increasing age suggesting worse diastolic function and alteration in LV relaxation (**Figure 73-4**). Some studies have attributed the age-related difference in LV diastolic function to greater intrinsic LV stiffness with a slowing in LV relaxation in early middle age and a significant reduction in diastolic LV function after the age of 65. Other studies have questioned the contribution of impairment in LV relaxation toward the age-related decline in LV diastolic function and implicated changes in the LA properties.

Age-related alterations in LV diastolic function are also evidenced by an atrial gallop (S4) physical examination findings in those older than 75 years. An atrial gallop is a manifestation of the increased contribution of LA systole to ventricular filling. The decrease in rapid cardiac relaxation during early diastole results in increased dependence on LA systole in late diastole for adequate LV cardiac filling. However, as things worsen, LA pressures increase, and early filling subsequently increases again. This pseudonormalization of LV filling is another marker that the aging process has tipped over to HF.

The age-related changes in diastolic function can also be modified and improved by exercise behavior and cardiorespiratory fitness levels. In old rats trained on treadmill exercise for 1 to 2 months, SR calcium uptake and cardiac relaxation improved to that seen in young sedentary rats. In mechanistic hemodynamic studies among humans, older individuals with greater lifetime exercise exposure have been shown to have more favorable LV diastolic function than sedentary individuals. Furthermore, recent exercise training studies in human participants have also demonstrated significant improvement in invasive measures of LV diastolic stiffness with intense, long-duration (up to 2 years) exercise training in middle-aged but not older age adults. Humans on caloric restriction diets have better diastolic function than age-matched controls, corroborating experiments in experimental animals. While this approach may not be highly practical, only 5 years of caloric restriction is needed to produce the change. Furthermore, intentional weight loss interventions have also demonstrated significant improvements (~20% reduction) in invasively assessed left-sided filling pressures. Taken together, these findings suggest that the age-related diastolic impairment may be modifiable, particularly, early in the course of the aging process, with lifestyle interventions.

Systolic function In healthy humans, no age-related changes in measurable, overall LV contractility, assessed at rest by the ejection fraction, fractional shortening, or mean velocity of circumferential fiber shortening, have been reported. (**Figure 73-4**). Wall motion abnormalities should not be considered normal, even in very old adults. In the CHS, the prevalence of unexpected wall motion abnormalities, in the absence of history and symptoms of coronary heart disease, was 0.4% in women and 0.5% in men.

The contraction and relaxation of the older LV are not uniform. In older people, segments of the heart have started to relax while others are still contracting. As LV pressure must be low before filling can start, this prolonged contraction shortens the time available for filling to occur.

Aging alters several Doppler measures of aortic outflow. Aortic peak flow velocity, time-velocity integral, and acceleration are reduced with advancing age. While these hemodynamic factors relate to LV systolic performance, they are also substantially affected by afterload, which increases with aging.

Right ventricular structure and function Autopsy studies of the RV have demonstrated a progressive loss of myocytes and increased myocyte volume per nuclei suggestive of cellular hypertrophy with increasing age. However, the magnitude of cellular hypertrophy is insufficient to make up for the loss of RV mass, which declines significantly with aging. In human cohort studies, cross-sectional comparison of echocardiographic RV parameters across different age groups of healthy individuals, aging was associated with

lower RV longitudinal systolic function as measured by the tricuspid annular plane systolic excursion. RV ejection fraction is relatively preserved with aging. Furthermore, studies have also demonstrated a decline in RV relaxation and increased right atrial pressure, as assessed by echocardiography, with aging. Doppler indices, reflective of flow pattern, demonstrate a reduced early RV diastolic filling, increased late filling, and reduced myocardial diastolic velocities. The abnormalities in RV systolic and diastolic function with aging have been attributed to increasing pulmonary artery pressure and RV afterload with aging, mostly secondary to increased pulmonary arterial stiffness and vascular resistance in the pulmonary vasculature. No significant differences in RV size were noted with aging in cross-sectional echocardiographic assessments.

Implications of the Age-Related Changes in Resting Cardiovascular Function

Aging is associated with a decline in resting oxygen uptake driven by decreases in cardiac output. The decline in cardiac output is related to the reduction in stroke volume. The resting peripheral oxygen extraction has been shown to increase with aging; however, its clinical significance is not well established (**Figure 73-5**).

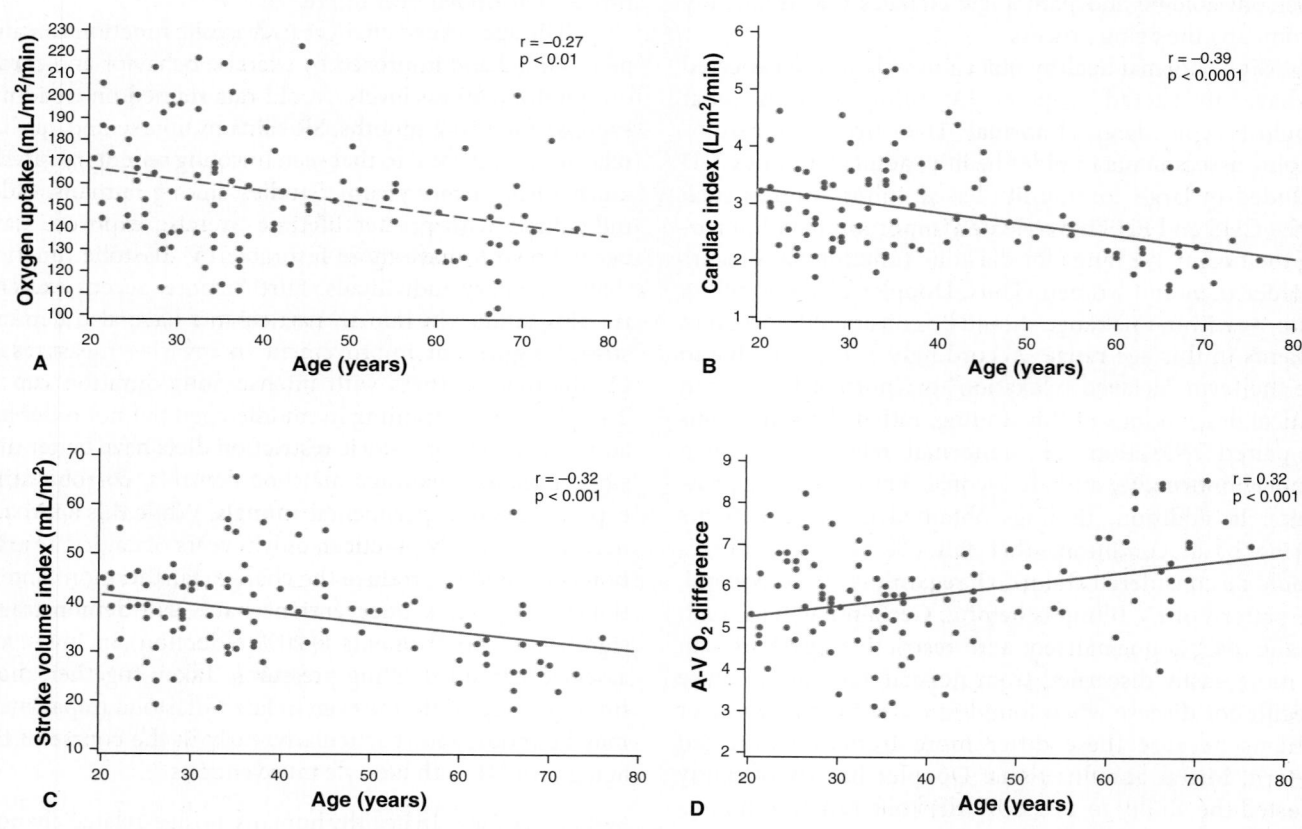

FIGURE 73-5. Correlation between age and resting measures of (**A**) oxygen uptake, (**B**) cardiac index, (**C**) stroke volume index, and (**D**) peripheral oxygen extraction among healthy, community-dwelling volunteers without cardiovascular disease. (Reproduced with permission from Pandey A, Kraus WE, Brubaker PH, et al. Healthy aging and cardiovascular function: invasive hemodynamics during rest and exercise in 104 healthy volunteers. *JACC Heart Fail.* 2020;8[2]:111–121.)

Aging decreases one's ability to tolerate challenges to homeostasis. This is most evident in the cardiovascular system. For example, the mortality and probability of developing HF after a myocardial infarction increase dramatically with age. While clearly, the pathogenesis of atherosclerosis and the myocardial infarction itself is not normal aging, the response to the systemic challenges produced by the infarction may well be impaired because of the aging process. Consistent with this, there is an age-related increase in mortality after experimental infarction in mice and rats. We suggest that homeostenosis, the depletion of reserves, may be the cost of invoking compensatory mechanisms to maintain homeostasis.

Similarly, acute hypertension is poorly tolerated in the old. Old (18 months) and adult (9 months) rats had afterload increased by constriction of the aorta. Immediate early response gene signals were attenuated in the old rats. Decreased skeletal actin expression after pressure overload was present, and skeletal actin expression precedes cardiac actin expression in most hypertrophy models. Atrial natriuretic peptide (ANP) stimulates the excretion of water and sodium by the kidney. The atria only express ANP in normal young hearts, but ANP is a marker of stress and compensation when seen in the ventricles. ANP is elevated in the ventricles at baseline in the old rat and could not be further stimulated after additional stress. This suggested that the hypertrophy response was already invoked as part of aging in the older rats and was less available to respond to acute stress.

While the normal heart is unlikely to ever be exposed to ischemia, ischemic preconditioning is an adaptation of the young heart that is not present in the old heart. If repeatedly exposed to brief episodes of ischemia, young hearts tolerate longer episodes well with less resultant damage by increasing heat-shock protein levels, opening ATP-gated potassium channels, stimulating the tumor necrosis factor-alpha (TNF-α) cascade, and activating antioxidant enzymes. Old hearts cannot make this adaptation, perhaps contributing to the increased mortality after myocardial infarct in the old. However, exercise training, caloric restriction, and certain growth factors may restore this adaptive capability.

The responsiveness is decreased to some cardioactive drugs, including atropine, dobutamine, and other β-adrenergic active agents, as noted above. These agents may require higher doses to reach a desired effect in the old. HF becomes increasingly common, reaching a prevalence of more than 10% and being the most common reason for hospitalization of Medicare beneficiaries. The syndrome of HFpEF, the most common form among older persons, is likely facilitated by the above- and below-discussed age-related changes in diastolic function, myocardial composition, and vasculature added to the arterial and myocardial changes caused by hypertension and other diseases. Findings from large epidemiological cohort studies have shown that risk of HFpEF increases with age.

Furthermore, age-related decline in exercise capacity and diastolic function are important predictors of HFpEF development. Age-related changes in vessels and the heart do not by themselves produce disease, but because of the changes in compliance, systolic hypertension is common. Finally, these changes make the old cardiovascular system more prone to decompensation in response to other insults.

Effect of Age on the Cardiovascular Response During Exercise

If aging affects cardiovascular performance even at rest or with moderate stress, one would expect this to be magnified and become even more apparent during exercise. This is indeed the case. Exercise capacity can be quantified objectively by measurement of maximal oxygen consumption (VO_2max) during exercise. It is solidly established that a reduction in VO_2max inescapably accompanies normal aging. While the age at which this decline begins is unclear, it is probably variable and begins early in adult life. The reduction in VO_2max is independent of gender and changes in body size. The magnitude of the decline is approximately 3% to 8% per decade, the rate of decline increasing with each decade and can be modified but not wholly halted or reversed by exercise training.

Initial studies from the BLSA in the 1980s had suggested a relatively small (~3%) decline in VO_2max with aging attributed largely to loss of muscle mass with a modest decline in exercise cardiac function. However, these findings were at substantial variance with other studies. At the time, the difference compared with prior studies was attributed to rigorous screening. A subsequent report from the BLSA in 2005, which examined a large number of subjects, both sedentary and well-conditioned by training, during 8 years of follow-up, thereby providing true longitudinal rather than cross-sectional data, showed that, in actuality, the decline in exercise capacity (VO_2max) among older persons was more accelerated and greater in magnitude than all previous estimates, with the rate of decline accelerating from 3% to 6% per decade till 40 years of age to more than 20% per 10 years among those older than 70 years. In addition, another subsequent report from the BLSA in 1995 showed that, in contrast to the original study in 1984, both men and women do indeed have substantial age-related declines in maximal exercise cardiac output, accompanying and contributing to a 40% decline in VO_2max. Similarly, in a recently reported study of 104 healthy, community-dwelling individuals aged 20 to 76 years who were rigorously screened for subclinical or clinical CVD, a 40% decline in VO_2max was observed across the six decades. This is in accord with reports from all other studies. Thus, there is now uniform agreement that aging, even in the absence of any identifiable disease, is associated with substantial declines in overall cardiovascular performance and reserve capacity, including maximal cardiac output (**Figure 73-6**).

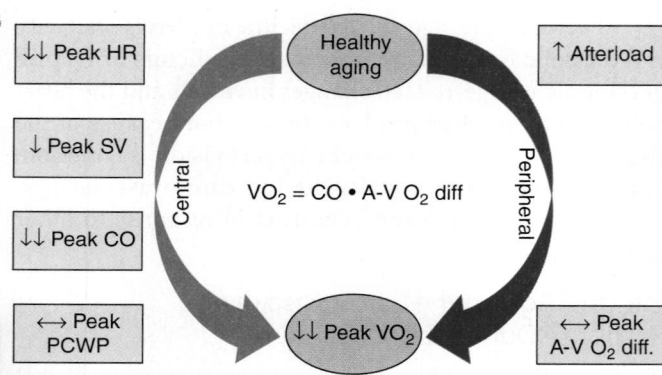

FIGURE 73-6. Mechanisms of decline in peak exercise oxygen uptake with aging. The key drivers of decline in peak exercise oxygen uptake are largely reductions in peak exercise heart rate and peak exercise stroke volume, which is driven by alterations in Frank-Starling mechanisms and reduced left ventricular contractility at peak exercise. (Reproduced with permission from Pandey A, Kraus WE, Brubaker PH, et al. Healthy aging and cardiovascular function: invasive hemodynamics during rest and exercise in 104 healthy volunteers. *JACC Heart Fail.* 2020;8[2]:111–121.)

By the Fick principle for oxygen, only a limited number of factors could be responsible for a decline in VO₂max. The following equations are pertinent to this discussion:

VO_2 = cardiac output × arteriovenous oxygen (A-VO₂ diff) difference

Cardiac output = stroke volume × heart rate

Stroke volume = end-diastolic volume – end-systolic volume

The A-VO₂ is determined by a number of noncardiac factors, including peripheral vascular and skeletal muscle mass and metabolic function. Thus, if VO₂max declines with aging, there must be a decline in peak cardiac output or A-VO₂ or both during exercise.

Measurement of cardiac output in healthy human subjects during exercise is challenging methodologically. Investigators have used various techniques, including direct Fick (probably the most reliable), dye dilution, equilibrium-gated radionuclide angiography, and gas rebreathing. Each of these methods uses multiple variables to derive the cardiac output measurement. Direct measurement of A-VO₂ by oximetry, however, is quite accurate and reliable. Most investigators who have measured A-VO₂ during maximal exercise have documented no difference or increased A-VO₂ in older compared with young subjects. By simple algebra, this suggests that the age-related decline in VO₂max must be because of reduced cardiac output. This has, indeed, been the finding reported by virtually all investigators. Accordingly, a decrease in the inotropic (contractility), chronotropic (heart rate), and as well as lusitropic (diastolic function) responses to dobutamine/exercise may all have a potential role in the age-related decline of VO₂max (**Table 73-3**).

The age-related decline in VO₂max appears to be driven primarily by reduced exercise cardiac output, stroke volume, and heart rate among older versus younger individuals, as shown in **Figure 73-7**. Specifically, the reduction in peak exercise stroke volume was most notable among individuals who were 60 years and older. Other studies using the direct Fick technique, dye dilution, or acetylene rebreathing to assess cardiac output have also demonstrated a decline in maximal cardiac output with aging. The primary mechanism of the age-related decline in exercise cardiac output is the age-related reduction in maximal heart rate. Reduced maximal exercise heart rate appears to be a universal observation and meets the basic biological aging phenomenon criteria. Future studies are needed to understand better the biological mechanisms underlying the age-related decline in maximal heart rate.

Although reduced maximal heart rate is the primary mechanism for reduced exercise cardiac output and oxygen

TABLE 73-3 ■ MEASURES OF CARDIAC PERFORMANCE AND LEFT VENTRICULAR DIMENSIONS AT REST, SUBMAXIMAL UPRIGHT EXERCISE (50 W), AND MAXIMAL UPRIGHT EXERCISE AMONG HEALTHY INDIVIDUALS ACROSS DIFFERENT AGE GROUPS

	RESTING			SUBMAX (50 W)			PEAK EXERCISE		
	<40 Y	40–60 Y	>60 Y	<40 Y	40–60 Y	>60 Y	<40 Y	40–60 Y	>60 Y
Peak oxygen uptake, mL/m²/min	160(29)	160 (24)	141 (25)	465 (75)	479 (55)	392 (46)	1226 (252)	1081 (282)	792 (179)
Heart rate, bpm	79 (13)	76 (12)	75 (16)	102 (16)	100 (1)	99 (18)	178 (10)	160 (13)	148 (11)
Stroke volume index, mL/m²	39 (10)	40 (10)	31 (10)	54 (11)	54 (11)	40 (7)	52 (11)	52 (10)	39 (6)
Cardiac index, L/m²/min	3.0 (0.8)	3.0 (0.9)	2.2 (0.6)	5.5 (1.3)	5.4 (1.1)	4.0 (0.7)	9.3 (1.9)	8.2 (1.6)	5.8 (1.1)
Ejection fraction (%)	64 (9)	65 (8)	65 (10)	71 (7)	72 (8)	71 (10)	78 (10)	73 (10)	71 (10)
PCWP, mm Hg	2 (2.6)	3 (2.3)	3 (3.3)	4.3 (3.3)	5.0 (2.7)	4.4 (3.3)	9 (3.8)	8 (3.4)	8(4.8)
A-V O₂ difference, (%)	5.5 (1.1)	5.8 (1.0)	6.7 (1.3)	8.6 (1.2)	9.2 (1.5)	10.1 (1.3)	13.5 (2.0)	13.2 (2.4)	13.4 (1.8)
LV EDV index, mL/m²	62 (18)	61 (14)	47 (14)	77 (17)	75 (11)	58 (11)	67 (17)	71 (15)	56(11)

Abbreviations: A-V O₂ difference, arteriovenous oxygen difference; bpm, beats per minute; EDV, end-diastolic volume; LV, left ventricle; PCWP, pulmonary capillary wedge pressure.
Adapted with permission from Pandey A, Kraus WE, Brubaker PH, et al. Healthy aging and cardiovascular function: invasive hemodynamics during rest and exercise in 104 healthy volunteers. JACC Heart Fail. 2020;8(2):111–121.

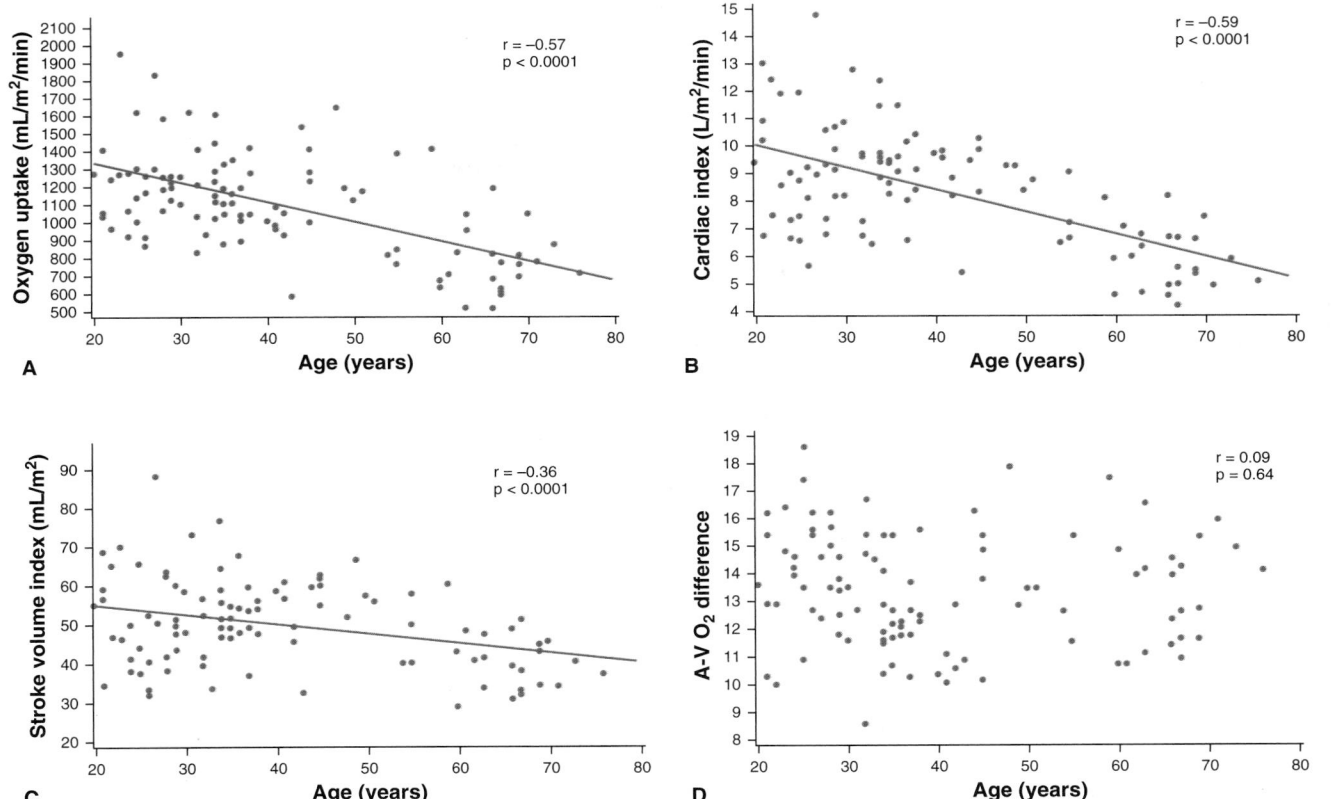

FIGURE 73-7. Correlation between age and peak exercise measures of (**A**) oxygen uptake, (**B**) cardiac index, (**C**) stroke volume index, and (**D**) peripheral oxygen extraction among healthy, community-dwelling volunteers without cardiovascular disease. (Reproduced with permission from Pandey A, Kraus WE, Brubaker PH, et al. Healthy aging and cardiovascular function: invasive hemodynamics during rest and exercise in 104 healthy volunteers. *JACC Heart Fail.* 2020;8[2]:111–121.)

consumption in older subjects, younger subjects in whom exercise heart rate is limited, either by congenital complete heart block or by a β-adrenergic blockade, stroke volume is increased and partially compensates for the reduced heart rate via the Frank-Starling response (increased end-diastolic volume). The effect of aging on the Frank-Starling mechanism and maximal stroke volume response to exercise depends on the age range examined. Specifically, studies limited to younger and middle-aged individuals (< 50 years) have failed to appreciate a significant decline in maximal exercise stroke volume with aging. The most recent and largest study of aging effects studied invasively in 104 well-screened, health healthy men and women reported by Kitzman and colleagues; there was a modest continuous decline in Frank-Starling from age 30 to age 80 (the oldest age studied), demonstrated by lower invasively measured end-diastolic and stroke volumes, lower LV ejection fraction, a trend toward higher pulmonary capillary wedge pressure during exhaustive upright exercise in the old (**Figure 73-8**).

Furthermore, the decline in end-diastolic and stroke volumes and ejection fraction were noted at both submaximal and maximal exercise levels with aging highlighting a consistent alteration in the Frank-Starling mechanisms in response to exercise (**Figure 73-9**). A lower exercise stroke

volume in older adults could be because of higher end-systolic volume or lower end-diastolic volume. LV end-systolic volume was higher, and ejection fraction was lower at peak exercise in the older subjects in most studies in which these were measured. Thus, systolic LV function reserve is reduced with aging as well. Reduced stroke volume could also result partially from increased afterload since systolic blood pressure, aortic impedance, and systemic vascular resistance are higher during exercise in old than in young, healthy subjects. When afterload is taken into account, maximal stroke work is fairly similar in young and old subjects.

When evaluating older patients for coronary heart disease, it should be recognized that in healthy older people, the LV ejection fraction does not increase as much from rest to peak exercise as it does in young, healthy subjects. In fact, a flat response in older men and a mild decline in older women should be considered normal. However, the development of wall motion abnormalities should be considered abnormal, even in the presence of a mild nonspecific decline in ejection fraction.

There has been less information regarding peripheral cardiovascular function with aging, including systemic arterial function, which is required to deliver oxygenated

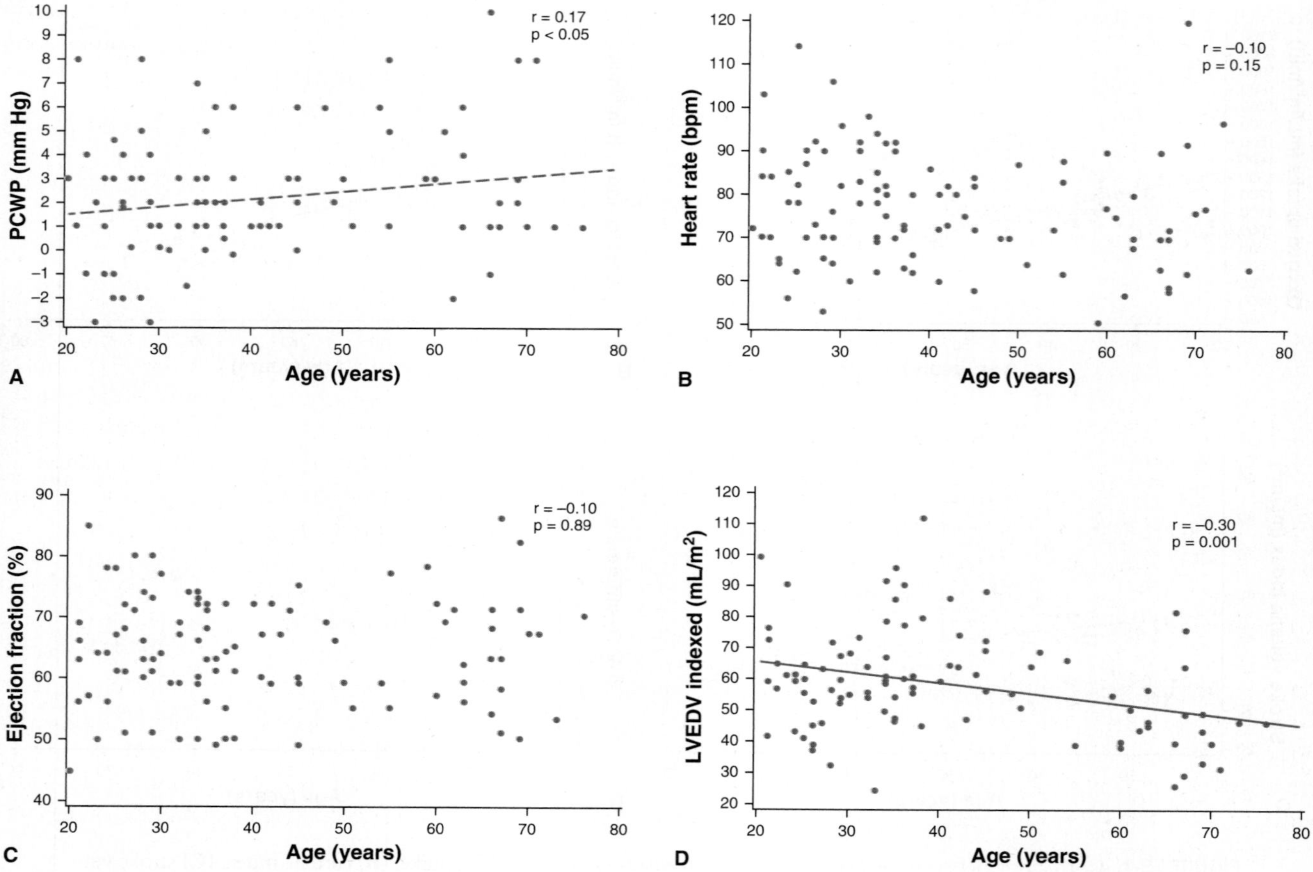

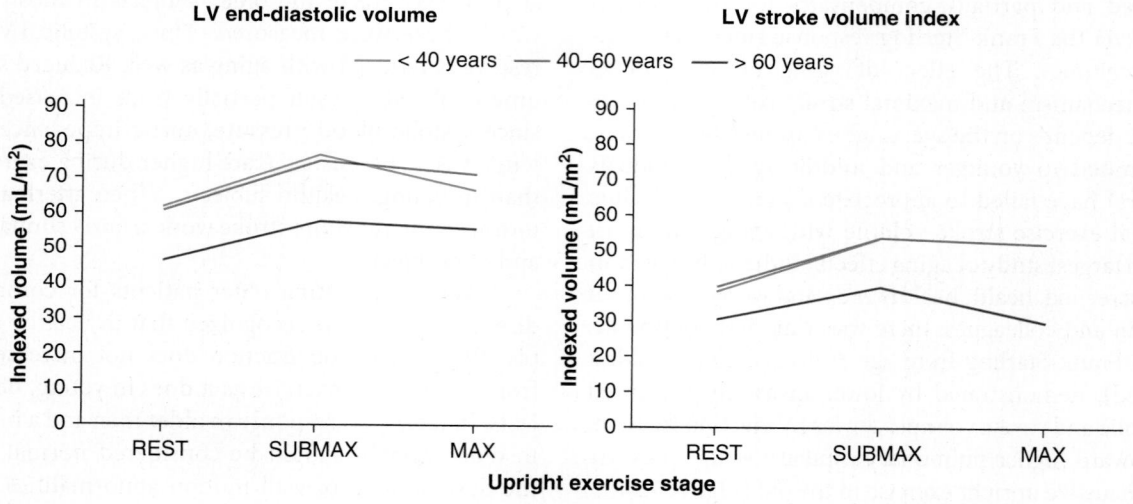

FIGURE 73-8. Correlation between age and peak exercise measures of (**A**) diastolic function assessed invasively using pulmonary capillary wedge pressure, (**B**) heart rate, (**C**) systolic function assessed as ejection fraction, and (**D**) left ventricular end-diastolic volume among healthy, community-dwelling volunteers without cardiovascular disease. (Reproduced with permission from Pandey A, Kraus WE, Brubaker PH, et al. Healthy aging and cardiovascular function: invasive hemodynamics during rest and exercise in 104 healthy volunteers. *JACC Heart Fail.* 2020;8[2]:111–121.)

FIGURE 73-9. Differences in left ventricular end-diastolic volume and stroke volume changes in response to exercise across different age groups as observed in a healthy, community-dwelling volunteers without cardiovascular disease. (Reproduced with permission from Pandey A, Kraus WE, Brubaker PH, et al. Healthy aging and cardiovascular function: invasive hemodynamics during rest and exercise in 104 healthy volunteers. *JACC Heart Fail.* 2020;8[2]:111–121.)

blood to working muscle efficiently and working muscle itself. Some studies have demonstrated a decline in exercise A-VO$_2$ with aging, while others have failed to observe this association. An invasive hemodynamic characterization of 104 healthy individuals at rest and peak exercise did not observe a significant association between A-VO$_2$ at peak exercise and age (**Figure 73-7**). However, a significant inverse association between age and A-VO$_2$ reserve (change from resting to peak exercise) with a smaller absolute increase in A-VO$_2$ from rest to peak exercise in older versus younger individuals was reported suggesting that reduced peripheral oxygen extraction ability in older age may contribute, to some degree, to the age-related decline in VO$_2$max (**Table 73-3**). In an invasive hemodynamic study of old and young individuals without CVD, Beere et al. demonstrated that in addition to reduced peak exercise cardiac output, older men had reduced exercise leg blood flow. The study also repeated the detailed measurements of central and peripheral cardiovascular functions following exercise training. Their results confirmed the findings of a number of previous investigators that exercise training could improve VO$_2$max by 15% or more and thereby "reverse" some of the age-related declines in physical work capacity. Furthermore, they found that the primary mechanism of improvement in exercise capacity following training in older subjects was a large improvement in leg arterial blood flow.

Skeletal muscle function is another potential contributor to the age-related reduction in VO$_2$max. There is a decline in skeletal muscle mass and increased fatty infiltration, a shift in fiber type, and variable alterations in mitochondrial density and function with aging. Each of these could contribute to reduced exercise capacity in older persons.

AGING OF THE VASCULATURE

Age-Related Changes in Arterial Structure

With age, a number of changes occur in the aorta, and all appear to contribute to increased stiffness (see **Table 73-4**). Elastin becomes fragmented in the internal elastic lamina and media, perhaps because of inappropriate activation of MMPs. The MMPs may also liberate proinflammatory signals such as NFκB. Calcification of the media is also seen. Collagen content increases and becomes increasingly cross-linked, making a stiff matrix, especially in the subendothelium.

Irregularities in size and shape of endothelial cells are seen at areas of turbulence, and high cellular turnover occurring at those sites suggests replicative or cellular senescence may occur at those sites. Further evidence of this "in situ" replicative senescence may be provided by manipulations that inhibit telomere shortening. In endothelial cells with persistently long telomeres, age-associated abnormalities may be significantly reduced. In contrast, senescent endothelial cells have upregulated adhesion molecules, proinflammatory cytokines, and decreased NO production. Senescence of endothelial progenitor cells is

TABLE 73-4 ■ COMPONENTS OF VASCULAR AGING

LAYER	MOLECULAR	CELLULAR	STRUCTURAL	DYNAMIC
Endothelium	• ↑ROS • NOS uncoupling from arginine • ↓Total and free NO • ↓SOD, FOXO, sirtuins, AMPK, mTOR activity • ↑Adhesion molecule expression	• ↓Angiogenesis • Endothelial cell senescence • Progenitor cell senescence	• ↑Permeability	• ↓Vasoreactivity • ↑Sheer stress and susceptibility to sheer stress
Intima	• ↑ROS • ↑MMP levels and activity • ↑Adhesion molecule expression • ↑ACE activity and AT-II activity • Switch in endothelin receptors • ↑TGF-β	• ↑SMC proliferation • SMC migration	• ↑Thickness (from SMC proliferation and matrix deposition) • ↑Luminal diameter • Basement membrane permeability	• ↑Susceptibility to mechanical stress
Media	• ↑Interleukins • ↑Advanced glycation end products • ↑Collagen and ↑cross linking • ↓Elastin (calcification and fragmentation) • ↑Fibronectin • ↑Glycosaminoglycans	• ↑SMC proliferation and migration • SMC hypertrophy • SMC senescence • Fibroblast senescence (resistance to apoptosis)	• ↑Thickness • ↑Luminal diameter • Collagen cross-linking • Elastin breakage • ↑Collagen fibrils • Fibrosis	• ↑Stiffness • ↓Elasticity and compliance

ACE, angiotensin-converting enzyme; AMPK, AMP-activated protein kinase; AT-II, angiotensin-II; FOXO, forkhead box O; MMP, matrix metalloproteinases; mTOR, mammalian target of rapamycin; NO, nitric oxide; NOS, nitric oxide synthase; ROS, reactive oxygen species; SMC, smooth muscle cell; SOD, superoxide dismutase; TGF-β, transcription growth factor beta.

associated with decreased angiogenesis and impairment of the complex vascular repair system intended to attenuate the chronic vascular injury and inflammation that may lead to atherosclerosis. In contrast to the endothelial senescence, pulsatile stretch stimulates vascular smooth muscle cell (SMC) proliferation and hypertrophy; SMCs may become increasingly polyploid with multiple sets of chromosomes. The proliferative SMCs may migrate from the media to the subintima.

Functional Changes of Aging Arteries

Multiple functional changes occur with aging in conduit arteries. For example, nitric oxide (NO) is a vasorelaxant and contributes to the balance that dictates resting arterial tone. Aortic strips isolated from older animals have higher NO synthase activity but produce less NO. Old aortas will relax appropriately when exposed to direct NO donors (nitroprusside) but are less responsive to agents whose effects are mediated by NO, such as acetylcholine. Similarly, forearm arterial blood flow is increased less in older individuals in response to acetylcholine compared to younger and athletically active older individuals. Flow-mediated dilation (FMD), the increase in artery diameter in response to blood pressure cuff-induced ischemia, is attenuated with age. The decline in endothelium-dependent dilation of conduit arteries is related to vascular dysfunction and occurs later in the aging process than the increase in arterial stiffness. As FMD is essentially NO-dependent and NO is produced from circulating arginine, with age, a relative increase in arginase (a scavenging enzyme that competes for arginine) results in reduced arginine availability for the endothelium. This explains, in part, the relatively poor efficacy of arginine supplementation. As the response to direct-acting agents, like nitroprusside, is unchanged by age, endothelial dysfunction must play a critical role. The integrity of the vessels is also dependent upon the endothelium and is less well maintained. Increased vascular permeability facilitates the transit of immune and inflammatory cells and signaling molecules into the vessel wall that stimulate MMP activity and, perhaps, atherosclerosis.

Tonically contracted arteries are partially due to an age-related increase in vasoconstricting (ETA) and loss of vasodilating (ETB) receptors for endothelin-1 and increased circulating levels of this potent vasoconstrictor. This results in a decreased maximum response to added endothelin in older persons. Exercise training appears to decrease basal endothelin-1 levels and restore its responsiveness.

Aging and the Microvasculature

The importance of the smallest blood vessels in age-related disease and dysfunction is increasingly recognized. The number of capillaries per volume of tissue (capillarity) is decreased, with aging in many organs, including skin, skeletal muscle, and brain. This is seen after a middle-age increase in capillarity in some tissues,

perhaps compensation for metabolic demands. Arterioles may play a larger role in oxygen and nutrient delivery in older age as compensation for the decreased capillarity. As arteriolar density is less homogeneous, this leads to disparities in oxygen available to regions of the aged brain and heterogeneous levels of oxygenation, including "hypoxic micropockets" clearly seen in the brains of awake, treadmill walking normal old, but not middle age or young, mice. Alteration in endothelial function is found in the small vessels of the aging brain leading to vascular dysregulation similar to that as described for the arteries, but the added fine vascular regulation of neurovascular coupling is also impaired in aging. The altered endothelial function is one of many age-associated changes that lead to changes in the blood-brain barrier, resulting in selective increases in permeability. These changes have potential implications since they are associated with cognitive dysfunction. A generalized age-related decrease in collateral vessels that lowers the threshold for damage during ischemia is seen in other organs.

Alterations in Angiogenesis with Aging

Angiogenesis is impaired in the old vascular tree in response to ischemia or chemical signals. Explants of arteries from old animals have decreased spouting of microvessels and decreased vascular invasion of implants. As noted above, there is no deficit of SMC proliferation, but endothelial cell proliferation is impaired. Endothelial cellular senescence, increased oxidative stress, reduced endothelial NO production, and reduced responsiveness to angiogenic growth factors contribute to lower angiogenesis in older individuals.

Clinical Implications of the Age-related Changes in Vascular Structure and Function

The aortic root and lumen diameter increase with age, as do vessel length and wall thickness. Because the aorta is fixed proximally and distally, the increase in length results in the tortuous, ectatic, and rightward-shifted aorta seen often on chest X-rays of older persons. Arterial wall stiffness can be assessed noninvasively as pulse wave velocity (PWV, the rate at which pressure travels in the artery wall), augmentation index (AI-central peak pressure/pulse pressure), distensibility, and systolic and pulse (systolic-diastolic) blood pressure. Aging is an important determinant of large artery stiffness with PWV increases twofold from age 20 to 80, independent of blood pressure. The age-related changes in large artery structure and function have been demonstrated in the absence of clinical CVD and CV risk factors highlighting the direct, more causal association between aging and vascular dysfunction.

A stiffer arterial wall allows pressure to reflect from the periphery to the heart while the aortic valve is still open, increasing the load on the heart. Thus PWV is a physiologically relevant parameter. In younger persons, PWV is relatively low. The reflected wave arrives back to the heart after the aortic valve closure, supporting diastolic pressure and improving coronary perfusion without contributing to LV afterload. With aging and arterial stiffening, PWV increases, and the reflected pressure waves are of greater amplitude and arrive back at the heart before aortic valve closure, resulting in increased LV afterload, LV hypertrophy, diastolic dysfunction, relative coronary hypoperfusion, lower diastolic blood pressure, and increased pulse pressure. Augmentation index, a more direct measure of the additive impact of the reflected pressure waves, increases fourfold from 20 to 80, contributing to the increase in systolic pressure that occurs with age. For men in the Framingham study, systolic BP increased 5 mm Hg per decade until the age of 60; then, the slope shifted to 10 mm Hg per decade. For women, systolic BP started lower but shifted to the higher slope earlier. Over the same age range, diastolic BP increases a little and then decreases. Thus the age-related arterial stiffening results in systolic hypertension.

Older athletes have lower systolic pressures and lower PWV than sedentary older adults, but higher than young people. In fact, PWV correlates inversely with maximum oxygen consumption (VO$_2$max) in healthy people across ages. VO$_2$max is strongly associated with measures of vessel stiffness, particularly PWV, suggesting a significant contribution to the age-related decline in exercise capacity via several mechanisms, including increased afterload on the LV and altered peripheral blood flow distribution.

The net result of these changes is reduced compliance and increased impedance, leading to increased systolic blood pressure and little, if any, effect on diastolic blood pressure, such that pulse pressure increases. The aorta and proximal large arteries act as an elastic buffering chamber, storing half the LV stroke volume delivered during systole in young adults and during diastole; the elastic forces of the aortic wall push this volume to the peripheral circulation, thus creating nearly continuous peripheral blood flow. The stiffer large arteries in older adults are less able to smooth out the flow, and thus smaller vessels are exposed to pulsatile flow and pressure. The age-related increases in arterial stiffening likely impact the prevalence and severity of a range of common disorders in older persons, including coronary, cerebrovascular, and peripheral artery disease, systolic hypertension, stroke, HF, particularly HFpEF, cognitive dysfunction, and renal disease.

Arterial stiffness is associated with frailty through CVD, but abnormal arterial structure and physiology may be independently associated with frailty. Cross-sectional studies show that markers of arterial stiffening are associated with frailty, as measured by both the Fried and Rockwood criteria. Increased PWV was associated with sarcopenia and slow gait speed as well.

As noted above, lifelong athletes have lower arterial stiffness than sedentary controls. Training for a marathon with thrice-weekly long runs resulted in lower arterial stiffness and modest blood pressure changes. This suggests that the aging changes may be reduced with aggressive exercise. Furthermore, novel therapies such as Alagebrium, a prototypical advanced glycosylation end-product collagen cross-link breaker, have effectively decreased PWV and augmentation index in older primates and people, highlighting this potential role in ameliorating age-related arterial stiffness. Pharmacologic therapies that reduce diastolic blood pressure appear able to arterial stiffness. While this may decrease the passive stretch when arterial stiffness is measured, studies focused on arterial stiffness showed no effect of classic anti-hypertensive drugs on PWV. RAAS antagonists reduce arterial collagen deposition. Renin-angiotensin blockers inhibit the expression of proinflammatory mediators and attenuate adverse vascular remodeling, but definitive studies in normotensive older people are not available.

SUMMARY

Normal aging is accompanied by substantial alterations in the anatomy and physiology of the heart and vasculature. There are declines in most cardiovascular function aspects, including cardiac output and blood flow distribution, and oxygen utilization, which create significantly reduced reserve capacity, which becomes more apparent during exercise and stress.

The age-related alterations in the anatomy and physiology of the heart likely have varying degrees of significance. Some may not have functional significance and are essentially epiphenomena of aging. Others, such as aortic sclerosis, ventricular septal thickening, and attenuated cardiac function response during exercise, may simulate disease. Some findings associated with age and are prevalent in older hearts, such as senile amyloid and calcified mitral annulus, are likely part of disease processes rather than aging.

Vascular aging also plays a critical role in the aging of the cardiovascular system, increasing the load on the heart and altering the perfusion of the target organs. While aging is a separate process from atherosclerosis, aging increases the risk of the development of atherosclerosis. The primary research focus has been large artery changes, but age-related alterations in the microvasculature may be just as important.

With the currently available information, it is not always possible to distinguish the effects of aging from the effects of the disease, particularly in very old persons. However, it is reasonable to propose that many of the age-related changes discussed may lower the threshold for clinical disease and, thus, predispose to a variety of cardiovascular disorders in older adults, including HF, hypertensive hypertrophic cardiomyopathy, valvular stenosis and regurgitation, systolic hypertension, supraventricular arrhythmias, and conduction disturbances. Awareness of these age-related changes and the principles of aging biology, in general, will help investigators avoid potential errors in research study design or interpretation and help clinicians tailor intelligent treatments to older adults. Since many of these age-related declines in cardiovascular and exercise performance are modifiable and have been shown to be partially preventable and reversible with exercise training, maintaining regularly scheduled physical activity and conditioning is a potentially important strategy to mitigate the potential adverse effects of aging on cardiovascular function.

FURTHER READING

Cieslik KA, Trial J, Entman ML. Defective myofibroblast formation from mesenchymal stem cells in the aging murine heart rescue by activation of the AMPK pathway. *Am J Pathol.* 2011;179:1792–806.

DeSouza CA, Shapiro LF, Clevenger CM, et al. Regular aerobic exercise prevents and restores age-related declines in endothelium-dependent vasodilation in healthy men. *Circulation.* 2000;102(12):1351–1357.

Hermeling E, Hoeks AP, Winkens MH, et al. Non-invasive assessment of arterial stiffness should discriminate between systolic and diastolic pressure ranges. *Hypertension.* 2010;55:124–130.

Jones MR, Ravid K. Vascular smooth muscle polyploidization as a biomarker for aging and its impact on differential gene expression. *J Biol Chem.* 2004;279(7):5306–5313.

Kawaguchi M, Hay I, Fetics B, Kass DA. Combined ventricular systolic and arterial stiffening in patients with heart failure and preserved ejection fraction: implications for systolic and diastolic reserve limitations. *Circulation.* 2003;107:714–720.

Lakatta EG, Levy D. Arterial and cardiac aging: major shareholders in cardiovascular disease enterprises: part II: the aging heart in health: links to heart disease. *Circulation.* 2003;107:346–354.

Lakatta EG, Sollott SJ. Perspectives on mammalian cardiovascular aging: humans to molecules. *Comp Biochem Physiol.* 2002;132:699–721.

Lee TM, Su SF, Chou TF, Lee YT, Tsai CH. Loss of preconditioning by attenuated activation of myocardial ATP-sensitive potassium channels in elderly patients undergoing coronary angioplasty. *Circulation.* 2002;105:334–340.

Leung DY, Boyd A, Ng AA, Chi C, Thomas L. Echocardiographic evaluation of left atrial size and function: current understanding, pathophysiologic correlates, and prognostic implications. *Am Heart J.* 2008;156:1056–1064.

Longobardi G, Abete P, Ferrara N, et al. "Warm-up" phenomenon in adult and elderly patients with coronary artery disease: further evidence of the loss of "ischemic preconditioning" in the aging heart. *J Gerontol A Biol Sci Med Sci.* 2000;55:M124–M129.

Matsushita H, Chang E, Glassford AJ, Cooke JP, Chiu CP, Tsao PS. eNOS activity is reduced in senescent human endothelial cells: preservation by hTERT immortalization. *Circ Res.* 2001;89(9):793–798.

Moeini M, Lu X, Avti PK, et al. Compromised microvascular oxygen delivery increases brain tissue vulnerability with age. *Sci Rep.* 2018;8(1):8219.

Nichols WW. Clinical measurement of arterial stiffness obtained from non-invasive pressure waveforms. *Am J Hypertens.* 2005;18(1 pt 2):S3–S10.

Novelli M, Pocai A, Skalicky M, Viidik A, Bergamini E, Masiello P. Effects of life-long exercise on circulating free fatty acids and muscle triglyceride content in ageing rats. *Exp Gerontol.* 2004;39(9):1333–1340.

Olsen H, Vernersson E, Lanne T. Cardiovascular response to acute hypovolemia in relation to age. Implications for orthostasis and hemorrhage. *Am J Physiol Heart Circ Physiol.* 2000;278:H222–H226.

Pandey A, Kraus W, Brubaker P, Kitzman D. Healthy aging and cardiovascular function: invasive hemodynamics during rest and exercise in 104 healthy volunteers. *JACC Heart Fail.* 2020;8(2):111–121.

Redfield MM, Rodeheffer RJ, Jacobsen SJ, et al. Plasma brain natriuretic peptide concentration: impact of age and gender. *J Am Coll Cardiol.* 2002;40:976–982.

Tanaka H, Monahan KD, Seals DR. Age-predicted maximal heart rate revisited. *J Am Coll Cardiol.* 2001;37:153–156.

Vaitkevicius PV, Lane M, Spurgeon H, et al. A cross-link breaker has sustained effects on arterial and ventricular properties in older rhesus monkeys. *Proc Natl Acad Sci USA.* 2001;98(3):1171–1175.

Wang M, Takagi G, Asai K, et al. aging increases aortic MMP-2 activity and angiotensin II in nonhuman primates. *Hypertension.* 2003;41:1308–1316.

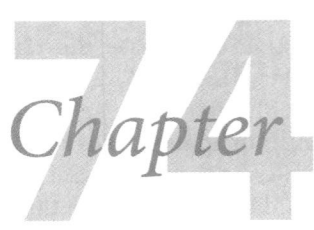

Chapter 74

Coronary Heart Disease and Dyslipidemia

Michael G. Nanna, Karen P. Alexander

INTRODUCTION

The spectrum of coronary heart disease (CHD) includes subclinical CHD, asymptomatic or stable ischemic heart disease, and acute coronary syndromes including unstable angina and acute myocardial infarction (MI). Atherosclerosis in the coronary circulation contributes to luminal narrowing and increases risk of vascular dysfunction and thrombosis. Clinical presentations of CHD result from insufficient oxygen supply for the demands of the myocardium. Dyslipidemia is a major risk factor for the development of CHD in individuals up to age 80. There are multiple available therapeutic options to reduce blood cholesterol levels, many of which also modify future risk of cardiovascular events.

EPIDEMIOLOGY

Despite declining mortality over the past three decades, CHD remains the leading killer of both men and women in the United States. More than 80% of deaths from CHD occur in those older than 65 years. In the United States, the prevalence of CHD, MI, and angina all increase with age in both men and women (**Figures 74-1** and **74-2**). The initial manifestation of CHD may be an acute MI, occurring in about 40% of cases, or sudden death in 10% to 20% of cases. The average age of first MI is 66 years for men and 72 years for women. In-hospital mortality following an MI also rises sharply with age: less than 1% in those younger than 50 years old, ~2.5% in those 60 to 69 years old, ~4% in those 70 to 79 years old, and ~8% among those 80 years or older. One-year mortality similarly increases with age. Furthermore, the majority of patients with CHD older than 75 years are women because of their longer life expectancy and the 10-year lag in CHD manifestations as compared with men.

Clinically evident CHD represents the tip of the iceberg with many older patients having asymptomatic and subclinical coronary disease. The Cardiovascular Health Study examined the prevalence of clinical and subclinical cardiovascular disease (CVD) in a large community-dwelling Medicare population. Using a composite measure of MI on electrocardiogram (ECG) or echocardiography and abnormal carotid artery wall thickness or

Learning Objectives

- Understand the prevalence of coronary heart disease (CHD) in older adults.
- Recognize the clinical aspects—including symptoms, signs, and diagnostic test results—that are common among older adults with CHD.
- Understand treatment of CHD, including treatment of dyslipidemias, in older adults.

Key Clinical Points

1. CHD is common and has high morbidity and mortality in older adults.
2. Many older patients have asymptomatic, stable, or subclinical ischemic heart disease.
3. Total cholesterol, low-density lipoprotein cholesterol (LDL-C), and triglyceride (TG) levels increase from the third to seventh decade of life. Typically, LDL-C remains stable or even declines in older age cohorts.
4. Dyslipidemia is a well-established risk factor for cardiovascular disease, but strength of this association is diminished with age and limited data exists for those older than age 80.
5. Typical angina is the most common presenting symptom of CHD regardless of age.
6. Delays in recognizing other symptoms such as dyspnea, fatigue, or epigastric discomfort may contribute to later presentations among older adults.
7. Evaluation for symptoms suggestive of CHD should be similar in older and younger patients. Functional testing is a valuable diagnostic and prognostic tool in older adults. Modified protocols or pharmacologic-based stress tests may be used for those who

(Continued)

experience difficulty with standard exercise protocols.

8. Management of CHD should be similar in older and younger patients prioritizing risk factor modification, symptomatic relief, and goals of care.

9. Revascularization is an effective method for relief of frequent angina particularly if symptoms remain despite optimally tolerated medical therapy.

ankle-brachial blood pressure index, they found that disease prevalence doubled from 22% in women aged 65 to 70 to 43% in those aged 85 or older. Similarly, the frequency of subclinical vascular disease in men increased from 33% to 45% in these age groups, respectively.

PATHOPHYSIOLOGY OF DYSLIPIDEMIA AND CHD

The development of CHD is associated with a variety of well-established risk factors, including the presence of dyslipidemia, hypertension, diabetes mellitus, tobacco use, obesity, chronic renal insufficiency, and genetic risk factors for CHD. Other risk factors, such as early menopause, connective tissue disease, and human immune deficiency virus, have also been linked with higher risk for future cardiovascular events. A complete discussion of these risk factors is beyond the scope of this chapter and is discussed elsewhere in this textbook. This chapter's focus is on the link between dyslipidemia and CHD.

Dyslipidemia and Age

Elevated total cholesterol and LDL-C increase the risk for atherosclerotic cardiovascular disease (ASCVD) in middle-aged men and women. Multiple cross-sectional studies have demonstrated changes in lipid patterns across age groups. In general, total cholesterol, LDL-C, and TG levels all increase in both men and women from the third to the seventh or eighth decades of life. Changes in LDL-C are accelerated in women starting at menopause with the reduction in systemic estrogen. Beyond the seventh and eighth decades of life, LDL-C and cholesterol levels plateau and often decline. Lower cholesterol levels in adults 75 years or older may be related to healthy survivorship bias with individuals with lower cholesterol levels more likely to survive to old age. The decline in cholesterol levels observed in older populations may also be related to a variety of other less favorable factors, including malnutrition, multimorbidity, inflammation, and frailty. The data supporting the association between LDL-C and the development of CHD in older adult populations is therefore less clear. For example, in a well-characterized cohort of US adults older than 75 years and free of CVD at baseline, LDL-C was not associated with 5-year CVD risk. In another analysis from the Copenhagen General Population Study, higher LDL-C was associated with future risk of MI among individuals aged 70 to 100. Comorbidities and frailty also confound the association between cholesterol and mortality. Older persons at both ends of the cholesterol curve, with the lowest and the highest cholesterol levels, may be at higher risk for cardiovascular events and mortality. Ultimately, regardless of the attributable risk associated with hypercholesterolemia in older adult populations, studies are ongoing to identify whether targeting lipids with pharmacologic therapies can improve cardiovascular

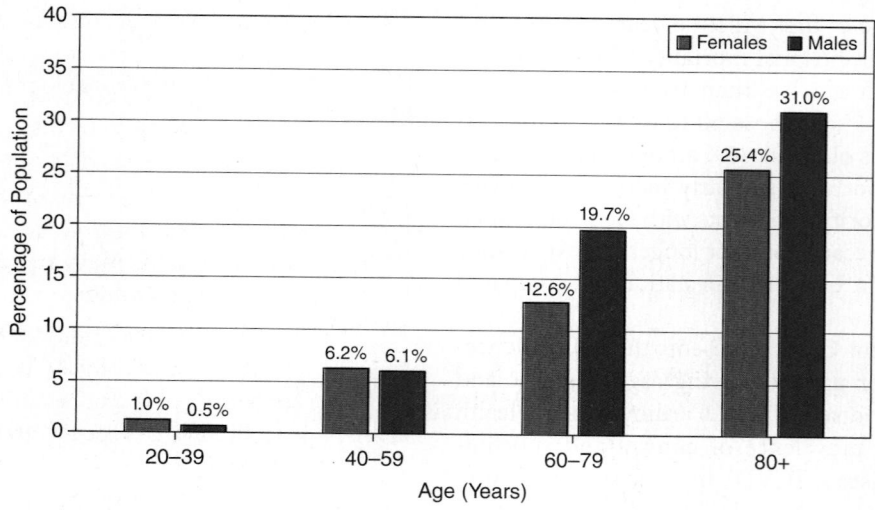

FIGURE 74-1. Prevalence of coronary heart disease by age and sex, United States. (Adapted with permission from NHANES, 2013–2016. National Heart, Lung, and Blood Institute. US Department of Health & Human Services.)

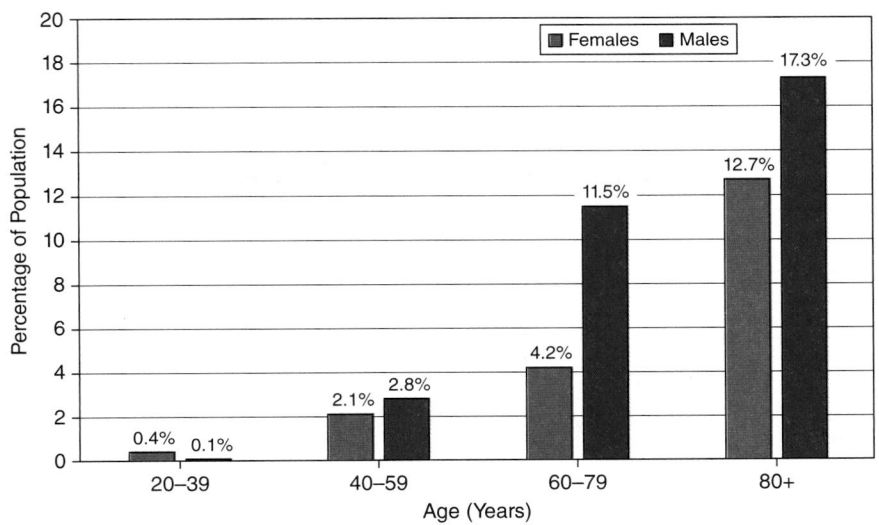

FIGURE 74-2. Prevalence of myocardial infarction (MI) by age and sex, United States. (Adapted with permission from NHANES, 2013–2016. National Heart, Lung, and Blood Institute. US Department of Health & Human Services.)

outcomes in older adults (which is discussed in more detail in the "Evaluation and Management" section).

There are five major subpopulations of lipoproteins that provide additional information on risk. These include chylomicrons, very low-density lipoproteins (VLDLs), intermediate-density lipoproteins (IDLs), low-density lipoproteins (LDLs), and high-density lipoproteins (HDLs). Each differs in composition, metabolic function, and atherogenic potential. Atherogenic lipid particles include apolipoprotein B (ApoB) and lipoprotein(a) (Lp[a]). ApoB is the primary lipoprotein for chylomicrons, VLDLs, IDLs, and LDLs and functions as the ligand for the LDL receptor. Lp(a) is a lipoprotein particle similar to LDL cholesterol (LDL-C) that binds to ApoB. While these subparticles are associated with risk, LDL-C remains the focus of existing therapies. The relationship between aging and changes in the concentration of these subparticles, as well as their association with cardiovascular risk, represents an important area for future investigation.

CHD and Age

Cardiovascular changes are common with age. Arterial stiffening is prevalent and results in isolated systolic hypertension with widened pulse pressures, factors known to increase risk of cardiovascular events. Heart failure with preserved ejection fraction (EF) is a prevalent and similar condition, which elevates end-diastolic pressures and impairs diastolic filling of the coronary circulation. Age-associated endotheliopathy, defined by progressive endothelial dysfunction and blunted responses to protective vasodilatory mediators, results in atherosclerotic plaques with increasing numbers and severity. The composition of these atherosclerotic lesions also changes with age, with reduction in the soft lipid core and an increase in calcification and fibrosis. While more advanced calcified plaques

are actually less likely to rupture, the sheer increase in lesion numbers is associated with a higher likelihood for CHD events in older adults.

The pathophysiology of MI involves atherosclerotic plaque rupture, platelet activation/aggregation, endothelial dysfunction, inflammation, and thrombus formation. If a clot completely occludes a coronary artery, the patient suffers an acute MI, and an injury pattern (eg, ST elevation) is often seen on the ECG. In contrast, patients with plaque rupture can also form a nonocclusive thrombus, resulting in subendocardial ischemia. The distinction between unstable angina and MI shifted with the advent of high-sensitivity troponins as they can now identify very low levels of circulating cardiac troponin. Even lowest levels of circulating troponin above the detection threshold are associated with increased risk. In practice, MI type is also often stratified by ECG findings of ST-segment elevation MI (STEMI) or nondiagnostic ECG considered non-ST–segment elevation MI (NSTEMI). Most recently, the fourth universal definition of MI provides updated definitions for myocardial injury and MI (**Figure 74-3**).

PRESENTATION

CVD may be diagnosed following an acute cardiovascular presentation, identification of ischemia on noninvasive testing, or finding obstructive coronary artery disease (CAD) on coronary imaging. Some examples of presentation types include evidence of prior silent MI on ECG, stable angina without ischemia on noninvasive testing, or asymptomatic ischemia found on noninvasive testing. The presence of obstructive CAD and angina may also vary across these presentations. Coronary calcifications, frequently noted on nongated chest imaging, identify the presence of atherosclerosis, and should trigger evaluation

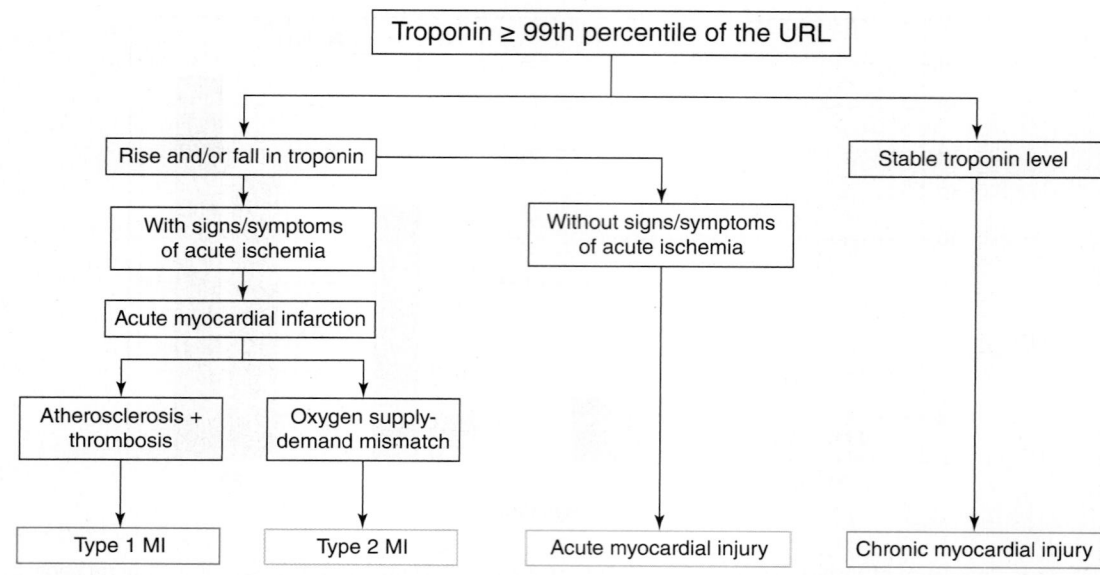

FIGURE 74-3. Fourth universal definition of myocardial infarction: a model for interpreting myocardial injury. URL, upper reference limit.

and management of risk factors and/or symptoms. An MI requires the presence of acute myocardial injury detected by abnormal cardiac biomarkers in conjunction with clinical evidence of acute myocardial ischemia. Abnormal cardiac biomarkers are generally defined as an elevated cardiac troponin value above the 99th percentile upper reference limit (URL). Signs of myocardial ischemia include clinical symptoms, ischemic ECG changes, pathological Q waves on ECG, imaging evidence of ischemia, or identification of coronary thrombus on angiography or autopsy. When patients present with a cardiac troponin level greater than or equal to the 99th percentile of the URL with a characteristic rise and fall and signs/symptoms of acute ischemia, they meet criteria for an acute MI. If the MI is due to atherosclerosis and thrombosis (with either complete or partial occlusion of a coronary artery), patients meet criteria for a type 1 MI. This is often triggered by plaque rupture or erosion. If, however, the findings are related to an oxygen supply and demand imbalance, such as due to fixed coronary atherosclerosis, coronary spasm, coronary embolism, coronary dissection, severe anemia, severe hypotension/hypertension or tachyarrhythmia, then the patient meets criteria for type 2 MI. When the patient has a characteristic rise and fall in troponin but without clinical signs of acute ischemia, they meet criteria for acute myocardial injury, which may be due to conditions such as acute heart failure or myocarditis. Finally, if troponin levels are stable without a characteristic rise and fall, this represents chronic myocardial injury. This can be seen with left ventricular hypertrophy, structural heart disease, or chronic kidney disease.

The prevalence of angina increases with age (**Figure 74-4**), but it is also the case that older individuals often have anginal equivalent symptoms such as dyspnea, epigastric pain, fatigue, confusion, or malaise that may be misinterpreted as consequences of aging or comorbid illness. Findings from the Global Registry of Acute Coronary Events, a large, prospective, multinational registry of ACSs, demonstrated that patients presenting with anginal-equivalent symptoms were less likely to receive appropriate cardiac medications, undergo cardiac catheterization, and were at higher risk of in-hospital morbidity and mortality. Older people can also have an impaired ischemia warning system. In a series of patients with CHD undergoing treadmill testing, researchers found that patients older than age 70 took more than twice as long as their younger counterparts to report angina after ECG-documented ischemia was noted.

Difficulty in recognizing symptoms contributes to later presentation of acute events in older patients. More than two-thirds of patients with MI, older than age 65, fail to reach an emergency department within 6 hours after the onset of their symptoms. The Rapid Early Action for Coronary Treatment study quantified delay time as an additional 14 minutes for every 10-year increment in age, beginning with the age of 30. While time to first medical contact has improved as community and state efforts have targeted improving MI systems of care, delays in MI presentation still have strong prognostic implications. Prehospital delays may result from atypical presentation, medical comorbidities, previous experiences within the health care system, socioeconomics, access to care, and cognitive and functional impairments. Thus, clinicians should advise that cardiac symptoms can vary and patients should seek rapid medical attention if concerning symptoms occur.

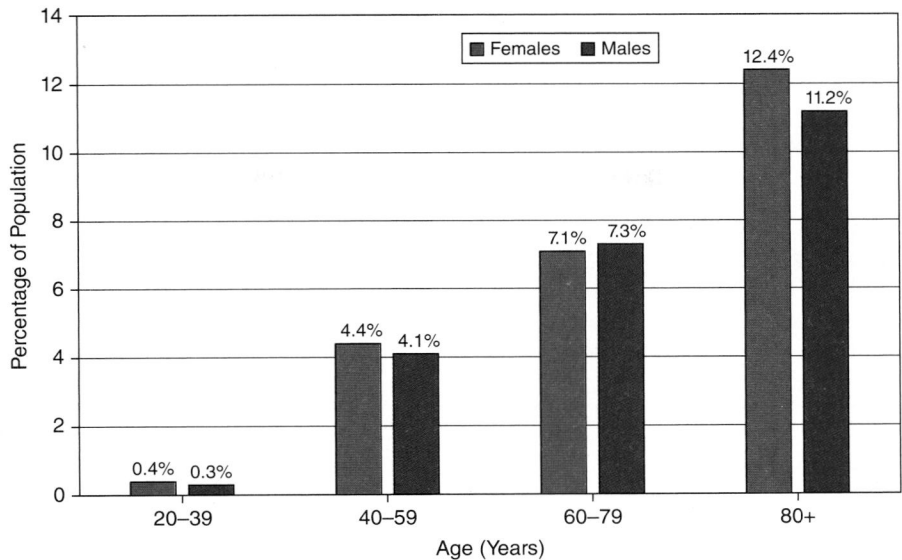

FIGURE 74-4. Prevalence of angina pectoris by age and sex, United States. (Adapted with permission from NHANES, 2013–2016. National Heart, Lung, and Blood Institute. US Department of Health & Human Services.)

EVALUATION

Evaluation of Stable CHD

Given the prevalence of CHD in older patients, clinicians must have a high index of suspicion to make the diagnosis. In taking a history, clinicians must consider risk factors as well as temporal course of symptoms suggestive of CHD. Patients with new, progressive, or refractory symptoms typically require an expedited—and possibly inpatient—evaluation.

A systematic approach to the physical examination may provide further clues to the presence of CHD. Some older patients develop calcific vascular disease, and pseudohypertension may be observed. Diminution of the femoral pulses or brachial-femoral delay may suggest the presence of atherosclerotic aorto-iliac disease, and these findings may accompany observed dermatologic changes with lower extremity hair loss. Performing ankle-brachial indices remains a useful and sensitive screening tool for identifying patients with peripheral vascular disease, a known risk factor for increased cardiovascular events. The cardiac examination may include signs of left- or right-sided heart failure (pulmonary edema, displaced point of maximal impulse, an S_3, or peripheral edema) or characteristic murmurs of valvular heart disease. Once a thorough history and physical has been completed, further diagnostic evaluation should be based on the patient's symptoms as outlined below. Risk factors, particularly blood pressure, should be measured. Obtaining a baseline ECG is also reasonable because of the high prevalence of silent MIs in older individuals. Beyond the standard history, physical examination, and laboratory tests, further diagnostic testing (carotid ultrasound, treadmill testing, echocardiography, or computed tomography) in the asymptomatic older patient to detect occult or subclinical CHD remains controversial and is not generally recommended.

Symptomatic older patients should undergo a similar assessment for obstructive coronary disease as younger patients based on algorithms that take into account symptom characteristics, including angina type (non-anginal, anginal-equivalent, or typical), its course (stable, progressive, or unstable), and its duration. This initial assessment of a patient's pretest probability of disease should guide diagnostic testing. In particular, clinicians need to be cognizant that, according to Bayesian theory, the predictive value of a test is influenced by the disease prevalence in the population tested. For example, clinicians may interpret a negative stress test in a high-risk older woman (pretest probability of disease 80%) as "ruling out" the presence of CHD, whereas this patient's posttest likelihood remains more than 60% (**Table 74-1**). For these reasons, older patients with high pretest likelihood for coronary disease should be considered for direct referral for cardiac catheterization (if revascularization is an appropriate option). At the other extreme, patients with a low pretest probability for CAD less than or equal to 20% (ie, no risk factors, normal ECG, and very atypical symptoms) can often be followed clinically and/or be assessed for other etiologies of their symptoms (gastrointestinal, pulmonary, musculoskeletal, etc). Older patients with an intermediate pretest probability for CHD (between 20% and 70%) are those in whom stress testing has its greatest impact on clinical decision-making.

When stress testing is indicated, guidelines recommend exercise ECG as a first strategy for patients with a normal baseline ECG. The exercise ECG provides important prognostic information (including exercise duration and hemodynamic response), as well as electrocardiographic indications of ischemia (ST depression). Older

TABLE 74-1 ■ INFLUENCE OF AGE ON PREDICTIVE VALUE OF STRESS TESTING (BAYES THEOREM)

HISTORY	AGE (Y)	PRETEST LIKELIHOOD OF SIGNIFICANT CAD[a] (%)	TREADMILL TEST[b]	POSTTEST LIKELIHOOD OF SIGNIFICANT CAD (%)
Female, typical CP	45	30	Positive	56
			Negative	16
↑ Lipids	75	80	Positive	92
			Negative	63
Female, non-anginal CP	45	5	Positive	12
			Negative	3
No RF	75	35	Positive	62
			Negative	18

CAD, coronary artery disease; CP, chest pain; RF, risk factor.
[a]Based on CAD risk nomogram for predicting significant CAD.
[b]Sensitivity of treadmill test = 68%, specificity = 77%.

patients, however, frequently experience difficulty with exercise testing because of deconditioning or disability and may need modified protocols starting at lower levels with slower stage progression. Alternatively, for patients who cannot exercise, a pharmacologic-based stress test (dobutamine, adenosine, or dipyridamole) can be performed. In older patients with baseline ECGs abnormalities (resting ST depression, left bundle branch block, left ventricular hypertrophy with strain, or paced rhythms), imaging modalities, such as nuclear perfusion or stress echocardiography, are required. While these modalities significantly add to the cost of the test, these improve the diagnostic accuracy beyond stress ECG alone and provide information as to the location and extent of coronary disease. Thus, the choice of diagnostic test should consider the clinical setting as well as local availability and expertise (**Figure 74-5**). In the PROMISE trial, functional testing was able to distinguish future risk of CV death/MI in individuals 65 years and older, whereas a positive result, defined as stenosis ≥ 70% or ≥ 50% left main stenosis, on anatomic testing (CCTA) did not correlate with future outcomes in older patients. There is likely a role for CCTA to exclude surgical disease in asymptomatic nonfrail older adults with low EF. There is no need to repeat stress tests without a change in symptoms. Guidelines advise against repeat testing within 2 years of percutaneous coronary intervention (PCI) and 5 years of coronary artery bypass graft (CABG).

Cardiac catheterization is as safe in contemporary practice in older patients as in younger patients, but it should always be performed based on a favorable risk-benefit ratio and in alignment with the patient's goals of care. Vascular injury, bleeding, MI, stroke, and even mortality can result, albeit rarely, and advanced age increases these risks. However, the risk to life remains less than 0.2%, and the risk of other serious adverse events is less than 0.5%, even in those aged 75 or older. Cardiac catheterization should be considered for those at high risk of severe coronary disease, or refractory ischemic symptoms despite maximally tolerated medical treatment. At the same time,

it is safe to defer cardiac catheterization for initial medical management in patients with stable ischemic heart disease. This is a helpful clarification particularly for older patients with multimorbidity and in those with even moderate to severe ischemia on stress testing as demonstrated in the International Study of Comparative Health Effectiveness with Medical and Invasive Approaches (ISCHEMIA) trial. In this study, there was no difference in the composite cardiovascular outcome or all-cause mortality with a conservative approach optimizing medical therapy compared to an initial invasive approach in patients with stable ischemic heart disease and EF greater than or equal to 35%. Revascularization does continue to provide important angina relief when frequent symptoms persist despite maximally tolerated medical therapy. It also improves survival for those with multivessel disease and EF less than 35%. In summary, if symptoms can be managed with medical therapy in stable patients, then a PCI is unlikely to add benefit and has not been shown to improve mortality. On the other hand, if patients are unable to tolerate antianginal therapies due to side effects, concerns around polypharmacy, or patient preferences, or if PCI can provide more effective symptom control and/or a more durable symptom relief, revascularization may be preferable. Given these complexities, person-centered decision-making around the management of CHD is of the utmost importance.

MI Evaluation

Older patients with MI often have an acceleration of chest pain symptoms and may have more subtle changes on the ECG (eg, flipped T waves or ST depression) or more dramatic changes (eg, ST elevation). There is some evidence that plasma levels of procoagulation markers and coagulation factors are elevated in older patients, but it remains unclear whether these findings alone are responsible for increased thrombotic tendencies in older patients or alter risk when accompanied by other traditional risk factors for thrombotic events. There are also significant proportions of older patients who develop MI secondary to exacerbations

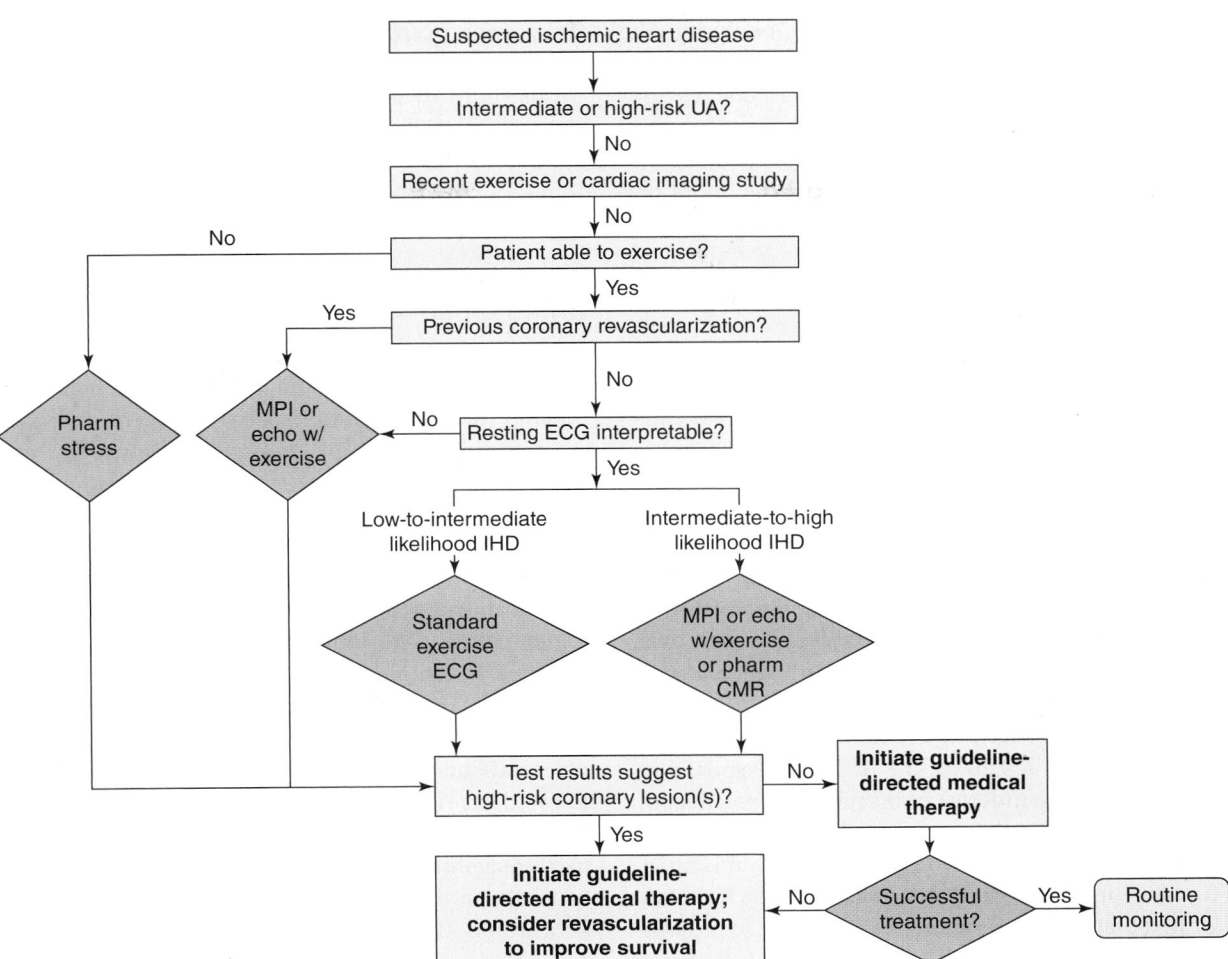

FIGURE 74-5. Work-up and management of suspected ischemic heart disease. CMR, cardiac magnetic resonance; IHD, ischemic heart disease; MPI, myocardial perfusion imaging; UA, unstable angina. (Reproduced with permission from Fihn SD, Gardin JM, Abrams J, et al. 2012 ACCF/AHA/ACP/AATS/PCNA/SCAI/STS guideline for the diagnosis and management of patients with stable ischemic heart disease: a report of the American College of Cardiology Foundation/American Heart Association task force on practice guidelines, and the American College of Physicians, American Association for Thoracic Surgery, Preventive Cardiovascular Nurses Association, Society for Cardiovascular Angiography and Interventions, and Society of Thoracic Surgeons. *Circulation*. 2012;126[25]:e354–e471.)

of chronic comorbid conditions or acute medical illnesses. These type 2 MIs occur in the setting of sepsis, acute blood loss or chronic anemia, pneumonia, pulmonary embolism, chronic obstructive pulmonary disease, congestive heart failure, dysrhythmias, or hypertensive urgencies. A retrospective study demonstrated that approximately 30% of patients present with an acute noncardiac condition concomitant with an MI, contributing to increased mortality and less use of cardiac medications and interventions. These secondary events usually occur in the context of increased myocardial oxygen demand or hemodynamic stress in patients with underlying CAD and represent a substantial number of cases. The distinction between a type 1, or spontaneous, MI and a type 2, or secondary, MI is helpful to determine best approach to management. In the latter, focus on supply-demand and risk stratification

is warranted, where as in the spontaneous MI group, a more typical approach with anticoagulation and cardiac catheterization is warranted.

MEDICAL MANAGEMENT

Antiplatelet Therapy

There is strong support for the benefit of aspirin in secondary prevention, and in select patients for primary prevention in the presence of risk factors. The Antithrombotic Trialists' Collaboration, which performed a meta-analysis of aspirin trials and included more than 135,000 patients, identified a 25% risk reduction in cardiovascular events. In the Physician's Health Study of 44,000 men without known CHD, those randomized to aspirin had a 44% lower risk for subsequent MI versus those taking placebo.

Observational data from the Nurse's Health Study suggest similar benefits of aspirin for primary CHD prevention in women. The reduction in nonfatal cardiovascular events and stroke was greater for secondary prevention than for primary prevention, particularly when at low risk. Recent randomized controlled trial data have cast more doubt on the benefit of aspirin for primary prevention. The ARRIVE (Aspirin to Reduce Risks of Initial Vascular Events) trial randomized nondiabetic individuals at moderate risk for CVD (men $\geq$ 55 years old, women $\geq$ 60 years old) to aspirin 100 mg/day versus placebo. At 5 years of follow-up, the composite CV outcome was the same in both groups with more gastrointestinal bleeding in the aspirin group. A limitation of ARRIVE was that event rates were generally lower than expected due to enrollment of a lower risk cohort than intended. The ASCEND (A Study of Cardiovascular Events in Diabetes) trial examined the effect of aspirin 100 mg versus placebo for primary prevention of cardiovascular events in patients with diabetes. ASCEND demonstrated that low-dose aspirin reduced cardiovascular events over a mean follow-up of 7 years in diabetic individuals (rate ratio 0.88; 95% confidence interval, 0.79–0.97, $p = 0.01$), while increasing major bleeding events compared with placebo (4.1% vs 3.2%; $p = 0.003$). The ASPREE (Aspiring in Reducing Events in the Elderly) trial evaluated the effect of aspirin versus placebo on disability-free survival, cardiovascular events, mortality, and bleeding in healthy adults older than 70 years (or $\geq$ 65 years among Blacks and Hispanics in the United States). Over 5 years, aspirin did not prolong disability-free survival but led to a higher rate of major hemorrhage compared with placebo. ASPREE also demonstrated a higher mortality among individuals receiving daily aspirin, attributed to cancer-related death. As a reflection of these data, the US Preventive Services Task Force recommends weighing the impact of aspirin therapy on primary vascular events versus bleeding when considering initiation of treatment within the broader context of health trajectory and individual patient priorities. Aspirin dose continues to be debated, but efficacy of aspirin does not appear to increase at doses greater than 150 mg/day, and higher doses increase the risk for bleeding. Thus, 81 mg of aspirin is the dose with the best evidence for secondary prevention.

Clopidogrel, a thienopyridine that inhibits ADP-dependent platelet aggregation, when added to aspirin in the setting on NSTEMI results in a 20% relative risk reduction in cardiovascular death, MI, or stroke as shown in the Clopidogrel in Unstable angina to prevent Recurrent Events (CURE) trial. The study found similar benefits in older patients; nevertheless, registry data suggest that the in-hospital use of clopidogrel in older patients after MI remains low. The use of clopidogrel is also recommended as an alternative to aspirin in the small subset of patients who are allergic or intolerant to aspirin. Newer ADP-dependent platelet aggregation inhibitors are used in patients following percutaneous interventions. Prasugrel has a black box warning against use in those age 75 or older or those with prior stroke or low body mass index due to increased risk of bleeding. Ticagrelor, with a different risk profile, seems safe for use in those age 75 or older based on current evidence. Patients who require long-term dual antiplatelet therapy (DAPT) or oral anticoagulation with warfarin are advised to take a reduced aspirin dose of 81 mg daily, and all older patients should be on reduced aspirin dose, regardless of other agents.

Antithrombotic Therapy

Consideration for the likelihood of a thrombotic process based on the type of MI and need for invasive management strategy should guide the approach to anticoagulation. Antithrombotic therapy reduces cardiovascular events in patients after an ACS, yet registry data show less use of antithrombotic therapy in older patients when compared to their younger counterparts. Unfractionated heparin, in conjunction with antiplatelet therapy, is associated with significant reduction in death or MI in patients with ACS. Older patients are more often susceptible to overdosing, reflected by an elevated partial thromboplastin time, and bleeding. Low-molecular-weight heparin also improves clinical outcomes for ACS with a greater relative benefit in older patients than younger patients, but caution is needed to avoid excessive dosing and bleeding complications due to its renal clearance. Bivalirudin, a direct thrombin inhibitor, is used frequently in invasively managed ACS patients, often in conjunction with oral antiplatelet loading. It has equivalent antithrombotic activity with less bleeding in several trials.

Newer oral antithrombotic therapies have been evaluated for safety and efficacy in reducing recurrent events in patients with ASCVD. The Apixaban for Prevention of Acute Ischemic Events 2 (APPRAISE-2) trial randomized high-risk patients following MI to apixaban 5 mg twice daily in addition to antiplatelet therapy. They found an increased risk of major bleeding without a significant reduction in recurrent ischemic events. The Cardiovascular Outcomes for People Using Anticoagulation Strategies (COMPASS) trial randomized a different population—patients with stable ASCVD—to a low dose of rivaroxaban (2.5 mg twice daily) plus aspirin versus aspirin alone. There was a reduction in cardiovascular events, but at the expense of more bleeding with rivaroxaban. Given the increased bleeding risk, oral anticoagulants are not recommended for acute or chronic CHD in the absence of another indication (eg, atrial fibrillation or deep venous thrombosis).

β-Blockers

β-Blockers lower myocardial oxygen demand and improve coronary blood flow with anti-hypertensive and anti-ischemic properties. Long-term benefits from β-blockers include management of ischemic symptoms, lowering blood pressure, or improving HF outcomes in those a depressed left ventricular function. Many patients, including older adults, are placed on β-blockers initially at the time of an acute MI. A meta-analysis of 25 randomized controlled trials of patients with prior MI showed β-blockers reduced all-cause mortality or MI by 25%. An observational analysis of older patients following acute MI showed those receiving β-blockers had a 33% reduction in 1-year mortality. The contemporary REACH registry analyzed use of β-blockers into three cohorts: CAD without MI, CAD with prior MI, and CAD risk factors only. There was no association between use of β-blockers and lower rates of death, nonfatal MI, or nonfatal stroke in any cohort. However, those with recent MI (≤ 1 year) had a 25% lower incidence of the composite which included cardiac rehospitalization with β-blocker use. This suggests the greatest benefit in the contemporary era for β-blockers is in the first year following an MI. Older patients are often vulnerable to drugs with hypotensive actions and have altered responses to β-blockers owing to conduction system deterioration and the physiologic desensitization of β-adrenergic receptor function, so this information is helpful in considering continuation after 1 year. Additionally, a recent trial found that early use of β-blockers in patients with MI could worsen risks for congestive heart failure and result in poorer outcomes. Thus, β-blockers should be administered to those with an identified potential for benefit, titrated with caution, and revisited based on tolerability and clinical stability over time.

Statins

Cholesterol is a key determinant of risk, reflected by levels of LDL-C and non–HDL-C. There are several classes of drugs for lowering serum cholesterol, including fibrates, bile acid sequestrants, niacin, fish oil, ezetimibe, hydroxymethylglutaryl coenzyme A (HMG-CoA) reductase inhibitors (statins), PCSK9-inhibitors, and bempedoic acid. Of these, only statins—alone or in combination with ezetimibe or PCSK9 inhibitors—have proven effective for secondary prevention of cardiovascular events.

There is no question that for secondary prevention of ASCVD, moderate-intensity statin use reduces major vascular events including in those aged 75 or older. Furthermore, the guideline states that it is reasonable to continue high-intensity statin in patients aged 75 or older if tolerated. Notably, an observational study from the Veterans Affairs health system identified a graded association between statin intensity and mortality in patients with ASCVD, with high-intensity statins conferring a small but significant survival advantage compared with moderate intensity statins in older adults (76–84 years old). Another large meta-analysis from the Cholesterol Treatment Trialists found no heterogeneity of treatment effect when high-intensity statin therapy was compared with moderate-intensity statin therapy across age groups.

In the immediate post-MI period, high-intensity lipid-lowering therapy has demonstrated benefit in older patients to prevent recurrent cardiovascular events. In fact, in a post hoc analysis of the Pravastatin or Atorvastatin Evaluation and Infection Therapy—Thrombolysis in Myocardial Infarction (PROVE IT-TIMI 22) trial, patients

age 70 years and older were found to derive greater benefit than younger counterparts in terms of absolute and relative reduction in cardiovascular events. A meta-analysis of age-specific outcome data from two primary prevention statin trials, JUPITER (Justification for Use of Statins in Prevention: An Intervention Trial Evaluating Rosuvastatin) and HOPE-3 (Heart Outcomes Prevention Evaluation), demonstrated a 26% relative risk reduction for those older than 70 years for the end point of nonfatal MI, nonfatal stroke, or cardiovascular death (HR, 0.74; 95% CI, 0.61–0.91; p = 0.0048). There was no heterogeneity of treatment effect by age observed but all included patients also had elevated C-reactive protein levels and most of the events were in those between age 70 and 75.

There is a paucity of RCT data supporting statin use for primary prevention in older adults (≥ 75 years old) as reflected in the guideline recommendation for clinical assessment of risk when deciding whether to continue or initiate statin treatment (Class IIa). Further compounding this uncertainty is the fact that the guideline emphasizes pretreatment risk stratification using the Pooled Cohort Equations 10-year ASCVD risk calculator to guide treatment decisions. However, the risk calculator was derived in populations only up to age 79 and multiple studies have demonstrated suboptimal performance of the risk calculator in older adult populations. The guideline states that a moderate-intensity statin in adults 75 years or older with an LDL-C level of 70 to 189 mg/dL may be reasonable (IIb), but balances that by stating it may be reasonable to stop statin therapy when functional decline (physical or cognitive), multimorbidity, frailty, or reduced life-expectancy limits the potential benefits of statin therapy (IIb).

A meta-analysis of data from patients included in randomized trials comparing statins to placebo (n = 134,537) demonstrated no statistically significant benefit in individuals older than 75 years for statin use in primary prevention (**Figure 74-6**). Observational evidence for primary prevention in US Veterans age 75 or older suggests new initiation of statin reduces all-cause and cardiovascular mortality. An observational subgroup analysis of healthy individuals age 70 or older in the Aspirin in Reducing Events in the Elderly (ASPREE) trial showed statin use at baseline was not associated with disability-free survival, all-cause mortality or dementia. However, those on statins at baseline had a lower risk of physical disability and adverse cardiovascular events. The question "Is statin therapy efficacious and safe in older patients (> 75 years of age)? If so, what is a net benefit of statin therapy in this age group?" was identified as an important question needing to be addressed by future RCTs in the most recent ACC/AHA cholesterol guideline. Two large, currently ongoing trials (A Clinical Trial of STAtin Therapy for Reducing Events in the Elderly, STAREE, ClinicalTrials.gov: NCT02099123 and Pragmatic Evaluation of Events and Benefits of Lipid-Lowering in Older Adults, PREVENTABLE, ClinicalTrials.gov: NCT04262206) are focused on this question.

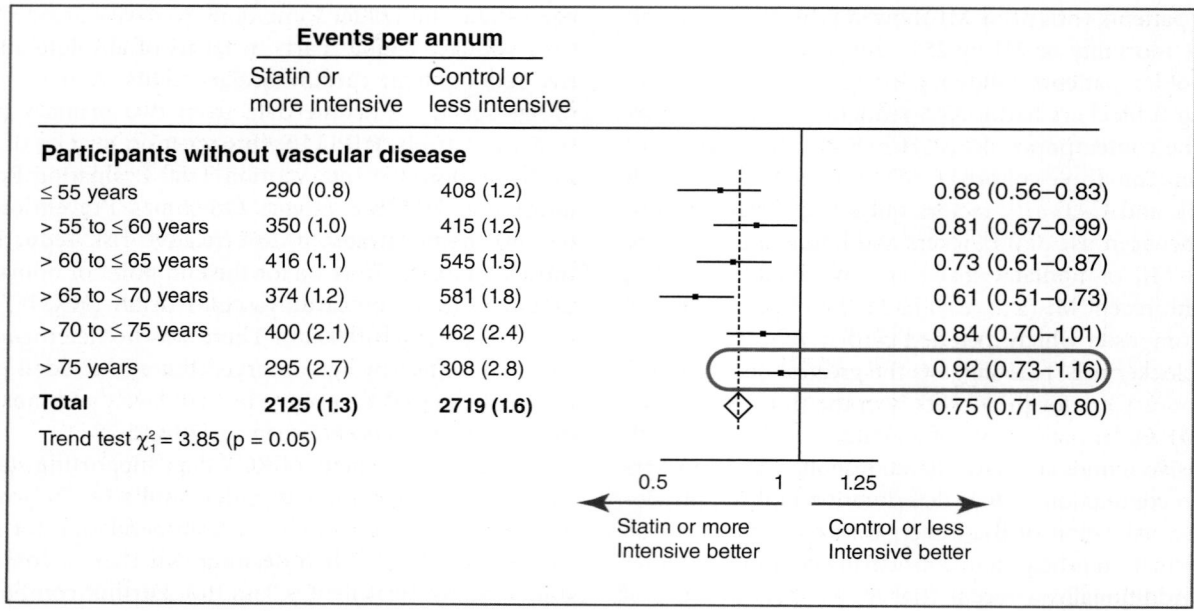

	Events per annum			
	Statin or more intensive	Control or less intensive		
Participants without vascular disease				
≤ 55 years	290 (0.8)	408 (1.2)		0.68 (0.56–0.83)
> 55 to ≤ 60 years	350 (1.0)	415 (1.2)		0.81 (0.67–0.99)
> 60 to ≤ 65 years	416 (1.1)	545 (1.5)		0.73 (0.61–0.87)
> 65 to ≤ 70 years	374 (1.2)	581 (1.8)		0.61 (0.51–0.73)
> 70 to ≤ 75 years	400 (2.1)	462 (2.4)		0.84 (0.70–1.01)
> 75 years	295 (2.7)	308 (2.8)		0.92 (0.73–1.16)
Total	**2125 (1.3)**	**2719 (1.6)**		0.75 (0.71–0.80)
Trend test $\chi_1^2 = 3.85$ (p = 0.05)				

0.5   1   1.25

Statin or more Intensive better   Control or less Intensive better

FIGURE 74-6. Forest plot of effect of primary prevention statin treatment on major vascular events stratified by age. (Adapted with permission from Cholesterol Treatment Trialists' Collaboration. Efficacy and safety of statin therapy in older people: a meta-analysis of individual participant data from 28 randomised controlled trials. *Lancet.* 2019;393[10170]:407–415.)

Older adults (≥ 75 years old) with ASCVD received high-intensity statins less often than younger patients in the Patient and Provider Assessment of Lipid Management (PALM) registry, highlighting a potential gap in care. While closing treatment gaps is important, identifying older populations where benefit is unlikely is important as well. A recent meta-analysis of randomized clinical trials of primary prevention in adults aged 50 to 75 found that the time to benefit for 100 adults treated with statin therapy to prevent one MACE was at least 2.5 years. An evaluation of US Medicare- and Medicaid-certified nursing home facilities demonstrated that more than one-third of nursing home residents aged 65 or older with a life-limiting illness remained on statin therapy. Time to benefit is an important consideration for initiating or discontinuing statin treatment in older individuals for primary or secondary prevention.

Statin intolerance is often a concern in older patients, however evidence on this is reassuring. The Effect of Statins on Skeletal Muscle Function and Performance (STOMP) study demonstrated that high-dose atorvastatin did not decrease muscle strength or exercise performance in healthy subjects, despite a mild increase in myalgias with statin treatment (9.4% vs 4.6%, $p = 0.05$). The Self-assessment Method for Statin Side Effects or Nocebo (SAMSON) trial was a recent double-blind n-of-1 trial of patients who had recently discontinued statins due to side effects. In this trial, 90% of symptom burden with statin treatment was elicited by placebo alone when compared to the statin months and no-tablet months—so many muscle symptoms attributed

to statins may be due to the "nocebo" effect. Reassuringly, half of the SAMSON trial participants were able to restart a statin after trial completion. Ofori-Asenso and colleagues also looked at switching, discontinuing, and reinitiating statins among adults aged 65 or older in a random sample of the Australian population. They also found that while statin discontinuation is common, most older individuals eventually restart a statin with improved persistent use. Importantly, older patients in the PALM registry reported tolerating statin therapy similarly to younger subjects. Taken together this evidence suggests older adults can tolerate statin therapy as well as younger populations. Ultimately, improving persistence and compliance with statin therapy in all age groups is a key priority.

Other Lipid-Lowering Agents

Ezetimibe, the first nonstatin lipid-lowering therapy demonstrated in a randomized controlled trial to improve cardiovascular outcomes in patients with ASCVD, targets the absorption of cholesterol from the diet. In the Vytorin Efficacy International Trial (IMPROVE-IT), 18,144 high-risk patients with an acute coronary syndrome in the preceding 10 days were randomized to simvastatin versus simvastatin plus ezetimibe. The addition of ezetimibe to statin treatment lowered LDL-C by 24%. There was also a modest 2% absolute risk reduction in the composite primary endpoint at 7 years of follow-up (cardiovascular death, MI, hospitalization for unstable angina, coronary revascularization, and nonfatal stroke). A secondary analysis of IMPROVE-IT set out to assess the effect of ezetimibe and simvastatin compared with simvastatin monotherapy among patients 75 years or older with recent acute coronary syndrome included in the trial. The authors determined that older adults in IMPROVE-IT actually derived the most benefit from the addition of ezetimibe to statin therapy, with the greatest absolute risk reduction observed in those 75 years or older without any increase in adverse safety events. There are also data for primary prevention treatment with ezetimibe. The Ezetimibe Lipid-Lowering Trial on Prevention of Atherosclerotic Cardiovascular Disease in 75 or Older (EWTOPIA 75), a multicenter, prospective, randomized, open-label, blinded trial in Japan, examined the preventive efficacy of ezetimibe for patients aged 75 or older, with elevated LDL-C without history of CAD. In EWTOPIA, ezetimibe treatment was associated with a lower rate of cardiovascular events, though the open-label nature of the trial and early termination somewhat limit interpretation of the results.

Monoclonal antibodies against the proprotein convertase subtilisin kexin 9 (PCSK9) are the latest addition to the lipid-lowering clinical arsenal. In recent years, two landmark trials have been published demonstrating the safety and efficacy of alirocumab and evolocumab, respectively, to lower LDL-C levels by up to 50% and improve clinical outcomes in individuals with ASCVD. These medications are recommended by the current ACC/AHA cholesterol guideline recommendations for patients with ASCVD deemed to be high-risk and with persistently elevated LDL-C levels. However, the impact of PCSK-9 inhibitors in high-risk multimorbid older adult populations has not been described. A prespecified secondary analysis of the ODYSSEY OUTCOMES trial demonstrated that the addition of PCSK9-inhibitor alirocumab reduced ischemic cardiovascular events in post-ACS patients on maximally tolerated statin intensive therapy across age groups, with increasing absolute benefit with advancing age and no significant safety concerns.

Other Secondary Prevention Strategies

Secondary prevention aims to lower the risk of recurrent cardiovascular events in patients with CHD. Since older patients with CHD face higher overall risk, the benefit of prevention in absolute terms rises with age and "number needed to treat" falls. Secondary prevention strategies target control of risk factors, such as hypertension and tobacco cessation. Exercise and lifestyle interventions should be similarly applied and are effective regardless of age. There is no upper age limit for the benefit of exercise, even if physical limitations modify the type of activity. Cardiac rehabilitation can be especially important following a cardiac event in assisting the older patient in selecting a sustainable exercise routine.

The renin-angiotensin-aldosterone system is a key determinant in hypertension, inflammation, atherosclerosis, and, ultimately, increased cardiovascular events. Angiotensin-converting enzyme (ACE) inhibitors have strong support for

safe and effective treatment of hypertension, and improving survival post-MI with depressed heart function, heart failure, or anterior MIs. The Heart Outcomes Prevention Evaluation (HOPE) study extended the benefits of ACE inhibitors to all patients with known CHD or at high risk of CHD. In HOPE, patients with CHD and other patients with high CHD risk (eg, diabetes plus one or more cardiac risk factor) were randomized to 10 mg of ramipril daily versus placebo. After 5 years, treated patients had 26% lower risk of CHD death than those who were not treated. Rates of MI, congestive heart failure, stroke, renal dysfunction, and even development of diabetes were lower in the ACE-treated patient group. The treatment effects of ACE inhibition were greater in those patients aged 65 or older than in younger patients. Current guidelines suggest consideration of ACE inhibitors in all patients having CHD with depressed ventricular function, diabetes, or hypertension. Some experts have suggested that these drugs be considered in all patients with known CHD regardless of other risk factors or left ventricular dysfunction, yet there remains conflicting evidence from clinical trials regarding this issue. Angiotensin receptor blockers (ARBs), similar to ACE inhibitors, are designed to produce antihypertensive and anti-inflammatory effects within the cardiovascular system, and recent studies demonstrate that these agents translate to decreased cardiovascular events. Several randomized control trials have shown that the ARBs can slow the progression of nephropathy in patients with diabetes and microalbuminuria in a fashion similar to ACE inhibitors. Overall, the data favor the use of established ACE inhibitors for primary and secondary prevention of cardiovascular events, with the consideration of ARB substitution in patients who are intolerant of ACE inhibitors (most commonly from troublesome cough). When used in older patients, one should monitor serum electrolytes and creatinine, as these drugs can cause decreased renal function and hyperkalemia.

CATHETERIZATION AND REVASCULARIZATION

Unstable Angina or Myocardial Infarction

Care guidelines recommend that all those diagnosed with an MI should have an assessment of both left ventricular function (via echocardiography or other means) and coronary disease severity. In patients with NSTEMI, the two options for assessment of post-MI risk are (1) routine angiography with revascularization as appropriate or (2) conservative strategy of medical therapy with selection for angiography based on refractory symptoms of ischemia ("ischemia-driven" approach). Recent clinical trials suggest that the early invasive approach might be preferable for patients at increased risk of recurrent cardiovascular events. With the introduction of contemporary trials, the Treat Angina with Aggrastat and Determine Cost of Therapy with an Invasive or Conservative Strategy—Thrombolysis in Myocardial Ischemia/Infarction (TACTICS-TIMI)-18 trial randomized patients with unstable angina/NSTEMI to one or the other of these strategies and found that those in the early invasive arm (within 48 hours) had nearly 20% lower rates of death, nonfatal MI, or rehospitalization at 6 months than conservatively treated patients. Interestingly, the successful enrollment of older patients (40% of patients were $\geq$ 65 years) allowed the identification of a 44% relative risk reduction in 30-day death or nonfatal MI among patients 65 years or older (invasive 5.7% vs conservative 9.8%; $p < 0.05$) and a 56% relative risk reduction in patients older than 75 years(invasive 10.8% vs conservative 21.6%; $p < 0.05$) with the early invasive strategy, findings consistent with a greater benefit in older relative to younger patients.

Multiple studies in older adult populations have demonstrated similar benefits to an early invasive strategy. In an open-label randomized controlled trial of patients 80 years or older with NSTEMI or unstable angina admitted to hospitals in Norway, an invasive strategy with early coronary angiography and immediate assessment for revascularization was superior to a conservative strategy of medical treatment alone for reducing cardiovascular events. In the Italian Elderly ACS Trial, a routine invasive strategy in NSTEMI patients 80 years or older was beneficial compared with a selective invasive strategy, though the trial did not meet its recruitment goal. One study of NSTEMI patients 80 years or older with chronic kidney disease found PCI offered a survival benefit regardless of eGFR but a higher risk of bleeding with eGFR less than 30 mL/min per 1.73 m². Similarly, a meta-analysis assessing the long-term outcome of a routine versus selective invasive strategy in patients with non–ST-segment elevation acute coronary syndromes demonstrated that increasing age is actually the strongest predictor for better outcomes with a routine invasive strategy. Taken together, a routine invasive strategy appears to be the appropriate approach in most older adults with NSTEMI.

Stable Ischemic Heart Disease

A major challenge in the care of older patients with stable CHD is related to who should undergo evaluation for coronary revascularization. In younger patients, randomized clinical trials have simplified this decision-making process by identifying subgroups in which PCI or CABG surgery improves survival and/or quality of life beyond medical therapy. However, patients older than 75 years were generally not represented in these pivotal trials, so clinicians and patients must rely on a careful comparison between the acute procedural risks and potential long-term benefits. Developments in the techniques of coronary catheterization, PCI, and CABG are changing the landscape for patient selection and outcomes for revascularization. Based on Medicare data, trends and outcomes in older patients after PCI were compared between the balloon

angioplasty era (1991–1995), the bare metal stents (BMS) era (1998–2003), and the drug-eluting stents (DES) era (2004–2006). Despite a significant increase in comorbidity, the number of post-PCI adverse cardiovascular events decreased over time, including less death and MI at 3-year follow-up. The improved outcomes were due to reductions in the need for repeat target vessel/lesion revascularizations and CABG, highlighting the efficacy of evolving technologies and techniques, as well as improving adjunctive therapy.

The use of fractional flow reserve (FFR < 0.8) to identify lesions contributing to ischemia has been shown to improve associated PCI outcomes. The use of third-generation stents has also improved the outcomes of PCI among those with multivessel disease, although CABG continues to demonstrate superior survival and fewer events at 5 years compared with PCI. The selection of patients for CABG as the optimal revascularization strategy should include those with reduced EF (< 35% with viable myocardium), left main CAD or its equivalent, and diabetes.

Age-associated risk in procedural mortality is not strictly linear but rises rapidly beyond the age of 75. Additionally, at any age, patients with CABG face two- to three-fold higher mortality risks compared to those undergoing angioplasty. However, technological advances have led to improved procedural success rates and lower risks for both procedures. Thus, despite the fact that procedures were performed on patients with higher risk, the risk of death after CABG in patients aged 65 or older in the Society for Thoracic Surgery database declined nearly 20% between 1990 and 1999 and now rests at just above 4%. The Society for Thoracic Surgery has devised risk models that can be used to guide the impact of patient risk factors on operative morbidity and mortality and can be used in patient management. The web-based risk calculator can be found at http://www.sts.org.

Nonfatal procedural complications (stroke, MI, and renal failure) also rise with age and are higher with CABG. Of major importance to many older patients are the procedural risks of stroke and loss in mental acuity. Patients with CABG aged 75 or older have a 3% to 6% incidence of stroke compared with less than 1% incidence of stroke with angioplasty. Additionally, by using highly sensitive neurocognitive testing, Newman and colleagues found that up to 50% of patients of all ages undergoing CABG had measurable impairments in neurocognitive function at hospital discharge. Although half of patients with initial impairment recovered by 6 months, cognitive deficits reappeared in many of them during long-term follow-up and portended an impaired functional status. However, one recent study that compared cognitive ability after CABG to angioplasty and age-matched controls noted no meaningful clinical deterioration of cognitive performance between groups. Similarly, the initial enthusiasm of improving neurocognitive outcomes by performing off-pump CABG versus traditional on-pump CABG has been tempered by findings from a recent randomized trial, which demonstrated comparable cognitive outcomes between the two groups, although long-term follow-up has yet to occur. While chronologic age is a major risk factor for procedural complications or mortality, it is biological age which is most important to consider. For example, by using published risk models, an octogenarian's likelihood for mortality with CABG ranges from 2% for a "healthy" patient without comorbidities, to less than 30% with multiple risk factors such as diabetes or preexisting CVD.

The risks of revascularization must be balanced against the potential benefits in terms of prolonged survival, improved functional outcomes, or both. The Alberta Provincial Project for Outcomes Assessment in Coronary Heart Disease registry examined the care and outcomes of more than 6000 patients aged 70 to 79 who underwent cardiac catheterization. Compared with medical therapy, those receiving CABG or PCI had significantly higher adjusted 4-year survival rates (CABG 87%, PCI 84%, medical therapy 79%, $p < 0.001$). These survival benefits of revascularization also held for octogenarians and increased in all aged patients in proportion with the number of diseased vessels and the degree of left ventricular dysfunction. Results from the Alberta Provincial Project for Outcomes Assessment in Coronary Heart Disease registry have been confirmed in other observational analyses. Together, these studies strongly suggest that older patients with multivessel coronary disease have higher survival rates if treated with optimal revascularization than if they are treated with medical therapy alone.

There is a growing body of literature to support the use of revascularization to reduce angina and improve functional outcomes of older patients with CHD. The Trial of Invasive Versus Medical Therapy in Elderly Patients with Chronic Symptomatic Coronary Artery Disease study randomized 305 patients with chronic angina, aged 75 or older, to diagnostic catheterization (followed by coronary revascularization as appropriate) or optimized medical therapy with intervention only for those with refractory symptoms. Of those randomized to catheterization and intervention as appropriate, 74% underwent CABG or PCI, while almost 33% of the conservative management arm crossed over to revascularization by 6 months. Patients in the early revascularization arm had significantly greater improvement in their symptoms, functional status and quality of life when compared with medically treated patients. However, there was a higher 6-month mortality rate but a lower incidence of nonfatal MI in the early invasive arm. While this randomized study had a small sample size and presented several methodological challenges, its results provide support for the consideration of revascularization in the very old patient with CHD. The Objective Randomised Blinded Investigation With Optimal Medical Therapy of Angioplasty in Stable Angina (ORBITA) trial randomized patients with stable angina and evidence of severe single-vessel stenosis 1:1 to either PCI or a placebo sham procedure ($n = 200$), demonstrating that PCI did not result in greater improvements in exercise times or angina frequency. However, the trial had a medical therapy run in period, and was powered for exercise treadmill-based endpoints. Both the COURAGE trial and the ISCHEMIA trial demonstrated improvements in angina with revascularization compared with medical therapy alone. In ISCHEMIA, patients with angina at baseline who underwent revascularization had improved symptom relief and quality of life compared with optimal medical therapy. Patients with more frequent angina (daily or weekly) were also more likely to be angina free at 1 year (50% of patients) compared with those on medical therapy alone (20%).

Fibrinolysis and Primary PCI

The primary management objective in patients with STEMI is to provide early reperfusion therapy by pharmacologic means (ie, fibrinolysis) or percutaneous intervention. Numerous studies have confirmed that reperfusion therapy (fibrinolytic therapy or primary angioplasty) in patients presenting with STEMIs improves survival if delivered in a timely fashion. Despite this, older adults may present differently from younger adults with STEMI, more frequently having abnormal baseline ECGs and atypical symptoms that may be attributed to multifactorial causes. This is reflected in multiple studies demonstrating more frequently delayed treatment (> 90 minutes door-to-balloon time) among older individuals, including lower use of invasive cardiac procedures and primary PCI despite higher risk features in older patients. Non-White race, atypical symptoms, and heart failure are all significantly associated with prehospital delays. Given that older adults are at the highest risk for mortality, they likely derive the highest magnitude of treatment benefit from early revascularization.

An overview of the major thrombolytic trials from the Fibrinolytic Therapy Trialists' Collaborative Group, a meta-analysis that included more than 58,000 patients, demonstrated a 15% relative risk reduction in death for patients 75 years or older with STEMI or bundle branch block treated with fibrinolytics. Despite older patients achieving a smaller relative reduction in death than younger patients, the trend toward absolute benefit in terms of lives saved with fibrinolytics was threefold greater in patients older than 75 years compared with those younger than 55 years.

In addition, an observational analysis from the ACTION Registry–GWTG found that approximately 6% of patients with STEMI treated in the community were 85 years or older (median age 88). Compared to younger patients, the oldest old patients were more likely to be women, had more hypertension, and were more likely to have prior heart failure and stroke. More than 42% of the oldest old patients were also cited as having contraindications to reperfusion, but absolute or relative contraindications were only reported in 10%. Patient preference was the most common reason indicated (45%). Even in reperfusion-eligible patients, the oldest old patients were less likely to receive it with neither mortality benefit nor harm in those who did receive it. Similarly, in the Nationwide Inpatient Sample, STEMI patients coming from a nursing home were compared to those coming from the community. Compared with their community-dwelling counterparts, nursing home residents are less likely to receive reperfusion therapy for STEMI and had higher in-hospital mortality.

The possible benefits of thrombolysis must be weighed carefully against the risks, especially in the older population. Data from the Fibrinolytic Therapy Trialists' meta-analysis showed that patients older than 70 years had nearly a threefold higher relative risk of intracranial hemorrhage, the most feared complication in the postlytic period, after fibrinolysis than those aged less than 60. Bearing this in mind, clinicians should realize that intracranial hemorrhage is a rare event and the absolute risk of this complication after fibrinolysis in those older than 70 years remains between 0.7% and 2.1% in major trials and nearing 3% in those older than 85 years. The risk factors for intracranial hemorrhage include low body weight, elevated blood pressures, facial or head trauma, and dementia. Dementia was found in one trial to significantly increase the risk for intracranial hemorrhage by threefold.

In contrast with mixed results for fibrinolysis, timely reperfusion for STEMI with PCI is almost universally associated with improved outcomes in all age groups. For example, a randomized study of primary PCI versus thrombolysis in patients with STEMI showed a 40% relative risk reduction for death, MI, and stroke in patients treated within 3 hours of presentation with PCI. In the ACTION Registry, primary PCI was associated with lower 30-day and 1-year mortality when compared to no therapy or thrombolysis among older patients with acute MI. Over the past decade, the use of primary PCI overall, and in older patients, has dramatically increased, in-hospital mortality has been reduced, and complications are lower with direct revascularization. However, when percutaneous intervention is not available in a timely manner, thrombolytic therapy may improve outcomes when given in the right window of time. Ultimately, an early invasive strategy aimed toward timely revascularization is a safe and effective approach for the majority of older adults presenting with acute MI with the purpose of improving survival.

SPECIAL CONSIDERATIONS

Multimorbidity and Frailty

The diagnosis and care of older CHD patients invokes an interplay of biological differences, comorbid conditions, functional status, drug pharmacology, and goals of care. The traditional approach of one disease at a time is of limited utility in the older population. Of Medicare beneficiaries, 68% have more than or equal to two chronic conditions,

and 14% have more than or equal to six chronic conditions. Among those Medicare beneficiaries with a diagnosis of ischemic heart disease, 81% have hypertension, 69% have hyperlipidemia, 42% have diabetes, 41% have arthritis, 39% have anemia, 36% have heart failure, and 30% have chronic kidney disease. Frailty is also a common occurrence in patients with CHD, including those presenting with acute MI, in part due to shared risk factors, and common end-organ manifestations. Frailty increases mortality and morbidity among those hospitalized with MI, with a twofold increased risk of mortality, rehospitalization, bleeding, stroke, or dialysis at 1 year. Similar increased risks are noted for frail elders following PCI and CABG. Frailty has been shown to be associated with longer hospital stays, higher rates of delirium, and increased resource utilization. Despite this increased risk, PCI still confers a survival benefit in frail older individuals presenting with acute MI and recent studies have not shown a significant difference in complication rates between frail and nonfrail older individuals. Thus, frail older adults with acute MI should safely undergo PCI assuming no other contraindications to treatment.

Guidelines are based on trials performed predominately in younger patients. Patients older than 75 years comprise approximately 9% of the population enrolled in clinical trials of ACS therapies, but account for more than 37% of patients with ACS in the community. Despite calls for inclusion, this trend has shown little improvement over the last two decades. There is good reason to believe that older adult populations with acute MI have key differences from younger populations that may impact treatment strategies and outcomes. Recently, the SILVER-AMI registry assessed older adults (≥ 75 years) presenting with acute MI, demonstrating a high prevalence of functional impairments, including deficits in cognition, strength, and sensory domains; interestingly, these functional impairments included some of the strongest predictors of 6-month mortality. In fact, hearing impairment, mobility impairment, recent weight loss, and lower patient-reported health status were all predictive of 6-month post-AMI mortality in this population. Given the current knowledge gaps as well as the inherent complexity of this population, the approach to cardiac care of the older patient requires a person-centered plan incorporating goals and health state.

Procedural Considerations

Despite the challenge of more complex anatomy from the right radial artery in particular, a transradial approach has a lower complication rate compared with the transfemoral approach (especially bleeding complications) and should be considered the first choice for arterial access in older patients. While BMS have been historically considered in older frail patients in order to shorten DAPT duration and reduce bleeding risk, recent data suggest that treatment with DES remains preferable. In the XIMA (Xience or Vision Stents for the Management of Angina in the Elderly) trial, a randomized trial of everolimus-eluting stents versus

BMS in octogenarians, DES were associated with a lower incidence of MI and target vessel revascularization without an increased risk of major hemorrhage. In another single-blind randomized trial of DES in older patients with CAD (SENIOR), a DES with short duration of DAPT improved the composite of all-cause mortality, MI, stroke, and ischemia-driven target lesion revascularization compared with BMS with a similar duration of DAPT. Thus, the use of DES is preferable to BMS in older patients who require PCI.

Role of Palliative Care

Treatment algorithms for CHD are ideally focused on symptom management—aligned with the goals of palliative care—but use of palliative care itself remains low in cardiology treatment algorithms. There is a subset of patients with CHD with poor prognosis related to their coronary disease or other multimorbid conditions who benefit from palliative care, and palliative care has been increasing among individuals hospitalized with AMI (from 0.2% in 2002 to 3.0% in 2016) particularly those with cardiogenic shock (from 0.6% in 2002 to 14.0% in 2016). Older age is strongly associated with increasing odds of palliative care use. When goals of care prioritize comfort, palliative care also can be initiated in the outpatient setting to avoid future hospitalizations and invasive procedures. Ultimately, increasing uptake of palliative care for select patients with CHD will benefit from defining the optimal integration of palliative care into the CHD treatment paradigm in older adults.

Patient Preferences

Cardiac treatment plans need to consider the patients' overall health, as well as their preferences and willingness to accept risk. While some older individuals engage in very active, independent lives well into their advanced years, others are frail and suffer disabling physical and/or mental illnesses. Beyond this variability in health and functional status, there is great diversity in the health values of older patients. Some consider illness and disability to be inevitable and have no interest in extensive medical or surgical intervention. However, many older patients favor longevity if coupled with good cognitive ability and lack of disability. In hospital settings, many older patients feel vulnerable and abdicate decision-making to family or physicians entrusted to act in the patient's best interest. Our group assessed the extent to which individual knowledge, preferences, and priorities explain lower use of invasive cardiac care among older versus younger adults presenting with acute coronary syndrome, demonstrating that age influences risk tolerance for CABG surgery, treatment goals and willingness to consider invasive cardiac care. It is incumbent on those caring for older patients to attempt to elicit preferences, while providing necessary information regarding potential risks and benefits of treatment options. Ethical mandates at the core of the shared decision-making include autonomy (goals of care) and nonmaleficence (do no harm).

Renal Function and Pharmacology

An individual's renal function remains a powerful predictor of cardiovascular morbidity and mortality. In the Cooperative Cardiovascular Project, renal dysfunction predicted adverse outcomes among an older post-MI population, such that 1-year mortality was 24% if serum creatinine was below 1.5 mg/dL and 66% if creatinine was above 2.5 mg/dL. The pitfalls attributed to using the serum creatinine as a surrogate for renal function are often compounded in the older population. Consistent with recommendations from the Panel on Acute Coronary Care in the Elderly, the creatinine clearance should be calculated on all patients 75 years or older who present with an ACS. In addition, the clinician should remain cognizant of changes in the creatinine clearance during the index hospitalization and after discharge, as several medications prescribed may have an impact on renal function. From the Global Registry of Acute Coronary Events study, a 10 mL/min decrease in creatinine clearance had the same impact on in-hospital mortality as a 10-year increase in age. The role of renal dysfunction in the management of older patients with ACSs cannot be overemphasized, as this entity plays a pivotal role at the interface of pharmacologic management.

Cardiovascular drugs are among the most commonly prescribed therapies in older patients, and altered pharmacokinetics (ie, drug distribution and metabolism) are frequently observed in older patients as a consequence of decreased lean body mass and volume of distribution. Combined, these factors lead to higher drug concentrations and prolonged half-lives. A drug's pharmacodynamics (ie, the effect of a drug on a target cell) can be considerably altered with age. For example, increased calcification of the cardiac conduction system can increase an older patient's sensitivity to atrioventricular nodal blocking agents and lead to profound bradycardia. Comorbid illness and frailty can also influence drug selection and safety. For instance, a frail older person may have a higher risk of falling, which can markedly increase the likelihood of bleeding complications with anticoagulants. Finally, polypharmacy is often a serious risk in older patients and can lead to life-threatening drug–drug interactions and poor adherence because of confusion over medications and/or prohibitive costs.

SUMMARY

Despite advances in prevention and treatment, CHD remains a major health problem for older patients. As the population ages, the need for evidence-based cardiac care for patients aged 75 or older will increase substantially. Older patients benefit as much, if not more, from existing therapies as do younger patients. However, the care of CHD in older patients is in the context of their multidimensional health status and requires awareness of atypical presentations of ACS, altered pharmacokinetics of therapy, and underlying cognitive and functional status. Bearing this in mind, treatment paradigms applied to younger patient groups are often appropriate when treating older patients, and adherence to guidelines translates into better outcomes. The classification of physiologic frailty may offer additional risk information for older patients considering revascularization. This information could identify a cohort who may benefit from a try at medical therapy optimization or geriatric intervention before revascularization, or for whom alternate treatment or palliative care is the preferred route. Despite the significant challenges in cardiovascular care of the oldest old patients, redirecting efforts to a person-centered model may provide the best opportunity to improve outcomes that matter most.

FURTHER READING

Armitage J, Baigent C, Barnes E, et al. Efficacy and safety of statin therapy in older people: a meta-analysis of individual participant data from 28 randomised controlled trials. *Lancet.* 2019;393:407–415.

Bach RG, Cannon CP, Giugliano RP, et al. Effect of simvastatin-ezetimibe compared with simvastatin monotherapy after acute coronary syndrome among patients 75 years or older: a secondary analysis of a randomized clinical trial. *JAMA Cardiol.* 2019;4: 846–854.

Dodson JA, Hajduk AM, Geda M, et al. Predicting 6-month mortality for older adults hospitalized with acute myocardial infarction: a cohort study. *Ann Intern Med.* 2020; 172:12–21.

Elgendy IY, Elbadawi A, Sardar P, et al. Palliative care use in patients with acute myocardial infarction. *J Am Coll Cardiol.* 2020;75:113–117.

Gencer B, Marston NA, Im K, et al. Efficacy and safety of lowering LDL cholesterol in older patients: a systematic review and meta-analysis of randomised controlled trials. *Lancet.* 2020;396:1637–1643.

Grundy SM, Stone NJ, Bailey AL, et al. 2018 AHA/ACC/AACVPR/AAPA/ABC/ACPM/ADA/AGS/APhA/ASPC/NLA/PCNA Guideline on the Management of Blood Cholesterol: A Report of the American College of Cardiology/American Heart Association Task Force on Clinical Practice Guidelines. *Circulation.* 2019;139: e1082–e1143.

Kumar S, McDaniel M, Samady H, Forouzandeh F. Contemporary revascularization dilemmas in older adults. *J Am Heart Assoc.* 2020;9:e014477.

Lowenstern A, Alexander KP, Hill CL, et al. Age-related differences in the noninvasive evaluation for possible coronary artery disease: insights from the Prospective Multicenter Imaging Study for Evaluation of Chest Pain (PROMISE) Trial. *JAMA Cardiol.* 2020;5:193–201.

McNeil JJ, Woods RL, Nelson MR, et al. Effect of aspirin on disability-free survival in the healthy elderly. *N Engl J Med.* 2018;379:1499–1508.

Nanna MG, Navar AM, Wang TY, et al. Statin use and adverse effects among adults >75 years of age: insights from the patient and Provider Assessment of Lipid Management (PALM) Registry. *J Am Heart Assoc.* 2018;7: e008546.

Nanna MG, Peterson ED, Wu A, et al. Age, knowledge, preferences, and risk tolerance for invasive cardiac care. *Am Heart J.* 2020;219:99–108.

Ofori-Asenso R, Ilomaki J, Tacey M, et al. Switching, discontinuation, and reinitiation of statins among older adults. *J Am Coll Cardiol.* 2018;72:2675–2677.

Orkaby AR, Driver JA, Ho YL, et al. Association of statin use with all-cause and cardiovascular mortality in US veterans 75 years and older. *JAMA.* 2020;324:68–78.

Ouchi Y, Sasaki J, Arai H, et al. Ezetimibe Lipid-Lowering Trial on Prevention of Atherosclerotic Cardiovascular Disease in 75 or Older (EWTOPIA 75). *Circulation.* 2019;140:992–1003.

Ouellet GM, Geda M, Murphy TE, Tsang S, Tinetti ME, Chaudhry SI. Prehospital delay in older adults with acute myocardial infarction: the ComprehenSIVe Evaluation of Risk Factors in Older Patients with Acute Myocardial Infarction Study. *J Am Geriatr Soc.* 2017;65: 2391–2396.

Rodriguez F, Maron DJ, Knowles JW, Virani SS, Lin S, Heidenreich PA. Association between intensity of statin therapy and mortality in patients with atherosclerotic cardiovascular disease. *JAMA Cardiol.* 2017; 2:47–54.

Sinnaeve PR, Schwartz GG, Wojdyla DM, et al. Effect of alirocumab on cardiovascular outcomes after acute coronary syndromes according to age: an ODYSSEY OUTCOMES trial analysis. *Eur Heart J.* 2019;41:2248–2258.

Tegn N, Abdelnoor M, Aaberge L, et al. Invasive versus conservative strategy in patients aged 80 years or older with non-ST-elevation myocardial infarction or unstable angina pectoris (after eighty study): an open-label randomised controlled trial. *Lancet.* 2016;387:1057–1065.

Thygesen K, Alpert JS, Jaffe AS, et al. Fourth universal definition of myocardial infarction (2018). *J Am Coll Cardiol.* 2018;72(18):2231–2264.

Zhou Z, Ofori-Asenso R, Curtis AJ, et al. Association of statin use with disability-free survival and cardiovascular disease among healthy older adults. *J Am Coll Cardiol.* 2020;76(1):17–27.

Valvular Heart Disease

Nikola Dobrilovic, Dae Hyun Kim, Niloo M. Edwards

INTRODUCTION

As the population ages, valvular heart diseases have become a significant public health problem. The prevalence of moderate or severe valvular heart disease increases with age, from less than 1% in 18- to 44-year-olds to 13% in the population 75 years or older. Without valve replacement, valvular heart disease is associated with decreased survival, functional limitations, and poor quality of life. Due to recent advances in surgical techniques, especially minimally invasive transcatheter valve procedures, older adults who were previously not considered for surgery are treated to improve survival and restore function and quality of life. However, challenges remain as to patient selection for surgical and transcatheter valve procedures, patient goal-directed shared decision-making, and optimization of health status prior to and after the procedure. This chapter summarizes latest evidence on evaluation and management of common valvular heart diseases in older adults, with a focus on the geriatrician's role in risk assessment and shared decision-making.

AORTIC STENOSIS

Definition

Aortic stenosis is the progressive narrowing of the aortic valve resulting in left ventricular (LV) outflow obstruction during systole. This is in distinction to aortic valve sclerosis, where the valve leaflets are calcified or thickened, but do not cause a meaningful outflow obstruction.

Epidemiology

Aortic stenosis is present in 2% to 9% of older patients and is the leading clinically significant valvular disorder in older adults. Risk factors for developing aortic stenosis include age, a bicuspid aortic valve, and rheumatic heart disease. In 90% of patients older than 65 years, aortic stenosis is caused by calcific degeneration of a tricuspid aortic valve. Although bicuspid valves are relatively common (~2% of the population), these patients present with stenosis earlier usually in the fourth to sixth decade of life. Similarly, rheumatic heart disease also presents earlier in life and often in association with concurrent mitral valve disease.

TABLE 75-1 ■ ECHOCARDIOGRAPHIC FINDINGS IN AORTIC STENOSIS			
	MILD	**MODERATE**	**SEVERE**
Aortic valve area (cm^2)	> 1.5	1.0–1.5	< 1.0
Velocity (m/s)	< 3	3–4	> 4
Mean gradient (mm Hg)	< 25	25–40	> 40

Pathophysiology

Although the causes of aortic valve calcification in aging are unclear, the process bears many similarities to atherosclerosis—both diseases are characterized by lipid deposition, inflammation, neoangiogenesis, and calcification. Bicuspid aortic valves are characterized by accelerated calcification and progressive outflow obstruction in the majority of patients. Rheumatic fever results in progressive fusion of the aortic valve leaflets causing both aortic valve stenosis and regurgitation. Aortic stenosis is classified as mild, moderate, or severe based on valve area, ejection velocity, and the pressure gradient that develops across the valve (**Table 75-1**).

Aortic valve sclerosis (valve thickening without outflow tract obstruction) is present in 25% of patients older than 65 years and 48% of those older than 75 years, and is associated with male gender, hypertension, smoking, diabetes, and lipid abnormalities. The rate of progression to frank stenosis occurs in approximately 10% within 5 years. The Cardiovascular Health Study has identified an increased incidence of adverse cardiovascular events in patients with sclerotic valves even when corrected for other cardiovascular risk factors. The mechanism for this association is unclear, and there are currently no guidelines for intervention.

On average, aortic valve stenosis progresses at an estimated increase in jet velocity of 0.3 m/s/year and a reduction in valve area of 0.1 cm^2/year. Despite these average rates of disease progression, the rate for each individual is difficult to predict, therefore asymptomatic patients with mild-to-moderate disease should be followed on a regular basis.

Clinical Presentation

Aortic stenosis has a long asymptomatic latency period, when the only finding is a harsh, late-peaking, crescendo-decrescendo systolic murmur that radiates to the carotids and is best heard over the right, second interspace. The second heart sound may be paradoxically split. Aortic stenosis is associated with "pulsus parvus et tardus," characterized by a weak and diminished pulse with a late upstroke that is most easily noted in the carotids. However, these physical findings may be less obvious in older adults, because of the effects of aging on the vascular bed.

Patients with aortic valve stenosis develop compensatory LV hypertrophy, which can be seen on echocardiogram, on electrocardiogram, and even on chest x-ray. The ventricular hypertrophy produces coronary malperfusion with subendocardial ischemia. Older women are prone to develop excessive ventricular hypertrophy, which may contribute to the higher perioperative morbidity and mortality in this patient cohort.

Once symptoms develop after a long latency period, the progression to death is rapid (**Figure 75-1**). The three classic symptoms are angina, syncope, and heart failure. While sudden death occurs in patients with aortic stenosis and may be considered a fourth symptom group, this is rarely seen in asymptomatic patients (< 1%). Unfortunately, older adults often move into the symptomatic phase of aortic stenosis undetected because of the overlap of these major symptom constellations with other changes associated with aging (eg, reduced exercise tolerance).

Two-thirds of patients present with angina, which may be caused by concomitant coronary artery disease,

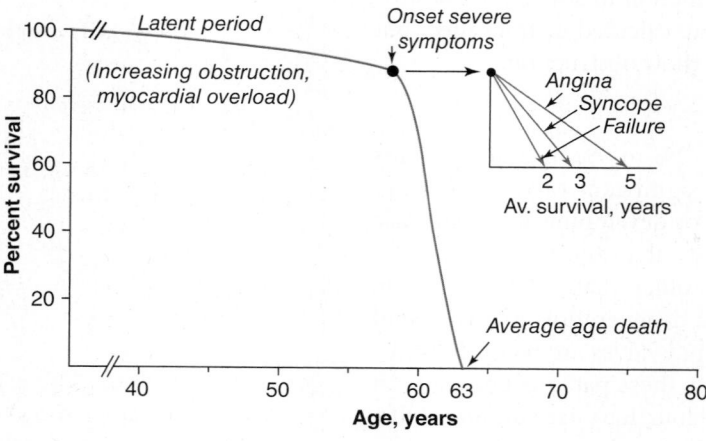

FIGURE 75-1. Valvular aortic stenosis in adults. Average course (postmortem data). (Reproduced with permission from Ross J Jr, Braunwald E. Aortic stenosis. *Circulation.* 1968;38[1 Suppl]:61–67.)

although 40% do not have significant coronary artery disease. The most likely etiology for angina in the absence of coronary artery disease is subendocardial ischemia and the increased oxygen demands of the hypertrophied ventricle together with decreased coronary flow reserve. Untreated patients with aortic stenosis and angina have a 50% 5-year survival.

Syncope due to aortic stenosis may be caused by inadequate cardiac output to meet demands, by a dysfunctional LV baroreceptor response, or by arrhythmias, and is associated with a 50% 3-year mortality without valve replacement.

Aortic valve stenosis presenting with congestive heart failure carries the worst prognosis—50% mortality at 2 years without valve replacement. Typical symptoms include paroxysmal nocturnal dyspnea, orthopnea, and dyspnea on exertion, which may be associated with signs of peripheral edema, pulmonary edema, and rales. Thickening of the left ventricle due to aortic stenosis as well as the changes associated with aging lead to diastolic dysfunction. Consequently, the older patient with aortic stenosis is more dependent on atrial contraction for ventricular filling. Therefore, these patients often present with exacerbated or new onset of symptoms if they develop atrial fibrillation.

Impaired platelet function and decreased levels of von Willebrand factor are also associated with severe aortic stenosis, and 20% of patients may present with epistaxis or ecchymoses. Patients can also develop Heyde syndrome (gastrointestinal bleeding due to colonic angiodysplasias). Interestingly, these abnormalities resolve with valve replacement.

Evaluation

The American Heart Association recommends evaluation of early systolic, mid-systolic grade 3 or greater, late systolic, or holosystolic murmurs with echocardiography. Older patients may present with ominous murmurs due to aortic valve sclerosis without significant valvular stenosis. Transthoracic echocardiography is the study of choice since it allows evaluation of valve morphology, severity of stenosis, and degree of LV hypertrophy and function. Echocardiography is also useful for following disease progression.

Stress echocardiogram can be utilized in asymptomatic patients with severe aortic stenosis to assess for physiologic changes that may indicate the need for earlier intervention. Computed tomography (CT) angiography is routinely used in patients being considered for transcatheter aortic valve replacement (TAVR) but is not helpful in assessing severity of aortic stenosis. Cardiac magnetic resonance imaging (MRI) is sometimes helpful in evaluating the severity of stenosis but is not widely used. Cardiac catheterization is routinely performed in older patients who are scheduled for valve replacement, in order to diagnose concomitant coronary artery disease and to measure transvalvular gradients if there is a question of severity of stenosis.

Management

Asymptomatic patients Survival of asymptomatic patients is the same as age-matched individuals without aortic stenosis. However, given the significant decline in survival once symptoms develop, it is essential to consider surgical intervention and to confirm the absence of symptoms in patients who do not appear symptomatic. If a careful history fails to elicit symptoms in patients with severe aortic stenosis, exercise testing may be considered. However, exercise testing in symptomatic patients is contraindicated because of the high risk of severe hemodynamic compromise.

Patients who are asymptomatic by history but who, on exercise testing, develop symptoms, fail to generate a 20 mm Hg increase in blood pressure, or develop ST-segment abnormalities, have a 19% 2-year symptom-free survival compared with 85% for patients who do not manifest these abnormalities on exercise testing. Exercise testing may elicit symptoms in as many as a third of patients thought to be asymptomatic by history alone. Close supervision and prompt termination of the study at any decline in blood pressure, significant ST-segment depression, or onset of arrhythmia is strongly advocated. On average, the probability of a patient with severe aortic stenosis remaining symptom-free at 5 years is only 50%, which has prompted some to recommend earlier surgery while the patient is "younger" and in better health.

If the patient is truly asymptomatic, continued frequent routine monitoring is reasonable, but patients should be instructed to report the development of angina, syncope, or any signs of congestive heart failure. Monitoring by echocardiography should include annual or biannual examinations for patients with severe aortic stenosis, whereas examinations should be performed every 1 to 2 years for patients with moderate aortic stenosis, every 3 to 5 years if the stenosis is mild, and as needed with referral for possible valve replacement if the patient develops symptoms. Patients who are demonstrated to be symptom-free need not restrict their activity and may exercise.

Symptomatic patients Once patients develop symptoms, they should be considered for valve replacement. Currently, there is no documented medical treatment that will delay or reverse aortic stenosis. Therefore, medical management is palliative and mainly reserved for patients with a remaining life expectancy less than 1 year even with a successful procedure or high chance of poor outcomes (death or no symptom reduction) due to advanced age, frailty, dementia, and other systemic conditions. Although standard guidelines for the management of hypertension are recommended, β-blockers are salutary in patients with concomitant coronary artery disease, and angiotensin-converting enzyme (ACE) inhibitors may have a beneficial effect in LV fibrosis. Diuretics are discouraged if the left ventricle is small due to the potential decrease in cardiac output. Statins have not demonstrated a regression of stenosis in randomized controlled trials, although they are indicated for patients with concomitant coronary artery disease or at high risk for atherosclerotic cardiovascular disease.

Aortic valve replacement—surgical aortic valve replacement (SAVR) or TAVR—should be considered for all symptomatic patients whose remaining life expectancy is at least 1 year (ie, no other significant life-limiting systemic disease) because of the improvement in both symptoms and survival. Current American College of Cardiology/ American Heart Association recommendations are listed in **Table 75-2**. Due to the increased risk of sudden death, replacement should be performed as soon as feasible after the development of symptoms.

Percutaneous aortic valvuloplasty Balloon aortic valvuloplasty (BAV) is not a substitute for valve replacement but it can be a useful tool in the treatment armamentarium for temporary palliation of symptoms for nonsurgical candidates or as a bridge for patients with hemodynamically unstable aortic stenosis. The procedure uses transvalvular balloon inflation to crack the calcified aortic valve. Unfortunately, the maximum enlargement rarely exceeds 1.0 cm² (severe-to-moderate aortic stenosis), carries a 10% risk of complications, and results in restenosis within 6 months to a year. One-year actuarial mortality is 35% to

---

TABLE 75-2 ■ AMERICAN COLLEGE OF CARDIOLOGY/ AMERICAN HEART ASSOCIATION RECOMMENDATIONS FOR VALVE REPLACEMENT IN AORTIC STENOSIS

Indications for valve replacement in aortic stenosis

- Symptomatic patients with severe aortic stenosis
- Asymptomatic patients with severe aortic stenosis and left ventricular dysfunction (ejection fraction < 50%)
- Asymptomatic patients with severe aortic stenosis undergoing other cardiac surgery
- Symptomatic patients with low-flow/low-gradient severe aortic stenosis with left ventricular dysfunction
- Symptomatic patients with low-flow/low-gradient severe aortic stenosis and LVEF > 50%, if clinical, hemodynamic, and anatomic data support valve obstruction as the most likely cause of symptoms

Considerations for valve replacement in aortic stenosis

- Asymptomatic patients with severe aortic stenosis, low surgical risk, and decreased exercise tolerance or a fall in blood pressure with exercise
- Asymptomatic patients with very severe aortic stenosis, defined by aortic velocity ≥ 5 m/s, and low surgical risk
- Asymptomatic patients with severe aortic stenosis, low surgical risk, and serum B-type natriuretic peptide level > 3 times normal
- Asymptomatic patients with severe aortic valve stenosis, low surgical risk, and rapid disease progression

Possible indication for valve replacement in aortic stenosis

- Patients with moderate aortic stenosis undergoing other cardiac surgery

LVEF, left ventricular ejection fraction.

50%, which is no better than untreated aortic stenosis, but it can result in significant temporary relief of symptoms and improvement in quality of life and can be a useful tool to optimize acutely decompensated patients prior to TAVR or SAVR. BAV is often a component of TAVR, used immediately preceding valve deployment. Currently, though, the BAV step is being skipped in favor of using a single step deployment technique.

Surgical aortic valve replacement Given long-term durability data (rate of primary structural deterioration is approximately 10% after 15–20 years), SAVR with a bioprosthetic valve can be considered for patients older than 65 years. Age alone is not a contraindication to SAVR, as numerous studies have demonstrated outcomes in carefully selected older patients to be comparable to those seen in younger patients. Operative mortality in older patients ranges from 3% to 4% to as high as 24%, depending on patient selection. Medicare outcomes data for 142,000 patients older than 65 years demonstrate an operative mortality of 8.8% overall, and 6.0% mortality in high-volume centers.

Operative risk associated with SAVR should be assessed using the Society of Thoracic Surgeons (STS) Predicted Risk of Mortality or EuroSCORE II risk calculator. Predictors of surgical mortality include emergency surgery, right heart failure, severity of symptoms (New York Heart Association [NYHA] class IV), renal insufficiency, female gender, depressed LV function, associated coronary bypass, or concomitant mitral valve surgery. Emergency surgery increases the surgical risk substantially and is often the result of not referring the patient for elective surgery because it is "too risky," but reconsidering surgery when the patient is critically ill and the medical options have dwindled to none. Unfortunately, the result is a self-fulfilling prophecy that older patients will not do well with surgery. A European study of older patients with aortic stenosis provocatively demonstrated that 41% of patients older than 70 years were not offered surgery despite severe valve stenosis and symptoms. These findings were corroborated in a second study of 1200 patients from 92 centers in 25 countries. In this study, 33% of patients older than 75 years with severe symptomatic aortic stenosis were not offered valve replacement.

Although many studies have found that concomitant coronary artery bypass or mitral valve surgery increases the surgical risk, there is clear support for performing concomitant aortic valve replacement for any patient with severe aortic stenosis, who is undergoing any other cardiac surgical procedure, regardless of symptoms. Similarly, in patients with moderate stenosis, it is "accepted practice" to replace the aortic valve at the time of other cardiac surgery. Simultaneous valve replacement in patients with mild aortic stenosis undergoing heart surgery is more controversial, although an argument can be made for concomitant replacement in patients with mild stenosis but moderate-to-severe valve calcification. However, some of the calculus of risk is changing with the availability of TAVR.

Transcatheter aortic valve replacement An alternative to SAVR is TAVR, in which a catheter-mounted bioprosthetic valve is deployed across the aortic valve. The valve can be introduced through the femoral artery, the apex of the heart, subclavian artery, carotid artery, or the aorta via small incisions. Alternatively, peripheral arteries such as femoral and subclavian can be accessed percutaneously and controlled using minimally invasive closure devices such as *Perclose Proglide* (Abbott Cardiovascular, Plymouth, MN).

Randomized controlled trials demonstrated that TAVR, particularly transfemoral TAVR, is as effective as SAVR in symptomatic older patients who are considered low, intermediate, and high operative risk, with different procedural risks of complications. TAVR is associated with lower rates of postoperative stroke, major bleeding, and atrial fibrillation, as well as faster recovery. However, the rates of paravalvular leak, vascular complications, and pacemaker implantation are higher with TAVR. Because durability of TAVR valves beyond 5 years is unknown, some patients may need a reintervention ("valve-in-valve" procedure). In symptomatic patients with prohibitive SAVR risk, defined as STS Predicted Risk of Morbidity and Mortality of over 50% due to comorbid disease or serious irreversible conditions, TAVR reduces mortality, hospitalizations, and symptoms, but causes higher rates of stroke and vascular complications, compared to medical management with or without percutaneous aortic valvuloplasty.

Surgical versus transcatheter aortic valve replacement The choice of SAVR versus TAVR should involve shared decision-making that carefully considers the patient's age, preferences, procedure-specific risk factors or contraindications, procedural complications, and durability of the value relative to the patient's remaining life expectancy (**Table 75-3**). A multidisciplinary team approach is invaluable for optimal procedure selection (TAVR vs SAVR). This approach to individualized risk assessment is described later in this chapter.

AORTIC INSUFFICIENCY

Definition

Aortic insufficiency occurs when the aortic valve fails to close during diastole resulting in blood flow from the aorta back into the left ventricle.

Epidemiology

Acute aortic regurgitation is uncommon and presents a surgical emergency. Chronic aortic insufficiency occurs in 20% to 30% of individuals older than 65 years and like aortic stenosis has a long asymptomatic latency period. However, even asymptomatic patients with normal LV function have a 0.2% incidence of sudden death, progress to symptomatic disease at a rate of approximately 3.5% per year, and develop either LV dysfunction or symptoms at a rate of approximately 6% per year. Once patients develop LV dysfunction, more than 25% each year will progress to symptomatic disease and, once symptomatic, the mortality rate for aortic regurgitation is more than 10% per year. Patients with NYHA class III or IV symptoms have an annual mortality rate of 25%, while patients with less severe symptoms (NYHA class II) have a 6% annual mortality rate.

Risk factors for the development of LV dysfunction, symptoms, or death include age, left ventricular end-systolic dimension (LVESD)/volume, left ventricular end-diastolic dimension (LVEDD)/volume, and LV ejection fraction with exercise. Each year 19% of patients with end-systolic size greater than 50 mm develop LV dysfunction and symptoms or die. The rate of development of these same end points was 6% per year for patients with end-systolic size between 40 and 50 mm.

Presentation

The findings and eponyms associated with aortic insufficiency are a delight to lovers of medical trivia (**Table 75-4**).

TABLE 75-3 ■ FACTORS FAVORING SAVR, TAVR, OR PALLIATIVE CARE

SAVR	TAVR	PALLIATIVE CARE
• Offers life prolongation and improvement in symptoms and quality of life • Lower risk of repeat intervention, permanent pacemaker, and vascular complications • Longer hospital stay	• Offers life prolongation and improvement in symptoms and quality of life • Accepts possible risk of repeat intervention and high risk of permanent pacemaker and vascular complications • Shorter hospital stay	• Offers temporary symptomatic relief but no life prolongation • Avoids risk of periprocedural stroke, permanent pacemaker, and vascular complications
Consider for patients with: • Longer life expectancy • No or few frailty markers • Patient-prothesis mismatch or anatomical challenges to TAVR • Concomitant coronary artery disease or valve disease	Consider for patients with: • Fewer years of life expectancy • Severe comorbidities (lung, liver, or renal disease) or mobility issue • Previous chest irradiation	Consider for patients with: • Limited life expectancy • Severe dementia, severe frailty, or multiorgan impairments • Valve anatomy or vascular access not amenable to TAVR • Goals of care to avoid futile or unnecessary procedures

PART V ORGAN SYSTEMS AND DISEASES

1153

TABLE 75-4 ■ EPONYMOUS SIGNS OF AORTIC INSUFFICIENCY

EPONYM	PHYSICAL FINDING
Austin Flint murmur	Low-pitched mid-diastolic rumble
Becker sign	Accentuated retinal artery pulsation
Corrigan pulses	Rapidly rising and falling pulse to palpation
de Musset sign	Bobbing of head
Duroziez sign	To-and-fro femoral artery murmur with compression
Gerhard sign	Pulsatile spleen
Hill sign	Higher BP in lower than upper extremity
Mayne sign	Decrease in blood pressure with arm elevated
Mueller sign	Pulsatile uvula
Quincke sign	Pulsatile nail beds
Rosenbach sign	Pulsatile liver
Traube sign	Double femoral artery pulse sound
Sherman sign	Dorsalis pedis pulse prominent in patients older than 75 y
Watson's water hammer pulse	Bounding peripheral pulse

TABLE 75-5 ■ SEVERITY OF AORTIC REGURGITATION

	MILD	MODERATE	SEVERE
Ratio of width of regurgitant jet to left ventricular outflow (%)	< 25	25–64	≥ 65
Vena contracta (cm)	< 0.3	0.3–0.59	≥ 0.6
Regurgitant volume (mL/beat)	< 30	30–59	≥ 60
Regurgitant fraction (%)	< 30	30–49	≥ 50
Effective regurgitant orifice area (mm²)	< 10	10–29	≥ 30

However, the most obvious physical findings are those of a diastolic murmur and a widened pulse pressure.

Patients with acute aortic regurgitation usually present dramatically in cardiogenic shock. The most common causes are infective endocarditis and acute aortic dissection. Data suggest a dramatically large, recent increase in opiate intravenous drug abuse as a cause for endocarditis. This effect is nationwide, although it seems to be disproportionately seen in younger adults and much less in the geriatric population. However, the geriatric patient still tends to be affected by more traditional etiologies of endocarditis, such as infected foreign bodies (dialysis catheters and access, other catheters, intravenous pacing leads), dental infection, remote abscesses, sepsis, and pneumonia.

Chronic aortic regurgitation progresses slowly and insidiously. Occasionally palpitations or awareness of each heartbeat may be the first signs owing to the large regurgitant volumes. Infrequently angina may develop due to coronary flow mismatch, and as the ventricle fails congestive heart failure develops with symptoms of dyspnea on exertion, orthopnea, paroxysmal nocturnal dyspnea, and lower extremity edema.

Evaluation

Echocardiography is the diagnostic modality of choice for both initial evaluation as well as routine follow-up. It provides both diagnostic confirmation, assessment of the severity of valve regurgitation, as well as evaluation of LV function and the aortic root. It can also help determine the etiology of the aortic regurgitation (eg, infective endocarditis or aortic dissection). The clinical stages and management recommendations are defined by symptomatic status, severity of the regurgitation, LV volume, and LV systolic function (**Table 75-5**). Transesophageal echocardiography may improve sensitivity and specificity.

Exercise testing may be reasonable for asymptomatic patients who wish to initiate an exercise regimen, but the results have not been consistently useful in predicting outcomes for asymptomatic patients with normal resting cardiac function. It may also be used to objectively assess exercise capacity in otherwise asymptomatic patients or patients with equivocal symptoms.

CT angiography is useful for the diagnosis and follow-up of patients with aortic dissections, aneurysms, or annuloaortic ectasia. Magnetic resonance angiography (MRA) similarly allows for evaluation and follow-up of aortic disease and also provides a quantitative assessment of aortic regurgitation, which can be helpful in patients with suboptimal echocardiographic images or if there is discordance between clinical assessment and noninvasive studies.

Cardiac catheterization is routinely performed in patients being evaluated for aortic valve replacement, and provides intraventricular pressure measurements, but is not recommended for routine quantification of aortic regurgitation. It is contraindicated in acute aortic dissection or when there are large mobile vegetations on the aortic valve.

Management

Medical management Surgery is indicated for patients who develop either angina or signs of congestive heart failure, since the mortality for patients with angina is more than 10% per year and for heart failure is more than 20% per year. Medical management in symptomatic patients results in poor outcomes even if the LV function is normal. Patients older than 75 years are more likely to develop either symptoms or ventricular dysfunction at earlier stages of the disease, and have a poorer prognosis once they develop ventricular dysfunction.

The medical management of aortic insufficiency is best achieved with vasodilators that reduce afterload and wall stress. Since symptomatic disease carries such a poor prognosis without surgery, medical management is primarily indicated for patients who are not surgical candidates because of comorbidities, to preoperatively optimize hemodynamics, or for asymptomatic hypertensive patients with normal ventricular function. Conflicting data exist as to the benefits of hydralazine, ACE inhibitors, and calcium channel blockers, which suggest that vasodilator therapy is not indicated for asymptomatic, normotensive patients with normal ventricular function. However, once symptoms or ventricular dysfunction develops, the patient should be considered and evaluated for surgery. Although β-blockers are not recommended as first-line medication for management of hypertension due to its bradycardic effect, they may benefit those patients who have LV dysfunction.

The absence of data indicating that exercise contributes to the progression of aortic insufficiency suggests, that the asymptomatic patient with normal LV function may participate in the full range of physical activities, with the exception of isometric exercises, which are contraindicated. However, it is prudent to exercise-test patients to the anticipated level of planned activity to assess tolerance prior to initiating an exercise regimen.

Patients with aortic regurgitation should have regularly scheduled follow-up. Mild regurgitation with normal ventricular function can be followed clinically on an annual basis with biennial or triennial echocardiograms; more severe valvular regurgitation should be followed with annual or even biannual echocardiograms depending on the presence of ventricular dilatation (60 mm). Asymptomatic patients with more severe dilatation (> 70 mm) should be followed with echocardiograms every 4 to 6 months because the likelihood of developing symptoms or ventricular dysfunction is as high as 20% per year. Asymptomatic patients with normal LV function and dilated ventricles (LVESD > 50 mm) may be candidates for early valve replacement.

The hospital clinician should also be aware that while intra-aortic balloon counterpulsation is an excellent adjunct to medical therapy in the appropriate patient, it is contraindicated in patients with aortic insufficiency.

Surgical management Surgery is not indicated for asymptomatic patients with normal ventricular function and minimal ventricular dilatation regardless of the severity of valvular regurgitation. However, once symptoms or LV dysfunction develop in patients with severe aortic regurgitation, the patient should be considered for surgery (**Table 75-6**). Patients with severe LV dysfunction have a high operative mortality (at least 10%) and a lower postoperative survival; therefore, asymptomatic patients should be closely followed for the development of LV dysfunction.

In older patients with severe compensated aortic insufficiency, the onset of symptoms can be hard to ascertain, since mild dyspnea on exertion and fatigue often mimic the effects of aging. However, once ventricular dysfunction develops, the older patient is more likely to have persistent postoperative ventricular dysfunction and symptoms, as well

TABLE 75-6 ■ RECOMMENDATIONS FOR SURGERY IN AORTIC INSUFFICIENCY

Indications for valve replacement in aortic insufficiency
- Symptomatic patients with severe aortic regurgitation regardless of LV function
- Asymptomatic patients with severe aortic regurgitation and left ventricular ejection fraction < 50%
- Patients with severe aortic regurgitation undergoing other cardiac surgery

Considerations for valve replacement in aortic insufficiency
- Asymptomatic patients with severe aortic insufficiency, normal left ventricular function, and dilated ventricle—LVESD > 50 mm
- Patients with moderate aortic insufficiency undergoing other cardiac surgery

Possible indication for valve replacement in aortic insufficiency
- Asymptomatic patients with severe aortic regurgitation, normal cardiac function, but progressive left ventricular dilatation > 65 mm if surgical risk is low

LVESD, left ventricular end-systolic dimension.

as decreased postsurgical survival. Therefore, in patients without comorbidities that contraindicate surgery, an earlier commitment to surgery is generally the preferred strategy.

If the patient is asymptomatic but the LVESD exceeds 65 mm, surgery should be considered if it is low risk, because of the high risk of sudden death. Although the surgical treatment of asymptomatic patients with severe aortic regurgitation and LV dilatation is controversial, if surgery is planned based on ventricular size or function, then two consecutive studies should confirm the findings.

Surgical valve replacement is the treatment of choice for symptomatic patients with aortic insufficiency. Patients with annuloaortic ectasia or concomitant ascending aortic aneurysms may be candidates for aortic valve repair and replacement of the ascending aorta (David procedure), although such procedures are usually reserved for experienced centers. This procedure should be judiciously used in older adults, in whom the operative risk is usually higher and aortic valve replacement alone is simpler and carries a more predictable result. Various new techniques in aortic leaflet repair and reconstruction have enjoyed recent popularity. They are mentioned here for completeness, although their application is likely more appropriate in a younger patient population. TAVR is currently not recommended in patients with aortic insufficiency.

MITRAL STENOSIS

Definition

Mitral valve stenosis is the progressive narrowing of the orifice of the mitral valve with a resultant increase in left atrial, pulmonary artery, and right ventricular pressures.

Epidemiology

The overwhelming majority of mitral stenosis is caused by rheumatic heart disease, which causes thickening and calcification of the leaflets and chordae as well as shortening of the chordae and fusion of the commissures. While this tends to occur in the younger patients and is rarely seen in older patients, the number of older patients may be increasing. In developed countries, most patients present in their forties and fifties, but some studies note that a third of patients are older than 65 years. Only 60% of patients presenting with mitral stenosis recall a history of rheumatic fever, the disease progresses very slowly, and it is estimated that mitral valve area, which normally measures 4.0 to 5.0 cm², decreases by 0.09 to 0.32 cm²/year. When the valve area is reduced to 2.5 to 1.5 cm², patients usually develop symptoms. Significant valvular disease lags the development of rheumatic fever by 20 to 40 years. However, once symptoms start, the 10-year survival is only 50% to 60%. Patients who are asymptomatic or with minimal symptoms have an 80% 10-year survival, and 60% have no progression of symptoms. Patients who meet criteria for surgery but do not get operated on have a 10-year survival below 30%. Patients with severe pulmonary hypertension usually live fewer than 3 years, and most patients will die from progressive pulmonary hypertension, congestive heart failure, systemic emboli, pulmonary emboli, or infection.

Senile calcific mitral stenosis is becoming more common in the United States. This is usually associated with mitral annular calcification that extends into the leaflets and is prevalent in patients with decreased renal function, elevated inflammatory markers, and in patients with senile aortic stenosis. Although not all patients develop progressive stenosis, the rate of progression, when it occurs, is accelerated compared to rheumatic disease.

Other rarer causes of mitral stenosis include intracardiac clot, intracardiac tumor (such as myxoma), or congenital malformations.

Presentation

Mitral stenosis often presents with new-onset atrial fibrillation or an embolic event; sometimes patients come to medical attention because of fatigue or dyspnea and rarely due to hemoptysis. The left recurrent laryngeal nerve can be compressed by the enlarged left atrium, causing hoarseness (Ortner syndrome). The onset of atrial fibrillation sometimes results in pulmonary edema and death. On physical examination an opening snap may be noted to the first heart sound as well as a diastolic rumble.

Diagnosis

Evaluation of patients with suspected mitral stenosis includes an echocardiogram, both to confirm the diagnosis and assess the severity of the disease and therapeutic options (**Table 75-7**). Patients have mild mitral stenosis if the valve area is greater than 1.5 cm², moderate if the valve area is 1.0 to 1.5 cm², and severe if the mitral valve area is

TABLE 75-7 ■ ECHOCARDIOGRAPHIC FINDINGS IN MITRAL STENOSIS

	MILD	MODERATE	SEVERE
Mitral valve area (cm²)	> 1.5	1.0–1.5	< 1.0
Pulmonary artery pressure (mm Hg)	< 30	30–50	> 50
Mean gradient (mm Hg)	< 5	5–10	> 10

less than 1.0 cm². Additionally, pulmonary pressures should be assessed, since this also determines the disease severity.

Transesophageal echocardiography is useful when transthoracic echocardiography provides limited images, when the presence of left atrial thrombus needs to be excluded, or when valvuloplasty is contemplated.

Cardiac catheterization is rarely used to facilitate assessment of mitral valve gradient. It is however recommended in assessing the coronaries as part of preoperative work-up, particularly in the older patient. Stress testing has a value when there is discrepancy between echocardiographic severity of mitral stenosis at rest and clinical symptoms. CT scanning is valuable in patients with senile mitral stenosis, especially those considered for surgical intervention as it complements the echocardiographic assessment of mitral annular and leaflet calcification.

Management

Medical management It should be emphasized that medical management cannot reduce a mechanical narrowing like mitral stenosis. However, increasing diastolic filling time by slowing the heart rate with β-blockade may be helpful in patients in sinus rhythm and exertional symptoms. The addition of sodium restriction and a diuretic ameliorates pulmonary edema. Antibiotic prophylaxis for infective endocarditis is reserved for patients at highest risk for developing infective endocarditis or experiencing complications (see General Considerations below). Asymptomatic patients should be followed closely for the development of symptoms, at which time they should be assessed by echocardiogram.

A substantial number of older patients (30%–40%) will present with atrial fibrillation. Both, age and left atrial size, are predictive of the developing atrial fibrillation. Unfortunately, atrial fibrillation carries a guarded prognosis, since only 25% of mitral stenosis patients with atrial fibrillation will survive 10 years compared to 46% of those who remain in sinus rhythm. Treatment includes anticoagulation, rate control, and electrical or chemical cardioversion, especially if associated with hemodynamic instability. Patients who remain in atrial fibrillation for more than 24 to 48 hours are at increased risk of embolic complications and should be promptly anticoagulated. Electrical cardioversion may be used but only after confirming the absence of a left atrial thrombus by echocardiogram. If a thrombus is present, treatment may include 3 weeks of anticoagulation, followed by confirmation of the absence of thrombus by repeat echocardiography and subsequent defibrillation. In this setting, transesophageal echocardiography is the diagnostic tool of choice.

Patients with paroxysmal or persistent atrial fibrillation, prior emboli or left atrial thrombus should be anticoagulated. Systemic emboli occur in 20% of patients and age and atrial fibrillation are predictive of embolization.

Exercise is not contraindicated in asymptomatic patients with mild mitral stenosis. In patients with more severe stenosis, exercise is often limited by symptoms. Therefore exercise regimens for patients with more symptomatic or severe disease should be individually tailored.

Percutaneous mitral valvuloplasty Percutaneous mitral valvuloplasty is successful in select patients and often doubles the valve area with a substantial decrease in valve gradient. The selection of patients for this treatment option is determined by echocardiographic assessment of the valve, and is based on leaflet mobility, subvalvular apparatus, leaflet thickening, and the presence of calcification (Wilkins Score). The lowest scores are assigned to valves with the greatest leaflet mobility, the least subvalvular thickening, the most normal leaflet thickness, and the least calcium deposition. Patients with these valve characteristics (lowest scores) have the best response to balloon valvuloplasty. The majority of patients (90%) will see symptomatic relief, with a freedom from valve-related complications or death of between 50% and 65% at 7 years and as high as 80% to 90% in patients with favorable (low) preprocedural echocardiographic scores.

Symptomatic patients or patients with pulmonary hypertension, those with favorable echocardiographic mitral valve scores and without atrial thrombi, should be referred for mitral valvuloplasty. The risks for percutaneous mitral valvuloplasty are low (**Table 75-8**). Therefore, even patients with less favorable echocardiographic scores who are at high surgical risk may be considered candidates for this approach. However, balloon valvuloplasty is contraindicated in patients with moderate-to-severe mitral regurgitation and/or the presence of left atrial clot. Unfortunately, patients older than 65 years have a lower success rate, higher incidence of complications, and shorter duration of symptom relief with this approach.

Surgical management As a result of the success of balloon valvuloplasty in patients with favorable valve morphology, surgery is usually indicated only if the patient has failed

percutaneous intervention or if the valve has unfavorable characteristics (high Wilkins Score) for balloon valvuloplasty. Patients with mitral stenosis ineligible for valvuloplasty are best treated surgically, as are patients with left atrial thrombus. Additionally, since balloon valvuloplasty requires a significant level of expertise and the outcomes are related to experience, the American Heart Association recommends surgery if this experience is not available.

Patients with mild symptoms, severe pulmonary hypertension, and moderate-to-severe mitral stenosis may also benefit from surgery if balloon valvuloplasty is not appropriate or available. Similarly, patients with recurrent systemic emboli despite therapeutic anticoagulation may benefit from surgical intervention if ineligible for percutaneous treatment (**Table 75-9**). Notably, surgery is not recommended for patients with isolated mild mitral stenosis.

The surgical options include open repair with commissurotomy or valve replacement with either a mechanical

TABLE 75-9 ■ SURGICAL RECOMMENDATIONS FOR MITRAL STENOSIS

Indications for valve intervention in mitral stenosis

- Percutaneous mitral balloon valvuloplasty is recommended in symptomatic patients with severe mitral stenosis, favorable morphology, and absence of contraindications
- Severely symptomatic patients (NYHA class III–IV) who are unable to undergo balloon valvuloplasty (owing to unavailability, contraindications, or unfavorable valve score) and are not high risk for surgery
- Patients with severe stenosis undergoing other cardiac surgery

Considerations for valve intervention in mitral stenosis

- Mildly symptomatic patients with severe mitral stenosis and severe pulmonary hypertension if ineligible for balloon valvuloplasty
- Percutaneous mitral balloon valvuloplasty is reasonable in asymptomatic patients with very severe mitral stenosis (MVA ≤ 1.0 cm^2), favorable morphology, and absence of contraindications

Possible indications for valve intervention in mitral stenosis

- Patients with moderate mitral stenosis undergoing other cardiac surgery
- Patients with severe mitral stenosis and recurrent emboli despite anticoagulation
- Percutaneous mitral balloon valvuloplasty may be considered in patients with severe mitral stenosis, new onset of atrial fibrillation with favorable morphology, and absence of contraindications
- Percutaneous mitral balloon valvuloplasty may be considered in symptomatic patients with severe mitral stenosis, suboptimal morphology who are not candidates for surgery or at high risk for surgery
- Percutaneous mitral balloon valvuloplasty may be considered in patients with mitral stenosis less than severe if there is evidence of hemodynamically significant stenosis during exercise

MVA, mitral valve area; NYHA, New York Heart Association.

TABLE 75-8 ■ COMPLICATIONS OF PERCUTANEOUS MITRAL VALVULOPLASTY

COMPLICATION	PROCEDURAL RISK (%)
Left ventricular perforation	0.5–4.0
Systemic embolization	0.5–3.0
Myocardial infarction	0.3–0.5
Death	1.0–2.0

or a bioprosthetic valve. The surgical risk increases with decreased preoperative functional status, older age, decreased cardiac function, pulmonary hypertension, and the presence of coronary artery disease. Operative mortality can be as high as 20% in the older patient with significant comorbidities and pulmonary hypertension. Nonetheless, it is not recommended to wait until the patient becomes severely symptomatic (NYHA class IV), since this results in a substantial increase in the surgical risk. Conversely, surgery should be considered despite severe symptoms, since both quality of life and survival are exceedingly poor without surgical intervention.

Patients with senile calcific mitral stenosis often present a surgical challenge, because the calcification involves the annulus and the base of the leaflets. Valve replacement is complex and often involves annular debridement with reconstruction, which significantly increases the operative risk. Therefore, intervention is often delayed until symptoms are severely limiting and cannot be managed medically.

Atrioventricular groove disruption is a rare but catastrophic complication of heart surgery. It is almost exclusively seen with mitral valve procedures and is most closely associated with two risk factors, age and mitral annular calcification.

MITRAL REGURGITATION

Definition

Mitral valve regurgitation is the inability of the mitral valve to close properly resulting in regurgitation of volume into the left atrium from the left ventricle during systole. It is important to distinguish between primary (organic) and secondary (functional) mitral regurgitation since this has implications in both treatment and prognosis.

Epidemiology

Significant mitral regurgitation occurs, equally in men and women—approximately 2% of the population. The most common cause is mitral valve prolapse, which is present in 1% to 2.5% of the population and can occur either spontaneously or as a familial disorder. The latter is associated with a low but significant incidence of sudden death, presumably due to ventricular arrhythmias.

Acute mitral regurgitation is caused by disruption of the valve apparatus (leaflet perforation, chordal rupture, or papillary muscle rupture) and is often caused by endocarditis or myocardial infarction.

Chronic mitral regurgitation can be either primary (organic) regurgitation, which can be caused by mitral valve prolapse, rheumatic heart disease, endocarditis, or coronary artery disease. Secondary (functional) regurgitation is due to LV dysfunction and annular dilation.

Chronic regurgitation is better tolerated, but when severe, especially in association with a flail leaflet, is associated with a 7% per year mortality. Patients with severe

mitral valve regurgitation and a low ejection fraction have a particularly poor prognosis. The 10-year survival for patients with ejection fractions less than 50% is 32%, compared to a 70% 10-year survival for patients with ejection fraction greater than 60%. Even patients with borderline normal ejection fraction (50%–60%) have a decreased 10-year survival (53%) if untreated.

Presentation

Patients with chronic mitral valve prolapse may present with palpitations, panic attacks, atypical chest pain, dyspnea, easy fatigue, volume overload, or congestive heart failure. Palpitations may be caused by the onset of atrial fibrillation. Cessation of caffeine, tobacco, alcohol, and other stimulants may help control the anxiety in some patients. Acute mitral regurgitation usually presents either with shock or respiratory distress.

Physical examination reveals a holosystolic murmur, which is best heard at the apex of the heart with radiation to the left axilla. If the mitral regurgitation is severe and the atrial and ventricular pressures start to equalize, the murmur may be diminished. With cardiac enlargement, a third sound may also be heard.

Evaluation

As with other cardiac valvular problems, the diagnosis is best confirmed and quantified by echocardiogram (**Table 75-10**), which allows assessment of the severity of regurgitation, putative causes of the valve dysfunction, as well as assessment of LV function. Transesophageal echocardiography often provides an even better assessment of the mitral valve. Cardiac catheterization, cardiac MRI, and viability studies can help identify those patients with functional ischemic MR who might benefit from surgical intervention.

Management

Medical management Asymptomatic patients with mild primary mitral regurgitation may be followed with

TABLE 75-10 ■ SEVERITY OF MITRAL REGURGITATION			
	MILD	MODERATE	SEVERE
Color Doppler jet area	Small central jet	Jet greater than small, but no criteria for severe mitral regurgitation	Large jet filling large portion of atrium or wall impinging jet
Vena contracta (cm)	< 0.3	0.3–0.69	≥ 0.7
Regurgitant volume (mL/beat)	< 30	30–59	≥ 60
Regurgitant fraction (%)	< 30	30–49	≥ 50
Regurgitant orifice area (cm²)	< 0.20	0.20–0.39	≥ 40

echocardiograms every 3 to 5 years while those with moderate mitral regurgitation should be followed every 1 to 2 years. Asymptomatic patients with severe organic regurgitation should probably undergo exercise testing to confirm the absence of symptoms, and if truly asymptomatic, should undergo restudy by echocardiogram every 6 to 12 months. The asymptomatic patient with organic mitral regurgitation, a normal ejection fraction without pulmonary hypertension, or LV dilation may exercise without restriction.

Medical management consists of blood pressure control with vasodilators and diuretics. Asymptomatic patients with normal blood pressure and LV function do not require treatment, and endocarditis prophylaxis is recommended for all patients with mitral valve prolapse and patients with moderate or severe organic mitral regurgitation.

Surgical management The surgical options consist of either repair or replacement (**Table 75-11**). All patients should be considered for valve repair because of the marked improvement in survival, LV function, and the avoidance of long-term anticoagulation with valve repair compared to replacement. Although durability of repair is excellent, with freedom from reoperation equaling that of valve replacement (7%–10% at 10 years), the freedom from reoperation is dependent on the adequacy of the repair, whether the

repair involved the anterior or the posterior valve leaflets, and whether chordal replacement was necessary. Patients with isolated posterior leaflet pathology are more likely to have long-term success compared to patients with anterior or bileaflet repairs.

When mitral replacement is necessary, the procedure should strive to retain as much of the mitral valve apparatus as possible. Preservation of these structures results in improved LV function, exercise tolerance, and survival. The choices for mitral valve replacement include bioprosthetic or mechanical valves. Bioprosthetic valves in the mitral position are not as durable as in the aortic position; however, this option avoids the risks of lifelong anticoagulation. Conversely, a mechanical valve has the advantage of durability but requires a commitment to lifelong anticoagulation.

Mitral valve repair or replacement is indicated for all patients with symptoms (NYHA class II–IV) and severe regurgitation even in the face of normal cardiac size and function. Asymptomatic patients benefit from surgical intervention if they develop atrial fibrillation, pulmonary hypertension, LV dysfunction (ejection fraction < 60%), or ventricular dilation (> 40 mm). In patients with atrial fibrillation, an intraoperative maze or modified maze procedure combined with suture closure of the left atrial

---

TABLE 75-11 ■ SURGICAL RECOMMENDATIONS FOR MITRAL REGURGITATION

Indications for valve repair or replacement in mitral regurgitation

- Symptomatic patients with chronic severe primary mitral regurgitation and left ventricular function > 30%
- Asymptomatic patients with severe regurgitation and decrease left ventricular dysfunction (EF 30%–60%) and/or ventricular dilatation (≥ 40 mm)
- Mitral repair is recommended in preference to replacement when surgery is indicated and regurgitation is limited to the posterior leaflet
- Mitral repair is recommended in preference to replacement when surgery is indicated and regurgitation involves the anterior leaflet or both leaflets and successful and durable repair can be accomplished
- Patients with severe primary mitral regurgitation undergoing other cardiac surgery
- Acute mitral regurgitation

Considerations for valve repair or replacement in mitral regurgitation

- Repair may be considered in asymptomatic patients with severe regurgitation and normal left ventricular size and function if the valve can be repaired with a high degree of certainty and low mortality
- Repair may be considered in asymptomatic patients with new-onset atrial fibrillation or pulmonary hypertension at rest with severe nonrheumatic regurgitation and normal left ventricular size and function
- Repair may be considered in patients with chronic moderate primary mitral regurgitation undergoing other cardiac surgery
- Patients with severe secondary chronic mitral regurgitation

Possible indications for valve repair or replacement in mitral regurgitation

- Symptomatic patients with chronic severe primary mitral regurgitation and EF ≤ 30%
- Repair may be considered in patients with rheumatic mitral valve disease if there are indications and durable repair is likely or long-term anticoagulation management is questionable
- Severely symptomatic patients (NYHA class III–IV) with chronic severe secondary mitral regurgitation
- Patients with chronic moderate secondary mitral regurgitation undergoing other cardiac surgery

Not indicated for valve replacement in mitral regurgitation

- Replacement should not be performed in patients with isolated primary mitral regurgitation limited to less than one-half of the posterior leaflet unless repair has been attempted and was unsuccessful

EF, ejection fraction; NYHA, New York Heart Association.

appendage should be considered, in order to reestablish sinus rhythm and possibly reduce the risk of systemic embolization, respectively. Once LV dysfunction develops, patient survival, even after repair or replacement, is compromised. Therefore, patients who are asymptomatic, with normal LV size and function, should be followed closely, and, if necessary, exercise testing should be considered to confirm the absence of symptoms. Surgical intervention may be warranted for asymptomatic patients with severe mitral regurgitation with none of the noted indications for surgery if and only if the mitral valve can be repaired.

Operative mortality varies based on the procedure. Mitral valve repair is associated with a 2% perioperative mortality compared to 6% for valve replacement. Patients with ischemic and functional mitral regurgitation do much worse than the patients with organic regurgitation. A study of 292 patients older than 70 years demonstrated an in-hospital mortality of 0.7% for mitral repair compared to 14% for replacement. A study comparing cohorts of patients older than 75 years, between 65 and 75 years, and younger than 65 years demonstrated an increased operative risk for older patients. However, restoration of life expectancy following surgery is the same for older as for younger patients. Current data suggest that in patients with functional mitral regurgitation there is no improvement in survival by performing a concomitant mitral repair with coronary artery bypass. Nonetheless, there may be an improvement in postoperative symptoms.

Percutaneous options Several percutaneous techniques for repair or replacement of the mitral valve are under investigation. Percutaneous approaches to the mitral repair include a clip that provides an edge-to-edge repair for both functional and organic mitral regurgitation. Other repair devices include a mitral annular constraint device placed into the coronary sinus and artificial cord implantation. There are several other repair devices as well as transcatheter valves that are at different phases of development that will broaden the armamentarium of treatment options available for the next generation of older patients.

GENERAL CONSIDERATIONS

Evaluation of Surgical Risk

Predicted risk of mortality (Table 75-12) Many older patients have multiple comorbidities that impact risk of surgery and the decision to operate. There are, however, a number of statistical models that can be helpful in weighing the impact of individual comorbidities on operative outcome. The two most widely used are the Society of Thoracic Surgeons Predicted Risk of Mortality (STS-PROM) score and the EUROpean Score for Cardiac Operative Risk Evaluation (EuroSCORE-II), which is derived from a European surgical population. The STS-PROM, derived from a rolling cohort of North American patients, analyzes the impact of preoperative variables of patients undergoing coronary artery bypass surgery and valve surgery (with or without concomitant coronary artery bypass) on 30-day mortality and postoperative complications. It is important to recognize that these data are derived only from patients who were operated on, and therefore do not provide insight into patients who were considered for surgery but did not undergo an operation. These risk models, though very informative, should not be relied on as the only indicator for surgery.

Frailty Traditionally physicians have guesstimated the probability of patient survival based on clinical judgment. In an attempt to quantify these parameters there has been an increasing study of frailty as a measure of survivability. For example, one frailty index that incorporates a combination of five domains (nutritional status, activity, mobility, strength, and energy) has been evaluated for its ability to predict postsurgical survival (see Chapter 42).

Multidisciplinary team approach As diagnostic methods and treatment options become more sophisticated, and patients present with more comorbidities, the optimal therapeutic choice is more complex and less clear. Assessing patients using a formal "heart valve team" has proven to improve outcomes. The heart valve team is comprised of a multidisciplinary team of clinicians that include cardiologists, cardiac surgeons, structural valve interventionalists, cardiovascular imaging specialists, anesthesiologists, nurses, and often a geriatrician. The team reviews the patient and collaboratively discusses the therapeutic options, and then works with the patient and their family to arrive at a decision tailored for each individual patient that is consistent with the patient's goals of care.

Endocarditis Prophylaxis

Although there is surprisingly a dearth of data supporting or refuting the use of antibiotic prophylaxis for patients

TABLE 75-12 ■ PREOPERATIVE RISK ASSESSMENT	LOW RISK	INTERMEDIATE RISK	HIGH RISK	PROHIBITIVE RISK
STS-PROM[a]	< 4% *and*	4%–8% *or*	> 8%	Surgical risk of death or major morbidity > 50%
Frailty	None *and*	1 index *or*	≥ 2 indices	
Major organ dysfunction that will not improve postoperatively	None *and*	1 organ system	No more than 2 organ systems	≥ 3 organ systems
Procedure-specific impediment	None	Possible	Possible	Severe

[a]Society of Thoracic Surgeons Predicted Risk of Mortality.

TABLE 75-13 ■ INDICATIONS FOR ENDOCARDITIS PROPHYLAXIS
Endocarditis prophylaxis is recommended
• Patients with any prosthetic valve—either mechanical or bioprosthetic
• Patients who have had valve repair procedures
• Patients with abnormal native valves—eg, bicuspid aortic valve
• Mitral valve prolapse with clinical findings of regurgitation or leaflet abnormalities by echocardiogram
Endocarditis prophylaxis is not required
• Mitral valve prolapse without regurgitation or abnormal leaflets
• Aortic valve sclerosis if jet velocity < 2 m/s
• Physiologic mitral regurgitation with normal valve leaflets
• Physiologic tricuspid regurgitation with normal valvular apparatus
• Physiologic pulmonary valve regurgitation with normal valvular apparatus

with valvular disease, the American Heart Association recommends antibiotic coverage for a variety of dental and surgical procedures.

Prophylactic antibiotics are recommended for patients with prosthetic cardiac valves, prior endocarditis, cardiac transplants with abnormal valves, and complex congenital repairs or defects (**Table 75-13**). Standard antibiotic prophylaxis is orally administered, penicillin-based, and given 1 hour before the procedure, but other regimens may be needed (see **Table 75-14**). Patients with repaired valves usually do not require endocarditis prophylaxis as the incidence of infective endocarditis is estimated to be very low. Patients at risk of endocarditis should be covered for dental procedures that involve manipulation of gingival tissue, the periapical region of teeth, or perforation of the oral mucosa. Nondental procedures in absence of active infection do not require prophylaxis.

Prior to any valve operation, all patients require dental clearance, and any potential infectious dental issues should be addressed prior to proceeding with surgery. When dental extractions are required, an interval of time is provided for recovery and to avoid bleeding before proceeding with surgery.

Anticoagulation

Anticoagulation has a significant associated morbidity particularly in the older patient. Consequently, the need for anticoagulation plays a pivotal role in the choice of valve. Patients with mechanical valves require lifelong anticoagulation, while patients with bioprosthetic valves are often anticoagulated for only 3 months (**Table 75-15**). If there is no contraindication to antiplatelet therapy, low-dose aspirin is also recommended for all patients with valve replacement.

Direct-acting oral anticoagulation agents are not approved for anticoagulation after mechanical valve replacement—therefore, chronic anticoagulation requires warfarin therapy. The recommended international normalized ratio (INR) for patients with mechanical aortic valves is between 2 and 3, although certain mechanical valves allow lower INRs of 1.5 to 2.0 after 3 months. However, if the patient has a history of prior thromboembolism, LV dysfunction, atrial fibrillation, or hypercoagulability, the INR should be maintained between 2.5 and 3.5. Patients with mechanical mitral valves should have their INR maintained between 2.5 and 3.5, and those with bioprosthetic valves are often anticoagulated (INR 2.0–3.0) for the first 3 months following implantation.

The risk of thromboembolism for anticoagulated patients with mechanical valves is approximately 1% to 2% per year. The risk is lower in bioprosthetic valves (0.7%), and lower in patients with aortic prosthetic valves compared to mitral valves, regardless of the type of prosthetic valve implanted.

Hemorrhagic complications are more likely if the INR is greater than 5. Patients with an INR between 5 and 10 can be treated by holding warfarin and administration of 1 to 2.5 mg of oral vitamin K. However, the INR should be monitored daily until the INR is below 5, at which time

TABLE 75-14 ■ ENDOCARDITIS PROPHYLAXIS ANTIBIOTIC RECOMMENDATIONS		
	ANTIBIOTIC	**DOSAGE**
Standard	Amoxicillin	2 g PO 1 h before procedure
Penicillin allergic	Clindamycin OR Cephalexin	600 mg PO 1 h before procedure / 2 g PO 1 h before procedure
Unable to take oral medicines	Ampicillin	2 g IV or IM 30 min before procedure
Unable to take oral medicines and penicillin allergic	Clindamycin OR Cefazolin	600 mg IV 30 min before procedure / 1 g IV or IM 30 min before procedure

TABLE 75-15 ■ ANTICOAGULATION FOR PROSTHETIC VALVES		
	MECHANICAL VALVE	**BIOPROSTHETIC VALVE**
Aortic	INR 2–3 Aspirin 75–325 mg daily	INR 2–3 *for 3 mo* Aspirin 75–100 mg daily
Aortic with risk factors[a]	INR 2.5–3.5 Aspirin 75–325 mg daily	INR 2–3 Aspirin 75–100 mg daily
Mitral	INR 2.5–3.5 Aspirin 75–325 mg daily	INR 2–3 *for 3 mo* Aspirin 75–100 mg daily
Mitral with risk factors[a]	INR 2.5–3.5 Aspirin 75–325 mg daily	INR 2.5–3.5 Aspirin 75–100 mg daily

[a]Risk factors: atrial fibrillation, prior thromboembolism, LV dysfunction (ejection fraction < 30%), and hypercoagulable condition.
INR, international normalized ratio.

warfarin can be reinitiated at adjusted doses. Of note, it is often harder to manage anticoagulation in the older patient as a result of polypharmacy in this patient population. An acute reduction in the INR for patients who are actively bleeding may be achieved by administering intravenous fresh frozen plasma. Vitamin K can also help reduce a dangerously high INR, but complicates reanticoagulation.

Temporary cessation of anticoagulation in patients with mechanical valves is sometimes medically necessary. Patients with mechanical aortic valves (without risk factors) can have warfarin held 48 to 72 hours preoperatively and restarted within 24 hours following surgery without the need for bridging heparin anticoagulation. However, patients with mechanical mitral or mechanical aortic valves and high-risk factors should be bridged with heparin when the INR falls below 2. The heparin may be held 4 to 6 hours before surgery and restarted as soon as possible when the immediate postoperative risk of bleeding allows. For emergency procedures, it is preferable to administer fresh frozen plasma to reverse the effects of warfarin, since the administration of vitamin K will make reanticoagulation difficult and increases the risk of a hypercoagulable state.

Prosthetic Valve Choices

Traditional, open-surgical, prosthetic valves fall into two broad groups: biological and mechanical valves. Mechanical valves have the advantage of durability but the disadvantage of requiring lifelong anticoagulation; bioprosthetic valves do not require anticoagulation but are limited by a finite durability. Of note, immediately following surgery, many surgeons will administer anticoagulants (or aspirin) for a limited interval (most commonly 3 months).

Notably the risk of embolization and the durability is determined, in part, by valve location. Biological aortic valves are more durable than the same valve in the mitral position, and mechanical valves in the aortic position have a lower risk of thromboembolism than in the mitral position.

Within each class of valve, mechanical and bioprosthetic, there are numerous types of prostheses; each type of valve is available in different forms (eg, porcine vs bovine pericardial or bileaflet vs tilting disc).

The choice of replacement valve is sometimes determined by the contraindication to anticoagulation (which would necessitate the implantation of a bioprosthetic valve). Otherwise, the choice resides with the patient. There are some data to suggest that the rate of bioprosthetic valve deterioration is attenuated in older patients, prompting many surgeons to recommend bioprosthetic aortic valves for patients older than 65 years and bioprosthetic mitral valves for patients older than 70 years. Valves such as On-X (Cryolife, Kennesaw, Georgia, USA) retain all the durability benefits of a mechanical valve while requiring considerably less anticoagulation (INR 1.5 to 2.0 with aspirin after 3 months).

Other indirect factors may impact the choice of valve: atrial fibrillation, multiple valve replacement, prior mechanical valve, prior cardiac surgery, and annulus size may argue in favor of a mechanical valve. Essentially, the risk of a mechanical valve is that of anticoagulation and embolization, while the risk of a bioprosthetic valve is that of valve failure and reoperation. In the end, the choice of valve—unless there are contraindications to anticoagulation—belongs to the patient, who ultimately must live with the perils of anticoagulation or the threat of reoperation.

Mechanical valves The original mechanical valve was the ball-caged design, which, while durable, had inefficient flow characteristics and required higher levels of anticoagulation than the current generation of valves. The bileaflet mechanical valve is the most commonly used valve in the aortic position because of its superior flow characteristics. The risk of thromboembolism with anticoagulation is approximately 1% to 2% per year.

Bioprosthetic valves Stented and nonstented porcine valves and bovine pericardial valves are available, and like homografts, do not require immunosuppression or anticoagulation. The risk of embolism for this class of valves is approximately 0.7% per year without anticoagulation. However, all the biological valves are prone to structural deterioration. The rate of deterioration is slower in older patients—at 15 to 20 years, patients at age 70 have a 90% freedom from structural valve deterioration and patients older than 75 years have freedom from reoperation of 90% to 95%. Stentless valves do not have the valve mounting and are therefore more hemodynamically efficient, but this does not increase survival in the older patient. Minimal aortic gradients can be achieved regularly with this type of valve.

Aortic homografts Cadaveric valves do not provide improved durability but are particularly useful in patients with endocarditis and tissue loss. The rate of thromboembolism is low, and, like the stentless porcine valves, they are hemodynamically efficient especially at small sizes. Although there is no need for antirejection medications, the valve has a propensity to become heavily calcified, making re-replacement much more challenging.

Pulmonary Valve Autotransplant (Ross Procedure)

Mr. Donald Ross devised an operation to excise the patient's own pulmonary valve, which is used to replace the aortic valve, and then to replace the pulmonary valve with a homograft or bioprosthetic valve. Conceptually, the lower-pressure pulmonary circuit will allow for longer durability of the homograft or bioprosthetic valve in this circuit, and the aortic valve, which is now an autologous valve, would, therefore, also have increased durability. The operative morbidity and mortality for this procedure, especially in inexperienced hands, are higher than bioprosthetic aortic valve replacement. The increased procedural risk and limited benefit in an older patient make it rarely indicated in this population.

A variation of this operation is also available for mitral replacement, but it is currently investigational and has the same limitations for use in an older patient.

Transcutaneous valves In the aortic position, various options are well-established and may be viewed from two broad categories, "balloon-expandable" and "self-expanding." No approved transcutaneous mitral valve currently exists, though multiple, multiple startup ventures are competing to fill this void. It is anticipated that a transcatheter option for the mitral valve will be available in the relatively near future.

Sutureless (aortic) valves Several "sutureless" valves are also currently available and offer a hybrid option. These valves are implanted through an open surgical approach and, therefore, still require cardiopulmonary bypass support. However, various features allow for a much quicker implantation—with no or considerably less suture—and a correspondingly larger aortic valve annular orifice area.

Valve repair Repair of the aortic or mitral valves is ideal. The ability to maintain ventricular geometry, to accommodate natural annular motion and the durability makes mitral valve repair the best option for suitable patients, since these advantages translate to lower operative mortality for mitral repair compared to replacement—1% to 2% versus 5.4% to 6.4%, respectively. Aortic valve repair for calcific disease is less durable and is rarely indicated; however, in the setting of normal leaflets, the aortic valve is repairable with excellent results (85% freedom from reoperation at 10 years).

1163

PART V

ORGAN SYSTEMS AND DISEASES

FURTHER READING

Afilalo J, Lauck S, Kim DH, et al. Frailty in older adults undergoing aortic valve replacement: the FRAILTY-AVR Study. *J Am Coll Cardiol.* 2017;70(6): 689–700.

Bonow RO. Chronic mitral regurgitation and aortic regurgitation. *J Am Coll Cardiol.* 2013;61(7):693–701.

Carabello BA. Clinical practice. Aortic stenosis. *N Engl J Med.* 2002;346(9):677–682.

Carabello BA. Modern management of mitral stenosis. *Circulation.* 2005;112(3):432–437.

Carabello BA. The current therapy for mitral regurgitation. *J Am Coll Cardiol.* 2008;52(5):319–326.

Enriquez-Sarano M, Tajik AJ. Clinical practice. Aortic regurgitation. *N Engl J Med.* 2004;351(15): 1539–1546.

Kim DH, Afilalo J, Shi SM, et al. Evaluation of changes in functional status in the year after aortic valve replacement. *JAMA Intern Med.* 2019;179(3):383–391.

Leon MB, Smith CR, Mack M, et al. Transcatheter aortic-valve implantation for aortic stenosis in patients who cannot undergo surgery. *N Engl J Med.* 2010;363(17): 1597–1607.

Otto CM, Nishimura RA, Bonow RO, et al. 2020 ACC/AHA Guideline for the Management of Patients With Valvular Heart Disease: A Report of the American College of Cardiology/American Heart Association Joint Committee on Clinical Practice Guidelines. *J Am Coll Cardiol.* 2021;77(4):e25–e197.

Rodes-Cabau J, Mok M. Working toward a frailty index in transcatheter aortic valve replacement. *JACC Cardiovasc Interv.* 2012;5(9):982–983.

Ross J Jr, Braunwald E. Aortic stenosis. *Circulation.* 1968;38(1s5):V61–V67.

Smith CR, Leon MB, Mack MJ, et al. Transcatheter versus surgical aortic-valve replacement in high-risk patients. *N Engl J Med.* 2011;364(23):2187–2198.

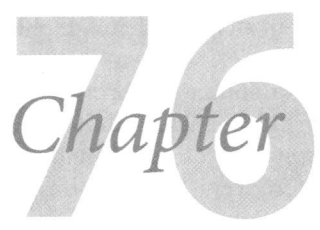

Chapter 76

Heart Failure

Mathew S. Maurer, Scott L. Hummel, Parag Goyal

INTRODUCTION

Heart failure is a complex clinical syndrome that can result from any structural or functional cardiac disorder that impairs the ability of the ventricle to fill with or eject blood. Heart failure is not a single disease but rather a syndrome, similar to falls and incontinence that have a diverse set of etiologies and multiple underlying mechanisms. Heart failure is among the most common cardiovascular conditions experienced by older adults due to a combination of normative age-related changes in cardiovascular structure and function as well as the rising prevalence of cardiovascular risk factors and diseases with advancing age and decline in premature cardiovascular deaths. Thus, although the clinical syndrome of heart failure has been recognized by physicians for more than two centuries, it has only been within the past four decades that it has been identified as a major public health concern, which is largely attributable to the aging of the population.

EPIDEMIOLOGY AND ECONOMIC IMPACT

Despite declines in age-adjusted mortality rates from coronary heart disease and stroke, both the incidence and the prevalence of heart failure are increasing, and these trends are projected to continue for the next several decades. As shown in **Table 76-1**, several factors have contributed to the rise in heart failure cases. Foremost among these is the increasing number of older adults who, by virtue of age-related changes in cardiovascular structure and function coupled with the high prevalence of hypertension, coronary heart disease, and valvular disease with advancing age, are predisposed to the development of heart failure. In addition, advances in the treatment of other acute and chronic cardiac and noncardiac conditions, most notably atherosclerotic heart disease, hypertension, renal failure, cancer, and infectious diseases, have paradoxically contributed to the increasing burden of heart failure. Indeed, individuals who might have died in middle age from acute myocardial infarction during a prior era are now surviving to older age and developing heart failure in their later years. Similarly, improved blood pressure control has led to a 60% decline in stroke mortality, yet these patients remain at risk for the development of heart failure due to hypertension and left ventricular hypertrophy.

Learning Objectives

- Understand the effects of aging on cardiovascular structure and function, and how these changes predispose to the development of heart failure.

- Describe the clinical features—including symptoms, signs, and results of diagnostic tests—that distinguish heart failure in older adults from heart failure occurring during middle age.

- Delineate nonpharmacologic aspects of care for older adults with heart failure.

- Understand current treatment of heart failure with reduced and preserved ejection fraction in older adults.

- Discuss management of heart failure in patients approaching the end of life.

Key Clinical Points

1. Cardiovascular aging is associated with significant changes in cardiac and vascular structure and function that predispose older adults to the development of heart failure.

2. The clinical features of heart failure, including symptoms, signs, and diagnostic test results, often differ in older adults with heart failure compared to those in younger patients.

3. Management of heart failure with reduced ejection fraction (HFREF) is generally similar in older and younger patients, but must be individualized in older patients given potentially reduced life expectancy and heterogeneity in patient priorities.

4. Although trials of many cardiovascular pharmacologic agents have not consistently found reduced mortality or substantially improved clinical outcomes in patients with heart failure and preserved ejection fraction (HFPEF), there has been some progress in recent trials. Nevertheless, effective treatment of this condition remains challenging.

(Continued)

5. Nonpharmacologic therapies, including lifestyle changes (eg, dietary interventions and exercise) and multidisciplinary care interventions, play a fundamental role in optimizing care and outcomes for older patients with heart failure.

6. The overall prognosis for heart failure in older adults is poor, and it is therefore essential to incorporate goals of care and end-of-life planning into the clinical decision-making process, especially as symptoms progress and quality of life declines.

Heart failure affects approximately 6.5 million Americans, and it is projected that by 2030 the prevalence of heart failure in the United States will exceed 8 million, largely due to the aging of the population. In addition, over 1 million new cases are diagnosed each year. Moreover, both the incidence and the prevalence of heart failure are strikingly age dependent (**Figures 76-1** and **76-2**). Indeed, heart failure prevalence doubles for each decade after 40 years of age and exceeds 10% in both men and women older than

TABLE 76-1 ■ FACTORS CONTRIBUTING TO THE RISING INCIDENCE AND PREVALENCE OF HEART FAILURE

Aging of the population

- Age-related cardiovascular changes in cardiac and vascular structure and function
- High prevalence of cardiovascular disease
- Age-related changes in body composition

Improved therapy for coronary heart disease and stroke

- Decline in coronary mortality
  - Fibrinolytic therapy and primary percutaneous coronary intervention
  - Coronary angioplasty, stents, and bypass surgery
  - Aspirin, β-blockers, and angiotensin-converting enzyme inhibitors
  - Statins
- Decline in stroke mortality
  - More widespread use of antihypertensive agents
  - Beneficial effects of treating hypertension
  - Fibrinolytic therapy

Improved therapy for other disorders

- Renal disease
- Diabetes and other metabolic disorders
- Cancer
- Pneumonia and other infections

Increased prevalence of metabolic disorders

- Obesity
- Diabetes

80 years. Similarly, heart failure mortality rates increase exponentially with advancing age in all major demographic subgroups of the US population.

Heart failure is also a major source of chronic disability and impaired quality of life in older adults, and it is the leading cause for hospitalization in individuals older than 65 years. In 2014, there were 1 million hospital admissions in the United States with a primary diagnosis of heart failure (**Table 76-2**). Of these, 71% were in patients older than 65 years, 53% were in patients 75 years or older, and 25% occurred in the 2% of the population aged at least 85 years (**Figure 76-3**). While the majority of heart failure patients younger than 65 years are males, women comprise more than half of heart failure hospitalizations after the age of 65, and the proportion of females continues to rise with advancing age. The prevalence of heart failure in older Caucasians and African-Americans is similar, and hospital admission rates are lower in Hispanics and Asians. Whether this represents a true difference in population prevalence or a difference in the likelihood that affected individuals will seek or receive medical attention is unknown. Heart failure is also a common reason for ambulatory care visits, with almost 2 million physician office visits with a primary diagnosis of heart failure occurring in 2016. In this regard, heart failure ranks second only to hypertension among cardiovascular reasons for outpatient physician visits.

As a result of its high prevalence and the need for intensive resource use in both the inpatient and the outpatient settings, the economic burden of heart failure is very high. Heart failure is one of the costliest diagnosis-related groups in the United States, with estimated total annual expenditures in excess of $35 billion. Projections suggest that by 2030, the total cost of heart failure will increase to $69.8 billion, amounting to ≈$244 for every US adult.

PATHOPHYSIOLOGY

Heart failure is the prototypical disorder of cardiovascular aging in that age-related changes in the cardiovascular system in concert with an increasing prevalence of cardiovascular risk factors and diseases at older age conspire to produce an exponential rise in heart failure prevalence with advancing age.

Aging is associated with extensive changes in cardiovascular structure and function (see Chapter 73). However, in the absence of coexistent cardiovascular disease, cardiac function at rest is well preserved even at very old age. Resting left ventricular ejection fraction and resting cardiac output are largely unaffected by age in healthy individuals.

From the clinical perspective, the changes associated with cardiovascular aging result in an impaired ability of the heart to respond to stress, be it physiologic (eg, exercise) or pathologic (eg, hypertension or myocardial ischemia). Four principal changes in the cardiovascular system

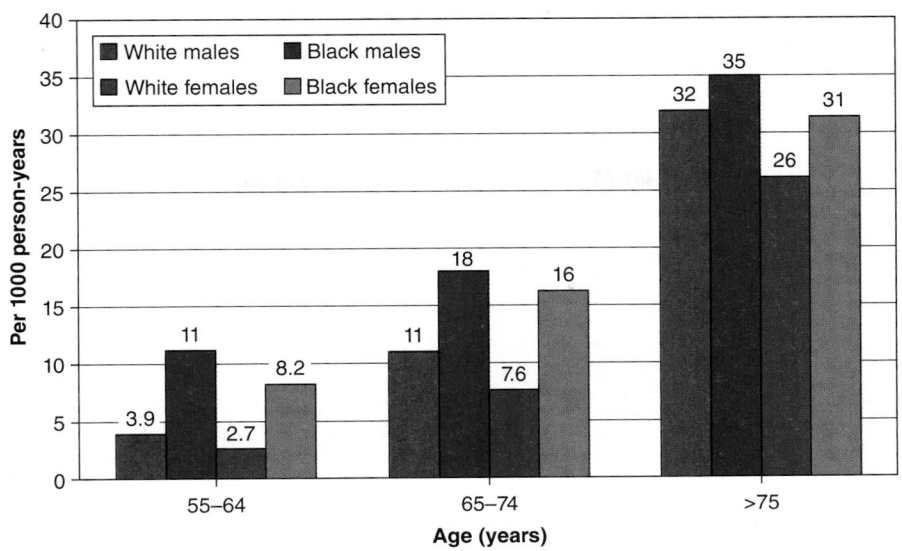

FIGURE 76-1. Incident heart failure hospitalizations in the United States by age, gender, and self-reported race, 2005–2011: the Atherosclerosis Risk in Communities Study. (Reproduced with permission from NHANES, 2013 to 2016. National Heart, Lung, and Blood Institute. US Department of Health & Human Services.)

contribute directly to the heart's attenuated capacity to augment cardiac output in response to stress. First, aging is associated with reduced responsiveness to β-adrenergic stimulation. This is related to increased sympathetic nervous system activity and circulating catecholamine levels resulting in β-adrenergic receptor desensitization, rather than decreased β-receptor density on cardiac myocytes or altered responsiveness to intracellular calcium. The diminished response to β-adrenergic stimulation limits the heart's capacity to maximally increase heart rate and contractility in response to stress, and β2-mediated peripheral vasodilatation is also impaired.

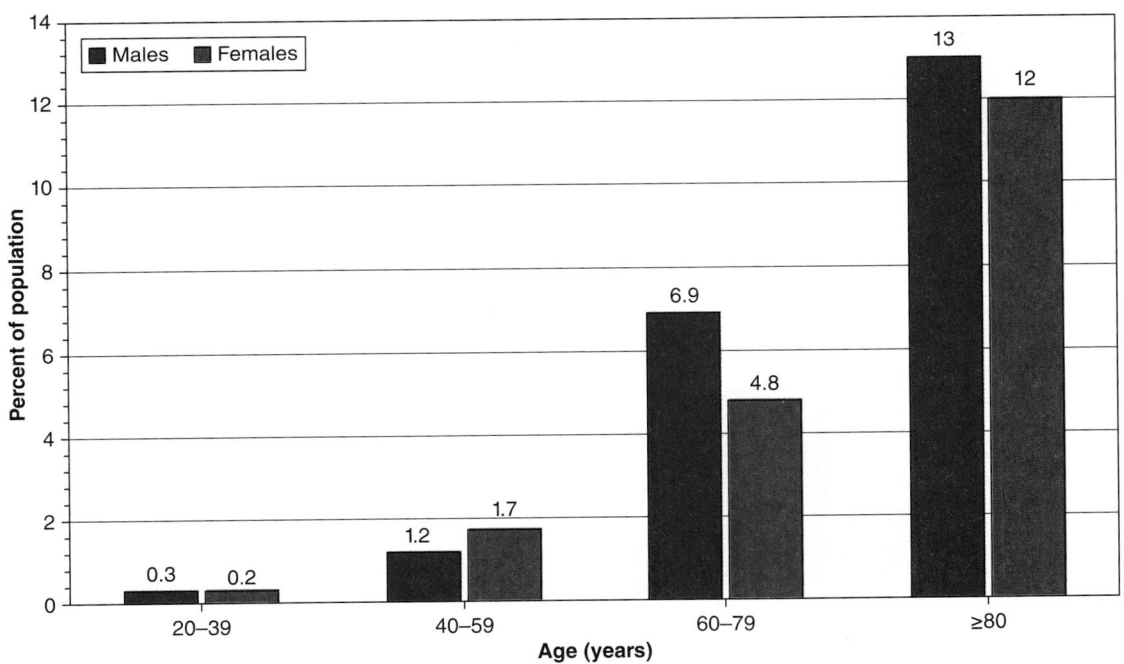

FIGURE 76-2. Prevalence of heart failure in the United States by age and gender: National Health and Nutrition Examinations Survey, 2009–2012. (Reproduced with permission from NHANES, 2013 to 2016. National Heart, Lung, and Blood Institute. US Department of Health & Human Services.)

TABLE 76-2 ■ EPIDEMIOLOGY OF HEART FAILURE IN THE UNITED STATES[a]

POPULATION GROUP	PREVALENCE (%), 2013–2016 (AGE ≥ 20)	INCIDENCE (CASES/ YEAR), 2014 (AGE ≥ 55)	ANNUAL MORTALITY, 2017 (ALL AGES)	HOSPITAL DISCHARGES (2016, ALL AGES)	COST[b]
Both sexes	6.0 million (2.1%)	1,000,000	80,480	809,000	$30.7
Men	3.4 million (2.5%)	495,000	36,824 (45.8%)	415,000	
Women	2.6 million (1.71%)	505,000	43,656 (54.2%)	394,000	
Race/ethnicity					
NH White men	2.4%	430,000	30,076		
NH White women	1.4%	425,000	36,004		
Black men	3.6%	65,000	4068		
Black women	3.3%	80,000	4863		
Hispanic men	2.4%	NA	1820		
Hispanic women	1.7%	NA	1960		

NA, not available; NH, non-Hispanic.
[a]Based on AHA 2020 report.
[b]Estimated for 2012, in billions of dollars.
Data from National Health and Nutrition Examination Survey 2015 to 2018; Atherosclerosis Risk in Communities study Community Surveillance, 2005 to 2014; National Vital Statistics System, 2018; Healthcare Cost and Utilization Project, 2016. US Department of Health & Human Services.

A second major effect of aging is increased stiffness of the large- and medium-sized arteries, primarily because of increased collagen deposition and cross-linking and degeneration of elastin fibers in the media and adventitia. Increased stiffness of the central conduit arteries results in increased impedance to left ventricular ejection (ie, increased afterload), and it also contributes to the increased propensity of older individuals to develop systolic hypertension (**Figure 76-4**).

A third major effect of aging is altered left ventricular diastolic filling. Diastole is characterized by four phases: isovolumic relaxation, early rapid filling, passive filling during mid-diastole, and late filling owing to atrial systole. The first two phases, isovolumic relaxation and early rapid filling, are largely dependent on myocardial relaxation, an active, energy-requiring process, whereas filling during the latter two phases is governed principally by intrinsic myocardial "stiffness," or compliance. Aging is associated

with impaired calcium release from the contractile proteins and reuptake by the sarcoplasmic reticulum, inhibiting early diastolic relaxation. In addition, increased interstitial connective tissue content and collagen cross-linking reduce ventricular compliance. Compensatory myocyte hypertrophy in response to increased ventricular afterload and myocyte loss due to apoptosis further compromises left ventricular compliance. Thus, normal aging is associated with important changes, adversely impacting all four phases of diastole and substantially altering the pattern of left ventricular diastolic filling.

Age-related changes in diastolic filling and atrial function can be evaluated noninvasively using Doppler echocardiography to examine diastolic inflow across the mitral valve (**Figure 76-5**). In healthy young persons, the transmitral inflow pattern is characterized by a large E-wave, with a rapid upstroke representing rapid filling of the ventricle immediately following the opening of the

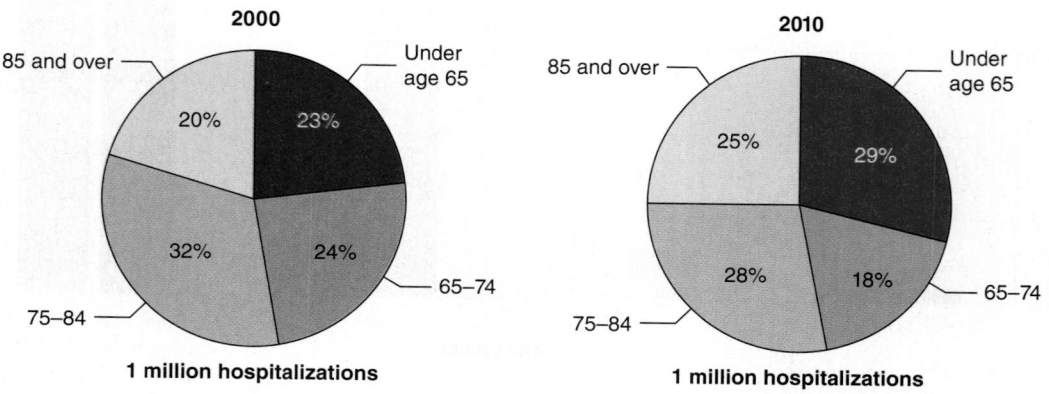

FIGURE 76-3. Distribution of hospitalizations for heart failure in the United States by age, 2000–2010. (Reproduced with permission from CDC/NCHS, National Hospital Discharge Survey, 2000–2010. US Department of Health & Human Services.)

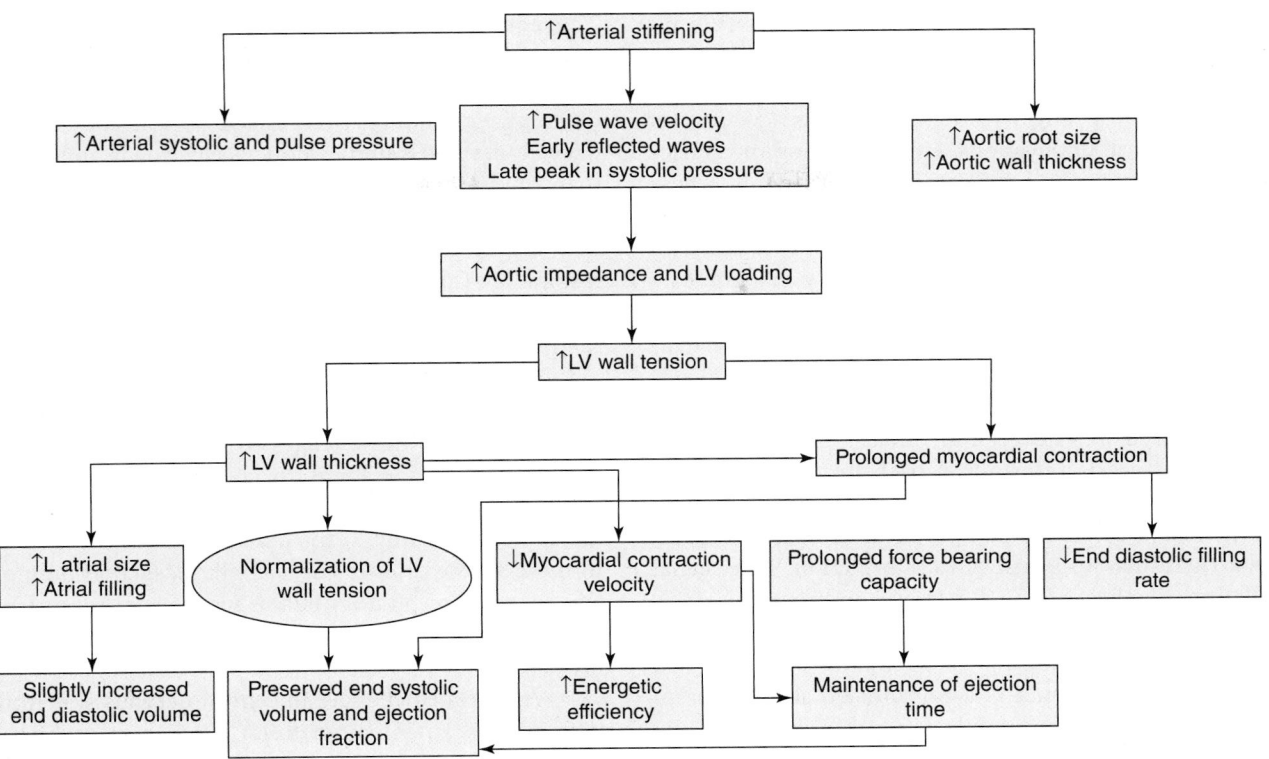

FIGURE 76-4. Age-related changes in central conduit arteries lead to numerous physiologic changes. (Reproduced with permission from Lakatta EG. Cardiovascular regulatory mechanisms in advanced age. *Physiol Rev.* 1993;73[2]:413–467.)

mitral valve and corresponding to active ventricular relaxation (**Figure 76-5A**). This is followed by a period in which the rate of filling slows (the downslope of the E-wave, called the deceleration time), mid-diastolic diastasis (in which left atrial and left ventricular pressures are essentially equal), and additional left ventricular filling at the end of diastole corresponding to atrial contraction (the A-wave, or atrial "kick"). Importantly, the majority of ventricular filling

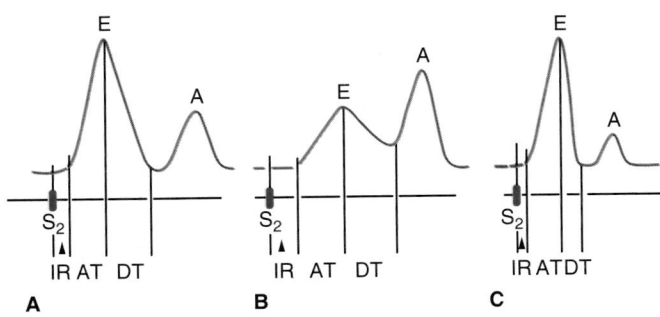

FIGURE 76-5. Schematic diagram of Doppler echocardiographic mitral valve inflow patterns. **A.** Normal pattern. **B.** Impaired filling pattern. **C.** Restrictive pattern. AT, acceleration time; DT, deceleration time; IR, isovolumic relaxation; S2, aortic valve closure. (Adapted with permission from Feigenbaum H. *Echocardiography*, 5th ed. Philadelphia, PA: Lea & Febiger; 1994.)

occurs in the first half of diastole in young individuals, with a relatively small contribution from atrial contraction.

In older persons, alterations in left ventricular relaxation and compliance result in characteristic changes in the pattern of diastolic filling (**Figure 76-5B**). Early filling is impaired, and the upstroke of the E-wave is delayed. Similarly, the downslope of the E-wave (deceleration time) is less steep. To compensate for increased resistance to emptying, the left atrium enlarges. This results in a more forceful left atrial contraction and an augmented A-wave and thus, a greater proportion of filling occurs in the latter period of diastole in older individuals. As much as 30% to 40% of left ventricular end-diastolic volume is attributable to atrial contraction. Thus, older individuals become increasingly reliant on the atrial "kick" to maximize left ventricular filling.

A third pattern of diastolic filling, referred to as the restrictive pattern, occurs when the left ventricle's ability to fill becomes severely compromised. In this situation (**Figure 76-5C**), very little flow occurs after the rapid filling phase in early diastole. This pattern is characterized by a tall, narrow E-wave with a rapid downslope, with diastasis achieved early in diastole. Little additional flow occurs during mid-diastole, and the A-wave is typically small, with an amplitude that is less than 50% of the E-wave. A restrictive pattern indicates marked elevation of the left ventricular diastolic pressure, and it tends to be associated with a poor prognosis. A restrictive filling pattern almost always occurs in patients with advanced cardiac disease and is not attributable to aging alone.

Age-related changes in diastolic filling have several important clinical implications. First, reduction in ventricular filling subverts the Frank-Starling mechanism (where increased preload volume results in a higher stroke volume), one of the cardinal adaptive responses (along with sympathetic activation) necessary to acutely increase cardiac output. Second, impaired diastolic filling results in a left-shift of the normal ventricular pressure-volume relationship; consequently, small increases in diastolic volume lead to greater increases in diastolic pressures among older compared to younger individuals. This increase in diastolic pressure is transmitted back to the left atrium. Over time this alters left atrial size and function which in turn, increases the likelihood of atrial ectopic beats and atrial arrhythmias, especially atrial fibrillation. Thus, atrial fibrillation, like heart failure, increases in prevalence with advancing age. Additionally, atrial fibrillation itself is a common precipitant of heart failure in older adults for two reasons. First, the absence of a coordinated atrial contraction substantially compromises left ventricular diastolic filling due to loss of the atrial "kick." Second, the rapid, irregular ventricular rate associated with acute atrial fibrillation shortens the diastolic filling period, which further attenuates ventricular filling.

A third effect of altered diastolic filling is an increased propensity for older adults to develop HFPEF, formerly called "diastolic heart failure." Because of the altered left ventricular pressure-volume relation, increases in left ventricular pressure from ischemia, venoconstriction, or multiple other factors can lead to pulmonary congestion and edema. Moreover, individuals with impaired diastolic function are often "volume sensitive"; that is, small increments in intravascular volume, as may occur with a dietary sodium indiscretion or intravenous fluid administration, result in abrupt rises in intraventricular pressure rises and consequently heart failure symptoms such as shortness of breath and/or exercise intolerance; while intravascular volume contraction, which may arise from poor oral intake or over diuresis, can cause marked falls in stroke volume, cardiac output, and blood pressure.

The fourth major effect of cardiovascular aging is altered myocardial energy metabolism at the level of the mitochondria. Under resting conditions, older cardiac mitochondria can generate enough adenosine triphosphate (ATP) to meet the heart's energy requirements. However, when stress causes an increase in ATP demands, the mitochondria are often unable to respond appropriately.

Aging is also associated with significant changes in other organ systems, which impact directly or indirectly on the development and/or management of heart failure. Aging is accompanied by a decline in glomerular filtration rate, which impairs regulation of intravascular volume and electrolyte homeostasis (see Chapters 39 and 82).

The reduced capacity of the kidneys to respond to intravascular volume overload or dietary sodium excess increases the risk of heart failure in older individuals. In addition, older patients are less responsive to diuretics and more likely to develop diuretic-induced electrolyte abnormalities than younger patients, which complicates the management of heart failure in the older age group.

Aging is also associated with numerous changes in respiratory function, which serve to diminish respiratory reserve (see Chapter 80). Some of these effects, such as ventilation:perfusion mismatching and sleep-related breathing disorders, may contribute directly to the development of heart failure by producing hypoxemia or pulmonary hypertension. Other changes in lung compliance reduce the capacity of the lungs to compensate for the failing heart by increasing tidal volume and minute ventilation, thereby contributing to the patient's sensation of dyspnea. In more severe cases of cardiac failure, such as pulmonary edema, acute respiratory failure may ensue, because of the inability of the lungs to maintain oxygenation and effective ventilation.

Age-related changes in central nervous system function include an impaired thirst mechanism, which may contribute to dehydration and intravascular volume contraction in patients treated with diuretics, and reduced capacity of the central nervous system's autoregulatory mechanisms to maintain cerebral perfusion in the face of changes in systemic arterial blood pressure. Aging is also associated with widespread changes in baroreflex responsiveness. For example, impaired responsiveness of the carotid baroreceptors to acute changes in blood pressure may cause orthostatic hypotension or syncope, and these effects may be further aggravated by many of the drugs used to treat heart failure.

Finally, as is well recognized, aging is associated with significant changes in the pharmacokinetics and pharmacodynamics of almost all drugs. When coupled with polypharmacy, which is nearly universal in adults with heart failure, the risk for adverse drug reactions is significant in older adults with heart failure. Strong consideration for drug-drug, drug-disease, and drug-person interactions thus remain paramount when prescribing medications to older adults with heart failure and should also be taken into consideration when developing pharmacotherapeutic strategies for older heart failure patients (see Chapter 22).

ETIOLOGY AND PRECIPITATING FACTORS

In general, the risk factors for heart failure are similar in older and younger patients (**Table 76-3**), but the etiology for heart failure in older individuals is more often multifactorial. Hypertension and coronary heart disease are the most common causes of heart failure, accounting for more than 70% of cases. The term cardiomyopathy, which refers to pathologic abnormalities of the heart, is a descriptor

TABLE 76-3 ■ COMMON ETIOLOGIES OF HEART FAILURE IN OLDER ADULTS

Coronary artery disease
- Acute myocardial infarction
- Ischemic cardiomyopathy

Hypertensive heart disease
- Hypertensive hypertrophic cardiomyopathy

Valvular heart disease
- Calcific aortic stenosis
- Mitral regurgitation
- Mitral stenosis
- Aortic insufficiency
- Prosthetic valve dysfunction

Other nonischemic cardiomyopathies
- Idiopathic
- Stress cardiomyopathy (takotsubo cardiomyopathy)
- Alcohol-related
- Chemotherapeutic agents (eg, anthracyclines, trastuzumab, immune checkpoint inhibitors)
- Hypertrophic
- Restrictive (especially wild type transthyretin amyloidosis)

Infective endocarditis

Myocarditis

Pericardial disease

High-output failure
- Chronic anemia
- Thiamine deficiency
- Hyperthyroidism
- Arteriovenous shunting
- Obesity

Age-related increase in arterial stiffness and diastolic dysfunction

frequently preceded by a modifier that indicates a potential cause of heart failure. For example, hypertensive hypertrophic cardiomyopathy represents a more severe form of hypertensive heart disease most commonly seen in older women and often accompanied by calcification of the mitral valve annulus. These patients often manifest severe diastolic dysfunction and may exhibit dynamic left ventricular outflow tract obstruction indistinguishable from that seen in hypertrophic cardiomyopathy due to sarcomere mutations.

Valvular cardiomyopathy is an increasingly common cause of heart failure at older age. Calcific aortic stenosis is now the most common form of valvular heart disease requiring invasive treatment, and aortic valve replacement is the second most common major cardiac procedure performed in patients older than 70 years (after coronary bypass grafting). Mitral regurgitation in older individuals may be caused by myxomatous degeneration of the mitral valve leaflets and chordae tendineae (mitral valve prolapse), mitral annular calcification, valvular vegetations, ischemic papillary muscle dysfunction, or altered ventricular geometry owing to ischemic or nonischemic dilated cardiomyopathy. Importantly, mitral regurgitation may be acute (eg, following acute myocardial infarction), subacute (eg, endocarditis), or chronic (eg, myxomatous degeneration), and the clinical manifestations may vary widely in each of these settings. In the United States, rheumatic mitral stenosis is a less common cause of heart failure in older adults. Functional mitral stenosis owing to severe mitral valve annulus calcification with narrowing of the mitral valve orifice is an uncommon cause of heart failure, but it is associated with a poor prognosis. Aortic insufficiency may be either acute (eg, because of endocarditis or type A aortic dissection) or chronic (eg, annuloaortic ectasia or syphilitic aortitis), but it is a relatively infrequent cause of heart failure in older adults. Finally, prosthetic valve dysfunction should be considered as a potential cause of heart failure in any patient who has undergone previous valve repair or replacement.

In older adults, ischemic cardiomyopathy from one or more prior myocardial infarctions is the most common cause of heart failure. Nonischemic dilated cardiomyopathy is less common in older than in younger individuals; when present, it is most often either idiopathic or genetic in origin or attributable to chronic ethanol abuse or cancer chemotherapy (eg, anthracyclines or trastuzumab). Stress cardiomyopathy (also known as takotsubo cardiomyopathy) is a cause of acute heart failure usually precipitated by physical or psychological stress. The majority of patients with Takotsubo cardiomyopathy are women. Sarcomeric hypertrophic cardiomyopathy, once thought to be rare in the older age group, has been increasingly recognized in adults older than 65 years. Similarly, restrictive cardiomyopathy, most commonly owing to transthyretin amyloid deposition, is an increasingly recognized cause of HFPEF in older adults. Clinical and autopsy series have shown an age-dependent prevalence of wild-type transthyretin cardiac amyloidosis (ATTRwt, formerly called senile cardiac amyloidosis), which is diagnosed in adults older than 60 years. Transthyretin cardiac amyloidosis is either due to the deposition of wild-type transthyretin protein (also known as prealbumin) or the result of a variant in the transthyretin gene (ATTRv), which are present in up to 4% of African-Americans, who are at increased risk for developing cardiac amyloidosis with advancing age. While the genetic defect is present from birth, penetrance is age dependent and clinical manifestations typically do not become apparent until after age 60. Wild-type transthyretin amyloidosis has been found in 13% of older adults hospitalized for HFPEF who have an increased left ventricular wall thickness of more than 12 mm. Novel therapies that inhibit production or promote stabilization of transthyretin amyloidosis, such as tafamidis, have been shown to reduce morbidity and mortality in this disease, though concerns about cost could limit access.

Infective endocarditis is an uncommon but important cause of heart failure in older patients because it is one of the few etiologies for which curative pharmacologic therapy is available. Endocarditis should be strongly suspected in any patient with persistent fever and either a prosthetic heart valve or a preexisting valvular lesion. It should also be considered in any patient with fever, recent dental work or other procedure, and a new or worsening heart murmur. It is important to recognize, however, that the clinical manifestations of endocarditis are often protean, and the absence of fever or a heart murmur does not exclude this diagnosis in older individuals.

Myocarditis is an uncommon cause of heart failure in older adults. It is most commonly infectious (eg, post-viral) but can be noninfectious (eg, owing to sarcoid or collagen vascular disease). Increasing cases are being described in the setting of cancer therapeutics, particularly immune checkpoint inhibitors. Pericardial effusions, for which there are numerous etiologies, occasionally present with heart failure symptomatology, including fatigue, exertional dyspnea, and edema. Constrictive pericarditis may be infectious (eg, tuberculous) or noninfectious (eg, postradiation), but it is a rare cause of heart failure in older patients.

High-output failure is cause of heart failure in older adults, but when present the diagnosis is frequently overlooked. Potential causes of high-output failure include chronic anemia, hyperthyroidism, thiamine deficiency, and arteriovenous shunting (eg, owing to a dialysis fistula or arteriovenous malformations) and morbid obesity.

Finally, in a small percentage of older heart failure patients, detailed investigation may fail to identify any primary cardiovascular pathology. In cases with a normal left ventricular ejection fraction, heart failure may be attributed to age-related diastolic dysfunction.

Precipitating Factors

In addition to determining the etiology of heart failure, it is important to identify coexisting factors that may have contributed to the acute or subacute exacerbation (**Table 76-4**). The most common precipitant in patients with preexisting heart failure is nonadherence to medications and/or diet. Indeed, nonadherence may contribute to as many as two-thirds of heart failure exacerbations. Older patients with cognitive impairment, depression, poor mobility, or limited social support may have particular difficulty following complex treatment plans, and this is important to remember when designing heart failure self-care and medication regimens.

Among cardiac factors, myocardial ischemia or infarction and new-onset or recurrent atrial fibrillation or flutter are the most common causes of an acute episode of heart failure. Other cardiac causes include ventricular arrhythmias, especially ventricular tachycardia, and bradyarrhythmias, such as marked sinus bradycardia or advanced atrioventricular block. Sick sinus syndrome, which is common in older adults, is a frequent cause of

TABLE 76-4 ■ COMMON PRECIPITANTS OF HEART FAILURE IN OLDER ADULTS

Dietary sodium excess

Medication nonadherence

Excess fluid intake

Myocardial ischemia or infarction

Iatrogenic volume overload
- Postoperative fluid administration
- Medication-related (such as NSAIDs and thiazolidinediones)

Arrhythmias
- Atrial fibrillation or flutter
- Ventricular arrhythmias
- Bradyarrhythmias, especially sick sinus syndrome

Associated medical conditions
- Fever
- Infections, especially pneumonia or sepsis
- Hyperthyroidism or hypothyroidism
- Anemia
- Renal insufficiency
- Thiamine deficiency
- Pulmonary embolism
- Hypoxemia from chronic lung disease
- Uncontrolled hypertension

Drugs and medications
- Alcohol
- β-Blockers (including ophthalmologic agents)
- Calcium channel blockers
- Antiarrhythmic agents
- Nonsteroidal anti-inflammatory drugs
- Corticosteroids
- Estrogen preparations
- Antihypertensive agents (eg, clonidine and minoxidil)

bradyarrhythmias in this population. In hospitalized patients, iatrogenic volume overload is also an important precipitant of heart failure.

As previously discussed, older patients have limited cardiovascular reserve and they are less able to compensate in response to increased demands. As a result, heart failure in older adults can be precipitated by acute or worsening noncardiac conditions. Patients with acute respiratory disorders, such as pneumonia, pulmonary embolism, or an exacerbation of chronic obstructive lung disease, are particularly prone to exhibit deterioration in cardiac function. Other serious infections, such as sepsis or pyelonephritis, may also lead to heart failure exacerbations. In patients with hypertension, inadequate blood pressure control is a common cause of worsening heart failure. Thyroid disease, anemia, and declining renal function may also contribute directly or indirectly to the development of heart failure. Substance abuse can also worsen heart failure. Alcohol is a cardiac depressant, and it may also precipitate arrhythmias, especially atrial fibrillation.

Finally, numerous drugs and medications may contribute to heart failure exacerbations. The American Heart Association issued a statement in 2016 enumerating medications that can cause or worsen heart failure. Approximately 30% to 50% of older adults with heart failure take at least one medication that can cause or worsen heart failure, an observation that likely relates to their high prevalence of multimorbidity and polypharmacy. Nonsteroidal anti-inflammatory drugs (NSAIDs) are one of the most commonly used offenders and can worsen heart failure by impairing renal sodium and water excretion and contributing to intravascular volume overload. In addition, NSAIDs antagonize the effects of angiotensin-converting enzyme (ACE) inhibitors, thereby limiting the efficacy of these agents. Corticosteroids and estrogen preparations can also cause fluid retention and an increase in plasma volume. Insulin-sensitizing thiazolidinediones (rosiglitazone and pioglitazone) can also cause fluid retention, and thus worsen heart failure. Cardiovascular medications can also potentially exert negative effects in heart failure. For example, the antihypertensive agent minoxidil also promotes fluid retention, and several other antihypertensive drugs (eg, clonidine) may have unfavorable hemodynamic effects. Even β-blockers (including ophthalmologic agents) and calcium channel blockers, which are widely used in older individuals with cardiovascular disease, when used in excess can exacerbate heart failure since they are negative inotropes. Class Ia (eg, quinidine, procainamide, and disopyramide) and Ic (eg, flecainide and propafenone) antiarrhythmic agents also have important myocardial depressant effects that may worsen cardiac function.

CLINICAL FEATURES

Symptoms

The most common symptoms of heart failure in older adults are exertional shortness of breath, orthopnea, edema, bloating, fatigue, and exercise intolerance. However, atypical symptoms are common in older patients, particularly those older than 80 years (**Table 76-5**). As a result, heart failure in older adults is paradoxically both over- and underdiagnosed. Thus, shortness of breath in an older individual may be attributed to heart failure when the underlying cause is chronic lung disease, pneumonia, or anemia. Similarly, fatigue and reduced exercise tolerance may be caused by anemia, hypothyroidism, depression, or deconditioning. On the other hand, sedentary individuals and those limited by arthritis or neuromuscular conditions may not report exertional dyspnea or fatigue, and atypical symptoms such as those listed in **Table 76-5** may be the first and only clinical manifestations of heart failure. In such cases, the clinician must maintain a high index of suspicion or the diagnosis of heart failure may be readily overlooked.

TABLE 76-5 ■ ATYPICAL MANIFESTATIONS OF HEART FAILURE IN OLDER PERSONS

Nonspecific systemic complaints
- Fatigue/anergia
- Malaise
- Weight loss
- Declining physical activity level

Neurologic symptoms
- Confusion
- Irritability
- Sleep disturbances

Gastrointestinal disorders
- Anorexia or early satiety
- Abdominal discomfort
- Abdominal bloating
- Nausea
- Diarrhea or constipation

Signs

The physical findings in older heart failure patients may be nonspecific or atypical. The classic signs of heart failure include pulmonary rales, an elevated jugular venous pressure, abdominojugular reflux, an S_3 gallop, and pitting edema of the lower extremities. However, rales in older individuals may be due to chronic lung disease, pneumonia, or atelectasis; and peripheral edema may be caused by venous insufficiency, renal disease, immobility, or medication (eg, calcium channel blockers). Conversely, older patients may have an unremarkable physical examination despite markedly reduced cardiac performance. Inversely, impaired sensorium or Cheyne-Stokes respirations may be the only findings to suggest the presence of heart failure.

DIAGNOSTIC EVALUATION

Heart failure is difficult to diagnose in older patients with multiple comorbid conditions and either vague or nonspecific symptoms and signs. Thus, clinicians need to perform a careful history and physical examination, giving due consideration to potential alternative etiologies for the patient's findings. While physical signs may be unreliable in older patients, certain findings, including pulsus alternans, an S_3 gallop, and the presence of jugular venous distension at rest or in response to the abdominojugular reflux maneuver, are highly specific signs of heart failure in older patients. In the absence of these findings, the diagnosis often remains in doubt, and additional laboratory studies are required.

To differentiate shortness of breath attributable to heart failure from other causes, the level of B-type natriuretic peptide (BNP—a 32-amino acid hormone released by the cardiac ventricles in response to increased wall tension) or its inactive fragment N-terminal pro-BNP (NT–pro-BNP) is the single most useful test. However, natriuretic peptide

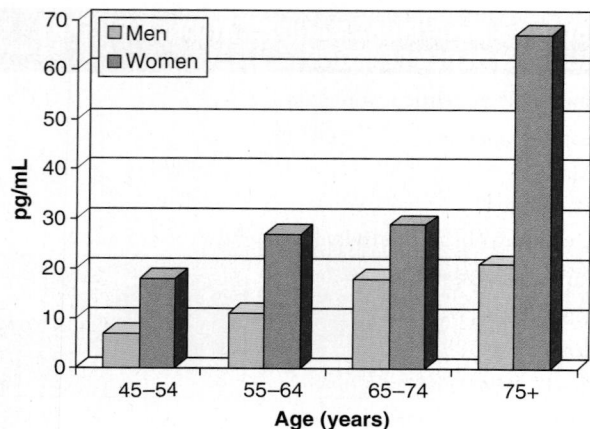

FIGURE 76-6. B-type natriuretic peptide levels by age and gender (mean values in healthy volunteers). (Data from Redfield MM, Rodeheffer RJ, Jacobsen SJ, et al. Plasma brain natriuretic peptide concentration: impact of age and gender. *J Am Coll Cardiol.* 2002;40[5]:976–982.)

levels increase modestly with age especially in women (**Figure 76-6**), declining renal function, and worsening anemia; and are generally lower with a higher BMI. Therefore, the specificity of an elevated natriuretic peptide level for identifying heart failure declines with age. BNP levels more than 500 pg/mL in the appropriate clinical context are highly suggestive of active heart failure, whereas a normal value (< 100 pg/mL) in a nonobese older adult makes the diagnosis of heart failure much less likely. In addition to the BNP level, the chest radiograph remains useful for establishing the presence of active pulmonary congestion. In patients with moderate or severe heart failure, the chest film will usually demonstrate typical findings of cardiomegaly, pulmonary vascular redistribution or edema, and pleural effusions. However, in patients with mild heart failure or coexisting pulmonary disease, the chest radiograph may be nondiagnostic.

Once heart failure has been diagnosed, the physician must address two crucial questions, the answers to which will serve as the basis for selecting appropriate therapy:

1. What is the underlying etiology and pathophysiology of heart failure (see **Table 76-3**)?
2. What additional factors, if any, contributed to or precipitated the development of heart failure (see **Table 76-4**)? Often, one or more precipitating factors can be identified, and alleviating these factors may significantly improve symptoms and reduce the likelihood of subsequent heart failure exacerbations.

In 2017, the American College of Cardiology and American Heart Association Task Force on Practice Guidelines published revised guidelines for the diagnosis and management of heart failure. **Table 76-6** outlines an appropriate initial diagnostic assessment for patients with

TABLE 76-6 ■ DIAGNOSTIC EVALUATION OF PATIENTS WITH HEART FAILURE

Class I (indicated in most patients)

- Complete blood count
- Blood chemistries: electrolytes, creatinine, blood urea nitrogen, glucose, magnesium, calcium, liver function tests, and lipid profile
- Thyroid-stimulating hormone (TSH)
- B-type natriuretic peptide (BNP) or N-terminal pro-BNP level
- Urinalysis
- Chest radiograph and electrocardiogram (ECG)
- Echocardiogram: two-dimensional with Doppler
- Cardiac catheterization and coronary angiography in patients with angina or significant ischemia unless the patient is not eligible for revascularization

Class II (acceptable in selected patients; see text)

- Serum iron and ferritin.
- If suspected, assessment for rheumatologic disease, human immunodeficiency virus, amyloidosis (kappa and lambda free light chains and serum and urine protein electrophoresis with immunofixation), or pheochromocytoma.
- Troponin in those with suspected myocardial ischemia or myocarditis.
- Screening for sleep-disordered breathing.
- Stress test to evaluate for ischemia in patients with unexplained heart failure who are potential candidates for revascularization.
- Coronary angiography if ischemia may be contributing to heart failure in patients who are potential candidates for revascularization.
- Invasive hemodynamic monitoring can be useful for carefully selected patients with acute HF who have persistent symptoms despite empiric adjustment of standard therapies and (a) whose fluid status, perfusion, or systemic or pulmonary vascular resistance is uncertain; (b) whose systolic pressure remains low, or is associated with symptoms, despite initial therapy; (c) whose renal function is worsening with therapy; (d) who require parenteral vasoactive agents; or (e) who may need consideration for mechanical circulatory support or transplantation.
- Endomyocardial biopsy when a specific diagnosis is suspected that would influence therapy.
- Technetium-99 scan if amyloidosis is suspected.

Class III (not routinely indicated)

- Routine repeat measurement of left ventricular function in stable patients
- Endomyocardial biopsy as a routine procedure in the evaluation of patients with heart failure

Data from Yancy CW, Jessup M, Bozkurt B, et al. 2017 ACC/AHA/HFSA Focused Update of the 2013 ACCF/AHA Guideline for the Management of Heart Failure: A Report of the American College of Cardiology/American Heart Association Task Force on Clinical Practice Guidelines and the Heart Failure Society of America. Circulation 2017;136(6):e137–e161.

new-onset heart failure. Class I studies are defined as those that are indicated in most patients, class II procedures are acceptable in some patients but are of unproven efficacy and may be controversial, and class III studies are not routinely indicated and, in some cases, may be harmful. Briefly, basic laboratory studies, a thyroid function test, a chest radiograph, an electrocardiogram, and an echocardiogram with Doppler are recommended in all patients. Cardiac catheterization and coronary angiography are appropriate in patients with angina or significant ischemia on noninvasive testing, and in those who require surgical correction of a valve lesion (eg, aortic stenosis), unless the patient is not a suitable candidate for coronary revascularization.

The recommendations outlined in **Table 76-6** are targeted toward a broad range of adult heart failure patients, and most are applicable even in patients at an advanced age. Nonetheless, in older patients it is appropriate to consider the potential risks and benefits of each diagnostic procedure on an individualized basis, considering comorbid conditions, the extent of cardiac and noncardiac disability, and the patient's goals of care. For example, in a frail 85-year-old individual with severe diabetic nephropathy, the risk of precipitating dialysis-dependent end-stage renal disease as a complication of coronary angiography must be carefully weighed against the potential benefits to be derived from a successful revascularization procedure. Similarly, patient autonomy must be respected in all cases, and it is inappropriate to exert pressure on an older patient to undergo a procedure that the patient clearly does not desire. In this regard, it is imperative to discuss the therapeutic implications of specific procedures (especially invasive procedures) with respect to the patient's subsequent care (eg, need for coronary bypass surgery) prior to performing the diagnostic assessment.

Heart Failure With Reduced Versus Heart Failure With Preserved Ejection Fraction

Current nomenclature distinguishes two forms of heart failure—HFREF, usually defined as ejection fraction less than 40% to 50% and HFPEF. The clinical manifestations of both forms of heart failure are similar. No single clinical feature can reliably distinguish patients with HFREF from those with HFPEF, although certain features tend to favor one form or the other (**Table 76-7**). The predictive accuracy of algorithms to predict HFREF versus HFPEF is modest, and additional testing is essential in order to reliably differentiate HFREF from HFPEF.

An important goal of the diagnostic evaluation is differentiating HFREF from HFPEF since the management of these two syndromes differs. As noted, it is difficult to make this distinction on clinical grounds alone, and it is therefore essential to evaluate left ventricular function directly by echocardiography, radionuclide angiography (commonly called a MUGA [multiple-gated acquisition] scan), magnetic resonance imaging, or contrast ventriculography. In general, transthoracic echocardiography is

TABLE 76-7 ■ CLINICAL FEATURES OF HEART FAILURE WITH REDUCED VERSUS PRESERVED EJECTION FRACTION

	HFREF	HFPEF
Demographics	Age < 60 y Male gender	Age > 70 y Female gender
Comorbid illnesses	Prior myocardial infarction Alcoholism Valvular insufficiency	Chronic hypertension Renal disease Obesity Diabetes Aortic stenosis Amyloidosis
Physical examination	May be normotensive or hypotensive Jugular venous distention Displaced PMI S_3 gallop Pitting edema	Often hypertensive Jugular venous distention often absent Preserved PMI S_4 gallop Peripheral edema often absent
Electrocardiogram	Q waves due to prior myocardial infarction	Left ventricular hypertrophy

HFPEF, heart failure with preserved ejection fraction; HFREF, heart failure with reduced ejection fraction; PMI, point of maximum impulse.

the most useful technique because it is noninvasive, widely available, and, in addition to providing information about systolic and diastolic function, it is helpful in evaluating chamber size, wall thickness and motion, valve function, pulmonary artery pressure, and pericardial disease. Thus, transthoracic echocardiography is appropriate in virtually all older patients with newly diagnosed heart failure and in those with an unexplained change in symptom severity. The principal limitation of echocardiography is that adequate visualization of the heart may be unobtainable in a small percentage of patients, although the availability of echo-contrast agents has reduced this problem. Alternatively, radionuclide angiography can provide an accurate assessment of left ventricular function, as well as information about cavity size and regurgitant valvular lesions. Magnetic resonance imaging provides more detail about myocardial characteristics (scar, inflammation, edema) than echocardiography but cannot assess diastolic function easily, is more expensive and less widely available, and some types of contrast administration are contraindicated in patients with impaired renal function.

Based on the results of echocardiography, radionuclide angiography, magnetic resonance imaging, or contrast ventriculography, heart failure may be classified as HFREF or HFREF (in the ensuing discussion HFREF is defined as ejection fraction < 45%, HFPEF is defined as ejection fraction ≥ 45%). However, it must be emphasized that systolic and diastolic dysfunction are not mutually exclusive.

Indeed, almost all patients with significant systolic dysfunction also have concomitant echo Doppler evidence of diastolic dysfunction. Conversely, systolic dysfunction may play a role in the development of heart failure even when the ejection fraction under resting conditions is normal or near normal. Despite these limitations, the classification of heart failure as HFREF or HFPEF is useful in guiding therapy.

MANAGEMENT

The primary goals of heart failure therapy are to improve quality of life, reduce the frequency of heart failure exacerbations, maximize independence and exercise capacity, enhance emotional well-being, and extend survival.

To achieve these goals, optimal therapy in older patients comprises three principal components: correction of the underlying etiology whenever possible (eg, aortic valve replacement for severe aortic stenosis or coronary revascularization for severe ischemia), attention to the nonpharmacologic and rehabilitative aspects of treatment, and the judicious use of medications and device-based therapies.

As will be discussed in the section on Prognosis, the outlook for patients with established heart failure is poor. Therefore, the importance of effectively treating the primary etiology and all comorbid conditions predisposing to heart failure cannot be overemphasized. Since coronary heart disease and hypertension are the most common causes of heart failure in older adults, primary and secondary prevention of these conditions are critical if the development of heart failure is to be forestalled. Indeed, it has now been shown in multiple clinical trials that effective treatment of hypertension can reduce the incidence of heart failure by more than 50%. Similarly, appropriate management of other coronary risk factors, particularly hyperlipidemia, sedentary lifestyle, and cigarette smoking, will undoubtedly further reduce the burden of heart failure through the primary prevention of coronary heart disease.

Nonpharmacologic Therapy

Despite recent advances in the pharmacotherapy of heart failure, recurrent heart failure exacerbations are common and are more often precipitated by behavioral and social factors than by either new cardiac events (eg, ischemia or an arrhythmia) or progressive deterioration in ventricular function. In one study, lack of adherence to prescribed medications and/or diet contributed to 64% of heart failure exacerbations, while emotional and environmental factors contributed to 26% of hospital readmissions. In another study involving 140 patients 70 years or older hospitalized with heart failure, 47% were readmitted at least once during a 90-day follow-up period. Behavioral and social factors contributing to readmission included medication and dietary nonadherence (15% and 18%, respectively), inadequate social support (21%), inadequate discharge planning (15%), inadequate follow-up (20%), and failure of the patient to seek medical attention promptly when symptoms recurred (20%). These findings suggest that interventions directed at behavioral and social factors could potentially reduce readmissions and improve quality of life in patients with heart failure, and this hypothesis has now been confirmed in numerous prospective randomized trials. In a meta-analytic review of 33 such trials, heart failure readmissions were reduced by 42%, all-cause readmissions were reduced by 24%, and mortality was reduced by 20% in patients with heart failure enrolled in a disease management program relative to conventional care.

Components of a comprehensive nonpharmacologic treatment program are listed in **Table 76-8**. As with other aspects of geriatric care, it is important to structure the treatment program to accommodate the needs of each individual patient. Not every patient will require all the components listed in the table. Similarly, the optimal intensity of any component, for example, patient education or follow-up care, will vary substantially. For these reasons, it is desirable to designate a single provider to coordinate all aspects of the patient's care.

By virtue of age and their preexisting cardiopulmonary syndrome, older adults with heart failure are particularly vulnerable to the adverse effects of pneumonia and respiratory viruses like influenza and SARS-CoV-2. Vaccinations have been shown to be effective and safe in older adults with heart failure and are thus recommended to prevent morbidity and mortality related to these conditions. Specifically, influenza vaccination is associated with reduced risk of death in patients with heart failure, and pneumonia vaccines are also recommended by current guidelines.

Nutrition and Diet

Dietary guidance for patients with heart failure has classically emphasized limiting sodium intake. This recommendation is based on the observation that patients with heart failure who consume excess sodium can retain fluid volume due to increased neurohormonal activation and renal sodium reabsorption. Due to increased consumption of restaurant and prepackaged foods sodium restriction is often difficult to implement in practice. Moreover, guideline recommendations for total daily sodium limit range from 1500 to 3000 mg/d and are based primarily on expert consensus rather than clinical trial data. In addition to uncertainty about appropriate targets, dietary sodium restriction can have potential harms in older patients with heart failure. First, aggressive reduction of sodium intake can lead to hypovolemia, orthostasis, decreased renal perfusion, and further activation of the neurohormonal axis. These issues can be mitigated through close clinical follow-up and adjustment of diuretics and other medications.

Less often appreciated is the relationship between sodium restriction and poor nutritional status. Malnutrition is a strong risk factor for death and hospitalization in

TABLE 76-8 ■ NONPHARMACOLOGIC ASPECTS OF HEART FAILURE MANAGEMENT

Patient education
- Symptoms and signs of heart failure
- Detailed discussion of all medications
- Emphasize importance of dietary and medical adherence
- Specific information about when to contact nurse or physician for worsening symptoms

Daily weight chart
- Specific directions on when to contact nurse or physician for changes in weight
- Self-management of diuretic dosage based on daily weights in selected patients
- Involve family/significant other when feasible

Dietary consultation
- Individualized and consistent with needs/lifestyle
- Avoidance of excess sodium intake (> 2–3 g/d)
- Avoidance of excess fluid intake (> 2 L/d, especially if Na < 130)
- Emphasize good nutrition while allowing flexibility
- Weight loss, if appropriate (consider frailty/sarcopenia in decision-making)
- Low fat, low cholesterol, if appropriate
- Adequate caloric intake (measure resting metabolic rate for most accurate determination)

Medication review
- Heart failure therapy in accordance with guidelines
- Eliminate unnecessary medications
- Simplify regimen whenever possible
- Consolidate dosing schedule

Social services
- Assess social support structure
- Evaluate emotional and financial needs
- Intervene proactively when feasible

Intensive follow-up
- Telephone and/or telemedicine contacts
- Home health visits as needed
- Frequent outpatient clinic visits
- Remote patient monitoring (including CardioMEMs)

Palliative care consultation in patients with advanced symptoms or frequent hospitalizations

Contact information
- Names and phone numbers of nurse and physician
- 24-hour availability

heart failure, particularly in older and/or frail individuals. Dietary sodium restriction has been associated with insufficient calorie intake and dietary deficiencies of critical micronutrients, both of which in turn predict poor clinical outcomes. Older patients with heart failure face a myriad of challenges in maintaining adequate nutrition, including age-related changes in taste and smell, symptoms such as shortness of breath, fatigue, bloating, and nausea, and psychological and logistical factors such as depression, cognitive impairment, poor mobility, and limited social support.

Despite these issues, few dietary intervention clinical trials have been completed in patients with heart failure. The SODIUM-HF pilot study (38 patients, mean age 65) demonstrated that individualized counseling with a dietitian could achieve dietary sodium restriction without compromising overall nutrient intake. The ongoing multinational SODIUM-HF trial (recruiting 1000 patients with stable heart failure) will clarify whether dietitian-guided aggressive sodium restriction (< 1500 mg/d) improves survival free of death or heart failure hospitalization versus usual care. The Spanish PICNIC trial (Nutritional Intervention Program in Hospitalized Patients with Heart Failure) studied intensive, highly individualized monthly dietary counseling in malnourished patients (mean age 79) who survived heart failure hospitalization. In 120 participants, the 6-month nutritional intervention markedly reduced death or heart failure hospitalization at 1-year postdischarge (27% vs 61%, $p < 0.001$).

The optimal dietary recommendations for older patients with heart failure have not been determined. The Dietary Approaches to Stop Hypertension (DASH) eating pattern and, to slightly lesser extent, the Mediterranean diet have been associated with lower long-term mortality in postmenopausal women with heart failure. Both options are reasonable, although guidance may need to be modified by food preference, economic concerns, or comorbidities (eg, potassium content of the DASH diet in the setting of chronic kidney disease). While obesity is a strong risk factor for heart failure (particularly HFPEF) and associated comorbidities, weight loss has been associated with poor outcomes in multiple heart failure cohorts. Weight loss is thus a controversial topic, and advice may need to be modified based on the presence of frailty or sarcopenia.

Physical Activity and Exercise

Historically, patients with heart failure were advised to restrict physical activity on the basis that exercise could potentially worsen cardiac function or precipitate arrhythmias. However, it is now recognized that excessive limitation of physical activity progressively worsens functional capacity because of deconditioning. In addition, several studies have demonstrated that participation in an appropriately structured exercise program may significantly improve functional capacity and quality of life in patients with heart failure. In the largest of these trials, HF-ACTION, 2331 patients with stable heart failure and an ejection fraction less than or equal to 35% were randomized to a supervised exercise program or usual care. The mean age was 59 (25% were ≥ 68 years) and 28% were women. After a median follow-up of 30 months, patients randomized to the exercise intervention experienced a 7% reduction in the primary end point of all-cause mortality or all-cause hospitalization, but the difference was not significant ($p = 0.13$).

After adjusting for highly prognostic baseline characteristics, exercise was associated with an 11% reduction in the primary end point ($p = 0.03$). In addition, exercise was associated with improved health status beginning at 3 months and persisting for up to 4 years. Based on these findings, current guidelines recommend regular exercise for most patients with heart failure. In addition, in 2014, the Centers for Medicare and Medicaid Services approved structured cardiac rehabilitation and exercise training for HFREF patients like those enrolled in the HF-ACTION trial.

While data on exercise training in older adults are limited, a randomized trial involving 200 patients 60 to 89 years (mean 72 years, 66% male) with New York Heart Association (NYHA) class II to III HFREF evaluated the effects of exercise prescription, education, occupational therapy, and psychosocial counseling. At 24 weeks of follow-up, intervention group patients experienced significant improvements in NYHA class, 6-minute walk distance, and quality of life, whereas control-group patients demonstrated no change from baseline in any of these parameters. Patients receiving the intervention also had significantly fewer hospital admissions relative to the control group. In addition, three small randomized trials in older patients with HFPEF have demonstrated that exercise training is safe and results in improved exercise capacity and quality of life. These data provide support for a beneficial effect of exercise and cardiac rehabilitation in older patients with either HFREF or HFPEF. Nonetheless, additional studies focused on traditional or remotely delivered therapy are needed to evaluate the safety and efficacy of regular exercise in older heart failure patients, especially those older than 75 years, with frailty or multiple comorbid conditions, and/or who have been recently hospitalized.

Exercise prescription A comprehensive exercise and conditioning program is appropriate for most older patients with mild-to-moderate heart failure symptoms and no other contraindications to exercise. **Table 76-9** enumerates specific contraindications that should be considered. **Table 76-10** outlines the basic components of such a program. In general, patients should try to exercise every day. A typical session should include some gentle stretching exercises as well as strengthening exercises using elastic bands

TABLE 76-9 ■ CONTRAINDICATIONS TO EXERCISE IN OLDER PATIENTS

Recent myocardial infarction or unstable angina (within 2 wk)
Severe, decompensated heart failure (New York Heart Association class IV)
Life-threatening arrhythmias not adequately treated
Severe aortic stenosis or hypertrophic cardiomyopathy
Any acute serious illness (eg, pneumonia)
Any condition precluding safe participation in an exercise program

TABLE 76-10 ■ EXERCISE PRESCRIPTION FOR OLDER PATIENTS WITH HEART FAILURE

Components of conditioning program
• Flexibility exercises
• Strengthening exercises/resistance training
• Aerobic conditioning
Frequency of exercise: daily, if possible, but not less than three times a week
Duration of exercise: individualized; start low, go slow
Intensity of exercise: low to moderate (see text for details)
Rate of progression: gradual over weeks to months
Monitoring: heart rate, perceived exertion (see text)

or light weights and targeting all the major muscle groups. Suitable forms of aerobic exercise for older patients include walking, stationary cycling, and swimming. The choice of aerobic exercise should be tailored to the patient's wishes and abilities. When initiating an exercise program, the duration and intensity of the aerobic activity should be well within the patient's comfort range. The activity should be enjoyable, not stressful, and after completing the activity the patient should feel "positive" about the experience and not unduly fatigued. For many older patients with heart failure, this may mean starting with as little as 2 to 5 minutes of slow-paced walking. Once the patient feels comfortable exercising, the duration of exercise can be gradually increased over a period of several weeks. Weekly increases of 1 to 2 minutes per session are appropriate for most patients. Once the patient can exercise continuously and comfortably for 20 to 30 minutes, the intensity of exercise may be increased, if desired. More recently, high-intensity interval training, in which short bursts of higher-intensity exercise are incorporated into the exercise regimen, has been shown to be safe and to result in more rapid increases in exercise capacity in heart failure patients. These findings, while encouraging, should be regarded as preliminary, and high-intensity training should only be initiated in a monitored setting.

The two most common techniques for monitoring exercise intensity are the target heart rate method and the patient's subjective assessment of perceived exertion. For patients not taking medications that lower heart rate (eg, β-blockers), the maximum attainable heart rate in beats/min can be estimated from the formula $208 - 0.7 \times age$). The patient's resting heart rate is then subtracted from this figure to determine the heart rate reserve. A suitable target heart rate for low-intensity exercise can be calculated as the resting heart rate plus 30% to 50% of the heart rate reserve. For moderate-intensity exercise, the target range is the resting heart rate plus 50% to 70% of the heart rate reserve.

For many older patients, calculating the target heart rate may be difficult. In addition, it may not be possible to accurately determine heart rate during exercise (unless a heart rate monitor is used). For these reasons, the patient's subjective assessment of perceived exertion is often the most practical method for monitoring exercise intensity. In addition, perceived exertion correlates reasonably well with exercise heart rate. A simple perceived exertion scale (Borg Scale) comprises five levels: very light, light, moderate, somewhat heavy, and heavy. Older patients with heart failure should begin with very light exercise, progressing to the light range as tolerated. After several weeks, some patients may wish to increase their perceived exertion level into the moderate range, but more strenuous exercise is not recommended for patients with heart failure.

Pharmacologic Treatment of Heart Failure With Reduced Ejection Fraction

In general, the treatment of HFREF in older patients does not differ substantially from that in younger patients. The primary goal of pharmacotherapy for HFREF is to reduce mortality and prevent events such as HF hospitalizations. Many patients who receive aggressive therapy can experience a substantial improvement in their ejection fraction. Relatedly, many of these agents can subsequently improve symptoms and improve quality of life. However, similar to any other medication prescribed to older adults, it is naturally important to weigh the risks and potential benefits in both the short and long term in conjunction with other comorbid conditions, geriatric syndromes like frailty and cognitive impairment, overall life expectancy, and health priorities.

β-Blockers As recently as 20 years ago, β-adrenergic blocking agents were considered contraindicated in patients with heart failure owing to their negative inotropic and chronotropic effects, both of which can diminish cardiac output. However, it is now recognized that persistent activation of the sympathetic nervous system is detrimental in patients with heart failure because it exacerbates ischemia, causes arrhythmogenesis, promotes β-receptor desensitization, and contributes to a progressive decline in ventricular function. Furthermore, several large prospective randomized clinical trials have now confirmed that long-term β-blockade improves left ventricular function and reduces both total mortality and sudden cardiac death in a broad spectrum of patients with HFREF.

In the Study of the Effects of Nebivolol Intervention on Outcomes and Rehospitalization in Seniors with Heart Failure trial (SENIORS), 2128 patients 70 years or older (mean age 76, 37% women) were randomized to nebivolol or placebo. During a mean follow-up of 21 months, the primary composite outcome of death or cardiovascular hospitalization was significantly lower in patients randomized to nebivolol, with similar results in younger and older patients, including those older than 85 years. Based on these studies, β-blockers are now recommended as a standard therapy in almost all patients with symptomatic HFREF in the absence of contraindications.

In the United States, carvedilol, bisoprolol, and metoprolol succinate have been approved for the treatment of heart failure. Among the many β-blockers on the market, it is worth noting that these are the only three drugs that were studied and subsequently demonstrated benefit in improving outcomes in heart failure. Therefore, these are the β-blockers that should be used for the purposes of treating heart failure. Starting dosages are carvedilol 3.125 to 6.25 mg BID, metoprolol tartrate 6.25 mg BID or QID (or metoprolol succinate 12.5–25 mg daily), and bisoprolol 1.25 to 2.5 mg daily. Of note, although metoprolol succinate (long-acting) is the evidence-based formulation of metoprolol for HFREF, metoprolol tartrate (short-acting) may be a reasonable alternative when titrating to target doses. Doses should be gradually increased at approximately 2-week intervals as tolerated to achieve maintenance dosages of carvedilol 25 to 50 mg BID, metoprolol succinate 100 to 200 mg daily, and bisoprolol 10 mg daily.

Contraindications to the use of β-blockers include severe decompensated heart failure, significant bronchospastic lung disease, marked bradycardia (resting heart rate < 50/min), systolic blood pressure less than 90 to 100 mm Hg, advanced heart block (> first degree), and known intolerance to β-blockade. It is important to monitor heart rate, blood pressure, clinical symptoms, and the cardiorespiratory examination during initiation and titration of therapy. Patients should be advised that they may experience a modest worsening in heart failure symptoms especially fatigue during the first few weeks of β-blocker therapy, but that in most cases these symptoms resolve, and the long-term tolerability of β-blockers is excellent. However, if severe adverse effects occur, dosage reduction or discontinuation of treatment may be necessary. Notably, hemodynamic intolerance to β-blocker may be suggestive of an advanced stage of heart failure and thus may warrant evaluation by a specialist if not already involved in the care of the patient.

ACE inhibitors Numerous prospective randomized clinical trials using multiple different angiotensin-converting enzyme (ACE) inhibitors in a variety of clinical settings have conclusively demonstrated that these agents significantly reduce mortality and hospitalization rates and improve exercise tolerance and quality of life in patients with impaired left ventricular systolic function, even in the absence of clinical heart failure. Although none of these studies included patients older than 80 years, available evidence indicates that ACE inhibitors are as effective in older patients as in younger ones.

In older patients, therapy should be initiated with a low dose (eg, captopril 6.25–12.5 mg TID or enalapril 2.5–5 mg BID), and the dose should be gradually increased as tolerated. In hospitalized patients who are hemodynamically stable, the dose may be increased daily; in outpatients, the dose should be increased weekly or biweekly. Throughout the titration period, blood pressure, renal function, and serum potassium levels should be monitored.

For maintenance therapy, ACE inhibitor dosages should be commensurate with those used in the clinical trials.

Recommended "target" doses for selected ACE inhibitors are as follows: captopril 50 mg TID, enalapril 10 to 20 mg BID, lisinopril 20 to 40 mg daily, ramipril 10 mg daily, trandolapril 4 mg daily, quinapril 40 mg BID, and fosinopril 40 mg daily. In patients unable to tolerate full therapeutic doses of ACE inhibitors, lower doses may be used; however, the clinical benefits may be attenuated with lower dosages. Clearly, the risks and benefits of higher doses must be weighed for each individual patient. Captopril and enalapril are excellent agents for use during the titration phase given its short half-life—but once the maintenance dose has been reached, it is desirable to change to a once-daily ACE inhibitor at equivalent dosage for reasons of increased convenience, potentially improved adherence, and lower cost.

The most common side effect from ACE inhibitors is a dry, hacking cough, which may be severe enough to require discontinuation of therapy in 5% to 10% of patients during long-term use. Less common but more serious side effects include hypotension, a decline in renal function, and hyperkalemia. These side effects tend to occur shortly after initiation of therapy and may be aggravated by intravascular volume contraction as a result of over diuresis. Indications for downward titration or discontinuation of an ACE inhibitor include symptomatic hypotension, persistent increase in serum creatinine of 1 mg/dL or greater, or a rise in the serum potassium level above 5.5 mEq/L. Note that asymptomatic low blood pressure does not necessarily mandate dosage reduction; but again, the risks and benefits must be weighed for each individual patient.

Angiotensin II receptor blockers The use of ARBs for the treatment of heart failure has been evaluated in several studies. In the second Evaluation of Losartan in the Elderly trial (ELITE-II), losartan 50 mg once daily was compared to captopril 50 mg TID in 3152 patients 60 years or older (mean age 71) with moderate heart failure and an ejection fraction of 40% or less, showing similar improvements in mortality. In the Candesartan in Heart Failure: Assessment of Reduction in Mortality and Morbidity (CHARM)—Alternative study, 2028 patients intolerant to ACE inhibitors were randomized to candesartan or placebo and followed for a median of 34 months. Compared to patients in the placebo group, patients randomized to candesartan experienced a significant 30% reduction in the composite end point of cardiovascular death or hospitalization for heart failure. All-cause mortality was reduced by 17%, which was of borderline statistical significance. The mean age of patients in the CHARM-Alternative study was approximately 66.5, and nearly one-fourth of patients were 75 years or older; however, subgroup analysis by age has not been reported. Accordingly, ARBs are approved for the treatment of heart failure with reduced ejection fraction. The recommended starting dose of valsartan is 20 to 40 mg BID, and the dose should be titrated to 160 mg BID as tolerated; the starting dose of candesartan is 4 to 8 mg once daily, with titration to 32 mg daily as tolerated; and the starting dose of losartan is 25 to 50 mg once daily, with titration up to 150 mg once daily as tolerated. For older adults, especially where significant concern for adverse effects, it may be reasonable to start at even lower doses (cutting the lowest dose pill in half) and slowly titrating based on tolerance. As with many drugs, especially among older adults, the adage of starting low and going slow applies.

It is important to note that combining ACEI and ARB is not recommended due to the adverse effects of using both agents concurrently. In the Valsartan in Acute Myocardial Infarction trial, 14,703 patients with heart failure and/or an ejection fraction less than 35% within 10 days of experiencing an acute myocardial infarction were randomized to receive valsartan, captopril, or both drugs. During a median follow-up of 25 months, there were no differences between groups with respect to all-cause mortality or the composite end point of fatal or nonfatal cardiovascular events. However, limiting side effects were more common in patients receiving both ACE and ARBs than in those receiving either drug alone. The median age was 65 years, and results were similar in older and younger patients.

The major side effects of ARBs are similar to ACEI and include hypotension, renal insufficiency, and hyperkalemia. Notably, ARBs bind directly to angiotensin II receptors on the cell membrane; thus, unlike ACE inhibitors, ARBs do not inhibit the breakdown of bradykinins, which eliminates the bradykinin-mediated side effects such as cough.

Angiotensin receptor neprilysin inhibitor (ARNi) Sacubitril inhibits a neprilysin, a neutral endopeptidase that degrades vasoactive peptides such as BNP thereby promoting the effects of natriuretic peptides. The combination of an angiotensin receptor antagonist (Valsartan) with a neutral endopeptidase inhibitor (sacubitril) has been shown superior to therapy with an ACE inhibitor (enalapril) reducing the composite endpoint of cardiovascular death or HF hospitalization significantly by 20% in the Prospective Comparison of ARNI with ACEI to Determine Impact on Global Mortality and Morbidity in Heart Failure (PARADIGM-HF) trial. The benefit was seen to a similar extent for both death and heart failure hospitalization and was consistent across subgroups including those <75 and >75 years. ARNi therapy increases the risk of hypotension and renal insufficiency and may lead to angioedema, but the risk of an elevation in creatinine and potassium were lower with ARNi therapy compared to ACEI therapy. Transition from ACE or ARB to ARNi therapy is recommended for all patients with HFREF with at least a 36-hour wash out from ACE Inhibitors to mitigate against angioedema. ARNi therapy is also recommended as first-line therapy for stable HFREF patients and after an acute decompensation based on the results of the PIONEER trial, which specifically studied the safety and short-term efficacy of in-hospital initiation of ARNi. Since systemic hypotension is common with ARNi therapy, caution is warranted among older adults with a low system blood pressure. Unless patients are transitioned to ARNi from high-dose ACE or ARBs, ARNi therapy should be initiated at low dosages (eg, 24/26 mg PO BID of sacubitril/valsartan) with uptitration over time.

Mineralocorticoid receptor antagonists (MRA) The MRAs spironolactone and eplerenone are relatively weak diuretics that are potassium-sparing and interfere with the effect of aldosterone. In the Randomized Aldactone Evaluation of Survival trial, spironolactone 12.5 to 50 mg once daily reduced mortality by 30% and heart failure hospitalizations by 35% in patients with NYHA class III or IV heart failure and a left ventricular ejection fraction less than or equal to 35%, when added to baseline therapy with an ACE inhibitor, digoxin, and loop diuretic. Moreover, the beneficial effects of spironolactone were at least as great in older as in younger patients. In the Eplerenone Post-Acute Myocardial Infarction Heart Failure Efficacy and Survival study, eplerenone 25 to 50 mg once daily significantly reduced mortality by 15% over a mean follow-up period of 16 months in patients with clinical evidence for heart failure and an ejection fraction of 40% or less within 3 to 16 days following acute myocardial infarction. Sudden death from cardiac causes and cardiovascular hospitalizations were also reduced in the eplerenone group. Compared to placebo, hyperkalemia occurred more commonly but hypokalemia occurred less frequently with eplerenone. The average age of patients in the Eplerenone Post-Acute Myocardial Infarction Heart Failure Efficacy and Survival study was 64, and although the relative benefit of eplerenone was somewhat less in older compared to younger patients, the difference was not statistically significant.

The EMPHASIS-HF trial randomized 2737 patients with NYHA class II heart failure and a left ventricular ejection fraction less than or equal to 35% to eplerenone at a dose of up to 50 mg or matching placebo. The mean age was 69 and 24% of patients were 75 years or older. The primary outcome was death from cardiovascular causes or hospitalization for heart failure. The study was stopped prematurely after a median follow-up of 21 months because eplerenone showed a marked reduction in the primary end point relative to placebo (18.3% vs 25.9%, hazard ratio 0.63, $p < 0.001$). Results were similar in patients over or under age 75. Eplerenone also reduced all-cause mortality, all-cause hospitalizations, and heart failure hospitalizations (hazard ratios 0.76, 0.77, and 0.58, respectively).

Based on the results of these studies, MRAs are recommended in patients with NYHA class II to IV heart failure symptoms and left ventricular ejection fraction less than or equal to 35%, and in patients with heart failure and an ejection fraction of 40% or less following myocardial infarction. These agents are contraindicated in patients with significant renal dysfunction (creatinine ≥ 2.5 mg/dL) or preexisting hyperkalemia. Older patients are at increased risk of adverse effects—accordingly, renal function and serum potassium levels should be monitored closely during initiation and titration of therapy (such as within 3–14 days of initiation or of increasing the dose). In addition, up to 10% of patients receiving long-term treatment with spironolactone may experience painful gynecomastia requiring discontinuation of the drug; this side effect occurs rarely with eplerenone.

Sodium-glucose cotransporter-2 inhibitors (SGLT2 inhibitors) Sodium-glucose cotransporter-2 (SGLT-2) inhibitors are agents that were developed initially to treat hyperglycemia. SGLT2 is the primary transport protein in the kidney that promotes reabsorption of glucose back into circulation after glomerular filtration. SGLT-2 is in the proximal tubule of the kidney and is responsible for approximately 90% of glucose reabsorption. Large cardiovascular outcome trials in patients with type 2 diabetes demonstrated that SGLT2 inhibitors improve cardiovascular and renal outcomes and reduce the risk of hospitalization for heart failure. Two subsequent randomized clinical trials of SGLT2 inhibitors in patients with existing HFREF (Study to Evaluate the Effect of Dapagliflozin on the Incidence of Worsening Heart Failure or Cardiovascular Death in Patients With Chronic Heart Failure [DAPA-HF] and Empagliflozin Outcome Trial in Patients With Chronic Heart Failure With Reduced Ejection Fraction [EMPEROR-Reduced]) confirmed that these agents reduce the risk of death and heart failure hospitalizations. Additionally, they reduce the risk of renal events defined as 50% or greater sustained decline in estimated glomerular filtration rate (eGFR), end-stage renal disease (ESRD), or death due to renal disease. The efficacy of SGLT-2 inhibitors appears similar in those older than 75 years compared with younger individuals, and, surprisingly, regardless of whether diabetes mellitus is present. The most common side effects of SGLT-2 inhibitors include genital yeast infections in men and women, urinary tract infections (UTIs), urinary frequency, and renal dysfunction. These adverse outcomes were similar in younger and older individuals. Rare but more severe side effects of diabetic ketoacidosis and amputation are more common with these agents in older adults.

Hydralazine/nitrates In patients who are unable to tolerate an ACE inhibitor or ARB, the combination of hydralazine with oral or topical nitrates provides an acceptable alternative. The African American Heart Failure Trial (A-HeFT) randomized 1050 Black patients with NYHA class III or IV heart failure to a fixed-dose combination of isosorbide dinitrate plus hydralazine or to placebo in addition to standard heart failure therapy. The study was stopped after an average follow-up of 10 months because of a significantly lower mortality rate in patients randomized to the intervention. Heart failure hospitalizations were also reduced, and quality of life was improved in patients randomized to hydralazine-nitrates relative to placebo. Based on the results of A-HeFT, the fixed-dose combination of isosorbide dinitrate and hydralazine has been approved for treatment of heart failure in Black patients in the United States. Although there was no upper-age restriction for the A-HeFT study, the average age of patients enrolled in the trial was 57, so the efficacy of this therapy in older Black patients remains unknown.

For older patients, treatment should begin with lower dosages (eg, hydralazine 12.5–25 mg TID–QID; isosorbide dinitrate 10 mg TID–QID), followed by gradual upward titration to achieve the doses used in the trials. The most common side effects associated with hydralazine/nitrates include headache and dizziness. A small percentage of patients developed arthralgias or other symptoms suggestive of hydralazine-induced lupus. The requirement for multiple doses over the course of the day, which may be inconvenient and contribute to increased pill burden and reduced overall nonadherence, should also be considered when prescribing to older adults.

Diuretics Diuretics are the most effective agents for relieving pulmonary congestion and edema, and for this reason they remain a key component of heart failure management. Although there is no data to suggest a mortality benefit, they are effective in reducing symptoms and improving many of the classic symptoms of heart failure including edema and dyspnea.

In patients with mild chronic heart failure, a thiazide diuretic may be sufficient for relieving congestive symptoms and maintaining fluid homeostasis. However, most patients will require a more potent agent, and the "loop" diuretics, including furosemide, bumetanide, and torsemide, are the drugs most widely used. For optimal effectiveness, patients should be instructed to avoid excessive sodium and fluid intake. Typical daily doses of "loop" diuretics range from 20 to 160 mg for furosemide, 0.5 to 5 mg for bumetanide, and 5 to 100 mg for torsemide. In patients hospitalized with an acute episode of heart failure, intravenous administration may be more effective than the oral route in promoting diuresis, in part due to bowel wall edema, which may decrease the drug's absorption. Patients who fail to respond adequately to a loop diuretic that has low bioavailability (eg, furosemide) may respond to a bioavailable loop diuretic (bumetanide or torsemide) or the addition of metolazone 2.5 to 10 mg daily.

The most common and important side effects of diuretics are electrolyte disturbances, including hypokalemia, hyponatremia, hypomagnesemia, and increased bicarbonate levels indicative of metabolic alkalosis. Owing to age-related changes in renal function as well as a higher prevalence of comorbid illnesses such as diabetes, older patients are at increased risk of serious diuretic-induced electrolyte abnormalities. For this reason, electrolytes should be monitored closely when diuretic therapy is being adjusted. This is particularly true when using metolazone, which can lead to a brisk diuretic response and cause life-threatening hyponatremia and hypokalemia even after relatively short-term use.

The relationship between diuretics and serum creatinine is complex. Patients with volume overload may have hemodilution, whereby serum creatinine will appear low and underestimate the extent of chronic kidney disease present. In such a situation, diuresis may be accompanied by increases in creatinine with the perception that the diuretic has worsened renal function. In older adults with heart failure, contributors to chronic kidney disease include other cardiovascular risk factors like hypertension and diabetes, as well as the chronic insult of heart failure which can adversely affect kidney perfusion through impaired cardiac output and/or chronically elevated filling pressures. Thus, by achieving and maintaining euvolemia with subsequent optimization of cardiac output, diuretics can theoretically mitigate heart failure-related kidney damage. Avoiding diuretic titration and instead opting for persistent congestion can occur at the expense of symptoms, worse quality of life, and/or increased risk for hospitalization. Thus, it may be reasonable to engage in shared decision-making regarding therapeutic options and inform patients of a possible increase in creatinine resulting from the resolution of hemodilution, rather than from diuretic-related injury. It is similarly important to counsel patients about symptoms of hypovolemia such as dizziness and lightheadedness as an indicator of overdiuresis, which can subsequently worsen cardiac output and cause kidney injury.

Digoxin Digoxin inhibits the sodium-potassium exchange pump located within the myocyte membrane, producing a rise in intracellular sodium concentration. This facilitates sodium-calcium exchange, leading to an increase in intracellular calcium. Calcium binds with troponin C, which initiates the process of contraction by allowing myosin to bind with actin. By increasing calcium availability, digoxin induces a modest increase in the force of myocardial contraction (positive inotropic effect). This effect occurs whether or not heart failure is present, and it does not appear to be affected by age.

The Digitalis Investigation Group (DIG) reported the results of a prospective randomized trial involving 6800 patients with HFREF. Patients were randomized to receive digoxin or placebo in addition to diuretics and an ACE inhibitor, and the average duration of follow-up was 37 months. Overall mortality did not differ between digoxin and placebo (34.8% vs 35.1%), but there were 28% fewer hospitalizations for heart failure in the digoxin group, and the combined end point of death or hospitalization for heart failure was significantly reduced. In addition, the beneficial effects of digoxin were similar in younger and older patients, including octogenarians. Subsequent analyses based on data from the DIG trial suggest that digoxin administered at low dosages to achieve serum concentrations in the range of 0.5 to 0.9 ng/mL may be associated with improved survival as well as a reduction in all-cause hospitalizations. These findings confirm that digoxin is beneficial in controlling heart failure symptoms and support the use of low-dose digoxin in patients who remain symptomatic despite appropriate dosages of an ACE inhibitor, β-blocker, MRA, and diuretic.

Side effects from digoxin include cardiac, neurologic, and gastrointestinal effects. In the DIG study, side effects that occurred more frequently in patients receiving digoxin included nausea and vomiting, diarrhea, visual disturbances, supraventricular and ventricular arrhythmias, and advanced atrioventricular heart block. Although not reported in the DIG trial, older patients may be at increased risk of digoxin toxicity, especially cardiac toxicity, in part owing to a decreased volume of drug distribution. Patients with chronic lung disease, amyloid heart disease, and other conditions may also be at increased risk of digoxin toxicity.

In most older patients with relatively normal renal function, a digoxin dose of 0.125 mg daily is usually sufficient to achieve a therapeutic effect. Patients with renal impairment or small body habitus may require a lower dose. Serum digoxin concentration should be measured 2 to 4 weeks after initiating therapy, and periodically thereafter, to ensure that the levels are not supratherapeutic which can be toxic given digoxin's narrow therapeutic index. It is worth noting that older adults can develop toxicity even at "therapeutic" levels of digoxin. It is therefore important to remain vigilant about signs and symptoms that may indicate digoxin toxicity such as worsening arrhythmias and/or heart block, gastrointestinal symptoms like nausea/vomiting, and/or confusion. Since diuretic-induced hypokalemia and hypomagnesemia potentiate digoxin's cardiotoxic effects, including proarrhythmia, it is important to maintain normal serum concentrations of these electrolytes in all patients receiving digoxin. All of these factors must be considered when weighing the risks and benefits of digoxin, especially among older adults with low body weight and fluctuating renal function.

Ivabradine Ivabradine is a new therapeutic agent that selectively inhibits the If current in the sinoatrial node, resulting in heart rate reduction. The SHIFT study, a double-blind randomized trial, demonstrated a reduction in the composite endpoint of cardiovascular death or HF hospitalization with ivabradine compared to placebo. The benefit of ivabradine was driven by a reduction in HF hospitalization and not by CV death. All subjects enrolled had a left ventricular ejection fraction (LVEF) less than or equal to 35% and were in sinus rhythm with a resting heart rate of more than or equal to 70 bpm. The target of ivabradine is heart rate slowing (the presumed benefit of action), but only 25% of patients studied were on optimal doses of β-blocker therapy. Given the well-proven mortality benefits of β-blockers, it is important to initiate and up titrate these agents to target doses, as tolerated, before assessing the resting heart rate for consideration of ivabradine.

Calcium channel blockers Non-dihydropyridine calcium channel blockers, including nifedipine, diltiazem, and verapamil, are contraindicated in patients with HFREF because each of these agents has been associated with adverse clinical outcomes. The third-generation calcium channel blockers amlodipine and felodipine have been studied in prospective randomized trials involving patients with HFREF. Although the Prospective Randomized Amlodipine Survival Evaluation (PRAISE) suggested that amlodipine might be beneficial in patients with nonischemic HFREF, this was not confirmed in PRAISE-2. Similarly, the V-HeFT-3 trial failed to demonstrate a significant benefit in patients with HFREF treated with felodipine. Thus, there are no approved indications for the use of calcium channel blockers in patients with HFREF, and their use in this condition is not recommended. However, in patients with heart failure and active anginal symptoms not controlled with β-blockers and nitrates, the addition of a long-acting calcium channel blocker is reasonable. Similarly, diltiazem or verapamil may be used in heart failure patients with rapid atrial fibrillation who do not respond adequately to β-blockers and other interventions.

Antithrombotic therapy Patients with left ventricular systolic dysfunction are at increased risk for thromboembolic events, including stroke. However, in the absence of atrial fibrillation, rheumatic mitral valve disease, or a history of prior embolization, the value of antithrombotic treatment for the prevention of embolic events is unproven. In the Warfarin and Antiplatelet Therapy in Chronic Heart Failure (WATCH) trial, 1587 patients with NYHA class II or III HFREF were randomized to receive aspirin 162 mg/day, clopidogrel 75 mg/day, or warfarin to maintain an international normalized ratio (INR) of 2.5 to 3.0. After a mean follow-up of 23 months, there were no differences between the three groups in the primary composite end point of death, myocardial infarction, or stroke. Hospitalizations for heart failure occurred more frequently in the aspirin group than with either clopidogrel or warfarin, whereas bleeding complications were more common with warfarin. The mean age of patients in the WATCH trial was 63; subgroup analysis by age has not been reported.

In the Warfarin versus Aspirin in Reduced Cardiac Ejection Fraction (WARCEF) study, 2305 patients with heart failure, a left ventricular ejection fraction less than or equal to 35%, and sinus rhythm were randomized to warfarin (target INR 2.0–3.5) or to aspirin 325 mg daily. The primary outcome was all-cause mortality, ischemic stroke, or intracerebral hemorrhage. The mean age was 61 and 80% of participants were men. After a mean follow-up of 3.5 years, there was no difference between groups in the primary outcome. Warfarin was associated with fewer ischemic strokes but more major bleeding events. Intracranial hemorrhage was infrequent and did not differ between groups. A subgroup analysis showed patients older than 60 years of age did not benefit from warfarin over aspirin on the primary outcome; and when major hemorrhage was included as part of a composite outcome, the adverse event rate was significantly higher for warfarin.

Based on currently available data, anticoagulation with warfarin to achieve an INR of 2 to 3 is recommended in heart failure patients with chronic or paroxysmal atrial fibrillation or atrial flutter, rheumatic mitral valve disease with left atrial enlargement, prior stroke or unexplained arterial embolus, a mobile left ventricular thrombus (as demonstrated by echocardiography or other imaging modality), or a left atrial appendage thrombus identified by transesophageal echocardiography. Routine use of warfarin in other circumstances is not recommended. In patients with nonvalvular atrial fibrillation, one of the newer oral anticoagulants (dabigatran, rivaroxaban, apixaban, edoxaban) may be used as an alternative to warfarin. Careful attention should be paid to recommended dosing adjustments for these drugs in the setting of renal insufficiency and/or advanced age to optimize benefits and risks. (See Chapters 22, 75, and 96 for more details.)

Aspirin is justified in patients with known coronary heart disease, particularly those with recent myocardial infarction, unstable angina, percutaneous coronary intervention, or bypass surgery. Aspirin is also recommended for older patients with peripheral arterial disease or diabetes. In addition, aspirin is appropriate in high-risk patients with atrial arrhythmias who are not suitable candidates for warfarin. As noted previously, additional study is needed to determine the value of aspirin in older patients with heart failure without established vascular disease or diabetes.

Device Therapy

Device therapy, including implantable cardioverter-defibrillators (ICDs) and cardiac resynchronization therapy (CRT) and the mitral clip, is playing an increasing role in the management of patients with HFREF. ICDs reduce mortality from sudden cardiac death in patients with NYHA class II to III HFREF and a left ventricular ejection fraction less than or equal to 35% (primary prevention), and in patients resuscitated from cardiac arrest attributable to ventricular tachyarrhythmias (secondary prevention). However, although current HF guidelines do not incorporate age into the recommendations for ICD therapy, very few patients greater than or equal to 75 years were enrolled in clinical trials evaluating these devices. In addition, a comprehensive meta-analysis suggested that the benefit of ICDs declines with age, most likely due to competing risks for mortality. Patients with life expectancies of less than 12 to 18 months are unlikely to benefit from an ICD, and patients greater than or equal to 80 years are twice as likely as younger patients to experience major complications related to device implantation. Thus, the benefit-to-risk relationship is modified by age, and consideration of ICD therapy must be individualized based on life expectancy, prevalent comorbidities, and patient goals of care using a process of shared decision-making. In patients who choose to undergo placement of an ICD, management of the ICD at end of life, including circumstances under which the patient would want to have the defibrillator portion of the device disabled in order to avoid painful shocks, should be clearly articulated prior to implantation and at routine clinic visits after implantation. Similarly, if a generator change is needed due to battery depletion, the option of foregoing the procedure, along with the implications of this decision, should be discussed.

In contrast to ICDs, which reduce the risk of sudden death but do not improve quality of life, CRT improves symptoms, exercise tolerance, quality of life, and survival in carefully selected patients with HFREF, including octogenarians. CRT involves placement of a biventricular pacemaker with one lead in the right ventricle and a second lead inserted into the coronary sinus in a retrograde fashion to pace the left ventricle. As the name implies, the goal of CRT is to "resynchronize" myocardial contraction, thereby increasing stroke work, ejection fraction, and cardiac output. CRT is indicated in patients with NYHA class II to IV HFREF, left ventricular ejection fraction less than or equal to 35%, and QRS duration greater than or equal to 150 milliseconds by electrocardiogram. Patients with left bundle branch block, which is present in 20% to 30% of patients with HFREF, derive the greatest benefit from CRT, and there is evidence that the benefits tend to be greater in women than in men. CRT can be performed with or without concomitant ICD therapy (CRT-D and CRT-P, respectively), and patients greater than or equal to 80 years are proportionately more likely than younger patients to receive a CRT-P device. As with ICDs, selection of patients for CRT should involve shared decision-making with appropriate consideration of the potential salutary effects on quality of life in older patients who are significantly limited by persistent heart failure symptoms despite optimal medical therapy.

The MitraClip is a transcatheter-based technology which grasps both the anterior and posterior mitral valve leaflets, thereby reducing mitral regurgitation (MR) by increasing the coaptation between the regurgitant valve leaflets. In the COAPT trial among patients with HFREF (n = 614) and moderate-to-severe or severe secondary mitral regurgitation who remained symptomatic despite the use of maximal doses of guideline-directed medical therapy, transcatheter mitral-valve repair resulted in a lower rate of hospitalization for heart failure and lower all-cause mortality than medical therapy alone. Many patients with HFREF have load-dependent mitral regurgitation that is no longer significant after optimization of medical therapy (diuretics and afterload reduction). Accordingly, such an intervention should only be performed after careful evaluation by a multidisciplinary heart team including a geriatrician.

Treatment of Heart Failure With Preserved Ejection Fraction

Even though more than 50% of older patients with heart failure have preserved left ventricular systolic function (ie, HFPEF), large-scale clinical trials have yet to clearly demonstrate major beneficial effects for any pharmacologic agents except for SGLT2 inhibitors (**Table 76-11**). As a result, therapy for HFPEF remains largely empiric, except for those with transthyretin cardiac amyloidosis as the cause.

TABLE 76-11 ■ TRIALS FOR HEART FAILURE WITH PRESERVED EJECTION FRACTION

		PHARMACOTHERAPY			
TRIAL[a]	PATIENTS	TREATMENT	LVEF(%) MEAN (SD OR RANGE)[b]	AGE MEAN (SD OR RANGE)	OUTCOMES COMPARED TO PLACEBO[c]
PEP-CHF	850	Perindopril	65 (56–66)	75 (72–79)	Death/hospitalization by 1 y—HR 0.69 (0.47–1.01, $p = 0.055$). HF hospitalization by 1 y—HR 0.63 (0.41–0.97, $p = 0.033$)
CHARM-Preserved	3023	Candesartan	54 ± 9	67 ± 11	CV death/HF admission—HR 0.89 (0.77–1.03, $p = 0.118$). HF admission—HR 0.85 (0.72–1.01, $p = 0.072$)
I-PRESERVE	4128	Irbesartan	60 ± 9	72 ± 7	Death/hospitalization—HR 0.95 (0.86–1.05, $p = 0.35$)
SENIORS (EF > 35% subgroup)	643	Nebivolol	49 ± 10	76 ± 5	All cause death/CV hospitalization—HR 0.81 (0.63–1.04)
TOPCAT	3445	Spironolactone	56 (51–62)	69 (61–76)	CV death/HF hospitalization/aborted SCD—HR 0.89 (0.77–1.04, $p = 0.14$). HF hospitalization—HR 0.83 (0.69–0.99, $p = 0.04$)
Aldo-DHF	422	Spironolactone	67 ± 8	67 ± 8	Reduced E/e' avg 1.5 ($p < 0.001$)
RELAX	216	Sildenafil	60 (56–65)	69 (62–77)	No difference in Δ VO₂ peak at 24 wk
ESS-DHF	192	Sitaxsentan	61 ± 12	65 ± 10	Median 43 s relative increase in Naughton treadmill time ($p = 0.03$)
DIG Ancillary	988	Digoxin	55 ± 8	67 ± 10	HF hospitalization—HR 0.79 (0.59–1.04, $p = 0.09$). Hospitalization for unstable angina—HR 1.37 (0.99–1.91, $p = 0.06$)
SWEDIC	113	Carvedilol	> 45	66 (48–84)	No effect on primary composite end point of diastolic function; improved E/A with carvedilol
RAAM-PEF	44	Eplerenone	62	70	No effect on 6-min walk distance; collagen turnover and E/e' improved with eplerenone
ELANDD	116	Nebivolol	62.6	66	No effect on 6-min walk distance, peak VO₂, or quality of life
INDIE-HFpEF	105	Inorganic nitrite	64	69	Did not result in significant improvement in exercise capacity
CAPACITY HFpEF	196	Praliciguat	64	70	Did not significantly improve peak VO₂ from baseline to week 12
PARAGON-HF	4822	Sacubitril-valsartan	57	73	Did not result in a significantly lower rate of total hospitalizations for heart failure and death from cardiovascular causes among patients with heart failure and an ejection fraction of 45% or higher
SOCRATES-PRESERVED	477	Vericiguat	≥ 45	73	Did not change NT-proBNP and left atrial volume at 12 wk compared with placebo but was associated with improvements in quality of life
EDIFY	179	Ivabradine	60	72	HR reduction with ivabradine did not improve outcomes
EMPEROR-Preserved	5988	Empagliflozin	>40	72	Reduced the combined risk of CV death or hospitalization
Preserved-HF	324	Dapaglifozin	≥ 45	70	12 wk of dapaglifozin significantly improved patient symptoms, physical limitations, and exercise function

(Continued)

TABLE 76-11 ■ TRIALS FOR HEART FAILURE WITH PRESERVED EJECTION FRACTION (CONTINUED)

		PHARMACOTHERAPY			
TRIAL[a]	PATIENTS	TREATMENT	LVEF(%) MEAN (SD OR RANGE)[b]	AGE MEAN (SD OR RANGE)	OUTCOMES COMPARED TO PLACEBO[c]
LIFESTYLE INTERVENTIONS					
TRAINING-HF	61	Inspiratory muscle training (IMT), functional electrical stimulation (FES), or a combination of both (IMT + FES)	67	74	IMT and FES were associated with a significant improvement in exercise capacity and quality of life
SECRET	100	Diet, exercise, or both for 20 wk	61	67	Among obese older patients with clinically stable HFPEF, caloric restriction or aerobic exercise training increased peak V̇O₂, and the effects may be additive. Neither intervention had a significant effect on quality of life as measured by the MLHF Questionnaire

[a]Trial acronyms: PEP-CHF, Perindopril in Elderly People with Chronic Heart Failure; CHARM-Preserved, Candesartan in Heart failure: Assessment of Reduction in Mortality and morbidity—Preserved LVEF; I-PRESERVE, Irbesartan in Heart Failure with Preserved Ejection Fraction study; SENIORS, Study of the Effects of Nebivolol Intervention on Outcomes and Rehospitalisation in Seniors with Heart Failure; TOPCAT, Treatment of Preserved Cardiac Function Heart Failure with an Aldosterone Antagonist; Aldo-DHF, Aldosterone Receptor Blockade in Diastolic Heart Failure; RELAX, Phosphodiesterase-5 Inhibition to Improve Clinical Status and Exercise Capacity in Heart Failure with Preserved Ejection Fraction; ESS-DHF, Effectiveness of Sitaxsentan Sodium in Patients with Diastolic Heart Failure; DIG Ancillary, Digitalis Investigation Group Ancillary Trial; SWEDIC, Swedish Doppler-echocardiographic Study; RAAM-PEF, Randomized Aldosterone Antagonism in Heart Failure with Preserved Ejection Fraction; ELANDD, Effects of the Long-term Administration of Nebivolol in Diastolic Dysfunction; INDIE-HFpEF, Inorganic Nitrite Delivery to Improve Exercise Capacity in HFpEF; CAPACITY-HFpEF, A Study of the Effect of IW-1973 on the Exercise Capacity of Patients With Heart Failure With Preserved Ejection Fraction (HFpEF); PARAGON-HF, Efficacy and Safety of LCZ696 Compared to Valsartan, on Morbidity and Mortality in Heart Failure Patients With Preserved Ejection Fraction) trial; SOCRATES-PRESERVED, Vericiguat in patients with worsening chronic heart failure and preserved ejection fraction: results of the Soluble guanylate Cyclase stimulatoR in heArT failurE patientS with PRESERVED EF study; EDIFY, The preserved left ventricular ejection fraction chronic heart Failure with ivabradine study; TRAINING-HF, Inspiratory Muscle Training and Functional Electrical Stimulation for Treatment of Heart Failure With Preserved Ejection Fraction Trial; SECRET, Exercise Intolerance in Elderly Patients With Diastolic Heart Failure.

[b]LVEF, left ventricular ejection fraction; E/e' avg, echocardiographic mitral inflow velocity/tissue Doppler velocity ratio; CV, cardiovascular; SCD, sudden cardiac death; HR, hazard ratio (with 95% confidence interval); HF, heart failure.
Age (in years) and LVEF (%) presented as mean ± SD or median (IQR).

[c]All-cause mortality was not significantly reduced in any trial.

At least 70% to 80% of older persons with HFPEF have hypertension, and coronary and valvular heart diseases are also highly prevalent in this population. Treatment for HFPEF begins with aggressive management of hypertension to target levels. Although there is limited data on the ideal blood pressure targets for patients with HFPEF, it may be reasonable to apply the recent observations from SPRINT and recommend systolic blood pressure less than 130 mm Hg and diastolic blood pressure less than 90 mm Hg for most ambulatory, community dwelling, older adults. This target should be personalized on an individual-level, however, accounting for the potential for increased risk of falls in older adults with HFPEF, a subpopulation with a high prevalence of frailty and who frequently take diuretics which can increase risk for orthostatic hypotension. Myocardial ischemia should be treated with antianginal medications and/or coronary revascularization as indicated. Resting and exercise heart rate should be adequately controlled in patients with atrial fibrillation. Patients with severe valvular heart disease should be considered for valve repair or replacement, and less severe regurgitant valvular lesions should be treated with vasodilators, such as ACE inhibitors. As with HFREF, nonpharmacologic aspects of therapy, including regular physical activity and exercise as described earlier, should be appropriately addressed. This, perhaps, is paramount in HFPEF given the paucity of data to date demonstrating beneficial effects from most of the pharmacologic approaches outlined below.

Diuretics Diuretics are an essential component of therapy for the relief of pulmonary and systemic venous congestion in most patients with HFPEF. However, such patients are often "volume sensitive." As a result, overly zealous diuresis can lead to a reduction in left ventricular diastolic volume, with a resultant decline in stroke volume and cardiac output, often manifested by increased fatigue, relative hypotension, and worsening prerenal azotemia. Thus, diuretics must be titrated judiciously to relieve congestion while avoiding over diuresis.

β-Blockers β-Blockers have little or no direct effect on diastolic function, but theoretically could improve symptoms in HFPEF by slowing heart rate and lengthening the diastolic filling period. However, chronotropic incompetence, or the inability to sufficiently increase the heart rate during exercise, is common in HFPEF and may be exacerbated by β-blockers. Effective blood pressure control may aid in the regression of left ventricular hypertrophy if present, but other antihypertensives may be more effective in this regard. When examining the effects of β-blockers on individuals with left ventricular ejection fraction of at least 50% from clinical trials to date, the benefits of β-blockers are not observed and in fact the data suggest an increase in all-cause mortality, although this was not statistically significant. A recent observational study of patients with HFPEF from the TOPCAT study also suggested harm from β-blockers, with increased rates of heart failure hospitalization observed in patients taking β-blocker at baseline. On the other hand, patients with HFPEF frequently contend with coronary artery disease and atrial fibrillation, where β-blockers have previously demonstrated benefit. Whether to continue/initiate a β-blocker is challenging; and deprescribing β-blockers in this setting is also not well-studied. Accordingly, until more data on this topic become available, decisions should be individualized based on the presence of other cardiovascular conditions where β-blockers are indicated, and consideration of the baseline heart rate, preexisting conduction disease, and possible side effects related to β-blocker use.

ACE inhibitors ACE inhibitors may improve symptoms in HFPEF both directly (by improving diastolic function) and indirectly (by promoting regression of left ventricular hypertrophy). The use of ACE inhibitors for the treatment of HFPEF in patients of advanced age is supported by findings from the Perindopril in Elderly People with Chronic Heart Failure study, in which 850 patients greater than or equal to 70 years (mean age 76, 55% women) with heart failure and estimated ejection fraction greater than or equal to 40 were randomized to perindopril 4 mg once daily or placebo and followed for an average of 2.1 years. Overall, there was no significant difference between groups with respect to the primary outcome of death or unplanned hospitalization for heart failure. However, heart failure hospitalizations were significantly reduced by 78% during the first 12 months of follow-up in patients randomized to perindopril. Relative to placebo, perindopril-treated patients also experienced significant improvements in NYHA class and exercise tolerance during the first year of therapy. Perindopril is not approved for the treatment of heart failure in the United States, and none of the other ACE inhibitors are approved for the treatment of HFPEF; however, given that the benefits of perindopril may be a class effect, the use of ACEI may be reasonable in HFPEF, especially when blood pressure is elevated and/or patients have other indications for an ACEI such as diabetes.

Angiotensin II receptor blockers ARBs lower blood pressure and may have salutary effects on diastolic function like those observed with ACE inhibitors. In the CHARM-Preserved Trial, 3024 patients with NYHA class II to IV heart failure and an ejection fraction greater than 40% were randomized to candesartan or placebo and followed for a median of 37 months. The mean age was 67, 27% were 75 years or older, and 40% were women. Mortality did not differ between groups, but patients randomized to candesartan experienced a significant 16% reduction in the risk of hospitalization for heart failure and 29% fewer total heart failure admissions. Subgroup analysis by age was not reported. In large part due to this study, ARBs are now considered reasonable for use to prevent hospitalizations for HFPEF as per the AHA/ACC heart failure guidelines (last updated 2017).

MRAs MRAs spironolactone and eplerenone reduce myocardial hypertrophy and fibrosis in laboratory animals and small studies indicate that they have a favorable effect on left ventricular diastolic function in humans. In addition, as discussed previously, both agents have been shown to improve mortality and other outcomes in patients with HFREF. In a recently published trial, 3445 patients with symptomatic heart failure and an ejection fraction greater than or equal to 45% were randomized to spironolactone or placebo and followed for a mean of 3.3 years. The average age was 69 and 52% were women. The primary outcome, a composite of cardiovascular death, aborted cardiac arrest, or hospitalization for heart failure, did not differ between patients randomized to spironolactone versus placebo. Similarly, total mortality and all-cause hospitalizations were not different between groups. However, hospitalizations for heart failure were reduced 17% among patients randomized to spironolactone ($p = 0.04$). Given some concerns about the study population and study conduct in Europe, post-hoc analyses have been conducted on patients from just North and South America. These data show that spironolactone was associated with a significant 18% reduction in the primary end point, as well as a 26% reduction in cardiovascular mortality and 18% reduction in heart failure rehospitalization. Thus, although additional research is needed, this study suggests that spironolactone may be beneficial for patients with HFPEF. In fact, the FDA is considering approval of MRA therapy for HFPEF based on these data.

Calcium channel blockers Calcium channel blockers decrease intracellular calcium and may have a modest beneficial effect on diastolic function. However, there have been no large clinical trials evaluating calcium channel blockers for the treatment of HFPEF. While calcium channel antagonists are not specifically indicated for the treatment of this condition, they may be helpful to treat other concurrent conditions common in adults with HFPEF such as atrial fibrillation. Caution should be exercised; however, given their potential to worsen cardiac output by impairing chronotropy and inotropy.

Nitrates In addition to relieving ischemia, nitrates are effective venodilators and thus lower pulmonary capillary wedge pressure. For these reasons, nitrates may serve as a useful adjunct to diuretics in relieving symptoms of pulmonary congestion, particularly orthopnea. However, nitrates also have the potential for decreasing venous return to the heart, thereby reducing left ventricular diastolic volume and stroke volume. In addition, tolerance to the hemodynamic effects of nitrates occurs in many patients. A randomized crossover trial of isosorbide mononitrate in subjects with HFPEF did not demonstrate better quality of life or submaximal exercise capacity and demonstrated that nitrates might lead to reduced activity among adults with HFPEF compared to placebo. As a result, use of nitrates for the routine management of HFPEF is not recommended.

Digoxin Digoxin, as well as other inotropic agents, may exert a favorable effect on diastolic function by accelerating calcium reuptake by the sarcoplasmic reticulum at the onset of diastole. In the original DIG trial, 988 patients with heart failure and an ejection fraction of more than 45% were randomized to digoxin or placebo in an ancillary study. As in the main trial, digoxin had no effect on mortality. Hospitalizations for heart failure were reduced in patients with HFPEF receiving digoxin, but this effect was counterbalanced by increased hospitalizations for acute coronary syndromes. Thus, digoxin does not appear to be beneficial in patients with HFPEF and is not recommended except as an adjunct for controlling heart rates in patients with atrial fibrillation.

ARNI While sacubitril/valsartan has demonstrated dramatic benefits in HFREF, its efficacy in HFPEF is less dramatic. In the prospective comparison of ARNI with ARB on management of heart failure with preserved ejection fraction (PARAMOUNT) trial of 301 HFPEF patients, ARNI therapy resulted in lower NTproBNP levels after 12 weeks than valsartan alone. However, in the phase III PARAGON trial among 4822 patients with NYHA class II to IV heart failure, ejection fraction of 45% or higher, elevated level of natriuretic peptides, and structural heart disease, sacubitril-valsartan did not result in a significantly lower rate of total hospitalizations for heart failure and death from cardiovascular causes. Notably in this large trial, there was heterogeneity of treatment effects with possible benefit with sacubitril-valsartan in patients with lower ejection fraction and in women. The FDA has recently approved sacubitril/valsartan therapy for patients with chronic heart failure regardless of ejection fraction, while noting that the drug is most effective in patients with a reduced ejection fraction.

Other agents For patients diagnosed with transthyretin cardiac amyloidosis, tafamidis, a TTR stabilizer, was approved by the FDA and EMU based on the ATTR-ACT trial which showed a lower all-cause mortality vs placebo (29.5% vs 42.9%) and a 32% lower risk of cardiovascular hospitalizations in those treated with tafamidis compared to placebo. Notably, subjects with NYHA class III symptoms in ATTR-ACT had higher rates of cardiovascular-related hospitalization with tafamidis therapy compared to placebo, emphasizing the importance of early diagnosis and treatment. In the ATTR-ACT trial, decline in the distance covered on 6-minute walk test and in the Kansas City Cardiomyopathy Questionnaire overall summary score was slowed with tafamidis therapy. Tafamidis has two formulations, tafamidis meglumine (20 mg capsules, dose 80 mg daily) and tafamidis free salt (61 mg capsule daily), the latter of which was formulated for patient convenience as a single-dose capsule. These formulations are bioequivalent, though are not substitutable on a per-milligram basis. The high cost (list price of $225,000 per year) could limit access.

Preliminary studies of phosphodiesterase 5 inhibitors suggested that these agents may have favorable effects on exercise capacity in patients with HFPEF. However, in the RELAX trial, which randomized 216 patients (mean age 69, 48% women) with heart failure and a left ventricular ejection fraction greater than or equal to 50% to sildenafil or placebo for 24 weeks, sildenafil did not result in significant improvements in exercise capacity or clinical status compared to placebo.

Endothelin type A receptor antagonists have also shown promise for treating HFPEF in preliminary studies. In the Effectiveness of Sitaxsentan Sodium in Patients with Diastolic Heart Failure (ESS-DHF) trial, 192 patients (mean age 65, 63% women) with HFPEF and a left ventricular ejection fraction greater than or equal to 50% were randomly assigned in a 2:1 ratio to receive sitaxsentan or placebo for 24 weeks. The primary outcome was change in treadmill exercise time; secondary outcomes included changes in left ventricular mass, diastolic function, symptom severity, and quality of life. Sitaxsentan therapy showed modest improvement in treadmill exercise time relative to placebo (37 seconds; $p = 0.03$), but there was no effect on any of the secondary outcomes. A recent study examining macitentan in adults with HFPEF and concurrent pulmonary hypertension was recently completed, with results anticipated in 2021.

SGLT2 inhibitors have been investigated in two large trials, DELIVER (evaluating dapagliflozin) and EMPEROR-Preserved (evaluating empagliflozin) in patients with HFPEF. Emperor-Preserved assigned 5988 patients with class II–IV heart failure and an ejection fraction of more than 40% to receive empagliflozin (10 mg once daily) or placebo. Over a median of 26.2 months, the primary endpoint of death or hospitalization for heart failure was lower in the empagliflozin arm (hazard ratio, 0.79; 95% confidence interval [CI], 0.69 to 0.90; P<0.001) mainly related to a lower risk of hospitalization for heart failure. The effects of empagliflozin appeared consistent in patients with or without diabetes.

Summary Studies published to date indicate that ACE inhibitors, ARBs, MRAs, and more recently ARNi may have favorable effects on some outcomes in patients with HFPEF, with only ARNi and SGLT2 therapy approved by the FDA for subjects with an EF greater than 50%. In subgroup analyses of randomized trials, ARNi therapy appears to have a more favorable effect in patients with EF of 40% to 50%, but this group may be more similar in pathophysiology and treatment responsiveness to HFREF. SGLT2 inhibitors can be considered to reduce the risk of hospitalization for heart failure. Consequently, management of HFPEF should include aggressive treatment of the underlying cardiac disease, and a diuretic should be administered at low-to-moderate doses to relieve congestion and edema. The addition of an ACE inhibitor, ARB, MRAs, ARNi, SGLT2 inhibitor, or β-blocker to improve symptoms and reduce the risk of hospitalization may be reasonable in some cases, but this will require individualization. Given lack of consistent data on its benefits, alternative treatment should be considered if/when these agents are not tolerated or lead to worse outcomes. Additional studies to evaluate novel therapies are ongoing and represent an important opportunity for older adults to participate and ensure that they are well-represented in these trials.

Isolated Right Heart Failure

While the most common cause of chronic right-sided heart failure is one or more abnormalities of left heart function, a small proportion of patients present with isolated right heart failure. Etiologies of isolated right heart failure in older adults include pulmonary arterial hypertension due to chronic lung disease, chronic pulmonary thromboembolic disease, sleep-disordered breathing, primary pulmonary vascular disease, and disorders of the tricuspid or (less commonly) pulmonic valve (eg, infectious endocarditis, carcinoid heart disease). Rarely, right heart failure in older patients may be attributed to congenital heart disease (eg, atrial septal defect), neoplasm (eg, right atrial myxoma or rhabdomyosarcoma), or a primary cardiomyopathy involving the right ventricle (eg, arrhythmogenic right ventricular dysplasia). Acute right heart failure may be due to right ventricular infarction, massive or sub-massive pulmonary embolism, or severe lung disease (eg, pneumonia, acute respiratory distress syndrome). Symptoms of right heart failure include dyspnea, impaired exercise tolerance, dependent edema, and, in severe cases, abdominal discomfort and swelling. The physical examination is notable for signs of elevated right-sided pressures (jugular venous distension, abdominojugular reflux, right ventricular heave, hepatomegaly), lower extremity edema, and possibly ascites. Depending on the etiology, other symptoms and signs may be present. Treatment is directed primarily at the underlying cause(s) and secondarily at alleviating systemic congestion through the judicious use of diuretics. The value of other pharmacologic agents, such as β-blockers and renin-angiotensin system inhibitors, for the treatment of isolated right heart failure is unknown.

Advanced Heart Failure

Refractory or advanced heart failure may be defined as heart failure not amenable to primary corrective measures (eg, valve replacement or revascularization) and not responsive to aggressive nonpharmacologic and pharmacologic therapy as described earlier. However, before designating heart failure as refractory, it is important to perform a careful search for potentially treatable causes, to carefully review the patient's medication regimen to ensure that therapy is optimal, and to discuss the patient's diet and medication habits in detail with the patient and family to ensure that an appropriate level of adherence is being maintained. The latter issue is of particular importance, since many cases of refractory heart failure can be traced to nonadherence to dietary restrictions, medications, or both.

In most cases, refractory or advanced heart failure simply represents the final common pathway of end-stage heart disease. Under these circumstances, the value of highly aggressive treatment is questionable, and decisions regarding the appropriateness of specific therapeutic interventions must be made on an individualized basis (see also Chapters 7 and 67).

In patients with persistent pulmonary congestion or peripheral edema, high-dose oral diuretics (eg, furosemide 200 mg BID or bumetanide 10 mg daily), alone or in combination with metolazone, may be effective. Alternatively, a continuous intravenous infusion of furosemide 5 to 40 mg/h or bumetanide 0.5 to 1 mg/h may facilitate diuresis.

The use of intravenous inotropic agents in the management of chronic heart failure is somewhat controversial since these agents have not been shown to improve outcomes and they may increase the risk of life-threatening arrhythmias. Nonetheless, extensive clinical experience indicates that continuous infusions of dobutamine or milrinone may reduce symptoms and improve quality of life in selected patients with refractory heart failure. The use of intravenous inotropic agents at home can also be used for select patients for the purposes of bridging them to advanced therapies or for the purposes of palliation.

As noted earlier, CRT has been shown to improve symptoms, quality of life, and survival in patients with advanced heart failure and left bundle branch block or marked intraventricular conduction delay on the 12-lead electrocardiogram. This procedure should, therefore, be considered in appropriately selected patients with persistent class III or IV heart failure symptoms.

An emerging therapy for patients with end-stage refractory heart failure (primarily HFREF) is mechanical circulatory support through implantation of a left ventricular assist device (LVAD). LVADs improve symptoms, exercise tolerance, quality of life, and survival in selected patients with severe heart failure, including patients in their 70s and early 80s. Although LVADs were originally developed as a bridge to heart transplantation, with technological advances they are now commonly implanted as "destination therapy" in patients who are not transplant candidates. As a result, an increasing number of older adults are receiving LVADs, and this trend is likely to continue as the technology evolves. Older adults are at increased risk for gastrointestinal bleeding following LVAD implantation; other potential complications include infection, stroke, and pump thrombosis. Optimal patient selection is critical, and patients with advanced comorbidities or frailty may not be suitable candidates. To this end, a thorough discussion of goals of care, facilitated by a palliative care team consultation, (which is required by CMS guidelines to be formally part of the LVAD team), is recommended as an integral component of the evaluation for LVAD therapy.

Heart transplantation is a highly effective therapy for patients with advanced heart failure, but its use is limited by the paucity of donor hearts. In part due to limited organ availability coupled with issues of immunosuppression in older adults and the increased risk of infection, most transplant centers exclude patients older than 70 to 75 years. Nonetheless, among carefully selected patients greater than or equal to 65 years undergoing heart transplantation, outcomes are favorable and generally similar to those in younger patients.

PROGNOSIS

The long-term prognosis in patients with established heart failure is poor, and the 5-year survival rate among older adults is less than 50%. In patients greater than or equal to 80 years old hospitalized with heart failure, fewer than 25% survive more than 5 years. In general, the prognosis is worse in men than in women and in patients with an ischemic rather than nonischemic etiology. Patients with more severe symptoms or exercise intolerance, as defined by the NYHA functional class or as assessed by a 6-minute walk test, also have a less favorable outlook. Other markers of an adverse prognosis include elevated BNP; low systolic blood pressure; hyponatremia; renal insufficiency; anemia; peripheral arterial disease; cognitive dysfunction; and the presence of atrial fibrillation or high-grade ventricular arrhythmias. In patients with chronic heart failure, 40% to 50% die from progressive heart failure, 40% die from arrhythmias, and 10% to 20% die from other causes (eg, myocardial infarction or noncardiac conditions). Notably, the proportion dying from noncardiac causes rises with advancing age owing to other comorbid conditions and the concurrence of geriatric conditions such as cognitive impairment and frailty. As a means to embed prognosis into medical decision-making, it may be reasonable to apply the domain management approach to caring for older adults with heart failure, where multiple domains of health across medical (multimorbidity, polypharmacy, malnutrition), mind/emotion (depression, anxiety, cognitive impairment), functional (frailty, impaired mobility, functional impairment, history of falls), and social environment (social support, financial means) are considered in the care of older adults.

ADVANCE CARE PLANNING AND END-OF-LIFE DECISIONS

Overall survival rates for patients with heart failure are lower than for most forms of cancer. In addition, once heart failure symptoms have reached an advanced stage (eg, NYHA class III or IV), quality of life is often severely compromised and therapeutic options are limited. Moreover, even patients with relatively mild or well-compensated heart failure are continually at risk of experiencing sudden cardiac arrest, and, if initial resuscitative efforts are successful, questions regarding life support and related issues may arise.

For these reasons, it is incumbent upon the physician to discuss the patient's wishes regarding the intensity of treatment and end-of-life care at a time when the patient is still capable of understanding the issues and making informed choices. In addition, since the patient's views may evolve over the course of illness, these issues should be readdressed at periodic intervals. The development of an advance directive and appointment of durable power of attorney should also be encouraged (see Chapters 7 and 26).

A related concern is the extent to which clinicians should offer aggressive or investigational therapeutic options that are unlikely to substantially alter the natural history of disease or significantly improve quality of life. This concern applies not only to many of the treatment modalities discussed in the Advanced Heart Failure section earlier, but also to such procedures as admission to an intensive care unit and endotracheal intubation. In many cases, these interventions not only fail to modify the clinical course but contribute to the patient's pain and suffering in the terminal stages of disease. Moreover, the suggestion that a given intervention may help stabilize the patient and slow disease progression may create false hopes in the minds of the patient and family, and subsequent failure of the intervention may compound the emotional suffering that both the patient and the family are forced to endure. For these reasons, it is essential that the clinician realistically appraise the potential benefits and attendant risks, both physical and emotional, prior to offering aggressive therapeutic options that may provide little or no hope of improving the patient's quality of life over a clinically important period of time. In this context, it is often appropriate to offer transition to a palliative care approach and to obtain consultation from a palliative care specialist.

Finally, as the patient approaches the terminal stages of disease, there should be discussions with the patient and family regarding where the patient would like to spend his or her final days. For many patients, the idea of dying at home surrounded by close family is comforting, and this desire should be honored whenever possible. Often home hospice affords optimal end-of-life care in the home environment by providing effective symptom control, as well as emotional, spiritual, and caregiver support. Home hospice is also associated with higher levels of patient and family satisfaction with care in most cases, though caregiver burden may be higher than in an inpatient setting. For some patients, the hospital or an inpatient hospice may be the preferred environment for terminal care, but an attempt should be made to secure a private room with open visitation hours. The intensive care unit, with its austere, "high-tech" facade, may be the least desirable place to die, and this should be avoided whenever possible.

PREVENTION

In view of the exceptionally poor prognosis associated with established heart failure in older adults, it is essential to develop and implement preventive strategies. Appropriate treatment of hypertension has been repeatedly shown to reduce the incidence of heart failure by 50% or more. In the Hypertension in the Very Elderly Trial, for example, treatment of hypertension was associated with a 64% reduction in incident heart failure among patients 80 years or older, and, similarly, the intensive, less than 120 mm Hg arm in the SPRINT study was found to result in a 36% lower rate of acute decompensated HF compared to the standard, 140 mm Hg arm. (Additional details are in Chapter 79.) The St. Vincent's Screening to Prevent Heart Failure (STOP-HF) and N-terminal Pro-brain Natriuretic Peptide Guided Primary Prevention of Cardiovascular Events in Diabetic Patients (PONTIAC) trials have shown that natriuretic peptide-based screening and targeted prevention can reduce heart failure and left ventricular dysfunction and other major cardiovascular events. Treatment of hyperlipidemia has also been shown to reduce the incidence of heart failure, most likely through prevention of myocardial infarction and other ischemic events. Likewise, smoking cessation and regular exercise reduce the risk of myocardial infarction and stroke in older adults and likely have similar effects on the development of heart failure. Unfortunately, despite abundant evidence that heart failure prevention is feasible through risk factor modification, such strategies are underused, especially in persons older than 80 years.

SUMMARY

Heart failure is a common and important clinical problem in older adults, owing, in large part, to the complex interplay between age-related changes in the cardiovascular system, the high prevalence of cardiovascular and noncardiovascular disorder in the older population, and the widespread use of certain drugs and other therapies that may adversely affect cardiovascular physiology. As the population continues to age, heart failure will have a progressively greater impact on health care delivery systems. The impact of heart failure on quality of life and independence in the growing number of older adults with this disorder is incalculable. Thus, there is a compelling need to develop and implement strategies for the prevention and treatment of heart failure, with particular emphasis on the geriatric population.

ACKNOWLEDGEMENT

This chapter was based on the many previous versions authored by our colleague, Dr. Mike Rich, who not only taught us much of what we know about Geriatric Cardiology but has been an inspiring leader and is considered by many as the founder of our field. His mentorship has fostered a new generation of cardiologists and geriatricians dedicated to the care of older adults with cardiovascular disease and benefited countless lives.

FURTHER READING

Afilalo J, Alexander KP, Mack MJ, et al. Frailty assessment in the cardiovascular care of older adults. *J Am Coll Cardiol*. 2014;63(8):747–762.

Anker SD, Butler J, Filippatos G, et al.; EMPEROR-Preserved Trial Investigators. Empagliflozin in heart failure with a preserved ejection fraction. *N Engl J Med*. 2021;385(16):1451–1461.

Beckett NS, Peters R, Fletcher AE, et al. Treatment of hypertension in patients 80 years of age or older. *N Engl J Med*. 2008;358:1887–1898.

Chaudhry SI, Wang Y, Gill TM, Krumholz HM. Geriatric conditions and subsequent mortality in older patients with heart failure. *J Am Coll Cardiol*. 2010;55:309–316.

Cleland JGF, Tendera M, Adamus J, Freemantle N, Polonski L, Taylor J. The perindopril in elderly people with chronic heart failure (PEP-CHF) study. *Eur Heart J*. 2006;27:2238–2245.

DeFilippis EM, Nakagawa S, Maurer MS, Topkara VK. Left ventricular assist device therapy in older adults: addressing common clinical questions. *J Am Geriatr Soc*. 2019;67(11):2410–2419.

Feltner C, Jones CD, Cene CW, et al. Transitional care interventions to prevent readmissions for persons with heart failure. A systematic review and meta-analysis. *Ann Intern Med*. 2014;160:774–784.

Flather MD, Shibata MC, Coats AJ, et al. Randomized trial to determine the effect of nebivolol on mortality and cardiovascular hospital admission in elderly patients with heart failure (SENIORS). *Eur Heart J*. 2005;26:215–225.

Forman DE, Arena R, Boxer R, et al. American Heart Association Council on Clinical Cardiology; Council on Cardiovascular and Stroke Nursing; Council on Quality of Care and Outcomes Research; and Stroke Council. Prioritizing functional capacity as a principal end point for therapies oriented to older adults with cardiovascular disease: a scientific statement for healthcare professionals from the American Heart Association. *Circulation*. 2017;135(16):e894–e918.

Gorodeski EZ, Goyal P, Hummel SL, et al. Domain management approach to heart failure in the geriatric patient: present and future. *J Am Coll Cardiol*. 2018;71(17):1921–1936.

Gurwitz JH, Magid DJ, Smith DH, et al. Contemporary prevalence and correlates of incident heart failure with preserved ejection fraction. *Am J Med*. 2013;126:393–400.

1192 Heidenreich PA, Albert NM, Allen LA, et al. Forecasting the impact of heart failure in the United States: a policy statement from the American Heart Association. *Circ Heart Fail*. 2013;6:606–619.

Homma S, Thompson JLP, Pullicino PM, et al. Warfarin and aspirin in patients with heart failure and sinus rhythm. *N Engl J Med*. 2012;366:1859–1869.

Jurgens CY, Goodlin S, Dolansky M, et al. Heart failure management in skilled nursing facilities: a scientific statement from the American Heart Association and the Heart Failure Society of America. *Circ Heart Fail*. 2015;8:655–687.

Lakatta EG, Levy D. Arterial and cardiac aging: major shareholders in cardiovascular disease enterprises: Part I: aging arteries: a "set up" for vascular disease. *Circulation*. 2003;107(1):139–146.

Lakatta EG, Levy D. Arterial and cardiac aging: major shareholders in cardiovascular disease enterprises: Part II: the aging heart in health: links to heart disease. *Circulation*. 2003;107(2):346–354.

Mentz RJ, Kelly JP, von Lueder TG, et al. Noncardiac comorbidities in heart failure with reduced versus preserved ejection fraction. *J Am Coll Cardiol*. 2014;64:2281–2293.

Nassif ME, Windsor SL, Borlaug BA, et. al. The SGLT2 inhibitor dapagliflozin in heart failure with preserved ejection fraction: a multicenter randomized trial. *Nat Med*. 2021;27(11):1954–1960.

Pitt B, Pfeffer MA, Assmann SF, et al. Spironolactone for heart failure with preserved ejection fraction. *N Engl J Med*. 2014;370:1383–1392.

Rich MW, Chyun DA, Skolnick AH, et al. Knowledge gaps in cardiovascular care of the older adult population: a scientific statement from the American Heart Association, American College of Cardiology, and American Geriatrics Society. *Circulation*. 2016;133(21):2103–2122.

Saczynski JS, Go AS, Magid DJ, et al. Patterns of comorbidity in older adults with heart failure: the Cardiovascular Research Network PRESERVE study. *J Am Geriatr Soc*. 2013;61:26–33.

Santangeli P, Di Blase L, Dello Russo A, et al. Meta-analysis: age and effectiveness of prophylactic implantable cardioverter-defibrillators. *Ann Intern Med*. 2010;153: 592–599.

Solomon SD, McMurray JJV, Anand IS, et al. PARAGON-HF Investigators and Committees. Angiotensin-neprilysin inhibition in heart failure with preserved ejection fraction. *N Engl J Med*. 2019;381(17):1609–1620.

Upadhya B, Stacey RB, Kitzman DW. Preventing heart failure by treating systolic hypertension: what does the SPRINT add? *Curr Hypertens Rep*. 2019;21(1):9.

Virani SS, Alonso A, Benjamin EJ, et al. American Heart Association Council on Epidemiology and Prevention Statistics Committee and Stroke Statistics Subcommittee. Heart Disease and Stroke Statistics-2020 Update: a report from the American Heart Association. *Circulation*. 2020;141(9):e139–e596.

Whelan DJ, Goodlin SJ, Dickinson MG, et al. End-of-life care in patients with heart failure. *J Cardiac Fail*. 2014; 20:121–134.

Yancy CW, Jessup M, Bozkurt B, et al. 2017 ACC/AHA/HFSA Focused Update of the 2013 ACCF/AHA Guideline for the Management of Heart Failure: A Report of the American College of Cardiology/American Heart Association Task Force on Clinical Practice Guidelines and the Heart Failure Society of America. *J Card Fail*. 2017;23(8):628–651.

Chapter 77

Cardiac Arrhythmias

Nway Le Ko Ko, Win-Kuang Shen

INTRODUCTION

This chapter is to provide an overview of conditions related to cardiac rhythm disorders with a focus on the older population. Terms used in this chapter such as "older patients" or "older population" are generally referring to patients older than 65 years unless otherwise stated based on specific referenced clinical investigations.

SYNCOPE

The incidence of syncope is high in the older population with a sharp increase in incidence after 70 years and is usually associated with poor outcome—there is a greater risk of hospitalization and death related to syncope in older adults. They are vulnerable to syncope due to age-related changes in cardiovascular and autonomic nervous system, comorbid conditions, polypharmacy, and decreased ability to conserve intravascular volume. In many instances, syncope is multifactorial in an older adult with many predisposing factors presenting simultaneously. Thence, a comprehensive multidisciplinary approach is often necessary for diagnosis and management. Guideline-directed evaluation and management of patients with syncope have been published by ACC/AHA/HRS (2017) and by ESC (2018). For the objectives of this chapter, pertinent conditions causing syncope in the older populations are discussed in this section.

Orthostatic Hypotension

Orthostatic hypotension (OH) is a common cause of syncope in the geriatric population, with a prevalence of 30% among those older than 75 years, and up to 50% among frail older adults living in nursing homes. OH is defined as a sustained decline of more than or equal to 20 mm Hg in systolic or more than or equal to 10 mm Hg in diastolic blood pressure upon standing. There are four types of OH (**Table 77-1**). OH can be caused by impaired autonomic reflexes resulting in pooling of blood upon standing, reduced vasoconstriction, and cerebral hypoperfusion with resultant syncope. An older adult has decreased heart rate responsiveness to postural changes and diminished baroreceptor sensitivity, which impair the ability to adapt to orthostatic stress. Also, reduced concentrations of plasma aldosterone, coupled with impaired thirst and

Learning Objectives

- Review guideline-directed management of syncope with a focus on conditions relevant to the older population.
- Understand the etiologies of bradyarrhythmia, indications for permanent pacemaker (PPM) placement, and selection of the PPM mode.
- Discuss the goals of rate and rhythm control and approach to anticoagulation in older patients with atrial fibrillation (AF).
- Summarize the management of supraventricular tachycardia (SVT) in the older population.
- Understand ventricular tachycardia (VT) in the older population along with indications for implantable cardioverter-defibrillator (ICD) for primary and secondary sudden cardiac death (SCD) prevention.
- Review indications for cardiac resynchronization therapy (CRT).

Key Clinical Points

1. Age-related changes throughout the heart and conduction system predispose older individuals to syncope, bradycardia, atrial fibrillation, and supraventricular and ventricular tachyarrhythmias.

2. Syncope is common in the older population. It is a clinical manifestation associated with cardiac arrhythmias or other conditions altering cerebral perfusion causing transient loss of consciousness.

3. The indications for a PPM for treatment of bradyarrhythmia are similar in older and younger patients. More than 80% of permanent PPMs are placed in patients 65 years or older, with sinoatrial dysfunction being the leading indication for PPM implantation in this age group.

(Continued)

(Cont.)

4. Compared with single-chamber ventricular pacing, dual-chamber pacing reduces the risk of AF but does not affect mortality or the risk of stroke.

5. Age greater than 65 years is a well-recognized risk factor for thromboembolism in patients with AF. Treatment for stroke prevention in patients with atrial fibrillation is based on the CHA_2DS_2-VASc risk stratification scheme.

6. In asymptomatic or mildly symptomatic patients with AF, a strategy of pharmacologic rate control and anticoagulation is associated with similar or better outcomes than a strategy of rhythm control.

7. In patients with symptomatic AF refractory to pharmacologic treatment, various catheter-based ablation procedures, as well as the surgical maze procedure, provide effective control of rate and/or arrhythmia in selected groups of older patients.

8. The indications for implantable cardioverter-defibrillator (ICD) and cardiac resynchronization therapy (CRT) are similar in older and younger patients, as are the benefits in terms of reducing mortality and improving symptoms. However, limited data are available on the outcomes from these devices in patients older than 80 years.

polypharmacy (diuretics and vasodilators), place older patients at risk of volume depletion. Underlying autonomic insufficiency such as autonomic neuropathy, diabetic neuropathy, amyloidosis, or neurologic disorders like Parkinson disease (Shy-Drager Syndrome) should be considered in older patients presenting with recurrent orthostatic syncope. Postprandial syncope is a subtype of orthostatic syncope occurring within 30 to 90 minutes of food consumption resulting from pooling of blood in splanchnic circulation. Treatments include withdrawing offending medications, liberalization of salt and fluid intake, slowly rising from a supine position, avoidance of prolonged standing, wearing compression stockings and physical countermeasures like crossing legs when standing. Pharmacologic therapy includes midodrine or fludrocortisone to improve hypotension. Small and frequent meals as well as cold water ingestion are recommended to alleviate postprandial syncope and octreotide may be beneficial to those with recurrent postprandial syncope. These treatment options need to be individualized due to the frequent presence of comorbid conditions in older patients.

Neurocardiogenic Syncope (Vasovagal Syncope or VVS)

Vasovagal syncope (VVS) is the most common form of syncope in younger population, but it occurs not infrequently in older patients. The pathophysiology of VVS results from a reflex causing hypotension and bradycardia, triggered by prolonged standing or exposure to emotional stress, pain, or medical procedures. It is typically associated with a prodrome of diaphoresis, warmth, and pallor, and with fatigue after the event. These clinical characteristics are often more subtle or absent in older patients. Three types of vasovagal response are summarized in **Table 77-2**. Conservative, nonpharmacologic management (such as counterpressure maneuvers, orthostatic training, liberalization of salt and fluid) may help, but no specific medical therapy has been proven widely effective. Pacemaker therapy may be beneficial in older patients with a predominant cardioinhibitory VVS. The 2017 ACC/AHA/HRS Guideline for the Evaluation and Management of Patients with Syncope recommends dual-chamber pacing as reasonable for patients older than 40 years with recurrent VVS and spontaneous pauses. Closed loop stimulation (CLS) is a new pacing technology that detects local impedance changes in the right ventricle (RV), which may be related to RV preload and contractility. Early detection of impedance changes from the RV pacemaker lead to initiate pacing that may

TABLE 77-1 ■ TYPES OF ORTHOSTATIC HYPOTENSION (OH)

Initial (immediate) OH	A transient BP decreases within 15 s after standing
Classic OH	A sustained reduction of systolic BP of ≥ 20 mm Hg or diastolic BP of ≥ 10 mm Hg within 3 min of assuming upright posture
Delayed OH	A sustained reduction of systolic BP of ≥ 20 mm Hg or diastolic BP of ≥ 10 mm Hg in > 3 min of assuming upright posture
Neurogenic OH	A subtype of OH that is due to dysfunction of the autonomic nervous system and not solely due to environmental triggers (eg, dehydration or drugs)

TABLE 77-2 ■ THREE TYPES OF VASOVAGAL RESPONSE

Cardioinhibitory response	Pauses of ≥ 3 s or heart rate < 40 bpm for more than 10 s
Vasodepressor response	Systolic BP falls by 50 mm Hg or more without symptoms or 30 to 50 mm Hg with symptoms of syncope or presyncope, and the heart rate does not decrease by more than 10%
Mixed response	Heart rate decreases but the ventricular rate does not fall below 40 bpm for more than 10 s, and there are no pauses > 3 s; BP usually decreases before the heart rate drop

prevent the activation of cardioinhibitory VV reflex. Preliminary data from two recent clinical trials demonstrated significant reduction of recurrent syncope in patients randomized to CLS pacing.

Carotid Sinus Syndrome

Carotid sinus hypersensitivity (CSH) is common in the older population with prevalence estimated to be as high as 30% among older individuals presenting with unexplained falls. It is defined as greater than or equal to 3-second pause or a decrease in systolic blood pressure greater than or equal to 50 mm Hg during carotid sinus massage (CSM). Carotid sinus syndrome (CSS) is defined when CSH is associated with symptoms of syncope or presyncope. CSM should be a routine part of examination in older patients presenting with syncope, unless there is a carotid bruit or transient ischemic attack, stroke, or myocardial infarction within the prior 3 months. Observational and randomized studies have shown that recurrent symptoms are significantly reduced after PPM implantation in patients with CSS. Dual-chamber pacing is recommended, although data are lacking from randomized trials. Newer pacing algorithms, such as the "rate-drop response" or "sudden-brady response," which accelerates the pacing rate when bradycardia is detected, are available. However, the clinical utility of these newer algorithms has not shown to be superior to conventional PPMs.

Cardiogenic Syncope

Cardiogenic syncope is caused by arrhythmia (bradyarrhythmia or tachyarrhythmia) or hypotension due to low cardiac index (cardiogenic shock, reduced cardiac filling from cardiac tamponade or restrictive cardiomyopathy, or infiltrative cardiomyopathy such as amyloidosis, etc.) or blood flow obstruction (flow obstruction from valvular stenosis or hypertrophic obstructive cardiomyopathy [HOCM]). Characteristics associated with increased probability of cardiac syncope are older age, male gender, presence of known heart disease (tachyarrhythmia, bradyarrhythmia, coronary artery disease [CAD], structural heart disease, reduced ventricular function, congenital heart disease), syncope with brief prodrome (eg, palpitation) or no prodrome, syncope during exertion or supine syncope, low number of previous syncopal episodes, and family history of sudden cardiac death (SCD). Treatments of syncope due to bradycardia or tachycardia are discussed in the following sections. Treatment of low cardiac output in the setting of structural heart disease or blood flow obstruction is beyond the scope of this chapter.

BRADYARRHYTHMIA

Bradycardia is common in older patients even without apparent cardiovascular disease. With advancing age, the number of cardiac myocytes declines, while residual myocytes enlarge with concurrent increased elastic and collagenous tissue in the interstitial matrix and conduction system. In addition to these age-related structural changes, prolongation of cellular action potential duration and diminished autonomic response further increase the propensity for bradycardia. Clinical bradycardia can be categorized by sinus node dysfunction (SND) and atrioventricular conduction block (AVB).

Sinus Node Dysfunction

Sinus node dysfunction (SND), historically known as sick sinus syndrome (SSS), is related to age-dependent progressive fibrosis of sinus nodal tissue, and surrounding atrial myocardium and hence, occurs more commonly in older patients. Extrinsic causes include myocardial ischemia or infarction, infiltrative diseases, collagen vascular disease, surgical trauma, endocrine abnormalities, autonomic effects, and neuromuscular disorders. Patients with SND may present with persistent sinus bradycardia, sinus arrest, or sinoatrial exit block (**Figure 77-1A-D**). The severity of symptoms such as lightheadedness, exercise intolerance, presyncope, or syncope generally correlates with the heart rate or the pause duration. In older patients with SND, paroxysmal atrial tachycardia (AT) or atrial fibrillation (AF) often are concurrently present (tachy-brady syndrome).

The benefit of PPM is to relieve symptoms and to improve quality of life (QOL) in patients with SND.

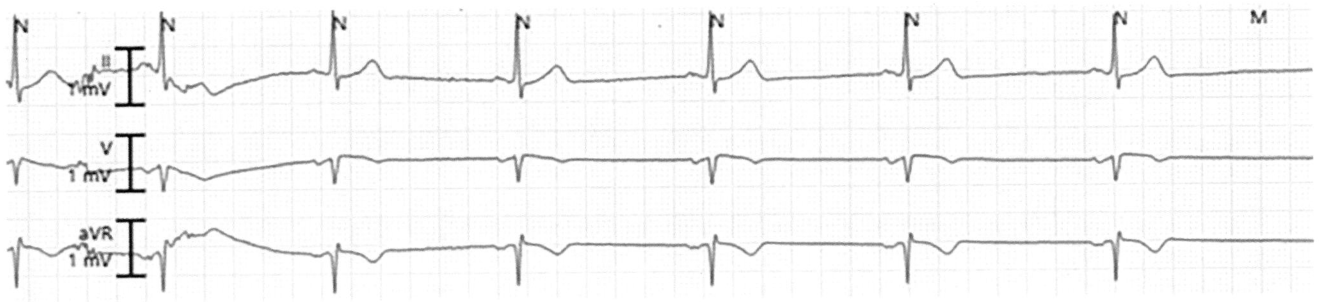

FIGURE 77-1A. Sinus bradycardia (sinus rate < 60 bpm). In this telemetry tracing, the heart rate is 42 bpm.

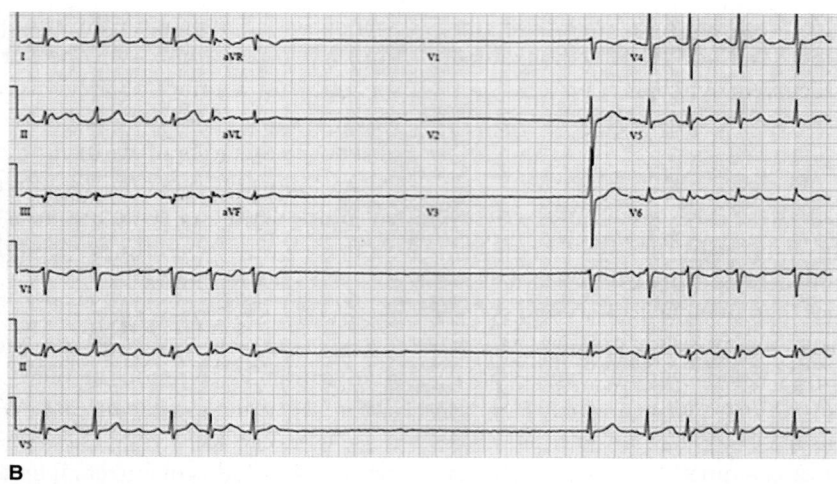

B

FIGURE 77-1B. Sinus arrest of 4.2 seconds in a patient with paroxysmal atrial fibrillation/flutter and sinus node dysfunction.

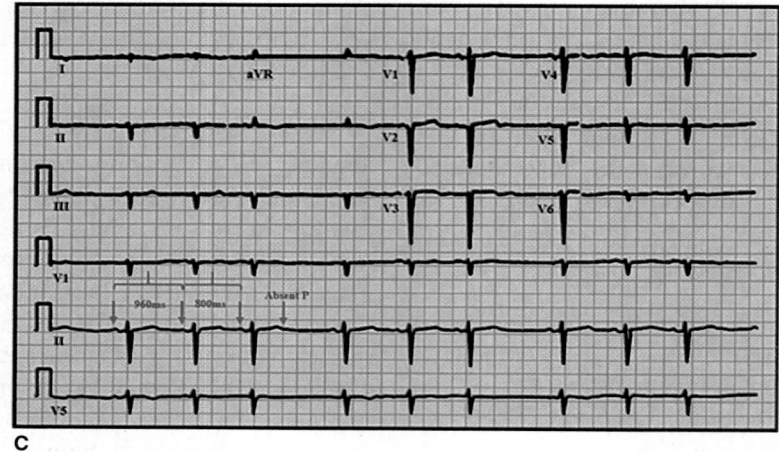

C

FIGURE 77-1C. Sinoatrial exit block, type I. There is progressive shortening of P-P interval before the absence of the next P wave.

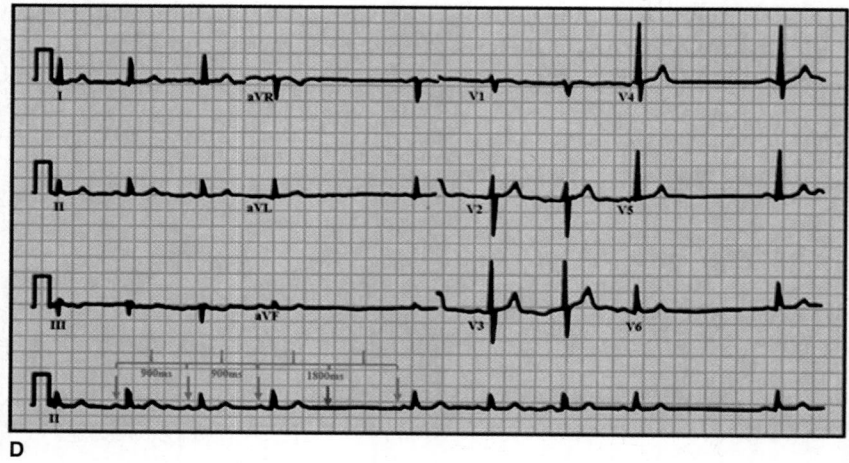

D

FIGURE 77-1D. Sinoatrial exit block type II. The P-P interval is constant before the absence of the next P wave. The pause, due to the absence of the next P wave (denoted by the red arrow), is exactly twice the previous P-P interval.

TABLE 77-3 ■ INDICATIONS AND SELECTION OF PACEMAKER (PPM) THERAPY IN SINUS NODE DYSFUNCTION (SND)

- PPM for symptomatic SND not attributable to reversible or physiologic causes
- PPM for symptomatic SND as a consequence of medication required for treating other coexisting conditions
- Single-chamber atrial-based PPM when there is no evidence of AV conduction abnormality
- Dual-chamber PPM when there is evidence of AV conduction abnormalities

Before PPM is considered, transient reversible causes should be corrected. The synopsis on indications and selection of PPM for SND from 2018 ACC/AHA/HRS bradyarrhythmia guideline can be found in **Table 77-3**. Based on randomized studies comparing atrial-based pacing (single-chamber AAI or dual-chamber DDD) versus single-chamber ventricular-based pacing (VVI), the incidence of AF is higher in ventricular-based pacing. The ventricular-based pacing causes pacemaker syndrome due to uncoordinated atrial and ventricular depolarization leading to valvular regurgitation and heart failure symptoms. However, for patients with symptomatic SND that is infrequent or in those who are frail/bedridden with limited functional capacity or unfavorable prognosis (survival <1 year), single-chamber ventricular pacing could be considered to reduce complications related to the pacemaker implantation. When single ventricular pacing is deemed appropriate, a leadless pacemaker could be considered in selected patients. A standard dual-chamber PPM is shown in **Figure 77-2A, B**; a contemporary single-chamber leadless PPM is shown in **Figure 77-3A, B**.

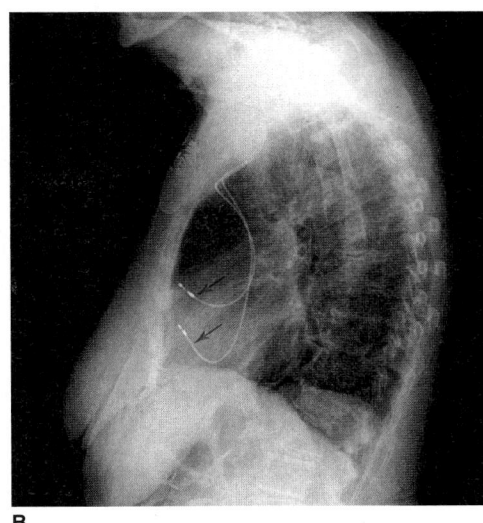

FIGURE 77-2B. Chest X-ray lateral view showing dual-chamber pacemaker with right atrial and right ventricular leads (green arrow indicates the atrial lead and red arrow indicates the right ventricular lead).

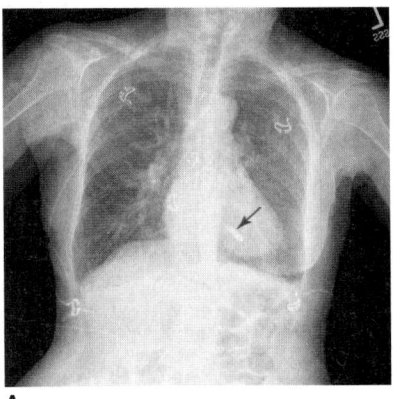

FIGURE 77-3A. Chest X-ray AP view showing a leadless pacemaker (arrowed).

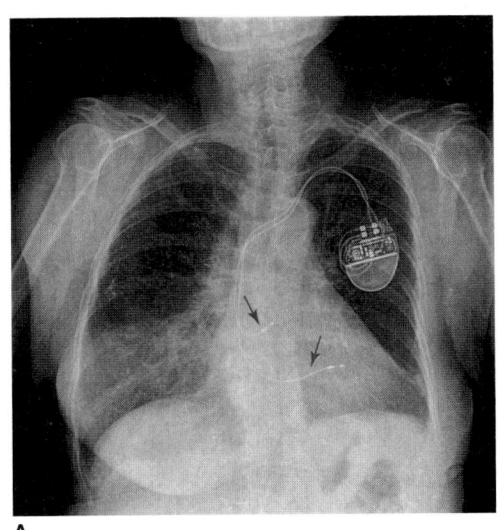

FIGURE 77-2A. Chest X-ray AP view showing dual-chamber pacemaker with right atrial and right ventricular leads (green arrow indicates the atrial lead and red arrow indicates the right ventricular lead).

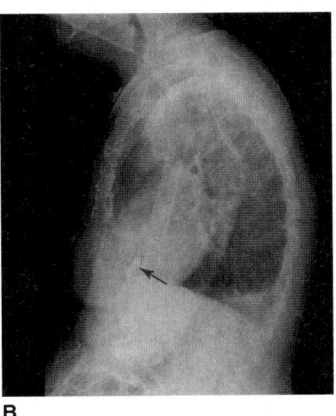

FIGURE 77-3B. Chest X-ray lateral view showing a leadless pacemaker (arrowed).

Atrioventricular conduction block (AVB) is mostly degenerative in nature due to fibrosis in the conduction system including the AV node, His bundle, bundle branches, and Purkinjie to myocardium connection. There are three degrees of AVB (first degree, second degree with Mobitz type I or type 2, and third degree AVB). The ECG characteristics of AVB are shown in **Figure 77-4A-F**.

In patients with AVB, transient reversible causes should be corrected before PPM is considered. A synopsis on indications and selection of PPM for AVB from the 2018 ACC/AHA/HRS bradyarrhythmia guideline can be found in **Table 77-4**.

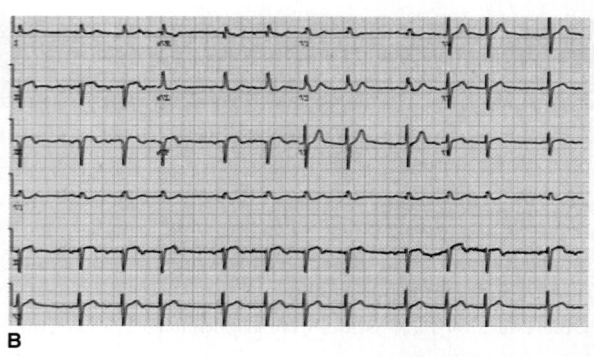

FIGURE 77-4B. Mobitz 1 AVB (P waves with a constant rate with a periodic single nonconducted P wave associated with progressive prolongation of PR interval before the nonconducted P wave – Wenckebach phenomenon).

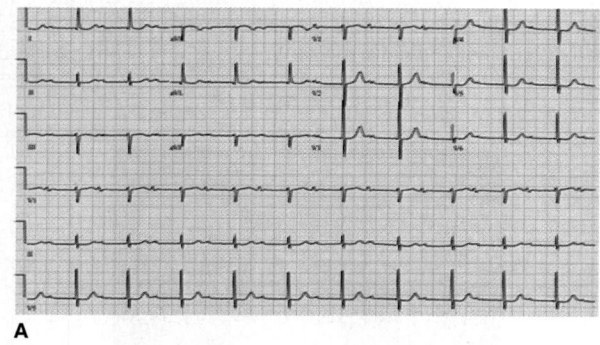

FIGURE 77-4A. First-degree AVB (P waves associated with 1:1 atrioventricular conduction and a PR interval > 200 ms). In this figure, PR interval is 460 ms.

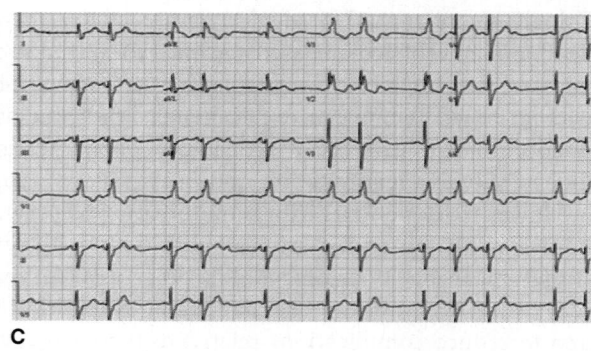

FIGURE 77-4C. Mobitz type II AVB (P waves with a constant rate with a periodic single nonconducted P wave associated with constant PR interval before and after the nonconducted P wave).

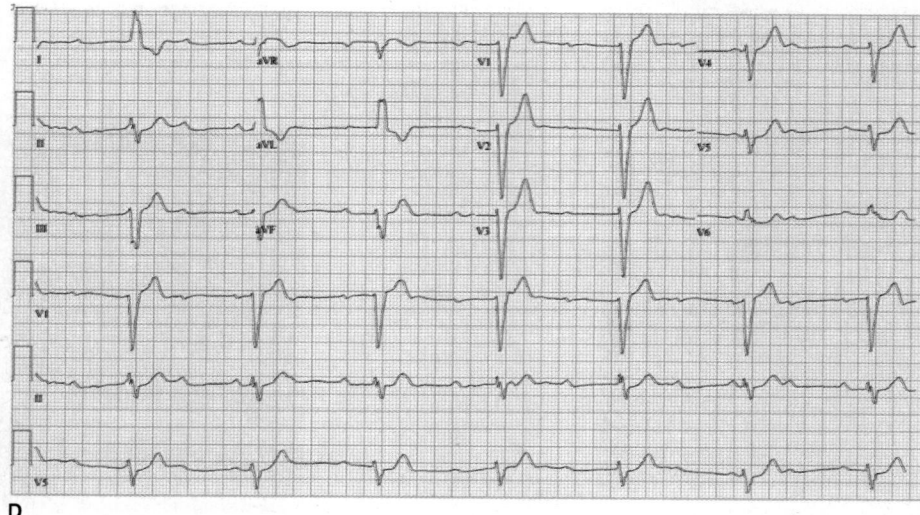

FIGURE 77-4D. Complete AVB (P waves with constant rate and QRS complexes with constant rate without evidence of AV conduction).

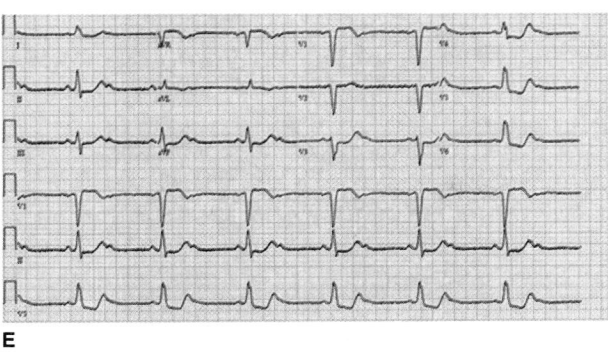

E

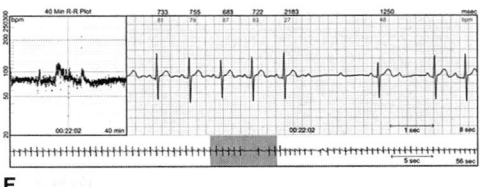

F

FIGURE 77-4F. Holter monitoring tracing showing high-grade AVB (≥ 2 consecutive P waves at a constant physiologic rate that do not conduct to the ventricles).

FIGURE 77-4E. 2:1 AVB (P waves with a constant rate where every other P wave conducts to the ventricles) with left bundle branch block (LBBB).

Physiologic Pacing (Cardiac Resynchronization Therapy)

RV pacing has been associated with negative physiologic and clinical consequences from ventricular dyssynchrony such as left ventricular (LV) chamber enlargement, worsening functional mitral regurgitation (MR), reduced left ventricular ejection fraction (LVEF), and increased inter and intraventricular dyssynchrony. The risk of RV pacing induced cardiomyopathy increases with increased RV pacing. The Mode Selection Trial showed that RV pacing greater than or equal to 40% of the time led to a 2.6-fold increase in HF hospitalizations. ACC/AHA/HRS guidelines on bradycardia (2018) suggest that it is reasonable to choose pacing methods that maintain physiologic ventricular activation such as cardiac resynchronization therapy (CRT) for patients with AVB who have LVEF less than 50% and are expected to require ventricular pacing more than 40% of the time. If ventricular pacing is expected to be less than 40%, it is reasonable to choose the conventional RV pacing.

In addition to the CRT in patients with AVB, CRT is indicated in patients with heart failure with New York Heart Association (NYHA) functional class II, III, and ambulatory class IV with left bundle brunch block (LBBB). Indications for CRT in patients with heart failure are summarized in **Table 77-5**. In patients meeting indication for CRT, clinical trials have consistently shown improvement of heart failure symptoms, exercise capacity, and survival.

Other physiologic pacing methodology is evolving such as HIS bundle pacing (HBP) and left bundle brunch area pacing (LBBAP). HIS bundle pacing can be considered to maintain physiologic ventricular activation for selected patients with AVB. Long-term outcome data pertaining to the older population are required for future guidelines. Chest X-rays of CRT PPM are shown in **Figure 77-5A, B**.

TABLE 77-4 ■ INDICATIONS AND SELECTION OF PACEMAKER (PPM) THERAPY IN ATRIOVENTRICULAR BLOCK (AVB)

- PPM for symptomatic acquired second-degree Mobitz type II AVB, high-grade AVB, or third-degree AVB not attributable to reversible or physiologic causes
- PPM for symptomatic acquired second-degree Mobitz type II AVB, high-grade AVB, or third-degree AVB as consequence of medication required for patient's other medical conditions
- Single-chamber ventricular PPM for patients with expected infrequent ventricular pacing

TABLE 77-5 ■ INDICATIONS FOR CARDIAC RESYNCHRONIZATION THERAPY (CRT)

Patients with highest likelihood to respond to CRT are those with:

- LVEF ≤ 35%, sinus rhythm, LBBB, QRS ≥ 150 msec, NYHA II, III, and ambulatory IV

Patients with moderate likelihood to respond to CRT are those with:

- LVEF ≤ 35%, sinus rhythm, LBBB, QRS 120–149 msec, NYHA II-ambulatory IV
- LVEF ≤ 35%, sinus rhythm, non-LBBB, QRS ≥ 150 msec, NYHA III-ambulatory IV
- LVEF ≤ 35%, AF with indications for CRT or requirement for ventricular pacing
- LVEF ≤ 35%, AF after AV nodal ablation with required 100% ventricular pacing
- LVEF ≤ 35% on PPM at the time of device change if RV pacing rate > 40%
- LVEF < 30%, ischemic, sinus rhythm, LBBB, QRS ≥ 150 msec, NYHA I
- LVEF ≤ 35%, sinus rhythm, non-LBBB, QRS 120–149 msec, NYHA III-ambulatory IV
- LVEF ≤ 35%, sinus rhythm, non-LBBB, QRS ≥ 150 msec, NYHA II

Patients who would not derive benefit from CRT are those with:

- NYHA I-II, non-LBBB, QRS < 150 msec
- Comorbidities and frailty that limit survival with good functional capacity to < 1 y

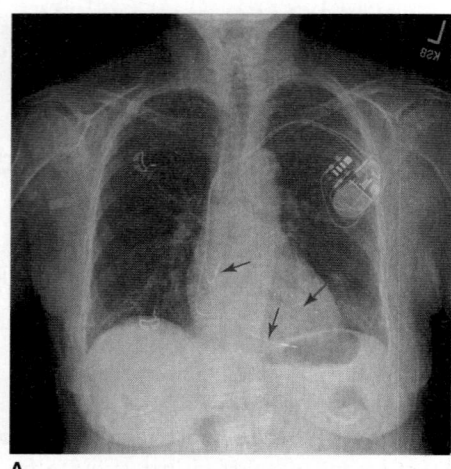

A

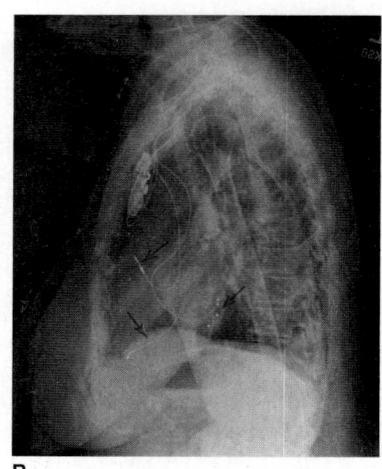

B

FIGURE 77-5A. Chest X-ray AP view showing CRT pacemaker with right atrial, right ventricular, and coronary sinus leads (the green arrow indicates the atrial lead; the red arrow right ventricular lead; and the blue arrow coronary sinus lead also known as left ventricular lead).

FIGURE 77-5B. Chest X-ray lateral view showing CRT pacemaker with right atrial, right ventricular, and coronary sinus leads (the green arrow indicates the atrial lead; the red arrow right ventricular lead; and the blue arrow coronary sinus lead also known as left ventricular lead).

Indications for PPM After Transcatheter Aortic Valve Replacement

Transcatheter aortic valve replacement (TAVR) is being increasingly performed in the older population (see Valvular Heart Disease, Chapter 75). Acquired AVB following TAVR commonly occurs. Predictors of PPM implantation are preexisting RBBB, increased left ventricular end-diastolic diameter, increased valve prosthesis to left ventricular outflow tract ratio, and new LBBB. Incidence of new LBBB is 19% to 55% and high-degree AVB is 10% after TAVR; however, half of these may resolve before discharge. PPM is indicated before discharge for patients with new and symptomatic AVB associated with hemodynamic instability. Indications for pacing in patients with persistent LBBB without symptoms are evolving. Studies have shown in up to 30% of patients with new LBBB, the first episode of high-degree AVB occurs after discharge with potential risk for syncope. Careful surveillance for bradycardia after discharge is recommended for those who develop prolonged PR interval or new BBB after TAVR.

PPM Management Near End of Life

Conversations related to end-of-life PPM management should be discussed at the time of implantation or at early stage of terminal illness. Patients should be encouraged to complete advanced directive early on to address device management and deactivation when patient becomes terminally ill. Like any other decision to withdraw treatments, the decision to deactivate PPM can be made by patient or the legal surrogate through shared decision-making process together with the physician. The role of physician is to inform patient, surrogate, and family member of the

consequences of deactivating the PPM. Death may immediately follow PPM deactivation in those who are dependent. Those who are not must be monitored for potential symptoms such as respiratory distress rendering intensification of comfort measures. After shared decision-making, written request to deactivate the PPM is required by the physician along with a do-not-resuscitate (DNR) order. Medical, ethical, and legal guiding principles on deactivation of PPM can be found in the Heart Rhythm Society 2010 Consensus Statement on this topic.

TACHYARRHYTHMIA

Atrial Fibrillation

Atrial fibrillation (AF) is the most common arrhythmia in the older population as its prevalence and incidence increase with age. Common symptoms of AF include palpitations, fatigue, lightheadedness, shortness of breath, chest discomfort or intolerance to activities, and severe symptoms including HF and syncope. Diagnostic studies involve ECG and echocardiogram to evaluate chamber size, valvular function, and filling pressures; laboratory tests such as complete blood count, comprehensive metabolic panel, thyroid function, and in select cases, cardiac biomarkers. If clinically warranted, ischemic evaluation or sleep study should be considered. Management of AF includes rate or rhythm control, stroke prevention, and modification of risk factors such as weight loss, blood pressure and diabetes control, reduction of alcohol consumption, diagnosis and treatment of obstructive sleep apnea (OSA), and regular exercise. The principles of AF management are the same between the younger and older population. However, the older population has higher prevalence of comorbidities in addition to higher stroke and bleeding risk, which makes them less tolerant to medications; they also have a lower success rate for interventional procedures and higher incidence of adverse events or complications.

Rate versus Rhythm Control

In the older population, neither rate nor rhythm control strategies by pharmacologic therapy was proven to be superior based on several studies including the AFFIRM (Atrial Fibrillation Follow-up Investigation of Rhythm Management) trial. Rate control appears safer with same efficacy to rhythm control in older patients especially if they are asymptomatic or only mildly symptomatic. Long-term rhythm control relies on antiarrhythmic drugs (AAD) or catheter ablation (CA). However, AAD are associated with increased incidence of adverse events in older patients due to variable pharmacokinetics, pharmacodynamics, drug interactions from polypharmacy, and impaired renal or hepatic function. In the AFFIRM study, subgroup analysis of population older than 70 years showed that AAD therapy was associated with higher all-cause mortality. Rate control is generally preferred in older patients with mild or no symptoms. Rhythm control is preferred in older patients with symptoms associated with AF.

Rate Control

β-Blockers (BB) and non-dihydropyridine calcium channel blockers (CCB) slow down the AV nodal conduction and are first-line agents for rate control. The optimal heart rate goal is between 80 and 110 bpm in the absence of significant symptoms such as palpitations, shortness of breath, lightheadedness, chest discomfort, or signs of HF. Although less effective, digoxin can also be considered for rate control, but caution must be taken due to narrowed therapeutic index, especially in the setting of unstable renal function. Rapid up-titration or use of higher doses of BB and CCB can be associated with adverse events related to hypotension, attenuation of baroreceptor reflex, impaired conduction, or autonomic function. CCB are related to higher mortality in patients with LVEF less than 40%. In patients with severe symptoms and in whom drug therapy fails for rate control, ablation of the AVN followed by implantation of PPM are effective for controlling ventricular rate. Although ablation of the AVN does not eliminate AF or the need for anticoagulation, it relieves symptoms and improves QOL, exercise tolerance, and LVEF in patients with tachycardia-induced cardiomyopathy. Biventricular pacing after AVN ablation is associated with improved 6-minute walk distance compared with conventional RV apex pacing in patients with preexisting HF symptoms.

Rhythm Control

Rate control alone may be insufficient to alleviate symptoms in some older patients. In those select patients, restoration of sinus rhythm can be beneficial. Approaches to

rhythm control includes AAD therapy, catheter ablation (CA), surgical ablation, and direct current electrical cardioversion (DCCV). In the acute setting, the efficacy of intravenous and oral AAD is highly variable, ranging from 30% to 75%. Efficacy also varies with the age of the patient, duration of the arrhythmia, underlying LVEF, and left atrial size. External DCCV can restore sinus rhythm in 75% to 90% of patients with AF. For maintenance of sinus rhythm in patients with recurrent AF, consideration for AAD can be given. AAD therapy for rhythm control is summarized in **Table 77-6**.

Role of Ablation

It has been shown in multiple randomized controlled trials that catheter ablation of AF is safe and superior to AAD in preventing recurrence of AF and maintaining sinus rhythm. The recent CABANA (Catheter Ablation versus Antiarrhythmic Drug Therapy in Atrial Fibrillation) trial (n = 2204 patients randomized to either catheter ablation or drug therapy) showed that catheter ablation was not superior to AADs for the primary endpoint of all cause of mortality, disabling stroke, serious bleeding, or cardiac arrest in 5 years. As a predefined secondary endpoint, catheter ablation did not reduce all-cause mortality alone but did reduce the combined all-cause death or cardiovascular hospitalization in comparison to AAD. AF recurrence was significantly less in patients randomized to catheter ablation. A recent metanalysis reported that catheter ablation resulted in a significant reduction in all-cause mortality in AF patients with HF and reduced EF and resulted in significantly fewer cardiovascular hospitalizations and fewer AF recurrences. The subgroup analyses from CABANA suggested that younger patients (age < 65 years) and men derived more benefit from catheter ablation compared with AAD in patients with HF. Such benefit was not evident in patients older than 75 years. Therefore, age and comorbidities are important factors in the decision-making for catheter ablation. Guidelines derived from clinical evidence recommend catheter ablation treatment is primarily for reduction of symptoms and improvement of QoL. There are currently no compelling data to support the use

---

TABLE 77-6 ■ SUMMARY OF ANTIARRHYTHMIC DRUG (AAD) THERAPY FOR RHYTHM CONTROL IN ATRIAL FIBRILLATION (AF)

1. Patients without heart disease
   a. Class Ic AAD (flecainide, propafenone) and class III AAD (sotalol, amiodarone, dronedarone, dofetilide)
2. Patients with CAD
   a. Class Ic AAD are contraindicated (flecainide, propafenone)
   b. Class III AAD can be used (sotalol, amiodarone, dronedarone, dofetilide)
3. Patients with reduced EF or HF
   a. Amiodarone and dofetilide can be used
   b. Dronedarone and class Ic AAD are contraindicated

of catheter ablation to reduce risk of stroke, especially in patients with high CHA_2DS_2-VASc score.

Cox maze procedure is another strategy of AF ablation that can be considered in patient with symptomatic AF undergoing cardiac surgery. The standalone surgical ablation with minimally invasive techniques is rapidly evolving. Limited data suggest it is reasonable for patients with persistent or long-standing persistent AF and paroxysmal AF who have failed one or more attempts of catheter ablation.

Stroke Prevention

The risk of stroke is five times higher in patients with AF. Anticoagulant therapy reduces stroke risk and mortality associated with AF. Although older patients are more vulnerable to stroke, less than two-thirds of octogenarians with AF are anticoagulated. One of the challenges is to maintain INR within the therapeutic range. The need for anticoagulation is determined by the validated CHA_2DS_2-VASc score (**Table 77-7A**). Risk of bleeding on anticoagulation is commonly assessed by the HAS-BLED score with a 0–2 score reflecting low, and a 3–9 score high risk (**Table 77-7B**). Advanced age is a major risk factor for stroke and for bleeding. Although stroke and bleeding risk coexist, benefits of anticoagulation outweigh bleeding risk in most scenarios. Before initiation of anticoagulation, a thorough assessment of frailty, cognitive function, life expectancy, polypharmacy/drug interaction, nutritional assessment, liver function, and renal function is warranted to ensure individualized optimal approach.

The available anticoagulation drugs include vitamin K antagonist (warfarin) and direct oral anticoagulants (DOACs). DOACs include factor Xa inhibitors (apixaban, rivaroxaban, edoxaban) and direct thrombin inhibitor (dabigatran). The disadvantages of warfarin therapy include the need for monitoring INR, narrow therapeutic range, interaction with different food and medications especially in the setting of polypharmacy in older patients, and there is increased tendency for unintentional overdose due to inter- or intraindividual variability in pharmacokinetics and pharmacodynamics. There have been four randomized controlled trials comparing DOACs with warfarin. Patients 75 years or older represent almost 40% of the population in these trials. There was consistent evidence of at least noninferiority for the combined endpoint of stroke or systemic embolism and superior safety profile with less intracranial bleeding risk compared to warfarin. DOACs are recommended as first-line therapy for stroke prevention in eligible patients with AF. For patients 75 years or older, there is lower risk of major bleeding especially with apixaban and edoxaban. However, full-dose dabigatran and rivaroxaban are significantly associated with an increased risk of gastrointestinal (GI) bleeding. A proton pump inhibitor is recommended when these two DOACs are used.

A bleeding risk assessment using the HAS-BLED score has been shown to be clinically useful. Older patients

TABLE 77-7 ■ SCORING SYSTEMS FOR STRATIFICATION OF STROKE AND BLEEDING RISK IN ATRIAL FIBRILLATION (AF)	
A: CHA_2DS_2-VASC SCORE AND STROKE RISK	
CHA_2DS_2-VASC SCORE	**POINTS**
Congestive heart failure	1
Hypertension	1
Age ≥ 65	1
Age ≥ 75	2
Diabetes mellitus	1
Stroke/TIA/thromboembolism	2
Sex category—female	1
Vascular disease (primary MI, PAD, or aortic plaque)	1
Maximum score	9
CHA_2DS_2-VASC SCORE	**ADJUSTED STROKE RISK (% PER YEAR)**
0	0
1	1.3
2	2.2
3	3.2
4	4.0
5	6.7
6	9.8
7	9.6
8	6.7
9	15.2
B: HAS-BLED SCORE AND BLEEDING RISK	
HAS-BLED SCORE	**SCORE**
Hypertension	1
Abnormal liver or renal function	1 point each
Stroke	1
Bleeding history	1
Labile INR	1
Elderly (> 65 y)	1
Drugs (antiplatelet or NSAIDs) or alcohol use	1 point each

with high-risk bleeding should be followed up frequently with routine labs such as cell count, liver, and renal function tests. With the use of DOAC, renal function should be evaluated before initiation and should be reevaluated at least annually or every 6 months or more frequently in those with renal insufficiency. To reduce the bleeding risk, modifiable risk factors must be addressed such as reduction of alcohol use, proper blood pressure control, and avoidance of NSAIDs and elimination of antiplatelet agents if possible. DOACs are contraindicated in advanced liver disease or liver failure with coagulopathy and should not be used in patients with Child-Pugh class C cirrhosis (Child-Pugh class B for rivaroxaban due to a more than a twofold increase in drug exposure). In patients with severe thrombocytopenia (< 50000/µL), the anticoagulation should be individualized and closely monitored given the lack of evidence from trials.

For those who have indication for anticoagulation but has contraindication for chronic anticoagulation but are able to tolerate short-term warfarin therapy, the percutaneously inserted left atrial appendage (LAA) occlusion device, the Watchman device, has been approved by FDA. Anticoagulation with warfarin to target INR between 2 and 3 is indicated for 45 days after the Watchman implantation and then discontinued if complete closure of LAA is confirmed by transesophageal echocardiogram (TEE). After warfarin, aspirin and clopidogrel are recommended for 6 months followed by long-term aspirin. For those with high bleeding risk, clopidogrel can be used for 6 months along with long-term aspirin therapy without oral anticoagulation. The surgical LAA amputation can also be considered for patients with AF undergoing cardiac surgeries.

The synopsis of recommendations for stroke prevention in AF is described in **Table 77-8** and summary of DOACs can be found in **Table 77-9**.

Cryptogenic Stroke, Embolic Stroke of Undetermined Source, and Atrial Fibrillation

The cause of embolic stroke may not be apparent in approximately 30% of patients many of whom are older with multiple comorbidities. Two randomized trials, NAVIGATE ESUS (Rivaroxaban Versus Aspirin in Secondary Prevention of Stroke and Prevention of Systemic Embolism in Patients with Recent Embolic Stroke of Undetermined Source) and RE-SPECT EUS (Dabigatran Etexilate for Secondary Stroke Prevention in Patients With Embolic Stroke of Undetermined Source), studied empiric anticoagulation with rivaroxaban and dabigatran, respectively, on the impact of recurrent stroke in ESUS patients comparing to aspirin. These studies found that empiric anticoagulation was not associated with lower rates of stroke recurrence than aspirin. Bleeding complications were higher with anticoagulation. Empirical anticoagulation in patients with cryptogenic stroke (CS) or embolic stroke of undetermined source (ESUS) is currently not recommended. In patients with CS and ESUS, long-term surveillance for subclinical AF can be accomplished by implantation of a cardiac monitor (loop recorder). Anticoagulation can be considered after AF is detected by the loop recorder.

Device Detected High-Rate Atrial Episodes

Older patients without a history of AF frequently have implanted cardiac devices such as a pacemaker or defibrillator with capabilities of continuous rhythm monitoring. Some patients have device detected intermittent

TABLE 77-8 ■ STROKE PREVENTION IN PATIENTS WITH ATRIAL FIBRILLATION (AF)
• Shared decision-making (risk of stroke vs bleeding, values, and preferences)
• CHA_2DS_2-VASc score stroke risk stratification for nonvalvular AF
• Warfarin for *valvular AF regardless of CHA_2D_2-VASc score (target INR 2–3)
• CHA_2DS_2-VASc ≥ 2 in men or ≥ 3 in women → anticoagulation
• DOACs over warfarin for *nonvalvular AF (monitor renal function)
• Switch to DOAC if unable to maintain therapeutic INR with warfarin
• Warfarin or apixaban (only for nonvalvular AF) when CrCl < 15 mL/min
• Reduce DOAC dose in moderate-to-severe CKD (serum creatinine ≥ 1.5 mg/dL [apixaban], CrCl 15 to 30 mL/min [dabigatran], CrCl ≤ 50 mL/min [rivaroxaban], or CrCl 15 to 50 mL/min [edoxaban])
• Percutaneous LAA occlusion for contraindications to long-term anticoagulation
• Surgical occlusion of the LAA for nonvalvular AF patients undergoing cardiac surgery
• No dabigatran, rivaroxaban, or edoxaban in end-stage CKD or dialysis
• DOACs should not be used in patients with mechanical valve
*Definitions
Valvular AF
• Valvular AF refers to AF in the setting of moderate to severe mitral stenosis (MS) or presence of mechanical valve.
Nonvalvular AF
• Nonvalvular AF is an AF in the setting of absence of moderate to severe MS or absence of mechanical valve.

atrial high-rate events (AHREs) with or without symptoms. Most devices detect AHREs when atrial rates exceed 180 to 190 bpm. An association between increased risk of stroke or systemic embolism and AHREs has been consistently observed. AHREs lasting a minimum of 5 to 6 minutes have been associated with an increased risk of ischemic stroke, cardiovascular events, and death. AHREs should prompt a careful review of the documented electrograms to confirm AF or to consider additional ambulatory monitoring if the data from the implanted device are equivocal. The data on the correlation between the risk of thromboembolic complications and AF burden (frequency, duration, and pattern) continue to evolve rapidly. At this time it is generally recommended that anticoagulation therapy should be considered when AF is confirmed in patients with AHRE greater than 6 minutes and CHA_2DS_2-VASc > 2 or > 24 hours with CHA_2DS_2-VASc > 1 after goals and risks of long-term anticoagulation are reviewed with the patient.

TABLE 77-9 ▢ SUMMARY ON DIRECT ORAL ANTICOAGULANTS (DOACS)

DOAC	MECHANISM OF ACTION	RTC	RESULTS (STROKE AND BLEEDING RISK)	COMMENTS	DOSAGE RECOMMENDATION	REVERSAL AGENTS
Dabigatran (Pradaxa)	Factor IIa inhibitor	RE-LY trial	**Primary outcomes (stroke or systemic embolism)** • 110 mg twice daily vs warfarin (1.53% vs 1.69% per year, RR 0.91; 95% CI, 0.74 to 1.11; $p < 0.001$ for noninferiority) • 150 mg twice daily vs warfarin (1.115% vs 1.69% per year, RR 0.66; 95% CI, 0.53 to 0.82; $p < 0.001$ for superiority). **Hemorrhagic stroke** • 110 mg twice daily vs warfarin (0.12% vs 0.38% per year, $p < 0.001$) • 150 mg twice daily vs warfarin (0.10% vs 0.38% per year, $p < 0.001$) **Major bleeding** • 110 mg twice daily vs warfarin (2.71% vs 3.36% per year, $p = 0.003$) • 150 mg twice daily vs warfarin (3.11% vs 3.36% per year, $p = 0.31$). **Mortality rate** • 110 mg twice daily vs warfarin (3.75% vs 4.13% per year, $p = 0.13$) • 150 mg twice daily vs warfarin (3.64% vs 4.13% per year, $p = 0.051$).	Dabigatran 150 mg twice daily reduced the rate of stroke or systemic embolism by 34% with a similar rate of major bleeds compared to warfarin Dabigatran 110 mg twice daily showed a similar rate of stroke or systemic embolism but reduced the rate of major bleeding by 20% compared to warfarin	150 mg twice daily 110 mg twice daily • With concomitant verapamil • Age ≥ 80 • Increased risk of GI bleeding	The monoclonal antibody **Idarucizumab** **Hemodialysis** **PCC or aPCC** (for severe or life-threatening bleeding if a specific reversal agent is not available) **Ciraparantag** (under investigation)
Rivaroxaban (Xarelto)	Factor Xa inhibitor	ROCKET AF trial	**Primary outcomes (stroke or systemic embolism)** • 20 mg daily vs warfarin (1.7% vs 2.22% per year, HR 0.79; 95% CI, 0.66 to 0.96; $p < 0.001$ for noninferiority) • Intention-to-treat: 20 mg daily vs warfarin (2.1% vs 2.4% per year, HR 0.88; 95% CI, 0.74 to 1.03; $p < 0.001$ for noninferiority; $p = 0.12$ for superiority) **Major and nonmajor clinical bleeding** • 20 mg daily vs warfarin (14.9% vs 14.5% per year, HR 1.03; 95% CI, 0.96 to 1.11; $p = 0.44$) **Intracranial bleeding** • 20 mg daily vs warfarin (0.5% vs 0.7% per year, $p = 0.02$) **Fatal bleeding** • 20 mg daily vs warfarin (0.2% vs 0.5% per year, $p = 0.003$)	Rivaroxaban is effective for prevention of stroke or systemic embolism with a similar rate of major bleeds to warfarin	20 mg daily 15 mg once daily (CrCl 30–49 mL/min)	**Andexanet alfa (Andexxa)** **PCC or aPCC** (for severe or life-threatening bleeding if a specific reversal agent is not available) **Ciraparantag** (under investigation)

Drug	Class	Trial	Outcomes	Summary	Dosing	Reversal
Apixaban (Eliquis)	Factor Xa inhibitor	ARISTOTLE	**Primary outcomes (stroke or systemic embolism)** • 5 mg twice daily vs warfarin (1.27% vs 1.6% per year, HR 0.79; 95% CI, 0.66 to 0.95; $p < 0.001$ for noninferiority; $p = 0.01$ for superiority) **Major bleeding** • 5 mg twice daily vs warfarin (2.13% vs 2.09% per year, HR, 0.69; 95% CI, 0.60 to 0.80; $p < 0.001$) **All-cause mortality** • 5 mg twice daily vs warfarin (3.52% vs 3.94% per year, HR 0.89; 95% CI, 0.80 to 0.99; $p = 0.047$). **Hemorrhagic stroke** • 5 mg twice daily vs warfarin (0.24% vs 0.47%, HR 0.51; 95% CI, 0.35 to 0.75; $p < 0.001$) **Ischemic or uncertain stroke type** • 5 mg twice daily vs warfarin (0.97% vs 1.05% per year, HR 0.92; 95% CI, 0.74 to 1.13; $p = 0.42$).	Apixaban reduced the rate of stroke or systemic embolism by 21% and the rate of major bleeding by 31% compared to warfarin	5 mg twice daily 2.5 mg twice daily (for at least two criteria) • Age ≥ 80 • Body weight < 60 kg • Serum creatinine ≥ 1.5 mg/dL	Andexanet alfa (Andexxa) PCC or aPCC (for severe or life-threatening bleeding if a specific reversal agent is not available) Ciraparantag (under investigation)
Endoxaban (Savaysa)	Factor Xa inhibitor	ENGAGE AF-TIMI 48	**Primary outcomes** • 60 mg once daily vs warfarin (1.18% vs 1.50% per year, HR 0.79; 97.5%; CI, 0.63 to 0.99; $p < 0.001$ for noninferiority) • Intention to treat: 60 mg once daily vs warfarin (HR 0.87; 97.5% CI, 0.73 to 1.04; $p = 0.08$) • 30 mg once daily vs warfarin (1.61% vs 1.50% per year, HR 1.07; 97.5% CI, 0.87 to 1.31; $p = 0.005$ for noninferiority). • Intention to treat: 30 mg once daily vs warfarin (HR 1.13; 97.5% CI, 0.96 to 1.34; $p = 0.10$) **Major bleeding** • 60 mg once daily vs warfarin (2.75% vs 3.43% per year, HR 0.80; 95% CI, 0.71 to 0.91; $p < 0.001$) • 30 mg once daily vs warfarin (1.61% vs 3.43%, HR 0.47; 95% CI, 0.41 to 0.55; $p < 0.001$) **Cardiovascular mortality** • 60 mg once daily vs warfarin (2.74% vs 3.17% per year, HR 0.86; 95% CI, 0.77 to 0.97; $p = 0.01$) • 30 mg once daily vs warfarin (2.71% vs 3.17% per year, HR 0.85; 95% CI, 0.76 to 0.96; $p = 0.008$) **Secondary end point (a composite of stroke, systemic embolism, or death from cardiovascular causes)** • 60 mg once daily vs warfarin (3.85% vs 4.43% per year, HR 0.87; 95% CI, 0.78 to 0.96; $p = 0.005$) • 30 mg once daily vs warfarin (4.23% vs 4.43% per year, HR 0.95; 95% CI, 0.86 to 1.05; $p = 0.32$)	Endoxaban is effective in preventing stroke or systemic embolism (nonsignificant reduction by 13%) and reduced major bleeding by 20% compared to Warfarin	60 mg once daily 30 mg once daily (for at least one criterion) • Estimated creatinine clearance 30–50 mL/min • Body weight ≤ 60 kg • Concomitant use: cyclosporine, dronedarone, erythromycin, or ketoconazole	Andexanet alfa (Andexxa) PCC or aPCC (for severe or life-threatening bleeding if a specific reversal agent is not available) Ciraparantag (under investigation)

Typical atrial flutter (AFL) is a reentrant tachycardia utilizing the inferior vena cava-tricuspid isthmus as the critical conduction pathway. It commonly coexists with AF. Rate control and cardioversion can be effective (electrical cardioversion or with use of class III antiarrhythmic). Ablation of cava-tricuspid isthmus is effective associated with greater than 90% to 95% success rate and less than 1% to 2% complications. Management for stroke prevention in patients with AFL is similar to patients with AF.

Supraventricular Tachyarrhythmia

Supraventricular tachyarrhythmia (SVT) is less common in older patients since most SVTs have been ablated when patients were young. AV nodal reentrant tachycardia (AVNRT) localized to the region of AV node is the most common type of SVT identified among older patients, followed by atrial tachycardia and atrioventricular reciprocating tachycardia (AVRT). The principles of drug and nondrug management of SVT are similar between younger and older patients as recommended in the ACC/AHA/HRS Guidelines 2015 (a synopsis is provided in **Table 77-10**). β-Blockers and CCBs are considered the first line of therapy for treating SVTs. Class I and III antiarrhythmic agents are effective for treating SVTs. Catheter ablation therapy is highly effective for the treatment of SVTs, even in older patients. Success rates for catheter ablation of SVT, regardless of age, range from 85% to better than 95%, depending primarily on the nature of the arrhythmia and the experience of the operator. The incidence of major complications associated with SVT ablation is less than 2% to 3%.

Ventricular Tachyarrhythmia

The management of ventricular arrhythmias in older patients is similar to that in younger patients. In patients with asymptomatic nonsustained ventricular tachyarrhythmia (NSVT), a careful evaluation for the presence of cardiac disease, including occult CAD, structural heart disease, and left ventricular dysfunction, is required. Premature ventricular contractions and NSVT are associated with a benign prognosis in the absence of any significant heart disease. The risk of SCD is increased in patients with compromised LVEF, whether due to ischemic or nonischemic heart disease. Preventing SCD entails optimizing therapy directed at the underlying disease and the use of ICD therapy in selected patients. Although none of the indications for ICDs exclude or allude to special considerations in older patients, individual assessment and determination of primary therapeutic objectives are particularly pertinent in this population because comorbid medical illnesses are frequently present and life expectancy is shorter in older patients.

Prevention of Sudden Cardiac Death

Indications for implantation of an ICD for primary SCD prevention include: (1) ischemic cardiomyopathy (> 40 days after MI or > 90 days after revascularization), LVEF of less

TABLE 77-10 ■ TREATMENT RECOMMENDATIONS FOR SUPRAVENTRICULAR ARRHYTHMIA (SVT)

- Vagal maneuver for acute SVT (education for future episodes recommended)
- Adenosine for acute SVT
- Synchronized cardioversion for acute SVT with hemodynamic instability
- Synchronized cardioversion for acute SVT refractory to adenosine
- Oral β-blocker or diltiazem/verapamil for ongoing SVT
- EPS with option of ablation for diagnosis and treatment of SVT
- Ibutilide or procainamide IV for pre-excited SVT
- IV β-blocker or diltiazem channel blocker for acute SVT
- IV Amiodarone for stable acute AVNRT
- Flecainide or propafenone for ongoing management of SVT with no structural heart disease or ischemia (if ablation not preferred)
- Pill in pocket β-blocker, diltiazem, or verapamil for well-tolerated AVNRT
- Sotalol for ongoing management of SVT (if ablation not preferred)
- Dofetilide for ongoing management of SVT (when other medications are not tolerated, contraindicated or not effective, and if ablation not preferred)
- Amiodarone for ongoing management of SVT (when other medications including dofetilide are not tolerated, contraindicated or not effective, and if ablation not preferred)
- Digoxin for ongoing management of SVT
- β-Blocker, diltiazem, verapamil, amiodarone, and digoxin are harmful for pre-excitation
- Treatment of SVT should be individualized in patients older than 75 years to incorporate age, comorbid illness, physical and cognitive functions, patient preferences, and severity of symptoms

than or equal to 35% with NYHA class II-III function class, or LVEF less than 30% with NYHA class I functional class on guideline-directed medical therapy (GDMT); (2) nonischemic cardiomyopathy, LVEF less than or equal to 35% with NYHA class II-III despite GDMT (benefit in patients with NYHA class I is not well established); (3) inducible sustained monomorphic ventricular tachyarrhythmia by electrophysiologic study (EPS) in patients with NSVT and EF less than or equal to 40% after MI. Indications for implantation of an ICD for secondary SCD prevention include: (1) cardiac arrest owing to VT or ventricular fibrillation (VF) not related to a transient or reversible cause (eg, acute myocardial infarction), (2) spontaneous sustained VT in association with structural heart disease, and (3) syncope of undetermined origin with clinically relevant, hemodynamically significant sustained VT or VF induced at EPS when drug therapy is ineffective, not tolerated, or not preferred. Randomized, prospective clinical trials comparing AAD therapy to ICD have demonstrated the usefulness of ICD in reducing the risk of SCD and total mortality for both primary and secondary prevention in selected populations.

Advanced age alone should not be a sole limiting factor for ICD implantation. However, data on survival benefit are limited from ICD trials in octogenarians and nonagenarians—the very old patient population. Individualized and shared decision with very old patients is important based on patient's preference, functional capacity, cognitive function, and underlying comorbidities.

ICD Management Near End of Life

During the shared decision-making process for initial ICD implantation, risks and benefits of device implantation and possible consequences of ICD therapy and shocks should be thoroughly discussed with the patient, family members, or caretakers. Studies showed that patients frequently do not completely understand the risks, benefits, and downstream burdens of their ICDs. Especially at the end of life, these repetitive shocks may cause additional distress to both patients and loved ones. Each patient or legal surrogate should be informed that they have a right to deactivate the ICD when the end-of-life decision is appropriate.

SUMMARY

The genesis of arrhythmia is the result of complex interactions amongst aging-related physiologic changes, disease-dependent substrate, risk factors, and genetic predisposition. Guidelines on the treatment of cardiac arrhythmias continue to evolve and are being updated regularly. Although many well-designed clinical trials have provided strong evidence for our clinical practice, these evidence-based recommendations need to be interpreted with caution in older patients (especially octogenarians and nonagenarians) as these patients are frequently underrepresented in clinical trials. Perhaps more so than survival rates, clinical outcomes such as symptoms, quality of life, functional capacity, independent living, and hospitalization need to be critically addressed when treating arrhythmias in this fastest growing segment of our population.

FURTHER READING

Al-Khatib SM, Stevenson WG, Ackerman MJ, et al. 2017 AHA/ACC/HRS Guideline for Management of Patients With Ventricular Arrhythmias and the Prevention of Sudden Cardiac Death: A Report of the American College of Cardiology/American Heart Association Task Force on Clinical Practice Guidelines and the Heart Rhythm Society. *J Am Coll Cardiol*. 2018;72:e91–e220.

Asad ZUA, Yousif A, Khan MS, Al-Khatib SM, Stavrakis S. Catheter ablation versus medical therapy for atrial fibrillation: a systematic review and meta-analysis of randomized controlled trials. *Circ Arrhythm Electrophysiol*. 2019;12:e007414.

Calkins H, Hindricks G, Cappato R, et al. 2017 HRS/EHRA/ECAS/APHRS/SOLAECE expert consensus statement on catheter and surgical ablation of atrial fibrillation. *Heart Rhythm*. 2017;14:e275–e444.

Connolly SJ, Ezekowitz MD, Yusuf S, et al. Dabigatran versus warfarin in patients with atrial fibrillation. *N Engl J Med*. 2009;361:1139–1151.

Friedman DJ, Piccini JP, Wang T, et al. Association between left atrial appendage occlusion and readmission for thromboembolism among patients with atrial fibrillation undergoing concomitant cardiac surgery. *JAMA*. 2018;319:365–374.

Giugliano RP, Ruff CT, Braunwald E, et al. Edoxaban versus warfarin in patients with atrial fibrillation. *N Engl J Med*. 2013;369:2093–2104.

Goyal P, Maurer MS. Syncope in older adults. *J Geriatr Cardiol*. 2016;13:380–386.

Goyal P, Rich MW. Electrophysiology and heart rhythm disorders in older adults. *J Geriatr Cardiol*. 2016;13:645–651.

Granger CB, Alexander JH, McMurray JJ, et al. Apixaban versus warfarin in patients with atrial fibrillation. *N Engl J Med*. 2011;365:981–992.

Hindricks G, Potpara T, Dagres N, et al. 2020 ESC Guidelines for the diagnosis and management of atrial fibrillation developed in collaboration with the European Association for Cardio-Thoracic Surgery (EACTS): the Task Force for the diagnosis and management of atrial fibrillation of the European Society of Cardiology (ESC) developed with the special contribution of the European Heart Rhythm Association (EHRA) of the ESC. *Eur Heart J*. 2020;42:373–498.

January CT, Wann LS, Calkins H, et al. 2019 AHA/ACC/HRS Focused Update of the 2014 AHA/ACC/HRS Guideline for the Management of Patients With Atrial Fibrillation: A Report of the American College of Cardiology/American Heart Association Task Force on Clinical Practice Guidelines and the Heart Rhythm Society in Collaboration With the Society of Thoracic Surgeons. *Circulation*. 2019;140:e125–e151.

Kusumoto FM, Schoenfeld MH, Barrett C, et al. 2018 ACC/AHA/HRS Guideline on the Evaluation and Management of Patients With Bradycardia and Cardiac Conduction Delay: A Report of the American College of Cardiology/American Heart Association Task Force on Clinical Practice Guidelines and the Heart Rhythm Society. *J Am Coll Cardiol*. 2019;74:e51–e156.

Ntaios G. Embolic stroke of undetermined source: JACC review topic of the week. *J Am Coll Cardiol.* 2020; 75:333–340.

Packer DL, Mark DB, Robb RA, et al. Effect of catheter ablation vs antiarrhythmic drug therapy on mortality, stroke, bleeding, and cardiac arrest among patients with atrial fibrillation: the CABANA Randomized Clinical Trial. *JAMA.* 2019;321:1261–1274.

Page RL, Joglar JA, Caldwell MA, et al. 2015 ACC/AHA/HRS Guideline for the Management of Adult Patients With Supraventricular Tachycardia: Executive Summary: A Report of the American College of Cardiology/American Heart Association Task Force on Clinical Practice Guidelines and the Heart Rhythm Society. *Circulation.* 2016;133:e471–505.

Patel MR, Mahaffey KW, Garg J, et al. Rivaroxaban versus warfarin in nonvalvular atrial fibrillation. *N Engl J Med.* 2011;365:883–891.

Schäfer A, Flierl U, Berliner D, Bauersachs J. Anticoagulants for stroke prevention in atrial fibrillation in elderly patients. *Cardiovasc Drugs Ther.* 2020;34:555–568.

Shen W-K, Sheldon RS, Benditt DG, et al. 2017 ACC/AHA/HRS Guideline for the Evaluation and Management of Patients With Syncope. A Report of the American College of Cardiology/American Heart Association Task Force on Clinical Practice Guidelines and the Heart Rhythm Society. *J Am Coll Cardiol.* 2017;70:e39–e110.

Sutton R, de Jong JSY, Stewart JM, Fedorowski A, de Lange FJ. Pacing in vasovagal syncope: physiology, pacemaker sensors, and recent clinical trials—precise patient selection and measurable benefit. *Heart Rhythm.* 2020;17:821–828.

Undas A, Drabik L, Potpara T. Bleeding in anticoagulated patients with atrial fibrillation: practical considerations. *Pol Arc Intern Med.* 2020;130:47–58.

Peripheral Vascular Disease

Jonathan R. Thompson, Jason M. Johanning

Peripheral vascular disease (PVD) is primarily a disease of aging and is strongly associated with impaired quality of life and increased cardiovascular mortality. The average age of patients seeking treatment is approximately 70 years. Various studies document a 15% to 20% prevalence rate over the age of 70 years. With the increasing age of the population, the diagnosis and treatment of PVD will become a priority. A working knowledge of the most common sites of disease, the initial diagnostic tests, options for treatment, and treatment outcomes in the geriatric population are necessary to provide optimal guidance for these patients. This chapter is organized by the most commonly encountered arterial and venous diseases of the geriatric patient. Although each subset of PVD has its unique presentation, the underlying atherosclerotic process is a systemic disease and should be treated similar to coronary atherosclerotic disease with regard to risk factor management (see Chapter 74 for additional information).

PERIPHERAL ARTERIAL DISEASE

Definition

Lower extremity arterial disease is commonly referred to as peripheral arterial disease (PAD). As a whole this disease encompasses atherosclerotic narrowing of arteries from the infrarenal aorta to the level of the tibial arteries at the foot.

Epidemiology

Risk factors for PAD are similar to those of coronary artery disease and include smoking history, advanced age, male gender, and positive family history. The prevalence of PAD increases with increasing age with up to 20% of people older than 75 years having some form of lower extremity arterial disease, although classic claudication symptoms are present in less than half of these individuals.

Presentation

The presentation of PAD includes a range of symptoms. The most common presentation is that of claudication, or cramping of the lower extremity muscles after walking a fixed distance. The cramping or aching is primarily in the calves and buttocks and is relieved within 10 minutes of cessation of activity. The above classic presentation of claudication has unfortunately been shown to be present

Learning Objectives

- Obtain a working knowledge of the most common sites of peripheral vascular disease (PVD), the initial diagnostic tests, and options for treatment as well as their outcomes.

- Understand the important role aging plays with regard to intervention in the PVD patient where the primary determination to intervene is based on risk-benefit ratio and the time to treatment equipoise.

- Describe the key indications with regard to intervention for the most common arterial disease presentations including claudication, critical limb ischemia, symptomatic and asymptomatic carotid artery stenosis, and abdominal aortic aneurysms (AAAs).

- Understand the role of minimally invasive endovascular intervention in comparison to open vascular surgery.

- Understand the key physiologic and nonphysiologic factors that affect surgical outcomes in vascular patients especially renal failure and functional status.

- Understand the presentation of chronic venous insufficiency including diagnosis and new treatment modalities.

Key Clinical Points

1. Peripheral arterial disease (PAD) is a common clinical condition in older adults with up to 20% of people older than 70 years having some form of PAD.

2. PAD can be diagnosed utilizing a simple and accurate test named the ankle-brachial index (ABI).

3. The decision to intervene in a patient with claudication is a lifestyle choice and should be pursued only after a trial of exercise therapy has been performed.

4. Intervention for patients with asymptomatic carotid artery stenosis utilizing carotid artery stenting (CAS) is not currently

(Continued)

(Cont.)

indicated due to the significant risk of perioperative stroke.

5. Carotid endarterectomy is the generally accepted intervention for older patients with both asymptomatic and symptomatic carotid artery stenosis with CAS acceptable for patients with specific indications.

6. Intervention of patients with AAA is generally accepted when aneurysmal diameter exceeds 5 to 5.5 cm.

7. Outcomes for patients with acceptable anatomy for open or endovascular repair of infrarenal AAAs are similar based on current randomized trials, although short-term mortality appears to benefit patients undergoing endovascular repair.

8. Long-term follow-up of patients undergoing endovascular repair of AAA using computed tomographic scanning is currently recommended based on changing morphology of the residual aneurysm.

9. Chronic venous disorders of the lower extremities are present in over 30% of the population and are generally treated first with graduated compression stockings.

10. Recent data support ablation of the saphenous vein as initial treatment in appropriate patients with venous stasis ulceration.

in less than half of patients with documented PAD and leg symptoms. Therefore, in the geriatric population, one must have a high index of suspicion for PAD as an underlying cause of ambulatory difficulties and leg symptoms. Additionally, in the older patient, coexisting conditions are common. The two most common conditions are osteoarthritis of the hip or knee and neurogenic claudication secondary to spinal stenosis. Osteoarthritis generally localizes to the joint, improves with pain medications, and has a varying course of improvement and worsening throughout the day. Neurogenic claudication is the most difficult to differentiate from vasculogenic disease because spinal stenosis is common in the older population. Neurogenic claudication most commonly presents with pain in the calves and posterior thigh and buttocks. In contrast to vasculogenic disease, neurogenic claudication has variable distance to onset, often takes 15 minutes to over hours to resolve, and claudication distance can be significantly increased with use of an assistive device such as a walker on which the patient can lean over and relieve the pressure on the spinal nerves.

A focused history of pain with ambulation is usually sufficient to confirm or provide high suspicion for the diagnosis of claudication in the majority of patients and provide a differential as to arterial, spinal, or muscular/joint etiology. The patient with true vasculogenic claudication will complain of pain with ambulation that starts after a known, relatively fixed, distance (two to three blocks are common as this interferes with activities of daily living). Upon cessation of ambulation and rest, the pain will subside and upon resuming ambulation will reoccur at a similar distance. This cycle in vasculogenic claudication can be repeated indefinitely. Often all three conditions (arterial, spinal, or muscular/joint) can coexist in the older patient and the diagnosis which is the primary limiting condition is of utmost concern to achieve an optimal outcome and maintain ambulatory independence.

Although claudication secondary to arterial disease can cause the patient significant distress, the rate of disease progression to rest pain (severe ischemic pain due to insufficient arterial inflow), critical limb ischemia (gangrene, ulceration, or tissue loss), and subsequent amputation is low—on the order of 10% over 10 years or 2.5% annually. Thus, patients presenting to providers worried about amputation should be reassured that amputation is unlikely with appropriate noninterventional or nonoperative management strategies (**Figure 78-1**).

Evaluation

A thorough lower extremity examination includes inspection of the legs to assess for lesions consistent with arterial ischemia. Arterial lesions are primarily located on the distal toes or distal foot and tend to be painful. Earlier presentation includes loss of hair on the toes and distal ankles. Palpation of pulses in the femoral, popliteal, and dorsalis pedis and posterior tibial distribution allows a gross determination of location of disease. Neuromotor functioning of the foot should be documented in the case of suspected acute or severe ischemia, as viability of the foot is determined not by pulse examination but retention of muscular and neurologic function.

The diagnosis of vascular disease relies heavily on the vascular laboratory. The initial and most important test is the ankle-brachial index (ABI). The ABI is a simple bedside examination that can be performed with a blood pressure cuff and handheld Doppler. It is defined as highest systolic blood pressure measured at each ankle divided by the highest systolic blood pressure measured in the arm (brachial artery).

The majority of the vascular system, including retroperitoneal vascular structures, can be imaged with high resolution using noninvasive techniques. Multiple radiologic studies can be used to assess the lower extremity arteries including duplex ultrasonography (DUS), computerized tomographic angiography (CTA) or magnetic resonance imaging (MRA), and conventional digital subtraction angiography (DSA). Each has utility in specific situations and should not be used interchangeably. However, DSA is

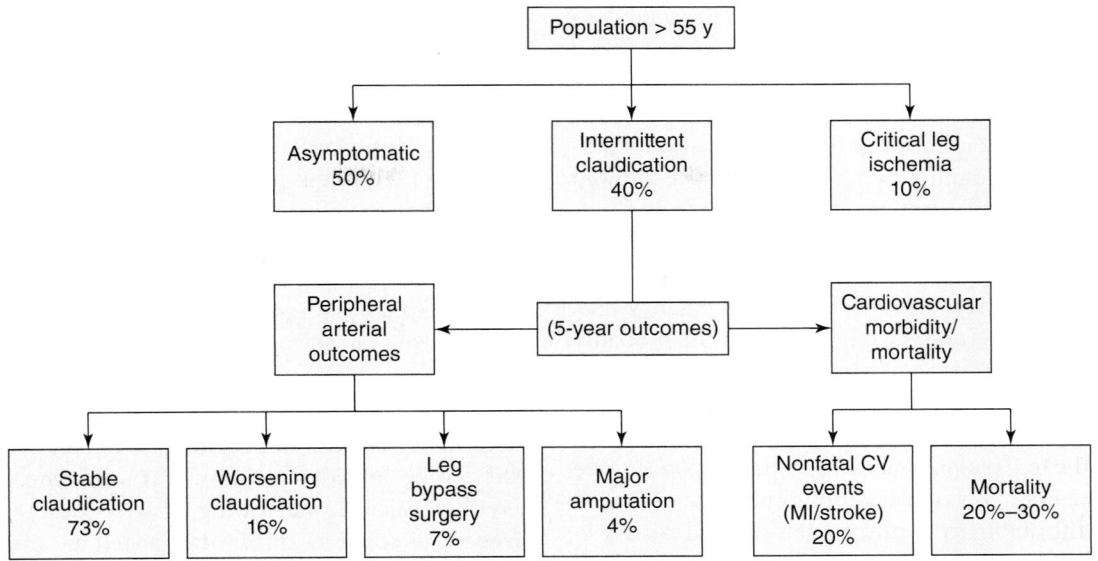

FIGURE 78-1. The natural history of patients with intermittent claudication including fate of the limb and the relationship to cardiovascular outcome. Note the benign nature of intermittent claudication with regard to the limb yet the high incidence of cardiovascular events. (Reproduced with permission from Weitz JI, Byrne J, Clagett GP, et al. Diagnosis and treatment of chronic arterial insufficiency of the lower extremities: a critical review. *Circulation.* 1996;94[11]:3026–3049.)

typically reserved for situations when an intervention is planned. Invasive procedures are not commonly used as the initial diagnostic study due to the improvements in resolution and lack of morbidity for noninvasive evaluations. The study of choice following an abnormal ABI varies based on historical use of specific modalities and is best ordered by the specialist treating the patient to avoid unnecessary tests and cost to the patient.

Management

Lifestyle modification The most important initial management strategies for patients with PAD are smoking cessation and continued ambulation. It has been shown that among patients who are smokers who subsequently stop smoking, the risk of amputation becomes exceedingly low with stabilization of PAD progression and often improvement of walking distance. Also, patients should be encouraged to ambulate even if they experience pain. There is no known negative impact of ambulation on the musculature. In fact, ambulation is the first-line treatment for patients presenting with symptomatic PAD. Supervised exercise therapy has been systematically shown to have a positive and sustainable improvement in ambulatory distances.

Exercise therapy Marked improvements in walking distances have been demonstrated in virtually all studies examining exercise therapy with supervised exercise therapy providing consistently increasing walking distances compared to baseline. Exercise therapy is classically performed by having patients walk beyond the onset of pain for as long as they can safely tolerate and repeating a series of walking trials with each session lasting 30 minutes occurring three times a week. Patients should be reassured that walking to and through the onset of pain will not have any adverse effect on their legs or muscles but, to the contrary, this will promote and increase walking distance by promoting collateral vessel formation. On average, walking distance can be increased on the order of 50% to 200% with a formal exercise program, and in many patients this increase in distance will allow them to accomplish the tasks of daily living that prompted their presentation at the outset. Medicare and many insurance carriers will pay for up to 12 weeks of supervised exercise therapy, although these programs generally only exist in large cities in conjunction with a robust cardiac rehab center. For those who don't have access to these formal programs, patient instructions and even smart phone applications exist to help patients with an exercise program.

Pharmacologic Medical management should consist of an antiplatelet agent in conjunction with a high-potency statin agent. Antiplatelet agents may be prescribed; however, these agents have known and not insignificant side effects and contraindications. These agents have been variably shown to improve ambulation in patients with claudication; however, the maximal gain in walking distance is marginal compared to exercise therapy. Cilostazol, a phosphodiesterase II inhibitor, inhibits smooth muscle cell contraction and platelet aggregation. It is FDA approved for the treatment of intermittent claudication. Caution should be used when administering to a patient with heart failure. Cilostazol has the most data supporting its use for intermittent arterial claudication with walking distances improved by up to 50%.

Interventional PAD treatment using a percutaneous endovascular approach has become the preferred initial treatment for those patients with both lifestyle-limiting claudication and rest pain or tissue loss. The approach is usually from the femoral arteries for both iliac and femoral/tibial lesions, although new technologies have allowed radial artery and pedal access to minimize complications. Short focal stenoses respond very well to angioplasty and stenting whereas long segment stenosis and occlusions are more challenging to treat and have a reduced patency rate, approaching 50% at 6 months, depending on the modality of treatment. Although generally believed to be less durable than open surgical approaches, the endovascular approach offers fewer major complications compared to open surgery especially in the frail patient and can be repeated two to three times after the initial revascularization procedure while still maintaining the ability to perform open surgical bypass in the future. This minimally invasive approach has resulted in a significant decrease in the number of open surgical procedures in older patients and has also been associated with a concomitant reduction in number of amputations nationwide. As a geriatrician one must focus on the goals of care in the patient with rest pain or tissue loss where pain relief, infection treatment, and sustaining or improving ambulatory function are often the primary end points.

Open surgical bypass of occluded or stenotic segments still remains the gold standard against which percutaneous interventions are gauged. Bypass surgeries using prosthetic or autogenous (vein) conduits are the most commonly performed procedures to provide pulsatile flow to the distal leg in the setting of ulcerated lesions or gangrene. The downside to open surgical revascularization is the definite risk of mortality and morbidity that accompanies these procedures. Contemporary quality databases have demonstrated that patients with advanced age greater than 80, renal failure, chronic obstructive pulmonary disease (COPD) requiring oxygen, and congestive heart failure are additive risk factors. Thus in high-risk patients, amputation may be the preferable option for treatment of pain and infection.

Complications associated with percutaneous intervention include vessel thrombosis, embolization, dissection, and rupture. The majority of these are tolerated due to the severity of the disease being addressed. Acute complications necessitating amputation can occur and the patient should be made aware of the potential for limb loss. Outcomes for percutaneous intervention are improving with patency rates of intervened segments approaching 80% at 2 years for iliac artery stents and 70% at 2 years for superficial femoral artery stents. Aortoiliac revascularization utilizing aortobifemoral bypass has a 90% 5-year patency while femoral popliteal and femoral tibial bypasses have 70% to 80% and 60% to 70% 5-year patency rates, respectively. More importantly, limb salvage is greater than 90% in the majority of patients at 2 years and this is confirmed by large-scale data documenting a reduction in amputation rates in population-based studies.

Knowledge of diagnosis and management of PAD is important for the geriatrician based on a high prevalence of the disease within the older population. A trend toward noninvasive diagnosis and minimally invasive approaches is noted. However, a treatment plan based on knowledge of current treatment paradigms with attention to provider and patient-specific factors should be taken into consideration to achieve optimal treatment outcome.

CAROTID ARTERY STENOSIS

Definition

Proper diagnosis, management, and treatment of carotid stenosis are critically important for reducing risk of ischemic stroke in older patients. Carotid stenosis is defined as atherosclerotic narrowing of the extracranial cervical arterial circulation primarily located at the bifurcation and extending into the proximal internal carotid artery. The stenosis and subsequent plaque rupture, embolism of plaque fragments, or platelet thrombi lead directly to the development of ischemic stroke primarily in the frontal and middle cerebral circulation.

Epidemiology

Stroke and its resultant disability are the third leading cause of death in the United States. In general, 80% of strokes are ischemic and 20% hemorrhagic. Among the ischemic strokes, 20% to 30% are attributed to atheroembolic disease due to carotid artery stenosis. The prevalence of asymptomatic carotid artery stenosis of moderate degree is 7.5% and severe stenosis is 3.1% in patients 80 years and older.

Presentation

A complete history is required to definitively classify patients as either symptomatic or asymptomatic as the treatment and aggressiveness of intervention for these two categories are markedly different. Neurologic symptoms including unilateral weakness, parasthesias, receptive or expressive aphasia, dysarthria, amaurosis fugax (transient unilateral loss of vision), as well as prior history of a documented transient ischemic attack (TIA) or stroke are significant findings to elicit. A clear understanding of the event's time course is key in determining symptomatic status. By definition, patients who experience any of the above symptoms in conjunction with an obstruction of 50% or greater of the corresponding carotid artery are considered symptomatic. Patients with confirmed amaurosis fugax, TIA, or stroke in the past 3 months are at greater risk for stroke. It is also important to note that the following symptoms are **not** usually associated with carotid stenosis—generalized weakness, vomiting, nausea, vertigo, ataxia, and diplopia.

Evaluation

Recommendations for screening of asymptomatic patients are in constant debate. Multiple societies and current guidelines recommend against the evaluation of the

TABLE 78-1 ■ OUTCOMES AFTER CAROTID ARTERY STENTING IN MEDICARE BENEFICIARIES, 2005 TO 2009

MORTALITY	1 Y	2 Y	3 Y	4 Y
Asymptomatic	6.20%	13.10%	19.80%	27.90%
Symptomatic	10.00%	18.80%	27.10%	36.30%

Data from Jalbert JJ, Nguyen LL, Gerhard-Herman MD, et al. Outcomes after carotid artery stenting in Medicare beneficiaries, 2005 to 2009. JAMA Neurol. 2015;72(3):276–286.

asymptomatic patient. In the case of the older patient, the "do no harm" imperative becomes even more pronounced, as older patients do not benefit from asymptomatic carotid intervention to the extent that younger patients may. The benefit of operative carotid treatment in the immediate postoperative period and in the long term in older and frail patients, particularly those with renal failure, is less pronounced. It is generally agreed upon that population screening examinations are not cost-effective for asymptomatic patients and only beneficial in highly selective patient populations such as patients undergoing coronary artery bypass grafting. Screening is not recommended for patients based solely on presence of an AAA, presence of a carotid bruit, or prior head and neck radiotherapy. In contrast, a patient with clear unilateral signs and symptoms of ischemia should undergo imaging of the cervical carotid circulation due to the change in risk-benefit equation that favors intervention based on symptomatic status and long-term survival. The need to ensure long-term survival in patients undergoing intervention should be emphasized with the recognition that the benefit of treatment accrues over time and patients on average should be expected to live 4 to 5 years after treatment (**Table 78-1**).

Complete physical examination is important to assess the potential subtle signs of neurologic ischemia. Focused physical examination includes auscultation of heart and detection of potential cardioembolic source from an arrhythmia, palpation of pulses, cranial nerve, and neurologic assessment to include examination of face for unilateral weakness or facial droop, and musculoskeletal examination for overall strength and symmetry. Ophthalmic consultation for detection of Hollenhorst plaques may be indicated especially in the setting of amaurosis fugax.

Multiple noninvasive imaging studies can assess the carotid arteries including DUS, CTA, or magnetic resonance angiography (MRA). Invasive conventional DSA is reserved for the rare situation when noninvasive imaging is equivocal or if the patient is in need of an intervention to treat the stenosis utilizing an endovascular approach. Each modality has utility in specific situations with each able to provide the degree of stenosis and characterization of the plaque's morphology and location. Even though DSA is considered the "gold standard," it is reserved only for questionable or contradictory findings on noninvasive imaging due to its inherent risk of stroke based on previous randomized trials.

DUS is an accurate, reliable, noninvasive imaging modality and is often the **initial** study to identify patients with disease. The degree of stenosis and plaque morphology of the carotids can be readily assessed but is operator dependent. CTA and MRA use contrast and can provide accurate imaging of the carotid arteries. Both tests are limited by allergic reactions with anaphylaxis or preexisting renal disease. However, both studies are very effective at imaging with high resolution both the cervical and intracranial carotid and vertebral circulation in addition to the brain itself. Both imaging modalities are more expensive than duplex imaging and both suffer from artifact such that an experienced interpretation is needed to accurately assess carotid plaque morphology and stenosis. DSA or catheter-based digital angiography provide excellent images which are easy to interpret regarding degree of stenosis, location, and plaque morphology. Again, it is reserved in patients with conflicting imaging prior to operation with limitations including risk of stroke, cost, and morbidity.

Management

Pharmacologic Initial management of both symptomatic and asymptomatic patients includes maximizing medical therapy with appropriate antiplatelet agents to prevent platelet aggregation and embolization in conjunction with lipid-lowering agents to stabilize the at-risk plaque in the carotid distribution. For patients who smoke, the risk of stroke nearly doubles with continuance and cessation will markedly reduce stroke risk. For the asymptomatic patient, aggressive medical management is thought to be equivalent to invasive intervention and ongoing trials are underway to address this issue. New data emphasize the additional need for tight blood pressure control (SBP < 120 mm Hg) and optimized diabetic management in stroke prevention. For symptomatic patients, in addition to medical management, the next step is confirming the presence of significant stenosis that would benefit from invasive intervention.

Interventional Once a diagnosis of carotid stenosis is made, several factors are taken into account when considering optimal treatment. One must consider multiple factors before embarking on interventional treatment including whether the stenosis is symptomatic or asymptomatic, degree of stenosis, anatomic ease of intervention, anticipated mortality rate over the upcoming years by assessment of medical comorbidities, frailty, and patient preferences regarding stroke risk reduction in the asymptomatic setting. Generally medical management is advised for low-grade stenoses (< 50%) in both asymptomatic and symptomatic patients. Intervention is recommended in symptomatic patients with more than 70% stenosis and in asymptomatic stenosis with more than 80% stenosis in centers with a track record of excellent outcomes and in patients with an anticipated life expectancy exceeding 5 years. In symptomatic patients with 50% to 69% stenosis, risk-benefit analysis should be given careful consideration prior to intervention as studies support intervention, but only in centers that have excellent perioperative outcomes.

Carotid artery stenting (CAS) via percutaneous approach is an acceptable approach to treating carotid stenosis in selected patients based on specific indications. CAS is less invasive allowing for intervention in poor surgical candidates, especially those with cardiac disease. CAS also allows for angiography, angioplasty, and stent placement all with one procedure. It is indicated in patients with prior neck radiation, prior surgical treatment of the carotid artery or neck lesions, contralateral vocal cord injury, significant coronary artery disease, or congestive heart failure. CAS can be anatomically challenging due to aortic arch anatomy, especially in older adults where calcific lesions and poor arch anatomy due to natural aortic remodeling are present. In addition, significant controversy exists on the benefit and outcomes in octogenarians and older patients as multiple studies have documented increased stroke rates in older patients such that trials to date have excluded this population from inclusion due to poor outcomes compared to younger patients. Carotid endarterectomy (CEA) is generally preferred in patients older than 80 years for this reason.

CEA is the gold standard operative procedure for treatment of high-grade carotid stenosis. It has been shown to reduce future stroke risk in multiple well-done randomized trials compared against medical management. For patients with asymptomatic stenosis, CEA is the currently indicated procedure except in select circumstances. A patient with a life expectancy of greater than 5 years should generally—except when there are neck anatomic concerns—be advised to undergo a CEA for asymptomatic disease with stenosis greater than 70% to 80%. Additionally, it is now becoming accepted that CAS in general carries a greater stroke risk compared to CEA. Newer techniques such as the Trans Carotid Artery Revascularization (TCAR) relies on a small neck incision for placement of a stent directly through the common carotid artery. The procedure uses a flow reversal system to limit embolization during the procedure which results in the lowest peri-operative stroke risk of any procedure. After intervention, patients are monitored overnight in the hospital and can be discharged the following day barring any complications or concerns. Antiplatelet agents are generally continued during the perioperative period to inhibit platelet adhesion and embolization as studies have shown decrease in stroke risk with an antiplatelet regimen.

Complications associated with CAS and CEA include stroke, hematoma, and death. CEA has the highest rate of cranial nerve injury compared to other revascularization techniques. However, complete recovery is typical and permanent injury with disability is rare. As noted above, risk of myocardial infarction is higher with CEA whereas perioperative stroke rates are higher in transfemoral CAS. Accepted 30-day stroke and death risk is less than 3% for asymptomatic patients and less than 6% for symptomatic patients. A major trial of open surgical versus endovascular treatment versus medical management is currently ongoing with results eagerly awaited to clarify the best option for management of carotid occlusive disease.

AORTIC ANEURYSM

Definition

AAA is a degenerative disease of the aorta characterized by inflammation and arterial wall degradation that lead to dilatation and possibly rupture. AAA is defined by increase in vessel diameter by more than 50%, generally over 3 cm in men. The majority of AAA remains asymptomatic until which time rupture or less commonly rapid expansion occurs leading to severe and unrelenting abdominal pain radiating to the back or a pulsatile abdominal mass.

Epidemiology

Aortic aneurysms occur 95% of the time in the infrarenal location and in 1% to 3% of people depending on the population screening criteria. Men commonly present starting at the age of 65 with women having a noted delay in presentation. This results in a male-to-female ratio of AAA in patients less than 80 years of 2 to 1, whereas in patients greater than 80 years, the incidence is equal. Racial differences are present too with Caucasians having a greater than threefold incidence of AAA compared to non-Caucasians.

Pathophysiology

AAA is often thought to be caused by atherosclerosis, but no specific cause and effect has been demonstrated; rather a strong correlation exists. In contrast, some inciting event—generally thought to be smoking since greater than 95% of patients have a smoking history—is believed to trigger an inflammatory state where there is an unchecked proinflammatory process that is present within the media and adventitia of the aortic wall that results in degradation of the wall's structure by matrix metalloproteinases (MMPs). The end result is loss of structural integrity of the aortic wall with dilation and weakening leading to rupture.

Presentation

Multiple studies have now documented that detection of AAA in men older than 65 years reduces overall AAA mortality and is cost-effective. A thorough history is required in determining a patient's risk for developing an AAA since the patient should ideally have their AAA detected when in the asymptomatic status as the risk of repair is markedly less than in patients with symptomatic unruptured and ruptured AAA. AAA risk factors include tobacco use (current or former), advanced age, coronary artery disease, atherosclerosis, high cholesterol, hypertension, first-degree relative affected, and male gender. Risk factors for expansion include advanced age, severe cardiac disease, prior stroke, and tobacco use. Independent risk factors for AAA rupture include female gender, large initial diameter, low forced expiratory volume in 1 second (FEV_1), current smoking, and elevated mean blood pressure. Patients with family history for inherited connective tissue disorders such as Marfan syndrome or Ehlers-Danlos are also at increased risk for developing AAA, albeit at younger age.

A complete physical examination is critical to assess overall patient function. Abdominal examination can be difficult especially with extreme obesity and may not reveal a pulsatile mass in the mid abdomen. AAAs over 5 cm can be detected on careful examination 76% of the time, whereas smaller AAAs between 3 and 3.9 cm are only detected 29% of the time thus reinforcing the need for screening examinations. In addition to abdominal examination, femoral and pedal pulses and cardiac and pulmonary examination should be performed at a minimum as these systems are commonly involved with atherosclerosis and end-organ dysfunction from long-term smoking.

Evaluation

Current screening recommendations are to obtain an abdominal ultrasound (US) examination on men older than 65 years who have any smoking history or older than 55 years with family history. Women should be screened with US at age 65 if there is a family history or smoking history. Currently Medicare offers US screening as part of their Welcome to Medicare Physical Examination to men who have smoked at least 100 cigarettes over their lifetime or any patient with a family history.

The Society for Vascular Surgery recommends the following surveillance algorithm once an AAA is detected. Surveillance imaging at 3-year intervals for AAAs between 3.0 and 3.9 cm, 12-month imaging for aneurysms between 4.0 and 4.9 cm, and imaging every 6 months for those patient with aneurysms between 5.0 and 5.4 cm. The above recommendations are based on an average growth rate of 0.1 to 0.4 cm per year for all aneurysms with smaller aneurysms growing at a lesser rate. Any symptoms potentially related to the aneurysm should prompt a repeat study to exclude rapid expansion. Recent studies seem to indicate a linear growth of aneurysms less than 5.0 cm in diameter.

As noted above, the initial screening study and the preferred method of surveillance is ultrasound. This is a simple, noninvasive, and painless test with no risk to the patient. However, the US is unable to fully image the aneurysm for screening purposes in many obese patients. Alternative modalities include both computed tomography (CT) and magnetic resonance imaging (MRI), which do not require dye to assess the presence of an aneurysm or its size.

Current CT imaging in the form of CT angiography provides excellent detail of the aortic aneurysm in addition to other potential intra-abdominal processes. CT is also more reproducible than US with more consistent measurements between examinations with operator variation removed. Additionally, if performed as an initial scan, CT also allows examination of the entire aorta from aortic root to bifurcation and provides for 3D reconstruction of vessels which is key for planning both open and endovascular intervention. As CT has become more accessible, it is more commonly used to follow patients after intervention but exposes the patient to contrast dye and radiation, hence the preference to use DUS whenever feasible. MRI can also be used to evaluate AAA; however, due to expense, time, and limited access, MRI should not be first-line imaging for AAA. Its use should be reserved for patients in whom a CT scan is otherwise contraindicated.

Management

Pharmacologic Optimal medical management is directed at controlling comorbidities in patients with AAA. This includes smoking cessation, hypertension control, lipid control, diabetes management, diet and exercise, lifestyle modifications, and regular primary care provider follow-up. It should be noted that exercise and transient increases in blood pressure are not predictors or causes of rupture and therefore patients with an AAA diagnosis should continue to be active while being monitored. Aerobic activity including walking, jogging, biking, and swimming should be encouraged. Standard medical therapy for atherosclerotic occlusive disease should be provided including antiplatelet agents and statin therapy when indicated. Although it would seem β-blockade would reduce vessel stress and thus rupture, this has not been the case and antihypertensive regimens should follow accepted guidelines. A recent trial to determine the efficacy of doxycycline to slow the growth of small aneurysms failed to show any benefit, therefore leaving the patient with AAA with only surgical management options to reduce mortality risk from rupture.

Interventional The single goal of AAA management is to reduce the chance of AAA rupture. As this is purely a risk-benefit analysis, knowledge of rupture and subsequent death risk at given AAA sizes is necessary to make appropriate recommendations for intervention. The size of the AAA is the major determining factor for risk of rupture and thus the major indicator dictating the timing of an intervention. Less commonly, rapid rate of expansion—generally agreed to be greater than 0.50 cm in 6 months—is an indication for intervention. The risk of rupture correlates directly with size. AAA less than 4 cm having a 0% to 0.5% yearly rupture risk, 4.0 to 4.9 cm having a 0.5% to 1.5% yearly rupture risk, 5 to 5.9 cm having a 1% to 11% yearly rupture risk, 6 to 6.9 cm having a 11% to 22% yearly rupture risk, and AAA greater than 7 cm having a 30% yearly rupture risk. It is generally accepted that AAAs greater than 5.5 cm for men and 5 cm for women have a high enough yearly risk for rupture that elective surgical intervention is indicated in good-risk patients. This recommendation is based on current data supporting a mortality risk of AAA repair of approximately 1% to 2% for both endovascular and open aneurysm repair.

Repair of infrarenal AAA is commonly approached by either endovascular or open surgical repair. Now three decades old, the endovascular approach uses femoral artery access for a graft placement under fluoroscopic guidance. Benefits of endovascular repair include less postoperative pain, shorter hospital stay, and lower 30-day mortality.

TABLE 78-2 ■ AAA SURVEILLANCE IMAGING RECOMMENDATIONS

AAA SIZE IN MAXIMUM DIAMETER (CM)	SCREENING INTERVAL	RECOMMENDATION LEVEL	QUALITY OF EVIDENCE
3.0–3.9	3 y	2 (weak)	C (Low)
4.0–4.9	1 y	2 (weak)	C (Low)
5.0–5.4	6 mo	2 (weak)	C (Low)

Data from Chaikof EL, Dalman RL, Eskandari MK, et al. The Society for Vascular Surgery practice guidelines on the care of patients with an abdominal aortic aneurysm. J Vasc Surg. 2018;67(1):2–77.e2.

Additionally, these benefits allow expansion to candidates who would not tolerate an open procedure. In spite of these immediate perioperative benefits, numerous studies have documented similar quality of life, and similar long-term morbidity and mortality comparing the endovascular to open repair. The gain of 6 to 8 weeks of pain-free recovery and similar outcomes has led to the utilization of the endovascular approach as the first-line treatment in the geriatric population, with over 90% of patients now anatomically suitable for graft placement.

Open repair of an AAA requires either a transperitoneal or retroperitoneal approach, with midline laparotomy common. The open approach is generally used for patients who do not meet anatomic specifications for endovascular aneurysm repair, specifically those with a poor segment of aorta immediately distal to the renal arteries. Thus, the patients undergoing open repair in today's era are generally at more risk than a standard AAA patient due to need for suprarenal clamping and concomitant risk of renal failure and complex anatomic characteristics that preclude endovascular repair. This generally includes renal artery involvement or complex pelvic anatomy that increases the risk of morbidity and mortality.

With proper diagnosis, surveillance, and medical management, patients can be monitored for years without needing surgical repair for their AAA, and with appropriate intervention, patients can have similar life expectancies compared to matched controls (**Table 78-2**).

CHRONIC VENOUS INSUFFICIENCY

Definition

Chronic venous insufficiency (CVI) is a condition of altered blood flow in the leg veins usually caused by functionally incompetent venous valves leading to increased pressure in the distal venous vasculature. Less likely in the older adult population is the presence of a proximal obstruction leading to venous hypertension. Regardless of the etiology, the increased venous pressure at the level of the lower leg results in the findings classic for CVI.

Epidemiology

The prevalence of venous insufficiency varies considerably between genders, ethnic backgrounds, and age groups.

In a general population, the age-adjusted prevalence for the whole population was 9.4% in men and 6.6% in women with increasing prevalence of CVI correlated closely with age and sex, being 21.2% in men greater than 50 years and 12.0% in women greater than 50 years. An important fact remains that the prevalence of CVI increases with age specifically in studies evaluating chronic leg ulceration.

Pathophysiology

Venous hypertension results from venous reflux due to valvular incompetence or obstruction due to thrombosis or narrowing of proximal veins. Superficial venous insufficiency is usually due to weakened valves or widened veins precluding normal valve coaptation. The most common location of the valvular incompetence is located at the saphenofemoral junction where the greater saphenous vein drains into the common femoral vein. Deep vein thrombosis (DVT) creates venous insufficiency by creating inflammation and adhesion of venous valves leading to resultant narrowing and valvular dysfunction.

Regardless of superficial or deep as the cause of venous hypertension, the constantly elevated hydrostatic pressure creates the findings of edema and venous microangiopathy. A common finding in older adults is lipodermatosclerosis and hemosiderin deposition at the malleolar level. Permanent skin hyperpigmentation occurs resulting from hemosiderin deposition as red blood cells extravasate and are deposited into the superficial tissues. Lipodermatosclerosis is the skin thickening and woody feeling which is due to fibrosis of subcutaneous fat. The ultimate outcome of this unopposed venous hypertension is the venous ulcer resulting from dysfunctional microcirculation and dermal weakness.

Presentation

The condition is characterized by symptoms including fatigue, discomfort, and a sensation of heaviness which worsen during the day. Physical examination findings such as swelling worsen as the day progresses and prior to ambulation. Late sequelae of chronic venous insufficiency includes lipodermatosclerosis, hyperpigmentation, stasis dermatitis, and venous ulceration. The diagnosis of CVI, similar to arterial conditions, can be challenging in the older patient due to coexisting conditions. In addition to neurologic complaints such as spinal stenosis, one must also consider vascular-related conditions such as congestive heart failure and chronic edema and lymphatic changes associated with joint replacement. A history focusing on the time course of swelling to include significant improvement when awakening in the morning after lying flat throughout the night with classic physical examination findings of lack of foot involvement and gaiter distribution of skin changes and associated varicosities will invariably be present. The history should also take into account conditions that may lead to valvular dysfunction such as previous deep venous thrombosis or superficial thrombophlebitis in addition to traumatic injuries to the superficial veins of the lower extremities. Particular attention should be paid to patients who are sedentary remaining in a sitting position for the majority of the day and night including those confined to a wheelchair or those who use a recliner to sleep at night for pulmonary and sleep apnea issues as this creates unrelieved pressure in the veins that will need to be addressed in conjunction with treatment of the venous insufficiency.

Evaluation

The gold standard for initial evaluation of CVI is duplex ultrasonography. Utilizing ultrasound images of the affected vein can be obtained to look specifically for valvular dysfunction and size changes consistent with narrowing or dilation. Additionally, ultrasound can be used to assess venous reflux. Reflux time of greater than or equal to 0.5 seconds is considered significant within a superficial venous segment. CT venogram can be obtained if one has a suspicion for a proximal obstructing process such as May Thurner or more commonly in older adults extrinsic compression from a tumor. Rarely is invasive venography utilized for diagnostic purposes and is usually based on findings of noninvasive studies leading to a therapeutic intervention. Venous plethysmography is still utilized in specific circumstances by physicians specializing in venous disease.

Management

Noninvasive The mainstay of treatment is relieving venous hypertension with elevation of the legs when not ambulating and the application of compression therapy.

The application of compression therapy has increased in recent times due to the ready availability of sufficient and inexpensive compression stockings not requiring a prescription or fitting. For patients with unusual lower leg anatomy, a formal fitting will likely provide a better compression result. In patients with ulcerations, compression is a must for ulcer healing and can take many forms including standard compressions stockings, ace wraps, and UNNA boots. With regards to ulcer healing, 90% of ulcers should heal given adequate compression compliance and normal arterial perfusion.

Invasive Recently treatment of superficial venous insufficiency has undergone a sea change in the ability to treat chronic insufficiency utilizing minimally invasive techniques. This ranges from in office sclerotherapy with or without ultrasound to the treatment of large vessel superficial incompetence of the saphenous system using advanced sclerosants, chemical sealing, and energy procedures aimed to obliterate the offending refluxing segment. Importantly, it has recently been shown that for patients with venous ulcerations and superficial reflux, early venous ablation of superficial incompetence resulted in faster healing of venous leg ulcers and more time free from ulcers than deferred endovenous ablation. Therefore in the older patient with a venous stasis ulcer, one should implement compression and confirm presence or absence of superficial venous reflux amenable to intervention since a truly cost-effective, minimally invasive office procedure is now available to speed ulcer healing and prevent ulcer recurrence.

FURTHER READING

Aronow WS, Ahn C, Gutstein H. Prevalence and incidence of cardiovascular disease in 1160 older men and 2464 older women in a long-term health care facility. *J Gerontol A Biol Sci Med Sci*. 2002;57(1):M45–M46.

Chaikof EL, Dalman RL, Eskandari MK, et al. The Society for Vascular Surgery practice guidelines on the care of patients with an abdominal aortic aneurysm. *J Vasc Surg*. 2018;67(1):2-77.e2.

Criqui MH, Aboyans V. Epidemiology of peripheral artery disease. *Circ Res*. 2015;116(9):1509–1526.

Daly KJ, Torella F, Ashleigh R, McCollum CN. Screening, diagnosis and advances in aortic aneurysm surgery. *Gerontology*. 2004;50(6):349–359.

De Martino RR, Goodney PP, Nolan BW, et al. Optimal selection of patients for elective abdominal aortic aneurysm repair based on life expectancy. *J Vasc Surg*. 2013;58(3):589–595.

Egorova NN, Guillerme S, Gelijns A, et al. An analysis of the outcomes of a decade of experience with lower extremity revascularization including limb salvage, lengths of stay, and safety. *J Vasc Surg*. 2010;51(4):878–885, 885.e1.

Ferguson GG, Eliasziw M, Barr HW, et al. The North American Symptomatic Carotid Endarterectomy Trial: surgical results in 1415 patients. *Stroke*. 1999;30(9): 1751–1758.

Hirsch AT, Criqui MH, Treat-Jacobson D, et al. Peripheral arterial disease detection, awareness, and treatment in primary care. *JAMA*. 2001;286(11):1317–1324.

Kwolek CJ, Jaff MR, Leal JI, et al. Results of the ROADSTER multicenter trial of transcarotid stenting with dynamic flow reversal. *J Vasc Surg*. 2015;62(5):1227–1234.

Lane R, Ellis B, Watson L, Leng GC. Exercise for intermittent claudication. *Cochrane Database Syst Rev*. 2014;7: CD000990.

Lederle FA, Freischlag JA, Kyriakides TC, et al. Outcomes following endovascular vs open repair of abdominal aortic aneurysm: a randomized trial. *JAMA*. 2009;302(14):1535–1542.

1218 LeFevre ML. U.S. Preventive Services Task Force. Screening for asymptomatic carotid artery stenosis: U.S. Preventive Services Task Force Recommendation statement. *Ann Intern Med.* 2014;161(5):356–362.

McDermott MM. Lower extremity manifestations of peripheral artery disease: the pathophysiologic and functional implications of leg ischemia. *Circ Res.* 2015; 116(9):1540–1550.

Melin AA, Schmid KK, Lynch TG, et al. Preoperative frailty risk analysis index to stratify patients undergoing carotid endarterectomy. *J Vasc Surg.* 2015;61(3): 683–689.

Muluk SC, Muluk VS, Kelley ME, et al. Outcome events in patients with claudication: a 15-year study in 2777 patients. *J Vasc Surg.* 2001;33(2):251–257; discussion 257–258.

Noorani A, Hippelainen M, Nashef SA. Time until treatment equipoise: a new concept in surgical decision making. *JAMA Surg.* 2014;149(2):109–111.

Oresanya L, Zhao S, Gan S, et al. Functional outcomes after lower extremity revascularization in nursing home residents: a national cohort study. *JAMA Intern Med.* 2015;175(6):951–957.

Qureshi AI, Chaudhry SA, Qureshi MH, Suri MF. Rates and predictors of 5-year survival in a national cohort of asymptomatic elderly patients undergoing carotid revascularization. *Neurosurgery.* 2015;76(1):34–40; discussion 40–41.

Savji N, Rockman CB, Skolnick AH, et al. Association between advanced age and vascular disease in different arterial territories: a population database of over 3.6 million subjects. *J Am Coll Cardiol.* 2013;61(16): 1736–1743.

Voeks JH, Howard G, Roubin GS, et al. Age and outcomes after carotid stenting and endarterectomy: the carotid revascularization endarterectomy versus stenting trial. *Stroke.* 2011;42(12):3484–3490.

CHAPTER 78 PERIPHERAL VASCULAR DISEASE

Chapter 79

Hypertension

Mark A. Supiano

INTRODUCTION

High blood pressure has the greatest impact on global attributable mortality of any risk factor. Compared with all other specific risks quantified in the Global Burden of Disease, Injuries, and Risk Factor studies, systolic blood pressure (SBP) of at least 110 to 115 mm Hg was the leading global contributor to preventable death in 2015. Three demographic changes—(1) the prevalence of elevated SBP ($\geq$ 110–115 and $\geq$ 140 mm Hg) has increased substantially in the past 25 years, (2) the age-associated increase in blood pressure, and (3) the worldwide demographic increase in the aging population—are conspiring to create an enormous, emerging public health impact. In addition to the well-ascribed hypertension risk for cardiovascular disease (CVD) and stroke, it is also a significant risk factor for chronic kidney disease, atrial fibrillation, congestive heart failure (CHF) with both reduced and preserved left ventricular ejection fraction, and cognitive impairment—each with a relative risk between 2.0 and 4.0. A reduction of 10 mm Hg systolic and 5 mm Hg diastolic at age 65 is associated with a reduction of up to 25% in myocardial infarction, 40% in stroke, 50% in CHF, and 10% to 20% overall decrease in mortality. Despite this knowledge, current rates of hypertension control are extremely low, especially among older women. In addition to illustrating the clinical importance of hypertension, these data are a compelling call to improve both our knowledge concerning the mechanisms that underlie the age-associated increase in blood pressure to aid in its prevention as well as to implement changes in the systems of care necessary to improve blood pressure control among those with hypertension.

EPIDEMIOLOGY

Although high blood pressure should not be construed to be a normal aspect of aging, there is clearly an age-associated increase in blood pressure and in the prevalence of hypertension. Data from the National Health and Nutrition epidemiologic survey from 2015 to 2018 documented that hypertension is a very prevalent condition among older Americans (**Figure 79-1**). Based on this study's updated definition of hypertension (discussed herein)—a self-report

Learning Objectives

- Understand what key age-related physiologic changes account for the progressive increase in the prevalence of hypertension with age.

- Explain the mechanisms for greater blood pressure variability with age, and understand why a hypertension diagnosis should never be based on a single elevated measurement.

- Determine the benefit-based systolic blood pressure (SBP) treatment goal based on age, comorbidities, and cardiovascular and cognitive impairment risk factors.

- Understand that arterial stiffness is an independent cardiovascular risk factor.

- Select the best thiazide-type diuretic and other medication classes to treat geriatric hypertension.

Key Clinical Points

1. The prevalence of hypertension increases steadily with age.

2. Older people develop systolic hypertension due to the age-related increase in arterial stiffness. SBP and pulse pressure, both closely associated with arterial stiffness, confer the greatest significance as cardiovascular and cognitive impairment risk factors.

3. Age-related changes in systems that regulate blood pressure result in greater blood pressure variability. Therefore, careful attention is needed to accurately measure and diagnose hypertension, as well as monitoring for adverse drug events—especially postural hypotension—throughout treatment.

4. The diagnosis of hypertension should be based on the average of a minimum of nine blood pressure readings that have been obtained on three separate office visits or derived from 24-hour ambulatory or home blood pressure monitoring results.

(Continued)

(Cont.)

5. Older hypertensive individuals commonly have physiologic characteristics that respond effectively to lifestyle modifications.

6. The focus of therapy should be on lowering the SBP to the patient's benefit-based target goal. Applying benefit-based therapy to the majority of adults age 65 or older who are at high cardiovascular disease or cognitive impairment risk favors a SBP goal of less than 130 mm Hg, and for some a goal of 120 mm Hg may be considered.

7. Thiazide-type diuretic drugs—notably chlorthalidone—are preferred as the initial drug class in most patients. Combination therapy with low doses of one or more agents should be considered if needed to achieve the target SBP level.

8. Current blood pressure control rates are inadequate. Systems approaches that incorporate geriatric approaches to team care combined with quality improvement strategies need to be adopted to improve treatment outcomes.

of BP result in excess of 130 mm Hg systolic and/or 80 mm Hg diastolic or those receiving an antihypertensive medication—the overall prevalence for hypertension among those aged 65 or older exceeds 65%. For women aged 75 and older, the prevalence is 85% and for men it is 84%. Of note, there is an age–gender interaction in hypertension prevalence across age. At younger ages, prevalence rates are higher among men, while above the age of menopause, the prevalence in women surpasses that of men.

Another perspective on epidemiology is to examine the lifetime risk of developing hypertension as has been done in participants in the Framingham Heart Study. This study identified that among men and women participants who had normal blood pressure readings at age 55, nearly 90% developed hypertension over the ensuing 20 to 25 years of follow-up.

CLASSIFICATION

The definitions for normal blood pressure and categories of hypertension were updated in 2017 with the publication of the revised American Heart Association High Blood Pressure Clinical Guideline. Importantly, the prior 140 mm Hg SBP threshold level that defined hypertension was lowered to 130 mm Hg. Contemporary definitions and categories of blood pressure are provided in **Table 79-1**. Of note, the blood

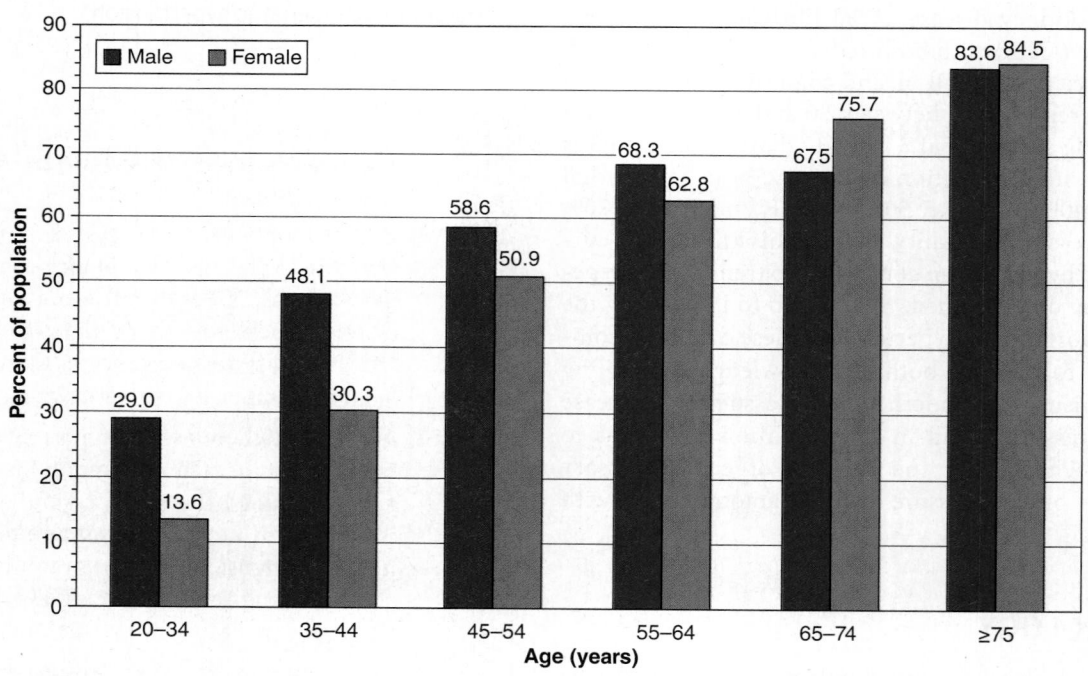

FIGURE 79-1. Prevalence of hypertension in US adults ≥ 20 years of age by sex and age (NHANES, 2015–2018). Hypertension is defined in terms of NHANES blood pressure measurements and health interviews. A person was considered to have hypertension if he or she had systolic blood pressure ≥ 130 mm Hg or diastolic blood pressure ≥ 80 mm Hg, if he or she said "yes" to taking antihypertensive medication, or if the person was told on two occasions that he or she had hypertension. NHANES indicates National Health and Nutrition Examination Survey. Source: Unpublished National Heart, Lung, and Blood Institute tabulation using NHANES, 2015 to 2018. (Reproduced with permission from NHANES, 2015 to 2018. National Heart, Lung, and Blood Institute. US Department of Health & Human Services.)

TABLE 79-1 ■ BLOOD PRESSURE (BP) CATEGORIES

	SYSTOLIC BP		DIASTOLIC BP
Normal	< 120 mm Hg	and	< 80 mm Hg
Elevated	120–129 mm Hg	and	< 80 mm Hg
Hypertension			
Stage 1	130–139 mm Hg	or	80–89 mm Hg
Stage 2	≥ 140 mm Hg	or	≥ 90 mm Hg

Reproduced with permission from Whelton PK, Carey RM, Aronow WS, et al. 2017 ACC/AHA/AAPA/ABC/ACPM/AGS/APhA/ASH/ASPC/NMA/PCNA Guideline for the Prevention, Detection, Evaluation, and Management of High Blood Pressure in Adults: A Report of the American College of Cardiology/American Heart Association Task Force on Clinical Practice Guidelines. Hypertension. 2018;71(6):e13–e115.

pressure categorizations make no adjustment for age. These definitions incorporate evidence that the cardiovascular risks associated with high blood pressure are continuous beginning at a level of 115/75 mm Hg. The definitions also emphasize that SBP is a more important CVD risk factor than diastolic blood pressure (DBP)—especially for individuals older than 50 years. Finally, since isolated diastolic hypertension is so uncommon among older patients, one may correctly classify an older patient's hypertension in almost all cases based entirely on the level of their SBP.

PATHOPHYSIOLOGIC CHARACTERISTICS

No single factor is likely to explain the cause of essential hypertension regardless of its age of onset. However, a number of age-related changes in physiology have been identified and summarized in **Table 79-2** that likely contribute to the age-associated increase in blood pressure and to the prevalence of hypertension. Lifestyle factors such as obesity, especially central adiposity, being sedentary, and eating a diet high in sodium content are also contributors commonly identified among older individuals.

Homeostatic regulation of blood pressure within its relatively narrow normal range while continuously maintaining adequate cerebral perfusion requires intricate and dynamic coordination of several complex interacting physiologic systems. Under resting conditions, despite age-related physiologic changes that occur in these systems, older individuals experience little difficulty maintaining their blood pressure and cerebral perfusion. However, when this balance is placed at risk by perturbations imposed by the intravascular volume shifts that occur with upright posture or following a meal, or the stimulus of exposure to one or more vasodilating medications, the older patient is less able to adapt and significant declines in blood pressure and inadequate cerebral perfusion may ensue.

Arterial stiffness, especially in the large central arteries, is the pathophysiologic characteristic that best exemplifies geriatric hypertension. The age-related increase in arterial stiffness is responsible for the type of hypertension most commonly encountered in older patients, namely, systolic hypertension with high pulse pressure (the difference between systolic and diastolic blood pressure). Moreover, several longitudinal studies have demonstrated that an individual's pulse wave velocity—a marker of arterial stiffness—is a predictor for the subsequent development of hypertension.

Beyond this structural change in the arteries, the regulation of vascular resistance is also affected by age-related changes in the autonomic nervous system and in the vascular endothelium. There is an age-associated decline in the sensitivity of the arterial baroreceptor. This affects the regulation of vascular resistance in two important ways. First, a larger change in blood pressure is required to stimulate the baroreceptor to invoke the appropriate compensatory response in heart rate. This contributes to the age-related increase in blood pressure variability and likely explains the greater prevalence of postural and postprandial hypotension observed in older individuals. Second, the decrease in baroreceptor sensitivity leads to relatively greater activation of sympathetic nervous system outflow for a given level of blood pressure.

Regulation of vascular resistance by the vascular endothelium is also changed in relation to age. Endothelial dysfunction demonstrated by a decrease in the production of endothelial-derived nitric oxide has been identified to accompany aging as well as hypertension. Impaired nitric oxide–mediated vasodilation is another potential contributor to the age-related increase in peripheral vascular resistance.

Age-related changes in renal function and in particular in renal regulation of sodium balance may also contribute to an increase in blood pressure. Decreased renal blood flow and glomerular filtration rate impair the aging kidney's ability to excrete a sodium load. These renal changes in the regulation of sodium balance create a tendency for sodium retention. This likely plays a part in the finding that a high proportion of older hypertensive individuals, perhaps as high as two-thirds, are characterized as having salt sensitivity. Salt sensitivity is operationally defined as an increase in mean arterial blood pressure, commonly 5 mm Hg or more, during a high compared to a low dietary sodium intake.

Aging also alters the renin-angiotensin-aldosterone system in ways that may contribute both to elevated blood pressure as well as sodium sensitivity. In general, older

TABLE 79-2 ■ AGE-RELATED PHYSIOLOGIC CHANGES THAT CONTRIBUTE TO ELEVATED BLOOD PRESSURE

- Arterial stiffness
- Decreased baroreceptor sensitivity
- Increased sympathetic nervous system activity
- Decreased α- and β-adrenergic receptor responsiveness
- Endothelial dysfunction
- Decreased ability to excrete sodium load (sodium sensitivity)
- Low plasma renin activity
- Resistance to insulin's effect on carbohydrate metabolism
- Central adiposity

hypertensive subjects are characterized by having low levels of plasma renin activity. A direct relationship between plasma aldosterone levels within the physiologic range of normal and the future development of hypertension has been shown in normotensive individuals. Since higher levels of aldosterone have also been linked with central obesity, vascular stiffness, blunting of baroreceptor sensitivity, impaired endothelial function, insulin resistance, and sodium sensitivity, it seems very possible that aldosterone may prove to be a unifying factor that accounts for many of the age-related changes in these physiologic features that also contribute to elevated blood pressure.

DIAGNOSTIC EVALUATION

Measurement Considerations

The first and most critical step in the diagnostic evaluation of hypertension among older individuals is the accurate measurement of blood pressure. In addition to the standard measurement instructions dictating patient preparation and positioning (minimum 5 minute rest in seated position with feet on floor), cuff size and type of instrument, several factors regarding appropriate blood pressure measurement deserve emphasis. As a result of the observation that blood pressure is more variable in older people, the dictum that "hypertension should never be diagnosed on the basis of a single blood pressure measurement" is especially true. Studies have documented that there is considerable overdiagnosis of hypertension among older people. For example, up to one-third of subjects who were receiving antihypertensive therapy when they enrolled in the Systolic Hypertension in the Elderly Program failed to meet entry blood pressure criteria for the study after their medications had been withdrawn. The diagnosis of hypertension should be based on the average of a minimum of nine blood pressure readings that have been obtained on three separate office visits or derived from 24-hour ambulatory or home blood pressure monitoring results.

Second, with respect to the appropriate measurement device, auscultatory methods are increasingly being supplanted by automated office blood pressure (AOBP) devices. These devices can record unattended BP readings over several minutes from which an average may be calculated. The limitations of auscultatory readings including challenges in accurately hearing the Korotkoff sounds, training requirements, and device calibration are all avoided with AOBP.

Third, while not directly related to the classification of hypertension, another important factor in blood pressure measurement is to always obtain supine and upright standing readings to determine if there is evidence for an orthostatic or postural decrease in blood pressure. The commonly used definition of postural hypotension is a decrease in SBP of 20 mm Hg or more from supine to upright positions within the first several minutes of standing. The presence of postural hypotension is an important risk factor for falls and may be exacerbated by almost all antihypertensive medication classes. During enrollment visits for the Systolic Blood Pressure Intervention Trial (SPRINT), nearly 10% of potential participants were found to have a SBP below 110 mm Hg and, as a result were excluded from the study. Clearly, identifying those patients with postural hypotension at the outset and throughout therapy is of critical importance.

Fourth, some individuals may have in-office blood pressure readings that are markedly elevated compared with their in-home, self-taken readings, commonly referred to as white coat hypertension. For these individuals, it is worth considering further evaluation with carefully taken home readings using an appropriately calibrated instrument or obtaining 24-hour ambulatory monitoring.

A final, fifth point concerning blood pressure measurement is to emphasize the primacy of systolic over diastolic blood pressure as the pressure that confers the most significance with respect to cardiovascular risk. Moreover, the pulse pressure, the difference between systolic and diastolic pressure, appears to outweigh either systolic or diastolic blood pressure as a cardiovascular risk factor.

Evaluation

Similar to younger patients, more than 90% of older hypertensive patients have essential hypertension. A diagnostic evaluation for secondary and potentially reversible causes of hypertension should be completed following the standard guidelines that have been developed for younger patients. There are several factors that deserve special attention in an older patient population. First, since the majority of hypertension in this population is systolic hypertension, older patients who present with primarily diastolic hypertension merit a careful evaluation with a focus on a renovascular cause. This is especially true for those who present with relatively abrupt onset of diastolic hypertension. Second, older patients are likely to be receiving a number of medications, some of which could be contributing to elevated blood pressure. A complete medication review is warranted to search for medications that may be implicated, for example, corticosteroids and nonsteroidal anti-inflammatory drugs including COX-2 inhibitors. Third, the prevalence of sleep apnea among older patients with hypertension is high and may be an important pathophysiologic explanation for their elevated blood pressure. Fourth, although the incidence of pheochromocytoma is rare, there is a suggestion from an autopsy study that the incidence of this condition increases with increasing age.

Target Organ Damage and Risk Factor Assessment

The evaluation should also include a determination of target organ damage, a cardiovascular risk factor assessment, and identification of comorbid conditions that may impact antihypertensive drug selection. Determining the extent of hypertension-related target organ damage may be complicated by the confounding effects of concurrent age- or disease-related changes. It is important to assess whether the patient has evidence of renal impairment, proteinuria, hypertensive retinopathy, electrocardiographic abnormalities, or left ventricular hypertrophy. An assessment of overall cardiovascular risk—smoking history, alcohol intake, dietary salt and fat intake, and level of physical activity—should also be completed. Finally, the presence of other comorbid conditions (eg, dementia, chronic kidney disease, chronic obstructive pulmonary disease [COPD]) and comorbidities such as frailty may influence antihypertensive medication selection as well as an individual's blood pressure target goal.

APPROACH TO TREATMENT

Treatment Effectiveness

Results from meta-analyses of numerous placebo-controlled randomized clinical trials that have been conducted in older hypertensive patients have confirmed that significant reductions in cardiovascular and cerebrovascular morbidity and mortality occur with antihypertensive therapy and that the treatments are also safe. Active treatment leads on average to a 12% to 25% decrease in the rate of death, a 35% reduction in stroke, and a 25% reduction in myocardial infarction in addition to significant decreases in the development of mild cognitive impairment, chronic kidney disease, and CHF. For these reasons, there is a clear consensus that treating hypertension in older patients is safe and effective.

Results published from the Systolic Blood Pressure Intervention Trial (SPRINT), which compared usual (< 140 mm Hg) with intensive (< 120 mm Hg) SBP targets (ClinicalTrials.gov, NCT01206062), suggest that a lower SBP target may be particularly effective for some patients with high CVD risk. SPRINT included 2636 community living subjects aged 75 and older (28% of the entire study population) who were assessed for frailty status including usual gait speed, orthostatic hypotension, adverse events including injurious falls and nursing home placement, and, in the SPRINT-MIND subset, comprehensive cognitive evaluations and brain imaging. In the group of older subjects randomized to the intensive arm there was a 34% reduction in the primary composite CVD outcome and a 33% reduction in all-cause mortality at 3.14 years of follow-up when the trial ended early due to its highly positive outcome (numbers needed to treat 27 and 41, respectively). These results did not differ for the most frail subgroup nor for those with impaired gait speed. While some adverse events were higher in the intensive group, there was no difference observed in serious adverse events including injurious falls and also no group difference in self-assessed health-related quality of life regardless of frailty status. The SPRINT Memory and Cognition in Decreased Hypertension (MIND) component was designed to address the hypothesis that the incidence of dementia would be lower with intensive SBP treatment. Although the 17% reduction in adjudicated all-cause probable dementia in the intensive

relative to the standard group did not achieve statistical significance, there were significant reductions of the same magnitude in the occurrence of mild cognitive impairment (MCI; 19%; $P = 0.01$) and in the composite outcome of MCI or dementia (15%; $P = 0.02$). The companion SPRINT-MRI study provided complementary results demonstrating that intensive therapy was associated with slower progression in the accumulation of white matter hyperintensity volume without significant differences in total brain volume. Longer term cognitive outcome data are currently being obtained in SPRINT MIND 2020 to further evaluate the dementia outcome as more cases accrue with extended follow-up.

Therapeutic Goals and Monitoring

In accordance with general geriatric principles, it is important to establish individualized patient treatment goals utilizing therapies that are least likely to produce adverse side effects or have a negative impact on quality of life. The inherent complexity and heterogeneity of older adults with multiple comorbidities that may include cognitive impairment and frailty who also have elevated SBP likely explains why it is proving to be so challenging to apply "one size fits all" treat-to-target therapy to this population.

The optimal SBP treatment goal for patients older than 65 years has evolved from the starting point of the seminal findings from the Systolic Hypertension in the Elderly Program (SHEP) study published in 1991 that for the first time demonstrated that treating what was then known as systolic hypertension was both safe and effective. Over time, subsequent clinical trials and guidelines have informed changes to the recommended SBP treatment goals for older individuals (**Figure 79-2**). Results from the SPRINT study have been incorporated into the most current, 2017, American Heart Association High Blood Pressure Clinical Practice Guideline. Its recommendation for ambulatory, community-living older adults is a SBP goal of 130 mm Hg. Its recommendation for those with "a high burden of comorbidity and limited life expectancy" is to utilize clinical judgment in a patient-informed discussion.

The most common treatment-related adverse side effect, shared by all antihypertensive medications, is the development of postural hypotension. Patients may present with atypical symptoms such as generalized weakness or fatigue rather than noting postural light-headedness or dizziness. For this reason, it is important not to treat blood pressure too aggressively and also to always determine supine and upright blood pressure measurements during monitoring of all older patients. If a patient's seated SBP cannot be lowered to below 130 mm Hg without the development of postural hypotension, it is prudent to consider modifying that patient's target blood pressure goal to instead focus on their standing blood pressure.

When patients present with markedly elevated blood pressures in the absence of a true hypertensive emergency (eg, signs of target organ damage, hypertensive

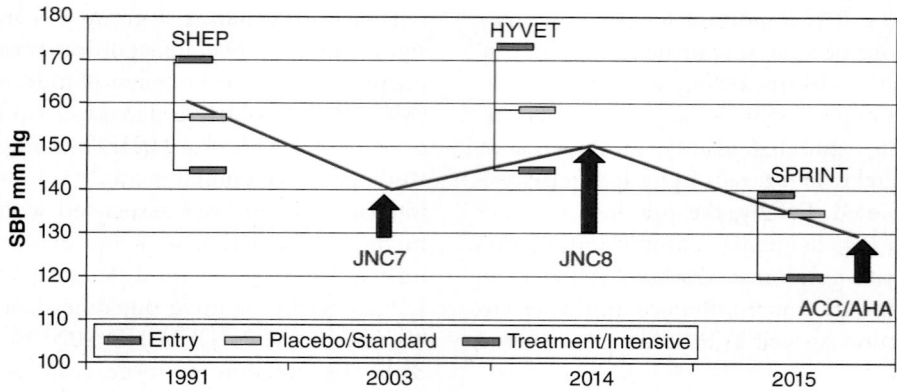

FIGURE 79-2. Recommended systolic blood pressure (SBP) treatment goals for older individuals. The red line illustrates the changes in the recommended systolic blood pressure (SBP) goal sequentially over time by the Joint National Committee on the Detection and Prevention of Hypertension's (JNC) 7 (published in 2003) and 8 (published in 2013) guidelines and the 2017 ACC/AHA guideline. The two major randomized controlled trials prior to the Systolic Blood Pressure Intervention Trial (SPRINT) that informed these changes—the Systolic Hypertension in the Elderly Project (SHEP) in 1991 and the Hypertension in the Very Elderly Trial (HYVET) in 2008—are superimposed with the entry SBP levels for their participants (red bar) and the achieved SBP for the placebo or standard (yellow bar) and active or intensive arms (green bars). It is important to recognize that the benefits observed with intensive therapy in SPRINT are relative to a standard arm whose SBP levels were below the level recommended in prior guidelines. (Reproduced with permission from Supiano MA, Williamson JD. New guidelines and SPRINT results: implications for geriatric hypertension. *Circulation.* 2019;140[12]:976–978.)

encephalopathy, intracranial hemorrhage, acute heart failure with pulmonary edema, dissecting aortic aneurysm, or unstable angina), it is not necessary and may in fact be deleterious to reduce blood pressure to normal values too rapidly. Setting an intermediate treatment goal of 160 mm Hg may be appropriate for these patients. Dosage adjustments or additions of new therapies should be made gradually over time to avoid overtreatment. Similarly, once patients have reached their therapeutic target and have been maintained on stable therapy, their need for continued treatment should be periodically reassessed. Many patients will tolerate a dosage reduction or medication discontinuation during a carefully monitored withdrawal period, especially if they have been successful in achieving lifestyle modifications.

Lifestyle Modifications

Based on the physiologic profile of the typical older hypertensive patient described in the preceding section—overweight, sedentary, and salt-sensitive—lifestyle modifications directed toward these characteristics would be predicted to be especially efficacious. Additional reasons to focus attention on lifestyle modification are that they will be adjunctive if medications are also needed, will lead to improvements in other cardiovascular risk factors, are associated with other salutary outcomes (notably exercise), and are associated with minimal adverse effects. For patients with stage 1 hypertension (systolic levels between 130 and 139 mm Hg) who do not have diabetes, a 6-month treatment intervention with appropriate lifestyle modifications is the recommended first step. Randomized controlled trials of multifactorial lifestyle interventions have

been conducted and demonstrated the benefit in blood pressure reduction that is achieved as well as sustained in the intervention groups. A meta-analysis of 105 such trials (although few were directed solely to older subjects), demonstrated the overall benefits of weight reduction, aerobic exercise, and decreased intake of sodium and alcohol. Each of these modifications was associated on average with a 5 mm Hg reduction in SBP, comparable to the reduction achieved with a single antihypertensive medication.

The Trial of Nonpharmacologic Intervention in the Elderly (TONE) targeted the effect of dietary sodium restriction and weight loss in older hypertensive patients. In this study, the intervention led to fairly modest declines in dietary sodium intake (average of 40 mmol/day) and body weight (average 4 kg), but there was a 30% decrease in the need to reinitiate antihypertensive therapy among the intervention group.

Pharmacologic Therapies

Overview Currently available evidence supports two general principles with respect to antihypertensive medication selection: one, that the level of blood pressure reduction achieved is more important than which drug is used, and two, that all classes of antihypertensive medications have been demonstrated to be equally efficacious in older patients. Following these principles, the initial antihypertensive drug selection should be based on patient-specific factors. For example, drug selection will depend on whether the patient's hypertension is simple or complicated by another comorbid condition. The presence of a coexisting condition will often dictate the optimal medication (eg, an ACE inhibitor for patients with type 2 diabetes or CHF). Beyond these factors, medications that are least likely to produce adverse effects should receive first priority. For this reason, as a general statement, centrally acting antihypertensive medications and direct vasodilators are best avoided in older hypertensive patients due respectively to concerns regarding central nervous system sedating effects and their association with marked postural hypotension. In addition, attention should be paid to selecting a once-daily medication to promote adherence and to avoiding any medication interactions with the patient's other medications.

General treatment recommendations for stage 1 hypertension are summarized in **Table 79-3**. For patients with stage 1 hypertension in whom a 6-month lifestyle modification intervention strategy has failed to lower blood pressure to the goal level, a thiazide-type diuretic is the most commonly recommended initial medication. Patients who present with stage 2 hypertension will almost certainly require at least two drugs to control their blood pressure— consequently, two antihypertensives should be initiated at the outset. Most often one of these two is a thiazide-type diuretic with the second agent selected either on compelling indications or on the basis of synergy with the initial agent (eg, combined with ACE inhibitor). It should be noted that regardless of the drug choice, in general the starting dose should be reduced in older patients and dosage titration be carried out gradually.

There are two additional general considerations to be made before a brief review of each of the major antihypertensive classes. (1) β-Receptor antagonists are not recommended as an appropriate choice for the initial antihypertensive drug, especially among older patients. Results from a meta-analysis concluded that unless there is a compelling indication for their use, β-blockers should not be considered as a first-line antihypertensive agent in older (60 years and older) patients. (2) Patient-specific factors

TABLE 79-3 ■ GENERAL TREATMENT RECOMMENDATIONS FOR STAGE 1 HYPERTENSION

- Begin with nonpharmacologic lifestyle modifications— weight loss, exercise, salt restriction for 6-mo period.
- Focus treatment goal on systolic blood pressure reduction to below 130 mm Hg.
- If target blood pressure is not met, consider low-dose thiazide-type diuretic—typically chlorthalidone—as initial drug selection.
- Base alternative drug selection on individual patient characteristics.
- Consider combination of low doses of one or more agents if goal blood pressure not met with a single drug.
- When initiating drug therapy, begin at half of the usual dose, increase dose slowly, and continue nonpharmacologic therapies.
- Aggressive therapy is not appropriate if adverse side effects (eg, postural hypotension) cannot be avoided.

that directly impact adherence also need to be taken into account. For example, thiazide diuretics are considered to be first-line agents, but persistence rates with their continued use are lower than with angiotensin receptor blockers. As with any prescribed medication, cost, simplicity of the regimen, and absence of side effects are important factors impacting rates of adherence.

Diuretics **Table 79-4** summarizes the advantages and disadvantages for each of the major drug classes from the geriatric patient perspective. There are several reasons why thiazide-type diuretics are considered to be the preferred initial antihypertensive agent for most older patients. The primary pathophysiologic explanation is that diuretic therapy has been noted to reduce SBP to a greater extent than diastolic blood pressure, and also achieves greater reductions in systolic pressure relative to other antihypertensive agents. Moreover, the majority of large-scale randomized controlled trials have utilized a thiazide-type diuretic in the treatment arm and there exist an abundance of outcome data demonstrating their therapeutic effectiveness in older hypertensive populations. Additional benefits include low cost, once-daily dosing, and a favorable side effect profile. The most common adverse drug events are metabolic abnormalities, especially hypokalemia, as well as hyperuricemia and impaired glucose intolerance; and urinary frequency or incontinence. However, these side effects are quite uncommon at lower doses. Within the thiazide diuretic class, chlorthalidone is the recommended medication. In addition to evidence of its efficacy from many randomized controlled trials, it has greater potency and a longer half-life than hydrochlorothiazide. When equipotent doses are compared, the incidence of hypokalemia is comparable. Finally, there is good synergy with most of the other commonly used medications, such that adding a second drug if needed to a thiazide-type diuretic is a reasonable approach.

Owing to the similarities observed between the physiologic effects of aldosterone and the age-related contributors to elevated blood pressure listed in **Table 79-2**, aldosterone receptor blockers (spironolactone or eplerenone) are other alternatives to consider.

Angiotensin-converting enzyme inhibitors and angiotensin receptor blockers ACE inhibitor agents and angiotensin receptor blockers are choices for initial therapy or as second agents in combination with a thiazide-type diuretic. Their advantages include the absence of central nervous system or metabolic side effects and overall favorable side effect profile. They are also often used owing to the recommendations for their use in the setting of coexisting type 2 diabetes or heart failure.

Calcium channel antagonists All three chemical classes of calcium channel antagonists have been shown to be effective in treating older hypertensive patients. Their mechanism of action—decreased peripheral vascular resistance—and lack of significant central nervous system or metabolic side

TABLE 79-4 ■ ADVANTAGES AND DISADVANTAGES OF ANTIHYPERTENSIVE MEDICATION CLASSES SPECIFIC TO OLDER PATIENTS

ANTIHYPERTENSIVE CLASS	POTENTIAL ADVANTAGES	POTENTIAL DISADVANTAGES	CLINICAL SITUATIONS TO RECOMMEND USE	CLINICAL SITUATIONS TO RECOMMEND AGAINST USE OR THAT REQUIRE MONITORING
Thiazide-type diuretics	• Documented benefit in clinical trials • Produce greater reduction in systolic than diastolic blood pressure • Improve bone mineral density • Inexpensive	• Metabolic abnormalities (eg, hypokalemia) • Urinary frequency	• Systolic hypertension	• Hyponatremia • Gout
ACE inhibitors and angiotensin receptor blockers	• Absence of CNS effects • Preservation of renal function • Decrease proteinuria	• Hyperkalemia, cough	• CHF, type 2 diabetes	• Renal insufficiency or renal artery stenosis
Calcium channel antagonists	• Benefit documented in clinical trials • Absence of CNS or metabolic effects	• Peripheral edema, constipation, heart block	• Systolic hypertension • Coronary artery disease	• Left ventricular dysfunction
β-Adrenergic receptor antagonists	• Not recommended as monotherapy	• May increase peripheral vascular resistance • Metabolic abnormalities • CNS effects	• Postmyocardial infarction	• COPD, peripheral vascular disease, heart block, glucose intolerance, type 2 diabetes, hyperlipidemia, depression
α-Adrenergic receptor antagonists	• Improve urinary symptoms in BPH	• Increased rate of CHF hospitalizations as monotherapy relative to thiazide-type diuretics	• Prostatism	• Left ventricular dysfunction

ACE, angiotensin-converting enzyme; BPH, benign prostatic hypertrophy; CHF, congestive heart failure; CNS, central nervous system; COPD, chronic obstructive pulmonary disease.

effects provide a good match with the characteristics of the geriatric patient. Age-related changes in the pharmacokinetics of these drugs (decreased clearance and increased plasma levels) mean that lower doses need to be used in older patients. The longer-acting agents in the dihydropyridine class of calcium channel antagonists have been the most widely studied in randomized controlled trials where their effectiveness in treating older patient populations has been demonstrated.

Adrenergic receptor antagonists As discussed previously, β-receptor antagonists are not an appropriate choice for monotherapy for older patients with uncomplicated hypertension. β-Receptor antagonists should be reserved for patients with a compelling indication for their use, namely, as secondary prevention for those patients who have had prior myocardial infarction or have coronary artery disease or in some patients with systolic dysfunction.

Several observations have limited the adoption of α_1-receptor antagonists as first-line treatment for older hypertensive patients. In addition to their predilection to

produce postural hypotension, subjects who received an α_1-receptor antagonist as monotherapy in the Antihypertensive and Lipid-Lowering Treatment to Prevent Heart Attack Trial (ALLHAT) were found to have a twofold higher risk of being hospitalized for heart failure relative to the subjects randomized to the diuretic arm of the study. Based on these observations, α_1-receptor antagonist therapy should be considered for use as monotherapy only in men in whom their use may be beneficial for symptoms related to benign prostatic hypertrophy, or in combination with another antihypertensive agent.

Barriers to Improving Blood Pressure Control

Since there is no cure for this chronic condition, effective treatment of hypertension requires a lifelong commitment to its management. For this reason, an approach that engages and sustains the patient's motivation and adherence over time is needed. Several methods may be recommended to promote the patient's efforts such as providing patient education materials appropriate for the patient's health literacy level, clear instructions for diet and exercise lifestyle recommendations, and prescribing once-daily medications to facilitate adherence. Some patients may benefit from the feedback and engagement that accompany home or self-taken blood pressure monitoring. Another patient factor is the likelihood that the older hypertensive patient will have two or more additional chronic conditions. The complexity imposed by concurrently managing these comorbid conditions becomes extremely challenging. This is especially the case when treating a frail older individual when it is not clear how to best prioritize which of several guidelines should take precedence or for that matter if the guideline is still applicable to the patient's clinical situation.

In addition to these patient-specific factors, a number of barriers have been identified in the health care system that may impede progress in achieving better success in blood pressure control rates in the older population. The underdetection, undertreatment, and inadequate control of hypertension, especially among older patients, are well documented. Some of these system factors are limited access, lack of a team approach to care, constraints imposed by limited patient visit times, access to and costs of treatment, and the reimbursement system. Physician factors—the failure to modify treatment when the patient's target blood pressure goal has not been achieved—also contribute to this situation. Many physicians overestimate their compliance with guidelines as well as the proportion of their patient populations who have blood pressure levels below their target. However, some quality improvement strategies have been demonstrated to be effective in improving hypertension management. The most effective strategies in this regard have involved a multidisciplinary team approach (assigning a nonphysician member of the team to assume responsibility for management), home blood pressure monitoring, and patient education. Thus, it appears that incorporating a geriatrics approach to hypertension management in the context of a quality improvement program is one effective way to eliminate some of the barriers to improving hypertension control in older patient populations.

The "Trial of Intensive Blood-Pressure Control in Older Patients with Hypertension," was conducted in China shortly after SPRINT (ClinicalTrials.gov NCT03015311).

8511 Chinese patients with hypertension (age range 60 to 80 years) were randomized to an intensive treatment goal (SBP 100 to < 130 mm Hg) or a standard goal (130 to < 150 mm Hg). In addition to the different racial composition, relative to SPRINT, participants in the Strategy of Blood Pressure Intervention in the Elderly Hypertensive Patients (STEP) trial were younger (mean age 66.2 years) and in general had lower CVD risk. There were also differences in the blood pressure measurement protocols, the achieved SBP in the two arms, and the anti-hypertensive drug regimens used to achieve the treatment goals. Nonetheless, similar to SPRINT, the trial ended early, at a follow-up of 3.3 years, when it was clear that its primary CVD outcome was met in favor of the intensive treatment goal. The STEP trial's major conclusion that "a reduction in the systolic blood pressure to less than 130 mm Hg resulted in cardiovascular benefits in older patients with hypertension in China" is confirmatory of the SPRINT results.

UNANSWERED QUESTIONS AND FUTURE RESEARCH DIRECTIONS

Future research directions should target our understanding of the mechanisms underlying the age-associated increase in blood pressure, with important implications for prevention and management. For example, it seems clear that understanding the predictors and modifiers of vascular stiffness is of critical importance in preventing the age-associated development of hypertension. Similarly, although none of the currently available antihypertensive agents specifically targets vascular stiffness, future advances in drug development aimed at preventing hypertension will likely address decreasing vascular stiffness as a mechanism of action. Balancing the competing risks between the SBP-related risk of stroke, heart failure, other cardiovascular events and cognitive impairment and the treatment-related risks, including adverse medication events, falls, and fall-related injuries, in a patient-centered approach remains a challenge that merits further research, particularly in the very frail older adult population. Finally, additional investigation will aim to elucidate why hypertension is a significant risk factor for cognitive impairment and dementia.

FURTHER READING

Beckett NS, Peters R, Fletcher AE, et al. Treatment of hypertension in patients 80 years of age or older. *N Engl J Med*. 2008;358:1887–1898.

Dickinson HO, Mason JM, Nicolson DJ, et al. Lifestyle interventions to reduce raised blood pressure: a systematic review of randomized controlled trials. *J Hypertens*. 2006;24:215–233.

Elliott WJ. Drug interactions and drugs that affect blood pressure. *J Clin Hypertens*. 2006;8:731–737.

Elmer PJ, Obarzanek E, Vollmer WM, et al. Effects of comprehensive lifestyle modification on diet, weight, physical fitness, and blood pressure control: 18-month results of a randomized trial. *Ann Intern Med*. 2006;144: 485–495.

1228 Forette F, Seux ML, Staessen JA, et al. Prevention of dementia in randomised double-blind placebo-controlled Systolic Hypertension in Europe (Syst-Eur) trial. *Lancet.* 1998;352:1347–1351.

Forouzanfar MH, Liu P, Roth GA, et al. Global burden of hypertension and systolic blood pressure of at least 110 to 115 mm Hg, 1990-2015. *JAMA.* 2017;317(2):165–182.

Gueyffier F, Bulpitt C, Boissel JP, et al. Antihypertensive drugs in very old people a subgroup meta-analysis of randomised controlled trials. *Lancet.* 1999;353: 793–796.

Kaess BM, Rong J, Larson MG, et al. Aortic stiffness, blood pressure progression, and incident hypertension. *JAMA.* 2012;308:875–881.

SPRINT MIND Investigators for the SPRINT Research Group. Effect of intensive vs standard blood pressure control on probable dementia: a randomized clinical trial. *JAMA.* 2019;321(6):553–561.

SPRINT MIND Investigators for the SPRINT Research Group. Association of intensive vs standard blood pressure control with cerebral white matter lesions. *JAMA.* 2019;322(6):524–534.

Staessen JA, Gasowski JG, Thijs L, et al. Risks of untreated and treated isolated systolic hypertension in the elderly: meta-analysis of outcome trials. *Lancet.* 2000;355: 865–872.

Steinman MA, Fischer MA, Shlipak MG, et al. Clinician awareness of adherence to hypertension guidelines. *Am J Med.* 2004;117:747–754.

Supiano MA, Williamson JD. New guidelines and SPRINT results. *Circulation.* 2019;140:976–978.

Vasan RS, Beiser A, Seshadri S, et al. Residual lifetime risk for developing hypertension in middle-aged women and men: the Framingham heart study. *JAMA.* 2002;287:1003–1010.

Walsh JM, McDonald KM, Shojania KG, et al. Quality improvement strategies for hypertension management: a systematic review. *Med Care.* 2006;44:646–657.

Whelton PK, Appel LJ, Espeland MA, et al. Sodium reduction and weight loss in the treatment of hypertension in older persons: a randomized controlled trial of nonpharmacologic interventions in the elderly (TONE). *JAMA.* 1998;279:839–846.

Whelton PK, Carey RM, Aronow WS, et al. 2017 ACC/AHA/AAPA/ABC/ACPM/AGS/APhA/ASH/ASPC/NMA/PCNA guideline for the prevention, detection, evaluation, and management of high blood pressure in adults: a report of the American College of Cardiology/American Heart Association Task Force on Clinical Practice Guidelines. *J Am Coll Cardiol.* 2018;71:e127–248.

Williamson JD, Supiano MA, Applegate WB, et al. Intensive vs standard blood pressure control and cardiovascular disease outcomes in adults aged ≥75 years: a randomized clinical trial. *JAMA.* 2016;315(24):2673–2682.

Wright JT Jr, Williamson JD, Whelton PK, et al. SPRINT Research Group. A randomized trial of intensive vs standard blood pressure control. *N Engl J Med.* 2015;373(22): 2103–2116.

Zhang W, Zhang S, Deng Y, et al. STEP Study Group. Trial of intensive blood-pressure control in older patients with hypertension. *N Engl J Med.* 2021;385(14):1268–1279

Chapter 80

Respiratory System and Selected Pulmonary Disorders

Daniel Guidot, Patty J. Lee, Laurie D. Snyder

INTRODUCTION

Respiratory function is the interplay between the functioning of the lung tissue itself, the airways, the muscles of respiration, and the bones and joints of the thorax. In addition, the respiratory system interacts closely with other organs like the heart. Changes in each and all of these different parts ultimately affect how one breathes. By understanding how each of these parts changes with aging, one can understand how the respiratory system as a whole changes with time.

Embryonic growth and development of the lung is a complex process, and after birth the development of the lung continues. Just as the normal body grows into young adulthood, the lungs and their function progress as well. Eventually, however, the lungs reach their peak capacity, usually well above the requirements needed for normal respiratory functioning. With normal aging, the pulmonary function declines as lung tissue, chest wall, and muscles change over time. For many patients, this decline never reaches the threshold of meaningful pulmonary disease (**Figure 80-1**). However, in other individuals, the accumulated insults and injuries lead to an accelerated aging process and pulmonary disease that can lead to breathlessness, decreased exercise capacity, and eventually death. Thus, when considering the aging process of a person's lung, one must take into account their childhood lung development, the cumulative burden of lung damage that they have incurred already, and any factors that may accelerate the decline in the lung function.

CELLULAR LUNG CHANGES WITH AGING

The lung undergoes many cellular changes over time. These changes are the result both of the natural aging process as well as the fact that the lung is continually exposed

Learning Objectives

- Identify the structural, physiologic, and cellular changes of the lung with age.
- Describe how aging processes relate to lung diseases in older patients.

Key Clinical Points

1. **Pulmonary function declines over time in healthy individuals leading to changes in oxygenation, ventilation, and the ability to fight infections.**
2. **Lung disease impacts pulmonary function and can accelerate pulmonary age-related decline.**
3. **Changes in the immune system with aging lead to decreased response to antigens and a proinflammatory state, which increases the risk for severe lung infections.**
4. **Best practices for pulmonary care of older patients includes avoidance of tobacco products and environmental pollution, maintaining ideal body weight, considering appropriate vaccinations, and if hypoxic, oxygen supplementation.**

to a range of stress insults, particularly from the external environment. Eventually the cells of the lung lose the ability to divide and differentiate in a process known as senescence. Senescent cells are characterized by arrested

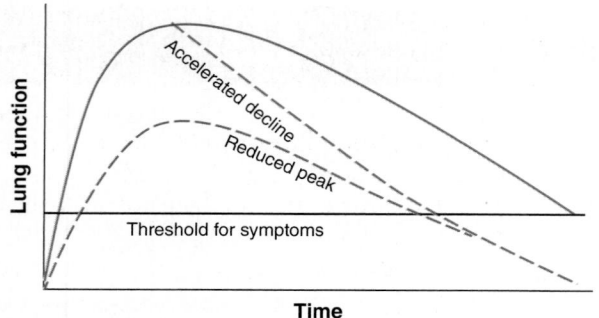

FIGURE 80-1. The figure shows lung function by time with a threshold below which patient experience symptoms. After reaching peak function, lung function declines with aging. Accumulated injuries lead to an accelerated aging process and pulmonary disease that can cause dyspnea, decreased exercise capacity, and death.

cell proliferation coupled with decreased apoptosis and a senescence-associated secretory phenotype (SASP) that is specific to the type of cell. While senescent cells can prevent the propagation of damaged cells, they also limit proliferation for tissue repair. Initially, the SASP may be immunosuppressive and promote wound healing, but persistence of the secretory phenotype leads to chronic inflammation and profibrotic processes.

Cellular senescence increases with aging and can be induced by a variety of insults, including oxidative stress, telomere shortening, DNA damage, inflammation, and mitochondrial stress. Environmental insults and disease states can increase oxidative stress to the lungs. Oxidative stress is the process by which highly reactive molecules arise inside cells, leading to damage to the structures within the cell. These molecules arise from the normal processes of oxygen metabolism within the cell. However, toxic environmental exposures and inflammatory states can increase oxidative stress and accelerate this process. With time, progressive oxidative stress can affect how effectively lung cells carry out their various functions and promote accumulation of senescent cells.

Cells are actively dividing and replenishing the tissues over time. With each cell replication, a small amount of genetic information is lost and discarded with each end of the DNA molecule. To protect against loss of vital information, chromosomes have segments of redundant DNA at each end, known as telomeres. However, after cells have undergone enough divisions, they can exhaust their telomeres, resulting in a process where each new cell division results in a cell with slightly less DNA than its parent cell. Genetic predispositions for short telomeres (known as short telomere syndromes) and cellular processes that require increased cell turnover can exacerbate the exhaustion of telomeres, leading to senescence.

In addition, changes in the immune system also occur with aging and impact the lung function and ability to respond to infections. Over time, the body acquires more memory T cells from previous antigen exposure.

In addition, the pool of naïve T cells declines over time. This results in an immune system with less capability to respond to new antigens, a state of immune senescence. Thus, when exposed to new infections, the adaptive immune system has less capacity to respond leading to increased innate immune response and increased inflammation and oxidative stress as well as reduced antigen clearance.

Cellular function can change with aging. The cells that line the surface of the alveoli and bronchi in the lungs have cilia, and the sweeping motion of the cilia are an important part of the clearance of debris and pathogens from the lungs. As the lungs age, the cilia have reduced movement, leading to reduced clearance of mucus. Cellular aging also affects the extracellular matrix of cells, the system of molecules on the surface of cells that help them maintain their normal structure and function. As cells age, the extracellular matrix changes to be composed less of elastin and more of collagen, a more rigid and less flexible molecule. This results in lung tissue that is stiff and has a reduced ability to return to its natural shape.

The end result of all of these cellular changes is that, with aging, the lung demonstrates reduced capacity to respond to stress, greater propensity toward proinflammatory cytokines, abnormal tissue repair, and increased susceptibility to infection.

MECHANICAL AND FUNCTIONAL LUNG CHANGES WITH AGING

Pulmonary function testing (PFT) is a widely used procedure in pulmonary medicine to measure lung volumes and lung mechanics. While many different studies can be performed, this chapter will focus on the three most commonly performed tests: spirometry, lung volumes, and diffusion capacity.

Spirometry

Spirometry measures the ability to move air in and out of the lungs. The patient maximally inhales and then maximally exhales into a closed-circuit tube, and the volume of air that they are able to exhale is measured. The total amount of air exhaled during this forced exhalation maneuver is called the forced vital capacity (FVC). The FVC can then be further subdivided over specific time points. The most clinically important subdivision is the amount of air exhaled within the first second of exhalation, called the forced expiratory volume in 1 second (FEV$_1$). By taking the ratio of FEV$_1$ to FVC, the clinician can evaluate for obstruction. The greater the airways obstruction, the longer it takes to exhale and the lower the FEV$_1$ to FVC ratio.

Lung Volumes

At the end of a full exhalation, there is no way to know how much air remains in the lungs. Thus, spirometry alone cannot measure total lung volumes. However, the PFT lab can use additional techniques to measure the volume in the lungs that can take advantage of gas exchange or plethysmography (change of pressure over volume). Using these methods, one can calculate the amount of air in the maximally inflated lung (total lung capacity or TLC) as well as the amount of air trapped in the lungs after maximal exhalation (residual volume or RV). These measures of TLC and RV provide additional insights into the lung function.

Diffusion Capacity

Finally, PFT can assess the ability of the lungs to extract oxygen from the air. Carbon monoxide (CO) is a toxic molecule with higher affinity for hemoglobin than oxygen. However, very low levels can be safely inhaled, and the body's ability to absorb carbon monoxide can be used as a surrogate for measuring the gas exchange of oxygen.

Several structural changes in the airways of the lungs occur as part of the normal aging process and can variably affect the spirometry measurements. In the airways, accumulated damage leads to bronchial thickening and hyperplasia, and increases in sympathetic tone over time result in increased smooth muscle tone. In addition, diaphragmatic weakness progresses with aging which reduces the maximal intake of air. The final result of all of these processes is that, with aging, the FEV_1 declines over time. Reduced diaphragmatic strength also reduces the FVC. Loss of elasticity of the lung results in more air residing in the lung at the end of maximum exhalation, resulting in more air trapping and therefore a reduced FVC. However, the reductions in FVC are less in the reductions in FEV_1. Thus, the FEV_1 to FVC ratio drops with aging. In other words, aging lungs develop progressive obstruction.

With aging, the lung elasticity changes. The inward pole of the lung tissues is reduced with aging, resulting in an increased tendency for the lungs to rest at a large volume and an increase in TLC with aging. At the same time, however, the chest wall itself becomes smaller with loss of vertebral height and calcification within the rib joint articulations, which increases the force required to expand the chest. These processes reduce TLC with age. The net result is that, with aging, TLC remains relatively constant.

With aging and the progressive accumulation of pulmonary insults, capillary destruction occurs over time. This results in a reduced body of small blood vessels that could absorb oxygen from the air. Additionally, reduced elasticity of the lung results in greater stretching of the lung at the apices due to the pull of the gravity. This results in greater amounts of air being at the top of the lung. Blood flow, which is greatest at the bases of the lung, goes to regions with the least amount of air, resulting in a ventilation–perfusion mismatch. The cumulative result of this is that, with aging, diffusion capacity for carbon monoxide (DLCO) declines.

AGING IN KEY DISEASE STATES

Idiopathic Pulmonary Fibrosis

As opposed to diseases that affect the airways (such as COPD and asthma), interstitial lung disease, also known as ILD, is a disease of the lung tissue itself. It is a group of rare disease subtypes with varying causes and clinical manifestations. The most common form of ILD is idiopathic pulmonary fibrosis, or IPF, a disease in which the lung tissue is slowly and progressively consumed by fibrous scar tissue. The exact etiology of IPF is unknown but it is more common in patients older than 60 years. This association with older individuals highlights that the aging lung is more prone to abnormal fibrosis.

Patients with IPF most commonly present with gradual and insidious onset of progressive dyspnea with exertion, and there are commonly significant delays in diagnosis. In any older patient who presents with progressive dyspnea on exertion, IPF should be in the differential. Patients can also have cough, fine crackles at the bilateral lung bases, and in advanced disease, hypoxia with possibly cyanosis or clubbing of the fingernails. PFT usually reveals reduced TLC and reduced DLCO. Ultimately, the most important diagnostic modality for suspected IPF is CT chest imaging. IPF does have a classical presentation on CT imaging, known as a usual interstitial pneumonia pattern with reticular changes, honeycombing, and traction bronchiectasis (**Figure 80-2**).

In patients with suspected or confirmed IPF, referral to pulmonologist is standard of care. Primarily a fibrotic disease, IPF treatment centers on antifibrotics, namely nintedanib and pirfenidone rather than immunosuppressive medications like chronic steroids or other immunosuppressants. The antifibrotic medications slow the progression of restriction in lung function studies, but do not reverse any scarring that has already occurred. As such, these medications may not lead to immediate improvements in the current symptoms and quality of life of patients. Additionally, the antifibrotics have significant gastrointestinal side effects including nausea and diarrhea, and discontinuation of these medications due to intolerance is not uncommon. Thus, the decision to initiate or maintain antifibrotics must also be tailored to each individual patient.

Even with therapies, IPF is a steadily progressive disease with high morbidity and mortality, with expected median survival from time of diagnosis on the order of only a few years. In addition, patients with IPF can have flares whereby known or unknown triggers (including infections and clots) can lead to life-threatening bouts of severe inflammation and scarring. As such, for suitable patients diagnosed with IPF, physicians should consider referral for lung transplantation evaluation.

COVID-19

The COVID-19 pandemic highlights how the immune system of the aging lung responds differently to infections. COVID-19 is a viral infection characterized by fever, cough, fatigue, loss of smell, and in some patients, shortness of breath. In patients with respiratory symptoms, chest imaging shows bilateral pulmonary infiltrates consistent with diffuse alveolar damage. Patients may progress to acute respiratory

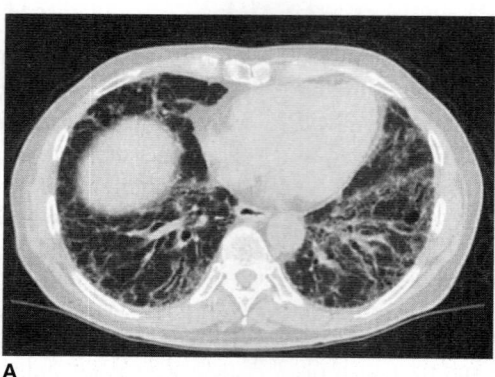

A

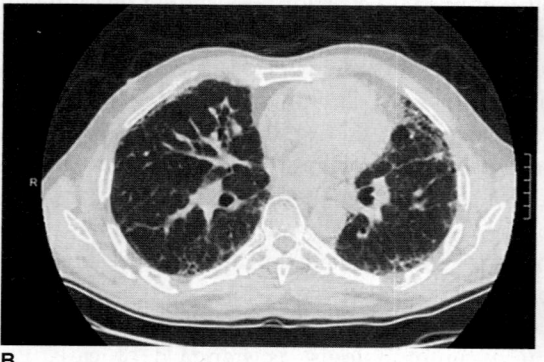

B

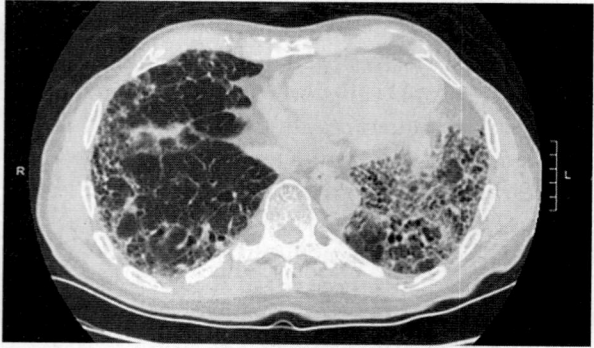

FIGURE 80-2. A. Idiopathic pulmonary fibrosis CT scan. In this image, there is traction bronchiectasis, septal thickening, and architectural distortion. There is honeycombing with subpleural distribution. **B.** Two images from same patient, different sections, same scan date. Image on left is mid-lung field slice with evidence of subpleural predominant honeycombing and reticulation. Image on right is lower lung fields showing subpleural involvement but more extensive disease, honeycombing, and traction bronchiectasis. (Reproduced with permission from Dr. Snyder.)

distress syndrome and require mechanical life support. This evolution to respiratory failure occurs in a highly proinflammatory state that drives activation of disseminated intravascular coagulation and subsequent multiorgan failure. Older patients with COVID-19 are particularly at risk for this proinflammatory state. The older patient's adaptive immune system limits viral clearance with the relative decrease in T and B cells and decreased ability to respond to specific antigens. This failure of the adaptive immune response combined with the proinflammatory response of the innate immune system sets the stage for an overwhelming immune response in the lungs, contributing to lung failure and systemic immune activation.

BEST PRACTICES IN PULMONARY MEDICINE TO COUNTER THE AGING PROCESS

The healthy aging lung's pulmonary function declines over time. That said, patients and clinicians can take important steps to mitigate both the aging process as well as the effects it has on lung health and function. One of the most important intervention is the avoidance of deleterious exposures

such as tobacco and air pollution. Exposures like these trigger a proinflammatory response and further direct damage to the lung tissue, accelerating the aging process and contributing to faster declines in lung function. For patients with respiratory disease at any age, avoidance of further damage to the lungs is key. This also includes preventing pulmonary infections. Older patients should receive vaccinations, specifically vaccinations against influenza, pneumococcal pneumonia (13-valent and 23-valent vaccines), and now COVID-19.

Maintaining an ideal body weight is also key to maintaining good lung health. Obesity not only increases the amount of work on the body during normal activities but also contribute to specific concerns of truncal obesity. Maintaining a healthy weight and minimizing abdominal fat make it easier for the respiratory muscles including the diaphragm to function. Ensuring good lung health with aging also requires maintaining the health systems that work with the lungs as part of respiratory function. This includes maintaining the health of the cardiovascular system and managing conditions like heart failure. Additionally, conditions like osteoporosis can lead to vertebral fractures, which can lead to loss of chest wall height and size and reduced ability to breathe. Treatment of osteoporosis and prevention of fractures can help promote lung health in the future.

Aging not only affects respiratory function but also the ability for the body to recover from stresses and illnesses. Especially for aging patients with chronic cardiac or pulmonary conditions, illnesses and exacerbations can lead to significant decline in function. With aging, the recovery process can be slow and incomplete. Cardiac and pulmonary rehabilitation is vital in mitigating and reversing functional declines that result from acute illnesses. Referral to these services should be considered for any aging patient with chronic heart or lung conditions recovering from an acute illness.

FURTHER READING

Bush A. Lung development and aging. *Ann Am Thorac Soc.* 2016;13:S438–S446.

Campisi J. Cellular senescence and lung function during aging. Yin and Yang. *Ann Am Thorac Soc.* 2016;13 Suppl 5: S402–S406.

Cho SJ, Stout-Delgado HW. Aging and lung disease. *Annu Rev Physiol.* 2020;82:433–459.

Cunha LL, Perazzio SF, Azzi J, Cravedi P, Riella LV. Remodeling of the immune response with aging: immunosenescence and its potential impact on COVID-19 immune response. *Front Immunol.* 2020;11:1748.

Faner R, Rojas M, Macnee W, Agusti A. Abnormal lung aging in chronic obstructive pulmonary disease and idiopathic pulmonary fibrosis. *Am J Respir Crit Care Med.* 2012;186(4):306–313.

Ito K, Barnes PJ. COPD as a disease of accelerated lung aging. *Chest.* 2009;135(1):173–180.

Liu R-M, Liu G. Cell senescence and fibrotic lung disease. *Exper Geront.* 2020;132:110836.

Lowery EM, Brubaker AL, Kuhlmann E, Kovacs EJ. The aging lung. *Clin Interv Aging.* 2013;8:1489–1496.

Murray MA, Chotirmall SH. The impact of immunosenescence on pulmonary disease. *Mediators Inflamm.* 2015: 692546.

Pardo A, Selman M. Lung fibroblasts, aging, and idiopathic pulmonary fibrosis. *Ann Am Thorac Soc.* 2016;13 Suppl 5: S417–S421.

Parikh P, Wicher S, Khandalavala K, Pabelick CM, Britt RD, Prakash YS. Cellular senescence in the lung across the age spectrum. *Am J Physiol Lung Cell Mol Physiol.* 2019;316:L826–L842.

Pellegrino R, Viegi G, Brusasco V, et al. Interpretative strategies for lung function tests. *Eur Respir J.* 2005; 26:948–968.

Thannickal VJ, Murthy M, Balch WE, et al. Blue Journal Conference: aging and susceptibility to lung disease. *Am J Respir Crit Care Med.* 2015;191(3)261–269.

Weyand CM, Goronzy JJ. Aging of the immune system: mechanisms and therapeutic targets. *Ann Am Thorac Soc.* 2016;13 Suppl 5:S422–S428.

Chapter 81

Chronic Obstructive Pulmonary Disease

Carolyn L. Rochester, Kathleen M. Akgün, Jennifer D. Possick, Jennifer M. Kapo, Patty J. Lee

INTRODUCTION

The population of adults older than age 65 is increasing in the United States and elsewhere in the world. Among older persons, respiratory symptoms are prevalent and associated with adverse outcomes. Dyspnea, for example, is reported in one-third of older persons and is associated with physical inactivity, impaired mobility, disability in activities of daily living, and death. Chronic bronchitis occurs in 15% of older persons and is associated with physical inactivity, reduced lung function, chronic obstructive pulmonary disease (COPD) exacerbations, and death. Wheezing occurs in 12% of older persons and is associated with physical inactivity and death.

The occurrence of respiratory symptoms frequently raises concerns regarding COPD. Currently the fourth leading cause of death in the United States, it is projected to be the fifth leading cause of disability and third cause of death worldwide by 2030. Older persons are at high risk of developing COPD, given both the age-related decline in physiologic capacity and the cumulative effect of frequent exposures to tobacco smoke, respiratory infections, air pollutants, and occupational exposures across the lifespan.

The prevalence of COPD varies across countries. A 2015 systematic review of population-based studies revealed an estimated global prevalence of 10% to 12% (up to 384 million cases) as of 2010. Epidemiologic surveys of COPD are often based on the symptoms of chronic bronchitis or physician-diagnosed emphysema/COPD, yielding prevalence rates of greater than or equal to 11.6% in US adults older than age 65. Alternatively, and more consistent with clinical guidelines, COPD is defined spirometrically as the presence of chronic airflow obstruction. When established by age-appropriate diagnostic thresholds, spirometry-confirmed COPD has a prevalence of 15.4% in US adults age 65 or older. It is estimated that half of adults with COPD will be 75 years or older by 2030. COPD prevalence in the United States is higher among adults with history of tobacco smoking, those with lower income, and those who use public insurance. Many individuals with COPD are never diagnosed or not diagnosed until they are hospitalized with severe respiratory symptoms or respiratory failure.

Learning Objectives

- Identify the most common clinical definitions of chronic obstructive pulmonary disease (COPD) and their limitations in older adults.

- Establish goals of care in older adults with COPD, most often directed at relieving symptoms, improving exercise tolerance and health status, reducing the risk of disease progression and exacerbations, as well as managing comorbidities.

- Define the palliative care needs of older adults with advanced COPD, including symptom management and potential indications for referral to hospice.

Key Clinical Points

1. Age is a major risk factor for respiratory symptoms and the development of COPD due to age-related changes in lung physiology, and a greater exposure to COPD risk factors, particularly a higher prevalence of "ever smoking" or other relevant exposures in the older adult population.

2. Although symptoms consistent with COPD (eg, cough, hypersecretion of mucus) are common among seniors, two-thirds of persons who have symptoms of chronic bronchitis and half of those with physician-diagnosed emphysema/COPD have normal spirometry (ie, do not have airflow obstruction, yet may be at risk for poor clinical outcomes).

3. A reduced FEV_1/FVC establishes a diagnosis of airflow obstruction and at least partial irreversibility is required to demonstrate chronic airflow obstruction, the hallmark of COPD. However, normal age-related airflow limitation is also characterized by a reduced FEV_1/FVC, and the threshold used to define

(Continued)

COPD in seniors must account for normal aging.

a. The most often used criteria for establishing and staging airflow obstruction are based on the Global Initiative for Obstructive Lung Disease (GOLD) criteria. The age-related limitations of the GOLD guidelines include two fundamental flaws: (1) GOLD defines a reduced FEV_1/FVC by a fixed ratio of 0.70, which does not distinguish between age-related airflow limitation and COPD (disease)-related airflow obstruction; and (2) GOLD expresses the FEV_1 as a percentage of predicted value, thus failing to account for age-related variability in spirometric performance. This leads to potential risk of overdiagnosis of COPD (ie, disease, as compared to age-related airflow obstruction, in older adults). The reduced FEV_1/FVC ratio among older adults for whom the ratio is normal for age is not associated with respiratory symptoms, exercise intolerance, impaired mobility, COPD hospitalization, or mortality.

b. The Global Lung Initiative (GLI) has recommended the lower limit of normal be instead defined as the fifth percentile distribution of Z-scores (Z-score of −1.64), and use reference equations that include Americans and many other ethnicities (worldwide), as well as age range of up to 95 years. Prior work has shown that airflow obstruction defined by an FEV_1/FVC Z-score less than −1.64 is associated with respiratory symptoms, impaired mobility, frailty status, COPD hospitalization, and mortality.

c. Reductions in FVC related to kyphosis/scoliosis, obesity, respiratory muscle weakness, and other factors may cause "pseudo-normalization" of the FEV_1/FVC ratio, and in turn mask the presence of COPD.

4. Treatment of COPD in seniors is complicated by difficulty with drug administration (eg, due to cognitive impairment, physical disability) and may require additional teaching/coaching and assessment to achieve optimal outcomes. Clinicians should be aware of potential adverse effects of COPD pharmacotherapies, including arrythmia, constipation, urinary retention, pneumonia, glaucoma, osteoporosis, compression fracture, thrush, and skin bruising.

5. COPD exacerbations are a major cause of worsening symptoms, disability, hospitalization, and death. Emphasis on prevention and early treatment of exacerbations is a key aspect of COPD care. Treatment of acute exacerbations includes:

a. Intensified bronchodilator therapy.

b. Corticosteroids should be considered for severe exacerbations, but side effects are common in seniors; for example, delirium is more common particularly at doses exceeding 60 mg daily.

c. Antibiotics should be considered for those exacerbations associated with increased sputum purulence and/or volume, especially for moderate or severe exacerbations. Older adult residents of skilled nursing facilities, or those who have spent time in acute-care or subacute rehab facilities within 90 days of exacerbation, and persons with severe airflow obstruction ($FEV_1 < 30\%$ predicted or FEV_1 Z-score < −2.55) are more likely to be colonized with resistant organisms (methicillin-resistant *Staphylococcus aureus* and multidrug-resistant gram-negative organisms [eg, *Pseudomonas aeruginosa*]). Thus, these latter risk factors together with local antibiotic resistance patterns should guide choice of empiric therapy. The duration of antibiotic therapy, in the absence of complicating factors such as pneumonia or bronchiectasis, is typically 3 to 7 days.

d. Discharge planning should consider referral for pulmonary rehabilitation, the need for home oxygen and/or noninvasive ventilation, and a recalibration of maintenance therapy; because new treatment regimens increase the likelihood of medication nonadherence or errors, formal medication reconciliation and pharmacist-based review should be implemented.

COPD DEFINITION

COPD is defined by the Global Initiative for Chronic Obstructive Lung Disease as "a common, preventable and treatable disease that is characterized by persistent respiratory symptoms and airflow limitation that is due to airway and/or alveolar abnormalities usually caused by significant exposure to noxious particles or gases and influenced by host factors including abnormal lung development."

RISK FACTORS FOR COPD

Advancing age is accompanied by a high frequency of COPD risk factors. The most important of these is tobacco smoke, accounting for the majority of COPD cases in the United States and other high-income countries. In recent cohorts of older Americans, the prevalence of ever-smokers was 56%, including 9% as current smokers, and, among never-smokers, 32% had exposure to second-hand smoke. The global prevalence of daily smoking was estimated at 15% in 2015. Although tobacco use has declined in many countries since the 1990s, active smoking contributed to an estimated 1.23 million deaths in 2017. Passive smoke exposure, particularly during childhood, also contributes to significant risk for COPD.

An estimated 20% to 40% of people with COPD worldwide are never smokers. Respiratory infections (bacterial and/or viral) further contribute to the onset and progression of COPD (see section on Acute Exacerbations below). About one-quarter of older Americans report a prior pneumonia, and those older than age 75 have a 10-fold increased rate of influenza hospitalization. Outdoor air pollution (especially fine particulate matter) is another major COPD risk factor worldwide. In 2009, 34% of older Americans lived in a major city, a surrogate for exposure to outdoor air pollution; wildfires related to climate change now pose an increasing threat. Other COPD risk factors include HIV infection, heroin use, and occupational exposures to dusts, vapors, fumes, and gases (eg, among freight, stock, and material handlers, and construction, metal and wood workers, miners, administrative support and information industry workers, healthcare workers, and others). Importantly, household air pollution related to use of biomass fuel for indoor cooking or heating is another key risk for COPD worldwide—the prevalence of these exposures are 12% and 18%, respectively, among older nonsmoking Americans, and is significantly higher (leading to an estimated 2 million deaths in 2017) in low- and middle-income countries.

Notably, not all COPD results from exposure to environmental agents during adulthood causing accelerated lung function decline. It is now clear that various trajectories of lung function exist; a substantial proportion of individuals develop COPD after having failed to reach optimal lung function early in life. This relates to several factors, including in utero exposures, bronchopulmonary dysplasia, prematurity and low birth weight, impaired nutrition, childhood asthma, tobacco smoke exposure and frequent childhood respiratory infections, and genetic predisposition (most notably α_1-antitrypsin deficiency). Environmental exposures later in life can further compound the risk of developing COPD in these persons.

PATHOPHYSIOLOGY OF THE AGING LUNG

Healthy aging is associated with structural and functional changes in the lungs and chest wall. As shown in **Table 81-1**, the aging lung is characterized by a reduced physiologic capacity, with multiple respiratory impairments that increase the vulnerability for developing COPD, including respiratory failure. Aging-related changes in the bony thorax including kyphosis, increased convexity of the sternum, stiffening of the ribcage, and decrease in respiratory muscle mass lead to a progressive increase in the rigidity of the chest wall (decreased chest wall compliance) and reduced curvature of the diaphragm, with resultant alterations in respiratory mechanics. Concurrently, in the lungs, degeneration of elastic fibers and alterations in collagen around the alveolar ducts result in homogeneous airspace enlargement, with a reduced total alveolar surface area but in the absence of alveolar wall destruction ("senile emphysema"). Surface tension is reduced due to increased alveolar size. These changes lead to decreased elastic recoil of the lung, further associated with a reduced diameter of the small airways. Collectively, these respiratory impairments lead to (1) airflow limitation: defined by a decreased spirometric ratio of forced expiratory volume in 1 second (FEV_1) to forced vital capacity (FVC); (2) air trapping and hyperinflation: defined by an increased residual volume (RV) and functional residual capacity (FRC), respectively; (3) decreased total lung capacity (TLC); (4) reduced maximum breathing capacity (MBC): defined by a decline in the maximal attainable minute ventilation, strongly correlating with a decrease in FEV_1 of ~30 mL/y; and (5) ventilation-perfusion mismatch: airway closing volume is increased (it approaches the FRC); this leads to premature closure of the small airways and widening of the alveolar-arterial oxygen gradient. Other age-related respiratory impairments that increase the vulnerability for developing COPD, including respiratory failure, relate to reductions in pulmonary capillary density and increased stiffness of pulmonary vasculature, alterations in the airway epithelium including reduced mucociliary clearance efficiency, decreased respiratory muscle strength, and reduced cerebrovascular responsiveness to carbon dioxide (CO_2) (tightly linked to the CO_2 ventilatory response). These age-related changes in the respiratory system also result in increased expiratory flow limitation, altered respiratory pattern (higher respiratory rate and lower tidal volume), increased dead space and increased work of breathing during exercise. Additional cellular and molecular changes in associated with aging include decreased lung progenitor cell populations, alterations in innate and adaptive immunity

TABLE 81-1 ■ RESPIRATORY IMPAIRMENTS OF THE AGING LUNG AND COPD

DOMAIN	AGING LUNG[a]	COPD[b]
Respiratory mechanics	• ↑ chest wall rigidity, kyphosis, ↓ elastic recoil of the lung, ↓ small airway diameter, "senile" emphysema *Contributing to:* • Airflow limitation (↓FEV_1/FVC and FEV_1) • ↓ mucociliary clearance efficiency • ↑ prevalence of chronic bronchitis • Air trapping (↑ RV) • Hyperinflation (↑ FRC, unchanged or decreased TLC) • ↑ closing volume (approaching FRC) • ↑ dead space ventilation[c] • ↓ maximum breathing capacity[d]	• Progressive small airways disease, emphysematous destruction of the alveolar-capillary interface *Contributing to:* • Airflow obstruction (↓↓ FEV_1/FVC and FEV_1) • ↓↓ mucociliary clearance • ↑↑ prevalence of chronic bronchitis • Air trapping (↑↑ RV) • Resting +/or dynamic hyperinflation (↑↑ FRC, ↑↑ TLC); low inspiratory capacity (IC) • ↑↑ closing volume (exceeding FRC) • ↑↑ dead space ventilation[c] • ↓↓ maximum breathing capacity[d]
Respiratory muscles	• Impaired respiratory mechanics/sarcopenia, leading to ↓ inspiratory and expiratory muscle strength	• Impaired respiratory mechanics/sarcopenia, leading to ↓↓ inspiratory and expiratory muscle strength
Ventilatory control	• ↓ cerebrovascular response to CO_2 (tightly linked to the CO_2 ventilatory response) *Other putative mechanisms:* • ↓ peripheral chemoreflex CO_2 sensitivity • ↓ feedback from peripheral mechanoreceptors • ↓ number of medullary ventral respiratory neurons	• Impaired respiratory mechanics leads to ↓↓ ventilatory responsiveness to elevations in CO_2 *Other putative mechanisms:* • ↓↓ central chemosensitivity (chronic hypercapnia) • ↓↓ intrinsic ventilatory drive
Gas exchange	• ↑ closing volume • ↓ alveolar surface area and density of lung capillaries • ↑ pulmonary vascular resistance • ↓ cardiac output response to exercise *Contributing to:* • ↑ ventilation-perfusion mismatch, including ↓$\dot{V}_a/\dot{Q}$ ratio and ↑ dead space ventilation • ↑ PA pressure, ↓D_{LCO}, ↓PaO_2, normal $PaCO_2$	• ↑↑ closing volume • ↓↓ alveolar surface area and density of lung capillaries • ↑↑ pulmonary vascular resistance • ↓↓ cardiac output response to exercise *Contributing to:* • ↑↑ ventilation-perfusion mismatch, including ↓↓ $\dot{V}_a/\dot{Q}$ ratio and ↑↑ dead space ventilation[c] • ↑↑ PA pressure, ↓↓ D_{LCO}, ↓↓ PaO_2, normal to ↑ $PaCO_2$
Exercise	• Reduced exercise capacity due to: • ↓ V_{Emax}, including flow and volume limited, dynamic hyperinflation with ↑ PEEPi • ↓ PaO_2,[e] ↑ dead space ventilation,[c] normal $PaCO_2$[f]	• Reduced exercise capacity due to: • ↓↓ V_{Emax}, including flow and volume limited, and dynamic hyperinflation with ↑↑ PEEPi • ↓↓ PaO_2, ↑↑ dead space ventilation,[c] normal to ↑ $PaCO_2$[g]

D_{LCO}, diffusing capacity of the lung for carbon monoxide; FEV_1, forced expiratory volume in 1 second; FRC, functional residual capacity; FVC, forced vital capacity; PA, pulmonary arterial; PEEPi, intrinsic positive end-expiratory pressure; RV, residual volume; TLC, total lung capacity; $\dot{V}_a/\dot{Q}$ ventilation to perfusion ratio; $\dot{V}_{Emax}$ minute ventilation at maximal exercise.

[a]The noted impairments occur in an otherwise healthy older person.

[b]The noted impairments occur most often in patients who have moderate-to-severe airflow obstruction.

[c]Dead space refers to wasted ventilation ($\dot{V}_d$) including regions that are ventilated but poorly perfused. This increases ventilatory demand (and dyspnea), as an increase in total ventilation ($\dot{V}_T$) is required to maintain alveolar ventilation ($\dot{V}_a$) where $\dot{V}_a = \dot{V}_T - \dot{V}_d$.

[d]Maximal attainable minute ventilation in liters/min, estimated as follows: $FEV_1 \times 40$ for men or $FEV_1 \times 35$ for women. It may also be directly measured by a 12-second maximum voluntary ventilation maneuver.

[e]PaO_2 declines from an average of 100 mm Hg in young adults (18–24 years) to 89 mm Hg in older adults (≥ 65 years).

[f]The $PaCO_2$ response to exercise remains normal, despite the increase in dead space, because the maximum breathing capacity remains adequate for a compensatory increase in total ventilation ($\dot{V}_T$) to maintain alveolar ventilation, where $\dot{V}_a = \dot{V}_T - \dot{V}_d$.

[g]A combined COPD-level increase in dead space and decrease in maximum breathing capacity, when severe, can lead to alveolar hypoventilation ($\downarrow\dot{V}_T - \uparrow\dot{V}_d = \downarrow\dot{V}_a$) resulting in higher $PaCO_2$ levels (normally decrease in response to exercise).

(immunosenescence) and other cell senescence, decreased proteostasis, altered mitochondrial function, reduced telomere length, and increased proinflammatory cytokines and oxidative stress. Collectively, these changes render the aging lung more prone to injury such as that conferred by exposure to tobacco smoke, with decreased capacity for tissue repair. These issues will be considered further below.

HISTOPATHOLOGY OF COPD

COPD is a heterogeneous disease characterized by several distinct histopathologic features, involving structural changes in the conducting airways and/or alveoli. The relative contribution of these features varies among individuals, and the differing features often coexist. The most important structural changes in COPD include (1) mucus hypersecretion and large airways inflammation, (2) inflammatory remodeling and fibrosis of small distal bronchioles 2 mm in diameter (or less), and (3) emphysema. Chronic bronchitis is defined as chronic cough and sputum production for at least 3 months per year for 2 consecutive years. Mucus hypersecretion is the hallmark of chronic bronchitis. These clinical features result from goblet cell hyperplasia in large and small airways, mucociliary dysfunction, and persistent neutrophil-predominant large airway inflammation. Mucus hypersecretion worsens airflow obstruction and predisposes to bacterial infection. Bronchiectasis, which is present in up to 30% of patients with COPD, is an additional mechanism that may underlie chronic cough and sputum production. A second key histopathologic feature of COPD is remodeling of small bronchioles < 2 mm in diameter. This is characterized by airway wall inflammation (CD8+T cell- CD20+B cell- and macrophage-predominant) and intralumenal mucus-containing inflammatory exudates as well as thickened airway walls and peribronchiolar fibrosis; collectively, these processes narrow the airway lumen. Emphysema, or loss of intact alveoli with enlargement of alveolar spaces, is the third key histologic feature of COPD. Emphysema may be centrilobular (the typical pattern related to tobacco smoke exposure), panacinar (typical in α_1-antitrypsin deficiency), or paraseptal in distribution. The distribution and severity of emphysema vary, and may worsen over time. A decrease in the number and total cross-sectional area of terminal bronchioles appears to precede emphysematous destruction. Some individuals develop "bullae"—large air-filled sacs greater than 1 to 2 cm in diameter.

PATHOGENESIS OF COPD

The pathogenesis of COPD is incompletely understood, especially in the context of the aging lung, varying environmental exposures, and different trajectories of acquiring the disease. The long-standing paradigms of COPD pathogenesis generally fall into three categories: (1) antioxidant/oxidant imbalance, (2) antiprotease/protease imbalance, and (3) inflammation. Early focus on these issues resulted from compelling animal models in which candidate gene identification included α_1-antitrypsin (α_1-AT), macrophage elastase, surfactant D, microsomal epoxide hydrolase, Nrf2, matrix metalloproteases, as well as cathepsins.

Most of these studies addressed the early, initiating phases of COPD development. However, COPD develops over decades despite smoking cessation, thought to be due to "progression" and "consolidation" phases of disease in genetically susceptible hosts. **Table 81-2** summarizes current understanding of COPD pathogenesis, in which, in addition to the three key mechanisms noted above, accelerated aging, aberrant immune responses, dysregulated tissue repair, and chronic viral infection have emerging

TABLE 81-2 ■ SUMMARY OF COPD PATHOGENESIS

PROCESS	GENES AND PROTEINS
Protease/antiproteases	• Neutrophil elastase • MMPs (1, 2, 9, 12) • Cathepsins (L, S, E) • Serpine2 • TIMPs
Oxidants/antioxidants	• General oxidants: OH^-, H_2O_2 • Intrinsic oxidant production: NADPH oxidase, xanthine oxidase, myeloperoxidase, mitochondrial oxidants • Antioxidants: NRF-2, HMOX-1, catalase, SOD2, SOD3, glutathione S-transferase
Immune responses	• Transcription factor NF-κB • Cytokines: TNF-α, IL-6, IL-8, IL-1α, IL-1β, IL-13, IL-17 • Chemokines: IL-8, MCP-2, MIP-1α, MIP-3α, CCL-18 • Toll-like receptors • Leukotrienes: LTE4, LTB4 • Autoreactive T cells • Antitissue antibodies
Growth and repair factors	• MIF • VEGF • HGF • MTOR
DNA damage, cellular senescence, and telomere shortening	• γ-H2AX • p16, p21, p53 • XRCC5 • FOXO3 • RORα • microRNA
Epigenetics	• HDAC2 • DNA methylation • Sirtuins
Cell death, metabolism, and organelle homeostasis	• Ceramides • Leptins/adiponectin • Autophagy • Mitochondrial fission-fusion
Genetic susceptibility	• α_1-antitrypsin • Multiple candidate susceptibility genes

CCL, chemokine (C-C motif) ligand; FOXO3, forkhead box O3; γ-H2AX, phosphorylated Histone 2A family member X; HDAC, histone deacetylase; HGF, hepatocyte growth factor; HMOX, heme-oxygenase; IL, interleukin; MCP, monocyte chemoattractant protein; MIF, macrophage migration inhibitory factor; MIP, macrophage inflammatory protein; MMP, matrix metalloproteases; MTOR, mammalian target of rapamycin; NRF-2, nuclear factor erythroid 2–related factor 2; RORα, retinoid orphan receptor alpha; Serpine, serpin peptidase inhibitor; SOD, superoxide dismutase; TIMP, tissue inhibitors of MMPs; TNF, tumor necrosis factor; VEGF, vascular endothelial growth factor.

roles. Genome-wide association studies have identified a wide array of genetic associations for COPD susceptibility and phenotypes beyond α_1-AT deficiency (see Further Reading).

Aspects of Biologic Aging Also Found in COPD

Telomere length, which is a biomarker of cell aging, is shorter in lung cells from COPD patients compared with age-matched individuals without COPD. Genetic mouse models of accelerated aging also show chronic lung disease. Mutant *Klotho* mice, which have a shortened lifespan and manifest signs of accelerated aging, exhibit emphysema despite normal lung development. Expression of the NAD-dependent deacetylase, SIRT1, a member of the sirtuin family that is implicated in caloric restriction-mediated lifespan extension and proinflammatory signaling, is decreased in emphysematous lungs. Cellular senescence and apoptosis are two age-related processes that also occur in COPD. Cellular senescence is increased by oxidative stress (such as that induced by tobacco smoke exposure and inflammation). Senescent cells can further active proinflammatory processes by activating the transcription factor NF-κB. Recent research has demonstrated that microRNAs (small noncoding RNA sequences) may play a role in cell senescence and impaired phagocytosis of apoptotic cells. Multiple studies have documented increased apoptosis in the lungs of patients with COPD and the resultant imbalance between apoptosis and tissue repair may underlie the development of emphysema.

Recent reports have identified innate immune molecules to be key regulators of age-related emphysema. There is functional overlap between immune responses to environmental and to invasive pathogens. The innate response constitutes the first phase of the immune response and is triggered by pattern-recognition receptors. Three main classes of recognition receptors activate the innate system: (1) the membrane-associated toll-like receptors (TLRs) recognize microbial components and ligands from damaged cells, (2) the NOD-like receptors (NLRs) are activated when stimuli enter the cytoplasm, and (3) the RIG-I-like receptors (RLRs) mediate cytoplasmic recognition of viral nuclei acids. Because immunosenescence contributes to susceptibility to infection and decreased vaccine responses in older adults, significant emphasis has been placed on immunology in understanding how aging affects the innate immune system. The roles of innate immune receptors in age-related lung disease have been reviewed elsewhere (see Further Reading).

Age-related loss of endogenous, protective immune molecules such as macrophage migration inhibitory factor (MIF) has recently been identified as a mechanism of emphysema in smokers and corroborated in mouse models. MIF exerts pleiotropic protective effects by modulating cellular senescence molecules, antioxidants (such as NRF-2), apoptosis, and key growth factors (such as VEGF). The loss of trophic factors (such as VEGF and Wnt signaling) found in lung samples from COPD patients are thought to lead to alveolar destruction and, potentially, the disappearance of the terminal airways in COPD. In addition to enhanced tissue destruction,

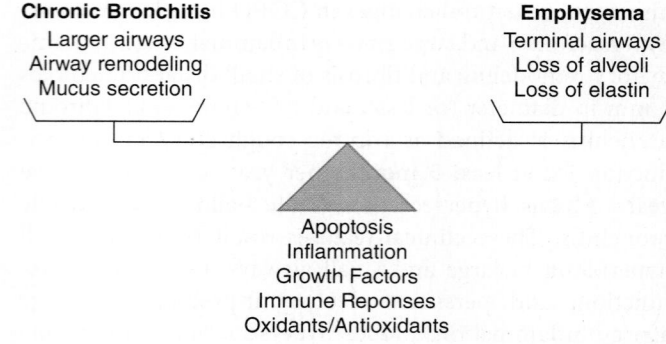

FIGURE 81-1. Cellular processes determining chronic bronchitis and emphysema.

the role of lung cell apoptosis has been highlighted by multiple studies. Enhanced cell death and inadequate regenerative responses including stem cell exhaustion, defective DNA repair, and decreased autophagy (removal of degraded proteins, damaged cells, or foreign pathogens) are pivotal to the progressive loss of gas exchange surface area in emphysema.

Most studies of COPD pathogenesis have focused primarily on emphysema rather than airway-predominant COPD and chronic bronchitis, but at least some of the same processes are likely involved (**Figure 81-1**). The paucity of animal models for chronic bronchitis has been a barrier. Mice, for instance, do not exhibit significant airway mucus secretion or airway remodeling typical of chronic bronchitis despite chronic cigarette exposure. However, studies of IL-13, VEGF, and IL-18 lung-targeted overexpressing mice in combination with clinical evidence of increased levels of these cytokines in smokers' lungs have provided new venues for further study.

Physiologic Impairments Resulting from Structural Changes in COPD

Several physiologic impairments result from the structural changes in the airways, alveoli, and chest wall in COPD. The respiratory impairments of COPD overlap with those of the aging lung, although in the presence of COPD (disease), they occur to a more severe extent (see **Table 81-1**). Each of the structural changes in the airways (airway wall inflammation, mucus, bronchoconstriction and/or small airway remodeling) and/or alveoli (emphysema) results in obstruction to the flow of air. Other key physiologic impairments include air trapping and hyperinflation and gas exchange abnormalities.

Chronic airflow obstruction is most often established by serial spirometry (confirming limited reversibility). The major site of airflow obstruction in COPD is the aforementioned inflamed and remodeled small airways less than 2 mm in diameter. In addition, emphysematous destruction of alveoli increases airflow obstruction, through loss of alveolar attachments (and in turn loss of outward tethering on small bronchioles) and a decrease in the elastic recoil of the lung. Bronchoconstriction is another contributor to airflow limitation, particularly during acute exacerbations of the disease.

Chronic airflow obstruction makes expiratory alveolar emptying increasingly difficult, resulting in air trapping and lung hyperinflation (measured clinically by helium dilution or whole-body plethysmography). Hyperinflation may be present at rest, particularly among those with severe airflow obstruction. Most individuals, even those with mild airflow obstruction, develop dynamic hyperinflation with exertion, when faster respiratory rates lead to insufficient time for exhalation to baseline end-expiratory lung volume. In combination, these impairments adversely affect (1) breathing patterns: flow and volume limited, with an increase in the intrinsic positive end-expiratory pressure (PEEPi); (2) respiratory muscle strength: the curvature of the diaphragm is reduced, altering length-tension relationships and thus decreasing the force generating capacity of the diaphragm; and (3) maximum breathing capacity (MBC): the maximal attainable minute ventilation is reduced, strongly correlating with a decrease in FEV_1. The net effect is exercise intolerance, symptom-limiting dyspnea, and an increased risk of respiratory failure. Of note, anything that increases respiratory rate or work of breathing, including anxiety, hypoxemia, pain, or concurrent congestive heart failure (CHF), can lead to dynamic hyperinflation and significant worsening of respiratory symptoms. Additional common symptoms in COPD include cough, sputum production, sense of chest tightness, sleep disturbances, and fatigue. Sleep disturbances may include nocturnal hypoxemia, alveolar hypoventilation with increase in $PaCO_2$, and/or concurrent obstructive sleep apnea (OSA).

Gas exchange abnormalities in COPD relate to ventilation-perfusion mismatch, owing to lung regions with a low ventilation-to-perfusion ratio or an increase in dead space (ventilated but underperfused)—these abnormalities relate to chronic airflow obstruction (leading to low V/Q areas) and alveolar-capillary destruction and air trapping (leading to high V/Q areas). Clinically, gas exchange abnormalities may be identified initially by a reduced diffusing capacity of the lung for carbon monoxide (DLCO) (adjusted for hemoglobin), suggesting emphysema when coexisting with airflow obstruction and hyperinflation. The reduced DLCO reflects loss of intact alveolar capillary surface area for gas exchange. In advanced COPD, based on the relative contributions of impairments in respiratory mechanics, respiratory muscle strength, and central chemosensitivity (see **Table 81-1**), gas exchange abnormalities may progress to hypoxemia and hypercapnia, yielding a reduction in arterial oxygen content and an acute/chronic respiratory acidosis—these abnormalities define the presence of respiratory failure.

In addition, destruction of the alveolar-capillary interface with loss of pulmonary capillaries and hypoxic pulmonary vasoconstriction (eg., resulting from resting, exertion, and/or sleep-related hypoxemia) and other mechanisms can lead to pulmonary hypertension and right ventricular failure (cor pulmonale). Moreover, ventricular interdependence (right ventricular pressure and volume overload) and marked intrathoracic pressure swings (increased work of breathing, hyperinflation, air trapping, and PEEPi) can decrease left ventricular preload and increase left ventricular diastolic dysfunction, ultimately reducing the cardiac output. The latter amplifies the ventilation-perfusion mismatch of COPD and reduces systemic oxygen delivery, and volume overload may develop, thus worsening exercise intolerance and increasing the risk of respiratory failure.

COMORBIDITIES AND COPD

COPD is also associated with several extrapulmonary impairments and comorbidities. Those involving the cardiovascular and musculoskeletal systems, in particular, overlap with those of normal aging (**Table 81-3**). Cardiovascular disease is one of the most common comorbidities seen. Hypertension, coronary artery disease, peripheral vascular disease, atrial fibrillation, and CHF (systolic and diastolic) occur frequently and in varying combinations. An estimated 40% of persons with COPD who require mechanical ventilation for hypercarbic respiratory failure due to COPD exacerbation have some (systolic and/or diastolic) left ventricular dysfunction. Skeletal muscle dysfunction, present in approximately 30% of people with COPD, is characterized by changes in muscle fiber structure and function (including reduction in type I endurance fibers with reduced oxidative enzyme capacity) that lead to reduced muscle mass, strength and endurance. Sarcopenia is present in an estimated 22% (up to 63% among those in nursing homes) and is associated with frailty. Older adults with COPD have an estimated twofold increased risk of frailty. Other common comorbidities include anxiety, depression, osteopenia and osteoporosis, arthritis, OSA, metabolic syndrome, anemia, respiratory infection, and lung cancer. Multiple pathogenic mechanisms underlie these comorbidities, including systemic inflammation, immune response, anorexia, deconditioning, and other factors. Importantly, several comorbidities typically coexist, and comorbidities increase the symptoms, functional disability, hospitalization, and mortality risk above that conferred by COPD alone. Clinicians should routinely assess individuals for these comorbidities.

Accordingly, the impairments imposed by advancing age and COPD (see **Tables 81-1** and **81-3**) collectively increase the risk of having respiratory symptoms (dyspnea, chronic bronchitis, and wheezing), exercise intolerance, disability, hospitalization, respiratory failure, and death.

TABLE 81-3 ■ CARDIOVASCULAR AND MUSCULOSKELETAL IMPAIRMENTS OF THE AGING PERSON AND COPD

DOMAIN	AGING PERSON[a]	COPD[b]	COMMENT
Cardiovascular	• ↓ heart rate • ↓ cardiac contractility • ↑ cardiac dilatation • ↑ arterial stiffness *Contributing to:* • ↓ cardiac output[c] • ↑ peripheral vascular resistance[d]	• Cor pulmonale • Ventricular interdependence • Intrathoracic pressure swings • Comorbid cardiovascular disease *Contributing to:* • ↓↓ cardiac output[c] • ↑↑ peripheral vascular resistance[d]	• Adverse effects on gas exchange at the lung and in (systemic) oxygen delivery • Leads to an earlier exercise-induced lactic acidosis (at a lower workload), increasing CO_2 flux (bicarbonate buffering of lactate) to the lung, ventilatory demand, and, ultimately, exercise intolerance and dyspnea
Musculoskeletal	• ↑ osteopenia • ↑ sarcopenia[e] *Contributing to:* • ↓ musculoskeletal capacity • ↓↓ peripheral oxygen extraction	• Osteoporosis • ↑↑ sarcopenia[e] *Contributing to:* • ↓↓ musculoskeletal capacity • ↓↓ peripheral oxygen extraction	• Adverse effects on mobility • Leads to earlier exercise-induced lactic acidosis (at a lower workload), increasing CO_2 flux (bicarbonate buffering of lactate) to the lung, ventilatory demand, and, ultimately, exercise intolerance and dyspnea

[a]The noted impairments occur in an otherwise healthy older person.
[b]The noted impairments occur most often in patients who have moderate-to-severe airflow obstruction.
[c]The predominant mechanism is an age-related reduction in sympathetic modulation, inclusive of adaptive cardiac structural and functional alterations in response to increased vascular stiffness.
[d]Includes less efficient redistribution of blood flow to the exercising muscle.
[e]Loss of skeletal muscle mass and function, accompanied by reduced physical performance.

DIAGNOSIS

The diagnosis of COPD requires a compatible history (symptoms and risk factors), and spirometry to confirm the presence of airflow obstruction. Given the heterogeneity of the disease with regard to symptoms, structural changes in the lungs, comorbidities, exacerbations, and disease trajectory, a comprehensive approach to patient assessment (see **Table 81-4**) and management is needed.

Epidemiologic Surveys

Epidemiologic surveys of COPD are often based on symptoms of chronic bronchitis or physician-diagnosed emphysema/COPD. Prior work has shown, however, that two-thirds of persons who have symptoms of chronic bronchitis and half of those with physician-diagnosed emphysema/COPD have normal spirometry (do not have airflow obstruction). This relates to overlap between symptoms of chronic bronchitis (cough in particular) and those of other conditions (postnasal drip, acid reflux, etc) or being drug-induced, and to low utilization of spirometry in primary care settings. Moreover, patients may underreport symptoms, due to assumptions that dyspnea, fatigue, and exercise intolerance may be due to aging alone. Also, many alternate conditions lead to symptoms similar to those of COPD, including but not limited to other forms of lung disease, cardiac disease, dynamic upper airway obstruction, pulmonary embolus, and others. As a result of these issues, COPD is frequently both underdiagnosed and misdiagnosed.

Spirometry Given the above concerns, and because pathologic confirmation is invasive and not routinely necessary or available, the clinical strategy for establishing a diagnosis of COPD is based on spirometry-confirmed chronic airflow obstruction (less than fully reversible). Spirometry can be performed conveniently with a portable, handheld device, using protocols from the American Thoracic and European Respiratory Societies (ATS/ERS). These protocols require performance of at least two FVC maneuvers that meet ATS/ERS acceptability criteria—FVC maneuver is defined as the maximal volume of air that is exhaled with maximal effort starting from maximal inspiration.

The most common spirometric measures of interest are the FEV_1 and FVC, and the ratio between the two (FEV_1/FVC). An additional measure is the forced expiratory volume in 6 seconds (FEV_6), used as an estimate of FVC. Although the FEV_6 is more reproducible and less physically demanding than the FVC, it is limited when distinguishing normal spirometry from a restrictive impairment, and predicted values are currently unavailable for those older than age 80.

Establishing airflow obstruction A reduced FEV_1/FVC ratio establishes the presence of *airflow obstruction*. However, given that healthy age-related *airflow limitation* is also characterized by a reduced FEV_1/FVC, the threshold that establishes *airflow obstruction* must account for normal aging, including increased variability in spirometric performance (at least 50% greater in healthy 80-year-olds than healthy 40-year-olds).

To account for age-related changes in lung function, the ATS/ERS recommend that airflow obstruction be established by a lower limit of normal (LLN) threshold for

TABLE 81-4 ■ COMPREHENSIVE ASSESSMENT OF THE COPD PATIENT

- COPD risk factors
- Pulmonary function testing
  - Spirometry (recommended annually)
  - Lung volumes and diffusing capacity
- Imaging—consider CT scan
  - Disease characterization (+/or lung cancer screening)
- Symptom assessment
  - MRC dyspnea score
  - COPD assessment test (www.catestonline.org)
  - Clinical COPD questionnaire (CCQ) (www.ccq.nl)
- Exercise tolerance: 6-minute walk test, shuttle walk test, or cycle/treadmill test
- Oxygenation/gas exchange
- Exacerbation risk (history): frequency, severity, possible triggers/causes
- α_1-Antitrypsin level and phenotype
- Comorbidities (CBC with differential [check also for blood eosinophilia], echocardiogram, stress testing, sleep, bone density, etc)
- Consider use of multidimensional disease assessment index, eg,
  - BODE Score (BMI, FEV_1% pred, MRC dyspnea, 6MWD) (Celli BR, Cote CG, Marin JM, et al. The body-mass index, airflow obstruction, dyspnea, and exercise capacity index in chronic obstructive pulmonary disease. *N Engl J Med.* 2004;350(10):1005–1012).
  - ADO Index (age, dyspnea, airflow obstruction) (Puhan MA, Garcia-Aymerich J, Frey M, et al. Expansion of the prognostic assessment of patients with chronic obstructive pulmonary disease: the updated BODE index and the ADO index. *Lancet.* 2009;374:704–711).
  - COTE Index (COPD Comorbidity Test) (deTorres JP, Casanova C, Marín JM et al. Prognostic evaluation of COPD patients: GOLD 2011 versus BODE and the COPD comorbidity index COTE. *Thorax.* 2014;69(9):799–804).

FEV_1/FVC. The ATS/ERS approach currently defines the LLN as the fifth percentile distribution of reference values, calculated in a population of healthy never-smokers matched for age, height, sex, and ethnicity (these predict normal lung function). In the United States, reference values are often based on equations from the Third National Health and Nutrition Examination Survey (NHANES III). Although these account for age-related declines in lung function, the NHANES III equations are limited to those age 80 or younger, and do not consider variability in spirometric performance. Hence, the GLI has recommended that the LLN be instead defined as the fifth percentile distribution of Z-scores (Z-score of –1.64) (**Table 81-5**). The GLI calculated Z-scores account for the age-related decline in lung function and increased variability in spirometric performance and use reference equations that include Americans and many other ethnicities (worldwide), as well as age range of up to 95. Prior work has shown that airflow obstruction defined by an FEV_1/FVC Z-score less than –1.64 is associated with respiratory symptoms, impaired mobility, frailty status, COPD hospitalization, and mortality. Moreover, Z-scores have a strong clinical precedence, given their use in bone mineral density testing and pediatric growth charts.

Assessing the severity of airflow obstruction After establishing a reduced FEV_1/FVC: Current practice stages the severity of airflow obstruction based on FEV_1 expressed as percent predicted (%Pred): [measured/predicted] × 100%. The ATS/ERS recommend the thresholds for FEV_1 of 70 and 50 %Pred when staging airflow obstruction (see **Table 81-5**). This approach has age-related limitations, however, since %Pred assumes incorrectly the equivalence of spirometric variability across the adult lifespan. To address this limitation, GLI-calculated FEV_1 Z-scores may be used to stage the severity of airflow obstruction (see **Table 81-5**). Prior work has shown that Z-score thresholds for FEV_1 have a graded association with respiratory symptoms, COPD hospitalization, and mortality.

The Global Initiative for Obstructive Lung Disease Despite age-related limitations in methodology, the most often used spirometric criteria for establishing and staging airflow obstruction are based on GOLD Report (see **Table 81-5**). The age-related limitations of the GOLD Report include two fundamental flaws. First, GOLD defines a reduced FEV_1/FVC by a fixed ratio less than 0.70, thus failing to distinguish between age-related airflow limitation (normal aging-related process) and COPD-related airflow obstruction (connoting the presence of disease). In particular, an FEV_1/FVC less than 0.70 is frequently seen in otherwise healthy, asymptomatic never-smokers who are age 65 or older. Second, GOLD expresses the FEV_1 as %Pred, thus failing to account for age-related variability in spirometric performance. It is therefore not surprising that the prevalence of airflow obstruction in older persons is more than twofold higher when defined by GOLD versus a Z-score approach (37.7% vs 15.4%, respectively). Prior work has shown that the overdiagnosis of airflow obstruction by GOLD is not associated with respiratory symptoms, exercise intolerance, impaired mobility, COPD hospitalization, or mortality. Third, several conditions such as kyphosis, weak respiratory muscles, obesity—all common among older adults—can lower the FVC, hence reduce the FEV_1/FVC ratio, and underlying COPD may be "masked" in such individuals.

Bronchodilator reversibility COPD is defined as chronic airflow obstruction that is less than fully reversible. However, up to two-thirds of individuals with COPD may have a partial component of bronchodilator (BD) reversibility. Clinical guidelines therefore recommend that spirometry should be performed before and after administration of an inhaled BD (pre- and post-BD, respectively) in order to establish (1) reversibility (pre- vs post-BD values) and (2) diagnosis of COPD (using post-BD values). Among older

TABLE 81-5 ■ SPIROMETRIC CRITERIA FOR ESTABLISHING AND STAGING CHRONIC AIRFLOW OBSTRUCTION

METHOD	CHRONIC AIRFLOW OBSTRUCTION[a,b]			COMMENT
	MILD	MODERATE	SEVERE	
AMERICAN THORACIC AND EUROPEAN RESPIRATORY SOCIETIES (ATS/ERS)				
FEV_1/FVC	< LLN[c]			• Accounts for age-related airflow limitation, but not age-related variability in spirometric performance
FEV_1	≥ 70 %Pred	50–69 %Pred	< 50 %Pred	• LLN and %Pred calculations are often based on NHANES III reference equations, which are limited to age < 80
				• Yields a COPD prevalence rate of 19.2%
GLOBAL LUNG INITIATIVE (GLI)				
FEV_1/FVC	Z-score < −1.64[d]			• Accounts for age-related airflow limitation and age-related variability in spirometric performance
FEV_1	Z-score[e]			• GLI reference equations include ages up to 95 and multiple ethnicities (worldwide)
	≥ −1.64	< −1.64 but ≥ −2.55	< −2.55	• Strong clinical precedence: Z-scores used in bone mineral density testing and pediatric growth charts
				• Novel, not yet widely applied
				• Yields a COPD prevalence rate of 15.4%
GLOBAL INITIATIVE FOR OBSTRUCTIVE LUNG DISEASE (GOLD)				
FEV_1/FVC	< 0.70			• Widely used in research and clinical practice
FEV_1	≥ 80 %Pred	50–79 %Pred	< 50 %Pred	• Does not account for age-related airflow limitation or age-related variability in spirometric performance
				• FEV_1/FVC fixed ratio of 0.70 will often misidentify COPD in aging populations
				• %Pred calculations are often based on NHANES III reference equations, limited to age < 80
				• Yields a COPD prevalence rate of 37.7%

FEV_1/FVC, ratio of forced expiratory volume in 1 second (FEV_1) to forced vital capacity (FVC); LLN, lower limit of normal; NHANES III, Third National Health and Nutrition Examination Survey; %Pred, percent predicted (measured/predicted × 100).

[a]Airflow obstruction is first established by FEV_1/FVC, with severity thereafter staged by FEV_1.

[b]The use of prebronchodilator spirometric measures provides a more reasonable approach when establishing and staging airflow obstruction in older persons, with reversibility best evaluated by serial spirometry over time.

[c]Defined by the fifth percentile distribution of reference values.

[d]Calculated as: [(measured FEV_1/FVC ÷ median FEV_1/FVC)^{Lambda} − 1] ÷ (lambda × sigma), wherein (1) median represents how the spirometric variable changes with a predictor variable (age and height); (2) sigma is the coefficient of variation, which models the spread of spirometric reference values; and (3) lambda, which models the departure from normality (skewness). GLI equations provide values for the median, lambda, and skewness, and are specific to sex and ethnicity. An FEV_1/FVC Z-score of −1.64 defines the LLN as the fifth percentile distribution of Z-scores.

[e]Calculated as: [(measured FEV_1 ÷ median FEV_1)^{Lambda} − 1] ÷ (lambda × sigma). An FEV_1 Z-score of −1.64 defines the LLN (fifth percentile), whereas −2.55 corresponds to the 0.5th percentile distribution of Z-scores.

persons, however, this approach has two disadvantages. First, older persons have limited capacity to perform multiple FVC maneuvers, and may have an adverse response to an inhaled BD. Second, post-BD values have limited clinical relevance in distinguishing COPD from asthma, and have low reproducibility over time. Hence, the use of pre-BD values provides a reasonable approach when diagnosing and staging COPD in older persons where necessary, with limited reversibility best established by serial spirometry over time.

Additional Considerations

Although chronic airflow obstruction is currently considered a necessary and sufficient criterion for defining COPD, there are additional problems with this approach. First, individuals with symptoms of chronic bronchitis and history of COPD-relevant exposures and other risk factors may lack spirometric airflow obstruction, yet have lower exercise capacity, increased risk of disease exacerbation, development of impaired lung function over time, and increased mortality risk. As such, these persons should be monitored over time. Second, as noted above, other individuals with COPD-relevant risk factors have preserved normal FEV_1/FVC ratio (owing to various factors), yet have radiologic features of COPD (including emphysema and/or chronically inflamed airways). Those with normal FEV_1/FVC ratio, with low FEV_1 and evidence of inflammatory airways disease are at risk of disease progression. The term PRISm (preserved ratio, impaired spirometry) is used to define this group of people.

Given the limitations of spirometry alone in establishing the diagnosis of COPD, some health care professionals advocate for an updated, alternate schema for establishing the diagnosis of COPD, in which symptoms,

TABLE 81-6 ■ RESPIRATORY IMPAIRMENTS THAT ARE COMMONLY EVALUATED TO ESTABLISH A DIAGNOSIS OF COPD

PHYSIOLOGIC IMPAIRMENT	CRITERIA	OUTCOMES
Chronic airflow obstruction	• See **Table 81-5** for spirometric criteria • Not fully reversible, as defined by serial spirometry over time • Necessary and sufficient criterion to establish a diagnosis of COPD	• ↑↑ respiratory symptoms • ↓↓ functional status • ↑↑ risk of respiratory failure
Hyperinflation	• Static lung volumes (helium dilution or whole-body plethysmography): ↑↑ TLC and ↑↑ FRC	
Air trapping	• Static lung volumes (helium dilution or whole-body plethysmography): ↑↑ RV and ↑↑ RV/TLC	
Pulmonary hypertension	• Echocardiography estimates of ↑↑ pulmonary arterial systolic pressure • Presence suggested by exercise-induced oxygen desaturation	
Gas exchange	• Reduced DLCO, adjusted for hemoglobin • Hypoxemia at rest, asleep, or with exercise: pulse oximetry • Hypercapnia while awake, asleep, or with exercise: arterial blood gases	

Exercise intolerance	• Reduced 6-minute walk distance
	• Maximal cardiopulmonary stress test with gas exchange:
	  ○ Pulmonary mechanical limitation: $V_{Emax} \geq 85\%$ of MBC,[a] expiratory flow limitation (over more than 80% of the tidal volume by peak exercise), inspiratory flow limitation (approach those available over higher lung volumes), volume limitation (↑↑ end-inspiratory lung volume relative to TLC), dynamic hyperinflation (↑↑ end-expiratory lung volume, ↑↑ PEEPi)
	  ○ Pulmonary vascular limitation: ↓↓PaO_2, ↑↑ dead space,[b] normal or ↑$PaCO_2$[c]	

D_{LCO}, diffusing capacity of the lung for carbon monoxide; FEV_1, forced expiratory volume in 1 second; FRC, functional residual capacity; MBC, maximum breathing capacity; PEEPi, intrinsic positive end-expiratory pressure; RV, residual volume; TLC, total lung capacity; V_{Emax}, minute ventilation at peak exercise.
[a]Maximal attainable minute ventilation in liters/min, estimated as follows: $FEV_1 \times 40$ for males or $FEV_1 \times 35$ for females. It may also be directly measured by a 12-second maximum voluntary ventilation maneuver.
[b]Dead space refers to wasted ventilation (V_d), including regions that are ventilated but poorly perfused. This increases ventilatory demand (and dyspnea), as an increase in total ventilation (V_T) is required to maintain alveolar ventilation (V_a), where $V_a = V_T - V_d$.
[c]A combined COPD-level increase in dead space and decrease in maximum breathing capacity, when severe, can lead to alveolar hypoventilation ($\downarrow V_T - \uparrow V_d = \downarrow V_a$), resulting in higher $PaCO_2$ levels (normally decrease in response to exercise).

relevant exposures, spirometry, and radiologic (CT scan) features all play a key role (see Further Reading). Use of such an approach leads to establishment of the diagnosis in a much larger population of people as compared with use of lung function testing alone. It would also have major implications for identification/selection/inclusion of participants for clinical trials of therapeutic interventions in COPD. Further research is needed to determine the impact of current therapies for COPD among those with chronic bronchitis and/or radiologic features of COPD without airflow obstruction, and those with PRISm. Currently, the diagnostic evaluation should assess additional respiratory impairments, as these further confirm COPD and are associated with adverse outcomes (**Table 81-6**).

Lastly, several subgroups ("phenotypes") of COPD with distinct features are recognized (**Table 81-7**). While the pathobiologic processes underlying these different groups is incompletely understood, combining the physiologic respiratory impairments with clinical and radiologic features further establishes clinical phenotypes and informs more personalized COPD-related treatment options and prognosis (**Table 81-7**). Additional assessments that should

be made routinely include measurement of peripheral blood eosinophil count and serum α_1-AT level (and phenotype), because these features both characterize patients and inform specific aspects of disease management.

CLINICAL MANIFESTATIONS

Because of shared risk factors (eg, tobacco smoke) and sequelae of progressive chronic disease, COPD is often associated with a high burden of symptoms and medical issues, as discussed above and as shown in **Table 81-8**. Typical symptoms of COPD include dyspnea, cough, sputum production, wheezing, fatigue, activity limitation, and sleep disturbances. The clinical course of COPD is further characterized by acute exacerbations that cycle between chronic and acute care settings, leading to accelerated declines in lung function and increases in medical burden (these are discussed further below). Importantly, spirometric measures and FEV_1 alone are insufficient to characterize the impact and burden of COPD on patients. Overall impact and prognosis of COPD are informed by the BODE Index, which includes the body mass index (B) as a measure of

TABLE 81-7 ■ COPD CLINICAL SUBGROUPS (PHENOTYPES)

CLINICAL PHENOTYPE[a]	CRITERIA	TREATMENT[b]
AIRWAY PREDOMINANT		
Airflow obstruction	• Airflow obstruction, without chronic bronchitis, bronchiectasis, or emphysema • ↑ small airway wall thickness on volumetric chest computed tomography • Variable reversibility, but lacks some features of COPD-asthma overlap (eg, sputum eosinophilia, high IgE)	Bronchodilator, anti-inflammatory[c]
Chronic bronchitis	• Airflow obstruction, with chronic cough and sputum production for at least 3 mo/y for 2 consecutive years, and with persistent airway inflammation and colonization/infection • ↑ small airway wall thickness on volumetric chest computed tomography	Bronchodilator, anti-inflammatory,[c,d] ± mucolytics[e]
Bronchiectasis	• Airflow obstruction (usually severe), with isolation of bacteria from sputum (especially *Pseudomonas*), increased sputum inflammatory markers, and at least one COPD exacerbation in the prior year • ↑ small airway wall thickness and bronchiectasis on volumetric chest computed tomography	Bronchodilator, airway-clearance techniques
COPD-asthma overlap	• Airflow obstruction, with enhanced response to inhaled corticosteroids (but not fully reversible), eosinophilia in respiratory secretions, high IgE • History of smoking (≥ 10 pack-years), asthma, and/or atopy • ↑ small airway wall thickness on volumetric chest computed tomography	Bronchodilator, anti-inflammatory,[c] consider biologics
EMPHYSEMA PREDOMINANT		
Emphysema	• Airflow obstruction, with alveolar-capillary destruction and airspace enlargement • Moderate-to-severe hyperinflation and air trapping, reduced DLCO (adjusted for hemoglobin), ± pulmonary hypertension, emphysema on volumetric chest computed tomography • Severe dyspnea and exercise intolerance, low BMI	Bronchodilator, anti-inflammatory,[c] lung volume reduction or transplantation surgery,[f] α₁-antiprotease[g]
Combined pulmonary fibrosis-emphysema syndrome (CPEFS)	• Includes both upper-lobe emphysema and lower-lobe fibrosis. Usually occurs in male smokers and associated with pulmonary hypertension, acute lung injury, and lung cancer.	Bronchodilator, anti-inflammatory,[c] other[h]
OTHER		
COPD with eosinophilia	• Airflow obstruction • Variable computed tomography features • Blood eosinophil levels > 200–300 cells/μL • Absent history of atopy or asthma	Bronchodilator, anti-inflammatory (ICS), consider biologics
Frequent exacerbator	• Defined by two or more symptom-defined exacerbations per year • ↓ health-related quality of life and accelerated decline in lung function	Bronchodilator, anti-inflammatory[c,d]
COPD-OSA overlap	• Worse nocturnal hypoxemia/hypercapnia than COPD and OSA alone • Severity of airflow obstruction and hyperinflation correlates with OSA severity	Positive airway pressure: may improve survival, pulmonary hypertension, hypoxemia, and risk of hospitalization

DLCO, diffusing capacity of the lung for carbon monoxide; OSA, obstructive sleep apnea.

[a]Although defined by the predominant clinical phenotype, patients may have multiple features (eg, combined chronic bronchitis, emphysema, and frequent exacerbator).

[b]Apply to stable COPD (see Management section for indications and comprehensive treatment considerations).

[c]Most often an inhaled corticosteroid and indicated in severe airflow obstruction, chronic bronchitis, and/or frequent exacerbator.

[d]In select cases, may also include roflumilast or a macrolide antibiotic.

[e]Includes thiols (eg, N-acetylcysteine), but indication limited to tenacious sputum production that is refractory to standard therapy.

[f]In selected patients (see Management section).

[g]Consider α₁-antitrypsin (AAT) deficiency as the underlying mechanism of emphysema, if the affected individual is aged ≤ 45, if a nonsmoker or minimal smoker, if the predominant distribution is basilar on chest imaging, if coexisting panniculitis or unexplained chronic liver disease, and/or if a family history of emphysema or liver disease. Treatment includes intravenous supplementation with pooled human α₁-antiprotease for those with a high-risk phenotype (PI*ZZ), a plasma AAT level < 11 micromol/L, persistent airflow obstruction, likely to comply with the treatment protocol, and aged ≥ 18.

[h]Immunosuppressive therapy for the fibrosis component is rarely indicated, as the pathology is typically end-stage usual interstitial pneumonia.

TABLE 81-8 ■ MEDICAL BURDEN OF COPD

- COPD patients average 3.7 chronic conditions and 35 filled prescriptions over a given year.
- Most frequent comorbidities in COPD are hypertension, diabetes mellitus, cardiovascular (heart failure, coronary artery disease, arrhythmias, stroke, and peripheral artery disease), psychiatric (depression and anxiety), sarcopenia (decreased skeletal muscle mass and function), osteoporosis, anemia, and lung cancer. Moreover, in response to untreated chronic hypoxemia, secondary erythrocytosis may also develop and contribute to pulmonary hypertension and reductions in cerebral and coronary blood flow.
- COPD-associated sequelae include severe deconditioning and weight loss (sarcopenia); disabling symptoms (dyspnea, chronic bronchitis, wheezing, and fatigue); multiple sensory, cognitive, and mobility impairments; limitations in activities of daily living; and social isolation. Regarding cognitive impairment, this is more prevalent in COPD patients who are oxygen dependent and have limitations in physical function (eg, difficulties in performing household chores).
- Clinical course of COPD is characterized by exacerbations that cycle between chronic and acute care settings, leading to progressive declines in lung function and further increases in medical burden.
- Advancing age further increases the likelihood of multimorbidity and polypharmacy, including the complicating sequelae of multifactorial geriatric health conditions.

COPD, chronic obstructive pulmonary disease; FEV$_1$, forced expiratory volume in 1 second.

nutritional status, FEV$_1$ as a measure of the severity of airflow obstruction (O), Medical Research Council score as a measure of the severity of dyspnea (D), and 6-minute walk distance as a measure of exercise (E) capacity.

Advancing age additionally increases the likelihood that comorbidities unrelated to chronic airflow obstruction will complicate the clinical course of COPD. For example, a postmortem examination of the cause of death in 43 older persons hospitalized for COPD exacerbation included heart failure in 16 (37%) and pulmonary thromboembolism in 9 (21%). The age-related predisposition for polypharmacy may also adversely affect COPD: (1) opiates and benzodiazepines may decrease ventilatory control and increase the risk of aspiration; (2) statins may have a myopathic effect on the muscles of respiration and ambulation; and (3) β-blockers may exacerbate underlying heart failure and bradycardia. The interaction between these adverse medication effects and age-related reductions in physiologic capacity, including respiratory and cardiovascular impairments (see **Tables 81-1** and **81-3**), may contribute to pneumonia (28%) and respiratory failure (14%), as additional causes of death among older persons hospitalized for COPD exacerbation.

Lastly, advancing age is characterized by multifactorial geriatric health conditions, such as cognitive and physical impairments (including delirium, balance impairment, and injurious falls), sleep disorders, incontinence, frailty (sarcopenia), malnutrition, and chronic pain and dyspnea. These frequently represent sequelae of multimorbidity, polypharmacy, sedentary status, psychologic disturbances, and social isolation. Importantly, polypharmacy and complex treatment regimens (which may include oxygen and/or noninvasive ventilation) may impact adherence to medications, in turn affecting disease control. Thus, a comprehensive approach is needed when managing COPD, particularly in older persons.

MANAGEMENT OF STABLE COPD

The goals of care for stable COPD are to relieve and minimize symptoms, optimize exercise/activity tolerance and health status, and reduce the risk of exacerbations, disease progression, and mortality. To achieve these goals, decisions regarding treatment strategies should consider the predominant clinical phenotype of COPD (see **Table 81-7**), including the severity of corresponding impairments (see **Tables 81-3** through **81-6**), as well as the accompanying medical comorbidities (see **Table 81-8**). Ultimately, treatment options are calibrated to patient preferences, needs, and advance directives, and appropriately modified when the clinical trajectory progresses to advanced COPD.

Pharmacologic Therapies

Treatment options Medication regimens should consider the patient's skills/abilities, peak inspiratory flow (PIF) rate, the questions in **Table 81-9**, and the algorithm in **Figure 81-2**. Prioritization is given to once-daily administration, self-contained inhaler devices, educating the patient/caregiver on medication administration, and ensuring the patient has adequate PIF rate to entrain the medication. **Table 81-10** summarizes currently available medications, emphasizing benefits, side effects, and complexity. In stable COPD, pharmacologic therapy should follow a stepwise approach that for some patients may lead

TABLE 81-9 ■ DEVICE SELECTION CONSIDERATIONS IN OLDER PERSONS WITH COPD

- Who will be administering the dose?
- Can the patient demonstrate proper "press and breathe" technique?
- Can delivery devices be easily confused?
- Does the product require a spacer or "valved holding chamber" device?
- Can the patient afford this medication?
- Does the patient have existing problems with medication adherence?
- Does the device require adequate dexterity or grip strength to use?
- Can the patient manage complex tasks?
- Is the patient capable of maintaining and cleaning the delivery device?
- Does the patient have a sufficient peak inspiratory flow?

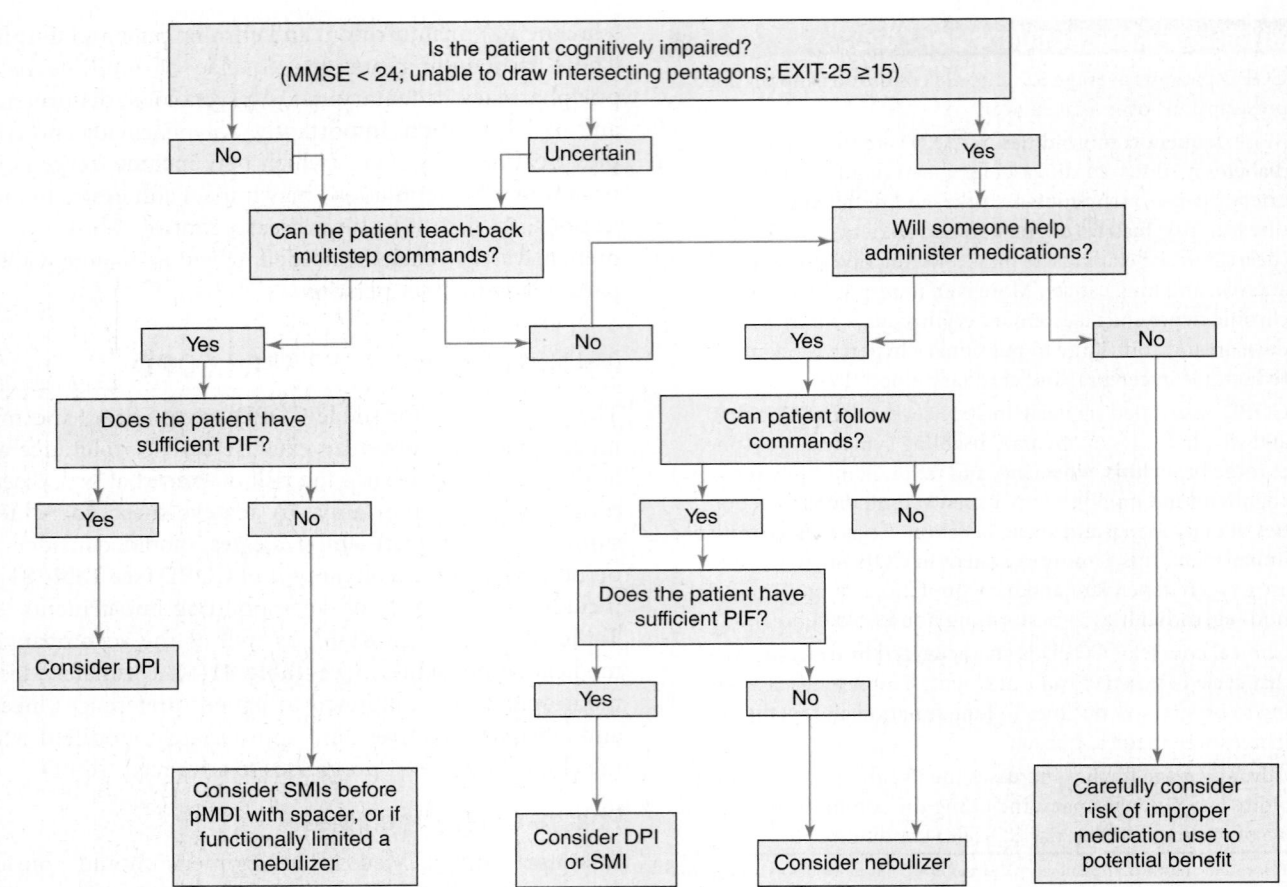

FIGURE 81-2. Algorithm for inhaler selection. DPI, dry powder inhaler; EXIT-25, a 25-item cognitive test (executive interview) that evaluates executive function (the higher the score, the worse the cognitive impairment); MMSE, Mini-Mental Status Examination (the lower the score, the worse the cognitive impairment); PIF, peak inspiratory flow; pMDI, pressurized metered-dose inhaler; SMI, soft-mist inhaler.

to use of triple-inhaler maintenance therapy, including two classes of long-acting inhaled bronchodilators (β_2-selective adrenergic agonist and anticholinergic) and an inhaled corticosteroid, as well as prn use of a rescue inhaler (short-acting β_2-agonist). Additional options include roflumilast, macrolides, vibratory positive expiratory pressure (PEP) devices, and mucolytics. Some individuals may also benefit from biologic monoclonal antibody therapies. A stepwise treatment approach to pharmacotherapy used commonly for those with confirmed airflow obstruction, based on symptom severity and disease exacerbations, is provided in the GOLD Report (see Further Reading).

Short-Acting Bronchodilators Bronchodilators are a mainstay of the treatment of stable COPD, irrespective of clinical phenotype, as they achieve improvements in symptoms, exercise capacity, and airflow obstruction. Inhaled bronchodilators are preferred over oral agents, based on efficacy and side effects, and aging itself does not reduce the bronchodilator response. Notably, bronchodilators are effective in spite of patients' fixed, irreversible airflow obstruction; they reduce dynamic hyperinflation and end-expiratory lung volume and improve inspiratory capacity and patients' breathing pattern.

Albuterol is an inhaled short-acting β_2-agonist (SABA) with a fast onset of action. It is usually the first bronchodilator used, serving primarily as *rescue therapy* (as needed, rather than regularly scheduled), and is commonly prescribed as a handheld pressurized metered-dose inhaler (pMDI). Albuterol is also available as a nebulizer, an alternative for older patients who have difficulties using handheld inhalers and/or who may benefit from the mucus-mobilizing properties of this therapy. Patients/caregivers should be advised to always have albuterol readily available in the event of acute worsening of symptoms (dyspnea) that does not improve with rest and use of slow, pursed lips breathing. Individuals with visual impairment should mark albuterol pMDIs to avoid confusion with other inhalers. Common side effects of SABAs are listed in **Table 81-10**, with concerns especially raised in people with COPD and concurrent cardiovascular disease (especially hypertension or tachyarrhythmias), coexisting asthma (mortality), and excessive dosing.

The anticholinergic ipratropium is a short-acting inhaled bronchodilator, with little systemic absorption. It is indicated as *maintenance therapy* (see **Table 81-10**), but adherence is problematic because it requires frequent dosing (4 times daily). Hence, ipratropium is often combined with

TABLE 81-10 ■ COPD PHARMACOLOGY[a]

MEDICATION (GENERIC/BRAND)	DOSAGE FORM/FREQUENCY	THERAPEUTIC BENEFITS	SIDE EFFECTS[b]	PATIENT TECHNIQUE INFLUENCES DRUG DELIVERY[c]	COMPLEXITY
SHORT-ACTING β₂-AGONIST (SABA) BRONCHODILATOR—RESCUE THERAPY					
Albuterol (ProAir HFA and Ventolin HFA)	pMDI 1–2 puffs Q4–6 h prn	Improve respiratory symptoms, exercise capacity, airflow obstruction	Class effect: tremor, headache, insomnia, palpitations, reflex tachycardia, arrhythmia, mortality, ± hypokalemia, ± hyperglycemia	++++ (inhaler alone) +++ (if spacer used)	Prime before first use and if not used in > 2 wk
Albuterol (Accuneb)	Nebulizer 1 vial 3–4× daily prn			+ (if mask is used) ++ (if mouthpiece used)	Vials need to be opened and placed inside nebulizer
Levalbuterol Tartrate (Xopenex HFA)	pMDI 2 puffs Q4–6 h prn			++++ (inhaler alone) +++ (if spacer used)	Prime before first use and if not used in > 3 d
Levalbuterol Hydrochloride (Xopenex)	Nebulizer 1 vial Q6–8 h prn (max 3× daily)			+ (if mask used) ++ (if mouthpiece used)	Vials need to be opened and placed inside nebulizer
LONG-ACTING β₂-AGONIST (LABA) BRONCHODILATOR—MAINTENANCE THERAPY					
Formoterol (Foradil Aerolizer)	DPI 1 capsule (12 μg) Q12 h	Improve respiratory symptoms, exercise capacity, and airflow obstruction in patients not controlled with a SABA	See class effect: Generally milder side effects than short-acting agents	+++	Capsules should be stored in blister pack and only removed before use
Arformoterol (Brovana)	Nebulizer 1 vial (15 μg) BID	Also improve adherence, improve health-related quality of life, and reduce exacerbations		+ (if mask used) ++ (if mouthpiece used)	Vials need to be opened and placed inside nebulizer
Formoterol (Peforomist)	Nebulizer 1 vial (20 μg) BID			+ (if mask used) ++ (if mouthpiece used)	Vials need to be opened and placed inside nebulizer
Indacaterol (Arcapta Neohaler)	DPI 1 capsule (75 μg) once daily			+++	Capsules should be stored in blister pack and only removed before use
Salmeterol (Serevent Diskus)	DPI 50 μg Q12 h			+++	Capsule has to be pierced before use
Olodaterol (Striverdi Respimat)	SMI 2 inhalations once daily			++	Prime prior to first use and if not used in > 21 d
Vilanterol	See combination inhalers below				

(Continued)

TABLE 81-10 ■ COPD PHARMACOLOGY[a] (CONTINUED)

MEDICATION (GENERIC/BRAND)	DOSAGE FORM/FREQUENCY	THERAPEUTIC BENEFITS	SIDE EFFECTS[b]	PATIENT TECHNIQUE INFLUENCES DRUG DELIVERY[c]	COMPLEXITY
SHORT-ACTING ANTICHOLINERGIC BRONCHODILATOR—*MAINTENANCE THERAPY*					
Ipratropium (Atrovent HFA)	pMDI 2 puffs 4× daily (not to exceed 12 puffs in 24 h)	Improve respiratory symptoms, exercise capacity, and airflow obstruction	Class effect: Headache, dry mouth, bad taste, pharyngitis, sinusitis, urinary retention, constipation, cardiovascular (arrhythmia, mortality), glaucoma, paradoxical bronchospasm	+++ (inhaler alone) +++ (if spacer used)	Prime prior to first use and if not used in > 3 d
Ipratropium (Atrovent)	Nebulizer 1 vial (500 μg) 3–4× daily			+ (if mask used) ++ (if mouthpiece used)	Vials need to be opened and placed inside nebulizer
COMBINED SHORT-ACTING ANTICHOLINERGIC + SABA BRONCHODILATOR—*MAINTENANCE THERAPY*					
Albuterol + Ipratropium (Combivent Respimat)	SMI 2 inhalations 4× daily	Additive improvement	See corresponding class effects	++	Prime prior to first use and if not used in > 21 d
Albuterol + Ipratropium (DuoNeb)	Nebulizer 1 vial (3 mL) Q4–6 h			+ (if mask used) ++ (if mouthpiece used)	Vials need to be opened and placed inside nebulizer
LONG-ACTING ANTICHOLINERGIC (LAMA) BRONCHODILATOR—*MAINTENANCE THERAPY*					
Aclidinium Bromide (Tudorza Pressair)	DPI 1 inhalation 2× daily	Improve respiratory symptoms, exercise capacity, airflow obstruction, adherence, and health-related quality of life; and reduce exacerbations	See class effect; generally milder side effects than short-acting agents *Note:* when LAMA is prescribed, the short-acting anticholinergic is discontinued	++	Need to press and release the green button prior to use; after correctly administering full dose, the button should turn red
Tiotropium (Spiriva Handihaler)	DPI 1 capsule (18 μg) once daily			+++	Capsule has to be pierced before use, may need to repeat inhalation in order to get full dose
Umeclidinium (Incruse Ellipta)	DPI 1 inhalation once daily			++	No
Glycopyrrolate (Lonhala Magnair)	Nebulizer 1 vial (25 μg) twice daily			++	Vials need to be opened and placed inside nebulizer
Revefenacin (Yupelri)	Nebulizer 1 vial (175 μg) daily			++	Vials need to be opened and placed inside nebulizer; requires use of mouthpiece
COMBINED LABA + LAMA BRONCHODILATOR—*MAINTENANCE THERAPY*					
Vilanterol + Umeclidinium (Anoro Ellipta)	DPI 1 inhalation once daily	Additive improvement, including increased adherence and decreased polypharmacy and caregiver burden	See corresponding class effects	++	No
Olodaterol + Tiotropium (Stiolto Respimat)	Fine mist 2 puffs once daily	Same as for vilanterol/umeclidinium above	See corresponding class effects	++	No

INHALED CORTICOSTEROID (ICS)—*MAINTENANCE THERAPY*

Beclomethasone (Qvar)	pMDI 1 inhalation BID	Improve symptoms, lung function, and health-related quality of life, and reduce exacerbations	+++	Prime before first use or if not used > 10 d. Rinse mouth after use
Ciclesonide (Alvesco)	pMDI 1 inhalation BID	*Note:* single therapy with ICS is not recommended in COPD, as it is less effective than ICS+LABA	+++	Prime before first use or if not used in 7–10 d. Rinse mouth after use
Flunisolide (Aerospan HFA)	pMDI 1 inhalation BID		+++	Prime before first use or if not used in 2 wk. Rinse mouth after use
Fluticasone (Flovent Diskus)	DPI 1 inhalation BID	Class effect: Dysphonia, oropharyngeal candidiasis, headache, skin bruising, pain in extremities, reduce bone mineral density, posterior subcapsular cataract, pneumonia	+++	Use in horizontal position. Rinse mouth after use
Fluticasone (Flovent HFA)	pMDI 1 inhalation BID		+++	Prime before first use, if not used in > 7 d, and if inhaler has been dropped. Rinse mouth after use
Mometasone (Asmanex Twisthaler)	pMDI 1 inhalation once daily in evening		+++	Twist to activate dose. Rinse mouth after use

COMBINED LABA BRONCHODILATOR + ICS—*MAINTENANCE THERAPY*

Formoterol + Budesonide (Symbicort)	pMDI 2 inhalations BID	Additive improvement, including increased adherence, and decreased polypharmacy and caregiver burden	++++ (inhaler alone) +++ (if spacer used)	Prime before first use, if not used in > 7 d, and if inhaler has been dropped, wait 1 min between doses. Rinse mouth after use
Formoterol + Mometasone (Dulera)	pMDI 2 inhalations BID	See corresponding class effects	++++ (inhaler alone) +++ (if spacer used)	Prime before first use and if not used in > 5 d, wait 30–60 s between doses. Rinse mouth after use
Salmeterol + Fluticasone (Advair Diskus)	DPI 1 inhalation Q12 h		+++	Use in horizontal position, have to slide lever to actuate dose. Rinse mouth after use
Vilanterol + Fluticasone (Breo Ellipta)	DPI 1 inhalation once daily		++	Rinse mouth after use

(Continued)

TABLE 81-10 ▮ COPD PHARMACOLOGY[a] (CONTINUED)

MEDICATION (GENERIC/BRAND)	DOSAGE FORM/FREQUENCY	THERAPEUTIC BENEFITS	SIDE EFFECTS[b]	PATIENT TECHNIQUE INFLUENCES DRUG DELIVERY[c]	COMPLEXITY
OTHER MEDICATIONS—*MAINTENANCE THERAPY*					
Roflumilast (Daliresp)	Oral tablets Take one 500 µg tablet once daily	Reduced exacerbations in chronic bronchitis and frequent exacerbators	Weight loss, decreased appetite, nausea, diarrhea, insomnia, headache, suicidal thoughts	+	N/A
Theophylline	Oral tablets, capsules, or solution; Aim for serum theophylline level of 8–12 mcg/mL	Third line bronchodilator: improve symptoms, exercise capacity, airflow obstruction, and quality of life	Headache, insomnia, nausea, diarrhea, seizure, arrhythmias	+	Take with water 1 h before meals or 2 h after meals. Monitor for drug interactions.
Azithromycin	Oral tablets Take one 250 mg tablet daily	Frequent exacerbators, not controlled by long-acting bronchodilators	QT prolongation; macrolide-resistant organisms, hearing decrements of 5%	+	Avoid coadministration with calcium supplements
TRIPLE-INHALER THERAPY: LAMA, LABA, AND ICS VIA A COMMON INHALATION DEVICE (ELLIPTA)[d]—*MAINTENANCE THERAPY*					
Umeclidinium (Incruse Ellipta)	DPI 1 inhalation once daily				
Vilanterol + Fluticasone (Breo Ellipta)	DPI 1 inhalation once daily				
Umeclidinium + Vilanterol + Fluticasone (Trelegy Ellipta)	DPI 1 inhalation once daily				

DPI, dry powder inhaler; HFA, hydrofluoroalkane; LABA, long-acting β$_2$-selective agonist; LAMA, long-acting muscarinic antagonist; pMDI, pressurized metered-dose inhaler; PIF, peak inspiratory flow; SABA, short acting β$_2$-agonist; SMI, soft-mist inhaler.

[a]Only medications FDA approved for use in COPD were included. Prescribing information obtained from package inserts.

[b]Limited to the most prominent and clinically concerning side effects (list is not comprehensive). When considering side effects, note that risk is substantially increased by concurrent multimorbidity and polypharmacy, and that disease severity may itself be an important underlying mechanism (eg, comorbid cardiovascular disease in the setting of a severe COPD exacerbation).

[c]Scaled as 1 + to 4+, where 1 + = little to no effect and 4+ = highest effect.

[d]Ellipta allows triple-inhaler therapy to be administered using the same device platform.

albuterol as a nebulized solution, particularly in long-term care and hospital settings. Combined ipratropium and albuterol is also available as a soft-mist inhaler (SMI). Common side effects of short-acting anticholinergics are listed in **Table 81-10**, with concerns especially raised in COPD patients with cardiovascular disease (especially bradyarrhythmias), narrow-angle glaucoma, benign prostatic hyperplasia with urinary retention, and severe constipation.

Long-Acting Bronchodilators Long-acting β_2-selective adrenergic agonists (LABA—formoterol, arformoterol, indacaterol, olodaterol, vilanterol) and long-acting anticholinergics (including the long-acting muscarinic antagonists [LAMA]—aclidinium, tiotropium, umeclidinium, glycopyrrolate, and revefenacin) are considered *maintenance therapy* (see **Table 81-10**) for persons whose symptoms are inadequately controlled with one or both classes of short-acting bronchodilator(s), and for those with frequent exacerbations or have moderate-to-severe airflow obstruction. Subsequent to initiating a long-acting bronchodilator, there is a continued role for a short-acting β_2-agonist (SABA) in the management of acute symptoms (rescue therapy). LAMA are typically used as the first-line long-acting bronchodilators due to their greater reduction in exacerbation risk as compared with LABA. Ultimately, however, the choice of initial class of LABD depends on patients' comorbidities, preferences (vis-à-vis symptom relief and side effects), and insurance coverage for the medication. For persons whose symptoms are inadequately controlled and/or who have disease exacerbations despite one class of LABD, the other class is typically added if safe to do so. Dual class BD treatment improves lung function, symptom control, and reduces exacerbation risk to a greater extent than that achieved with single BD agents.

Long-acting BD are usually delivered by handheld inhalers. Long-acting nebulized BD (eg, twice-daily β_2-selective adrenergic agonist [arformoterol, formoterol]) and/or long-acting anticholinergics (glycopyrrolate, revefenacin) are an option for persons who are unable to use or gain benefit from handheld inhaler devices (see treatment barriers, discussed further below). Of note, an increased risk of cardiovascular events was demonstrated in a large cohort study within 30 days of new initiation of LABA and/or LAMA therapy; hence, patients should be monitored especially carefully during this period.

Inhaled Corticosteroids Oral corticosteroids are not indicated in stable COPD due to multiple side effects. Long-term treatments with inhaled corticosteroids (ICS) have an important role in patients with frequent exacerbations not adequately managed by a long-acting β_2-selective adrenergic agonist (LABA) and/or anticholinergic (LAMA), who have been hospitalized for COPD exacerbation or who have concomitant asthma. Some people with COPD (nearly 40% in the ECLIPSE Study Cohort) have peripheral blood eosinophilia in the absence of atopy, allergy or asthma. Recent evidence suggests ICS combined with LABA are also an important component of treatment, reducing exacerbations and hospitalizations for those with absolute eosinophil count greater than or equal to 300 cells/mL and a high symptom burden and frequent exacerbations (GOLD Group D). However, in contrast to asthma, the use of ICS as single therapy is not advised in stable COPD, since in general, airway inflammation in COPD is less steroid-responsive than in asthma, and where used in COPD, it is more effective when combined with inhaled LABA. For those with COPD who experience exacerbations despite dual class LABD, addition of ICS improves respiratory symptoms, lung function, and health-related quality of life, (QOL) as well as reduces exacerbations. Recent data from two large randomized controlled trials (RCTs) also show a survival benefit of "triple therapy" (LABA/LAMA/ICS) among individuals with frequent exacerbations (eg, > 2 per year).

The adverse effects of ICS are dose- and duration-dependent, and influenced by patient-specific factors, specifically inhaler technique. While ICS doses are lower than oral corticosteroids, the duration of therapy is often lifelong, leading to longer exposures. Significant localized deposition of ICSs occurs in the oropharynx (60%–90% of dose) and may lead to dysphonia, oropharyngeal candidiasis, and allergic contact dermatitis of the mouth, nostrils, and eyes. Poor inhaler technique and suboptimal mouth care may increase the risk for these localized adverse drug effects. For example, older adults who forget to rinse, gargle, and spit after using their ICS are more likely to develop dysphonia and/or oral and/or esophageal candidiasis. Once swallowed, the remaining ICS is absorbed from the gastrointestinal tract, undergoes first-pass metabolism, and the majority of the dose is inactivated. What is not inactivated is available systemically and contributes to potential adverse effects. Predicting the degree of systemic glucocorticoid activity from ICS is difficult. Factors that influence risk from systemic glucocorticoid activity include advanced age, sex, cigarette smoking, activity level, and dietary calcium and vitamin D intake.

The systemic adverse effects of ICS are well described. Several have unique implications in older COPD patients. In particular, ICS are associated with decreased bone mineral density and posterior subcapsular cataract development, both of which can increase the risk of injurious falls in older adults. While studies examining the impact of ICSs on the risk of osteoporosis are mixed, doses above 1000 mcg/day of fluticasone or equivalent appear to be associated with accelerated loss of bone mineral density, and increased risk of fracture. Hence, osteoporosis prevention therapy should be considered for any patient receiving long-term ICS. Though subcapsular cataracts are clearly linked to systemic glucocorticoids, causality with ICS is less clear (with advancing illness, patients are more likely to receive both oral and ICS). In addition to increasing the risk of falls, visual impairment due to cataracts can also contribute to medication errors and difficulty with proper inhaler technique. Capillary fragility, with easy bruising of the skin and risk of skin tears, is also associated with long-term ICS use.

Importantly, meta-analyses of RCT and a large case-control study have observed an increase (1.2–1.6-fold) in the risk of pneumonia associated with ICS; although prior work showed that the use of ICS did not increase mortality in veterans hospitalized with COPD and pneumonia, it remains prudent to consider discontinuation of ICS among COPD patients who develop pneumonia. The pneumonia risk is greatest among those with older age, frailty and low BMI, high ICS dose and blood eosinophils < 100 cells/mL. Long-term ICS use in COPD has also been associated with increased incidence of atypical mycobacterial infection (such as mycobacterium avium intracellulare), which can lead to symptom exacerbation (including cough, sputum production), worsening airflow obstruction (due to airway inflammation and mucus plugging), bronchiectasis, pulmonary infiltrates, and worse gas exchange. Clinicians should be aware of this association and obtain sputum samples for AFB stain and culture where needed. Lastly, chronic ICS use is associated with tracheobronchomalacia (TBM), with dynamic central airway obstruction. This can mimic symptoms and spirometric features of COPD, but does not respond to typical bronchodilator therapy; consideration of noninvasive ventilation may be needed. Otherwise, whether a specific ICS or delivery device poses greater risk has been inconclusive. Withdrawal of ICS can be considered for persons with blood eosinophils < 300 cells/mL (and especially if < 100 cells/mL, or those who demonstrate prolonged periods of time (eg, > 1 year) free of exacerbations.

Combination Inhalers **Table 81-10** presents inhalers that combine (1) a β_2-selective adrenergic agonist and an anticholinergic, (2) a β_2-selective adrenergic agonist and ICS, or (3) a β_2-selective adrenergic agonist, anticholinergic, and ICS. Combination therapy provides additional benefit on lung function, symptoms, exercise capacity, and exacerbation risk as compared with its components, particularly in patients who have severe airflow obstruction and/or who have frequent exacerbations. Triple LABA/LAMA/ICS further improves lung function, reduces moderate to severe exacerbations, improves QOL, and as noted above, may confer a mortality benefit for those with frequent exacerbations despite taking dual class LABA/LAMA therapy.

Roflumilast Roflumilast is a once-daily oral phosphodiesterase-4 inhibitor, serving as maintenance therapy to prevent COPD exacerbations in patients with severe airflow obstruction (FEV$_1$ < 50% of predicted), chronic bronchitis, and a history of exacerbations (despite standard inhaled bronchodilator therapy). Common side effects include nausea, diarrhea, and weight loss, occurring at higher rates in those aged greater than or equal to 65. It is not effective in reducing exacerbations amongst those with emphysema-predominant COPD.

Macrolides Azithromycin (250 mg once daily or three times weekly) is a macrolide antibiotic that has been shown to decrease the frequency of COPD exacerbations when added to usual care among former tobacco smokers. This effect is accompanied by an improved QOL, but also an increased incidence of macrolide-resistant organisms and hearing decrements. Maintenance azithromycin therapy may be considered for frequent exacerbators whose symptom escalation is thought primarily due to bouts of worsened airflow obstruction and airway inflammation (rather than other processes such as unrecognized hypoxemia or "dyspnea crisis"), who are maximized on triple-inhaler therapy and do not have a hearing impairment, resting tachycardia or other arrythmia, apparent risk of QTc prolongation, or clinical/radiographic evidence of nontuberculous mycobacterial infection. Since macrolide resistance can complicate treatment for nontuberculous mycobacteria (when needed), careful assessment for possible nontuberculous mycobacteria infection is warranted prior to considering regular use of macrolide therapy for routine COPD exacerbation prevention.

Mucolytics Based on low efficacy and increased risk of adverse effects, there is little evidence to support mucolytics (eg, N-acetylcysteine) as routine care for stable COPD. Hence, mucolytic use is limited to management of tenacious sputum production that is refractory to standard therapy (smoking cessation, inhaled BD and corticosteroid, antibiotics, and/or roflumilast). Although not proven to improve lung function or reduce exacerbations, some patients report symptom relief and increased ease of sputum clearance with regular or intermittent use of guaifenesin. Persons with severe airflow obstruction with chronic mucus production and those with bronchiectasis may benefit from a regular "airway clearance" routine, with nebulized albuterol (and/or hypertonic saline), followed by use of a vibratory PEP device. This can improve symptoms (dyspnea, cough, sputum production, and wheezing) and airflow and reduce frequency and/or severity of infectious exacerbations.

Biologic Monoclonal Antibody Therapies Owing to their success in the management of severe eosinophilic asthma, recent clinical trials have investigated the role of monoclonal antibody therapies (eg., omalizumab, benralizumab, mepolizumab, etc) in the treatment of COPD. A modest reduction in exacerbations has been found among individuals with COPD with elevated peripheral blood eosinophil counts, and history of frequent exacerbations despite triple LABA/LAMA/ICS treatment. Results have varied across trials, and further work is needed to determine which patients may be best suited to receive these therapies.

Theophylline Theophylline is a nonselective phosphodiesterase inhibitor, available in multiple oral formulations. While it has small BD effect, affords symptom relief for some persons, and was formerly used commonly in the management of stable COPD, it is now usually NOT recommended for routine management of COPD or COPD exacerbations, given the narrow therapeutic dose range, lack of efficacy, and high likelihood of side effects, which may include tremor, tachyarrhythmia, nausea, vomiting, jitteriness, and/or seizures. If used as a third or fourth line treatment, theophylline requires therapeutic drug monitoring with a goal serum level in older adults of 8 to 12 mcg/mL. Levels can increase significantly in the presence of cirrhosis, heart failure, hypothyroidism, and cimetidine. In older adults patients treated with theophylline, coadministration of ciprofloxacin (CYP1A2 inhibitor) is associated with a twofold increased risk of hospitalization. Conversely, theophylline levels decrease when hepatic enzymatic activity is increased as in hyperthyroidism, smoking, use of phenytoin, phenobarbital, and carbamazepine, or consumption of cruciferous vegetables and charbroiled meats.

Treatment barriers Medication nonadherence is reported in 50% to 60% of COPD patients. Nonadherence is associated with more frequent exacerbations, worsening of disease, and difficulty in reconciling medications. The causes of nonadherence include cognitive and physical impairments, cost, medication complexity, lack of perceived benefit, and adverse drug effects.

Cognitive and physical impairments leading to improper inhaler technique are considered further below.

Cognitive Impairment A Mini-Mental Status Examination (MMSE) score less than 24, inability to perform intersecting pentagons, and/or an EXIT-25 cognitive test score greater than or equal to 15 is associated with impaired ability to learn inhaler techniques. Requiring patients to "teach-back" inhaler technique may further identify those with difficulty performing multistep commands. Cognitive impairment often leads to uncoordinated "press and breathe" use of inhalers, as well as nonadherence. Consequently, nebulizers often replace handheld inhalers in cognitively impaired patients. Recently, electronic devices attached to inhalers have been introduced; these may help promote adherence by providing sound and/or light-based prompts.

Physical Impairment Many handheld inhalers require both fine-motor skills and adequate grip strength to actuate. This is especially problematic for certain pMDIs, dry powder inhalers (DPIs), and newer SMIs. Decreased hand strength, for example, is a predictor for incorrect use of a pMDI. The presence of arthritis, joint pain, or neuromuscular diseases may prevent proper use of handheld inhalers, by reducing grip strength or impairing dexterity. Impaired manual dexterity prevents patients from properly priming or preparing the inhaler/nebulizer, particularly if devices require removing capsules from foil packaging, mixing diluents with active agents, and puncturing capsules prior to inhalation.

Visual impairment can make distinguishing between products difficult (rescue inhaler versus maintenance inhaler) and negate the adherence feedback mechanisms built into certain devices (dosage counters). Individuals with impaired hearing may have difficulty understanding

inhaler training, and several inhaler/valved-chamber devices (VCD) use auditory cues for proper inhalation technique, to which the hearing impaired older adult is unable to respond.

DPIs require a sufficient PIF of > 45 L/min to disaggregate the dry powder from the container. Reduced respiratory muscle strength due to aging and progressive COPD (severe airflow obstruction) may explain the variability in DPI drug–lung deposition in older adults. While DPIs result in higher drug–lung deposition (10%–40%) when compared to pMDIs (10%–20%), the increased PIF required to disaggregate the product also results in up to 80% oropharyngeal deposition. The use of pMDIs may be also adversely affected by a low PIF, since these require a slow, deep inhalation, preferably through a spacer device, to allow for maximal drug–lung deposition. In contrast, SMI require a gentle breathing maneuver, thus offering an advantage over DPIs and pMDIs for patients with reduced PIF or who struggle with "press and breathe" coordination. When performed correctly, SMIs can achieve 40% to 60% drug–lung deposition. Importantly, patients/caregivers should be reminded that inhalation technique varies with DPI, pMDI, and SMI. Poor inspiratory effort and/or coordination can result in suboptimal medication delivery to the lungs, and in turn may result in suboptimal treatment effects.

When cognitive or functional impairments limit the use of handheld inhalers, a nebulizer is the easiest delivery device to use. Moreover, patients who have severe dyspnea, severe airflow obstruction, or frequent exacerbations may also find nebulizers more effective. Lastly, as discussed below, nebulizer therapy may be a cost-effective alternative in patients with high Medicare Part D health care costs. Unfortunately, nebulizers have disadvantages, requiring a power source, are not easily portable, must be carefully maintained/cleaned, and generally take longer to administer.

Cost Payers often seek lower cost therapies, potentially compromising efficacy, complexity, and patient adherence, or they require prior authorization for certain products (COPD prescription fill rates decline when patients perceive barriers to obtaining medications). In addition, because older adult patients regularly experience polypharmacy, they may have significant out-of-pocket expenses due to a coverage gap ("the donut hole") in their Medicare Part D annual provider and prescription expenses. This increased cost impacts handheld inhalers, as these are covered under Medicare Part D. However, nebulizers, compressors, and medications that are available as inhalation solutions are covered under Medicare Part B. Hence, any premiums, deductibles, and copayments for these items do not count toward Medicare Part D costs, potentially helping older patients avoid gaps in coverage.

Nonpharmacologic Therapies

Vaccination Annual influenza vaccination is a well-established safe and efficacious means of reducing complications related to the flu, including COPD exacerbations. Older adult patients can elect to receive either the regular dose influenza vaccine or newer high-dose influenza vaccine designed for persons aged 65 and older. Evidence supports recommending older adults receive the high-dose quadrivalent vaccine. This vaccine is associated with a higher immune response in older adults and was 24.2% more effective in preventing flu when compared to the standard-dose vaccine. The Centers for Disease Control and Prevention (CDC) and its Advisory Committee on Immunization Practices have not expressed a preference for either vaccine.

Pneumococcal vaccination has been shown to reduce COPD exacerbations, community-acquired pneumonia, and bacteremia. Patients should therefore be vaccinated according to CDC guidelines, which recommend use of polysaccharide pneumococcal vaccine (PPV23; pneumovax) for all adults with COPD or who are current smokers. The 13-valent conjugate vaccine (PCV-13) is recommended for people with COPD older than age 65 and those who are immunocompromised, have history of invasive pneumococcal vaccine, or have a history of cochlear implant.

Smoking cessation Abstinence from tobacco smoking is important for all persons with COPD, irrespective of age or disease severity. Smoking cessation, even undertaken in older age, has been associated with better preservation of general daily functioning in older adult years. Smoking status should be addressed at every office visit and during hospitalizations, including number of cigarettes per day, triggers for smoking, time to first cigarette use following morning awakening, details of prior quit attempts, and patient-identified barriers to quitting. Smoking cessation attenuates the rate of decline in lung function, improves the response to inhaled BD therapy, and reduces the risk of COPD exacerbation, cardiovascular disease, cancer, and death.

Several methods are available to assist patients with smoking cessation. The combination of behavioral counseling and pharmacotherapy is most effective in achieving long-term abstinence. Importantly, available interventions for smoking cessation have comparable efficacy among older adults to those seen for younger persons. Therefore, a nihilistic approach based on advanced patient age should not be taken. The "5 A's" algorithm (developed by the US Public Health Service)—Ask, Advise, Assess, Assist, and Arrange—is an effective behavioral counseling strategy for use in the clinic setting. Referral to a smoking cessation program should be offered, and information regarding the US nationwide toll-free telephone counseling service (1-800-QUIT-NOW) should be provided. Recently developed mobile phone apps, text messaging, and computer-based interventions are effective for some persons. For patients ready to make a quit attempt, a quit date should be set, an action plan for managing cravings and triggers for smoking should be created, and a plan for follow-up with the health care provider must be arranged. The three pharmacologic treatments with the best efficacy include nicotine replacement (NRT) (especially the combination

of nicotine patch and a faster-acting agent such as gum or lozenges to address urges), varenicline, and bupropion. No single strategy has proven to be better than the other. Patient preference, comorbidities, and previous experience with quit attempts influence the choice of first-line treatment. Nicotine replacement therapy is generally safe, even for persons with underlying cardiovascular disease, but should be avoided in the setting of recent MI or stroke. Bupropion may be the best first-line agent for persons with depression or schizophrenia, but NRT may be preferable for persons with bipolar disorder, since antidepressant agents can trigger manic episodes. Patients taking bupropion or varenicline must also be monitored for development of neuropsychiatric symptoms, including suicidal ideation. Close partnering with patients' mental health care providers is important in choosing pharmacotherapy for smoking cessation, especially since some patients may already be taking other antidepressants. Combination therapy can be considered when single class pharmacotherapy has failed. The combination of NRT and varenicline has thus far demonstrated the highest rates of short-term success. Nicotine replacement should be provided as needed during hospitalizations, to prevent nicotine withdrawal symptoms. Other pharmacologic therapies for smoking cessation are the subject of active research.

Long-term oxygen therapy Requirement for long-term oxygen therapy (LTOT) is a poor prognostic feature of COPD. The indications for LTOT are shown in **Table 81-11**. A formal oxygen prescription specifying the indications for treatment, conditions for use (rest, exercise, and/or sleep), and type of oxygen system(s) is required. LTOT worn more than 16 hours per day improves survival for patients with severe resting hypoxemia ($PaO_2 \le 60$ mm Hg) with COPD. Among persons with resting hypoxemia, LTOT can also improve exercise capacity, dyspnea, sleep quality, cognition,

TABLE 81-11 ■ INDICATIONS FOR LONG-TERM OXYGEN THERAPY

Daily use (at least 16 h/d):
- Resting arterial PO_2 (PaO_2) ≤ 55 mm Hg, or pulse oxygen saturation (SpO_2) $\le 88\%$
- $PaO_2 \le 59$ mm Hg or $SpO_2 \le 89\%$, concurrent with CHF/cor pulmonale, pulmonary hypertension, or erythrocytosis (hematocrit > 55%) at rest, during exertion, +/or sleep

Nocturnal use:
- $PaO_2 \le 55$ mm Hg or $SpO_2 \le 88\%$ during sleep for > 5 min OR
- Decrease in $PaO_2 > 10$ mm Hg or in $SpO_2 > 5\%$ during sleep with symptoms or signs of nocturnal hypoxemia such as disrupted sleep, morning headaches, impaired cognitive function, or insomnia

Use with exertion:
- Decrease in $PaO_2 \le 55$ mm Hg or in $SpO_2 \le 88\%$ during exercise and documented improvement in hypoxemia with O_2 administration

depression, cardiovascular comorbidity, and QOL, as well as reduce the frequency of hospitalizations. However, a recent RCT did not find clear benefits of supplemental oxygen in regard to lung function, exercise capacity, QOL, time to first hospitalization, or mortality among people with moderate resting or exercise-induced oxygen desaturation alone. It may still be used for those who desaturate less than 88% or PaO_2 less than 55 mm Hg during exertion AND who have improvements in dyspnea and/or exercise capacity with its use. The role of isolated supplemental O_2 during sleep for those without CHF, pulmonary hypertension, OSA, or concurrent lung disease who lack daytime hypoxemia is also unclear.

Practical issues and potential risks associated with providing LTOT must be considered, particularly among older adult persons. Patients often perceive a reduction in their mobility and/or QOL based on requirement for supplemental O_2. Long oxygen tubing attached to oxygen concentrators in the home can pose a fall risk. Cigarette smoking, cooking flames, and other heating systems can pose the risk of explosion or fire. Lightweight portable O_2 systems maximize the likelihood that the older adult patient will be physically capable of using their O_2 with exertion, but may not be available and/or may not sufficiently maintain an adequate SaO_2 (eg, for those with high liter flow rates). Rollator walkers with handbrakes, seat, and basket assist debilitated patients in carrying their O_2 systems and maintaining mobility both in and outside the home. Patient cognition and home layout and safety should also be assessed. Education about oxygen equipment and safety should be provided to patients and their caregivers.

Noninvasive positive pressure ventilation Noninvasive positive pressure ventilation (NPPV) is indicated for the management of some patients with COPD. First, OSA is a common comorbidity of COPD; persons with both conditions are considered as having COPD-OSA overlap syndrome. Individuals with COPD-OSA overlap syndrome have worse gas exchange disturbances, increased risk of pulmonary hypertension, and a higher mortality risk than those with either condition alone. Continuous positive airway pressure (CPAP) therapy is indicated for the management of OSA, when present. Second, NPPV (usually bilevel positive airway pressure [BPAP]) is indicated for persons with acute exacerbations of COPD associated with acute hypercarbia ($PaCO_2 > 45$–50 mm Hg) and respiratory acidosis (who lack contraindications as noted below). In this setting, NPPV improves gas exchange, improves breathing pattern, and provides support to the respiratory muscles, while allowing time for medical therapy such as BD, antibiotics, and corticosteroids to improve airflow and reduce the work of breathing. High-quality RCTs have shown that, as compared with medical therapy alone, NPPV for acute hypercarbia related to COPD exacerbations reduces intubation rates, shortens hospital length of stay, reduces the risk of ventilator-associated pneumonia, and improves

survival. Addition of NIV to home supplemental O_2 among those with persistent hypercarbia ($PaCO_2 > 53$ mm Hg) within 4 weeks of an acute COPD exacerbation with acute on chronic hypercarbic respiratory failure have a longer time to readmission and a reduced risk of death over the subsequent 12 months.

The role of "chronic" NPPV for long-term management of stable patients with COPD and hypercarbia is less certain. Uncontrolled case series suggest that nocturnal NPPV can improve daytime gas exchange and daytime walking activity (postulated to be related to respiratory muscle rest and reduction in hyperinflation), but randomized trials have not consistently shown these effects. Recent RCTs suggest chronic NPPV can reduce dyspnea and improve QOL, and may have very slight benefit with regard to reducing hospitalizations and improving mortality rate for those with stable COPD and chronic hypercarbia. It has been shown in research settings to facilitate exercise training in pulmonary rehabilitation (PR) for some persons. However, patient intolerance and poor acceptance of NPPV commonly limit its long-term use. Chronic NPPV is considered for nocturnal use in persons with daytime hypercarbia ($PaCO_2 \geq 50$ mm Hg), in those with sustained alveolar hypoventilation for more than 5 continuous minutes during sleep despite supplemental oxygen therapy greater than or equal to 2 L/min, or in those who have episodes of hypercarbic respiratory failure requiring assisted ventilation. In these individuals, chronic NPPV may provide symptomatic relief, particularly if there is coexisting sleep disruption and daytime fatigue. Noninvasive ventilation settings should be adjusted to target reduction in $PaCO_2$.

Contraindications to NPPV include cardiorespiratory arrest, unstable vital signs, inability to tolerate the face mask (discomfort, skin breakdown, or claustrophobia), facial trauma, inability to protect the airway, combative behavior, severely impaired consciousness, need to clear purulent secretions, high aspiration risk, and recent gastric or esophageal surgery. Caution is also urged regarding NPPV in persons with giant bullae or very severe bullous emphysema, given the risk of inducing a pneumothorax with a resultant nonhealing bronchopleural fistula.

Pulmonary rehabilitation People with COPD are less active than healthy age-matched persons. Exertional dyspnea, leg fatigue, anxiety, depression, impaired balance, and fear may all contribute to a low physical activity level. Other contributory factors include skeletal muscle dysfunction (including sarcopenia), which is common in COPD, and the increased dyspnea and gas exchange abnormalities that result from acute exacerbations. Importantly, because it can lead to deconditioning, sarcopenia, and other aspects of muscle dysfunction, decreased endurance, and exercise intolerance, physical inactivity is itself associated with an earlier onset of lactic acidosis at low work rates, yielding a greater ventilatory demand and dyspnea at any given activity level. Moreover, as physical inactivity progresses, there is increased physical disability, social isolation, anxiety, and depression, as well as risk of COPD exacerbation (hospitalization), obesity, diabetes, cardiovascular disease, and death.

PR is "a comprehensive intervention based on a thorough patient assessment followed by patient-tailored therapies that include, but are not limited to, exercise training, education and behavior change, designed to improve the physical and psychological condition of people with chronic respiratory disease and to promote the long-term adherence to health-enhancing behaviors." PR reduces dyspnea and leg fatigue, improves exercise tolerance and patient-reported QOL, decreases the risk of hospitalizations and other urgent health care utilization, and reduces anxiety and depression. It can also improve balance, reduce the risk of falls, and improve physical activity levels.

Participation in PR within 90 days of hospitalization for COPD exacerbation is also associated with improved survival. The process of PR includes patient assessment, supervised exercise training and reconditioning, patient education, and outcome assessment. Exercise training typically includes aerobic and strength training of the lower and upper extremities, using a treadmill or hallway walking, cycling, arm ergometry, stair climbing, and light weight lifting. Nordic walking and interval-type exercise, balance training, and Tai chi are also effective. Walking aids such as rollator walkers can assist in improving tolerance of walking in severely disabled persons. The education component of PR is geared toward helping patients understand and manage their condition (including early recognition of exacerbations), as well as promotion of a healthy and active lifestyle. Emphasis is also typically placed on training patients with pacing, energy conservation, and pursed lips breathing techniques, as well as strategies for management of anxiety and prevention of "dyspnea crisis." PR also affords the opportunity to counsel and educate patients regarding advance care planning and educate them regarding life support interventions.

All patients who remain symptomatic despite optimized pharmacologic therapy (including those with severely impaired lung function) should be referred for PR. Persons older than age 70, even those with severe lung function impairment and comorbidities, benefit to the same degree as younger persons. Close partnering between patients' health care providers and PR staff is important to ensure patient safety.

Surgical therapies Surgical therapies for COPD include lung volume reduction surgery (LVRS) and lung transplantation. LVRS is a procedure wherein areas of lung that are virtually functionless (not contributing to ventilation or perfusion) are removed, thereby reducing hyperinflation and improving elastic recoil and diaphragm positioning and function. LVRS can be accomplished by surgical resection of regions of lung (typically upper lung zones), or bronchoscopic placement of coils, valves, or other devices that lead to atelectasis of targeted lung zones. When used in carefully selected patients, LVRS can lead improvements in exercise tolerance, oxygenation, lung function,

QOL, and survival. LVRS can also serve as a bridge to lung transplantation for some patients. Ideal candidates for surgical LVRS are those with severe emphysema-predominant COPD (heterogeneous distribution, upper lung zone predominant) with FEV_1 less than 50% predicted, lung hyperinflation (eg, RV > 150–200% of predicted), who lack features of chronic bronchitis, are not at extremes of body weight, lack other unstable medical comorbidity, do not require regular treatment with systemic corticosteroids, and who remain symptomatic with low exercise tolerance despite optimized pharmacologic therapy and PR, and have maintained long-term abstinence from tobacco use. Those whose FEV_1 or diffusing capacity (DLCO) is less than 20% of predicted and homogeneous distribution of emphysema have higher mortality following surgical LVRS and should not undergo the procedure. Patients must be selected carefully also for bronchoscopic LVRS, as it is associated with complications including pneumothorax (in up to 30%) and infection. Bronchoscopic LVRS can be considered in those with variable distribution of emphysema (including homogeneous pattern), as long as evaluation demonstrates complete lobar fissures without collateral ventilation to areas targeted for decompression.

Single or double lung transplantation may be considered for selected older adult persons with very severe COPD. Although lung transplantation can improve exercise tolerance, QOL, and survival of some individuals, anticipated survival benefit should exceed the short-term and long-term risks of undergoing the procedure, including surgical and perioperative morbidity and mortality, and potential complications related to long-term immunosuppressive therapy. Since median survival following lung transplantation is 5 to 6 years, and since surgical risk is high among older adult persons with multimorbidity, referral for lung transplantation should be undertaken only when anticipated survival related to the COPD is lower than that related to age and/or comorbidities. Given the variable rate of progression of COPD over time, this is difficult to predict. Current guidelines suggest lung transplantation referral for COPD patients who have FEV_1 and diffusing capacity (DLCO) less than 25% of predicted, $PaCO_2$ greater than 50 mm Hg and/or PaO_2 less than 60 mm Hg, pulmonary hypertension and/or cor pulmonale, BODE Index score greater than 5, are worsening clinically despite optimized medical therapies (including PR), had one or more hospitalizations for exacerbation with acute hypercapnia or at least three severe exacerbations in the prior year, and have demonstrated long-term complete abstinence from tobacco or other substance use. They must also lack other contraindications as indicated in the 2014 lung transplantation guidelines, including recent cancer, other unstable medical or psychological conditions, BMI greater than 35 kg/m², inadequate social support, inability to adhere to medical therapies, uncorrectable bleeding disorder, active tuberculosis infection, or significant spinal/chest wall distortion. Although older than age 65 is a relative, rather than absolute contraindication to lung transplantation, recent studies have shown that those older than age 70 have an increased risk of 30-day and 1-year mortality and are less likely to return to prior baseline functional status, as compared to younger persons.

ACUTE COPD EXACERBATION

The GOLD Report defines an acute exacerbation of COPD as a change in sputum volume or purulence, and/or an increase in dyspnea beyond usual day-to-day variation that warrants a change in therapy. However, not all exacerbations leading to escalation of symptoms lead to a change in therapy; in particular, patients may underreport symptoms, attributing them to aging or other conditions. The frequency of exacerbations increases with severity of airflow obstruction, with older persons likely to have more severe disease. It is estimated that the average older person with COPD experiences two to three exacerbations per year, each lasting up to 2 weeks. Each of these events presents a risk for respiratory failure and death, but more commonly results in tangible impacts on symptoms, increased airflow obstruction and related respiratory impairments, disability, and QOL. COPD exacerbations also increase the risk of myocardial infarction, pulmonary emboli, and stroke; are responsible for up to 20% of hospitalizations in individuals 75 years or older; and are a major source of health care costs. Moreover, institutions are now financially penalized for all-cause readmissions following admissions for COPD exacerbations.

Risk Factors

Risk factors for acute exacerbations include advanced age, severe airflow obstruction, chronic bronchitis, comorbid diseases (particularly cardiovascular disease, diabetes mellitus, and gastroesophageal reflux), and prior exacerbations. Those with history of two or more exacerbations in a year, or an exacerbation requiring hospitalization are at particular increased risk of subsequent exacerbation events. In the aging patient, the weakening of thoracic muscles, degenerative changes of the spine, and impairment of mucociliary clearance make secretion clearance and cough less effective. Older adult patients are therefore less able to manage the increased secretions resulting from even a mild exacerbation. Age-related changes to both adaptive and innate immune systems make responses to infection less robust, and the inflammatory responses to acute illness more discordant. Protective immunity from prior immunization may be waning or frankly incompetent. The previously discussed changes to overall respiratory function with both age and COPD limit underlying pulmonary reserve. Comorbid conditions may make it more difficult to tolerate the stress of acute illnesses. For all these reasons, the presentations of and outcomes from acute exacerbations in older adults may be more severe than those in middle-aged individuals of similar spirometric severity.

Etiologies

Respiratory infection accounts for approximately 70% of COPD exacerbations. Viruses, typically detected using direct fluorescent antibody (DFA) or polymerase chain reaction (PCR)-based methods, can be found in up to two-thirds of individuals with acute exacerbations. Common viral pathogens, of which rhinoviruses are the most prevalent, are shown in **Table 81-12**. However, a positive PCR does not definitively indicate causality, as positive results can also be found in asymptomatic, stable individuals with COPD. The exceptions to this are influenza and SARS-CoV-2, which should always be considered causative pathogens and treated accordingly.

Bacteria are responsible for 40% to 60% of COPD exacerbations, and may coinfect with viral pathogens. As shown in **Table 81-12**, *Haemophilus influenzae, Moraxella catarrhalis*, and *Streptococcus pneumoniae* are the most common, but *Pseudomonas aeruginosa* and enteric gram-negative bacteria and *Staphylococcus aureus* (including MRSA) are frequently isolated in more severe COPD and in residents of skilled nursing facilities and/or those who have received frequent courses of antibiotics; the contribution of atypical pathogens is more difficult to estimate accurately given the infrequency with which titers or accurate cultures are obtained. Acquisition of new strains of common pathogens plays a much more important role in acute exacerbations of COPD than changes in the load of colonizing bacteria. This is supported by observations that new bacterial strains are associated with more robust humoral immunity and inflammatory responses, and clearance of these strains correlates with resolution of acute illness. Other common causes of COPD exacerbation include exposure to environmental irritants (including pollutants, environmental smoke, strong odors such as floor cleansers or perfumes), GERD, allergens, and changes in ambient air temperature and/or humidity. Chronic aspiration is another consideration in older persons. Hypogammaglobulinemia is another recently recognized risk for COPD exacerbation that is also associated with increased risk of hospitalization and mortality.

TABLE 81-12 ■ COMMON INFECTIOUS PATHOGENS IN ACUTE EXACERBATIONS OF COPD	
VIRAL	**BACTERIAL**
Rhinovirus	*H. influenzae*
Influenza	*M. catarrhalis*
Parainfluenza	*S. pneumoniae*
Adenovirus	*P. aeruginosa*
Coronavirus	Enterobacteriaceae
Respiratory syncytial virus	*M. pneumoniae*
Human metapneumovirus	*C. pneumoniae*
	Legionella spp.
	Staphylococcus spp.

COPD exacerbation is a clinical diagnosis. COPD exacerbations are typically associated with worsened airflow obstruction over and above that present at the patient's baseline. The worsened airflow obstruction may relate to increased airway mucus, airway wall inflammation, and/or bronchoconstriction. Other triggers for worsening symptoms in people with COPD include episodes of hypoxemia (with associated increase in ventilatory demand), unrecognized ventilatory insufficiency (with acute and/or chronic hypercarbia with need for NPPV support), and "dyspnea crises" related to episodes of dynamic hyperinflation above baseline with worsened mechanical disadvantage of the respiratory muscles and reduced inspiratory capacity. The latter typically result from exertion or other causes of faster respiratory rate (with less time for exhalation and lung emptying), such as anxiety, pain, or other causes of tachypnea. Importantly, several other conditions including pneumonia, pulmonary embolus, CHF (systolic and/or diastolic), pulmonary hypertension/cor pulmonale, sepsis, anemia, variable dynamic upper airway obstruction (intrathoracic—such as TBM; or extrathoracic—such as vocal cord dysfunction) can lead to escalation of symptoms and/or worsened gas exchange among individuals with COPD, but are not COPD exacerbations per se.

These conditions are not, therefore, expected to respond to typical treatment for COPD exacerbation (considered further below). Moreover, treatments that are crucial to COPD exacerbations may exacerbate comorbidities or cause potentially dangerous drug interactions. These comorbidities may additionally complicate or prolong recovery from COPD exacerbation. Individuals with COPD are particularly vulnerable to cardiovascular morbidity and mortality both during exacerbations and in the recovery period. Rigorous attention to detection and individualized treatment of these conditions is needed among persons in whom COPD and COPD exacerbation are suspected.

For those with true COPD exacerbation, in many cases, sputum culture does not differentiate between colonizing flora and true infectious pathogen, and underestimates the most common bacterial culprits; therefore, sputum culture is not necessary in routine COPD exacerbations. However, sputum culture may be helpful in detecting worrisome pathogens or resistant strains, if an individual has failed empiric outpatient treatment strategies or has risk factors for *Pseudomonas aeruginosa* (hospitalization in the past 3 months, ≥ 4 courses of antibiotics in the past year, or severe airflow obstruction). DFA, with or without PCR, is important during influenza season, as specific antiviral therapy may be initiated.

Treatment of COPD Exacerbations

Most exacerbations can be treated as an outpatient. Patients with more severe airflow obstruction, significant comorbidities, inadequate home support, new/worsening gas exchange abnormalities, prior treatment failure and/or diagnostic uncertainty should be admitted to the hospital for further evaluation (labs, chest x-ray, ECG, arterial blood gas, and other testing as indicated); however, depending on home-based resources, a few such patients may still be candidates for intensive home care. Those with impending respiratory failure are admitted to the intensive care unit (ICU).

Escalation of inhaled medications Escalation of BD therapy is required for all COPD exacerbations and may be sufficient to treat mild cases. The preferred BD is a short-acting inhaled β_2-agonist with or without a short-acting anticholinergic. Nebulized delivery may be more effective and comfortable than metered dose inhalers, particularly for patients with significant dyspnea, cognitive impairment, or severe airflow obstruction. Usual maintenance therapies, such as long-acting BD and inhaled corticosteroids, should be continued during mild exacerbations. For those with severe exacerbations requiring frequent regular dosing with nebulized BD, it may be advisable to withhold LABD temporarily to prevent risk of arrythmia, tremulousness and other adverse effects. As recovery ensues, the patient is transitioned back to a maintenance regimen, but a step-up in inhaled therapy may be warranted to reduce the risk of subsequent exacerbations. For example, a second class of long-acting BD may be added for those previously receiving single class maintenance BD, and addition of ICS may be considered for those who exacerbate despite taking dual class maintenance BD (see algorithm in GOLD Report in Further Reading). If clinical improvement is thereafter achieved, attention is given to streamlining the number of inhaled medication devices to improve self-efficacy and compliance.

Antibiotics General antibiotic recommendations for COPD exacerbations are presented in **Table 81-13**. Antibiotics used for treatment of exacerbations associated with increased volume and/or purulence of sputum are associated with reduced treatment failure and increased time between exacerbations. Procalcitonin, a peptide

TABLE 81-13 ■ SUGGESTED ANTIBIOTIC REGIMENS FOR ACUTE EXACERBATION OF COPD

EXACERBATION SEVERITY	ANTIBIOTICS
Mild	None
Moderate[a,b]	Macrolide, doxycycline, cephalosporin, amoxicillin/clavulanate, bactrim, fluoroquinolone
Severe[c,d]	Fluoroquinolone, antipseudomonal penicillin, cephalosporin (third generation), vancomycin (if concern for MRSA)

[a]Moderate exacerbations are accompanied by at least two of the following: increased dyspnea, sputum volume, and sputum purulence—in the absence of respiratory failure.
[b]Severe exacerbations are accompanied by at least two of the following: increased dyspnea, sputum volume, and sputum purulence—concurrent with respiratory failure.
[c]If risk factors for *Pseudomonas*, use ciprofloxacin and obtain sputum culture.
[d]If risk factors for *Pseudomonas*, use pipercillin-tazobactam or ceftazidime, and obtain sputum culture. If risk factors for MRSA, check nasal MRSA swab and obtain sputum culture.

precursor that increases in the serum in response to bacterial toxins, has been advocated as a potential biomarker to guide antibiotic use. One Cochrane meta-analysis demonstrated that procalcitonin guidance could reduce antibiotic exposure without increase in treatment failure or mortality. However, procalcitonin is not currently recommended to guide antibiotic use in COPD exacerbations, since the level may not be elevated in persons with bronchitis (rather than pneumonia), and its use to guide antibiotics among patients requiring ICU care for acute exacerbation of COPD demonstrated an increase in adverse outcomes. In contrast, recent evidence suggests that serum C-reactive protein (CRP) levels may have utility in guiding which individual will benefit from antibiotic therapy, and for whom antibiotics can be avoided.

Choice of antibiotic is driven by a number of factors (history, tolerance, disease severity, comorbidities, medication interactions, prior treatment failure, local patterns of resistance), and complicated by the fact that sputum culture data is unreliable in guiding decisions. Older adult residents of skilled nursing facilities, or those who have spent time in acute-care or subacute-rehab facilities within 90 days of exacerbation, and persons with severe airflow obstruction are more likely to be colonized with resistant organisms (methicillin-resistant *Staphylococcus aureus*, *Pseudomonas aeruginosa*, and multidrug-resistant gram-negative organisms). These latter risk factors should guide choice of empiric therapy. The duration of antibiotic therapy, in the absence of complicating factors such as pneumonia or bronchiectasis, is typically 3 to 7 days. Those with bronchiectasis may require longer treatment (10–14 days).

Corticosteroids The acute use of systemic corticosteroid for treatment of moderate to severe COPD exacerbation is associated with improved symptoms, faster improvement in lung function, decreased treatment failure, and shorter duration of hospitalization. However, systemic steroids can cause side effects, particularly in older persons with multimorbidity. Common side effects include hyperglycemia, delirium, fluid retention, myopathy, and/or thrush. In addition, because older COPD patients often have atrial fibrillation requiring anticoagulation, and because systemic corticosteroids can cause skin thinning and purpura, this combination of medications may also lead to greater bruising and bleeding. Frequent use of systemic corticosteroids can lead to acquired hypogammaglobulinemia and worsen immune suppression.

The adverse effects of systemic corticosteroid are dose- and duration-dependent. For example, delirium is more likely to occur with doses greater than 60 mg of prednisone per day. As such, dose and duration of therapy should be as conservative as possible. The optimal dose and duration of corticosteroids is unknown; however, a study of individuals hospitalized with COPD exacerbations (most of whom had severe disease) demonstrated that a 5-day course of oral prednisone (40 mg/day) was noninferior to a more conventional 7- to 14-day steroid taper in terms of event resolution and time to next exacerbation. In fact, those on the shorter course had a reduced length of stay, though reasons for this were unclear.

Supplemental oxygen: Supplemental oxygen should be provided as needed to achieve $SaO_2 > 88\%$ at rest, during exertion, and sleep. Those with history of hypercarbia should be monitored closely for any worsening CO_2 retention while receiving oxygen therapy. High flow nasal cannula O_2 can reduce work of breathing post-extubation among those recovering from acute hypercarbic respiratory failure requiring mechanical ventilation.

Invasive and noninvasive ventilation Many patients admitted to the hospital with impending respiratory failure in the setting of COPD exacerbation can be managed effectively with noninvasive ventilation, though less so in the case of concomitant pneumonia. Intubation and mechanical ventilation may be required in the case of severe respiratory failure, if consistent with an individual's goals of care.

Discharge planning Discharge planning should consider referral for PR and/or tobacco cessation counseling, the need for home oxygen, and a recalibration of maintenance therapy (see Management section) above. Because new treatment regimens increase the likelihood of medication nonadherence or errors, this may be addressed by a formal medication reconciliation and pharmacist-based review. Patient and caregiver education regarding the discharge treatment plan is likewise essential, as are interventions to support safe and prompt transition back to routine care by the primary care provider or specialist. Furthermore, advance care planning should be initiated or reviewed in the wake of hospitalization, as history of a severe exacerbation increases the risk of future events.

COVID-19 (SARS-CoV-2) and COPD

The emergence of COVID-19 posed new, unprecedented challenges for people with COPD. Prior to the widespread availability of vaccines, fear of contracting COVID-19 led most individuals to remain homebound, which led to further reduction in daily physical activity levels, worsened functional disability, increased social isolation, fear, anxiety, and depression. Most PR programs had to close at least temporarily due to the pandemic. Ironically, social distancing mandates, use of masks, avoidance of crowds, and home isolation as well as increased adherence to prescribed medical therapies (eg, related to anxiety and fear) contributed to an overall reduction in acute COPD exacerbation events and community-based management of many exacerbations that did occur, for many with COPD. While to date, there is no clear evidence that individuals with COPD are more susceptible to contracting SARS-CoV-2, worse clinical outcomes have been noted among those with COPD who became infected, including increased risk of hospitalization, ICU admission, respiratory failure, and possibly also death. Older age and cardiovascular morbidity further increase the risk of poor outcomes. Evidence to date suggests those with COPD who contract COVID-19 should continue their usual COPD treatment, that they should be considered for standard COVID-19 therapies (eg, monoclonal antibody, remdesivir, dexamethasone, etc) as appropriate, and close attention should be paid to their oxygen levels and work of breathing. SARS-CoV-2 mRNA vaccines appear to be safe and effective in older adults; however, limited data exist among older persons with multiple comorbidities and frailty.

PALLIATIVE CARE

Palliative care is an important and beneficial component of the overall integrated care of people with COPD. Average life expectancy for COPD from time of diagnosis is shorter compared with other chronic conditions such as heart disease or stroke (14 years for COPD compared with 21 years for heart disease). The health trajectory for aging persons with COPD is variable. While for many, disease progression is gradual, some have a more rapid and progressive decline in lung function resulting in increased disability, intermittent exacerbations requiring hospitalizations, and death. Respiratory symptoms of dyspnea, cough, and sputum production are frequently reported by patients with advanced COPD, affecting up to 98% of patients (**Table 81-14**). Dyspnea may be more pronounced in older persons with COPD due to coexisting respiratory muscle weakness and comorbidities including cardiovascular disease, sarcopenia, and generalized frailty. Chest tightness and wheezing are also common. Older persons with advanced COPD may also suffer from nonrespiratory symptoms, including fatigue and weakness, likely secondary to shortness of breath and progression of underlying disease and comorbidities including frailty. Pain is also present in 20% to 70% of persons with advanced COPD. Finally, psychological and spiritual distress such as anxiety, depression, and spiritual worries are common in COPD. These chronic physical, psychological, and spiritual symptoms typically persist over many years, and contribute to a poor QOL. Moreover, COPD has impact and poses demands on family members and caregivers. The needs of these persons are often not assessed or addressed in the context of patients' routine health care visits.

Despite growing evidence of the substantial palliative care needs of patients with COPD (particularly those with advanced disease), optimal timing for referral to palliative care or hospice is difficult to predict, given the chronic nature and variable progression of the disease. Very severe airway obstruction (FEV$_1$ < 30% predicted or FEV$_1$ Z-score < −2.55) can help identify patients at risk for uncontrolled symptoms from advanced COPD. However, FEV$_1$ alone is not sufficient to identify patients who would benefit from palliative care. Gas exchange impairments (hypoxemia or

hypercarbia) and weight loss also suggest advanced COPD. Health care utilization, including frequent emergency department visits, hospitalizations, or ICU admissions, may be a marker of those with COPD who would benefit from palliative care involvement. Patients who face declining functional status with difficulty completing activities of daily living, or those with impaired mobility due to progressive dyspnea, have a considerably higher mortality rate than those with normal functional status.

Given the complexities of prognostication, some palliative care specialists suggest asking, "Would you be surprised if this patient were to die in the next 12 months?" If the answer is "no," this statement may help identify patients in need of palliative care. However, as with all serious life-limiting conditions, palliative treatment and support can be beneficial when provided longitudinally to older patients with COPD. In addition, since the definition of palliative care has evolved to include patients and families facing serious and/or life-threatening diseases, as well as having physical, spiritual, or psychosocial sources of suffering, the population who might benefit from a palliative care team's involvement has expanded significantly. Hence, rather than focusing on prognosis or end of life as the key criterion for referral to palliative care, medical providers could identify which COPD patients would benefit from assistance managing severe, refractory, disabling symptoms, and/or those who need an "extra layer of support" by an interdisciplinary team consisting of doctors, nurses, social workers, respiratory therapists, care managers, and chaplains.

The goal of palliative treatment for patients with advanced COPD is to reduce symptoms, maintain independence and dignity, and improve overall QOL. To this end, in addition to optimized pharmacotherapy, supplemental oxygen should be provided to older persons with severe COPD who are chronically hypoxemic. Of note, among patients with COPD, the level of measured peripheral oxygen saturation often does not correlate with the level of perceived breathlessness. Education regarding the causes of dyspnea and use of pursed lips breathing to minimize dynamic hyperinflation are important. For patients with more advanced disease and respiratory insufficiency resulting in gas exchange abnormalities and/or chronic respiratory failure, NPPV should be considered for nighttime support and as needed for uncontrolled daytime symptoms (dyspnea). NPPV is also a key tool to consider for patients presenting with acute respiratory failure, including those who have declined endotracheal ventilation. Palliative care and hospice teams recognize the value of NPPV in the end-stage COPD population, and many programs are able to provide this treatment, although its availability in these settings is highly variable.

Inhaled BD, inhaled and systemic corticosteroids (where appropriate), and other adjuvant therapies that relieve symptoms should be continued during palliative treatment for patients with advanced COPD (see **Table 81-14**). However, it is important to consider

TABLE 81-14 ■ SYMPTOM BURDEN AND MANAGEMENT IN ADVANCED COPD

SYMPTOM	PREVALENCE	THERAPIES	NOTES
PHYSICAL			
Dyspnea	94%	Blowing fan/air	See **Table 81-10**, and text on pharmacologic and nonpharmacologic management sections
		Bronchodilators	
		Inhaled corticosteroids	
		Mucolytics (glycopyrrolate)	
		Pulmonary rehabilitation	
		Opioids	Monitor for respiratory depression, delirium, and constipation
		Benzodiazepines	Monitor for respiratory depression and delirium
Pain	54%	Acetaminophen, NSAIDs, opioids	Monitor for liver and renal dysfunction, delirium, and see above opioid note
GASTROINTESTINAL			
Anorexia	67%	Dietary counseling, food fortification, mirtazapine (if depressed)	Monitor for underlying cause, particularly medication-related adverse effects
Nausea/vomiting		Haloperidol	
Constipation	44%	Bowel regimen, increased mobility, careful hydration, dietary modification as tolerated	Routinely required when using opioids
Fatigue/weakness	68%	Dietary counseling, food fortification, pulmonary rehabilitation	Monitor for underlying cause, particularly medication-related adverse effects
PSYCHOLOGICAL			
Depression	> 90%	Antidepressants, supportive counseling	Palliative care social worker and physicians discuss with patient and family future treatment and needs
Anxiety	> 90%	Benzodiazepines, behavioral interventions	
Delirium		Antipsychotics and behavioral interventions	Monitor for underlying cause, including medication-related, infection, etc
SLEEP DISTURBANCES			
	40%	• Symptom management (COPD-specific and psychological treatments), with judicious use of hypnotics (trazodone, Z-meds[a]) • Nocturnal supplemental oxygen • Continuous positive airway pressure (CPAP) • Cognitive-behavioral: reduce light and noise, comfortably cool temperature in bedroom; may benefit from hospital bed and relaxation techniques (muscle relaxation, imagery, meditation)	• Sleep efficiency and quality in COPD • COPD and obstructive sleep apnea (OSA) overlap syndrome • Poor sleep contributes to fatigue and low quality of life

[a]Z-meds include eszopiclone, zaleplon, and zolpidem (nonbenzodiazepine GABA receptor agonists).

deprescribing medications for COPD patients whose care is shifting toward palliation and comfort measures only. In addition, smoking cessation counseling and treatments should be offered, even during palliative-only stages of COPD treatment. Smoking cessation at any stage of disease can reduce exacerbation risk and improve QOL. Nicotine replacement and non-nicotine-based therapies can usually be safely prescribed in older smokers with COPD. Screening for and treatment of symptoms of anxiety, depression, and pain are additional components of optimal care. In addition to pharmacologic therapies, clinicians should also offer nonpharmacologic interventions, such as cognitive behavioral therapy, written action plans, and advanced relaxation techniques (eg, guided imagery training). PR can also improve symptom management for patients with COPD through training in breathing techniques and improving exercise capacity. Finally, simple environmental changes may help decrease the sensation of dyspnea, including use of a fan or opening windows and doors to increase air movement, maintaining a relativity cool temperature, and providing humidified air. Education and support for caregivers are essential.

For patients with uncontrolled symptoms despite maximal supportive and medical therapy, opioids may be considered for symptom relief. The American Thoracic Society guidelines support their use in refractory dyspnea at any stage of illness, chronic and end of life. Opioids are thought to be effective in relieving dyspnea by several mechanisms including decreasing respiratory drive through a direct effect on respiratory centers in the brain stem, by altering the perception of dyspnea and anxiety (central effect), and by direct action on peripheral mu-receptors in the lung (bronchioles). Early studies of oral, sustained-release morphine in opioid-naive patients with advanced COPD (doses 10–30 mg orally) and a recent Cochrane Review suggest significant relief of dyspnea. Subsequent studies have not reported data to suggest the efficacy of one opioid (eg, morphine) over another opioid (eg, oxycodone). As COPD progresses and patients near the end of life, swallowing may be impaired or the patient may experience episodes of worsening dyspnea. In this setting, intravenous or subcutaneous opioids may be indicated. Studies of nebulized morphine have failed to prove efficacy compared to placebo, although case studies report improvement in dyspnea. Safety in the end-stage COPD population is clearly a concern given the risk of CO_2 retention in this population. While some data suggest that carefully monitored patients who are given low-dose opioids in this setting are at low risk for opioid-induced respiratory failure, a recent analysis of the US Medicare database demonstrated increased risk of hospitalization for respiratory conditions among those taking opioids, and in a Canadian study, new incident use of opioids was associated with increased respiratory-related and all-cause mortality. If used, opioids should be titrated carefully to patient reported dyspnea. Importantly, also, although benzodiazepines may afford relief of anxiety, they pose risk of dependency and do not consistently relieve dyspnea. The risk of respiratory failure also increases with concurrent use of benzodiazepines and opiates and requires close monitoring, consistent with the overall goals of care. Constipation, cognitive impairment, somnolence, and delirium are the most frequently experienced adverse drug events. The latter can be anticipated and managed prophylactically with close monitoring, careful use of low-dose antipsychotics, opioid dosage adjustment in response to adverse cognitive effects, and the prescription of a laxative regimen to prevent constipation in any patient who requires daily opioids.

Finally, data suggest that patients and families facing serious illnesses such as COPD value clear and honest communication about their disease process. The majority of patients want all information, both positive and negative, but also value statements of "hope" integrated into the shared information. Patients and families also desire the opportunity to discuss options for care, especially near the end of life. Several communication guidelines are available to assist medical providers in discussing distressing news, such as the results of medical tests that reveal progression of their disease. One widely shared framework is called SPIKES, created by Dr. Robert Buckman. In summary, these steps include:

S Setting: Ensuring that the setting is appropriate to provide patient comfort and privacy and that adequate support is provided as needed/desired by the patient.

P Perception: Assessing the patient's and/or family's understanding of illness.

I Invitation: Obtaining the patient's invitation or permission to discuss distressing news (and respecting their choice not to discuss such news).

K Knowledge: Giving knowledge and information to patient and family in a clear and concise manner, avoiding complex technical/medical terminology.

E Empathy: Addressing patient's emotions with empathic responses.

S Strategy and summary: Creating a care plan for the next steps in treatment and follow-up, as well as providing contact information for future concerns.

Once information is shared, the medical provider can begin to discuss goals of care by asking patients what is most important to them. For example, a clinician may say to a patient with COPD: "We discussed that time may be short given this is your third admission to the ICU in 2 months and, each time you come to the hospital, your ability to care for yourself deteriorates significantly. Given this reality, what is most important to you? What do you hope for? What has been left undone?" Once the patient's and/or family's goals are elucidated, clinicians can help guide the medical decision-making toward treatments that will likely achieve patient-centered goals, while refusing treatments that are unlikely to meet such stated goals. Ideally, these discussions occur in the outpatient setting, with medical providers that the patient knows well and trusts, when the patient is not in a crisis, and when time is not limited. Advance directive completion and identification of proxy decision maker are two key outcomes of these discussions, particularly in the ambulatory setting. While patient-centered palliative care benefits patients with COPD and their families across a spectrum of needs, access to it currently remains limited. Health care professionals and societies should advocate for more resources for palliative care services for patients with advanced lung disease, even in the absence of cancer.

CONCLUSION

COPD presents a major public health challenge, projected worldwide to be a leading cause of disability (fifth) and death (third) by 2030. This is concurrent with a demographic shift toward an aging population, further amplifying the public health challenge. In particular, older persons are at high risk of developing COPD, given the age-related decline in respiratory physiology and the cumulative effect of frequent exposures to tobacco smoke, respiratory infections, air pollutants, and occupational exposures across the adult lifespan. Moreover, both advancing age and COPD are associated with increasing multimorbidity, polypharmacy, and functional decline, as well as recurrent hospitalizations and end-of-life decisions. Hence, the management of COPD in older persons requires an approach that considers the interactions between aging and disease and includes a multidisciplinary team of heath care providers.

ACKNOWLEDGMENT

The authors would like to formally acknowledge the important contributions of authors who contributed substantially to the previous version of this chapter, including Dr. Carlos A. Vaz Fragoso and Dr. Sean M. Jeffery.

FURTHER READING

Agusti A, Hogg JC. Update on the pathogenesis of chronic obstructive pulmonary disease. *N Engl J Med.* 2019;381(13):1248–1256.

Balte PP, Chaves PHM, Couper DJ, et al. Association of nonobstructive chronic bronchitis with respiratory health outcomes in adults. *JAMA Intern Med.* 2020;180(5):676–686.

Barnes PJ. Pulmonary diseases and ageing. In: Harris JR, Korolchuk VI, eds. *Biochemistry and Cell Biology of Ageing: Part II, Clinical Science, Subcellular Biochemistry 91.* Singapore: Springer Nature Singapore Pte Ltd; 2019:45–74.

Barrons R, Pegram A, Borries A. Inhaler device selection: special considerations in elderly patients with chronic obstructive pulmonary disease. *Am J Health-Syst Pharm.* 2011;68:1221–1232.

Celli BR, Wedzicha JA. Update on clinical aspects of chronic obstructive pulmonary disease. *N Engl J Med.* 2019;381(13):1257–1266.

Global Initiative for Chronic Obstructive Lung Disease: 2021 Report. www.goldcopd.org. Accessed June 30, 2021.

Halpin DMG, Criner GJ, Papi A, et al. Global Initiative for the Diagnosis, Management and Prevention of Chronic Obstructive Lung Disease: The 2020 GOLD Science Committee report on COVID-19 and chronic obstructive pulmonary disease. *Am J Respir Crit Care Med.* 2021;203(1):24–36.

Leuppi JD, Schuetz P, Bingisser R, et al. Short term vs conventional glucocorticoid therapy in acute exacerbations of chronic obstructive pulmonary disease. *JAMA.* 2013;309:2223–2231.

Lindenauer PK, Stefan MS, Pekow PS, et al. Association between initiation of pulmonary rehabilitation after hospitalization for COPD and 1-year survival among Medicare beneficiaries. *JAMA.* 2020;323(18):1–11.

Lowe KE, Regan EA, Anzueto A, et al. COPD Gene 2019: redefining the diagnosis of chronic obstructive pulmonary disease. *Chron Obst Pulm Dis.* 2019;6(5):384–399.

Macrea M, Oczkowski S, Rochwerg B, et al. Long-term noninvasive ventilation in chronic stable hypercapnic chronic obstructive pulmonary disease. An Official American Thoracic Society Clinical Practice Guideline. *Am J Respir Crit Care Med.* 2020;202(4):e74–e87.

Maddocks M, Lovell N, Booth S, et al. Palliative care and management of troublesome symptoms for people with chronic obstructive pulmonary disease. *Lancet.* 2017;390:988–1002.

Murphy PB, Rehal S, Arbane G, et al. Effect of home noninvasive ventilation with oxygen therapy vs oxygen therapy alone on hospital readmission or death after an acute COPD exacerbation: a randomized clinical trial. *JAMA.* 2017;317(21):2177–2186.

Quanjer PH, Stanojevic S, Cole TJ, et al. Multi-ethnic reference values for spirometry for the 3–95 year age range: the global lung function 2012 equations. *Eur Respir J.* 2012;40(6):1324–1343.

Ritchie AI, Wdezicha JA. Definition, causes, pathogenesis, and consequences of chronic obstructive pulmonary disease exacerbations. *Clin Chest Med.* 2020;41(3):421–438.

Schneider JL, Rowe JH, Garcia-de-Alba C, et al. The aging lung: physiology, disease and immunity. *Cell.* 2021;184:1990–2019.

Silverman EK. Genetics of COPD. *Annu Rev Physiol.* 2020;82:413–431.

Spruit MA, Singh SJ, Garvey C, et al. An official American Thoracic Society/European Respiratory Society statement: key concepts and advances in pulmonary rehabilitation. *Am J Respir Crit Care Med.* 2013;188:e13–e64.

Strnad P, McElvaney NG, Lomas DA. Alpha-1-antitrypsin deficiency. *N Engl J Med.* 2020;382(15):1443–1455.

Vaz Fragoso CA, Gill T. Respiratory impairment and the aging lung: a novel paradigm for assessing pulmonary function. *J Gerontol Med Sci.* 2012;67:264–275.

Aging of the Kidney

Jocelyn Wiggins, Abhijit S. Naik, Sanjeevkumar R. Patel

CLINICAL RELEVANCE

Data on individuals reaching end-stage kidney disease (ESKD) are collected by the US Renal Data System (USRDS). As a condition for coverage, all dialysis units receiving Medicare funding must file data with the Centers for Medicare and Medicaid Services (CMS). The 2020 USRDS annual data report shows that approximately 1.27 in 1000 persons aged 65 to 69 initiate treatment for ESKD each year. For the 70- to 75-year-old age group, the incidence rate of ESKD is 1.43 per 1000 persons, and this incidence peaks in the 80 to 84 age group to 1.82 per 1000. Over the last 10 years, the number of older individuals receiving renal replacement therapy has increased by 35% in those 75 years or older and by 43% in those older than 80 years. In contrast, the incidence of ESKD in the 20- to 44-year-old age group has remained flat over the last 10 years, with only modest growth in the 45- to 64-year-old age group. Although some of the increase in renal replacement therapy for the older population indicates a greater willingness to offer treatment to older individuals, much of the growth is owing to people surviving to experience the chronic changes that occur with aging. The kidney undergoes significant age-related change. Other common, age-related diseases such as hypertension and diabetes accelerate these changes.

THE AGING PROCESS

Aging in the kidney is characterized by changes in both structure and function. It must be emphasized that many of the aging studies have been performed on laboratory animals, particularly rodents, demonstrate quite different patterns of aging from humans. For example, kidney weight increases throughout life in rats, while kidney mass and size in humans peak in the fourth decade and decline

Learning Objectives

- Understand normal kidney aging.
- Classify kidney disease using the estimated glomerular filtration rate (eGFR).
- Recognize environmental factors that impact the rate of decline in kidney function.
- Recognize that genetic factors play a role in the age-related decline of kidney function.
- Understand the general guidelines for managing patients with chronic kidney disease (CKD).
- Understand the implications of aging on organ donation and receiving an organ transplant.

Key Clinical Points

1. All older adults have some decline in renal function.
2. Older patients can typically maintain normal physiologic homeostasis but are compromised in their ability to respond to challenges.
3. Kidneys become more susceptible to injury with advancing age.
4. Rates of decline in renal function in aging are quite variable and impacted by genetic and environmental factors.
5. Preventing people from reaching end-stage renal disease reduces care costs and dramatically improves the quality of life.

thereafter. Care should be taken when reading the literature to keep in mind that changes observed in animal models may not reflect parallel changes seen in humans. Historical data from human postmortems describing changes in the kidney made no effort to exclude patients with kidney disease or significant comorbidities. More recently, data on aging have been developed from longitudinal studies, such as the Baltimore Longitudinal Aging Study, in which the medical histories of the study volunteers are well documented. There are also data accumulating from older living kidney donors that undergo rigorous work-up of their kidney function and detection of comorbid conditions. Such individuals are presumed to have undergone healthy aging and thus allow the acquisition of normal kidney aging data. The aging kidney is generally characterized by a spontaneous progressive decline in renal function accompanied by thickening of the basement membrane, mesangial expansion, and progressive glomerulosclerosis.

Functional Changes

Changes in renal function with age are well documented both in human and animal models. Although baseline homeostasis of fluids and electrolytes is maintained with normal aging, there is a progressive decline in renal reserve. This results in a compromise in the kidney's ability to respond to either a salt or water load or deficit. This manifests clinically in patients being vulnerable to superimposed renal complications during acute illnesses. Chronic conditions such as hypertension accelerate this age-related loss of renal reserve, and increased vulnerability in these patients should be anticipated. Age-related changes in function will be considered by separate functional domains within the kidney.

Renal blood flow Average renal blood flow decreases about 10% per decade, dropping from 600 mL/min/1.73 m^2 to 300 mL/min/1.73 m^2 by the ninth decade. This is accompanied by increasing resistance in both afferent and efferent arterioles. These changes occur independently of a decline in cardiac output or reductions in renal mass. This decline in renal blood flow contributes to the decrease in efficiency with which the aging kidney responds to fluid and electrolyte load and loss.

Glomerular filtration rate Newer data have shown a wide variation in the rate and extent of changes in the kidney within the older population. Approximately 30% of the population shows no measurable decline in renal function with normal aging. The bulk of the population loses about 10% of the glomerular filtration rate (GFR) and 10% of renal plasma flow per decade after the fourth decade of life. Between 5% and 10% of the population shows an accelerated loss, even in the absence of identifiable comorbidities. Since there is also a steady loss of muscle mass with age, with a concomitant reduction in creatinine production, serum creatinine should remain relatively constant. Elevations in serum creatinine should therefore be taken

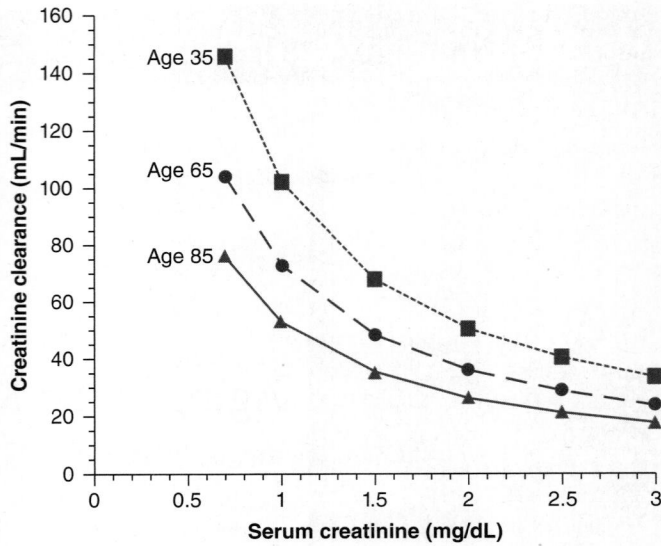

FIGURE 82-1. Relationship between serum creatinine and calculated creatinine clearance for men aged 35, 65, and 85. Calculations are based on a 70-kg man.

seriously and not dismissed as normal aging. As can be seen in **Figure 82-1**, serum creatinine at the upper limit of the "normal range" in an older individual represent significant decline in renal function, and thought should be given to renal dosing of medications. These curves were calculated using the Cockcroft-Gault equation for a 70-kg man:

$$\text{Creatinine clearance} = \frac{(140 - \text{age})(\text{weight [kg]})}{72 \times \text{serum creatinine (mg/dL)}}$$

Results for women should be multiplied by 0.85, which shift the curves downward. In frail older women with very little residual muscle mass, this equation probably overestimates GFRs. This steady decline in renal function with age manifests itself clinically as impaired ability to excrete a salt or water load. Extra care should be taken when replacing fluids in an older individual to prevent extracellular fluid overload and its consequences.

In 1999, an improved formula for estimating GFR was developed known as the MDRD formula (because it was developed as part of the Modification of Diet in Renal Disease study). Many routine laboratories now automatically calculate an MDRD glomerular filtration estimate when a basic or a comprehensive metabolic panel is ordered. In some institutions, it is necessary to order a "renal panel" for the calculation to be done. It is essential to understand that this formula was based on data from community-dwelling volunteers aged 18 to 70. It has never been validated in a very old or frail population. Several investigators have studied its performance in older patients and compared its efficacy with Cockcroft Gault, creatinine clearances based on 24-hour urine or iothalamate clearances, or a combination of these methods. All of the studies have shown significant discrepancies between these methods in patients with advanced age and at both extremes of the weight spectrum. These limitations should be kept in mind when using the formula in clinical geriatric practice. Although iothalamate clearance is the gold standard, it is expensive and impractical for routine use. The most reliable results come from calculating creatinine clearances based on 24-hour urine collection. This will always be an overestimate of the GFR, since some creatinine is actively excreted into the urine from the proximal tubule, not all of the urinary creatinine is filtered. It is however more reliable than the formula estimations in the very old and frail people. In 2009, a new modification of MDRD—the CKD-EPI equation—was developed. This is more accurate than the original formula and is now used in routine clinical practice reported by most clinical labs. Using cystatin C as a measure of GFR circumvents the problem of the decline in creatinine production with age, and its use has gained popularity in many clinical settings.

Classification of kidney disease The classification of kidney disorders has undergone a significant revision over the past few years. A consensus committee, sponsored by the National Kidney Foundation, published clinical practice guidelines in 2002. The traditional chronic renal insufficiency has become chronic kidney disease (CKD), and end-stage renal disease (ESRD) has become kidney failure. CKD is defined as either kidney damage or decreased kidney function for 3 or more months. Kidney failure is defined as a GFR of less than 15 mL/min or the need to start kidney replacement therapy. Along with renaming kidney disease, the committee also developed a system of staging. It was felt that having a structure would help with standardizing diagnosis and opportunities for preventative management. CKD is now classified into five stages, regardless of underlying diagnosis. The classification defines stage 1 as kidney damage (primarily proteinuria) with preserved GFR and progresses to stage 5 kidney failure (**Table 82-1**). Declines in GFR are accompanied by a broad range of complications (**Table 82-2**). In 2007, the classification was revised and stage 3 CKD was subdivided into 3A and 3B. This was done because this is by far the category with the largest number

TABLE 82-2 ■ COMPLICATIONS OF CHRONIC KIDNEY DISEASE

Hypertension
Anemia
Increased cardiovascular mortality and morbidity
Disorders of calcium and phosphorus metabolism
Compromised nutritional status
Metabolic bone disease
Neuropathy
Impaired functioning and well-being
Depression

of patients and there was significant heterogeneity in complications that develop within this group. Early recognition of impaired kidney function allows the physician to screen for and manage these complications and thus prevent comorbidities and declines in quality of life. National Kidney Foundation guidelines recommend referral to a nephrologist when a patient reaches stage 4 CKD for management of the complications of impaired function such as acidosis, phosphorus retention, and anemia. An informed discussion regarding kidney replacement therapy should also begin during stage 4.

Proteinuria Despite the significant decline in GFR that occurs with aging, proteinuria is not a normal feature of the aging process. Proteinuria is always a pathological finding and requires a full work-up. In contrast, in most rodent models, particularly in the rat, proteinuria is a normal feature of the aging kidney. This difference between humans and rodents should be kept in mind when reading the aging literature.

Tubular function Older individuals are more susceptible to acute renal failure. Much of the information on tubular function comes from animal studies, particularly rat models. Rats spontaneously develop proteinuria with aging, and this protein load is believed to be toxic to the tubule. Since proteinuria is not a feature of normal aging in humans, these animal studies may not paint an accurate picture of changes in tubular function in humans. There are also large numbers of studies in experimental animals looking at vasoconstrictive and vasodilatory responses in the older kidney. Impaired response to ANP, acetylcholine, and blunted responses of cAMP to β-adrenergic stimulus has all been implicated. Virtually none of these findings have been confirmed in humans. Functional magnetic resonance imaging (MRI) in older volunteers has demonstrated decreased ability to modulate renal medullary oxygenation. Whether this is caused by fixed vascular changes or changes in renal autocrine systems such as prostaglandins, dopamine, nitric oxide (NO), natriuretic peptides, or endothelin is not clear. The clinical result is increased sensitivity to acute ischemic renal failure.

Animal and human studies have shown impaired concentrating ability in the older kidney. Whether this is

TABLE 82-1 ■ NATIONAL KIDNEY FOUNDATION CLASSIFICATION OF CHRONIC KIDNEY DISEASE

STAGE	DESCRIPTION	GFR (ML/MIN/1.73 M²)
1	Kidney damage with normal or increased GFR	> 90
2	Kidney damage with mild reduction in GFR	60–89
3	Moderate decrease in GFR	30–59 3A: 45–59 3B: 30–44
4	Severe decrease in GFR	15–29
5	Kidney failure	< 15 (or dialysis)

caused by intrinsic defects in the tubular epithelium or impaired response to antidiuretic hormone (ADH) is not clear. Studies have also demonstrated impaired capacity to acidify urine manifested clinically as reduced excretion of an acid load. Whatever the underlying mechanism, older individuals are less likely to be able to maintain normal homeostasis when challenged. Although there is an age-related decline in tubular functions such as glucose and amino acid transport, these declines closely parallel the decline in GFR and are believed to correlate with the loss of nephrons rather than age effects in the tubule. Older individuals are also more sensitive to nephrotoxic injury. Careful thought should be given to the choice and dosing of antibiotics and other nephrotoxic drugs including the use of iodinated contrasts.

Age-related changes in sodium and water handling are discussed in Chapter 39. An overview of potassium disorders in the older adults is presented below.

Physiologic Regulation of Potassium Balance

As the major determinant of transmembrane potential, and therefore neural, muscular, and neuromuscular currents, both total body potassium homeostasis and the extracellular-to-intracellular potassium gradient are strongly defended. Potassium is the major intracellular cation and the vast majority of body potassium stores are located in the skeletal muscle cells. Thus, serum potassium concentration reflects total body stores imperfectly, especially under stress conditions. Serum potassium is influenced by two separate sets of factors: those related to kidney function and those related to the transmembrane movement of potassium in and out of cells. In the setting of relatively well-preserved kidney function, older individuals have a normal serum potassium under unstressed conditions, but as the GFR declines, the fractional excretion of potassium does not rise as much as in young individuals in part due to lower aldosterone levels and/or aldosterone resistance in older adults. Several factors will regulate the movement of potassium in and out of cells including the glucoregulatory hormones insulin and glucagon, adrenergic stimulation of either α- or β-receptors, acid-base balance, and alterations in serum osmolality.

Hypokalemia, defined as a serum potassium less than 3.5 mEq/L, occurs rarely in healthy adults. However, because older individuals frequently are taking medications that alter potassium homeostasis such as diuretics or have a diet low in potassium, the frequency of hypokalemia can be as high as 5%. Hypokalemia associated with medications, underlying disease processes, or diet has been reported in 21% of hospitalized patients. Although many individuals with hypokalemia are clinically asymptomatic, hypokalemia is associated with a wide variety of clinical manifestations including muscle weakness—including proximal muscle weakness and intestinal ileus—cardiac arrhythmias, polyuria, and fatigue. Hypokalemia is frequently accompanied by multiple electrolyte abnormalities including hyper- or

hyponatremia, metabolic acidosis or alkalosis, and hypomagnesemia. Individuals with very poor nutrition such as those with alcoholism or eating disorders may present with normal or minimally decreased potassium that belies the extent of their potassium deficiency. The potassium level may plummet with refeeding, leading to potentially catastrophic cardiac events, especially if this has occurred in the setting of underlying organic heart disease. A similar dramatic fall in potassium can occur with aggressive insulin therapy or aggressive bicarbonate replacement. For these reasons, it is recommended that potassium replacement, parenteral, enteral, or both, be initiated immediately when these therapies are anticipated. Avoidance of dextrose-containing parenteral fluids should be considered in the setting of severe hypokalemia, until it can be at least partially corrected.

Hypokalemia can result from poor intake (eating disorders, alcoholism), increased losses (diuretics, mineralocorticoid excess, diarrhea), or shift of potassium from the extracellular to the intracellular compartment (insulin therapy). Often, the history alone will alert the clinician to the most likely cause of hypokalemia, but additional testing of the urine for potassium, creatinine, and osmolality can effectively narrow the differential diagnosis by establishing whether there are excessive urinary potassium losses. An isolated urine potassium of greater than 40 mEq/L suggests excessive renal losses.

The safest method for potassium replacement is orally, through potassium-rich foods or potassium supplements, as overdose is unlikely. For severe hypokalemia or hypokalemia associated with acute cardiac arrhythmias, however, parenteral potassium may be required. Determining the amount of potassium needed to replace losses may be calculated, but administration of relatively small doses such as 10 or 20 mEq at a time with frequent repeat measures is the safest approach. For patients who require continuous diuretic therapy, addition of a potassium-sparing diuretic in low dose may blunt potassium losses. However, these agents need to be used carefully in individuals with CKD or those who are already taking a medication that blunts renal potassium excretion.

Hyperkalemia rarely occurs in the setting of normal kidney function because of the tremendous capacity of the kidneys to excrete the daily potassium load. Older patients are more susceptible to hyperkalemia because of the loss of kidney function, the loss of muscle mass, the changes in regulation of muscle ion content described earlier, lower levels of renin and aldosterone, and the use of many medications for chronic conditions which are associated with hyperkalemia such as angiotensin-converting enzyme (ACE) inhibitors, angiotensin receptor blockers, and potassium-sparing diuretics. Older individuals also are more likely to have glucose intolerance, which may blunt the ability of potassium to be translocated to the intracellular compartment and type IV renal tubular acidosis which will diminish renal potassium excretion even in the presence of relatively normal kidney function. Hyperkalemia is seen in up to 10% of hospitalized patients. Despite the theoretical predisposition to hyperkalemia, it has been difficult to show that older patients using inhibitors of the renin-angiotensin-aldosterone system, singly or in combination, have a higher incidence of hyperkalemia than do younger patients.

The definition of hyperkalemia varies from laboratory to laboratory and from clinical report to clinical report. Generally, a potassium of greater than 5.3 mEq/L is accepted as hyperkalemia. Spurious hyperkalemia, where the measured potassium is elevated but the ambient serum potassium is normal, can occur in the setting of hemolysis of the blood sample associated with difficult phlebotomy or deterioration of the sample, severe thrombocytosis, severe leukocytosis, or red cell disorders. If this is suspected, obtaining a plasma potassium would be the next appropriate step. Hyperkalemia is frequently asymptomatic but muscle weakness and fatigue are the most common symptoms. The heart is the major target of significant hyperkalemia as increasingly greater potassium concentrations result in varying degrees of heart block progressing to cardiac arrest. Unfortunately, the electrocardiographic manifestations of hyperkalemia may be subtle and missed; conversely, the same level of hyperkalemia may produce vastly different effects on the electrocardiogram (ECG) including sinus bradycardia, complete heart block, wide QRS tachycardia, or the classic sine wave pattern. The widely taught progression of the ECG manifestations of hyperkalemia such as peaked T waves, prolonged PR interval, absence of P wave, and QRS prolongation is seldom seen. Thus, the absence of ECG findings in the presence of a high potassium level should not lead the clinician to conclude that the hyperkalemia is erroneous or insignificant. The physical examination may show muscle weakness, a reduction in deep tendon reflexes, and bradycardia.

The causes of hyperkalemia are numerous. Older patients are generally more prone to hyperkalemia primarily due to the reduction in kidney function. Most cases of significant hyperkalemia are multifactorial due to a reduction of kidney function coupled with excessive potassium intake, use of medications that reduce potassium excretion or movement into cells, or occurrence of acute kidney injury superimposed on CKD. A complete history can generally identify these factors. Recent studies have identified particularly high-risk situations for severe hyperkalemia in older adults including the use of trimethoprim/sulfamethoxazole in patients on spironolactone, the use of two inhibitors of the renin-angiotensin-aldosterone axis, the use of nonsteroidal anti-inflammatory drugs, and the presence of type 2 diabetes. One additional diagnosis to consider when an older patient presents with unexpected hyperkalemia is adrenal insufficiency. Modest adrenal insufficiency in the geriatric population may present episodically with recurrent volume depletion and acute kidney injury with varying degrees of hyponatremia and hyperkalemia which correct easily with the administration of parenteral sodium chloride. Often, the only symptom is fatigue.

Treatment of hyperkalemia is determined by the severity and the presence or absence of significant cardiac effects. Asymptomatic, non–life-threatening hyperkalemia can be approached in the outpatient setting through elimination of medications that cause hyperkalemia, improving hydration status, and addressing any reversible causes of reduction in kidney function such as medications and volume depletion. Severe hyperkalemia manifested as advanced degrees of conduction delays or bradycardia will require, in addition to the above measures, more immediate interventions. Intravenous calcium gluconate will stabilize the myocardial cell membrane, decreasing the potential for cardiac arrest. This effect is essentially immediate, but transient, and does not lower potassium levels. Intravenous insulin, inhaled β-agonists, and, if the individual also has a metabolic acidosis, intravenous bicarbonate, will enhance potassium entry into the cells, thus lowering serum potassium and diminishing the risk of a fatal cardiac event. Insulin works fastest, within 15 minutes, but is more transient than the β-agonists. All of these interventions are transient, and ultimately treatment is directed toward removal of excessive potassium from the body. The three options listed in order of aggressiveness are forced diuresis with loop diuretics, the use of exchange resins such as sodium polystyrene sulfonate, or dialysis. The choice of which modality or modalities to employ is dependent on the severity of hyperkalemia, the level of kidney function, the presence or absence of any intestinal disease, and patient/physician preference. Without doubt, the least invasive approach, forced diuresis, is highly effective in the presence of preserved kidney function. When kidney function is impaired, exchange resins and/or dialysis can be considered. For severe hyperkalemia, the immediate therapies as well as oral exchange resins would be required.

Underlying Structural Changes

There are at least 100 years of meticulous research describing the anatomical changes that underlie the functional changes that are observed in patients as they age.

Gross anatomy Kidneys grow vigorously from birth through adolescence, reaching their maximum weight and volume during the third decade of life. In humans, although not in most laboratory animals, renal mass starts to decline after the fourth decade and continues its decline throughout the remaining lifespan. Most of the decrease in weight and volume appears to happen in the cortex, with relative sparing of the medulla.

Glomerulus The young healthy human kidney contains roughly 1 million nephrons. There is no evidence for postnatal nephrogenesis. This underlies the hypothesis that low birth weight babies might have fewer initial nephrons and as a result are more susceptible to renal failure in later life. Although there are some observational data to support this hypothesis, no causal relationship has been proved. There is a steady decline in nephron number with age that starts around the fourth decade. This appears to be driven by podocyte loss. These specialized cells are postmitotic and if damaged in any way, cannot be replaced. This decline is believed to underlie the reduction in GFR discussed above. Kidneys obtained at autopsy from patients with no known history of renal disease have been studied. Light microscopy showed the development of a focal sclerosing process, accompanied by thickening of the glomerular basement membrane. There was a steady progression with age in the percentage of glomeruli that were scared. By age 50, all subjects examined had some evidence of sclerosis, with the percentage of sclerotic glomeruli increasing steadily with age.

Age-related glomerulosclerosis Sclerotic glomeruli typically first appear in the fourth decade of life. This starts as a segmental process with one part of a glomerulus becoming acellular and the normal architecture being replaced by extracellular matrix. The glomerular tuft becomes adherent to Bowman capsule (**Figure 82-2**). Gradually an entire glomerulus becomes sclerosed and shrivels down with resultant loss of that nephron and its filtration capacity. It is not known what triggers this pattern of focal sclerosis, which is apparently randomly scattered throughout the cortex. The glomerular tuft increases in size with age. Concomitant with this expansion is an increase in endothelial and mesangial cells, such that the ratio of cells to glomerular area remains constant. Podocytes, the specialized cells that form the filtration barrier in the glomerulus, are postmitotic. They are not able to multiply in response to the increase in tuft volume and become a progressively smaller percentage of the total cells making up the glomerular tuft. As the filtration area that they have to cover increases, it is believed that they may detach from the basement membrane, leaving a denuded area behind. It is this area of bare basement membrane that acts as the trigger for the sclerosing process. Many different experimental models of glomerulosclerosis have concluded that loss of the podocyte and its inability

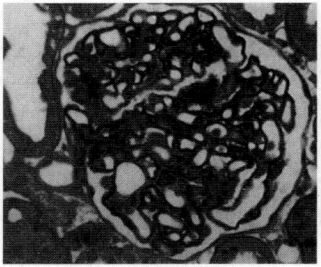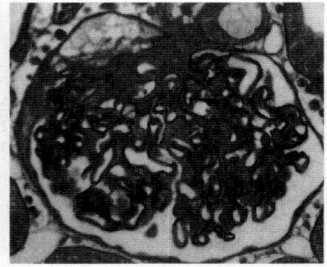

FIGURE 82-2. Renal glomeruli from a 24-month Fischer 344 rat stained with a podocyte marker, GLEPP1, and counterstained with PAS. Left panel: normal glomerulus showing normal architecture of the glomerular tuft. Right panel: age-related glomerulosclerosis showing normal cellular architecture replaced by extracellular matrix and adherence to Bowman's capsule.

to be replaced are the sentinel events that trigger sclerosis. A transgenic rat model that expresses the diphtheria toxin receptor on the podocyte has been developed to deplete podocytes in a dose-dependent manner. This model has shown that the loss of podocytes precedes the appearance of sclerosis, and podocytes markers can be detected in the urine prior to the development of global sclerosis.

Models of induced glomerular injury, of course, do not exist in humans. However, research has shown selective loss of podocytes in the kidneys of people with type 1 diabetes as diabetic nephropathy progresses. Podocyte number per glomerulus is the best predictor of progression of diabetic nephropathy in Pima Indians with type 2 diabetes. Studies of the aging process in rat kidneys noted that a decline in podocyte counts is accompanied by the appearance of glomerulosclerosis. Studies to address this in aging humans are currently being conducted.

Some authors have suggested a role for the mesangial cell in initiating the sclerosis process. Certainly with aging, there is an increase in mesangial matrix and in mesangial cell numbers. However, this increase is just as marked in strains of rat that do not develop age-related glomerulosclerosis, as it is in strains that do. Several investigators have studied mesangial cell activation in rat models of glomerulosclerosis and found little or none. This suggests that mesangial expansion is a benign manifestation of the aging process rather than a pathological one.

Tubule With the loss of the glomerulus, the tubular section of the nephron usually degenerates and is replaced by connective tissue. Tubular hypertrophy then occurs in the remaining nephrons, principally in the proximal convoluted tubule. This appears to result from both hypertrophy and hyperplasia. With thinning of the cortex, there is a decrease in tubule length and development of diverticuli in the distal convoluted tubule. As nephrons are lost, there is generalized tubular interstitial fibrosis. The structure of the distal tubule does not appear to change significantly with age.

Vasculature Renal arteries undergo age-related thickening, similar to that seen throughout the circulation. Smaller arteries may become tortuous and show luminal irregularities. When a glomerulus becomes sclerosed, there is frequent formation of an arteriovenous shunt as the afferent and efferent arterioles develop a direct connection when the glomerular capillary is lost. This shunt is very important in maintaining medullary blood flow. Physiologic studies in both animals and humans have documented a decline in renal blood flow and an increase in vascular resistance with age. Studies of renal perfusion in healthy older individuals from a pool of potential kidney donors have shown steady declines in renal perfusion with age that exceeded the reduction in renal mass, suggesting that declines in blood flow were a significant factor in the changes seen in renal function with age. The age-related increase in central arterial stiffness (discussed in Chapter 73) leads to increased forward transmission of a larger forward wave exposing the small arteries and microvessels in the renal parenchyma to damaging levels of pressure pulsatility and may contribute to kidney injury in aging. Taken together, these changes contribute to the susceptibility of older individuals to acute renal failure, volume overload, and electrolyte abnormalities.

Infarcts may occur in the kidney, just as they do in other tissues of the body. Since one-fifth of the circulating volume passes through the kidney each minute, the kidney is also particularly susceptible to embolization. If other signs of embolization are visible clinically, it is highly probable that the kidney is also undergoing embolization, and embolic disease should certainly be kept in mind in an older individual with widespread vascular disease who demonstrates accelerated loss of renal function.

MECHANISMS UNDERLYING THE DECLINE IN KIDNEY FUNCTION

There is no clear-cut consensus about what mechanisms may underlie the structural and functional changes occurring in the kidney in the older population. It is fairly clear, however, that there are both predisposing genetic and environmental factors that play a role.

Genetic Predisposition

There are as yet no genes known to cause age-related glomerulosclerosis, although several podocyte genes have been identified as causative in childhood focal segmental glomerulosclerosis. Accumulating evidence from animal studies, combined with evidence of genetic predisposition in humans, has led to a concerted effort to seek genes that may increase susceptibility to renal failure. Many of the genes identified as playing a role in the aging process, such as IGF-1 and target of rapamycin (TOR), also seem to play a role in kidney aging. Rodent studies using rapamycin to slow the aging process are currently ongoing that are likely to produce information on renal aging.

Animal models Rats are particularly susceptible to kidney failure and much of the work with models of renal disease has been carried out in laboratory rat strains. There are very marked strain differences in susceptibility to age-related glomerulosclerosis. Since these rats are maintained in pathogen-free environments and are fed uniform scientifically developed diets, this strongly suggests a genetic basis for the development of age-related glomerulosclerosis. The appearance of glomerulosclerosis has been reported as early as 5 months in the Milan normotensive rat, with extensive disease by 10 months of age. This occurs in the total absence of hypertension and is not ameliorated by administration of ACE inhibitors. Wistar rats were used as controls in this study and showed no significant disease during the same time period. In Sprague-Dawley rats, spontaneous age-related glomerulosclerosis first becomes apparent around 9 months of age, and disease became

widespread by 18 months of age. In studies of aging in Fischer 344 rats, little glomerulosclerosis is seen until almost 2 years of age with fairly rapid progression thereafter. Other rat strains appear remarkably resistant to renal disease. Brown Norway rats show minimal sclerosis, even at 32 months of age, an advanced age in rat lifespan.

Human studies Clearly, these kinds of studies cannot be duplicated in humans. However, there are observational data that would support a similar variation in genetic susceptibility in humans. Cross-sectional studies, donor organ data, and longitudinal studies clearly show a wide variation in kidney function with age. Around 5% to 10% of the population show accelerated loss of kidney function with age even in the absence of accelerating factors such as hypertension, while 30% show no measurable decline. In the presence of predisposing comorbidities, there is also wide variation in the development of kidney disease. Some people with diabetes may never develop nephropathy, while others develop rapidly progressive kidney disease early in the course of their diabetes, suggesting an underlying genetic susceptibility. Within the African-American population, rates of kidney disease are much higher than in the Caucasian population independent of the precipitating cause. Within an ethnic group, there are also distinct differences in vulnerability. An African-American who develops any predisposing disease, be it hypertension, diabetes, or lupus, who has a first-degree relative on renal replacement therapy has a ninefold increased risk of developing kidney disease compared to another African-American with the same disease burden who has no family history of kidney disease. Similarly, human immunodeficiency virus (HIV)-associated glomerulosclerosis occurs almost exclusively in the African-American population, while HIV-associated mesangial hyperplasia and immune-complex glomerular nephritis occur equally in all ethnic groups. Much of this disparity can now be attributed to genetic variants in the apoL1 (APOL1) gene found only in individuals with recent African ancestry. These variants greatly increase rates of hypertension-associated ESKD, focal segmental glomerulosclerosis, HIV-associated nephropathy, and other forms of nondiabetic kidney disease. Thus, there is evidence for a genetic predisposition with respect to the development of glomerulosclerosis. Considerable effort and resources are currently being directed toward identifying genes that predispose to kidney disease.

Environmental Predisposing Factors

Several diseases predispose to kidney failure and accelerate the progress of age-related glomerulosclerosis. By far the most prevalent of these are hypertension and diabetes, both common disorders in the older population. There are, however, several other mechanisms that have been postulated to underlie the aging changes in the kidney.

Diet One of the most striking aspects of rodent models of age-related nephropathy is its complete reversal with caloric restriction. Both the anatomical and functional changes related to aging in the kidney are completely abolished in animals that are fed two-thirds of the calories given to their ad libitum-fed litter mates. Even though these animals live one-third longer than their ad libitum-fed littermates, they do not develop age-related glomerulosclerosis. Several explanations have been proffered to account for this observation.

Free radicals and lipid peroxides One possible explanation for the profound effects of caloric restriction is a reduction in the generation of free radicals and lipid peroxides. There is a wide body of literature discussing the damaging effects of free radicals on cellular systems and the role that this plays in aging (refer to Chapters 1 and 40). The main consequence of free radical production is lipid peroxidation, which results in damage to cellular proteins, lipids, and nucleic acids. Increased caloric intake is believed to fuel increased free radical production with accelerated aging damage. This hypothesis has generated interest in the role of antioxidants in slowing the aging process. The effects of supplementing the diets of Sprague-Dawley rats with vitamin E have been studied. Although there were reductions in markers of oxidative stress and the rate of decline in GFR slowed, glomerulosclerosis still developed. Vitamin E supplement studies in humans have also been disappointing.

Protein restriction The benefits of caloric restriction have been attributed to concomitant reductions in dietary protein. There is a large body of older literature on protein restriction in experimental animal models of kidney disease. In many of these studies, experimental and control animals were not fed isocaloric diets, and protein restriction also meant caloric restriction. Many of these studies have shown a slowing in the progression of established kidney disease; however, the results were not corrected for total calorie content. Studies of spontaneous age-related glomerulosclerosis in Fischer 344 rats have shown that protein restriction was much less effective than caloric restriction in preventing age-related declines in kidney function. Modest benefits from protein restriction when rats were fed isocaloric diets have been demonstrated, as have some benefits when the type of protein in the diet was changed from casein to soy. In contrast, caloric-restricted animals had little or no decline in kidney function and they were not able to show significant glomerulosclerosis despite significantly increased longevity. Rats that were fed a high-protein diet, but restricted to 60% caloric intake compared to their ad libitum-fed litter mates, also showed dramatic reductions in age-related glomerulosclerosis. Clearly, protein restriction does have some benefit in the prevention of age-related nephropathy, but that advantage is small compared to that achieved with caloric restriction. Very few of the studies examined changes in sodium, phosphate, and calcium content of the experimental diets. Many of the results of protein restriction can be duplicated by phosphate restriction. The relevance of these studies in humans remains unclear. An observational study that included individuals up to 80 years of age compared healthy vegetarians who consume an average of 30 g/day of protein with nonvegetarians who consume an average of 100 g/day and showed no differences in kidney function between these groups. There is evidence to support protein restriction in patients with established renal disease to reduce symptoms of uremia, but none to support the role of protein restriction to prevent age-related changes in the human kidney.

Lipids There is a well-established link between lipids and cardiovascular disease, and restriction of fat intake accompanied by treatment of hyperlipidemia has been shown to be efficacious in preventing or slowing the progress of the cardiovascular disease. Certainly, protecting the integrity and function of the vascular supply to the kidney is important to maintaining normal function. Evidence for benefits from the manipulation of lipids in kidney disease comes mainly from animal models of diabetes. Animal studies using high-fat diets have shown accelerated progress of kidney disease, but in most cases, diets were not corrected for total caloric intake. Lipogenic diets fed to Sprague-Dawley rats resulted in an earlier appearance of widespread glomerulosclerosis compared to standard fed animals. The use of lipid-lowering agents in a variety of animal models of glomerulosclerosis has shown reductions in the incidence of glomerular damage. Patients with an established renal disease with or without diabetes have more rapid deterioration of kidney function in the presence of hyperlipidemia. The relevance of lipids to the age-related decline in kidney function remains to be established, but it would certainly be reasonable to recommend a low-fat diet and lipid management in patients with declining renal function.

Hyperfiltration The term hyperfiltration is used to describe putative glomerular injury from long-term increases in intraglomerular pressure. The age-related loss of glomeruli causes intraglomerular hypertension with hypertrophy of remaining glomeruli. Persistent intraglomerular hypertension causes pressure-mediated renal injury. Most of the supporting evidence for this mechanism comes from animal models where one kidney and part of the remaining kidney are removed, leaving a partial kidney remnant. These animals develop a pattern of renal damage in the remnant indistinguishable from age-related glomerulosclerosis but over an accelerated time course. Long-term follow-up in humans for older than 20 years has not shown accelerated declines in renal function in people who have donated one of their kidneys for transplantation, even though the remaining kidney does undergo hypertrophy. Nutrition may also play a part in hyperfiltration. After a meal of protein, increases in both renal blood flow and GFR in animals as well as in humans have been demonstrated. Excessive intake, particularly of animal proteins, therefore could cause constant hyperperfusion in the kidney, leading to intraglomerular hypertension and accelerated glomerulosclerosis. This would certainly help to explain the

TABLE 82-3 ■ LIFE EXPECTANCIES FOR SELECTED AGE GROUPS, COMPARING DIALYSIS PATIENTS WITH GENERAL POPULATION STATISTICS

AGE (Y)	DIALYSIS POPULATION (Y)	US POPULATION (Y)
40–44	6.7–9.2	30.1–40.8
50–54	5.1–6.9	22.5–31.5
60–64	3.7–5.1	16.0–22.8
70–74	2.7–3.5	10.8–15.2
80–84	2.0–2.4	6.9–8.8

Numbers are shown as ranges to accommodate differences by gender and ethnic group.

benefits so clearly seen with caloric restriction in laboratory animals.

The efficacy of ACE inhibitors in preventing renal hyperperfusion damage early in the course of diabetes and hypertension would also lend support to the hyperfiltration hypothesis. Angiotensin II appears to be important in maintaining glomerular filtration pressure by vasoconstricting the efferent arteriole. ACE inhibition is believed to preserve renal function by blocking the vasoconstriction of the efferent arteriole and reducing intraglomerular pressure. Long-term ACE inhibition dramatically reduces the incidence of age-related glomerulosclerosis in Munich-Wistar rats. However, a sufficient dose of an ACE inhibitor to significantly lower systolic blood pressure was administered in the treatment group as compared to the control animals. Whether low doses of ACE inhibitors would help to maintain normal renal function in humans and prevent the appearance of age-related glomerulosclerosis is a matter for speculation. There is no doubt about their efficacy in preventing a progressive decline in renal function when there is an underlying disease. It remains to be seen whether they have any role in modifying age-related changes.

CONSEQUENCES OF IMPAIRED KIDNEY FUNCTION

Patients who show signs of significantly diminished kidney function should be managed aggressively, regardless of their age. Individuals who reach dialysis have a mortality rate four to five times that of age-matched controls (**Table 82-3**) and are at 10 times the risk of a cardiovascular event. It costs more than $80,000 per year to maintain someone on dialysis without including the cost of treatment for any other health problems. Transplantation is also expensive and requires patients to remain on toxic immunosuppressive regimens for the rest of their lives. Patients who show signs of impaired kidney function should be managed with the idea of preventing them from reaching end-stage disease. Aggressive measures should be taken to reduce blood pressure with a target systolic blood pressure goal of less than 120 mm Hg. A regimen should be used

that includes an ACE inhibitor or an angiotensin receptor blocker, particularly in patients who have albuminuria. However, it should be kept in mind that neither of these classes of the drug will confer significant renal protection in the absence of good blood pressure control. Lipids should also be aggressively managed, as should blood sugar and other potential accelerators of renal decline. The novel SGLT2 inhibitors reduce the risk of kidney disease progression among patients with diabetic kidney disease who are already taking ACE inhibitors, as well as the incidence of cardiovascular disease. Overweight patients should be encouraged to lose weight. Great care should be taken to avoid potential renal toxins, such as aminoglycoside antibiotics, nonsteroidal anti-inflammatory drugs (NSAIDs), and radiocontrast dyes. Medications excreted by the kidney should be appropriately dosed in amount and frequency. Maintaining residual renal function confers on the patient a greatly superior prognosis when compared to those on renal replacement therapies. Hopefully, the current emphasis on finding genes that predispose to declines in kidney function and the development of age-related glomerulosclerosis will help us to identify those at greatest risk before major losses of function have occurred. As with recent gains in the prevention of cardiovascular disease through control of risk factors, we anticipate that similar guidelines will be available for the prevention of age-related declines in kidney function.

Kidney Donation

Kidneys from older donors have lower life expectancy in recipients compared to those from younger donors. However, the ever-increasing demand and supply mismatch in organ transplantation has led to an increase in the utilization of organs from older live and deceased donors. For example, utilization of living donors older than 55 years has increased from approximately 13% in 2008 to 22% in 2020. At the same time the use of kidneys from older deceased donors has remained constant. This difference is in part due to concerns of accentuation of age-related changes when these organs are exposed to peri-donation and peri-transplant ischemia and reperfusion injury. Furthermore, in recipients these organs undergo additional immune and nonimmune stresses that likely cause further progression of age-related structural abnormalities and early graft loss or recipient death. The increased concern for utilizing older deceased donor organs is in part driven by concerns of being penalized by regulatory bodies for poor transplant outcomes. This is despite studies showing that kidney transplant recipients receiving such kidneys on average still do better than those who remained on dialysis.

Kidney Transplantation

The proportion of individuals older than 65 years who are now on the waitlist has increased from 18% in 2009 to 24% in 2019 suggesting an increasing burden of kidney disease in this age group, an increase in willingness by transplant centers to list such patients, as well as reduction in wait-listing mortality. Many transplant programs are routinely offering transplantation to people in their late sixties and early seventies if they are otherwise in good health. This is reflected in the fact that donor transplant rates among those older than 65 years has increased from approximately 10 (per 100 waitlist years) in 2015 to 17 (per 100 waitlist years) in 2019.

In summary, kidney disease and failure are predominantly diseases of the older population. All older patients should have an estimate made of their GFR. If a deficit in their kidney function is identified, they should be managed aggressively to prevent progression to kidney failure. As CKD progresses, special attention should be paid to the choice of drugs and their dosing and to the use of contrast dyes for imaging.

FURTHER READING

Anderson AH, Yang W, Hsu CY, et al. CRIC Study Investigators. Estimating GFR among participants in the Chronic Renal Insufficiency Cohort (CRIC) Study. *Am J Kidney Dis.* 2012;60(2):250–261.

Bowling CB, Sharma P, Fox CS, O'Hare AM, Muntner P. Prevalence of reduced estimated glomerular filtration rate among the oldest old from 1988–1994 through 2005–2010. *JAMA.* 2013;310(12):1284–1286.

Fukuda A, Chowdhury MA, Venkatareddy MP, et al. Growth-dependent podocyte failure causes glomerulosclerosis. *J Am Soc Nephrol.* 2012;23(8):1351–1363.

Glassock RJ. An update on glomerular disease in the elderly. *Clin Geriatr Med.* 2013;29(3):579–591.

Naik AS, Afshinnia F, Cibrik D, et al. Quantitative podocyte parameters predict human native kidney and allograft half-lives. *JCI Insight.* 2016;1(7):e86943.

National Kidney Foundation. K/DOQI clinical practice guidelines for chronic kidney disease: evaluation, classification, and stratification. *Am J Kidney Dis.* 2002; 39:S1–S246.

Organ Procurement and Transplantation Network (OPTN) and Scientific Registry of Transplant Recipients (SRTR). OPTN/SRTR 2019 Annual Data Report. Rockville, MD: Department of Health and Human Services, Health Resources and Services Administration; 2021. Abbreviated citation: OPTN/SRTR 2019 Annual Data Report. HHS/HRSA.

O'Hare AM. Measures to define chronic kidney disease. *JAMA.* 2013;309(13):1343.

O'Hare AM, Armistead N, Schrag WL, Diamond L, Moss AH. Patient-centered care: an opportunity to accomplish the "three aims" of the national quality strategy in the Medicare ESRD program. *Clin J Am Soc Nephrol.* 2014;9(12):2189–2194.

O'Hare AM, Hotchkiss JR, Kurella-Tamura M, et al. Interpreting treatment effects from clinical trials in the context of real-world risk information: end-stage renal disease prevention in older adults. *JAMA Intern Med.* 2014;174(3):391–397.

Rule AD, Glassock RJ. Chronic kidney disease: classification of CKD should be about more than prognosis. *Nat Rev Nephrol.* 2013;9(12):697–698.

Rule AD, Glassock RJ. GFR estimating equations: getting closer to the truth? *Clin J Am Soc Nephrol.* 2013; 8(8):1414–1420.

Treit K, Lam D, O'Hare AM. Timing of dialysis initiation in the geriatric population: toward a patient-centered approach. *Semin Dial.* 2013;26(6):682–689.

United States Renal Data System. 2020 annual data report: an overview of the epidemiology of kidney disease in the United States. National Institutes of Health, National Institute of Diabetes and Digestive and Kidney Diseases, Bethesda, MD, 2020.

Wiggins JE, Patel SR, Shedden KA, et al. NFkappaB promotes inflammation, coagulation, and fibrosis in the aging glomerulus. *J Am Soc Nephrol.* 2010;21(4): 587–597.

Yaffe K, Ackerson L, Kurella-Tamura M, et al. Chronic Renal Insufficiency Cohort Investigators. Chronic kidney disease and cognitive function in older adults: findings from the chronic renal insufficiency cohort cognitive study. *J Am Geriatr Soc.* 2010;58(2):338–345.

Chapter 83

Kidney Diseases

Mark Unruh, Nitin Budhwar

INTRODUCTION

Given the relationship of kidney disease with age and chronic conditions, older adults have a higher frequency of both chronic kidney disease (CKD) and acute kidney injury (AKI). The older adult with kidney injury should be systematically evaluated and treated for AKI and CKD. As the population ages, there will be an increased number of patients with advanced CKD and kidney failure. The older patient with kidney failure now has a multitude of choices for renal replacement therapy (RRT) including hemodialysis, peritoneal dialysis, conservative management, palliative care, and kidney transplantation. Primary care physicians and geriatricians should identify CKD in older patients and have their care managed by a multidisciplinary team. The geriatrics team remains in the key role of addressing advance directives and planning long-term care and continued management of their nonrenal problems. Older patients with CKD will remain an economic and medical challenge, and a multidisciplinary approach to care for these patients will provide the best long-term outcomes.

AGING KIDNEYS

The kidneys undergo anatomic and physiologic changes that are not only the consequences of normal organ senescence but also of specific diseases that occur with greater frequency in older individuals. Structural changes that occur at an increasing rate with age include glomerular hypertrophy and glomerulosclerosis, tubular atrophy, and interstitial fibrosis as well as arteriolosclerosis. Functionally, several longitudinal studies have shown that glomerular filtration rate (GFR) declines in the majority of people with older age independent of other chronic diseases. Additional details are provided in Chapter 82, Aging of the Kidney.

CHRONIC KIDNEY DISEASE (CKD)

Definition

CKD is a general term for heterogeneous disorders affecting the kidney's structure and function. CKD is now recognized as a worldwide public health problem. Its management in early stages is tasked to the general practitioners

Learning Objectives

- Recognize that chronic kidney disease (CKD) is most often caused by common systemic diseases, including diabetes and hypertension.
- Understand that diabetic nephropathy is a chronic progressive kidney disease that requires treatment with angiotensin-converting enzyme inhibitor (ACEI) or angiotensin receptor blockers (ARBs) if tolerated, optimization of blood pressure and blood glucose levels, and management of comorbidities. SGLT2 inhibitors and GLP-1 receptor agonists show benefits in treatment of diabetes and substantial reduction of risk of kidney disease progression.
- Assess acute kidney injury (AKI) for pre-, post-, and intrarenal causes among the older adult. Even episodes of mild AKI can increase the risk for future CKD and the etiology of AKI is often related to the sex, age, and location of the patient.
- Understand the prognosis of older adults with kidney failure.
- Characterize the approaches to managing end-stage kidney disease (ESKD) among older adults.
- Describe the influence of multiple chronic health conditions on quality of life and functioning among older adults with kidney failure.
- Recognize the challenges in providing care to older patients with kidney failure and concurrent cognitive impairment and frailty.
- Discuss the role of clinicians and care teams in advance care planning for patients with ESKD.

Key Clinical Points

1. In patients with CKD, management of elevated blood pressure and avoidance of nephrotoxins can delay progression to ESKD.
2. Complications of CKD include iron-deficient anemia and secondary hyperparathyroidism.
3. Proteinuria in the absence of hematuria is a sign of kidney damage, is a risk factor for progression of CKD to ESKD, and requires evaluation.

(Continued)

4. In patients with renovascular disease, intervention is usually only indicated if conservative management fails.

5. Clinical guidelines suggest that patients with progressive CKD should be managed in a multidisciplinary setting. Nephrologist referral should be considered under the following circumstances: AKI, urinary red cell casts, CKD and refractory hypertension, persistent abnormalities of potassium, recurrent or extensive nephrolithiasis, hereditary kidney disease, CKD stages 4 and 5, and patients with severely increased albuminuria.

6. Older patients with kidney failure have a multitude of choices for kidney replacement therapy including hemodialysis, peritoneal dialysis, conservative management, palliative care, and kidney transplantation.

7. There are no age restrictions on access to kidney transplantation in the United States. Older kidney transplant patients tend to have less kidney allograft rejection and a higher complication rate from infections.

8. Kidney failure is associated with a markedly high mortality rate among older patients initiating dialysis—average 1-year survival rate is 50% for octogenarians and nonagenarians who start dialysis.

and geriatricians. The presentation of patients with CKD can vary and is related to disease etiology, severity, and rate of progression. CKD is classified into stages of disease severity, which are based on GFR described in clinical practice guidelines (**Figure 83-1**).

The criteria for CKD include an estimated GFR less than 60 mL/min/1.73 m² (normal GFR in young adults is about 125 mL/min/1.73 m²; GFR < 15 mL/min/1.73 m² is defined as kidney failure), albuminuria (urinary albumin-to-creatinine ratio > 30 mg/g), hematuria (any degree on urine dipstick), presence of urinary casts in the urine sediment (seen by microscopy of urinary sediment), and abnormalities on kidney imaging for a duration of more than 3 months.

It should be mentioned that some in the field have raised concerns that this classification overestimates the CKD burden in the older adult population when considering clinical outcomes. The equations estimating GFR have relied on creatinine, sex, age, and race as factors to predict kidney function. It has been determined that low estimated GFR (eGFR) and high albuminuria are independently associated with increased mortality and risk to develop end-stage kidney disease (ESKD) regardless of age across a wide range of populations. In addition, even smaller decreases in eGFR (such as < 30% reduction over 2 years) were strongly and consistently associated with increased mortality and risk of ESKD. Thus, CKD contributes significantly to increased morbidity and mortality. However, patients with CKD are a very heterogeneous group and eGFR and albuminuria alone may not be sufficient to predict outcomes, especially in the older adult population. Therefore, care should be provided in context of the individual situation and needs.

Epidemiology

Even though the prevalence and incidence of kidney failure treated with dialysis and kidney transplantation is monitored closely in many countries, the estimation of the burden of early stages of kidney disease remains difficult. In the United States, the prevalence of CKD based on estimated GFR and albuminuria was about 11.5% (4.8% in stages 1–2 and 6.7% in stages 3–5) in the general population but was 47% in people older than 70 years. Therefore, CKD constitutes a major health concern in particular in older adults.

Pathophysiology (Classification)

Many systemic diseases can result in CKD, in particular diabetes mellitus and hypertension. Diabetic nephropathy (DN) and glomerular and tubule-interstitial diseases with defined etiologies and presentations will also be described. Hypertension can contribute to CKD (hypertensive nephropathy) and also accelerate progression of CKD due to other etiologies.

Presentation

CKD is usually asymptomatic until GFR falls below approximately 15 to 20 mL/min/1.73 m² when patients may report early signs and symptoms of uremia. Initial symptoms are nonspecific and include decreased energy levels and appetite, metallic taste, worsening of lower extremity edema, and new onset or worsening of nocturia. Some patients notice bubbly or dark urine as a sign of proteinuria or hematuria, respectively.

Evaluation

Kidney function is usually assessed by serum creatinine and blood urea nitrogen (BUN) levels, electrolytes, urinalysis, and urine protein-creatinine protein ratio (or quantitative albuminuria). If there are situations that may limit the accuracy of creatinine, one could use cystatin C to provide another estimate of GFR. If these tests are abnormal, further evaluation may include a kidney ultrasound with Doppler to determine kidney size (enlarged kidneys can be seen in patients with polycystic kidney disease [PKD], infiltrative processes, amyloidosis, and diabetic and HIV nephropathy; small kidneys can be congenital or due to long-standing CKD), echogenicity (increased in long-standing CKD and infiltrative processes), renal blood flow (decreased with long-standing CKD or with occlusion of renal arteries

Prognosis of CKD by GFR and Albuminuria Categories: KDIGO 2012			Persistent albuminuria categories Description and range		
			A1	A2	A3
			Normal to mildly increased	Moderately increased	Severely increased
			< 30 mg/g < 3 mg/mmol	30–300 mg/g 3–30 mg/mmol	> 300 mg/g > 30 mg/mmol
GFR categories (mL/min/1.73 m²) Description and range	G1	Normal or high	≥ 90			
	G2	Mildly decreased	60–89			
	G3a	Mildly to moderately decreased	45–59			
	G3b	Moderately to severely decreased	30–44			
	G4	Severely decreased	15–29			
	G5	Kidney failure	< 15			

Green, low risk (if no other markers of kidney disease, no CKD); yellow, moderately increased risk; orange, high risk; red: very high risk.

FIGURE 83-1. Prognosis of chronic kidney disease (CKD) by glomerular filtration rate (GFR) and albuminuria category. (Reproduced with permission from Kidney Disease: Improving Global Outcomes (KDIGO) Diabetes Work Group. KDIGO 2020 Clinical Practice Guideline for Diabetes Management in Chronic Kidney Disease. *Kidney Int.* 2020;98[4S]:S1–S115.)

including after renal infarct), and renal pelvis dilatation (in ureteral or severe bladder outflow obstruction).

Previous blood, urine, and imaging test results should be obtained if available to determine duration and rate of change. A detailed medical and surgical history should be obtained, including childhood diseases, in particular edema and proteinuria in the past and history of rheumatic fever or other severe conditions. The family history can point toward inheritable kidney diseases (including PKD and focal segmental glomerular sclerosis [FSGS]). Social history may identify exposure to toxins and herbal remedies. Additionally, the history can help to identify risk factors for progression of CKD to ESKD. A comprehensive physical examination can detect elevated blood pressure, obesity, signs of heart failure, pulmonary and peripheral edema, liver disease, vasculitis/autoimmune disease, etc.

Management

Significant progress has been made in establishing approaches that target underlying specific diseases with the goal of improving disease-related outcomes. However, features of geriatric populations such as complex comorbidities, life expectancy, functional state, and health priorities may limit the utility of disease-oriented models of care. Individualized patient-centered approach to care may have more to offer than a traditional disease-based approach to CKD in many older adults.

Attention should be given to cardiovascular disease, which is not only a risk factor for CKD, but also for progression of CKD. Blood pressure control has been shown to limit the progression of CKD. There are a number of guidelines that address target blood pressure goals in CKD with the recommendations aiming for systolic blood pressures between 120 and 130 mm Hg and diastolic under 90. Given the complexity of the geriatric patient, numerous factors need to be considered such as tolerance, cost, side-effect profile, polypharmacy, competing chronic conditions, and goals of care.

Pharmacologic Choice of antihypertensive medications should be guided not only for blood pressure control, but also for benefits related to delaying CKD progression and controlling proteinuria, with an acceptable side-effect profile.

Blockade of the renin-angiotensin system (RAS) using ACEIs or ARB lowers blood pressure and also decreases proteinuria and is therefore the mainstay in patients with diabetes in whom DN is suspected. Combination of ACEI and ARB is associated with increased complications and is in general not advised. Two FDA-approved diabetes medications have also been shown to have significant reduction of risks associated with CKD—SGLT2 inhibitors and GLP-1 receptor agonists.

Medications from these classes should be considered for patients with type 2 diabetes and CKD and the indications for use of SGLT2 may be expanding to other etiologies of kidney disease such as IgA nephropathy. They may also be of benefit in nondiabetics with CKD—but the data to support this is still emerging. In addition, management of hyperlipidemia with statins or statins plus ezetimibe is recommended for older adults with eGFR less than 60 mL/min/1.73 m^2.

Nonpharmacologic Patients with CKD are more likely to experience AKI, and AKI is a risk factor for progression to ESKD. Thus, preventing AKI is important to delay CKD progression. Avoidance of nephrotoxins is a mainstay of CKD management. In particular, nonsteroidal anti-inflammatory drugs (NSAIDs) can have detrimental effects especially if the patient is also taking ACEIs or ARBs, by decreasing glomerular perfusion and filtration rate. Contrast dye can cause tubular cell damage and AKI possibly leading to CKD. Many antibiotics can have nephrotoxic effects and cause AKI.

Obesity is associated with compensatory glomerular hypertrophy, which causes podocyte hypertrophy that may progress to podocyte dysfunction, decreased podocyte density, and accelerated loss of kidney function. CKD is associated with salt retention and a low-salt diet may slow progression of CKD independent of improving hypertension.

Prevention

Prevention is the ideal approach to prevent ESKD and its associated morbidity and mortality. High-risk patient subgroups may particularly benefit from implementation of measures to detect and prevent CKD. Patients with diabetes mellitus should be screened regularly for albuminuria and elevations in serum creatinine levels. Similarly, patients with hypertension, peripheral vascular occlusive disease, reduced kidney mass (ie, after a nephrectomy), or a family history of kidney disease should be regularly evaluated. Patients with risk factors for CKD should be monitored for optimal blood pressure control, avoidance of nephrotoxins, polypharmacy, and episodes of AKI.

Protein in the Diet

In nondiabetic patients with CKD with less advanced disease (CKD stage 3 or lower), low-protein diets do not appear to reduce the progression to ESKD compared with normal-protein diets.

There is some evidence that low-protein diets (0.5–0.6 g per kg per day) or very low-protein diets (0.3–0.4 g per kg per day) may reduce the number of patients with advanced kidney disease (CKD stage 4 or 5) who progress to ESKD. This should be done with regular monitoring to prevent malnourishment.

Special Issues

Patient preference Once the eGFR falls below approximately 20 mL/min/1.73 m^2, the risk to develop ESKD requiring dialysis support increases significantly and a discussion about patient preferences regarding dialysis should be initiated. In this context, the comorbidities and functional status of the patient should be considered, because quality of life and functional status may not improve or could be worsened after initiation of dialysis in patients with high comorbidity burden and low functional status.

Comorbidity Management of comorbidities is important in the care of patients with CKD. One of the most important comorbidities is hypertension. With worsening kidney function secondary hyperparathyroidism can develop due to retention of phosphate and decreased activation of vitamin D causing parathyroid hormone (PTH) to increase. Therefore, serum phosphate, 25-OH-vitamin D, and PTH levels should be monitored. Hyperphosphatemia can be managed by low-phosphate diet. Oral phosphate binders, such as calcium acetate, sevelamer, or lanthanum carbonate, may have to be given if diet is not successful in maintaining normal phosphate levels. Decreased 25-OH-vitamin D levels should be treated with supplementation of cholecalciferol or ergocalciferol. Significantly, elevated PTH levels unresponsive to vitamin D supplementation may require treatment with active vitamin D analogs, including calcitriol, but have to be used with great care due to the risk of hypercalcemia and hyperphosphatemia. Patients with PTH levels unresponsive to vitamin D supplementation may be evaluated for tertiary hyperparathyroidism.

Care settings CKD is primarily managed in an outpatient setting.

ACUTE KIDNEY INJURY

Definition

AKI is defined by an increase in creatinine (decrease in eGFR) within a few days or even hours, but it is important to understand that rising creatinine levels are likely not very sensitive. AKI is further classified as nonoliguric (> 400 mL/day), oliguric (100–400 mL/day), and anuric (< 100 mL/day). This has prognostic implications as nonoliguric AKI is associated with better outcomes. AKI can be further distinguished by etiology such as prerenal, intrarenal, and postrenal.

Epidemiology

The incidence of AKI increases with age, with the majority of patients who develop AKI being older than 65 years. When AKI does occur in this age group, it is associated with significant morbidity and mortality. However, the epidemiology of AKI is difficult to determine consistently and detailed information about long-term outcomes is often lacking. Studies have shown that even modest increases (< 50%) of serum creatinine levels are associated with significantly higher risk of long-term CKD.

Pathophysiology (Classification)

Etiologies of AKI can be categorized into prerenal, postrenal (obstructive), and intrarenal (intrinsic) causes (summarized in **Table 83-1**). Prerenal etiologies include

TABLE 83-1 ■ ACUTE RENAL FAILURE IN OLDER ADULTS

PRERENAL (ACUTE REVERSIBLE RENAL HYPOPERFUSION)	RENAL OR INTRINSIC	OBSTRUCTIVE
Hypovolemia	**Acute glomerulonephritis**	**Ureteral and pelvic**
Fluid loss	Mesangiocapillary	Intrinsic obstruction
Gastrointestinal	Postinfectious	Blood clots
Diarrhea	Rapidly progressive	Fungus balls
Fistulas	Goodpasture syndrome	Sloughed papillae
Vomiting	Idiopathic	Diabetics
Renal	SLE	Analgesic abusers
Diuretic intake	**Vasculitis**	Stones
Salt wasting	Hypersensitivity angiitis	Extrinsic obstruction
Redistribution of the extracellular volume	Classic	Fecal impaction
Shock (septic, cardiogenic)	Hemolytic-uremic syndrome	Malignancy
Hypoalbuminemia	Henoch-Schönlein	Retroperitoneal fibrosis
Nephrotic syndrome	Mixed cryoglobulinemia	**Bladder**
Liver diseases	Scleroderma	Bladder carcinoma
Malnutrition	Serum sickness	Blood clots
Hemorrhage	Wegener granulomatosis	Neuropathic
Inappropriate fluid restriction	Polyarteritis nodosa	Prostatic hypertrophy
Interference with renal autoregulatory mechanisms	**Tubulointerstitial nephropathies**	Stones
ACEIs	Drugs	**Urethra**
Cyclosporine	ACEIs	Phimosis
NSAIDs	Allopurinol	Strictures
Cardiac failure	Ampicillin	
Acute	Analgesics (including NSAIDs)	
Acute myocardial infarction	Cimetidine	
Arrhythmias	Diphenylhydantoin	
Cardiac tamponade	Methicillin	
Malignant hypertension	Thiazides	
Chronic: ischemic and hypertensive cardiomyopathies	**Infectious:** acute pyelonephritis	
Valvulopathies	**Infiltrative**	
	Leukemia	
	Lymphoma	
	Sarcoidosis	
	Idiopathic	
	Intratubular obstruction	
	Myeloma proteins	
	Myoglobin	
	Sulfonamides	
	Urates	
	Hypercalcemia	
	Hepatorenal syndrome	

(Continued)

TABLE 83-1 ■ ACUTE RENAL FAILURE IN OLDER ADULTS (*CONTINUED*)

PRERENAL (ACUTE REVERSIBLE RENAL HYPOPERFUSION)	RENAL OR INTRINSIC	OBSTRUCTIVE
	Vascular obstruction	
	Arterial	
	Aneurysms	
	Atheroembolic disease	
	Venous: thrombosis of vena cava	
	Tubule cell damage	
	Nephrotoxin-related	
	Antibiotics (aminoglycosides)	
	Iodinated contrast media	
	IV immunoglobulin G	
	Metals (Hg, Ag, Pt, Bi)	
	Organic solvents	

ACEI, angiotensin-converting enzyme inhibitor; ARF, acute renal failure; NSAIDs, nonsteroidal anti-inflammatory drugs; SLE, systemic lupus erythematosus.
Modified with permission from Macías-Núñez JF, López-Novoa JM, Martínez-Maldonado M. Acute renal failure in the aged. Semin Nephrol. 1996;16(4):330–338.

intravascular volume depletion due to fluid loss with decreased total body volume (ie, diarrhea, vomiting, and active bleeding) or low intravascular oncotic pressure (hypoalbuminemia secondary to nephrotic syndrome [NS], liver dysfunction, or malnutrition). Decreased cardiac output can also lead to a prerenal state even if the patient has peripheral and pulmonary edema. Patients with preexisting renal vascular disease are also at increased risk for prerenal AKI with milder degree of hypovolemia or hypotension.

Postrenal etiologies for AKI include bladder outflow or ureteral obstruction. Obstruction of one ureter usually does not cause markedly elevated creatinine levels except in patients with some degree of preexisting CKD or only one functional kidney. In older adults, benign prostate hypertrophy and malignancies, including prostate cancer and cancer of cervix and uterus, have to be considered. In particular, bilateral ureteral obstruction without bladder retention is highly suspicious for a malignant mass in the lower abdomen.

Intrarenal causes of AKI can be caused by acute glomerular nephritis (GN) or tubule-interstitial nephropathies. Acute GN can be caused by rapidly progressive GN due to systemic vasculitis or autoimmune complex deposition in the kidney (see below). Tubulointerstitial nephropathies can be secondary to nephrotoxins, which cause acute tubular necrosis (ATN), intratubular obstruction, interstitial infiltration, or inflammation. ATN can be caused by a large number of nephrotoxins, including IV contrast dye, chemotherapeutic agents, and antibiotics, which are taken up by tubular epithelial cells leading to acute tubular cell damage. In the setting of trauma or hemolysis, free hemoglobin and myoglobin can cause ATN (pigment nephropathy). Tumor lysis

syndrome is seen during treatment of cancer, in particular lymphomas and leukemias and is characterized by hyperkalemia, hyperphosphatemia, and hyperuricemia. Contrast-induced acute kidney injury (CI-AKI) represents a common form of iatrogenic AKI. Major risk factors for CI-AKI include old age, presence of CKD, diabetes, heart failure, volume depletion, and concomitant exposure to other nephrotoxins. There has been research into the best strategies to mitigate the risk for CI-AKI when administering IV contrast. The primary approach is to avoid the exposure if possible and confirm that a study with iodinated contrast generates adequate benefit to assume the risk. In higher-risk patients, approaches to attenuate the risk of CI-AKI include stopping any nephrotoxins, use of intravenous isotonic saline for volume expansion, and use of a low or iso-osmolar contrast agent.

Polypharmacy and drug toxicity exacerbate the susceptibility of older adults to AKI. Drugs commonly associated with AKI include NSAIDs, diuretics, ACEIs, ARBs, and antibiotics. Moreover, NSAID use doubles the risk for AKI in adults older than age 65. Older adults are also at increased risk for renal injury in particular due to hypovolemia, sepsis, and iatrogenic complications related to drug toxicity.

Presentation

Patients with AKI can be asymptomatic and detected solely by elevated creatinine levels or present with symptoms that result from various disturbances of kidney function. Patients may have decrements in urine output and signs of volume overload. In patients with more advanced stages of AKI, accumulation of substances cleared by the kidney can lead to uremic symptoms characterized by fatigue, loss of appetite, headache, nausea and vomiting, metallic taste, shortness of breath, asterixis, lethargy, and seizure. Potassium levels can increase and lead to cardiac arrhythmias, which can be life threatening.

Evaluation

Kidney function should be examined in every patient at risk for AKI based on presenting symptoms. If creatinine is found to be elevated, values from previous tests are helpful to determine duration of renal dysfunction. Urine output has to be monitored accurately and catheterization of the bladder should be considered if clinically indicated as in case of bladder outflow obstruction. An ultrasound of the kidneys may be performed to evaluate for hydronephrosis and kidney size as well as echogenicity, which can be increased in both CKD and ATN. Doppler of the kidneys can determine blood flow (decreased or absent in renal artery or vein thrombosis) and resistive indices (increased in CKD and ATN). Urinalysis findings including casts, crystals, and tubular cells can be suggestive of tubular necrosis. Prerenal volume depletion is supported by clinical examination, including hypotension, tachycardia, decreased skin turgor, and dry oral mucosa.

Management

The management of AKI is focused on treating the underlying cause and supportive medical management. Prerenal volume depletion is treated with volume repletion using isotonic solutions with careful monitoring of fluid status, respiratory function, and urine output. Postrenal causes acutely require placement of a bladder catheter for bladder outflow obstruction or placement of ureteral stents or nephrostomy for ureteral obstruction. The mainstay in the management of patients with intrarenal AKI is close monitoring of renal function, electrolytes, volume status, and urine output as well as signs or symptoms of uremia in order to determine need for dialysis support. Diuretics can be used if needed to manage volume status and potentially avoid respiratory failure, but maintaining urine output above oliguric levels does not improve the outcome of AKI. Thus, diuretics should be used to address volume overload, and prevent respiratory failure. Hyperkalemia can often be managed nonacutely with low-potassium diet and diuretics. Dialysis support may be required in patients with AKI. Dialysis initiation is determined by the development of indications for dialysis, including electrolyte, acid–base and fluid volume abnormalities that are life-threatening and cannot be managed medically, and symptoms related to uremia.

Prevention

Older adults are at increased risk for AKI due to polypharmacy, high prevalence of preexisting CKD, and decreased oral intake (decreased thirst). Limiting polypharmacy is already a mainstay of geriatric care, but a particular focus is necessary for AKI prevention.

Special Issues

Patient preference AKI may require temporary dialysis support or lead to ESKD and permanent chronic dialysis dependence. It is important to discuss the patient's preferences toward dialysis with sufficient time prior to initiation of dialysis, especially among older adults who initiate dialysis in the intensive care (ICU) setting due to a decreased survival rate.

Comorbidity Almost half of Medicare beneficiaries age 65 or older have three or more chronic conditions, and the number of preventable hospitalizations per 1000 beneficiaries increases with the number of chronic conditions. Comorbidities that increase the risk for AKI are common among older patients. Patients with both CKD and AKI tend to be older, have ischemic heart disease, and be less likely to recover kidney function than patients with AKI alone.

Care settings AKI is very common in the inpatient setting owing to the complications of an acute illness and resulting acute interstitial nephritis (AIN) and ATN. The underlying etiologies of AKI in the outpatient setting are different with obstruction and polypharmacy as more likely causes in the geriatric population.

GLOMERULONEPHRITIS (GN)

Some GN conditions have a second peak in the geriatric population such as small-vessel vasculitis and postinfectious glomerulonephritis (PIGN). GN can be classified into groups based on course, histopathologic findings, and disease etiology. Rapidly progressive GN (RPGN) can be associated with autoimmune processes, infectious diseases, and systemic diseases, in particular vasculitides, malignancies, and medications (**Table 83-2**). The most common primary GN worldwide is immunoglobulin A (IgA) nephropathy. It can have a highly variable course with some patients presenting with RPGN, approximately 30% to 40% of patients progressing to ESKD within 20 years and other patients only having persistent hematuria without proteinuria or changes in GFR. The incidence of ESKD in older patients with IgA nephropathy (older than age 50) is almost two times higher than that in younger patients. PIGN is considered primarily a childhood disease, but more recently its occurrence in older patients is becoming recognized. PIGN presents typically with hematuria and proteinuria 10 to 14 days after an infection. Hypocomplementemia was present in more than 70% and almost half of patients required acute dialysis. Only about 20% achieved complete recovery, half had persistent renal dysfunction, and about 30% progressed to ESKD. In summary, the epidemiology of PIGN is shifting as the population ages. Older men and patients with

TABLE 83-2 ■ CLASSIFICATION OF RAPIDLY PROGRESSIVE GLOMERULONEPHRITIS

Primary diffuse crescentic glomerulonephritis
  Type I: anti–GBM-mediated disease without pulmonary hemorrhage (with anti-GBM)
  Type II: immune complex–associated disease (without anti-GMB or ANCA)
  Type III: pauci-immune (with ANCA)
  Type IV: mixed pattern (with anti-GBM and ANCA)
  Type V: pauci-immune (without ANCA or anti-GBM)
  Fibrillary and immunotactoid glomerulonephritis
  Focal sclerosis (rare)
  IgA nephropathy
  Mesangiocapillary glomerulonephritis (especially type II)
  Membranous glomerulonephritis (with or without anti-GBM)
  Superimposed on another primary glomerular disease

Associated with infectious disease
  Hepatitis B and C
  Histoplasmosis
  Infective endocarditis
  Influenza (?)
  Mycoplasma infection
  Poststreptococcal glomerulonephritis
  Visceral abscesses

Associated with multisystem disease
  Carcinoma (lung, bladder, prostate)
  Goodpasture disease (anti-GBM with pulmonary hemorrhage)
  Lymphoma
  Mixed (IgG/IgM) cryoimmunoglobulinemia (hepatitis C)
  Relapsing polychondritis
  Henoch-Schönlein purpura
  Systemic lupus erythematosus
  Systemic polyangiitis
    Churg-Strauss syndrome
    Microscopic polyangiitis (with ANCA)
    Wegener granulomatosis (with ANCA)
    Other variants

Associated with medications
  Allopurinol
  Bucillamine
  D-Penicillamine
  Hydralazine
  Rifampin

ANCA, antineutrophil cytoplasmic antibodies; GBM, glomerular basement membrane. *Modified with permission from Massry SG, Glassock RJ. Textbook of Nephrology, 4th ed. Baltimore, MD: Williams and Wilkins; 2000.*

fever, and weight loss. Occasionally hemoptysis, rash, and joint pain are noted. Some patients do not have any systemic symptoms, but rather develop hematuria, variable degree of proteinuria, and rising creatinine. In those patients, a kidney biopsy may show pauci-immune GN.

Presentation

Patients with GN report constitutional symptoms, including decreased energy, general malaise, decreased appetite, fever and weight loss, and muscle aches. These symptoms are nonspecific and some patients attribute those symptoms to viral infections like upper respiratory infections. Any of those symptoms should prompt examination of kidney function and urine. The presence of hematuria and proteinuria should immediately raise concern for GN.

Evaluation

The evaluation of a patient with suspected glomerular disease depends primarily on the acuity of the presentation. If the patient presents with acute kidney failure and has hematuria and proteinuria, RPGN has to be suspected. In emergent and urgent presentations, the prompt consultation of nephrology may help to guide both diagnostics and therapeutic approaches.

The decision whether and when to perform a kidney biopsy depends on the overall condition and status of each individual patient. Increased frailty and decreased functional status at baseline, preexisting baseline CKD with decreased eGFR, and small echogenic kidneys on ultrasound, limited life expectancy as well as anemia, thrombocytopenia, and coagulopathy increase the risk for complications after kidney biopsy.

If the patient has stable renal function but a glomerular disease is suspected because of hematuria and proteinuria, the patient should first undergo serologic evaluation. Depending on those results a kidney biopsy can be considered. If the creatinine is rising and pre- and postrenal causes of AKI have been excluded, an urgent kidney biopsy may be considered.

Management

The diagnosis of RPGN may justify empiric immunosuppressive therapy. Even with stable kidney function, it is important to establish specific disease etiologies to guide therapy.

Pharmacologic Corticosteroids are the mainstay in the treatment of acute and chronic GN. Patients need to be monitored closely for any signs or symptoms of recurrence of disease in particular during tapering prednisone dose and after its discontinuation.

Cytotoxic therapy with agents such as cyclophosphamide is considered in patients with crescentic and proliferative GN detected on biopsy or in the setting of other potentially life-threatening complications (ie, hemoptysis, severe hemolytic anemia, and thrombocytopenia). Whether to use IV or oral Cytoxan and length

diabetes or malignancy are particularly at risk, and the sites of infection and causative organisms differ from the typical childhood disease.

Small-vessel vasculitis is rare and often presents with systemic symptoms, including fatigue, malaise, loss of appetite, of therapy depends on the specific disease, severity of initial presentation, and degree of response. Anti-CD20 antibodies (rituximab) can be considered with equivalent potency compared to Cytoxan as suggested by recent studies. Maintenance therapy is usually required to prevent disease recurrence. The goal is to maintain the patient on the lowest dose of corticosteroids and steroid-sparing agents without flare of the disease or significant complications of therapy.

Supportive medical management is critical for patients with GN, in particular management of blood pressure (hyper- and hypotension), intravascular and total body fluid volume, electrolyte abnormalities, and unwanted effects and complications of therapy.

Special Issues

Patient preference Treatment of GN is associated with significant side effects and complications, which need to be balanced with side effects and complications of renal failure and ESKD. Risks and benefits of all options with specific consideration of the underlying condition, renal and overall survival prognosis with and without treatment, comorbidities, functional status, and expectations should be discussed. Furthermore, treatment with immunosuppressive medications often requires frequent office visits and laboratory tests, which may significantly affect quality of life or may even not be feasible.

NEPHROTIC SYNDROME (NS)

Definition

NS is defined as the presence of nephrotic range proteinuria (> 3 g/day), hypoalbuminemia, edema, and dyslipidemia. It is caused by different diseases affecting primarily the glomerular structure, in particular podocytes and the slit diaphragm that spans between the foot processes of podocytes. Thus, patients with NS always have glomerular and podocyte damage detected on kidney biopsy. Patients in all age groups can develop NS and the incidence and prevalence of NS in older adults is not clear. NS is likely to be missed in older adults who often have edema and low serum albumin caused by other etiologies. Minimal change disease (MCD) is most common in children and has a second peak in adults older than age 50. DN may be the most common cause of NS in adults.

Pathophysiology (Classification)

The differential diagnosis in older adult patients presenting with NS includes most diseases that are seen in younger adults. A kidney biopsy may be needed to define the cause of NS and estimate the degree of fibrosis in this age group, and thereby greatly aid in focusing the diagnostic evaluation and in planning treatment. Many clinicians recommend deferring additional laboratory or imaging procedures until the histopathologic diagnosis of NS has been made by renal biopsy.

The most common diseases identified by kidney biopsy are membranous nephropathy (MN), MCD, and amyloidosis, with approximately 60% of all cases accounted for by these three conditions. Less common causes among older patients undergoing a biopsy for diagnosis of NS are FSGS, proliferative GN, and DN. A membranoproliferative pattern of injury can be seen in association with a monoclonal deposition disease, such as light-chain deposition disease, which is more common in older adults. DN is less commonly encountered on biopsies, largely because patients with diabetes and NS seldom undergo renal biopsy unless "atypical" features are present such as onset of NS fewer than 5 years from discovery of diabetes, rapid progression of renal impairment, or absence of proliferative retinopathy and other microvascular complications of diabetes.

MCD is encountered in approximately 15% and MN in approximately 30% to 40% of renal biopsies in older adult with isolated NS. Both MN and MCD can be primary idiopathic glomerular diseases or secondary to extra renal conditions such as neoplasia, drugs, or infection. Approximately 10% of renal biopsies in older patients believed to have primary idiopathic NS on clinical grounds will reveal amyloidosis. Amyloidosis in the older adult is most often of the primary variety.

Presentation

The most common symptom is lower extremity edema and sometimes patients also notice facial or upper extremity swelling or increased abdominal girth from ascites. Often, patients are asymptomatic and albuminuria is detected. Occasionally, patients are found to have hyperlipidemia as the first presenting abnormality. Rarely patients with NS present with an arterial or venous thrombotic event. Renal vein thrombosis should especially raise the concern for NS.

Evaluation

New onset of lower extremity edema should always warrant a urinalysis, which is cheap, noninvasive, and can quickly guide further diagnostic interventions. If the urinalysis shows albuminuria, renal function, serum albumin, and lipid levels should be determined. At the point of diagnosing a NS in a patient, a nephrology consultation is indicated for work-up and therapeutic recommendations. A kidney ultrasound is used to evaluate for kidney size, which can be increased in patients with NS due to diabetic and HIV nephropathy, amyloidosis, and infiltrative diseases that can also cause MN. A kidney biopsy should be considered in all patients with new onset of NS. Because some etiologies of NS, including MCD and MN, are paraneoplastic syndromes, a malignancy work-up should be considered.

Management

Pharmacologic Treatment of the underlying etiology of NS is usually divided into immunosuppressive and nonimmunosuppressive therapies. Immunosuppressive therapy usually includes induction and maintenance regimen. Which regimen is recommended depends on the specific disease etiology, risk for progression, presence of comorbidities, and risk of complications. Disease-specific immunosuppressive regimens usually include pulse-dose corticosteroids, followed by oral steroids very similar to patients with GN as described earlier. The rate of steroid taper often is guided by response to therapy. Additional therapeutic strategies may include B-cell depletion using anti-CD20 antibodies, calcineurin inhibitors, and mycophenolate mofetil.

Non-immunosuppressive therapies target mainly proteinuria and edema. The mainstay of interventions to lower proteinuria is blockade of the RAS with either ACEI or ARB, which lower intraglomerular pressure and also exhibit direct beneficial effects on podocytes. Peripheral edema and ascites require sodium restriction (< 2 g/day) and loop diuretics, it should be reversed slowly to avoid hypovolemia and AKI. Hyperlipidemia usually resolves with resolution of NS. In patients who experience a thrombotic event due to hypercoagulopathy in NS, anticoagulation may have to be considered.

Prevention

Management of diabetes attenuates the likelihood of developing DN and subsequent NS.

Special Issues

Patient preference NS is a potentially life-threatening disease due to cardiovascular and infectious complications. In addition, NS can lead to AKI, potentially requiring dialysis support, but is potentially reversible. On the other hand, NS can lead to CKD and progression to ESKD even with treatment. Therefore, patients need to be educated about the overall prognosis and a discussion of goals of care should be initiated early during the course.

DIABETIC NEPHROPATHY

Definition

Diabetic kidney disease or DN is a progressive microvascular complication due to long-standing diabetes mellitus that can lead to ESKD.

Epidemiology

About 30% of patients with diabetes mellitus develop DN during their lifetime. In the general adult population in the United States, DN is the most common cause of NS and ESKD requiring dialysis. DN is more common in patients with other microvascular complications, in patients with neuropathy and retinopathy, and in patients with a family history of kidney disease, including DN.

Pathophysiology (Classification)

DN is a microvascular complication of patients with diabetes mellitus. DN has several distinct phases and complex molecular mechanisms are involved in the development of the disease and its outcomes. A significant proportion of patients exhibit accelerated loss of kidney function once eGFR is below 45 mL/min/1.73 m². Hyperglycemia appears to contribute significantly to development of DN because DN is a complication of both types 1 and 2 diabetes.

Presentation

Patients are usually diagnosed with DN because of routine screening tests for renal function and albuminuria, as is standard of care. Patients with earlier stages of DN can be found to hyperfiltrate with eGFR above 120 mL/min/1.73 m², and/or albuminuria, often below the detection limit of standard urinalysis tests requiring testing for "microalbuminuria." At later stages, patients may present with "macroalbuminuria" and NS. In all patients with DM and eGFR below 60 mL/min/1.73 m², DN is the likely underlying etiology. Absence of or less than nephrotic range proteinuria does not exclude DN.

Evaluation

All patients with DM should be regularly evaluated for development of albuminuria and changes in eGFR. Even though a kidney biopsy may not be necessary in many patients with suspected DN, it has to be considered in the presence of any concern for other etiologies. Patients have to be evaluated for electrolyte abnormalities because type IV renal tubular acidosis (RTA) may lead to hyperkalemia, and serum albumin and lipid levels need to be determined to diagnose NS and its associated complications.

Management

The main goals in patients with DN are optimization of blood glucose levels, blood pressure, and use of kidney-protective medications. In addition, complications of CKD as well as timely preparation for dialysis have to be managed.

Pharmacologic The development of agents to protect kidney function among those with DN has been a dramatic success in the prevention of ESKD. Blockade of the RAS and tight glycemic control have been shown to improve outcomes in patients with DN. The medications used to achieve these goals should be tailored specifically toward an individual patient's comorbidities. ACEI, ARBs, SGLT2 inhibitors, and GLP-1 receptor agonists delay progression of CKD to ESKD and should be started in all patients with diabetes mellitus and any stage of CKD and/or hypertension if tolerated. If sodium retention and edema are present, diuretics may be used. The blood pressure goal for patient with diabetes and CKD is generally agreed by various organizations to be kept below 130/80 mm Hg.

Special Issues

Patient preference Patients with diabetes who require dialysis have a higher complication rate and mortality.

Comorbidities Many patients with DN suffer from other complications of DM, including neuropathy and retinopathy, hyperlipidemia, macrovascular disease (coronary artery disease [CAD]), and obesity. Management of these comorbidities can potentially delay progression of CKD to ESKD. Diabetic patients with ESKD receiving dialysis are also at increased risk for cardiovascular and infectious complications.

INTERSTITIAL NEPHRITIS

Definition

Interstitial nephritis is characterized by inflammation of the tubulointerstitial area of the kidney causing tubular dysfunction and thereby proteinuria and decrease in renal function.

Epidemiology

The number of patients with acute interstitial nephritis (AIN) is very difficult to assess with confidence, as many episodes are likely undiagnosed and/or self-limited. In patients with AKI, AIN is an important cause. In studies, 80% of older patients showed partial or complete recovery within 6 months.

Pathophysiology (Classification)

The most common cause of AIN is secondary to drug therapy, but autoimmune diseases or other systemic diseases, infections, and tubulointerstitial nephritis with uveitis (TINU) syndrome can also cause AIN. In older adults most cases of AIN are due to drugs. Even though virtually any drug can cause AIN, the most common culprits are antibiotics (especially penicillins, cephalosporins, and ciprofloxacin), proton pump inhibitors, NSAIDs, and diuretics.

Presentation

AIN presents with nonspecific signs and symptoms, including nausea, vomiting, and malaise, unless the patient has systemic signs of an allergic drug reaction such as fever or rash. Hematuria is rare and proteinuria is usually not significant, with the exception of NSAID-induced AIN, which can be accompanied by NS. Atypical presentations with minimal symptomatology require a higher index of suspicion seen in older adults—NSAIDs and proton pump inhibitors are frequent offenders.

Evaluation

In addition to the physical examination, serum creatinine levels have to be monitored. In the urine, sediment white cells, red cells, and white cell casts are typically seen. Eosinophilia may be present, but lacks sensitivity and specificity to help in the diagnosis of AIN. Glucosuria, high fractional excretion of sodium (> 1%), and RTA may be present indicating renal tubular cell damage. A kidney biopsy may be considered in situations where the diagnosis of AIN would change management.

Management

The most important intervention when drug-induced AIN is suspected is to stop the offending agent. Consider medications that have been recently initiated, but in the absence of recent exposure to a new drug, medications to consider among those that have been used for a longer periods include proton pump inhibitors.

Drugs Corticosteroid therapy has been shown to improve outcomes if initiated within 14 days after first symptoms. Even though the recommended dose is equivalent to treatment of GN or vasculitis, lower doses used for allergic dermatitis should have the same effect in the kidney.

Prevention

To prevent AIN, medications with known higher-than-average risk of AIN—in particular proton pump inhibitors—should only be prescribed if and for as long as needed.

Special Issues

Patient preference To limit complications, the use of corticosteroids in AIN treatment regimens should be limited in length and to the lowest effective dose, even if the efficiency of lower doses remains uncertain.

Comorbidity AIN can present with systemic symptoms, in particular skin rash and peripheral eosinophilia. In rare cases, involvement of the airways in the allergic reaction can cause bronchospasm.

RENOVASCULAR DISEASE

Definition

Renovascular disease is anatomic narrowing of a main renal artery (renal artery stenosis) or its branches and can cause secondary hypertension and progressive renal insufficiency. Renal artery stenosis may be asymptomatic or cause hypertension and ischemic nephropathy. Renovascular hypertension is defined as the elevation of blood pressure secondary to compromised arterial circulation of the renal parenchyma causing chronic renal hypoperfusion. Ischemic nephropathy can be defined as a reduction in kidney function resulting from a partial or complete luminal obstruction of the preglomerular renal arteries of any caliber.

Epidemiology

Renovascular hypertension is a common cause of potentially remediable secondary hypertension in older patients with an estimated prevalence of 2% to 3% in the general hypertensive population and perhaps as much as 40% of those with refractory hypertension.

Pathophysiology

Atherosclerosis accounts for almost 90% of cases in the geriatric population, with fibrous dysplasia comprising the rest, but the spectrum of diseases that can cause renovascular

TABLE 83-3 ■ CATEGORIES OF RENAL ARTERY DISEASE

Aneurysms
Arteriovenous malformations
Atherosclerosis
Dissection of the aorta
Embolic disease
Fibrous dysplasia
Kawasaki disease
Neurofibromatosis
Other systemic necrotizing vasculitides
Polyarteritis nodosa
Takayasu arteritis
Thromboangiitis obliterans
Thrombotic diseases
Trauma
Vasculitis involving the renal artery

Modified with permission from Greco BA, Breyer JA. The natural history of renal artery stenosis: who should be evaluated for suspected ischemic nephropathy? Semin Nephrol. 1996;16(1):2–11.

disease includes many different diseases (**Table 83-3**). Atheroembolic renal disease falls into the category of renal insufficiency induced by preglomerular ischemia. This entity has been usually described in patients with clinical evidence of atheromatous occlusive disease following invasive intra-aortic diagnostic or therapeutic procedures, although spontaneous embolic episodes have been reported.

Presentation

Findings that might prompt the clinicians to consider renal artery stenosis are onset of hypertension after the age of 50, notably diastolic hypertension, accelerated or difficult-to-control hypertension, coexisting diffuse atherosclerotic vascular disease and decreased GFR, acute or subacute increase in serum creatinine levels after initiation of therapy with ACEIs or ARBs, recurrent pulmonary edema, grades III to IV hypertensive retinopathy, abdominal or flank bruit, hypokalemia in the absence of diuretic use, erythrocytosis, microangiopathic hemolytic anemia, and hyperuricemia.

Acute or subacute fall in GFR (rise in serum creatinine) can be precipitated by treatment of hypertension with ACEIs or ARBs during a period of days to weeks after initiating therapy. It is associated with hypoperfusion of the kidneys caused by inhibition of angiotensin II–dependent autoregulatory pathways in the glomerulus. Even so many patients with renovascular disease tolerate these agents and do not require additional noninvasive studies. The role of direct-renin inhibitors and renal artery stenosis has not been defined. Patients with suspected or documented renovascular hypertension and poorly controlled hypertension may present with progressive azotemia or with recurrent pulmonary edema (23% prevalence in some series).

Azotemia in an older patient that cannot be explained by other renal diseases—in particular in the setting of worsening renal failure, bland urinary sediment, proteinuria

(< 1 g/day), hypertension, and evidence of peripheral vascular disease—should prompt an evaluation for renovascular disease. It is not clear what proportion of the dialysis population have renovascular disease as the underlying cause of ESKD.

Evaluation

The diagnosis of renovascular hypertension is based on the demonstration of renal artery stenosis (usually by angiography or CT angiography), pathophysiologic significance of the stenotic lesion, and correction of the hypertension by an intervention that relieves the stenosis.

Duplex ultrasound scanning also allows scanning of the renal arteries and measurement of kidney size and is not affected by medications or the level of GFR. The reported sensitivity and specificity values are in the low- to mid-90% range. The disadvantage of this test is that it is technically demanding and has a steep learning curve for each center that performs this test.

Magnetic resonance angiography (MRA) has been effective in screening for the presence of renal artery stenosis with the advantage of having less exposure to contrast media and less invasive than the arteriogram. However, patients with CKD exposed to gadolinium and developing nephrogenic systemic fibrosis (NSF) have been described in case series. Therefore, MRA for defining renal artery stenosis in patients with CKD is infrequent and carefully considered. Another highly accurate noninvasive study for screening for renal artery stenosis is the spiral (helical) CT scan with CT angiography. However, there is a risk of contrast nephropathy with the spiral CT scan in patients with CKD.

ACEI radionuclide scintirenography using technetium-99m diethylenetriamine penta-acetic acid (^{99m}Tc-DTPA) has shown high sensitivity and specificity for renovascular hypertension. Two limitations should be kept in mind: (1) these tests have not been evaluated in patients with azotemia, and (2) while a positive test predicts an improvement in blood pressure, it is not known whether it also predicts an improvement in renal function.

The gold standard for diagnosing renal artery stenosis is renal angiography. Intra-arterial digital subtraction angiography (IA-DSA) or a CO_2 angiogram also provides excellent anatomic detail and requires less contrast than conventional angiography. The technique of intravenous DSA, although less invasive, does not provide comparable resolution to the aforementioned tests because of the high degree of bowel gas and motility artifacts, and usually requires a significantly larger amount of nephrotoxic contrast material.

The second step in making the diagnosis of renovascular hypertension is to determine the pathophysiologic significance of the lesion. Some of the diagnostic tests already mentioned are also used to assess this issue. Selective renal vein renin measurement is the gold standard for establishing the functional nature of the stenotic lesion and helps predict the blood pressure response to revascularization. In general, a renal vein renin ratio of greater than or equal to 1.5 between the two renal veins is predictive of a beneficial blood pressure response following surgery or angioplasty, but failure to lateralize does not predict a negative response. Overall, the blood pressure response to revascularization cannot be determined with confidence by using renal vein renin measurements.

Management

Renovascular disease can remain stable or worsen over time. Of patients with renal artery stenosis, up to 50% can expect their stenosis to worsen, with reports of up to 5% per year. In general, the rate of progression of renal insufficiency and the likelihood of deterioration of renal function correlates with the extent of stenosis at the time of diagnosis. Older adult patients who develop ESKD secondary to progressive atherosclerotic renal artery obstruction have poor survival.

Medical therapy is universally accepted first-line treatment for renal artery stenosis. The approach to patients with RAS should address hypertension, as well as anti-platelet, hyperlipidemia, and hyperglycemia therapies. ACE inhibitors and ARBs have improved the likelihood of blood pressure control among patients with RAS. Therapy must be further individualized and based on the general status of the patient, the presence of any concomitant disease, and the local surgical or angiographic experience of the center.

In the presence of unilateral renal artery stenosis and at least moderately decreased GFR, the latter is usually not improved by intervention. In the Cardiovascular Outcomes in Renal Atherosclerotic Lesions (CORAL) trial, which included 947 patients, there was no benefit to revascularization versus medical management. Those patients assigned to revascularization in CORAL had similar primary composite outcomes after a median follow-up of 3.6 years. The meta-analysis of the trials comparing revascularization to medical management also demonstrates no benefit.

In bilateral stenosis, there are a number of possible clinical presentations and the approaches are informed by scarce data given that the revascularization trials for RAS were largely unilateral and stable disease. The first clinical presentation is bilateral occlusion of the renal arteries. This situation does not necessarily imply irreversible damage because the viability of the kidneys may be maintained by a collateral blood supply. This is particularly true in patients who have a gradual onset of arterial occlusion. Clinical findings suggesting parenchymal salvageability include the following: angiographic demonstration of retrograde filling of the distal renal arterial system by collateral vessels; renal biopsy showing preserved glomerular architecture; kidney size greater than 9 cm by ultrasound; and function of the involved kidney on renal scintigraphy. Some centers perform kidney biopsies in surgical candidates if their serum creatinine is higher than 4 mg/dL. In patients with serum creatinine less than 3 mg/dL, improved renal function (defined as a reduction in serum creatinine of > 20% from the baseline value) can be expected post-revascularization in nearly half of patients undergoing this procedure.

The second scenario is bilateral stenosis without total occlusion or stenosis in a solitary kidney. Improvement in renal function is frequently seen after reconstructive surgery in 75% to 89% of these patients. Unlike cases with total renal occlusion, revascularization to preserve renal function is not worthwhile in patients with severe renal insufficiency (serum creatinine > 4 mg/dL) because they usually have advanced underlying renal parenchymal disease (nephrosclerosis and/or atheroembolic disease), which is not improved by revascularization. In older patients, atherosclerosis of large vascular structures poses additional challenges to bypass procedures. Considering the significant risks of progressive renal occlusive disease and renal failure that are associated with medical management of this condition, surgical options for treatment may be considered.

Initially percutaneous transluminal renal angioplasty (PTRA) had a limited role in older patients because of the concomitant presence of aortic atherosclerotic disease, making any endovascular procedure hazardous and technically difficult. Restenosis following dilatation of atheromatous lesions was quite common and a significant number of older patients present with ostial lesions, which are not amenable to PTRA. PTRA with the use of endovascular stenting devices have come into vogue with improved outcome of the revascularization of these ostial lesions. Surgical intervention is presently recommended for more complicated lesions, or angioplasty failures. One advantage of angioplasty over surgery is that it can be undertaken in patients who have prohibitively high surgical risks that are related to systemic atherosclerosis.

Prevention

Renovascular disease can be prevented by the same measures that prevent atherosclerosis, in particular smoking cessation, exercise, and control of hyperlipidemia.

Special Issues

Patient preference Even though interventions have not provided benefits in outcome, in specific patients an intervention may be considered if it improves quality of life to reduce side effects of antihypertensive medications.

END-STAGE KIDNEY DISEASE (ESKD)

Definition

End-stage kidney disease (ESKD), or kidney failure, has been defined as having kidney function less than 15 mL/min/1.73 m^2. Causes of ESKD are usually progression of a CKD or by AKI. It is associated with the inability to excrete waste products, control serum electrolytes, handle the daily dietary and metabolic acid load, and maintain fluid balance. In addition, kidney failure causes inadequate production of erythropoietin, deranged calcium and phosphorous metabolism, high blood pressure, and accelerated progression of cardiovascular disease.

Most etiologies of CKD demonstrate a progression to kidney failure and variability in rate and trajectory of progression among individuals with kidney disease. The rates of decline in kidney function vary by underlying nephropathy, by severity of hypertension and albuminuria, by modifying factors, and between individuals. Historically, the rate of decline could be estimated as 7 to 10 mL/min/year in those with untreated chronic nephropathies such as DN. However, chronic nephropathies have similar effects on electrolyte homeostasis, causes of progressive decline in function, and manifestations of kidney failure so that classification by severity permits a better understanding of underlying routes to progression, symptoms, and hopefully, treatments of CKD.

Epidemiology

The prevalence of kidney failure is substantial worldwide; approximately 10% to 13% of the adult population in North America, Europe, and Asia are estimated to have some form of CKD based on meta-analysis and meta-regression. The majority of those with CKD stages 1 and 2 may not be aware of their kidney disease. The number of patients at risk for developing kidney disease will increase with the increasing prevalence of diabetes and the aging of the population.

The prevalence of older people with kidney failure has been driven by an increased incidence of kidney failure, greater access to renal replacement therapy (RRT), and improved survival of both dialysis patients and kidney transplant recipients. A substantial proportion of patients in the United States receiving hemodialysis are aged 65 and older (**Figure 83-2**). This has been a worldwide phenomenon with a marked increase in the rate of incident dialysis patients older than 75 years over the past two decades. Similar rates of increase of kidney failure in older adults have been noted in Europe and Japan with a marked increase in octogenarian hemodialysis patients in Japan. Once referred for kidney failure, older patients have been surviving longer with RRT as dialysis treatment and kidney transplant outcomes have improved. As a result of improvements in technology and greater access to dialysis, the increased prevalence of older adults undergoing RRT generally mirrors the aging trend of the general population.

Referral of Patients to Nephrology

The Kidney Disease: Improving Global Outcomes (K/DIGO) guidelines recommend that patients with progressive CKD should be managed in a multidisciplinary setting. These guidelines advise involvement of a nephrologist under the following circumstances: AKI, GFR less than 30 mL/min/1.73 m^2, consistent findings of significant albuminuria, progression of CKD, urinary red cell casts, CKD and refractory hypertension, persistent abnormalities of potassium, recurrent or extensive nephrolithiasis, and hereditary kidney disease. The aim is to provide time for the nephrology team to provide an individualized care plan consistent with the goals of the older patient with CKD. Older patients with worsening CKD have a wide spectrum of choices for the treatment of kidney failure. Once therapy has been selected, some of the treatments require lead time prior to the development of an indication for dialysis, hence the need for early nephrology involvement.

CKD and Management of Chronic Health Conditions

Since liberalizing access to dialysis and kidney transplantation, there has been a steady shift for this population

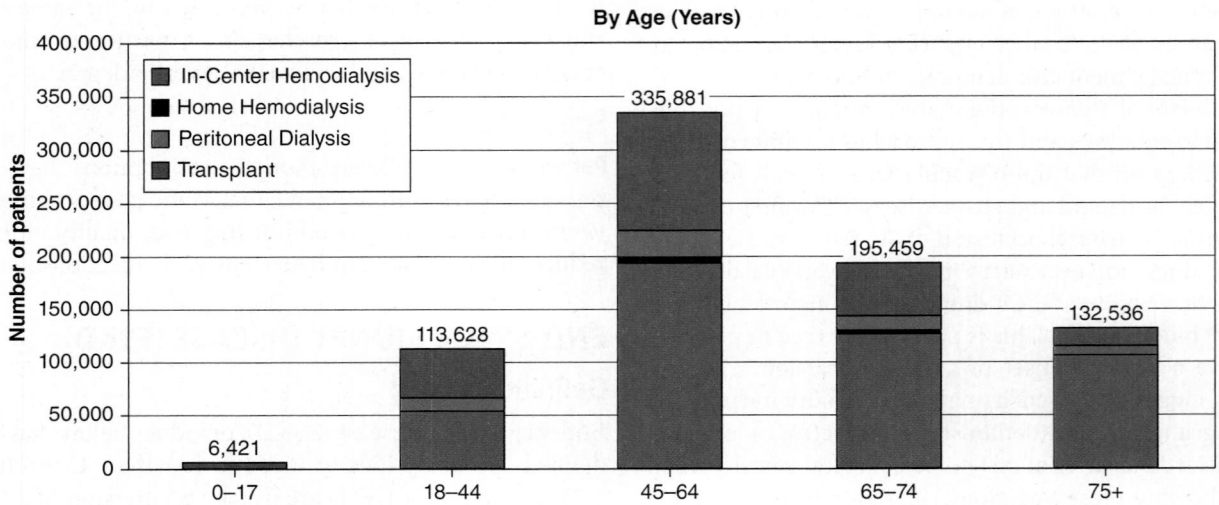

FIGURE 83-2. Distribution of treatment modality among prevalent ESRD patients by age. (Reproduced with permission from United States Renal Data System. *2020 USRDS Annual Data Report: Epidemiology of kidney disease in the United States.* National Institutes of Health, National Institute of Diabetes and Digestive and Kidney Diseases. Bethesda, MD, 2020.)

to include not only older patients, but also to those with multiple chronic conditions. Given the complexity of managing older patients with a high burden of comorbid disease, the primacy care/geriatrics team has the opportunity to play a crucial role in the care of these patients. Patients with advanced CKD often have been shown to have gaps in their primary health care, diabetes care, and cardiovascular disease care. There are also gaps in nutrition, fall prevention, management of depression, and frailty among older patients undergoing dialysis.

Indications for Initiation of Dialysis

The most common symptoms that present before initiation of maintenance dialysis in older patients tend to be anorexia, weight loss, fatigue, nausea, and vomiting. The recognition of uremia in the older patient, however, may prove difficult. Behavioral changes, unexplained impaired cognition, "adult failure to thrive," unexplained worsening of congestive heart failure, or a change in sense of well-being may be a manifestation of uremia in the geriatric patient.

While timely initiation of RRT avoids the need for urgent dialysis, clinical trials of earlier initiation of dialysis (GFR 10–15 mL/min/1.73 m^2) have shown no significant benefit compared to later initiation (GFR 7 mL/min/ 1.73 m^2). A strong correlation between "baseline" serum albumin just prior to initiation of dialysis and patient survival has been demonstrated. Although hypoalbuminemia itself does not necessarily indicate protein-energy malnutrition, it is believed to be a major contributing factor. Analysis of the Modification of Diet in Renal Disease (MDRD) study showed that patients tend to adapt to their declining GFR and associated uremic symptoms by reducing their protein intake. Nevertheless, approximately 60% of American ESKD patients experience nausea and vomiting at the time dialysis is initiated.

Contraindications to Renal Replacement Therapy

It may be reasonable not to start or to stop dialysis for older patients with a very poor prognosis or who cannot be dialyzed safely. For the practitioner, there are few absolute medical contraindications to RRT. Some propose that advanced dementia, metastatic cancer, heart failure with marked hypotension, and advanced liver diseases are reasons for withholding RRT. However, progressive dementia can be confused with uremia-induced delirium in a patient with advanced kidney dysfunction, and a "trial" of dialysis may be justified. It may take as long as 3 to 4 weeks to clear uremic symptoms with dialysis. The patient's family should be aware that if the patient's mental status fails to improve, RRT may be inappropriate. Similarly, providing dialysis for a patient with metastatic cancer or end-stage liver disease may allow the patient to get their affairs in order and spend some important time with friends and family. Cognitive and behavioral contraindications may play an even larger role in older patients than medical contraindications. Dialysis units are communities where a patient with inappropriate,

unsafe, or violent behavior may adversely affect care provided to others at that unit.

Health-Related Quality of Life (HRQOL)

Maintaining health-related quality of life (HRQOL) is very meaningful for older patients with chronic illness. Studies of older patients undergoing dialysis have shown markedly lower functional status compared to older community-dwelling adults. However, hemodialysis has improved since these early studies and there have been advances in technology, treatment of comorbidities such as anemia and hyperparathyroidism, and quality improvement initiatives that have improved the HRQOL of patients on dialysis. As shown in **Figure 83-3**, there is evidence of both decrements in physical and mental well-being associated with dialysis compared to the general population across regions. While there is a marked decrement in physical well-being with older age, there are similar scores for physical well-being across age groups. These findings may be informative to older patients and health care providers and they also underline the need to improve HRQOL among all patients undergoing dialysis. Interventions aimed at preserving residual kidney function, monitoring HRQOL, treatment of anemia, engaging the patient in physical therapy and rehabilitation, applying palliative care principles, and perhaps more frequent and longer hemodialysis treatments may preserve HRQOL among older patients undergoing hemodialysis.

CHOICE OF RENAL REPLACEMENT THERAPY

When faced with kidney failure, the older patient has a number of choices to make regarding therapy consistent with their overall level of well-being and goals of care. The most common forms of kidney replacement in the United States are three-times weekly outpatient hemodialysis, peritoneal dialysis (PD), and renal transplantation. There has also been a proliferation of home therapies and therapies tailored to older patients such as nursing home–based dialysis units. The older patient may also choose conservative management and thereby avoid dialysis or opt for palliative care. The patients should have time to develop a relationship with the nephrologist and team in order to have discussions of goals for care and how RRT may be tailored to meet those goals.

Hemodialysis

Hemodialysis removes excess fluids and solutes from the blood in order to maintain euvolemia and homeostasis. The conventional hemodialysis schedule requires three treatments per week for approximately 4 hours per treatment. In order to perform hemodialysis, the patient must have an access placed to circulate the blood through the hemodialysis filter. The three options for hemodialysis access include arteriovenous (AV) fistula, AV graft, and temporary hemodialysis catheters. Permanent hemodialysis

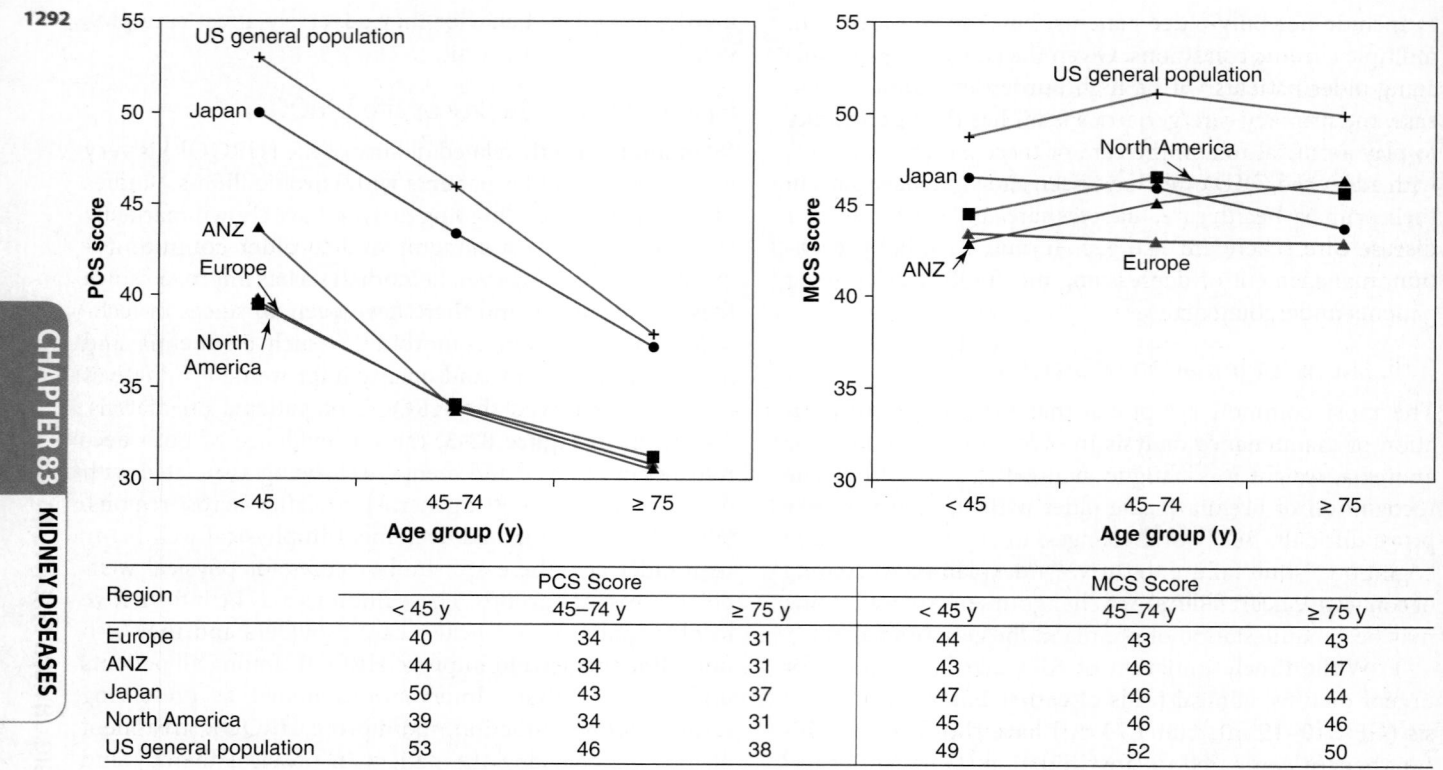

Region	PCS Score			MCS Score		
	< 45 y	45–74 y	≥ 75 y	< 45 y	45–74 y	≥ 75 y
Europe	40	34	31	44	43	43
ANZ	44	34	31	43	46	47
Japan	50	43	37	47	46	44
North America	39	34	31	45	46	46
US general population	53	46	38	49	52	50

FIGURE 83-3. Kidney disease quality of life (KDQOL) physical component summary (PCS) and mental component summary (MCS) scores by age categories across Dialysis Outcomes and Practice Patterns Study (DOPPS) regions versus US population norm. Cross-section of participants in DOPPS III (2005–2007; *n* = 8161). Europe includes United Kingdom, France, Germany, Italy, Spain, Belgium, and Sweden; North America includes United States and Canada; ANZ represents Australia and New Zealand. (Adapted from Canaud B, Tong L, Tentori F, et al. Clinical practices and outcomes in elderly hemodialysis patients: results from the Dialysis Outcomes and Practice Patterns Study (DOPPS). *Clin J Am Soc Nephrol.* 2011;6[7]:1651–1662.)

access requires minor surgery in the arm or leg. The AV fistula, which creates a connection between the native artery and the AV fistula vein, matures and thickens to handle the higher blood flow rates and permit the use of a needle for access after approximately 3 months. The use of an AV fistula has been associated with better access survival, fewer infections, fewer hospitalizations, and longer patient survival. The AV graft uses a synthetic bridge between the artery and the vein. The graft has been used in a broader population than the AV fistula but has the major limitations of shorter access survival as well as more infections and hospitalizations. For patients who have been referred late or who have acute kidney failure, hemodialysis is performed using a dialysis catheter. This is typically a large-bore catheter placed in a major vessel such as the superior vena cava. In the outpatient setting, these catheters are usually tunneled under the skin and treated with sterile precautions by the dialysis unit when accessing the catheters for blood. They have been associated with high rates of bacteremia, catheter malfunction, venous stenosis, and increased costs. Despite the increased rate of complications with grafts and catheters, the older adult should participate

in shared decision-making to select an access as the delayed maturation of a fistula may prove unsatisfactory to someone with a limited life expectancy. By far, in-center hemodialysis remains the predominant form of dialysis in the United States. While most patients maintain a certain quality of life on hemodialysis, the drawbacks include pain, fatigue, depression, loss of freedom, dietary and fluid restrictions, and concern about burden to caregivers.

Peritoneal Dialysis

PPD permits older patients to maintain more control over their schedule and play a larger role in the management of their kidney failure. PD uses the peritoneal membrane as a dialysis membrane by drawing excess fluid and toxins from the blood and into the peritoneal cavity where the fluid will then be drained through a plastic catheter that has been placed into the abdomen. Depending on the dialysis prescription, the peritoneal cavity is filled with fluid and drained a number of times over the course of the day or night. The advantages to using PD include a less-restrictive diet and avoiding the need to travel to a dialysis unit for treatment. The disadvantages of PD include back pain, peritonitis, hyperglycemia, obesity, and hernia formation. PD has been successfully used in older patients, but its use in patients with poor functional status depends on a caregiver willing to commit to performing the daily therapy. PD can also be performed safely and effectively in a long-term care facility by staff with specialized training and with assistance of medical staff or caregiver. The preferred mode of PD in this setting is continuous cyclic PD or nocturnal PD, which requires less nursing time, allows patients to be more fully integrated into social activities, and allows interruption-free intensive rehabilitation.

Kidney Transplantation

Kidney transplantation is a potential therapy for patients with ESKD, and the percentage of patients awaiting kidney transplantation has increased among older adults compared to all other age groups. As shown in **Figure 83-4**, among those older than 75 established on a kidney-transplant waitlist, fewer than 40% receive either a living or deceased kidney transplant in the subsequent 5 years. Overall life expectancy increases for older patients post kidney transplantation compared to those who are on dialysis and on the waitlist for a kidney transplant. Older patients with comorbidities such as diabetes and hypertension also have a survival advantage with kidney transplantation compared to those who remain on the waitlist on dialysis.

Health-related quality of life also improves for older patients after kidney transplant. Transplant patients older than age 65 have been shown to have significantly higher scores in physical functioning, general health perception, and mental health compared to hemodialysis patients. The older individual is not the only one to benefit from kidney transplant—health care systems also benefit, as the cost of care decreases.

Older individuals may have less rejection after kidney transplantation secondary to changes in both adaptive and innate immunity. However, as both T- and B-cell immunities are dampened with aging, transplantation is associated with a higher risk of infection in older adults.

For the older patient seeking a kidney transplant, screening for cognitive function and physical performance tests to better assess frailty should be part of the evaluation process. Physical performance tests can help screen older patients for the risk of falls, hospitalizations, and death posttransplantation.

The degree to which comorbidity influences graft and patient outcomes is significantly less in recipients of living donor kidneys compared to recipients of deceased donor kidneys. A living donor kidney may offset some of the risk of increased comorbidity in the older recipient and highlights living donor kidney transplantation as an opportunity for older patients with kidney failure to receive optimal treatment.

Time-Limited Trial of Dialysis

One of the options for older patients with ESKD would be to have a trial of hemodialysis to assess the extent to which the treatment is consistent with the life goals of the patient. The approach of a time-limited trial is reasonable when the patient, family, or physician is unsure about the prognosis or the impact that dialysis will have upon the patient's quality of life. If a trial of dialysis is to be conducted, it is important to predetermine a time period (usually 4–6 weeks) and to inform all the members of the dialysis team. Such measures will ease the appropriate withdrawal from dialysis and may also help to resolve conflicts when a consensus cannot be reached for the best approach to managing an older patient with ESKD.

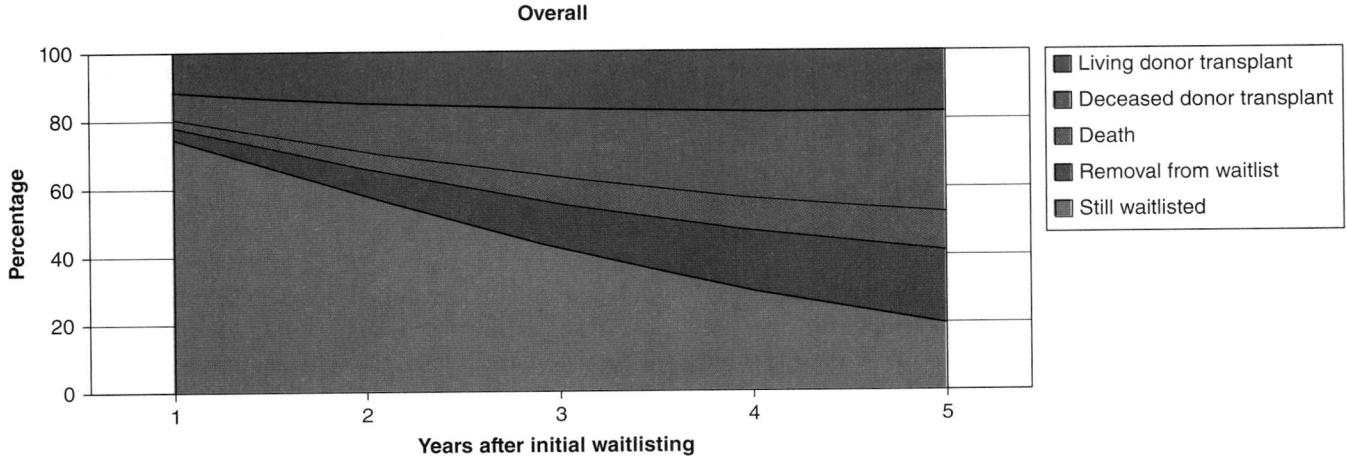

FIGURE 83-4. Yearly distribution of living donor transplantation, deceased donor transplantation, death, and removal from the waitlist after initial waitlisting for those greater than 75 years of age, 2009 to 2013. (Reproduced with permission from United States Renal Data System. *2020 USRDS Annual Data Report: Epidemiology of kidney disease in the United States.* National Institutes of Health, National Institute of Diabetes and Digestive and Kidney Diseases, Bethesda, MD, 2020.)

Conservative Management (Nondialytic Treatment) and Palliative Care

The approach to managing older adults who chose to forgo RRT is twofold. Comprehensive conservative therapy or nondialytic treatment is focused on maximal medical management of CKD and the metabolic complications of advanced CKD. While this aspect of care is focused on slowing the progression of kidney disease, palliative care or supportive care treats symptoms and addresses the psychological, spiritual, and social needs of the patient. In very old patients and in frail older patients, there may be similar outcomes in terms of mortality and quality of life between those getting dialysis and conservative management.

Conservative management should aim to maintain quality of life while keeping in mind the shared decision to avoid dialysis therapy. In addition to continuing to manage fluid status, anemia, electrolytes, and bone metabolism, symptoms should be addressed by the geriatric, nephrology, and palliative care teams. Between both groups of patients undergoing dialysis and receiving palliative care, symptoms should be treated since pain, dry itchy skin, poor sleep, and fatigue impact mood and quality of life. A nutritional approach to avoiding dialysis therapy has shown that the dietary intervention can provide an additional 6 to 12 months off dialysis. This suggests that nutrition and palliative approaches play an important role in managing patients who elect to avoid dialysis.

MANAGEMENT OF END-STAGE RENAL DISEASE COMPLICATIONS

Anemia

Anemia is a common problem with CKD and kidney failure. The cause of anemia may be multifactorial and due to both CKD and other chronic conditions. In addition to CKD, one should consider iron deficiency due to loss of blood from the gastrointestinal (GI) tract or hematologic etiologies. Among older patients with CKD, the fall in hematocrit correlates roughly with the severity of the renal disease, although individual variation is considerable. In general, anemia develops when the GFR is around 35 mL/min. The bone marrow is hypoproliferative while peripheral blood (red cell) indices are normal unless there is superimposed deficiency of iron or folic acid. Thus, the anemia seen with kidney failure is typically a normochromic, normocytic anemia. The lack of erythropoietin production is the primary cause of anemia with kidney failure. Erythropoietin levels are inadequate with CKD, thus depriving the bone marrow of the stimulus necessary for production of red blood cells. The isolation of human erythropoietin and subsequent production of recombinant erythropoietin has been a major advance in the care of those with CKD. Since 1989, synthetic erythropoietin has been available and effectively treats the anemia of chronic renal failure. Darbepoetin permits less frequent dosing regimens and other agents are under investigation. Hypoxia-inducible factor prolyl hydroxylase inhibitors (HIF PHI) are a class of oral agents that stabilize HIF and promote red blood cell production. A growing number studies have demonstrated noninferiority compared to erythropoietin-based therapies for correction of hemoglobin and mixed results when examining the impact of HIF PHI on cardiovascular events.

Correction of anemia has been associated with improved quality of life, reduced the need for transfusions, improved cognitive performance, and decreased left ventricular hypertrophy. There are adverse effects of using erythropoietin in the CKD patient, including iron deficiency (the stimulation of red blood cell production outstrips iron stores), hypertension, cardiovascular events, and vascular thrombosis.

The optimal hemoglobin target for patients with anemia caused by CKD remains somewhat unclear. The current conservative target is a hemoglobin level near 11.5 mg/dL. In addition to close attention to erythropoietin dosing and hemoglobin levels, adequate anemia management requires routine analysis and treatment of iron deficiency. Iron levels tend to drop in patients on erythropoietin therapy because of increased iron utilization. Iron-deficient ESKD patients usually receive intravenous replacement iron at the end of their dialysis treatments. Because they absorb oral iron poorly, ESKD patients have "functional" iron deficiency when their ferritin falls below 500 ng/mL or their iron saturation is less than 30%.

Cardiovascular Disease

Many more patients have CKD compared to the numbers receiving RRT. The disparity between the number receiving RRT and the number with CKD is explained in part by the high mortality from cardiovascular disease prior to needing dialysis in the CKD population. While on dialysis, the risk of death from cardiovascular disease remains 10 to 100 times higher than the risk of a person from the general population. While traditional risk factors account for only a portion of the increased risk associated with kidney disease, the etiology of the increased cardiovascular risk is unclear. There are a number of potential factors that represent classical risk factors shared between atherosclerosis and kidney disease such as age, hypercholesterolemia, hypertension, diabetes mellitus, smoking, and obesity. In addition, there are a number of factors specific to kidney failure such as anemia, hyperhomocysteinemia, hypervolemia, and hyperparathyroidism. These factors can act to promote both cardiomyopathy and ischemic heart disease. The current treatment recommendations focus on optimizing management of known cardiovascular risk factors and on recognizing harbingers of active cardiovascular disease. While guidelines recommend using statins among patients with CKD, a reasonable course would be to individualize cardiovascular disease care for older patients with ESKD. Those caring for patients with CKD should consider cardiovascular disease management as an important part of their care.

Calcium, Phosphorous, Hyperparathyroidism, and Bone Disorders

Kidney failure is associated with abnormalities of divalent ions (Ca^{2+}, P) and of the hormones that regulate the concentration of these minerals in body fluids. One of the earliest detectable abnormalities in kidney failure is a rise in PTH, which can occur at a GFR of 40 mL/min. Secondary hyperparathyroidism is a major cause of bone disease in patients with kidney failure. Two inhibitors of PTH are ionized calcium (the active form of calcium) and 1,25-$(OH)_2D_3$, which has an independent inhibitory effect on PTH release. No difference has been found in hyperphosphatemia or severity of renal osteodystrophy in older dialysis patients as compared with younger dialysis patients, and there is no correlation between plasma 1,25-dihydroxyvitamin D_3 levels and age in patients with kidney failure. Older female dialysis patients have significantly lower bone mineral content and bone width when compared with younger dialysis patients matched for duration of dialysis. There is a higher incidence of pathologic fracture, vascular or metastatic calcification, and bone pain in older patients on dialysis than in younger patients. The overall result of these disturbances is that patients with ESKD may develop a complex form of bone disease—renal osteodystrophy. Furthermore, there has been a strong association of disordered bone and mineral metabolism and risk of cardiovascular disease. This association between calcium and phosphate metabolism has been most striking when images of the heart demonstrating extensive calcification have been related to levels of both calcium and phosphate.

The management of bone disorders among older patients with ESKD is complicated by other bone diseases found among this age group. For example, osteoporosis and renal osteodystrophy may both present in the older patient with ESKD. Treatment of renal osteodystrophy and secondary hyperparathyroidism in the geriatric renal patient is similar to the younger patients. Hyperphosphatemia is treated with a low-phosphate diet and with various phosphate binders. Refractory hyperparathyroidism can be treated with parathyroidectomy or with a trial of a calcimimetic. While the agents used to regulate calcium and phosphate levels remain controversial, the goals of normalizing calcium and phosphate levels and improving bone health are widely accepted as important in the management of CKD patients.

Cognitive Impairment

Cognitive impairment is prevalent among patients with ESKD, especially as patients age. The potential causes of cognitive impairment in patients with CKD might be explained by two hypotheses. The vascular hypothesis states that the brain and the kidneys are low-resistance end organs exposed to highly pulsatile blood flow which is exacerbated by CKD and thus are susceptible to microvascular damage that contributes to the cognitive impairment in CKD patients. The neurodegenerative hypothesis states that the accumulation of uremic toxins in ESKD patients impairs the functions of the central nervous system in this population.

Cognitive impairment in ESKD is associated with decreased quality of life, suboptimal medical care, decreased adherence to medication regimens and dietary modifications, more frequent and prolonged hospitalizations, and decreased decision-making capacity, especially in making very important health-related decisions. This underlines the need for periodic screening to accurately identify ESKD patients with cognitive impairment in order to improve their clinical care. Recognizing and addressing cognitive impairment in ESKD may lead to improved adherence to treatment, increased ability to make informed medical decisions, decreased rate and length of hospitalization, decreased morbidity and mortality, and improved health-related quality of life.

Malnutrition

Nutrition plays an important role in the health and well-being of patients with kidney failure. Poor nutrition in older patients can be linked to dietary restrictions for ESKD patients, compounded with challenges of access to foods, difficulty with food preparation, medication side effects, and decrements in appetite. Patients with kidney failure benefit from close monitoring of nutritional status. The recommended assessments include but not limited to periodic check of body weight, dietary interviews, and serum albumin levels. A renal dietician may offer alternative foods and recommendations to patients that feel limited by fluid, sodium, potassium, and phosphate restrictions. Weight loss and inability to maintain nutritional status are indications for initiating hemodialysis and adequacy of dialysis therapy should be evaluated to avoid anorexia and nausea. Dietary supplements and vitamin and mineral supplements, such as zinc or oral pyridoxine (50 mg/day), might be helpful. Adherence to a regimented diet, in the older patient should be balanced against adequate protein and calorie intake.

Physical Functioning and Frailty

Most older individuals with ESKD have some degree of functional decline or frailty which are associated with high risk for falls, disability, hospitalization, and mortality. Among patients initiating dialysis, frailty has been associated with increased risk of death and shorter time to first hospitalization. Several potential mechanisms have been suggested to explain the association of ESKD with poor functional status and frailty. Elevated inflammatory markers, poor nutritional status, weight loss, and sarcopenia as well as complications related to ESKD such as electrolyte and acid–base disturbances, hyperphosphatemia, anemia, and bone and mineral disorders are also linked to frailty in ESKD population. Management includes evaluation and treatment of reversible conditions attributable to frailty such as neglect, alcohol abuse, and depression. Resistance exercise training, improvement in nutritional status, and treatment of complications of CKD such as anemia are also suggested to address frailty.

Pruritus

Itching has been reported in up to 40% of patients with kidney failure and can adversely affect sleep and quality of life. The causes of itching in older patients with kidney failure include xerosis, uremic itching, and medication sensitivity. Pruritus is also common in the older dialysis patient, possibly because of skin changes seen with aging. As a part of an approach to managing uremic pruritis, it has been recommended to optimize dialysis treatment by increasing dialysis dose, treating anemia and iron deficiency, and maintaining a low serum phosphate. Treatment of itching caused by xerosis or uremia has been largely symptomatic local treatment consisting of keeping the skin protected and moist with standard skin care recommendations. In addition to these symptomatic approaches, topical capsaicin and pramoxine lotions may also be effective. Low-dose gabapentin has been shown to reduce uremic pruritus among patients with advanced CKD on hemodialysis. Kappa-opioid agonists have demonstrated efficacy reducing itch in randomized placebo-controlled trials among patients undergoing thrice-weekly hemodialysis. Finally, antihistamines such as diphenhydramine or hydroxyzine should be avoided if at all possible due to increased anti-cholinergic adverse events in this age group.

SPECIAL ISSUES

Prognosis and Survival

Kidney failure is associated with a decrease in life expectancy for all age groups when compared to age-matched patients. The survival of older patients undergoing dialysis has been recently assessed showing a 1-year survival rate for octogenarians and nonagenarians after dialysis initiation of 54%. The characteristics strongly associated with death were older age, nonambulatory status, comorbid conditions, and frailty. In addition to survival, it is important to convey the impact of dialysis on quality of life. It is important to convey the limited life expectancy of those patients who are not transplant candidates, and particularly those with limited functional status and comorbidity. Ultimately it remains up to the individual whether to pursue dialysis or palliative therapy.

There have been increasingly successful attempts to develop and test predictive survival models for outcomes of older patients with ESKD that could be used for shared decision-making. As one example, residing in a nursing home conveys a high risk of death in the first year of dialysis. As shown in **Figure 83-5**, 87% of nursing home residents died or experienced decreased

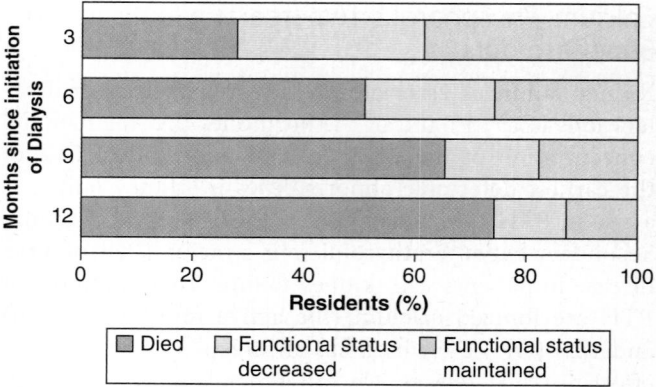

FIGURE 83-5. Change in functional status after initiation of dialysis. (Reproduced with permission from Kurella Tamura M, Covinsky KE, et al. Functional status of elderly adults before and after initiation of dialysis. *N Engl J Med*. 2009;361[16]:1539–1547.)

functional status within 1 year of starting hemodialysis. In addition to place of residence, clinicians can use functional status, other chronic health conditions, and frailty to improve their estimate of prognosis. Integrated prognostic models can provide additional precision by taking into account laboratory values, comorbidities, changes in clinical factors over time, functional status, frailty, quality of life, and either the patient's or clinician's prediction of survival. The "surprise question"—Would you be surprised if your patient died within the next 6 months?—is a strong indicator of mortality, and when combined with serum albumin, age, and two comorbid factors (dementia and peripheral vascular disease) results in an instrument with clinically adequate sensitivity and specificity. The application of prediction tools will help to overcome practitioner uncertainty about prognosis and increase the likelihood of meaningful dialogues between clinicians, older patients, and their families. However, there remains a critical gap among the existing predictive instruments since they uniformly assess only survival. Other issues such as quality of life, functional status, and independence are critical factors for older patients when deciding whether to proceed with RRT.

Withdrawal from Dialysis

Stopping dialysis has become a common reason for death in the dialysis population, especially for older patients. Up to one-third of patients are withdrawn or voluntarily withdraw from dialysis therapy annually. The factors associated with dialysis discontinuation in the United States include White race, diabetes, female sex, symptoms, and older age. The reasons cited for withdrawal from dialysis include failure to thrive and medical complications. While dialysis patients should understand that they have the right to stop treatment, the health care team should ensure that the patient is not withdrawing because of an underlying depression or "burdens" that can be ameliorated. It is important to document the decisional capacity of the older adult on dialysis wishing to withdraw and involve family and friends. While the end-of-life issues in renal failure have received increasing attention, there remain many barriers to management of these issues, as underscored by the fivefold lower use of hospice among patients undergoing hemodialysis compared to those older patients not using dialysis. In order to overcome the barriers to a good death for those on dialysis, it is important to have a multidisciplinary approach to advance care planning and an awareness of hospice services.

Advance Care Planning

Practice guidelines underscore that a complete review of treatment options, prognosis, and quality of life should be included when discussing advance directives of a patient with CKD stages 4 and 5. Having the patient's wishes expressed prior to starting dialysis makes the burden of decision-making much easier for the families and physicians should the patient become critically ill. It is crucial to involve the family and surrogates in the advance directives process and to fully document the directives in order to avoid a change in direction with an unplanned hospitalization. Patients who decide not to undergo dialysis should have clear documentation in their medical records. There

should be similar documentation of do-not-resuscitate orders, wishes regarding artificial nutrition and other measures, and identification of their health care surrogate.

SUMMARY

Providers of older adults face many challenging chronic conditions and CKD can be a primary kidney disease or a cotraveler with diabetes and hypertension. Similar to CKD, AKI is often found in older hospitalized patients and may be related to the primary illness such as sepsis or heart failure. The management of a patient with CKD can be optimized with the use of a multidisciplinary team and appropriate consultation. In most cases, medical management of CKD serves to delay kidney failure and avoid the need for dialysis. For those patients progressing to kidney failure, the management of complications such as anemia and nutrition can help sustain quality of life and functioning. In addressing the treatment options for kidney failure, the older patient faces a range of options from conservative medical management to transplantation and these decisions should be informed by shared decision-making. Primary care and geriatric teams will play a key role in addressing the long-term care and management of these complex medical problems.

FURTHER READING

Burns RB, Waikar SS, Wachterman MW, Kanjee Z. Management options for an older adult with advanced chronic kidney disease and dementia: grand rounds discussion from Beth Israel Deaconess Medical Center. *Ann Intern Med.* 2020;173(3):217–225.

Chertow GM, Pergola PE, Farag YMK, et al. Vadadustat in patients with anemia and non-dialysis-dependent CKD. *N Engl J Med.* 2021;384(17):1589–1600.

Cooper BA, Branley P, Bulfone L, et al. A randomized, controlled trial of early versus late initiation of dialysis. *N Engl J Med.* 2010;363(7):609–619.

Cooper CJ, Murphy TP, Cutlip DE, et al. Stenting and medical therapy for atherosclerotic renal-artery stenosis. *N Engl J Med.* 2014;370(1):13–22.

Hill NR, Fatoba ST, Oke JL, et al. Global prevalence of chronic kidney disease—a systematic review and meta-analysis. *PLoS One.* 2016;11(7):e0158765.

Kurella Tamura M, Covinsky KE, Chertow GM, Yaffe K, Landefeld CS, McCulloch CE. Functional status of elderly adults before and after initiation of dialysis. *N Engl J Med.* 2009;361(16):1539–1547.

Navaneethan SD, Zoungas S, Caramori ML, et al. Diabetes management in chronic kidney disease: synopsis of the 2020 KDIGO Clinical Practice Guideline. *Ann Intern Med.* 2021;174(3):385–394.

Vilaca T, Salam S, Schini M, et al. Risks of hip and non-vertebral fractures in patients with CKD G3a-G5D: a systematic review and meta-analysis. *Am J Kidney Dis.* 2020;76(4):521–532.

Wheeler DC, Stefánsson BV, Jongs N, et al. Effects of dapagliflozin on major adverse kidney and cardiovascular events in patients with diabetic and nondiabetic chronic kidney disease: a prespecified analysis from the DAPA-CKD trial. *Lancet Diabetes Endocrinol.* 2021;9(1):22–31.

Chapter 84

Aging of the Gastrointestinal System and Selected Lower GI Disorders

Karen E. Hall

Gastrointestinal (GI) symptoms are common in patients aged 65 and older and can range from mild self-limited episodes of constipation or acid reflux to life-threatening episodes of infectious colitis or bowel ischemia. According to data from the US Census Bureau in 2005, 45 to 50 million people older than age 65 had at least one GI complaint that impacted their daily life and might result in a medical visit. In older adults, GI disorders, especially those of the large intestine, account for a significant proportion of physician visits, inpatient hospitalizations, and health care expenditure in the United States. Not only are large intestinal disorders common, but in older adults their presentations, complications, and treatment may be different than in younger people. This chapter focuses on changes in the GI tract with aging, and diagnosis and treatment of a variety of intestinal diseases, including diverticular disease, *Clostridium difficile*–associated diarrhea, microscopic colitis, inflammatory bowel disease, colonic ischemia, colonic obstruction, and lower GI bleeding. Other chapters cover disorders of the upper GI tract (Chapter 85); hepatic, biliary and pancreatic diseases (Chapter 86); and constipation (Chapter 87). GI malignancies, such as gastric cancer and colonic cancer screening and treatment, are covered in Chapter 92.

AGING OF THE GASTROINTESTINAL SYSTEM

Older adults may present with unusual or subtle symptoms of serious GI disease due to alterations in physiology with aging. For example, a patient with a GI perforation or colitis may not have guarding or significant abdominal tenderness due to decreased visceral sensitivity.

Learning Objectives

- Understand the effects of aging on GI function.
- Recognize common presentations of GI dysfunction in older adults.
- Understand key differences in diagnosis and treatment for a variety of disorders of the large intestine between younger and older patients.
- Determine the most suitable evaluation and management plans for disorders of the large intestine frequently encountered in clinical practice.

Key Clinical Points

1. Dysmotility in the colon is common in older adults and is often due to a combination of effects of aging and superimposed disease.

2. Older patients with serious GI disease, such as intestinal ischemia or perforation, may present with subtle symptoms due to age-related visceral hyposensitivity. Thus, the severity of the condition may be underestimated.

3. The aging process per se has clinically significant effects on GI immunity and GI drug metabolism.

4. Advanced age is not a contraindication to gastrointestinal endoscopic procedures, and diagnostic testing is relatively high yield.

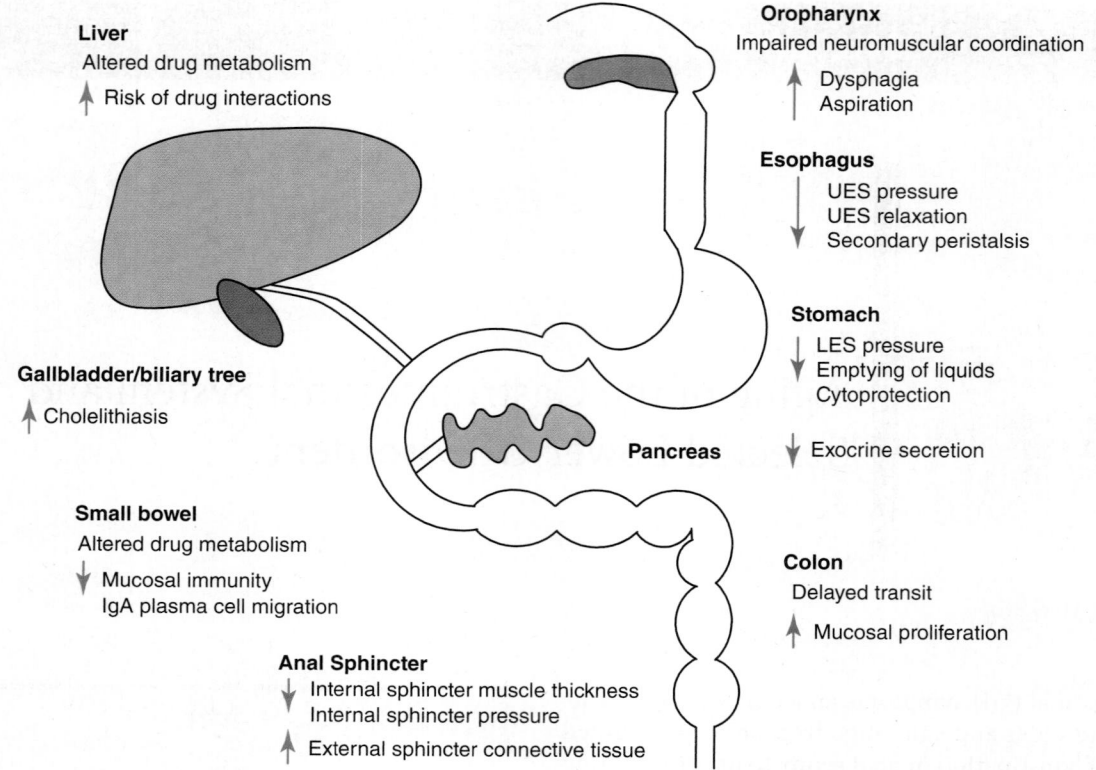

FIGURE 84-1. Effects of physiologic aging on the gastrointestinal tract. This schematic diagram summarizes significant effects of aging on various divisions of the gastrointestinal tract. *Key: up arrow,* increased; *down arrow,* decreased. LES, lower esophageal sphincter; UES, upper esophageal sphincter.

Some GI dysfunction in older patients can be attributed to the superimposed effects of chronic diseases and environmental/lifestyle exposures (medications, alcohol, tobacco). A modest decline in function with aging, such as mild constipation, may be significant when side effects of certain medications or concurrent disease are superimposed. The aging process per se has clinically significant effects on oropharyngeal and upper esophageal motility (see Chapter 31), colonic function, GI immunity, and GI drug metabolism (**Figure 84-1**). On the other hand, because the GI tract exhibits considerable reserve capacity, many aspects of GI function, such as intestinal secretion and absorption, are preserved with aging. A modest decline in gastric mucosal cytoprotection or esophageal acid clearance may become significant when superimposed side effects of certain medications or concurrent disease are also present. Common age-related changes in GI function, such as constipation, can be due to multiple causes such as medications, pelvic floor dysfunction, or comorbidities such as progressive neurodegenerative disorders. Additional research is needed on the effects of aging on the pathophysiology of swallowing disorders, esophageal reflux, dysmotility syndromes, GI immunobiology and microbiome, and the cellular mechanisms of neoplasia in the GI tract. Animal studies provide important insights into the cellular physiology of aging, despite the issue of species variation.

Small Intestinal Function

Small bowel function appears to be relatively preserved in normal human aging. The small intestine has a large functional reserve capacity, because of the substantial mucosal surface area available for secretion and absorption. Changes in small bowel epithelial development and intestinal absorption with aging have been described and are summarized in **Table 84-1**.

In the absence of significant small bowel damage or surgical resection, these changes are unlikely to result in significant weight loss or malnutrition.

Colonic Function

Aging is associated with diverse effects on the large intestine including alterations in mucosal cell growth, differentiation, metabolism, and immunity (**Table 84-2**).

These changes likely contribute to the observations of increased constipation and risk of malignancy in older adults.

Gastrointestinal Immunity

The GI tract is the largest immunological system in mammals. Older people appear to be more susceptible to infections that enter the body via the GI tract, suggesting that aging may impair mucosal immunity. The GI mucosal immune response in the small intestine is a

TABLE 84-1 ■ SMALL INTESTINAL FUNCTION

AGING EFFECTS ON SMALL INTESTINAL FUNCTION	CLINICAL IMPLICATIONS
Mucosal epithelial cell regeneration ↑ Crypt cell proliferation ↑	Uncertain
Maturation and expression of brush border enzymes ↓	May affect absorption during recovery from epithelial damage due to infection or inflammation
Specific activity of disaccharidases, aminopeptidases unchanged	Absorption of lactose, mannitol and lipid unaffected in age > 60 years
Rapidly absorbed proteins (eg, whey) ↑	Possible greater net protein gain
Specific micronutrient absorption ↓	Decreased uptake of vitamin D, folic acid, vitamin B_{12}, calcium, copper, zinc, fatty acids, cholesterol
Iron absorption ↓	Dietary iron content usually more than adequate to replace losses
Visceral chemosensitivity and hormone responsiveness ↑	Increased satiety

complex process that involves a series of events: antigen uptake and presentation of antigen at the mucosal surface by specialized epithelial cells (M cells) overlying Peyer patches in the small intestine; differentiation and migration of immunologically competent lymphocytes to the lamina propria; regulation of local antibody production in the intestinal wall; and mucosal epithelial cell receptor–mediated transport of antibodies to the intestinal lumen. **Table 84-3** summarizes the effect of aging on intestinal immunity.

Gastrointestinal Drug Metabolism

Older patients are at increased risk for drug interactions and adverse drug reactions, primarily because of the large number of drugs and known side effects of drugs prescribed in this age group. While most drug metabolism occurs in the liver, usually via the cytochrome P450 system, there is expression of the CYP3A subfamily in the GI tract. This subclass oxidizes a wide variety of drugs and toxins including procarcinogens such as aflatoxins, calcium channel antagonists, immunosuppressant agents, cholesterol-lowering agents, benzodiazepines, nonsedating antihistamines, and macrolide antibiotics. CYP3A activity is reduced by 25% to 50% in aged individuals, explaining some of the risk for adverse drug effects.

COMMON INTESTINAL DISORDERS

Diagnosis of GI disorders in an older adult patient poses several challenges to the physician. First, comorbid illnesses are frequent and often numerous, and some such as dementia and depression may impair adequate communication between patient and caregiver. Second, medications and their side effects may cloud the clinical picture as polypharmacy is common in older adults.

Differences in usual diagnosis for common presenting lower GI symptoms among older adults are summarized in **Table 84-4**. For example, rectal bleeding in a young person is most commonly from hemorrhoids or inflammatory bowel disease (IBD). In older adults, diverticulosis, ischemic colitis, or colon cancer more commonly cause rectal bleeding. A complete and thorough history is imperative in older adults. Subtle clues to the diagnosis are sometimes dismissed as physiologic aspects of aging. Physical

TABLE 84-2 ■ COLONIC FUNCTION

AGING EFFECTS ON COLONIC FUNCTION	CLINICAL IMPLICATIONS
1. Mucosal epithelial cell growth and differentiation altered	Increased risk of colonic mucosal dysplasia and cancer
2. Release of acetylcholine in myenteric neurons ↓ 3. Calcium entry into ↓ myenteric neurons 4. Colonic muscle cells ↓	Higher prevalence of constipation older than age 60
5. Nitric oxide-containing neurons in myenteric plexus ↓	Impaired relaxation of colonic muscle predisposing to development of colonic diverticulosis

TABLE 84-3 ■ GASTROINTESTINAL IMMUNITY

AGING EFFECTS ON GASTROINTESTINAL IMMUNITY

- Antigen presentation and uptake in small bowel +/−
- Gastrointestinal T-cell immunity and recruitment ↓
- Gastrointestinal B-cell immunity and recruitment ↓

- Number of Peyer patches in small bowel +/−
- ↓ Number of rectal T lymphocytes
- ↓ IL-2 release
- ↓ Recruitment of IgA-producing B lymphocytes in small bowel
- ↓ IgA production

TABLE 84-4 ■ INFLUENCE OF AGE ON LIKELY DIAGNOSIS OF LOWER GASTROINTESTINAL SYMPTOMS

SYMPTOM	YOUNGER PATIENT	OLDER PATIENT
Rectal bleeding	Hemorrhoids Inflammatory bowel disease Colonic polyp	Diverticulosis Vascular ectasia Colon cancer
Constipation	Irritable bowel syndrome	Obstructing lesion
Anal stricture	Inflammatory bowel disease	Neoplasm Radiation-induced injury

examination and some laboratory tests including tests of liver function are unaffected by aging, and any abnormality should be evaluated for the presence of a disease state and not dismissed as an age-related change.

Colonoscopy Colonoscopy in older adults is safe and well tolerated. Several studies of indications and outcomes of patients older than 80 years having elective and emergency endoscopic procedures found those tests to be safe. Moreover, the yield for diagnostic testing with colonoscopy in older adults is relatively high. Colonoscopy is often done for colon cancer screening (see Chapter 92).

Adequate bowel preparation is critical to a successful colonoscopic examination. Bowel cleansing in older adults should be performed with care. Preparation with standard doses of polyethylene glycol–based lavage solutions (PEG-ELS) in older adults is well tolerated and produces satisfactory bowel cleansing in more than 95% of all cases. Split dose regimens, where a part of the preparation is given 6 to 8 hours before the procedure, are recommended for optimal bowel cleansing. Sodium phosphate osmotic laxative preparations should not be used in older adults, as they cause significant fluid shifts and may cause electrolyte abnormalities or phosphate nephropathy and renal failure in this subset of patients.

Most colonoscopies are performed under moderate sedation. Sedation for colonoscopy usually includes a combination of a benzodiazepine (midazolam or diazepam) and a narcotic (meperidine or fentanyl), or may include a short-acting anesthetic agent such as propofol. As older adults may be more sensitive to these agents, small incremental doses should be given and the patient monitored closely for signs of cardiopulmonary compromise.

Endoscopic ultrasound Endoscopic ultrasound (EUS) can be used to diagnose and manage disease of the anorectum and usually does not require sedation. EUS may be helpful in evaluating the layers of the rectal wall, the internal and external anal sphincters, and the pelvic floor muscles in patients with fecal incontinence. EUS is frequently used to stage rectal malignancy, providing information about the depth of tumor invasion and the status of regional lymph nodes. Direct tissue sampling is available through fine needle aspiration and biopsy at the time of the EUS.

Capsule endoscopy Wireless capsule endoscopy is an increasingly important test in the evaluation of obscure GI bleeding. The capsule transmits images of the small bowel to a hard drive that the patient wears, and following the completion of the study the images are downloaded to a computer for review. Common findings in older adults being evaluated for obscure bleeding or iron deficiency anemia include angioectasias and ulcers.

Contrast studies Contrast studies of the large intestine involve coating the colonic mucosa with a contrast medium, usually barium sulfate, following thorough colonic preparation. Barium enemas may be performed by either the single- or double-contrast method; in the latter, air is insufflated as well as barium. The single-contrast technique often is used to diagnose colonic strictures, fistula, obstruction, or diverticulitis. Double-contrast barium enema more commonly is used to detect polyps or mucosal abnormalities.

CT colonography CT colonography (virtual colonoscopy) is a radiographic technique that combines helical CT and graphics software to create a three-dimensional view of the colonic lumen. This technology was developed to detect colonic polyps. In clinical trials of CT colonography, detection rates for polyps greater than 5 mm are similar to those for optical colonoscopy. Specific recommendations for use in colon cancer screening are covered in Chapter 92.

Diverticular Disease

Colonic diverticula are herniations of colonic mucosa through the smooth muscle layers of the colon. Strictly speaking, because colonic diverticula do not involve the muscle layer but rather are herniations of the mucosa and submucosa, they are actually pseudodiverticula. Diverticulosis has been increasingly recognized in Western society, and prevalence in the descending and sigmoid colon increases with age. Diverticula are present in approximately one-third of persons by age 50 and in approximately two-thirds by age 80. In Western society, the majority of diverticula occur on the left side of the colon, specifically the sigmoid colon, although diverticula can occur anywhere in the colon.

Pathophysiology There are three factors implicated in the pathogenesis of colonic diverticulosis. First, altered colonic motility results in increased luminal pressure along segments of the colon, and the resulting high-pressure areas cause outpouchings at areas of weakness. Second, low intake of dietary fiber may contribute because low stool weights and slower stool transit times allow for relative increases in colonic intraluminal pressure. Third, with age the structural integrity of the colonic muscular wall decreases, and diverticula are more likely to form.

Asymptomatic diverticulosis Diverticulosis is usually an incidental finding in patients undergoing radiographic studies or colonoscopy for other reasons. There is no indication for therapy or follow-up in such patients. Large cohort studies suggest that complications of diverticular disease may be prevented by intake of a high-fiber diet.

Painful diverticular disease Some patients with diverticulosis have left lower quadrant pain, and when examined, do not have evidence of inflammation. These patients may have painful diverticular disease. Pain often is described as crampy, located in the left lower abdomen, and may be associated with diarrhea or constipation as well as tenderness over the affected area. The pain is often exacerbated by eating and diminished by defecation or the passage of flatus. The symptoms of painful diverticular disease often overlap with those of irritable bowel syndrome, and therefore painful diverticular disease is considered part of the spectrum of functional bowel disorders. It is important to consider other causes of left lower quadrant pain such as diverticulitis, colonic obstruction, and incarcerated hernias in such patients.

Diverticulitis Diverticulitis, defined as having diverticulosis in association with inflammation, infection, or both, is probably the most common clinical manifestation of diverticular disease. Diverticulitis develops in approximately 10% to 25% of individuals with diverticulosis who are followed for 10 years or more; however, less than 20% of these patients require hospitalization.

The process by which a diverticulum becomes inflamed has been compared to appendicitis, in which the diverticulum becomes obstructed by stool in its neck. The resulting obstruction eventually leads to micro- or macroperforation of the diverticulum. Fever, leukocytosis, and rebound tenderness often ensue. Due to decreased visceral sensation, older patients may have reduced rebound, and the white blood cell (WBC) may not be elevated; therefore, an aggressive evaluation is indicated if this diagnosis is suspected. Segmental colitis associated with diverticulitis (SCAD) has also been increasingly recognized as a cause of abdominal pain. Unlike diverticulitis, inflammation in SCAD involves the mucosa between diverticuli, and spares the diverticular orifice. The symptoms include chronic diarrhea, intermittent bleeding, and pain. There is evidence this entity may be an overlap with IBD.

Clinical guidelines recommend abdominal and pelvic CT scan for diagnosis. Colonoscopy should also be performed in older patients, but should be delayed until inflammation has improved because of an increased risk of colonic perforation. Patients with severe pain, nausea, and vomiting often require hospitalization. Antibiotics should be used selectively rather than routinely in older patients who are immune-competent and who have mild disease. Most patients with diverticulitis will improve within 48 to 72 hours. Selected patients with relatively mild symptoms and who are able to tolerate oral intake may be managed with close outpatient monitoring and intake of clear fluids. Given the high incidence of complicated disease and effects of dehydration in older adult patients with diverticulitis, there should be a low threshold for hospitalization.

Patients with complicated disease, such as abscesses, may need drainage by surgery or interventional radiology. Surgery is recommended for patients with diverticulitis who fail to respond to medical therapy within 72 hours, and for those with refractory abscess, obstruction, or when the inflammatory process involves the bladder. Elective segmental resection of the colon should not be based on number of episodes of diverticulitis, but should be customized based on severity of disease, patient preference, and risks and benefits.

Diverticular hemorrhage Three to five percent of patients with diverticulosis have hemorrhage from a diverticulum. Diverticular hemorrhage is the most common identifiable cause of significant lower GI bleeding, accounting for 30% to 40% of cases with confirmed sources.

Bleeding associated with diverticula is typically brisk and painless. While the majority of diverticula are located in the left colon, bleeding from diverticular disease usually arises from the right colon. Bleeding is said to arise from arterial rupture of the vasa recta as it courses over the dome of a diverticulum. Bleeding ceases spontaneously in 70% to 80% of patients, and rebleeding rates range from 22% to 38%. Rebleeding is more likely when the initial bleed is severe.

The initial step in the management of patients with hemodynamically significant bleeding from diverticulosis is stabilization with intravenous fluid and blood products as necessary. Stable patients with suspected diverticular hemorrhage may undergo colonoscopy following rapid colonic purge. Colonoscopy in this setting can identify a diverticular source, exclude alternative diagnoses, and provide therapy of actively bleeding lesions.

In patients with recurrent bleeding, nuclear tagged red blood cell scans (scintigraphy) or CT angiography may localize the bleeding site. A positive bleeding scan may lead to angiography, which may allow for nonsurgical management of diverticular hemorrhage. Patients who require more than three units of packed red cell transfusions over 24 hours, have bleeding refractory to treatment, or are hemodynamically unstable may require surgical management. Preoperative nuclear red blood cell scans or angiography often help localize the diseased segment and allow for limited bowel resections. Blind total colectomy is rarely indicated.

Diarrhea

Diarrhea, while less common than constipation, causes significant morbidity in older adults. The etiology of acute diarrhea (lasting < 2 weeks) is similar in older versus younger adults, with a few exceptions. Most cases of acute diarrhea are related to viral or bacterial infection, but it can also be caused by medications, medication interactions, or dietary supplements.

Chronic diarrhea, lasting more than 2 weeks, may result from fecal impaction, medications, irritable bowel syndrome, microscopic or lymphocytic colitis, IBD, obstruction from colon cancer, malabsorption, small bowel bacterial overgrowth, thyrotoxicosis, or lymphoma. Many of these conditions are not due to changes with aging per se, but due to superimposed disease. Older patients may present with new-onset fecal urgency and frequency that is similar to diarrhea-predominant irritable bowel syndrome. The onset may coincide with an acute diarrheal illness caused by viral or bacterial infection. However, many patients continue to have distressing fecal urgency for weeks or months, resulting in considerable lifestyle impairment. Many curtail their travel and social activities outside the home for fear of fecal incontinence. The etiology is often multifactorial. Side effects of medications that alter small bowel and colonic motility should always be considered. Decreased rectal compliance occurs with aging, and may contribute to sensations of fecal urgency in these patients. Screening for fecal impaction resulting in constipation is always warranted in older patients, as it is often overlooked. Diarrhea and fecal urgency should not be attributed simply to aging as it is often due to superimposed disease or other potentially treatable causes.

Clostridium Difficile Colitis

C difficile, an anaerobic gram-positive, spore-forming toxigenic bacillus was first isolated in 1935. It was not until 1978 when the association between the toxin elaborated by this bacterium and antibiotic-associated pseudomembranous colitis was made. The organism is now recognized as the single most important cause of nosocomial infectious diarrhea in the United States. **C difficile colitis is more prevalent in older adults because of more frequent hospitalizations, increased antibiotic use, and increased time in institutional settings. C difficile colonization in long-term care facilities has been estimated to be at least 50% in the United States.** Pathogenesis often involves exposure to an agent that alters normal colonic flora such as an antibiotic. While the most common antibiotics associated with C difficile colitis are ampicillin, amoxicillin, cephalosporins, and clindamycin, virtually all antibiotics (including those used to treat C difficile colitis) have been implicated in causing disease.

For this reason, efforts to decrease infection have focused on decreasing the reflexive or routine use of antibiotics in high-risk populations such as residents of nursing facilities. C difficile infection may result in an asymptomatic carrier state, or patients may develop diarrhea and colitis. Patients with intact immune systems and an ability to mount an early antibody response to C difficile toxin usually become asymptomatic carriers of the organism. On the other hand, patients lacking sufficient ability to mount an adequate immune response develop diarrhea and colitis.

Risk factors for the development of C difficile colitis are summarized in **Table 84-5**.

C difficile infection disproportionally affects older patients. Approximately two out of three infections occur in patients aged 65 or older, and older people are also at

TABLE 84-5 ■ RISK FACTORS FOR *CLOSTRIDIUM DIFFICILE* INFECTION
Antimicrobial therapy
Older age
Use of nasogastric tube
Gastrointestinal procedures
Acid antisecretory medications
Intensive care unit stay
Length of hospitalization

high risk for recurrent infection. Risk factors that may especially predispose older patients include exposure to systemic antibiotics used to treat other diseases, contact with bacterial spores as a result of frequent health care exposure, and age-related changes in the immune system. Decreased functional status is also an independent risk factor for severe infection.

Clinical manifestations of C difficile infection range from asymptomatic carriage to mild to moderate diarrhea to life-threatening pseudomembranous colitis (**Figure 84-2**). While there is no evidence that age per se is a risk for asymptomatic carriage of C difficile, older patients appear to be at risk for developing severe disease including complications such as colonic ileus or toxic dilation.

Diagnostic tests There are several tests for diagnosing C difficile colitis, which appear to be equally effective in older versus younger patients. The most widely used is enzyme-linked stool immunoassay directed against one of the two C difficile toxins. While the main advantages are speed, cost, ease of testing, and high specificity, this immunoassay has relatively low sensitivity. Polymerase chain reaction tests that detect bacterial antigens or toxin genes are available; however, these tests may be positive in asymptomatic carriers and use varies by institution. Other diagnostic tests including C difficile stool culture and tissue culture cytotoxic assay are less commonly used because of

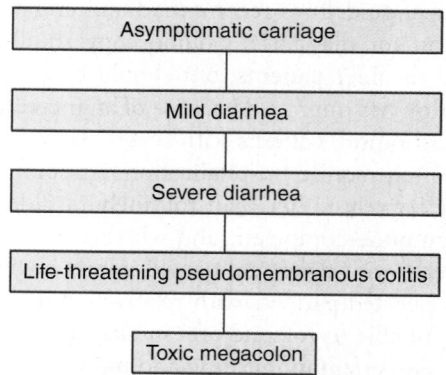

FIGURE 84-2. Clinical manifestations of *Clostridium difficile* infection.

their high cost, need for specialized laboratory techniques, and length of time to make the diagnosis, but may be helpful if stool toxin assay results are equivocal.

Colonoscopy, or more often flexible sigmoidoscopy, may be helpful in making the diagnosis of *C difficile* colitis, but is usually not necessary. Endoscopy is most useful when the diagnosis is in doubt or when disease severity demands rapid diagnosis. The finding of colonic pseudomembranes in a patient with antibiotic-associated diarrhea is almost pathognomonic for *C difficile* colitis (**Figure 84-3**).

Treatment Therapy for *C difficile* colitis begins with withdrawal of the precipitating antibiotics if possible. Older patients treated with metronidazole appear to have a high risk of treatment failure and disease recurrence. Thus, guidelines from the Infectious Diseases Society of America recommend use of oral vancomycin or fidaxomicin to treat *C difficile*–associated disease rather than metronidazole. The usual initial therapy in mild-moderate disease is a 10-day course of either oral vancomycin 125 mg four times daily or oral fidaxomicin 200 mg twice daily. This is effective in treating the majority of patients. Patients who are very ill should receive oral vancomycin 500 mg four times daily and IV metronidazole 500 mg every 8 hours. Vancomycin retention enemas (500 mg in 100 mg normal saline every 6 hours) can be used in patients who cannot tolerate oral medications. Intravenous vancomycin does not penetrate the colonic lumen and is not effective in treating *C difficile* colitis. Probiotic agents such as *Lactobacillus* GG and *Saccharomyces boulardii* have been used to reconstitute the colonic microflora, and are occasionally added to metronidazole or vancomycin to treat *C difficile* colitis, but their effectiveness has not been demonstrated in well-designed trials. Bezlotoxumab, a monoclonal antibody targeting *C difficile* toxin B, offers an option for treatment in patients with disease refractory to other treatments, although experience in older patients is limited.

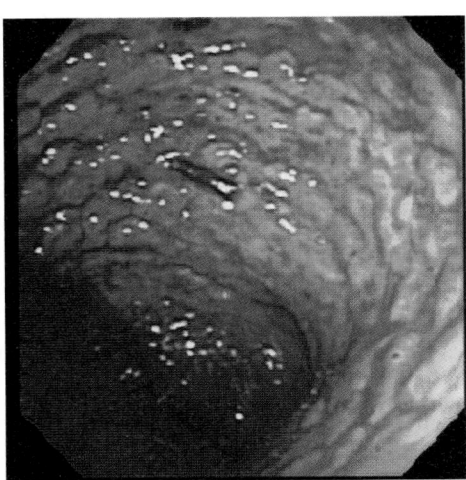

FIGURE 84-3. Pseudomembranes.

TABLE 84-6 ■ VANCOMYCIN TAPER FOR SECOND RELAPSE OF *CLOSTRIDIUM DIFFICILE* COLITIS
Vancomycin 125 mg po QID for 7 d
Vancomycin 125 mg po BID for 7 d
Vancomycin 125 mg po QD for 7 d
Vancomycin 125 mg po QOD for 7 d
Vancomycin 125 mg po Q 3 d for 7 d

Unfortunately, recurrent *C difficile* infection is a common problem, and older patients are at increased risk. Symptomatic recurrence may result from relapse of the same strain (usually within 28 days) or reinfection with a different strain of *C difficile*. Resistance to initial treatment is seldom an important factor in recurrence. Therefore, patients with recurrent *C difficile* colitis generally are given another trial with the antibiotic used to treat the initial infection. In some patients, a prolonged taper of vancomycin may be needed to prevent further recurrence (**Table 84-6**). Fecal microbiota transplantation is highly effective in the treatment of recurrent *C difficile* infection in older patients with disease refractory to usual vancomycin taper and use of oral probiotics, and is also very effective therapy for selected patients with severe or fulminant disease (**Table 84-7**).

Microscopic Colitis

The term *microscopic colitis* refers to two distinct clinical entities with similar presentation, namely lymphocytic and collagenous colitis. They are characterized by chronic watery diarrhea and feature histologic evidence of chronic mucosal inflammation in the absence of endoscopic or radiological abnormalities of the large intestine. They differ principally by the presence or absence of a thickened collagenous band, which when present in collagenous colitis is located in the colonic subepithelium.

Both lymphocytic and collagenous colitis occur most commonly in people in their sixth to eighth decade with a strong female predominance. Most patients present with chronic watery stools for months to years. The pattern of symptoms in patients with microscopic colitis fluctuates

TABLE 84-7 ■ INDICATIONS FOR FECAL MICROBIOTA TRANSPLANTATION FOR RECURRENT *CLOSTRIDIUM DIFFICILE* INFECTION
• ≥ 3 episodes of mild-to-moderate *Clostridium difficile* (CDI) and failure to respond to a 6- to 8-wk taper of vancomycin ± alternative antibiotic
• ≥ 2 episodes of CDI resulting in hospitalization and associated with significant morbidity
• Moderate CDI with no response to standard therapy for at least 1 wk
• Possibly severe (even fulminant) CDI with no response to standard therapy for 48 h

TABLE 84-8 ■ TREATMENT OF MICROSCOPIC COLITIS

- Review medications and consider elimination of those associated with microscopic colitis (NSAIDs, lansoprazole, acarbose, ranitidine, sertraline, ticlopidine)
- Recommend discontinue smoking
- Antidiarrheals (Kayopectate, Pepto-Bismol, loperamide). Avoid lomotil, which contains atropine
- Stool bulking agents such as psyllium
- Corticosteroids (budesonide best due to low systemic absorption)
- Other anti-inflammatory medications: mesalamine, sulfadiazine, immunomodulators, anti-TNF therapies

TABLE 84-9 ■ DIFFERENTIATING CROHN DISEASE AND ULCERATIVE COLITIS

	CROHN DISEASE	ULCERATIVE COLITIS
Distribution	Throughout the GI tract, with skipped segments	Continuous disease from the rectum involving only the colon
Rectum	Relatively spared	Typically involved
Mucosal lesions	Aphthous ulcers, cobblestoning	Micro ulcers, linear ulcers
Rectal bleeding	Uncommon	Common
Depth of inflammation	Transmural	Mucosal
Fistulas	Present	Not present

and consists of exacerbations and remissions over years. Crampy abdominal pain is common, and symptoms often improve with fasting. Patients are more likely to be active smokers and use drugs such as NSAIDs and acid-suppressing medications for heartburn. Physical examination is usually unremarkable, and occult blood in the stool is uncommon. Colonoscopy is usually normal. It is important to exclude infectious causes of diarrhea by testing the stool for ova and parasites, bacterial pathogens, and *C difficile* toxin prior to making the diagnosis of microscopic colitis. The diagnosis relies on histopathologic evaluation of biopsied material from the diseased colon.

Treatment **Table 84-8** summarizes treatment options for microscopic colitis. One-third of patients respond to antidiarrheal agents such as loperamide as well as stool bulking agents like psyllium or methylcellulose; however, these agents do not improve the subepithelial inflammation or reduce the thickness of the collagen band. American Gastroenterology guidelines (2016) recommend the oral steroid budesonide 9 mg daily to induce remission, as several clinical trials showed benefit versus no treatment or treatment with mesalamine. Budesonide reduces inflammation in the bowel and is used to treat IBD such as ulcerative colitis (UC) or Crohn disease. Budesonide is also the first-line agent recommended to continue remission of microscopic colitis. If budesonide is contraindicated or is not affordable, other medications listed in **Table 84-8** can be used as second-line treatments. Oral prednisone, while effective in treating symptomatic microscopic colitis, is less optimal due to its many adverse effects in older people. In severe refractory patients, diverting ileostomy or proctocolectomy is a treatment of last resort.

Inflammatory Bowel Disease

Crohn disease and UC comprise the vast majority of IBD (**Table 84-9**). They are characterized by inflammation within the GI tract. IBD commonly has its onset in the young adult population, but is found with increasing frequency in older adults. As discussed in the section on diverticulitis, inflammation may present as segmental colitis, usually in the left colon, associated with diverticuli (SCAD)

but involving the interdiverticular mucosa. The older patient may present with new-onset diarrhea, abdominal pain, intermittent bleeding, or symptoms of chronic complications of IBD such as anemia, weight loss, or obstruction in small bowel or colon. There is considerable overlap between these symptoms and other conditions such as bowel ischemia and cancer that are more common in older patients; therefore, work-up requires imaging of the bowel and endoscopy of the affected bowel if possible. An increasing cohort of older patients with IBD were diagnosed with IBD at a younger age and have been aging with disease. They are at risk for development of long-term complications such as colonic cancer and require additional surveillance compared to low-risk older patients. Most patients will have long-term involvement of a gastroenterologist; however, geriatricians and other primary care providers should be aware of common issues affecting IBD patients.

There appears to be a bimodal distribution of the age of onset, with the peak incidence of IBD occurring in the second and third decades, and a second smaller peak in older adults between the ages of 60 and 70. "Late-onset" IBD accounts for approximately 12% cases of UC and 16% cases of Crohn disease.

Crohn disease Crohn disease is a chronic inflammatory process of unknown etiology, which most often affects the distal ileum, but can affect any segment of the GI tract from mouth to anus. It is characterized by transmural inflammation of the bowel wall, the presence of aphthae and ulcers, and the interspersing of segments of involved bowel with uninvolved bowel (skip lesions). Fissures, fistulas, and strictures are common in Crohn disease. Crohn disease of the colon, also known as Crohn colitis, is more common in older than in younger adults.

Symptoms and Signs The presentation of Crohn disease may be subtle and varies considerably. In older adults, Crohn disease often primarily involves the colon. Consequently, features usually associated with small bowel disease such as intestinal obstruction, perforation, and fistula are less common. The majority of older adult patients with Crohn disease have abdominal pain, weight loss, fever, and diarrhea. The diarrhea, typically watery in Crohn disease of the small bowel, can be bloody when the colon is involved.

Laboratory abnormalities such as anemia, leukocytosis, thrombocytosis, hypoalbuminemia, elevated erythrocyte sedimentation rate, and C-reactive protein vary with the severity of the illness. Interestingly, anemia in Crohn disease can be because of either iron deficiency from chronic GI blood loss or from vitamin B_{12} deficiency if the Crohn disease involves a large segment of the distal ileum, the site for vitamin B_{12} absorption in the small bowel.

Unfortunately, no single symptom, sign, or diagnostic test definitively establishes the diagnosis of Crohn disease, and prolonged delays in diagnosis may occur more frequently in older adults. In the end, a constellation of suggestive symptoms and laboratory abnormalities should prompt further evaluation. Common intestinal infections should be excluded by stool cultures, stool examination for ova and parasites, and assays for *C difficile* toxin.

Ultimately, the diagnosis of Crohn disease is confirmed by findings from CT or MR enterography, colonoscopy, and histopathology. These studies can identify the characteristic linear ulcers, skip lesions, and mucosal edema in Crohn disease. Enterography can identify pyogenic complications like abscesses and perforations, and also can detect other intra-abdominal pathology that might mimic the presentation of Crohn disease, such as appendicitis or nephrolithiasis.

Management The principles of IBD management are the same regardless of the age of the patient and are summarized in **Table 84-10**. The most commonly used medications in the treatment of Crohn disease include sulfasalazine, mesalamine (5-aminosalicylic acid), and corticosteroids; all of these are well tolerated in the older adult population. However, corticosteroid use confers a higher risk of complications.

Immunomodulators such as azathioprine, 6-mercaptopurine, and methotrexate can be used effectively to maintain remission of Crohn disease. Although these agents are usually well tolerated in older adults, their use in older patients is low compared to younger patients. Concerns include increased risk of infection or malignancy such as nonmelanoma skin cancers associated with their use. Biologic agents, such as anti-Tumor Necrosis Factor (TNF) drugs infliximab and adalimumab, have been used to manage moderate to severe Crohn disease; however, their use is also less common in older adults. Anti-TNF agents are contraindicated in patients with class III and IV heart failure. Other newer agents such as integrin antagonists, interleukin antagonists, and Janus Kinase inhibitors have shown benefit in treating both Crohn disease and UC; however, use in older patients is very limited.

Antibiotics such as metronidazole and ciprofloxacin are effective in inducing and maintaining remission, as well as for healing perineal fistulas, in patients with Crohn disease. The long-term use of antibiotics typically is limited by the occurrence of significant side effects. Specifically, irreversible peripheral neuropathy can occur with the use of metronidazole, while antibiotic-associated diarrhea may be a complication of prolonged ciprofloxacin use.

Older adults with ileal or ileal–colonic Crohn disease occasionally require intestinal resection, but generally tolerate surgery well and appear to have low rates of postoperative recurrence. Proctocolectomy with ileostomy is a common surgical option for patients with extensive Crohn colitis. In older adult patients who are debilitated or malnourished, an initial subtotal colectomy with ileostomy is less debilitating and permits weight gain and improved physical well-being. If proctocolectomy is subsequently required, it can be done with a low complication rate, but may not be necessary at all if rectal disease is absent. A conventional ileostomy is generally favored in older patients following colectomy, because anal sphincter sparing surgical procedures, such as an ileal pouch–anal anastomosis, often have poor functional results in older patients.

TABLE 84-10 ■ DOSES AND ADVERSE REACTIONS WITH COMMONLY USED MEDICATIONS TO TREAT INFLAMMATORY BOWEL DISEASE

MEDICATION	DOSE	ADVERSE REACTIONS
Sulfasalazine	4–6 g/d	Nausea, folate deficiency, hemolytic anemia with glucose-6-phosphatase dehydrogenase deficiency
Mesalamine	Up to 4.8 g/d	Headaches
Prednisone	Up to 60 mg/d	Cushingoid appearance, glucose intolerance, osteoporosis, avascular necrosis, proximal myopathy, irritability, hypertension, cataract, glaucoma
6-Mercaptopurine, azathioprine	6-MP 1.5 mg/kg, AZA 3 mg/kg	Pancreatitis, pancytopenia, hepatitis
Metronidazole	Up to 1 g/d	Anorexia, nausea/vomiting, disulfiram-like effect, peripheral neuropathy
Ciprofloxacin	Up to 1 g/d	Nausea/vomiting, rash, hepatitis, spontaneous tendon rupture
Infliximab	5–10 mg/kg IV	Headache, nausea, vomiting, infections, induction and lupus-like syndrome, malignancy then maintenance

Ulcerative colitis UC is a chronic inflammatory disorder of the GI tract of unknown etiology that affects the mucosa and submucosa of the large intestine in a continuous fashion. The inflammatory process invariably involves the rectum and extends proximally to variable distances, but does not involve the GI tract proximal to the colon. For many older patients, UC is a relatively mild illness, because colonic inflammation often is limited to the rectum or sigmoid colon. This distribution of disease is generally associated with less systemic manifestations, better response to medical therapy, and less need for surgery than more extensive UC.

Symptoms and Signs The severity of UC may be subjectively classified as mild, moderate, or severe and is generally proportional to the extent of colonic inflammation. Symptoms in older adults are similar to those seen in young patients, and include bloody diarrhea, rectal pain, tenesmus, urgency, and abdominal pain. In comparison to Crohn disease, the diarrhea in UC almost always is bloody. Fecal urgency, a sensation of incomplete evacuation, and fecal incontinence also are common. Unfortunately, older patients appear to be more likely than younger patients to present with a severe initial attack, and that first severe manifestation is associated with a relatively high fatality rate.

Laboratory findings in UC are nonspecific and reflect the severity of the underlying disease. In patients with limited distal disease, laboratory abnormalities may be absent except perhaps for mild anemia. In patients with extensive disease, severe iron deficiency anemia, hypoalbuminemia, leukocytosis, and thrombocytosis are common.

Toxic megacolon is a feared complication of UC, and it occurs more frequently in older patients. One should be suspicious of toxic megacolon in a patient whose diarrhea improves but whose abdomen is distended and tympanic. Other markers of worsening systemic inflammation, such as fever and leukocytosis, will also be present. The diagnosis is usually made by abdominal radiography or CT imaging. Colonoscopy should not be attempted when there is a suspicion for toxic megacolon, as perforation may ensue.

Similar to the situation in Crohn disease, there is no single test that can definitively diagnose UC with acceptable sensitivity and specificity. In older adults, it is important to exclude other diseases that may mimic UC, such as ischemic colitis, radiation proctocolitis, diverticulitis, malignancy, and infectious colitis.

Endoscopic examination can demonstrate the classic findings of diffuse erythema, mucosal edema, granular mucosa, and ulcerations starting in the rectum without intervening areas of normal mucosa (**Figure 84-4**). In the proper clinical setting, flexible sigmoidoscopy with biopsy is usually sufficient to establish a diagnosis of UC. Complete colonoscopy with ileoscopy is necessary to determine the extent of disease and to exclude Crohn disease. However, complete colonoscopy is not recommended in patients with active UC for fear of perforation; the procedure can be safely performed once active disease has been controlled.

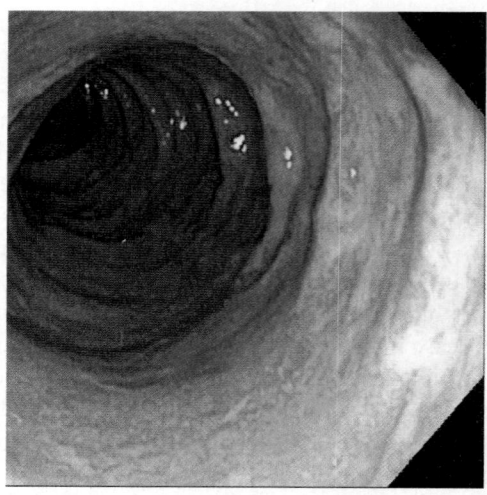

FIGURE 84-4. Ulcerative colitis as seen on colonoscopy.

Management Most older adult patients with UC respond favorably to medical management. Once in remission, relapse occurs less frequently in older adults regardless of the severity of the initial attack. The mainstays of treatment for UC are aminosalicylates, and they may be administered orally or rectally. Formulations designed either for enema or suppositories are reasonable choices when treating distal disease. Unfortunately, distal disease in older patients can be refractory to topical therapy, and so older subjects with distal disease may require oral formulations of aminosalicylates to achieve and maintain remission.

In addition to aminosalicylates, corticosteroids are effective in achieving remission. As steroid use is associated with frequent side effects, they should only be used temporarily in UC as a means to induce remission. Steroids have not been shown to be effective at preventing relapses, and their side effect profile makes prolonged use unsatisfactory.

In patients who do not respond to aminosalicylates, immunomodulators such as azathioprine or 6-mercaptopurine should be used. Patients may require up to 6 to 12 weeks to see an effect from these agents. However, once a response is achieved, they are effective at maintaining remission. Use of other immune agents and biologics, as discussed above for Crohn disease, should be individualized as there is limited data on efficacy and tolerance in older adults.

Surgery for UC is indicated in patients who fail medical therapy, have acute fulminant disease, are steroid dependent, or develop a dysplastic lesion or cancer. UC is cured following total proctocolectomy. In older adults, total proctocolectomy with ileostomy remains a popular choice, because restorative procedures like ileo–anal anastomosis are limited by functional morbidity. An alternative surgical procedure is a subtotal colectomy, which leaves a rectal stump that provides the patient with an improved chance for fecal continence. Such patients, however, continue to have colonic mucosa, and thus have an ongoing increased risk for colon cancer to develop in the diseased segment. Practitioners with older patients that have had subtotal colectomy need to be aware of the need for continued frequent cancer surveillance of the rectal stump.

Colon cancer in IBD The risk of colorectal cancer (CRC) in older patients with long-standing IBD is a significant complication of the disease, with rates of early and missed CRC up to three times that of non-IBD older patients. Colon cancer rates generally are higher in patients with UC than those with Crohn disease; it appears to be the degree and extent of ongoing inflammation in the colon that confers an increased risk of colon cancer. Patients with Crohn colitis are believed to have an equally high risk of developing colon cancer as their UC peers. Cumulative risk of CRC increases with disease duration in UC from 2% after 10 years to 18% after 30 years of disease. The older IBD patient with long-standing colonic disease should be considered at high risk for CRC. Surveillance for CRC includes colonoscopy with random mucosal biopsies of the entire colon every 1 to 3 years starting 8 to 10 years after onset of disease. During surveillance, patients found to have low- or high-grade dysplasia or carcinoma generally are offered proctocolectomy. No specific age recommendations for discontinuing IBD cancer surveillance are available. However, discontinuing routine CRC surveillance is generally recommended when life expectancy falls below 10 years. A study in 2019 found that patients with long-standing IBD and two consecutive negative screening endoscopies had no advanced colorectal neoplasia with an average follow up of 4 years. Therefore, it may be possible in future to identify a lower risk IBD cohort that could be followed less frequently.

Small Bowel Ischemia

Small bowel ischemia is uncommon and is usually due to superior mesenteric artery (SMA) obstruction. Sudden obstruction by clots results in complete ischemia of the majority of the small bowel and presents as a catastrophic event. Usually patients are unstable, and older patients have a very poor prognosis. Slowly progressive obstruction presents with increasing cramping pain with eating, termed intestinal angina, and in later stages with diarrhea after eating. Patients often lose weight due to food avoidance. The diagnosis is often overlooked due to the nonspecific symptoms early on. Angiography is needed; however, CT angiography is increasingly used as it is safer and less invasive. Angioplasty can often be performed and is a safer option than vascular surgery in older patients.

Colon Ischemia

Colon ischemia (CI) is the most common intestinal vascular disorder in older adults. CI encompasses a spectrum of injury. The specific conditions resulting from ischemic injury to the colon are classified as reversible or irreversible, and then can be characterized further as reversible

TABLE 84-11 ■ CAUSES OF COLONIC ISCHEMIA	
• Inferior mesenteric artery thrombosis	• Volvulus
• Arterial embolus	• Strangulated hernia
• Cholesterol emboli	• Vasculitis
• Cardiac arrhythmia	• Inherited and/or acquired hypercoagulable states
• Shock	• Medications

ischemic colonopathy, reversible or transient ischemic colitis, chronic ulcerative ischemic colitis, ischemic colonic stricture, colonic gangrene, and fulminant universal ischemic colitis.

Pathophysiology The colon receives its blood supply from branches of the SMA and inferior mesenteric artery. The colon is protected from ischemia by an abundant collateral circulation formed by the marginal arterial complex of Drummond, central anastomotic artery, and arc of Riolan. Occlusion of a major vessel results in opening of collateral pathways in response to arterial hypotension distal to the occlusion. Increased blood flow through collateral pathways maintains adequate perfusion for a variable but brief period of time. If blood flow is diminished for a prolonged period, vasoconstriction develops in the affected bed and may persist after the primary cause of the mesenteric ischemia is reversed.

In most cases, the cause of an episode of CI cannot be established with certainty, and no vascular occlusion can be identified. The causes of CI are vast (**Table 84-11**) and include thrombosis, embolus, shock, volvulus, hematologic disorders, infections, trauma, surgery, as well as several medications (**Table 84-12**). The colon is particularly susceptible to ischemia, perhaps owing to its relatively low blood flow during periods of functional activity and its sensitivity to autonomic stimulation.

Clinical features Many cases of transient or reversible ischemia still are missed because diagnostic studies are not performed early enough in the course of disease. This is because patients may not seek medical advice for a disease that is self-limited, or the initial symptoms may be confused with other conditions such as IBD.

Approximately 90% of persons with CI are older than age 60 and have widespread evidence of atherosclerosis. Up to 10% of patients may have a potentially obstructing

TABLE 84-12 ■ MEDICATIONS ASSOCIATED WITH COLON ISCHEMIA	
• Digitalis	• Vasopressin
• Gold	• Pseudoephedrine
• Sumatriptan	• Cocaine
• Methamphetamine	• Nonsteroidal anti-inflammatory drugs
• Imipramine	• Saline laxatives
• Estrogens	• Psychotropic drugs

lesion of the colon, including carcinoma, benign stricture, and diverticulitis. Patients with CI usually are not critically ill at the time of diagnosis, and their abdominal pain typically is mild. Mesenteric angiography plays little role in the diagnosis and management of this condition, since colonic blood flow usually has normalized by the time of presentation. In contrast to small bowel ischemia, the prognosis is often excellent.

Typically, CI presents with the sudden onset of mild crampy left lower quadrant abdominal pain. The pain frequently is accompanied, or followed within 24 hours, by bloody diarrhea or bright red blood per rectum. In most cases, blood loss is minimal; hemodynamically significant bleeding should prompt consideration of other diagnoses, such as diverticular bleeding. Severe pain is unusual and may indicate irreversible transmural necrosis. The differential diagnosis of CI includes infectious colitis, IBD, pseudomembranous colitis, diverticulitis, and colon carcinoma. In all patients suspected of having colonic ischemia, infection with organisms such as *Salmonella, Shigella, Campylobacter*, and *Escherichia coli* O157:H7 should be excluded. In fact, *E coli* O157:H7 infection induces a colitis that mimics or may even cause CI.

American College of Gastroenterology guidelines from 2015 recommend that an older patient who presents with the sudden onset of abdominal pain and rectal bleeding or bloody diarrhea should undergo abdominal and pelvic CT with intravenous and oral contrast as this will demonstrate colonic wall abnormalities such as bowel wall thickening, edema, thumbprinting, or pneumatosis. If acute mesenteric ischemia (AMI) is suspected due to severe wall abnormalities, laboratory evidence of inflammation and renal impairment, or cardiovascular instability, then multiphasic CT angiography should be performed rapidly. If CT angiography is not diagnostic, then conventional angiography can be attempted. Early surgical consultation should be considered for older patients, as delayed surgery results in much poorer outcomes compared to younger patients. Colonoscopy should be avoided acutely due to increased risk of perforation. Colonoscopy can be performed 24 to 48 hours later if safe to do so to demonstrate mucosal abnormalities and obtain histopathologic mucosal samples. Conventional sigmoidoscopy has some risk of perforation and is of value only if the segment of involved bowel is within reach of the sigmoidoscope; CI involves the sigmoid in 50% to 60% of patients and the rectum in less than 10% of cases. At the outset, purplish blebs representing mucosal and submucosal hemorrhage may be seen. As hemorrhage is absorbed, varying degrees of necrosis, inflammation, ulceration, and mucosal sloughing occur, resembling UC or Crohn disease.

Management Treatment of CI is based on early diagnosis and continued monitoring, with special attention to the radiologic or colonoscopic appearance of the colon for diagnosis and to demonstrate either improvement or progression to chronic ischemic colitis or stricture. Guidelines recommend staging patients into mild, moderate and severe disease to guide management (**Table 84-13**).

Management includes stabilization of the patient, optimization of cardiac function, and bowel rest. Systemic antibiotics are administered in moderate or severe cases. Systemic glucocorticoids are of no proven value and increase the risk of perforation.

Colonic Obstruction

Colonic obstruction results in dilation of the colon, abdominal distention and in some cases, colonic perforation. The majority of colonic obstructions are the result of mechanical obstruction from cancer, volvulus, stricture, impacted stool, surgical adhesion, or bowel intussusception. While patients of any age can develop obstruction, the condition is more common in older patients due to increased prevalence of underlying conditions that predispose to obstruction. Patients with acute colonic obstruction can develop megacolon, the diagnosis of which is based on a cecal diameter of 12 cm or greater. Cecal distension is critical, because the cecum is the part of the colon that is most susceptible to ischemia and perforation. With obstruction, as fluid and gas accumulate in the colon and intraluminal pressure increases, the radius of the colon increases. Wall tension is the greatest, and hence the risk for perforation most acute, at the area of greatest radius, which is generally in the cecum.

Acute colonic pseudo-obstruction Acute colonic pseudo-obstruction, also known as Ogilvie syndrome, usually presents as intestinal ileus with massive bowel dilation postoperatively or in the setting of a severe intercurrent illness. The mechanism is a relative increase in sympathetic neuronal inhibitory motor input that results in colonic ileus and acute colonic pseudo-obstruction.

Clinical features Acute colonic pseudo-obstruction usually presents in patients with severe underlying illness such as stroke, myocardial infarction, sepsis, or after surgical procedures. It is most common in older people after abdominal surgery or orthopedic procedures of the pelvis, hips, or knees. The presentation of acute colonic pseudo-obstruction may be subtle and variable, although the most characteristic clinical feature is severe abdominal distention and failure to pass flatus or stool. Some patients report only mild distention and minimal pain. Indeed, a high level of suspicion is necessary to make the diagnosis, because patients often have perioperative bowel cleansing prior to surgery and early passage of stool is not expected.

The hallmark of the disease is colonic dilation on standard abdominal radiography. The entire colon can be affected, although in some cases just the right-sided segments can be dilated. The presence of air in the rectum implies that there is no mechanical obstruction, and is therefore important to note before making a diagnosis of acute colonic pseudo-obstruction.

TABLE 84-13 ■ CLASSIFICATION OF COLON ISCHEMIA (CI) SEVERITY AND MANAGEMENT

DISEASE SEVERITY	CRITERIA	TREATMENT
Mild	Typical symptoms of CI with a segmental colitis not isolated to the right colon and with none of the commonly associated risk factors for poorer outcome that are seen in moderate disease	Observation Supportive care
Moderate	Any patient with CI and up to three of the following factors: Male gender Hypotension (systolic blood pressure < 90 mm Hg) Tachycardia (> 100 bpm) Abdominal pain without rectal bleeding BUN > 20 mg/dL Hgb < 12 g/dL Serum LDH > 350 U/L Serum sodium > 136 mEq/L (mmol/L) WBC 15 cells/mm³ (×10⁹/L) Colonic mucosal ulceration identified by colonoscopy	Correction of cardiovascular abnormalities (eg, volume replacement) Broad-spectrum antibiotic therapy Surgical consultation
Severe	Any patient with CI and more than three of the criteria for moderate disease or any of the following: Peritoneal signs on physical examination Pneumotosis or portal venous gas on radiologic imaging Gangrene on colonoscopy Pancolonic distribution or IRCI on imaging or colonoscopy	Emergent surgical consultation (treatment is likely to be surgical) Transfer to intensive care unit Correction of cardiovascular abnormalities (eg, volume replacement) Broad-spectrum antibiotic therapy

BUN, blood urea nitrogen; CI, colon ischemia; Hgb, hemoglobin; IRCI, isolated right colon ischemia; LDH, lactate dehydrogenase; WBC, white blood cell count.
Reproduced with permission from Brandt LJ, Feuerstadt P, Longstreth GF, et al. ACG clinical guideline: epidemiology, risk factors, patterns of presentation, diagnosis, and management of colon ischemia (CI). Am J Gastroenterol. 2015;110(1):18–44.

Management Initial management of acute colonic pseudo-obstruction involves correcting reversible causes of colonic ileus such as electrolyte imbalances, hypoxemia, hypovolemia, and removal of medications that can exacerbate the problem. The vast majority of patients are successfully treated with these relatively simple measures. Bowel rest and intravenous hydration are imperative.

Neostigmine, a cholinesterase inhibitor, given in doses of 1 to 2 mg IV or SC is effective in patients with acute colonic pseudo-obstruction. There are several relative contraindications to the use of neostigmine listed in **Table 84-14**. Following neostigmine administration, patients should be monitored closely. A second administration of neostigmine can be attempted if there is partial or no response to the first trial.

TABLE 84-14 ■ CONTRAINDICATIONS TO USE OF NEOSTIGMINE IN ACUTE COLONIC PSEUDO-OBSTRUCTION

ABSOLUTE	RELATIVE
Hypersensitivity to neostigmine Mechanical urinary or intestinal obstruction	Recent myocardial infarction Acidosis Asthma Bradycardia Peptic ulcer disease Therapy with β-blockers

In selected patients who fail conservative and medical management, colonoscopic decompression of the unprepped bowel can be attempted. However, care is required since during colonoscopy air is insufflated into an already dilated colon and the risk of colon perforation is increased. Surgical decompression, sometimes via placement of a cecostomy tube, remains another option for patients who do not respond to medical and endoscopic interventions.

The overall prognosis of patients with acute colonic pseudo-obstruction is poor, with an in-hospital mortality approaching 30%, attributable primarily to the severity of the underlying illness. The most significant complication of acute dilatation is colonic perforation, which occurred in 3% of cases in one retrospective series.

Lower Gastrointestinal Bleeding

Lower GI bleeding is defined as that which arises distal to the ligament of Treitz. Lower GI bleeding occurs less frequently and usually is less severe than upper GI bleeding. The incidence of lower GI bleeding increases significantly with age. The majority of lower GI bleeding in older adults is the result of diverticula, vascular ectasias, and CI, but there are many other causes (**Table 84-15**). This section will focus on the approach to the patient with lower GI bleeding and bleeding from vascular ectasias.

Acute lower GI bleeding presents with bright red blood per rectum, hematochezia, or melena depending on

TABLE 84-15 ■ CAUSES OF LOWER GI HEMORRHAGE

Diverticulosis
Ischemic colitis
Vascular ectasia
Hemorrhoids
Neoplasm
Postpolypectomy
Inflammatory bowel disease
Infectious colitis
NSAID-induced colopathy
Radiation colopathy
Dieulafoy lesion
Colonic ulcerations
Meckel diverticulum
Rectal varices
Aortoenteric fistula
Small bowel sources

the location of the bleeding. Bright red blood per rectum usually indicates a distal colonic source or rapidly bleeding upper source. Melena usually indicates a right-sided colonic lesion or a source in the upper GI tract.

The first goal in the management of a patient with lower GI bleeding is resuscitation and hemodynamic stabilization. This may include administration of crystalloid intravenous fluids and blood products. Initial testing usually includes complete blood count, blood chemistry, coagulation profile, and blood type and cross-match, and the results help guide further management. For example, a low mean corpuscular volume often is a sign of chronic blood loss; a BUN-to-creatinine ratio of greater than 20:1 usually indicates an upper GI source; an elevated INR requires consideration of reversal in the face of hemodynamically significant bleeding. Older patients are more susceptible to complications from hypotension and anemia, and rapid stabilization and monitoring are essential. There should be a low threshold to recommend emergency room evaluation and hospitalization of these patients.

Approximately 12% of patients thought to have lower GI bleeding have an upper GI bleeding source. It is important to exclude upper GI bleeding in patients with presumed lower GI bleeding. This can be accomplished with passage of a nasogastric tube and analysis of the gastric aspirate. Bilious fluid without blood in the nasogastric tube aspirate usually confirms the suspicion of lower GI bleeding. If an upper GI source is still in question, urgent upper endoscopy may be performed.

Although urgent upper endoscopy for the diagnosis and treatment of upper GI bleeding is predicated on sound data, urgent colonoscopy in lower GI bleeding has been practiced less consistently. Colonoscopy has the advantage of allowing for the diagnosis and immediate treatment of actively bleeding lesions. A number of reports have shown that "urgent colonoscopy" is safe and yields a specific diagnosis in a high

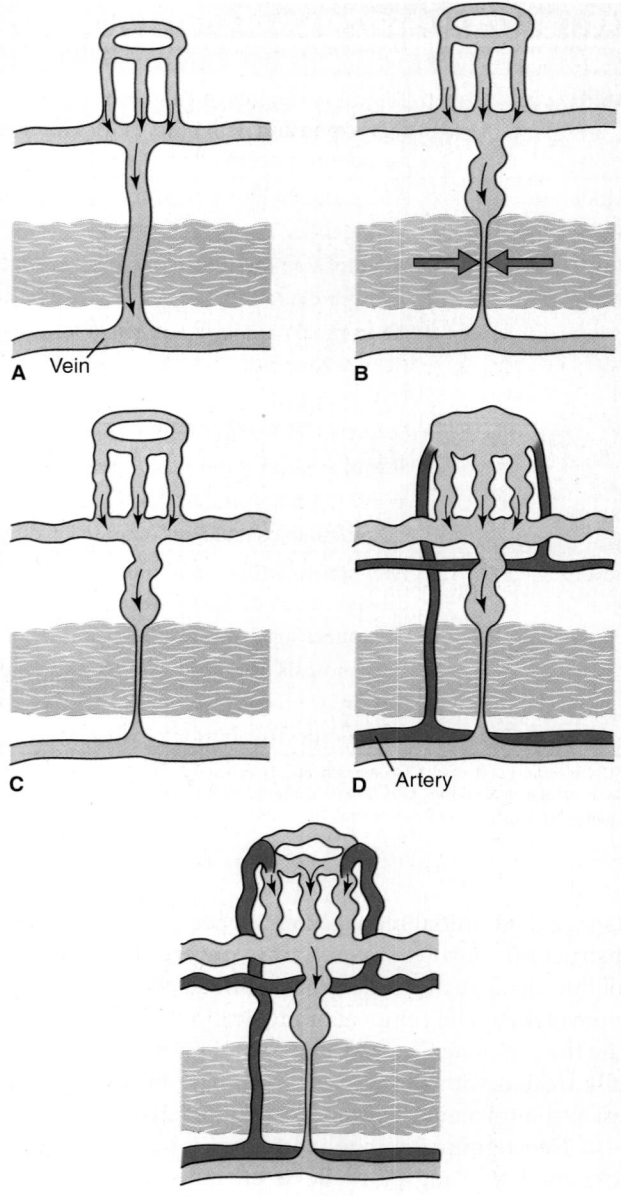

FIGURE 84-5. Proposed concept of the development of cecal vascular ectasias. **A.** Normal state of vein perforating muscular layers. **B.** With muscle contraction or increased intraluminal pressure, the vein is partially obstructed. **C.** After repeated episodes over many years, the submucosal vein becomes dilated and tortuous. **D.** Later, the veins and venules draining into the abnormal submucosal vein become similarly dilated and tortuous. **E.** Ultimately, the capillary ring becomes dilated, the precapillary sphincter becomes incompetent, and a small arteriovenous communication is present through the ectasia.

proportion of older patients with lower GI bleeding. On the basis of a high diagnostic yield, low rate of complications, and theoretical therapeutic potential, urgent colonoscopy following a rapid colonic purge has been recommended as the diagnostic procedure of choice in most patients with hemodynamically significant lower GI bleeding.

Other diagnostic tests in patients with active lower GI bleeding include scintigraphy (nuclear tagged red blood cell scans), CT angiography, and conventional angiography. Approximately 45% of patients with lower GI bleeding have positive red blood cell scintigraphy. Tagged red blood cell scans can detect bleeding at a rate greater than 0.1 mL/min and are useful to localize the site of bleeding, but unfortunately offer no option for therapy. If a patient has a positive bleeding scan or CT angiography, traditional angiography with selective embolization can be performed to attempt to stop the bleeding. In order to detect active bleeding, angiography requires a higher rate of bleeding than scintigraphy, 0.5 mL/min compared to 0.1 mL/min. Transcatheter embolization of a lower GI bleeding source is effective in 70% to 90% of patients. If bleeding cannot be stopped with angiography, surgery to remove the bleeding colonic segment may be necessary. If a specific bleeding site can be localized with the above studies, a limited surgical resection can be performed rather than a subtotal colectomy.

Vascular ectasias Vascular ectasias, which arise from an age-related degeneration of previously normal blood vessels, typically occur in the cecum and proximal ascending colon. Along with diverticular bleeding, they are responsible for the majority of significant lower GI bleeding episodes in older adults. Ectasias are found in up to 25% of persons older than 60 years who do not have symptoms; they typically are multiple and less than 5 mm in diameter. Vascular ectasias probably arise as a result of repeated episodes of incomplete, low-grade obstruction of submucosal veins caused by increased tension in the colonic wall. The ultimate result is tortuosity and dilation of the venules and the arteriolar–capillary unit that feeds it, resulting in a small arteriovenous communication (**Figure 84-5**).

Lower GI bleeding caused by a vascular ectasia may be clinically indistinguishable from diverticular bleeding and is characterized by painless hematochezia. Bleeding from vascular ectasias may be hemodynamically significant, and a variety of treatment options exists including electrocoagulation, injection therapy, heater probe application, or argon plasma coagulation.

ACKNOWLEDGMENT

Many thanks to Richard Saad, MD, for his review and very helpful comments and to David A. Greenwald, MD, for his contributions to the chapter Common Large Intestinal Disorders in earlier editions of this book. Material from that chapter, including tables and figures, has been incorporated into this one.

FURTHER READING

Asempa TE, Nicolau DP. *Clostridium difficile* infection in the elderly: an update on management. *Clin Interv Aging.* 2017;12:1799–1809.

Brandt LJ, Feuerstadt P, Longstreth GF, Boley SJ. American College of Gastroenterology clinical guideline: epidemiology, risk factors, patterns of presentation, diagnosis, and management of colon ischemia (CI). *Am J Gastroenterol.* 2015;110(1):18–44.

Broens RM, Pennickx FM. Relation between anal electrosensitivity and rectal filling sensation and the influence of age. *Dis Colon Rectum.* 2005;48:127–133.

Comparato G, Pilotto A, Franze A, et al. Diverticular disease in the elderly. *Dig Dis.* 2007;25:151–159.

Drekonia D, Reich J, Gezahegn S, et al. Fecal microbiota transplantation for *Clostridium difficile* infection: a systematic review. *Ann Intern Med.* 2015;162:630–638.

Gispert JP, Chaparro M. Systematic review with meta-analysis: inflammatory bowel disease in the elderly. *Aliment Pharmacol Ther.* 2014;39:459–477.

Greenwald DA, Brandt LJ, Reinus JF. Ischemic bowel disease in the elderly. *Gastroenterol Clin.* 2001;30(2):445–473.

Hall KE, Proctor DD, Fisher L, Rose S. AGA future trends committee report: effects of aging of the population on gastroenterology practice, education and research. *Gastroenterology.* 2005;129:1305–1338.

Jafri SM, Monkemuller K, Lukens FJ. Endoscopy in the elderly: a review of the efficacy and safety of colonoscopy, esophagogastroduodenoscopy, and endoscopic retrograde cholangiopancreatography. *J Clin Gastroenterol.* 2010;44:161–166.

Jain A, Vargas HD. Advances and challenges in the management of acute colonic pseudo-obstruction (Ogilvie syndrome). *Clin Colon Rectal Surg.* 2012;25:37–45.

McDonald CL, Gerding DN, Johnson S, et al. Clinical practice guidelines for *Clostridium difficile* infection in adults and children: 2017 Update by the Infectious Diseases Society of America (IDSA) and Society for Healthcare Epidemiology of America (SHEA). *Clin Infect Dis.* 2018;66(7):e1–e48.

Nguyen GC, Smalley WE, Vege SS, Carrasco-Labra A; Clinical Guidelines Committee. American gastroenterological association Institute guideline on the medical management of microscopic colitis. *Gastroenterology.* 2016;150(1):242–246.

Pardi DS. Microscopic colitis. *Clin Geriatr Med.* 2014;30:55–65.

Peery AF, Shaukat A, Strate LL. AGA Clinical practice update on medical management of colonic diverticulitis. *Gastroenterology.* 2021;160(3):906–911.e1.

Rezapour M, Stollman N. Diverticular disease in the elderly. *Curr Gastroenterol Rep.* 2019;21(9):46.

Schembri J, Bonello J, Christodoulou DK, Katsanos KH, Ellul P. Segmental colitis associated with diverticulosis: is it the coexistence of colonic diverticulosis and inflammatory bowel disease? *Ann Gastroenterol* 2017;30(3):257–261.

Shaukat A, Kahi CJ, Burke CA, Rabeneck L, Sauer BG, Rex DK. ACG clinical guidelines: colorectal cancer screening 2021. *Am J Gastroenterol.* 2021;116(3):458–479.

Stepaniuk P, Bernstein CN, Targowink LE, et al. Characterization of inflammatory bowel disease in elderly patients: a review of epidemiology current practices and outcomes of current management strategies. *Can J Gastroenterol Hepatol.* 2015;29:327–333.

Ten Hove JR, Shah SC, Shaffer SR, et al. Consecutive negative findings on colonoscopy during surveillance predict a low risk of advanced neoplasia in patients with inflammatory bowel disease with long-standing colitis: results of a 15-year multicentre, multinational cohort study. *Gut.* 2019;68(4):615–622.

Tran V, Limketkai BN, Sauk JS. IBD in the elderly: management challenges and therapeutic considerations. *Curr Gastroenterol Rep.* 2019;21(11):60.

Travis AC, Plevsky D, Saltzman JR. Endoscopy in the elderly. *Am J Gastroenterol.* 2012;107:1495–1501.

Wang YR, Cangemi JR, Loftus EV Jr, Picco MF. Rate of early/missed colorectal cancers after colonoscopy in older patients with or without inflammatory bowel disease in the United States. *Am J Gastroenterol.* 2013;108(3):444–449.

Chapter 85

Upper Gastrointestinal Disorders

Alberto Pilotto, Marilisa Franceschi

INTRODUCTION

Upper gastrointestinal disorders (UGIDs) are highly prevalent in the aging population and may influence greatly nutrition, general well-being, and quality of life of older people. This chapter discusses the pathophysiology, clinical features, diagnostic approaches, and treatments of UGIDs, focusing on gastroesophageal reflux disease (GERD), peptic ulcer disease (PUD) including considerations on *Helicobacter pylori* infection and its eradication, and upper gastrointestinal bleeding (UGIB). Particular attention is given to pharmacology of UGIDs, both as a causal mechanism, as in the use of nonsteroidal anti-inflammatory drugs (NSAIDs) alone or in combination with anticoagulants/antiplatelet agents, but also in the treatment of acid-related disorders. Special attention is given to situations when deprescription of widely used antisecretory drugs, mainly proton pump inhibitors, is warranted. UGIDs may present insidiously in older adults, who often have nonspecific symptoms, independently of whether esophageal and/or gastroduodenal lesions are demonstrated on instrumental diagnostic evaluations. Since UGIDs often require an interdisciplinary approach including endoscopists, radiologists, gastroenterologists, and surgeons, scenarios when referral to a specialist is recommended are also described.

GASTROESOPHAGEAL REFLUX DISEASE

Definition

GERD is defined by symptoms and/or histopathologic alterations (esophagitis) caused by reflux of gastric contents into the esophagus. Manifestations of GERD range from mild episodes of heartburn and acid regurgitation without esophagitis, commonly defined as nonerosive reflux disease (NERD), to chronic mucosal inflammation with erosive esophagitis and ulceration, complicated in severe cases by stricture and bleeding.

Epidemiology

GERD is a frequent condition with worldwide distribution. The prevalence of GERD is estimated to be 12% in Australia, 7.8% in East Asia, 8.8% to 26% in Europe, 8.7% to 33% in the Middle East, 18% to 28% in North America, and 23% in South America. A large US nationwide cohort

Learning Objectives

- Identify the presentation of gastroesophageal reflux disease (GERD) in older adults and select the most appropriate therapeutic strategies.

- Employ management strategies that reduce the risk of peptic ulcer disease (PUD) in older adults including limiting the use of nonsteroidal anti-inflammatory drugs and eradicating *H pylori* when indicated.

- Ascertain the mechanisms that ensure proper use of proton pump inhibitors (PPI) in preventing PUD and UGIB with appropriate discontinuation of PPI therapy when not needed, making use of good clinical practice guidelines including multidimensional approach and noninvasive gastric function tests.

Key Clinical Points

1. **GERD is common in older adults with an incidence of 5 per 1000 person years in the United Kingdom and United States. Symptoms may not correlate with the severity of esophageal findings on endoscopy so a trial of proton pump inhibitors (PPIs) should rarely be done without endoscopy for suspected GERD in older adults. PPIs are more effective than H$_2$-blockers, but prokinetic agents have not been shown to be superior to placebo.**

2. **The prevalence of PUD increases with age, likely due to *H pylori* infection, use of mucosa-damaging drugs, and an imbalance between mucosal erosive and protective factors. Treatment of *H pylori* reduces PUD relapse, but many older adults go untested and untreated. *H pylori* eradication after treatment should be documented with a breath test or stool antigen.**

(Continued)

(Cont.)

3. Upper GI bleeding (UGIB) occurs in older adults due to the same pathologies as seen in young adults, but may present with exacerbation of underlying disease (eg, cardiac disease) or non-GI symptoms such as syncope.

4. PPIs interact with many drugs prescribed for older adults, and long-term PPI use has been associated with multiple adverse outcomes, especially in frail older adults. Thus, long-term PPI use should be avoided unless there are clear indications, and deprescription should be enacted whenever possible.

TABLE 85-1 ■ PATHOPHYSIOLOGIC CHANGES AFFECTING THE ESOPHAGUS WITH AGING

FUNCTIONAL	ANATOMICAL
Impaired motility of the esophagus	Hiatus hernia
Reduced LES pressure and length	Difficulty in maintaining an upright position
Normal or slightly reduced gastric acid secretion	
Delayed gastric emptying transit time	
Reduced salivary secretion	
Decreased tissue resistance as a result of impaired epithelial cell regeneration	
Duodenogastroesophageal reflux of bile salts	

LES, lower esophageal sphincter.

study reported that the prevalence of GERD is increasing overall, but seemingly this increase is not seen in subjects older than 70 years, whose proportion of GERD patients remains stable around 15% during the time period from 2006 to 2016. Indeed, GERD prevalence remains higher amongst subjects older than 70 years, but as prevalence of GERD in those age 30 to 39 is increasing, the proportion of GERD patients older than 70 years is decreasing.

While it is still unclear whether the incidence and the prevalence of GERD symptoms increase with advancing age, the frequency of esophagitis is higher in older versus younger adults. Indeed, older age was found to be a significant risk factor in the development of severe forms of GERD in both epidemiologic and clinical studies from the United States, Japan, and Europe. Consistently, GERD was the sixth most common disorder in a retrospective cross sectional study of almost 20,000 long-term care residents of nursing homes older than 65 years, with an overall prevalence of 23%. In summary, GERD is a highly prevalent disorder in older adults, and associated with more severe and advanced disease than in young adults.

Pathophysiology

Pathophysiologic changes in esophageal function that occur with aging, the so-called presbyesophagus, are summarized in **Table 85-1** and may be responsible, at least in part, for the high prevalence of GERD in old age. Older patients have a high prevalence of other risk factors that predispose the aging esophagus to lesions (also see **Table 85-1**): (1) difficulty in maintaining an upright position after meals due to the modifications of the thorax anatomy linked to the dorsal kyphosis and collapse of the dorsal vertebrae; and (2) hiatus hernia associated with both repeated episodes of acid reflux and with more severe diseases such as Barrett esophagus. Older adults often use drugs that may have a directly damaging effect on esophageal mucosa or an indirect effect on reducing lower esophageal sphincter (LES) pressure (**Table 85-2**). Delayed esophageal transit time of many drugs in older

people creates a potentially dangerous situation when it coexists with acid reflux, as reported for alendronate and NSAIDs.

Presentation

Particular attention has been given to the clinical presentation of GERD in older adults since important differences have been reported when compared to younger individuals. Older patients report fewer typical symptoms of heartburn, acid regurgitation, and epigastric pain (**Figure 85-1**). Atypical symptoms also are relatively rare in older adults (**Table 85-3**). In contrast, the prevalence of nonspecific symptoms of vomiting, anorexia, weight loss, and anemia increase with age (**Figure 85-2**). Reflux esophagitis in older adults may thus be missed, and a substantial number of patients may suffer subclinical relapses of the disease. The cause of such a different clinical expression of GERD in older adults is not clear, but a diminished sensitivity to visceral pain has been documented in older adults. Moreover, 24-hour esophageal pH monitoring and endoscopy examinations demonstrate an age-related reduction in acid chemosensitivity and a reduced symptom severity despite a

TABLE 85-2 ■ DRUGS THAT MAY INCREASE THE RISK OF SEVERE GERD

DIRECT EFFECT ON ESOPHAGEAL MUCOSA	REDUCTION IN LES PRESSURE
Aspirin	Theophylline
NSAIDs	Nitroderivates
Potassium salts	Calcium channel blockers
Ferrous sulfate	Benzodiazepines
Corticosteroids	Dopaminergics
Alendronate	Tricyclic antidepressants
	Anticholinergics

LES, lower esophageal sphincter.

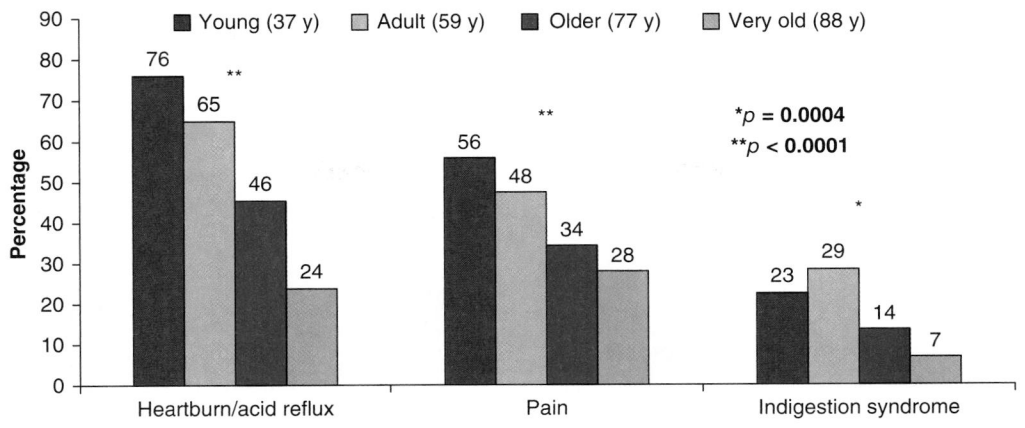

FIGURE 85-1. Prevalence of typical symptoms in 840 subjects with reflux esophagitis divided according to age. (Adapted with permission from Pilotto A, Franceschi M, Leandro G, et al. Clinical features of reflux esophagitis in older people: a study of 840 consecutive patients. *J Am Geriatr Soc.* 2006;54[10]:1537–1542.)

tendency toward increased severity of esophageal mucosal injury.

Evaluation

Since the presentation of GERD is often nonspecific in older adults, *endoscopy* should be undertaken early as the initial diagnostic test in any older patient suspected of having GERD. Early endoscopy is very useful in diagnosing the presence and the grade of severity of esophagitis **(Figure 85-3)** and/or hiatus hernia, which are important prognostic factors to be considered in long-term treatment, especially if the hernia is greater than 3 cm. Endoscopy also identifies GERD complications, especially esophageal strictures and Barrett esophagus, and concomitant gastroduodenal diseases including gastric or duodenal ulcers and/or *H pylori* infection. *Barium radiography* of the esophagus is a useful test to establish the presence of a hiatus hernia and is indicated as part of the evaluation of the patient with suspected motility abnormalities or peptic stricture.

A barium study may also identify rings, webs, or other obstructive lesions. The barium swallow test is also a key test in studying older patients with dysphagia, and it should be performed in conjunction with endoscopy in all older patients with this symptomatology. Moreover, coupled with videofluoroscopic swallowing studies, barium swallow (esophagram) allows the identification of Zenker diverticulum and cricopharyngeal dysfunction. Barium studies are widely available and usually well tolerated by older people. *Esophageal 24-hour pH testing* is helpful before antireflux surgery and in those patients not responsive to medical treatment. In the patient with persistent symptoms and a negative endoscopy, an abnormal esophageal pH test may suggest the need for more aggressive drug therapy, whereas a normal test may indicate the presence of a functional disorder. In the patient with persistent esophagitis, a normal test could differentiate pathophysiologic mechanisms, that is, a drug-induced esophagitis from acid reflux disease or biliary reflux. *Esophageal manometry* is useful in identifying abnormalities of LES pressure or esophageal motility. In older patients, its major use in GERD is reserved for the localization of LES before pH testing and for obtaining preoperative information on esophageal peristalsis.

A therapeutic trial with PPI has been suggested as a useful diagnostic test in patients with GERD. Meta-analyses of clinical studies demonstrated that an empiric PPI trial has 78% sensitivity and 54% specificity in confirming the diagnosis of GERD when compared with endoscopy or 24-hour esophageal pH monitoring. In patients with noncardiac chest pain, sensitivity and specificity are reported to be 80% and 74%, respectively. Since typical (heartburn, acid regurgitation) and extraesophageal symptoms (pulmonary, otorhinolaryngeal, noncardiac chest pain) of GERD are less frequent in older than in younger patients, the older patient's history is less reliable, and there is a high prevalence of severe esophagitis despite mild symptoms; a trial of PPIs should be used with great caution

TABLE 85-3 ■ TYPICAL AND ATYPICAL SYMPTOMS OF GASTROESOPHAGEAL REFLUX DISEASE	
TYPICAL SYMPTOMS	**ATYPICAL SYMPTOMS**
Heartburn	Pulmonary symptoms:
Acid regurgitation	Bronchial asthma
Epigastric pain	Bronchiectasis
	Chronic bronchitis
	Chronic cough
	Otorhinolaryngeal symptoms:
	Hoarseness
	Chronic laryngitis
	Odynophagia
	Noncardiac chest pain

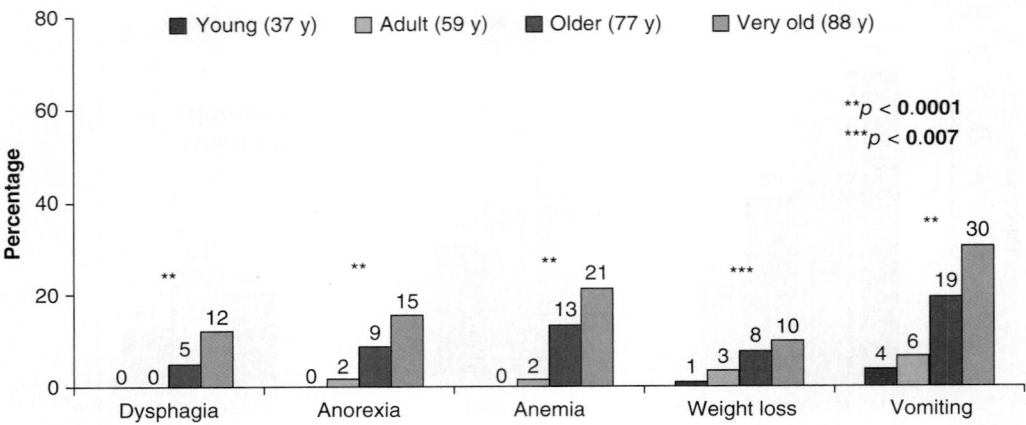

FIGURE 85-2. Prevalence of nonspecific symptoms in 840 subjects with reflux esophagitis divided according to age. (Adapted with permission from Pilotto A, Franceschi M, Leandro G, et al. Clinical features of reflux esophagitis in older people: a study of 840 consecutive patients. *J Am Geriatr Soc.* 2006;54[10]:1537–1542.)

in older patients, possibly only after endoscopy as a first diagnostic test.

Management

The objectives of GERD treatment are (1) relief of symptoms, (2) esophagitis healing, (3) prevention of relapse, and (4) prevention of complications.

Nonpharmacological Although there is clinical and physiologic evidence that smoking, alcohol, chocolate, peppermint, coffee, fatty, or citrus intake may adversely affect symptoms or esophageal pH, there is little evidence that cessation of these agents will improve GERD variables.

Elevation of the head of the bed and weight loss, however, have been associated with improvement in GERD variables in case-control studies. Medications that decrease LES pressure and promote gastroesophageal reflux as well as drugs that may cause direct esophageal injury (see **Table 85-2**) should be avoided when possible or used with caution in older patients with GERD. In any case, these drugs must be taken while maintaining an upright position and with a full glass of water.

Drugs

Short-Term Therapy Antacids and alginic acid provide symptomatic relief in mild, nonerosive esophagitis. Possible

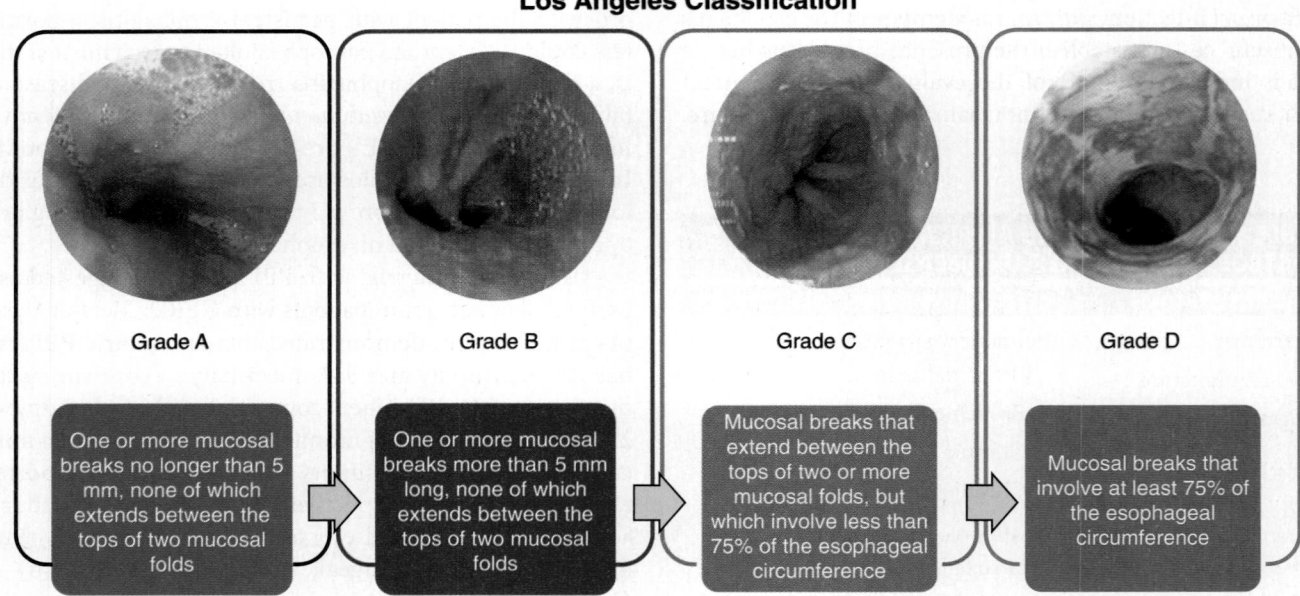

FIGURE 85-3. Endoscopic classification of esophagitis (according to the Los Angeles Grading System). (Data from Lundell LR, Dent J, Bennett JR, et al. Endoscopic assessment of oesophagitis: clinical and functional correlates and further validation of the Los Angeles classification. *Gut.* 1999;45[2]:172–180.)

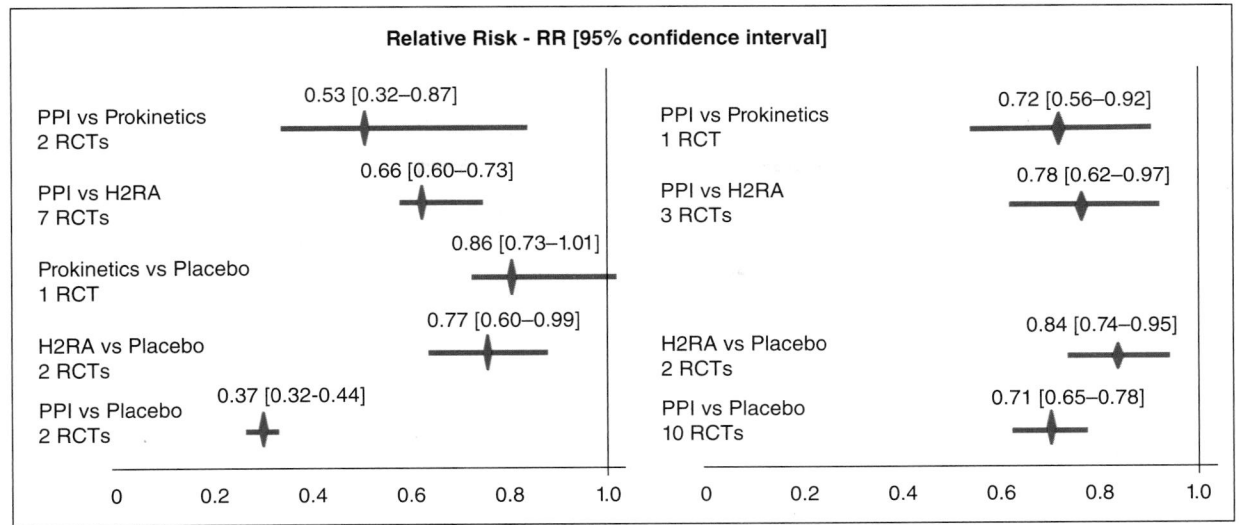

FIGURE 85-4. Efficacy of short-term use of proton pump inhibitors (PPI), H_2-receptor antagonists (H2RA), and prokinetics in adults with GERD treated empirically (left) and in those with endoscopy-negative reflux disease (ENRD) (right). (Data from Sigterman KE, van Pinxteren B, Bonis PA, et al. Short-term treatment with proton pump inhibitors, H2-receptor antagonists and prokinetics for gastro-oesophageal reflux disease-like symptoms and endoscopy negative reflux disease. *Cochrane Database Syst Rev.* 2013;31[5]:CD002095.)

side effects of antacids include salt overload, constipation, hypercalcemia, and interference with the absorption of other drugs, particularly antibiotics such as tetracycline, azithromycin, and quinolones. Caution is warranted in patients with chronic kidney disease or liver failure, not only because of reduced clearance but also because of modified electrolyte metabolism.

Prokinetic drugs, including metoclopramide, clebopride, domperidone, and levosulpiride, either alone or in combination with antisecretory drugs, are only moderately effective in GERD. Unfortunately, no controlled clinical trials have evaluated the role of these drugs specifically in the treatment of GERD in older adults. However, older patients treated with prokinetic drugs are more likely than younger subjects to have adverse events such as tardive dyskinesia, mental confusion, drowsiness, and age-related renal dysfunction, which may require dose reduction and close clinical monitoring. Thus, antireflux therapy is focused largely on suppressing gastric acid secretion with H_2-blockers and PPIs.

A series of meta-analyses of 34 trials including 1314 participants demonstrated that PPIs were more effective than H_2-blockers and prokinetics in relieving heartburn both in patients with GERD who were treated empirically and in patients with endoscopy-negative reflux disease (ENRD) (**Figure 85-4**). Moreover, a meta-analysis of 134 trials involving 35,978 patients with esophagitis demonstrated benefit for standard dose PPI therapy and H_2-blockers but not prokinetics compared to placebo in healing of esophagitis. In addition, 26 trials evaluating 4032 participants reported that there was benefit for PPI therapy compared to H_2-blockers or H_2-blockers plus prokinetics in healing of esophagitis. Thus, PPI is the most effective therapy

for heartburn relief and healing of esophagitis, and H_2-blocker therapy is also effective. However, the effectiveness of prokinetics over placebo is marginal (**Figure 85-5**).

Currently, six PPIs are available: omeprazole, lansoprazole, dexlansoprazole (lansoprazole's R-enantiomer), rabeprazole, pantoprazole, and esomeprazole. Some age-associated differences in pharmacokinetics and pharmacodynamics of PPIs have been reported. However, it is unknown if these differences are associated with different clinical effects, particularly in older patients. Indeed, a series of meta-analyses evaluating acute therapy of esophagitis reported that the PPIs were superior to ranitidine and placebo in healing erosive esophagitis, without differences in efficacy between omeprazole 20 mg daily and lansoprazole 30 mg daily or pantoprazole 40 mg daily or rabeprazole 20 mg daily. A systematic review and meta-analysis of randomized controlled trials comparing effectiveness and acceptability of the FDA-licensed PPIs for esophagitis reported that esomeprazole 40 mg provided higher healing rates than omeprazole 20 mg, lansoprazole 30 mg, pantoprazole 40 mg, and rabeprazole 20 mg at 4 weeks and omeprazole 20 mg, lansoprazole 30 mg, and rabeprazole 20 mg at 8 weeks (**Figure 85-6**). In terms of acceptability, only dexlansoprazole 60 mg had significantly more all-cause discontinuation than omeprazole 20 mg, pantoprazole 40 mg, and lansoprazole 30 mg (**Figure 85-7**).

Long-Term Maintenance Therapy GERD is a chronic disease with a 70% to 90% annual relapse rate after the interruption of an effective antisecretory regimen. Risk factors for relapse are shown in **Table 85-4**. Maintenance therapy with antisecretory drugs reduces relapse of GERD in older patients. Also PPIs have higher efficacy than H_2-blockers

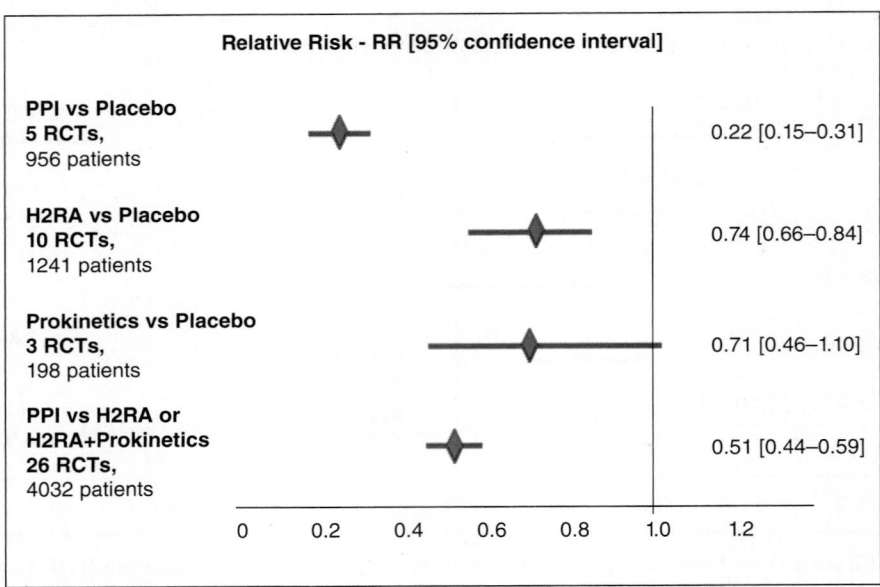

FIGURE 85-5. Effectiveness of proton pump inhibitors (PPIs), H₂-receptor antagonists (H2RAs), prokinetic therapy, sucralfate, and placebo in healing esophagitis. (Data from Khan M, Santana J, Donnellan C, et al. Medical treatments in the short term management of reflux oesophagitis. *Cochrane Database Syst Rev.* 2007;[2]:CD003244.)

and prokinetics in maintaining mucosal healing after an episode of esophagitis. There are two main approaches to maintenance drug therapy for GERD: step-up and step-down. In the step-up approach, therapy is initiated with weak inhibition of gastric acid (eg, an H₂-blocker or half dosage of a PPI), and progresses to a higher degree of acid inhibition (standard and then escalating doses of PPI), until adequate symptom control is obtained. The step-down approach involves starting with the most effective regimen (full dosage of a PPI) and switching to lower doses of PPI for maintenance therapy once symptoms are under control. This latter approach is perhaps more rational, based on evidence showing superior efficacy of PPIs over H₂-blockers across all grades of severity of GERD. Withdrawal of maintenance therapy with PPI after 6 months reduces the remission rate of esophagitis at 1 year from 95% to 33% in patients

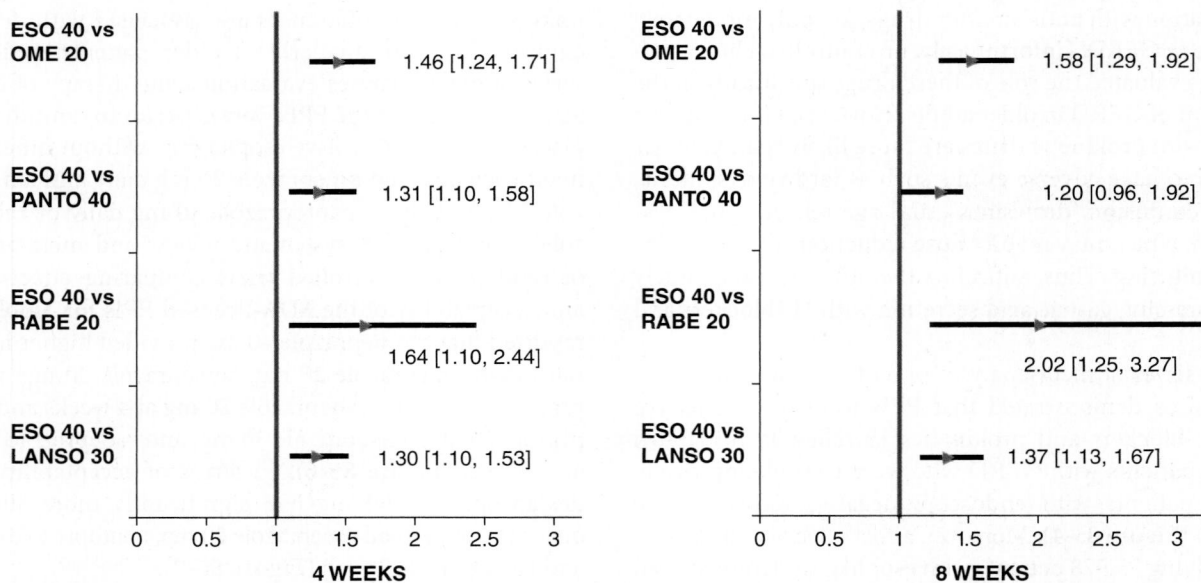

Omeprazole (OME), Pantoprazole (PANTO), Lansoprazole (LANSO),
Rabeprazole (RABE), Esomeprazole (ESO)

FIGURE 85-6. Healing rates of erosive esophagitis at 4 and 8 weeks. (Data from Li MJ, Li Q, Sun M, et al. Comparative effectiveness and acceptability of the FDA-licensed proton pump inhibitors for erosive esophagitis: a PRISMA-compliant network meta-analysis. *Medicine (Baltimore).* 2017;96[39]:e8120.)

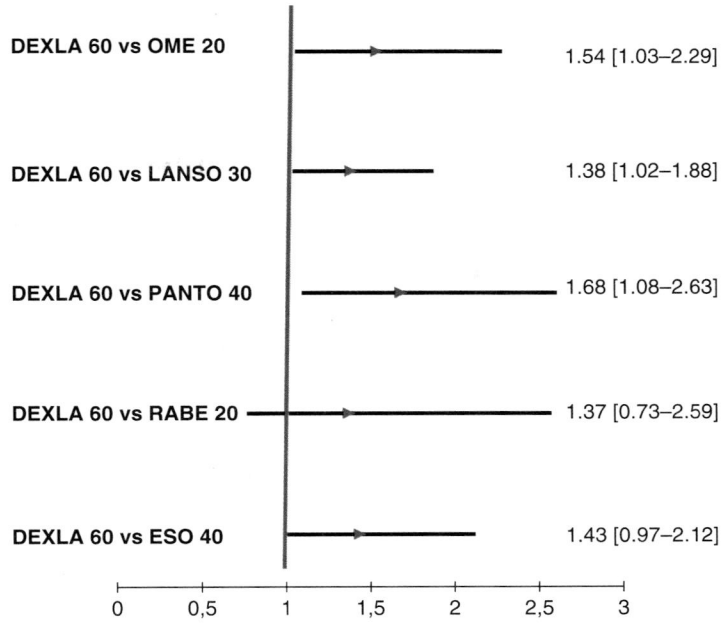

Omeprazole (OME), Pantoprazole (PANTO), Lansoprazole (LANSO),
Rabeprazole, (RABE), Esomeprazole (ESO), Dexlansoprazole (DEXLA)

FIGURE 85-7. Acceptability (risk of discontinuation) of the FDA-licensed proton pump inhibitors for erosive esophagitis. (Data from Li MJ, Li Q, Sun M, et al. Comparative effectiveness and acceptability of the FDA-licensed proton pump inhibitors for erosive esophagitis: a PRISMA-compliant network meta-analysis. *Medicine (Baltimore).* 2017;96[39]:e8120.)

older than 65 years (**Figure 85-8**). Presently, no comparative studies have been carried out to evaluate which strategy (step-down vs step-up) is more cost-effective in older subjects. As chronic PPI use without reassessment contributes to polypharmacy and puts subjects at risk of experiencing drug interactions and adverse events (see below), deprescribing should be a goal of treatment. A Cochrane review, however, found that although effectively reducing costs and medication intake, deprescription strategies including on-demand PPI intake versus continuous indefinite use, are associated with patient dissatisfaction due to symptomatic disease relapse. Unfortunately, studies carried out specifically in older people are lacking. **Figure 85-9** summarizes the therapeutic schemes for short-term and

TABLE 85-4 ■ RISK FACTORS FOR RELAPSE OF ESOPHAGITIS
Patient characteristics
Old age
High body mass index (BMI)
Clinical features
Long history of reflux symptoms
Latency prolonged between appearance of symptoms and therapy
Persistence of symptoms after the healing of esophagitis
Endoscopic characteristics
Severity of the esophagitis at baseline
Presence of a large hiatus hernia
Pathophysiology features
Reduced pressure of the lower esophageal sphincter (manometry)
Modified curve of 24-h ph-metry

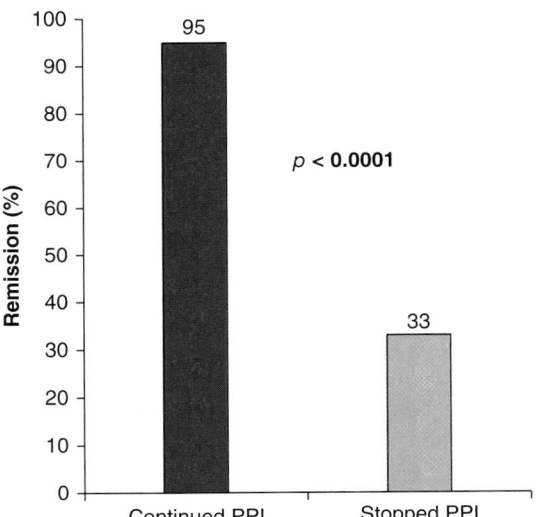

FIGURE 85-8. Remission at 12 months in older patients with esophagitis who continued versus stopped proton pump inhibitor (PPI) maintenance treatment after 6 months. (Data from Pilotto A, Leandro G, Franceschi M, et al. Short- and long-term therapy for reflux oesophagitis in the elderly: a multi-centre, placebo-controlled study with pantoprazole. *Aliment Pharmacol Ther.* 2003;17[11]:1399–1406.)

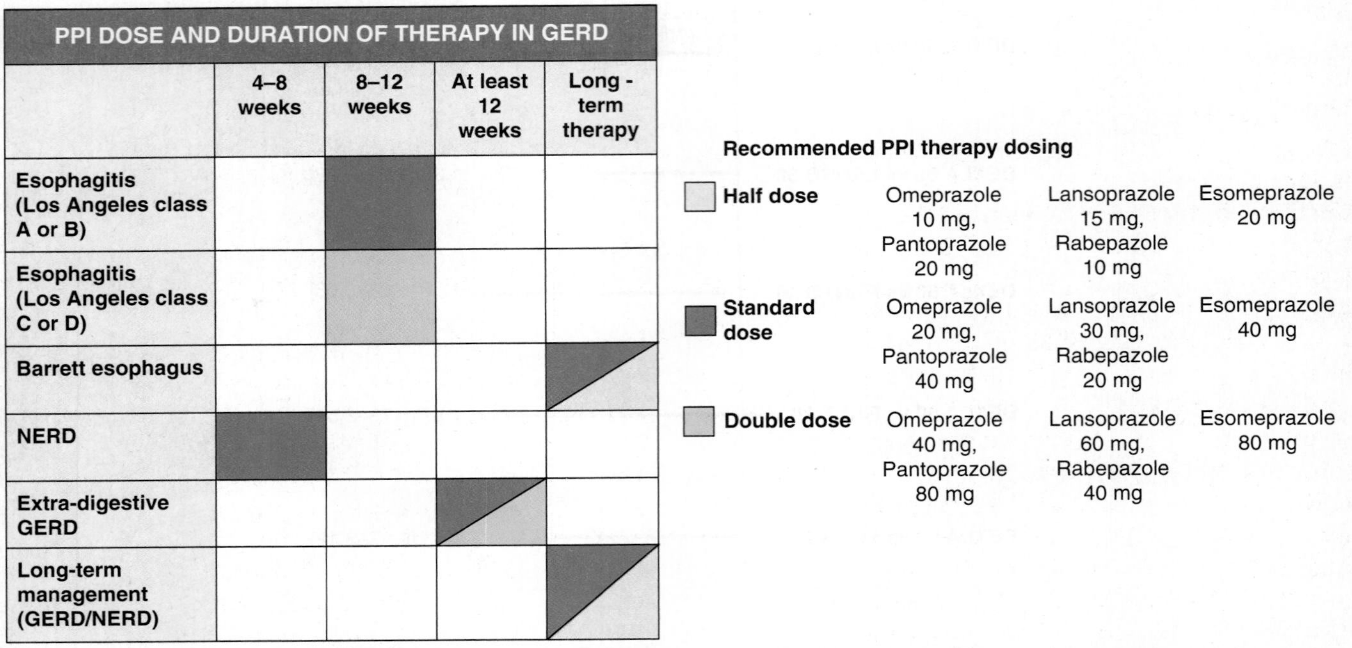

FIGURE 85-9. Therapeutics schemes for short-term and long-term proton pump inhibitor (PPI) treatments in older people with gastroesophageal reflux disease (GERD) and nonerosive reflux disease (NERD).

long-term PPI treatment in older people with GERD and NERD.

Safety of Long-Term Antisecretory Treatment PPIs represent a very effective class of drugs widely prescribed in all age populations, including older subjects, and often for prolonged periods of time. The potential adverse effects of long-term PPI use are widespread, as illustrated in **Figure 85-10**. Thus, safety evaluation of long-term treatment with PPIs is emerging as a major topic in clinical practice.

PPIs AND ESOPHAGEAL AND GASTRIC HISTOLOGIC CHANGES. There is presently no evidence supporting the hypothesis that long-term PPI therapy may increase the risk of neoplastic degeneration in patients with Barrett esophagus. Conversely, based on meta-analysis of observational studies, the long-term use of PPIs was associated with a decreased risk of esophageal adenocarcinoma and/or high-grade dysplasia in patients with Barrett esophagus. As regards PPI long-term use and the risk of gastric cancer, conflicting data have been reported. A positive association between fundic gland polyps (FGPs) and acid suppression has been reported. Although this constitutes a frequent endoscopic finding, it is not associated with risk of neoplastic disease and lacks clinical significance.

PPIs AND HYPERGASTRINEMIA. The physiologic role of gastrin is to stimulate gastric enterochromaffin-like (ECL) cells to secrete histamine, which in turn stimulates the secretion of hydrochloric acid from gastric parietal cells. Since PPIs inhibit the final step of gastric acid secretion by irreversible binding to the parietal cell $H^+K^+ATPase$ (the proton pump), secondary hypergastrinemia may occur in subjects

treated long-term with PPIs. Indeed, an increase in the average serum gastrin level as well as a diffuse (simple) or linear/micronodular (focal) ECL-cell hyperplasia has been observed in patients continuously using PPIs. The clinical relevance of these findings is currently uncertain.

PPIs AND IRON AND VITAMIN B_{12} DEFICIENCIES. While gastric acid suppression may decrease iron absorption, it remains uncertain whether iron-deficiency anemia may result from chronic PPI therapy.

Long-term use of gastric acid suppressant drugs, particularly PPIs, is associated with the development of vitamin B_{12} deficiency, especially in older subjects. Thus, it is appropriate to assess vitamin B_{12} status in long-term users of PPIs, especially in older subjects who may have poor nutrition (and therefore low vitamin B_{12} intake) and/or in patients requiring life-long PPI treatments, such as those with Zollinger-Ellison syndrome.

PPIs AND MAGNESIUM. Long-term PPI use can be associated with a subclinical magnesium deficiency, as has been observed in hospitalized adult patients. Thus, the FDA has suggested monitoring serum magnesium levels in patients on PPI therapy.

PPIs, BONE METABOLISM, OSTEOPOROSIS, AND RISK OF FRACTURES. Antisecretory drugs may interfere with calcium absorption through induction of hypochlorhydria; PPIs, moreover, may reduce bone resorption through inhibition of the osteoclastic vacuolar proton pump. Indeed, long-term PPI therapy has been associated with an increased risk of hip, wrist, or spine fractures. The risk of fracture is higher in patients who receive multiple daily doses of PPIs and when therapy is prolonged for a period of 1 year or longer. Additional risk factors for osteoporosis, such as old age and female gender, may also contribute to increase the risk of fractures in long-term acid suppression drug users.

PPIs and enteric infections. Inhibition of acid secretion may induce an increase of the bacterial flora at the gastrointestinal level with potential to increase the incidence of systemic infections particularly in immune depressed older subjects. Indeed, the use of antisecretory drugs has been associated with an increased risk of infections of the lower gastrointestinal tract, mainly because of *Salmonella* species and *Clostridium difficile*. In a large population-based study, subjects treated with acid-lowering drugs had a threefold higher risk of developing bacterial diarrhea than those taking hypotensive or antiasthmatic medications. In older patients this susceptibility is increased, particularly for *Salmonella* and *Campylobacter* infections. Some data suggest that widespread use of PPIs, especially in the hospital setting, may contribute to the current in-hospital epidemic of *C difficile* infections. Indeed, a meta-analysis of 56 studies involving 356,683 patients provided strong evidence that PPI use is associated with a double risk for development of *C difficile* infection without differences in subgroup analyses for age less than 65 years versus equal or more than 65 years.

PPIs and community-acquired pneumonia. A series of observational studies have suggested that the use of PPIs could increase the risk of hospitalization for community-acquired pneumonia (CAP), particularly in older subjects. The potential presence of confounding factors, however, seems to limit the conclusions of these studies. Indeed, meta-analyses have demonstrated that PPI and H_2-blocker long-term use is not associated with an increased risk of hospitalization for CAP.

PPIs and COVID-19. The recent pandemic due to SARS-CoV-2 has prompted examination of PPI use and risk of adverse outcomes of COVID-19. Two meta-analyses found that PPI use is associated with higher risk for becoming infected with COVID-19, but not significantly (5 studies; odds ratio [OR], 1.33) and with significantly higher risk for severe outcomes of COVID-19, including intensive care unit admission or death (9 studies; OR, 1.67). In another meta-analysis, PPI use was associated with significantly higher risk for severe outcomes of COVID-19 (3 studies; OR, 1.46) and for developing secondary infections (2 studies; OR, 2.91). Although a causal relation between PPI use and susceptibility to COVID-19 or worse COVID-19 outcomes has not been proven, a plausible biological mechanism might involve facilitated gut viral entry due to abated acidic gastric production.

PPIs and microbioma/microbiota. As it is becoming more evident that gut microbiota is markedly different at different life stages and in health versus in the presence of diseases, the association between medications and the microbiome is

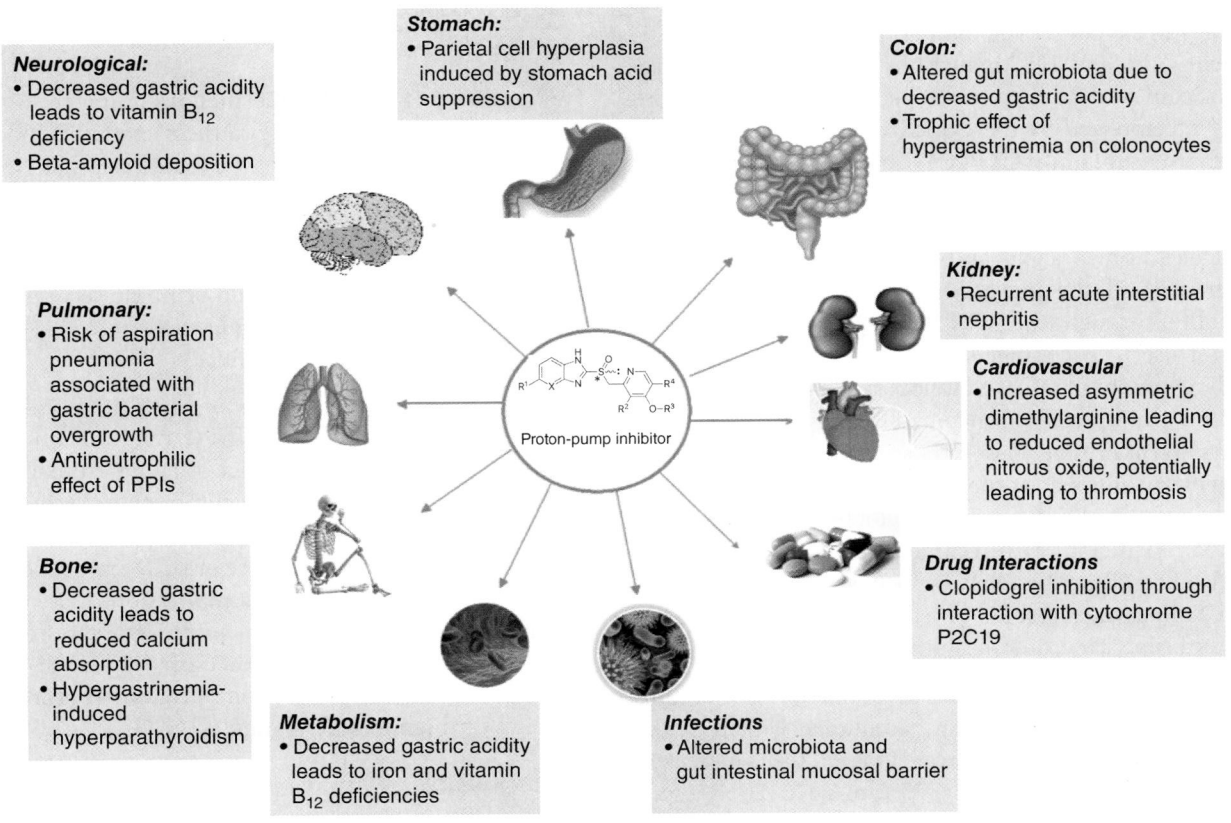

FIGURE 85-10. Possible mechanisms of adverse events associated with long-term use of proton pump inhibitors (PPIs).

being explored. It is becoming clear that greater diversity of gut microbiota is associated with good health, and that the predominance of certain bacterial species over others is a hallmark of certain conditions. Among older hospitalized patients compared to healthy subjects, polypharmacy was significantly associated with gut microbiota dysbiosis, that is, reduction in species richness and significant variations in the average relative abundance of a large number of taxa, including *Helicobacter*. Importantly, dysbiosis also exhibited a significant association with mortality at follow-up. Healthy-active older subjects without polypharmacy did not exhibit dysbiosis. Of note, among specific drug classes, PPIs, antipsychotics, and antidepressants had the strongest associations with gut microbiota composition.

PPIs, FRAILTY, AND MORTALITY. Chronic use of PPIs has been reported to be associated with a higher risk of functional decline in frail older subjects. Moreover, in older patients discharged from acute care hospitals, the use of high-dose PPIs was associated with increased 1-year mortality. Although further studies are needed, these data suggest caution when continuing PPIs following an episode of hospitalization in older adults.

BIOAVAILABILITY AND METABOLISM OF OTHER AGENTS. Due to the profound and long-lasting elevation of intragastric pH, it is not surprising that PPIs interfere with the absorption of concurrent medications, as drug solubility may be substantially reduced at neutral pH compared with acidic conditions. PPIs reduce the bioavailability of many drugs (eg, ketoconazole, atazanavir) by 50% or more compared with the control values. Moreover, omeprazole has been associated with 30% and 10% reductions in systemic clearance of diazepam and phenytoin, respectively. Since PPIs are mainly metabolized by the cytochrome P450 (CYP), particularly the subfamily CYP2C19, clinically relevant drug interactions may occur in case of concomitant administration of CYP2C19-metabolized drugs.

Due to omeprazole' and esomeprazole's competitive interference with the conversion of clopidogrel to its active metabolite through the CYP2C19 pathway, their concomitant use is discouraged. Although evidence of safety regarding concomitant use of clopidogrel and other PPIs including pantoprazole, rabeprazole, and lansoprazole is still lacking, at present these drugs are not contraindicated in patients on antiplatelet therapy, but caution is warranted, and an individualized approach which assesses the real need for PPI therapy is recommended. Drug interactions have also been described between PPIs and warfarin, phenytoin, ledipasvir, sofosbuvir, methotrexate, digoxin, nelfinavir, and rilpivirine, amongst others.

Overutilization of acid inhibitors. Acid inhibitors are among the most commonly used pharmaceuticals. United States trends in PPI prescriptions indicate that PPI users increased from 5.70% in 2002–2003 to 6.73% in 2016–2017, especially in adults aged 65 and older, and those who were obese. A previous study of 946 PPI users showed that 35% were prescribed PPI for a documented upper GI disorder, 10% for empirical symptomatic treatment, and 18% for gastric protection while on NSAIDs or antiplatelet drugs, while up to 36% of subjects had no documented appropriate indication for PPI therapy. Other studies have reported that PPIs are frequently prescribed during hospitalization, especially in older adults, and that as many as 50% of such prescriptions may be continued after discharge without clear indications. All these data suggest that older patients on long-term PPI therapy should be periodically evaluated for the indications for continued therapy.

The role of surgery The role of surgery in the treatment of GERD is controversial. Laparoscopic fundoplication has greatly reduced the morbidity and mortality of antireflux surgery, and this is also true for older adults. Indications for surgery are evolving; at present, evidence suggests that surgery may be indicated in older patients who (1) are medical treatment failures; (2) have severe complications, such as strictures not treatable by endoscopy; (3) have severe dysphagia, aspiration, or atypical symptoms associated with a large hiatal hernia; and/or (4) have preneoplastic lesions, that is, Barrett esophagus with high-grade dysplasia. Randomized clinical studies are needed to compare the outcome of antireflux surgery with that of medical therapy in older adults. Furthermore, surgery for GERD should be centralized to units specialized in these techniques to reduce surgical complications and improve successful clinical outcomes.

PEPTIC ULCER DISEASE

Definition

Peptic ulcer is a break of the mucosa lining the stomach or the duodenum. According to their anatomical location, peptic ulcers are divided into *gastric ulcers*, that is, peptic ulcers of the gastric fundus, body, or antrum; *prepyloric and pyloric ulcers,* that is, located within 3 cm from the pyloric ring and in the pyloric ring, respectively; and *duodenal ulcers*, that is, located in the bulb or in the second portion of the duodenum (**Figure 85-11**).

Epidemiology

The prevalence of PUD worldwide ranges from 0.1% to 4.7%, with an annual incidence ranging from 0.19% to 0.3%. Duodenal ulcers are most common in Western populations, and gastric ulcers are more frequent in Asia. Overall, the prevalence and incidence of PUD are declining, but the incidence of PUD and its complications increases with advancing age (**Figure 85-12**). Indeed, the rates of hospitalization for complicated peptic ulcer (**Figure 85-13**) and mortality rates for upper GI complications (**Figure 85-14**) remain very high in older patients.

Pathophysiology and Classification

Two main factors that might explain the observed increase in PUD in older patients are the high prevalence

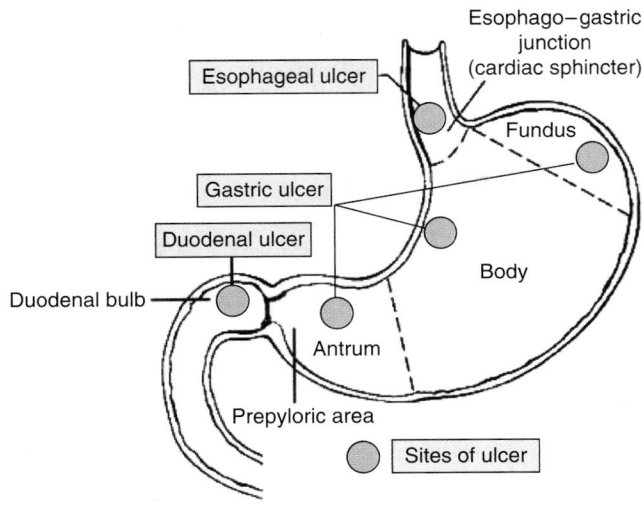

FIGURE 85-11. Anatomical location of peptic ulcers.

of *H pylori* infection and the frequent use of mucosa-damaging drugs, such as NSAIDs and aspirin. Nevertheless, in older subjects, around 20% of all peptic ulcers are not associated with either of these risk factors (**Figure 85-15**). The pathophysiology of "idiopathic" non-NSAID, non-*H pylori* peptic ulcers is still uncertain, but a critical disequilibrium between protective and erosive factors in the gastric or duodenal mucosa seems to be involved. Advancing age is associated with a reduction of the gastric mucosal barrier, that is, the capacity to resist external damage owing to secretion of gastric mucus, bicarbonate secretion, mucosal prostaglandins, gastric mucosal proliferation, and/or mucosal blood flow. Moreover, in older patients with PUD, normal or high levels of gastric acid and pepsin secretions have been observed. Although advancing age is independently

related to chronic atrophic gastritis and a functional status of hypo/achlorhydria, the atrophic changes of the gastric mucosa appear to be associated with *H pylori* infection rather than with aging. Emotional stress, smoking tobacco, and/or alcohol use are potential risk factors that may contribute to the development of PUD in predisposed subjects.

H pylori–associated peptic ulcer disease Approximately, 70% of older peptic ulcer patients are *H pylori* positive (see **Figure 85-15**). Treatment of *H pylori* infection heals ulcers in more than 95% of older patients and improves symptoms in more than 85%. Moreover, the eradication of *H pylori* infection improves clinical outcomes, reducing ulcer recurrences and symptoms. Health programs leading to widespread eradication of *H pylori* infection in symptomatic patients have reduced the prevalence of PUD, particularly of duodenal ulcer, both in Europe and in the Far East. Unfortunately, the percentage of older patients with PUD who are treated for their *H pylori* infection is still quite low. In one US study, only 40% to 56% of patients older than 65 years who were hospitalized for PUD were tested for *H pylori* infection; among the *H pylori* positive patients, only 50% to 73% were treated with specific antibiotic-based anti-*H pylori* therapy.

NSAID/aspirin-associated peptic ulcer disease In older patients, approximately 25% of duodenal ulcers and 40% of gastric ulcers are associated with the use of NSAIDs and/or aspirin (see **Figure 85-15**). The risk of NSAID-related peptic ulcers and their severe complications tends to increase linearly with age and becomes particularly high in the presence of disability, comorbidity, and polypharmacy. A case-control study performed in more than 3000 older patients who underwent an endoscopy documented that subjects undergoing treatment with NSAIDs and/or aspirin had a higher prevalence of gastric and duodenal ulcers compared

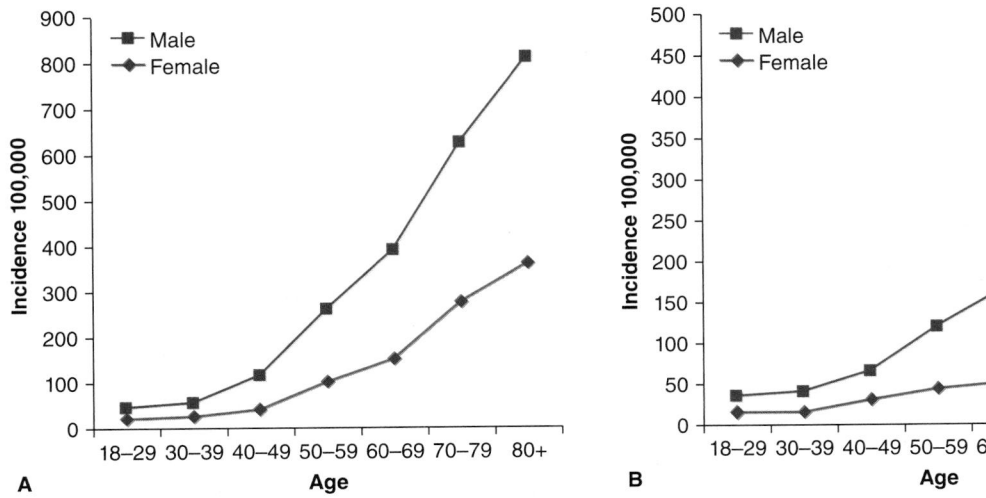

FIGURE 85-12. Age- and gender-specific annual incidence of peptic ulcer disease (**A**) and severe complications (**B**) (per 100,000) during 2000 to 2008 in Finland. (Adapted with permission from Malmi H, Kautiainen H, Virta LJ, et al. Incidence and complications of peptic ulcer disease requiring hospitalisation have markedly decreased in Finland. *Aliment Pharmacol Ther.* 2014;39[5]:496–506.)

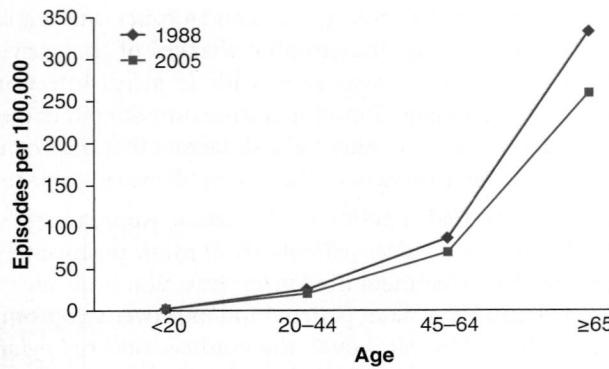

FIGURE 85-13. Trends in hospitalizations for peptic ulcer disease in United States according to age. (Data from Feinstein LB, Holman RC, Yorita Christensen KL, Steiner CA, Swerdlow DL. Trends in hospitalizations for peptic ulcer disease, United States, 1998–2005. *Emerg Infect Dis.* 2010;16[9]:1410–418.)

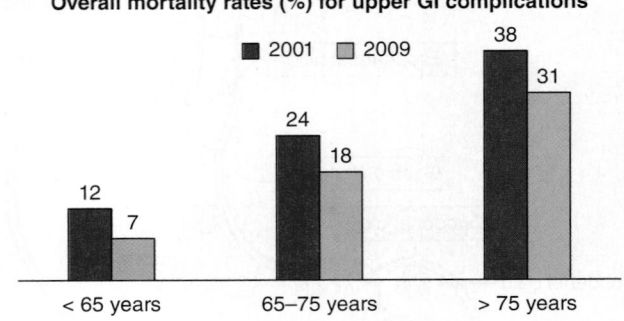

FIGURE 85-14. Mortality rates (%) for upper GI complications in the different age groups in United States in 2001 and 2009. (Data from Laine L, Yang H, Chang SC, et al. Trends for incidence of hospitalization and death due to GI complications in the United States from 2001 to 2009. *Am J Gastroenterol.* 2012;107[8]:1190–1195.)

to nonuser control subjects. Moreover, the risk of PUD is significantly higher in acute than chronic users of NSAIDs or aspirin (**Figure 85-16**). The injurious gastroduodenal effects of NSAIDs and aspirin are mainly caused by the inhibition of COX-1 and its role in mucosal defense mechanisms, but also through the inhibition of thromboxane A2, which reduces platelet function, resulting in a higher risk of bleeding. However, a direct effect on gastroduodenal mucosal surface cannot be excluded especially by those NSAIDs that have a high acid/base pK ratio.

Different NSAIDs are associated with distinct GI adverse events; nevertheless, none of them shows an absolutely safe profile. Drug-related pharmacodynamic and pharmacokinetic properties may explain the individual variability observed in terms of adverse effects on the upper GI tract. A genetic predisposition due to polymorphism of cytochrome P4502C9 that reduces the metabolism of some NSAIDs with a prolonged duration of drug

levels, enhancing the risk of GI mucosal damage, has been reported as a potential factor influencing the ulcerogenic effect of the different NSAIDs.

Presentation

In older adults, PUD is often difficult to diagnose, as symptoms may be atypical. The patient's concomitant diseases and treatments may cause symptoms that mask those of the ulcer. In patients older than 60 years, only one-third suffered from typical epigastric pain, and two-thirds experienced vague abdominal pain as a main symptom. Moreover, the intensity of pain may be less severe in older subjects and therefore may not receive the full attention of the physician or may not be taken seriously by the patient. Frequently, symptomatology includes nausea, vomiting, weight loss, and/or anorexia as the first, or even the only, symptom of PUD in older adults. Unfortunately, the first symptom might be a severe complication, especially bleeding or stenosis. Because of the insidious clinical presentation of the disease in older patients, the

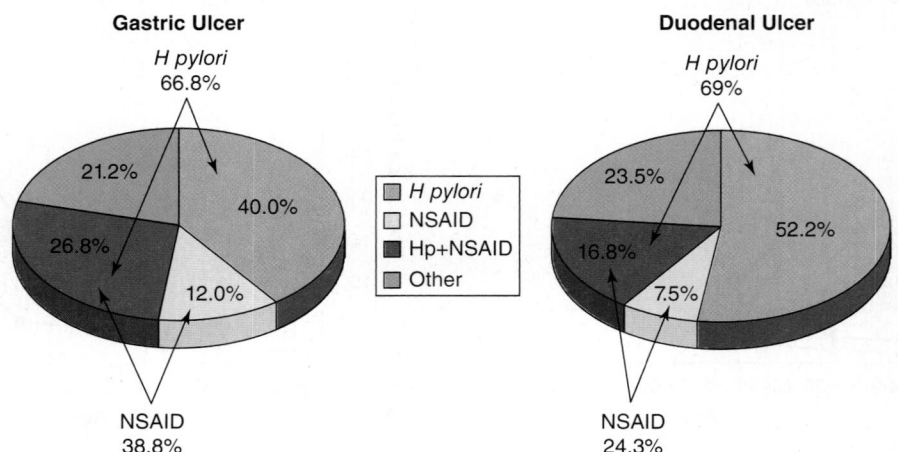

FIGURE 85-15. Prevalence of gastric and duodenal ulcer in older patients divided according to the presence of *H pylori* infection and/or NSAID use. (Data from Pilotto A. Helicobacter pylori-associated peptic ulcer disease in older patients: current management strategies. *Drugs Aging.* 2001;18[7]:487–494.)

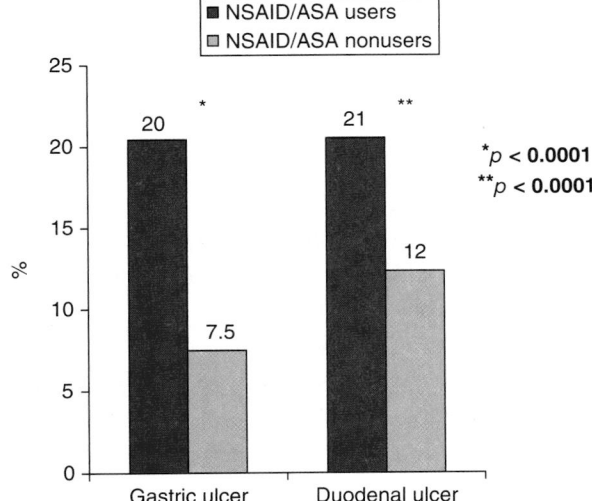

	NSAID Acute Users		NSAID Chronic Users	
	OR	95% CI	OR	95% CI
Gastric ulcer	4.47	3.19–6.26	2.80	1.97–3.99
Duodenal ulcer	2.39	1.73–3.31	1.68	1.22–2.33

FIGURE 85-16. Prevalence of gastric ulcer and duodenal ulcer in NSAID users and NSAID nonusers. ASA, aspirin. (Data from Pilotto A, Franceschi M, Leandro G, et al. Proton-pump inhibitors reduce the risk of uncomplicated peptic ulcer in elderly either acute or chronic users of aspirin/non-steroidal anti-inflammatory drugs. *Aliment Pharmacol Ther.* 2004;20[10]:1091–1097.)

consequences of PUD are more serious than those in younger subjects.

Evaluation

Upper GI endoscopy is always indicated for older subjects with new abdominal symptoms because of the high prevalence of serious gastric diseases in this age group. Upper GI endoscopy is safe and well tolerated in older adults. By direct visual identification, the location and size of an ulcer can be described. Peptic ulcer is a round to oval mucosal defect, from 5 mm to even 4 cm in diameter, with a smooth base and perpendicular borders. A series of biopsies to exclude malignancy is mandatory both in the center and on the borders of the gastric ulcer, even if they are not elevated or irregular as in ulcerative forms of advanced gastric cancer. Gastric *biopsies* allow for identifying the presence and the severity of chronic gastritis and/or the presence of *H pylori* infection. Endoscopic healing is the gold standard for evaluating treatment success in clinical trials. The surrounding mucosa may present radial folds, as a consequence of the parietal scarring.

Barium radiography of the stomach and duodenum is indicated as part of second-line evaluation of the patient with suspected motility disorders, peptic strictures, or fistulas in which gastrografin may be used as an alternative to barium in contrast studies. Radiography is contraindicated

in the presence of bleeding, severe vomiting with a high risk of pulmonary aspiration, or in cases of suspected gastric or duodenal perforation. If a peptic ulcer perforates, air will leak from the inside of the gastrointestinal tract to the peritoneal cavity. This leads to "free gas" within the peritoneal cavity that may be observed underneath the diaphragm on an erect or supine lateral *abdominal x-ray.*

Testing for *H pylori* infection *Helicobacter pylori* infection may be diagnosed by means of either histology evaluation, rapid urease test, or culture performed on gastric biopsies taken during endoscopy (**Table 85-5**). However, the biopsy site needs to be selected with care, since *H pylori* may only be found in the fundus or body and not in the antral mucosa of older patients who are taking antisecretory drugs. Moreover, the presence of chronic atrophic gastritis as a result of a past colonization of *H pylori* may be associated with a lower prevalence of the bacterium in the gastric biopsy specimens in older than in younger patients. For the same reasons, the rapid urease test performed on gastric biopsies has lower sensitivity in subjects 60 years and older compared with younger patients.

The presence and severity of histologically proven gastritis can be investigated through the histological evaluation of morphological parameters of the gastric mucosa at two sites. All these findings suggest that in older adults (1) it is advisable to perform gastric biopsies from both the antrum and the body of the stomach; and (2) a second test for *H pylori* should be performed in this age group if a urease-based or histologic test is negative.

Posttreatment *H pylori* evaluation Successful eradication should always be confirmed by a noninvasive or an invasive test if endoscopy is clinically indicated. Older patients with a diagnosis of peptic ulcer (especially gastric ulcer), gastric mucosa-associated lymphoid tissue, lymphoma, or severe gastritis should be evaluated by endoscopy and gastric mucosal histology after completion of anti-*H pylori* therapy. Most experts agree that this evaluation must be carried out at least 1 month after completion of therapy in order to minimize false-negative results. Older patients with mild or moderate forms of chronic gastritis may be evaluated after therapy by a noninvasive test. The ^{13}C-urea breath test demonstrated higher sensitivity, specificity, and diagnostic accuracy than serology (IgG anti-*H pylori* antibodies) in older subjects. An *H pylori*–stool antigen (HpSA) test for the detection of *H pylori* has been suggested as a valuable option with a high-potential role in the diagnosis after eradication therapy. In hospitalized frail older patients, the HpSA was less accurate than the ^{13}C-urea breath test, while antibiotic therapy and corpus atrophy decreased the positivity rate.

Other noninvasive tests Serum pepsinogen I and II levels (sPGI, sPGII), which are biomarkers of inflammation, are known to increase in the presence of *H pylori*-related non-atrophic gastritis. sPGII levels are higher in subjects with both gastric and duodenal ulcer, and levels correlate with the

TABLE 85-5 ■ TESTING FOR *H PYLORI*

TEST	PROS	LIMITS
Histology	• Establishes the presence and severity of *H pylori* gastritis at different sites of the stomach • High sensitivity/specificity (95%–98%)	• Invasive (requires EGD) • Sensitivity reduced by acute peptic bleeding and use of PPIs • Interobserver variability • Unequal distribution of *H pylori* upon different gastric sites
Rapid urease test	• Rapid (1 h) • High sensitivity/specificity (90%–95%)	• Invasive (requires EGD) • False-negative related to acute upper GI bleeding, use of PPIs, antibiotics or bismuth-containing compounds
Culture	• High specificity • Antibiotic sensitivity testing (antibiogram)	• Invasive (requires EGD) • Long response times (> 7 d) • Difficult to culture (low sensibility)
Serology	• Easy to perform • Local prevalence of *H pylori* affects the positive predictive value of antibody testing	• Low specificity and sensitivity (85%–79%) • Cannot distinguish between active and past infection • Inaccurate in older people
***H pylori* stool antigen**	• Noninvasive • High sensitivity/specificity (94%–97%) • Indicates the presence of active infection • Useful for monitoring after *H pylori* treatment	• Less acceptable in some patients • Active bleeding reduces specificity (but not sensitivity)
^{13}C-urea breath test	• Noninvasive • High sensitivity/specificity (91%–92%) • Indicates the presence of active infection • Useful for monitoring after *H pylori* treatment	• False-negative related to PPIs, bismuth, antibiotics, or active peptic ulcer bleeding

EGD, esophagogastroduodenoscopy; PPI, proton pump inhibitors.

severity of inflammation. A study in older people reported that sPGII levels decreased significantly after a successful *H pylori* cure. Moreover, sPGI or the ratio of sPGI/sPGII measurements may be useful to identify atrophic gastritis of the gastric corpus. Assays for gastrin (particularly gastrin-17) could be an indicator of the morphological status of the antral mucosa.

Management

Eradication of *H pylori* infection There is currently a worldwide consensus that the first-line therapy for eradication of *H pylori* infection should be triple therapy with a PPI twice daily combined with clarithromycin 500 mg twice daily and amoxicillin 1 g twice daily or nitroimidazole 500 mg twice daily for a minimum of 7 days. The cumulative results of clinical trials evaluating anti-*H pylori* therapies in older subjects confirmed that PPI-based triple therapies for 1 week were highly effective and well tolerated. Adverse event rates of less than 13% were reported, with less than 6% of patients discontinuing therapy owing to these effects (**Table 85-6**). In older patients, a reduction of the dosage of the PPI from a twice to once daily standard dose did not influence cure rates of the PPI-triple therapies. Since aging may modify the pharmacokinetic distribution of clarithromycin, independent of renal function, clinical trials evaluated the efficacy of PPI-based triple therapies including clarithromycin at a low dose of 250 mg twice daily in older patients. Results demonstrated no significant differences in cure rates and tolerability between clarithromycin 250 mg versus 500 mg twice daily. All these findings suggest that in older patients, 1-week PPI-based triple therapies should include low doses of both PPIs and clarithromycin, in combination with standard doses of either amoxicillin or a nitroimidazole, to obtain excellent cure rates and tolerability. Increasing the duration of treatment from 7 days to 14 days is associated with higher eradication rates. At present, however, no studies have evaluated the clinical usefulness of these 2-week triple therapy regimens specifically in older patients. Studies of a 10-day sequential regimen of 5 days of PPI plus amoxicillin followed by five additional days with PPI plus clarithromycin and tinidazole have reported higher eradication rates in comparison with standard triple therapy in both geriatric and adult patients.

Low compliance and antibiotic resistance are the two major reasons for treatment failure. Primary resistance to amoxicillin remains uncommon, but the frequency of clarithromycin resistance has reached rates above 70% in some countries including China, nearly 50% in Portugal and Iran, and approximately 16% in the United States. Metronidazole resistance ranges between 20% and 30%, and is more frequent among women and in developing countries. Consensus exists in using clarithromycin and metronidazole for *H pylori* eradication therapies when prevalence of antibiotic resistance is lower than 15% and 40%, respectively.

Because failure of therapy is often associated with secondary antibiotic resistance, retreatment should ideally

TABLE 85-6 ■ CUMULATIVE RESULTS OF CLINICAL TRIALS EVALUATING 1-WEEK PPI-BASED TRIPLE THERAPIES, SEQUENTIAL THERAPIES, AND QUADRUPLE THERAPIES AGAINST *HELICOBACTER PYLORI* INFECTION IN OLDER PATIENTS

	PATIENTS (N)	ERADICATION		DROP OUTS (%)	SIDE EFFECTS (%)
		ITT (%)	PP (%)		
TRIPLE THERAPY					
PPI + C + M or T	296	88	91	3.0	3.4
PPI + Aª + C	253	84	89	5.5	7.1
PPI + Aª + M	154	80	84	4.5	7.1
PPI + Aª + C	90	80	83	3.3	12
SEQUENTIAL THERAPY					
PPI + A, PPI C + Tᵇ	89	94	97	2.2	10
QUADRUPLE THERAPY					
PPI + TE + M + BS	95	91	95	4.2	28

ITT, intent-to-treat analysis; PP, per-protocol analysis; PPI, proton pump inhibitors, that is, omeprazole 20 mg daily or twice daily, lansoprazole 30 mg twice daily, pantoprazole 40 mg daily, or esomeprazole 20 mg daily or twice daily; R, rabeprazole 20 mg twice daily; A, amoxicillin; BS, bismuth subcitrate 240 mg twice daily for 10 days; C, clarithromycin 250 mg twice daily; M, metronidazole 250 mg four times a day or 500 mg twice daily; T, tinidazole 500 mg twice daily; TE, tetracycline 500 mg.
ª1 g twice daily or 500 mg three times a day.
ᵇFor 5 days followed by 5 additional days.
Data from Pilotto A, Franceschi M. Helicobacter pylori infection in older people. World J Gastroenterol. 2014;20(21):6364–6373.

be guided by data on susceptibility. Since such information is often unavailable, the choice of a second-line treatment depends on which treatment was used initially. Indeed, eradication of *H pylori* infection is more difficult when a first treatment attempt has failed, and the optimal strategy for retreatment has not yet been established in older patients. Thus, specialist referral should be made in this situation.

NSAID-related PUD

Drug Treatment NSAID- or aspirin-associated peptic ulcers usually heal after 4 to 8 weeks of treatment with a PPI. Healing rates are higher if NSAID or aspirin treatments are stopped. Presently, no consensus exists on the clinical usefulness of maintenance therapy with antisecretory drugs in patients who stopped NSAID or aspirin treatment after healing an NSAID-related peptic ulcer.

Prevention The following strategies have been suggested to prevent NSAID- or aspirin-related gastroduodenal peptic ulcer in older adults (**Figure 85-17**).

IDENTIFYING HIGH-RISK PATIENTS (MULTIDIMENSIONAL ASSESSMENT). Current strategies to reduce ulcer relapse and/or complications are considered cost-effective in high-risk patients. Great importance is placed, therefore, on defining those patients who are at high risk for peptic ulcer and its complications when they are treated with gastro-damaging drugs. A history of upper GI symptoms, PUD, and/or bleeding; the presence of multimorbidity and concomitant medications, particularly oral steroids, antiplatelet drugs, antithrombotic therapies (ie, low-molecular-weight heparins), and oral anticoagulants increase the risk of NSAID-related PUD and its complications. Moreover, functional and cognitive impairment, malnutrition, immobilization, and social factors, that is, the main determinants of multidimensional

frailty, may negatively influence the outcomes and trajectories of drug-related PUD and its complications. Thus, a comprehensive geriatric assessment may be useful in the evaluation of the multidimensional risk of older patients.

REDUCE DOSAGE AND USE OF LESS GI-TOXIC NSAIDS. The risk of peptic ulcer and its complications appears to be directly related to the dose of the given NSAID or coxib. Lower risk of upper GI damage has been reported with NSAIDs with a short plasma half-life versus those with a prolonged plasma half-time. Furthermore, slow-release formulations present an augmented risk of ulcer complications.

CO-TREATMENT WITH GASTROPROTECTIVE DRUGS. Misoprostol and PPIs are more effective than H₂-blockers in preventing severe gastric and duodenal damage. However, misoprostol administered at effective doses of 200 μg four times daily has higher adverse effects, particularly diarrhea, than PPIs. PPIs are very effective in preventing gastroduodenal injuries in both acute and chronic older users of NSAIDs (**Figure 85-18**). Similarly, PPIs prevent PUD and its complications in older patients treated with low-dose aspirin as antiplatelet therapy, independent of the presence of *H pylori* infection.

ERADICATION OF *H PYLORI* INFECTION. NSAID use and *H pylori* infection are independent risk factors for PUD and gastroduodenal bleeding in older subjects. In *H pylori*–positive patients who are starting long-term treatment with NSAIDs, the cure of *H pylori* infection reduces the 6-month risk of PUD. In older high-risk patients, however, the use of PPIs concomitantly with the NSAID reduces the occurrence of both acute and chronic NSAID-related gastroduodenal damage more effectively than the eradication of *H pylori* infection alone. Moreover, after the eradication of *H pylori*, maintenance treatment with a PPI is effective in the prevention of ulcer bleeding in older patients. All these findings suggest

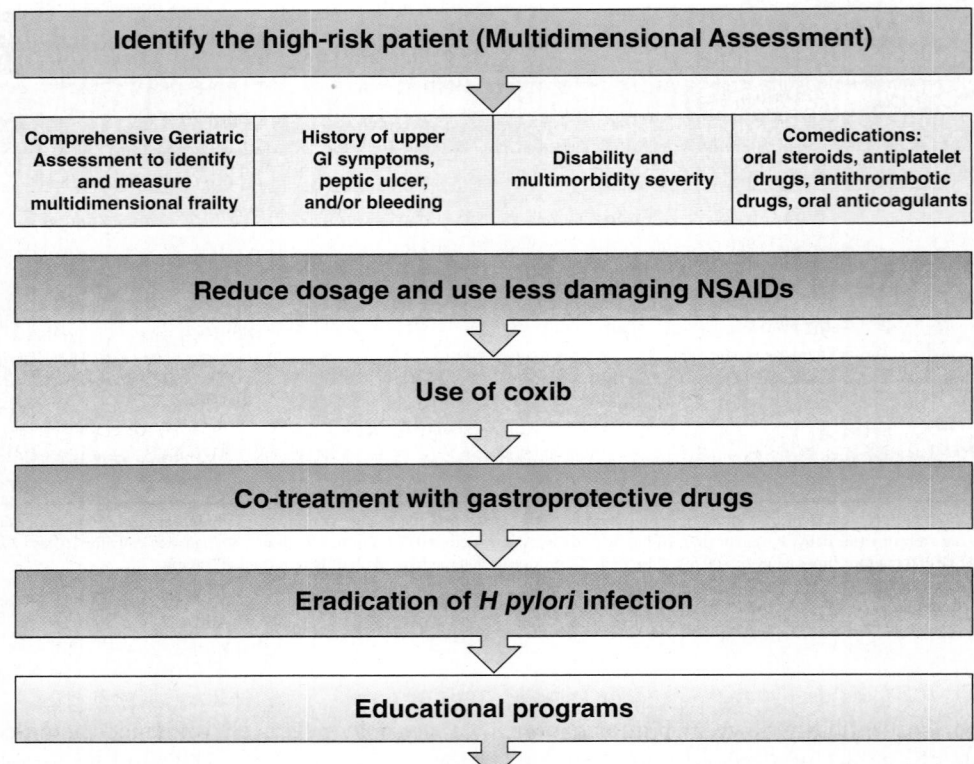

FIGURE 85-17. Strategies for the prevention of NSAID- or aspirin-related gastroduodenal peptic ulcer in older patients.

that *H pylori* eradication may be a useful strategy to prevent NSAID-related peptic ulcer. Consequently, *H pylori* infection should be tested for and treated in older people in whom prolonged NSAID use is anticipated.

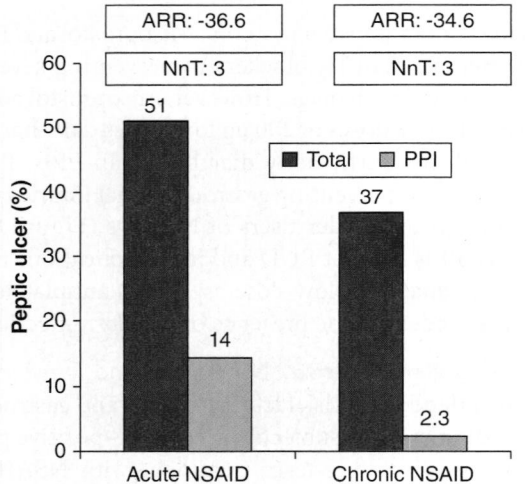

FIGURE 85-18. Absolute risk reduction (ARR) of peptic ulcer and the number needed to treat (NnT) in older acute and chronic users of nonsteroidal anti-inflammatory drugs (NSAIDs) and/or aspirin concomitantly treated with proton pump inhibitors (PPIs). (Data from Pilotto A, Franceschi M, Leandro G, et al. Proton-pump inhibitors reduce the risk of uncomplicated peptic ulcer in elderly either acute or chronic users of aspirin/non-steroidal anti-inflammatory drugs. *Aliment Pharmacol Ther.* 2004;20[10]:1091–1097.)

EDUCATIONAL PROGRAMS. A crucial strategy in the prevention of NSAID-related adverse events is the discontinuation of NSAID therapy. Indeed, studies from Canada and the United States reported an estimated 37% to over 50% of unnecessary, that is, inappropriate, NSAID prescriptions in older patients with osteoarthritis. Active interventions to improve appropriateness of drug prescription, particularly in older adults, demonstrated a reduction in NSAID prescriptions. For example, a significant reduction in rehospitalization rates for PUD as well as mortality rates within 1 year was observed in older subjects who participated in a quality improvement project in the United States that involved counseling of patients and their caregivers about NSAID toxicity.

Non-NSAID, non–H pylori PUD Antisecretory therapy remains the cornerstone of treatment to promote ulcer healing. Standard doses of PPIs should be prescribed at least for 4 weeks in patients with duodenal ulcers and for 8 weeks in patients with gastric ulcers. Generally, patients respond well to these therapies, and no established evidence supports the need for a longer duration or higher dose of antisecretory therapy in uncomplicated idiopathic ulcer. Older nonresponders should be investigated for any possible underlying pathophysiology, including medication noncompliance, acid hypersecretory state, or use of damaging drugs. Noninvasive evaluation of gastric function tests and referral to a specialist in gastroenterology are advised in case of *H pylori*-unrelated, persistent ulcers unresponsive to optimized PPI treatment.

PPI DOSE AND DURATION OF THERAPY IN GASTRIC DISEASES

	7–14 days	4–8 weeks	Intensive Cure Unit stay	Long-term therapy
H pylori eradication (1)	■			
Non *H pylori*-related PU disease		■		
Stress ulcer prophylaxis (2)			■	
Peptic ulcer bleeding (3)			■	

1. In combination with antimicrobials
2. Standard dose by intravenous route
3. Intravenous bolus of 80 mg of the available injectable PPIs, followed by 8 mg/h for 72 hours

A

PPI DOSE AND DURATION OF THERAPY IN DRUG-RELATED DAMAGE

	8 weeks	Long-term therapy	
NSAID prevention of gastroduodenal lesions		◪	Starting from the very first dose of NSAIDs
NSAID treatment of gastroduodenal lesions	■		
Antiplatelet therapy		◪	Starting from the very first dose of antiplatelet agents
Steroid therapy	No need for gastroprotection unless used in combination with NSAIDs		
Anticoagulant therapy	No need for gastroprotection unless used in combination with antiplatelet therapy		

B

Recommended PPI therapy dosing

☐ **Half dose**	Omeprazole 10 mg, Pantoprazole 20 mg	Lansoprazole 15 mg, Rabepazole 10 mg	Esomeprazole 20 mg
■ **Standard dose**	Omeprazole 20 mg, Pantoprazole 40 mg	Lansoprazole 30 mg, Rabepazole 20 mg	Esomeprazole 40 mg
☐ **Double dose**	Omeprazole 40 mg, Pantoprazole 80 mg	Lansoprazole 60 mg, Rabepazole 40 mg	Esomeprazole 80 mg

PART V ORGAN SYSTEMS AND DISEASES

FIGURE 85-19. (**A**) Therapeutic schemes for older people to treat *H pylori* infection, stress ulcer prophylaxis, and peptic ulcer disease and its bleeding complication. (**B**) Therapeutic schemes for older people to treat and/or prevent drug-related gastroduodenal damage.

Figures 85-19A and B summarize the therapeutic schemes for older people with PUD and its bleeding complication and drug-related gastroduodenal damage.

UPPER GASTROINTESTINAL BLEEDING

Definition

Upper gastrointestinal bleeding (UGIB) is defined as bleeding derived from a source proximal to the ligament of Treitz, and can be categorized as variceal or nonvariceal hemorrhage. UGIB can be classified as acute (presenting with hematemesis, melena and/or hematochezia) or chronic, suspected because of the detection of occult gastrointestinal blood loss or anemia.

Epidemiology

There has been a decrease in both the incidence and mortality rates due to UGIB across all age groups in the United States. However, UGIB remains a significant cause of hospital admission and mortality in older subjects. Indeed, the rates of admission for acute UGIB increase 30-fold between the third and ninth decades, and 70% of acute UGIB episodes occur in subjects older than 60 years. Moreover, in older US residents, the risk of hospitalization for UGIB is associated with age above 80 years, limited instrumental activities of daily living, multiple comorbidities, and polypharmacy.

The mortality of patients who present with variceal hemorrhage has historically exceeded 30%, but

TABLE 85-7 ■ CAUSES OF UPPER GASTROINTESTINAL BLEEDING

ENDOSCOPIC DIAGNOSIS	%
Peptic ulcer	31–67
Erosive gastritis	7–31
Variceal bleeding	4–20
Esophagitis	3–12
Mallory-Weiss tear	4–8
Neoplasm	2–8
Other	2–8
None	3–19

Data from Holster IL, Kuipers EJ. Management of acute nonvariceal upper gastrointestinal bleeding: current policies and future perspectives. World J Gastroenterol. 2012;18(11):1202–1207.

has decreased over time, possibly as a result of advances in medical and endoscopic therapy; however, these data come from cohorts of patients with a mean age well below 65 years, and extensive data about older patients with variceal bleeding are lacking.

Pathophysiology

UGIB can be caused by peptic ulcers, gastric erosions, esophageal varices, and other causes such as gastric cancer (**Table 85-7**).

Peptic ulcer disease PUD is the most frequent cause of major, life-threatening acute UGIB. Significant hemorrhage results from erosion of an underlying artery, and the magnitude of bleeding is related to the size of the arterial defect and the diameter of the artery. Consequently, bleeding may be particularly severe from large posterior duodenal ulcers which erode the gastroduodenal artery as well as from lesser curve gastric ulcers involving branches of the left gastric artery.

The high incidence of acute UGIB in older people has been attributed to many factors, including an increase in the use of NSAIDs as well as a high prevalence of upper GI disorders including GERD and PUD. Moreover, advanced age has been consistently identified as a risk factor for mortality among patients presenting with UGIB, presumably because of the high prevalence of frailty, comorbid illnesses, and polypharmacy in older adults as compared with younger patients.

Esophageal varices and portal hypertensive gastropathy Esophageal and gastric varices are caused by increased venous collateral flow from the portal circulation through the gastric coronary veins, usually because of portal hypertension. Variceal hemorrhage can occur when the hepatic venous pressure gradient exceeds 12 mm Hg. Features predictive of variceal hemorrhage include large variceal size and the presence of red "wale" marks on varices. The vessels may leak blood or even rupture, causing life-threatening bleeding. Portal hypertensive gastropathy results from venous congestion of the gastric mucosa; in most patients, this is caused by portal hypertension from cirrhosis.

Esophagitis and erosive gastritis These are superficial mucosal injuries in the esophagus and stomach, respectively. These lesions are most commonly caused by hypersecretion of gastric acid and/or erosive medications, such as NSAIDs and alendronate (see GERD section).

Mallory-Weiss tears These occur at the esophagogastric junction and are due to prolonged retching. Alcohol abuse is the usual cause, but other causes including vomiting (eg, chemotherapy, digoxin toxicity, renal failure, advanced malignancy) may be responsible. Bleeding usually stops spontaneously, and active endoscopic or surgical intervention is seldom required.

Presentation

Hematemesis, bloody gastric aspirate, or melena usually indicates bleeding from the upper GI tract. Older people with UGIB may have specific aspects of clinical presentation that need a comprehensive clinical approach. Indeed, an UGIB may initially present with symptoms such as light-headedness, syncope, or postural hypotension; neurologic symptoms including transient ischemic attack and/or stroke; cardiovascular symptoms, including ischemic heart disease; or even a delirium episode or behavioral disorders due to the UGIB-related acute anemia or hypotension. These general symptoms are more frequent in frail, comorbid, and multitreated older subjects.

Evaluation

The initial evaluation of the older patient presenting with features of acute UGIB includes a complete medical history, physical examination, and laboratory assessment including serum electrolyte and coagulation parameters, liver biochemical tests, and a complete blood count with the goal of assessing the severity of the bleeding. Details should be documented of prior UGIB episodes, previous abdominal surgery and current medication use, particularly aspirin, NSAIDs and oral anticoagulants, that is, warfarin or the newer oral anticoagulants (NOACs). Life-threatening peptic ulcer bleeding, with all-cause mortality rates as high as 12%, has been observed in patients on NOACs, especially in the presence of comorbidities such as coronary artery disease, stroke, peripheral vascular disease, and heart failure. High-dose dabigatran (150 mg bid), rivaroxaban, and high-dose edoxaban (60 mg daily) are associated with a higher risk of UGIB than warfarin. Other risk factors for NOAC-related UGIB include concomitant use of ulcerogenic agents, older age, renal impairment, H pylori infection, and previous history of UGIB. UGIB in cirrhotic patients has a nonvariceal origin in over 50% of cases. Physical findings of chronic liver disease are suggestive of underlying portal hypertension.

Upper GI endoscopy has three main purposes: (1) to provide an accurate diagnosis, (2) to give prognostic

	Endoscopic images	Forrest classification	Endoscopic findings	Re-bleeding rate (%)	Mortality rate (%)
Type II: Active bleeding		1a	Spurting arterial vessel	55	11
		1b	Oozing hemorrhage	55	11
Type II: Recent bleeding		2a	Nonbleeding visible vessel	43	11
		2b	Adherent clot	22	7
Type 3: Lesion without bleeding		2c	Flat pigmented spot	10	3
		3	Clean ulcer base	5	2

FIGURE 85-20. Forrest classification of nonvariceal UGIB. (Data from Gralnek IM, Dumonceau JM, Kuipers EJ, et al. Diagnosis and management of nonvariceal upper gastrointestinal hemorrhage: European Society of Gastrointestinal Endoscopy (ESGE) Guideline. *Endoscopy.* 2015;47[10]:a1–a46.)

information, and (3) to carry out endoscopic therapy. Early endoscopic examination allows precise identification of the site and nature of the bleeding, and provides prognostic information. Indeed, stigmata of recent hemorrhage, according to endoscopy Forrest classification, predict risk of further bleeding and guide management decisions (**Figure 85-20**).

Endoscopy performed within 24 to 48 hours from the bleeding episode reveals an actual or potential site of bleeding in the majority of patients; 15% to 30% of all lesions are actively bleeding at the time of endoscopy. In any case, endoscopy should not be carried out until the patient is adequately resuscitated and in stable clinical conditions. Routine second-look endoscopy, in which repeated endoscopy is performed 24 hours after initial endoscopic hemostatic therapy, is not recommended. A second-look endoscopy however should be performed in patients with clinical evidence of recurrent bleeding.

Management

General management Hemodynamic status should be assessed immediately upon presentation and resuscitative measures begun as needed. Blood transfusions should always be carried out with hemoglobin levels less than or equal to 8 g/dL. In older patients with higher hemoglobin levels, blood transfusions should be performed when clinical evidence of intravascular volume depletion or severe comorbidities, such as coronary artery disease, pulmonary diseases, and renal insufficiency, are present. Risk assessment should be performed to stratify patients into higher and lower risk categories, which may assist in initial decisions such as timing of endoscopy, time of discharge, and level of care.

Peptic ulcer bleeding The best management of acute bleeding ulcer includes a combination treatment with endoscopy (eg, bipolar electrocoagulation, heater probe, clips, and/or injection of sclerosant or vasoactive drugs) and intravenous PPI with a bolus followed by continuous infusion. These treatments reduce the rates of rebleeding and surgical interventions, but short- and long-term mortality rates are not reduced (**Table 85-8**). Endoscopic therapy for peptic ulcer hemorrhage seems to be well tolerated in older adults.

Pre-endoscopic PPI (80 mg omeprazole or pantoprazole bolus followed by 8 mg/h infusion) seems to decrease the need for endoscopic therapy but does not improve the final clinical outcome. After successful endoscopic hemostasis, continuous intravenous PPI therapy for 72 hours should be administered to patients who have an ulcer with active bleeding, a nonbleeding visible vessel, or an adherent clot. However, a meta-analysis found that oral and IV PPIs have similar efficacy after endoscopic treatment in controlling recurrent bleeding, the requirement for surgery, and mortality in patients with peptic ulcer bleeding. Thus, oral PPIs may be a useful and cost-saving alternative.

Recurrent bleeding after endoscopic therapy is treated with a second endoscopic treatment; if bleeding persists or recurs, treatment with surgery or interventional radiology is undertaken. In case of NOAC-related UGIB, initial management includes withholding the anticoagulant, followed by delayed endoscopic treatment. In severe bleeding, additional measures include the use of specific reversal agents such as idarucizumab for dabigatran and andexanet alfa for factor Xa inhibitors (rivaroxaban, apixaban, edoxaban), and urgent endoscopic management.

Variceal bleeding Endoscopic variceal band ligation has supplanted injection sclerotherapy under endoscopy, due to a lower rate of complications. The use of nonselective β-blockers seems to be effective for primary prophylaxis of variceal hemorrhage; however, older patients should be monitored closely for adverse effects, which include

TABLE 85-8 ■ PPI THERAPY AND OUTCOME OF ENDOSCOPIC HEMOSTASIS IN BLEEDING PEPTIC ULCER

	REBLEEDING	SURGERY	MORTALITY
EndoTx + PPI vs PPI alone	0.2 (0.09–0.4)	0.17 (0.06–0.4)	NS
EndoTx + PPI vs EndoTx alone	0.5 (0.37–0.7)	NS	NS
EndoTx + PPI bolus vs infusion	NS	NS	NS
PPI after EndoTx vs EndoTx alone	0.52 (0.4–0.7)	0.53 (0.35–0.8)	NS
Oral PPI	0.32 (0.2–0.5)	0.38 (0.2–0.6)	NS
Intravenous PPI	0.57 (0.4–0.7)	0.67 (0.5–0.9)	NS

EndoTx, endoscopic treatment; NS, not significant.
Data from Andriulli A, Annese V, Caruso N, et al. Proton-pump inhibitors and outcome of endoscopic hemostasis in bleeding peptic ulcers: a series of meta-analyses. Am J Gastroenterol. 2005;100:207–219 and Leontiadis GI, Sharma VK, Howden CW. Systematic review and meta-analysis of proton pump inhibitor therapy in peptic ulcer bleeding. BMJ. 2005;330:568–570.

orthostasis, fatigue, and affective disturbance. Vasoactive drugs (somatostatin or its analogue, octreotide; vasopressin or its analogue, terlipressin) should be initiated as soon as variceal hemorrhage is suspected. Selected patients at high risk of liver failure or rebleeding may be considered for an "early" (within 72 hours) trans-jugular intrahepatic portosystemic shunt (TIPS). However, TIPS placement for control of variceal bleeding may be associated with higher mortality and hospitalization rates in older compared to younger patients. Thus, the decision regarding use of TIPS should be made in consultation with a gastroenterologist.

UGIB in patients affected by portal hypertensive gastropathy is usually chronic and occult rather than overt and hemodynamically significant. Reduction of portal venous pressure with a nonselective β-blocker might be beneficial for these patients; however, the data to support this indication are limited, especially in older subjects.

Prognostic evaluation of the older patient with UGIB Early stratification of patients into groups with different risk of rebleeding and mortality may be useful to support clinicians in the management of UGIB and in the choice of the most appropriate treatment, that is, medical, endoscopic, or surgical interventions. Indeed, prognostic scores have been developed that include endoscopy-based analysis of bleeding lesions, preendoscopic clinical scores, and combined clinical and endoscopic evaluation.

The Forrest classification is an endoscopy-based tool useful to stratify patients with UGIB into high- and low-risk categories for mortality and rebleeding, and it has been used to evaluate the endoscopic intervention modalities.

It is increasingly evident, however, that the prognosis of older patients with UGIB is strongly affected by a multiplicity of factors, including functional status, cognition, nutrition, multimorbidity, and polypharmacy, which are not directly related to the UGIB itself, suggesting that any prognostic model for these patients should be multidimensional in nature. Three such models are described below and a summary is provided in **Table 85-9**.

The Glasgow-Blatchford score (GBS) is a screening tool to assess the likelihood that a patient with UGIB will need blood transfusion or endoscopic intervention. A score of 0 identifies low-risk patients who might be suitable for outpatient management; a patient with a GBS greater than 0 is considered at high risk, and should receive clinical evaluation and surveillance.

The Rockall score (RS) categorizes patients into risk groups. Patients with clinical RS (ie, before endoscopy) greater than 0 and patients with complete RS (ie, after endoscopy) greater than 2 are considered to be at intermediate or high risk for developing recurrent bleeding and death.

The Multidimensional Prognostic Index (MPI) is a prognostic tool based on a standard comprehensive geriatric assessment that predicts short- and long-term mortality in older subjects. As shown in **Table 85-9**, the MPI values range from 0 (low risk) to 1 (severe risk of mortality). The MPI can also be expressed as three grades of risk. Patients with higher MPI grades have higher risk of in-hospital stay and institutionalization after hospital discharge.

Prevention

Long-term prevention of recurrent bleeding peptic ulcers Prevention is based on the etiology of the bleeding ulcer. Patients with *H pylori*-associated, NSAID-associated, or idiopathic bleeding ulcers should receive therapy as outlined in the previous section. In patients who must resume NSAIDs, a COX-2–selective NSAID at the lowest effective dose plus daily PPI is recommended.

In patients with low-dose ASA-associated bleeding ulcers, the need for aspirin should be assessed. If given for secondary prevention (ie, established cardiovascular disease), aspirin should be resumed as soon as possible after bleeding ceases in most patients: ideally within 1 to 3 days and certainly within 7 days. Long-term daily PPI therapy should also be provided. If given for primary prevention (ie, no established cardiovascular disease), antiplatelet therapy likely should not be resumed in most patients.

Long-term prevention of recurrent variceal bleeding Although β-blockers have an established role as primary prophylaxis (ie, reducing the risk of variceal bleeding in patients who have never bled), their use as secondary prophylaxis (preventing variceal rebleeding) is not established, and

TABLE 85-9 ■ CLINICAL PROGNOSTIC SCORES IN ACUTE UPPER GASTROINTESTINAL BLEEDING

	GLASGOW BLATCHFORD SCORING SYSTEM	ROCKALL SCORING SYSTEM	MULTIDIMENSIONAL PROGNOSTIC INDEX (MPI)
Variable	1. Blood urea nitrogen 2. Hemoglobin 3. SBP 4. Pulse (HR/bpm) 5. Presence of melena 6. Syncope 7. Hepatic disease 8. Cardiac failure	1. Age 2. Presence of shock 3. Comorbidity (CHF, IHD, major morbidity, renal failure, liver failure, metastatic cancer) 4. Endoscopic diagnosis nonmalignant, non-Mallory-Weiss diagnosis, upper GI tract malignancy 5. Evidence of bleeding adherent clot, active bleeding	1. ADL 2. IADL 3. SPMSQ 4. CIRS 5. MNA 6. ESS 7. Number of drugs 8. Cohabitation status
Items	8	5	8 domains
Score ranges	0–23	0–11	0–1
Score risk	Low risk (0) High risk (> 0)	Low risk (0–2) Intermediate risk (3–7) High risk (8–11)	MPI risk class: MPI class 1 (low risk): MPI value < 0.33 MPI class 2 (moderate risk): MPI value 0.34–0.66 MPI class 3 (high risk): MPI value > 0.66
Type	Pre-endoscopic clinical score	Clinical and endoscopic score	Multidimensional, comprehensive, geriatric assessment-based
Evaluation	Management and timing of endoscopy for upper GI bleeding	Risk of rebleeding and mortality	Risk of mortality Risk of hospitalization Length of in-hospital stay

ªFor each domain, a tripartite hierarchy was used, ie, 0 = no problems, 0.5 = minor problems, and 1 = major problems. The sum of the calculated scores from the eight domains was divided by 8 to obtain a final MPI score ranging from 0 = no risk to 1 = highest risk. MPI tool is available for free download at multiplat-age.it /index.php/en/tools/.
ADL, activities of daily living; CHF, congestive heart failure; CIRS, cumulative illness rating scale; ESS, Exton-Smith scale; GI, gastrointestinal; HR, heart rate; IADL, instrumental-ADL; IHD, ischemic heart disease; MNA, mini nutritional assessment; SBP, systolic blood pressure; SPMSQ, short portable mental status questionnaire.

endoscopic variceal ablation by a program of repeated variceal banding is the treatment of choice.

AUTOIMMUNE ATROPHIC GASTRITIS

Autoimmune atrophic gastritis (AAG) may be found during endoscopic evaluation of patients for PUD or UGIB. It is a chronic progressive inflammatory condition that results in the replacement of the normal cell mass by atrophic and metaplastic mucosa. It represents an insidious condition that may go undiagnosed for many years, especially in older people. AAG is more common in women than men (3:1 ratio). There is an age-related increase in the prevalence of AAG, from 2.5% in the third decade to 12% in the eighth decade. Although the trigger for this disease is incompletely understood, autoantibodies against parietal cells and against intrinsic factor result in achlorhydria and pernicious anemia, respectively. Diagnosis of AAG is based on the presence of mucosal atrophy of the gastric corpus/fundus in biopsy histological samples obtained during esophago-gastro-duodenoscopy. A composite serological test using serum levels of gastrin-17, pepsinogen I and II, and antibodies against *H pylori* has been reported to be useful to identify AAG, demonstrating a negative predictive value of over 95% and a positive predictive value of above 95%. After serological diagnosis of atrophic gastritis, endoscopic evaluation with biopsy sample obtainment allows for exclusion of eventual neoplastic lesions, which are more frequent in patients with AAG.

AAG has been reported in approximately 20% to 30% cases of iron-deficiency anemia refractory to iron supplementation and vitamin B$_{12}$ deficiency. Concerning clinical features of AAG, nearly half of subjects are asymptomatic, especially in the initial phases. However, when present, symptoms tend to be nonspecific and often misleading such as early satiety, postprandial fullness, and also reflux symptoms, most probably linked to nonacid reflux. Importantly, PPIs are frequently prescribed in these patients, representing a clear case of inappropriate prescription.

Once the diagnosis of AAG has been established, endoscopic surveillance is suggested at 3-year intervals, with the goal of early gastric cancer detection, and referral to a gastroenterologist for follow-up is recommended. Concomitant autoimmune diseases including thyroiditis and diabetes must be excluded, and parenteral supplementation of vitamin B$_{12}$ must be ensured.

FURTHER READING

Barkun AN, Almadi M, Kuipers EJ, et al. Management of nonvariceal upper gastrointestinal bleeding: guideline recommendations from the International Consensus Group. *Ann Intern Med.* 2019;171:805–822.

Boghossian TA, Rashid FJ, Thompson W, et al. Deprescribing versus continuation of chronic proton pump inhibitor use in adults. *Cochrane Database Syst Rev.* 2017;3(3):CD011969.

Costable NJ, Greenwald DA. Upper gastrointestinal bleeding. *Clin Geriatr Med.* 2021;37(1):155–172.

Coxib and Traditional NSAID Trialists' (CNT) Collaboration, Bhala N, Emberson J, Merhi A, et al. Vascular and upper gastrointestinal effects of non-steroidal anti-inflammatory drugs: meta-analyses of individual participant data from randomised trials. *Lancet.* 2013;382:769–779.

Deutsch D, Romegoux P, Boustière C, et al. Clinical and endoscopic features of severe acute gastrointestinal bleeding in elderly patients treated with direct oral anticoagulants: a multicentre study. *Therap Adv Gastroenterol.* 2019;12:1756284819851677.

Kamada T, Satoh K, Itoh T, et al. Evidence-based clinical practice guidelines for peptic ulcer disease 2020. *J Gastroenterol.* 2021;56(4):303–322.

Kurin M, Fass R. Management of gastroesophageal reflux disease in the elderly patient. *Drugs Aging.* 2019;36(12):1073–1081.

Malfertheiner P, Megraud F, O'Morain CA, et al. European Helicobacter and Microbiota Study Group and Consensus panel. Management of *Helicobacter pylori* infection-the Maastricht V/Florence Consensus Report. *Gut.* 2017;66(1):6–30.

Mishuk AU, Chen L, Gaillard P, et al. National trends in prescription proton pump inhibitor use and expenditure in the United States in 2002-2017. *Science Pract Res.* 2021;61(1):87–94.

Pilotto A, Custodero C, Maggi S, et al. A multidimensional approach to frailty in older people. *Ageing Res Rev.* 2020;60:101047.

Pilotto A, Franceschi M. *Helicobacter pylori* infection in older people. *World J Gastroenterol.* 2014;20:6364–6373.

Tursi A, De Bastiani R, Franceschi M, et al. Non-invasive assessment of gastric secretory function in centenarians. *Geriatric Care.* 2017;3:6682.

Yamasaki T, Hemond C, Eisa M, et al. The changing epidemiology of gastroesophageal reflux disease: are patients getting younger? *J Neurogastroenterol Motil.* 2018;24(4):559–569.

Hepatic, Pancreatic, and Biliary Diseases

Dylan Stanfield, Mark Benson, Michael R. Lucey

INTRODUCTION

The liver and pancreas are remarkable in their ability to preserve function despite advanced age. Older patients are at an increased risk of more severe hepatic injury when exposed to hepatic insults. This increased risk is likely related to the liver's age-related decrease in regenerative capacity. The aging pancreas can alter its morphology and function, but often times this can be asymptomatic in the older individual. Throughout this chapter we will review the hepatobiliary and pancreatic changes that are known to occur with aging and their pathologic consequences of disease in older patients.

As will be discussed multiple times in this chapter, most of the therapies available for younger patients are safe and appropriate for use in the geriatric population. However, older patients with advanced pancreatic, liver, or biliary disease may not be eligible for curative treatments in some circumstances. For example, due to comorbid disease, few patients older than 70 years meet entry criteria for liver transplantation. Similarly, geriatric patients with newly diagnosed neoplasms of the pancreas or hepatobiliary system may not tolerate the extensive surgery that may be appropriate in a younger patient. Palliative care for patients with advanced pancreatic and hepatobiliary disease has become a well-recognized subspecialty and provides valuable therapies and counseling to alleviate suffering near the end of life.

LIVER DISEASE

Liver Morphology

For a number of years, liver volume was thought to decrease with age. More recently, it was determined that liver volume remains unchanged over time when adjusting for body surface area. Tagged albumin scans have shown that while corrected liver volume remains constant with age, functional hepatocyte volume decreases significantly. There is also a contemporaneous decrease in hepatic blood flow by approximately 35% to 40%. The cause of decreased blood flow is likely multifactorial—as a result of changes in cardiovascular output, diminished splanchnic blood flow, reduced portal vein blood flow, and increased resistance to

- Learn aging-associated changes in hepatic function, epidemiology, genetics, pathogenesis, and pathology of common hepatic diseases in older adults.

- Understand the prevalence, common clinical presentations, diagnosis, and treatment of hepatotropic viruses, autoimmune liver diseases, chronic fatty liver diseases, and drug-induced injury in older patients.

- Appreciate the challenges older persons encounter when living with chronic liver disease, including consideration of liver transplantation in older adults.

- Learn the epidemiology, genetics, etiology, and pathogenesis of common biliary and pancreatic diseases in older adults.

- Understand the common and atypical manifestations, and tests to diagnose common gallbladder and pancreatic diseases in older patients.

- Learn state-of-the-art and emerging treatments for biliary and pancreatic disorders in older population.

- Acquire knowledge about the symptoms, diagnosis, and treatment of gallbladder and pancreatic cancers in older adults.

Key Clinical Points

1. Older adults are more prone to hepatic injury due to aging-associated changes, including a reduction in regenerative capacity, functional hepatocyte volume, and hepatic blood flow.

2. Patients with metabolic syndrome are at high risk for developing nonalcoholic fatty liver disease (NAFLD).

3. Drug-induced liver injury occurs more frequently in older patients and tends to be more severe.

4. Chronic fatty liver diseases, alcohol-related and non-alcohol-related, are the two most

(Cont.) common causes of end-stage liver disease in older patients in the developed world. The advent of direct-acting antiviral agents for the treatment of hepatitis C virus (HCV) has changed the landscape of chronic liver disease.

5. Age is a major risk factor for gallstones, which are more common among older adults, especially women.

6. Acute cholecystitis may present atypically in older patients without fever, nausea, vomiting, or severe abdominal pain.

7. Ultrasound is the initial diagnostic test of choice, and incidental discovery of gallstones is not an indication for treatment. When appropriate, early laparoscopic cholecystectomy is the treatment of choice in older patients.

8. In the absence of gallstones and alcohol use disorder, the most common cause of acute pancreatitis in older adults is malignancy.

9. Alcohol use disorder is the most common cause of chronic pancreatitis in older patients.

10. The significance of alcohol use disorder in patients presenting with alcohol-related liver or pancreatic disease is frequently not recognized, and the opportunity to intervene with treatment of alcohol use disorder is missed.

portal flow. On the cellular level, both hepatocytes and the mitochondria of hepatocytes become hypertrophied, but decrease in overall number with age. Hepatocytes accumulate lipofuscin with age while undergoing a decrease in the concentration of smooth endoplasmic reticulum (SER), telomere length, and the activity of several liver microsomal enzymes.

Liver Function

Despite the observed changes in functional hepatocyte volume and blood flow, age-related changes to hepatic function are less evident in clinical practice (**Table 86-1**). The capacity to sustain liver function during aging is reflected in the ability to successfully transplant livers from older deceased donors. Traditional liver chemistry tests, including serum aminotransferases, bilirubin, alkaline phosphatase, and gamma-glutamyl transpeptidase, do not change with age. Likewise, there are no significant changes in coagulation factors. Serum albumin slightly decreases with age, but typically remains within the normal range. Serum cholesterol

TABLE 86-1 ■ EFFECTS OF AGE ON THE LIVER

Liver chemistry tests and coagulation factors: unaffected

Serum albumin: slightly decreased but within the normal range

Serum cholesterol and triglycerides: increased

Phase I drug metabolism: decreased

Phase II metabolism: unaffected

Hepatic proliferation after surgical resection: decreased

Hepatotoxicity (hepatitis viruses, drug reactions): more severe

and triglycerides increase with age since there is a gradual decline in the metabolism of low-density lipoprotein (LDL) cholesterol.

There are age-related changes in the hepatic metabolism of certain medications, which is important since more than 30% of prescription drugs are prescribed to older men and women. The incidence of adverse drug reactions significantly increases with increasing age. Phase I drug metabolism relies on microsomal enzymes and results in metabolism by oxidation, reduction, demethylation, and hydrolysis. Phase II drug metabolism relies on cytosolic enzymes and results in metabolism by conjugation with several different polar ligands. Phase I reactions are usually catalyzed by the cytochrome P450 system in the hepatocyte SER. There is a significant decrease in the phase I metabolism of several medications by as much as 50% with increasing age. Interestingly, medications that undergo phase II metabolism remain unaffected by aging. The activity of phase I metabolism is dependent on oxygen delivery. Thus, some of the age-related decreases in phase I metabolism could be explained by decreased hepatic blood flow as well as by decreased SER concentration. Medications with known phase I metabolism should be started at a low dose and titrated slowly in order to circumvent the problems associated with adverse drug reactions in older patients (**Table 86-2**).

Another important aspect of the effects of aging on hepatic function is the diminished ability of the liver to

TABLE 86-2 ■ DRUGS WITH EXTENSIVE PHASE I METABOLISM

Alprazolam, diazepam, midazolam, triazolam

Amitriptyline, imipramine

Atorvastatin, lovastatin, simvastatin

Carbamazepine, phenytoin

Clozapine, olanzapine

Corticosteroids

Cyclosporine, tacrolimus

HIV protease inhibitors

Sildenafil, tadalafil, vardenafil

Theophylline

Warfarin

TABLE 86-3 ■ DRUG-INDUCED LIVER INJURY

DRUG	TYPE OF LIVER INJURY	UNIQUE FEATURES
Acetaminophen	Marked hepatocellular necrosis	Dose-dependent injury; fatal doses 15–25 g; thiol therapy within 12 h often prevents significant toxicity
Amoxicillin-clavulanic acid	Cholestasis	Small percentage affected, but common cause of liver injury since medication is used so frequently
Isoniazid	Hepatocellular necrosis	Hepatitis in 21 of 1000, 5%–10% of cases are fatal; increased ALT in 10%–36% in first 10 wk; second only to acetaminophen as indication for LT for DILI
Methotrexate	Macrovesicular steatosis, periportal fibrosis	Patients on methotrexate require regular monitoring of LFTs and avoidance of alcohol
Amiodarone	Phospholipidosis (similar to steatosis)	Widespread effects, liver damage among most serious, abnormal LFTs in 15%–80%; progression may occur despite discontinuation
Tetracyclines	Mixed; necrosis and microvesicular steatosis	Toxicity is rare with newer forms of oral tetracyclines
Tamoxifen	Mixed; cholestasis, peliosis hepatis, necrosis, steatosis	Steatosis occurs in 30% of women
Phenytoin	Histiocytic granulomas, cholestasis, multifocal necrosis	Pathology also shows lymphocyte beading in sinusoids (similar to mononucleosis)
Nitrofurantoin	Mixed; eosinophils seen in one-third	8:1 female predominance for chronic hepatitis; mortality rate for chronic hepatitis is 20% vs 5%–10% for acute hepatitis
TMP-sulfa, griseofulvin, terbinafine, ketoconazole	Cholestasis	Hepatic toxicity of antifungal drugs is enhanced by alcohol

ALT, alanine aminotransferase; DILI, drug-induced liver injury; LFT, liver function test; LT, liver transplantation; TMP, trimethoprim.

PART V

ORGAN SYSTEMS AND DISEASES

recover and regenerate in response to injury. There is an age-related proliferative decline in the rate at which partial living donor livers regenerate. Also, there is a higher mortality in older patients after partial hepatic resection. Lastly, the hepatotoxic effects of hepatitis viruses and medications like acetaminophen and amoxicillin-clavulanate are more pronounced in older adults. Drug-induced liver injury will be discussed later. Refer to **Table 86-3** and **Figure 86-1** for information on patterns of drug injury and pathology findings, respectively.

Fatty Liver Disease

Nonalcoholic fatty liver disease Older persons have not been spared from the rising prevalence of obesity seen throughout the developed world. In 2010, the predicted prevalence of obesity in Americans, 60 years and older was 37%. This tsunami of obesity has gone hand in hand with rising prevalence of metabolic syndrome, which is comprised of systemic hypertension, insulin resistance, central adiposity, elevated BMI, and dyslipidemia. Patients with metabolic syndrome are at high risk for developing nonalcoholic fatty liver disease (NAFLD). NAFLD is defined as the presence of more than 5% hepatic steatosis on imaging or liver histology without evidence of steatohepatitis or fibrosis and after other causes of liver injury have been ruled out. A minority of patients with NAFLD have nonalcoholic steatohepatitis or NASH which is defined as the presence of greater than 5% hepatic steatosis *plus* inflammation with hepatocyte injury. Whereas NAFLD *without* NASH is a relatively benign condition, NASH may progress to fibrosis and ultimately cirrhosis, portal hypertension, and liver failure. Patients with NASH may develop hepatocellular carcinoma (HCC), which is usually associated with cirrhosis, although NASH-associated HCC in the absence of cirrhosis does occur. In one cross-sectional multicenter study from the United States, when compared to younger patients with NAFLD, older NAFLD patients had a higher prevalence of NASH (56% vs 72%) and advanced fibrosis (25% vs 44%).

NAFLD and NASH have the same presentation in older and younger persons, often as elevated liver-related chemistries and increased fat observed on liver imaging in the setting of metabolic syndrome. The keys to evaluation are the exclusion of secondary causes of liver injury (eg, heavy alcohol use, drug-related, viral hepatitis, metabolic disease), and the discrimination of NASH from NAFLD without NASH. The latter determination can start with noninvasive testing based on blood tests such as the FIB-4 test, followed by estimates of liver fibrosis using elastography.

Patients with fibrosis in the NASH setting are candidates for therapy. In patients with metabolic syndrome and elevated BMI, weight loss is the most effective way to reverse fibrosis and improve liver chemistries. Although diet, exercise, and risk factor modification are widely advocated, they are difficult to accomplish. Weight loss of more than 10% improves insulin sensitivity and liver tests. Although not yet demonstrated unequivocally, weight

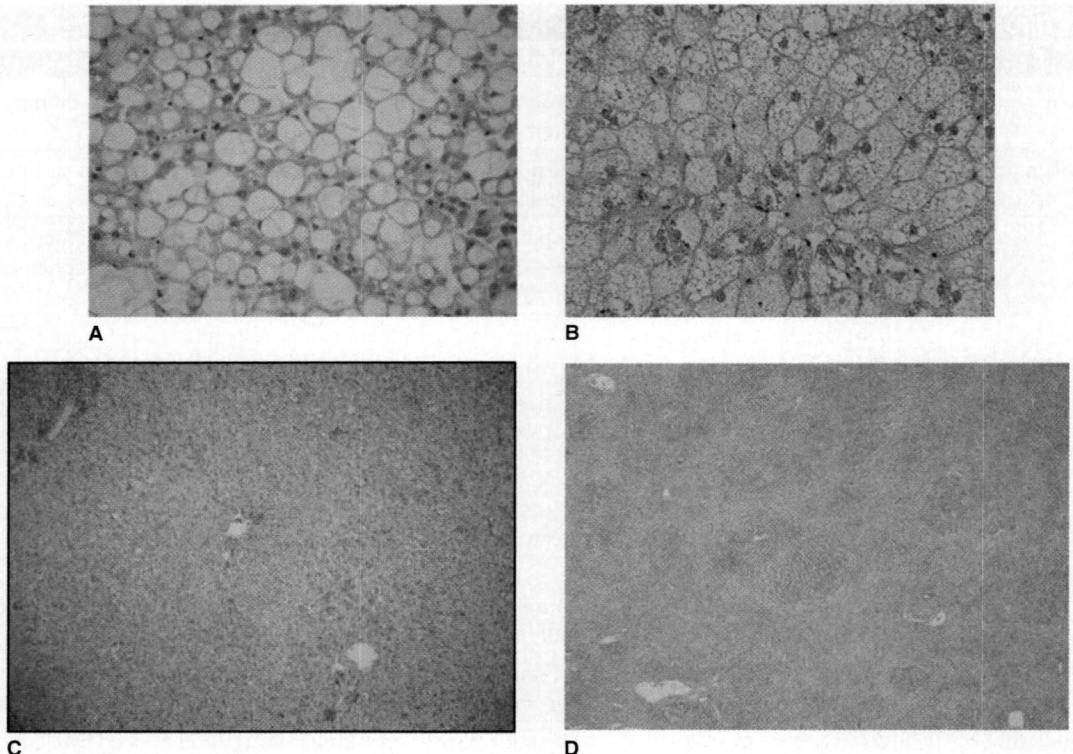

FIGURE 86-1. Examples of drug-induced liver injury. **A.** Macrovesicular steatosis—methotrexate. **B.** Microvesicular steatosis indicating mitochondrial injury: valproate, tamoxifen, tetracyclines. **C.** Hepatocellular necrosis in acetaminophen toxicity in zone 3. **D.** Necrosis due to isoniazid.

loss may also reverse fibrosis. Bariatric surgery is appropriate in selected patients with NASH-associated liver fibrosis.

NASH cirrhosis has become the second most common indication for liver transplantation in the United States, and the most common in women. The specific issues related to liver transplantation in older persons is discussed elsewhere.

Alcohol-associated liver disease Almost 50% of the adults older than 65 years and almost 25% of persons older than 85 years drink alcohol. Alcohol use disorder (AUD) in older persons has been called "the silent epidemic." AUDs afflict 1% to 3% of older subjects and represent a cause of physical and psychiatric morbidity and social distress. In addition, up to 30% of older patients hospitalized in divisions of general medicine, and up to 50% of those hospitalized in psychiatric divisions present AUDs. Unfortunately, AUD is often underreported or even unrecognized in these clinical settings. Questionnaires such as AUDIT and AUDIT-C are simple tools that when used on a regular basis will greatly increase the recognition of underlying AUD.

Alcohol-associated liver disease (ALD) refers to a continuum of liver injury ranging from benign deposition of fat to cirrhosis, portal hypertension, and liver failure. In common with NAFLD, ALD causing cirrhosis is associated with HCC. In contrast with NAFLD, ALD may also present with an acute form of liver failure called alcoholic hepatitis. Alcoholic hepatitis is a syndrome of jaundice and a systemic inflammatory reaction in the setting of recent consumption of alcohol. When severe, AH can result in multisystem organ failure (sometimes referred to as acute on chronic liver failure) and death.

Abstinence from alcohol is the *sine qua non* of all treatment of ALD. Unfortunately, ALD patients, whether younger or older, rarely receive formal treatment for AUD. Sustained abstinence can result in remarkable improvements in ALD, even after decompensating events such as ascites or variceal hemorrhage. Brief courses of corticosteroids offer a modest, albeit short-term, improvement for severe AH. ALD is the most common indication for liver transplantation in North America and Europe.

Viral Hepatitis

Unvaccinated older adults are susceptible to viral hepatitis, which can cause severe illness. Key aspects of the different types of viral hepatitis are summarized in **Table 86-4**. This section will focus on the three most common types of viral hepatitis occurring in older people.

Hepatitis A Hepatitis A virus (HAV) is an RNA virus spread via fecal-oral transmission. Acute HAV infection is diagnosed by the demonstration of HAV IgM antibodies within the serum in symptomatic patients. As the acute illness resolves, anti-HAV IgG antibodies develop conferring lifelong immunity. With the development of improved

TABLE 86-4 ■ HEPATOTROPIC VIRAL DISEASE

	GENOME	ROUTE OF TRANSMISSION	OUTCOME	SEROLOGIES	SEROLOGY INTERPRETATION	PREVENTION; TREATMENT
HAV	RNA	Fecal-oral	Acute only	HAV IgG and IgM	(+) IgM = acute infection (+) IgG = prior exposure or vaccination and immunity	HAV vaccine; supportive
HBV	DNA	Parenteral	Acute and chronic	HBV core Ab, surface Ag, surface Ab, quantitative DNA	(+) core Ab only = prior exposure (+) surface Ab only = immunity (+) core Ab and surface = prior exposure and immunity (+) surface Ag = infection	HBV vaccine; entecavir, adefovir, tenofovir, telbivudine
HCV	RNA	Parenteral	Acute and chronic	HCV Ab, quantitative RNA	(+) Ab = infection; check RNA with negative Ab and high suspicion for HCV	No vaccine; sofosbuvir and other new agents
HDV	RNA	Parenteral	Acute and chronic	HDV Ag, IgM Ab, IgG Ab, quant. RNA	(+) Ag = infection	HBV vaccine; PEG-IFN-α +/− HBV meds
HEV	RNA	Fecal-oral	Acute and chronic	HEV IgM Ab, IgG Ab, quant. RNA	HEV RNA most reliable marker of infection	Supportive; PEG-IFN-α and ribavirin with chronic HEV

sanitation, the proportion of adults lacking immunity to HAV has increased. There is a safe and effective vaccine for HAV. Providers should screen and vaccinate older patients traveling to endemic areas. No outbreaks of hepatitis A have been reported at nursing facilities to date. While HAV vaccination is not required for most geriatric patients, it is safe and simple, and providers should have a low threshold for vaccinating susceptible patients of any age.

Hepatitis B Hepatitis B virus (HBV) is a DNA virus and blood-borne pathogen. Nearly 1.2 million people in the United States and over 350 million people worldwide are infected with chronic hepatitis B. Less than 5% of acute HBV infections arising de novo in adults living in the United States will lead to chronic infections. Acute HBV infection is relatively rare in older adults, as the primary risk factors associated with transmission are intravenous drug use and high-risk sexual behavior. There is an increased risk of becoming a chronic HBV carrier with increasing age at acquisition, which is possibly related to an age-related decline in cellular immunity. Chronic HBV infection is a risk factor for hepatocellular carcinoma, and this risk increases with age. With regards to therapy, entecavir and adefovir are safe to use irrespective of age. Lastly, there is a significant age-related decreased antibody response rate after immunization with the HBV vaccine. Older patients might require an additional injection in order to improve immunogenic HBV vaccine response.

Hepatitis C Hepatitis C virus (HCV) is an RNA virus and blood-borne pathogen. Prevalence data varies widely, but it is estimated 71 million people are infected with chronic hepatitis C worldwide. Acute HCV infections in the United States are almost exclusively confined to persons injecting street drugs. Chronic HCV infection develops in 50% to 80% of infected individuals with the subsequent development of cirrhosis in a significant proportion of these patients. Chronic HCV-related cirrhosis is associated with the development of hepatocellular carcinoma, and this risk is increased significantly with age. Also, the severity of liver disease among patients with chronic HCV infection is worse with increasing age. Similarly, the progression to cirrhosis is faster in older patients, and the serum HCV viral load is significantly higher when compared to younger adults. The older population should be screened for HCV, especially patients who used intravenous or intranasal drugs or received blood products prior to 1992.

In the developed world, the landscape of HCV has been changed radically by the development of highly effective, direct-acting, oral antivirals. These agents are easy to use, often for as little as an 8-week course, and have few side effects in most patients. The AASLD-IDSA clinical guideline is an excellent resource for practitioners who are not familiar with using these agents. Eradication of HCV is achieved in more than 90% of patients. The presence of cirrhosis is one factor that impairs responsiveness. Eradication of HCV in patients with established cirrhosis diminishes but does not remove the risk of development of HCC, and surveillance should be continued (see HCC below). Global challenges to the goal of HCV eradication include educating patients and treatment providers on the need to screen for HCV, increasing screening and diagnosis, as well as ensuring these efficacious medications are accessible and available.

Older patients consume the largest portion of both prescription and over-the-counter medications. Both age and polypharmacy are risk factors for drug-induced hepatotoxicity. Older patients often have altered pharmacokinetics and pharmacodynamics caused by changes in renal, hepatic, cardiovascular, and pulmonary function and decreased body mass. Drug-induced liver toxicity occurs more frequently in older patients and tends to be more severe. Clinically, drug-induced hepatotoxicity presents with nonspecific symptoms or subclinically, reflected only in serum laboratory abnormalities. Some medications have a well-recognized increased risk of liver toxicity with age. For example, isoniazid frequently causes some evidence of liver toxicity in patients older than 50 years, yet, rarely causes liver damage in patients younger than 20 years. Health care providers taking care of older patients should be aware of this increased risk of drug-induced hepatotoxicity and should be vigilant in assessing for hepatic inflammation. Medications that are heavily metabolized by the liver, some of which are listed in **Table 86-2**, should be initiated at a dose 30% to 40% lower than average doses used in middle-aged adults. LiverTox is a very helpful website sponsored by the National Institutes of Health for drug-specific information (http://livertox.nih.gov/). Refer to **Table 86-3** and **Figure 86-1** for information on patterns of drug injury and pathology findings, respectively.

Primary Biliary Cholangitis

Primary biliary cholangitis (PBC) is characterized by an immune-mediated destruction of the intralobular biliary system. It is predominantly regarded as a disease affecting middle-aged women, but since many patients with PBC live into old age, it is seen both as a new diagnosis or a continuing diagnosis in older patients. Many patients remain asymptomatic and are diagnosed on the basis of an incidentally found elevated alkaline phosphatase level, though pruritus or lassitude may present as early symptoms. Patients with PBC have a higher incidence of other autoimmune conditions such as thyroiditis, Sjögren syndrome, and celiac disease. Disruption of the metabolism of the fat-soluble vitamins leads to an increased risk for developing osteoporosis. The antimitochondrial M2 antibody is a highly sensitive and specific serologic test for PBC, so that liver biopsy is rarely required for diagnosis. PBC is a slowly progressive disease that leads to portal hypertension and cholestatic liver failure in some patients. Treatment is directed to symptom management of pruritus, correction of malabsorption of fat-soluble vitamins, and arresting progression using ursodeoxycholic acid. A small minority of patients may benefit from adding obeticholic acid to ursodeoxycholic acid, although this agent exacerbates pruritus and is contraindicated in patients with decompensated liver failure. Liver transplantation remains the ultimate therapy and should be considered in well-selected geriatric patients.

Autoimmune Hepatitis

Autoimmune hepatitis is a condition of unknown etiology leading to chronic hepatic inflammation and destruction, with resultant cirrhosis in untreated patients (see Mack et al. for a recent comprehensive review). Autoimmune hepatitis has a bimodal onset, with a second peak of presentation in persons in their sixth decade or older. While autoimmune hepatitis may be present with elevated serum aminotransferases that are discovered incidentally in an otherwise healthy older person, it has a wide spectrum of presentation including new-onset severe liver injury with markedly elevated aminotransferases. Initial serologic workup should include IgG antibody level, antinuclear antibody, and anti-smooth muscle antibody, and exclusion of other causes of liver injury. Liver biopsy is essential for making the diagnosis. Autoimmune hepatitis generally responds well to immunosuppressive therapy. Patient who have features of both autoimmune hepatitis and PBC or PSC, so-called "cross-over syndromes," present a diagnostic and therapeutic challenge. For years, prednisone and azathioprine have been the cornerstones of treatment. More recently, budesonide has replaced prednisone in many cases for both initiation and maintenance therapy, thereby limiting the systemic side effects of corticosteroids. Budesonide is not recommended in patients with established cirrhosis. Older patients receiving chronic therapy with corticosteroids need to be monitored closely for serious side effects such as osteoporosis, glucose intolerance, and cataract formation. Prognosis is likely similar between older patients and younger adults.

Primary Sclerosing Cholangitis (PSC)

PSC is a chronic condition of inflammation and scarring of medium and large-sized bile ducts. Up to 70% of patients with PSC involving both large and medium-size ducts have accompanying chronic inflammatory bowel disease, usually ulcerative colitis, whereas 10% of persons with IBD of the colon will have PSC at some point in their clinical illness. Some other variants are often included under the rubric of PSC including IgG4 cholangiopathy, and cross-over syndromes autoimmune hepatitis. Chronic inflammation and structuring of the smaller bile ducts are sometimes called "small duct PSC." It is not associated with IBD and may represent a form of AMA-negative PBC. PSC should be distinguished from forms of secondary biliary sclerosis, which may have vascular, infectious, malignant, or drug-induced origin. Typically, PSC presents in younger persons, but presentation in older age occurs also. Pruritus' may be a prominent symptom. Elevation of the serum markers of cholestasis (alkaline phosphatase and later total bilirubin) is chrematistic. In contrast to PBC and autoimmune hepatitis, autoantibodies are of little clinical utility. Diagnosis is made by cholangiography, initially MRCP. ERCP may be both diagnostic and therapeutic. While PSC causes characteristic changes in the liver (peribiliary sclerosis or "onion skinning"), small intralobular bile ducts are often less affected, and the liver biopsy features are often nonspecific and are rarely required to make the diagnosis. There is no approved medical treatment for PSC. The keys to management are:

1. Control of symptoms, particularly itching
2. Recognition and treatment of episodic ascending cholangitis
3. Endoscopic management of dominant biliary strictures, when possible
4. Surveillance for cholangiocarcinoma

Approximately half of all patients with PSC will develop dominant biliary strictures leading to clinically significant obstructions. The specter of cholangiocarcinoma hangs over all patients with PSC and most cholangiocarcinomas develop within dominant bile duct strictures. Interventional endoscopists are able to treat dominant strictures through endoscopic dilation and stenting, and to survey suspicious strictures with cytology, ERCP-guided trans-papillary biopsy, endoscopic ultrasound with fine needle aspiration, and cholangioscopy with direct biopsy. There is no established guideline for interval surveillance, but annual MRI/MRCP (where available) is a good option. Ultimately, liver transplantation is the treatment of choice in selected individuals.

Living With Chronic Liver Disease

Cirrhosis of the liver results in derangements in three interconnected clinical aspects of liver physiology: liver blood flow, hepatic metabolism, and the formation and secretion of bile. Perturbations to these functions may cause greater problems for older patients than for their younger counterparts. Nowadays, many patients with established liver disease survive past 70 years and experience a combination of frailty and portal hypertension with recurrent ascites or hydrothorax, encephalopathy, and fatigue. Often, the process of injury to the liver continues unabated while the patient experiences these decompensating symptoms. Excessive alcohol consumption, or increased body mass in the setting of metabolic syndrome are just two common explanations for how liver injury can progress despite clinical deterioration. The resistance to portal blood flow due to pre- and intrasinusoidal injury in cirrhosis proceeds silently at first. The asymptomatic cirrhotic patient may have porto-systemic varices, splenomegaly, and thrombocytopenia. The most common first clinical manifestation of portal hypertension is ascites, or its variant portal hypertensive hydrothorax. The consequences of portal hypertension and liver failure which are called "decompensation" (ie, ascites, hydrothorax, encephalopathy, variceal hemorrhage, slow gastrointestinal hemorrhage from gastropathy) can prove difficult to manage in an older patient, particularly if he or she has other systemic diseases such as impaired kidney function or COPD. There has been an increasing recognition of the adverse effects of advancing cirrhosis on muscle mass.

The first and most important step in assisting older patients with decompensated liver disease is to have a frank discussion with them and their caregivers about the prospects for improvement in symptoms and prognosis, and then to set their goals of therapy. Wherever possible, we advocate that the injurious process be arrested, for example by institution of robust abstinence from alcohol in alcohol-associated liver failure.

Next, we aim to find a balance between the symptoms and the distress caused by treatment. A brief review of treatment of recurrent ascites or encephalopathy in an older patient illustrates the special challenges posed by the combination of liver failure and advanced age. Recurrent ascites due to portal hypertension with or without hydrothorax causes pain, dyspnea, and immobility and carries the risk of spontaneous bacterial peritonitis. Many older patients find it difficult to adhere to dietary salt restriction. The standard next step is to increase free water clearance with diuretics. Older patients may not tolerate diuretics because of urinary incontinence or impaired kidney function. When diuretics fail or induce rising creatinine, or electrolyte disturbance (hyponatremia, hyperkalemia), the choices are limited and unsatisfactory: intermittent large-volume paracentesis which requires transport, is painful, and may lead to infection; or a transjugular intrahepatic portosystemic shunt (TIPS), which is confounded by encephalopathy. In a comfort-directed clinical plan, placement of an indwelling intraperitoneal catheter is reasonable, but should be viewed as an option for no more than a few final weeks.

Hepatic encephalopathy in an older patient is both difficult to improve and to live with. It complicates other forms of age-related changes in memory and mental acuity, making it difficult to determine the contribution of progressive dementia and what is metabolic. Hepatic encephalopathy shows capricious variability. One of the biggest issues for some patients is the recommendation that they stop driving. Each new episode of encephalopathy necessitates a search for a precipitating event: variceal hemorrhage, electrolyte disturbance, inadvertent misuse of sedatives or other medicines that alter the sensorium, clandestine intracranial hemorrhage, and infection (such as SPB). Treatment of hepatic encephalopathy is less than satisfactory. Many patients find lactulose to be unpalatable, and they dislike the accompanying loose stools. Other patients may choose to stop lactulose on account of the taste or to avoid flatulence and fecal incontinence.

Frail patients with recurrent ascites or encephalopathy may be too ill to manage at home and require skilled nursing. Liver transplantation is an appropriate consideration in carefully selected patients, and age alone is not a contraindication. However, a careful assessment of comorbidities typically shows that many older patients, particularly after age 70, are not suitable candidates for liver transplantation. When in doubt, it is always appropriate for the primary care provider or geriatrician to contact their liver transplant center and discuss referring their patient. Similarly, other interventions such as TIPS are more hazardous in the over-70 cohort. There is a growing consensus that palliative care directed at improving symptom management and quality of life needs to become a priority in the care of patients with chronic liver disease.

HEPATOBILIARY CANCER

Hepatocellular Carcinoma

In Western Europe and North America, hepatocellular carcinoma (HCC) usually occurs in older patients, although the age of presentation is lower in communities where hepatitis B viral infection is endemic. HCC arises typically as a consequence of chronic inflammation of the liver that has resulted in cirrhosis. Consequently, in the individual patient, the prognosis of HCC is intertwined with the clinical stage and prognosis of cirrhosis (see the discussion of living with cirrhosis). Patients with cirrhosis should undergo surveillance for HCC with serial imaging and measurement of serum alpha feto protein (AFP). While controversial, we recommend sonography and AFP every 6 months, until clinical judgement suggests that further surveillance lacks utility. Treatment of carefully selected geriatric patients with HCC, whether by surgical resection, liver transplantation, or by anticancer therapies such as radiofrequency ablation, chemoembolization (TACE), radioembolization (yttrium-90), or chemotherapy, appears to have a similar morbidity and mortality as compared to similar treatment given to younger patients. Thus, age should not be a contraindication for therapy for HCC in the appropriate older patient. In many tertiary centers, management of HCC is conducted in a team approach involving the subspecialties of hepatology, medical and radiation oncology, surgical oncology, surgical transplantation, and interventional radiology.

Cholangiocarcinoma

Cholangiocarcinoma may arise de novo, in association with PSC, or more rarely with secondary forms of chronic biliary inflammation. Cholangiocarcinoma affecting the large bile ducts may be discovered on surveillance in PSC or on presentation of ascending cholangitis or biliary obstruction. It is often difficult to make the diagnosis of cholangiocarcinoma since the tumor is hypocellular, arises in a desmoid scar, and usually is difficult to access. Treatment for cure is also challenging, although a minority of cases respond to surgery (Whipple procedure, or liver transplantation after extensive directed radio- and chemotherapy).

Gallbladder Cancer

Cancer of the gallbladder is uncommon in the United States and carries a poor prognosis. Often, this diagnosis is not made until late in its course. The 5-year survival for local disease is 42%, but drops to 0.7% with distant spread of disease. SEER data show that gallbladder cancer occurs primarily in older adults. Approximately 75% of cases occur in patients older than 65 years. It has been noted that 80% of patients with gallbladder cancer have a history of cholelithiasis. Chronic inflammation from gallstones is thought to induce metaplasia of the gallbladder. Prophylactic cholecystectomy in certain higher risk groups is controversial. Among those who may benefit from this procedure include patients with a porcelain gallbladder, gallbladder polyps greater than or equal to 1 cm and patients with a congenital defect in the junction of the pancreatobiliary duct.

BILIARY DISEASE

Cholelithiasis

Table 86-5 outlines the risk factors associated with gallstone formation. Age is a major factor, although the reasons are unclear. By the ninth decade of life, the prevalence of gallstones is 38% in women and 22% in men. The prevalence of gallstones in the US population increases by 1% per year in women and by 0.5% per year in men after age 15. The increase in risk in women is related to increased biliary cholesterol excretion by estrogen. Approximately 500,000 people in the United States develop symptomatic gallstones each year. The incidence of gallstones is increasing within the United States due to the increasing incidence of obesity.

The majority of patients with gallstones are asymptomatic, and the gallstones are found incidentally when a patient undergoes abdominal imaging. It is often a challenge to determine whether symptoms such as chronic nonsevere abdominal pain are causally related to the newly discovered gallstones. Serious complications that may arise from cholelithiasis include severe abdominal pain ("biliary colic"), acute cholecystitis, chronic cholecystitis, or cancer of the gallbladder. These complications can be especially problematic in older patients with comorbid conditions.

Choledocholithiasis

With gallbladder contraction, gallstones can enter and potentially obstruct the common bile duct. Such obstructions can lead to pain, jaundice, ascending cholangitis, liver abscess, and acute pancreatitis. The prevalence of stones in the common bile duct increases with age. Although dilatation of the common bile duct correlates with choledocholithiasis, the common bile duct may become dilated as a result of the normal aging process or following a cholecystectomy due to the reservoir effect. Comparison to previous imaging studies to evaluate for interval change is important when available.

The classical signs and symptoms of biliary obstruction are called biliary colic and include epigastric or right

TABLE 86-5 ■ RISK FACTORS FOR GALLSTONE FORMATION
Increasing age
Female sex
Obesity
Dyslipidemia
Rapid weight loss
Medications
Ethnicity—White, Native American, and Hispanic

upper quadrant pain, nausea, vomiting, and pruritus. Patients may develop dark urine and acholic stools. The presence of fever and jaundice is concerning for ascending cholangitis. The constellation of abdominal pain, jaundice, and fever, known as Charcot triad, is helpful in making the diagnosis of ascending cholangitis.

Acute Cholecystitis

Approximately 50% to 70% of cases of acute cholecystitis occur in the geriatric population. This condition is characterized by prolonged obstruction of the cystic duct by one or more gallstones. This leads to ischemia, inflammation, and possibly infection of the gallbladder. Acalculous cholecystitis, which occurs in 5% to 10% of cases, refers to inflammation of the gallbladder in the absence of gallstones. It is usually idiopathic, but tends to occur in debilitated and or vasculopathic patients. The severity of cholecystitis varies from mild gallbladder wall edema to severe inflammation and, at its most catastrophic, necrosis or perforation of the gallbladder.

Acute cholecystitis has several classic clinical manifestations. The usual symptoms include abdominal pain, especially in the right upper quadrant or epigastrium, which may radiate to the back or shoulder. It is typically continuous and severe. Patients may notice the onset of such pain after eating a fatty meal. Fevers, chills, nausea, and vomiting are common as well.

Acute cholecystitis may present atypically in older adults and with delayed recognition results in a greater risk of complications. Older patients usually have right upper quadrant or epigastric pain and tenderness, but other signs and symptoms may be lacking. Older patients present without fever, nausea, or vomiting in more than 50% of acute cases. These signs may not be present in 33%, even in the setting of gallbladder gangrene or perforation. Acalculous cholecystitis is more common in older adults, and diagnosis of such cases may be more difficult because of the lack of stones on imaging studies.

Chronic Cholecystitis

Chronic cholecystitis refers to biliary pain caused by recurrent episodes of cystic duct obstruction or direct irritation of the gallbladder wall due to stones leading to a chronic inflammatory response. Ultimately this may lead to scarring, fibrosis, and gallbladder dysfunction. On ultrasound or CT imaging, chronic cholecystitis has a more subtle appearance than acute cholecystitis. As with acute cholecystitis, elective cholecystectomy is the treatment of choice.

Investigations

In acute cholecystitis, ultrasound typically shows gallstones and pericholecystic fluid and/or edema. A sonographic Murphy sign is helpful in establishing the diagnosis. Ultrasonography will demonstrate the presence of stones with an accuracy of 90%. A HIDA (^{99m}technetium-N-substituted hepatoiminodiacetic acid) scan will show opacification of the bile ducts, but not of the gallbladder, in cholecystitis.

Ultrasound is the usual initial diagnostic test of choice for choledocholithiasis with a sensitivity of 20% to 38% and specificity of 80% to 100% (**Table 86-6**). It has the advantage of being noninvasive, easily tolerated by the patient, widely available, and inexpensive. Abdominal CT has higher sensitivity than ultrasound (50%–88%), but often fails to identify stones less than 5 mm. Magnetic resonance cholangiopancreatography (MRCP) allows for visualization of biliary anatomy as well as stones and has sensitivity of 57% to 100% and specificity of 73% to 100% for common bile duct stones. It also has the advantage of being noninvasive, but its disadvantages include cost and potential patient discomfort from claustrophobia.

Endoscopic ultrasound (EUS) is a useful imaging modality in cases where the presence of stones in the common bile duct is suspected, but remains uncertain. EUS has sensitivity and specificity of 94% and 95%, respectively, and sedation needs are similar to an upper endoscopy. Endoscopic retrograde cholangiopancreatography (ERCP) is a therapeutic modality for treatment of choledocholithiasis. The injection of contrast into the biliary tree to obtain a cholangiogram allows visualization of all but very small stones. A biliary sphincterotomy is routinely performed to remove common bile duct stones and to prevent recurrent obstruction. In the case of cholangitis, a stent may be left in the common bile duct to drain purulent material, stones,

TABLE 86-6 ■ IMAGING AND THERAPIES FOR CHOLEDOCHOLITHIASIS

TEST	SENSITIVITY	SPECIFICITY	ADVANTAGES	DISADVANTAGES
Ultrasound	20%–38%	80%–100%	Noninvasive, low cost	Low sensitivity, nontherapeutic
CT	50%–88%	84%–98%	Ease for patient	Expensive, nontherapeutic
MRCP	57%–100%	93%–97%	Highly sensitive	Expensive, nontherapeutic, may cause claustrophobia
EUS	94%	95%	High precision	Expensive, nontherapeutic, sedation
ERCP	57%–100%	73%–100%	Therapeutic	Expensive, may cause pancreatitis
PTC			Therapeutic	Bleeding, pain (especially in the absence of dilated bile ducts)

ERCP, endoscopic retrograde cholangiopancreatography; EUS, endoscopic ultrasound; MRCP, magnetic resonance cholangiopancreatography; PTC, percutaneous transhepatic cholangiography.

and sludge. The disadvantages of ERCP include the potential for procedural complications such as acute pancreatitis, technical and infrastructural requirements to complete the procedure, and cost. However, ERCP poses no greater risk in older adults than in the younger population. One study of ERCP in the geriatric population showed no difference in the rate of therapeutic ERCP complications in patients older than 80 years (6.8%) versus those younger than 80 years (5.1%). In a retrospective cohort between 2002 and 2005, there were no significant differences in successful biliary drainage, complications, or mortality in a group of 178 patients older than 75 years compared to 159 patients less than 75 years. Another study evaluated the safety of ERCP in patients older than 90 years, and the complication rate in this age group was 6.3% compared to 8.4% in patients aged 70 to 89. Therefore, ERCP is a safe procedure even in those with very advanced age. The rate of recurrence of symptomatic CBD stones after ERCP was higher in patients older than 80 years (20%) versus 4% in patients 50 years old or younger. Thus, older adults are at higher risk for needing a repeat ERCP. Despite this increased procedural burden, the American Society of Gastrointestinal Endoscopy (ASGE) does not list advanced age as an independent risk factor for the development of post-ERCP pancreatitis, infection or higher bleeding rates. Refer to **Figure 86-2** for review of multiple ERCP images.

Treatment

Incidental discovery of gallstones is not an indication for therapy. Because asymptomatic gallstones tend to follow a benign course, cholecystectomy should be considered primarily in those with symptoms or complications.

Prompt treatment of acute cholecystitis is warranted to prevent clinical deterioration, complications, and progression to chronic cholecystitis. In addition to intravenous fluids, antibiotics, and pain control, surgery is the mainstay of treatment. Each patient's clinical status and comorbidities must be considered in the decision to proceed with general anesthesia and surgery. Laparoscopic cholecystectomy has several advantages over open cholecystectomy including less discomfort, shorter hospital stay, and lower cost. Complications from this procedure often involve biliary trauma. Age and comorbidities are predictors of surgical outcomes. Timing of intervention is also important with better outcomes in patients who undergo early laparoscopic cholecystectomy for acute cholecystitis. Whenever possible, this should be performed within the same hospital stay for definitive treatment of gallstone disease.

As discussed above, in older patients with acute cholecystitis who are felt to be suitable surgical candidates, laparoscopic cholecystectomy is a reasonable option. However, for older patients who are very ill or have significant comorbidities, gallbladder drainage prior to surgery may be a viable alternative. Percutaneous cholecystostomy drainage is an effective and often definitive treatment for both acute cholecystitis as well as acalculous cholecystitis in select cases. Patients with symptomatic gallstone who

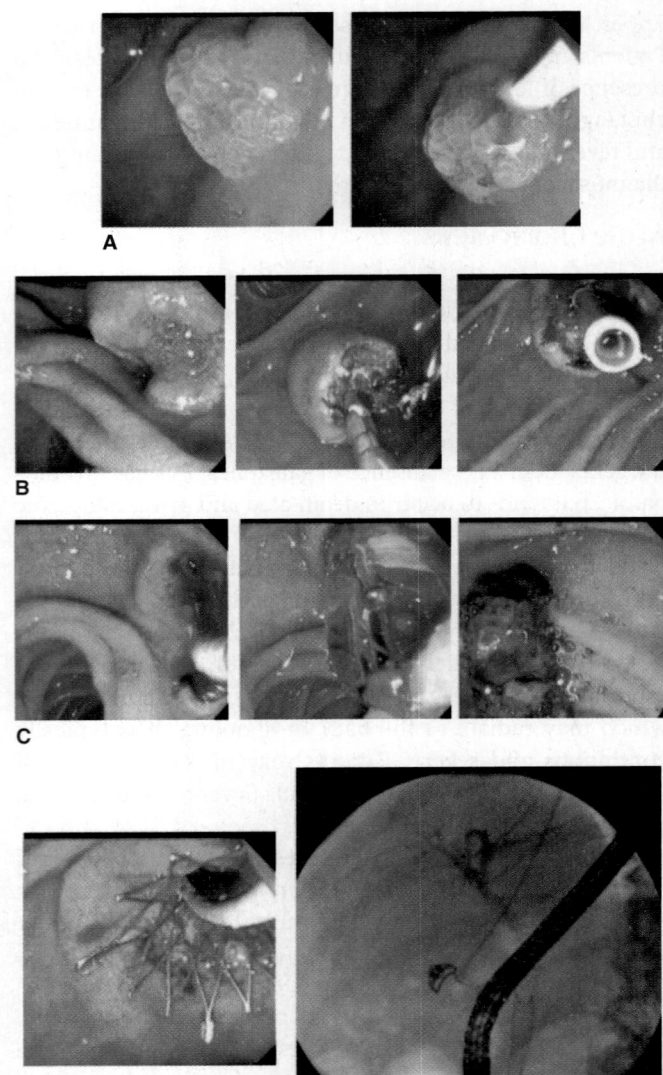

FIGURE 86-2 A–D. Multiple ERCP images. **A.** Normal ampulla with cannulation. **B.** Bulging, ulcerated ampulla found to be adenocarcinoma s/p sphincterotomy and plastic biliary stent placement. **C.** Common bile duct stone removed with balloon. **D.** Common hepatic duct stricture due to cholangiocarcinoma. Endoscopic and fluoroscopic images s/p metal biliary stent placement. (Reproduced with permission from Deepak Gopal, MD, University of Wisconsin, Madison, WI.)

cannot or do not wish to undergo invasive procedures may benefit from dissolution of gallstones with ursodiol. This medication is only useful in the setting of cholesterol gallstones. However, at least 50% of patients treated with ursodiol for gallstones will have recurrent stone formation.

PANCREATIC DISEASE

Anatomy and Physiology

Figure 86-3 shows the gross anatomy of the pancreas. The pancreas can be divided into the endocrine and the

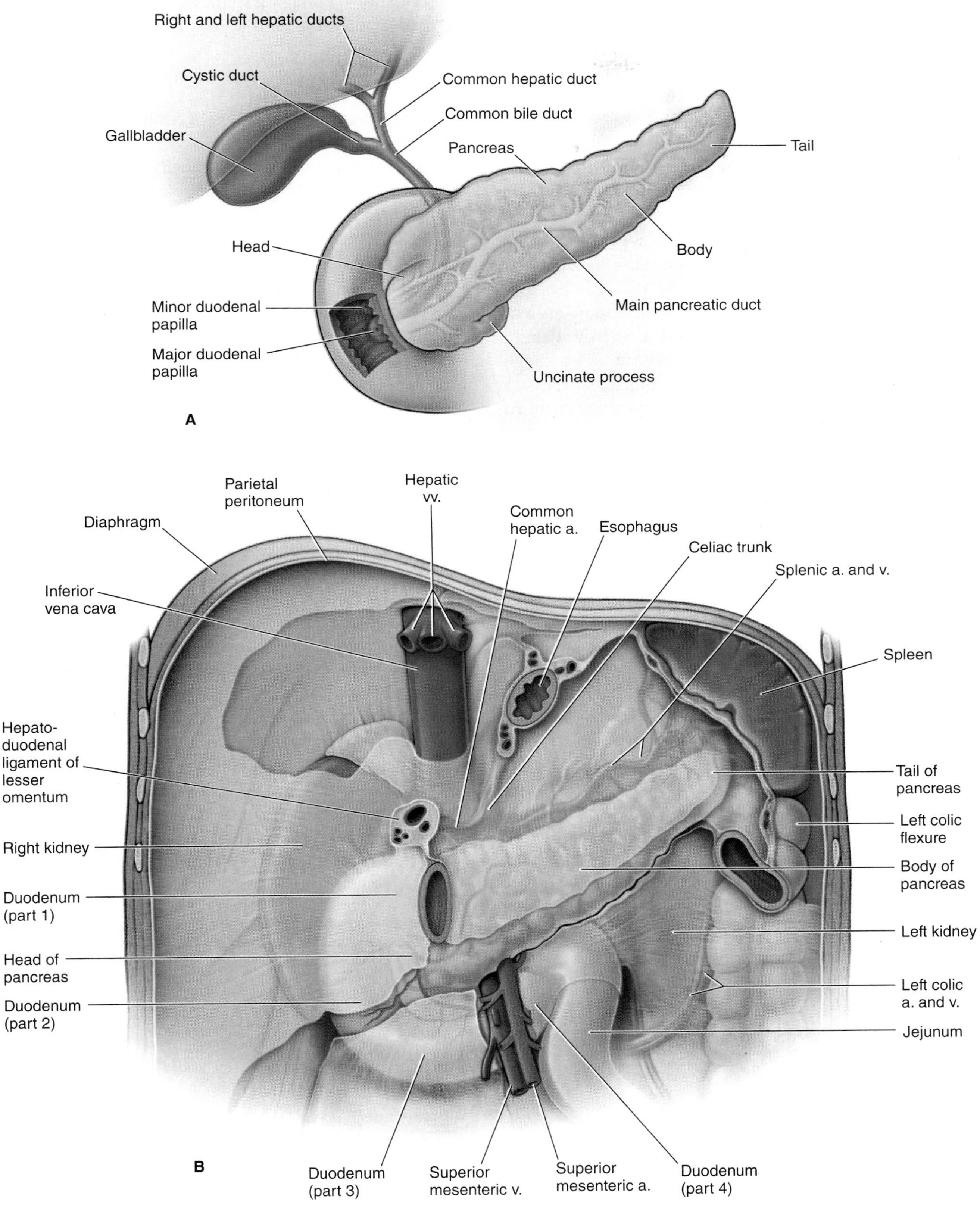

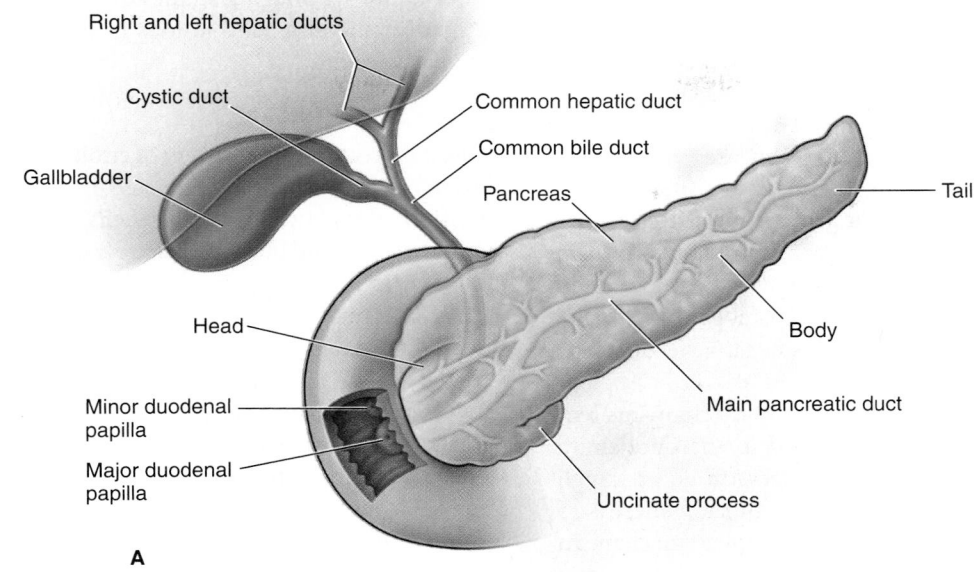

A

Right and left hepatic ducts
Cystic duct
Gallbladder
Head
Minor duodenal papilla
Major duodenal papilla
Common hepatic duct
Common bile duct
Pancreas
Tail
Body
Main pancreatic duct
Uncinate process

B

Diaphragm
Parietal peritoneum
Hepatic vv.
Common hepatic a.
Esophagus
Celiac trunk
Splenic a. and v.
Inferior vena cava
Spleen
Hepato-duodenal ligament of lesser omentum
Tail of pancreas
Left colic flexure
Right kidney
Body of pancreas
Duodenum (part 1)
Left kidney
Head of pancreas
Duodenum (part 2)
Left colic a. and v.
Jejunum
Duodenum (part 3)
Superior mesenteric v.
Superior mesenteric a.
Duodenum (part 4)

FIGURE 86-3. Normal anatomy of the pancreas. (Reproduced with permission from Morton DA, Foreman KB, Albertine KH. *The Big Picture: Gross Anatomy.* New York, NY: McGraw Hill; 2011.)

exocrine pancreas. Four different types of islet cells comprising the endocrine pancreas produce hormones such as insulin, glucagon, pancreatic polypeptide, and somatostatin. The exocrine pancreas is composed primarily of acinar cells and duct cells. The acinar cells produce the digestive enzymes. The key enzyme is trypsinogen. The duct cells produce the bicarbonate-rich fluid for secretion. The exocrine pancreas has proteases, lipases, glycosidases (amylase), and nucleases. Most proteases and the nucleases are stored in an inactive form. Trypsinogen, the primary protease, is activated to trypsin in the duodenum by enterokinase. Trypsin subsequently activates the other digestive enzymes and, in the presence of calcium, activates trypsinogen to trypsin. In the absence of calcium, trypsin has negative feedback by degrading other trypsin molecules.

There are two additional important mechanisms regulating pancreatic function. First, acid in the duodenum stimulates secretion of the hormone secretin and through vagal mediation leads to the duct cells of the pancreas to secrete bicarbonate. The second regulatory mechanism involves the cholecystokinin (CCK) feedback loop. Human pancreatic acini lack CCK receptors. The presence of protein in the duodenum effectively increases cholecystokinin releasing factor (CCK RF), which stimulates CCK release. The elevated CCK level is recognized by the brain, leading to vagal stimulation of the acinar cells of the pancreas to secrete more digestive enzymes.

Aging and the Pancreas

Table 86-7 outlines the age-related changes of the pancreas. The maximal volume of pancreatic juice excreted in response to secretin and CCK stimulation increases until the fifth decade and thereafter decreases steadily. Bicarbonate decreases steadily after the fourth decade of life. Also, in ERCP studies, a slight increase in size of the pancreatic duct in the head and body but not the tail has been noted with aging. Despite these anatomic and physiologic changes, only rare cases of pancreatic exocrine deficiency are clinically apparent in healthy older adults.

Over and above the normal changes of aging, advanced age poses other threats to pancreatic structure and function. Pancreatitis secondary to alcohol tends to be a disease of middle age, while gallstone disease continues to have a relatively high incidence in older cohorts.

TABLE 86-7 ■ AGING AND THE PANCREAS

Fat, fibrosis, and reduced weight after seventh decade

Bicarbonate decreases steadily after the fourth decade of life

Pancreatic exocrine deficiency: rare in older people without underlying pathology

Alcoholic pancreatitis: a disease of middle age

Gallstone prevalence, and therefore gallstone pancreatitis, increases with age

Increased incidence of malignancy, particularly adenocarcinoma

The biggest risk in the older population is an increased incidence of malignancy, particularly adenocarcinoma. In addition, during imaging studies of the abdomen, incidental small cystic and solid lesions of the pancreas are now frequently found.

Acute Pancreatitis

Acute pancreatitis has a variety of etiologies, but all eventually lead to activation of the digestive enzymes particularly trypsin in the pancreatic acinar cells. The most common etiologies for acute pancreatitis are gallstones and alcohol. However, in an older patient without gallstones or a history of chronic excessive use of alcohol, the suspicion for underlying malignancy needs to be especially high. Inherited defects in the trypsinogen to trypsin pathway may lead to rare forms of acute pancreatitis, termed "hereditary pancreatitis." Obstruction of the pancreatic duct by a gallstone is an important mechanism of initiating pancreatic injury. Alcohol, on the other hand, causes mitochondrial dysfunction, which allows for increased levels of intracellular calcium and subsequent activation of trypsin. Hypertriglyceridemia is often overlooked as a cause of acute pancreatitis. Triglycerides should be measured on admission to hospital because levels will often quickly decrease with bowel rest and fluids. Although many medications may cause acute pancreatitis, medication-induced acute pancreatitis is uncommon. See **Table 86-8** for etiologies of acute pancreatitis.

The incidence of acute pancreatitis is increasing in the United States. The predominant symptom of acute pancreatitis is epigastric pain, commonly with radiation into the back. Nausea and vomiting are also frequently present. Acute pancreatitis is a clinical diagnosis with support from elevated serum amylase and lipase. Serum amylase or lipase levels at least 3 times the upper limit of normal are typical of acute pancreatitis. Lipase is more sensitive than amylase and will stay elevated for a longer period of time. Many other conditions cause minor elevations in amylase or lipase. Radiographic studies have little role in diagnosis, but

TABLE 86-8 ■ ETIOLOGIES FOR PANCREATITIS

Gallstones

Alcohol

Hypertriglyceridemia

Medications/toxins

Hereditary pancreatitis

Cystic fibrosis gene mutation

Autoimmune pancreatitis

Pancreatic divisum

Trauma

Post-ERCP

Tumors

Elevated calcium

Idiopathic

do play important roles in evaluating etiology (gallstones, neoplasia, pancreatic calcification indicating chronic pancreatitis) and complications such as necrosis, and pseudocysts. Acute pancreatitis can be divided clinically into mild (absence of organ failure or local complications), moderate (transient organ failure), and severe (persistent organ failure). The range of disease can be from self-limited mild disease to multiorgan failure and death. Approximately 20% of patients with acute pancreatitis will have severe disease due to pancreas necrosis. The overall mortality for patients with acute pancreatitis is 5%. Older patients with comorbid cardiopulmonary diseases are at increased risk of clinical complications due to acute pancreatitis. A variety of grading prognostic systems including Ranson criteria, Apache score, Glasgow score, and the Baltazar CT grade ± necrosis do correlate with morbidity and mortality.

Treatment of mild pancreatitis is accomplished with bowel rest, intravenous fluids, and pain control. Intravenous fluids, when given within the first 72 hours of presentation, can lead to improved clinical outcomes. Gallstone pancreatitis is treated with ERCP, biliary sphincterotomy, and stone extraction if cholangitis or evidence of biliary obstruction is present. However, the routine use of urgent ERCP is not recommended in patients with acute biliary pancreatitis without cholangitis. In patients with severe pancreatitis due to gallstones, cholecystectomy should be undertaken during the initial hospital admission.

Severe pancreatitis often becomes management of multiorgan failure within an ICU setting. Although the use of prophylactic antibiotics is not advised solely because of predicted severe AP and necrotizing pancreatitis, evidence of infected necrosis on CT scan warrants intravenous antibiotics with good pancreatic penetration such as imipenem. Patients who develop sepsis in the setting of pancreatic necrosis should be surveyed by interventional radiology or interventional gastroenterology for biopsy, gram stain, and culture of the necrotic area to help tailor antibiotic therapy. Evidence of infected pancreas necrosis may require temporary percutaneous or endoscopic drain placement or surgical debridement. In patients with acute alcohol-related pancreatitis, brief intervention to address alcohol use disorder is appropriate during admission, and follow-up referral to a formal addiction program is recommended.

The presentation of acute pancreatitis due to alcohol is an opportunity to initiate therapy for alcohol use disorder. Unfortunately, AUD is often overlooked, and this is a particular risk for older persons. The patient with combined pancreatitis and alcohol use disorder should be offered brief therapeutic intervention for AUD while an inpatient and referred for formal treatment of AUD on discharge.

Pseudocyst formation is an important complication of acute pancreatitis. Approximately 10% of patients with acute pancreatitis proceed to formation of these fluid collections. Most pseudocysts resolve with time; however, if symptoms are present (early satiety, pain, infection, bleeding), then drainage via interventional radiology, endoscopic cystogastrostomy, or surgery may be necessary.

Chronic Pancreatitis

Since 2016, the major pancreas societies have adopted a new "mechanistic definition" of chronic pancreatitis that affirms the characteristics of end-stage disease as pancreatic atrophy, fibrosis, pain syndromes, duct distortion and strictures, calcifications, pancreatic exocrine dysfunction, pancreatic endocrine dysfunction, and dysplasia, but also addresses the disease mechanism as a pathologic fibroinflammatory syndrome of the pancreas in individuals with genetic, environmental, and/or other risk factors who develop persistent pathologic responses to parenchymal injury or stress. Alcohol use disorder accounts for approximately 70% of chronic pancreatitis. Idiopathic causes are the second most common cause of chronic pancreatitis. In older adults, it is important to evaluate for tumors compressing the pancreatic duct as a possible etiology.

The diagnosis of chronic pancreatitis can be challenging to make in the early stages of the disease. Approximately 85% of patients will have epigastric postprandial pain. Amylase and lipase can be mildly elevated or normal. Structural changes, such as pancreas atrophy, ductal dilation, and calcifications, can be detected by ultrasound, x-ray, or CT scan and are found in 30% to 40% of cases, leading to a diagnosis. Often, more advanced imaging studies such as ERCP, MRCP, or EUS are used to evaluate the anatomy of the pancreas and give a diagnosis. The major features of chronic pancreatitis include pain, malabsorption, and frequently diabetes.

Treatment is based on resolving malabsorption with pancreatic enzyme replacement. Narcotic pain medication is often needed. If a dilated main pancreatic duct is present, a pancreaticojejunostomy (Puestow procedure) can be helpful. In some cases, near total pancreatectomy is needed with or without islet cell transplantation.

Pancreatic Cancer

Approximately 34,000 new cases of pancreatic cancer will be diagnosed, and 33,000 patients will die secondary to pancreatic cancer each year. Approximately 87% of patients will be older than age 55 at diagnosis with the median age being 72. The overall 5-year survival is 5%. Unfortunately, little progress has been made to change the mortality from this disease over the last several decades. The genetics have now been further elucidated showing that 85% of adenocarcinomas of the pancreas have an activating point mutation in the K-ras oncogene. In addition, 95% have an inactivated p16 tumor-suppressor gene. Genetic changes and new knowledge about the cytokine milieu are continued areas of active research.

More than 70% of adenocarcinomas arise in the head of the pancreas, which leads to common presentations including jaundice, gastric outlet obstruction, and pain. Approximately 15% of lesions do not have vasculature

TABLE 86-9 ■ IMAGING FEATURES OF PANCREATIC CYSTS AND CYST FLUID ANALYSIS

	PSEUDOCYST	SCN	MCN	IPMN
Imaging features	Often occurs in setting of pancreatitis	Hypodense cysts with central scar	Peripheral calcification, no communication with pancreatic duct	Irregular, polycystic, communicates with pancreatic duct
Malignancy risk	None	Extremely low	Up to 20%	Main duct IPMN 50%; branch duct IPMN 10%
Cystic fluid characteristics	Inflammatory cells	Glycogen-containing cells	Mucin-producing cells, possible dysplasia	Mucin-producing cells, possible dysplasia
Cyst amylase	> 250 U/L	< 250 U/L	< 250 U/L	< 250 U/L
Cyst CEA	< 192 ng/mL	< 10 ng/mL	> 192 ng/mL	> 192 ng/mL

CEA, carcinoembryonic antigen.

invasion or metastatic disease on presentation making surgical resection possible, with curative intent. The 5-year survival in this population is approximately 20%. Staging with CT scans and EUS to evaluate for metastatic disease and vascular invasion is thus important.

Other tumors exist in the pancreas including neuroendocrine tumors and many types of cystic lesions of the pancreas. Neuroendocrine tumors of the pancreas are typically solid tumors. Evaluation by EUS with or without FNA and surgical resection are often performed except in multiple endocrine neoplasia (MEN) 1, where the pancreatic lesions are often multifocal in nature.

Pancreatic Cysts

Cystic lesions of the pancreas are becoming increasingly recognized because of more widespread abdominal imaging (**Table 86-9**). Incidental pancreatic cysts are noted on 1% of abdominal CT scans obtained for any reason. These lesions include pseudocysts, congenital cysts (also known as simple cysts), and cystic neoplasms including serous cystadenomas (SCN), mucinous cystic neoplasms (MCN), cystadenocarcinomas, and intraductal papillary mucinous neoplasm (IPMN). According to guidelines from the American Society of Gastrointestinal Endoscopy, cystic lesions of the pancreas, even when found incidentally, may represent malignant or premalignant neoplasms and require diagnostic evaluation regardless of size. Pancreatic pseudocysts and congenital cysts have no malignant potential. Serous cystadenomas represent nearly 30% of pancreatic cystic neoplasms and are most commonly found in women older than 70 years. After a lesion is identified on imaging studies, EUS with FNA is used to obtain fluid for cytologic evaluation and for tumor markers and amylase in order to classify pancreatic cystic lesions (see **Table 86-9** and **Figure 86-4**). Given the high malignant potential, mucinous cystic neoplasms and main duct IPMNs are managed with surgical resection in geriatric patients who are healthy enough to tolerate surgery. Branch duct IPMNs may be surgically resected as well, though serial imaging is often appropriate based on current guidelines.

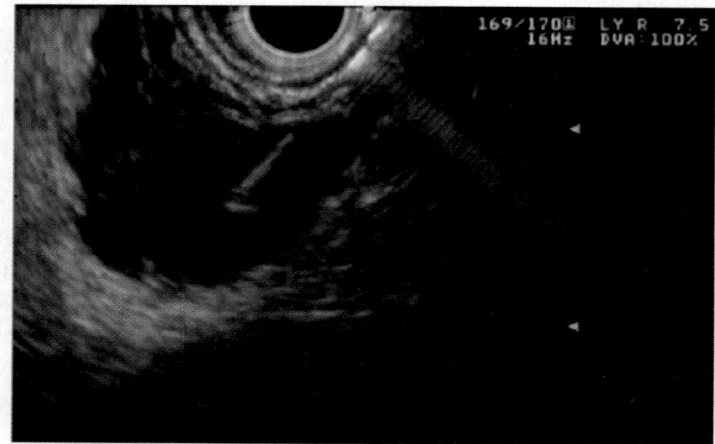

FIGURE 86-4. Endoscopic ultrasound with fine needle aspiration in pancreatic cyst. This cyst proved to be a serous cystadenoma. (Reproduced with permission from Deepak Gopal, MD, University of Wisconsin, Madison, WI.)

FURTHER READING

Agarwal PD, Phillips P, Hillman L, et al. Multidisciplinary management of hepatocellular carcinoma improves access to therapy and patient survival. *J Clin Gastroenterol.* 2017;51(9):845–859.

ASGE Standards of Practice Committee, Buxbaum JL, Abbas Fehmi SM, et al. ASGE guideline on the role of endoscopy in the evaluation and management of choledocholithiasis. *Gastrointest Endosc.* 2019;89(6): 1075–1105 e15.

Blazer DG, Wu LT. The epidemiology of at-risk and binge drinking among middle-aged and elderly community adults: National Survey on Drug Use and Health. *Am J Psychiatry.* 2009;166(10):1162–1169.

Caputo F, Vignoli T, Leggio L, Addolorato G, Zoli G, Bernardi M. Alcohol use disorders in the elderly: a brief overview from epidemiology to treatment options. *Exp Gerontol.* 2012;47(6):411–416.

Chalasani N, Younossi Z, Lavine JE, et al. The diagnosis and management of nonalcoholic fatty liver disease: practice guidance from the American Association for the Study of Liver Diseases. *Hepatology.* 2018;67(1):328–357.

Crabb DW, Im GY, Szabo G, Mellinger JL, Lucey MR. Diagnosis and treatment of alcohol-associated liver diseases: 2019 Practice Guidance From the American Association for the Study of Liver Diseases. *Hepatology.* 2020;71(1):306–333.

Crockett SD, Wani S, Gardner TB, Falck-Ytter Y, Barkun AN, American Gastroenterological Association Institute Clinical Guidelines Committee. American Gastroenterological Association Institute Guideline on Initial Management of Acute Pancreatitis. *Gastroenterol.* 2018;154(4):1096–1101.

Gardner TB, Adler DG, Forsmark CE, Sauer BG, Taylor JR, Whitcomb DC. ACG Clinical Guideline: chronic pancreatitis. *Am J Gastroenterol.* 2020;115(3):322–339.

Ghany MG, Morgan TR, AASLD-IDSA Hepatitis C Guidance Panel. Hepatitis C Guidance 2019 Update: American Association for the Study of Liver Diseases-Infectious Diseases Society of America recommendations for testing, managing, and treating hepatitis C virus infection. *Hepatology.* 2020;71(2):686–721.

Lindor KD, Bowlus CL, Boyer J, Levy C, Mayo M. Primary biliary cholangitis: 2018 Practice Guidance from the American Association for the Study of Liver Diseases. *Hepatology.* 2019;69(1):394–419.

Mack CL, Adams D, Assis DN, et al. Diagnosis and management of autoimmune hepatitis in adults and children: 2019 Practice Guidance and Guidelines From the American Association for the Study of Liver Diseases. *Hepatology.* 2020;72(2):671–722.

Mathus-Vliegen EM. Obesity and the elderly. *J Clin Gastroenterol.* 2012;46(7):533–544.

Noureddin M, Yates KP, Vaughn IA, et al. Clinical and histological determinants of nonalcoholic steatohepatitis and advanced fibrosis in elderly patients. *Hepatology.* 2013;58(5):1644–1654.

Tandon P, Montano-Loza AJ, Lai JC, Dasarathy S, Merli M. Sarcopenia and frailty in decompensated cirrhosis. *J Hepatol.* 2021;75 (Suppl 1):S147–S162.

Tandon P, Walling A, Patton H, Taddei T. AGA clinical practice update on palliative care management in cirrhosis: expert review. *Clin Gastroenterol Hepatol.* 2021;19(4): 646–656 e3.

Terrault NA, Lok ASF, McMahon BJ, et al. Update on prevention, diagnosis, and treatment of chronic hepatitis B: AASLD 2018 Hepatitis B Guidance. *Clin Liver Dis* (Hoboken). 2018;12(1):33–34.

Vege SS, Ziring B, Jain R, Moayyedi P, Clinical Guidelines Committee; American Gastroenterology Association. American gastroenterological association institute guideline on the diagnosis and management of asymptomatic neoplastic pancreatic cysts. *Gastroenterol.* 2015;148(4):819–822; quize12-3.

Zeeh J, Platt D. The aging liver: structural and functional changes and their consequences for drug treatment in old age. *Gerontology.* 2002;48(3):121–127.

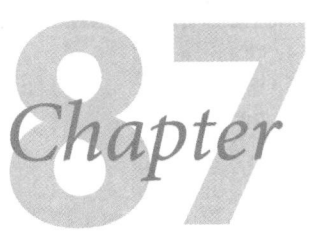

Chapter 87

Constipation

Gerardo Calderon, Andres Acosta

INTRODUCTION

Constipation is a frequent health concern for older people in every health care setting. Primary care visits for constipation increase markedly in people older than 60 years, as does regular use of laxatives. Self-reported constipation in older people is associated with anxiety, depression, and poor health perception, while clinical constipation in vulnerable individuals may lead to complications such as fecal impaction, overflow incontinence, sigmoid volvulus, and urinary retention. Constipation is an expensive condition, with high costs ranging from laxative expenditure to nursing time. For instance, it is estimated that 80% of community nurses working with older people in the United Kingdom are managing constipation (particularly fecal impaction). An Australian study used in-depth, semi-structured interviews to explore older individuals' experiences with constipation, and their findings largely summed up feelings and problems, no doubt, shared by many older people across the developed world:

- They feel "not right" in themselves when they are constipated.
- Physicians can have a dismissive attitude about constipation and do not consider the problem seriously.
- Patients are keen to find a solution, but feel useful and empathic advice and information are generally unavailable.
- At the same time, they have a strong imperative for self-management including use of over-the-counter laxatives.
- There are some barriers to lifestyle approaches, for example, expense of fruit and vegetables, fear of urinary incontinence with increased fluid intake, or reluctance to walk out alone.
- One-quarter still need to do self-manual removal despite measures taken.

This chapter will describe the definition, epidemiology, risk factors, clinical presentation, assessment, and treatment of constipation in older adults. Data sources were searched of the English language literature (1966–2020), systematic review including the Cochrane database, reference lists from recent systematic reviews and book chapters, and expert committee reports, society guidelines, and

Learning Objectives

- Define and identify the prevalence of constipation in the older adult.
- Describe the pathophysiology of constipation in the older adult.
- Understand how to diagnose and classify constipation in the older adult.
- Explain the assessment and management of constipation in the older adult.
- List complications of constipation in the older adult.

Key Clinical Points

1. Constipation is a common problem in the older adult.
2. Constipation is an expensive condition, with high costs ranging from laxative expenditure to nursing time.
3. Health care providers should routinely inquire about constipation symptoms in older people and be alert to the presence of clinical constipation in individuals unable to communicate.
4. In many older people with constipation symptoms, lifestyle advice (diet, fluids, exercise, toileting habits) will preempt the need for laxative therapy.
5. In higher-risk patients, a stepwise approach to prescribing laxatives, suppositories, or enemas should be used, with the goal of achieving comfortable and regular evacuation.
6. Rectal evacuation difficulties should be specifically addressed in order to identify conditions that may require additional interventions.

expert opinion. Levels of evidence are as used by the US Preventive Services Task Force:

- Good evidence, Level 1: consistent results from well-designed, well-conducted studies
- Fair evidence, Level 2: results show benefit, but strength limited by number, quality, or consistency of studies
- Poor evidence, Level 3: insufficient because of limited number, power, or quality of studies

DEFINITIONS

Definitions of constipation in older people in medical and nursing literature have been inconsistent. Studies of older people have tended to define constipation subjectively by self-report, according to specific bowel-related symptoms, or by daily laxative usage. Constipation is a syndrome of difficulty moving bowels, characterized as difficulty or infrequent passage of stool, hardness of stool, or a feeling of incomplete evacuation that may occur in isolation or secondary to another underlying disorder. However, the definition of constipation can be broader and referred to as any condition that changes the bowel functions such as reduced stool frequency, straining to defecate, hard stool, or inability to defecate. Patients and their physicians have vastly different perceptions on what constitutes constipation and a patient-centered approach generally takes them at their word. Use of the Bristol Stool Scale also puts the patient and their practitioner on the same page (**Figure 87-1**). However,

TABLE 87-1 ■ DEFINITIONS OF CONSTIPATION

Constipation (Rome IV Criteria)
Two or more of the following symptoms present on more than 25% of occasions for at least 12 wk in the last 12 mo:
Two or less bowel movements per week
Straining at stool
Hard stools (Bristol Stool Form Scale 1-2)–See **Figure 87-1**
Sensation of incomplete evacuation
Sensation of anorectal obstruction
Manual maneuvers to facilitate defecations
Loose stools are rarely present without the use of laxatives
Insufficient criteria for irritable bowel syndrome
Clinical Constipation
Large amount of feces (hard or soft) in rectum on digital examination *and/or*
Colonic fecal loading on abdominal radiograph

the study of constipation in a more scientific manner requires specific criteria.

The Rome IV symptom criteria are useful in defining constipation in older people (**Table 87-1**). The Rome criteria overlap with constipation-predominant irritable bowel syndrome (IBS-C). Diagnostic criteria for IBS require recurrent abdominal pain at least one day per week in the last three months, associated with two or more of the following: abdominal pain related to defecation, change in frequency of stool toward infrequent, or change in form of stool toward harder stools. IBS-C subtype includes more than one-fourth of the defecations with Bristol stool types 1 or 2 and less than one-fourth of defecations with Bristol stool types 6 or 7 (**see Figure 87-1**).

PREVALENCE OF CONSTIPATION

Constipation prevalence is between 12% to 19% in North America and the prevalence increases with age. A systematic review reported that approximately 63 million people in North America meet the Rome II criteria for constipation with a disproportionate number being older than 65. **Table 87-2** provides practice guidance screening and identifying risk factors based on evidence from epidemiological studies (prevalence, symptomatology, and risk factors) of constipation in older people.

Self-Reported Constipation

One older community-based study of 3166 persons aged 65 and older asked the question, "Do you have recurrent constipation?" and found a prevalence of 26% in women and 16% in men; in the 84+ years age group, prevalence was 34% and 26%, respectively. Age was a strong independent risk factor for self-reported constipation. Other community studies support this relationship with age and show prevalence rates of up to 34% of women and 30% of men older than age 65.

Bristol Stool Chart

Type 1		Separate hard lumps, like nuts (hard to pass)
Type 2		Sausage-shaped but lumpy
Type 3		Like a sausage but with cracks on the surface
Type 4		Like a sausage or snake, smooth and soft
Type 5		Soft blobs with clear-cut edges
Type 6		Fluffy pieces with ragged edges, a mushy stool
Type 7		Watery, no solid pieces, **entirely liquid**

FIGURE 87-1. Bristol Stool Scale chart. (Reproduced with permission from Lewis SJ, Heaton KW. Stool form scale as a useful guide to intestinal transit time. *Scand J Gastroenterol.* 1997;32[9]:920–924.)

TABLE 87-2 ■ PRACTICE GUIDANCE BASED ON EPIDEMIOLOGICAL EVIDENCE

Screening

Constipation symptoms should be routinely asked about in patients aged 65+ in view of the high prevalence of the condition in this population [2].

Men and women in their eighth decade and beyond should be regularly screened for constipation symptoms, as prevalence increases with advancing age [2].

Periodic objective assessment for constipation in older nursing home residents should be incorporated into routine nursing and medical care [2]. Patients unable to report symptoms owing to cognitive or communication difficulties should be especially targeted [3]. Such an assessment should occur at minimum every 3 mo (the 3-monthly incidence rate of new-onset constipation is 7% in nursing home residents), and optimally monthly [3].

Identifying Risk Factors

The identification of risk factors for constipation in older people is critical to effectively managing the condition [2].

Systematic identification of multiple risk factors in vulnerable older people with constipation should be incorporated into good practice guidelines in all health care settings [3].

Patients at increased risk of constipation from recognized comorbidities (eg, Parkinson disease, diabetes) should be regularly assessed for the condition [2].

Assessment

Identifying specific bowel symptoms in older individuals reporting constipation is important to guide appropriate management of this common complaint [2].

Reduced bowel movement frequency is not a sensitive clinical indicator for constipation in older people [2], though it is specific [3].

Difficulty with evacuation and rectal outlet delay are primary symptoms in older individuals [2].

An objective assessment should be undertaken in frail older people with constipation as these patients are at increased risk of developing complications [2].

Older patients being prescribed laxatives on a daily basis should be regularly reviewed for symptoms of constipation and the appropriateness of long-term laxative therapy [3].

Level [1] indicates good evidence, that is, consistent results from well-designed, well-conducted studies.
Level [2] indicates fair evidence, that is, results show benefit, but strength limited by number, quality, or consistency of studies.
Level [3] indicates poor evidence, that is, insufficient because of limited number, power, or quality of studies.

The preponderance of women over men reporting constipation tends to equalize after the age of 80 years. The incidence rate of new-onset constipation is 7% in nursing home residents with screening every 3 months.

Infrequent Bowel Movements

Two or fewer bowel movements per week are below normal range and tend to signify slow-transit constipation. Weekly frequency of bowel movements is not changed with age, in contrast to self-reporting of constipation. In community-based studies:

- Only 1% to 7% of both younger and older community-dwelling individuals report two or fewer bowel movements a week.
- This consistent bowel pattern across age groups persists even after statistical adjustment for the greater number of laxatives used by older people.
- Among older people complaining of constipation, less than 10% report two or fewer weekly bowel movements, and more than 50% move their bowels daily.

Difficult Evacuation

Symptoms other than infrequent bowel movements drive self-reporting of constipation in older people. These symptoms are predominantly straining and passage of hard stools. Of older people reporting constipation in a US community study, 65% had persistent straining and 39% had passage of hard bowel movements. Difficult rectal evacuation is a primary cause of constipation in older people. Twenty-one percent of community-dwelling people aged 65 and older had rectal outlet delay (according to Rome II criteria), and many describe the need to self-evacuate. Among frailer individuals, difficult evacuation can lead to rectal impaction and fecal soiling.

Constipation in the Acute Care Setting

According to the updated 2019 report from the Bowel Interest Group, 71,430 people in England were admitted to hospital with constipation between 2017 and 2018, which is equivalent to 196 people a day. The cost of treating constipation was £162 million. Also, the prescription cost of laxatives in England during this same period of time was £91 million, without considering over-the-counter laxatives.

Constipation in the Long-Term Care Setting

Long-term care residents are at increased risk of developing complications of constipation (**Table 87-3**) that may precipitate acute hospital admissions. Physical frailty in older persons does increase the prevalence of infrequent bowel movements, with 17% of nursing home residents reporting two or fewer bowel movements a week. Among the total population of long-term care residents self-reporting constipation, 33% have two or fewer bowel movements a week. A Finnish study showed the prevalence of chronic constipation and/or rectal outlet delay to be 57% in women and 64% in men living in residential homes, and 79% and 81% respectively in the nursing home setting. A UK study found that 64% of nursing home residents taking laxatives still reported straining on more than one in four occasions. This and the fact that 50% to 74% of long-term care residents use daily laxatives suggest that rectal evacuation difficulties are not being well managed in this population.

TABLE 87-3 ■ COMPLICATIONS OF CONSTIPATION IN OLDER PEOPLE

Fecal incontinence [1]
Fecal impaction [1]
Stercoral perforation [3]
Urinary retention [2]
Sigmoid volvulus [2]
Acquired megacolon [2]
Rectal prolapse [3]
Diverticular disease [2]
Impaired quality of life [3]
Agitation in patients with dementia [3]

Level [1] indicates good evidence, that is, consistent results from well-designed, well-conducted studies.

Level [2] indicates fair evidence, that is, results show benefit, but strength limited by number, quality, or consistency of studies.

Level [3] indicates poor evidence, that is, insufficient because of limited number, power, or quality of studies.

PATHOPHYSIOLOGY

Physiologic studies suggest that changes in the lower bowel predisposing toward constipation in older people are not primarily age-related. This is compatible with the epidemiology showing that (1) bowel movement frequency does alter with aging, and (2) constipation symptoms are more prevalent in older people with comorbidities. Extrinsic causes such as reduced mobility, reduced fluid intake and dietary fiber, medical comorbidities, and related medications all impact colonic motility and transit and influence the pathophysiology of constipation.

Colonic Function

Colonic motility depends on the integrity of the central and autonomic nervous systems, gut wall innervation and receptors, circular smooth muscle, and gastrointestinal hormones. Propagating motor complexes in the colon are stimulated by increased intraluminal pressure generated by bulky fecal content. Studies of total gut transit time (passage of radiopaque isotope from mouth to anus, normally less than 72 hours), colonic motor activity, and postprandial gastrocolic reflex show no differences between healthy older and younger people. Older people with chronic constipation do, however, tend to have a prolonged total gut transit time, ranging from 4 to 9 days. Radiologic markers pass especially slowly through the left colon with striking delay in the recto-sigmoid, suggesting that total transit time is prolonged due to a decline in propulsive activity in the colon. This may be secondary to a reduction in colonic enteric neurons producing nitric oxide and acetylcholine. The prolongation in transit time is even greater in institutionalized or bedridden patients with constipation, with total gut transit time ranging from 6 to more than 14 days. Slow transit results in a cycle of worsening colonic

dysfunction by reducing water content of stool (normally 75%) and shrinking fecal bulk, which then diminishes the intraluminal pressures, and hence the generation of propagating motor complexes and propulsive activity.

Intrinsic Mechanisms for Colonic Dysfunction in Older People With Constipation

Certain intrinsic mechanisms for altered colonic function in older persons with constipation have been postulated from physiologic studies (**Table 87-4**). The colonic epithelia decrease the secretion of water and electrolytes with aging due to a decrease of numbers of crypts and nongoblet epithelial cells. Overall collagen deposition in the left side of the colon increases with aging, and this could alter colonic compliance and motility. Direct electrophysiologic measurement of colonic motor activity in older subjects has shown that the sigmoid motor response to intraluminal bisacodyl (a direct stimulant of the myenteric plexus) is diminished in patients who are constipated, implying a deficit in intrinsic innervation. Myenteric plexus dysfunction may partially account for impaired gut motility in older persons with constipation. The total number of neurons in the myenteric plexus decreases with increasing age, and this neuronal loss bears no relation to the presence of pseudomelanosis coli cells, implying that use of anthraquinone laxatives is not the primary cause. Interestingly, these aging effects on the colon are not present in caloric restricted mice.

Another possible intrinsic factor is age-related deficit in the density of inhibitory nerves, or in the binding sites on smooth muscle for inhibitory gut neuropeptides. In vitro studies of colons across age groups showed an

TABLE 87-4 ■ PATHOPHYSIOLOGICAL MECHANISMS FOR CONSTIPATION IN OLDER PEOPLE

Chronic Constipation
Intrinsic myenteric plexus dysfunction
Increased collagen deposit in colon (age-related)
Reduced inhibitory nerve input to circular muscle (age-related)
Increased binding of plasma endorphins to gut receptors (age-related)
Prolonged transit owing to extrinsic factors (immobility, diet, drugs, comorbidity)
Rectal Outlet Delay
Rectal dysmotility
Rectal dyschezia secondary to suppression or disregard of urge to pass stool
Sacral cord dysfunction
Pelvic floor descent
Pelvic floor dyssynergia (paradoxical contraction of pelvic floor muscles and external sphincter)
Irritable bowel disease
Weak abdominal musculature

age-related reduction in the amplitude of inhibitory junction potentials, but no decrease in the levels of inhibitory gut neuropeptides. This age-related decline occurs earlier in women as compared with men. Such a decrease in inhibitory nerve input to the circular smooth muscle could result in segmental motor incoordination, which may lengthen transit time and promote constipation in older persons with other predisposing risk factors. Individuals older than age 60 have higher plasma concentrations of beta-endorphin with increased binding to opiate receptors in the gut wall and myenteric plexus. Higher opiate binding has the effect of relaxing colonic tone, reducing motility, and inhibiting the gastrocolic reflex. Constipation is more prevalent in patients with nonulcer dyspepsia, as both conditions involve gastrointestinal hypomotility.

Anorectal Function

In normal defecation, colonic activity propels stool into the rectal ampulla causing distension and intrinsically mediated relaxation of the smooth muscle of the internal anal sphincter (or anal canal). This is followed promptly by reflex contraction of the external anal sphincter and pelvic floor muscles, which are skeletal muscles innervated by the pudendal nerve. The brain registers a desire to defecate, the external sphincter is voluntarily relaxed, and the rectum is evacuated with assistance from abdominal wall muscle contraction.

Age-Related Changes in Anorectal Function

There is a tendency toward an age-related decline in internal sphincter tone, particularly in the eighth decade onward. Clinically, this predisposes older individuals to fecal incontinence, particularly with loose stools. There is a more definite age-related decline (greater in women than men) in external anal sphincter and pelvic muscle strength, which can contribute toward evacuation difficulties. Failure of the anorectal angle to open and excessive perineal descent in older women can lead to constipation. In simulated defecation studies, 37% of non-constipated older subjects were unable to evacuate a small solid sphere. Consequent prolonged straining may compress the pudendal nerve, further exacerbating any preexisting weakness. There appears to be a reduction in rectal motility with normal aging, again in oldest age groups. Rectal sensation does not alter with normal aging.

Anorectal Dysfunction in Older Persons

The most common form of anorectal dysfunction in older people is *rectal dysmotility,* characterized by reduced rectal motility, increased rectal compliance with a variable degree of rectal dilatation, and impaired rectal sensation such that the urge to pass stool is blunted (see **Table 87-4**). Over time, an increasing degree of rectal distension is required to reflexly trigger the defecation mechanism. These patients have rectal retention of hard or soft stool on digital examination of which they may be unaware. The resulting rectal distension leads to relaxation of the internal sphincter and hence to fecal soiling. One study showed that rectal contractions could be elicited in only 14% of older people with a history of rectal impaction. One postulated cause for rectal dysmotility is diminished parasympathetic outflow as a result of impaired sacral cord function, for example, from ischemia or spinal stenosis. Rectal dysmotility can also develop through a persistent disregard or suppression of the urge to defecate that can occur with dementia, depression, immobility, or painful anorectal conditions. Voluntary increase in intra-abdominal pressure during defecation could overcome rectal dysmotility to produce enough of an increase in rectal pressure for evacuation to occur, but older people often have weakened abdominal musculature, limiting their ability to compensate in this way.

Pelvic floor dyssynergia, though more common in younger women, can cause rectal outlet delay in older people (**Figure 87-2**). This is caused by paradoxical contraction or failure to relax the pelvic floor and external anal sphincter muscles during defecation. Manometric studies show paradoxical increases in anal canal pressure on straining. This abnormal expulsion pattern occurs in individuals with severe and long-standing symptoms of rectal outlet delay and in patients with Parkinson disease.

RISK FACTORS FOR CONSTIPATION IN OLDER PEOPLE

Both the epidemiology and pathophysiology of constipation in older people point to the enormous importance of identifying predisposing causes for the condition in each affected individual. One prospective study examined baseline characteristics predictive of new-onset constipation in older nursing home residents, using the US Minimum Data Set. Seven percent (*n* = 1291) developed constipation over a 3-month period. Independent predictors were White race, poor consumption of fluids, pneumonia, Parkinson disease, allergies, decreased bed mobility, arthritis, greater than five medications, dementia, hypothyroidism, and hypertension. The authors postulated that allergies, arthritis, and hypertension were associated primarily because of the constipating effect of drugs used to treat these conditions. Other studies have shown that institutionalization itself is an independent risk factor for symptom-based constipation in older people. **Table 87-5** summarizes evidence-based risk factors of constipation in the older population.

Reduced Mobility

Impaired mobility is a common risk factor for constipation in older people. Greater physical activity (including regular walking) is associated with less self-reported and symptom-specific constipation in older people living both at home and in long-term care. Reduced mobility is the strongest independent correlate of heavy laxative use among nursing

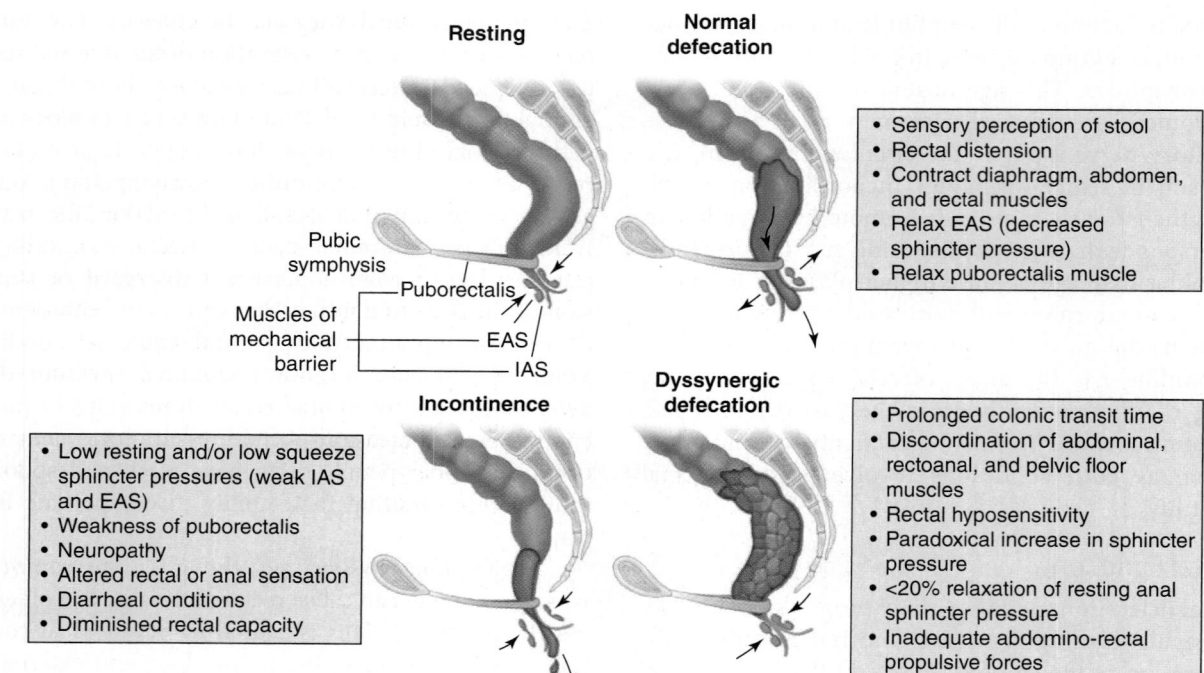

Resting

Normal defecation

Pubic symphysis

Puborectalis

Muscles of mechanical barrier

EAS

IAS

- Sensory perception of stool
- Rectal distension
- Contract diaphragm, abdomen, and rectal muscles
- Relax EAS (decreased sphincter pressure)
- Relax puborectalis muscle

Incontinence

Dyssynergic defecation

- Low resting and/or low squeeze sphincter pressures (weak IAS and EAS)
- Weakness of puborectalis
- Neuropathy
- Altered rectal or anal sensation
- Diarrheal conditions
- Diminished rectal capacity

- Prolonged colonic transit time
- Discoordination of abdominal, rectoanal, and pelvic floor muscles
- Rectal hyposensitivity
- Paradoxical increase in sphincter pressure
- <20% relaxation of resting anal sphincter pressure
- Inadequate abdomino-rectal propulsive forces

FIGURE 87-2. A series of schematic diagrams that reveal the normal anatomy and physiology of the pelvic floor in the sagittal plane at rest, during defecation, and the key pathophysiologic changes in subjects with fecal incontinence and dyssynergic defecation. EAS, external anal sphincter; IAS, internal anal sphincter. (Reproduced with permission from Rao SS. Advances in diagnostic assessment of fecal incontinence and dyssynergic defecation. *Clin Gastroenterol Hepatol.* 2010;8[11]:910–919.)

home residents, following adjustment for age, comorbidity, and other relevant clinical factors. Gut transit time in older subjects was 3 days in ambulant patients and 3 weeks in bedridden patients, although comorbid factors were likely to be contributory. A study of healthy young male volunteers showed that after only 1 week of bed rest, both transit through the sigmoid colon and stool frequency were reduced. It is well documented that exercise increases colonic propulsive activity ("joggers diarrhea"), especially when measured after eating. In a population survey of younger women (36–61 years), daily physical activity was associated with less constipation (defined as two or fewer bowel movements per week), and the association strengthened with increased frequency of physical activity. This suggests that increasing physical activity in adulthood may reduce the likelihood of constipation problems in older age.

Drug Side Effects

Polypharmacy increases the risk of constipation in older patients, particularly in nursing homes where each individual takes an average of six to nine prescribed medications per day. *Anticholinergic medications* reduce contractility of the smooth muscle of the gut via an antimuscarinic effect at acetylcholine receptor sites, and in some cases (eg, patients with schizophrenia taking neuroleptics), long-term use may result in chronic megacolon. In two cross-sectional studies of nursing home residents, anticholinergic antidepressants

were independently associated with daily laxative use following adjustment for age, gender, function, and cognition. Anticholinergic neuroleptics and antihistamines were also independently associated in one of the studies; non-anticholinergic sedatives, however, were not found to be constipating. A study of 532 community-dwelling older US veterans found that among the 27% using anticholinergic drugs, the rate of constipation (42%) was significantly greater than among those not using the drugs.

While older people are very susceptible to the constipating effects of *opiate analgesia*, a study of nursing home residents with persistent nonmalignant pain found that there was no increased rate of constipation in chronic opiate users over a 6-month period compared to those not taking opiates. They also observed a general improvement in functional status and social engagement. Constipation in chronic opiate users can be effectively managed (by diet and laxative or suppository co-prescription where needed)—an important finding as chronic pain is often undertreated in older people perhaps owing to fear of the adverse effects of analgesic drugs. Community-based studies of adults receiving opiates for chronic pain have shown equal constipation risk for all sustained-release oral preparations. Transdermal patches (eg, fentanyl), however, are associated with lower risk of constipation than oral preparations.

All types of *iron supplements* (sulfate, fumarate, and gluconate) cause constipation, the constipating factor being

TABLE 87-5 ■ RISK FACTORS FOR CONSTIPATION IN OLDER PEOPLE

Medications
  Polypharmacy (≥ 5 medications) [2]
  Anticholinergic drugs (tricyclics, antipsychotics, antihistamines, antiemetics, drugs for detrusor hyperactivity) [1]
  Opiates [2]
  Iron supplements [3]
  Calcium channel antagonists (nifedipine and verapamil) [2]
  Calcium supplements [2]
  Nonsteroidal anti-inflammatory drugs [2]

Impaired mobility [2]

Nursing home residency [2]

Neurologic conditions
  Dementia [2]
  Parkinson disease [1]
  Diabetes mellitus [1]
  Autonomic neuropathy [2]
  Stroke [3]
  Spinal cord injury or disease [1]

Depression [3]

Dehydration [2]

Low dietary fiber [3]

Metabolic disturbances
  Hypothyroidism
  Hypercalcemia
  Hypokalemia
  Uremia
  Patients receiving renal dialysis [3]

Mechanical obstruction (eg, tumor, rectocele)

Lack of privacy or comfort

Poor toilet access [3]

Level [1] indicates good evidence, that is, consistent results from well-designed, well-conducted studies.
Level [2] indicates fair evidence, that is, results show benefit, but strength limited by number, quality, or consistency of studies.
Level [3] indicates poor evidence, that is, insufficient because of limited number, power, or quality of studies.

the amount of elemental iron absorbed. Slow-release preparations have a lesser impact on the large bowel, but this is because they tend to carry the iron past the first part of the duodenum into an area of the gut where elemental iron absorption is poorer. Administration of iron sulfate in doses greater than 325 mg per day does not substantially increase iron absorption in older people and may significantly increase gastrointestinal side effects. Intravenous iron does not cause constipation and may be an alternative in patients with chronic anemia (eg, chronic kidney disease) who have symptomatic constipation on oral iron.

In a 5-year study of *calcium supplementation* in older women, the only side effect was constipation (treatment 13% vs placebo 9.1%). The study showed that calcium supplementation reduced bone loss and turnover and fracture rates in older women who took it, but long-term compliance was poor, and constipation may have contributed to this.

Calcium channel antagonists impair lower gut motility, particularly in the rectosigmoid, by inhibiting calcium uptake into smooth muscle cells and altering intraluminal electrolyte and water transportation. Severe constipation has been reported in older patients taking calcium channel antagonists, with nifedipine and verapamil being the most potent inhibitors of gut motility in this class of drugs.

Nonsteroidal anti-inflammatory drugs (NSAIDs) increase the risk of constipation in older people, most likely through prostaglandin inhibition. In a large case-controlled primary care study, constipation and straining were more common reasons for stopping NSAIDs than dyspepsia. NSAIDs have also been implicated in causing stercoral perforation in patients with chronic constipation.

Aluminum antacids have been associated with constipation in older people living in both nursing homes and in the community.

Dietary Factors

Fiber Low consumption of wheat bran, fiber, vegetables, fruit, rice, and calories can all predispose toward constipation. A UK survey showed that consumption of fruit, vegetables, and bread decreases with advancing age. The prevalence of constipation is likely rising in part because modern food processing produces refined food with low roughage. Community studies of older Europeans who eat a Mediterranean diet rich in fruit, vegetables, and olive oil show a low prevalence of constipation (4.4% in people aged 50+). Conversely, a German questionnaire survey of adults with and without constipation reported that chocolate, white bread, and bananas were the foodstuffs most strongly perceived to harden stools.

Calories Low calorie intake in older people (adjusted for fiber intake) is associated with constipation. One study looked at nutritional factors across all nursing homes in Finland and found that malnutrition and constipation were associated. This may be a two-way association in that marked constipation or fecal impaction can cause anorexia, while low calorie intake can promote constipation.

Enteral nutrition Constipation is a recognized problem in patients receiving enteral nutrition. A recent prospective multicenter longitudinal study from Spain followed adult patients (mean age 70 in males, 72 in females) receiving home enteral nutrition for a 4-month period and identified an IR of 1.9 and 1.1 in males and females, respectively. Another common complication seen in this study was diarrhea (IR 1.6 in males, 0.6 in females), although not as frequent as constipation. Diarrhea is usually associated due to the feed volume or its osmolarity.

Fluid Intake

Amount Low fluid intake in older adults has been associated with symptomatic constipation in epidemiologic surveys and to slow colonic transit. In patients with Parkinson disease, low water has been associated with severity of constipation. Withholding fluids over a 1-week period in young male volunteers significantly reduces stool output. Older people are at greater risk of dehydration and resulting constipation because of:

- Impaired thirst sensation
- Less effective hormonal responses to hypertonicity
- Limited access to drinks because of coexisting physical or cognitive impairments
- Voluntary fluid restriction in an attempt to control urinary incontinence

Alcohol and coffee A large Japanese survey of constipation symptoms found that alcohol consumption was a preventive factor in men. A population survey of middle-aged women in the United States showed that daily alcohol consumption (exceeding 12 g/d) and low-moderate caffeine intake were independently inversely related to infrequent bowel movements. Black coffee has been shown to increase colonic motility specifically in the rectosigmoid within 4 minutes of ingestion in young healthy volunteers (a reaction not observed with ingestion of hot water), implying that caffeine triggers the gastrocolic reflex.

Parkinson Disease

Patients with Parkinson disease suffer from three primary pathologies that lead to constipation:

- Primary degeneration of dopaminergic neurons in the myenteric plexus resulting in prolonged colorectal transit
- Pelvic dyssynergia causing rectal outlet delay and prolonged straining
- Small increases in intra-abdominal pressures on straining (compared with age-matched controls)

Constipation can become prominent early in the course of the disease, even 10 to 20 years prior to motor symptoms. In a 24-year longitudinal study in Honolulu, less than one bowel movement a day was associated with a threefold risk of future Parkinson disease in men. A study of patients at a Parkinson disease clinic found that 59% were constipated according to the Rome criteria (vs 21% in age-matched control group without neurologic disease), and 33% were very concerned by their bowel problem. Antiparkinsonian drugs can further exacerbate constipation. Pelvic dyssynergia affects 60% of people with Parkinson disease and may be hard to treat. Botulinum toxin injected into the puborectalis muscle has been used to improve rectal emptying in Parkinson disease patients with good effect, though repeat injections every 3 months are required to maintain clinical benefit.

Dementia

Dementia predisposes individuals to rectal dysmotility, partly through ignoring the urge to defecate. A study in which young men deliberately suppressed defecation resulted in prolonged transit through the rectosigmoid with a marked reduction in frequency of bowel movements. Epidemiological studies show a significant association between cognitive impairment and nurse-documented constipation in nursing home residents. Patients with non-Alzheimer dementias (Parkinson disease, Lewy body, vascular dementia) compared to those with Alzheimer dementia are more likely to suffer from autonomic symptoms, including constipation.

Mood-Related Disorders

Depression, psychological distress, and anxiety are all associated with increased self-reporting of constipation in older persons. In certain cases, the symptom of constipation is a somatic manifestation of psychiatric illness. A careful assessment is required to differentiate subjective complaints from clinical constipation in depressed or anxious patients.

Stroke

Constipation affects 60% of those recovering from stroke while undergoing rehabilitation, and a high number of these have combined rectal outlet delay and slow-transit constipation. For stroke survivors living in the community, difficulties accessing the toilet due to residual functional impairment can worsen problems with bowel evacuation. Weakness of abdominal and pelvic muscles following stroke also contributes to problems with evacuation.

Spinal Cord Injury/Disease

Constipation affects the majority of people with spinal cord disease or injury. Age and duration of injury interact to promote complications of chronic constipation such as acquired megacolon, which affects more than half of patients with spinal cord injury. Lumbar stenosis in older people caused by degenerative joint disease may lead to cauda equina problems with severe rectal outlet delay. One study in younger people showed that an average of 27 of rectosigmoid emptying was achieved with each defecation in patients with cauda equina syndromes, versus 81% in healthy controls.

Diabetes Mellitus

A Turkish study of outpatients with type 2 diabetes showed that 56% complained of constipation (vs 30% of controls). Neuropathy symptom scores are correlated with laxative usage and straining. Diabetic patients with autonomic neuropathy are more likely to be constipated because of markedly slowed transit throughout the colon and impairment of the gastrocolic reflex. However, one-third of diabetic patients with constipation do not have neuropathic symptoms, so additional potentially reversible factors should be considered particularly in older people (eg, drugs, mobility, fluids). For example, a US community study found that constipation and/or laxative use was increased in type 1 versus type 2 diabetic men, but this difference was associated with use of calcium channel blockers rather than with neuropathy symptoms. Acute hyperglycemia inhibits the gastrocolic reflex and colonic peristalsis, so glycemic control may be an important factor in the genesis of constipation. Colonic transit time in immobile older people with diabetes is extremely prolonged at 200 ± 144 hours. An Israeli study showed that this very long transit time in long-term care residents with diabetes can be significantly reduced by administering acarbose, an alpha-glucosidase inhibitor with a potential adverse effect of causing diarrhea. Overall, gut dysmotility can lead to bacterial overgrowth and the clinical problem of explosive diarrhea; treatment with erythromycin and long-term motility agents such as metoclopramide should be considered in these individuals. The risk of developing tardive dyskinesia, a known adverse reaction from metoclopramide, is increased in the older individual. In order to decrease the risk, older adults should be advised to avoid continuous treatment for longer than 12 weeks. A drug holidays of 2 weeks or a decrease of metoclopramide dose as tolerated, with tight blood glucose control, is encouraged whenever clinically possible.

Metabolic Disorders

Hypokalemia produces neuronal dysfunction that minimizes acetylcholine stimulation of gut smooth muscle and so prolongs transit through the gut. Hypokalemia should be excluded in cases of colonic pseudo-obstruction and sigmoid volvulus. *Hypercalcemia* causes conduction delay within the extrinsic and intrinsic innervation of the gut. Surgical treatment of hyperparathyroidism reverses the neuromuscular bowel dysfunction seen with this condition. Patients with *myxedema* have been observed to have edema of the gut wall with mucopolysaccharide deposition, although whether this contributes to the colonic hypomotility seen commonly in *clinical hypothyroidism* is uncertain. Patients on *long-term renal dialysis* have prolonged age-adjusted transit time, more so in hemodialysis than peritoneal dialysis. In a questionnaire study in Japan, 63% of hemodialysis patients complained of constipation. Important contributors to this problem were high (49%), including use of resin to avoid hyperkalemia, suppression of the defecation urge while undergoing dialysis, and low fiber intake. Resin administration also places older inpatients at risk of fecal impaction.

Colorectal Cancer

Colorectal cancer has been associated with both constipation and use of laxatives, although this risk association is likely to be confounded by the influence of underlying habits. One study, adjusted for age and potential confounders, found that having fewer than three reported bowel movements a week was associated with a greater than twofold risk of colon cancer, with the association being most strong in Black women. As the prevalence of colorectal cancer increases with age, index of suspicion should be higher in older adults. Constipation alone, however, is not an indication for proceeding to colonoscopy (see below).

Rectocele

Posterior vaginal wall prolapse and rectocele are common in older multiparous women. These individuals have an increased risk of rectal outlet delay, particularly incomplete emptying and need for digital evacuation. This is presumably caused by mechanical obstruction, as this association is not seen in women with anterior pelvic prolapse.

COMPLICATIONS OF CONSTIPATION IN OLDER PEOPLE

Fecal Incontinence

Constipation is a common, treatable, preventable, and often overlooked cause of fecal incontinence in older people (see **Table 87-4**). Few medical symptoms are as distressing and social isolating for older people as fecal incontinence, a condition that places them at greater risk of morbidity, mortality, dependency, and nursing home placement. All too often, untreated overflow leads to hospitalization of vulnerable older patients. Many older individuals in the community with fecal incontinence will not volunteer the problem to their physician and, regrettably, physicians and nurses do not routinely inquire about the symptom. This "hidden problem" therefore leads to social isolation and a downward spiral of psychological distress, dependency, and poor health. Even when health care professionals identify older people with fecal incontinence, it is often poorly assessed and passively managed, especially in the long-term care setting where it is most prevalent.

In one study, overflow (continuous fecal soiling and fecal impaction on rectal examination) was the underlying problem in 52% of frail nursing home residents with long-standing fecal incontinence. A therapeutic intervention consisting of enemas until no further response followed by lactulose achieved complete resolution of incontinence in 94% with full treatment adherence. Notably, this study showed that only 4% of nursing home residents with long-standing fecal incontinence had been referred for further assessment, reflecting a tendency toward unnecessarily conservative nursing management (eg, use of pads and undergarments only). Another nursing home study found that daily lactulose and suppositories plus weekly enemas only effectively resolved overflow incontinence when complete rectal emptying was consistently achieved over a period of 2 months. An effective therapeutic program for overflow incontinence depends on the following:

- Regular toileting (ideally every 2 hours, which also promotes mobility)
- Monitoring of treatment effect by rectal examination and bowel chart
- Responsive stepwise drug and dosage changes
- Prolonged treatment (at least 2 weeks)
- Subsequent maintenance regimen to prevent recurrences

Fecal impaction is an important cause of comorbidity in older patients, increasing the risk of hospitalization and of potentially fatal complications. A survey of patients admitted to acute geriatric units in the United Kingdom over 1 year reported that fecal impaction was a primary reason for hospitalization in 27%. In frail patients, fecal impaction may present as a nonspecific clinical deterioration; specific symptoms may include anorexia, vomiting, and abdominal pain. Findings on physical examination may include fever, delirium, abdominal distension, reduced bowel sounds, arrhythmias, and tachypnea secondary to splinting of the diaphragm. The mechanism for the fever and leukocytosis response is thought to be microscopic stercoral ulcerations of the colon. A plain abdominal radiograph will show colonic or rectal fecal retention associated with lower bowel dilatation. Presence of fluid levels in the large or small bowel suggests advanced obstruction; the closer the fecal impaction is to the ileocecal valve, the greater the number of fluid levels seen in the small bowel. People with fecal impaction may also be predisposed to vasovagal reactions when the bowel is evacuated, which can cause complications such as syncope, vomiting, and aspiration.

Urinary Retention/Lower Urinary Tract Symptoms

Rectosigmoid fecal loading may impinge on the bladder neck causing some degree of urinary retention. Two Finnish studies of older women and men showed an independent association between constipation and lower urinary tract symptoms (LUTS) in both genders. A case-control study in hospitalized women aged 65 and older found that after adjustment for relevant confounders, constipation was the primary predictor of urinary retention, increasing the risk of retention fourfold as measured by portable ultrasound postvoid residual (PVR) > 100 mL (other predictors were urinary tract infection and previous urinary retention). Urinary symptoms of difficult voiding were unreliable in diagnosing retention in this study, suggesting that it is good practice to do screening PVRs in hospitalized older women with constipation, particularly in the context of coexisting urinary tract infection. A prospective cohort study examined the impact of treating chronic constipation on coexisting urinary symptoms in older people (mean age 72). After 4 months, there was a significant improvement in constipation, as well as urgency, frequency, and voiding difficulty, mean PVR (reduced from 85–30 mL), and fewer urinary tract infections. There are also case reports in frail older people of bilateral hydronephrosis associated with renal failure that resolved following fecal disimpaction. Other urinary symptoms, including those of overactive bladder may be caused by stimulation of pelvic nerves by the distended rectum. Thus, bowel management is a key aspect of managing urinary incontinence in older people.

Stercoral Perforation

Fecal impaction increases the risk of stercoral perforation of the wall of the colon (usually sigmoid) secondary to ischemic necrosis. Stercoral perforation can also occur in chronically constipated persons where pressure from a hard fecaloma produces an ulcer with characteristically necrotic and inflammatory edges; these individuals tend to present with sudden onset of acute abdominal pain. Prompt surgical intervention and rigorous treatment of peritonitis are needed to prevent the high mortality rate associated with this condition. A case-control study found that the most prevalent risk factor for colon ischemia in 700 cases was the use of drugs that cause constipation (one in three cases compared to only one in nine controls).

Sigmoid Volvulus

Chronic constipation in frail older people is the leading cause of sigmoid volvulus in the developed world. Volvulus is:

- The third most common cause of large bowel obstruction in the United States
- More likely in constipated patients with Parkinson disease and neuropathic colon (eg, from spinal cord disease or long-term neuroleptic treatment)
- Associated with hypokalemia
- Treated initially by sigmoidoscopic deflation but with a high recurrence rate
- Managed surgically, usually by partial colectomy, when sigmoidoscopic deflation fails

Colonic Pseudo-Obstruction

Acute colonic pseudo-obstruction (Ogilvie syndrome) is most likely to occur in hospitalized frail older people with a history of chronic constipation who are acutely medically ill, or in postoperative phase. It presents with abdominal distension and colonic dilatation on x-ray, with a cecal diameter of 10 cm or more. Nothing by mouth, flatus tube, and correction of electrolyte imbalances (particularly potassium and magnesium) are initial treatments, progressing to neostigmine (if no cardiac contraindications), and then endoscopic decompression if dilatation persists. Administration of polyethylene glycol after initial resolution of colonic dilatation has been shown to reduce the likelihood of recurrence requiring escalation of therapy.

Rectal Prolapse

Prolonged straining at stool in constipated patients can result in rectal prolapse of varying degrees, and older people are more at risk from developing fecal soiling as a result. Surgery should be considered for full-thickness prolapses, and laparoscopic versus transabdominal repair is now an effective treatment (including improving bowel-related symptoms) with a low recurrence rate.

Diverticular Disease

Left-sided diverticulosis coli affects 30% to 60% of people older than 60 in developed countries. The etiology has been attributed to high intraluminal pressures while straining at stool in people who have a low fiber diet. A case-control study of patients mean age 68 with acute uncomplicated diverticulitis showed 74% to have prolonged transit (longest in those with constipation symptoms), and 59% had small intestinal bacterial overgrowth. Newer approaches to preventing recurrence of symptomatic flare-ups of diverticular disease are use of mesalazine and *Lactobacillus casei*, separately or in combination.

Impact on Quality of Life

Functional bowel symptoms in older people can impair quality of life, even following adjustment for other chronic illnesses. Patients with constipation generally have an impaired quality of life compared with the general population, though few studies have looked at this specifically in older people. A Hong Kong study of community-living people aged 70 and older showed an independent association between constipation and low morale as measured by the Philadelphia Geriatric Morale Scale. A Canadian study of the general population found an association between constipation and a low SF-36 score, with the rate of physician visits for constipation being strongly associated with the physical component of the SF-36. The Patient Assessment of Constipation Quality of Life questionnaire is a validated tool for assessing quality of life over time in older adults in long-term care; scores correlate with abdominal pain and constipation severity. Patients whose constipation is associated with abdominal pain or other irritable bowel symptoms score even lower on quality of life measures, plus have poor general health perception. Constipation in long-term care residents unable to communicate because of dementia has been linked to physically aggressive behavior. A US study of almost 9000 nursing home residents examined characteristics associated with the development of wandering behavior over a 1-year period and found that constipation increased the risk almost twofold. The authors postulated that residents with dementia may wander to alleviate constipation-related discomfort, and nursing home health professionals should be alert to this.

CLINICAL EVALUATION

General Assessment

Older patients with constipation should have an assessment focusing on predisposing causes. In addition to bowel symptoms, the history should include over-the-counter medications, diet, and fluid intake. Physical examination should include cognition, mood, and function in addition to abdominal and rectal examinations. Laboratory tests when indicated include complete blood count; plasma electrolytes; calcium; glucose; and liver and thyroid function tests.

Figure 87-3 illustrates a recommended approach to the patient with chronic constipation.

History

Table 87-6 lists the important aspects of the bowel history in older people who complain of constipation. It is essential to identify rectal evacuation difficulties in order to manage the patient effectively. Although constipation may be underestimated in older patients with dementia and depression, studies have shown that adults complaining of constipation frequently underestimate the number of bowel movements. Thus it may be helpful to have them keep a stool chart for a week to document frequency and characteristics of their bowel movements and associated symptoms. The Bristol Stool Form Scale, a validated tool to assess for stool consistency, may be used when the duration of constipation is not clear during history taking (see **Figure 87-1**). Bristol stool type 1 and 2 indicate hard or lumpy stool consistency respectively and may be a more reliable indicator of colonic transit than stool frequency. Patients may also complain of straining, use of manual maneuvers, and incontinence.

A recent history of altered bowel habit should prompt an exploration of precipitants (eg, new medications, changes in diet), and where unexplained, an evaluation for colorectal cancer. Family history of colorectal cancer should be obtained. Abdominal pain, rectal bleeding, and certainly any systemic features such as weight loss and anemia should prompt further investigations for underlying neoplasm.

Perianal fecal soiling is a common and embarrassing symptom that patients are reluctant to volunteer. In one large nursing home study, 38% of older individuals who complained of constipation reported fecal soiling of undergarments. Overflow fecal incontinence typically presents as frequent passive leakage of watery stool, sometimes confusing patients and caregivers who think they have "diarrhea" rather than constipation. Fecal impaction must be ruled out in the presence of fecal soiling or incontinence. The other important diagnoses to consider in older people are loose stools caused by inappropriate laxative use, other drug side effects, or undiagnosed bowel disease.

IBS should be a diagnosis of exclusion in older people and only made in those with a many-year history of intermittent symptoms such as abdominal distension or pain relieved by defecation, passage of mucus, and feeling of incomplete emptying (Rome criteria). Rectal pain associated with defecation should alert the physician to rectal ischemia as well as to other more common anorectal conditions. Rectal bleeding should prompt further evaluation for an underlying tumor, unless examination clearly reveals bright red blood from anal fissure or hemorrhoids. Lower urinary tract symptoms may be exacerbated by constipation and should be documented.

A person's attitude toward their bowel problem (positive, acceptance, denial, distress, apathy) and the impact on their quality of life should be included when

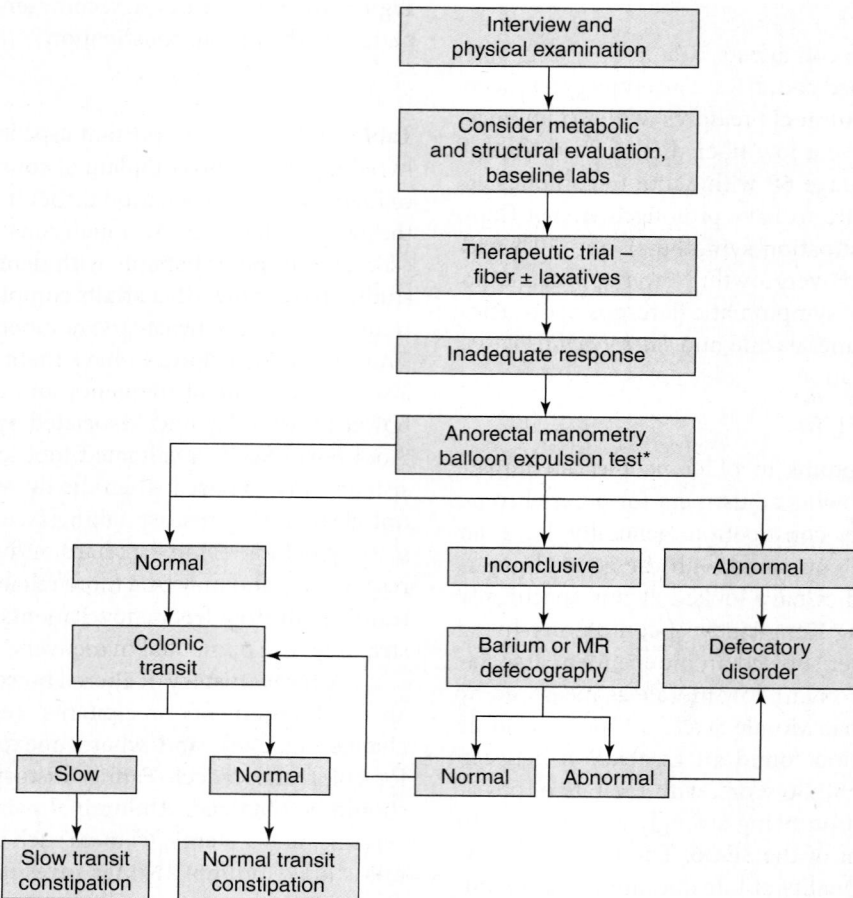

Figure 87-3. A practical approach to assessment of constipation in older people. *Because anorectal manometry and rectal balloon expulsion test may not be available in all practice settings, it is acceptable in such circumstances to proceed to assessing colonic transit with the understanding that delayed colonic transit does not exclude a defecatory disorder. (Reproduced with permission from American Gastroenterological Association, Bharucha AE, Dorn SD, et al. American Gastroenterological Association medical position statement on constipation. *Gastroenterology*. 2013;144[1]:211–217.)

taking a history. Some health care providers share the generally held belief that constipation is an inevitable consequence of aging, and patients may feel that their problem is not taken seriously. A thorough clinical history and assessment is an important first step in developing a sound patient–physician partnership, which enhances successful outcomes in managing what is usually a chronic condition.

Digital Rectal Examination

Digital rectal examination is required in all patients who report constipation to reveal rectal impaction, rectal dilatation, hemorrhoids, anorectal disease, and perianal fecal soiling. Retained stool in rectal impaction does not have to be hard; loading with soft stool is common in older people taking laxatives who have problems with rectal outlet delay. Absence of stool on rectal examination does not exclude the diagnosis of constipation. A dilated rectum with diminished sensation and retained stool suggests rectal dysmotility. External sphincter tone is assessed by asking the patient to "squeeze and pull up" around the examining finger. Indicators of reduced internal anal tone are easy insertion of the finger into the anal canal and gaping of the anus on applying gentle traction to the anal margin. Anal sphincter weakness should prompt (1) careful prescribing to avoid causing fecal leakage though excessive laxative-induced softness of stool, and (2) instruction in exercises to strengthen the anal sphincter (**Table 87-7**). Absent cutaneous-anal reflex (gentle scratching of the anal margin should normally induce a visible contraction of the external sphincter) and, in particular, perianal anesthesia point to significant sacral cord dysfunction with associated rectal dysmotility. Proctoscopy is a simple, quick, and useful test for diagnosing internal hemorrhoids and abnormalities of the rectal wall.

Pelvic Floor and Rectal Prolapse

Excessive perineal descent can be observed by asking the patient to "bear down" while lying in the lateral position.

TABLE 87-6 ■ DIAGNOSIS OF CONSTIPATION IN OLDER PEOPLE

Bowel History
Number of bowel movements per week
Stool consistency
Straining/symptoms of rectal outlet delay
Duration of constipation
Fecal incontinence/soiling
Irritable bowel syndrome symptoms (abdominal pain, bloating, passage of mucus)
Rectal pain or bleeding
Laxative use, prior and current
Psychological and quality of life impact of bowel problem
Urinary incontinence/lower urinary tract symptoms

General History
Mood/cognition
Symptoms of systemic illness (weight loss, anemia)
Relevant comorbidities (eg, diabetes, neurologic disease)
Mobility
Diet
Medications
Toilet access (location of bathroom, manual dexterity, vision)

Specific Physical Examination
Digital rectal examination including external and internal sphincter tone
Perianal sensation/cutaneous anal reflex
Rectal prolapse/hemorrhoids
Pelvic floor descent/rectocele
Abdominal palpation, auscultation
Neurologic, cognitive, and functional examination

Tests
Indications for plain abdominal radiograph
   Empty rectum with clinical suspicion of constipation
   Evaluation for fecal impaction
   Persistent fecal incontinence despite clearing of any rectal impaction
   Evaluation of abdominal distension, pain, or acute discomfort
   Persisting complaints of constipation with increasing laxative usage
Indications for colonoscopy
   Systemic illness (weight loss, anemia, etc.)
   Bleeding per rectum
   Recent change in bowel habit without obvious risk factors
Indications for anorectal function tests
   Severe or persistent symptoms of rectal outlet delay
   Persistent fecal incontinence with clinical evidence of anal sphincter weakness

Normal perineal descent is less than 4 cm (can be eyeballed by drawing an imaginary line between that ischeal prominences). Rectal prolapse may also be observed in this manner, though lesser degrees of prolapse may only be identified by having the patient strain while sitting on a toilet or commode. An examination for posterior vaginal prolapse (bearing down in the gynecological position) is appropriate in all women with constipation, especially those reporting incomplete rectal emptying and the need to manually evacuate their rectum.

Plain Abdominal X-Ray

Clinical diagnosis can often be made by a thorough history and examination. However, a plain abdominal radiograph is useful in patients without rectal impaction in whom colonic loading is suspected because of a high-risk profile, constipation-related symptoms, or fecal incontinence. In those patients who continue to report troublesome constipation-related symptoms despite regular laxative use, it can guide management by showing the following:

- No stool—patient may require education about what constitutes a normal bowel habit and no increase and possibly a reduction in laxative usage.
- Colonic fecal loading—patient requires education on lifestyle measures and a change in type or increased dose of laxative.
- Rectal loading with a clear colon—patient requires suppositories or enemas, and no increase and possibly a reduction in laxatives.

Rectal air with marked fecal loading in the descending colon may correlate with normal-transit constipation or an evacuation disorder (**Figure 87-4A**). Marked fecal loading in the ascending and transverse colon correlates well with prolonged transit time, or slow-transit constipation, as does the presence of feces rather than air in the cecum (**Figure 87-4B**). Dilatation of the colon (> 6.5 cm maximum diameter) in the absence of acute obstruction points toward megacolon (**Figure 87-4C**). Rectal dilatation (> 4 cm) implies dysmotility and evacuation problems. Finally, in patients with abdominal distension and/or pain, an abdominal radiograph is necessary to rule out acute problems such as sigmoid volvulus and small bowel obstruction secondary to severe impaction.

Anorectal Function Tests

Anorectal function tests should be considered in assessment of constipation in older people if a rectal evacuation disorder is suspected (see **Figure 87-2**). Anorectal manometry and balloon expulsion should be considered as initial assessment in patients who have not responded to fiber. They may be indicated in patients with severe and persistent rectal outlet delay, in order to diagnose pelvic dyssynergia, which is more effectively treated by biofeedback than laxatives. Another indication is fecal incontinence of formed stool that persists despite clearing of fecal impaction. Balloon expulsion is a simple procedure that evaluated the ability to defecate a water-filled balloon. During the balloon expulsion, the time required to expel the balloon

TABLE 87-7 ■ PATIENT EDUCATION[a]

Toilet Habits and Positioning

Do not delay having a bowel movement when you feel the urge.

Put aside a particular time each day (we would advise after breakfast) when you can sit on the toilet without being in a hurry.

A relaxed attitude to bowel evacuation will especially help if you have problems with straining or a feeling of anal blockage.

If straining is a problem, it is helpful to have a footstool under your feet while sitting on the toilet as this increases the ability of your abdominal muscles to help evacuation of stool.

Abdominal Massage

Lie on the bed with pillows under your head and shoulders.

Your knees should be bent up with a pillow underneath them for support.

Cover your abdomen with a light sheet.

Massage your abdomen with firm but gentle circular movements starting at the right side and working across to the left side.

Continue the massage for approximately 10 min.

This massage should be a pleasant experience—if you feel any discomfort then stop.

Diet

To help prevent constipation you should eat more of the foods from List A and less of the foods from List B. Foods in List A tend to make the stool softer and easier to pass, because they are high in fiber. Foods in List B tend to make the stool harder, because they bind together the contents of the bowel.

List A: Fresh fruit, prunes and other dried fruit, whole meal bread, bran cereals and porridge, salad, cooked vegetables (with skin where possible), beans, lentils.

List B: Milk, hard cheese, yogurt, white bread or crackers, refined cereals, cakes, pancakes, noodles, white rice, chocolate, creamed soups.

You should increase your fiber intake gradually because sudden change in fiber content may cause temporary bloating and irregularity. It is important to eat the foods that contain fiber all through the day and not just at one meal such as breakfast.

Increase the amount of fluid that you drink gradually up to 8–10 glasses a day. Try to drink more water, fruit juices, and fizzy drinks.

Sphincter Strengthening

Learning to do your exercises

Sit in a comfortable position with your knees slightly apart. Now imagine that you are trying to stop yourself passing wind from the bowel. To do this you must squeeze the muscle around the back passage. Try squeezing and lifting that muscle as tightly as you can. You should be able to feel the muscle move. Your buttocks, abdomen, and legs should not move at all. You should be aware of the skin around the back passage tightening and being pulled up and away from your chair. Really try to feel this. You are now exercising your anal sphincter muscles. (You do not need to hold your breath when you tighten the muscles!)

Practicing your exercises

Tighten and pull up the anal sphincter muscles as tightly as you can. Hold tightened for at least 5 seconds, then relax for at least 10 sec.

Repeat this exercise at least 5 times. This will work on the strength of your muscles.

Next, pull the muscles to approximately half of their maximum squeeze. See how long you can hold this for. Then relax for at least 10 sec.

Repeat at least 5 times. This will work on the endurance or staying power of your muscles.

Pull up the muscles as quickly and tightly as you can and then relax and then pull up again, and see how many times you can do this before you get tired. Try for at least 5 quick pull-ups. Try this quick pull-up exercise at least 10 times each day.

Do all these exercises as hard as you can and at least 5 times a day. As the muscles get stronger, you will find that you can do more pull-ups each time without the muscle getting tired.

It takes time for exercises to make muscle stronger. You may need to exercise regularly for several months before the muscles gain their full strength.

Instructions for Using Suppositories

These may be inserted into your rectum (back passage) by your nurse or caregiver or yourself if you are physically able to do it.

If necessary go to the toilet and empty your bowels if you can.

Wash your hands.

Remove any foil or wrapping from the suppository.

(Continued)

TABLE 87-7 ■ PATIENT EDUCATION^a (*CONTINUED*)

Either lie on your side with your lower leg straight and your upper leg bent toward your waist or squat.

Gently but firmly insert the suppository, narrow end first, into the rectum using a finger. Push far enough (approximately 1 inch) so that it does not come out again.

You may find your body wanting to push out the suppository. Close your legs and keep still for a few minutes.

Try not to empty your bowels for at least 10–20 min.

^aSee Constipation (Aftercare Instructions)—What You Need to Know. https://www.drugs.com/cg/constipation-aftercare-instructions.html.

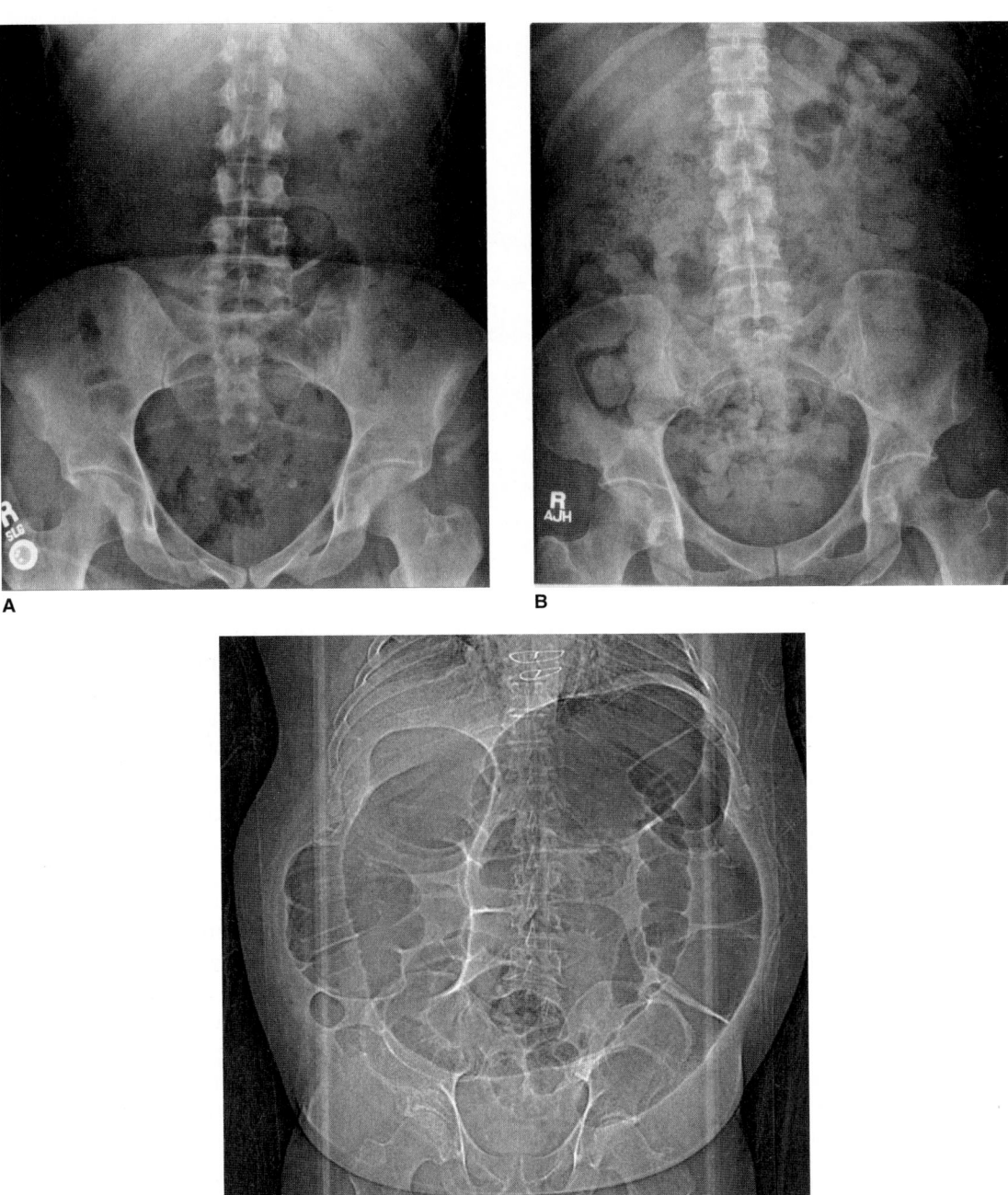

FIGURE 87-4. Plain radiographs of patients with constipation. **(A)** Colonic or rectal fecal retention associated with air in rectum and cecum. **(B)** Large amount of fecal material in the entire colon with no evidence of bowel obstruction or no free intraperitoneal air. **(C)** Megacolon: Dilatation of the colon (> 6.5 cm maximum diameter) in the absence of acute obstruction.

should be recorded, with normal range between 1 to 5 minutes. Alternatively, if spontaneous evacuation is not possible, the other outcome is to measure the additional weight added to assist in expelling the balloon. Anorectal tests (including endoanal ultrasound) can measure the integrity of the anal sphincters and thus guide management of incontinence toward conservative treatment (sphincter strengthening exercises and biofeedback therapy) or surgical intervention (sphincter reconstruction).

Defecography

There are several modalities to assess the defecatory movements and anatomy. Traditionally, barium and scintigraphy defecographies have been used and more recently, magnetic resonance defecography were developed to identify anatomic abnormalities with higher resolution, visualization, and without radiation. Defecography should be used when the anorectal manometry and balloon expulsion are inconclusive or when there is a high suspicion for an anatomic disorder. The most relevant findings in defecography are inadequate or excessive perineal descent during defecation, excessive straining, internal intussusception, solitary rectal ulcers, rectoceles, and rectal prolapse. Unfortunately, these tests are not widely available.

Colonic Transit

Colonic transit is the rate at which fecal residue moves through the colon. There are several approved methods to measure colonic transit. The most common and inexpensive measurement is using radiopaque markers (sitzmarks), which consist of the Hinton Technique. A capsule containing 24 radiopaque markers is swallowed and in 5 days, five or less markers should remain in the colon on an abdominal radiograph. Radionucleotide gamma scintigraphy or wireless pH-pressure capsule are other well-validated methods but less commonly used. The benefit of scintigraphy is that results can be obtained in 48 hours when compared to radiopaque markers. Colonic transit studies are useful to differentiate patients with slow-transit constipation versus normal-transit constipation (**Figure 87-5**).

Colonoscopy

Chronic constipation alone is not an appropriate indication for colonoscopy; the range of neoplasia found is similar to that in asymptomatic patients undergoing primary colorectal cancer screening. A meta-analysis showed that the presence of constipation as the primary indication for colonoscopy was associated with a significantly lower prevalence of colorectal cancer. Further investigation is warranted in the context of systemic illness or laboratory abnormalities. Barium enema is no longer used as the first line of testing. Colonoscopy causes significantly less discomfort than does a barium

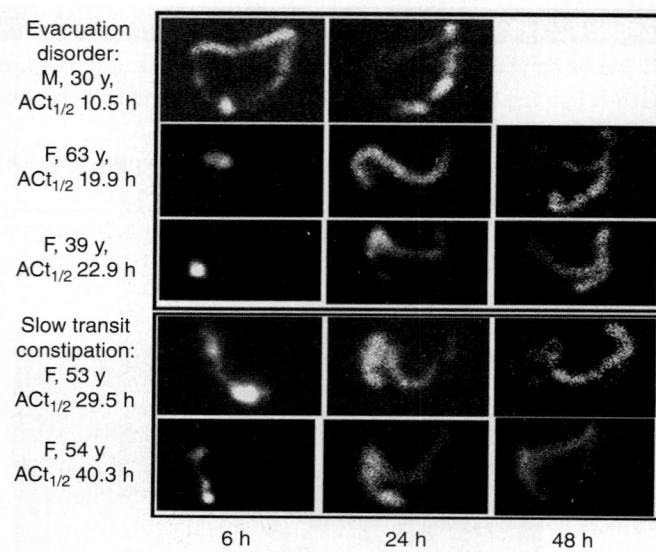

Evacuation disorder:
M, 30 y, $ACt_{1/2}$ 10.5 h

F, 63 y, $ACt_{1/2}$ 19.9 h

F, 39 y, $ACt_{1/2}$ 22.9 h

Slow transit constipation:
F, 53 y, $ACt_{1/2}$ 29.5 h

F, 54 y, $ACt_{1/2}$ 40.3 h

6 h   24 h   48 h

FIGURE 87-5. Examples of scintiscans at 6, 24, and 48 hours in patients with evacuation disorder and slow-transit constipation (STC); note the delayed transit is also demonstrated at 48 hours in the patients with STC and the retention of isotope in the left colon in patients with evacuation disorder. (Reproduced with permission from Nullens S, Nelsen T, Camilleri M, et al. Regional colon transit in patients with dys-synergic defaecation or slow transit in patients with constipation. *Gut.* 2012;61[8]:1132–1139.)

enema and is diagnostically more sensitive. A review of 400 colonoscopies in octogenarians and upwards showed a good safety profile but low cancer detection rate for symptoms (eg, constipation, abdominal pain) other than bleeding (2% vs 12%). Inadequate colonoscopies are common in older people because of poor bowel preparation. Older age, constipation, reported laxative use, tricyclic antidepressants, stroke, and dementia have been associated with inadequate preparation and thus taking longer to instrument the cecum. Clear instruction (such as booklets, visual aids, cell phone apps), split preparations instructions added by pharmacy to the product, pre-procedure phones calls, and availability of at least two alternative bowel preparation options are methods used to reduce poor bowel preparation and improve compliance in the older adults. There are no specific bowel preparation regimens for older patients recommended by the current guidelines. The most common ones in the general population include polyethylene glycol electrolyte lavage solution or sodium phosphate type laxatives. Magnesium citrate should be used cautiously in the older adults given age-related electrolyte derangement (increased levels of sodium, potassium, and magnesium). Older patients with cardiovascular disease may have increased risk of ischemic colitis when taking bisacodyl. Lastly, older patients with reduced renal function should avoid sodium phosphate as it has been associated with tubular toxicity from calcium phosphate.

NONPHARMACOLOGIC MANAGEMENT

Nonpharmacologic treatments for constipation are underused as first-line management in constipation that is not acute or severe, and as adjunctive treatment even when laxatives are deemed necessary. Symptoms of difficult evacuation may be particularly amenable to nonpharmacologic management such as stool softening and bulking through increasing fiber and fluid intake, pelvic muscle strengthening exercises, and footstool elevation of the legs during evacuation (see below). A systematic review examining nonpharmacologic treatment of chronic constipation in older people found no studies evaluating the effect of exercise therapy and only a few nonrandomized trials examining fiber and fluid supplementation, and there has been little further research in this area since then. However, a study of older patients from two nursing homes in Ismailia, Egypt, reported that lifestyle modification (fluid intake included, with 87% taking > 1.5 L compared to 39% pre-intervention) improved symptoms and quality of life. Available data, expert opinion, and practical recommendations are summarized below.

Education

Educating patients as to what constitutes normal bowel habit should be one of the first steps in managing self-reported constipation. Patients with no or mild symptoms of constipation should be encouraged to discontinue chronic laxative therapy. Patients who require laxative treatment for constipation should be told to aim for regular, comfortable evacuation rather than daily evacuation, which is often their preconceived norm. Educational interventions promoting lifestyle changes for patients with chronic constipation should focus on exercise and diet. In order to persuade older people with constipation to change their lifestyle, they need to be convinced that:

- Their current behaviors are "bad for their bowels."
- Bowel-related and general health improvements associated with recommended measures are worth the trouble and expense of changing.
- It is they who are responsible for what they eat and how much exercise they engage in.
- They have the skills and knowledge to modify their own lifestyle to improve their constipation, if they choose to do so.

It is important to provide people with clearly written educational materials. A randomized controlled trial in stroke survivors with constipation evaluated the impact of a one-off nurse-led assessment (with feedback to primary care physician) and an educational session including provision of a booklet (Bowels and bladder | Heart and Stroke Foundation from https://www.heartandstroke.ca/stroke/recovery-and-support/physical-changes/bowels-and-bladder). At 6 months after intervention, subjects reported improved bowel function in terms of number and normality of bowel movements; at 1 year, they were more likely to be altering their diet and fluid intake to control their bowel problem. **Table 87-7** illustrates some of the patient-centered instructions from this study booklet, which are relevant to all older people with constipation.

Other trials have sought to influence fiber intake at a population level. Nutrition newsletters sent to older Americans in their homes significantly improved their dietary fiber intake. Another community intervention used media and social marketing in educational targeting of small retirement communities under the theme "Bread: It's a Great Way to Go," and reported a result of a 49% decrease in laxative sales and 58% increase in sales of whole meal and whole grain bread.

Educating caregivers on maintaining fecal continence in patients with dementia (with focus on constipation and other contributing factors) is crucial, and the same applies for patients with chronic neurologic diseases other than dementia, such as Parkinson disease, stroke, and neuropathic bowel (Constipation-Medical and physical issues-Caring for someone with dementia-Living with dementia-Alzheimer Europe [alzheimer-europe.org] from https://www.alzheimer-europe.org/Living-with-dementia/Caring-for-someone-with-dementia/Medical-and-physical-issues/Constipation#fragment1; Constipation and Faecal Impaction - Information Sheet IS41 [alzscot.org] from https://www.alzscot.org/sites/default/files/images/0000/0175/constipation-and-faecal-impaction.pdf).

DIET

Fiber increases stool frequency either by accelerating time or by increasing stool bulk. A systematic review of six randomized controlled trials (four with soluble fiber, and two with insoluble fiber) showed that soluble fiber led to improvements of global symptoms, straining, pain on defecation, and stool consistency. Also, there was an increase in stool frequency per week. Mixed fiber and psyllium were compared in a randomized controlled trial with both equally improving constipation and quality of life; mixed fiber was more effective in relieving flatulence, bloating and dissolved better. A meta-analysis of 20 nonrandomized studies in younger adults with constipation associated additional wheat bran with increased stool weight and decreased transit time. Evidence for the effectiveness of fiber in treatment of constipation in older people is more equivocal. In one community study, higher fiber intake was associated with lower laxative use among older women, but in another study, higher intake of bran was associated with no reduction in constipation symptoms and greater fecal loading in the colon on abdominal radiography. In older hospitalized patients, daily bran supplementation increased weekly bowel movement frequency and improved overall symptoms as compared with placebo. There have been several "before and after" studies in nursing home residents reporting that addition of dietary fiber (ranging from bran to processed pea hull) or fruit mixtures (apple puree to fruit porridge) to the daily diet improved bowel movement frequency and consistency and reduced laxative intake and the need for nursing intervention. Bias cannot be excluded from these nursing home studies, including that of concomitant increased fluid intake contributing to these positive results. Despite these reservations, these observational studies emphasize the usefulness of increasing dietary fiber, fluid, and fruit in older people at high risk of constipation. Additional benefits may be observed; for instance, adding oat bran to the diet in one study reduced cholesterol levels more markedly in older versus younger women.

The recommended daily fiber intake is 20 to 35 g per day with patients starting at a low dose of 3 to 4 g daily and increasing gradually as tolerated. While coarse bran rather than refined fiber is more effective in increasing stool fluid weight, it is far less palatable, and is more likely to cause initial symptoms of increased bloating, flatulence, and irregular bowel movements. Fiber should therefore be recommended to older individuals in the form of foods such as whole meal or whole grain bread, porridge, fresh fruit (preferably unpeeled), seeded berries, raw or cooked vegetables, beans, and lentils. A crossover trial in subjects aged 60 and older that entailed taking a daily kiwi fruit resulted in bulkier and softer stools and increased bowel movement frequency. Fiber supplementation should also be culturally appropriate. Chinese food is typically low in fiber, and dietary additives such as konjac glucomannan can serve as "natural laxatives." Other examples of natural laxatives are aloe vera and rhubarb, both of which contain stimulant anthraquinone derivatives similar to senna.

Fluids

A randomized controlled trial in adults aged 18 to 50 with chronic constipation showed that the beneficial effect of increased dietary fiber was significantly enhanced by increasing fluid intake to 1.5 to 2 L daily. This level of fluid intake is often not practical or acceptable to frail older patients, many of whom restrict fluid intake because of overactive bladder symptoms. Upping fluid intake by two 8-ounce beverages a day for 5 weeks in dependent nursing home residents significantly increased bowel movement frequency and reduced laxative use. This "hydration program" used a colorful beverage cart and four beverage choices to stimulate residents' interest in drinking. Caffeine is known to increase both bowel and bladder smooth muscle activity, though its impact on constipation in older people is not documented.

Physical Activity

A randomized controlled trial in middle-aged inactive patients with chronic constipation showed that regular physical activity (30-min brisk walk and 11-min home exercises a day) decreased colonic and rectosigmoid transit time and improved defecation. A systematic review and meta-analysis of eight studies involving aerobic exercise and one study involving anaerobic exercise indicated that exercise may be an effective treatment for constipation. A review of physical activity interventions in older adults concluded that incorporating exercise naturally into a person's day tends to provide the most effective means for increasing activity levels. Studies conducted in older nursing home patients showed the following outcome:

- Six months of moderate-intensity exercise training had no impact on constipation symptoms or habitual physical activity randomized controlled trial (RCT).
- Six months of 2 hourly prompted toileting improved measures of daily physical activity and functional performance but did not alter bowel movement frequency (RCT).
- Daily exercise in bed and the use of abdominal massage reduced laxative and enema use in chair-fast patients, although transit time was unaffected (non-RCT).

Existing evidence would tend to support exercise programs to influence constipation in nursing home residents and older community-dwelling people within the context of addressing other risk factors also. For some frail older people, exercise is difficult, but even short time periods of walking or other mobility exercises may be feasible and helpful.

Abdominal Massage

Abdominal massage added to the standard bowel regimen in spinal cord patients has been shown to shorten colonic transit time and increase weekly bowel movement frequency. A vibrating device that applied kneading force to the abdomen once a day for 20 minutes was evaluated in older constipated nursing home residents, and after 12 weeks resulted in softening of stool, increased bowel movement frequency, and a 47% reduction in transit time. Case reports show that physiotherapists can incorporate daily 10-minute abdominal massage into home activity programs for community-dwelling people suffering from constipation with good effect.

Biofeedback: Pelvic Floor Rehabilitation and Sphincter Strengthening Exercises

Biofeedback focuses on sensory and muscular retraining of the rectum and pelvic floor with the goals of improving sensation, muscular relaxation or strengthening, and improving the defecation dynamics (see **Figure 87-2**). Biofeedback is not well standardized and the best approach is unclear. A Cochrane review of 17 eligible studies with a total of 931 participants showed that because of the heterogeneity of the different samples and large range of different outcome measures, meta-analysis was not possible. However, the larger studies are summarized here:

- 70% (21/30) of biofeedback patients had improved constipation compared to 23% (7/30) of diazepam patients at 3-month follow-up (relative risk [RR] 3.00, 95% CI 1.51–5.98).
- In a 52-patient study, patients receiving manometry biofeedback had 4.6 complete spontaneous bowel movements (CSBM) per week compared to 2.8 CSBM for sham biofeedback or standard therapy consisting of diet, exercise, and laxatives at 3 months (mean difference 1.80, 95% CI 1.25–2.35; 52 patients).
- In a study of EMG biofeedback reported at both 6 and 12 months, 80% (43/54) of biofeedback patients reported clinical improvement compared to 22% (12/55) of laxative-treated patients (RR 3.65, 95% CI 2.17–6.13).

The evidence recommended for these studies overall is low because the majority of trials are of poor methodologic quality and subject to bias.

A randomized controlled trial showed that home-based biofeedback improved the number of CSBM per week and quality of life with similar efficacy to office-based biofeedback and was a cost-effective treatment.

Where rectal outlet delay and/or persistent straining is associated with excessive pelvic floor descent, pelvic strengthening exercises should be employed. In women, it is helpful to do the teaching while undertaking a pelvic examination (with the examining hand resting on the posterior vaginal wall), so that positive verbal feedback can be given when the patient correctly contracts the pelvic floor. Pelvic floor retraining can help rectal outlet symptoms, but a greater degree of perineal descent is predictive of poorer treatment responses. Patients with fecal soiling and/or weak external sphincter should be taught sphincter-strengthening exercises (see **Table 87-7**).

Biofeedback and pelvic strengthening exercises are not a feasible option for older patients with significant cognitive impairment, as executive dysfunction can interfere with cooperating and learning the exercises, and memory impairment can interfere with practicing and using the exercises.

Visceral Manipulation

Visceral manipulation can be used in patients who have failed feedback. This approach, which is commonly used by osteopaths, consists of the mobilization of the bowels through gentle manipulation to normalize their mechanical, vascular, and neurologic dysfunction with subsequent function improve improvement. The benefit of this therapy in constipation may be related to the loss of resilience in structures surrounding the peritoneal bowels. A randomized, controlled, double-blind, clinical trial including 30 patients with a mean age of 66 years and recent history of stroke compared visceral manipulation versus standard physical therapy. Significant improvements in frequency of bowel movements, difficulty defecating, and sensation of incomplete bowel movement were seen in the visceral manipulation group.

Toileting Habits and Access

Small nonrandomized studies show that regular toileting habits (scheduled evacuation) restores comfortable evacuation in stroke survivors (with the assistance of digital stimulation) and in older postoperative inpatients. The preservation of the gastrocolic reflex with aging supports the rationale for postprandial toileting. Hemorrhoids and other uncomfortable anorectal conditions that interfere with toileting should be identified and treated. Expert opinion supports the use of footstools during evacuation in individuals with weakened abdominal and pelvic muscles to optimize the Valsalva maneuver.

Toilet access should be assessed and facilitated, particularly in patients with mobility, visual, or dexterity impairments. Bathroom comfort and privacy must be considered, particularly for individuals in institutional settings. Reluctance to use the toilet in institutional settings has been linked to residents developing fecal impaction in case reports. **Table 87-8** summarizes basic but important recommendations relating to toileting and maintaining privacy and dignity.

TABLE 87-8 ■ TOILETS AND TOILETING—MAINTAINING PRIVACY AND DIGNITY

A multidisciplinary assessment should be made of older person's ability to access and use the toilet [3].

Commodes/sani-chairs/shower chairs
- should be available to residents in institutional settings [3];
- should provide a safe seated position for prolonged use by older people with skin vulnerability and trunk support problems (eg, padded seat, footstool if feet are unsupported, back and arm support, grab rails, etc.) [3].

Older people should be given the opportunity to use the toilet (either directly or by using a sani-chair or shower chair) rather than a bedside commode [3].

Bedpans should be avoided for defecation purposes.

Transportation to the toilet and use of the toilet or commode should be carried out with due regard to privacy and dignity.

A direct method of calling for assistance should be provided when an older person is left on the toilet/commode.

When using a commode
- methods to reduce noise and odor should be offered;
- methods to facilitate bottom wiping should be available;
- in living area and cannot be emptied immediately, a chemical toilet should be offered instead [3].

Level [1] indicates good evidence, that is, consistent results from well-designed, well-conducted studies.
Level [2] indicates fair evidence, that is, results show benefit, but strength limited by number, quality, or consistency of studies.
Level [3] indicates poor evidence, that is, insufficient because of limited number, power, or quality of studies.
Data from Potter J, Norton C, Cottenden A. Bowel Care in Older People. London, United Kingdom: Royal College of Physicians of London; 2002.

Laxative and Enema Use and Abuse in Older People

A Food and Drug Administration (FDA) Advisory Panel has registered concern over the widespread overuse of over-the-counter (OTC) laxatives; laxatives are second only to analgesics as the most commonly used OTC medications by older people. OTC laxative use is common in the United States and Europe, and is encouraged by advertising and popular ignorance of adverse effects. Only 38% of OTC laxative users in Italy were guided in their choice of laxative by a physician. The remainder were influenced by pharmacists (21%), relatives or friends (16%), and advertisements (12%). Six percent of users reported adverse effects. One-fifth to one-third of regular laxative users do not consider themselves to be constipated, and many people take them through a misguided belief in the benefits of regular purgation. One study showed that 78% of older people who used laxatives regularly had never gone for more than 3 days without a bowel movement. Habitual rather than surreptitious abuse is more likely in older individuals; repeated purging empties the colon of stool that would normally descend into and distend the rectal ampulla, thereby removing the urge to defecate, and prompting the patient to take further laxatives.

Although patients in hospitals and nursing homes are at higher risk for constipation, this does not entirely justify the very high levels of cathartic prescribing in these settings. Seventy-six percent of hospitalized older patients are prescribed at least one type of laxative. A prospective study of 2355 nursing home residents in the Netherlands showed that over the course of 2 years, 47% were started on laxatives, with 79% of these continuing with the long-term treatment. Prescribing rates in US nursing homes are high at 54% to 74%, with almost half of these users prescribed more than one agent. Most commonly prescribed agents are stool softeners (26%), magnesium salts (18%), and stimulants (16%). Two contributing factors may lead to overprescribing of laxatives to older patients: lack of objective confirmation of the diagnosis by the prescribing physician or nurse, and prescribing patterns of laxatives that are clinically ineffective. In US nursing homes, docusate (a fecal softener with little or no laxative effect) is the predominantly prescribed agent. Docusate prescription should be discouraged, and other more effective methods of softening the stool should be prescribed.

Evidence-Based Summary of Laxative, Suppository, and Enema Treatment in Older Persons

Many reported trials of laxative and enema treatment in older people are low quality, limited by unclear definitions for constipation, inconsistent outcome measurement, and underreporting of potential confounding factors during the trial period (eg, fiber intake). The absence of good level evidence may in part underlie the somewhat empirical way in which laxatives are prescribed to older people.

The following conclusions are drawn from meta-analytical reviews (1997, 2001, 2002, 2004, 2010, 2011, 2018) of efficacy of laxatives in treating chronic constipation in adults:

- Availability of published evidence is poor for many commonly used agents including senna, magnesium hydroxide, bisacodyl, and stool softeners.
- In trials conducted in older people, significant improvements in bowel movement frequency were observed with a stimulant laxative (cascara) [3] and with lactulose [2], while psyllium [2] and lactulose [2] were individually reported to improve stool consistency and related symptoms in placebo-controlled trials.
- Level [1] evidence supports the use of polyethylene glycol (PEG) in adults.
- Level [2] evidence supports the use of lactulose and psyllium in adults.
- None of the currently available trials include quality of life outcomes.
- A systematic review of older adults (68–85 years) at long-care facilities concluded there were insufficient data to evaluate the safety and efficacy of laxatives. Senna in combination with bulking agents had greater efficacy than lactulose based on two trials. One trial showed that senna with psyllium was found to be more effective in adult ambulatory patients than psyllium alone.
- A stepped approach to laxative treatment in older people is justified, starting with cheaper laxatives before proceeding to more expensive alternatives.

Tables 87-9 and **87-10** summarize the onset of action, mechanisms of action, potential side effects, and benefits of selected laxatives in current usage, and the following discussion describes efficacy and safety.

Stimulant Laxatives

Senna is a cheap and safe agent for use in older patients. A trial of cascara (a similar plant-derived stimulant laxative) in older hospitalized patients increased bowel movement frequency by an average of 2.6 bowel movements per week as compared to placebo. Administration of 20 mg of senna daily for 6 months to patients older than 80 years did not cause any significant losses of intestinal protein or electrolytes, and repeated studies in mice show no evidence of myenteric nerve damage resulting from its use. *Senna* generally induces evacuation 8 to 12 hours following administration, and should therefore be taken at bedtime. Some patients may require several weeks of daily use before achieving a regular bowel habit. Maintenance therapy with *Senna* is appropriate in patients with chronic constipation, and it can be used in higher doses for short-term treatment of fecal impaction. In patients with weak anal sphincters, the *Senna* alone may be sufficient to treat constipation without causing or exacerbating fecal incontinence through excess stool softening.

TABLE 87-9 ■ MEDICATIONS USED IN OLDER PEOPLE WITH CONSTIPATION

TYPE	GENERIC NAME	TRADE NAME	DOSAGE	SIDE EFFECTS	TIME TO ONSET OF ACTION (H)	MECHANISM OF ACTION
Fiber	Bran	—	1 cup/d	Bloating, flatulence, iron and calcium malabsorption	—	Stool bulk increases, colonic transit time decreases, gastrointestinal motility increases
	Psyllium	Metamucil Konsyl	1 tsp up to 3 times daily	Bloating, flatulence	—	
	Methylcellulose	Citrucel	1 tsp up to 3 times daily	Less bloating	—	
	Calcium polycarbophil	FiberCon	2–4 tablets once daily	Bloating, flatulence	—	
Stool softener	Docusate sodium	Colace	100 mg twice daily		12–72	
Hyperosmolar agents	Sorbitol	—	15–30 mL once daily or twice daily	Sweet tasting, transient abdominal cramps, flatulence	24–48	Nonabsorbable disaccharides metabolized by colonic bacteria into acetic acid and other short-chain fatty acids
	Lactulose	Chronulac	15–30 mL once daily or twice daily	Same as sorbitol	24–48	
	PEG	Golytely Colyte Miralax	8–32 oz once daily	Incontinence due to potency	0.5–1	Osmotically increases intraluminal fluids
Stimulant	Glycerin		Suppository; up to once daily	Rectal irritation	0.25–1	Evacuation induced by local rectal stimulation
	Bisacodyl	Ducolax	10 mg suppositories or 5–10 mg by mouth up to 3 times/wk	Incontinence, hyperkalemia, abdominal cramps, rectal burning with daily use of suppository form	0.25–1	Bisacodyl and sodium picosulfate are prodrugs that are hydrolyzed by colonic bacteria (sodium picosulfate) or intestinal and colonic brush border enzymes (bisacodyl) to the active metabolite, bis-(p-hydroxyphenyl)-pyridyl-2-methane, which has antiabsorptive/secretory and prokinetic effects
	Picosulfate					Similar to bisacodyl

(*Continued*)

TABLE 87-9 ■ MEDICATIONS USED IN OLDER PEOPLE WITH CONSTIPATION (CONTINUED)

TYPE	GENERIC NAME	TRADE NAME	DOSAGE	SIDE EFFECTS	TIME TO ONSET OF ACTION (H)	MECHANISM OF ACTION
Stimulant (continued)	Anthraquinones (senna, cascara)	Senokot Perdiem (plain) Peri-Colace	2 tablets once daily to 4 tablets twice daily 1–2 tsp once daily 1–2 tablets once daily	Degeneration of Meissner and Auerbach plexus (unproven), malabsorption, abdominal cramps, dehydration, melanosis coli	8–12 8–12 8–12	Electrolyte transport altered by increased intraluminal fluids; myenteric plexus stimulated; motility increases
Saline laxative	Magnesium	Milk of magnesia Haliey's M-O (with mineral oil)	15–30 mL once daily or twice daily 15–30 mL once daily or twice daily	Magnesium toxicity, dehydration, abdominal cramps, incontinence	1–3 1–3	Fluid osmotically drawn into small bowel lumen; cholecystokinin stimulated; colon transit time decreases
Lubricant	Mineral oil	—	15–45 mL	Lipid pneumonia, malabsorption of fat-soluble vitamins, dehydration, incontinence	6–8	Stool lubricated
Enemas	Mineral oil retention enema	—	199–250 mL once daily per rectum	Incontinence, mechanical trauma	6–8	Stool softened and lubricated
	Tap water enema	—	500 mL per rectum	Mechanical trauma	5–15 min	Evacuation induced by distended colon; mechanical lavage
	Phosphate enema	Fleet	1 unit per rectum	Accumulated damage to rectal mucosa, hyperphosphatemia, mechanical trauma	5–15 min	
	Soapsuds enema	—	1500 mL per rectum	Accumulated damage to rectal mucosa, mechanical trauma	2–15 min	

Adapted with permission from Locke GR 3rd, Pemberton IH, et al. AGA technical review on constipation. American Gastroenterological Association. Gastroenterology. 2000;119(6):1766–1778.

TABLE 87-10 ■ NEWER MEDICATIONS FOR TREATMENT OF CONSTIPATION

GENERIC NAME (TRADE NAME)	MECHANISM OF ACTION	METABOLISM, BIOAVAILABILTY	PHARMACODYNAMIC EFFECTS	CLINICAL TRAILS	COMMON SIDE EFFECTS	CARDIOVASCULAR SAFETY[a]
SECRETAGOGUES						
Lubioprostone (Amitiza)[b]	Stimulate instestinal chloride and fluid secretion by activating chloride channels	Intestinal degradation, minimal oral bioavailability	Accelerated small bowel and colonic transit in health	Phases 2 and 3 in CC, IBS-C	Diarrhea, nausea	No arrhythmic effects
Linaclotide (Linzess)[b]	Stimulate instestinal chloride and fluid secretion by activating CFTR	Intestinal degradation, minimal oral bioavailability	Dose-related acceleration of colonic transit in IBS-C	Phases 2 and 3 in CC, IBS-C	Diarrhea	No arrhythmic effects
SEROTONIN 5-HT$_4$ RECEPTOR AGONISTS						
Prucalopride[c] (Resolor)	High selectivity and affinity for 5-HT$_4$ receptors; much weaker affinity for human D4 and s1 and mouse 5-HT$_3$ receptors	Limited hepatic, not CYP3A4	Accelerated colonic transit in health and CC	Phases 2 and 3 in CC	Diarrhea, headache	No arrhythmic activity in atrial cells; inhibits hERG at very high μmol/L concentration; no clinically relevant adverse cardiac effects in large trials (> 4000 subjects)

Note: Only agents that have been tested in phase 3 clinical trials are included.

CC, chronic constipation.

[a]In addition to the listed effects, none of the agents shown in this table affect QTc in healthy subjects.

[b]Approved by the FDA

[c]Approved by the European Agency for Evaluation of Medical Products.

Bisacodyl is a useful alternative stimulant laxative to *Senna*. Bisacodyl 10 mg daily improved stool frequency and consistency without side effects in a randomized, controlled trial among outpatients with a mean age of 62.

Phenolphthalein and *castor oil* should not be used in older people because of a high risk of side effects including malabsorption, dehydration, lipoid pneumonia, and, with heavy prolonged use, cathartic colon.

Bulk Laxatives

Bulk laxatives are generally under-prescribed to older people, despite evidence that they increase bowel movement frequency (by a mean of 1.4 bowel movements per week as compared to placebo), and improve consistency and ease of evacuation. This may partly be because of intolerance in the form of bloating and unpredictable bowel habit in the first weeks of taking them, and also of caution on the part of prescribers because of the documented risk of impaction with these agents in patients with poor fluid intake. Psyllium has been shown to increase stool frequency in people with Parkinson disease, but did not alter transit time.

Bulking agents are generally useful in older individuals with mild to moderate constipation who are able to tolerate them and who drink sufficient fluids. They have the additional benefit of reducing abdominal pain in patients with IBS, limiting flare-ups of diverticulitis, and facilitating painful defecation associated with hemorrhoids.

Furthermore, psyllium significantly lowers serum cholesterol by binding bile acids in the intestine. Available preparations are natural non-wheat fibers such as psyllium and ispaghula husk, and synthetic compounds such as calcium polycarbophil and methylcellulose. The synthetic compounds tend to be cheaper and are available in more easily administrated tablet forms, as compared to reconstituted powder, which can be hard for older patients to swallow. The synthetic bulking agents and the natural fibers are equally effective in increasing stool frequency and volume. Bran in tablet form is considerably cheaper than bulk laxatives, but the former may cause even more bloating and unpredictability of bowel habit and may also predispose to malabsorption of iron or calcium in older people.

Magnesium Salts

Magnesium salts are commonly prescribed to older hospitalized patients, and magnesium hydroxide is popular as an over-the-counter laxative. There is only one published study evaluating magnesium hydroxide in older people—a small trial in nursing home residents, which suggested that this laxative was more effective than a bulking agent in increasing bowel movement frequency and softening stool. Magnesium salts may be favored by physician and patient alike because of their rapid action, but in general, a gradual catharsis is preferable to restore regular bowel habit in older persons. Their potent catharsis increases the risk of fluid and electrolyte losses and of fecal incontinence in less-mobile people, or in those with weak sphincters. Furthermore, magnesium levels should be monitored in all older people who are using magnesium hydroxide on a regular basis, as hypermagnesemia can occur even with normal serum creatinine levels. Long-term use of magnesium hydroxide is contraindicated in chronic kidney disease. The more potent salt magnesium citrate carries an even greater risk of side effects, including promoting colonic pseudo-obstruction, and is therefore not recommended for use in the older population. Based on evidence and known side effects, there is no clear role for using magnesium salts in treatment of chronic constipation in older people.

Hyperosmolar Laxatives

Hyperosmolar laxatives are the most rigorously studied laxative group in the current literature. The following summarizes findings from nursing home studies:

- Lactulose (or the related agent lactitol) versus placebo shortened transit time, increased bowel movement frequency (by an average of 1.9 bowel movements per week), and improved stool consistency.
- In a comparison study with a bulking/stimulant combination agent, lactulose was a little less effective in influencing bowel pattern and consistency.
- Lactulose and sorbitol were equally effective in mostly eliminating the use of other laxatives and enemas in residents with dementia and chronic constipation, with sorbitol being considerably cheaper.

A well-designed trial in ambulatory older veterans with severe constipation also showed lactulose and sorbitol to be equally efficacious. Lactulose and sorbitol are effective agents in treating chronic constipation in older people in all health care settings, with sorbitol being the cheaper option.

Polyethylene glycol (PEG) is a more potent hyperosmolar laxative than lactulose as demonstrated by its impact on transit time in normal subjects. In a randomized controlled trial in hospitalized patients with a mean age of 55, PEG produced a greater increase in bowel movement frequency and a greater reduction in straining than lactulose, but at the expense of a higher mean number of liquid stools. A similar efficacy and side-effect profile plus a reduction in laxative expenditures were shown with use in long-stay residents of a mental health institution. PEG treatment of fecal impaction (in combination with daily enemas) showed greater efficacy than lactulose, without the dehydration or hemodynamic side effects in older nursing home residents. Another trial in adults aged 17 to 88 with fecal loading on x-ray or rectal examination, and bowels not open for 3 to 5 days showed that 1 L (or 8 sachets) a day of PEG plus electrolytes for 3 days resolved impaction in 89% of patients, with few adverse effects. The current evidence base suggests that the role of PEG in older people is for acute disimpaction (ensuring that easy toilet access is guaranteed) and for regular use as a laxative only in high-risk people whose constipation has proved resistant to milder and cheaper alternatives.

Stool Softeners

Docusate sodium has been shown experimentally to have no effect on colonic motility, and little or no laxative action, even at doses of 300 mg/day. Current evidence suggests that docusate is not effective in the treatment of constipation or rectal outlet delay in older people. In a randomized controlled trial in adults with severe constipation docusate proved significantly inferior to psyllium for both softening stools and increasing bowel movement frequency. A systematic review of prospective controlled trials evaluating oral docusate in chronically ill people (though hampered by poor data) showed only a small trend toward increased stool frequency, and concluded that there was insufficient evidence to support its use in this population.

Nevertheless, docusate is frequently recommended and used in older people as a laxative as well as fecal softener. This is of particular concern in the nursing home and hospital settings, where constipation may as a result be undertreated with an increased risk of fecal impaction. Furthermore, docusate (in combination with the stimulant danthron) increases the risk of fecal incontinence in nursing home residents. As stated earlier, docusate prescription should be discouraged, and other more effective methods of softening the stool should be prescribed.

Enemas

Enemas have a role in both acute disimpaction and in preventing recurrent impactions in susceptible patients. They induce evacuation as a response to colonic distension, as well as by plain lavage; the commonest reason for a poor result from an enema is inadequate administration. In one study of nursing home residents with overflow incontinence associated with fecal impaction on rectal examination, daily phosphate enemas continued until no further results were effective in completely resolving incontinence in 94% of patients. Some patients with poor mobility or neurogenic bowel dysfunction may have recurrent stool impactions despite regular laxative and suppository use, and they will benefit from weekly enemas.

Tap water enemas are the safest type for regular use, although they take more nursing administration time than phosphate enemas, and are not available in certain countries. Regular use of phosphate enemas should be avoided in patients with renal impairment as dangerous hyperphosphatemia has been reported. Soapsuds enemas should never be administered to older patients. Arachis oil retention enemas are particularly useful in loosening colonic impactions. In patients who have a firm and large rectal impaction, manual evacuation should be performed before inserting enemas or suppositories, using local anesthetic gel if needed to reduce discomfort.

Suppositories

The predominance of rectal outlet delay (including manual evacuation) in older people, many of whom take regular laxatives, is likely associated with the underuse of suppositories. Although research data are lacking, clinically suppositories are very useful in treatment of rectal outlet delay, and when symptoms of prolonged straining are prominent. Regular suppository administration (usually three times a week, and ideally after breakfast) can effectively control symptoms in these patients. A study of nursing home patients with overflow incontinence found that a regimen of daily lactulose and suppositories plus weekly enemas was only effective in restoring continence when long-lasting and complete rectal emptying was achieved. Regular use of suppositories is indicated in older patients with impaired rectal motility and/or recurrent rectal impactions. With appropriate education, many older people can self-administer suppositories; they are easier to insert and more effective if used blunt end first, and people with impaired dexterity may be able to use suppository inserters designed for spinal cord injured patients. First-line suppository use is with glycerin, a hyperosmolar laxative used solely in suppository form. If ineffective, *bisacodyl* suppositories (in PEG base) should be used, although daily use can sometimes cause symptoms of rectal discomfort or burning. *Bisacodyl* suppositories have been shown to be effective in treating severe constipation in patients with spinal cord injuries. The onset of action of suppositories varies by individual from 5 to 45 minutes (most likely influenced by the state of the rectal innervation); thus patients should be advised to set a quiet time aside for effective evacuation. Postprandial use of suppositories can also potentially take advantage of the gastrocolic reflex.

Secretagogues

Lubriprostone is approved in the United States for the treatment of chronic constipation. It is classified as a prostone, a bicyclic fatty acid compound derived from a metabolite of prostaglandin E1, which acts locally in the small intestinal mucosa, inducing secretion of fluid and electrolytes through the activation of the type-2 chloride channels in the intestinal apical cell membrane. A secondary analysis of one trial showed that 24 µg twice daily *lubriprostone* significantly improved the number of spontaneous bowel movements, consistency and straining rate compared to placebo in a 4-week trial among 57 patients age 65 and older, and was well tolerated with less side effects than placebo. In another secondary analysis of 163 older adults, *lubriprostone* showed significant improvement in constipation severity, abdominal bloating, and discomfort compared to placebo.

Linaclotide activates guanylate cyclase C on the intestinal mucosa, resulting in increased levels of intracellular and extracellular cyclic guanosine monophosphate, which results in increased luminal secretion of chloride and bicarbonate via the cystic fibrosis transmembrane conductance regulator. A meta-analysis of seven trials in patients with IBS or chronic constipation showed that *linaclotide* increases the number of complete spontaneous bowel movements per week and was associated with a 30% or more reduction from baseline in the weekly average of daily worst abdominal pain scores for 50% of the treatment weeks. *Linaclotide* also improved stool form and reduced abdominal pain, bloating, and overall symptom severity. Trials are lacking in the older population, and this drug, like lubriprostone, is expensive and not covered as a first-line agent by most insurance plans in the United States.

Plecanatide is another guanylate cyclase C agonist, similar to linaclotide. Multiple placebo-controlled trials showed the efficacy of *plecanatide* 3 and 6 mg when compared to placebo; *plecanatide* improved bowel symptoms (stool frequency, stool consistency, cramping, discomfort fullness) and had a major percentage of responders. Mean weekly CSBM frequency also increased from baseline. Most recently, an analysis including data from phase III trials in chronic idiopathic constipation and IBS-C with patients older than 65 years (451 patients of whom 287 were randomized to *plecanatide*) showed that *plecanatide* improved stool consistency from baseline at week 12 and was well tolerated.

Enterokinetic Agents

Altered serotonin (5-HT) signaling may predispose to chronic constipation, and 5-HT4 agonists (eg, *prucalopride*) have been shown to stimulate gastrointestinal motility and increase stool water content. The efficacy and safety of 5-HT4 agonists in treating chronic constipation were evaluated in a recent meta-analysis of 13 randomized controlled trials where 5-HT4 agonists were superior for all outcomes: mean $\geq$ 3 SCBM/week (RR = 1.85; 95% CI 1.23–2.79); mean $\geq$ 1 SCBM over baseline (RR = 1.57; 95% CI 1.19–2.06). Two of these studies were done in older populations and *prucalopride* was superior to placebo. Although previous 5-HT4 agonists (cisapride and tegaserod) were associated with cardiac ischemia, strokes, cardiac arrhythmias, and QTc prolongation, *prucalopride* is not associated with major adverse cardiovascular events and has been approved in the United States. *Tenapanor* is a selective sodium/hydrogen exchanger isoform 3 (NHE3) inhibitor. It induces increased water secretion due to a decrease in sodium absorption in the intestines. A phase III, placebo-controlled clinical study in 629 patients with IBS-C reported an increase from in baseline in average weekly number of CSBM in the *tenepanor* group compared to placebo. Unfortunately, mean age was 45 years and data for outcomes in the older population are unknown.

Treatment Options for Opioid-Induced Constipation

Constipation is the most common gastrointestinal effect of opioids, with development in 41% to 94% of users. Activation of enteric µ-opioid receptors induces a decrease in bowel tone and contractility and an increase in colonic fluid absorption and anal sphincter tone leading to increased difficulty to pass stool. No treatment guidelines in the older population are available, but it has been suggested to use nonpharmacologic interventions and laxatives as first-line therapy. In case of refractory constipation, peripherally acting μ-opioid receptor antagonists (PAMORA), such as naldemedine, naloxegol, alvimopan, and methylnaltrexone, are strongly recommended.

Four RCTs demonstrated that naldemedine increased the rate of patients having greater than 3 CSBM when compared to placebo (52% vs 35%; relative risk, 1.51; 95% CI, 1.32–1.72), with also statistically significant changes in straining, stool consistency, and quality of life. Naloxegol was associated with a higher rate of response to therapy measured by greater than or equal to 3 CSBM per week (42% vs 29%; relative risk, 1.43; 95% CI, 1.19–1.71). Regarding methylnaltrexone, the evidence of five RCTs demonstrated an improvement in bowel movement frequency compared with placebo but was considered low quality.

Treatment Option for Refractory Constipation

Transanal irrigation (TAI) consists of the instillation of water into the rectum using a rectal catheter or a cone that can be self-administered. A systematic review and meta-analysis identified seven studies (two uncontrolled, five retrospective) with a total of 254 patients with chronic constipation. A total of 128 patients reported a positive response to irrigation therapy, either subjectively or using a visual-analogue score. A fixed effect analysis of proportions gave a pooled response rate of 50.4% (95% CI: 44.3%–56.5%). Retrospective evaluation of 102 patients with refractory chronic idiopathic constipation treated with TAI reported improvement in general well-being (65%), rectal clearance (63%), bloating (49%), abdominal pain (48%), bowel frequency (42%), and SCBMs (22%). Unfortunately, these two studies included mostly patients less than 65 years; therefore, benefits in the older population are unknown.

Surgery is reserved for a small proportion of patients with medically refractory chronic constipation. Surgical interventions include colonic resection, rectal suspension, rectal wall excision, and rectovaginal reinforcement. Patients with slow-transit constipation reported a global satisfaction rate of 86% after colectomy. Surgical intervention in older patients should be considered carefully given the lack of studies assessing benefits and complication rates.

Novel Therapies

Bilateral transcutaneous tibial nerve stimulation (TENS) was studied in 44 patients aged 65 or older with chronic refractory constipation for 12 weeks. Inadequate defecation, obstructive defecation, colonic inertia, and pain improved at 6 weeks, with pain score continuing to decrease at 12 weeks. Other therapies, such as sacral nerve stimulation and vibrating capsule, have not been tested in the older population.

TREATMENT GUIDANCE

Table 87-11 represents a combination of evidence-based and expert opinion in providing treatment guidance, which can be summarized as follows:

- In ambulatory older patients with chronic constipation, a daily bulk laxative is appropriate for both rectal outlet delay and slow-transit constipation. Patients

TABLE 87-11 ■ PHARMACOLOGIC TREATMENT OF CONSTIPATION IN OLDER PEOPLE—A STEPWISE APPROACH

Chronic constipation

In ambulant older people
  Bulk laxative (psyllium) 1–3 times daily with fluids as required
  If symptoms persist, add senna 1–3 tablets at bedtime
  In individuals with questionable fluid intake or those intolerant of bulk laxatives, start with senna 1–2 tablets at bedtime
  If symptoms persist, add sorbitol or lactulose 15 mL daily as needed, titrating the dose to achieve regular (≥ 3 times a week) and comfortable evacuation

In high-risk patients (bedridden individuals, patients with neurologic disease, and patients with history of fecal impaction)
  Senna 2–3 tablets at bedtime and sorbitol or lactulose 30 mL daily, titrating upward as needed
  If symptoms persist, give PEG (half to two sachets daily)

Colonic fecal impaction

Clinical or radiological obstruction
  Daily retention enemas (eg, arachis oil) until obstruction resolves, before starting oral laxatives

Colonic disimpaction
  Daily enemas (preferably tap water) until no further washout result
  PEG (0.5–2 L daily or 2–3 sachets of Movicol) with fluids
  Ensure that patient has easy access to toilet to avoid fecal incontinence
  When impaction resolves, give laxative regimen for chronic constipation in high-risk patients for long-term treatment to avoid recurrence

Rectal outlet delay

Rectal disimpaction
  Manual disimpaction where necessary, followed by phosphate enema(s) for initial complete clearance of rectal impaction

Regular treatment
  Glycerine suppositories at least once a week and as required to relieve symptoms
  For persistent symptoms, use bisacodyl suppositories instead of glycerine suppositories
  In patients at high risk of rectal impaction (rectal dysmotility, neurologic disease) give regular enemas (usually once weekly) and daily suppositories
  If stool is hard or infrequent, add daily laxative as for chronic constipation

must be able to drink adequate amounts of fluid to avoid further constipation and fecal impaction.

- If the bulking agent is not tolerated, or proves ineffective, then senna may be substituted (1–3 tablets at night) with prn sorbitol (or lactulose) if needed to achieve patient-centered goals of comfortable regular evacuations.
- In less-mobile older people at higher risk of impaction, a combination of regular senna and sorbitol (or lactulose) should be used with dosage titration.
- In patients with colonic impaction, oil retention enemas should be administered daily until there are no clinical or radiologic signs of obstruction, and then tap

water enemas continued regularly until they produce no further result.

- Where the patient has easy access to a toilet, PEG 0.5 to 2 L daily should be given as long as is needed to clear the impaction, followed by a regular maintenance laxative regimen of senna and sorbitol (or lactulose) to avoid recurrence of fecal impaction.
- In cases where toilet access is not easy (eg, at home with stairs), a more gradual clear-out using higher-dose senna and sorbitol or lactulose is appropriate to limit problems with incontinence.
- For rectal outlet delay or a predominant complaint of straining, the first-line approach should be regular

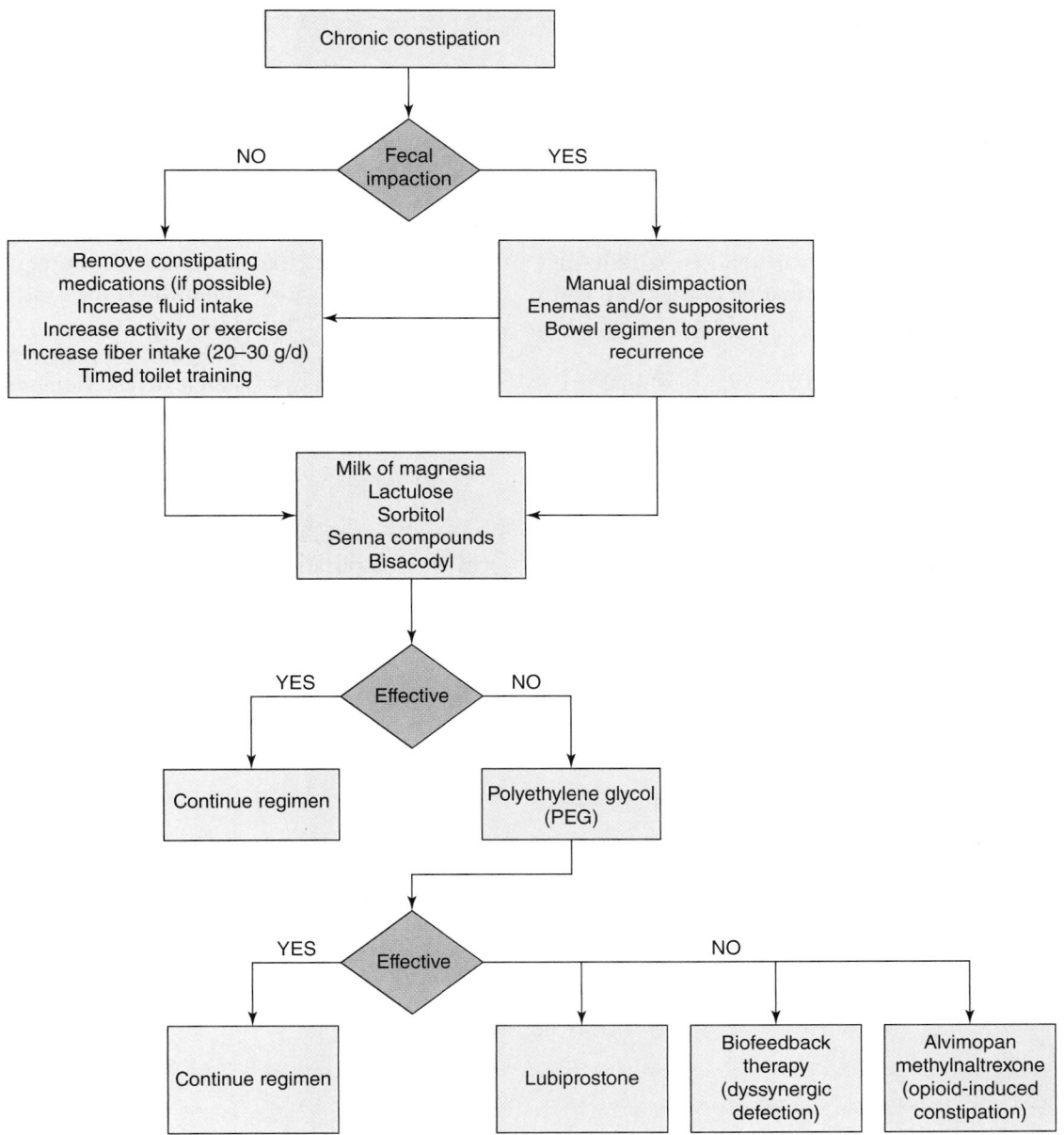

FIGURE 87-6. Treatment algorithm for the management of chronic constipation in the older adults. (Reproduced with permission from Rao SS, Go JT. Update on the management of constipation in the elderly: new treatment options. *Clin Interv Aging.* 2010;5:163–171.)

use of suppositories, and laxatives should only be given for coexisting symptoms of hard or infrequent bowel movements.

- Interventions for constipation such as senna, osmotic laxatives, and suppositories should be supplemented by regular toileting after breakfast as the food and caffeine intake may help take advantage of the gastrocolic reflex.

CONCLUSIONS

A practical algorithmic approach to assessment and treatment of constipation in older people is illustrated in **Figures 87-3** and **87-6**. Health care professionals should routinely inquire about constipation symptoms in older people and be alert to the presence of clinical constipation in individuals unable to communicate. In many older people with constipation symptoms, lifestyle advice (diet, fluids, exercise, toileting habits) will preempt the need for laxative therapy. In higher-risk patients, a stepwise approach to prescribing laxatives, suppositories, or enemas should be used, with the goal of achieving comfortable and regular evacuation. Rectal evacuation difficulties should be specifically addressed in order to identify conditions that may require additional interventions.

FURTHER READING

Brenner DM, Fogel R, Dorn SD, et al. Efficacy, safety, and tolerability of plecanatide in patients with irritable bowel syndrome with constipation: results of two phase 3 randomized clinical trials. *Am J Gastroenterol.* 2018;113:735–745.

DeMicco M, Barrow L, Hickey B, et al. Randomized clinical trial: efficacy and safety of plecanatide in the treatment of chronic idiopathic constipation. *Therap Adv Gastroenterol.* 2017;10:837–851.

Emmett CD, Close HJ, Yiannakou Y, et al. Trans-anal irrigation therapy to treat adult chronic functional constipation: systematic review and meta-analysis. *BMC Gastroenterol.* 2015;15:139.

Erdogan A, Rao SS, Thiruvaiyaru D, et al. Randomised clinical trial: mixed soluble/insoluble fibre vs. psyllium for chronic constipation. *Aliment Pharmacol Ther.* 2016;44:35–44.

Menees SB, Franklin H, Chey WD. Evaluation of plecanatide for the treatment of chronic idiopathic constipation and irritable bowel syndrome with constipation in patients 65 years or older. *Clin Ther.* 2020;42:1406–1414 e4.

Miner PB Jr, Koltun WD, Wiener GJ, et al. A randomized phase III clinical trial of plecanatide, a uroguanylin analog, in patients with chronic idiopathic constipation. *Am J Gastroenterol.* 2017;112:613–621.

Nullens S, Nelsen T, Camilleri M, et al. Regional colon transit in patients with dys-synergic defaecation or slow transit in patients with constipation. *Gut.* 2012;61:1132–1139.

Vijayvargiya P, Camilleri M. Use of prucalopride in adults with chronic idiopathic constipation. *Expert Rev Clin Pharmacol.* 2019;12:579–589.

Wanden-Berghe C, Patino-Alonso MC, Galindo-Villardon P, et al. Complications associated with enteral nutrition: CAFANE Study. *Nutrients.* 2019;11.

Chapter 88

Cancer and Aging: General Principles

Carolyn J. Presley, Harvey Jay Cohen, Mina S. Sedrak

INTRODUCTION

This chapter discusses many of the general relationships of cancer and aging. It focuses on the epidemiologic, basic etiologic, and biological relationships between the processes of aging and neoplasia and the generalizable aspects of management of cancer in the older patient. The approach to specific malignancies is covered in subsequent chapters related to the appropriate organ system. Cancer is a major problem for older adults. It is the second leading cause of death after heart disease in the United States and age is the single most important risk factor for developing cancer. Over 60% of all newly diagnosed malignant tumors and 70% of all cancer deaths occur in persons 65 years or older according to the National Cancer Institute (NCI). If one examines incidence and mortality data obtained from the NCI's Surveillance, Epidemiology, and End Results (SEER) Program (**Figure 88-1**), one sees that age-specific cancer incidence and mortality rise progressively throughout the age range. While the rate of incidence increase diminishes somewhat in the oldest age groups, and the rate actually falls slightly in the very oldest (perhaps a survivor effect), the overall risk for developing cancer is certainly greatest in the later years. Because the number of people in this country older than age 65 is rising rapidly and the oldest of the old, that is, those older than age 85, are increasing at the greatest rate, geriatricians, generalists, and internists will be encountering an increasing number of older adults with cancer in their practices and within the entire health care system.

Data from the SEER Program show that 5-year survivals for most types of cancer decrease with advancing age. Possible explanations include an altered natural history of some cancers, competing comorbid medical conditions, decreased physiologic reserve compromising the

Learning Objectives

- Identify risk factors inherent in the aging process that may promote neoplasia.
- Apply an understanding of lifespan and patient-centered choice to cancer screening recommendations.
- Integrate the concept of comprehensive geriatric assessment (CGA) and personal choice into cancer treatment decisions and individual management plans.
- Become aware of age-related factors that influence the risk of toxicity from cancer treatment such as radiation, surgery, or systemic treatment (eg, chemotherapy, immunotherapy).

Key Clinical Points

1. Aging is associated with an increasing risk of developing cancer, with a number of mechanisms likely contributing including duration of exposure to carcinogens, susceptibility to DNA and other cellular damage with impaired repair mechanisms, a proneoplastic environment (eg, low-level inflammation), and impaired immune surveillance.

2. The 5-year survival rate for most cancers decreases with advanced age; many factors may contribute including altered tumor biology (ie, more aggressive tumor behavior), tolerance to therapy, and the presence of multiple comorbidities.

(Continued)

(Cont.)

3. Age bias in diagnostic and treatment decisions for older adults with cancer exists. Older adults are continually underrepresented in clinical trials.

4. Although performance status (eg, Eastern Cooperative Oncology Group [ECOG] performance score) is routinely applied to patients with cancer, a CGA that includes assessment tools to predict functional age based on physical function, comorbidities that may interfere with cancer therapy, nutritional status, polypharmacy, psychological and cognitive status, socioeconomic issues, and geriatric syndromes has been shown to add substantial prognostic information for older adults.

5. Patients and their caregivers should continually discuss goals of care throughout the course of their disease with the treating oncologist and primary care physician.

ability to tolerate therapy, physicians' reluctance to provide aggressive therapy, and barriers in the older person's access to care. Communication between health care providers and older patients may be hampered by deficits in hearing, vision, and cognition. The older cancer patient often has an older caregiver, and the diagnosis of cancer often affects the health-related quality of life of both individuals. Thus, not only does cancer occur at an increased rate in older individuals, but it makes a significant impact on such people's lives, from the standpoint of both increasing morbidity and mortality. All of these challenges contribute to defining "geriatric oncology" as a true subspecialty and has

led to the development of guidelines by the National Comprehensive Cancer Network (NCCN) that addresses special considerations in older patients with cancer.

RELATIONSHIP BETWEEN AGING AND NEOPLASIA

The processes resulting in the evolution of neoplasia and those resulting in aging involve many of the same biological mechanisms, known respectively as the Hallmarks of Cancer and the Hallmarks of Aging (eg, genetic instability, proteostasis, stem cell function, metabolism, intercellular communication), but generally working in opposite directions. In the genesis of neoplasia, they result in accumulation of damage leading to increased cell proliferation, while in aging, they result in reduced cell proliferation or cellular senescence. Thus cancer and aging have often been referred to as opposite sides of the same coin. Both are multistage processes. Neoplasia proceeds through a series of changes known as initiation, or the first "hit"; promotion, where cell proliferation increases; and progression, itself a multistage step, resulting in the transformation of a cell from a premalignant to a malignant state. Local invasion and/or distant metastasis may then ensue but the mechanisms governing these processes are less well understood. As described elsewhere (see Chapter 1), aging also involves sequential accumulation of alterations in similar mechanisms but in what appears to be a less distinctly separated set of events.

Gene regulation is a particularly important aspect of neoplastic evolution. Broadly there are two types of genes involved; oncogenes, which when mutated transform cells from pre-malignant to malignant, and suppressor genes which generally prevent uncontrolled cell growth. Oncogene activation or suppressor gene inactivation can result in malignant tumor formation. It is generally felt that multiple genetic alterations are required for the progression to malignancy, with each subsequent "hit" increasing the

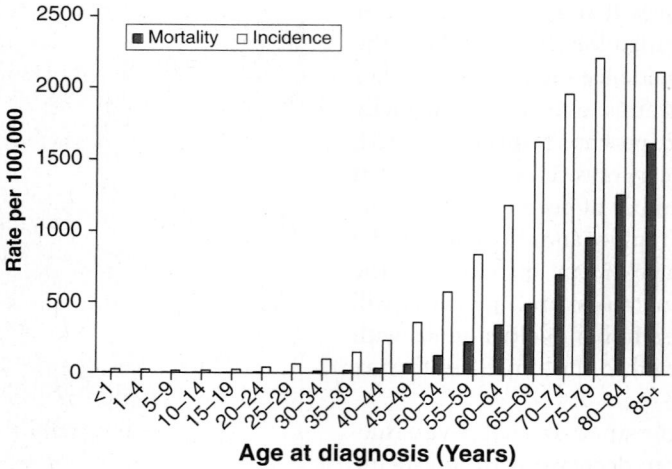

FIGURE 88-1. Comparison of the percentage of total cancer incidence and mortality by age with age-specific incidence and mortality. (Data from SEER Cancer Statistics Review; 2013–2017: National Center for Health Statistics; 2014–2018.)

likelihood of malignancy. It has become apparent in recent years that while gene alterations are important in this process, changes in the environment in which these cells live plays a critical role in neoplastic evolution. This may be of particular importance in the aging/cancer relationship as will be discussed further below.

There are several theories on how the aging process influences the process of neoplastic transformation to result in the markedly increased rates of cancer in older adults. These include the following:

1. Longer duration of carcinogenic exposure: It is possible that aging simply allows the time necessary for the accumulation of cellular events to develop into a clinical neoplasm. There is evidence for age-related accumulation and expression of genetic damage. Somatic mutations are believed to occur at the rate of approximately 1 in 10 cell divisions, with approximately 10 cell divisions occurring in a lifetime of a human being. Certainly, the complex set of events required in the multistep process of carcinogenesis, for example, as described for colon cancer in humans, does occur over time. The passage of time alone, however, is not likely to explain the entire cancer phenomenon. The time required for a mutated cell to become a malignant cell and then subsequently to become a detectable tumor has been estimated to be approximately 10% to 30% of the maximum lifespan for a given animal species, which may vary from just a few years to more than 100 years.

2. Altered susceptibility of aging cells to carcinogens: Data regarding carcinogen exposure are contradictory. In some cases, the incidence of skin tumors in mice produced with benzpyrene has been more related to dose than to age, whereas in other models, accelerated carcinogenesis as a function of age has been demonstrated, as, for example, when dimethylbenzanthracene (DMA) was applied to skin grafts of young and old mice. An age-related increase in the sensitivity of lymphocytes to cell-cycle arrest and chromosome damage after radiation has been demonstrated. It is also possible that there are alterations in carcinogen metabolism with age, but the findings from such studies have also been contradictory.

3. Decreased ability to repair DNA: It is possible that damage, once initiated, is more difficult to repair in older cells. A number of studies demonstrate decreased DNA repair as a function of age following damage by carcinogens as well as radiation. Such repair failures may also be reflected in increased karyotype abnormalities in aged normal cells as well as in older patients with neoplastic disease.

4. Oncogene activation or amplification or decrease in tumor-suppressor gene activity: These processes might be increased in the older adult, resulting either in increased action or promotion or in differential clonal evolution. Although evidence is currently limited, there have been observations of increased amplification of proto-oncogenes and their products in aging fibroblasts in vitro as well as evidence for increased c-myc transcript levels in the livers of aging mice. Alternatively, such factors as genetic alterations or DNA damage could lead to inactivation of cancer-suppressor genes. Given that age-related mutations frequently appear to result in the loss of function, alterations in tumor-suppressor genes may prove to be an important mechanism.

5. Telomere shortening and genetic instability: The function of telomeres and the enzyme telomerase appears to be intimately involved in both the senescence and neoplasia processes. Telomeres, the terminal end of all chromosomes, shorten progressively as cells age. This functional decline begins at age 30 and continues at a loss of approximately 1% per year. Because the major function of telomeres is to protect the stability of the more internal coding sequences, that is, allow cells to divide without losing genes; the loss of this function may lead to genetic instability, which may promote mutations in oncogenic or tumor-suppressor gene sequences. Without telomeres, chromosome ends could fuse together and degrade the cells' genetic blueprint, making the cell malfunction, become cancerous, or even die.

6. Cellular senescence and the microenvironment: Older adults have been shown to accumulate senescent cells as shown by β-galactosidase staining and other methods. A number of factors in the tumor microenvironment are critical for the development of the malignant phenotype, especially invasion and metastasis. There is accumulating evidence showing that senescent cells can have deleterious effects on the tissue microenvironment. The most significant of these effects is the acquisition of a "senescence-associated secretory phenotype" (SASP) that turns senescent fibroblasts into proinflammatory cells (secreting factors such as inflammatory cytokines like IL-1 and IL-6) and epithelial growth factors (eg, heregulin and matrix metalloproteinases like MMP-3), which can have the ability to promote tumor progression. A variety of stresses can provoke cellular senescence and include telomere dysfunction resulting from repeated cell division (termed replicative senescence), mitochondrial deterioration, oxidative stress, severe or irreparable DNA damage and chromatin disruption (genotoxic stress), and the expression of certain oncogenes (oncogene-induced senescence). These stresses can be induced by external or internal chemical and physical insults encountered during the course of the lifespan, during therapeutic interventions (eg, radiation or chemotherapy), or as a consequence of endogenous processes such as oxidative respiration and mitogenic signals.

In early life, cellular senescence suppresses cancer by arresting cells at risk of malignant transformation. However, their ability to promote carcinogenesis in later life as described above suggests that the senescence response is antagonistically pleiotropic. Thus, a function important for the organism in early life (through the reproductive period) will be selected for, despite the fact that it may be quite injurious in later life. In this sense senescence could be viewed as the price we pay in later life for the rigorous attempt to control proliferation to avoid neoplasia early on. Recently drugs that destroy or inhibit senescent cells (senolytics) have been studied for their potential to delay aging and age-related diseases such as cancer.

7. Decreased immune surveillance: A decrease in immune surveillance, or immunosenescence, could contribute to the increased incidence of malignancies. In animal models there is a considerable amount of evidence for a loss of tumor-specific immunity with progressive age. This includes the altered capacity of old mice to reject transplanted tumors, the close relationship between susceptibility to malignant melanomas and the rate of age-related T-cell–dependent immune function decline, and the ability by immunopharmacologic manipulation to increase age-depressed tumoricidal immune function and to decrease the incidence of spontaneous tumors. The evidence linking such data to age-associated immune deficiency and the rise of cancer incidence in humans, however, is mainly circumstantial and not likely to be fully explanatory, as the types of tumors seen in the most striking examples of immune deficiency are very different from those seen in the usual aging human.

Figure 88-2 summarizes in a schematic fashion the potential interaction of these many factors that may be

of importance in the increase of cancer with age. It indicates the interface of time- and age-related events, such as free radical and other carcinogenic exposure, resulting in initiation, then cumulative promoting events, including mutations and other alterations in critical genes, which ultimately exceed a threshold of host resistance factors, which have been progressively reduced during the aging process.

CLINICAL PRESENTATIONS AND DISEASE BEHAVIOR

Screening in Asymptomatic Individuals

Older adults continue to be both underscreened and thus underdiagnosed with cancer, as well as overscreened and placed at increased risk of overtreatment. It is well known that mammography and Papanicolaou (Pap) tests are underutilized in certain older racial and ethnic minority groups, and in those who have less than high school education or live below the poverty level. On the other hand, there is general agreement that routine cancer screening has little likelihood to result in a net benefit for individuals with limited life expectancy. Despite this a number of studies have continued to show that screening is common in individuals with less than 5-year life expectancy, and even in many in nursing homes with severe disability who could likely not benefit from treatment. Cancer screening in such patients not only has implications for utilization of health care resources in a setting unlikely to result in net benefit but may also cause net patient harm owing to subsequent

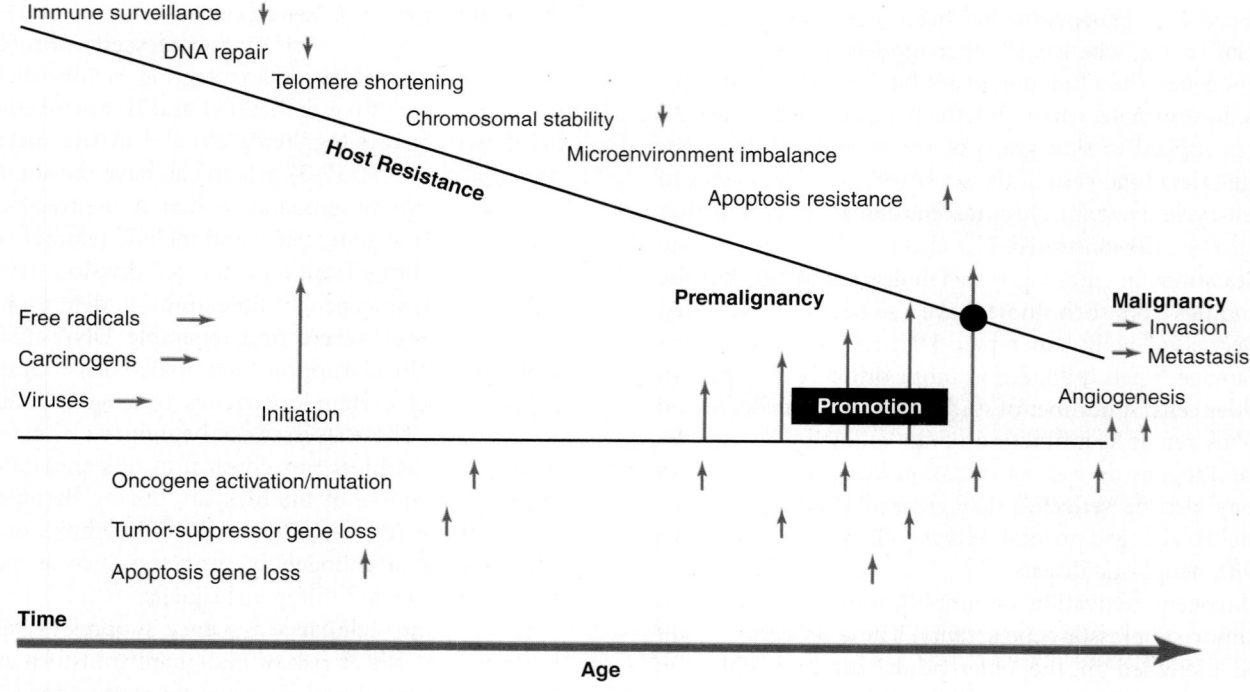

FIGURE 88-2. Age and cancer susceptibility. This figure presents a model incorporating the various factors that may play a role in the increased incidence of cancer with age.

diagnostic procedures and overtreatment. A general approach to screening that may help avoid these problems is discussed in Chapter 12, and approaches in specific tumor types are discussed in Chapters 38 and 89 to 93.

Initial Presentation

As an extension of the screening concept, the goal for initial cancer detection is to make the diagnosis as early as possible, with the hope that treatment at the earliest stages of disease would yield the best survival rates. It is, therefore, of great importance that both patient and physician pay attention to symptoms that may herald the onset of the neoplastic process. Current evidence suggests that once having noticed a symptom that appears to be related to cancer, most older individuals do not delay appreciably in seeking medical help. In one study from New Mexico of 800 patients over 65 years, only 29% of the subjects were asymptomatic when cancer was detected, and 48% presented within 2 months of symptom onset. However, 19% of the subjects delayed seeking care for at least 12 weeks and 7.4% delayed at least 1 year. Older women, who are at greater risk of developing breast cancer, are also more likely to delay their presentation. Physicians may also play a role in delaying further diagnostic pursuits in older patients. Part of the problem may lie in a failure to recognize some of the new signs and symptoms in patients with multiple disease processes. It is easy to attribute such symptoms as anorexia, weight loss, or decrease in performance status to social or psychological changes. The increasing prevalence of findings such as anemia in older patients may lower the index of suspicion for attributing the factor to a new specific neoplastic process. Hence, symptom awareness and appraisal by patients and doctor is an important determinant of timely presentation and investigation, although it must be balanced by judgment concerning the risk-benefit ratio for diagnostic evaluations in individual patients depending on their other medical status. For example, the initial discovery of a new symptom in a previously totally well, active 80-year-old may be pursued rather differently than a similar discovery in a severely demented, bedbound individual with severe congestive heart failure, diabetes, and pulmonary failure.

Biological Behavior of Tumors in the Older Host

The effect of the aging process on the clinical course of cancer, or to put it another way, whether cancer behaves differently in the older individual, is not clear cut. Although the SEER data noted previously suggested that in many cancers the 5-year survival rate is lower for older people, it is possible that this is related more to comorbid disease and other factors rather than simply to aging per se. On the other hand, there is a widespread belief that cancers may behave more indolently in older patients. These are important issues because they may to a considerable degree, affect decisions regarding treatment. Both clinical and experimental evidence support both sides of this issue, and it is likely that there is a spectrum of responses dependent on initial tumor types as well as individual host status. One indicator of the phenomenon is the extent of disease at presentation. For most cancers examined, there has been no consistent difference in the stage of disease or presentation for different age groups. For those that have been determined, the directions are not always the same. For malignant melanoma, older patients have been consistently found to have more advanced-stage local disease with deeper penetrating lesions at presentation. For breast cancer, some studies show a greater proportion of older patients with distant metastatic spread at presentation, whereas for lung cancer the opposite has been found, and older patients have been noted to present with localized disease in a greater proportion of cases. Uterine and cervical cancers have in some cases been noted to be later in the course of disease at presentation in older individuals. Of course, even these differences might be related to such phenomena as delay in the patient's presenting for diagnosis, delay in pursuing the diagnosis, intensity of diagnostic endeavors, or a combination of these factors, or, on the other hand, a greater chance for a serendipitous finding because of more frequent visits to physicians.

Another biological factor that may influence neoplastic behavior in differently aged hosts is the histologic subtype of the tumor. Thus, while thyroid cancer overall appears to behave more aggressively in the older host, it is also true that a larger proportion of thyroid neoplasia in older patients is made up by anaplastic carcinoma, which at any age has more aggressive behavior. Similarly, for malignant melanoma, although there is an increased proportion of older people who have melanomas of poor prognostic histologic type and location at presentation, older individuals have a poorer prognosis for survival than do younger ones independent of this phenomenon even for localized disease. Such biological differences may be manifested in other ways, as in the case of breast cancer, in which older women have an increased frequency of estrogen receptor–positive breast cancer, probably related to hormonal influences of the postmenopausal state. An additional factor is the longer tumor doubling time seen in breast cancer cells from older women. Because estrogen receptor (ER) positivity and longer doubling times are associated with better prognosis, with more slow-growing tumors, and with longer disease-free survivals, these phenomena, rather than age per se, might provide the reason why this cancer appears to behave more indolently in an older individual. Despite this, overall cancer-related survival is lower in older women, emphasizing the complex interactions of tumor and host that must be considered.

Acute myelogenous leukemia (AML) has a much poorer prognosis in older patients and the biology underlying the poor prognosis and poor treatment outcome of AML in the older adult has been extensively studied. Among the findings to date are a high incidence of poor-prognosis karyotypes (5q-, 7q-), high frequency of preceding myelodysplastic syndromes, and an increased expression of proteins involved in intrinsic resistance to chemotherapeutic agents.

Compared to younger patients, leukemic blasts from older patients with AML had a lower propensity to apoptosis following traditional remission-induction treatment with ara-C and daunorubicin. Gene-expression studies have demonstrated that older AML patients tend to have worse survival compared to their younger counterparts which may be driven in part by an increased expression of ras, src, and tumor necrosis factor (TNF) pathways in the bone marrow of older patients.

Experimental data in animal models likewise show this spectrum in rate of tumor growth and progression as a function of age. In these studies, the ability to contain tumor growth depends on the particular host tumor system used, thus mimicking the clinical situation to some extent. A proposed explanation for the situation in which the older host more effectively controls the rate of tumor is a paradoxical effect of decreasing immune function with age, that is, decreased activity of those cells in the old host's immune system, which, under the stimulation of the neoplastic process, produce tumor-enhancing factors such as angiogenesis factor. When this occurs, tumor growth might be expected to be diminished. To what extent these various factors play a role in the biological behavior of neoplasia in the human aging host remains a fascinating puzzle to be unraveled.

MANAGEMENT

General Principles

Balancing the benefits and risks of cancer treatment in older patients is challenging because of the dearth of high-quality, evidence-based studies. Older adults, especially those with age-associated vulnerabilities, remain vastly underrepresented in research that sets the standards for the safety and efficacy of cancer treatments. This lack of evidence puts this group at high risk of clinical uncertainty that leads to both under- and overtreatment.

To help inform treatment decisions, expert panels and guidelines have been developed regarding the practical assessment and management of older patients with cancer. In this section, we will review the general approach that treating physician should consider when caring for older patients with cancer. We discuss the Comprehensive Geriatric Model framework, which accounts for biological, psychological, social, and treatment factors involved in the patient's well-being, and highlight the need to individualize treatment decisions. We also review use of biological and clinical markers in the evaluation of older adults with cancer and discuss the role of aging-directed interventions in improving treatment for this rapidly growing population.

The Comprehensive Geriatric Model

Physicians cannot rely on chronological age alone when making decisions related to the treatment of older patients with cancer. Aging is a heterogeneous process that is not captured by chronological age. There is substantial heterogeneity in the physiologic and functional characteristics of older persons. We proposed one framework in which the general aspects of treatment decision-making can be considered for the individual older patients with cancer. This is shown in **Figure 88-3** and is called the Comprehensive Geriatric Model. It graphically presents a number of the concepts critical to the care of the older adult, that is, that there is a decreased functional reserve and that, as an extension of Engel's Bio-Psycho-Social Model, all of these various aspects of the individual's background must be taken into account when making decisions about the new process, that is, the cancer. Each of these levels, for example, biological or psychosocial, can create interactions that influence both the cancer and the host, and, likewise, any intervention directed at the cancer may influence both the cancer and each of these levels of the host's function. Conversely, each of these levels of function, when compromised by the aging process or other comorbid diseases, may influence the ability to deliver these various interventions. Thus, in a sense, a conceptual checklist is presented in which a four-way interaction of various factors can be systematically considered when making decisions. Examples of ways in which physiologic changes occurring with age can impact on cancer treatment are shown in **Table 88-1**.

Biological Markers of Aging

Attempts to characterize or measure the cellular and molecular level of change that occurs with aging and that might be usefully applied in the context of cancer have been explored. However, it has been difficult to identify biological measurements that accurately reflect individual's physiological or functional age. Many biomarkers of aging have been studied, although no single biomarker or combination of biomarkers has been sensitive or specific enough to accurately assess the physiologic aging process.

The most widely studied biomarkers of aging have been markers of inflammation. Aging is associated with increased levels of circulating cytokines and proinflammatory markers. Age-related changes in the immune system, that is, immunosenescence, and increased secretion of cytokines by adipose tissue, can lead to a state of chronic inflammation or "inflammaging." High levels of IL-6, IL-1, TNF-α, and C-reactive protein in older adults are associated with increased risk of morbidity and mortality. In particular, cohort studies in older subjects have indicated that increased TNF-α and IL-6 levels are associated with frailty as well as several cancer-related symptom complexes including cachexia, fatigue, poor performance status, and cognitive issues.

Markers of cellular senescence, such as p16INKa, a component of the cell cycle, has been shown to increase with chronological age and chemotherapy exposure in patients with breast cancer. This may represent a promising biomarker that links aging, cancer, and cancer treatment.

Epigenetic age or clock, an estimation of biological age using DNA-methylation based biomarkers, may also

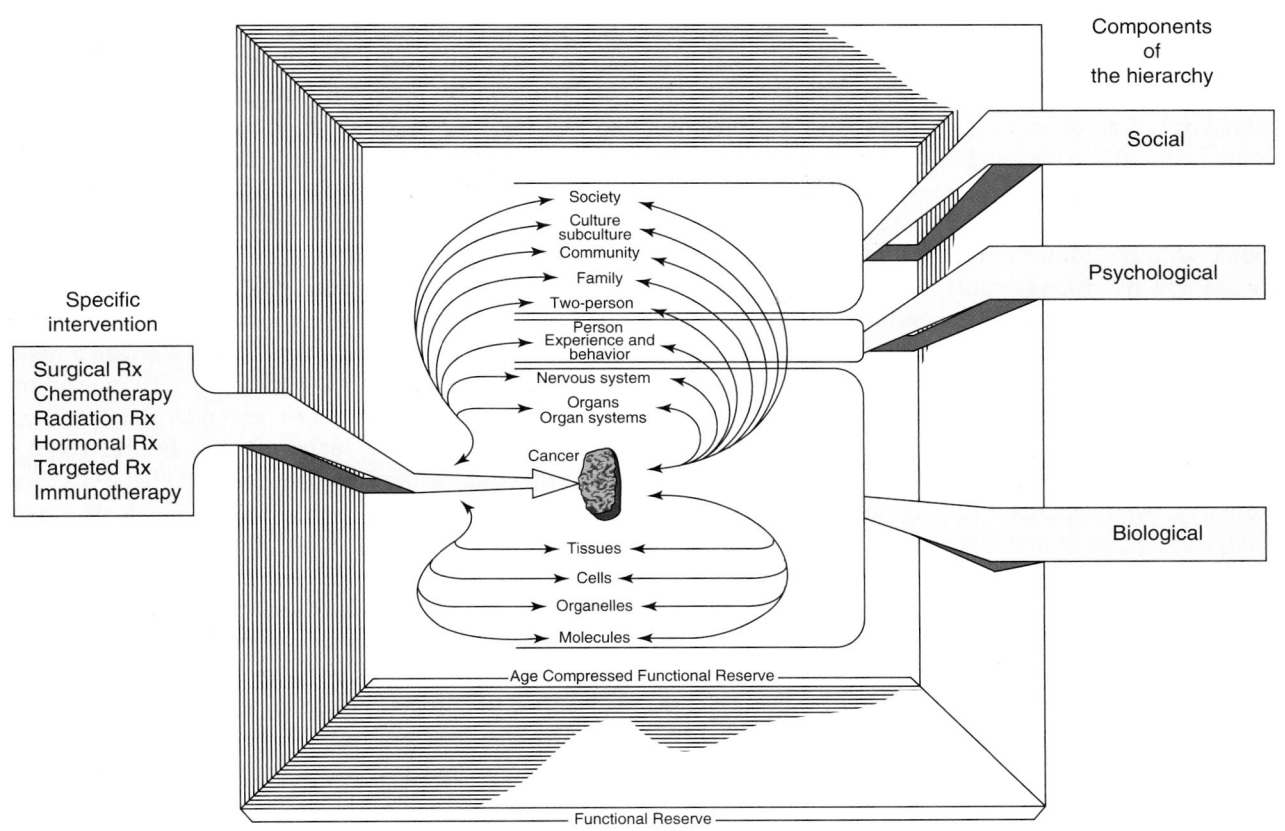

FIGURE 88-3. The Comprehensive Geriatric Model. (Modified with permission from Lazlo J. *Physician's Guide to Cancer Care Complications*. New York, NY: Dekker; 1986.)

be an important assessment of biological aging in cancer. Individuals with epigenetic age that surpasses their chronological age have an increased risk of all-cause mortality, even after adjusting for other risk factors. However, more research is needed, to enhance our understanding of biological measures of aging that are clinically meaningful, reliable, and feasible to obtain in older patients with cancer.

Clinical Markers of Aging

In the absence of an easily measurable or precise marker of aging, clinical tools remain the gold standard for evaluating an individual's functional and physiologic status in older patients with cancer. The multidimensional CGA (as described in detail in Chapter 8) has been demonstrated to be feasible in both daily clinical practice and oncology clinical trials, and the American Society of Clinical Oncology (ASCO), the National Comprehensive Cancer Network (NCCN), and the International Society of Geriatric Oncology (SIOG) have all recommended performing a CGA in all older patients with cancer receiving systemic therapy.

Traditionally in oncology, performance status (PS) is used as an attempt to quantify cancer patients' general well-being and is also utilized to determine whether they can receive chemotherapy. The most commonly used measure, the Eastern Cooperative Oncology Group (ECOG) PS runs from 0 to 5, with 0 denoting perfect health and 5, death. However, in the geriatric oncology population, it has been demonstrated that ECOG PS alone is not sufficient, and CGA adds substantial information to the functional

TABLE 88-1 ■ AGING PHYSIOLOGY AND CANCER	
AGING PHYSIOLOGY	**CANCER RELEVANCE**
Cardiopulmonary ↓ Max CO, VO$_2$ max ↓ Elasticity	Surgery C/P toxic drugs
Skin—↓ wound healing	Surgery
CNS—↓ brain weight, cerebral blood flow	Patient interactions CNS toxic drugs
Special senses—↓ taste, smell, salivary flow	Nutrition radiation therapy
Hematopoiesis—↓ response under stress	Chemotherapy and radiation therapy
Immune system—↓ response	Infection
Body composition—↓ lean, ↑ fat	Drug distribution
Liver—↓ mass and flow	Hepatic drug metabolism
Kidney—↓ GFR	Renal drug excretion

CNS, central nervous system; C/P, cardiopulmonary; GFR, glomerular filtration rate.

assessment of older cancer patients, including patients with a good ECOG PS.

The CGA has proved very useful in assessing the functional age of an older adult. It can uncover problems that would not otherwise be identified by routine history and physical or by the traditional oncology performance status tools. A CGA comprises several domains, including functional status, comorbidities that may interfere with cancer therapy, nutritional status, polypharmacy, psychological and cognitive status, socioeconomic issues, and geriatric syndromes. The CGA identifies clinically significant aging-related problems, such as risk for falls and cognitive impairment.

The CGA can identify patients age 65 or older at increased risk of experiencing chemotherapy toxicity. In one study, by the Cancer and Aging Research Group (CARG), geriatric assessment variables along with sociodemographics, tumor/treatment variables, and laboratory test results were incorporated into a model that would predict for chemotherapy toxicity in older adults. This model identified older adults at low (0–5 points; 30%), intermediate (6–9 points; 52%), or high risk (10–19 points; 83%) of chemotherapy toxicity ($p < 0.001$). In another study the Chemotherapy Risk Assessment Scale for High-Age Patients (CRASH) determined that patients with low-risk scores had only a 7% chance of hematologic and 33% chance of nonhematologic toxicity compared to high-risk patients, who had a 100% risk of hematologic and 93% risk of nonhematologic toxicity from chemotherapy.

To identify patients who are likely to benefit from undergoing a CGA, a series of screening instruments have been designed and evaluated in older cancer patients as listed in **Table 88-2**. These screening tools can be easily performed by health care providers in a busy clinical setting. A complete assessment can be performed after screening and one that is increasingly being used in North America in clinical trials performed by cooperative groups, includes measures reflecting the domains of a CGA. The geriatric assessment tool primarily consisted of self-reported measures, which were completed by the patient. Three items were completed by the health care professional. The median time to complete the CGA tool was 22 minutes, and 87% of patients completed their portion without assistance.

CGA-Guided Interventions

Although high-quality data support the use of the CGA to identify geriatric syndromes and to predict mortality and chemotherapy toxicity, evidence supporting the implementation of CGA-guided processes for informing cancer treatment has been limited. Recent randomized clinical trials have assessed the effectiveness of CGA-guided interventions for older adults with cancer. In one study, a cluster randomized controlled trial in community practices, investigators analyzed the effect of providing oncologists CGA-guided recommendations on treatment-related

toxicity in patients aged 70 or older with advanced cancers and at least one geriatric deficit or syndrome. Forty-one practices, which included 718 patients, were randomized to the CGA intervention or to usual oncologist-directed care alone. Findings revealed that the intervention arm had an absolute reduction in toxicity of 20% when compared with the usual care arm. Another study, a single-center randomized controlled trial, examined the effect of a multidisciplinary team (MDT) CGA-guided intervention on treatment-related toxicity in patients 65 years or older with solid tumors (any stage) starting a new line of chemotherapy. Patients in the intervention arm underwent a CGA that was then reviewed by the MDT, which implemented tailored interventions. In the usual care arm, the treating oncologist received the CGA results, but no interventions were implemented. In the 620 patients randomized, a 10% reduction in chemotherapy toxicity was observed in the intervention arm compared with the usual care arm. These studies demonstrate that CGA-guided interventions can in fact lead to decreased treatment toxicity and improve key outcomes for older patients with cancer. However, more effort is needed to address the barriers to widespread implementation of geriatric oncology care, including health care system-level organizational issues, lack of time, limited staffing, lack of training and familiarity with available tools, and unclear reimbursement rules.

MAJOR THERAPEUTIC MODALITIES

Surgery

Surgery and other invasive procedures are frequently involved in initial diagnostic as well as in therapeutic approaches to the older adult with cancer. An increased number of comorbid medical conditions, decreased wound healing, and lack of physiologic reserve contribute to both prolonged hospital stay and rehabilitation following operative treatment. All phases of healing are compromised by the aging process. Both the inflammatory and proliferative responses are decreased, remodeling occurs to a lesser degree, and the collagen formed is qualitatively different from that in younger individuals. Normally, the repair process initiated by inflammation requires intact sensory nerves that stimulate increased blood flow and growth factor production. The loss of sensory neurons and the coexistence of other medical conditions, such as diabetes and vascular disease, contribute to delayed wound healing. Additionally, complications are more common when surgical intervention is performed on an emergency basis. Often, it is more appropriate to perform an operation as a preventive measure when dealing with older populations; for example, a hemicolectomy may be performed—even for patients with advanced colorectal cancer—to prevent the need for an emergency operation to treat bowel perforation or obstruction. Increasingly CGA and geriatric comanagement are being applied to the evaluation and preparation

TABLE 88-2 ■ COMPARISONS OF VARIOUS SCREENING COMPREHENSIVE GERIATRIC ASSESSMENT (CGA) METHODOLOGIES

INSTRUMENT	METHOD	SCORING	INTERPRETATION	REMARKS
G8	Interview	Total score 17	Score 0–14 = presence of geriatric risk profile Score > 14 = absence of geriatric risk profile	Takes 2–3 min to complete screening
Groningen Frailty Indicator (GFI)	Conducting screening tests on patient	Total score 15	Score 0–3 = absence of geriatric risk profile Score 4–15 = presence of geriatric risk profile	Circle answers and use specific scoring rules set by the test
Vulnerable Elders Survey 13 (VES-13)	Self-report and interview	Total score 10	Score 0–2 = absence of vulnerability Score 3–10 = presence of vulnerability	Takes less than 5 min to complete
Senior Adult Oncology Program 2 (SAOP2)	Self-report and interview	N/A	If one item is positive: respective specialist consulted If several items impaired: geriatric referral for MDT	Clinic staff administers last page of interview
Abbreviated CGA (aCGA)	Interview 3 questions about ADLs 4 questions about IADLs 4 questions from the MMSE 4 questions from the GDS		GDS score ≥ 2: complete full 15-item GDS ADLs: any impairment: complete full ADLs IADLs: any impairment: complete full IADLs Cognitive screening score ≤ 6: complete full MMSE	

ADLs, activities of daily living; GDS, Geriatric Depression Scale; IADL, instrumental activities of daily living; MDT, multidisciplinary team; MMSE, Mini Mental State Examination.

PART V — **ORGAN SYSTEMS AND DISEASES**

of older patients for surgery as well as to guide postoperative management. Geriatric comanagement can lead to improved 90-day postoperative mortality. The American Geriatrics Society Task Force and the American College of Surgeons provide general guidelines for older adults undergoing surgery and these may be applied to older patients with cancer undergoing surgery.

Radiation Therapy

Radiation therapy (RT) can be used in the older adults with cancer with both curative and palliative intent. RT is also used as an effective adjunct to surgery or chemotherapy or both. The International Society of Geriatric Oncology (SIOG) Task Force has put forth guidelines for best practices in radiation oncology in older adults. Per these guidelines, patient selection should include comorbidity and geriatric evaluation. In older adults with breast cancer, shorter courses of hypofractionated whole breast RT are safe and effective. In patients with non-small-cell lung cancer (NSCLC), conformal radiotherapy and involved field techniques without elective nodal irradiation have improved outcomes without increasing toxicity. If comorbidities preclude surgery, stereotactic body radiotherapy (SBRT) is an option for early stage NSCLC and pancreatic cancer. For patients with lymphoma, involved field radiotherapy (IFRT) may be based on pretreatment positron emission tomography (PET) data to reduce toxicity. For patients with intermediate-risk prostate cancer, 4 to 6 months of hormonal therapy combined with external-beam radiotherapy (EBRT) may be an option. Short-course EBRT is an alternative to combined modality therapy in older patients with rectal cancer without significant comorbidities. Endorectal RT may be an option for early stage disease. For primary brain tumors shorter courses of postoperative RT following maximal debulking provides equivalent survival to longer schedules. Stereotactic RT provides an alternative to whole-brain RT in patients with limited brain metastases. Intensity-modulated radiotherapy provides an excellent technique to reduce dose to the carotids in head and neck cancer and improves locoregional control in esophageal cancer. It is crucial to monitor older patients receiving radiation since the effects of radiation on normal tissue may be enhanced by 10% to 15% in the older patient. Radiation to the oral pharynx and oral cavity can produce a loss of taste, dryness of mucous membranes, and involution of salivary glands, which when combined with a precarious nutritional intake in a frail and older individual might be lethal, or certainly contribute a considerable amount of morbidity, if not recognized. Moreover, if daily treatment is tolerated poorly, owing to nausea or weakness, treatment may be compromised because of the decreased daily doses, the patient's unscheduled absences, or decrease in the total planned dose. Pulmonary complications such as severe radiation pneumonitis have been noted to occur more frequently in older adults with lung cancer versus younger patients, regardless of radiation field size and concurrent therapies. Depression, disabling fatigue, and cognitive decline are potential side effects of whole-brain RT.

Systemic Therapy

Chemotherapy A thorough discussion of the principles of pharmacology in older adults can be found in Chapter 22. Although still understudied, in recent years there have been more direct studies of the effect of age on the pharmacokinetics of orally or parenterally administered chemotherapeutic agents. Changes in organ function with age and the declining ability of senescent cells to repair DNA damage increase the incidence and severity of chemotherapy-related toxicity. For example, increased destruction of and lower numbers of rapidly renewing mucosal stem cells increase susceptibility to mucositis. Reduced hematopoietic stem cell reserve may both worsen the severity and slow recovery of cytopenias.

When oral agents are used, despite delayed gastric emptying, absorption is adequate but one must pay attention to concomitant medications like H_2 blockers, antacids, and proton pump inhibitors. Caution must be exercised when administering cytotoxic drugs like methotrexate, bleomycin, cisplatin, and ifosfamide. Both decreases in the number of nephrons and a decline in the glomerular filtration rate may contribute to excess toxicity. Also, there is a decrease in lean body mass in the older adult, thus, adjusting the dose based on a creatinine clearance and not merely the creatinine is very important. In addition, concomitant administration of drugs like nonsteroidal anti-inflammatory drugs may compromise renal function. Although the reasons are unclear, acute toxicities like nausea and vomiting occur less frequently in older patients; however, the lack of functional reserve can lead to catastrophic outcomes quickly, that is, dehydration and renal insufficiency. Neurotoxicity secondary to taxanes, platinum agents, vincristine, high-dose cytarabine, and bortezomib; cardiotoxicity from doxorubicin; and mucositis from 5-fluorouracil are all more common and severe in older patients.

Despite this knowledge, there is a persistent lack of prospective data for older patients, particularly for those patients older than 80 years, in cancer treatment clinical trials. However, the SIOG Task Force has published guidelines for dose modification of chemotherapy in older patients with renal insufficiency and has reviewed the use of certain classes of drugs: alkylators, antimetabolites, anthracyclines, taxanes, camptothecins, and epipodophyllotoxins. As described previously, a CGA is helpful when incorporated with other parameters to predict for the risk of toxicity in older adults.

Hormonal therapy Older women are more likely to have ER-positive tumors and approximately 70% to 80% of all breast tumors in older patients express ER. Thus, tamoxifen,

and aromatase inhibitors like anastrozole and letrozole have been used widely in the neoadjuvant, adjuvant, and metastatic setting. These drugs each have their own side effects. The well-known higher risk of thromboembolic events and cerebrovascular accidents reported with tamoxifen should be taken into account when proposing this treatment to a patient already suffering from severe peripheral venous insufficiency, hypertension, and/or atrial fibrillation. On the other hand, because of the increased risk of osteoporosis and bone fractures with aromatase inhibitors, fracture risk should be assessed and recommendation with regard to exercise and calcium/vitamin D supplementation given. Bone-directed therapy should be given to all patients with a T score less than −2.0 standard deviations (SD), or with a T score less than −1.5 SD with one additional risk factor, or with two or more risk factors (without bone mineral density). Androgen-deprivation therapy with luteinizing hormone–releasing hormone (LHRH) agonists and antiandrogens is used in older men with prostate cancer. Side effects of impotence, breast tenderness, hot flashes, osteoporosis, and memory decline are common with these agents.

Targeted Therapies

There has been an exponential increase in both the approval and use of targeted therapeutic agents in the past decade due to "precision medicine." Precision medicine aims to target a specific genetic alteration with a specific drug. This tailored approach includes many drugs that are oral including tyrosine kinase inhibitors, mammalian target of rapamycin inhibitors, drugs targeted to the human epidermal growth factor receptor 2, and BRAF-mutation targeted drugs. While, there have not been dedicated clinical trials for use among older adults, the data have been extrapolated from larger trials in which older patients generally were a fraction of the participants. Many of these agents are orally administered, and older patients with comorbidities often are on many other medications, which may be metabolized by the cytochrome P450 liver enzymes. Thus, the treating oncologist, geriatrician, and primary care physician should be aware and prepare for significant drug interactions when these new agents are taken concomitantly with P450 inhibitors or inducers. One study has demonstrated that comorbidities and polypharmacy impacted cytogenetic response rates in older adults with chronic myeloid leukemia being treated with imatinib. In addition, while these drugs have a favorable safety profile compared to parenteral chemotherapy, there is still a risk of toxicity, leading to a higher rate of dose reduction and discontinuation among older versus younger patients.

Immunotherapy

Immunotherapy is one of the newest treatments that has revolutionized cancer care. Immunotherapy uses the body's own immune system to recognize and kill cancer cells. Cancer cells manipulate immune checkpoints evading cell death. One of the main types of immunotherapy are immune checkpoint inhibitors (ICIs, eg, pembrolizumab, nivolumab, ipilimumab, atezolizumab). ICIs block the checkpoint between the tumor cells and regulatory T cells that would result in downregulation of activated T cells, thereby upregulating T-cell activity. ICIs treat many cancer types including melanoma and lung, bladder, colorectal, and renal cell carcinoma, among others. While there are many new ICIs available, clinical trials predominantly include younger and the most healthy adults, limiting the generalizability of outcomes to older adults. The most common side effects are fatigue, rash, itching, diarrhea, and elevated liver function tests. One main issue is the occurrence of immune-related adverse events (irAEs). irAEs can affect almost every organ in the body due to dysregulation of the immune system causing colitis, pneumonitis, hepatitis, rash, thyroiditis, arthritis, myocarditis, and hypophysitis among others. While some irAEs can be mild, a subset can be severe requiring high-dose steroids and hospitalizations. Due to a proinflammatory aging host environment, termed "inflammaging", the concern is that older adults are at higher risk for irAEs. Recent data demonstrate equivalent incidence of high-grade irAEs, but worse overall survival among older adults regardless of cancer type who experience high-grade irAEs versus young adults with metastatic cancer. This may be due to side effects from the treatment of high-grade irAEs (steroids and hospitalization), which are often much less tolerated in older adults. Though a potential risk, the use of immunotherapy in general is producing durable long-term survival for some patients with advanced cancer.

Hematopoietic Stem Cell Transplantation

Hematopoietic stem cell transplantation (HSCT) is a widely utilized treatment modality for high-risk hematologic malignancies. Historically, the associated morbidity and mortality limited the use of allogeneic SCT to individuals age less than 50. However, autologous SCT for lymphoma and myeloma has been performed in fit patients older than 70 years. There are no guidelines for HSCT in older adults so, patient selection, choice of conditioning regimen, immunosuppression, stem cell source is arbitrary and may be based on cardiopulmonary and hepatorenal function. Risk-assessment tools such as a CGA, and comorbidity measures have recently been applied to facilitate decisions regarding HSCT eligibility and tolerance. Reduced-intensity conditioning (RIC) for allogeneic HCT, has led to improved tolerance and decreased mortality and removed traditional age barriers. RIC regimens may vary in the degree of immunosuppression and myeloablation and transplant-related mortality is typically lower than myeloablative approaches. Another important issue is donor selection for older recipients. Older patients tend to have older human leukocyte antigen (HLA)-matched siblings, raising issues about the upper age or health limitations for donor collection since older donor age slightly diminishes

hematopoietic stem cell yields. Numerous other geriatric domains such as nutrition, caregiver support, and cognitive assessment have not been evaluated in the setting of HSCT. For example, delirium occurs in up to 50% of allogeneic HSCT recipients and likely more often among older adults and needs further study.

Palliative and Supportive Care

Palliative care focuses on providing patients with relief from the symptoms caused by the cancer itself or cancer treatment with the goal of improving quality of life for both the patient and caregiver. Older adults frequently underreport their symptoms, which requires routine and early symptom assessment by the treating cancer team. In fact, routine symptom assessment and intervention can improve overall survival upwards of 5 months without any change to cancer treatment. Many of the specific aspects of supportive care are covered in other chapters and are only mentioned here to stress its importance in the comprehensive management of the older adults with cancer. These include the extreme importance of effective pain management (Chapter 68); maintenance of appropriate nutritional support (Chapter 32); the supportive role of nursing (Chapter 14); the importance of patient, physician, and family discussions regarding end-of-life care and other issues (Chapters 67, 71, and 72); and the utility of hospice care (Chapter 70).

Nausea and vomiting One complication frequently seen in treatment of the older adult with cancer is nausea and vomiting. These side effects can seriously compromise the ability to deliver effective chemotherapy, but also cause significant morbidity (eg, dehydration and renal insufficiency). All older adults on chemotherapy should focus on hydration and environmental factors, such as food and other odors that may trigger vomiting. Patients can try eating smaller portions of food but more frequently to meet caloric needs and drinking clear, cooler beverages. Patients can try saltier rather than sweet foods and those that are low in fat for easier digestion. Antiemetic drugs have improved substantially and are routinely given for all types of chemotherapy, many types of oral targeted treatments, radiation depending on location, and surgery. Corticosteroids are a useful adjunct to most antiemetic regimens that include benzamides (eg, metoclopramide), butyrophenones (eg, haloperidol), benzodiazepines (eg, lorazepam), and serotonin ($5HT_3$) antagonists such as ondansetron, palonosetron, and dolasetron. One recent study evaluated the comparative efficacy and tolerability of palonosetron and ondansetron/dolasetron in a retrospective post hoc analysis using pooled data from 171 older adults (age $\geq$ 65) with cancer enrolled in two randomized, double-blind, phase III clinical studies comparing single intravenous doses of these antiemetic agents given prior to receipt of moderately emetogenic chemotherapy. Palonosetron was more effective in controlling chemotherapy-induced nausea and vomiting in older adults. Avoidance of constipation is also a key component of both prevention and management of nausea and vomiting. Chemotherapeutic drugs like vincristine, vinblastine, thalidomide, and opioids can also cause severe obstipation necessitating a good bowel regimen with stool softeners and laxatives.

Pain Cancer-related pain is experienced by 50% to 90% of patients with advanced disease and in about 60% to 70% patients who are receiving active treatment for their tumors. The Hospitalized Elderly Longitudinal Project (HELP) showed that one out of three patients in this study died in severe pain. Older patients are at risk for undertreatment of pain because of underestimation of their sensitivity to pain, the expectation that they tolerate pain well, and misconception about their ability to benefit from the use of opioids. The approach to pain management in older adults described in Chapter 68 can be applied to the older patient with cancer. Comprehensive geriatric care involving other geriatric team members and palliative care early, demonstrates not only improved pain management and symptom control but also improved survival. Moreover, an educational intervention (patients watched a 14-minute video that presented information on "Managing Cancer Pain" aimed at older patients with cancer) was effective in prevention and management of cancer pain in older adults.

Fatigue This is one of the most common and debilitating symptoms from cancer and cancer treatment. It significantly affects a patient's quality of life. In one systematic review, the prevalence of fatigue was 40% to 90% during treatment and 19% to 80% after completion of treatment. The etiology of fatigue is multifold ranging from immobility and deconditioning, to anemia, depression, pain, poor nutrition, drugs, and metabolic causes. Treatment of fatigue is to treat the underlying cause if found, for example, treat anemia as appropriate with hematinics, iron, B_{12}, folate, transfusions. There are both pharmacologic and nonpharmacologic approaches for the treatment of cancer-related fatigue. Pharmacologic interventions include antidepressants and stimulants such as modafinil, corticosteroids, or methylphenidate. More commonly, nonpharmacologic interventions are used such as psychosocial interventions, exercise, sleep therapy, and acupuncture. Though counter-intuitive, increasing physical activity and exercise programs is one of the most effective treatments for cancer-related fatigue. Additional research is needed to treat cancer-related fatigue particularly among older adults.

Anxiety and depression

Recent studies indicate that the prevalence of depression among patients with cancer is between 17% and 25%. Patients at greatest risk are those with lung cancer, older age, unmarried men, women with severe illness, poor performance and functional status, and advanced cancer. Among patients with cancer, there is a strong relationship between pain and depression. Before making the diagnosis in older adults, it is important to exclude other causes. We recommend checking thyroid-stimulating hormone

(TSH), B_{12}, calcium, and liver function tests. For depression treatment, selective serotonin reuptake inhibitors like citalopram, fluoxetine, paroxetine, and sertraline are first-line choice of drugs in older adults, especially if patients have ischemic heart disease or conduction heart defects, prostatic hypertrophy, or uncontrolled glaucoma. Venlafaxine, mirtazapine, and bupropion are considered second-line drugs. However, for patients with cancer, mirtazapine is useful for mood, appetite, and sleep with minimal side effects. Nortriptyline or desipramine are used as third-line drugs and for severe melancholic depression and they can be difficult to tolerate because of side effects or, in the case of monoamine oxidase inhibitors, because of dietary and medication restrictions.

Anorexia and cancer cachexia An older adult's nutritional status can be compromised in direct response to tumor-induced alterations in metabolism. Cachexia is characterized by advanced protein-calorie malnutrition, involuntary weight loss, muscle wasting, and decreased quality of life. Tumor-induced weight loss occurs frequently in patients with solid tumors of the lung, pancreas, and upper gastrointestinal tract and less often in patients with breast cancer or lower gastrointestinal cancer. Conditions that may cause poor intake and that can be easily treated—gastritis, constipation, oral candidiasis, pain, and nausea—should be treated. Several agents have been tried in clinical trials (not specifically in older patient) to stimulate the patient's appetite. These include oral corticosteroids, progestational agents like megestrol acetate, cannabinoids like dronabinol, antidepressants like mirtazapine, olanzapine, and omega-3-fatty acids. Anorexia and cachexia are common among dying patients. For family members, accepting their loved one is not eating is often difficult because it means accepting that the patient is dying. It is important to educate family members in advance that if a patient is close to death, neither food nor hydration is necessary to maintain the patient's comfort. Intravenous fluids, total parenteral nutrition (TPN), and tube feedings do not prolong the life of dying patients, and in fact may even increase discomfort and hasten death. Adverse effects of artificial nutrition in dying patients can include pulmonary congestion, pneumonia, edema, and pain associated with inflammation. Conversely, dehydration and ketosis due to caloric restriction correlate with analgesic effects and absence of discomfort. The only reported discomfort due to dehydration near death is xerostomia, which can be prevented and relieved with oral swabs or ice chips.

Survivorship

We are in the midst of an unprecedented increase in the number of older adults diagnosed with, and surviving from, cancer. By 2030, 70% of patients with cancer will be 65 years or older, and the cancer incidence in this group will increase nearly 70% from 2010 to 2030. There are 16 million cancer survivors in the United States, and approximately 60% are age 65 or older. By 2040, it is estimated that the number of cancer survivors will grow to 26 million, with 73% age 65 or older and almost 50% age 75 or older. Despite this substantial growth in the number of older adult cancer survivors, there are many knowledge gaps regarding how cancer and cancer treatment impact the aging process.

In some individuals, cancer and its treatments contribute to an accelerated or accentuated aging phenotype. The majority of these data come from pediatric literature, where cancer survivors are predisposed to the development of frailty and comorbid conditions, such as myocardial infarction and congestive heart, compared to their peers without a history of cancer. There is a smaller yet growing body of literature pointing toward similar findings in the geriatric population. Compared to adults without a history of cancer, older cancer survivors are more likely to report physical and mental health-related quality of life. Cancer and cancer treatments are associated with second malignancies and late effects that can affect any organ system. Given that older cancer survivors are more likely to have limitations in performing activities of daily living, mobility limitations, and increased number of comorbidities, it is imperative to understand the aging-related consequences of cancer and cancer treatments. Strategies such as exercise, diet, nutrition, therapies targeting immune senescence, and supportive care interventions are under further investigation to examine their potential to address the long-term effects of cancer and cancer treatment.

Caregiver Assessment and Interventions

Older adults with cancer often require additional care at home. In the United States, 63% of home care for older adults with cancer is provided by informal caregivers, who are often family members, and as the population ages, the number of informal caregiver is expected to increase. Caregivers of older adults with cancer tend to be older, with studies showing that nearly 40% have comorbidities and are likely to report their health as fair or poor. These caregivers experience substantial physical and emotional challenges leading to increased caregiver burden. Compared with non-caregivers of the same age, caregivers of older adults with cancer are more likely to experience deterioration in physical health, report symptoms of anxiety and depression, and to have poor health-related behaviors (including decreased exercise, sleep, and poor eating habits). Moreover, caregiver burden is associated with increased all-cause mortality in patients as well as increased risk of hospitalizations and inappropriate end-of-life care.

CONCLUSION

Cancer is the leading cause of death in men and women aged 60 to 79 years. The biology of certain tumors is different in older versus younger adults. In addition, older patients have a lower physiologic reserve with decreased tolerance to intensive chemotherapy or other modalities of cancer treatment. Chronological age is not a reliable estimate of life expectancy, functional reserve, or risk of treatment-related complications. A CGA is increasingly being utilized in clinical trials of several tumor types and aids in decision-making and prediction of chemotherapy toxicity, and should be incorporated in the care of older adults with cancer. The patient and their caregivers should continue discussions with the treating oncologist with respect to goals of care throughout the course of their disease.

FURTHER READING

Aunan J, Cho W, Soreide K. The biology of aging and cancer: A brief overview of shared and divergent molecular hallmarks. *Aging Dis.* 2017;5(8):628–642.

Champiat S, Lambotte O, Barreau E, et al. Management of immune checkpoint blockade dysimmune toxicities: a collaborative position paper. *Ann Oncol.* 2016;27(4): 559–574.

Colloca G, Di Capua B, Bellieni A, et al. Biological and functional biomarkers of aging: definition, characteristics, and how they can impact everyday cancer treatment. *Curr Oncol Rep.* 2020;22(11):115.

Extermann M, Boler I, Reich RR, et al. Predicting the risk of chemotherapy toxicity in older patients: the Chemotherapy Risk Assessment Scale for High-Age Patients (CRASH) score. *Cancer.* 2012;118(13):3377–3386.

Fane M, Weeraratna A. How the ageing microenvironment influences tumor progression. *Nat Rev Cancer.* 2020;20(2):89–106.

Hurria A, Cirrincione CT, Muss HB, et al. Implementing a geriatric assessment in cooperative group clinical cancer trials: CALGB 360401. *J Clin Oncol.* 2011;29(10):1290–1296.

Hurria A, Togawa K, Mohile SG, et al. Predicting chemotherapy toxicity in older adults with cancer: a prospective multicenter study. *J Clin Oncol.* 2011;29:3457–3465.

Institute of Medicine. Delivering high quality cancer care. Charting a new course for a system in crisis. Institute of Medicine (IOM) 2013 Report. https://www.nap.edu/read/18359/chapter/1. Accessed January 14, 2022.

Kadambi S, Loh KP, Dunne R, et al. Older adults with cancer and their caregivers – current landscape and future directions for clinical care. *Nat Rev.* 2020;17(12):742–755.

Klepin HD, Geiger AM, Tooze JA, et al. Geriatric assessment predicts survival for older adults receiving induction chemotherapy for acute myelogenous leukemia. *Blood.* 2013;121(21):4287–4294.

Mohile SG, Dale W, Somerfield MR, et al. Practical assessment and management of vulnerabilities in older patients receiving chemotherapy: ASCO Guideline for Geriatric Oncology. *J Clin Oncol.* 2018;36(22):2326–2347.

Muhandiramge J, Orchard S, Haydon A, et al. The acceleration of ageing in older patients with cancer. *J Geriatr Oncol.* 2021;12(3):343–351.

National Comprehensive Cancer Network (NCCN) guidelines for Senior Adult Oncology version 1.2020. http://www .nccn.org/professionals/physician_gls/f_guidelines.asp#age.

Peterson LL, Hurria A, Feng T, et al. Association between renal function and chemotherapy-related toxicity in older adults with cancer. *J Geriatr Oncol.* 2017;8(2):96–101.

Postow MA, Sidlow R, Hellmann MD. Immune-related adverse events associated with immune checkpoint blockade. *N Engl J Med.* 2018;378(2):158–168.

Presley CJ, Krok-Schoen JL, Wall SA, et al. Implementing a multidisciplinary approach for older adults with cancer: geriatric oncology in practice. *BMC Geriatrics.* 2020;s12877-020-01625-5.

Rowland JH, Bellizzi KM. Cancer survivorship issues: life after treatment and implications for an aging population. *J Clin Oncol.* 2014;32(24):2662–2668.

Shahrokni A, Tin A, Saman S, et al. Association of geriatric comanagement and 90-day postoperative mortality among patients aged 75 years and older with cancer. *JAMA Netw Open.* 2020;e209265-e209265.

Smith GL, Smith BD. Radiation treatment in older patients: a framework for clinical decision making. *J Clin Oncol.* 2014;32(24):2669–2678.

Wyld L, Bellanton I, Tchkonia T, et al. Senescence and cancer: a review of clinical implications of senescence and senotherapies. *Cancers (Basel).* 2020;12(8):2134.

Chapter 89

Breast Disease

Mina S. Sedrak, Hyman B. Muss

EPIDEMIOLOGY

Breast cancer is the most common cancer in women, and the American Cancer Society has estimated that in 2020 it will account for 30% of all newly diagnosed malignancies (276,000 new breast cancer cases) and remain the second leading cause of cancer-related death (42,000 deaths, ie, 15%). Moreover, current US incidence and mortality data show that 12.8% of all women (1 in 8) will be diagnosed with breast cancer during their lifetime and that 2.6% (1 in 39) will die from it.

The incidence of breast cancer, like most other human cancers, increases dramatically with age. In the United States the median age at which breast cancer is diagnosed is 62 years and the median age of dying from breast cancer is 69, with highest percent of breast cancer deaths occurring between ages 65 and 74. National Vital Statistics indicate that the dramatic increase in incidence and mortality with age (**Figure 89-1**) from an invasive breast cancer rate of approximately 1 in 5000 in women aged 15 to 39 to about 1 in 200 in women aged 64 to 74. Of equal concern, although breast cancer–related mortality has been decreasing for several decades, older age has been associated with a lower breast cancer–specific survival rates (**Figure 89-2**), possibly reflecting less screening or poorer treatment.

Breast cancer is a major health concern in the United States and will become of greater importance since the size of the older population is growing dramatically. Although breast cancer is more common in older women, they are less likely to be appropriately screened, more likely to present for care at a more advanced stage, more likely to receive inferior surgical and postoperative management, and are less likely to be entered into clinical trials. This has resulted in older breast cancer patients sharing less in the dramatic decline in breast cancer mortality rates in the last two decades as compared with younger women.

PATHOPHYSIOLOGY

The specific cause of breast cancer is unknown. Many factors associated with increased risk have been identified. These include the following: increasing age, family history of breast cancer (especially in a first-degree relative) or known

Learning Objectives

- Describe the key principles regarding breast cancer, including epidemiology, screening, risk factors, presentation, and initial evaluation of disease.
- Understand the basic local and systemic therapy for early, nonmetastatic breast cancer.
- Understand the basic approaches to treatment of metastatic breast cancer.
- Describe the usual surveillance recommended for patients with breast cancer.
- Understand potential prevention strategies.
- Become aware of special (understudied) populations with breast cancer, including men, racial/ethnic minorities, and those with advanced comorbidity.
- Become aware of survivorship and palliative care issues.

Key Clinical Points

1. Breast cancer in the older patient is common and will become more common as our population ages.
2. Although many older patients die from causes other than breast cancer, it remains a deadly disease for many, especially those with higher-risk cancers.
3. Older patients typically benefit from treatments (such as endocrine therapy and chemotherapy) as much as younger patients do but may experience more toxicity with chemotherapy.
4. Geriatric assessments and estimates of life expectancy (exclusive of breast cancer) can help optimize treatment decisions.
5. When discussing treatment, screening, and surveillance strategies with older patients,

(Continued)

(Cont.)

it is important to be mindful of each patient's competing medical issues, risk for cancer recurrence and cancer-related death, and functional status.

6. Older patients with breast cancer are often understudied. How to best optimize care with regard to treatment, comorbidity, functional status, and outcomes remains a priority for future research.

genetic predisposition, early menarche, late age at birth of first child (older than 30 years), late menopause, dense breast tissue, history of benign breast disease (hyperplasia or atypical hyperplasia), heavy radiation exposure, obesity, high endogenous hormone levels (postmenopausal estrogen replacement therapy), moderate-to-excessive alcohol use, and possibly cigarette smoking history. Most of these factors are associated with relative risks in the range of 1.1 to greater than 4 times the risk in the general population. A breast cancer risk assessment tool, based on the Gail Model, can be used to calculate the 5-year and lifetime risk of breast cancer in a patient (https://bcrisktool.cancer.gov/).

A family history of breast cancer, implying a genetic defect, has been found in from 5% to 20% of all cases of breast cancer and is particularly important in breast cancer diagnosed before age 50. *BRCA1, BRCA2,* and *PALB2* are the most common genes involved in hereditary predisposition. Other, rarer mutations are also associated with breast cancer that include *ATM, TP53, PTEN,* and *CHEK2.* In addition to inherited disease-causing genetic variations, there are many modifying factors, including genetic, hormonal, and environmental, that may determine whether a genetic mutation will lead to cancer.

Most breast cancers originate from ductal epithelium. Comparisons of older and younger patients with breast cancer reveal that infiltrating ductal carcinoma is the most common histologic type in both groups, accounting for 75% to 80% of cases, with lobular carcinoma accounting for approximately 5% to 10% and other subtypes accounting for the remaining cancers. Compared to younger patients, older patients are more likely to be well differentiated and moderately differentiated, be estrogen and progesterone receptor (PR)-positive (60%–70% of patients), have lower rates of tumor proliferation (the number of cells synthesizing deoxyribonucleic acid [DNA]), and less frequently express the human epidermal growth factor receptor 2 (HER2) oncogene. These data suggest that breast cancer in older patients is biologically less aggressive than it is in younger women. Mortality from breast cancer, however, is not lower in older women, leading us to explore issues associated with treatment choice and other patient- and tumor-related factors that might affect disease-specific survival.

SCREENING

The majority of breast cancers in the United States are diagnosed as a result of an abnormal screening study, although a significant number are first brought to attention by the patient. Breast cancer screening in a postmenopausal woman includes mammography and a physical examination. After menopause, estrogen levels diminish, breast glandular tissue and ductal tissue decrease, fat tissue increases, and there are fewer cysts and fibroadenomas. These age-related changes in breast tissue, especially the increased percentage of fat tissue, allow for improved contrast between small foci of malignancy and the surrounding breast tissue, resulting in fewer false-negative mammographic examinations.

Several randomized trials show that the routine use of screening mammography in women aged 50 through

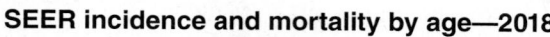

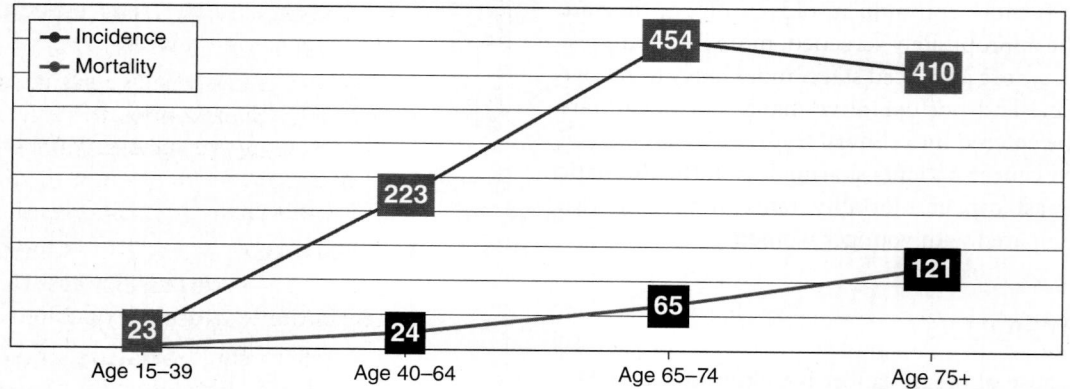

FIGURE 89-1. Breast cancer incidence and mortality rates by age. (SEER*Explorer: An interactive website for SEER cancer statistics [Internet]. Surveillance Research Program, National Cancer Institute. [2021 September]. Available from https://seer.cancer.gov/explorer/.)

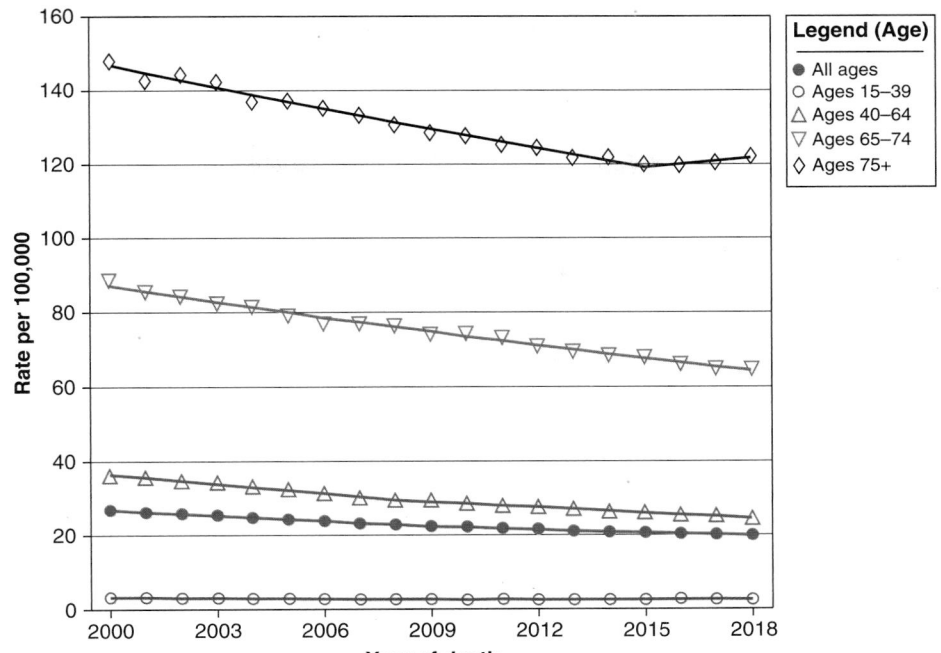

FIGURE 89-2. SEER age adjusted mortality rates (2000–2018). (SEER°Explorer: An interactive website for SEER cancer statistics [Internet]. Surveillance Research Program, National Cancer Institute. [2021 September]. Available from https://seer.cancer.gov/explorer/.)

75 improves survival by detecting breast carcinoma at an earlier stage and before metastatic dissemination. Only limited data are available to provide guidance for screening in women older than 75 years. Guidelines differ among experts; we suggest consideration of annual or biennial screening in women age 75 and older if their estimated life expectancy is at least 10 years. For women in this age group with life expectancies between 5 and 10 years, screening is not likely to be of value in improving breast cancer–related mortality; however, shared decision-making should be used in discussing screening and decided upon on an individualized basis. Decision aids can be helpful when discussing the patient's risk of developing breast cancer, the potential benefits and harms of screening, and the patient's values. Physical examination by health professionals remains an essential and complementary adjunct to mammographic screening and is especially important in women who decline or are not likely to benefit by mammographic screening. **Table 89-1** presents our recommendations for the screening of older women.

PRESENTATION

Breast cancer usually presents either as a breast mass or a suspicious finding on a mammogram. The discovery of a breast mass in a postmenopausal woman requires prompt attention, as the majority of palpable masses in this age group are malignant and all require biopsy. Mammography can help define the nature of a mass and detect other nonpalpable lesions if present and should be performed when a breast mass is found. A small percent (up to 15%) of palpable breast cancers in women may not show on mammogram (false negatives) but require biopsy.

Locally advanced breast cancer can present with axillary adenopathy (suggesting locoregional disease) or skin findings such as erythema, thickening, or dimpling of the overlying skin (peau d'orange), suggesting inflammatory breast cancer. Symptoms of metastatic breast cancer can be nonspecific (eg, weight loss, fatigue, or loss of appetite) or can depend on the organs involved, with the most common sites of involvement being the bone (eg, back or leg pain), liver (abdominal pain, nausea, jaundice), and lungs (eg, shortness of breath or cough).

DIAGNOSIS

Typically, a stepwise process of diagnosis and definitive surgery is followed, as depicted in **Figure 89-3**. This allows for pathologic confirmation of cancer and time to decide surgical treatment choice.

For palpable or mammographically detected lesions, core needle biopsy is preferable to fine-needle aspiration biopsy, because it can distinguish invasive from in situ lesions and also allows better ascertainment of hormone receptor and HER-2 status. If the core biopsy is negative or inconclusive, unless the mass proves to be a cyst and resolves after aspiration, further biopsy, preferably excision, is necessary. If atypical ductal hyperplasia is found on core biopsy, excisional biopsy is required, because a small proportion of suspicious lesions for which core biopsy finds

TABLE 89-1 ■ SCREENING GUIDELINES FOR BREAST CANCER IN WOMEN OLDER THAN 70 YEARS

	FREQUENCY	COMMENT
Breast self-examination	Monthly	Value uncertain, but many breast cancers are still detected by the patient
Physical examination	Yearly	By physician or other health professional; detects 15% of cancers *not* discovered on screening mammogram
Mammography	Every 1–2 y	Value in improving survival in women older than 75 y is unproven. We suggest screening in those with life expectancy of at least 10 y and discussion with patients about the pros and cons if life expectancy is 5–10 y

only atypical hyperplasia may also contain in situ or invasive cancer when excised.

The diagnosis of breast cancer is defined by the presence of malignant epithelial cells (carcinoma) on biopsy. When biopsy is diagnostic of malignancy, preoperative evaluation typically includes a complete history and physical examination, a complete blood count and chemistry profile, and a chest x-ray. Magnetic resonance imaging (MRI) of the breasts may also be helpful in the management of older women in specific settings but is not recommended for routine screening or diagnostic purposes. However, bilateral mammography should be performed on all patients during their diagnostic work-up to evaluate both the ipsilateral breast and the contralateral breast for other nonpalpable lesions.

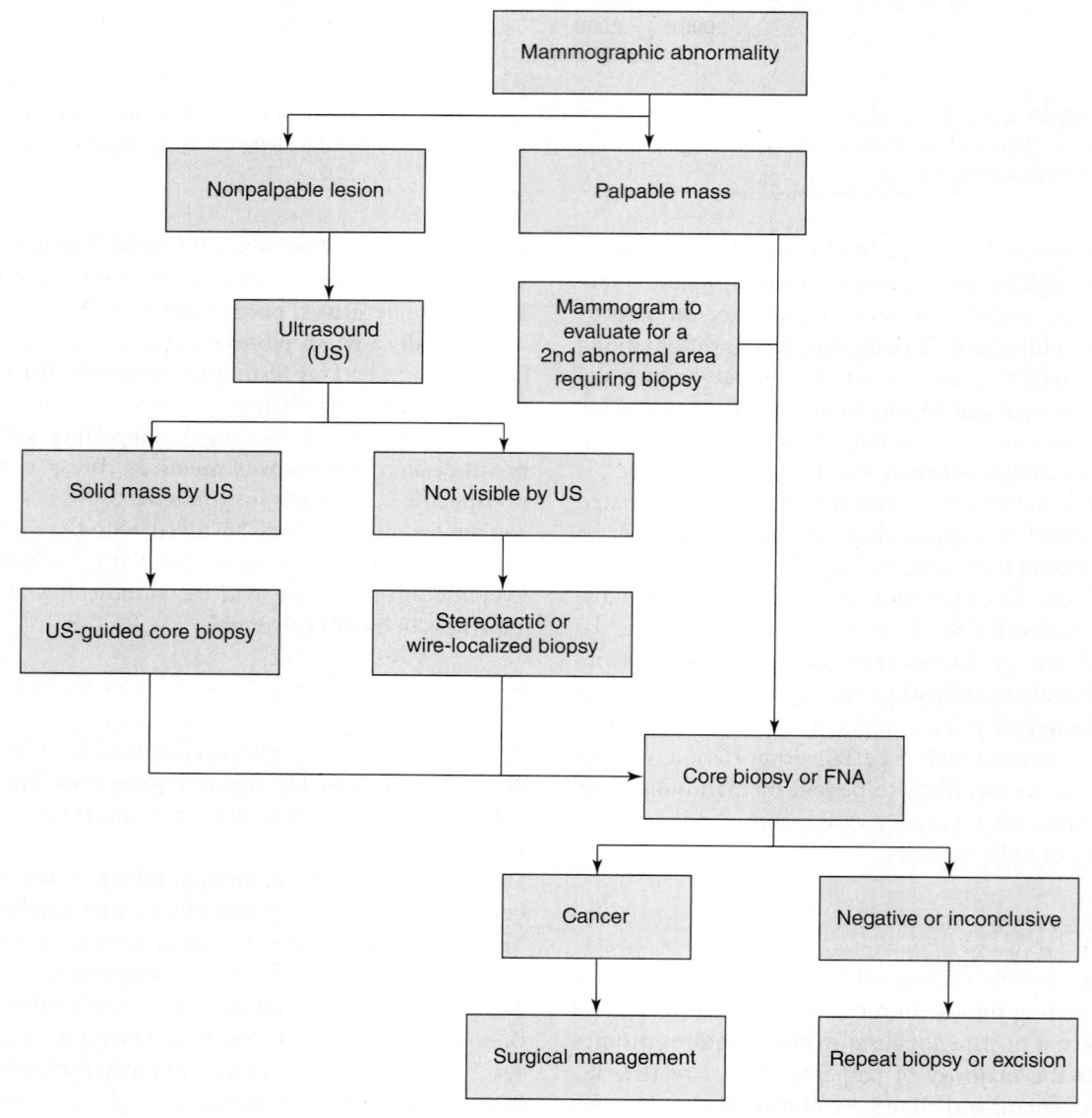

FIGURE 89-3. Stepwise evaluation of suspicious breast finding. FNA, fine-needle aspiration.

POSTDIAGNOSIS EVALUATION

Once a patient is diagnosed with breast cancer, specific receptor testing is performed and appropriate staging work-up is necessary to determine local and distant extent of disease.

Breast Cancer Receptor Testing

Newly diagnosed breast cancer must be tested for estrogen receptor (ER), PR, and overexpression of HER2 receptor status. This information is critical for both prognostic and therapeutic purpose because breast cancer is characterized into different subtypes by whether they express ER, PR, and HER2 receptors. The majority (80%) of cases are hormone receptor (ER and/or PR positive), followed by HER2 overexpression. ER-, PR-, and HER2-negative (triple-negative) cancers compromise approximately 10% of cases.

Staging

The American Joint Committee on Cancer (AJCC) guidelines set the standard for breast cancer staging. This system categorizes the extent of malignancy according to the size of the primary lesion (T), the extent of nodal involvement (N), and the occurrence of metastasis (M). Tumor size (the largest diameter of the infiltrating component) and the extent of nodal involvement (the number positive) are determined from pathologic examination and are included in the pathology report and ascertainment of staging. Nodal assessment is done either by sentinel lymph node biopsy or by axillary dissection. Sentinel lymph node mapping and sampling is preferred as it allows identification and assessment of the one to four nodes most likely to contain cancer. If an axillary lymph node dissection is completed, a sample of at least six nodes (if possible) is ideal in order to reflect the prognosis accurately.

Most patients presenting with breast cancer have stage I or II disease (confined to the breast) with no or limited (ie, less than three) nodes involved and do not routinely undergo additional work-up for metastatic disease in the absence of signs or symptoms suspicious for distant spread. Patients with stage III breast cancer or inflammatory breast cancer and those with signs or symptoms worrisome for metastatic disease should have imaging with computerized tomography of chest, abdomen, and pelvis and a radionuclide bone scan or a positron emission tomography–computed tomography (PET-CT) scan to rule out metastases. The use of tumor markers (such as the carcinoembryonic antigen [CEA] and mucin antigens CA27.29 and CA15.3) and circulating tumor cells is not recommended as part of the staging evaluation.

TREATMENT

The vast majority of patients with newly diagnosed breast cancer in the United States have no evidence of metastatic disease. For these patients, the treatment approach depends on stage at presentation, prognostic receptor status, and, in some cases, biomarker testing. The general treatment principles of carcinoma in situ, early (nonmetastatic) breast cancer, and metastatic breast cancer will be reviewed here.

Carcinoma In Situ

Ductal carcinoma in situ (DCIS) of the breast represents a heterogenous group of neoplastic lesions confined to the breast ducts. The goal of therapy for DCIS is to prevent the development of invasive cancer and therapeutic approaches include surgery, radiation therapy (RT), and adjuvant endocrine therapy. Mastectomy cures almost all patients, but breast-conserving procedures followed by breast irradiation are as effective for patients with smaller lesions. Axillary dissection or sentinel node biopsy finds metastases in less than 1% of patients and is generally not recommended. Excision alone, without local RT, may be appropriate for patients with lesions less than 2.5 cm with generous (> 1 cm) margins of normal tissue surrounding the in-situ component. Most DCIS lesions are ER- and PR-positive and clinical trials on tamoxifen have been shown to decrease the risk of recurrence and contralateral breast cancer in women with DCIS but without improvements in survival. For older women with DCIS, the risks of tamoxifen are likely to exceed the benefits in many women and we recommend consideration of tamoxifen use on an individual basis.

Lobular carcinoma in situ (LCIS) is more common in premenopausal patients, lacks clinical and mammographic signs, is bilateral in 25% to 35% of cases, and is usually an incidental finding at breast biopsy. It is not a palpable lesion. Treatment options range from observation to bilateral mastectomy, but observation is preferred. Of note, 20% to 40% of patients with LCIS subsequently develop infiltrating ductal cancer, with both the ipsilateral breast and the contralateral breast at similar risk. LCIS serves as a high-risk marker for subsequent invasive cancer, and treatment selection must rest on the desires of the patient. Most experts recommend close follow-up of these patients, without aggressive surgery. Tamoxifen dramatically decreases the risk of subsequent invasive breast cancer in patients with LCIS and should be considered on an individual basis.

Early-Stage, Nonmetastatic Breast Cancer

In general, patients with early-stage breast cancer undergo primary surgery (lumpectomy or mastectomy) to the breast and regional nodes with or without RT. Following definitive local treatment, patients should be offered adjuvant systemic therapy based on primary tumor characteristics, such as tumor grade, size, lymph node involvement, and ER, PR, and HER2 receptor status. However, some patients with early-stage disease, particularly those with HER2-positive or triple-negative breast cancer, may benefit from upfront (neoadjuvant) chemotherapy first, followed by surgery. Although the field is constantly changing, there are several key principles of surgical, radiation, and systemic treatment, which we will review here.

Breast-conserving therapy The breast-conserving approach to breast cancer management involves removing the tumor mass with a clear margin of surrounding normal breast tissue (lumpectomy, partial mastectomy, quadrantectomy, etc), assessing axillary lymph nodes when indicated, and for many, delivering local breast irradiation (discussed below) after surgery. Breast-conserving therapy results in virtually identical relapse-free and overall survival compared with more extensive surgical treatment, including simple, modified-radical, and radical mastectomy. It allows patients to preserve their breast without sacrificing oncologic outcomes. Criteria that preclude breast-conserving surgery include: two or more gross tumors in separate quadrants of the breast, large tumor/breast size ratio (mass > 5 cm in size), which interferes with cosmesis, diffuse indeterminate or malignant-appearing microcalcifications, a history of therapeutic irradiation to the chest (eg, radiation for Hodgkin disease), and persistently positive margins despite attempts at re-excision. For patients who desire breast conservation therapy but are not candidates at the time of presentation, an alternative approach is the use of neoadjuvant therapy (discussed below), which may allow for desired surgical management without compromising survival outcomes.

Mastectomy A mastectomy is indicated for patients who are not candidates for breast conserving therapy and those who prefer a mastectomy. Reasonably healthy older women tolerate simple or modified mastectomies as well as younger women do and should be offered the option when clinically appropriate.

Axillary assessment Tumor size and axillary nodal status are the most consistent predictors of the risk of recurrence and key in making decisions about the risk/benefit ratio of adjuvant systemic treatment. The evaluation of the regional nodes depends on whether axillary involvement is suspected prior to surgery. For patients with clinically suspicious axillary nodes, a preoperative work-up including biopsy to confirm nodal involvement is recommended to determine the best surgical approach (eg, upfront axillary node dissection at the time of breast surgery) and whether neoadjuvant therapy should be considered. For patients with a clinically negative axillary examination, sentinel lymph node mapping and sampling at the time of surgery is recommended. When one or two sentinel lymph node(s) are positive (pathologically involved), further axillary dissection can be omitted without any detrimental effects on local recurrence or survival. For patients with three or more sentinel nodes involved, axillary dissection is indicated.

In older women, the role of assessing axillary nodes is quite controversial because of the risk of arm morbidity. If adjuvant chemotherapy is not a consideration because of physician or patient choice, the risk of axillary dissection is not worth its prognostic yield, regardless of the primary tumor size. It is generally acceptable to omit axillary assessment in older women (age 70 or older) with small (2 cm or less), clinically node-negative, ER-positive breast cancer, who will take adjuvant endocrine therapy for at least 5 years.

Breast reconstruction For older women who have had a mastectomy, breast reconstruction represents another option for restoring body image. Many physicians, because of personal bias, are unlikely to discuss reconstruction with older patients. However, this procedure can be done safely in older patients and should be discussed, with subsequent surgical consultation if desired.

Adjuvant Radiation

Radiation after mastectomy The likelihood of local recurrence is directly proportional to both the size of the primary lesion and the number of involved axillary nodes. Postoperative adjuvant irradiation is generally recommended for patients with primary lesions greater than 5 cm or with four or more positive nodes. It is also considered reasonable for any woman with breast cancer that involves lymph nodes to receive postmastectomy "adjuvant" irradiation therapy to the chest wall and the contiguous regional lymph nodes (internal mammary, supraclavicular, and upper axilla), because it reduces the likelihood of local recurrence (recurrence in the mastectomy site or contiguous nodal areas) by 70% and improves overall breast cancer–specific survival.

Radiation after lumpectomy Breast irradiation after removal of tumor mass reduces the likelihood of recurrence in the affected breast from 30% to 40% to less than 10% and may improve survival in women with higher-risk breast cancers. Although radiation after breast conservation is standard therapy in younger women, older women with smaller, hormone receptor–positive breast cancers (≤ 3 cm in largest dimension) may be spared breast irradiation if they are willing to take adjuvant endocrine therapy. In such patients, survival is identical, although there is a somewhat higher risk of breast recurrence over a 10-year period (about 10% without radiation and 2%–3% with radiation). Most breast relapses occur in or in close proximity to the previously resected lesion. Other techniques, such as brachytherapy (localized RT), may prove to be as effective as whole-breast RT and can be completed over a period of days to weeks. For healthy older patients at high risk for in-breast recurrence (tumors 3 cm or greater or positive lymph nodes) and reasonable life expectancy, breast radiation is recommended.

Adjuvant Systemic Therapy

Systemic therapy refers to the medical treatment of breast cancer using chemotherapy, endocrine therapy, and/or biologic therapy. Tumor characteristics predict which patients are likely to benefit from specific types of systemic therapy in early-stage breast cancer. These therapies can be given preoperatively (neoadjuvant) or postoperatively (adjuvant). The goal of systemic therapy in early breast cancer is to reduce risk of and delay relapse as well as improve survival. Such treatment is aimed at eradicating occult, clinically undetectable metastasis. **Figure 89-4** shows the

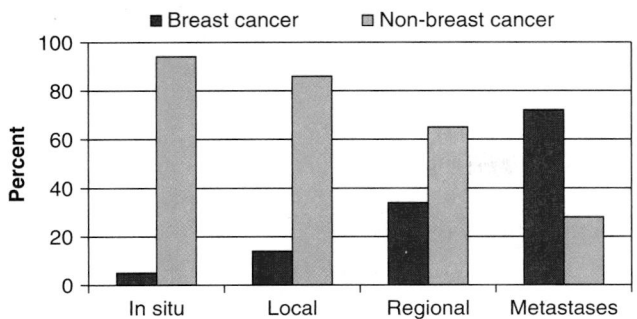

FIGURE 89-4. Cause of death after approximately 28-year follow-up for White women age greater than or equal to 70 with breast cancer. SEER data, *n* = 395,000; during 1973–2000. (Data from Schairer C, Mink PJ, Carroll L, et al. Probabilities of death from breast cancer and other causes among female breast cancer patients. *J Natl Cancer Inst.* 2004;96[17]:1311–1321.)

cause of death for women with breast cancer by stage of disease and **Figure 89-5** shows the overall survival of older women by breast cancer stage. As demonstrated in these figures, women, and in particular older women, mostly die of non–breast cancer causes in the setting of early-stage disease. Treatment considerations should therefore be individualized based on general prognostic tumor-related markers (biology and extent of disease), global health status (providing information on life expectancy and treatment tolerance), and patient preference, and not on chronological age.

Chemotherapy Adjuvant chemotherapy is generally recommended for older women who are fit and where chemotherapy in addition to other treatment will improve survival by at least a few percent. Data suggest that standard combination regimens (two or more chemotherapy drugs) are efficacious in older patients, with acceptable toxicity. Indeed, studies have shown a survival benefit for women aged 50 to

70 with regimens that are also well tolerated in healthy women older than 70 years. However, prior to making decisions regarding chemotherapy, a risk-stratified approach should be done to take into account patient and tumor characteristics to select which older patients should receive adjuvant chemotherapy. The decision to proceed with adjuvant chemotherapy is thus chosen on the basis of the risk to benefit ratio: the anticipated risk reduction for metastatic disease is weighed against the risk of toxicity from treatment.

Tools to predict the benefit of chemotherapy are available. These include genomic expression profiles of the tumor (Oncotype Dx), which are used in routine practice to determine the specific benefit of chemotherapy in given subsets of patients with hormone receptor–positive breast cancer. Online calculators, such as PREDICT, can also be used as a starting point to estimate overall survival benefits with and without chemotherapy.

Tools to predict the patient's life expectancy (exclusive of their breast cancer diagnosis), general health status, and risk for chemotherapy toxicity should be used to assess the older patient. There is vast heterogeneity in function and comorbidity in older patients at any given age. **Table 89-2** presents a list of key websites and resources for providers who care for older patients with cancer.

An online tool, ePrognosis (https://eprognosis.ucsf. edu/), estimates life expectancy based on medical history and has been validated for use among women with early-stage breast cancer. By providing an estimate of noncancer mortality risk, the ePrognosis tool can help frame treatment decisions for adjuvant chemotherapy and provide a starting point for conversation with the patient about their own preferences.

Additionally, we recommend that patients older than 70 years and/or with multiple comorbid conditions should be screened for geriatric syndromes using a

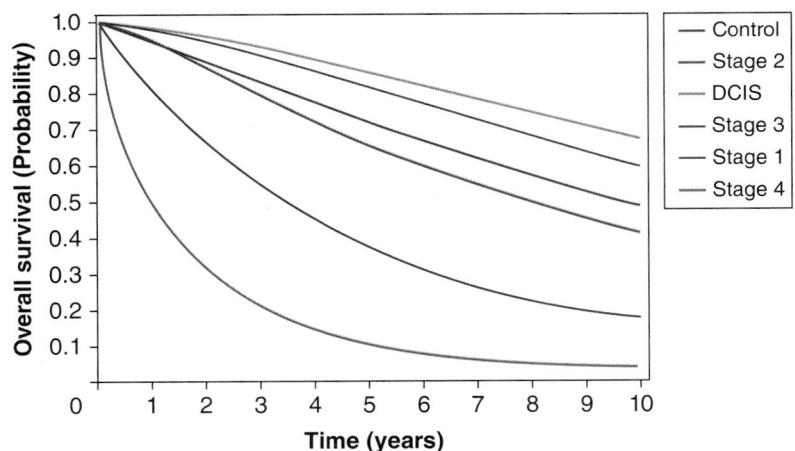

FIGURE 89-5. Overall survival of women age 67 and older by breast cancer stage and of their controls. (Reproduced with permission from Schonberg MA, Marcantonio ER, Ngo L, et al. Causes of death and relative survival of older women after a breast cancer diagnosis. *J Clin Oncol.* 2011;29[12]:1570–1577.)

TABLE 89-2 ■ KEY WEBSITES AND RESOURCES FOR HELP IN CARING FOR OLDER PATIENTS WITH CANCER

ORGANIZATIONS	DESCRIPTION	URL/LINK
American Society of Clinical Oncology (ASCO)	ASCO University modules explore treatment options for older patients with cancer. Also has Maintenance of Certification (MOC) Course on Geriatric Oncology.	http://university.asco.org/geriatric-oncology
International Society of Geriatric Oncology (SIOG)	Website has links to geriatric oncology guidelines and other educational materials.	http://www.siog.org/
Portal of Geriatrics Online Education (POGOe)	Comprehensive site with free access to expert-contributed geriatrics materials.	http://www.pogoe.org/about
Cancer and Aging Research Group (CARG)	A group of researchers with major interest in geriatric oncology research. Opportunities for mentoring. Also online chemotherapy toxicity calculator and geriatric assessment tools.	http://www.mycarg.org/
Lineberger Comprehensive Cancer Center Geriatric Oncology	Free core lectures, resources, links in geriatrics.	http://unclineberger.org/geriatric
ONLINE TOOLS AND CALCULATORS	DESCRIPTION	URL/LINK
ePrognosis	A series of calculators based on systematic review of literature that allows for estimation of life expectancy in older adults (not specific to cancer).	http://eprognosis.ucsf.edu/default.php
Moffitt Cancer Center Senior Adult Oncology Program Tools	Online tools for estimating chemotherapy toxicity ("CRASH" score) and other geriatric calculators.	http://moffitt.org/cancer-types—treatment/cancers-we-treat/senior-adult-oncology-program-tools

brief geriatric screening tool, such as VES-13 or G8. Based on the results of the screening, a comprehensive geriatric assessment (GA)—which includes evaluations of functional status, comorbid medical conditions, cognitive status, psychological state, social support, nutritional status, and a review of the medication list—may help to uncover age-related deficits that are not routinely obtained in a history and physical examination. This cancer-specific, comprehensive GA, developed by Dr. Arti Hurria and colleagues, was shown to identify older adults who have diminished life expectancy and/or are at risk for hospitalization and functional decline. Findings from the GA may guide interventions that can improve the ability to undergo cancer treatment, with emerging evidence showing that these GA-driven interventions can reduce chemotherapy toxicity and improve the quality of life of older patients with cancer. Several national and international organizations now recommend incorporating data from a GA for optimizing treatment in older patients who are planned to receive systemic therapy.

Recently, a new risk prediction model was developed predict chemotherapy-related toxicities in patients older than 65 years with early-stage breast cancer receiving neoadjuvant or adjuvant chemotherapy. The Cancer and Aging Research Group–Breast Cancer (CARG-BC) risk score is derived by combining eight disease and patient-reported predictors, including: use of an anthracycline chemotherapy, stage II or III breast cancer, planned treatment duration, abnormal liver function, low hemoglobin, falls, limited walking ability, and lack of social support (**Table 89-3**).

The total score classifies patients age 65 and older with early breast cancer into low, intermediate, or high risk for severe, debilitating, or deadly side effects to chemotherapy. The CARG-BC score was also validated and outperformed other tools, including a general risk prediction model for older adults with cancer (nonbreast cancer–specific) and physician-rated performance status (ie, "eyeball test").

Endocrine therapy Almost all patients with hormone receptor–positive breast cancer should be offered adjuvant endocrine therapy to reduce the risk of breast cancer recurrence and breast cancer-related mortality, regardless of age. Although older adults may have more comorbidities that predispose them to increased toxicities related to endocrine treatment, the benefits of adjuvant endocrine therapy on reducing the risks of recurrence and death from breast cancer are similar to younger patients. We recommend that patients at risk for treatment-related toxicities due to adjuvant endocrine therapy should be managed appropriately, with care coordinated between their oncology team and primary care clinician or geriatrician. Patients at increased risk of major toxicities, such as those with preexisting history of thrombosis, cerebrovascular disease, osteoporosis, or fractures should have shared discussions with their medical team to make the most informed decisions.

Endocrine therapy as initial (or primary) treatment Although surgical resection reduces the risk of local recurrence and its associated morbidity, for many older patients, especially those with advanced but localized lesions (T3 and T4) and those with significant comorbidity or frailty (where

TABLE 89-3 ■ CANCER AND AGING RESEARCH GROUP-BREAST CANCER (CARG-BC) SCORE CALCULATOR

RISK PREDICTOR	RESPONSE	SCORE
Breast cancer stage	II or III	3
	I	0
Planned use of anthracyclines	Yes	1
	No	0
Planned treatment duration	> 3 months (12 weeks)	4
	≤ 3 months (12 weeks)	0
Hemoglobin	≤ 12 g/dL (female)	3
	≤ 13 g/dL (male)	3
	> 12 g/dL (female)	0
	> 13 g/dL (male)	0
Liver function	Abnormal LFTs, outside reference range	3
	Normal LFTs, within reference range	0
How many times have you fallen in the last 6 months?	≥ 1	4
	0	0
Does your health limit you in walking more than 1 mile?	Somewhat or very limited	3
	Not limited at all	0
How often is someone available to give you good advice about a crisis?	None, little, or some of the time	3
	Most or all of the time	0

LFTs, liver function tests.

Scoring. The total CARG-BC risk score is the sum of each point(s) derived from the eight independent clinical and geriatric assessment predictors of grade 3–5 chemotherapy toxicity in patients age 65 and older with early stage breast cancer. Each patient's total CARG-BC score can then be classified into three risk groups: low (0–5 points), intermediate (6–11 points), or high (≥ 12 points).

Reproduced with permission from Magnuson A, Sedrak MS, Gross CP, et al. Development and validation of a risk tool for predicting severe toxicity in older adults receiving chemotherapy for early-stage breast cancer. J Clin Oncol. 2021; 39(6):608–618.

anesthesia is contraindicated), initial treatment with endocrine therapy is appropriate in patients with hormone receptor–positive tumors. Tumor shrinkage occurs in 40% to 70% of patients and tumor control usually is maintained for 18 to 24 months. The majority of patients treated initially with endocrine therapy do not achieve complete tumor regression and will need surgery or other treatments to control the primary lesion if their life expectancy is longer than several years. Although surgery is more likely to be effective (and potentially curative) in patients with small lesions, several randomized trials comparing surgery with endocrine treatment for initial therapy suggest that long-term survival is not changed by using endocrine therapy as the initial treatment and reserving surgical management for patients with tumor progression. Radiation therapy also can be used as "salvage" treatment after endocrine therapy fails, but large tumor masses, especially those greater than 3 cm and those with extensive skin involvement, frequently

respond only partially. For patients treated with endocrine therapy because comorbidity precludes surgical therapy, radiation therapy should be considered when tumor shrinkage is maximal to try to prolong the duration of local tumor control. In the authors' opinion, older women with localized breast cancer amenable to surgery should be offered surgical treatment at diagnosis unless they are extremely frail or have dramatically reduced life expectancy.

Metastatic Breast Cancer

Management of metastatic breast cancer in older women follows the same principles as in younger women, with few exceptions. Like younger women, older patients with metastatic breast cancer are currently incurable and have a median survival of approximately 2 to 7 years after the discovery of recurrence with about 20% of those with hormone receptor positive tumors surviving 5 years. The goal of therapy is palliation rather than cure and patients may derive considerable palliative benefit from judiciously chosen therapy. Bone, soft tissue (skin and lymph nodes), pleural, and pulmonary metastases are the most common sites of breast cancer recurrence. Women with localized, symptomatic lesions in brain, skin, lymph nodes, and bone should also be considered for palliative radiation therapy, which relieves symptoms in the majority of patients.

Patients with disseminated metastases should be considered for palliative systemic treatment and consideration for clinical trial enrollment should occur at every line of therapy. **Table 89-4** describes endocrine and cytotoxic agents used in the treatment of breast cancer and their common and major side effects. Endocrine therapy usually is associated with minimal toxicity, while the toxicity associated with chemotherapy is frequently substantial and, in a small percent of patients, may be life-threatening. Provided that metastases are not rapidly progressive or life-threatening, all women with hormone receptor–positive, metastatic breast cancer should have an initial trial of endocrine therapy. The combination of a cyclin-dependent kinase (CDK) 4/6 inhibitor and an aromatase inhibitor appears to be effective and of comparable tolerability in older patients as in younger patients; however, older adults should be carefully monitored for myelosuppression or diarrhea, depending on the choice of CDK4/6 inhibitor used.

Once breast cancer is deemed refractory to endocrine therapy or in the setting of triple negative disease (breast cancers without estrogen, progesterone expression, and HER2 overexpression), chemotherapy is usually the treatment of choice. Chemotherapy may also be a first-line therapy if life-threatening or rapidly progressive (visceral) disease is present. Chemotherapy should not be withheld solely on the basis of older age and decisions on the administration of chemotherapy in older women should be individualized based on the extent of their tumor, symptoms, and the potential benefits and risks of treatment. Sequential single-agent therapy as opposed to combination chemotherapy as in most patients, regardless of age, is equally

TABLE 89-4 ■ ENDOCRINE AND CYTOTOXIC AGENTS USED IN THE TREATMENT OF BREAST CANCER

CLASS	COMMON AND MAJOR TOXICITIES
ENDOCRINE THERAPY	
Selective estrogen receptor modulators (SERMs)	
Tamoxifen	Hot flashes; vaginal effects; rare: thrombosis, endometrial hyperplasia/
Toremifene	carcinoma
Aromatase inhibitors	
Anastrozole	Hot flashes, arthralgias, bone mineral density loss
Letrozole	
Exemestane	
Pure antiestrogen	
Fulvestrant	Injection site pain, hot flashes, malaise, nausea
Progestin	
Megace	Weight gain, gastrointestinal side effects
CYTOTOXIC AGENTS	
Alkylating agents	
Cyclophosphamide	Myelosuppression (M), N + V, cystitis
Carboplatin or cisplatin	M, N + V (mild)
Antitumor antibiotics	
Doxorubicin, epirubicin, liposomal doxorubicin	M, N + V, mucositis (MS), alopecia, cardiomyopathy, vesication
Antimetabolites	
Methotrexate	M (uncommon), nephrotoxicity, MS
Fluorouracil	M (uncommon), N + V (uncommon), rash (rare)
Capecitabine	Diarrhea, "hand-foot" syndrome
Gemcitabine	M, N + V (mild)
Taxanes and antimicrotubule agents	
Paclitaxel	M, hypersensitivity reactions (HR), neuropathy, MS, arthralgia/myalgia, alopecia, MS (rare)
Docetaxel	M, HR (rare), neuropathy, fluid retention, rash, alopecia
Nanoparticle albumin-bound paclitaxel	M, neuropathy, arthralgia/myalgia, alopecia
Ixabepilone	M, neuropathy, arthralgia/myalgia, alopecia
Eribulin	M, fatigue, neuropathy
Vincas	
Vinorelbine	Peripheral neuropathy, alopecia, M (rare), vesication
HER2 TARGETED	
Trastuzumab	Cardiomyopathy, infusion reactions
Lapatinib	Diarrhea, rash, decrease in left ventricular function
Pertuzumab	Diarrhea, rash, decrease in left ventricular function
Ado-trastuzumab emtansine	Transaminitis, thrombocytopenia, fatigue
Fam-trastuzumab deruxtecan	Alopecia, fatigue, interstitial lung disease
Tucatinib	Hepatoxicity, "hand-foot" syndrome, fatigue

M, myelosuppression; N + V, nausea and vomiting.

effective and less toxic. Osteoclast inhibition with bisphosphonates or denosumab significantly reduces the risk of skeletal-related events in women with bone metastases.

Older patients with metastatic disease, whose general health is otherwise satisfactory, display response and toxicity profiles to chemotherapy similar to those of their younger counterparts. Most cytotoxic drugs are metabolized in the liver with only a select few dependent on renal excretion (methotrexate, carboplatin, and cisplatin); major liver dysfunction probably is required to alter drug metabolism significantly. Chemotherapy-related myelosuppression is more common in older patients due to diminished bone marrow reserve with aging; nausea and vomiting are seen less frequently than they are in younger patients. Of importance, psychosocial adjustments to chemotherapy appear to be better for older than for younger patients. Complete and partial responses to most single chemotherapy agents range from 20% to 30%, while responses to combination chemotherapy average 50% to 70%. Responses generally last an average of 6 to 12 months; response rates to subsequent "salvage" regimens are generally low and last only several months.

SPECIAL ISSUES AND SPOPULATIONS

Prevention

There is no simple strategy to prevent breast cancer in older women. As the pathogenesis of breast cancer is likely to be related to interactions of estrogens, other hormones, and breast tissue, agents that lower breast tissue estrogen exposure, such as selective estrogen receptor modulators (SERMs) and aromatase inhibitors, have been studied and found to be effective in breast cancer prevention lowering the incidence by about half. None of these large trials, even after long term follow have shown any survival advantage in spite of decreased breast cancer occurrences in the treated patients. At present, we believe that only a few older high-risk patients should be considered for preventive therapy and that these patients should have an estimated life expectancy of at least 10 years. Like younger patients, older patients should be encouraged to maintain an ideal body mass and engage in exercise. In addition, prophylactic, contralateral surgery as a method for prevention is not recommended. In older women with *BRCA1* or *BRCA2* mutations prophylactic surgery should be considered on a case by case basis.

Follow-Up for Women With Early Breast Cancer

There is good evidence that close follow-up after diagnosis or adjuvant therapy does not result in improved overall survival, but that detection of early skin or lymph node (soft tissue) recurrence may result in more effective palliation. Mammography is an exception, and in women with life expectancies of at least 5 to 10 years, should be performed yearly or every other year to detect new primary lesions.

Because a history of breast cancer is a risk factor for another breast cancer, follow-up visits do provide an opportunity for patients to express concerns and for physicians to give them reassurance. Extensive laboratory and radiologic procedures are now available for the detection of metastatic disease, but trials have indicated that a brief, focused history and a limited physical examination (skin, chest, breast, and abdominal examination) detect more than 75% of metastases. Even when mammography is not recommended, an annual breast exam should be part of the patient's care. National guidelines suggest that optimal follow-up consists of periodic clinic visits and annual screening mammography in asymptomatic patients with a history of breast cancer. Available data do not support the use of routine laboratory work, imaging, or tumor markers for routine follow-up and should not be used in asymptomatic patients (**Table 89-5**).

Male Breast Cancer

Male breast cancer accounts for less than 1% of all breast cancer incidence and has a similar natural history as female breast cancer. Males usually present at a later stage, probably because of a delay in diagnosis. Almost all cases are sporadic, except for males with Klinefelter syndrome (sex chromosomes XXY)—in which the prevalence of breast cancer ranges from 3% to 6%—or men with the *BRCA2* gene, which is associated with a 5% to 10% risk. Men with a *BRCA2* are also at higher risk for prostate and other cancers. A careful family history is mandatory in all males with breast cancer. Mastectomy with axillary dissection is the standard approach to treatment but breast-conserving surgery and irradiation are appropriate for males with small tumors. Histologically, most lesions are infiltrating ductal carcinomas, and the frequency of ER-positive lesions is 70% to 80%. Because of the rarity of male breast cancer, there are few data on the role of adjuvant systemic therapy, and it is unlikely that large randomized trials will be undertaken. We suggest using the same guidelines for adjuvant therapy in men that are used in women with a similar stage and receptor status. Uncontrolled trials suggest that such treatment is similar in

TABLE 89-5 ■ FOLLOW-UP OF EARLY BREAST CANCER AFTER DIAGNOSIS AND INITIAL TREATMENT			
	FREQUENCY OF EXAMINATION		
	1–3 Y	3–5 Y	5+ Y
History and physical examination	Every 3–6 mo	Every 6–12 mo	Yearly
Breast self-examination	Monthly	Monthly	Monthly
Mammogram[a]	Yearly	Yearly	Yearly
Gynecologic examination[b]	PRN	PRN	PRN
Other[c]	PRN	PRN	PRN

[a]Breast MRI is not currently recommended as part of routine screening unless jn the setting of a known genetic predisposition or other higher-risk condition.
[b]Yearly gynecologic examinations are recommended, for older women on tamoxifen who have an intact uterus.
[c]Tumor marker studies, complete blood count, automated chemistry studies, chest and skeletal x-rays, ultrasound, and radionuclide, computed tomographic, and positron emission tomographic scans are not recommended in asymptomatic patients. Appropriate studies should be obtained for patients with signs or symptoms of recurrence only.
Data from Recommended Breast Cancer Surveillance Guidelines. American Society of Clinical Oncology; 2013.

efficacy in men to that in women, although tamoxifen is the preferred adjuvant endocrine therapy in men.

Men with metastatic breast cancer are incurable but frequently respond to endocrine therapy, including tamoxifen and androgen deprivation with LHRH agonists and aromatase inhibitors if they are hormone receptor positive. The results with systemic chemotherapy are similar to those in females.

Palliative Care, End-of-Life Care, and Hospice

For many patients and families with cancer, palliative care is synonymous with end-of-life care. This certainly is not the case and especially in the care of older patients with symptoms, early palliative care at the time of diagnosis of metastases or even for some patients with potentially curable disease, palliative care can make the cancer journey much more tolerable for both the patient and their family. Studies have shown that integrating palliative care with standard cancer treatment, including chemotherapy, can lead to significant improvements in quality of life and even survival. Although many oncologists are capable of managing the complex array of symptoms related to cancer and its treatment, partnering with a trained team of palliative care experts results in better outcomes and relieves the oncologist from providing the extensive array of supportive services needed for their patients. We suggest that a palliative care consultation be considered for all older patients with metastatic breast cancer and symptomatic patients with early breast cancer early in their course and preferably at the time of diagnosis.

For those with metastasis, the vast majority of older patients will succumb to their breast cancer. Those receiving palliative care can be easily transitioned to end-of-life care and hospice care. For those who have not had palliative care interventions, end-of-life care provided by palliative care experts and transition to hospice is recommended.

Disparities

Racial and age disparities in breast cancer care and outcomes have been well documented and have persisted over time,

despite increasing awareness of this issue. Past examinations of receipt of care and outcomes for women have consistently demonstrated lower rates of treatment and worse outcomes for Black and older patients compared to their White and younger counterparts. Furthermore, studies within cohorts of older patients also demonstrate racial disparities, including more delays to treatment, less standard therapy, shorter durations in therapy, and higher mortality rates for older Black versus White women. Patients with less access to care, those who are underinsured, and those from lower socioeconomic groups also suffer from worse outcomes from breast cancer. Assurance that all patients receive guideline-concordant care is a national priority and rigorous interventions to better understand optimal ways of delivering care to all women are desperately needed. Patients felt to be at risk for problems with system navigation and social issues should be referred for patient navigation, social work, and resource assistance whenever possible.

CONCLUSION

Breast cancer is a major gerontologic problem. Both physician and patient education concerning screening, early diagnosis, and management of breast cancer in this age group are required. Available data indicate that optimal treatment of breast cancer in older women results in outcomes similar to those from treatment of younger women. The GA should be used to optimize treatment decisions and those older patients with satisfactory function and good life expectancy should be managed with judicious "state-of-the-art" therapy. Palliative care should be initiated early in almost all symptomatic patients. Barriers to the treatment of breast cancer in older women are generic to the treatment of all illnesses in this age group and include access to care, transportation, adequate family and social support, physician bias, racial inequities, and treatment costs. Changes in health care policy, as well as focused research related to cancer in the geriatric population, will be needed to overcome these obstacles.

FURTHER READING

Amin MB, Edge S, Greene F, et al (eds). *AJCC Cancer Staging Manual (8th edition)*. Springer International Publishing: American Joint Commission on Cancer; 2017.

Early Breast Cancer Trialists' Collaborative Group (EBCTCG). Effects of chemotherapy and hormonal therapy for early breast cancer on recurrence and 15-year survival: an overview of the randomised trials. *Lancet*. 2005;365(9472):1687–1717.

Early Breast Cancer Trialists' Collaborative Group (EBCTCG), Peto R, Davies C, et al. Comparisons between different polychemotherapy regimens for early

breast cancer: meta-analyses of long-term outcome among 100,000 women in 123 randomised trials. *Lancet*. 2012;379(9814):432–444.

ePrognosis. Estimating prognosis for elders. http://eprognosis.ucsf.edu/.

Helson HD, Smith ME, Griffin JC, Fu R. Use of medications to reduce risk for primary breast cancer: a systematic review for the U.S. Preventative Services Task Force. *Ann Intern Med*. 2013;158(8):604–614.

Hughes KS, Schnaper LA, Bellon JR, et al. Lumpectomy plus tamoxifen with or without irradiation in women age 70 years or older with early breast cancer: long-term follow-up of CALGB 9343. *J Clin Oncol.* 2013;31(19): 2382–2387.

Hurria A, Naylor M, Cohen HJ. Improving the quality of cancer care in an aging population: recommendations from an IOM report. *JAMA.* 2013;310(7):1795–1796.

Hurria A, Togawa K, Mohile SG, et al. Predicting chemotherapy toxicity in older adults with cancer: a prospective multicenter study. *J Clin Oncol.* 2011;29(25): 3457–3465.

Khatcheressian JL, Hurley P, Bantug E, et al. Breast cancer follow-up and management after primary treatment: American Society of Clinical Oncology clinical practice guideline update. *J Clin Oncol.* 2013;3(7):961–965.

Lichtman SM. Chemotherapy in the elderly. *Semin Oncol.* 2004;31(2):160–174.

Lyman GH, Temin S, Edge SB, et al. Sentinel lymph node biopsy for patients with early-stage breast cancer: American Society of Clinical Oncology Clinical Practice Guideline Update. *J Clin Oncol.* 2014;32(13):1365–1386.

Magnuson A, Sedrak MS, Gross CP, et al. Development and validation of a risk score for predicting severe toxicity in older adults receiving chemotherapy for early-stage breast cancer. *J Clin Oncol.* 2021;39(6):608–618.

Mandelblatt JS, Sheppard VB, Hurria A, et al. Breast cancer adjuvant treatment decisions in older women: the role of patient preference and interactions with physicians. *J Clin Oncol.* 2010;28(19):3146–3153.

Mohile SG, Dale W, Somerfield MR, et al. Practical assessment and management of vulnerabilities in older patients receiving chemotherapy: ASCO Guideline for Geriatric Oncology. *J Clin Oncol.* 2018;36(22):2326–2347.

Muss HB, Berry DA, Cirrincione CT, et al. Adjuvant chemotherapy in older women with early-stage breast cancer. *N Engl J Med.* 2009;360(20):2055–2065.

Muss HB, Woolf S, Berry D, et al. Adjuvant chemotherapy in older and younger women with lymph node-positive breast cancer. *JAMA.* 2005;293(9):1073–1081.

Schonberg MA, Breslau ES, McCarthy EP. Targeting of mammography screening according to life expectancy in women aged 75 and older. *J Am Geriatr Soc.* 2013;61(3):388–395.

Schonberg MA, Marcantonio ER, Ngo L, Li D, Sillman RA, McCarthy EP. Causes of death and relative survival of older women after a breast cancer diagnosis. *J Clin Oncol.* 2011;29(12):1570–1577.

Walter LC, Schonberg MA. Screening mammography in older women: a review. *JAMA.* 2014;311(13):1336–1347.

Wildiers H, Heeren P, Puts M, et al. International Society of Geriatric Oncology consensus on geriatric assessment in older patients with cancer. *J Clin Oncol.* 2014;32(24):2595–2603.

Yancik R, Wesley MN, Varicchio CG, et al. Effect of age and comorbidity in postmenopausal breast cancer patients aged 55 years and older. *JAMA.* 2001;285(7):885–892.

Prostate Cancer

Liang Dong, Mark C. Markowski, Kenneth J. Pienta

EPIDEMIOLOGY AND RISK FACTORS

Prostate cancer remains the most common noncutaneous malignancy diagnosed in American men and is the second leading cause of cancer-related deaths. Currently about 248,000 US men per year are diagnosed with prostate cancer and about 34,000 US men per year die of the disease.

The only undisputed risk factors for prostate cancer are older age, African-American race, and positive family history. Prostate cancer is generally a disease of older men; risk increases exponentially with age, with a median age at presentation of 66 years. More than half of prostate cancer diagnoses and 90% of prostate cancer deaths occur in men older than 65. The incidence rates of the disease among African-American men are higher than rates for men in *any* other racial or ethnic background. African-American men are more likely to be diagnosed with prostate cancer and to die from it than their White counterparts. The estimated lifetime risk of prostate cancer is 17.6% for White and 20.6% for African-Americans, while the estimated lifetime risk of death is 2.8% and 4.7%. Early-onset prostate cancer may be inherited in an autosomal dominant fashion. Approximately 10% of all prostate cancer cases are hereditary, with an onset 6 to 7 years earlier than nonhereditary cases. Several germline mutations such as *BRCA1/2*, *HOXB13*, or *ATM* may also identify families at high risk. *BRCA1/2* germline mutations are present in up to 6% of unselected prostate cancer patients. The prospective Identification of Men With a Genetic Predisposition to Prostate Cancer targeted screening study confirmed a higher incidence of prostate cancer, at a younger age and with more clinically significant tumors, only in *BRCA2* mutation carriers compared with noncarriers.

Additional factors such as diet, obesity, hormones, inflammation and sexually transmitted diseases, and occupational exposure have all been implicated in prostate carcinogenesis, but without consistent results. Dietary fat may be a risk factor for prostate cancer. Multiple epidemiologic, case-control, and cohort studies have suggested a moderate-to-strong increased risk of developing prostate cancer, particularly advanced disease, associated with total dietary fat, saturated fat, α-linolenic fatty acid, and cooked red meat. Two large prospective studies and a smaller case-control study suggest that fish intake may be

Learning Objectives

- List the risk factors for the development of prostate cancer.
- Understand the screening recommendations for prostate cancer in older men.
- Describe the treatment options for localized and advanced prostate cancer in older patients.

Key Clinical Points

1. There is no Food and Drug Administration (FDA)-approved treatment shown to reduce the risk of developing prostate cancer.
2. Life expectancy and comorbidities should be considered before initiating prostate cancer screening.
3. Localized prostate cancer in an older patient can be effectively treated with a range of therapies including watchful waiting, active surveillance, surgery, and/or radiation.

protective, possibly owing to marine omega-3 fatty acids—known antagonists of arachidonic acid, which suppress the production of proinflammatory cytokines. Evidence for the association with dietary fat is further correlated with worldwide incidence patterns; prostate cancer is more common in the United States and northern European countries and is relatively rare in Asia and Africa. When Asian men migrate to the West and change from a low-fat to a high-fat diet, their risk of prostate cancer increases. However, many of the men migrating from low-fat diet areas also consume green tea and soy products, which contain isoflavones and estrogen that may act as antioxidants and chemoprotectants against prostate-specific carcinogenesis. There appears to be an inverse relationship between soy intake and prostate cancer risk.

There is no consistent association between obesity and prostate cancer incidence. However, there are associations between obesity and aggressive prostate cancer, recurrence after primary therapy, and death from prostate cancer.

Data from the Prostate Cancer Prevention Trial (PCPT) suggest that obesity increases the risk of higher-grade cancers, but decreases the risk of low-grade prostate cancer. These findings suggest that obesity may somehow play a role in the progression from latent to clinically significant prostate cancer. Data from a prospective study of 3398 African-American and 22,673 non-Hispanic White men who participated in the Selenium and Vitamin E Cancer Prevention Trial (SELECT) demonstrated that obesity was more strongly associated with increased prostate cancer risk among African-American than non-Hispanic White men and that reducing obesity among African-American men could reduce the racial disparity in cancer incidence. Although the specific role of obesity in prostate cancer risk is unclear, it may be linked to other risk factors such as dietary fat and meat intake, hormone metabolism, and insulin metabolism. The prevalence of obesity also correlates with prostate cancer risk across populations and may provide a link between the increased risk of prostate cancer with westernization.

A diet rich in fruits and vegetables is associated with reduced risk for several cancers, but their effect on prostate cancer risk is unclear. There is an inverse association with use of tomatoes and tomato products, presumably owing to the effects of lycopene, the most common carotenoid in the human body and one of the most potent carotenoid antioxidants. The Health Professionals Follow-Up Study (HPFS) found that frequent consumption of tomato products is associated with a decreased risk of prostate cancer, and in a meta-analysis of 21 case-control and cohort studies, a significant 10% to 20% risk reduction was associated with high versus low intake of tomatoes. The majority of these studies also show a stronger effect for cooked versus raw tomatoes.

Although it seems intuitive that testosterone levels may influence the incidence of prostate cancer, no evidence confirms this association. Dihydrotestosterone, the active hormone produced from the conversion of testosterone by the enzyme 5α-reductase, is associated in some studies with increased risk. A prospective, population-based study of 1156 men showed no correlation between 17 different hormones and prostate cancer development, with the possible exception of androstanediol glucuronide. Importantly, no dose-response relationships were seen, suggesting that serum hormone levels may not be useful even in risk stratification.

There is some evidence that chronic inflammation may increase prostate cancer risk. One meta-analysis of 11 studies on prostatitis and prostate cancer showed an overall relative risk of 1.6. A prospective study of men without biopsy indication (PCPT participants who had a negative end-of-study biopsy and who subsequently enrolled in the SELECT) demonstrated that benign tissue inflammation was positively associated with prostate cancer. Population studies have suggested an increased risk of prostate cancer in patients with sexually transmitted diseases (STDs), including syphilis, recurrent gonorrhea, human papilloma

virus (HPV), and HIV. A meta-analysis of 17 studies of prostate cancer and sexual patterns suggested that an increased number of sexual partners is associated with an increased prostate cancer risk, possibly through an increased exposure to STDs. There are currently no strong data to suggest a link between benign prostate hypertrophy (BPH) and prostate cancer risk.

PREVENTION

Chemoprevention is an area of ongoing research, and in many ways, prostate cancer is an ideal disease for this approach—relatively slow growing, centered in the older adult population, yet with devastating effects and difficult management after the onset of metastasis. To date, many promising agents have failed to show a protective benefit against developing prostate cancer, and no drugs or food supplements have been approved for prostate cancer prevention.

5α-Reductase Inhibitors

Finasteride blocks the actions of 5α-reductase, the enzyme that converts testosterone to dihydrotestosterone. The PCPT and the Reduction by Dutasteride of Prostate Cancer Events (REDUCE) trials investigated the role of 5α-reductase in prostate cancer prevention. These trials were based on two observations: androgens are required for prostate cancer development and men with congenital 5α-reductase deficiency develop neither BPH nor prostate cancer. Both of these randomized, double-blind, placebo-controlled trials showed prostate cancer risk reduction with finasteride. However, both trials also found an apparent increase in high-risk cancers in the intervention groups. High-grade prostate cancers are associated with a poorer prognosis after definitive therapy. Both the PCPT and REDUCE trials led the FDA to issue a safety announcement that 5α-reductase inhibitors may increase the risk of more serious prostate cancers and so are not approved for chemoprevention.

Vitamin E and Selenium

Oxidative stress may play a role in the development of prostate cancer. Reactive oxygen species can damage deoxyribonucleic acid (DNA), lipids, and proteins. The association of prostate cancer and a high-fat diet may be secondary to the generation of increased fatty acids, which can cause lipid peroxidation. Selenium is an essential trace nutrient with antioxidant properties. α-Tocopherol is the most active and abundant source of vitamin E, and its antioxidant properties have been studied extensively in a variety of prostate cell lines and animal models. One trial of male smokers with a primary lung cancer end point included α-tocopherol (50 mg daily). Because groups taking α-tocopherol may have had decreased prostate cancer incidence and mortality, the role of antioxidants in prostate cancer prevention was studied further.

SELECT was a large, randomized, prospective, double-blind trial designed to determine whether selenium and vitamin E decrease the risk of prostate cancer in healthy men. In 2008, the trial was stopped early when an interim analysis demonstrated no evidence of clinical benefit of either agent. In addition to the lack of benefit of either agent alone or combined, there was a nonsignificant increased risk of prostate cancer in the vitamin E alone group. With additional follow-up in 2011, the number of prostate cancers in patients treated with vitamin E alone was significantly increased compared to the placebo arm. Thus, although there was great excitement about antioxidant supplementation for prostate cancer prevention, particularly in older people, randomized prospective trial data has shown no overall benefit.

PRESENTATION/SCREENING

Most men who present with prostate cancer are asymptomatic, particularly in the era of prostate-specific antigen (PSA) testing, which detects many cancers long before they are clinically apparent. Patients rarely have urinary symptoms, as the majority of cancers arise in the posterior aspect of the prostate. Most men undergo evaluation after routine screening reveals either an elevated PSA or abnormal digital rectal exam (DRE). Since the advent of PSA testing and regular screening, in the United States the majority of patients have clinically localized, intermediate-risk prostate cancer at diagnosis. A minority of patients are diagnosed when they present with symptomatic metastatic disease, usually manifested as bony pain. For example, in 1988, 14% of new prostate cancer patients presented with metastatic disease, but that number had fallen to 3.3% by 1998 and has remained stable since that time. Although screening has strongly influenced this downward stage migration, there is still a debate as to whether it has significantly decreased prostate cancer–specific mortality.

Two large-scale, long-term, randomized clinical trials were designed to evaluate whether screening decreases mortality. The Prostate, Lung, Colorectal, and Ovarian Cancer (PLCO) trial was based in the United States and randomized over 76,000 men (age 55–74) to either an annual screening arm or control group. Those patients randomized to get screened had an annual PSA value for 6 years as well as a DRE for 4 years. After 7 years, screening was associated with a 22% relative increase in prostate cancers diagnosed with no difference in prostate cancer–specific mortality after both 7 and 10 years. The European Randomized Study of Screening for Prostate Cancer (ERSPC) trial randomized over 180,000 men (age 50–74) to screening versus control. In contrast to the PLCO trial, PSA screening resulted in a significant 20% relative reduction in prostate cancer–specific mortality after a median follow-up of 13 years (the number of men needed to be invited for screening to prevent one prostate cancer death was 742). The updated findings from the follow-up of the ERSPC trial (maximum of 16 years) corroborate earlier results that PSA screening significantly reduces prostate cancer–specific mortality.

However, it also reconfirms that PSA screening does not reduce all-cause mortality.

The results of the Cluster Randomized Trial of PSA Testing for Prostate Cancer (CAP) in men aged 50 to 69 suggested that a single PSA test did not improve prostate cancer–specific mortality after a median follow-up of 10 years. However, the optimal time intervals for PSA testing and when to stop screening is still unknown and under debate. One study predicted a 27% relative decrease in the probability of lives saved if the stopping age for PSA screening was changed from 74 to 69. This was tempered with a 50% relative decrease in overdiagnosis. A comparison of systematic and opportunistic screening suggested a reduction in overdiagnosis and cancer-specific mortality by systematic screening, while opportunistic screening resulted in a higher overdiagnosis rate with a marginal survival benefit. The National Comprehensive Cancer Network (NCCN) suggested that PSA screening after age 75 should be done only in very healthy men with little or no comorbidity to detect the small number of aggressive cancers that pose a significant risk if left undetected.

A summary of the various screening recommendations is provided in **Table 90-1**. These recommendations do not apply for men at higher risk for prostate cancer. In the absence of unified guidelines, a difficult task for primary care physicians is thus deciding which patients should undergo screening for prostate cancer. In the absence of definitive data, a reasonable approach to screening should involve an active discussion between the physician and patient, taking into consideration the patient's overall health and treatment preferences. Men with a life expectancy of

TABLE 90-1 ■ PSA SCREENING RECOMMENDATIONS IN OLDER ADULTS[a]	
ORGANIZATION	**RECOMMENDATIONS**
NCCN	> Age 75: PSA screening should be done only in very healthy men with little or no comorbidity to detect the small number of aggressive cancers that pose a significant risk if left undetected.
USPSTF 2018	Age 55–69: individualized and informed decision-making regarding PSA screening (grade C)
	> Age 70: PSA screening not recommended (Grade D)
AUA 2018	Age 55–69: Shared decision-making and review of risks/benefits prior to PSA screening. If electing PSA screening, an interval of 2 or more years may be preferred over annual screening.
	> Age 70: No PSA screening with less than 10–15 years of life expectancy

[a]Not applicable to men at higher risk for prostate cancer.
AUA, American Urological Association; NCCN, National Comprehensive Cancer Network; PSA, prostate-specific antigen; USPSTF, US Preventative Services Task Force.

less than 10 to 15 years (owing to age or comorbidities) should be informed that screening may not be beneficial. Younger men with a family history of prostate cancer or *BRCA2* mutation and African-American men should be encouraged to undergo screening, as the disease prevalence is high in these groups. Any patient with symptoms that may be attributable to prostate cancer (bone pain, hypercalcemia, symptomatic pelvic lymphadenopathy) warrants a PSA evaluation as a part of his initial evaluation, since symptomatic patients can enjoy significant improvement with the institution of hormonal therapy.

EVALUATION

Once the decision to do screening for prostate cancer is made, the appropriate examinations include a serum PSA and DRE. PSA is a protein produced and secreted by both normal prostate and prostate cancer cells. It provides a sensitive but not highly specific screening test, as it is also elevated with BPH, inflammation, and infection of the prostate. The usual cutoff is 4 ng/mL, but 15% of men with normal PSA levels will have prostate cancer and 2% will have high-grade prostate cancer. PSA is, however, more sensitive than DRE, detecting more cancers at earlier stage and smaller-sized cancers than rectal examination alone. The free-to-total PSA ratio stratifies the risk of prostate cancer in men with 4 to 10 ng/mL total PSA. PSA-doubling time is also a factor in prostate assessment, and any patient with a rapid PSA-doubling time should be sent for further evaluation, even if the absolute value of the PSA is below the normal cutoff level. On the basis of an elevated PSA or an abnormal DRE, the patient should be referred for a transrectal or transperineal ultrasound-guided prostate biopsy. In general, six to 12 cores are taken for evaluation; areas that are abnormal on DRE may receive more biopsy attempts. Multiparametric magnetic resonance imaging (mpMRI) is a major tool for biopsy optimization with pooled sensitivity of greater than 0.90 and specificity of greater than 0.35. When mpMRI has shown a suspicious lesion, MR-targeted biopsy can be obtained through cognitive guidance, ultrasound/magnetic resonance fusion software, or direct in-bore guidance. In biopsy-naïve patients, the addition of targeted biopsy increases the number of detected prostate cancers by 20% to 30%.

If the biopsy is positive, a Gleason score is assigned. This score is one of the most important determinants of prognosis. The pathologist assigns a numerical value (on a scale of 1–5) to the most prevalent and the second most prevalent grades of cancer seen in the specimens. The score is then reported on a scale of 2 to 10, with 10 being the most aggressive cancer. Gleason scores should be reported separately, for example, 3 + 4 = 7, as the primary pathology has prognostic implications. Risk stratification plays an important role in both the selection and timing of treatment and is an important part of the initial evaluation. After

diagnosis, the natural course of prostate cancer can be estimated from tumor volume, aggressiveness, PSA level, and extent of disease. Tumor volume assessment includes local stage, the number of positive biopsy cores, and the extent of cancer in affected cores. Gleason score is currently the standard measurement of aggressiveness with grade group 1 tumors being Gleason score ≤ 6, grade group 2 being Gleason score 3 + 4, grade group 3 being Gleason score 4 + 3, grade group 4 being Gleason score 8, and grade group 5 being Gleason score 9 to 10. Taking all of these prognostic factors into account, newly diagnosed patients are classified as having very low-, low-, intermediate-, or high-risk disease. The patients in the intermediate risk group can be further stratified to favorable and unfavorable subgroups. A summary of the risk stratification and recommendations on staging is provided in **Table 90-2**. In addition to these broad risk groups, multiple nomograms are available to help clinicians estimate an individual patient's probability of localized disease, risk of progression without intervention, and risk of recurrence after definitive therapy. Several of these tools are available online, and they can sometimes be more helpful than the broad categories in assessing an individual's risk, as they allow integration of discordant factors (eg, high PSA with low Gleason score). PSA velocity prior to diagnosis may also provide valuable information in risk assessment; a PSA velocity greater than or equal to 2 ng/mL in the year prior to radical prostatectomy (RP) is predictive of greater risk of biochemical recurrence, cancer-specific mortality, and overall mortality.

The conventional staging evaluation for men with known prostate cancer or symptoms that could be attributable to metastatic prostate cancer includes serum chemistries, PSA, bone scan, and computed tomography (CT) scan of the abdomen and pelvis. These initial tests provide evaluation of the most likely sites of metastatic disease to avoid inappropriate surgical intervention or radiation therapy. As described in **Table 90-2**, the extent of evaluation for metastatic disease relates to the likelihood of finding disease. However, advanced imaging technologies have been dramatically changing this field. For example, choline positron emission tomography (PET)/CT, prostate-specific membrane antigen (PSMA) PET/CT, and whole-body MRI provide more sensitive detection of lymph nodes and bone metastases than the conventional tools. **Figure 90-1** illustrates a stepwise approach to evaluation, monitoring, and treatment.

MANAGEMENT

After an initial diagnosis of prostate cancer, treatment decisions should take into consideration a number of factors including the individual patient's remaining life expectancy if known, comorbidities, baseline quality of life (QoL), treatment preferences, and disease characteristics/risk factors.

TABLE 90-2 ■ GUIDELINES FOR STAGING IMAGING EVALUATION

RISK	PARAMETERS			IMAGING EVALUATION
Very low	• T1c AND • Grade group 1 AND • PSA < 10 ng/mL AND • Fewer than 3 prostate biopsy cores positive, ≤ 50% cancer in each core AND • PSA density < 0.15 ng/mL			Not indicated
Low	• T1-T2a AND • Grade group 1 AND • PSA < 10 ng/mL			Not indicated
Intermediate	Has no high- or very high-risk features and has one or more of these: • T2b-T2c • Grade group 2 or 3 • PSA 10–20 ng/mL	Favorable	• 1 intermediate risk factor AND • Grade group 1 or 2 AND • < 50% biopsy core positive	Bone scan is not recommended. Perform pelvic/abdominal imaging.
		Unfavorable	• 2 or 3 intermediate risk factor AND/OR • Grade group 3 AND/OR • ≥ 50% biopsy core positive	Bone scan is recommended if T2 and PSA > 10 ng/mL. Perform pelvic/abdominal imaging.
High	• T3a OR • Grade group 4 or 5 OR • PSA > 20 ng/mL			Perform bone scan and pelvic/abdominal imaging.
Very high	• T3b-T4 OR • Primary Gleason pattern 5 OR • > 4 cores with grade group 4 or 5			Perform bone scan and pelvic/abdominal imaging.

PSA, prostate-specific antigen; T, tumor size based on the standard TNM classification.

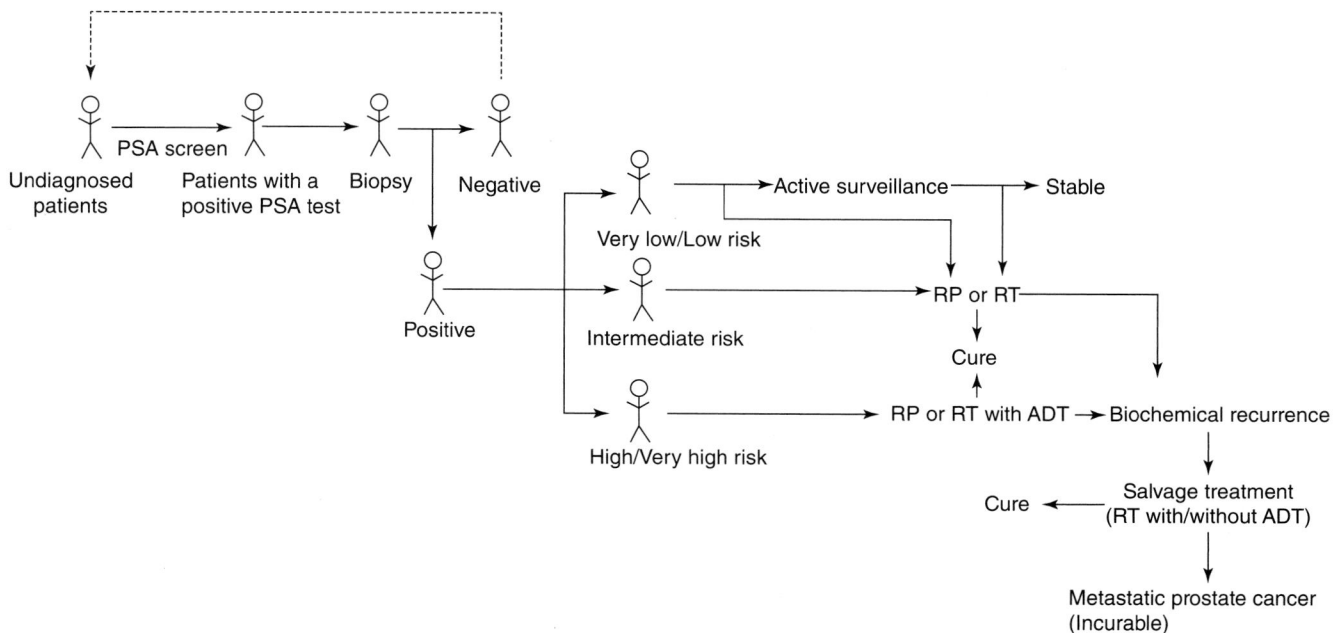

FIGURE 90-1. Prostate cancer evaluation and management flowchart. ADT, androgen deprivation therapy; PSA, prostate-specific antigen; RP, radical prostatectomy; RT, radiation therapy.

Watchful Waiting

The concept of observation or watchful waiting involves deferring treatment until patients develop symptomatic disease. It was first proposed in the 1970s when research suggested that delaying therapy until the onset of symptoms did not increase prostate cancer–specific mortality in patients with locally advanced or metastatic disease. However, a subsequent study found that overall survival was longer in patients treated immediately, and the rate of complications, such as bone pain, pathologic fractures, spinal cord compression, and ureteral obstruction was higher in the deferred group. Because PSA testing allows detection of cancers some 5 to 15 years earlier than DRE, men with T1c (PSA detected) tumors treated with watchful waiting may have better than 20-year disease-specific survival. Among a prospective cohort of 300 men (mean age 72) with localized disease, an equivalent 15-year overall survival was observed in those who deferred therapy versus those who received initial treatment. Watchful waiting, either at the time of initial diagnosis or at the time of progression, may be applicable in older men without metastatic disease. In the AUA guideline, watchful waiting is recommended for men with a life expectancy greater than or equal to 5 years with low- or intermediate-risk localized prostate cancer. In patients with high-risk disease, watchful waiting should only be considered in asymptomatic men with limited life expectancy ($\leq$ 5 years).

Active Surveillance

Active surveillance or expectant management differs from watchful waiting in the intensity of monitoring and the expectation of delayed but successful definitive, potentially curative therapy. This strategy is based on the observation that there is tremendous heterogeneity in the natural history of prostate cancer, and a significant number of men may be "overdiagnosed" in the sense that diagnosis and treatment may not improve either QoL or survival. The selection criteria for active surveillance remain controversial, so should be made by the patient with his urologist. Active surveillance involves regular monitoring with PSA every 3 months, clinical examination with DRE every 6 months, and repeat biopsies as warranted by PSA and DRE (which can occur as frequently as once a year). An increase in PSA velocity (doubling time fewer than 3 years), primary Gleason pattern of 4 or 5 on repeat biopsy, or an increased number or extent of positive biopsy cores suggests progression of disease, and intervention with appropriately selected therapy should be initiated. Many experts feel that this is a reasonable approach for men with low-risk disease and may represent a practical compromise between radical treatment for all patients and watchful waiting with palliative treatment only (a strategy that undertreats aggressive disease). Although active surveillance may avoid overtreatment and allow patients to maintain their baseline QoL, the strategy carries with it a risk of local or metastatic progression before active treatment is initiated. It is important, therefore, that patients are made aware that even the most careful monitoring may miss the window for administering curative therapy.

Local Therapy: Surgery, Radiation, or Brachytherapy

Radical prostatectomy RP involves removal of the prostate and seminal vesicles, and is an appropriate therapy for any patient with disease confined to the prostate, a life expectancy more than 10 years, and no contraindications to surgery. Data have shown that outcomes are generally better with high-volume surgeons within high-volume medical centers. Laparoscopic and robotic prostatectomies have been refined and moved into mainstream care. Outcome data to date suggest that in the hands of an experienced surgeon, these approaches are comparable to open surgery and may involve less morbidity. Randomized clinical trials have shown no benefit for neoadjuvant hormonal therapy with RP. Pathologic examination after surgery allows for verification of organ confinement and margin status as well as complete histologic examination. Almost 50% of patients with biopsy Gleason 6 disease are upgraded to Gleason 7 or higher once the entire gland is removed and evaluated.

External beam radiation therapy External beam radiation therapy (EBRT) in most centers is now delivered using intensity-modulated radiation therapy (IMRT) or stereotactic body radiotherapy (SBRT). IMRT is a form of external beam photon therapy that uses multiple radiation beam and/or arcs to provide a highly conformal treatment of the prostate with normal tissue sparing of adjacent organs. SBRT generally utilizes photon-based IMRT treatment to deliver hypofractionated radiation treatment usually in five or fewer fractions of treatment. Often gold fiducial markers are implanted in the prostate prior to EBRT to provide landmarks for accurate daily dosing.

Radiation dosing is currently based on risk of recurrence. Patients with low-risk prostate cancer are generally treated with 70 to 75 Gy in 35 to 41 fractions. Higher doses of 75 to 80 Gy are recommended for patients with intermediate- and high-risk features. In addition, intermediate-risk patients benefit from 4 to 6 months of neoadjuvant and adjuvant androgen deprivation therapy (ADT), while high-risk patients should receive neoadjuvant and adjuvant ADT for a total of 2 to 3 years. Because the prostate is not removed with EBRT, there is no pathologic confirmation of the extent of disease or adjustment of the biopsy Gleason score. Relative contraindications to EBRT include active collagen vascular disease, inflammatory bowel disease, and microvascular damage from hypertension or diabetes.

Brachytherapy Brachytherapy involves radioactive iodine (^{125}I) or palladium (^{103}Pd) implants, which are placed in the prostate under general anesthesia. They emit short-range radiation within the prostate, generally avoiding the bladder and rectum, and lose their radioactivity gradually.

Prostate brachytherapy as monotherapy is indicated for patients with low-risk disease and small prostate volume (< 60 g). For intermediate-risk patients, brachytherapy is frequently combined with EBRT (40–50 Gy). High-risk patients are generally considered poor candidates for this treatment modality.

Although there are no good randomized data comparing local treatment modalities, a review of 2991 patients treated at the Cleveland Clinic and Memorial Sloan Kettering Cancer Center showed similar 5-year biochemical relapse-free survival rates for RP, EBRT, and brachytherapy, leading the authors to conclude that intrinsic tumor characteristics rather than treatment modality play the larger role in determining progression after definitive therapy. Given similar outcomes between EBRT and prostatectomy, logistics and potential side effects may play a significant role in treatment decisions. Some men may not be candidates for major pelvic surgery, and therefore prostatectomy may not be an option. Others may find the 8 to 9 weeks of daily radiation treatments unacceptable and opt for prostatectomy or brachytherapy, which is completed in a single surgical procedure. Incontinence is the primary side effect noted after prostatectomy, though reported rates vary significantly from surgeon to surgeon. EBRT causes short-term irritative bladder symptoms; long-term incontinence is rare. Bowel dysfunction is a potential short and/or delayed side effect of radiation therapy. Impotence occurs in as many as 50% of patients treated with any of the three local approaches, though it tends to occur later with EBRT than with prostatectomy. Primary care providers may want to refer patients to both urology and radiation oncology in order to fully educate patients about their choices.

Primary Androgen Deprivation

Patients with unfavorable prognostic factors, or those patients who are not interested in the risk-benefit ratio of local therapy, may choose primary hormonal therapy. Approximately 12.5% of the 3486 men in the Prostate Cancer Outcomes Study chose hormonal treatment as initial therapy, considered to be a surprisingly high number. Clearly, there is no chance of cure with this modality, but for some patients the risk of relapse may be too high to pursue aggressive local therapy. There is also scant evidence about the outcomes associated with this approach. In the European Association of Urology (EAU) guideline, ADT monotherapy is not recommended for asymptomatic patients. In patients with locally advanced disease, ADT monotherapy is only recommended for those patients unwilling or unable to receive any form of local treatment if they have a PSA-doubling time of less than 12 months and a PSA value of greater than 50 ng/mL, a poorly differentiated tumor, or troublesome local disease-related symptoms.

Adjuvant Therapy

At this time, there is no standard adjuvant chemotherapy for patients at high-risk of recurrence, although there are several intergroup trials examining the role of adjuvant chemotherapy with both RP and EBRT. Adjuvant hormonal therapy, as noted earlier, is now standard of care with EBRT in patients with intermediate- and high-risk disease; after RP, it is recommended only for patients with node-positive disease. Patients whose PSA levels do not fall to an undetectable level after surgery should be evaluated for adjuvant salvage therapy, including EBRT with or without ADT, or ADT alone.

POSTTREATMENT SURVEILLANCE

The scheduled follow-up after definitive local therapy depends on the risk of recurrence and the potential for curative salvage therapy. Patients at high risk of recurrence who would be good candidates for further intervention should have regular PSA testing (every 1–3 months) and DRE at least annually. Patients at low risk of recurrence or poor intervention candidates are more appropriately followed with evaluations every 4 to 6 months for the first 5 years and annually thereafter. Forty-five percent of patients who recur after prostatectomy do so within 2 years. Seventy-seven percent of recurrences occur within the first 5 years after prostatectomy and 96% within 9 years. Any patient with symptoms referable to local or systemic relapse (particularly new bone pain) should be evaluated with repeat serum and radiologic tests.

Biochemical Recurrence

Biochemical recurrence after RP is defined as a PSA level greater than or equal to 0.2 ng/mL and rising on two or more determinations. Recurrence after EBRT has been redefined by consensus as nadir PSA plus 2. The pattern of local recurrence is usually 1 to 3 years after primary therapy, with a slowly rising PSA or new finding on DRE; these patients should be followed closely and referred for local salvage therapy, if appropriate. The need for biopsy of radiologically proven disease in this setting is controversial. Patients who relapse quickly after local therapy (< 6 months) are more likely to have metastatic disease that was not discovered prior to definitive local therapy and are therefore unlikely to respond to local salvage therapy. As mentioned above, new PET imaging tracers appear more accurate in the assessment of prostate cancer. In 2019, the EAU guidelines for imaging in patients with recurrence recommend performing a PSMA PET/CT early after initial treatment if the result will influence subsequent treatment decisions.

Patients with a rising PSA and no clinical, symptomatic, or radiographic evidence of disease present a therapeutic dilemma, as there is no clear consensus as to the timing of further therapy. Some men with biochemical recurrence will eventually die of prostate cancer, while others will have indolent disease and ultimately die of other causes. Prognosis is best estimated by considering initial stage, Gleason grade, and PSA in addition to the absolute value of the

TABLE 90-3 ■ COMMONLY USED HORMONAL THERAPY OPTIONS

TREATMENT	MECHANISM	EXAMPLE	ADMINISTRATION
Orchiectomy	Removal of major source of testosterone		Surgical
LHRH agonist/antagonist	Stops the pulsatile secretion of LHRH from the pituitary and production of testosterone by the testes	Zoladex, Lupron, Trelstar	By depot injection, every 3–4 mo
First-generation antiandrogen	Androgen receptor antagonist	Casodex, Eulexin, Nilandron	Daily pill
CYP17 inhibitors	Inhibit synthesis of adrenal and testicular androgens	Abiraterone acetate	Daily pill
Second-generation antiandrogen	Androgen receptor antagonist	Enzalutamide, apalutamide, darolutamide	Daily pill

LHRH, luteinizing hormone–releasing hormone.

PSA at the time of recurrence and the PSA-doubling time. PSA-doubling time has been shown to be a useful parameter for monitoring patients and deciding when to initiate treatment after biochemical recurrence. PSA-doubling time of fewer than or equal to 3 months predicts cancer-specific mortality among patients with biochemical recurrence after either RP or EBRT.

Salvage Local Therapy

Approximately 20% to 25% of men with local recurrence postprostatectomy can be cured with early salvage EBRT. Several factors predict long-term response to salvage ERBT: Gleason score less than or equal to 7, positive surgical margins at RP, negative nodal or seminal vesicle involvement, and post-RP PSA kinetics consistent with local failure. Patients who recur immediately after definitive radiation therapy are candidates for ADT, observation, or, in selected cases, salvage prostatectomy.

ADVANCED DISEASE

A positive bone scan and pain in a weightbearing area correlating to the scan should prompt an x-ray to assess for impending pathologic fractures. Patients should be made nonweightbearing and immediately referred for both surgical and radiation consultation. The possibility of cord compression should be suspected in any man with a history of prostate cancer and new-onset back pain. Pain from spinal cord compression is often severe and generally predates neurologic symptoms. A negative neurologic examination should not delay a definitive radiologic study (preferably MRI or CT myelogram), and patients with suspected cord compression should be initiated and maintained on steroids until compression is ruled out.

Hormonal Therapy

First-line hormonal therapy Patients with advanced disease at presentation, or patients who relapse after definitive local therapy are initially treated with some form of ADT. The timing of hormonal therapy for a biochemical recurrence after definitive therapy is controversial. Early initiation of ADT in these patients reduced prostate cancer–specific mortality (17% relative risk) when compared to symptom-driven initiation. However, overall mortality was similar in both groups. Without clear guidelines, ADT is typically initiated based on PSA-doubling time, Gleason score, and patient preferences. Hormonal therapy for patients with advanced disease is usually initiated at presentation.

The goal of ADT is to decrease the level of testosterone available to potentiate growth of the prostate cancer cells. A variety of treatments can achieve this goal; **Table 90-3** outlines the spectrum of drugs, which either alone or in combination are used as ADT. Currently, the majority of men on ADT are treated with luteinizing hormone–releasing hormone (LHRH) agonists or antagonists alone (monotherapy) or in combination with an antiandrogen (combined androgen blockade). Although some physicians routinely use combination therapy, others prefer LHRH monotherapy, and there are no clear data showing benefit of one strategy over the other. Patients with known metastatic disease, however, need to be on an antiandrogen for at least 30 days, starting 7 to 10 days prior to initiation of LHRH agonist therapy to avoid the initial testosterone flare associated with LHRH therapy.

Orchiectomy (surgical castration) is an underused and underappreciated form of hormonal treatment. Morbidity associated with the procedure currently is minimal and barring unforeseen complications, it is an outpatient procedure. Data from the Prostate Cancer Outcomes Study provided an update on QoL issues for patients receiving hormonal therapy. Men who chose LHRH agonist therapy reported greater problems than orchiectomy patients did with their overall sexual functioning, despite both groups having similar levels of function prior to beginning treatment. LHRH patients were also less likely to perceive themselves as free of cancer, likely because of the need for ongoing injections.

The duration of response to first-line ADT is typically 18 to 24 months, although patients who initiate therapy for biochemical relapse alone may show PSA responses for much longer. The continuation of ADT in the setting of hormone-refractory disease is a subject of some controversy.

Given the potential for improved survival for patients remaining on testicular androgen suppression, many physicians continue to administer LHRH agonists for the duration of treatment with secondary hormonal therapies and chemotherapy.

Side effects from hormonal therapies include hot flashes, insomnia, decreased libido, erectile dysfunction, weight gain/fluid retention, diabetes, increased risk of cardiovascular events, and breast enlargement/nipple tenderness. Breast enlargement can be curtailed, although not reversed, by a few treatments of electron beam radiation directly to the breast stem cells underneath the areola. This low-risk treatment can provide significant physical and psychological benefit. Antiandrogen treatment can lead to hepatic dysfunction, requiring monitoring of liver function tests (LFTs) after the initial month of therapy, and every 3 months thereafter. Antiandrogens are also associated with gastrointestinal effects, including nausea, diarrhea, and constipation. Estrogens can predispose patients to thromboembolic complications, including deep vein thrombosis, pulmonary embolism, and myocardial infarction.

Patients with decreased testosterone caused by orchiectomy or ADT also have a significantly increased risk of bone loss. Most studies have demonstrated a 2% to 3% decrease per year in bone mineral density (BMD) of the hip and spine during initial testosterone suppressing therapy, and BMD continues to decline during long-term therapy. Fracture rates are also higher in patients on ADT. Three large, claims-based studies have shown that LHRH treatment is independently associated with fracture risk. Patients on testosterone suppressing therapy should, therefore, be encouraged to take daily calcium (500 mg) and vitamin D (400 IU) supplements to prevent bone loss. In addition, patients may benefit from BMD testing to evaluate overall bone health. Men with osteopenia or osteoporosis should be considered for treatment with oral bisphosphonates (see section on "Supportive Care").

Intermittent androgen deprivation Intermittent androgen blockade has been advocated as a way to decrease side effects from ADT and also to, potentially, increase the time to androgen independence. With this strategy, patients are cycled on and off hormonal therapy based on PSA response. Once patients achieve an undetectable PSA in response to ADT, they are taken off therapy and monitored; treatment is reinitiated based on absolute PSA value and/or PSA-doubling time. Two prospective trials found that intermittent therapy was noninferior to continuous treatment for the primary outcome of overall survival. Additionally, QoL indicators were better in the intermittent treatment group in one trial.

Second-line hormonal therapy Castration-resistant prostate cancer (CRPC) is defined as a rising PSA (or radiographic progression) with a castrate level of serum testosterone (< 50 ng/dL) and after withdrawal or addition of an antiandrogen. For instance, if the CRPC patient is receiving combined androgen blockade (ie, a gonadotropin-releasing

hormone [GnRH] agonist and antiandrogen), the next step is antiandrogen withdrawal. The maximum duration of response is approximately 5 months. To date, there have been no identified predictors of androgen withdrawal response, although a longer duration of treatment with flutamide has been associated with response in two larger trials.

Since 2010, there have been several new antineoplastic agents that have shown a survival benefit in metastatic CRPC (mCRPC). In the majority of instances, a medical oncologist will manage the treatment regimens described below. However, recognizing the side effects of each treatment is paramount in the care provided by the geriatrician, which may require a dose adjustment or cessation of therapy. Abiraterone acetate and enzalutamide are approved for the treatment of mCRPC, both of which target androgen signaling. Abiraterone acetate is an irreversible inhibitor of the cytochrome P450 isoform-17 (CYP17), a key enzyme for androgen synthesis in the testes and adrenal glands. The precursor to abiraterone acetate, ketoconazole, can inhibit multiple P450 enzymes resulting in off-target effects and toxicities. In combination with prednisone, abiraterone acetate increases overall survival. Its ability to inhibit androgen synthesis can lead to mineralocorticoid excess, resulting in edema (31%), hypokalemia (17%), and hypertension (10%). Less common side effects are LFT elevations and cardiac abnormalities (tachycardia, atrial fibrillation). In addition to the survival benefit, abiraterone acetate delayed the use of opioids for pain and skeletal-related events. Enzalutamide, apalutamide and darolutamide are androgen receptor antagonists, which prevent androgen from binding to the receptor and also inhibit nuclear translocation of the receptor. Similar to abiraterone acetate, enzalutamide increased overall survival regardless of chemotherapy status. Common side effects include fatigue, headaches, and hot flashes. Seizures were observed in approximately 1% of patients so these drugs should be used with caution in patients with a known seizure disorder. Since enzalutamide is used without prednisone, the side effects of mineralocorticoid excess are not seen. The most effective sequence of abiraterone acetate and enzalutamide is not known and may be dictated by the side effect profile of each medication or physician preference.

Estrogens, such as diethylstilbestrol, have shown promise both singly and in combination, although estrogen therapy is associated with side effects such as edema and thromboembolic complications. Judicious use of prophylactic agents, such as warfarin or low-dose aspirin, has been included in estrogen trials, but not prospectively. With the development of next-generation androgen signaling antagonists, use of estrogens has fallen out of favor.

The decision to pursue secondary hormonal manipulations will likely depend on several factors. Available data suggest that patients with a significant and prolonged response to initial hormonal therapy, or a significant antiandrogen withdrawal response, may be good candidates for a trial of secondary hormonal therapy. Poor functional status and the presence of other medical problems may render attempts at further hormonal manipulation an attractive option, as these patients are often intolerant of the side effects associated with chemotherapy. Patients with rapid PSA-doubling times are likely to have more aggressive disease and may receive more benefit from chemotherapy or a clinical trial with a novel agent.

Chemotherapy

Chemotherapy still has an important role in mCRPC after progressing through the multiple lines of hormonal therapy. Although mCRPC was once labeled "chemotherapy resistant," a number of agents now show great promise in both palliative and response end points. Docetaxel is the first chemotherapeutic agent with demonstrated survival benefit in prostate cancer and has become standard of care for first-line therapy in castration-resistant disease. Mitoxantrone with prednisone has demonstrated palliative benefits in patients with bone metastases and is generally well tolerated. However, mitoxantrone has been supplanted by cabazitaxel as second-line chemotherapy. Cabazitaxel is a semisynthetic taxane with a similar mechanism to docetaxel. It increased overall survival when compared to mitoxantrone in the post-docetaxel setting. Mitoxantrone is currently third-line chemotherapy and used less frequently due to side effects and lack of survival benefit.

Radium-223

Radium-223 dichloride is an α-particle emitter, and it is the only bone-specific FDA-approved drug for mCRPC that is associated with a survival benefit. It selectively targets bone metastases, as it gets built into hydroxyapatite as a calcium substitute. In one trial, radium-223 improved median survival by 3.6 months, prolonged time to first skeletal event, and improved pain scores and QoL. However, in a more recent trial, the addition of radium-223 to abiraterone acetate plus prednisone or prednisolone did not improve symptomatic skeletal event-free survival in patients with mCRPC, and was associated with an increased frequency of bone fractures compared with placebo.

Sipuleucel-T

Sipuleucel-T was the first active cellular immunostimulant approved as a first-line therapy for non- to minimally symptomatic mCRPC. Mononuclear blood cells are harvested through leukapheresis. Antigen-presenting cells are activated with the antigen prostatic acid phosphatase and granulocyte-macrophage colony-stimulating factor ex vivo. The autologous, activated product is reinfused three times. One sipuleucel-T trial demonstrated a 4.1-month increase in survival. However, no PSA decline was observed, and there was no difference in the progression-free survival (PFS) in the treatment group compared to placebo.

Poly (ADP Ribose) Polymerase Inhibitors

Poly (ADP ribose) polymerase (PARP) inhibitors have shown high rates of response in men with somatic and/or germline homologous recombination repair (HRR) deficiency. There are two PARP inhibitors that have been approved by the US FDA. Olaparib is approved for patients with deleterious or suspected deleterious germline or somatic HRR gene-mutated mCRPC, who have progressed following prior treatment with enzalutamide or abiraterone. The most common adverse events of olaparib are anemia, nausea, decreased appetite, and fatigue. Rucaparib is approved for patients with a germline and/or somatic deleterious *BRCA* mutation-associated mCRPC who have been treated with AR-directed therapy and a taxane-based chemotherapy.

SUPPORTIVE CARE

Bisphosphonates/RANKL Inhibitors

Bisphosphonates are synthetic analogues of inorganic pyrophosphates with high avidity for calcium and areas of bone mineralization (see Chapter 51 for a full discussion of these drugs). Although various bisphosphonates have been tested in multiple clinical trials in the setting of advanced prostate cancer, only zoledronic acid- has a demonstrated effect on bone metastases in this population. Intravenous zoledronic acid is generally well tolerated, though patients should have regular creatinine assessment as renal insufficiency is a contraindication for zoledronic acid and renal toxicity is a known, but relatively uncommon, side effect. In addition, bisphosphonate use is rarely associated with osteonecrosis of the jaw—so patients should have a dental examination prior to initiating therapy, and clinicians should ask patients regularly about their dental health.

As both increasing age and ADT place men at higher risk of osteoporosis, bisphosphonates may also be useful in prevention of secondary fractures in this population. Furthermore, bone is a major target for prostate cancer metastases. Thus, bone protection should be paramount, especially in the early stages of the disease. Zoledronic acid is commonly used in the outpatient setting in patients with bone metastases.

Denosumab is a monoclonal antibody directed against the RANK ligand to prevent pathologic fracture and osteopenia/osteoporosis. Denosumab was shown to be noninferior to zoledronic acid with respect to preventing skeletal-related events in men with mCRPC. Denosumab can be administered as a subcutaneous injection and used safely in patients with renal insufficiency.

Pain Control

The majority of men with advanced prostate cancer have bone metastases, which are frequently very painful. Pain control is thus a critical issue in these patients and needs to be frequently monitored. Bone pain generally responds well to treatment with both nonsteroidal anti-inflammatory drugs and opioids, used alone or in combination. Although some older patients are very tolerant of narcotic analgesics, as a rule they should be started on low doses with careful dose titration and individualized treatment plans to achieve maximal analgesia and maintain QoL. Constipation, the most common side effect of pain medications, should be aggressively addressed, but is generally well controlled with laxatives.

Palliative Radiation and Systemic Radioisotopes

Palliative radiation therapy can provide significant pain relief for symptomatic bone metastases and is also used to prevent impending pathologic fracture. Thus, patients with one or two areas of severe bone pain, which is either inadequately controlled with narcotics or which requires unacceptably high doses of narcotics, should be referred to radiation oncology for consultation. Most palliative radiation is given in one to 10 dose fractions, and 80% to 90% of prostate cancer patients who receive palliative radiation for bone metastases experience significant and durable pain relief. The onset of pain relief may be as soon as 48 hours after the initiation of therapy, although some patients will not experience maximal relief for up to 2 weeks after therapy is complete. Systemic radioisotopes can deliver high-dose radiation to bone lesions without significantly affecting normal bone and can provide palliative benefit to patients with widespread, painful bone metastases, which are refractory to palliative chemotherapy or narcotic analgesia. Strontium-89 and samarium-153 are both β-emitters that are FDA-approved for palliation and pain relief. These agents have the potential to cause significant myelosuppression and thrombocytopenia. More recently, the calcium mimetic radium-223 was shown to increase overall survival as well as provide pain relief, making it an attractive treatment for castration-resistant, symptomatic, bony metastases. Radium-223 is an α-emitter, which can transmit higher energy over shorter distances compared to β-emitters, making this treatment more effective with less side effects.

FURTHER READING

Andriole GL, Crawford ED, Grubb RL 3rd, et al. Mortality results from a randomized prostate-cancer screening trial. *N Engl J Med.* 2009;360(13):1310–1319.

Aus G, Robinson D, Rosell J, et al. South-East Region Prostate Cancer Group. Survival in prostate carcinoma—outcomes from a prospective, population-based cohort of 8887 men with up to 15 years of follow-up: results from three countries in the population-based National Prostate Cancer Registry of Sweden. *Cancer.* 2005;103(5):943–951.

Barrington WE, Schenk JM, Etzioni R, et al. Difference in association of obesity with prostate cancer risk between US African American and non-Hispanic white men in the Selenium and Vitamin E Cancer Prevention Trial (SELECT). *JAMA Oncol.* 2015;1(3):342–349.

Cornford P, van den Bergh RC, Briers E, et al. EAU-EANM-ESTRO-ESUR-SIOG Guidelines on Prostate Cancer. Part II-2020 update: treatment of relapsing and metastatic prostate cancer. *Eur Urol.* 2021;79(2):263–282.

Crook JM, O'Callaghan CJ, Duncan G, et al. Intermittent androgen suppression for rising PSA level after radiotherapy. *N Engl J Med.* 2012;367(10):895–903.

de Bono J, Mateo J, Fizazi K, et al. Olaparib for metastatic castration-resistant prostate cancer. *N Engl J Med.* 2020;382:2091–2102.

Epstein JI, Egevad L, Amin MB, Delahunt B, Srigley JR, Humphrey PA. The 2014 International Society of Urological Pathology (ISUP) consensus conference on Gleason grading of prostatic carcinoma: definition of grading patterns and proposal for a new grading system. *Am J Surg Pathol.* 2016;40:244–252.

Fenton JJ, Weyrich MS, Durbin S, Liu Y, Bang H, Melnikow J. Prostate-specific antigen-based screening for prostate cancer: evidence report and systematic review for the US Preventive Services Task Force. *JAMA.* 2018;319:1914–1931.

Fizazi K, Shore N, Tammela TL, et al. Darolutamide in nonmetastatic, castration-resistant prostate cancer. *N Engl J Med.* 2019;380:1235–1246.

Hofman MS, Lawrentschuk N, Francis RJ, et al. Prostate-specific membrane antigen PET-CT in patients with high-risk prostate cancer before curative-intent surgery or radiotherapy (proPSMA): a prospective, randomised, multicentre study. *Lancet.* 2020;395:1208–1216.

Hoskin P, Sartor O, O'Sullivan JM, et al. Efficacy and safety of radium-223 dichloride in patients with castration-resistant prostate cancer and symptomatic bone metastases, with or without previous docetaxel use: a prespecified subgroup analysis from the randomised, double-blind, phase 3 ALSYMPCA trial. *Lancet Oncol.* 2014;15:1397–1406.

Hugosson J, Roobol MJ, Mansson M, et al. A 16-yr follow-up of the European randomized study of screening for prostate cancer. *Eur Urol.* 2019;76:43–51.

Hussain M, Fizazi K, Saad F, et al. Enzalutamide in men with nonmetastatic, castration-resistant prostate cancer. *N Engl J Med.* 2018;378:2465–2474.

Kantoff PW, Higano CS, Shore ND, et al. Sipuleucel-T immunotherapy for castration-resistant prostate cancer. *N Engl J Med.* 2010;363(5):411–422.

Klein EA, Thompson IM Jr, Tangen CM, et al. Vitamin E and the risk of prostate cancer: the Selenium and Vitamin E Cancer Prevention Trial (SELECT). *JAMA.* 2011;306(14):1549–1556.

Martin RM, Donovan JL, Turner EL, et al. Effect of a low-intensity PSA-based screening intervention on prostate cancer mortality: the CAP randomized clinical trial. *JAMA.* 2018;319:883–895.

Mottet N, van den Bergh RC, Briers E, et al. EAU-EANM-ESTRO-ESUR-SIOG Guidelines on Prostate Cancer—2020 Update. Part 1: screening, diagnosis, and local treatment with curative intent. *Eur Urol.* 2021; 79(2):243–262.

Neal DE, Metcalfe C, Donovan JL, et al. Ten-year mortality, disease progression, and treatment-related side effects in men with localised prostate cancer from the ProtecT randomised controlled trial according to treatment received. *Eur Urol.* 2020;77:320–330.

Nicolosi P, Ledet E, Yang S, et al. Prevalence of germline variants in prostate cancer and implications for current genetic testing guidelines. *JAMA Oncol.* 2019;5:523–528.

Nyberg T, Frost D, Barrowdale D, et al. Prostate cancer risks for male *BRCA1* and *BRCA2* mutation carriers: a prospective cohort study. *Eur Urol.* 2020;77:24–35.

Palapattu GS, Sutcliffe S, Bastian PJ, et al. Prostate carcinogenesis and inflammation: emerging insights. *Carcinogenesis.* 2004;26:1170–1181.

Pienta K, Bradley D. Mechanisms underlying the development of androgen-independent prostate cancer. *Clin Cancer Res.* 2006;12(6):1665–1671.

Potosky AL, Knopf K, Clegg LX, et al. Quality-of-life outcomes after primary androgen deprivation therapy: results from the prostate cancer outcomes study. *J Clin Oncol.* 2001;17:3750–3757.

Rouviere O, Puech P, Renard-Penna R, et al. Use of prostate systematic and targeted biopsy on the basis of multiparametric MRI in biopsy-naive patients (MRI-FIRST): a prospective, multicentre, paired diagnostic study. *Lancet Oncol.* 2019;20:100–109.

Ryan CJ, Smith MR, de Bono JS, et al. Abiraterone in metastatic prostate cancer without previous chemotherapy. *N Engl J Med.* 2013;368(2):138–148.

Saad F, Gleason DM, Murray R, et al. Long-term efficacy of zoledronic acid for the prevention of skeletal complications in patients with metastatic hormone-refractory prostate cancer. Zoledronic Acid Prostate Cancer Study Group. *J Natl Cancer Inst.* 2004;96:879–882.

Schroder FH, Hugosson J, Roobol MJ, et al. Screening and prostate-cancer mortality in a randomized European study. *N Engl J Med.* 2009;360(13):1320–1328.

Smith M, Parker C, Saad F, et al. Addition of radium-223 to abiraterone acetate and prednisone or prednisolone in patients with castration-resistant prostate cancer and bone metastases (ERA 223): a randomised, double-blind, placebo-controlled, phase 3 trial. *Lancet Oncol.* 2019; 20:408–419.

Smith MR, Saad F, Chowdhury S, et al. Apalutamide treatment and metastasis-free survival in prostate cancer. *N Engl J Med.* 2018;378:1408–1418.

Tannock IF, de Wit R, Berry WR, et al. Docetaxel plus prednisone or mitoxantrone plus prednisone for advanced prostate cancer. *N Engl J Med.* 2004;351:1502–1512.

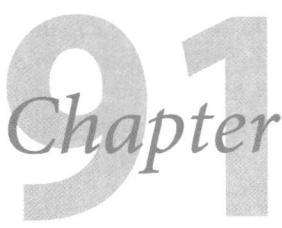

Lung Cancer

Asrar Alahmadi, Ajeet Gajra, Carolyn J. Presley

EPIDEMIOLOGY AND RISK FACTORS

Lung cancer remains the second most common cancer diagnosis, and the most common cause of cancer-related deaths among men and women in the United States. More patients die from lung cancer than from colon, breast, and prostate cancers combined. In 2021, it is estimated there will be 235,760 new cases of lung cancer with 69,410 men and 62,470 women dying from their disease. Lung cancer–associated deaths have been declining and have contributed to the overall decline in the cancer-related death rate from 2014 to 2018. This decline in the lung cancer death rate is attributable to several changes: (1) a decrease in smoking rates, (2) the advent of new therapies in lung cancer, and (3) the introduction of screening for high-risk populations. The risk of lung cancer increases with age. The median age at diagnosis is 71 years. By the year 2034, it is projected that there will be 77 million people 65 years or older, an almost 80% increase since 2012. This combination of a burgeoning geriatric population and newly recommended annual low-dose computed tomography (LDCT) scan screening will increase the number of older adults needing evaluation and treatment for lung cancer. Despite advances in screening for high-risk individuals, the majority (75%) of lung cancer is diagnosed with either spread to regional lymph nodes or distant sites (ie, stage III or IV).

The major modifiable risk factor for the development of lung cancer is tobacco use, accounting for approximately 80% of lung cancer cases. Smokers and nonsmokers are at risk for lung cancer; however, the risk is much higher (10-fold) among patients who have smoked cigarettes. The risk is directly proportional to the number of pack-years and tar content. Patients exposed to passive tobacco smoke are also at risk, accounting for 25% of lung cancer cases. Men or women who smoke cigars and pipes are at an increased risk as well; however, their risk may be less than that of cigarette smokers. Smoking cessation even in long-time smokers decreases the risk of lung cancer development and is a major public health priority.

Lung cancer in never-smokers accounts for approximately 13% of patients with lung cancers in the United States, disproportionately affecting women. Never-smokers are more likely to have activating genetic alterations such as the epidermal growth factor receptor (*EGFR*) or

Learning Objectives

- Become familiar with the general principles of lung cancer evaluation and its inherent need for a multidisciplinary approach to management.
- Identify the broad treatment paradigms for different stages of lung cancer, including more recent developments in therapeutics and their potential side effects.
- Discern geriatric issues in the multidisciplinary care of older adults with lung cancer and apply geriatric assessment and palliative care principles to their care trajectory.

Key Clinical Points

1. Lung cancer remains a cancer of older adults and confers substantial morbidity and mortality in an aging patient population.
2. Although major advances have been made in molecular diagnostics and therapeutics for a significant proportion of patients with advanced non–small-cell lung cancer (NSCLC), the side effects of cytotoxic chemotherapy, targeted therapy, and immunotherapy, among other modalities, have to be apprised on an individual basis.
3. Given the trade-offs of various lung cancer treatment options and poor prognosis in most patients with advanced disease, geriatricians play a key role in helping older adults with lung cancer and their caregivers define goals of care, optimize the management of geriatric syndromes and comorbid conditions, and better assess functional, cognitive, and psychosocial reserve to undergo an expanding menu of treatments.
4. Early integration of palliative and supportive care improves mood and quality of life and may prolong survival in patients with advanced disease, and such interventions may be particularly relevant for older adults.

chromosomal rearrangements in anaplastic lymphoma kinase (ALK). These patients are treated with oral tyrosine kinase inhibitors targeting the specific mutation. Aside from the activating mutations in oncogenes, other possible pathogenic theories for lung cancer in never-smokers include exposure to environmental or occupational etiologic factors such as asbestos or radon. Occupational and environmental exposures are important questions to ask patients particularly if they have worked in construction, naval shipyards, or live in areas with high air pollution, diesel exhaust, or smoke from cooking and heating. Prior radiation therapy to the chest for other malignancies also increases the risk of a second primary lung cancer, particularly among smokers.

SCREENING

Despite smoking cessation efforts and declining rates of heavy cigarette smoking, millions of Americans remain at increased risk for the development of lung cancer. Two randomized trials have reported statistically significant reductions in lung cancer mortality associated with LDCT screening. The National Lung Screening Trial (NLST) in the United States demonstrated that screening higher-risk persons (30+ pack-years and either current smokers or quit within the past 15 years) aged 55 to 74 years annually for 3 years with LDCTs reduced lung cancer mortality by 20% (95% confidence interval [CI], 6.8%–26.7%; $p = .004$) and all-cause mortality by 6.7% (95% CI, 1.2%–13.6%; $p = .02$) over screening with chest radiographs. An updated analysis showed that the estimated reduction in lung cancer mortality was 16% (95% CI, 5%–25%). The NELSON Netherlands trial reported that among high-risk current and former smokers, men who were randomly assigned to four rounds of LDCT screening had a 24% reduction (95% CI, 6%–39%) in lung cancer mortality compared with men who were randomly assigned to no screening. These two large randomized trials (NLST and NELSON) found that the average false-positive rate per screening round was 23.3% and 10.4%, respectively. Using a more recent definition of a positive LDCT screening on the basis of the Lung-RADS criteria yields a false-positive rate that may be somewhat lower than that seen in the NLST. A total of 0.06% of all false-positive screening results in the NLST led to a major complication after an invasive procedure was performed as a diagnostic follow-up to the screening. Over three screening rounds, 1.8% of NLST participants who did not have lung cancer had an invasive procedure after a positive screening result. An extended follow-up analysis of the NLST reported data after a median of 12.3 years of follow-up for mortality. The estimated number needed to screen with LDCT to prevent one lung cancer death was 303.

Based on the decrease in lung cancer–associated mortality in screening trials, in December 2013, the US Preventive Services Task Force (USPSTF) released its updated recommendations to perform annual screening for lung cancer with LDCT scans in adults aged 55 to 80 who have a 30-pack-year smoking history and currently smoke or have quit within the past 15 years. Ideally, most cancers would be diagnosed at an early stage; however, among older adults with increasing comorbidity, it is critical to understand the impact of undergoing screening as they may be more likely to die from other comorbid conditions and not from cancer. The impact of these screening guidelines remains to be determined with regard to the diagnosis and treatment of early-stage lung cancers. The Centers for Medicare and Medicaid Services and the Veterans Administration (VA) have approved health care coverage for this screening recommendation. The issues of lead-time bias and additional morbidity and mortality are particularly relevant in the population of older adults in whom competing causes of death and multiple comorbidities are frequently encountered. In addition to the overdiagnosis of small tumors detected during screening, which could otherwise remain silent until the patient dies from other causes, screening for lung cancer with LDCT could potentially cause harm secondary to morbidity and mortality associated with biopsies and surgery, since lung tumors often appear as noncalcified nodules. In the NLST trial, only 25% of patient enrolled in the screening arms were age 65 to 74 and less than 1% were 75 years or older. Over 96% of the patients with a positive screen had a false-positive result after further work-up. This has important implications for screening among the oldest old patients with comorbid conditions. Among older adults, there is a higher risk for false-positive LDCT screening findings. Despite screening being endorsed as a new standard of care (SOC) for high-risk individuals, the regional utilization of LDCT screening for lung cancer varies considerably within the United States. Adults aged 65 to 74 seem somewhat more likely to utilize it in addition to those with prior cancer diagnoses as well as underlying respiratory illnesses. In another report, age was not associated with lung cancer screening, but retired status and presence of a personal physician were associated with receipt of screening. Other barriers may include a lack of physician awareness and resources as well as the requirement of a shared decision-making visit prior to screening.

PATHOLOGY

Lung cancer is broadly characterized into non–small-cell lung cancer (NSCLC) versus small-cell lung cancer (SCLC) (**Table 91-1**). Distinguishing between these two histopathology subtypes is critical as the subtype dictates treatment course. For example, SCLC is more responsive to chemotherapy and radiation, may require prophylactic cranial irradiation (PCI), and often has a more aggressive clinical course compared to NSCLC. NSCLC is the most common subtype accounting for up to 85% of diagnoses. Among

TABLE 91-1 ■ OVERVIEW OF LUNG CANCER STAGING, EPIDEMIOLOGY, AND TREATMENT

STAGE	8TH TNM STAGING	DEFINITION	% CASES AT DIAGNOSIS	% 5-YEAR SURVIVAL	MANAGEMENT STRATEGY
NON–SMALL-CELL LUNG CANCER					
I	T1a–T2a N0 M0	Localized	15%	54% (68%–92%)	Surgery +/– postoperative chemotherapy Stereotactic body radiation therapy (SBRT): nonsurgical candidate patients
II	T1a–T2a, N1 T2b, N0–1 T3, N0	Spread to regional lymph nodes	22%	53%–60%	Surgery + postoperative chemotherapy RT +/– chemotherapy TKI targeted therapy if EGFR mutated
III	Any T, N2–N3 T3, N1–N2 All T4 disease	Spread to regional lymph nodes	22%	13%–36%	Most IIIA/all IIIB: concurrent or sequential chemoradiation followed by consolidative ICI Select IIIA: preoperative chemotherapy/radiation + surgery if potentially resectable TKI targeted therapy if EGFR mutated
IV	Any T Any N M1a or M1b	Distant spread	57%	< 10%	ICI Combination of chemotherapy and ICI Single-agent chemotherapy Targeted therapy (if applicable) Clinical trial
SMALL-CELL LUNG CANCER					
Limited stage (stages I–IIIB)		Primary tumor and involved lymph nodes can be safely encompassed in a single radiation port	35%–40%	10%–15%	Concurrent chemoradiation (Occasionally detected after surgical resection for small lesion; then postoperative chemotherapy) Prophylactic PCI Clinical trial
Extensive stage (stage IV)		Usually metastatic	60%–65%	≤ 2%	Combination of chemotherapy and ICI

EGFR, epidermal growth factor receptor; ICI, immune checkpoint inhibitor; PCI, prophylactic cranial irradiation; RT, radiation therapy; TKI, tyrosine kinase inhibitor; TNM, tumor, node, metastasis.

NSCLC, adenocarcinoma accounts for the most common histologic type followed by squamous cell carcinoma. Less prevalent subtypes recognized by the World Health Organization (WHO) include large-cell carcinoma, adenosquamous carcinoma, sarcomatoid carcinoma, and carcinoid tumors. Bronchoalveolar carcinoma is currently classified under adenocarcinoma. Multiple conceptual changes have been incorporated within the updated pathological classification. These include the use of immunohistochemistry throughout the classification, an emphasis on genetic studies, and in particular, the integration of molecular testing to help personalize treatment strategies for patients with advanced lung.

Adenocarcinoma is classically a peripheral, solitary lung nodule, often associated with malignant pleural effusion and early development of metastases frequently involving the brain and bone. Squamous cell carcinoma classically is central in location, endobronchial in nature, sometimes with central cavitation, and commonly associated with lobar collapse, obstructive pneumonia, or hemoptysis, with relatively late development of distant metastases. SCLC has the strongest association with smoking and commonly forms rapidly growing, central masses. The pathologic classification of lung cancer is evolving due to new sampling and radiologic techniques, molecular biomarkers, and histologic/pathologic advances. In 2011, the International Association for the Study of Lung Cancer, American Thoracic Society, and European Respiratory Society International (IASLC/ATC/ERSI) developed a multidisciplinary international team to iteratively incorporate advances in the molecular and histologic lung cancer subtypes of resection specimens, small biopsies, and cytology into a new, separate classification schema from the WHO. Mutational analysis is now routinely done on adenocarcinomas as oral targeted therapies exist for multiple actionable mutations (see Molecular Markers).

CLINICAL PRESENTATION

The initial clinical presentation of lung cancer patients is evolving. With new screening guidelines and regular use of chest CT scans for several medical indications, many new lung cancers are diagnosed during evaluation of incidental pulmonary nodules that require serial follow-up CT scans.

Despite these practice changes, patients still present with classic symptoms of cough, unintentional weight loss, and/or hemoptysis. Symptoms related to the primary tumor depend on the location of the tumor. Central tumors produce cough, dyspnea, hoarseness, stridor, hemoptysis, and postobstructive pneumonia. Superior sulcus tumors may produce shoulder pain, arm pain, brachial plexopathy, or Horner syndrome. Peripheral lesions may cause pleuritic chest pain due to pleural involvement. Symptoms related to mediastinal disease include hoarseness caused by the involvement of the left recurrent laryngeal nerve with left-sided tumors and obstruction of the superior vena cava (SVC) with right-sided tumors or associated lymphadenopathy.

Because more than half of patients have metastases at presentation, initial symptoms related to a metastatic site are frequent, particularly in patients with adenocarcinoma or small-cell carcinoma. Often, the initial presentation is due to symptomatic brain metastases and associated vasogenic edema causing seizures, new headaches, or neurologic deficits. Subsequent metastases from lung cancer are common. Sites of spread include the brain, pleura, bone, liver, adrenal glands, and contralateral lung. Rarely, lung cancer is diagnosed due to a paraneoplastic syndrome such as hypertrophic pulmonary osteoarthropathy leading to hypercalcemia in squamous cell carcinoma. SCLCs are known to cause syndrome of inappropriate secretion of antidiuretic hormone, Cushing syndrome, and various neurologic syndromes such as Eaton-Lambert reverse myasthenia syndrome, among others. More commonly in advanced disease, hypercoagulability results in venous thromboembolic disease either concomitantly at the time of diagnosis or during the disease trajectory.

Special Presentation Issues

Lung cancer is unique in that it can present in several ways including but not limited to superior sulcus (Pancoast) tumors, chest wall tumors, or solitary brain metastases. Superior sulcus tumors are carcinomas that develop in the apex of the lung with invasion into the thoracic inlet. The most common initial symptom is shoulder pain due to invasion of the brachial plexus. This invasion into the sympathetic chain and stellate ganglion is termed Horner syndrome, the classic triad of miosis, ptosis, and anhidrosis. Chest wall tumors are bulky primary lung tumors that directly invade the chest wall. Treatment options for both superior sulcus and chest wall tumors include combinations of surgery, radiation, and chemotherapy. A third unique presentation is SVC syndrome in which edema develops in the face and neck with dilated veins in the neck and torso due to compression of the SVC outlet. SCLC is a common histology encountered with this presentation. Urgent treatment measures include chemotherapy, radiation therapy, and/or a vascular stent to relieve the obstruction. Lastly, patients who present with solitary brain metastases after curative treatment intent for early-stage NSCLC, are eligible for resection of the solitary metastases, achieving prolonged disease-free survival in the absence of other distant metastatic disease. Performance status (PS), extent of extracranial disease, and age are key prognostic factors in this scenario. If the metastasis is not causing symptoms, stereotactic radiosurgery (SRS) is the preferred modality but for symptomatic patients, or if histologic evaluation is warranted, surgical resection followed by radiation in the form of whole-brain radiation therapy (WBRT) or SRS is appropriate. Notably, one-half of patients treated with resection and postoperative radiation therapy will develop recurrence in the brain. SRS is preferred over WBRT as it spares late cognitive side effects of WBRT and can be performed on more than one intracranial site in the event of subsequent metastases. However, if SRS is not an option due to presence of multiple larger tumors or multiple areas previously treated with SRS, then WBRT can be considered as a palliative measure.

EVALUATION

Diagnostic Approaches

Although patients may present with symptoms outlined above, it is becoming increasingly common for solitary pulmonary nodules (SPNs) being detected on chest x-ray and/or CT scans of the chest that are ordered for other indications. The pretest probability of SPNs being benign or malignant depends on several factors, including the size and appearance of the nodule, as well as patient risk factors including smoking exposure. Assessing for dynamic changes of an SPN over serial CT imaging may be recommended at first if there is a low or intermediate level of suspicion. If the clinical suspicion is high and CT imaging supports an early-stage process, patients may be eligible for video-assisted thoracoscopic surgery (VATS) via wedge resection or lobectomy that may be both diagnostic and therapeutic if lung cancer is confirmed. Otherwise transthoracic imaging-guided biopsies or transbronchial biopsies of SPN or thoracic lymph nodes via bronchoscopy and endobronchial ultrasound (EBUS), respectively, may be indicated to obtain a tissue diagnosis. The general principles of diagnostic evaluation include electing the least invasive biopsy with the likelihood for highest yield as the first biopsy. Patients with central masses are best addressed via bronchoscopy while peripheral nodules (outer third) will likely benefit from navigational bronchoscopy, radial EBUS, or transthoracic needle aspiration. Patients with suspected nodal involvement by imaging may be biopsied using EBUS, endoscopic ultrasound (EUS), navigational bronchoscopy, or mediastinoscopy. Lymph node sampling is essential for accurate pathologic staging. Certainly, if more distant lesions are noted in the liver or elsewhere that may be more accessible to a percutaneous approach, this ought to be considered as well. Finally, in patients with a suspected malignant pleural effusion, thoracentesis with cytologic evaluation may provide sufficient material to render a diagnosis. A single negative cytology result does not exclude pleural involvement, and in the presence of an effusion, additional thoracentesis or thoracoscopic evaluation should be performed.

Staging Work-Up

When there is strong clinical suspicion for lung cancer and/or whenever a diagnosis of lung cancer is confirmed, CT staging imaging of the chest and abdomen (ie, liver and adrenal glands) is needed. Current guidelines also warrant brain imaging even among patients with suspected early-stage disease, preferably with magnetic resonance imaging (MRI), and especially for those with confirmed SCLC. Integrated positron emission tomography (PET)/CT is mostly incorporated in the evaluation of patients with potentially resectable early-stage NSCLC (stages I–II) and some cases of stage IIIA, for which a noninvasive evaluation of the mediastinal lymph nodes (ie, N2 disease) can be important in surgical and nonsurgical treatment planning. EBUS and EUS are less invasive approaches to evaluating hilar and mediastinal lymphadenopathy on staging imaging to guide treatment planning and are becoming more readily adopted into pathologic staging approaches. However, patients may still need mediastinoscopy (ie, surgical staging) prior to surgery if there are concerns about accessibility or yield by EBUS/EUS, particularly in NSCLC arising from the left upper lobe.

If metastatic disease is identified on initial CT staging imaging, a PET/CT is unlikely to change management. Evaluation for brain metastases with MRI or contrast-infused CT is indicated for any SCLC diagnosis, and patients with stage III or IV NSCLC, or in any patient with suggestive signs or symptoms regardless of stage. Since SCLC is still conventionally staged into limited versus extensive stage (see "Small-Cell Lung Cancer"), this distinction invariably can be made with staging imaging alone since the treatment of choice is nonsurgical with the rare exception of resection of early-stage SPNs.

Once the diagnosis and stage have been established, in addition to a comprehensive history and physical examination with special focus on antecedent weight loss, PS, and comorbid conditions, it is essential to assess whether an older adult is a candidate for cancer treatment based on overall life expectancy. It is essential to assess decision-making capacity given the complexity of risk-benefit decisions of choosing cancer treatment options as well as the patient's goals and preferences. If a decision is made to proceed with cancer treatment, then side effects and potential toxicities are addressed.

Molecular Markers

The past decade has seen the emergence of molecular testing that has furthered our understanding of lung cancer biology and accelerated the development of targeted therapies against identified oncogenic driver mutations. A significant proportion of patients have tumors with a therapeutically targetable molecular abnormality, the vast majority of which occur in lung adenocarcinomas. Multiple organizations, including

the IASLC, the American Society of Clinical Oncology, the College of American Pathologists, and the National Comprehensive Cancer Network, have issued guidelines for molecular testing as an important first step to determining therapy in NSCLC. Mutational testing of genes including EGFR, ALK, ROS1, RET, MET, NTRK, and BRAF is currently standard for all patients with advanced NSCLC. Further testing is encouraged to include ERBB2 and KRAS, given it informs tumor biology, prognosis, and systemic therapy. Due to the ever-growing number of recommended molecular tests for lung cancer, multigene panel testing using next-generation sequencing is cost-effective compared with sequential individual gene testing and is covered by the Centers for Medicare and Medicaid Services.

TREATMENT OF NON–SMALL-CELL LUNG CANCER

Early Stages (I and II)

Stage I and II patients account for approximately 30% of NSCLC cases, corresponding to a 5-year overall survival rate of 53% to 92%. Depending on a patient's comorbidity burden and pulmonary function status, a curative treatment approach with either radiation or surgery is pursued for those with NSCLC (see **Table 91-1**). For fit patients, the treatment of choice is surgical resection of the tumor, resulting in cure for many patients, and preferably done by lobectomy, as a more limited resection (segmentectomy or wedge resection) is associated with increased local recurrence and decreased survival. Either open thoracotomy or video-assisted thoracoscopic surgery access can be considered, although the latter is a more attractive approach for patients because of a reduced postoperative pain and improved quality of life.

For patients with coexisting medical conditions, such as severe chronic obstructive pulmonary disease, diabetes, or heart disease, thoracic surgery is often not an option and is considered medically inoperable disease. Historically, the 3-year overall survival for medically inoperable disease remains low (20%–35%) with conventional radiation treatment or observation alone. However, the more recent use of stereotactic body radiotherapy (SBRT) over conventional radiotherapy allows the delivery of focused and ablative radiation doses over a few fractions to the primary lung tumor with lower toxicity. Prospective trials of SBRT in medically inoperable candidates showed local control rates exceeding 92% with limited toxicity, and a 3-year disease control rate and overall survival of 48% to 76% and 56% to 60%, respectively. Population studies showed a significant reduction of untreated early-stage NSCLC with the introduction of SBRT among older adults, translating to a survival benefit. Recently, a pooled analysis from two randomized studies, StereoTactic Radiotherapy versus Surgery (STARS) and Radiosurgery or Surgery for Operable Early-Stage Non–Small-Cell Lung Cancer (ROSEL), compared lobectomy to SBRT in medically operable patients and found no difference in local control but a statistically significant 3-year overall survival of 79% for surgery versus 95% for SBRT (hazard ratio [HR] 0.14; 95% CI 0.017–1.190; $p = 0.037$). This observed overall survival benefit could be attributed to postsurgical mortality.

Even with excellent local control rates after curative-intent surgery or SBRT, the risk of systemic failure is high and varies considerably by disease stage. Patients with stage II NSCLC (including tumor size > 4 cm and/or ipsilateral hilar lymph node) are at higher risk for recurrence than those with stage I, and are most likely to derive benefit from postoperative (ie, adjuvant) chemotherapy to improve cancer-specific mortality. Adjuvant chemotherapy utilizing cisplatin-based doublets has improved cancer-related and overall survival, but no single preferred regimen has been established. Preoperative (ie, neoadjuvant) chemotherapy may allow the delivery of more cycles of chemotherapy without interruption or delay due to toxicities but has not been shown to improve outcomes compared to postoperative administration. However, many of these seminal trials evaluating postoperative chemotherapy enrolled patients with a median age of 60 to 65 years, excluding those 75 years or older, or incorporated cisplatin-based regimens, which may be more difficult for older adults to tolerate, particularly those with age- and/or comorbidity-related renal dysfunction. To date, large, prospective trials evaluating carboplatin-based regimens remain sparse. Regardless of chemotherapy regimen choice, a clinical benefit still remains in selecting older adults with stage II disease who experienced a proper recovery from surgery, good PS, and no significant comorbidities. While older adults may be slower to recover from surgery and face a higher risk for postoperative complications, a recent analysis of the National Cancer Database showed that delayed adjuvant chemotherapy administration upon recovery after surgery remains efficacious. Unlike for surgery, currently, there are no data to support adjuvant chemotherapy after SBRT in early-stage NSCLC.

Routine incorporation of postoperative radiation after curative resection has been shown to benefit overall survival. Postoperative radiation therapy should be considered in patients with a positive surgical margin. However, for those upstaged to IIIA disease due to mediastinal nodal (ie, N2) involvement, the LungART study showed higher cardiopulmonary toxicity related to postoperative radiation therapy delivery with no 3-year disease-free survival and overall survival advantage. The publication from this trial is pending, yet some institutions have started to change their current practice.

Stage III

Patients with stage III NSCLC remain a clinically heterogeneous patient population necessitating a multidisciplinary approach to navigate the multiple surgical, radiation, and chemotherapy treatments available. Patients with stage III NSCLC due to chest wall involvement with limited or no

nodal involvement should be assessed for surgical resection because of improved local control. However, stage III is usually attributable to mediastinal nodal involvement and thus precludes upfront surgical resection. Therefore, accurate mediastinal staging is essential in clinically appearing early-stage disease with the incorporation of PET/CT imaging for staging and pathologic confirmation by tissue either by EBUS-guided biopsy and/or surgically by mediastinoscopy when appropriate. Preoperative chemotherapy or concurrent chemoradiation for potentially resectable disease has led to conflicting results in cancer-related survival. Those patients able to undergo lobectomy (as opposed to pneumonectomy) after preoperative chemoradiation can achieve a median overall survival rate of 2 to 3 years, depending on pathologic mediastinal nodal response, as opposed to 12 to 18 months typically reported with definitive chemoradiation alone.

For unresectable IIIA disease or stage IIIB disease (due to contralateral hilar or mediastinal nodal disease), more functionally fit patients are usually offered definitive concurrent chemoradiation therapy. However, concurrent chemoradiation significantly increases the risk of short-term radiation toxicities such as esophagitis as well as neutropenia that may be more difficult to tolerate in vulnerable older adults. Although the absolute benefit of concurrent versus sequential therapy is relatively small in younger adults, it can still be seen in select older adults (ie, age ≥ 70) as evidenced in several subset analyses of phase III clinical trials. Consolidation chemotherapy after chemoradiation remains a controversial area, but data are accumulating that older adults with stage III NSCLC may not benefit from this additional treatment. There were two significant advances, namely consolidation with immune checkpoint inhibitor (ICI) after concurrent chemoradiation and the use of a tyrosine kinase inhibitor (TKI), osimertinib, for EGFR mutant resected NSCLC.

In the PACIFIC trial, 713 patients with unresectable stage III NSCLC who had disease control after concurrent chemoradiation were randomized 2 to 1 to durvalumab (an ICI) 10 mg/kg every 2 weeks or placebo for 12 months. After a median follow-up of 25.2 months, durvalumab significantly prolonged progression-free survival from 16.8 months to 5.6 months (HR 0.52; 95 % CI, 0.42 to 0.65: $p < 0.001$). In an updated analysis after 3 years of follow-up, the median overall survival was not reached with durvalumab compared to 29.1 months with placebo (HR 0.69; 95% CI, 0.55 to 0.86; $p = 0.0025$). Grade 3 or 4 adverse events were noted in 29.9% of patients in the durvalumab arm compared to 26.1% in the placebo arm. Given acceptable tolerability and the survival benefit, durvalumab has become the new SOC.

The other major breakthrough is the introduction of targeted therapy to early-stage and locally advanced NSCLC. In the ADAURA study, 682 patients with resected IB, II, or III NSCLC were randomized 1:1 to osimertinib or placebo for 3 years. The disease-free survival in stage II–IIIA patients, the primary endpoint, was not reached in the osimertinib arm compared with 20.4 months in the placebo arm (HR, 0.17; 95% CI, 0.12–0.23; $p < .0001$). Results showed that the EGFR-targeted therapy with osimertinib reduced the risk of disease recurrence or death by 83% in this patient population. Although adapting the results of this study is still under debate, given the lack of overall survival benefit and concerns about long-term toxicity and financial burden, it highlights the importance of performing molecular testing in all stages of NSCLC cases to identify candidates for targeted therapy.

Because of the treatment intensity involved, among older adults, geriatric assessments play an important clinical role in the selection of those patients who are most likely to benefit from more intensive combined modality treatment since no prospective data exist to guide decision-making. Optimization of comorbidities, functional status, cancer symptoms, social support, and geriatric syndromes would prove useful because of the increased morbidity of these therapeutic approaches employed in stage III NSCLC.

Stage IV

Over half of patients with NSCLC will have distant metastases at the time of diagnosis, for which the goal of treatment is palliative, not curative. Platinum-based doublets have been the SOC as first-line therapy, showing improved survival and quality of life among fit older patients. In the last decade, the identification of activating molecular alterations and the development of new targeted therapies and ICI have changed the treatment of advanced NSCLC. Initial molecular testing of the tumor sample to determine therapy in NSCLC is endorsed by multiple organizations and considered a SOC. In the absence of molecular alteration, early incorporation of immunotherapy guided by the tumor proportion score of programmed death-ligand 1 (PD-L1) improves overall survival. In addition, the early introduction of palliative and supportive care remains a main cornerstone of lung cancer treatment.

When a molecular alteration is identified (ie, EGFR, ALK), targeting the mutation results in better disease control, improved quality of life, and longer progression-free survival compared to standard chemotherapy. Molecular alterations are usually mutually exclusive and more common in patients identified as either never-smokers, longtime ex-smokers, or light smokers (< 15 packs per year), but they can be found among patients with a smoking history. Association between molecular alteration and age is not strongly established, yet MET skip mutation tends to have a higher prevalence in older women. There are currently multiple biomarkers with effective matched targeted therapy approved by the FDA in the settings of advanced NSCLC. Due to the high efficacy and favorable toxicity profile of those agents, clinical trials have frequently included older adults. The evidence of efficacy among older adults can be retrieved from subgroup analysis, with key trials of first-line therapy in advanced NSCLC summarized in **Table 91-2**.

Epidermal growth factor receptor (EGFR) is the most established genomic biomarker in NSCLC, with multiple effective EGFR tyrosine kinase inhibitors (TKIs), including gefitinib and erlotinib (first-generation), afatinib and dacomitinib (second-generation), and osimertinib (third-generation). The two main sensitizing mutations are EGFR L858R and EGFR exon 19 deletion. Multiple studies compared first-generation EGFR TKIs with chemotherapy, and later with second-generation TKIs showing superior results. In subgroup analyses, these trials showed that TKIs had comparable benefits in older adults (aged > 65 years), but analyses of toxicities specific to older adults were not reported. Retrospective studies showed that although generally well tolerated, older adults treated with first-generation TKIs encountered more adverse events requiring dose reduction. Osimertinib is a third-generation TKI that selectively inhibits EGFR-sensitizing mutation and EGFR Thr790Met (T790M) mutation, which is the most common acquired resistance to first- and second-generation TKIs. Recently, osimertinib was approved as an initial therapy for EGFR-mutant NSCLC, based on the FLAURA trial that showed superior outcomes, improved overall survival, and efficacy in patients with central nervous system (CNS) metastases. Around 46% of the enrolled patients were 65 years or older, and the benefit of osimertinib was maintained. Unlike first-generation TKIs, osimertinib is more tolerable with a favorable toxicity profile. Further NSCLC FDA-approved matched therapies to actionable mutations in NSCLC are listed in **Table 91-2**.

The introduction of ICIs targeting the PD-1 or PD-L1 changed the treatment paradigm of advanced NSCLC without molecular alteration. The KEYNOTE-024 trial established pembrolizumab (a PD-L1 inhibitor) as an initial therapy for patients with a PD-L1 score of 50% or greater who did not have EGFR mutations or ALK gene rearrangements. More than 50% of patients enrolled in the study were older than 65 years. Pembrolizumab showed a superior response and overall survival benefit compared to systemic chemotherapy in all age subgroups (**Table 91-3**). It also has a lower frequency of severe adverse events (27%) compared to chemotherapy (53%). Unlike conventional chemotherapy, immunotherapy-related adverse events (irAEs) are associated with nonspecific autoimmune reactions or inflammation to any given organ, and occur mostly in the skin, colon, thyroid, lung, pituitary gland, and liver. The majority of irAEs can be managed successfully with steroids and discontinuation of ICI. Two ongoing phase II clinical trials (CheckMate 153 and CheckMate 171) evaluated the safety and efficacy of nivolumab (a PD-1 inhibitor) in patients older than 75 years and showed similar rates of irAE between younger versus older adults.

After the introduction of pembrolizumab in biomarker-selected patients (PD-L1 > 50%), randomized trials with a regimen of ICI and systemic chemotherapy showed that this combination was an effective strategy. The KEYNOTE-189 trial demonstrated that

TABLE 91-2 ■ FIRST-LINE TREATMENT FOR PATIENTS WITH METASTATIC NON–SMALL-CELL LUNG CANCER WITH TARGETABLE MOLECULAR ALTERATIONS

BIOMARKER/ MOLECULAR ALTERATION	TREATMENT REGIMENS	CLINICAL TRIAL AND/OR FIRST AUTHOR	CLINICAL EFFICACY			COMMON ADVERSE SIDE EFFECTS
			AGE	HR (95% CI)	OVERALL CLINICAL EFFICACY	
EGFR sensitizing mutation	Osimertinib	FLAURA trial Osimertinib (3rd-generation TKI) vs 1st-generation TKI therapy	< 65 = 298/556 (53.6%)	PFS 0.44 (0.33–0.58)	ORR 80% mPFS of 18.9 m vs 10.2 m (HR, 0.46; 95% CI, 0.64–0.96; *p* = 0.02) mOS of 38.6 m vs 31.8 m (HR, 0.80; 95% CI, 0.64 to 1.00; *p* = 0.046)	Dry skin, diarrhea, lymphopenia, thrombocytopenia, pneumonitis, cardio-myopathy, prolonged QT interval
			≥ 65 = 258/556 (46.4%)	PFS 0.49 (0.35–0.67)		
ALK rearrangement	Alectinib	ALEX trial Alectinib vs Crizotinib	< 65 = 233/303 (77%)	PFS 0.48 (0.34–0.70)	ORR 82.9% mPFS of 34.8 m vs 10.9 m (HR, 0.43; 95% CI, 0.32–0.58)	Nausea, hyperbiliru-binemia, increased AST/ALT, anemia, diarrhea, pneumoni-tis, renal impairment
			≥ 65 = 70/303 (23%)	mPFS 0.45 (0.24–0.87)		
	Brigatinib	ALTA-1L trial Brigatinib vs Crizotinib	< 65 = 93/137 (68%)	PFS 0.44 (0.26–0.74)	ORR 71% 12-month PFS of 67% vs 43% (HR, 0.49; 95% CI, 0.33-0.74; *p* < 0.001)	Nausea, increased AST/ALT, diarrhea, creatinine kinase elevation, lipase ele-vation, pneumonitis, bradycardia, visual disturbance
			≥ 65 = 44/137 (32%)	PFS 0.59 (0.3-1.18)		
ROS1 gene rearrangement	Crizotinib	Shaw et al. *NEJM* 2014 Crizotinib (phase I study)	NR		ORR 72% mPFS of 19.2 m (95% CI, 14.4 to not reached)	Diarrhea, edema, visual disturbance, increased AST/ALT, asymptomatic brady-cardia, pneumonitis
	Entrectinib	Drilon et al. *Lancet Oncol.* 2020 Entrectinib (Phase I study)	Excluded		ORR 77% mPFS of 19.0 m (95% CI, 12.2–36.6)	Dizziness, constipa-tion, diarrhea, elevated AST/ALT, elevated weight, peripheral edema, elevated crea-tinine kinase
BRAF V600E mutation	Dabrafenib plus trametinib	Planchard et al. *Lancet Oncol.* 2017 *J Thorac.* 2021 Dabrafenib plus trametinib	< 65 = 29/57 (51%) ≥ 65 = 28/57 (49%)		Treatment Naïve: ORR 63.9% mPFS of 10.8 m (95% CI, 7.0–14.5) Pretreated: ORR 68.4% mPFS of 10.2 m (95% CI, 6.9–16.7)	Fever, rash, hyper-glycemia, hypophos-phatemia, elevated AST/ALT, cardio-myopathy, uveitis, cutaneous squamous cell cancers
RET rearrangement	Selpercatinib	Drilon et al. *NEJM.* 2020 LIBRETTO trial Selpercatinib (Phase I/II study)	NR		Treatment Naïve: ORR 85% 90% DoR at 6 m Pretreated: ORR 64% mDoR of 17.5 m (95% CI, 12.0 to could not be estimated)	Dry mouth, increased AST/ALT, hypertension, diar-rhea, fatigue

(Continued)

TABLE 91-2 ■ FIRST-LINE TREATMENT FOR PATIENTS WITH METASTATIC NON–SMALL-CELL LUNG CANCER WITH TARGETABLE MOLECULAR ALTERATIONS *(CONTINUED)*

BIOMARKER/ MOLECULAR ALTERATION	TREATMENT REGIMENS	CLINICAL TRIAL AND/OR FIRST AUTHOR	CLINICAL EFFICACY			COMMON ADVERSE SIDE EFFECTS
			AGE	HR (95% CI)	OVERALL CLINICAL EFFICACY	
MET exon 14 skipping mutations	Capmatinib	GEOMETRY trial Capmatinib Wolf et al. *NEJM.* 2020	NR		Treatment-naive: ORR 68% mDoR of 12.6 m (95% CI, 5.6 to could not be estimated) Pretreated: ORR 41% mDoR of 9.7 m (95% CI, 5.6 to 13.0)	Peripheral edema, nausea, fatigue, vomiting, dyspnea, decreased appetite, interstitial lung disease, hepatotoxicity, photosensitivity
NTRK 1-3 fusion	Larotrectinib	Drilon et al. *NEJM* 2018	NR		ORR 75% 71% DoR at 12 m 55% PFS at 12 m	Anemia elevated AST/ALT, weight increase, decrease in the neutrophil count, fatigue, vomiting, dizziness, arthralgia
	Entrectinib	Doebele et al. *Lancet Oncol.* 2020	NR		ORR 57.4% mDoR of 10 m (95% CI, 7.1 to not estimable)	Dizziness, constipation, diarrhea, elevated AST/ALT, elevated weight, peripheral edema, elevated creatinine kinase

ALK, anaplastic lymphoma kinase; ALT, alanine aminotransferase; AST, aspartate aminotransferase; CI, confidence interval; EGFR, epidermal growth factor receptor; HR, hazard ratio; m, months; mDoR, median duration of response; mOS, median overall survival; mPFS, median progression-free survival; NR, not reported; ORR, objective response rate; TKI, tyrosine kinase inhibitor.

the combination of pembrolizumab and platinum-based chemotherapy offers a significant survival advantage to patients with nonsquamous histology (adenocarcinoma) over platinum-based systemic chemotherapy alone, including patients with a PD-L1 tumor proportion score of 1% to 49% and less than 1%. KEYNOTE-189 included patients older than age 65, constituting approximately 49% of the study population. The ICI combination group had a slightly higher frequency of grade 3 to 4 adverse events in comparison to the doublet chemotherapy group (67.2%–65.8%, respectively). Different combinations of ICI and doublet chemotherapy were tested based on the tumor histology (squamous vs nonsquamous), and all showed superior outcomes (**Table 91-3**). Thus ICI and platinum-based chemotherapy became the standard regimen for treating advanced-stage NSCLC without an actionable mutation, yielding superior survival and clinical outcomes. Contraindications to ICI include autoimmune diseases such as systemic lupus erythematosus, rheumatoid arthritis, connective tissue disease, inflammatory bowel disease, and interstitial lung disease. For patients with contraindications to ICI, a histology-appropriate systemic chemotherapy may be used.

Although data are limited, age is not a contraindication for chemotherapy. Historically, the phase III Elderly Lung Cancer Vinorelbine Italian Study (ELVIS) established that single-agent chemotherapy improves survival and quality of life among older adults compared to supportive care alone. Subsequent clinical trials demonstrated the superiority of platinum-based chemotherapy versus single-agent chemotherapy among older adults, establishing four to six cycles of doublet platinum-based chemotherapy as the current SOC for fit older adults. Patient selection is key as older adults are more likely to have comorbidities such as cardiopulmonary disease, physiological changes in body composition and drug metabolism, decline in cognitive function, and/or poor PS. Several novel platinum combinations have been studied. Scagliotti et al. demonstrated that a pemetrexed-based regimen has better clinical outcomes in nonsquamous histology NSCLC, making it the first treatment of choice when indicated. On the other hand, a study by Socinski et al., a weekly dose of albumin-bound paclitaxel (nab-paclitaxel) was compared to solvent-bound paclitaxel administered in combination with carboplatin every 3 weeks. In a subgroup analysis of patients aged 70 or older, the overall survival improved in the nab-paclitaxel arm

TABLE 91-3 ■ FIRST-LINE TREATMENT FOR PATIENTS WITH METASTATIC NON–SMALL-CELL LUNG CANCER WITHOUT TARGETABLE MOLECULAR ALTERATIONS

| BIOMARKER | TREATMENT REGIMENS | CLINICAL TRIAL AND FIRST AUTHOR | CLINICAL EFFICACY | | | COMMON ADVERSE SIDE EFFECTS |
			AGE	HR (95% CI)	OVERALL CLINICAL EFFICACY	
PD-L1 tumor proportion score (TPS) ≥ 50%	Pembrolizumab (ICI)	KEYNOTE-024 trial Pembrolizumab vs platinum-based chemotherapy	< 65 = 141/305 (46.2%)	PFS 0.61 (0.40–0.92)	ORR 45% mPFS of 10.3 m vs 6 m (HR, 0.50; 95% CI, 0.37–0.68; $p < 0.001$) mOS of 30 m vs 14.2 m (HR, 0.60; 95% CI, 0.41 to 0.89; $p = 0.005$)	ICI: diarrhea, fatigue, colitis, pneumonitis, hypothyroidism, dermatitis, nephritis, transaminitis, myocarditis, myositis, arthralgia
			≥ 65 = 164/305 (53.8%)	PFS 0.45 (0.29–0.70)		
Nonsquamous NSCLC with PD-L1 TPS < 50%	Platinum-based chemotherapy pemetrexed and pembrolizumab (ICI)	KEYNOTE-189 trial Pembrolizumab and platinum-based chemotherapy and pemetrexed vs platinum-based chemotherapy followed by maintenance pemetrexed +/– pembrolizumab	< 65 = 312/616 (50.6%)	OS 0.43 (0.31–0.61)	ORR 48% mOS of not reached vs 11.3 m (HR, 0.49; 95% CI, 0.38–0.64; $p < 0.001$)	Carboplatin: fatigue, nausea, myelosuppression (particularly thrombocytopenia) Pemetrexed: fatigue, nausea, rash, myelosuppression (anemia most common) ICI: diarrhea, fatigue, colitis, pneumonitis, hypothyroidism, dermatitis, nephritis, transaminitis, myocarditis, myositis, arthralgia
			≥ 65 = 304/616 (49.4)	OS 0.64 (0.43–0.95)		
	Carboplatin, paclitaxel, atezolizumab (ICI), and bevacizumab	IMpower 150 trial Atezolizumab, bevacizumab, platinum-based chemotherapy, and paclitaxel vs bevacizumab, platinum-based chemotherapy, and paclitaxel followed by maintenance atezolizumab +/ placebo	< 65 = 375/692 (54%)	PFS 0.65	ORR 64% mOS 19.2 m vs 14.7 m (HR, 0.78; 95% CI, 0.64–0.96; $p = 0.02$)	Carboplatin: fatigue, nausea, myelosuppression (particularly thrombocytopenia) Paclitaxel: alopecia, neuropathy, infusion reactions, myelosuppression, myalgias/arthralgias Bevacizumab: hypertension, proteinuria, bleeding/hemorrhage, thrombotic events, impaired wound healing ICI: diarrhea, fatigue, colitis, pneumonitis, hypothyroidism, dermatitis, nephritis, transaminitis, myocarditis, myositis, arthralgia
			65–74 = 248/692 (36%)	PFS 0.52		
			75–84 = 64/692 (9%)	PFS 0.78		
Squamous NSCLC with PD-L1 TPS < 50%	Carboplatin and paclitaxel or nab-paclitaxel, and pembrolizumab (ICI)	KEYNOTE-407 trial Pembrolizumab and platinum-based chemotherapy vs platinum-based chemotherapy followed by maintenance placebo +/– pembrolizumab	< 65 = 254/559 (45.4%)	PFS 0.50 (0.37–0.69)	ORR 58% mOS of 15.9 m vs 11.3 m (HR, 0.64; 95% CI, 0.49–0.85; $p < 0.001$)	Carboplatin: fatigue, nausea, myelosuppression (particularly thrombocytopenia) Paclitaxel: alopecia, neuropathy, infusion reactions, myelosuppression, myalgias/arthralgias ICI: diarrhea, fatigue, colitis, pneumonitis, hypothyroidism, dermatitis, nephritis, transaminitis, myocarditis, myositis, arthralgia
			≥ 65 = 305/559 (54.6%)	PFS 0.63 (0.47–0.84)		

CI, confidence interval; HR, hazard ratio; ICI, immune checkpoint inhibitor; m, months; mOS, median overall survival; mPFS, median progression-free survival; NR, not reported; ORR, objective response rate; PD-L1, programmed death ligand 1; TPS, tumor proportion score.

(19.9 vs 10.4 months). The improved clinical outcome with nab-paclitaxel among older adults may be related to better tolerability of the weekly schedule, suggesting that the weekly nab-paclitaxel combination might be the preferred approach in this population. To date, only one trial (Elderly Selection on Geriatric Index Assessment [ESOGIA]) has incorporated a geriatric assessment into treatment decision-making among older patients with stage IV NSCLC (see Geriatric Assessment below).

For second-line therapy or beyond for NSCLC, approved treatment options usually include docetaxel, erlotinib, and, based on histology, pemetrexed and gemcitabine if not already employed as first-line treatment. Ramucirumab, an antibody directed against vascular endothelial growth factor receptor 2, has been approved in combination with docetaxel based on a phase III trial. However, the combination's survival advantage over docetaxel monotherapy is relatively small. Based on subset analysis, no survival benefit over docetaxel monotherapy was seen in the few patients aged 70 or older compared to those younger than age 70 (HR 0.96 vs 0.74, respectively). Furthermore, meta-analysis and retrospective studies demonstrated that the addition of angiogenesis to chemotherapy among older adults is associated with more toxicity with no survival benefit. For patients who did not receive immunotherapy in the first-line settings, three ICIs are currently approved for second-line treatment of advanced NSCLC: nivolumab (PD-1), pembrolizumab (PD-1), and atezolizumab (PD-L1). All three ICIs were compared to docetaxel in the second-line settings and showed superior overall survival with better tolerability. Furthermore, second-line or beyond therapy trials specifically in older or functionally vulnerable patients with metastatic NSCLC remain elusive. Goals-of-care discussions including the patient's and caregivers' preferences about relative risks and benefits are even more significant at the time of disease progression for metastatic lung cancer.

Maintenance chemotherapy is an evolving treatment strategy for select patients with stage IV NSCLC with a good response to initial platinum-based doublet chemotherapy to delay recurrence. Pemetrexed-based maintenance therapy for patients with adenocarcinoma histology has been shown in several studies to improve progression-free survival and, in at least one major study (PARAMOUNT), demonstrated an overall survival benefit over placebo. In the PARAMOUNT trial, patients older than 70 years comprised 17% of the study population. In a subgroup analysis, this group met the primary endpoint and had a significant reduction in the risk of disease progression with maintenance pemetrexed (HR 0.35; 95% CI 0.20–0.63) but failed to demonstrate an overall survival advantage. How maintenance chemotherapy strategies versus "drug holidays" should be employed in older and/or frailer patients with NSCLC remains unclear. For those with squamous cell carcinoma, the evidence for gemcitabine- or erlotinib-based maintenance chemotherapy is less robust. In addition, the optimal duration of ICI is not yet determined.

Different durations are currently being used for different ICIs, based on the original clinical trial design, ranging from treatment until progression or toxicity versus a fixed duration of 2 years.

SMALL-CELL LUNG CANCER

SCLC is less common than NSCLC (< 15% of all lung cancer cases), but is associated with smoking exposure and duration. SCLC has a rapid growth and, unlike NSCLC, patients with SCLC tend to be symptomatic at the time of diagnosis, with common symptoms including chest pain, dyspnea, hemoptysis, SVC syndrome, hyponatremia/the syndrome of inappropriate antidiuretic hormone (SIADH), or symptoms related to brain metastases. Although the same tumor, node, metastasis (TNM) staging system for NSCLC is applied to SCLC, cancer providers frequently still utilize the older clinical staging of limited-stage (LS) (ie, disease that can be confined to a radiation port, ie, up to stage IIIB) versus extensive-stage (ES) disease (ie, stage IVA–B). Because of SCLC's higher penchant for CNS involvement, all patients with SCLC should undergo brain imaging as part of their initial staging evaluation. SCLC is a chemo- and radiosensitive disease, with high response rates to chemotherapy, which leads to rapid symptomatic relief in first-line therapy. Unfortunately, SCLC has a high rate of recurrence, and it is much more refractory to treatment in the second line. Median overall survival rates associated with treatment for LS- and ES-SCLC range from 12 to 18 months and 8 to 12 months, respectively.

Platinum-based chemotherapy with etoposide is the cornerstone of SCLC treatment. Limited-stage SCLC (LS-SCLC) represents less than a third of SCLC cases. The standard treatment for these patients is concurrent chemoradiation. Early administration of concurrent chemoradiation is associated with a better disease control and survival over a sequential approach but with higher rates of esophagitis and toxicity. Although data in older adults are lacking, different factors such as PS, pulmonary function, and comorbidities should be considered in the treatment plan. Based on a large meta-analysis, carboplatin can be incorporated in lieu of cisplatin for older adults or other patients in whom cisplatin may not be well tolerated for either limited- or extensive-stage SCLC.

ES-SCLC accounts for the majority of cases diagnosed with SCLC. The first treatment strategy to demonstrate an improvement is overall survival in first-line ES-SLCL was the addition of ICI to platinum-based chemotherapy. The IMpower 133 trial demonstrated that the combination of atezolizumab and platinum-based chemotherapy followed by maintenance atezolizumab offers a significant survival advantage to patients with ES-SCLC over platinum-based systemic chemotherapy alone, regardless of the PDL1 tumor proportion score, with a median overall survival of 12.3 versus 10.3 months (HR, 0.70; 95% CI, 0.54–0.91; $p = 0.007$). Patients aged 65 or older comprised

46% of the study population, and they showed a significant improvement in overall survival with the addition of atezolizumab (HR 0.53; 95% CI, 0.36–0.77). Durvalumab, another ICI, has also been investigated in the first-line settings with platinum-based chemotherapy in the CAPSIAN trial, showing similar results of superior clinical outcomes that were maintained in older adults. Both ICIs are currently FDA-approved in combination with platinum etoposide combination in the first-line settings of ES-SCLC.

Because of the risk of CNS involvement and as a site of relapse in patients with limited- or extensive-stage SCLC, PCI has been evaluated in patients with SCLC who have exhibited a clinical response to initial cancer therapy and remain free of obvious brain metastases. Multiple studies in LS-SCLC have demonstrated its benefit in lowering the risk and time of development of brain metastases, with a recent metanalysis showing a 5.4% 3-year survival benefit. Older adults (ie, 70–80 years) with LS-SCLC may still derive a survival advantage with PCI but are at increased risk of treatment-related adverse events. Any form of WBRT may confer risk of later-term neurocognitive effects, which may particularly be of concern for LS-SCLC patients whose prognosis is generally better than that of those with ES-SCLC. Data for older adults with LS-SCLC who may have subclinical mild cognitive impairment at baseline may be at higher risk for these complications. Hippocampal-sparing radiation therapy planning techniques and the use of neuroprotectants such as memantine have shown some initial promise in patients undergoing WBRT for known brain metastases that may help reduce this risk in patients undergoing PCI in the future. On the contrary, a recent study by Takahashi et al. evaluated the role of PCI in ES-SCLC patients who received brain imaging at baseline and during close surveillance. PCI was associated with detrimental effect on survival, making the role of PCI controversial.

Upon relapse, disease is usually divided into sensitive relapse (> 3 months after completing first-line chemotherapy) or resistant relapse (< 3 months). Platinum-based chemotherapy plus etoposide remains a very good option for sensitive disease. For decades, treatment for refractory disease apart from camptothecins (ie, topotecan, irinotecan) has been limited. Topotecan is associated with a response rate of 15% to 30% and survival of 4 to 8 months (depending on platinum-sensitivity status to initial treatment) and comes with a very high cost of hematological and nonhematological toxicity. A new major breakthrough is the FDA approval for lurbinectedin in both sensitive and refractory relapse settings based on a single-arm phase II study ($N = 105$). After a median follow-up of 17.1 months, lurbinectedin had a high response rate of 35.2% with manageable safety profile. Common side effects include hematological toxicity, transaminitis, elevated creatinine, nausea, and fatigue. Although the outcome of older adults was not reported, lurbinectedin can be a reasonable option given its acceptable toxicity profile that can be managed with granulocyte colony-stimulating factor (G-CSF) prophylaxis. Patients with platinum-refractory SCLC whose disease progresses on or fails to respond to additional therapy are unlikely to benefit from further therapy.

THE ROLE OF PALLIATIVE AND SUPPORTIVE CARE

Palliative care is gaining acceptance as essential cancer care, particularly for patients with advanced lung cancer. A randomized controlled study evaluated the effect of early palliative care after a new diagnosis of metastatic NSCLC on patient-reported outcomes and end-of-life compared to SOC. Of the 151 patients who underwent randomization, 27 died by 12 weeks and 107 (86% of the remaining patients) completed assessments. Patients assigned to early palliative care experienced improved quality of life versus SOC (mean score on the Functional Assessment of Cancer Therapy-Lung [FACT-L] scale [in which scores range from 0–136, with higher scores indicating better quality of life] 98.0 vs 91.5; $p = 0.03$). In addition, fewer patients in the palliative care group than in the SOC group had depressive symptoms (16% vs 38%, $p = 0.01$). Despite the fact that fewer patients in the early palliative care group received less aggressive end-of-life care (33% vs 54%, $p = 0.05$), median overall survival was longer (11.6 vs 8.9 months, $p = 0.02$) compared to SOC.

Older adults may have goals or expectations different from those of younger patients, which is particularly relevant in the setting of advanced lung cancer. In a multi-institutional, prospective, observational cohort study that included 710 patients with advanced lung cancer treated with palliative-intent chemotherapy, 69% gave answers that were not consistent with understanding that chemotherapy was very unlikely to cure their cancer. Using multivariable logistic regression, factors that were associated with a greater likelihood of this apparent misunderstanding were non-White race or ethnic group as compared with White race (odds ratio [OR] for Hispanic patients, 2.82; 95% CI, 1.51–5.27; OR for Black patients, 2.93; 95% CI, 1.80–4.78). Educational level, functional status, and the patient's role in decision-making were not associated with such inaccurate beliefs about chemotherapy. However, there was a strong trend of worse understanding with increasing age (OR 1.68 for patients in the age group 70–79; 95% CI, 1.10–2.59). Thus, goals of chemotherapy need to be conveyed clearly to older adults as there is a high prevalence of misconceptions about the role of chemotherapy. Furthermore, in the above-cited prospective study evaluating the role of early integration of palliative care, participants completed baseline and longitudinal assessments of their perceptions of prognosis and the goals of cancer therapy over a 6-month period. Despite having terminal cancer, a third of patients reported that their cancer was curable at baseline, and a majority (69%) endorsed eradicating the cancer as a goal of therapy. A greater proportion of patients who were assigned to early palliative care in this study developed an accurate assessment of their prognosis over time (83% vs 60%; $p = 0.02$) compared to SOC. Patients receiving early palliative care who reported an accurate perception of their prognosis were less likely to receive intravenous chemotherapy near the end of life (9.4% vs 50%; $p = 0.02$). This study has not been replicated with newer treatments such as targeted therapies and immunotherapy.

Every patient with lung cancer, whether they are receiving treatment or not, should receive full supportive care. Among treatment patients, supportive care includes but is not limited to transfusions of blood and blood products, nutritional support, growth factor support (eg, G-CSF), antibiotics, antiemetics, and antidiarrheal agents.

Nausea, vomiting, and diarrhea are the typical non-hematologic adverse side effects of many chemotherapeutic agents; however, antiemetics have significantly improved. Extreme caution and aggressive management is undertaken with both oral and intravenous medications, particularly with the use of cisplatin (highly emetogenic). Prophylactic use of dexamethasone, 5-HT$_3$ antagonists (ondansetron and granisetron), and NK1 receptor antagonists (fosaprepitant, IV, or aprepitant, oral) is common. Both acute and delayed nausea and vomiting are more easily prevented and controlled with the use of these combinations.

Mucositis and esophagitis are particularly common during receipt of concurrent chemoradiation. Several topical and oral medications are available for use; however, nutritional support becomes of utmost importance, particularly with combined modality use. Anorexia, weight loss, and dysgeusia are also very common, requiring close monitoring of weight and hydration status. Management with a nutritionist/dietician is advised. Fatigue, pain control, and stress also require supportive care. Steroids have been found to be more effective for fatigue than usual care or methylphenidate. Pain control often requires long- and short-acting narcotics, nonsteroidal anti-inflammatory drugs (NSAIDs), or gabapentin for neuropathic pain. Neuropathic pain is often associated with taxane-containing chemotherapy regimens used in both curative- and palliative-intent regimens. Bisphosphonates are also used for bony metastatic disease. See the Palliative and Supportive Care section of the Cancer and Aging: Genera Principles chapter (Chapter 88) for further information.

Currently in clinical practice, physicians use age, PS, and an overall "gestalt" of how fit an older adult is leading to both under- and overtreatment. Identifying appropriate treatment for a potentially vulnerable patient population is not straightforward in the absence of evidence-based guidelines. Moreover, chronological age does not capture the physiologic and functional status in older adults with advanced lung cancer. There has been a great reliance on ECOG performance status as a measure of physical function in lung cancer clinical trials. However, this test is an oversimplification for the assessment of function in older adults with lung cancer. Comorbidity, polypharmacy, nutrition, cognitive function, and psychosocial factors should be taken into account when caring for older adults with lung cancer. A comprehensive geriatric assessment (CGA) would serve as a uniform and reproducible instrument to guide therapy and optimize treatment decisions. The ESOGIA trial is the largest phase III randomized clinical trial using a CGA-directed approach among older adults with stage IV NSCLC. It was a multicenter study comparing older adults ($\geq$ 70 years) with stage IV NSCLC randomized to either a standard strategy of treatment allocation (carboplatin-based doublet chemotherapy or monotherapy with docetaxel) based on PS and age with an experimental strategy allocating the same regimen or best supportive care (BSC) without cancer treatment according to the CGA-directed arm. There was no significant difference in overall survival between the two treatment arms but decreased toxicity and adverse events in the CGA-directed arm. In the United States, the Cancer and Leukemia Group B (CALGB) set a precedent and completed a feasibility study of incorporating CGA into cancer treatment trials. Patients older than age 65 with cancer, who enrolled on cooperative group cancer treatment trials, were eligible to enroll. They completed the CGA tool prior to initiation of protocol therapy, consisting of valid and reliable GA measures, which are primarily self-administered and require minimal resources and time by health care providers. This brief, primarily self-administered CGA large prospective study across several tumor types of over 500 patients using the same CGA process, predicted toxicity of chemotherapy in adults receiving chemotherapy better than MD-rated PS. More recently, randomized clinical trials including all cancer types demonstrate the effectiveness of CGA-directed cancer care and interventions to improve treatment toxicity (see Chapter 88). Future studies using a CGA among patients with lung cancer are needed.

FURTHER READING

Aberle DR, Adams AM, Berg CD, et al. Reduced lung-cancer mortality with low-dose computed tomographic screening. *N Engl J Med.* 2011;365(5):395–409.

Antonia SJ, Villegas A, Daniel D, et al. Durvalumab after chemoradiotherapy in stage III non–small-cell lung cancer. *N Engl J Med.* 2017;377(20):1919–1929.

Arbour KC, Riely GJ. Systemic therapy for locally advanced and metastatic non–small cell lung cancer: a review. *JAMA.* 2019;322(8):764–774.

Chang JY, Senan S, Paul MA, et al. Stereotactic ablative radiotherapy versus lobectomy for operable stage I non-small-cell lung cancer: a pooled analysis of two randomised trials. *Lancet Oncol.* 2015;16(6):630–637.

Coughlin JM, Zang Y, Terranella S, et al. Understanding barriers to lung cancer screening in primary care. *J Thorac Dis.* 2020;12(5):2536–2544.

De Koning HJ, van der Aalst CM, de Jong PA, et al. Reduced lung-cancer mortality with volume CT screening in a randomized trial. *N Engl J Med.* 2020;382(6):503–513.

Gandhi L, Rodríguez-Abreu D, Gadgeel S, et al. Pembrolizumab plus chemotherapy in metastatic non–small-cell lung cancer. *N Engl J Med.* 2018;378(22):2078–2092.

Goldstraw P, Chansky K, Crowley J, et al. The IASLC lung cancer staging project: proposals for revision of the TNM stage groupings in the forthcoming (eighth) edition of the TNM classification for lung cancer. *J Thorac Oncol.* 2016;11(1):39–51.

Horn L, Mansfield AS, Szczęsna A, et al. First-line atezolizumab plus chemotherapy in extensive-stage small-cell lung cancer. *New Engl J Med.* 2018:379(23):2220–2229.

Hurria A, Mohile S, Gajra A, et al. Validation of a prediction tool for chemotherapy toxicity in older adults with cancer. *J Clin Oncol.* 2016;34(20):2366–2371.

Kalemkerian GP, Narula N, Kennedy EB, et al. Molecular testing guideline for the selection of patients with lung cancer for treatment with targeted tyrosine kinase inhibitors: American Society of Clinical Oncology endorsement of the College of American Pathologists/International Association for the study of lung cancer/association for molecular pathology clinical practice guideline update. *J Clin Oncol.* 2018;36(9):911.

Mohile SG, Dale W, Somerfield MR, et al. Practical assessment and management of vulnerabilities in older patients receiving chemotherapy: ASCO guideline for geriatric oncology. *J Clin Oncol.* 2018;36(22):2326–2347.

Moyer VA; US Preventive Services Task Force. Screening for Lung Cancer: U.S. Preventive Services Task Force recommendation statement. *Ann Intern Med.* 2014;160(5):330–338.

Pollock Y, Chan CL, Hall K, et al. A novel geriatric assessment tool that predicts postoperative complications in older adults with cancer. *J Geriatr Oncol.* 2020;11(5):866–872.

Rule WG, Foster NR, Meyers JP, et al. Prophylactic cranial irradiation in elderly patients with small cell lung cancer: findings from a North Central Cancer Treatment Group pooled analysis. *J Geriatr Oncol.* 2015;6(2):119–126.

Siegel RL, Miller KD, Fuchs HE, et al. Cancer statistics, 2021. *CA Cancer J Clin.* 2021;71(1):7–33.

Socinski MA, Bondarenko B, Karaseva NA, et al. Weekly nab-paclitaxel in combination with carboplatin versus solvent-based paclitaxel plus carboplatin as first-line therapy in patients with advanced non-small-cell lung cancer: final results of a phase III trial. *J Clin Oncol.* 2012;30(17):2055–2062.

Temel JS, Greer JA, Muzikansky A, et al. Early palliative care for patients with metastatic non-small-cell lung cancer. *N Engl J Med.* 2010;363(8):733–742.

Trigo J, Vivek S, Besse B, et al. Lurbinectedin as second-line treatment for patients with small-cell lung cancer: a single-arm, open-label, phase 2 basket trial. *Lancet Oncol.* 2020;21(5):645–654.

Weeks JC, Catalano PJ, Cronin A, et al. Patients' expectations about effects of chemotherapy for advanced cancer. *N Engl J Med.* 2012;367(17):1616–1625.

Chapter 92

Gastrointestinal Malignancies

Ryan D. Nipp, Nadine J. McCleary

INTRODUCTION

Gastrointestinal (GI) cancers are primarily diseases of persons in their sixth, seventh, and eighth decades of life. GI cancers are expected to account for 18% of new cancer cases and 28% of cancer-related deaths in the United States in 2020. Both incidence and mortality of GI cancers increase with advancing age (**Figures 92-1, 92-2,** and **92-3**). Despite overall decreases in incidence of some GI malignancies, older age is associated with higher prevalence of GI malignancies. Many older persons, however, have additional medical conditions, functional limitations, and social isolation that almost certainly contribute to inferior survival and morbidity outcomes. This chapter will explore the epidemiology, presentation, treatment options, and disparities in the care of older persons with GI malignancies.

In general, the symptoms and presentation of GI cancers in older adults appear similar to those of younger adults. Although treatments for these cancers have been developed primarily in younger adults, greater expertise over time has permitted similarly safe and efficacious therapy to be extended to older age groups. Since the greatest percentage of GI cancers are located in the colon and rectum, most of the information regarding older persons focuses on colorectal cancer (CRC). Unfortunately, there is a paucity of information concerning the treatment of older adults with other GI malignancies. Where we lack data specific to efficacy of individual therapies for older adults, attention should be paid to the toxicities of the treatments, with consideration of adults' concurrent medical conditions, functional status, and/or social support. Additionally, early referral to an oncologist to facilitate decision-making is advised. In this chapter, GI malignancies are ordered by incidence in the US population.

CLINICAL TRIALS

Older adults are disproportionately underrepresented in clinical trials by which treatment standards are derived. The US Food and Drug Administration evaluated the proportion of older adults participating in registration trials for new drugs or new indications for existing drugs. Adults older than 65, 70, or 75 represent 36%, 20%, and 9% of those participating in cancer clinical trials compared to 60%, 46%, and 31% of older adults diagnosed with cancer in the

Learning Objectives

■ Identify effective methods of colorectal cancer (CRC) screening.

■ Integrate appropriate CRC screening recommendations into health maintenance models of care for older adults, including potential discontinuation of screening when expected lifespan is fewer than 5 to 10 years.

■ Recognize the overwhelming need to enroll older adults with gastrointestinal (GI) cancers in clinical trials.

Key Clinical Points

1. Older adults remain underrepresented in clinical trials from which treatment standards are defined. The Food and Drug Administration stipulates inclusion of Geriatric Use prescribing information pertinent for older adults because limited guidance can be drawn from product labeling.

2. CRC accounts for approximately 9% of all cancer-related deaths in the United States; it causes more deaths than prostate cancer in men 60 to 79 years and falls just short of breast cancer in women 80 years or older. Noncancer deaths account for a sizeable percentage of deaths in older adults with CRC; congestive heart failure, chronic obstructive pulmonary disease, and diabetes account for 9.4%, 5.3%, and 3.9% of deaths, respectively, in older adults with localized disease.

3. Medicare covers surveillance fecal occult blood testing (FOBT) plus sigmoidoscopy or barium enema or colonoscopy for all beneficiaries; it may be reasonable to discontinue screening when life expectancy is shorter than the time a polyp progresses to a cancer, that is, 5 to 10 years.

4. Early genomic testing of advanced cancers can identify opportunities for use of novel

(Continued)

targeted therapies or immunotherapy and identify adults eligible for clinical trial.

5. Perioperative mortality is lower for CRC surgery in high-volume centers versus low-volume centers. Further, less aggressive surgical intervention is more likely in low-volume centers and in older adults, and increases the risk of recurrence and cancer-related death. Finally, laparoscopic procedures have lower mortality and equivalent outcomes in older adults.

6. Morbidity and mortality for surgery to treat resectable pancreatic or gastric cancer are similar in young and older adults.

7. A large number of expanded options in chemotherapy (eg, targeted antibodies, kinase inhibitors, immunotherapy) that are generally tolerated by older adults are now available and should prompt clinicians caring for older adults to seek medical oncology consultation even in those with advanced GI cancer.

8. In those with esophageal cancer, African-American adults 65 years and older were noted to have a lower rate of surgical consultation and half the rate of curative surgery as their older adult Caucasian counterparts—very likely contributing to worse outcomes in minorities with esophageal cancer.

9. African-American adults age 65 or older are approximately 44% more likely to die from colon cancer despite better reduction in mortality among those receiving oxaliplatin-based therapy compared to Caucasian counterparts.

United States. Whereas 70% to 75% of CRCs are diagnosed in adults older than 65 years, only 40% to 48% of adults enrolled in National Cancer Institute (NCI)-sponsored or cooperative group trials are drawn from the age group. Similar data are not available for the less common GI malignancies.

Plausible explanations for the lack of participation of older adults in clinical trials may include lack of social and home care support, physician reluctance to offer research protocols to older individuals, difficulties with access to clinics and hospitals, potential noncoverage of investigational treatments by Medicare, patient refusal, increasing concomitant medication usage and comorbidities with advancing age, and fewer trials specifically aimed at older adults. The North Central Cancer Treatment Group (NCCTG) attempted a prospective study in collaboration with Cancer and Leukemia Group B (CALGB) (now combined with other clinical trial groups as the alliance) evaluating the benefit of oxaliplatin added to 5-FU/capecitabine and bevacizumab among untreated older adults with metastatic colon cancer (N0949). This study was terminated early due to poor accrual, which may be related to the concern oncologists have about the use of oxaliplatin in older adults.

An unintended consequence of limited efficacy, tolerance, and benefit data, older adults are less likely to be referred for oncology consultation, receive standard therapy or be offered clinical trial. Barriers to clinical trial participation for older adults are multifactorial. The Cancer and Aging Research Group (CARG) issued a call to action to increase older adult participation in cancer clinical trials. Following a detailed systematic literature review of 11,094 studies discussing system, provider, patient, and caregiver level barriers to and interventions to improve clinical trial participation for older adults, the authors detailed a qualitative evaluation of 13 studies included for final analysis. Key barriers included restrictive eligibility criteria, provider bias, limitations of patient/caregiver knowledge, social determinants of health, and caregiver burden. In a separate qualitative analysis, barriers to clinical trial participation

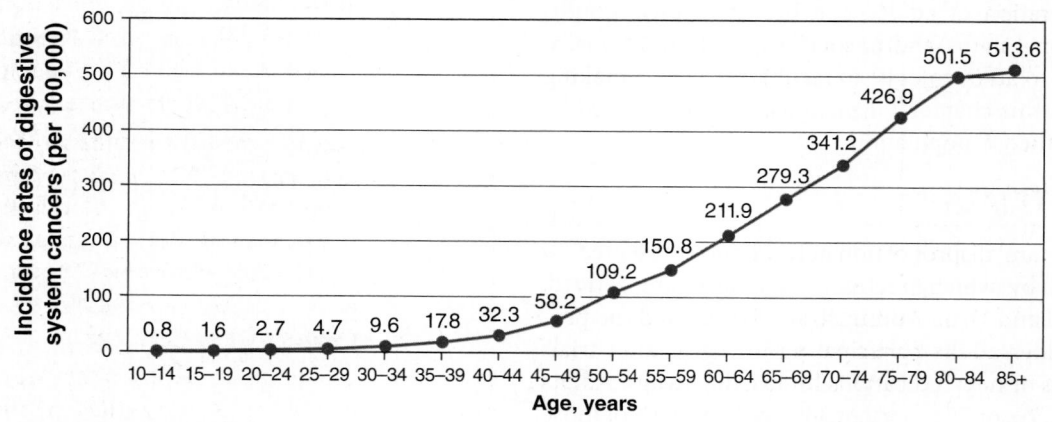

FIGURE 92-1. Incidence rates of digestive system cancers by age at diagnosis, 2013 to 2017 (all races, both sexes).

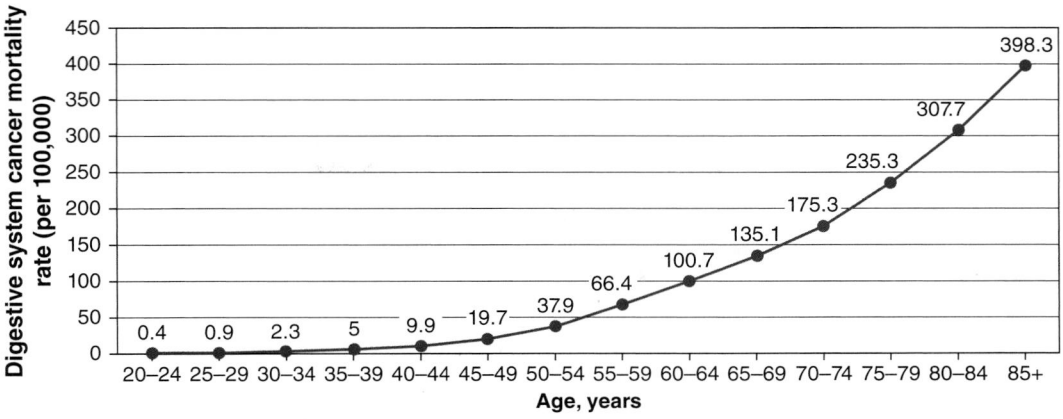

FIGURE 92-2. Mortality rates of digestive system cancers by age at death, 2014 to 2018 (all races, both sexes).

for older adults differed by provider practice setting with academic provider citing physician bias and time limitations while community providers acknowledged patient perception and caregiver burden. The authors provide key recommendations for expanding inclusion of older adults in cancer clinical trials. Some of these recommendations are in place in cooperative clinical trial groups, pooled analyses of key studies and secondary analyses of large real-world data sets.

COLORECTAL CANCER

CRC accounts for approximately 8% of all new cancer cases and 9% of all cancer-related deaths in the United States. In fact, CRC causes more deaths than prostate cancer in men 60 to 79 years and falls just short of breast cancer in women 80 years or older. In 2020, 104,610 new cases of colon cancer and 43,340 new cases of rectal cancer will be diagnosed, accounting for approximately 53,200 deaths. Nearly one-third of cases diagnosed occur in adults age 80 or older and 40% of deaths from colon cancer occur in octogenarians.

Incidence is decreasing by 4% annually for older adults, largely attributed to recommendations for earlier screening and detection of CRC. The probability of developing CRC increases from 0.4% in the first four decades of life to 3.0% for women and to 3.3% for men in the seventh decade of life (**Figure 92-4**). Median age at diagnosis of CRC is 68 years for men and 72 years for women. The overall 5-year relative survival is 64% with this cancer. It is 69% for persons younger than age 65 and declines to 61% for persons older than age 65 (**Figure 92-5**).

Studies suggest that older adults present at the time of diagnosis with the same probability of having localized, regionalized, or advanced colon cancer as younger adults. In randomized studies, older adults are reported to have the same performance status and incidence of tumor-related symptoms as younger adults but tend to have more disease-related weight loss. Older adults also appear to have a greater incidence of right-sided (proximal) tumors, and higher rates of obstruction and perforation. This in turn results in a greater likelihood of acute presentations, leading to a higher perioperative mortality rate in this older age group.

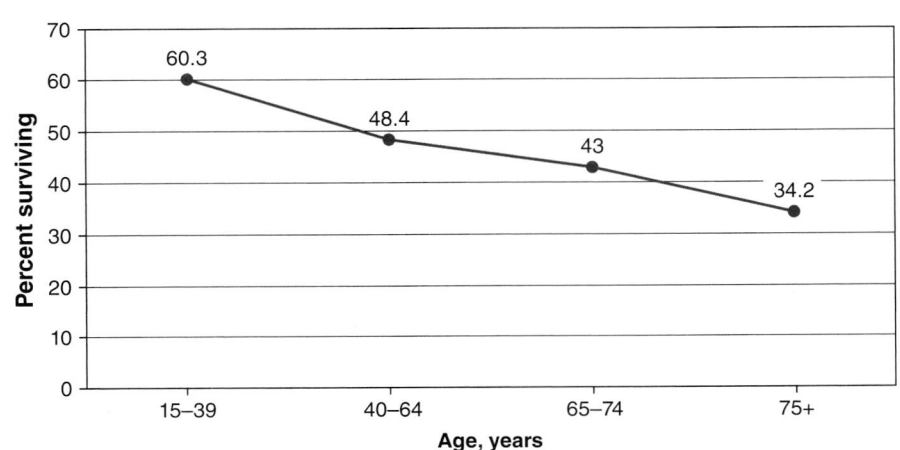

FIGURE 92-3. Digestive system cancer, SEER 5-year relative survival rates by age group, 2010 to 2016 (all races, both sexes).

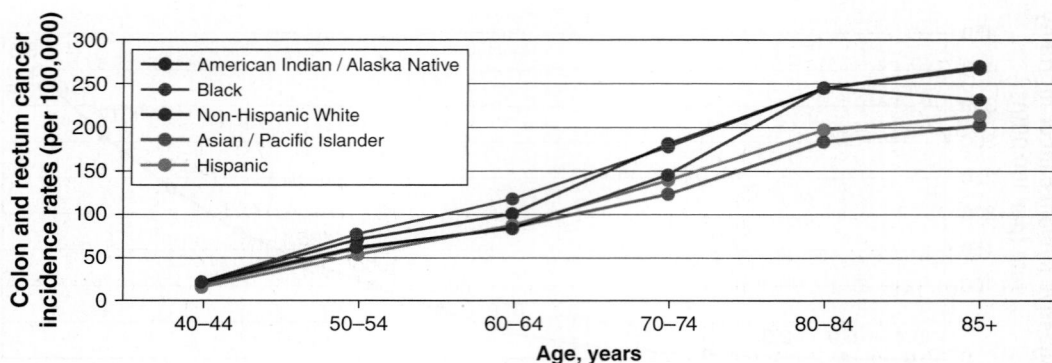

FIGURE 92-4. Colon and rectum cancer, SEER incidence rates by age at diagnosis, 2013 to 2017 (both sexes).

While some investigators have noted that overall survival (OS) is shorter in older adults, this difference is not significant if noncancer deaths are excluded. In fact, comorbid illnesses account for a substantial number of deaths among older adults with CRC. In one study of 29,733 adults 67 years and older with localized CRC in the Surveillance, Epidemiology, and End Results (SEER)/Medicare database, congestive heart failure, chronic obstructive pulmonary disease, and diabetes accounted for 9.4%, 5.3%, and 3.9% of deaths, respectively.

Risk Factors of CRC

Most older adults have no clearly defined risk factors for the development of CRC beyond the process of aging. Hereditary syndromes, such as familial adenomatosis polyposis or hereditary nonpolyposis CRC, have less impact in this older age group, since the majority of hereditary cases are diagnosed before the age of 65. There is one risk factor specific to men who were curatively treated with radiation for localized prostate cancer. These men have a 70% increased risk of developing cancer in previously irradiated portions of the bowel and could potentially benefit from more frequent CRC screening.

Chemoprevention of CRC

Various dietary supplements and drugs have been proposed as chemopreventive agents for colorectal neoplasia. Of these, aspirin has been the most widely studied; the regular use of this drug appears to confer a significant risk reduction (relative risk 0.56–0.68). In a study of 536 adults age 70 or older, aspirin use began after colon cancer diagnosis in 20% and was associated with longer OS (adjusted relative risk 0.59, 95% confidence interval 0.44–0.81, $p = 0.001$).

In at least two prospective cohort studies, the use of postmenopausal estrogens has been shown to reduce the risk of CRC by approximately 30%. Estrogen supplementation, however, has been associated with an increased risk for coronary heart disease, breast cancer, thromboembolic events, and early mortality in at least one large randomized study of postmenopausal women, thereby limiting its use as a chemopreventive agent in older women.

Additionally, it has been reported that cholesterol-lowering statins can significantly reduce the risk of CRC. As compared to individuals who did not use statins, individuals who used these agents for at least 5 years were able to reduce their relative risk of CRC by one-half.

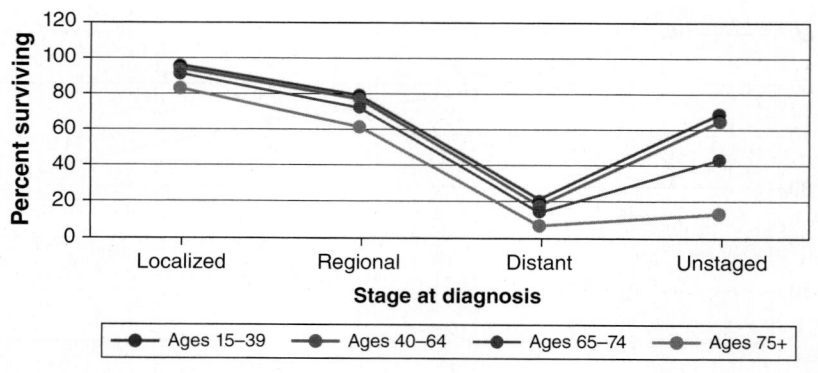

FIGURE 92-5. Colon and rectum cancer, 5-year relative survival rates by stage at diagnosis, 2010 to 2016 (all races, both sexes).

Screening of CRC

Approximately, one in two persons will have an adenomatous polyp in their colon by the age of 70. In a Veteran's Affairs cohort of 17,732 men, prevalence of advanced neoplasia was noted in 13% of those age 70 to 75 compared to 5.7% of men age 50 to 59 undergoing colonoscopy ($p < 0.001$). Odds of neoplastic transformation from adenoma to invasive carcinoma increases with age by 1.78 per additional decade, with rates of advanced neoplasia and CRC (14.3% and 2.6%, respectively) for adults age 75 or older double that of adults age 50 to 75. Older adults are also more likely to have metachronous advanced neoplasia. The risk of sporadic CRC can be reduced by 50% to 90% if adenomatous polyps are implicated by direct visualization (sigmoidoscopy, colonoscopy, computed tomography [CT] colonography, or capsule endoscopy) or stool-based testing (FOBT or stool-based DNA) and are then removed before they transform into a malignancy over a 5- to 10-year period. Colonoscopy is the most invasive CRC screening option, associated with a 50% reduction in CRC incidence in older adults. The number needed to screen to prevent 1 CRC case in older adults is 126 for men and 98 for women age 75 to 79. Sigmoidoscopy is associated with a 20% reduction in CRC incidence and 35% reduction in CRC death for adults age 70 or older based on the Prostate, Lung, Colorectal, and Ovarian Cancer Screening Trial of 20,726 older adults. The number needed to screen using sigmoidoscopy to prevent one CRC case is 282. Capsule endoscopy, while less invasive, still requires bowel preparation with secondary risk of electrolyte imbalance and poor prep, and requires colonoscopy if screen is positive. CT colonography also requires bowel preparation and insufflation with risk of bowel perforation. Colonography has sensitivity of 82% to 92% to detect adenomas 1 cm or larger, but still requires colonoscopy for polyps greater than 0.6 cm.

Noninvasive screening modalities risk false positives and ultimate recommendation for colonoscopy to evaluate initial screening finding. FOBT is associated with an 11% to 16% reduction in CRC death with number needed to screen to prevent one CRC-related death of 525 in men and 408 in women age 75 to 79. However, false-positive rates are high with FOBT at 86% to 98%. Randomized trials have demonstrated that routine FOBT can diminish colon cancer mortality by 15% to 20% during an 8- to 18-year follow-up period. While there appears to be a slightly lower mortality benefit to FOBT for older adults (10%–16% compared to 19%–23% for younger adults), this was not observed for immunochemical FOBT such as stool-based DNA testing. In fact, sensitivity of fecal immunochemical testing (FIT) does not differ significantly by age. Sensitivity of FIT to detect CRC or precancerous lesions is higher for stool DNA than FIT (stool DNA: 73.8% or 23.8% vs FIT: 92.3% or 42.4%). Despite better sensitivity, stool DNA testing is not recommended for adults age 85 or older given limited data in that subgroup. Blood testing for methylated septin 9 is not recommended given high false-positive rate with increasing age.

Case-control studies suggest that lower endoscopy and removal of polyps may decrease the incidence and mortality of CRC by 50% to 80%. However, screening extends life to a lesser degree with advancing age. Although colonoscopy appears to be particularly beneficial in older adults who have a higher incidence of proximal neoplasms, which are beyond the view of a flexible sigmoidoscopy, the risk of perforation and serious bleeding from colonoscopy is higher than from sigmoidoscopy (3–5 compared to 0.2 per 10,000 procedures and 16 compared to 0.5 per 10,000 procedures, respectively). Older adults are also more likely to have an incomplete colonoscopy, ranging from 78% to 86% for those 70 or older to 52% to 95% for those age 80 or older. While sigmoidoscopy offers lower risk of complications, it should be noted that older adults are more likely to present with proximal tumors, which will be missed on sigmoidoscopy. Prevalence of proximal neoplasia increased from 2% for men age 50 to 59 to 5.9% for those age 70 to 75 in a large Veterans Affairs cohort. This risk increases with advancing age and number of comorbidities. Therefore, screening decisions must be individualized for every older adult.

Guidelines from the American Cancer Society, US Multisociety Task Force on Colorectal Cancer, and the American Radiological Society suggest the following regarding the screening of average-risk men and women beginning at age 50: flexible sigmoidoscopy to 40 cm or splenic flexure every 5 years, colonoscopy every 10 years, double-contrast barium enema every 5 years, or CT colonography every 5 years. These guidelines also review screening and surveillance for CRC in increased-risk and high-risk persons, with accompanying recommendations. Those at increased risk include those individuals with a personal history of adenomatous polyps or CRC and adults with a family history of colon neoplasia. The US Preventive Services Task Force suggests discussing risk and benefits of CRC screening in adults age 76 to 85 and discontinuing screening for those age 86 or older. However, reduced rates of screening in older adults are likely associated with increased rates of unplanned admissions for colorectal surgery among older adults resulting in longer hospital stays, need for rehabilitation, and less opportunity for preoperative interventions to improve functional outcomes such as prehabilitation.

Since only a small percentage of persons at risk for colorectal neoplasia undergo routine screening in the United States, Medicare provides reimbursement for surveillance FOBT (including stool DNA) plus sigmoidoscopy or barium enema or colonoscopy for all beneficiaries. This has increased the prevalence of "screening within 1 year" for FOBT from 20% in persons younger than 65 years to 26% in persons 65 years and older and the prevalence of "endoscopy within 5 years" from 37% in persons younger than 65 years to 48% in persons 65 years or older.

Most older adults have a stated preference to continue CRC screening, feeling that their own life expectancy does not factor into this decision. Since the risk of advanced neoplasia and CRC is highest in older adults, it seems doubtful that screening should be arbitrarily discontinued after a certain age. In the United States, an individual who reaches the age of 80 has an average life expectancy of an additional 10 years for women and 8 years for men. At age 85, average survival is 7 years for women and 6 years for men. This estimate must be adjusted for the number and severity of chronic diseases affecting the individual, as well as his or her functional status. Prognostic tools, such as ePrognosis, incorporate actuarial data along with baseline health, cognition, and comorbid medical conditions. It may be reasonable to discontinue screening when life expectancy is shorter than the time a polyp progresses to a cancer, that is, 5 to 10 years.

Localized CRC

Surgery—localized colon cancer Cancers of the colon are typically resected with a hemicolectomy. Whether older age is an adverse prognostic factor in resection of localized colon cancer is controversial. Data on 20,862 adults undergoing surgery in 1997 for colon cancer from the Nationwide Inpatient Sample, a claims-based database, suggested that perioperative mortality increases gradually with advancing age until the age of 80, after which a substantial increase in mortality is seen (6.9 for adults older than 80 years). Older adults in the Nationwide Inpatient Sample from 1997 had lower mortality rates at high-volume hospitals than at low-volume institutions: 3.1% versus 4.5% for adults older than 65 years ($p = 0.03$). This effect was even more pronounced for adults older than 80 years, where 4.6% of adults died at high-volume centers compared to 7.3% at smaller institutions ($p = 0.04$). Therefore, it may be preferable to send the very oldest adults with colon cancer to high-volume hospitals for their resections. Yet a recent study of 24,426 adults (44% age $\geq$ 75) from the New York State Cancer Registry and the Statewide Planning and Research Cooperative System showed that older adults tended to have surgery in community hospitals rather than academic medical centers. Older age was associated with higher rate of death at 1-year (2.8% for those < 65, 13.9% for those age $\geq$ 75, $p < 0.0001$) and postoperative complication (22.6% vs 35.5%, $p < 0.0001$). Mortality rates in the older age group in this US cohort were like the 11.9% to 14% rates noted in European studies. Following death from CRC (45.6%), most frequent cause of death among the 2171 who died was cardiovascular disease (24.5%) and another primary cancer (7.4%).

A tendency to perform less aggressive surgery in older adults may be evident from an analysis of 116,995 adults with localized CRC in the SEER database (1988–2001). This retrospective study revealed that adults 71 years or older were half as likely to receive adequate lymph node evaluation (examination of at least 12 lymph nodes) as younger adults. Multiple studies have now demonstrated that inadequate lymph node evaluation correlates with inferior survival. These data would suggest that less aggressive surgical intervention predisposes older adults to a higher risk of recurrence and cancer-related death.

Increasingly, laparoscopic-assisted colectomies are being performed in the United States and elsewhere. Randomized studies indicate that adults undergoing this procedure have a similar outcome to adults undergoing an "open" colectomy, with slightly less postoperative pain and a 1-day shorter hospital stay. Persons 75 years or older tolerate laparoscopic-assisted colectomy equally as well as younger individuals. One study compared 51 adults ages 70 years or older who underwent laparoscopic colectomy to 102 age-matched adults who underwent open colectomy. Older adults had less overall morbidity with laparoscopic colectomy (17.6%) than with open surgery (37.3%), suggesting that laparoscopic surgery may lessen surgical morbidity for frail, older individuals ($p = 0.013$).

Surgery—localized rectal cancer A radical resection with anastomosis or ostomy is the standard surgical procedure for cancers of the rectum. A Veteran's Administration study of 7243 adults who underwent surgery for their rectal cancer during the period of 1990 to 2000 revealed that 30-day mortality following resection for rectal cancer was 2.1% for adults younger than 65 years compared with 4.9% for adults 65 years or older ($p < 0.0001$). Five-year survival was 60% versus 48%, respectively ($p < 0.0001$). French investigators reviewed the records of 92 surgical adults who were 80 years or older and matched these to records of 276 younger adults who underwent resection during the same time interval. Although not statistically significant, older adults had a higher operative mortality than younger adults (8% vs 4%, respectively). Among elective surgeries, the operative mortality was nearly identical (3%–4%). Although 5-year OS was greater for younger adults, 5-year cancer-specific survival was comparable for the two groups.

Adjuvant therapy—localized colon cancer Since the publication of a National Institutes of Health (NIH) consensus statement in 1990, 5-fluorouracil (5-FU)-based adjuvant therapy has represented the standard of care for adults in the United States following the complete resection of colon cancer that has spread to regional lymph nodes (stage III disease). A benefit for postoperative chemotherapy has not been prospectively demonstrated in adults with fully resected, muscle-invasive, lymph node–negative (stage II) colon cancer. However, stage II cancers with high-risk features for recurrence (eg, presentation with obstruction, perforation, or invasion into adjacent organs—stage IIB) are often treated by medical oncologists and are included in many randomized adjuvant trials.

For stage III colon cancer, single-agent 5-FU (with leucovorin [LV]) adjuvant chemotherapy became the standard of care after the publication of multiple studies in the 1990s highlighting its superior survival benefits compared to observation alone. The benefit of adding oxaliplatin to 5-FU/LV was first suggested in the Multicenter International Study of Oxaliplatin/5-Fluorouracil/Leucovorin in the Adjuvant Treatment of Colon Cancer (MOSAIC) trial, which randomly assigned 2246 adults with resected stage II (40%) or III colon cancer to a 6-month course of 5-FU/LV plus oxaliplatin compared to 5-FU/LV. Adults receiving FOLFOX (5-fluorouracil and oxaliplatin) experienced improved survival. The data are less clear concerning the optimal adjuvant treatment of stage II disease. For adults with stage II tumors with mismatch repair enzyme deficiency (dMMR) or microsatellite instability (MSI-H), an oxaliplatin-based regimen should be considered superior to a fluoropyrimidine-alone regimen.

In 2013, an updated analysis of the Adjuvant CC End Points (ACCENT) database (including seven randomized trials of newer adjuvant chemotherapy, such as MOSAIC, National Surgical Adjuvant Breast and Bowel Project [NSABP] C-07, and NO16968) showed no disease-free survival (DFS) or OS benefit among older adults receiving oxaliplatin-based adjuvant chemotherapy. In 2012, Sanoff et al. published an updated SEER-Medicare analysis of receipt and effectiveness of adjuvant chemotherapy which looked at the differences based on age for colon cancer adults. The data showed trend toward a marginal survival benefit with oxaliplatin use in adults age 75 or older. Another study performed a subpopulation analysis of 315 adults age 70 to 75 enrolled onto the MOSAIC trial. This study demonstrated that age did not alter the impact of treatment on survival outcome. Although the previously observed survival benefit of fluoropyrimidine persisted in the older subgroup, there was no survival advantage with the addition of oxaliplatin to fluoropyrimidine chemotherapy. Additionally, a subgroup analysis of adults 70 years or older from the phase III RCT NSABP C-07 trial showed no benefit to the addition of oxaliplatin to fluoropyrimidine chemotherapy, despite the risk of added toxicity. There are other studies that also question the use of oxaliplatin in the postoperative setting for older adults, but prospective studies are needed. Until then, the current data need to be considered when planning treatment, and caution taken when considering the addition of oxaliplatin for older adults. Currently, oxaliplatin can be considered for fit adults with minimal comorbidities.

The International Duration Evaluation of Adjuvant therapy (IDEA) collaboration evaluated DFS and overall survival of noninferiority of 3 versus 6 months adjuvant chemotherapy following resection of colon cancer. This prospective pooled analysis of six randomized clinical trials (CALGB/SWOG 80702, IDEA France, SCOT, ACHIEVE, TOSCA, and HORG) included 12,835 adults from 12 countries diagnosed with stage III colon cancer enrolled from June 2007 through December 2015. Age-specific data have not yet been published. The analysis established similar 5-year overall survival for 3 versus 6 months oxaliplatin-based chemotherapy (82.4% vs 82.8%, respectively), establishing noninferiority of short duration therapy. Many oncologists recommend

continuing 6-month IV-based FU combined with oxaliplatin for those with T4 or N2 disease. Shorter duration adjuvant therapy is particularly appealing for older adults with potential to reduce toxicity and confirm completion of planned therapy, often curtailed in this subgroup.

Data have shown that the receipt of oxaliplatin is inversely related to advancing age, and older adults are more likely to prematurely discontinue this therapy. The addition of oxaliplatin to fluoropyrimidine adjuvant therapy in some older adults may also exacerbate underlying comorbidities and unmask frailty. For example, oxaliplatin-induced peripheral neuropathy may increase the risk of falls and limit functional status in some older adults with colon cancer. Falls and impaired functional status are both associated with a poorer prognosis in this population.

Older adults receive adjuvant chemotherapy less often than their younger counterparts. A retrospective cohort study from 2012 utilized multiple data sets, including the SEER database, to identify 5489 adults 75 years or older with resected stage III colon cancer from 2004 to 2007. Overall, over 40% of adults received adjuvant chemotherapy. The likelihood of receiving treatment declined steeply with increasing age. Similar results were noted in an Italian study of 1014 adults with resected stage II/III colon cancer.

The reason for this age-related disparity in management is not entirely clear. In one study utilizing the California Cancer Registry, oncologists cited patient refusal, comorbid illness, or advanced age as the most common reasons for not providing chemotherapy to older adults with resected colon cancer. Financial considerations and logistical problems may also prevent some older adults from seeking care. Additionally, treatment for older adults is more frequently discontinued, suggesting reluctance by physicians to treat older adults who have experienced some degree of side effects to chemotherapy.

A pooled analysis of 3351 adults in the United States, stratified by decade of life, from seven randomized trials evaluated the benefit of adjuvant chemotherapy in older persons with stage II or III colon cancer. The primary conclusion of this pooled analysis was that older adults derive the same clinical benefit from postoperative chemotherapy as younger adults. Treatment-related toxicity was somewhat higher for older adults, yet not statistically significant. Another US study, however, could not extend this observation to adults 75 years and older, given limitations in the data.

African-American adults age 65 or older are approximately 44% more likely to die from colon cancer. However, a large cohort study of 1162 adults diagnosed with stage III colon cancer between January 2004 and December 2006 in the SEER-Medicare database (477 receiving oxaliplatin) demonstrated that African-Americans receiving oxaliplatin experienced a greater reduction in CRC mortality compared to Caucasians (adjusted HR 0.31, 95% CI 0.12–0.82 vs adjusted HR 0.83, 95% CI 0.62–1.09). Reasons for improved effectiveness of oxaliplatin in African-Americans is unknown but supports the notion that removal of insurance barriers to access in this Medicare population can lead to improved outcomes for historically undertreated populations.

In conclusion, it appears that postoperative chemotherapy in stage III colon cancer is as beneficial in older adults as it is in younger individuals. A slight increase in toxicity should not prevent the clinician from treating these older adults, although increased vigilance during chemotherapy is warranted. Shorter duration of adjuvant therapy is feasible for patients diagnosed with stage III cancer; age-related data for those with T4 or N2 disease are pending.

Neoadjuvant/adjuvant therapy—localized rectal cancer Chemoradiation before or after surgery reduces the local recurrence rate and increases DFS in adults with deeply invasive (T3–T4) or lymph node–positive rectal cancer. Although there are few data to suggest that older adults respond any differently to chemoradiotherapy than younger adults, they are less frequently referred to oncologists for this treatment. Analysis of the SEER database identified adults 65 years or older with stage II or III rectal cancer who underwent surgical resection between 1992 and 1996. Increasing age corresponded inversely with the percentage of adults who received adjuvant therapy. Overall, chemoradiation therapy was associated with a 17% reduced risk of death among all cases, with a 29% reduced risk of death in stage III adults, but no statistically significant improvement in stage II cases, similar to the results reported in younger adults. More recently, three studies (PROSPECT, PRODIGE23, RAPIDO) examined the role of radiation therapy in perioperative management of localized rectal cancer, age-specific data pending. PROSPECT examined replacement of preoperative chemoradiation therapy with oxaliplatin-based chemotherapy for those diagnosed with stage II or III rectal cancer; analyses are pending at this time. PRODIGE23 evaluated total neoadjuvant therapy with FOLFIRINOX versus chemoradiation therapy for those diagnosed with T3 or T4 rectal cancer. Disease-free and metastasis-free survival at 3 years was improved in those receiving total neoadjuvant therapy (HR 0.69 [95% CI 0.49, 0.97]; HR 0.64 [95% CI 0.44, 0.93], respectively) with improved pathologic complete response (27.5% vs 11.7%, $p < 0.001$). RAPIDO also evaluated total neoadjuvant therapy, comparing short-course radiation therapy (5×5 Gy) compared to chemoradiation therapy ($25–28 \times 2.0–1.8$ Gy), followed by oxaliplatin-based chemotherapy then surgical resection. Disease-related treatment failure a composite endpoint of locoregional failure, disease recurrence, metastasis or death, was the primary outcome. Disease-related treatment failure was improved among the short-course group with reduction in distant metastasis but not locoregional failure. All three studies have potential to reduce toxicity and DFS for subsets of older adults, particularly where overall survival benefit may be limited due to competing risk of death from comorbidities.

Postoperative surveillance—localized CRC There is general agreement that all adults with resected CRC should undergo regular surveillance screening with colonoscopy, carcinoembryonic antigen (CEA) testing, and possibly an annual CT scan. Analysis of 52,283 Medicare beneficiaries treated for locoregional CRC between 1986 and 1996 suggested that younger adults are more likely to undergo periodic surveillance endoscopies and that the median time to first follow-up endoscopy is significantly shorter ($p < 0.0001$) for adults at younger ages.

Advanced CRC

Surgery—advanced CRC Removal of the primary cancer is indicated in adults who have an (impending) obstruction, uncontrollable bleeding, or oligometastatic disease that may potentially be cured with aggressive therapy. In spite of these restrictive criteria, a recent pattern of care study, utilizing the SEER database revealed that the majority of adults 65 years or older with stage IV CRC undergo resection of their primary tumor. Overall, 72% of adults underwent this primary cancer–directed surgery. The percentage of adults undergoing surgery declined gradually from 76% in adults 65 to 69 years old to 70% in adults 80 to 84 years old, and then dropped to 62% in adults 85 years or older.

In this pattern of care study, the 30-day mortality was 10% for all adults. However, higher perioperative mortality rates for older adults with advanced CRC have been reported elsewhere. In adults 70 to 79 years, the mortality may be as high as 21% and in octogenarians it may reach 38%. Overall, improvements in surgical technique and postoperative care have led to a decrease in operative mortality particularly in older adults, so that current operative survival figures for older adults now approach those reported for younger adults a decade ago.

Older adults with oligometastatic disease or isolated recurrences of their CRC may be candidates for a "curative-intent" resection. In a series from the Memorial Sloan Kettering Cancer Center, 128 adults 70 years or older underwent liver resection for metastatic CRC between 1985 and 1994. While these adults experienced a 4% perioperative mortality rate and a 42% complication rate, their median survival was 40 months and 5-year survival rate was 35%. These older adults had a similar outcome to 449 adults less than 70 years old who underwent comparable liver resections during the same time period. In a retrospective analysis of adults age 65 and older in the SEER database, only 6.1% of the 13,599 adults identified with colorectal metastases limited to the liver underwent hepatic resection. The 30-day mortality rate was 4.3%. Five-year survival for resected adults was superior to those who did not undergo resection (32.8% vs 10.5%; $p < 0.0001$). Additionally, investigators have reported that appropriately selected older adults can tolerate resection of colorectal lung metastases with similar outcome as younger adults, with acceptable morbidity and mortality.

Chemotherapy—advanced CRC

5-Fluorouracil Until the early 1990s, the only active treatment for advanced CRC was 5-FU, a thymidylate synthase inhibitor. Multiple studies have now demonstrated that this agent, given as a bolus with LV or as an infusion with or without LV, is effective and well tolerated in the older adult population, with similar response rates and overall survival compared to younger cohorts.

Folprecht and colleagues carried out a pooled analysis of 22 randomized European trials in which adults received palliative 5-FU-based therapy. In this retrospective analysis, OS (10.8 months for younger adults vs 11.3 months for older adults; $p = 0.31$) and response rate (20.8% for younger adults vs 17.6% for older adults; $p = 0.14$) were nearly identical in younger and older adults. Infusional 5-FU proved to be superior to bolus 5-FU in all age groups. Similar results were obtained in a meta-analysis of four large trials of 5-FU-based therapy to examine the efficacy and toxicity of 5-FU in adults 70 years and older ($n = 303$) compared to younger individuals ($n = 1181$). While severe neutropenia (40.4% vs 33.6%) and stomatitis (10% vs 4.6%) were significantly increased in older adults, overall response rate (39.5% vs 33.1%) and OS (15.9 vs 15.4 months) were similar to that of younger adults.

The NCCTG conducted another pooled analysis of 1748 adults with advanced CRC treated with 5-FU-based therapy. No significant differences in response rate ($p = 0.90$) or OS ($p = 0.42$) were observed between adults younger than 56 years and older than 70 years. Adults 65 years or older had more overall severe toxicity than their younger counterparts (53% vs 46%; $p = 0.01$). Statistically significant differences in severe diarrhea and stomatitis were reported. Other studies have also noted higher rates of 5-FU-related palmar-plantar erythrodysesthesia in older adults.

Capecitabine The oral 5-FU prodrug, capecitabine, has similar efficacy to monthly intravenous 5-FU and LV (Mayo Clinic Regimen) in the metastatic and adjuvant setting. In adults 70 years or older with metastatic CRC, the overall response rate with capecitabine was 24% and the OS time was 11 months. In adults 70 years and older with resected colon cancer, capecitabine offered the same DFS advantage as standard 5-FU and LV. In this adjuvant trial, severe capecitabine-related toxicity was noted in only 12% of adults. Overall, the results with capecitabine in older adults appear similar to those seen in younger individuals.

Irinotecan Irinotecan, a topoisomerase I inhibitor, is another active drug in metastatic CRC. A multi-institutional phase II study found similar rates of severe toxicity in adults 65 years or older and those younger than 65 years receiving a weekly schedule of this agent. In a trial comparing the weekly and the triweekly dosing regimens of this drug as second-line therapy for metastatic disease, more than one-third of 291 adults were at least of 70 years. Age greater than 70 did not affect survival or time to progression but was associated with an increased risk of severe neutropenia and diarrhea compared to adults younger than 70 years.

Various trials have evaluated irinotecan-based chemotherapies in older adults with metastatic CRC. These have included combinations of irinotecan, bolus 5-FU and leucovorin (IFL), irinotecan, infusional 5-FU and leucovorin (FOLFIRI), irinotecan and capecitabine (CAPIRI), and irinotecan and oxaliplatin (IROX). These trials uniformly revealed that response to chemotherapy, median survival times, and degree of toxicity in these older adults appear to be similar to those observed in younger adults.

Oxaliplatin Oxaliplatin is a third-generation platinum analogue, which induces platinum-DNA adducts, inhibiting the replication of DNA. Although it has limited activity as a single agent in CRC, oxaliplatin has notable synergy with 5-FU and LV (FOLFOX). In metastatic CRC, the toxicity following treatment with FOLFOX was evaluated for adults 70 years and older in a pooled analysis of four randomized clinical trials. Although severe hematologic toxicity was increased in older adults, there was no difference in other severe toxicities or 60-day mortality.

For adults with resected colon cancer, a randomized adjuvant trial, in which 35% of adults were 65 years or older, has suggested that DFS can be enhanced if oxaliplatin is added to 5-FU and LV. Subgroup analysis suggested a similar benefit for older adults as for the group as a whole. For those older adults with resectable liver metastases, preoperative FOLFOX therapy may be superior to 5-FU therapy. In this study, 2-year OS was prolonged in the FOLFOX group compared to the 5-FU group or to the no chemotherapy group (84% vs 60% vs 23%).

The combination of capecitabine and oxaliplatin (CAPOX) has been evaluated in 76 adults 70 years and older with metastatic CRC. Overall response was 41%, median progression-free survival (PFS) was 8.5 months, and median OS was 14.4 months with little severe toxicity (3% peripheral neuropathy and 13% palmar-plantar erythrodysesthesia). A recent randomized study has suggested that the FOLFOX and CAPOX regimens have similar efficacy and rates of toxicity.

The FOCUS2 trial investigated reduced-dose chemotherapy for frail and older adults. A total of 459 adults were randomized to treatment with 5-FU, FOLFOX, capecitabine, or CAPOX all starting at 80% of standard doses with discretionary adjustment as appropriate. Median survival for the groups ranged from 10 to 12 months. The addition of oxaliplatin showed nonsignificant improvement in PFS (5.8 vs 4.5 months). Capecitabine did not improve quality of life compared with 5-FU.

Bevacizumab The humanized monoclonal antibody, bevacizumab, binds to the vascular epidermal growth factor (VEGF), reducing the vascularity of tumors, leading to hypoxia and necrosis. It also appears to lower interstitial fluid pressure in cancer nodules, promoting diffusion of other chemotherapeutic agents into these tumors. Three pivotal studies in adults with advanced CRC have established that this agent consistently enhances the efficacy of 5-FU-based therapy with either irinotecan or oxaliplatin for adults of all age groups. A fourth study compared bolus 5-FU and LV alone or in combination with bevacizumab in adults 65 years and older or in adults of poor performance status. This study demonstrated that bevacizumab could significantly improve survival by 4 months in "suboptimal" adults without significantly increasing toxicity.

Bevacizumab may increase the risk of arterial thrombosis, that is, myocardial infarction, stroke, or peripheral arterial thrombotic event. In multivariate analysis, persons 65 years or older increased their risk of arterial thrombosis from 2.3% with chemotherapy alone to 7.1% with chemotherapy plus bevacizumab. This risk increased further to 17.9% if the patient had a history of prior arterial thrombosis. However, progression-free and OS was better for those receiving the bevacizumab combination than for those receiving chemotherapy alone. Therefore, bevacizumab was felt to potentially provide a benefit in carefully selected older adults with a history of atherosclerosis-related disease.

Prospective studies evaluating the clinical benefit of combining bevacizumab with 5-FU or capecitabine as first-line therapy for older adults with metastatic colon cancer have been promising. A phase II study evaluating treatment with 5-FU with or without bevacizumab among adults age older than 65 demonstrated a statistically significant increase in PFS and a nonsignificant improvement in OS. The prospective, randomized phase III Avastin in Elderly With Xeloda (AVEX) study was recently published, comparing capecitabine alone or in combination with bevacizumab. PFS was longer in the combination arm, and a trend was seen toward improved OS. The NCCTG attempted a prospective study evaluating the benefit of oxaliplatin added to 5-FU/capecitabine and bevacizumab among untreated older adults with metastatic colon cancer (N0949). This study was terminated early due to poor accrual, which may be related to the concern oncologists have about the use of oxaliplatin in older adults.

Cetuximab/Panitumumab Cetuximab and panitumumab are monoclonal antibodies to the epidermal growth factor receptor (EGFR). Blockade of this receptor in CRC cells induces apoptosis and cell death. In individuals with extensively treated metastatic CRC, these agents can induce significant tumor regressions in 8% to 11% of adults; cetuximab in combination with irinotecan has a response rate of 23%. The most common severe toxicities of these agents include dyspnea, asthenia, and an acneiform rash. Cetuximab may also cause a hypersensitivity reaction. In one phase II study of 114 adults 65 years and older with metastatic CRC refractory to irinotecan, oxaliplatin, and 5-FU, cetuximab achieved a response rate of 9.6% compared to a 12.5% response rate in 232 adults younger than 65 years ($p > 0.05$).

In a randomized trial for adults with chemotherapy-refractory metastatic CRC, panitumumab resulted in partial response rate of 8% and a 46% reduction in risk of tumor progression compared to best supportive care (BSC). Similar to cetuximab, rash is the predominant adverse effect of panitumumab therapy. A severe rash early in the treatment course is predictive of enhanced response and survival with either agent. Based on systematic reviews of the relevant literature, the American Society of Clinical Oncology (ASCO) released a provisional clinical opinion in 2009 stating that all adults with metastatic CRC who are candidates for anti-EGFR antibody therapy should have their tumor tested for KRAS mutations. For adults with metastatic CRC, if KRAS mutation in codon 12 or 13 is found, they should not receive anti-EGFR antibody therapy as part of their treatment.

Cetuximab and bevacizumab along with FOLFOX or FOLFIRI were compared in a phase III Cancer and Leukemia Group B (CALGB)/Southwest Oncology Group (SWOG) 80405 trial presented at the 2014 ASCO Annual Meeting. The targeted agents had comparable benefits as first-line treatment with chemotherapy for metastatic CRC, suggesting that the selection of the targeted agent does not impact the outcomes, as long as 5-FU is used, and the biomarkers are appropriately considered. Biomarker data are likely to be increasingly used to help guide treatment decisions for CRC adults. Recent papers, including an analysis of ARCAD data, showed that the distribution of age and the prognostic effect of age did not differ according to KRAS or BRAF mutational status. The data regarding use of biomarkers in routine clinical practice are likely to evolve and further relationships between age and these biomarkers will be explored.

Regorafenib Regorafenib is an oral multikinase inhibitor that blocks the activity of several protein kinases, including kinases involved in the regulation of tumor angiogenesis, oncogenesis, and the tumor microenvironment. In the phase III international CORRECT trial, adults with metastatic CRC who had progressed on previous therapies were randomized to regorafenib or BSC. The adults receiving regorafenib had a median survival of 6.4 months, compared to a 5-month median survival for those who received BSC.

Aflibercept Aflibercept is a recombinant fusion protein containing VEGF-binding portions from the extracellular domains of human VEGF receptors that blocks the activity of VEGF. A phase III trial published in 2012 demonstrated that aflibercept in combination with FOLFIRI showed a survival benefit over FOLFIRI combined with placebo in adults with metastatic CRC previously treated with oxaliplatin.

Pembrolizumab Checkpoint inhibitor therapy has been approved as first-line treatment for MSI-H or dMMR advanced CRC based on findings from KEYNOTE 177. Pembrolizumab was associated with a doubling in median time to progression (16 months vs 8 months) and 2-year PFS (48% vs 19%)

while reducing incidence of moderate-severe toxicity (grade ≥ 3 adverse event 66% vs 22%) compared to provider's choice of palliative systemic chemotherapy. A minority of older adults present with MSI-H/dMMR disease; however, first-line immunotherapy provides added advantage of reducing toxicity and assessing potential to tolerate more aggressive cytotoxic therapy in the future.

HER2/neu Targeted Therapy Trastuzumab deruxtecan is an antibody-drug conjugate composed of an anti-HER2 antibody (trastuzumab), a cleavable tetrapeptide-based linker, and a cytotoxic topoisomerase I inhibitor. The DESTINY CRC01 study noted remarkable rates of overall response (45.3%) and disease control (83%) for this combination in third-line for HER2/neu 3+ patients, one-third of whom received anti-HER2 therapy previously. Patients with known interstitial lung disease were excluded given the known toxicity of this regimen.

PANCREATIC CANCER

In the United States, the number of expected new cases and the number of anticipated deaths for pancreas cancer in 2020 are 57,600 and 47,050, respectively. Overall, the probability of 5-year survival for this cancer has historically been under 10%. The median age at presentation is 70 years and thus a significant proportion of patients are older adults. A tissue confirmation of pancreas cancer is established less frequently in older individuals. Thus, a disproportionate number of older patients may be misdiagnosed with this malignancy and may be incorrectly given a poor prognosis to spare them the discomfort of an accurate pathologic diagnosis.

A study published in 2018 demonstrated that almost 10% of adults harbored inherited genetic variations or mutations that may have increased their susceptibility to the disease. Based on data from this and other studies, many oncologists now offer genetic testing to all adults with pancreatic cancer regardless of age and family history.

Treatment—Localized Pancreas Cancer

Older patients are more likely than younger patients to present with early-stage pancreas cancer. Surgical resection represents the only potentially curative therapy for this malignancy. Ample evidence suggests that surgical resection can be performed safely in carefully selected older adults. For example, in 206 adults older than 70 years who underwent surgery at the Mayo Clinic between 1982 and 1987, operative morbidity and mortality rates were 28% and 9%, respectively. Overall median survival was 19 months and 5-year survival were 4%. Similarly, the operative mortality in 138 adults older than 70 years who underwent pancreatic resection at Memorial Sloan-Kettering Cancer Center was 6% and the major complication rate was 45%. These results are virtually identical to those of younger patients. However, the probability of 5-year survival was slightly lower in this

group of older adults (21% vs 29%; $p = 0.03$), possibly because of an enhanced risk from comorbid diseases.

Adults with resected pancreas cancer or locally unresectable pancreas cancer may benefit from chemotherapy and/or chemoradiation therapy. In 2017, the ESPAC-4 trial was published, which compared adjuvant gemcitabine plus capecitabine to gemcitabine alone. With over 700 adults enrolled, the median OS for adults in the gemcitabine plus capecitabine group was 28.0 months compared with 25.5 months in the gemcitabine group (hazard ratio 0.82, $p = 0.032$). The average patient age in this study was 65 years, with a range of 37 to 80. In 2018, a study published in the *New England Journal of Medicine* randomly assigned 493 adults with resected pancreatic ductal adenocarcinoma to receive a modified FOLFIRINOX regimen or gemcitabine for 24 weeks, and demonstrated a median OS was 54.4 months in the modified-FOLFIRINOX group and 35.0 months in the gemcitabine group. The age range for adults in this study was 30 to 81 years, with about one-fifth of adults age 70 and older.

Neoadjuvant chemotherapy has emerged as a potential option for adults with locally advanced or borderline resectable pancreas cancer to help enhance long-term outcomes. Studies are underway to investigate the role and efficacy of neoadjuvant FOLFIRINOX or gemcitabine/abraxane to try to improve the R0 resection rates and thereby help more patients achieve cure.

Treatment—Advanced Pancreas Cancer

Gemcitabine has typically been considered the standard initial therapy for adults with metastatic pancreas cancer who are not candidates for a more intensive first-line chemotherapy regimen. Adults treated with gemcitabine have a median survival time of 5 to 7 months and a 1-year survival rate of 20%. In the pivotal trial of this agent, median age was 62 years and individuals as old as 79 years of age were enrolled, indicating tolerance of such treatment in older adults. Although the addition of erlotinib, an EGFR inhibitor, to gemcitabine demonstrated a small survival benefit in younger patients, no such advantage was demonstrated in the 268 adults 65 years or older.

In 2013, a phase III trial (the ACCORD 11 trial) enrolled 342 adults who were chemotherapy-naïve with metastatic pancreatic cancer (10% of adults were age ≥ 75 years). Patients were randomly assigned to gemcitabine alone versus FOLFIRINOX. The response rate was significantly higher with FOLFIRINOX (32% vs 9%). Median PFS (6.4 vs 3.3 months) and OS (11.1 vs 6.8 months) were both better in the FOLFIRINOX arm. A multivariate analysis of this data revealed that age greater than 65 years correlated with worse OS. The side effects of FOLFIRINOX include febrile neutropenia, thrombocytopenia, diarrhea, and sensory neuropathy, whereas gemcitabine can cause liver enzyme elevations and rarely hemolytic uremic syndrome (HUS).

An alternative to FOLFIRINOX for metastatic pancreatic cancer would be gemcitabine plus nanoparticle albumin bound (nab)-paclitaxel. Phase III trial data from 2013 showed significant improvements in nab-paclitaxel-gemcitabine as compared with gemcitabine alone. Median OS was 8.5 months in the nab-paclitaxel-gemcitabine group as compared with 6.7 months in the gemcitabine. Median PFS was 5.5 months in the nab-paclitaxel-gemcitabine group, as compared with 3.7 months in the gemcitabine group; the response rate was 23% versus 7% in the two groups. Over 40% of the adults in this trial were older than 65 years. The added toxicity of nab-paclitaxel includes peripheral neuropathy, nausea, and cytopenias.

In 2019, the *New England Journal of Medicine* published the Pancreas Cancer Olaparib Ongoing (POLO) trial, which sought to evaluate the efficacy of maintenance therapy with olaparib in adults with a germline BRCA mutation and metastatic pancreatic adenocarcinoma that had not progressed during first-line platinum-based chemotherapy. Following at least 16 weeks of continuous first-line platinum-based chemotherapy for metastatic pancreatic cancer, adults were randomly assigned, in a 3:2 ratio, to receive maintenance olaparib tablets (300 mg twice daily) or placebo. The median PFS was significantly longer in the olaparib group than in the placebo group (7.4 months vs 3.8 months; hazard ratio for disease progression or death, 0.53; 95% CI, 0.35 to 0.82; $p = 0.004$). However, an interim analysis of OS, at a data maturity of 46%, showed no difference between the olaparib and placebo groups (median, 18.9 months vs 18.1 months; hazard ratio for death, 0.91; 95% CI, 0.56 to 1.46; $p = 0.68$).

Palliative Care

Pancreatic cancer patients may require treatment of biliary and gastric outlet obstruction, pain, depression, cachexia, and malnutrition. Stents or percutaneous biliary drainage may be necessary to alleviate patients' symptoms from biliary obstruction. Cachexia, anorexia, and weight loss occur in up to 80% of pancreatic cancer patients and pancreatic insufficiency can contribute to this problem. Microencapsulated lipase supplements can alleviate these symptoms. For pain management, celiac plexus neurolysis may help.

A study published in 2017 evaluated the impact of early integrated palliative care in adults with newly diagnosed lung and GI cancer (mean age of 64.8). The study enrolled 87 adults with pancreatic cancer. In this study, patients who received early palliative care experienced improved quality of life and lower depression at week 24 compared with patients who received usual care alone.

GASTRIC CANCER

Gastric cancer is the fifth most common cancer in the world with nearly 1 million new cases per year accounting for 8% of all cancer cases. The median age at diagnosis is 68. Over 60% of new cases are diagnosed in adults older than age 65 and nearly one-third of gastric cancer patients are age 75 or older. In the United States, the predicted number of new cases for 2020 was 27,600, with 11,010 deaths expected. The results of a German study have suggested that cancers with diffuse histology are more common in younger adults than in adults 70 years or older. In Japan, adults 80 years or older are found to have more advanced disease than younger adults, perhaps because of a later time to diagnosis.

Treatment—Localized Gastric Cancer

Gastrectomy is the only curative treatment for gastric cancer. In adults who undergo the resection of all macroscopic and microscopic disease, the long-term survival is approximately 20% to 35% with surgery alone. Addition of perioperative chemotherapy, postoperative chemotherapy, or chemoradiation can further improve survival outcomes. A prospective review of 310 older adults with gastric cancer found that surgery in this group was reasonably well tolerated and led to a survival duration comparable to the results obtained in younger adults. In contrast, a multicenter retrospective study of 1465 adults following surgery for gastric cancer found a statistically significant lower 5-year OS for adults age 70 or older vs adults younger than age 70 (38.9% vs 58.9%, $p < 0.001$) while 5-year cancer-specific survival was comparable. Most, but not all, studies suggest a similar perioperative morbidity and mortality risk for gastrectomy in older and younger adults. Japan has the highest proportion of older adults worldwide and a significant number of gastric cancer cases. In a retrospective case control study of 95 adults age 80 or older compared to 366 adults age 60 to 69, there was no statistically significant difference in postoperative complication by age (both groups 23.2%). Type and extent of surgical resection also did not differ by age group with 82.1% of older adults receiving an R0 resection, 69.5% receiving a distal gastrectomy, and 29.5% receiving total gastrectomy. However, a lower proportion of older adults received D2 dissection (37.9% vs 50.3%, $p = 0.03$). While length of hospital stay did not differ, older adults were twice as likely to require rehabilitation stay following hospital discharge despite no statistical difference in postoperative complications. Still, older adults were less likely to receive adjuvant chemotherapy (9.5% vs 29%, $p = 0.05$), in part due to increased number of comorbid medical conditions in the older age group (proportion with at least one comorbid medical condition 74.7% vs 49.5%, $p < 0.05$). Older adults with stage II or III disease experience lower 5-year OS compared to younger adults (II: 17% vs 83%; III: 28% vs 54%), although survival was similar among older adults regardless of receipt of adjuvant chemotherapy.

A British multicenter prospective cohort study showed that surgical morbidity and mortality did not differ significantly by age. Of the 955 adults who underwent esophagectomy or gastrectomy, morbidity for adults younger than 70 years and older than 70 years was 50% and 48%, respectively. Mortality was also similar at 10% and

14%, respectively, for those two age groups. In Italy, age was found to be an independent predictor of recurrence in 536 adults following gastric cancer resection. It appears that short-term benefit from surgical resection is feasible for older adults; however, options for postoperative therapy are key to sustained benefit.

The CRITICS trial evaluated 788 adults (172 [22%] age 70 or older) randomized to perioperative chemotherapy or preoperative chemotherapy with postoperative chemoradiation therapy. In an unplanned posthoc analysis by age, chemotherapy grade 3 to 5 toxicity was greater in older adults (77% vs 62%, $p < 0.001$) and older adults were less likely to complete planned preoperative therapy despite 10% lower dose intensity for epirubicin, cisplatin, oxaliplatin, and capecitabine compared to younger adults. While most adults proceeded to curative surgery regardless of age (80% older adults vs 81% younger adults, $p = 0.74$), fewer older adults went on to receive planned postoperative therapy (64% vs 78%, $p < 0.001$). Again, older adults receiving postoperative chemotherapy did so at a significantly lower dose intensity than younger adults, in some cases 20% lower dosing and fewer older adults completed planned postoperative therapy (68% vs 79%) despite similar grade 3 to 5 toxicities. For the subset randomized to postoperative chemoradiotherapy, radiotherapy dosing, toxicity, and completion rates were similar. Despite differences in treatment receipt and dose intensity, 2-year OS and event-free survival (EFS) were similar regardless of age (2-year OS: 59% vs 61%; 2-year EFS: 53% vs 51%). In a randomized controlled trial of perioperative chemotherapy for resectable esophageal, gastroesophageal junction, and gastric cancers, two cycles of combination chemotherapy administered before and after surgical resection provided a 4-month improvement in median survival compared with surgical resection alone. In another study of 556 adults with resected gastric or gastroesophageal junction cancer, individuals who received adjuvant chemoradiotherapy had a 9-month increase in OS compared to those who underwent surgery alone. It is currently uncertain which one of these two approaches is better tolerated and offers a superior survival advantage. Although prospective data specific to older adults are not currently available, the unplanned posthoc analysis by age from the CRITICS and other trials suggests that adults with localized gastric cancer be considered for perioperative chemotherapy or postoperative chemoradiation.

Treatment—Advanced Gastric Cancer

The efficacy of chemotherapy programs for gastric cancer has not been specifically analyzed by age. Single-agent therapy generally results in less toxicity than is observed with platinum-based combinations and may be better suited for older individuals. Platinum analogues must be carefully dosed, since renal platinum clearance declines with increasing age. Single agents commonly used in gastric cancer include 5-FU, capecitabine, the taxanes, and irinotecan. Trials including combinations of 5-FU, LV, and oxaliplatin, capecitabine and oxaliplatin, irinotecan and cisplatin (IC), and 5-FU, LV, and irinotecan have included adults 65 years or older. However, subgroup analyses evaluating response and toxicity in these older adults have not been performed. However, two pooled analyses provide some insight into treatment response among older adults. Pooled analysis of three United Kingdom studies of advanced esophagogastric cancer in 257 adults age 70 or older (160 age 70–74, 78 age 75–74, 19 age 80 or older) compared to 823 adults younger than 70. Age was not predictive of survival, overall response rate, OS, or risk of severe toxicity. Pooled analysis of eight North Central Cancer Treatment Group trials evaluating treatment tolerance for 154 older adults age 65 or older compared to 213 younger adults diagnosed with esophagogastric cancer demonstrated comparable OS and PFS outcomes despite higher frequency of severe toxicities among older adults (73% vs 66%, $p = 0.02$). Small, single-institution trials have shown a benefit for combination therapy in selected, fit older adults. One such study of cisplatin, LV, and FU in 58 adults 65 years and older with metastatic gastric cancer noted significant responses in 43% of adults. Investigators noted that the therapy was well tolerated. Another study comparing epirubicin, cisplatin, and fluorouracil (ECF), IC, and FOLFOX found that ECF and FOLFOX both had similar response rates and OS (better than IC), but that FOLFOX was less toxic. More recently, FLOT was shown to improve overall response rate and PFS in younger adults but not those with metastatic disease or older than age 70. Further FLOT was associated with increased severe toxicity and inferior quality of life across all groups suggesting older adults are unlikely to benefit from this regimen. Given the paucity of data about the older adults in studies of gastric cancer, this may represent an appropriate time to weigh the toxicities of the chemotherapy regimens when selecting the treatment of older adults with gastric cancer.

Human epidermal growth factor receptor 2 Human EGFR 2 (HER2; also known as ERBB2), a member of a family of receptors associated with tumor cell proliferation, apoptosis, adhesion, migration, and differentiation, is a biomarker in gastric cancer showing amplification or overexpression in 7% to 34% of tumors. In 2010, the phase III ToGA trial demonstrated that trastuzumab, a monoclonal antibody against HER2, in addition to chemotherapy benefits adults with gastric cancer (median survival of 13.8 months in those assigned to trastuzumab plus chemotherapy compared to 11.1 months to the control group).

Ramucirumab Published in 2014, the phase III REGARD trial demonstrated significant improvements in OS (5.2 vs 3.8 months) in adults receiving ramucirumab, a human immunoglobulin G1 (IgG1) receptor targeted antibody. In this trial, 36% of the adults were older than age 65. Ramucirumab resulted in similar improvements for OS and PFS between adults younger than 65 years and those age 65 and older. Adverse effect profiles were also similar between age groups.

Results were released from the RAINBOW trial in 2014, an international phase III, randomized, double-blind study of ramucirumab plus paclitaxel versus placebo plus paclitaxel in the treatment of metastatic gastroesophageal junction and gastric adenocarcinoma following disease progression on first-line platinum- and fluoropyrimidine-containing combination therapy. The authors found a statistically significant and clinically meaningful OS benefit of more than 2 months for the adults treated with ramucirumab plus paclitaxel versus placebo plus paclitaxel. There is currently no documented data regarding the outcomes of the older adults from this trial.

PRIMARY LIVER CANCER

Primary liver cancer—hepatocellular carcinoma (HCC) and intrahepatic cholangiocarcinoma (ICC)—is the second most common cause of cancer death in the world, leading to over half a million deaths annually. In contrast, the annual incidence in the United States has been relatively low, with 42,810 new cases and 30,160 deaths expected in 2020. In the United States, the incidence of HCC levels is higher among Blacks than Whites (10.9 vs 6.9 per 100,000 population) as is mortality (13.5 vs 8.4 for men; 4.9 vs 3.5 per 100,000 population for women). Incidence of HCC has increased for older adults by 8% for those age 65 to 69 years and 3% for those age 70 or older. The risk factors for primary liver cancer are potentially related to aging including comorbid medical conditions, fatty liver disease, and acquired hepatitis.

Treatment—Primary Liver Cancer

Treatment options for older adults with HCC restricted to the liver include liver resection, liver transplant, nonsurgical tumor ablation, transarterial chemoembolization, selective internal radiation therapy, or stereotactic body radiotherapy. Surgery and chemoembolization in the geriatric population have been found to be tolerable in some but not all experiences. Older adults are more likely to receive ablative therapy than resection or chemoradiation therapy. In a review of the 2696 Medicare adults with HCC between 1992 and 1999, 13% had procedures with curative intent (0.9% transplant, 8.2% resection, 4.1% local ablation), 4% underwent transarterial chemoembolization, 57% received palliative therapy, and 26% did not get treatment. Only 34% of adults with solitary lesions or lesions less than 3 cm in diameter received therapy with curative intent, suggesting underutilization of curative interventions in eligible older adults. Three-year survival for transarterial chemoembolization or local ablation was less than 10%. While recurrence-free survival appeared similar with surgery versus radiofrequency ablation among older adults participating in the SURF study, the cohort was limited to those younger than age 80. Similarly, transarterial chemoembolization increased survival at 1 and 3 years following procedure with similar 5-year survival and rate of complication

for adults age 75 or older compared to younger adults. Considering life expectancy of older adults diagnosed with HCC and risk of morbidity following surgical resection, an ablative or embolization approach is reasonable for older adults as an alternative to resection.

In a retrospective, multicenter study by the Italian Liver Cancer Group evaluating a 20-year cohort of 614 older adults age 70 or older and 1104 younger adults, survival outcomes for older adults appeared like that of younger adults following surgical resection (52 months vs 47 months, respectively). Surgical resection of liver tumors is well tolerated in older adults. In a European study, cirrhotic adults with HCC older than 70 years were compared to adults younger than 70. The operative morbidity and liver failure rates were lower in the subset of older adults (23.4% vs 42.4% and 1.6% vs 12.9%, respectively). Operative mortality and 5-year survival rates were not significantly different between the two groups. In a smaller study of less than 300 patients, older adults were observed to have higher frailty based on a modified Frailty Index, higher mortality rates (8% vs 2%, $p = 0.011$) but similar overall and DFS at 5 years compared to younger adults (5-year OS 62% vs 68.5%, DFS 30.4% vs 38.8%, respectively). One measure of frailty, G8, was independently predictive of postoperative complications among older adults suggesting that geriatric assessment, among other preoperative factors such as comorbid medical conditions, nutritional status, and cognition, can help select older adults for surgical resection.

While few transplants are offered to older adults (3.1% in the United States in 2014), studies suggest that older adults with preserved synthetic function experience similar survival benefit and graft loss rates to younger adults following liver transplantation. The use of cytotoxic chemotherapy has shown modest benefits for adults with HCC, and the durations of these benefits are commonly short. No single regimen has proven superior to any other. Molecularly targeted agents, particularly sorafenib, offer the potential for improved survival for advanced HCC. The phase III multicenter European SHARP trial randomly assigned 602 adults with inoperable HCC and Child-Pugh A cirrhosis to sorafenib versus placebo. OS was significantly longer in the sorafenib-treated adults (10.7 vs 7.9 months), as was time to radiologic progression (5.5 vs 2.8 months). The average age for adults on this trial was approximately 65.

Systemic therapy options for treatment of HCC have increased to include first- and second-line tyrosine kinase inhibitors as well as immunotherapy; however, few prospective studies included specific analyses regarding older adults, frailty, and/or comorbid medical conditions. Retrospective analysis of sorafenib following approval from the SHARP study demonstrates similar survival outcomes for older adults. The REFLECT study of lenvatinib demonstrated similar survival among the 43% of participants age 65 or older compared to younger adults. Hand-foot syndrome appears higher for older adults prescribed sorafenib versus higher rates of hypertension for those receiving lenvatinib. Second-line therapy for HCC now includes regorafenib for those for whom sorafenib is no longer effective based on the RESORCE study. Cabozantinib also appears to have a similar overall and PFS benefit regardless of age. Lastly, the REACH-2 study demonstrated OS benefit of ramucirumab, although age-specific data have not yet been published. Thus far, age-specific data are not available for checkpoint inhibitors, nivolumab or pembrolizumab, both demonstrating a survival benefit following sorafenib for treatment of HCC. Optimal treatment for HCC in older adults should include consideration of potential toxicities, ability to consistently take oral medications, and possible interaction with other medications or comorbid conditions.

ESOPHAGEAL CANCER

Squamous cell carcinomas and adenocarcinomas of the esophagus are the eighth leading cause of cancer death worldwide. In the United States, esophageal cancer is less common, with 18,440 new cases and 16,170 deaths anticipated in 2020. Median age of diagnosis is 68 with 41% of cases occurring in adults age 75 or older. Highest incidence rates occur in men age 85 to 89 and women age 90 or older. Between 1974 and 1994, the appearance of adenocarcinomas of the esophagus increased substantially, particularly in White men between 65 and 74 years, while the incidence of squamous cell carcinomas declined slightly. The epidemiologic pattern of esophageal carcinoma does not appear different in older adults. Most studies report similar clinical symptoms at the time of presentation, as well as similar distribution of histology, stage, and location of tumors for adults older and younger than 70 years. In these series, approximately 50% to 75% of the older adults were found to have adenocarcinoma and 25% to 50% had squamous cell carcinoma.

It is unclear if the incidence of Barrett-associated adenocarcinoma increases with advanced age. Although one study has suggested a higher incidence in older adults, another study suggested this incidence is not age-dependent. The location of tumors in the esophagus does not differ between older and younger adults—distal esophageal tumors predominate in all groups. A similar distribution in early- and late-stage cancers has also been reported.

Treatment—Localized Esophageal Cancer

At this time, there is no prospective study evaluating outcome of preoperative chemoradiation therapy followed by esophagectomy for older adults. Extrapolating from subgroup and retrospective analyses, most, but not all studies suggest that age is not a limiting factor in surgery of the esophagus. Although older adults tend to have a higher incidence of respiratory and cardiovascular complications than younger adults, this does not appear to have a significant effect on operative mortality or survival. In one study, 50 adults older than 70 years were compared to 89 adults younger than 70 years; postoperative complications and in-hospital mortality occurred in 38% and 3% of younger adults and in 44% and 0% of older adults. The mean duration of hospitalization was 17.9 days for younger adults and 18.6 days for older adults. The severity of postoperative dysphagia and weight loss was similar for both groups. The likelihood of survival after 8 years was identical at 20%.

In a second study of 60 adults 70 years and older, no difference was observed in the rate of resection with curative intent, surgical complications, or hospital mortality rate in comparison to a younger population. This was confirmed in another study, demonstrating equivalent surgical morbidity and mortality for older adults stratified by performance status and overall fitness in comparison to younger adults. A contradictory study suggested that age was predictive of morbidity and mortality following esophagectomy in multivariate analysis ($p = 0.002$). Age and comorbidity were also noted to be significant predictors of outcome in a simple risk score developed to predict surgical mortality for esophageal cancer.

Although the rate of surgical complications may not be significantly increased in older adults, the presence of such complications significantly worsens survival. This was the conclusion in a review of 510 adults who underwent resection of esophageal or gastroesophageal junction carcinoma at the Memorial Sloan Kettering Cancer Center from 1996 to 2001. Surgical complications occurred in 31.8% of the 173 adults 65 to 74 years and in 34.8% of the 66 adults 75 years and older. Although survival at 30 days did not differ significantly between patient groups who did and did not experience surgical complications, there was a notable decline in 1-year survival for adults 65 years and older who had suffered a perioperative complication. In a separate study at the same institution, octogenarians were noted to have more than a threefold higher mortality rate than adults 50 to 79 years, although they experienced similar rates of operative complications (blood loss, cardiopulmonary complications, infection, and anastomotic leak).

A review of 945 adults in the Veterans Administration National Surgical Quality Improvement Program found no difference in 30-day surgical mortality and morbidity between transthoracic and transhiatal esophagectomies. Age did significantly impact the overall mortality rate for both surgical techniques, with increasing age associated with an increased risk of surgical mortality. The same age-related surgical mortality risk was also noted in a French study of gastroesophageal junction adenocarcinomas.

Although age may not be a significant factor in the rate of curative resection, curative surgery is still underutilized in older racial minority adults. African-American adults 65 years and older were noted to have a lower rate of surgical consultation and half the rate of curative surgery as their older adult Caucasian counterparts (70% vs 78%; $p < 0.001$ and 25% vs 46%; $p < 0.001$, respectively).

Chemoradiation therapy appears equally effective in adults 70 years and older as in younger individuals. Furthermore, there appears to be no association between age and toxicity in adults of good performance status. At Memorial Sloan Kettering Cancer Center, 24 older adults (median age 77) with locally advanced esophageal cancer were treated with 5040 cGy of radiation and infusional 5-FU plus mitomycin C over a 6-week period. Nine of these individuals (38%) required hospitalization for toxicity and three required dose reductions. Sixteen adults achieved a clinical remission and 10 remained without evidence of disease after a median follow-up of 1.2 years, suggesting that selected chemoradiation therapy is a feasible and well-tolerated alternative to esophagectomy in older adults.

The CROSS trial, published in 2012, compared surgery alone to neoadjuvant carboplatin and paclitaxel and concurrent radiotherapy followed by surgery. The chemoradiotherapy group had higher rates of complete resection (92% vs 69%) and OS (49.4 vs 24 months). The median age of adults in this trial was 60. Subsequent analysis using the National Cancer Database evaluated 4099 older adults age 76 or older who would have been excluded from the CROSS trial based on age. Most older adults underwent definitive chemoradiotherapy (73%) while 14% received neoadjuvant chemoradiotherapy followed by surgery and 12% underwent surgery alone. Median OS was highest for those receiving trimodality therapy (26.7 months) compared to 20.3 months for surgery alone and 17.8 months for definitive chemoradiotherapy ($p < 0.05$). Attempting to control for selection bias, propensity matching demonstrated a trend toward improved OS, lower hospital 30-day readmission, and improved 30- and 90-day mortality with trimodality therapy compared to surgery alone ($p = 0.08$); OS of definitive chemoradiotherapy was comparable to surgery alone ($p = 0.67$).

Recognizing the predictive value of platelet-to-lymphocyte ratio (PLR) and neutrophil-to-lymphocyte ratio (NLR) as markers of systemic inflammation, frailty, disability, and poor outcomes in other cancer, Jain et al. conducted a retrospective analysis of PLR and NLR for 125 adults ($n = 67$ age ≥ 65) receiving neoadjuvant chemoradiotherapy at a single academic medical center from 2002 through 2014. While older age was not associated with significant differences in treatment-related toxicity, relapse-free survival, OS, or pretreatment PLR in multivariate analysis, older age was associated with high pretreatment NLR ($p = 0.01$), which in turn was associated with reduced relapse-free survival ($p = 0.002$). Neither NLR nor PLR was associated with toxicity or OS.

Treatment—Advanced Esophageal Cancer

Single agents, such as the taxanes, irinotecan, 5-FU, capecitabine, and vinorelbine, have some efficacy in palliating metastatic esophageal cancer and represent management options for older adults, particularly for those with lower performance status or significant comorbidities.

Combination chemotherapy regimens tend to have more side effects and have not been systematically evaluated in older adults with esophageal cancer. Preliminary results of one study in adults 70 years or older suggested that the combination of weekly docetaxel and infusional 5-FU is well tolerated in this age group. Toxicities were primarily neutropenia and mucositis. The advances in gastric cancer frequently apply to the esophageal population; thus, the promising results from the REGARD trial and the RAINBOW trial discussed in gastric cancer may also extend to this population.

BILIARY TRACT CANCERS

Cancers of the biliary tract (gallbladder, cholangiocarcinoma) occur infrequently in the United States. The incidence increases with age and reaches its peak in the seventh decade of life. Yearly, under 5000 new cases of gallbladder cancer and under 12,000 new cases of cholangiocarcinoma are diagnosed in the United States. The presentation and clinical features of this cancer do not appear to differ appreciably between older and younger adults. Endoscopic retrograde cholangiopancreatography (ERCP) is often used in the diagnosis of biliary tract cancers and is well tolerated in older adults—even the very old. In a study of 126 adults 90 years and older who underwent a total of 147 ERCP procedures, 9.5% were noted to have malignant stenosis. The overall morbidity and mortality rates were low at 2.5% and 0.7%, respectively.

Treatment—Biliary Tract Cancers

Surgery is the only potentially curative treatment for this disease. A retrospective single institution study from Japan reviewed the cases of 54 adults who were 75 years or older and compared them to 152 adults less than 75 years. Approximately 58% of adults in both age groups underwent a radical resection (rather than a simple cholecystectomy). Operative mortality and survival rates were similar between the two age groups. The investigators noted that the likelihood of 5-year survival was better for those older adults who had undergone a radical resection, compared to those who had undergone a simple cholecystectomy (61% vs 14%; $p = 0.0098$). These uncontrolled results have not been validated through a randomized trial. For adults with localized disease who undergo surgical resection, adjuvant therapy for all adults following resection is often recommended. Options for adjuvant treatment in bile duct cancer include capecitabine for 6 months, or four cycles of capecitabine plus gemcitabine followed by concurrent radiation plus oral capecitabine, as was used in Southwest Oncology Group (SWOG) S0809, or 6 months of single-agent LV-modulated FU. Notably, clinical trials in biliary tract cancers have not been age-specific nor always included age subgroup analysis. However, secondary analyses of trials and retrospective data suggest equivalent survival benefit, regardless of patient age.

Although advanced biliary tract cancer is highly resistant to chemotherapy, single agents such as gemcitabine, 5-FU, and capecitabine are generally well tolerated in older adults and may offer some palliation in this disease. Trial data to date suggest that gemcitabine and gemcitabine-based platinum regimens offer a slight advantage over other regimens for gallbladder cancer. Studies have shown that adding fluoropyrimidines, cisplatin, oxaliplatin, and irinotecan to gemcitabine can yield similar results, but the toxicity and tolerability data tend to favor gemcitabine-oxaliplatin combinations. Thus, while several combinations have been tried, single agents appear to be better for older adults. In a small study of advanced biliary tract cancers and gallbladder cancer treated with the combination of gemcitabine and cisplatin, no difference in response rate was noted between 10 adults 60 years and older and 30 younger adults, although the older adults had higher rates of hematologic toxicity.

Recently, growing evidence supports the use of targeted agents in biliary tract cancers. For example, studies in adults with previously treated advanced cholangiocarcinoma whose tumors harbor fibroblast growth factor receptor 2 (FGFR2) gene rearrangements/fusions or an isocitrate dehydrogenase 1 (IDH1) mutation demonstrate promise for agents specifically targeting these alterations: pemigatinib (FIGHT-202 trial) and ivosidenib (ClarIDHy phase 3 trial), respectively. Although not specifically tested in older adults, analyses across different age groups for the FGFR agent seemed to suggest similar benefits for older and younger patients.

ANAL CANCER

Squamous cell carcinoma of the anal canal is one of the least common but most treatable of the GI malignancies. Anal cancer represents only 2.7% of all GI malignancies in the United States, with under 10,000 new cases diagnosed annually. The risk factors for anal cancer and genital malignancies are similar. Increased risk of anal cancer has been associated with female gender, infection with human papillomavirus (HPV), lifetime number of sexual partners, genital warts, cigarette smoking, receptive anal intercourse, infection with HIV, and other causes of chronic immunosuppression. The risk of HPV-related anal cancer increases with age. Older age at first receptive intercourse was associated with increased prevalence of both low- and high-grade squamous dysplasia, the precursor lesions to anal cancer. The higher incidence of anal cancer is more pronounced in adults 65 years and older than in younger age groups. Five-year survival does not differ significantly by gender or age.

Treatment—Anal Cancer

Since the 1970s, the standard treatment for localized anal cancer has been the combination of 5-FU, mitomycin, and radiation therapy. With this technique, 60% to 73% of

adults will remain free of disease recurrence and a colostomy at 4 years. Age has not been associated with either tumor-related or therapy-related rates of colostomy. A small study evaluating this nonsurgical strategy in adults 75 years or older demonstrated similar complication rates to those seen in younger adults, suggesting that sphincter-conserving treatment is feasible in older adults with anal carcinoma. In an Australian study of 62 adults, treated with chemoradiation (mitomycin C and 5-FU) and anal sphincter preservation surgery, the local control rate was 86% and the colostomy-free survival at 2 years was 83%. This study included 38 adults 60 years and older.

Radiation used in the treatment of anal cancer in women 65 years or older can lead to a threefold increased risk of pelvic fracture. These women are at greater risk for fracture than women treated with radiation therapy for cervical or rectal cancer. Therefore, older women treated with chemotherapy and radiation therapy for anal cancer should undergo regular bone densitometry screening and bisphosphonate therapy.

Systemic therapy represents the standard approach for treatment of advanced, metastatic anal cancer. The regimen of cisplatin plus FU represents the most widely published active regimen for the treatment of advanced anal cancer. Recent evidence from the InterAACT trial demonstrated the efficacy of paclitaxel plus carboplatin for anal cancer, although the maximum patient age in this study was 75 years, and we lack subgroup analyses by age for this regimen.

Notably, for adults with advanced anal cancer, immune checkpoint inhibitors that target the PD-1 pathway, such as nivolumab and pembrolizumab, may represent viable options. Currently, limited data exist about the safety and efficacy of these agents for older adults with anal cancer.

NEXT-GENERATION SEQUENCING (NGS)

Next-generation sequencing (NGS), a form of DNA sequencing technology that uses parallel sequencing of multiple fragments of DNA to determine sequence, provides a "high-throughput" method for increasing the speed of sequencing an individual's genome. NGS can be used to sequence a patient's entire genome or smaller portions of the genome. In GI cancer, NGS gene panels can be used clinically to guide screening, preventive options, and cancer treatment, including the use of a cancer gene panel that includes *BRCA1* and *BRCA2* if there is a personal or family history of pancreatic cancer, even in the absence of breast or ovarian cancer. Additionally, in CRC, screening for inherited causes may consider the use of NGS panels that include *APC, BMPR1A, EPCAM, MLH1, MSH2, MSH6, MUTYH, PMS2, PTEN, SMAD4, STK11, TP53, BLM, CHEK2, GALNT12, GREM1, POLD1,* and/or *POLE.*

Importantly, NGS can provide both predictive and prognostic information for adults with cancer. Specifically,

NGS could help identify possible targets for therapies, which could potentially represent less toxic and more effective options for older adults with cancer. Additionally, NGS can help to identify markers with prognostic significance. For example, microsatellite instability high status often correlates with better survival, while *BRAF* mutations correlate with worse survival outcomes, regardless of patient age. Recently, growing evidence supports the use of noninvasive genomic profiling of tumors with NGS from blood-derived circulating tumor DNA (ctDNA). Collectively, NGS can help as a strategy to guide treatment discussions for older adults with cancer, yet NGS-enabled precision oncology can add complexity to clinical decision-making and additional work is needed to understand the optimal tissue on which to perform NGS (primary tumor or metastasis, tumor DNA or circulating tumor DNA, etc) and the optimal timing for when to obtain NGS (at initial diagnosis, following a predefined amount of therapy, or when the disease is refractory).

FURTHER READING

Introduction

McCleary NJ, Hubbard J, Mahoney MR, et al. Challenges of conducting a prospective clinical trial for older patients: lessons learned from NCCTG N0949 (alliance). *J Geriatr Oncol.* 2018;9(1):24–31.

Nee J, Chippendale RZ, Feuerstein JD. Screening for colon cancer in older adults: risks, benefits, and when to stop. *Mayo Clin Proc.* 2020;95(1):184–196.

Sedrak MS, Freedman RA, Cohen HJ, et al. Older adult participation in cancer clinical trials: a systematic review of barriers and interventions. *Cancer J Clin.* 2020;71:78–92.

Sedrak MS, Mohile SG, Sun V, et al. Barriers to clinical trial enrollment of older adults with cancer: a qualitative study of the perceptions of community and academic oncologists. *J Geriatr Oncol.* 2020;11(2):327–334.

Talarico L, Chen G, Pazdur R. Enrollment of elderly patients in clinical trials for cancer drug registration: a 7-year experience by the US Food and Drug Administration. *J Clin Oncol.* 2004;22(22):4626–4631.

The American Cancer Society. Cancer Facts & Figures 2020: Revised June 2020. https://www.cancer.org/content/dam/cancer-org/research/cancer-facts-and-statistics/annual-cancer-facts-and-figures/2020/cancer-facts-and-figures-2020.pdf.

Colorectal Cancer

André T, Meyerhardt J, Iveson T, et al. Effect of duration of adjuvant chemotherapy for patients with stage III colon cancer (IDEA collaboration): final results from a prospective, pooled analysis of six randomized, phase 3 trials. *Lancet Oncol.* 2020;21(12):1620–1629.

André T, Shiu K-K, Kim T W, et al. Pembrolizumab in microsatellite-instability–high advanced colorectal cancer. *N Engl J Med.* 2020;383:2207–2218.

Ayanian JZ, Zaslavsky AM, Fuchs CS, et al. Use of adjuvant chemotherapy and radiation therapy for colorectal cancer in a population-based cohort. *J Clin Oncol.* 2003;21(7):1293–1300.

Conroy T, Lamfichekh N, Etienne P-L, et al. Total neoadjuvant therapy with mFOLFIRINOX versus preoperative chemoradiation in patients with locally advanced rectal cancer: final results of PRODIGE 23 phase III trial, a UNICANCER GI trial. *J Clin Oncol.* 2020;38(15):4007.

ePrognosis. Colorectal Screening Survey. http://cancer-screening.eprognosis.org/screening/.

Goldberg RM, Rabah-Fisch I, Bleiberg H, et al. Pooled analysis of safety and efficacy of oxaliplatin plus fluorouracil/leucovorin administered bimonthly in older adult patients with colorectal cancer. *J Clin Oncol.* 2006;24(25):4085–4091.

Gross CP, Andersen MS, Krumholz HM, McAvay GJ, Proctor D, Tinetti ME. Relation between Medicare screening reimbursement and stage at diagnosis for older adults with colon cancer. *JAMA.* 2006;292(23):2815–2822.

Gross CP, Guo Z, McAvay GJ, Allore HG, Young M, Tinetti ME. Multimorbidity and survival in older persons with colorectal cancer. *J Am Geriatr Soc.* 2006;54:1898–1904.

Hospers G, Bahadoer RR, Dijkstra EA, et al. Short-course radiotherapy followed by chemotherapy before TME in locally advanced rectal cancer: the randomized RAPIDO trial. *J Clin Oncol.* 2020;38(15):4006.

Hurria A, Dale W, Mooney M, et al. Designing therapeutic clinical trials for older and frail adults with cancer: U13 conference recommendations. *J Clin Oncol.* 2014;32(24):2587–2594.

Iwashyna TJ, Lamont EB. Effectiveness of adjuvant fluorouracil in clinical practice: a population-based cohort study of older adults with stage III colon cancer. *J Clin Oncol.* 2002;20(19):3992–3998.

Kozloff MF, Berlin J, Flynn PJ, et al. Clinical outcomes in older adult adults with metastatic colorectal cancer receiving bevacizumab and chemotherapy: results from the BRiTE observational cohort study. *Oncology.* 2010;78(5–6):329–339.

Lieu CH, Renfro LA, de Gramont A, et al. Association of age with survival in adults with metastatic colorectal cancer: analysis from the ARCAD Clinical Trials Program. *J Clin Oncol.* 2014;32(27):2975–2984.

McCleary NJ, Dotan E, Browner I. Refining the chemotherapy approach for older adults with colon cancer. *J Clin Oncol.* 2014;32(24):2570–2580.

Reimers MS, Bastiaannet E, van Herk-Sukel MPP, et al. Aspirin use after diagnosis improves survival in older adults with colon cancer: a retrospective cohort study. *J Am Geriatr Soc.* 2012;60(12):2232–2236.

Sanoff HK, Carpenter WR, Stürmer T, et al. Effect of adjuvant chemotherapy on survival of adults with stage III colon cancer diagnosed after age 75 years. *J Clin Oncol.* 2012;30(21):2624–2634.

Sargent DJ, Goldberg RM, Jacobson SD, et al. A pooled analysis of adjuvant chemotherapy for resected colon cancer in older adult adults. *N Engl J Med.* 2001;345(15):1091–1097.

Seymour MT, Thompson LC, Wasan HS, et al; FOCUS2 Investigators; National Cancer Research Institute Colorectal Cancer Clinical Studies Group. Chemotherapy options in older adults and frail adults with metastatic colorectal cancer (MRC FOCUS2): an open-label, randomised factorial trial. *Lancet.* 2011;377(9779):1749–1759.

Gastroesophageal Cancer

Fuchs CS, Tomasek J, Yong CJ, et al; REGARD Trial Investigators. REGARD: a phase III, randomized, double-blind trial of ramucirumab (RAM) and best supportive care (BSC) versus placebo (PL) and BSC in the treatment of metastatic gastric or gastroesophageal junction (GEJ) adenocarcinoma following disease progression (PD) on first-line platinum- and/or fluoropyrimidine-containing combination therapy: age subgroup analysis. *J Clin Oncol.* 2014;32(suppl 5):4057.

Slagter AE, Tudela B, van Amelsfoort RM, et al. Older versus younger adults with gastric cancer receiving perioperative treatment: results from the CRITICS trial. *Eur J Cancer.* 2020;130:146–154.

Trumper M, Ross PJ, Cunningham D, et al. Efficacy and tolerability of chemotherapy in elderly patients with advanced oesophago-gastric cancer: a pooled analysis of three clinical trials. *Eur J Cancer.* 2006;42:827–834.

Primary Liver Cancer

El-Serag HB, Siegel AB, Davila JA, et al. Treatment and outcomes of treating of hepatocellular carcinoma among medicare recipients in the United States: a population-based study. *J Hepatol.* 2006;44(1):158–166.

Pancreaticobiliary Cancer

Gourgou-Bourgade S, Bascoul-Mollevi C, Desseigne F, et al. Impact of FOLFIRINOX compared with gemcitabine on quality of life in adults with metastatic pancreatic cancer: results from the PRODIGE 4/ACCORD 11 randomized trial. *J Clin Oncol.* 2013;31(1):23–29.

Makary MA, Winter JM, Cameron JL, et al. Pancreaticoduodenectomy in the very older adults. *J Gastrointest Surg.* 2006;10:347–356.

McNamara MG, de Liguori Carino N, Kapacee ZA, et al. Outcomes in older patients with biliary tract cancer. *Eur J Surg Oncol.* 2021;47(3 Pt A):569-575.

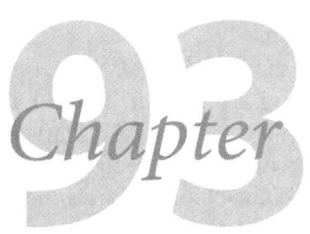

Chapter 93

Skin Cancer

Shreya A. Sreekantaswamy, Suzanne Olbricht, Jonathan Weiss, Daniel C. Butler

INTRODUCTION

More than 5 million new cases of skin cancer are diagnosed annually, making it the most common malignancy in the United States. Despite these staggering numbers, statistics on the incidence and prevalence of skin cancer are thought to be underestimated since many cancer registries do not collect data on all types of cutaneous carcinomas. As with most cancers, skin cancer places a disproportionate burden on older adults, particularly since skin photoaging from cumulative ultraviolet (UV) exposure is a major risk factor. One in five Caucasian Americans develops skin cancer by age 70, and the incidence of cutaneous carcinoma has been rising in older adults, exemplified by a 100% increase in the incidence of skin cancer from 1992 to 2012 in data from Medicare fee-for-service patients. As incidence rises, so too do associated costs. From 2002 to 2006, skin cancer treatment costed $3.6 billion, and from 2007 to 2011, this rose by 126% to $8.1 billion.

There are three main types of cutaneous carcinomas: basal cell carcinoma (BCC), squamous cell carcinoma (SCC), and melanoma. Collectively, BCCs and SCCs are referred to as nonmelanoma skin cancer or keratinocyte carcinomas. BCCs are the most common form of skin cancer (79% of skin cancers), followed by SCCs (14%), melanoma (5%), and then other forms of cutaneous carcinoma. Despite accounting for only 5% of skin cancer diagnoses, melanoma is responsible for a significant proportion of skin cancer–related deaths; 2018 global data from the World Health Organization estimated 65,155 deaths from keratinocyte carcinomas and 60,172 deaths from melanoma. In the United States, it is estimated that one person dies from melanoma every hour. While BCCs and SCCs are typically less lethal, they are instead associated with significant morbidity. Given skin cancer's increasing prevalence, cost to the healthcare system, and morbidity and mortality, it is important for providers to understand this disease, and with its predilection for older adults, it is especially important for geriatricians to not only have a working knowledge of skin cancer, but also of the special considerations that come with diagnosing and treating cutaneous carcinoma in this population.

Learning Objectives

- To recognize different types of skin cancer including basal cell carcinoma (BCC), squamous cell carcinoma (SCC), melanoma, and Merkel cell carcinoma (MCC).
- To understand available treatment modalities for different types of skin cancer.
- To determine when referral to a dermatology specialist is indicated.

Key Clinical Points

1. Skin cancers are common in older adults, and the vast majority of skin cancers in this population are BCCs and SCCs.
2. Malignant melanoma and MCC are more aggressive than BCCs and SCCs and carry a higher risk of lymph node and distal metastasis.
3. Overall, definitive treatment of skin cancers is well tolerated by older adults.
4. When determining appropriate treatment for skin cancers in older adults, it is important to discuss the risks versus benefits of the various treatment modalities available, while assessing the mortality and morbidity risk of the lesion in the context of the patient's goals for treatment.

ETIOLOGY

The major underlying risk factor across all forms of skin cancer is cumulative exposure to UV radiation including sunlight, artificial tanning devices (tanning booths), and sunburns. Blistering sunburns, in particular, have a strong association with skin cancer. Caucasian women with at least five blistering sunburns between ages 15 and 20 have been found to have a 68% increased risk for keratinocyte carcinoma and an 80% increased risk for melanoma. This increased risk, however, is not just limited to adolescent or childhood sunburn history; it is found with adult and cumulative lifetime sunburns as well. Skin cancer is therefore more predominant in older adults whose age lends to greater cumulative UV exposure compared to younger patients.

UV radiation is part of the electromagnetic radiation that is released by the sun. It is subclassified by wavelength, with UVC ranging from 200 to 280 nm, UVB from 290 to 320 nm, and UVA from 320 to 400 nm. A majority of UVC is blocked by the ozone layer, but both UVA and UVB reach the Earth's surface in significant amounts and are absorbed by the skin. UVB is responsible for much of the actinic skin damage, erythema, and sunburns caused by sunlight. On the other hand, the longer wavelengths of UVA penetrate deeper into the skin, and while it has a reduced risk of sunburn compared to UVB, UVA still contributes to photoaging and cutaneous carcinogenesis. UV radiation induces skin cancer via a variety of mechanisms, including direct DNA damage, damage to DNA repair systems, and alteration of the local cutaneous immune system. Cumulative UV exposure will therefore be greatest in patients whose occupational and recreational activities (eg, farming, sailing) lead them to spend more time in the sun. Geographic location can also play a role in increased UV exposure. UV at the Earth's surface is affected by the number of atmospheric particles it must pass through, and therefore it is highest in areas which are more directly hit by the sun, including the equator and higher altitudes. Lastly, while many patients' UV exposure is obtained from spending time outdoors, indoor tanning beds are also significant sources of UV radiation. Studies show that UV output in these salons can be up to 10 times more potent than sunlight. When assessing risk for skin cancer, it is therefore important to ask patients about their prior occupations, recreational activities, and history of tanning bed use. Screening questions for these risk factors are summarized in **Table 93-1**, with additional

TABLE 93-1 ■ SCREENING QUESTIONS TO ASSESS RISK FOR SKIN CANCER

FOR ALL TYPES OF SKIN CANCER

Do you have a history of skin cancer? What type of skin cancer was it and how was it treated?

What is/was your occupation? Do/did you spend a lot of time outdoors for work?

What are/were your hobbies? Do/did you spend a lot of time outdoors for recreational activity?

Do you currently use tanning beds? Have you ever in the past?

Have you had sunburns? How many were blistering sunburns?

What type of sun-protective measures do you use (hat, clothing, sunscreen, shade-seeking)?

FOR SCC

Do you have a history of solid-organ transplant or other immunosuppression?

FOR MELANOMA

Does anyone in your family have a history of melanoma?

discussion of unique risk factors for each cutaneous carcinoma under its appropriate sections.

Not every patient with the same history of UV exposure has an equal risk of developing skin cancer. The risk is greatest in patients who are most sensitive to UV radiation, that is, light-skinned individuals with blue or green eyes and red, blonde, or light brown hair. Light-colored skin is more likely to burn than tan on UV exposure, and as epidermal melanin increases, individuals instead tend to tan and are less likely to burn. This association between UV sensitivity and skin pigmentation is illustrated by the Fitzpatrick Phototyping Scale, which categorizes skin into six phototypes, with each successive type having increased UV resistance and epidermal melanin. Individuals with darker skin tones therefore have reduced skin cancer risk compared to those with lighter skin. For example, in the case of melanoma, while non-Hispanic Whites have an annual incidence rate of 28 cases of melanoma per 100,000 individuals, and this decreases to 5 per 100,000 for Hispanics and 1 per 100,000 in non-Hispanic Blacks and Asians/Pacific Islanders.

Chronic solar damage from UV exposure leads to "photoaging" of the skin. The skin changes of photoaging are distinct from changes caused by chronologic aging. In photoaging, UV radiation induces an inflammatory cytokine cascade that leads to collagen degradation. Over time, this degradation manifests as cutaneous atrophy, mottled pigmentation, wrinkling, dryness, telangiectasia, and decreased skin elasticity. In comparison, chronologic aging is characterized by fine lines and decreased skin elasticity. Given that darker pigmentation attenuates the effect of UV radiation on skin, patients with darker skin tend to experience delayed and less severe photoaging.

Adverse effects of UV radiation can be prevented via photoprotective behaviors including topical sunscreen, wearing protective clothing, avoiding the sun at noon, and seeking shade. Providers should ask patients about their current sun-protective habits and encourage them to pursue these measures.

NONMELANOMA SKIN CANCER (KERATINOCYTE CARCINOMA)

Actinic Keratoses

Definition Actinic keratoses (AK) are precancerous lesions classically found in sun-exposed areas of the body. AKs develop when exposure to chronic UV radiation leads to dysplasia of keratinocytes in the epidermis.

Risk factors AKs are extremely common in older light-skinned individuals who have had significant chronic sun exposure. Refer to the *Etiology* section for a thorough discussion on factors contributing to increased UV exposure.

Clinical presentation AKs present as ill-defined, rough papules often with adherent scale in areas that are chronically exposed to the sun, such as the scalp (especially if bald),

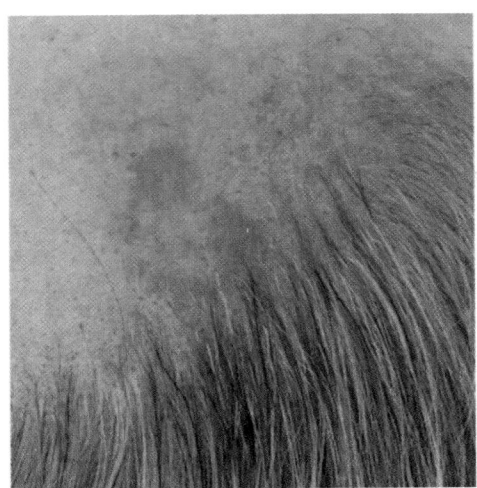

FIGURE 93-1. Actinic keratosis of the scalp. Erythematous ill-defined plaque.

face, upper chest, and dorsum of the hands and forearms. They can coalesce to form plaques, and their color can vary from skin-colored, to erythematous, pink, or brown (**Figure 93-1**). The overlaying scale is typically white or yellow, and adherent during palpation or light pressure. AKs are classically described as feeling "gritty" or "sandpaper-like" to the touch. In many cases, AKs might be more easily discernable via palpation than visual inspection.

AKs are diagnosed clinically and do not require biopsy. A biopsy should be obtained, however, to rule out keratinocyte carcinoma if the lesion is thick, indurated, or has not responded to appropriate treatment.

Differential diagnosis Several lesions may present similarly to an AK. Of these, it is most important to differentiate AKs from SCCs and superficial BCCs. It is clinically difficult to make this distinction with certainty if the lesion is indurated or hypertrophic, in which case a biopsy should be performed to confirm the diagnosis. Other common confounders include seborrheic keratoses (differentiated by well-defined borders and a "stuck on" appearance) and solar lentigo (a dark brown macule with an irregular outline). AKs can also be confused with eczema, dry skin, or guttate psoriasis.

Course and complications While most AKs remain stable or undergo spontaneous remission, a small percentage of them develop into cutaneous SCCs. This change, if it does occur, happens over the course of several years in immunocompetent individuals. The cumulative risk for malignant change depends on the number of lesions and their chronicity.

Basal Cell Carcinoma

Definition BCC is the most common type of skin cancer. It originates from tumor progenitor cells that are typically within the basal layer of the epidermis, or less commonly,

from the hair follicle. There are three major types of BCCs based on clinical presentation and histopathology: (1) nodular, (2) superficial, and (3) morpheaform (scarring, sclerotic).

Risk factors BCCs can either be sporadic—resultant from UV damage (refer to *Etiology* for a thorough discussion on UV radiation) or ionizing radiation (x-ray)—or hereditary, associated with a genetic syndrome or mutation. Over 90% of both sporadic and hereditary BCCs display uncontrolled Hedgehog (Hh) signaling. The Hh pathway is essential to normal skin development, playing a role in both cell growth and keratinocyte proliferation. Both inactivating mutations of the tumor-suppressor patched (*PTCH*) gene and activating mutations of the proto-oncogene smoothened (*SMO*) have been shown to play a role in the pathogenesis of BCCs. These mutations result in the unregulated activation of the Hh pathway, leading to promotion of growth and cancer development in tumor progenitor cells within the epidermis and hair follicle.

Clinical presentation

Nodular The most common BCC subtype is the well circumscribed or nodular variant. This typically begins as a small translucent or waxy flesh-colored or pink, pearly papule or nodule with arborizing vessels on the surface and a translucent, sometimes rolled, border (**Figure 93-2**). With time, the nodule increases in size and can undergo central ulceration. Although pigmentation can be seen in all BCC subtypes, it is most common in nodular BCCs. Nodular BCCs tend to present on the head and neck.

Superficial Superficial BCCs are the second most common BCC subtype. They present as ill-defined pink to red, flat, scaly lesions, sometimes with a fine, thread-like translucent border (**Figure 93-3**). The middle of the lesion can erode over time, leaving an atrophic central clearing. As their name suggests, superficial BCCs grow with peripheral extension,

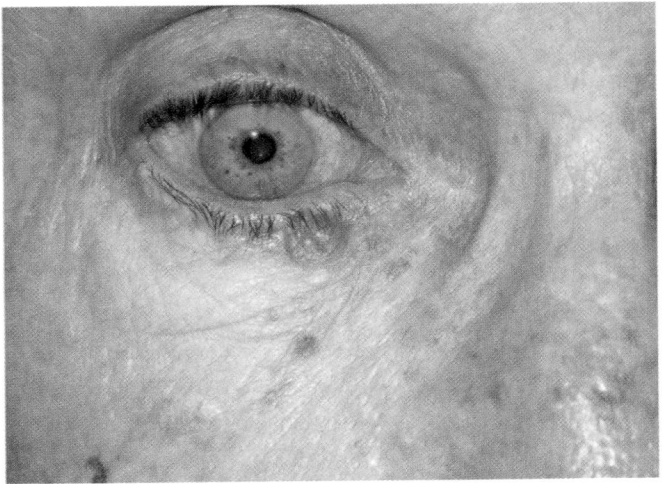

FIGURE 93-2. Nodular BCC on the lower eyelid. Small pearly papule with telangiectatic blood vessel visible at superior aspect of lesion.

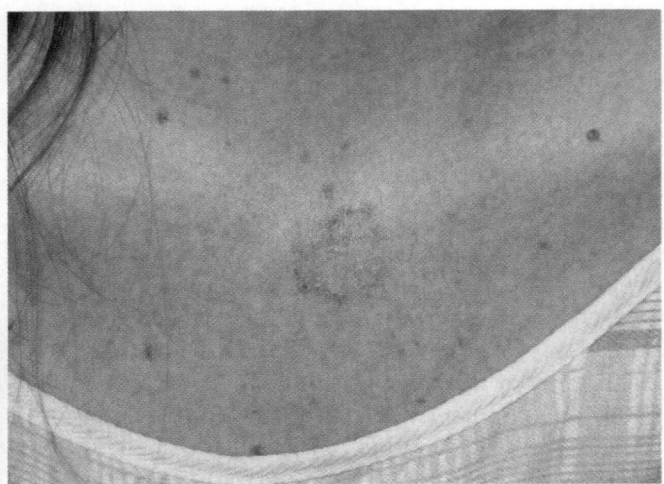

FIGURE 93-3. Superficial BCC occurring on the chest. Pink, flat lesion with slightly raised scaly borders.

which can lead to significant superficial subclinical involvement. BCC of the trunk tends to be superficial BCC.

Morpheaform The morpheaform BCC subtype is also referred to as aggressive, infiltrating, sclerosing, sclerotic, or fibrotic. It usually presents as a flat, firm, indurated, pale, white-to-yellow papule or plaque with ulceration, indistinct clinical borders, and a "scar-like" appearance (**Figure 93-4**). Morpheaform BCCs may exhibit subclinical extension widely beyond (> 1 cm) their apparent borders with distant, small finger-like projections of tumor cells that may invade deep into the dermis, subcutis, and muscle, skating along fascial planes, cartilage, and bone. These projections can be missed with standard histologic margin control and therefore morpheaform BCCs have a higher rate of recurrence following standard treatment modalities.

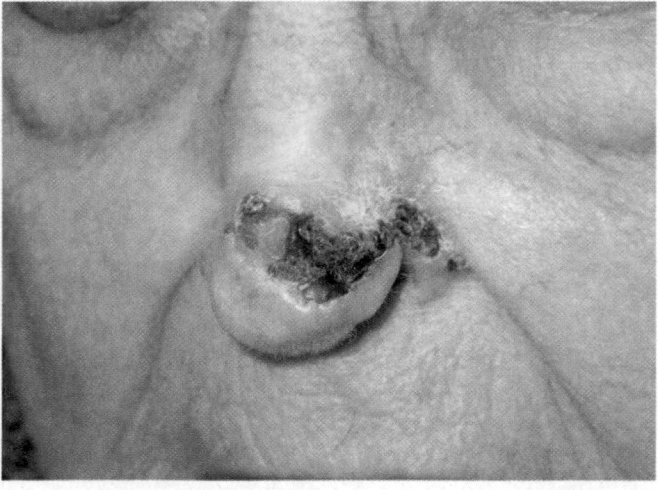

FIGURE 93-4. Aggressive BCC on the nose. Note the indurated plaque central ulceration. This lesion is likely to have wide subclinical extension present.

Differential diagnosis There are several dermatologic lesions that can present similarly to BCCs. Sebaceous hyperplasia can be confused with a nodular BCC due to its presentation as a yellow papule with overlaying telangiectasias and a central pore. Other lesions on the differential for BCCs include skin-colored nevi and benign hair follicle tumors of the face. Of note, superficial BCCs can be mistaken for eczema or other erythematous, well demarcated rashes, which should be considered if a patient has a plaque that is not responsive to standard therapies. It is most important, however, to ensure differentiation between the three main types of skin cancer: BCCs, SCCs, and melanoma. Any lesion suspicious for cutaneous carcinoma should be biopsied. Histologic processing will be able to differentiate between the three.

Course and complications BCCs typically grow indolently for years but are capable of sudden exponential growth. Occult local invasion may be deep and asymmetric with root-like extensions sometimes several centimeters beyond the lesion's clinically apparent borders. If left untreated, relentless growth can lead to extensive local destruction, ulceration, drainage, bleeding, infection, and disfigurement. Depending on the tumor's location, it can invade bone and even impair function of vital structures such as the eyes, nose, or ears. Neglect of BCCs until they present with significant morbidity can be particularly prevalent among older adults, where factors such as functional and cognitive impairment, low socioeconomic status, and lack of social support can all delay their presentation to the health care system.

Metastasis is rare, however does occur, particularly if the lesion is larger than 2 cm in diameter, on the head and neck, and invades beyond fat. The estimated incidence of BCC metastasis ranges from 0.0028% to 0.55%. Recurrence is more likely than metastasis, even though the risk of recurrence is small after any standard treatment. Since BCCs grow slowly, recurrence is more likely several years after treatment of the initial tumor, with studies finding that 56% of recurrences occurred 5 years or more after the primary tumor was definitively treated. The risk of a new primary skin cancer is higher than either metastasis or recurrence, for example, for men with SCC, 28% will develop a BCC. Regular follow-up should therefore be provided to these patients, generally in the form of a skin check once a year.

Squamous Cell Carcinoma

Definition SCC is the second most common type of skin cancer. The majority of cutaneous SCCs develop from AKs; yet, while AKs are considered to be precancerous lesions, not every AK develops into an SCC. Most SCCs are low-risk lesions that have high cure rates following treatment. It should be noted, however, that SCCs do have the potential to metastasize.

Risk factors Just as with other skin cancers, SCCs occur most often in patients with high levels of chronic sun exposure (refer to the *Etiology* section for a thorough discussion on UV radiation). SCCs also have several additional unique risk factors. Conditions that can predispose patients to SCC development include ionizing radiation (x-ray), arsenic exposure, scarring from a previous injury such as a burn, and chronic inflammatory processes like wounds or ulcers, osteomyelitis sinuses, or discoid lupus. Viruses, in particular the human papillomavirus (HPV), are also implicated. Although HPV is classically associated with cervical SCC, it has also been linked to cutaneous SCC. This association was first reported in the genetic disorder epidermodysplasia verruciformis. Patients with this disorder develop hundreds of warts, and those warts that are caused by HPV-5 in sun-exposed areas frequently become cutaneous SCC.

The biggest risk factor for SCC, however, is immunosuppression. SCC is the most common skin cancer in immunosuppressed solid organ transplant recipients, occurring 65 to 250 times more frequently in these patients than in the general population. Light-skinned, immunosuppressed individuals can quickly develop large numbers of AKs which tend to behave aggressively and transform into invasive, rapidly growing SCCs with an increased risk for metastasis. It has been shown that the development of cutaneous SCCs in solid organ transplant recipients is proportional to the intensity of their immunosuppressive regimen, with an increased number of immunosuppressive agents correlating to higher rates of cutaneous SCC formation. Of note, transplant patients with skin of color also develop SCC at high rates, but their lesions are more likely to be found in non–sun-exposed sites, necessitating a careful and thorough skin examination.

Clinical presentation A majority of cutaneous SCCs (80%) develop in chronically sun-exposed areas on the head and neck. Clinical presentation varies, but most often SCCs are 0.5 to 1.5 cm firm, sometimes tender, hyperkeratotic pink to red papules, nodules, or plaques that may bleed (**Figures 93-5, 93-6**, and **93-7**). The center of the lesion can become ulcerated or crusted and has the potential for rapid and deep invasion. In darker skinned patients, SCC may present in

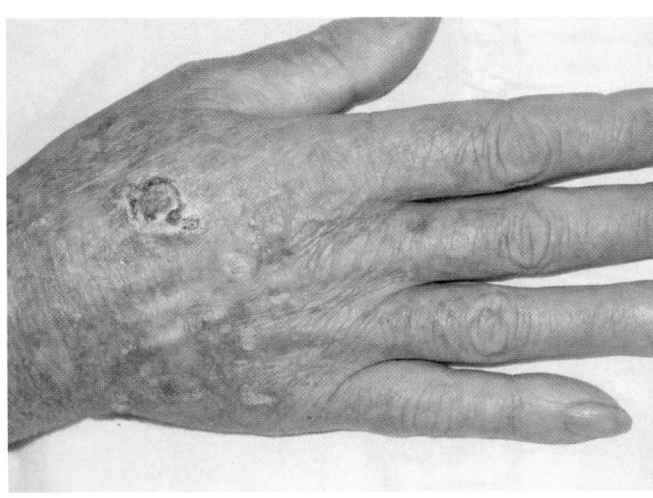

FIGURE 93-6. Invasive SCC on the dorsal hand. Crusted lesion on the hand with surrounding actinic damage.

non–sun-exposed areas and be associated with chronic inflammatory or scarring processes.

Several clinical and histologic SCC subtypes exist, of which perhaps the subtype of the most consequence is keratoacanthoma. Keratoacanthomas tend to grow rapidly, usually over the course of 4 to 6 weeks. They present as a flesh-colored nodule with a central hyperkeratotic crater (**Figure 93-8**). Although they may spontaneously involute, excision is often recommended for keratoacanthomas since their clinical course is difficult to predict.

Differential diagnosis The differential diagnosis for SCCs includes hypertrophic AKs, warts, seborrheic keratoses, lichenoid keratosis (erythematous or violaceous inflamed

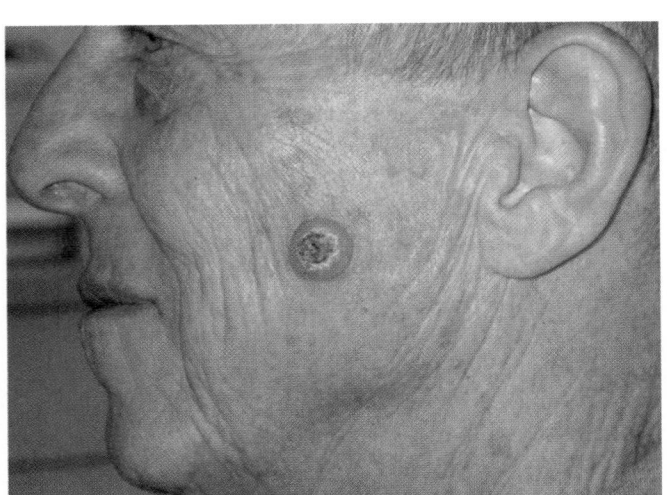

FIGURE 93-5. Invasive SCC on the cheek. Large ulcerated nodule with central core filled with hyperkeratotic material.

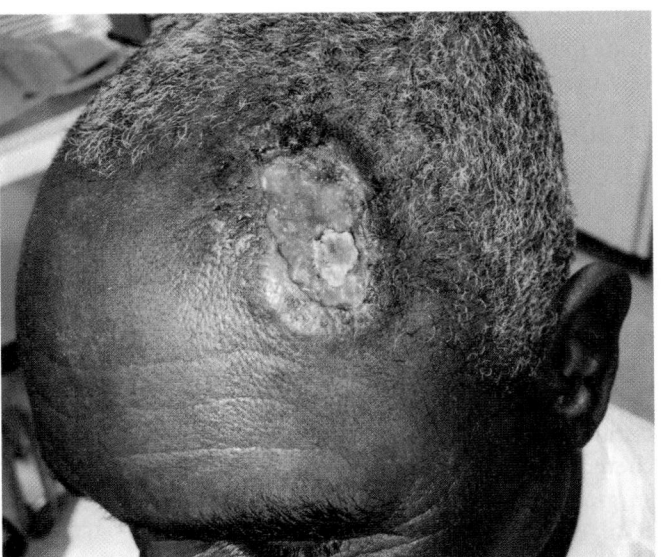

FIGURE 93-7. Squamous cell carcinoma on the scalp of a Haitian man. Ulcerated plaque with raised borders.

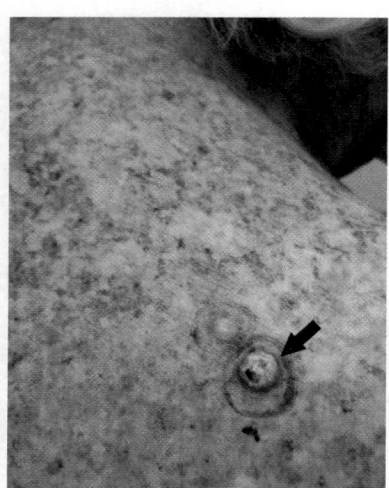

FIGURE 93-8. Keratoacanthoma on the back (black arrow). Flesh-colored nodule with a central hyperkeratotic crater.

TABLE 93-2 ◼ BASAL CELL CARCINOMA (BCC) AND SQUAMOUS CELL CARCINOMA (SCC) HIGH-RISK FACTORS FOR OCCULT SUBCLINICAL INVASION AND RECURRENCE
FOR BOTH TUMORS
Recurrent tumor

High-risk location
  Mask areas of face (eyelid, eyebrow, periorbital, nose, lip, chin, mandible, temple, ear, in front/behind ear)
  Genitalia
  Hands
  Feet

Size
  Lesions > 5 mm on high-risk areas: mask areas of face, genitalia, hands, feet
  Lesions > 9 mm on medium-risk areas: cheeks, forehead, scalp, neck
  Lesions > 19 mm on low-risk areas: trunk and extremities (excluding pretibial, hands, feet, ankles)

Ill-defined clinical borders
Perineural invasion or vascular involvement
Immunosuppression
Development in site of prior radiation, scar, chronic inflammatory process
FOR BCC
Histology   Aggressive growth (morpheaform, fibrosing, sclerosing, infiltrating, micronodular)
FOR SCC

Histology
  Poorly differentiated
  Subtypes: adenoid, adenosquamous, desmoplastic
  Depth of invasion ≥ 2 mm or Clark level IV or V

Rapid growth
Neurologic symptoms

macule), and BCC. Any lesion suspicious for cancer, including persistent ulcers, should be biopsied.

Course and complications Although the majority of cutaneous SCCs are low-risk lesions that have high cure rates when treated, SCCs do have the potential to metastasize. Lesions that are more likely to metastasize tend to have a diameter > 2 cm, invade deep into the dermis and can have perineural involvement, are recurrent or occur at high-risk sites (eg, ear, lips), develop in scarred skin, or are in immunosuppressed patients. The regional lymph nodes are often the first site of metastasis, involved in approximately 85% to 90% of metastatic cases. Around 10% to 15% of metastases involve distant sites such as the lungs, liver, brain, bone, and skin. The prognosis for patients with metastatic SCC is poor, with 10-year survival rates of less than 20% for patients with advanced regional lymph node involvement and less than 10% for patients with distant metastases.

Treatment for AKs and Keratinocyte Carcinoma

AKs do not require biopsy. Biopsy is, however, mandatory to confirm the diagnosis in lesions suspicious for keratinocyte carcinoma. Numerous surgical and nonsurgical modalities are effective in treating BCC and SCC. The selection of therapy is based on several clinical and histologic risk factors noted in **Table 93-2**. The majority of lesions are relatively low-risk and can be treated effectively with control rates greater than 90% for low-risk tumors treated by techniques such as cryosurgery, topical chemotherapy, electrodessication and curettage (ED&C), surgical excision, or radiation. Additional field destruction procedures such as photodynamic therapy (PDT) can also be used. For lesions complicated by high-risk factors, noted in **Table 93-2**, the control (cure) rate drops precipitously. High-risk lesions are usually treated with Mohs micrographic surgery (MMS) or surgical excision with comprehensive margin control.

Cryotherapy Cryotherapy with liquid nitrogen is the gold standard treatment for isolated AKs. Liquid nitrogen (–196°C) is directly sprayed on the lesion, destroying it via intracellular and extracellular ice formation. The spraying, or "freezing," should last about 10 seconds, during which the patient will feel a burning or stinging at the site. The lesion is then allowed to thaw, and a repeat freeze-thaw cycle should be performed. Although generally reserved for AKs, cryotherapy can be a highly effective treatment for BCCs or SCCs when timed and performed under local anesthesia or done with thermocouples to measure temperature. Cryotherapy is generally well tolerated by older adults.

Topical chemotherapy (5-fluorouracil, imiquimod) The two main topical chemotherapeutic agents available are topical 5-fluorouracil (5-FU) and imiquimod. Both are used to treat large areas with multiple AKs where localized cryotherapy would be impractical. The 5% strength versions of 5-FU and imiquimod can also be used to treat select biopsy-confirmed low-risk superficial BCCs. Although both topical agents have similar indications, they work via different mechanisms: imiquimod is a toll-like receptor-7 agonist that induces an immune response against atypical keratinocytes, and 5-FU is a pyrimidine analog that blocks DNA synthesis by inhibiting the enzyme thymidylate synthetase. In head-to-head comparisons, 5-FU is thought to be more effective for the treatment of AKs than imiquimod. Clinical trials for both 5-FU and imiquimod did not find any significant differences in the safety and efficacy of the topical agents between older and younger adults. Patients should be warned though, that both topical therapies can cause significant skin irritation, dryness, and burning. 5-FU should be applied to AKs once a day for up to 4 weeks, whereas imiquimod should be applied two times per week for 16 weeks. If using either agent for BCCs, refer to the Food and Drug Administration (FDA) labels for appropriate dosing. 5-FU and imiquimod can also be used off-label to treat SCC in situ.

Photodynamic therapy PDT can be used to treat AKs and keratinocyte carcinomas. It is a two-step process: a photosensitizing agent is applied to the area being treated, and then light irradiation is administered to the same area to activate the drug. The two traditional photosensitizing agents used are methyl aminolevulinate (MAL) (no longer available in the United States) and 5-aminolevulinic acid (ALA). Both agents are absorbed by neoplastic cells and then converted into porphyrins. Porphyrins are particularly efficient at absorbing visible light, and when activated by light in the presence of oxygen, the resultant chemical reactions lead to cell death. In order to allow for an adequate buildup of porphyrins, photosensitizing agents may be left on the skin for several hours prior to irradiation. The irradiating light source is typically red, blue, or broadband, but pulsed dye laser can also be used. Although surgical excision is more likely to result in complete clearance and reduced recurrence rates compared to PDT, PDT may be associated with a better cosmetic outcome.

PDT is a good option to consider in older adults who are not appropriate surgical candidates or who are unable or unwilling to apply daily topical medications. It is generally well tolerated, with the main adverse effect being pain or burning at the site of treatment. This burning can be particularly severe if the lesion is located on the head. In practice, pain is often the most cited cause of PDT discontinuation among older patients, so providers should consider administering analgesics, anesthetics, or cold air when treating extensive lesions, particularly if on the head.

Electrodessication and curettage ED&C is a common, effective treatment option for thick AKs as well as low-risk keratinocyte cancers in low-risk areas. Results are operator-dependent. Reported 5-year cure rates range from 91% to 97% for both cutaneous SCC and BCC. ED&C is quickly performed in the office with local anesthesia. First, a curette is used to remove the gross tumor, which is soft and friable. This is followed by electrodessication of the periphery and base of the wound to destroy residual tumor cells. Depending on the size and feel of the lesion, this process is repeated for two to four cycles. The resulting wound heals by granulation with a hypopigmented, atrophic, or sometimes depressed, scar. ED&C can be first choice treatment for small superficial lesions or SCC in situ but may also be considered for older patients who are otherwise not good surgical candidates.

Radiation therapy Fractionated radiation therapy (RT) may be used for both BCC and SCC, with 5-year cure rates for both types of keratinocyte carcinoma ranging from 90% to 96%. RT should be used to treat patients in whom surgery is contraindicated or in whom surgical excision would result in a poor functional outcome. Radiotherapeutic modalities include interstitial brachytherapy, superficial x-rays, electrons, and megavoltage photons. Each treatment session of RT is considered a fraction, and these fractions are summated to calculate a total dose. Fractionation allows for normal tissue to repair cellular damage prior to the next RT session; malignant cells, however, have limited capability to do so. Although RT is associated with "late effects" of hypopigmentation and epidermal atrophy after multiple treatments, these cosmetic issues are typically not a major concern for older adults. Therefore, while younger patients usually receive 2 to 2.5 Gy (RT units) over 4 to 5 weeks in order to minimize late effects, treatment for older adults instead aims to decrease course length, with a typical schedule involving 3 to 4 Gy over 2 to 3 weeks. Hypofractionation, or less frequent administration of greater Gy, is recommended for older adults (eg, 5–7 Gy in 5–6 fractions). Compared to normal fractionation, where patients need to receive daily treatment, hypofractionation can allow for older patients with significant comorbidity or poor overall status to receive treatment on alternating days or even just once a week. Even with hypofractionation though, RT still requires multiple visits, which can make it difficult for older adults to attend, especially if they rely on a caregiver to bring them to the doctor. Providers should also be aware that there is an increased likelihood of developing skin cancer secondary to RT 15 years after completion of therapy, and it is therefore not ideal for patients with a life expectancy greater than 15 years.

Surgical excision Surgical excision is the standard of care for an older adult who has a skin cancer that does not have any concerning features (eg, large size or aggressive pathology) and is not in the head/neck region or in an area that has compromised vascular supply (eg, the lower legs in patients with venous stasis). It is an effective treatment modality for all types of keratinocyte carcinoma and possesses the advantage of supplying a tissue specimen for histologic assessment of margins. Five-year disease-free rates with surgical excision are 98% for low-risk BCC and higher than 91% for low-risk SCC. When compared to destructive techniques, excisions tend to heal rapidly and with superior cosmetic results. Most excisional procedures can be performed in a treatment room with local anesthesia, but rarely, an extensive procedure may require intravenous sedation or general anesthesia in the operating room. Recommended margins for keratinocyte carcinoma excision generally range from 4 to 10 mm, with the deep margin in mid fat. High-risk lesions require wider margins to ensure clearance and achieve high control rates. If histopathologic processing indicates that the lesion was incompletely excised, then additional therapeutic intervention should be sought, or re-excision should be performed via MMS.

Mohs micrographic surgery MMS is considered the gold standard for removal of high-risk keratinocyte carcinoma. Factors to take into consideration in determining if a lesion is high risk include the type and subtype of cancer, the location, whether the tumor is primary or recurrent, its size, and the patient's health status. Cure rates with MMS for high-risk primary cutaneous SCCs that have a high likelihood of recurrence with other treatments have been reported as up to 96%. Primary BCCs treated with MMS have only a 1% recurrence rate.

MMS is a specialized form of dermatologic surgery that involves serial tangential excisions with real-time microscopic evaluation of the entirety of the surgical margins to ensure that the tumor is excised completely. Each excision involves removing cancerous tissue with 1 to 3 mm margins per stage and then microscopically examining the entire undersurface and edges of the specimen (the entire true margin) cut as en face horizontal sections. If residual cancer cells are noted at a margin, the precise location is mapped and identified on the patient. Then, another layer of tissue at the corresponding site of the residual tumor is excised and examined microscopically for cancer cells. This process continues layer by layer in stages until no detectable cancer cells remain at the surgical margin. MMS aims to preserve the maximum amount of normal tissue possible, and since nearly 100% of the margin is examined, it results in exceedingly high rates of local control. Reconstruction is usually performed without delay after tumor-free margins are confirmed. Rarely, adjuvant RT may be indicated in cases of extensive perineural spread and cases with a higher risk of local recurrence, but the ability to achieve clear margins surgically is the single best indicator of successful cure. MMS is performed by experienced surgeons who have undergone advanced postgraduate ACGME (Accreditation Council for Graduate Medical Education) fellowship training and are adept at microscopic interpretation of

horizontally cut frozen sections and local flap and graft soft tissue reconstruction techniques. It is often the extensive repair that follows MMS which contributes to morbidity in older adults, rather than the serial excisions of MMS itself. In cases involving large defects or very complex tumors, it is important to have a collaborative, multidisciplinary team approach.

Providers can use the free Mohs Surgery Appropriate Use Criteria app to determine their patient's suitability for MMS. Even though it may be appropriate, the procedure can be long and tedious and therefore is perhaps not the most desired treatment for all older adults. It is important to consider the patient's functional status and any physical or cognitive limitations that would make them poor candidates for this form of surgery. Patients who do pursue MMS tend to be highly functioning, or if they are lower functioning, have large symptomatic tumors that severely negatively impact their quality of life. As with any surgical procedure, MMS presents with risk of wound dehiscence, bleeding, pain or tenderness at the surgical site, and infection. Large scale studies have reported no difference in incidence of postsurgical complications between older and younger adults (7% across both patients ≥ 80 and < 80), with one study even reporting that the mean postoperative pain score in adults younger than 66 was significantly greater than in those who were older. While many in the dermatologic community have concluded that MMS is a safe and effective treatment for keratinocyte carcinoma in older adults, it is important for providers to have a thorough discussion with older patients and their families on the risks and benefits of this procedure, as well as expectations for the day of surgery.

Treatment of nodal disease with keratinocyte carcinoma If keratinocyte carcinoma metastasizes to involve the regional lymph nodes (more commonly seen with SCC), then nodal disease is treated with complete lymph node dissection. If indicated by the number of involved nodes and the status of extranodal extension, adjuvant local RT can be administered.

Systemic therapy for BCC Systemic therapy should be considered for patients who have exhausted other therapeutic modalities. Although a few trials have reported that SCC responds to systemic cytotoxic therapy, there is currently no standard accepted systemic treatment for SCC, though PD-1 inhibitors are gaining in popularity. BCCs, on the other hand, have two accepted systemic therapeutic options: vismodegib and sonidegib.

Vismodegib (brand name Erivedge) and sonidegib (brand name Odomzo) are Hh pathway inhibitors that bind and inhibit smoothened (SMO). Erivedge was approved by the FDA in 2012 and Odomzo in 2015. Both drugs are indicated for the treatment of metastatic BCC or locally advanced inoperable BCC in patients who are not candidates for RT. Vismodegib's reported objective response rates approach 33% for metastatic disease and 48% for locally advanced BCC, with sonidegib similarly at 15% for metastatic disease and 43% for locally advanced BCC. Common adverse effects for both drugs include muscle spasms, alopecia, weight loss, fatigue, dysgeusia, nausea/vomiting, constipation, and diarrhea. Unfortunately, clinical studies of Erivedge did not include a sufficient number of older adults to determine whether safety and efficacy differ between older and younger patients. Trials of Odomzo, however, did—reporting that 54% of patients in Study 1 were 65 and older. Although no difference in efficacy was observed between older and younger patients, older adults who took Odomzo were found to have a higher incidence of serious adverse events, grade 3 (severe but not immediately life-threatening) and grade 4 (urgently life-threatening) adverse events, and events that required dose disruption or medication discontinuation. Adverse reactions that led to discontinuation included muscle spasms and dysgeusia, asthenia, increased lipase, and nausea. Given this risk of severe musculoskeletal adverse events, creatinine kinase levels should be obtained prior to initiating sonidegib therapy and should be monitored throughout the therapeutic course, with discontinuation if indicated.

Prescribers should also be aware of several key drug interactions with the Hh pathway inhibitors. Drugs that inhibit vismodegib's drug transporter such as clarithromycin, erythromycin, and azithromycin increase systemic exposure to vismodegib and the risk of adverse events. Vismodegib's FDA label also cautions that proton pump inhibitors, H2-receptor antagonists, antacids, and other drugs that alter the pH of the digestive system may potentially reduce the bioavailability of vismodegib, though this has not been evaluated in clinical trials. Increasing the dose of vismodegib in patients on these medications, however, might not compensate for its potentially reduced bioavailability. Although sonidegib is not noted to have the same interactions with pH-altering drugs, concomitant administration with moderate and strong CYP3A inhibitors (eg, ketoconazole, diltiazem) should be avoided.

Follow-Up

Thirty to fifty percent of patients with keratinocyte carcinoma will develop another primary carcinoma within 5 years and are at increased risk of developing melanoma. Therefore, it is important that patients with keratinocyte carcinoma have regular skin examinations and receive education on utilizing sun protection and performing monthly self-skin examinations. For SCC in particular, recurrence most often happens within the first 2 years, so close follow-up during this time frame is indicated for SCC patients. Providers should observe the primary site of the initial lesion for signs of recurrence, and regional lymph nodes should be evaluated for lymphadenopathy indicative of metastatic disease. These patients should be taught to perform self-examinations of their lymph nodes in concordance with their self-skin examinations. For BCCs in

patients with limited life expectancy, some providers also consider active surveillance appropriate when lesions are in low-risk areas without other risk factors. Since BCCs are generally indolent and slow-growing, active surveillance can help patients avoid unnecessary treatments while closely monitoring for tumor growth or development of symptoms. Although active surveillance is not the standard of care, it is an option that providers can discuss with their patients when managing low-risk lesions.

MELANOMA

Definition

Melanoma results from the malignant transformation of melanocytes usually located at the dermal-epidermal junction. When confined to the epidermis, melanoma is termed melanoma in situ. With time, melanoma invades vertically into the dermis where it can metastasize to the regional lymph nodes and other distant organs via the lymphatic or vascular systems. The deeper the melanoma invades, the greater the risk of metastasis and advanced systemic disease.

The incidence of melanoma has been steadily rising over the years. In 2010, the American Cancer Society estimated that 68,130 patients would be diagnosed with melanoma that year. This number jumped to 100,350 estimated cases in 2020. When comparing data across 2007 to 2016, it has been found that the incidence of melanoma has increased 2.2% per year in adults over 50, yet during the same timeframe has decreased by 1.2% in individuals younger than 50. Older adults with melanoma also have a higher mortality rate compared to younger patients. Although new treatments have led to decreased mortality across age groups, trends for younger adults started to dip beginning in the mid-1980s but have only been going down for older adults in the past decade. Data from 2013 to 2017 show a decline in melanoma-related mortality by 7.0% in adults younger than 50, but only 5.7% in older adults. Melanoma's higher mortality rate and worse prognosis in older patients are thought to be because they often present with more aggressive prognostic features, such as thicker depth and higher mitotic rates.

Risk Factors

As with the keratinocyte carcinomas, the main risk factors for melanoma are UV exposure, a history of blistering sunburns, and light complexion. Patients with congenital nevi (CN), or nevi that are present at birth or appear within the first 6 months of life, also have an increased risk for developing melanoma. Large (≥ 20 cm) CN tend to progress to melanoma prior to age 10, and since melanoma may originate deep in the lesion, melanoma nested within CN tends to be detected late. Personal and family history of melanoma are also important risk factors. Five to fifteen percent of melanoma patients endorse a positive family history of melanoma and 5% to 10% of individuals with a personal history of prior melanoma develop a second primary melanoma.

Genetics also play a large role in melanoma risk. CDKN2A, CDK4, BAP1, and TERT are considered melanoma predisposition genes, and are implicated in both somatic and familial mutations leading to melanoma. Of these, mutations in CDKN2A and CDK4 are the most common in familial melanoma and are found in 45% of cases. Familial occurrence of melanoma is also seen with the familial atypical multiple mole-melanoma syndrome, which is due to a germline mutation in CDKN2A. Criteria for diagnosis of this syndrome include cutaneous melanoma in at least one first- or second-degree relative and greater than 50 total body nevi with multiple atypical nevi that have specific histologic features (eg, subepidermal fibroplasia). It should be noted, however, that dysplastic nevi are not technically considered as "premelanoma" because the melanoma in these patients may arise de novo in normal skin.

The genetic discoveries that have perhaps been the most critical to shaping our understanding and treatment of melanoma are those in the MAPK signaling pathway. The MAPK pathway (also known as the Ras-Raf-MEK-ERK pathway) transfers extracellular signaling intracellularly via a phosphorylation cascade, influencing cell growth, proliferation, and differentiation. One of the kinases in this pathway is BRAF, a proto-oncogene that when mutated can become constitutively activated, leading to unopposed cellular growth, a forebearer of neoplastic transformation. BRAF mutations have been discovered in 50% to 70% of melanomas, and 90% of those mutations are missense point mutations which result in the substitution of glutamic acid for valine at amino acid 600, known as BRAF^{V600E}. This has led to the development of BRAF inhibitors, vemurafenib and dabrafenib (further discussed under *Systemic Therapy*).

Clinical Presentation

Melanoma can arise anywhere on the skin surface. Approximately one-third of melanomas arise from a melanocyte within a preexisting pigmented lesion, and two-thirds arise within scattered melanocytes, developing on clinically normal-appearing skin. The most frequent site for melanoma in men is the trunk, particularly the upper back and shoulders. In women, the most frequent site of melanoma is on the legs. Although rare, it should also be noted that melanoma can occur in the mucosa, genitals, nail beds, and ocular sites. In dark skinned individuals, melanoma is most common on the palms and soles of the feet.

The earliest clinical features of melanoma include a change in the size, shape, or color of a lesion. Persistent itching of a lesion can also occasionally be an early clinical feature of melanoma. Later features include ulceration, bleeding, and tenderness. The clinical changes associated with melanoma can be remembered by the ABCD rule (**Table 93-3, Figure 93-9**). "A" stands for asymmetry—one half of the lesion is not a mirror image of the other half. "B" stands for irregular borders—the edges of the lesion might appear ragged, notched, jagged, scalloped, or fuzzy. "C" stands for color, since the lesion will typically lack homogenous pigmentation

TABLE 93-3 ■ ABCDS OF MELANOMA

CHARACTERISTIC	DESCRIPTION
Asymmetry	One-half of the lesion is not the mirror image of the other
Border	The border of the lesion is irregular, ragged, notched, jagged, scalloped, or fuzzy
Color	There are varying colors within the lesion
Diameter/ Difference	Diameter > 6 mm Or the "ugly duckling sign"—it does not look like other moles the patient has
Evolution	Changing in size, shape, or color

throughout; varying and mottled shades of tan, dark brown to jet-black, or shades of red, white, and/or blue may be present. Historically, "D" stood for a diameter greater than 6 mm; however, this has proven to be relatively insensitive as an independent factor. Therefore, in many melanoma centers, "D" stands for difference. This could be interpreted as any change or difference in an individual lesion, especially with respect to size, shape, color, or persistent itching. "Difference" could also refer to being suspicious of a lesion that *looks* different from others, which is known as the "ugly duckling sign." This means that in patients with multiple normal or slightly abnormal-appearing nevi, any isolated lesion that appears different from the overwhelming majority should be regarded with suspicion and biopsied for further testing. "D" can also stand for dark since melanoma is typically heavily pigmented even when very small. The ABCD rule has now been expanded to include "E," denoting how evolution or change in any of the ABCD characteristics is what can be most concerning for melanoma.

Providers, however, should be aware that not all melanomas will display every ABCD characteristic, and that early melanomas can even lack all of these classic features. Therefore, any changing pigmented lesion or new atypical lesion should be evaluated with a low threshold for biopsy,

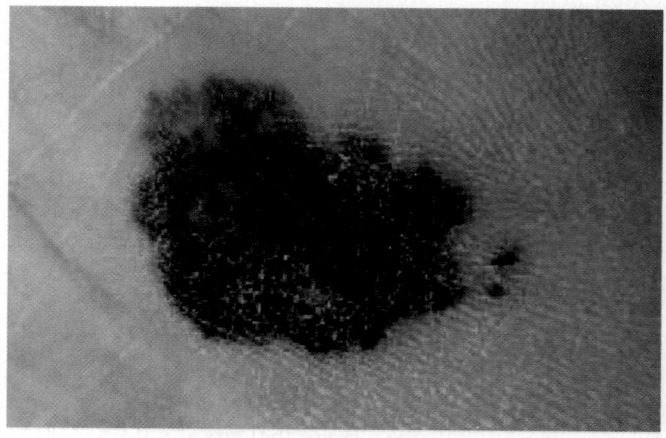

FIGURE 93-9. Melanoma displaying the typical ABCD characteristics—asymmetry, irregular borders, varying colors, and diameter > 6 mm.

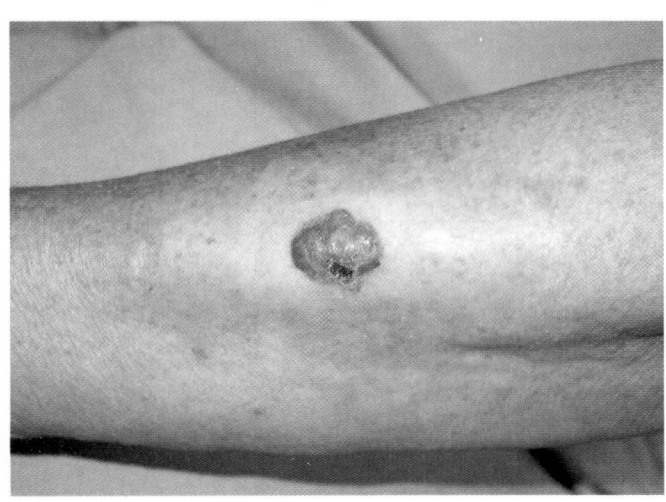

FIGURE 93-10. Amelanotic melanoma. Pink nodule on the lower leg.

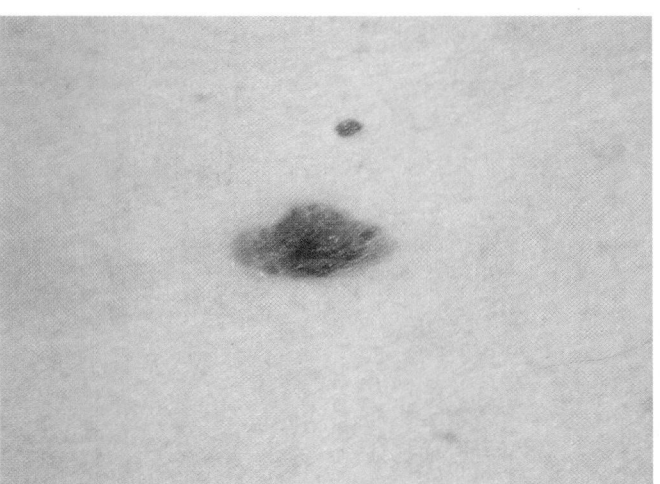

FIGURE 93-12. Superficial spreading melanoma showing all of the ABCD features. Breslow depth 3.5 mm.

especially if the patient has risk factors for melanoma. Since only 33% of melanomas develop within preexisting nevi though, there is no indication for prophylactic removal of preexisting nevi. It should also be noted that 3% to 4% of melanomas completely lack pigmentation; these amelanotic melanomas are understandably often detected at later stages of development than pigmented lesions (**Figure 93-10**).

Superficial spreading (low cumulative sun damage) Superficial spreading melanoma, also known as low cumulative sun damage melanoma, is the most common melanoma subtype, representing approximately 60% to 70% of melanomas. It typically develops as a spreading pigmented plaque with irregular borders and variation in color and surface contour (**Figures 93-11** to **93-13**). Regression might result in pink to white areas within the black or brown tumor.

As its name suggests, this subset of melanoma initially grows horizontally, and invasion is typically not seen until the lesion is 2.5 cm in diameter.

Lentigo maligna (high cumulative sun damage melanoma) Approximately 10% to 15% of all melanomas are categorized under the lentigo maligna, or high cumulative sun damage, subtype. This type of melanoma is particularly common in older adults and is most often located on sun-damaged skin, for example, the head and neck. It usually begins as a pigmented macular lesion with variation in black and brown color. It typically has an irregular outline, and over the course of several years it can darken and enlarge (**Figures 93-14** and **93-15**). The in situ phase of this lesion is known as lentigo maligna. Once histologic invasion is documented, it is termed lentigo maligna

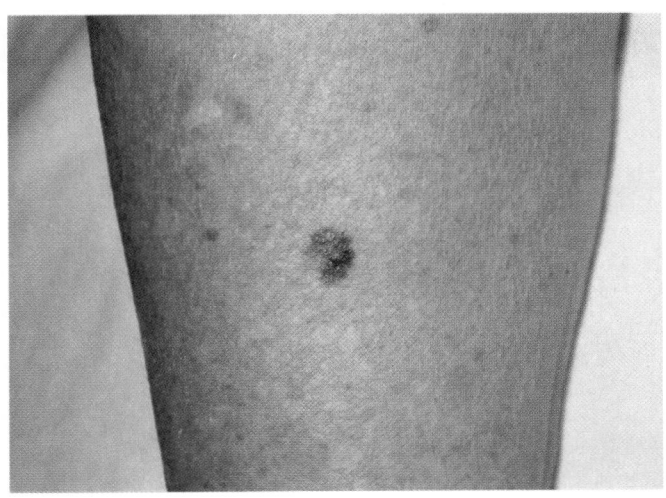

FIGURE 93-11. Early superficial spreading melanoma. Note asymmetry and irregular border.

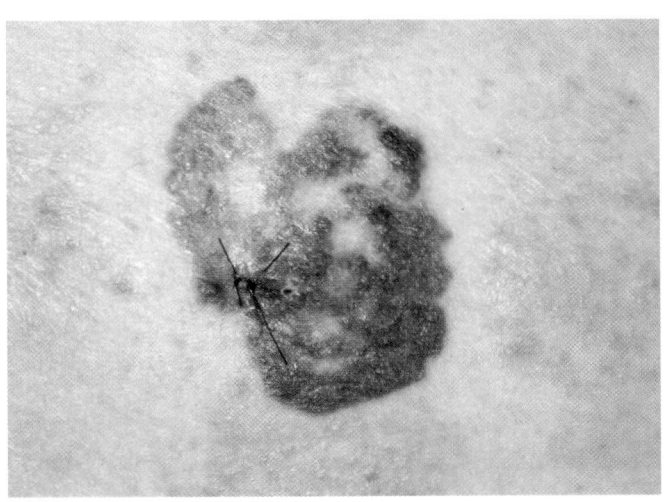

FIGURE 93-13. Superficial spreading melanoma. Breslow depth 1.1 mm.

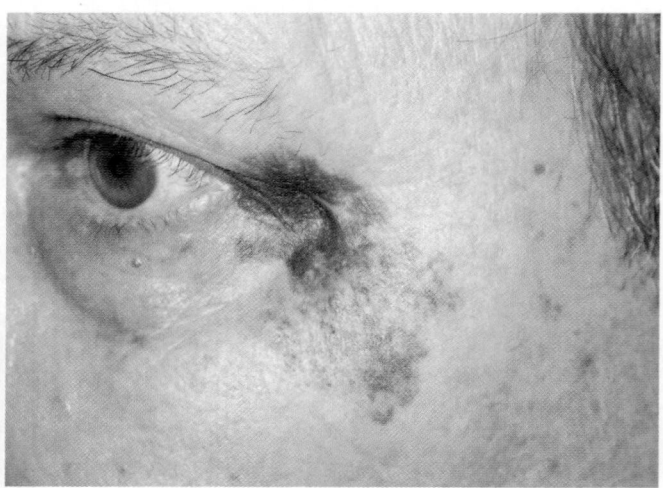

FIGURE 93-14. Lentigo melanoma (melanoma in situ) on the left lateral canthus and cheek. Large, asymmetric, irregularly pigmented flat patch.

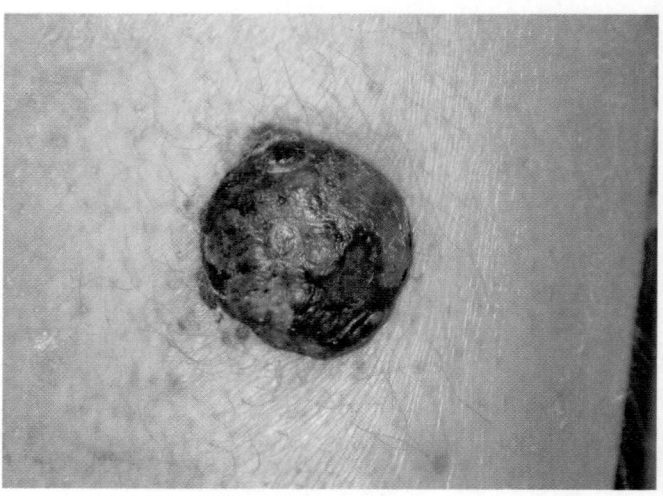

FIGURE 93-16. Large nodular melanoma. Breslow depth 11.5 mm with ulceration associated with 45% 5-year survival (stage IIc).

melanoma. Malignant cells may asymmetrically reach several centimeters beyond the clinical lesion, extending down hair follicles and other skin appendages.

Nodular Nodular melanoma constitutes approximately 15% to 30% of melanomas. It often arises without evidence of a preexisting lesion. Nodular melanoma has a minimal lateral growth phase, and instead grows vertically early in the course of the disease. Due to this early vertical growth, nodular melanoma typically has invaded substantially by the time of detection, leading to a worse prognosis. Clinically, nodular melanoma appears as a raised, nodular, or polypoid lesion with relatively uniform color and regular borders (**Figure 93-16**). Nodular melanoma may ulcerate with rapid growth and can lack classic melanoma features.

Acral lentiginous Acral lentiginous melanoma represents approximately 2% to 8% of melanomas in Caucasians, but 35% to 60% in people of color. As its name suggests, it usually occurs in acral sites, that is, the hands, feet, fingers, toes, and under the nails. It presents as a brown or black macule or patch with irregular borders (**Figures 93-17** and **93-18**). Subungual melanoma may present as an irregular, tan-brown longitudinal streak in the nail without a visible tumor. It is generally under the proximal nailfold in the nail matrix (**Figure 93-19**). Unfortunately, given this presentation, subungual melanomas are often misdiagnosed as subungual hematomas.

Differential Diagnosis

The differential diagnosis of melanoma encompasses several benign etiologies. For superficial spreading melanoma

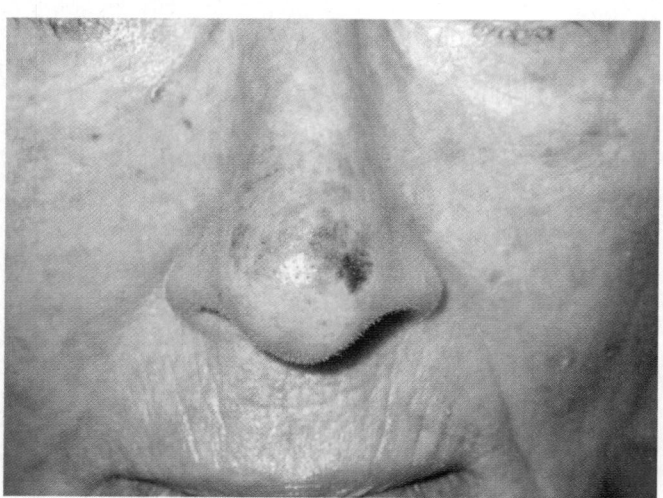

FIGURE 93-15. Lentigo melanoma (melanoma in situ) on the dorsum of the nose. Irregularly pigmented flat macule that had been slowly enlarging over a number of years.

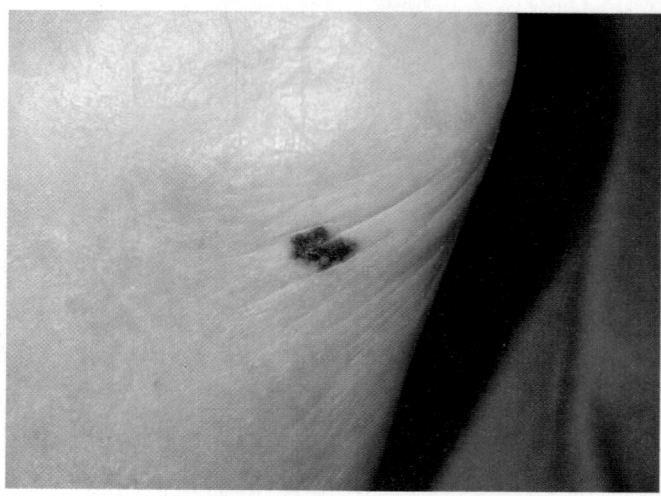

FIGURE 93-17. Acral lentiginous melanoma. Black, irregularly shaped macule on the sole of the foot.

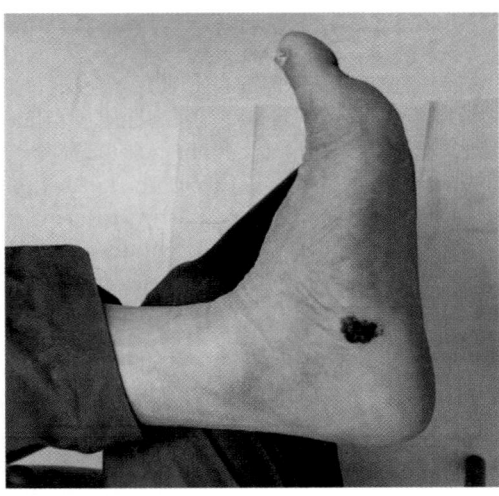

FIGURE 93-18. Acral lentiginous melanoma on the lateral aspect of the foot. Black patch with irregular borders.

that list includes atypical nevi, pigmented BCC, and seborrheic keratoses; for nodular melanoma—angiokeratoma, blue nevi, and dermatofibroma. Nevi and the rare fungal infection tinea nigra palmaris should be considered in the differential for acral lentiginous melanoma.

Course and Complications

The American Joint Committee on Cancer (AJCC) classifies melanoma based on the tumor thickness (T), nodal status (N), and metastatic disease (M) staging system. There are five stages, with each successive stage associated with a worse prognosis and deeper invasion into the dermis (Breslow depth): stage 0 (in situ melanoma), stage I (local disease with no evidence of spread), stage II (local disease with deeper invasion into the dermis but still no evidence

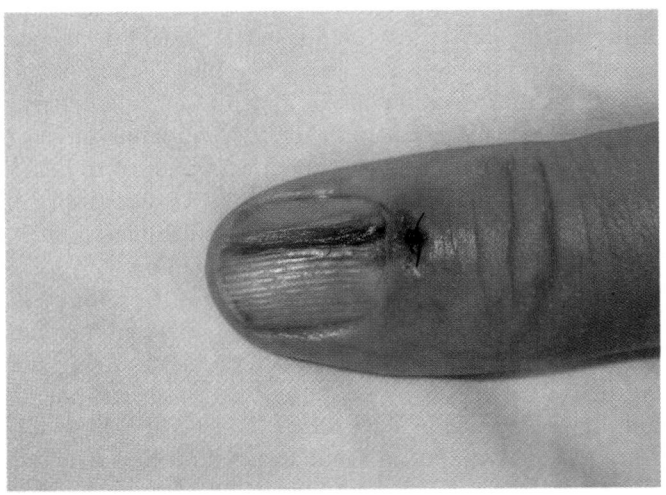

FIGURE 93-19. Subungual melanoma. Longitudinal dark brown streak along nail plate with associated brown pigmentation on the proximal nail fold and nail dystrophy. Suture identifies biopsy site of the nail matrix.

of spread), stage III (evidence of spread to regional lymph nodes or skin), and stage IV (distant metastases). The more distal the metastases, the poorer the prognosis. Frequent sites of metastases include the lymph nodes, skin, and subcutaneous tissue. Visceral metastases most commonly involve the lungs, liver, brain, bone, and intestines, though they may occur in any organ.

Clinically, node-negative patients with significant risk of regional nodal disease at the time of diagnosis are staged via a sentinel lymph node biopsy (SLNB), ideally performed at the time of definitive treatment of the primary site. The lymph node status and nodal tumor burden (based on SLNB) are incorporated into the current AJCC staging system. A thorough description of prognosis based on Breslow depth and other prognostic factors is found in a seminal article by Balch et al.

Treatment of Melanoma

Biopsy considerations All lesions clinically concerning for melanoma should be biopsied via a full-thickness excision with narrow margins (2 mm) oriented parallel to the lines of lymphatic drainage, or a deep saucerization shave biopsy of the complete lesion. The goal of biopsy is to remove the entire clinical lesion for comprehensive histologic evaluation. A superficial shave biopsy is never recommended for a lesion suspicious for melanoma; if the melanoma is transected with a shave biopsy then it will be difficult to accurately determine the thickness of the tumor. For suspicious lesions too large for complete excision, a full-thickness incisional biopsy deep enough to avoid transecting the lesion at the deep margin may be performed using an ellipse, deep saucerization shave, or punch. Incisional biopsies of melanoma do not increase the risk of metastasis. Formalin-fixed, paraffin-embedded, permanent sections are required for accurate microstaging and diagnosis of the primary lesion.

Surgical excision of the primary tumor Surgical excision of the primary tumor is the standard therapy for melanoma to prevent local recurrence caused by persistent disease. The National Comprehensive Cancer Network (NCCN) guidelines include recommendations for lateral margins, which are based on the depth of invasion of the lesion. The deep margin of the excision should be in the deep fat or in the tissue plane above the fascia. Excision specimens are sent to the pathologist for confirmation or change of the histologic stage of disease, as well as evaluation of the surgical margins. Since lentigo maligna, or the superficial portions of the lentigo maligna melanoma, can extend subclinically, excision with 5 mm margins often yields tumor at the margin, leading to recurrence. For these lesions, excision with margin control is necessary. A modification of the MMS procedure with permanent sections is often used, having an excellent success rate of less than 2% recurrence in many studies with long-term follow-up. A comparison study at the Mayo Clinic of wide local excision versus frozen section MMS for lentigo maligna had 5.9% versus 1.9% recurrence rates, respectively.

Lentigo maligna without evidence of invasive melanoma can also be treated with imiquimod cream used five times a week for 12 or more weeks to the point of inflammation, or with RT. An older patient with limited life expectancy could have the lesion observed, utilizing follow-up examination, lesion photography, dermoscopy, or possibly confocal laser microscopy.

Sentinel lymph node biopsy and regional lymph node management Melanoma's spread to the regional nodal basin typically begins with initial metastasis to one lymph node, referred to as the sentinel lymph node (SLN). The SLN can be identified by use of radiolabeled colloid lymphatic tracers plus blue dye injected intradermally at the site of the primary lesion. The tracers and dye then drain from the primary lesion, traveling through the lymphatic vessels and collecting in the SLN. This node (or nodes if multiple collect dye) is then removed for careful histologic evaluation with immunohistochemical staining. The entire process is termed the SLNB and is performed as an outpatient procedure. The accuracy of SLNB requires injection of tracers at the site of the primary lesion, so ideally SLNB is completed concurrently with wide local excision, ensuring that tracers are injected at the most appropriate site. If the SLNB is negative for melanoma, no further treatment is indicated. If instead, the SLNB is positive for melanoma, then patients should consider regional therapeutic lymphadenectomy and may be eligible for adjuvant therapy.

The NCCN melanoma guidelines recommend considering SLNB in patients with high-risk stage IB (Breslow depth > 1 mm or 0.76–1.0 mm thick lesions with high-risk features) or stage II melanoma, for whom SLN status is the strongest independent predictor of survival. High-risk features for regional metastasis warranting SLNB in thin melanoma (0.76–1.0 mm thick) include young patient age, ulceration of the primary lesion, angiolymphatic invasion, a mitotic rate of greater than or equal to 1 mitosis/mm^2, or a positive deep margin on the initial biopsy. SLNB is not recommended for stage 0 melanoma, or very thin (≤ 0.75 mm) lesions that are stage IA or 1B.

Although SLNB is generally well tolerated, reported complication rates vary from 5% to 10%. Old age is one of the known risk factors for complications associated with SLNB, so it is important that older adults considering SLNB are well-educated on the risks and benefits of the procedure. Complications that are most likely to occur include wound dehiscence and infection, seroma/hematoma, and lymphedema. Other reported risks include allergic reactions to the dye used, nerve injury and thrombophlebitis, deep vein thrombosis, and hemorrhage. Given these risks, SLNB has remained controversial in older adults, and especially in the very old. A study at the University of Michigan, however, of 952 melanoma patients 75 years or older concluded that in patients with good functional status who were appropriate surgical candidates, SLNB should be strongly considered; it was found to be associated with improved outcomes, even after factoring in age and comorbidities.

SLNB allows for early identification of patients with nodal disease and for immediate intervention with completion lymph node dissection (CLND). Although data on improved clinical outcomes with CLND are conflicting, the procedure is still recommended by the NCCN for patients with stage III disease or a positive SLNB. The NCCN panel determined, however, that there was insufficient evidence to detail a specific number of lymph nodes that have to be removed in lymph node basins in order for CLND to be considered adequate.

Adjuvant therapy

Adjuvant radiation therapy NCCN guidelines recommend considering adjuvant RT following surgery for patients with desmoplastic melanoma, or melanoma that involves nerve fibers, otherwise known as neurotropic melanoma. These tumors are at high risk of recurrence, which can be ameliorated by adjuvant RT. For patients with positive nodes and a high risk of nodal basin relapse, however, the expert panel was unable to reach a consensus to recommend adjuvant RT. Although high-level evidence displays that adjuvant RT can delay relapse in these patients, some experts noted that this benefit could be outweighed by late RT-related toxicity. Therefore, the use of adjuvant RT in these patients should be determined on a case-by-case basis.

Adjuvant systemic therapy Historically, interferon-α was used as adjuvant systemic therapy in surgical patients with no known metastases. Data have now shown that interferon-α is ineffective as a therapeutic for melanoma, with the field instead embracing targeted therapy and immune checkpoint inhibitors. These therapeutics were initially only used for stage IV disease; however, they are now often considered as adjuvant therapy in stage II disease.

Systemic therapy

Targeted therapies Targeted therapeutics for melanoma include the BRAF inhibitors vemurafenib (brand name Zelboraf) and dabrafenib (brand name Tafinlar), developed to counteract the constitutively active BRAF kinase resultant from the mutation BRAF^{V600E}. BRAF^{V600E} mutations must be confirmed in patients prior to initiating targeted therapy. The kinase immediately downstream from BRAF is MEK, and therefore constitutive BRAF activation in BRAF^{V600E} leads to constitutive MEK activation. As such, BRAF inhibitors are often given in conjunction with MEK inhibitors (trametinib) for further efficacy. Clinical studies of vemurafenib did not include a sufficient number of adults older than 65 years to determine the safety and efficacy of the drug in this population. Trials of dabrafenib did, however, include older adults. When dabrafenib was administered as a single agent for melanoma, no differences were observed in the safety and efficacy of the drug between older and younger patients. When given in conjunction with trametinib, efficacy remained the same across patient age, but older patients had an increased incidence of peripheral edema (26% vs 12%) and anorexia (21% vs 9%) when compared to younger adults. It should be noted that trials of trametinib as a single agent did not include sufficient numbers of older adults. Common adverse reactions for both vemurafenib and dabrafenib include arthralgias, alopecia, and skin papilloma, with vemurafenib additionally displaying photosensitivity, and dabrafenib hyperkeratosis and palmar-plantar erythrodysthesia syndrome. When dabrafenib was given in conjunction with trametinib as adjuvant treatment for melanoma or for unresectable or metastatic melanoma, common adverse reactions included pyrexia, rash, chills, and headache. Providers should additionally be aware that dabrafenib can decrease systemic exposure of warfarin, and the label recommends that during the initiation or discontinuation of dabrafenib in patients who receive warfarin, providers should frequently monitor the international normalized ratio (INR).

Immunotherapies Immunotherapeutic treatment options for melanoma include ipilimumab (CTLA-4 inhibitor), nivolumab (PD-1 inhibitor), and pembrolizumab (PD-1 inhibitor). Both CTLA-4 and PD-1 are involved in immune checkpoints, which are inhibitory pathways that deter autoimmunity by preventing immune cells from indiscriminately attacking all cells and tissue that they come across. CLTA-4 decreases T-cell activity, and PD-1 inhibits T-cell proliferation and cytokine production. Inhibiting these checkpoints effectively switches "on" T-cell activity against melanoma, inducing an antitumor immune response.

Although insufficient numbers of older adults were included in trials for adjuvant melanoma treatment with Yervoy (ipilimumab) and in some of the trials for Opdivo (nivolumab), those trials across Yervoy, Opdivo, and Keytruda (pembrolizumab) that did include sufficient numbers of older adults, did not find any significant differences in the safety and efficacy of the drugs between younger and older adults. Common adverse reactions across CTLA-4 and PD-1 therapeutics include nausea, vomiting, fatigue, rash, and diarrhea, but providers should be aware that severe and fatal immune-mediated adverse reactions can occur with these medications. Such reactions include immune-mediated hepatitis, pneumonitis, endocrinopathies, and renal dysfunction.

Role of imaging in melanoma diagnosis In the case of an unremarkable history and physical examination in a patient with recently diagnosed melanoma, the NCCN recommends against routine imaging studies (computed tomography [CT], positron emission tomography [PET] scan, and magnetic resonance imaging [MRI]) and lab tests for patients with stage I melanoma. These imaging modalities may be used for symptom-directed work-up for patients with stage II disease. Imaging for asymptomatic patients with stage III disease is generally felt to be low yield but may be performed at the discretion of the treating physician. Stage IV metastatic disease should be confirmed by tissue biopsy (either fine needle aspiration or open biopsy) when possible and it is recommended to perform additional staging with imaging and blood serum lactate dehydrogenase (LDH).

There are a number of less common cutaneous tumors that are beyond the scope of this chapter. Of these, the geriatrician should be familiar with Merkel cell carcinoma (MCC) given that it is a highly aggressive tumor with a predilection for older adults. For readers interested in discussion of other tumors, please refer to a standard dermatology text.

Merkel Cell Carcinoma

Definition MCC is a rare, highly aggressive cutaneous neuroendocrine carcinoma. As its name suggests, the tumor develops from Merkel cells, which are responsible for the sensation of light touch and are found in the basal layer of the epidermis. Approximately 1600 cases are diagnosed annually in the United States, and 81.7% of patients who are diagnosed are older than 70. The 5-year overall survival after diagnosis ranges from 51% for patients with local disease to 14% for those with distal metastases.

Risk factors As with other skin cancers discussed in this chapter, the major risk factor for MCC is extensive UV exposure, with the typical patient being an older adult with light-colored skin (refer to the *Etiology* section for a thorough discussion on UV exposure). Other important risk factors include chronic immunosuppression and infection with the Merkel cell polyomavirus (MCV). Although MCV is typically a benign virus to which much of the world's population is exposed to as children, MCV is found in the cells of eight out of 10 MCCs, suggesting that it has a significant oncogenic role in the development of this cancer.

Clinical presentation and histology MCC commonly occurs on the sun-exposed skin of the head and neck in older adults. In younger patients, however, the trunk is the most common site of occurrence. On examination, patients present with a red-to-purple bump or nodule that grows rapidly over 3 months (**Figures 93-20** and **93-21**).

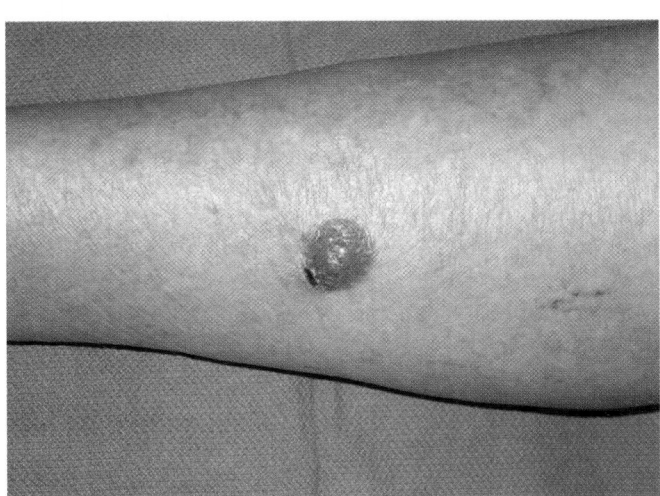

FIGURE 93-20. Merkel cell carcinoma. Red-to-purple 2.3-cm nodule on the lower leg.

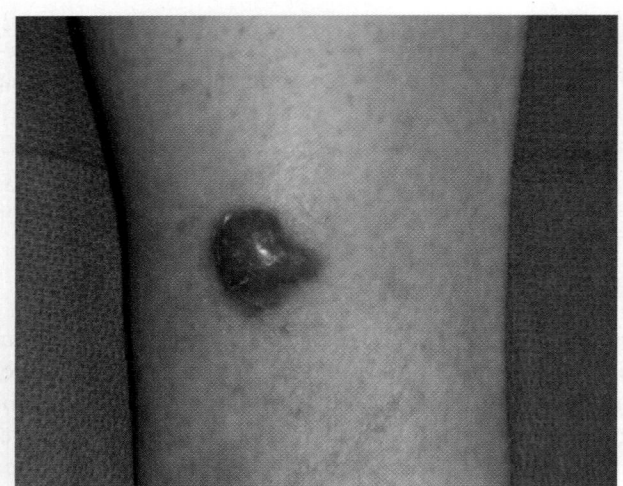

FIGURE 93-21. Merkel cell carcinoma presenting as a red nodule.

Differential diagnosis Initially, MCC may be misdiagnosed as an inflamed hair follicle, boil, or cyst. Rapid growth of the lesion often prompts biopsy and accurate diagnosis.

Course and complications As an aggressive tumor, MCC presents with a high risk of recurrence and metastases. The first consensus staging system for MCC was introduced in 2010 by the AJCC. The system follows the primary tumor (T), nodal status (N), and distant metastases (M) structure. Four stages exist, stage I (local disease with primary tumor < 2 cm), stage II (local disease with larger tumor size), stage III (regional nodal disease), and stage IV (distant metastatic disease). Although MCC is capable of metastasizing to distal viscera, it commonly affects the regional nodal basin, with studies showing that even the smallest clinical tumors have at least 15% to 20% risk for occult metastatic disease in the regional lymph node basin.

Given its aggressive nature and risk for metastasis, it is critical to identify and treat MCC early. Yet, in a study of more than 26,000 patients from the National Cancer Database, it was found that even after diagnosis, time to definitive surgical treatment for stage I to III MCC was significantly longer for Black patients (58.9 days) than it was for non-Hispanic Whites (46.3 days). Of note, these disparities persisted for Medicare and private insurance, but not for Medicaid or uninsured patients, and occurred despite Black patients living closer to the hospital than non-Hispanic Whites. These findings highlight some of the many disparities in health care, bringing to attention the fact that minority patients often do not just experience delays in diagnosis, but unacceptable delays in treatment.

Treatment for MCC The treatment of MCC is based on the staging and spread of the disease. Wide local excision can be used for management of the primary tumor, with radiation administered to the tumor bed and any regionally involved lymph nodes. Successful treatment has also been documented with a combination of narrow margin excision and RT, or even with just radiation alone. Distant metastases can be treated with chemotherapy, PD-1 immune checkpoint inhibitors, or other targeted molecular therapies.

NUANCES IN TREATMENT

Throughout this chapter, multiple modalities of treatment have been discussed for skin cancer. While each treatment presents with its own data on efficacy and cure rates, ultimately, if an individualized approach is taken to choose the right treatment, it is possible to cure every local lesion. Yet, if the wrong treatment is chosen, then the cure rate diminishes. For example, while a 5-mm well-demarcated nodular BCC on the back should have a 99% cure rate via any treatment, this is not the case if the same tumor is in a more high-risk location, like the nasal ala. Such a tumor might require a procedure like MMS with very careful margin control. Another common situation is a 6 mm ulcerated nodular BCC on the lower nose. ED&C in this site has a less than 50% cure rate. Radiation treatment has a 90% cure rate but would require multiple visits. For a 95+% cure rate with a one stage excision with delayed standard histologic evaluation, the procedure entails an excision through fat (to fascia) with at least 4 mm margins and requires reconstruction, likely with a flap and sutures. MMS with a 98% cure rate for this lesion will take place in 1 day, often without even a previous appointment for consultation, and generally result in a smaller and thinner defect that can heal by second intention, removing most of the morbidity and risk of complication from the surgical procedure. Providers must therefore be aware of all of the implications that come with discussing treatment. When patients and families hear the word "surgery," they are often reflexively hesitant since they may picture a big operation in the operating room. On the other hand, they might be told that a procedure is minor and may not anticipate the need for a large reconstructive flap or graft. Care should therefore be taken to educate patients on the exact procedure that they will undergo, and thorough discussions between the treatment team and the patient should include details regarding the day of surgery, potential options for repair, and their implications. The patient's concerns should be addressed, and they should have appropriate expectations for the procedure and ensuing recovery. Ultimately, the decision of which treatment to pursue is extremely nuanced and individualized. Several considerations particularly important in the geriatric population are discussed below.

GERIATRIC PRINCIPLES APPLIED TO DERMATOLOGY

Given that skin cancer increasingly presents with advanced age, providers must be comfortable with triaging these lesions. For older adults, it is important to assess the mortality risk of the lesion (eg, concern for melanoma versus concern for superficial BCC) as well as the morbidity risk (eg, a long-standing 2 cm BCC that constantly bleeds versus a new 5-mm lesion concerning for early BCC). These considerations can help when assessing appropriateness of treatment within the conceptual framework of principles such as life expectancy, functional status, and lag time to benefit. Biopsies should always be performed for lesions concerning for high-risk skin cancer, for example SCC in concerning locations or in immunosuppressed patients, melanoma, or MCC. Once a lesion is biopsied and diagnosed, treatment recommendations should be tailored to the individual. Factors to consider include patient preferences, as well as if the patient presents at the end of life, has multiple comorbidities, or the morbidity of treatment outweighs the benefits. While treatments are often well tolerated for skin cancers that are not considered "high risk," active nonintervention can be reasonably considered in patients who are near the end of life, particularly if the lesion is asymptomatic. Palliative surgery, however, should still be an option for low-functioning adults if they have symptomatic lesions that significantly impair their quality of life (eg, pain, bleeding, pungent odor). For older adults, it is particularly important for dermatologists and geriatricians or primary care providers to collaborate and involve both the patient and their family in treatment discussions, utilizing shared decision-making to marry medical advice with the patient's desire for or against treatment of their lesion. Ultimately, when determining appropriate treatment in the aging population, it is crucial to weigh the patient's overall status and their wishes over their chronological age.

FURTHER READING

Ad Hoc Task Force, Connolly SM, Baker DR, et al. AAD/ACMS/ASDSA/ASMS 2012 appropriate use criteria for Mohs micrographic surgery: a report of the American Academy of Dermatology, American College of Mohs Surgery, American Society for Dermatologic Surgery Association, and the American Society for Mohs Surgery. *J Am Acad Dermatol.* 2012;67(4):531–550.

Balch M, Gershenwald JE, Soong SJ, et al. Final version of the American Joint Committee on Cancer melanoma staging and classification. *J Clin Oncol.* 2009;27(36):6199–6206.

Bichakjian C, Armstrong A, Baum C, et al. Guidelines of care for the management of basal cell carcinoma. *J Am Acad Dermatol.* 2018;78(3):540–559.

Coggshall K, Tello TL, North JP, Yu SS. Merkel cell carcinoma: an update and review: pathogenesis, diagnosis, and staging. *J Am Acad Dermatol.* 2018;78(3):433–442.

Jung JY, Linos E. Adding active surveillance as a treatment option for low risk skin cancers in patients with limited life expectancy. *J Geriatr Oncol.* 2016;7(3):221–222.

Morgan FC, Ruiz ES, Karia PS, Besaw RJ, Neel VA, Schmults CD. Factors predictive of recurrence, metastasis, and death from primary basal cell carcinoma 2 cm or larger in diameter. *J Am Acad Dermatol.* 2020;83(3):832–838.

National Comprehensive Cancer Network. Basal Cell Skin Cancer (Version 1.2020). 2019; https://www.nccn.org/professionals/physician_gls/pdf/nmsc.pdf. Accessed November 23, 2020.

National Comprehensive Cancer Network. Cutaneous Melanoma (Version 4.2020). 2020; https://www.nccn.org/professionals/physician_gls/pdf/cutaneous_melanoma.pdf. Accessed November 23, 2020.

National Comprehensive Cancer Network. Squamous Cell Skin Cancer (Version 2.2020). 2020; https://www.nccn.org/professionals/physician_gls/pdf/squamous.pdf. Accessed November 24, 2020.

Regula CG, Alam M, Behshad R, et al. Functionality of patients 75 years and older undergoing Mohs micrographic surgery: a multicenter study. *Dermatol Surg.* 2017;43(7):904–910.

Siegel JA, Korgavkar K, Weinstock MA. Current perspective on actinic keratosis: a review. *Br J Dermatol.* 2017;177(2):350–358.

Tripathi R, Bordeaux JS, Nijhawan RI. Factors associated with time to treatment for Merkel cell carcinoma. *J Am Acad Dermatol.* 2021;84(3):877–880.

Wu S, Han J, Laden F, Qureshi AA. Long-term ultraviolet flux, other potential risk factors, and skin cancer risk: a cohort study. *Cancer Epidemiol Biomarkers Prev.* 2014;23(6):1080–1089.

Chapter 94

Aging of the Hematopoietic System and Anemia

Jiasheng Wang, Changsu Park, Jino Park, Robert Kalayjian, William Tse

INTRODUCTION

The hematopoietic system is composed of short-lived blood cells that require continuous replenishment in a process called hematopoiesis. Adult hematopoiesis occurs in the bone marrow, where hematopoietic stem cells (HSCs) self-renew and differentiate into progenitor cells, with the latter further developing into mature blood cells (**Figure 94-1**). Three key changes occur in the aged hematopoietic system: (1) HSC functional decline, (2) increased clonal hematopoiesis, and (3) myeloid skewing and impaired lymphopoiesis. These changes respectively lead to three well-described manifestations of the dysfunctional hematopoietic system in older adults: the deficiency in stress-induced hematopoiesis, increased incidence of myeloid malignancy, and compromised innate and adaptive immunity. The mechanisms of HSC aging can be intrinsic and extrinsic. Intrinsic changes of the HSC range from DNA damage and epigenetic changes to alteration of proteins and signaling pathways. Cell-extrinsic mechanisms are related to the aging of the microenvironment where HSCs reside. This chapter will focus on the phenotypes and mechanisms of the aged hematopoietic system.

HALLMARKS OF THE AGED HEMATOPOIETIC SYSTEM

Given that HSCs are at the apex of the hematopoietic differentiation, changes of the aged hematopoietic system can be traced back to alterations of the HSCs. While most HSCs are quiescent under homeostasis, in demand situations such as inflammation or infection, HSCs become active and differentiate into blood cells to compensate for these reactive processes. Upon aging, their functions are impaired and their regenerative capacity is reduced, leading to relative cytopenia and slow blood-count recovery when

Learning Objectives

- Understand the integral knowledge of the aging mechanism and process of the hematopoietic system.
- Identify the actionable targets and signal pathways that can be physiologically modified as part of the treatment of medical conditions.
- Become aware of other nonhematologic medical conditions that can directly or indirectly affect the hematologic system's aging process.
- Understand the clinical and societal burden of anemia in the older population and its management.

Key Clinical Points

1. The hematopoietic system's aging is associated with a complex process that includes molecular biology, signal transduction profiles, and epigenetics.
2. The aging process of the hematopoietic system can be potentially modifiable with the current medical technologies. However, such short-sighted attempts outside of the context of medical treatment should be made with greater caution.
3. Anemia among older adults will be a significant medical and financial burden on the incoming "Silver Tsunami." It is unknown if anemia in older adults without medical causes is pathological versus physiological. Although some anemia treatment recommendations in this chapter are proposed, readers are encouraged to apply good medical judgment for an individual patient.

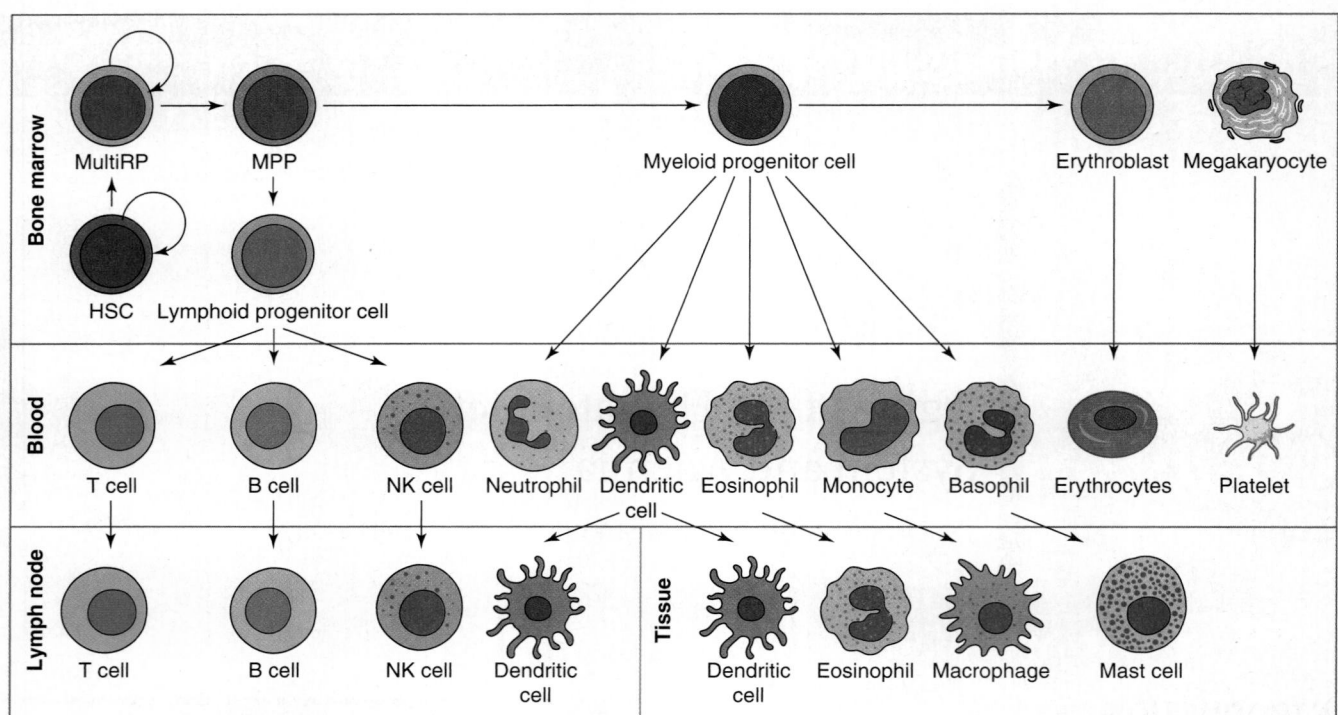

FIGURE 94-1. Model of hematopoietic stem cell (HSC) self-renewal and lineage differentiation. HSCs constitute only a small number of hematopoietic cells and undergo limited cycles of self-renewal during the whole life. The multipotent repopulating progenitors (MultiRP) derived from HSC can also self-renew and are the main source of daily hematopoiesis. Multipotent progenitors (MPP) lose self-renewal ability, but can differentiate into myeloid and lymphoid progenitor cells, which further differentiate into various blood cells residing in peripheral blood, lymph nodes, and tissues. Aging is associated impaired HSC function, leading to reduced differentiation and repopulation capabilities.

encountering bone marrow stress. Furthermore, as a type of stem cells, HSCs have the capacity to propagate themselves through symmetrical divisions. However, if somatic mutations of leukemia-associated driver genes occur during the process, a genetically identical, hematological malignancy precursor clone would expand predominantly and indefinitely. This phenomenon, known as the clonal hematopoiesis of indeterminate potential (CHIP), is associated with an increased risk of myeloid malignancy in the older adult. Lastly, recent advances in single-cell sequencing revealed that the population of HSCs are heterogeneous with various differentiation potentials. Aging is associated with preferentially increased myelopoiesis and decreased lymphopoiesis, which would impair innate and adaptive immunity, leading to high infection rate in older adults (**Figure 94-2**).

Hematopoietic Stem Cell Functional Decline

HSCs represent a rare and highly quiescent population of cells, which divide very infrequently. Early in vivo studies in mice showed that marrow donors can repopulate blood cells in serial hematopoietic transplantation experiments spanning multiple lifetimes, prompting the hypothesis that HSCs are "effectively immortal." Moreover, in patients receiving HSC transplantation, advanced donor age does not place the recipient at an increased risk of delayed engraftment or prolonged cytopenia. However, using

competitive transplantation assay, where young and aged HSCs are mixed and transplanted into the same recipient, aged HSCs exhibit a functional decline in their repopulation capacity. Indeed, in a landmark study by Bernitz et al. in 2016 when the authors used in situ genetic labeling, they showed that HSCs can only undergo four self-renewal divisions in their lifetimes before entering a dormancy state, with long-term regenerative potential and differentiation ability lost upon a fifth division. Further studies showed that progenitor cells downstream of HSCs serve as the major self-renewing source of day-to-day hematopoiesis, whereas HSCs themselves represent a dormant compartment which can only be called on demand into an active compartment. This is probably why although aged HSCs have multilevel dysfunction, clinically significant anemia and thrombocytopenia only occur in situations of bone marrow stress, such as bleeding, infection, or inflammation. Indeed, an underlying cause of chronic anemia can be found in the majority of older patients, while only a minority of unexplained anemia is likely due to HSC functional decline. In summary, HSC functional decline leads to deficiency in stress-induced hematopoiesis.

Clonal Hematopoiesis

Aging is associated with the accumulation of somatic mutations in HSCs. However, the vast majority of these

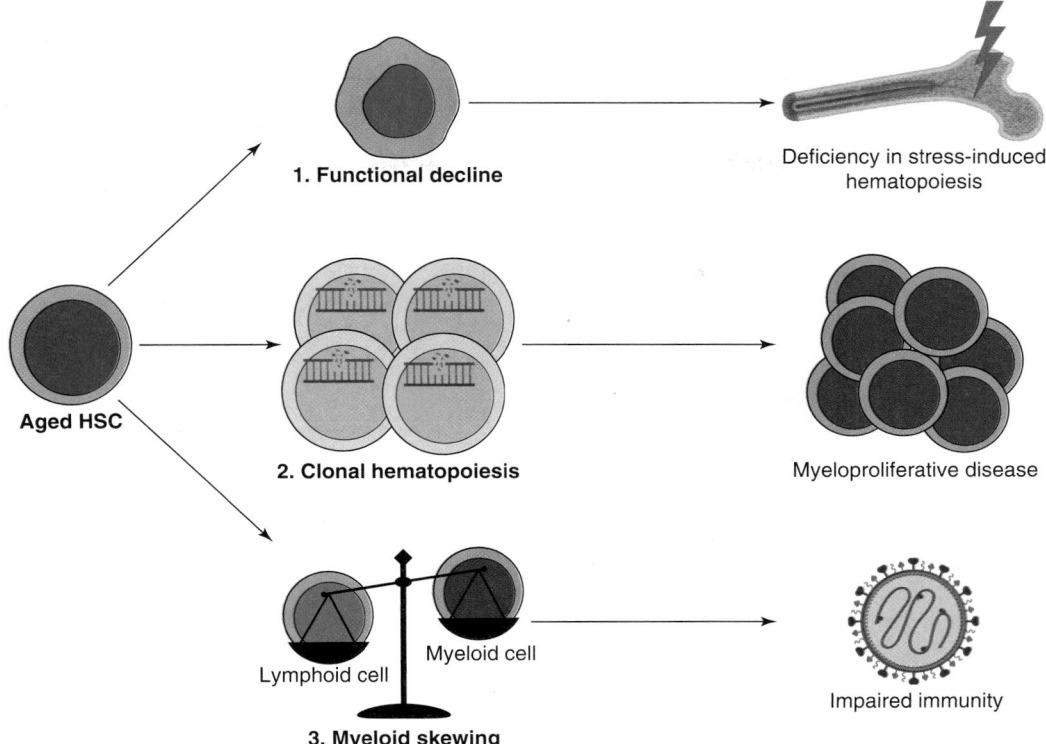

1. Functional decline

Deficiency in stress-induced hematopoiesis

Aged HSC

2. Clonal hematopoiesis

Myeloproliferative disease

Lymphoid cell

Myeloid cell

Impaired immunity

3. Myeloid skewing

FIGURE 94-2. Hallmarks of aged hematopoietic system. The aged hematopoietic system is characterized by three key changes: functional decline, clonal hematopoiesis, and myeloid skewing. These changes lead to deficiency in stress-induced hematopoiesis, myeloproliferative disease, and impaired immunity.

mutations are silent and have no effect on the phenotype. Rarely, mutations occur at the loci of the leukemia-associated driver genes, conferring a selective growth advantage to the mutated cell. As a result, a substantial proportion of mature blood cells harboring the same mutation are produced—a process known as clonal hematopoiesis. Once the clonal outgrowth reaches a certain threshold, the process is then termed CHIP. Contradictory to its name, CHIP is generally regarded as the "first hit" for malignant transformation, and the presence of CHIP is associated with a 10-fold increased relative risk of myeloid malignancies. In addition, emerging evidence also associates CHIP with nonhematologic conditions, such as cardiovascular disease, chronic obstructive lung disease (COPD), autoimmune disorders, and death.

Myeloid malignancies, such as acute myeloid leukemia (AML) and myelodysplastic syndrome (MDS), are predominantly diagnosed in older adults and the incidence increases with age. Indeed, the median ages of diagnosis are 65 and 70 years for AML and MDS, respectively. Similarly, the prevalence of CHIP also rises sharply in older adults, reaching 15% in their 70s and 20% in their 90s. The most common mutations associated with CHIP involve *DNMT3A, TET2,* and *ASXL1,* which are also commonly found in AML and MDS, further supporting a causal correlation between CHIP and myeloid malignancies.

Intriguingly, all three of these genes are key players in epigenetic remodeling of chromatin in HSC, which will be explored later in this chapter.

Myeloid Skewing and Impaired Lymphopoiesis

Aging is associated with immune remodeling and dysfunction, affecting both innate and adaptive immunity, a phenomenon that is known as immunosenescence. The effects of age on adaptive immunity include lymphopenia with declines in B-cells and naïve T-cells, but expansion of inhibitory regulatory (Tregs) and terminally differentiated, senescent T-cells. These cellular imbalances result in impaired responses to immunization and increased susceptibility to new infections; increased rates of autoimmune disorders; and increased risk of reactivation by chronic, latent infections. Innate immune changes are more complex and less well studied; they involve multiple myeloid cell lines including monocytes, macrophages, and neutrophils.

The causes of immunosenescence are multifactorial. However, one important association is aging-related myeloid skewing and impaired lymphopoiesis. Single-cell sequencing has revealed that HSCs' differentiation potential is not homogenous—a subgroup of myeloid-restricted progenitors resides in the young HSC compartment, which expands dramatically with aging, leading to myeloid skewing. However, even though the numbers of myeloid cells are

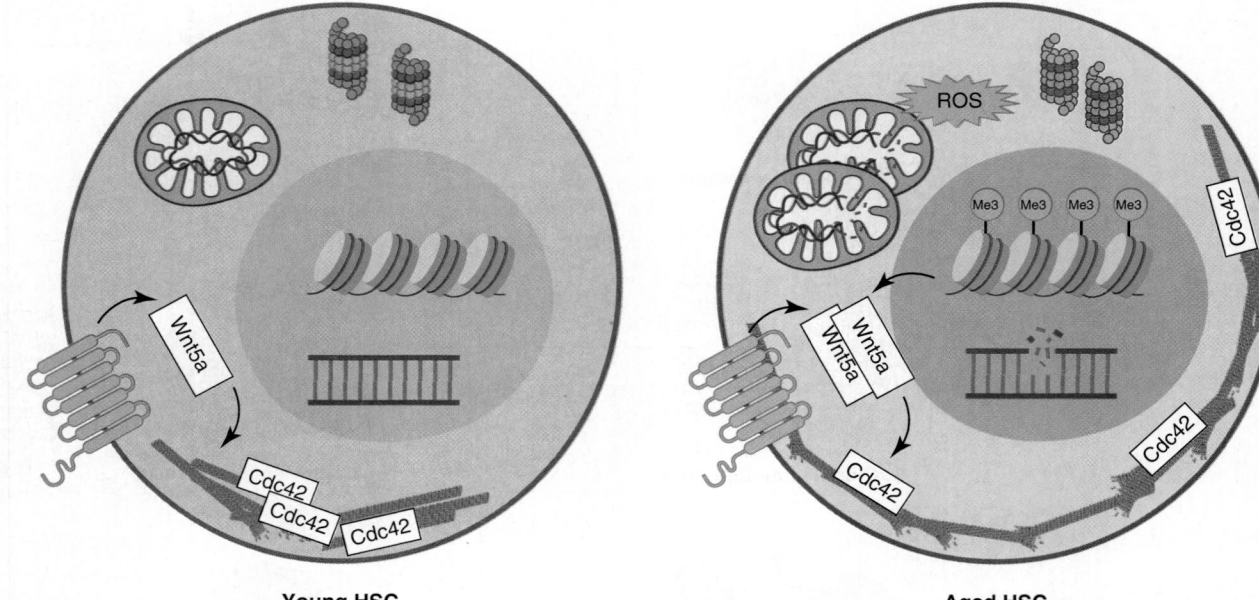

FIGURE 94-3. Intrinsic changes of aged HSC comparing to young HSC. Mutations in the DNA accumulate during the aging process, leading to clonal hematopoiesis and predisposing the older adult to myeloid malignancies. Epigenetic drift in the aged HSC affects gene expression including molecules in the Wnt signaling pathway, leading to its noncanonical activation and cell loss of polarity. In the meantime, mutations of mitochondrial DNA (mtDNA) also accumulate, causing excessive reactive oxygen species (ROS) production.

higher, their functions are compromised, leading to impaired innate immunity. Conversely, the number of lymphoid precursors is reduced, resulting in impaired lymphopoiesis and adaptive immunity. Clinically, about a quarter of the older population have lymphopenia at baseline, and lymphopenia itself is an independent risk factor for mortality.

INTRINSIC MECHANISMS OF HSC AGING

Intrinsic changes of the HSCs on the molecular and phenotypic level have long been identified. Alterations range from DNA damage, metabolic alterations, loss of cell polarity, and impaired autophagy to changes of the intrinsic signaling pathway (**Figure 94-3**). Historically, DNA damage was deemed as the driver for HSC aging and responsible for all the phenotypic changes. However, recent studies have shown that epigenetic changes and mitochondrial dysfunction might have played bigger roles in the aged phenotype. Current research is trying to decipher the link between the molecular alterations and the phenotypic changes.

DNA Damage

DNA damage is common in mammalian cells and originates from normal cellular activities such as metabolism and DNA replication or external factors such as drug exposure and irradiation. A conserved signaling cascade to prevent accumulation of mutations called DNA damage response (DDR) results in DNA repair, cell-cycle arrest, cellular senescence, and cell death. Nevertheless, DNA

mutations still accumulate with aging, which are especially pronounced in cells with a long lifespan such as HSCs. Therefore, HSCs rely heavily on the damage-response mechanism to maintain genomic stability. Earlier studies using DDR-deficient mice demonstrated a phenotype of premature aging, raising the concern of defective DNA repair mechanism in aged HSCs. However, recent research found that aged HSCs are as effective as young HSCs in repairing DNA. While HSCs possess an effective DNA repair mechanism throughout the aging process, point mutations in epigenetic regulators can still occur leading to clonal hematopoiesis and predisposing older adults to myeloid malignancies.

Historically, DNA damage in HSCs is deemed as the driver for both HSC functional decline and myeloid malignancies in older people. However, the former notion has been challenged in recent years as the function of aged HSCs could be restored by a variety of rejuvenation methods. For example, aged HSCs can be reversed to young phenotypes through induced pluripotent stem cell (iPSC) generation and redifferentiation, which would be impossible if dysfunction originates from the genomic level. On the other hand, although DNA damage and CHIP predispose the older adult to myeloid malignancies, the majority of CHIP does not evolve into MDS and AML, and not all myeloid malignancies have CHIP-associated gene mutations. Therefore, DNA damage and CHIP is only one of the many mechanisms leading to myeloid malignancies and may only partially explain HSC functional decline with aging.

Epigenetic Drift

Young and aged HSCs have a drastically different gene expression pattern. For example, aged HSCs have augmented platelet gene expression at the expense of lymphopoietic genes, leading to the myeloid skewing feature of aged HSCs. Such genome-wide transcriptional differences can only occur at the epigenetic level, which includes DNA methylation, histone modification, and chromatin architecture. Epigenetic mechanisms encompass chromatin-based regulation of gene expression without altering the DNA sequence. These pathways are more dynamic and responsive to the environment and stress disease can serve as a form of cellular memory to previous insults. Given that the phenotype of the aged hematopoietic system can be reversed by iPSC generation and redifferentiation, it is likely that most aging-associated changes are not at the durable genetic code but originate from the epigenetic level.

DNA methylation is an epigenetic signaling mechanism via covalent modification of cytosine moieties by a class of enzymes called DNA methyltransferases (DNMT) to produce 5-methylcytosine (5mC). These modifications are highly restricted to cytosine phosphate guanine (CpG) dinucleotides and are traditionally viewed as a repressive signal, which is associated with transcriptional inactivation of nearby promoter sequences. Intriguingly, the most common single nucleotide mutation found in aging HSCs is the transition from C to T at CpG dinucleotides. Spontaneous deamination of cytosine results in uracil, which is recognized as an error and converted back to cytosine by DNA repair. However, 5mC deamination yields thymine, which can surpass DNA repair and results in a CpG to TpG mutation. Given that CpGs are highly methylated, this transition suggests an interplay between epigenetic regulation and DNA mutations throughout aging. Although global hypomethylation occurs in most somatic cells during aging, aged HSCs demonstrate local hyper- and hypomethylation, indicating a pattern of differential gene expression. Indeed, such alterations in CpG methylation patterns can be modeled to accurately predict chronological age in healthy people and identify apparent discrepancies between chronological and biological age in conditions that have been associated with accelerated aging, including Down syndrome and chronic HIV infection. Furthermore, such modeling also predicted increased mortality in persons with age-related comorbidities.

The mechanism of dysregulation of DNA methylation in aged HSCs is still under investigation. However, DNA mutations in epigenetic regulators, such as *DNMT3A*, *TET2*, and *ASXL1*, can only lead to clonal hematopoiesis and myeloid skewing without the phenotypic changes seen in aged HSCs. Considering DNA methylation being the terminal step of signaling pathways, it is likely that the cause of epigenetic drift comes from outside in (environmental changes leading to epigenetic drift), rather than inside out (DNA damage leading to epigenetic drift).

Histone modification is an additional layer of epigenetic signaling that dictates the availability of specific gene loci to regulatory proteins. The N-terminal tail of histones serve as a robust platform for a myriad of modifications, which in concert lead to transcriptional activation or repression. Various histone code writers, readers, and erasers have been identified but the diversity of these modifications and permutations, especially in the context of neoplasia and senescence, have made clinical interpretation challenging. Nevertheless, both local and global changes in histone modifications have been reported in the aging bone marrow. For example, histone methyltransferase SUV39H1 experiences significant functional loss during aging, leading to decreased H3K9me3 level in HSCs. Accumulation of these changes within the histone code provides a dynamic epigenetic landscape for sophisticated gene regulation superimposed on the static DNA code.

Loss of Mitochondrial Homeostasis

Loss of mitochondrial homeostasis is an important mechanism for HSC aging. Just like genomic DNA, mutations of mitochondrial DNA (mtDNA) also accumulate during aging. Indeed, in murine models using the proofreading-deficient mtDNA polymerase, premature aging phenotypes were observed. However, it is still unclear as to whether mtDNA mutations directly lead to aging. Nonetheless, it is well known that accumulations of mtDNA mutations increase with age and lead to mitochondrial dysfunction.

HSCs reside in the relatively hypoxic bone marrow niches because they are exquisitely sensitive to reactive oxygen species (ROS). The oxidative stress imposed by ROS can lead to DNA structural modification and impaired HSC function. Not surprisingly, aging is associated with incremental levels of ROS. As mitochondria is a major source of ROS production, young HSCs have a significantly lower number of mitochondria. Therefore, oxidative stress is an important cause of HSC dysfunction during the aging process.

Changes of Intrinsic Signaling Pathways

Signaling pathways are bridges connecting extracellular stimuli and intracellular response. However, intrinsically altered expression of signaling molecules could also lead to aberrant cellular response, conferring the cells the aging phenotypes.

The Wnt5a-Cdc42 axis is one of the most well identified pathways in HSC aging. The Wnt pathway is a highly conserved pathway across animal species; it regulates gene transcription, cytoskeleton shaping, and calcium homeostasis. Intrinsically increased Wnt5a expression, possibly secondary to epigenetic drift, leading to the activation of Cdc42, a known regulator of cytoskeleton, results in the loss of cellular polarity along with other aging phenotypes. Moreover, genetically modified mice lacking Wnt5a have attenuated aging, and Cdc42 inhibitor CASIN is able to reverse the aging phenotypes in aged HSCs.

Tse's group found a small acidic protein AF1q, originally discovered in patients with AML with chromosomal abnormality t(1;11) (q21;q23), is a critical cofactor in the Wnt signaling pathway. The expression of AF1q is bimodal—significantly upregulated AF1q expression is seen in the early and aged HSC compartment. Activation of AF1q simultaneously enhances multiple signaling pathways closely related to HSC aging, including the Notch pathway and the phosphatidylinositide 3-kinases (PI3k)/Akt (protein kinase B) pathway. AF1q boosts Akt phosphorylation at Thr308 specifically through activation of the signaling of platelet-derived growth factor receptor (PDGFR) with resultant enhanced PDGF-BB expression. The imbalance of PI3k/Akt signaling is associated with aging in various tissues. Taken together, it is hypothesized that AF1q is involved in the aging process through enhanced Akt phosphorylation via PDGFR activation by AF1q-induced PDGF-BB. In addition, the Cdc42-binding protein, SPEC1, shares the same bidirectional transcriptional promoter as AF1q. Therefore, it is also possible that one of the important mechanisms of HSC aging is associated with the switch of the transcriptional direction of the bidirectional promoter (**Figure 94-4**).

EXTRINSIC MECHANISMS OF HSC AGING

In 1978, Schofield first proposed the "niche" concept to describe the microenvironment that maintains and regulates HSCs. In recent years, a growing body of evidence is supporting the hypothesis that HSC aging is not only an autonomous process, but also influenced by the functional changes of the HSC niches. Upon aging, alterations such as imbalanced mesenchymal stromal cell (MSC) differentiation and adrenergic signaling remodeling coordinately

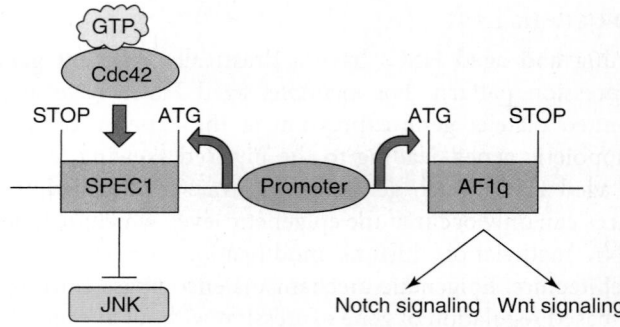

FIGURE 94-4. Illustration of the bidirectional promoter. A bidirectional promoter regulates AF1q and SPEC1, which are actively involved in Wnt and Cdc42 signaling pathways for the hematopoietic stem cell aging process.

regulate the fate of HSCs, leading to myeloid skewing and impaired lymphopoiesis.

The Bone Marrow Niches

During embryonic development, the arteries are responsible for the emergence of HSCs. Similarly, the bone marrow niches for HSCs are also located in the perivascular regions. The bone marrow space is uniformly occupied by sinusoids. However, the peri-endosteal region is highly vascularized by arterioles, which ultimately connect with sinusoids through arterial capillaries. Therefore, the bone marrow consists of two functionally distinct niches, the arteriolar and the sinusoidal niches (**Figure 94-5**). The arteriolar niche is in the periendosteal region; dormant HSCs are predominantly found in this region, where lymphopoiesis preferentially occurs. On the contrary, the sinusoidal niche is highly innervated by sympathetic nerve fibers and

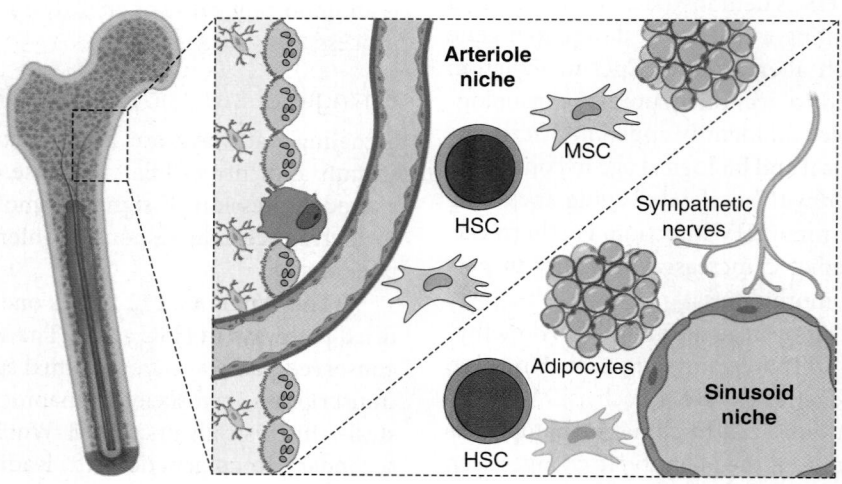

FIGURE 94-5. HSC niches in bone marrow. Two distinct perivascular niches, the arteriole niche and the sinusoidal niche, exist in the bone marrow. The arteriole niche contains dormant HSCs where lymphopoiesis preferentially occurs. The sinusoidal niche is highly innervated by sympathetic nerve fibers and contains less quiescent HSCs, and myelopoiesis mostly takes place in this region. HSC, hematopoietic stem cell; MSC, mesenchymal stem cell.

contains less quiescent HSCs; myelopoiesis mostly takes place in this region.

Location Shift Between Niches During Aging

HSCs redistribute within the bone marrow niches upon aging. It has been well recognized that aged HSCs locate further away from the bone surface than young HSCs. This represents the migration of aged HSCs from the periendosteal arteriolar niche where they remain quiescent, to the sinusoidal niche where they become active in myelopoiesis. Therefore, the aging-related redistribution of HSCs contributes to the impaired lymphopoiesis in older adults.

Mesenchymal Stromal Cell Dysfunction

The cellular components of bone marrow niches consist of endothelial cells, osteoblasts, adipocytes, neuro-glial cells, as well as MSCs. MSCs are multipotent precursors that can differentiate into osteoblasts, adipocytes, and chondrocytes to support HSCs within the niches; they can also secrete inhibitory cytokines and chemokines to help maintain HSCs in the quiescent state. Similar to HSCs, MSCs also experience aging-related dysfunctional changes, such as DNA damage, telomere shortening, elevated ROS, and cell-signaling alterations. These changes lead to impaired osteoblasts differentiation and increased adipogenesis, which are responsible for the increased fat tissues in the bone marrow among the older people.

Sympathetic Nervous System Remodeling

The bone marrow niche is heavily innervated by the sympathetic nervous system. The release of adrenergic neurotransmitter provides a stress signal to the bone marrow, regulating the functions and mobilization of HSCs. In fact, the sympathetic activity is universally elevated in older adults, manifesting as an increased concentration of noradrenaline in the plasma. In the bone marrow, the aging-dependent increase of sympathetic activity can cause myeloid skewing of aging HSCs through activation of a specific type of β-adrenergic receptor.

Immunosenescence, Inflammaging, and Extrinsic Signaling Pathway Changes

Normal aging is associated with systemic, chronic inflammation known as inflammaging. Characterized by low-grade and persistent inflammation in response to physical, chemical, or metabolic noxious stimuli, inflammaging also may develop in response to chronic infections including cytomegalovirus, Epstein–Barr virus, hepatitis C virus, and HIV. These inflammatory responses may damage tissues and organs over time, and contribute to the emergence of multiple comorbidities including cardiovascular disease and autoimmune and neurodegenerative disorders, while also contributing to hematopoietic dysfunction.

The mechanisms of inflammaging are diverse and incompletely understood but may include the expansion of immunosenescent populations of helper (CD4+) and

effector (CD8+) T-cells. These cells are characterized by telomere shortening and a reduced capacity to proliferate, defective mitochondrial function, and increased ROS formation; in addition, they activate proinflammatory pathways including p38 MAP kinase (MAPK) and NF-κB.

Telomeres are repeating hexameric sequences of nucleotides that protect against DNA damage. Located at the ends of chromosomes, telomeres shorten with each replicative cycle, but may be partially restored by enzymatic telomerase activity. DNA damage ensues when telomere shortening exceeds a critical threshold, at which time cells lose their ability to replicate. Senescent T-cells exhibit shortened telomeres with reduced telomerase activity, and they lose their surface expression of CD27 and CD28. CD8+/CD28− cells that reexpress CD45RA (T_{EMRA}) identify a subset of terminally differentiated immunosenescent memory CD8+ T-cells that more specifically associate with age-related adverse clinical outcomes. For example, Alzheimer disease patients have decreased percentages of naïve T-cells, elevated memory cells, and expansion CD28− CD4+ and CD8+ T-cell populations, particularly including CD45RA (T_{EMRA}) cells, compared to healthy young or older adults.

In the hematopoietic system, interleukin-1 (IL-1) induces HSC myeloid skewing and IL-6 promotes thrombopoiesis leading to thrombosis. These cytokines exert their functions through extrinsic signaling pathways. Among them, the NF-κB pathway is involved in the cellular response of a variety of cytokines. Constitutive NF-κB activation in older people, possibly due to inflammaging, leads to hyperproliferation of HSCs with resultant exacerbated myelopoiesis and increased myeloproliferative disorders.

ANEMIA IN THE OLDER ADULT

Burden of Anemia in Older Adults

Anemia, defined by the World Health Organization (WHO) as hemoglobin less than 13 g/dL in men and less than 12 g/dL in women, becomes more common as people age. More than 10% of community-dwelling adults 65 years or older have anemia, and the prevalence grows above 20% in those 85 years or older. Although usually mild, anemia in older adults is associated with a significant increase in mortality and morbidity, such as decreased physical performance, increased falls, impaired cognition, restricted quality of life, and more frequent hospitalization. One would argue if a lower limit of normal hemoglobin should be proposed for older adults. However, large surveillance databases (eg, the NHANES-III database and the Scripps-Kaiser database) have shown that when excluding patients with iron deficiency anemia, elevated creatinine, and elevated ESR or CRP, the mean hemoglobin remains unchanged across different age groups regardless of gender or race. This indicates that although anemia is more common in older adults, the majority is associated with an underlying cause, such as iron deficiency or chronic inflammation. Indeed, as mentioned above, most aged HSCs remain dormant, and can only turn into active states under demand or stress. Therefore, aging is associated with defective stress-induced hematopoiesis, which would not be apparent under normal situations.

Causes of Anemia in the Older Adult

The prevalence of different causes of anemia varies in different studies. Nevertheless, the major causes of anemia include iron deficiency anemia (12%–20%), anemia of chronic inflammation (6%–20%), chronic kidney disease (4%–8%), folate or vitamin B_{12} deficiency (0%–14%), MDS (9%–16%), or malignant hematologic disorder (0%–2%). If none of the above causes can be found, the anemia is defined as unexplained anemia of the elderly (UAE), which ranges from 34% to 44% in different studies. It has been questioned whether UAE represents a real entity or is just the result of an unidentified underlying cause. Indeed, smaller studies with more extensive work-up find a significant portion of UAE is due to insufficient erythropoietin (EPO) production without impaired excretory renal function or chronic kidney disease. To date, the cause of insufficient EPO production older adults is yet to be discovered. Recently, there has been increasing enthusiasm to study the correlation between clonal hematopoiesis and anemia. However, although clonal hematopoiesis is more frequently detected in individuals with anemia, the relative difference is small between anemic people and controls, suggesting that the mutations do not account for the majority of UAE. Lastly, UAE may occur after an unidentified bone marrow stress, and anemia develops as a result of aging-related impaired stress-induced hematopoiesis.

Evaluation of Anemia

Initial work-up for anemia in older adults includes a complete blood count with differential, reticulocyte count, ferritin, iron studies, creatinine, vitamin B_{12}, red blood cell folate, thyroid function test, and liver function test. These tests help clinicians rule out the most common causes of anemia, including iron deficiency, nutritional deficiency, and chronic kidney disease. If the above tests are nonrevealing, further work-ups such as EPO level, copper, zinc, C-reactive protein, lactate dehydrogenase, haptoglobin, and serum electrophoresis could be pursued to rule out more rare causes. At last, if a hematological malignancy is suspected, bone marrow aspiration and biopsy are mandatory to exclude disorders such as MDS or leukemia.

Management of Anemia in Older Adults

Treatment for anemia should be "age-adjusted" with recognition of potential side effects and impact on the quality of life. For frail patients, even a weekly clinic visit for injection could be burdensome and significantly affect their quality of life.

In patients with iron deficiency anemia, oral iron substitution would be sufficient in most cases. However, the efficacy of daily dosing of oral iron has been questioned as iron supplements increase hepcidin level for up to 24 hours and are associated with lower iron absorption on the following day. Thus, every-other-day dosing of oral iron is generally

preferred over daily dosing. In situations when oral iron does not ameliorate anemia or the patient does not tolerate oral iron, intravenous iron is an effective alternative. Different formulations of intravenous iron exist, such as iron sucrose, ferric gluconate, and ferric carboxymaltose, which are all generally well tolerated.

Erythropoiesis-stimulating agents (ESAs) are analogs of EPO and widely used in end-stage renal disease–related anemia and patients with MDS with moderate to severe anemia. Data on application of ESAs in other causes of anemia including UAE are limited.

Blood transfusion is the most effective treatment for acute symptomatic anemia. For the transfusion threshold, we generally use the cutoff hemoglobin level recommended by the AABB—7 g/dL for the general population and 8 g/dL for patients with symptoms of end-organ ischemia. However, older anemic patients should always be transfused with the recognition of comorbidities. Transfusion threshold and frequency may differ based on many factors and should be evaluated on a case-by-case basis. For example, in a patient with chronic hemolytic anemia who is otherwise asymptomatic from a baseline hemoglobin of 6 g/dL, aiming a higher hemoglobin goal of 7 g/dL would only increase the frequency of transfusion without improving quality of life.

CONCLUSION

Clearly, there are biological features and properties that distinguish young and aged HSCs (**Table 94-1**). These differences provide insights into pathogenic mechanisms

TABLE 94-1 ■ PROPERTIES OF YOUNG AND AGED HEMATOPOIETIC STEM CELLS (HSCS)

PROPERTIES	YOUNG HSCS	AGED HSCS
Hematopoietic skewing	Balanced	Myelopoiesis skewing
Clonal hematopoiesis	Minimal	Common
Self-renewal	Brisk	Restricted
Intrinsic changes		
DNA damage	Minimal	Accumulated
Epigenetic modification	Normal	Local hypo- or hypermethylation
Mitochondria	Normal	mtDNA mutation, ROS production
Signaling pathway	Canonical Wnt signaling	Non-canonical Wnt signaling
Extrinsic changes		
Niche switch	Arteriole niche	Sinusoidal niche
MSC function	Normal	Dysfunctional
Sympathetic activity	Suppressed	Activated
Proinflammatory cytokine	Reduced	Elevated

MSC, mesenchymal stem cells; mtDNA, mitochondrial DNA; ROS, reactive oxygen species.

of diseases, especially the increased risk of immunologic, hematologic, myelodysplastic, and HSC-proliferative disorders that so frequently accompany aging. Furthermore, aging affects not only the cellular or the HSC compartment, but also the bone marrow microenvironment. With improved understanding of the fundamental molecular events contributing to these pathogenic changes, there have been prospects to develop mechanism-based therapeutic interventions to preserve and maintain normal hematopoiesis. This may provide opportunities to prevent these diseases and further identify, in a more rational manner, novel therapeutic approaches in treating these disorders in older adults.

FURTHER READING

Barbe-Tuana F, Funchal G, Schmitz CRR, Maurmann RM, Bauer ME. The interplay between immunosenescence and age-related diseases. *Semin Immunopathol.* 2020;42(5):545–557.

Furman D, Campisi J, Verdin E, et al. Chronic inflammation in the etiology of disease across the life span. *Nat Med.* 2019;25(12):1822–1832.

Gate D, Saligrama N, Leventhal O, et al. Clonally expanded CD8 T cells patrol the cerebrospinal fluid in Alzheimer's disease. *Nature.* 2020;577(7790):399–404.

Gross AM, Jaeger PA, Kreisberg JF, et al. Methylome-wide analysis of chronic HIV infection reveals five-year increase in biological age and epigenetic targeting of HLA. *Mol Cell.* 2016;62(2):157–168.

Henson SM, Lanna A, Riddell NE, et al. p38 signaling inhibits mTORC1-independent autophagy in senescent human CD8(+) T cells. *J Clin Invest.* 2014;124(9): 4004–4016.

Horvath S. DNA methylation age of human tissues and cell types. *Genome Biol.* 2013;14(10):R115.

Horvath S, Garagnani P, Bacalini MG, et al. Accelerated epigenetic aging in Down syndrome. *Aging Cell.* 2015;14(3):491–495.

Horvath S, Levine AJ. HIV-1 infection accelerates age according to the epigenetic clock. *J Infect Dis.* 2015; 212(10):1563–1573.

Larbi A, Pawelec G, Witkowski JM, et al. Dramatic shifts in circulating CD4 but not CD8 T cell subsets in mild Alzheimer's disease. *J Alzheimers Dis.* 2009;17(1):91–103.

Marioni RE, Shah S, McRae AF, et al. DNA methylation age of blood predicts all-cause mortality in later life. *Genome Biol.* 2015;16:25.

Salminen A, Kauppinen A, Suuronen T, Kaarniranta K. SIRT1 longevity factor suppresses NF-kappaB -driven immune responses: regulation of aging via NF-kappaB acetylation? *Bioessays.* 2008;30(10):939–942.

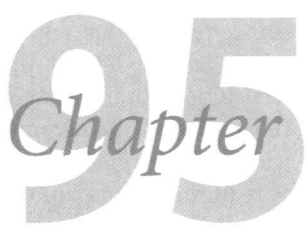

Chapter 95

Hematologic Malignancies (Leukemia/Lymphoma) and Plasma Cell Disorders

Anita J. Kumar, Tanya M. Wildes, Heidi D. Klepin, Bayard L. Powell

INTRODUCTION

Hematologic malignancies represent varied diseases ranging from indolent to aggressive. Symptoms, treatments, and natural history vary widely. Hematologic malignancies include myeloid malignancies (ie, myelodysplastic syndromes, acute myeloid leukemia, myeloproliferative disorders) and lymphoid malignancies (chronic lymphocytic leukemia, lymphomas, and plasma cell neoplasms). Older adults make up a large proportion of incident and prevalent cases of these diseases as well as those dying from these conditions. As the population ages, the burden of these diseases will rise affecting older adults disproportionately.

The effectiveness of treatments has improved substantially over recent decades for most hematologic malignancies. Unfortunately, the response rates and cure rates for older patients have lagged behind for a number of reasons, including in some cases: more resistant tumor biology, presence of multiple chronic conditions, and functional impairments that decrease treatment tolerance. Underrepresentation of older adults in clinical trials remains a limitation. With the increased focus on clinical trials designed specifically for older adults and the ongoing development of less toxic, targeted therapies, opportunities for effective treatment of older adults with hematologic malignancies continue to improve.

MYELODYSPLASTIC SYNDROMES

Myelodysplastic syndromes (MDS) are a heterogenous group of clonal hematopoietic disorders characterized by ineffective hematopoiesis and peripheral blood cytopenias. In these diseases, cells of the affected lineage are unable to undergo maturation and differentiation, resulting in cytopenias. MDS can be indolent or progress rapidly to bone marrow failure. The major clinical significance of these disorders is the morbidity associated with profound cytopenias and the potential to evolve into acute myeloid leukemia (AML). MDS is associated with impaired quality of life and high health care utilization with an estimated 3-year survival rate of 45%. Approximately 15,000 to 20,000 new cases are diagnosed annually in the United States, and about 80% of these are among adults older than age 70.

Learning Objectives

- Recognize presentation, workup, and management of common hematologic malignancies in older adults.
- Recognize the value of geriatric assessment to personalize care for older adults with hematologic malignancies.
- Recognize treatment approaches for older adults diagnosed with common hematologic malignancies.

Key Clinical Points

1. Older adults make up a large proportion of incident and prevalent hematologic disorders, as well as those dying from these conditions.

2. The response rates and cure rates for older patients with hematologic disorders have lagged behind those of young adults for a number of reasons: more resistant tumor biology, presence of multiple chronic conditions, and functional impairments that decrease treatment tolerance. Underrepresentation of older adults in clinical trials remains a limitation as well.

3. Myelodysplastic syndromes can be indolent or progress rapidly to bone marrow failure; treatment should be risk-adapted based on disease and patient characteristics.

4. Antileukemic therapy improves survival for most older adults with acute myeloid leukemia.

5. Oral tyrosine kinase inhibitors provide long-term disease control for older adults with chronic myelogenous leukemia.

6. Chronic lymphocytic leukemia (CLL) is the most common leukemia in the Western Hemisphere and may be expected to be encountered in a geriatric practice. Older symptomatic patients with and without comorbidity can benefit from targeted therapy regimens.

(Cont.)

7. Modern classification systems for lymphomas are evolving rapidly and incorporate immunophenotyping and genetics.

8. Comorbidity and frailty are strong modifiers of prognosis and must be incorporated into treatment planning.

9. Immunotherapies play an increasing role in treatment of some lymphomas; consider life expectancy and potential toxicity when planning treatment.

10. Plasma cell disorders (PCDs) are among the few neoplasms where routine laboratory testing other than by tissue biopsy can detect a clonal population by detection of monoclonal protein in the serum or urine.

11. Male gender and African-American race are risk factors for all PCDs.

12. All patients with PCDs require evaluation for associated abnormalities, that is, "CRAB" criteria: hypercalcemia, renal insufficiency, anemia, or bone lesions.

13. Prevention of complications in those with multiple myeloma includes intravenous bisphosphonates to reduce the risk of pathologic fractures or painful lytic lesions requiring radiation; and infection prophylaxis with pneumococcal vaccine, annual influenza vaccine, and, for patients receiving certain treatments, herpes zoster prophylaxis with acyclovir or valacyclovir.

Diagnosis and Work-Up

Diagnosis of MDS relies mainly on peripheral blood and bone marrow findings. The diagnosis should be suspected in older individuals presenting with cytopenia. In clinical studies, the majority of patients have a hemoglobin of less than 11, platelet count less than 100,000, and an absolute neutrophil count less than 1000 at the time of diagnosis. However, careful attention should be paid to consistent decreases in blood counts over time in an older adult, which may signify early developing MDS. A frequent presentation is progressive macrocytic anemia in an older adult followed by developing pancytopenia. Many patients are asymptomatic at the time of diagnosis. However, careful history-taking should include questions regarding recurrent infections, bruising, and bleeding. The differential diagnosis for suspected MDS includes AML, aplastic anemia, megaloblastic anemia (B_{12} and folate deficiency), copper deficiency, viral infections (HIV), large granular lymphocytic leukemia, and heavy metal poisoning.

The initial serologic work-up includes a complete blood count (CBC) with differential, reticulocyte count, RBC folate, serum B_{12}, iron studies, and review of the peripheral smear. Classic peripheral blood findings associated with MDS include macrocytosis and hypogranular, hypolobated (dysplastic) neutrophils. A bone marrow biopsy with cytogenetic analysis is required to confirm the diagnosis. The bone marrow is typically hypercellular and demonstrates evidence of dysplasia. Cytogenetic abnormalities play a critical role in the diagnosis and natural history of MDS. Common cytogenetic abnormalities involve chromosomes 5, 7, 8, 17, or 20.

Risk Stratification

The World Health Organization (WHO) classification scheme incorporates evolving knowledge of the biology of disease including the significance of cytogenetic abnormalities and highlights the heterogeneity of MDS. The International Prognostic Scoring System (IPSS) was developed to risk stratify patients at the time of diagnosis based on cytogenetic, morphologic, and clinical data. The IPSS for MDS was derived from an analysis of 816 patients, 75% of whom were older than 60 years. The IPSS incorporates specific cytogenetic abnormalities, the percentage of marrow blasts in the bone marrow, and the number of hematopoietic lineages involved in the cytopenia. Risk scores are determined based on these variables, and a categorization of low risk, intermediate-1, intermediate-2, and high risk is assigned. These categories can differentiate patients with median survival of more than 5 years at diagnosis (low risk) from those with less than 1-year survival (high risk). Another risk stratification system proposed by the WHO includes additional variables shown to add prognostic information including multilineage dysplasia, severe anemia, or transfusion dependency. This system can be used both at diagnosis and after progression to predict survival. A five-category revised IPSS was developed using over 7000 patients (median age 71) that differs by further subdividing cytogenetic abnormalities and increasing the weight of higher blast percentages. In the development cohort, age was a prognostic factor for survival but not for progression to AML, having more impact in lower- versus higher-risk disease. The revised IPSS is commonly used and represented in **Tables 95-1** and **95-2**.

Selection of treatment for patients with MDS depends not only on disease risk stratification but on assessment of a patient's overall fitness and competing comorbid conditions. Most patients with MDS have additional comorbidity, and higher comorbidity burden has been associated with shorter survival independent of age or disease risk. A prospective study investigating the predictive utility of a geriatric assessment among older adults treated nonintensively for MDS ($N = 51$) and AML ($N = 69$) found that requiring assistance with activities of daily living (ADLs) and high fatigue rating were independently associated with shorter survival. Another study showed that

TABLE 95-1 ■ REVISED INTERNATIONAL PROGNOSTIC SCORING SYSTEM (IPSS) FOR MYELODYSPLASTIC SYNDROMES

PROGNOSTIC VARIABLE	SCORE						
	0	0.5	1.0	1.5	2.0	3.0	4.0
Cytogenetics[a]	Very good		Good		Intermediate	Poor	Very poor
Bone marrow blasts (%)	< 2		> 2 to < 5		5–10	> 10	
Hemoglobin (g/dL)	> 10		8 to < 10	< 8			
Platelets (cells/μL)	≥ 100	50–100	< 50				
Absolute neutrophil count (cells/μL)	≥ 0.8	< 0.8					

[a]Very good: −Y, del (11q); Good: Normal, del(5q), del(12p), double including del (5q); Intermediate: del (7q), +8, +19, i(17q), and other single or double independent clones; Poor: −7, inv(3)/del(3q), double including -7/del(7q), complex: 3 abnormalities; Very poor: complex: > 3 abnormalities.
Data from Greenberg PL, Tuechler H, Schanz J, et al. Revised international prognostic scoring system for myelodysplastic syndromes. Blood. 2012;120(12):2454–2465.

requiring assistance with instrumental activities of daily living (IADLs), impaired cognition, or mobility limitation were associated with higher likelihood to discontinue therapy early. Studies evaluating strategies for assessing frailty among MDS patients are presented in **Table 95-3**. Use of geriatric assessment and frailty screening can assist in treatment decision-making and guide supportive care.

Treatment

Treatment strategies emphasize targeting higher-risk MDS and subgroups defined by specific cytogenetic abnormalities. Current treatment recommendations involve a risk-adapted therapeutic approach (outlined in **Table 95-4**). Supportive care, aimed at controlling symptoms related to cytopenias, is indicated for all patients and is the mainstay of treatment for lower-risk patients or frail patients. Supportive care often includes red cell and platelet transfusions and antibiotics for infection. Hematopoietic growth factors such as erythropoietin are used to try to minimize transfusion requirements in responding patients. Those most likely to benefit have lower risk IPSS-R scores, serum erythropoietin level less than 500 mU/mL, low transfusion requirement, and shorter interval between diagnosis and treatment. A subcutaneously administered recombinant fusion protein targeting Smad2/3 signaling, luspatercept-aamt, decreased transfusion requirements for patients with low-/intermediate-risk MDS with ringed sideroblasts that failed to respond to erythropoiesis stimulating agents. Many MDS patients are also at risk for iron overload due to transfusion dependence. Iron chelation therapy should be initiated for those with lower-risk MDS, ongoing transfusion dependence, and expected survival greater than 1 year.

Patients in the higher-risk IPSS categories are more likely to experience morbidity related to cytopenias and to progress to acute leukemia in a shorter time interval from diagnosis. Hypomethylating agents which inhibit DNA methyltransferases (azacitidine and decitabine) represent the mainstay of treatment for most patients. Randomized studies with azacitidine compared to placebo have shown improvements in survival, quality of life, and a longer time to progression to acute leukemia, in patients with MDS. A survival advantage exists even for those greater than 75 years. The Food and Drug Administration (FDA) also approved decitabine for the treatment of higher-risk MDS. Decitabine decreases transfusion requirements and symptoms although has not shown a definitive survival benefit in randomized trials. A challenge for older adults using hypomethylating agents is myelosuppression which often worsens for several months before response is detectable. The duration of treatment can be challenging as well with most clinical trials treating for more than 6 months for all patients and more than 12 months for responders.

TABLE 95-2 ■ OVERALL SURVIVAL AND RISK OF AML EVOLUTION BY REVISED IPSS SCORE

RISK GROUP	IPSS-R SCORE	MEDIAN OVERALL SURVIVAL (YEARS)	MEDIAN TIME TO 25% AML EVOLUTION (YEARS)
Very low	< 1.5	8.8	> 14.5
Low	< 1.5–3.0	5.3	10.8
Intermediate	> 3–4.5	3.0	3.2
High	> 4.5–6	1.6	1.4
Very high	> 6	0.8	0.7

Data from Greenberg PL, Tuechler H, Schanz J, et al. Revised international prognostic scoring system for myelodysplastic syndromes, Blood. 2012;120(12):2454–2465.

TABLE 95-3 ■ FRAILTY MEASURES FOR MYELODYSPLASTIC SYNDROMES

FRAILTY MEASURE	MEASURE DESCRIPTION	OUTCOME
Clinical frailty scale	9-item descriptive scale based on physician judgment	Overall survival
MDS-specific frailty index	42-item deficit accumulation index (DAFI)	Overall survival
MDS-specific frailty index	15-item DAFI-weighted toward available labs and fatigue, assistance with food preparation, and 4-m walk time	Overall survival

TABLE 95-4 ■ TREATMENT OPTIONS FOR OLDER ADULTS WITH MDS BASED ON DISEASE AND PATIENT CHARACTERISTICS

DISEASE CHARACTERISTICS (REVISED IPSS)	GOAL OF THERAPY	PATIENT CHARACTERISTICS	TREATMENT CONSIDERATIONS
Very low, low risk and asymptomatic	Improve QOL	Any	Observation
Very low/low/intermediate risk and symptomatic			
5q deletion	Improve QOL	Any	Lenalidomide
Absence of 5q– with erythropoietin level < 500	Improve QOL	Any	Erythropoietin+/– GCSF Consider luspatercept if erythropoietin fails Consider lenalidomide
	Improve QOL	Good performance status/ minimal comorbidity	Consider hypomethylating agents
Intermediate/high/very high risk	Delay progression, extend life	Any age, good performance status, absence of major comorbidity	Hypomethylating agents (ie, azacitidine)
	Cure	Age 60–75, excellent performance status, absence of major comorbidity	Consider referral for RIC HSCT versus hypomethylating agents. Comprehensive geriatric assessment may help inform "fitness"
	Delay progression, extend life	Poor performance status and/ or major comorbidity	Consider hypomethylating agents versus supportive care

GCSF, granulocyte colony-stimulating factor; HSCT, hematopoietic stem cell transplantation; RIC, reduced-intensity conditioning; QOL, quality of life.
Adapted with permission from Klepin HD, Rao AV, Pardee TS. Acute myeloid leukemia and myelodysplastic syndromes in older adults, J Clin Oncol. 2014;32(24):2541–2552.

Patients with the 5q– syndrome, defined by a deletion of the long arm of chromosome 5 as the sole abnormality, tend to present with refractory, severe anemia, and a relatively normal platelet count. It is considered a more favorable MDS subset because a large percentage of patients do not progress to acute leukemia. Lenalidomide, an oral immunomodulatory drug, significantly decreases transfusion requirements and demonstrates reversal of cytogenetic abnormalities in patients with 5q– syndrome, which may translate into improved quality of life. The primary toxicity is myelosuppression which can result in dose reductions and dose delays. Careful attention to dosing is required with adjustments needed for mild impairment in renal function which is common among older adults. This drug is a standard of care treatment for transfusion-dependent patients with 5q– syndrome and reinforces the clinical and therapeutic importance of cytogenetic evaluation in MDS. Studies suggest it also has efficacy in patients with low-risk MDS without 5q deletion and may be considered for these patients as well if they are transfusion dependent.

Higher-intensity therapy such as allogeneic stem cell transplantation, to date the only curative therapy for MDS, is generally restricted to younger adults with acceptable donors because of the high morbidity and mortality associated with therapy. However, with use of reduced-intensity conditioning regimens (RIC), stem cell transplantation is considered for selected adults between ages 60 to 80 with good functional status and minimal comorbidity. Hematopoietic stem cell transplantation (HSCT) can result

in appreciable survival rates among patients with high-risk disease. However, most older adults in this context are age less than 70 with minimal data for those greater than 75. The real-world applicability of transplantation for most older adults with high-risk MDS will require refined definitions of "fitness" and collection of outcomes such as quality of life, functional independence, and health care utilization to inform treatment decisions. Evidence supports the use of geriatric assessment to identify vulnerabilities that increase morbidity associated with transplant (functional dependence and cognitive impairment) and to inform supportive care optimization to enhance resilience.

ACUTE MYELOID LEUKEMIA

AML refers to a group of clonal hematopoietic disorders that are characterized by proliferation of immature myeloid cells in the bone marrow. Accumulation of leukemic cells impairs the normal hematopoietic function of the bone marrow, resulting in cytopenias with or without leukocytosis.

AML is a disease of older adults, with a median age at diagnosis between 68 and 72; approximately one-third are greater than or equal to 75 years. Risk factors for the development of AML include a history of preceding MDS, exposure to certain chemotherapy drugs (alkylating agents, topoisomerase 2 inhibitors, and nitrosoureas), radiation or benzene exposure, and a history of Down syndrome. The majority of diagnosed cases of AML, however, are not linked to any known risk factor.

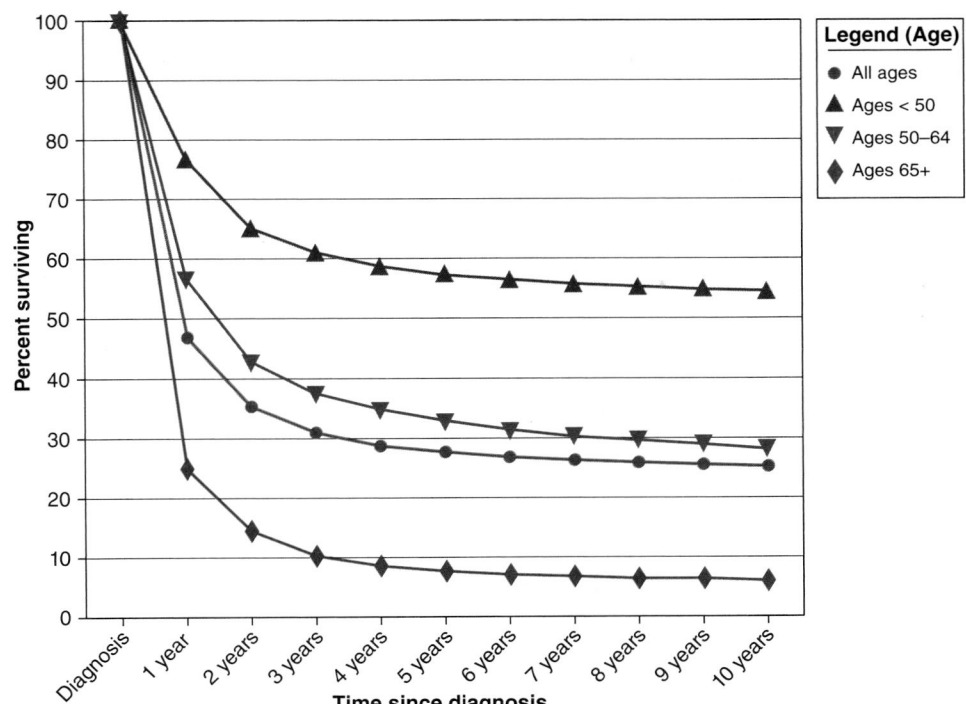

FIGURE 95-1. Acute myeloid leukemia (AML) SEER survival rates by time since diagnosis, 2000–2017. All stages by age, both sexes, all races (includes Hispanic). (Reproduced with permission from SEER: Surveillance, Epidemiology, and End Result.)

The clinical signs and symptoms of AML can be varied and nonspecific. Patients usually present with evidence of bone marrow failure: anemia, thrombocytopenia, granulocytopenia. Fatigue, dyspnea, bleeding, fever, and infection are common upon presentation. Leukemic infiltration of tissues outside the bone marrow such as liver, spleen, skin, lymph nodes, and central nervous system (CNS) can produce a variety of other symptoms specific to the site of involvement. Some patients present with severe leukocytosis, which can produce symptoms of leukostasis as a result of a large blast fraction in the peripheral blood. Peripheral blood findings range from pancytopenia with or without circulating blasts cells to severe leukocytosis with circulating blasts typically with anemia and thrombocytopenia.

Diagnosis

The diagnosis of AML depends primarily on detection of leukemic blasts of myeloid lineage (≥ 20%) in the bone marrow. Morphologic evaluation can be aided by immunohistochemical and flow cytometry techniques to confirm myeloid versus lymphoid origin. The WHO classification of AML incorporates morphologic, immunophenotypic, genetic, and clinical features. Identification of genetic and molecular abnormalities have highlighted the heterogeneity of AML and identified subsets associated with better or worse prognosis. For example, the core binding factor leukemias [inv 16, t(8;21), t(16;16)] and acute promyelocytic leukemia [t(15;17)] are associated with better prognosis.

The presence of mutations in *FLT-3* in tumors with normal karyotype is associated with worse overall survival. Risk-adapted treatment strategies have been developed to maximize clinical outcomes and minimize toxicity based on cytogenetic classification. In addition, molecular abnormalities are increasingly identified as treatment targets.

Treatment

If untreated or unresponsive to chemotherapy, AML may be rapidly fatal (median survival < 2 months). The major causes of death are overwhelming infection and hemorrhage related to the disease-associated cytopenias. AML is one of the most dramatic examples of age-related outcome disparity in oncology (**Figures 95-1 and 95-2**). In general, older adults (commonly defined as age ≥ 60) experience higher morbidity and mortality rates with treatment compared with those younger than 60 years. Concerns regarding the efficacy and toxicity of therapies have resulted in a large proportion of older adults in the United States receiving no therapy for the disease. However, it is clear from both clinical trial and population-based data that chemotherapy can provide a survival benefit over supportive care for many older adults.

Age-related treatment disparity is due to both disease and patient-related factors. The biology of AML differs among older adults compared to younger patients. Cytogenetic abnormalities are the most important prognostic factor in AML. As a group, older patients with

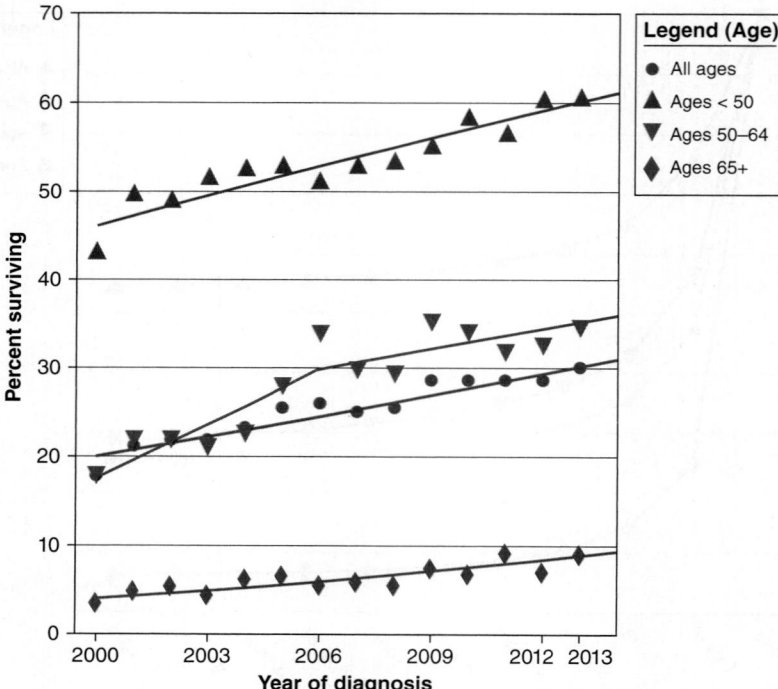

FIGURE 95-2. Acute myeloid leukemia (AML) trends in SEER relative 5 year survival rates, 2000–2013. All stages by age, both sexes, all races (includes Hispanic). (Reproduced with permission from SEER: Surveillance, Epidemiology, and End Result.)

AML have a higher percentage of unfavorable cytogenetic abnormalities and a lower percentage of favorable cytogenetic abnormalities compared to younger patients. Unfavorable cytogenetic abnormalities are associated with decreased rates of remission and shortened overall survival. In addition, expression of MDR1, which confers resistance to chemotherapeutic agents, is more common in older AML patients. Older patients are more likely to have a secondary AML arising from underlying MDS, which is less responsive to standard therapy. Finally, age-related changes in the bone marrow microenvironment influence outcomes for older adults. Overall, AML in older patients is more resistant to available therapies, resulting in lower remission rates and higher chance of relapse after achieving remission. In addition, patient-factors such as comorbidity and functional limitations influence treatment tolerance. While older age (particularly > 75 years) is consistently associated with worse outcomes, treatment toxicity and benefit are inadequately predicted by age alone.

For nonacute promyelocytic AML, treatment strategies include intensive therapy, less intensive therapy, or best supportive care (BSC). Randomized studies have shown consistent survival advantage for antileukemic therapy over BSC. Currently BSC alone should be considered for the minority of older adults who have pre-existing frailty, limited non-AML life expectancy, or express a preference to forgo therapy in favor of hospice after informed discussion. Treatment at specialized leukemia centers should be prioritized when possible.

In general, intensive induction chemotherapy (inclusive of anthracycline and cytarabine) is recommended for those older adults with minimal comorbidity and good functional status who also have favorable or intermediate risk disease. For those patients with *FLT3* mutated AML, the multitargeted kinase inhibitor midostaurin should be added given the survival advantage seen in the pivotal trial despite the lack of inclusion of older adults. The goal of treatment is to achieve remission and proceed to tailored post-remission therapy to render long-term disease-free survivorship. Another advance for older adults is the availability of CPX-351, a dual-drug liposomal encapsulation of cytarabine and daunorubicin, which improved survival for older adults (aged 60–75) with secondary AML (ie, therapy-related, antecedent MDS), a group with historically poor outcomes.

Many older adults may not be considered "fit" for treatment with intensive chemotherapy or may prefer an alternate approach. Single-agent DNA hypomethylating agents (eg, azacitidine and decitabine) and low-dose cytarabine have both been shown to improve outcomes compared to BSC. Recently, the addition of the BCL-2 inhibitor venetoclax to azacitidine, decitabine, or low-dose cytarabine has become a standard of care option with improved remission rates and survival compared to single-agent therapy. In the registration trial, which defined "unfit" for intensive therapy by age greater than or equal to 75 or 60 to 74 years with comorbidity (ie, congestive heart failure, creatinine clearance 30–45 mL/min, pulmonary disease, or other comorbidity per physician judgement), the median overall survival improved from 10 to 15 months. Side effects of cytopenias and infections were more common on the combination arm.

Patients who achieve remission should be evaluated for post-remission therapy in an attempt to prevent or delay relapse. Optimal post-remission therapy in older patients remains poorly defined. Oral azacitidine maintenance provides a survival advantage for patients who are not candidates for allogeneic transplantation. An increasing number of older adults who achieve remission are being referred for reduced-intensity allogeneic transplantation in an effort to improve longer-term disease-free survival and cure rates.

Geriatric assessment can be feasibly performed in the setting of AML therapy and it adds information to standard clinical assessment. For example, in a prospective study of adults age greater than or equal to 60 who received intensive therapy, pretreatment geriatric assessment detected significant impairments: cognitive impairment, 24%; depression, 26%; distress, 50%; ADL impairment, 34%; impaired physical performance, 31%; and comorbidity, 40%. Importantly, most patients on study were impaired in one (92.6%) or more (63%) measured characteristics. Impaired cognition (modified Mini Mental Status Examination < 77) and physical performance (short physical performance battery < 9) were independently associated with worse survival. Geriatric assessment measures including dependence in ADLs and higher comorbidity burden have also been predictive of survival among older adults receiving lesser intensive therapy. Similarly, a role for geriatric assessment is emerging to identify older adults who may tolerate allogenic transplantation as post-remission therapy. Understanding specific patient vulnerabilities is imperative to help to predict tolerance to standard therapies and identify targets for intervention to improve treatment tolerance.

Treatment recommendations differ for patients with acute promyelocytic leukemia (APL). APL is characterized by a translocation between chromosomes 15 and 17 leading to the fusion of the promyelocytic leukemia (PML) gene with the retinoic acid receptor α (RARα) gene, resulting in disruption of normal cell differentiation. While less common among older adults, this disease has a very high response and cure rate with current therapies that include use of all-trans retinoic acid (ATRA), which overcomes the differentiation block. A unique clinical feature of APL is presentation with bleeding secondary to disseminated intravascular coagulation and requires emergent treatment. Hemorrhage is a frequent cause of early mortality, particularly if untreated. When suspected, treatment with ATRA should begin immediately. Curative treatment includes induction with ATRA with either arsenic trioxide (ATO) for patients with WBC less than or equal to 10,000/μL, or plus an anthracycline for patients with WBC greater than 10,000/μL. Induction therapy is followed by consolidation with ATRA plus ATO-based therapy, with remission and disease-free survival rates of approximately 90%. In addition, relapsed patients may respond to ATO, with a high proportion achieving a second remission. This subtype of AML should be treated aggressively in older adults given the high probability of response. Effective non-chemotherapy regimens extend therapeutic options to the extremes of age and for vulnerable and frail older adults.

CHRONIC MYELOGENOUS LEUKEMIA

Chronic myelogenous leukemia (CML) is a myeloproliferative disorder characterized by excess production of mature granulocytes that eventually progresses to a clinical picture similar to acute leukemia with an overgrowth of immature cells (blast crisis). CML is associated with the fusion of two genes: BCR (on chromosome 22) and ALB1 (on chromosome 9). It accounts for a little over 10% of all leukemias. The incidence increases with age, and the average age at diagnosis is approximately 65 years.

Diagnosis is suspected by the demonstration of granulocytosis in the peripheral blood with a predominance of segmented neutrophils and myelocytes, increased basophils and eosinophils, and increased bone marrow cellularity. The presence of the Philadelphia chromosome t(9;22) and/or its products (BCR/ABL fusion mRNA, Bcr/Abl protein) are required to confirm the diagnosis. Diagnosis can be made on peripheral blood using PCR or fluorescent in situ hybridization (FISH) techniques. Bone marrow biopsy is still required for complete cytogenetic evaluation.

The disease characteristically proceeds through three phases: chronic (present in ~ 85% at diagnosis), accelerated, and terminal (blastic) phase (**Table 95-5**). The length

TABLE 95-5 ■ CHRONIC MYELOGENOUS LEUKEMIA CLASSIFICATION		
CHRONIC PHASE	**ACCELERATED PHASE**	**BLAST PHASE**
< 10% blasts	Any of the following: 10%–19% blasts Thrombocytopenia < 100,000/mcL Thrombocytosis > 1,000,000 unresponsive to therapy Peripheral basophilia > 20% Appearance of additional cytogenetic abnormality Increasing spleen size or progressive leukocytosis on therapy	Any of the following: ≥ 20% blasts Extramedullary blasts or large foci/clusters of blasts in the bone marrow

of the chronic phase is highly variable. In the chronic phase, the disease is easily controlled without aggressive therapy. Many patients are asymptomatic (diagnosis prompted by leukocytosis), common symptoms include fatigue, weight loss, and abdominal fullness or pain related to splenomegaly. The accelerated phase begins with gradual increases in white cells, platelets, and spleen size. Initially good maturation persists, but eventually more blasts are seen in the peripheral blood. The terminal phase of the disease is indistinguishable from acute leukemia. The blasts have myeloid surface markers in 85% of the patients and lymphoid markers in the remaining 15%.

Treatment for CML has changed dramatically in the past decades, altering the natural history of this disease. Imatinib mesylate (Gleevec; STI-571), a targeted tyrosine kinase inhibitor (TKI), designed specifically for the treatment of CML (in oral formulation), proved to have significant activity in the blast phase and accelerated phase of CML. In chronic phase CML, imatinib mesylate yielded marked improvements in clinical and cytogenetic responses, rates of disease progression, and treatment-related toxicity compared to previously used IFN-α plus low-dose ara-C in a randomized clinical trial. Based on these results, imatinib mesylate replaced interferon regimens as the standard of care for patients with chronic phase CML. Imatinib is very well tolerated, which is particularly relevant for the older adult population. Responses are durable with many patients maintaining response now after well over a decade of therapy. More potent, second-generation, tyrosine kinase inhibitors (ie, dasatinib, nilotinib, bosutinib) produce more rapid and better responses than imatinib in first-line treatment although no difference in overall survival has been demonstrated to date. These drugs are also active in patients who have progressed on imatinib providing sequential treatment options prior to consideration of cytotoxic therapy. Adherence to daily administration is critical for successful treatment of CML with careful monitoring of response to determine when other therapies should be considered. PCR techniques provide a highly sensitive and reliable method to monitor response to treatments. Long-term follow-up data from imatinib clinical trials show that cytogenetic and molecular responses are durable and there are low rates of cumulative or late toxic effects. Choice if first line therapy for CML for older adults is informed by concurrent comorbid conditions such as heart failure, risk of cardiotoxicity, QT prolongation, and thrombosis. Imatinib has the longest term safety data and remains an appealing standard for many older adults.

Allogeneic stem cell transplantation in the chronic phase remains a consideration for curative treatment for younger patients, primarily those with suboptimal response to TKIs. It has minimal role in older patients because of the morbidity and mortality of this treatment and availability of therapies to control disease. TKIs should be the initial treatment for both the accelerated and blastic phases of

CML if not already used during the chronic phase of the disease although responses are often short lived. Treatment of the blastic transformation (after TKI therapy) depends on the cell origin of the blasts. Myeloid blastic states respond poorly to standard AML therapies, and no standard therapy is available. Lymphoid blastic states can be controlled for 6 to 12 months, with standard combination regimens as used for de novo acute lymphoblastic leukemia.

CHRONIC LYMPHOCYTIC LEUKEMIA

Chronic lymphocytic leukemia (CLL) is the most common leukemia in the Western Hemisphere and may be commonly encountered in a geriatric practice. CLL is a disorder of clonal proliferation of mature lymphoid cells in the peripheral blood, bone marrow, and lymphoid organs. CLL occurs predominantly in older adults, with median age at diagnosis of approximately 70. About 21,250 new cases were estimated in the United States for 2021 by the American Cancer Society. This may be an underestimate because many patients are asymptomatic for years. There is no racial difference in the United States, and a slight male predominance. Current diagnostic studies, especially immunophenotyping, allow for differentiation of the chronic lymphoid malignancies: B-cell CLL, T-cell CLL, prolymphocytic, circulating non-Hodgkin lymphomas, and hairy cell leukemia.

B-Cell CLL

B-cell CLL accounts for over 95% of all CLL. Approximately 25% of such patients are identified with asymptomatic lymphocytosis during evaluation for other medical problems. Symptomatic patients may present with weight loss, fatigue, recurrent infections, fevers, or pain associated with hepatosplenomegaly or bulky lymphadenopathy. In most patients, the disease has a gradual progression spanning several years and the extent of the lymphoid burden at diagnosis correlates well with length of preexisting disease. In some patients, the disease has a more aggressive course, and progression to advanced clinical stages may occur within a few months of diagnosis. Identification of molecular and protein markers are beginning to explain the heterogenous natural history observed in this disease.

The diagnosis of CLL requires presence of monoclonal B lymphocytes greater than or equal to 5×10^9/L with a specific immunophenotyping pattern (coexpression of CD5 and CD20/23 with weak expression of surface immunoglobulin) by flow cytometry. Diagnosis and staging of CLL can usually be established by history, physical examination (careful evaluation for lymphadenopathy and splenomegaly), CBC with review of the blood smear, and immunophenotyping of the peripheral blood using flow cytometry. Classic findings on the peripheral smear include increased mature-appearing lymphocytes and smudge cells (peripheral smear artifact reflecting the fragility of the B-CLL cells to mechanical manipulation). Bone marrow studies are usually not needed for diagnosis.

TABLE 95-6 ■ IMMUNOPHENOTYPE OF MATURE B-CELL NEOPLASMS

DIAGNOSIS	SIG	CD5	CD10	CD23	CD43	CD103
B-CLL	+/−	+	−	+	+	−
Mantle cell lymphoma	+	+	−	−	+	−
B-cell prolymphocytic leukemia	++	+/−	−	−	−	−
Splenic marginal zone lymphoma	+	−	−	−	−	−
Hairy-cell leukemia	+	−	−	−	−	++

The differential diagnosis for B-CLL includes other mature B-lymphoproliferative disorders such as mantle cell lymphoma, prolymphocytic leukemia, hairy cell leukemia, and splenic lymphoma with villous lymphocytes. The clinical course and treatments differ widely for these disorders, particularly mantle cell lymphoma. Evaluation of clinical presentation, morphology, and immunophenotype is necessary to arrive at the correct diagnosis (**Table 95-6**). Inclusion of flow cytometric evaluation for cyclin D1 or FISH analysis for t(11:14) is essential to rule out mantle cell lymphoma.

The original Rai classification (**Table 95-7**) implied an orderly progression from lymphocytosis alone to the successive development of adenopathy, organomegaly, and, eventually, anemia and thrombocytopenia. The prognostic importance of these variables has been confirmed although survival patterns differ primarily by the low-, intermediate-, and high-risk categories. Specific cytogenetic abnormalities correlate with prognosis. A 13q deletion is associated with a better prognosis, compared to deletions of 11q and 17p, which confer a worse prognosis.

Therapy for B-cell CLL is not considered curative and therefore has been reserved for patients who are symptomatic or who progress to develop cytopenias. Leukocytosis alone (stage 0) does not require therapy, because the prognosis of these patients is excellent in the absence of the other poor prognostic factors. The rate of increase of leukocytosis is a better indicator of disease activity than the absolute count. Leukostasis, associated with high circulating blast counts in acute leukemias, does not generally occur in this condition because most of the lymphocytes are mature, small cells.

Treatment with systemic therapy or local radiation can be used to control symptoms in patients with stage I or II disease; however, symptomatic improvement does not appear to prolong survival. In contrast, patients with stage III or IV CLL have an improved survival with treatment.

Treatment options for older adults have expanded significantly in the past several years. In general, initial systemic treatment options are determined by disease characteristics (del 17p, TP53 mutation, and IGVH mutation status) as well as functional status and comorbid conditions.

Most regimens utilize targeted therapies as a single agent or in combination. Standard first-line regimens for older adults include use of Bruton tyrosine kinase (BTK) inhibitors (ie, ibrutinib or acalabrutinib) as a single agent or in combination with monoclonal antibodies (ie, rituximab or obinutuzumab) or the BCL2 inhibitor venetoclax as single agent or in combination with obinutuzumab. Chemoimmunotherapy regimens may be considered in some settings for fit older adults with standard risk disease by those willing to undergo more intensive therapy for the potential of longer treatment-free intervals compared to BTK inhibitors, which are given as continuous oral therapy.

Clinical trials in older adult populations have shown that ibrutinib improves outcomes compared to single-agent chlorambucil and chemoimmunotherapy using bendamustine plus rituximab. Overall, the totality of the evidence supports use of single-agent BTK inhibitor for many older adults as a first-line therapy. While well tolerated, there is an increased risk of bleeding, and caution is advised for patients who require anticoagulation. Cardiovascular toxicities are also a known risk including arrhythmias such as atrial fibrillation, heart failure, and hypertension. Frequently, presence of comorbid conditions and associated medications may determine choice of initial treatment regimen. For frail patients, or those with multiple chronic conditions, use of monoclonal antibody therapy is a reasonable choice. For example, a phase 3 randomized trial compared the efficacy of adding obinutuzumab (a humanized glycoengineered type 2 antibody to CD20) to chlorambucil versus rituximab specifically in patients with comorbidity. This study population had a median age of 73 and required a meaningful comorbidity burden (cumulative illness rating scale > 6) for eligibility. The median progression-free

TABLE 95-7 ■ CLL RAI CLINICAL CLASSIFICATION

STAGE	RISK[a]	CLINICAL FINDINGS
0	Low	Lymphocytosis only
1	Intermediate	↑ Lymphs plus ↑ nodes
2	Intermediate	↑ Lymphs plus ↑ spleen and/or liver ± ↑ Nodes
3	High	↑ Lymphs plus ↓ Hgb (< 11 g/dL) ± ↑ Nodes, ↑ liver, ↑ spleen
4	High	↑ Lymphs plus ↓ platelets (<100, 000/mcL) ± ↑ Nodes, ↑ liver, ↑ spleen, ↓ Hgb

[a]Data from Rai classification.

survival was improved from 11.1 months to 26.7 months when comparing the anti-CD20 combination therapy arms with chlorambucil alone. Treatment with the obinutuzumab combination resulted in improved overall survival compared to chemotherapy alone and was superior to Rituxan combination therapy for progression-free survival and response. This study was a landmark trial by both demonstrating efficacy of a novel therapeutic combination but also doing so in an older patient population with comorbidity.

Autoimmune manifestations of CLL are common and include development of antibodies to platelets and red cells (IgG and C3 on direct antiglobulin test) and to erythroid precursors, resulting in red cell aplasia. For anemic patients, reticulocyte counts and direct Coombs testing should be obtained to help differentiate hemolysis from decreased bone marrow production. All of the autoimmune complications are indications for therapy with steroids or intravenous gamma globulin for refractory cases of red cell aplasia.

Recurrent infections are the most common complications leading to death in CLL. Patients with stage 0 CLL have minimal increased risk of infection. In anticipation of gradual deterioration in immune response, however, pneumococcal vaccine and boosters should be administered while the potential for response is still intact. All other patients have higher risks for infection. As the disease advances clinically, immune function becomes progressively compromised, with increased susceptibility to viral, bacterial, and fungal infection. The subset of patients presenting with recurrent bacterial infections may benefit from administration of intravenous gamma globulin.

NON-HODGKIN AND HODGKIN LYMPHOMAS

Introduction

The lymphoid malignancies comprise over 100 heterogeneous and complex entities as identified in the 2016 World Health Organization (WHO) classification of lymphoid malignancies (**Table 95-8**). Non-Hodgkin lymphomas (NHLs) are the most common lymphoid malignancy, representing a heterogeneous group of lymphoproliferative disorders that originate from cells of the immune system, including B lymphocytes, T lymphocytes, or natural killer (NK) cells. In the United States, the B-cell lymphomas predominate, making up 80% to 85% of lymphoma diagnoses, with T-cell histologies representing 15% to 20% of the balance; NK-cell lymphomas are rare at less than 1%. Broadly speaking, lymphomas can be characterized as either indolent, behaving with median survivals measured in up to decades, or aggressive, with life-threatening consequences in weeks to months if untreated.

Indolent lymphomas are more often identified incidentally during routine physical examination or laboratory evaluation, particularly with increased reliance on routine blood testing and imaging in the modern era. Often, these entities present with slowly progressive lymphadenopathy, splenomegaly, and potential cytopenias from bone marrow involvement. Examples include the prototypic follicular lymphoma (FL), marginal zone lymphomas, and small lymphocytic lymphoma (SLL).

In contrast, aggressive lymphomas are more likely to present with acute or subacute symptoms including a rapidly growing mass, systemic B symptoms (see next paragraph), elevated serum lactate dehydrogenase, hypercalcemia, and hyperuricemia. Examples include diffuse large B-cell lymphoma (DLBCL), peripheral T-cell lymphomas (PTCL), and Burkitt lymphoma (BL).

Clinical characteristics of lymphomas include "B" symptoms, defined as fever greater than 38°C, unexplained weight loss greater than 10% of body weight over the past 6 months, and drenching night sweats. Up to 40% of patients with NHL may have B symptoms; more commonly evident in aggressive or biologically transformed disease (approaching 50%) than in low-grade lymphomas (< 25%). Less common presenting features include skin rash, pruritus, fatigue, fever of unknown origin, effusions, and hypersensitivity to insect bites. Extranodal presentations occur in 10% to 35% of patients at initial diagnosis, with extranodal sites developing in half of patients over the course of their disease. As lymphocytes naturally transit through blood and can be found in any tissue compartment, lymphomas have been reported in essentially all conceivable sites.

Epidemiology

In 2021, an estimated 90,390 individuals will be diagnosed with lymphoma in the United States, 81,560 NHL and 8,830 Hodgkin lymphoma (HL), with 21,680 individuals dying from a lymphoid malignancy. To put this in perspective, NHL and HL together account for 4.3% and 0.5% of all new cancer diagnoses, and NHL is the eighth leading cause of cancer death in the United States.

With the aging of the population, the United States is projected to witness increases in incidence of NHL by 67% and HL by 70% in older adults by the year 2030. This fact is evidenced as well by the increasing median age of individuals with NHL over the last two decades. Consequently, the interplay between aging biology, comorbidity, and competing risks is ever more prevalent for the treating oncologist.

Non-Hodgkin Lymphoma

World health organization classification system Although lymphoma classification has remained a complicated endeavor, iterative changes in the classification systems over the past 30 years have increasingly integrated cell of origin (B, T, NK), morphology, immunophenotype, and genetic and clinical features to define disease. The recent WHO updates have more broadly integrated new diseases and subtypes identified in the past, affirmed the importance of detecting viral entities in some diagnoses (eg, EBV, HHV8,

TABLE 95-8 ■ 2016 WORLD HEALTH ORGANIZATION (WHO) CLASSIFICATION OF MATURE LYMPHOID NEOPLASMS[a]

Mature B-cell neoplasms

Chronic lymphocytic leukemia/small lymphocytic lymphoma

Monoclonal B-cell lymphocytosis

B-cell prolymphocytic leukemia

Splenic marginal zone lymphoma

Hairy-cell leukemia

Splenic lymphoma/leukemia, unclassifiable

    Splenic diffuse red pulp small B-cell lymphoma

    Hairy-cell leukemia-variant

Lymphoplasmacytic lymphoma

    Waldenström macroglobulinemia

Monoclonal gammopathy of undetermined significance (MGUS), IgM

Heavy chain diseases

    α Heavy chain disease

    γ Heavy chain disease

    μ Heavy chain disease

Plasma cell myeloma

Solitary plasmacytoma of bone

Extraosseous plasmacytoma

Monoclonal immunoglobulin deposition diseases

Extranodal marginal zone B-cell lymphoma of mucosa-associated lymphoid tissue (MALT lymphoma)

Nodal marginal zone B-cell lymphoma (MZL)

    Pediatric-type nodal MZL

Follicular lymphoma

    In situ follicular neoplasia

    Duodenal-type follicular lymphoma

Pediatric type follicular lymphoma

Large B-cell lymphoma with IRF4 rearrangement

Primary cutaneous follicle center lymphoma

Mantle cell lymphoma

    In situ mantle cell neoplasia

Diffuse large B-cell lymphoma (DLBCL), not otherwise specified

    Germinal center B-cell type

    Activated B-cell type

T-cell/histiocyte-rich large B-cell lymphoma

Primary DLBCL of the central nervous system (CNS)

Primary cutaneous DLBCL, leg type

    Epstein-Barr virus (EBV)+ DLBCL, NOS of older adults

EBV+ mucocutaneous ulcer

DLBCL associated with chronic inflammation

Lymphomatoid granulomatosis

Primary mediastinal (thymic) large B-cell lymphoma

Intravascular large B-cell lymphoma

ALK+ large B-cell lymphoma

Plasmablastic lymphoma

Primary effusion lymphoma

HHV8+ DLBCL, NOS

Burkitt lymphoma

Burkitt-like lymphoma with 11q aberration

High-grade B-cell lymphoma, with MYC and BCL2 and/or BCL6 rearrangements

High-grade B-cell lymphoma, NOS

B-cell lymphoma, unclassifiable, with features intermediate between DLBCL and classic Hodgkin lymphoma

Hodgkin lymphoma

Nodular lymphocyte-predominant Hodgkin lymphoma

Classic Hodgkin lymphoma

    Nodular sclerosis classic Hodgkin lymphoma

    Lymphocyte-rich classic Hodgkin lymphoma

    Mixed cellularity classic Hodgkin lymphoma

    Lymphocyte-depleted classic Hodgkin lymphoma

[a]Only B-cell and Hodgkin lymphoma included here. See Swerdlow et al, Blood. 2016 for full classification.

Italics indicate provisional entities for which there was thought to be insufficient evidence to classify as distinct entities.

and HTLV1), as well as increased the use of genetic features in diagnosis, such as cytogenetics and FISH in defining specific NHL entities.

Etiology Despite an increasing understanding of biology, the cause of most lymphomas remains unknown. Mutational events inherent in the normal cell division process of lymphocytes are expected to result in a continuous random event rate. Increased incidences are associated with a personal family history of lymphoma, past radiation or chemotherapy treatment, immunosuppressive agents, smoking, and obesity. Environmental exposures to agricultural pesticides, hair dyes (prior to the 1980s), agent orange, and other dioxins accounted for an increased incidence of lymphoma in the central United States. Dysregulation of the immune system may precede a lymphoma diagnosis, with increased risk associated with autoimmune diseases (eg, rheumatoid arthritis, lupus, Sjögren syndrome, Hashimoto thyroiditis), solid organ transplantation, chronic immunosuppression, and celiac sprue. A number of infections have also been implicated in the pathogenesis of lymphomas, either as a consequence of immune dysregulation or chronic antigenic drive. Examples include human immunodeficiency virus (HIV), human T lymphoma atrophic virus type I (HTLV-I), Epstein-Barr virus (EBV), hepatitis C, hepatitis B virus, *Helicobacter pylori*, and human herpesvirus 8 (HHV8).

EBV in Lymphoma and Older Adults In the most recent WHO classification iteration of 2016, a provisional entity termed EBV (+) DLBCL, NOS was specified. In previous versions (2008) this had been EBV+ DLBCL of older adults, but has since been reframed to reflect younger patients who may experience this diagnosis, which consists of an EBV-positive monoclonal large B-cell proliferation with no known history of immunodeficiency. Most patients have an activated B-cell (ABC) phenotype, strong NF-κβ activation, increased extranodal distribution at diagnosis, and inferior survival. Optimal treatment strategies are not defined. EBV has also been implicated in the pathogenesis and outcome of HL, with a negative impact on outcome in advanced age as distinct from younger patients.

Genetic Factors—Translocations NHLs are frequently characterized by balanced translocations, resulting in functional fusions that confer a survival advantage for the affected cell population (**Table 95-9**). Such translocations often involve the immunoglobulin heavy chain region on chromosome 14, leading to constitutive activation of the translocated partner and consequently to increased signaling for the translocated gene, such as the antiapoptotic pathways (*BCL2*), cell cycle proteins (*CCND1*), and cellular proliferation (*cMYC*).

Evaluation and staging Evaluation of a patient with suspected lymphoma includes a careful history and physical examination, with close attention to lymphatic sites including Waldeyer ring and the spleen. Extranodal sites of involvement to consider on examination include the skin, CNS abnormalities, testes, breasts, and bone. Standard

TABLE 95-9 ■ LYMPHOMAS WITH KNOWN TRANSLOCATIONS

LYMPHOMA HISTOLOGY	COMMON TRANSLOCATION	GENE PARTNERS
Mucosa-associated lymphoid tissue lymphoma	t(11;18)(q21;q21)	AP12/MALT, BCL-10
Mantle cell lymphoma	t(11;14)(q13;q32)	BCL-1, IgH
Follicular lymphoma	t(14;18)(q32;q21)	BCL-2, IgH
Diffuse large-cell lymphoma	t(3;-)(q27;-) t(17;-)(p13-) t(14;18))(q32;q21) t(8;14)(q24;q32)	BCL-6 P53 BCL-2 C-MYC
Burkitt lymphoma	t(8;14)(q24;32) t(8;22)	C-MYC, IGH
Anaplastic large-cell lymphoma	t(2;5)(p23;q35)	ALK
Lymphoplasmacytoid lymphoma	t(9;14)(p13;q32)	PAX5, IgH

blood work includes a CBC, comprehensive metabolic panel, calcium, uric acid, lactate dehydrogenase (LDH), serum protein electrophoresis, β_2 microglobulin (indolent lymphomas), and serologic testing for HIV and hepatitis B and C.

A biopsy is required for diagnosis and classification of NHL and HL. Generally, an excisional or incisional core lymph node biopsy is preferred given the requirements for increasingly complex pathologic diagnostic evaluations. Fine-needle aspiration is often helpful as an initial discriminator between reactive adenopathy, carcinoma, and lymphoma but is not adequate for identifying lymphoma subtype. Studies needed include morphologic assessment, immunohistochemical (IHC) staining, flow cytometry, FISH testing, cytogenetics, polymerase chain reaction (PCR) studies for clonality (immunoglobulin gene rearrangement studies for B-cell clonality, T-cell receptor gene rearrangements for T-cell lymphomas), and increasingly gene expression profiling (GEP). Functional imaging (eg, positron emission tomography [PET] scan) may direct the site of biopsy when discordant fluorodeoxyglucose (FDG) avidity is present, with the most metabolically active lesions generally representing the most aggressive biology.

Ann Arbor Staging System Originally developed in 1974 for HL, the Ann Arbor staging system was the equivalent of the TNM (tumor-lymph node-metastasis) staging system for lymphoid malignancies. This staging system defines disease location and extent and prognostic information, permitting cross-study comparisons, and establishes baseline disease extent to allow for response comparison. Modified in 1988, the Cotswold classification formally included CT scans and designations for bulky disease (X), dividing HL patients in four stages, with A and B subclassifications based on the absence or presence of B symptoms. Universally accepted response criteria in NHL and HL were published in 1999 by the NCI Working Group and revised in 2007 by the International Working Group (IWG) to incorporate PET and bone marrow immunohistochemistry (IHC)/flow in response assessment. This has formed the foundation for staging and response evaluations for NHL and HL over the last decades, acknowledging certain histologies have warranted their own staging and response assessment given varied clinical course (eg, CLL/SLL, Waldenström macroglobulinemia, cutaneous T-cell lymphoma).

Of note, in contrast to many solid tumors, it is important to realize stage alone is often a poor arbiter of outcome in NHL. Clinical and biologic prognostic models, generally including stage as one of the risk factors, are better predictors of outcome. For instance, a substantial number of DLBCL patients with advanced-stage III/IV disease will be cured, and for indolent lymphoma patients, stage IV disease is the norm, but survival is measured in decades.

Updated Lugano Classification 2015 The Lugano classification was published in 2014 in an effort to modernize

	STAGE	SITES	EXTRANODAL (E) STATUS
TABLE 95-10 ■ REVISED STAGING SYSTEM FOR PRIMARY NODAL LYMPHOMAS			
Limited stage	I	One node or a group of adjacent nodes	Single extranodal lesions without nodal involvement
	II[a]	Two or more nodal groups on the same side of the diaphragm	Stage I or II by nodal extent with limited contiguous extranodal involvement
Advanced stage	III	Nodes on both sides of the diaphragm; nodes above the diaphragm with spleen involvement	Not applicable
	IV	Additional noncontiguous extralymphatic involvement	Not applicable

Extent of disease determined by PET/CT for FDG-avid lymphomas and CT for nonavid lymphomas. Tonsils, Waldeyer ring, and spleen are considered nodal sites. Bulky disease is defined as 10 cm or greater on CT or greater than 1/3 transthoracic diameter at any level of thoracic vertebrae.
[a]Stage II bulky disease is considered limited or advanced based on histology and prognostic factors.

recommendations for evaluation, staging, and response assessment for patients with HL and NHL (**Table 95-10**). The most salient changes included formal integration of PET scanning into initial staging for FDG-avid lymphomas, modification of the Ann Arbor terminology eliminating A/B qualifiers except for HL, and departure from routine bone marrow biopsy in DLBCL and HL based on functional imaging. FDG-PET utilizing the Deauville 5-point scale was integrated into response assessment. The Lugano revision of the staging criteria has suggested that bone marrow biopsy may not be necessary in most DLBCL or any HL if functional imaging fails to identify osseous lesions. One must acknowledge, however, that bone marrow involvement with indolent lymphoma is generally not evident on FDG-PET. A bone marrow biopsy should be performed if this knowledge alters clinical management (eg, identification of transformed biology).

Clinical Risk Prognostic Models

IMPACT OF AGE ACROSS ALL PROGNOSTIC MODELS. The most frequently utilized model is the international prognostic index (IPI) that identifies five clinical factors as prognostic variables for progression-free survival (PFS) and OS in DLBCL (**Table 95-11**). Importantly, chronologic age remains an integral part of many lymphoma clinical risk predictors, including the IPI, the follicular lymphoma IPI (FLIPI), the mantle cell IPI (MIPI), and the HL international prognostic score (IPS). However, the populations from which these prognostic indices were developed may not have uniformly included older patients. For example, the IPS included patients up to 65 years old, with ages 55 to 65 representing only 9% of the study population. It is well appreciated that age is a continuous variable and that a more clinically relevant cutoff above which patients are likely to require treatment modifications exists between 70 and 75 years in the current era.

From a clinical decision-making standpoint, distinctions in older populations among those age 65 to 74 years, 75 to 84 years, and 85 years or older are somewhat arbitrary but have clinical utility in minimizing heterogeneity when devising treatment guidelines. Ultimately, however, the variable nature of the aging process mandates thinking beyond chronologic age.

Biological Risk Factors In the modern era, with targeted therapies an increased reality, biomarkers to guide therapeutic decision making will be essential. The Ki67 proliferative index, a measure of cellular division, has been demonstrated to have prognostic impact in DLBCL and MCL, and in predicting increased risk of indolent NHL transformation.

In DLBCL, the putative cell of origin as identified on GEP is prognostic, with germinal center-derived DLBCL enjoying a better outcome than non-GC (ABC phenotype). The concurrent presence of the antiapoptotic t(14;18) BCL2 translocation and a cMYC t(8;14) cellular proliferation signal (or less frequently BCL6 translocations) has been termed a "double hit" biology (DH). Roughly 10% of patients with DLBCL will have DH biology, a finding associated with very aggressive disease, older age, higher CNS risk, and no current standard of care recommendation. A larger population (~1/3) of DLBCL patients may have protein overexpression of BCL and MYC, termed double expressers, and have increased disease risk as well, but to a more variable degree.

CNS Risk Assessment CNS evaluation with lumbar puncture and analysis of cerebrospinal fluid (CSF) is important in patients with a clinical suspicion of nervous system involvement or those at high risk for CNS involvement at presentation. CSF investigation should include cell count, glucose, protein, cytology, as well as the more sensitive flow cytometry. This is generally a consideration in aggressive lymphomas and high-grade disease, with involvement rare in mantle cell or indolent lymphomas. Increased risk of CNS involvement historically has been associated with higher clinical risk factors, anatomic sites of involvement such as the testes, breast, multiple extranodal sites, and bone marrow.

Recently, a predictive model for DLBCL risk of CNS relapse was reported. This validated model comprises six factors (age, PS, LDH, stage, extranodal sites, and kidney/adrenal involvement) with stratification of CNS relapse based on number of risk factors. Although the optimal method (intrathecal or high-dose methotrexate) and the actual magnitude of risk reduction in CNS prophylaxis remain debated, this predictive model is useful when considering the pros and cons in older adults.

TABLE 95-11 ■ VARIOUS PROGNOSTIC SCORES FOR LYMPHOMAS

PROGNOSTIC FACTOR					
IPI	**FLIPI**	**FLIPI2**	**MIPI**	**PIT**	**IPS**
Age > 60	Age > 60	Age > 60	Age	Age > 60 or (≤ 60)	Age > 45
Stage III/IV	Stage III/IV	BM involvement	Ki67	BM involvement	Stage IV
PS > 1	Hgb < 12 g/L	Hgb < 12 g/L	PS	PS	Hgb < 10.5 g/L
LDH > ULN	LDH > ULN	B2M > ULN	LDH compared ULN	LDH > ULN	Albumin < 4 g/dL
ENS > 2	> 4 nodal sites	LN diameter > 6 cm	WBC		WBC > 15 ALC < 600 or < 8% of total WBC count Male gender
Low (0–1) 2 y OS 84%, 5 y OS 73%	Low (0–1) 5 y OS 91%, 10 y OS 71%	Low (0) 3 y PFS 91%, 5 y PFS 80%	Low 5 y OS 81%	Low (0) 5 y OS 62.3%, 10 y OS 54.9%	0 factors 5 y FFP 84%, 5 y OS 89%
Low-Int (2) 2 y OS 66%, 5 y OS 51%	Int (1–2) 5 y OS 78%, 10 y OS 51%	Int (1–2) 3 y PFS 69%, 5 y PFS 51%	Int 5 y OS 63%	Low–Int (1) 5 y OS 52.9%, 10 y OS 38.8%	1 factor 5 y FFP 77%, 5 y OS 90%
High-Int (3) 2 y OS 54%, 5 y OS 43%	High (≥ 3) 5 y OS 53%, 10 y OS 36%	High (3–5) 3 y PFS 51%, 5 y PFS 19%	High 5 y OS 35%	High-Int (2) 5 y OS 32.9%, 10 y OS 18%	2 factors 5 y FFP 67%, 5 y OS 81%
High (4–5) 2 y OS 34%, 5 y OS 26%				High (≥ 3) 5 y OS 18.3%, 10 y OS 12.6%	3 factors 5 y FFP 60%, 5 y OS 78% 4 factors 5 y FFP 51%, 5 y OS 61% ≥ 5 factors 5 y FFP 42%, 5 y OS 56%

B2M, β₂-microglobulin; BM, bone marrow; FFP, failure-free progression; FLIPI, follicular lymphoma international prognostic index; IPI, international prognostic index; IPS, international prognostic score; LDH, lactate dehydrogenase; MIPI, mantle cell international prognostic index; OS, overall survival; PIT, prognostic index for T-cell lymphoma; PFS, progression-free survival; ULN, upper limit of normal; WBC, white blood cell.

Treatment In the older patient, establishing clinical and disease-associated risk predictors is an essential part of the assessment, but this evaluation still represents an incomplete clinical picture for the treating oncologist. With increasing age, the patient may have aging-associated risk factors that may be equally or more profound than the aforementioned lymphoma factors and ultimately define the range of therapeutic options. The oncogeriatric factors of life expectancy, comorbidity, frailty, and geriatric syndromes independently predict treatment-associated morbidity and mortality, and consequently become essential considerations when deriving a treatment strategy. Ultimately, these clinical concerns are most weighty when there is an aggressive histology that is potentially curable, but therapy is associated with very real risks. In recent years, several studies have identified frailty as a predictor of chemotherapy tolerance and survival. Geriatric assessments provide physicians with a tool to individualize decision-making based on factors beyond age and documented comorbidity. Further, there are modified chemotherapy regimens geared toward older or more frail patients, with the goal of reducing toxicity while optimizing survival. One example is a reduced dose version of the common combination of cyclophosphamide,

doxorubicin hydrochloride (hydroxydaunorubicin), vincristine sulfate (Oncovin), and prednisone, or CHOP.

Comorbidity and Frailty Assessments Comorbidity is prevalent in older patients, with 60% to 70% of NHL patients older than 60 years possessing some comorbidity. Frequently used measures include the Charlson comorbidity score and the Cumulative Illness Rating Scale for Geriatrics, both of which capture information distinct from lymphoma-specific prognostic indexes and are independently associated with risk. The presence of comorbidity in NHL and HL patients has been associated with increased treatment-related mortality (TRM), treatment toxicity, lower dose intensity, and higher treatment failure.

Frailty is a distinct syndrome from comorbidity and has its own impact on outcomes (see Chapter 42). Frailty is often defined practically, with suggested criteria including age greater than 80 or 85, dependence in ADL, exhaustion, slow gait speed, decreased hand grip, unintentional weight loss, and decreased physical activity. Frail patients have shorter life expectancies than nonfrail patients and have a higher likelihood of toxicity with interventions such as chemotherapy. Thus, frailty identifies a group of patients at greatest risk given lack of functional reserves, and palliative chemotherapy approaches are generally recommended in this setting.

Comprehensive Geriatric Assessment Performance status and clinical judgment alone are insufficient to identify at-risk older individuals and may misclassify a significant percent of patients, exposing them to harm or denying curative intent. In this vein, the National Comprehensive Cancer Network (NCCN), American Society of Clinical Oncology (ASCO), and International Society of Geriatric Oncology (SIOG) guidelines recommend performance of comprehensive geriatric assessment (CGA) in older patients. Instructively, Tucci and colleagues demonstrated that a CGA applied in 173 DLBCL patients older than 69 years segregated fit (46%), unfit (16%), and frail (38%) patients with significantly different outcomes (OS 84% fit vs 47% nonfit, $p < .0001$) and a lack of clinical benefit from curative intent therapy in the frail category.

The Fondazione Italiana Linfomi (FIL) integrated a CGA tool into a trial treatment paradigm that stratified 334 DLBCL patients older than 65 years as either fit (68%) or frail (29%). Fit patients were randomized on a trial between RCHOP and R-mini-CEOP and had excellent and equivalent outcomes, while frail patients were treated per investigator choice. Frail patients were more frequently older (median age 78, range 65–93), with advanced stage (62%) and high risk, and reported a 5-year estimated OS of 28% despite polychemotherapy administration in three-fourths of patients. TRM was 18% in this group compared with only 8% in the fit group. Most recently, this group completed a prospective project on older patients with DLBCL using a simplified version of their original geriatric assessment. The simplified assessment included age greater than or equal to 80, Cumulative Illness Rating Scale for Geriatrics comorbidity assessment, ADLs and IADLs. They identified 55% fit, 28% unfit, and 18% frail patients. Future prospective trials will need to build upon this work to help optimize treatment decisions for older patients with DLBCL.

Pharmacologic Considerations for Older NHL Patients

NEUROPATHIC AGENTS: VINCA ALKALOIDS (VINCRISTINE, VINBLASTINE), CISPLATIN, OXALIPLATIN, BRENTUXIMAB VEDOTIN, BORTEZOMIB. A number of approved agents for the treatment of NHL are associated with peripheral and autonomic neuropathy. In the older individual, although grade 3 neuropathy generally provokes drug modification or cessation, grade 2 neuropathy may interfere with ADL/IADLs, increase the risk of falls, and impact quality-of-life (QOL). Dose reductions and omissions need to be balanced against the potential benefit in a given scenario.

ANTHRACYCLINE. Doxorubicin is one of the most active and essential agents in the treatment of aggressive histologies such as DLBCL and HL. The anthracyclines are associated with a defined risk of anthracycline-induced cardiomyopathy that is related to cumulative dose (although rarely idiopathic), with risk increasing significantly with doxorubicin equivalents in excess of 400 mg/m² lifetime. Hypertension is an established risk factor. Infusional doxorubicin

and liposomal doxorubicin may have an increased safety margin, and a variety of non-anthracycline regimens exist when there is an absolute contraindication that may still preserve a curative intent.

Small Molecule Inhibitors Ibrutinib is a small molecule inhibitor of Bruton tyrosine kinase (BTK), FDA approved for the treatment of CLL and MCL. With longer follow-up, propensity toward bleeding has been identified with consideration for risk-versus-benefit in patients requiring antiplatelet or anticoagulation therapies. Concurrent warfarin is generally contraindicated given interactions with CYP3A inhibitors and inducers. New-onset atrial fibrillation has also been occasionally reported (< 5%).

Idelalisib is a small molecule inhibitor of PI3 kinase-δ that is FDA approved for patients with CLL/SLL and refractory FL. This drug has been associated with fatal and/or serious hepatotoxicity, severe diarrhea or colitis, pneumonitis, and intestinal perforation. Hepatic abnormalities typically resolve with interruption of drug dosing; patients can frequently resume therapy.

Diffuse Large B-Cell Lymphoma

Introduction Diffuse large B-cell lymphoma (DLBCL) is the most common subtype of NHL both in the United States and globally, representing roughly 30% of all new diagnosis. With a median age at diagnosis of greater than or equal to 65 years, DLBCL is in many ways a disease of older individuals. With the aging population, there is a pressing need to understand age-related host and disease factors, how they impact therapeutic choices and outcomes, and to develop specific strategies to address these factors.

Treatment DLBCL is an aggressive entity with the natural history characterized by rapid progression and death within weeks to months in the absence of treatment. Based on randomized controlled trials (RCTs), frontline therapy with anthracycline-based chemoimmunotherapy for DLBCL (eg, rituximab-CHOP) results in overall survival rates of 60% to 70% and represents the best chance for cure, as the majority of patients with relapsed or refractory disease will die of lymphoma. However, older patients frequently have comorbidities and functional impairment limiting feasibility of standard therapy. The initial decision regarding the feasibility of anthracycline-based chemotherapy is consequently paramount and must integrate assessments of organ function, clinical judgment, comorbidity, and performance status as previously discussed. Chemotherapy may extend survival, even among patients where curative intent cannot be achieved.

Early-stage DLBCL (stage I/II without bulk) may be treated with fewer cycles of chemotherapy followed by radiation. Whether or not to include radiation consolidation may be informed by disease location, associated RT toxicity, comorbidity, and life expectancy. Radiation should be considered for definitive therapy in patients who cannot tolerate chemotherapy. The standard of care for initial treatment of DLBCL in both older and younger patients is chemoimmunotherapy comprised of rituximab, cyclophosphamide, doxorubicin, vincristine, and prednisone (RCHOP 21) given every 21 days for 6 to 8 cycles. Ongoing efforts to improve outcomes in groups at higher risk for relapse based on unfavorable disease biology are exploring regimens such as dose-adjusted R-EPOCH (rituximab, etoposide phosphate, prednisone, vincristine, cyclophosphamide, and doxorubicin) regimen or adding novel agents such as bortezomib, ibrutinib, and lenalidomide.

Patients who relapse following RCHOP chemotherapy have a poor prognosis, even when second-line therapy and subsequent high-dose therapy and autologous stem cell rescue (HDT/ASCR) are utilized. For the vast majority of older individuals, this intensive strategy is not feasible due to age-related comorbidity and increased TRM associated with transplant approaches. In this setting, goals of care shift to disease control and palliation. Several novel agents are being explored for relapsed/refractory disease for patients ineligible for transplant.

Prephase Concept and Reduced Intensity Often at initial presentation, disease-related factors impair host performance status and are associated with treatment-associated morbidity and mortality. The German NHL high-grade study group has utilized a concept termed "prephase" to mitigate the impact of decreased functional status initially. Employing a week of corticosteroid and a single dose of vincristine before the initiation of therapy, the RICOVER60 study suggested there was a 50% reduction in cycle 1 and 2 TRM as a consequence of this maneuver.

Reduced Dose or Nonanthracycline-Based Curative Intent In clinical scenarios where RCHOP is not deemed feasible, there exist a variety of dose-reduced regimens, with relative dose intensities of 50% to 70% standard dosing, and nonanthracycline regimens that maintain curative potential (**Table 95-12**). In general, the trade-off includes a reduction in efficacy with the advantage of reduced toxicity and TRM. Direct comparative data are frequently lacking in

this area, with data more frequently culled from retrospective cohorts or phase II trials.

DLBCL patients older than age 80 or with geriatric syndromes and/or frailty are underrepresented in clinical trials. Typically, full-dose chemotherapy is not feasible in these patients, but curative regimens can still be considered with modifications designed to mitigate serious toxicity. Some clinical trials have been completed, specifically enrolling adults aged 80 and older with DLBCL, examining protocols such as R-mini-CHOP, which have resulted in about half of patients being alive without progression at 2 years.

Therapy for Relapse and CAR-T Therapy If patients with DLBCL do not have a complete response or experience a relapse of disease following initial therapy, subsequent options can include further chemotherapy and/or high-dose therapy/ autologous stem cell transplant (ASCT), for which many older adults will not be eligible. In the past decade, chimeric antigen receptor T-cell therapy (CAR-T therapy) has been approved for patients with relapsed refractory B-cell non-Hodgkin lymphomas. CAR-T therapy uses a patient's own T lymphocytes that are genetically modified to encode a chimeric antigen receptor that in turn directs the modified T cells against cancer cells. Several pivotal studies led to approvals for CAR-T use among patients whose B-cell NHL has progressed after more than or equal to two lines of previous therapy.

It is important to recognize the potential toxicity for CAR-T infusions. The complications of cytokine release syndrome (CRS) and immune effector cell-associated neurotoxicity syndrome among the two commercial CAR-T products have been well-described. As the modified cells encounter native CD-19 expressing cells, they proliferate and release cytokines resulting in an inflammatory response and CRS. This often manifests as systemic signs and symptoms mimicking sepsis (fever, hypotension, coagulopathy, multiorgan failure), and can occur within hours to a few days after drug infusion. A post hoc analysis of the ZUMA-1 trial with axicabtagene ciloleucel for relapsed/

TABLE 95-12 ■ REDUCED DOSE OR NONANTHRACYCLINE THERAPY

REGIMEN	N	PLANNED RDI	AGE MEDIAN (RANGE)	ORR (CR/PR)	EFS	OS	TRM
Reduced dose regimens							
RCHOP21 (phase III)	N = 202	100%	69 y (60–80)	83% (75%/7%)	57% @ 2 y	70% @ 2 y	6%
RCHOP21 (retrospective)	N = 61	70%	76 y	87% (79%/8%)	57% @ 2 y	68% @ 3 y	NR
R-mini-CHOP (phase II)	N = 149	~50%	83 y (80–95)	74% (63%/11%)	47% @ 2 y (PFS)	59% @ 2 y	8%
DRCOP (phase II)	N = 80	NA	69 y (61–92)	86% (75%/11%)	60% @ 3 y	74% @ 3 y	5%
Nonanthracycline regimens							
R-miniCEOP (phase III)	N = 114	100%	73 y (64–84)	81% (68%/13%)	54% @ 2 y	~74% @ 2 y	6%
R-GCVP (EF ≤ 55%) (phase II)	N = 61	NA	76 y (52–90)	61% (39%/23%)	50% @ 2 y (PFS)	56% @ 2 y	NR
R-Bendamustine (phase II)	N = 14	NA	85 y (80–95)	69% (54%/15%)	40% @ 2 y (PFS)	40% @ 2 y	0%

CR, complete response; EF, ejection fraction; EFS, event-free survival; NR, not reported; ORR, overall response rate; OS, overall survival; PFS, progression-free survival; PR, partial response; RDI, reduced dose intensity; TRM, treatment-related mortality.

refractory DLBCL found that outcomes of response and survival were similar to slightly better for older versus younger patients (patients 65 years or older made up one-quarter of the trial cohort). However, the incidence of grade more than or equal to 3 neurologic toxicity was higher (44% vs 28%) in the older age cohort. Future studies are needed to identify which older patients are optimal candidates for CAR-T therapy through understanding of patient preferences, risk of toxicity, and functional status.

Follicular Lymphoma/Indolent Lymphomas

Introduction Follicular lymphoma (FL) is the second most common NHL histology in the United States, accounting for approximately 30% of new cases. FL is the prototypical indolent or slow-growing lymphoma, characterized by systemic disease with a protracted disease course associated with waxing and waning adenopathy that is frequently asymptomatic and may not require therapy. Average survival can exceed 15 years.

Most patients with FL will present with painless adenopathy, with bone marrow involvement in up to 70%. FL remains a chronic illness that is characterized by the need for intermittent therapy with generally shorter and shorter response intervals. Marked heterogeneity does exist in disease course, with perhaps 10% to 15% of patients experiencing a more aggressive disease course with shorter survival.

Indications for therapy Many patients will present with advanced-stage disease but will not require immediate intervention. Asymptomatic patients with low burden of disease may be expectantly monitored with no detrimental effect on overall survival. Randomized studies have shown that the early initiation of therapy did not improve long-term disease-specific or overall survival, supporting an expectant monitoring approach. The median time from diagnosis to treatment in controlled settings has generally been about 3 years. Spontaneous regression of adenopathy in FL may occur in 10% to 15% of patients. Indications for therapy, which is generally chemoimmunotherapy in the modern era, are derived from clinical trial criteria established by the French in the context of clinical trials (termed the GELF criteria) and adopted by the NCCN guidelines. These criteria generally relate to tumor burden (**Table 95-13**).

Therapy—Localized disease While expectant monitoring may be reasonable in some patients with localized indolent lymphoma, others will require therapy. Radiation alone may be an option for 5% to 10% of patients who present with localized disease (stage I or II), with roughly 50% of patients remaining long-term disease free. Patients with bulky FL are generally managed according to advanced-stage strategies.

Therapy—Advanced-stage disease

Chemoimmunotherapy Therapy for advanced-stage FL is generally indicated when there are criteria indicating increased tumor burden and symptomatic disease. Current therapies

TABLE 95-13 ■ INDICATIONS FOR THERAPY IN FOLLICULAR LYMPHOMA

HIGH TUMOR BURDEN INDICATIONS FOR THERAPY
At least one of the following:
3 distinct nodal sites, each ≥ 3 cm
Single nodal site ≥ 7 cm
Symptomatic splenomegaly
Cytopenias (WBC < 1 and/or PLT < 100 × 10⁹/L)
Leukemic disease (circulating cells > 5 × 10⁹/L)
Pleural effusion, peritoneal ascites
B symptoms (fever, drenching night sweats, weight loss)
LDH elevated or B2M ≥ 3 g/dL
PS ≥ 1

B2M, beta 2 microglobulin; LDH, lactate dehydrogenase; PLT, platelet count; PS, performance status; WBC, white blood cell count.

are not curative, so the goal of treatment is resolution of disease symptoms and maintenance of remission, balanced with toxicity. FL are very responsive to immunotherapy alone and in combination with chemotherapy, as well as radiation, with a rapid expansion of available agents in the current era. In almost all instances, the addition of rituximab to a chemotherapy backbone has consistently resulted in improved response rates and increased PFS, as well as of evidence of increased OS. Alkylator-based regimens (eg, RCHOP and R-CVP), purine analogue regimens (eg, R-FCM), and rituximab-bendamustine have all been evaluated in the frontline treatment of symptomatic FL. Overall response rates are generally in the 80% to 95% range, with median response durations over 2 years. For older frail patients, low-dose targeted radiation or single-agent rituximab may provide effective palliation.

Relapsed Disease At relapse, the selection of salvage regimens depends on the efficacy and tolerability of prior therapies. Rituximab is generally included if the benefit from initial therapy was more than 6 months, and data support maintenance rituximab in the relapsed setting as well. Radioimmunotherapy with ⁹⁰Y-ibritumomab tiuxetan and ¹³¹I-tositumumab represents an effective approach and is a particular consideration in older patients with comorbidities not appropriate for chemotherapy. The oral phosphatidylinositol 3-kinase (PI3K) inhibitor idelalisib has proven safety and efficacy in relapsed indolent NHL refractory to rituximab and alkylators. Other aggressive options as used in relapsed/refractory DLBCL, such as ASCT or CAR-T therapy may be considered for select patients with short remission duration (< 2 years) from initial chemoimmunotherapy induction.

Risk of transformation Up to half of patients may experience transformation to a more aggressive biology that approximates DLBCL in appearance. Clinically, transformation is often heralded by a rapidly growing nodal mass, new-onset B symptoms, hypercalcemia, elevated

LDH, increased Ki67%, and higher standardized uptake values (SUVs) on FDG-PET. Once transformation is documented, treatment generally follows DLBCL paradigms to eradicate the aggressive life-threatening clone. Median survival following transformation is reported at less than 2 years.

Hodgkin Lymphoma

While HL median age of diagnosis is 39 years, there is a bimodal age peak of distribution, with peaks of incidence in the 20s to 30s and again in the 60s to 70s. Older patients pose a particularly difficult dynamic for the treatment team. If therapy can be given safely, these patients can be cured. However, many patients are not given dose-intense chemotherapy due to perceived or actual risk of toxicity. Older patients are also less represented in clinical trials (< 5% of HL trial demographics are older) leaving less guidance and fewer advancements in the treatment of older patients. Hence, there remains a significant gap in curability for older patients due to disease biology, aging-associated vulnerabilities, and therapy administered.

Biology and outcomes in older patients HL is characterized by the presence of malignant multinucleated giant cells, termed "Reed-Sternberg" cells, that have a typical immuno-histochemical profile with expression of CD15 and CD30. Four histologic subtypes are recognized: nodular sclerosis, mixed cellularity, lymphocyte-rich, and lymphocyte-depleted classical HL. Another subtype of HL, nodular lymphocyte-predominant Hodgkin lymphoma (NLPHL), is even rarer, both in terms of incidence (only 5% of all HL) and presentation at advanced age.

Older patients with HL, typically defined as older than or equal to 60 years, have poorer outcomes compared to younger patients. The reasons for these disparities are many, including disease biology, comorbidity, functional status, relative chemotherapy intensity, and toxicity. A recent population analysis evaluated first-line treatment patterns in adults 65 years or older with incident HL in the United States. Less than one-quarter of patients received "full regimen" dose-intense chemotherapy, and 26% of patients received no treatment within 4 months of diagnosis. This study highlighted the heterogeneity of treatment practices and patient characteristics in this particularly vulnerable population. Further, there is a lack of prognostic tools for this population. The IPS developed by Hansenclever is the most widely used prognostic score, but there were no patients older than 65 years at diagnosis, making the IPS difficult to apply to older individuals. Retrospective assessments have suggested comorbidity and ADLs are important predictors in older HL patients.

Early-stage disease (stage I-IIA) The standard of care for early-stage patients is the chemotherapy combination of adriamycin, bleomycin, vinblastine, and dacarbazine (ABVD), with or without radiation, depending on location of disease and initial response to treatment. Recently, trials in early-stage favorable patients have integrated interim PET into the treatment paradigm, allowing omission of radiation based on initial response. Additionally, the toxicity of bleomycin outweighs its benefits after more than two cycles of bleomycin. Thus, it is now recommended that after two cycles, older patients receive AVD without bleomycin to protect from pulmonary toxicity.

Advanced-stage disease (stage III/IV) For patients with advance stage HL, ABVD is the standard of care in the United States. Alternate regimens, such as Stanford V and BEACOPP, are associated with increased toxicity in older adults. The SHIELD study was specifically designed for adults with HL older than age 60; they prospectively studied the VEPEMB (vinblastine, cyclophosphamide, procarbazine, etoposide, mitoxantrone, bleomycin, prednisolone) program in this cohort, with phase II data demonstrating 3-year PFS and OS of 58% and 66%, respectively, for advanced-stage patients. For early-stage patients, 74% of patients achieved CR with PFS at 3 years of 87%.

Novel approaches to older adults with Hodgkin lymphoma In recent years, there has been a shift to exploring non-chemotherapeutic options that may be less toxic for older patients. Brentuximab vedotin (Bv) is an anti-CD30 antibody that disrupts microtubule networks, resulting in cell cycle arrest and apoptosis of HL cells. Bv was first FDA approved for relapsed/refractory HL, and has since been approved in combination with AVD (A-AVD) for advanced-stage HL. Since then, several trials are being completed to assess combination therapy of Bv with additional agents for treatment of newly diagnosed HL. A multicenter phase II study used sequential Bv prior to and after AVD for patients older than or equal to 60 years at diagnosis. They found an 82% and 95% overall response rate after the lead-in Bv cycles and then six cycles of ABVD, respectively. Two year progression-free and overall survival rates were 84% and 93%, respectively, with patients with lower geriatric comorbidity score experiencing higher PFS rates. Additional studies have assessed Bv as a single agent or in combination with nivolumab or dacarbazine as potential therapeutic options.

Relapsed/refractory disease At the time of relapsed/refractory disease, understanding suitability for autologous stem cell transplant (ASCT) is an important early step for older patients. For younger patients, standard treatment is second-line chemotherapy followed by ASCT for chemosensitive disease; over 60% of patients may be cured. However, ASCT is not appropriate for many older patients, who should be evaluated for fitness for ASCT in the context of comorbidity, frailty, and life expectancy.

For patients not eligible for ASCT, goals of care include achieving disease control balanced with toxicity. Patients may be treated with single agents or novel combinations. Patients may be treated with single-agent Bv or gemcitabine with or without radiation therapy when appropriate. Additionally, novel approaches, such as immunotherapy may be considered. Further studies are being conducted to assess treatment options for older patients with relapsed/refractory disease, but this population remains a challenge to treat.

Follow-Up and Survivorship in NHL and HL

PET-CT scan should generally be utilized at the end of treatment to assess response, which may reveal complete metabolic response or be indeterminate, requiring integration of clinical context. A complete metabolic response, even with persistent mass, is considered complete remission and has been associated with similar outcomes. CT imaging is preferred in low or variable FDG-avid histologies.

Surveillance imaging in remission is increasingly discouraged, given the lack of evidence demonstrating improvement in survival and concerns over exposure to medical radiation. The clinical context is important to consider when making these decisions, as risk of relapse is greatest in the 1 to 2 years following completion of therapy for aggressive histologies. Given the long natural history of indolent lymphomas, judicious use of follow-up scans can be considered, particularly when intra-abdominal retroperitoneal disease is present. The risks of secondary malignancies from medical radiation exposure may have less impact in patients diagnosed at older age, given the latency period.

PLASMA CELL DISORDERS

Plasma cell disorders (PCDs) encompass a range of clonal conditions, ranging from monoclonal gammopathy of undetermined significance (MGUS), which is by definition asymptomatic and requires no treatment, through multiple myeloma, wherein the clonal plasma cells cause end-organ damage, require therapy, and will ultimately cause the patient's death if left untreated. The incidence of PCDs increases with age, and the presence of multimorbidity may make it a challenge to distinguish between end-organ damage (ie, anemia, renal insufficiency, or vertebral compression fractures) related to a PCD versus another underlying comorbid condition. **Table 95-14** summarizes key aspects of the PCDs.

Laboratory Evaluation

PCDs are among the few neoplasms where routine laboratory testing other than tissue biopsy can detect the "fingerprint" of a clonal population, in this case detection of a monoclonal protein in the serum or urine. This protein may be referred to as a paraprotein, M-component/M-spike or restricted peak. The monoclonal protein may be an intact immunoglobulin (comprising both heavy and light chains), light chain only or, rarely, heavy chain only. Advances in laboratory technology have allowed more sensitive and specific detection and identification of a paraprotein and have improved our ability to monitor response to treatment in those PCDs that require treatment.

Serum protein electrophoresis In serum protein electrophoresis (SPEP), the serum proteins are separated by an electric field on an agarose gel and stained with Amido black, and quantitated by densitometer tracing of the gel. An alternate, more sensitive SPEP method, involves separation of serum proteins in a capillary tube in a liquid phase buffer by a high-voltage current and quantitation by light absorbance. The latter mechanism is more accurate as it does not rely on uptake of dye. Monoclonal proteins are named for the protein region in which they migrated, such as α_1, α_2, β, or γ (eg, "γ-restricted peak").

Serum immunofixation Immunofixation is more sensitive than is SPEP, allowing for confirmation of monoclonality and determination of the type of immunoglobulin heavy and light chain class of the involved protein. However, it is purely qualitative and does not allow quantitation. In this test, the separated serum proteins are tested with specific antibodies (eg, anti-γ, anti-μ, anti-α, anti-κ, anti-λ) and stained.

Urine protein electrophoresis Urine protein electrophoresis (UPEP) is performed in a similar manner as described for SPEP. It allows quantitation of the types of protein found in the urine. Generally the percentage of each type of protein is reported, allowing distinction between proteinuria caused primarily by albumin versus light chain production. Coupled with the total amount of protein in a 24-hour urine collection, this allows quantitation of the total amount of monoclonal protein eliminated in the urine.

Urine immunofixation Urine immunofixation, like serum immunofixation, is more sensitive for the presence of a paraprotein. Given that only the light chains are freely filtered at the glomerulus, generally only kappa or lambda light chains are detected on immunofixation of the urine, though occasionally heavy chain fragments are detectable. Urine immunofixation is a qualitative test only.

Serum-free light chain assay The serum-free light chain is a quantitative measure of excess kappa or lambda light chains produced by a plasma cell clone. Under normal circumstances, a slight excess of light chains is produced relative to heavy chains in the production of intact immunoglobulins, resulting in small quantities of kappa and lambda light chains free in the serum. The ratio of kappa to lambda light chains is roughly 1:1, with the normal range of ratios of kappa to lambda ranging from 0.26 to 1.65. In a clonal PCD, the ratio will either be greater than the upper limit of normal with a kappa paraprotein, or less than the lower limit of normal with a lambda paraprotein. Notably, as the light chains are renally cleared, the absolute level of kappa and lambda light chains may be elevated in patients with renal impairment, but the ratio will remain close to normal.

Monoclonal Gammopathy of Undetermined Significance

Definition MGUS is an asymptomatic premalignant condition characterized by the presence of a monoclonal protein in the serum or urine. The 2014 International Myeloma Working Group (IMWG) criteria defined that a diagnosis of MGUS requires a total serum M-component less than

TABLE 95-14 ■ PLASMA CELL DISORDERS: DIAGNOSTIC CRITERIA

DISORDER	SERUM MONOCLONAL PROTEIN	BONE MARROW PLASMA CELLS	END-ORGAN DAMAGE				PROGRESSION RATE AND DIAGNOSIS
			HYPERCALCEMIA	RENAL INSUFFICIENCY	ANEMIA	BONE LESIONS	
Non-IgM MGUS	< 30 g/L	< 10%	Absent	Absent	Absent	Absent	1% per year to multiple myeloma, solitary plasmacytoma, or amyloidosis
IgM MGUS[a]	< 30 g/L	< 10%	NA[a]	NA[a]	Absent	NA[a]	1.5% per year to Waldenström macroglobulinemia or amyloidosis
Light chain MGUS	No serum heavy chain by immunofixation. Abnormal free light chain ratio. Urinary monoclonal protein 500 mg/24 h	< 10%	Absent	Absent	Absent	Absent	0.3% per year to light chain multiple myeloma or amyloidosis
Solitary plasmacytoma	Negative or small monoclonal protein	No clonal plasma cells	Absent	Absent	Absent	Single, biopsy-proven lesion of bone or soft tissue; otherwise normal imaging	10% in 3 y progress to multiple myeloma
Solitary plasmacytoma with minimal marrow involvement	Negative or small monoclonal protein	< 10%	Absent	Absent	Absent	Single, biopsy-proven lesion of bone or soft tissue; otherwise normal imaging	60% (bone) or 20% (soft tissue) in 3 y progress to multiple myeloma
Smoldering myeloma	Serum monoclonal protein (IgA or IgG) ≥ 30 g/L or urinary monoclonal protein ≥ 500 mg/24 h	10%–60%	Absent	Absent	Absent	Absent	10%/y for first 5 y; 70% at 10 y progress to multiple myeloma
Multiple myeloma	Generally detectable in serum or urine with modern techniques; nonsecretory myeloma is rare	Any or > 60% if CRAB criteria absent	May be present	May be present	May be present	May be present	NA

[a]As IgM paraprotein is essentially never associated with multiple myeloma, signs or symptoms of Waldenström macroglobulinemia rather than the "CRAB" criteria for myeloma should be ruled out prior to diagnosis of IgM MGUS: constitutional symptoms, hyperviscosity, lymphadenopathy, hepatosplenomegaly; or other findings attributable to underlying lymphoproliferative disorder.

Adapted with permission from Rajkumar SV, Dimopoulos MA, Palumbo A, et al. International Myeloma Working Group updated criteria for the diagnosis of multiple myeloma. Lancet Oncol. 2014;15(12):e538–e548.

30 g/L, with bone marrow plasma cells (or lymphoplasmacytic cells in the case of an IgM paraprotein) less than 10% and no end-organ damage related to the monoclonal protein (eg, "CRAB" criteria: hyper*c*alcemia, *r*enal insufficiency, *a*nemia, or *b*one lesions) or amyloidosis (see **Table 95-14**).

Epidemiology The prevalence of MGUS in the United States is approximately 3% and ranges from 1% to 5% in other countries throughout the world. It increases in prevalence with age, and is more common in men and African-Americans. Additional risk factors include having a primary relative with a history of MGUS or myeloma, exposure to pesticides, rural residence, and possibly obesity.

Pathophysiology (classification) MGUS may be classified as IgG, IgA, light chain MGUS, or IgM MGUS. MGUS may progress to multiple myeloma, solitary plasmacytoma, or primary amyloidosis. IgM MGUS generally does not progress to multiple myeloma, but to Waldenström macroglobulinemia or amyloidosis. The rate of progression to symptomatic myeloma is about 1% per year; high-, high-intermediate, low-intermediate, and low-risk groups are defined based on the type of monoclonal protein, level of the M-spike, and whether the serum-free light chain ratio is normal.

Presentation MGUS may be discovered when the patient is undergoing evaluation for another disorder and is found to have a monoclonal protein. This may include evaluation for anemia, renal insufficiency, proteinuria, osteoporosis or fractures, hypergammaglobulinemia, or peripheral neuropathy.

Evaluation The identification of a monoclonal protein requires evaluation for the presence of end-organ damage. The history and physical examination should focus on symptoms suggestive of CRAB criteria. A CBC should be obtained to rule out anemia; a basic metabolic panel estimates renal function and rules out hypercalcemia. In the presence of concomitant explanations for anemia (eg, iron deficiency) or renal insufficiency (eg, established diagnosis of diabetic nephropathy with stable renal function), the criterion for end-organ damage is not satisfied. Finally, bone imaging is required. The traditional skeletal survey is being replaced by more sensitive bone imaging, including 15-fluorodeoxyglucose positron emission tomography (PET), magnetic resonance imaging (MRI) (either whole body or spine), or low-dose whole-body computed tomography (CT).

Management MGUS does not require treatment. Patients identified as having MGUS are followed at 6- to 12-month intervals for progression to a malignant disorder, with monitoring for anemia, renal insufficiency, hypercalcemia, or bone lesions.

Smoldering Myeloma

Definition Smoldering myeloma is intermediate between MGUS and symptomatic multiple myeloma, defined as the presence of an IgG or IgA monoclonal protein greater than or equal to 30 g/L or urinary monoclonal protein greater than or equal to 500 mg per 24 hours and/or clonal bone marrow plasma cells 10% to 60%. End-organ damage related to the paraprotein (hypercalcemia, renal insufficiency, anemia, bone lesions, or amyloidosis) must be absent.

Pathophysiology (classification) Only 50% of patients with smoldering myeloma progress to require therapy in 5 years (10% risk per year), and 30% are free of progression to myeloma at 10 years. Because of this heterogeneity, subgroups of patients at highest risk for progression from smoldering to overt myeloma were identified, in order to not subject the patient to end-organ damage before initiation of treatment. About 90% of patients with more than 60% plasma cells in their bone marrow progress to multiple myeloma requiring treatment within 2 years, leading to the recent change in myeloma diagnostic criteria: These patients previously diagnosed with smoldering myeloma are now categorized as having multiple myeloma requiring treatment.

Evaluation Evaluation should be as for MGUS earlier, but also requires a bone marrow biopsy to determine the percentage of plasma cells in the bone marrow. As with MGUS, bone imaging such as whole-body CT, PET-CT, or whole body MRI to detect lytic lesions is required

Management

Nonpharmacologic Patients with smoldering myeloma should be followed at 3- to 6-month intervals for history and physical examination and laboratory evaluation including CBCs, a basic metabolic profile, and quantitation of the monoclonal protein.

Drugs Previously, only observation was recommended for patients with smoldering myeloma. Data are emerging demonstrating a benefit to treatment with the immunomodulatory agent lenalidomide in individuals with intermediate or high-risk smoldering myeloma, with delay of progression to myeloma and the development of myeloma-related end organ damage.

Multiple Myeloma

Definition Multiple myeloma is the malignant clonal proliferation of plasma cells with related end-organ damage, including hypercalcemia caused by lytic bone lesions, anemia, and renal insufficiency, which may be caused by hypercalcemia or light chain nephropathy.

Epidemiology Multiple myeloma is the second most common hematologic malignancy, with an estimated 34,920 new diagnoses in 2021 in the United States. Current evidence supports the fact that all cases of multiple myeloma are preceded by MGUS. As with MGUS, male gender, African-American race, and advancing age are all associated with increased incidence of multiple myeloma. With the aging of the population, there will be a 57% increase in the incidence of myeloma, and more strikingly, a 77% increase in the incidence of myeloma in people older than age 65.

Presentation The most common presenting symptom is bone pain, present in three out of five patients. Back pain is generally of less than 1 year in duration. Fatigue is present in one-third of patients. Other symptoms may include altered mental status or constipation due to hypercalcemia, recurrent infections, or weight loss. Patients who have developed cord compression may present with paresis. Some patients may present with abnormal laboratory findings alone, including anemia, renal insufficiency, hypercalcemia, or an elevated total serum protein level with hypoalbuminemia (an elevated "protein gap").

Evaluation Evaluation includes a thorough history and physical examination, seeking evidence of end-organ damage. Examination may reveal pallor, indicative of anemia, kyphosis related to vertebral compression fractures, or mental status changes due to hypercalcemia. Laboratory evaluation includes CBCs, comprehensive metabolic profile, serum protein electrophoresis and immunofixation, urine protein electrophoresis and immunofixation, quantitative immunoglobulins, serum-free light chains, lactate dehydrogenase, and β_2-microglobulin. Radiographic evaluation begins with advanced bone imaging, such as low-dose whole body CT, PET-CT, or whole body MRI. Skeletal survey alone is no longer considered adequate for detection of myeloma bone lesions. Notably, nuclear medicine bone scans are generally negative in multiple myeloma, given that myeloma bone lesions are purely lytic. Finally, pathologic confirmation of the diagnosis is obtained with bone marrow core biopsy and aspirate. The bone marrow aspirate is also sent for cytogenetics and FISH for chromosomal abnormalities commonly seen in multiple myeloma.

Pathophysiology (classification) The current staging system used for multiple myeloma is the Revised-International Staging System. This system, replacing the older Durie-Salmon staging system and its precursor International Staging System, requires the serum albumin, β_2-microglobulin, and lactate dehydrogenase levels as well as the presence or absence of higher risk chromosomal abnormalities, including t4;14, t14;16, and del 17p.

Management The management of multiple myeloma in older adults can be complex.

Nonpharmacologic As a systemic disease, multiple myeloma essentially categorically requires systemic therapy. However, radiation or surgery may have a role in the management of skeletal lesions or the oncologic emergency spinal cord compression. Patients who present with cord compression may undergo surgical decompression followed by radiation with a goal of preserving or restoring function. Patients who present with pathologic fractures or lesions of the long bones at risk for pathologic fracture may undergo surgical stabilization to preserve or restore function; such lesions are generally irradiated postoperatively to facilitate healing and decrease pain. Other painful bone lesions may be irradiated for pain relief.

Drugs The therapeutic options for multiple myeloma have improved dramatically in the past 20 years, resulting in a near-doubling of the average overall survival times. For adults aged 65 to 74, the 5-year survival rate improved from 27% in 1998 to 2004 to 39% in 2005 to 2009 then to 48% in 2010 to 2014. For adults aged 75 to 90, the 5-year survival rate improved from 16% in 1998 to 2004 to 23% in 2005 to 2009 then to 31% in 2010 to 2014. Continued advances promise continuing improvement in the duration of survival.

MELPHALAN. For over three decades, oral melphalan was the standard of care for patients with multiple myeloma. When melphalan is combined with prednisone, about 50% of patients will have at least a partial response to therapy. The main toxicity of melphalan is myelosuppression. Melphalan is still used in some regimens for older adults, but has largely been supplanted by newer more effective treatment options.

CORTICOSTEROIDS. Corticosteroids are incorporated into essentially every antimyeloma regimen. Corticosteroids have rapid direct antimyeloma efficacy and act synergistically with other agents. Corticosteroids are often used when patients present acutely and highly symptomatically with a new diagnosis of multiple myeloma. High-dose corticosteroids (eg, dexamethasone 40 mg orally × 4 days) can be used to rapidly ameliorate hypercalcemia or significant bone pain. However, corticosteroid dosing should be chosen cautiously for longer-term management. In a randomized trial of lenalidomide with high-dose versus low-dose dexamethasone (lenalidomide plus dexamethasone 40 mg orally on days 1–4, 9–12, and 17–20 [RD] versus lenalidomide plus dexamethasone 40 mg weekly), RD was associated with a higher response rate but *poorer overall survival* due to increased toxicity (primarily venous thromboembolic events and infections). Thus, high-dose corticosteroids should be avoided in older patients due to increased risk of treatment-related mortality. Further, a recent randomized trial demonstrated that in intermediate-fit older adults, discontinuation of steroids after the first 9 months of the initial therapy resulted in superior event-free survival, indicating less toxicity with preserved antimyeloma efficacy. Similar studies have not been conducted in the setting of relapsed/refractory myeloma, and steroids remain an anchor in the treatment of myeloma.

THALIDOMIDE. The antimyeloma efficacy of the immunomodulatory agent thalidomide was first reported in 1999, heralding a revolution in the treatment of multiple myeloma. Over the first decade of the new century, thalidomide was utilized in a number of combinations, including with melphalan and prednisone (MPT) and bortezomib, melphalan, and prednisone (VMPT). The toxicities of thalidomide include sedation, constipation, peripheral neuropathy, and venous thromboembolic events. It is used less frequently now in preference for more effective and less toxic options.

LENALIDOMIDE. Lenalidomide, another immunomodulatory agent, has largely supplanted thalidomide due to improved tolerability and efficacy. Lenalidomide's toxicities include venous thromboembolism and cytopenias. A randomized trial demonstrated that continuous lenalidomide with dexamethasone improves progression-free and overall survival over MPT or lenalidomide and dexamethasone of a fixed duration (18 months), establishing this regimen as a standard of care in older adults with multiple myeloma. Dose must be adjusted for renal insufficiency.

POMALIDOMIDE. Pomalidomide is approved in the United States for patients with relapsed or refractory myeloma who have previously been treated with bortezomib and lenalidomide.

BORTEZOMIB. Bortezomib is a proteasome inhibitor administered parenterally for initial therapy or at relapse. It was initially administered intravenously and twice weekly, a regimen which was found to be excessively toxic in older adults. Once-weekly subcutaneous administration of bortezomib is tolerated much better in older adults, with similar efficacy. The main toxicities of bortezomib are peripheral neuropathy, cytopenias, and herpes zoster. Bortezomib is administered in combination with dexamethasone, and may be used in combination with another agent, such as lenalidomide or cyclophosphamide. Bortezomib does not require dose adjustment for renal impairment.

CARFILZOMIB. Carfilzomib is the second-in-class proteasome inhibitor, approved in the United States for patients with relapsed or refractory multiple myeloma who have received bortezomib and an immunomodulatory agent (either lenalidomide or thalidomide). Its toxicities include cytopenias and dyspnea. Cardiotoxicity is an increasingly recognized adverse effect of particular concern in older adults.

IXAZOMIB. Ixazomib is an orally administered proteasome inhibitor with efficacy and toxicity similar to bortezomib. It is approved in combination with lenalidomide and dexamethasone in patients with relapsed myeloma, but there is interest in its use in the initial therapy setting, particularly for older adults.

MONOCLONAL ANTIBODIES. Elotuzumab is a monoclonal antibody directed against SLAMF7, a marker found on both selected normal hematopoietic cells and myeloma cells. It is approved for use in combination with lenalidomide and dexamethasone for patients with relapsed myeloma. Daratumumab is a monoclonal antibody directed against CD38, present on plasma cells. It is available in both intravenous and subcutaneous formulations, with its main toxicities being infusion reactions and risk of infection. It is approved for use in combination with lenalidomide and dexamethasone for older adults who will not be undergoing stem cell transplant, as well as in the relapsed setting.

COMBINATION REGIMENS. Numerous combinations of the above agents have been examined in clinical trials. Generally, combination regimens result in higher response rates, but also in greater toxicity; whether the combination improves outcomes like overall survival depends on the balance of efficacy and toxicity. The IMWG recommends that older adults with multiple myeloma deemed more frail receive either well-tolerated three-drug combinations or only two-drug combinations (lenalidomide and dexamethasone).

HIGH-DOSE THERAPY AND AUTOLOGOUS STEM CELL TRANSPLANTATION. Select, fit older adults, generally under age 75 but occasionally older, may be candidates for high-dose therapy and autologous stem cell transplantation. Even with the tremendous advances in treatment, the approach of induction therapy, high-dose therapy/autologous stem cell transplant, followed by maintenance therapy, continues to produce the longest durations of myeloma control of all therapeutic options.

EMERGING THERAPIES. The entire wealth of emerging treatments, either approved in relapsed settings or still investigational, is beyond the scope of this chapter. Among the newest options approved are selinexor, belantamab mafodotin-blmf, isatuximab, and melphalan flufenamide. A paucity of data on the toxicity of the newest drugs in older patients presents a challenge for clinicians and patients considering these approaches. Chimeric antigen receptor T cells are a still-investigational approach expected to emerge in practice in 2021.

Prevention of complications

Skeletal-Related Events Intravenous bisphosphonates are effective for primary or secondary prevention of skeletal-related events (including pathologic fractures or painful lytic lesions requiring radiation). Zoledronic acid and pamidronate are utilized in the United States. Denosumab, the RANK ligand inhibitor, is approved for patients with multiple myeloma and utilized in patients with renal impairment in whom bisphosphonates are contraindicated.

Infection Prophylaxis Patients with multiple myeloma should receive the pneumococcal vaccine and annual influenza vaccinations. Patients receiving certain treatments should receive herpes zoster prophylaxis with acyclovir or valacyclovir. One randomized trial demonstrated a reduction in fever or early death in patients treated with levofloxacin for the first 3 months after diagnosis.

Special issues

Frailty Given that the majority of patients with myeloma are older than age 65, there has been great interest in developing an easily implemented measure of frailty. The International Myeloma Working Group developed a frailty score based on age greater than 80, dependence in ADL/IADL, and comorbidities that predict toxicity of therapy and survival. Studies selecting patients based on their frailty level (fit, intermediate, or frail) or adjusting treatment based on the same are emerging and underway, promising improved means to tailor treatment to the health of older adults.

Comorbidity The presence of comorbidities is prognostic in older adults with multiple myeloma. Comorbidities may also limit treatment options or influence the rates of toxicity. For example, underlying peripheral neuropathy may limit the use of bortezomib. Diabetes may limit the dose of corticosteroids due to hyperglycemia. Patients and clinicians may have concerns about using carfilzomib in the presence of underlying cardiac disease given risk for dyspnea.

Solitary Plasmacytomas

Definition Solitary plasmacytomas are malignant proliferations of plasma cells located either in bone or soft tissue, in the absence of other evidence of end-organ damage, and with no or minimal (< 10%) plasma cells in the bone marrow (see **Table 95-14**).

Epidemiology Plasmacytomas are a relatively rare PCD, with an incidence rate of 0.34 cases per 100,000 person-years. Similar to multiple myeloma, plasmacytomas are more common among males and those of Black race.

Presentation Solitary plasmacytomas of bone occur most commonly in the axial skeleton, including the vertebrae or pelvis. Solitary extramedullary plasmacytomas occur most commonly in the upper aerodigestive tract, including the nasal cavity, nasopharynx, oral cavity, or sinuses. Presentation is generally related to local symptoms of the mass.

Evaluation Evaluation of plasmacytomas proceeds as the evaluation for multiple myeloma, with the goal of ruling out multiple myeloma.

Management

Nonpharmacologic The treatment for solitary plasmacytoma is radiation therapy, with curative intent. Radiation is highly effective at establishing local control of the plasmacytoma, and relapses within the radiation field are unusual. If the patient experiences recurrence, it is generally progression to multiple myeloma rather than a local recurrence or persistence of the plasmacytoma.

Drugs Systemic therapy as for multiple myeloma is utilized in the setting of a radiation-refractory solitary plasmacytoma or progression to multiple myeloma.

Primary Amyloidosis

Definition Amyloidosis is a heterogenous group of rare disorders characterized by the deposition of amyloid fibrils in soft tissues. Nearly 30 different amyloidogenic proteins have been implicated; herein we focus exclusively on AL amyloidosis, where a monoclonal PCD results in the formation of amyloidogenic kappa or lambda light chains.

Epidemiology AL amyloidosis is extremely rare, with only 10 patients diagnosed per 1,000,000 person-years. It coexists with multiple myeloma in 10% of cases.

Presentation Presenting symptoms may be diverse given the range of organs potentially involved in AL amyloidosis. Symptoms may include fatigue, dyspnea, edema, or neuropathy.

Evaluation History may reveal fatigue, dyspnea on exertion or orthopnea suggestive of heart failure, lower extremity edema, or paresthesias or abnormal bruising. Examination may reveal periorbital purpura, macroglossia, signs of heart failure, hepatosplenomegaly, ecchymosis, or sensory neuropathy. Laboratory evaluation includes CBCs and a comprehensive metabolic profile, serum and urine electrophoresis, and immunofixation and serum-free light chain assay. A 24-hour urine collection for electrophoresis will demonstrate that proteinuria is largely albuminuria rather than light chain excretion. A bone marrow biopsy may demonstrate a small clonal plasma cell population and amyloid deposition. Echocardiography or cardiac MRI may demonstrate evidence of cardiac involvement. Serum N-terminal pro-brain natriuretic peptide (NT-proBNP) and troponin-T levels are prognostic and should be obtained. A periumbilical fat pad aspiration may provide the patient with pathologic confirmation of amyloid deposition without subjecting the patient to a more invasive endomyocardial, renal, or hepatic biopsy.

Pathophysiology (classification) Distinguishing AL amyloidosis from other forms of amyloidosis can be challenging; a monoclonal protein may coexist with another form of amyloid. Amyloid typing can be accomplished through direct immunofluorescence microscopy or immunohistochemistry. Staging is based on NT-proBNP levels, troponin-T levels, and serum-free light chain levels. Cardiac involvement portends a particularly poor prognosis, with a median survival of fewer than 6 months in patients with elevated cardiac markers and involved serum light chains. In patients with no high-risk factors, the median survival is nearly 8 years.

Management Management of AL amyloidosis is essentially entirely pharmacologic. There is no role for surgery or radiation aside from skeletal issues if there is overlap with multiple myeloma. Treatment is directed at the malignant plasma cell clone. A small minority of patients is eligible for high-dose therapy and autologous stem cell transplantation and may experience complete responses and long-term survival (> 10 years). The systemic therapeutic options utilized in multiple myeloma have activity in amyloidosis, though some require lower doses for tolerability.

Conclusion

The PCDs share in common a clonal proliferation of plasma cells, which are detectable via a monoclonal protein in the serum or urine. MGUS is a premalignant, asymptomatic laboratory finding, which progresses to a malignant disorder at a rate of 1% per year. Solitary plasmacytomas are potentially curable with radiation therapy. Multiple myeloma remains an incurable plasma cell malignancy, but therapeutic options have substantially improved in the past two decades. Amyloidosis remains a therapeutic challenge, though improved risk stratification and the use of novel agents developed in myeloma are improving the landscape.

FURTHER READING

Coiffier B, Lepage E, Briere J, et al. CHOP chemotherapy plus rituximab compared with CHOP alone in elderly patients with diffuse large B-cell lymphoma. *N Engl J Med*. 2002;346:235–242.

Cook G, Larocca A, Facon T, et al. Defining the vulnerable patient with myeloma-a frailty position paper of the European Myeloma Network. *Leukemia*. 2020;34(9):2285–2294.

Delarue R, Tilly H, Mounier N, et al. Dose-dense rituximab-CHOP compared with standard rituximab-CHOP in elderly patients with diffuse large B-cell lymphoma (the LNH03-6B study): a randomised phase 3 trial. *Lancet Oncol*. 2013;14(6):525–533.

DiNardo CD, Jonas BA, Pullarkat V, et al. Azacitidine and venetoclax in previously untreated acute myeloid leukemia. *N Engl J Med*. 2020;383(7):617–629.

Gertz MA. Immunoglobulin light chain amyloidosis: 2020 update on diagnosis, prognosis, and treatment. *Am J Hematol*. 2020;95(7):848–860.

Goede V, Fischer K, Busch R, et al. Obinutuzumab plus chlorambucil in patients with CLL and coexisting conditions. *N Engl J Med*. 2014;370(12):1101–1110.

Greenberg PL, Tuechler H, Schanz J, et al. Revised international prognostic scoring system for myelodysplastic syndromes. *Blood*. 2012;120(12):2454–2465.

Hochhaus A, Larson RA, Guilhot F, et al. Long-term outcomes of imatinib treatment for chronic myeloid leukemia. *N Engl J Med*. 2017;376(10):917–927.

Klepin HD, Geiger AM, Tooze JA, et al. Geriatric assessment predicts survival for older adults receiving induction chemotherapy for acute myelogenous leukemia. *Blood*. 2013;121(21):4287–4294.

Kornblith AB, Herndon JE, Silverman LR, et al. Impact of azacytidine on the quality of life of patients with myelodysplastic syndrome treated in a randomized phase III trial: a Cancer and Leukemia Group B study. *J Clin Oncol*. 2002;20(10):2441–2452.

List A, Dewald G, Bennett J, et al. Lenalidomide in the myelodysplastic syndrome with chromosome 5q deletion. *N Engl J Med*. 2006;355(14):1456–1465.

Lo-Coco F, Avvisati G, Vignetti M, et al. Retinoic acid and arsenic trioxide for acute promyelocytic leukemia. *N Engl J Med*. 2013;369(2):111–121.

Mikhael J, Ismaila N, Cheung MC, et al. Treatment of multiple myeloma: ASCO and CCO Joint Clinical Practice Guideline. *J Clin Oncol*. 2019;37(14):1228–1263.

Morrison VA, Hamlin P, Soubeyran P, et al. Approach to therapy of diffuse large B-cell lymphoma in the elderly: the International Society of Geriatric Oncology (SIOG) expert position commentary. *Ann Oncol*. 2015;26(6):1058–1068.

Palumbo A, Rajkumar SV, San Miguel JF, et al. International Myeloma Working Group consensus statement for the management, treatment, and supportive care of patients with myeloma not eligible for standard autologous stem-cell transplantation. *J Clin Oncol*. 2014;32(6):587–600.

Peyrade F, Jardin F, Thieblemont C, et al. Attenuated immunochemotherapy regimen (R-mini-CHOP) in elderly patients older than 80 years with diffuse large B-cell lymphoma: a multicentre, single-arm, phase 2 trial. *Lancet Oncol*. 12(5):460–468, 2011.

Rajkumar SV, Dimopoulos MA, Palumbo A, et al. International Myeloma Working Group updated criteria for the diagnosis of multiple myeloma. *Lancet Oncol*. 2014;15(12):e538–548.

Rosko AE, Cordoba R, Abel G, et al. Advances in older adults with hematologic malignancies. *J Clin Oncol*. 2021;39(19):2102–2114.

Sekeres MA, Guyatt G, Abel G, et al. American Society of Hematology 2020 guidelines for treating newly diagnosed acute myeloid leukemia in older adults. *Blood Adv*. 2020;4(15):3528–3549.

Starkman R, Alibhai S, Wells RA, et al. An MDS-specific frailty index based cumulative deficits adds independent prognostic information to clinical prognostic scoring. *Leukemia*. 2020;34(5):1394–1406.

Woyach JA, Ruppert AS, Heerema NA, et al. Ibrutinib regimens versus chemoimmunotherapy in older persons with untreated CLL. *N Engl J Med*. 2018;379(26):2517–2528.

Chapter 96

Coagulation Disorders

Ming Y. Lim

OVERVIEW OF COAGULATION

Hemostasis typically refers to the process of thrombus formation at areas of endothelial or vascular wall injury (**Figure 96-1**). Under normal physiologic conditions, this process is localized to the site of injury and is rapid, dynamic, and highly regulated. Phases of this response include initial formation of the platelet plug following endothelial injury, activation of the coagulation cascade for further hemostatic control, regulation of coagulation by endogenous anticoagulants to limit thrombus formation, and finally, fibrinolysis for thrombus removal.

Platelets

Platelets are integral directors and mediators of hemostatic responses. Following activation by collagen, laminin, microfibrils, and other elements in the exposed subendothelium, platelets are activated and bind to von Willebrand factor (VWF) and fibrinogen via the platelet glycoprotein 1b-alpha and platelet glycoprotein IIb/IIIa receptor (also referred as integrin $\alpha IIb\beta_3$), respectively. This leads to enhanced platelet adhesion and aggregation, resulting in a platelet plug.

Coagulation Cascade

While the clotting cascade is a complex series of pathways, several key events are briefly reviewed here. Classically, the coagulation cascade has been divided into the intrinsic and extrinsic pathways, as illustrated in **Figure 96-2**. In recent years, investigators have proposed a cell-based model of coagulation that occurs on the cell surface in four overlapping steps: (1) initiation, (2) amplification, (3) propagation, and (4) termination (**Table 96-1**). The primary event for initiation of the clotting cascade and subsequent thrombus formation is interactions of activated factor VII (FVIIa) with exposed tissue factor, an integral membrane glycoprotein, at areas of endothelial or tissue injury. The TF-FVIIa complex (also known as the extrinsic tenase complex) then activates factor IX (FIX) and factor X (FX). Activated factor X (FXa) converts a small amount of factor II (FII, also known as prothrombin) to thrombin (FIIa). The small amount of thrombin generated during the initiation phase then activates platelets, factor V (FV), factor VIII (FVIII), and factor XI (FXI) (amplification phase). During the propagation phase, activated FXI (FXIa) generates activated

Learning Objectives

- Understand how aging alters hemostatic pathways to increase the risk of both bleeding and thrombosis.
- Review the evaluation of older adults with bleeding disorders.
- Understand the pathophysiology, diagnosis, and treatment of venous thromboembolism (VTE) in older adults.
- Review the strategies to reduce bleeding risk in older adults on anticoagulation.

Key Clinical Points

1. The risk of bleeding rises with age and is most commonly due to acquired bleeding disorders and disorders of platelet number or function.
2. Aging is associated with an increased risk of VTE.
3. Direct oral anticoagulants (DOACs) are safe and effective in carefully selected older adults for the treatment of VTE.
4. A careful consideration of the net clinical benefit of anticoagulation in older adults is integral to the selection and management of oral anticoagulants in this high-risk population.

FIX (FIXa), which binds to activated (FVIIIa) to form the intrinsic tenase complex. This complex (FIXa:FVIIIa) results in large production of FXa, which in combination with its cofactor, FVa, forms the prothrombinase complex (FXa:FVa), which cleaves prothrombin to thrombin. The efficiency of both the intrinsic tenase complex and prothrombinase complex is enhanced by their co-localization on the surface of activated platelets recruited to the site of endothelial or tissue injury, resulting in a burst of thrombin formation. Thrombin then converts fibrinogen to fibrin and overlapping fibrin strands are cross-linked and stabilized by activated factor XIII (FXIIIa).

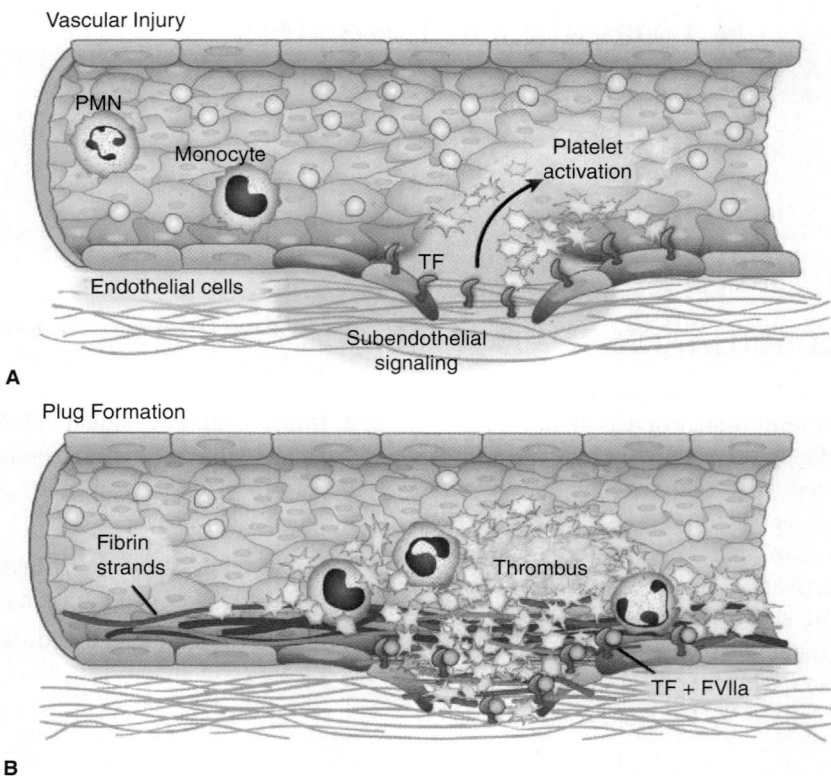

FIGURE 96-1. Thrombus formation may occur at areas of endothelial or vascular wall injury. Under normal physiologic conditions, this rapid, dynamic process is localized to the site of injury. **A.** Upon exposure of tissue factor (TF) in the exposed endothelium, there is initial platelet activation and adhesion with binding of platelets to the damaged vessel. **B.** As formation of the hemostatic plug continues, additional platelets, monocytes, polymorphonuclear cells (PMNs), and other cells migrate to and become incorporated within the hemostatic plug. Deposition of fibrin strands additionally helps seal the injured area.

Endogenous anticoagulants, including antithrombin (AT), protein C, protein S, and tissue factor pathway inhibitor (TFPI), act to limit coagulation at the site of injury. AT binds and inactivates thrombin, as well as FXa. Activated protein C, in complex with its cofactor protein S, inactivates FVa and FVIIIa. TFPI inhibits the extrinsic tenase complex (TF-FVIIa) and FXa. Together, these reactions limit further thrombin generation.

Fibrinolytic System

The formed fibrin clot undergoes fibrinolysis which is initiated by the release of tissue plasminogen activator (tPA) from endothelial cells. tPA converts plasminogen to plasmin, which cleaves fibrin into soluble fibrin degradation products, including D-dimer. Fibrinolysis is regulated by plasminogen activator inhibitor-1 (PAI-1) and α2-antiplasmin (α2AP), which inhibit tPA and plasmin, respectively.

BLEEDING DISORDERS

Epidemiology and Pathophysiology

The risk of bleeding rises with age and is most commonly due to acquired bleeding disorders affecting coagulation factors and/or platelet number and function. For example, bleeding due primarily to disorders of coagulation factors may be seen in older patients with sepsis and disseminated intravascular coagulation (DIC), liver disease, acquired hemophilia with inhibitors to FVIII, acquired von Willebrand syndrome, or due to anticoagulant use. Disorders in older adults that may primarily affect platelet number and/or function include immune thrombocytopenia (ITP), chronic kidney disease, myeloproliferative neoplasms, drug-induced thrombocytopenia, and use of antiplatelet agents. The precise incidence and prevalence of these vary depending on the patient and clinical situation studied. Some of these disorders are described in more detail below.

In addition, and while still incompletely understood, aging itself—devoid of any comorbid influences or anticoagulant/antiplatelet use—has been associated with dysregulation of coagulation factors, fibrinolytic proteins, and activation molecules, which increases bleeding risk. Conversely, the plasma concentrations of many coagulation factors increase with aging. While these age-related changes are not uniform, the net effect seemingly results in a tendency toward thrombosis, rather than bleeding.

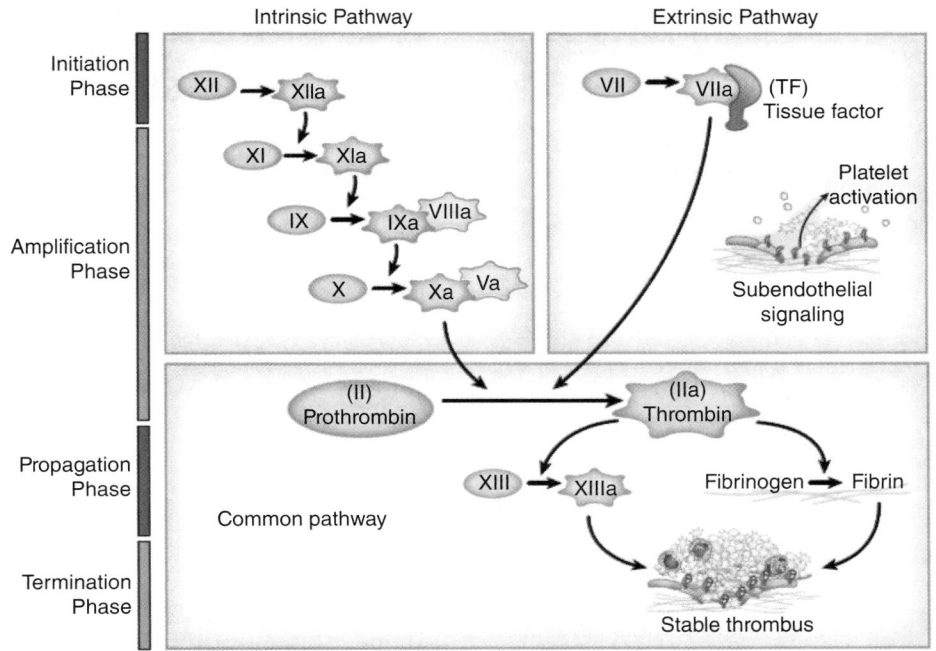

FIGURE 96-2. The clotting cascade is a complex series of pathways and key events. The coagulation cascade may be divided into the intrinsic and extrinsic pathways and, in parallel, also considered in the context of a cell-based model of coagulation that occurs on the cell surface in four sequential phases, as illustrated on the left side of this panel and described in Table 96-1: (1) initiation, (2) amplification, (3) propagation, and (4) termination. The primary event for initiation of the extrinsic pathway is the interaction between activated factor VII (FVIIa) and exposed tissue factor (TF), often at areas of endothelial or tissue injury. The intrinsic pathway begins with activation of factor XII, driving subsequent activation of factors XI, IX, and X. Both the intrinsic and extrinsic pathways result in the conversion of prothrombin (FII) to thrombin (FIIa), in the final common pathway. Thrombin then converts fibrinogen to fibrin, and overlapping fibrin strands are cross-linked and stabilized by activated factor XIII (FXIIIa), resulting in stable thrombus formation.

For example, plasma fibrinogen levels, which correlate with an increased risk of cardiovascular disease, increase with age, with an approximate 10 mg/dL incremental rise per decade in healthy subjects. Similarly, vWF levels increase approximately 10% to 20% per decade of life and are associated with an increased risk of cardiovascular disease.

Components of the fibrinolytic pathway are also altered in older adults. Plasma levels of PAI-1, the major inhibitor of fibrinolysis, increase with aging, resulting in an age-dependent decrease in fibrinolytic activity. Age-related increases of plasmin-antiplasmin complex and D-dimer have also been reported suggesting enhanced hyperfibrinolysis.

Presentation and Diagnosis

The initial steps to evaluating bleeding in older adults, like many assessments in medical practice, begin with a careful history and physical examination. Identifying and integrating key components of the patient's history and physical examination with laboratory data allows providers to more precisely diagnose the underlying etiology of a bleeding diathesis. Patients should be asked about the initial onset and site of bleeding, prior bleeding episodes (spontaneous and/or postsurgery or trauma), a history of iron deficiency anemia, prior blood transfusions, and a history of heavy menstrual bleeding and/or postpartum hemorrhage (in women).

The presence of other family members with similar bleeding tendencies, particularly in the presence of bleeding that began after birth or during childhood, may suggest an inherited bleeding diathesis. A thorough medication history, including the use of anticoagulants, herbal agents, and over-the-counter (OTC) products, should be obtained. Patients may need to be asked specifically about the use of aspirin, nonsteroidal anti-inflammatories, or other OTC antiplatelet agents. To assess for the possibility of dietary vitamin K deficiency, providers should inquire about the patient's dietary habits, and whether there have been any changes recently to the diet.

Physical Examination

The physical examination is typically normal, but can vary considerably. Petechiae (small capillary hemorrhages most commonly seen on the legs), epistaxis or gingival bleeding may be seen if there is a disorder of platelet number/function or blood vessels. Older adults with an acquired coagulation disorder can present with large, palpable ecchymoses, soft tissue hematomas, hemarthrosis, and extensive postprocedural bleeding.

TABLE 96-1 ■ KEY PHASES OF THE CELL-BASED MODEL OF COAGULATION[a]

PHASE OF COAGULATION	DESCRIPTION OF KEY EVENT(S)	LOCATION OF KEY EVENT(S)
Initiation	Extrinsic tenase complexes activate factors V, IX, and X resulting in conversion of prothrombin to thrombin	TF-expressing cells, including monocytes, endothelial cells, and platelets
Amplification	Small amounts of thrombin generated during the initiation phase activate platelets, factors V, VIII, and XI	The surface of activated platelets
Propagation	Activated platelets co-localize the intrinsic tenase complexes and prothrombinase complexes to generate a burst of thrombin and form stable fibrin plugs	The surface of activated platelets
Termination	Endogenous anticoagulants, such as TFPI, PC, PS, and AT limit widespread thrombotic occlusion	The site of injured endothelium or vasculature

AT, antithrombin; PC, protein C; PS, protein S; TF, tissue factor; TFPI, tissue factor pathway inhibitor.
[a]This is a complex series of pathways that is still actively studied, but critical events during each phase of this model are described.

Laboratory Evaluation of Coagulation Pathways in Older Adults

Laboratory evaluation includes routine tests available through most laboratories as well as more specialized tests that may require a reference laboratory and the expertise of a hematologist for interpretation. General screening tests include a platelet count, hemoglobin and/or hematocrit, prothrombin time (PT), and activated partial thromboplastin time (aPTT). The PT assay measures the function of the extrinsic and common pathways (see **Figure 96-2**) and detects deficiencies in the vitamin K–dependent coagulation factors: factors II, VII, IX, and X. If a deficiency in factor VII is suspected, the PT is the most sensitive test available. The aPTT measures components of the intrinsic and common pathways and can detect deficiencies of—or inhibitors to—factors II, V, VIII, IX, X, XI, and XII (see **Figure 96-2**). Both the PT and aPTT can also be prolonged in patients with fibrinogen disorders. Examination of any abnormalities in the PT and/or aPTT can help guide clinicians as to the differential diagnostic and appropriate management steps (**Table 96-2**). Other routine testing (eg, liver or renal function panels, peripheral smears, DIC panel, mixing study etc.) may be indicated depending on the patient's clinical presentation, history, and physical examination.

Causes of a prolonged PT with a normal aPTT Causes include warfarin or other vitamin K antagonist (VKA) use, vitamin K deficiency, systemic heparin exposure, factor VII deficiency (inherited or acquired), early liver disease, and in some early cases of DIC. PT prolongation is commonly seen in older hospitalized patients who, unable to eat or have reduced dietary intake of food rich in vitamin K, become deficient in vitamin K.

Causes of a normal PT with a prolonged aPTT Causes include anticoagulant use (eg, heparin), deficiencies in factor VIII and/or VWF (hemophilia A, von Willebrand disease), factor IX (hemophilia B), and factor XI (hemophilia C). The use of subcutaneous heparin for venous thromboembolism (VTE) prophylaxis is the most common cause for an isolated prolonged aPTT in hospitalized patients. Von Willebrand disease is the most common inherited bleeding disorder affecting up to 1% of the general population and typically presents with mucocutaneous bleeds (epistaxis, heavy menstrual bleed, easy bruising, and postpartum hemorrhage). Patients with hemophilia usually present in childhood or young adulthood with recurrent soft tissue and joint bleeding and postprocedural bleeding. Factor XI deficiency has a more variable bleeding history, often following surgical procedures.

A prolonged aPTT may also be due to the presence of a circulating acquired inhibitor. The most common acquired inhibitor is the lupus anticoagulant, although this inhibitor causes thrombosis instead of bleeding. Acquired hemophilia A (AHA) is a rare autoimmune disorder, with an incidence of approximately 1.5 cases per million per year, that is caused by the production of IgG autoantibodies against endogenous FVIII. It is predominantly a disease of older adults (median age 64–78), but can be associated with malignancies, rheumatological conditions, and pregnancy in younger patients. In up to 50% of patients, there may be no underlying, identifiable etiology. Older adults presenting with an acute onset of subcutaneous bleeding, gastrointestinal bleeding, or muscle bleeding without a history of trauma or prior known bleeding diathesis should prompt evaluation for AHA as it is associated with a high mortality rate of more than 20% if diagnosis is delayed or misdiagnosed.

Causes of a prolonged PT and aPTT Patients with prolongation of both the PT and aPTT should be suspected of having either an inherited disorder of the common pathway or an acquired disorder that affects the intrinsic, extrinsic, and/or common pathways in combination. In older adults, the most common causes of a prolonged PT and aPTT include supratherapeutic anticoagulation with a VKA or anticoagulation bridging therapy with a VKA and heparin that occurs during the initial treatment of acute VTE. Rarely, accidental rodenticide (brodifacoum) poisoning is a cause for significantly prolonged PT and aPTT. Other possible causes include end-stage liver

TABLE 96-2 ■ PATTERNS AND EVALUATION OF A PROLONGED PROTHROMBIN TIME (PT) AND/OR ACTIVATED PARTIAL THROMBOPLASTIN TIME (aPTT)*

PT RESULT	aPTT RESULT	POTENTIAL ETIOLOGY
Prolonged	Normal	Intended or surreptitious VKA use Dietary vitamin K deficiency Factor VII deficiency[a] Early liver disease Early DIC Heparin exposure (high doses)
Normal	Prolonged	Lupus anticoagulant Factor VIII, IX, XI, XII deficiency[a] von Willebrand disease[a] Heparin exposure
Prolonged	Prolonged	Supratherapeutic anticoagulation Concomitant heparin and VKA therapy End-stage liver disease Disseminated intravascular coagulation Systemic fibrinolytic therapy Inherited disorder of common pathway Deficiency or inhibitor of factor II, V, X[a] Deficiency or inhibitor to fibrinogen[a] Accidental rodenticide poisoning

DIC, disseminated intravascular coagulation; VKA, vitamin K antagonist.

[a]May be inherited or acquired.

*This list represents common causes of PT/aPTT prolongations. Other less common causes may also exist and the reader is referred to more comprehensive reviews on this subject.

disease, DIC, or administration of systemic fibrinolytic agents (eg, tPA). Additional diagnostic measures in this setting may include measurements of fibrinogen and fibrinogen degradation products.

Abnormal Platelet Number in Older Adults

The normal half-life of circulating platelets in healthy humans is 8 to 10 days. Any process that disrupts this, leading to reductions in platelet number, may increase the risk of, or cause, bleeding in older adults. Quantitative disorders of platelet number in older adults are numerous and some of the more common of these are outlined in **Table 96-3**. Broadly, the causes of thrombocytopenia in older adults can be due to decreased platelet production, increased platelet destruction or consumption, increased platelet sequestration, dilutional effects, and spurious thrombocytopenia.

Decreased production of platelets is most often encountered in patients with disorders that impair bone marrow thrombopoiesis. These disorders commonly include nutrient deficiencies, myelodysplastic syndromes, and acute or chronic infectious syndromes. These are particularly common in older adults. For example, vitamin B_{12} and folate deficiency can be found in up to 24% and 10% of older adults, respectively. Similarly the median age at diagnosis for patients with myelodysplastic syndromes exceeds 65 in most studies, with an onset of disease earlier than 50 being very uncommon. Finally, older adults are at markedly increased risk of infection from bacterial, viral, and fungal causes—many of which may result in bone marrow suppression and associated thrombocytopenia. Many of these disorders are covered in more detail in other chapters within this book. Increased destruction or consumption can be a result of an autoimmune process,

TABLE 96-3 ■ COMMON CAUSES OF THROMBOCYTOPENIA IN OLDER ADULTS

ETIOLOGY OF THROMBOCYTOPENIA[a]	POSSIBLE DISORDER(S)
Decreased platelet production	Nutrient deficiencies (B_{12} or Folate) Myelodysplastic syndrome Bone marrow failure (eg, aplastic anemia, PNH) Bone marrow infiltration (eg, solid tumor malignancy, TB, sarcoidosis) Prescription or over-the-counter medications Chronic alcohol abuse Acute or chronic infection[b]
Increased platelet destruction	Immune thrombocytopenia Systemic lupus erythematosus Antiphospholipid syndrome Heparin-induced thrombocytopenia Drug-induced thrombocytopenia Acute or chronic infection[b] Disseminated intravascular coagulation Mechanical prosthetic valve Thrombotic thrombocytopenic purpura
Platelet sequestration/ other	Chronic liver disease Hypersplenism Spurious (eg, pseudothrombocytopenia) Dilutional (eg, in setting of trauma with massive transfusion)

PNH, paroxysmal nocturnal hemoglobinuria; TB, tuberculosis.

[a]There may be more than one mechanism leading to thrombocytopenia.

[b]Thrombocytopenia in the setting of infection is most commonly due to bone marrow suppression. Nevertheless, immune-mediated processes during infectious syndromes may also result in thrombocytopenia.

sepsis or an accelerated, antibody-mediated clearance from medications.

Immune thrombocytopenia ITP is an autoimmune disorder characterized by isolated thrombocytopenia (platelet count < 100 × 10⁹/L) and occurs as a result of platelet autoantibodies causing platelet destruction and impaired platelet production. It has an incidence of 2 to 5 per 100,000 and increases with age.

Primary ITP is diagnosed in the absence of other causes or disorders that may be associated with thrombocytopenia. The clinical presentation is highly variable, ranging from incidental asymptomatic thrombocytopenia discovered on an annual physical examination to life-threatening bleeding events. Patients typically come to clinical attention when they present with mild petechial or purpuric lesions on the extremities and epistaxis. This usually occurs when the platelet count is less than 30 × 10⁹/L but many patients remain asymptomatic even in the 10 to 30 × 10⁹/L range.

Although there is no test that can reliably diagnose primary ITP, the evaluation in older adults should include a thorough history and physical, complete blood cell count, reticulocyte count, comprehensive metabolic panel, peripheral blood smear, human immunodeficiency virus (HIV), and hepatitis C serology. The peripheral blood smear is usually normal except for the identification of low numbers of platelets with occasional large-appearing platelets. Depending on the history, other diagnostic tests can be helpful in excluding other potential etiologies of the thrombocytopenia. A bone marrow examination is not routinely required but may be undertaken in selected patients if there is other unexplained cytopenia.

For adults with newly diagnosed primary ITP (diagnosed within the preceding 3 months) and a platelet count of less than 30 × 10⁹/L who are asymptomatic or have minor mucocutaneous bleeding, first-line treatment includes either prednisone (0.5–2.0 mg/kg per day) or dexamethasone (40 mg per day for 4 days). Given the potential side-effects of corticosteroids, especially in older adults, close monitoring of the patient for hypertension, hyperglycemia, insomnia, depression, gastric irritation, myopathy, and osteoporosis is recommended.

Secondary ITP Secondary ITP is defined as any form of ITP other than primary. This includes drug-induced thrombocytopenia, which is the most common cause of thrombocytopenia in older adults. While the timing, severity, and duration of drug-induced thrombocytopenia can vary substantially, thrombocytopenia is usually evident within the first week of initiation of the causative drug (**Figure 96-3**). Common drugs known to definitely or probably cause thrombocytopenia are shown in **Table 96-4**, and an exhaustive list of drugs linked to low platelet counts can be accessed online (http://www.ouhsc.edu/platelets/ditp.html). Providers may also consider reporting cases of drug-induced thrombocytopenia to the US FDA (or similar organizational bodies in

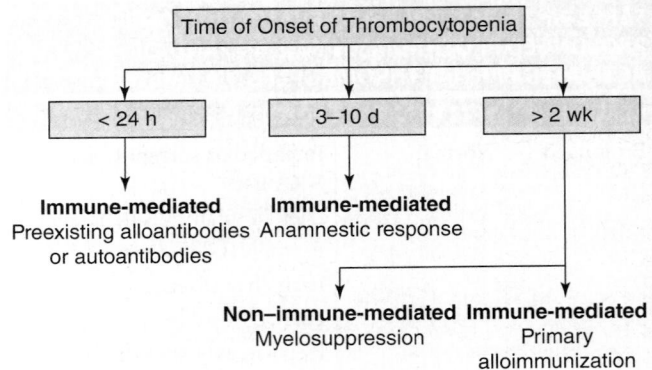

FIGURE 96-3. Categorization of drug-induced thrombocytopenia by time of onset of the thrombocytopenia. (Adapted with permission from Kenney B, Stack G. Drug-induced thrombocytopenia. Arch Pathol Lab Med. 2009;133[2]:309–314.)

other countries) Adverse Event Reporting System at www.fda.gov/medwatch.

In hospitalized patients, heparin-induced thrombocytopenia (HIT) is a severe complication that increases the risk of both arterial and venous thrombosis. Antibodies targeting platelet factor 4 increase platelet activation and consumption, activating the coagulation cascade, with resultant arterial and venous thrombi. HIT is associated with morbidity and mortality if undiagnosed and not treated promptly. The diagnosis of HIT can be challenging and providers are encouraged to use validated clinical prediction tools, such as the 4T Score or the HIT Expert

TABLE 96-4 ■ MEDICATIONS IMPLICATED AS DEFINITE OR PROBABLE CAUSES OF DRUG-INDUCED THROMBOCYTOPENIA	
Abciximab	Furosemide
Daptomycin/actinomycin	Gentamicin
Eptifibatide	Hydrochlorothiazide/triamterene
Hepatitis B vaccine	Inamrinone
Quinine	Influenza vaccine
Tirofiban	Melperone
Acetyldigoxin	Meropenem
Captopril	Molsidomine
Cilastatin/imipenem	Phenytoin
Clopidogrel	Piperacillin
Digoxin	Spironolactone
Dipyridamole	TNF alpha/INF gamma
Drospirenone/ ethinylestradiol	Trimethoprim/sulfamethoxazole
Famotidine	Vancomycin
Fluconazole	

Data from http://www.ouhsc.edu/platelets/WEB%20Table%20Group%202018.pdf.

Probability Score, in combination with the results of serologic testing and/or functional platelet assays.

Acute and chronic infections, including hepatitis C, HIV, influenza, and *Helicobacter pylori*, may also cause secondary ITP, although precise mechanisms and pathways remain incompletely understood. In some of these infectious syndromes, thrombocytopenia can also result from ineffective thrombopoiesis as a result of bone marrow infiltration and/or megakaryocyte infection. Finally, secondary ITP can also be a complication of rheumatologic and autoimmune disorders, including systemic lupus erythematosus (SLE), antiphospholipid antibody syndrome, IgA deficiency, and common variable immunodeficiency (CVID).

Nonautoimmune thrombocytopenia In addition to immune-mediated thrombocytopenia, low platelet counts in older adults can be the result of other nonimmune causes. One of the most commonly encountered causes is spurious thrombocytopenia, also referred to as pseudothrombocytopenia, being identified in about 0.1% of all blood samples in adults. Spurious thrombocytopenia is due to exogenous platelet clumping in the presence of ethylenediaminetetraacetic acid (EDTA), which is found within some vacutainer tubes. This can be identified by examining the blood film for platelet clumping and repeating a platelet count using blood drawn into an alternative anticoagulant such as citrate buffer. In addition, enhanced platelet consumption can occur in processes such as DIC and thrombotic microangiopathies such as thrombotic thrombocytopenia purpura. Dilutional thrombocytopenia may be seen in trauma patients who have undergone massive fluid resuscitation protocols that include large number of packed red blood cells transfusions.

Abnormal Platelet Function in Older Adults

Bleeding in older adults may also occur due to inhibition of normal platelet functions (eg, activation, adhesion, and aggregation) that impairs hemostasis. Traditional antiplatelet agents, including aspirin, nonsteroidal anti-inflammatories, clopidogrel, ticagrelor, dipyridamole, and cilostazol, may all increase the risk of bleeding in older adults. The relative risk increase for bleeding varies among different agents and between different patients. A number of other medications commonly prescribed to older adults may also inhibit platelet activation or aggregation. These include nitrates, calcium channel blockers, and selective serotonin reuptake inhibitors (SSRIs). Many of the mechanisms underlying these drugs' effects on platelet function remain incompletely understood.

Acquired abnormalities of platelet function in older adults may be due to their underlying co-morbidities. Chronic liver disease may cause abnormalities in platelet aggregation even in the absence of absolute thrombocytopenia. Similarly, acute and chronic kidney disease have been associated with various pathophysiologic effects on platelet function, including abnormal platelet aggregation responses to adenosine diphosphate (ADP) and epinephrine as well as impaired platelet adhesion.

VENOUS THROMBOEMBOLISM

Background

Deep vein thrombosis (DVT) and pulmonary embolism (PE), collectively referred to as venous thromboembolism (VTE), are common and, in many cases, preventable causes of in-hospital death. Age and accumulation of comorbidities markedly increase the risk of VTE in older adults. Yet, the diagnosis of VTE remains underrecognized in older adults. Clinical suspicion is essential for a prompt diagnosis in older adults who may have an atypical presentation; autopsy studies demonstrate PE is frequently not suspected, nor identified, despite being a common cause of death in older persons. Anticoagulants are the mainstay of VTE treatment given their substantial risk reductions in VTE recurrence and mortality. However, the benefit of anticoagulants may be offset in older adults by their age-related increased risk of bleeding, as described earlier. Balancing the risks of recurrence with bleeding is important to guide treatment duration.

Epidemiology and Pathophysiology

Incidence of VTE In the general population, the annual incidence of VTE approximates 2 to 3 in 1000 persons and appears to be increasing over time. Notably, the incidence rises with age with an approximate 7 per 1000 persons in those over the age of 70.

Risk factors One or more clinical risk factors are usually identifiable at the time of VTE diagnosis in older adults. In patients presenting with a first episode of VTE, recent hospitalization is the most common risk factor. Additional known risk factors include recent surgical procedures, malignancy, acute infection, impaired mobility, heart failure exacerbation, chronic lung disease, central venous catheter placement, inflammatory bowel disease, obesity, hormonal therapy, and prior VTE. Major orthopedic procedures such as elective hip and knee arthroplasty, or surgical repair of a hip fracture, are additional major VTE risk factors in older adults. Less commonly occurring risk factors include antiphospholipid syndrome, nephrotic syndrome, myeloproliferative neoplasms, HIT and inherited thrombophilias (factor V Leiden mutation, prothrombin G20210A gene mutation, protein C or S deficiency, AT deficiency).

Aging is considered a nonmodifiable risk factor; as patients age they accumulate VTE risk factors with additive risk. Impaired mobility, malignancy, and medical comorbidities (ie, heart failure, chronic lung disease, chronic kidney disease, obesity) are common in older adults and highlight the importance of VTE awareness in this patient population.

Pathophysiology of venous thrombosis Venous thrombi are comprised of red blood cells, white blood cells, and platelets enmeshed in a fibrin lattice (see **Figure 96-1**). The Virchow's triad of vascular endothelial injury, impaired blood flow (stasis), and hypercoagulability predisposes to venous thrombus formation. Typically, venous thrombi form in an area of blood vessel injury or venous stasis. Endothelial injury activates the clotting cascade shifting the natural balance between blood coagulation and fibrinolysis toward thrombus formation. Vessel injury from inflammation, surgery, trauma, or malignancy exposes subendothelial proteins, specifically tissue factor and collagen. Tissue factor precipitates initial thrombin generation and subsequent coagulation cascade (see **Figure 96-2**). Exposed collagen acts as binding sites for platelet activation and aggregation. Venous stasis lengthens the time coagulation factors are exposed to sites of vascular injury, further propagating clot formation.

Impaired venous blood flow is attributable to several factors commonly found in older adults. Reduced mobility leads to venous pooling in the legs, development of venous varicosities, and associated venous valvular incompetence. The sinuses behind venous valve cusps represent particularly vulnerable areas for thrombus formation due to disturbed blood flow and stasis. Polycythemia from dehydration, chronic hypoxemia or a myeloproliferative neoplasm, or hypergammaglobulinemia related to chronic inflammation or multiple myeloma results in blood hyperviscosity, further altering blood flow and increasing thrombotic risk. Venous outflow obstruction from incompletely resolved DVT or extrinsic venous compression from solid tumors may worsen venous stasis and promote thrombosis.

Blood coagulation is carefully regulated by inhibitors of thrombin generation and subsequent fibrin formation and the fibrinolytic system. Disruptions in these counterregulatory systems may be inherited or acquired. The circulating natural anticoagulants, including proteins C and S, and AT are essential to prevent unabated fibrin formation. Inherited proteins C and S, and AT deficiencies are uncommon, occurring in 0.02% to 0.3% of the population. The most commonly inherited thrombophilia is factor V Leiden (FVL) mutation, with a prevalence of 5% in an unselected Caucasian population. A point mutation in the FV gene at amino acid 506 (substitution of arginine to glutamine) renders FVa less susceptible to inactivation by activated protein C, which leads to a three- to fivefold increased risk of VTE. Even so, due to incomplete penetrance of FVL, many individuals with the mutation will never develop a VTE. The prothrombin *G20210A* gene mutation, the second most commonly inherited thrombophilia, is a point mutation in the FII gene that results in a 30% increase in prothrombin levels. It occurs in about 2% of an unselected White population and confers a threefold increased risk of VTE.

Acquired thrombophilias in older adults include antiphospholipid syndrome, HIT, hormone replacement therapy, myeloproliferative neoplasms, and malignancy. Antiphospholipid syndrome is defined by persistent circulating antiphospholipid antibodies (aPL) and the presence of arterial or venous thrombosis, or pregnancy-related complications. The clinically significant aPL are immunoglobulin G (IgG) or immunoglobulin M (IgM) anticardiolipin antibodies, IgG or IgM β_2-glycoprotein I antibodies, or the lupus anticoagulant. These antibodies target multiple sites resulting in monocyte, platelet, complement, and endothelial cell activation; tissue factor production; and cytokine production, contributing to arterial and venous thrombotic events, thrombocytopenia, pregnancy complications, and cardiac valvular disease. aPL titers at the time of an acute thrombotic event may be transiently positive. As such, guidelines recommend that an initial positive aPL test be repeated after at least 12 weeks to confirm a diagnosis of antiphospholipid syndrome. The prevalence of aPL increases with age, yet many patients remain asymptomatic without any evidence of arterial or venous thrombosis. As the clinical significance of aPL in older adults remains uncertain, routine screening is not recommended.

Hormone replacement therapy to treat postmenopausal symptoms increases VTE risk nearly threefold, especially in the first year of use. Myeloproliferative neoplasms including polycythemia vera and essential thrombocythemia are frequently associated with both arterial and venous thrombosis. These patients, especially those who have the gain-of-function mutation of the Janus kinase-2 (JAK2) enzyme, the *JAK2* V617F mutation, are particularly prone to thrombosis of the splanchnic veins (hepatic, portal, splenic, and mesenteric).

Patients with malignancy have a four- to sevenfold increased risk of VTE, with up to 20% of all VTEs occurring in cancer patients. The molecular mechanisms of cancer-associated thrombosis remain an area of research. Cancer cells can directly activate the coagulation cascade and platelets through the expression and secretion of tissue factor, platelet agonists, inflammatory cytokines, and PAI-1. In addition, many anticancer therapies are prothrombotic themselves (eg, lenalidomide, cisplatin, L-asparaginase), thus further promoting thrombus formation.

Clinical Presentation

Acute venous thromboembolism Venous thrombi in the legs may originate in the superficial (greater and lesser saphenous veins) or deep veins. For the deep veins, involvement of the popliteal, femoral, or iliac vein is classified as a proximal DVT, whereas a distal DVT involves the calf veins only (gastrocnemius, soleal, peroneal, or posterior tibial). The deep intramuscular calf veins are frequent sites of thrombus initiation; distal DVTs represent up to 50% of leg DVTs. When confined to the calf veins, patients may be asymptomatic or minimally symptomatic. Proximal leg DVT typically results in asymmetrical leg swelling, diffuse tenderness, erythema, and engorgement of collateral veins if the thrombus is occlusive. These symptoms of DVT can occur suddenly or subacute over days to weeks. In the upper extremities, the deep venous system includes the brachial, axillary, subclavian, and brachiocephalic vein, whereas the superficial veins include the antecubital, cephalic, and basilic veins. Patients with upper extremity DVT can present similarly as leg DVT with asymmetrical arm swelling, pain, and erythema. Symptoms of acute superficial venous thrombosis (SVT) of the upper and lower extremities are easily recognized by localized tenderness over the affected veins, swelling, erythema, warmth, and often a palpable thrombus within the vein. PE can range from asymptomatic, to mild chest discomfort and dyspnea, to severe pleuritic pain and breathlessness, or sudden death with massive PE. Additional signs and symptoms include hemoptysis, cough, tachypnea, tachycardia, syncope, fatigue, and hypoxemia.

Chronic venous thromboembolism Although acute VTE is associated with significant morbidity and mortality, chronic symptoms may develop following an acute event. Post-thrombotic syndrome (PTS) is the most frequent complication of DVT, affecting 20% to 50% of patients 1 to 2 years after the event. Due to chronic venous occlusion from incompletely cleared thrombus and incompetent venous valves that were damaged by the acute DVT, patients with PTS present with chronic symptoms of leg pain, heaviness, swelling, skin induration, hyperpigmentation, and venous ulcerations in the most severe cases (5%–10%). In the United States, the annual cost of PTS treatment is estimated at ≈$7000 per patient per year. Given the prevalence and chronicity of the disease, PTS is associated with a large socioeconomic burden to patients and the health care system.

Chronic thromboembolic pulmonary hypertension (CTEPH) is a complication of PE with a reported incidence ranging from 0.4% to 6.2%. CTEPH is characterized by chronically occluded pulmonary arteries, which is thought to result from nonresolving pulmonary emboli. These patients typically present with chronic dyspnea and fatigue. If left untreated, it can lead to right heart failure and death.

Diagnosis of Deep Vein Thrombosis

Clinical prediction models Asymmetrical leg swelling, pain, erythema, and warmth should prompt evaluation for DVT. However, clinical assessment alone cannot accurately identify DVT, and it is estimated that of all patients evaluated, only 20% have the disease. The integration of clinical prediction models with laboratory assays and noninvasive imaging allows for accurate DVT diagnosis in the majority of patients. Several clinical scoring systems exist (eg, Wells, Oudega, Hamilton, Geneva) that have been validated in the outpatient adult population for accuracy and reproducibility. The Wells DVT model remains the best validated and most utilized for determining the likelihood of DVT. Points are assigned based on clinical signs and symptoms, medical and surgical history, and clinician judgment regarding the likelihood of DVT (**Table 96-5**). Using a dichotomized score, patients are stratified into two pretest probability categories: DVT likely or DVT unlikely. The subjectivity involved with the clinician estimating DVT likelihood is a

TABLE 96-5 ■ WELLS DVT MODEL—A DVT CLINICAL PROBABILITY SCORE

VARIABLES	POINTS[a]
Active cancer (treatment ongoing or within previous 6 mo or palliative)	1
Paralysis, paresis, or recent plaster immobilization of the lower extremities	1
Recently bedridden > 3 d or major surgery within the past 4 wk	1
Localized tenderness along the distribution of the deep venous system	1
Entire leg swollen	1
Calf swelling by > 3 cm when compared with the asymptomatic leg (measured 10 cm below the tibial tuberosity)	1
Pitting edema (greater in the symptomatic leg)	1
Collateral superficial veins (nonvaricose)	1
History of DVT	1
Alternative diagnosis is as likely as or more likely than deep vein thrombosis	−2
Total points	

[a]Total score < 2 indicates DVT is unlikely; score ≥ 2 indicates DVT is likely.

major criticism of the Wells DVT model. However, several studies have shown that when pretest probability is objectively assessed, the accuracy of DVT diagnosis is enhanced, minimizing unnecessary testing.

Laboratory testing D-Dimer is a cross-linked fibrin degradation product generated when mature thrombus is cleaved by plasmin. Levels of D-dimer are typically elevated not only in patients with acute DVT but also in other nonthrombotic conditions including advanced age, inflammation, infection, malignancy, and recent surgery, thus limiting its positive predictive value. In addition, multiple D-dimer assays exist and there is a lack of standardization with the assays, with some assays highly sensitive and some less so. Also, as D-dimer levels increase with age, older adults are more likely to have false-positive results, which lead to lower specificity for DVT diagnosis in the aging population. An age-adjusted D-dimer threshold has been proposed to improve the diagnostic accuracy in older adults, and is currently being validated prospectively before adoption into clinical practice (ClinicalTrials.gov identifier: NCT02384135).

At this time, D-dimer levels alone are insufficient to diagnose or exclude DVT and must be combined with a clinical prediction model (eg, Wells DVT model) and ultrasonography, if warranted. A low clinical probability (DVT unlikely) with a negative D-dimer result safely excludes the presence of DVT, and no further imaging study is required (**Figure 96-4**). A positive D-dimer result in patients with a low clinical probability for DVT necessitates further imaging to safely exclude DVT. Patients with a high clinical

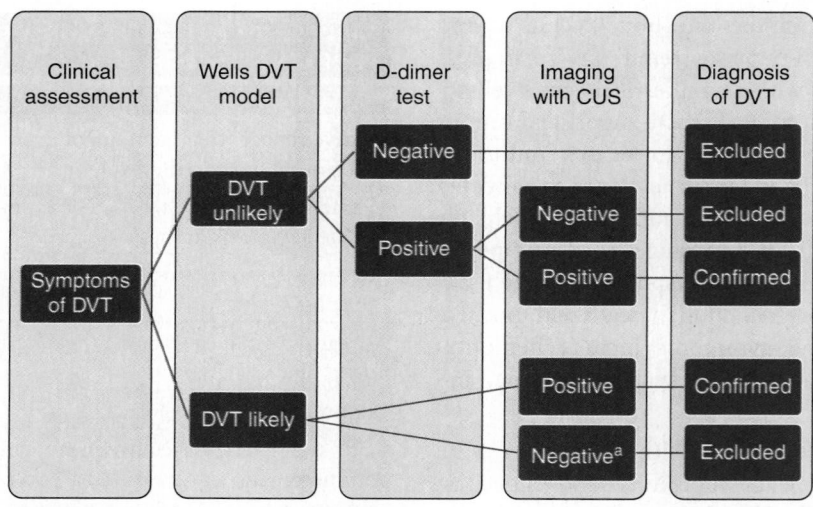

aIf negative, a D-dimer should be measured. If the D-dimer result is negative, then DVT is essentially ruled out, but if the D-dimer is positive, then repeat CUS in 1 week is recommended to safely exclude DVT, especially if the initial imaging was not whole-leg CUS.

FIGURE 96-4. Diagnostic management of outpatients with suspected DVT using the Wells DVT Model. CUS, compression ultrasonography.

probability (DVT likely) should initially undergo compression ultrasonography (CUS); if negative, then a D-dimer should be measured. If the D-dimer result is negative, then DVT is essentially ruled out, but if the D-dimer is positive, then repeat CUS in 1 week is recommended to safely exclude DVT, especially if the initial imaging was not whole-leg CUS.

Imaging

Compression Ultrasonography Noninvasive imaging with CUS is the most widely used study to diagnose DVT. Whole-leg CUS involves imaging the entire venous network from the common femoral vein distally to the deep calf veins with external pressure applied through the ultrasound transducer to visualize complete vessel collapse. Incompressibility or partial vessel collapse anywhere along the venous network is the hallmark of an intraluminal filling defect, representative of a thrombus. Supplementary imaging techniques including color Doppler and augmentation (manually squeezing the limb) allow visualization of venous blood flow, or the lack thereof, suggestive of thrombus. Benefits of whole-leg CUS are the ability to image proximal and distal veins in a single study, eliminating the need for follow-up imaging. However, whole-leg CUS is time-consuming and highly operator dependent. A simplified, two-point CUS involves only imaging the common femoral and popliteal veins. Patients with low clinical probability (DVT unlikely) and a positive D-dimer result can safely forego anticoagulation therapy following a negative two-point CUS. However, patients with a high clinical probability (DVT likely) and a positive D-dimer should undergo serial two-point CUS approximately 1 week apart to safely exclude proximal DVT.

While whole-leg CUS is a more comprehensive examination and frequently identifies distal DVT, the majority of distal DVT will not extend proximally and will

resolve spontaneously. The overdiagnosis and overtreatment of clinically insignificant findings may increase the risk of bleeding, especially in older patients.

Magnetic Resonance Venography Magnetic resonance (MR) venography of the leg is a sensitive test to detect DVTs. However, it is not recommended for routine use as it is expensive and not widely available. It is a valuable alternative test for those in whom CUS are inconclusive or in whom CUS is not feasible, such as morbidly obese patients.

Diagnosis of Pulmonary Embolism

Clinical prediction models The most common symptoms of acute PE reported in older adults can be nonspecific and include dyspnea, tachypnea, tachycardia, and chest pain. Symptoms of DVT (leg pain and swelling) are present in more than 40% of patients with acute PE, and simultaneous DVT is identified in up to 60% of patients diagnosed with a PE. Clinical signs including rales, accentuated pulmonic second heart sound, and jugular venous distension may be identified at presentation. Similar to DVT, these signs and symptoms are insufficient to diagnose PE, but are useful to estimate the clinical probability and guide additional testing.

Probability estimation of PE can be accomplished through several clinical prediction models, including the Wells or Geneva scores, or even clinical gestalt. The Wells score for PE has been validated in the outpatient adult population and utilizes different clinical signs and symptoms than the DVT prediction model, although still incorporating the subjective assessment of likelihood of PE, a potential limitation. The Wells PE model stratifies patients as "likely" or "unlikely" (**Table 96-6**) and, when combined with a D-dimer assay and computed tomographic pulmonary angiography (CTPA), provides an effective diagnostic strategy for PE.

TABLE 96-6 ■ WELLS PE MODEL—A PE CLINICAL PROBABILITY SCORE

VARIABLES	POINTS[a]
Signs or symptoms of DVT	3.0
Alternative diagnosis is less likely than PE	3.0
Heart rate > 100 beats/min	1.5
Immobilization or surgery in the previous 4 wk	1.5
History of DVT or PE	1.5
Hemoptysis	1.0
Active cancer	1.0
Total points	

[a]Total score ≤ 4 indicates PE is unlikely; score > 4 indicates PE is likely.

Laboratory testing Similar to its role in DVT evaluation, a negative D-dimer result combined with a low clinical probability (PE unlikely) can safely exclude the diagnosis of PE. Conversely, a positive D-dimer result must be followed up with an imaging study. The use of an age-adjusted D-dimer threshold has been prospectively validated in outpatients 50 years or older and was found to increase the diagnostic utility of the test. The age-adjusted threshold is equal to age (in years) × 10 μg/L (using D-dimer assays with a cutoff of 500 μg/L). Depending on the type of D-dimer assay used at each institution, this may not be generalizable for use.

Imaging

Chest Radiography The diagnostic utility of chest radiography in suspected PE is primarily to exclude other causes of dyspnea and hypoxemia (ie, pneumothorax or pneumonia), as most chest radiographs are normal with an acute PE. Identifiable signs of PE on chest radiography include oligemia (Westermark sign), a focal area of decreased perfusion of pulmonary vessels distal to the PE; wedge-shaped pleural-based opacity (Hampton hump) representative of a pulmonary infarct; and hilar enlargement, due to thrombus impaction and pulmonary artery engorgement.

Ventilation-Perfusion Lung Scanning Prior to widespread adoption of computed tomographic pulmonary angiography (CTPA), ventilation-perfusion (V/Q) lung scanning was the most reliable noninvasive imaging modality to diagnose PE. Many factors have contributed to its declining use including lack of availability at some institutions, time needed to perform an examination, and frequently encountered nonspecific test results. However, V/Q lung scanning remains clinically useful in older patients with renal insufficiency or contrast allergy, or when attempting to minimize external beam radiation to the chest of young women.

In suspected PE, the performance characteristics of lung scanning improve when paired with a normal chest radiograph and pretest probability assessment. For example, a patient with high clinical probability (PE likely) and a high probability scan has a 96% likelihood of having PE, whereas a low clinical probability (PE unlikely) paired with a low probability scan has a 4% likelihood of having PE; a normal perfusion scan essentially excludes PE. Unfortunately, the majority of patients presenting with suspected PE will have nondiagnostic imaging and require additional evaluation. The increased prevalence of abnormal chest radiographs and high clinical probability of PE in older adults further limit the utility of V/Q lung scanning.

Computed Tomographic Pulmonary Angiography Widespread availability and technological advances have made CTPA the primary imaging modality for suspected PE, except when contraindicated (severe renal insufficiency or contrast allergy). The advent of multidetector CT scanners' spatial and temporal resolution has improved, increasing the sensitivity for PE diagnosis. Although the increased use of CTPA and the addition of more detectors have resulted in greater recognition of PE, a corresponding decline in mortality has not been seen, raising doubts about the clinical significance of subsegmental PE.

To minimize the number of unnecessary imaging studies and potential overtreatment of clinically insignificant PE, CTPA should be paired with clinical prediction models and D-dimer testing. Outpatients with low clinical probability (PE unlikely) and a negative D-dimer can safely avoid further imaging. Outpatients with a low clinical probability for PE and a positive D-dimer test and any patient with a high clinical probability for PE (PE likely) need to undergo imaging studies.

Additional benefits of CTPA over other imaging modalities are its abilities to simultaneously diagnose PE and detect right ventricular dilation (useful in risk stratification) and to identify alternative diagnoses when PE is not present, which is especially useful in older adults with atypical presentations.

Treatment of Venous Thromboembolism

Home treatment vs hospital treatment For patients with newly diagnosed uncomplicated DVT, home treatment is generally recommended. As compared to hospital treatment, treating patients with DVT at home was demonstrated to reduce the risk of PE, subsequent DVT, and major bleeding. However, older patients with multiple comorbidities that may require hospitalization, or at high risk for anticoagulant-related bleeding, may be more appropriately treated in the hospital. Socioeconomic factors, such as limited financial or home support, may also require hospital treatment for the initial management.

Similarly, patients with newly diagnosed PE at low risk for complications may be treated at home effectively and safely. The difficulty is in determining which patients are appropriate for outpatient treatment. The Pulmonary Embolism Severity Index (PESI) and simplified PESI, both clinical prediction score for PE severity, are the best-validated scoring systems. Points are assigned based on age, vital signs, and medical history to determine risk of 30-day mortality. Yet, clinical judgement is needed as other factors, including comorbidities, high risk for anticoagulant-related bleeding, and socioeconomic factors, may require inpatient management for the initial phase of treatment.

Choice of anticoagulant therapy Initial VTE treatment requires an anticoagulant with a rapid onset of action to reduce thrombus extension, recurrence, or embolization. This can be accomplished through parenteral anticoagulants such as unfractionated heparin (UFH) or low-molecular-weight heparin (LMWH), or the use of selected direct oral anticoagulants (DOACs) (rivaroxaban and apixaban).

UFH use is declining for VTE treatment; however, it remains useful in patients with renal insufficiency or high bleeding risk where rapid reversal may be needed, conditions commonly encountered in older adults. UFH may be administered as a continuous infusion or subcutaneously in doses sufficient to achieve therapeutic levels. Intravenous administration typically begins with a bolus dose of 80 U/kg followed by a continuous infusion of 18 U/kg/h. Close laboratory monitoring (every 6 hours until stable) is essential to ensure the desired therapeutic effect and to minimize bleeding. Monitoring is done with either the activated partial thromboplastin time (aPTT) or an antifactor Xa (anti-Xa) activity assay. Expert consensus recommends a therapeutic heparin range of 0.35 to 0.7 U/mL measured by anti-Xa activity, which is typically 1.5 to 2.5 times the control aPTT. Alternatively, and less commonly used, short courses of fixed-dose subcutaneous UFH (333 U/kg load, then 250 U/kg every 12 hours) may be safely used in some patients for initial treatment and without laboratory monitoring.

Subcutaneous LMWH has more predictable pharmacology than UFH infusions. This allows outpatient VTE treatment with fixed, weight-based doses without routine laboratory monitoring in select patients. When compared to UFH for VTE treatment, LMWH is associated with fewer thrombotic complications, less major bleeding, and a mortality benefit.

Oral anticoagulant therapy with warfarin (a vitamin K antagonist) was the cornerstone of VTE treatment for nearly 60 years, until the introduction of DOACs. Warfarin initiation must be overlapped with a parenteral anticoagulant (UFH or LMWH) for a minimum of 5 days, and until the international normalized ratio (INR) is greater than 2.0 for at least 24 hours, due to its delayed anticoagulant effect. Warfarin's narrow therapeutic window (INR 2.0–3.0) and numerous food and drug interactions necessitate routine INR monitoring for the duration of therapy. Close INR monitoring is especially important in older adults. Aging is associated with alterations in some vitamin K–dependent coagulation factors, and older adults typically have increased sensitivity to the anticoagulant effects of warfarin. In addition, older adults usually have a higher prevalence of polypharmacy which can increase the risk of major bleeding.

DOACs represent a new class of anticoagulants targeting specific sites within the coagulation cascade (**Table 96-7**). Dabigatran is a direct thrombin inhibitor that

TABLE 96-7 ■ DOAC DOSING FOR MANAGEMENT OF VTE

DOAC TYPE	TREATMENT DOSE	RENAL DOSING (ML/MIN)
Dabigatran	150 mg BID AFTER 5 d of parenteral anticoagulation	CrCl < 30: Avoid
Apixaban	10 mg BID for 7 d, then 5 mg BID	No dose adjustment
Rivaroxaban	15 mg BID for 21 d, then 20 mg daily	CrCl < 30: Avoid
Edoxaban	60 mg daily AFTER 5 d of parenteral anticoagulation	CrCl 15–50: 30 mg CrCl < 15: Avoid

BID, twice daily.

competitively binds to soluble and fibrin-bound thrombin, inhibiting the conversion of fibrinogen to fibrin and subsequent thrombus formation. Rivaroxaban, apixaban, and edoxaban are factor Xa inhibitors that selectively block the active site of factor Xa, inhibiting the coagulation cascade without the use of a cofactor (antithrombin). Both dabigatran and edoxaban require an initial 5-day course of parenteral anticoagulant (UFH or LMWH) prior to DOAC initiation, whereas rivaroxaban and apixaban can be initiated immediately. Although there are no dedicated randomized trials in the older adult population, a meta-analysis of data extracted from the landmark phase III trials (RE-COVER I-II, EINSTEIN DVT-PE, AMPLIFY and HOKUSAI) for a subgroup of patient 75 years or older demonstrated that DOACs were more effective in preventing VTE recurrence (risk ratio for recurrence 0.55, 95% confidence interval [CI] 0.38–0.82) and were associated with a reduced risk of major bleeding (relative risk ratio 0.39, 95% CI 0.17–0.90) compared to warfarin. Additional appealing attributes of the DOACs compared to warfarin include fewer drug interactions and more predictable pharmacokinetics, thus eliminating the need for routine laboratory monitoring.

Thrombolytic therapy Given the high mortality in patients presenting with acute PE with hemodynamic compromise, defined as a systolic blood pressure less than 90 mm Hg or a decrease in systolic blood pressure greater than or equal to 40 mm Hg from baseline, the use of systemic thrombolysis may be warranted. Catheter-directed thrombolysis (CDT) is an alternative for patients with an intermediate risk for bleeding as the total dose of thrombolytic delivered by CDT is lower. The role of thrombolytics for patients with submassive PE (evidence of right ventricular dysfunction without hemodynamic compromise) is less clear. The PEITHO study found a reduction in hemodynamic decompensation without a mortality benefit, but at the cost of marked increases in major bleeding and hemorrhagic strokes. Particularly, patients older than 75 years suffered significantly more major bleeding events than younger patients. Additionally, as age greater than 75 is considered a relative contraindication to thrombolytic therapy in general, thrombolytics currently have a limited role in older adults.

Typically, CDT of acute proximal DVT to reduce the risk of PTS is not recommended. In the ATTRACT trial, the addition of CDT to anticoagulation for acute proximal DVT did not result in a lower risk of PTS (risk ratio, 0.96; 95% CI, 0.82 to 1.11), but did result in a higher risk of major bleeding within 10 days (1.7% vs 0.3% of patients). A subgroup analysis of patients with acute iliofemoral DVT in the ATTRACT trial also showed no difference in PTS occurrence at 2 years but found that CDT led to greater reduction in leg pain and swelling, and improved quality of life. In contrast, the CaVenT study found that patients with iliofemoral DVT and low bleeding risk who underwent CDT demonstrated an absolute risk reduction of 14.4% in development of PTS at 2 years. No difference in clinical symptoms was evident at 6 months. This highlights the importance of proper patient selection as CDT may be reasonable in selected younger patients at low risk of bleeding with symptomatic iliofemoral DVT. Additionally, as both studies excluded patients older than 75 years, further studies are needed to determine the relative safety and efficacy of these strategies in older adults.

Duration of anticoagulant therapy The duration of anticoagulant therapy is determined by balancing the thromboembolic risk with the bleeding risk. In general, VTE provoked by a transient (ie, reversible) risk factor such as surgery or trauma is associated with a low risk of recurrence, and a 3-month treatment course is sufficient. VTE without identifiable risk factors (ie, unprovoked) is associated with nearly 20% risk of recurrence at 2 years, and 30% risk of recurrence at 8 years. As such, extended anticoagulant therapy (> 3 months) is reserved for unprovoked VTE with low-moderate bleeding risk and recurrent unprovoked VTE with high bleeding risk. The decision to continue long-term anticoagulant therapy must be periodically revisited (ie, annually) to determine the net clinical benefit, especially in older patients who are at increased risk for VTE and bleeding complications.

Anticoagulant Use in Older Adults

The use of anticoagulants in the management of VTE increase the risk of bleeding. Older adults who are anticoagulated have a 3% to 5% risk per year of having a major bleeding event as compared to younger subjects (1%–2% per year). This relative risk increase depends to some degree among the patient group being studied, the anticoagulant class, and most importantly, the presence or absence of comorbidities such as chronic kidney disease, uncontrolled hypertension, a history of bleeding, liver disease, concomitant antiplatelet agent or nonsteroidal anti-inflammatory drug (NSAID) use, and others. This increased bleeding risk presents a challenging clinical dilemma for practitioners as older patients, while having an increased bleeding risk, also have a significantly higher risk of VTE recurrence. As such, a baseline assessment of bleeding risk, measurement

TABLE 96-8 ■ THE HAS-BLED BLEEDING RISK SCORE

	RISK FACTORS	SCORE
H	Hypertension[a]	1
A	Abnormal liver[b] or kidney function[c]	1 or 2
S	Stroke	1
B	Bleeding[d]	1
L	Labile INR[e]	1
E	Elder[f]	1
D	Drugs[g] or alcohol[h]	1 or 2

[a]> 160 mm Hg systolic.
[b]Cirrhosis, bilirubin > 2 × ULN (upper limit of normal), Aspartate aminotransferase/alanine aminotransferase/alkaline phosphatase > 3 × ULN.
[c]Renal dialysis, history of renal transplant or serum creatinine ≥ 2.26 mg/dL.
[d]Requiring hospitalization, decrease in hemoglobin > 2 g/L or requiring blood transfusion.
[e]Time in therapeutic range < 60%.
[f]Age > 65.
[g]Use of antiplatelet agents or nonsteroidal anti-inflammatory drugs.
[h]> 8 drinks per week.

of renal and liver function and platelet count, and a thorough medication review are essential prior to anticoagulation initiation and periodically while on anticoagulation.

Assessment and Management of Bleeding Risk in Older Adults on Anticoagulants

Various bleeding risk prediction tools (eg, ACCP risk table, VTE-BLEED, RIETE, HAS-BLED) have been published, and the reader is referred to several recent reviews for more detailed information on the topic. The HAS-BLED score is probably the best validated and most utilized risk estimation tool for major bleeding, particularly for patients with atrial fibrillation (AF) treated with VKA (**Table 96-8**). Evaluation of HAS-BLED in the VTE population and in patients treated with DOACs has been limited to small cohort studies. Additionally, the HAS-BLED score includes the item "labile INR," which is not relevant if DOACs are the choice of anticoagulant. As a result, these bleeding risk prediction tools should not be used to exclude patients from anticoagulant therapy, but rather to identify and eliminate modifiable bleeding risk factors (**Table 96-9**).

Other strategies to reduce the risk of bleeding in older adults prescribed anticoagulants include a thorough medication reconciliation to identify concomitantly prescribed medications that might interact with an anticoagulant or increase the risk of bleeding. In addition, patients, family members, and caregivers should receive comprehensive education on anticoagulants as insufficient education may increase the risk of bleeding. Referral to a Thrombosis Clinic for education and monitoring may improve compliance and the therapeutic time in range (if on a VKA) while also preventing avoidable medication interactions. These specialty anticoagulation clinics may also have a valuable role in following patients on DOACs by providing regular patient follow-up, counseling, education, and laboratory monitoring (eg, for early identification of renal dysfunction where a switch in choice of anticoagulant may be needed).

TABLE 96-9 ■ MODIFIABLE BLEEDING RISK FACTORS IN OLDER ADULTS PRESCRIBED ANTICOAGULANTS AND POTENTIAL STRATEGIES TO REDUCE THE RISK

RISK FACTOR	POSSIBLE INTERVENTION(S)
Concomitant NSAID use	Replace NSAID with acetaminophen or selective COX-2 inhibitor
Concomitant use of an antiplatelet agent	Eliminate antiplatelet agent if not indicated
Highly variable time in therapeutic range (TTR)[a]	Consider referral to anticoagulation clinic, if available, or switch to DOAC
Frequent falls or high risk of falls	Consider evaluation by Faint and Fall Clinic or geriatric specialist
Uncontrolled hypertension	Control blood pressure to appropriate goal
History of gastrointestinal bleeding	Consider proton pump inhibitor (PPI) or H_2 antagonist
Poor adherence or compliance	Education; referral to anticoagulation clinic if available

COX-2, cyclooxygenase 2; NSAID, nonsteroidal anti-inflammatory drug; TSOAC, target-specific oral anticoagulant.
[a]In patients treated with a VKA.

TABLE 96-10 ■ MODEL FOR DETERMINING A RISK OF VENOUS THROMBOEMBOLISM (VTE) IN HOSPITALIZED MEDICAL PATIENTS

VARIABLES	POINTS[a]
Malignancy (ongoing treatment or within previous 6 mo)	3
Previous deep vein thrombosis/pulmonary embolism	3
Immobilization (≥ 3 d)	3
Known thrombophilic disorder	3
Recent surgery and/or trauma	2
Age ≥ 70 y	1
Respiratory and/or cardiac failure	1
Acute ischemic stroke or myocardial infarction	1
Acute infection and/or rheumatologic disease	1
Obesity (BMI > 30)	1
Active hormonal treatment	1

[a]High risk of development of VTE is defined as total score ≥ 4 points.

Reversal Agents for Anticoagulants

Heparin and to some extent, LMWH can be reversed with protamine. The anticoagulant effect of warfarin can be reversed using vitamin K (takes ~24 hours) or four-factor prothrombin complex concentrates (PCC) (eg, KCentra) if immediate reversal is required. Idarucizumab is a humanized monoclonal antibody fragment that binds to dabigatran with a higher affinity than its affinity to thrombin, thus effectively neutralizing its anticoagulant effect. It was approved by the Food and Drug Administration (FDA) in 2015 for use in patients treated with dabigatran presenting with life-threatening or uncontrolled bleeding, or those requiring emergency surgery or urgent procedures. Andexanet alfa, a modified human factor Xa decoy protein that binds and sequesters factor Xa inhibitors, received accelerated FDA approval in 2018 for the reversal of rivaroxaban or apixaban due to life-threatening or uncontrolled bleeding. Despite its regulatory approval, andexanet alfa is not yet widely available in hospital formularies due to concerns about its efficacy and financial cost. Given the uncertainty of its clinical benefit, the FDA mandated a postmarketing randomized clinical trial of andexanet alfa against usual care (typically four-factor PCC) that is currently recruiting (ClinicalTrials.gov identifier: NCT03661528).

Primary VTE Prophylaxis

Extensive clinical practice guidelines have been published by professional societies addressing a wide range of indications for VTE prophylaxis and should be referenced for detailed guidance. In general, all hospitalized patients should be evaluated for VTE prophylaxis on an individualized basis. Clinical scoring systems exist to guide these decisions for medical and surgical patients. For example, in medical patients, the Padua Prediction Score (**Table 96-10**) incorporates intrinsic factors and acute physiologic condition, with points assigned on a weighted scale. A cumulative score greater than or equal to 4 points is considered high risk and is associated with a 32-fold increased incidence of VTE compared to a low-risk score, which is less than 4 points. When the VTE risk is high and pharmacologic prophylaxis is being considered, bleeding risk must also be estimated. Although, bleeding risk scoring systems to guide VTE prophylaxis are not well developed or validated, active peptic ulcer disease, thrombocytopenia (platelets < 50 k/μL), and age greater than 85 are considered to carry excessive bleeding risk and may preclude pharmacologic prophylaxis.

The choice of pharmacologic and/or mechanical prophylaxis depends on the clinical situation and provider assessment. Pharmacologic agents are generally more effective than mechanical devices and currently approved regimens include low-dose UFH, LMWH, fondaparinux, dose-adjusted warfarin, apixaban, rivaroxaban, and aspirin. Mechanical prophylaxis relies on intermittent pneumatic compression devices or graduated compression stockings to minimize venous stasis and is either used in conjunction with pharmacologic agents for high-risk indications (ie, post–total hip/knee arthroplasty or hip fracture surgery) or as a stand alone method when bleeding risk is high and pharmacologic prophylaxis is contraindicated.

Conclusion

Age-related physiologic changes and accumulation of comorbidities increase both the risk of bleeding and VTE in older adults. As anticoagulant therapy remains the cornerstone of VTE treatment, screening for and targeting of modifiable risk factors for major bleeding is essential. Given the advantages of DOACs compared with warfarin, and the availability of DOAC-specific reversal agents, it is anticipated that the use of DOACs in older adults will continue to rise. Dedicated anticoagulation clinics play a valuable role in mitigating the risk of bleeding in older adults prescribed anticoagulants by providing regular follow-up, counseling, and education.

ACKNOWLEDGMENTS

The author acknowledges Dr. Stacy Johnson and Dr. Matthew Rondina for their prior contributions to this chapter in the 7th edition of this textbook.

FURTHER READING

Anderson DR, Morgano GP, Bennett C, et al. American Society of Hematology 2019 guidelines for management of venous thromboembolism: prevention of venous thromboembolism in surgical hospitalized patients. *Blood Adv.* 2019;3(23):3898–3944.

Bethishou L, Gregorian T, Won K, et al. Management of venous thromboembolism in the elderly: a review of the non-vitamin K oral anticoagulants. *Consult Pharm.* 2018;33:248–261.

Brown JD, Goodin AJ, Lip GYH, et al. Risk stratification for bleeding complications in patients with venous thromboembolism: application of the HAS-BLED bleeding score during the first 6 months of anticoagulant treatment. *J Am Heart Assoc.* 2018;7(6):e007901.

Chan NC, Eikelboom JW. How I manage anticoagulant therapy in older individuals with atrial fibrillation or venous thromboembolism. *Blood.* 2019;133(21):2269–2278.

Chopard R, Albertsen IE, Piazza G. Diagnosis and treatment of lower extremity venous thromboembolism: a review. *JAMA.* 2020;324(17):1765–1776.

Donze J, Clair C, Hug B, et al. Risk of falls and major bleeds in patients on oral anticoagulation therapy. *Am J Med.* 2012;125(8):773–778.

Engbers MJ, van Hylckama Vlieg A, Rosendaal FR. Venous thrombosis in the elderly: incidence, risk factors and risk groups. *J Thromb Haemost.* 2010;8(10):2105–2112.

Favaloro EJ, Franchini M, Lippi G, et al. Aging hemostasis: changes to laboratory markers of hemostasis as we age—a narrative review. *Semin Thromb Hemost.* 2014;40(06):621–633.

Geldhof V, Vandenbriele C, Verhamme P, et al. Venous thromboembolism in the elderly: efficacy and safety of non-VKA oral anticoagulants. *Thromb J.* 2014;12:21.

Hisada Y, Mackman N. Cancer-associated pathways and biomarkers of venous thrombosis. *Blood.* 2017;130:1499–1506.

Kahn SR, Comerota AJ, Cushman M, et al. The postthrombotic syndrome: evidence-based prevention, diagnosis, and treatment strategies: a scientific statement from the American Heart Association. *Circulation.* 2014;130:1636–1661.

Kearon C. Natural history of venous thromboembolism. *Circulation.* 2003;107(23 suppl 1):I22–I30.

Kearon C, Akl EA. Duration of anticoagulant therapy for deep vein thrombosis and pulmonary embolism. *Blood.* 2014;123(12):1794–1801.

Klok FA, Huisman MV. How I assess and manage the risk of bleeding in patients treated for venous thromboembolism. *Blood.* 2020;135(10):724–734.

Kruse-Jarres R, Kempton CL, Baudo F, et al. Acquired hemophilia A: updated review of evidence and treatment guidance. *Am J Hematol.* 2017;92:695–705.

Lim W, Le Gal G, Bates SM, et al. American Society of Hematology 2018 guidelines for management of venous thromboembolism: diagnosis of venous thromboembolism. *Blood Adv.* 2018;2(22):3226–3256.

Neunert C, Terrell DR, Arnold DM, et al. American Society of Hematology 2019 guidelines for immune thrombocytopenia. *Blood Adv.* 2019;3(23):3829–3866.

Ortel TL, Neumann I, Ageno W, et al. American Society of Hematology 2020 guidelines for management of venous thromboembolism: treatment of deep vein thrombosis and pulmonary embolism. *Blood Adv.* 2020;4(19):4693–4738.

Righini M, Van Es J, Den Exter PL, et al. Age-adjusted D-Dimer cutoff levels to rule out pulmonary embolism: The ADJUST-PE Study. *JAMA.* 2014;311(11):1117–1124.

Rodeghiero F, Stasi R, Gernsheimer T, et al. Standardization of terminology, definitions and outcome criteria in immune thrombocytopenic purpura of adults and children: report from an international working group. *Blood.* 2009;113(11):2386–2393.

Schünemann HJ, Cushman M, Burnett AE, et al. American Society of Hematology 2018 guidelines for management of venous thromboembolism: prophylaxis for hospitalized and nonhospitalized medical patients. *Blood Adv.* 2018;2(22):3198–3225.

Tritschler T, Kraaijpoel N, Le Gal G, et al. Venous thromboembolism: advances in diagnosis and treatment. *JAMA.* 2018;320(15):1583–1594.

van Belle A, Buller HR, Huisman MV, et al. Effectiveness of managing suspected pulmonary embolism using an algorithm combining clinical probability, D-dimer testing, and computed tomography. *JAMA*. 2006;295(2):172–179.

Warkentin TE. Laboratory diagnosis of heparin-induced thrombocytopenia. *Int J Lab Hematol*. 2019;41 (Suppl 1): 15–25.

Wells PS, Anderson DR, Rodger M, et al. Evaluation of D-dimer in the diagnosis of suspected deep-vein thrombosis. *N Engl J Med*. 2003;349(13):1227–1235.

Wells PS, Ihaddadene R, Reilly A, et al. Diagnosis of venous thromboembolism: 20 years of progress. *Ann Intern Med*. 2018;168:131–140.

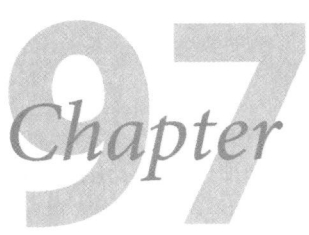

Chapter 97

Aging of the Endocrine System and Non-Thyroid Endocrine Disorders

Bradley D. Anawalt, Alvin M. Matsumoto

GERIATRIC ENDOCRINOLOGY

The clinical presentation, laboratory confirmation, and treatment of endocrine disorders may present challenges in older compared to young persons.

Clinical Presentation

The symptoms and signs of endocrine disorders are often nonspecific and attributed to "old age" by geriatric patients. Clinical manifestations may also be altered, muted, or masked by age-associated comorbid illnesses and increased use of medications. For example, cardiovascular (eg, heart failure and atrial fibrillation) and neurobehavioral (eg, cognitive impairment and depression) manifestations of thyroid disease occur more frequently and are often the most prominent features in older patients compared to younger patients (see Chapter 98 for details). Clinically significant endocrinopathies may present with atypical manifestations and physical examination findings may differ in older patients (the best examples are thyroid diseases per Chapter 98). Older patients with endocrine disorders may present with geriatric syndromes (eg, falls or functional or cognitive impairment) and some disorders occur almost exclusively in older patients, for example, nonketotic diabetic hyperosmolar hyperglycemia and anaplastic thyroid cancer.

Laboratory Confirmation

Confirmation of endocrine diagnoses in older persons relies on laboratory measurements of hormone concentrations. Most clinical studies of endocrine dysfunction in older patients are defined as hormone values above or below reference ranges in healthy young individuals, rather than age-specific ranges. For example, hypogonadism in older men is defined by serum testosterone concentrations

Learning Objectives

- Understand the presenting manifestations of common endocrinopathies in older patients.
- Describe the initial diagnostic evaluation and fundamentals of management of common endocrinopathies in older patients.
- Identify when to consult and how to optimize the collaboration with endocrinologists.

Key Clinical Points

Pituitary Disorders

1. Mild hyperprolactinemia (serum prolactin 20–50 ng/mL) is common in older people and seldom needs treatment, but primary hypothyroidism should be excluded.

2. Patients with moderate to severe hyperprolactinemia should be referred to an endocrinologist.

3. Serum pituitary hormone concentrations may be inappropriately or even slightly elevated in patients with hypopituitarism.

4. Older patients with diabetes insipidus often have concomitant impaired thirst and are best managed in collaboration with an endocrinologist.

Adrenal Disorders

1. Older patients are particularly prone to suffer fragility fractures and sarcopenia due to Cushing syndrome.

(Continued)

2. The most common cause of Cushing syndrome in older patients is iatrogenic.

3. The most common cause of adrenal insufficiency in older patients is a rapid discontinuation of chronic glucocorticoid therapy.

4. The sole or primary manifestation of adrenal insufficiency in older patients may be weakness, weight loss, anorexia, or chronic nausea.

5. It is essential that patients with adrenal insufficiency take the equivalent of 60 mg hydrocortisone daily (triple the usual daily replacement dosage) for a febrile illness and are able to administer intramuscular hydrocortisone if they cannot take oral medications due to illness.

6. Patients on chronic corticosteroid therapy (3 months or more) must have their corticosteroid dosage reduced slowly to avoid acute adrenal insufficiency. An endocrinologist may be helpful to manage this taper.

7. Patients with an adrenal incidentaloma should be evaluated for pheochromocytoma and malignancy.

8. Older patients with hypertension that requires three or more antihypertensive medications or with hypertension and spontaneous hypokalemia should be evaluated for primary aldosteronism with measurement of plasma aldosterone and renin.

Gonadal Disorders

1. The diagnosis of male hypogonadism requires symptoms or signs of androgen deficiency as well as low testosterone concentrations measured in two or more blood samples obtained between 7 AM to 10 PM on different days.

2. Older men on testosterone therapy should be assessed for erythrocytosis 3 to 6 months after any increased dosage and annually thereafter.

Calcium and Bone Disorders (also see Chapter 51)

1. Parathyroid surgery should be considered in older patients with symptoms of hypercalcemia, serum calcium greater than 1 mg/dL above the upper limit of normal, chronic kidney disease, nephrolithiasis, or hypercalciuria.

2. Vitamin D deficiency is defined by serum 25-hydroxyvitamin D less than 30 ng/mL in older patients.

3. Paget disease should be considered in patients with isolated elevated serum alkaline phosphatase concentrations or characteristic radiographic findings of focal lytic and sclerotic areas. Patients with significant bone pain or (potential) complications including joint involvement or potential neurologic sequelae may be treated with zoledronic acid (often as a single dose).

below those of healthy young men. In contrast, the distribution of serum thyrotropin concentrations is higher in older persons (see Chapter 98), suggesting that the upper limit of thyrotropin concentrations is higher, for example, 7 to 8 mIU/L, (particularly in those 80 years and older) than in younger individuals.

The clinical significance of mild abnormalities of serum hormone concentrations, subclinical endocrine dysfunction, is common in older patients but their clinical significance is unclear. It is important that geriatricians recognize that hormone levels may be affected transiently by illnesses (eg, slight thyrotropin elevation during recovery from acute illness) and medications (eg, suppression of gonadotropin and testosterone levels by opioids). Therefore, it is crucial to repeat hormone testing in older patients with mild endocrine laboratory abnormalities when baseline health status is restored fully.

Treatment

In older patients with clinical endocrine deficiency, the dosage of hormone replacement may be lower than in young patients because the metabolic clearance of some hormones is reduced with aging (eg, thyroid hormone, hydrocortisone, and testosterone). It is important to appreciate that underlying age-related conditions may be worsened by hormone overtreatment (eg, worsening of osteoporosis with excessive glucocorticoid or thyroid hormone therapy). For hormone replacement, starting treatment at slightly lower than full hormone replacement dosages is appropriate (eg, lower dosages of testosterone to avoid erythrocytosis that occurs more frequently with full replacement dosages). Multimorbidity and polypharmacy may predispose older patients to poor medication adherence and adverse drug effects or interactions.

The management of older persons with endocrine disorders should focus on improvement in function and quality of life within the social context of the patient; this might require multidisciplinary care in consultation with an endocrinologist. Some older patients may request hormone therapy (eg, testosterone, growth hormone, dehydroepiandrosterone [DHEA]) as a rejuvenation remedy to reverse the symptoms and signs of aging. It is important for geriatricians to dispel this myth, educate patients about realistic goals of treatment, and avoid initiation of hormone therapy trials for mild or subclinical endocrine dysfunction with the false expectation of dramatic clinical improvements.

In this chapter, we review the geriatrician's approach to the evaluation and management of the most common non-thyroid endocrine disorders that occur in patients 65 years or older. Even when the geriatrician refers a patient to an endocrinologist for recommendations, the geriatrician plays an indispensable role in providing information about the goals of therapy based on the patient's quality of life, functional status, other comorbidities, and personal/family preferences.

ANTERIOR PITUITARY

The two most common anterior pituitary endocrine disorders that geriatricians will encounter or manage are hyperprolactinemia and pituitary incidentalomas. In addition, the geriatrician may occasionally have a patient with an established or new diagnosis of hypopituitarism. The geriatrician should understand the basic management of these disorders and when to consult an endocrinologist.

Hyperprolactinemia

Physiology and presentation Prolactin has two established physiologic effects: induction of lactation and suppression of gonadotropin secretion from the pituitary. Lactation requires estrogen, and only premenopausal women typically have high enough circulating estradiol concentrations for lactation. Thus, lactation due to hyperprolactinemia is very rare in men and postmenopausal women. Prolactin is tonically secreted from the anterior pituitary, and it is regulated primarily by negative feedback from dopamine that is secreted by the hypothalamus into the hypothalamic-pituitary portal venous system. Any process that stimulates the nipple or the peri-areolar chest wall (rubbing, suckling, or infectious processes) may induce prolactin release via a neurologic pathway. Finally, exercise, sleep, and acute physiologic or psychological stress may stimulate prolactin secretion and may result in mildly elevated serum prolactin concentrations.

There are three common settings when a geriatrician may encounter hyperprolactinemia in older patients. Older men commonly have low to low-normal serum testosterone concentrations and inappropriately normal serum FSH and LH concentrations, a biochemical pattern consistent with secondary hypogonadism. Serum prolactin is often measured in that setting, and it might be elevated. Older women and men may present with pituitary tumors that are discovered during brain imaging, and evaluation may include measurement of serum prolactin. Finally, serum prolactin is sometimes measured and found to be elevated in some clinical settings when serum prolactin measurement is not

indicated (eg, erectile dysfunction without any evidence of endocrinopathy).

Epidemiology and causes There are not good data on the prevalence of hyperprolactinemia in the general population or in older people, but the overall incidence of hyperprolactinemia appears to be about 0.1 per 100 patient-years in people 65 years or older. The incidence and prevalence appear to be increasing over the past three decades, but that likely reflects increased testing of serum prolactin. The data are based on surveys of patients at higher risk of hyperprolactinemia (eg, cohorts of patients taking psychoactive drugs or retrospective studies of databases that include patients who have had a serum prolactin measured). The prevalence of hyperprolactinemia is similar in older women and men.

The causes of hyperprolactinemia may be categorized by the physiology of prolactin secretion and clearance (**Table 97-1**). Conditions that disrupt the normal negative feedback of dopamine on prolactin secretion include antidopaminergic drugs and large pituitary tumors that impinge on the pituitary stalk and pituitary portal venous system. Thyrotropin-releasing hormone (TRH) also stimulates the release of prolactin from the anterior pituitary. Moderate to severe primary hypothyroidism that results in high portal venous TRH concentrations (and high peripheral circulating thyrotropin [TSH] concentrations) may cause hyperprolactinemia. Because prolactin is cleared from the circulation by the kidney, moderate to severe kidney injury is a cause of hyperprolactinemia. Another cause of decreased clearance of prolactin is the presence of antibodies that aggregate with prolactin; this aggregation of antibodies and prolactin is known as "macroprolactin." The prevalence of anti-prolactin antibodies and macroprolactinemia is common and increases with age, and there are assay methodologies for detecting macroprolactin. Because the

TABLE 97-1 ■ COMMON CAUSES OF HYPERPROLACTINEMIA
Loss of inhibition of negative feedback on prolactin secretion
Drugs (eg, psychoactive drugs)
Pituitary disorders (eg, pituitary tumor ≥ 1 cm)
Increased prolactin secretion due to increased production
Primary hypothyroidism
Prolactinoma
Increased prolactin secretion due to decreased clearance of serum prolactin
Kidney injury
Idiopathic
Physiological causes of hyperprolactinemia[a]
Physical or psychological stress
Exercise
Sleep
Nipple stimulation

[a]Physiologic causes are associated mild hyperprolactinemia (< 50 ng/mL).

measurement of macroprolactin does not alter the management of hyperprolactinemia in most older patients, it is not useful to measure macroprolactin routinely in the evaluation of hyperprolactinemia in older people.

There are no known adverse effects of hyperprolactinemia per se in postmenopausal women. Although there has been some speculation about direct adverse effects of prolactin on sexual function independent of effects on gonadal function, there has been no convincing evidence to support this hypothesis. Thus, measurement of prolactin is generally performed in older men with suspected hypogonadotropic hypogonadism and older men and women with a large pituitary mass (to determine if the tumor is a prolactinoma).

Evaluation and management The key factors for the evaluation and management of hyperprolactinemia in patients 65 years or older are the overall health and likely longevity of the patient, male sex, the presence or absence of hypogonadotropic hypogonadism, and whether the hyperprolactinemia is mild, moderate, or severe.

Patients 65 years or older with mild hyperprolactinemia (20–50 ng/mL) will not generally benefit from therapy directed at lowering the serum prolactin. As noted above, hypogonadotropic hypogonadism (causing testosterone deficiency and reduced fertility) is the single significant adverse sequela known to be directly related to hyperprolactinemia. Women and eugonadal men 65 years or older therefore will not benefit from resolution of mild hyperprolactinemia, but they should be assessed for primary hypothyroidism with a serum TSH. Serum prolactin measurement should be repeated when the patient has been sitting quietly for 15 minutes because mild hyperprolactinemia might be due to the stress of venipuncture. The patient's medication list should be reviewed for prescription and over-the-counter medications associated with hyperprolactinemia, but it is not necessary to discontinue a medication that is suspected to be the cause of mild hyperprolactinemia (**Table 97-2**). Mild hyperprolactinemia rarely causes hypogonadotropic hypogonadism in men. In men 65 years or older with hypogonadotropic hypogonadism and mild hyperprolactinemia, another cause of hypogonadotropic hypogonadism should be considered, and the geriatrician should refer those men to an endocrinologist.

TABLE 97-2 ■ MEDICATIONS ASSOCIATED WITH HYPERPROLACTINEMIA IN OLDER PATIENTS

Antipsychotics: phenothiazines, haloperidol, and risperidone
- Most of the newer (atypical) antipsychotics are not associated with hyperprolactinemia

Metoclopramide and domperidone

Tricyclic antidepressants (particularly clomipramine)

Verapamil but not other calcium channel blockers

Opioids

Estrogen products

Patients 65 years or older with modest hyperprolactinemia (serum prolactin 50–250 ng/mL) typically have a prolactinoma or more than one cause of hyperprolactinemia (eg, two medications that are associated with hyperprolactinemia). These patients should be referred to an endocrinologist who may evaluate other anterior pituitary function including the thyroid and gonadal axes and may order sellar imaging to ensure that the patient does not have a large pituitary tumor or other disease that affects prolactin secretion.

Virtually all patients 65 years or older with severe hyperprolactinemia (serum prolactin > 250 ng/mL) have a large prolactinoma. These patients should be referred to an endocrinologist to assess anterior pituitary function and sellar imaging. As with the evaluation of moderate hyperprolactinemia, the most important element of the evaluation of severe hyperprolactinemia is to determine if there is a large sellar mass or other pituitary pathology that requires treatment. It is not the hyperprolactinemia per se that requires management.

Optimal management of hyperprolactinemia necessitates collaboration between the geriatrician and an endocrinologist. The treatment of hyperprolactinemia depends upon whether the patient has hypogonadotropic hypogonadism and whether there is a large sellar mass that needs treatment with medication or surgery to reduce the size of the tumor. In general, women 65 years or older need treatment if there is a large sellar mass that is impinging on the optic tract or important intracranial structures. Men 65 years or older with hypogonadotropic hypogonadism may be treated with androgen replacement therapy (or gonadotropin replacement therapy if fertility is desired), and testosterone replacement therapy is likely to be tolerated and more uniformly effective in normalizing serum testosterone than medical therapy with dopamine agonists (eg, cabergoline) to lower prolactin. Similar to women 65 or older, men 65 years or older with a large sellar mass should be evaluated to determine whether it benefits the patient to have medical or surgical therapy to reduce the size of the mass. In general, prolactinomas are treated with medical therapy (ie, dopamine agonists) if tumor shrinkage is deemed beneficial. Other pituitary masses and disease require therapies specific to the etiology of the mass.

Pituitary Incidentaloma

Physiology and presentation Pituitary tumors are commonly found during brain imaging with CT or MRI that is performed for a different indication than evaluation for pituitary disease. These lesions are called pituitary incidentalomas.

Epidemiology and causes The prevalence of pituitary incidentaloma is about 10% to 20% in autopsy and imaging series. Because patients 65 years or older may have brain imaging performed because of concerns about cognition dysfunction, head trauma due to falls or evaluations for possible strokes, geriatricians need to be aware of the following: most solid-appearing pituitary incidentalomas are nonsecretory benign pituitary adenomas, and most cystic incidentalomas are Rathke cleft cysts that represent benign remnants of embryological development of the pituitary.

Evaluation and management The geriatrician should generally refer patients with a pituitary incidentaloma to an endocrinologist. The minimum evaluation for a solid pituitary incidentaloma is a history and examination for evidence of a pituitary hormonal excess syndrome (eg, Cushing syndrome or acromegaly) and serum prolactin measurement. For a large (≥ 1 cm) pituitary macroincidentaloma (solid or cystic), a careful evaluation for pituitary hormone deficiency syndrome (eg, testosterone, LH and FSH; free T4 and TSH; and morning cortisol concentrations) should be done. The treatment of pituitary hormone deficiencies and pituitary hormonal excess syndromes is generally done by endocrinologists. Pituitary macroincidentalomas that are impinging on vital intracranial structures may need to be treated with medical therapy, radiation therapy, or surgery depending on the specific etiology of the mass. Pituitary macroincidentalomas are surveilled with serial sellar images (usually MRI) at 1- to 2-year intervals. There is some controversy about whether smaller tumors require surveillance and the most appropriate interval between imaging studies.

Chronic Hypopituitarism

Physiology and presentation The anterior pituitary produces growth hormone, FSH, LH, TSH, adrenocorticotropic hormone (ACTH), and prolactin. Hypopituitarism is defined by deficiency in two or more of the hormones. Prolactin deficiency is not clinically relevant in older adults, and growth hormone deficiency has minimal clinical relevance because most patients with chronic hypopituitarism do not have a significant benefit with growth hormone replacement therapy. The physiology of chronic hypopituitarism is characterized by which pituitary hormones are affected, and the presentation of untreated or undertreated hypopituitarism depends on which hormones are deficient. A characteristic of hypopituitarism is that the affected pituitary hormone(s) may be circulating at low, inappropriately normal, or even slightly elevated concentrations. In pituitary disease, the pituitary hormones that are detected by immunoassay are generally not fully bioactive due to the lack of normal post-translation modification.

Epidemiology and causes Chronic hypopituitarism is very uncommon (incidence < 0.5 per 100,000 annually), but the geriatrician may provide care for patients who have been already diagnosed with chronic hypopituitarism because these patients may live for many years after the diagnosis. In chronic hypopituitarism, there is end-organ atrophy and deficiency due to inadequate stimulation by affected anterior pituitary hormones. The most common causes of chronic hypopituitarism are a large (> 1 cm) benign pituitary macroadenoma, cranial radiation, and severe head trauma. Chronic hypopituitarism usually occurs years after cranial radiation.

Evaluation and management The most common deficiencies of hypopituitarism are secondary hypogonadism and secondary hypothyroidism, but secondary hypoadrenalism, although less common, may be life-threatening. All patients with secondary hypoadrenalism should wear an alert bracelet or necklace. It is generally not beneficial to treat growth hormone deficiency in older people, and this expensive therapy should be initiated and monitored by an endocrinologist. Prolactin deficiency also does not require treatment in older people. The treatment of secondary hypogonadism is covered in the male hypogonadism section below and the menopause section in Chapter 36. The treatment of secondary hypoadrenalism (including sick day coverage) is reviewed in the adrenal section below. The treatment of secondary hypothyroidism is reviewed in Chapter 98.

POSTERIOR PITUITARY

Physiology

Antidiuretic hormone (also known as ADH or arginine vasopressin) is synthesized in hypothalamic neurons and released from nerve terminals in the posterior pituitary gland. ADH promotes water reabsorption from the kidney in response to increased plasma osmolality and also to large reductions in arterial volume and blood pressure. ADH and thirst are both regulated by hypothalamic osmoreceptors and by cardiovascular and intrathoracic baroreceptors, and are the main physiologic regulators of free water balance. ADH secretion and thirst preserve total body water and protect against dehydration and resultant hypernatremia as well as hypovolemia. ADH is regulated by small changes in serum osmolarity, and suppression of ADH secretion protects against hyponatremia due to excessive water intake. It is important that geriatricians recognize age-related alterations in the homeostatic mechanisms that affect water balance.

Aging is associated with relative ADH excess with increased to normal basal (unstimulated) ADH concentrations and increased ADH response to osmotic stimuli, as well as decreased renal free water excretion are attributed mainly to an age-associated decrease in glomerular filtration rate (GFR). These physiologic changes with age predispose older persons to developing hyponatremia.

Hyponatremia and Syndrome of Inappropriate ADH

Hyponatremia or water excess is the most common electrolyte disorder experienced by older persons. In addition to a decrease in free water clearance due mostly to reduced GFR with age, aging is associated with a decrease in lean body mass and total body water (see Chapter 39). Also, older people are more likely to have severe heart failure or liver disease that are each associated with appropriate increases of ADH secretion.

More common than the latter, other age-associated comorbidities (such as brain and pulmonary disease, malignancy, and hypothyroidism) and use of medications that cause syndrome of inappropriate ADH ([SIADH] such as selective serotonin and serotonin-norepinephrine reuptake inhibitors, tricyclic antidepressants, phenothiazines, and carbamazepine) are the main contributors to the increased prevalence of hyponatremia in older patients. Hyponatremia due to SIADH in older patients is usually mild with serum sodium concentrations as low as 130 mmol/L and asymptomatic. However, such hyponatremia is associated with increased mortality, gait instability, falls, fractures, cognitive impairment, hospitalization, and nursing home placement. Management of hyponatremia is discussed in Chapter 39.

Risk of Hypernatremia

Reduced thirst and fluid intake in response to fluid deprivation, hypovolemia, and hyperosmotic stimuli contribute to the increased risk of dehydration (water deficiency) and hypernatremia in older patients. Older patients with immobility or dementia who have limited access to or have reduced intake of water or other liquids are especially at risk for hypernatremia. ADH deficiency due to central diabetes insipidus (idiopathic or secondary to hypothalamic-pituitary disease) is a rare cause of hypernatremia and dehydration in older persons. Loss of the thirst response to dehydration that normally protects against hypernatremia makes diabetes insipidus difficult to manage in older patients who are treated with an ADH analog, desmopressin (diamino-D-arginine vasopressin, DDAVP). As such, older patients with diabetes insipidus should be referred to an endocrinologist for management. Management of hypernatremia is discussed in Chapter 39.

Nocturnal Polyuria

Age-related blunting of nocturnal circadian ADH concentrations in addition to nighttime increases in atrial natriuretic hormone levels predispose older persons, particularly those with dementia including Alzheimer disease, to nocturnal polyuria. In contrast, patients with diabetes insipidus have daytime as well as nocturnal polyuria.

In older patients with age-related mobility impairment and bladder dysfunction, ADH dysregulation may contribute to urinary incontinence (see Chapter 47). Older patients with nocturnal polyuria and incontinence may benefit from administration of desmopressin in addition to behavioral interventions and detrusor muscle relaxants, as causes of incontinence are often multifactorial. In older patients being treated with desmopressin, geriatricians should monitor serum sodium for the development of hyponatremia that might occur with excessive desmopressin dosage and/or excessive water intake while taking desmopressin.

ADRENAL

The geriatrician will most commonly comanage three adrenal endocrinopathies: Cushing syndrome, adrenal insufficiency, and adrenal incidentaloma.

Cushing Syndrome

Cushing syndrome is a constellation of symptoms and signs of glucocorticoid excess and evidence of supraphysiologic exposure to glucocorticoids. Older patients are particularly susceptible to Cushing syndrome and its adverse effects because of decreased metabolism of glucocorticoids and a high prevalence of baseline frailty, sarcopenia, and osteopenia.

Physiology and presentation Glucocorticoids are generally catabolic, and glucocorticoid excess results in muscle wasting and weakness, bone resorption and osteoporosis, thin skin and easy bruisability, and body composition and metabolic changes. The average daily production of cortisol in a normal person is about 10 to 12 mg/m² body surface, and that is equivalent to about 15 to 20 mg daily of exogenous hydrocortisone. Supraphysiologic replacement dosages suppress secretion of corticotropin releasing hormone from the hypothalamus and result in reduced synthesis of ACTH in the anterior pituitary.

The most suggestive symptoms of Cushing syndrome are easy bruisability, broad (> 1 cm) purple striae found typically on the abdomen and proximal muscle weakness and wasting. These symptoms are much less specific in older people who tend to have thin skin, particularly in areas that have had chronic sun exposure, and they also tend to have sarcopenia and weakness. In older people, thin skin and easy bruisability in body regions without extensive sun exposure may be a sign of glucocorticoid excess. Low-trauma fractures and osteoporosis with densitometry Z score of worse than −2.0 (2 standard deviations worse than age-matched peers) may by an indication of Cushing syndrome.

Epidemiology and causes The most common cause of Cushing syndrome is iatrogenic. There are no accurate estimates of the prevalence of iatrogenic Cushing syndrome, but prescription of supraphysiologic dosages of corticosteroids is very common, and the effect of these excessive dosages may cause adverse effects within weeks. Commonly prescribed oral formulations of hydrocortisone, prednisone, and dexamethasone do not reproduce the normal diurnal cyclicity of serum cortisol (with peaks in the early morning and a nadir at about midnight). Daily dosages of prednisone as low as 5 mg or dexamethasone of 0.75 mg are supraphysiologic for many older patients.

Evaluation and management Because Cushing syndrome may significantly impair the function of frail, older patients and significantly worsen the risk of major osteoporotic fractures, the geriatrician must be vigilant in collaborating with specialists who prescribe corticosteroids to discontinue corticosteroid therapy as quickly as feasible. In addition, the geriatrician has an essential role in collaborating with specialists and endocrinologists to use the lowest possible dosages of glucocorticoids if replacement or continual maintenance therapy is required. High dosages of inhaled or topical corticosteroids may also cause Cushing syndrome. Geriatricians who suspect Cushing syndrome should ask the patient about "natural remedies" and nonprescription medications because some of these health supplements contain adrenal extracts with glucocorticoids. If the geriatrician suspects endogenous Cushing syndrome, a rare and often difficult-to-diagnose disorder, then an endocrinologist should be consulted.

Adrenal Insufficiency

Physiology and presentation Glucocorticoids are essential hormones for normal, healthy living. In addition to being "stress hormones" that are important for survival during severe illness or other physiologic stress, glucocorticoids are important for normal function of many organ systems such as the brain, gut, and the cardiovascular system. In severe glucocorticoid deficiency, patients may report fatigue, loss of appetite, nausea, diffuse abdominal pain, weight loss, and dizziness, and they may have postural hypotension. Patients with long-standing primary adrenal insufficiency may have hyperpigmentation of the palmar creases, bite line of the buccal mucosa, gingivae, and nipples. These symptoms and signs may appear as a constellation or a patient may present with one or few of these as the predominant or sole presenting manifestation of adrenal insufficiency.

Compared to patients with secondary hypoadrenalism, patients with primary adrenal insufficiency due to adrenal disease are more likely to report dizziness and hypotension, and they are likely to have hyperkalemia because they have both glucocorticoid and mineralocorticoid deficiency. Patients with secondary adrenal insufficiency due to hypothalamic or pituitary disease (with loss of normal ACTH secretion) have glucocorticoid deficiency, but they typically do not have mineralocorticoid deficiency because aldosterone synthesis and secretion are primarily regulated by the renin-angiotensin system that remains intact in secondary hypoadrenalism.

Epidemiology and causes The incidence of adrenal insufficiency in patients 65 years or older is about 100 per 100,000, and the incidence might be higher in patients 85 years or older . As with Cushing syndrome, the most common cause of glucocorticoid deficiency (adrenal insufficiency or hypoadrenalism) is iatrogenic due to prescription of chronic corticosteroids. The most common cause of primary adrenal insufficiency in industrialized countries, autoimmune adrenalitis (Addison disease), rarely occurs in older patients. Primary adrenal insufficiency due to tuberculosis remains common worldwide, but it is very rare in older people who reside in industrialized countries. On the other hand, primary hypoadrenalism secondary to bilateral adrenal hemorrhage may be more common in older adults who are more likely to be using one or more systemic anticoagulants than younger people.

Evaluation and management In general, the geriatrician's role in the evaluation and management of adrenal insufficiency is to recognize that an older patient with weight loss, nausea,

and nonspecific abdominal or back pain and weakness might have primary or secondary adrenal insufficiency. Secondary hypoadrenalism due to iatrogenic suppression of the hypothalamic-pituitary-adrenal axis by prolonged corticosteroid therapy is the most common and important cause of adrenal insufficiency in older patients: for example, abrupt discontinuation of chronic corticosteroid therapy for an inflammatory disorder such as polymyalgia rheumatica. The key questions for the geriatrician to ask when considering adrenal insufficiency in this setting are the following: (1) Has the patient been on topical, inhaled, oral, or injectable corticosteroids in the past year and then recently stopped them abruptly? (2) Has the patient been on systemic anticoagulants and had an episode of significant hypotension in the past year (suggesting the possibility of bilateral adrenal hemorrhage)?

The definitive diagnosis of adrenal insufficiency is based on a stimulation test using corticotropin administered intramuscularly or intravenously. This test is usually done by an endocrinologist. In a properly executed corticotropin (Cosyntropin) stimulation test, the serum cortisol should exceed 18 mg/dL 30 to 60 minutes after the administration of corticotropin.

The management of chronic adrenal insufficiency is best done in collaboration with an endocrinologist, but the geriatrician should recall that oral hydrocortisone taken one to three times daily is generally the optimal glucocorticoid replacement therapy (**Table 97-3**). The usual replacement dosage of hydrocortisone is a total dosage of 15 to

---

TABLE 97-3 ■ KEY POINTS IN THE MANAGEMENT OF ADRENAL INSUFFICIENCY IN OLDER PATIENTS

Avoid excessive glucocorticoid replacement

- Total of 15–20 mg hydrocortisone in divided doses daily
- Typical regimens:
  - 20 mg once daily OR
  - 15 mg in the morning (when arising for the day) and 5 mg at lunchtime

Avoid hydrocortisone in the late afternoon or evening

- A late dose may cause insomnia

Patient should wear an alert bracelet or necklace

- Example language: "Adrenal insufficiency. Give hydrocortisone 100 mg IM"

Sick day glucocorticoid coverage and use of IM hydrocortisone

- If fever of 101.5°F or higher, triple the daily hydrocortisone dose
- If fever persists for > 3 d, seek medical attention
- Review whether the patient has IM glucocorticoid at home and someone to administer it if the patient cannot take oral meds or has severe vomiting
  - Sample prescription: 100 mg hydrocortisone succinate (Solu-Cortef) IM prn vomiting and inability to take or keep down hydrocortisone tabs
  - Renew prescription of Solu-Cortef annually

20 mg daily; higher dosages may cause adverse effects of Cushing syndrome. The geriatrician should remind the patient of the importance of wearing an alert bracelet with clear language such as "Adrenal insufficiency. Give hydrocortisone 100 mg IM." The geriatrician should also reinforce the "sick day" management of glucocorticoids that requires tripling the usual daily replacement glucocorticoid dosage (ie, 60 mg of hydrocortisone or the equivalent) for 3 days when the patient has a fever of 101.5°F or higher. The patient should take 100 mg of hydrocortisone intramuscularly if unable to take oral glucocorticoid therapy due to illness. The patient should seek medical evaluation if not feeling significantly better after 3 days. Short-term administration of stress dosages of glucocorticoids generally should be given for all patients with adrenal insufficiency for severe systemic illness that requires care in an intensive care unit or for major surgeries. Consultation with an endocrinologist is useful to determine the dosage and duration.

For patients with primary adrenal insufficiency due to destruction of all or part of both adrenal cortices, mineralocorticoid replacement with fludrocortisone is indicated if the patient has hyperkalemia or hypotension despite adequate glucocorticoid therapy. Patients with secondary hypoadrenalism do not need mineralocorticoid replacement therapy.

For patients that are on chronic corticosteroids (and likely have iatrogenic secondary hypoadrenalism), the geriatrician should educate the patient and family about the same principles of care including wearing an alert bracelet. The management of "sick days" is similar to above, but patients on chronic corticosteroids greater than 10 mg prednisone daily (or > 1 mg dexamethasone) do not need to increase their dosage for "sick days." When a decision is made to discontinue chronic (> 1 month) corticosteroid therapy, a tapering of the dosage over days to months is necessary in order to allow the hypothalamic-pituitary-adrenal axis to recover and to avoid adrenal crisis. The duration of the taper is related to the dosage and duration of chronic glucocorticoid therapy. Collaboration with an endocrinologist is often beneficial.

Adrenal Incidentaloma

Physiology and presentation By definition, adrenal incidentaloma presents as a radiologic finding on an imaging study ordered for an indication other than suspected adrenal pathology.

Epidemiology and causes Adrenal masses are common and are found in about 4% of high-resolution CT abdominal scans. The prevalence is higher in older patients with obesity, hypertension, and/or diabetes mellitus. The majority are benign adenomas that are nonsecretory. The most common secretory adrenal incidentalomas produce cortisol, often at levels just above normal physiologic amounts. Adrenal incidentalomas are rarely catecholamine-producing pheochromocytomas, but these tumors can be fatal.

Evaluation and management The evaluation of an adrenal incidentaloma is generally performed by an endocrinologist, but the geriatrician should know certain basic principles. All patients with an adrenal incidentaloma must be evaluated for a pheochromocytoma and for malignancy. Low radiodensity due to fat content on CT imaging (< 10 Hounsfeld units) excludes malignancy and pheochromocytoma. Masses greater than 4 cm are more likely to be malignant.

Adrenal incidentalomas of higher density must be assessed for pheochromocytoma with a 24-hour urine collection for catecholamine metabolites or measurement of plasma-free metanephrines. Assessment for other hormone-secreting tumors is based on clinical suspicion by history and physical examination. For example, a patient with adrenal incidentaloma and spontaneous hypokalemia or hypertension should be evaluated for primary hyperaldosteronism. Finally, there is controversy about the value of assessment for mild or subclinical Cushing syndrome (also known as "autonomous cortisol secretion") in adrenal incidentaloma. There is no consensus on follow-up imaging of adrenal incidentaloma, but most experts and guidelines recommend periodic follow-up until lack of significant growth (≥ 5 mm in longest diameter in ≤ 12 months) makes malignancy very unlikely. Given the controversies, collaboration between the geriatrician and an endocrinologist is advised, as the geriatrician's knowledge of the patient's functional status, quality of life, and personal preferences are important to guide decision-making.

Endocrine Hypertension

There are multiple endocrinopathies that may raise blood pressure, but, for the geriatrician, the two most clinically important endocrine causes of hypertension are primary hyperaldosteronism and pheochromocytoma. Primary hyperaldosteronism and pheochromocytoma present with blood pressure elevation as a primary manifestation, but the other endocrine causes of hypertension (eg, thyrotoxicosis, acromegaly or Cushing syndrome) tend to cause modest increases in blood pressure and have other findings that are much more prominent.

Physiology and presentation Primary hyperaldosteronism causes hypertension by increased renal sodium reabsorption with passive water reabsorption, resulting in increased intravascular volume and blood pressure. Primary hyperaldosteronism also results in increased renal potassium excretion and is often associated with hypokalemia. Geriatricians should suspect primary hyperaldosteronism in older patients who have difficulty managing hypertension despite confirmation of adherence to a regimen for three or more antihypertensive medications or in patients with hypertension and spontaneous hypokalemia. Pheochromocytomas cause hypertension and tachycardia by the direct cardiovascular effects of catecholamines. In addition, catecholamines activate the renin-angiotensin pathway causing hypertension via the vasoconstrictive effects of angiotensin II and by sodium retention due to secondary hyperaldosteronism. A pheochromocytoma should be considered in patients with new onset of severe headaches or unexplained paroxysmal chest pain, diaphoresis, or tachycardia.

Epidemiology of primary hyperaldosteronism and pheochromocytoma Primary hyperaldosteronism occurs in 5% to 10% of patients with hypertension, but pheochromocytomas are very rare with an incidence of less than 5 per million per year. On the other hand, primary hyperaldosteronism is less likely to contribute to hypertension in older people, but pheochromocytoma appears to be more common after age 50.

Evaluation and management of primary hyperaldosteronism and pheochromocytoma The initial evaluation of primary hyperaldosteronism is a plasma aldosterone to renin (plasma renin activity) ratio (ARR). Ideally, the blood sample is drawn in the morning after the patient has been out of bed for at least 2 hours. The patient should be instructed to be on a liberal sodium diet for a few days before testing. The only medication that must be stopped prior to the ARR assessment is spironolactone (for 4 weeks). Hypokalemia (that inhibits aldosterone and stimulates renin secretion) should be corrected before the test. Also, assessment of serum potassium on the same sample as the plasma aldosterone and renin is useful. The specificity of an elevated aldosterone to renin ratio is lower in older patients. The primary explanation for decreased specificity of this screening test is age-related decreases in basal and stimulated plasma-renin concentrations. In patients with primary hyperaldosteronism, the plasma aldosterone is generally greater than 10 ng/dL and the plasma-renin activity is undetectable or markedly suppressed (< 1 ng/mL/hour). Because older patients are less likely to have a significant benefit with adrenalectomy than younger patients, the geriatrician may opt to commence aldosterone antagonist therapy (eg, spironolactone or eplerenone). In the occasional patient with a very high ARR, plasma aldosterone greater than 20, severe hypertension and spontaneous hypokalemia, consultation with an endocrinologist might be indicated for further evaluation for potential surgical excision of a unilateral adrenal aldosterone-secreting adenoma or asymmetric hypersecretion of aldosterone.

Screening for pheochromocytoma is done by measurement of 24-hour urine catecholamines or plasma-free metanephrines when the patient is at baseline health and not under stress. There are a number of causes of false positives including psychological stress, acute illness, and certain medications. A patient with a positive screening test

for a pheochromocytoma should be referred to an endocrinologist. The treatment of pheochromocytoma includes localizing the source of excess catecholamine production and surgical extirpation.

TESTES

Physiology

Aging is associated with a gradual and progressive decline in serum total and free testosterone and increase in sex hormone-binding globulin (SHBG, the main binding protein for testosterone) concentrations. The decrease in testosterone concentrations is due both to an age-related decline in testosterone production by the testes (partially counterbalanced by a decrease in testosterone catabolism) and lack of an appropriate increase of pituitary gonadotropin production (to compensate for the lower blood testosterone concentration) due to altered hypothalamic gonadotropin-releasing hormone secretion.

Hypogonadism

With the age-related decline in serum testosterone, an increasing proportion of older men have serum testosterone concentrations in the hypogonadal range, that is, below the normal range for young men. Aging is also associated with a parallel decline in sexual function, mood, muscle mass and strength, and bone mineral density that can all be manifestations of testosterone deficiency. However, the cause of these age-related changes is usually multifactorial, and these changes have numerous other etiologies that occur commonly in older persons.

Diagnosis According to Endocrine Society clinical practice guidelines, the diagnosis of hypogonadism in men of any age requires symptoms and signs of testosterone deficiency and a consistently low morning serum testosterone on at least two occasions, preferably fasting. However, the symptoms and signs of testosterone deficiency (**Table 97-4**) are nonspecific; also, low testosterone levels may be associated with age-associated comorbidities and medications, which can suppress gonadotropin and testosterone production. Therefore, geriatricians should consider other causes

TABLE 97-4 ■ COMMON NONSPECIFIC SYMPTOMS AND SIGNS OF TESTOSTERONE DEFICIENCY IN OLDER MEN		
SEXUAL	**PSYCHOLOGICAL**	**PHYSICAL**
↓ Libido (sex drive)	↓ Vitality, fatigue	↓ Male hair
↓ Spontaneous erections	Depressed mood, irritability	↓ Muscle mass and strength
↓ Sexual activity	↓ Concentration, memory	↓ Bone mineral density
Erectile dysfunction (ED)	Sleep disturbance, hot flashes	↓ Hemoglobin, anemia
		↑ Breast size

↓ = Decreased; ↑ = Increased.

of clinical manifestations and low testosterone before making a diagnosis of hypogonadism.

Testosterone assays used in most local laboratories are not standardized. As a result, serum testosterone concentrations measured in different assays and their reference ranges vary considerably from assay to assay. If possible, testosterone should be measured using a testosterone assay that is CDC-standardized for accuracy and reliability; testosterone assays used in most commercial reference laboratories are CDC certified. Also, because older age and age-associated comorbidities (eg, obesity) and use of certain medications (eg, anticonvulsants) may increase or decrease SHBG, guidelines recommend that an accurate free testosterone measurement, that is, calculated free testosterone or free testosterone by equilibrium dialysis, be measured to confirm a diagnosis of hypogonadism in older men.

Serum luteinizing hormone (LH) and follicle-stimulating hormone (FSH) concentrations should be measured together with testosterone to determine whether the source of low testosterone is the testes (ie, primary hypogonadism indicated by low testosterone and high LH and FSH levels) or the hypothalamus or pituitary (ie, secondary hypogonadism indicated by low testosterone and low or inappropriately normal LH and FSH levels).

Prior to considering testosterone replacement therapy for hypogonadism, it is important to determine the etiology of hypogonadism and whether low testosterone is due to organic or functional hypogonadism. Organic hypogonadism is caused by a congenital, structural, or destructive disease of the hypothalamus, pituitary, or testes and is irreversible. Functional hypogonadism is caused by a nondestructive gonadotropin suppression that is potentially reversible with treatment of the underlying causative condition or discontinuation of the offending medication and may not require testosterone treatment (**Table 97-5**).

Once the diagnosis of hypogonadism is confirmed whether organic or functional and prior to or in conjunction with initiating testosterone treatment, geriatricians should consider alternative or adjunctive treatments of clinical manifestations of hypogonadism (eg, phosphodiesterase type 5 inhibitor for ED; exercise and weight loss for low energy, depressed mood and muscle weakness; or bisphosphonates for osteoporosis). Also, treatment or

management of potentially reversible functional causes of testosterone deficiency (eg, discontinuation of opioids) should be considered prior to or in addition to starting testosterone therapy. In many instances however, the cause of functional hypogonadism might not be treatable (eg, older patients taking opioids for chronic pain or morbidly obese older men who have failed attempts to lose weight and are not candidates for bariatric surgery). Older men with severe clinical and biochemical testosterone deficiency due to organic hypogonadism should be referred to an endocrinologist for further evaluation and management.

Contraindications to testosterone treatment are active prostate cancer and breast cancer, as these malignancies might be stimulated by testosterone and its active metabolite, estradiol, respectively. Testosterone should be used with caution in older patients with an abnormal digital rectal examination or prostate-specific antigen (PSA) greater than 4.0 ng/mL, hematocrit greater than 50, untreated obstructive sleep apnea, severe lower urinary tract symptoms (LUTS), for example, International Prostate Symptom Score (IPSS) greater than 19, uncontrolled heart failure, myocardial infarction or stroke within the last 6 months, and thrombophilia.

Prior to initiation of testosterone therapy, geriatricians should discuss the potential short-term benefits and risks of treatment (**Table 97-6**) and patient-specific goals of therapy. The Testosterone Trials (T Trials), a coordinated set of seven double-blind, placebo-controlled studies, provided evidence of short-term benefits and risks of testosterone treatment in 790 older men (average age 72) with unequivocal hypogonadism (symptoms and signs of testosterone deficiency and two morning total testosterone levels [by mass spectrometry] < 275 ng/dL) for no apparent reason other than age. The T Trials evaluated the effect of testosterone versus placebo treatment for 1 year on sexual function, physical function, vitality, bone density, anemia, cognitive function, and coronary artery disease outcomes. Moreover, validated outcome measures were used, and testosterone dosages were adjusted to maintain serum concentrations between 500 and 800 ng/dL. Therefore, the design of the T Trials addressed all the major limitations of previous testosterone treatment studies.

TABLE 97-5 ■ COMMON CAUSES OF FUNCTIONAL HYPOGONADISM IN OLDER MEN DUE TO POTENTIALLY REVERSIBLE SUPPRESSION OF GONADOTROPINS AND TESTOSTERONE

Obesity

Medications (opioids, glucocorticoids, megestrol)

Hyperprolactinemia (usually drug-induced)

Malnutrition, energy deficit (energy intake < expenditure)

Chronic systemic illness (eg, malignancy)

Organ failure (lung, heart, liver, kidney failure)

TABLE 97-6 ■ SHORT-TERM BENEFITS AND RISKS OF TESTOSTERONE TREATMENT

BENEFITS	RISKS
↑ Sexual function	Erythrocytosis
↑ Mood, ↓ depressed mood	↑ Prostate biopsy (with excessive monitoring)
↑ Muscle mass and strength	Gynecomastia (uncommon)
↑ Bone mineral density	Formulation-related adverse effect
↑ Hemoglobin	Obstructive sleep apnea (rare)

↑ = Increased; ↓ = Decreased.

In the T Trials, compared to placebo, testosterone was associated with a moderate improvement in sexual function (libido, sexual activity, and erectile function) and hemoglobin concentration and correction of anemia; slight improvement in walking distance, vitality, mood and depression, and bone density and strength; no improvement in cognitive function; slight increase in noncalcified and total coronary artery plaque of unclear significance; erythrocytosis in some men; and an increase in PSA and referral for urologic evaluation.

In discussing the benefits and risks of testosterone, geriatricians should acknowledge that long-term effects of testosterone treatment on clinically important outcomes, such as disability, frailty, depression, dementia, fractures, major adverse cardiovascular events (myocardial infarction, stroke, and cardiovascular death) and prostate cancer are not known; results of observational correlation studies have been conflicting (different studies showing beneficial, no and adverse effects of testosterone treatment on these outcomes).

Testosterone treatment Numerous formulations are approved for testosterone treatment of organic hypogonadism and used off-label for irreversible functional hypogonadism, including intramuscular, subcutaneous, transdermal, transbuccal, transnasal, and oral pellet testosterone preparations. Choice of specific testosterone formulations depends on acceptability, dosage regimen, patient preference, cost, and preparation-specific adverse effects. Short-acting intramuscular testosterone esters (testosterone cypionate and enanthate) and transdermal testosterone preparations are most often used to treat hypogonadism (**Table 97-7**). A short-acting

testosterone ester (testosterone enanthate) administered subcutaneously using an autoinjector was approved recently; it has the advantage of not needing intramuscular injection but requires weekly injections which may be less desirable for some older men. Long-acting testosterone formulations (intramuscular testosterone undecanoate or testosterone pellets) cannot be withdrawn rapidly if an adverse effect develops and should be avoided in older men. Transbuccal, transnasal, and oral testosterone formulations that require administration two or three times daily are less practical for testosterone replacement therapy of older men, particularly those on multiple medications.

Monitoring of both efficacy and safety should be performed during testosterone treatment. Change in symptoms and signs of testosterone deficiency should be evaluated for 3 to 12 months and then yearly after starting testosterone therapy. Improvement in sexual function, vitality, mood, and hemoglobin occur within 3 months but improvement in muscle strength and bone mineral density, takes longer, up to 12 months. If symptomatic improvement does not occur by 6 months of testosterone therapy in the presence of acceptable hormone compliance and normal serum testosterone concentrations, testosterone treatment should be stopped and other causes of symptoms should be considered.

Patients treated with testosterone should have a hematocrit measured at baseline, 3 to 6 months after initiation of treatment, and then yearly to detect the occurrence of erythrocytosis that can be induced by testosterone. If a hematocrit greater than 54% occurs during treatment, the dosage should be reduced or testosterone should be

TABLE 97-7 ■ MOST USED FORMULATIONS FOR TESTOSTERONE TREATMENT IN OLDER MEN

FORMULATION	DOSAGE	ADVANTAGES	DISADVANTAGES
INTRAMUSCULAR INJECTION			
Testosterone enanthate or cypionate	150–200 mg IM every 2 wk or 75–100 mg IM weekly	Reliable dose delivery Inexpensive Some dose flexibility	Discomfort with IM injection Large fluctuations of T level and symptoms More erythrocytosis vs transdermal T
TRANSDERMAL			
Testosterone gel or solution	1% gel: 5–10 g daily 1.62% gel: 20.25–81.00 mg daily 2% gel: 40–70 mg daily 2% solution: 30–120 mg daily	Low-normal to high-normal T levels No injections Dose flexibility Short duration if adverse effect	Potential contact transfer of T to women and children Daily application Expense Skin dry or sticky with gel; dripping with solution; musk odor with one gel
Testosterone patch	2–6 mg daily	Low-normal to mid-normal T levels Less erythrocytosis vs IM injections No injections Dose flexibility Short duration if adverse effect	Frequent skin irritation Two patches may be needed Poor skin adhesion with excessive sweating Daily application Expense

IM, intramuscular; T, testosterone.

stopped until the hematocrit normalizes, after which testosterone can be restarted at a lower dosage. Patients who develop erythrocytosis should be evaluated for disorders that cause hypoxia, for example, obstructive sleep apnea or chronic lung disease.

Monitoring of prostate-specific antigen (PSA) and performance of DRE to detect prostate cancer is not recommended in testosterone-treated men 70 years or older, or with a life expectancy less than 10 years due to comorbid illnesses. In men younger than 70 years on testosterone, PSA monitoring should be a shared decision between the physician and patient after a discussion of the benefits and risks of prostate cancer screening. In men who desire prostate cancer screening, PSA should be measured at baseline, 3 to 12 months after starting testosterone treatment, and then according to accepted guidelines. In patients who develop a confirmed PSA greater than 4.0 ng/mL at any time, a PSA increase greater than 1.4 ng/mL within 12 months of treatment, palpable nodule or induration on DRE, or severe LUTS (IPSS >19), testosterone should be discontinued and patients referred for a urologic evaluation.

OVARY

Ovarian failure (menopause) is universal in older women. As serum estrogen concentrations decrease with ovarian failure, the classic symptoms and signs of menopause ensue. Clinical management of menopause symptoms is discussed in Chapter 36 and effects on sexual function in older women in Chapter 35. Menopausal hormone loss results in a rapid decline in bone mineral density during the first 3 to 5 years, followed by a slower decline in bone mineral density after estrogen production has reached a nadir. The most important systemic endocrine effect of menopause is the increased risk of osteoporosis and low-trauma fractures. It is essential to query women 65 years or older about a history of low-trauma fracture, family history of low-trauma fracture, personal history of height loss greater than or equal to 4 inches, and other risk factors for osteoporotic fracture. Osteoporosis is reviewed extensively in Chapter 51.

CALCIUM, PARATHYROID, AND VITAMIN D

Physiology

In the circulation, calcium is 40% bound to serum proteins (primarily albumin), 15% bound to inorganic and organic anions, and 45% is free (ionized calcium), the physiologic active fraction in serum. In states of hypoalbuminemia (eg, malnutrition or chronic systemic illness) or hyperalbuminemia (eg, volume depletion) that occur commonly in older persons, serum total calcium concentration may be low or high, respectively, but ionized calcium is normal.

Ionized calcium is regulated by parathyroid hormone (PTH) and vitamin D. However, ionized calcium is acutely and rapidly decreased by alkalosis (eg, respiratory alkalosis caused by hyperventilation) and increased by acidosis (eg, metabolic acidosis caused by chronic kidney disease [CKD]). Therefore, ionized calcium may not always reflect the state of chronic calcium balance. Furthermore, blood specimens must be collected anaerobically and processed within 1 hour; if incorrectly handled, acidosis (decrease in pH) results in a falsely elevated ionized calcium.

The interactions of serum calcium, PTH, and vitamin D are summarized in **Figure 97-1**. Ionized calcium binds to the calcium-sensing receptor (CaSR) on parathyroid glands to regulate PTH secretion by a negative feedback mechanism; hypercalcemia inhibits and hypocalcemia stimulates PTH secretion. PTH has direct actions on kidney and bone and indirect actions mediated by vitamin D on the intestines to maintain serum calcium within a relative narrow range. PTH decreases urinary calcium and phosphate excretion by the kidney causing retention of calcium and phosphate in blood; stimulates osteoclastic bone resorption and release of calcium and phosphate into blood; and stimulates conversion of 25-hydroxyvitamin D to 1,25-dihydroxyvitamin D in the kidney and the latter stimulates absorption of calcium and phosphate from the intestines.

Primary Hyperparathyroidism

Background Primary hyperparathyroidism is caused by an abnormality in the parathyroid glands that results in autonomous pathologic hypersecretion of PTH and hypercalcemia; occasionally, serum calcium may be normal (normocalcemic primary hyperparathyroidism). The etiology of primary hyperparathyroidism is a single parathyroid adenoma in 80%; diffuse parathyroid hyperplasia in 10% to 15%; multiple parathyroid adenomas in less than 5%; and parathyroid carcinoma in less than 1% of cases.

In contrast to primary hyperparathyroidism, serum calcium is low-normal or normal in secondary hyperparathyroidism which is physiologic PTH hypersecretion in response to hypocalcemia (eg, caused by vitamin D deficiency or CKD). Tertiary hyperparathyroidism is caused by parathyroid hyperplasia induced by chronic severe secondary hyperparathyroidism (eg, in patients with CKD stage 5) resulting in autonomous PTH hypersecretion and hypercalcemia.

Epidemiology The annual incidence of primary hyperparathyroidism is ~1/1000 person-years and increases with age (peak annual incidence 6.3/1000 person-years at age 65–74). It is more common in women (2:1) versus men and in Black people. The prevalence of asymptomatic primary hyperparathyroidism has increased since serum calcium was included in chemistry panels. Primary hyperparathyroidism is the most common cause of hypercalcemia in outpatients, whereas malignancy-associated hypercalcemia is the most common cause of hypercalcemia in hospitalized patients.

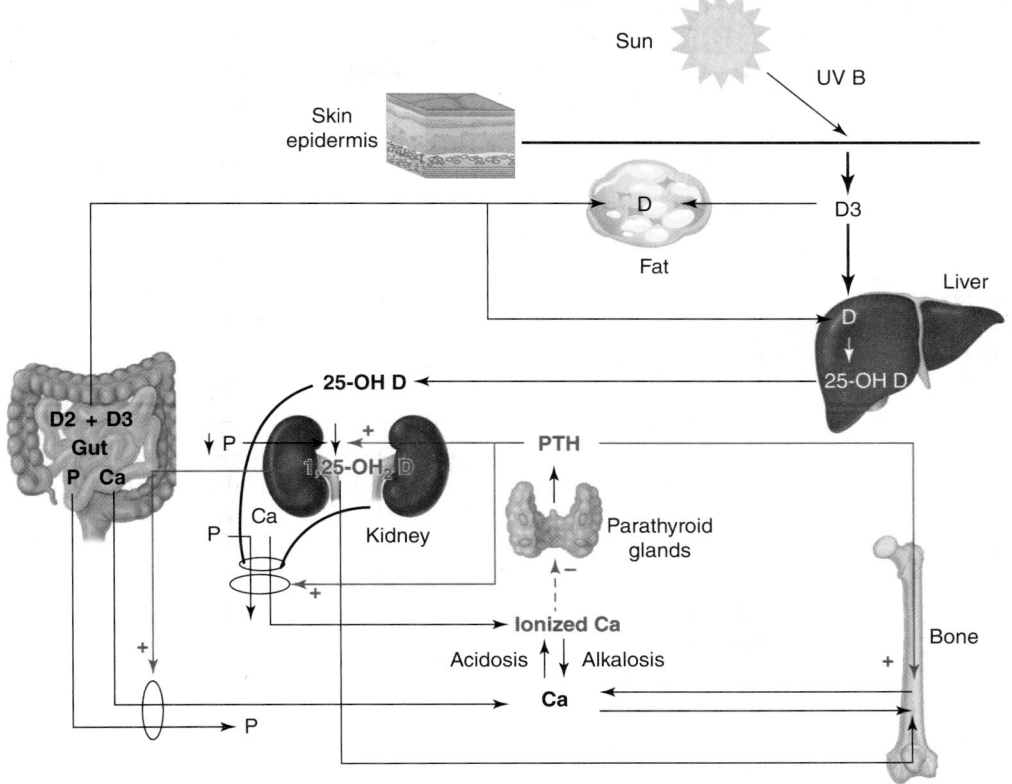

FIGURE 97-1. Schematic representation of the hormonal regulation of calcium homeostasis by parathyroid hormone (PTH) and vitamin D (D). A reduction in serum calcium (Ca) below normal reduces negative feedback suppression of the parathyroid glands and prompts a proportional increase in PTH secretion. PTH stimulates osteoclastic bone resorption and mobilizes calcium (and phosphate [P]) from bone; increases conversion of 25-hydroxyvitamin D (25-OH D) to 1,25-dihydroxyvitamin D (1,25 OH₂ D) in the kidney, which in turn stimulates calcium (and phosphate) absorption from the intestines and stimulates distal tubular reabsorption of calcium (and inhibits proximal tubular reabsorption of phosphate) from the kidney. These actions of PTH restore serum calcium, which then exerts negative feedback suppression of PTH secretion.

Clinical presentation The majority (80%) of patients with primary hyperparathyroidism are asymptomatic, and they have mild hypercalcemia detected incidentally on routine measurement of serum total calcium in a chemistry panel. Some older patients with mild to moderate chronic hypercalcemia caused by primary hyperparathyroidism may exhibit gradual onset of low energy, fatigue, proximal (leg > arm) muscle weakness, and functional impairment, especially in those with a high burden of comorbidities and medications.

The classical clinical manifestations of primary hyperparathyroidism are less common and characterized by the following:

- Nephrolithiasis occurs in 20% of patients with primary hyperparathyroidism. Uncommonly, nephrocalcinosis or calcium pyrophosphate deposition in joints (chondrocalcinosis), tendons, skin, conjunctiva, or cornea (band keratopathy) may also occur.

- Older patients may demonstrate low bone mineral density, osteopenia or osteoporosis, in cortical bone sites (ie, 1/3 distal radius) and have an increased fracture risk. Rarely, osteitis fibrosa cystica (osteopenia, subperiosteal bone resorption, brown tumors, bone cysts, and diffuse lytic foci ["salt and pepper"] skull) may occur with long-standing, severe primary hyperparathyroidism.

- Some patients with primary hyperparathyroidism may experience diffuse abdominal pain, nausea, vomiting, anorexia, constipation, or pancreatitis.

- Polyuria, polydipsia, or nephrogenic diabetes insipidus may also occur.

- In older patients, development or worsening of cognitive impairment or depression ("psychiatric overtones") may occur. With rapid onset of severe hypercalcemia, lethargy, stupor, and coma may occur; this is uncommon, however, unless there is a predisposing condition (eg, immobility or severe volume depletion), or another cause of hypercalcemia (eg, malignancy).

TABLE 97-8 ■ DIAGNOSTIC EVALUATION FOR PRIMARY HYPERPARATHYROIDISM IN OLDER PATIENTS

- Review medical records for previous high serum calcium concentrations
- Review for excessive calcium intake
- Serum calcium, albumin, corrected total calcium or ionized calcium, phosphate, and PTH (by second- or third-generation assay)
- 24-hour calcium and creatinine to rule out familial hypocalciuric hypercalcemia
- Serum 25-OH vitamin D to rule out coincident vitamin D deficiency

25-OH vitamin D, 25-hydroxyvitamin D; PTH, parathyroid hormone.

A palpable neck mass in a patient with primary hyperparathyroidism is more likely to be caused by a non-parathyroid source (eg, thyroid nodule or lymph node) and rarely by parathyroid carcinoma.

Diagnosis Recommended laboratory and imaging studies to diagnose patients with primary hyperparathyroidism are summarized in **Table 97-8**. Initial laboratory evaluation of hypercalcemia should include a serum total calcium, albumin, and calculated corrected total calcium (total calcium corrected for serum albumin concentration) or ionized calcium. The corrected total calcium (preferred vs ionized calcium) = total calcium in mg/dL + 0.8 (4.0 − albumin in g/L) is usually elevated, but may be high-normal (known as normocalcemic primary hyperparathyroidism). Ionized calcium requires anaerobic serum collection and analysis within 1 hour of collection. Therefore, ionized calcium is more susceptible to falsely abnormal values, for example, acidosis associated with delay in processing of samples, prolonged tourniquet use, or excessive muscle contraction with blood sampling will increase ionized calcium; and alkalosis associated with hyperventilation during blood sampling will decrease ionized calcium. Finally, 24-hour urine calcium and creatinine will exclude familial hypocalciuric hypercalcemia, and 25-hydroxyvitamin D will detect vitamin D deficiency that may accompany primary hyperparathyroidism.

It is useful to search laboratory records for previous serum calcium measurements because chronic hypercalcemia suggests primary hyperparathyroidism rather than malignancy. Corrected serum total calcium should be repeated to confirm hypercalcemia and serum intact PTH (using second- or third-generation immunoassay) should be measured to determine whether hypercalcemia is due to a PTH-dependent or PTH-independent cause (**Table 97-9**). If PTH-dependent hypercalcemia is established with high serum calcium and high or inappropriately high-normal serum PTH concentrations, the most likely diagnosis is primary hyperparathyroidism. However, further evaluation is needed to exclude other causes of PTH-dependent hypercalcemia and determine whether indications for surgical intervention are present. Geriatricians

TABLE 97-9 ■ PTH-DEPENDENT AND PTH-INDEPENDENT CAUSES OF HYPERCALCEMIA IN OLDER PATIENTS

PTH-DEPENDENT	PTH-INDEPENDENT
High Calcium and High or High-Normal PTH	High Calcium and Low PTH
Common • Primary hyperparathyroidism	Common • Malignancy-associated hypercalcemia • Local osteolytic hypercalcemia (eg, multiple myeloma, metastatic breast, or lung cancer) • Humoral hypercalcemia of malignancy (PTHrp-mediated, eg, squamous cell lung, renal, breast, bladder, ovarian cancer) • 1,25 $(OH)_2$-vitamin D-dependent (lymphoma)
Uncommon • Tertiary hyperparathyroidism • Lithium-induced hypercalcemia • Familial hypocalciuric hypercalcemia • Ectopic PTH secretion (rare)	Uncommon • Thiazide diuretics • Acute kidney injury • Parenteral nutrition • Immobilization with malignancy or Paget's disease • Granulomatous disease [1,25 $(OH)_2$-vitamin D-dependent hypercalcemia] • Endocrine disorder (eg, hyperthyroidism, adrenal insufficiency) • Vitamin D or A intoxication • Milk-alkali syndrome • Hyperproteinemia

1,25 (OH)2-vitamin D, 1,25-dihydroxyvitamin D; PTH, parathyroid hormone; PTHrp, parathyroid hormone-related peptide.

should consider referring patients to an endocrinologist for further evaluation of PTH-dependent and PTH-independent hypercalcemia.

Treatment Management of older patients with asymptomatic primary hyperparathyroidism should include maintenance of euvolemia with adequate fluid and solute intake, avoidance of thiazides and immobilization that could exacerbate hypercalcemia, careful maintenance of adequate calcium and vitamin D intake to avoid vitamin D deficiency and secondary hyperparathyroidism, and avoidance of excessive calcium or vitamin D intake.

Guidelines for surgery in older patients with primary hyperparathyroidism are summarized in **Table 97-10**. They include severity of hypercalcemia, evidence of significant osteoporosis, and renal complications. Off-guidelines, surgery is considered for some older patients with symptoms that may be attributable to primary hyperparathyroidism (eg, functional or cognitive impairment) or for patient preference after discussion of benefits and risks of

TABLE 97-10 ■ INDICATIONS FOR PARATHYROIDECTOMY IN OLDER PATIENTS WITH PRIMARY HYPERPARATHYROIDISM

Hypercalcemia

- Symptoms and/or patient preferences
- Serum total calcium > 1 mg/dL above the upper limit of normal

Skeletal

- Bone mineral density by DXA T-score < −2.5 at any site (lumbar spine, total hip/femoral neck, and radius)
- Clinical or radiographic vertebral compression fracture (especially with minimal trauma history)

Renal

- Creatinine clearance < 60 mL/min
- 24-hour urine calcium > 400 mg/24 h (nephrolithiasis risk)
- Radiographic nephrolithiasis or nephrocalcinosis (by x-ray, ultrasound, or CT)

CT, computed tomography; DXA, dual energy x-ray absorptiometry.

surgery. Referral to an experienced parathyroid surgeon is the most important factor that determines successful management of primary hyperparathyroidism without complications.

For selected older patients with symptomatic primary hyperparathyroidism who are not surgical candidates, medical treatment could be considered in collaboration with an endocrinologist. Cinacalcet, a CaSR agonist (calcimimetic), may be used to lower PTH and calcium in selected patients (eg, to assess if there is potential for improved symptoms with parathyroidectomy). However, cinacalcet has not been shown to decrease fracture risk and may cause gastrointestinal upset (abdominal pain, nausea, vomiting, diarrhea), dizziness, myalgias, and muscle weakness, and is poorly tolerated by older patients. Bisphosphonates may be used to improve bone mineral density (BMD), although there is no evidence of fracture prevention in these patients.

Active surveillance may be appropriate in older patients with contraindications to surgery. In these patients, monitoring should include serum calcium, creatinine, and eGFR yearly; three-site DXA BMD every 1 to 2 years; and abdominal imaging to detect an asymptomatic kidney stone.

Vitamin D Deficiency

Background and epidemiology There is not a consensus definition of vitamin D sufficiency and deficiency. Based on 25-hydroxyvitamin D concentrations that are optimal for bone health in the general population, the Institute of Medicine defined vitamin D sufficiency as a serum 25-hydroxyvitamin D greater than 20 ng/mL (50 nmol/L); vitamin D insufficiency as a 25-hydroxyvitamin D of 12 to 20 ng/mL (30–50 nmol/L); and vitamin D deficiency as a 25-hydroxyvitamin D less than 12 ng/mL (30 nmol/L). Based on the minimal 25-hydroxyvitamin D concentrations needed for fracture and fall prevention in frail, high-risk

community-dwelling older patients, the American Geriatrics Society defined vitamin D sufficiency as a serum 25-hydroxyvitamin D greater than 30 ng/mL (75 nmol/L).

Prevalence of vitamin D deficiency in community-dwelling older persons is 40% to 50%. Vitamin D deficiency is common in older, dark-skinned and obese persons, hospitalized patients and nursing home residents, and individuals taking medications that increase the metabolism of vitamin D (eg, phenytoin).

Physiology The main source of vitamin D is synthesis of vitamin D3 (cholecalciferol) in skin in response to UVB exposure in sunlight (see **Figure 97-1**). Dietary sources of vitamin D3 (animal sources) and D2 (ergocalciferol, plant sources) are limited, for example, fatty fish (eg, salmon, cod liver oil) and small amounts in fortified food. As a fat-soluble vitamin, vitamin D is stored in adipose tissue, and fat represents a large reservoir of vitamin D.

Vitamin D is metabolized in the liver where it is converted to 25-hydroxyvitamin D. The latter is further metabolized in the kidney to 1,25-dihydroxyvitamin D, the biologically active form of vitamin D. Conversion of 25-hydroxyvitamin D to 1,25-dihydroxyvitamin D is increased by PTH and phosphate. Vitamin D deficiency that results in secondary hyperparathyroidism increases conversion of 25-hydroxy- to 1,25-dihydroxyvitamin D. Therefore, 25-hydroxyvitamin D is a better biomarker of vitamin D deficiency than the biological active 1,25-dihydroxyvitamin D. 1,25-Dihydroxyvitamin D binds to vitamin D receptors in the intestines and enhances calcium and phosphate absorption. Vitamin D, 25-hydroxy-, and 1,25-dihydroxyvitamin D circulate bound largely to serum proteins, mainly vitamin D-binding protein (VDBP).

The causes and risk factors for vitamin D deficiency may be categorized according to disorders of vitamin D production, metabolism, and action (**Table 97-11**). Older persons demonstrate numerous risk factors for vitamin D deficiency, including inadequate sunlight exposure (eg, individuals who are home-bound or live in a nursing home); heavy use of high-sun protection factor (SPF) sunscreen (advised for skin cancer prevention); decreased vitamin D substrate and synthesis in skin (independent of sunlight exposure); decreased 1-hydroxylation (conversion of 25-hydroxy-, to 1,25-dihydroxyvitamin D) in the kidney (proportional to reduction in GFR); resistance to 1,25-dihydroxyvitamin D action in the intestines; and comorbidities and medications that affect vitamin D metabolism.

Clinical manifestations Most patients with mild to moderate vitamin D deficiency (25-hydroxyvitamin D as low as 15–20 ng/mL or 38–50 nmol/L) are asymptomatic. Secondary hyperparathyroidism occurs in 40% and 50% of patients with 25-hydroxyvitamin D levels of 20 and 10 ng/mL (50 and 25 nmol/L) and increases the risks of BMD loss and low-trauma fractures. Patients with chronic severe vitamin D deficiency (25-hydroxyvitamin D < 15 ng/mL)

TABLE 97-11 ■ CAUSES/RISK FACTORS FOR VITAMIN D DEFICIENCY RELATED TO VITAMIN D PRODUCTION AND METABOLISM

↓ Vitamin D synthesis in the skin

- Dark skin
- Sunscreen use (SPF > 8)
- Inadequate sunlight (UVB) exposure (living in latitude > 40 degrees north)
- Age

↓ Dietary intake or absorption of vitamin D from the gut

- Inadequate dietary vitamin D intake
- Malabsorption
- Bariatric surgery, gastrectomy
- Small bowel disease (inflammatory bowel disease, celiac disease)
- Pancreatic insufficiency

↑ Adipose tissue storage

- Obesity

↓ 25-Hydroxylation or ↑ 25 OH-vitamin D catabolism in the liver

- End-stage liver disease (cirrhosis)
- Anticonvulsants

↓ 1-Hydroxylation of 25 OH-vitamin D in the kidney

- Age (proportional to ↓ in GFR)
- End-stage kidney disease (CKD stage 4–5)
- Hypoparathyroidism

↑ Renal loss of 25-OH vitamin D (↓ vitamin D-binding protein)

- Nephrotic syndrome

↓ 1,25 (OH)$_2$-vitamin D action in the gut (vitamin D resistance)

- Age
- Glucocorticoids

↓ = Decreased; ↑ = Increased; 1,25 (OH)$_2$-vitamin D = 1,25-dihydroxyvitamin D; 25 OH-vitamin D = 25-hydroxyvitamin D; CKD = chronic kidney disease; GFR = glomerular filtration rate; SPF = sun protection factor; UVB = ultraviolet B.

with secondary hyperparathyroidism may have cramps and tetany due to hypocalcemia; bone pain, pseudofractures, and fractures due to osteomalacia (impaired bone mineralization); worsening of osteoporosis and fracture risk; muscle aches and weakness; difficulty walking and functional impairment; and increased fall risk.

Diagnosis Diagnosis of vitamin D deficiency is confirmed by measurement of serum 25-hydroxyvitamin D concentration. However, 25-hydroxyvitamin D assays are highly variable and many are not standardized. If possible, diagnosis of vitamin D deficiency should be confirmed using an assay that is standardized for accuracy and reliability, for example, by the CDC standardization program.

Older patients with 25-hydroxyvitamin D concentrations less than 20 ng/mL (50 nmol/L) have a diagnosis of or are at risk for osteoporosis or have sustained falls or are at risk for falls should undergo further evaluation. This evaluation should include serum calcium, phosphate, PTH,

and alkaline phosphatase to detect secondary hyperparathyroidism and increased bone turnover; tissue transglutaminase to rule out celiac disease; and BMD by DXA, if not already performed, to assess fracture risk.

Treatment The treatment of vitamin D deficiency should include both adequate amounts of calcium intake in addition to vitamin D supplementation to prevent or treat secondary hyperparathyroidism. The combination of dairy intake and calcium supplementation (if needed) should total 1000 mg to 1200 mg daily. The calcium content of dairy foods can be estimated by the number of dairy equivalents (cup of milk = slice of cheese = cup of ice cream or yogurt = approximately 250 mg of calcium, accounting for intake of smaller amounts of calcium in other fortified foods and drinks).

In addition to calcium, patients with vitamin D deficiency should be treated with vitamin D2 or D3 (cholecalciferol). Older patients with mild to moderate vitamin D deficiency should be treated with vitamin D2 or D3 800 to 1000 international units (IU) daily. Patients with severe vitamin D deficiency (serum 25 hydroxyvitamin D concentration < 15 or < 20 ng/mL [<38 or <50 nmol/L] if patient is at high risk for fractures or falls) should be treated with higher dosages of vitamin D3, for example, 2000 IU daily for 6 to 12 months. Alternatively, severely vitamin D deficient patients may be treated with vitamin D2 50,000 IU weekly for 8 to 12 weeks, then vitamin D3 800 to1000 IU daily.

Individuals with gastrointestinal malabsorption require much higher calcium supplementation and dosages of vitamin D3 treatment. Patients with CKD stage 5 may require calcitriol (1,25-dihydroxyvitamin D) treatment and should be referred to a nephrologist or endocrinologist.

The risk of vitamin D toxicity is rare using the dosages mentioned above and has not been reported to occur with prolonged use of vitamin D3 up to 4000 IU daily, the safe upper limit defined by the Institute of Medicine. The first indication of over-treatment with vitamin D is hypercalciuria which predisposes individuals to nephrolithiasis, and subsequently, hypercalcemia. Early biochemical indications of vitamin D toxicity have been reported to occur when 25-hydroxyvitamin D levels exceeded 90 ng/mL (225 nmol/L), but severe toxicity has not occurred until concentrations exceeded 150 ng/mL (375 nmol/L).

PAGET DISEASE

Background

Paget disease is a chronic local bone disorder characterized by osteoclast hyperactivity resulting initially in excessive bone resorption and subsequently disordered bone formation. The resulting disorganized bone architecture and enlargement contributes to bone fragility that is associated with an increased risk of fractures and bone deformities (eg, bowing of long bones with weight-bearing), as illustrated in **Figures 97-2** and **97-3**. With time, bone turnover

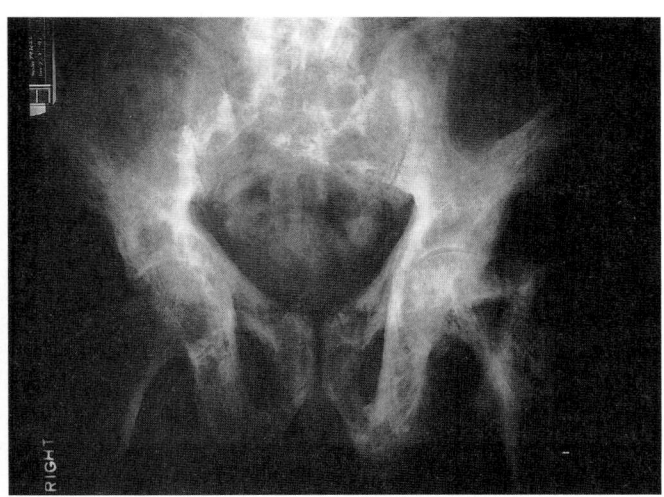

FIGURE 97-2. Anteroposterior pelvis radiograph from a 72-year-old man with Paget disease of bone involving the entire pelvis. Femurs are not involved, but the right side of the pelvis has marked protrusion of the acetabulum.

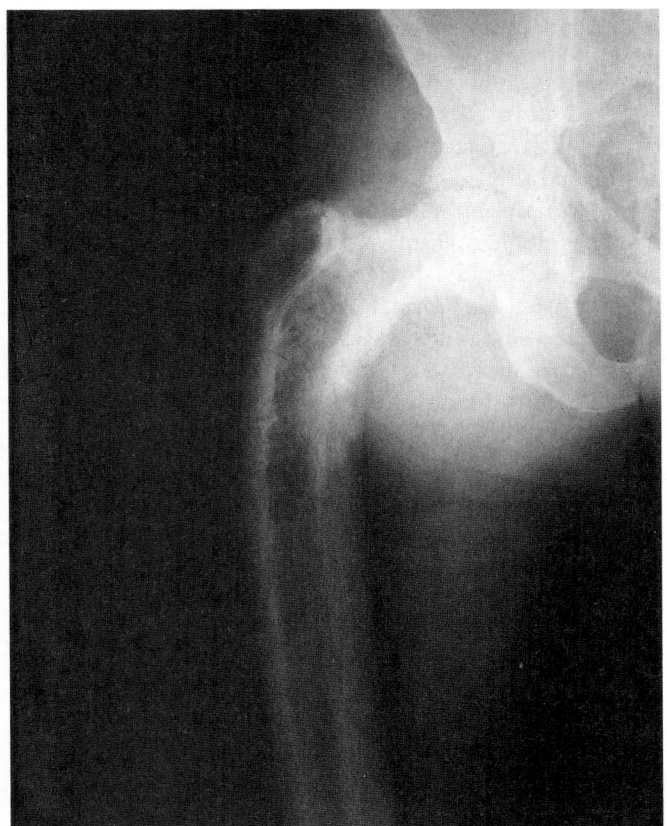

FIGURE 97-3. Right proximal femur and pelvis radiograph of a 68-year-old man with Paget disease of bone involving both the femur and ileum. The angles of the femoral neck and femur are decreased as the bone is weaker (coxa vara deformity). Note the lateral bowing of the femur with stress fractures on the convex side of the femur.

declines and bone becomes sclerotic. The etiology of Paget disease is unknown, but it is thought to occur in individuals with a genetic predisposition who subsequently develop a viral infection that causes the disease to become manifest in middle to late life.

Epidemiology

Paget disease is most common in North America, Western Europe, Australia, and New Zealand; it rarely occurs in Asia and Scandinavia. In the United States, the prevalence of Paget disease is 2% to 3% in persons 55 years or older and has been decreasing in the last two decades. The disease predominantly affects White people and slightly more men than women.

Clinical Presentation

Paget disease most commonly affects the pelvis (~70%), lumbar spine and proximal femur (~50%), skull (~40%), and proximal tibia and humerus (~30%), that is, the axial skeleton. Most patients are asymptomatic. Paget disease is usually discovered incidentally on x-rays performed for other reasons or during an evaluation for an isolated high serum alkaline phosphatase. Constant aching bone pain (due to periosteal stretching and increased bone vascularity) or periarticular and joint pain (due to osteoarthritis secondary to periarticular bone enlargement and altered force transmission in affected joints) that is worse with weight-bearing and at night develops in 40% of patients. Bone pain may affect ambulation, physical functioning, and fall risk in older patients.

Bones affected by Paget disease may become enlarged grossly and deformed (eg, bowed), and there may be increased warmth over affected bones due to increase blood flow associated with high bone turnover. Patients may also develop osteoarthritis in an unaffected joint as a result of favoring the joint affected by Paget disease. Pain may also be due to fractures that can occur with minimal trauma. There is also a higher rate of nonunion, secondary skeletal deformities, and pseudo-fractures (transverse bands of demineralization).

Bone involvement and enlargement by Paget disease may be associated with neurologic complications. For example, skull involvement may cause hearing loss, vertigo, tinnitus from cochlear damage, cranial nerve impingement and rarely, hydrocephalus; and vertebral Paget disease may cause spinal stenosis or ischemic steal syndrome that may rarely result in paraplegia or quadriplegia. Jaw involvement may cause loosening of teeth and ill-fitting dentures that may affect adequate nutritional intake in older persons.

In patients with a high burden of disease involving multiple bones (polyostotic Paget disease), high rates of bone turnover and release of calcium from bone may result in hypercalcemia and nephrolithiasis with immobilization. Rarely, polyostotic Paget disease increases the risk of osteosarcoma, other primary and secondary bone

TABLE 97-12 ■ CAUSES OF INCREASED SERUM BONE-SPECIFIC ALKALINE PHOSPHATASE IN OLDER PATIENTS
Paget disease
Metastatic neoplasm to bone (eg, sclerotic metastatic prostate or mixed sclerotic and lytic breast cancer)
Osteomalacia
Primary hyperparathyroidism with osteitis fibrosis cystica
Bone fracture and/or surgery

malignancies, benign giant cell bone tumors, and high-output heart failure.

Diagnosis

Paget disease of bone is a radiographic diagnosis. Typically, plain radiographs (eg, **Figures 97-2** and **97-3**) reveal a mixture of focal lytic areas (eg, flame-shape in long bones and punched out lesions in the skull) and sclerotic areas with coarse trabeculae, cortical thickening, and bone enlargement; sclerosis becomes predominant in late-stage disease with decline in bone turnover ("burnt out" Paget disease).

Serum alkaline phosphatase, (a marker of osteoblast activity), is elevated in 90% of patients with Paget disease; the degree of elevation correlates with the extent of bone involvement and activity of disease. Alkaline phosphatase may be normal or slightly elevated in monostotic Paget disease. In patients with normal alkaline phosphatase or liver disease, serum bone-specific alkaline phosphatase (see **Table 97-12** for other causes of elevation) or procollagen type 1 N-terminal propeptide (P1NP), another marker of osteoblast function, can be used to confirm the diagnosis and monitor disease activity. A radionuclide bone scan should be performed to assess the extent of bone involvement by Paget disease and asymptomatic sites. CT or MRI is not necessary unless there is suspicion for malignancy on plain radiographs.

Further evaluation of patients with Paget disease should include measurement of serum calcium to detect hypercalcemia that would require further evaluation and treatment and serum 25-hydroxyvitamin D to detect vitamin D deficiency that could contribute to elevated serum alkaline phosphatase.

Treatment

Treatment is not needed for asymptomatic patients with mild Paget disease who have minimal risk for complications. Indications for treatment include: symptoms of Paget disease or complications (eg, bone or joint pain, headache, neurologic complications, heart failure); prior to elective surgery at or adjacent to bone involved by Paget disease (eg, joint replacement, osteotomy for bone deformity, fracture fixation, resection of malignancy); active Paget disease in bone that has the potential of future complications (eg, risk of fracture in weight-bearing bone, hearing loss from skull involvement, paraplegia or quadriplegia from vertebral involvement with spinal stenosis); and hypercalcemia associated with immobilization.

The bisphosphonate zoledronic acid 5 mg IV over 15 to 20 minutes is the treatment of choice for Paget disease. It is more potent than other bisphosphonates and results in a longer duration of response. Bisphosphonates are contraindicated in patients with creatinine clearance less than 35 mL/min. These patients should be referred to an endocrinologist or metabolic bone specialist for management (usually with reduced dosages of zoledronic acid or denosumab). Zoledronic acid causes a rapid and sustained reduction in bone resorption and turnover; decreases alkaline phosphatase and bone scan activity; and improves bone pain and strength, physical function, and quality of life. In most patients, clinical remission following a single administration is sustained for 5 to 6 years and sometimes longer. Before administering zoledronic acid, patients should receive adequate calcium and vitamin D supplementation (as summarized earlier in this chapter) to avoid hypocalcemia.

Zoledronic acid may induce a transient flu-like symptoms (fever, chills, fatigue, myalgias, arthralgias, bone pain, nausea). Acetaminophen treatment prior to and a few days after administration may reduce the likelihood of this adverse effect. Osteonecrosis of the jaw occurs rarely with zoledronic acid treatment of Paget disease.

Acetaminophen, physical therapy, and other non-pharmacologic measures are often needed for joint and bone pain. In older patients, physical and occupational therapy are useful for gait training, fall prevention, shoe lifts, orthotics, cane, assistive devices for patients with gait disturbance, bone deformities, and spinal stenosis. Audiology evaluation for patients with hearing impairment and dental examination for those with jaw-bone involvement should be considered. In some patients with Paget disease, surgery might be necessary, for example, for bone deformities, prevention or treatment of fractures and spinal stenosis. If surgery is needed, immobilization should be avoided to reduce the risk of hypercalcemia. Preoperative zoledronic acid should be considered for orthopedic procedures on bones and joints affected by Paget disease.

ACKNOWLEDGMENT

Many thanks to Christine Swanson, Kenneth Lyles, and Eric Orwoll for their contributions to the hyperparathyroidism and Paget disease components of this chapter in earlier editions of this book.

FURTHER READING

American Geriatrics Society Workgroup on Vitamin D Supplementation for Older Adults. Recommendations abstracted from the American Geriatrics Society consensus statement on vitamin D for the prevention of falls and their consequences. *J Am Geriatr Soc.* 2014;62:147–152.

Berends AMA, Buitenwerf E, de Krijger RR, et al. Incidence of pheochromocytoma and sympathetic paraganglioma in the Netherlands: a nationwide study and systematic review. *Eur J Intern Med.* 2018;51:68–73.

Bhasin S, Brito JP, Cunningham GR, et al. Testosterone therapy in men with hypogonadism: an Endocrine Society clinical practice guideline. *J Clin Endocrinol Metab.* 2018;103:1715–1744.

Bilezikian JP. Primary hyperparathyroidism. *J Clin Endocrinol Metab.* 2018;103:3993–4004.

Bilezikian JP, Brandi ML, Eastell R, et al. Guidelines for the management of asymptomatic primary hyperparathyroidism: summary statement from the Fourth International Workshop. *J Clin Endocrinol Metab.* 2014;99:3561–3569.

Bornstein SR, Allolio B, Arlt W, et al. Diagnosis and treatment of primary adrenal insufficiency: an Endocrine Society clinical practice guideline. *J Clin Endocrinol Metab.* 2016;101:364–389.

Bovio S, Cataldi A, Reimondo G, et al. Prevalence of adrenal incidentaloma in a contemporary computerized tomography series. *J Endocrinol Invest.* 2006;29:298–302.

Cowan LE, Hodak SP, Verbalis JG. Age-associated abnormalities of water homeostasis. *Endocrinol Metab Clin North Am.* 2013;42:349–370.

Fassnacht M, Arlt W, Bancos I, et al. Management of adrenal incidentalomas: European Society of Endocrinology Clinical Practice Guideline in collaboration with the European Network for the Study of Adrenal Tumors. *Eur J Endocrinol.* 2016;175:G1–G34.

Freda PU, Beckers AM, Katznelson L, et al. Pituitary incidentaloma: an Endocrine Society clinical practice guideline. *J Clin Endocrinol Metab.* 2011;96:894–904.

Funder JW, Carey RM, Mantero F, et al. The management of primary aldosteronism: case detection, diagnosis, and treatment: an Endocrine Society clinical practice guideline. *J Clin Endocrinol Metab.* 2016;101(5):1889–1916.

Gallagher JC. Vitamin D and aging. *Endocrinol Metab Clin North Am.* 2013;42:319–332.

Grossmann M, Matsumoto AM. A perspective on middle-aged and older men with functional hypogonadism: focus on holistic management. *J Clin Endocrinol Metab.* 2017;102:1067–1075.

Imran SA, Yip CE, Papneja N, et al. Analysis and natural history of pituitary incidentalomas. *Eur J Endocrinol.* 2016;175:1–9.

Isidori AM, Arnaldi G, Boscaro M, et al. Towards the tailoring of glucocorticoid replacement in adrenal insufficiency: the Italian Society of Endocrinology Expert Opinion. *J Endocrinol Invest.* 2020;43:683–696.

Leese GP. The epidemiology of hyperprolactinaemia over 20 years in the Tayside region of Scotland: the Prolactin Epidemiology, Audit and Research Study (PROLEARS). *Clin Endocrinol (Oxf).* 2017;86:60–67.

Lenders JW, Duh QY, Eisenhofer G, et al. Pheochromocytoma and paraganglioma: an Endocrine Society clinical practice guideline. *J Clin Endocrinol Metab.* 2014;99:1915–1942.

Maas M, Nassiri N, Bhanvadia S, Carmichael JD, Duddalwar V, Daneshmand S. Discrepancies in the recommended management of adrenal incidentalomas by various guidelines. *J Urol.* 2021;205:52–59.

Matsumoto AM. Testosterone replacement in men with age-related low testosterone: what did we learn from The Testosterone Trials. *Curr Opin Endocr Metab Res.* 2019;6:34–41.

Melmed S, Casanueva FF, Hoffman AR, et al. Diagnosis and treatment of hyperprolactinemia: an Endocrine Society clinical practice guideline. *J Clin Endocrinol Metab.* 2011;96:273–288.

Mulatero P, Burrello J, Williams TA, Monticone S. Primary aldosteronism in the elderly. *J Clin Endocrinol Metab.* 2020;105(7):dgaa206.

Samson SL, Hamrahian AH, Ezzat S; AACE Neuroendocrine and Pituitary Scientific Committee; American College of Endocrinology (ACE). American Association of Clinical Endocrinologists, American College of Endocrinology Disease State Clinical Review: Clinical relevance of macroprolactin in the absence or presence of true hyperprolactinemia. *Endocr Pract.* 2015;21:1427–1435.

Singer FR. The evaluation and treatment of Paget's disease of bone. *Best Prac Res Clin Rheumatol.* 2020;101506.

Singer FR, Bone HG 3rd, Hosking DJ, et al. Paget's disease of bone: an Endocrine Society clinical practice guideline. *J Clin Endocrinol Metab.* 2014;99:4408–4422.

West CD, Brown H, Simons EL, Carter DB, Kumagai LF, Englert E Jr. Adrenocortical function and cortisol metabolism in old age. *J Clin Endocrinol Metab.* 1961;21:1197–1207.

Chapter 98

Thyroid Diseases

Anne R. Cappola

Thyroid hormone has widespread systemic effects and plays a critical role in metabolism at all ages. Both excess and deficiency can have severe physiologic consequences. The hypothalamic-pituitary-thyroid axis ensures tight regulation of thyroid hormone concentrations, even in advanced age. In addition, the thyroid gland has evolved to have sufficient redundancy so that only a minority of the gland is required for normal thyroid function. Nevertheless, the prevalence of all forms of thyroid disease, both functional and structural, increases in older people. An astute clinician is required, as recognition and management are more challenging in this age group.

CHANGES IN THYROID FUNCTION WITH AGE

Thyroid Physiology

The thyroid gland produces two thyroid hormones, thyroxine (T_4) and triiodothyronine (T_3), which differ only in the number of iodines (**Figure 98-1**). T_4 is the major hormone secreted by the thyroid gland, at an amount that is 11 times the secretion of T_3. Additional T_3 is produced peripherally by deiodination of T_4 in the liver, kidney, and brain. Within the cell, T_3 is the more potent hormone, binding to thyroid hormone receptors with higher affinity. However, because T_4 levels act as a reservoir of thyroid hormone, with a longer half-life and circulating concentrations 100 times higher than T_3, T_4 concentrations are more commonly measured in the clinical setting.

In addition, both T_4 and T_3 are highly protein bound. Only 0.04% of T_4 and 0.4% of T_3 circulate in the biologically active free state, with the remainder bound to thyroxine-binding globulin (TBG), thyroxine-binding prealbumin, and albumin. A variety of conditions can affect levels of these binding proteins. Therefore, measurement of free T_4 is preferable to total T_4 when T_4 assessment is required.

Thyroid hormone levels are tightly regulated by TSH through a classic endocrine feedback loop (**Figure 98-2**). Thyrotropin-releasing hormone (TRH) released from the hypothalamus stimulates pituitary production of TSH, which in turn stimulates thyroidal production of T_4 and T_3. T_4 and T_3 exert feedback control on the hypothalamus and pituitary to regulate TRH and TSH release. In essence, the pituitary and hypothalamus act as a thermostat to maintain

Learning Objectives

- Understand age-related changes in thyroid function and structure.
- Recognize the symptoms of thyroid dysfunction in older people.
- Interpret thyroid function tests in the context of concurrent medication use and illness.
- Describe the evaluation and treatment of thyroid disease in older people.
- Identify thyroid nodules that require evaluation via fine-needle aspiration (FNA).
- Summarize therapy for papillary thyroid carcinoma in older people.

Key Clinical Points

1. Aside from a slight increase in thyroid-stimulating hormone (TSH) with age, changes in thyroid function and structure are not considered normal aging and require assessment of medications or conditions that affect thyroid function and investigation for thyroid disease.

2. Overt hyperthyroidism and overt hypothyroidism may be difficult to recognize in older people and always require treatment.

3. Treatment should be considered for subclinical hyperthyroidism in older people and for patients with subclinical hypothyroidism who have higher concentrations of TSH.

4. The evaluation of thyroid nodules does not differ with age. Any nodule meeting criteria should undergo FNA, preferably with ultrasound guidance.

5. Papillary thyroid carcinoma is the most common thyroid cancer and may be more aggressive in older people. Thyroid surgery should be performed, and additional management should be tailored to the health status of the individual.

6. Anaplastic thyroid carcinoma presents almost exclusively in older people and has a poor prognosis.

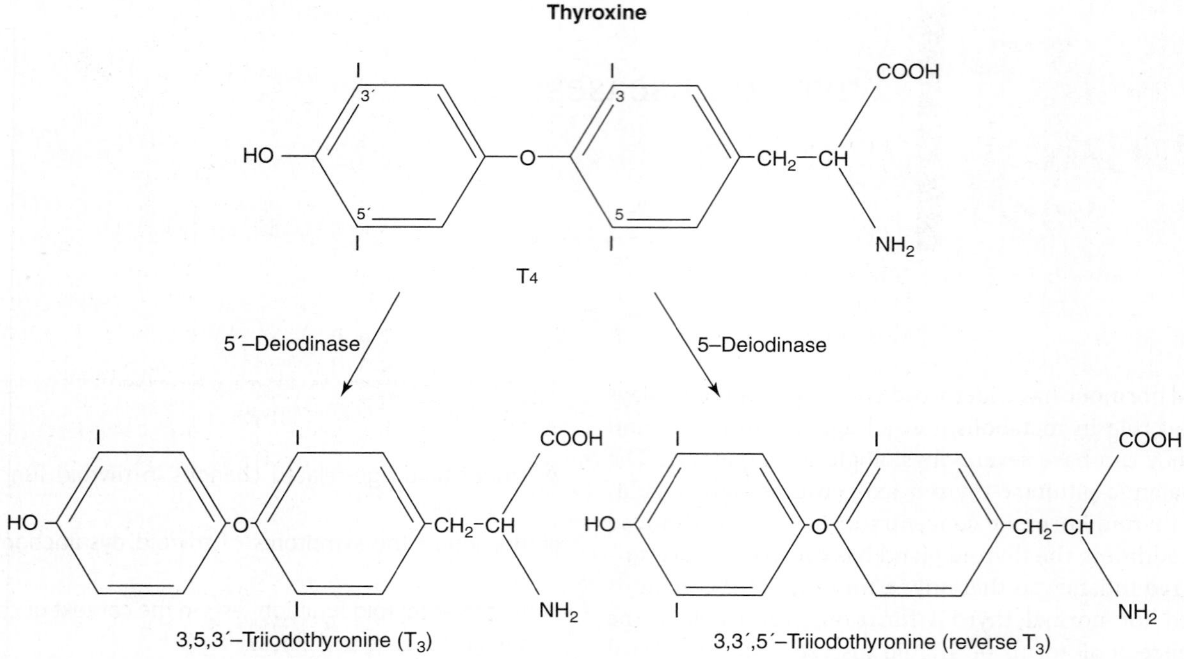

Thyroxine

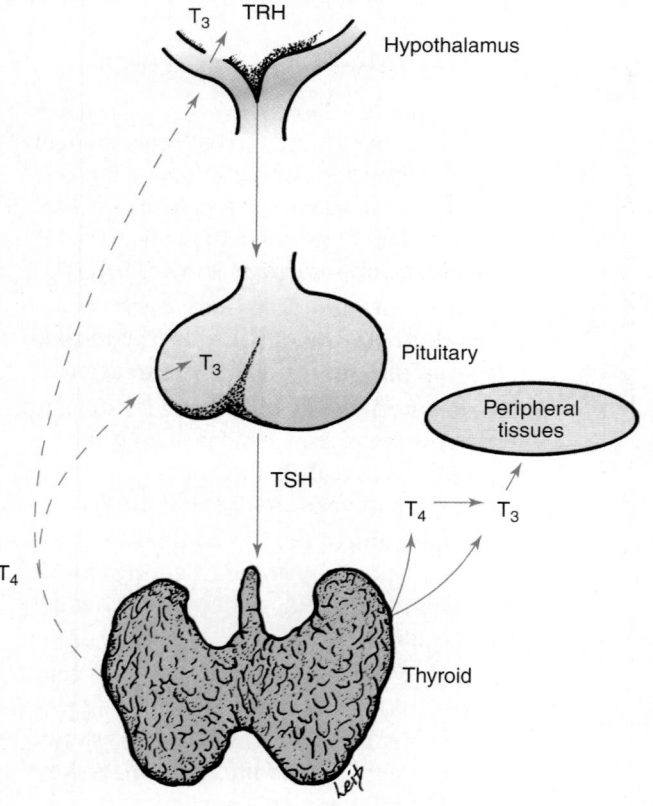

FIGURE 98-1. Structures of T_4 and the enzymatic pathways for deiodination of T_4 to its major active metabolite, T_3, and to reverse T_3 in peripheral tissues.

FIGURE 98-2. Feedback regulation for control of thyroid function that involves the hypothalamus-pituitary-thyroid axis. Arrows represent positive feedback; dashed lines denote the inhibitory feedback of T_4 and T_3 on pituitary thyroid-stimulating hormone (TSH) and hypothalamic thyrotropin-releasing hormone (TRH) secretion.

thyroid hormone levels within a narrow range. Because of variation between individuals in thyroid hormone set point and the sensitivity of the pituitary to perturbations in the set point, TSH levels are used clinically to screen for thyroid problems, rather than levels of T_4 or T_3.

Physiologic Changes with Age

TSH concentrations gradually increase with increasing age, without change in free T_4 levels, in euthyroid individuals without underlying thyroid autoimmunity or thyroid disease. The increase in TSH with normal aging does not indicate occult thyroid failure, since free T_4 levels do not decline. Instead, there may be changes in the bioactivity of TSH or thyroidal sensitivity to TSH. Lower T_3 levels have been documented in healthy centenarians compared to younger people and may reflect a decrease in deiodinase activity with aging.

Clearance of T_4 and T_3 decreases with age, leading to an increase in the half-life of T_4. There is a compensatory decline in T_4 and T_3 secretion, resulting in stability in thyroid hormone concentrations with age. Production of T_4 declines from 80 to 60 μg/day, and T_3 production declines from 30 to 20 μg/day. The half-life of T_4 increases from 7 days up to 9 days in those aged 80 and older. TBG concentrations do not change with age.

The prevalence of thyroid autoantibodies increases in older people, particularly in women, consistent with an increase in autoimmune thyroid disease with age. Therefore, aside from a slight increase in TSH concentrations with age, deviations in thyroid function tests are not due to normal aging. Thus, when the TSH is abnormal in an older person, investigation of thyroid disease and exogenous processes that affect thyroid function should be pursued.

Impact of Drugs and Medical Conditions

Iodine status, medications, and comorbid conditions can each affect thyroid function, either transiently or chronically (**Table 98-1**). All thyroid hormones contain iodine (see **Figure 98-1**). The optimal iodide intake is 150 µg/day, with no changes in this recommendation for older people. Thyroidal uptake of iodine is tightly regulated by the sodium-iodide symporter (NIS) to allow adaptations to variations in dietary supply and ensure that thyroid hormone synthesis does not fluctuate with changes in iodine status. Low iodide increases NIS, and high iodide decreases NIS. The effect of an iodine load on the thyroid gland depends on the underlying state of the gland, that is, whether it is normal or abnormal. When a normal thyroid is exposed to an iodine load, such as iodinated radiographic contrast, thyroid hormone synthesis is temporarily inhibited, followed by escape from this inhibitory effect and recovery, a phenomenon known as the Wolff-Chaikoff effect. These changes are usually clinically insignificant. In patients with underlying thyroid pathology, an iodine load can precipitate hypo- or hyperthyroidism.

Amiodarone is a highly effective antiarrhythmic that can alter thyroid function in numerous ways. Some of these effects are mediated by the iodine content of amiodarone, which is 37% organic iodide by weight. In patients with a normal underlying thyroid, amiodarone administration may cause transient TSH elevation and chronically higher free T_4 and lower T_3 concentrations that do not require intervention. Occasionally, a destructive thyroiditis may occur and present as new-onset thyrotoxicosis, with increase in release of preformed thyroid hormone, as a result of a direct toxic effect of amiodarone. This can be treated acutely with corticosteroids. In patients with underlying thyroid nodular disease or Graves disease who receive amiodarone, increased thyroid hormone production may occur, which can be treated with methimazole. It can be difficult to distinguish among these etiologies of thyrotoxicosis at the time of presentation. Radioactive iodine scanning is not possible

TABLE 98-1 ■ DRUGS THAT AFFECT THYROID FUNCTION

Decrease TSH secretion	**Increase serum TBG**
Dopamine	Estrogen
Glucocorticoids	Tamoxifen and raloxifene
Octreotide	Clofibrate
Bexarotene	Fluorouracil and capecitabine
Increase thyroid hormone secretion	Mitotane
Iodine and iodine-containing compounds	Heroin
Amiodarone	Methadone
Lithium	**Decrease serum TBG**
Interferon-α and IL-2	Androgen
Checkpoint inhibitors	Anabolic steroids (danazol)
Decrease thyroid hormone secretion	Glucocorticoid
Thionamides (propylthiouracil, methimazole)	**Inhibit thyroid hormone binding to transport proteins**
Lithium	Phenytoin and carbamazepine
Iodine and iodine-containing compounds	Furosemide
Amiodarone	Salicylates and salsalate
Aminoglutethimide	Fenclofenac and meclofenamate
Interferon-α and IL-2	Heparin
Thalidomide	Sulfonylureas
Decrease T_4 absorption	**Decrease T_4 5′-deiodinase activity**
Calcium	Propylthiouracil
Proton pump inhibitors	Amiodarone
Cholestyramine, colestipol	Glucocorticoids
Aluminum hydroxide, sevelamer	**Increase hepatic T_4 and T_3 metabolism**
Ferrous sulfate	Phenobarbital
Sucralfate	Rifampin
Raloxifene	Phenytoin
	Carbamazepine
	Sertraline
	Increase T_3 metabolism
	Tyrosine kinase inhibitors

due to competition from the nonlabeled iodide in amiodarone, and so patients may initially be treated with both corticosteroids and methimazole. Patients with underlying Hashimoto thyroiditis may develop hypothyroidism, which is often reversible with cessation of amiodarone. In most cases, amiodarone should not be stopped when thyroid function abnormalities occur. The half-life of amiodarone is long, fat solubility is high, and the iodine load is large. It takes months for the effects of amiodarone to wear off, and thyroid dysfunction can generally be managed while continuing amiodarone treatment.

Several oncology drugs can cause thyroid dysfunction. Tyrosine kinase inhibitors and checkpoint inhibitor immunotherapy can each cause hypothyroidism that may be preceded by a destructive thyroiditis. Hypothyroidism also occurs with thalidomide use.

High doses of corticosteroids and dopamine may each lower TSH levels without affecting thyroid function. This effect is important to remember when interpreting TSH testing in hospitalized patients who are administered either of these medications.

In addition, numerous medications and conditions affect production of thyroid-binding proteins. Estrogens, tamoxifen, and acute hepatitis increase TBG concentrations. This effect is compensated by increased thyroid hormone production in a normally functioning thyroid, to keep free thyroid hormones stable, but may result in changes in total T_4 concentrations. Conversely, androgens, chronic liver disease (through decreased synthesis of TBG), nephrotic syndrome, and severe systemic illness may decrease TBG concentrations. High-dose furosemide, heparin, and high doses of aspirin or salsalate decrease TBG binding to thyroid hormones without affecting TBG. When TBG concentration or binding is reduced, the thyroid produces less thyroid hormone to avoid elevation in free T_4 concentrations.

Nonthyroidal Illness Syndrome

In the setting of severe, nonthyroidal illness, alterations in thyroid function may occur, called the "nonthyroidal illness syndrome." Alternative names are "low T_3 syndrome" and "euthyroid sick syndrome." This altered pattern of thyroid function occurs in reaction to acute illness and may represent an adaptive slowing of metabolism as a physiologic response to systemic illness. It is likely that reduced caloric intake and cytokines play an important role in the pathogenesis of these changes in thyroid function. The first testing abnormality to manifest is low T_3 levels. These are a consequence of decrease in deiodination of T_4 to T_3. In addition, there is a decrease in deiodination of reverse T_3 (see **Figure 98-1**), which has no activity at thyroid hormone receptors, to its metabolite, leading to increased concentrations of reverse T_3. Subsequent changes include a decrease in free T_4 levels, followed by a mild decrease in TSH levels in those with the most critical illnesses. Patients taking high-dose corticosteroids or dopamine

may have completely suppressed TSH levels. The pattern of low TSH and low thyroid hormones is identical to that of central hypothyroidism. Central hypothyroidism is a rare cause of hypothyroidism and does not present without other manifestations of pituitary or hypothalamic disease. Additional diagnostic testing does not need to be pursued if the clinical picture supports nonthyroidal illness as the cause of thyroid testing abnormalities. Measurement of reverse T_3 concentrations is not indicated. Patients with the full constellation of thyroid testing abnormalities have a high mortality rate, at 80%. Thyroid hormone replacement with T_4 or T_3 results in no benefit in the nonthyroidal illness syndrome. During recovery from nonthyroidal illness, TSH levels appropriately rise in order to stimulate thyroid hormone production, which may be interpreted as overt or subclinical hypothyroidism. In this setting, when the patient is also improving clinically, repeat thyroid function testing as an outpatient is preferred over initiation of levothyroxine.

THYROID DYSFUNCTION

Classification

When thyroid dysfunction is suspected clinically, the first step is to measure a TSH level. A low TSH is consistent with pituitary efforts to slow thyroid hormone production, as in hyperthyroidism, and a high TSH is consistent with pituitary efforts to stimulate thyroid hormone production, as in hypothyroidism (**Figure 98-3**). Further discrimination, based on measurement of free T_4 levels, can be made to distinguish between what have been termed "subclinical" (normal free T_4) and "overt" (abnormal free T_4) dysfunction. These unfortunate historical terms frequently cause confusion, since they suggest a role for symptoms in the assignment of thyroid status when, in fact, the distinction is made solely on the basis of thyroid function testing.

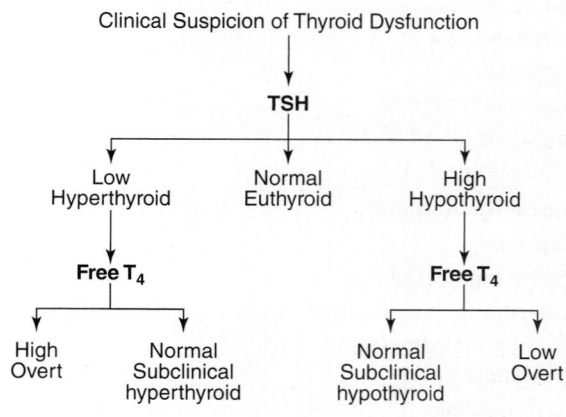

FIGURE 98-3. Classification of thyroid dysfunction based on thyroid-stimulating hormone (TSH) and free thyroxine (free T_4) testing.

Hyperthyroidism

Overt hyperthyroidism is defined as a low TSH with elevated free T_4 or T_3. The prevalence is 1% to 2% in older people. The prevalence in women is higher than in men, though this difference is only twofold in older people, compared to 10-fold at younger ages.

Symptoms Consistent with the myriad and widespread molecular effects of thyroid hormone, there are multiple symptoms associated with hyperthyroidism (**Table 98-2**). As with younger individuals, cardiovascular, psychiatric, gastrointestinal, and musculoskeletal symptoms predominate. Unfortunately, there is no single "defining" symptom that is specific to hyperthyroidism. Overt hyperthyroidism usually causes at least one symptom, albeit nonspecific. One or more of the symptoms should prompt evaluation by TSH testing. **Table 98-3** displays myriad symptoms and their frequency in a study of 84 overtly hyperthyroid patients aged 70 or older and 50 or younger. Of the 19 signs examined, the three signs found in more than 50% of older patients were tachycardia, fatigue, and weight loss. These data also show the paucity of classical symptoms of hyperthyroidism in older people, particularly hyperadrenergic symptoms, due to diminished physiologic response or concomitant β-blocker use, and increased prevalence of nonclassical symptoms such as apathy and anorexia. This presentation has been referred to as "apathetic hyperthyroidism" and can be mistaken for a chronic wasting illness. In addition, the classic symptoms associated with Graves disease, a goiter and ophthalmopathy, are often absent in older people.

Thyroid storm describes the most severe symptomatic presentation of thyrotoxicosis. In thyroid storm, central nervous and cardiovascular systems may be particularly compromised, and patients may present with delirium,

TABLE 98-3 ■ COMPARISON OF CLINICAL FEATURES OF HYPERTHYROIDISM IN OLDER VERSUS YOUNG PATIENTS

SYMPTOMS AND SIGNS	OLDER, ≥ 70 Y (%)	YOUNG, ≤ 50 Y (%)
Tachycardia	71	96
Fatigue	56	84
Weight loss	50	51
Tremor	44	84
Dyspnea	41	56
Apathy	41	25
Anorexia	32	4
Nervousness	31	84
Hyperactive reflexes	28	96
Weakness	27	61
Depression	24	22
Increased sweating	24	95
Diarrhea	18	43
Muscular atrophy	16	10
Confusion	16	0
Heat intolerance	15	92
Constipation	15	0

psychosis, coma, extreme tachycardia, or heart failure. Such patients usually require hospitalization and management by an endocrinologist. Although diagnostic criteria have been proposed for the diagnosis of thyroid storm, any patient whose clinical status is compromised from the effects of hyperthyroidism should be managed aggressively to remove the impact of thyroid dysfunction from the clinical picture.

Etiology and diagnosis The term "hyperthyroidism" refers to overproduction of thyroid hormone by the thyroid gland, whereas "thyrotoxicosis" is a broader term that encompasses any clinical situation with thyroid hormone excess, including thyroiditis or excess exogenous thyroid hormone. The majority of endogenous thyrotoxicosis is due to overproduction of thyroid hormone, either from autoimmune stimulation of the thyroid in Graves disease or an autonomous thyroid nodule within a nodular thyroid gland. These are usually permanent conditions. In younger people, Graves disease is the most common cause of hyperthyroidism, whereas with increasing age, multinodular toxic goiter increases in prevalence. Nodules within multinodular glands may become autonomous over time. Acute worsening of thyrotoxicosis can be precipitated by an iodine load in a patient with autonomous thyroid nodules, which are lacking a normal regulatory response to iodine. Less commonly, leakage of thyroid hormone due to autoimmune or viral thyroiditis can cause transient thyrotoxicosis that resolves within several weeks. The diagnosis of thyrotoxicosis does not require elevations in both free T_4

TABLE 98-2 ■ CLINICAL FEATURES OF HYPERTHYROIDISM IN OLDER PATIENTS

Cardiovascular
  Palpitations
  Chronic or intermittent atrial fibrillation
  Congestive heart failure
Psychiatric and behavioral
  Depression
  Apathy
  Lethargy
  Irritability
Gastrointestinal
  Decreased appetite
  Weight loss
  Nausea
  Constipation
Musculoskeletal
  Proximal muscle weakness
  Muscle atrophy

and T_3 concentrations. "T_3 toxicosis" may occur with normal free T_4 levels, particularly with autonomous nodules; conversely, only free T_4 levels may be elevated with concomitant nonthyroidal illness syndrome.

The process of assessment of the etiology of thyrotoxicosis does not require invasive testing and does not differ between young and old adults. Although there are some clues from thyroid testing (T_4 and T_3 levels tend to be higher in Graves disease than in other etiologies) and physical examination (the presence of proptosis, skin findings of pretibial myxedema, or thyroid bruit are specific for Graves disease), additional testing may be required. Measurement of thyroid receptor antibodies (TRAb) can be used to distinguish Graves disease from other causes. Radioiodine scanning is the definitive way to discriminate among thyrotoxicosis etiologies. NIS is highly expressed in the thyroid, with low levels in salivary glands, lactating breast, and placenta. It allows radioactive iodine scanning in a selective manner. It does not provide valid results in the setting of recent high unlabeled iodide intake, such as from iodinated contrast. Otherwise, it is a useful test to discriminate between high uptake (Graves disease and autonomous nodule) and low uptake (autoimmune or viral thyroiditis) states. Concomitant imaging may discriminate between diffuse uptake in Graves disease and focal uptake by an autonomous nodule. Thyroid ultrasonography may be useful when correlated with a radioiodine scan.

Management The metabolic derangements of thyrotoxicosis can complicate the care of any coexisting condition in an older patient. Furthermore, there are multiple causes of thyrotoxicosis and multiple treatment options. Therefore, management should involve close collaboration between the geriatrics or primary care team and an endocrinologist. β-Blocking drugs are useful in the management of tachycardia and other hyperadrenergic symptoms from thyrotoxicosis of any etiology. Nonsteroidal anti-inflammatory drugs can be useful for treating patients with subacute or silent thyroiditis. Patients who do not respond may require prednisone. Since the thyrotoxicosis is due to release of preformed thyroid hormone in these conditions, antithyroid drugs are not indicated.

Antithyroid drugs are useful in the management of thyrotoxicosis due to overproduction of thyroid hormone from autonomous thyroid nodules and in Graves disease. The antithyroid drugs decrease thyroid hormone production by acting directly on the thyroid to interfere with thyroid hormone synthesis. Methimazole is the preferred drug due to a longer half-life and fewer adverse effects. Propylthiouracil (PTU) has the advantage of decreasing T_4 to T_3 conversion, but its use has been limited by reports of fulminant hepatic failure. However, even in good candidates (Graves disease with mild to moderate hyperthyroidism and a small thyroid gland) recurrence exceeds 60%, and concerns about how well the older patient may tolerate a recurrence of hyperthyroidism should be considered prior to taking this approach. The most common side effects of either methimazole or PTU are skin reactions, which occur in 4% to 6% of patients. The most serious side effect is agranulocytosis, which occurs in 0.1% to 0.5% of patients. Rarely, methimazole can cause cholestasis, and both methimazole and PTU can cause antineutrophil cytoplasmic antibody (ANCA)-positive vasculitis or severe polyarthritis. Because of these risks, an endocrinologist should be involved in the selection and dosage of antithyroid drug therapy over time.

Radioactive iodine is the preferred therapeutic option in patients who have persistent thyrotoxicosis due to overproduction of thyroid hormone. Radioiodine emits γ-rays and β-particles. It is used in low doses for diagnostic purposes and at higher doses for therapy. The effects are dose dependent, and the degree of uptake and size of the thyroid gland are considerations in determining the correct dose (as defined by nuclear medicine). Any antithyroid drug should be stopped 3 to 5 days prior to treatment, though β-blocking drugs should be continued. Radioactive iodine induces necrosis of thyroid follicular cells followed by disappearance of colloid and fibrosis of the gland over months. Contact precautions must be observed for 5 days after treatment, and, if necessary, antithyroid drugs may be resumed 5 days after treatment. A plan for managing contact precautions must be devised before treatment for patients who are caregivers of young children or who have caretakers who are in close contact. Radioactive iodine that is not taken up by the thyroid is cleared in the urine, and patients with urinary incontinence must have a plan for disposal of contaminated absorptive pads. Older patients may benefit from pretreatment with methimazole to achieve euthyroidism more quickly and "cool" down before radioactive iodine or surgery.

Autonomous nodules can be treated definitively with radioactive iodine. If the autonomous nodule is the source of thyrotoxicosis, the remaining normal gland will be unaffected by radioactive iodine therapy, resulting in normal thyroid function after ablation of the affected thyroid nodule. Radioactive iodine therapy is commonly used in the long-term management of thyrotoxicosis due to Graves disease. The goal of radioactive iodine therapy in Graves disease is ablation of all functioning thyroid tissue, with resultant hypothyroidism. Incomplete ablation increases the risk of recurrence due to regrowth of thyroid tissue secondary to persistent stimulation by antibody binding to the TSH receptor. The advantage of radioactive iodine ablation is the permanency of treatment without the risks associated with thyroidectomy, though contact precautions must be observed for 5 days after treatment, ophthalmopathy may be exacerbated, and thyroid function monitoring is required every 4 to 6 weeks after treatment until the patient is taking a stable dose of thyroid hormone replacement.

Thyroidectomy is the fastest way to achieve euthyroidism, but because of increased operative risk in older patients, it is reserved for select cases, such as concomitant thyroid cancer or severe ophthalmopathy. Only an experienced thyroid surgeon should perform the thyroidectomy. Potential complications include transient or permanent recurrent laryngeal nerve paralysis and hypoparathyroidism.

Subclinical Hyperthyroidism

Subclinical hyperthyroidism is defined as low TSH with normal levels of free T_4 and T_3. The prevalence of subclinical hyperthyroidism on a single test is 1% to 6% in an older population. Repeat testing is recommended 3 to 6 months later, and persistence is high, at more than 50%. The etiologies of subclinical hyperthyroidism are the same as those causing overt hyperthyroidism.

Untreated subclinical hyperthyroidism is associated with increased cardiovascular, musculoskeletal, and neurocognitive risk compared to euthyroidism. Subclinical hyperthyroidism in older people increases the risk of atrial fibrillation, heart failure, and overall cardiovascular mortality. It is also associated with increased risk of fracture and dementia. Current recommendations support treatment of older people with subclinical hyperthyroidism to achieve euthyroidism by laboratory testing. The therapeutic options are the same as those for overt hyperthyroidism.

Hypothyroidism

Overt hyperthyroidism is defined as a high TSH with low free T_4 concentrations. The prevalence is 1% to 2% in older people. It is not useful to measure T_3 concentrations when assessing hypothyroidism.

Symptoms Thyroid hormone insufficiency affects multiple organs, often with insidious onset. Symptoms of hypothyroidism are often, but not always, opposite to those of hyperthyroidism, and manifest as a generalized slowing of metabolic processes (**Table 98-4**). Cognitive changes and functional decline are late manifestations of unrecognized hypothyroidism. As with younger individuals, cardiovascular, psychiatric, gastrointestinal, and musculoskeletal symptoms predominate. Unfortunately, there is no single defining symptom that is specific to hypothyroidism. One or more of the myriad symptoms should prompt evaluation by TSH testing. **Table 98-5** displays symptoms of hypothyroidism and their frequency in a study of 121 overtly hypothyroid young and old patients. Of the 24 signs examined, fatigue and weakness were the two signs found in more than 50% of older patients. The usual clinical signs were not well represented in older people. Since the effects of hypothyroidism are reversible with treatment, clinicians caring for older patients should measure TSH at the earliest indication of hypothyroid symptoms.

Etiology and diagnosis The etiologies of hypothyroidism are similar in older and younger adults. Primary hypothyroidism from thyroid failure is the most common source of thyroid dysfunction; central hypothyroidism from pituitary or hypothalamic failure is rare. Primary hypothyroidism is largely due to autoimmune destruction of the thyroid (chronic autoimmune thyroiditis; Hashimoto thyroiditis),

TABLE 98-4 ■ CLINICAL FEATURES OF HYPOTHYROIDISM IN OLDER PATIENTS

Dry skin

Hair loss

Edema of face and eyelids

Cold intolerance

Neurologic
    Paresthesia (carpal tunnel syndrome)
    Ataxia
    Dementia

Psychiatric and behavioral
    Depression
    Apathy or withdrawal
    Psychosis
    Cognitive dysfunction

Metabolism
    Weight gain
    Hypercholesterolemia
    Hypertriglyceridemia
    Peripheral edema

Musculoskeletal
    Myopathy
    Arthritis/arthralgia

Cardiovascular
    Bradycardia
    Pericardial effusion
    Congestive heart failure

TABLE 98-5 ■ COMPARISON OF CLINICAL FEATURES OF OVERT HYPOTHYROIDISM IN OLDER VERSUS YOUNG PATIENTS

SYMPTOMS AND SIGNS	OLDER, ≥ 70 Y (%)	YOUNG, ≤ 55 Y (%)
Bradycardia	12	19
Fatigue	68	83
Weight gain	24	59
Cold intolerance	35	65
Depression	28	52
Disorientation	9	0
Hypoactive reflexes	24	31
Weakness	53	67
Paresthesia	18	61
Dry skin	35	45
Hair loss	12	28
Reduced hearing	32	25
Muscle cramps	20	55
Snoring	18	22
Constipation	33	41

TABLE 98-6 ■ CAUSES OF HYPOTHYROIDISM IN OLDER PEOPLE

Primary hypothyroidism
  Chronic autoimmune thyroiditis (Hashimoto thyroiditis)
  Radiation
    ^{131}I therapy for hyperthyroidism
    Radiation therapy for head and neck cancer
  Surgical thyroidectomy
  Drugs
    Iodine-containing drugs: amiodarone, radiocontrast agents containing iodine
    Antithyroid drugs (propylthiouracil, methimazole)
    Other drugs that decrease TSH or thyroid hormone secretion (see **Table 98-1**)

Central hypothyroidism
  Hypothalamic tumors or infiltrative lesions
  Pituitary tumors or infiltrative lesions
  Pituitary surgery
  Radiation

though exogenous destruction of the thyroid from surgery or radiation (including radioactive iodine therapy) and drugs are also common (**Table 98-6**). All compounds containing iodine, including amiodarone and lithium, as well as interferon-α, interleukin 2 (IL-2), tyrosine kinase inhibitors such as sunitinib, and checkpoint inhibitors such as pembrolizumab, may accelerate hypothyroidism in a gland with underlying Hashimoto thyroiditis (see **Table 98-1**). Transient hypothyroidism can also occur during recovery from thyroiditis or acute, nonthyroidal illness. Bexarotene and octreotide can cause secondary hypothyroidism. A serum TSH is the initial diagnostic test for detection of hypothyroidism; both TSH and free T_4 should be measured if central hypothyroidism is a clinical consideration. Antithyroid antibody measurement is not indicated for diagnostic assessment of hypothyroidism.

Management The aim of therapy for hypothyroidism is hormone replacement, not cure. Levothyroxine therapy should be used, and therapy is usually lifelong. Tissue deiodination of ingested levothyroxine to T_3 allows physiologic thyroid hormone replacement without the need for additional T_3 replacement. T_3 or dessicated thyroid hormones should not be used for thyroid hormone replacement in older people due to risk of adverse cardiac effects from supraphysiologic T_3 concentrations. Levothyroxine is available in 12 to 25 μg increments to allow precise titration. Side effects are largely from inappropriate dosing.

Considerations for initial dosing include the age of the patient and degree of thyroid failure. In patients aged 65 or older who have cardiac disease, it is usually recommended to "start low, go slow." It should be noted that the benefit of this approach, compared with starting with a full estimated starting dose, has not been tested in a clinical trial. The smallest available doses, 25- and 50-μg tablets,

are reasonable starting doses in older people. TSH testing usually occurs 6 weeks (six half-lives of levothyroxine) after initiation of treatment, but older people may benefit from 7 to 8 weeks to achieve steady state, given lower clearance of thyroid hormone. Dose increments initially may be as high as 25 μg, but finer titrations in 12 μg increments are preferred once the dose is above 75 to 100 μg. The target TSH is toward the upper limit of the normal range and could be as high as 4 to 6 mU/L in those older than age 80. While there is individual variation, full replacement of thyroid hormone is often required, regardless of the severity of hypothyroidism initially. The usual full replacement dose in older adults is lower than the 1.6 μg/kg/day recommended in younger patients. Care should be taken to avoid overreplacement, which may have adverse effects. If given intravenously, 75% of the oral dose should be administered.

The pace of progression of thyroid failure is variable, though once TSH levels stabilize, TSH testing need only be performed on an annual basis. When variability in TSH levels occurs, difficulty with adherence should be considered first. For example, a patient taking 112 μg of levothyroxine daily who misses one dose per week will have an average daily dose of 96 μg, which could be sufficient to cause TSH elevation. If an increase in TSH occurs after concentrations have stabilized, drugs or conditions that decrease levothyroxine absorption, increase levothyroxine metabolism, or increase TBG should be considered (**Table 98-7**). These situations may require an increase in levothyroxine dose. After exclusion of these drugs and conditions, it is reasonable to consider progression of endogenous thyroid disease if TSH increases. If a decrease in TSH occurs after concentrations have stabilized, factors that decrease TBG levels should be considered (**Table 98-7**).

Thyroid hormone replacement has a narrow therapeutic window, and iatrogenic hyperthyroidism should be avoided. As many as 40% of older individuals taking thyroid hormone replacement may have a low TSH. Potential risks from iatrogenic hyperthyroidism parallel those of endogenous hyperthyroidism, most notably atrial fibrillation and bone loss. Careful initial titration and subsequent monitoring should reduce the risk of overreplacement.

Myxedema coma Myxedema coma is a serious medical condition that occurs almost exclusively in older people. Despite the name, the patient does not have to be in coma, though an altered mental status is common. The usual presentation is long-standing untreated hypothyroidism, with decompensation often precipitated by infection, cold exposure, alcoholism, or use of narcotics, sedatives, or antipsychotic medication. It is characterized by profound slowing across systems, including hypothermia, bradycardia, and hypoventilation. A thermometer capable of reading low temperatures may be required. Close monitoring is required, and headaches, erratic behavior, and neurologic symptoms such as ataxia, nystagmus, and muscle spasms may be harbingers of impending coma. Hyponatremia and

TABLE 98-7 ■ DRUGS/CONDITIONS AFFECTING LEVOTHYROXINE DOSAGE

Decreased levothyroxine absorption
- Increased GI tract binding of levothyroxine
  - Iron (as supplements and in multivitamins)
  - Calcium carbonate
  - Aluminum hydroxide
  - Sucralfate
  - Cholestyramine
- Proton pump inhibitors
- Small intestinal diseases
  - Celiac disease
  - *Helicobacter pylori*-associated gastritis
  - Atrophic gastritis
  - Crohn disease
  - Short bowel

Increased levothyroxine metabolism
- Phenobarbital
- Carbamazepine
- Phenytoin
- Rifampin

Increased thyroid-binding globulin
- Estrogens
- Hepatitis

Decreased thyroid-binding globulin
- Androgen use
- Progressive liver failure
- Nephrotic syndrome
- Severe systemic illness

hypoglycemia as well as elevated creatinine phosphokinase of muscle origin may also be present.

Treatment of precipitating factors and supportive therapy for any associated metabolic disturbances is as important as initiation of thyroid hormone replacement. Serum should be obtained for cortisol measurement, and then intravenous hydrocortisone should be initiated to treat impaired adrenal reserve that may be present in profound hypothyroidism. Treatment with thyroid hormone without hydrocortisone can precipitate adrenal crisis. Hydrocortisone may be stopped if the cortisol level is found to be adequate. An initial dose of 200 to 400 μg of levothyroxine should be initiated, followed by 75 to 100 μg daily. The addition of a T_3 preparation, which has more immediate effects than levothyroxine, has the risk of acute cardiac effects, and is generally discouraged in an older patient. Metabolism of all medications is diminished in profound hypothyroidism, and sedatives should be especially avoided.

Subclinical hypothyroidism Subclinical hypothyroidism is defined as a high TSH with a normal level of free T_4. The prevalence of subclinical hypothyroidism is 4% in the general population. The prevalence increases with age, to approximately 10% of those aged 65 or higher, and it is more common in women. Follow-up testing and indications for treatment are based on the degree of TSH elevation and patient age, as summarized in **Figure 98-4**. TSH elevations may be transient, due to recovery from silent thyroiditis or from the nonthyroidal illness syndrome. Therefore, repeat testing is recommended in 1 to 3 months if the initial TSH is 4.5 to 14.9 mIU/mL and in 1 to 2 weeks if the initial TSH is 15.0 mIU/mL or higher. The etiologies of subclinical hypothyroidism are the same as overt hypothyroidism, though many older patients without any risk factors for hypothyroidism or antithyroid antibodies are found to have subclinical hypothyroidism. Studies in overt hypothyroidism underscore the difficulty with using symptoms to define the severity of thyroid dysfunction in an older person. The milder physiologic abnormalities of subclinical hypothyroidism result in an even greater diagnostic challenge, particularly given the frequency of hypothyroidism-like symptoms in older people without thyroid disease.

Potential effects of mild thyroid deficiency include hypercholesterolemia, decreased systemic vascular resistance, and diminished cardiac contractility. There is a dose-response relationship between the degree of TSH elevation and incident risk of cardiovascular disease and heart failure in people with untreated subclinical hypothyroidism. Independently of age, a TSH concentration of 10 mIU/L or higher predicts increased cardiovascular mortality, coronary heart disease, and heart failure. A TSH concentration of 7 mIU/L or higher predicts cardiovascular mortality. However, subclinical hypothyroidism is not associated with fractures, dementia, or depression. Although skeletal muscle function is impaired in hypothyroidism, one study found older individuals with subclinical hypothyroidism to have better physical function than their euthyroid counterparts, and another showed decreased mortality in older individuals with subclinical hypothyroidism. Treatment of subclinical hypothyroidism did not improve fatigue or hypothyroid symptoms in a randomized trial of individuals aged 60 or older. However, no randomized trials with clinical endpoints have been performed.

Per **Figure 98-4**, levothyroxine therapy at 25 to 50 μg daily should be initiated for patients aged 65 and older if the TSH is persistently 10.0 mU/mL or higher, and treatment should be considered if the TSH is 7.0 to 9.9 mU/mL. The average replacement dose in subclinical hypothyroidism is 1 μg/kg/day, which is lower than that of overt hypothyroidism, though the treatment goals are the same. The risks of iatrogenic subclinical or overt hyperthyroidism should be avoided when initiating levothyroxine therapy in this age group. There are no adverse consequences to following older patients who have TSH levels less than 7 mIU/L with annual testing. As the rate of progression to overt hypothyroidism is low in this range, no treatment is recommended.

Screening

Because the adverse effects of overt hyperthyroidism and hypothyroidism are reversible with treatment, the symptoms are often less pronounced or atypical in older people,

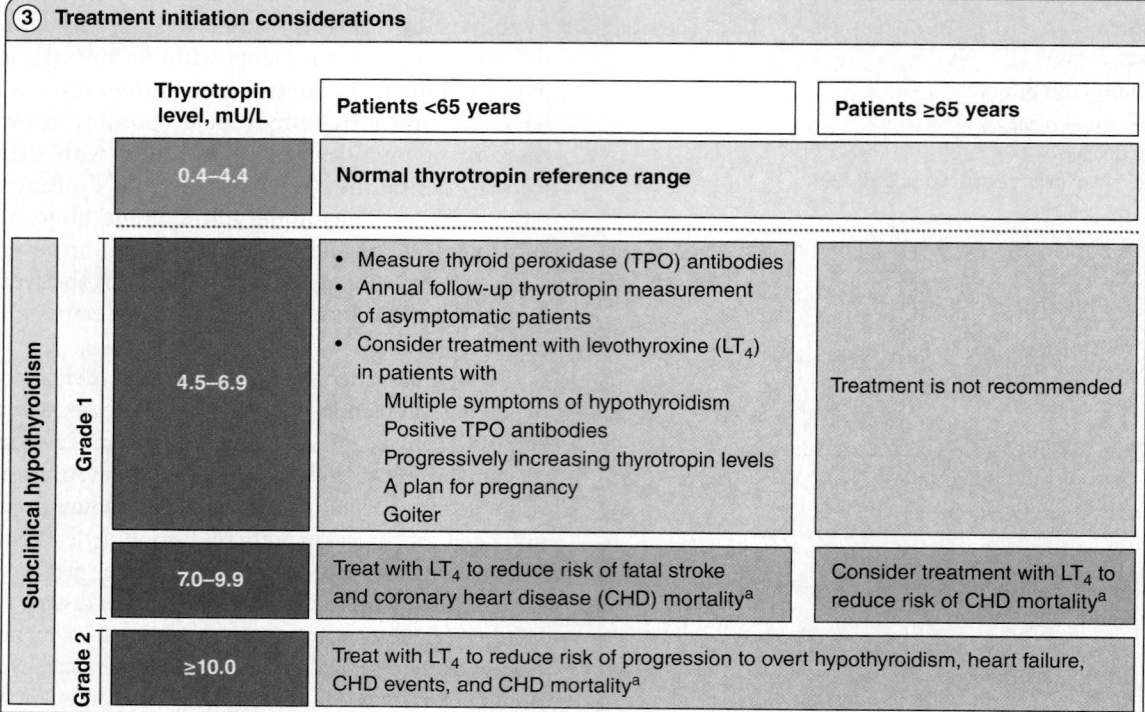

① **Diagnosis of an elevated serum thyrotropin (TSH) level in a nonpregnant adult**

② **Confirmation of persistent subclinical hypothyroidism**

- Initial thyrotropin level 4.5–14.9 mU/L, repeat measurement and document normal free thyroxine level in 1–3 months.
- Initial thyrotropin level ≥15 mU/L, repeat measurement and document normal free thyroxine level in 1–2 weeks.

③ **Treatment initiation considerations**

Thyrotropin level, mU/L	Patients <65 years	Patients ≥65 years
0.4–4.4	Normal thyrotropin reference range	

4.5–6.9 (Grade 1)	• Measure thyroid peroxidase (TPO) antibodies
	• Annual follow-up thyrotropin measurement of asymptomatic patients
	• Consider treatment with levothyroxine (LT$_4$) in patients with
	  Multiple symptoms of hypothyroidism
	  Positive TPO antibodies
	  Progressively increasing thyrotropin levels
	  A plan for pregnancy
	  Goiter
		Treatment is not recommended

7.0–9.9	Treat with LT$_4$ to reduce risk of fatal stroke and coronary heart disease (CHD) mortality[a]	Consider treatment with LT$_4$ to reduce risk of CHD mortality[a]
≥10.0 (Grade 2)	Treat with LT$_4$ to reduce risk of progression to overt hypothyroidism, heart failure, CHD events, and CHD mortality[a]	

(Subclinical hypothyroidism)

④ **Treatment follow-up**

- If treatment is initiated, measure thyrotropin level in 6 weeks and adjust LT$_4$ dose if necessary.
- Once target thyrotropin level is reached, perform annual measurement to confirm that it remains within the target range.

FIGURE 98-4. General therapeutic approach to the management of subclinical hypothyroidism in nonpregnant adults. [a]Recommendation is based on an association of subclinical hypothyroidism with increased rates of the outcomes listed and is not based on clinical trial evidence that treatment can reduce these outcomes. (Reproduced with permission from Biondi B, Cappola AR, Cooper DS. Subclinical hypothyroidism: a review. *JAMA.* 2019;322[2]:153–160.)

and TSH is a readily available test, screening older people for thyroid dysfunction has been proposed. However, the management of subclinical thyroid dysfunction, which is more common than overt disease, is not sufficiently supported by clinical trial data. Furthermore, the definition of the reference range may differ between older and younger people. If the 95% confidence interval is applied to a population free of thyroid disease, the upper limit of the reference range is 3.6 mIU/L for 20 to 29 year olds, but 7.5 mIU/L for those aged 80 and older. The US Preventive Services Task Force has concluded that there is insufficient evidence to recommend routine screening for thyroid dysfunction. This recommendation is unlikely to change until there is clear evidence to support management of any TSH concentration found on screening.

NODULAR THYROID DISEASE AND THYROID CANCER

Thyroid Anatomy

Thyroidal size is similar in older and younger individuals, and the volume of the thyroid correlates more with body weight than with age. Pathologic evaluation shows increased frequency of lymphocyte infiltration, fibrosis, and diminished colloid and follicle size in older people. Palpation of the thyroid gland may be more difficult in older individuals in the setting of pulmonary disease or kyphosis. With increasing age, there is an increase in the frequency of both thyroid nodules and thyroid cancer. The higher incidence with age is not entirely due to detection bias from increased frequency of radiologic testing, such as computed tomography (CT) scans or carotid ultrasounds, though the initial presentation of a thyroid nodule in an older person is often an incidental finding.

Evaluation of Thyroid Nodules

In autopsy series, 50% of thyroid glands have one or more thyroid nodules. Multinodular glands are more common in people from areas of iodine insufficiency. Patients with a history of childhood radiation to the neck or childhood exposure to ionizing radiation have an increased risk of developing thyroid nodules. The majority of these nodules are benign, though these nodules have an increased risk of thyroid cancer, which declines starting four decades after initial exposure.

The evaluation of a thyroid nodule does not differ by age. The main consideration is detecting the malignancy present in 7% to 9% of thyroid nodules. Men have a higher risk of malignancy than women. Nonpalpable nodules discovered incidentally have the same risk of malignancy as palpable nodules of the same size. Patients with multiple nodules have the same risk of malignancy as patients with a solitary nodule. Any palpable thyroid abnormality or one found through an imaging modality should be examined via a dedicated thyroid ultrasound. In addition to size in three dimensions, high-risk nodule characteristics such as hypoechogenicity, irregular margins, taller-than-wide shape, intranodular vascularity, and microcalcifications, as well as low-risk characteristics, such as spongiform appearance or noncalcified, mixed cystic and solid composition, should be documented. The presence and characteristics of lymph nodes should be assessed. A TSH should also be measured. Patients who have a low TSH should undergo a radionuclide thyroid scan to assess for thyroid nodule functioning;

TABLE 98-8 ■ FINE-NEEDLE ASPIRATION (FNA) OF A THYROID NODULE

FNA indicated
- Abnormal cervical lymph nodes
- Nodules ≥ 1 cm that are solid and hypoechoic
- Nodules ≥ 1.5 cm that are isoechoic or hyperechoic solid

FNA or observation
- Mixed cystic-solid nodules or spongiform nodules ≥ 2 cm

FNA not required/indicated
- Purely cystic nodules
- Nodules < 1 cm

functioning "hot" nodules rarely harbor malignancy and do not require cytologic evaluation.

All other patients meeting the criteria in **Table 98-8** should undergo fine-needle aspiration (FNA) with ultrasound guidance, which improves the accuracy. For multinodular goiters, any nodule that meets criteria for aspiration should undergo FNA. Categories of FNA results are summarized in **Figure 98-5**. Nodules with either atypia of undetermined significance or follicular lesions of undetermined significance should have additional analysis of aspirates using molecular analysis, using either an mRNA classifier system or mutational analysis. Nodules determined to be benign should have ultrasound follow-up, and those at high risk of malignancy should be removed surgically, usually a total thyroidectomy.

Benign Nodular Disease

Nodules that did not meet initial criteria for FNA or underwent FNA with benign pathology have a low likelihood of a later diagnosis of thyroid cancer. Current understanding

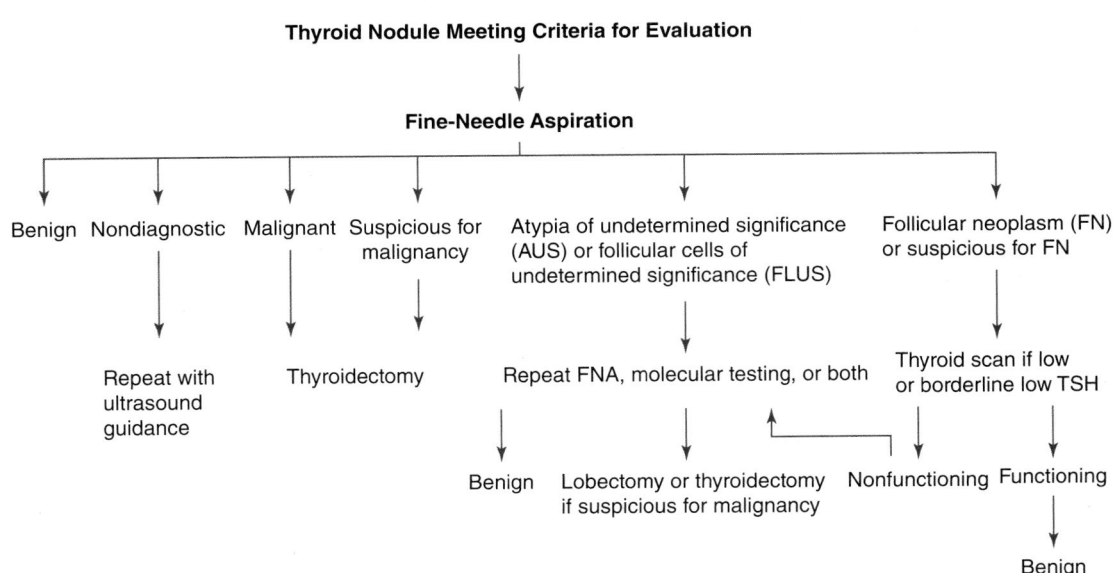

FIGURE 98-5. Algorithm for management of patients presenting with nodular thyroid disease, based on results of fine-needle aspiration (FNA).

of thyroid cancer biology suggests that a cancerous nodule develops as a cancerous nodule, and that benign nodules do not become cancerous over time. However, because false negatives do occur, periodic ultrasound surveillance is advised for nodules that did not meet initial criteria for FNA, either due to size or sonographic characteristics, or whose FNA results indicated a benign diagnosis. On follow-up ultrasounds, each nodule should be evaluated for the development of size or ultrasound characteristics that meet criteria for FNA. Benign nodules should be followed up with a repeat thyroid ultrasound in 12 to 18 months, and continued ultrasound surveillance every 2 to 5 years, with FNA for development of sonographically suspicious features or significant growth. Any nodule that has undergone FNA twice does not need additional aspirations, due to the vanishingly small likelihood of two false-negative FNAs.

Nodular goiters may grow to the point of causing compressive symptoms, including dyspnea or wheezing from tracheal narrowing or disturbances of swallowing from esophageal impingement. These goiters often have a substernal component which can be evaluated by CT scan of the neck. Flow-volume loop evaluation through pulmonary function testing can be used to evaluate extrinsic compression in the neck, and barium swallow evaluation can demonstrate the degree of thyroidal extension abutting the esophagus. Even if FNA confirms benign nodular disease, thyroid surgery may be indicated to relieve mass effect from an enlarged nodular goiter.

Thyroid Cancer

The incidence of thyroid cancer increases with age, peaking at age 65 to 69 at 29.6 per 100,000. Thyroid cancer can be of follicular cell origin (papillary, follicular, or anaplastic) or C-cell origin (medullary thyroid cancer). Thyroid lymphoma and metastases to the thyroid can also occur. The majority of thyroid cancers are papillary thyroid carcinomas. Older patients are more likely to present with more aggressive disease, higher recurrence rates, and multicentricity. However, the prognosis of thyroid cancer is excellent and improving, with 5-year survival rates of 98% in those aged 50 to 64, 97% in those aged 65 to 74, and 88% in those aged 75 or older.

The diagnosis of thyroid cancer is made via cytologic interpretation of FNA specimens. Surgery is the primary modality for management of thyroid cancer, irrespective of age. For patients with tumors of 1 to 4 cm without extrathyroidal extension and no lymph node involvement, lobectomy may be performed instead of total thyroidectomy. This surgery should be performed by an experienced thyroid surgeon, with lymph node sampling as indicated. For thyroid cancer confined to the thyroid gland, no additional initial therapy is required. Thyroid hormone replacement is required after total thyroidectomy. Since TSH has a trophic effect on the thyroid, a high levothyroxine dose is recommended in high-risk patients to suppress TSH levels. In low-risk patients, maintaining a TSH in the lower half of the normal range is acceptable. Cardiac effects of high levothyroxine doses can be mitigated by β-blockers and bisphosphonates attenuate effects on bone.

A subset of patients requires additional therapy, such as radioactive iodine ablation of residual disease in the neck or metastatic outside the neck, capitalizing on the retention of NIS in the majority of differentiated cancers of follicular origin. Radioactive iodine scanning for residual disease can be performed with recombinant TSH treatment, avoiding the physiologic consequences associated with withdrawal-induced hypothyroidism. Multitargeted kinase inhibitors are available for patients with metastatic disease that does not respond to radioactive iodine therapy.

Medullary thyroid carcinoma should be treated with total thyroidectomy, and residual disease can be monitored through assessment of calcitonin and carcinoembryonic antigen levels. Since the C-cells do not contain NIS, radioactive iodine therapy has no effect on medullary thyroid carcinoma. For extensive nodal disease or local disease in the neck, external beam therapy can be considered. Tyrosine kinase inhibitors have been used in progressive systemic disease. All patients with medullary thyroid carcinoma should undergo genetic testing for a *RET* germline mutation.

Anaplastic thyroid carcinoma is an undifferentiated thyroid cancer that is typically found in older people, with a mean age at diagnosis of 65. It has the worst prognosis of any thyroid cancer, due to rapid growth and local invasiveness, and the treatment team should include palliative care expertise. Patients with anaplastic thyroid carcinoma often have a multinodular goiter or history of papillary thyroid carcinoma. The presentation of anaplastic thyroid carcinoma is as a rapidly enlarging neck mass. Thyroidectomy, radiotherapy, and chemotherapy have limited benefit, and median survival from diagnosis is 5 months.

Thyroid lymphoma is also rapid growing, and usually arises in a background of Hashimoto thyroiditis. Like anaplastic thyroid carcinoma, it presents as a rapidly growing mass that may cause compressive symptoms, but the response to treatment is better. A characteristic asymmetrical pseudocystic pattern is present on ultrasound. Large needle or surgical biopsy is required to establish the diagnosis. Treatment with radiation and chemotherapy and prognosis parallel other non-Hodgkin lymphomas, and thyroidectomy is not indicated.

ACKNOWLEDGMENTS

Drs. Jerome Hershman, Sima Hassani, and Mary Samuels wrote this chapter in the 6th edition. **Tables 98-1** through **98-6** and **Figures 98-1** and **98-2** from that chapter have been retained in this edition.

FURTHER READING

Bible KC, Kebebew E, Brierley J, et al. 2021 American Thyroid Association guidelines for management of patients with anaplastic thyroid cancer. *Thyroid*. 2021; 31(3):337–386.

Biondi B, Cappola AR, Cooper DS. Subclinical hypothyroidism: a review. *JAMA*. 2019;322(2):153–160.

Burch HB. Drug effects on the thyroid. *N Engl J Med*. 2019; 381(8):749–761.

Chaker L, Cappola AR, Mooijaart SP, Peeters RP. Clinical aspects of thyroid function during ageing. *Lancet Diabetes Endocrinol*. 2018;6(9):733–742.

Doucet J, Trivalle C, Chassagne P, et al. Does age play a role in clinical presentation of hypothyroidism? *J Am Geriatr Soc*. 1994;42(9):984–986.

Garber JR, Cobin RH, Gharib H, et al. Clinical practice guidelines for hypothyroidism in adults: cosponsored by the American Association of Clinical Endocrinologists and the American Thyroid Association. *Thyroid*. 2012;22(12):1200–1235.

Haugen BR, Alexander EK, Bible KC, et al. 2015 American Thyroid Association management guidelines for adult patients with thyroid nodules and differentiated thyroid cancer: the American Thyroid Association guidelines task force on thyroid nodules and differentiated thyroid cancer. *Thyroid*. 2016;26(1):1–133.

Jonklaas J, Bianco AC, Bauer AJ, et al. Guidelines for the treatment of hypothyroidism: prepared by the American Thyroid Association task force on thyroid hormone replacement. *Thyroid*. 2014;24(12):1670–1751.

LeFevre ML, US Preventive Services Task Force. Screening for thyroid dysfunction: U.S. Preventive Services Task Force recommendation statement. *Ann Intern Med*. 2015;162(9):641–650.

Ross DS, Burch HB, Cooper DS, et al. 2016 American Thyroid Association guidelines for diagnosis and management of hyperthyroidism and other causes of thyrotoxicosis. *Thyroid*. 2016;26(10):1343–1421.

SEER*Explorer: An interactive website for SEER cancer statistics [Internet]. Surveillance Research Program, National Cancer Institute. [Cited 2021 April 15]. Available from https://seer.cancer.gov/explorer/.

Stott DJ, Rodondi N, Kearney PM, et al. Thyroid hormone therapy for older adults with subclinical hypothyroidism. *N Engl J Med*. 2017;376(26):2534–2544.

Trivalle C, Doucet J, Chassagne P, et al. Differences in the signs and symptoms of hyperthyroidism in older and younger patients. *J Am Geriatr Soc*. 1996;44(1):50–53.

Wells SA, Asa SL, Dralle H, et al. Revised American Thyroid Association guidelines for the management of medullary thyroid carcinoma. *Thyroid*. 2015;25(6):567–610.

Diabetes Mellitus

Pearl G. Lee, Jeffrey B. Halter

Diabetes mellitus is a common metabolic disorder affecting older people. Although it is recognized by its effects on carbohydrate metabolism to cause hyperglycemia, diabetes usually also affects lipid and protein metabolism. With time, effects of diabetes on the cardiovascular system, the kidneys, the retina, and the peripheral nervous system, often referred to as long-term complications of diabetes, substantially increase mortality and morbidity in older adults. Furthermore, diabetes may accelerate the risk and contribute to worse outcomes for other common age-related conditions, including physical function decline, cognitive impairment, and geriatric syndromes. Older adults with diabetes are highly heterogeneous in their health and functional status. Many older adults who are relatively healthy and have good functional status may benefit from the same aggressive, often complex diabetes care regimen that is recommended for younger adult diabetes patients. However, the risks and difficulties of implementing such a diabetes care regimen may lead to more harm than benefit for some older adults, especially those who have many comorbidities. Therefore, diabetes management and goals of care for older adults should be individualized to address the heterogeneity of this population. More research is needed to identify optimal care for older patients with diabetes, improve their functional outcomes, and preserve their long-term independence.

DEFINITION

Diabetes mellitus is a heterogeneous set of disorders affecting multiple body systems; however, diabetes diagnostic criteria are based on documentation of elevated blood glucose levels. While glucose levels vary during the course of the day, the diagnostic criteria for diabetes mellitus are based on standardized values that predict poor outcomes in population studies. The challenge of establishing appropriate diagnostic criteria for older adults is made more difficult by well-described effects of aging on glucose metabolism (summarized later in this chapter in the section on "Effects of Aging"). **Table 99-1** summarizes the currently accepted diagnostic criteria published by the American Diabetes Association (ADA), which were most recently updated in 2021.

Type 1 Diabetes

Type 1 diabetes is a condition characterized by destruction of the insulin-producing β-cells of the endocrine pancreas, resulting in absolute deficiency of insulin. While evidence

Learning Objectives

- Understand the epidemiology of diabetes and the heterogeneity of its complications and comorbidities in older adults, including geriatric conditions.
- Describe preventive strategies and initial management strategies for diabetes in older adults.
- Determine appropriate diabetes management goals and regimens for older adults, based on their individual functional status, cognition, and available social support.

Key Clinical Points

1. Older adults, as a result of interactions among genetics, lifestyle, and aging, are at high risk of developing prediabetes and diabetes.
2. Intensive lifestyle interventions, including diet and physical activity to achieve weight loss, are effective strategies for prevention of progression from prediabetes to diabetes and for management of diabetes in older adults.
3. Treatment of diabetes in the older adult, particularly drug therapy, should involve consideration of patient and caregiver preferences, and other coexisting medical and geriatric conditions.

of cell-mediated autoimmunity is a hallmark of type 1 diabetes, some patients develop a type 1 diabetes phenotype with evidence of severe insulin deficiency and episodes of diabetic ketoacidosis (DKA) with no detectable autoimmunity. Such individuals have idiopathic type 1 diabetes. Although the incidence of new-onset type 1 diabetes in older adults is very low, effective treatment of type 1 diabetes may prevent or delay the development of long-term complications and increased mortality. Thus, people who develop type 1 diabetes earlier in life now often live to old age and therefore become a part of the spectrum of diabetes mellitus in an older adult population.

TABLE 99-1 ■ THREE METHODS TO DETERMINE DYSGLYCEMIA AND DIAGNOSTIC CRITERIA[a] FOR DIABETES IN ALL ADULTS, REGARDLESS OF AGE

GLYCEMIC STATUS	A1C	FPG	OGTT (2-H GLUCOSE)
Diabetes	≥ 6.5%	≥ 126 mg/dL (7 mmol/L)	≥ 200 mg/dL (11.1 mmol/L)
Prediabetes	5.7%–6.4%	100–125 mg/dL (5.6–6.9 mmol/L)	140–199 mg/dL (7.8–11.0 mmol/L)
Normal	< 5.7%	< 100 mg/dL (5.5 mmol/L)	< 140 mg/dL (7.8 mmol/L)

FPG, fasting plasma glucose, glucose measurement after no caloric intake for at least 8 hours; A1C, glycosylated hemoglobin A1C; OGTT, oral glucose tolerance test, 2 hours.
[a]Any of these criteria should be confirmed on a separate day to establish a diagnosis of diabetes.

Type 2 Diabetes

Approximately 90% of older adults with diabetes have type 2 diabetes. Hyperglycemia, often asymptomatic, is the hallmark and DKA is not part of the clinical syndrome. Type 2 diabetes is associated with a progressive insulin secretory defect, but severe absolute insulin deficiency is usually not present. Coexisting obesity is common, and resistance to insulin's metabolic effects is usually a characteristic feature. While there is a strong genetic predisposition to development of type 2 diabetes, its etiology remains unknown and is likely to be both highly heterogeneous and multifactorial. The interaction between genetics, lifestyle factors, and aging in the development of type 2 diabetes is discussed later in this chapter in the section on "Pathophysiology."

Other Specific Types of Diabetes

The ADA classification for diabetes mellitus identifies a number of specific conditions that lead to development of diabetes, each of which is relatively uncommon. One group of disorders includes genetic defects of the pancreatic β-cell. The clinical phenotype for these genetic disorders is maturity-onset diabetes of youth (MODY). These genetic disorders have autosomal dominant inheritance with first presentation of asymptomatic hyperglycemia early in life. Patients with MODY can live to old age, however, and therefore become part of the spectrum of diabetes in an older adult population. The metabolic disorder in some affected individuals may be mild, whereas others may develop symptomatic hyperglycemia and long-term complications of diabetes mellitus similar to patients with typical type 2 diabetes. Another type of genetic defect has been identified in a few families in which insulin processing prior to secretion is impaired, which can predispose to development of hyperglycemia.

Other families have genetic defects affecting insulin action. Severe insulin resistance results, and when it is not adequately compensated for by increased insulin secretion, hyperglycemia occurs. Diseases of the exocrine pancreas can lead to damage to pancreatic β-cells, diminished

TABLE 99-2 ■ DRUGS THAT MAY INCREASE GLUCOSE LEVELS

Diuretics
α-Adrenergic agonists
β-Adrenergic blockers
Alcohol
Ca²⁺ channel blockers
Caffeine
Clozapine
Glucocorticoids
Growth hormone
Nicotine
Nicotinic acid
Nonsteroidal anti-inflammatory drugs
Female sex steroids (estrogen/progesterone)
Pentamidine
Phenytoin

insulin secretion, and hyperglycemia. Hyperglycemia also can occur in patients with excessive secretion of hormones that adversely affect carbohydrate metabolism, such as in acromegaly, Cushing syndrome, glucagonoma, and pheochromocytoma. Similarly, tumors making aldosterone can cause hyperglycemia as a result of hypokalemia-induced inhibition of insulin secretion. A number of drugs or toxins can impair insulin secretion or insulin action and lead to the development of hyperglycemia. **Table 99-2** lists such drugs. Several genetic neuromuscular disorders are associated with diabetes mellitus, but they are rare in the older adult population.

Gestational Diabetes Mellitus

Gestational diabetes mellitus (GDM) refers to the first identification of an alteration in glucose metabolism during pregnancy. While GDM per se is not part of the spectrum of diabetes in older adults, a history of GDM may be part of the background of an older woman presenting with type 2 diabetes. GDM has been aggressively screened for and treated, thus increasing numbers of women reaching the geriatric age group will have this history, as GDM affects approximately 4% of all pregnancies in the United States. After pregnancy, 5% to 10% of women with GDM continue to have type 2 diabetes. Women who have had GDM have a 20% to 50% chance of developing diabetes in the next 5 to 10 years.

Diagnostic Criteria

The rationale for the circulating glucose level criteria shown in **Table 99-1** is based on prediction of risk for diabetes-related complications. For example, a 2-hour value during the oral glucose tolerance test (OGTT) greater than or equal to 200 mg/dL is a strong predictor of diabetes complications, even when the fasting glucose level (FPG) is less than 126 mg/dL. The term "isolated postchallenge hyperglycemia"

(IPH) is sometimes used for individuals who meet the 2-hour OGTT criterion for diabetes, but who do not meet the fasting glucose criterion. There is no age adjustment in the recommended criteria for the diagnosis of diabetes mellitus because the same glucose level cut points that predict complications appear to apply regardless of age.

Since 2010, diagnostic criteria for diabetes include a hemoglobin A1C level of 6.5% or higher. An A1C of 6.5% or higher predicts diabetic retinopathy at approximately the same rate (ie, 10%) as in individuals who are diagnosed on the basis of the fasting and postchallenge glucose criteria.

Adding A1C as a diagnostic criterion for diabetes can improve the identification of asymptomatic diabetic patients. About 20% of people who meet criteria for diabetes, or 8 million of the US population, are undiagnosed. The A1C test does not require the patient to be fasting; it can be done at any time that a clinical visit is scheduled, is simpler to perform than the OGTT, and is less dependent on the patient's health status at the time a blood sample is obtained. On the other hand, the A1C level will be falsely lowered by any health condition that shortens red blood cell survival such as acute or chronic blood loss, hemoglobinopathies, hemolytic anemia, thalassemia, spherocytosis, and severe hepatic and renal disease. Among certain ethnic populations such as African-Americans, the A1C level is slightly higher than in White Americans when matched for actual degree of glycemia.

The three different criteria shown in **Table 99-1** are not entirely concordant in diagnosing diabetes. For example, in a sample of adults aged 70 to 79 years without known diabetes, 36% of them met the criteria for diabetes using both A1C and FPG test; another 36% met the criteria using A1C only and 28% using FPG only. When comparing FPG, OGTT, and A1C tests to diagnose diabetes, A1C identified the fewest individuals as having diabetes. Such studies suggest that A1C, FPG, and OGTT measure different aspects of glycemia. Furthermore, the discordance among these tests is particularly significant in older adults. At this time, unless there are clear clinical hyperglycemic symptoms, the ADA recommends verifying with two diagnostic tests for confirmation (eg, both FPG > 125 mg/dL and A1C ≥ 6.5%). If a patient has discordant results on two different tests, then the test with the result higher than the diagnostic threshold should be repeated to confirm the diagnosis. For example, if FPG is less than 126 mg/dL (7 mmol/L) but A1C is greater than or equal to 6.5%, then A1C should be repeated, and if the repeat A1C is greater than or equal to 6.5%, then the person would be considered to have diabetes.

The ADA criteria shown in **Table 99-1** also define prediabetes, an earlier stage in the development of diabetes. People with prediabetes do not meet the criteria for diabetes, but have glucose levels that are higher than normal. These people are at increased risk for developing diabetes and cardiovascular disease (CVD). People with prediabetes include those with impaired glucose tolerance (IGT), impaired fasting glucose (IFG), or an A1C range of 5.7%

TABLE 99-3 ■ CRITERIA FOR ANNUAL SCREENING FOR DIABETES OR PREDIABETES IN HIGH-RISK OLDER ADULTS

- Presence of overweight or obesity (BMI ≥ 25 kg/m²)
- First-degree relative with diabetes
- High-risk race/ethnicity (eg, African American, Latino, American Indian, Asian, Pacific Islander)
- History of CVD
- Hypertension (≥140/90 mm Hg or on therapy for hypertension)
- HDL cholesterol level < 35 mg/dL (0.90 mmol/L) and/or a triglyceride level > 250 mg/dL (2.82 mmol/L)
- Women with polycystic ovary syndrome or history of GDM
- Physical inactivity
- Other clinical conditions associated with insulin resistance (eg, glucocorticoid therapy, acanthosis nigricans)
- Prior diagnosis of prediabetes
- HIV on antiretroviral therapies

CVD, cardiovascular disease; GDM, gestational diabetes mellitus; IFG, impaired fasting glucose; IGT, impaired glucose tolerance.
Data from American Diabetes Association. 2. Classification and Diagnosis of Diabetes: Standards of Medical Care in Diabetes-2021. Diabetes Care. 2021;44(Suppl 1):S15–S33.

to 6.4%. IGT is based on results of an OGTT, and IFG is defined from FPGs. The IFG category allows easy identification of some, but not nearly all, of the older individuals who would meet criteria for IGT if an OGTT were performed. There is no recommended age adjustment for the criteria for either IGT or IFG, as these criteria predict risk for subsequent diabetes and CVD similarly in older people.

Diagnostic Testing for Older Adults

The ADA 2021 Standards of Medical Care in Diabetes and the 2019 Endocrine Society Guideline on Treatment of Diabetes in Older Adults (both evidence-based) recommend screening all individuals older than age 65 with FPG and/or A1C level to detect prediabetes or diabetes. The Endocrine Society Guideline further suggests obtaining a 2-hour glucose post–OGTT measurement in older people with prediabetes values to identify those who meet diabetes criteria (ie, IPH), especially in high-risk populations. The rationale for such screening includes the high rate of undetected diabetes mellitus in population studies and the strong evidence that early intervention delays the progression to diabetes in people with prediabetes, including those older than 60. The ADA standards and the Endocrine Society Guideline recommend follow-up screening every 2 to 3 years based on the patient's situation. However, yearly follow-up testing of people at high risk should be considered (see **Table 99-3** for high risk factors), especially those who meet criteria for prediabetes.

EPIDEMIOLOGY

Type 2 diabetes is a growing worldwide problem, becoming the 10th leading cause of death globally in 2017. Although the death rate (deaths/100,000 persons) fell slightly in North America and most of Europe between 2007 and

2017, it has increased steadily in Asia, India, Mexico, and northern Africa. Both the prevalence of diabetes and the rate of new cases of diabetes are projected to increase in the next three decades. These projected increases are attributable to aging of the world's population, increasing numbers of higher-risk ethnic groups, and people with diabetes living longer due to falling rates of cardiovascular deaths.

Diabetes was the seventh leading cause of death in the United States in 2019 based on death certificate records. In fact, diabetes may be underreported as a cause of death. Only 35% to 40% of people who died with diabetes had it listed anywhere on the death certificate, and only 10% to 15% had it listed as the underlying cause of death. Overall, risk for death among those with diabetes is about twice that of people with similar age but without diabetes. Over 70% of diabetes attributed deaths occurred among people age 70 and older.

Figure 99-1 describes the prevalence of diabetes (diagnosed and undiagnosed) by age groups in the United States in 2013 to 2016, along with the prevalence of people with prediabetes (https://www.cdc.gov/diabetes/pdfs/data/statistics/national-diabetes-statistics-report.pdf, accessed 5/31/2021). Among people aged 65 or older in the United States, the total prevalence of diabetes is about 27% and the prevalence of prediabetes is nearly 50%, both higher than younger age groups. About 20% of people meeting criteria for diabetes are undiagnosed. The incidence rate of newly diagnosed diabetes is the highest among those aged 45 to 64 and 65 to 79, estimated at 10 new cases/1000 people and 9 new cases/1000 people in 2017 to 2018, respectively.

Older adults with diabetes mellitus are susceptible to all the usual complications of diabetes. Rates of end-stage renal disease (ESRD), loss of vision, myocardial infarction, stroke, peripheral vascular disease (PVD), and peripheral neuropathy all increase with age in the absence of diabetes, and their incidence and co-occurrence are all exaggerated by the

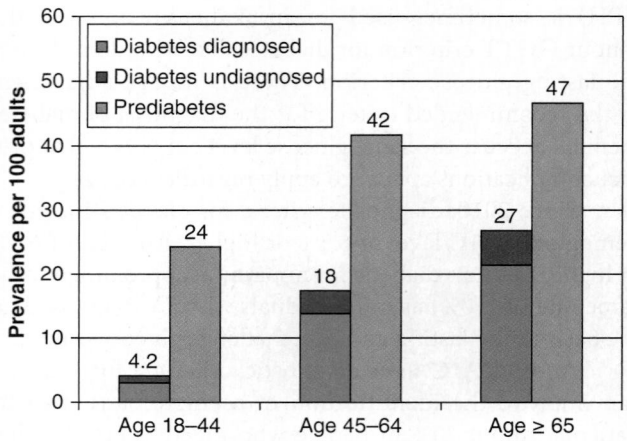

FIGURE 99-1. Diabetes (diagnosed and undiagnosed) and prediabetes prevalence in the United States in adults aged 18 or older, 2013–2016. (Diabetes defined by A1C, fasting blood glucose, or 2-h OGTT; Data from National Diabetes Statistics Report 2020. Estimates of Diabetes and Its Burden in the United States. US Department of Health and Human Services. Centers for Disease Control and Prevention.)

presence of diabetes in older adults, as shown in **Figure 99-2**. Patients with diabetes are at very high risk for CVD, and this risk increases dramatically with age. In 2011, the percentage of US adults with diabetes reporting heart disease or stroke was 28% among those aged 35 to 64, 43% among those aged 65 to 74, and 55% among those aged 75 or older.

Diabetic kidney disease (DKD) is the leading cause of chronic kidney disease (CKD) in the United States. Identification of DKD involves assessment of kidney function, usually with an estimated glomerular filtration rate (eGFR) less than 60 mL/min/1.73 m^2, and kidney damage, usually by estimation of albuminuria greater than 30 mg/g creatinine. Approximately 50% of individuals with diabetes older than age 65 have DKD, manifested as albuminuria, impaired GFR, or both (**Figure 99-3**). **Figure 99-3** also shows that the

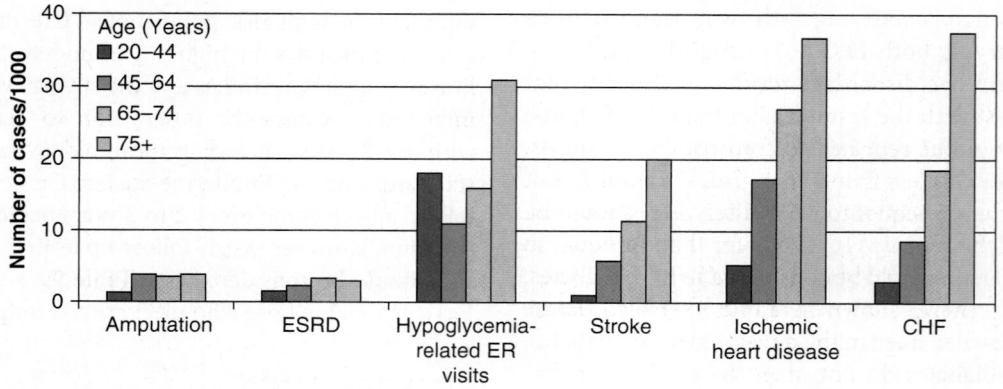

FIGURE 99-2. Incidence (per 1000) of major diabetes complications among adults with diabetes, by age, 2009. CHF, congestive heart failure; ER, emergency room; ESRD, end-stage renal disease. (Data from National Diabetes Statistics Report 2020. Estimates of Diabetes and Its Burden in the United States. US Department of Health and Human Services. Centers for Disease Control and Prevention.)

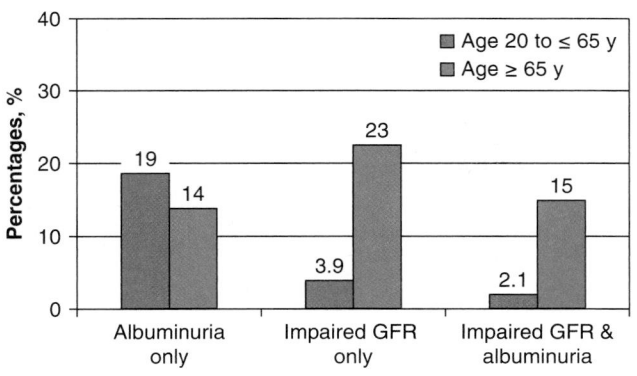

FIGURE 99-3. Prevalence of diabetic kidney disease in the United States, 2005–2008. GFR, glomerular filtration rate. (Data from de Boer IH, Rue TC, Hall YN, et al. Temporal trends in the prevalence of diabetic kidney disease in the United States. *JAMA*. 2011;305[24]:2532–2539.)

prevalence of combined albuminuria and impaired GFR is much higher in older people. This is especially important as combined albuminuria and impaired GFR is a strong predictor of future risk of CVD in this population. DKD accounts for nearly half of all incident cases of ESRD in the United States, and the rate is highest among those aged 75 or older. Five-year survival for patients with ESRD is less than 40%; therefore, prevention of DKD is important to improve health outcomes of older persons with diabetes.

Diabetic retinopathy may be the most common microvascular complication of diabetes. It is responsible for approximately 10,000 new cases of blindness every year in the United States alone. Retinopathy may begin to develop as early as 7 years before the diagnosis of diabetes in patients with type 2 diabetes.

Diabetic neuropathy is usually defined by the presence of symptoms and/or signs of peripheral nerve dysfunction in people with diabetes after the exclusion of other causes. Diabetic neuropathy is highly correlated with the duration of diabetes, and it is estimated that approximately 50% of patients with diabetes will eventually develop neuropathy. Clinical and subclinical neuropathies have been estimated to occur in 10% to 100% of diabetic patients, depending on the diagnostic criteria and patient populations examined.

In an older adult population, the presence of hyperglycemia and diabetes mellitus should be viewed as a risk factor for these complications, analogous to hypertension or hypercholesterolemia. The level of increased relative risk may appear modest on an individual level. However, since older people have by far the highest rates of these conditions, the increase in absolute risk is substantial. Thus a twofold relative risk increase as occurs for myocardial infarction, stroke, and ESRD, represents a very large number of added adverse outcomes in an older adult diabetes population. The risk for lower-extremity amputation is dramatically increased in older people with diabetes mellitus, approximately 10-fold greater than that for older people without diabetes.

As a result of the growing number of older people with diabetes and their high risk for diabetes complications, diabetes is costly for the US health care system. Over $300 billion were spent on patients with diabetes in the United States in 2017, and the majority of these costs were for older adults with long-standing diabetes and severe complications. On average, people with diagnosed diabetes have medical expenditures approximately 2.3 times higher than those without diabetes: approximately $1 in $5 health care dollars is spent caring for someone with diagnosed diabetes and approximately $1 in $10 health care dollars is attributed to diabetes. The annual attributed health care cost per person with diabetes increases with age, primarily as a result of increased use of hospital inpatient and nursing facility resources, physician office visits, and prescription medications. For example, 63% of the inpatient hospital costs for diabetes are attributed to utilization by adults aged 65 or older compared to 30% and 6% by adults aged 45 to 64 and younger than 45, respectively.

PATHOPHYSIOLOGY

Although the rate of new onset of type 1 diabetes is relatively low in older people, the mechanism for type 1 diabetes does not appear to be different in this population. Usually, patients with type 1 diabetes have markers of immune destruction of pancreatic β-cells such as islet cell antibodies, antibodies to insulin, or other pancreatic β-cell–specific antibodies. There are also strong human leukocyte antigen associations.

Type 2 diabetes is by far the most prevalent form in older adults. Autoimmune destruction of pancreatic β-cells is rarely observed. Limited pathologic investigation suggests that total β-cell mass may be moderately reduced, but severe loss of β-cell mass is uncommon. The pathophysiology of type 2 diabetes is unknown, but it appears to occur as a result of a complex interaction among genetic, lifestyle, and aging influences, as illustrated in **Figure 99-4**. The heterogeneity of type 2 diabetes likely reflects the varying contributions of each of multiple factors to the development of hyperglycemia in a given individual or family.

Effects of Aging

Many studies have demonstrated age-related glucose intolerance in humans. In normal people who do not meet criteria for either diabetes mellitus or IGT, there is a slight age-related increase in FPGs and a more dramatic slowing of return to normal of glucose levels following an oral glucose challenge.

Insulin Resistance

There is a decline in sensitivity to the metabolic effects of insulin with age. An age-related impairment of intracellular insulin signaling reduces insulin-mediated mobilization of glucose transporters, which are critical to glucose uptake and metabolism in insulin-dependent tissues such as muscle and fat. There is currently little evidence for an age-related impairment of insulin effects on protein or fat metabolism.

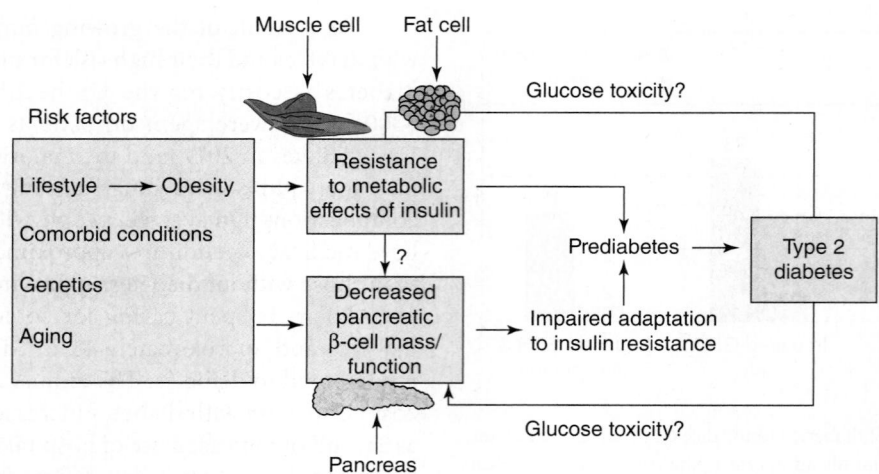

FIGURE 99-4. Model for age-related hyperglycemia. Biological changes associated with risk factors give rise to alterations in both insulin secretion and insulin sensitivity.

An absolute or relative increase of body adiposity, particularly central body adiposity, has been well-documented with advancing age and appears to account in large part for the age-related increase in insulin resistance. Decreased physical activity (PA) is associated with insulin resistance, and exercise training can improve insulin sensitivity. Thus, diminished PA in an older individual can also contribute to decreased insulin sensitivity. Both in animal studies and in humans, it has been difficult to demonstrate a residual effect of aging on insulin action when the changes in body composition and PA are controlled for.

Impaired Insulin Secretion

The progression from normal glucose tolerance to prediabetes and type 2 diabetes in aging is characterized by progressive defects in pancreatic β-cell function. Animal studies have demonstrated an age-related decline in β-cell function. However, there has been great variability in previous studies examining insulin secretion in older people. These human studies, however, may have failed to address adequately the importance of the normal adaptive response to insulin resistance. As most older individuals demonstrate insulin resistance, a compensatory increase of insulin secretion, leading to increased circulating insulin levels, would be expected. However, both basal and stimulated insulin levels in older adults are similar to those of insulin-sensitive young people, suggesting an inadequate adaptive response to insulin resistance in older subjects. Furthermore, when older and younger people are carefully matched for degree of insulin sensitivity, absolute impairments in β-cell function are evident with normal human aging, as shown in **Figure 99-5**. Such defects are even greater in older people with prediabetes. Thus, impaired pancreatic β-cell adaptation to insulin resistance is an important contributing factor to age-related glucose intolerance and risk for diabetes.

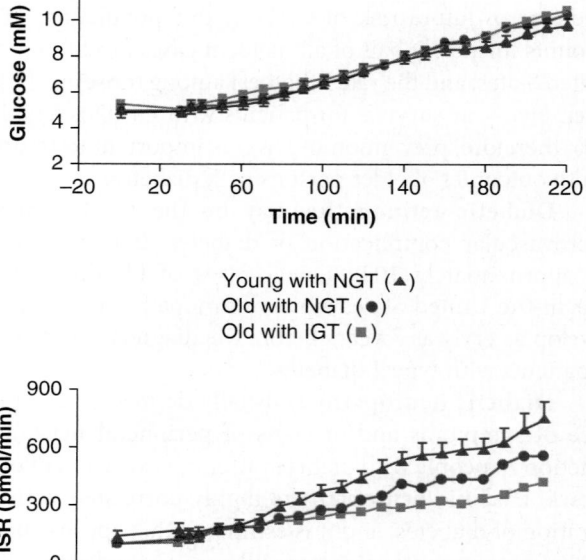

FIGURE 99-5. Effect of age on insulin secretion rate (ISR) in humans with normal glucose tolerance (NGT) or impaired glucose tolerance (IGT) by American Diabetes Association criteria. Plasma glucose concentrations and ISR are shown over time during intravenous glucose infusions, comparing young with NGT ($n = 15$, mean age = 26), old with NGT ($n = 16$, mean age = 70), and old with IGT ($n = 14$, mean age = 70). Glucose levels during variable rate glucose infusion begun at time 0 were well matched in the three study groups, and degree of insulin resistance was also similar in the three study groups. ISR was significantly and progressively decreased in the two older groups, with the greatest impairment in old IGT ($p = 0.0002$, old IGT vs young and old IGT vs old NGT; and old NGT vs young NGT). Data are means ± SE. (Adapted with permission from Chang AM, Smith MJ, Galecki AT, et al. Impaired beta-cell function in human aging: response to nicotinic acid-induced insulin resistance. *J Clin Endocrinol Metab.* 2006;91[9]:3303–3309.)

Interaction Between Impaired Insulin Secretion and Insulin Resistance

As summarized in **Figure 99-4**, in the setting of impaired β-cell function, there is a maladaptive response leading to impaired insulin secretion and progression to prediabetes and type 2 diabetes. Hyperglycemia, in turn, is known to contribute directly to insulin resistance and to impair pancreatic β-cell function, thereby setting up a vicious cycle of maladaptive mechanisms.

Coexisting illness is another factor affecting both insulin sensitivity and insulin secretion in an older person. Both hypertension and hyperlipidemia are common in older people and have been associated with diminished insulin sensitivity. In fact, a metabolic syndrome has been described that includes coexisting hypertension, hyperlipidemia, central obesity, and glucose intolerance. Some have proposed that insulin resistance is a unifying feature linking the components of this metabolic syndrome; however, there is uncertainty about whether the insulin resistance in these circumstances is primary or a secondary result of these other conditions. Furthermore, any acute illness can precipitate hyperglycemia because of effects of stress hormones to cause insulin resistance combined with the α-adrenergic effects of catecholamines released during stressful illness to inhibit insulin secretion. Drugs that may be used by older people may also contribute to hyperglycemia by causing insulin resistance (see **Table 99-2**).

A pathogenetic sequence common to many syndromes in old age can be readily illustrated by diabetes in an older patient: asymptomatic hyperglycemia over time becomes symptomatic, leading to acute complications and such syndromes as hyperosmotic nonketotic coma or, with time, to microvascular or macrovascular complications such as renal disease, stroke, or myocardial infarction. These events may in turn lead to superimposed drug treatment–induced aggravation of impaired glucose regulation and to decreased PA, progressive disability, and functional decline: that is, a downward spiral of mutually reinforcing conditions perhaps triggered by an event such as influenza or a fall that would be readily withstood by a younger person, especially a younger person without diabetes.

Genetics

There is a strong genetic predisposition to type 2 diabetes mellitus. For example, the concordance rate for type 2 diabetes in identical twins is 75% or higher. However, the genetic susceptibility to type 2 diabetes is polygenic, involving a number of variants, where each allele has a modest effect on the risk of disease in an individual person. Genome-wide association studies, linkage analysis, a candidate gene approach, and large-scale association studies have already identified approximately 70 loci conferring susceptibility to type 2 diabetes. These genetic alleles appear to affect the risk of type 2 diabetes primarily through impaired pancreatic β-cell function, reduced insulin action, or obesity risk.

A goal of genetic testing would be to improve clinical prediction of an individual's risk for developing diabetes, but this goal remains elusive.

Mechanisms for Diabetes Complications

Chronic exposure to hyperglycemia may contribute directly to the development of diabetes complications in a number of ways. One mechanism may be the interaction of glucose with proteins to cause protein glycosylation and subsequent formation of advanced glycosylation end (AGE) products. The AGE products can accumulate in proteins of slow turnover such as collagen, potentially leading to tissue damage and injury. Tissue exposure to high concentrations of glucose can also lead to accumulation of metabolic products of the aldose reductase system including nonmetabolized molecules such as sorbitol. Such accumulation can potentially affect cellular energy metabolism and contribute to cell injury and death. Given the complexity of the genetic background contributing to type 2 diabetes, the possibility also exists that some of the genetic background of an individual may directly contribute to the risk for one or more long-term complications of diabetes (eg, nephropathy) independent of the effects of hyperglycemia. However, such a possibility remains speculative. Interactions between diabetes and other comorbidities may contribute to the manifestation and severity of diabetes-related complications. Diabetic patients who also have hypertension are at greater risk for renal disease, retinopathy, and macrovascular disease than diabetic patients without hypertension. Similarly, neuropathy is more likely in a diabetic patient who is exposed to a neurotoxic agent. Growth factors, including vascular endothelial growth factor, growth hormone, and transforming growth factor β, have been postulated to play important roles in the development of diabetic retinopathy.

PREVENTION

Type 2 diabetes is a gradually progressive disorder of carbohydrate metabolism that develops over a long period of time. It has been estimated that abnormalities of glucose regulation can be detected 8 to 10 years before the clinical diagnosis of type 2 diabetes is made. Older adults have a high rate of prediabetes and other risks for progressing to type 2 diabetes in the next few years (eg, see **Table 99-3**).

Effective means to delay progression to type 2 diabetes in high-risk people, such as those with prediabetes, have been identified. Intensive lifestyle interventions, which include weight loss and increased PA, can substantially reduce the rate of progression to type 2 diabetes in such high-risk people. Lifestyle intervention appears to be especially beneficial in prevention of progression to diabetes among older adults. For example, in the multicenter Diabetes Prevention Program (DPP) in the United States, a lifestyle intervention program including both caloric restriction and exercise was remarkably effective in reducing the rate of progression to type 2 diabetes, even though only 5% to 7% weight reduction was achieved. During the

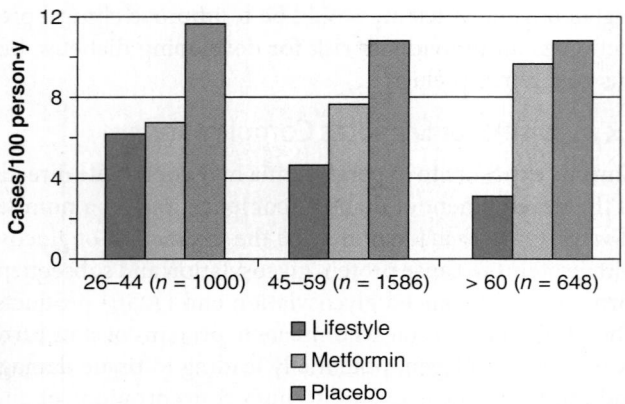

FIGURE 99-6. Diabetes incidence rates by age, Diabetes Prevention Program. (Reproduced with permission from Diabetes Prevention Program Research Group, Crandall J, Schade D, et al. The influence of age on the effects of lifestyle modification and metformin in prevention of diabetes. *J Gerontol A Biol Sci Med Sci.* 2006;61[10]:1075–1081.)

3 years of active treatment in DPP, the lifestyle intervention program was more effective in people older than age 60 than in younger people, reducing progression to diabetes by more than 70% as compared to a control group, as shown in **Figure 99-6**. Metformin was also used in the DPP and was effective in slowing progression in younger adults, but had somewhat less effect in people older than age 60.

The benefit of lifestyle intervention appears to be long term among older adults, as they had reduced frequency of developing type 2 diabetes during 15 years of follow-up after the original lifestyle intervention, associated with maintenance of over 5% weight loss by nearly half of lifestyle intervention participants. Overall, onset of diabetes was delayed by about 4 years by lifestyle intervention compared with placebo. Given the benefits observed in the DPP and other similar studies, both the ADA 2021 Standards of Medical Care in Diabetes and the 2019 Endocrine Society Guideline recommend a lifestyle program similar to the DPP to delay progression to diabetes in patients aged 65 years and older who have prediabetes. Since 2018, a DPP-like lifestyle intervention is a covered benefit for Medicare beneficiaries in the United States who meet the criteria for prediabetes.

PRESENTATION

The finding of an elevated glucose level on routine laboratory testing is the most common presentation for type 2 diabetes in an older person. The classical clinical hallmarks of diabetes are symptoms associated with marked hyperglycemia, including polydipsia, polyuria, polyphagia, and weight loss. Older patients with type 2 diabetes may present with such symptoms, although it is relatively uncommon for them to do so, and the rate of emergency department visits by older adults for severe hyperglycemia have been declining. Some older patients may have sufficient hyperglycemia to cause mild classical symptoms, while others may have had gradual unexplained weight loss. Other older patients may present with atypical symptoms from hyperglycemia such as falls, urinary incontinence, fatigue, or confusion. Because type 2 diabetes may go undetected for years, some older adults first present with symptoms or findings related to diabetes complications, such as visual loss with classic retinopathy on examination, proteinuria, or symptomatic peripheral neuropathy.

With the profound insulin deficiency of type 1 diabetes, mobilization of fatty acids occurs leading to accelerated production of ketoacids, potentially resulting in life-threatening DKA. Although type 1 diabetes usually occurs in early life, it can occur at any age, including first presentation in an older patient. Development of DKA is the classic form of presentation for a patient with type 1 diabetes, but it is now recognized that people with type 1 diabetes may have long periods of abnormal circulating glucose levels before the development of DKA. Furthermore, with early detection of such hyperglycemia and appropriate diabetes management, an episode of DKA might never occur. An older person with type 1 diabetes may be particularly more likely to present with an indolent course.

EVALUATION

Diabetes mellitus is a complex disorder that can have effects on many body systems, and its treatment requires a complex program including lifestyle changes (eg, increase PA, healthy diet) and medications. The choice of intervention strategies and the patient's capability to adhere to a treatment program may be limited by the presence of other health problems such as cognitive impairment, as well as by the patient's living environment, economic status, availability of caregiver support, and the like. A comprehensive geriatric assessment (Chapter 8) is highly appropriate to provide the basis for developing a treatment plan for an older person with diabetes mellitus. Both the ADA and Endocrine Society Guidelines recommend assessing the overall health and personal values of older patients with diabetes, including multiple domains of health status and screening for geriatric syndromes, consistent with a Medicare annual wellness exam, as summarized in **Table 99-4**.

Medical Evaluation

Once a diagnosis of diabetes is established, a thorough medical evaluation is needed. Because the risk for developing diabetes complications is related to the duration of hyperglycemia, effort should be made to pinpoint the time of onset. Unless patients at risk have been followed up carefully with yearly measurement of an FPG, as currently recommended, it may be difficult to establish a time of onset for type 2 diabetes in a given patient. Given the uncertainty about time of onset, a careful search for

TABLE 99-4 ■ EVALUATION OF OLDER PATIENTS WITH DIABETES

GENERAL HEALTH ASSESSMENT[a]	GENERAL HEALTH TESTS[b]	DIABETES-SPECIFIC HEALTH[c]
Functional status (ADLs/IADLs[d])	ECG	Retinopathy (dilated retinal examination)
Depression	Lipid panel	Nephropathy (urine albumin, eGFR)
Cognition	Bone mineral density	Neuropathy (micro-filament test and tuning fork)
Fall risk	AAA ultrasound	
Weight (kg)/ height (m)² = BMI		
Blood pressure		Medical nutrition therapy
Tobacco use		Diabetes management
Alcohol use		
Medication review		Diabetes self-management training
Cancer screening		
Hearing		
Comorbid conditions		
Visual acuity		
Frailty/physical performance		

Abbreviations: AAA, abdominal aortic aneurysm; ADL, activity of daily living; BMI, body mass index; IADL, instrumental activity of daily living.

[a]All items are required services to qualify for Medicare coverage of annual wellness examinations for people in the United States > 65 y, except for frailty/physical performance. These are generally conducted by primary care providers.

[b]All items are services covered by Medicare for people in the United States > 65 y as part of annual wellness examinations at intervals varying from annually to once per lifetime.

[c]All items are services covered by Medicare for people in the United States > 65 y as part of standard diabetes care. These are covered annually except for diabetes management visits, which are covered as recommended by the diabetes care team.

[d]Functional status is based on assessment of independence or dependency (having difficulty and receiving assistance) of five ADLs (bathing, dressing, eating, toileting, and transferring) and five IADLs (preparing meals, shopping, managing money, using the telephone, and managing medications).

Reproduced with permission from LeRoith D, Biessels GJ, Braithwaite SS, et al. Treatment of diabetes in older adults: an Endocrine Society® clinical practice guideline. J Clin Endocrinol Metab. 2019;104(5):1520–1574.

existing diabetes complications is warranted even when a new diagnosis is made in an older adult. Such an evaluation is even more justified in a patient with a multiyear history of diabetes mellitus who is establishing a new relationship with a health care system or primary care provider. The evaluation for **eye complications of diabetes** should be carried out by an ophthalmologist with a detailed retinal examination, as early signs of diabetic retinopathy can easily be missed.

Evaluation of **DKD** should include a screening urine albumin and serum creatinine level, which should be followed at least annually. An elevated serum creatinine is a poor prognostic sign, suggesting that substantial kidney damage has already occurred and that an irreversible course of progressive renal insufficiency has already started. Albuminuria is a marker for kidney/glomerular disease as well as for CVD risk and is often the first clinical indicator of the

presence of DKD. It is a clinically useful tool for predicting prognosis and for monitoring response to therapy. To confirm a diagnosis of increased albuminuria, it should be measured more than once and two of three samples should be elevated over a 3- to 6-month period. The relationship of albuminuria to ESRD and CVD risk is a continuum, starting from "normal" levels less than 30 mg/g creatinine. Therefore, there is a trend to no longer refer to categorical nomenclature of "microalbuminuria" (30–300 mg/g creatinine) and "macroalbuminuria" (> 300 mg/g creatinine). Depending on the patient's overall situation, referral to a nephrologist may be warranted to assess other potential causes of renal insufficiency.

A careful neurologic examination should be carried out for signs of **diabetic neuropathy**. The 2021 ADA Guideline recommends that patients should be assessed for diabetic peripheral neuropathy starting at diagnosis of type 2 diabetes and at least annually thereafter. Assessment for distal symmetric polyneuropathy should include a careful history and assessment of either temperature or pinprick sensation (small fiber function) and vibration sensation using a 128-Hz tuning fork (for large-fiber function). Annual 10-g monofilament testing should be done to identify feet at risk for ulceration and amputation. The neuropathy evaluation should be carried out in conjunction with a careful foot examination to identify possible structural abnormalities that might contribute to risk for skin breakdown and damage.

The medical evaluation of an older patient with diabetes should also include information about other **coexisting risk factors** including hypertension, hyperlipidemia, and use of cigarettes. These conditions interact with diabetes to increase CVD risk and therefore need to be addressed in an overall patient management program. Blood pressure should be assessed both in the supine position and with upright posture, as an orthostatic drop in blood pressure may be another marker of diabetic neuropathy and is often associated with supine hypertension. The genitourinary system should also be assessed, as patients with diabetes may be prone to bladder dysfunction associated with autonomic neuropathy, thereby increasing the risk for urinary tract infection and kidney damage. Sexual dysfunction has been reported in a high percentage of older men with diabetes, suggesting an interaction between aging, neuropathy, and vascular disease in this population.

A thorough evaluation of **the cardiovascular system** also should be carried out, given the high rate of CVD in older people with diabetes mellitus. The history and physical examination should carefully assess evidence for CVD, coronary heart disease (CHD), and PVD. Suggestive history or physical findings should be documented with more in-depth testing including Doppler evaluation for carotid artery stenosis or extremity blood flow, or cardiovascular stress testing if there is any suggestion of coronary artery disease. Silent ischemia and myocardial infarction appear to be more common in people with diabetes mellitus. Thus, the threshold for stress testing should be rather low.

The **pharmacological history** of an older patient with diabetes is important both to identify drug therapy that may be contributing to the patient's hyperglycemia (see **Table 99-2**), as well as to identify potential drug interactions that may affect diabetes management. The initial assessment should also include a diet history, a review of potential nutritional problems, and an oral health assessment, as dietary intervention is a key component of a treatment program for virtually all patients with diabetes. The assistance of a nutritionist who has a particular interest in diabetes is often very helpful for this part of the evaluation. Particular attention should be paid to dietary habits, ethnic food preferences, and meal patterns.

Other Evaluation Components

Diabetes knowledge Because of the complexity of diabetes management, usually requiring both lifestyle and medication interventions, the patient and/or caregivers must be actively involved in their own care and take responsibility for its many aspects. It is particularly important to review the patient's knowledge base regarding diabetes and its complications. Standardized diabetes knowledge tests are available, or an interview with a diabetes educator or suitably trained nurse can establish the status of the patient's knowledge base. The diabetes education program that becomes part of the treatment plan can then provide this base for new patients or fill in needed gaps for existing patients.

Cognitive function Since diabetes and aging are each independently associated with increased risk of cognitive impairment, older adults with diabetes are especially at high risk. Dementia, including both Alzheimer type and vascular type, is approximately twice as likely to occur in those with diabetes compared with age-matched nondiabetic people. Subtler impairments of cognition such as mild cognitive impairment (MCI) are also common. Cognitive impairment is associated with poorer glycemic control in clinical trials, and study participants with cognitive impairment had a higher risk for severe hypoglycemia. Hypoglycemia is also associated with higher risk for dementia. Therefore, both the ADA and Endocrine Society Guidelines recommend that older patients with diabetes should have periodic screening for cognitive impairment: at the time of diagnosis, then annually for those with borderline results initially or every 2 to 3 years when initial screening is normal. A positive screening test should be followed up by an appropriate diagnostic evaluation for dementia or MCI.

While advanced dementia may be identified in a routine clinical encounter, moderate cognitive impairment or MCI may be missed. Formal neuropsychological testing demonstrates that patients with diabetes frequently have unrecognized deficits in psychomotor efficiency, global cognition, and memory. They also frequently have abnormalities in cognitive function mediated by frontal lobes (executive function), which can affect their ability to perform complex behaviors such as attention, planning, organization, insight, reasoning, and problem solving. Such complex cognitive functions are necessary for diabetic patients to manage the complex treatment regimens for their disease. Early identification of cognitive impairment will help patients, their families, and health providers to individualize diabetes care regimens to set achievable diabetes goals without causing harm to the patients.

Functional status Both aging and diabetes are risk factors for functional impairment, and people with diabetes have more functional impairment than those without diabetes. Both the ADA and Endocrine Society Guidelines recommend that review of activities of daily living and instrumental activities of daily living should be a part of the comprehensive assessment of an older patient with diabetes mellitus (**Table 99-4**). The presence of functional limitations must be considered in developing a diabetes treatment program, as described below. In addition to general assessment of functional status, the ability of the patient and caregiver to carry out diabetes-specific functional tasks needs to be evaluated. For example, the ability to carry out home glucose monitoring or self-injection of insulin requires certain functional abilities.

Overall health status The presence of other medical problems needs to be documented, as decisions about the extent of intervention for diabetes should be made in the context of the patient's overall health situation, disease burden, and prognosis in terms of functional status and estimated longevity. The presence of psychiatric disorders such as depression or bipolar disorder could have a major impact on the decision about diabetes treatment interventions. The relationship between depression and diabetes appears to be bidirectional. Depression is associated with increased risk of type 2 diabetes (up to 60% higher per one meta-analysis). Individuals with diabetes have twice the rate of depression as those without diabetes, and older patients have higher mortality risk if they have both diabetes and depression. Other coexisting illnesses such as congestive heart failure or uncontrolled cancer may substantially limit a patient's life expectancy, and thus may influence the decision about intensity of diabetes management.

MANAGEMENT

General Approach

The complexity of diabetes and its management requires a collaborative effort by a team of health providers, which may include physicians, nurse practitioners, nurses, dietitians, pharmacists, and mental health professionals. Patients and family members must also assume an active role. There is increasing recognition of the importance of active collaboration between the patient's geriatrics-oriented primary

TABLE 99-5 ■ ROLES OF THE PRIMARY CARE TEAM AND ENDOCRINOLOGIST IN CARE OF OLDER PATIENTS WITH DIABETES

1. In patients aged 65 and older with newly diagnosed diabetes, an endocrinologist should work with the primary care provider, a multidisciplinary team (potentially including a pharmacist, a nurse, a diabetes educator, and a social worker), and the patient in the development of individualized diabetes treatment goals.

2. When feasible, an endocrinologist should be primarily responsible for diabetes care in patients aged 65 and older with diabetes who:
   - Have type 1 diabetes
   - Require complex hyperglycemia treatment to achieve treatment goals
   - Have recurrent severe hypoglycemia
   - Have multiple diabetes complications
   - Require hyperglycemia management during hospitalization

Data from LeRoith D, Biessels GJ, Braithwaite SS, et al. Treatment of diabetes in older adults: an Endocrine Society' clinical practice guideline. J Clin Endocrinol Metab. 2019;104(5):1520–1574.

care team and an endocrinologist who focuses on diabetes care, with the role of each varying depending on the needs of the patient (see **Table 99-5**).

The first key step in developing a diabetes management program for an older patient is to establish the treatment goals. Basic treatment goals for any patient with diabetes are to prevent metabolic decompensation and to control other risk factors that may contribute to long-term complications. Control of hyperglycemia as a means to reduce what some have termed glucose toxicity as a contributing factor to long-term diabetes complications is one part of an overall strategy of risk reduction. Such a strategy must include intensive effort at identifying and controlling hypertension, lipid disorders, and cigarette smoking among other risk factors (see section below on CVD risk reduction). Thus, a complex, multifaceted treatment program is important for many older patients with diabetes. As other chapters cover the management of hypertension (Chapter 79) and lipid disorders (Chapter 74), these will be referred to only briefly in this chapter. This chapter will focus on management of hyperglycemia. However, control of the traditional CVD risk factors is absolutely critical to successful diabetes management. Unfortunately, many studies have documented the overall lack of success of standard clinical practice in achieving these goals.

Any decision about the level of intensity for a treatment program must take into account coexisting conditions and the overall complexity of the patient's medical regimen. For example, the existence of advanced diabetes complications in an older patient may provide a rationale for less strict goals for hyperglycemia or dyslipidemia. A significant psychiatric or cognitive disorder may also preclude an intensive management program. The target for hyperglycemia control might need to be higher for a patient at risk for

severe hypoglycemia (see the section on "Hypoglycemia" later in this chapter). On the other hand, some older adults are able to devote a substantial amount of time to their own health care and are able to manage complex multidrug interventions for multiple health problems. Based on the initial comprehensive patient assessment as described here, many older adults with diabetes may fit in a category for which intensive treatment goals are appropriate.

It may be neither feasible nor appropriate to attempt to implement a complex diabetes management program for some patients. It is true that a limited remaining life expectancy shortens the time for long-term complications to develop and progress. However, given the increasing life expectancy of older adults, only the very oldest segment of the population or those with coexisting illness that markedly shortens remaining life expectancy should be excluded from consideration for an aggressive treatment program. For example, it would be hard to justify abandoning risk reduction goals in an otherwise healthy 75-year-old woman with a recent diagnosis of type 2 diabetes, as such a person's remaining life expectancy may be 15 years or more. Given the potential complexity of treatment programs designed to minimize diabetes risks, the commitment on the part of an adequately informed patient is clearly critical. Availability of a supportive environment including a strong diabetes treatment team and adequate economic support for an intensive treatment program are also important. Such a treatment goal is also difficult to achieve without commitment of the health care team, which must believe that achievement of the treatment goal will really make a difference in the patient's long-term health.

Information about a diabetic patient's cognitive status, socioeconomic and living situation can also help guide the care plan for an older adult. Limitations in cognition and economic support may affect the patient's ability to adhere to the medical regimen. The health provider may need to simplify the diabetes regimen or loosen the glycemic and/or blood pressure targets to minimize risks for hypoglycemia and/or hypotension. The health provider may need to enlist the patient's caregivers to be more involved in the patient's care. The availability of caregivers in the home or nearby can compensate for some limitations in the patient's self-care abilities and influence lifestyle factors that can affect diabetes management. For patients who have moderate or advanced cognitive impairment, support for basic home care will be needed either from family or more formal home care services or both, including the tasks of obtaining daily meals, administering medications and monitoring home glucose levels. Some patients may need to be transitioned from the home setting to assisted living facilities or long-term care facilities to receive necessary care. This decision will be influenced by their financial resources and the support of family members. The availability of a social worker or suitably trained nurse to assist in this aspect of the patient's care program can be extremely helpful.

Several approaches have been proposed by diabetes specialists and geriatricians to better identify older adults who would benefit from more strict diabetes control versus less stringent management. Age alone is not a good marker, as age is a poor predictor of overall disease complexity and mortality risk. In **Figure 99-7**, a group of nationally representative older adults with diabetes were grouped by their comorbidities, physical function status, and cognitive status. While the oldest age group includes many people with very complex/poor health, over 50% of people older than 75 were relatively healthy by these criteria. Thus, a classification based on a patient's comorbidities, physical function status, cognitive status, social support, history of hypoglycemia, etc can provide the basis for individualized goals to optimize the risk and benefit of diabetes treatments for a given patient. **Table 99-6** provides such a framework to guide setting treatment goals for hyperglycemia in older adults with diabetes, published in the 2019 Endocrine Society Guideline (a similar framework is in the ADA 2021 Standards of Care). Based on the patient's comorbidities, cognitive status, and physical function (as determined from the overall patient evaluation per **Table 99-4**), s/he may be categorized into one of the three groups. The Good Health group will likely benefit from more stringent glycemic management. The Intermediate Health group will likely have some difficulty in achieving stricter goals for glycemia. The Poor Health group of very complex patients will likely not benefit greatly from intensive treatment of hyperglycemia so a less aggressive goal is more appropriate.

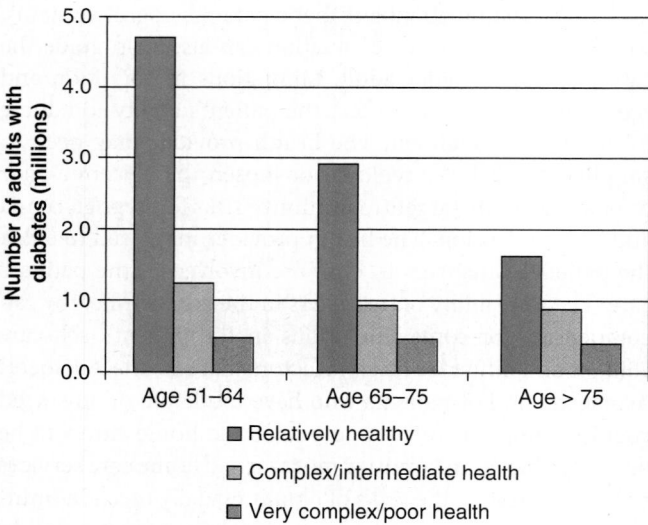

FIGURE 99-7. Health status by age group of people over age 50 in the United States who have diabetes, based on data from the Health and Retirement Study. Definitions of the three health status categories illustrated are as stated in **Table 99-6**. (Data from Blaum C, Cigolle CT, Boyd C, et al. Clinical complexity in middle-aged and older adults with diabetes: the Health and Retirement Study. *Med Care.* 2010;48[4]:327–334.)

Diabetes Education and Support

A key component of diabetes care is to educate the patient and their caregivers about the complications associated with diabetes, how to manage diabetes through lifestyle modification and various medications, how to monitor and treat complications associated with diabetes, and the risks and benefits of various medications that may be prescribed. People with diabetes benefit from receiving diabetes self-management education and support (DSMES) when diabetes is diagnosed and as needed thereafter, such as when not meeting treatment targets. DSMES is an ongoing process of facilitating the knowledge, skills, and ability necessary for diabetes self-care. This process is evidence-based, and can be individualized for each patient, incorporating the needs, goals, and life experiences of the individual. DSMES is associated with improved diabetes knowledge and self-care behavior, improved quality of life, lower A1C, and lower health care costs.

Recognizing the effectiveness and the need for DSMES, the Centers for Medicare and Medicaid Services (CMS) and most insurance provide reimbursement for DSMES when the service meets the national standards and is accredited by either the ADA or the American Association of Diabetes Care and Education Specialists (ADCES). Yet, despite reimbursement, only 5% to 7% of individuals eligible for DSMES through Medicare or a private insurance plan actually receive it. The increased availability in telemedicine and internet-based health care may be an opportunity to reduce the barrier for patients to obtain DSMES.

Cardiovascular Disease Risk Reduction

Some of the risk factors for CVD among diabetic patients include hyperglycemia, dyslipidemia, hypertension, cigarette use, and age-related changes of the cardiovascular system including diminished vascular responsiveness (**Table 99-7**). Additional risk factors include obesity, insulin resistance, autonomic dysfunction, and inflammation. Individuals with diagnosed diabetes are at higher risk for CHD, and CHD risk also is elevated modestly among individuals with prediabetes.

Hyperglycemia Initial interventions targeting hyperglycemia had limited or no benefit on CVD risk reduction for older adults with diabetes. In fact, the ACCORD trial was terminated early due to a higher rate of mortality in the intensively treated glycemic group. However, the results of cardiovascular outcome trials (CVOTs) required by the US FDA since 2008 (and later adopted by the European Medicines Agency) for new glucose lowering drugs have been much more encouraging. The required CVOTs must include higher risk patients including older adults and those with a history of CVD or other diabetes complications. As a result, the average age of study pwarticipants has been over 60. The CVOTs have established the CVD safety of three major newer classes of glucose-lowering drugs: dipeptidyl peptidase-4 (DPP-4) inhibitors, glucagon-like peptide-1 (GLP-1) agonists, and

TABLE 99-6 ■ CONCEPTUAL FRAMEWORK FOR CONSIDERING OVERALL HEALTH AND PATIENT VALUES IN DETERMINING CLINICAL TARGETS IN ADULTS AGED 65 AND OLDER

OVERALL HEALTH CATEGORY		GROUP 1: GOOD HEALTH	GROUP 2: INTERMEDIATE HEALTH	GROUP 3: POOR HEALTH
Patient characteristics		No comorbidities **or** 1–2 non-diabetes chronic illnesses[a] **and** No ADL[e] impairments and ≤1 IADL impairment	3 or more non-diabetes chronic illnesses[a] **and/or** Any one of the following: Mild cognitive impairment or early dementia ≥2 IADL impairments	Any **one** of the following: End-stage medical condition(s)[b] Moderate to severe dementia ≥2 ADL impairments Residence in a long-term nursing facility
		Reasonable glucose target ranges and HbA1C by group — Shared decision-making: individualized goal may be lower or higher		
Use of drugs that may cause hypoglycemia (eg, insulin, sulfonylurea, glinides)	No	Fasting: 90–130 mg/dL Bedtime: 90–150 mg/dL <7.5%	Fasting: 90–150 mg/dL Bedtime: 100–180 mg/dL <8%	Fasting: 100–180 mg/dL Bedtime: 110–200 mg/dL <8.5%[d]
	Yes[c]	Fasting: 90–150 mg/dL Bedtime: 100–180 mg/dL ≥7.0 and <7.5%	Fasting: 100–150 mg/dL Bedtime: 150–180 mg/dL ≥7.5 and <8.0%	Fasting: 100–180 mg/dL Bedtime: 150–250 mg/dL ≥8.0 and <8.5%[d]

Note: While glucose targets are highlighted for each group in this framework, overall health categories can also be considered for other treatment goals, such as blood pressure and dyslipidemia. See Appendix A on "How to use the conceptual framework."

[a]Coexisting chronic illnesses may include osteoarthritis, hypertension, chronic kidney disease stages 1–3, or stroke, among others.

[b]One or more chronic illnesses with limited treatments and reduced life expectancy. These include metastatic cancer, oxygen-dependent lung disease, end-stage kidney disease requiring dialysis, and advanced heart failure.

[c]As long as achievable without clinically significant hypoglycemia; otherwise, higher glucose targets may be appropriate. Note also that the lower HbA1C boundary was included, as data suggesting increased hypoglycemia and mortality risk at lower HbA1C levels are strongest in the setting of insulin use. However, the lower boundary should not reduce vigilance for detailed hypoglycemia assessment.

[d]HbA1C of 8.5% correlates with an average glucose level of approximately 200 mg/dL. Higher targets than this may result in glycosuria, dehydration, hyperglycemic crisis, and poor wound healing.

[e]ADLs include bathing, dressing, eating, toileting, and transferring, and IADLs include preparing meals, shopping, managing money, using the telephone, and managing medications.
Includes data from Cigolle CT, Kabeto MU, Lee PG, Blaum CS. Clinical complexity and mortality in middle-aged and older adults with diabetes. J Gerontol A Biol Sci Med Sci 2012; 67(12); 1313-1320 (39); and from Kirkman MS, Jones Briscoe V, Clark N, et al. Diabetes in older adults. Diabetes Care 2012; 35(12); 2650–2664 (40).

Abbreviations: IADL, instrumental activity of daily living; ADL, activity of daily living; SU, sulfonylurea.
Reproduced with permission from LeRoith D, Biessels GJ, Braithwaite SS, et al. Treatment of diabetes in older adults: an Endocrine Society' clinical practice guideline. J Clin Endocrinol Metab. 2019;104(5):1520–1574.

sodium glucose transporter (SGLT)-2 inhibitors. Furthermore, benefits for important CVD outcomes such as CVD deaths and new events, including subanalyses of the oldest age cohorts, were found in trials of three SGLT-2 inhibitors (empagliflozin, canagliflozin, and dapagliflozin) and three GLP-1 agonists (liraglutide, semaglutide, and dulaglutide) currently in use in the United States. As all of these drugs result in modest weight loss (especially the GLP-1 agonists) and lower BP, the positive CVD outcomes observed cannot be ascribed solely to their glucose-lowering effects.

Dyslipidemia (see Table 99-8) There are no large trials of lipid-lowering interventions specifically in older adults with diabetes. Trials of older adults at risk for CVD that include but are not limited to those with diabetes have shown consistent CVD benefits across the age spectrum. Several trials in adults with diabetes have demonstrated a beneficial effect of statins on lipid profiles and a reduction in CVD events, including subanalyses of the oldest age cohorts. As CVD prevention with statins, especially in

people with prior CVD, is apparent within 1 to 2 years, statins may be indicated for nearly all older adults with diabetes except those with an end-stage disease and very limited life expectancy. For patients aged 75 years or older without atherosclerotic CVD, the benefit of statin therapy is still being studied.

Hypertension (see Table 99-8) Lowering blood pressure from very high levels (eg, systolic blood pressure [SBP] 170 mm Hg) to moderate targets (eg, SBP 150 mm Hg) reduces CVD risk in older adults with diabetes. However, the ACCORD-BP trial showed no benefit on major CVD events of an SBP target less than 120 mm Hg compared with less than 140 mm Hg, but found a significant reduction in stroke. Other studies found no benefit when lowering SBP to less than 140 mm Hg, and low diastolic blood pressure (DBP) (eg, < 70 mm Hg) may actually be a risk factor for mortality in older adults. These findings contrast with those of SPRINT and other studies in older people without diabetes indicating added CVD protection with

TABLE 99-7 ■ CARDIOVASCULAR DISEASE RISK FACTORS AMONG OLDER ADULTS WITH DIABETES, IN ADDITION TO FASTING PLASMA GLUCOSE LEVEL

Elevated systolic blood pressure

Cigarette use

Obesity

Elevated total cholesterol

High non-HDL cholesterol

Long duration of diabetes

Elevated 2-h plasma glucose concentration during an oral glucose tolerance test

Age-related changes to the cardiovascular system

 Heart

  Slowing kinetics of diastolic filling

  Left ventricular wall thickening

  Left atrial enlargement

  Augmentation in the atrial contribution to diastolic ventricular filling

  Decreased cardiovascular reserve function

  Increased risk for arrhythmia

  Altered regulation of cardiomyocyte calcium homeostasis

 Arterial system

  Diffuse intimal thickening

  Stiffening of the aorta and carotid arteries

  Endothelial dysfunction

TABLE 99-8 ■ INTERVENTIONS TO REDUCE CARDIOVASCULAR DISEASE RISK IN OLDER ADULTS WITH DIABETES, IN ADDITION TO GLYCEMIC MANAGEMENT

1. Dyslipidemia
   ○ Statin therapy and an annual lipid profile are recommended to achieve levels for reducing absolute CVD events and mortality.
   ○ If statin therapy is inadequate for reaching the LDL-C reduction goal, then alternative or additional drugs (such as ezetimibe or proprotein convertase subtilisin/kexin type 9 inhibitors) should be initiated.
   ○ In patients with fasting triglycerides > 500 mg/dL, the use of fish oil and/or fenofibrate is recommended to reduce the risk of pancreatitis.

2. Hypertension
   ○ A target BP of < 140/90 mm Hg is recommended to decrease the risk of CVD outcomes, stroke, and progressive CKD.
   ○ An angiotensin-converting enzyme inhibitor or an angiotensin receptor blocker is recommended as first-line therapy for hypertension in patients with nephropathy.

3. Use of aspirin
   ○ Low-dosage aspirin (75–162 mg/d) is recommended for secondary prevention of cardiovascular disease after careful assessment of bleeding risk and collaborative decision-making with the patient, family, and other caregivers.

BP, blood pressure, CKD, chronic kidney disease; CVD, cardiovascular disease; LDL-C, low-density lipoprotein cholesterol.

Data from LeRoith D, Biessels GJ, Braithwaite SS, et al. Treatment of diabetes in older adults: an Endocrine Society clinical practice guideline. J Clin Endocrinol Metab. 2019;104(5):1520–1574.*

lower SBP targets (see Chapter 79). Thus, the ideal BP target for older people with diabetes is controversial. However, both the 2021 ADA and 2019 Endocrine Society Guidelines recommend lowering BP to less than 140/90 for most older diabetes patients, with adjustments based on patient preference and overall health status. For example, a higher SBP target may be appropriate for some patients with poor health per **Table 99-6**. Conversely, some high-risk patients (eg, previous stroke or progressing CKD) could be considered for a lower BP target such as 130/80 mm Hg. If a lower BP target is selected, the patient should be carefully monitored to avoid orthostatic hypotension. Both the 2021 ADA and 2019 Endocrine Society Guidelines recommend an angiotensin-converting enzyme (ACE) inhibitor or angiotensin receptor blocker (ARB) as first-line therapy for hypertension in older diabetes patients with evidence of nephropathy.

Aspirin (see Table 99-8) As diabetes and aging both are associated with high CVD risk, and aspirin has well-known benefits for secondary prevention of CVD, aspirin therapy (75–162 mg) is recommended in both the 2021 ADA and 2019 Endocrine Society Guidelines for older adults with diabetes and known CVD. However, aspirin use remains controversial for primary prevention of CVD events in older adults with diabetes, as the benefits of aspirin may not outweigh the risk of adverse events such as bleeding.

Prevention and Treatment of Microvascular Complications

Older adults are particularly overrepresented among those with microvascular complications due to diabetes. The risk of developing microvascular complications is thought to be proportional to the duration and magnitude of exposure to hyperglycemia and hypertension.

Diabetic kidney disease Due to the high prevalence of DKD in older people with diabetes (see Epidemiology section and **Figure 99-3**), both the 2021 ADA and 2019 Endocrine Society Guidelines recommend annual screening with an eGFR and urine albumin-to-creatinine ratio. Assessment of renal function is important both for prevention of progression from early nephropathy to ESRD and for adjusting drug dosages of glucose lowering and other agents used in overall diabetes management. Lowering blood glucose levels reduces the risk of developing albuminuria and other microvascular diabetes complications. There is no evidence that age of the patient limits this beneficial effect of glucose lowering. As ACE inhibitors and ARBs reduce the rate of progression from microalbuminuria to overt proteinuria and diabetic nephropathy, one of them should be added to a treatment program for any patient who has evidence of nephropathy. Also, rigorous blood pressure control is particularly important for such individuals. However, as discussed above, for older adults with diabetes and nephropathy, the optimal blood pressure target remains unclear. CVOTs of two SGLT-2 inhibitors (empagliflozin and canagliflozin) and two GLP-1 agonists (liraglutide and semaglutide) found lower rates of nephropathy, as secondary outcomes; and one large canagliflozin trial focused primarily on nephropathy has reported positive outcomes. Thus, there is growing interest in use of these drugs both for treatment of hyperglycemia and for protection from progression of nephropathy.

Diabetic retinopathy (Figure 99-8) As close surveillance for the existence or progression of retinopathy in patients with diabetes is crucial, both the 2021 ADA and 2019 Endocrine Society guidelines recommend an annual comprehensive eye examination by an ophthalmologist. Retinopathy is generally classified as either nonproliferative or proliferative. Nonproliferative retinopathy is characterized by nerve fiber layer infarcts (cotton wool spots), hard exudates, intraretinal hemorrhages, and microvascular abnormalities (microaneurysms, dilated, or tortuous vessels). Proliferative retinopathy is characterized by the formation of new

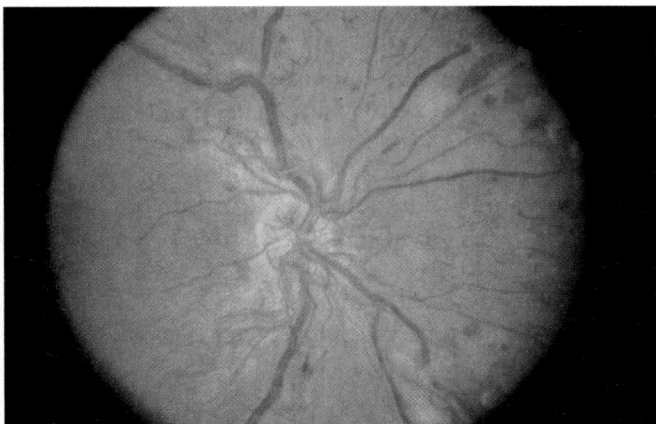

A

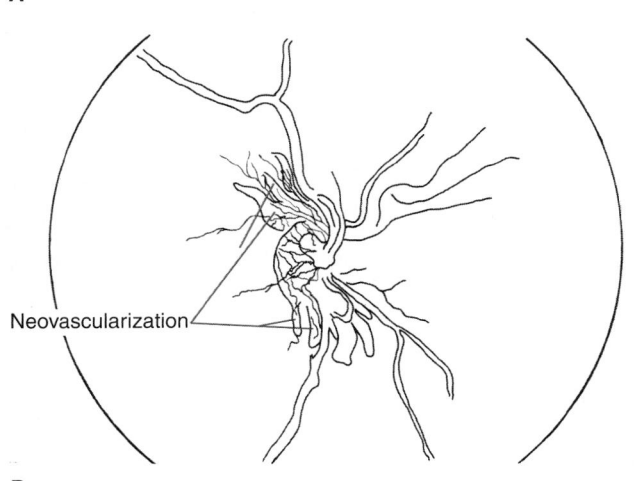

Neovascularization

B

FIGURE 99-8. Proliferative diabetic retinopathy (**A**). In addition to the signs seen in background and preproliferative diabetic retinopathy, neovascularization is seen here coming off the disk (shown schematically in **B**). (Reproduced with permission from Knoop K, Stack L, Storrow A, et al. *The Atlas of Emergency Medicine*, 3rd ed. New York, NY: McGraw Hill; 2010. Photo contributor: Richard E. Wyszynski, MD.)

blood vessels on the surface of the retina and can lead to vitreous hemorrhage. If proliferation continues, blindness can occur through vitreous hemorrhage and traction retinal detachment. With no intervention, visual loss may occur including progression to blindness. Laser photocoagulation and intravitreal injections of the anti–vascular endothelial growth factor (anti-VEGF) ranibizumab appear to be equally effective in prevention of visual loss in diabetic retinopathy. Macular edema may occur at any stage of diabetic retinopathy, especially in older adults. It is characterized by retinal thickening and edema involving the macula. Retinal edema may require intervention because it is sometimes associated with rapid visual deterioration. Intravitreal anti-VEGF agents (bevacizumab, ranibizumab, and aflibercept) provide effective treatment for central-involved diabetic macular edema and have largely replaced laser photocoagulation. Despite clear evidence of efficacy of retinopathy screening by ophthalmologic examination and appropriate intervention, many older diabetic patients do not receive recommended annual screening for retinopathy.

Diabetic neuropathy, present in 50% to 70% of older patients with diabetes, can lead to substantial morbidity, including foot ulcerations, infections, and potentially amputations. In addition, diabetic neuropathy increases the risk of postural instability, balance problems, and muscle atrophy, limiting PA and increasing the risk of falls. Therefore, neuropathy screening, vigilant foot care, and fall prevention are critically important for older diabetic patients. Patients with foot neuropathy should be referred to a podiatrist. Patients with neuropathy should be screened regularly for falls and if positive referred to physical therapy or a fall management program.

Diabetic neuropathy is classified into distinct clinical syndromes: distal symmetric polyneuropathy; autonomic neuropathy; thoracic and lumbar nerve root disease, causing polyradiculopathies; individual cranial and peripheral nerve involvement causing focal mononeuropathies, especially affecting the oculomotor nerve (cranial nerve III) and the median nerve; and asymmetric involvement of multiple peripheral nerves, resulting in a mononeuropathy multiplex. Diabetic autonomic neuropathy may affect many organ systems and can be manifested by gastroparesis, constipation, diarrhea, anhidrosis, bladder dysfunction, erectile dysfunction, exercise intolerance, resting tachycardia, silent ischemia, and even sudden cardiac death. Cardiovascular autonomic dysfunction is associated with increased risk of silent myocardial ischemia and mortality.

There is no specific treatment of diabetic neuropathy. Management primarily consists of controlling hyperglycemia, which has been shown to be effective in clinical trials, pain control, fall risk reduction, and vigilant foot care. The 2021 ADA Guideline recommends pregabalin, gabapentin, and duloxetine for initial treatment of diabetic neuropathy pain. Other agents that are probably effective include amitriptyline, venlafaxine, tramadol, and local capsaicin. Lidocaine patch is possibly effective.

Management of Hyperglycemia

The A1C level is the primary tool for setting goals for hyperglycemia management and monitoring progress toward the goal for most patients. A major challenge in diabetes management is that there is no single best A1C goal for all older adults with diabetes. The relationship between A1C and mortality appears to be U-shaped, rather than linear. Older patients with diabetes have lower risk for death or other complications at an A1C between 6% and 9%, but higher risk at both lower or higher A1C. As older adults with diabetes are highly heterogeneous with respect to their health status, the A1C goal should be individualized. The 2019 Endocrine Society Guideline provides a framework to begin individualizing the goals (see **Table 99-6**). This framework also provides glucose level targets throughout the day. An important recommendation of the Endocrine Society Guideline is that outpatient diabetes regimens be designed specifically to minimize hypoglycemia. Thus, this framework takes into account hypoglycemia risk, with lower limits set for A1C targets in at risk patients (eg, avoiding an A1C < 7.5% for someone with Intermediate Health treated with insulin or a sulfonylurea drug). Providers should measure the A1C at least two times a year in patients who are meeting treatment goals, and more frequently for those not meeting glycemic goals or who have changes in their therapy. Providers should recognize that certain medical conditions can affect the usefulness of the A1C measurement (see discussion of the A1C test in the section on diagnostic criteria). Periodic measurement of glucose levels throughout the day complements the A1C test and allows detection of hypoglycemia in at-risk patients. Continuous glucose monitoring (CGM) has been increasingly used to improve glycemic control and reduce hypoglycemia for younger patients with type 1 diabetes. However, more recently CGM use showed benefit in people with type 1 diabetes older than age 60 and also in patients with type 2 diabetes.

Essential components of hyperglycemia management include patient self-monitoring of blood glucose (SMBG), CGM for selected patients, and recognition and self-treatment of hypoglycemia. The ability to perform these tasks is especially important for those individuals at risk for hypoglycemia (ie, being treated with insulin or a sulfonylurea drug). Coexisting geriatric syndromes and comorbidities may create difficulties for older adults to handle these tasks. For example, individuals with hand arthritis may have difficulty operating the SMBG instruments, individuals with vision impairment may have difficulty reading the results, or individuals with cognitive impairment may have difficulty in reacting appropriately to treat hypoglycemia. Therefore, providers should routinely assess the patient's ability to perform SMBG or CGM and to appropriately recognize and treat hypoglycemia.

Nonpharmacologic approaches

Exercise An exercise program is an important part of diabetes management, particularly for older patients. Exercise programs can be beneficial by helping to control hyperglycemia, improve physical functioning, reduce CVD risk factors, contribute to weight loss, and improve well-being. The ADA recommends that all adults with diabetes should perform at least 150 min/week of moderate-intensity aerobic PA, spread over at least 3 days/week with no more than 2 consecutive days without exercise. As part of the exercise routine, resistance training should be performed at least twice per week. Flexibility and balance exercises are also important in older adults with diabetes to maintain range of motion, strength, and balance. However, over 60% of adults with type 2 diabetes are not physically active. Older adults are especially likely to be sedentary; only 12% of adults aged 75 or older engage in 30 minutes of PA 5 or more days per week, and 65% report no leisure PA. While many barriers to PA exist, health providers can also leverage motivators to improve exercise participation among older adults (**Table 99-9**). Many different PA intervention approaches currently exist, but no single type of intervention has been shown to be superior. Furthermore, many older adults with chronic medical conditions and geriatric syndromes have been excluded from studies of PA interventions. Additional research on PA is needed to target older adults with diabetes who have functional limitations.

Although exercise training alone has not had consistent effects to improve circulating glucose levels in patients with diabetes mellitus, it is a useful adjunct to drug therapy and may well contribute to enhanced effectiveness of glucose-lowering agents. Given the high prevalence of CHD and diabetic autonomic neuropathy in older patients with diabetes mellitus, which may be asymptomatic or atypical in symptoms, it is important for such patients to have medically supervised stress testing before entering any challenging

TABLE 99-9 ■ COMMONLY REPORTED PHYSICAL ACTIVITY BARRIERS AND MOTIVATORS BY OLDER ADULTS

BARRIERS	MOTIVATORS
1. Poor health	1. Pleasure from exercise
2. Exercise is not motivating	2. Positive attitude toward exercise
3. Emotions	3. Health
4. Lack of knowledge about exercise	4. Enhanced self-regulatory skills
5. Lack of awareness of being inactive	5. Tools for monitoring own exercise
6. Lack of social support	6. Social support and encouragement
7. Lack of facilities for exercise	
8. Religious and cultural barriers	
9. Weather	

exercise training program. Even PA at levels lower than usually recommended for cardiorespiratory conditioning (eg, < 50% VO_2max) may enhance glucose tolerance, improve coronary risk factor profile, and reduce CVD-related mortality. Furthermore, patients with lower baseline PA status are likely to experience greater health benefit with a given increase in PA, especially with longer and/or more frequent exercise sessions. Thus, adults with diabetes may benefit from PA of lower intensity but longer duration and/or greater frequency.

Additional issues to consider in an older person participating in an exercise program include the potential for foot and joint injury with upright exercise such as jogging, unstable comorbidities, autonomic neuropathy, peripheral neuropathy or foot lesions that may predispose to injures, and the ability to promptly identify and treat hypoglycemia. Therefore, each patient's exercise prescription needs to be individualized based on their capability to safely participate in an exercise program. A more detailed discussion of the effects of exercise training in older individuals is provided in Chapter 54.

Obesity/Diet As part of diabetes management, the ADA recommends that overweight older adults with type 2 diabetes lose 5% to 7% of body weight through lifestyle changes. However, the benefits versus risks associated with weight loss in older patients with diabetes remain unclear. Among nondiabetic severely obese adults aged 65 or older, individuals who lost weight by caloric restriction and exercise had less reduction in lean muscle mass, increased bone density, and more improvement in physical function than individuals who lost weight by calorie restriction alone or by exercise alone. Therefore, a combination of calorie restriction and exercise may be the best approach for obese older adults with type 2 diabetes.

Dietary intervention has long been a cornerstone of hyperglycemia management. However, there are many challenges with diet programs in older people (see Chapter 30). The ADA currently recommends that medical nutrition therapy be included in any diabetes care program, but that it should be tailored for each patient. Fundamental to any dietary recommendation is ensuring that essential dietary needs are met with adequate provision of vitamins and minerals. Over the years, dietary supplements have been proposed to assist in diabetes treatment such as vitamins C, E, or B complex, or minerals such as zinc or chromium to replace possible diabetes-related losses, thereby improving the metabolic state and possibly reducing the rate of various complications. There is, however, no convincing evidence that any of these dietary supplements improves hyperglycemia control or influences diabetes complications. Two aspects of diet need to be addressed in any dietary program: the total caloric intake, which is a key to maintenance of body weight or weight reduction; and dietary composition, or the distribution of fat, carbohydrate, and protein calories.

CALORIC INTAKE. Caloric restriction is usually part of the initial approach to management of overweight patients with

diabetes mellitus. Because it is generally desirable to maintain muscle and bone mass, the target of caloric restriction is reduction in adiposity, particularly the central adiposity that seems to be critical in mediating obesity-related insulin resistance. The widely accepted definition for obesity is a body mass index (BMI) over 30 kg/m² and for overweight is a BMI of 25 to 30 kg/m². A serious effort at weight reduction should be considered for any obese, older diabetic patient and for many who are overweight as well. Because of an age-related decline in lean body mass, older individuals may have increased adiposity and central adiposity without being overweight or obese by usual BMI criteria. Documentation of central adiposity by waist measurement or computed tomography may suggest a role for caloric restriction in such individuals. Relatively normal-weight people with central adiposity likely already have diminished lean body mass, which will be further threatened by caloric restriction. For individuals who are not overweight and who do not have central adiposity, caloric restriction should not be part of the hyperglycemia treatment program.

Although many types of diets are successful in the short term in achieving weight reduction, long-term maintenance of weight reduction continues to be a major challenge. Some individuals are able to lose a significant amount of weight and maintain it. Therefore, patients should be offered assistance with caloric restriction and supported for a weight loss program. In general, behavioral modification to change dietary habits is the most successful approach long term. Relatively modest weight reduction can have a significant impact on the degree of insulin resistance and on control of glucose levels. Part of the approach should be to set a realistic goal of no more than 5% to 10% reduction of body weight, even if that will not achieve a normal BMI. The role for medications to assist weight loss in an older person with diabetes mellitus is uncertain. With the current explosion of knowledge about regulation of food intake in relation to obesity, it is likely that new medications will appear in the future to assist in weight reduction. For example, the GLP-1 agonist oral semaglutide reduces caloric intake and was approved by the US FDA in 2021 for weight loss.

DIET COMPOSITION. The average American diet includes approximately 45% of calories as carbohydrate, 40% as fat, and 15% as protein. Limited research exists concerning the ideal amount of fat for individuals with diabetes. People with diabetes should follow the guidelines for the general population for the recommended intakes of saturated fat, dietary cholesterol, and trans fat. Increased consumption of foods containing long-chain omega-3 fatty acids is recommended.

Consistency of dietary intake in terms of meal composition, carbohydrate intake, and timing is particularly an issue in patients treated with insulin. The ADA's diet exchange program is one means of providing guidance to such patients to maintain consistency of dietary intake.

Nutritional counseling can be particularly helpful in assisting patients to adhere to a dietary program.

DIETARY ISSUES IN OLDER PEOPLE. Caloric restriction is appropriate for healthier overweight and obese older patients as part of diabetes management. However, it is not appropriate for some older patients who are in a catabolic state due to undernutrition and comorbidities, meet criteria for frailty, or are generally in poor health (see **Table 99-6**). For such persons, more pressing dietary issues are eating regularly and coordinating food intake with administration of glucose-lowering agents appropriately to avoid hypoglycemia. Both the 2019 Endocrine Society and 2021 ADA guidelines recommend diets rich in protein and energy to prevent malnutrition and weight loss in older diabetes patients who meet criteria for frailty. As summarized in **Table 99-10**, there are a number of special issues that increase an older adult's vulnerability to poor dietary habits. Older adults with a significant mobility limitation and/or lacking transportation are likely to have limited access to healthy and fresh food. Thus, convenient pre-prepared foods with high calorie, high cholesterol, and high sodium levels may become staples of an older patient's diet, thereby interfering with good diabetes management. Older persons, especially men living alone, may have limited food preparation skills. The presence of impaired cognitive function may make following a dietary prescription particularly difficult. Furthermore, dietary habits established for a lifetime and often with a cultural background may be particularly difficult to modify. Problems with taste and oral health, including xerostomia and periodontal disease, are common in older adults (see Chapter 32), can be exacerbated by diabetes, and may further limit adaptation to a prescribed diet. Social isolation (ie, living alone, eating alone), poverty, and functional reliance on others to purchase food are all risk factors for decreased food intake. A social worker may be able to help older adults to access resources from local community social services organizations and involve the patient's caregivers to improve the dietary support.

TABLE 99-10 ■ DIETARY THERAPY: SPECIAL CONSIDERATIONS FOR OLDER ADULTS WITH DIABETES MELLITUS

Access to food
- Functional disability
- Poor meal preparation skills
- Lack of formal or informal support to obtain food

Limited financial resources

Decreased food intake
- Decline in taste and smell appreciation
- Poor dentition and/or xerostomia

Ingrained dietary habits

Past experience and ethnic food preference

Impaired cognitive function

Depression

Glucose-lowering drugs A growing range of therapeutic options enables the treatment program to be tailored to the specific situation of the individual patient, as determined in part by the initial comprehensive assessment carried out. A summary of currently available glucose-lowering drugs is provided in **Tables 99-11** and **99-12**. Note that among the 12 classes of drugs available, only insulin and sulfonylureas pose a significant risk for hypoglycemia. In older adults with type 2 diabetes at increased risk of hypoglycemia, medication classes with low risk of hypoglycemia are preferred. However, high cost may be a barrier for patients to obtain newer classes of medications such as SGLT-2 inhibitors, DPP4 inhibitors, GLP-1 agonists, or long-acting insulin.

Noninsulin Agents A growing number of medications other than insulin are available for hyperglycemia management of older adults with diabetes mellitus. **Table 99-11** lists the available drugs with their common dosages, mechanism of action, and advantages and disadvantages.

As the different classes of drugs have different mechanisms of action, there is increasing opportunity to individualize therapy as more is learned about the heterogeneity of type 2 diabetes. All of these agents are effective in lowering glucose levels in clinical trials of patients with type 2 diabetes mellitus. Some of them may also assist in lowering glucose levels as an adjunct to insulin therapy in patients with type 1 diabetes. The potential risks associated with these agents must be considered in relation to the patient's comorbidities and their hypoglycemia risks.

BIGUANIDE. Metformin is widely recommended as the first-line oral medication for hyperglycemia in type 2 diabetes unless there is a specific contraindication. Metformin primarily suppresses hepatic glucose production and may also enhance peripheral sensitivity to insulin. Metformin rarely causes hypoglycemia when used alone. The most common side effect of metformin is gastrointestinal (GI) discomfort, which in some patients can be associated with decreased appetite and modest weight loss. While some have viewed this as a potential benefit for a patient on a weight-reduction program, this effect needs to be balanced against the degree of symptoms and the appropriateness of decreased caloric intake and weight loss in a given individual. The biguanide class of drugs is also known to be associated with development of life-threatening lactic acidosis under some circumstances. Although this complication appears to be very rare in patients using metformin, this drug should be avoided in situations that may put people at risk for development of lactic acidosis: unstable congestive heart failure and during acute hospitalization for any major illness that could result in decreased tissue perfusion as a precipitating factor for lactic acidosis. Metformin is contraindicated in patients with eGFR below 30 mL/min/1.73 m². Monitoring of renal function and perhaps dose adjustment of metformin to account for reduced renal clearance is highly appropriate for older diabetes patients with CKD.

SULFONYLUREA DRUGS. Sulfonylurea drugs have been on the market for many years and are still commonly used in

TABLE 99-11 ■ NONINSULIN GLUCOSE-LOWERING AGENTS FOR TREATMENT OF TYPE 2 DIABETES

CLASS	ROUTE OF ADMINISTRATION AND USUAL DAILY DOSAGE	PRIMARY PHYSIOLOGIC ACTION	ADVANTAGES	DISADVANTAGES
Biguanide • Metformin • Metformin ER	Oral • 500–1000 mg BID • Max 2500 mg/d • 500–2000 mg qd	• ↓ Hepatic glucose production, possible ↑ insulin-mediated uptake of glucose in muscles	• No weight gain • Minimal hypoglycemia • Likely ↓ in both microvascular and macrovascular events • Extensive clinical experience • Lower cost	• Gastrointestinal side effects (diarrhea and abdominal discomfort; less GI side effects with metformin ER) • Lactic acidosis (rare) • Contraindicated in presence of progressive liver, kidney, or cardiac failure • Contraindicated if eGFR < 30 mL/min/1.73 m²
Sulfonylureas • Glipizide • Glyburide • Glimepiride • Gliclazide[a]	Oral • 2.5–10 mg qd BID • 2.5–20 mg qd • 1–4 mg qd • 40 mg qd–160 mg BID	• ↑ Insulin secretion from pancreatic β-cells	• ↓ Microvascular events • Extensive clinical experience • Lower cost	• Hypoglycemia (esp. with longer half-life: glyburide) • Weight gain • Skin rash (including photosensitivity)
DPP-4 inhibitors • Sitagliptin • Saxagliptin • Vildagliptin[a] • Linagliptin • Alogliptin[c]	Oral • 100 mg qd • 2.5 5 mg qd • 50 mg qd BID • 5 mg qd • 25 mg qd	• ↑ Insulin secretion (glucose-dependent) • ↑ Glucagon secretion (glucose-dependent)	• Minimal hypoglycemia • Well tolerated • Once a day dosing • OK to use in renal impairment • No renal dose adjustment (Linagliptin)	• Urticaria/angioedema • Renal dose adjustment (sitagliptin, saxagliptin, alogliptin) • ? ↑ risk of pancreatitis • ? ↑ Heart failure hospitalization • Higher cost
GLP-1 receptor agonists • Exenatide • Exenatide extended release • Liraglutide • Dulaglutide • Lixisenatide • Semaglutide • Insulin glargine/lixisenatide • Insulin degludec/liraglutide 100/3.6	Injection • 5–10 µg SC bid • 2 mg SC qwk • 0.6–1.8 mg SC qd • 0.75 mg/0.5 mL SC qwk • 10–20 µg SC qd • Oral 3–14 mg qd • 0.25–1 mg SC qwk • 15–60 units SC qd • 16–50 units SC qd	• ↑ Insulin secretion (glucose-dependent) • ↓ Glucagon secretion (glucose-dependent) • Slows gastric emptying • ↑ Satiety	• Minimal hypoglycemia risk (lower risk for the fixed combination with insulin than insulin alone) • Weight reduction (weight neutrality for the fixed combination with insulin) • ↓ Blood pressure • ↓ Postprandial glucose excursions • No renal dose adjustment (liraglutide, semaglutide, and dulaglutide) • ↓ CVD events (liraglutide, semaglutide, and dulaglutide) • May ↓ CKD progression (liraglutide, semaglutide, dulaglutide)	• Gastrointestinal side effects (nausea, vomiting) • ↑ Heart rate • ? Acute pancreatitis • Thyroid C-cell hyperplasia/tumors in rodents (human relevance uncertain) • Avoid if eGFR < 30 mL/min/1.73 m² (exenatide, lixisenatide) • Higher cost

(Continued)

TABLE 99-11 ■ NONINSULIN GLUCOSE-LOWERING AGENTS FOR TREATMENT OF TYPE 2 DIABETES (CONTINUED)

CLASS	ROUTE OF ADMINISTRATION AND USUAL DAILY DOSAGE	PRIMARY PHYSIOLOGIC ACTION	ADVANTAGES	DISADVANTAGES
SGLT-2 inhibitors • Canagliflozin • Empagliflozin • Dapagliflozin • Ertugliflozin	Oral • 100–300 mg qd • 10–25 mg qd • 5–10 mg qd • 5–15 mg qd	• ↓ Glucose reabsorption by the kidney • ↑ Urinary glucose excretion	• Minimal hypoglycemia • Weight reduction • ↓ Blood pressure • Once-a-day dosing • ↓ CVD events (empagliflozin, canagliflozin, and dapagliflozin) • ↓ CKD progression	• Renal dose adjustment and avoid if eGFR < 25–30 mL/min/1.73 m² • Genitourinary infections • Genital yeast infections • Polyuria • Hyperkalemia • Orthostatic hypotension • DKA (rare in T2DM) • ↑ fractures (canagliflozin) • Higher cost
α-Glucosidase inhibitors • Acarbose • Miglitol	Oral • 25–100 mg TID with meals • 25–100 mg TID with meals	• Slows intestinal carbohydrate digestion or absorption	• Minimal hypoglycemia • ↓ Postprandial glucose excursions • ? ↓ CVD events • Lower cost (acarbose)	• Generally modest A1C reduction • Flatulence • Abdominal discomfort • Contraindicated in cirrhosis • Frequent dosing schedule (with meals)
Thiazolidinediones • Pioglitazone • Rosiglitazone[b]	Oral • 15–45 mg qd • 2–8 mg qd or divided BID	• ↑ Insulin sensitivity	• Minimal hypoglycemia • ↑ HDL-C • ↓ Triglycerides (pioglitazone) • Lower cost (pioglitazone)	• Weight gain • Edema/heart failure (avoid in renal impairment • Bone fractures • ↑ LDL-C (rosiglitazone) • ? ↑ MI
Meglitinides • Repaglinide • Nateglinide	Oral • 0.5–4 mg QAC • 60–120 mg QAC	• ↑ Insulin secretion from pancreatic β-cells	• ↓ Postprandial glucose excursions • Dosing flexibility (before meals)	• Hypoglycemia • Weight gain • Frequent dosing schedule • Intermediate cost
Amylin-like • Pramlintide[c]	Injection • 60–120 µg SC QAC	• ↓ Glucagon secretion • Slows gastric emptying • ↑ Satiety	• ↓ Postprandial glucose excursions • Weight reduction	• GI side effects (nausea; vomiting) • ↑ Hypoglycemic risk of insulin • Frequent dosing schedule • Higher cost
Bile acid sequestrant • Colesevelam[d]	Oral • 3750 mg qd (or 1875 mg BID) with meals	• Unclear • ? ↓ Hepatic glucose production • ? ↑ Incretin levels	• Minimal hypoglycemia • ↓ LDL-C	• Generally modest A1C efficacy • Constipation • ↑ Triglycerides • Reduce absorption of fat soluble vitamins • Higher cost
Dopamine-2 agonist • Bromocriptine, immediate-release form[c]	Oral • 1.6–4.8 mg QAM	• Modulates hypothalamic regulation of metabolism • ↑ Insulin sensitivity	• Minimal hypoglycemia	• Nausea; headache; orthostatic hypotension; potential exacerbation of psychosis • Higher cost

BID, twice a day; CKD, chronic kidney disease; CVD, cardiovascular disease; DKA, diabetic ketoacidosis; DPP-4, dipeptidyl peptidase-4; eGFR, estimated glomerular filtration; GLP-1, glucagon-like peptide 1; HDL-C, high-density lipoprotein cholesterol; LDL-C, low-density lipoprotein cholesterol; MI, myocardial infarction; QAC, before meals; QAM, every morning; qd, once daily; SC, subcutaneous injection; SGLT2 inhibitors, inhibitors of sodium glucose cotransporter 2; T2DM, type 2 diabetes mellitus; TID, three times a day.
[a]Not licensed in United States.
[b]Prescribing highly restricted in the United States; withdrawn in Europe.
[c]Not licensed in Europe.
[d]Limited use in the United States/Europe.

TABLE 99-12 ■ INSULIN FOR TREATMENT OF TYPE 2 DIABETES

INSULIN AGENTS	ONSET OF ACTION	PEAK EFFECT	DURATION OF ACTION
Long-acting			
• Glargine 100	• About 2 h	• No peak	• 20–> 24 h
• Detemir	• About 2 h	• 3–9 h	• 6–24 h (duration of action is dose-dependent; at ≥ 0.8 units/kg, mean duration of action is longer and less variable—22–23 h)
Ultra-long acting			
• Degludec	• About 2 h	• No peak	• > 40 h
• Glargine 300	• About 6 h	• No peak	• 28–36 h
Intermediate acting			
• Human NPH	• About 2 h	• 4–12 h	• 18–28 h
• Neutral protamine lispro[a]	• About 2 h	• 6 h	• 15 h
Short acting			
• Human regular	• About 30 min	• 2–4 h	• 5–8 h
Rapid acting			
• Lispro	• 5–15 min	• 45–75 min	• 2–4 h
• Aspart			
• Glulisine			
Inhalation powder			
• Human insulin[b]	• 5–15 min	• 50 min (wide variation)	• 2–3 h
Premixed insulins			
• NPH/Regular 70/30	• About 30 min	• 4–12 h	• 18–24 h
• Lispro 50/50 (lispro protamine and lispro)	• 5–15 min	• 1– 5 h	• 11– 22 h
• Lispro 75/25 (Lispro protamine and lispro)	• 5–15 min	• 1–6 h	• 13–22 h
• NovoLog Mix 70/30 (aspart protamine and aspart)	• 5–15 min	• 1–4 h	• Up to 24 h

The insulin agents lead to increased glucose disposal and decreased hepatic glucose production. They are nearly universally responsive and likely lead to decreased microvascular risk (UK Prospective Diabetes Study [UKPDS]). Disadvantages are hypoglycemia risks, which vary based on the individual agent's dose and its course of the action.

[a]Only available in the United States in a premixed combination with insulin lispro.

[b]Inhaled human insulin (Afrezza) is contraindicated in patients with chronic lung disease such as asthma or chronic obstructive pulmonary disease (COPD).

older adults with type 2 diabetes. As first-generation sulfonylureas are rarely used, **Table 99-11** only includes second-generation agents. Because of their long history, there is a substantial body of knowledge about the mechanism of action and side effect profile of sulfonylureas. Their primary mechanism of action is to enhance insulin secretion by the β-cells of the endocrine pancreas.

Sulfonylurea drugs have established a long record of safety, with hypoglycemia being the main adverse effect. Conservative dosing is recommended for older people. Glyburide has been associated with a higher risk for hypoglycemia in older patients due to its long half-life, so is not recommended in this population. Glipizide may be safer to use in older patients, but all of these drugs should be avoided if there is concern about hypoglycemia. These drugs should not be used in patients with renal insufficiency or with significant liver disease, as they depend on the liver for metabolism and the kidney for excretion. Hyponatremia has also been observed as a complication in some patients. Because of similar risk with use of thiazide diuretics, the combination of thiazide and sulfonylurea drugs should be avoided if hyponatremia is a concern.

GLUCAGON-LIKE PEPTIDE-1 (GLP-1) AGENTS. GLP-1 is an incretin, an intestinal hormone that is released with meals and causes glucose-dependent insulin secretion. Two classes of GLP-1 drugs are used clinically.

Dipeptidyl peptidase-4 (DPP-4) inhibitors Native incretin hormones such as GLP-1 have very short half-lives as they are degraded by the enzyme, DPP-4, and thus cannot be used therapeutically. Inhibitors of DPP-4 are orally effective agents that increase and prolong the action of endogenous incretin hormones, and several are now available. These agents are used once daily and result in modest reductions of A1C. Used alone, they rarely cause hypoglycemia, as GLP-1's effect on insulin secretion is reduced as glucose levels fall. They do not cause weight loss, but may have a few nonspecific side effects including nasopharyngitis and headache. Safety and efficacy studies in older people show no overall differences compared to use in younger patients.

GLP-1 agonists are analogs of GLP-1 that are much less susceptible to DPP-4 and so provide prolonged GLP-1 effects. When they are used in pharmacologic doses, they are potent enhancers of glucose-dependent insulin secretion. They also suppress glucagon secretion, slow gastric emptying, and reduce food intake, usually resulting in some loss of body weight. Overall, they usually lead to greater reductions of A1C than DPP-4 inhibitors. Like DPP-4 inhibitors, they rarely cause hypoglycemia. Current GLP-1 agonists require injection, except semaglutide, which is also available for oral use. Exenatide is a peptide derived from frog skin that has GLP-1 agonist activity. There is now a long-acting form of exenatide that can be administered once a week. More recent GLP-1 agonists are actual modifications of GLP-1 itself. There are now fixed injectable combinations available of insulin with a GLP-1 agonist (insulin glargine/lixisenatide and insulin degludec/liraglutide), see **Table 99-11**.

Given the clinically significant cardiovascular and possibly nephropathy benefits of some GLP-1 agonists (see **Table 99-11**), they are recommended for patients who have not achieved adequate glycemic control with metformin alone, especially among patients with previous CVD or CKD. Side effects of GLP-1 agents include nausea, vomiting, increased heart rate, and weight loss, which may be particularly undesirable for some older adults. There are reports of possible associated acute pancreatitis with GLP-1 agents, and development of C-cell hyperplasia or medullary thyroid tumors in animals.

SGLT-2 INHIBITORS. Two sodium glucose transporters (SGLT) cause glucose reabsorption: SGLT-1 and SGLT-2. SGLT-2 is found only in the proximal tubule of the kidney, and accounts for 90% of the reabsorption of glucose. SGLT-1 is found in the gut and other tissues, and accounts for approximately 10% of glucose reabsorption. SGLT-2 inhibitors are oral agents that lower glucose levels in patients with diabetes by increasing urinary excretion of glucose. They are used once daily, result in modest lowering of A1C, and rarely cause hypoglycemia. These agents have cardiovascular benefits in patients with established atherosclerotic CVD and heart failure, and slow the progression of CKD, including in older patients per secondary analyses of CVOTs. However, they are contraindicated if the eGFR is below 30 mL/min/1.73 m². Use when the eGFR is 30 to 60 mL/min/1.73 m² varies with the specific product but may be best to avoid until more data are available. These agents increase urine volume and sodium excretion, so usually lower BP modestly, but may cause volume depletion. This volume effect may contribute to increased risk for DKA in susceptible patients. There is increased risk for genital yeast infection and urinary tract infection, likely due to the induced glucosuria. Because of these side effects and relatively high cost, some older patients may not be able to use these agents.

α-GLUCOSIDASE INHIBITORS. These agents work by inhibiting the key GI enzyme responsible for breakdown of carbohydrates prior to absorption. They are particularly helpful to reduce postprandial increases of glucose levels and may be a useful adjunct to therapy with other agents. The major side effects are local to the GI tract (flatulence, diarrhea, abdominal pain) because these drugs are not absorbed to any significant degree. These agents may be useful and relatively safe in older people with fairly well-controlled diabetes. One can expect an approximate 0.5% decrease in hemoglobin A1C.

THIAZOLIDINEDIONES. This class of drugs appears to work primarily by enhancing peripheral and hepatic sensitivity to insulin. This mechanism of action complements that of the other drug classes available. As peripheral resistance to insulin is a key part of the metabolic syndrome that predisposes to development of diabetes, use of a drug that targets this abnormality is attractive. These drugs have been shown to have similar efficacy and adverse events in older adults. However, they can cause fluid retention, peripheral edema, weight gain, and increase the risk for congestive heart failure, so should not be used in patients with heart failure. Use of these agents should also be avoided in patients at risk for osteoporosis, falls or fractures, and/or macular edema.

MEGLITINIDE AND D-PHENYLALANINE DERIVATIVE. Both repaglinide and nateglinide act directly on pancreatic β-cells to rapidly stimulate insulin secretion, but by a mechanism that differs from the sulfonylureas. Both drugs were designed to be used immediately before meals and both improve postprandial glucose levels. No dose adjustments are necessary in older people. Repaglinide should not be combined with gemfibrozil because of increased repaglinide levels. Nateglinide has no known drug interactions, and can be used in patients with renal insufficiency.

Other Drugs Three other types of drugs are approved for lowering glucose levels: the bile acid sequestrant colesevelam, the dopamine-2 agonist bromocriptine, immediate-release form (Cycloset), and pramlintide acetate (Symlin), an injectable analog of the peptide amylin available in the United States that reduces postprandial glucose in conjunction with mealtime insulin. Because of limited experience with these drugs (especially in older adults) and modest glucose lowering, they are rarely used.

Combination Therapy Combinations of oral agents or a combination of one or more of these oral/injectable agents with insulin are theoretically attractive because of the different modes of action of the various classes of drugs. Thus, combination therapy addresses various aspects of the pathophysiology of hyperglycemia in diabetes, offering the possibility of synergism in therapeutic efficacy without synergism in toxicity. For older patients, the logic of combination therapy must be balanced against incremental costs and incremental risks of side effects with each additional drug. Furthermore, the potential for polypharmacy for multiple coexisting conditions such as hypertension, hyperlipidemia, osteoarthritis, and coronary artery disease needs to be considered. The overall treatment goal for the patient must also be kept in mind. Adding a second or third oral or injectable agent without achieving the glycemic goal can be an indication to proceed to use of insulin.

Insulin Therapy Use of insulin is required in patients with type 1 diabetes mellitus. Insulin also may be needed in patients with type 2 diabetes either as part of an outpatient glucose-lowering regimen or to maintain reasonable glucose control in the hospital setting (usually managed by an inpatient diabetes care team) during acute stressful illness or in the perioperative period when oral agents may be less acceptable or useful.

ADVANTAGES OF INSULIN. There are now more than 100 years of clinical experience with use of insulin since its discovery in 1922 and the dramatic demonstration of its effectiveness to save the lives of patients with type 1 diabetes in DKA. Many formulations of insulin with varying duration of action allow individualization of treatment plans. Insulin is the natural hormone that is deficient in relative or absolute terms in diabetes, so its use fits with the overall concept of hormone replacement for endocrine deficiency syndromes. Virtually all forms of insulin currently in use are identical to human insulin or with only slight molecular modifications, so the incidence of allergic reactions is very small. There are virtually no known pharmacokinetic drug interactions and virtually no absolute contraindications to insulin use.

With appropriate dosage modification and monitoring of glucose levels, insulin can be used safely for patients with renal or hepatic insufficiency, patients unable to eat, and during major illness. Insulin itself is relatively inexpensive. However, the overall program of insulin treatment, including use of modern insulin analogs and frequent glucose monitoring, may be expensive. While appropriate insulin use can be a challenge, it encourages active self-care by the patient and/or caregivers. Finally, and perhaps most important from the point of view of achieving treatment objectives, insulin can effectively lower glucose levels in virtually any patient and, in sufficient dosage, has at least the potential to normalize circulating glucose levels if the regimen intensity is sufficient.

DISADVANTAGES OF INSULIN. One disadvantage of insulin is that it requires injection to be effective, although approval of Afrezza (human insulin) Inhalation Powder provides a rapid-acting insulin option for patients unable or unwilling to perform injections. Injection may represent an insurmountable psychological barrier for a small number of patients. For others, insulin injections may not be feasible owing to functional limitations or insufficient caregiver support. Most older adults can, however, be trained to use insulin appropriately. Insulin is a potent agent, and so the dose must be carefully measured to minimize risk of hypoglycemia. Accidental overdose is also a risk. The most common issue to address with insulin management is risk for hypoglycemia, which is discussed below.

INSULIN REGIMENS. Before prescribing any insulin, the provider should have a good understanding of the different duration of each agent's glucose-lowering effect. As described in **Table 99-12**, insulin agents have variable onset of action, peak effect, and duration of action; these characteristics are important when selecting which agent to prescribe. Long-acting agents are modified to slow degradation, and have a stable time course of action over 24 hours, so can be given once daily for basal insulin replacement. These long-acting insulin analogs can improve management of diabetic patients, with a relatively low incidence of nocturnal hypoglycemia (especially the two ultra–long-acting agents), no pronounced peak, a long duration of action, and little interpatient absorption variability. Insulin glargine can be dosed as 0.2 units/kg/day subcutaneously once daily or initiated at 10 units once daily and adjusted as needed. Insulin detemir (Levemir) can be initiated at 0.2 to 0.5 unit/kg/day (0.1 to 0.2 unit/kg/day for insulin-naïve patients) with one injection daily in the evening or at bedtime.

Insulin aspart (NovoLog), insulin lispro (Humalog), and insulin glulisine (Apidra) were developed as agents with a very rapid onset and short duration of action. These insulins are used for injection just prior to meals and are less likely to result in postmeal hypoglycemia than human regular insulin. They can even be given within 20 minutes after starting a meal. Thus, a combination of once-daily, long-acting insulin analog plus premeal injections of a rapid-acting insulin analog may be used for intensive insulin therapy. Similar results can be achieved with such a regimen as with use of a subcutaneous insulin pump system delivering a continuous basal insulin infusion plus bolus injections with meals. Intensive insulin therapy of selected older adults with uncomplicated type 2 diabetes using either of these two regimens achieved an average hemoglobin A1C of 7% over a period of 1 year with minimal adverse effects.

INITIATION OF INSULIN THERAPY. In developing an insulin treatment regimen for an older adult, it is useful to keep in mind a target total dose range per 24 hours, even though the initial starting dose may be substantially lower. The total daily insulin dose required for a thin patient with type 1 diabetes is typically 0.5 to 1.0 units/kg. The total daily insulin dose for a type 2 diabetes patient with insulin resistance may vary considerably, but up to 1.0 to 2.0 units/kg may be needed to achieve the glucose control target selected. For most such patients, insulin should be initiated at a much lower dose, such as 0.1 to 0.2 units/kg/day. Of course, there will be substantial variation among individuals in total dose needed, depending on the target treatment goal, patient adherence to lifestyle modification recommendations, degree of insulin resistance, and individual variation of insulin dose pharmacokinetic patterns. Thus, a low starting dose of a single injection of long-acting insulin 10 to 20 units daily, depending on the degree of obesity, is reasonable. Initiation of insulin treatment is usually done as an outpatient and in conjunction with a diabetes education program for the patient and family members.

Frequent follow-up should be provided initially to ensure that the treatment program is progressing smoothly and that hypoglycemia does not occur early on. Given the metabolic stability of most older patients with type 2 diabetes, there is no need to escalate the insulin dose rapidly. Doses can be adjusted in 2- to 5-unit increments every 3 to 5 days (or every 7 days for long-acting insulin analogs) while glucose levels are being monitored. Patients should be prepared from the outset to progress to at least two injections per day, although some patients may achieve the treatment goal with a single dose.

As insulin doses continue to be gradually adjusted upward, an obese patient with type 2 diabetes may need a total of more than 100 units/day to achieve an aggressive treatment goal. Also, as doses are increased, it makes sense to add use of a rapid-acting insulin to help cover meal-related increases of glucose levels.

As glucose levels are reduced, insulin sensitivity will likely improve owing to amelioration of the direct effects of hyperglycemia. Thus, an overweight older patient who appears relatively unresponsive to a moderate dose of insulin initially may begin to respond dramatically to modest further increases of insulin dose. In fact, the patient may progress to having episodes of hypoglycemia even with reduction to a total insulin dose that previously was not very effective. It is apparent that close follow-up with the diabetes care team, careful attention to glucose monitoring, and coaching about symptoms of hypoglycemia are all critical to a successful treatment program. A suitably trained diabetes nurse educator can play a particularly critical role during this phase of treatment.

COMBINATION OF INSULIN AND NONINSULIN AGENTS. Insulin therapy can be combined with use of one or more other classes of glucose-lowering drugs, although there are little data on such regimens specifically in older adults. One option is use of an evening or bedtime injection of a long-acting insulin analog to target control of the FPG plus use of another drug for daytime use.

There are theoretical advantages to combining insulin with a drug that induces weight loss such as a GLP-1 agonist or with an agent that reduces meal-related glucose excursions. However, insulin regimens alone with dose adjustments can achieve remarkably similar control of hyperglycemia as combinations of lower doses of insulin with another class of drug. Given the limited incremental cost of additional insulin to a patient already on insulin and the potential for adverse drug reaction with any addition of a different therapeutic agent, the practical gain of such combination therapy remains unclear.

Another theoretical advantage of combination therapy is that lower doses of insulin can be used to achieve similar glycemic control. It has been argued that high doses of insulin may have adverse cardiovascular effects, but no convincing data links dose of insulin in patients with diabetes to adverse cardiovascular effects. A concern about using a high dose of insulin is the potential for weight gain. For patients for whom the indication for insulin is a period of substantial weight loss caused by decompensated diabetes, insulin therapy should be expected to cause weight gain back toward baseline with accompanying restoration of lean body mass. For other patients, it may be necessary to balance the potential risk of weight gain versus the benefit of substantial lowering of circulating glucose levels. In general, weight gain with insulin therapy is modest (in the range of a few kilograms) except for those individuals who have lost substantial weight prior to insulin therapy. By emphasizing and reinforcing lifestyle modifications as insulin therapy is instituted, substantial weight gain can generally be avoided.

Follow-up care and quality indicators Diabetes mellitus is a complex disease that requires long-term follow-up and involves multidisciplinary health providers. Key items to document in routine diabetes follow-up care are summarized in **Table 99-13**. For patients with type 1 diabetes or with type 2 diabetes who have an aggressive treatment goal or with multiple diabetes complications, participation by a specialized diabetes care team in the overall management program should be carefully considered. As a means to standardize and improve the quality of health care for diabetic patients, a number of health insurance providers, including the CMS, have adopted measurements to assess the quality of diabetes care. These measures

---

TABLE 99-13 ■ KEY COMPONENTS OF ROUTINE FOLLOW-UP CARE (USUALLY EVERY 1–3 MONTHS) FOR OLDER PATIENTS WITH DIABETES[a]

Pertinent history:

- Home glucose monitoring/CGM data
- Hypoglycemia review (potential cause, appropriate management)
- Interim health and psychosocial changes (especially access to food, physical activity, falls, cognition, functional status, and social support)
- Medication reconciliation

Physical examination:

- Body weight
- Blood pressure
- Focused examination

Laboratory data:

- Hemoglobin A1C
- Renal function (if nephropathy present)
- Others as appropriate (eg, serum potassium if patient is on an ACE inhibitor or diuretic)

Assessment and plan:

- Adjustments in the overall treatment plan
- Review of lifestyle components of the treatment program (diet, physical activity)

[a]Annual evaluation should be done per **Table 99-4**.
ACE, angiotensin-converting enzyme; CGM, continuous glucose monitoring.

are designed to assess the care of groups of patients in a given care setting, not the care of individual patients. Furthermore, these quality measures do not include all older patients, some measures are not appropriate for patients with poor health status, and measures that may have a larger impact on an older adult's safety are not included. For example, patients older than age 75 are traditionally excluded from such quality assessment. While the quality measures routinely include the proportion of patients with poor glycemic or blood pressure control (ie, A1C > 9% or blood pressure > 135/90 mm Hg), virtually none of them currently assess the proportion of patients with hypoglycemia events or hypotension events. Diabetes quality measures that are based on the health status of the patient rather than age may be more appropriate for older patients given their heterogeneous health status.

SPECIAL ISSUES

Hypoglycemia

Hypoglycemia is the primary short-term risk of a hyperglycemia treatment program that includes a sulfonylurea drug or insulin, particularly one that is targeted at achieving near-normal control of glucose levels. In the absence of a sulfonylurea drug or exogenous insulin, neither metformin nor the newer classes of glucose lowering drugs cause hypoglycemia. The GLP-related drugs stimulate significant insulin secretion only when glucose levels are elevated. Similarly, the SGLT-2 antagonists enhance renal excretion of glucose primarily when glucose levels are elevated and are minimally effective as glucose levels approach the normal range.

Multiple mechanisms exist to maintain adequate circulating glucose levels because glucose is a fuel particularly targeted to meet the needs of the brain and other tissues that are not dependent on insulin for glucose uptake. Muscle and fat, the major peripheral tissues, have a glucose transport system that primarily depends on insulin for activation. Brain cells, however, have a different type of glucose transporter molecule that is continually expressed on the cell surface and does not depend on insulin for activation. After an overnight fast, when insulin levels are low, the brain does not have to compete with other major tissues for access to glucose. This is in contrast to fat-related fuel such as free fatty acids and ketones, which have ready access to muscle and fat tissue and therefore are less available to the brain. Because of the brain's dependency on glucose as a fuel, it is particularly vulnerable to injury from hypoglycemia, a fact that must be carefully considered as the overall benefits and risks of a diabetes treatment program are reviewed. Thus, an older diabetic adult on a glucose-lowering regimen that includes a sulfonylurea drug or insulin must be counseled to always carry glucose tablets or food. An older adult on insulin therapy and their family or caregiver should be given a glucagon emergency kit and teaching on its use.

TABLE 99-14 ■ FACTORS AFFECTING RECOVERY FROM HYPOGLYCEMIA
Hepatic glucose production
Glucose uptake by tissues
Degree of hypoglycemia
Wearing off of drug effect
Counterregulatory hormone responses
Behavioral responses

Hypoglycemia counterregulation Hypoglycemia can be the result of absolute therapeutic hyperinsulinemia alone, but more commonly is the result of compromised physiologic and behavioral defenses against falling plasma glucose concentrations in the presence of unregulated insulin levels due to a sulfonylurea drug or exogenous insulin. **Table 99-14** lists factors that are important in recovery from hypoglycemia by increasing the glucose level either from endogenous sources or from ingestion of glucose. The major source of endogenous glucose is the liver. The liver contributes to recovery from hypoglycemia by increasing glucose production under the influence of counterregulatory hormones. As the insulin effect fades during insulin-induced hypoglycemia, there is a decline in peripheral glucose uptake, preserving more circulating glucose for recovery. The degree of fall of glucose levels determines the magnitude of counterregulatory responses and the speed with which normal glucose levels can be restored. Normally, there is a hierarchy of responses to hypoglycemia with release of counterregulatory hormones such as epinephrine and glucagon occurring before a patient becomes symptomatic and aware of hypoglycemia. The initial symptoms are caused by autonomic nervous system activation with tachycardia, nervousness, and a sweating response, all of which can alert the patient to the need to seek exogenous sources of glucose to facilitate recovery. Hunger is often a part of this behavioral response. However, as glucose levels fall lower and brain cell function becomes compromised, confusion, lethargy, and progression to coma can occur. Fortunately, the response to glucose administration is quick, and dramatic recovery normally occurs.

It is now recognized that the history of the glucose level that the brain is exposed to influences the counterregulatory response mechanisms, perhaps by affecting the brain glucose transport system. For example, there appears to be adaptation to chronic hyperglycemia in patients with diabetes, with resulting elevation of the glucose level at which counterregulatory responses begin to occur. Thus, a patient with diabetes may begin to develop symptoms of hypoglycemia at a glucose level in the range of 80 to 100 mg/dL, well above the symptomatic threshold in nondiabetic individuals of 50 to 60 mg/dL. Conversely, the brain appears to adapt to low glucose levels as well, with a shift downward of the glucose threshold for activation of counterregulatory responses. Prior exposure to hypoglycemia leads to diminished counterregulatory hormone responses.

This can set up a vicious cycle by which patients are less able to counterregulate hypoglycemia and have more recurrent episodes. A key issue seems to be that as the glucose threshold for counterregulation drops, it becomes perilously close to glucose levels that can adversely affect brain function. Thus, a patient may have a very narrow margin for error, proceeding from relatively normal function without symptoms to profound hypoglycemia and loss of consciousness. This so-called hypoglycemia unawareness syndrome is in part iatrogenic in origin and generally responds to strict avoidance of hypoglycemia.

Hypoglycemia in older patients with diabetes Hypoglycemia is dangerous for older patients as it is associated with increased risks for falls and dementia, and it can be fatal. Therefore, episodes of hypoglycemia should be ascertained and addressed at routine visits for any patient receiving a sulfonylurea drug or insulin. A self-reported history of severe hypoglycemia (requiring the assistance of another person) predicts increased mortality 5 years later. ED visit rates for hypoglycemia are highest among adults with diabetes aged 75 or older, almost three times as high as in patients aged 45 to 64 (see **Figure 99-2**). Thus, prevention of hypoglycemia among older adults should be an important priority in the management of diabetes. **Table 99-15** summarizes the risk factors for hypoglycemia in an older patient with diabetes. The primary risk factor is iatrogenic: prescription of insulin or a sulfonylurea. Other risk factors are physiologic changes associated with aging, which may be difficult to prevent, and health behaviors that can be modified through targeted interventions.

Impairment of autonomic nervous system reflexes can contribute to risk for hypoglycemia. Aging is associated with a decrease in β-adrenergic receptor function, which is an important part of the body's counterregulation to combat hypoglycemia. As a result, the sympathoadrenal system that stimulates catecholamine secretion to induce the rapid elevation of blood glucose levels is less effective. Some older patients may have autonomic neuropathy because of long-standing diabetes or other causes, and many older patients are treated with antiadrenergic agents for CVD. For example, β-adrenergic blocking drugs can potentially interfere with counterregulation of hypoglycemia. Given the substantial benefit of β-adrenergic blockade to patients with CVD, combination with insulin or a sulfonylurea should be avoided and other glucose-lowering drugs used if possible.

Fortunately, the counterregulatory system is redundant. Glucose counterregulation can be maintained quite well as long as there is an adequate glucagon response even when the adrenergic nervous system is blocked. However, normal aging is associated with reduced glucagon responses to hypoglycemia, and older adults with type 2 diabetes have further impairment in glucagon responses to hypoglycemia when compared to age-matched control subjects. The growth hormone response to hypoglycemia is reduced with normal aging, and it is also further impaired in older adults with type 2 diabetes. Epinephrine and cortisol responses are similar or reduced in older adults with type 2 diabetes.

Patients who have relatively poor nutrition and an irregular meal pattern are at increased risk of hypoglycemia, in part because of inadequate maintenance of muscle and liver glycogen stores. Use of alcohol or a sedating agent should be avoided in patients receiving hypoglycemic agents, particularly if an aggressive treatment program is being pursued. Clearly, a cognitive disorder will interfere with recognition of hypoglycemia and possibly affect decisions about responding to hypoglycemia. Patients with underlying renal or hepatic insufficiency may have problems eliminating insulin or a sulfonylurea. Insulin is partly cleared by the kidney, and the insulin dose must often be reduced substantially in patients with renal insufficiency. A patient with severe hepatic insufficiency may have difficulty mobilizing a counterregulatory increase of glucose production. Finally, any complex drug regimen may include agents that influence the pharmacokinetics of insulin or a sulfonylurea, or counterregulatory or behavioral responses to hypoglycemia, and therefore should be an issue when considering risk for hypoglycemia. Older adults often have impairments in vision, dexterity, and mobility, which may limit their ability to self-monitor for hypoglycemia and react quickly to avoid more disastrous consequences.

Despite all these issues and concerns, the availability of newer drug classes means that many older patients with diabetes can be treated aggressively with low risk for hypoglycemia. Even if insulin or a sulfonylurea must be part of the regimen, the risk for hypoglycemia may be reduced by assessing the patient's overall health and social support status thoroughly on a regular basis, providing a strong educational program focused on hypoglycemia recognition and treatment, and considering and perhaps intervening on the risk factors outlined in **Table 99-15**.

TABLE 99-15 ■ RISK FACTORS FOR HYPOGLYCEMIA IN OLDER DIABETIC PATIENTS
Therapeutic
Insulin
Sulfonylurea
Physiologic
Impaired autonomic nervous system function
Diminished glucagon secretion
Kidney or liver failure
Cognitive disorder
Sensory impairment (vision, hearing)
Functional impairment (mobility, hand dexterity)
Behavioral
Poor or irregular nutrition
Use of alcohol or another sedating agent
Others
Polypharmacy

Hyperosmolar Coma and Diabetic Ketoacidosis

DKA and hyperosmolar coma are the extreme examples of impaired metabolism in patients with diabetes mellitus. DKA is relatively uncommon in older people, but it can occur in an older patient with type 1 diabetes mellitus. As in younger people, the hallmarks of DKA are substantial hyperglycemia, hyperosmolarity, and volume depletion, and the presence of systemic acidosis caused by marked elevation of ketoacids. Ketoacids result from metabolism of elevated free fatty acids released by lipolysis as a result of severe insulin deficiency. DKA can occur in a patient with type 1 diabetes when insulin is inappropriately discontinued, but in an older adult, DKA may be a result of a major underlying illness that interferes with the patient's self-care capability. In the setting of severe coexisting major illness in an older individual and decreased tissue perfusion, lactic acidosis may occur in the setting of hyperglycemia. Thus, it is important to document the presence of significant ketonemia to ensure that DKA is contributing to the systemic acidosis observed. Treatment of DKA should focus on immediate insulin replacement to inhibit lipolysis and reverse the ketoacidosis, vigorous replacement of fluids and salt to replace losses, and a thorough evaluation to identify underlying illness. Careful monitoring is required to ensure response and particularly to monitor the cardiovascular system for signs of failure.

Hyperosmolar coma, which occurs primarily in older people, is characterized by marked hyperglycemia, hyperosmolality, severe volume depletion, and associated renal insufficiency. The mortality rate is high because there is often a severe underlying illness such as pneumonia or a cerebrovascular accident. Metabolic acidosis is notably absent, or, if present, it is caused by lactic acid rather than ketoacids. The reason for failure to mobilize fatty acids despite severe insulin deficiency in these patients is unclear. While insulin should be provided as part of the initial therapy, the focus should be on volume and sodium replacement and on identification and intervention for major underlying illness. In fact, as volume status is corrected, in the presence of recovering renal function, glucose levels can fall precipitously. Therefore, attention must be paid to avoidance of hypoglycemia.

Diabetes in Long-Term Care Facilities

Diabetes mellitus is very common among nursing home residents. Based on national surveys the prevalence of diabetes mellitus in nursing homes is 26% in men and 22% in women. Residents in nursing homes who have diabetes, compared to those without diabetes, tend to have a greater disease burden, are more likely to be frail and have cognitive decline, and have an increased risk for aspiration pneumonia and fecal incontinence. Because of the degree of disability and limited life expectancy of these patients, basic diabetes care should usually be the goal, rather than a stringent set of goals for A1C, BP, or lipids. In fact, based

on several observational studies, residents in long-term care facilities have better survival if their A1C levels are higher, between 8% and 9%. This goal is consistent with the recommendations for those in poor health listed in **Table 99-6.**

When prescribing medications, particularly hypoglycemic and hypotensive agents, several limitations common among nursing facilities should be considered: non-RN aides (eg, licensed practical nurse or pharmacy technician) usually administer the medications, low staff to resident ratio, and staff may be less trained to understand the risks associated with these agents and have limited ability to recognize and treat hypoglycemia rapidly. The staff may also have limited ability to provide residents' meals in a timely fashion after administration of rapid-acting insulin. Except for residents who have type 1 diabetes, few nursing home residents with diabetes require frequent insulin injections as tight glucose control is not recommended. However, a simple short-acting insulin regimen may be safer for those patients who require insulin but whose nutrient intake is irregular. For example, short-acting insulin can be given immediately **after** nutrient ingestion, which allows adjustment for the actual intake.

As undernutrition may be a much more important health problem than obesity for nursing home patients, diet therapy should focus on matching caloric intake to meet nutritional needs rather than restriction of calories. Nursing home residents may lose weight for a variety of reasons, and weight loss in older adults is associated with increased risk of death. Some common causes of weight loss in nursing home residents are depression, swallowing problems, poor dentition, restrictive diet (eg, low-salt, and low-cholesterol diet), and occult infection. Thus, assessment for preventable causes of weight loss should be performed. Furthermore, for a nursing home patient with limited remaining life expectancy, the priority should be to stimulate the patient's appetite and take advantage of opportunities for the patient to enjoy life, rather than introduction of unnecessary dietary restrictions. Consistency of caloric intake is important for a patient treated with insulin and may be a particular challenge for a disabled nursing home resident. The facility dietician can play a key role by educating facility aides and nurses in appropriate estimates of consumption.

Similarly, regular physical activities should be provided for residents in a safely monitored environment. Both aerobic and resistance exercise may improve physical function, decrease injurious falls, decrease depression, improve cognition, and decrease agitated behavior in this setting.

In nursing home patients already at high risk for developing urinary tract infection, diabetes may further increase this risk because of bladder dysfunction secondary to autonomic neuropathy. Particular attention should be paid to keeping the bladder free of infection and carrying

TABLE 99-16 ■ RECOMMENDED PRINCIPAL GOALS FOR DIABETES CARE OF PATIENTS AT THE END OF LIFE

Be respectful and supportive

- Provision of an appropriate level of intervention according to stage of illness, symptom profile, and respect for dignity
- Supporting the individual patient (in diabetes self-management) and caregivers to the last possible stage

Avoid pain or discomfort

- Provision of a painless and symptom-free death
- Tailoring glucose-lowering therapy and monitoring to minimize burden of the treatment and adverse treatment effects
- Avoiding metabolic decompensation and diabetes-related emergencies such as frequent and unnecessary hypoglycemia, diabetic ketoacidosis, hyperosmolar hyperglycemic state, or persistent symptomatic hyperglycemia
- Glucose target between 6 mmol/L (108 mg/dL) and 15 mmol/L (270 mg/dL)
- Avoiding foot complications in frail, bed-bound patients with diabetes
- Avoiding symptomatic clinical volume depletion

Tailoring treatment plan according to four stages of the end of life

- Stage A—Diagnosis stable with year plus prognosis
  ○ Evaluate the time to benefit of some cardioprotective therapies, and consider withdrawal or dose reductions on some therapies (eg, ACE inhibitors/ARBs, aspirin, statins)
  ○ Evaluate oral intake and weight stability, and consider dose reduction of antiglycemic agents to avoid hypoglycemia

- Stage B—Unstable/advanced disease with months prognosis
  ○ Simplify antiglycemic regimens
  ○ Relax dietary restrictions, particularly among patients with poor oral intakes
- Stage C—Deteriorating with weeks prognosis
  ○ Discuss with caregivers and patients, consider relaxing glucose targets
  ○ Avoid long-acting sulfonylureas
- Stage D—Final days/terminal care with days prognosis
  ○ For patients with type 2 diabetes and diet controlled/metformin treated → stop monitoring glucose
  ○ For patients with type 2 diabetes on other oral antiglycemics/insulin/GLP-1 agonists → stop pills and GLP-1 injections and consider stopping insulin depending on dose
    - If insulin stopped, urinalysis for glucose daily → if over 2+ glucose, check capillary blood glucose
      - If blood glucose over 20 mmol/L (360 mg/dL) → 6 unit rapid-acting insulin and recheck glucose after 2 h
      - If > 2 doses of rapid-acting insulin per day → consider daily long-acting insulin (eg, glargine)
    - If insulin to continue → once-daily morning dose of glargine based on 25% less than total previous daily insulin dose
      - Check daily blood glucose after an afternoon snack → ↓ insulin by 10%–20% if < 8 mmol/L (144 mg/dL) or ↑ insulin by 10%–20% if > 20 mmol/L (360 mg/dL)
  ○ For patients with type 1 diabetes, continue insulin at reduced dose and monitor and adjust dose as above

Data from Diabetes UK: End of life diabetes care: clinical care recommendations. 2nd ed. October 2013.

out intermittent catheterization as needed. Careful attention to skin and foot care is important to avoid problems with healing and infection.

Palliative and End-of-Life Care

When an older adult with diabetes is transitioning to palliative care or end-of-life care, the patient and the provider may choose to modify the diabetes treatment goals and intensity of care. Strict glucose, lipid, and blood pressure control may no longer be appropriate, and deprescribing of some drugs may be considered. For example, withdrawal of lipid-lowering therapy may be reasonable. Appropriate diabetes care for patients at the end of life currently lacks quality standards and guidance on best clinical practices. Diabetes UK (formerly British Diabetes Association) commissioned a panel of professional groups and developed recommendations on diabetes care at the end of life. These recommendations are endorsed by the UK National Health Service. The panel recognized that no published evidence justifies specific glucose or hemoglobin A1C targets for end-of-life diabetes care management. The optimal glucose

range will vary according to the stage of illness, ability of the patient to eat and drink normally, the presence of hypoglycemia, the nutritional status, and the treatment given. The panel recommended glucose control target ranges between 6 mmol/L (108 mg/dL) to 15 mmol/L (270 mg/dL). Several principal goals for diabetes care of patients at the end of life were recommended as described in **Table 99-16**.

Based on the prognosis, the panel made detailed recommendations on different approaches to control glucose. Patients with diabetes near the end of life may still require hypoglycemic drugs and monitoring in order to stay comfortable. Severe hyperglycemia such as 350 mg/dL or higher may impair comfort if it leads to thirst, dehydration, infections, urinary incontinence, and falls. A more complicated glucose-lowering regimen that requires more monitoring may be appropriate if the prognosis is several months to a year, whereas minimizing glucose-lowering treatment and monitoring needs would be appropriate if the prognosis is days to weeks. The UK Diabetes recommendations were last updated in November, 2021.

American Diabetes Association. Standards of medical care in diabetes—2021. *Diabetes Care.* 2021;44(suppl 1): Classification and diagnosis of diabetes (S15-S33), prevention or delay of type 2 diabetes (S34-S39), and older adults (S168–S179).

Blaum C, Cigolle CT, Boyd C, et al. Clinical complexity in middle-aged and older adults with diabetes: the Health and Retirement Study. *Med Care.* 2010;48: 327–334.

Booth GL, Kapral MK, Fung K, Tu JV. Relation between age and cardiovascular disease in men and women with diabetes compared with non-diabetic people: a population-based retrospective cohort study. *Lancet.* 2006;368:29–36.

Cefalu WT, Kaul S, Gerstein HC, et al. Cardiovascular outcomes trials in type 2 diabetes: where do we go from here? Reflections from a *Diabetes Care* editors' expert forum. *Diabetes Care.* 2018;41(1):14–31.

Centers for Disease Control and Prevention. National Diabetes Statistics Report, 2020. Atlanta, GA: Centers for Disease Control and Prevention, US Dept of Health and Human Services; 2020.

Chang AM, Halter JB. Aging and insulin secretion. *Am J Physiol Endocrinol Metab.* 2003;284:E7–E12.

Cigolle CT, Blaum CS, Halter JB. Diabetes and cardiovascular disease prevention in older adults. *Clin Geriatri Med.* 2009;25:607–641.

Cigolle CT, Kabeto MU, Lee PG, Blaum CS. Clinical complexity and mortality in middle-aged and older adults with diabetes. *J Gerontol A Biol Sci Med Sci.* 2012;67(12):1313–1320.

de Boer IH, Bangalore S, Benetos A, et al. Diabetes and hypertension: a position statement by the American Diabetes Association. *Diabetes Care.* 2017;40(9):1273–1284.

Diabetes Prevention Program Research Group. Long-term effects of lifestyle intervention or metformin on diabetes development and microvascular complications over 15-year follow-up: the Diabetes Prevention Program Outcomes Study. *Lancet Diabetes Endocrinol.* 2015;3(11):866–875.

Geijselaers SL, Sep SJ, Stehouwer CD, Biessels GJ. Glucose regulation, cognition, and brain MRI in type 2 diabetes: a systematic review. *Lancet Diabetes Endocrinol.* 2015;3(1):75–89.

Halter JB. Diabetes mellitus in an aging population: the challenge ahead. *J Gerontol A Biol Sci Med Sci.* 2012;67(12):1297–1299.

Halter JB, Musi N, McFarland Horne F, et al. Diabetes and cardiovascular disease in older adults: current status and future directions. *Diabetes.* 2014;63:2578–2589.

Holman RR, Paul SK, Bethel MA, et al. 10-year follow-up of intensive glucose control in type 2 diabetes. *N Engl J Med.* 2008;359(15):1577–1589.

Huang ES, Zhang Q, Gandra N, Chin MH, Meltzer DO. The effect of comorbid illness and functional status on the expected benefits of intensive glucose control in older patients with type 2 diabetes: a decision analysis. *Ann Intern Med.* 2008;149:11–19.

Inzucchi SE, Bergenstal RM, Buse JB, et al. Management of hyperglycemia in type 2 diabetes, 2015: a patient-centered approach. Update to a position statement of the American Diabetes Association and the European Association for the Study of Diabetes. *Diabetes Care.* 2015;38:140–149.

James J, Hicks D, Sinclair A. https://trenddiabetes.online/portfolio/end-of-life-guidance-for-diabetes-care/ [trenddiabetes.online]. Accessed January 28, 2022.

Kirkman MS, Briscoe VJ, Clark N, et al. Diabetes in older adults: a consensus report. *J Am Geriatr Soc.* 2012; 60(12):2342–2356 and *Diabetes Care.* 2012;35(12): 2650–2664.

Laiteerapong N, Huang ES. Chapter 16. Diabetes in older adults. In: Cowie CC, Casagrande SS, Menke A, et al., eds. *Diabetes in America*, 3rd ed. Bethesda, MD: National Institute of Diabetes and Digestive and Kidney Diseases (US); 2018 Aug.

Lee P, Halter JB. The pathophysiology of hyperglycemia in older adults: clinical considerations. *Diabetes Care.* 2017;40(4):444–452.

LeRoith D, Biessels GJ, Braithwaite SS, et al. Treatment of diabetes in older adults: an Endocrine Society clinical practice guideline. *J Clin Endocrinol Metab.* 2019;104(5): 1520–1574.

Lipska KJ, Krumholz H, Soones T, Lee SJ. Polypharmacy in the aging patient: a review of glycemic control in older adults with type 2 diabetes. *JAMA.* 2016;315(10): 1034–1045.

Munshi MN, Florez H, Huang ES, et al. Management of diabetes in long-term care and skilled nursing facilities: a position statement of the American Diabetes Association. *Diabetes Care.* 2016;39:308–318.

Pratley RE, Kanapka LG, Rickels MR, et al. Wireless Innovation for Seniors With Diabetes Mellitus (WISDM) Study Group. Effect of continuous glucose monitoring on hypoglycemia in older adults with type 1 diabetes: a randomized clinical trial. *JAMA.* 2020;323:2397–2406.

Punthakee Z, Miller ME, Launer LJ, et al. Poor cognitive function and risk of severe hypoglycemia in type 2 diabetes: post hoc epidemiologic analysis of the ACCORD trial. *Diabetes Care.* 2012;35(4):787–793.

Rejeski WJ, Ip EH, Bertoni AG, et al.; Look AHEAD Research Group. Lifestyle change and mobility in obese adults with type 2 diabetes. *N Engl J Med.* 2012;366: 1209–1217.

Resnick HE, Heineman J, Stone R, Shorr RI. Diabetes in U.S. nursing homes, 2004. *Diabetes Care.* 2008; 31:287.

Seaquist ER, Anderson J, Childs B, et al. Hypoglycemia and diabetes: a report of a workgroup of the American Diabetes Association and the Endocrine Society. *Diabetes Care.* 2013;36(5):1384–1395.

Tuttle KR, Bakris GL, Bilous RW, et al. Diabetic kidney disease: a report from an ADA Consensus Conference. *Diabetes Care.* 2014;37:2864–2883.

Villareal DT, Chode S, Parimi N, et al. Weight loss, exercise, or both and physical function in obese older adults. *N Engl J Med.* 2011;364(13):1218–1229.

Whitmer RA, Karter AJ, Yaffe K, Quesenberry CP Jr, Selby JV. Hypoglycemic episodes and risk of dementia in older patients with type 2 diabetes mellitus. *JAMA.* 2009;301(15):1565–1572.

Wray LA, Ofstedal MB, Langa KM, Blaum CS. The effect of diabetes on disability in middle-aged and older adults. *J Gerontol Med Sci.* 2005;60A:1206.

Myopathies, Polymyalgia Rheumatica, and Giant Cell Arteritis

Vivek Nagaraja

Healthy muscle contributes to metabolic processes and functional status in humans. Myopathies are not uncommon in older adults, and when present, magnify the effects of age-related decline in muscle structure, mass, and function. This chapter reviews the common myopathies seen in older people as well as polymyalgia rheumatica and giant cell arteritis. Please see Chapter 49 for age-related changes in muscle and sarcopenia.

CLINICAL EVALUATION OF MUSCLE DISEASE SYMPTOMS IN OLDER PEOPLE

The age-unrestricted list of conditions that can cause muscle disease symptoms is extensive. Candidate conditions are typically categorized as either acquired (autoimmune, endocrine disorder-related, toxin or drug-associated, amyloid, infectious, cancer-related, and others) or inherited (muscular dystrophies, metabolic myopathies, muscle channelopathies). The approach to the individual with myopathic symptoms is not age-specific, but the results must account for age-related variations within each component of the evaluation (see **Figure 100-1**). Most importantly, it is essential to factor in the coexistent medical conditions, impact on the activities of daily living (ADL) and instrumental activities of daily living (IADL), and the risks versus benefits of initiating the treatments for the underlying medical condition.

History

As most extremity muscle bulk is proximal, symptoms of myopathic weakness tend to be associated with shoulder and hip girdle motions. Patients may report the inability to perform a specific task due to weakness or poor stamina in performing tasks once readily accomplished. Independence with ADLs, maintenance of balance and gait, and freedom from falling should be addressed as all are sustained in part

Learning Objectives

- Be able to characterize common muscle disorders of aging.
- Contrast the clinical presentation and management of polymyalgia rheumatica and giant cell arteritis.

Key Clinical Points

1. Most myopathies tend to present with proximal (large) muscle group involvement.
2. Inclusion body myositis (IBM), a gradual and insidious loss of muscle mass and strength, is associated with characteristic histology and normal to mildly elevated muscle enzyme levels. It is the most common form of inflammatory myositis in older adults.
3. Older adults are at risk for multiple drug-induced myopathies, including those related to corticosteroids, heavy ethanol use, and lipid-lowering agents.

by maintaining muscle strength. Muscle pain is an uncommon symptom of primary myopathy in older people. It can be seen in polymyalgia rheumatica (PMR) or a regional or generalized musculoskeletal disorder, such a rotator cuff tendinopathy, subacromial or trochanteric bursitis, or fibromyalgia syndrome.

Examination

Documenting the severity of initial and serial assessments of muscle strength should be based on the MRC grading scale of 0 to 5. The healthy older person should sustain

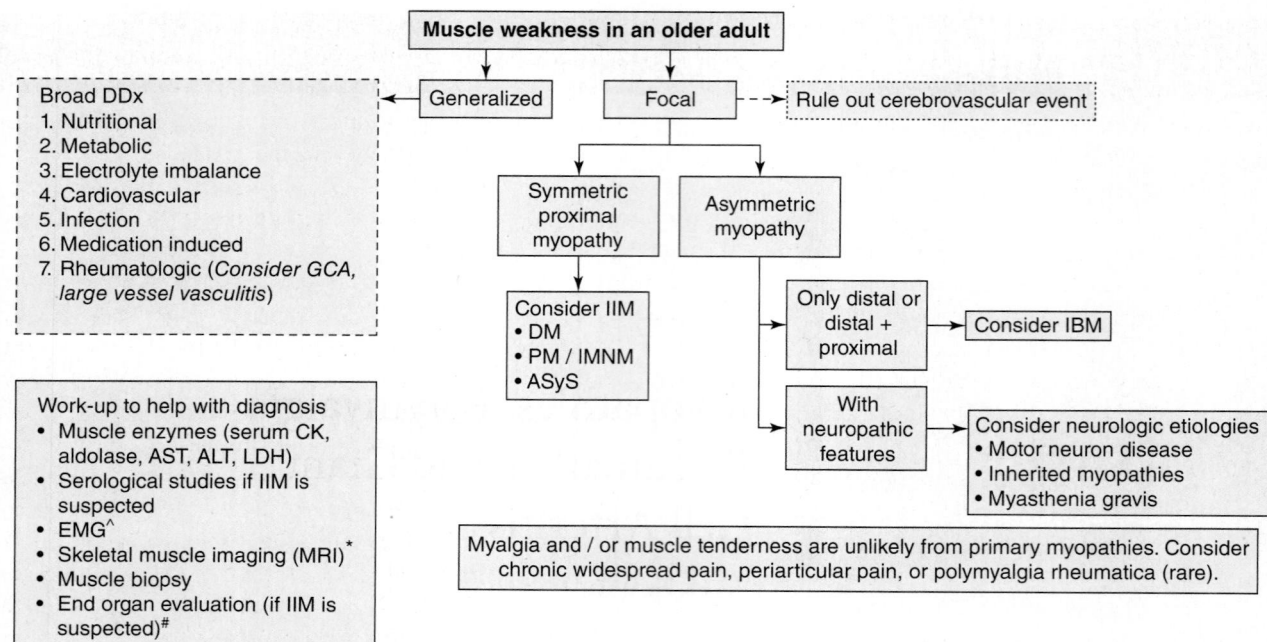

ALT, alanine aminotransferase; AST, aspartate aminotransferase; ASyS, anti-synthetase syndrome; CK, creatine kinase; DDx, differential diagnosis; DM, dermatomyositis; EMG, electromyography; GCA, giant cell arteritis; IBM, inclusion body myositis; IIM, idiopathic inflammatory myopathy; IMNM, immune-mediated necrotizing myopathy; LDH, lactate dehydrogenase; MRI, magnetic resonance imaging; PM, polymyositis.
^EMG and skeletal muscle MRI can help in localizing a site for muscle biopsy.
*MRI can demonstrate areas of muscle inflammation, edema with active myositis, fibrosis, and calcification.
#IIM can be associated with skin, lung, joint, and can sometimes overlap with other systemic rheumatic diseases.

FIGURE 100-1. Approach to evaluation of myopathy in older adults.

muscle contraction against full resistance for 2 to 4 seconds, usually allotted to test individual muscles. More physiologically complex yet standard functional assessments, such as arising from a chair without the use of the arms, measuring the time necessary to perform this maneuver 5 to 10 times, or squatting from the standing position then arising without assistance, should be accomplished without difficulty by normal younger adults but may be difficult even for the healthy older person. The distribution of weakness may provide clues as to broad categorical etiologies: symmetric proximal extremity weakness with a normal neurologic exam suggests a myopathy, whereas distal weakness, distal and proximal weakness, or asymmetric weakness, suggests an underlying neuropathic problem or inclusion body myositis (IBM). Compared with objective muscle weakness, muscle tenderness is a less common finding in most primary myopathies. Muscle tenderness in older people, without demonstrated significant weakness, may be seen with fibromyalgia (chronic widespread pain), regional musculoskeletal disorders (focal findings), and rarely in some patients with PMR (symmetric proximal extremities).

Laboratory Markers

Routine laboratory measurements of electrolytes (sodium, potassium, calcium, magnesium, and phosphorous) and muscle enzymes (primarily creatine kinase [CK] and aldolase, secondarily AST, ALT, and LDH) are essential components of muscle disease evaluation. Older people have an age-related decrease in CK and aldolase-specific activity per unit DNA in muscle. Despite this fall in mean CK levels with age, the diagnostic accuracy of an elevated CK level in patients older than age 65 with histologically proven myopathy is equal to that in patients younger than age 65 in two retrospective studies.

Electromyography

Electromyogram (EMG) assessment can identify myopathic changes that help to distinguish myopathy from neuropathic causes of motor weakness such as motor neuron disease, peripheral polyneuropathy, or myasthenia gravis. Changes in the voluntary motor unit action potentials (MUAP) and spontaneous muscle electrical activity on EMG can categorize muscle symptoms as arising primarily from either muscle or nerve and provide information on the distribution and severity. If done serially, the progression of myopathic changes can be tracked. MUAP duration best distinguishes between myopathy and neuropathy: total duration increases in neuropathies but decreases in myopathies. Other myopathic findings include MUAPs of small amplitude and polyphasic composition. Increased needle insertional activity (increased in damaged muscles, decreased in muscles replaced by fat or scarring) and spontaneous activity (fibrillation potentials [a degenerating muscle fiber with an unstable membrane fires spontaneously at a regular rate] and positive sharp waves [needle touching damaged, degenerating fibers]) are features of inflammatory myopathy. Older people have a slight tendency toward prolonged MUAP duration and a small increase in the proportion of polyphasic potentials. These changes are due to denervation followed by intramuscular axonal spouting from neighboring axons and reinnervation as described above. This process occurs slowly, and thus the typical features of active degeneration—fibrillations and positive sharp waves—are not seen with aging alone. EMG assessment of a cool limb will also produce a higher percentage of increased duration, polyphasic potentials, and reduced spontaneous activity. During EMG testing, this must be considered in older people, who are at increased risk for cool limbs from circulatory insufficiency and reduced insulation (subcutaneous fat). EMG can be used to identify the muscle group that is likely to provide helpful information on biopsy. However, muscle biopsy should not be performed on a muscle that has recently undergone EMG testing.

Imaging of the Skeletal Muscles

Magnetic resonance imaging (MRI) can demonstrate muscle inflammation, edema with active myositis, fibrosis, and calcification. Unlike muscle biopsy, MRI can assess large areas of muscle (eg, both thighs and both arms), thereby avoiding problems with sampling error. However, MRI is nonspecific and may not distinguish the changes of myositis from those that occur in rhabdomyolysis, muscular dystrophy, or metabolic myopathy. To minimize the sampling error from muscle biopsy and to increase the yield of diagnostic information, MRI can be a noninvasive option to identify the muscle group for biopsy. Musculoskeletal ultrasound is a less expensive and less time-consuming technology than MRI. However, there is not as much experience with ultrasound as MRI, and skeletal muscle ultrasound remains operator-dependent.

Muscle Biopsy

Clinical features—history, exam, laboratories, EMG, and MRI—infrequently provide a diagnosis of a specific muscular disorder. Therefore, muscle biopsy is often necessary to confirm a diagnosis and to provide a basis for therapy. In most clinical circumstances, satisfactory muscle samples for evaluation can be provided by either open or percutaneous techniques. Complimentary tissue stains are chosen to evaluate general muscle morphology and fiber typing and distribution, and screening tests are chosen to evaluate enzyme deficiencies and storage diseases. Based on autopsy and muscle biopsy studies, muscle biopsy specimens from older people show an increased frequency of type II muscle fiber atrophy, type II fiber-specific decline in muscle satellite cell content, neurogenic changes (including fiber type grouping, angular atrophic fibers, target or "targetoid" fibers), and changes indicating mitochondrial dysfunction (ragged red fibers, and fibers staining negative for cytochrome c oxidase

[COX] with concomitant increase in succinate dehydrogenase [SDH] activity). In addition, findings of necrosis, cytoplasmic bodies, ring-fibers, and fibers with increased central nuclei have been noted in muscle specimens from those older than age 70. Clinically, the diagnostic accuracy of muscle biopsy findings for inflammatory myopathy in patients aged 65 and older approximates younger adults.

MYOPATHIES IN OLDER PEOPLE

Table 100-1 provides a more specific list of conditions that should be considered in the older patient suspected of having a myopathy. These diseases, both primary muscular diseases, and diseases or drug-related syndromes with symptomatology in the muscular system, represent a more focused list of inflammatory and noninflammatory conditions and assume a comprehensive evaluation has excluded electrolyte disturbances, organ failure syndromes and rhabdomyolysis as causes of weakness. These disorders can also be separated into those causing primarily proximal muscle weakness or spinal weakness. The discussion to follow will survey these diseases, highlighting clinical findings of presentation or therapy that are more distinctive in older patients.

TABLE 100-1 ■ MYOPATHIES MORE SPECIFIC FOR THE OLDER PERSON

Acquired Myopathies
- *Idiopathic inflammatory myopathies*
  - Dermatomyositis
  - Polymyositis
  - Immune-mediated necrotizing myopathy
  - Anti-synthetase syndrome
  - Sporadic inclusion body myositis
- *Endocrine/metabolic diseases*
  - Thyroid disease
  - Osteomalacia
- *Amyloid myopathy*
- *Drug-induced myopathies*
  - Corticosteroids
  - Alcohol
  - Colchicine
  - Lipid-lowering agents
  - Immune checkpoint inhibitors
  - Hydroxychloroquine

Inherited Myopathies
- *Late-onset muscular dystrophies*
  - Facioscapulohumeral dystrophy
  - Oculopharyngeal dystrophy
  - Late-onset limb girdle dystrophy
- *Late-onset mitochondrial myopathy*
- *Paraspinal myopathies*
  - Bent spine syndrome (camptocormia)
  - Dropped head syndrome

Idiopathic Inflammatory Myopathies

The idiopathic inflammatory myopathies (IIM) are the most common cause of primary myopathy in older people. These conditions share to varying degrees findings of slowly progressive muscle weakness, which is usually symmetric and proximal, elevated serum levels of muscle enzymes, and characteristic changes of an inflammatory myopathy on muscle histopathology. In addition, extramuscular manifestations may include constitutional symptoms, dysphagia, cutaneous features, arthritis, and cardiopulmonary involvement. In 2017, the European League Against Rheumatism (EULAR) and the American College of Rheumatology (ACR) developed and validated revised classification criteria for adult IIMs and their significant subgroups.

The EULAR/ACR criteria classify patients as having "definite," "probable," and "possible" disease based on a score and corresponding probability of disease. This classification approach identifies up to 16 distinct clinical, serologic, and muscle biopsy variables. The broad categories of the IIMs based on their antibody subsets and clinical phenotypes are described in **Table 100-2**.

Dermatomyositis (DM), Polymyositis (PM), Immune-Mediated Necrotizing Myopathy (IMNM), and Anti-Synthetase Syndrome (ASyS)

Patients with classic **dermatomyositis (DM)** typically present with symmetric proximal muscle weakness, elevated muscle enzymes, and characteristic cutaneous findings.

TABLE 100-2 ■ ASSOCIATIONS OF MYOSITIS-SPECIFIC AUTOANTIBODIES IN INFLAMMATORY MYOPATHIES

AUTOANTIBODY	TARGET AUTOANTIGEN AND FUNCTION	FREQUENCY IN IDIOPATHIC INFLAMMATORY MYOPATHIES, %	CLINICAL PHENOTYPE
Anti-ARS	ARS—intracytoplasmic protein synthesis		Antisynthetase syndrome myositis, mechanic's hand, Gottron papules, arthritis, fever, high frequency of interstitial pneumonitis; sometimes clinically amyopathic
Anti-Jo-1	Histidyl	15–20	
Anti-PL-7	Threonyl	5–10	
Anti-PL-12	Alanyl	< 5	
Anti-EJ	Glycyl	5–10	
Anti-OJ	Isoleucyl	< 5	
Anti-KS	Asparaginyl	< 5	
Anti-Ha	Tyrosyl	< 1	
Anti-Zo	Phenylalanyl	< 1	
Anti-200/100	HMGCR (3-hydroxy-3-methylglutaryl-coenzyme A reductase)	40% of necrotizing myopathy	Immune-mediated necrotizing myopathy, frequently associated with prior statin use
Anti-SRP	SRP—intracytoplasmic protein translocation (six polypeptides and RNP 7SLRNA)	5–10	Acute-onset necrotizing myopathy (severe weakness, high CK, frequent myocardial involvement); may be refractory to treatment
Anti-Mi-2	Helicase protein—nuclear transcription (forms the NuRD complex)	5–30	Adult DM and JDM (classical DM, often sudden onset, generally without ILD or malignancy, milder muscle disease with good response to treatment)
Anti-p155/140	TIF1-γ (p155)—nuclear transcription + cellular differentiation	15%–25% adult DM 40%–75% cancer-associated DM 30% juvenile DM	CAM in adult DM; severe cutaneous disease in adult DM and JDM
Anti-MJ	NXP-2—nuclear transcription + RNA metabolism	< 5; 25% juvenile DM	JDM with calcinosis
Anti-SAE	SAE—posttranslational modification (targets include transcription factors)	5	Adult DM; may present with CADM first
Anti-CADM-140	Intracytoplasmic MDA5—innate immune	50% of CADM	CADM; rapidly progressive interstitial pneumonia
Anti-PMS1	Subunit of a DNA-binding protein complex	7.5	Rare DM and PM

ARS, aminoacyl-tRNA synthetase; CADM, cancer-associated dermatomyositis; CAM, cancer-associated myositis; ILD, interstitial lung disease; JDM, juvenile dermatomyositis; MDA5, melanoma-differentiation associated gene 5; NA, not applicable; NuRD, nucleosome remodeling histone deacetylase; NXP-2, nuclear matrix protein NXP-2; SAE, small-ubiquitin-like modifier activating enzyme; SRP, signal recognition particle; TIF1- γ, transcriptional intermediary factor 1-gamma.

Adapted with permission from Lazarou IN, Guerne PA. Classification, diagnosis, and management of idiopathic inflammatory myopathies. J Rheumatol. 2013;40(5):550–564.

Patients presenting with weakness and elevated muscle enzymes in the absence of characteristic cutaneous findings of DM present a more complex diagnostic challenge. There are no specific cutaneous findings of other IIMs, and diagnostic serologic tests are less likely to be present. Historically, such patients were diagnosed with PM if the muscle weakness involved proximal muscle groups. With the newer classifications of IMNM and ASyS, and some overlaps with IBM, the existence of PM as a distinct entity is being questioned. In an older study, before the EULAR/ACR classification, the estimated annual incidence for the clinically amyopathic subtype of DM was 0.2 per 100,000 persons, with a higher incidence in women.

The cardinal manifestation of DM is a symmetric proximal weakness of subacute onset. In some patients, the cutaneous or pulmonary features could precede the onset of muscle weakness. Several dermatologic features are described in DM: *Gottron's papules* (erythematous to violaceous papules that occur symmetrically over bony prominences, particularly the extensor [orsal] aspects of the metacarpophalangeal [MCP] and interphalangeal [IP] joints), *Heliotrope eruption* (erythematous to violaceous eruption on the periorbital skin, sometimes accompanied by eyelid edema), *facial erythema, shawl, Holster,* and *V-signs* (skin that demonstrates both hyperpigmentation and hypopigmentation, as well as telangiectasias and epidermal atrophy, over the neck, upper chest, upper back, and lateral aspect of the thighs), and *nail fold abnormalities* (cuticular hypertrophy, periungual erythema, and dilated/dropped out capillary loops). In a subtype of DM called clinically amyopathic DM (CADM), associated with antimelanoma differentiation-associated gene 5 (anti-MDA5) antibody, additional cutaneous features can be seen, namely diffuse hair loss, panniculitis, oral ulcers, and ulcers at the digital pulp/periungual region (30). Interstitial lung disease (ILD) can be present in varying frequencies (20%–80%) in DM and can sometimes precede the onset of myositis. Often, the presenting symptom is dyspnea, which, when present with underlying myositis, could be compounded by myopathy due to the involvement of the diaphragm or respiratory muscles. In evaluating cardiopulmonary symptoms in an older patient with DM, it is essential to utilize studies such as pulmonary function tests with maximum inspiratory and expiratory pressure assessments and high-resolution CT scan of the chest. Cardiac manifestations can be present in IIM and may include arrhythmia, congestive heart failure, myocarditis, pericarditis, angina, and fibrosis. Early myocardial involvement can be identified using cardiac magnetic resonance imaging techniques in IIM patients without any overt baseline left ventricular dysfunction by an echocardiogram.

The muscle biopsy specimens from patients with DM show evidence of injury to capillaries and perifascicular myofibers in the forms of myofiber necrosis, perifascicular atrophy, fibrosis, and regeneration in perifascicular regions near areas of connective tissue pathology. The earliest abnormality observed is the deposition of the membrane attack complex around small blood vessels. There may be suggestions of microinfarction mediated by blood vessel dysfunction, evident as abnormal muscle fibers are grouped in one portion of the fascicle. The predominant inflammatory infiltrate is seen in the perimysial and perivascular regions and comprises CD4+ T-cells, B-cells, dendritic cells, and macrophages. A pathognomonic feature is the increased expression of major histocompatibility complex (MHC) I on the muscle fibers (diffuse staining in PM, perifascicular staining in DM)—differentiating these conditions from dystrophies and certain metabolic myopathies causing mononuclear cell infiltrates. Advances in autoantibody detection have identified clinical subgroups of patients with either DM or myositis associated with malignancy. These myositis-specific autoantibodies define more homogeneous populations within the spectrum of the IIM, each with distinct clinical findings and immunogenetic associations (**Table 100-2**). The syndromes marked by these autoantibodies are more commonly seen in younger adults, with a mean age at diagnosis between 36 and 46, but can be seen in older people.

There is a strong association with specific malignancies in patients with DM, including ovarian, lung, pancreatic, stomach, and colorectal cancer. Approximately 15% of adult DM patients, especially those older than 40 years, have either a preexisting malignancy or will develop a malignancy in the future. In addition, the literature supports an association, based mainly on case-control and cohort studies, of DM with malignancy: up to 15% of patients with DM will have or develop an internal malignancy. Thus, in older people with DM, heightened awareness of the possibility of an underlying malignancy must be maintained. Although an intensive clinical evaluation to exclude an occult malignancy is not without patient risk. In addition, it is not cost-effective for all patients. Therefore, patients should complete gender-specific health care maintenance evaluations and investigations directed to determine the source of any abnormal sign or symptom uncovered through a comprehensive review of systems and physical examination.

Polymyositis (PM) Polymyositis is a term that was used traditionally to denote all IIMs that were not DM or sIBM. However, it is now a controversial entity with questionable specificity. PM is frequently misdiagnosed as it lacks a unique clinical phenotype. Common myopathies that have been misdiagnosed as PM include sIBM, DM, IMNM, overlap syndrome associated with a connective tissue disease (like systemic sclerosis), muscular dystrophies, myalgia syndromes, or toxic and endocrine myopathies. In the future, the term polymyositis could likely become obsolete as there is a refinement of the clinic-sero-pathologic classifications of IIMs.

Immune-mediated necrotizing myopathy IMNM is a group of inflammatory myopathies distinguished from PM in 2004.

Most IMNMs are associated with anti-signal recognition particle (anti-SRP) or anti-3-hydroxy-3-methylglutaryl-CoA reductase (anti-HMGCR) myositis-specific autoantibodies, although ~20% of patients with IMNM remain seronegative. Anti-SRP-positive IMNM tends to have a rapidly progressive proximal myopathy associated with high CK levels. Patients can frequently have dysphagia, ILD, and myocarditis. The prevalence of anti-HMGCR-positive IMNM ranges from 6% to 10% of IIMs, and anti-HMGCR-positive IMNM occurs more frequently in women older than 40 years. In patients positive for anti-HMGCR antibodies, the target of these autoantibodies is also the target of statins. Therefore, it has been hypothesized that statins may be a trigger of the disease. The percentage of statin exposure in these patients ranges from 15% to 65% depending on their geographic origin and age (90% of patients with anti-HMGCR-positive IMNM and older than 50 years have been exposed to statins). The presence of the MHC class II allele DRB1*11:01 confers a strong immunogenetic predisposition to anti-HMGCR-positive IMNM. Patients with anti-HMGCR-positive IMNMs tend to have proximal muscle involvement mainly in the lower extremities and often precedes upper extremity involvement. They tend not to have extramuscular features.

On muscle histopathology in patients with IMNM, the characteristic finding is the presence of necrotic muscle fibers. Necrotic myofibers exhibit the characteristics of different stages of necrotic and regenerating myofibres (ie, hyalinized, granular, myophagocytic, lytic, and regenerative). MHC class I on the sarcolemma is usually multifocal, whereas MHC class II is consistently absent from the sarcolemma. The inflammatory infiltrate is often minimal and, when present, tends to be CD 8+ T-cells with macrophages. Therefore, it is important to obtain a muscle biopsy from a muscle group with mild to moderate weakness. Muscle biopsies in patients who are chronically ill with myopathy will be of a low yield.

The disease course is often prolonged, and the main concerns are residual disability and mortality. In seropositive IMNM, muscle atrophy, residual weakness, and sarcopenia are quite profound due to the severity of the muscle damage. In older people, recovery can be expected to be prolonged as a consequence. Patients with seronegative and anti-HMGCR-positive IMNM must be screened for cancer. Patients with anti-SRP-positive IMNM must be screened for myocarditis, as these conditions have been associated with reduced survival for patients with these subclasses of IMNM.

Anti-synthetase syndrome ASyS is a complex autoimmune disorder characterized by the presence of autoantibodies against one of the aminoacyl-transfer (t)RNA synthetases, commonly anti-Jo1. It is a clinical syndrome including variable expression of myositis, ILD, polyarthritis, mechanic's hands (roughening and cracking of the skin of the tips and sides of the fingers), Raynaud's phenomenon, and fever. Both anti-PL7 and anti-PL12 are associated with more prevalent and severe ILD, whereas anti-Jo1 is associated with more intense muscle involvement. Independent of the autoantibody status, Black race is a significant prognostic factor for ILD severity in the United States. The severity of the myopathy tends to be milder compared to other DM subtypes. The anti-Ro-52 antibody can be commonly present with anti-Jo-1 and is associated with an increased tendency to cause arthritis, mechanics hands, and DM-specific skin findings. The 5-year mortality rate reported in different cohorts ranges from 88% to 97%, and the co-existence of ILD increases this risk.

Treatment for IIM remains a challenge, especially in older people. The low prevalence, wide phenotypic heterogeneity, and variable clinical course complicate the assessment of different treatment approaches, hence the absence of standardized therapeutic guidelines. Management needs to be multidisciplinary with experienced clinicians and rehabilitation therapists. Tailored rehabilitation programs under the supervision of a physical therapist are safe in all types of IIMs and are generally recommended to increase strength and reduce disability. There are no current FDA-approved treatments for IIM and few randomized controlled trials to guide treatment. Current treatment approaches are primarily empirical and based on large observational cohorts, case series, and expert opinion. Once the diagnosis is confirmed and co-existent medical conditions are carefully reviewed, systemic glucocorticoid therapy is the initial treatment of choice. However, it is rarely used as monotherapy because of its side effects, such as osteoporosis, hypertension, or weight gain. The route of administration (oral versus intravenous) is based on the acuity and severity of clinical presentation, need for hospitalization, and severity of extramuscular manifestations (for example, certain forms of ILD, arthritis, overlap with another systemic rheumatic disease). Glucocorticoid therapy is started at a high dose and gradually tapered over many weeks to months based on the physician's clinical judgment. Steroid-sparing therapies are initiated early in treatment to limit the cumulative dose of glucocorticoid, reduce glucocorticoid-related side effects, and maintain remission. These therapies include methotrexate, azathioprine (in patients with normal thiopurine methyltransferase activity), mycophenolate mofetil, ciclosporin, tacrolimus, and intravenous immunoglobulin. Special considerations in older people before initiating these therapies include coexistent medical conditions (especially liver or kidney disease to avoid drug toxicities), medication interactions, and certain unique aspects of the disease like ILD (where methotrexate is not preferred). Intravenous immunoglobulin has shown efficacy in DM and IMNM. For refractory forms of IIM, rituximab (a monoclonal antibody targeting the CD20 antigen on B lymphocytes) is preferred over cyclophosphamide due to decreased toxicity and better tolerance.

In recent years, few studies have addressed the differences in clinical manifestations, response to therapy, and prognosis between older and younger adults with IIM. In a comprehensive review of an older cohort, Marie and colleagues retrospectively analyzed 79 consecutive patients with PM-DM presenting to a university's clinic or hospital over 14 years. It is important to note that this study was conducted many years before identifying the newer IIM variants. Twenty-three (29%) of the patients were 65 years or older (9 men and 14 women, median age 69), 11 with DM, and 12 with PM. In comparing older with younger patients, there were no differences in the duration of symptoms prior to diagnosis or in frequencies of myositis diagnoses, Raynaud phenomenon, dysphonia, cardiac impairment, ILD, and peripheral neuropathy. There was a statistically higher frequency ($p < 0.05$) in the older cohort of esophageal dysfunction (35% vs 16%) and bacterial pneumonia (21% vs 5%), as well as a trend ($p = 0.12$) toward ventilatory insufficiency. Aspiration from esophageal dysfunction, combined with ventilatory insufficiency, were postulated factors leading to the higher frequency of pneumonia. The diagnostic accuracy of an elevated CK or aldolase, myopathic EMG findings, and characteristic inflammatory changes on muscle biopsy were similar to that in younger patients. However, older patients had a statistically higher frequency of elevated acute phase reactants and lower hemoglobin levels, total protein, and albumin. These latter findings may be owing to concurrent malignancy.

The response to therapy and outcome of older patients with PM-DM is poorer than in younger adults. Despite a similar distribution of most therapeutic modalities (steroids, azathioprine, intravenous immunoglobulin, methotrexate) between younger and older adults in the study of Marie, only 13.6% of older patients achieved complete remission of PM-DM versus 41% of younger patients. This trend is supported in previous reports. The age-specific mortality rate is also higher in older patients with PM-DM. Older age is but one of many described poor prognostic factors in PM-DM, including malignancy, gender, disease severity, ILD, dysphagia, bacterial pneumonia, delays in initiating therapy, and resistance to complications from therapy. It is therefore not surprising that older patients reported by Marie, who overall had a higher frequency of malignancy, dysphagia, bacterial pneumonia, and inability to induce remission with therapy versus younger patients, had a higher mortality rate as well: 48% versus 7%. Malignancies were directly responsible for six of the 11 deaths (54%) in older patients and bacterial pneumonia for four (36%). As the development of aspiration and ventilatory insufficiency is associated with bacterial pneumonia, an early assessment of esophageal and lung involvement in patients presenting with PM-DM can detect subclinical muscle involvement and early intervention, which may reduce subsequent morbidity and mortality.

Sporadic IBM and the hereditary inclusion body myopathies

The term IBM was first used in 1971 to describe patients with IIM whose muscle biopsies displayed degenerating muscle fibers with rimmed vacuoles and unique, tubulofilamentous nuclear and cytoplasmic inclusions. Patients with IBM are now separated into two distinct sets based on patterns of inheritance, clinical findings, muscle biopsy changes at the light- and electron-microscopic levels, and immunoreactivities demonstrated in the filaments: sporadic IBM (s-IBM) and the hereditary inclusion body myopathies (h-IBM). These two patient subsets share similar features on muscle biopsy. However, unlike in s-IBM, there is an absence of inflammatory change in muscle biopsy specimens from patients with h-IBM, hence the term inclusion body "myopathy," not "myositis."

S-IBM is the most common inflammatory myopathy in patients older than age 50, with a reported median age of 65 years at the time of diagnosis. The prevalence estimates range from five to seven cases per million, with more recent reports of up to 70 per million from Scandinavia. Older age of onset has been associated with a faster progression of weakness. As contrasted against PM and DM, s-IBM affects men two to three times more frequently than women and is more common in Caucasians than other races. The course of painless, proximal muscle weakness and atrophy develops insidiously, commonly over the years, often leading to a delay between the onset of symptoms and diagnosis. Unlike PM and DM, distal limb muscle involvement is seen in 50%, occurs early, and may predominate in up to one-third of patients. Quadriceps weakness, an early manifestation, is manifested as difficulty in climbing up or (more frequently) down a flight of stairs. Eventually, with progressing muscle weakness, getting out of a chair is difficult. Quadriceps weakness and knee giving-way may lead to an increased frequency of falling. The fall risk may be accentuated by co-existent medical conditions and polypharmacy in older adults. The tibialis anterior is frequently involved, leading to asymmetric and subtle foot drop further contributing to falls. In the clinic, "hopping on one leg" or "heel walk" can identify the early weakness of the tibialis anterior. A characteristic pattern of (often asymmetric) finger and wrist flexor, knee extensor, and ankle dorsiflexor weakness have been described. It may be specific enough to diagnose even when rimmed vacuoles and other characteristic histologic muscle biopsy findings are absent. Although interosseous muscles of the hand are generally spared, characteristic involvement of the flexor digitorum profundus and the flexor pollicis longus impairs the ability to oppose the thumb and index finger and perform fine motor movements, leading to significant disability. The prominent involvement of the quadriceps muscles may be severe enough in some patients that patellar reflexes are diminished, simulating an underlying neuropathy.

Rarely, cricopharyngeal involvement may lead to dysphagia and can precede limb weakness by years. The risk of aspiration is the highest in this group. Muscle enzymes are normal in approximately 20% and elevated no more than 12 times normal in most patients. A recently described autoantibody against cytosolic 5′-nucleotidase 1A (cN1A) has been recognized in patients with s-IBM. While not a diagnostic test, early studies have described good sensitivity (72%) and high specificity (92%). EMG findings are atypical in 30%, including the absence of inflammatory changes or the presence of a prominent neuropathic component. A small percentage of patients may have an associated autoimmune, infectious (most commonly viral), or another systemic inflammatory disease. There are at least 12 published criteria sets for s-IBM, which encompass at least 24 diagnostic categories. Categories include age threshold, symptom duration and progression, strength assessment, CK level, EMG findings, and histologic and immunoreactivity assessments on muscle pathology. A data-driven assessment of these patient variables demonstrated that the combination of (1) finger flexion or quadriceps weakness, (2) endomysial inflammation on biopsy, and (3) either invasion of nonnecrotic muscle fibers or rimmed vacuoles had 90% sensitivity and 96% specificity as diagnostic criteria.

The mechanisms that underlie the pathogenesis of s-IBM are not well understood. It should no longer be considered a myodegenerative disorder solely, and often cited reports of intramuscular accumulation of β-amyloid and tau proteins have been refuted. Current evidence suggests a more complicated pathophysiologic process that involves a genetic contribution (strong association with the HLADRB1 and the MHC8.1 haplotypes), immunologic activity (autoantibody to cN1A, T and B cells surrounding and displacing myofibers, B cell maturation, and differentiation within muscle in the absence follicles, active myeloid dendritic cells), and other abnormalities of unclear relationship to the immune system (nuclear degeneration, sarcoplasmic accumulation of normally nuclear nucleic acid-binding proteins, and loss of fast-twitch sarcomeric proteins).

Rehabilitation strategies, more so than medical treatments, play critical roles in disease management. A physical therapy program of strength training should be prescribed for all patients with s-IBM and will not elevate serum CK levels. The presence of foot drop or knee instability requires splinting or bracing, respectively, to prevent contractures and aid in ambulation. Dysphagia should prompt evaluation to assess the need for intravenous immunoglobulin (IVIg), esophageal dilation, botulinum toxin injections, or cricopharyngeal myotomy. Standard medical therapy for IIM—corticosteroids with or without immunosuppressive agents—does not stop disease progression. Immunosuppressive therapy in IBM has been helpful in IBM only in specific subgroups, such as those with rapid progression and creatine phosphokinase > 15 × upper limit of normal, or overlap with other autoimmune conditions. The use of steroids is associated with accelerated atrophy of type II fibers in IBM. This lack of improvement with medical therapy has been described as a clinical hallmark of the disease. Furthermore, corticosteroids decrease CK levels if even the underlying pathophysiology is not autoimmune, and CK level changes do not always correlate with changes in strength. A recent study demonstrated that those treated with immunosuppressive medication developed difficulty walking faster than untreated patients.

Endocrine/Metabolic Diseases

Thyroid disease Thyroid disease is prevalent in the older population. Hypothyroidism is more prevalent than hyperthyroidism (approximately 7% vs 2%, respectively), both conditions are more common in women than men, and either condition can lead to myopathic symptoms.

The diagnosis of hypothyroidism in older people can be difficult, as they present with fewer signs and symptoms and a diminished frequency of the classical signs of chilliness, paresthesias, weight gain, and cramps compared to younger patients. The prevalence of neuromuscular symptoms in patients with hypothyroidism is reported to be high (up to 80%) and includes weakness, muscle fatigue, and muscle cramps. Weakness is a common sign and symptom in older people with hypothyroidism, occurring in 53% of patients older than age 70 in one prospective study. Myopathic symptoms may rarely be the sole presenting feature of hypothyroidism. The spectrum of muscle involvement in hypothyroidism is broad. Symptomatic patients may present with myalgias without CK elevation, muscle hypertrophy with stiffness, weakness, and cramps, a myopathy that may simulate polymyositis with CK elevation. Pain and stiffness, when predominant, may suggest PMR or fibromyalgia. Rhabdomyolysis has been reported in hypothyroidism and is associated with muscle weakness; myalgia markedly elevated CK, and myoglobinuria. In hypothyroid myopathy without rhabdomyolysis, serum CK can vary from normal to markedly elevated. A delay in muscle relaxation after handgrip or muscle percussion—pseudomyotonia—may be seen. The severity of the myopathy parallels the degree and duration of the hormone deficiency. CK levels are usually elevated, and electromyography may either be normal or show myopathic features. Muscle biopsy may be normal, may show focal necrosis and mild inflammatory infiltrates, or demonstrate nonspecific morphologic changes, including fiber size variation, type I fiber predominance, and type II fiber atrophy. Thyroid hormone replacement therapy leads to rapid improvement of myopathic signs and symptoms, with complete recovery over several weeks or months. However, weakness may take longer to improve than chemical and EMG abnormalities. Most patients have recovered by 6 months, but up to 10% have weakness on examination 1 year after initiation of treatment.

Hyperthyroidism may also cause proximal myopathy. The reported prevalence of hyperthyroidism in older people is up to 4%, but those over 60 accounts for 10% to 17% of all hyperthyroid patients and 35% of all patients with thyrotoxicosis. Like patients with hypothyroidism, one prospective cohort study of hyperthyroid patients older than age 70 demonstrated a paucity of clinical signs compared with a younger adult population, emphasizing the difficulty of making a diagnosis. Clinically, the proximal myopathy of hyperthyroidism develops insidiously and progresses slowly but may lead to marked weakness. Rarely, an acutely progressive form of muscle weakness is described. Weakness is not uncommonly greater than the degree of muscle atrophy. Paradoxically, serum CK levels are usually normal or minimally elevated. EMG and muscle biopsy features may show a myopathic process. As with hypothyroid patients, therapy is directed at correcting the underlying thyroid dysfunction.

Osteomalacia Osteomalacia is a metabolic bone disease of the under mineralized collagen matrix in which an unmineralized matrix (osteoid) accumulates at bone surfaces. This disease most often affects older people whose most common etiology is vitamin D deficiency, superimposed on the age-related decrease in muscle vitamin D receptor number and function. In this way, the presentation may mimic that of osteoporosis. Nonspecific bone pain and tenderness with or without fractures are the dominant symptoms, but muscle weakness is not uncommon. Patients with severe weakness may mimic the presentation of PM. The myopathy is characteristically proximal in distribution, and the lower limbs may produce a waddling gait. CK levels are typically normal, and a myopathic pattern may be seen on EMG. Minimal inflammatory infiltrates may be found with other myopathic features on muscle biopsy. Myopathy usually responds to vitamin D administration, with or without supplemental calcium or phosphate, depending on the etiology of osteomalacia.

Amyloid Myopathy

Muscle involvement in patients with amyloidosis is a common finding in this rare disorder. Typical manifestations in skeletal muscle include pseudohypertrophy, palpable nodular masses within the muscle, and a "wooden consistency" firmness of muscles. These abnormalities may be severe enough to lead to weakness, pain, and immobility. Amyloid myopathy may present without these more typical features but rather with progressive proximal muscle weakness and dysphagia, elevated serum CK levels, and EMG changes of inflammatory myopathy. In addition, muscle biopsies may reveal extracellular amyloid deposits around muscle fibers and some small vessels. This proximal myopathy from amyloid is rare but should be considered in the older patient with a proximal myopathy without pseudohypertrophy.

Drug-Induced Myopathies

Although the exact percentage is unknown, the prevalence of drug-induced myopathy in older people is not trivial. Older people are at risk for drug-induced myopathies. The medications commonly causing myopathic symptoms are given for diseases that themselves have an increased incidence with age. Such drugs usually require a cofactor (eg, renal or hepatic insufficiency), some of which are age-related. A drug-induced myopathy may present as a necrotizing myopathy (eg, autoimmune necrotizing myopathy from statins), inflammatory myopathy (eg, procainamide), mitochondrial myopathy, antimicrotubular myopathy (eg, colchicine), lysosomal storage myopathy (eg, amiodarone), myofibrillar myopathy, or as type II muscle fiber atrophy (eg, corticosteroids). The scope of this chapter does not allow for an in-depth discussion of all possible toxic myopathies, but the awareness of this important category is essential. The reader is referred to recent reviews. Summary comments below are limited to selected drugs with risk for toxic myopathy in older people.

Corticosteroids Myopathy is a well-known side effect of corticosteroids. Myopathy is generally seen with larger doses, longer duration, and more frequent dosing. The likelihood is also higher with the use of fluorinated steroids. The dichotomy exists when treating older patients with IIM, PMR, giant cell arteritis (GCA), or another systemic rheumatic disease that needs a prolonged duration of treatment with systemic steroids. The benefits of such prolonged steroid therapy should be weighed against the risk of causing steroid-induced myopathy. Proximal hip girdle muscles are mainly affected, but shoulder girdle and diffuse muscle involvement may be seen. Respiratory muscles can be affected, even when limb muscles remain strong. Typical findings include normal serum CK levels, a myopathic EMG without inflammatory changes, and muscle biopsy findings of excessive type II (IIb) muscle fiber atrophy or normal changes for age. Steroids induce a decrease in muscle protein synthesis and an increase in protein degradation. Antianabolic effects include inhibition of amino acid transport into muscle, inhibition of the ability of insulin, insulin-like growth factor I (IGF-I) and certain amino acids to stimulate the initiation of mRNA translation, and downregulation of myogenin and the degradation of MyoD, transcription factors required for differentiation of satellite cells into muscle fibers. Catabolic effects of steroids are mediated by stimulating proteolysis of muscle contractile proteins through ubiquitin-proteasome, lysosomal (cathepsins), and calcium-dependent (calpains) systems. Muscle wasting leads to increased urinary creatine excretion, detected as an increase in % creatinuria; urine creatine divided by the sum of urine creatine plus creatinine in a 24-hour specimen should be less than 6%, but is elevated in a steroid myopathy. This test is useful when trying to distinguish steroid myopathy from myalgias without myopathy in a normal CK level setting. Therapy for steroid myopathy involves steroid taper and reconditioning exercises, with exercise additionally beneficial for reducing glucocorticoid receptors in muscle.

Alcohol Older people are not immune to alcohol-related health problems. See Chapter 23 for details of aging and alcohol use. Alcoholic myopathy may present in three forms. First, a subclinical form is manifested solely by the elevation of muscle enzymes that return to normal during abstinence. Second, acute alcoholic myopathy is associated with acute intoxication. There may be a profound weakness, myalgias, and rhabdomyolysis, with marked elevation of CK and myoglobinuria. Findings of an inflammatory myopathy are seen on EMG, and biopsy shows necrosis with varying degrees of inflammation. There is also a high risk of falls with acute intoxication that may cause rhabdomyolysis or a fracture. With conservative care, the CK may rapidly drop over days to a week. This observation is essential to keep in mind so that the patient may be kept from the inappropriate early use of corticosteroids. Third, the syndrome may mimic severe polymyositis at the onset. Finally, alcohol more commonly causes a chronic proximal myopathy. Chronic alcohol use may lead to muscle atrophy, more in the legs than arms, with evaluation showing normal CK levels, noninflammatory myopathic EMG, and type II fiber atrophy on muscle biopsy.

Colchicine Colchicine is used to manage acute gouty arthritis and less often for chronic management of chronic calcium pyrophosphate deposition disease. It is an uncommon cause of drug-induced myopathy. Colchicine can cause toxicity by preventing the extension of myotubules in the myocyte due to the binding of the drug to tubulin dimers. Patients present with proximal muscle weakness, elevated CK, and a nonspecific vacuolar myopathy on biopsy. Renal insufficiency is a major risk factor, making even low daily prophylactic doses (eg, in the treatment of gout) in this situation prone to causing neuromyotoxicity. Therefore, colchicine dose should always be adjusted for the degree of renal function.

Lipid-lowering agents All lipid-lowering agents, except for bile acid sequestrants (resins) and plant sterols, may cause myalgias or myopathy. Nicotinic acid, uncommonly, may cause myalgias and elevated CK levels. Ezetimibe (an inhibitor of the intestinal intraluminal sterol transporter) has been documented in case reports to cause tendinopathy and myopathy, either alone or when given with statins. Fibric acid derivatives can cause muscle cramps, acute or painful subacute myopathy, and elevated CK levels with or without signs of myoglobinuria. Myopathy from fibrates is more likely to occur in a patient with renal insufficiency. Among the lipid-lowering therapies, fibrates appear to have a higher relative risk for myopathy than do statins.

Statin drugs have been associated with myalgias (cramping, aching or stiffness, transient or persistent, with normal CK level) in 5% to 10%, myositis (elevated CK) in approximately 1%, and rhabdomyolysis in approximately 0.1% of treated patients. Statins have also been reported to cause tendon-associated pain, and it is estimated that up to 25% of statin users may develop exercise-induced muscle pain, cramping, or fatigue. Older people are at higher risk for the development of statin-induced myopathy. Other risk factors include patient characteristics (female sex, renal insufficiency, hepatic dysfunction, hypothyroidism, biliary tract obstruction, underlying muscle disease, grapefruit juice intake) and properties of the statin (higher dose, lipophilicity, and potential for drug-drug interactions with other medications metabolized by cytochrome P450 [especially CYP3A4] pathways, eg, amiodarone, fibrates, cyclosporine, HIV protease inhibitors and numerous antibiotics including erythromycin, clarithromycin, rifampin). The median duration of statin therapy before symptom onset is 6 months but maybe as long as 4 years. The myopathy is self-limited, with a median duration of myalgias and resolution of CK elevation following cessation of statin therapy of 2 to 3 months. Persistent symptoms and/or elevated

CK level despite statin discontinuation may indicate an underlying other myopathy or the development of a statin-induced necrotizing myopathy. There is no agreed-upon case definition for statin-induced myopathy, contributing to the inconsistent recommendations from national organizations (ACC/AHA/NHLBI, FDA, National Lipid Association) to screen for statin-related toxicity management symptoms. There is agreement that the statin be discontinued if the CK is more than 10-fold the upper limit of normal but differing recommendations as to when to measure CK (at baseline +/− at regular follow-up intervals, or just with symptoms) and how to manage statin therapy at lower levels of CK elevation. Treatment strategies include reducing the statin dose, changing to nondaily statin dosing, changing to a statin metabolized by a route other than by the CYP3A4 pathway, changing to a nonstatin lipid-lowering agent, and adding supplemental coenzyme Q10. The precise mechanisms of statin-induced myopathy are incompletely understood. However, they may include induction of apoptosis, induction of atrogin-1 (a ubiquitin ligase active in proteolysis), instability of myocyte membranes from decreased cholesterol content, depletion of isoprenoids (isoprenylation being responsible for the posttranslational modification of up to 2% of cellular proteins) or coenzyme Q10, mitochondrial dysfunction, and increased hepatic uptake of statins in individuals heterozygous (odds ratio for myopathy of 4.4) or homozygous (odds ratio 17.4) for the C-allele variant of the *SLCO1B1* gene.

As mentioned above, persistent myopathic symptoms and/or hyperCKemia following discontinuation of statin therapy may indicate the development of a medication-triggered immune-mediated necrotizing myopathy. Statins not only inhibit HMG-CoA reductase (HMGCR) but lead to a compensatory increase in HMGCR levels. Detection of an autoantibody (anti-200/100) against HMGCR is found in those patients with a progressive myopathy despite discontinuation of statin therapy. However, this antibody may also be detected in patients without prior statin exposure who presumably have sustained muscle damage (eg, from a toxin or infectious agent), leading to increased HMGCR expression from regenerating muscle cells. In statin-exposed patients, this autoimmune myopathy shows no gender bias, but the risk for developing anti-HMGCR antibodies is strongly associated with the HLA-DRβ1*11:01 gene allele. Several statins have been associated with this syndrome. Before the onset of myopathy, the duration of statin therapy could range from 31 months to as long as 7 years. Muscle biopsy shows a necrotizing myopathy without significant inflammation, similar to that seen in patients with anti-SRP antibodies. In contrast to those with no prior statin exposure, statin-exposed patients with this immune-mediated necrotizing myopathy respond to immunosuppressant therapy. However, aggressive therapy may be required, and the course of treatment may be prolonged.

Immune Checkpoint Inhibitors

The past decade has seen the emergence of a revolutionary approach to cancer therapy using checkpoint inhibitors, called immunotherapy. These are immunomodulatory antibodies used to enhance the immune system and have substantially improved the prognosis for patients with advanced malignancy. Multiple antibodies against programmed cell death receptor 1 (PD-1) and programmed cell death ligand 1 (PD-L1) are in development and have shown great promise in multiple malignancies. Nivolumab, pembrolizumab, cemiplimab, and dostarlimab, all of which target PD-1, and atezolizumab, avelumab, and durvalumab, all of which target PD-L1, have been approved in various indications (for example, melanoma, renal cell carcinoma, non–small cell lung cancer, head and neck cancer, urothelial carcinoma, Hodgkin lymphoma, Merkel cell carcinoma, and endometrial cancer). Ipilimumab, an anti-CTLA-4 antibody, is approved for use in patients with advanced melanoma based on a significant improvement in overall survival. However, with their increasing use, there are a growing number of reports on immune-related adverse events from immunotherapies. Immune-mediated neuromuscular side effects of checkpoint inhibitors greatly vary in presentation and differ from IIM. These side effects can be life-threatening and may result in permanent sequelae. In a multicenter cancer registry, myositis was the most frequent neuromuscular adverse event. In 32% of cases, myositis was complicated by concomitant myocarditis. Furthermore, cases of isolated myocarditis, myasthenia gravis, PMR, neuro-radiculopathy, and asymptomatic CK elevation were reported.

Hydroxychloroquine

Hydroxychloroquine (HCQ) is an antimalarial medication with immunomodulatory properties. It is a mainstay of the medication regimen in systemic lupus erythematosus. It is also used in some patients with rheumatoid arthritis, inflammatory arthritides, IIMs with cutaneous manifestations, and Sjogren's disease with joint involvement. The long-term use of HCQ can be associated with muscle toxicity, mainly described as a proximal myopathy with evidence of lysosomal dysfunction on muscle biopsy. Symptom onset has been reported anywhere from 6 months to 21 years of using HCQ. In a single-center study, the median age of presentation was 66 years. The clinical presentation could include proximal limb muscle weakness, dysphagia, axial weakness, heart failure due to myocardial involvement, and, rarely, respiratory failure. On electrocardiogram, QT interval prolongation can be seen in patients with cardiac involvement. However, the diagnosis is often delayed as it is a rare association. Muscle histopathology shows a myopathy with rimmed vacuoles and marked acid phosphatase reactivity and curvilinear bodies on electron microscopy. The mainstay of treatment is to stop HCQ, which can result in variable improvement in muscle weakness.

Late-Onset Muscular Dystrophies

Muscular dystrophies are genetically determined degenerative myopathies that usually present before adulthood. These diverse groups of inherited muscle protein disorders are characterized by their patterns of inheritance and penetrance, age of onset, progression, severity, and muscles involved. Weakness proceeds slowly, and the arrest of progression has been described. Depending on the particular disease, some patients may proceed into older adulthood with minimal or undetectable symptoms before the cumulative effects of muscle degeneration lead to functional decline. Three late-onset muscular dystrophies are described, each causing proximal limb weakness: facioscapulohumeral dystrophy, oculopharyngeal dystrophy, and late-onset limb-girdle dystrophy. These dystrophies are associated with normal or mild elevations of serum CK and a nonspecific myopathic pattern on EMG. Muscle biopsy findings are nondiagnostic and can show loss of muscle fibers, variation in fiber size, and degrees of muscle fiber necrosis. Therapy is limited to patient and family education, palliative measures to prevent aspiration, and empiric physical therapy.

Facioscapulohumeral dystrophy is an autosomal dominant disease that typically begins with facial muscle weakness (eg, inability to tightly close eyes or whistle), sparing the extraocular and pharyngeal muscles. Weakness tends to proceed caudally, involving muscles of the shoulder (scapular winging) then pelvic girdles, although early tibialis anterior involvement is characteristic. Extramuscular features include sensorineural hearing loss and retinal vasculopathy. Diagnosis can be made by molecular genetic testing of blood.

Oculopharyngeal dystrophy is also inherited through an autosomal dominant pattern with complete penetrance and is the only dystrophy that presents more commonly in older people. It is classified as a polyalanine disorder, with the mutation in poly (A) binding protein 1 (PABPN1). Symptoms begin in the fifth or sixth decade of life. Proximal upper and lower extremity weakness is a late finding, following the onset of symptoms with ptosis (bilateral, but can be asymmetric) and dysphagia. Supportive care includes surgery to correct ptosis and cricopharyngeal myotomy for severe dysphagia. The pathologic hallmark is unique, filamentous intranuclear inclusions that have been shown to contain aggregations of mutated PABPN1. Diagnosis is made through molecular genetic testing.

Limb-girdle dystrophy represents disorders with heterogeneous phenotypes but with predominant scapular and pelvic girdle involvement (legs earlier and more severely than the arms). The presence of dysrhythmia or contractures suggests laminopathy. Mutations in at least 19 genes have been described, encoding proteins for calpain 3, caveolin, dysferlin, lamin, sarcoglycans, and telethonin. Autosomal dominant (with incomplete penetrance) and recessive inheritance patterns are observed; thus, the clinical phenotype does not accurately predict the genotype. A specific diagnosis is based on the combination of results from DNA mutation testing and muscle protein analysis.

Late-Onset Mitochondrial Myopathy

Ragged red fibers are the histologic hallmark of mitochondrial dysfunction and represent the result of a diverse set of conditions, including normal aging, sporadic IBM and other neuromuscular diseases, and myopathies from drugs that cause mitochondrial damage. The mitochondrial myopathies/encephalomyopathies are a heterogeneous group of disorders displaying specific clinical manifestations, maternal inheritance, excessive ragged red fibers on muscle biopsy, the altered energy state of resting muscle, mutations in mitochondrial DNA (mtDNA), and deficiencies in the activities of oxidative phosphorylation enzymes. Most patients present symptomatically within the first three decades of life. A syndrome of late-onset mitochondrial myopathy has been described. Patients have progressive proximal muscle weakness of insidious onset and limb muscle fatigability, mainly in the lower limbs. Serum levels of CK are mildly elevated, and myopathic changes can be seen on EMG. Excessive ragged red fibers are noted on muscle biopsy. This condition represents an exaggerated form of the accumulation of mtDNA mutations that occurs with aging, which manifests clinically as a proximal myopathy.

Paraspinal Myopathies of Older People

Severe weakness isolated to paraspinal muscles is uncommon and usually a manifestation of another underlying neurologic disease, muscular dystrophy, or myopathy. Weakness is evident when in the erect position, and the postural abnormality resolves when supine or with passive extension. Conditions reported to be associated with this finding include inflammatory and noninflammatory myopathies (including polymyositis, IBM, and certain endocrine/metabolic myopathies), facioscapulohumeral and limb-girdle dystrophies, neurologic diseases of the motor neuron (ALS, postpolio syndrome), and peripheral nerves (chronic inflammatory polyneuropathy), Parkinson disease, and as a paraneoplastic phenomenon. Involvement of the cervical spine is termed dropped head syndrome, while the phenotype of thoracolumbar spinal weakness is referred to as bent spine syndrome.

Although kyphosis is a frequent finding in older people, it is usually limited to the thoracic spine and rarely involves the lumbar spine. Bent spine syndrome, or camptocormia (from the Greek for active forward trunk bending), is the consequence of chronically progressive lumbar and thoracic kyphosis in the absence of an architectural abnormality of the vertebral column to account for the postural change. The majority of cases of muscular origin are due to idiopathic, late-onset, axial myopathy. Those affected are predominately older women, and a positive family history of similar symptoms is reported in up to three-fourth of patients. CK levels are normal or mildly elevated. EMG testing can reveal myopathic and/or neuropathic changes in paravertebral muscles and mild myopathic changes (some with inflammatory infiltrates) with a marked increase in connective tissue and fatty infiltration is seen in muscle biopsy specimens from affected patients. Radiographic, computerized tomographic, and magnetic resonance scanning analyses show diffuse muscle atrophy limited to the spinal muscles, without evidence of significant bony changes, in a pattern of muscle involvement

distinct from that caused by spinal stenosis. Treatment for this primary axial myopathy is mainly supportive, including exercise therapy, orthoses, and assistive devices for ambulation. Patients with secondary forms or with myositis on biopsy may respond to corticosteroids.

A more limited form of spinal weakness of the neck extensors causes dropped head syndrome. Weakness leads to the inability to keep the head from dropping on the chest. CK is usually normal but may be elevated, and EMG testing of affected muscles shows myopathic changes. Muscle biopsy may reveal inflammatory infiltrates as well as nonspecific mild myopathic abnormalities. Dropped head syndrome from isolated myositis may respond to steroid therapy.

POLYMYALGIA RHEUMATICA AND GIANT CELL ARTERITIS

PMR and GCA are discussed together as they share similar epidemiologic, clinical, laboratory, and treatment findings. Each is a systemic inflammatory disease that probably forms the ends of a spectrum of illnesses. Thus, individual patients may be affected by one disease or both conditions simultaneously. The reported frequency of GCA occurring in patients with PMR ranges from 0% to 80% and varies according to how aggressively an approach to temporal artery biopsy is undertaken. A more realistic estimate is that GCA occurs in 15% to 20% of PMR patients.

Conversely, PMR occurs in 40% to 60% of patients with GCA and is the presenting symptom in 25%. Thus, the incidence of PMR is higher than that of GCA, and prevalence estimates are at least three times higher. Apart from the approach taken as to the clinical timing and size of temporal artery biopsy, differences in these prevalence data likely reflect selection bias of the populations studied and the use of different diagnostic criteria.

Polymyalgia Rheumatica

PMR is a clinical syndrome of the neck and limb-girdle aching of older adults. Patients have laboratory evidence of systemic inflammatory response, an excellent response to low-dose corticosteroids and no evidence to support other causes of a systemic illness such as malignancy or another connective tissue disease.

Epidemiology and pathogenesis PMR is seen in patients aged 50 and older, and 90% of cases occur in those older than 60. The female-to-male ratio is 2:1, and Caucasians are the most commonly affected subgroup. The condition is especially prevalent among those from northern European ancestry. The incidence rate is 50 cases per 100,000 persons over the age of 50 per year, rises with increasing age, and is two- to threefold higher than the rate for GCA. The corresponding prevalence rate for PMR is 600 per 100,000. Lifetime risk is 2.4% for women and 1.7% for men.

The etiology of PMR is unknown, and the source of pain symptoms is not clearly defined. Evidence from studies of the shoulder, hip, and surrounding tissues using radioisotopes, ultrasound, and fat-suppressed magnetic resonance imaging with gadolinium enhancement has demonstrated combinations of nonerosive synovitis at the phenotypic level, bursitis, tenosynovitis, and muscle edema in patients with active PMR. On musculoskeletal ultrasound, subdeltoid bursitis, biceps tenosynovitis, and/or glenohumeral/hip synovitis are characteristic findings in PMR. The diffuse distribution of these findings—particularly the presence of abnormalities outside synovial compartments—may explain the generalized pain felt by patients and reflects a pattern of inflammatory changes distinct from that seen in rheumatoid arthritis. Microscopically, arthroscopic biopsy studies have documented the presence of synovitis. In the synovial lesion, vascular proliferation is accompanied by an inflammatory infiltrate composed primarily of macrophages, CD4+ T-cells, and scarce neutrophils. A relative absence of B-cells and γδ T-cells differentiate the synovitis of PMR from that seen in rheumatoid arthritis. The cellular milieu parallels that seen in the temporal arteries of patients with GCA (see further). This finding and the presence of GCA histology and proinflammatory cytokines without typical histologic changes in temporal artery biopsy specimens of PMR patients without GCA symptoms further strengthen the association between the two diseases. There is a reported association of PMR at the genetic level with the markers HLA-DRB1*0401 and HLA-DRB1*0404. Cases occurring in family members support a possible genetic component to the disease. However, the event that triggers disease in the setting of potential genetic risk is unknown. Seasonal outbreaks of cases have suggested an infectious etiology, but no specific, causal pathogen has been identified to date. PMR, unlike certain IIM, is not associated with malignancy.

Clinical features and diagnostic criteria An abrupt onset or slowly progressive, symmetric pain (of at least 1 month) and stiffness develop in the neck and proximal limb-girdle areas. Symptoms may be difficult to localize and can be severe enough to limit activity analogous to proximal myopathy or impingement syndrome. Shoulder pain (75%–90%) is more common than hip pain (50%–70%). Constitutional symptoms include fever, malaise, night sweats, and weight loss in a third of patients, but high fever is uncommon. Other associated symptoms include prolonged morning stiffness upon awakening of affected areas, daytime gelling with inactivity, and arthralgias. Symptoms of GCA (see below) are noted in 15% to 20% of patients. A thorough history, including an extensive review of systems, and general physical examination, is essential to exclude conditions that may present with similar complaints, including sources of myopathy (see section Myopathies in Older People), occult malignancy, other connective tissue diseases, chronic infections, and spinal and regional musculoskeletal disorders.

Physical examination is usually unrevealing. Palpable muscular tenderness, when present, is not dramatic. Shoulder and hip motion may be limited by pain, but true weakness is usually not present. A mild, symmetric, nonerosive polyarthritis of the hands, wrists, and knees may be seen in a third of patients and be difficult to distinguish from the presentation of late-onset rheumatoid arthritis, especially when symptoms are confined to the large joints. Synovitis of the glenohumeral joint and tenosynovitis of the long head of the biceps tendon can be present in more than half of patients. Synovitis of small foot joints is less common than in older patients with rheumatoid arthritis. Steroid-responsive, dorsal hand pitting edema occurs with hand and wrist synovitis, similar to that seen in RS3PE (remitting seronegative symmetric synovitis with pitting edema) syndrome is seen in up to 8%.

An elevated acute-phase reactant is present in at least 80% to 90% of cases at presentation. The Westergren ESR is greater than 40 mm/h and not uncommonly as high as 100 mm/h. C-reactive protein is also elevated, but no specific cutoff is universally used to support the clinical diagnosis. In addition, test results are occasionally discordant because one test may perform better in certain persons than others. Using the height of serum IL-6 level elevation as a marker for adjusting initial corticosteroid therapy and monitoring response to treatment has been investigated but is not a standard of care.

Similarly, some have suggested that the height of ESR at presentation correlates with severity and prognosis. Normochromic, normocytic anemia during active disease may be seen in two-thirds of patients, and abnormal liver function tests in up to a third. Rheumatoid factor and antinuclear antibody testing are negative. To evaluate late-onset rheumatoid arthritis, it is important to obtain rheumatoid factor and anticyclic citrullinated protein levels. CK levels are normal, but EMG testing on rare occasions may show changes of inflammatory myopathy.

PMR is a clinical diagnosis based on a combination of clinical and laboratory findings, as no single manifestation is pathognomonic for the disease. The American College of Rheumatology (ACR) and the European League Against Rheumatism (EULAR) have proposed provisional classification criteria for PMR (**Table 100-3**).

Treatment The mainstay therapy for PMR is systemic glucocorticoids. Additional treatment with immunosuppressive agents may be considered individually, as suggested in the 2015 EULAR/ACR recommendations for PMR management. The minimum effective dose from a range of 12.5–25 mg prednisone equivalent daily should be used. Patients at high risk for relapse or prolonged therapy should receive the higher dose; those at lower risk should receive the lower dose. Clinical improvement should be noted after 2 weeks, with a nearly complete response at 4 weeks. For initial glucocorticoid tapering, the oral dose should be gradually reduced to 10 mg prednisone equivalent daily within 4 to 8 weeks; during therapy for relapse, the dose should be decreased gradually (within 4–8 weeks) after the relapse occurs. Once remission is achieved (after initial and relapse therapies), oral prednisone should be tapered by 1 mg every 4 weeks (or similar, eg, 2.5 mg every 10 weeks)

TABLE 100-3 ■ PROVISIONAL CLASSIFICATION CRITERIA FOR POLYMYALGIA RHEUMATICA

REQUIRED FINDINGS: AGE ≥ 50, BILATERAL SHOULDER ACHING, ABNORMAL CRP AND/OR ESR		
VARIABLE FINDINGS (ODDS RATIO [95% CI])	**POINTS WITHOUT ULTRASOUND (0–6)**	**POINTS WITH ULTRASOUND (0–8)**
Morning stiffness duration > 45 min (5.0 [2.8, 9.1])	2	2
Hip pain or limited range of motion (1.4 [0.8, 2.6])	1	1
Absence of rheumatoid factor or anticitrullinated peptide antibody (eg, CCP) (5.2 [2.1, 12.6])	2	2
Absence of other joint involvement (2.2 [1.3, 4.0])	1	1
At least: *1 shoulder*: subdeltoid bursitis and/or biceps tenosynovitis and/or glenohumeral synovitis AND *1 hip*: synovitis and/or trochanteric bursitis (2.6 [1.3, 5.3])	Not applicable	1
Both shoulders with subdeltoid bursitis, biceps tenosynovitis, or glenohumeral synovitis (2.1 [1.2, 3.7])	Not applicable	1
SCORE TO BE CATEGORIZED AS PMR	**≥ 4**	**≥ 5**
Sensitivity of criteria	68%	66%
Specificity of criteria	78%	81%

CRP, C-reactive protein; ESR, erythrocyte sedimentation rate.

Reproduced with permission from Dasgupta B, Cimmino MA, Kremers HM, et al. 2012 Provisional classification criteria for polymyalgia rheumatica: a European League Against Rheumatism/American College of Rheumatology collaborative initiative. Arthritis Rheum. 2012;64(4):943–954.

until discontinuation, as long as remission is maintained. Lack of initial response should prompt an evaluation for an alternate diagnosis. Despite rapid clinical improvement, further tapering of the dose is done slowly in order to prevent relapse. Once the ESR normalizes and symptoms resolve, but usually after 4 to 8 weeks, the dose is reduced in small decrements: by 2.5 mg every 2 to 4 weeks until 10 mg QD is reached, then by 1 mg every 4 weeks. The lowest dose that controls symptoms should always be used. If exacerbations occur during the taper (approximately 25% of patients), the dose can be increased (although not necessarily to the starting level), and the tapering recommenced. Patient symptoms rather than the ESR level alone are the main parameter to follow. Alternate-day dosing of steroids is less effective than a daily schedule.

A course of steroids under these guidelines may take a minimum of 12 to 18 months to complete. Three-quarters of patients are off steroid therapy by 2 years. Persistent elevation of the ESR, rise of the ESR after initial fall and symptom improvement during therapy, or failure to improve with low-dose corticosteroids, may indicate the presence of GCA and the consideration for temporal artery biopsy or an alternate diagnosis. Patients should be evaluated for signs and symptoms of GCA at every visit, and if present, referred for temporal artery biopsy even while on corticosteroid therapy. All patients receiving corticosteroids should be started on measures to prevent osteoporosis and be closely monitored for other metabolic side effects. A percentage of patients, ranging from 10% to 30% depending on the reported series, may require longer corticosteroid courses or chronic daily doses (eg, prednisone at 5 mg or less per day) to maintain symptom control. The benefits of such prolonged therapy should be weighed against the serious risk of steroid-induced side effects in older people. Conclusive clinical trials do not well support alternative therapies.

Methotrexate is the only immunosuppressive agent that has proved efficacious for PMR in randomized controlled trials and should be considered early in treatment of patients at increased risk of PMR relapse or glucocorticoid-related side effects. Other steroid-sparing therapies like HCQ, azathioprine, and other cytotoxics have been used, albeit with only limited success. While there are case reports and open-labeled studies indicating benefit with tocilizumab (an interleukin-6 inhibitor) in PMR, due to the lack of approval of tocilizumab for PMR and because of the absence of placebo-controlled trials, it should be considered only in individual cases as a second-line immunosuppressive agent. Analgesics may be added to improve pain symptoms. An NSAID or COX-2 inhibitor may be used as initial therapy in very mildly affected patients but should be changed over to corticosteroids if the marked improvement is not seen in 2 to 4 weeks. NSAIDs do not alter ESR levels or suppress subclinical GCA if present. More frequently, these agents are used to provide adjunctive anti-inflammatory therapy to ongoing steroid therapy. Their use must be balanced against the risk of eliciting renal, cardiovascular, gastrointestinal, and hematologic side effects.

Giant Cell Arteritis

GCA is a systemic, granulomatous, segmental, and focal panarteritis usually focused along the internal elastic lamina of medium- and large-sized extracranial arteries. The aorta and branch vessels from the aortic arch are most frequently involved. Disease manifestations are generally the result of tissue-organ ischemia or necrosis downstream from the site of vascular occlusion. Certain disease manifestations are steroid-responsive but require higher doses at the initiation of therapy as contrasted against treatment for PMR.

Epidemiology and pathogenesis As in PMR, GCA is seen in patients older than 50 years, most commonly in Caucasians, women, and in those from northern Scandinavian ancestry, with an incidence rate of approximately 17 to 27 cases per 100,000 persons older than age 50, and prevalence rate of about 200 per 100,000. The disease is rare in the United States in those of African and Asian descent, with an associated incidence rate of approximately 1 case per 100,000 persons.

The cause of GCA is unknown, but histologic and biochemical evaluations of affected arteries suggest that it is an antigen-driven disease with a cell-mediated immune response. Like PMR, GCA shares genetic risk factors (such as susceptibility to HLA-DRB1*01 and HLA-DRB1*04 genotypes) and pathogenetic pathways involving both the innate and adaptive immune system. The cellular infiltrate throughout the vessel wall mirrors that seen in the synovium of patients with active PMR. Destruction of the arterial wall is centered on the elastic fibers of the internal elastic lamina. The process is thought to begin in the adventitia, where activated dendritic cells recruit CD4+ T-cells coexpressing CD161 into the vessel wall. Based on the cytokine milieu secreted by dendritic cells, these ultimate T-effector cells (1) following exposure to IL-1β, IL-6, and IL-23, differentiate into IL-17 producing Th17 cells, or (2) following exposure to IL-12 and IL-18, differentiate into interferon-gamma (IFN-γ) producing T-helper-1 (Th1) cells. Research implicates these two independent inflammatory cytokine pathways in driving disease pathogenesis: the IL-17 axis thru activation of endothelial cells, vascular smooth muscle cells, and fibroblasts and associated with IL-6–mediated systemic/constitutional symptoms, and the IFN-γ axis activating macrophages, endothelial cells, and cytotoxic cells and associated with vascular occlusion and ischemic complications. The IL-17–mediated pathway is steroid-sensitive, whereas the IFN-γ pathway is steroid-resistant and is the predominant cell type in intramural infiltrates. The activity of both pathways characterizes the early disease, but the chronic disease is characterized by persistent Th1-inducing signals, independent of IL-17–mediated inflammation. In combination with proteolytic enzymes and growth factors, a granulomatous reaction develops in the vessel wall, while secondary smooth muscle and matrix proliferation contributes to vascular occlusion.

Clinical features and diagnostic criteria Most patients have clinical findings attributable to involved arteries during the illness. The most prevalent symptoms include headache (65%) in the distribution of either the temporal or occipital arteries, visual disturbance (30%), permanent visual loss (15%), jaw claudication symptoms (eg, from chewing or talking; 45%), dysphagia or swallowing claudication (8%), tongue claudication (6%), limb (usually arm) claudication (4%), and persistent cough or sore throat (4%). Rare manifestations include tinnitus and ischemia of the scalp or tongue. Headaches may be severe, acute, and associated with scalp sensitivity in temporal and or occipital artery distributions. Typical PMR is seen in 40% to 60% and maybe the presenting finding in 25%. In approximately 25% of patients, nonerosive arthritis may be present, typically involving the metacarpophalangeal joints, wrists, and knees. Constitutional symptoms are common and may exist as the sole manifestation of disease. These include weight loss or anorexia (50%), fever (which may be prolonged and meet the criteria for fever of unknown etiology; 45%), fatigue (40%), and depression symptoms. Overall, the nonspecific nature of many of the symptoms mentioned above contributes to the delay, which on average can be weeks before the diagnosis is made. **Table 100-4** lists the test characteristics of individual symptoms and their combinations as expressed by likelihood ratios.

Examination reveals signs related to affected arteries in up to two-thirds of patients. Scalp artery tenderness (27%) is a less frequent finding than a decreased temporal pulse (46%) in one study. Care should be taken to differentiate temporal artery findings from the signs of radiating pain from ipsilateral C2 radiculopathy (tenderness in the paraspinal area of the ipsilateral upper cervical spine, pain exacerbated by head position or motion), or scalp pain radiating from a myofascial pain emanating from the suboccipital muscles at the base of the skull (focal muscular tenderness, which may "trigger" radiating pain into the temporal scalp). A swollen, nodular or erythematous scalp artery is detected with equal frequency as a large artery bruit (20%). Large vessel vasculitis occurs in 25% of patients. Involvement of the thoracic or abdominal aorta may lead to aneurysmal dilation and possibly rupture, usually occurring years after the onset of disease during a time when most patients are not otherwise thought to have active disease. Hypertension from renovascular involvement is rare. Involvement of the ophthalmic, central retinal, and posterior ciliary arteries to the eye can cause optic nerve ischemic lesions (either anterior or posterior ischemic optic neuropathy, the former the commonest lesion and associated with partial or complete visual loss) or retinal ischemic lesions (either central retinal or cilioretinal artery occlusions which may also lead to severe visual

TABLE 100-4 ■ LIKELIHOOD RATIOS FOR SINGLE SYMPTOMS AND IN COMBINATION FOR GIANT CELL ARTERITIS

	LIKELIHOOD RATIO (LR)	
	LR+ (95% CI)	LR− (95% CI)
SINGLE SYMPTOMS		
Jaw claudication	6.9 (5.0–9.5)	0.64 (0.59–0.70)
Diplopia	3.7 (1.5–9.2)	0.97 (0.95–0.99)
Scalp tenderness	3.1 (2.4–4.0)	0.75 (0.70–0.81)
Myalgia/arthralgia	2.2 (1.6–3.1)	0.90 (0.86–0.95)
New headache	1.7 (1.5–1.9)	0.54 (0.46–0.63)
Decreased vision	1.5 (1.0–2.1)	0.95 (0.91–0.99)
Weight loss	1.3 (1.0–1.6)	0.93 (0.87–0.99)
COMBINATIONS OF SYMPTOMS		
Jaw claudication + decreased vision	44 (5.9–322)	0.98 (0.97–0.99)
Jaw claudication + diplopia	30 (1.7–519)	0.98 (0.97–0.99)
New headache + jaw claudication + scalp tenderness	19 (8.1–42)	0.86 (0.82–0.90)
Jaw claudication + scalp tenderness	18 (8.3–39)	0.84 (0.80–0.88)
New headache + jaw claudication	8.7 (5.8–13)	0.71 (0.66–0.76)
New headache + decreased vision	6.2 (2.7–14)	0.95 (0.93–0.98)
New headache + scalp tenderness	3.9 (2.9–5.3)	0.77 (0.72–0.82)

CI, confidence interval; LR+, positive likelihood ratio; LR−, negative likelihood ratio.
Data from Simel DL, Rennie D. The Rational Clinical Examination: Evidence-Based Clinical Diagnosis. Chicago, IL: American Medical Association; 2009.

loss). Fundoscopic exam revealing a chalky white edematous optic disc suggests infarction of the optic nerve head, whereas optic disc cupping is a late finding. Visual loss occurs in 10% to 15% of patients, may be sudden and without warning, with the risk for permanent loss increased in patients with prior transient loss. Warning signs include symptoms of amaurosis fugax, visual disturbance with postural change, or diplopia. Vision loss for more than a few hours only very rarely returns. Less common findings in patients with GCA include peripheral neuropathy, scalp necrosis, cerebral infarction, and lesions that may mimic CNS vasculitis, tinnitus, and deafness.

The ESR is usually markedly elevated, not uncommonly to 80 to 100 mm/h or higher. A normo to hypochromic anemia may be seen and can be accompanied by reactive thrombocytosis. Other acute phase reactants such as C-reactive protein, haptoglobin, and alpha-2 globulin can be elevated; however, these measures, including an elevated ESR, should not be the only indication to begin immunosuppressive medication. A mild hepatic transaminitis and/or an elevated alkaline phosphatase can occur. The presence of anticardiolipin antibodies at presentation may be a poor prognostic marker for the subsequent development of vascular complications.

Radiographic investigations can help define the extent of disease but alone are rarely sufficient to diagnose GCA. The combination of positron emission tomography (PET) with computed tomography (CT) using 18F-fluorodeoxyglucose (18F-FDG) can detect hypermetabolic activity in vascular walls but cannot reliably distinguish between vasculitis and atherosclerotic changes. Therefore, PET/CT is most useful in patients with GCA with suspected involvement of the aorta and its major branches or when other diagnoses that mimic GCA should be ruled out. Some disadvantages of PET/CT are the high cost of the test, radiation exposure, and the intrinsic limitation of resolution to approximately 2.4 mm. Magnetic resonance (MR) or CT angiography of the aorta and its proximal major branches can demonstrate the vascular occlusion or dissection responsible for limb claudication, or clinically suspected aortic involvement, but wall thickening or delayed enhancement of the arterial wall may not change with treatment and is not a reliable measure of disease status. Doppler ultrasonography (US) of the temporal arteries may show hypoechoic changes representing edema of the vessel wall ("halo sign") and decreased blood flow and velocity as noninvasive diagnostic signs of active inflammation. However, Doppler US is neither sufficiently sensitive nor specific to routinely replace diagnostic arterial biopsy.

As clinical features are not specific, temporal artery biopsy remains the gold standard diagnostic test. The yield is increased when the artery to be biopsied is palpably or visibly abnormal. As the pathologic changes in an involved artery tend to occur as skip lesions along its length, a biopsy specimen of a minimum of 1 cm, preferably greater than 2 cm, is preferred. The artery should be sectioned at 3- to 5-mm intervals before microscopic examination. The need for biopsy should not delay steroid therapy, but biopsy performance should preferably occur within the first few days of steroid use. Prior or ongoing therapy with steroids (eg, in a patient with PMR) should not prevent a decision to confirm the diagnosis by biopsy if the patient has active signs and symptoms of GCA. The temporal artery is the preferred site for biopsy, although a diagnosis can be confirmed by biopsy from a symptomatic occipital artery. A positive biopsy demonstrates evidence of vasculitis centered at the intima-media junction with a predominance of mononuclear cell infiltrates or granulomatous inflammation, usually with multinucleated giant cells. However, multinucleated giant cells are found in only 50% of specimens. Rarely is the inflammation restricted to the vasa vasorum or periadventitial small vessels. Histologic changes of GCA need to be distinguished from the normal changes in aging vessels, although distinguishing between "healed arteritis" and senescent changes may be difficult at best due to a significant overlap in the microscopic findings. Normal senescent changes in the temporal artery include progressive and relatively regular intimal thickening, medial degeneration and thinning with occasional calcium deposition, focal internal elastic fiber fracture, and fibrosis.

An initial negative biopsy occurs in up to one-third of patients and should first lead to a careful reevaluation of the specimen. Biopsy of the contralateral artery infrequently provides pathologic confirmation when the initial biopsy is negative but may be pursued in a patient for whom the diagnosis remains in doubt, especially if systemic symptoms predominate and there is a very high clinical suspicion for GCA. The diagnostic sensitivity of a temporal artery biopsy remains high even if steroid therapy was begun preoperatively, but biopsy is ideally not delayed for more than 1 week. A negative biopsy does not preclude a diagnosis of GCA if sufficient other clinical findings are present. It is a situation more commonly seen in patients who have predominately subclavian artery involvement.

The 1990 American College of Rheumatology classification criteria for GCA have become de facto diagnostic criteria in clinical practice (**Table 100-5**). These criteria provide structure to diagnose if artery biopsy is either not available or temporal artery abnormality is not present. In the original derivation, the criteria had a sensitivity of 94% and a specificity of 91%.

Treatment

The risk of acute visual loss mandates that corticosteroid therapy be initiated in anyone suspected of having GCA, even before the temporal artery biopsy. Initial doses of 1 mg/kg (eg, 40–60 mg) of prednisone per day in a single morning dose, higher than starting doses for PMR, are standard. Even higher doses of 15 mg/kg (eg, 1000 mg given intravenously) per day are suggested for patients with active visual symptoms. The initial dose is maintained for 4 to 8 weeks to suppress clinical symptoms and normalize the ESR and/or CRP, slowly tapered over months. Most patients require an average of 2 years of therapy to control symptoms. One suggested schedule for tapering is to reduce the initial dose by 10 mg every 2 to 4 weeks until 40 mg daily is reached, then by 5 mg every 2 to 4 weeks until 20 mg daily, followed by a reduction

TABLE 100-5 ■ CLASSIFICATION CRITERIA FOR GIANT CELL ARTERITIS

CRITERION	DEFINITION
1. Age at onset ≥ 50 years	Development of symptoms or findings beginning at age ≥ 50
2. New headache	New onset of or new type of localized pain in the head
3. Temporal artery abnormality	Temporal artery tenderness to palpation or decreased pulsation, unrelated to arteriosclerosis of cervical arteries
4. Elevated ESR	Erythrocyte sedimentation rate (ESR) ≥ 50 mm/h by the Westergren method
5. Abnormal artery biopsy	Biopsy specimen with artery showing vasculitis characterized by a predominance of mononuclear cell infiltration or granulomatous inflammation, usually with multinucleated giant cells

For purposes of classification, a patient shall be said to have GCA if at least three of the five criteria are present.
Reproduced with permission from Hunder GG, Bloch DA, Michel BA, et al. The American College of Rheumatology 1990 criteria for the classification of giant cell arteritis. Arthritis Rheum. 1990;33(8):1122–1128.

of 2.5 mg every 2 to 4 weeks until 10 mg/day. After that, the dose is tapered following the pattern for patients with PMR, by 1 mg every 2 to 4 weeks. Disease exacerbations during tapering of steroids or after completion of therapy occur in up to two-thirds of patients, are more commonly manifested as PMR than ischemic complications, and require a transient increase or resumption in dose followed by further attempts at weaning. There are no clinical predictors for those at risk for relapse. The ESR is an imperfect indicator of disease activity and must be used in combination with clinical symptoms to assess disease and adjustment of therapy. Persistent elevation of ESR despite the absence of clinical disease activity may indicate silent large vessel disease (eg, aortitis) or be associated with another condition such as an unrecognized infection masked by steroid use.

The efficacy and glucocorticoid-sparing effects of tocilizumab, an interleukin-6 receptor α inhibitor, in GCA were recently demonstrated in the GiACTA trial. Based on the results of this study, which included 251 patients with GCA, the US Food and Drug Administration approved the use of tocilizumab in GCA. For patients with new-onset GCA who are at increased risk of developing glucocorticoid-related adverse effects or complications, relapse, or prolonged therapy and in patients who experience relapse, tocilizumab should be instituted early on in the course of treatment. A clinical trial involving 41 patients with GCA showed that more patients treated with abatacept (selective T-cell costimulation inhibitor) had relapse-free survival at 12 months (compared to placebo) but did not make a difference on the overall frequency and severity of adverse events. There may be a modest benefit from methotrexate as a steroid-sparing agent to lower relapse rates and total cumulative steroid dose, but steroid-associated side effects are not reduced. Infliximab was not effective as a steroid-sparing agent, and only anecdotal reports of utility for this purpose are described for trials of dapsone, adalimumab, leflunomide, HCQ, and azathioprine. Low-dose aspirin has been demonstrated to reduce the incidence of cranial ischemic events (particularly anterior ischemic optic neuropathy), and aspirin is known to reduce IFN-γ levels. All patients beginning steroids should be started on bone-protective therapy. Prophylaxis against infection from *Pneumocystis jirovecii* should be considered for those on a daily prednisone dose of 20 mg or higher. As aortic aneurysms occur more frequently in patients with GCA within 10 years of diagnosis, a yearly chest radiograph should be performed, with more sensitive studies such as chest CT reserved for patients with equivocal plain radiographic findings.

Although the life expectancy of patients with GCA is similar to that of the age-matched general population, unless severe aortitis is present, morbidity from the disease itself and its therapy may be substantial. Twenty to fifty percent of patients develop toxicities from corticosteroids. Thus, the impact of disease manifestations and the side effects of therapy cannot be underestimated in older people.

FURTHER READING

Aggarwal R, Bandos A, Reed AM, et al. Predictors of clinical improvement in rituximab-treated refractory adult and juvenile dermatomyositis and adult polymyositis. *Arthritis Rheumatol.* 2014;66(3):740–749.

Alemo Munters L, Dastmalchi M, Andgren V, et al. Improvement in health and possible reduction in disease activity using endurance exercise in patients with established polymyositis and dermatomyositis: a multicenter randomized controlled trial with a 1-year open extension followup. *Arthritis Care Res (Hoboken).* 2013;65(12):1959–1968.

Allenbach Y, Benveniste O, Stenzel W, Boyer O. Immune-mediated necrotizing myopathy: clinical features and pathogenesis. *Nat Rev Rheumatol.* 2020;16(12):689–701.

Balakrishnan A, Aggarwal R, Agarwal V, Gupta L. Inclusion body myositis in the rheumatology clinic. *Int J Rheum Dis.* 2020;23(9):1126–1135.

Buttgereit F, Matteson EL, Dejaco C. Polymyalgia rheumatica and giant cell arteritis. *JAMA.* 2020;324(10):993–994.

Cortese A, Machado P, Morrow J, et al. Longitudinal observational study of sporadic inclusion body myositis: implications for clinical trials. *Neuromuscul Disord.* 2013;23(5):404–412.

Dasgupta B, Cimmino MA, Kremers HM, et al. 2012 provisional classification criteria for polymyalgia rheumatica: a European League Against Rheumatism/American College of Rheumatology collaborative initiative. *Arthritis Rheum.* 2012;64(4):943–954.

Dejaco C, Singh YP, Perel P, et al. 2015 recommendations for the management of polymyalgia rheumatica: a European League Against Rheumatism/American College of Rheumatology collaborative initiative. *Arthritis Rheumatol.* 2015;67(10):2569–2580.

Doran MF, Crowson CS, O'Fallon WM, Hunder GG, Gabriel SE. Trends in the incidence of polymyalgia rheumatica over a 30 year period in Olmsted County, Minnesota, USA. *J Rheumatol.* 2002;29(8):1694–1697.

Feng C, Liu W, Sun X, et al. Myocardial involvement characteristics by cardiac MR imaging in patients with polymyositis and dermatomyositis. *Rheumatology (Oxford).* 2021; 20:keab271.

Katzberg HD, Kassardjian CD. Toxic and endocrine myopathies. *Continuum (Minneap Minn).* 2016;22(6, Muscle and Neuromuscular Junction Disorders):1815–1828.

Lundberg IE, Tjärnlund A, Bottai M, et al. 2017 European League Against Rheumatism/American College of Rheumatology Classification Criteria for Adult and Juvenile Idiopathic Inflammatory Myopathies and Their Major Subgroups. *Arthritis Rheumatol.* 2017;69(12): 2271–2282.

Mammen AL, Chung T, Christopher-Stine L, et al. Autoantibodies against 3-hydroxy-3-methylglutaryl-coenzyme A reductase in patients with statin-associated autoimmune myopathy. *Arthritis Rheum.* 2011;63(3):713–721.

Mariampillai K, Granger B, Amelin D, et al. Development of a new classification system for idiopathic inflammatory myopathies based on clinical manifestations and myositis-specific autoantibodies. *JAMA Neurol.* 2018;75(12):1528–1537.

Matteson EL, Dejaco C. Polymyalgia rheumatica. *Ann Intern Med.* 2017;166(9):ITC65–ITC80.

Moreira A, Loquai C, Pföhler C, et al. Myositis and neuromuscular side-effects induced by immune checkpoint inhibitors. *Eur J Cancer.* 2019;106:12–23.

Motomura K, Yamashita H, Yamada S, Takahashi Y, Kaneko H. Clinical characteristics and prognosis of polymyositis and dermatomyositis associated with malignancy: a 25-year retrospective study. *Rheumatol Int.* 2019;39(10):1733–1739.

Naddaf E, Paul P, AbouEzzeddine OF. Chloroquine and hydroxychloroquine myopathy: clinical spectrum and treatment outcomes. *Front Neurol.* 2020;11:616075.

Pinal-Fernandez I, Casal-Dominguez M, Huapaya JA, et al. A longitudinal cohort study of the anti-synthetase syndrome: increased severity of interstitial lung disease in black patients and patients with anti-PL7 and anti-PL12 autoantibodies. *Rheumatology (Oxford).* 2017;56(6):999–1007.

Stone JH, Klearman M, Collinson N. Trial of tocilizumab in giant-cell arteritis. *N Engl J Med.* 2017;377(15): 1494–1495.

Rheumatoid Arthritis and Other Autoimmune Diseases

Jiha Lee, Raymond Yung

The past decade has witnessed tremendous strides in our understanding of the pathogenesis and approach to treatment of autoimmune diseases. This is mirrored by a growing knowledge of the many immune system changes in aging, and clinicians' experience in administration of biological therapies in older adults with rheumatic diseases. While the field of rheumatology continues to focus on individual rheumatic illnesses, there is also a greater appreciation of the corresponding risks and side effects of these powerful agents on older patients with polypharmacy and multiple comorbid illnesses. This chapter summarizes recent key advances, with specific references to the geriatric population.

RHEUMATOID ARTHRITIS

Definition

Rheumatoid arthritis (RA) is a chronic systemic inflammatory disease that preferentially affects diarthrodial joints. The American College of Rheumatology (ACR), in collaboration with the European League Against Rheumatism (EULAR), updated the classification criteria of RA in 2010 (**Table 101-1**). The impetus for updating the original 1987 criteria was the recognition of the importance of early diagnosis and treatment of this disease. The new classification criteria therefore no longer include late sequelae of RA such as rheumatoid nodules or radiographic evidence of bony erosions. The new set of criteria should allow the study and treatment of patients with earlier stages of the disease. It should be noted that the new classification criteria apply to patients with objective evidence of synovitis in at least one joint, and the synovitis is not better explained by another disease such as lupus, psoriatic arthritis, or crystal-associated arthritis. It is also important to understand that the mean age of patients in the nine arthritis cohorts used to develop the new classification criteria ranges from 46 to 58 years. While the criteria set is useful for diagnosing early and active disease in younger patients, its usefulness in detecting community late-onset (> 60 years old) rheumatoid arthritis (LORA) has not been established. This is important because the disease presentation in LORA may be distinct from that of young-onset RA (YORA).

One important change in the 2010 classification criteria for RA is the inclusion of blood circulating anticyclic citrullinated peptide (anti-CCP) antibodies as equal to

Learning Objectives

- To relate the consequence of aging to the clinical manifestations of rheumatoid arthritis (RA) and other autoimmune diseases.

- To understand the effects of age-associated physiologic changes and comorbidities on the use of common anti-rheumatic disease drugs.

- To identify the use and limitations of current rheumatic disease classification and treatment guidelines in older patients with autoimmune diseases.

Key Clinical Points

1. Patients with various autoimmune diseases exhibit evidence of accelerated aging.

2. Recent rheumatoid arthritis classification criteria focus on early disease diagnosis; their usefulness is untested in older patients with the disease.

3. Injectable and oral biologic therapies targeting multiple immune system pathways represent major advances in the treatment of autoimmune diseases, but these therapies are all associated with significant risk of side effects in older patients, particularly those with multiple comorbidities.

4. Functional and social assessments are important components in the management of autoimmune diseases in older adults.

5. It is important to exclude iatrogenic causes of rheumatic symptoms in older patients, as polypharmacy is a common issue in this age group.

6. Paraneoplastic rheumatic syndromes occur in many malignancies prevalent in older patients.

rheumatoid factor (RF) in its scoring system. Citrullination is a posttranslational modification of protein-bound arginine into the nonstandard amino acid citrulline, and many

TABLE 101-1 ■ THE 2010 AMERICAN COLLEGE OF RHEUMATOLOGY/EUROPEAN LEAGUE AGAINST RHEUMATISM CLASSIFICATION CRITERIA FOR RHEUMATOID ARTHRITIS

Patients who (1) have at least 1 joint with definite clinical synovitis, (2) with the synovitis not better explained by another disease. A patient with a score of > 6 is classified as having definite disease.

	SCORE
A. Joint involvement	
1 large joint	0
1–3 large joints	1
1–3 small joints (with or without involvement of large joints)	2
4–10 small joints (with or without involvement of large joints)	3
> 10 joints (at least 1 small joint)	5
B. Serology (at least 1 test result is needed for classification)	
Negative RF and negative ACPA	0
Low-positive RF or low-positive ACPA	2
High-positive RF or high-positive ACPA	3
C. Acute-phase reactants (at least 1 test result is needed for classification)	
Normal CRP and normal ESR	0
Abnormal CRP or abnormal ESR	1
D. Duration of symptoms	
< 6 weeks	0
≥ 6 weeks	1

ACPA, anti-citrullinated protein antibodies; CRP, C-reactive protein; ESR, erythrocyte sedimentation rate; RF, rheumatoid factor.

Reproduced with permission from Aletaha D, Neogi T, Silman AJ, et al. 2010 Rheumatoid arthritis classification criteria: an American College of Rheumatology/European League Against Rheumatism collaborative initiative. Arthritis Rheum. 2010;62(9):2569–2581.

citrullinated proteins have been found to be expressed in inflamed joints. Anti-CCP antibodies are as sensitive (70%–78%) as, and more specific (88%–96%) than IgM RF in early and fully established disease. Furthermore, the presence of these antibodies is a marker for erosive disease and may predict the eventual development of RA in patients presenting with undifferentiated arthritis. These antibodies may also be detected in healthy individuals, years before the onset of clinical RA. Anti-CCP antibodies may be helpful in assessing arthritis symptoms in high-risk groups, such as those with a strong family history of RA. Unlike classical RF, the incidence of anti-CCP antibodies does not appear to increase with normal aging, making it a particularly useful marker for this disease in older patient population.

In addition to classification criteria for the diagnosis of RA, the ACR has established criteria for functional status and for determining clinical remission in RA. The usefulness of these classification systems in older patients who often suffer functional disability from concomitant osteoarthritis, soft-tissue rheumatism, and cardiovascular or neurologic diseases is unclear.

Epidemiology

The overall incidence of RA has been declining for a few decades. Interestingly, a long-term study from Mayo Clinic suggests that this may no longer be true. The study examined medical records in Olmsted County, Minnesota between 1985 and 2014, and found a steady incidence of age, sex, and race-adjusted RA. However, incidence of RF-positive RA decreased and incidence of RF-negative RA increased in 2005 to 2014 as compared with previous decades. The authors speculated that changing prevalence of environmental factors such as smoking, obesity, and others may have contributed to this trend.

The disease affects approximately 0.8% of the population in the United States and in many Western developed countries. Lower prevalence rates of 0.2% to 0.3% have been observed in China, Japan, some regions in Greece, and Africa. Southern Europeans may have a milder disease, with less extra-articular complications and less evidence of radiographic damage. Conversely, a much higher prevalence rate (up to 7%) and a more aggressive clinical course have been reported in several American-Indian and Alaska native populations. Gender and age are important factors in RA. Overall, women are affected by the disease two to three times more than men. However, this gender parity disappears in old age. The prevalence of RA increases with age and is commonest in the oldest group studied (often 65 years and older or 70 years and older). Approximately 5% of women older than 55 are affected by the disease. The incidence of RA also increases with age, with the peak incidence occurring in the sixth to eighth decades (**Figure 101-1**). The reason for the age-associated increase in disease susceptibility is currently unknown.

Pathophysiology

There has been marked progress in our understanding of the pathogenesis of RA. In the future, RA and other autoimmune disease may be subclassified based on the individual's genetic and molecular signatures, helping clinicians select the most appropriate treatment(s). RA is characterized by the activation and recruitment of T cells to the synovium, which set into motion a complex cascade of inflammatory responses (**Figure 101-2**). These responses result in further accumulation of inflammatory cells, panus formation, localized osteoporosis, bony erosions, and destruction of periarticular structures, which are characteristic of this disease. Rheumatoid synovitis is accompanied by the accumulation of inflammatory joint fluid with white cell count typically in the range of 2000 to 20,000 cells/mL. Soluble proteins that have been implicated in the inflammatory process include a number of proinflammatory cytokines (interleukin [IL]-1, IL-6, IL-13, IL-15, and tumor necrosis factor [TNF]), metalloproteinases (stromelysin, collagenases, and gelatinases), transforming growth factor-β,

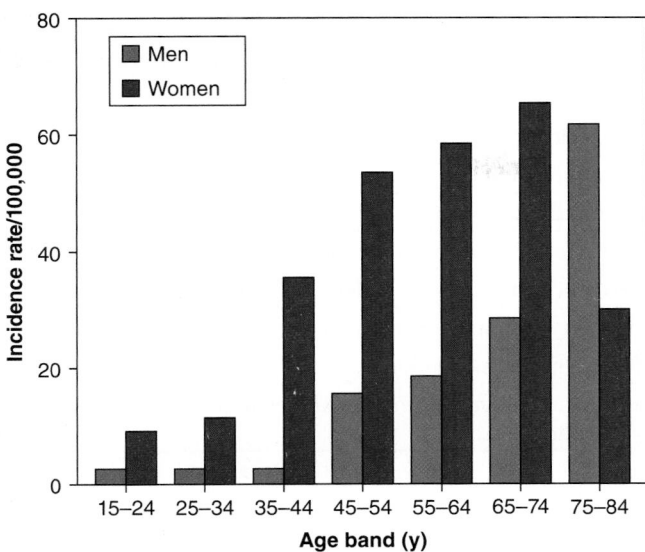

FIGURE 101-1. Age-related incidence of rheumatoid arthritis. (Reproduced with permission from Symmons DP, Barrett EM, Bankhead CR, et al. The incidence of rheumatoid arthritis in the United Kingdom: results from the Norfolk Arthritis Register. Br *J Rheumatol*. 1994;33[8]:735–739.)

granulocyte colony-stimulating factor, and activated complement components.

Genetic factors play an important role in RA susceptibility. The association between RA and human leukocyte antigen (HLA) has been refined to alleles coding for a "shared" epitope (the sequences QRRAA or QKRAA) on the HLA-DRB1 genes. The presence of the DRB1*04 (DR4) allele is a marker for increased susceptibility and severe disease. Population differences in the prevalence of the "shared epitope" may help to explain in part the geographic variation in the prevalence of RA. Genome-wide association studies (GWAS) have identified over 50 genetic susceptibility loci, including the HLA-DRB1 allele, and. may help explain racial and geographical differences in RA susceptibility. Importantly, GWAS have identified new and exciting pharmaceutical targets for this disease.

An infectious etiology for RA has been postulated for more than half a century. Acute and chronic "reactive" arthritis can follow specific gastrointestinal (GI) or genital urinary infection. A transient RA-like illness can be seen in viral infections including parvovirus B19, Epstein-Barr virus, and human T-lymphotropic virus type 1. Accumulating evidence suggests that "dysbiosis" of the oral and intestinal microbiomes may be important in RA pathogenesis. *Porphyromonas gingivalis*, which causes periodontal diseases and contains the citrullination enzyme peptidyl-arginine deiminase, has been linked to RA autoantibody formation and joint inflammation. Dysbiosis in older adults, usually referred to as inflammaging, contributes to the chronic low-grade proinflammatory state, and may influence characterization of RA in older adults.

RA had been considered to be primarily a Th (T helper) 1-mediated disease based on the cytokine and chemokine receptor profile of T cells in synovial joints. The related

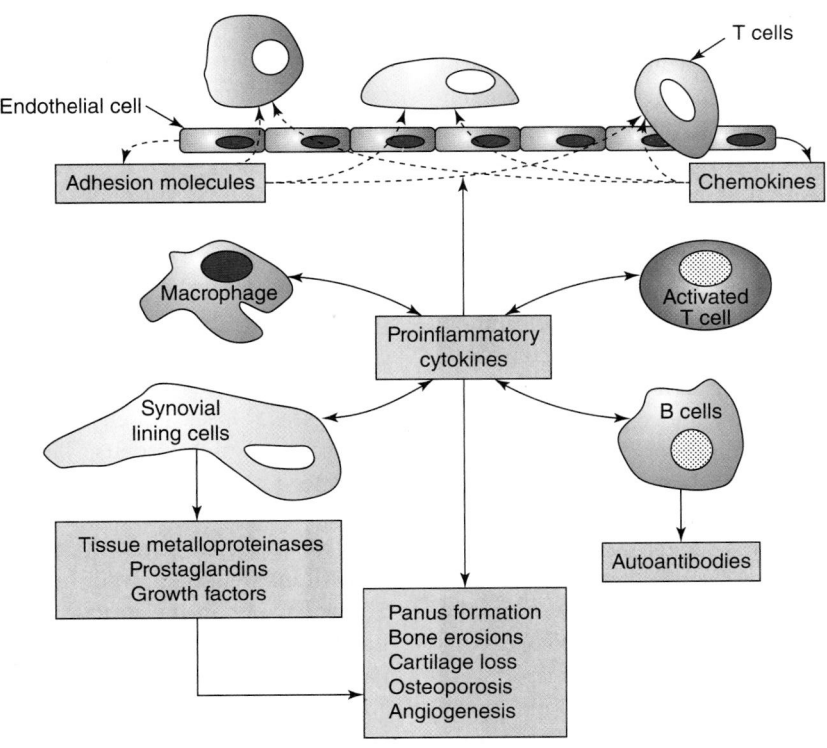

FIGURE 101-2. The inflammatory cascade in rheumatoid arthritis.

Th 17 (IL-23/IL-17) pathway may also be important in driving disease chronicity and joint destruction, although targeting the IL-23/IL-17 pathway has only modest success in RA compared to other forms of inflammatory arthritis. Although it is tempting to postulate that RA-associated DRB1 epitope triggers disease by presenting an arthrogenic peptide to T cells, extensive search of unique peptides that are displayed selectively by RA-associated HLA molecules has so far been unsuccessful. Costimulatory molecules, including CD28 and CD60, may play a role in activating T cells in RA joints. Dysfunctional T and non-T cell immune signaling has been increasingly recognized to be important in RA pathogenesis. This has resulted in the successful development of tofacitinib, a Janus kinase inhibitor (JAK inhibitor), as a novel therapy for RA. The precise contribution of B cells in RA pathogenesis is less well defined. The recent success of B cell depletion therapy has refocused attention on the role of these immune cells beyond autoantibody production, including plasma cells differentiation, and their immunomodulating effects on proinflammatory cytokines such as IL-6 and IL-17.

Aging effects The reason for the age-associated increase in RA susceptibility is unclear. The traditional view that aging is associated with a "decline" in immune response does not explain the high incidence and severe onset of this autoimmune disease that is commonly seen in older adults. Decline in sex hormone production also cannot account for the high incidence of RA in postmenopausal women. Age-related decline in thymic function has been suggested as a possible mechanism in autoimmunity in aging. While features of accelerated immune system aging are prevalent in RA patients, it is unclear if these represent primary or secondary events. Unlike in their younger counterparts, LORA occurs with equal frequency in men and women. Again, the rising incidence of RA in postmenopausal women suggests that reproductive hormones may influence the disease manifestation. However, they are unlikely to play a major pathogenic role in older adult population.

A central role of T cells in RA pathogenesis is well established, and enhanced production of proinflammatory cytokines in aging, including IL-6, TNF-α, and IL-1, important in the recruitment of T cells to RA joints may contribute to the increased susceptibility and severity of RA in older patients. Aging-associated obesity and changes in the gut microbiota may be important sources of chronic low-grade inflammation in older patients, which in turn may play a role in age-related diseases such as coronary artery disease, metabolic syndrome, Alzheimer disease, and cancer.

Presentation

Whether LORA is a different disease from YORA is controversial. The clinical studies that address the issue were mostly descriptive or cross-sectional studies done in the 1950s and 1960s that have significant methodologic problems. The older definition of RA used in these studies also allowed terms such as "classical," "definite," and "probable"

TABLE 101-2 ■ CLINICAL FEATURES OF OLDER ADULT-ONSET RHEUMATOID ARTHRITIS
Age of onset > 60 years
Male: female ~1:1
Acute presentation
Oligoarticular (2–6 joints) disease
Involvement of large and proximal joints
Systemic complaints, eg, weight loss
Absence of rheumatoid nodules
Sicca symptoms common
Laboratory: high erythrocyte sedimentation rate; often negative rheumatoid factor

RA, which are no longer used today. As mentioned before, the most current RA classification criteria have not been validated in older patients.

Table 101-2 summarizes the features of LORA. In general, patients with LORA have a more equal gender distribution. The large joints, including the shoulder joint, are more often involved at presentation in LORA. Whether this is a result of concomitant rotator cuff disease that is prevalent in this age group is unclear. Symptoms in the proximal girdles have led to the belief that LORA may present with a polymyalgia rheumatica-like illness. Erythrocyte sedimentation rate (ESR) normally increases with age, especially in women. Elevated ESR is also more common in LORA. The prevalence of RF similarly increases after the age of 60 years, reaching 30% by the age of 90 years. Earlier reports suggest a lower frequency of RF in LORA than YORA. However, this has not been confirmed in more recent studies. As in younger patients, patients with LORA who are seropositive for RF have more severe clinical disease, more bony erosions on x-ray, worse functional outcome, and increased mortality. Whether patients with LORA who are seropositive have worse prognosis than do their younger counterparts is unclear. It is possible that the poor prognosis of LORA reported in some studies reflects the greater number of comorbid conditions that are present in older patients.

"Benign polyarthritis in older adults" occurs in up to a third of patients with LORA. They have a more explosive disease onset associated with systemic features such as fever and night sweats. The clinical features have led some to describe the disease as "infectious like." The disease is called benign because its general prognosis is good, with most people going into remission within 1 year with or without treatment. Within this group can be included a peculiar syndrome unique to older patients called the RS₃PE (remitting, seronegative, and symmetric synovitis with pitting edema) syndrome. This typically affects older adult men (2–3:1, male to female ratio) and is characterized by acute onset of symmetric polyarthritis/tenosynovitis with pitting edema involving both upper and lower extremities. As the name implies, these patients generally have negative RF and antinuclear antibody (ANA). They often have high ESR and respond to low-dose prednisone. The association with HLA-B7 has been reported inconsistently. RS$_3$PE may occasionally be associated with other rheumatic diseases, including polymyalgia rheumatica, spondyloarthropathies, psoriatic arthritis, RA, and sarcoid, and, rarely, malignancies.

Evaluation

The assessment of RA in older adults is different from that of the younger age group. The nonspecific symptoms and signs of RA are prevalent in older patients. Rheumatic diseases that can mimic LORA, such as polymyalgia rheumatica, osteoarthritis, and crystal-induced arthritis, are prevalent in the older patient population. Anti-CCP antibody measurement may be useful in distinguishing LORA from polymyalgia rheumatica. In one small study, 65% of patients with LORA were anti-CCP antibody positive, but none of the patients with PMR or aged healthy subjects had the antibodies. Arthritis associated with malignancy can be misdiagnosed as RA before the correct diagnosis is made months or years later. Other differential diagnoses of RA in older population include inflammatory (erosive) osteoarthritis, late-onset spondyloarthropathy, endocrinopathy (eg, hypothyroidism, hyperparathyroidism, and diabetic cheiroarthropathy), amyloidosis, and the edematous phase of scleroderma. Conditions such as sarcoidosis, adult Still disease, hemochromatosis, and glycogen storage diseases can mimic RA but are unlikely to present for the first time so late in life. In addition to the above considerations, the initial evaluation of an older patient with RA should include a careful assessment of the patient's living condition, social support, and cognitive and functional status. Many older patients have the misconception that there is no effective treatment for arthritis, and they should accept their physical suffering as part of normal aging. Older adults may feel embarrassed about or minimize their symptoms of arthritis by using terms such as "aching" and "stiff" instead of pain. Unfortunately, many clinicians also do not take their symptoms seriously, resulting in older adults receiving less aggressive treatment and the patients frequently feeling that their care resembles "a lick and a promise." Because pain is, by far, the commonest presenting symptom of RA, pain assessment should be an integral part of the patient's evaluation at presentation and in subsequent office visits. This can be difficult in older patients who have significant cognitive or verbal impairment. Information from caregivers, nonverbal pain behavior, physical and radiographic evidence of active joint inflammation, and decline in function are important clues that more aggressive therapy may be necessary.

The ACR classification system for assessing the functional status of patients with RA is shown in **Table 101-3**. However, use of this classification for an older patient may be difficult because of functional disability from other coexisting diseases. This quick assessment tool is useful for

TABLE 101-3 ■ AMERICAN COLLEGE OF RHEUMATOLOGY 1991 REVISED CRITERIA FOR THE CLASSIFICATION OF GLOBAL FUNCTIONAL STATUS IN RHEUMATOID ARTHRITIS	
Class I	Completely able to perform usual activities of daily living (self-care, vocational, and avocational)
Class II	Able to perform usual self-care and vocational activities, but limited in avocational activities
Class III	Able to perform usual self-care activities, but limited in vocational and avocational activities
Class IV	Limited in ability to perform usual self-care, vocational, and avocational activities

Reproduced with permission from Hochberg MC, Chang RW, Dwosh I, et al. The American College of Rheumatology 1991 revised criteria for the classification of global functional status in rheumatoid arthritis. Arthritis Rheum. 1992;35(5):498–502.

describing the global functional status and allows patients to be grouped for studies. Patients with RA with the worst (class IV) functional status were reported to have extremely poor prognosis, with survival similar to patients with multiple vessel coronary artery disease and stage IV Hodgkin lymphoma. More recently the ACR recommended five RA disease activity measures including the Disease Activity Score in 28 Joints (DAS28) with ESR or C-reactive protein (CRP), Clinical Disease Activity Index (CDAI), and Simplified Disease Activity Index (SDAI), along with three patient-reported functional status assessment measures including the Patient-Reported Outcomes Measurement Information System (PROMIS) physical function 10-item short form and the Health Assessment Questionnaire (HAQ) for routine use in clinical practice in patients with RA. These composite measures containing patient, provider, laboratory, and/or imaging data have been used to evaluate physical, mental, and social health in older adults. Many clinicians now feel that the prognosis for RA has improved with the advent of better therapeutic regimens for RA in the past two decades. Whether this translates into prolonged survival remains to be determined. Concomitant medical conditions affecting the patient's hearing, eyesight, continence, and balance need to be addressed to optimize functional ability and to prevent falls. Current and past medical histories are important elements of the initial evaluation. This information is needed for the selection of specific treatment (see "Management" section). In contrast, family history is not as clinically helpful in assessing older patients with RA.

In addition to excluding the diseases mentioned above, a new patient suspected of having RA should be tested for the presence of anemia, cytopenia, liver or renal dysfunction, RF, anti-CCP, and elevated inflammatory markers of ESR and CRP. The presence of extremely high RF should prompt the clinician to consider the possible diagnosis of cryoglobulinemia. Some patients have negative RF but positive ANA. These patients tend to have more severe disease, similar to the patients with positive RF. A work-up for secondary Sjögren syndrome should be done in patients with concurrent sicca symptoms (dry eye and dry mouth). In general, ESR is a better indicator of disease activity than changes in the titer of RF. For some patients CRP level may more closely parallel their clinical course than ESR. Anti-CCP titer is not useful in following RA disease activity, although patients with reduced anti-CCP antibodies may have less joint damage in the long run. Anti-mutated citrullinated vimentin (MCV) antibodies have been touted as potentially new biomarkers for RA; early studies suggest the test could be a better predictor of aggressive disease and bone erosion than the anti-CCP test. Age does not appear to impact anti-MCV antibody titer, although this has not been demonstrated to be true in older RA population. A multibiomarker blood test of 12 proteins, Vectra DA, for determining RA disease activity has been approved by the US Food and Drug Administration (FDA). The test has good correlation with traditional clinical assessment of RA disease activity. The test is intended to complement, and not replace, sound clinical judgment. The test could be a useful objective tool in older RA patients who are unable to provide reliable feedback to the clinician because of impaired cognitive function or other comorbidities. "Cytokine panel" can be measured to examine for individual patient's proinflammatory cytokine profile, but its role in personalized medicine (eg, choosing between anti-TNF versus another class of biologic therapy) and improving clinical outcomes has not been established.

Radiographic joint examination is an integral part of the evaluation of patients with RA. Older patients with RA for more than 10 years are at particular risk of cervical spine disease and atlantoaxial joint instability. This is an important consideration before a patient is intubated, as overextension of the cervical spine may compromise

the brainstem or spinal cord. Early x-ray changes include soft-tissue swelling and regional osteoporosis around the joint. Typical erosions in hands and feet involve the juxta-articular "bare areas" of bone not covered with cartilage (**Figure 101-3**). Isolated erosions in the first and second metacarpophalangeal joints may prompt the clinician to search for occult calcium pyrophosphate depositive disease, hyperparathyroidism, or hemochromatosis. Erosions are less common in the knee and hip joints. At these sites, RA typically causes cartilage loss and joint-space narrowing. Joint-space narrowing occurring predominantly in the lateral compartment of the knee and diffusely in the hip without bony proliferation is helpful for distinguishing RA from osteoarthritis. To assess joint-space narrowing of the knees, clinicians should request semiflexed weight-bearing films.

Because of the limitation of clinical examination in detecting subtle signs of inflammation, peripheral joint ultrasound and magnetic resonance imaging have been increasingly used for detecting early or mild synovitis. The majority of patients with treated disease and considered by their physicians to be in remission continue to have evidence of active synovitis in advanced imaging such as ultrasound and magnetic resonance imaging. The unanswered question is whether more aggressive treatments of patient with clinically inactive disease but imaging evidence of ongoing synovitis affect patient outcomes such as overtreatment (and drug side effects), and long-term disability. Moreover, older patients with RA have additional facets that need to be taken into consideration, such as a more limited lifespan and greater infection risk with immunosuppression. Although embraced by many rheumatologists, the utility of these sensitive imaging modalities in clinical practice remains incompletely defined. The ACR "Choosing Wisely" recommendations recommend that MRI of the peripheral joints should not be used to routinely monitor

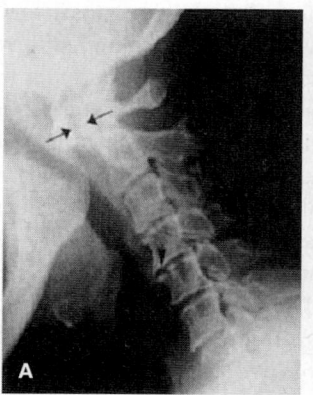 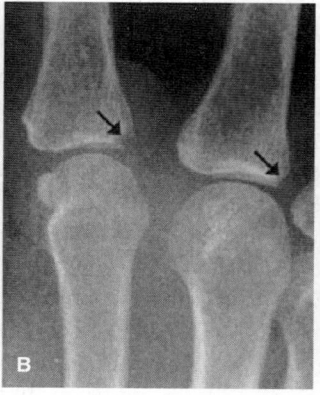 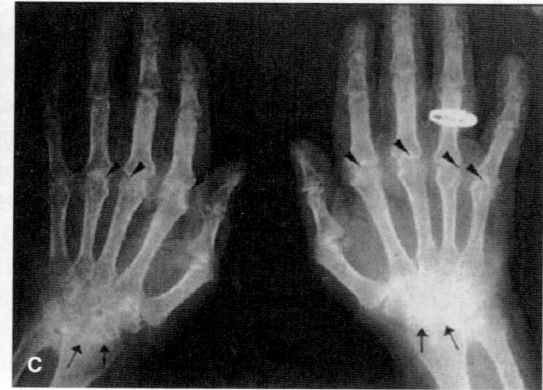

FIGURE 101-3. Radiographic changes of rheumatoid arthritis. (**A**) An x-ray of the cervical spine in the flexed position showing severe atlantoaxial joint subluxation in a patient with chronic rheumatoid arthritis, with *arrows* highlighting the abnormal distance between the posterior surface of the anterior arch of the atlas and the anterior surface of the odontoid process. *Arrowhead* points to the erosion on the surface of C5. (**B**) Early erosive changes in the metacarpal phalangeal joints affecting the "bare area" of the bone not protected by cartilage. (**C**) Bilateral hand x-ray with advanced rheumatoid arthritis. Some of the features include juxta-articular osteoporosis, collapse of the carpal bones, radial deviation of the radiocarpal joint of the wrist (*arrows*), and erosion and destruction of metacarpal phalangeal joints (*arrowheads*). Note also the symmetric nature of the disease. (Reproduced with permission from Curtis Hayes, MD, University of Michigan.)

inflammatory arthritis. And the ACR Musculoskeletal Ultrasound Committee recognizes that the imaging modality may be reasonable to use in many clinical scenarios in rheumatology practice, but lacks cost-effectiveness data.

There is no evidence that patients with LORA are more likely to develop extra-articular disease, as compared to those with YORA. However, older patients may be disproportionately affected because extra-articular manifestations are more common in chronic RA. High titer of RF is a risk factor for extra-articular RA, especially in male patients. Rheumatoid nodules are the most characteristic extra-articular manifestation of RA and are present in up to 40% of seropositive White patients. These are most commonly found in areas of pressure such as the elbows, heels, and sacrum. Their presence does not correlate with disease activity and may increase in number during methotrexate therapy when synovitis is improving. Rheumatoid vasculitis affects vessels of all sizes. This complication may present as cutaneous vasculitis, mononeuritis multiplex, nail fold infarcts, or deep "punched-out" ulcers at atypical sites that fail to respond to conventional therapy. Pleuritis and pericarditis are found in 20% to 30% of patients with RA and do not usually cause any symptoms. Other respiratory complications of RA include pulmonary granuloma (often in the upper lobes), Caplan syndrome, fibrosing alveolitis, and bronchiolitis obliterans. Felty syndrome (RA with splenomegaly and neutropenia) typically occurs in White patients with long-standing, chronic erosive RA. These patients are at increased risk of developing lymphoproliferative malignancies. Thrombocytopenia may occur, in part, because of splenic sequestration. Mild-to-moderate normochromic, normocytic anemia is extremely common in patients with chronic RA. Iatrogenic causes (eg, nonsteroidal anti-inflammatory drugs [NSAIDs] and methotrexate) of anemia need to be excluded in all patients with RA who have anemia.

Management

A number of treatment concepts and standards have emerged in RA clinical management. There is increasing recognition of the benefits of early and aggressive therapies in improving the long-term outcomes of RA. Outdated treatment goals have focused on improving patient symptoms by 25% or 50%. The concept of "treat-to-target" has long been embraced by clinicians treating diseases such as hypertension, hyperlipidemia, and diabetes. A similar "treat-to-target" approach has gained wide acceptance in RA management, utilizing composite disease activity indexes that have traditionally been confined to research, such as the DAS-28 or CDAI. The advent of biological therapies has allowed clinicians to aim for disease remission in many RA patients. And patients with poor prognostic factors of female sex, seropositive for RF and anti-CCP, increased inflammatory markers, functional limitations, and erosive changes on radiography have benefited from early initiation of biologic therapy. Nevertheless, there are unanswered questions about this aggressive management approach. These include lack of consensus on what disease activity measurements should be used and frequency of monitoring. And important issues to be addressed in future research include treatment burden (including cost and side effects), and benefits in remaining life (prognostication) in older patients with multi-comorbid diseases.

Nonpharmacologic therapies Successful management of RA involves patient participation in his/her care. In addition, family, social, and psychological supports are particularly critical in maintaining the older RA patient's independence. Older patients diagnosed with the disease may be particularly fearful of what it means to their independence or may become depressed. Establishing a good rapport, gaining the trust of the patient and the family, providing information about the nature of the disease, and setting realistic goals are all important elements of the initial management of RA. Many patients and their relatives also find it helpful to seek out support groups in their local area. Increasingly, older patients and their families are turning to the Internet, health magazines, and other nontraditional sources for information about treatment options, including over-the-counter complementary therapies. There is a need for health care professionals to become knowledgeable in web and social media medical resources. Unexpected side effects of over-the-counter medications are increasingly being recognized. The latest information is often not available in traditional textbooks. Directing the patients to reputable websites such as those offered by the National Institute on Aging, the National Center for Complementary and Integrative Health, the Natural Medicines Comprehensive Database, the Cochrane Reviews, the American College of Rheumatology, or the Arthritis Foundation can be useful for more up-to-date information.

Nonpharmacologic therapies are crucial components of the total care of the patient with RA, which should be emphasized throughout the treatment course. In addition to their inherent usefulness, participation in these treatment modalities often provides the patients and their families with a sense of control over their chronic illness. The interprofessional team approach that typifies geriatric medicine is eminently suitable for treating older patients with chronic arthritis. Physical and occupational therapy should be offered to every patient with RA, including those with mild and early disease. Education about rest/activity, use of cold/heat, massage, and adaptive devices (to improve function and to prevent/correct joint deformity) are important. Performing exercises to strengthen muscles and ligaments for joint protection, gait training, and fall prevention can make a big difference in the life of patients with RA. Community-based exercise programs, such as the Centers for Disease Control and Prevention (CDC)-endorsed Arthritis Foundation Exercise Program (AFEP), are a good resource for those who are able to participate. Psychological counseling and support groups are often helpful, especially to those who are socially isolated because of their arthritis. Depression is increasingly recognized as a common problem in older patients and in those with chronic illness. Adequate treatment will help break the vicious cycle of pain, depression, and disability. Although nonpharmacologic therapies do not affect the progression of RA joint destruction, they can improve the patient's quality of life and help to reduce the requirement for pain medications that have significant potential for side effects in this vulnerable population.

Pharmacologic therapies There is an explosion of new drugs available for the treatment of RA. In particular, the number of biological response modifiers available to clinicians has expanded considerably, and many more are in the late stages of clinical development. The success of these agents, which target soluble inflammatory proteins, T cells, and B cells, suggests that targeting the downstream mediators may be sufficient to modulate the disease. The mechanism of action, monitoring considerations, and common side effects of conventional synthetic disease-modifying antirheumatic drugs (csDMARDs), targeted synthetic DMARDs (tsDMARDs), and biologic DAMRDs (bDMARDs) are summarized in **Table 101-4**.

The gradualism of the "pyramid approach" to RA treatment in the 1980s has been replaced with the widespread "treat-to-target" approach that aims to suppress RA

TABLE 101-4 ■ PHARMACOTHERAPY AGENTS FOR THE MANAGEMENT OF RA

MEDICATION	MECHANISM/BENEFITS	SIDE EFFECTS/ADVERSE EVENTS/CONSIDERATIONS
CONVENTIONAL-SYNTHETIC DMARDs (csDMARDs)		
Methotrexate	• Potent inhibitor of dihydrofolic acid reductase • Most commonly prescribed for RA • Subcutaneous with better bioavailability than oral administration	• Side effects: cytopenia (anemia), liver toxicity (fibrosis and cirrhosis), hypersensitivity pneumonitis, infections, mucosal ulcerations, alopecia • Daily folic acid supplementation
Antimalarials (hydroxylchloroquine, quinacrine, chloroquine)	• Unclear, may change intracellular pH and affect Ag presentation by immune cells • Recommended hydroxychloroquine dose: 5 mg/kg • Annual ocular screening, preferably with optical coherence tomography (OCT)	• Retinal (macular) toxicity and reversible corneal deposits, may be lower with hydroxychloroquine compared to chloroquine • Avoid in older adults with macular degeneration or inoperable dense cataracts • May prolong QT interval
Sulfasalazine	• Unclear, may reduce Ig levels, suppress T- and B-cell proliferative response, and cytokine inhibition	• Side effects: cytopenia (leukopenia), GI symptoms, skin rashes • Avoid in those with sulfa drug allergy
Leflunomide	• Inhibitor of pyrimidine synthesis • Equal in efficacy to MTX	• Side effects: diarrhea, reversible alopecia, elevated LFTs • Half-life of 14 days, chelate with cholestyramine
BIOLOGIC DMARDs (bDMARDs)		
TNF inhibitors Etanercept	• Recombinant soluble p75TNF receptor fused to the Fc portion of human IgG • Subcutaneous once or twice a week	• Increased risk of serious infections • Screen for infections: TB quant, hepatitis panel, fungal serology every 1–2 years
Infliximab	• Chimeric (mouse-human) anti-TNF monoclonal antibody • IV every 4–8 weeks	• Increased risk of malignancy • May exacerbate NYHA class III/IV heart failure
Adalimumab	• Fully human anti-TNF antibody • Subcutaneously every 2 weeks	• Rare cases of demyelinating disorders, aplastic anemia, lupus-like illness, depression
Certolizuman pegol	• Monoclonal antibody with an extended half-life • Subcutaneously every 4 weeks	
Golimumab	• IV anti-TNF, every 8 weeks	
Abatacept	• Recombinant fusion protein combining extracellular domain of human CTLA-4 and Fc domain of human IgG1 • Modified to avoid complement fixation • IV or subcutaneous administration	• Contains maltose and can give falsely elevated glucose readings in some glucose monitors

(Continued)

TABLE 101-4 ■ PHARMACOTHERAPY AGENTS FOR THE MANAGEMENT OF RA (*CONTINUED*)

MEDICATION	MECHANISM/BENEFITS	SIDE EFFECTS/ADVERSE EVENTS/CONSIDERATIONS
BIOLOGIC DMARDs (bDMARDs) *(Cont.)*		
Anakinra	• IL-1 receptor antagonist • Subcutaneous daily	• High incidence of local skin injection site reaction • Adjust dose based on renal function
Tocilizumab	• Humanized monoclonal antibody targeting IL-6 • IV or subcutaneous administration	
Rituximab	• Chimeric anti-CD20 antibody • B-cell depletion therapy approved for use of RA patients with inadequate response to anti-TNFs or other biologics	• Has nonhuman protein sequence and should be used with another agent such as methotrexate • Increased risk of infection • Consider PJP prophylaxis
TARGETED-SYNTHETIC DMARDs (tsDMARDs)		
JAK inhibitor	• 3 agents are FDA-approved: tofacitinib, baracitinib, and upadacitinib • Oral administration	• Increase in cholesterol levels • Early reports of increased risk of cardiovascular disease and cancer compared to anti-TNF agents • Increase risk of gastrointestinal perforation
OTHER MEDICATIONS		
Glucocorticoids	• May be "disease modifying" in early disease	• Dose-dependent increased risk of serious infection • Consider prophylaxis of osteoporosis; CV risk factors, diabetes, and GI complications are important
NSAIDs	• Anti-inflammatory	• Age-dependent increased risk of upper GI bleed • Nephrotoxicity
COX-2 inhibitors	• Analgesics	• Increased incidence of cardiac events

CV, cardiovascular; GI, gastrointestinal; LFT, liver function test; MTX, methotrexate; NYHA, New York Heart Association; PJP, *Pneumocystis jirovecii* pneumonia; TNF, tumor necrosis factor.
Data from Fraenkel L, Bathon JM, England BR, et al. 2021 American College of Rheumatology Guideline for the Treatment of Rheumatoid Arthritis. Arthritis Care Res (Hoboken). 2021;73(7):924–939.

disease activity as completely and as soon as possible once the diagnosis is confirmed. This change in philosophy is, in part, a result of the recognition that joint damage occurs much sooner than was previously believed. Results of well-designed clinical trials have persuaded many that this new standard is attainable with more aggressive and early initiation of drug regimens. The 2021 ACR Guideline for the Treatment of Rheumatoid Arthritis provides updated recommendations for the pharmacologic management of RA, taking into consideration current disease activity, prior therapies used, and the presence of comorbidities **(Table 101-5)**. For DMARD-naïve RA patients with moderate-to-high disease activity, methotrexate monotherapy is recommended over other csDMARD (as dual or triple therapy), bDMARD, or tsDMARD therapy. Oral methotrexate is recommended at initiation, and those not at target may switch to subcutaneous methotrexate for better bioavailability. For RA patients not at target despite maximal tolerated methotrexate use, addition of bDMARD or tsDMARD is recommended, over triple therapy of methotrexate, hydroxychloroquine, and sulfasalazine. If patients have inadequate response to a bDMARD or tsDMARD, they may switch to a different class of biologic-modifying DMARD.

Clinicians are often reluctant to use csDMARDs such as methotrexate and leflunomide as monotherapy because of their limited efficacy, high dropout rate, and potential serious side effects, especially in older patients. Great caution and dose adjustment are often needed when using these drugs to treat older adults with RA, especially in those with a history of renal and liver failure. The use of bDMARD or tsDMARDs in combination with or without methotrexate can boost the therapeutic efficacy of selected biologics. However, whether older patients tolerate combination therapies as well as monotherapy is uncertain.

Rituximab may be of benefit in patients with RA refractory to other biologic therapy and extra-articular manifestations such as rheumatoid vasculitis and interstitial lung disease. The main advantage of using combination of csDMARD therapy over the anticytokine biologic treatments is cost. Many European countries and US insurance companies continue to require patients to have a trial of methotrexate before receiving biologic therapies. An important advantage of biologic agents is rapid onset of action, with many patients experiencing improvement within a few weeks of treatment. These agents appear to be effective in patients with both seropositive and seronegative RA. The author has also found in his own practice that biologics

TABLE 101-5 ■ 2021 ACR GUIDELINES FOR PHAMACOLOGIC MANAGEMENT OF RA

CLINICAL CONTEXT/PRESENTATION	RECOMMENDATIONS
DMARD-NAÏVE PATIENTS	
Moderate-to-high disease activity	• Methotrexate monotherapy strongly recommended • Initiate csDMARD, without short- or long-term glucocorticoids
Low disease activity	• Hydroxychloroquine recommended over other csDMARDs • Sulfasalazine recommended over methotrexate • Methotrexate recommended over leflunomide
csDMARD treated but methotrexate-naïve patients with moderate-to-high disease activity	• Methotrexate monotherapy recommended over combination of methotrexate plus a bDMARD or tsDMARD
DMARD MODIFICATION FOR PATIENTS NOT AT TARGET	
On maximally tolerated dose of methotrexate	• Addition of bDMARD or tsDMARD recommended over triple therapy with methotrexate, hydroxychloroquine, and sulfasalazine
On bDMARD or tsDMARD	• Switching to a different class of bDMARD or tsDMARD recommended over switching to another in the same class
TAPERING/DISCONTINUING DMARDs	
At target for at least 6 months	• Continuation of all DMARDs at current dose recommended over dose reduction • Dose reduction recommended over discontinuation • Gradual discontinuation recommended over abrupt discontinuation
SPECIFIC PATIENT POPULATION	
With subcutaneous nodules	• Methotrexate recommended over alterative DMARDs
Mild and stable pulmonary disease	• Methotrexate recommended over alterative DMARDs
With NYHA class III or IV heart failure and inadequate response to csDMARDs	• Addition of non-TNF inhibitor bDMARD or tsDMARD recommended
On TNF inhibitor and develop heart failure	• Switching to a non-TNF inhibitor bDMARD or tsDMARD recommended
With lymphoproliferative disorder	• Rituximab recommended over other DMARDs
Hepatitis B infection	• Prophylactic antiviral therapy recommended over frequent monitoring
Nonalcoholic fatty liver disease without LFT abnormality or evidence of fibrosis	• Methotrexate recommended over alternative DMARDs
Persistent hypogammaglobulinemia without infection	• Continuation of rituximab for patients at target
Serious infection within previous 12 months	• Addition of csDMARD recommended over bDMARD or tsDMARD if not at target • Avoid initiation/dose escalation of glucocorticoids
Nontuberculosis mycobacterial (NTM) lung disease	• Addition of csDMARD recommended over bDMARD or tsDMARD if not at target • Use of lowest possible dose of glucocorticoids (discontinuation if possible) • Abatacept recommended over other bDMARDs and tsDMARDs

Data from Fraenkel L, Bathon JM, England BR, et al. 2021 American College of Rheumatology Guideline for the Treatment of Rheumatoid Arthritis. Arthritis Care Res (Hoboken). 2021;73(7):924–939.

are more efficacious in reducing specific symptoms such as fatigue in RA patients, compared to csDMARDs.

As new data emerge and new therapies become available, it is anticipated that updated treatment guidelines will be available much more frequently than in the past. However, older adults are often excluded from clinical trials, leaving a gap in knowledge on the efficacy and safety of RA treatment with DMARDs. It will be important to draw from limited clinical trial data and observational studies to understand how the new guidelines apply to older RA patients, especially in those with multiple medical conditions. Pharmaceutical companies have increasingly included older adults in pre- and postmarketing clinical trials. Additionally, there are an increasing number of rheumatology research consortia and registries that have provided "real world" data on the benefits and side effects of new treatments on older RA patients. Knowing that these agents may be efficacious in older patients provides some reassurance to clinicians. However, it is important to remember that subjects participating in these studies rarely mirror the patients geriatricians see in their clinic who have multiple comorbidities and who already suffer from polypharmacy. The decision as to which biological modifier to use will depend on individual patient characteristics such as comorbidity, patient preferences such as administration schedule, physician experience, and insurance coverage owing to the high cost of these drugs. Because of the complexity of modern treatment regimens, coupled with the need to monitor many potentially serious side effects, drug therapy for RA should ideally be instituted in consultation with a rheumatologist. Involvement of physicians experienced in the use of immunosuppressive therapies (eg, hematologists and oncologists, or a gastroenterologist in the case of infliximab) will be helpful in patients living in isolated communities where there may not be a local rheumatologist.

Safety and Other Issues with Biologics While there is little doubt about the potential efficacy of the biologics in RA, there remains significant concern about their side effects, especially in vulnerable populations such as older patients with RA having multiple comorbidities. One useful acronym for the safe use of biologics is CONSIDER, outlined in **Table 101-6**. TNF is involved in host defense against foreign pathogens and in tumor surveillance. The most important risk associated with anticytokine therapy for older patients with RA is the increased incidence of fungal infections, tuberculosis, and atypical mycobacterial infections. The incidences of infections and serious infection were higher among older adults with RA compared to younger patients enrolled in the community-based Consortium of Rheumatology Researchers of North America (CORRONA) registry. Moreover, infection risks associated with tofacitinib were comparable to that of other biologic DMARDs such as anti-TNF therapies. As tuberculosis is usually caused by reactivation of latent infection, tuberculosis skin testing or interferon-gamma release assay and a chest x-ray should be done prior to starting these agents. Whether yearly tuberculosis screening and chest x-ray to detect new exposure are necessary in countries with a low incidence of tuberculosis is unclear. Yearly screening is recommended for selected patients who are at risk, such as those who travel regularly to TB endemic areas and nursing home residents.

Rare cases of demyelinating disorders, aplastic anemia, lupus-like illnesses, and depression have also been associated with anti-TNF therapies. The long-term consequences of anticytokine suppression are unknown. One meta-analysis reported a fourfold higher rate of malignancies in patients treated with TNF inhibitors.

Rituximab dramatically lowers the peripheral blood B-cell count for months after the infusion, and these patients also have lower IgG and IgM levels. The use of rituximab has been associated with the reactivation of JC polyomavirus infection, resulting in the disease progressive multifocal leukoencephalopathy. This complication, although very rare, highlights the potential for the development of all B-cell–dependent viral diseases in patients receiving the drug. Interestingly, progressive multifocal leukoencephalopathy has also been reported in patients with multiple sclerosis receiving natalizumab, a chimeric anti-α4 integrin antibody. Patients on rituximab are at risk for hepatitis B reactivation, and should be screened

for the virus before initiation of therapy. Interestingly, rituximab has been successfully used in hepatitis C virus (HCV)-associated cryoglobulinemia without worsening of HVC-associated liver disease.

Are biologics "cost effective" in the treatment of older adults with rheumatic diseases? Cost effectiveness for young patients with RA is based on remaining in the workforce, but there are no such data for the geriatric cohort of retirees, and it is hard to define the economic value of improved functional status or quality of life. Wide variability has been observed in the prescription of biologics for older adults and their economic impact is all the more elusive. Changes in frailty, falls, fractures, hospitalization for serious infections, and potentially inappropriate medication use may provide alternative measures of cost effectiveness of RA treatment in older adults. The US FDA approved several "biosimilars" for adalimumab, infliximab, and rituximab, and increasing competition among the growing number of biologics is anticipated to help drive down the cost. Additionally, lower doses (than FDA guidelines) and, in some cases, reducing dose frequencies or duration of biologic treatments may be acceptable in selected patients to reduce risk of side effects and cost without adversely affecting outcomes.

As in other populations, cardiovascular disease is the single largest cause of death in patients with autoimmune inflammatory disorders. However, after accounting for the known traditional risk factors for heart diseases, patients with RA and lupus are at greater risk of developing coronary artery disease and stroke than those without these conditions. The reason for the increased incidence of cardiovascular disease in patients with these disorders of autoimmunity is not clear. Furthermore, a patient with RA who has a myocardial infarction has a similar prognosis as that of a diabetic patient with a similar event. Conventional therapies, such as the use of lipid-lowering agents, may not reverse the cardiovascular risk associated with these inflammatory conditions. While not proven, it is hoped that use of more aggressive immunosuppressive regimens will help reduce the cardiovascular morbidity and mortality in these patients. Aging per se has been described by some as a state of chronic low-grade inflammation that has been termed "inflamm-aging," which may play a role in frailty and sarcopenia in both normal aging and chronic inflammatory conditions such as RA. Current data do not support an increased risk of major adverse cardiovascular events in tocilizumab-treated RA patients, despite the drug's propensity to increase lipid levels.

A disease-associated inflammatory state, chronic use of steroids, and the lack of exercise owing to arthritis-associated disability may all contribute to the high incidence of osteoporosis in older patients with rheumatic diseases. Since these are chronic conditions, aggressive treatment with antiresorptive agents, adequate calcium intake, and vitamin D to prevent and treat osteoporosis and fracture is critical.

Many RA therapies involve significant immunosuppression that may affect the patient's ability to mount an antibody response to immunization, worsening the

TABLE 101-6 ■ CONSIDER THE FOLLOWING WHEN USING IMMUNOMODULATORY THERAPY IN OLDER ADULTS

Comorbidities: The patient's underlying conditions such as cancer, unhealing pressure ulcers, chronic lung diseases, frequent urinary tract infections, hypercholesterolemia, or diverticulitis can increase the risk of complications when using immunosuppressive medications. Cognitive issues may also result in noncompliance and increase the risk for side effects.

Opportunistic infections: The older and more frail patients are at an even greater risk of developing opportunistic infections when exposed to biologics, such as reactivation and new acquisition of tuberculosis, viral (eg, herpes zoster, cytomegalovirus, viral hepatitis), or fungal infections.

Novel presentation of side effects: Older adults often have novel or atypical presentation of infection complications. For example, the patient may present with altered mental status and be unable to mount a fever or adequate white cell count elevation.

Screening: The physician should ensure that the older rheumatic disease patient be appropriately screened for cancer, infection, dental health, and heart disease. There should be a low threshold for re-screening for health conditions and to initiate early treatment as necessary.

Immunization: If at all possible, older adults should receive vaccinations against infections before they are started on an immunomodulatory agent.

Drug dosing and interactions: Older patients are more likely to suffer from polypharmacy. While there is a paucity of information regarding drug interactions with biologics, old age has an effect on pharmacokinetics of selected biologics. In addition, it may be prudent to select shorter acting biologics in the older adult population who are at risk for severe infection complications.

Evaluate: Physicians need to aggressively evaluate and monitor older patients for early sign of adverse events, including more frequent follow-up, than younger patients.

Remaining lifespan: The potential benefit of biologics should be considered in the context of a patient's life expectancy. Frail older patients with limited remaining lifespan are at high risk of side effects from biological therapies.

already-impaired immune reaction as a result of immune senescence in older patients. It is, therefore, important that these patients are given their age-appropriate immunizations such as pneumococcal and flu vaccines preferably prior to receiving therapy with biologics. Patients already on biologics should avoid receiving any live vaccines.

Glucocorticoid Use in Treatment of RA Clinicians continue to debate the role of glucocorticoids in the management of RA, despite intriguing data showing that in early disease it may be "disease modifying," because of frequent difficulty tapering and negative impacts associated with unintended prolonged glucocorticoid use. There is general consensus that high-dose chronic oral glucocorticoids should not be used in RA. Low-dose glucocorticoid may be considered for short-term (< 3 months) symptom control in patients with active RA. Unfortunately, older patients commonly develop significant side effects and become functionally dependent on the drug. Medicare beneficiaries older than age 75 with RA receiving less than or equal to 5 mg, more than 5 to 10 mg, or more than 10 mg of glucocorticoid per day had a 20%, 32%, and 47% increased risk for serious infection, respectively, compared to 13% risk in nonglucocorticoid users. In addition to dose-dependency, the risk of serious infection increases with prolonged use of glucocorticoids even at low dose. Older RA patients in Canada (mean age 74) taking as little as 5 mg prednisolone had a 30%, 46%, or 100% increased risk of serious infection when used continuously for the prior 3 months, 6 months, or 3 years, respectively, compared to nonsteroid users. Overall, it is important to use the lowest dose of glucocorticoids, with alternate day dosing if possible, for the shortest duration of time possible in this population, and to discontinue the drug when it is feasible. Interestingly, provider preference is one of the strongest predictors of RA patients receiving long-term glucocorticoids use. Assessment, prophylaxis, and treatment of osteoporosis, cardiovascular risk factors, diabetes, and GI complications are important. Judicious use of intra-articular steroid injections may provide local (and systemic) symptom relief and may be safer than oral glucocorticoids in older patients with poorly controlled diabetes, severe osteoporosis, and congestive heart failure. A time-release prednisone formulation has been approved by the US FDA, and the drug can be taken at night to improve morning symptoms in RA patients.

Prevention

A major problem in attempting to prevent RA is identifying those who are at risk of developing the disease in the first place. Although genetic studies provide some clues as to which segment of the population may be at risk, the available information is not precise enough to be of practical use. Conversely, epidemiologic data suggest that smoking is a strong risk factor for RA, as well as more active and difficult to control disease, and developing RA-related interstitial lung disease. Smoking cessation is associated with lower RA disease activity, and may delay or even prevent development of seropositive RA. Along with environmental factors, preclinical anti-CCP positivity is associated higher risk of developing erosive RA, and ongoing studies are examining the early use of DMARDs such as hydroxychloroquine to determine if such approaches will prevent development of the full-blown chronic disease.

Special Issues

Patient preference and comorbidity The choice of therapy should be made in conjunction with the patient and the caregivers. Although exercises are important to maintain joint and muscle functions in patients with RA, some older patients are unable to perform regular exercises because of their other medical conditions, or if they have lived an inactive lifestyle for many years and are reluctant to adopt any change. In these situations, emphasizing the positive aspects of exercise (physical, psychological, and social), setting realistic goals, and recommending exercise programs specially tailored for the older population are helpful. In this regard, finding a physical and occupational therapist accustomed to working with older adults is important. Too often the author has seen patients who refuse to return to their therapist because of unrealistic short-term exercise goals.

The importance of assessing a patient's risk of developing GI, renal, or cardiac complications, and osteoporosis prior to starting NSAIDs and corticosteroids has already been emphasized. Patient preference is important when deciding on a specific DMARD. Older patients with poor eyesight are often reluctant to begin antimalarials out of fear of potential ocular complications, however small the risk may be. These drugs are contraindicated in older patients who cannot be monitored for retinal toxicity, including individuals with macular degeneration or untreated cataract. Older adults who do not want to give up drinking alcohol may choose not to take methotrexate. Some older women have refused to take methotrexate because the drug was part of their breast cancer chemotherapy in the distant past. Intramuscular or subcutaneous methotrexate can be used in older patients who experience dyspepsia or who have difficulty swallowing. Methotrexate and biological response modifiers must be used with extreme caution or not at all in patients with chronic or active infection. Whether older patients with chronic lung disease taking DMARDs should receive *Pneumocystis carinii* prophylaxis is unclear. Assessment of the patient's tuberculosis status should be done prior to beginning anticytokine therapy. The appropriate use of biologics has already been discussed extensively.

Older patients on biologic therapies are faced with several important questions about immunization. Older patients with RA should have their immunization history thoroughly reviewed, and ideally have received all the appropriate immunizations prior to receiving DMARDs and biologic therapies (particularly rituximab). Influenza and pneumococcal vaccines should be given as they are in the general population. Short-term discontinuation of methotrexate for 2 weeks after influenza vaccination may improve vaccine response without significant increase in RA disease activity or transient risk of arthritis flare. Those who have not received the pneumococcal 13-valent vaccine (Prevnar 13) should receive the vaccination. The use of tetanus toxoid should be as per normal guidelines except for patients who have received rituximab within the previous 24 weeks, when passive immunization with tetanus immunoglobulin is recommended. Current recommendation is against the use of live vaccines in patients on biologic therapies. However, two studies suggest that RA patients on biologics may be safely vaccinated with the attenuated live herpes zoster vaccine, particularly if their disease is under good control. In recent years, a recombinant zoster vaccine was approved by the FDA offering a safer option for biologics-exposed patients. High rheumatoid disease activity and the use of biologics, prednisone, or hydroxycholoroquine are all risk factors for zoster in RA patients.

One study examined the influence of comorbidities on clinical outcomes of over 1500 DAMRD/biologics-treated RA patients in the CORRONA registry. As expected, older patients have more comorbidities than the younger cohort. Although disease activity measures at entry to the registry were similar across age categories, older patients have less improvement in their disease and functional measures over time, and were less likely to attain remission at follow-up. Importantly, the age difference can be largely accounted for by the number of comorbidities in the older patient population.

Care settings The physician's choice of therapy has to take into account the patient's overall state of health and mobility, and the care setting. In most cases, home laboratory monitoring for DMARD toxicity can be arranged for patients with significant mobility problems. Instead of DMARDs, the use of corticosteroids (oral, intra-articular, or parenteral; low- or high-dose "pulse" treatment) may be a good option in patients with RA with active disease in the end stages of their lives. Therapeutic goals may also be different in a patient near the end of life, when either long-term treatment outcome or side effects may not be important considerations. An example is a patient with RA who has end-stage dementia, when judicious use of corticosteroid rather than high-dose immunosuppression for active disease may be more appropriate. Biologic therapies achieve their therapeutic effect much sooner than DMARDs, such as methotrexate, and may therefore be a reasonable choice in DMARD-naïve patients whose disease is not controlled by corticosteroids and who are near the end of life.

SYSTEMIC LUPUS ERYTHEMATOSUS

Systemic lupus erythematosus (SLE) is a prototypic auto-immune disease that predominantly affects the female population. The incidence of lupus has been increasing with an estimated quarter of a million patients now with the disease in the United States. Late-onset lupus (LOL) is defined as symptoms beginning after the age of 55, representing approximately 10% of all cases of lupus. However, the United Kingdom General Practice Research Database (a population database covering 5% of the United Kingdom) has surprising data that the peak incidence of lupus in women occurs at age 50 to 54 years and for men it is 70 to 74 years. Improved therapies and greater appreciation of the importance of treating comorbid conditions such as coronary artery disease have resulted in more patients with lupus surviving into old age. An ongoing CDC–sponsored study in Southeast Michigan in the United Sates showed that there are substantial racial disparities in the burden of SLE, with Black patients experiencing earlier age at diagnosis and a twofold increase in SLE incidence and prevalence compared to White (**Figure 101-4**).

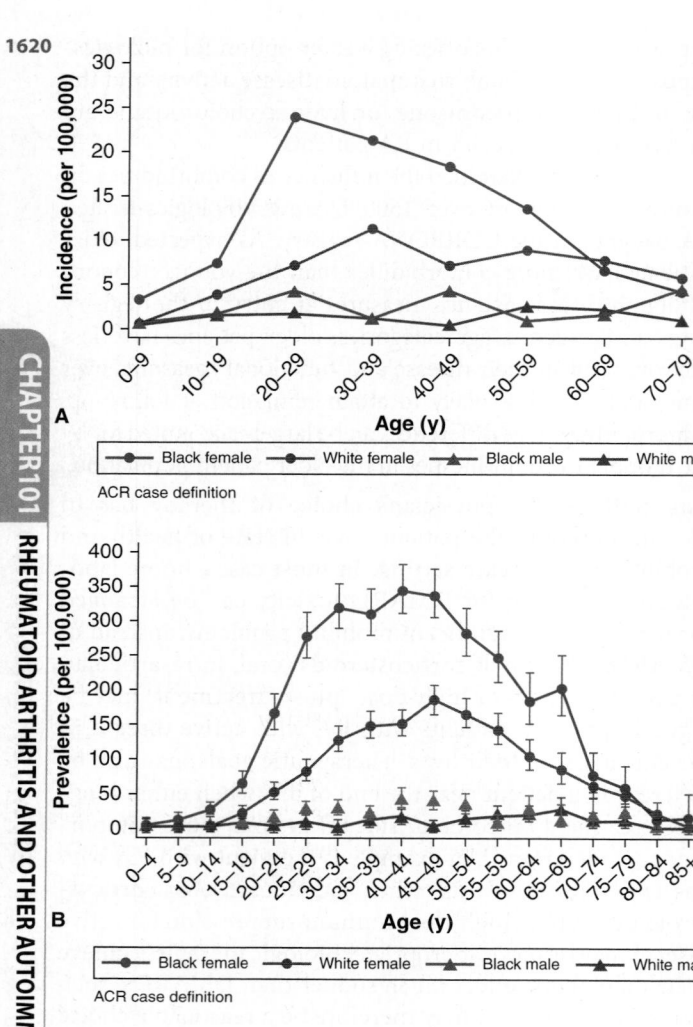

FIGURE 101-4. Age-specific annual incidence (**A**) and prevalence (**B**) rates (per 100,000 persons) of systemic lupus erythematosus in southeastern Michigan, United States, 2002–2004 (Reproduced with permission from Somers EC, Thomas SL, Smeeth L, et al. Incidence of systemic lupus erythematosus in the United Kingdom, 1990–1999. *Arthritis Rheum.* 2007;57[4]:612–618.)

TABLE 101-7 ■ 2019 EULAR/ACR CLASSIFICATION CRITERIA FOR SYSTEMIC LUPUS ERYTHEMATOSUS (SLE)

ANA	≥ 1:80 TITER ON HEP-2 CELLS OR AN EQUIVALENT POSITIVE TEST
Fever	Temperature > 38.3°C
Hematologic abnormalities	Hemolytic anemia, leukopenia/lymphopenia, or thrombocytopenia
Neuropsychiatric illness	Seizures or psychosis
Oral or nasal ulceration	Oral ulcers are often painless and occur in unusual parts of the oral cavity
Cutaneous manifestations	Subacute/acute cutaneous or discoid lupus
Serositis	Pleuritis, acute pericarditis, or peritonitis, pleural or pericardial effusion
Arthritis	Nonerosive polyarthritis involving the small joints
Renal disease	Proteinuria (> 0.5 g/d), lupus nephritis on biopsy according to ISN/RPS 2003 classification
Immunologic abnormalities	Anti-dsDNA, anti-Sm, or antiphospholipid antibody
Low complement	Low C3 and/or low C4

ANA, antinuclear antibody; dsDNA, double-stranded deoxyribonucleic acid; Sm, Smith (antigen).
Data from Aringer M, Costenbader K, Daikh D, et al. 2019 European League Against Rheumatism/American College of Rheumatology Classification Criteria for Systemic Lupus Erythematosus. Arthritis Rheumatol. 2019;71(9):1400–1412.

Diagnosis

The diagnosis of SLE is based on the presence of signs, symptoms, and laboratory features of autoimmunity. The 1982 ACR Classification Criteria for SLE were revised to include the presence of antiphospholipid antibodies. And the most recent 2019 EULAR/ACR Classification Criteria for SLE use ANA as an entry criterion and include noninfectious fever (**Table 101-7**). These criteria were designed for research purposes and have not been validated in LOL. Low-titer ANA may be present in up to one-third of older adults. Positive ANAs (titer ≥ 1:80) have high sensitivity but poor specificity for SLE when measured by indirect immunofluorescence using the standard Hep-2 substrate. In contrast, the presence of anti-dsDNA (double-stranded deoxyribonucleic acid) or anti-Sm (Smith) antibodies is highly specific for SLE. However, these antibodies are only detected in 31% to 86% and 0% to 24% of patients with LOL, respectively.

Pathogenesis

The cause of SLE is unknown. The concordance rate of SLE in monozygotic twins is between 25% and 50%, suggesting that genetic and environmental factors are both important. Hormonal factors are important in the pathogenesis of SLE as the disease often affects women of childbearing age. Similar to other autoimmune diseases, an inciting role for microbial organisms has been postulated but not proven. Human SLE is a polygenic disease. At least 50 susceptibility or resistance loci have been identified in human and murine lupus (eg, *sle*1, 2, 3). A defect or deficiency in gene product(s) regulating immune complex clearance, such as in some cases of inherited complement (C1, C4, and C2) deficiencies, is associated with a high likelihood of the development of SLE. Variability in the Fcγ receptor alleles is believed to play a role in determining the susceptibility to SLE in some racial and ethnic populations.

In addition to changes in the adaptive arm of the immune system, there is a pathogenic role for aberrant innate immune responses in lupus. Immune cells such as dendritic cells, macrophages, and other myeloid cells all participate in both the adaptive and innate arms of immune responses. Interferon alpha, a key mediator of innate immunity, may also be important in lupus pathogenesis. A Toll-like receptor 7 (TLR7) signaling defect may be important in sustaining the inflammatory response in this disease.

It is not clear whether LOL is a different disease from younger onset lupus. Many older adults have a low level of circulating autoantibodies. Additionally, measures of various markers of immunosenescence suggest that patients with autoimmune diseases have accelerated aging of the immune system. Given the apparent high incidence of lupus in middle-aged and late life, a better understanding of how immune senescence can affect the normally tightly regulated process that prevents the development of autoimmunity is needed. One hypothesis is that defective T-cell activation in aging may result in a suboptimal immune response to foreign antigen, which, in turn, may allow these cells to cross-react with self-antigens. Secondly, thymic involution and the accumulation of memory T cells in aging may "force" the proliferation of naïve T cells with high affinity for self-antigen. Thirdly, epigenetics, which refers to the regulation of gene expression through cellular processes including DNA methylation, histone modification, and RNA interference, is affected by aging. Both DNA methylation and histone acetylation are important mechanisms for the development of lupus and potentially other autoimmune diseases. Whether the age-dependent epigenetic changes also affect genes that are important in the development of autoimmunity in aging is unknown. Finally, it has been postulated that age-related DNA methylation changes may "reawaken" X-chromosome genes that have previously been inactivated in females. This, in turn, may help to explain the gender differences in lupus in the older adult population.

Presentation

Because of the lack of awareness of this disease in older people, the average time it takes from the onset of symptoms to the diagnosis of LOL is long, averaging between 2 and 3 years. The female to male ratio of LOL is approximately 4:1, much lower than the 9:1 ratio in the younger age group. The high prevalence of SLE in younger African-Americans is not so apparent in LOL. However, whether this merely reflects the demographics of the study locations is unclear.

The clinical features of patients with LOL are quite different from those of patients who develop lupus at a younger age (**Table 101-8**). The patients with LOL tend to have a milder disease and are less likely to develop alopecia, malar rash, photosensitivity, oral/nasal ulceration, glomerulonephritis, and lymphadenopathy. Patients with LOL may be more prone to develop cytopenias, serositis, and interstitial pneumonitis. Interestingly, the incidence of cancer, with the exception of non-Hodgkin lymphoma, may be lower in LOL than in younger patients with lupus. The cause of death in patients with LOL is usually related to complications of treatment such as infections, cardiovascular disease, and stroke.

Management

The choice of therapy is largely dictated by the specific disease manifestations. Antimalarials (see above) are useful for many lupus symptoms including arthritis, serositis, mucositis, and

TABLE 101-8 ■ THE FREQUENCY OF SYMPTOMS AND SIGNS OF LATE-ONSET SLE

SYMPTOMS/SIGNS	FREQUENCY (%)
Arthritis/arthralgia	60
Rash	47
Cytopenias	45
Interstitial pneumonitis	41
Serositis	32
Raynaud phenomenon	28
Neuropsychiatric	25
Peripheral neuropathy	25
Glomerulonephritis	24

Adapted with permission from Kammer GM, Mishra N. Systemic lupus erythematosus in the elderly. Rheum Dis Clin North Am. 2000;26(3):475–492.

skin disease. Available evidence strongly supports the long-term use of antimalarials in patients with lupus. Quinacrine, available from many compounding pharmacists, does not cause retinal damage and may be used in older patients who cannot take potentially retinotoxic drugs. NSAIDs are used by the majority of patients with lupus for symptomatic relief of arthralgia, myalgia, serositis, fever, and headaches. Their use in older patients must be weighed against their potential side effects. NSAIDs are best avoided in patients with lupus having renal involvement.

Local corticosteroid treatments such as (short-term) topical or intradermal injections can be helpful in cutaneous lupus. Systemic steroids are often reserved for more severe diseases such as lupus pneumonitis, carditis, hemolytic anemia, or new-onset renal disease. Intravenous "pulse" methylprednisolone in doses of 1 g/day for up to 3 consecutive days can be lifesaving in rapidly progressive or fulminant disease.

The use of cytotoxic drugs such as cyclophosphamide has significantly reduced morbidity and mortality associated with lupus nephritis. Monthly intravenous pulse cyclophosphamide is generally well tolerated and has fewer side effects than daily oral administration of the drug. Azathioprine, mycophenolate mofetil, or rituximab may be used in lupus patients with renal disease who are unable to tolerate high-dose corticosteroids or cyclophosphamide. Cytotoxics should not be withheld from older patients with lupus who have major organ involvement. The use of alkylating agents is associated with an increased risk of future cancer development. However, this may be a more important consideration in younger patients with a longer life expectancy. Gonadal toxicity is not a very important issue in the older adult population.

There has been an explosion of interest in clinical treatment trials of newer drugs in lupus. Promising preliminary data include drugs that target the interferon pathway, including anifrolumab. In 2011, belimumab, a human monoclonal antibody that inhibits soluble B-lymphocyte activating factor (BAFF), became the first lupus drug in its class to receive US

FDA approval and its indication was expanded to include the treatment of active lupus nephritis in 2021. Vovlosporin, an oral calcineurin inhibitor, in combination with other background immunosuppression, has recently been approved by the FDA for adult patients with active lupus nephritis but the role in older lupus patients remained untested.

SJÖGREN SYNDROME

Definition

Sjögren syndrome is a chronic inflammatory autoimmune disease characterized by progressive lymphocytic and plasma cell infiltration of the exocrine glands, leading to dry mouth (xerostomia) and dry eye (keratoconjunctivitis sicca). The syndrome can occur in isolation (primary) or in association with other autoimmune diseases (secondary) such as RA, SLE, or polymyositis. In addition to the sicca symptoms (dry eyes and dry mouth), serologic evidence of autoimmunity and objective assessment of oral and ocular involvement need to be documented before the diagnosis of Sjögren syndrome is made. The Schirmer test, in which a strip of Whatman No. 41 filter paper is placed in the lower conjunctival sac, is considered positive if less than 5 mm of the paper is wet after 5 minutes. Ocular involvement can also be documented by staining the conjunctiva with 1% Rose Bengal stain and slit-lamp eye examination. Minor salivary gland biopsy is the most commonly performed test used in diagnosing salivary gland involvement in Sjögren syndrome. The test is considered positive when there is more than one focus (aggregate of ≥ 50 lymphocytes) per 4 mm^2 of biopsy specimen. Biopsy of the parotid, rather than of a minor salivary gland, should be done in patients complaining of parotid gland swelling. Saliva production is measured after overnight fasting without oral stimulation (brushing of teeth, smoking, etc). A normal person should produce at least 1.5 mL of saliva in 15 minutes. Parotid sialography and salivary gland scintigraphy are alternate procedures for documenting salivary gland involvement.

Epidemiology

Depending on the definition and the age of the population studied, the prevalence of Sjögren syndrome has been estimated to be between 0.04% and 4.8%, making it the second commonest autoimmune disease after RA. The disease is likely underdiagnosed as patients often fail to discuss their symptoms with their physicians or believe that the symptoms are part of the inevitable consequence of aging. One study on a geriatric population suggests that subclinical disease may occur in up to 3% of the nursing home population. Although the prevalence of sicca symptoms increases with age, the peak incidence of primary Sjögren syndrome occurs in the fourth and fifth decades of life, with a 9:1 female:male ratio.

Pathogenesis

Most cases of Sjögren syndrome occur sporadically, although there are examples of familial aggregation. An association with HLA antigens has been reported, including HLA-DR3, HLA-DR2, and HLADRw52 in White populations. In addition, HLA-DR3 and HLADQw2.1 are linked to the development of anti-Ro antibodies. Like most other autoimmune diseases, an environmental or viral trigger has been proposed for Sjögren syndrome. One theory suggests that autoimmune lymphocytes are "homed" to salivary and lacrimal glands. This is followed by clonal expansion of the autoreactive cells in the glands, upregulation of major histocompatibility complex and adhesion molecules by epithelial cells, and secretion of proinflammatory cytokines by lymphocytes and epithelial cells. Defective apoptosis causing the failure to delete autoreactive cells has been proposed as a central mechanism explaining the lymphoid aggregates seen in the exocrine glands. α-Fodrin, a cytoskeletal protein, was recently identified as a candidate autoantigen in Sjögren syndrome. Interestingly, neonatal immunization with this antigen can prevent the development of the disease in an animal model of Sjögren syndrome.

Presentation and Clinical Features

Most patients with Sjögren syndrome have a slowly progressive and benign course. The onset of the disease is insidious, and it may take up to 10 years for the full-blown disease to develop. Older patients with Sjögren syndrome usually present with sicca symptoms. They may complain of difficulty chewing and swallowing dry foods, the frequent need to drink liquid especially at night, difficulty wearing dentures, abnormal taste, sore/burning sensation in the mouth, and intolerance to spicy foods. Xerostomia also predisposes these patients to dental decay and the development of oral candidiasis. Instead of the classical white candida plaque, patients with Sjögren syndrome may have erythematous oral candidiasis. In addition to the feeling of dryness in the eyes, patients with ocular involvement may complain of an itching or burning sensation, the feeling that there is a foreign body in the eye, and photosensitivity. Unilateral or bilateral parotid gland swelling occurs in one-third of all patients with primary Sjögren syndrome and is more commonly seen in the younger age group. The differential diagnosis of unilateral or bilateral parotid gland swelling includes viral (including HIV-1) and bacterial infections, sarcoidosis, salivary gland ductal obstruction, and neoplasm. Immunoglobulin G4-related disease (IgG4-RD) is increasingly being recognized to have clinical features that overlap with Sjögren syndrome. This heterogeneous collection of disorders shares features of tumor-like swelling of involved organs such as salivary and parotid glands, a lymphoplasmacytic infiltrate of IgG4-positive plasma cells, and elevated serum IgG4 levels in 60% to 70% of affected patients. This disease should be considered in patients with sicca symptoms but who have negative autoantibodies.

Approximately 60% of patients with Sjögren syndrome develop extraglandular disease (**Table 101-9**). Nonerosive arthritis/arthralgia is the commonest extraglandular manifestation and may precede sicca symptoms. Any part

TABLE 101-9 ■ EXTRAGLANDULAR MANIFESTATIONS OF SJÖGREN SYNDROME

Cutaneous	Xerosis (including dryness of nasal passage, skin, and vagina); Raynaud phenomenon; cutaneous vasculitis
Pulmonary	Desiccation of the tracheobronchial tree; lymphocytic infiltration (alveolitis, interstitial pneumonitis, pseudolymphoma, lymphoma); pleuritis/pleural effusion; vasculitis; pulmonary hypertension
Gastrointestinal	Dysphagia; atrophic gastritis; malabsorption; pancreatic dysfunction and pancreatitis; hepatomegaly and hepatitis; primary biliary cirrhosis
Renal	Interstitial nephritis; glomerulonephritis; distal renal tubular acidosis; kidney stones
Hematologic	Anemia; cryoglobulinemia
Neuromuscular	Sensory and trigeminal neuralgia; vasculitis; mononeuritis multiplex; neuropsychiatric disorders; seizures; encephalopathy; myelitis; aseptic meningitis; dementia; myopathy and myositis
Endocrine	Autoimmune thyroid disease

of the pulmonary tree from the trachea to the pleural lining may be involved, causing cough, hoarseness, and shortness of breath. Pseudolymphoma and lymphoma should be suspected when an unexplained pulmonary nodule or lymphadenopathy is seen on chest radiograph. Patients with Sjögren syndrome may experience dysphagia because of dryness of the oral pharynx or abnormal esophageal motility. Chronic atrophic gastritis, gastric lymphoma, vitamin B_{12} deficiency, and antibodies to parietal cells have all been described in this disease. Autoimmune thyroid disease is present in 13% to 45% of patients with Sjögren syndrome. Patients with Sjögren syndrome often have an elevated liver enzyme profile, especially if antimitochondrial antibodies are present. Interestingly, sicca symptoms are present in 50% of patients with primary biliary cirrhosis. Renal disease occurs in approximately 10% of patients with Sjögren syndrome. Lymphocytic infiltration and immune complex deposition, proximal renal tubular acidosis with Fanconi syndrome, renal stones, electrolyte imbalance, and cryoglobulinemia have all been reported.

The association of RA and Sjögren syndrome was first described by Henrik Sjögren in 1933. Although it is believed that RA is the commonest cause of secondary Sjögren syndrome, its true prevalence in RA is unknown. Patients with secondary Sjögren syndrome have milder disease with primarily sicca symptoms (dry eyes and dry mouth). Systemic complications such as salivary gland swelling, central nervous system disease, renal disease (interstitial nephritis or glomerulonephritis), and lymphoproliferative disease are uncommon.

Patients with Sjögren syndrome often have polyclonal hypergammaglobulinemia, as well as selective increased production of specific autoantibodies. ANA and RFs are present in more than 75% and 66% of patients with Sjögren syndrome, respectively. Anti-Ro and anti-La antibodies are detected in 70% and 40% of the affected patients. Interestingly, anti-La antibodies are less common in the secondary form of the disease.

Management

Simple lifestyle changes such as air humidification and avoidance of cigarette smoke are helpful. Nasal dryness can be treated with saline drops or gel. Vaginal dryness can be reduced using water-soluble lubricants and estrogen cream. Dry skin can be improved by using moisturizers and bath oil. Lipstick and lip balm can be used to reduce lip dryness. Meticulous oral hygiene and frequent dental visits are important to prevent dental decay and oral candidiasis. Frequent fluid replacement, topical fluoride treatment, the use of non-alcohol-based or water-soluble vitamin-based mouthwash, and sugarfree chewing gum can all be helpful. Unfortunately, artificial saliva substitutes that are currently available are not very helpful. Oral candidiasis can be treated with a prolonged course (1–4 months) of a noncariogenic antifungal drug (eg, nystatin vaginal tablets 100,000 units two to three times a day), with separate treatment of dentures.

The mainstay of treatment for dry eye remains artificial tears. Preparations now available can penetrate into the epithelial cell layer, extending duration of action. However, these may occasionally cause blurring and leave residue on eye lashes. Because patients with Sjögren syndrome generally require long-term tear replenishment, preservative-free artificial tears should be used. Topical low-dose cyclosporine can be used for Sjögren eye disease. Tear drainage can also be reduced by the placement of occlusive elements (eg, silicon implants) in the puncta or permanently by laser or thermal cautery. Soft contact lenses may be used to protect the cornea, especially in the presence of keratitis filamentosa. Because the contact lenses require wetting, the patient needs to be careful not to introduce infection to the eyes. Plastic wrap or swimming goggles can be used at night to reduce tear evaporation.

Whenever possible, drugs with significant cholinergic side effects should be discontinued. Muscarinic agonists (pilocarpine and cevimeline) may be helpful in alleviating dry mouth symptoms in patients with Sjögren syndrome. In 2016, the Sjögren's Syndrome Foundation provided clinical practice guidelines on the use of biologic agents. Anti-TNFs are not recommended to treat sicca symptoms in primary Sjögren syndrome. For musculoskeletal symptoms, hydroxychloroquine should be considered first line, and if ineffective, methotrexate, leflunomide, sulfasalazine, azathioprine, cyclosporine, and corticosteroids can be prescribed. For extraglandular disease, azathioprine may be more beneficial than leflunomide or sulfasalazine, and

Rituximab may be considered for severe systemic manifestations such as interstitial pneumonitis, interstitial nephritis, and vasculitis. Unfortunately, while treatments are helpful for symptomatic relief, the destruction of exocrine gland continues despite best current effort.

DRUG-INDUCED RHEUMATIC SYNDROMES

Polypharmacy and iatrogenic diseases are important geriatric issues. Medications are also increasingly recognized as common causes of rheumatic syndromes. These can be broadly categorized into drug-induced lupus (DIL), drug-induced myopathy/myositis, and drug-induced vasculitis. Drug-induced myopathy/myositis will be discussed in detail in the myopathy chapter.

Drug-Induced Lupus

More than 100 drugs have now been implicated in DIL (**Table 101-10**), although a much smaller number have a strong association. The average age of onset is between 50 and 70 years. However, specific criteria for the diagnosis of DIL have not been established. Compared to the idiopathic

TABLE 101-10 ■ DRUGS IMPLICATED IN DRUG-INDUCED LUPUS

Acebutolol	Interferon (α, γ)	Phenylacetylurea
Aminoglutethimide	Interleukin-2	*Phenytoin*
Amiodarone	*Isoniazid*	Practolol
Amoproxan	Labetalol	Prazosin
Anthiomaline	Lamotrigine	Primidone
Atenolol	Leuprolide acetate	Prinolol
Benoxaprofen	Levodopa	*Procainamide*
Canavanine (L-)	Levomeprazone	Promethazine
Captopril	Lithium carbonate	Propylthiouracil
Carbamazepine	Lovastatin	Psoralen
Chlorpromazine	Mephenytoin	Pyrathiazine
Chlorprothixene	Mesalazine	Pyrithoxine
Cimetidine	Methimazole	*Quinidine*
Cinnarizine	*Methyldopa*	Quinine
Clonidine	Methysergide	Rifamycin
Clozapine	Methylthiouracil	*Sulfasalazine*
COL-3	Metrizamide	(5-Amino) salicylic acid
Danazol	*Minocycline*	Simvastatin
Diclofenac	Minoxidil	Spironolactone
1,2-Dimethyl-3-hydroxypyride-4-1 (Ll)	Nalidixic acid	Streptomycin
Disopyramide	Nitrofurantoin	Sulindac
Estrogens	Nomifensine	Sulfadimethoxine
Etanercept	Oral contraceptives	Sulfamethoxypyridazine
Ethosuximide	Olsalazine	Terbinafine
Flutamide	Oxyphenisatin	Tetracycline
Fluvastatin	Para-aminosalicylic acid	Tetrazine
Gold salts	*Penicillamine*	Thioamide
Griseofulvin	Penicillin	Thioridazine
Guanoxan	Perazine	Timolol eye drops
Hydralazine	Perphenazine	Tolazamide
Hydrazine	Phenelzine	Tolmetin
Ibuprofen	Phenopyrazone	Trimethadione
Infliximab	Phenylbutazone	Zafirlukast

Drugs with the strongest associations are in italic.
Data from Yung RL, Richardson BC. Drug-induced rheumatic syndromes. Bull Rheum Dis. 2002;51(4):1.

disease, patients with "classical" DIL have a milder illness and a more restricted autoantibody profile. Antihistone antibodies are present in high frequencies in DIL associated with drugs such as procainamide or hydralazine but are not as frequently seen in patients with drugs such as minocycline or anti-TNF agents. The incidence of DIL has been estimated to be approximately 15,000 to 20,000 per year, with between 30,000 and 50,000 patients currently affected in the United States.

Procainamide (procainamide-induced lupus, PIL) and hydralazine (hydralazine-induced lupus, HIL) are drugs historically associated with DIL and are well-defined DIL models. Patients with DIL are usually older and more likely to be men, reflecting the age and sex of the population receiving these drugs. One-third of patients receiving procainamide for more than a year will develop symptoms, and almost all will become ANA-positive after 2 years. In contrast, fewer than 20% of hydralazine-treated patients will develop DIL. The risk for developing HIL is dose-dependent and is highest in patients taking more than 200 mg/day and in those who have taken more than 100 g cumulative dose. Compared to patients with idiopathic lupus, patients with PIL and HIL have fewer renal, neuropsychiatric, and skin manifestations. Pleuropulmonary complaints are particularly common in PIL, while immune cytopenias are uncommon in DIL in general. By definition, all patients with DIL are ANA-positive (mostly homogenous pattern). More than 90% of patients with PIL and HIL have antihistone antibodies, and 20% to 40% are RF-positive.

Up to 19% of patients treated with IFN-α develop some form of autoimmunity. Approximately 12% of patients receiving this drug develop positive ANA, and between 0.15% and 0.7% will develop a lupus-like illness. Anti-dsDNA antibodies occur in 8%, and almost all the patients with IFN-α-induced lupus have elevated anti-dsDNA antibodies. The development of autoimmunity appears to be dependent on the dose and duration of treatment. Other rheumatic syndromes associated with IFN-α include RA, polymyositis, psoriatic arthritis, Reiter syndrome, and sarcoidosis. Autoimmune thyroid diseases are common following IFN-α treatment. It is important to differentiate this from idiopathic hypothyroidism that is prevalent in the older adult population.

Patients receiving TNF antagonists often develop serologic evidence of autoimmunity. In one study, new ANA and anti-dsDNA antibodies were found in 33% and 9% of infliximab recipients, respectively. However, there is clear discordance between the development of autoantibodies and clinical autoimmunity, with only a handful of symptomatic patients reported, mostly with skin diseases. Approximately 13% of patients exposed to infliximab develop infliximab-specific antibodies. Patients receiving concurrent immunosuppressants such as methotrexate or azathioprine are less likely to develop these antibodies. The presence of antibodies to infliximab increases the likelihood of an infusion reaction but does not predict the development of autoantibodies or DIL.

Clinicians are often concerned that a patient's rheumatic complaints may represent the early systemic presentation of an occult tumor. Patients with autoimmune diseases are also at higher risk of developing cancers. Many cancer therapies are complicated by rheumatologic side effects. Finally, immunosuppressive therapies used for treating autoimmune diseases may predispose the patients to malignancies.

Musculoskeletal Symptoms Associated with Cancer

Although the mechanisms for paraneoplastic rheumatologic complications are often poorly understood, many are believed to be endocrine or immune-mediated. An extensive search for an occult malignancy is not recommended in patients with most rheumatic syndromes unless there are specific symptoms or findings suggesting the possible presence of a tumor. Nevertheless, the possibility of metastatic disease should be considered in an older patient presenting with severe pain in or around a joint. Metastatic joint disease caused by lung or breast cancer is usually monoarticular or oligoarticular (two to five joints). Pain and synovitis are caused by synovial inflammation in response to tumor cells in and around the joint. Large joints (eg, knee and hip) are most commonly affected. However, asymmetric polyarthritis can occur at the late stages of cancer. The vertebral column is a common place for metastatic disease. A malignancy work-up should be done if an older patient presents with intractable or nocturnal back pain that is increasing in severity and if the patient has constitutional symptoms such as fever or weight loss. Multiple myeloma frequently causes lytic lesions and pathologic fractures. Light-chain amyloidosis occurs in 15% of these patients and is associated with a symmetric small-joint arthropathy. In addition, amyloid infiltration in the shoulder joint produces the classical "shoulder pad sign." Hyperuricemia and gout may develop in patients with large tumor bulk, especially during chemotherapy. Raynaud phenomenon with or without panniculitis in older adults has been described in occult malignancy including cutaneous manifestations of myeloma.

Hypertrophic osteoarthropathy is the most common rheumatic syndrome associated with malignancy and is almost always caused by metastatic lung cancer in the Western world. Ankles, wrists, knees, and fingers are the sites most frequently affected. The cause is unknown, but a neurally mediated mechanism is suggested by improvement with vagotomy and atropine. Carcinomatous polyarthritis can precede or follow the diagnosis of the underlying cancer, most commonly breast in women and lung in men. The classical description is an acute-onset asymmetric seronegative polyarthritis in an older patient that resembles LORA. The arthritis often improves with cancer therapy and may relapse with tumor recurrence. A polymyalgia rheumatica-like disease has been linked to metastatic cancer. This is suggested by a younger age of onset, prominent constitutional symptoms, asymmetric involvement of proximal muscle groups, a relatively low sedimentation rate, and an incomplete response to prednisone. The Lambert-Eaton syndrome is characterized by an antibody-mediated defect in acetylcholine release at the neuromuscular junction. It is most commonly associated with small cell carcinoma of the lung. Ptosis, distal muscle involvement, and characteristic electromyogram findings distinguish the disease from common inflammatory myopathies. Bilateral palmar fasciitis with or without polyarthritis is associated with gynecologic tumors, in particular, ovarian carcinoma. This is usually associated with late metastatic disease and carries a poor prognosis. Panniculitis with synovitis and serositis is a well-known accompaniment of pancreatic cancer. POEMS syndrome (polyneuropathy, organomegaly, endocrinopathy, M-[monoclonal] protein, and skin abnormalities) is associated with plasma cell dyscrasias, including multiple myeloma. Finally, there are sporadic reports of steroid-resistant eosinophilic fasciitis associated with hematologic malignancies.

Rheumatic Diseases and Cancer

Patients with autoimmune diseases are at an increased risk of the development of a variety of malignancies. This tendency may be exacerbated by the use of specific immunosuppressive drugs. Patients with RA have a two- to fivefold increased risk of developing hematologic malignancies, including Hodgkin and non-Hodgkin lymphomas. The risk is even higher if secondary Sjögren syndrome or a serum paraprotein is present. An increased risk for oral-pharyngeal cancers has been described in geographic locations where these tumors are prevalent. Interestingly, patients with RA may be at a lower risk of developing colorectal cancer. Whether the lower risk is related to the regular use of NSAIDs in this population is unknown. Patients with Sjögren syndrome are 44 times more likely to develop lymphoma than are age-, sex-, and race-matched normal subjects. The risk may be higher if the patient is anti-Ro or anti-La positive. In some of these patients, there appears to be a progression from benign exocrinopathy to pseudolymphoma to lymphoma. These tumors are almost exclusively B-cell lymphomas with a high frequency of a t(14;18) chromosomal translocation. The malignant transformation is likely the result of chronic B-cell stimulation. The presence of a monoclonal IgM spike on serum protein electrophoresis may herald the transformation to malignant lymphoma. Hypogammaglobulinemia and loss of autoantibodies may eventually occur when the lymphoma cells replace the normal antibody-producing plasma cells.

Patients with polymyositis have a twofold increased risk of developing cancer, particularly in the 1 to 5 years following the diagnosis of the muscle disease. The risk of cancer in patients with dermatomyositis is much higher (four to five times), and the cancer may be discovered years before or after the muscle disease is diagnosed. Older age, the presence of digital vasculitis, and normal serum creatinine kinase levels have all been cited as possible risk factors for cancer development in patients with inflammatory myositis. Patients with overlap syndromes and those with myositis-specific antibodies do not appear to have a higher incidence of cancer than other patients with polymyositis or dermatomyositis. The cancers associated with inflammatory myositis are those that are commonly seen, including breast, lung, gynecologic, and GI malignancies. Interestingly, nasopharyngeal carcinomas are the dominant cancers associated with myositis in countries that have a high prevalence of these malignancies.

It is controversial whether patients with other autoimmune diseases are more likely to develop cancer. Some reports have described an increased risk of lymphoma (particularly non-Hodgkin lymphoma) and possibly lung, breast, and cervical cancers in patients with SLE. Patients with scleroderma may be predisposed to skin cancer, and patients with systemic sclerosis who have pulmonary fibrosis are at risk of developing lung cancer.

Risk of Cancer with Immunosuppression

Patients with RA treated with methotrexate may be at increased risk of developing cancer and lymphoma. The actual risk is unclear, however, because the relative risk has been compared to that of the general population. Nevertheless, there are a large number of case reports or case series linking the occurrence of lymphoma (mostly diffuse large-cell non-Hodgkin lymphomas) in patients with RA receiving low-dose weekly methotrexate. In most cases, cessation of therapy is associated with complete regression of the lymphoid cancer, suggesting a causative relationship. DNA analysis shows that approximately 50% of these lymphomas harbored the Epstein-Barr virus genome. It is, therefore, possible that the drug regimen may promote the malignant transformation of normal lymphoid tissue by the oncogenic virus. Patients with RA on azathioprine and cyclosporin A have a twofold increased risk of lymphoma relative to control patients with RA. A real association between the use of immunosuppressive therapy and the development of lymphoproliferative disorders also occurs with organ transplantation. The incidence of non-Hodgkin lymphoma is 50-fold greater in patients with renal transplant, especially if they receive cyclosporin A as part of their immunosuppressive regimen.

The issue of cancer risk in patients on anti-TNF agents has already been discussed. Early results from a safety clinical trial comparing tofacitinib and anti-TNF agents suggest there may be increased risk of cancer associated with the JAK inhibitor. Cyclophosphamide is commonly used to treat severe lupus manifestations, including nephritis and cerebritis. Patients with lupus on cyclophosphamide are more likely to develop bladder cancer, lymphoma (primarily non-Hodgkin lymphoma), and possibly skin cancer.

Chemotherapy-Associated Rheumatologic Complications

As many as half of women receiving aromatase inhibitors for breast cancer experience subjective joint achiness or pain, but these symptoms rarely translate to frank arthritis. Taxanes (eg, paclitaxel and docetaxel) are used for many breast and gynecologic cancers, as well as for HIV-related Kaposi sarcoma. These drugs may cause myalgias and arthralgias, as well as skin rashes with histologic features of subacute cutaneous lupus. Rapid cell turnover from chemotherapy, particularly in cases of lympho- and myeloproliferative malignancies, can result in an acute gout attack if the patients are not given adequate prophylactic treatment. Bisphosphonates are increasingly used as part of chemotherapeutic regimens in metastatic bone disease, and their use is associated with a number of musculoskeletal complications including complications of hypocalcemia, osteonecrosis of the jaw, and atypical femur fractures. Bleomycin use has been linked to Raynaud phenomenon and scleroderma-like skin diseases.

In recent years, immune checkpoint inhibitors (ICIs) such as CRLA-4/PD-1 inhibitors and anti-PD-1 or anti-PD-L1 monotherapy have been increasingly utilized to treat malignancies. The use of ICIs is associated with immune-related adverse events (IRAEs), and a wide spectrum of rheumatic manifestations including arthralgia/arthritis, myalgia/myositis, polymyalgia rheumatica, rheumatoid arthritis (RA), Sjögren's syndrome, lupus and vasculitis have been reported. In addition, ICIs may exacerbate underlying rheumatic diseases. Rheumatic-IRAEs should be recognized early and the approach to management should be transdisciplinary in conjunction with oncology. The musculoskeletal side effects may be transient and regress after stopping ICIs. Corticosteroids are most commonly used to treat rheumatic spectrum IRAEs and, if unresponsive, immunosuppressive medications such as hydroxychloroquine, methotrexate, TNF-inhibitors and anti-IL-6 are preferred treatments.

COVID-19 AND RHEUMATIC DISEASES

On March 11, 2020, the World Health Organization declared the novel SARS-CoV-2 (COVID-19) outbreak a global pandemic. COVID-19 is thought to be transmitted through respiratory droplets and aerosols and have an incubation period exceeding 14 days. Although most recover from COVID-19, some experience severe disease and complications including acute respiratory failure, shock, multiorgan dysfunction, and thromboembolic events. There was concern from the outset whether patients with rheumatic disease, and especially those receiving immunotherapy, may be more susceptible to COVID-19 infection. Several registries including the Global Rheumatology Alliance were established to track the impact of COVID-19 on rheumatic disease patients. Early epidemiologic data suggest multimorbidity, older age, and high doses of glucocorticoid may be associated with more frequent hospitalization and worse outcomes among patients with rheumatic diseases. Based on limited available data, the ACR recommends caution

with initiation of new biologic therapy and continued use of established immunosuppressive therapy for patients with rheumatic diseases during the COVID-19 pandemic.

Early in the pandemic, hydroxychloroquine and chloroquine garnered international attention and controversy for their potential role in the prevention and treatment of COVID-19 given in vitro inhibition of severe SARS-CoV-2. A national drug shortage ensued, limiting the availability of drugs for patients reliant on these medications for treatment of many rheumatic conditions. Then, multiple rigorous studies showed no benefit of hydroxychloroquine as postexposure prophylaxis or COVID-19 treatment. Subsequently in June 2020, the FDA revoked emergency use authorization (EUA) on the use of hydroxychloroquine to treat COVID-19 in certain hospitalized patients. Another immunosuppressive medication tocilizumab emerged as a potential alternative treatment for COVID-19 after early observational data from China showed increased risk of death in COVID-19 patients with elevated IL-6 levels. In addition, nonrandomized trials suggested possible benefit in the treatment of cytokine storms from severe COVID-19 and off-label use of tocilizumab was for a time considered standard of care in the United States. In February 2021, the National Institutes of Health and Infectious Diseases Society of America recommended against the use of tocilizumab for the treatment of COVID-19 except in clinical trials after preliminary results from several randomized studies including the largest of its kind, the Multifactorial Adaptive Platform Trial of Community-Acquired Pneumonia (REMAP-CAP), showed insufficient data to support its use in hospitalized patients.

A number of COVID-19 vaccines have been developed, and as of early 2022, two nonlive mRNA COVID-19 vaccines developed by Pfizer and Moderna and one viral-vector vaccine developed by Johnson and Johnson (JJ) are FDA authorized for use in the United States. A rare but serious syndrome of thrombosis with thrombocytopenia has been reported at an incidence of 1 in 7 million with the JJ vaccine, as has been reported with another viral-vector AstraZeneca vaccine in Europe. The ACR recommends patients with rheumatic diseases to receive and be prioritized for COVID-19 vaccination as they are at higher risk for hospitalization for COVID-19 and worse outcomes compared to the general population. Either of the mRNA vaccines is recommended over the J&J vaccine for patients with rheumatic diseases, and immunosuppressed patients who previously completed the 2-dose mRNA series should receive an additional COVID-19 vaccine dose at least 28 days after the completion of the primary vaccine series. Increasingly studies are showing immunosuppressed patients have lower response rates to available COVID-19 vaccines, and the ACR provided clinical guidance on immunomodulatory medication use and timing of COVID-19 vaccination to optimize vaccine response as outlined in **Table 101-11**.

TABLE 101-11 ■ USE AND TIMING OF COVID-19 VACCINATION IN RMD PATIENTS

IMMUNOMODULATORY THERAPY	TIMING CONSIDERATIONS FOR VACCINATION	LEVEL OF CONSENSUS
Abatacept IV	One week prior to next dose of IV abatacept	Moderate
Abatacept SQ	Hold for 1–2 weeks (as disease activity allows) after each dose	Moderate
Acetaminophen, NSAIDs	Hold for 24 hours prior to vaccination. No restrictions on use post vaccination once symptoms develop	Moderate
Belimumab SQ	Hold for 1–2 weeks (as disease activity allows) after each COVID-19 vaccine dose	Moderate
TNFi, IL-6R, IL-1R, IL-17, IL-12/23, IL-23, and other cytokine inhibitors[a]	The Task Force failed to reach consensus on whether or not to temporarily interrupt these following each COVID-19 vaccine dose, including both primary vaccination and supplemental (booster) dosing	Moderate
Cyclophosphamide IV	Time CYC administration so that it will occur approximately 1 week after each vaccine dose, when feasible	Moderate
Hydroxychloroquine	No modifications to either immunomodulatory therapy or vaccination timing	Strong
Rituximab or other anti-CD20 B-cell depleting agents	Provide vaccine 2–4 weeks before next anticipated rituximab dose (e.g., at month 5.0 or 5.5 for patients on every 6-month rituximab dosing schedule)	Moderate
All other conventional and targeted immunomodulatory or immuno-suppressive medications (e.g., JAKi, MMF) except those listed above§	Hold for 1–2 weeks (as disease activity allows) after each COVID-19 vaccine dose	Moderate

CYC, cyclophosphamide; IL, interleukin; IV, intravenous; IVIG, intravenous immunoglobulin; JAKi, janus kinase inhibitor; MMF, mycophenolate mofetil; NSAID, non-steroidal anti-inflammatory drugs; RMD, rheumatic and musculoskeletal disease; RTX, rituximab; SQ, subcutaneous; TNFi, tumor necrosis factor inhibitor; JAKi, baricitinib, tofacitinib, upadacitinib.
[a]Examples of specific cytokine inhibitors are as follows: IL-6R, sarilumab; tocilizumab; IL-1R. anakinra, canakinumab; IL-17, ixekizumab, secukinumab; IL-12/23, ustekinumab; IL-23, guselkumab, rizankizumab..
Data from Curtis JR, Johnson SR, Anthony DD, et al. American College of Rheumatology Guidance for COVID-19 Vaccination in Patients With Rheumatic and Musculoskeletal Diseases: Version 1. Arthritis Rheumatol. 2021;73(7):1093–1107.

FURTHER READING

2010 Rheumatoid Arthritis Classification Criteria: An American College of Rheumatology/European League Against Rheumatism Collaborative Initiative. *Arthritis Rheum.* 2010;62:2569–2581.

American College of Rheumatology COVID-19 Vaccine Clinical Guidance Summary for Patients with Rheumatic and Musculoskeletal Disease (updated April 28, 2021), https://www.rheumatology.org/Portals/0/Files/COVID-19-Vaccine-Clinical-Guidance-Rheumatic-Diseases-Summary.pdf.

Cappelli LC, Gutierrez AK, Bingham CO, et al. Rheumatic and musculoskeletal immune-related adverse vents due to immune checkpoint inhibitors: a systematic review of the literature. *Arthritis Care Res.* 2017;69:1751–1763.

Fraenkel L, Bathon JM, England BR, et al. 2021 American College of Rheumatology Guideline for the Treatment of Rheumatoid Arthritis. *Arthritis Care Res.* 2021;73(7): 924–939.

Furer V, Rondaan C, Heijstek MW, et al. 2019 update of EULAR recommendations for vaccination in adult patients with autoimmune inflammatory rheumatic diseases. Ann Rheum Dis. 2020;79:39–52.

George MD, Baker JF, Winthrop K, et al. Risk for serious infection with low-dose glucocorticoids in patients with rheumatoid arthritis: a cohort study. *Ann Intern Med.* 2020;173:870–878.

Kammer GM, Mishra N. Systemic lupus erythematosus in the elderly. *Rheum Dis Clin North Am.* 2000;266: 475–492.

Manasson J, Blank RB, Scher JU. The microbiome in rheumatology: where are we and where should we go? *Ann Rheum Dis.* 2020;79:727–733.

Mohan C, Putterman C. Genetics and pathogenesis of systemic lupus erythematosus and lupus nephritis. *Nat Rev Nephrol.* 2015;11(6):329–341.

Ranganath VK, Maranian P, Elashoff DA, et al. Comorbidities are associated with poorer outcomes in community patients with rheumatoid arthritis. *Rheumatology.* 2013;52:1809–1817.

Somers EC, Marder W, Cagnoli P, et al. Population-based incidence and prevalence of systemic lupus erythematosus: the Michigan Lupus Epidemiology and Surveillance program. *Arthritis Rheumatol.* 2014;66(2):369–378.

Vivino FB, Carsons SE, Foulks G, et al. New treatment guidelines for Sjögren's disease. *Rheum Dis Clin North Am.* 2016;42(3):531–551.

Yung RL, Richardson BC. Drug-induced rheumatic syndromes. *Bull Rheum Dis.* 2002;51(4):1–5.

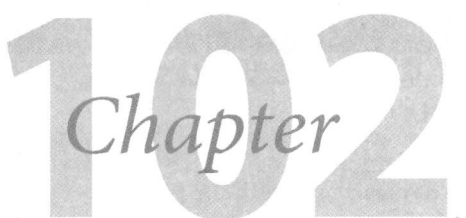

Chapter 102

Back Pain and Spinal Stenosis

Owoicho Adogwa, Una E. Makris, M. Carrington Reid

EPIDEMIOLOGY

Low back pain in older adults is a major public health problem with significant consequences. Prevalence estimates range from 27% to 86% depending on the population evaluated, the study design, and criteria employed to identify back pain. One study conducted in Israel found that 44% of 70-year-olds and 58% of 77-year-olds reported back pain. In the Framingham Heart Study cohort (ages 68–100), 22% of participants reported back pain on most days. As the second most common reason for visiting a physician, annual all-cause medical costs related to back pain exceeded $350 billion and are expected to rise as the population continues to age. Over the past decade, health care–related spending on low back pain diagnostic and "therapeutic" procedures has skyrocketed, yet patient outcomes (in all age groups) have not improved.

A longitudinal study demonstrated that older adults are more likely to develop recurrent episodes of back pain if they are female, suffer from depressive symptoms, have two or more chronic conditions, or self-report arthritis. Back pain in older adults is associated with dependence in activities of daily living, mobility impairment, and poor self-reported health. The association of back pain and physical function has been quantified; the number of months with back pain (resulting in restricted activity) is associated with such markers of frailty as gait speed, chair stands, and foot tap performance. In a study of Medicare beneficiaries 65 years and older, back pain was second only to shortness of breath while climbing stairs in its association with impaired general physical health status. Cross-sectional data from the Framingham Heart Study have shown that back symptoms account for a large percentage of functional limitations in older adults, especially in women. Psychosocial factors, including comorbid depression or anxiety as well as pain-related fear avoidance and pain catastrophizing, play an important role in the experience/reporting of back pain and potentially mediate the relationship with subsequent disability.

While low back pain is a common problem in older adults, its etiology, natural history, and methods for effective management are not fully understood nor well defined.

Learning Objectives

- Review the epidemiology of back pain in older adults, including associated psychosocial factors.
- Understand how back pain is classified and review its clinical course.
- Recognize the broad differential of back pain etiology in older adults.
- Understand the value of history, physical examination, and observation when evaluating an older adult with back pain and the indications for imaging in this population.
- Learn how to select age-appropriate methods to manage back pain in older adults that combine pharmacologic and nonpharmacologic (including behavioral, activity-based) modalities, as well as surgical interventions as appropriate.

Key Clinical Points

1. Back pain is one of the most common complaints among older adults leading to considerable morbidity and cost.
2. Diagnostic and therapeutic costs have increased; however, outcomes have not improved.
3. Back pain must be assessed in the context of comorbid conditions (including mental health conditions and potentially other sites of pain) as multimorbidity impacts management.
4. Psychosocial factors (such as depression and pain-related fear avoidance and/or pain catastrophizing) play an important role in the experience of back pain and potentially mediate the relationship with subsequent outcomes (such as disability).
5. Infection, malignancy, and compression fractures must be ruled out prior to characterizing nonspecific mechanical back pain.

(Continued)

6. Imaging of the spine often demonstrates anatomic abnormalities in asymptomatic older adults and should only be ordered when red flags are present.

7. A combination of pharmacologic, nonpharmacologic, and rehabilitative approaches (including physical therapy, occupational therapy, and/or spinal manipulation) in addition to a strong therapeutic alliance between the patient and physician is essential in setting, adjusting, and achieving realistic goals of therapy.

8. Multimodal management programs for back pain should be tailored to the older adult's preferences and abilities.

9. Surgery may be indicated in patients with symptomatic compression of neural structures, progressive deformity, or mechanical low back pain, who fail conservative measures.

CLASSIFICATION

Back pain is often categorized as acute (lasts < 4 weeks), subacute (lasts between 4 and 12 weeks), or chronic (lasting > 3 months; some definitions require > 6 months). While much of the literature evaluates chronic symptoms, research shows that low back pain is *not* likely constant, but rather, recurrent or episodic. Understanding the various patterns of back pain in older adults, including what precipitates recurrent episodes, is important as prevention and treatment planning may differ.

ETIOLOGY/PRESENTATION OF BACK PAIN

A number of discrete conditions manifest as back pain in older adults (**Table 102-1**). These conditions include mechanical causes, lumbar spinal stenosis, sciatica, osteoarthritis of the hip, vertebral compression fractures, osteoporotic sacral fractures, tumors, and infections. Systemic conditions such as malignancy and infections, although rarely the cause of back pain, are more common in older compared to younger age groups. One of the most challenging aspects of assessing and managing back pain is identifying the source(s) of pain in the older adult who often has multiple musculoskeletal comorbidities (eg, trochanteric bursitis, hip osteoarthritis, multilevel lumbar degenerative changes and lumbar stenosis). These conditions rarely occur in isolation, and pinpointing which one contributes most to the patient's pain may be difficult but is vital.

The vast majority of low back pain seen in primary care settings is labeled "nonspecific low back pain" as there is no specific attributable disease or spinal pathology. The

TABLE 102-1 ■ DIFFERENTIAL DIAGNOSES FOR BACK PAIN IN OLDER ADULTS
NONSYSTEMIC/MECHANICAL CAUSES OF BACK PAIN
Lumbar strain (muscle)
Spinal stenosis
Degenerative disease: spondylosis (discs and facet joints), osteoarthritis of hip (referred)
Spondylolisthesis
Spondylolysis
Sciatica
Piriformis syndrome
Herniated disc
Osteoporotic vertebral or sacral compression fractures
Diffuse idiopathic skeletal hyperostosis (DISH)
Congenital disease: kyphosis, scoliosis
SYSTEMIC CAUSES OF BACK PAIN
Malignancy: multiple myeloma, metastatic disease, lymphoma, spinal cord tumors, retroperitoneal tumors
Infection: osteomyelitis, septic discitis, paraspinous abscess, or septic emboli (sometimes related to bacterial endocarditis)
Inflammatory arthritis: ankylosing spondylitis, psoriatic arthritis, reactive arthritis, inflammatory bowel disease
Osteochondrosis
Paget disease
Visceral: aortic aneurysm, prostatitis, nephrolithiasis, pyelonephritis, perinephric abscess, pancreatitis, cholecystitis, penetrating ulcer, fat herniation of lumbar space

natural history, associated features, and etiology of back pain in older adults remain poorly characterized. Assessment of back pain in older adults includes evaluation of the historical, physical, and diagnostic imaging features of the affected patients for the conditions listed below, and then to make a diagnosis of nonspecific low back pain after these conditions have been ruled out.

Tumor

The clinician must always be alert to nonmechanical, either referred or systemic, causes of low back pain. Visceral causes of back pain, such as abdominal aortic aneurysms or pancreatic cancer, are usually nonpositional, progressive, and associated with a normal examination of the lumbar spine and hip. Older adults with spinal column tumors often believe that their pain is temporally related to an event or trauma in the recent past. This usually indicates a pathological fracture which occurs as a result of minor trauma. However, acute onset of pain that starts in the absence of recent trauma should also be considered a possible pathological fracture. Tumors usually present with a gradual onset and progressive course, usually worse at night with persistent worsening of the pain over weeks and months. Additionally, tumor pain is often nonpositional, lasts longer than 4 weeks, and is associated with systemic/constitutional symptoms. The pain associated with spinal column tumors can occur for several reasons. Vertebral column tumors cause bone remodeling, thinning of the cortical rim which leads to pathological fractures. In the early stages of the disease, the stretched periosteum is the cause of pain; however, after development of the pathological fracture, pain secondary to neural compression, radiculopathy, and instability (micromotion) predominates.

Infection

Although a rare cause of back pain, vertebral and disc infections can be difficult to distinguish from a mechanical cause of back pain; disc infections can cause the same abrupt onset, positional changes, and L4, L5 and L5, S1 neurologic abnormalities seen in mechanical disc disease. Unremitting back pain not relieved by rest is the most common presenting complaint. Back pain is the most common musculoskeletal complaint reported by patients with endocarditis, due to metastatic infection (abscess or septic emboli). Because the disc is often involved in this condition, the signs and symptoms can mimic mechanical disc disease. Pain may be accompanied by other constitutional symptoms, such as weight loss, fever or poor appetite; fever can be absent in older patients with infection. The clinician must be alert to a possible infectious cause of back pain for patients with a high risk of endovascular infection (artificial heart valves, indwelling venous catheters, intravenous drug abuse, etc) and in patients with systemic symptoms and signs of inflammation. When osteomyelitis or discitis is discovered, it is imperative to image the entire neural axis with a magnetic resonance imaging (MRI) scan with and without contrast of the cervical, thoracic, and lumbar spine, to rule out tandem, noncontiguous areas of infection.

Vertebral Compression Fractures

The abrupt onset of severe back pain, especially in a patient with risk factors for osteoporosis, with or without a history of falls, should always call for a spinal x-ray to rule out a vertebral compression fracture (**Table 102-2**). Vertebral compression fracture is the most common type of osteoporotic fracture. Those that occur slowly (especially in the mid and upper thoracic spine) are often asymptomatic. Only approximately 30% to 40% of all vertebral compression fractures are symptomatic. Most symptomatic fractures are in the lower thoracic and lumbar spine. Height loss and kyphosis should heighten suspicion for the presence of a vertebral fracture.

TABLE 102-2 ■ CHARACTERISTICS OF VERTEBRAL COMPRESSION FRACTURE

Severe mechanical pain with lower thoracic and lumbar fracture
High and mid-thoracic fracture often asymptomatic
Pain resolves in 4–6 weeks
Increased risk for subsequent fracture

At times, the initial x-ray is normal and the changes of vertebral collapse appear several days to weeks after the onset of pain. As there is no dislocation with osteoporotic vertebral fractures, neurological signs and symptoms are rare. Pain is usually localized to the midline spine but may be referred, however, into the chest, abdomen, or leg. Any movement, including rolling in bed, bending, coughing, or lifting, usually exacerbates the pain. Pain, and muscle spasm if present, then gradually improves over the next several weeks and typically resolves in 4 to 6 weeks. Persistent severe pain (symptoms that continue despite the expected normal period of healing) may suggest additional fractures or an alternative diagnosis.

The presence of a vertebral fracture increases the risk of a subsequent vertebral and nonvertebral (ie, hip) fractures. Studies suggest that over 20% of patients who sustain a fracture will have another fracture within 5 years. The relationship between osteoporosis and vertebral fracture and chronic back pain and disability is still under investigation. Osteoporotic compression fractures that develop slowly over time are often asymptomatic and may not lead to deleterious sequelae. While some studies have shown increased disability in patients with vertebral fractures, a British population–based study found no correlation between minor vertebral deformities and back pain. Functional impairment from vertebral compression fracture appears to be comparable to that related to hip fracture.

Osteoporotic Sacral Fractures

There have been a number of reports of "sacral/pelvic insufficiency fractures" as a cause of back pain. Older patients, usually women, may report persistent pain in the low back, groin, or buttock area, occasionally lasting weeks to months. The application of pressure to the sacrum is very painful. Associated neurologic sequelae are rare; however, if present, they often manifest as a sacral radiculopathy. Leg length discrepancy, abnormal positioning of the leg, focal tenderness around the hip/pelvis, or limited range of motion of the leg should raise suspicion for pelvic injury. The pain usually resolves spontaneously in 4 to 6 weeks. Approximately 50% of these patients had a preceding fall, and the majority of patients have old pelvic and vertebral compression fractures on x-ray.

A sacral insufficiency fracture should be considered especially in older adults with risk factors for fracture (ie, osteoporosis, low body weight, glucocorticoid therapy) and with sudden pain in the low back and buttock with sacral tenderness. Plain radiographs of the pelvis, despite low sensitivity for small fractures, should be obtained to evaluate for the possibility of a hip, pelvic, or lumbosacral spine fracture. If plain films are negative but clinical suspicion is high, MRI or CT scan may be useful to document minor pelvic fractures. Some advocate for treating patients symptomatically without advanced imaging so long as other important diagnoses have been ruled out and appropriate follow-up has been arranged.

Sciatica is usually defined as pain radiating down one leg below the gluteal fold. It is often felt in the buttock area, radiating into the posterior aspect of the leg down to the ankle. It may, however, be incomplete, as in the calf pain seen in the "pseudoclaudication" syndrome with lumbar spinal stenosis. The natural history of this condition is well defined in younger adults. Fifty percent of these patients have full resolution of symptoms within 6 weeks. Sciatica in older adults, which develops abruptly and occurs in all positions, usually has a good natural history, similar to that seen in younger individuals. Patients who develop sciatica as part of the lumbar spinal stenosis syndrome, with gradual progression of pain with shorter and shorter periods of standing and walking, may have a more prolonged and persistent natural history.

Lumbar Spinal Stenosis

Lumbar spinal stenosis can be acquired or congenital. Congenital stenosis results from congenitally shortened pedicles and affects patients in their 30s to 50s. Acquired stenosis is more common and typically seen in patients 50 years and older. A good understanding of the normal anatomy of the lumbar spine is necessary to understand how spinal stenosis causes symptoms. The anterior border of the spinal canal is formed by the vertebral body, the disc, and posterior longitudinal ligament. The pedicle, lateral ligamentum flavum, and neural foraminal comprise the lateral border. The posterior border is formed by the facet joints, laminar, and ligamentum flavum. The shape of the spinal canal can be trefoil or oval, with the trefoil having the smallest cross-sectional area. Narrowing of the intraspinal (central) vertebral canal, lateral recess, and/or neural foramina is frequently seen on diagnostic imaging causing compression of the thecal sac and nerve roots. These abnormalities, often caused by spondylosis or degenerative arthritis affecting the spine, have clinical significance only if the typical history of lumbar spinal stenosis is present (**Table 102-3**). Spinal stenosis is associated with increased vascular disturbance, neuroinflammation, and electrophysiologic alteration, all of which contribute to the lower extremity pain

TABLE 102-3 ■ CHARACTERISTICS OF LUMBAR SPINAL STENOSIS

Pain with extended spine
Prolonged standing
Walking
Walking down hill
Pain relieved on flexing spine
Sitting
Leaning on walker or grocery cart
Sciatic pain on walking
Incomplete sciatica—"pseudoclaudication"

experienced by patients. In addition to the aforementioned static factors, the degenerative cascade can lead to translational and rotational abnormalities, which contribute to segmental instability and pain. Changes in spinal dynamics with movement explain some of the clinical features of lumbar spinal stenosis. Flexion of the lumbar spine decreases the intraspinal protrusion of the disc, decreases the bulge of the yellow ligaments within the canal, and stretches and decreases the cross-sectional area of nerve roots, resulting in an increase in spinal canal volume in relation to nerve root bulk. Extension of the lumbar spine causes bulging of the disc into the canal, enfolding and protrusion of the yellow ligaments into the spinal canal, and a relaxation and increase of the cross-sectional diameter of nerve roots. Extension of the canal thus produces a decreased volume of the spinal canal in relation to nerve root bulk.

These changes in dynamics explain the clinical picture of lumbar spinal stenosis. Positions that extend the spine (standing, walking down hill, prone lying, and extending the back) worsen symptoms, while positions that flex the spine (sitting, bending forward, placing weight on a walker or cart, and lying in a flex position) relieve the symptoms.

Patients with lumbar spinal stenosis most commonly present with leg pain. The leg pain presents either as neurogenic claudication or radicular leg pain. With neurogenic claudication, patients report a feeling of lower extremity heaviness, numbness, cramping, burning, and infrequently weakness. Both legs are typically involved, although not infrequently one leg may be worse than the other. Rarely do lower extremity symptoms follow a dermatomal distribution, and are usually exacerbated by prolonged standing and walking. These symptoms are usually worse with extension, hence individuals with this condition often lean forward (lumbar flexion) with ambulation to minimize discomfort and maximize function (ie, shopping cart sign). Lying supine, flexion, or squatting helps ameliorate symptoms. In contrast to neurogenic claudication, which arises from compression of the thecal sac, radiculopathy occurs as a result of lateral recess or foraminal compression. Since lumbar stenosis is most commonly observed at L4-L5, followed by L3-L4 and L5-S1, the L5 nerve root is most commonly involved from lateral recess stenosis causing an L5 radiculopathy.

Lumbar spinal stenosis should not produce pain when going from lying to sitting and should not produce severe pain with bending, stooping, or lifting objects. New back pain/leg symptoms in an older patient and/or neurologic deficits usually warrant imaging to determine structural narrowing of the lumbosacral spine. Plain radiographs, MRI, and CT scans are important to fully characterize the degree of stenosis/spondylosis.

Severe neurological symptoms, such as profound lower extremity weakness, and bowel or bladder changes, are uncommon but when present mandate that a careful history is performed to exclude other nonspinal causes. Neurogenic bladder dysfunction is usually associated with

TABLE 102-4 ■ CHARACTERISTICS OF MECHANICAL LOW BACK PAIN
Intermittent sharp back pain
Pain comes on and subsides rapidly
Pain going from supine to sitting or upright positions and with bending
Weakness of L4, L5, and S1 innervated muscles from dynamic instability and compression

perianal sensory disturbance, longer duration of symptoms, and higher postvoid residual volumes.

Mechanical Low Back Pain

The majority of older adults with low back pain do not have tumors, infections, vertebral compression fractures, or lumbar spinal stenosis (**Table 102-4**). They are best described as patients with mechanical back pain of uncertain etiology.

A good deal of back pain in younger individuals is probably caused by displacement of the outer annulus fibrosis or inner nucleus pulposus of the intervertebral disc. The disc does not contain pain fibers: the periverterbral structures with the most sensitive pain fibers are the posterior longitudinal ligament and the dura mater, which lie posterior to the vertebrae and discs. The sinuvertebral nerve innervates these structures. Irritation of this nerve causes reflex spasms of the paravertebral muscles of the lumbar spine. It is, thus, logical to assume that soft-tissue displacement in this area will cause pain and limitation of some, but not all, of the planes of movement of the lumbar spine, spasm of the paravertebral muscles, and subtle weakness of the muscles innervated by the appropriate nerve roots (L4, L5, and S1—in most cases).

In a young adult's lumbar spine, the central nucleus pulposus often herniates outside the annulus fibrosis and indents the pain-sensitive posterior longitudinal ligament and dura mater, producing pain that often lasts for several weeks and occasionally causing sciatica owing to nerve root irritation. Because the nucleus pulposus loses water content with aging, herniation of this structure is less common beyond the age of 55.

Older patients often have a syndrome of sharp pain in the lumbar area, worsened with bending movements, which comes on and subsides rapidly but recurs frequently. On physical examination, these patients often have asymmetric loss of range of motion in the lumbar spine, paravertebral muscle spasm, weakness of the L4-, L5-, and S1-innervated muscles, and pain going from the flexed to the erect position. Clinicians often use the term "unstable lumbar spine" to describe this syndrome, although the evidence for specific mechanical instability is lacking. Patients with this condition often have one intervertebral disc space narrowed and sclerotic changes out of proportion to other disc spaces, and anterior displacement of one vertebra on another (spondylolisthesis). Maneuvers such as going from lying to sitting and bending forward often produce pain. Before considering major interventions, it is important

to distinguish this condition, in which pain results from movement of the lumbar spine (eg, lying to sitting), from lumbar spinal stenosis, in which pain results from prolonged extension of the spine (standing and walking).

Diffuse Idiopathic Skeletal Hyperostosis

Diffuse idiopathic skeletal hyperostosis (DISH) is characterized by calcification of prevertebral and peripheral ligaments. Ossification of spinal ligaments is often confused with osteophytes, and the condition is frequently mislabeled as disc degeneration or osteoarthritis. Spinal involvement is characterized by the following: (1) the presence of flowing calcification and ossification along the anterolateral aspect of at least four contiguous vertebral bodies, (2) relative preservation of intervertebral disc height in the involved area, and (3) the absence of apophyseal joint bony ankylosis or other features of ankylosing spondylitis.

Most studies have not found any association with DISH and back pain, while other studies have noted an increase in ligamentous tenderness, stiffness, and immobility of the cervical, thoracic, and lumbar spine in individuals with this condition. The condition should be distinguished from disc disease with vertebral osteophytes and is a cause of significant spinal immobility in older individuals.

EVALUATION

The evaluation of the older adult with back pain should rely heavily on the history, physical examination, and direct observation. The history and physical examination remain the most helpful tools in the assessment of back pain in older adults, particularly because of the high false-positive rate of spinal diagnostic imaging tests in this age group. Laboratory tests and diagnostic imaging studies have a secondary role in the assessment of these patients. The clinician must verify that the clinical presentation of the patient fits the results of the diagnostic imaging tests before proceeding with interventions.

The role of the clinician in assessing and managing back pain in older individuals focuses on (1) identifying those conditions that require immediate attention (eg, infections and tumors), (2) recognizing the usual patterns of pain for defined causes of back pain, (3) assisting the patient to engage in therapy that mitigates pain and associated symptoms, (4) educating the patient on the natural history, precipitating events, and therapeutic approaches to nonspecific mechanical low back pain, and (5) establishing realistic expectations, identifying goals of management, and assessing progress toward these goals over time.

History

Patients with a mechanical cause for pain usually have intermittent, positional pain, often with the peak intensity of pain at the episode onset (**Table 102-5**).

Pain that is worse on going from lying to sitting and with bending, that occurs when one suddenly changes

TABLE 102-5 ■ HISTORY ITEMS THAT HELP DIFFERENTIATE CAUSES OF BACK PAIN
Abrupt onset of pain
Intervertebral disc herniation
Muscle strain
Vertebral compression fractures
Mechanical low back pain
Insidious onset, progressive course, nonpositional pain
Tumor
Infection
Nonspinal visceral pain
Degenerative disc disease
Osteoarthritis
Positional attributes
Pain when lying to sitting or bending
Mechanical low back pain
Pain when standing and walking, relieved with sitting
Lumbar spinal stenosis
Nonpositional
Tumor
Infection

TABLE 102-6 ■ PHYSICAL EXAMINATION FINDINGS THAT HELP DIFFERENTIATE CAUSES OF BACK PAIN
Paravertebral muscle spasm
Mechanical low back pain
Vertebral compression fracture
Asymmetric loss of range of motion of lumbar spine
Mechanical low back pain
Weakness of great toe extensor and hip abductor (L4, L5) and hip extensors (L5, S1)
Mechanical low back pain
Lumbar spinal stenosis

position, and that resolves quickly but recurs frequently, suggests mechanical disease of the lumbar spine as a result of soft-tissue displacement. Severe pain in any position, which comes on abruptly and is aggravated by even rolling over in bed, suggests a vertebral compression fracture. A woman with sacral and buttock pain, sacral tenderness, and osteoporosis should be evaluated for a sacral insufficiency fracture. Gradually worsening progressive pain, lasting more than a month, which is nonpositional and associated with systemic symptoms and signs, might suggest the possibility of a tumor as a cause of the pain. Hip disease can often mimic back problems. Pain that is worse when going from sitting to standing, that causes a limp, or that radiates into the groin indicates possible hip disease.

Physical Examination

A good physical examination of patients with lumbar pathologies should start with observation. It is important to note whether patients are sitting flexed forward on a chair or laying down on the examination table. This provides clues on the possible etiology of the patient's complaints. In patients where the supine position is preferred, mechanical back pain may be the predominant complaint. Next, the clinician must determine whether the problem is in the hip or back. It can be difficult to distinguish these conditions, as both can present with buttock and low back pain. Pain that occurs when going from the supine to sitting position is more apt to be from the back, while groin pain, worsened with weight bearing, favors the hip as the cause of the pain. A complete examination of the passive range of motion of the hip, done with the patient in the supine position, should reveal 40 degrees of hip abduction, more than 100

degrees of flexion, 50 to 60 degrees of external rotation, and 20 degrees of internal rotation. In addition, a manual muscle examination of the lower extremities, which demonstrates mild weakness of the L4, L5 (hip abductor and great toe extensor) and L5, S1 (hip extensors) innervated muscles of the lower extremities, favors the back as the cause of pain. One study demonstrated that the presence of groin pain, a limp, and limited internal rotation of the hip all favored the hip as the cause of pain.

Several findings on physical examination can be useful in determining discrete causes of back pain (**Table 102-6**).

The physical examination of the lumbar spine is an essential component of the assessment of a patient with back pain (**Figure 102-1**). This is best done while standing. The examiner observes the patient for kyphosis or scoliosis and then palpates for paravertebral muscle spasm. The patient is then brought through the four ranges of motion of the lumbar spine, side flexion to the right, side flexion to the left, forward flexion, and extension, observing for asymmetric limitation of motion or reproduction of the patient's pain by these maneuvers (see **Figure 102-1**). In the supine position, straight leg raise tests can indicate nerve root irritation if positive, but a negative test does not exclude any condition. The hips should be examined by testing the passive range of motion. The examiner should be able to abduct the leg to 40 degrees before the pelvis tilts. There should be 60 degrees of external rotation (heel toward the midline) and 20 degrees of internal rotation (heel away from the midline) of each hip (**Figure 102-2**).

Manual muscle testing of the lower extremity gives much useful information, as subtle L4, L5 and L5, S1 weakness is common in patients with mechanical back pain. L4, L5 is tested by resisting the patient's abducted leg at the lateral upper thigh (gluteus medius muscle) (see **Figure 102-2**), by resisting the patient's ability to dorsiflex the foot (tibialis anterior muscle), and by resisting the great toe extensor (extensor hallucis longus) (**Figure 102-3**). L5, S1 (gluteus maximus muscle) is tested by trying to overcome hip extension (trying to pull the leg off the examining table, when the patient has been instructed to hold the leg firmly on the table). One can also test L5, S1 by resisting the patient's ability to evert the foot (peroneus longus and peroneus brevis).

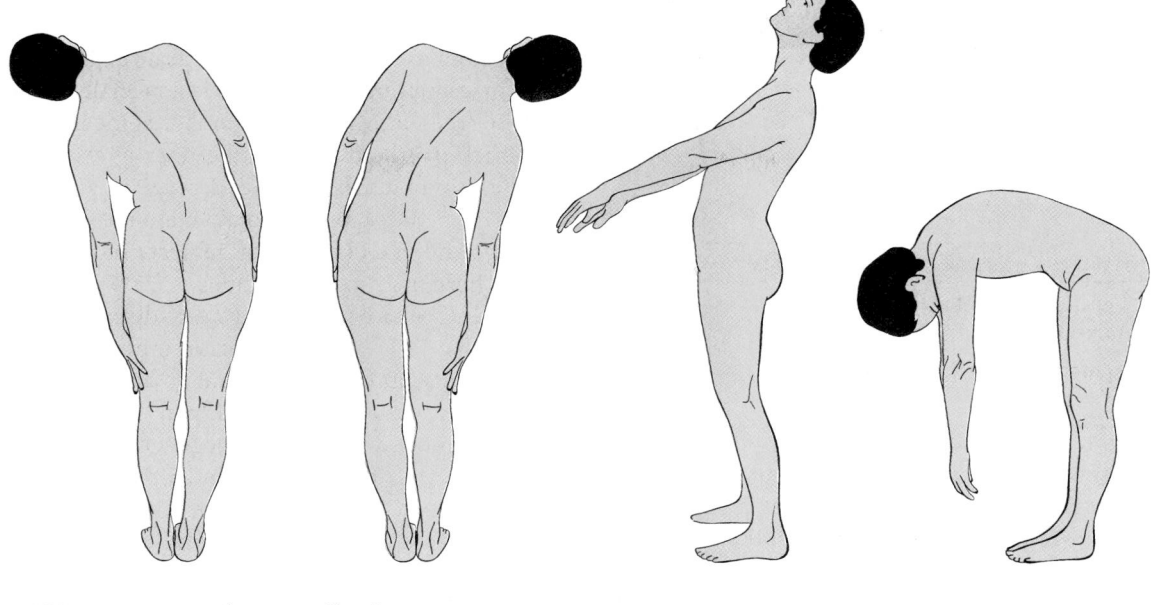

FIGURE 102-1. Range of motion of lumbar spine.

Most patients with lumbar disc disease or lumbar spinal stenosis will have some abnormalities of the examination of the lumbar spine or of the muscles innervated by L4, L5 or L5, S1. Patients with vertebral compression fractures may have a good deal of tenderness in the lumbar spine but should have no neurologic abnormalities. Patients with osteoporotic sacral fractures will have sacral tenderness, but a normal lumbar spine examination and no lower extremity muscle weakness. Those with sciatica almost always have L4, L5 and L5, S1 weakness. A patient with persistent, severe back pain, but with a normal examination of the lumbar spine, sacrum, and hips and no evidence of L4, L5 or L5, S1 muscle weakness, should be evaluated thoroughly for a possible neoplasm or infection.

New neurologic abnormalities (dermatomal sensory deficits, focal weakness, clonus) associated with abrupt onset back pain may suggest retropulsed bone fragments in the spinal canal or foraminae which should be further evaluated with urgent MRI or CT scan and urgent consultation with a spine surgeon.

Laboratory Tests and Imaging

The interpretation of diagnostic tests in older patients with back pain is a challenge, given the high rate of abnormal tests in asymptomatic individuals in this age group. A complete blood count and erythrocyte sedimentation rate/C-reactive protein are reasonable screening tests if the patient's history and physical examination suggest a tumor or infection. While routine imaging for low back pain in younger

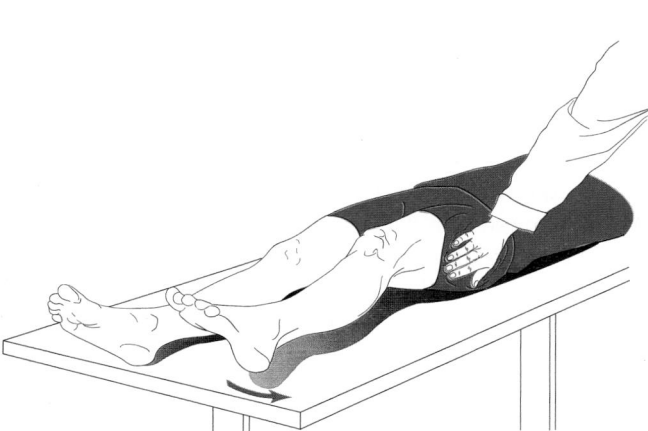

FIGURE 102-2. Resisting abduction of the leg.

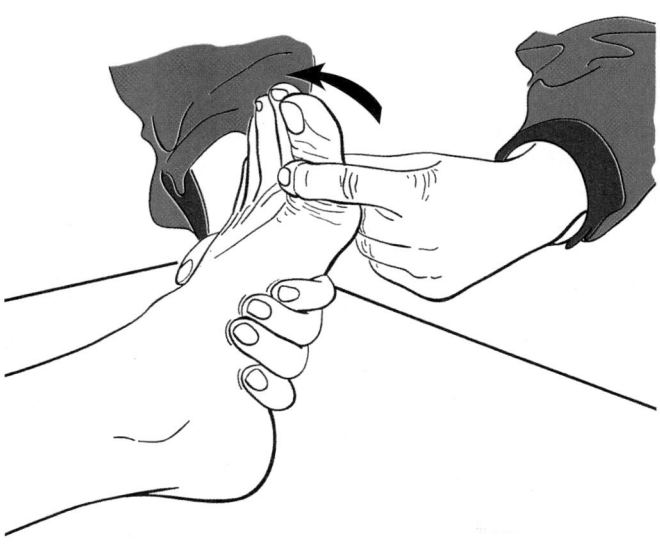

FIGURE 102-3. Resisting great toe extensor.

TABLE 102-7 ■ RED FLAGS FOR BACK PAIN DUE TO SYSTEMIC DISEASE

Age > 70
Recent significant trauma or milder trauma (age > 50)
Unexplained weight loss or fever
Immunosuppression (such as diabetes mellitus)
History of cancer
Osteoporosis or prolonged use of glucocorticoids
Focal neurologic deficits that are progressive or produce disabling symptoms
Duration of symptoms > 6 wk or more (subacute or chronic)
IV drug use

populations is not recommended, plain films of the spine may be appropriate in older adults with back pain. A plain x-ray of the lumbar spine is more helpful in the evaluation of older patients than younger ones, as it may demonstrate a vertebral compression fracture, DISH, or spondylolisthesis.

According to the American College of Radiology, the criteria listed in **Table 102-7** should be used to determine who is at higher risk for systemic disease-related back pain and when imaging is appropriate.

The clinician must be aware that changes in the lumbar spine are ubiquitous in older individuals and not well correlated with back pain. Kellgren and Lawrence's classic epidemiological study in Leigh, England, found that 89% of the men and 57% of the women aged 55 to 64 had disc degeneration of the lumbar spine. Proper radiographic evaluation of the lumbar spine includes obtaining static and dynamic views. Anterior-posterior, lateral and flexion-extension views should be obtained. Specific findings notable on plain films include narrow interpedicular distance, sagittal canal diameter, and evidence of spondylotic changes such as facet hypertrophy, osteophytosis, disc collapse, or deformity. Additionally, vacuum disc phenomenon "air in disc space" can be noted on plain radiographs, and is a sign of advanced degeneration and instability. A study of lumbar sacral spine x-rays found no association between back pain and Schmorl nodes, the disc vacuum sign, traction spurs, and disc space narrowing between the third and fourth lumbar vertebrae, or between the fifth lumbar and first sacral vertebrae. There was an association between acute low back pain and disc space narrowing, and traction spurs between the fourth and fifth lumbar vertebra. Another study found no correlation between vertebral osteophytes and low back pain but did find increased back pain in individuals with spondylolisthesis (pars interarticularis defect and frontal slippage of one vertebra on an adjacent vertebra).

MRI is considered the standard imaging modality for patients with lumbar spinal stenosis. It is used to identify central and lateral recess stenosis, annular tears, facet degeneration, and diastasis, because it provides excellent contrast between fat, neural tissue, and epineural vessels.

A disadvantage of MRI is its ability to detect degenerative changes that may not be associated with symptoms. MRIs of the lumbar spine often demonstrate anatomic abnormalities in asymptomatic individuals, especially in older adults. In one study of MRIs of the lumbar spine in patients without back pain, only 36% had a normal examination; 52% of these individuals had a disc bulge in at least one level, and 27% had disc protrusions. In another study of asymptomatic individuals, 36% of subjects older than 60 years had a herniated nucleus pulposus, 21% had spinal stenosis, and 93% had degenerative disc disease. Another study found that 56% of asymptomatic individuals had tears of the annulus fibrosis of the lumbar disc. In a study of 198 veterans who had had no back pain for at least 4 months, 83% had moderate-to-severe degeneration of the disc, 64% had at least one bulging disc, and 32% had at least one disc protrusion. In individuals older than 65 years, 100% had disc degeneration and desiccation, 83% had a disc bulge, and 38% had facet joint degeneration.

CT scans are also useful for evaluation of lumbar stenosis. CT offers greater detail than plain films, with ability to obtain images in various planes—axial, coronal, and sagittal. Other potential causes of back pain such as pars interarticular defects and spondylosis can be easily identified with CT scans. In stenotic patients, hypertrophy of the facet joints and articular processes contribute to the trefoil shape of the central canal. Because a significant portion of the stenosis comes from soft tissue pathology, visualization of the soft tissues is a top priority. A CT scan is a poor modality for detailed analysis of soft tissue. The diagnostic utility of CT scan can be improved by combining it with myelography. CT myelography is infrequently used for routine evaluation of spinal stenosis; however, this modality can be useful in patients with lumbar deformity, such as scoliosis or those unable to tolerate an MRI. Central stenosis presents as a hourglass constriction of the thecal sac. Areas of complete contrast block represent severe central or foraminal stenosis. While CT myelography provides useful information on areas of central or foraminal stenosis, invasiveness of the myelogram and radiation associated with the CT scans are the two biggest drawbacks of this diagnostic modality.

Bicycle and treadmill tests help to differentiate between neurogenic claudication and vascular claudication. Patients with neurogenic claudication present with symptoms including pain, cramping, and lower extremity paresthesias, which are also common in older patients with underlying vascular claudication. With neurogenic claudication, patients have worse symptoms during the treadmill test that is relieved during the bicycle test. This is because the flexion of the spine that occurs during the bicycle test increases the diameter of the central canal. In contrast, patients with vascular claudication have persistent difficulty with both treadmill and bicycle test.

Electromyography (EMG) and nerve conduction velocity (NCV) can be helpful when evaluating patients with a history that is not classic for neurogenic claudication or radiculopathy. EMG identifies lower motor neuron dysfunction and can be useful in differentiating chronic changes from active ongoing denervation.

The above findings indicate that the clinician cannot depend on imaging studies alone to diagnose the cause of back pain in older adults. These studies are used to confirm a diagnosis, indicated by the history, physical examination, and the clinician's knowledge of applied anatomy.

MANAGEMENT

Back pain in older adults is often inadequately treated for several reasons including: a limited evidence base to guide management, lack of physician education, physician concerns about the potential for treatment-related harm, and older adults' beliefs about pain and pain treatments. Other treatment barriers specific to geriatric populations include *age-related* physiologic changes resulting in altered drug absorption and decreased renal excretion; sensory impairments; polypharmacy; and multimorbidity. Additional attitudinal, access, and system-level barriers have been identified that also contribute to undertreated pain in vulnerable populations, including older adults.

Management of back pain should begin with a combination of nonpharmacologic and rehabilitative approaches, as described below, along with pharmacologic and then more invasive management strategies if indicated, depending on the circumstance (listed by specific etiology).

Nonpharmacologic Approaches (General Principles)

Interest in nonpharmacologic approaches for managing back pain in older adults is increasing. Nonpharmacologic approaches include cognitive behavioral therapy for chronic pain, acupuncture, mindfulness, massage, self-management programs and/or behavioral (eg, goal setting, exercise, tai chi, yoga) techniques that constitute well-established methods for treating pain (in general). Existing evidence suggests that these therapies are safe, can reduce pain, and in many cases improve patient function. Nearly all studies of nonpharmacologic interventions conducted to date, however, have been for short term (< 6 months). The long-term efficacy and ability of older adults to sustain their use over time remain inadequately defined. Despite this, temporary relief from back pain may offer an opportunity to develop positive expectations and commitments from the patient and provider.

It is important to communicate to older patients that using both nondrug and drug therapies is the standard of care and can be productive, particularly with individuals who may hesitate to engage in nonpharmacologic treatments. Recommending a specific nonpharmacologic modality will depend upon its availability, affordability (eg, Medicare does not cover many of the approaches listed, however), patient preferences, and the physician's ability to accurately describe its benefits and risks. As there are no head-to-head comparisons evaluating the nonpharmacologic approaches, recommending a modality that is accessible and affordable is essential.

Rehabilitative Approaches

Addressing function and fall risk is critically important for all older patients, particularly in those with persistent pain, including chronic back pain. Rehabilitative therapies, including physical therapy (PT) and occupational therapy (OT), can help maintain and possibly enhance functional independence. Geriatric pain management guidelines recommend that all older patients with persistent pain (including back pain) adopt physical activity regimens that include strengthening, flexibility, balance, and endurance exercises. PTs/OTs can help older adults implement individualized home-based treatment programs. Home-based services directed at improving safety and mobility could potentially facilitate involvement in out-of-home activities; these services might indirectly yield dividends such as more time spent socializing with family and friends. Physical therapists can play an important role in developing "function-enhancing interventions" in older adults with mobility limitations.

In addition, PTs can conduct an inventory of existing equipment (eg, does the patient have a functional walker?) and make recommendations about new assistive/mobility devices. OTs can directly observe a patient's ADL functioning in the home and make recommendations about assistive devices that may help to improve ADL functioning. Both paid and family caregivers, especially of older adults with cognitive impairment, can reinforce patients' ongoing use of rehabilitative techniques and should be engaged and empowered to do so. Finally, PTs/OTs can also train caregivers to reinforce concepts learned during treatment sessions, including coaching on fall risk, safety, body mechanics, and pacing.

Rehabilitation health care specialists often use various modalities including both therapeutic exercise and spinal manipulation. There is growing popularity and interest in spinal manipulation (often defined as [low to] high velocity and low amplitude thrust and/or manual mobilization of vertebral joints and/or soft tissue manipulation, performed by either a chiropractor, physiotherapist, or other manual health care practitioner) for both acute and chronic back pain. As of yet, there are no studies proving the mechanism underlying the benefit of spinal manipulation. There are strongest data for patients with acute low back pain (without radiculopathy); however, this population has a favorable prognosis even without manipulation. Most studies have focused on chronic back pain, and often exclude subjects with spinal stenosis, spondylolisthesis (second degree or more), lumbar scoliosis (> 20 degrees or more), osteoporosis and previous vertebral fractures (seen more often in older adults), systemic causes of chronic back pain (including ankylosing spondylitis, infection, or metastatic disease), or psychiatric or cognitive comorbidities. In the general population (including younger adults), spinal manipulative therapy and spinal stabilization have shown improvements in both pain and function as compared to various treatments (back school—education, relaxation techniques, postural and tailored back exercises, individual physiotherapy—mobilization, active exercise, massage, education, or general exercise), especially in the short term. While data suggest there is a statistically significant improvement with spinal manipulation, its clinical importance remains uncertain.

ETIOLOGY-SPECIFIC MANAGEMENT

Therapy of tumors and infectious causes of low back pain is straightforward albeit often difficult. Appropriate management of vertebral compression fractures, lumbar spinal stenosis, and mechanical low back pain is less clear.

Vertebral Compression Fractures

The traditional treatment for vertebral compression fractures is activity modification and pain control at the onset of symptoms. Oral analgesics are usually needed for acute pain relief. These include acetaminophen, nonsteroidal anti-inflammatory drugs (NSAIDs), mild opioids combined with acetaminophen, tramadol, or medications that block serotonin or norepinephrine reuptake. Calcitonin (2- to 4-week course) does have some additional analgesic effect in the acute stage. The choice of first-line agent depends on severity of symptoms and the patient's comorbidities. Muscle relaxants have not been rigorously evaluated in this setting and given the high rate of adverse effects in older adults should be used cautiously, if at all. Opioids, when necessary, should be used cautiously given known side effects particularly in older adults (sedation/altered mental status, constipation, nausea). For severe pain, hospitalization for pain management may be warranted.

Complete bed rest is not recommended, patients should resume physical activity as soon as possible (as pain permits). Physical therapy should focus on gait and core strengthening. Aquatic therapy has been shown to accelerate pain relief and physical activities. In several studies, exercise programs have reduced analgesic use and improved quality of life in older adults with vertebral fractures. Education including management of expectations (eg, that it can take several months for the pain to improve) is essential. Bracing is not usually needed for pain management from osteoporotic compression fractures, although it has been shown to be helpful in acute management of patients with traumatic vertebral compression fractures. Long-term use of bracing should be avoided as its use may lead to immobility of the spine, weakening of paraspinal and core muscles, as well as potential for disuse osteoporosis.

Long-term management of vertebral compression fractures, related to osteoporosis, focuses on improving low bone density (ie, antiresorptive therapy). Underlying conditions that are present and may contribute to development of vertebral compression fractures (hyperthyroidism, granulomatous diseases, infections) require further, specific management beyond the scope of this chapter. Lifestyle modification, namely, smoking cessation and reducing alcohol use, are important. Fall prevention education is effective and essential especially in older adults who have already experienced a traumatic fall or at risk for falls.

There is much interest in vertebral augmentation (the techniques of vertebroplasty and kyphoplasty) in the management of vertebral compression fractures. In a vertebroplasty, extension positioning opens the cleft within a fractured vertebral body, and bone cement is injected into the vertebral body and stabilizes the fracture in this position. In a kyphoplasty, an inflated bone balloon displaces vertebral trabelate and elevates the superior end plate, allowing some restoration of the height of the vertebral body. The balloon is then removed and bone cement is injected into the vertebral space.

The indications and timing for the use of these augmentation procedures remain controversial. Current evidence supporting use of these procedures is of low quality. In the acute setting, although uncontrolled studies show encouraging relief of pain with vertebroplasty, the favorable natural history of the pain from compression fractures, and the potential complications and expense of this procedure, should lend caution to its use. In one nonrandomized trial, the control patients were those who elected not to have the procedure. The pain score was significantly decreased in the vertebroplasty group as compared to the conservative therapy group in the first few days, but there were no significant differences in clinical outcomes at 6 weeks or 6 to 12 months. In a study of patients who had pain for greater than 1 year associated with compression fractures, kyphoplasty was performed on 40 patients, with 20 control patients who elected not to have the procedure. At 1 year, the patients with kyphoplasty had fewer new fractures, fewer back pain–related physicians' visits, and greater improvement in pain scores. Again, neither of these studies were randomized controlled trials. Most experts in this field suggest analgesics, calcitonin, and exercise in the acute phase, and moving on to vertebroplasty or kyphoplasty only if patients have persistent severe pain despite conservative management (and the pain is thought to arise from the fracture).

Lumbar Spinal Stenosis

Conservative nonsurgical therapies, alone and in combination, are warranted prior to attempting surgical treatment. Physical therapy is advocated for this condition, but there is little evidence to justify advocating one treatment regimen over another. The goal of therapy is to increase muscular stabilization (often via strengthening of abdominal muscles) and correction of posture (reduce or prevent lumbar lordosis). In general, stretching, strengthening, and aerobic fitness are advocated. Along with physical therapy, analgesic and anti-inflammatory medications (as monotherapy or in combination) are often used.

The choice of nonsurgical treatment is difficult, as there are few randomized controlled trials of these therapies. Epidural steroid injections have been used for more than 50 years for sciatica. While there are a number of uncontrolled studies suggesting a good outcome with these injections for lumbar spinal stenosis, randomized controlled trials have produced inconsistent results. A randomized trial of 400 older adults with lumbar spinal stenosis and moderate-to-severe leg pain and disability showed minimal or no short-term benefit in outcomes (disability and leg pain intensity) between the group who received epidural steroid injections of glucocorticoids plus lidocaine versus injection with lidocaine alone. A placebo group was not included in this study.

The decision to proceed with spine surgery in an older patient is always a difficult one. An increasing number of studies support surgical decompression for symptomatic lumbar stenosis. Evidence-based guidelines now recommend surgery for patients with moderate to severe spinal stenosis. The Spine Patient Outcomes Research Trial (SPORT), a multicenter randomized control trial (with younger patients, average age in the 40s), one of the largest and well-known studies to date, demonstrated significant advantages associated with surgery compared to nonoperative treatment at 3 months that remained significant and durable through the 2-year duration of the study. It is unclear how results would differ among older adults with comparable spine pathology. At 8-year follow-up, 52% of patients randomized to nonoperative treatment had undergone surgery. A Cochrane review of surgery for degenerative lumbar spondylosis found that "there is still insufficient evidence of the effectiveness of surgery to draw any firm conclusions." On the other hand, the Maine Lumbar Spinal study did show that spinal surgery can be effective. This study is an observational analysis of patients treated by orthopedic surgeons and neurosurgeons in community-based practices throughout Maine. This study followed patients treated surgically or medically, at the choice of the patient and surgeon. In this cohort, patients initially treated surgically demonstrated better outcomes in all measures than those treated nonsurgically. After 10 years, however, the relative difference between surgery and conservative therapy was no longer significant. A randomized controlled multicenter trial of an interspinous process decompression system did find that patients who underwent this procedure had a statistically significant improvement in neurogenic intermittent claudication versus controls.

For patients who have failed maximum nonsurgical management (physical therapy, pharmacotherapy, activity modification, injections) and require surgery, patient selection is critical to optimize the likelihood of a successful outcome. Patients with symptomatic neurogenic claudication, with primary complaints of lower extremity pain, numbness, and paresthesias with prolonged ambulation are ideal

candidates for surgery. An observational study from four surgical centers found that the most powerful predictors of good outcomes of greater walking capacity, milder symptoms, and greater satisfaction were the patient's report of good or excellent health before surgery, as well as low cardiovascular comorbidity. A variety of surgical options exist including decompressive laminectomy with or without fusion, laminotomy, or placement of interspinous devices. Surgical decompression can be performed through traditional open techniques or newer minimally invasive approaches. The majority of these procedures are performed on an outpatient basis with patients usually discharged home on the day of surgery. Prior to surgical intervention, a thorough review of the static and dynamic radiographs, MRI, and CT scans is important. Preoperative identification of spinal instability, preferably by flexion-extension radiographs, is critical to avoid procedures that further destabilize the spine.

Surgery in older adults is associated with higher adverse events rates, which should be discussed with the patient along with the understanding of long-term outcomes from surgery. Complication rates of lumbar decompressive surgeries range from 1.8% to 18% and include wound infection, durotomy, nerve root injury, vascular complications, epidural hematoma, implant failures, adjacent segment degeneration, and nonunion.

In summary, lumbar spinal stenosis should be treated first with a conservative approach including physical therapy, perhaps manipulative therapy, analgesics, and possibly epidural steroid injections. If this approach does not give relief in a reasonable period of time, then a surgical approach, decompressing the stenotic canal space, should be considered. Those patients with high self-reported health and low cardiovascular morbidity seem to achieve the best surgical results.

Mechanical Low Back Pain

The management of back pain in older persons requires a logical, if not yet evidence-based, approach based on both an anatomical understanding of the most likely cause and precipitants of the older adult's pain. For pain that is exacerbated by spinal movement (lying to sitting, bending, etc), spinal instability is the most likely explanation, and thus attempts to stabilize the spine make the most sense. Stabilization may be achieved by isometric abdominal strengthening exercises, lumbar sacral corsets (avoid using for extended periods of time due to muscle disuse/deconditioning), and back protection maneuvers (lifting with one's knees with the back straight, etc). Spinal fusion is reserved for intractable cases of severe low back pain where there is radiographic evidence of progressive deformity, dynamic instability, or pars interarticularis defects.

There is no therapy needed or indicated for DISH. The pain from sacral insufficiency fractures resolves in 4 to 6 weeks, and analgesics should suffice. Antiresorptive therapy for osteoporosis should be initiated to prevent future fractures.

Spontaneous sciatica usually improves without therapy in most older adults. Epidural steroids may be helpful in the management of sciatica. Surgery should be considered only if the pain persists despite trials of conservative therapy.

Prolonged bed rest should be avoided in older adults, given the complications of this intervention in this age group. Patients should, however, avoid those activities that appear to precipitate their pain. Firm corsets may be considered to allow patients to stay mobile and active.

Analgesics should be used, though cautiously, in the management of pain, especially if used chronically. There is little evidence that anti-inflammatory drugs are any better than simple analgesics, and these are associated with a high incidence of complications in this age group. Pain that occurs only with movement often does not respond well to analgesics. While opioid medications may be very helpful with severe pain, the older patient should be watched closely for confusion and constipation. Adjunctive pain therapy, with such agents as tricyclic antidepressants with limited anticholinergic side effects (nortriptyline and disimpramine) and anticonvulsants (gabapentin, pregabalin), may also be helpful but can produce unwanted side effects that limit therapeutic benefit in older adults. The use of combinations of multiple analgesic classes (at the lowest effective dose) may be effective at reducing pain while keeping side effects to a minimum.

PREVENTION

Since back pain in older adults is often recurrent and, while chronic back pain is often reported in the literature, the symptoms often wax and wane. The older adult can usually identify a precipitating event or certain activities or movements that make the back pain worse or prompt a recurrent episode. Once aware of these movements, the clinician can work with the patient to modify behavior and activity to minimize or avoid such movements. Further, it is important to recognize certain risk factors for developing more disabling back pain: being female, having multiple comorbid conditions (including arthritis), reporting depressive symptoms, and having poor grip strength (this may serve as a marker for global muscle weakness) or hip weakness. Obesity is also considered a risk factor for back pain. Several of these risk factors, namely depressive symptoms, muscle weakness, and body mass index are potentially modifiable and amenable to intervention via primary care interventions. Back pain is also associated with psychosocial repercussion, including anxiety, depression, and social isolation. Expanding the evaluation and management of back pain from physical to include psychosocial aspects of daily life may provide benefits for older adults who suffer from these conditions.

SPECIAL ISSUES

While back pain in older adults is prevalent, costly, and leads to considerable morbidity, much of the literature has focused on younger populations with this condition. Few trials comparing efficacy and safety of different treatments have included older adults with back pain. Pain management and treatment are particularly challenging because clinical guidelines do not currently exist for back pain in older adults; moreover, guidelines for back pain in younger populations fail to account for decision-making complexities that occur commonly in older populations, such as multiple comorbid conditions, polypharmacy, frailty, and fragmented social support systems.

Therapeutic Alliance and Patient Preference

The patient-physician relationship lies at the center of treatment for older adults with (chronic) back pain. Therapeutic alliance is defined as a constructive collaboration between the patient and provider. Although few studies have addressed the specific contribution of the therapeutic alliance to treatment outcomes in patients with back pain, a positive patient-physician relationship has been associated with improved treatment outcomes among patients receiving general and rehabilitative medical care. Devoting the time to establish mutually agreed-upon treatment goals is an important step in building a therapeutic alliance. Other core elements of the therapeutic alliance include (1) setting realistic expectations about what can and cannot be accomplished, taking into account such immutable factors as patient age, etiology, and duration of the pain; (2) availability of the physician for advice, reassurance, and support during back pain flares; (3) tenacity and commitment on the part of both provider and patient; (4) mutual respect; and finally, (5) a reciprocal bond of warmth generated by both parties having an emotional investment in the outcomes of treatment.

Discussing and listening to patient preferences regarding management and goals of care are essential. Management programs can be tailored to the older adult's preferences and abilities; preferably, the patient has identified aspects of the program that are most desirable, realistic, and feasible, thus increasing likelihood of adherence. To motivate older adults to engage with a management program, the environment in which the older patient completes therapeutic activity should be appropriate and accessible. In order to reinforce treatment initiation and maintenance, the physician can leverage social supports, for example, family members, home attendants, and community-based agencies.

Comorbidity As noted above, multimorbidity and medical complexity often seen in older adults make management decisions more difficult and sometimes limit treatment options. Further, it is important to recognize that older adults often have multiple sites of pain. Clinicians should inquire about different concomitant locations of pain (eg, spine, knee, hand, hip, peripheral neuropathy) as this may impact management options, patient priorities, treatment expectations, and ultimately achieving outcomes of interest. Mental illness (eg, depression and anxiety) often co-occurs with chronic (back) pain and must be acknowledged and managed optimally (and simultaneously) for pain outcomes to also improve.

Care settings Multiple resources exist to help both clinicians and patients manage back pain. We advocate for clinicians to seek out/learn about resources that exist within their respective communities by contacting the local Area Agency on Aging (AoA) to find out if they have lists of relevant programs. Also, for example, many continuing care retirement communities offer wellness/exercise programs that are run by trained staff.

ACKNOWLEDGMENT

Leo Cooney, Jr., MD, authored this chapter in the sixth edition, and some material from that chapter has been retained here.

FURTHER READING

Abdulla A, Adams N, Bone M, et al. Guidance on the management of pain in older people. *Age Ageing.* 2013;42(suppl 1):i1–i57.

Adogwa O, Carr RK, Kudyba K, et al. Revision lumbar surgery in elderly patients with symptomatic pseudarthrosis, adjacent-segment disease, or same-level recurrent stenosis. Part 1. Two-year outcomes and clinical efficacy: clinical article. *J Neurosurg Spine.* 2013;18(2):139–146.

Adogwa O, Rubio DR, Buchowski JM, D'Souza A, Shlykov MA, Jennings JW. Spine-specific skeletal related events and mortality in non-small cell lung cancer patients: a single-institution analysis. *J Neurosurg Spine.* 2020:1–8.

AGS Panel on Persistent Pain in Older Persons. Pharmacological management of persistent pain in older persons. *J Am Geriatr Soc.* 2009;57(8):1331–1346.

Anderson DB, Luca K, Jensen RK, et al. A critical appraisal of clinical practice guidelines for the treatment of lumbar spinal stenosis. *Spine J.* 2021;21(3):455–464.

Brown CJ, Flood KL. Mobility limitation in the older patient: a clinical review. *JAMA.* 2013;310(11):1168–1177.

Carley JA, Karp JF, Gentili A, et al. Deconstructing chronic low back pain in the older adult: tep by tep evidence and expert-based recommendations for evaluation and treatment: part IV: depression. *Pain Med.* 2015;16(11):2098–2108.

Chou R, Deyo R, Friedly J, et al. Nonpharmacologic therapies for low back pain: a ystematic review for an American College of Physicians Clinical Practice Guideline. *Ann Intern Med.* 2017;166(7):493–505.

Deyo RA, Dworkin SF, Amtmann D, et al. Report of the NIH task force on research standards for chronic low back pain. *Spine J.* 2014;14:1375–1391.

Ebeling PR, Akesson K, Bauer DC, et al. The efficacy and afety of vertebral augmentation: a second ASBMR Task Force Report. *J Bone Miner Res.* 2019;34(1):3–21.

Ferreira PH, Ferreira ML, Maher CG, Refshauge KM, Latimer J, Adams RD. The therapeutic alliance between clinicians and patients predicts outcome in chronic low back pain. *Phys Ther.* 2013;93(4):470–478.

Freburger JK, Holmes GM, Agans RP, et al. The rising prevalence of chronic low back pain. *Arch Intern Med.* 2009;169:251–258.

Fridley J, Gokaslan ZL. The evolution of surgical management for vertebral column tumors. *J Neurosurg Spine.* 2019;30(4):417–423.

Gregori F, Grasso G, Iaiani G, Marotta N, Torregrossa F, Landi A. Treatment algorithm for spontaneous spinal infections: a review of the literature. *J Craniovertebr Junction Spine.* 2019;10(1):3–9.

Hartvigsen J, Hancock MJ, Kongsted A, et al. What low back pain is and why we need to pay attention. *Lancet.* 2018;391(10137):2356–2367.

Institute of Medicine. *Relieving Pain in America: A Blueprint for Transforming Prevention, Care, Education, and Research.* Institute of Medicine (US) Committee on Advancing Pain Research, Care, and Education. Washington, DC: National Academies Press; 2011.

Kanda Y, Kakutani K, Sakai Y, et al. Prospective cohort study of surgical outcome for spinal metastases in patients aged 70 years or older. *Bone Joint J.* 2020;102-B(12):1709–1716.

Lai MKL, Cheung PWH, Cheung JPY. A systematic review of developmental lumbar spinal stenosis. *Eur Spine J.* 2020;29(9):2173–2187.

Leveille SG, Jones RN, Kiely DK, et al. Chronic musculoskeletal pain and the occurrence of falls in an older population. *JAMA.* 2009;302(20):2214–2221.

Lisi AJ, Breuer P, Gallagher RM, et al. Deconstructing chronic low back pain in the older adult—step by step evidence and expert-based recommendations for evaluation and treatment: part II: myofascial pain. *Pain Med.* 2015;16:1282–1289.

Lo J, Chan L, Flynn S. A systematic review of the incidence, prevalence, costs, and activity and work limitations of amputation, osteoarthritis, rheumatoid arthritis, back pain, multiple sclerosis, spinal cord injury, stroke, and traumatic brain injury in the United States: a 2019 update. *Arch Phys Med Rehabil.* 2021;102(1):115–131.

Makris UE, Abrams RC, Gurland B, Reid M. Management of persistent pain in the older patient: a clinical review. *JAMA.* 2014;312(8):825–837.

Makris UE, Fraenkel L, Han L, Leo-Summers L, Gill TM. Restricting back pain and subsequent mobility disability in community-living older persons. *J Am Geriatr Soc.* 2014;62:2142–2147.

1642 Makris UE, Fraenkel L, Han L, Leo-Summers L, Gill TM. Risk factors for restricting back pain in older persons. *J Am Med Dir*. 2014;15:62–67.

Makris UE, Higashi RT, Marks EG, et al. Physical, emotional, and social impacts of restricting back pain in older adults: a qualitative study. *Pain Med*. 2017;18:1225–1235.

Martin BI, Deyo RA, Mirza SK, et al. Expenditures and health status among adults with back and neck problems. *JAMA*. 2008;299:656–664.

Morone NE, Lynch CS, Greco CM, Tindle HA, Weiner DK. "I felt like a new person." The effects of mindfulness meditation on older adults with chronic pain: qualitative narrative analysis of diary entries. *J Pain*. 2008;9(9):841–848.

Nordin C, Gard G, Fjellman-Wiklund A. Being in an exchange process: experiences of patient participation in multimodal pain rehabilitation. *J Rehabil Med*. 2013;45(6):580–586.

Park J, Hughes AK. Nonpharmacological approaches to the management of chronic pain in community-dwelling older adults: a review of empirical evidence. *J Am Geriatr Soc*. 2012;60(3):555–568.

Qaseem A, Wilt TJ, McLean RM, Forciea MA; Clinical Guidelines Committee of the American College of Physicians. Noninvasive treatments for acute, subacute, and chronic low back pain: a clinical practice guideline from the American College of Physicians. *Ann Intern Med*. 2017;166(7):514–530.

Reid MC, Bennett DA, Chen WG, et al. Improving the pharmacologic management of pain in older adults: identifying the research gaps and methods to address them. *Pain Med*. 2011;12(9):1336–1357.

Spitz A, Moore AA, Papaleontiou M, Granieri E, Turner BJ, Reid MC. Primary care providers' perspective on prescribing opioids to older adults with chronic non-cancer pain: a qualitative study. *BMC Geriatr*. 2011;11:35.

Thielke S, Sale J, Reid MC. Aging: are these 4 pain myths complicating care? *J Fam Pract*. 2012;61(11):666–670.

Weiner DK. Introduction to special series: deconstructing chronic low back pain in the older adult: shifting the paradigm from the spine to the person. *Pain Med*. 2015;16:881–885.

Weiner DK, Fang M, Gentili A, et al. Deconstructing chronic low back pain in the older adult—step by step evidence and expert-based recommendations for evaluation and treatment: part I: hip osteoarthritis. *Pain Med*. 2015;16:886–897.

Whitney SL, Marchetti GF, Ellis JL, Otis L. Improvements in balance in older adults engaged in a specialized home care falls prevention program. *J Geriatr Phys Ther*. 2013;36(1):3–12.

Chapter 103

Fibromyalgia and Myofascial Pain Syndromes

Cheryl D. Bernstein, Simge Yonter,
Aishwarya Pradeep, Jay P. Shah, Debra K. Weiner

Fibromyalgia and myofascial pain syndromes (MPSs) are among the most common musculoskeletal disorders from which older adults suffer. Clinically, these disorders represent opposite ends of the pain spectrum with the discrete character of MPS at one extreme and the widespread symptoms of fibromyalgia at the other. Health care professionals have been poorly educated about these common and treatable conditions, and they are often confused with each other. We discuss them in the same chapter to highlight their distinct characteristics. Because MPSs are so commonplace, patients with fibromyalgia often have coexisting MPS. MPS may be acute or chronic and is associated with regional pain syndromes, taut muscle bands, and hypersensitive areas called trigger points. Fibromyalgia syndrome includes symptoms of sleep disruption, fatigue, and psychological distress in addition to widespread pain. Both fibromyalgia and MPS may result in significant functional impairment and cause suffering and disability comparable to that of rheumatoid arthritis and osteoarthritis. Diagnosis of these disorders is grounded in appropriately targeted history and physical examination; these are the tools required to avoid unnecessary ordering of "diagnostic" tests and foster implementation of appropriate management strategies.

FIBROMYALGIA SYNDROME

Fibromyalgia Criteria: Historical Perspective

The gold standard for diagnosing fibromyalgia (FM) is clinical evaluation by a specialist. In 1990, the American College of Rheumatology (ACR) developed criteria to help distinguish FM from other rheumatologic disorders associated with widespread pain (eg, systemic lupus erythematosus, rheumatoid arthritis), and these criteria require the performance of a physical examination to identify tender points. In 2010, Wolfe and colleagues put forth new criteria that did not require a tender point exam and queried symptoms other than pain. These criteria were revised in 2011, then converted into a self-report questionnaire useful for epidemiological research (**Figure 103-1**). Scoring instructions are found in the legend of **Figure 103-1** and scores of greater than or equal to 13 are 96.6% sensitive and 91.8%

Learning Objectives

- Know the distinguishing elements of the history and physical examination for older adults with fibromyalgia as compared with myofascial pain.

- Describe the three-pronged approach to treating myofascial pain syndromes.

- List the nonpharmacologic and pharmacologic treatments for fibromyalgia that are supported by strong evidence and have an acceptable safety profile for older adults.

Key Clinical Points

1. **Fibromyalgia and myofascial pain are distinct syndromes that may occur independently or coexist.**

2. **Myofascial pain syndromes are diagnosed by eliciting a characteristic history coupled with identification of active trigger points on physical examination.**

3. **Myofascial pain syndromes may present with neuropathic symptoms such as paresthesias and burning sensations and can mimic radiculopathy. As they are treated best using nonpharmacologic strategies, their diagnosis can prevent exposing frail older adults to multiple potential adverse drug effects and unnecessary procedures.**

4. **Older adults presenting with widespread pain should undergo a comprehensive history and physical examination including careful review of their medications. If a potential cause is not elicited fibromyalgia screening should ensue. Revised criteria allow for disease screening without the need for a tender point examination.**

(*Continued*)

(Cont.)

5. Fibromyalgia syndrome (FMS) is common in older adults and may be the sole cause of pain or a key pain comorbidity. Axial pain is common in FMS, and in older adults with neck, upper, or low back pain, FMS should be screened routinely.

6. FMS is associated with a number of non-pharmacologic and pharmacologic treatments with strong efficacy evidence. Older adults should be encouraged about the wide range of available effective treatments.

specific, compared with the 1990 ACR criteria, which are 81% sensitive and 88% specific.

In 2016, Wolfe et al. further modified their survey to include a generalized pain requirement and eliminate wording on "absence of another disorder to explain pain." The authors suggest these changes will reduce misdiagnosis of regional pain syndromes and allow for both clinical and research application.

In 2019, an international working group of experts published new fibromyalgia criteria as part of a novel pain diagnostic system. Known as the ACTTION-APS Pain Taxonomy (AAPT), this screen requires pain in 6 of 9 body regions and the presence of moderate fatigue and/or sleep disturbances. **Table 103-1** compares the various fibromyalgia criteria.

Despite good sensitivity, specificity, and concordance between 1990, 2010, and 2011 criteria, the authors do not recommend using screening methods to diagnose fibromyalgia. The practitioner must evaluate for other causes of widespread pain and obtain a careful history and physical examination to that end.

EPIDEMIOLOGY

Estimates of fibromyalgia prevalence vary widely from 1.7% using the 1990 ACR criteria to 5.4% in studies using the modified 2011 scale. According to these original criteria, women are four to seven times as likely to have fibromyalgia compared to men, with the greatest prevalence in those 60 to 79 years of age. When using the 2011 survey, the female-to-male ratio drops to 1.8:1 overall and 3.4:1 in those aged 60 and older. Experts suggest that elimination of the tender point examination and addition of the somatic symptoms scale improves the identification of fibromyalgia in men. Patients with fibromyalgia are estimated to have a two- to sevenfold greater risk of suffering from depression, anxiety, headache, irritable bowel syndrome, chronic fatigue syndrome, systemic lupus erythematosus, and rheumatoid arthritis compared to healthy individuals. Fibromyalgia patients display comorbid pain disorders, known as

chronic overlapping pain conditions, which are listed in **Table 103-2**. This heterogeneous group of pain conditions tend to occur more frequently in women and are associated with sleep disturbances, anxiety, depression, and poor physical function.

PATHOGENESIS

While recent studies have added to our understanding of fibromyalgia's pathogenesis, the exact cause is still unknown and considered to be multifactorial. Most experts believe that abnormal pain regulation, known as central sensitization, plays a crucial role in fibromyalgia pathogenesis. Sensitization likely stems from a variety of neuroendocrine and biochemical abnormalities. Potential environmental triggers include acute pain and trauma, viral infections (Epstein-Barr virus, Lyme disease, Q fever, viral hepatitis), and psychological stress. Studies also suggest a "central pain-prone phenotype," which includes factors such as female sex, early life trauma, and family history of pain or mood disorders. The various proposed mechanisms of fibromyalgia pathogenesis and their supportive findings are summarized in **Table 103-3**.

CLINICAL PRESENTATION

Patient history

Fibromyalgia patients often report that they feel pain "all over." Pain diagrams, on which patients are asked to shade painful areas of a human figure, help make the diagnosis. For fibromyalgia patients, these diagrams show diffuse shading on the right and left sides of the body as well as above and below the waist. We observe that some fibromyalgia patients shade, circle, or put an X through the entire figure. Patients generally rate their pain as moderate to severe in intensity. Over time, pain will fluctuate in severity but typically does not resolve completely. Pain descriptions vary widely from deep and aching to mildly tender or sharp. Symptoms are generally constant throughout the day but often are worse in the morning and the evening. Triggers, including stress, cold weather, illness, and unaccustomed exertion, will likely increase pain. In addition to pain, 75% of patients report stiffness, and over 50% report a sensation of swelling. Low back pain and chronic whiplash are relatively common and affect 20% to 30% of fibromyalgia patients.

Fibromyalgia patients are likely to describe a wide variety of nonmusculoskeletal symptoms, most commonly fatigue and difficulty sleeping. Sixty percent of patients report psychological and neuropsychological symptoms, including anxiety, mental distress, and cognitive dysfunction. Thirty percent of patients report current depression, with over 50% of patients reporting a history of depression. Headaches are also common. Uncommon symptoms (< 20% prevalence) include tinnitus, dizziness,

This is a self-report questionnaire based on the modification of the 2010 ACR preliminary diagnostic criteria for fibromyalgia (0–31 points).

1. Widespread pain index (0–19 points)

Check all areas of pain or tenderness during the past 7 days

- ○ Right jaw
- ○ Left jaw
- ○ Neck
- ○ Right shoulder
- ○ Left shoulder
- ○ Upper back
- ○ Chest
- ○ Right upper arm
- ○ Left upper arm
- ○ Right lower arm
- ○ Left lower arm
- ○ Lower back
- ○ Abdomen
- ○ Right hip or buttocks
- ○ Left hip or buttocks
- ○ Right upper leg
- ○ Left upper leg
- ○ Right lower leg
- ○ Left lower leg

2. Severity of symptoms other than pain, part 1

For each symptom indicate the severity of the symptom during the past 7 days.

	No Problem (0 points)	Slight or Mild Problem (1 point)	Moderate Problem (2 points)	Severe Problem (3 points)
A. Fatigue				
B. Trouble thinking or remembering				
C. Waking up tired or unrefreshed				

3. Severity of symptoms other than pain, part 2

During the past six months have you had the following symptoms?

	No (0 points)	Yes (1 point)
A. Pain or cramps in the lower abdomen		
B. Depression		
C. Headache		

4. Symptoms duration ≥ 3 months? 0 points
- ○ Yes
- ○ No

5. Absence of another disorder to explain pain? 0 points
- ○ Yes
- ○ No

FIGURE 103-1. Modified Fibromyalgia Criteria 2011: A Survey. This is a self-report questionnaire based on the modification of the 2010 ACR preliminary diagnostic criteria for fibromyalgia (0–31 points). A patient satisfies diagnostic criteria for fibromyalgia if the following conditions are met: (1) Widespread pain index (WPI) ≥ 7 and symptom severity scare (SS) score ≥ 5 or WPI 3-6 and SS scale score ≥ 9; (2) Symptoms have been present at similar level for at least 3 months, and (3) The patient does not have a disorder that would otherwise explain the pain.

TABLE 103-1 ■ COMPARISON OF FIBROMYALGIA DIAGNOSTIC CRITERIA

CRITERIA	ACR 1990	ACR 2011 MODIFIED	ACR 2011 WITH 2016 PROPOSED CHANGES	ACTTION-APS TAXONOMY INITIATIVE (AAPT)
Duration of symptoms	≥ 3 months	≥ 3 months	≥ 3 months	≥ 3 months for pain and fatigue/sleep
Pain	11/18 tender points on exam	Widespread pain index (WPI)	WPI and generalized pain (pain in ≥ 4 of 5 body regions: upper left, upper right, lower left, lower right, and axial)	≥ 6 of 9 pain site of map (head, left arm, right arm, chest, abdomen, upper back, lower back/buttocks, left leg, right leg)
Fibromyalgia Symptom (FS) score (widespread pain index and symptom severity score [SSS] of non-musculoskeletal symptoms such as headache, depression, fatigue, and abdominal pain)	Not used as part of ACR 1990 criteria	WPI score ≥ 7 and SSS ≥ 5 or WPI score 4–6 and SSS ≥ 9	WPI score ≥ 7 and SSS ≥ 5 or WPI score 4–6 and SSS ≥ 9	Not used as part of the AAPT criteria
Fatigue/sleep	Not used as part of ACR 1990 criteria	Not used as part of ACR 2011 modified criteria	Not used as part of 2016 criteria	Moderate to severe sleep problems or fatigue
Comments	Pain not attributable to another cause	Pain not attributable to another cause	Diagnosis of fibromyalgia valid regardless of other diagnoses	Additional features support diagnosis but not required (tenderness, cognitive problems, muscle stiffness, environmental sensitivities, hypervigilance)

Reproduced with permission from Bair MJ, Krebs EE. Fibromyalgia, Ann Intern Med. 2020;172(5):ITC33-ITC48.

vertigo, and Raynaud phenomenon. Studies demonstrate that fibromyalgia may coexist in 17% of patients with osteoarthritis, 21% of patients with rheumatoid arthritis, and 37% of patients with systemic lupus erythematosus. **Table 103-2** lists the symptoms and syndromes commonly associated with fibromyalgia.

Up to 80% of fibromyalgia patients report debilitating fatigue. This complaint encompasses mental fatigue and impaired concentration, commonly referred to as "fibro fog," physical fatigue after exertion, and general sleepiness. In fibromyalgia patients, these symptoms most often occur in the absence of other medical illnesses. Neuropsychological performance testing demonstrates objective deficits in patients with fibromyalgia, most notably inhibitory control and short-/long-term memory. It is important, therefore, that neuropsychological performance testing results in the older adult with fibromyalgia are interpreted in the context of typical neuropsychological performance deficits related to fibromyalgia.

Poor sleep quality seen in fibromyalgia patients is known as nonrestorative sleep. A number of sleep abnormalities have been documented in fibromyalgia patients and are listed in **Table 103-4**. A recent large epidemiologic study found that improvements in restorative sleep correlate with the resolution of chronic widespread pain.

CLINICAL ASSESSMENT

When evaluating the older adult with widespread chronic pain, the practitioner should be mindful of fibromyalgia-associated rheumatologic disorders such as generalized osteoarthritis, pseudogout, gout, rheumatoid arthritis, systemic lupus erythematosus, and polymyalgia rheumatica, as summarized in **Table 103-5**. A careful history and thorough physical examination for synovial and extrasynovial findings can help differentiate these conditions from fibromyalgia. **Table 103-5** lists many key features on history and physical examination that help diagnose fibromyalgia. Other diagnostic considerations include hypothyroidism, vitamin D deficiency, demyelinating polyneuropathies, and paraneoplastic syndromes. A targeted laboratory panel may help tease out these differential diagnostic considerations.

The practitioner should review all medications when assessing the older adult with widespread pain. Toxic myopathy is a well-documented and dose-related side effect of HMG-CoA reductase inhibitors and high-dose corticosteroids (30 mg of prednisone equivalents per day). The antiretroviral agent zidovudine, the antifungal agent voriconazole, and several immunosuppressant medications, including interferon, cyclosporin, and tacrolimus, may cause painful myopathies. Commonly abused drugs, including cocaine, heroin, amphetamines, and alcohol, also cause painful myopathies. Symptoms typically begin

TABLE 103-2 ■ FIBROMYALGIA-ASSOCIATED SYMPTOMS AND DISORDERS

Musculoskeletal

Stiffness

Sensation of joint swelling

Nonmusculoskeletal

Fatigue

Difficulty sleeping

Dysesthesias

Paresthesias

Depression

Anxiety

Stress

Dyspnea

Palpitations

Difficulty concentrating

Tinnitus

Dizziness

Vertigo

Pelvic pain

Restless leg syndrome

Chronic overlapping pain conditions that may co-occur with fibromyalgia

Vulvodynia

Temporomandibular disorders

Myalgic encephalomyelitis/chronic fatigue syndrome

Irritable bowel syndrome

Interstitial cystitis/painful bladder syndrome

Endometriosis

Chronic tension-type headache

Chronic migraine headache

Chronic low back pain

Associated rheumatological disorders

Systemic lupus erythematosus

Rheumatoid arthritis

Sjögren syndrome

---

within weeks to months of drug exposure and resolve with discontinuation.

TREATMENT

A variety of pharmacologic and nonpharmacologic interventions are available for the treatment of fibromyalgia. There are not first-line fibromyalgia treatments, and evidence-based guidelines vary. Most experts agree that effective treatment starts with patient education and integrates both pharmacologic and nonpharmacologic therapies, as illustrated in **Figure 103-2**. Although the response is likely to be modest, we have successfully employed a number of management approaches in our older adult patients with fibromyalgia. Patients may benefit from treatment

with antidepressants and some antiseizure medications, especially if they report associated symptoms such as disrupted sleep, depression, and/or anxiety (**Table 103-6**). Experts recommend a tailored treatment approach that addresses the patient's most bothersome symptoms.

Medications

Antidepressants Antidepressants are among the most widely studied medications for the treatment of fibromyalgia. The analgesic effect of antidepressants may result from increased central nervous system serotonin and norepinephrine, which block pain signals from the periphery. In addition to reducing pain, antidepressants may improve sleep and emotional well-being. Those used most commonly are the tricyclic antidepressants (TCAs) and serotonin norepinephrine reuptake inhibitors (SNRIs). Selective serotonin reuptake inhibitors (SSRI) may be less effective than the SNRIs for treating chronic pain. However, some practitioners find SSRIs more effective for treating depression. Fibromyalgia treatment guidelines recommend TCAs in doses ranging from 10 to 50 mg at night. A comparative review of amitriptyline versus other FDA-approved fibromyalgia medications found similar improvements in pain and fatigue. Cyclobenzaprine, a muscle relaxant with structural similarity to the tricyclics, has shown efficacy in several short-term clinical trials.

Even in low doses, TCAs have significant side effects that limit use. This class's anticholinergic effects are responsible for most of the adverse effects, including sedation, confusion, constipation, and palpitations. TCAs may contribute to impaired mobility and cause falls in older adults. TCAs may also prolong the QT interval, which results in torsade de pointes and death. Practitioners should obtain a baseline electrocardiogram to assess cardiac rhythm prior to starting TCAs and monitor periodically during use. According to FDA guidelines for QTc prolongation with antidepressant use, QTc increases of greater than 10 ms over baseline are of "increasing concern" and greater than 20 ms are of "definite concern." FDA guidelines caution against prescribing/continuing TCAs when QTc intervals are greater than 500 ms or have increased 60 ms or more over baseline. Secondary tricyclic amines, desipramine, and nortriptyline have fewer side effects but are not as well studied.

Practitioners may favor SNRIs compared to TCAs for fibromyalgia as they have fewer adverse effects. Duloxetine (60 mg daily) and milnacipran (100–200 mg daily) are FDA-approved for fibromyalgia. Both duloxetine and milnacipran improve pain, depression, and quality of life. Compared to duloxetine, milnacipran is a more potent inhibitor of norepinephrine reuptake and may be more effective for patients with fatigue and cognitive symptoms. SNRIs may elevate blood pressure in some patients, and vital signs should be monitored routinely. Common side effects are nausea and orthostatic hypotension and may be reduced by taking the medication with food and using slow titration.

TABLE 103-3 ■ PROPOSED MECHANISMS IN FIBROMYALGIA PATHOGENESIS

PROPOSED MECHANISM	SUPPORTIVE EVIDENCE IN FIBROMYALGIA PATIENTS VERSUS CONTROLS	COMMENTS
Peripheral tissue abnormalities	Minimal evidence to support peripheral mechanisms	
Muscle	High muscle nitric acid levels	High nitric acid may be associated with increased cell death
	Low muscle phosphocreatine and ATP. Increased muscle substance P, DNA fragmentation, interleukin-1, and perfusion deficits	May suggest abnormal muscle metabolism in fibromyalgia patients
Peripheral nerve	Reduced epidermal nerve fiber density on skin biopsy	Reduced nerve density similar to that found in small fiber neuropathy. Nonspecific finding and relationship to pain is unclear
Sensitization and pain amplification	Abnormalities of pain processing are well established in fibromyalgia	See Phillips and Clauw, Sluka and Clauw, and Sarzi-Puttini et al. references in Further Reading section
Peripheral sensitization	Increased neuronal excitability and nociceptive fields	Contributes to peripheral pain sensitization
Central sensitization	Increased pain sensitivity after repeated exposure to noxious stimuli	Increased pain after repeated exposure to painful stimuli is known as "windup" or temporal summation and is an example of central sensitization. Diminished endogenous pain inhibition also contributes to sensitization
Neuroendocrine and autonomic abnormalities	Dysregulation of the hypothalamic-pituitary axis (HPA) and autonomic system	
Neuroendocrine abnormalities	Abnormal levels of ACTH and cortisol	HPA may be less responsive to stress in fibromyalgia patients compared to controls
Autonomic system abnormalities	Abnormal heart rate variability and peripheral blood flow suggesting high levels of sympathetic activity	Autonomic nervous system dysregulation is also found in disorders that overlap with fibromyalgia, ie, chronic fatigue syndrome, interstitial cystitis and irritable bowel syndrome
	Attenuated orthostatic challenge and cold pressor response suggests sympathetic dysfunction	
	Reduced plasma and CSF catecholamines	
Functional imaging of pain	Functional imaging demonstrates central nervous system involvement in fibromyalgia	
Functional MRI	Increased activation in the anterior cingulate cortex, insula, and secondary somatosensory cortex	Functional MRI demonstrates increased blood flow after exposure to noxious, positive and negative stimuli
Voxel-based morphology	Decreased gray matter volume in areas involved in pain processing	Reduced gray matter volume found in a variety of chronic pain disorders and is similar to that found in the aging process
		Reduced brain volume may reflect abnormal pain processing and cognitive function
SPECT scanning	Reduced blood flow in selective brain regions	
Genetics	Suggests fibromyalgia is a heritable disorder	
	Familial aggregation, ie, siblings 14× as likely to develop fibromyalgia	
	Lower pain threshold in first-degree relatives of fibromyalgia patients	
	Linkage to chromosome 17	
	Genetic polymorphisms in promoter region of the serotonin transporter gene (5HTT)	
	Epigenetic changes such as histone modification and DNA methylation	Epigenetic changes are modifications of DNA without alteration of DNA sequence
		These changes are believed to occur as a response environmental stress such as childhood abuse

TABLE 103-4 ■ SLEEP ABNORMALITIES IN FIBROMYAGLIA

FINDINGS	COMMENTS
Insomnia	Delayed sleep onset in fibromyalgia patients versus controls. Sleep hygiene education may be helpful, ie, keeping regular schedules, eliminating daytime naps, establishing a restful sleep environment, and excluding caffeine
Frequent awakenings	Overall sleep time reduced in fibromyalgia patients
Abnormalities of sleep architecture Alpha intrusion	Alpha waves (usually present in light sleep) are present during slow wave, deep sleep Alpha intrusion may be associated with reduced growth hormone and insulin growth factor production
Rapid eye movement sleep (REM) deficiency	REM sleep considered restorative sleep

Increased prevalence of primary sleep disorders
   Sleep apnea
   Restless legs syndrome
   Periodic limb movement disorders
	Recommend screening and diagnostic polysomnography if needed

We recommend starting duloxetine at 20 mg daily and increasing to 60 mg slowly over at least several weeks. If the practitioner decides to discontinue the drug, this also must be done slowly to avoid SNRI withdrawal syndrome. We recommend slowly decreasing the dose by no more than 50% at 1 to 2 weeks intervals. Standard recommendations for milnacipran are to start with 12.5 mg daily and slowly titrate to 50 mg bid. The authors of this chapter do not prescribe milnacipran for older adults because of lack of data in this age group.

Antiepileptics Aside from the antidepressants, very few drug classes have evidence for efficacy in the treatment of fibromyalgia. Some studies support using the antiepileptic drugs gabapentin (currently available in generic form) and pregabalin. Research suggests that antiepileptic drugs reduce neuronal excitability, decrease ectopic neuronal discharge, and modulate various neurotransmitter levels. A large study of pregabalin, which binds to the alpha(2)-delta subunit of the voltage-gated calcium channel, found that fibromyalgia patients experienced significant improvement in pain, fatigue, social functioning, vitality, and general health perception compared to controls. Pregabalin, in doses ranging from 300 to 450 mg daily, was the first medication approved for fibromyalgia syndrome. A recent meta-analysis of anticonvulsants for fibromyalgia found mild improvements with pregabalin in pain, sleep, and fatigue compared to placebo. Despite the lack of conclusive evidence to support gabapentin for fibromyalgia, our clinical experience suggests that low doses (eg, 100–600 mg/day) may help reduce pain and improve sleep. Sedation and dizziness are common side effects of both medications and may contribute to falls in older adults. These are minimized by starting with low bedtime doses and slowly titrating upward. **Table 103-7** compares the benefits and side effects of the three FDA-approved fibromyalgia medications.

Analgesics Except for tramadol, there are no data to support the efficacy of analgesics for fibromyalgia treatment. Tramadol, a weak mu receptor agonist with dual serotonin and norepinephrine reuptake inhibition, is unique in its mechanism and was effective for fibromyalgia symptoms in three randomized controlled trials.

Hormonal supplements and other agents Studies of hormonal supplements for patients with fibromyalgia have had mixed results. Randomized growth hormone studies demonstrate some improvement in pain and fatigue but do not support routine use. Several other hormonal supplements, including thyroid hormone, dehydroepiandrosterone, and calcitonin, have been tried anecdotally but are not widely accepted for fibromyalgia treatment. Similarly, rigorous data do not support the use of nutritional supplements, herbal medications, guaifenesin, or vitamin therapy. In a few small uncontrolled studies, low-dose naltrexone demonstrated improved inflammation, pain, and function in patients with fibromyalgia.

For patients with fibromyalgia and vitamin D deficiency, repletion of vitamin D may reduce pain and improve function. Given the other risks associated with vitamin D deficiency in older adults (eg, falls, osteoporosis), 25-OH vitamin D levels should be checked routinely, not just in those with chronic pain.

There is growing interest in the use of cannabinoid molecules for the treatment of chronic pain. Because data from rigorous randomized controlled trials are lacking, treatment recommendations related to medical cannabis are currently informed by clinical experience and uncontrolled studies (see **Table 103-6**).

Nonpharmacologic Therapies

Nonpharmacologic therapies for fibromyalgia include cognitive-behavioral techniques, exercise, acupuncture, balneotherapy (ie, bathing), and massage. Systematic review

TABLE 103-5 ■ DIFFERENTIATION OF OSTEOARTHRITIS FROM OTHER COMMON RHEUMATOLOGIC DISORDERS: HISTORY, PHYSICAL EXAMINATION, AND OTHER DIAGNOSTIC FEATURES

| DISORDER | HISTORY | | PHYSICAL EXAMINATION | | OTHER DIAGNOSTIC FEATURES/COMMENTS |
	AM STIFFNESS	LOCATION OF PAIN	SYNOVITIS	EXTRASYNOVIAL DISEASE	
Osteoarthritis	Generally short-lived, eg, < 30 min	Weight-bearing appendicular joints, cervical and lumbar spine, DIPs, PIPs, and first CMC. MCP and wrist involvement go against OA	Absent or mild	None related to arthritis itself	Since OA is ubiquitous in older adults, x-rays should be used to rule out other disorders, not to diagnose OA.
Pseudogout	Pseudorheumatoid pattern may be associated with prolonged AM stiffness	Knee and wrist are most common locations; disease is often symmetrical	Acute flares are intensely inflammatory	Chondrocalcinosis on x-rays; eye deposits, bursitis, tendonitis, carpal, and cubital tunnel syndromes may occur. Tophaceous soft tissue deposits uncommon	Chondrocalcinosis may be asymptomatic. Identification of intracellular CPPD crystals offers a definitive diagnosis in acute flares. Acute and chronic forms occur.
Gout	Pseudorheumatoid pattern may be associated with prolonged AM stiffness	Joints of the lower extremities are most often involved, especially first MTP; disease is typically asymmetrical	Acute flares are intensely inflammatory	Tophi may deposit in soft tissues	Hyperuricemia may be asymptomatic. Serum uric acid cannot diagnose gout. Identification of intracellular monosodium urate monohydrate crystals offers a definitive diagnosis in acute flares.
Rheumatoid arthritis	Prolonged, eg, > 30 min. Duration of stiffness is used as one parameter of disease activity	Any synovial joint. The lumbar spine is typically spared.	Present	Not uncommon; rheumatoid nodules can develop in soft tissues. Many other possible manifestations including anemia, vasculitis (skin lesions, peripheral neuropathy, pericarditis, visceral arteritis, palpable purpura), pulmonary disease, etc	Patients may be seronegative. If disease is suspected, patient should promptly be referred to a rheumatologist to retard disease progression.
Systemic lupus erythematosus	Not a prominent feature	Depends on tissues involved—may or may not be limited to joints. Comorbid fibromyalgia is not uncommon	Generally absent; arthralgias are more common than arthritis	Common—eg, anemia, skin rash, pleuritis, peritonitis, pericarditis, nephritis, meningitis, etc	Anyone with suspected SLE should promptly be referred to a rheumatologist.
Fibromyalgia syndrome	Generally short-lived, eg, < 30 min	Typically diffuse. Worst symptoms often involve the axial skeleton	Absent. Joints themselves are not involved, although patients experience pain in joints and soft tissues	Many other disorders may coexist (see **Table 103-2**)	Fibromyalgia syndrome is not a diagnosis of exclusion, but one based upon careful history (see text).

Polymyalgia rheumatica	May be prolonged, lasting several hours	Typically proximal—eg, shoulder girdle, hip girdle, neck. If headaches, jaw claudication, and/or prominent systemic symptoms (eg, fever), consider temporal arteritis	May occur, especially in small joints of hands	Occurs if comorbid temporal arteritis and relates to involvement of arteries (eg, Raynaud phenomenon, bruits, claudication)	Because the erythrocyte sedimentation and C-reactive protein are very nonspecific, these tests should be used to assist with confirmation of a suspected diagnosis. Note that cases of PMR and TA with a normal ESR/CRP have been reported.
Vitamin D deficiency	Absent	Typically described as diffuse, deep pain. Bony pain is often present	Absent	Fatigue is a common feature with proximal muscular weakness (pelvic-girdle myopathy). Tenderness with palpation of bony structures	Fatigue and difficulty climbing stairs are common complaints. Gait imbalance and falls may be seen. In severe cases, the profound weakness results in need for a wheelchair. Radiologic findings include fractures and Looser-Milkman pseudofractures (osteomalacia giving a striped appearance to bones). Direct measurement of serum 25(OH)D is the best marker for vitamin D deficiency.
Hypothyroidism	Absent	Diffuse myalgias and arthralgias	Joint swelling may be present with noninflammatory joint effusions. Hand, knee, and wrist involvement. Avascular necrosis, gout, and/or pseudogout may coexist	Myalgias, generalized weakness, and carpal tunnel may exist	Fatigue, mental slowing, and depression often seen. Associated symptoms include hair loss, edema, cold intolerance, dry skin, constipation, and weight gain.

CMC, carpometacarpal joint; CPPD, calcium pyrophosphate dehydrate; DIP, distal interphalangeal joint; ESR, erythrocyte sedimentation rate; MCP, metacarpophalangeal joint; MTP, metatarsophalangeal; OA, osteoarthritis; PIP, proximal interphalangeal joint; PMR, polymyalgia rheumatica; SLE, systemic lupus erythematosus; TA, temporal arteritis.

Reproduced with permission from Weiner DK. Office management of chronic pain in the elderly. Am J Med. 2007;120(4):306–315.

PART V

ORGAN SYSTEMS AND DISEASES

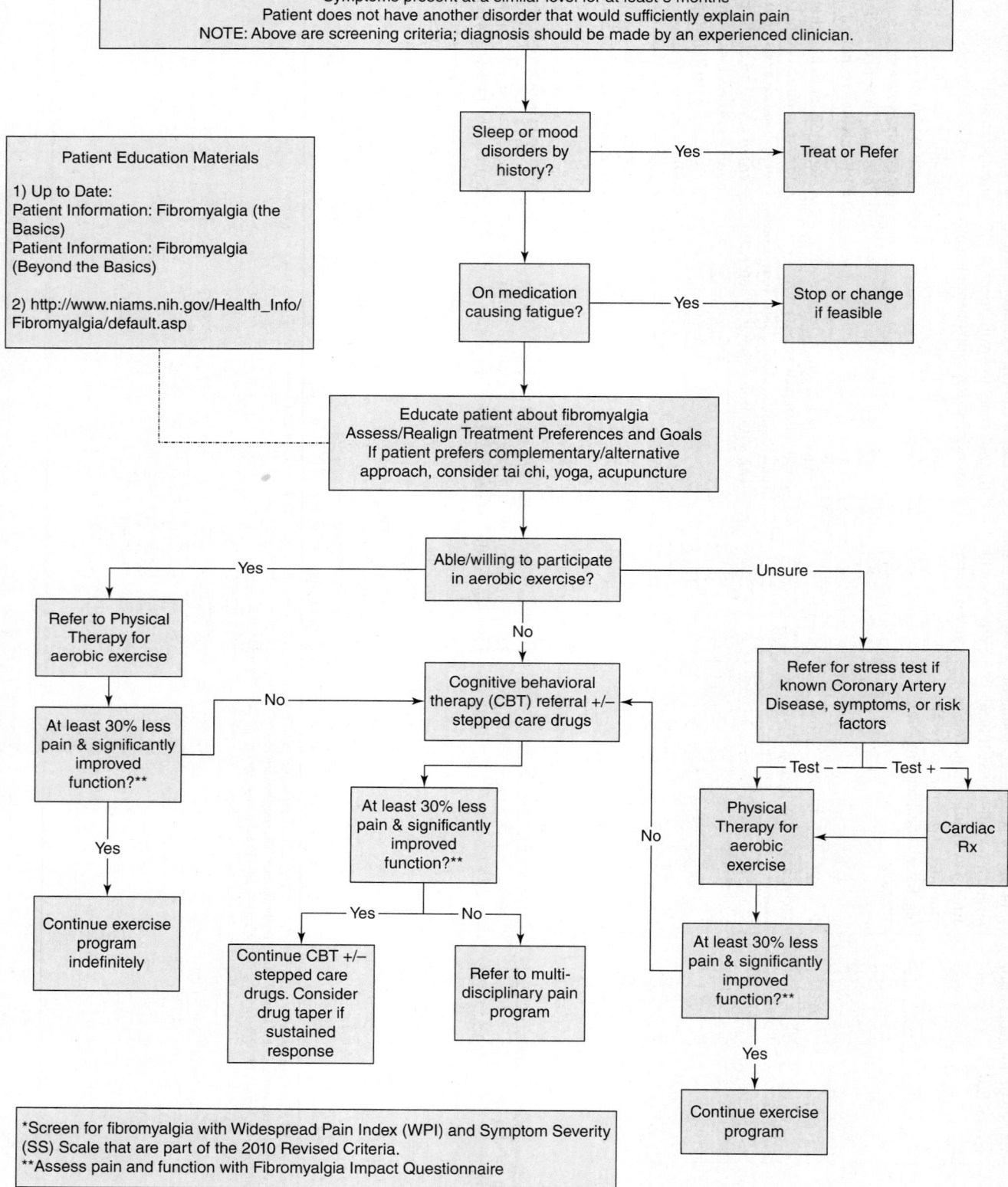

FIGURE 103-2. Algorithm for the management of fibromyalgia in the older adult. (Reproduced with permission from Fatemi G, Fang MA, Breuer P, et al. Deconstructing chronic low back pain in the older adult—step by step evidence and expert-based recommendations for evaluation and treatment part III: fibromyalgia syndrome. *Pain Med.* 2015;16[9]:1709–1719.)

TABLE 103-6 ■ MEDICATIONS USED IN FIBROMYALGIA TREATMENT

DRUG	RECOMMENDED DOSE	COMMENTS
Antiepileptic medications Gabapentin Pregabalin	100–600 mg daily Max dose 1800 mg daily 150–300 mg daily Max dose of 450 mg	Titrate slowly May cause sedation or dizziness Dose adjustment for renal failure
Tricyclic antidepressants (TCA) Nortriptyline	10–50 mg nightly	Sedation and confusion Avoid in narrow angle glaucoma Recommend baseline ECG to evaluate QT prolongation; if present, avoid use
Selective serotonin reuptake inhibitors (SSRI) Fluoxetine Citalopram	20–80 mg daily 20–40 mg daily	SSRIs have superior tolerability compared to TCAs
Serotonin norepinephrine reuptake inhibitors (SNRI) Venlafaxine Duloxetine Milnacipran	75–100 mg daily 30–60 mg daily 100–200 mg daily	Avoid in those with uncontrolled hypertension Avoid in patients with liver disease Avoid in those with narrow angle glaucoma More potent for inhibition of norepinephrine reuptake than duloxetine
Analgesics Tramadol	50–100 mg every 6 h as needed	May cause sedation and confusion Avoid in patients with seizures May cause serotonin syndrome in combination with SSRIs or other antidepressants Dose adjustment for renal failure
Muscle relaxants Cyclobenzaprine	5–10 mg nightly	Likely to cause sedation Similar side effects to tricyclic antidepressants

of regular aerobic exercise for fibromyalgia (20 minutes daily, 2–3 times a week) demonstrated improvements in pain, function, aerobic capacity, and well-being. Most therapists recommend individualizing programs based on patient abilities and symptoms. During pain flares, which may occur after physical exertion, exercise and daily routines should be modified but not ceased. Water aerobics may benefit those who have difficulty with traditional physical therapy. The evidence supporting strength training is not as robust as that for aerobic exercise. Strength training is beneficial for fibromyalgia patients who may be deconditioned and up to 30% weaker than control subjects.

Data support the benefits of coupling exercise programs with educational sessions and cognitive-behavioral techniques. Lectures on fibromyalgia and the benefits of

TABLE 103-7 ■ SUMMARY COMPARISON OF FDA-APPROVED DRUGS FOR THE TREATMENT OF FIBROMYALGIA

DRUG	EFFICACY OF SX RELIEF					SAFETY/TOLERABILITY
	PAIN	SLEEP	FATIGUE	MOOD	HRQOL	
Pregabalin	++	++	++	+	++	Dizziness Somnolence Weight gain
Duloxetine	++	++	+	++	++	Headache Nausea Diarrhea Hepatotoxicity
Milnacipran	+	+	++	+	++	Headache Nausea

HRQOL, health-related quality of life.

exercise improve treatment outcomes. Cognitive-behavioral therapy (CBT) is useful for fibromyalgia patients who tend to catastrophize their painful symptoms. We have found that CBT performed via telemedicine is an effective option for those who have trouble traveling or wish to avoid in-person appointments. Studies of internet-based CBT for fibromyalgia demonstrate improvements in pain, depression, and patient satisfaction. Mindfulness-based therapy, such as meditation, may improve sleep, symptom severity, and stress. Cognitive approaches to pain management are most useful as part of an interdisciplinary program that includes education and exercise.

Complementary medicine treatments for fibromyalgia may be beneficial. Several randomized controlled trials of acupuncture have shown effectiveness for relieving fibromyalgia symptoms, although none have been performed exclusively in older adults. These data are encouraging, however, given the overall safety of this treatment modality. Mind-body movement techniques such as yoga, qigong, and tai chi are promising as fibromyalgia therapies. Two controlled trials of tai chi for fibromyalgia showed improvements in pain, sleep, and function. Fibromyalgia patients participating in an 8-week yoga program had similar symptomatic improvements compared to those receiving standard care. Weak evidence supports chiropractic treatment, massage therapy, interferential current, and ultrasound to treat fibromyalgia syndrome. Further studies are needed to determine the potential impact of all these modalities and identify potential long-term treatment benefits.

Treatment for Refractory Cases

Several factors limit the effectiveness of fibromyalgia treatment, including medication under-prescribing, under-dosing, and/or patient noncompliance. One fibromyalgia study demonstrated that only 31% of patients received at least one medication listed on the ACR treatment guidelines. Those patients treated with appropriate medicines did not necessarily achieve the recommended dose or adhere to the prescribed regimen. Optimal treatment may require combining several medications, which increases the risk of severe side effects. Patients with refractory pain may benefit from consultation with a specialist for medication adjustment, multidisciplinary rehabilitation, or interventional procedures for comorbid pain conditions. Patients with severe mood disorders are prone to fail traditional treatments and may benefit from psychiatric comanagement.

Assessing Response to Treatment

Several standardized questionnaires are available to assess response to treatment. One of the most efficient and useful is the 20-question Fibromyalgia Impact Questionnaire (FIQ), which takes only a few minutes to complete and quantifies physical function, painful symptoms, and emotional well-being specifically in fibromyalgia patients (**Figure 103-3**).

MYOFASCIAL PAIN SYNDROME

Background and Epidemiology

Myofascial pain syndrome (MPS) arises from muscle as well as surrounding fascia and is characterized by the presence of taut bands of skeletal muscle, which may contain palpable nodules (myofascial trigger points [MTrPs]; **Figure 103-4**). MPS can be an acute or chronic condition, and the pain is often regional, compared to widespread pain characteristic of fibromyalgia.

MPS is prevalent in older adults with one study demonstrating a 95.5% prevalence in those older than 60 years with chronic low back pain. MPS may exist alone or in combination with other pain conditions, such as temporomandibular joint dysfunction, visceral pain syndromes, radiculopathy, and fibromyalgia.

PATHOPHYSIOLOGY

While substantial advances have been made, a full understanding of the etiology and pathophysiology of MPS and the role of MTrPs in this is still lacking. Several hypotheses have prevailed in providing an explanation for gaps in knowledge of MPS pathophysiology, two of which include the integrated hypothesis and neurogenic hypothesis. According to the integrated hypothesis, MPS arises from direct (eg, whiplash, muscle injury) or indirect (eg, through muscle overuse or misuse) muscle trauma. This leads to a release of proinflammatory substances that maintain the perception of pain, as well as a dysfunctional motor endplate that ultimately leads to a group of contraction knots in the muscle, forming an MTrP. A traumatic event itself can additionally open ion channels along the membranes of free nerve endings, resulting in cation influx and subsequent excessive, persistent nociceptor depolarization. The neurogenic hypothesis accounts for the occurrence of MPS and MTrPs in patients with no signs of muscle trauma but suffer from visceral or somatic diseases such as irritable bowel syndrome, chronic pelvic pain, and osteoarthritis, deemed as the **primary pathology**. The primary pathology leads to the constant activation of afferent nociceptors, which connect to the thinly myelinated (group III) and unmyelinated (group IV) nerve fibers that synapse onto dorsal horn neurons in the spinal cord, thereby initiating the process of persistent nociceptive bombardment, leading to central and peripheral sensitization. Central sensitization, a core concept of the neurogenic hypothesis, involves neuroplastic changes in the dorsal horn, resulting in sensitized dorsal horn neurons, apoptosis of inhibitory neurons, operation of previously ineffective synapses, and the expansion of receptive fields to nearby segments in the spinal cord. Several biochemicals such as calcitonin gene-related peptide and substance P are released antidromically by dorsal root ganglion via the activated nociceptors in the periphery, leading to neurogenically mediated inflammation. Surrounding alpha motor neurons in the spinal cord

Name: _____   Date: /   /

Directions: For questions 1 through 11, please circle the number that best describes how you did overall for the *past week*. If you don't normally do something that is asked, cross the question out.

Were you able to:	Always	Most	Occasionally	Never
Do shopping?	0	1	2	3
Do laundry with a washer and dryer?......	0	1	2	3
Prepare meals?	0	1	2	3
Wash dishes/cooking utensils by hand?....	0	1	2	3
Vacuum a rug?..	0	1	2	3
Make beds?	0	1	2	3
Walk several blocks?	0	1	2	3
Visit friends or relatives?	0	1	2	3
Do yard work?..	0	1	2	3
Drive a car?	0	1	2	3
Climb stairs?	0	1	2	3

12. *Of the 7 days in the past week, how many days did you feel good?*

0   1   2   3   4   5   6   7

13. *How many days last week did you miss work, including housework, because of fibromyalgia?*

0   1   2   3   4   5   6   7

Directions: For the remaining items, mark the point on the line that best indicates how you felt overall for the past week.

14. *When you worked, how much did pain or other symptoms of your fibromyalgia interfere with your ability to do your work, including housework?*

No problem with work   •___|___|___|___|___|___|___|___|___•   Great difficulty with work

15. *How bad has your pain been?*

No pain   •___|___|___|___|___|___|___|___|___•   Very severe pain

16. *How tired have you been?*

No tiredness   •___|___|___|___|___|___|___|___|___•   Very tired

17. *How have you felt when you get up in the morning?*

Awoke well rested   •___|___|___|___|___|___|___|___|___•   Awoke very tired

18. *How bad has your stiffness been?*

No stiffness   •___!___!___!___!___!___!___!___!___•   Very stiff

19. *How nervous or anxious have you felt?*

Not anxious   •___!___!___!___!___!___!___!___!___•   Very anxious

20. *How depressed or blue have you felt?*

Not depressed   •___!___!___!___!___!___!___!___!___•   Very depressed

FIGURE 103-3. Fibromyalgia Impact Questionnaire (FIQ).

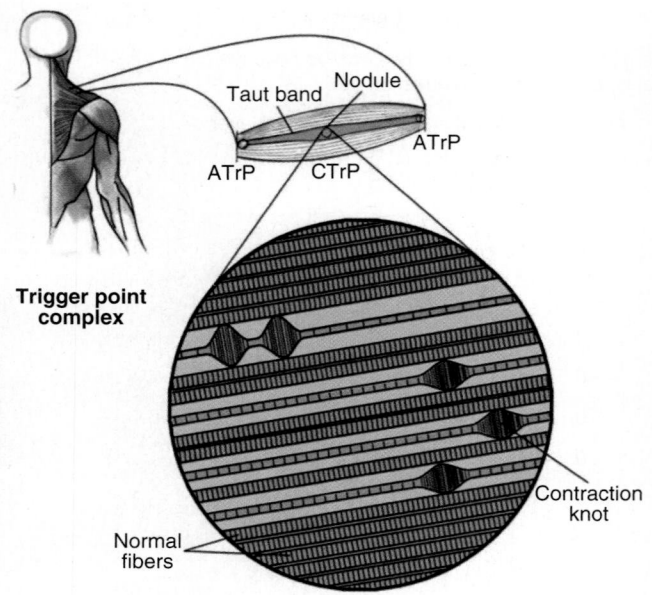

FIGURE 103-4. Schematic of a trigger point complex. CTrP identifies the central trigger point that is found in the endplate zone and contains numerous contraction knots and electrically active loci among normal fibers. A taut band of muscle fibers extends from the trigger point to the attachment (ATrP) at each end of the involved fiber. (Reproduced with permission from Simons DG, Travell JG, Simons LS. *Travell & Simons' Myofascial Pain and Dysfunction: The Trigger Point Manual.* 2nd ed. Baltimore, MD: Williams & Wilkins; 1998.)

are also excited, leading to the formation of an MTrP. Other hypotheses that emphasize dysfunctional recruitment of muscle fibers, such as prolonged contraction periods of small fibers due to submaximal loads (Cinderella hypothesis) or decreased relaxation times for postural muscles working in "shifts" (Shift hypothesis), have been proposed as well. **Table 103-8** expands on the underlying mechanisms elucidated by the prevailing hypotheses on MPS pathogenesis.

Despite being distinct conditions, both chronic MPS and fibromyalgia share the process of central sensitization as part of their underlying pathophysiology. Many researchers have proposed a role for MTrPs in initiating and maintaining the chronic, widespread pain found in patients with fibromyalgia. However, several studies have shown that not all patients with fibromyalgia present with MTrPs, casting doubt upon the need for active MTrPs to drive both syndromes. Further, most patients presenting with active MTrPs report regional pain that may or may not refer to other areas, but they do not report widespread pain characteristic of fibromyalgia. Nevertheless, deactivation of MTrPs should be incorporated as part of the treatment plan for the patients with fibromyalgia that also have MTrPs.

CLINICAL PRESENTATION AND EVALUATION

MPS may occur in virtually any body location, and the accompanying pain may be relatively discrete or cover a large area, spreading from the MTrP. MPS can present abruptly due to acute overload, exercise (overexercise, improper body mechanics that can cause muscle sprain and strain), direct trauma, and chilling (exposure to cold temperatures especially when the muscle is fatigued). MPS also can present gradually due to chronic overload from poor posture, stress, and overuse of muscles while performing work activities using improper body mechanics that can lead to muscle fatigue, sustained muscular contraction in a shortened position, and repetitive stress injuries. It can also manifest secondary to visceral, viral, metabolic, and endocrine diseases, arthritic joints, nutritional deficiencies, anxiety, and emotional distress. We commonly treat older adults with myofascial low back pain that is perpetuated by multiple coexisting factors such as anxiety, leg length inequality, axial spondylosis, and spinal malalignment.

Taking the History

Patients with MPS may use a variety of pain descriptors—dull, aching, sharp, stabbing, burning, etc. Factors that commonly exacerbate pain in these patients are: (1) excessive physical activity, (2) firm pressure over the painful muscle, (3) cold exposure, (4) psychological stress, and (5) acute illness (eg, viral infection). Those that tend to alleviate pain include: (1) mild activity, (2) gentle stretching, (3) gentle pressure (eg, massage), (4) moist heat, and (5) a brief rest period following activity. Common accompanying neurologic and motor signs and symptoms include weakness, paresthesias, changes in gait, limitations in range of motion, and autonomic phenomena, such as piloerection, sweating, and temperature changes. As with other chronic pain disorders, changes in appetite, mood, sleep, and cognitive function can occur.

Diagnosing Myofascial Pain: Performing the Physical Examination

Diagnosing MPS requires an accurate physical examination that relies on palpation and identification of (1) taut bands—groups of taut muscle fibers extending from MTrPs to the muscle attachments, (2) exquisitely tender, hyperirritable nodules (MTrP) in taut bands (note that taut bands may not always contain MTrPs), and (3) reproduction of the patient's spontaneous pain with sustained pressure that may radiate distal to the MTrP (**Figure 103-5**). MTrPs may be latent (ie, painful only upon compression) or active (ie, spontaneously painful). Latent MTrPs may occur in a muscle group contralateral to the site of pain because of a compensatory response. Active MTrPs are those that are responsible for clinical symptoms. In addition to pain with compression of MTrPs, a "jump sign" may be elicited—a pain behavior response that may include verbal as well as nonverbal expression (eg, crying out, grimacing, withdrawing). The examiner may also appreciate a *local twitch response* (LTR), which is an involuntary, transient contraction of a taut band that traverses a MTrP and occurs in response to stimulation of the MTrP (eg, with needling or snapping palpation).

TABLE 103-8 ■ THEORIES OF MTRP PATHOGENESIS

HYPOTHESIS	MECHANISM	SUPPORTING STUDIES
Integrated	Energy crisis – muscle injury → aberrant ACh release in neuromuscular junction → excessive Ca^{2+} released from sarcoplasmic reticulum and ATP depletion → sustained fiber contracture and capillary compression → tissue distress, development of MTrP, production of inflammatory substances	EMG—spontaneous electrical activity (SEA) in MTrP vs silence in healthy muscle; SEA is linked to dysfunctional motor endplates (uncoordinated, excessive, prolonged release of ACh); SEA is correlated highly with decreased pain threshold and increased pain intensity Biochemical milieu—inflammatory substances found in the area of MTrP such as SP, CGRP, BK, 5-HT, TNF-α, IL-1b, IL-6, IL-8, H^+. These are by-products of tissue distress following the cascade of events in energy crisis
Cinderella	Small fiber recruitment in recurring low- to mid-level exertion and small fibers are last to be deactivated after the movement has occurred. Large fibers in the same region will rarely be activated. Disequilibrium with muscle fiber recruitment leads to tissue damage and pain	Office workers engaged in 30 min of typing developed MTrPs in upper trapezius muscles, exemplifying relation between low-level, continuous muscle contractions and MTrP formation. Poor posture also can facilitate MTrP formation
Neurogenic	Selective fiber overuse, decreased muscle perfusion, and inflammatory biochemical milieu set stage for **peripheral sensitization** of nociceptive terminals (decrease in threshold for nociceptive activation). **Central sensitization** also occurs with persistent nociceptive bombardment to dorsal horn neurons and increased activity in specific brain regions associated with hyperalgesia, maintaining the MTrPs	MPS/MTrPs described in patients with no signs of muscle trauma but those who suffered from visceral or somatic diseases (IBS, chronic pelvic pain, osteoarthritis), deemed as primary pathology. Primary pathology leads to persistent nociceptive bombardment fMRI studies—MTrP stimulation demonstrates increased activity of brain regions associated with hyperalgesia, such as primary and secondary somatosensory cortices, mid and anterior insula, and inferior parietal cortex. Decreased activity of right dorsal hippocampus, involved in descending pain modulation, also has been observed
Shift	Challenges Cinderella hypothesis by delineating differences in recruitment patterns between postural (tonic) and phasic muscles. While phasic muscles follow the Cinderella pattern (small fibers first, large fibers last), postural muscles recruit by **rotation** instead of size, allowing fibers to contract in sequential "shift-like" patterns of relaxation and contraction. MPS onset is predicted by a reduced relaxation time for fibers → less time for blood flow and oxygen replenishment. The weaker the muscle, the more fibers recruited and the lesser the time for relaxation	Phasic muscle studies—Phasic muscles predominantly contain fast-twitch fibers and are more adapted to short contractions under higher loads. Here, motor units are recruited in a hierarchal pattern. Postural (antigravity) muscles involved with keeping individuals upright (lesser loads, prolonged periods of work) work in shifts. In pathological conditions, the relaxation/contraction ratio is below a threshold value

Ach, acetylcholine; ATP, adenosine triphosphate; BK, bradykinin; Ca²⁺, calcium ions; CGRP, calcitonin gene-related peptide; EMG, electromyography; fMRI, functional magnetic resonance imaging; H⁺, protons; IBS, irritable bowel syndrome; IL, interleukin; MPS, myofascial pain syndrome; MTrP, myofascial trigger point; SP, substance P; 5-HT, serotonin; TNF-α, tumor necrosis factor alpha.

Accurate diagnosis of MPS requires the use of precise physical examination technique, summarized in **Table 103-9**. Before examining the painful muscles, a general physical examination including comprehensive musculoskeletal, neurologic, and mobility examinations must be performed. These examinations must be carried out with an eye toward identifying abnormalities that create muscular dysfunction. Examples in the musculoskeletal examination include decreased motor strength, abnormal muscle tone, decreased range of motion of the hips, knees, cervical spine, and shoulders; congenital or acquired deformities such as scoliosis; kyphosis; and functional or actual leg length discrepancy. Inspection of the patient's gait allows for an integrated assessment of body mechanics.

Prior to palpating the musculature, the examiner should assess the movement of the skin over the subcutaneous tissues using very light palpation and simply gliding the skin in a direction that is perpendicular to the orientation of the involved muscle fibers. Patients with chronic MPS commonly have reduced skin movement over the involved region. After palpating the skin, the muscles should be examined. MTrPs are associated with the finding of a "nodule." The MTrP may be large and easily palpable or small and difficult to identify; regardless, the muscle should be palpated thoroughly to search for the area of greatest tenderness. Sweeping hand motion is needed to appreciate taut bands and better elicits the radiating pain that is a pathognomonic feature of MTrPs.

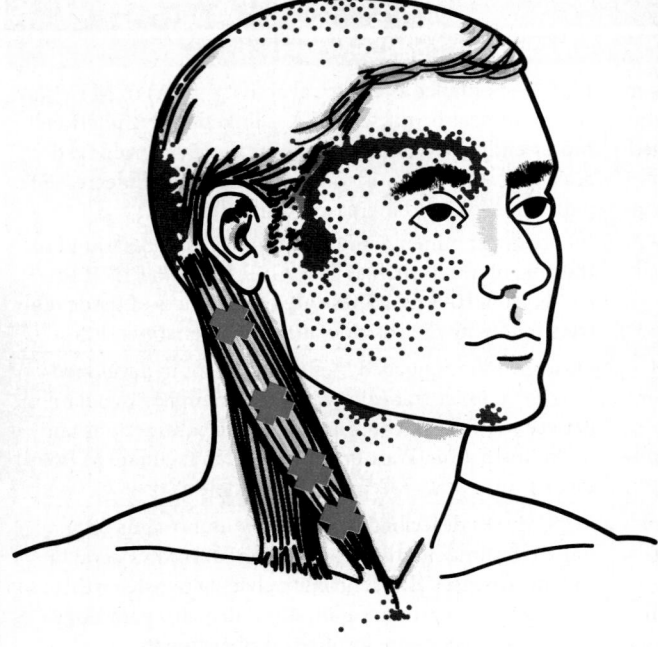

FIGURE 103-5. Schematic of referred pain patterns. Stimulation of MTrPs (X's) in the right sternocleidomastoid muscle produces major pain referral patterns as indicated by the shaded areas, as well as minor patterns as indicated by the dotted areas. (Reproduced with permission from Simons DG, *Travell JG, Simons LS. Travell & Simons' Myofascial Pain and Dysfunction: The Trigger Point Manual.* 2nd ed. Baltimore, MD: Williams & Wilkins; 1998.)

While physical examination remains the procedure of choice for diagnosing MPS, it is difficult to standardize, and a number of other techniques have been evaluated. Intramuscular needling, surface electromyography-guided assessment, infrared thermography, ultrasound imaging, elastography, color Doppler, and laser Doppler flowmetry have been examined but all have drawbacks, and none is routinely used in clinical practice for the diagnosis of MPS.

COMMON MYOFASCIAL PAIN SYNDROMES IN ADULTS

Common presentations of MPS include cervicogenic headaches, piriformis MPS, trapezius MPS (sometimes associated with "tension neckache"), pseudotrochanteric bursitis, upper and lower back pain, and postherpetic pain. These syndromes are discussed below.

Cervicogenic Headache

Cervicogenic headaches are characterized by neck and pericranial pain and are often associated with structural abnormalities of the cervical spine, including osteoarthritis and facet arthrosis. Typically, cervicogenic headaches are unilateral in location and range from moderate to severe in intensity. While cervicogenic headaches lack the pulsating quality of migraine headaches, they may have migraine-associated features such as photophobia, phonophobia,

---

TABLE 103-9 ■ PHYSICAL EXAMINATION TECHNIQUE FOR EXAMINING THE PATIENT WITH MYOFASCIAL PAIN

1. Perform a general musculoskeletal examination looking for contributors to myofascial pain (eg, spinal malalignment, leg length discrepancy, arthritis).
2. Place the patient in a comfortable and relaxed position.
   a. When examining the upper body, the patient should be sitting with forearms resting in lap.
   b. When examining the lower back, the patient may be standing, sitting, or lying prone. If none of these positions are comfortable, examine side-lying.
   c. When examining the lower extremities, the patient should be lying supine or prone.
3. Place yourself in a comfortable and relaxed position.
   a. When examining the upper body, the examiner should be standing squarely in front of the patient.
   b. When examining the lower back, the examiner should be standing to the side of the patient, allowing for the use of one arm to brace the patient from the front and the other hand to palpate. If the patient is lying, stand beside the patient. If the patient is sitting, stand to the side of the exam table and behind the patient.
   c. When examining the lower extremities, the examiner should be standing at the bedside.
4. When there is unilateral pain, always palpate the nonpainful side first.
5. Assess the movement of the skin over the subcutaneous tissue before palpating the muscles.
6. When palpating taut bands, sweep the examining hand firmly across the involved muscle, in a direction that is perpendicular to the orientation of the muscle fibers and in the same plane as the fibers.
7. When palpating trigger points, palpate firmly over the muscle in a direction that is perpendicular to the orientation of the muscle fibers and in a plane that is perpendicular to the fibers.
8. Physical examination targeting potential visceral pathology of the abdomen and/or pelvis should be performed if myofascial pain of these regions is diagnosed.

---

nausea, vomiting, and dizziness. Triggers include specific neck postures and movements especially in extension, extension with rotation toward the side of pain, on applying digital pressure to the involved facet regions, over the ipsilateral greater occipital nerve, or pressure applied to the cervical spine. Palpation of these neck muscles including paraspinal muscles, suboccipital muscles, and trapezius also may produce pain, which usually radiates through the head and may extend to the ipsilateral shoulder. MTrPs are usually found in the suboccipital, cervical, and shoulder musculature, and can also refer pain to the head when manually or physically stimulated. There are no neurologic findings of cervical radiculopathy, though the patient might report scalp paresthesia or dysesthesia.

Making the diagnosis for cervicogenic headaches may be difficult especially if structural lesions of the cervical spine are not present. A careful history and examination that clearly implicate the cervical spine and its musculature as the sources of the pain are essential for diagnosis. Diagnostic imaging such as radiography, MRI, and computed tomography (CT) myelography can be used as supportive diagnostic tools. Zygapophyseal joint, cervical nerve, or medial branch blockades are used to confirm the diagnosis of cervicogenic headache and may predict effective treatment modalities.

Deep Gluteal Pain Syndrome

When MPS occurs in the pelvic and buttock regions, the resulting pain and associated limitations in muscle function may mimic that of sciatica. The piriformis muscle originates from the pelvic surface of the sacrum, passes through the greater sciatic foramen, and inserts into the medial side of the upper end of the greater trochanter. The fibers of the sciatic nerve course through the piriformis. Piriformis syndrome describes the occurrence of sciatica in association with piriformis MPS that results from nerve entrapment by the myofascial taut bands in the piriformis. Patients with piriformis MPS describe intense gluteal discomfort. Because the piriformis acts to externally rotate the thigh at the hip joint, patients with piriformis MPS sometimes demonstrate external rotation of the leg when standing or laying supine. Palpation of the piriformis can be performed with the patient standing or laying supine. The technique recommended for examining the patient in the supine position is described in **Table 103-10**. Piriformis MPS may involve the lower back, buttock, and posterior thigh. Typically, this form of MPS is increased by sitting, standing, and walking.

The gluteus minimus is another muscle in which MPS symptoms may mimic sciatica, and, therefore, this muscle should be carefully examined. The fibers of this fan-shaped muscle extend from the outer surface of the pelvis and converge onto a tendon, which is attached to the anterior surface of the greater trochanter. The gluteus minimus fibers work with the gluteus medius to abduct the thigh during extension and stabilize the pelvis during ambulation. Patients with MPS arising from the gluteus minimus typically complain of hip pain during ambulation, often present with a limp, and may also have trouble rising from a sitting position. Because the gluteus minimus is the deepest of the gluteal muscles, it may be difficult for the examiner to palpate taut bands. However, if the patient lays in the supine position or on their side and relaxes the gluteal muscles, MTrPs may be located by identifying the areas of greatest localized tenderness. Palpation of MTrPs in the gluteus minimus may also induce a thigh jerk.

Trapezius MPS

The trapezius is a large muscle; as a result, associated MPS can have a number of presentations. The fibers originate from the occiput, the ligamentum nuchae, and the vertebral spinous processes of the seventh cervical vertebra and all of the 12 thoracic vertebrae. They insert onto the distal third of the clavicle, the acromion, and the length of the spine of the scapula. The upper fibers elevate the scapula, the middle fibers pull the scapula medially, and the lower fibers pull the medial border of the scapula downward. The upper and lower fibers also assist the serratus anterior muscle in rotating the scapula when the arm is raised above the head.

Patients with trapezius MPS typically do not complain of limitations in movement, but full rotation of the head and neck to the opposite side is often painful, and lateral bending contralaterally may be restricted. Radiating pain patterns vary according to the trapezius fibers that contain MTrPs (ie, upper, middle, or lower). MTrPs that occur in the upper trapezius may cause pain that radiates up the posterolateral part of the neck to the mastoid process, causing so-called "tension neckache." Sometimes this pain may radiate to the angle of the jaw and/or the temple and back of the orbit. Dizziness also may occur. MTrPs of the middle fibers of the trapezius may be associated with a superficial burning pain very close to the spinous processes of the seventh cervical and the third thoracic vertebrae or with aching on the top of the shoulder or acromion process. MTrPs of the lower fibers of the trapezius, typically located along the lower border of the muscle, may refer pain to the high paracervical spinal musculature, the mastoid and the acromion, as well as aching and tenderness of the suprascapular region. Perpetuating factors include anything that causes abnormal biomechanics of the upper body such as a whiplash injury or prolonged computer work in an ergonomically unfriendly workspace.

Levator Scapulae MPS

The levator scapulae muscle extends from the upper medial border of the scapula to the transverse processes of the first four cervical vertebrae. The levator scapulae muscle, in conjunction with the other shoulder muscles, has an important action in stabilizing and moving the scapula and is associated with movement of the shoulder. Levator scapulae pain could be at the angle of the neck, the medial border of the scapula, or out to the posterior aspect of the shoulder joint. It causes restriction of neck movements and pain on stretching the levator scapulae muscle, such as with contralateral bending and rotation of neck. Tenderness is maximal over the angle of the neck along the line of the muscle and most prominent close to attachment at medial border of scapula. It is often precipitated by a prolonged abnormal position and with neck rotation.

Upper and Lower Back Pain

These syndromes may be caused by MPS in the thoracolumbar paraspinal musculature. Numerous muscles constitute the paraspinal group, including superficial and deep muscles. The superficial group is collectively referred to as the erector spinae and is the largest muscular mass of the back. It originates from the sacrum, the iliac crest, and the spinous processes of most of the lumbar and the last two thoracic vertebrae, and inserts into the ribs, the transverse

TABLE 103-10 ■ PHYSICAL EXAMINATION IN OLDER ADULTS WITH LOW BACK AND LEG PAIN: DETECTION OF MTrPS, BIOMECHANICAL PERPETUATING FACTORS, AND OTHER PAIN GENERATORS

FINDING	OPERATIONAL DEFINITION	EXAMINATION TECHNIQUE
Functional leg length discrepancy	Pelvic asymmetry	Have patient stand with both feet on floor, shoes removed. Ask him to stand with feet together, and as erect as possible. Kneel behind patient. With palms parallel to floor, and fingers extended, place lateral surface of index finger of both hands atop pelvic brim bilaterally. Level of eyes doing the examination should be level with hands. Determine if right and left hands are at different heights.
Scoliosis (lateral/rotational)	Lateral/rotational curvature of thoracolumbar spine	Have patient stand on floor with shoes removed. Stand behind patient. Run index finger along spinous processes (do not lift hand between vertebrae) a series of 3 times. If you do not detect scoliosis, then: Ask patient to bend forward. Determine if there is asymmetry in height of paraspinal musculature.
Sacroiliac joint pain	Pain with direct palpation of sacroiliac joint or with Patrick test	*Direct palpation:* Have patient stand on floor with shoes removed. Stand behind patient. Exert firm pressure over sacroiliac joint, first on one side, then the other. Palpate right joint with right thumb, standing to left side of patient; palpate left joint with left thumb, standing to right of patient. *Patrick (FABER) test*—Have the patient lie supine on the examining table and place the foot of involved side on opposite knee. Then slowly lower the test leg in abduction toward the examining table. If patient reports pain in back (*not* groin, buttocks, or leg), then test is positive. Other commonly performed SI provocation tests include supine distraction and compression; compression in side-lying; Gaenslen maneuver; thigh thrust
Myofascial pain, piriformis	Presence of pain on deep palpation of piriformis	Have patient lay supine on examination table. Have patient flex right hip and knee, keeping sole of foot on table. Cross bent leg over opposite leg; again place sole on table and exert mild medially directed pressure on lateral aspect of knee to put piriformis in stretch. Exert firm pressure (4 kg) over middle extent of piriformis. Repeat examination on opposite side.
Myofascial pain, TFL ± iliotibial (IT) band pain	Presence of pain on deep palpation of tensor fascia lata and/or IT band	Have patient lying supine on examination table. Using thumbs of both hands, exert firm pressure (4 kg) over full extent of TFL and IT band. Repeat examination on opposite side.
Kyphosis	Deformity of thoracic spine creating forward flexed posture	Have patient stand on floor with shoes removed. Ask him to stand fully erect. Inspect posture from the side.
Myofascial pain of paralumbar musculature	Presence of pain on deep palpation of paralumbar musculature	Have patient stand on floor with shoes removed. Stand behind and to left of patient and brace him in front with left arm and palpate full extent of right paravertebral musculature with right thumb. Exert approximately 4 kg of force. Repeat, palpating the left paravertebral musculature.
Myofascial pain of gluteus medius	Presence of pain on deep palpation of gluteus medius	Have the patient either prone or side-lying. Palpate just distal to the iliac crest, following its course on either side of the hip joint.
Vertebral body pain	Presence of pain on firm palpation of lumbar spinous processes	Position yourself behind patient, as for examination of paravertebral musculature above. Using dominant thumb, firmly palpate spinous processes
Hip disease	Pain and restricted motion of hip	*Hip internal rotation*—measure with patient sitting and leg dangling, OR have patient lie supine on examining table with hip and knee bent to 90 degrees. Put the hip into maximum internal rotation and ask patient if he experiences pain. *Hip flexion*—have patient lie supine and pull knee to chest; then have patient let go and examiner should hold leg in maximum flexion, ensuring that pelvis is flush with exam table. American College of Rheumatology clinical criteria for hip OA, ie, self-reported pain in hip + exam consistent with hip OA • Internal hip rotation < 15° + hip flexion < 115° OR • Internal hip rotation > 15° and painful + hip AM stiffness < 60 min *Patrick test*—as above.

Adapted with permission from Weiner DK, Sakamoto S, Perera S, et al. Chronic low back pain in older adults: prevalence, reliability, and validity of physical examination findings. J Am Geriatr Soc. 2006;54(1):11–20.

processes of the cervical vertebrae, thoracic vertebrae, and mastoid process. The deep group comprises the semispinalis, multifidus, and rotatores. The primary function of the paraspinal musculature is spinal extension. Patients with parathoracic MPS may experience pain that radiates to the region of the scapula or more medially, and sometimes to the anterior lower chest; patients with paralumbar MPS may experience pain that radiates to the buttocks or lower abdomen. Precipitation of MPS may be caused by sudden muscular overload (eg, when lifting objects using poor body mechanics) or associated with a vertebral compression fracture. Multiple vertebral compression fractures may also accumulate to cause hyperkyphosis and associated muscular strain. Physical examination typically reveals diminished spinal range of motion.

Upper and lower back pain in older adults often relates to the presence of axial spondylosis. This spondylosis causes aberrant neuronal input by injuring spinal nerves, disrupting generation of neurotrophic factors, and resulting in muscle shortening and pain. This condition, formally described by Chan Gunn et al., is referred to as neuropathic MPS. Axial spondylosis is ubiquitous in older adults; thus, it is not surprising that MPS commonly occurs in older adults with axial arthritis, even in the absence of frank radiculopathy (eg, MPS of the sternocleidomastoid and trapezius in patients with cervical spondylosis).

Techniques used to examine the lower back to identify MTrPs and associated perpetuating factors are described in **Table 103-10**. Treatment of postural abnormalities is an important component of treating paraspinal MP. Physical therapy geared toward strengthening of core muscles is a key component of treatment, not only for the pain itself, but also for reducing the risk of future vertebral compression fractures.

Pseudotrochanteric bursitis

This syndrome is caused by MPS that involves the tensor fasciae latae (TFL) muscle. The TFL originates from the outer edge of the iliac crest between the anterior superior iliac spine and iliac tubercle and inserts into the iliotibial tract. It assists the gluteus maximus in maintaining the knee in extension when a person stands and also flexes the hip. Patients with TFL MPS experience pain in the region of the hip and lateral thigh, sometimes extending to the knee along the iliotibial band. The pattern of pain radiation is sometimes confused with trochanteric bursitis and is referred to as pseudotrochanteric bursitis. Patients may also complain of poor sitting tolerance, difficulty walking rapidly, and laying on the involved side. They may also have difficulty laying on the opposite side unless a pillow is placed between the knees because of the tight iliotibial band. Physical examination may reveal restricted hip extension and adduction and TFL MTrPs. When standing, patients with TFL MPS tend to maintain the hip in slight flexion. Other disorders that should be considered in the differential diagnosis include L4 radiculopathy and meralgia paresthetica.

Postherpetic MPS

This is likely caused by a combination of axial spondylosis and the varicella-zoster virus (VZV) mainly in older adults. Both VZV and spondylosis-related MPS sensitize dorsal horn neurons and contribute to postherpetic neuralgia. We hypothesize that a spinal nerve already vulnerable from spondylosis that has caused muscle shortening may be particularly prone to the generation of MPS following an acute insult such as VZV. The myofascial pathology may then further exacerbate neuropathic pain by entrapping the spinal nerves as they course through the taut bands of the muscles. This results in a feedback loop.

MPS pathology may also develop in the setting of postherpetic neuralgia as a result of guarding behavior. The pain associated with reactivation of VZV can cause patients to move their body in ways to protect the painful area. When this type of behavior occurs over a prolonged period of time, muscles may develop contraction knots that are characteristic of MPS. The mechanism by which postherpetic neuralgia occurs may be complicated by the development of MPS pathology. Treatment of both the MPS pathology and the neuropathy may be needed to afford optimal pain relief.

Other Myofascial Pain and Dysfunction Syndromes

Since muscles cover virtually the entire body, any region may be affected by MPS. Thus, MPS should always be included in the practitioner's list of differential diagnoses for regional pain syndromes. Furthermore, the practitioner must be aware that MPS may occur in response to visceral disease; when myofascial dysfunction is identified in the abdomen and pelvis, the possibility of underlying visceral pathology must be kept in mind. Sometimes, even after the visceral pathology has been eradicated, MPS may persist, which further complicates evaluation and treatment.

Some less common causes of MPS include pelvic floor myofascial dysfunction causing chronic pelvic pain in both men and women, pelvic myofascial dysfunction causing urologic pain (eg, interstitial cystitis and the urgency-frequency syndrome), masticatory myofascial dysfunction causing toothache, abdominal wall myofascial dysfunction causing chronic abdominal pain (eg, following abdominal surgery or a gastrointestinal illness), intercostal myofascial dysfunction causing postthoracotomy pain, and TMJ dislocation/arthritis causing jaw locking and severe pain.

As noted earlier in this chapter, myofascial dysfunction is not always associated with complaints of pain (ie, in the case of latent MTrPs). For example, masticatory myofascial dysfunction has been associated with tinnitus and myofascial dysfunction of the trapezius with dizziness. Cervical myofascial dysfunction may also be associated with dizziness, a sense of imbalance and tinnitus, and treatment (as outlined below) may alleviate these symptoms. For a more extensive discussion of these and other MPS and dysfunction syndromes, as well as diagrams of common MTrPs and their radiating pain patterns, the reader is referred to

Travell and Simons' *Myofascial Pain and Dysfunction: The Trigger Point Manual.* Another less detailed but very useful introductory text that practitioners may want to consider is *Trigger Point Therapy for Myofascial Pain: The Practice of Informed Touch,* 2005, edited by Finando and Finando; www.InnerTraditions.com.

TREATMENT

An overview of MPS treatment is provided in **Table 103-11** and **Figure 103-6.** Effective treatment of MPS involves a three-pronged approach. First, it is important to identify and address perpetuating factors that maintain the pain/muscle dysfunction, and precipitating factors that initiate the syndrome. In the older adult, these may lie along a continuum. Second, the MTrPs should be treated. Third, muscle resilience should be addressed through a home exercise program. Treatments should focus not only on resolving the MTrP but also on the health of the surrounding environment (eg, fascia, connective tissue) that may contribute to MPS. In addition, the presence of biochemical markers of pain are very important. This thinking has led clinicians to try to reduce the size of the MTrP, correct underlying contributors to the pain, and restore the normal working relationship between the muscles and surrounding connective tissues of the affected functional units. There are two phases for effective treatment: a pain-control phase and a deep conditioning phase. During the pain-control phase, MTrPs are deactivated, improving blood circulation, decreasing pathological nociceptive activity, and eliminating the abnormal biomechanical force patterns. During the deep conditioning phase, the intra- and inter-tissue mobility of the functional unit is improved, which may include specific muscle stretches, neurodynamic mobilizations, joint mobilizations, orthotics, and strengthening muscle.

Addressing Precipitating and Perpetuating Factors

The factors that *perpetuate* MPS are typically multiple and develop over a long period of time, and each should be addressed to afford an optimal treatment. Lower back pain, for example, could be perpetuated by lumbar spondylosis, degenerative scoliosis, and hip arthritis. The physical factors that *precipitate* MPS may be overt such as a fall with direct trauma to the piriformis that causes piriformis syndrome or may be more subtle, such as a flare of knee osteoarthritis that alters gait and initiates TFL pain. Psychological stressors may also precipitate flares of MPS or act as perpetuating factors.

The correction of perpetuating factors is arguably one of the most important aspects of MPS treatment. Even if precipitating factors are addressed, the presence of perpetuating factors may reactivate the patient's original MPS complaint, preventing resolution of pain and dysfunction. Perpetuating factors typically persist over time, and often require behavioral and lifestyle adjustments. As part of the search for perpetuating factors, the practitioner should identify any contributing vitamin deficiencies (eg, B_1, B_6, B_{12}, C, D, folic acid) or hormonal imbalances. Repetitive movements that contribute to muscular dysfunction, such as those in wheelchair users and computer operators, also should be identified. Proper body mechanics during sitting, standing, walking, and sleeping should be taught by an occupational or physical therapist and efforts to modify repetitive movements and/or other mechanical stressors should be instituted.

Patients who spend prolonged periods resting in static positions (eg, sitting, reclining) may perpetuate their MPS through inactivity. Efforts should be made to incorporate

---

TABLE 103-11 ■ APPROACH TO TREATING MPS

1. Identify and treat perpetuating factors (eg, correct leg length discrepancy, optimize treatment of underlying pathology such as rotator cuff tendinitis, osteoarthritis, prescribe assistive devices and adaptive equipment if needed, correct vitamin and electrolyte deficiencies).

2. Refer to a physical therapist or other manual therapist (eg, chiropractic, massage) who is experienced in treating patients with MPS with gentle stretching, strengthening, and education regarding postural correction, activity pacing, flare self-management techniques, and home exercise programs.

3. Treat MTrPs:
   ○ Noninvasive techniques: Manual therapies including myofascial release and myofascial manipulation. Other nonpharmacological interventions include manual therapies, which continue to include postisometric relaxation, counterstrain method MTrP compression, muscle energy techniques, and myotherapy
   ○ Invasive techniques:
     ▪ Dry needling with the insertion of a small-caliber needle (eg, acupuncture needle or small-caliber hypodermic needle) directly into the MTrP, to either a superficial or deep level. The goal of deep dry needling is to induce an LTR.
     ▪ MTrP injections with a local anesthetic (wet needling): no added benefit to dry needling
     ▪ Steroid injections into MTrPs: controversial, not enough evidence, higher risk for systemic and local side effects
     ▪ Botulinum toxin A (BTA) for deactivating MTrPs: is not superior to dry needling, causes muscle weakness, and is very expensive

4. If psychological stressors are identified as a perpetuating factor, refer for CBT and treat underlying mood and sleep disorders.

5. Prescribe aerobic exercise for cardiovascular fitness and prevention of pain flares.

6. Prescribe oral medications only as adjunctive therapy, not as the primary mode of treatment.

7. Refer patients who do not respond to these treatments to interdisciplinary management in a pain clinic for trial of alternative modalities including acupuncture, massage, electrotherapy, laser, ultrasonography, and more invasive treatments such as nerve blocks and dorsal rhizotomy.

CBT, cognitive behavioral therapy; LTR, local twitch response; MPS, myofascial pain syndrome; MTrP, myofascial trigger point.

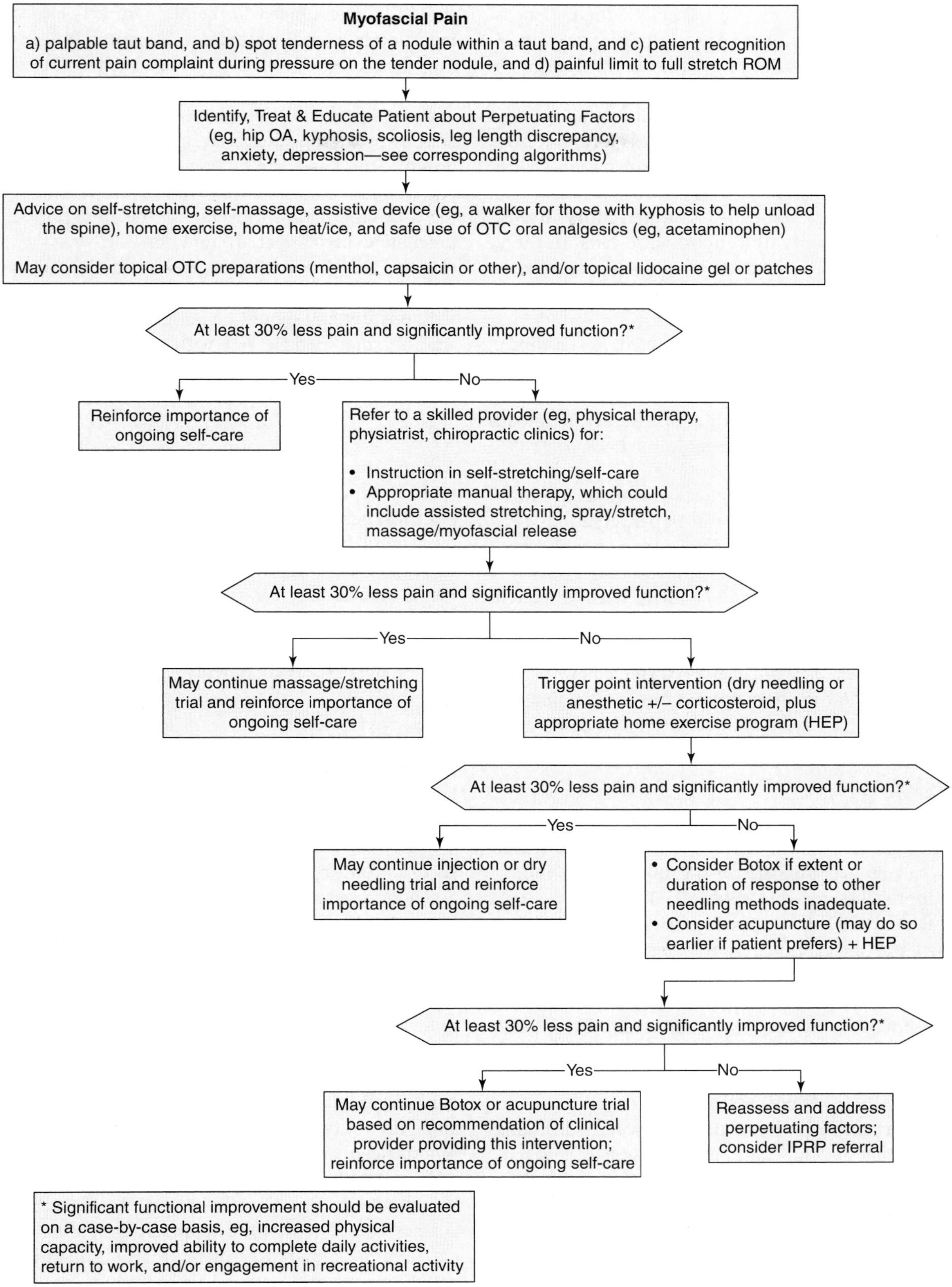

Myofascial Pain

a) palpable taut band, and b) spot tenderness of a nodule within a taut band, and c) patient recognition of current pain complaint during pressure on the tender nodule, and d) painful limit to full stretch ROM

Identify, Treat & Educate Patient about Perpetuating Factors (eg, hip OA, kyphosis, scoliosis, leg length discrepancy, anxiety, depression—see corresponding algorithms)

Advice on self-stretching, self-massage, assistive device (eg, a walker for those with kyphosis to help unload the spine), home exercise, home heat/ice, and safe use of OTC oral analgesics (eg, acetaminophen)

May consider topical OTC preparations (menthol, capsaicin or other), and/or topical lidocaine gel or patches

At least 30% less pain and significantly improved function?*

Yes → Reinforce importance of ongoing self-care

No → Refer to a skilled provider (eg, physical therapy, physiatrist, chiropractic clinics) for:
- Instruction in self-stretching/self-care
- Appropriate manual therapy, which could include assisted stretching, spray/stretch, massage/myofascial release

At least 30% less pain and significantly improved function?*

Yes → May continue massage/stretching trial and reinforce importance of ongoing self-care

No → Trigger point intervention (dry needling or anesthetic +/– corticosteroid, plus appropriate home exercise program (HEP)

At least 30% less pain and significantly improved function?*

Yes → May continue injection or dry needling trial and reinforce importance of ongoing self-care

No →
- Consider Botox if extent or duration of response to other needling methods inadequate.
- Consider acupuncture (may do so earlier if patient prefers) + HEP

At least 30% less pain and significantly improved function?*

Yes → May continue Botox or acupuncture trial based on recommendation of clinical provider providing this intervention; reinforce importance of ongoing self-care

No → Reassess and address perpetuating factors; consider IPRP referral

* Significant functional improvement should be evaluated on a case-by-case basis, eg, increased physical capacity, improved ability to complete daily activities, return to work, and/or engagement in recreational activity

FIGURE 103-6. Algorithm for the management of myofascial pain in the older adult. IPRP, interdisciplinary pain rehabilitation program; OA, osteoarthritis; OTC, over the counter; ROM, range of motion. (Reproduced with permission from Lisi AJ, Breuer P, Gallagher RM, et al. Deconstructing chronic low back pain in the older adult-step by step evidence and expert-based recommendations for evaluation and treatment: Part II: Myofascial pain. *Pain Med.* 2015;16[7]:1282–1289.)

intervals of light movement or stretching if the patient is able to tolerate such activities in order to minimize overuse of small muscle fibers (ie, the Cinderella hypothesis).

Direct or indirect acute trauma should also be identified. For example, if a patient has a sudden leg length discrepancy following total hip replacement, prescription of a shoe lift may be helpful. For patients with long-standing leg length discrepancy, a shoe lift may disrupt the patient's established compensatory strategies and lead to mobility dysfunction and falls. In these patients, the muscle dysfunction of the pelvis and lower extremities should be first addressed before considering an orthotic device.

Abnormal posture should be corrected. For instance, in older adults with severe kyphosis related to multiple vertebral compression fractures, restoration of normal posture may not be possible and prescription of a walker to unload the spine (ie, alleviate strain on the lower back musculature) should be considered.

To the extent that psychological stressors such as anxiety and depression are playing a role in perpetuating MPS, cognitive behavioral therapy and/or other nonpharmacological and pharmacological treatments may be useful. Vitamin D deficiency also should be identified and treated given its association with musculoskeletal pain, although randomized controlled clinical trials evaluating its efficacy in patients with MPS have not been performed. For patients who do not respond to these approaches in combination with MTrP treatment, referral to an interdisciplinary pain clinic can be considered.

Treating MTrPs

The second prong of MPS treatment is to directly treat MTrPs. The goal of treating MTrPs is to *deactivate* them, and this can be accomplished using noninvasive and/or invasive approaches, listed in **Table 103-11.**

Oral medications are often considered as potential supplements to the aforementioned treatments for MPS, such as nonsteroidal anti-inflammatory drugs (NSAIDs), benzodiazepines, TCAs, and thiocolchicoside, but these generally should be avoided in older adults because of their risk profile. We have had some success with low-dose gabapentin (eg, 300 mg twice a day) for the treatment of neuropathic MPS in patients with cervical spondylosis and MPS in the paracervical musculature. Topical medications such as diclofenac and lidocaine patches as well as capsaicin and EMLA cream also may have limited efficacy. Medications that target perpetuating factors such as anxiety and insomnia should be considered routinely.

Home Exercise Program

The third prong of MPS treatment is maintaining muscular health through a home exercise program. Many factors that contribute to MPS in older adults cannot be eliminated (eg, axial spondylosis, scoliosis); therefore, active pain self-management is key to sustaining improvement. Patients should be encouraged to maintain an active lifestyle and incorporate a cardiovascular and aerobic fitness program into their routine. Aerobic exercise such as water aerobics may reduce generalized pain and the number of MTrPs, whereas isometric strengthening can increase pain tolerance by providing additional sustenance to affected muscle groups. Pain flares can be prevented by educating patients regarding exercise that includes targeted muscular stretching and eliminating movements that may perpetuate or precipitate myofascial dysfunction. Self-massage also is effective for MPS self-management that involves applying pressure in a rolling motion through the MTrPs. These methods initially should be performed under the supervision of a qualified (ie, one with specific expertise in MPS management) physical therapist, chiropractor, or massage therapist before transitioning into a home exercise program.

Other Treatments

A number of other treatments have been tried for MPS such as repetitive magnetic stimulation, transcutaneous electrical nerve stimulation (TENS), biofeedback, massage, ultrasound, hydrocortisone/diclofenac phonophoresis, laser therapy, traditional Chinese and Japanese acupuncture, nerve blocks, and cervical spine dorsal root rhizotomy for the treatment of cervicogenic headaches. The quality of evidence at the present time cannot recommend for or against any of these treatments.

CONCLUSION

Fibromyalgia and MPS are common causes of chronic pain in older adults. Fibromyalgia is a central sensitivity syndrome with patients demonstrating increased sensitivity to a variety of stimuli, especially pain. While the pathogenesis of fibromyalgia needs further study, there seems to be a genetic predisposition and a clear familial aggregation. Lower levels of central neurotransmitters and nociceptive chemicals are believed to be involved with fibromyalgia pathogenesis. Data on the pathophysiology of MPS support both central and peripheral sensitization. The biochemical milieu of muscles affected by MPS is distinct from that of normal musculature.

For both fibromyalgia and MPS, individualized approaches to treatment are recommended. Medications alone do not typically improve function, but may improve mood, sleep, and pain. Stretching and local modalities as well as identification and treatment of perpetuating factors should be considered first line for MPS and aerobic exercise is a key component of the approach to treating fibromyalgia. Interdisciplinary treatment programs that include education, cognitive behavioral therapy, and exercise may be effective for both fibromyalgia and MPS. Further studies are needed to advance treatment for older adult patients with these disorders, reduce the associated risk of functional compromise and unnecessary health care expenditure, and improve overall quality of life.

FURTHER READING

Bell T, Trost Z, Buelow MT, et al. Meta-analysis of cognitive performance in fibromyalgia. *J Clin Exp Neuropsychol.* 2018;40(7):698–714.

Borg-Stein J, Iaccarion MA. Myofascial pain syndrome treatments. *Phys Med Rehabil Clin N Am.* 2014;25:357–374.

Clauw, DJ. Fibromyalgia: a clinical review. *JAMA.* 2014; 311(15):1547–1555.

Dommerholt J, Bron C, Franssen J. Myofascial trigger points: an evidence-informed review. *J Man Manip Ther.* 2006;14(4):203–221.

Fernández-de-las-Peñas C, Dommerholt J. International consensus on diagnostic criteria and clinical considerations of myofascial trigger points: a Delphi study. *Pain Medicine.* 2018;19:142–150.

Gerwin RD. Classification, epidemiology, and natural history of myofascial pain syndrome. *Curr Pain Headache Rep.* 2001;5(5):412–420.

Gerwin RD. Diagnosis of myofascial pain syndrome. *Phys Med Rehabil Clin N Am.* 2014;25:341–355.

Giamberardino MA, Affaitati G, Fabrizio A, Costantini R. Myofascial pain syndromes and their evaluation. *Best Pract Res Clin Rheumatol.* 2011;25(2):185–198.

Gunn CC. Neuropathic myofascial pain syndromes. In: Loeser JD, Butler SH, Chapman CR, Turk DC, eds. *Bonica's Management of Pain.* Philadelphia: Lippincott Williams & Wilkins; 2001.

Hauser W, Walitt B, Fitzcharles M, Sommer C. Review of pharmacological therapies in fibromyalgia syndrome. *Arthritis Res Ther.* 2014;16(1):201.

Jones GT, Atzeni F, Beasley M, et al. The prevalence of fibromyalgia in the general population: a comparison of the American College of Rheumatology 1990, 2010, and modified 2010 classification criteria. *Arthritis Rheumatol.* 2015;67(2):568–575.

Macfarlane GJ, Kronisch C, Dean LE, et al. EULAR revised recommendations for the management of fibromyalgia. *Ann Rheum Dis.* 2017;76(2):318–328.

Nuesch E, Hauser W, Bernardy K. Comparative efficacy of pharmacological and non-pharmacological interventions in fibromyalgia: network meta-analysis. *Ann Rheum Dis.* 2013;12:955–962.

Phillips K, Clauw DJ. Central pain mechanisms in the rheumatic diseases: future directions. *Arthritis Rheum.* 2013;65(2):291–302.

Sarzi-Puttini P, Giorgi V, Marotto D, et al. Fibromyalgia: an update on clinical characteristics, aetiopathogenesis and treatment. *Nat Rev Rheumatol.* 2020;16(11): 645–660.

Shah JP, Thaker N, Heimur J, Aredo JV, Sikdar S, Gerber LH. Myofascial trigger points then and now: a historical and scientific perspective. *PM R 7.* 2015;746–761.

Simons DG, Travell JG, Simons LS. *Travell & Simons' Myofascial Pain and Dysfunction: The Trigger Point Manual,* 2nd ed. Baltimore: Williams & Wilkins; 1999.

Sluka KA, Clauw DJ. Neurobiology of fibromyalgia and chronic widespread pain. *Neuroscience.* 2016;338: 114–129.

Srbely JZ. New trends in the treatment and management of myofascial pain syndrome. *Curr Pain Headache Rep.* 2010;14:346–352.

Weiner DK. Office management of chronic pain in the elderly. *Am J Med.* 2007;120(4):306–315.

Chapter 104

Infection and Appropriate Antimicrobial Selection

Kevin P. High

PREDISPOSITION OF OLDER ADULTS TO INFECTION

Risk factors for infection in older adults are both intrinsic to the host due to aging itself and comorbid illness, as well as extrinsic due to medications, availability of proper nutrition, and living conditions.

Intrinsic Changes

The older adult host is a very different being than a healthy, young adult. The most important risk factor for infection in seniors is the accumulation of comorbid disease with age (eg, diabetes, chronic pulmonary disease, vascular disease, heart failure, functional decline, and immobility). These conditions alter immune response, reduce blood flow, impair mucociliary clearance mechanisms, and alter drug distribution and metabolism. Cognitive decline and comorbid illness can alter presentation of illness, delay diagnosis, or reduce adherence to medical regimens. Comorbid disease also reduces physiologic reserve and thus is an important predictor for adverse outcomes when infection occurs.

While comorbidities substantially influence the risk and outcome of infection, the immune response itself—both innate and adaptive immunity—changes with advancing age (detailed in **Figure 104-1** and Chapter 3). These changes are collectively termed *immune senescence* and are not simply a universal reduction in response; on the contrary, some responses are actually overactive or prolonged and can lead to tissue destruction or aggravated symptoms.

The components of innate immunity that are frequently impaired include physical barriers (skin integrity, cough/gag reflex, mucociliary clearance, and gastric acid) and polymorphonuclear neutrophil (PMN) functions—migration to the site of infection and ingestion/killing

Learning Objectives

- Identify and address modifiable risk factors for infection in older adults.

- Appropriately order and use culture data in older adults, including knowing when NOT to order cultures of urine and skin.

- Distinguish function-based options for management of prosthetic joint (PJ) infections and link the appropriate risk factors that influence option selection.

- Recognize the most common causes of fever of unknown origin (FUO) and modify the work-up as appropriate for the differential diagnosis of FUO in older adults.

Key Clinical Points

1. Multiple risk factors including comorbidity, malnutrition, immune senescence, and social determinants of health (eg, nursing home residence, poor access to care) increase the risk of infection in older adults versus young adults.

2. The adage of "start low, go slow" should NOT be used to guide initial antibiotic dosing for serious infections in older adults—time to therapeutic antibiotic blood levels is a major determinant of outcome. Full initial dosing of antibiotics is critical with subsequent doses adjusted accordingly for renal or hepatic function and drug interactions.

(Continued)

(Cont.)

3. Because colonization in the absence of infection (eg, asymptomatic bacteruria) is common in seniors, it is prudent to adopt a practice of "culture stewardship" (ie, limiting the collection of samples to only those clinical conditions where culture data are of clear benefit, greatly reducing inappropriate antibiotic use). Almost universally, cultures should NOT be obtained from skin surface swabs or urine in the presence of a long-term indwelling catheter; cultures in these settings are more often misleading than helpful and should NOT guide antibiotic selection.

4. Baseline and anticipated long-term functional outcomes drive the management of seniors with prosthetic device infections, particularly PJ infections. In those with limited function, control of initial infection followed by long-term antibiotic suppression with the device in place may be a prudent alternative to attempting cure through device removal. Specific risk factors of stability of the prosthesis, susceptibility of the organism, and the presence of comorbid conditions help guide clinical decision making.

5. The causes of FUO differ in old versus young adults; giant cell arteritis (GCA) accounts for nearly one in every six cases of FUO in those 60 years and older, but is absent in published FUO series of adults younger than 50 years.

6. Specific strategies for novel vaccines are beginning to overcome immune senescence; recent examples include the high-dose influenza vaccine, novel adjuvants in influenza and recombinant zoster protein vaccines, and mRNA-based strategies for SARS-CoV-2. These strategies result in greater efficacy even in frail, older adults.

of organisms. The slower PMN response leads to more prolonged inflammatory phase in many infections, slower microbial clearance, enhanced tissue damage, and often worse disease outcomes. There are even more profound changes in adaptive immunity. Decreases in naïve T-cell subsets with accumulation of memory T cells substantially reduce the diversity of the T-cell pool and impair responses to specific antigen. These changes are linked to the risk of tuberculosis, zoster, and impaired vaccine responses in older adults.

The overall clinical impact of immune senescence is an area of intense study. While it is clear that age itself is associated with reduced responses to vaccines as early as the third or fouth decade (eg, human papillomavirus vaccine, hepatitis B vaccine), the most critical deficits appear later in life. Disability-adjusted life-years lost due to vaccine preventable illness shows a major inflection point at about age 70. Specific vaccine formulations and strategies developed to overcome immune senescence include higher antigen concentration (eg, high-dose influenza vaccine), adding specific adjuvant to a protein subunit vaccine (eg, zoster subunit vaccine), and most recently the mRNA and viral carrier strategies employed to produce the SARS-CoV-2 vaccines. The adjuvanted zoster and mRNA-based SARS-CoV-2 vaccine strategies resulted in remarkably enhanced efficacy, greater than or equal to 90% for most seniors and even more than 80% in frail older adults, with tolerable increases in reactogenicity/side effects.

Extrinsic Factors

Major external dynamics impact infection risk and outcomes in older adults. Physiologic and medication-induced effects on appetite, taste, and absorption/clearance, as well as inconsistent access to nutritious food sources, can result in protein–energy malnutrition (PEM). Thirty to sixty percent of adults older than 65 years admitted to the hospital have PEM, which is linked to delayed wound healing, pressure ulcer formation, risk of pneumonia and other nosocomial infections, longer hospital stays and increased mortality. In the outpatient setting, even mild PEM (ie, seniors with a serum albumin of 3.0–3.5 g/dL) has reduced vaccine responses. Despite this, high protein/high calorie nutritional supplements have not consistently shown benefit for preventing infection or boosting immune responses. Specific micronutrient deficiencies in older adults are also linked to infection risk (eg, vitamin D deficiency and risk for tuberculosis (TB), Clostridiodes difficile and SARS-CoV-2 infection). Patients identified with true micronutrient deficiencies should receive supplementation to reverse the deficiency. However, in otherwise healthy adults with normal or even "insufficient" (low but not to the level of true deficiency) vitamin levels, very thin data support supplementation.

Additional "social determinants of health" combine to influence infection risk in seniors. Lower socioeconomic status (SES) is associated with higher rates of community-acquired pneumonia (CAP) and invasive pneumococcal infections in older adults, perhaps due to reduced access to care, but other factors are in play as well. Low SES is associated with increased exposure to pollution and tobacco exposure, infectious agents (eg, grandparents raising young children more often), and poor nutrition, as well as an increased rates of comorbid disease (eg, asthma, diabetes).

Living condition/setting also plays a major role for many seniors. Long-term care (ie, nursing home) residents have a particularly high incidence of respiratory,

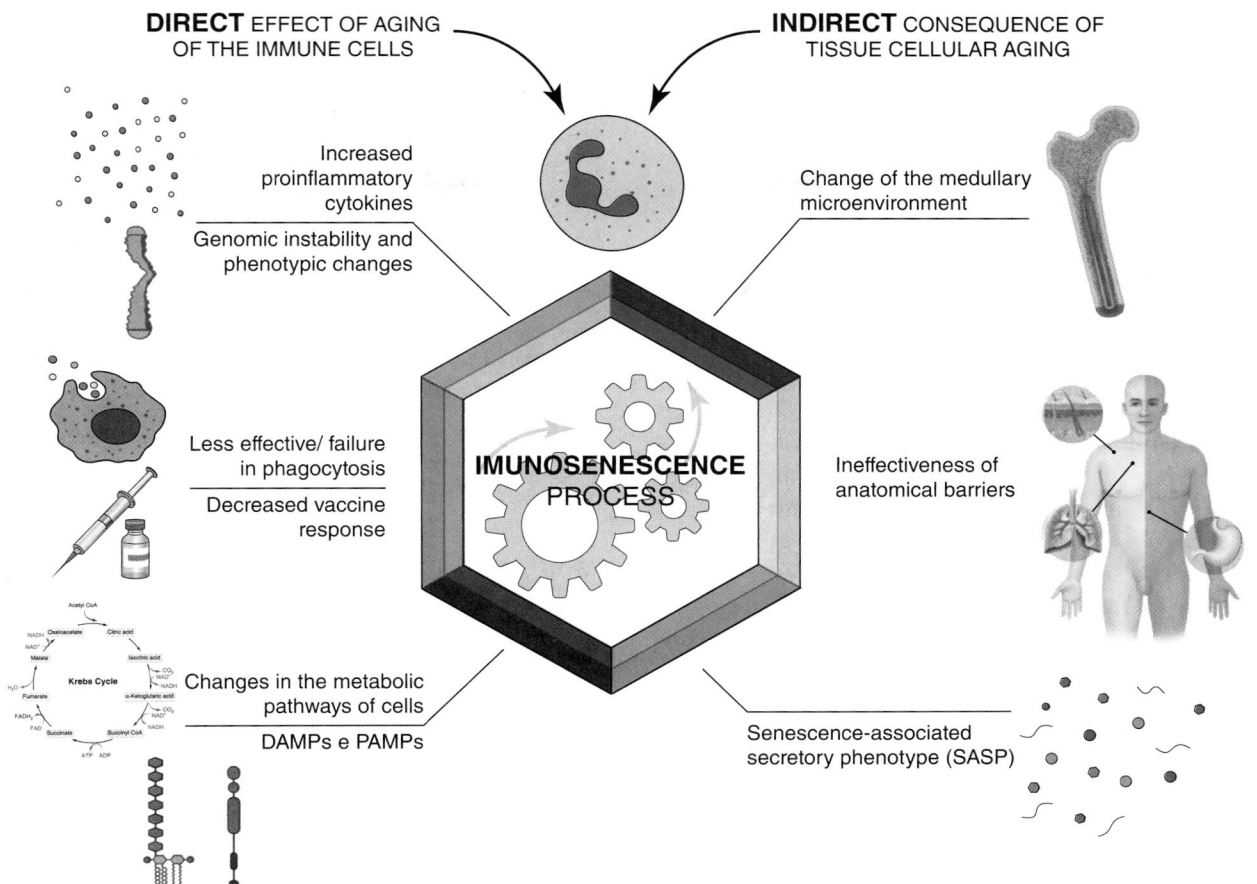

FIGURE 104-1. Cytokines, phagocytosis, metabolic pathways, SASP, anatomical barriers, and medullary microenvironment are associated with the immunosenescence process in immune cells and tissues. DAMPs, damage-associated molecular patterns; PAMPs, pathogen-associated molecular patterns. (Reproduced with permission from Rodrigues LP, Teixeira VR, Alencar-Silva T, et al. Hallmarks of aging and immunosenescence: connecting the dots. *Cytokine Growth Factor Rev.* 2021;59:9–21.)

genitourinary, gastrointestinal (GI), and skin infections, and unique infection control challenges exist in the long-term care setting. Close contact between residents and staff plays a key role in the spread of respiratory infections (eg, influenza, RSV) or infections transmitted by contact (eg, *Streptococcus pyogenes, C difficile*). The setting of frail older adults in a confined space can lead to severe outbreaks with high mortality rates; never was this more evident than in the recent COVID-19 pandemic in which long-term care facilities were a major site of transmission and mortality.

PRESENTATION OF INFECTION IN SENIORS

Even serious, life-threatening infection often presents atypically in older adults. Exacerbations of underlying illness or nonspecific declines in function or mentation may lead older adult patients to seek medical attention for symptoms related to comorbidity rather than infection. The predominant indicator of infection, fever, is absent in up to one-third of older adults with serious infection. Older adults, particularly frail older adults, have lower baseline body temperatures than the "normal" 98.6°F (37°C). Further, temperature increases in response to inflammatory stimuli are dampened with advanced age, and the combination of lower basal temperature and a blunted response makes it less likely that an older adult will reach the definition of fever (≥ 100.4°F/38°C) delaying diagnosis and treatment.

Cognitive impairment may also contribute to the difficulty of diagnosing infection in older adults. While a high index of suspicion for infection is warranted in such patients, clinicians should be cautioned to thoughtfully order tests and interpret results carefully. For example, subtle symptoms often lead to overdiagnosis when ill-advised cultures identify colonization (eg, asymptomatic bacteriuria) rather than true infection. Those positive cultures are assumed to be causing the nonspecific symptoms, when dehydration, medication changes, and other factors may truly be the cause. Further, the utility of culture data in some situations is very poor (eg, swab cultures of skin surface wounds or urine cultures when catheters are present), leading to overdiagnosis and overtreatment (see specific syndromes below).

Antimicrobial Treatment

Drug distribution, metabolism, excretion, and interactions change with age and comorbid illness. Antibiotic dose adjustments are needed commonly in seniors due to reduced renal function or increased sensitivity to side effects. Polypharmacy can make antibiotic selection and dosing particularly challenging due to drug interactions. These factors often lead clinicians to the maxim of "start low, go slow" when treating geriatric patients. However, for antibiotics, this is *not* an appropriate strategy. Early, therapeutic antibiotic levels are particularly important in older adults—much more important than in young adults—perhaps due to the slower initial innate immune response previously discussed and poor physiologic reserve. Outcomes of serious infection in seniors depend on reaching adequate drug levels quickly, particularly for antibiotics with a concentration-dependent mechanism of action (eg, fluoroquinolones), so aggressive first-dose strategies are appropriate (eg, loading doses) in serious infection. Slowed gastric motility, decreased absorption, increased adipose tissue, and coadministration of other drugs can also decrease blood levels of antimicrobials in older adults. Adherence may be limited by poor cognitive function, inadequate understanding of the drug regimen, impaired hearing or vision, and polypharmacy. Studies suggest that any regimen requiring greater than twice daily dosing is associated with reduced adherence rates. Finally, antibiotics can only reach tissues that are well-perfused; poor blood flow due to macro- or microvascular disease can impair drug delivery and lead to clinical failures even when the organism is susceptible.

Outpatient Parenteral Antibiotic Therapy

Outpatient parenteral antibiotic therapy (OPAT) is commonly used for infections that occur in older adults (eg, endocarditis, osteomyelitis, PJ infection), but this modality is underused in older adults in the United States. Instead, patients are often admitted to nursing homes to achieve insurance/Medicare "coverage." Medicare Part D, however, does cover OPAT at home, although navigating the system to obtain reimbursement for both the antibiotic and the necessary supplies/home health assistance for drug administration takes considerable skill. OPAT is safe and effective therapy in seniors that have adequate support and monitoring and can often avoid long-term care admission. In addition, oral regimens with high bioavailability and reliable pharmacokinetics can be used in specific situations—an infectious disease consultation may help avoid the need for long-term IV therapy.

Antibiotic and Culture Stewardship

Older adults, particularly long-term care residents, have some of the highest rates of multidrug resistant organism (MDRO) colonization and infection. Patients with indwelling devices (eg, urinary catheters, G-tubes) and those with marked functional impairment are at highest risk. Widespread antibiotic use in long-term care is sometimes viewed as inevitable, but it can be studied and unnecessary use greatly reduced. Residents in long-term care facilities with higher rates of antibiotic use are more susceptible to antibiotic-related adverse events *even if the individual resident doesn't receive antibiotics.* Just being in a high-risk environment increases the risk of adverse consequences (*C difficile* infection [CDI], non-CDI diarrhea, MDRO colonization and infection, allergic reactions, or general medication adverse events) (**Figure 104-2**).

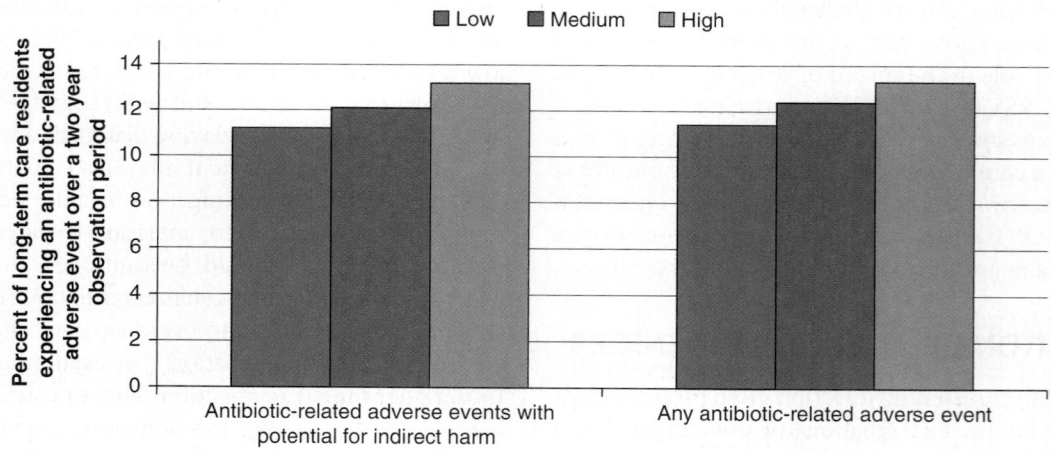

FIGURE 104-2. Percent of long-term care residents experiencing antibiotic-related adverse events with potential for indirect harm (*C difficile*, diarrhea/gastroenteritis, multidrug-resistant organism infection) or any antibiotic-related adverse event (including antibiotic allergic reaction and general adverse medication event). All differences were statistically significant. (Data from Daneman N, Bronskill SE, Gruneir A, et al. Variability in antibiotic use across nursing homes and the risk of antibiotic-related adverse outcomes for individual residents. *JAMA Intern Med.* 2015;175[8]:1331–1339.)

Though comprehensive educational programs and in-nursing home consultation by infectious diseases specialists reduce antibiotic use, system approaches are likely to be most effective. The Centers for Disease Control and Prevention (CDC) has an excellent resource center on antibiotic stewardship in long-term care facilities (https://www.cdc.gov/longtermcare/prevention/antibiotic-stewardship.html). One of the most effective approaches is culture stewardship—limiting unnecessary cultures (eg, swab cultures of pressure ulcers, urine cultures with indwelling catheters). Cultures from pressure ulcers and urine in the presence of an indwelling catheter will *always* be positive, but the information does not correlate with infection. Culture stewardship, using preset criteria to obtain cultures, can markedly reduce antibiotic use in this setting.

Antibiotics at the End of Life

Since 1998, the American Medical Association Council of Ethical and Judicial Affairs has included antibiotics as "life-sustaining" treatment to be discussed as part of advanced directive and end-of-life care. Many clinicians, however, feel antibiotics are not sufficiently "invasive" to warrant discussion in scope of care orders. While every clinical situation is unique, and no comprehensive recommendation made for withholding antibiotics in the terminally ill, it seems prudent to include antibiotic administration in advanced directives just as one would for any medical intervention such as surgery, mechanical ventilation, or administration of food/fluids. Antibiotics may be palliative in some situations (vs prolongation of life) when symptoms are due to infection itself and readily reversible with treatment—an excellent example is severe, painful oral or esophageal candidiasis. Otherwise, limiting diagnostic testing for infection in palliative care situations is prudent when it will not alter longer-term outcomes or provide symptom relief that cannot be achieved with other measures (eg, antipyretics).

SPECIFIC CLINICAL SYNDROMES

A complete review of all the clinical infectious syndromes experienced by older adults is beyond the scope of this chapter, and several chapters in this textbook cover individual conditions in detail. **Table 104-1** provides a summary of treatment for common infections in older adults. Key aspects of prevalent syndromes not discussed in other chapters are discussed below. Older adults were the most common patient group affected by COVID-19, and this viral illness had devastating effects in US nursing homes that are likely to result in changes in the way institutional care is provided over the next several decades. COVID-19 is discussed in Chapter 16.

Bacteremia and Sepsis

Early sepsis mortality (within 30 day) is 50% higher for adults older than 65 years versus younger adults primarily due to poor physiologic reserve and multimorbidity in the former. In addition, gram-negative bacilli—usually from GI or genitourinary (GU) sources—are more common in seniors and antibiotic management should emphasize the importance of initially broad coverage. This is particularly true when MDRO risk is high (eg, indwelling device present in a nursing home patient, known MDRO colonization). Early sepsis is very challenging to identify and manage in the nursing home setting because of the nonspecificity of its presentation and lack of resources such as stat labs, intravenous antibiotics, and pharmacy services.

When older adults survive sepsis they are more likely than young adults to suffer long-term impairment of physical or cognitive function. In one study, seniors surviving sepsis had a risk of moderate to severe cognitive impairment of 6% prehospitalization, but nearly 17% after hospitalization. Those same patients also experienced a decrease in activities of daily living (ADLs) and instrumental ADLs (IADLs), and about 40% of those older than 65 years require admission to a long-term care facility versus only 15% in those younger than 65 years.

Infective Endocarditis

Fever and leukocytosis in infective endocarditis (IE) are less common (55% and 25%, respectively, in those 65 years and older versus 80% and 60%, respectively, in younger adults). Transthoracic echocardiography (TTE) sensitivity is lower in older adults due to calcified valves, more turbulent blood flow, and shadows off prosthetic valves (when present). Transesophageal echocardiography (TEE) is more sensitive and improves the diagnostic yield by 45% in seniors over that of TTE. Native valve IE is typically caused by streptococci and staphylococci in both young and older adults. However, as noted for bacteremia above, GI and GU organisms such as enterococci and gram-negative rods become more common with increasing age, and initial antibiotic treatment may need to be broader until a specific organism is isolated. IE prophylaxis recommendations do not differ based on age.

Prosthetic Device Infections

Infection of implanted prosthetic devices (joints, cardiac pacemakers/heart valves, intraocular lens implants, vascular grafts, etc) is common in older adults. Foreign material creates an environment for bacterial biofilms, and bacteria embedded in these biofilms are often more difficult for antibiotics or immune mechanisms to clear. Skin flora—coagulase-negative staphylococci, *S aureus* and diphtheroids—are the predominate causative organisms for early (< 60 days after implantation) infections. The source is presumably due to contamination of the surgical site or occult bacteremia with skin organisms from incision sites/IV sites. Gram-negative bacilli, fungi, and polymicrobial infection are rare causes of early infection, but can be seen in some situations that increase the risk of occult bacteremia (eg, GU instrumentation). Late (beyond day 60 postimplantation) infections are more likely due to asymptomatic

TABLE 104-1 ■ SUGGESTED EMPIRIC ANTIMICROBIAL THERAPY FOR COMMON INFECTIONS IN OLDER ADULTS

INFECTION	THERAPY	COMMENTS
COMMUNITY ACQUIRED		
Outpatient Therapy		
Acute sinusitis	Antibiotics rarely needed; if symptoms > 10 days: Amoxicillin-clavulanate	Oral cephalosporin if penicillin allergic (except anaphylaxis); levofloxacin if refractory
Acute exacerbations of chronic bronchitis	Mild-Mod: Amoxicillin, doxycycline, TMP-SMX Severe: Amoxicillin-clavulanate or resp-FQ	Infectious exacerbations only; resp-FQs have been shown to extend the time between acute exacerbations and therefore may be preferable in those with frequent, infectious exacerbations. Short course of oral corticosteroids (5 days) for severe, acute exacerbations
Pneumonia	[Azithromycin or clarithromycin + 2nd gen cephalexin or amox/clav] *or* resp-FQ	Five days adequate therapy. Review and update immunization status
Cellulitis	Amox/clav *or* cephalexin	If pustules/skin abscesses *S aureus* more likely than *Streptococcus* spp. About half of all *S aureus* will be community-acquired MRSA; include TMP-SMX or minocycline if suspected
Infected neuropathic ulcer with deep tissue inflammation	[Amox/clav + TMP-SMX] or [FQ + linezolid]	If inflammation superficial, may use TMP-SMX, doxycycline, or clindamycin alone; if no inflammation, NO ANTIBIOTICS
Symptomatic UTI (cystitis)	Nitrofurantoin, TMP-SMX	Beware asymptomatic bacteriuria—only treat if symptoms clearly new/indicative of infection. For refractory symptoms, culture warranted to guide directed therapy
Bacterial diarrhea	FQ	Oral rehydration is key—most will resolve without antibiotics. DO NOT USE ANTIBIOTICS IF SHIGA TOXIN IS POSITIVE (due to risk of HUS/TTP)
C difficile diarrhea	Vancomycin	Fidaxomicin is FDA approved and is equivalent to vancomycin for cure, but reduces relapse rate (cost is a major consideration keeping fidaxomicin from being first-line therapy); metronidazole no longer first-line therapy except in serious disease *with* vancomycin Recurrent disease: vancomycin followed by taper; consider fecal microbiota transplantation if multiple recurrences Prophylaxis: in patient with recent *C difficile* colitis needing antibiotics—vancomycin prophylaxis reduces risk to 4% from 26%; monoclonal antibody treatment protects for up to 6 months; insufficient data for/against probiotics
Inpatient Therapy		
Pneumonia	Moderate: [Ceftriaxone or ceftaroline + azithromycin or clarithromycin] *or* resp-FQ alone Severe: [Ceftriaxone or ceftaroline + azithromycin or clarithromycin or respiratory FQ]	Consider *Legionella*, MRSA, and severe viral pathogens (SARS-CoV-2, influenza, RSV); consider *Pseudomonas* if severe COPD (FEV$_1$ < 30% predicted) or structural lung disease First dose: improved survival if within 6 hours of presentation Duration of therapy: 5–7 days clearly efficacious, emerging data suggest only 3–5 may be necessary
Pyelonephritis (no catheter)	3rd gen cephalosporin *or* FQ	High risk for resistant bacteria (recent inpatient, history of MDRO) consider carbapenem, particularly if seriously ill
Sepsis from urologic source (with catheter)	3rd gen cephalosporin + ampicillin or vancomycin	Catheter-related sepsis due to urologic source is often polymicrobial; have to consider enterococcal species, in addition to gram-negative bacilli. Early catheter exchange improves outcome
Acute bacterial meningitis	Ampicillin + ceftriaxone + vancomycin	Vancomycin needed because of small percentage of ceftriaxone-resistant *S pneumoniae*; give dexamethasone with or prior to antibiotics. For severe penicillin allergy use vancomycin + aztreonam + trimethoprim/sulfamethoxazole

(Continued)

TABLE 104-1 ■ SUGGESTED EMPIRIC ANTIMICROBIAL THERAPY FOR COMMON INFECTIONS IN OLDER ADULTS (*CONTINUED*)

INFECTION	THERAPY	COMMENTS
COMMUNITY ACQUIRED (Cont.)		
Intraabdominal infection	[Ampicillin/sulbactam + gentamicin] *or* [ampicillin + gentamicin + metronidazole] *or* pip/tazo *or* carbapenem	Surgery nearly always indicated for ischemic colitis, abscess drainage, but rarely required for diverticulitis; increasing data that appendicitis without fecolith on ultrasound may be managed medically in high surgical risk patients; cholecystitis usually requires surgery, but may be delayed if rapidly responds to antibiotics and/or gallbladder can be drained percutaneously; tigecycline for patients with significant β-lactam allergy
C difficile colitis/toxic megacolon	Vancomycin (oral or via enema) + metronidazole IV (if ileus or toxic megacolon)	Colectomy may be necessary for toxic megacolon; early surgical consultation prudent
Native valve endocarditis	Vancomycin + ceftriaxone	Substitute gentamicin for ceftriaxone or use daptomycin alone for severely penicillin-allergic patient
Prosthetic valve endocarditis	Vancomycin + gentamicin +/− rifampin	May wait until pathogen identified and level of bacteremia reduced to add rifampin (may decrease development of rifampin resistance). Treat pacemaker and implantable defibrillator devices similarly. Recent data suggest $_{18}$F-FDG-PET/CT can be helpful to confirm PV involvement when blood cultures positive, but TTE/TEE nondiagnostic.
Infected diabetic foot ulcer	[Ampicillin/sulbactam or ertapenem] + vancomycin	3rd gen ceph and clinda for penicillin allergy; tigecycline for significant β-lactam allergy; if patient septic with this as primary source, use vancomycin + [pip/tazo or carbepenem]
Cellulitis	Ampicillin/sulbactam	Add clinda if high suspicion for GAS or vancomycin if MRSA suspected; vancomycin + FQ for β-lactam allergy; many options for single dose parental therapy without hospitalization rather than admission for mild/moderate illness—dalbavancin/oritavancin/etc
Prosthetic joint infection	Empirical therapy NOT recommended; base treatment on culture results	In the very rare circumstance of sepsis due to prosthetic joint infection, treatment is the same as that when there is no obvious focus (see below)
Septic shock syndrome; with no obvious focus	Vancomycin + [carbepenem or pip/tazo]	Aggressive supportive care—sepsis bundles/protocols; consider intravenous immunoglobulin and addition of clindamycin if streptococcal toxic shock syndrome
HOSPITAL ACQUIRED		
Pneumonia	Low MRSA risk: cefepime or pip/tazo or meropenem or levofloxacin Add vancomycin if: MRSA colonized or suspected	If severe disease, vancomycin + [cefepime or pip/tazo or meropenem]; add azithromycin or levofloxacin if legionellosis suspected. Linezolid can substitute for vancomycin. ID consult for MDRO
Catheter-associated urosepsis	Vancomycin plus 3rd gen ceph or FQ	Culture to guide subsequent therapy
Intravenous catheter-associated infection (cellulitis, phlebitis, abscess, bacteremia)	Vancomycin	If immunocompromised, add cefepime or ceftazidime; surgery required for septic thrombophlebitis
Postoperative wound infection; incision/deep with cellulitis, abscess, or bacteremia	Mild infection: Amox/clav (especially if GI/GU surgery) or cefazolin or TMP-SMX or clindamycin Severe infection: Vancomycin + [3rd gen ceph or pip/tazo or carbepenem]	Reopen and explore wound; empiric therapy can be driven by Gram stain; definitive therapy guided by cultures

2nd gen, second generation; 3rd gen, third generation; amox/clav, amoxicillin-clavulanate; carbepenem, imipenem-cilastatin or meropenem; ceph, cephalosporin; clinda, clindamycin; COPD, chronic obstructive pulmonary disease; FQ, fluoroquinolone; GAS, group A streptococci (*S pyogenes*); HUS/TTP, hemolytic uremic syndrome/thrombotic thrombocytopenia purpura; MRSA, methicillin-resistant *S aureus*; MDRO, multidrug-resistant organism; pip/tazo, piperacillin-tazobactam; resp-FQ, respiratory fluoroquinolone (levofloxacin, moxifloxacin); ticar/clav, ticarcillin-clavulanate; TMP-SMX, trimethoprim-sulfamethoxazole; vanco, vancomycin; UTI, urinary tract infection.

episodes of bacteremia seeding the implant and subject to a wider array of organisms, including GI and GU sources of bacteremia as noted previously, but skin organisms (staphylococci) still predominate. Empirical therapy of prosthetic device infections is NOT recommended unless there is an overt clinical justification (eg, sepsis). In clinically stable patients, there is almost always time to safely obtain cultures without antibiotics—for example in PJ infection—to base treatment on culture data.

Anticipated functional outcomes and patient/infection characteristics determine the approach to prosthetic device infection—particularly PJ infection (**Figure 104-3**). Cure may be difficult with the device in place, but in some instances—short duration of symptoms or early after primary implantation—aggressive surgical debridement and antibiotic therapy may result in cure with the device in situ. The highest cure rates are achieved with removal/replacement of the infected implant either in a one- or two-step procedure particularly if the device is unstable or the organism is not highly susceptible to well-absorbed oral antibiotics. However, cure using these methods requires an extended period of very limited mobility that may lead to

further functional decline. When future ambulation is not likely even if the infection is cured or life expectancy is relatively short and surgical risk high, it may be reasonable to control the infection initially with joint aspiration and IV antibiotics followed by long-term antibiotic suppression. Thus, clinical judgment is critical in devising a comprehensive plan for therapy. Although many factors may mitigate enthusiasm to attempt cure, age alone should *not* be a reason to withhold curative therapy—function at baseline and the likely long-term outcome should drive the decision, not age.

Antimicrobial prophylaxis to reduce the risk of device infection around dental, GI, and GU procedures is hotly debated. While recommended for prosthetic heart valves, and by extrapolation vascular grafts, particularly within the first 12 to 24 months after placement, supportive evidence for prophylaxis is thin even in these clinical situations. There is even weaker evidence for prophylaxis in patients with PJs, intracoronary artery stents, and many other less-commonly implanted prostheses. Despite this, the American Dental Association (ADA) recommends "considering" antibiotic prophylaxis for patients with a PJ

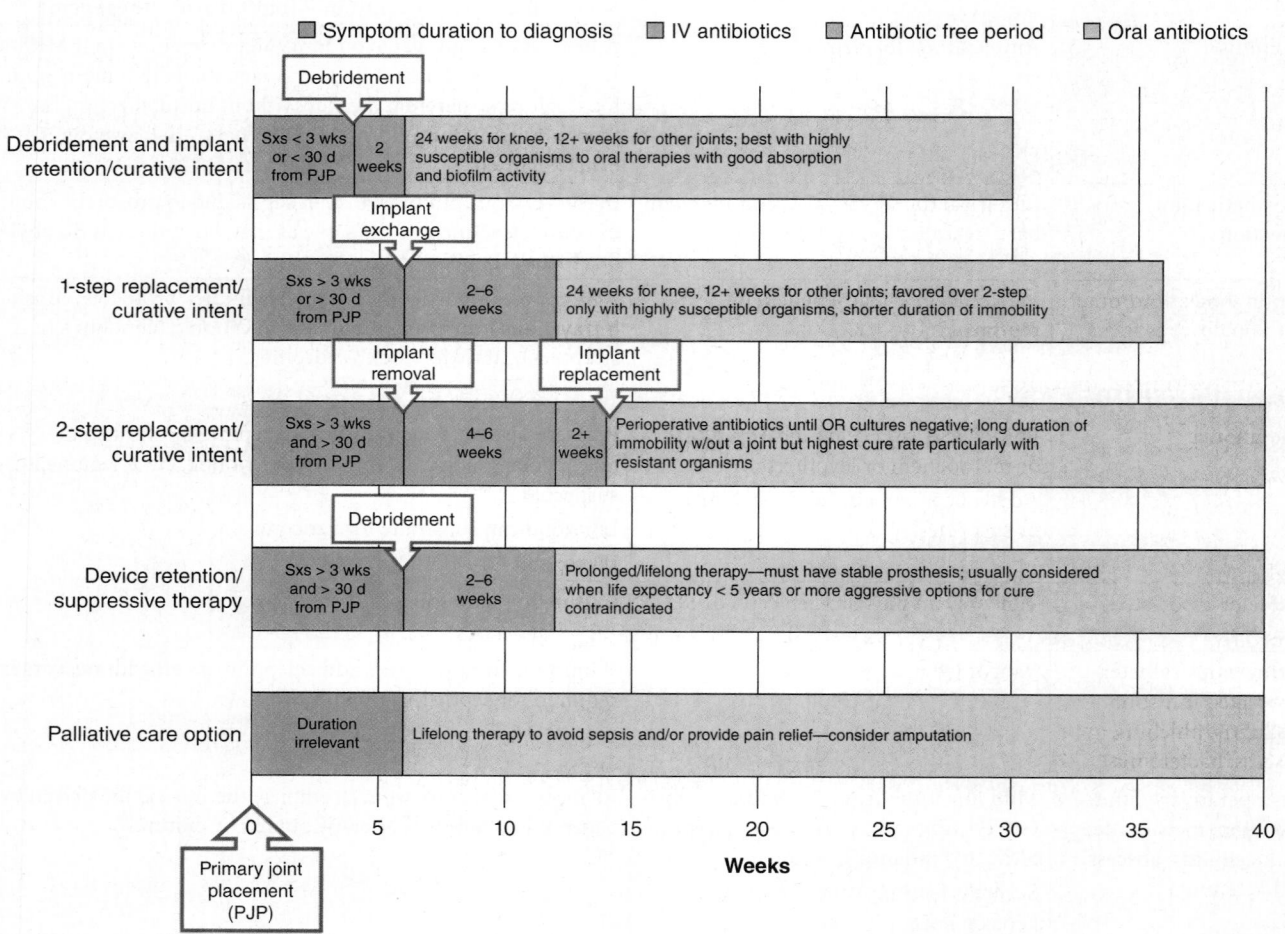

FIGURE 104-3. Summary of management of prosthetic joint infections based on clinical characteristics, most appropriate strategy, and intended outcome of treatment.

at "high risk"—defined as PJs placed within 2 years or in immunosuppressed patients (including those with diabetes mellitus, rheumatoid arthritis, or malnourishment), or in patients with a history of prior joint infection.

Gastrointestinal Infections

Altered transit time, achlorhydria, diverticular disease, immune senescence, altered GI microbiota, and comorbid diseases predispose seniors to GI infection. Diagnosis and management of most GI infections are similar regardless of age; however, a number of aspects deserve further comment.

Viral GI pathogens (eg, norovirus) are common causes of gastroenteritis in older adults and can lead to marked dehydration and/or exacerbation of underlying comorbid disease. Further, such pathogens are commonly the cause of gastroenteritis outbreaks in long-term care facilities—even one or two cases in residents or staff should prompt rapid infection control interventions in such settings.

CDI disproportionately affects older adults and results in greater morbidity and mortality. Asymptomatic carriage of *C difficile* is not relatively common in seniors; 2% in the community, 10% in community dwellers with outpatient health care exposure, and 20% to 50% in hospital or long-term care settings. Symptomatic CDI occurs in about 15% of asymptomatic carriers after antibiotics. Older adults with CDI are more likely to develop severe sequelae (sepsis, hypotension, renal failure, toxic megacolon), but even mild-moderate CDI can have major consequences in advanced age. The need to use the bathroom six to eight times daily is not trivial for mobility-limited, visually impaired, or demented older adults, and even mild-moderate CDI may result in loss of independence for such seniors.

Guideline-driven therapy for CDI does not differ specifically by age, but the risk of relapse after treatment is much greater in older adults than in those yonger than age 65. Prolonged taper of vancomycin is commonly used in patients who relapse with high rates of success. However, refractory relapse may require fecal microbiota transplantation (FMT) that has become standard in recent years. FMT using donated stool or oral capsules of commercially available preparations is safe and effective with success rates of 80% to 90%. Prevention of CDI in high risk, older adults who require another course of antibiotics benefit from passive antibody administration prior to receiving antibiotics. Vancomycin prophylaxis is also be effective.

Tuberculosis

Advanced age is a long-established, major risk factor for clinical tuberculosis. Fever, night sweats, cough, and hemoptysis are less likely to be present than in young adults; older adults are more likely to present with nonspecific symptoms of dizziness, generalized pain, or mental "dullness." Older adults are more likely to have widespread lung infiltrates, whereas young adults are more likely to have isolated upper lobe infiltrates/cavities, and older adults are more likely to have evidence of malnutrition (ie, reduced serum albumin).

Tuberculin skin test (TST) sensitivity to detect latent infection declines with age. Newer diagnostic tests for tuberculosis (eg, interferon-γ release assay [IFGRA] from blood measured after ex vivo *Mycobacterium tuberculosis* antigen exposure) are minimally more sensitive (~ 70% for TST vs ~ 75% for IFGRAs). However, IFGRA requires a single blood draw (rather than a second visit 48 to 72 hours later to assess a TST), does not require two-step testing in nursing home residents, and has greater interrater reliability and specificity than TST. Therefore, most latent tuberculosis testing is now done by IFGRA. The treatment of tuberculosis in older adults does not differ from that of young adults, but drug side effects are more common than in young adults.

Fever of Unknown Origin

FUO is classically defined as temperature more than 101°F (38.3°C) for at least 3 weeks and undiagnosed after 1 week of medical evaluation. The cause of FUO can be determined in about 90% of cases and approximately one-third will have treatable infections, most often intraabdominal abscess, bacterial endocarditis, tuberculosis, or occult osteomyelitis (see **Table 104-2**). In contrast to young adults, autoimmune disease is a more frequent cause of FUO in adults older than 60 years accounting for nearly one of every four FUOs. Systemic lupus erythematosus (SLE), the most common autoimmune cause of FUO in young adults, is essentially absent in published cohorts of FUO in older adults, and replaced by GCA and polyarteritis nodosa (PAN). Neoplastic disease accounts for another 20%, most often a result of hematopoietic malignancies (eg, lymphoma and leukemia). Drug fever is a common cause in older adults

TABLE 104-2 ■ FEVER OF UNKNOWN ORIGIN (FUO) IN OLDER PATIENTS

MAJOR CAUSES	% OF CASES[a]
Infections	35
Intraabdominal abscess	12
Tuberculosis	6
Infective endocarditis	10
Other	7
Inflammatory disorders	28
Temporal arteritis/polymyalgia rheumatica	19
Polyarteritis nodosa	6
Other	3
Malignancy	19
Lymphoma/other hematologic	10
Solid tumors	9
Other (pulmonary emboli, drug fever)	5
No diagnosis	13

[a]Percentages represent pooled data from multiple studies of FUO in the older patient.

and deep venous thrombosis with or without recurrent pulmonary emboli occasionally causes the syndrome.

The diagnostic algorithm for older adults is influenced by the age-varied differential diagnosis in FUO. A thorough history and physical examination; basic laboratory evaluations of complete blood counts with differential, serum chemistries and hepatic enzymes, thyroid function studies, erythrocyte sedimentation rate (ESR), C-reactive protein (CRP), IFGRA for TB, HIV serology, creatinine kinase, antinuclear antibodies (ANAs), serum protein electrophoresis (SPEP), urinalysis, chest x-ray, and blood (x3) and urine cultures should begin the search. If initial work-up does not provide a clearer direction, chest/abdominal/pelvic computed tomography (CT) is most likely to provide assistance and is the next suggested test. However, if the ESR is elevated, temporal artery biopsy even in the absence of typical history or objective physical findings should be considered in older adults.

Another potentially valuable modality, $_{18}$F-FDG-PET/CT is superior to tagged WBC scans or gallium scans in FUO and its earlier use in the work-up can be cost-effective when one considers the avoidance of other tests. This is particularly important in older adults—several small studies estimate $_{18}$F-FDG uptake in the temporal, maxillary, or vertebral arteries occurs in 64% to 82% of patients with GCA with very high specificity. This has led some authors to conclude that temporal artery biopsy may be avoided in patients with absent $_{18}$F-FDG uptake in the cranial arteries. In both $_{18}$F-FDG-PET/CT and temporal artery biopsy corticosteroid administration for more than a few days can markedly reduce sensitivity.

IMMUNIZATION AND TRAVEL RECOMMENDATIONS FOR OLDER ADULTS

The most widely used vaccines in seniors for influenza, pneumococcus and zoster are covered in those specific chapters. Comprehensive immunization recommendations for adults are provided by the CDC by age or comorbid illness category and updated annually (https://www.cdc.gov/vaccines/ for the most recent updates).

Immune senescence has presented a major obstacle to effective vaccinations in seniors. However, three recently approved vaccines (high-dose influenza vaccine, adjuvanted recombinant zoster vaccine, and the SARS-CoV-2 mRNA-based vaccines) provide higher protection rates than earlier, standard vaccines—even in frail older adults—outlining future strategies to advance future vaccine development. Another strategy to address immune senescence is to "cocoon" older adults from exposure by immunizing family members, caregivers, and others who regularly come into contact with seniors. This has been demonstrated in many settings (eg, immunizing nursing home staff to protect residents, conjugate pneumococcal vaccines in children reduce pneumonia risk in older adults).

Active, older adults travel frequently raising additional vaccine issues. Many countries require yellow fever vaccine; however, the live, yellow fever vaccine requires great caution in seniors. Older adults are six times more likely than young adults to experience a serious adverse events after yellow fever vaccine and adults 60 years and older are cautioned to discuss risk/benefit carefully prior to vaccination (https://www.cdc.gov/vaccines/hcp/vis/vis-statements/yf.html). Yellow fever risk in travelers is very low, particularly when travel is limited to urban areas, and a physician's letter of exemption is often acceptable for countries that require proof of yellow fever vaccination for entry.

Other major issues in traveling seniors include malaria chemoprophylaxis. Side effects are more common for many agents (eg, mefloquine may produce dizziness, change in mental status, and bradycardia or prolonged QT intervals), and coadministration may be difficult in those taking cardiac medications or with significant heart disease. Alternative regimens are available, but recognition of current resistance patterns is critical (see CDC website [www.cdc.gov/travel] for up-to-date information). Diarrhea occurs in 25% to 50% of travelers to developing countries. Primary treatment consists of fluid and electrolyte replacement, but antimicrobial therapy with a quinolone is indicated when diarrhea is accompanied by fever or bloody stools or is prolonged. Antimotility agents are safe in this situation when coadministered with antibiotics.

FURTHER READING

Baghban A, Juthani-Mehta M. Antimicrobial use at the end of life. *Infect Dis Clin North Am.* 2017;31(4):639–647.

Benson JM. Antimicrobial pharmacokinetics and pharmacodynamics in older adults. *Infect Dis Clin North Am.* 2017;31(4):609–617.

Cassone M, Mody L. Colonization with multi-drug resistant organisms in nursing homes: scope, importance, and management. *Curr Geriatr Rep.* 2015;4(1):87–95.

Chakhtoura NEG, Bonomo RA, Jump RLP. Influence of aging and environment on presentation of infection in older adults. *Infect Dis Clin N Am.* 2017:31(4): 593–608.

Connors J, Bell MR, Marcy J, Kutzler M, Haddad EK. The impact of immuno-aging on SARS-CoV-2 vaccine development. *Geroscience.* 2021;43(1):31–51.

Cunningham AL, Lal H, Kovac M, et al. Efficacy of the herpes zoster subunit vaccine in adults 70 years of age or older. *N Engl J Med.* 2016;375(11):1019–1032.

Cunningham AL, McIntyre P, Subbarao K, Booy R, Levin MJ. Vaccines for older adults. *BMJ.* 2021;372:n188.

Daneman N, Bronskill SE, Gruneir A, et al. Variability in antibiotic use across nursing homes and the risk of antibiotic-related adverse outcomes for individual residents. *JAMA Intern Med*. 2015;175(8):1331–1339.

DiazGranados CA, Dunning AJ, Kimmel M, et al. Efficacy of high-dose versus standard-dose influenza vaccine in older adults. *N Engl J Med*. 2014;371(7):635–645.

Donskey CJ. *Clostridium difficile* in older adults. *Infect Dis Clin North Am*. 2017;31(4):743–756.

Dumyati G, Stone ND, Nace DA, Crnich CJ, Jump RL. Challenges and strategies for prevention of multidrug-resistant organism transmission in nursing homes. *Curr Infect Dis Rep*. 2017;19(4):18.

Jump RLP, Crnich CJ, Mody L, Bradley SF, Nicolle LE, Yoshikawa TT. Infectious diseases in older adults of long-term care facilities: update on approach to diagnosis and management. *J Am Geriatr Soc*. 2018;66:789–803.

Marion C, High KP. Tuberculosis in older adults in infectious disease in the aging. In: Yoshikawa TT, Norman DC, eds. *Infections in aging: a clinical handbook*. Totoway, NJ: Humana Press; 2010:97–110.

McDonald LC, Gerding DN, Johnson S, et al. Clinical practice guidelines for *Clostridium difficile* infection in adults and children: 2017 update by the Infectious Diseases Society of America (IDSA) and Society for Healthcare Epidemiology of America (SHEA). *Clin Infect Dis*. 2018;66(7):e1–e48.

McElligott M, Welham G, Pop-Vicas A, Taylor L, Crnich CJ. Antibiotic stewardship in nursing facilities. *Infect Dis Clin North Am*. 2017;31(4):619–638.

Nair R, Schweizer ML, Singh N. Septic arthritis and prosthetic joint infections in older adults. *Infect Dis Clin North Am*. 2017;31(4):715–729.

Nikolich-Žugich J. The twilight of immunity: emerging concepts in aging of the immune system. *Nat Immunol*. 2018;19(1):10–19.

Olsho LE, Bertrand RM, Edwards AS, et al. Does adherence to the Loeb minimum criteria reduce antibiotic prescribing rates in nursing homes? *J Am Med Dir Assoc*. 2013;14(4):309.e1–7.

Rodrigues LP, Teixeira VR, Alencar-Silva T, et al. Hallmarks of aging and immunosenescence: connecting the dots. *Cytokine Growth Factor Rev*. 2021;59:9–21.

Schrank G, Branch-Elliman W. Breaking the chain of infection in older adults: a review of risk factors and strategies for preventing device-related infections. *Infect Dis Clin North Am*. 2017;31(4):649–671.

Tal S, Guller V, Gurevich A, et al. Fever of unknown origin in the older adults. *Clin Geriatr Med*. 2007;23: 649–668.

Talbird SE, La EM, Carrico J, et al. Impact of population aging on the burden of vaccine-preventable diseases among older adults in the United States. *Hum Vaccines Immunother*. 2021;17(2):332–343.

Tinelli M, Tiseo G, Falcone M for the ESCMID Study Group for Infections in the Elderly. Prevention of the spread of multidrug-resistant organisms in nursing homes. *Aging Clin Exp Res*. 2021;33(3):679–687.

Wilcox MH, Gerding DN, Poxton IR, et al. Bezlotoxumab for prevention of recurrent *Clostridium difficile* infection. *N Engl J Med*. 2017;376:305–317.

Youngster I, Russell GH, Pindar C, et al. Oral, capsulized, frozen fecal microbiota transplantation for relapsing *Clostridium difficile* infection. *JAMA*. 2014;312: 1772–1778.

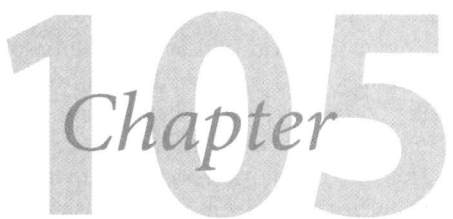

Chapter 105

Bacterial Pneumonia and Tuberculosis

Juan González del Castillo,
Francisco Javier Martín Sánchez

INTRODUCTION

In developed countries, pneumonia is a major cause of mortality and the most frequent cause of infectious death, as well as the leading cause of severe sepsis and septic shock. The incidence of pneumonia increases with age and is associated with high morbidity, mortality, and health care costs. Pneumonia in older adults affects a heterogeneous spectrum of patients; the assessment of clinical, cognitive, functional, and social issues is key to achieving correct ascertainment of most likely pathogens and thus initial antibiotic management, clinical decision making, and subsequent care planning.

DEFINITION

Pneumonia can be defined from three different points of view: the clinician, researcher, and pathologist. Pneumonia is clinically defined as the combination of symptoms (fever, chills, cough, pleuritic chest pain) and signs (hyper- or hypothermia, increased respiratory rate, dullness upon percussion, crackles, wheezing, pleural rub) associated with an opacity (or opacities) on a chest x-ray. In epidemiological or clinical trials, the presence of two or more of these symptoms, one or more of the physical signs, and a new opacity on the chest x-ray not due to other conditions (such as congestive heart failure, vasculitis, pulmonary infarction, drug reactions or atelectasis) is typically required for a diagnosis of pneumonia. From the pathologist point of view, pneumonia is an acute inflammatory process of the lung parenchyma in response to an infectious agent that affects the structures of the distal airways. The pneumonic process can predominantly develop in the alveoli (alveolar pneumonia), the interstitial space (interstitial pneumonia), or both (mixed pneumonia or diffuse alveolar damage). Alveolar pneumonia is predominantly exudative inflammation. Interstitial pneumonia is normally referred to as proliferative or productive, with inflammation in the stromal space and production of fibrous tissue, respectively. The histology of pneumonia depends on the state of progression, etiological agent, and host conditions, such as immune deficiency.

Pneumonia can also be defined in terms of the characteristics of the host, place of acquisition, and severity. As these circumstances are related to the etiology, we will address them in the etiology section.

Learning Objectives

- Identify the critical differences in presentation, etiology, and management of pneumonia in older adults versus young adults.
- Determine risk factors for infection due to antibiotic-resistant organisms.
- Integrate pneumonia prevention measures into routine care of older adults.

Key Clinical Points

1. The diagnosis of pneumonia in older adults may be more complex due to the physiologic changes that occur with age and accumulation of comorbidity. Both promote subtle and/or atypical clinical presentations with fever, productive cough, and other classic signs being less common in older adults.

2. It is important to categorize older patients with pneumonia based on functional status, which predicts severity of illness and changes the likelihood of specific pathogens, including multidrug-resistant organisms.

3. Known risk factors for infection due to resistant pathogens include functional impairment, recent hospitalization, previous antibiotic treatment, the presence of indwelling devices, and severe illness. It is important to know local resistance rates to adapt antibiotic treatment choices.

4. An interdisciplinary approach to management is critical with a goal of preserving and/or recovering function. Shorter courses of therapy (5–7 days) have demonstrated effectiveness similar to longer courses for most patients with pneumonia including older adults.

5. Prevention measures, which diminish the incidence and severity of pneumonia in older adults, should be employed; these include immunization versus influenza and pneumococcal disease and optimized management of comorbidities.

The epidemiology of pneumonia is difficult to determine and even more so in older population; data differ across continents, states, and hospitals. It is estimated that pneumonia has an incidence of 2 to 10 cases per 1000 inhabitants per year. The risk is higher in males, and in both sexes increases dramatically with age. According to European and American registries, the incidence of pneumonia is 25 to 40 cases per 1000 inhabitants per year with a mortality rate of 7% to 35% in patients older than 65 years. This increased vulnerability associated with age is presumed to be due to physiologic changes in the immune response that occur during aging and a higher burden of associated chronic diseases that are cumulative with age.

Pneumonia causes more than 4 million annual outpatient visits in the United States. There are more than 1 million hospitalizations due to pneumonia each year and 600,000 occur in adults older than 65 years. Between 10% and 20% of hospitalized patients require admission to the intensive care unit (ICU). The mean length of stay in the hospital is 5 days, and the overall 30-day mortality rate is 23%. Mortality depends on the severity of the pneumonic episode, as well as age and associated risk factors. This ranges from 1% to 2% in young patients without comorbidity, to 25% to 50% in older adults with a severe comorbidity. The 30-day mortality rate is three times higher among those older than 85 years, compared to the group of patients aged 65 to 74. In the United States, more than 50,000 deaths per year are attributed to pneumonia and 85% occur in patients older than 65 years. The 30-day readmission rate is approximately 20%. Total cost of care for patients with pneumonia is over 17 billion dollars a year in the United States. The cost of treatment is mainly in seniors as total cost is primarily driven by hospitalization—responsible for 80% of economic resources devoted to this disease.

The presence of indwelling devices (nasogastric tube, urinary catheter), comorbidity (chronic obstructive pulmonary disease [COPD], diabetes, cancers, liver disease, heart disease, renal disease), tobacco use, malnutrition, splenectomy, and age extremes (older patients or children < 5 years) is associated with an increased risk of pneumonia. In older adults, other risk factors have also been described, such as swallowing disorders, use of sedatives, and the presence of disability and baseline functional status. Vaccination and the use of angiotensin-converting enzyme inhibitors (which may protect by stimulating cough mechanisms) are protective factors.

Summarizing briefly, when compared to young adults, pneumonia in older adults is associated with increased risk of morbidity, mortality, and functional impairment, with a higher percentage of admissions, more often to the ICU, a longer length of hospital stay, and increased use of health resources.

PATHOPHYSIOLOGY

Pneumonia is most frequently produced by the microaspiration of flora that colonizes the oropharynx and sinuses. A high percentage of silent oropharyngeal microaspiration has been demonstrated in older adults with community-acquired pneumonia (CAP). This microaspiration occurs in up to half of older patients hospitalized for pneumonia. A systematic review showed microaspiration risk factors include male gender, dementia, lung disease (COPD), and administration of certain drugs (antipsychotics, proton pump inhibitors); angiotensin-converting enzyme inhibitor use was protective. Taylor et al. simplified aspiration risk factors as the presence of chronic neurologic disorders, esophageal disease, decreased level of consciousness, and history of vomiting.

Other less common forms of infection are (1) direct inhalation of the infectious agent, as with the tubercle bacillus, influenza, and other respiratory viruses and fungi; (2) hematogenous spread, except in the case of staphylococcal pneumonia after a viral influenza infection; (3) contiguous spread of infection from a subphrenic abscess, esophageal rupture, or other anatomic breach; and (4) iatrogenic contamination (eg, through an endotracheal tube).

The probability of infection depends on the aspiration volume, the virulence of the bacteria and the host's defense mechanisms. Several factors have been described as causing a higher risk of pneumonia in older adults, such as physiologic changes associated with age, increase and severity of underlying diseases, and an increase in the number of hospitalizations. Age-associated changes in the respiratory system are a decrease in rib cage mobility and respiratory muscle strength, increases in "dead" space and residual volume, a decrease in the sensitivity of the respiratory centers to hypoxemia and hypercapnia, and modifications in the airway receptors. Changes in the immune system associated with aging, or immunosenescence, consist of a progressive reduction in the immune response that affects all components of both the innate and adaptive immune system (see Chapter 3). The most significant changes are alterations in mucosal barriers, favoring invasion by microorganisms; reduction of native T cells and the differentiation and proliferation of T cells; alteration of T-cell subtypes ($\downarrow$CD4+/$\uparrow$CD8+); B-lymphocyte deficiency and impaired production of specific antibodies; and cytokine imbalance ($\downarrow$ IL-2, IL-1, and IFN and $\uparrow$ IL-4, IL-6, IL-8, IL-10, and TNF). These modifications involve a greater risk for infection and rapid progression of infection, a poor response to vaccines, a lesser subjective sensation of shortness of breath, and increased susceptibility to bronchial and respiratory failure.

ETIOLOGY

A microbiologic diagnosis is generally difficult to establish, even when complex and invasive diagnostic methods are employed. The etiology is usually monomicrobial and, overall, the most common agent is *Streptococcus pneumoniae* (20%–65%) and should always be taken into account when choosing initial antibiotic coverage. With an increase in age, there is a reduction in the frequency of microorganisms conventionally known as *atypical (Legionella pneumophila, Mycoplasma pneumoniae,* and *Chlamydophila pneumoniae),* and there is a relative increase in the incidence of pneumonia due to *Haemophilus influenzae* and gram-negative bacilli (GNB). In a smaller percentage of cases, it appears that viruses are involved (12%–18%), and the strongest causative associations have been drawn with particularly influenza virus, respiratory syncytial virus (RSV), and human metapneumovirus (HPV); these three organisms may account for 8% to 14% of pneumonias in older adults—particularly during seasonal outbreaks.

Pneumonias are often classified by the etiologic agent (pneumococcal pneumonia, staphylococcal pneumonia, etc), but this approach is not very practical from a clinical point of view, as the causative pathogen is generally unknown at the time of diagnosis and is often never established. Therefore, initial treatment must be established empirically and may not be modifiable based on a microbiologic diagnosis. In clinical practice, it is more useful to consider other aspects to select initial therapy such as the immunocompetence of the host, the place of acquisition, the presence of risk factors for resistant microorganisms, and the severity of the acute episode.

Differentiation depending on the immunocompetence of the host is essential, as this frequently points to a totally different etiologic spectrum. The type of immunosuppression, intensity, and duration influence the etiology, management, and prognosis. Neutropenia favors pneumonia due to *Staphylococcus aureus* (SA), enteric GNB such as *Pseudomonas aeruginosa* (Ps), and fungi (especially *Aspergillus* spp, *Mucor,* or *Candida*). Cellular immunodeficiency, as in an advanced HIV infection, transplant patients, or those receiving immunosuppressive therapy, predisposes to bacterial pneumonia with a much larger spectrum than in immunocompetent patients, including Ps, SA, *L pneumophila,* tuberculosis, invasive fungal infections, *Pneumocystis jiroveci,* viral pneumonia due to *cytomegalovirus* or RSV, helminths, or protozoa.

Depending on the place of acquisition, pneumonia is classified as either CAP or hospital-acquired pneumonia (HAP). CAP is pneumonia that presents outside the hospital setting (and may be further differentiated into health care–associated pneumonia [HCAP]—see commentary below). HAP occurs after more than 48 hours of hospital stay or during 10 to 14 days after a hospital discharge. This differentiation is important due to the spectrum in microbial etiology. The microorganisms most frequently isolated in HAP are enteric GNB (*Klebsiella pneumoniae, Escherichia coli,* Ps, *Serratia marcescens,* and *Enterobacter* spp), followed by gram-positive cocci (SA). In severe HAP, Ps and *Acinetobacter* spp are the most common among gram-negative bacteria. Viruses and fungi are isolated less

frequently, but must be taken into account in immunocompromised patients. The etiology may vary depending on the period of time pneumonia develops. In early HAP (within 5 days), the most common etiology is enteric GNB (*E coli, K pneumoniae, Proteus,* and *Serratia*), *H influenzae,* SA, and *S pneumoniae.* In late HAP (more than 5 days), *Acinetobacter* spp, Ps, and methicillin-resistant SA (MRSA) increase in frequency. There are additional, specific risk factors associated with certain microorganisms that can guide the clinician toward a specific diagnosis in HAP. These risk factors can be useful when deciding the antibiotic treatment to establish (**Table 105-1**).

TABLE 105-1 ■ SPECIFIC RISK FACTORS FOR HOSPITAL-ACQUIRED PNEUMONIA	
	ASSOCIATED RISK FACTORS
Multidrug-resistant pathogen	• Previous antibiotic treatment • Hospitalization > 5 d in the previous 90 d • Increased resistance rate in the hospital • Residence in a nursing home • Home intravenous treatment (including antibiotics) • Chronic dialysis • Active wound care • Contact with a patient infected by a multidrug-resistant pathogen • Immunosuppressive disease and/or immunosuppressive therapy
Bacilli gram negative	• Underlying disease • Functional impairment
Pseudomonas, multidrug-resistant bacilli	• Recent intensive care unit admission • Previous antibiotic treatment • Chronic corticosteroid therapy • Structural lung disease • Late-onset nosocomial pneumonia
Legionella spp	• Chronic corticosteroid therapy • Hematologic cancer • Contact with contaminated water • Previous cases of nosocomial pneumonia caused by *Legionella* spp
Staphylococcus aureus	• Recent intensive care unit admission • Previous influenza • Colonization or prevalence of methicillin-resistant strains • Traumatic brain injury • Coma • Diabetes mellitus • Renal failure
Aspergillus spp	• Chronic corticosteroid therapy
Anaerobic organisms	• Poor oral hygiene • Decreased level of consciousness • Manipulation of the airway • Recent abdominal surgery

Health care–associated pneumonia (HCAP) can be defined as pneumonia that occurs in patients who meet one of the following criteria: (1) hospitalization for 2 days or more in the preceding 90 days; (2) residence in a nursing home or extended care facility; (3) home infusion therapy (including antibiotics); (4) chronic dialysis within 30 days; (5) home wound care; or (6) family member with multi-drug-resistant pathogen. However, this concept is currently under some scrutiny. Evidence provided by two large retrospective observational studies that included patients from the United States showed that those who met one of these criteria had a higher prevalence of pneumonia caused by MRSA or resistant GNB, such as Ps. These results have not been confirmed in studies carried out in European countries. Further, it has been documented that up to 50% of patients with pneumonia attending the emergency department may met criteria for HCAP and only 10% to 30% of these patients have infections caused by resistant bacteria. Therefore, the use of such criteria with high sensitivity and limited specificity may lead to excessive utilization of broad spectrum antimicrobials, unnecessary costs and an increased prevalence of resistant bacteria. Finally, the concept of HCAP does not take into account the severity of the disease, and it is well known that resistant bacteria appear most frequently in patients with severe disease. In conclusion, though widely employed and specifically identified in many guidelines, the HCAP concept lacks the necessary precision to identify a profile of patients at risk of infection by resistant organisms, and therefore an etiologic approach is recommended by many authors based on individual risk factors for infection caused by resistant organisms and severity of disease.

The etiology of CAP is influenced by comorbidities, basal functional status, severity of the acute episode, antimicrobial treatment received and contact with the hospital setting or place of residence. Therefore, an etiologic approach can also be recommended according to risk factors for resistant microorganisms and severity of disease. Several scales have been developed to rule out infection by multidrug-resistant microorganisms (MDRO). Shorr et al. proposed a scale that includes four items: recent hospitalization (4 points), admission from long-term care (3 points), hemodialysis (2 points), and critical illness (1 point). When the total score is zero, there is a high negative predictive value (84%) for MDRO. Aliberti et al. documented that independent MDRO risk factors were living in a nursing home and previous hospitalization in the last 90 days. Another study found that patients with clinical signs of severe pneumonia and presence of two risk factors (immunosuppression, hospitalization in the previous 90 days, severe dependence quantified with a Barthel index less than 50, and taking antibiotics within the previous 6 months) were associated with a higher frequency of MDRO (2% vs 27%).

It has been published that the probability of Ps or MRSA infection is increased in severe CAP, defined as a pneumonia that requires admission to an ICU or has a risk class V according to the Pneumonia Severity Index (PSI). If we consider the approach proposed by Ewig in Europe and by Brito and Niederman in the United States, when making an empirical treatment decision, the key would be the initial clinical severity status and the prior functional status. Thus, when there are at least two factors for multidrug resistance (severe pneumonia, hospitalization in the previous 90 days, residence in a nursing home, severe basal dependence for daily living activities, immunosuppression, or taking antibiotics during the previous 6 months), empiric coverage of MDRO is warranted.

Risk Factors for Uncommon Microorganisms

Colonization of the oropharynx may favor pneumonia due to unusual microorganisms through microaspiration. This is more common in older adults compared to younger patients. Risk factors for less common pathogens are shown in **Table 105-2**.

TABLE 105-2 ■ RISK FACTORS FOR INFECTION BY LESS COMMON PATHOGENS

MICROORGANISM	RISK FACTORS
Pseudomonas aeruginosa	• Severe COPD with $FEV_1 < 35\%$ • COPD > 4 cycles of antibiotic treatment in the last year • Bronchiectasis with previous colonization • Nasogastric enteral feeding • Intensive care unit admission
Enterobacteriaceae and/or anaerobic organisms	• Functional impairment • Risk factors for aspiration • Dysphagia • Gastroesophageal reflux • History of vomiting • Cerebrovascular diseases • Dementia • Periodontal disease • Poor oral hygiene
Extended-spectrum β-lactamase–producing *Enterobacteriaceae*	• Previous antibiotic • Hemodialysis • Long-term indwelling urinary catheter • Residence in long stay center • Recent hospitalization • Diabetes mellitus • Recurrent urinary tract infections
S aureus resistant to methicillin	• Undergoing care for bedsores or wounds • Clinically serious illness + recent hospitalization + prior intravenous antibiotics + institutionalization • Previous colonization • Superinfection of pneumonia virus influenza during influenza epidemic

Bacterial colonization depends on multiple factors such as age, comorbidity, basal functional status, bacterial load, antimicrobial use, presence of devices, indwelling devices, and prior contact with health centers or nursing homes. Etiologic studies show an increased incidence of pneumonia due to *Enterobacteriaceae* in relation to age. El-Solh et al. identified *Enterobacteriaceae* and anaerobes as the most frequently isolated pathogens in institutionalized patients with aspiration pneumonia with the basal functional status as main determining factor. This study concluded that functional impairment is associated with more frequent colonization by GNB, especially *Enterobacteriaceae*. Another important aspect to consider in suspected infection by *Enterobacteriaceae* is whether they may produce extended-spectrum β-lactamase (ESBL). A recent study with the aim to determine the sensitivity of strains isolated from patients hospitalized with pneumonia, in both the United States and Europe, showed that 20% and 35% of isolated *Klebsiella* spp (the main *Enterobacteriaceae* involved in pneumonia) were ESBL-producing in each geographical area.

Despite recognized classical risk factors for anaerobic infection, the role of anaerobes in pneumonia in seniors is not well known because anaerobic cultures or other detection methods are rarely used in studies.

The frequency of Ps in older adults is low (1%–2%). Chronic respiratory disease and nasogastric tube use stand out as the main risk factors. This microorganism should be suspected in severe COPD (FEV$_1$ < 35% predicted), multiple previous antibiotic treatments, admission to ICU and/or presence of bronchiectasis, and prior colonization with this organism.

Finally, it is known that colonization by SA is more frequent when there has been a prior episode of influenza. The probability of MRSA is more frequent in patients admitted in the ICU, with a history of intravenous antibiotic treatment at home or undergoing ulcer care. Shorr et al. proposed a scale to predict MRSA infections with low risk if the score is less than or equal to 1 (2 points: recent hospitalization or ICU admission; 1 point for each of the following: < 30 or > 79 years of age, prior exposure to intravenous antibiotics, dementia, cerebrovascular disease, being a female with diabetes, coming from a residential care home). MRSA infection should be suspected with the presence of pneumonia with bilateral radiological infiltrates with cavitation or in the presence of risk factors, and primarily in patients with severe disease. If the older patient has been living in a nursing home during the previous year, it is important to know the prevalence of MRSA in that institution.

Viral etiologies are increasingly recognized with wider utilization of PCR-based respiratory virus panels. In particular, influenza and RSV cause substantial morbidity and mortality in older adults. In the context of outbreaks in institutionalized patients, pneumonia can be caused either by primary viral agents or by a bacterial superinfection

TABLE 105-3 ■ CLINICAL AND EPIDEMIOLOGIC CONDITIONS RELATED TO SPECIFIC PATHOGENS

CLINICAL AND EPIDEMIOLOGIC CONDITION	ETIOLOGY
COPD, tobacco addiction	*S pneumoniae, H influenzae, C pneumoniae, L pneumophila*
Bronchiectasis, cystic fibrosis	*P aeruginosa, S aureus*
Alcohol intoxication	*S pneumoniae, K pneumoniae,* anaerobes, *S aureus*
Prison inmates	*S pneumoniae, M tuberculosis*
Contact with birds, fowl, and farm animals	*Chlamydophila psittaci*
Contact with rabbits	*Coxiella burnetii*
Contact with bats or residence in an endemic area	*Histoplasma capsulatum*
Flu epidemic	Virus influenza, *S pneumoniae, H influenzae, S aureus*
Septic mouth, aspiration	Polymicrobial, anaerobes
Advanced HIV infection	*S pneumoniae, H influenzae, P jiroveci, M tuberculosis*
Intravenous drug users	*S aureus,* anaerobes
Steroid treatment	*S aureus, Aspergillus* spp, *L pneumophila*
Comorbidities (diabetes, liver disease, renal failure)	*S pneumoniae, H influenzae,* gram-negative bacilli
Recent antibiotic use	*S pneumoniae* resistant, *P aeruginosa*
Exposure to air conditioning, cooling towers	*L pneumophila*
Travel to Southeast Asia	*B pseudomallei,* avian influenza virus

COPD, chronic obstructive pulmonary disease.

from *S pneumoniae*, SA, and *H influenzae*. Other respiratory viruses, such as parainfluenza, metapneumovirus, adenovirus, rhinovirus, and coronavirus (except for SARS-CoV-2), usually cause less severe respiratory infections in immunocompetent adults.

Finally, there are a number of epidemiologic factors that predispose patients to CAP caused by certain specific agents (**Table 105-3**). **Figure 105-1** depicts an etiologic approach for older patients based on severity of illness, risk factors, and basal functional status to help guide the most appropriate empiric selection of antibiotic coverage.

PRESENTATION

Clinical diagnosis of pneumonia in older adults is complex and may be subtle. Symptoms and signs of infection in older adults differ from younger patients. Asymptomatic or atypical clinical presentations such as exacerbation of chronic diseases are more frequent presenting manifestations in older adults. Absence of fever, hypoxemia, or respiratory

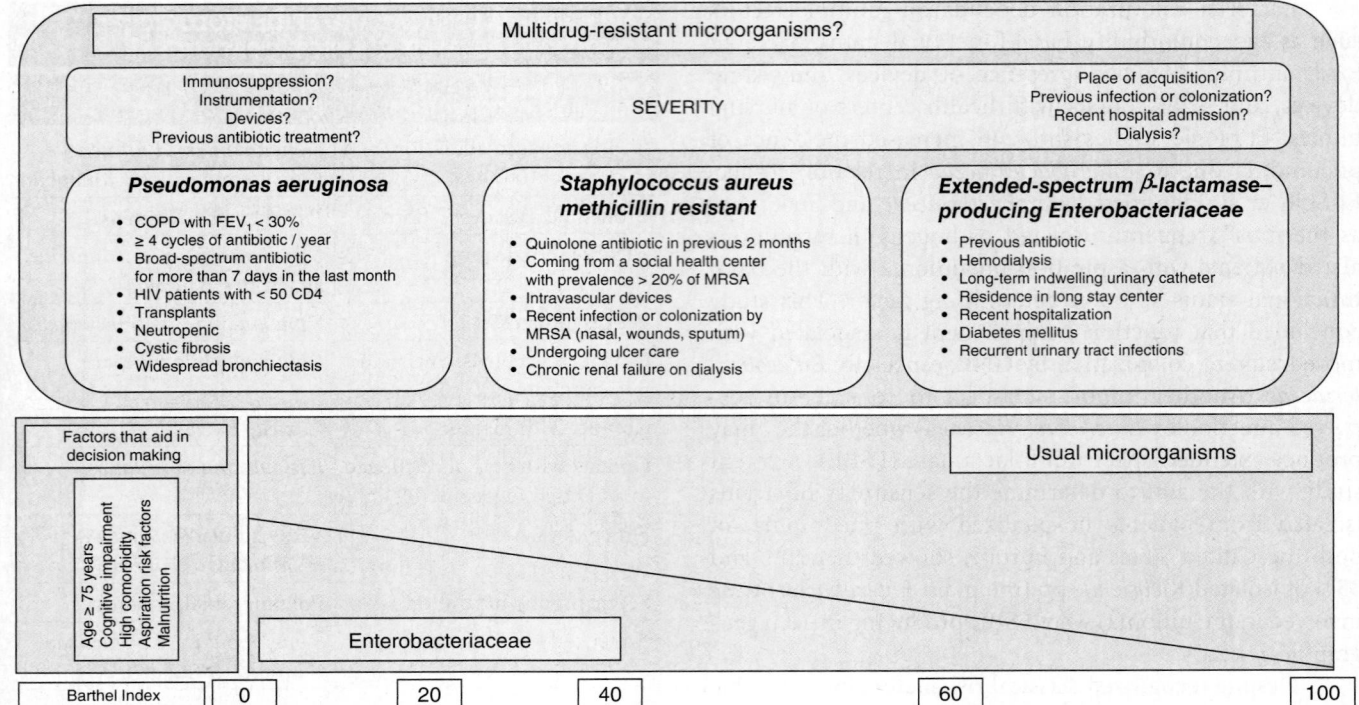

FIGURE 105-1. The Pneumonia Severity Index (PSI) is used to calculate the need for admission and probability of death due to pneumonia based on specific patient characteristics, physical examination, and laboratory findings at presentation. Age is a major driver of the PSI.

symptoms do not rule out a pneumonia diagnosis. The most common atypical manifestations are altered mental status or behavior, acute functional impairment, falls, dizziness, loss of consciousness, generalized weakness, anorexia, dehydration, or incontinence. Such presenting symptoms are most frequently associated with the presence of cognitive impairment.

EVALUATION

Initial Evaluation

At the time of initial assessment of the older patient with pneumonia stratification by severity of illness should be performed based on the level of consciousness, respiratory, and hemodynamic parameters, taking into account medical, functional, and/or cognitive situations. Nonspecific complaints or atypical clinical presentation are associated with a lower level of acuity and therefore a delay in the initial assessment and early antibiotic administration in the emergency department. Older adults less frequently have fever, tachycardia, and/or elevation of leukocytes compared with younger patients. These changes may hinder an appropriate diagnosis of sepsis and impact adequate early therapeutic treatment. A recent study has shown that the undisturbed vital signs such as normal heart rate and temperature in older patients with suspected infection delay antibiotic administration and increase the likelihood of hospitalization with the need for intensive care. Therefore, respiratory

rate and altered level of consciousness may be the only initial signs of severity in older patients with suspected infection and should trigger evaluation for pneumonia.

Diagnostic Evaluation

After the initial stratification of severity status, tests should be performed to diagnose pneumonia and its etiology. The diagnosis of pneumonia based on physical examination has poor sensitivity and specificity; therefore, the diagnosis should be confirmed by performing a chest x-ray.

The diagnostic tests performed in older adults should not differ from those in younger patients. In daily clinical practice, the chest x-ray is usually enough to rule in the diagnosis of pneumonia in most older patients. However, radiologic signs may not be obvious in up to 30% of the cases and this is more frequent in patients with dehydration and neutropenia. Therefore, in patients with suspected pneumonia and first chest x-ray without pathologic signs, a second study is recommended after 24 to 48 hours. Computed tomography (CT) is very accurate for the diagnosis of pneumonia, although it is usually reserved either for patients with atypical chest x-ray patterns or as a second step in those cases without response to initial treatment. The role of other imaging tests is evolving. Bedside ultrasound can support suspicion of pneumonia and allows evaluation of suspected pleural effusion as well as guidance for a possible thoracentesis. Other procedures, such as bronchoscopy, CT-guided biopsy, biopsy by thoracotomy, or videothoracoscopy, do not differ from indications in younger adults, except for the logical consideration of the patient's life expectancy, desires, and the risks and contraindications related to comorbidities.

Regarding laboratory tests, C-reactive protein and white blood cell counts are not helpful for assessing the severity of illness in older patients with pneumonia. The inflammatory response may be impaired as a consequence of immune senescence and thus may underestimate the severity of the process. Procalcitonin (PCT) has not shown good sensitivity in older populations for the diagnosis of acute bacterial infection, although it may be useful for severity assessment.

Serum lactate value greater than or equal to 2 mmol/L is a predictor of 30-day mortality in older adults. MR-pro-ADM is a peptide produced by the endothelium, derived from proadrenomedullin, which is released in a state of physiologic stress. It has been evaluated in observational studies and seems to perform well as a prognostic marker in respiratory infection.

A microbiologic diagnosis should be sought in older adults with pneumonia via blood cultures, Gram stain and culture of respiratory samples, and the detection of bacterial antigens in urine (pneumococcal and *Legionella* immunochromatographic test). European guidelines recommend the performance of blood cultures in all hospitalized patients. US guidelines reserve blood cultures for the most severe patients, such as those with cavitary infiltrates, leukopenia, alcoholism, severe liver disease, asplenia, positive antigenuria test for pneumococcus, or pleural effusion. Blood cultures have low clinical impact when performed in unselected patients with CAP. However, given the high frequency of atypical clinical presentation in older patients, blood cultures may contribute both to the confirmation of diagnostic suspicions, when potential pulmonary pathogens are isolated, and to the reconsideration of the patient's primary causative agent and therefore it is the opinion of this author that blood cultures should be obtained in all older adults with pneumonia. Adequate sputum cultures can be obtained in about a third of patients, even higher when performed by invasive methods. The importance of Gram stain and sputum culture is reflected in its influence in the modification of the initial antibiotic treatment. The presence of SA, *Klebsiella pneumoniae*, or Ps in Gram stain of the purulent sputum requires consideration when choosing the antibiotic treatment. Likewise, absence of organisms with the morphology of these agents in high-quality respiratory samples has a high negative predictive value, allowing the narrowing of antimicrobial therapy. In older patients with significant functional impairment, it is often difficult to obtain quality sputum specimens, and an increase in frequency of oropharyngeal colonization by GNB, SA, and MDRO suggests there may be lower specificity of Gram stain and culture of respiratory specimens from such patients.

Detecting pneumococcal and *L pneumophila* bacterial antigens in urine by immunochromatographic techniques has been an important advance in the identification of these two microorganisms. The sensitivity of pneumococcal antigen is estimated at over 60%, with a specificity greater than 90% in adult patients, including patients with chronic bronchitis and pneumococcal colonization. It also has diagnostic value in the pleural fluid and test performance is not altered by prior antibiotic treatment or pneumococcal vaccination. However, the test remains positive until 3 months after the resolution of pneumonia, which limits the utility in patients with recurrences or in the assessment of treatment response. The urinary antigen test for legionellosis only detects *L pneumophila* serogroup I, with a sensitivity greater than 90%. This is recommended in all patients with suspected clinical or epidemiologic concern for legionellosis or in the case of severe pneumonia without another clear etiology.

Test for viral detection in nasopharyngeal aspirates should be used in epidemiologic studies and in those patients diagnosed with influenza who are candidates for antiviral treatment. The best use of these tests has not been defined as many viruses that can cause illness are not represented on widely used viral panels (decreasing sensitivity) and a positive test may not provide sufficient evidence of an alternate diagnosis to allow the clinician to stop antibacterial therapy (limited specificity).

Risk Stratification

The assessment of severity status is essential to designing an individualized care plan for older patients with pneumonia; age, comorbidity, microbial etiology, and early administration of appropriate antibiotic therapy all influence mortality. Previous studies have showed that older pneumonia patients with moderate-severe basal functional dependence have an increased risk of mortality in the short- and long-term compared to those who are independent.

Several short-term prognostic scales have been published that are helpful for assessing severity status and therefore the decision making for hospital admission. The PSI (**Figure 105-2**) and CURB-65 (**Table 105-4**) are risk stratification scales with similar predictive power for 30-day mortality, although they have certain limitations. The PSI gives excessive weight to age and relative to hypoxemia and it does not take into account other factors associated with adverse outcomes such as COPD, functional status, social factors, proper oral intake of the patient, or the capacity for good adherence. CURB-65 has the limitation of not including the evaluation of hypoxemia and functional status. In fact, studies have suggested oxygenation as the best prognostic indicator in older adults. Neither of these two scales is very useful in assessing the need for ICU admission.

In clinical decision making related to ICU admission, other scales have been developed, such as Severity of Community-Acquired Pneumonia (SCAP), SMART-COP, or the American Thoracic Society/Infectious Diseases Society of America (ATS/IDSA) scale (**Tables 105-5 to 105-7**). SCAP identifies patients who require monitoring and more aggressive treatment and it is very useful for

Age > 50 years	NO	YES
Cancer	NO	YES
Liver disease	NO	YES
Cardiac failure	NO	YES
Cerebrovascular disease	NO	YES
Kidney disease	NO	YES
Confusion	NO	YES
Systolic BP < 90 mm Hg	NO	YES
HR ≥ 125 bpm	NO	YES
RR ≥ 30 bpm	NO	YES
TA < 35 or > 40°C	NO	YES

If any answer is yes calculate PSI using the following:
(The arrow points to the table that the reader should use.)

Group	Score	Mortality rate (%)
I	≤ 50 years and without risk predictors[1]	0.1
II	≤ 70	0.6
III	71–90	2.8
IV	91–130	8.2
V	> 130	29.2

Patient characteristics	Points assigned
Demographic factors	
Age (men)	Number of years
Age (women)	Number of years − 10
Nursing home resident	Number of years + 10
Comorbidity	
Cancer	+ 30
Liver disease	+ 20
Cardiac failure	+ 10
Cerebrovascular disease	+ 10
Nephropathy	+ 10
Physical examination	
Altered level of consciousness	+ 20
Respiratory rate ≥ 30 bpm	+ 20
Systolic BP < 90 mm Hg	+ 20
TA < 35°C or > 40°C	+ 15
HR ≥ 125 bpm	+ 10
Laboratory findings	
Arterial pH < 7.35	+ 30
Urea > 60 mg / dl or creatinine > 1.5 mg/dl	+ 20
Na < 130 mEq/l	+ 20
Glucose > 250 mg/dl	+ 10
Hematocrit < 30%	+ 10
PaO_2 < 60 mm Hg or $SatO_2$ < 90%	+ 10
Pleural effusion	+ 10

[1] Predictors of risk: cancer, cardiac failure, cerebrovascular disease, liver or kidney disease.
BP: blood pressure; HR: heart rate; RR: respiratory rate; TA: axillary temperature.

FIGURE 105-2. Pneumonia severity should be assessed according to the clinical situation, biomarkers, and risk stratification scales. In severe cases, the possibility of infection by resistant microorganisms is increased; therefore, expanded antimicrobial therapy should be considered, especially when a risk factor is present. Infection by resistant pathogens should be considered, and likelihood of infection by *Pseudomonas aeruginosa*, methicillin-resistant *Staphylococcus aureus*, or extended-spectrum β-lactamase–producing *Enterobacteriaceae* specifically assessed to choose antibiotic coverage. Colonization of the oropharynx by *Enterobacteriaceae* is more likely in those with severe functional dependence.

predicting hospital mortality and/or the need for mechanical ventilation or inotropic support. SMART-COP is useful to decide on a more aggressive treatment, without necessarily predicting ICU admission.

The detection of frailty and vulnerability by screening scales, such as Identification of Seniors at Risk (ISAR) or Triage Risk Screening Tool (TRST), or comprehensive geriatric assessment is particularly valuable to predict short-term adverse outcomes and decision making about diagnostic and therapeutic procedures and the most appropriate site of care.

There are other independent and dynamic factors that influence prognosis regarding the infection itself and

TABLE 105-4 ■ PROGNOSTIC SCALES: CURB-65

A POINT IS APPLIED FOR EACH ITEM PRESENT

C	Confusion
U	Urea plasmatic > 44 mg/dL (BUN > 20 mg/dL)
R	Respiratory rate ≥ 30 bpm
B	Systolic BP < 90 mm Hg or diastolic BP ≤ 60 mm Hg
65	Age ≥ 65
Score	Stratification
0 or 1	Low mortality (0.7%–2.1%). Possible outpatient treatment
2	Intermediate mortality (9.2%). Consider hospital treatment
3	High mortality (15%). Hospital admission.
4–5	Mortality of > 40%. Admission. Consider intensive care unit

TABLE 105-5 ■ PROGNOSTIC SCALES: SEVERITY OF COMMUNITY-ACQUIRED PNEUMONIA (SCAP)

MAJOR CRITERIA	MINOR CRITERIA
pH < 7.30 (13 points)	C: confusion (5 points)
	U: BUN > 30 mg/dL (5 points)
Systolic blood pressure < 90 mm Hg (11 points)	R: breaths per minute > 30 (9 points)
	X: multilobar/bilateral chest x-ray (5 points)
	O: PaO_2 < 54 mm Hg or PaO_2/FiO_2 < 250 mm Hg (6 points)
	80: Age ≥ 80 (5 points)

Low risk: 0–1 (< 10 points); intermediate risk: 2 (10–19 points); high risk: 3–4 (> 20 points).

TABLE 105-6 ■ PROGNOSTIC SCALES: SMART-COP

S Systolic BP < 90 mm Hg (2 points)	**C** Confusion (1 point)
M Multilobar affectation (1 point)	**O** Oxygenation age-adjusted[b] (2 points)
A Albumin < 3.5 g/dL (1 point)	**P** pH < 7.35 (2 points)
R RR age-adjusted[a] (1 point)	
T Tachycardia ≥ 125 (1 point)	

[a] < 50 years: ≥ 25/min; ≥ 50 years: ≥ 30/min.
[b] < 50 years: PaO_2 < 70 Hg or oxygen saturation ≤ 93% or PaO_2 / FiO_2 < 333; ≥ 50 years: PaO_2 < 60 mm Hg or oxygen saturation ≤ 90% or PaO_2/FiO_2 < 250.
0–2 points: low risk for vasopressor support or intensive respiratory support.
3–4 points: moderate risk for vasopressor support or intensive respiratory support.
5–6 points: high risk for vasopressor support or intensive respiratory support.
≥ 7 points: very high risk for vasopressor support or intensive respiratory support.

the systemic inflammatory response. Therefore, the probability of bacteremia, the presence of sepsis, severe sepsis or septic shock, and the inclusion of biomarkers should be taken into account in the decision-making process. As discussed previously, sepsis may be underdiagnosed in older adults due to physiologic changes with aging.

Site of Care

Clinical guidelines recommend the use of prognostic scales, mainly PSI and CURB-65, for admission decision making. Patients with PSI greater than or equal to III or CURB-65 greater than or equal to 2 meet criteria for hospital admission. The SCAP, SMART-COP, or ATS/IDSA scales can be helpful when deciding on ICU admission. In addition, other issues should be considered regarding site of care such as functional, cognitive, and social factors that may affect the final location.

TABLE 105-7 ■ PROGNOSTIC SCALES: ATS/IDSA

MAJOR CRITERIA
Need for mechanical ventilation
Septic shock

MINOR CRITERIA
Systolic blood pressure < 90 mm Hg requiring fluid
Multilobar involvement (≥ 2 lobes) or progression
Respiratory rate ≥ 30 bpm
Confusion
Urea ≥ 45 mg/dL
PaO_2/FiO_2 ≤ 250
Leukopenia < 4000/mm³
Thrombocytopenia < 100,000/mm³
Hypothermia (temperature < 97°F or 36°C)
Metabolic acidosis
Lactate > 3 mmol/L or > 27 mg/dL
Hyponatremia
Hyperglycemia in nondiabetic
Alcohol intake

ICU admission if one major or three minor criteria are met.

Alternatives to Conventional Hospitalization

There are different units that can treat patients with CAP. A short stay unit (SSU) is a safe and cost-effective alternative to conventional hospitalization for patients with CURB-65 of 2 or PSI of III. In those seniors living in a nursing home, site of care depends on the characteristics of the center, but if appropriate care can be rendered without moving the patient, it is preferable. Several studies have shown the same mortality, adjusted by functional status, among patients treated in the hospital or in nursing home. Transfer to hospital should be under the following circumstances: worsening of underlying disease, immunosuppression, clinical signs of severe pneumonia, oral intolerance, difficulties in completing the treatment in the facility, complications evident on radiography, or individual assessment (eg, need for specific isolation or high risk of morbidity and mortality without advanced directive).

Considerations for Discharge

Clinical stabilization is considered present when vital signs have normalized, mental status is baseline, and oxygen requirements have improved. The criteria that should be met to discharge the patient include heart rate less than 100 bpm, respiratory rate less than 24 breaths per minute, axillary temperature less than 37.2°C (< 98.96°F), systolic blood pressure greater than 90 mm Hg, oxygen saturation greater than 90%, good awareness, and tolerance of oral therapy. Most patients with pneumonia usually stabilize between the third and fourth hospital day. However, this period of time may increase up to 7 days in the frail older adults.

Specific Recommendations for Antibiotic Selection in Older Adults

Table 105-8 outlines empirical treatment recommendations according to site of care, functional status, and severity. **Table 105-9** reflects the treatment of choice depending on the suspected etiology. Regarding HAP, treatment depends on start time (early or late) and the patient's individual risk factors (**Table 105-10**). **Table 105-11** shows the dosing information for the main antimicrobials used to treat pneumonia.

Given the heterogeneity of older patients and individual risk factors for specific microorganisms, two questions should drive antibiotic treatment choice. First, does the patient have a severe pneumonia or risk factors for unusual microorganisms? And second, does the patient meet the definition of frailty? If the answer to both questions is "no," therapeutic regimens commonly used in younger adults apply; if the patient has severe pneumonia and/or risk factors for less common pathogens, resistant microorganisms are more likely, and broadening antimicrobial treatment should be considered.

The issue of frailty is more complex. Mildly frail seniors (ie, independent or nearly independent for all basic ADLs) at baseline may suffer acute functional and/or cognitive impairment with pneumonia. In this case,

TABLE 105-8 ■ TREATMENT OF COMMUNITY-ACQUIRED PNEUMONIA IN OLDER ADULTS

	SCENARIO	TREATMENT
Patient without frailty	Outpatient treatment	Amoxicillin/clavulanate or second-generation cephalosporin + Azithromycin or fluoroquinolone
	Inpatient treatment	Amoxicillin/clavulanate or ceftriaxone or cefotaxime or ceftaroline + Azithromycin or fluoroquinolone
	Severe pneumonia	Ceftriaxone or cefotaxime or ceftaroline or ertapenem + Azithromycin or fluoroquinolone ± Linezolid[a] or vancomycin[a] ± Antipseudomonal β-lactam[b] ± Oseltamivir[c]
Patient with frailty	Prefrailty[d]	Amoxicillin/clavulanate or ceftriaxone or cefotaxime or ceftaroline + Azithromycin or fluoroquinolone
	Frail	Ertapenem or Amoxicillin/clavulanate[e] or Ceftriaxone + clindamycin[e]

[a]If there are risk factors for *Staphylococcus aureus*.
[b]If there are risk factors for infection by *Pseudomonas aeruginosa*.
[c]Assess if influenza is epidemic in the community.
[d]Be particularly cautious rating risk factors of microaspiration and multiresistant bacteria.
[e]Consider local resistance rates of *Enterobacteriaceae* to amoxicillin/clavulanate and ceftriaxone; and anaerobes to clindamycin.

TABLE 105-9 ■ DIRECTED ANTIBIOTIC TREATMENT IN PNEUMONIA FOR SPECIFIC PATHOGENS

MICROORGANISMS	TREATMENT
Enterobacteriaceae/ anaerobes	Ertapenem or Amoxicillin/clavulanate[a] or Ceftriaxone + clindamycin[a]
Extended-spectrum β-lactamase–producing *Enterobacteriaceae*	Ertapenem
Staphylococcus aureus methicillin resistant	Add linezolid or vancomycin to chosen treatment
Pseudomonas aeruginosa	Piperacillin/tazobactam or Imipenem or meropenem or Cefepime + Levofloxacin or ciprofloxacin or Amikacin or tobramycin

[a]Consider local resistance rate of *Enterobacteriaceae* to amoxicillin/clavulanate and ceftriaxone and anaerobes to clindamycin.

monitoring of clinical, functional, and cognitive areas and interventions to restore function to the previous baseline should be paramount and part of the overall treatment plan. The same antibiotic choices as those used for independent patients suffice.

In moderate-severe frailty, the invasive diagnostic and therapeutic procedures depend on individual goals and the site of care. Furthermore, these patients usually have severe

TABLE 105-10 ■ EMPIRICAL ANTIBIOTIC TREATMENT FOR HOSPITAL-ACQUIRED PNEUMONIA (HAP)

Group I early HAP (< 5 d) without risk factors	Ceftriaxone or cefotaxime or ceftaroline or Fluoroquinolone
Group II late HAP (≥ 5 d) or with risk factors	Ceftazidime or cefepime or imipenem or meropenem or piperacillin/tazobactam + Ciprofloxacin or levofloxacin or amikacin or tobramycin ± Linezolid or vancomycin

TABLE 105-11 ■ DOSAGE OF THE MAIN ANTIBIOTICS USED IN PNEUMONIA

ANTIBIOTIC	DOSE	DOSE IN RENAL INSUFFICIENCY (mL/min)	
Amikacin	15–20 mg/kg/24 h	60–80: 9–12 mg/kg/24 h 30–40: 4.5–6 mg/kg/24 h 10–20: 1.5–3 mg/kg/24 h	40–60: 6–9 mg/kg/24 h 20–30: 3–4.5 mg/kg/24 h < 10: 1–1.5 mg/kg/24 h
Amoxicillin/clavulanate IV	2 g/6–8 h	30–50: 1 g/8 h < 10: 500 mg/24 h	10–30: 500 mg/12 h
Amoxicillin/clavulanate PO	2/0.125 g/12 h	30–50: 500 mg/8 h < 10: 500 mg/24 h	10–30: 500 mg/12 h
Azithromycin IV/PO	500 mg/24 h	No adjustment required	
Cefditoren PO	400 mg/12 h	30–50: 200 mg/12 h	< 30: 200 mg/24 h
Cefepime IV	2 g/8 h	30–50: 2 g/12 h < 10: 1 g/24 h	10–30: 2 g/24 h
Ceftriaxone IV	1–2 g/12–24 h	> 10: not required	< 10: maximum 2 g/24 h
Ciprofloxacin IV	400 mg/12 h	30–50: not required	< 30: 200 mg/12 h
Ciprofloxacin PO	500 mg/12 h	30–50: not required	< 30: 250 mg/12 h
Ertapenem IV/IM	1 g/24 h	< 30: 500 mg/24 h	
Imipenem IV	1 g/6–8 h	30–50: 250–500 mg/6–8 h	< 30: 250–500 mg/12 h
Levofloxacin IV/PO	500 mg/12–24 h	20–50: 250 mg/12–24 h < 10: 125 mg/24 h	10–20: 125 mg/12–24 h
Linezolid IV/PO	600 mg/12 h	No adjustment required	
Meropenem IV	1 g/8 h	30–50: 1 g/12 h < 10: 500 mg/24 h	10–30: 500 mg/12 h
Moxifloxacin IV/PO	400 mg/24 h	No adjustment required	
Piperacillin/tazobactam IV	4/0.5 g/6–8 h	20–50: 2/0.25 g/6 h	< 20: 2/0.25 g/8 h
Tobramycin IV	4–7 mg/kg/24 h	60–80: 4 mg/kg/24 h 30–40: 2.5 mg/kg/24 h 10–20: 1.5 mg/kg/24 h	40–60: 3.5 mg/kg/24 h 20–30: 2 mg/kg/24 h

IM, intramuscular; IV, intravenous; PO, oral.

comorbidity and polypharmacy, making them more vulnerable to the occurrence of adverse drug reactions. In addition, there may be important risk factors that determine specific etiologic risk (MDRO or MRSA colonization, aspiration risk, etc). Antibiotic choices in such patients must include broader coverage in addition to routine pathogens.

The first antibiotic dose should be administered as soon as possible because a shorter interval to effective therapy is associated with decreased length of hospital stay and mortality, both in nonsevere patients and in those who present with severe sepsis or septic shock. Combination therapy is indicated in patients that meet criteria for ICU admission; β-lactam and a macrolide or fluoroquinolone are superior to fluoroquinolone monotherapy. If influenza is circulating in the community, oseltamivir should be added, even if more than 48 hours have passed since symptom onset, and treatment against *S aureus* provided until cultures suggest otherwise. In patients with risk factors, empiric MRSA treatment is advisable while awaiting conventional cultures and nasopharyngeal swabs—specific treatment against MRSA should be suspended if these are negative.

Intracellular pathogens are less common in older patients compared to younger patients, and the need for coverage of atypical pathogens is currently a point of discussion. In some studies, the incidence of "atypical pneumonia" can reach 50% and mixed infections may represent 10% to 15% of cases. There is some controversy, except for *L pneumophila*, regarding the benefit of atypical pathogen coverage; American guidelines recommend adequate coverage of atypical pathogens in all cases, while the British guidelines limit it to patients requiring hospitalization. For *L pneumophila*, recent studies show similar rates of causality in nonsevere pneumonia and those requiring hospitalization. Therefore, if it is not possible to rule out infection due to *Legionella*, a macrolide or respiratory quinolone should be given with a β-lactam. In case of suspected pulmonary tuberculosis, quinolones should not be prescribed due to their tuberculostatic activity and the possibility of delaying the diagnosis of pulmonary tuberculosis.

Finally, it should be emphasized that aging produces certain pharmacokinetic and pharmacodynamic modifications of drugs. Doses and intervals must be adapted to the older patient's body weight (or body mass index) and renal function, and modified by drug interactions. Underdosing antibiotics have severe consequences and should be avoided as vigorously as overdosing to ensure the best outcome and reduce the risk of emergence of antibiotic-resistant pathogens.

Switch From Intravenous to Oral Antibiotics and Duration of Therapy

After reaching clinical stability, a switch from intravenous to oral antibiotic formulations is safe and reduces length of hospital stay with equivalent outcomes. The presence of bacteremia does not extend the required duration of intravenous antibiotic therapy. Isolation of a causative organism should prompt de-escalation to specific, narrowed coverage, but when no organism is isolated, it is advisable to complete therapy using and oral equivalent with respect to the spectrum of activity.

Meta-analyses suggest 5 to 7 days of antibiotic treatment is sufficient to cure pneumonia even in older adults. However, there are exceptions, and treatment should be extended in cases of infection by *Legionella*, resistant GNB, or MRSA. In addition, there are clinical situations that may also involve an extension of the duration, such as persistent fever over 72 hours, persistence of more than one criterion of clinical instability, inadequate initial coverage, or the occurrence of complications.

Treatment Failure

Treatment failure is defined as the absence of clinical stability after 3 to 4 days of antibiotic treatment or the occurrence of clinical deterioration, respiratory failure, or septic shock in the first 72 hours. This situation is associated with a five-fold increase in mortality. However, reaching clinical stability may take longer without implying a therapeutic failure in older patients with severe pneumonia or concomitant serious comorbidity such as severe COPD or untreated heart failure.

Possible causes of treatment failure include resistant microorganisms, involvement of unusual pathogens, lack of optimized treatment for comorbidity, or the existence of an undiagnosed concomitant process (eg, pulmonary embolism, neoplasm).

When treatment failure is suspected antibiotics should be changed if culture data suggest a pathogen resistant to antibiotics being given, comorbidity treatment optimized, and new imaging studies may be of value. Broadening the antimicrobial spectrum should follow, and risk factors for unusual pathogens reevaluated or the possibility of infection by fungi, mycobacteria, *Nocardia*, and other unusual pathogens reconsidered.

Concomitant Treatment

In conjunction with antibiotic treatment, other therapeutic measures should be carried out such as proper oxygenation (including initial appraisal of noninvasive mechanical ventilation, especially in patients with respiratory failure), fluid balance, and the correction of electrolyte disturbances, glycemic control, management of associated comorbidities, nutritional support if needed, and the prevention of thromboembolic events. Early physical and cognitive stimulation is very important, even for inpatients; early mobilization is recommended, if possible from the first day of admission, seating the patient out of bed for a minimum of 20 minutes and subsequent progressive mobilization recommended.

Palliative Treatment

Pneumonia is a common complication in older patients with advanced dementia and limited life prognosis, often being the final cause of death. The identification of these patients is very important in order to provide adequate palliative treatment, since in this patient profile clear benefits of intravenous antibiotic therapy have not been proven. Withholding antibiotics may be very appropriate for some patients and palliative treatment only considered individually.

PREVENTION

Given the high incidence, morbidity, and mortality of pneumonia in older adults, preventive measures, especially vaccination, are critical. This becomes even more important in institutionalized older adults, where "herd" immunity plays a major role in reducing risk. Vaccination against influenza and pneumococcus is recommended for all patients aged 65 and older. Despite the existence of a reduced response to vaccination, particularly in frail seniors, risk of infection, mortality, and associated complications is lower in patients vaccinated against influenza and pneumococcus compared with those unvaccinated. Recently, conjugate vaccine (PCV13) has been recommended in addition to polysaccharide for all adults aged 65 and older. According to the Advisory Committee for Immunization Practices (ACIP), PCV13 should be given first with PPS given at least 8 weeks later.

In older adults at risk of aspiration pneumonia, oral care may reduce pneumonia, though efficacy in the highest risk groups (eg, nursing home residents) was not demonstrated in a high-quality, randomized study. Oral hygiene should be performed daily by mechanical cleaning (brushing and sponging of the mucosa and lips twice a day and floss once a day), rinsing with chlorhexidine gluconate in cases of gingivitis, saliva substitutes if there is xerostomia, and weekly oral evaluation. If partial or full dental prostheses are present, they should be brushed and left in a cleaning solution for 10 minutes and rinsed using the same procedure as in patients with teeth. Postural measures for feeding (elevation of the head of the bed and remaining in that position until 2 hours after completion of the intake) make sense, but have not been proven to reduce risk in rigorous trials.

There is increasing data on pharmacological interventions that act on the swallowing reflex such as those involved in the thermoregulatory centers and the cough reflex. It is important to avoid all medications that could potentiate aspirations, such as sedatives, and especially antipsychotics. The use of proton pump inhibitors that produce achlorhydria and stomach bacteria is an issue of debate, but should be clearly justified if given. Treatment of hypertension and heart failure may include the use of angiotensin-converting enzyme inhibitors, and in seniors at risk for pneumonia, the stimulated cough reflex may reduce risk. Other preventive measures that can reduce infections in seniors include optimizing treatment of comorbidities (eg, diabetes mellitus, heart failure) and improving nutritional status.

PULMONARY TUBERCULOSIS

Epidemiology

Mycobacterium tuberculosis causes tuberculosis (TB) and is a leading infectious cause of death in adults worldwide. More than 1.7 billion people (about 25% of the world population) are estimated to be infected with *M tuberculosis*. The highest rates (100 per 100,000 or higher) are observed in sub-Saharan Africa, India, the islands of Southeast Asia, and Micronesia. Low rates (< 25 cases per 100,000 inhabitants) occur in the United States, Western Europe, Canada, Japan, and Australia. TB continues to be an important social and health problem in our environment today, given that the geriatric contingent represents a considerable part of the population, doubly exposed to suffering from the disease, either due to the reactivation of an old form, or due to exogenous disease, and their forms of presentation seem to differ from those usually seen. The disease has two waves of higher incidence, one between 15 and 35 years old and another after 65 years of age. TB can be activated during the course of life, especially as a consequence of the alterations in immune response in old age. Long-term facilities, especially those related to geriatric care, represent an increase in bacillary transmission.

Etiology

Mycobacteria are slow-growing aerobic bacilli. Their distinctive characteristic is a complex cell envelope rich in lipids, responsible for their classification as acid-alcohol resistant, and their relative resistance to Gram staining. Tuberculosis really only designates the disease caused by *M tuberculosis*, the main reservoir of which is humans. A similar disease can occasionally be found due to infection with closely related mycobacteria, such as *M bovis*, *M africanum*, and *M microti*, which, in conjunction with *M tuberculosis*, are known as the *Mycobacterium tuberculosis* complex.

Pathophysiology and Immunological Aspects

With age there is a decline in immunological protection both in the production of high-affinity antibodies as well as a decrease in immune memory in response to vaccination and delayed hypersensitivity. In senescence, in addition to the response of T cells, which contribute to defense against infections with the production of specific cytokine patterns, other frequent and negative extrinsic factors associated with age and tuberculosis must be taken into account, such as inappropriate diet, poor nutritional status, low physical activity, and comorbidity. In the immune system, by displaying antigens, macrophages, give rise to clonal proliferation of T lymphocytes that differentiate into memory T lymphocytes, cytotoxic and suppressor T helper lymphocytes (CD4+), and T lymphocytes (CD8+). When suppressor CD8+ T lymphocytes show high activity with little response to CD4+, as can occur with age, large numbers of bacilli are released and severe forms of the disease appear.

Asymptomatic parasitic infections have been described that, when associated with TB and other immunosuppressive states, can lead to genetic activation of type 2 cytokines, instead of type 1 cytokine response, which would be adequate against TB, and could explain cases with extensive TB disease. In the same way, a decrease in previously elevated cytokine levels may be indicative of good response to treatment.

Older adults are at greater risk of suffering therapeutic failure and adverse drug reactions due to pharmacokinetic and pharmacodynamic alterations produced by physiologic changes secondary to aging, associated chronic diseases and drug interactions as a consequence of polypharmacy.

TB can occur in three stages: primary infection, latent infection, and active infection. Initially, the *M tuberculosis* bacillus causes a primary infection that does not usually lead to acute disease. Most primary infections (about 95%) do not produce symptoms and in the end enter a latent phase. A variable percentage of latent infections are reactivated with signs and symptoms of the disease. The infection is not usually transmitted during the primary stage and is not contagious in the latent phase.

Primary infection TB infection requires the inhalation of particles small enough to pass through the upper respiratory defenses and settle in the deep regions of the lungs, usually in the subpleural air spaces of the middle or lower lobes. Larger droplets tend to lodge in the more proximal airways and do not cause infection. To initiate infection, alveolar macrophages must ingest *M tuberculosis* bacilli. Then, bacilli not destroyed by macrophages replicate within and ultimately kill the macrophages that host them (with the cooperation of CD8 lymphocytes); inflammatory cells are attracted to the area, where they cause localized pneumonitis that coalesces to form the characteristic tubercles observed on histological examination. During the first weeks of infection, some infected macrophages migrate to regional lymph nodes (eg, hilar, mediastinal), where they enter the bloodstream. The microorganisms then spread hematogenously to any part of the body, especially the apicoposterior portion of the lungs, the epiphyses of long bones, the kidneys, the vertebral bodies, and the meninges. Hematogenous spread is less likely in patients with partial immunity due to vaccination or previous natural infection with *M tuberculosis* or environmental mycobacteria.

Latent infection Latent infection occurs after most primary infections. After about 3 weeks of unlimited growth, in about 95% of cases, the immune system inhibits bacillary replication, usually before the appearance of signs or symptoms. Bacilli foci in the lungs or other sites develop into epithelioid cell granulomas, which may have caseous and necrotic centers. Tubercle bacilli can survive in this material for years, and the balance between host resistance and virulence of the organism determines the possibility that the infection will resolve without treatment, remain latent, or become active. Infectious foci can leave fibronodular scars on the apices of one or both lungs (foci of Simon, which generally occur as a result of hematogenous arrival from another site of infection) or small areas of consolidation (foci of Ghon). A Ghon focus with lymph node involvement is a Ghon complex, which, if calcified, is called a Ranke complex. The tuberculin test and interferon-γ release assays (IGRAs) are positive during the latent phase of infection. Latent infection sites are dynamic processes, not entirely inactive as previously believed.

Less commonly, the primary focus progresses immediately and causes acute illness with pneumonia (often cavitary), pleural effusion, and significant enlargement of the mediastinum or hilar lymph nodes (which, in children, can compress the bronchi). Small pleural effusions are primarily lymphocytic, typically contain few organisms, and resolve within a few weeks. This sequence is more frequently seen in young children and in recently infected or reinfected immunocompromised patients.

Extrapulmonary TB can appear anywhere and manifest without evidence of pulmonary involvement. Tuberculous lymphadenopathy is the most common extrapulmonary presentation; however, meningitis is the most feared due to its high mortality rate at the extremes of life.

Active disease Healthy people who are infected with TB have a 5% to 10% risk of developing active disease during their lifetime, although the percentage varies significantly based on age and other risk factors. In 50% to 80% of people with active disease, TB reactivates within the first 2 years, but it can also manifest several decades later. Any organ seeded by the primary infection can host a focus of reactivation, although these foci are most frequently identified in the pulmonary apexes, which may be due to more favorable conditions, such as elevated oxygen tension. Foci of Ghon and involved hilar lymph nodes are less likely to reactivate. Pathologies that impair cellular immunity (which is essential for defense against TB) significantly facilitate reactivation. Therefore, HIV coinfected patients who do not receive appropriate antiretroviral treatment have a 10% annual risk

of developing active disease, diabetes, head and neck cancer, gastrectomy, jejunoileal bypass surgery, dialysis-dependent chronic kidney disease, and significant weight loss, which are conditions that facilitate reactivation. Patients who require immunosuppression after solid organ transplantation are at increased risk, but other immunosuppressants, such as corticosteroids and tumor necrosis factor (TNF) inhibitors, can also cause reactivation. Smoking is also a risk factor.

In some patients, active disease develops when they are reinfected, rather than when latent disease reactivates. Reinfection is more likely to be the mechanism in areas where TB is prevalent and patients are exposed to a large inoculum of bacilli. Reactivation of latent infection predominates in low prevalence areas. In a given patient, it is difficult to determine whether active disease is the result of reinfection or reactivation.

Clinical Characteristics

In the immunocompetent population, the usual form of presentation of TB is pulmonary. However, TB in older patients acquires a series of special characteristics with respect to other age groups. Thus, there is a high risk of disseminated forms, or less radiological evidence of cavitation in its pulmonary presentation. Consequently, this can lead to a high morbidity and mortality in this group, perhaps derived from a delay in diagnosis and the frequent association with other intercurrent diseases in this population group.

From a clinical point of view, if TB has been defined as the great simulator, this is particularly true in immunosuppressed patients and in those older than 65 years. In patients older than 65 years with pulmonary disease, the forms of radiological presentation are different from those described in individuals younger than 65 years, but the most prominent is the presentation of extrapulmonary disease, as well as infrequent, cryptic, or disseminated forms. All of this, together with the high comorbidity of this population, can lead to diagnostic delays with high morbidity and mortality, and it is not uncommon for the final diagnosis to be given in the autopsy report.

TB damages tissues through a delayed hypersensitivity reaction (DHT), which causes typical granulomatous necrosis with the histological appearance of caseous necrosis. Pulmonary lesions are usually cavitary, especially in immunocompromised patients with compromised delayed hypersensitivity. Pleural effusion is found less frequently than in primary progressive TB, but it can appear as a result of direct spread of infection or hematogenous spread. The rupture of a large tuberculous lesion in the pleural space can cause an empyema with or without a bronchopleural fistula, and sometimes pneumothorax. In the prechemotherapy era, tuberculous empyema could complicate the treatment of a drug-induced pneumothorax and lead to rapid death, and so could massive sudden hemoptysis secondary to erosion of the pulmonary artery by a proliferating cavity. The course of TB varies greatly depending on the virulence of the microorganism and the defenses of the host. Evolution can be rapid in members of isolated populations who, unlike many Europeans and their American descendants, have not experienced centuries of selective pressure to develop innate or natural immunity to disease. In European and American populations, evolution is more silent and slower.

Sometimes an acute respiratory distress syndrome appears due to the development of hypersensitivity to antigens of the tubercle bacillus and occurs after rapid hematogenous spread or rupture of a large cavity with intrapulmonary bleeding.

Reactivation of the disease in older adults can involve all organs, although those most frequently affected are the lungs, brain, kidneys, long bones, vertebrae, or lymph nodes. Reactivation may cause few symptoms and go unnoticed for weeks to months, delaying proper evaluation. The frequent finding of other diseases in older adults further complicates the diagnosis. Regardless of their age, nursing home residents are at risk of contracting the disease due to recent transmission, which can cause apical, middle lobe, or lower lobe pneumonia, as well as pleural effusion. Pneumonia may not be recognized as TB and may persist and also spread to others, while being erroneously treated with ineffective broad-spectrum antibiotics. In the United States, miliary TB and tuberculous meningitis, which in the past were believed to mainly affect young children, are more common in older adults.

Diagnosis

TB is a frequently overlooked diagnosis in older patients. A high index of suspicion is crucial for the identification of infected individuals.

Tuberculin skin test The Mantoux method of the tuberculin skin test (TST) remains the diagnosis modality of choice despite its potential for fast negative results. In older patients, there is an increase in anergy to cutaneous antigens. Therefore, the two-step tuberculin test is suggested for initial geriatric assessment in order to avoid potential false negative reactions. This means that after a negative response to the TST (induration of < 10 mm) other tests must be performed after 2 weeks. A positive TST reaction is a skin test of 10 mm or more and an increase of 6 mm or more over the first skin test reaction.

Conversion must not be confused with the previously described booster phenomenon. Conversion occurs in persons previously uninfected but with a true negative TST who become infected within 2 years as demonstrated by a positive TST. Decreased skin test reactivity is associated with waning delayed-type hypersensitivity over time, disseminated TB, corticosteroids, and other drugs, and the elimination of TB infections. A false positive TST occurs with cross-reactions with nontuberculous mycobacteria and in persons receiving the bacillus Calmette-Guerin (BCG) vaccine.

Chest radiography Chest x-ray is indicated in all individuals with suspected TB infection. Although reactivation of tuberculosis disease characteristically involves the apical and posterior segments of the upper lobes of the lungs, many older patients manifest the pulmonary infection in either the middle or lower lobes of the pleura, and also present with interstitial, patchy, or cavitary infiltrates that may be bilateral. Primary TB can involve any lung segment but more often tends to involve the middle or lower lobs, as well as mediastinal or hilar lymph nodes.

Laboratory diagnosis Sputum samples must be collected from all patients with pulmonary symptoms or chest radiography changes compatible with TB disease. Other diagnostic techniques, such as sputum induction or bronchoscopy, should be considered in patients unable to expectorate sputum. Flexible bronchoscopy to obtain bronchial washings and to perform bronchial biopsies has diagnostic value in older adults. However, in frail and very old patients, the risk of such a procedure must be carefully balanced against the potential benefit of making a definite diagnosis of TB.

Sputum samples must initially be examined by smear before and after concentrations and then cultured for *M tuberculosis*. Smear tests for *M tuberculosis* are designed to detect acid-fast bacilli (AFB) and require a minimum of 10^{4-5} AFB per mm to be seen by light microscopy. Culture methods may require up to 6 weeks for growth, and therefore, many laboratories use radiometric procedures for the isolation and susceptibility testing of *M tuberculosis*. Radiometric systems can identify the organisms in as few as 8 days.

Histologic examination of tissue from various sites, such as the liver, lymph nodes, bone marrow, pleura, or synovium, can show the characteristic tissue reaction (caseous necrosis with granuloma formation) with or without AFB, which also strongly supports the diagnosis of TB.

The IGRA test (interferon-γ release assay) was designed to improve latent TB infection diagnosis and increase the sensitivity and specificity by means of quantifying interferon-γ produced by sensitized T lymphocytes in response to contact with specific *M tuberculosis* antigens. The specificity of IGRA test for mycobacterium complex diagnosis is much higher than that of the tuberculin skin tests, maintaining the same sensitivity, with the exception of the immunosuppressed patients and those under 5 years in which is lower. Gamma interferon is an important molecule for the control of TB infection, and its participation is essential in the protective immune response against this microorganism. This cytokine is produced by CD4+, CD8+, and NK T lymphocytes and activates infected macrophages, with the consequent release of IL-1 and TNF-γ, which limit the growth and multiplication of mycobacteria.

However, the IGRA test is still incapable of discriminating either previous from current *M tuberculosis* infection or differentiating between latent and active TB. A positive IGRA test result indicates infection with TB bacteria. However, more tests are needed to determine if a person has latent TB infection or TB disease. A negative IGRA test result indicates little likelihood of having latent TB infection or disease. Clinical efficacy is affected in immunocompromised individuals owing to a reduced and fluctuant interferon-γ synthesis in these patients. Factors such as immunosuppression contribute to obtaining indeterminate results, which must be taken into account when interpreting the test.

Treatment

The treatment of TB in older adults does not differ from that in the adult population, although it must be taken into account that adverse effects increase with age. The goals of TB treatment include eradication of *M tuberculosis* infection, and prevention of transmission, disease relapse, and the development of drug resistance.

The risks and benefits of preventive treatment must be carefully evaluated before treating the older adult. Isoniazid causes hepatotoxicity in up to 4% to 5% of patients older than 65 years (compared to < 1% in those < 65 years old).

Risk factors for treatment failure and relapse include inadequate adherence to treatment, high burden of clinical disease (presence of cavitary disease, bilateral disease, and/or extrapulmonary disease), drug resistance, malabsorption, malnourishment, and mistakes in diagnosis.

Chemoprophylaxis

Due to the possible appearance of adverse events in older adult, chemoprophylaxis is generally administered only if the induration of the Mantoux TST increases by ≥ 15 mm following a previous negative reaction. In close contacts of patients with active TB and other individuals at high risk with negative TST or interferon-γ release tests, preventive treatment should also be considered, unless contraindicated.

Intensive Phase

First-line drugs include isoniazid, rifampin, pyrazinamide, and ethambutol. Drug doses are summarized in **Table 105-12**. The drugs should be administered on an empty stomach if tolerated, but dosing with food is acceptable to ameliorate gastrointestinal upset and is preferable to dividing doses or changing to second-line agents.

The intensive phase usually consists of four drugs (isoniazid, rifampin, pyrazinamide, and ethambutol) administered for 2 months. The use of this regimen is intended to minimize the likelihood of developing secondary resistance to rifampin in regions with a high rate of primary resistance to isoniazid (≥ 4%). If susceptibility data become available before the end of the intensive phase and demonstrate that the isolate is sensitive to isoniazid, rifampin, and pyrazinamide, ethambutol may be discontinued.

If pyrazinamide must be excluded from the intensive phase of treatment (due to hepatotoxicity, gout, or pregnancy), the intensive phase should consist of isoniazid, rifampin, and ethambutol administered daily for 2 months, and the continuation phase should be extended to 7 months (total duration of treatment extended to 9 months).

Continuation Phase

The continuation phase usually consists of two drugs (isoniazid and rifampin) administered for at least 4 additional months for a total of 6 months. The continuation phase should be extended to 7 months (total duration of treatment 9 months) for patients in the following circumstances:

a. Patients with both cavitary pulmonary TB on initial chest radiograph and positive sputum culture after the 2-month intensive-phase treatment. The decision to prolong the continuation phase for patients with either cavitation or positive cultures (but not both) should be made on an individual basis.

b. Patients in whom the intensive treatment phase did not include 2 months of pyrazinamide.

Drug-Resistant TB

Drug-resistant TB varies according to the pattern of resistance. In general, multidrug-resistant TB requires treatment for 18 to 24 months with a regimen containing four or five active drugs. The presumed activity is based on the results of susceptibility tests, previous exposure to antituberculosis drugs, or patterns of drug susceptibility in the community. The regimen should include all remaining active first-line drugs, including pyrazinamide if the strain is susceptible, plus second-line drugs. Fluoroquinolones are alternative antituberculous agents that should only be used with other second-line drugs as needed to achieve a four-dose regimen or five drugs in patients with drug intolerance or resistance to first-line agents. Designing a treatment regimen for super-resistant TB is even more challenging, often requiring the use of highly toxic and unproven drugs such as clofazimine and linezolid.

Treatment of Latent TB

Treatment of latent TB is primarily indicated in people with a negative TST result, which became positive in the previous 2 years, and people with radiological changes compatible with previous TB but without evidence of active TB. Other indications for preventive treatment are people who, if infected, would be at high risk of developing active TB (HIV-infected, drug-induced immunodeficiency) and all children older than 5 years who are in close contact with a person with a positive TB smear, regardless of whether they present TST conversion. Other individuals with an incidental positive TST or IGRA test but without these risk factors are usually treated with the drugs indicated for latent TB. However, clinicians must consider the individual risks of drug toxicity and compare these with the benefits of treatment.

Treatment is usually based on the administration of isoniazid for 9 months, unless resistance is suspected. An alternative for isoniazid-resistant or intolerant patients is rifampin for 4 months. Therapy with isoniazid plus rifapentine for 12 weeks was also shown to be effective.

TABLE 105-12 ■ TREATMENT OF PULMONARY TUBERCULOSIS

INTENSIVE PHASE (2 MONTHS)		CONTINUATION PHASE (6 MONTHS)		
DRUGS	DAILY DOSE	DRUGS	DAILY DOSE	COMMENT
Isoniazid	5 mg/kg (300 mg)	Isoniazid	5 mg/kg (300 mg)	Isoniazid can cause peripheral neuropathy due to pyridoxine deficiency in certain situations (alcoholic, malnourished, diabetic, kidney failure). Prophylactic administration of pyridoxine supplements (10–50 mg/day) is recommended in these cases. If isoniazid cannot be used (toxicity or infection by a resistant strain): treatment can be carried out with rifampin, pyrazinamide, ethambutol, and moxifloxacin 400 mg/day for 6 months or, after the initial 2 months, continue with rifampin and ethambutol until complete 12 months.
Rifampin	10 mg/kg (600 mg)	Rifampin	10 mg/kg (600 mg)	If rifampicin cannot be used (toxicity or infection by a resistant strain): treatment can be carried out with isoniazid, pyrazinamide, and ethambutol for 12 months. During the first 2 months, moxifloxacin 400 mg/day or streptomycin (< 40 kg, 15 mg/kg; 40–90 kg, 750 mg/day) can be added in patients with extensive lesions. In AIDS patients receiving protease inhibitors or other drugs that are metabolized in cytochrome P-450, consider substituting rifampicin for rifabutin (5 mg/kg/day—maximum dose 300 mg /day); assess the possibility of antiretroviral treatment with a regimen compatible with the use of rifampin (two non-nucleoside reverse transcriptase inhibitors with efavirenz or raltegravir).
Pyrazinamide	20–25 mg/kg 1000 mg 40–55 kg 1500 mg 46–75 kg 2000 mg 76–90 kg			If pyrazinamide cannot be used (liver disease): treatment can be carried out with isoniazid and rifampin, associated with ethambutol or streptomycin (< 40 kg, 15 mg/kg; 40–90 kg, 750 mg/day) for 2 months. If the bacillary load is potentially high (existence of radiological cavitation), the addition of a fluoroquinolone may be considered. From the second month on, isoniazid and rifampin are continued until 9 months are completed.
Ethambutol	20 mg/kg 800 mg 50–55 kg 1200 mg 56–75 kg 1600 mg 76–90 kg			

(1) Patients with noncavitated pulmonary tuberculosis, caused by a susceptible strain, if they do not have HIV infection, can receive treatment in both phases for 3 days a week under direct observation. In this case, isoniazid is used at a dose of 15 mg/kg (usually 900 mg); rifampin 10 mg/kg (usually 600 mg); pyrazinamide 1500 mg for patients 40–55 kg, 2500 for patients 56–75 kg, and 3000 for patients with 76–90 kg; and ethambutol 1200 mg for patients 40–55 kg, 2000 mg for patients 56–75 kg, and 2400 mg for patients 76–90 kg.

(2) Patients with a positive sputum culture at month 2 (10% of cases) and cavitated lesions on the initial chest x-ray have a high risk of recurrence. In these cases, it is advisable to prolong the treatment with isoniazid and rifampin for up to 9 months. In the presence of only one criterion (cavitation or positive sputum at month 2), it is advisable to prolong treatment in patients with diabetes, HIV infection, immunosuppression, extensive lung disease, silicosis, or smokers.

(3) If isoniazid and pyrazinamide cannot be used (severe liver disease or infection by a resistant strain): treatment can be carried out with rifampin, ethambutol, and levofloxacin 500 mg/day or moxifloxacin 400 mg/day or cycloserine 10–15 mg/kg/day in one or two doses for 12–18 months.

(4) If isoniazid, rifampicin, or pyrazinamide cannot be used (severe liver disease or infection by a resistant strain): treatment should be done with the combination of at least four active drugs according to the antibiogram, administered for at least 18–24 months. The combination of a fluoroquinolone (levofloxacin 750 mg/day or moxifloxacin 400 mg/day), an aminoglycoside (amikacin 1 g/day), a polypeptide (capreomycin 15 mg/kg/day), ethambutol, and at least one other active drug (linezolid [300–600 mg/day], ethionamide [15 mg/kg/day—maximum dose 1 g/day], or prothionamide and cycloserine [15 mg/kg/day—maximum dose 1 g/day] can be used.

(5) Pulmonary tuberculosis in HIV-infected patients: if the patient is receiving antiretroviral treatment (ART), they can be treated for 6 months with the same recommended regimen for non-HIV-infected patients. In exceptional cases, in which the patient does not receive ART during the entire tuberculostatic treatment, the second phase of treatment should be extended to 9 months. If the patient was not receiving ART, it should be started within the first 2 weeks of tuberculosis treatment, if the CD4 count is < 50 cells/µL and there is no CNS involvement, and between 8 and 12 weeks of treatment if CD4 is ≥ 50 cells/µL or < 50 cells/µL and the CNS is involved. The initiation of ART during antituberculous treatment can cause a temporary paradoxical worsening (10–30 days) with fever and increased infiltrate and/or adenopathies. In patients with AIDS-associated enteropathy, absorption of tuberculostatics may be irregular. If the patient receives protease inhibitors, substitute rifampin for rifabutin 150–300 mg/day.

(6) Treatment failure is defined as the persistence of a positive sputum culture after 4–5 months of treatment. Perform an antibiogram from the last isolation. If it is possible, determine the serum concentration of the tuberculostatics used. Until this information is available, add 2–3 new drugs, administered under direct observation.

Patients under treatment for a latent infection should be advised to stop taking the drug if they develop new symptoms, particularly unexplained tiredness, loss of appetite, or nausea. Monitoring the onset of symptoms and encouraging patients to complete treatment are considered to be part of appropriate standard clinical and public health practice.

Adverse Events

Antituberculous drugs are associated with a broad array of adverse effects. Hepatotoxicity is an important adverse effect that warrants careful clinical care. In both curative and preventive treatments, the possible development of isoniazid-induced hepatitis increases with age, with no differences between men and women. Despite this and other adverse effects, the benefits versus harm of the treatment have been clearly demonstrated. More than one antituberculous drug in a treatment regimen may be associated with hepatotoxicity, and in some cases the most significant contributor may be identified and eliminated without loss of the other drugs in the regimen. Among the first-line antituberculous drugs, hepatotoxicity may be caused by isoniazid, rifampin, and pyrazinamide.

Patients receiving antituberculous therapy should undergo baseline measurement of liver function tests (serum bilirubin, alkaline phosphatase, and transaminases). An asymptomatic increase in aspartate transaminase concentrations occurs in approximately 20% of patients treated with the standard four-drug regimen. In most patients, asymptomatic aminotransferase elevations resolve spontaneously over days to weeks.

In general, hepatitis attributed to antituberculous drugs should prompt discontinuation of all hepatotoxic drugs if serum bilirubin values are ≥ 3 mg/dL or serum transaminases are more than five times the upper limit of normal (or, in individuals with symptoms of hepatitis, serum transaminases more than three times the upper limit of normal). Thereafter, once liver function tests return to baseline (or fall to less than twice normal), potentially hepatotoxic drugs can be restarted one at a time with careful monitoring between resumption of each agent.

Alternative regimens for the treatment of TB disease due to susceptible strains in the setting of drug intolerance include the following:

a. For patients who cannot tolerate isoniazid, a regimen of rifampin, pyrazinamide, and ethambutol may be administered for 6 months. Alternatively, rifampin and ethambutol may be given for 12 months, preferably with pyrazinamide during at least the initial 2 months.

b. For patients who cannot tolerate rifampin, isoniazid, and ethambutol may be given for 12 to 18 months, with pyrazinamide during at least the first 2 months. An agent may be added for the first 2 to 3 months in individuals with extensive disease or to shorten the overall treatment duration to 12 months.

c. For patients who cannot tolerate pyrazinamide, isoniazid, and rifampin should be administered for 9 months (supplemented by ethambutol until isoniazid and rifampin susceptibility is demonstrated).

d. For patients who require a regimen with no hepatotoxic agents, potential agents include ethambutol, levofloxacin, or moxifloxacin, an agent, and other second-line oral drugs. The optimal choice of agents and duration of treatment (at least 18 to 24 months) are uncertain.

FURTHER READING

Aliberti S, Di Pasquale M, Zanaboni AM, et al. Stratifying risk factors for multidrug-resistant pathogens in hospitalized patients coming from the community with pneumonia. *Clin Infect Dis.* 2012;54:470–478.

Arias Guillén M. Advances in the diagnosis of tuberculosis infection. *Arch Bronconeumol.* 2011;47(10):521–530.

Brito V, Niederman MS. Healthcare-associated pneumonia is a heterogeneous disease, and all patients do not need the same broad-spectrum antibiotic therapy as complex nosocomial pneumonia. *Curr Opin Infect Dis.* 2009;22:316–325.

Cabré P, Serra-Prat M, Palomera E, Almirall J, Pallares R, Clavé P. Prevalence and prognostic implications of dysphagia in elderly patients with pneumonia. *Age Aging.* 2010;39:39–45.

Chalmers J, Taylor JK, Singanayagam A, et al. Epidemiología, antibiotic therapy and clinical outcomes in health care-associated pneumonia: a UK cohort study. *Clin Infect Dis.* 2011;53:107–113.

El-Solh A, Pietrantoni C, Bhat A, et al. Microbiology of severe aspiration pneumonia in institutionalized elderly. *Am J Respir Crit Care Med.* 2003;167:1650–1654.

Ewig S, Welte T, Chastre J, Torres A. Rethinking the concepts of community-acquired and health-care-associated pneumonia. *Lancet Infect Dis.* 2010;10:279–287.

González-Castillo J, Martín-Sánchez FJ, Llinares P, et al. Guidelines for the management of community-acquired pneumonia in the elderly patient. *Rev Esp Quimioter.* 2014;27:69–86.

Jung YEG, Schluger NW. Advances in the diagnosis and treatment of latent tuberculosis infection. *Curr Opin Infect Dis.* 2020;33(2):166–172.

Kikuchi R, Watabe N, Konno T, Mishina N, Sekizawa K, Sasaki H. High incidence of silent aspiration in elderly patients with community-acquired pneumonia. *Am J Respir Crit Care Med.* 1994;150:251–253.

Kollef MH, Shorr A, Tabak YP, Gupta V, Liu LZ, Johannes RS. Epidemiology and outcomes of health-care-associated pneumonia: results from a large US database of culture-positive pneumonia. *Chest.* 2005;128:3854–3862.

Lim WS, Baudouin SV, George RC, et al; Pneumonia Guidelines Committee of the BTS Standards of Care Committee. BTS guidelines for the management of community acquired pneumonia in adults: update 2009. *Thorax.* 2009;64:S1–S55.

Metlay JP, Waterer GW, Long AC, et al. Diagnosis and treatment of adults with community-acquired pneumonia. An Official Clinical Practice Guideline of the American Thoracic Society and Infectious Diseases Society of America. *Am J Respir Crit Care Med.* 2019;200(7): e45–e67.

Musher DM, Thorner AR. Community-acquired pneumonia. *N Engl J Med.* 2014;371:1619–1628.

Sader HS, Farrell DJ, Flamm RK, Jones RN. Antimicrobial susceptibility of Gram-negative organisms isolated from patients hospitalised with pneumonia in US and European hospitals: results from the SENTRY Antimicrobial Surveillance Program, 2009-2012. *Int J Antimicrob Agents.* 2014;43:328–334.

Salgueiro Rodríguez M. Tuberculosis en pacientes ancianos [Tuberculosis in elderly patients]. *An Med Interna.* 2002; 19(3):107–110.

Self WH, Courtney DM, McNaughton CD, Wunderink RG, Kline JA. High discordance of chest x-ray and computed tomography for detection of pulmonary opacities in ED patients: implications for diagnosing pneumonia. *Am J Emerg Med.* 2013;31:401–405.

Shorr AF, Myers DE, Huang DB, Nathanson BH, Emons MF, Kollef MH. A risk score for identifying methicillin-resistant *S. aureus* in patients presenting to the hospital with pneumonia. *BMC Infect Dis.* 2013;13:268.

Shorr AF, Zilberberg MD, Reichley R et al. Validation of a clinical score for assessing the risk of resistant pathogens in patients with pneumonia presenting to emergency department. *Clin Infect Dis.* 2012;54:193–198.

Stucker F, Herrmann F, Graf JD, Michel JP, Krause KH, Gavazzi G. Procalcitonin and infection in elderly patients. *J Am Geriatr Soc.* 2005;53:1392–1395.

Taylor JK, Flemming GB, Singanayagam A, Hill AT, Chalmers J. Risk factors for aspiration in community-acquired pneumonia: analysis of hospitalized UK cohort. *Am J Med.* 2013;126:995–1001.

van der Maarel-Wierink CD, Vanobbergen JN, Bronkhorst EM, Schols JM, de Baat C. Risk factors for aspiration pneumonia in frail patient. *J Am Med Dir Assoc.* 2011;12:244–254.

von Baum H, Welte T, Marre R, Suttorp N, Ewig S. Community-acquired pneumonia through *Enterobacteriaceae* and *Pseudomonas aeruginosa*: diagnosis, incidence and predictors. *Eur Respir J.* 2010;35:598–605.

UpToDate. https://www-uptodate-com.m-husc.a17.csinet. es/contents/treatment-of-drug-resistant-pulmonary-tuberculosis-in-adults?search=tuberculosis&source= search_result&selectedTitle=8~150&usage_type= default&display_rank=8.

Chapter 106

Urinary Tract Infections

Muhammad S. Ashraf, Mandy L. Byers

INTRODUCTION

Urinary tract infection (UTI) is the most frequently encountered bacterial infection in older adults. While the presence of bacteria in the urine in older adults is usually asymptomatic and considered a colonization state, symptomatic infection is associated with morbidity and, rarely, mortality. Optimal management of UTI in this population is challenging in the face of diagnostic uncertainty, concerns with excess antimicrobial use, and increasing antimicrobial resistance in the community and postacute/long-term care (PALTC) settings. In addition, the heterogeneity of the older adult population means approaches may vary for different groups. The impact and management of urinary infection differs for older adults in the community and in those residing in PALTC settings. There are also unique considerations for the subgroup of older adults with chronic indwelling catheters and those who are in hospice care toward the end of their life. The discussion in this chapter is relevant to individuals without long-term indwelling catheters, unless otherwise stated.

DEFINITIONS

UTI is both one of the most commonly diagnosed infections in older adults and one of the most difficult infections to accurately diagnose. The uncertainty surrounding the definition of UTI, particularly in older adults, poses significant diagnostic challenges for providers caring for this population. Definitions of bacteriuria, pyuria, and ASB are more universally agreed upon. Bacteriuria implies the presence of bacteria in the urine. Pyuria is generally defined by the presence of 10 or more white blood cells (WBC/mm^3) per high-power field (hpf) in a urine sample, suggesting inflammation of the genitourinary tract. ASB is broadly defined as the presence of bacteria in the urine, with or without pyuria, in the absence of localizing (genitourinary) signs or symptoms. In asymptomatic women, the accepted definition for ASB is defined as two consecutive voided urine specimens with isolation of the same uropathogen in quantitative counts greater than or equal to 10^5 colony forming units/milliliter (cfu/mL). In asymptomatic men, ASB is defined as a single clean-catch voided urine specimen with one uropathogen isolated in quantitative counts

Learning Objectives

- Differentiate asymptomatic bacteriuria (ASB) and symptomatic urinary tract infection (UTI) in older adults.

- Apply specific considerations and guidelines for evaluation of UTI in older adults residing in postacute/long-term care (PALTC) settings.

- Recognize the recommendations and limitations of current guidelines for diagnosis and treatment of UTI in both community-dwelling older adults and residents of PALTC settings.

- Utilize strategies to limit unnecessary antibiotic use in older adults with suspected UTI.

- Understand antimicrobial stewardship principles and how to apply those in management of UTI both in outpatient and PALTC settings.

Key Clinical Points

1. ASB and UTI are the most common reasons antibiotics are prescribed for older adults in both the community and health care settings.

2. Distinguishing ASB and symptomatic UTI is problematic. Many older adults do not present with localized genitourinary symptoms required by guidelines to diagnose a symptomatic infection, and the baseline prevalence of bacteriuria is high.

   a. Clinicians should NOT screen older adults for ASB and those with ASB should NOT be treated with antibiotics; the only exception being older adults undergoing invasive urologic procedures.

   b. In older adults with vague, nonspecific symptoms in either community-dwelling or PALTC settings (eg, behavioral changes exclusive of delirium, functional decline, falls, anorexia), a short period

(Continued)

(Cont.)

of observation for the evolution of symptoms along with hydration and evaluation for alternative diagnoses should be the first management strategy as it does NOT lead to worse outcomes in those eventually proven to have UTI when compared to empiric, immediate antibiotic therapy.

3. Clinicians in outpatient and inpatient settings often do not use guidelines aimed at reducing unnecessary antibiotic prescriptions.

4. Use (and overuse) of antibiotics to treat UTI is associated with the development of uropathogens with higher rates of resistance to commonly used antibiotics.

5. Implementing culture and antibiotic stewardship programs (ASPs) to reduce inappropriate cultures and promote appropriate antibiotic prescribing in PALTC settings for UTI decreases inappropriate antibiotic use for UTI and rates of *Clostridioides difficile* infection without increasing hospitalizations or deaths.

greater than or equal to 10^5 cfu/mL. A single *catheterized* urine specimen with one uropathogen isolated in a quantitative count greater than or equal to 10^2 cfu/mL defines ASB in both asymptomatic women and men.

Symptomatic UTI refers to an infection anywhere in the genitourinary tract. It can be further divided into acute simple cystitis (or uncomplicated cystitis), complicated UTI and catheter-associated UTIs. Acute simple cystitis is most commonly encountered UTI syndrome which is diagnosed when pyuria and bacteriuria are accompanied by urinary symptoms confined to the bladder. These symptoms include dysuria, frequency, gross hematuria, suprapubic pain, and new or worsening urinary incontinence or urgency. Complicated UTI is diagnosed when pyuria and bacteriuria are accompanied by signs and symptoms that indicate that infection has extended beyond the bladder. Acute pyelonephritis refers to infection involving renal parenchyma; therefore, it is also considered a complicated UTI. The signs and symptoms that usually suggest infection is extending beyond the bladder include fever, chills/rigors, marked fatigue/malaise, nausea/vomiting, flank pain, costovertebral angle tenderness, or pelvic or perineal pain in men (that may suggest accompanying prostatitis). Usually signs and symptoms of systemic illness in complicated UTI will accompany localizing signs and symptoms of UTI. However, complicated UTI (including acute pyelonephritis) may sometimes present without symptoms of cystitis.

Catheter-associated UTI (CAUTI) refers to patients with an indwelling urethral, suprapubic, or intermittent catheterization with signs or symptoms compatible with UTI (ie, fever, rigors/chills, clear-cut delirium with no other identified cause, suprapubic tenderness, flank pain/costovertebral angle tenderness, pelvic or perineal discomfort/pain); **OR** signs or symptoms localizing to genitourinary tract (eg, dysuria, urgency, frequency, gross hematuria, suprapubic tenderness, or flank pain/costovertebral angle tenderness) in patients whose catheters have been removed within the previous 48 hours with no other identified source of infection, **ALONG WITH** greater than or equal to 10^5 cfu/mL of one or more bacterial species in a single catheter urine specimen. It is important to note that even though most patients with CAUTI have higher colony counts ($\geq 10^5$ cfu/mL), some patients may have lower colony counts ($\geq 10^2$ cfu/mL). Recurrent UTI is defined as three or more symptomatic UTIs within a 12-month period or two or more symptomatic UTIs in a 6-month period following clinical resolution of each UTI with antimicrobial treatment **(Table 106-1)**.

EPIDEMIOLOGY

UTIs are both common and costly in the United States. They account for more than 8 million outpatient and emergency department visits, and are responsible for over 100,000 hospitalizations with cost of $1.6 billion annually. It is one of the most frequently listed diagnoses among hospitalized patients 50 years or older in the United States, and the incidence of hospital admissions for UTIs has increased dramatically since the late 1990s. UTIs are also the most commonly diagnosed infections in the PALTC settings. A 1-day point prevalence survey of antimicrobial use performed between April and October 2017 involving 161 nursing homes found that one in 38 residents was receiving an antibiotic for UTI and a quarter of antibiotic use was for UTI prophylaxis.

ASB in Older Adults

The prevalence of ASB increases with age and is more prevalent in those residing in PALTC settings. In healthy, older adult women, ASB ranges from approximately 5% to 20% in women aged 65 to 90, but increases to nearly 45% in women older than 90 years. Bacteriuria is uncommon in younger men, but increases significantly with age, especially in men with prostatic hypertrophy. The rate of ASB is approximately 5% in men living in the community, but increases to 20% in men older than 80 years. ASB is highly prevalent in long-term care (LTC) settings, with multiple studies documenting rates for men and women to be approximately 15% to 50%. The rate of ASB in this population is likely to be higher than current estimates, as adults with urinary incontinence and dementia are more likely to have ASB, but also more likely not to be included in research studies given the difficulty of obtaining a urine specimen. Essentially 100%

TABLE 106-1 ■ COMMON DEFINITIONS

Asymptomatic bacteriuria	Broadly defined as a urinary pathogen isolated in appropriate quantitative counts from a urine culture in adults without genitourinary tract signs or symptoms.
	In older women: Two consecutive clean-catch midstream urine samples growing at least 10^5 colony-forming units (cfu)/mL with no more than two species of microorganisms or a single *catheterized* urine specimen with one uropathogen isolated in a quantitative count $\geq 10^2$ cfu/mL.
	In older men: One clean-catch midstream urine sample growing at least 10^5 cfu/mL with no more than two species of microorganisms or a single *catheterized* urine specimen with one uropathogen isolated in a quantitative count $\geq 10^2$ cfu/mL.
Pyuria	Presence of ≥ 10 white blood cells (WBC/mm^3) per high power field (hpf) in a urine specimen.
Leukocyte esterase	Component of a urinary dipstick that is used to detect a substance that suggests there are white blood cells in the urine.
Nitrite	Component of a urinary dipstick used to indicate that bacteria may be present in significant numbers in the urine.
Acute simple cystitis (or uncomplicated cystitis)	A UTI syndrome in which pyuria and bacteriuria are accompanied by urinary symptoms confined to the bladder (eg, dysuria, frequency, gross hematuria, suprapubic tenderness, and new or worsening urinary incontinence or urgency).
Complicated UTI[a]	A UTI syndrome with signs and symptoms indicating extension of UTI beyond the bladder (eg, fever, chills/rigors, marked fatigue/malaise, nausea/vomiting, flank pain, costovertebral angle tenderness, or pelvic or perineal pain in men).
Recurrent UTI	≥ 3 confirmed urinary tract infections within a 12-mo period or ≥ 2 symptomatic UTIs in a 6-mo period following clinical resolution of each infection with antimicrobial treatment.
Catheter-associated UTI[b]	Signs or symptoms of a UTI in adults who have an indwelling urethral or suprapubic catheter, perform intermittent catheterization, or in those whose catheters have been removed within the previous 48 h *and* $\geq 10^5$ cfu/mL of ≥ 1 bacterial species in a single catheter urine specimen.

UTI, urinary tract infection.

[a]Usually signs and symptoms of systemic illness in complicated UTI will accompany localizing signs and symptoms of UTI. However, complicated UTI (including acute pyelonephritis) may sometimes present without symptoms of cystitis.

[b]Even though most patients with catheter-associated UTI have higher colony counts (> 10^5 cfu/mL) of bacteria, some patients may have lower colony counts (10^2–10^3 cfu/mL).

of chronically catheterized older adults develop bacteriuria within 1 month of catheterization.

ASB often resolves spontaneously, without antibiotic treatment. A large cohort study evaluating the prevalence of ASB in older men and women living in the community reported that almost 30% of individuals with ASB at baseline had negative urine cultures at 6 months, whereas among those adults that were negative for ASB at baseline, 6% developed bacteriuria at 6 months.

UTI in Older Adults

The incidence of UTI in postmenopausal women is 0.07 per person-year according to a large population-based study. Irrespective of gender, the incidence of clinically diagnosed UTI increases with age. Accurately estimating the prevalence of UTI, however, is challenging, as the definition of UTI varies significantly across the literature. For example, a prospective population-based study of healthy older adult women in Brazil described the prevalence of UTI to be approximately 17% over a 2-year period; however, "foul-smelling urine" was included as a symptom in their definition of UTI, even though recent guidelines do not consider it as a diagnostic criterion for UTI. In residents of PALTC settings, the rate of UTI appears to remain high with an estimated rate of 0.15 per patient-year for

older women and 0.11 per patient-year for older men. One study of nursing home residents with advanced dementia reported that 27% of older adults were diagnosed with UTI over a 2-year period.

PATHOPHYSIOLOGY

The urinary tract (ie, urethra, bladder, ureters, and kidneys) is presumed to be sterile in a normal host. However, this premise particularly changes in older adults as those with increasing disability tend to become colonized, therefore leading to the high rates of ASB. In most adults, a variety of host factors prevent contamination of the urinary tract from pathogenic organisms. The process of urination is the most effective defense mechanism for preventing bacterial invasion of the urinary tract from gastrointestinal microorganisms. Other mechanisms include acidity of urine, peristaltic activity of ureters, a competent vesicoureteral valve, and a variety of other mucosa and immunologic barriers. UTI most often occurs by an ascending route. Organisms colonize the periurethral area and ascend the urethra into the bladder, and sometimes kidneys. Renal infection is determined by virulence characteristics of the infecting organism or the presence of genitourinary abnormalities, such as obstruction or reflux in the host. Rarely, infection may be hematogenous rather than ascending, with urinary infection secondary to bacteremia from a nonurinary source (this is particularly a consideration when *Staphylococcus aureus* is isolated in patients without an indwelling catheter).

Risk Factors in Older Adults for UTI

Older adults may be at higher risk for development of UTI due to a variety of host factors associated with aging, such as a decline in B- and T-cell function. Environmental factors play a large role, as older adults are more likely to have been exposed to the health care system, either through hospitalization or residence in a LTC facility (LTCF), increasing their exposure to virulent nosocomial organisms. Hospitalization often leads to genitourinary instrumentation, and placement of an indwelling catheter has consistently been shown to be a strong risk factor for development of symptomatic UTI in both men and women. Older adults are more likely to have structural or functional abnormalities (eg, benign prostatic hypertrophy in men and cystoceles in women), which lead to urinary stasis by impairing normal voiding and, thus, inhibit the host from "flushing" pathogenic organisms. However, having a high postvoid residual (PVR) has not consistently been shown to increase the risk of developing a symptomatic UTI in either ambulatory women or in PALTC residents. A case-control study in an outpatient setting comparing 149 postmenopausal women who had a history of recurrent UTI with 53 age-matched women without a history of UTI identified three urologic risk factors for recurrent UTI including incontinence (41% vs 9.0%, $p < 0.001$), presence of a cystocele (19% vs 0%; $p < 0.001$), and postvoiding residual urine (28% vs 2.0%; $p < 0.001$). However, a large prospective cohort study of ambulatory women aged 55 to 75 did not find PVR greater than 200 mL to be significantly associated with developing UTI compared to women with residuals less than 50 mL. Another prospective surveillance study in both male and female residents of six Norwegian nursing homes did not find a significant difference in mean PVR between residents who developed UTI compared to those that did not (79 vs 97 mL, $p = 0.26$). They also concluded that having a PVR of 100 mL or greater was not associated with an increasing risk of developing UTI.

The most common risk factor associated with developing UTI in older adults is having a history of UTI. A case-controlled study of postmenopausal women found over a fourfold increase in developing UTI in those women with at least one infection before menopause compared to those with no prior history (odds ratio [OR] 4.20; 95% confidence interval [CI], 3.25–5.42). In postmenopausal women, sexual activity, urinary incontinence, and estrogen deficiency have all been associated with developing UTI, although the extent to which they increase the risk is debated, as studies have demonstrated conflicting results. Declining estrogen levels is associated with increased colonization of the vagina with potential uropathogens.

Postmenopausal women are less likely to have lactobacilli colonizing the vagina, and more likely to have *Escherichia coli* and *Enterococci* spp. These changes in vaginal flora, together with the higher pH in the absence of lactobacilli, are similar to changes observed in younger women with recurrent UTI, and have been suggested to facilitate urinary infection in older women. Certain comorbidities have been linked to developing UTI in older adults. Diabetes mellitus appears to have the strongest association across all age groups. In a cohort of postmenopausal women, those with a diagnosis of diabetes mellitus were almost three times as likely to develop UTI compared to women without diabetes (OR, 2.78; 95% CI, 1.78–4.35). Older adults with diabetes are also at an increased risk for having UTI from a more uncommon uropathogen (eg, *Pseudomonas* spp, *Proteus* spp) and more likely to develop upper tract disease (eg, pyelonephritis). In a cohort of outpatient male veterans with UTI, the most common comorbidities were diabetes mellitus (35%), prostate hypertrophy (33%), and history of prior UTI (31%). Other comorbidities that have been associated with UTI include cerebrovascular disease, Alzheimer disease, and Parkinson disease.

PRESENTATION AND EVALUATION

Asymptomatic Bacteriuria

It has been well documented that clinicians should not screen older adults for ASB and those with ASB should not be treated with antibiotics. Four prospective randomized studies evaluating treatment of ASB in older adults demonstrated no differences in morbidity or mortality in those treated with antibiotics compared to those who did not receive treatment. Furthermore, persistent asymptomatic colonization of the urinary tract is not associated with an increased risk of development of renal failure or hypertension. Thus, the US Preventative Services Task Force (USPSTF), Society for Healthcare Epidemiology of America (SHEA), Infectious Diseases Society of America (IDSA), AMDA—the Society for Post-Acute and Long-Term Care Medicine's UTI consensus statement, and the American Geriatrics Society's Choosing Wisely campaign all recommend against screening and treating for ASB in this population. Only in older adults undergoing invasive urologic procedures should ASB screening and treatment be considered (**Table 106-2**).

Presentation and Evaluation of Symptomatic UTI

The presentation of UTI varies significantly in the older population and is particularly dependent on a person's age, medical comorbidities (eg, diabetes, cerebrovascular disease, Parkinson disease, etc), structural or functional urinary tract abnormalities, demographics (ie, PALTC settings or community-dwelling), and presence of a urinary catheter (eg, urethral or suprapubic). The wide variety of presentations and uncertainty in the definition of what constitutes a symptomatic UTI make it one of the most challenging infections to accurately diagnose and effectively treat.

TABLE 106-2 ■ SUMMARY OF RECOMMENDATIONS FOR SCREENING AND TREATMENT OF ASB IN OLDER ADULTS

PROFESSIONAL SOCIETY	RECOMMENDATION
Infectious Diseases Society of America	• Screening for or treatment of ASB is NOT recommended for the following persons: (1) healthy postmenopausal women, (2) older, community-dwelling men and women who are functionally impaired, (3) older adults residing in long-term care facilities, (4) patients with diabetes, (5) renal transplant recipients > 1 month posttransplant, (6) nonrenal solid organ transplant recipients, (7) patients with spinal cord injury, (8) patients with indwelling catheters, (9) patients undergoing elective nonurologic surgery, and (10) patients living with implanted urologic devices or planning to undergo surgery for an artificial urine sphincter or penile prosthesis implantation (although they should still receive standard perioperative antimicrobial prophylaxis prior to device implantation). • Screening for and treatment of ASB is recommended for patients who will undergo endoscopic urologic procedures associated with mucosal trauma.
US Preventative Services Task Force	• Recommends against screening for and treatment of ASB in nonpregnant adults.
American Geriatrics Society, Choosing Wisely	• Recommends against using antimicrobials to treat bacteriuria in older adults unless specific urinary tract symptoms are present.
AMDA—The Society for Post-Acute and Long-Term Care Medicine's UTI Consensus Statement	• Screening for and treatment of ASB is not recommended for older adults residing in postacute and long-term care settings except before undergoing transurethral resection of the prostate or other urologic procedures associated with mucosal trauma.

ASB, asymptomatic bacteriuria.

Community-Dwelling Older Adults

Presentation In older, cognitively intact adults, the presentation of a symptomatic UTI is similar to that of younger adults and generally begins with the presence of new or worsening genitourinary symptoms. Acute simple cystitis is the most common presentation of symptomatic UTI, and usually manifests as dysuria with or without frequency, urgency, suprapubic pain, or hematuria. Older adults are often suspected for having a UTI when they manifest nonspecific signs and symptoms (eg, confusion, falls, anorexia, functional decline). However, evidence is building that unless more specific localizing signs and symptoms for UTI are present, clinicians should NOT initiate UTI treatment for these symptoms. A prospective cohort study studied older adults who were admitted to the hospital with delirium to determine the association of treating asymptomatic UTI (defined as suspected UTI without concurrent infectious or urinary symptoms) with functional recovery. They defined poor functional recovery as either death, new permanent long-term institutionalization, or decreased ability to perform activities of daily living. Treatment for asymptomatic UTI was associated with poor functional recovery compared to other older inpatients with delirium (RR 1.30; 95% CI, 1.14–1.48 overall). It is important to carefully evaluate the etiology for various nonspecific symptoms as they may have noninfectious etiologies. Patients with upper tract disease (eg, pyelonephritis) typically have additional symptoms such as fever, chills, nausea/vomiting, and flank pain. Presence of warning signs (such as fever, rigors, acute delirium, or unstable vital signs) should also alert clinicians to evaluate a resident for possible infection. Delirium should be carefully distinguished from other behavioral changes. In addition, alternative etiologies for delirium should also be considered before attributing it to UTI, especially in the absence of additional signs and symptoms of UTI.

Evaluation and diagnosis In younger women, the diagnosis and treatment of UTI is usually based on urinary symptoms alone, without the need for confirmation with laboratory testing. Use of a urinary dipstick (to evaluate for leukocyte esterase and nitrite), urinalysis, and urine culture is not routinely recommended in patients with reliable histories. In older adults, this is problematic because of the high prevalence of chronic urinary symptoms (eg, incontinence, urgency, nocturia), which may complicate the diagnosis. Diagnosing and treating UTI with antibiotics without further evaluation for bacteriuria and pyuria in this age group often lead to overtreatment with antimicrobials, especially in those with known chronic urinary symptoms.

A study evaluated five different management strategies for evaluation and treatment of UTI in adult women aged 18 to 70 including empirical antibiotics, empirical delayed (by 48 hours) antibiotics, targeted antibiotics based on a symptom score, performing dipstick and offering antibiotics based on result and prescribing symptomatic treatment until microbiology results became available followed by targeted antibiotics. The investigators found that all management strategies achieve similar symptom control. In another prospective cohort study, which included women up to the age of 89, outpatient adult women presenting with a possible UTI were asked to delay antibiotic treatment for as long as possible. Over half of women who delayed antibiotic treatment did not ultimately require antibiotic therapy, and 71% of them reported clinical improvement or cure without any antibiotic therapy. No adults in this study developed worsening disease (pyelonephritis or bacteremia) as a consequence of delaying antibiotic treatment. An older meta-analysis of five randomized controlled trials (RCTs) involving nonpregnant, nonimmunocompromised adult women with clinically and microbiologically documented acute uncomplicated cystitis concluded that antibiotics are superior to placebo in achieving symptom resolution but also reported no difference in development of pyelonephritis. More recent meta-analysis evaluated four RCTs comparing the use of nonsteroidal anti-inflammatory drugs (NSAIDs) with antibiotic treatment of uncomplicated UTI in nonpregnant women 18 years or older. Antibiotic treatment was found to be more effective than NSAIDs in achieving symptom resolution. The odds of developing upper UTI complications with use of NSAIDs were significantly higher according to this study. However, it has been postulated that the reason for higher upper UTI complications compared to what have been seen in placebo-controlled studies may be related to NSAIDs causing interference with the inflammatory element of the host's defenses.

Based on above-mentioned evidence, it is reasonable to delay empiric antibiotics in women whose diagnosis of UTI is unclear while continuing further evaluation. On the other hand, it is recommended to initiate empiric antibiotics in patients with UTI-specific presentation without further delay after obtaining urine specimens for urinalysis and culture. When UTI is suspected in older adults due to nonspecific clinical presentation without evidence of systemic infection, routine urinary testing should not be performed. Instead, providers should encourage hydration, review medications for potential side effects (eg, diuretics, antipsychotics), and consider other etiologies. If nonspecific clinical symptoms persist, a urinary dipstick can then be performed. If urinary dipstick is positive, and further testing with a urinalysis and urine culture reveals bacteriuria plus pyuria, treatment with antimicrobials for symptomatic UTI may be indicated (**Figure 106-1**). In all cases, a clean catch voided urine specimen collected to minimize

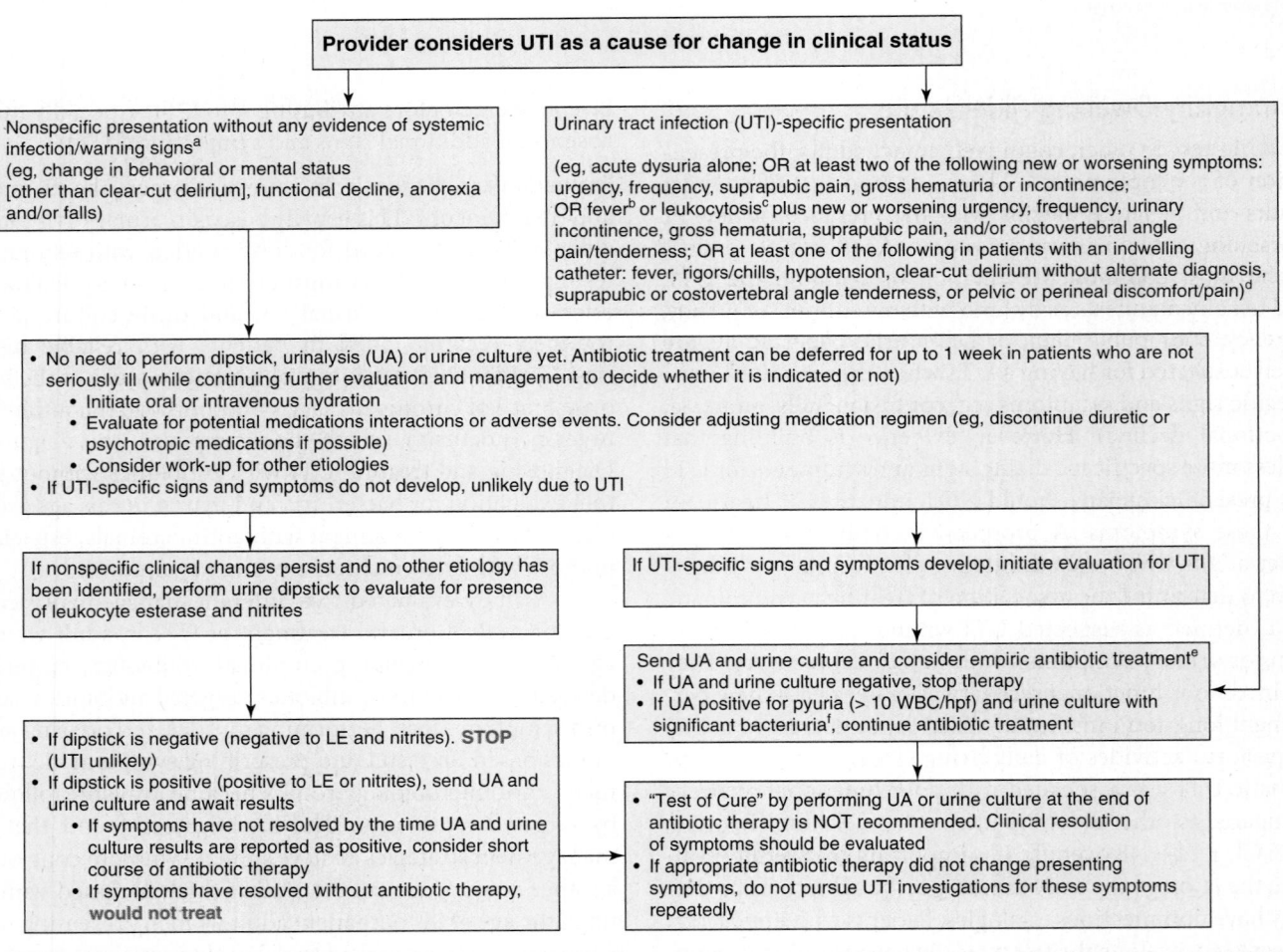

FIGURE 106-1. Urinary tract infection (UTI) assessment and treatment algorithm for older adults.

contamination is preferred. Women should use an antiseptic cloth to first clean the inner folds of the labia, wiping from front to back. A second wipe should then be used to clean the opening of the urethra. Attempts should be made to collect a midstream urine sample, if possible. Although uncommon, symptomatic sexually active women who present with dysuria without pyuria and/or bacteriuria should be evaluated for a sexually transmitted infection (STI). If history is suggestive of a possible STI, screening for chlamydia, gonorrhea, trichomoniasis, HSV, and HIV is warranted.

Postacute and Long-Term Care Residents

Presentation The presentation of symptomatic UTI in PALTC residents is much more elusive. Residents in these settings often do not present with typical signs or symptoms of a genitourinary tract infection (eg, dysuria, frequency, flank pain) and, similar to community-dwelling older adults, many have chronic urinary symptoms such as urinary incontinence, frequency, nocturia, and urgency making it difficult for providers to distinguish which patients have a symptomatic UTI that would benefit from treatment. Furthermore, residents in PALTC settings often suffer from advance cognitive impairment and are unable to verbally communicate genitourinary symptoms suggestive of a symptomatic UTI. It is recommended that in the absence of specific urinary signs or symptoms, behavioral change (exclusive of delirium), decline in functional status, falls, or anorexia should NOT prompt further evaluation for UTI. Furthermore, change in character of the urine is not sufficient to indicate a UTI and may instead reflect mild dehydration or changes to diet or medication.

Evaluation and diagnosis The absence of an agreed-upon definition for symptomatic UTI in PALTC residents makes the diagnosis particularly challenging. Several consensus-based criteria have been published in attempts to help clinicians appropriately prescribe antibiotics for UTI in this population. The McGeer and Loeb criteria, published in 1996 and 2001, respectively, recognized the differences in establishing a diagnosis of infection in LTCFs compared to other settings. The McGeer criteria identified criteria for infection surveillance purposes and the Loeb criteria were developed to help clinicians identify patients that would benefit from empiric antimicrobial therapy. In 2012, an expert consensus panel for SHEA proposed revised guidelines for infection surveillance definitions in LTCFs. The new guidelines (revised McGeer criteria) expanded the definition of UTI and included a new requirement for microbiologic confirmation with urine culture **(Table 106-3)**.

Both original McGeer and revised McGeer criteria were developed to perform surveillance in nursing homes and therefore are not recommended for clinical decision-making. Loeb minimum criteria were specifically developed for clinical decision-making and require presence of localizing signs and symptoms making these challenging for clinicians to proceed with decision-making when nonspecific signs and symptoms are present. As in community-dwelling

TABLE 106-3 ■ 2012 SHEA SURVEILLANCE DEFINITIONS FOR UTI IN LTC RESIDENTS WITHOUT AN INDWELLING CATHETER

≥ 1 of the following signs or symptoms:

1. Acute dysuria or acute pain, swelling, or tenderness of the testes, epididymis, or prostate

or

2. Fever[a] or leukocytosis[b] and ≥ 1 of the following:
   a. Acute costovertebral angle pain or tenderness
   b. Suprapubic pain
   c. Gross hematuria
   d. New or marked increase in incontinence
   e. New or marked increase in urgency
   f. New or marked increase in frequency

or

3. ≥ 2 of the following:
   a. Suprapubic pain
   b. Gross hematuria
   c. New or marked increase in incontinence
   d. New or marked increase in urgency
   e. New or marked increase in frequency

AND

At least 10^5 cfu/mL of ≤ 2 species of microorganisms in a voided urine sample or at least 10^2 cfu/mL of any number of organisms in a specimen collected by an in-and-out catheter.

[a]Single oral temperature > 37.8°C or repeated oral temperatures > 37.2°C or rectal temperatures > 37.5°C or single temperature > 1.1°C over baseline from any site (oral, tympanic, axillary).
[b]Neutrophilia > 14,000 leukocytes/mm³ or left shift (> 6% bands or ≥ 1500 bands/mm³).

older adults, LTC residents with vague, nonspecific symptoms should first be observed for the evolution of symptoms, hydration should be optimized, and alternative diagnoses should be considered. Providers should consider holding medications such as antipsychotics and/or diuretics, if possible, to see if symptoms improve. In PALTC settings, these observation, evaluation, and intervention measures can be combined in an order set which is usually referred to as "active monitoring" protocol. An active monitoring protocol usually consists of an order set that specifies frequent monitoring intervals for vital signs, hydration status (eg, fluid intake), and clinical signs and symptoms. This helps nursing home staff to identify any further change in condition. The protocol also includes orders on how to maintain hydration status of the resident (eg, by specifying the amount of fluid the resident should be offered at predefined intervals). Finally, the protocol outlines when a physician should be notified (eg, if signs and symptoms worsen or do not resolve, if new signs and symptoms arise, or if fluid intake is less than a certain predefined amount).

More recent consensus-based criteria incorporate the use of active monitoring protocol. These consensus-based criteria/guidance include the Agency for Healthcare Research and Quality (AHRQ) decision tool, Improving Outcomes of UTI (IOU) Consensus Guideline, and International Delphi Consensus decision tool **(Table 106-4)**.

TABLE 106-4 ■ CONSENSUS-BASED CRITERIA FOR EVALUATION OF SUSPECTED UTI IN POSTACUTE AND LONG-TERM CARE SETTINGS

CONSENSUS-BASED CRITERIA	COMMENTS
Loeb minimum criteria	Established minimum criteria for the initiation of antibiotics in residents of long-term care facilities.
	For residents without an indwelling urinary catheter, the minimum criteria to initiate antibiotics are described as presence of acute dysuria alone OR fever (100°F or 2.4°F over baseline) and at least one or more of the following new or worsening signs and symptoms: urgency, frequency, gross hematuria, suprapubic tenderness, costovertebral angle tenderness, or urinary incontinence.
	For residents with an indwelling urinary catheter, the minimum criteria to initiate antibiotics are described as presence of at least one of the following: fever, rigors, new-onset delirium, or costovertebral angle tenderness.
AHRQ decision tool for suspected UTI	A decision aid tool for diagnosis of UTI that incorporated standard communication guidance and an order set including option for initiating active monitoring protocol,[a] when applicable.
	For residents without an indwelling catheter, the protocol criteria to initiate antibiotics require the presence of (1) acute dysuria alone, OR (2) fever (100°F) with any of the following new or worsening signs and symptoms: urgency, frequency, back or flank pain, suprapubic pain, gross hematuria, or urinary incontinence, OR (3) two or more of the following signs and symptoms in absence of fever: urgency, frequency, back or flank pain, suprapubic pain, gross hematuria, or urinary incontinence.
	For residents with an indwelling catheter, the protocol criteria to initiate antibiotics require presence of one or more of the following: (1) fever (100°F or repeated temperatures of 99°F or 2°F above the baseline), (2) back or flank pain, (3) acute pain, (4) rigors/shaking chills, (5) new dramatic change in mental status, or (6) hypotension (significant change from baseline BP or a systolic BP < 90).
IOU Consensus Guidelines for the Diagnosis of Uncomplicated Cystitis	Identified five signs and symptoms likely indicative of uncomplicated cystitis in nursing home residents and developed a diagnostic algorithm that can be used to promote antibiotic stewardship in nursing homes.
	Also described warning signs and symptoms that can suggest possible complicated UTI including fever, flank pain, rigors/chills, prostatic/scrotal pain, urinary catheter, hypotension, and elevated serum WBC.
	Uncomplicated cystitis diagnosis is considered to be likely if resident has: (1) dysuria along with one of the following: gross hematuria, suprapubic pain, or urinary frequency/urgency, OR (2) hematuria and suprapubic pain.
	Active monitoring and evaluation for other causes are recommended if no warning signs or symptoms are present and uncomplicated cystitis criteria are not met.
International Delphi Consensus decision tool	A decision tool for suspected UTI in frail older adults that emphasizes that the majority of nonspecific signs and symptoms should be evaluated for causes other than UTI. Active monitoring is also recommended in those clinical scenarios.
	For frail older adults without an indwelling catheter, prescribing antibiotics for suspected UTI is recommended (unless urinalysis shows negative nitrite and leukocyte esterase) in any one of the following scenarios: (1) recent onset of any one of the following localizing signs/symptoms: dysuria, urgency, frequency, incontinence, or visible urethral purulence AND presence of systemic signs/symptoms (fever,[b] rigors/shaking chills, and/or clear-cut delirium[c]); (2) recent onset of ≥ 2 of the aforementioned localizing signs/symptoms OR one very bothersome localizing sign and symptom with no other cause; (3) recent onset of any one of the localizing signs and symptoms AND presence of costovertebral angle pain/tenderness and/or suprapubic pain; (4) recent onset of costovertebral angle pain/tenderness AND presence of systemic signs/symptoms without another infectious focus. Clinicians are recommended to consider obtaining urine culture to evaluate empiric antibiotic choice when diagnostic criteria for UTI are met.
	For frail older adults with an indwelling catheter, prescribing antibiotics for suspected UTI is recommended when fever[b] (lasting for ≥ 24 hours), rigors/shaking chills, or clear-cut delirium (after excluding urinary retention as a possible cause) is present in the absence of other infectious focus. Discontinuation of catheter and obtaining a urine specimen for culture are recommended before prescribing antibiotics. If discontinuation of catheter is not possible, replacing the catheter and obtaining a urine specimen for culture from the new catheter are recommended.

AHRQ, Agency for Healthcare Research and Quality; BP, blood pressure; IOU, improving outcomes of UTI; UTI, urinary tract infection; WBC, white blood cell.
[a]An active monitoring protocol usually consists of an order set that specifies (1) frequency for repeated clinical assessments including vital signs, other signs/symptoms for infection, and hydration status (eg, fluid intake); (2) amount of fluid a resident should be offered at predefined intervals; and (3) triggers for physician notification.
[b]Fever in International Delphi Consensus decision tool is defined as single oral temperature > 37.8°C or repeated oral temperatures > 37.2°C or rectal temperatures > 37.5°C or a 1.1°C increase over the baseline temperature.
[c]International Delphi Consensus decision tool recommended *Diagnostic and Statistical Manual of Mental Disorders-V* definition for delirium.

If upon active monitoring symptoms persist and no other identifiable cause is found, further evaluation is required. A urinary dipstick testing for the presence of leukocyte esterase and nitrite may be performed in that scenario. In patients with nonspecific symptoms and a negative dipstick for leukocyte esterase and nitrites, clinicians should consider other potential etiologies and suspend further evaluation of UTI. If either leukocyte esterase or nitrites are positive, additional testing in with urinalysis and urine culture may be appropriate (see **Figure 106-1**). Every attempt to obtain a clean catch urine is recommended. In patients with severe dementia or urinary incontinence, and whom clinicians determine have a high probability of UTI, in-and-out catheterization for urine collection should be performed if a voided specimen cannot be obtained.

Older Adults With Indwelling Urinary Catheters

Presentation CAUTI is the most common health care–associated infection. CAUTI is difficult to accurately diagnose in older adults, as older adults with catheters often present with nonspecific symptoms such as fever (33%) and mental status changes (13%). Furthermore, almost all adults with a chronic catheter will have bacteriuria and pyuria making it difficult to distinguish between catheter-associated asymptomatic bacteriuria (CA-ASB) and CAUTI in patients with nonspecific symptoms.

Evaluation and diagnosis In 2009, the IDSA updated its current guidelines for diagnosis, treatment, and prevention of CAUTI in adults in an effort to reduce the amount of unnecessary antibiotic treatment in this population. These guidelines include patients with indwelling urethral catheters, indwelling suprapubic catheters, or intermittent catheterization. According to the guidelines, CAUTI is defined as patients with a catheter who develop symptoms or signs compatible with UTI, such as new onset or worsening of fever, rigors, altered mental status, malaise, or lethargy with *no* other identifiable cause; flank pain; costovertebral angle tenderness; acute hematuria; pelvic discomfort; OR dysuria, urgency, or frequency in patients whose catheters have been removed in the previous 48 hours with no other identified source of infection, along with greater than or equal to 10^3 cfu/mL of one or more bacterial species in a single catheter urine specimen or in a midstream voided urine specimen from a patient whose catheter has been removed in the previous 48 hours. AMDA UTI consensus statement describes some of the same signs and symptoms but recommends using greater than or equal to 10^5 cfu/mL threshold while making clinicians aware that even though most persons with CAUTI will have the higher colony counts, CAUTI can be present with lower colony counts of bacteria ($\geq 10^2$ cfu/mL). The 2012 SHEA surveillance definitions for CAUTI also require the presence of a urinary catheter specimen culture with at least 10^5 cfu/mL of any organism(s). Similar to residents without a catheter, CA-ASB should not be screened for, except in patients undergoing urologic instrumentation or procedures. The presence or absence of odorous or cloudy urine should not be used to differentiate CA-ASB from CAUTI (**Table 106-5**).

MANAGEMENT

Microbiology of UTI

The most frequent organism isolated from urinary cultures in both asymptomatic and symptomatic ambulatory elderly women is *E coli*, accounting for 75% to 95% of infections. Other organisms occasionally isolated from this population include other *Enterobacteriaceae* (eg, *Klebsiella pneumoniae, Proteus mirabilis)* and *Enterococcus* spp. Rarely, *Pseudomonas aeruginosa* or group B and D streptococci will be isolated. Common skin flora in this group usually signify contamination, especially if multiple organisms are present. In uncomplicated UTI, over 95% of infections are due to a single organism. Risk factors for non-*E coli* UTIs in community-dwelling older adults include male gender, severe clinical presentation (eg, symptoms more than 7 days, documented or reported fever, nausea or vomiting, flank pain), those with a history of UTI in the past 12 months, history of diabetes mellitus, previous failure of trimethoprim-sulfamethoxazole (TMP/SMX) for treatment of UTI, or patients with functional or anatomical abnormalities. Similar to community-dwelling older adults, *E coli* remains the most frequent organism isolated from urine specimens in residents of LTCFs followed by *Proteus* spp, *Klebsiella* spp, *Enterococcus* spp, *Staphylococcus* spp and *Pseudomonas* spp. Less common causes of UTI in this group include *Acinetobacter, Candida* spp, and methicillin-resistant *S aureus* (MRSA). In older adults with MRSA detected in urine culture, staphylococcal bacteremia as a potential source should be considered. LTC residents, especially those with a chronic urinary catheter, are also more likely to have polymicrobial bacteriuria, with more than one organism isolated in 10% to 25% of bacteriuric subjects. More recently published data described antibiotic resistance in pathogens causing UTI reported by 243 nursing homes to the National Healthcare Safety Network (NHSN) between January 2013 and December 2017. The three most frequently identified pathogens in this dataset are similar to previous reports (*E coli*, 41%; *Proteus* species, 14%; and *K pneumoniae/oxytoca*, 13%). More than a third (36%) of the UTIs were associated with a resistant pathogen. Among *E coli*, fluoroquinolone (FQs) and extended-spectrum cephalosporin resistances were most prevalent (50% and 20%, respectively).

Treatment for UTI

Pharmacologic therapy for ASB in older adults In general, ASB does not require treatment in older adults. However, screening for ASB along with short course of antibiotic treatment (one or two doses) is recommended prior to endoscopic urologic procedures associated

TABLE 106-5 ■ DEFINITIONS FOR UTI IN RESIDENTS WITH AN INDWELLING CATHETER

IDSA GUIDELINES 2009	SHEA SURVEILLANCE DEFINITION 2012	AMDA UTI CONSENSUS STATEMENT 2019
≥ 1 of the following:	≥ 1 of the following:	≥1 of the following:

1. New onset of ≥ 1 of the following with no other identifiable cause:
  a. Worsening fever
  b. Rigors
  c. Altered mental status[a]
  d. Malaise
  e. Lethargy
2. Flank pain
3. Costovertebral angle tenderness
4. Acute hematuria
5. Pelvic discomfort
6. Dysuria, urgent, or frequent urination, or suprapubic pain or tenderness in those whose catheters have been removed
	1. Fever,[b] rigors, or new-onset hypotension, with no alternate site of infection
	2. Either acute change in mental status[a] or acute functional decline,[c] with no alternate diagnosis and leukocytosis[d]
	3. New-onset suprapubic pain or costovertebral angle pain or tenderness
	4. Purulent discharge from around the catheter or acute pain, swelling, or tenderness of the testes, epididymis, or prostate
		1. Systemic or nonspecific signs and symptoms such as fever, rigors/chills, or new-onset clear-cut delirium with no other identified cause
		2. Signs and symptoms localizing to genitourinary tract such as suprapubic or costovertebral angle tenderness; or acute pain swelling or tenderness of the testes, epididymis, or prostate (in men)
		3. If a catheter was removed in the previous 48 hours, presence of signs and symptoms that localize to the genitourinary tract such as urgency, frequency, dysuria, gross hematuria, suprapubic tenderness, or costovertebral angle tenderness

Plus	*Plus*	*Plus*
≥ 10³ cfu/mL of ≥ 1 bacterial species in a single catheter urine specimen *or* in a midstream voided urine specimen from a patient whose catheter has been removed within the previous 48 h	≥ 10⁵ cfu/mL of ≥ 1 of any organism from a urinary catheter specimen	≥10⁵ cfu/mL of ≥ 1 species of bacteria[e]

CDC, Centers for Disease Control and Prevention; IDSA, Infectious Diseases Society of America; SHEA, Society for Healthcare Epidemiology of America.
[a]Acute onset of inattention, disorganized thinking, altered level of consciousness, or fluctuating changes in mental status from baseline.
[b]Single oral temperature > 37.8°C (100°F) or repeated oral temperatures > 37.2°C (99°F) or rectal temperatures > 37.5°C (99.5°F) or single temperature > 1.1°C (2°F) over baseline from any site (oral, tympanic, axillary).
[c]New ≥ 3 point increase in total activities of daily living score from baseline (bed mobility, transfer, locomotion within long-term care facility, dressing, toilet use, personal hygiene, eating).
[d]Neutrophilia > 14,000 leukocytes/mm³ or left shift (> 6% bands or ≥ 1500 bands/mm³).
[e]AMDA UTI consensus statement also alerted clinicians that CAUTI can present with lower colony counts of bacteria (10²–10³) but most will have higher colony counts.

with mucosal trauma. The antibiotic course should be targeted based on the organism identified from the screening urine culture. The therapy should be initiated 30 to 60 minutes before the procedure.

Pharmacologic therapies for community-dwelling older adults
Treatment of UTI for community-dwelling older adults generally follows the same diagnostic algorithm used in younger adults. However, a urine culture should be obtained to guide treatment, as older adults are at higher risk for harboring multidrug-resistant organisms (MDROs). For acute simple cystitis, the International Clinical Practice Guidelines issued by the European Society for Microbiology and Infectious Diseases and the IDSA recommend as first-line treatment either nitrofurantoin monohydrate/macrocrystals, 100 mg twice daily for 5 days, OR TMP/SMX, 160/800 mg twice daily for 3 days. Fosfomycin (3 g as a single dose) is an acceptable alternative, although few studies have demonstrated inferior efficacy compared to nitrofurantoin or TMP/SMX for treatment of uncomplicated UTI. Fosfomycin continues to have activity against many multidrug-resistant isolates. However, there are concerns that overuse of fosfomycin may result in increasing rates of resistance. Therefore, current recommendations are to use fosfomycin when

suspecting infection with multidrug-resistant pathogens or when other first-line agents cannot be used (**Table 106-6**).

It is important to consider prior culture data (if available) or local resistance pattern when choosing antibiotics empirically. In one study, three-quarters of empiric antibiotics provided adequate coverage for the current UTI when clinicians chose the regimen based on susceptibility results from the urine cultures in the preceding 6 to 24 months. In contrast, when the chosen antibiotics were not effective against previously identified pathogens, only one-third of empiric antibiotics provided adequate coverage for UTI. When previous culture results are not available, clinicians should consider looking at local resistance pattern before prescribing the antibiotics. The 2010 guidelines recommend avoiding using TMP/SMX for acute simple cystitis if local resistance rates of uropathogens exceed 20%. Nitrofurantoin is listed on the American Geriatric Society's Beers Criteria for potentially inappropriate medication use in older adults due to potential for pulmonary toxicity, hepatotoxicity, and peripheral neuropathy, especially with long-term use. It recommends avoiding using nitrofurantoin in individuals with creatinine clearance less than 30/mL/min or for long-term suppression. However, nitrofurantoin has consistently lower rates of resistance to

TABLE 106-6 ■ COMMONLY USED ORAL ANTIBIOTICS FOR TREATMENT OF UTI

ANTIBIOTIC	STANDARD DOSE FOR CRCL[a] > 60 mL/min	SIDE EFFECTS	COMMENTS
Trimethoprim + sulfamethoxazole	Acute simple cystitis: 800/160 mg orally twice daily for 3 d Complicated UTI: 800/160 mg orally twice daily for up to 14 d	GI intolerance Elevation in serum creatinine (~ 20%)	First-line treatment for acute simple cystitis, although avoid empiric use if local resistance rates to uropathogens exceed 20% If used for empiric treatment of complicated UTI, then patient should at least receive an initial dose of long-standing parenteral agent and clinicians may consider waiting for the culture and susceptibility result before switching to oral trimethoprim + sulfamethoxazole Significant interaction with warfarin (increases international normalized ratio) and sulfonylurea (increases risk of hypoglycemia)
Nitrofurantoin monohydrate/macrocrystals	Acute simple cystitis: 100 mg orally twice daily for 5 d	GI intolerance Pulmonary toxicity (rare)	First-line treatment for acute simple cystitis, *E coli* resistance remains low (< 10%) Not appropriate for treatment of complicated UTI Avoid if CrCl[a] < 30
Fosfomycin trometamol	Acute simple cystitis: 3 g single oral dose	GI intolerance (diarrhea ~ 10%) Headache, dizziness Vaginitis	First-line treatment for acute simple cystitis but generally reserved for infections with highly resistant pathogens (including to ESBL[b] gram-negative rods and VRE[c]) or when other first-line agents cannot be used Not recommended for complicated UTI Additional doses of fosfomycin will be administered every 2–3 d if intended treatment duration is > 3 d
Amoxicillin + clavulanate	Acute simple cystitis: 500/125 mg orally twice daily for 5–7 d Complicated UTI: 875 mg twice daily for 10–14 d	GI intolerance Rash	Second-line treatment due to high resistance rates Avoid in complicated UTI and, if used for treatment of complicated UTI, should follow appropriate parenteral therapy
Ciprofloxacin	Acute simple cystitis: 250 mg orally twice daily for 3 d Complicated UTI: 500 mg orally twice daily for 5–7 d	Higher risk of *C difficile*-associated colitis Tendinopathy and tendon rupture Peripheral neuropathy Aortic aneurysm/aortic dissection Hyperglycemia and hypoglycemia CNS side effects QT prolongation	Second-line treatment for acute simple cystitis due to high resistance and significant side effects Only oral antibiotic recommended for empiric treatment for complicated UTI, although use is limited in clinical settings due to increasing resistance rates and significant side effects If used for treatment of complicated UTI in areas where local resistance rates to common uropathogens exceeds 10%, it should follow an initial dose of long-acting parenteral agent Significant interactions with antacids and vitamins, may decrease absorption

[a]Creatinine clearance.
[b]Extended spectrum β-lactamase.
[c]Vancomycin-resistant enterococci.

E coli (the most commonly identified pathogen in urine cultures), and when given for 5 to 7 days has been shown to have similar effectiveness as other antimicrobials for treatment of acute simple cystitis. Therefore, nitrofurantoin remains a good option for treatment of acute simple cystitis in older adults with creatinine clearance greater than or equal to 30 mL/min.

Second-line antibiotics for empiric treatment of acute simple cystitis or for patients whose organisms are sensitive to the following antibiotics include (1) amoxicillin/clavulanate 500/125 mg orally twice daily for 5 to 7 days; (2) cefpodoxime 100 mg orally twice daily for 5 to 7 days; or (3) cefixime 400 mg orally for 5 to 7 days. FQs are no longer considered first-line treatment of acute simple cystitis because of increasing resistance against gram-negative pathogens and serious side effects associated with its use. These side effects include prolongation of the QT interval, tendon rupture, hypoglycemia, rupture of an aortic aneurysm, peripheral neuropathy, and other central nervous system side effects.

In general, evidence supports that for older adults with acute simple cystitis a shorter course of antibiotics

(< 7 days) has similar efficacy as compared to a longer course (≥ 7 days). Further, longer antibiotic course may be associated with more side effects. One of the double blinded RCT compared 3-day course of ciprofloxacin to 7-day course in older women with uncomplicated UTI. They found similar cure rates (98% vs 83%, $p = 0.16$) 2 days after the course, along with similar reinfection (14% vs 18%, $p = 0.54$) and relapse (15% vs 13%, $p = 0.83$) rates at 6 weeks posttreatment in both groups. However, adverse events were significantly less in the 3-day versus 7-day group both at day 5 (0.9 vs 1.6, $p = 0.001$) and day 9 (1.2 vs 2.1, $p = 0.001$) of treatment. There are several underlying factors that may increase the risk of complications in patients who are being treated for acute simple cystitis (**Table 106-7**). These factors include obstructions, instrumentation, impaired voiding, metabolic abnormalities, and immunocompromised status. In past, acute simple cystitis in patients who may have some of these underlying conditions have been treated for longer (10- to 14-day) duration. However, it has been shown that shorter duration of treatment may also be sufficient in patients who are at high risk of recurrence or complications. A retrospective study evaluated the relationship between antibiotic regimen and the cure rate of febrile UTI among patients with neurogenic bladder. The patients were divided into less than 10 days, 10 to 15 days and greater than 15 days groups. One month after the end of treatment, there were no significant differences in the cure rates (71%, 54%, and 57%, $p = 0.34$). Treatment decision for acute simple cystitis in patients who are at higher risk for recurrence or complications should be based on response to the treatment. For most of these patients, 7 days of antibiotic treatment should be adequate if they respond promptly to antibiotic (within 72 hours). Longer (10- to 14-day) durations are reasonable for those patients who have delayed response to treatment or were found to have more complicated infections (eg, bacteremia).

In men, all UTI episodes have been considered as complicated in the past. However, it is not the best way to classify UTI episodes since men can also have acute simple cystitis. The first-line antimicrobial agents for treatment of acute simple cystitis in men are the same as for women (TMP/SMX, nitrofurantoin, and fosfomycin). However, older men with urologic abnormalities or other immunocompromising conditions are more likely to be at higher risk for complicated infection. Therefore, careful evaluation is always needed to rule out any signs and symptoms indicating extension of infection beyond the bladder before treating acute simple cystitis. In general, men with UTI

TABLE 106-7 ■ FACTORS THAT MAY PREDISPOSE OLDER ADULTS WITH A UTI TO TREATMENT FAILURE OR COMPLICATIONS

COMPLICATING FACTORS	CLINICAL EXAMPLES	CONSIDERATIONS
Obstruction	Ureteric or urethral strictures Tumors of the urinary tract Urolithiasis Prostatic hypertrophy Diverticulae Pelvicalyceal obstruction Renal cysts Congenital abnormalities	A history of obstruction, by itself, is not a complicating factor unless the obstruction is still ongoing. Older male patients have been historically considered to be at high risk as many presenting with UTI may also have underlying urologic abnormalities like prostate hypertrophy. More recent evidence indicates that 7 d of antibiotic is sufficient to treat cystitis in men (see text). Prostatitis (which requires longer length of therapy) should be suspected in residents with recurrent cystitis or if resident also has fever or pelvic or perineal pain. Management of obstruction is also a key component of UTI treatment
Instrumentation	Indwelling urethral catheter Intermittent catheterization Ureteric stent Nephrostomy tube Urological procedures	Frequently reassess the need for an indwelling catheter and if deemed unnecessary, remove the catheter.
Impaired voiding	Neurogenic bladder Cystocele Vesicoureteral reflux Ileal conduit	Risks of complication may depend on severity of the voiding impairment.
Metabolic abnormalities	Nephrocalcinosis Medullary sponge kidney Renal failure (eCrCl <30 mL/min) Diabetes mellitus	Risks of complications in patients with diabetes with good glycemic control and without long-term diabetes complications will be lower than those with poor glycemic control and presence of diabetic compications.
Immunocompromised	Renal transplant	

Reproduced with permission from Rodrigues LP, Teixeira VR, Alencar-Silva T, et al. Hallmarks of aging and immunosenescence: connecting the dots. Cytokine Growth Factor Rev. 2021;59:9–21.

are usually treated with a 7- to 14-day antibiotic course. A study conducted in male veterans found shorter-course treatments for UTI (< 7 days) to be as effective compared to longer duration of treatment (> 7 days). Another study compared 7- and 14-day courses for patients with febrile UTI. In men, 7 days of antibiotics was inferior to 14 days in achieving short-term (10–18 days posttreatment) clinical cure. However, the long-term clinical cure rates were similar indicating no difference in outcomes at 70 to 84 days posttreatment. Therefore, for most older men with acute simple cystitis 7 days of antibiotic treatment should be adequate if they respond promptly to antibiotics (within 72 hours).

Management of complicated UTI (infection extending beyond the bladder including pyelonephritis) varies depend on the severity of the illness. Although age more than 60 years has been described to be a relative indication for hospitalization in patients with acute pyelonephritis, outpatient management in those with mild to moderate illness, adequate social support, and clinical stability is likely to be as safe and as effective compared to hospitalization. Older adults with complicated UTI (including pyelonephritis) who present with severe symptoms (eg, persistent vomiting), suspected sepsis, uncertain diagnosis, evidence of urinary tract obstruction, and have significant frailty should be hospitalized. FQs are the only oral antibiotic recommended for empiric treatment of complicated UTI. However, increasing resistance of FQ and concerns of side effects limit the use of this drug in many clinical settings. Experts do not recommend empiric FQ use in areas with local resistance noted to be higher than 10%. Similarly, FQ use should also be avoided if patient at high risk for infection with MDROs or adverse events are secondary to its use. If FQ is being used for treatment of complicated UTI in areas with more than 10% resistance, then the patient should receive an initial dose of long-acting parenteral agent (eg, ceftriaxone, ertapenem, etc) before starting FQ. Similarly, if using any other oral antibiotic (eg, TMP-SMX) for empiric treatment of complicated UTI, patients should receive one dose of long-acting parenteral agent before starting the oral antibiotic. Clinicians may consider continuing parenteral treatment and wait for the culture and susceptibility results before switching to oral antibiotics especially if the patient is at higher risk of infection secondary to MDROs or severe illness. Oral beta-lactam agents are usually less effective than FQ and TMP-SMX for treatment of complicated UTI including acute pyelonephritis and should be avoided when other treatment options are available. Nitrofurantoin and fosfomycin should not be used for complicated UTI because of inadequate renal penetration. When choosing parenteral agent for the initial dose, aminoglycosides (such as gentamicin or tobramycin) are usually avoided because they are more toxic than other available parenteral antibiotics (eg, ceftriaxone, ertapenem, etc), although the risk of ototoxicity and nephrotoxicity with aminoglycoside therapy is very low when therapy duration is limited to 48 to 72 hours (see **Table 106-6**).

Pharmacologic therapies for postacute and LTC residents In general, pharmacologic therapies for postacute and LTC residents are usually similar to what have been described above for community-dwelling older adults. Some of the factors that usually influence decision-making for treatment of UTI may need additional attention in postacute and LTC settings. First, antibiotic resistance is generally much higher in these settings compared to the community population. Thus, it is imperative that clinicians become familiar with local resistance rates and guide empiric antibiotic regimens based on resistance patterns. Urine culture results should always help adjust antibiotic choices. Second, alterations in antimicrobial pharmacokinetics such as increased volume of distribution and decreased renal clearance are often observed in older adults; thus, providers should be cognizant of a patient's glomerular filtration rate (GFR) when dosing antimicrobials. Third, older adults in these settings often must manage polypharmacy and drug–drug interactions should always be evaluated. For instance, TMP/SMX, along with many other antibiotics, has significant interactions with anticoagulants and thus, close international normalized ratio (INR) monitoring is recommended in patients receiving warfarin. In most cases, warfarin dosages will need to be decreased by at least 50% through the entire duration of antimicrobial therapy.

Finally, establishing a diagnosis of UTI is very challenging in frail and medically complex residents of postacute and long-term settings, some of whom may not be able to verbalize any symptoms. In order to avoid initiating unnecessary antibiotic treatment, AMDA's consensus statement recommends that clinicians in PALTC setting use standard clinical algorithms to guide the diagnosis and decision to initiate antibiotics for residents with suspected UTI.

Several consensus-based criteria have been published to assist with diagnosis and treatment of suspected UTI in residents of PALTC settings (see **Table 106-4**). Loeb minimum criteria describe the clinical signs and symptoms that should be present prior to initiating antibiotics in nursing home residents suspected of having infection. AHRQ also developed a set of criteria, which were incorporated into a standard communication and decision aid tool. The UTI SBAR tool developed by AHRQ aims to assist in better assessment of resident signs and symptoms by the nursing home staff, effective communication of those findings with prescribing clinicians, and differentiating between when a resident needs to be started on antibiotic versus on an active monitoring protocol. International Delphi Consensus decision tool consists of separate clinical algorithms for management of suspected UTI in frail older adults with and without indwelling catheters. The decision tool describes which specific and nonspecific signs and symptoms are associated with UTI and when the antibiotic prescribing is justified. The IOU consensus statement also used the Delphi procedure to provide guidance on which clinical signs and symptoms to consider when making decision on empiric treatment of uncomplicated cystitis. There has been no head-to-head comparison for the clinical impact of the above-mentioned consensus-based criteria. Therefore, the AMDA UTI consensus statement has suggested that PALTC settings should choose one of the consensus-based criteria that seems most closely aligned with their current practices to facilitate the implementation.

Older adults including residents of postacute and LTC settings may manifest acute illness with atypical signs and symptoms that can also be nonlocalizing. Clinicians should perform careful evaluation to differentiate between infectious and noninfectious etiologies for change of condition in residents of PALTC settings. SHEA has published an expert guidance that outlines those signs and symptoms that should and should not prompt further evaluation for infection in these settings. According to this guidance, clinicians should evaluate residents with fever, hypothermia, hypotension, hyperglycemia, and/or unequivocal delirium for an infection while considering the possibility of noninfectious causes for these symptoms. The guidance recommends against further evaluation for infection in residents who present with a fall, functional decline, or anorexia. Furthermore, it recommends using Confusion Assessment Method (CAM) to identify the presence of delirium in a resident of a nursing home with behavioral/mental status changes. Delirium in residents of PALTC settings may be precipitated by a number of infectious and noninfectious conditions, including medications and metabolic disorders. If delirium has been excluded, further evaluation for infection is not necessary unless additional, more specific signs and symptoms are present. The AMDA UTI consensus statement also

recommends against initiating empiric treatment for UTI when clinical criteria for UTI are not met and there are no warning signs (ie, evidence of systemic infection, such as fever, rigors/chills, unstable vitals, or new-onset, clear-cut delirium). In those situations, if clinicians are still concerned for UTI, the AMDA consensus statement recommends responding to this diagnostic uncertainty with an "active monitoring" protocol. If the resident condition improves with the supportive care (including hydration), that will obviate the need for treating suspected UTI. The approach to management of suspected UTI in PALTC settings is summarized in **Figure 106-2**.

Shorter length of therapy, similar to what is described for community-dwelling older adult, is also sufficient for treatment of UTI in residents of PALTC settings. The recently published AMDA consensus statement recommended fewer than 7-day antibiotic course to PALTC residents with acute simple cystitis who are not severely ill and not at high risk for developing complications. For those residents who are at higher risk of treatment failure or who have complicated UTI, the length of antibiotic is recommended to be based on the severity of the illness and response to treatment. For most of these residents, 7 days of antibiotic treatment should be adequate if they respond promptly to antibiotics (within 72 hours). Longer (10–14 days) durations are reasonable for residents with severe illness, such as bacteremia, or a delayed response to treatment. The choice of antibiotics also impacts the duration of treatment. For example, when treating complicated UTI, FQs are usually prescribed for 5 to 7 days, TMP-SMX for 7 to 14 days, and oral beta-lactams for 10 to 14 days.

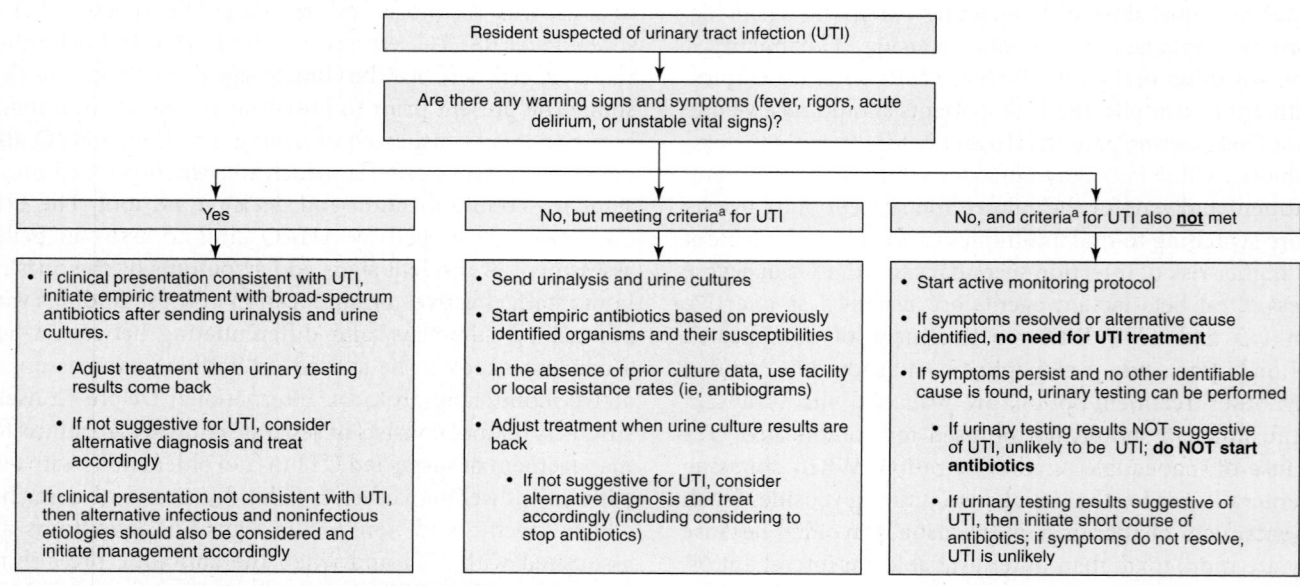

^aSeveral consensus-based criteria have been published to assist with diagnosis and treatment of suspected UTI (see text). Postacute and long-term care settings may choose a consensus-based criteria that seem most closely aligned with their current practices to facilitate the implementation.

FIGURE 106-2. Approach to management of suspected UTI in postacute and long-term care settings.

PREVENTION

Cranberry Formulations

Cranberry juice has been used as a home remedy for prevention and treatment of UTI for decades, although the evidence to support this intervention as a prevention strategy is still debated. Cranberry proanthocyanidin (PAC) is the active ingredient in cranberry that is thought to inhibit adherence of P-fimbriated *E coli* to uroepithelial cell receptors. However, a Cochrane review evaluating use of cranberry containing products (ie, juice, tablets, or capsules) did not find significant evidence that any of these products prevented UTI in women compared to placebo, water, or no treatment. Another study examining cranberry capsules containing 36 to 108 mg of PAC found a trend toward a decrease in bacteriuria plus pyuria in LTC residents, suggesting formulations with higher doses of PAC may be beneficial. A systematic review and meta-analysis of only RCTs did conclude that cranberry products reduced UTI recurrence in women with at least three UTIs in a 1-year period (risk ratio [RR] 0.53; 95% CI, 0.33–0.83). However, because of the substantial heterogeneity across trials, the authors mention that this conclusion should be interpreted with great caution. A more recent systematic review and meta-analysis of seven randomized trials came to similar conclusion. They found cranberry reduced the risk of UTI by 26% (pooled RR: 0.74; 95% CI, 0.55–0.98; $I^2 = 54\%$) in healthy women at risk for UTI. However, most of the studies had small sample size and there were significant limitations due to which the authors noted that larger high-quality studies are needed to confirm these findings. Given the issues of volume and glucose load for a cranberry juice supplement and size and cost of cranberry capsules, further investigation of cranberry supplements in older adults is warranted prior to recommending either product as a prevention strategy. Even though more recent urology guidelines stated that clinicians may offer cranberry prophylaxis for recurrent UTI (while acknowledging the limitations), AMDA UTI consensus statement for PALTC setting concluded that current evidence does not support the use of cranberry products for the prevention of UTI.

Vaginal Estrogen

In older adults, declining estrogen levels are thought to lead to declining levels of lactobacilli in the vaginal tract and thus, increase colonization of the perineal area with organisms such as *E coli*. Topical estrogen appears to be a safe and potentially effective method for prevention of UTI in postmenopausal women. A systematic review and meta-analysis evaluated the evidence regarding use of vaginal estrogens as a prevention strategy for recurrent UTI in postmenopausal women. Both RCTs included in this study found that vaginal estrogen (vaginal cream containing 0.5 mg of estriol or vaginal ring with 2 mg estradiol) significantly reduced the risk of UTI in postmenopausal women (RR 0.25; 95% CI, 0.13–0.50; and RR 0.64; 95% CI,

0.47–0.86, respectively). However, their pooled effect was not significant (RR 0.42; 95% CI, 0.16–1.10). In one of the study that described significant decrease in incidence of UTI in the vaginal estriol group as compared to placebo group (0.5 vs 5.9 episodes per-patient year, $p < 0.001$), reported side effects of vaginal estrogen use included vaginal irritation, burning or itching. However, the side effects were described as mild and self-limited. As benefits of vaginal estrogens appear to outweigh potential minor side effect concerns most experts including recent urology guidelines and AMDA UTI consensus statement for PALTC settings recommend considering vaginal estrogen therapy for prevention of recurrent UTI in older women. Vaginal estrogen has not been demonstrated to increase the risk of estrogen-dependent cancer (eg, breast cancer). However, clinicians are recommended to coordinate with patients' oncologists when considering vaginal estrogen therapy for those who either have personal history or are at high risk for estrogen-dependent cancer.

Suppressive Antibiotics

In general, prolonged suppressive antimicrobial therapy for prevention of UTI in older adults should be avoided. It may be considered when there is persistent or recurrent morbidity attributable to UTI. Such circumstances are uncommon, but might include recurrent invasive infection in the presence of an underlying genitourinary abnormality that cannot be corrected, persistent infected stones where suppressive therapy may prevent further stone enlargement, frequent symptomatic recurrences from a prostatic source, or with chronic renal failure. Antimicrobial selection for suppressive therapy is individualized, based on susceptibilities of the infecting organism and tolerance. Deciding whether to use antibiotic prophylaxis must be determined based on the frequency of UTI, severity of symptoms, and possibility of adverse effects of chronic antimicrobial use such as development of *Clostridioides difficile* colitis, selection of multidrug-resistant organisms and various other adverse drug reactions. Patients should also be made aware of the risks and benefits for choosing suppressive antibiotics for prevention of UTI. For many older adults, these risks are likely to outweigh any benefit and suppressive therapy is seldom indicated. More recently, a matched cohort study compared older adults with UTI receiving antibiotic prophylaxis (defined as antibiotic treatment for at least 30 days) that was started within 30 days after a positive urine culture to those who did not receive prophylaxis (but received the treatment). Antibiotic prophylaxis recipients were at higher risk of emergency department visits or hospitalizations for UTI, sepsis or bloodstream infection (HR, 1.33; 95% CI, 1.12–1.57), acquisition of antibiotic resistance to any urinary antibiotics (HR, 1.31; 95% CI, 1.18–1.44), developing *C difficile* infections (HR, 1.56; 95% CI, 1.05–2.23), and experiencing general medical adverse events (HR, 1.62; 95% CI, 1.11–2.29). Recent urology guidelines state that clinicians may prescribe antibiotic prophylaxis to decrease the risk of future UTI but emphasize that all antibiotics have potential risk and the decision to prescribe should follow the discussion of the risks, benefits, and alternatives with the patients. Recent AMDA UTI consensus statement acknowledges that antibiotic prophylaxis may reduce the risk of recurrent uncomplicated cystitis but points out that the potential harms associated with long-term use, coupled with the prevalence of multidrug-resistant organisms among PALTC residents, argue against long-term antibiotic prophylaxis in these settings.

Other Antimicrobial Sparing Agents

In addition to the cranberry products and vaginal estrogens, several other agents have been used in clinical practice for prevention of UTI but their benefits remain uncertain. These agents include methenamine salts, probiotics, ascorbic acid, and D-Mannose. A structured review published in 2019 evaluated the available evidence for the use of several nonantibiotic agents to prevent UTI in women 45 years or older concluded that there is a lack of evidence to make recommendations for or against the use of ascorbic acid, cranberry juice, cranberry capsules with high proanthocyanidin content, D-mannose, *Lactobacillus*, and methenamine hippurate. Further studies are needed to clarify the roles of these antimicrobial sparing agents in prevention of UTI among older adults.

Prevention of Catheter-Associated UTI

The most effective strategies for prevention of CAUTI are to avoid catheterization and, when an indwelling catheter is indicated, to discontinue the catheter as soon as possible. The Healthcare Infection Control Practices Advisory Committee as part of the Centers for Disease Control (CDC), issued guidelines in 2009, aimed to help providers with the prevention, diagnosis, and management of persons with CAUTI, particularly hospitalized patients and residents of LTCFs. In older adults that require catheter placement, recommendations include insertion of catheters aseptically by trained personnel, use of the smallest diameter catheter as possible, hand washing before and after catheter manipulation, maintenance of a closed catheter system, avoiding irrigation unless anticipating obstruction (eg, after prostatic or bladder surgery), keeping the collecting bag below the bladder, and maintaining good hydration in residents. The guidelines also recommend against changing indwelling catheters or drainage bags at routine, fixed intervals. Instead, it is suggested to change catheters and drainage bags based on clinical indications such as infection, obstruction, or when the closed system is compromised. The catheter should only be replaced if still indicated. Use of antimicrobial-coated catheters has been shown to delay bacterial colonization and thus reduce the incidence of bacteriuria. However, an RCT evaluating the use of two antibiotic-coated catheters did not find significant benefit in prevention of CAUTI. These catheters are more expensive and thus are likely not beneficial in most clinical settings. Use of a computerized clinical decision support intervention for reducing the duration of catheter use has been shown to be effective in limiting the duration of catheters and CAUTIs in hospitalized patients, although this intervention may be more difficult to implement in LTCFs.

As CAUTIs are the most common health care–associated infection, there have been regulatory changes directed toward incentivizing CAUTI reduction in both hospitals and nursing homes. PALTC settings are paying special attention to incorporating strategies for CAUTI prevention including making sure that residents have an indwelling catheter only when indicated. In one of the observational cohort studies including 228 long-stay residents with an indwelling catheter, 86% had a documented indication for the catheter. Of those 193 residents with a documented indication, 99% had one or more indications deemed appropriate, including urinary retention (83%), pressure ulcer (21%), hospice care (10%), and need for accurate measurement of input and output (6%). Evidence suggest that implementing intervention bundles that incorporate technical strategies (focusing on aseptic insertion, catheter maintenance, regular assessments, prompt removal when no longer indicated, and incontinence care planning) and socioadaptive strategies (focusing on effective communication and engaging nursing home leadership, staff, residents and their families in CAUTI prevention efforts) can result in significant reductions in CAUTI especially in those facilities struggling with higher CAUTI rates. When such intervention was implemented in 404 community nursing homes, their adjusted CAUTI rates decreased from 6.42 to 3.33 infections per 1000 catheter days (incidence rate ratio, 0.46; 95% CI, 0.36–0.58; $p < .001$). However, a similar intervention in Veterans Affairs nursing homes did not result in significant change (2.26–3.19 infections per 1000 catheter days; incidence rate ratio, 0.99; 95% CI, 0.67–1.44). The lack of success in further reduction of CAUTI rate was thought to be secondary to lower baseline CAUTI rate in this setting. Therefore, it is important for the nursing home leaders to evaluate their baseline CAUTI rates before dedicating resources specifically to a CAUTI-reduction bundle. Another study evaluated the impact of a multimodal targeted infection prevention program implementation in 12 community nursing homes. The program included active surveillance for infections, ongoing educational programs for staff, hand hygiene promotion, and preemptive barrier precautions for all residents with indwelling devices. This intervention resulted in both decreased MDRO prevalence density and CAUTIs. It provides evidence that CAUTI reduction effort can also be incorporated into more comprehensive infection prevention and control bundle in PALTC settings.

SPECIAL ISSUES

Outcomes

Most healthy older adults with symptomatic UTI respond well to antibiotic therapy. However, bacteriuria is associated with significant morbidity, often related to antibiotic use, which promotes the development of multidrug-resistant bacteria and overgrowth of organisms such as *C difficile*. Presence of an indwelling catheter, age, and medical comorbidities influence outcomes. CAUTI was associated with a significantly higher mortality in hospitalized adults aged 65 or older compared to UTI in noncatheterized patients (19% vs 11%, $p < 0.05$). In a retrospective cohort study of residents with UTI in LTCFs in the United States, risk factors that appeared to increase the risk of hospitalization included advancing age, Hispanic or African-American race/ethnicity, diabetes mellitus, Parkinson disease, dementia, and stroke. Factors that decreased the risk of hospitalization in this same cohort included the ability to walk, physician visit at the time of admission to a LTCF, and maintaining or improving mobility in those with severe mobility problems. One of the most serious complications of UTI is the development of bacteremia as a consequence of persistent infection causing hematologic spread. Older adults are more likely than younger adults to develop gram-negative bacteremia as a consequence of UTI. The mortality in patients with bacteremic UTI has been described to be between 14% and 33%. However, adults with bacteremia as a result of UTI compared to bacteremia from other etiologies tend to have better outcomes.

Antibiotic Resistance

Antibiotic resistance is a large problem in all health care settings including outpatient, PALTC and acute hospital settings. UTI remains the most common reason antibiotics are prescribed in older adults, despite increased awareness of emerging resistance as a result of overtreatment. A substantial proportion of antibiotics are prescribed for asymptomatic infection or presentations without localizing urinary symptoms, fostering the development of increasingly resistant organisms.

Antibiotic resistance in the community Antibiotic resistance is no longer limited to the hospital setting. Primary care providers are responsible for a significant number of antimicrobial prescriptions in community-dwelling older adults and recent antibiotic use in the primary care setting has been shown to be the most important risk factor for development of an infection with a resistant organism. Adults who receive an antibiotic for UTI are over four times more likely to develop a resistant organism within 1 month compared to adults not prescribed an antimicrobial agent. Although the risk is greatest at 1 month, resistance persists for up to 12 months in many patients. A population-based cohort study in Minnesota found the incidence of resistant *E coli* urinary isolates to FQ plus TMP/SMX in adults aged 80 or older to nearly double over a 4-year period (274–512 per 100,000 person-years, $p < 0.05$). Despite the increasing awareness of drug-resistant pathogens in the community, overuse with antimicrobials for treatment of UTI remains. Community-dwelling older adults may believe that antibiotic resistance is a hospital-acquired condition and may not fully understand the risks associated with each antibiotic prescription. Primary care providers may feel that

increasing resistance to antibiotics is largely out of their control. Further studies assessing patient and community physician understanding of antibiotic resistance, particularly as it relates to UTI, are needed.

Antibiotic resistance in PALTC settings Over the past several years, increased awareness has been placed on infection control practices and ASPs in LTCFs, although inappropriate use of antibiotics remains high in this setting. Prevalence rates of colonization with antibiotic-resistant bacteria have been reported to be higher than 50% in some LTCFs. Among all urinary isolates of residents in five nursing homes in Connecticut, 26% were resistant to TMP/SMX, 40% were resistant to FQs, and 25% were resistant to cefazolin. The resistance rates to FQ in only *E coli* isolates were much higher at nearly 60%. *E coli* isolates were highly sensitive to nitrofurantoin (93%), although its sensitivity to all organisms was much lower at 68%. Similar to the community setting, high antibiotic prescriptions driving increasing resistance rates continue to be prevalent despite increased awareness. Qualitative studies have characterized some variables, which drive inappropriate antimicrobial use in this setting. When antimicrobial therapy is prescribed, often, nursing personnel are evaluating patients and communicating their findings to physicians. Physicians may not assess patients directly. Nursing personnel (ie, nurses and nurses' aides) are critical to identifying patients that are suspected of having UTI, requesting urine studies to be sent, and suggesting that antibiotic therapy may be warranted. Interventions focused on educating nursing staff to perform detailed assessment of a resident when a UTI is suspected and improving communication with physicians after assessment have resulted in decreased antibiotic use for the UTI in PALTC settings.

Antimicrobial Stewardship Programs

UTIs are major driver of antibiotic use and inappropriate antibiotic prescribing related to UTI is common in various health care (including acute-care, outpatient, and PALTC) settings. ASPs are designed to promote appropriate antibiotic prescribing while reducing the adverse events associated with antibiotic use. CDC has published core elements of antibiotic stewardship programs for different health care settings. For hospitals and nursing homes, there are seven recommended core elements including (1) leadership commitment, (2) accountability, (3) pharmacy expertise (for hospitals)/drug expertise (for nursing homes), (4) action, (5) tracking, (6) reporting, and (7) education. For outpatient antibiotic stewardship, they outlined four core elements including (1) commitment, (2) action for policy and practice, (3) tracking and reporting, and (4) education and expertise. CDC's core elements of antibiotic stewardship provide a framework that clinicians and health care facilities can use to put in place comprehensive set of interventions that involves reviewing antimicrobial stewardship related data (eg, antibiotic use and outcome data), identifying opportunities for improvement, implementing action plan for improvement in antibiotic prescribing practices, and providing periodic updates and feedback to health care workers on the progress. If the initial evaluation of the data points toward UTI as the major driver of the inappropriate antibiotic prescribing in the facility, then ASP should consider focusing its attention on interventions that can promote appropriate antibiotic use for UTIs. The exact intervention needed may depend on underlying reason for inappropriate prescribing. For example, if antibiotics are being initiated for UTI in scenarios where the patients are not meeting the clinical criteria for the diagnosis of UTI, then introducing an assessment or decision-aid tool prompting clinicians to look for those criteria during initial evaluation will be a good intervention. If the reason for inappropriateness is unnecessary use of broad-spectrum antibiotics or use for longer than recommended duration, then introducing facility-specific guidance for clinicians outlining the preferred empiric regimen and duration will be helpful. **Figure 106-3** highlights some examples of UTI-focused interventions that can be implemented in various health care settings. Depending on the identified challenges, a combination of interventions might be necessary for reducing inappropriate antibiotic prescribing and improving patient outcomes. One of the recent studies conducted in 25 nursing homes (12 intervention and 13 control) implemented a multifaceted antimicrobial stewardship program focused on reducing unnecessary antibiotic use for uncomplicated cystitis. Intervention nursing homes were randomized to receive a 1-hour introductory webinar, posters and pocket-sized educational cards with the diagnostic and treatment guidelines, tools for system change (eg, standardized physician order set forms; and an active monitoring sheet), and educational clinical vignettes addressing the diagnosis and treatment of suspected uncomplicated cystitis. Monthly web-based coaching calls were held for staff of intervention nursing homes and the facilities received quarterly feedback reports regarding management of uncomplicated cystitis. Overall antibiotic use was lower and fewer unlikely cystitis cases were treated in the intervention group without any increase in all-cause hospitalizations or death. Furthermore *C difficile* infection rates were also lower in the intervention as compared to the control nursing homes.

Evaluation and Management of UTI Near End of Life

Antimicrobials are usually overused at end-of-life and in the setting of advanced dementia, often without a known source of infection. That being said, UTIs can carry a heavy symptom burden. Thus, the decision to evaluate symptoms and subsequent management of a confirmed UTI are influenced greatly by the goals of care and life expectancy of the individual. If a patient is able to reliably report symptoms, and is expected to survive long enough to benefit from antimicrobial treatment, it would be appropriate to consider routine care. Enrollment in hospice alone should not be a barrier to receiving work-up and treatment of UTIs. However, antibiotic therapy has risks along with the potential benefits for a patient and should not be presented as a benign treatment plan. A discussion of potential side effects, risk for infection with resistant organisms, and any medical monitoring that is required for the selected antibiotic

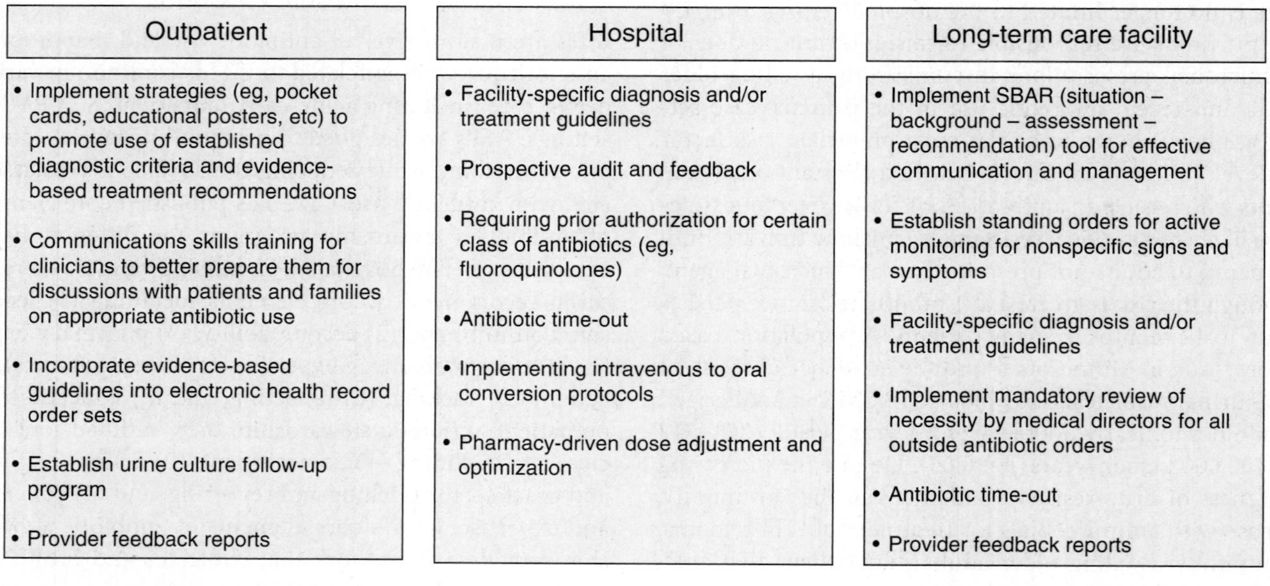

Outpatient	Hospital	Long-term care facility
• Implement strategies (eg, pocket cards, educational posters, etc) to promote use of established diagnostic criteria and evidence-based treatment recommendations • Communications skills training for clinicians to better prepare them for discussions with patients and families on appropriate antibiotic use • Incorporate evidence-based guidelines into electronic health record order sets • Establish urine culture follow-up program • Provider feedback reports	• Facility-specific diagnosis and/or treatment guidelines • Prospective audit and feedback • Requiring prior authorization for certain class of antibiotics (eg, fluoroquinolones) • Antibiotic time-out • Implementing intravenous to oral conversion protocols • Pharmacy-driven dose adjustment and optimization	• Implement SBAR (situation – background – assessment – recommendation) tool for effective communication and management • Establish standing orders for active monitoring for nonspecific signs and symptoms • Facility-specific diagnosis and/or treatment guidelines • Implement mandatory review of necessity by medical directors for all outside antibiotic orders • Antibiotic time-out • Provider feedback reports

FIGURE 106-3. Examples of interventions that can be implemented by healthcare settings as part of antibiotic stewardship program.

should be presented so patients can make a well-informed decision.

Advanced dementia, aphasia, or any disease process which interferes with a patient's ability to provide a reliable history can confound efforts to assess symptoms of infection, such as dysuria. If a UTI is suspected, it is important for clinicians to have a good understanding of the patient's wishes for their care prior to further investigation. Patients or their surrogate decision-makers may have set limits on what treatments they would want in such circumstances. If the goal is comfort, then it may be most appropriate to defer a work-up and focus on palliation of symptoms alone. If no limits have been set, or there is confusion about what a patient may or may not have wanted in this clinical setting, factors such as evidence of the seriousness of the infection, overall life expectancy and likelihood of survival benefit from antimicrobial treatment should be discussed with the medical decision-makers. When deciding against additional work-up and antibiotic treatment for a suspected UTI, focus can be directed toward symptom management strategies.

CONCLUSION

UTI is the most common infection occurring in older populations. The management of UTI for older ambulatory individuals is similar to younger populations, and determined by the presentation as either acute simple cystitis, complicated UTI or CAUTI. Treatment of symptomatic UTI requires optimal use of urine culture for diagnosis, appropriate antimicrobial selection, and appropriate duration of therapy. In PALTC settings, the very high prevalence of ASB interferes with ascertainment of symptomatic infection, especially in residents without localizing genitourinary symptoms. Bacteriuric older individuals who present with clinical decline without localizing findings should not be assumed to have a urinary source, despite a positive urine culture. A critical approach to diagnosis, investigation, and treatment is necessary. Further characterization of symptomatic presentations of urinary infection in the functionally disabled older population, together with evaluation of management approaches such as nontreatment with observation compared with empiric antimicrobial treatment, is needed.

FURTHER READING

Arinzon Z, Shabat S, Peisakh A, Bemer Y. Clinical presentation of urinary tract infection (UTI) differs with aging in women. *Arch Gerontol Geriatr*. 2012;55(1):145–147.

Ashraf MS, Gaur S, Bushen OY, et al. Diagnosis, treatment, and prevention of urinary tract infections in post-acute and long-term care settings: a consensus statement from AMDA's Infection Advisory Subcommittee. *J Am Med Dir Assoc*. 2020;21(1):12–24.e2.

Centers for Disease Control and Prevention. Core Elements of Antibiotic Stewardship. https://www.cdc.gov/antibiotic-use/core-elements/index.html. Accessed August 29, 2021.

D'Agata E, Loeb MB, Mitchell SL. Challenges in assessing nursing home residents with advanced dementia for suspected urinary tract infections. *J Am Geriatr Soc*. 2013;61(1):62–66.

Drekonja DM, Rector TS, Cutting A, Johnson JR. Urinary tract infection in male veterans: treatment patterns and outcomes. *JAMA Intern Med*. 2013;173(1):62–68.

Eure TR, Stone ND, Mungai EA, Bell JM, Thompson ND. Antibiotic-resistant pathogens associated with urinary tract infections in nursing homes: summary of data reported to the National Healthcare Safety Network Long-Term Care Facility Component, 2013–2017. *Infect Control Hosp Epidemiol*. 2021;42(1):31–36.

Falagas ME, Kotsantis IK, Vouloumanou EK, Rafailidis PI. Antibiotics versus placebo in the treatment of women with uncomplicated cystitis: a meta-analysis of randomized controlled trials. *J Infect*. 2009;58(2):91–102.

Gordon LB, Waxman MJ, Ragsdale L, Mermel LA. Overtreatment of presumed urinary tract infection in older women presenting to the emergency department. *J Am Geriatr Soc*. 2013;61(5):788–792.

Gould CV, Umscheid CA, Agarwal RK, Kuntz G, Pegues DA; Healthcare Infection Control Practices Advisory Committee. Guideline for prevention of catheter-associated urinary tract infections 2009. *Infect Control Hosp Epidemiol*. 2010;31(4):319–326.

Gupta K, Hooton TM, Naber KG, et al. International clinical practice guidelines for the treatment of acute uncomplicated cystitis and pyelonephritis in women: a 2010 update by the Infectious Diseases Society of America and the European Society for Microbiology and Infectious Diseases. *Clin Infect Dis*. 2011;52(5):e103–e120.

High KP, Bradley SF, Gravenstein S, et al. Clinical practice guideline for the evaluation of fever and infection in older adult residents of long-term care facilities: 2008 update by the Infectious Diseases Society of America. *Clin Infect Dis*. 2009;48(2):149–171.

Hooton TM, Bradley SF, Cardenas DD, et al. Diagnosis, prevention, and treatment of catheter-associated urinary tract infection in adults: 2009 International Clinical Practice Guidelines from the Infectious Diseases Society of America. *Clin Infect Dis*. 2010;50(5):625–663.

Huang AJ, Brown JS, Boyko EJ, et al. Clinical significance of postvoid residual volume in older ambulatory women. *J Am Geriatr Soc*. 2011;59(8):1452–1458.

Juthani-Mehta M, Malani PN, Mitchell SL. Antimicrobials at the end of life: an opportunity to improve palliative care and infection management. *JAMA*. 2015; 314(19):2017–2018.

Juthani-Mehta M, Quagliarello V, Perrelli E, Towle V, Van Ness PH, Tinetti M. Clinical features to identify urinary tract infection in nursing home residents: a cohort study. *J Am Geriatr Soc*. 2009;57(6):963–970.

Juthani-Mehta M, Tinetti M, Perrelli E, Towle V, Van Ness PH, Quagliarello V. Diagnostic accuracy of criteria for urinary tract infection in a cohort of nursing home residents. *J Am Geriatr Soc*. 2007;55(7):1072–1077.

Knottnerus BJ, Geerlings SE, Moll van Charante EP, ter Riet G. Women with symptoms of uncomplicated urinary tract infection are often willing to delay antibiotic treatment: a prospective cohort study. *BMC Fam Pract*. 2013;14:71.

Krein SL, Greene MT, King B, et al. Assessing a National Collaborative Program to Prevent Catheter-Associated Urinary Tract Infection in a Veterans Health Administration Nursing Home Cohort. *Infect Control Hosp Epidemiol*. 2018;39(7):820–825.

Little P, Moore MV, Turner S, et al. Effectiveness of five different approaches in management of urinary tract infection: randomised controlled trial. *BMJ*. 2010;340:c199.

Loeb M, Bentley DW, Bradley S, et al. Development of minimum criteria for the initiation of antibiotics in residents of long-term-care facilities: results of a consensus conference. *Infection Control Hosp Epidemiol*. 2001; 22(2):120–124.

Mody L, Greene MT, Meddings J, et al. A national implementation project to prevent catheter-associated urinary tract infection in nursing home residents. *JAMA Intern Med*. 2017;177(8):1154–1162.

Nace DA, Hanlon JT, Crnich CJ, et al. A multifaceted antimicrobial stewardship program for the treatment of uncomplicated cystitis in nursing home residents. *JAMA Intern Med*. 2020;180(7):944–951.

Nace DA, Perera SK, Hanlon JT, et al. The Improving Outcomes of UTI Management in Long-Term Care Project (IOU) Consensus Guidelines for the Diagnosis of Uncomplicated Cystitis in Nursing Home Residents. *J Am Med Dir Assoc*. 2018;19(9):765–769.e3.

Nicolle LE, Gupta K, Bradley SF, et al. Clinical Practice Guideline for the Management of Asymptomatic Bacteriuria: 2019 Update by the Infectious Diseases Society of America. *Clin Infect Dis*. 2019;68(10):e83–e110.

Ong Lopez AMC, Tan CJL, Yabon AS 2nd, Masbang AN. Symptomatic treatment (using NSAIDS) versus antibiotics in uncomplicated lower urinary tract infection: a meta-analysis and systematic review of randomized controlled trials. *BMC Infect Dis*. 2021;21(1):619.

Perrotta C, Aznar M, Mejia R, Albert X, Ng CW. Oestrogens for preventing recurrent urinary tract infection in postmenopausal women. *Cochrane Database Syst Rev*. 2008(2):CD005131.

Rogers MA, Fries BE, Kaufman SR, Mody L, McMahon LF Jr, Saint S. Mobility and other predictors of hospitalization for urinary tract infection: a retrospective cohort study. *BMC Geriatr*. 2008;8:31.

Rowe TA, Jump RLP, Andersen BM, et al. Reliability of nonlocalizing signs and symptoms as indicators of the presence of infection in nursing-home residents. *Infect Control Hosp Epidemiol*. 2020;1–10.

Stone ND, Ashraf MS, Calder J, et al. Surveillance definitions of infections in long-term care facilities: revisiting the McGeer criteria. *Infect Cont Hosp Ep*. 2012; 33(10):965–977.

Thompson ND, Penna A, Eure TR, et al. Epidemiology of antibiotic use for urinary tract infection in nursing home residents. *J Am Med Dir Assoc*. 2020;21(1):91–96.

Thompson ND, Stone ND, Brown CJ, et al. Antimicrobial use in a cohort of us nursing homes, 2017. *JAMA*. 2021;325(13):1286–1295.

Toolkit 1. Start an Antimicrobial Stewardship Program. Agency for Healthcare Research and Quality. Available at: https://www.ahrq.gov/nhguide/toolkits/implement-monitor-sustain-program/toolkit1-start-program.html. Accessed August 29, 2021.

van Buul LW, Vreeken HL, Bradley SF, et al. The development of a decision tool for the empiric treatment of suspected urinary tract infection in frail older adults: a Delphi consensus procedure. *J Am Med Dir Assoc*. 2018;19(9):757–764.

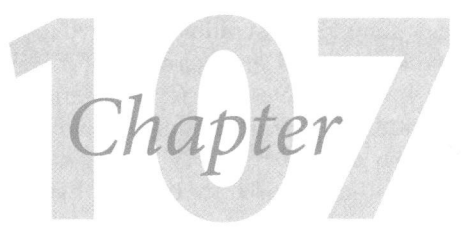

Chapter 107

Other Viruses: Human Immunodeficiency Virus Infection and Herpes Zoster

Kristine M. Erlandson, Kenneth Schmader

HUMAN IMMUNODEFICIENCY VIRUS INFECTION

Learning Objectives

- Recognize the shift in the epidemiology of human immunodeficiency virus (HIV) over the last three decades.
- Identify older adults at risk for HIV infection and include HIV testing in routine care.
- Recognize that some comorbidities may present earlier or have a higher prevalence among older adults with HIV.
- Integrate the principles of geriatrics (eg, management of multimorbidity and polypharmacy) into the care of older adults with HIV.

Key Clinical Points

1. Antiretroviral therapy (ART) has turned HIV into a chronic disease that one ages with over many decades. More than 50% of all people living with HIV in the United States are age 50 or older.

2. HIV is often unrecognized in older adults because of subtle or nonspecific presentation (anemia, fatigue, weight loss, pneumonia) and provider bias that older adults are not at risk.

3. While AIDS-associated conditions have declined markedly, comorbid illnesses occur more frequently than in age-matched, HIV-uninfected control populations leading to early multimorbidity, polypharmacy, and functional decline even in those with HIV controlled by ART.

DEFINITION

HIV is the virus that causes acquired immunodeficiency syndrome (AIDS). HIV destroys CD4+ T cells vital to defense of infections, and when untreated, leads to a progressively immunocompromised state with an increased risk for opportunistic infections, cancers, and other complications.

EPIDEMIOLOGY

One of the most amazing success stories of our lifetime is the transformation of HIV infection from a rapidly fatal disease that manifested in the first AIDS cases in early 1980s to a chronic health condition, with this shift driven in part by the tremendous advocacy of the HIV community. With early initiation of effective ART, HIV-1 RNA can now be quickly reduced to undetectable levels. Not only does this decrease the risk of immune suppression and associated comorbidities, but effective ART essentially eradicates between person transmission of HIV. This discovery that Undetectable = Untransmittable (or U = U) has resulted in a transformative experience for many people living with HIV, as they can now live without the fear of transmitting HIV to partners or close contacts. Unfortunately, despite early initiation of ART, we have yet to fully eradicate HIV, with rare exceptions occurring in the setting of bone marrow transplantation. As a result, a growing number of people are now living, and aging, with HIV. In the United States and Europe, as of 2018, over 50% of people living with HIV are age 50 or older, with approximately 20% age 65 or older.

In addition to aging with HIV, many older adults continue to become newly infected with HIV: more than 15% of new HIV diagnoses in the United States are in adults aged 50 or older. Those aging with HIV are more likely than other aging individuals to use psychoactive substances including alcohol, marijuana, and opioids, which can both interfere with antiretroviral adherence and increase higher-risk sexual encounters. Use of medications to treat erectile dysfunction and enhance sexual performance may also increase sexual risk behavior. Additionally, older men are less likely to use condoms and postmenopausal women may be less likely to request barrier protection without the risk of pregnancy. Age-associated erectile changes may make condom use difficult, and age-associated declines in immunity and changes in mucosal barriers may place older individuals at higher risk of transmission with each exposure. Finally, older individuals often present later in the course of HIV disease, extending the period of highest infectivity due to unsuppressed HIV-1 RNA.

While uptake of pre-exposure prophylaxis (PrEP) is less common among older versus younger adults, PrEP is an extremely effective tool for prevention of HIV transmission among patients at risk of HIV acquisition. Efficacy is presumed to be similar among older adults; however, few studies have included older adults, and the risk of adverse events and toxicity may be higher. A combination of strategies (barrier protection, ensuring viral suppression among people with diagnosed HIV, and providing PrEP to people at risk for HIV) has decreased and can continue to decrease transmission of new cases of HIV.

EVALUATION

Screening

No one is immune to HIV infection, and nearly 15% of people with HIV (PWH) in the United States and approximately 45% of persons worldwide are unaware of their diagnosis, presenting the greatest transmission risk. The nonspecific or asymptomatic presentation of new HIV may lead to a missed diagnosis for months or even years, as physicians and their patients are both likely to underestimate the risk of HIV infection among older adults. Prompt diagnosis and treatment of HIV decreases transmission and improves outcomes across the age spectrum. U = U has also led to a greater emphasis on the HIV care continuum: ensuring that each person living with HIV is diagnosed, linked to and receives care, is retained in care overtime, and achieves viral suppression.

The Centers for Disease Control and Prevention and the US Preventive Services Task Force (USPSTF) currently recommend that adolescents and adults aged 13 to 64 (CDC) or 15 to 65 (USPSTF) and all pregnant women should have HIV screening at least once; other expert panels (including the American College of Physicians) recommend screening up to age 75. More frequent annual testing is recommended for adults with higher risk, including persons who use injection drugs; have sex with a partner who has HIV or unknown HIV status, or uses injection drugs; and men who have sex with men. An individual in a monogamous relationship may present with a sexually transmitted disease because their partner

has more than one partner; any patient with a sexually transmitted disease (gonorrhea, syphilis, chlamydia, or trichomonas) should be screened (or rescreened) for HIV. Older patients may not spontaneously report sexual or drug use behaviors, and physicians seldom ask. Notably, some older patients may assume that HIV testing is part of routine blood work, thus incorrectly believe they are regularly tested. Annual wellness visits or hospitalizations are opportunities to ensure that HIV testing is up-to-date and repeated if indicated. Specific signed consent is no longer required for HIV testing though verbal consent may be required in some states.

In addition to routine testing, HIV testing should be conducted as part of a diagnostic work-up in any patient with unexplained laboratory results (anemia, leukopenia, pancytopenia, transaminitis, hyperproteinemia); new diagnoses of peripheral neuropathy, oral candidiasis, herpes zoster, recurrent bacterial pneumonia, anal cancer; or any AIDS-associated conditions (*Pneumocystis jiroveci* pneumonia, Kaposi sarcoma, atypical mycobacterial infection, tuberculosis, non-Hodgkin lymphoma). Finally, any patient presenting with debilitating fatigue, weight loss, or cognitive changes should be tested for HIV.

HIV Testing

In most clinical settings, the prior two-step ELISA (antibody) and Western blot testing strategy has been replaced by a fourth-generation combination HIV-1/2 immunoassay that tests for both HIV-1 and HIV-2 antibodies and the HIV p24 antigen. If positive, a confirmatory immunoassay will distinguish between HIV-1 and HIV-2 (primarily found in Africa). If there is any concern for recently acquired HIV infection, based on recent exposure or symptoms (fever, malaise, lymphadenopathy), the immunoassay should be combined with a PCR test for HIV-1 viral load as the p24 antigen will not turn positive until approximately 5 to 7 days after the HIV-1 viral load is detectable. Both false-negative and false-positive tests are now extremely rare with the combined antibody/antigen test. Rapid screening tests (including home kits) detect antibody only and have a higher rate of false negative results.

MANAGEMENT

Selection and Initiation of Antiretroviral Treatment

Patients with a new HIV diagnosis should be connected to HIV care as quickly as possible. ART is recommended for any patient regardless of CD4+ T-cell count, with greatest benefit on long-term prognosis seen if the CD4+ count remains more than 500 cells/μL. Rapid treatment of HIV offers immediate benefit by preventing declines in CD4+ count and decreasing HIV transmission. Indeed, some HIV programs have instituted rapid start programs with initiation of ART on the same day of HIV testing. Data also suggest that rapid initiation of ART with lower peak HIV-1 viral loads may decrease the "reservoir" of HIV that is difficult to eradicate and may have added benefits on long-term inflammation and immune alterations with aging. Older adults appear to adhere more effectively to ART and are quite successful at achieving HIV-1 RNA suppression, but experience a slower improvement in CD4+ cell count, thus even more emphasis is placed on early initiation. Without treatment, the natural history of HIV infection is usually one of progressive immunodeficiency, with development of symptomatic AIDS approximately 8 to 12 years after infection. Prognosis is poorer among those who present late for care, fail to adhere to their treatment regimen, and/or develop widely resistant virus.

Standard ART regimens require medications from at least two different classes, most commonly an integrase strand transferase inhibitor (INSTI) combined with one or two nucleoside reverse transcriptase inhibitors (NRTIs). Compared to older antiretrovirals, contemporary regimens have less adverse effects, fewer drug–drug interactions, rapid viral suppression, and are generally tolerant of minor variations in adherence. Furthermore, many of the regimens are available in a single coformulated tablet once a day. Long-acting injectable drugs also have promising data on adherence and acceptability, though with very limited data among older populations. Notably, while ART appears safe in older populations and is essential in the prevention of disease progression, very few adults older than age 60 were included in clinical trials.

There are many antiretrovirals from which to choose, and this selection should be informed by consultation with an experienced HIV care provider. Selection of a regimen incorporates likelihood of resistance (and HIV-1 genotyping if available), cost, patient preference, comorbidities, preexisting organ system injury and anticipated toxicity, and concomitant medications. Patients are followed closely for the first several months of therapy to ensure tolerability, safety, and HIV-1 viral load suppression. After the first 6 to 12 months of therapy, if viral suppression is achieved and the patient has a CD4+ count above 350 to 500 cells/mL, HIV-1 viral load monitoring can occur approximately every 6 months and CD4+ count annually or less. While selection of antiretroviral regimens should be informed by an experienced HIV provider, once patients have achieved HIV-1 viral load suppression, care could be managed by a primary care provider or geriatrician with consultation as needed.

Many toxicities with ART are predictable. Weight gain is common with any regimen, but appears to be more common and significant with newer antiretroviral regimens. While some weight gain may be beneficial among those who are underweight, in many, weight gain is associated with incident hypertension, hyperlipidemia, diabetes, and hepatic steatosis. Thus, all patients initiating ART should be provided general nutrition and physical activity recommendations to avoid excess weight gain. Physical activity prescriptions specific for adults with HIV have been developed and can be given at the time of ART to provide strategies to maintain adequate levels of physical activity.

General Care Considerations for the Older Adult With HIV

After antiretroviral initiation, the incidence of AIDS conditions drops dramatically, but ongoing and consistent therapy is imperative. The Strategies for Management of Antiretroviral Therapy (SMART) trial demonstrated that continued viral suppression decreases incident non-AIDS conditions including liver disease, kidney disease, lung disease, and cardiovascular disease. Even with early initiation of ART, PWH experience some comorbidities many years before their uninfected peers (accelerated), or with a much higher prevalence than their uninfected peers (accentuated). This concept of accelerated versus accentuated aging is particularly important for diseases that might occur earlier and require a change in screening recommendations (eg, low bone density, falls, frailty, some cancers), and for diseases that occur more frequently and may require particular vigilance for monitoring and aggressive management (eg, cardiovascular disease and certain cancers). With the earlier manifestation of many diseases, a threshold of 50 years has been used for characterizing "aging" with HIV. As the population of people older than 60 or 65 years continues to grow, it will be important to also study effects of HIV among those of more advanced age.

Potential mechanisms underlying accelerated or accentuated aging in PWH include immune dysfunction, dysregulation, and suppression; chronic inflammatory stimulation due to reservoirs of HIV-1 RNA replication and chronic microbial translocation; hypercoagulability; and direct effects of viral proteins, modifiable lifestyle factors, and social or structural determinants of health. Many of the immune system changes of senescence in aging mirror the changes seen with HIV. Furthermore, markers of aging such as DNA methylation patterns and shortened telomere length indicate that PWH are approximately 5 years older, biologically, than their HIV-uninfected peers. Those who acquire HIV infection often have had years of struggle with structural inequalities (homelessness; biases due to race, ethnic, and gender minority populations; employment; insurance), contributing to additional stress-related immune responses.

While these mechanistic changes may occur to some extent among almost all PWH, the disease process, immune system alterations, and comorbidities of someone who has lived with HIV for over 30 years may be much different than someone diagnosed more recently and started on therapy immediately. The "legacy" effect of immune suppression, opportunistic infections, and exposure to older, toxic ART may be long-lasting. In contrast, those that survived the early years of HIV, while experiencing the stress and trauma of the AIDS epidemic, may also have a unique "survivor" effect. Individuals who are diagnosed early in their disease process, achieve and maintain excellent HIV-1 RNA suppression, do not gain excess weight after ART initiation, and avoid ongoing substance use are likely to experience a very different aging trajectory from those who do not.

Models of Geriatric HIV Care

Accompanying an increasing number of older adults with HIV is, unfortunately, a shortage of both HIV and geriatric medicine clinic providers. In addition to routine clinic-based care, people aging with HIV are substantially more likely to be hospitalized than their HIV-uninfected peers. How these patients and their many transitions between inpatient and outpatient care, general medical care and specialty care, and skilled nursing facility care will best be managed in the future remains to be seen. Incorporation of telehealth or telephone consultation for geriatric, HIV, or other subspecialty care may be an important component of care in the future. Similarly, HIV providers should have appropriate training in geriatric medicine, and geriatric care providers in HIV medicine. What is nearly certain is that older PWH will place new demands on parts of the health care system, including short- and long-term nursing facilities that have previously not managed those with HIV infection in any substantial numbers.

While the management of most diseases will be the same among older PWH, providers should be cognizant of diseases that occur more frequently or manifest differently in HIV. As in other geriatric populations, consideration of the 5 M's approach to care can prioritize key clinical issues among many PWH, with a focus on Mind, Multimorbidity, Medications, Mobility, and (what) Matters most. We have proposed adding a sixth M for modifiable, emphasizing the importance of addressing the still *modifiable* factors in a population that might be younger than the typical geriatric population.

Mind incorporates cognitive impairment, mood disorders, the impact of substance use, and the added impact of stressors such as HIV stigma, loneliness, and depression. PWH have almost a fivefold risk for developing cognitive impairment independent of age, and may experience both HIV-related impairments and age-associated cognitive disorders such as Alzheimer disease, mild cognitive impairment, and vascular dementia. Up to 50% of PWH (of any age) will have evidence of HIV-associated neurocognitive impairment on neuropsychiatric testing, and approximately one-quarter experience an impact on daily function. Importantly, the Mini-Mental State Examination may miss the executive function impairment most common in HIV-associated neurocognitive disorders; the Montreal Cognitive Assessment is a more sensitive screening tool, though

formal neuropsychiatric testing is generally recommended. Although HIV disease severity (low CD4+ count, high HIV-1 RNA) is strongly linked to HIV-associated neurocognitive disorder, the impairments have changed minimally despite early and consistent ART; comorbidities, medication toxicity, psychiatric disease, and substance use also play an important role. Depression, anxiety, and severe mental illnesses such as psychosis and posttraumatic stress disorder are more common among older PWH infection than among the general population, with depression occurring in over 50% of PWH in some cohorts. Mood disorders can overlap with and confound the diagnosis of cognitive impairment, thus teasing out the diagnosis of both can be challenging. PWH who are aged 50 or older are also more likely than uninfected demographic counterparts to consume hazardous amounts of alcohol, use illicit drugs (especially marijuana, cocaine, and opioids), and smoke cigarettes. Lastly, social isolation, loneliness, and HIV-related stigma are highly prevalent among older PWH and may contribute to both poor cognition and mental health.

PWH experience a greater burden of *multimorbidity* at a given age than other populations, particularly in regard to clusters of cardiovascular and metabolic diseases, including diabetes, hypertension, hyperlipidemia, and nonalcoholic fatty liver disease. These disease clusters may be linked to toxicities of older ART, weight gain associated with newer therapy, and chronic inflammation. Kidney disease and loss of bone density are particularly common with some ART regimens and may occur as a consequence of coinfection with hepatitis B or C. The risk of some cancers is heightened due to coinfection with oncogenic viruses (human papilloma virus and anal cancer), exposure to carcinogens (lung cancer and smoking), or immunosuppression (some lymphomas). When referring to specialists, it is important to recognize that many older PWH continue to experience stigma related to HIV, gender, sexual preference, and age, and may be resistant to evaluation in a new clinic with a new provider.

With the initiation of ART, *multiple medications* or polypharmacy becomes the "norm" among PWH, often at least a decade before those without HIV experience polypharmacy. In addition to the burden of daily medications and pill fatigue, many antiretroviral agents are associated with significant drug–drug interactions. The protease inhibitors are particularly problematic, increasing levels of some concomitant medications (such as atorvastatin) by over 800%. With the introduction of newer ART, treatment guidelines have emphasized a shift away from certain medication classes, particularly among older PWH, to avoid these often dangerous drug interactions. Interactions with food, vitamins, and both prescription and nonprescription medications can still occur with almost any of the HIV medications and careful attention to possible drug interactions should be considered with any new prescription or change in dose. Further, due to preexisting organ system injury among those with HIV, those with HIV infection may be particularly susceptible to the harms associated with polypharmacy. These harms include decreased medication adherence and increased serious adverse drug events including organ system injury, hospitalization, geriatric syndromes (falls, fractures, and cognitive decline), and all-cause mortality. Utilizing pharmacists and drug–drug interactions programs (eg, HIV-druginteractions.org) can be extremely helpful.

Mobility tends to decline at a faster rate among PWH compared to uninfected controls, with differences apparent as early as age 50. Even among those with early initiation of ART, impairments in measures of grip strength, lower extremity function (repeat chair stands), and balance are common. The effects of ART on mitochondria, inflammation, neuropathy, obesity, and sarcopenia are heightened further by the impact of comorbidities, socioeconomic factors, and physical inactivity. Importantly, mobility impairments in middle-aged and older PWH are linked strongly to poor outcomes, including increased morbidity, mortality, and risk of falls. Indeed, people aged 45 to 65 with HIV experience fall rates similar to populations aged 65 and older without HIV. Many of the mobility impairments can be attenuated with cardiovascular and strength training. Thus physical activity counseling and fall risk reduction should be an important component of the care of PWH, regardless of age.

Ultimately, care should address what *Matters Most* to the patient. Recommendations should be informed by prognosis and the added risk/benefit ratio. Greater comorbid burden, frailty, and cognitive impairment among a relatively younger PWH may limit the added benefit of a screening procedure or intervention; other older adults with HIV may have robust health with few comorbidities. For example, patients need to live at least 5 to 7 years after screening for the benefit of the screening (decreased mortality) from colon cancer to outweigh the risk of perforation and the pain and discomfort of the procedure. Conversely, more aggressive screening for anal cancer may be indicated, particularly among those with good health, because of the increased incidence of this condition among those with HIV infection. Thus, "age appropriate" primary care guidelines for those without HIV may differ among PWH—careful consideration for the individual's prognosis, preferences for care, and personal

risk of these conditions should be incorporated in the conversation. What matters most in the care of an older PWH may be impacted considerably by loss, trauma, and stigma. Importantly, these conversations and designated decision makers should be carefully documented. Less than half of patients in most HIV clinics have completed any form of advanced care planning. Many PWH in the United States have estranged relationships with family and have same sex partners or close friends that they would prefer to designate as a medical power of attorney. As the recognition of these decision makers can differ by state, addressing advanced directives and designating medical power of attorney among older PWH is even more important to ensure the right person can help to make the right choices at the end of life.

Lastly, *modifiable* risk factors should be a key component of the care of PWH throughout the lifespan. Some older PWH may continue to engage high-risk sexual behaviors and have frequent exposures to sexually transmitted infections (STIs); safer sex and decreasing long-acting consequences of STIs, including syphilis, hepatitis B, and hepatitis C. Food insecurity is up to six times more common in older adults with HIV, and loneliness occurs in nearly 60% of older adults with HIV: ensuring access to nutritious food and connecting with social resources may improve multiple domains of health. As previously mentioned, consistent ART adherence and adequate levels of physical activity remain key components of care for all PWH.

In summary, people aged 50 or older now account for a majority of PWH as a consequence of improved lifespan of those with HIV and increased acquisition of HIV at older ages. Older adults should be screened for HIV at least once, and more often if sexual risk is unknown or the patient has nonspecific symptoms. As a consequence of biobehavioral factors, HIV or ART-associated factors, structural inequalities, and the impact of aging-related factors, PWH experience a greater burden of comorbidities and develop geriatric syndromes, often at a much earlier age than their HIV-uninfected peers. A 6 M's approach to the older PWH may guide providers in prioritizing care components (**Figure 107-1**). Importantly, the study of HIV infection among aging individuals may provide a template for improving the management of complex chronic disease more generally, especially among special populations of aging individuals—people of color, sexual minorities, and those with limited socioeconomic resources.

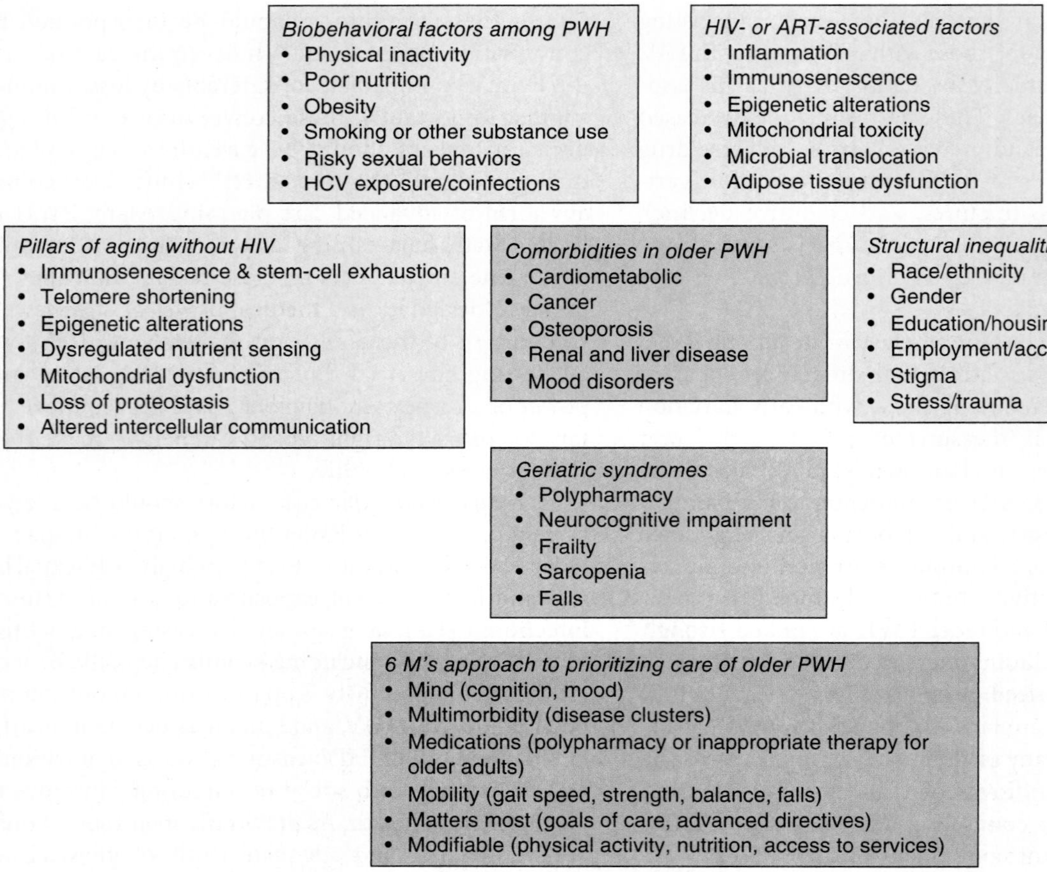

Biobehavioral factors among PWH
- Physical inactivity
- Poor nutrition
- Obesity
- Smoking or other substance use
- Risky sexual behaviors
- HCV exposure/coinfections

HIV- or ART-associated factors
- Inflammation
- Immunosenescence
- Epigenetic alterations
- Mitochondrial toxicity
- Microbial translocation
- Adipose tissue dysfunction

Pillars of aging without HIV
- Immunosenescence & stem-cell exhaustion
- Telomere shortening
- Epigenetic alterations
- Dysregulated nutrient sensing
- Mitochondrial dysfunction
- Loss of proteostasis
- Altered intercellular communication

Comorbidities in older PWH
- Cardiometabolic
- Cancer
- Osteoporosis
- Renal and liver disease
- Mood disorders

Structural inequalities among PWH
- Race/ethnicity
- Gender
- Education/housing
- Employment/access to insurance
- Stigma
- Stress/trauma

Geriatric syndromes
- Polypharmacy
- Neurocognitive impairment
- Frailty
- Sarcopenia
- Falls

6 M's approach to prioritizing care of older PWH
- Mind (cognition, mood)
- Multimorbidity (disease clusters)
- Medications (polypharmacy or inappropriate therapy for older adults)
- Mobility (gait speed, strength, balance, falls)
- Matters most (goals of care, advanced directives)
- Modifiable (physical activity, nutrition, access to services)

FIGURE 107-1. Underlying factors influencing development of comorbidities and geriatric syndromes and considerations to the approach of care of the older adult with HIV. Numerous factors contribute to the development of comorbidities and geriatric syndromes among older adults with HIV (blue boxes) including the pillars of aging, behavioral factors, HIV, or antiretroviral therapy (ART) associated, and structural inequalities that may be more common among people with HIV (PWH). Many comorbidities (green box) and geriatric syndromes (orange box) appear to occur earlier or more common among PWH. These contributing factors, comorbidities, and geriatric syndromes may be best approached through a 6 M's approach to care, as summarized in the purple box. HCV, hepatitis C virus.

HERPES ZOSTER

Learning Objectives

- Understand the impact of aging on the incidence of herpes zoster.

- Recognize typical and atypical presentations of herpes zoster in older adults.

- Know when to order microbiological testing for the diagnosis of herpes zoster and what tests to order.

- Employ the appropriate use of different treatments for the management of herpes zoster.

- Summarize Advisory Committee on Immunization Practices (ACIP), Centers for Disease Control and Prevention (CDC), recommendations for the use of the recombinant zoster vaccine.

Key Clinical Points

1. All cases of herpes zoster are caused by the reactivation of endogenous varicella-zoster virus (VZV) from latent infection of dorsal sensory or cranial nerve ganglia and not by exogenous transmission of VZV from an individual with herpes zoster or varicella.

2. Increasing age and impaired cellular immunity are the strongest risk factors for herpes zoster.

3. Although the diagnosis can be made on clinical grounds in the majority of cases with a typical dermatomal vesicular rash and pain, laboratory diagnostic testing is indicated when differentiating herpes zoster from

(Continued)

(Cont.) HSV, for suspected organ involvement, and for atypical presentations, particularly in the immunocompromised host; polymerase chain reaction (PCR) of vesicular fluid is the preferred diagnostic test.

4. The goal of the treatment of herpes zoster in older adults is to decrease the length of the acute attack and to reduce pain by the use of early antiviral therapy (acyclovir, famciclovir, valacyclovir), scheduled analgesia, and if the pain is not adequately controlled, adjunctive agents.

5. The recombinant zoster vaccine is recommended for all immunocompetent adults 50 years and older by ACIP for the prevention of herpes zoster.

DEFINITION

Herpes zoster is a neurocutaneous disease that is caused by the reactivation of VZV from a latent infection of dorsal sensory or cranial nerve ganglia following primary infection with VZV earlier in life. Herpes zoster is characterized by unilateral, dermatomal pain and rash. Postherpetic neuralgia (PHN) is pain 90 or more days after rash onset.

EPIDEMIOLOGY

VZV Transmission

VZV is a double-stranded DNA herpesvirus that is transmitted from person to person via direct contact or airborne or droplet nuclei when a virus-naive individual is exposed to the vesicular rash of varicella or herpes zoster. These exposed individuals may then develop varicella. Health care workers and staff in nursing homes and hospitals and children who have not received the varicella vaccine may not have had VZV primary infection and are potentially at risk for varicella. However, nearly all older adults are seropositive and latently infected with VZV. The exposure of a latently infected individual to herpes zoster does not cause herpes zoster or varicella. All cases of herpes zoster are caused by the reactivation of endogenous VZV.

Herpes Zoster Incidence and Risk Factors

In general population studies from North America and Europe, the estimated incidence of herpes zoster in persons older than age 65 varies from approximately 10 to 14 cases per 1000 per year. The lifetime incidence of herpes zoster is estimated to be about 30% in the general population and may be as high as 50% among those surviving to 85 years or older. Current population figures and herpes zoster incidence data yield estimates of about 1 million new cases of herpes zoster each year in the United States.

The cardinal epidemiological feature of herpes zoster is its increase in incidence with aging and with diseases and drugs that impair cellular immunity. The increase in the likelihood of herpes zoster with aging starts around 50 to 60 years of age and increases into late life in individuals older than 80 years (**Figure 107-2**). Immunocompromised patients at risk for herpes zoster include persons with HIV infection, Hodgkin disease, non-Hodgkin lymphomas, leukemia, hematopoietic stem cell or solid organ transplant, systemic lupus erythematosus, and those taking immunosuppressive medications. Other risk factors

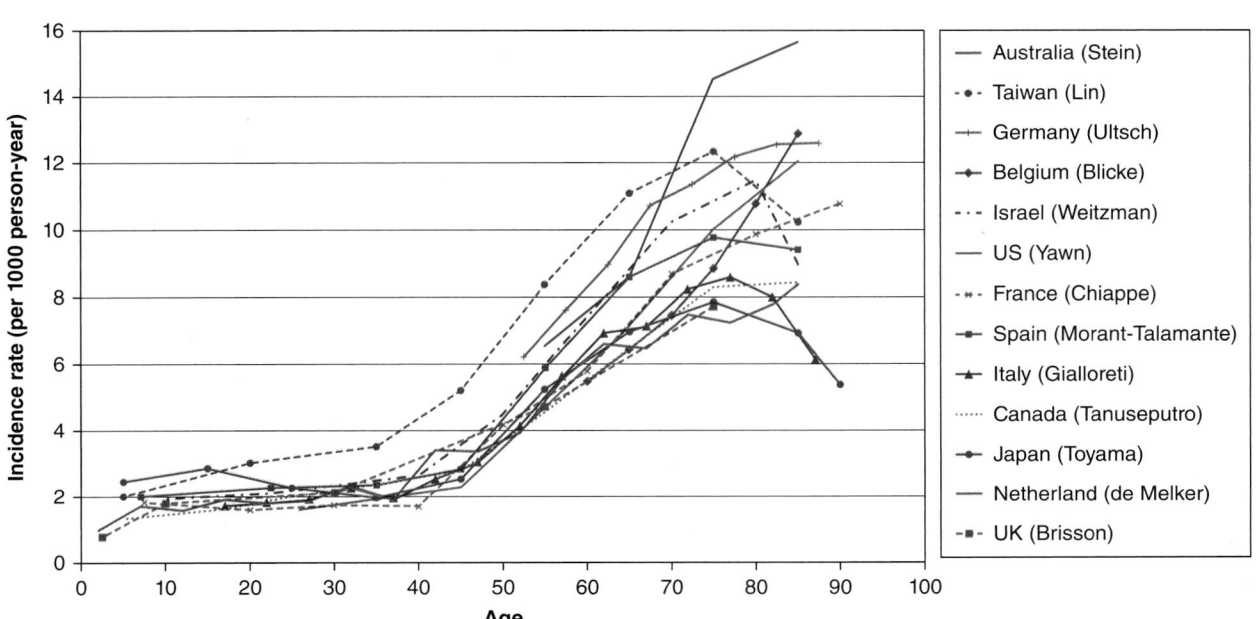

FIGURE 107-2. Age-specific incidence rate of herpes zoster in North America, Europe, and Asia-Pacific.

include White race, female sex, psychological stress, and physical trauma.

PRESENTATION

VZV reactivates in the affected sensory ganglion and spreads in the peripheral sensory nerve, causing prodromal symptoms that frequently precede the rash by several days. These prodromal symptoms are located in the involved dermatome and range from a superficial itching, tingling, or burning to severe, deep, boring, or lancinating pain, paresthesia, or hyperesthesia. The pain can be constant or intermittent. The prodrome may be mistaken for many other conditions in older adults, including pleurisy, a myocardial infarction, cholecystitis, appendicitis, renal colic, a collapsed intervertebral disk, glaucoma, trigeminal neuralgia, or unappreciated trauma. The prodromal symptoms usually last a few days, although they have been reported to last more than a week. Zoster sine herpete is a condition when patients experience acute dermatomal neuralgia without ever developing a skin eruption.

When VZV reaches the dermis and epidermis, the initial cutaneous presentation of herpes zoster occurs as a unilateral, dermatomal, red, maculopapular eruption. Vesicles generally form within 24 hours and evolve into pustules, which dry and crust in 7 to 10 days. The rash usually heals over in 2 to 4 weeks. In normal individuals, new lesions may continue to appear for 1 to 4 days and occasionally for as long as 7 days. The T1 to L2 or V1 dermatomes are most commonly involved (**Figure 107-3**). Atypical rashes may occur in older persons. The atypical rash may be limited to a small patch located within a dermatome or may remain maculopapular without ever developing vesicles.

Herpes zoster–associated acute neuritis produces dermatomal neuralgic pain in many older adults. Some older patients never develop pain, while others may experience the delayed onset of pain days or weeks after rash onset. The neuritis is described as burning, deep aching, tingling, itching, or stabbing. A subset of patients may develop severe pain, especially those with trigeminal nerve involvement. Acute herpes zoster pain can interfere with all activities of daily living (ADLs), but interference is greatest for instrumental ADLs, as well as sleep, general physical activity, and leisure activities. As overall pain burden increases, patients experience poorer physical, role, and emotional functioning.

The most feared complication of herpes zoster among older adults is PHN. PHN patients describe the quality of their pain as burning, throbbing, stabbing, shooting, sharp, aching, gnawing, tiring, or tender. The pain may be spontaneous and/or stimulus-evoked. Spontaneous pain may be constant aching or burning and/or brief, intermittent shock-like sensations. Stimulus-evoked pain consists of allodynia or hyperpathia. Allodynia is pain elicited by an innocuous stimulus and is particularly problematic. A cold wind, clothes, or bed sheets against the allodynic skin may cause debilitating pain. Hyperpathia is an exaggerated pain after a mildly painful stimulus. A minor bump of the affected dermatome against an object can cause severe pain that lasts for hours. Patients may experience discomfort that is not described as pain such as numbness or itching. Postherpetic itch can be maddening and appears to be mediated by damage and dysfunction of peripheral and central itch-specific neurons.

PHN greatly interferes with the functional status and quality of life of older adults. Patients can suffer from a variety of constitutional symptoms including chronic fatigue, anorexia, weight loss, and insomnia. PHN is associated with depression and social isolation in older adults. Reduced quality of life and interference with ADLs increase significantly as pain severity increases. Instrumental and basic ADLs are all compromised by PHN. For example, the patient with allodynic skin may be forced to avoid bathing or clothing around the affected area. Instrumental ADLs commonly affected include traveling, shopping, cooking, and housework. Studies using standardized pain scales and measures of function and quality of life such as the SF-36, SF-12, EuroQol, and Nottingham Health Profile have shown that PHN significantly interferes with multiple ADLs, reduces health-related quality of life (HRQL), and impairs mental and physical health.

Other complications include ocular inflammation in the setting of ophthalmic herpes zoster, cranial neuropathies, myelitis, visceral involvement, and motor paralysis. VZV-induced damage to the cornea and uvea and other eye structures can cause corneal anesthesia and ulceration, glaucoma, optic neuritis, eyelid scarring and retraction, visual impairment, and blindness in patients who did not receive antiviral therapy. Ophthalmic herpes zoster is also associated with stroke occurring weeks to months after the onset of the rash. Involvement of the third division of cranial nerve V can produce lesions and pain in the mandibular

Herpes zoster rash

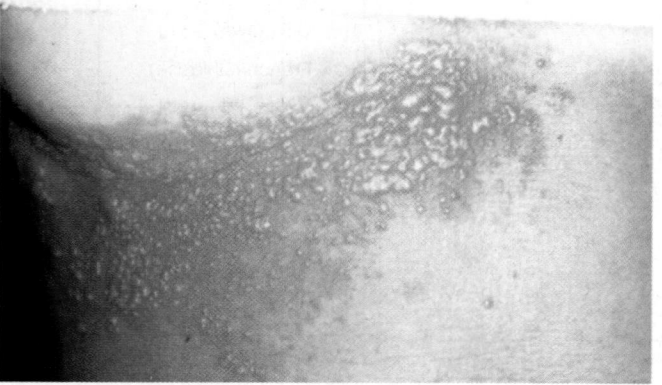

FIGURE 107-3. A patient with herpes zoster illustrates a range of lesions (eg, vesicles, populates, and crusting).

area of the face and in the mouth. Cranial nerve VII and VIII involvement, or Ramsey Hunt syndrome, is characterized by facial palsy in combination with herpes zoster lesions of the ipsilateral external ear, ear canal, tympanic membrane, or hard palate. Symptoms include tinnitus, vertigo, deafness, problems with balance, and facial paresis. Involvement of cranial nerves IX and X may produce pharyngeal or laryngeal lesions and resulting pharyngitis or laryngitis. Motor paralysis, from VZV-induced destruction of motor neurons in the anterior spinal horn or motor radiculitis corresponding to the extension of VZV infection from the involved sensory ganglion, involves muscle groups with innervation that is contiguous with that of the affected dermatome. Painful Bell palsy in an older adult strongly suggests herpes zoster.

EVALUATION

In patients who present with prodromal pain and no rash, herpes zoster is often confused with other causes of unilateral, localized pain in older adults. One diagnostic clue to the presence of prodromal pain is localized cutaneous sensory abnormalities (eg, hyperesthesia, dysesthesia) in the affected dermatome. Herpes zoster is easily diagnosed when an older adult patient presents with the typical dermatomal vesicular rash and pain. During the rash phase, herpes simplex has the most similar presentation to herpes zoster. Evidence supporting herpes simplex includes a presentation in a younger population, multiple reoccurrences of lesions, and the absence of chronic pain. The lesions themselves are more difficult to distinguish, particularly when herpes zoster occurs in areas commonly affected by simplex (eg, oral, genital, buttock lesions). The differential diagnosis also includes contact dermatitis, burns, and vesicular lesions associated with fungal infections, but the history and examination usually make the distinction clear.

The diagnosis of herpes zoster may need laboratory diagnostic testing when differentiating herpes zoster from HSV infection is necessary, for suspected organ involvement, and for atypical presentations, particularly in the immunocompromised host. The preferred diagnostic test is PCR because it is highly sensitive and specific, and results are available within hours of specimen receipt. The best specimen is vesicle fluid, which contains abundant VZV. Lacking vesicle fluid, acceptable specimens include lesion scrapings, crusts, tissue biopsy, or cerebrospinal fluid.

MANAGEMENT

Acute Herpes Zoster

The principal goal of the treatment of herpes zoster in older adults is to decrease the length of the acute attack and to reduce or eliminate pain. Patients should be instructed to keep the rash clean and dry to decrease the chances of developing bacterial superinfection. Cool compresses, calamine lotion, cornstarch, or baking soda may help to reduce local symptoms and speed the drying of the vesicles.

Antiviral Therapy

The guanosine analogs acyclovir, famciclovir, and valacyclovir are phosphorylated by viral thymidine kinase to a triphosphate form that inhibits VZV DNA polymerase and VZV replication (**Table 107-1**). Valaciclovir and famciclovir are prodrugs, which have greater bioavailability, resulting in higher blood levels and a less frequent dosing schedule. Randomized controlled trials indicate that oral acyclovir (800 mg five times a day for 7 days), famciclovir (500 mg every 8 hours for 7 days), and valaciclovir (1 g three times a day for 7 days) reduce acute pain and the duration of chronic pain in older patients with herpes zoster who are treated within 72 hours of rash onset. The most common adverse effects are nausea, vomiting, diarrhea, and headache. The effectiveness of antiviral agents has not been evaluated for treatment after 72 hours have elapsed since the onset of rash. An exception to the 72-hour threshold for treatment is made for patients who have ophthalmic zoster or patients that continue to have new vesicle formation. Topical antiviral therapy is not an effective treatment regardless of when started.

Analgesics

Acute herpes zoster pain requires the use of standardized pain measures, scheduled analgesia, and close monitoring

TABLE 107-1 ■ ANTIVIRAL TREATMENT OF HERPES ZOSTER IN IMMUNOCOMPETENT AND IMMUNOCOMPROMISED PERSONS

IMMUNE STATUS	TREATMENT
Immunocompetent	
Age ≥ 50 years, and patients of any age with cranial nerve involvement (eg, ophthalmic zoster)	Famciclovir 500 mg PO every 8 hours for 7 days or Valacyclovir 1 g PO every 8 hours for 7 days or Acyclovir 800 mg PO five times a day for 7 days[a]
Immunocompromised	
Mild compromise	Famciclovir 500 mg PO every 8 hours for 7–10 days or Valacyclovir 1 g PO every 8 hours for 7–10 days or Acyclovir 800 mg PO five times a day for 7–10 days[a]
Severe compromise	Acyclovir 10mg/kg every 8 hours for 7–10 days[a]
Acyclovir resistant	Foscarnt 40 mg/kg IV every 8 hours until healed

[a]Adjust acyclovir dosing for renal function.

to adjust dosing and detect adverse effects. Opioid and nonopioid analgesia are a standard of care for the acute pain syndrome. The choice of treatment will depend on the patient's pain intensity, comorbidities, and preferences. Patients with mild pain may be managed with acetaminophen or nonsteroidal agents. Patients with moderate to severe pain usually require treatment with an opioid analgesic (eg, oxycodone).

Corticosteroids

The anti-inflammatory effects of corticosteroids have been postulated to reduce herpes zoster symptoms but there remains controversy over their use. Randomized, controlled clinical trials demonstrated that corticosteroids do not prevent PHN when compared to placebo or acyclovir. These findings, the risk of VZV dissemination, and the adverse effects of corticosteroids in older adults argue against the routine use of these agents in herpes zoster. However, clinical trials have shown reductions in acute pain and one randomized controlled trial showed benefits in improvement in time to uninterrupted sleep, return to routine activities, and cessation of analgesic medications among patients with no relative contraindications to corticosteroids. In the trial, prednisone was administered orally at 60 mg/day for days 1 to 7, 30 mg/day for days 8 to 14, and 15 mg/day for days 15 to 21. Therefore, corticosteroids may be useful in reducing moderate to severe acute pain unrelieved by antiviral agents and analgesics. Corticosteroids are used to treat VZV-induced facial paralysis and cranial polyneuritis to improve motor outcomes and provide pain relief. If prescribed, corticosteroids should always be used in conjunction with antiviral agents.

Adjuvant Agents

If moderate-to-severe herpes zoster pain is inadequately relieved by antiviral agents in combination with oral analgesic medications and/or corticosteroids, then other therapies to consider include gabapentin or pregabalin or neural blockade. The use of these anticonvulsant agents must be balanced against adverse effects of sedation, dizziness, ataxia, and peripheral edema. A randomized controlled trial of antiviral therapy, oral analgesics, and a single epidural block with bupivacaine and methylprednisolone compared to antiviral therapy and oral analgesics alone showed that neural blockade reduces acute pain but does not prevent PHN.

Ophthalmic zoster with ocular involvement requires ophthalmological consultation. Oral antiviral and analgesic therapy is the mainstay of treatment as it is for herpes zoster presenting on the rest of the body but other ocular therapies may be necessary. These treatments are best managed by an ophthalmologist and include antibiotic ophthalmic ointment to prevent bacterial infection of the ocular surface, topical steroids to reduce ocular inflammation, mydriatics as needed for iritis, and ocular pressure-lowering drugs as needed for glaucoma.

PREVENTION

Recombinant Zoster Vaccine

The adjuvanted recombinant zoster vaccine (RZV; Shingrix©) is a powerful tool to prevent herpes zoster and PHN in older adults. It contains two components: recombinant VZV surface glycoprotein E (gE) antigen and the AS01B adjuvant system. AS01B adjuvant contains monophosphoryl lipid A (MPL) and QS-21, a saponin, combined in a liposomal formulation. VZV gE elicits an immune response against VZV, while the adjuvant strongly potentiates the immune response by enhancing the innate immune response to the antigen.

Efficacy

The efficacy of RZV was demonstrated in over 30,000 immunocompetent community-dwelling elders in the randomized, blinded, placebo-controlled Zoster Efficacy Study in Adults 50 Years of Age or Older (ZOE-50) and Zoster Efficacy Study in Adults 70 Years of Age or Older (ZOE-70) (**Figure 107-4**). The intervention was two doses of RZV at a 2-month interval. The median follow-up time was 3.2 years in the ZOE-50 study and 3.7 years in the ZOE-70 study. The vaccine efficacy (VE) for the prevention of herpes zoster was 97% (95% confidence interval [CI] = 89.6–99.3) in persons aged 50–59 and 97% (95% CI = 90.1–99.7) in persons aged 60–69 (see **Figure 107-3**). The VE against herpes zoster was 91% (95% CI = 86.8–94.5) in participants aged 70 years or older using pooled data from the ZOE-50 and ZOE-70 studies.

VE in the first year after vaccination was 98% (95% CI = 90.9–99.8). It was 85% (95% CI = 69.0–93.4) or higher for the remaining 3 years of the study in persons aged 70 or older.

Safety and Reactogenicity

The only contraindication to RZV is a history of a severe allergic reaction to any component of the vaccine or after a previous dose of RZV. Serious adverse events, potential immune mediated diseases, and deaths were reported at similar rates in vaccine and placebo groups in the clinical trials.

Using pooled data from the ZOE-50 and ZOE-70 trial from all participants, the most common solicited adverse reactions after RZV administration were injection site pain (78%), myalgia (45%), fatigue (45%), headache (38%), shivering (27%), fever (21%), and gastrointestinal symptoms (17%). **Table 107-2** shows the frequency of adverse reactions by age group. The frequency of adverse reactions decreased with increasing age. Grade 3 reactions are defined as those that prevented normal activity. **Table 107-2** shows the frequency of grade 3 reactions by age group, which also decreased with increasing age. About 16% of participants 50 years and older experienced any grade 3 reaction.

To better characterize the impact of reactogenicity on functional status and quality of life in older adults, a separate study of 401 adults age 50 and older who received RZV

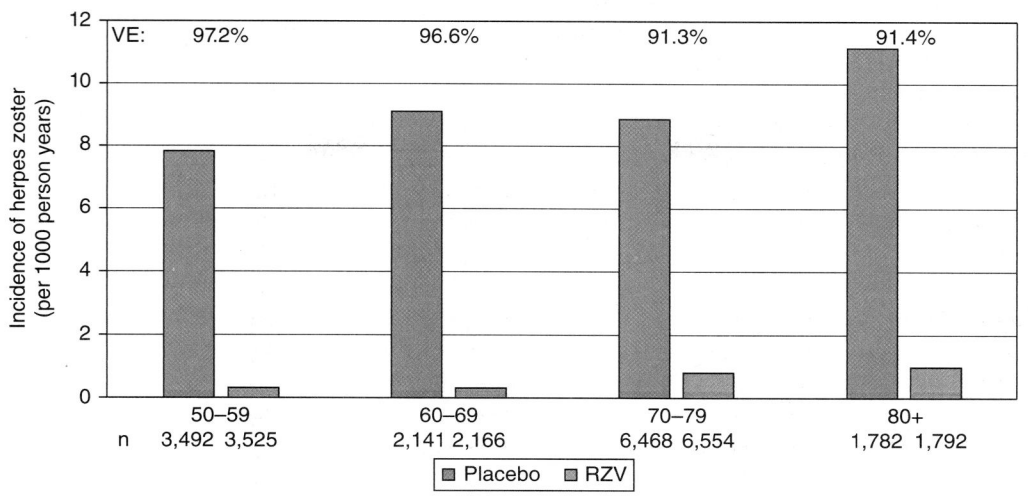

FIGURE 107-4. Recombinant zoster vaccine efficacy (VE) against herpes zoster from Zoster Efficacy 50 (ZOE-50) and Zoster Efficacy 70 (ZOE-70) pooled analyses. (Data from the US Food and Drug Administration. https://www.fda.gov/downloads/BiologicsBloodVaccines/Vaccines/ApprovedProducts/UCM581605.pdf.)

found that overall the physical functioning and quality of life of older adult were not affected by the first or second dose of RZV over 7 days postvaccination. However, participants who experienced a grade 3 reaction after either dose had a transient clinically important decrease in physical functioning and quality of life, affecting activities such as walking distances, carrying groceries, climbing stairs, lifting items, and moderate to vigorous activities. The impact was noted on days 1 to 2 post vaccination and resolved by day 3.

Given that frailty is strongly associated with adverse health outcomes, investigators studied how frailty impacts RZV VE, immunogenicity, reactogenicity, and safety. In secondary analyses of ZOE-50 and ZOE-70 studies, a baseline frailty index (FI) was created retrospectively following previously validated methods using preexisting comorbidities and patient reported outcomes. Participants were categorized as nonfrail (FI ≤ 0.08), prefrail (FI = 0.08–0.25), or frail (FI ≥ 0.25) for stratified analyses. RZV VE against HZ was consistently above 90% for all frailty categories (nonfrail: 96% [95% CI: 91.6–98.2], prefrail: 90% [84.4–94.4], frail: 90% [75.4–97.0]). The RZV group demonstrated robust antibody responses postdose 2 across frailty categories. In the RZV group, the percentage of participants reporting postvaccination reactions decreased with increasing frailty.

Clinical Guidance

The Advisory Committee on Immunization Practices (ACIP) at the CDC recommends RZV for the prevention of herpes zoster and related complications in immunocompetent adults aged 50 or older including individuals who previously received zoster vaccine live (ZVL; Zostavax©). RZV is included in the routine adult immunization schedule for older adults.

The lyophilized VZV gE antigen is reconstituted with the liquid adjuvant to comprise the vaccine and administered as a 0.5 mL intramuscular (IM) injection. RZV is administered in a 2-dose series. Screening for a prior history of varicella or herpes zoster before administration of the first dose is not necessary. After the first dose, the second dose should be administered 2 to 6 months later. If the patient does not return within that time window, then the second dose should be administered at the next available opportunity. It is not necessary to restart the series. RZV may be coadministered with influenza, pneumococcal, and Tdap vaccines.

TABLE 107-2 ■ RZV LOCAL AND GENERAL ADVERSE EVENTS (%) BY AGE[a]

EVENT	50–59 YEARS	60–69 YEARS	≥ 70 YEARS
Injection site reaction, pain	89	83	69
Grade 3[b]	10	6.9	4.0
Myalgia	57	49	35
Grade 3	8.9	5.3	2.8
Fatigue	57	46	37
Grade 3	8.5	5.0	3.5
Headache	51	40	29
Grade 3	6.0	3.7	1.5
Shivering	36	30	20
Grade 3	6.8	4.5	2.2
Fever	28	24	14
Grade 3	0.4	0.5	0.1

[a]Reactogenicity subgroup within 7 days after vaccination, vaccine n = 4884.
[b]Grade 3—prevented normal activity.
Data from the US Food and Drug Administration.
https://www.fda.gov/downloads/BiologicsBloodVaccines/Vaccines/ApprovedProducts/UCM581605.pdf.

It is essential to counsel the patient about potential injection site and systemic reactions before administering both doses of RZV. They may feel pain, redness swelling at the injection site or muscle pain, tiredness, headache, chills, fever or nausea. About one in six persons have reactions that transiently prevent them from doing normal activities. Most symptoms resolve in 1 to 3 days. Patients should be counseled to avoid strenuous activities for a few days after vaccination. Reactions to the first dose do not strongly predict reactions to the second dose.

The ACIP provides no recommendation, either for or against, the use of RZV in immunocompromised populations. The FDA label does not list immunocompromised as a contraindication or precaution so administering RZV to immunocompromised individuals is not off-label prescribing to persons 50 years and older; it is off-label for persons younger than 50 years. Currently, best practice is to allow for RZV use in immunocompromised persons on a case-by-case basis if potential benefit is judged to outweigh the risk, using shared decision. Current information from randomized controlled trials indicate that RZV was immunogenic and had no safety concerns in small numbers (100–1000) of different immunocompromised populations including hematopoietic stem cell transplant (HSCT), kidney transplant, hematologic malignancies, solid cancers on chemotherapy, HIV, and immune-mediated disease. RZV VE was demonstrated prospectively in HSCT (VE = 68%) and in post-hoc analyses in hematologic malignancies (VE = 87%) and immune-mediated diseases (VE = 91%).

FURTHER READING

HIV

American Academy of HIV Medicine: HIV & Aging Clinical Recommendations. Available at: https://aahivm-education.org/hiv-age/contents. Updated May 13, 2020. Accessed December 1, 2020.

Back D, Marzolini C. The challenge of HIV treatment in an era of polypharmacy. *J Int AIDS Soc.* 2020;23(2):e25449.

CD4+ Count-Guided Interruption of Antiretroviral Treatment. *N Engl J Med.* 2006;355(22):2283–2296.

Centers for Disease Control and Prevention. HIV and Older Americans. Available at: https://www.cdc.gov/hiv/group/age/olderamericans/index.html. Updated September 14, 2020. Accessed January 6, 2021.

Costagliola D. Demographics of HIV and aging. *Curr Opin HIV AIDS.* 2014;9(4):294–301.

Deeks SG. HIV infection, inflammation, immunosenescence, and aging. *Annu Rev Med.* 2011;62:141–155.

Deeks SG, Lewin SR, Havlir DV. The end of AIDS: HIV infection as a chronic disease. *Lancet.* 2013;382(9903):1525–1533.

Erlandson KM, Karris MY. HIV and aging: reconsidering the approach to management of comorbidities. *Infect Dis Clin North Am.* 2019;33(3):769–786.

Freiberg MS, Chang CC, Kuller LH, et al. HIV infection and the risk of acute myocardial infarction. *JAMA Intern Med.* 2013;173(8):614–622.

Greene M, Covinsky KE, Valcour V, et al. Geriatric syndromes in older HIV-infected adults. *J Acquir Immune Defic Syndr.* 2015;69(2):161–167.

Hasse B, Ledergerber B, Furrer H, et al. Morbidity and aging in HIV-infected persons: the Swiss HIV cohort study. *Clin Infect Dis.* 2011;53(11):1130–1139.

High KP, Brennan M, Clifford DB, et al. HIV and aging: state of knowledge and areas of critical need for research. A report to the NIH Office of AIDS Research by the HIV and Aging Working Group. *J Acquir Immune Defic Syndr.* 2012;60(suppl 1):S1–18.

Jones A, Cremin I, Abdullah F, et al. Transformation of HIV from pandemic to low-endemic levels: a public health approach to combination prevention. *Lancet.* 2014;384(9939):272.

Mahale P, Engels EA, Coghill AE, Kahn AR, Shiels MS. Cancer risk in older persons living with human immunodeficiency virus infection in the United States. *Clin Infect Dis.* 2018;67(1):50–57.

Montoya JL, Jankowski CM, O'Brien KK, et al. Evidence-informed practical recommendations for increasing physical activity among persons living with HIV. *AIDS.* 2019;33(6):931–939.

Pahwa S, Deeks S, Zou S, et al. NIH Workshop on HIV-Associated Comorbidities, Coinfections, and Complications: Summary and Recommendation for Future Research. *J Acquir Immune Defic Syndr.* 2021;86(1):11–18.

Pathai S, Bajillan H, Landay AL, High KP. Is HIV a model of accelerated or accentuated aging? *J Gerontol A Biol Sci Med Sci.* 2014;69(7):833–842.

Panel on Antiretroviral Guidelines for Adults and Adolescents. Guidelines for the Use of Antiretroviral Agents in Adults and Adolescents with HIV. Department of Health and Human Services. Available at https://clinicalinfo.hiv.gov/sites/default/files/inline-files/AdultandAdolescentGL.pdf. Accessed December 20, 2020.

Piggott DA, Erlandson KM, Yarasheski KE. Frailty in HIV: epidemiology, biology, measurement, interventions, and research needs. *Curr HIV/AIDS Rep.* 2016;13(6):340–348.

Sangarlangkarn A, Merlin JS, Tucker RO, Kelley AS. Advance care planning and HIV infection in the era of antiretroviral therapy: a review. *Top Antivir Med.* 2017;23(5):174–180.

Schouten J, Wit FW, Stolte IG, et al. AGEhIV Cohort Study Group. Cross-sectional comparison of the prevalence of age-associated comorbidities and their risk factors between HIV-infected and uninfected individuals: the AGEhIV cohort study. *Clin Infect Dis.* 2014;59(12):1787–1797.

Siegler EL, Brennan-Ing M. Adapting systems of care for people aging with HIV. *J Assoc Nurses AIDS Care.* 2017;28(5):698–707.

Singh HK, Del Carmen T, Freeman R, Glesby MJ, Siegler EL. From one syndrome to many: incorporating geriatric consultation into HIV care. *Clin Infect Dis.* 2017;65(3):501–506.

Smit M, Brinkman K, Geerlings S, et al. Future challenges for clinical care of an ageing population infected with HIV: a modelling study. *Lancet Infect Dis.* 2015;15(7):810–808.

HERPES ZOSTER

Cohen JI. Herpes zoster. *N Engl J Med.* 2013;369:255–263.

Cunningham AL, Lal H, Kovac M, et al. ZOE-70 Study Group. Efficacy of the herpes zoster subunit vaccine in adults 70 years of age or older. *N Engl J Med.* 2016;375: 1019–1032.

Curran D, Kim JH, Matthews S, et al. Recombinant zoster vaccine is efficacious and safe in frail individuals. *J Am Geriatr Soc.* 2021;69(3):744–752.

Dooling KL, Guo A, Patel M, et al. Recommendations of the advisory committee on immunization practices for use of herpes zoster vaccines. *MMWR Morb Mortal Wkly Rep.* 2018;67:103–108.

Forbes HJ, Bhaskaran K, Thomas SL, et al. Quantification of risk factors for postherpetic neuralgia in herpes zoster patients: a cohort study. *Neurology.* 2016;87(1):94–102.

Johnson RW, Rice ASC. Postherpetic neuralgia. *N Engl J Med.* 2014;371:1526–1533.

Kawai K, Gebremeskel BG, Acosta CJ. Systemic review of incidence and complications of herpes zoster: towards a global perspective. *BMJ Open.* 2014;4(6):e004833.

Lal H, Cunningham AL, Godeaux O, et al. ZOE-50 Study Group. Efficacy of an adjuvanted herpes zoster subunit vaccine in older adults. *N Engl J Med.* 2015;372:2087–2096.

Schmader KE, Levin MJ, Grupping K, et al. The impact of reactogenicity after the first dose of recombinant zoster vaccine upon the physical functioning and quality of life of older adults: an open phase III trial. *J Gerontol A Biol Sci Med Sci.* 2019;74:1212–1224.

Yawn BP, Saddier P, Wollan PC, St Sauver JL, Kurland MJ, Sy LS. A population-based study of the incidence and complication rates of herpes zoster before zoster vaccine introduction. *Mayo Clin Proc.* 2007;82:1341–1349.

Chapter 108

Influenza, COVID-19, and Other Respiratory Viruses

Lauren Hartman, H. Keipp Talbot

INFLUENZA

Viruses are an important threat to the health of older adults. Each year, it is estimated that influenza alone is associated with the death of 36,000 older adults in the United States. Despite immunization, outbreaks of influenza occur regularly in nursing homes and other long-term care facilities. This section of the chapter summarizes the biological, epidemiological, and clinical features of influenza that are relevant to older adults, with a particular emphasis on prevention.

Clinically Relevant Biological Characteristics of Influenza Virus

To understand the impact of influenza in older adults, it is important to be familiar with several key characteristics of the virus. The structure of influenza consists of an envelope with a central nucleic acid core composed of single-stranded RNA that encodes key structural proteins of the virus including hemagglutinin and neuraminidase. There are three types of influenza viruses: A, B, and C. However, only A and B are clinically relevant. Influenza A viruses are characterized by the structure of the hemagglutinin, a surface protein that binds glycoprotein on the surface of respiratory epithelial cells, allowing the virus to enter by forming an endosome and then using the protein-making machinery of the cell to replicate itself. Each year, new mutations occur resulting in small changes in the hemagglutinin ("antigenic drift") hence the reason why influenza vaccine needs to be reformulated and given annually. The other surface projection, neuraminidase, cleaves terminal sialic acid residues from carbohydrate moieties on surfaces of infected cells, promoting the release of virions that go on to infect other cells. As discussed below, this is a key target for neuraminidase inhibitors, thus preventing the influenza virus from replicating.

An important feature of influenza is the segmented structure of the RNA at the core of the virus, with each of eight segments coding for a structural or enzymatic component of the virus. This gives the virus the potential to recombine with influenza viruses of animal origin, forming a virus with a novel genotype and hemagglutinin to which there is no preexisting immunity. This is known as "antigenic shift" and was responsible for pandemics in

Learning Objectives

- Understand the biology of influenza virus that leads to "drift" and "shift" in surface protein structure and their impact on vaccine formulation and the emergence of influenza pandemics.

- Recognize clinical situations where there is a need for diagnostic testing to confirm a specific viral etiology in symptomatic older adults and recommend the specific tests appropriate in different clinical scenarios.

- Identify appropriate interventions to control outbreaks of influenza, respiratory syncytial virus (RSV), and severe acute respiratory syndrome coronavirus-2 (SARS-CoV-2) in a nursing home.

- Recognize the appropriate use of antiviral therapies for influenza in seniors.

- Review the biological and other features of SARS-CoV-2 infection that contribute to pandemic spread.

Key Clinical Points

1. The influenza virus has a segmented RNA core that encodes key proteins on the viral surface including hemagglutinin and neuraminidase. Annual mutations in the RNA lead to "drift" in these proteins requiring annual reformulation and administration of the vaccine.

2. When entire segments of the influenza RNA recombine in animals, it can lead to an antigenic "shift" and may result in a pandemic as there may be little or no immunity in the population.

3. Detection of influenza virus by direct antigen testing is insensitive in older adults, and a negative test does not rule out influenza infection. Reverse transcriptase polymerase chain reaction (RT-PCR) is more than 90% sensitive. Similarly, RSV is best detected by RT-PCR.

(Continued)

(Cont.)

4. RSV is clinically indistinguishable from influenza in older adults—both may present subtly or primarily as an exacerbation of underlying chronic illnesses.

5. Antiviral therapy with neuraminidase inhibitors is indicated for treatment of influenza and as chemoprophylaxis for nursing home outbreaks. Supportive care is currently the only treatment for RSV.

6. Influenza immunization is recommended for all older adults. Enhanced influenza vaccines are more effective than a standard-dose vaccine in seniors.

7. Immunization of staff reduces influenza mortality for nursing home residents.

8. Transmission of SARS-CoV-2 is highest at the beginning of infection, often prior to the onset of symptoms.

9. Symptomatic cases of SARS-CoV-2 present with fever, cough, fatigue, and dyspnea, though older adults may have atypical presentations.

10. Older adults, particularly those residing in nursing homes, are at high risk of complications, hospitalization, and death as a result of influenza, RSV, and SARS-CoV-2 infections.

1957–1958, 1968–1969, and 2009. Of note, the highest mortality rates occurring in the 1918–1919 and the 2009 pandemics were not in older adults but in younger adults, perhaps due to cross protection from the many influenza strains to which older adults were exposed over a lifetime. However, mortality in interpandemic periods is highest in those at the extremes of age. At present, there are only three hemagglutinins (H1, H2, and H3) and two neuraminidases (N1 and N2) that have developed a stable lineage in humans.

General Epidemiology of Influenza

Epidemics of influenza occur annually between November and April in the Northern Hemisphere. In any given season, there may be several strains circulating, hence the annual influenza vaccine contains multiple influenza strains.

Important Host Considerations in Older Adults

During the interpandemic period, older adults and particularly residents of long-term care facilities are equally likely to contract influenza as young, healthy adults, but are among those at highest risk for complications of influenza. Rates of hospitalization for influenza in older persons range from 136 to 508 per 100,000 persons versus 10 to 25 for those 5 to 49 years of age. The presence of chronic conditions, such as chronic lung disease, congestive heart failure, conditions that predispose to aspiration, and metabolic disease, increases the risk for complications following infection with influenza. Many of these conditions occur predominately in older age groups. Moreover, studies that have assessed complications have found that age older than 65 is independently associated with increased risk for influenza complications.

Based on our current understanding, the causes of death as a result of influenza in older adults in the interpandemic period include viral pneumonia, a bacterial infection complicating the influenza infection, myocardial infarction, stroke, and exacerbation of underlying comorbid conditions. Infection with influenza virus predisposes to *Streptococcus pneumoniae* or *Staphylococcus aureus* infection, which most often results in bacterial pneumonia. Deficits in innate immunity (phagocytes, natural killer cells) and acquired immunity (T-cell function, cytokine activity, antibody response) are all felt to play a role, as discussed in Chapter 3.

Clinical Presentation

Young, healthy individuals with influenza characteristically present with a sudden onset of fever, cough, myalgia, sore throat, and headache. Fever and cough have been shown in a systematic review to be the best predictors of influenza in the general population. In older adults, however, the presentation may be more subtle with cough and change in baseline temperature predominating. Often, older adults present with worsening of comorbid conditions such as a chronic obstructive pulmonary disease or congestive heart failure exacerbation. One of the most important factors in making the diagnosis of influenza, whether on clinical grounds or through diagnostic testing, is the local influenza activity. That is, if a community is experiencing an outbreak of influenza, particularly if the incidence of influenza is at its peak, fever and cough in an older person increase the likelihood of infection with influenza. In the nursing home setting, it is essential to obtain prompt diagnostic testing because the clinical presentation is nonspecific. Even when there are peaks of influenza in the community, RSV or other respiratory viruses can circulate. Additionally, an outbreak of influenza in a nursing home warrants chemoprophylaxis (see further discussion) as well as immunization of nonimmunized residents in whom it is safe to do so.

Specific Diagnostic Tests

The traditional method to detect influenza has been viral culture, which is limited by moderate diagnostic accuracy and delay in obtaining results (**Table 108-1**). Rapid tests include direct fluorescent antigen (DFA), or direct immunofluorescence, where monoclonal antibodies labeled with fluorescent material are directed to influenza cell coat antigens. A result can be reported within hours. Rapid enzyme-linked immunosorbent assay (ELISA) tests are

TABLE 108-1 ■ SUMMARY OF TEST CHARACTERISTICS OF DIFFERENT DIAGNOSTIC TESTS FOR VARIOUS RESPIRATORY VIRAL PATHOGENS IN OLDER ADULTS

	CULTURE	RAPID EIA	DFA/IFA	PCR	SEROLOGY
Influenza A	++	+	+	+++	++[a]
Influenza B	++	+	+	+++	++[a]
RSV	+	+/−	+/−	+++	+++

+/−, available but poor sensitivity; +, fair sensitivity; ++, good sensitivity; +++, optimal sensitivity.
[a]Interpretation complicated by vaccination.

commercially available but are very insensitive in older adults, with sensitivities as low as 20%. Nucleic acid amplification testing, such as RT-PCR, is the most promising test since it is over 95% sensitive and specific and the turnaround time can be rapid. The drawback, however, is that not all laboratories are capable of performing PCR daily.

Infection Control Aspects

The incubation period of influenza, the period of time from initial infection to development of symptoms, is typically 2 days but can range from 1 to 4 days. An infected individual becomes contagious 1 day prior to the onset of symptoms. In adults, viral shedding at levels high enough to cause transmission occurs over 5 or 6 days. The majority of spread of influenza is large droplet caused by coughing and sneezing and hence medical workers should wear a mask to prevent infection and spread. In terms of practical implications, use of "respiratory etiquette," coughing, and sneezing into tissues, for example, may help prevent spread to older adults who are susceptible to complications, although supporting epidemiologic evidence is limited.

Immunization

Many influenza vaccine formulations are now available in the United States. The most well-known influenza vaccine is the standard-dose quadrivalent inactivated vaccine, abbreviated as SD-IIV4, which contains components of an H1N1, an H3N2, and two B strains.

For the same reasons that older adults are more likely to have complications due to influenza infection, older adults respond less well to influenza immunizations. A 2014 systematic review summarized 35 influenza vaccine effectiveness studies performed in 15 countries. Cases were influenza positive; controls were patients who also had an acute respiratory illness but who tested negative for influenza. Vaccine effectiveness for the prevention of medically attended acute respiratory illness was found to be 38% to 70% during seasons of vaccine and circulating strain match and 15% to 59% during seasons of mismatch. These data show that influenza immunization plays an important but modest role in prevention.

Due to decreased immune responses and poorer clinical responses when SD-IIV4 is administered in seniors (compared with young adults), enhanced influenza vaccines have been developed and approved for use. A high dose vaccine quadrivalent formulation (HD-IIV4) has four times the dose of each component versus the standard dose. This high dose formulation has been shown to generate higher antibody levels in older adults than SD-IIV4 and is more effective for the prevention of illness and hospitalization due to influenza. The MF59 adjuvanted influenza vaccine, abbreviated aIIV4, also demonstrates increased immunogenicity and effectiveness in older adults compared to the SD-IIV4. Observational studies show MF59 adjuvanted influenza vaccines are associated with reduced hospitalization risk for not only influenza, but also pneumonia and cardiovascular diagnoses—common complications of influenza infection. The quadrivalent, recombinant influenza vaccine (RIV4) also shows promise in preventing intensive lifestyle intervention in older adults. At this time, the Advisory Committee on Immunization Practices recommends the use of any of these vaccines in older adults.

Influenza and Long-Term Care

Residents of nursing homes and other long-term care facilities are at high risk for complications of influenza, including pneumonia, hospitalization, and death. This is likely because there is close contact between residents and staff in these facilities, increasing the exposure to and transmission of influenza, and because the majority of residents have comorbidities, including cognitive impairment, chronic lung disease, and stroke. Outbreaks of influenza are well characterized in nursing homes, often described as "explosive" in that the onset is relatively abrupt. Such outbreaks are usually first detected by nursing home staff who notice a higher incidence of respiratory symptoms than usual on specific units, although at least one surveillance study has shown that such outbreaks are commonly missed even when active surveillance by trained nurses is performed. Such outbreaks are best managed using a multifaceted approach that includes the following: cohorting residents, increasing adherence to hand hygiene, chemoprophylaxis with antiviral agents, and immunization of those not previously vaccinated. It should be noted that because of space and staffing limitations, it is usually not feasible to cohort ill residents together as a means of separating them from noninfected residents in long-term care facilities. Administering neuraminidase inhibitors as chemoprophylaxis to noninfected residents helps to reduce further spread. In one randomized controlled trial where long-term units were randomized to zanamivir or to rimantadine, the risk of influenza was 3% in the zanamivir arm versus 8% in the rimantadine arm ($p = 0.038$). More recent data suggest that immunizing nursing home staff against influenza benefits residents. There have been four cluster-randomized controlled trials showing that immunizing health care workers against influenza reduces mortality in residents of long-term care facilities. Vaccinating nursing home staff against influenza may prevent influenza-like illness, use of health services, and deaths in nursing home residents, even more so than immunizing residents.

Use of Antivirals to Prevent and Treat Influenza in Older Adults in the Community

There are six antivirals that are approved for treating influenza: amantadine (oral), rimantadine (oral), zanamivir (inhaled), oseltamivir (oral), peramivir (IV), and baloxavir marboxil (oral). Amantadine and rimantadine are only active against influenza A, and currently circulating influenza A strains are predominantly resistant to both; their use is no longer recommended. The neuraminidase inhibitors, zanamivir and oseltamivir, are active against influenza A and B. They are 70% to 90% effective for prophylaxis in preventing influenza and when used as treatment to reduce clinical severity if given within 48 hours of symptom onset. However, the feasibility of using these agents for treatment is reduced since the majority of patients in the community present over 48 hours following symptom onset. It is important to note that the doses of treatment and prophylaxis are different; hence, it is important to use treatment doses if a patient is symptomatic. Zanamivir and oseltamivir are associated with few adverse effects. Zanamivir may worsen or provoke respiratory distress in those with underlying obstructive disease. Oseltamivir should be dosed based on renal function. In early 2015, the Food and Drug Administration (FDA) approved a third neuraminidase inhibitor, peramivir, for the treatment of influenza that is only available in an IV formulation. Baloxavir marboxil, a polymerase inhibitor, was approved in 2018 for treatment of uncomplicated cases of both influenza A and B. Similar to the neuraminidase inhibitors, it must be used within 48 hours of symptom onset. Unfortunately, viruses develop resistance to baloxavir very quickly, limiting its use.

Indirect Benefit of Immunization in Children to Protect Older Adults

There is observational data to suggest that children play an important role in the spread of influenza in the community. For example, data from a 3-year longitudinal surveillance study of children and adults in New York State demonstrated that children were about twice as likely to acquire and shed influenza compared to adults. In a longitudinal study conducted in Seattle from 1968 to 1974, elementary and junior high school students had the highest rates of influenza during epidemics, reaching 54%. In the Tecumseh, Michigan, studies from 1976 to 1981, over one-third of children between the ages of 5 and 14 had influenza virus isolated from specimens, and the highest rate was among persons with febrile respiratory illness. Serological data revealed similar results; from 1977 to 1978, children in 5 to 9, 10 to 14, and 15 to 19 age groups had an approximately 30% infection rate with H3N2. This was over twice the rate seen in adults. There were similar infection rates with influenza B in children aged 5 to 14, rates 14-fold higher than those in adults older than 20 years.

Given that school-aged children appear to play an important role in introducing and transmitting influenza into households and hence into the community, immunizing these children may interrupt spread to older adults who are at high risk for complications. In the Tecumseh studies, selectively immunizing 86% of children in this 7500-person community with inactivated influenza vaccine reduced influenza in adults by a third when compared to an adjacent community where children were not immunized. More evidence for the potential benefit of immunizing children with inactivated vaccine has been derived from an analysis of the effect of influenza vaccination in Japan. Japan began a program of immunizing school-aged children in 1962 and continued this policy until 1994. The effect of this policy was to dramatically reduce excess mortality rates to values similar to those in the United States. The fact that there was a rapid increase in excess deaths after 1994, the year in which mass immunization formally ended, supports the conclusion that the effects observed in earlier years were because of vaccine-induced herd immunity, although it is possible that social factors may have amplified the effects of this program. The authors explain their findings by hypothesizing that the high levels of vaccination in school children protected transmission of influenza to their grandparents. There have been several more recent observational studies where children have been immunized showing a reduced attack rate of influenza in adults. However, randomized clinical trial evidence of immunizing children to prevent influenza in older adults is limited.

RESPIRATORY SYNCYTIAL VIRUS

RSV has been long recognized as a major cause of bronchiolitis in children. Since the 1970s, there have been numerous reports about the burden of RSV in older adults, particularly those residing in nursing homes. RSV is now recognized as an important contributor to morbidity in both community-dwelling older adults as well as in residents of long-term care facilities. This section will describe the epidemiology of RSV in both settings including clinical, diagnostic, and management issues.

Characteristics of Respiratory Syncytial Virus

RSV is an enveloped RNA virus that can be classified into two major groups, A and B, based on antigenic and genetic properties. An important feature of RSV is that reinfections occur frequently throughout life and into older age. Because RSV infection does not produce robust immunity, developing a vaccine has been a major challenge. In addition, RSV is a very labile virus, meaning it can be difficult to grow if it is not transported carefully, making traditional diagnostic methods such as culture and antigen less sensitive outside of the hospital setting.

General Epidemiology

Like influenza, RSV circulates during winter months in temperate climates roughly beginning in October and lasting until early spring. Often, clinical cases precede influenza epidemics. The incubation period of RSV is 3 to 5 days. The majority of those who are infected show respiratory symptoms. In contrast to infants who shed higher titers (10^{5-6} plaque-forming units/mL of secretion) for longer time periods (10–14 days), adults tend to shed lower titers of the virus (10^{2-3} plaque-forming units/mL of secretion for 3–6 days). RSV is spread primarily by large droplets and fomites.

Community-Dwelling Older Adults and Respiratory Syncytial Virus

The best data about RSV in older persons living in the community are derived from a cohort study conducted in Rochester, New York, from 1999 to 2003. This cohort was composed of 608 healthy people aged 65 and older. Forty-six (8%) of the 608 participants developed RSV, compared to 56 (10%) of high-risk older participants (defined as having congestive heart failure or chronic pulmonary disease). The impact of RSV infection was important in both the healthy older adults group and in the high-risk group: 17% and 23%, respectively, of these groups made physician office visits. Morbidity was greater in the high-risk group, where 16% required hospitalization. The study was also useful because it allowed for a comparison to influenza: 42% of healthy older participants and 60% of high-risk participants required office visits for influenza, rates statistically significantly higher than for RSV. Since then, RSV has been shown in other studies to cause similar if not higher hospitalization rates than influenza in older adults.

Epidemiology of Respiratory Syncytial Virus in Long-Term Care Facilities

RSV attack rates during nursing home outbreaks have been reported to be variable, ranging from 2% to 90%. However, most involved relatively small numbers of residents and included the use of diagnostic assays with varying levels of sensitivity. In one prospective study conducted in Rochester, where a sensitive enzyme immunoassay was used, the overall attack rate was 7% and the virus was identified as a cause of 27% of illness. One retrospective cohort study estimated the burden of illness in nursing homes in Tennessee by linking cardiopulmonary hospitalization, medical utilization, and death to viral activity in the general community during a period of 88,581 person-years. According to these data, RSV accounted for 15 hospitalizations and 17 deaths per 1000 residents.

Clinical Features of Respiratory Syncytial Virus in Older Adults

The clinical features of RSV cannot definitively be distinguished from those of other viruses, though fever is typically less pronounced than for influenza and wheezing more pronounced. The nonspecific nature of the clinical presentation indicates the need for diagnostic testing. Signs and symptoms include rhinorrhea, nasal congestion, sore throat, cough, and dyspnea. Similar to patients infected with influenza, patients with RSV may present with exacerbation of underlying conditions.

Diagnosis

This can be done by viral culture, antigen detection in respiratory secretions, nucleic acid amplification, or serology. For diagnosis in real time, only the first three tests are appropriate. It is important to note that viral culture is only 50% sensitive. Similarly, detection of RSV antigens using immunofluorescence is very insensitive in older adults. In contrast, RT-PCR is relatively sensitive and specific. As the use of multiplex PCR systems increases, RSV will likely be recognized more often as the causative agent in the clinical setting.

Therapy

Care is mainly supportive in the older adult with RSV infection. The only licensed antiviral with activity versus RSV is ribavirin, but there are sparse data on which to base treatment recommendations in adults. Practical considerations surrounding ribavirin include that the administration of this aerosolized drug to older adults using face masks may be difficult, and that ribavirin is teratogenic, which is important for the health care provider who is delivering care and the family that is entering the patient's room.

Prevention

Transmission of RSV is believed to be caused by large droplets and fomites. Strategies such as increasing hand hygiene, particularly in nursing homes, may help to reduce spread. Isolation practices for RSV include gowning and gloving when taking care of a patient with RSV. At the present time, there are no licensed RSV vaccines.

SARS-COV-2 AND OTHER CORONAVIRUSES

Coronaviruses are a large family of enveloped, positive-strand RNA viruses that are endemic in animals and typically cause mild upper respiratory symptoms in humans, known as "the common cold." In the past two decades, however, three novel coronaviruses have transitioned from their animal hosts to cause severe disease in humans: SARS-CoV in 2002, Middle East respiratory syndrome (MERS-CoV) in 2012, and SARS-CoV-2 in 2019, the cause of pandemic coronavirus disease known as COVID-19. The COVID-19 pandemic has had global impact unparalleled in this generation, and like influenza, disproportionately impacts older adults. This section will review SARS-CoV-2 transmission, clinical manifestations, diagnosis, and infection control measures.

Characteristics of Coronaviruses and SARS-CoV-2

Coronaviruses were named for their spike-like surface projections that resemble a crown. Bats are an important ecological host of coronaviruses and likely serve as reservoirs. Zoonotic transmission—the spread of pathogens from animals to humans—leads to human disease. The virus must first acquire mutations that allow it to begin replicating in human cells. These mutations typically arise randomly in the natural reservoir. Transmission of the virus to a human host can occur directly, via saliva, bites, or through the air, or by way of an intermediate species. Intermediate hosts—palm civets for SARS-CoV and dromedary camels for MERS-CoV—contributed to zoonotic transmission of these viruses. There is no conclusive evidence regarding when and where SARS-CoV-2 transitioned to humans. Bats and pangolins have been linked to SARS-CoV-2 as possible zoonotic reservoirs, and it is not known whether an intermediate host was involved. Adaptation to a human host is necessary but not sufficient to cause disease outbreak; human-to-human transmission must also occur.

Transmission of SARS-CoV-2

Similar to SARS-CoV, SARS-CoV-2 binds to the angiotensin-converting enzyme 2 receptor to enter human respiratory epithelial cells and replicates rapidly throughout the respiratory tract. While SARS-CoV and MERS largely reproduce in the lower respiratory tract, high viral loads of SARS-CoV-2 are found in the upper respiratory tract. Though SARS-CoV and influenza transmission occur largely after symptoms begin and peak with severity of disease, pharyngeal shedding of SARS-CoV-2 is highest at the beginning of infection. This means transmission may occur prior to the onset of symptoms and before a person knows they are infected. Transmission through asymptomatic or pre-symptomatic cases is thought to be a major contributor to pandemic spread, estimated in one study as accounting for up to 79% of documented cases. Its tropism for the upper respiratory tract and asymptomatic spread makes SARS-CoV-2 a highly transmissible pathogen. Case detection is challenging and spread difficult to prevent without widespread public health measures.

The main mechanism of transmission is via respiratory droplets and airborne particles that are directly inhaled while in close contact with an infected person. It is hypothesized that some people, deemed "super spreaders," shed more infectious particles in speech and respiratory droplets than others, leading to high numbers of new infections related to large gatherings. Evidence for transmission via droplet contact with the conjunctiva has led to the recommendation for eye protection for all those caring for patients infected with SARS-CoV-2.

Coronaviruses have higher stability than the enveloped influenza virus, including stability on surfaces, and fomite transmission of SARS-CoV-2 is possible. Viable virus has been demonstrated to persist on inanimate surfaces for several days; however, the inoculum required to spread from touching surfaces is not known. Fomites are thus thought to be a possible, though not major source of viral transmission. Though prolonged viral shedding in

fecal samples has been demonstrated, there is no evidence for fecal-oral spread of disease at this time.

Clinical Features of SARS-CoV-2

Coronaviruses have a longer incubation period—time from infection to symptom onset—compared to influenza. Various estimates of the incubation period of SARS-CoV-2 have been proposed. Most recent data estimates symptom onset at around 5 days after infection, with most people demonstrating symptoms within 12 days. There is evidence that older adults experience a longer incubation period, with symptoms typically occurring at 7 days after infection.

Clinical manifestations of COVID-19 disease range from asymptomatic or mild symptoms in the majority of cases, to severe respiratory failure and multiorgan dysfunction, which occur in a small proportion of infections. For those who develop symptoms, fever, cough, fatigue, and dyspnea are most common. However, atypical presentations are also common, particularly in older adults. One study found that 40% of patients with a mean age of 81 presented with atypical symptoms such as falls, generalized weakness, and delirium. A wide variety of symptoms, including myalgias, headache, diarrhea, nausea, vomiting, sore throat, and loss of sense of smell and/or taste have been associated with SARS-CoV-2 infection. Other notable clinical features include lymphopenia and other cytopenias, elevated inflammatory markers, and ground-glass opacities on chest imaging in those who develop respiratory symptoms.

Though the majority of cases are mild, the proportion of cases requiring respiratory support is higher than that of 2009 pandemic influenza. It is hypothesized that the rapid replication of SARS-CoV-2 in the respiratory tract can lead to recruitment of inappropriately high levels of pro-inflammatory cytokines and cells, referred to as a "cytokine storm." This excessive inflammatory response is thought to underlie more severe cases of SARS-CoV-2 infection.

Epidemiology of SARS-CoV-2

All ages are susceptible to SARS-CoV-2 infection. While early in the pandemic COVID-19 incidence was highest in adults age 50 and older, the median age of SARS-CoV-2 infection has decreased as testing has become more available to those with asymptomatic or mild cases of infection, who tend to be younger. While all ages are susceptible, severity of disease increases with increasing age. Severe illness occurs in a minority of patients, with the highest rate in those older than 70 years, and is rare in children. Variable case fatality rates have been reported, largely due to differences in testing; however, fatal illness occurs primarily in those older than 50 years, and up to 80% of deaths from SARS-CoV-2 have been in adults 65 years and older.

Frailty has been proposed as a means to capture the heterogeneity of older adults with SARS-CoV-2 infection and guide decisions regarding prognosis and treatment. One observational cohort study demonstrated an association between frailty, measured using the clinical frailty scale, and 7-day mortality in adults hospitalized with SARS-CoV-2 infection. In this study, frailty was a better predictor of disease outcome than age or comorbidity alone. In addition to frailty, many common comorbidities are associated with increased risk of severe illness, progression to acute respiratory distress syndrome, and death, including type 2 diabetes, chronic obstructive pulmonary disease, heart failure, chronic kidney disease, obesity, cancer, and solid organ transplant.

SARS-CoV-2 is notable for its ability to cause outbreaks in congregate settings. Early outbreaks were reported on several cruise chips and later affected institutions like meat-packing plants, where employees work in close quarters, and college dormitories. Nursing homes, however, have been most critically affected by the COVID-19 pandemic. The combination of the close quarters of congregate living, a frail population with high personal care needs, and the conditions leading to chronic understaffing and lack of resources for nursing homes created a setting ripe for uncontrolled spread of infection and high mortality. Over a quarter of deaths have occurred in the postacute and long-term care sector, despite accounting for only 2% of the total confirmed cases as of November 2020.

The impact of physical distancing, loneliness, and social isolation on behavioral health and mortality, particularly for older adults and those who reside in nursing homes, has yet to be fully expounded. In one pre-pandemic study, social isolation, loneliness, and living alone corresponded to an average of 29%, 26%, and 32% increased likelihood of mortality, respectively, in older adults. This is comparable to the risk of unhealthy diet, physical inactivity, alcohol misuse, and smoking. The loss of social interaction may have particular negative consequences for those with dementia.

Though a smaller proportion of people infected with SARS-CoV-2 require hospitalization compared to those with SARS-CoV, as well as to those infected with 2009 pandemic influenza, the overall number of people infected is much higher. This has placed strain on health system resources, at times exceeding hospital and ICU capacity and leading to higher mortality in many areas of the world.

Diagnosis

RT-PCR for detection of viral RNA in a sample from the nasopharynx is the cornerstone of testing for active SARS-CoV-2 infection. Compared to other diagnostic tests, it has the highest sensitivity at early stages of infection, and specificity is also high; however, appropriate sample collection is vital. Turnaround time ranges from 15 minutes to several days. RT-PCR is time- and labor-intensive and requires a well-equipped laboratory, which also impacts turnaround time, particularly for facilities like nursing homes and rural hospitals that must send tests to a central laboratory.

Development of point-of-care (POC) testing has been a priority during the pandemic in order to provide rapid results that can guide clinical management, allocation of personal protective equipment (PPE), and activation of isolation protocols. Currently available POC devices automate multiple steps of lab-based immunoassay methods to detect viral antigens in nasal specimens in under an hour. Sensitivity is lower than RT-PCR, particularly early in the course of infection, with high specificity; however, these devices have been tested and received authorization for use on symptomatic persons only, and test characteristics for screening and testing asymptomatic persons are unknown.

While there is no role for serologic testing for antibodies to SARS-CoV-2 in diagnosing active infection, the immunology of SARS-CoV-2, including the course of antibody production and protection against future infection, is an active area of study.

Treatment

The global impact of the COVID-19 pandemic has stimulated an exceptional period of research and development of not only diagnostics but also a myriad of potential therapeutics. Several medications have shown benefit in specific populations—for example, the steroid dexamethasone reduces mortality in hospitalized patients requiring oxygen or mechanical ventilation, though confers no benefit in those not requiring respiratory support. Though several have been approved for emergency use in the United States, antivirals and monoclonal antibodies, as well as convalescent plasma, have yet to be evaluated in phase 3 trials; availability is also limited, and expense high, for these treatments. Hundreds of drugs continue in development or clinical trials; however, no treatment has demonstrated general prophylactic or therapeutic benefit against SARS-CoV-2.

Infection Control Aspects of the COVID-19 Pandemic

Without broadly effective therapeutics, infection control measures are paramount in mitigating the adverse health outcomes of the pandemic. Basic measures including hand hygiene and masks to reduce the spread of respiratory droplets, identical to those recommended for other respiratory viruses including influenza, have been demonstrated to reduce transmission. Cities and states across the United States also implemented restrictions on public gatherings to encourage social distancing and limit the spread of infection.

As discussed in a previous section, rapid, accurate, and readily available diagnostic tests are essential to identifying cases and isolating infected patients. SARS-CoV was mitigated in part due to rigorous contact tracing and case isolation measures, and countries able to implement similarly robust public health measures were able to rapidly control the spread of SARS-CoV-2. Gaps in diagnostics exist, most notably accurate tests for screening asymptomatic persons to identify those in the incubation phase of infection. Detection of these cases is critical to control asymptomatic and presymptomatic transmission.

Nursing home best practices have developed to include regular testing of staff and residents along with appropriate PPE and hand hygiene. Increases in nursing home cases and deaths are associated with increases of cases in the community, and staff testing frequencies are based on community positivity rates. Contract tracing and isolation of positive residents, as well as cohorting staff so that different groups care for positive and negative residents, are ideal but often unattainable due to staffing and resource limitations in this setting.

In addition to limiting spread of infection, a crucial approach to pandemic mitigation is to reduce the number of susceptible people via immunization. Promising vaccine candidates have demonstrated more than 90% effectiveness in preventing infection, and immunization can also have a role in reducing transmission and attenuating illness. Large-scale production and global vaccine deployment remain an ongoing challenge in combating the COVID-19 pandemic.

Concerns about emerging coronaviruses have been growing even prior to the COVID-19 pandemic. The global experience of encountering a novel virus with pandemic spread and an impact far beyond health care has highlighted the need for ongoing research into emerging infectious diseases. The need for coordinated international response and cooperation, not only in combating the COVID-19 pandemic but also in preparing for future pandemics, has become more evident than ever.

FURTHER READING

Darvishian M, Bijlsma MF, Hak E, van den Heuvel ER. Effectiveness of seasonal influenza vaccine in community-dwelling elderly people: a meta-analysis of test-negative design case-control studies. *Lancet Infect Dis.* 2014;14:1228–1239.

Elis SE, Coffey CS, Mitchel EF Jr, et al. Influenza and respiratory syncytial virus-associated morbidity and mortality in the nursing home population. *J Am Geriatr Soc.* 2003;51:761–767.

Falsey AR, Hennessey PA, Formica MA, Cox C, Walsh E. Respiratory syncytial virus infection in elderly and high-risk adults. *N Engl J Med.* 2005;352:1749–1759.

Falsey AR, Walsh EW. Respiratory syncytial virus infection in adults. *Clin Microbiol Rev.* 2000;13:371–384.

Fox JP, Hall CE, Cooney MK, Foy HM. Influenza virus infections in Seattle families, 1975–1979. Study design, methods and the occurrence of infections by time and age. *Am J Epidemiol.* 1982;116:212–227.

Glezen WP, Keitel WA, Taber LH, Piedra PA, Clover RD, Couch RB. Age distribution of patients with medically-attended illnesses caused by sequential variants of influenza A/H1N1: comparison to age-specific infection rates, 1978–1989. *Am J Epidemiol.* 1991;133:296–304.

Hall CB. Respiratory syncytial virus and parainfluenza virus. *N Engl J Med.* 2001;344:1917–1928.

Hayward AC, Harling R, Wetten S, et al. Effectiveness of an influenza vaccine programme for care home staff to prevent death, morbidity, and health service use among residents: cluster randomised controlled trial. *BMJ.* 2006;333:1241.

Hewitt J, Carter B, Vilches-Moraga A, et al. The effect of frailty on survival in patients with COVID-19 (COPE): a multicentre, European, observational cohort study. *Lancet Public Health.* 2020;5(8):e444–e451.

Hu B, Guo H, Zhou P, Shi ZL. Characteristics of SARS-CoV-2 and COVID-19. *Nat Rev Microbiol.* 2020;6:1–14.

Jackson LA, Jackson ML, Nelson JC, Neuzil KM, Weiss NS. Evidence of bias in estimates of influenza vaccine effectiveness in seniors. *Int J Epidemiol.* 2006;35:337–344.

Long CE, Hall CB, Cunningham CK, et al. Influenza surveillance in community-dwelling elderly compared with children. *Arch Fam Med.* 1997;6:459–465.

Martines RB, Ritter JM, Matkovic E, et al. Pathology and pathogenesis of SARS-CoV-2 associated with fatal coronavirus disease, United States. *Emerg Infect Dis.* 2020;26(9):2005–2015.

Monto A, Davenport FM, Napier JA, Francis T. Modification of an outbreak of influenza in Tecumseh, Michigan by vaccination of schoolchildren. *J Infect Dis.* 1970;122:16–25.

Monto AS, Koopman JS, Longini IM Jr. Tecumseh study of illness. XIII. Influenza infection and disease, 1976–1981. *Am J Epidemiol.* 1985;121:811–822.

Palese P. Influenza: old and new threats [review]. *Nat Med.* 2004;10(12 suppl):S82–S87.

Petersen E, Koopmans M, Go U, et al. Comparing SARS-CoV-2 with SARS-CoV and influenza pandemics. *Lancet Infect Dis.* 2020;20(9):e238–e244.

Petric M, Comanor L, Petti CA. Role of the laboratory in diagnosis of influenza during seasonal epidemics and potential pandemics [review]. *J Infect Dis.* 2006;194(suppl 2):S98–S110.

Reichert TA, Sugaya N, Fedson DS, et al. The Japanese experience with vaccinating school children against influenza. *N Engl J Med.* 2001;344:889–896.

Talbot HK, Falsey AR. The diagnosis of viral respiratory disease in older adults. *Clin Infect Dis.* 2010;50:747–751.

Index

Note: Page numbers followed by f indicate figures; those followed by t indicate tables.

INDEX